Diseases of the Heart

Diseases of the Heart

Edited by

Desmond G. Julian
Consultant Medical Director
The British Heart Foundation
Emeritus Professor of Cardiology,
University of Newcastle upon Tyne, UK

A. John Camm
Professor of Clinical Cardiology
Department of Cardiological Sciences
St. George's Hospital Medical School
London, UK

Kim M. Fox
Consultant Cardiologist
National Heart Hospital
London, UK

Roger J.C. Hall
Consultant Cardiologist
University Hospital of Wales
Cardiff, Wales, UK

and

Philip A. Poole-Wilson
Professor of Cardiology
The National Heart and Lung Institute
London, UK

Baillière Tindall
London   Philadelphia   Toronto   Sydney   Tokyo

Baillière Tindall   24–28 Oval Road
W.B. Saunders   London NW1 7DX

The Curtis Center
Independence Square West
Philadelphia, PA 19106–3399, USA

1 Goldthorne Avenue
Toronto, Ontario M8Z 5T9, Canada

Harcourt Brace Jovanovich (Australia) Pty Limited
32–35 Smidmore Street
Marrickville, NSW 2204, Australia

Harcourt Brace Jovanovich Japan Inc.
Ichibancho Central Building, 22–1 Ichibancho
Chiyoda-ku, Tokyo 102, Japan

© 1989 Baillière Tindall

British Library Cataloguing in Publication Data
Diseases of the Heart
1. Man. Heart. Diseases
I. Julian, Desmond G. (Desmond Gareth)
616.1′2

ISBN 0-7020-1260-2

Typeset by MC Typeset Limited, Gillingham.
Printed in Great Britain by Mackays of Chatham PLC, Chatham, Kent.

Contents

Other Conditions Affecting the Heart

Contributors

Robert H. Anderson
Joseph Levy Professor of Paediatric Cardiac Morphology, Cardiothoracic Institute, University of London; Honorary Consultant, Brompton Hospital, London; Visiting Professor of Pediatrics, Children's Hospital of Pittsburgh, Pittsburgh, PA.

Stephen G. Ball
Professor of Cardiovascular Studies, University of Leeds, Leeds.

Martin Been
Senior Registrar in Cardiology, Regional Cardiothoracic Centre, Freeman Hospital, Newcastle-upon-Tyne.

Christopher P. Bennett
Research Registrar, Division of Human Genetics, University of Newcastle upon Tyne.

David H. Bennett
Consultant Cardiologist, Regional Cardiac Centre, Wythenshawe Hospital, Manchester.

Ronald D. Bradley
Consultant Physician, Intensive Therapy Unit, St. Thomas's Hospital, London.

Nicholas Brooks
Consultant Cardiologist, Regional Cardiothoracic Centre, Wythenshawe Hospital, Manchester.

Robert E. Bullock
Consultant in Anaesthesia and Intensive Care, General Hospital, Newcastle-upon-Tyne.

John Burn
Consultant Clinical Geneticist, Department of Human Genetics, Regional Genetics Advisory Centre, Royal Victoria Infirmary, Newcastle-upon-Tyne.

Ghazwan S. Butrous
Consultant Cardiologist, St. George's Hospital Medical School, London.

A. John Camm
Professor of Clinical Cardiology, St. George's Hospital Medical School, London.

Stuart M. Cobbe
Walton Professor of Medical Cardiology, University of Glasgow, Glasgow.

Henry J. Dargie
Consultant Cardiologist, Western Infirmary, Glasgow.

John H. Dark
Consultant Cardiothoracic Surgeon, Regional Cardiothoracic Centre, Freeman Hospital, Newcastle-upon-Tyne.

Graham J. Davies
Senior Lecturer in Cardiovascular Medicine, Royal Postgraduate Medical School, London; Consultant Cardiologist, Hammersmith Hospital, London.

Michael J. Davies
British Heart Foundation Professor of Cardiovascular Pathology, St. George's
Hospital, Medical School, London.

Tom Evans
Consultant Cardiologist and Honorary Senior Lecturer, Royal Free Hospital and
School of Medicine, London.

Kim M. Fox
Consultant Cardiologist, National Heart Hospital, London.

Leisa J. Freeman
Formerly Medical Registrar, The National Heart Hospital, London.

Roger Freeman
Reader in Bacteriology, Newcastle University and Honorary Consultant
Microbiologist, Freeman Hospital, Newcastle-upon-Tyne.

C.F. George
Professor of Clinical Pharmacology, University of Southampton, Southampton.

Derek G. Gibson
Consultant Cardiologist, Brompton Hospital, London.

Gerald J. Gibson
Consultant Physician, Freeman Hospital, Newcastle-upon-Tyne.

Ian R. Gray
Consultant Cardiologist, Coventry and South Warwickshire (Retired).

Roger J.C. Hall
Consultant Cardiologist, University Hospital of Wales, Cardiff.

Sheila G. Haworth
Professor of Experimental Paediatric Cardiology, Institute of Child Health, London
and Honorary Consultant in Paediatric Cardiology, Hospital for Sick Children,
Great Ormond Street, London.

Stewart Hunter
Consultant Paediatric Cardiologist, Regional Cardiothoracic Center, Freeman
Hospital, Newcastle-upon-Tyne.

Stephen J. Hutchinson
Lecturer in Cardiology, University of Wales, College of Medicine, Department of
Cardiology, Cardiff.

Desmond G. Julian
Consultant Medical Director, British Heart Foundation, London.

Michael Joy
Consultant Cardiologist, St. Peter's Hospital, Chertsey, Surrey and The Civil
Aviation Authority Medical Branch, Gatwick Airport, Crawley, Sussex.

David P. Lipkin
Consultant Cardiologist, Royal Free Hospital, London; Honorary Senior Lecturer,
Hammersmith Hospital, London.

W.A. Littler
British Heart Foundation Professor of Cardiovascular Medicine, University of
Birmingham and East Birmingham Hospital, Birmingham.

Anthony Martin
Consultant Physician, Jersey General Hospital.

Christopher G.A. McGregor
Consultant Cardiothoracic Surgeon and Director of Cardiothoracic
Transplantation, Mayo Clinic, Rochester, MIV 1, USA.

William J. McKenna
Senior Lecturer and Honorary Consultant, St. George's Hospital, Medical School,
London.

A.L. Muir
Reader in Medicine, University of Edinburgh, Consultant Physician, Royal
Infirmary, Edinburgh.

Celia Oakley
Consultant Cardiologist, Hammersmith Hospital and The Royal Postgraduate
Medical School, London; Honorary Consultant Cardiologist, St. Mary's Hospital,
London.

G.D.G. Oakley
Consultant Cardiologist, Northern General Hospital, Sheffield.

Olusola Odemuyiwa
Registrar in Cardiology, Freeman Hospital, Newcastle-upon-Tyne.

Lionel H. Opie
Professor of Cardiology, University of Capetown, South Africa.

Michael C. Petch
Consultant Cardiologist, Papworth Hospital, Papworth Everard.

Philip A. Poole-Wilson
Professor of Cardiology, National Heart and Lung Institute, London.

M.J. Raphael
Consultant Radiologist, National Heart Hospital, London.

J.I.S. Robertson
Janssen Research Foundation, Beerse, Belgium.

Derek J. Rowlands
Consultant Physician, Manchester Royal Infirmary, Manchester.

Michael B. Rubens
Consultant Radiologist, National Heart Hospital and London Chest Hospital,
London; Honorary Senior Lecturer, Cardiothoracic Institute, University of London,
London.

A.G. Shaper
Professor of Clinical Epidermiology, Royal Free Hospital School of Medicine,
London.

Leonard M. Shapiro
Consultant Cardiologist, Papworth Hospital, Papworth Everard, Addenbrookes
Hospital, Cambridge and HCA Cambridge Lea Hospital, Impington.

Man Fai Shiu
Senior Lecturer/Consultant in Cardiovascular Medicine, Queen Elizabeth Hospital,
Birmingham.

Elspeth B. Smith
Reader in Chemical Pathology, University of Aberdeen, Aberdeen.

George R. Sutherland
Director of Clinical Echocardiography, Thorax Centre, Erasmus University, Rotterdam, The Netherlands.

George C. Sutton
Consultant Cardiologist, Hillingdon Hospital, Uxbridge, Middlesex.

Richard Sutton
Consultant Cardiologist, Westminster Hospital, London.

E. Malcolm Symonds
Foundation Professor, Department of Obstetrics and Gynaecology, University Hospital, Nottingham.

K.M. Taylor
British Heart Foundation Professor of Cardiac Surgery, University of London, London; Professor and Chief of Cardiac Surgery, Royal Postgraduate Medical School, London.

Gilbert R. Thompson
External Staff, Medical Research Council, Honorary Senior Lecturer in Medicine, Royal Postgraduate Medical School, London; Honorary Consultant Physician, Hammersmith Hospital, London.

Charles R.V. Tomson
Lecturer in Medicine, University of Leicester, School of Medicine, Leicester.

Michael Tynan
Joseph Levy Professor of Paediatric Cardiology, United Medical and Dental Schools of Guy's and St. Thomas's Hospitals, London.

D.G. Waller
Senior Lecturer in Clinical Pharmacology, University of Southampton, Southampton.

David E. Ward
Consultant Cardiologist, Regional Cardiothoracic Centre, St. George's Hospital, London.

David J. Wheatley
British Heart Foundation Professor of Cardiac Surgery, University of Glasgow, Glasgow.

David Zideman
Consultant in Anaesthesia, Hammersmith Hospital, London; Honorary Senior Lecturer in Anaesthesia, Royal Postgraduate Medical School, London.

Preface

Diseases of the heart and circulation predominate as causes of morbidity and death in the developed parts of the world, and are becoming of increasing importance in developing countries. They are the commonest form of disorder seen in the medical wards of hospitals, and a cardiac operation (coronary bypass surgery) is the most frequently performed of all major surgical procedures. A detailed knowledge of modern cardiology is, therefore, a prerequisite for any physician, as well as for the increasing number of those who specialize in cardiac medicine and surgery. This book is written both for those training in medicine and cardiology and for those, already trained, who wish to consult an up-to-date text that covers the whole field of clinical cardiology while providing the necessary background of anatomy, physiology, biochemistry and pathology.

There have been those who have doubted the necessity of textbooks, but their continuing popularity confirms the existence of a need to encapsulate the present state of knowledge in a readily accessible form. Whilst reading original articles and reviews in journals is a more certain way of keeping abreast with the latest research, these do not provide comprehensive coverage of a subject nor can they be so easily consulted by the doctor at home. Inevitably, a textbook is only as up-to-date as the time when the chapters were written, but it does provide perspective as well as knowledge and this should compensate to some extent for any "out-of-dateness" that may exist.

"*Diseases of the Heart*" is deliberately shorter and easier to handle than some of the very large textbooks that are available. The editors have attempted to marry readability with comprehensiveness and, in doing so, have had in mind the great success of Paul Wood's unrivalled text which combined lucidity with erudition. His book also had the virtue of single authorship, but it would be impossible today for any one person to cover the whole field of cardiology with authority. The editors have tried to overcome the problem of multiple authorship by maintaining close contact with the experts in the various subjects addressed. We believe that this has led to a consistency of style and approach that would otherwise have been difficult to achieve.

The practice of cardiology has undergone enormous changes in recent years as has our understanding of the cardiovascular system. Nowhere is this more evident than in the area of heart failure. In the past, students who have tried to grapple with this difficult topic have been confused by the apparent gap between the definitions provided and the clinical manifestations. A better appreciation of the circulatory and hormonal responses to impaired cardiac performance has changed the concepts of heart failure and has improved the correlations between pathophysiology on the one hand and the symptoms and signs on the other; these are reflected in the section on this subject by Philip Poole-Wilson.

The problems presented by congenital heart disease as seen by the physician have altered greatly in recent years. Today, they are concentrated either in disorders of the neonatal period or in the residual defects that are present in those who have undergone palliative or corrective surgery in earlier years. Because the readers of this book will be mainly concerned with the latter, Robert Anderson and Michael Tynan have paid particular attention to it, but it was thought that the classification of complex congenital disorders in which they have played such an important part in developing should be explained in some detail.

Although coronary heart disease remains the major problem in cardiology, there have been very substantial advances in our understanding of its pathology and epidemiology, to which the authors of the respective chapters, Michael Davies and Gerald Shaper, have made outstanding contributions. Other subjects of contemporary interest which are addressed in detail by Kim Fox and his fellow contributors are silent ischaemia, therapy by thrombolytic agents and antiplatelet drugs, and angioplasty.

Arrhythmology is, perhaps, in danger of becoming a superspecialty, understood only by a few cognoscenti. John Camm and his associates have sought to make the subject comprehensible to all, while providing the latest information on such matters as invasive electrophysiology, catheter ablation of arrhythmias and arrhythmia surgery.

Hypertension is one of the major causes of cardiovascular disease, yet in recent years it has been relatively neglected by cardiologists and become virtually a specialty on its own. Ian Robertson and Stephen Ball have contributed a chapter designed to integrate well with the more "cardiological" topics to which it relates, whilst providing an authoritative overview of contemporary knowledge of the causes, effects and management of high blood pressure.

From the practising physician's point of view, the rapid developments in non-invasive investigation have extended diagnostic capability immensely. Roger Hall and his colleagues have described and profusely illustrated such techniques as Doppler echocardiography, nuclear cardiology and magnetic resonance imaging.

The availability of several new classes of drugs, each with many members, makes cardiac pharmacology a complex topic. We have attempted to deal with this not only by devoting a chapter to the principles of pharmacology, and describing the use of the drugs in the relevant clinical chapters, but also by including an appendix in which the salient features of each drug are summarized.

The many other subjects dealt with in this book help to make it, we hope, a ready and comprehensive source of information, which both students and postgraduates will enjoy consulting.

The successful completion of a book of this size requires the support and co-operation of many people. We are very grateful to the many experts who found the time in their busy lives to contribute to this volume. We would also like to thank Sean Duggan for his helpful guidance throughout this book's gestation, and also Erica Ison for the final polish she has given to each chapter.

Desmond G. Julian
A. John Camm
Kim M. Fox
Roger J.C. Hall
Philip A. Poole-Wilson

Acknowledgement

The editors and the publishers gratefully acknowledge permission granted from Churchill Livingstone to reproduce many of the illustrations appearing in Chapters 28, 29, 31 and 32. These illustrations first appeared in *Diseases of the Cardiac Valves* by Roger Hall and Desmond Julian, 1989, published by Churchill Livingstone.

Chapter 1

Cardiac Morphology

Robert H. Anderson

INTRODUCTION

Although the details of cardiac morphology have been known for centuries, at no time have studies conducted using the simplest techniques of gross observation been more important than the present. Recent techniques such as cross-sectional echocardiography, magnetic resonance or computed tomographic imaging reveal the nuances of cardiac structure with such precision that the cardiologist can often appreciate the anatomy with greater facility than the morphologist, especially as the anatomy can be appreciated during the heart's motion and, hence, at various stages of the cardiac cycle. Such information is denied to the pathologist. Maximization of this newly available information requires a firm understanding of basic cardiac morphology. Most importantly, this information must be acquired in the setting of the heart as it is positioned within the body. It makes little sense for the cardiologist to learn anatomy as though the heart was balanced on its apex with the atriums* above the ventricles and the right-sided chambers pictured as though they were truly to the right of their left-sided counterparts. Yet, with few exceptions, this is how cardiac anatomy is usually displayed. The intention within this chapter is to satisfy the need of the cardiologist to understand the structural features of the heart in a functional and clinical context. Therefore, in the opening section, the position of the heart within the thorax will be reviewed and the location of the various cardiac structures relative to the silhouettes projected to the body will be described. Thereafter, the important relationships of the heart to the mediastinal structures will be outlined. In the next section, the detailed features of the various cardiac chambers and great vessels will be reviewed, and those of particular clinical significance will be highlighted.

* Anglicized version of atria.

Sections will then be devoted to the important clinico-anatomical features of the coronary arteries, veins and lymphatics, the conduction system and the nervous components of the heart.

THE HEART WITHIN THE CHEST

The heart is the largest component of the mediastinum, occupying an eccentric mid position so that, in frontal projection, its mass extends two-thirds to the left and one-third to the right of the mid-line (Fig. 1.1). Although conventionally described in terms of a triangle, the shape of the frontal silhouette seems to be more that of a rounded but lop-sided trapezoid (Fig. 1.1, inset). The upper border is much shorter than the lower, the latter lying on the diaphragm. The two lateral borders then diverge markedly, with the right border being more or less vertical whereas the left border extends sharply out to the so-called apex. This apex is the point of a triangle in which the sides are the lower and left borders of the overall silhouette. It is a line joining the left upper and right lower corners that forms the cardiac base. This line is important, because it marks the plane in which the atriums join the ventricles at the atrioventricular junction. Incorporated within the plane are the arterial valves marking the origin of the great arterial trunks. The line is obliquely situated across the orthogonal planes of the body, as is the long axis of the heart. Therefore, cross-sectional cuts along the coronal, sagittal and short axes of the body section the cardiac structures obliquely. To demonstrate the particular inter-relationship of the cardiac structures themselves, it makes more sense to consider the heart within its own orthogonal planes (Fig. 1.2). As with the body, these are best considered as two series of long axis and one of short axis planes. The long axis plane through the heart, which is equivalent to the coronal or frontal plane of the

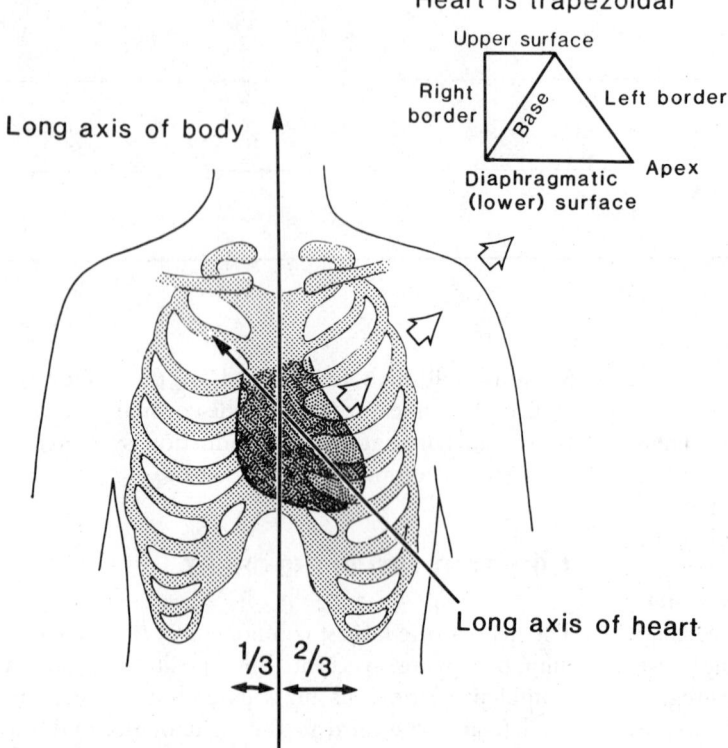

Heart is trapezoidal

Upper surface

Right border

Base

Left border

Apex

Diaphragmatic (lower) surface

Long axis of body

Long axis of heart

1/3   2/3

Fig. 1.1. Diagram showing the usual location and borders of the heart within the chest. The inset shows the trapezoidal arrangement, itself containing the cardiac triangle.

body, can show, in one particular cut, the four basic cardiac chambers. For this reason, it is conventionally known as the 'four chamber plane' (Fig. 1.3a). The other long axis plane, at right angles to the four chamber plane, is akin to a sagittal section of the body but, owing to the considerable discrepancy between the long axes of the heart and the body, is considerably angled relative to the verticle.

This plane is conventionally described simply as the 'long axis plane'. This should not obscure the fact that the four chamber plane is also in one long axis of the heart. In comparison with the 'four chamber' appearance, the reciprocal long axis plane can be considered as a 'two chamber plane' (Fig. 1.3b).

The heart also presents a lateral silhouette, which is of less value clinically. Nonetheless, the projec-

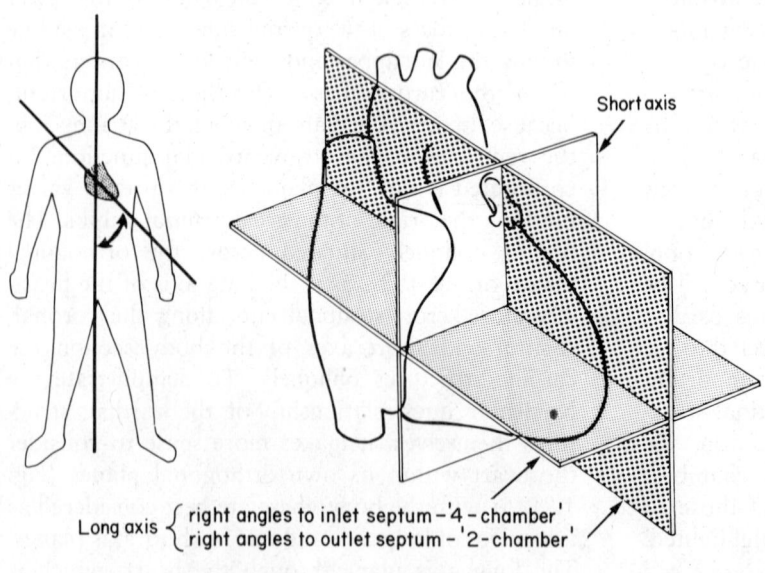

Short axis

Long axis { right angles to inlet septum – '4 – chamber'
            right angles to outlet septum – '2 – chamber'

ORTHOGONAL PLANES OF HEART

Fig. 1.2. Diagram showing how the heart has its own orthogonal planes which are at a considerable angle relevant to the orthogonal planes of the body.

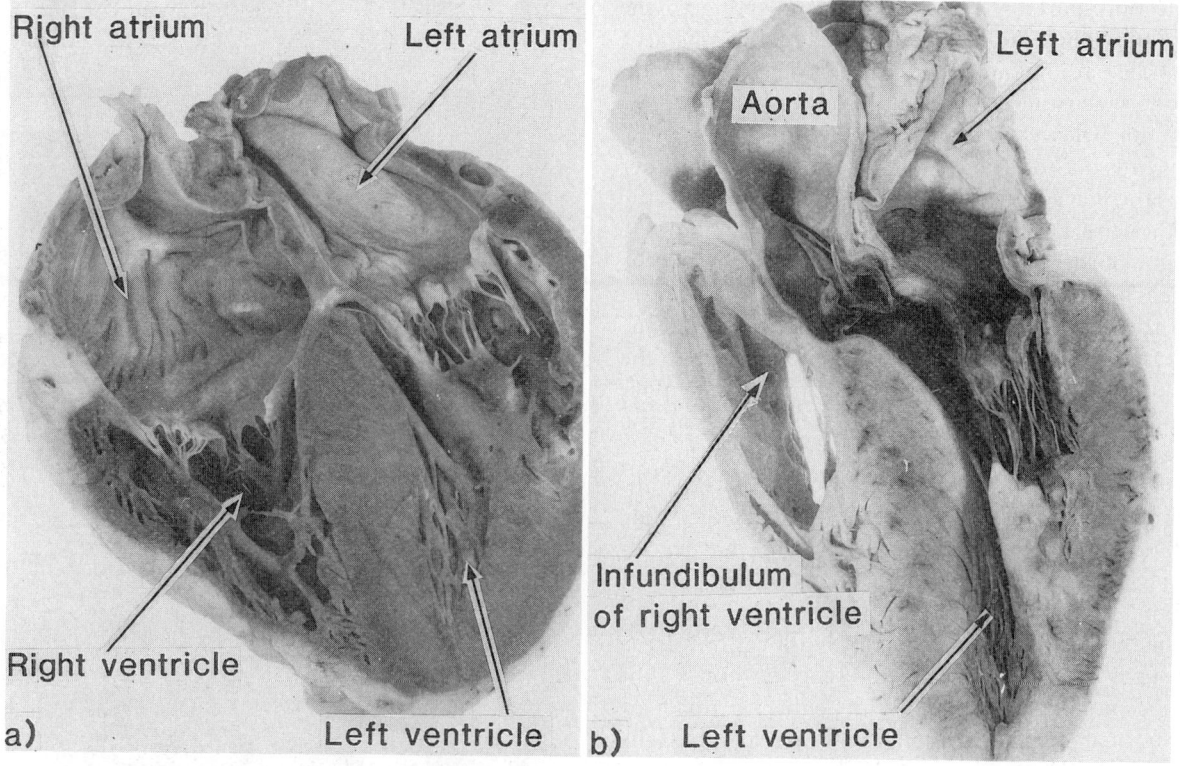

Fig. 1.3. Characteristic long axis planes of the heart (a) at right angles to the inlets (so-called four chamber plane) and (b) at right angles to the outlets. Although the latter plane is more-or-less a two chamber one, the spiralling outflow tracts result in part of the right ventricle being incorporated within the section.

tion shows that the heart occupies the area which anatomists call the middle mediastinum. This is surprising, as the anterior margin of the cardiac mass seen in this silhouette is directly applied to the chest wall. More superiorly, the base of the heart and the atriums recede from the wall, although there are no major structures to be found in the anterior mediastinum apart from the thymus. In contrast, several important structures descend through the posterior mediastinum, notably the oesophagus and the descending aorta. It is the intimate relationship between the left atrium (the most posterior part of the heart) and the oesophagus that gives the lateral projection its most significant clinical value. Radiographs taken in lateral projection with a barium-filled oesophagus can demonstrate enlargement of the left atrium.

There is considerably more information to be derived from the frontal projection of the cardiac silhouette, as this is the one seen most regularly in the chest radiograph. The diameter of the cardiac shadow in health and at its widest makes up less than half the diameter of the thoracic cage, so this ratio is a useful guide for estimating enlargement of

the heart. More importantly, knowledge of the nature of the chambers making up the margins of the silhouette permits inferences to be drawn when the outline itself is abnormal. The top of the silhouette is formed by the aortic arch bending back on itself, having sprung from the middle of the base to descend in left-sided position. Right-sided rather than left-sided descent of the aortic arch can readily be distinguished in the normal chest radiograph. An indentation is seen on the left border of the shadow below the bulge of the aortic knob, and then a second bulge is visible behind the second left costal cartilage. This second impression is formed by the pulmonary trunk which, although a component of the right heart, springs from the left border of the cardiac silhouette. This bulge is enhanced when the pulmonary trunk is enlarged (as, for example, in pulmonary hypertension). Conversely, the bulge is replaced by a concavity when the trunk is underdeveloped or atretic as occurs frequently in the presence of cyanotic congenital heart disease. In the normal silhouette, the area of the pulmonary trunk is reinforced by the left atrial appendage although not so much as to provide a visible feature. This is the only part of the left atrium projecting to the frontal silhouette. An unusual shadow in this area can be pathognomonic for herniation of the appendage when there is partial absence of the pericardium. Below the pulmonary knob, the shadow extends out to the apex and is formed by the border of the left ventricle. The inferior border of the silhouette then runs along the diaphragm to the right border of the sternum and is formed by the right ventricle and atrium, respectively. The right border then peeps out just beyond the border of the sternum and is made up of the right atrium with the superior and inferior caval veins joining at its upper and lower extremities. The precise shape of the silhouette changes not only in the setting of disease, as discussed above, but also varies among individuals. Tall and thin people have elongated cardiac shadows whereas short and squat people have fatter ones. The shape also changes in the presence of some congenital diseases of heart and lungs and some acquired ones. An abnormal location of the heart is a good guide to the presence of disease, but it is not a diagnosis. With either cardiac or pulmonary abnormalities, the heart can be left-sided, mid-line or right-sided. The orientation of the apex can be to the left, to the middle or to the right.

Of equal significance to the location of the cardiac chambers relative to the frontal shadow is knowledge of the position of the four valves. All four are located within the single plane referred to previously as the base. This plane drops obliquely from the left upper to the right lower border of the silhouette. The view that the anatomist tends to show of these valves, taken from their atrial aspect (Fig. 1.4, lower), is important for understanding cardiac anatomy but does not give a good indication of their position within space. The pulmonary valve is the most superior, the most leftward and the most anterior of the four valves (Fig. 1.4, upper). It is situated almost horizontally at the left upper border of the shadow. From it, the other three valves cascade down to the tricuspid valve which is rightward, inferior but again anterior. Between the two right-sided valves, but located more posteriorly within the heart (see Fig. 1.4b), are the aortic and mitral valves, the aortic valve being located more superiorly. The key to understanding this complex arrangement is the central location of the aortic valve within the cardiac base, wedged deeply between the mitral and tricuspid valves yet positioned immediately behind the pulmonary valve.

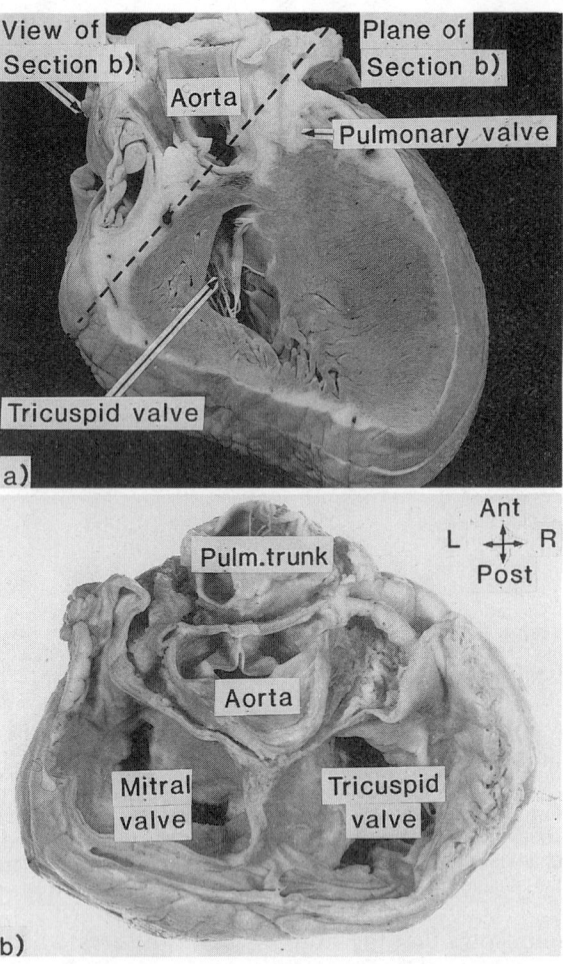

Fig. 1.4. The upper panel (a) shows how the pulmonary valve is the most superior and leftward of the cardiac valves. The lower panel (b) shows the short axis of the cardiac base from a different heart viewed from its atrial aspect. Note the 'wedged' position of the aortic valve. (Fig. 1.4a is reproduced by kind permission of Professor Anton Becker.)

RELATIONSHIPS OF THE HEART

Located in its mediastinal position, the heart has significant relations to most of the important thoracic organs or to the conduits that pass to and from the abdomen. In this respect, it is more accurate to state that the pericardium has these relationships, because the heart is tightly encased within the pericardial sack. Arguably, this is the heart's most important relationship. Considered developmentally, the pericardium consists of a tough outer sack* (the fibrous pericardium) and a finer double membranous layer (the serous pericardium). In reality, the two layers of serous pericardium (the parietal and visceral components) are

* Anglicized version of sac.

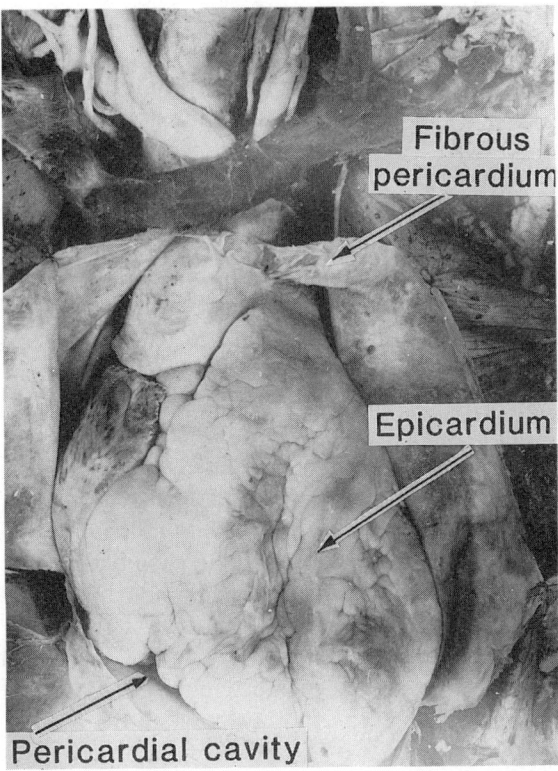

Fig. 1.5. The opened pericardial cavity, showing how the space is between the fibrous pericardium and the epicardium, the opposing surfaces of these layers being the two components of the serous pericardium.

fused with the fibrous pericardium and the surface of the heart, respectively (Fig. 1.5). The pericardial cavity, in consequence, lies between the fibrous wall of the sack (itself a composite of fibrous and parietal serous pericardial layers) and the epicardium (the visceral layer of the serous membrane). This tough fibrous sack which encloses the mass of the heart has been accurately and graphically characterized as the cardiac seat-belt. Inferiorly, it is firmly adherent to the upper surface of the diaphragm, providing fixation for the cardiac structures. The sack is closed at the base of the heart by fusion of the fibrous pericardium to the adventitial linings of the various venous and arterial trunks that enter and leave the heart. These fibrous junctions extend along the vessels for a short distance away from the heart. In contrast, the serous layer is reflected back from the epicardium at the margins of the heart chambers. It is customary to describe two compartments within the overall pericardial cavity. One of these is of considerable surgical significance, because it provides a track within the overall cavity at the site of the inner heart curvature. This is known as the transverse sinus; it lies between the posterior aspect of the arterial pedicle and the anterior interatrial wall (Fig. 1.6a). The other component is simply the recess in the postero-inferior surface of the cardiac cradle between the left pulmonary veins to one side and the right pulmonary and the caval

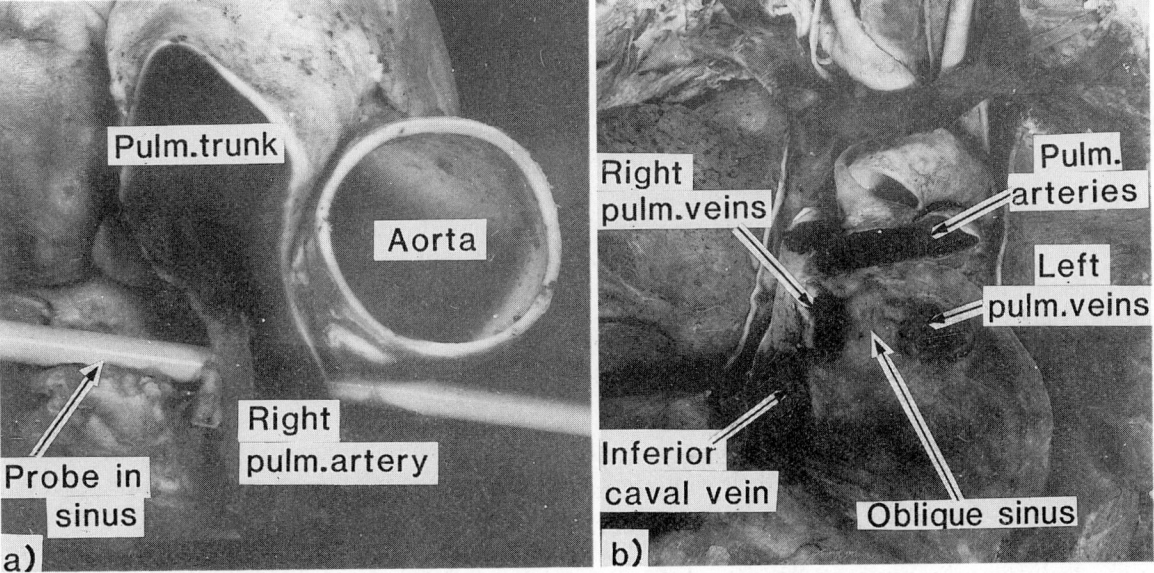

Fig. 1.6. The two sinuses within the pericardium: (a) the transverse sinus lies between the great arteries and the atriums; and (b) the oblique sinus lies posteriorly between the orifices of the right and left pulmonary veins.

veins to the other (Fig. 1.6b). This pouch, known as the oblique sinus, is of clinical significance because it is relatively indistensible and, therefore, it tends not to expand in the presence of a pericardial effusion.

The major nerve trunks coursing through the mediastinum have important relationships to the pericardium. On each side, the phrenic nerve (accompanied by the pericardiacophrenic vessels) courses in front of the hilum of the lung whereas the vagus nerve passes posteriorly. The vagus nerves give off their important recurrent laryngeal branches in relation to the aortic arch and its own branches. Thus, the left nerve recurs round the arterial ligament and runs back along the trachea, whereas the right nerve turns at a much higher level around the right subclavian artery. The subclavian sympathetic loop (ansa subclavia) also turns round the right subclavian artery. The anterior surface of the pericardial sack at the cardiac base is itself covered by the thymus gland. This reticulo-endothelial organ, made up of two lobes joined by an isthmus, is at its most prominent during infancy. Thereafter, it regresses, becoming inconspicuous by adulthood. On either side, the heart within its pericardial sack is intimately related to the lungs, the left lung in particular because the cardiac apex occupies the corresponding notch within the left lung. The pulmonary vessels cross from heart to lung in the posterior aspects of the cardiac base. Also in this area, the trachea branches into its two bronchi which run into the lung together with the pulmonary vessels (see Fig. 1.12). The mode of tracheal branching is of some importance, because the distance from bifurcation to lungs is such that the left-sided bronchus is almost twice as long as the right. This disproportion in bronchial size is readily distinguished on penetrated radiographs of the chest, and is a much better guide to the arrangement of the thoracic organs than is lung lobation (almost always the morphologically right lung has three lobes whereas the left has only two). Without exception, the morphologically left bronchus is long and the morphologically right is short. As will be shown (see Chapter 25), this arrangement is crucial in diagnosis of those infants and children with congenitally malformed hearts who have gross abnormalities in the arrangement of their thoracic and abdominal organs (so-called 'splenic syndromes'). It is also important to note that the inferior caval vein normally pierces the diaphragm to the right side of the spine whereas the aorta descends from thorax to abdomen in left-sided

position. In reaching this left-sided location, the aorta ascends from the cardiac base and arches over the left bronchus. This is the criterion for definition of a left aortic arch rather than the position of the descending aorta. The oesophagus runs down, along the spine, immediately behind the left atrium. As discussed previously, this means that barium within the oesophagus can outline the size of the left atrium. The oesophagus also provides a portal whereby an echocardiographic transducer can be brought into immediate contact with the heart chambers.

THE STRUCTURE OF THE HEART

In this section the important structural characteristics of the atrial and ventricular chambers of the heart together with the aortic and pulmonary arterial pathways will be discussed. As the major venous channels connect directly to the atrial chambers, they will be included in the description of atrial morphology.

THE MORPHOLOGICALLY RIGHT ATRIUM

The term 'morphologically' has been used several times in this chapter. The reason for this will become more obvious in Chapter 25. The chamber with the morphological characteristics associated with the structure seen in the normal heart does not always occupy its anticipated position. For example, in the individual with complete mirror-image arrangement of the organs (so-called 'situs inversus'), the chamber with the morphological characteristics of the normal right atrium is found in left-sided position. Because of this, it is most accurately described as the *morphologically* right atrium. The same can be applied to the other chambers. In this chapter, such detail is unnecessary, because only the normal heart is being described. However, it should be noted that, whenever the adjective 'right' or 'left' is applied to a cardiac chamber, it denotes morphological rightness or leftness.

Applying these considerations to the right atrium, it occupies the right and anterior portion of the heart, receiving the superior and inferior caval veins at its upper and lower extremities (Fig. 1.7). The superior caval vein is formed by fusion of the right and left brachiocephalic veins, which in turn are formed by union on each side of the subclavian and jugular veins. These various venous channels are the

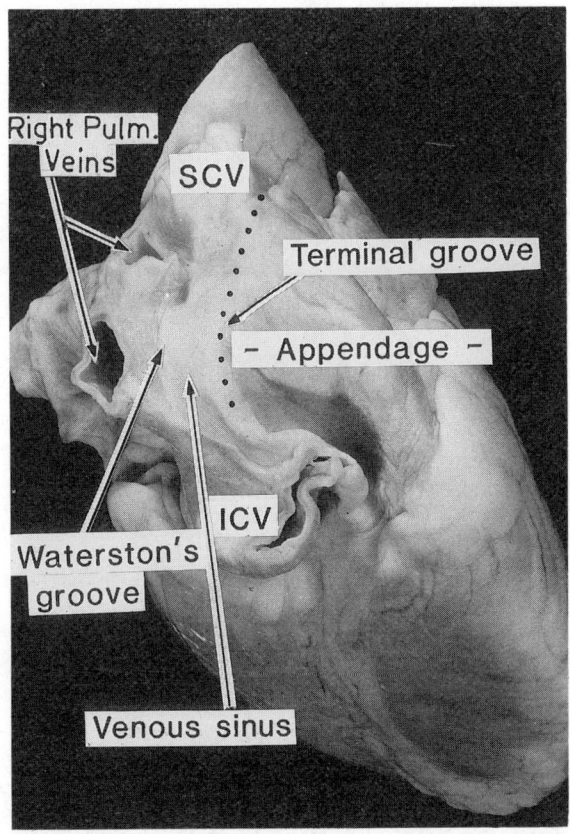

Fig. 1.7. View of the heart taken from the right and posteriorly showing the cavo-atrial junctions and the site of the terminal and Waterston's grooves. (Reproduced by kind permission of Professor Anton Becker.)

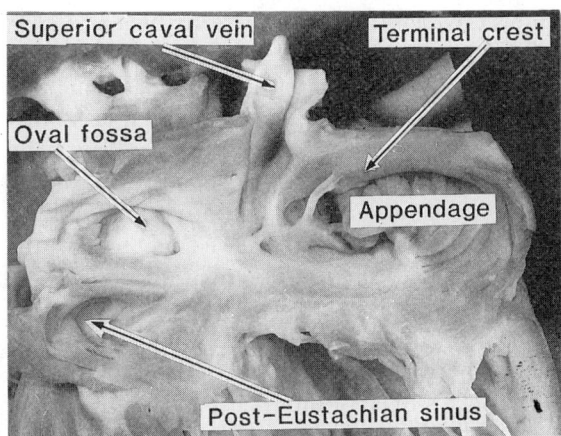

Fig. 1.8. The internal aspect of the right atrium seen through a posterior incision.

most anterior structures found within the superior mediastinum. The inferior caval vein, in contrast, has a particularly truncated course within the thorax, entering the right atrium almost as soon as it has pierced the diaphragm. The two caval veins join to form the posterior, smooth-walled, venous component of the right atrium. When viewed from behind, this venous portion can be seen to be separated from its neighbouring structures by two grooves. The right-sided and anterior groove is more prominent and is situated laterally at the right margin of the atrial chamber. This groove, the terminal groove ('sulcus terminalis'), separates the venous component of the right atrium from its prominent appendage. The appendage is much redder than the whitish venous sinus, because it has multiple trabeculations on its inner aspect. These trabeculations take origin from a prominent bar of muscle marking the internal aspect of the terminal groove (Fig. 1.8). The muscle bar is described as the terminal crest ('crista terminalis'); the muscles, owing to their comb-like appearance, are known as

pectinate muscles. When viewed externally, the appendage has a characteristic blunt and triangular shape, with the terminal groove forming the exterior base of the triangle (Fig. 1.9). It is this arrangement of the appendage that is the best marker of morphological rightness of the atrial chamber. The other groove demarcating the external extent of the venous component of the right atrium is left-sided, and separates it from the left

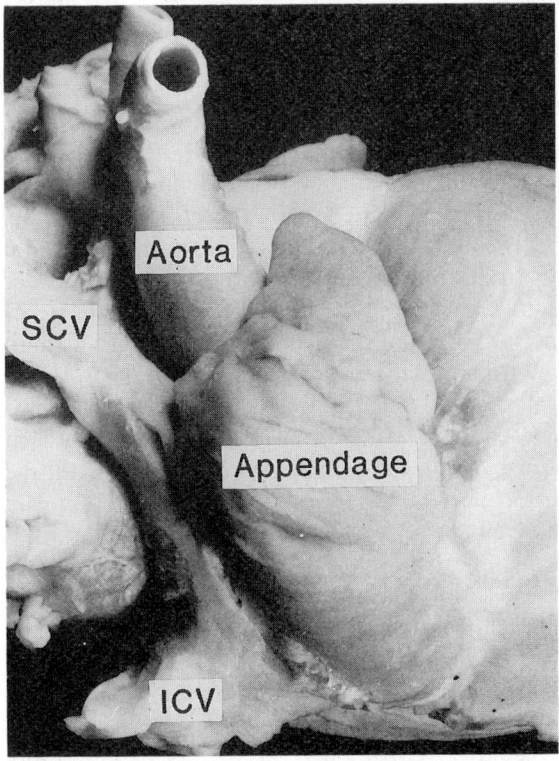

Fig. 1.9. The lateral aspect of the right atrium showing the characteristic shape of the appendage.

atrium. It is most obvious superiorly, where it is an infolding of the atrial roof between the right pulmonary veins and the superior caval vein. It is known as Waterston's groove. Although it is often considered to represent the atrial septum, it is really an infolding of the atrial walls, and it can be dissected for a considerable distance prior to reaching its base. When viewed internally, the predominant feature of the right atrium is the terminal crest marking the junction of the smooth venous and the trabeculated appendage components of the atrium. The floor of the atrium is taken up by the vestibule of the tricuspid valve, which is dealt with most appropriately as a ventricular component. The rest of the atrium is made up of the 'septal' surface, which appears to be an extensive area. Careful dissection shows that this appearance is deceptive (Fig. 1.10). The true atrial septum (that part of the wall separating the cavities of the right and left atrial chambers) is limited in its extent, being confined to the floor and immediate surrounds of the oval fossa ('fossa ovalis'). The fossa functions during fetal life as a communication to convey to the left atrium the richly oxygenated blood entering the heart from the placenta via the umbilical vein, the venous duct ('ductus venosus') and the inferior caval vein. As such, it is situated immediately opposite the orifice of the inferior vein. Often, a thin fold of tissue extends from the terminal crest as a curtain to deflect blood away from the tricuspid valve and towards the oval fossa. This fold, the Eustachian valve, is best developed during fetal life and regresses gradually with ageing. Its insertion into the terminal crest usually persists and is continued along the inferior rim of the oval fossa. This muscle rim also forms the upper border of the coronary sinus, which opens at the postero-inferior corner of the 'septal' surface of the atrium. Only the muscle rim separating its origin from the oval fossa is a true septal structure. The sinus is also guarded by a valve (the Thebesian valve) which springs from the muscle rim. It fuses with the Eustachian valve and, from their junction, an important structure then runs forward to bury itself in the inferior rim of the oval fossa. This structure, composed of fibrous tissue, runs through the atrial musculature to reach the fibrous skeleton of the heart in the aortic root. It is the tendon of Todaro. Inferior to the tendon of Todaro, the atrial musculature runs down to insert into the septal leaflet of the tricuspid valve. Although this area is unequivocally septal, it is not part of the atrial septum since the mitral valve leaflets are attached more proximally

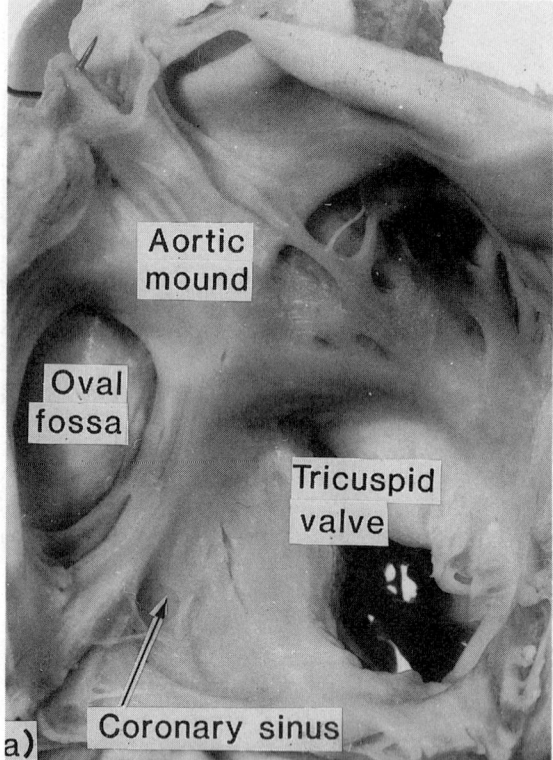

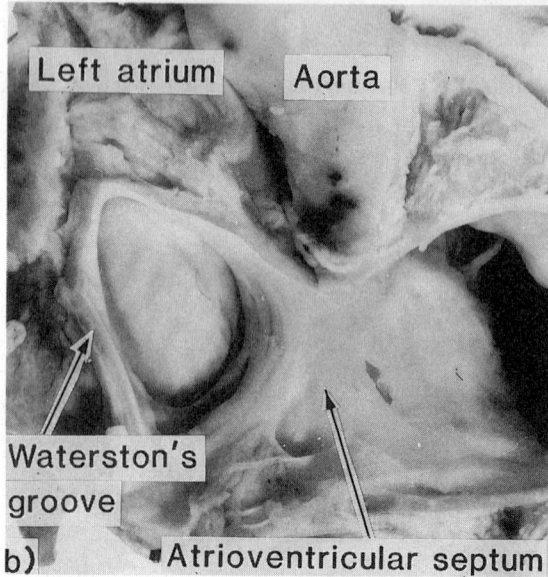

Fig. 1.10. Views of the right atrium before (a) and after (b) the removal of non-septal wall, showing the minimal extent of the true septum.

than those of the tricuspid valve. As a consequence, the atrial and ventricular structures overlap obliquely, producing the muscular component of the atrioventricular septum (see below). The atrial aspect of this area is important because it contains the atrioventricular node. The area is demarcated by a triangle having as its base the orifice of the coronary sinus. The tendon of Todaro, together with the attachment of the tricuspid valve, form the sides that join at the apex. The triangle is known eponymously for Koch (Fig. 1.11). A broad sweep of atrial wall is seen antero-superiorly relative to the apex. This also seems to be 'septal', but is simply the wall surrounding the centrally located aortic root. It is well described as the aortic mound. In the roof of the atrium behind and above the mound can be seen the orifice of the superior caval vein. This is sandwiched between the terminal crest and the superior rim of the oval fossa. As described, the superior rim is often considered to be septal. Rather, it is the infolded wall marking the site of Waterston's groove. The true atrial septum is the smooth floor of the oval fossa together with its immediate rim. The terminal crest swings round anteriorly to become continuous with the superior rim. Often a conspicuous muscular trabeculation extends at right angles from this junctional area into the roof of the atrial appendage. This is simply one of the pectinate muscles. It is not septal and is correctly described as the 'septum spurium'. One further feature of the right atrium warrants description. It is the often extensive cavitation found in the postero-inferior corner of the atrium behind and beneath the coronary sinus. This is a simple diverticulum often described as the post-Eustachian sinus of Keith (Fig. 1.8).

THE MORPHOLOGICALLY LEFT ATRIUM

Although having the same components as the right atrium (venous portion, appendage and vestibule), the structure of the left atrium is much simpler. The

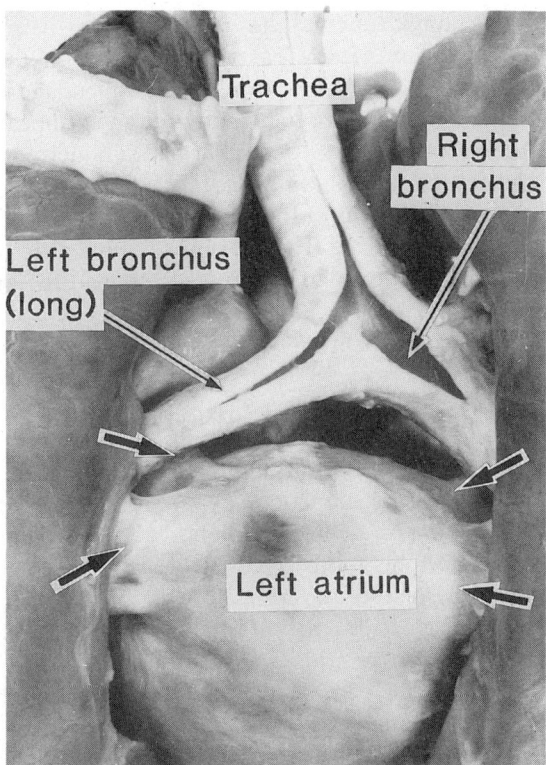

Fig. 1.12. The posterior aspect of the left atrium, showing the 'tethering' effect of the four pulmonary veins (arrows). Note the asymmetric arrangement of the bronchi.

venous component is the most posterior part of the heart, sitting between the bronchi and on top of the oesophagus, spine and descending aorta. It is tightly anchored by the entrance of the pulmonary vein at each of its four corners (Fig. 1.12). The lining is very smooth and leads directly into the vestibule supporting the mitral valve. The appendage has a narrow junction with the left upper margin of the

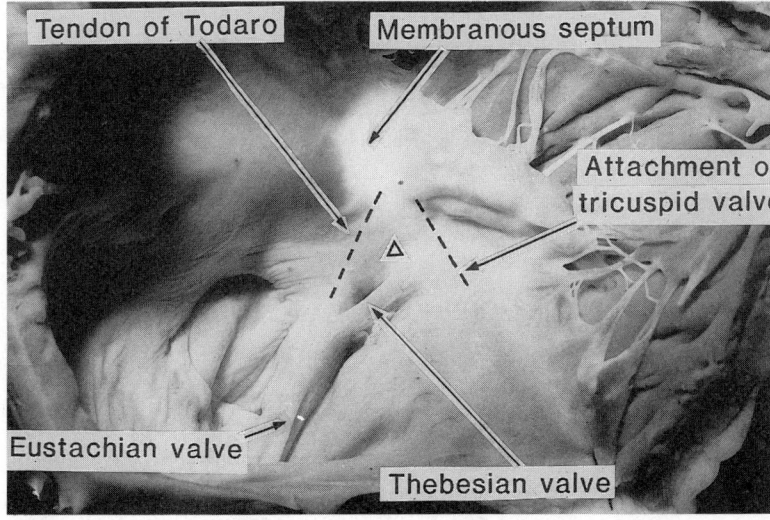

Fig. 1.11. The septal aspect of the right atrium with transillumination of the membranous septum showing the landmarks of the triangle of Koch. (Reproduced by kind permission of Professor Anton Becker.)

venous compartment, the junction not being marked by any muscle bar comparable with the terminal crest of the right atrium. The appendage is itself tubular and narrow, hooking round to appear on the anterior surface of the cardiac silhouette to the left of the pulmonary trunk (Fig. 1.13). Almost all the trabeculations of the left atrium are confined within the appendage. The left surface of the atrium is wrinkled and overlaps the rim of the oval fossa, such that no evidence is seen of the fossa from the left atrial aspect.

THE ATRIOVENTRICULAR JUNCTION

Although not manifest as an area in its own right, the atrioventricular junction is so significant to the understanding of cardiac anatomy that it warrants separate consideration. The region can be well studied by isolating the 'rings' of the four cardiac valves. This is easily achieved by removing the atrial chambers and great arteries at the base and sectioning across the ventricular mass. The junctional segment remaining can then be studied from its atrial and ventricular aspects. The atrial view (Fig. 1.14a) clearly shows how the aortic valve is deeply wedged between the mitral and tricuspid valves, at the same time separating the pulmonary and tricuspid orifices. Removal of the leaflets of the aortic valve (Fig. 1.14b) demonstrates the deep posterior extension of the outflow tract which 'lifts' the mitral valve such that only a small part of the left atrioventricular junction abuts against the ventricular septum. In reality, because the tricuspid valve is attached more distally in this area, it constitutes a muscular atrioventricular septum (Fig. 1.15). The atrioventricular node is buried within the atrial

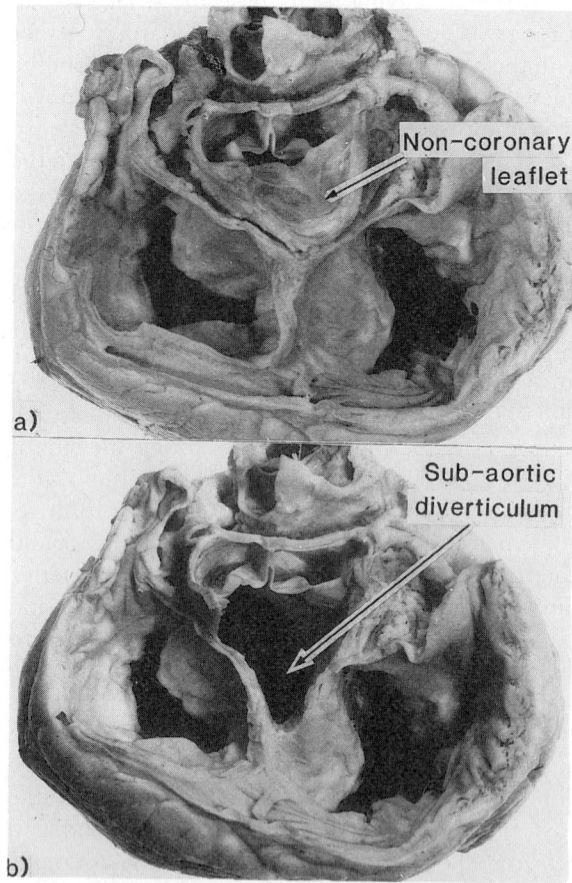

Fig. 1.14. The atrial view of the cardiac short axis (see Fig. 1.4) before (a) and after (b) the removal of the non-coronary leaflet of the aortic valve.

surface of this septal area. Forming the medial wall of the posterior extension of the left ventricular outflow tract is another atrioventricular septum, which is fibrous (Fig. 1.16). This is part of the membranous septum, itself a component of the central fibrous body, the keystone of the cardiac skeleton. The atrial view of the junctional region shows well the arrangement of the leaflets of the various valves. This is seen also from the ventricular aspect, notably the fibrous continuity between aortic and mitral valves in contrast to the separation of the tricuspid and pulmonary valves (Fig. 1.17).

THE MORPHOLOGICALLY RIGHT VENTRICLE

Although conventionally described in terms of 'sinus' and 'conus' (or inflow and outflow tracts), it is more sensible to describe the ventricles in terms of three components, namely the inlet, apical trabecular and outlet portions. These radiate around the area of the membranous septum (Fig. 1.18). The

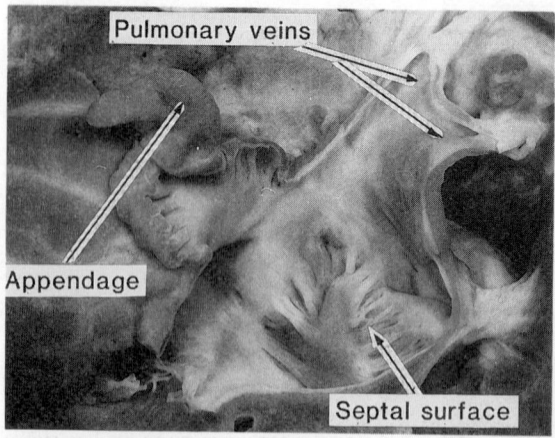

Fig. 1.13. The internal aspect of the left atrium, showing the characteristic septal appearance and the shape of the appendage.

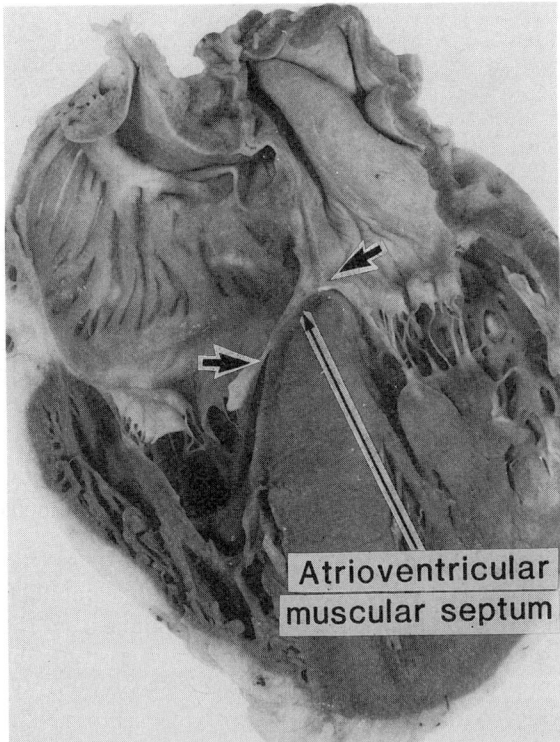

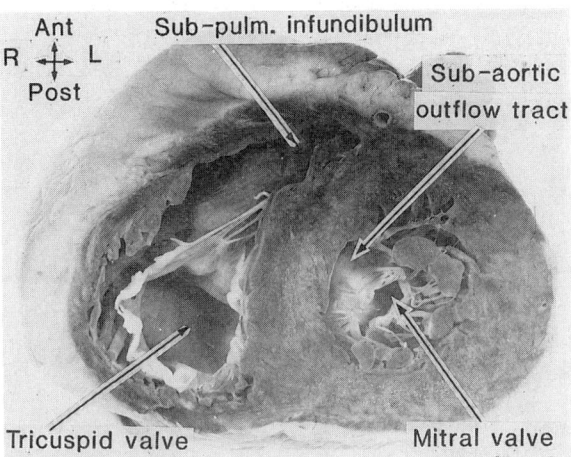

Fig. 1.17. Short axis section through the ventricular mass viewed from the ventricular aspect.

inlet component surrounds and supports the tricuspid valve, extending from the atrioventricular junction to the insertion of the papillary muscles. The valve has three leaflets situated in septal, antero-superior and inferior (or mural) positions. The septal leaflet is supported distally by multiple cords attached to the inlet part of the ventricular septum (Fig. 1.19). The extent of this 'inlet' septum is deceptive because, as a consequence of the wedged

Fig. 1.15. Four chamber section through the heart showing the muscular component of the atrioventricular septum as a consequence of offsetting (arrows) of the septal attachments of the atrioventricular valves.

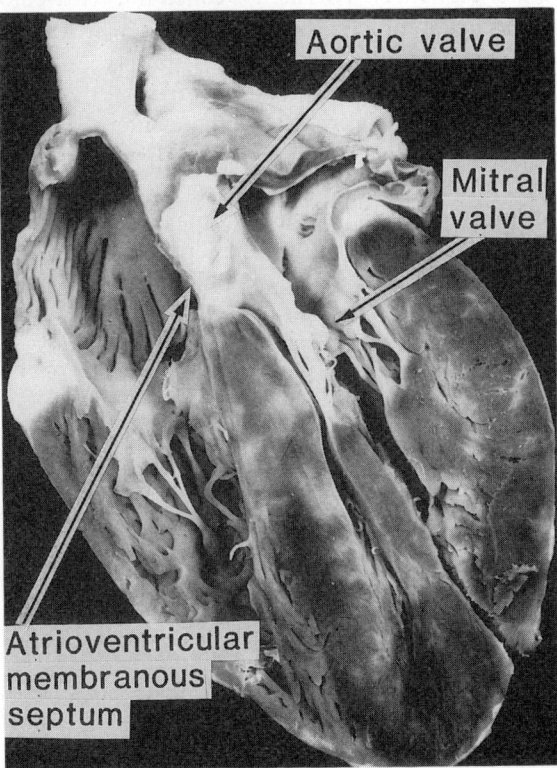

Fig. 1.16. Four chamber section showing the membranous component of the atrioventricular septum.

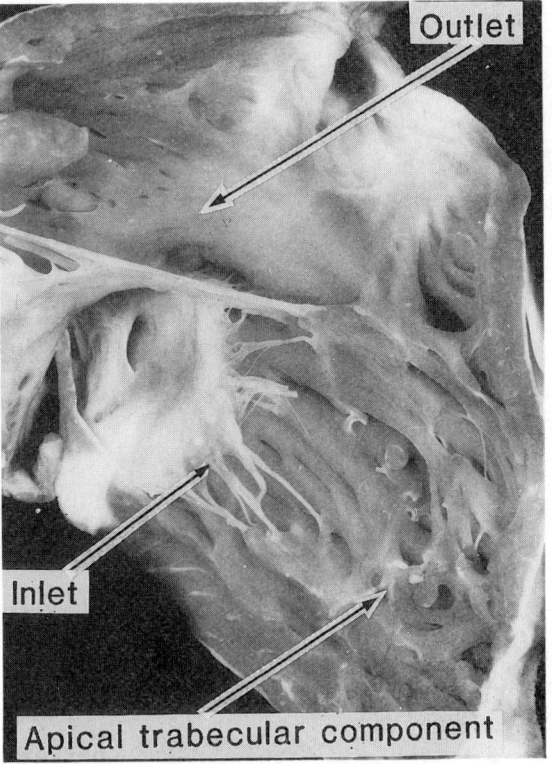

Fig. 1.18. The right ventricle opened to show its component parts.

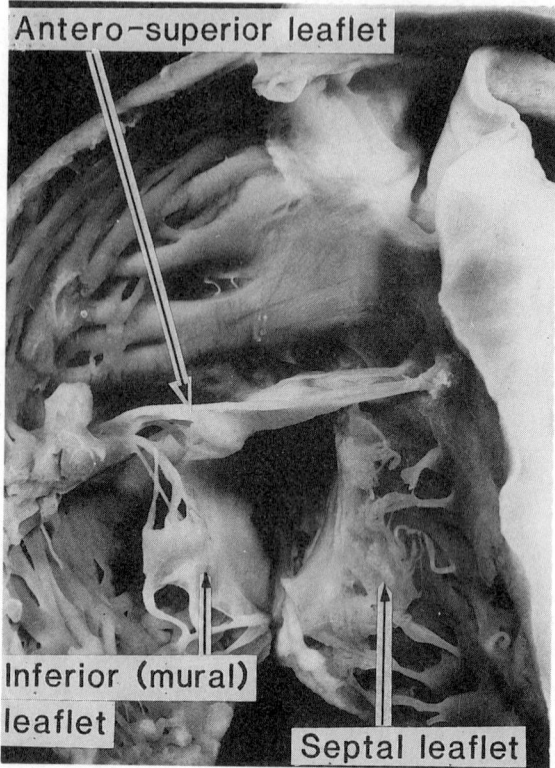

Fig. 1.19. The leaflets of the tricuspid valve viewed from their ventricular aspect.

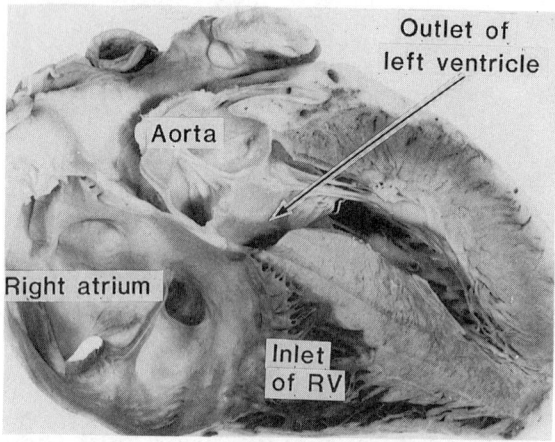

Fig. 1.20. Oblique section through the inlet of the right ventricle to show how the septum separates this component from the outlet of the left ventricle.

sub-aortic outflow tract, it mostly separates inlet of right ventricle from outlet of left (Fig. 1.20). The commissure between the septal and antero-superior leaflets is supported by the medial papillary muscle complex. Used in a morphological sense, the term 'commissure' describes the point at which the breaches in the skirts of leaflet tissue of the valves reach their circumferential and marginal attachments. This is the case for both atrioventricular and arterial valves. In the case of the atrioventricular valves, this point is supported by characteristic fan-shaped cords from the tips of the prominent papillary muscles. The point of insertion of these fan-shaped commissural cords is then taken by the morphologist as the criterion for the site of the commissure. However, the word commissure means a site of junction. In functional terms, the commissures in the valves could be considered as the lines of apposition of the leaflets during ventricular systole (for the atrioventricular valves) or diastole (for the arterial valves). Such 'commissures' would exist for only part of the cardiac cycle, whereas the point defined by the morphologist is present throughout the cardiac cycle as a junction between adjacent leaflets. The antero-septal commissure, as defined in this morphological sense, is supported by

commissural cords arising from the medial papillary muscle complex, these muscles springing from the posterior aspect of an extensive muscle strap, the septomarginal trabeculation, or 'septal band', which reinforces the surface of the septum. The antero-superior leaflet is dependent from the inner heart curvature, this latter structure being seen as a muscle bar separating the tricuspid and pulmonary valves (Fig. 1.21). This area is called the ventriculo-infundibular fold. The inferior leaflet, which is the least conspicuous, takes origin from the parietal component of the right atrioventricular junction. The commissure between it and the antero-superior leaflet is supported by a prominent papillary muscle, the apical or anterior muscle, which takes origin from the apical part of the septomarginal trabeculation. The commissure with the septal leaflet springs from the inferior papillary muscle.

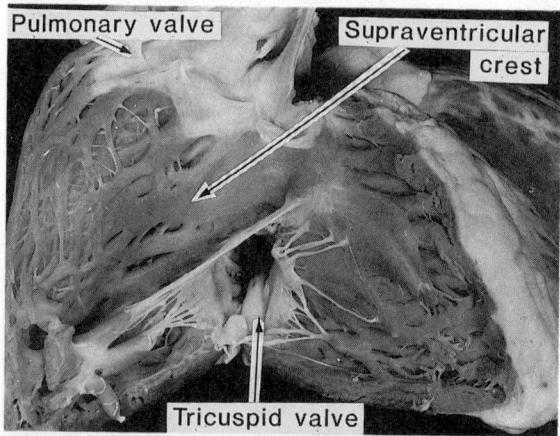

Fig. 1.21. This preparation reveals the extensive supraventricular crest of the right ventricle separating the tricuspid and pulmonary valves.

The apical trabecular component is the most characteristic part of the right ventricle, having much coarser trabeculations than the corresponding zone of the left ventricle. Its septal surface is dominated by the septomarginal trabeculation which runs up into the outlet component. The outlet portion itself, the infundibulum, is a complete sleeve of muscle which supports the leaflets of the pulmonary valve. Part of this muscular funnel is often described as 'septal', although very little, if any, of the musculature separates the cavities of the right and left ventricles. Indeed, the entire sleeve of sub-pulmonary infundibulum can be removed as a free-standing structure (Fig. 1.22). The extensive area separating the tricuspid and pulmonary valves in the ventricular roof (the supraventricular crest or 'crista supraventricularis') is almost exclusively made up of the ventriculo-infundibular fold. It is fallacious to think of the pulmonary valve as having a 'ring' or annulus. The anatomy of both arterial valves is conditioned by the semilunar attachments of the leaflets. In the case of the pulmonary valve, these simply take origin from the muscular outlet component (Fig. 1.21). The zeniths of commissural attachment extend onto the fibrous wall of the pulmonary trunk. The uppermost extent of the infundibulum is thus of tricorn pattern and bounded by the fibrous arterial wall rather than pulmonary infundibular musculature. A similar arrangement is seen in the sub-aortic outflow tract (see below).

THE MORPHOLOGICALLY LEFT VENTRICLE

Like the right ventricle, the left ventricle has three components, although their arrangement is fun-

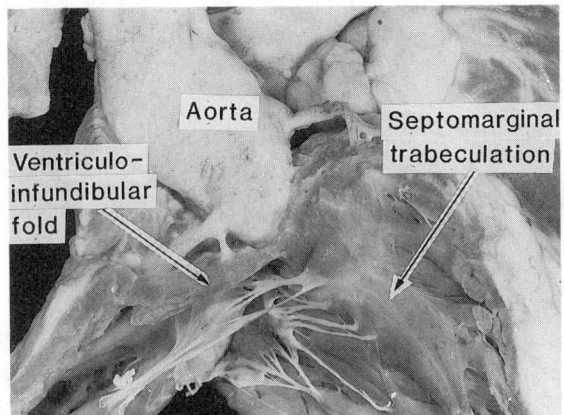

Fig. 1.22. This dissection of the heart seen in Fig. 1.21 shows how virtually all of the sub-pulmonary infundibulum can be removed without touching the left ventricle.

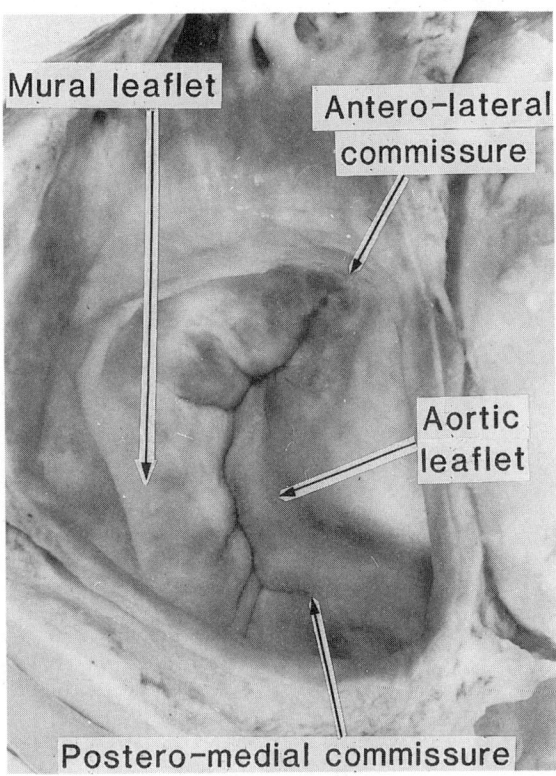

Fig. 1.23. The left atrial aspect of the mitral valve, to show the extent of circumferential attachment of the mural and aortic leaflets.

damentally different. The inlet component surrounds the leaflets of the mitral valve, extending from the atrioventricular junction to the insertion of the papillary muscles. Unlike the right ventricular arrangement, the inlet overlaps the outlet because of the deeply wedged location of the aortic valve (Fig. 1.17). The characteristic feature of the left ventricle is the fibrous continuity between aortic and mitral valves together with the complete lack of attachment of papillary muscles to the ventricular septum. The mitral valve has two leaflets of markedly different appearance. They take up one- and two-thirds of the annular circumference, respectively (Fig. 1.23). The shorter leaflet has considerably more depth when compared with the longer leaflet which is more shallow (Fig. 1.24). The longer leaflet is divided into subunits (usually three) which are termed 'scallops'. There are problems in naming the leaflets because they are neither anterior nor posterior, nor is one leaflet 'septal'. It is most accurate to call them *mural* and *aortic*, respectively, because one is attached to the parietal junction whereas the other is in fibrous continuity with the aortic valve. The commissures between the leaflets are supported by paired papillary muscles located postero-

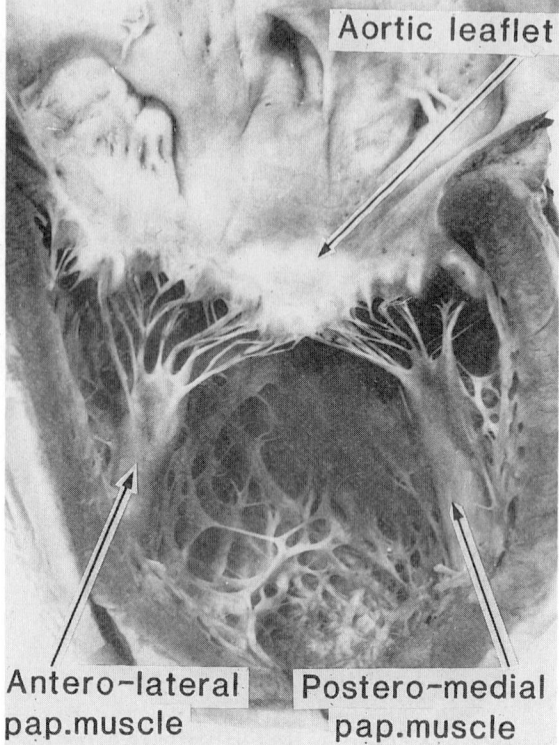

Fig. 1.24. The structure of the mitral valve demonstrated by 'spreading' a posterior incision through the atrioventricular junction.

medially and antero-laterally. The apical trabecular part of the left ventricle is much more finely trabeculated than that of the right ventricle and has a particularly smooth septal surface, in distinction to the coarser right ventricle with the septomarginal trabeculation. The morphology of the outlet component of the left ventricle is conditioned by the semilunar attachments of the three leaflets of the aortic valve. These are attached in part to muscle and in part to the fibrous skeleton of the heart. This is primarily composed of the area of the fibrous continuity between the aortic and mitral valves, thickened at each end to give the right and left fibrous trigones. The right trigone is then incorporated with the membranous part of the septum to give the central fibrous body. This forms the roof and right-sided border of the extensive posterior extension of the left ventricular outflow tract. Within the outflow tract, the apices of the semilunar attachments are considerably higher than the troughs. Indeed, as with the sub-pulmonary outlet, the tips of the commissures are attached in tricorn fashion to the aortic wall rather than to the ventricular myocardium. At each commissure, there is then a small triangular area through which the left ventricular outflow tract is in potential communication with the pericardial cavity (Figs. 1.25–1.27). The posterior triangle is located along the region of aortic–mitral continuity. Incisions through the triangle provide the facility for posterior enlargement of the sub-aortic area by the surgeon. The apex of this triangle separates the left ventricular outlet from the transverse sinus of the pericardium (Fig. 1.26a). The medial fibrous triangle, located between the right coronary and non-coronary leaflets of the aortic valves, is an integral part of the central fibrous body. Its base is part of the interventricular membranous septum. It is crossed on its right ventricular aspect by the insertion of the ventriculo-infundibular fold. The apex of the triangle separates the cavity of the left ventricle from the right margin of the transverse

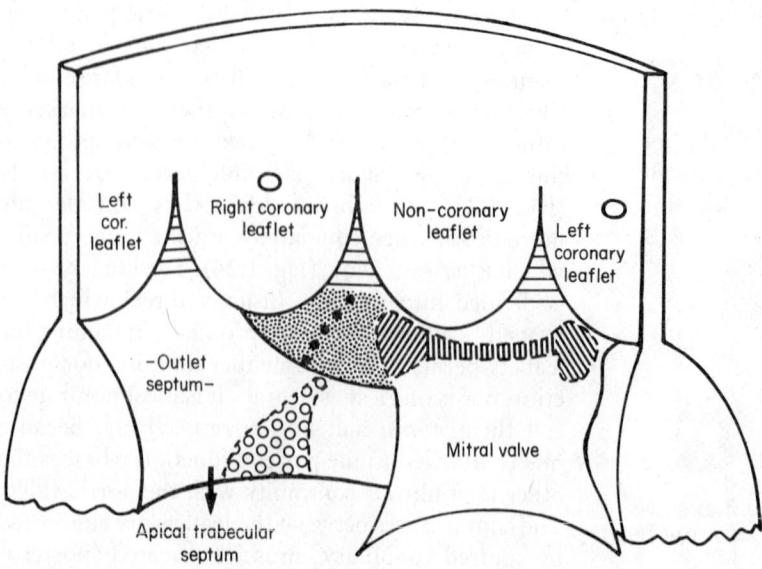

Fig. 1.25. Diagram to show how the morphology of the sub-aortic outflow tract is conditioned by the semilunar attachment of the valve leaflets.

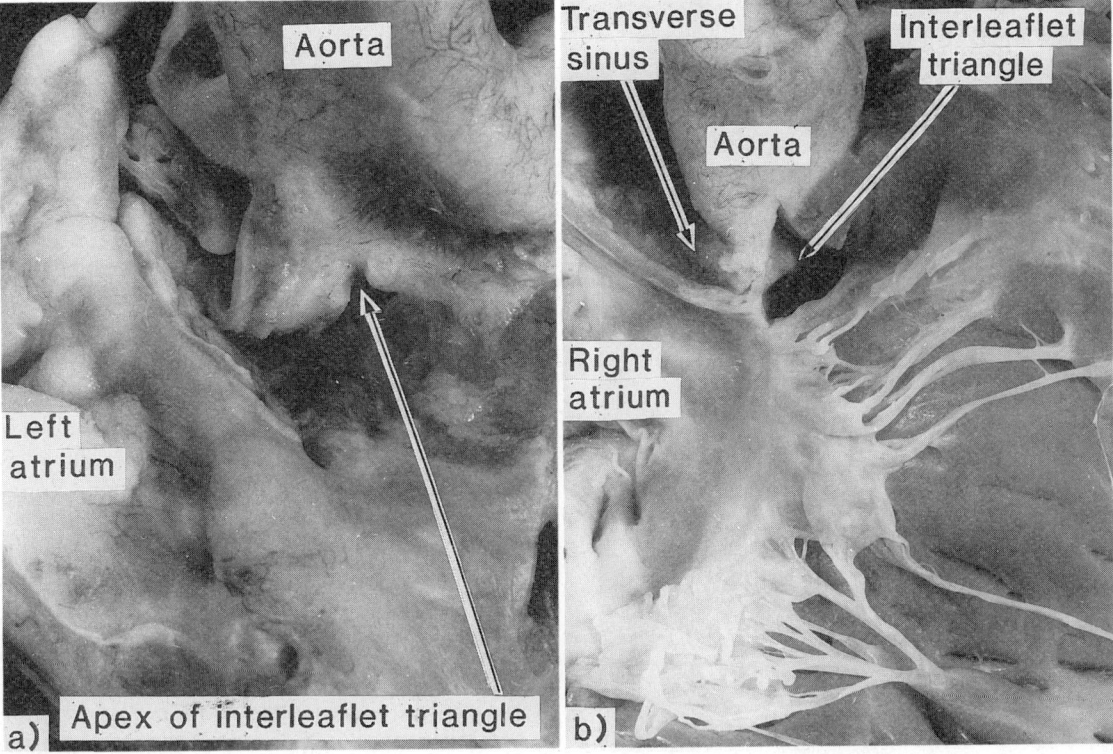

Fig. 1.26. This dissection of the interleaflet triangles between (a) the non- and left coronary leaflets and (b) the non- and right coronary leaflets shows how they separate the left ventricular outflow tract from the transverse sinus.

sinus (Fig. 1.26b). This area is intimately related to the origin and initial course of the right coronary artery. The third triangle, between the right and left coronary leaflets of the aortic valve, is of significance to the surgeon who undertakes an anterior enlargement of a restrictive sub-aortic outflow tract. The base of the triangle is supported by septal musculature. Deep incisions through this area reach the right ventricle. Incisions through the fibrous triangle lead to the tissue plane between the anterior surface of the aorta and the posterior aspect of the muscular sub-pulmonary infundibulum (Fig. 1.27). It is possible for the surgeon to make an incision from the apex of the left ventricle outlet between the right and left coronary leaflets and to reach the sub-pulmonary infundibulum. The incision passes outside the heart in order to connect the two ventricles.

THE ARTERIAL TRUNKS

Both arterial trunks commence at the sinuses of Valsalva, the expanded tricorn arrangements of the aortic and pulmonary walls that accommodate the arterial valve leaflets during ventricular systole. At the junction of the leaflets of the arterial valves with the ventricular myocardium, there is an abrupt change from the myocardial structure of the ventricle to the fibrous structure of the elastic arteries. As emphasized above, there is no 'ring' of collagen supporting the leaflets of the arterial valves. Instead both valve leaflets and arterial walls take origin from the ventricular myocardium (or the area of fibrous continuity in the case of the aortic valve). Furthermore, as described above, at the tips of the commissures between the leaflets part of the fibrous walls of the arterial trunks form boundaries of the outflow tracts of both right and left ventricles. At this point, the walls of the trunks separate the inside of the heart from the pericardial cavity. In reality, the sinuses together with the ventricular outflow tracts and the leaflets of the arterial valves constitute a 'complex' that must function in concert to ensure adequate opening and closure of the valves. This arterial valvar complex can be likened to the constellation of structures such as tension apparatus and papillary muscles recognized as being necessary for appropriate working of the atrioventricular valves.

At the top of the sinuses in both arterial trunks, there is a marked constriction which indicates the origin of the ascending portions of aorta and

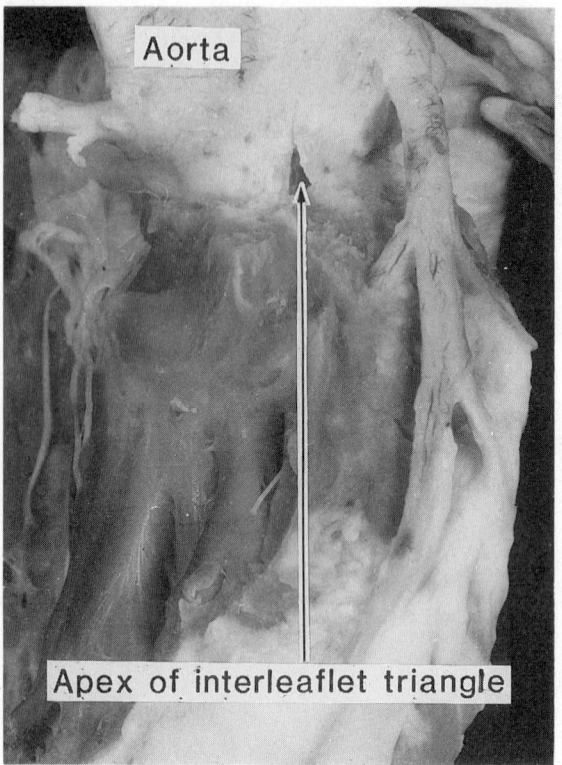

Fig. 1.27. Dissection of the interleaflet triangle between the two coronary leaflets of the aortic valve leads to the tissue space between the aorta and the pulmonary trunk.

pulmonary trunk. In the aorta, this circumferential structure is known as the aortic bar. The ascending portion of the aorta runs from this bar superiorly and slightly forwards toward the sternum with a mild inclination to the right. It is contained within the fibrous pericardium so its surface is covered by serous pericardium, the sleeve of pericardium encircling adjacent portions of both aorta and pulmonary trunk and forming posteriorly one border of the transverse sinus. The short ascending aortic component becomes the arch at the superior attachment of the pericardial reflection. The arch then continues to ascend for a short distance before giving rise to the brachiocephalic (innominate) artery. It then turns posteriorly and to the left, crossing the left bronchus, and giving rise superiorly to the left common carotid and subclavian arteries. The arch terminates on the left lateral aspect of the vertebral column where it turns inferiorly to become the descending aorta. Anteriorly at this position the aorta is tethered to the bifurcation of the pulmonary trunk by the arterial ligament, the fibrous remnant of the arterial duct ('ductus arteriosus'). The segment of aortic arch between the origin of the left subclavian artery and the insertion of the ligament is known as the isthmus. In the child and the adult, this segment is of comparable dimensions to the rest of the arch. During fetal life, it is narrower than the descending aorta. The recurrent laryngeal branch from the left vagus nerve passes round the arterial ligament before running superiorly along the trachea to supply the laryngeal musculature. On the right side, the comparable recurrent nerve turns around the right subclavian artery along with the sympathetic loop ('ansa subclavia'). The descending thoracic aorta continues down the left lateral aspect of the vertebral bodies gradually becoming more anterior before passing into the abdomen between the limbs of the diaphragm. Throughout its course, it gives off multiple branches to the thoracic organs along with the lower nine pairs of intercostal arteries. The upper two intercostal arteries are derived from branches of the subclavian arteries. The most significant branches to thoracic organs are probably the bronchial arteries, which may also arise from the underside of the aortic arch.

The pulmonary trunk is a short vessel completely contained within the pericardium and enclosed within the sleeve of serous pericardium, which also incorporates the ascending aorta. The arterial ligament marks the very end of the pulmonary trunk at the point where it bifurcates into right and left pulmonary arteries. These branches then extend on each side to enter the hilums* of the lungs. During fetal life, the arterial duct is the major flow pathway from pulmonary trunk to descending aorta, the pulmonary arteries then being relatively minor branches. All this, along with remodelling of the aortic isthmus, changes within the first six weeks or so of independent life.

THE CARDIAC SUB-SYSTEMS

THE CORONARY ARTERIES

The right and left coronary arteries are the first branches from the aorta. As there are almost always three aortic sinuses and only two coronary arteries, this permits the sinuses along with their arterial valve leaflets to be nominated as right coronary and left coronary, respectively. The third sinus, which does not carry a coronary artery, is then termed the non-coronary sinus. This convention circumvents the use of terms such as 'anterior' or 'posterior', which are invalidated in the normal heart because

* Anglicized version of hila.

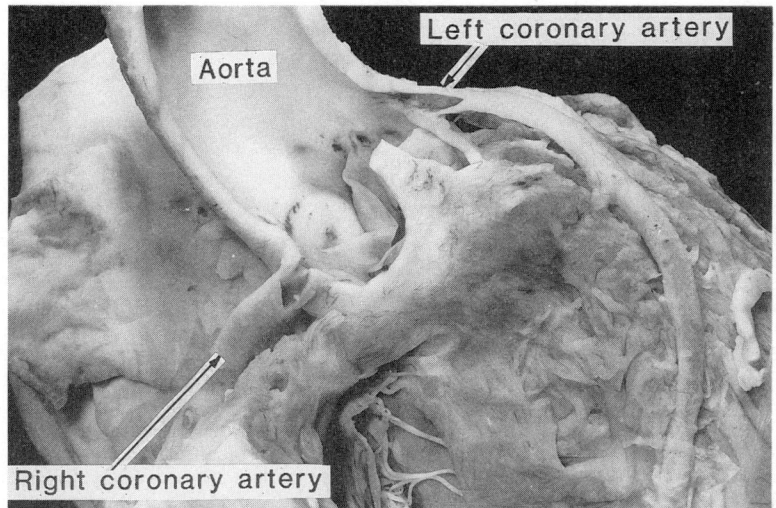

Fig. 1.28. This dissection of the aorta shows the origin of the coronary arteries from the sinuses of Valsalva. (Reproduced by kind permission of Professor Anton Becker.)

of the oblique location of the leaflets of the aortic valve. The coronary arteries almost always arise within the sinuses of Valsalva, i.e. below the aortic bar (Fig. 1.28). Origin from the ascending aorta is considered a minor congenital malformation of little clinical significance. Of more importance is an origin close to a commissure with oblique course of the artery through the aortic wall. The latter arrangement has been implicated as a possible cause of sudden death. The coronary arteries emerge from the aortic sinuses into the lateral margins of the transverse sinus. In this position, they are related to the anterior extent of both right and left atrioventricular grooves (Fig. 1.29). The right coronary artery enters the atrioventricular groove and encircles the tricuspid orifice, giving atrial branches superiorly and ventricular branches inferiorly. The most prominent atrial branch in over half the population (about 55%) runs through the interatrial groove to become the artery to the sinus node. The most prominent ventricular branch arises at the acute margin of the ventricular mass and, hence, is termed the acute marginal branch (Fig. 1.30). The artery also gives off important infundibular (or conal) branches from its proximal course. The left coronary artery, entering the lateral margin of the transverse sinus beneath the left atrial appendage, has a very short course. Almost immediately it divides into the anterior interventricular (descending) and circumflex arteries. It is these two arteries, together with the right coronary artery, that comprise the three vessels whose disease is the territory of so many physicians and surgeons. The anterior interventricular artery runs forward and inferiorly within the interventricular groove. It gives off a series of significant penetrating arteries which pass

perpendicularly backwards into the ventricular septum. It also gives rise to one or more diagonal branches which supply the anterior part of the obtuse marginal surface of the left ventricle along with smaller branches to the infundibular area of the right ventricle (Fig. 1.31). The circumflex artery is much more variable in its morphology. It gives rise superiorly to several atrial arteries, one of which, in just under half the population (45%), becomes the artery to the sinus node. The circumflex artery also gives rise to the important obtuse marginal arteries. One of these obtuse branches may arise directly from the left coronary artery, producing a tri- rather than a bifurcation. Although previously it was considered to be an intermediate branch, it is now the practice to name this as the first obtuse marginal artery. The extent of the circumflex artery relative to the mitral orifice is

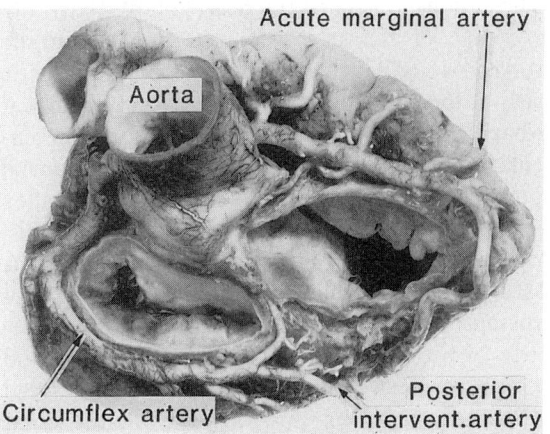

Fig. 1.29. This dissection of the short axis shows the relationship of the right and circumflex coronary arteries to the atrioventricular valves in a heart with left coronary arterial dominance.

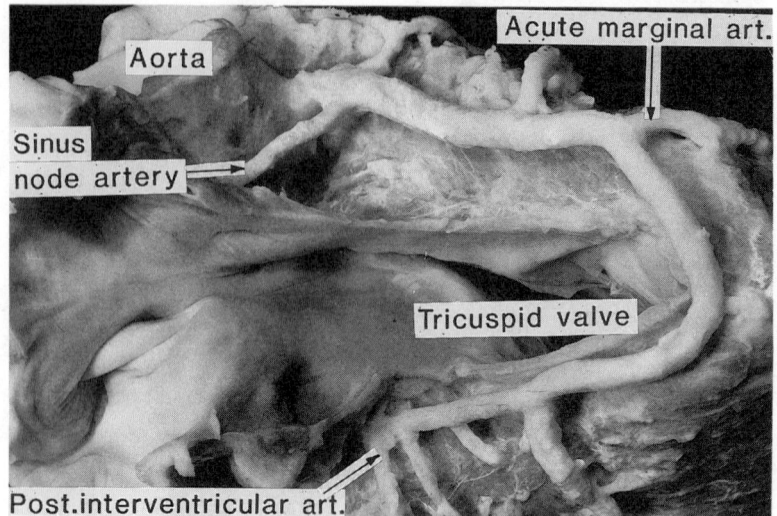

Fig. 1.30. This dissection of the right atrioventricular junction shows the course of a right coronary artery which is dominant. (Reproduced by kind permission of Professor Anton Becker.)

reciprocal with the extent of the right coronary artery. One or other of these arteries gives rise to the posterior interventricular (descending) artery, producing either right or left dominance. The interventricular artery itself gives rise to several inferior septal perforating branches which are important in the context of anastomotic networks. In about 90% of cases, it is the right coronary artery that supplies the posterior interventricular branch, often then continuing across the crux to supply the diaphragmatic surface of the left ventricle (Fig. 1.32). In these circumstances, the circumflex artery terminates at the obtuse margin of the ventricular mass. In about 10% of cases, the circumflex artery continues around the mitral orifice and gives rise to the posterior interventricular artery, at the same time supplying the diaphragmatic surface of the left ventricle (Fig. 1.29).

The venous system of the heart follows basically the course of the arteries but terminates in the coronary sinus which occupies the diaphragmatic aspect of the left atrioventricular groove. The great cardiac vein runs along with the anterior interventricular artery and then turns beneath the left atrial appendage, following the course of the circumflex artery and expanding to become the coronary sinus. It is guarded along its length by several valves, the most significant of which is described as the valve of Vieussens. The middle cardiac vein follows the course of the posterior interventricular artery and joins the coronary sinus at the crux. The small cardiac vein also runs into the sinus at the crux, having accompanied the right coronary artery. The sinus also accepts smaller venous tributaries along its length and empties into the right atrium, its orifice being guarded by the Thebesian valve. Many

smaller venous channels open directly into the cavity of the right atrium. These are termed the Eustachian veins.

There is an extensive lymphatic system within the

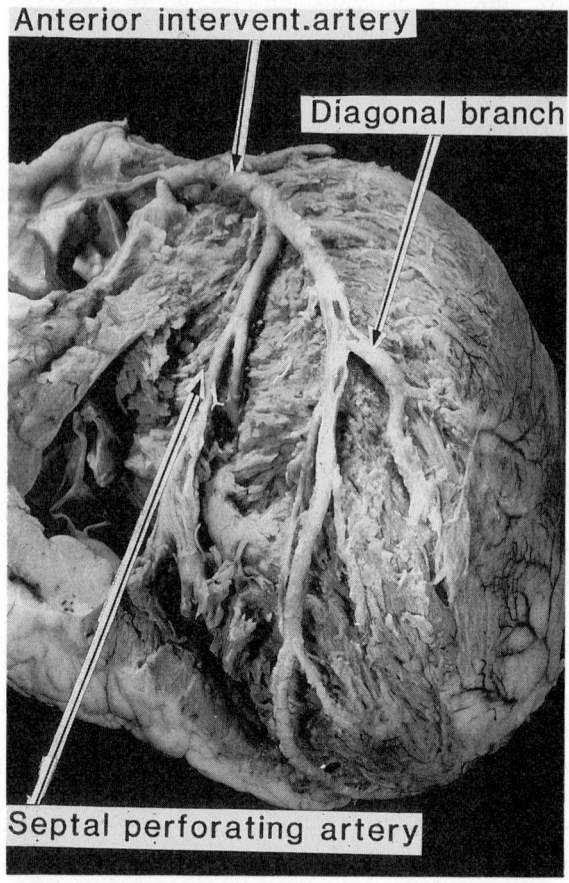

Fig. 1.31. This dissection shows the course of the anterior interventricular coronary artery. (Reproduced by kind permission of Professor Anton Becker.)

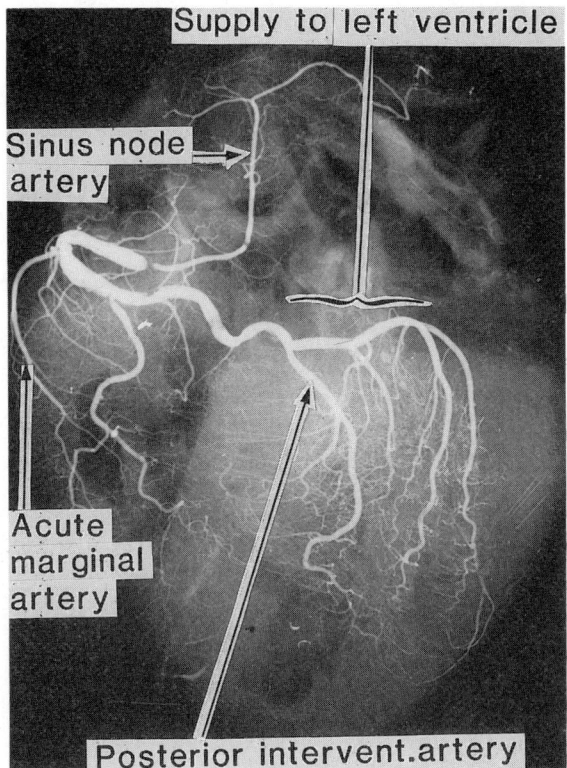

Fig. 1.32. Postmortem angiogram showing a dominant right coronary artery which supplies most of the diaphragmatic aspect of the left ventricle.

heart, but its morphology and function, as yet, are far less well understood in comparison to its arterial and venous counterparts. The lymphatics percolate throughout the myocardial structure, the major lymph channels running with the coronary vessels and terminating in either the thoracic duct or the collecting lymphatic channel of the right chest.

THE CONDUCTION SYSTEM

The conduction system is the network of modified cardiac muscle that initiates the cardiac impulse and transmits it through the ventricular myocardium to ensure synchronized action of the heart. It is important to emphasize that the nodal and conduction tissues are made up of muscle rather than nervous tissue, although the atrial components are richly supplied with terminals of autonomic nerves. The overall conduction system consists of the sinus node and the atrioventricular conduction axis. Equally significant for normal cardiac contraction is the arrangement of the insulating mechanism of the atrioventricular junction which, in the normal heart, ensures that only at the penetrating atrioventricular bundle (of His) is the cardiac impulse able to pass from atrial to ventricular muscle masses (Fig. 1.33).

The sinus node is a small cigar-shaped structure located immediately sub-epicardially within the terminal groove. The node is nearly always found inferiorly and laterally to the crest of the atrial appendage (Fig. 1.34), although in about 10% of hearts the node may extend across the crest and into the interatrial groove in horseshoe fashion (Fig. 1.34, inset). The important artery to the sinus node is derived from the right coronary artery in about 55% of individuals and from the circumflex artery in almost all the remainder. However, in about 1% of normal individuals but perhaps 10% of those with congenitally malformed hearts, the artery arises more distally from either parent vessel and either crosses laterally across the right atrial appendage or courses over the dome of the left atrium. With the more usual pattern, the nodal artery arises

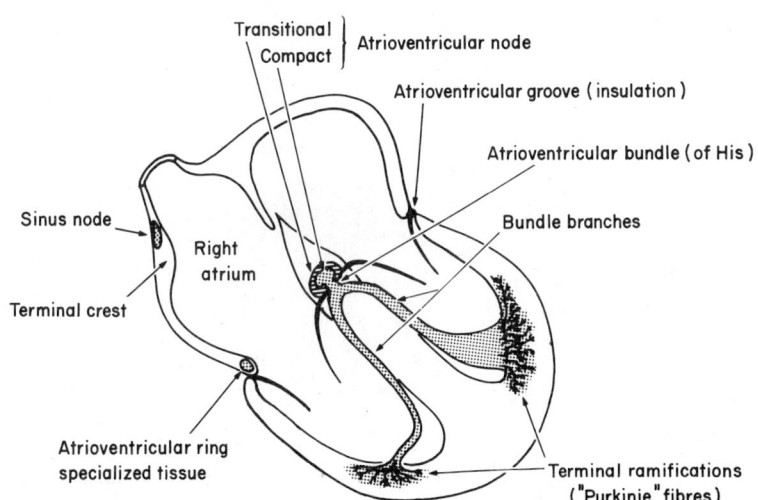

Fig. 1.33. Diagram of the components of the cardiac conduction system.

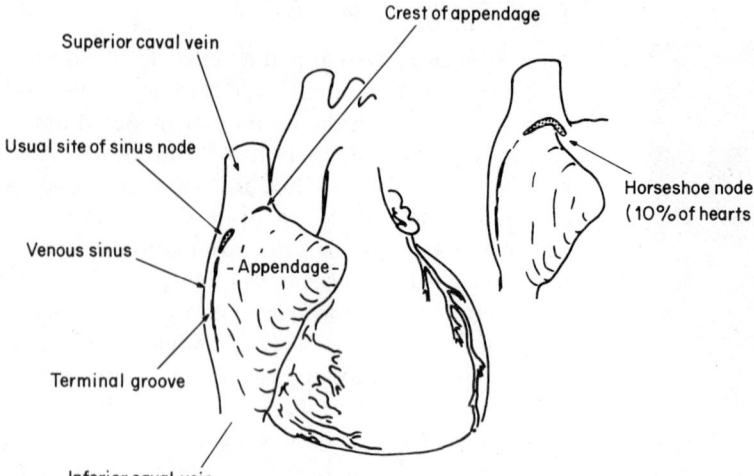

Fig. 1.34. Diagram to show the site of the sinus node. The inset shows the variation found with a 'horseshoe' node.

from the proximal segments of the parent artery and runs up through the interatrial groove to the superior cavo-atrial junction. The artery to the node can then pass precavally or retrocavally to enter the node within the terminal groove. Alternatively, it may divide to form an arterial circle around the superior caval vein.

The specialized atrioventricular junctional area is responsible for delay of the sinus impulse, thus permitting the ventricles to fill during diastole. It is made up of several segments: the transitional cell and compact areas of the atrioventricular node within the atriums; the penetrating atrioventricular bundle (of His); and the branching bundle together with the bundle branches and the ventricular conduction network (Purkinje fibres) within the sub-endocardial area of the ventricular mass. Although it is described in several components, the system is a continuous axis of cells extending from the atrial septum to the ventricular apexes* (Fig. 1.35). The atrial components, both the transitional cell zones and the compact node, are contained exclusively within the triangle of Koch. This zone of the atrial septum is limited superiorly by the tendon of Todaro (the continuation into the septum of the fibrous commissure between the Eustachian and Thebesian valves) and inferiorly by the attachment of the septal leaflet of the tricuspid valve. These borders converge to meet at the atrioventricular membranous septal component of the central fibrous body, while the coronary sinus forms a rather distant base to the triangle. The compact node penetrates into the central fibrous body at the apex of the triangle, running a short course through

* Anglicized version of apices.

the insulating fibrous tissue as the bundle of His. It emerges into the sub-aortic outflow tract beneath the commissure between the non- and right coronary leaflets of the aortic valve, although distant from the commissure as the bundle is sandwiched between the membranous and muscular components of the ventricular septum. In this position, the bundle usually branches astride the ventricular septum. In some hearts, branching may occur on the left ventricular aspect of the septal crest. The branching pattern is grossly eccentric: the left

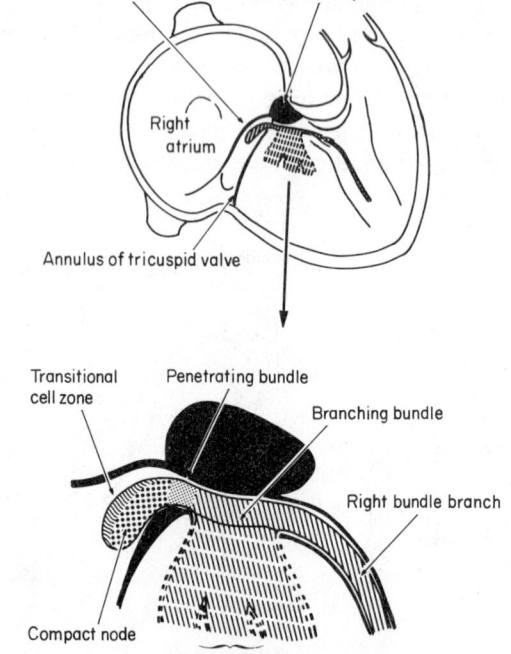

Fig. 1.35. The site and components of the atrioventricular conduction axis.

bundle branch radiates down as a fan of sheet-like fibres whereas the right bundle is a continuation of the major axis of the bundle, descending somewhat as it pierces the septum in cord-like fashion to pass beneath the medial papillary muscle of the tricuspid valve. The fan-like left bundle branch has a common stem which descends down the upper third of the smooth left ventricular aspect of the septum. It then radiates in interlinking tripartite fashion, the anterior and posterior radiations running towards the bases of the paired left ventricular papillary muscles. There is no anatomical evidence to support the concept of a bifascicular left bundle branch in the human heart. The right bundle branch descends as a narrow cord through the substance of the septomarginal trabeculation to the apex of the right ventricle. Both bundle branches presumably ramify extensively within the ventricular apexes, although little is known of the transition to ventricular myocardium in the human heart because of the difficulty at this level of distinguishing between the populations of conducting and working myocardial cells. Indeed, within all the segments of conduction tissue described above, accurate delineation of their course and position can be achieved only with histological examination. Although the approximate site of the nodes and the bundle branches can be recognized with the eye of faith, the anatomical markers are a much better guide to their precise location. The blood supply to the atrioventricular axis is derived from two sources. The atrial component is supplied by the atrioventricular nodal artery, a branch of the posterior interventricular artery which, having supplied the node, penetrates into the ventricles to varied extent. The major supply to the ventricular conduction segments, however, comes from the septal perforating branches of the anterior interventricular artery.

The ability to distinguish cells of the conduction system histologically has underscored one of the major controversies concerning conduction of the heart beat. Since the discovery of the cardiac nodes, some individuals have suggested that tracts of cells with 'conduction' characteristics are to be found connecting them. These contentions were largely discounted prior to 1963, as the evidence was less than convincing. However, one early claim did stimulate extensive debate within the German Pathological Society. It was pointed out that the major anatomical feature distinguishing the ventricular conduction pathways was their insulation from the working myocardial mass rather than their specific staining characteristics; it was clear that no

insulated tracts of cells separate from the myocardial mass were, or are, to be found in the atrial tissues. Had these criteria been followed subsequent to 1963, there would be no contention over these pathways. In 1963, it was again suggested, on questionable grounds, that discrete tracts did indeed exist traversing the right atrial walls. Although this concept was accepted so enthusiastically by the cardiological world that, in several circles, it has become conventional wisdom, there is neither anatomical nor electrophysiological evidence to support the concept of the atrial impulse being conducted over narrow tracts in advance of the activation sequence of the adjacent atrial myocardium. In short, there are *no* specialized internodal pathways. There is certainly preferential conduction along the major muscle bundles, but this is more than adequately explained by the overall geometric arrangement of the atrial muscle fibres.

Although there are no histologically distinct conduction structures to be found in the region of the purported internodal pathways, there are other segments of node-like tissue present within the atrial myocardium. These are found in the terminal segments of atrial myocardium at their insertion into the leaflets of the tricuspid valve. The node-like structures are scattered around the right atrioventricular junction, particularly at the acute point. Significantly, this is the precise site at which Stanley Kent, an English physiologist working at the turn of the century, claimed to have demonstrated in normal hearts pathways of conduction different to those provided by the atrioventricular conduction axis discovered by His and clarified by Tawara. Examination of Kent's illustrative material shows that he was certainly demonstrating node-like remnants, but never muscular atrioventricular connections. Furthermore, the structures found by Kent bear no resemblance to the accessory muscular atrioventricular connections now known to be responsible for the Wolff–Parkinson–White variant of ventricular pre-excitation, and so often described in his name. Thus, in the normal heart, the atrial myocardium (including the node-like remnants) is always separated from the ventricular myocardial mass by the atrioventricular tissue plane. Although this is not always a firm ring-like collagenous structure (a complete ring is only rarely found around the mitral orifice and never around the tricuspid orifice), the fibro-fatty atrioventricular groove does separate the muscle masses at all points except around the penetrating atrioventricular bundle.

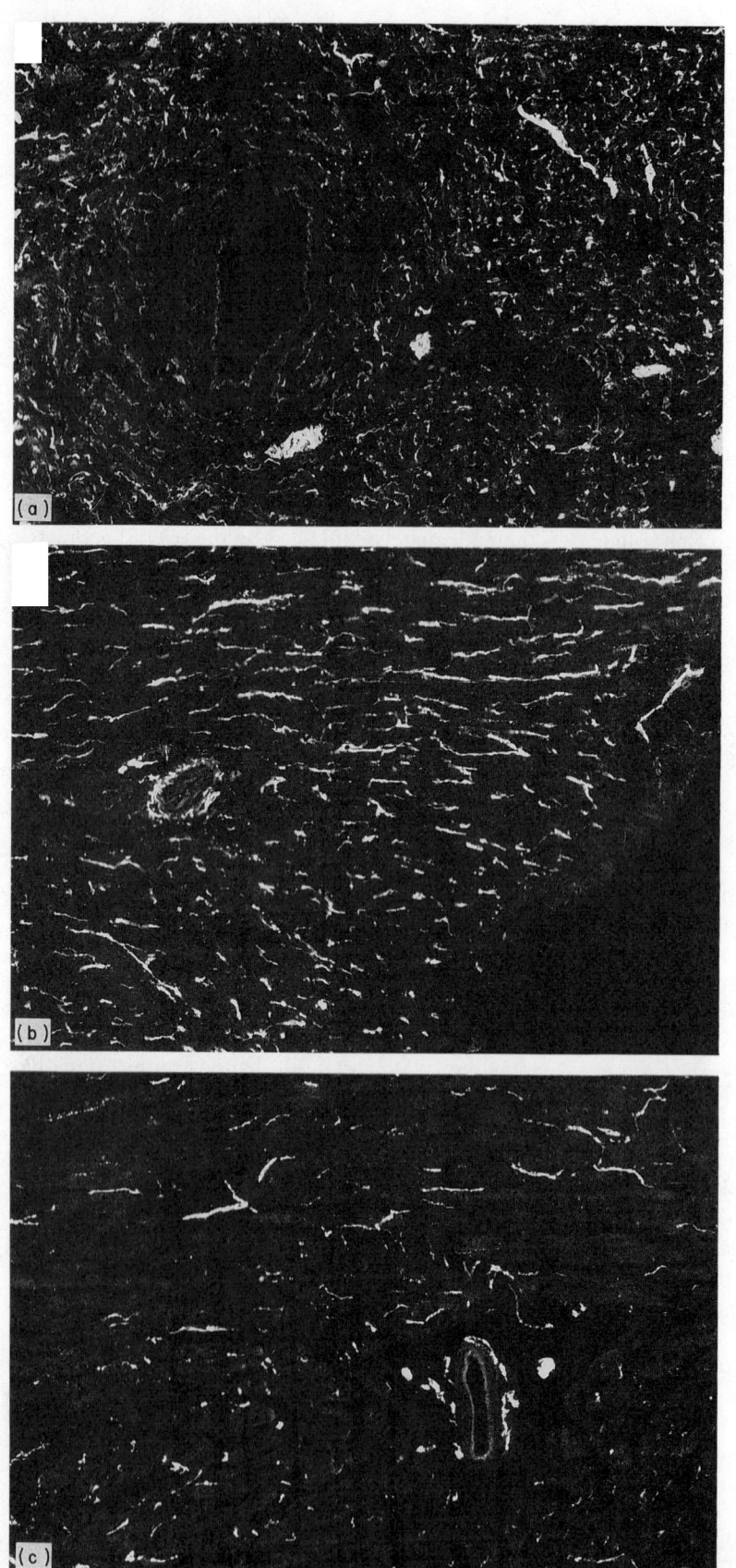

Fig. 1.36. Nerves in the human heart displayed by a fluorescence technique which identifies antibodies to the protein gene product 9.5. This demonstrates all autonomic nerves. The upper panel shows the dense innervation of the sinus node, the middle panel the less dense innervation of the right atrial myocardium and the lower panel the sparse innervation of the ventricular myocardium. Different antibodies can be used to demonstrate the sympathetic and parasympathetic components of this innervation. (By courtesy of Dr John Wharton from unpublished work.)

INNERVATION OF THE HEART

The heart receives nerves from both sympathetic and parasympathetic sources. The precise anatomical distribution of these two networks has yet to be fully established, but with the advent of developments whereby nerves can be labelled with antibody, this will be clarified in the near future. The parasympathetic component reaches the heart through the vagus nerves. These carry both preganglionic fibres, which have their cell bodies in the dorsal vagal nucleus, and sensory fibres from the heart, which extend to cell bodies in the nodose ganglion of the vagus. The vagus itself also carries fibres that supply many other organs. Those nerves running to and from the heart branch from the vagal nerves in their cervical and thoracic course. The sympathetic nerves take origin from the superior, middle and inferior cervical along with the upper five ganglions* of the sympathetic chains. These sympathetic branches also carry both efferent and afferent fibres. Thus, autonomic nerves from both sympathetic and parasympathetic sources run from the neck and upper thorax to reach the heart. At the heart, the fibres from both sources intermingle to form the cardiac plexus, which is arbitrarily divided into superficial and deep parts although the two are extensively linked. The superficial part of the plexus lies below the arch of the aorta in front of the right pulmonary artery. It is formed mostly by branches from the left vagus and the sympathetic trunks. The deep component of the plexus is found in front of the tracheal bifurcation. It receives the upper cervical branches of the vagus

* Anglicized version of ganglia.

along with branches from the sympathetic trunks. From the plexus, the intrinsic cardiac nerves run to supply the coronary arteries, the conduction tissues, the musculature and the pericardium, epicardium and endocardium (Fig. 1.36). In general, the vagal nerves are confined to the atrial chambers, with particularly rich innervation of the sinus node. The sympathetic nerves give branches to the atrioventricular node, with minimal supply to the sinus node, but they also form dense networks around the coronary arteries with a contributory innervation to the ventricular myocardium.

ACKNOWLEDGEMENTS

In compiling this chapter, I have drawn extensively on previous collaborations with Professor Anton Becker, University of Amsterdam, and Dr Siew Yen Ho, National Heart and Lung Institute, University of London. I am grateful to both of them, the more so since Professor Becker permitted me to use illustrative material from our previous studies and Dr Ho contributed my line diagrams. Many of the other photographs were taken during collaborative studies performed with Dr James R. Zuberbuhler of the Children's Hospital of Pittsburgh, and I am indebted to him for his hospitality and on-going support. The photomicrographs of the innervation of the heart are from the work, as yet unpublished, of Dr John Wharton, Department of Histochemistry, Royal Postgraduate Medical School, London, and I thank him for permission to include them. Finally, I am indebted to Rachel Marinos for secretarial assistance and Christine Anderson for considerable help in completing the manuscript.

Chapter 2

A Brief Account of the Physiology of the Heart and Circulation

P.A. Poole-Wilson

INTRODUCTION

The contraction of the heart, the vasomotor tone of the veins and arteries and the intravascular volume are carefully controlled in the body in order to supply substrates to and remove metabolites from the body organs. The critical substrate is oxygen provided through the lungs. The total body oxygen consumption of an average 70-kg person is approximately 3–5 ml/min/kg and this can increase on exercise to 40 ml/min/kg or above. The cardiovascular system adjusts to maintain an adequate cardiac output on exercise and in the event of trauma or haemorrhage. In addition, the system is able to respond rapidly to demands for increased flow in stressful situations. This latter requirement is necessary for survival and is the probable reason why the blood pressure in man and other mammals is high in the resting state.

FUNCTION OF THE NORMAL CIRCULATION AT REST

The heart of a normal 70-kg person contracts at a rate of 70–75 beats/min at rest and pumps 5.5 l/min. Arterial blood is 97% saturated (Po_2 100 mmHg) and the content is 190 ml/l when the haemoglobin is 14 g/dl ($19 = 14 \times 1.36 \times 0.97$). Mixed venous blood (blood in the pulmonary artery after mixing in the chambers of the right side of the heart) has a saturation in normal man at rest of 70% and the content is 145 ml/l. The oxygen content is made up of the oxygen bound to haemoglobin and a small additional amount of oxygen in solution. The binding of oxygen to haemoglobin depends on pH, Pco_2, temperature and concentration of 2,3-diphosphoglycerate in the red cell.

The Fick equation states that in a steady state:

total body oxygen consumption = cardiac output × (arterial oxygen content − mixed venous oxygen content)

which becomes at rest:

total body oxygen consumption = $5.5 \times (190 - 145) = 3.5$ ml/min/kg.

The fuels for the body depend on diet, prandial state, exercise and other factors. In normal man, the carbon dioxide production is lower than the oxygen consumption so that the respiratory quotient (oxygen consumption/carbon dioxide production) is approximately 0.82. If glucose were the sole substrate, the respiratory quotient would be 1.0, if fat, 0.72 and if protein 0.80.

DISTRIBUTION OF BLOOD VOLUME AND FLOW IN THE BODY

The distribution of blood volume in the body is shown in Table 2.1. Two-thirds of the blood volume is in the veins. The distribution of the cardiac output and the oxygen consumption of body organs at rest are shown in Table 2.2. Blood flow to an organ is not simply determined by the

Table 2.1. **Blood volume.**

	% of total	ml
Left heart	4	220
Right heart	4	220
Capillaries	4	220
Lungs	10	550
Arteries	12	660
Veins	66	3630
Total	100	5500

Table 2.2. Distribution of the cardiac output, and oxygen consumption of the body organs at rest.

	Blood flow			Oxygen consumption			a-v O$_2$ difference (ml/100 ml)	Ratio of % CO to O$_2$ consumption
	ml/min	ml/min/100 g	% total CO	ml/min	ml/min/100 g	% of total		
Brain	825	59	15	45	3	19	6	0.8
Heart	275	92	5	25	8	10	10	0.5
Liver/GI tract	1100	28	20	75	2	30	6	0.7
Kidneys	1100	370	20	15	5	5	1.3	4
Muscle	1100	3	20	50	0.1	20	5	1
Skin	275	14	5	5	0.2	2	2.5	2.5
Skeleton/bone/fat	825	3	15	35	0.1	15	5	1
Total	5500		100	250		100		

oxygen consumption. Some organs, such as the heart, extract almost all the oxygen in arterial blood and depend for an increase of supply on increased blood flow. The liver and brain extract rather less oxygen. The kidney and skin extract relatively little oxygen so that ratio of percentage cardiac output to percentage oxygen consumption is high; these organs have special roles, that of the kidney to control fluid balance and excrete nitrogen and acid, and that of the skin to thermoregulate the body. The primary role of blood flow in these two organs is not simply to supply substrate and oxygen.

EXERCISE

On exercise the cardiac output can increase to 20 l/min (Table 2.3). The higher cardiac output is partly attributable to the increase of heart rate which may reach 200 beats/min but also due to an increase in the stroke volume from a normal value of 75 to 150 ml/beat. Peak oxygen consumption on exercise in a normal person is approximately 40 ml/min/kg. This represents an elevenfold increase from rest and is achieved not just by increasing cardiac output but also by widening of the arterio-venous difference for oxygen, as a result of a decrease in the venous content due to greater extraction.

On exercise, blood is diverted from tissues such as the skin, splanchnic circulation and kidney to skeletal muscle (Table 2.3). Blood flow to the heart increases in proportion to the increase of cardiac output. Blood flow to the brain remains the same on exercise so that the proportion of the cardiac output to the brain decreases. Somewhat similar changes occur in heart failure.

PRESSURES IN THE CIRCULATION

To sustain the circulation the heart develops pressure. The pressures in the chambers of the heart and in the circulation are shown in Table 2.4. The timing of the pressure changes in the heart with each beat is shown in Fig. 2.1. Systole is made up of three time-periods: isovolumic contraction, rapid ejection and late systole. Diastole has four time-periods: isovolumic relaxation, rapid filling, passive filling and atrial systole. Each of these periods correspond to different biochemical and physiological events in the heart.

Table 2.3.
(a) Oxygen consumption and cardiac output.

	Rest	Maximum exercise	Ratio of exercise/rest
Cardiac output (l/min)	5.5	20	3.6
Total body oxygen consumption (ml/min/kg)	3.5	40	11

(b) Blood flow to body organs (as a percentage of cardiac output).

	Rest	Maximum exercise	Ratio of flow on exercise/flow at rest
Brain	15	4	0.96
Heart	5	5	3.6
Liver/GI tract	20	3	0.54
Kidneys	20	3	0.54
Muscle	20	81	15
Skin	5	1	0.72
Skeleton/bone/fat	15	3	0.72
Total	100	100	

Table 2.4. Pressures in the circulation (mmHg).

	Systolic	Diastolic	Mean	'a' wave	'v' wave
Right atrium	—	—	0–8	2–10	2–10
Right ventricle	15–30	2–10	—	—	—
Pulmonary artery	15–30	8–8	—	—	—
Left atrium	—	—	1–10	3–15	3–12
Left ventricle	100–140	3–12	—	—	—
Aorta	100–140	60–90	70–105	—	—

THE HEART

CHARACTERISTICS OF THE HUMAN HEART

The global characteristics of the human heart are
listed in Table 2.5. The heart is made of muscle
which is critically dependent on oxygen supply and
the muscle contains numerous mitochrondria to

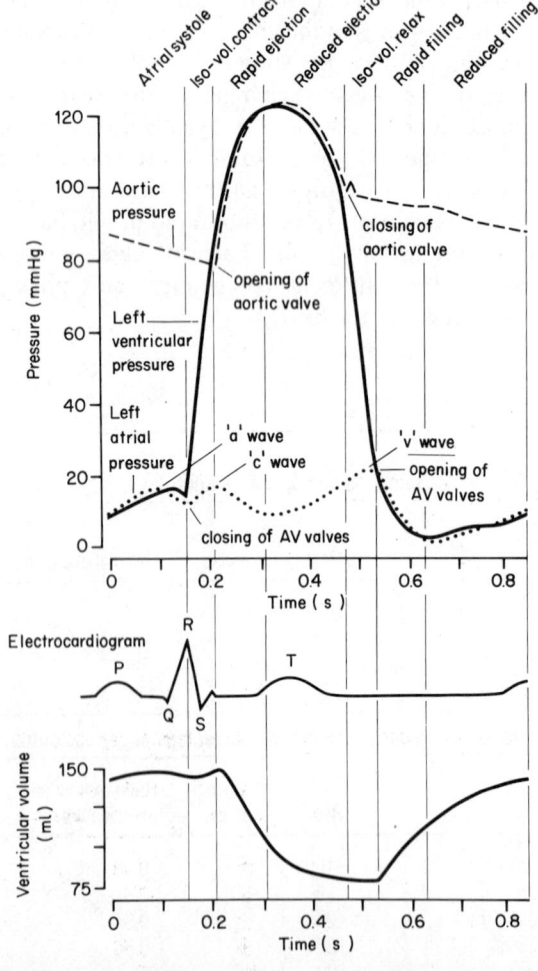

Fig. 2.1. The relation of pressure changes in the various
cardiac chambers to opening and closing of the heart valves,
the electrocardiogram and ventricular volume. Left ventricular
systole extends from closing of the mitral valve to closing of the
aortic valve. Diastole is the remainder of the cycle.

Table 2.5. Characteristics of the human heart.

Heart rate	72 beats/min
Cardiac output	5.5 l
Stroke volume	75 ml/beat
Left ventricular end-systolic volume	75 ml
Left ventricular end-diastolic volume	150 ml
Ejection fraction	50%
Cycle time	830 ms
Ventricular systole	300 ms
Ventricular diastole	530 ms
Weight	300 g
Coronary blood flow	0.8 ml/min/g
Coronary arterial oxygen content	190 ml/l
	(P_{O_2} 100 mmHg, Hb = 14 g/dl, saturation 97%)
Coronary venous oxygen content	68 ml/l
	(P_{O_2} 25 mmHg, Hb = 14 g/dl, saturation 37%)
Oxygen consumption of heart	27 ml/min
Basal oxygen consumption of the heart	6 ml/min (22%)
Oxygen consumption per gram of heart	0.09 ml/min/g
Basal oxygen consumption per gram of heart	0.02 ml/min/g (22%)
Oxygen consumption of electrical activation	0.0004 ml/min/g
Efficiency at rest (using total oxygen consumed)	15%
Efficiency at rest (subtracting basal oxygen consumption)	20%

permit oxidative phosphorylation. The heart extracts almost all the oxygen from the arterial blood.
The ability of the heart to increase oxygen availability by increased extraction is small. Indeed, decrease
of the coronary sinus oxygen is usually a feature of
myocardial ischaemia. The reason that the coronary
sinus oxygen saturation is low remains uncertain
but may represent the minimum value that permits
the optimum flux of oxygen across the tissue to the
mitochondria in the myocytes.

ULTRASTRUCTURE

The heart is made up of many different cell types.
Some cells such as those in the sino-atrial node, the
atrioventricular node, the bundle of His and Purkinje fibres are specialized for the purpose of
initiating a heart beat and transmitting this signal in
a regular and co-ordinated manner to the heart
muscle in atria and ventricles. By volume, the most
common cells are myocardial cells (myocytes).
These provide the contractile force needed for the
ejection of blood from the right and left ventricles.

The myocardial cell is 100 μm long and 15 μm
wide (Fig. 2.2). The cell branches and interdigitates
with adjacent cells and is surrounded by a rich

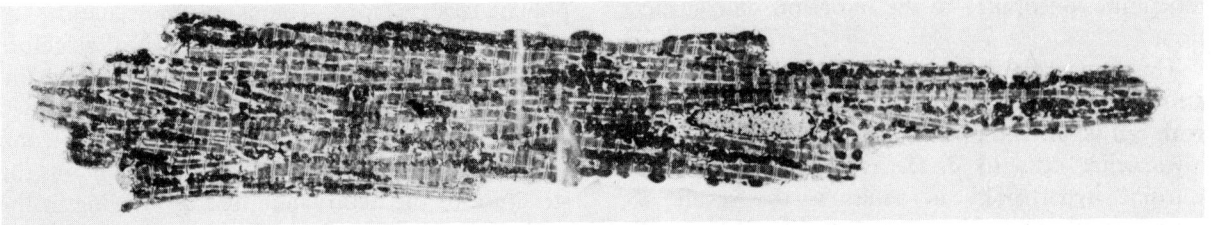

Fig. 2.2. Electron-micrograph of a cross-section of a single myocardial cell from a rat. Note the nucleus, the large number of mitochondria and the alignment of the sarcomeres.

capillary network. At their ends and sides, each cell has contact with other cells. At the cell ends is an area of specialized cell membrane, the intercalated disc. The intercalated disc contains several structures, the fascia adherens, macula adherens (desmosome) and gap junctions (nexus). The fascia adherens are mechanical links so that force can be transmitted between cells when the heart contracts. The macula adherens (desmosome) are the sites where cytoplasmic filaments, which provide a lattice structure for the cell, link to the cell membrane. The gap junctions are the areas of the intercalated disc where the membranes of adjacent cells are particularly close and the permeability of the cell membrane to ions is low so that an electrical signal can pass easily between cells. Myocytes are contained in a complex mesh of fibres in the extracellular space.

The basic unit of contraction, the sarcomere (Figs 2.2 and 2.3), is 2 μm in length at rest. The sarcomeres in adjacent myofibrils are aligned at the Z-line. This gives heart muscle its striated appearance under both the light and electron microscope.

The myocardial cell is surrounded by a cell membrane (the sarcolemma). The sarcolemma is made up of a trilaminar membrane (10 nm in thickness) and an outer layer (70 nm in thickness) called the surface coat or glycocalyx. The trilaminar membrane consists of two layers of lipid molecules which align themselves so that the polar heads of the molecules are facing outwards and the lipid tails are within (the meat in the sandwich). The trilaminar membrane is not a static structure but has liquid properties. Numerous proteins are located in the cell membrane and move freely in the membrane. These are the channels for the passage of ions through the membrane and receptor sites for hormones and pharmacologically active substances. Attached to the cell membrane is the glycocalyx made up of glycoproteins, glycolipids and polysacharrides.

Most of the volume of a myocardial cell is taken up by cell water, myofibrils and mitochondria (30% of the volume). The mitochondria provide the energy for contraction in the form of adenosine triphosphate (ATP).

The myocardial cell has wide T-tubules and an extensive sarcoplasmic reticulum (Fig. 2.3) The T-tubules are invaginations from the cell surface with openings up to 200 nm in diameter. The tubules are regularly spaced (approximately 2 nm apart) so that one T-tubule goes down to each Z-line in each myofibril. The T-tubules allow the electrical signal for contraction and the passage of calcium across the cell membrane to be in close proximity to the Z-line. The sarcoplasmic reticulum is a lace-like tubular structure (30 nm in diameter) spreading over the myofibrils and throughout the whole cell. Where the sarcoplasmic reticulum comes close to the surface membrane of T-tubules, swellings develop called lateral cysternae. Feet, seen as dark opacities under the electron microscope, connect the lateral cysternae to the trilaminar membrane. The sarcoplasmic reticulum is a sink for the uptake of calcium within the cell, thus maintaining the low intracellular calcium concentration in diastole. The release of calcium from the sarcoplasmic

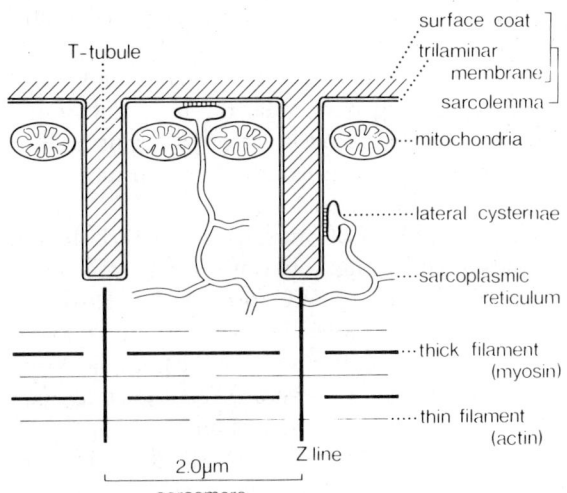

Fig. 2.3. Diagram of the relation between the cell membrane, T-tubules, sarcoplasmic reticulum and the contractile proteins.

reticulum contributes to the initiation of contraction.

The myocardial cell has a nucleus, Golgi apparatus and ribosomes. These structures are concerned with cell repair and protein synthesis. The ability of myocardial cells to divide is lost early in life. Cardiac hypertrophy in adults is the result of protein synthesis and increase in the size of each cell not cell division.

THE SARCOMERE AND CONTRACTILE PROTEINS

Contraction of the heart is brought about by shortening of the sarcomeres within each cell. The contraction requires energy generated by the mitochondria in the form of ATP and is triggered by increase of the calcium concentration in the region of the myofibrils.

The sarcomere at rest is between 2.0 and 2.2 μm in length from Z-line to Z-line. The sarcomere is made up of two interdigitating filaments (Figs 2.3 and 2.4). The thick filament is made of the protein myosin and the thin filament is made of actin. Each myosin molecule is 160 nm in length. The molecule has a body consisting of two intertwining alpha-helical peptide molecules (heavy chains). At the end of each peptide is a head composed of heavy chains with the addition of two further peptide chains (light chains). The heads of the myosin molecule extend laterally from the thick filament in opposed pairs every 14.3 nm and are staggered around the filament repeating every 43 nm. Six myosin heads connect every 43 nm with the actin molecules of the thin filaments. The myosin head contains the enzyme myofibrillar ATPase (on the heavy chain) which breaks down ATP thus providing the energy for contraction.

The thin filament is a more complex structure. The actin molecule is a small globular protein which polymerizes to form chains of molecules. Two chains of actin molecules form a helical structure such that one revolution occurs every 39 nm and contains seven actin molecules in each of the two strands. In the grooves of the helix runs a second molecule tropomyosin. Tropomyosin maintains the structure of the actin chain and by moving in the groove transmits information to all seven actin molecules in each revolution of the molecule. Attached to every seventh actin molecule is a further protein troponin. This protein has three parts. Troponin C binds calcium with a high affinity and initiates contraction. Troponin I prevents an interaction between actin and myosin and is under the control of troponin C. Troponin T binds the troponin complex to tropomyosin.

The exact mechanism by which movement occurs between actin and myosin molecules in cardiac muscle is still uncertain. Contraction is initiated by the binding of calcium to troponin C which then no longer causes troponin I to inhibit the interaction between actin and myosin. The muscle shortens and ATP is broken down to ADP and phosphate. A mechanical change in the angle at which the myosin head is attached to the body of the myosin molecule causes the two filaments to move. Muscle shortening is brought about by a ratchet mechanism.

ENERGY FOR CONTRACTION OF THE HEART

Oxygen is utilized in the mitochondria by the process of oxidative phosphorylation to generate ATP. The heart has a limited facility for anaerobic metabolism. The major substrates for the heart are fatty acids, glucose and lactate. At rest and in the fasting state, 60% of the total oxygen consumption of the heart is utilized in the metabolism of fatty acids, 30% by glucose, 9% by lactate and 1% by pyruvate. During ischaemia, the main substrate is either glucose of extracellular origin or intracellular glycogen, whereas on exercise the consumption of fatty acids is increased.

The metabolism of fatty acids and carbohydrate is efficient, releasing between 40 and 60% of the potential free energy in the form of ATP. Fatty acids generate 8 ATP molecules per carbon atom and glucose 6 ATP molecules. Per weight, the breakdown of fatty acids generates 2.5 times as many ATP molecules as glucose metabolism.

Energy in the form of ATP is used to maintain the integrity of cell structures, to fuel the pumps for maintenance of ionic gradients and to provide energy for muscle shortening. The overall efficiency

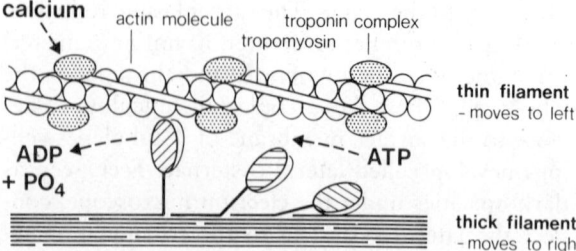

Fig. 2.4. Diagram of the contractile proteins. Shortening comes about by movement of the heads of myosin molecules (thick filament) in relation to the thin filament with the breakdown of adenosine triphosphate (ATP).

of the heart is the energy required to eject a volume of blood against the arterial pressure expressed as a percentage of energy which could be released from the uptake of oxygen in a given time. Approximately 22% of the oxygen consumption of the heart at rest is basal energy consumption necessary for processes other than contraction. If this part of the oxygen consumption is excluded, the efficiency of the heart is 20%.

ELECTROPHYSIOLOGY

Each heart beat is initiated by a spontaneous electrical depolarization of cells making up the sino-atrial node. The electrical signal passes across the atria to the atrioventricular node, through the bundle of His and down the Purkinje fibres to the ventricular myocardium. The electrical depolarization of the atria and ventricles are recorded on the surface of the chest as the electrocardiogram. The electrocardiogram is the sum of all the electrical events in the heart.

Within a ventricular cell the concentrations of potassium and sodium ions are 140 and 10 mmol/l of cell water, respectively (Fig. 2.5). Negative charges are found on proteins which cannot perme-

ate the cell membrane. In the extracellular fluid, the concentrations of potassium and sodium are 5.0 and 140 mmol/l, respectively; the major negatively charged ions are chloride (110 mmol/l) and bicarbonate (24 mmol/l). In the resting state, the cell membrane is more permeable to potassium than any other ion. Potassium passes down the concentration gradient to the outside of the cell. As potassium is positively charged and proteins remain in the cell, the inside of the cell becomes negatively charged. An equilibrium is reached where the electrical forces retaining potassium in the cell are balanced by the tendency to diffuse out of the cell down the concentration gradient. The electrical potential is then the equilibrium potential for that ion. The equilibrium for any ion can be calculated from the Nernst equation:

$$E = \frac{RT \text{ (concentration outside)}}{ZF \text{ (concentration inside)}}$$

where E is the equilibrium potential in millivolts, T the absolute temperature, R the gas constant, F the Faraday and Z the valency.

For potassium,

$$E_{K^+} = 61.5 \log \frac{5}{140} = -89 \text{ mV}.$$

The calculated equilibrium potential for potassium is -89 mV, for sodium $+70$ mV and for calcium $+120$ mV.

In resting cardiac muscle (diastole), the membrane is permeable to potassium and the intracellular potential is -80 mV. The difference between this value and the equilibratium potential for potassium (-89 mV) is accounted for by a small leakage of other ions, particularly sodium, and differences between activity and concentration of intracellular ions. The sodium pump (3 Na$^+$ for 2 K$^+$) is electrogenic and also contributes to the resting membrane potential. The pump maintains the intracellular ion concentrations despite small leakage currents. When a cell is electrically excited, the cell membrane allows sodium ions to enter the cell. The potential increases to approximately $+20$ mV (phase 0). The rate of change of the potential is related to the propagation velocity of the action potential across the heart. The increase in sodium conductance lasts only a few milliseconds ('fast' channel current) and is followed by a transient outward current probably carried by potassium (phase 1). Phase 2 is caused in part by the 'slow' inward current. This current is predominantly made

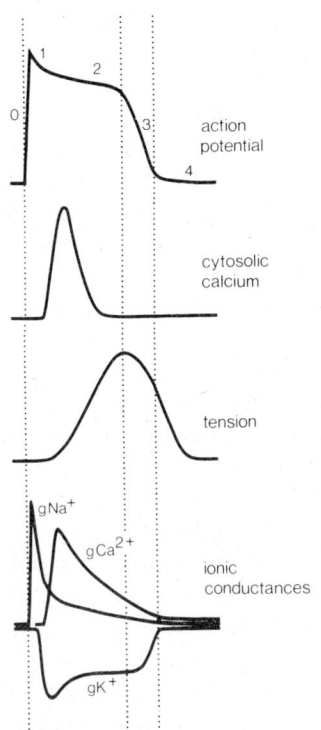

Fig. 2.5. The temporal relation between the action potential, the cytosolic calcium concentration, tension development and ionic conductances.

up of calcium ions but some sodium ions are present. At the same time, the conductance to potassium is reduced so that despite depolarization a large outward potassium current does not occur (anomalous rectification). Phase 2 of the cardiac action potential is referred to as the plateau and is not present in skeletal muscle which has a much shorter action potential. Finally, the cell repolarizes (phase 3). Repolarization occurs because of an increase in potassium conductance and termination of the calcium current.

In specialized cardiac tissue (sino-atrial node, atrioventricular node) and in damaged myocardial cells, the resting membrane spontaneously depolarizes (phase 4) mainly due to a decrease of potassium conductance, although sodium and calcium conductance may increase. When the membrane potential reaches a value of approximately −50 mV (threshold voltage), the cell spontaneously depolarizes and an action potential is initiated.

CONTROL OF CONTRACTION—CALCIUM

Contraction of cardiac muscle is brought about by changes in the concentration of calcium within the cell. As the calcium concentration in the region of the myofibrils rises from 10^{-7} M to 3×10^{-6} M, calcium binds to troponin C causing contraction. Later, calcium is released and tension declines. For the development of half maximal tension, the concentration must rise to 10^{-6} M. Such a concentration change requires only one µmole of calcium per litre of cell water. The total amount of calcium required to bring about contraction is substantially greater because an appreciable quantity of calcium is bound to troponin C. The total calcium needed for half maximal tension is 40 µmoles per kilogram wet tissue.

The calcium for contraction arises from the inward calcium current, from the release of calcium by the sarcoplasmic reticulum and, under special conditions, from sodium–calcium exchange (Fig. 2.6). During the action potential, calcium enters the cell as the inward calcium current which accounts for 10 µmol/kg wet tissue. In order to maintain a steady state, an equal quantity of calcium must be ejected from the cell during diastole. The extracellular space contains 400–1200 µmol/kg and the sarcoplasmic reticulum 150–350 µmol/kg. Calcium (80–200 µmol/kg wet tissue) is also bound to the cell membrane, some of it to the carbohydrate in the glycocalyx and some to the lipids in the trilaminar membrane. Calcium enters the myocardial cell as

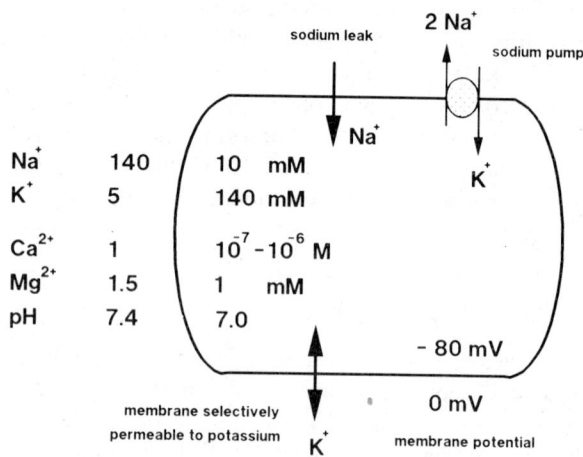

RESTING MYOCYTE

Na^+	140	10	mM
K^+	5	140	mM
Ca^{2+}	1	10^{-7}-10^{-6} M	
Mg^{2+}	1.5	1	mM
pH	7.4	7.0	

Fig. 2.6. Intra- and extracellular concentrations of ions in cardiac muscle at rest. The increase of the calcium concentration causes contraction.

the inward calcium current of the action potential and causes an increase of the cytosolic calcium concentration. This increase triggers further release of calcium from the sarcoplasmic reticulum. During relaxation, calcium is taken up again by the sarcoplasmic reticulum.

In recent studies, it has been demonstrated that the calcium concentration in the cell rises rapidly after the start of the action potential and returns to the resting value before the end of the action potential and before tension starts to fall. Relaxation of cardiac muscle is not determined, therefore, simply by the rate of fall of the cytosolic calcium concentration but by other factors, such as the rate of release of calcium from troponin C.

A sodium–calcium (3 Na^+ for 1 Ca^+) exchange mechanism in the cell membrane is an important mechanism for the extrusion of calcium from the cell and functioning in the reverse direction may under some exceptional circumstances contribute to the inward movement of calcium (Fig. 2.7). Calcium can also be pumped out of the cell by a calcium ATPase. Such mechanisms are necessary to maintain the large gradient between the extracellular calcium concentration (10^{-3} M) and the intracellular concentration (10^{-7} M), and to remove the small amount of calcium entering the cell with each heart beat.

TIMING OF EVENTS IN THE HEART

The timing of events in the heart and the relation to volume changes are shown in Fig. 2.1. The relation

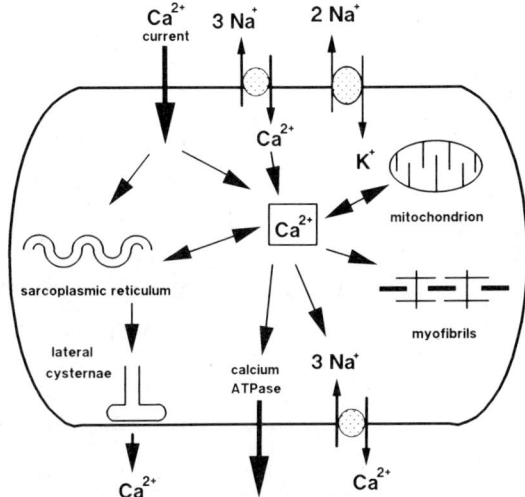

Fig. 2.7. The pathways for calcium in the cardiac cell. Calcium for contraction arises from the calcium current, from the sarcoplasmic reticulum and from sodium–calcium exchange. Calcium is removed by the sarcoplasmic reticulum, by sodium–calcium exchange, functioning in the other and more usual direction, and by a calcium pump sited in the membrane (calcium ATPase). The mitochondria act largely as buffers.

between cytosolic calcium concentration, the action potential and contraction is shown in Fig. 2.7. In recent studies, it has been shown that the calcium concentration rises rapidly and reaches a maximum before the end of the action potential and before peak tension has been reached. The cytosolic calcium concentration declines before muscle relaxation. Thus, the decline of tension in diastole is not simply related to the cytosolic calcium concentration but probably also to the release of calcium from troponin C.

HAEMODYNAMICS

The basic unit of contraction in cardiac muscle is the sarcomere. In resting muscle, the sarcomere length is between 1.8 and 2.0 μm. If the pressure at the end of diastole (the left ventricular filling pressure) is increased, as in acute heart failure, the volume of the ventricle is increased and the sarcomere lengthens to a maximum of 2.3 μm. Only when acute dilatation of the ventricle occurs, for example by accident during cardiac surgery, is the sarcomere length increased beyond 2.3 μm. This is associated with tearing of the muscle and irreversible damage. The enlargement of the heart that occurs in severe chronic heart failure is due to slippage of the myofibrils and adjacent myocardial cells and is not due to excessive elongation of the sarcomere.

The extent to which the sarcomere can shorten determines the stroke volume. During severe exercise, or in the presence of powerful inotropic drugs, the sarcomere length at end-systole may be only 1.4 μm. At this length, cardiac muscle recoils. A negative pressure is present during early diastole and filling of the ventricle is partly due to suction. With zero filling pressure, the sarcomere length is about 1.6 μm. Under normal resting conditions in man, the ventricle is filled by a positive pressure and the sarcomere length is between 1.8 and 2.0 μm.

The cardiac output of the intact heart is determined by the heart rate and the stroke volume. Increase of heart rate in addition to being an immediate determinate of cardiac output also increases the contractility of the myocardium, although in man this is a small effect. Stroke volume is determined by the preload (end-diastolic pressure) and the afterload (almost synonymous with blood pressure). The increase of stroke volume resulting from an increase of end-diastolic pressure (Fig. 2.8). (Starling's Law) is partly due to increased overlap of the contractile proteins and partly due to an increased activation of the excitation–contraction mechanism. The relation between stroke volume and afterload is less well known. Reduction of the blood pressure allows the heart muscle to shorten more and thus to increase cardiac output. The third factor determining cardiac output is the contractile state of the myocardium. This can be modified by neuro-endocrine mechanisms (notably the sympathetic system) and by numerous reflexes.

The response observed to a drug such as a vasodilator in intact man depends on the effect on preload, afterload and the reflex response (Fig. 2.9). For example, in normal man, nitroglycerine results in a reduction of cardiac output or no change. The fall of cardiac output due to a fall of preload is counteracted by an increase of cardiac output as a result of a fall of afterload and reflex stimulation of the heart. By contrast, in patients with heart failure, cardiac output increases with administration of nitroglycerine because the effect of the fall of afterload is greater than the effect of the reduction of preload.

The function of the intact heart is often described by the pressure–volume loop (Fig. 2.8). The line relating end-systolic pressure to volume has been shown to reflect with some limitations the inotropic state of the heart. The relation between pressure and volume in diastole reflects the biochemical mechanisms of relaxation, the compliance of the

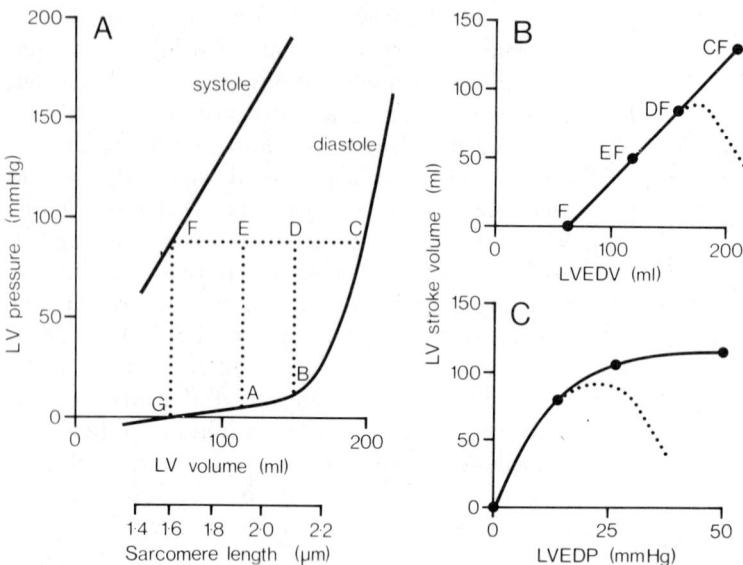

Fig. 2.8. (A) Pressure–volume relationship. BDFG represents a cardiac cycle. Without a change in contractility, the end-systolic pressure–volume relationship remains relatively constant. (B) A linear relation exists between stroke volume and left ventricular end-diastolic volume (LVEDV) unless ischaemia occurs at high end-diastolic volumes. (C) A curvilinear relation exists between stroke volume and left ventricular end-diastolic pressure (LVEDP). The relations in (B) and (C) can be deduced from (A).

myocardium and incoordinate relaxation and geommetrical properties of the ventricle.

CORONARY FLOW

The heart increases the supply of oxygen by an increase of coronary blood flow. Arteriovenous difference cannot widen greatly because the oxygen content of coronary sinus blood is low. Coronary blood flow can increase by up to five times. The relation between flow and oxygen consumption is almost linear under a wide variety of different conditions.

The factors regulating coronary flow are autoregulation, metabolic regulation and neuroendocrine factors. Autoregulation is the process by which coronary flow is maintained constant over a wide range of perfusion pressure (Fig. 2.10). The underlying mechanism is uncertain but is partly attributable to the myogenic reflex. Metabolic regulation is the process by which at constant perfusion pressure blood flow increases in response to an increase of

work (Fig. 2.10). One mechanism is the release of adenosine after the breakdown of ATP associated with the increased work. Other mechanisms for metabolic regulation include changes in pH, P_{CO_2}, P_{O_2} and extracellular potassium concentration. The response to increased work is rapid and can be demonstrated to occur after one beat. In man, an increase of cardiac work due to an increase of heart rate is accompanied by a fall in coronary sinus oxygen content which returns to normal within 5 s as blood flow increases. The third factor controlling coronary blood flow relates to the neural and hormonal control of coronary resistance.

Extravascular contraction of the myocardium has an important effect on coronary flow in the left ventricle but less of an effect in the right ventricle (Fig. 2.11). This is because the forces in the myocardium are greater in the left ventricle.

The coronary resistance is determined by the arterioles. Drugs and hormones have different or varying effects on large conduit arteries, on the epicardium of the heart and on the arterioles.

Heart failure

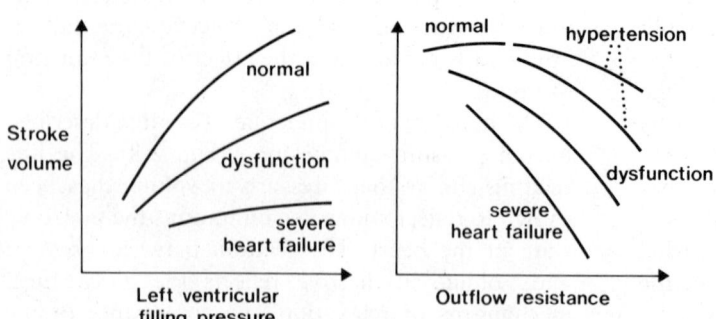

Fig. 2.9. In heart failure, the relation between stroke volume and end-diastolic pressure becomes flatter; the relation between stroke volume and outflow resistance becomes steeper.

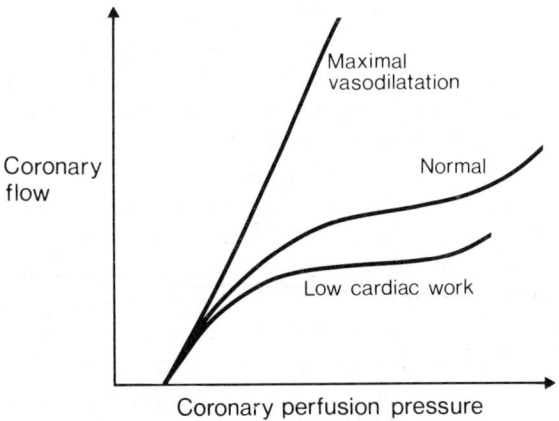

Fig. 2.10. Autoregulation is a mechanism whereby over a limited range of perfusion pressure coronary flow is relatively unchanged. Metabolic regulation is a process whereby at a given perfusion pressure coronary flow increases in relation to the work done by the heart.

Coronary vessels are innervated by the sympathetic and parasympathetic systems. Stimulation of alpha-receptors causes vasoconstriction. Beta-2 receptors stimulated largely by circulating adrenaline bring about vasodilatation. Beta-1 receptors are localized mainly on the myocytes, and beta-1 stimulation has only limited effects on the coronary circulation. Stimulation of sympathetic nerves causes vasodilatation because the increased cardiac work brings about metabolic vasodilatation which overrides any effect of alpha- or beta-constriction. Parasympathetic stimulation causes modest vasodilatation. Intracoronary acetylcholine causes a substantial vasodilatation by stimulating the release of endothelial relaxing factor, which has been shown to be nitric oxide. In patients with coronary atheroma, acetylcholine causes vasoconstriction by a direct effect on smooth muscle in the absence of endothelial relaxing factor due to endothelial cell damage. The release of endothelial relaxing factor is also sensitive to flow and may be a mechanism maintaining an optimal distribution of flow in tissues.

MECHANISM OF ACTION OF DRUGS

POSITIVE INOTROPIC DRUGS

No drug currently used in clinical practice increases the force of contraction by a direct effect on the myofibrils or troponin complex. Caffeine and other phosphodiesterase inhibitors affect the ability of the sarcoplasmic reticulum to sequester calcium and this may account for part of their clinical effect. All other drugs act primarily on the cell membrane.

Cardiac glycosides (e.g. digoxin) inhibit the sodium pump (the sodium–potassium ATPase). The intracellular sodium rises, which causes a decrease in calcium efflux and probably increases calcium influx. Calcium accumulates in the cell and is taken up by the sarcoplasmic reticulum. More calcium is available during each heart beat (entering as the inward calcium current and released from the sarcoplasmic reticulum) and an increased force of contraction results. An increase of heart rate also increases intracellular sodium because more sodium enters with each beat. Contractility is increased by the same mechanism as for cardiac glycosides.

Catecholamines (adrenaline and isoprenaline) react with beta-1 receptors which interact with a modulator protein causing stimulation of the enzyme adenyl cyclase (Fig. 2.11). Adenyl cyclase brings about the conversion of ATP to cyclic-AMP. Cyclic-AMP has many effects in the cell, three of which are to increase calcium influx during the action potential (increase contractility), to augment calcium uptake by the sarcoplasmic reticulum (increase relaxation) and to phosphorylate the contractile proteins (reduce contractility). The increase of calcium influx is due to an increase of the

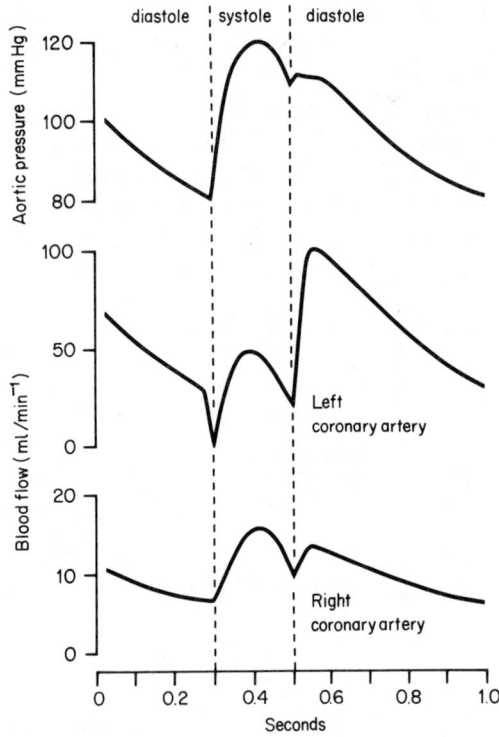

Fig. 2.11. Aortic pressure and coronary flow in the left and right coronary arteries. In the left coronary artery, flow occurs mainly during diastole, whereas in the right coronary artery flow occurs in both systole and diastole.

number of channels opening and the frequency of opening in a single channel rather than the rate of movement of calcium through the channel. The overall effect of catecholamines is that both contraction and the rate of relaxation of cardiac muscle are increased.

NEGATIVE INOTROPIC DRUGS

The 'calcium antagonists' (verapamil, nifedipine, diltiazem) have the property of inhibiting the slow calcium channel of the action potential and thus causing a fall in contractility. The calcium antagonists also bring about relaxation of arterial smooth muscle (vasodilatation) and reduce conduction in the atrioventricular node.

ARRHYTHMIAS

Electrical disequilibrium in the heart leads to arrhythmias. There are at least three cellular mechanisms. The first is called 'automaticity'. Injured myocardial cells or Purkinje fibres develop spontaneous phase 4 depolarization. Conditions that make the resting membrane potential less negative, the threshold voltage more negative or increase the rate of phase 4 depolarization favour automaticity.

The second mechanism is 're-entry'. The requirements for re-entry are undirectional block of an electrical impulse and slow propagation of the action potential. Under these circumstances, the electrical wavefront may pass round diseased tissue where the passage of the electrical wave is blocked.

The wavefront can approach the diseased tissue from the reverse direction, pass through the block retrogradely and stimulate cells which have had sufficient time to repolarize and not be refractory. A circus movement is established.

The third mechanism relates to after-potentials and the slow calcium current. Injured cells are often partly depolarized. This is particularly common in ischaemic tissue where the extracellular potassium can be high (up to 18 mmol/l) due to leakage of the ion out of the cell. Under these circumstances spontaneous depolarization can occur and is often caused by calcium currents. Depolarization may also be initiated by mechanical stretching of injured myocardium. If the phenomenon occurs in a sufficient number of cells, the current density can be large enough to cause depolarization of adjacent healthy cells and initiate an ectopic heart beat.

The precise cause of an arrhythmia in an individual patient is rarely known, and the classification of anti-arrhythmic drugs is based on electrophysiological and pharmacological observations. At present, a complete understanding of the interrelation between the aetiology of arrhythmias, the electrophysiological properties of drugs in single cells and the effectiveness of the drug as an anti-arrhythmic agent is only possible under special circumstances.

ISCHAEMIA

DEFINITION

Myocardial ischaemia is regarded as the state that

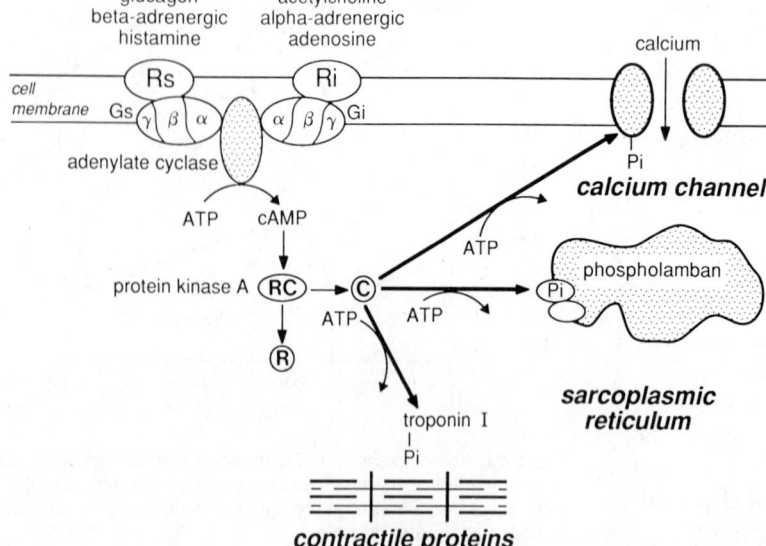

Fig. 2.12. The sympathetic cascade by which catecholamines and other substances affect contraction of cardiac muscle.

exists when myocardial oxygen supply is less than demand. Oxygen demand is more accurately the rate of consumption of ATP and oxygen supply is related to blood flow. Furthermore, blood flow not only provides a source of oxygen and substrate for heart muscle but also removes the product of metabolism. Two key products are heat and carbon dioxide. Ischaemia is better defined as an imbalance between ATP consumption and blood flow or as the state that exists when anaerobic metabolism occurs because of a low blood flow.

CAUSE OF CONTRACTILE FAILURE

Whatever the initiating mechanism for acute myocardial ischaemia, the three important consequences are a failure of contraction, arrhythmias and cell death. Total ischaemia results in cessation of contraction within 60 s. Important mechanisms are the rapid development of an intracellular acidosis and the rise in the intracellular concentration of phosphate. Acidosis results from the breakdown of ATP and metabolism of intracellular glycogen. Phosphate is formed from the breakdown of creatinine phosphate and ATP. Both acidosis and the phosphate ion reduce the response of the contractile proteins to calcium. Total tissue ATP does not decline within 60 s, but the rapid fall of tissue creatine phosphate suggests that energy availability is reduced. A low cytosolic ATP as opposed to total tissue ATP might affect contraction if insufficient ATP were available to maintain the normal functioning of ionic channels in the cell membrane or to allow shortening of the contractile proteins.

MECHANISM OF CELL DEATH

The exact sequence of events leading to cell death is at present controversial. Under normal resting conditions, the myocardium will recover almost completely after 10–15 min of ischaemia. More prolonged periods of ischaemia are associated with less than full recovery of myocardial contractility. If a small residual blood flow is present from collateral coronary arteries or from 'stuttering' ischaemia in the native coronary artery, the time before recovery is complete is lengthened. After 60–90 min of total ischaemia, the cell membrane is destroyed. This can be attributed to a low tissue ATP, acidosis, activation of phospholipases and lysosomal activity. In the presence of permanent occlusion of a coronary artery, cell death is inevitable unless residual flow is sufficient to maintain the integrity of the cell until

flow increases or new collaterals develop. New collaterals take at least 48 h to develop. Different animal species vary in the existence of collaterals. The dog has many collaterals, whereas the rabbit and pig have almost none. Man has few collaterals in the absence of atheromatous coronary artery disease. In patients with severe obstruction to their coronary arteries, collaterals may have formed over many years. These will affect the consequences of an acute occlusion of a native artery.

Recovery of myocardial function is impossible without the restoration of flow by some mechanism. Controversy still exists as to whether the ultmate survival or death of myocardial tissue is dependent solely on events during ischaemia, on events at the time of reperfusion or both. Certainly, cell necrosis is inevitable when the cell membrane is destroyed. Furthermore, it seems that necrosis is preceded by alterations in the function of the cell membrane which result in such gross changes in the intracellular environment that the homeostatic mechanisms of the cell are overwhelmed. A key ion in this respect is calcium, see 'Reperfusion'.

REPERFUSION

Reperfusion of ischaemic heart muscle is associated with the signs of cell damage ('reperfusion damage'). There is an immediate swelling of the cell, release of intracellular enzymes and a large influx of calcium. Calcium is taken up by the mitochondria and can be seen as dark granules under the electron microscope. A large gain of calcium is an indicator of cell death since it prevents the normal functioning of mitochondria and the regeneration of ATP. Many theories exist to explain the sudden influx of calcium. A popular hypothesis is that the reintroduction of oxygen causes an increased generation of oxygen radicals which damage the cell membrane and in particular render the membrane permeable to calcium. The normal mechanisms within the cell for the removal of radicals are partly destroyed during the period of ischaemia. The cell membrane may be sensitized to the harmful effects of radicals by the action of phospholipases during the period of ischaemia. Phospholipases are activated by acidosis and raised cytosolic calcium, and modify the lipids of the cell membrane. An alternative mechanism for the influx of calcium is stimulation of sodium–calcium exchange.

The determinants of infarct size in man are the duration of the period of ischaemia, the pre-existing coronary anatomy, the presence of collaterals, residual flow in the native coronary artery ('stuttering ischaemia') and the myocardial oxygen consumption at the onset of ischaemia.

Recovery from a period of ischaemia is slow. Full recovery of contractile function after 5 min of ischaemia may take many hours and 60 min of low flow ischaemia days or even weeks. This is partly because the myocardium loses nucleotides. ATP is broken down to ADP and AMP, which, in turn, are broken down to inosine and adenosine, which are then lost from the cell. The regeneration of nucleotides takes several days. Abnormalities of the excitation–contraction system also persist for hours or weeks. This condition has been called the 'stunned' or 'hibernating' myocardium.

At present, drugs used in an attempt to reduce the size of a myocardial infarction act either by reducing ATP consumption (cardioplegic solutions, hypothermia, afterload reduction, negative inotropic agents) or by increasing coronary flow (coronary vasodilators) through collaterals or the native coronary. The recent introduction of thrombolytic therapy for selected patients with myocardial infarction should reduce infarct size if the occlusion is due to thrombus, if the thrombus can be dissolved and if the occlusion has not been present for more than one hour. If collateral flow is possible or the occlusion is only transient, the period of ischaemia before cell death becomes inevitable may be extended up to 6 h. No drug has been shown to benefit the ischaemic myocardial cell by a mechanism that acts directly on the cell structure or cell metabolism, with the possible exceptions of insulin, glucose and potassium therapy, corticosteroids and hyaluronidase. Hypothermia is effective partly because metabolic pathways are inactivated. Cardioplegia, nitrates, calcium antagonists and possibly beta-adrenergic blockers have actions on myocardial contractility (cardioplegia associated with a reduction of oxygen consumption) or on coronary flow.

FURTHER READING

Folkow B., Neil E. *Circulation*. Oxford: Oxford University Press, 1971.

Hearse, D.J., Yellon S.M. *Therapeutic approaches to myocardial infarct size limitation*. New York: Raven Press, 1984.

Katz A.M. *Physiology of the heart*. New York: Raven Press, 1977.

Noble D. *The initiation of the heart beat*. Oxford: Clarendon Press, 1979.

Opie L. *The Heart*. New York: Grune and Stratton, 1985.

Parratt J.R. *Control and manipulation of calcium movement*. New York: Raven Press, 1985.

Kalsner S. *The Coronary Artery*. London: Croom Helm, 1982.

Marcus M. *The coronary circulation in health and disease*. New York: McGraw-Hill, 1983.

Chapter 3

Acute Heart Failure

R.D. Bradley

HEART FAILURE AND CIRCULATORY FAILURE

The term heart failure is confined to states in which there is a demonstrable abnormality of function of the heart. Circulatory failure has a wider context, and includes entities such as pulmonary embolism, overtransfusion and nephritis. These entities may occur in patients who have normal hearts and the response is that of a normal heart with an unimpaired ability to generate work;[1] impairment of cardiac function and the advent of true heart failure is frequently the terminal destabilizing influence leading rapidly to death. Some of the topics dealt with in this section are better thought of as manifestations of circulatory failure. Confusion arises because these conditions share the abnormal physical signs that are regarded as the classic hallmarks of heart failure.

Major acute derangements, such as anterior or inferior myocardial infarction, and pulmonary embolism, give rise to recognizable syndromes relating not merely to the function of the heart, but to the response of the entire circulation. Understanding these patterns of response allows insight into those manoeuvres that are likely to destabilize the circulation, and those that may improve it. Patients with a pulmonary embolus have an obstructed circulation, those who have acute nephritis or who have sustained overtransfusion, have an overexpanded circulation, and those with cor pulmonale have the circulatory consequences of underventilation. None of these can be or should be equated with heart failure, whereas the circulatory instability with septicaemia is frequently associated with heart failure, and myocardial infarction invariably so, irrespective of the presence or absence of the accepted physical signs of heart failure.

The descriptions that follow are confined to patients who have major disturbances of the circulation.

OVERTRANSFUSION

Overtransfusion allows the description of the impact of a relatively simple disturbance upon a normal heart, and contrasts well with the findings in more complex abnormalities to be described later. Patients commonly have the physical signs of heart failure, namely, raised venous pressure, loud third and fourth heart sounds, diffuse lung crepitations, pulmonary oedema on the chest X-ray but a normal electrocardiogram.

The feature that poses the most serious threat to the patient is pulmonary oedema which if untreated may be life-threatening. The critical value of the left atrial or pulmonary wedge pressure (measured from the sternal angle as zero) for the formation of pulmonary oedema is approximately 0.57 times the plasma albumin concentration ($0.57 \times 42 = 24$ mmHg). The greater the margin by which this value is exceeded, the faster the rate at which the pulmonary oedema appears.[2] Conversely, the greater the reduction of the left atrial pressure below this value, the faster the reabsorption of the oedema into the circulation.

The treatment of pulmonary oedema due to overtransfusion in the presence of a normal heart requires the removal of a much larger quantity of fluid from the circulation than is the case with pulmonary oedema generated by a failing heart. This difference is due to the increased compliance of the capacity vessels and the 2:1 relationship of the slopes of the equations relating stroke volume to filling pressure in the two ventricles. The stroke volume equations in Fig. 3.1 show that a reduction of the left atrial pressure from 17 to 3 mmHg (from 5 mm above the critical pressure to 9 mm below), corresponds to a reduction of right atrial pressure from 4 to −3 mmHg, and a fall of stroke output from 130 to 70 ml, or of cardiac output from 12.5 to 6.5 l/min. The relative compliance of the overfilled capacity vessels (330 ml/mmHg) indicates that

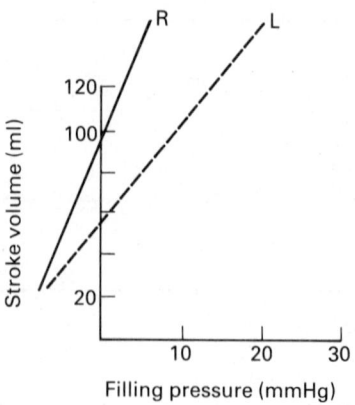

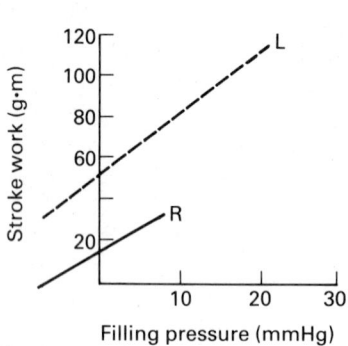

Fig. 3.1. Overtransfusion. Venous compliance = 330 ml/mmHg; systemic vascular resistance = 6–18–21 units (*or* 480–1440–1680 dyn·s/cm⁵); pulmonary vascular resistance = 0.2–1–1.8 units (*or* 16–80–144 dyn·s/cm⁵).

this change will require the removal of 2300 ml from the circulation. This is in the region of 10 times the volume that commonly has to be removed to control the pulmonary oedema generated by a failing left ventricle.

Two further facts of importance emerge from consideration of Fig. 3.1. First, volume expansion inevitably lowers the vascular resistances. Initially, the patient's systemic resistance was only 480 dyne s/cm⁵, and the pulmonary resistance 16 dyne s/cm⁵; these values rose to normal with the removal of sufficient volume to render the atrial pressures normal. Second, at normal atrial pressures, this patient's heart generated normal values of stroke work, and had a high stroke volume in response to high atrial pressures.

The pattern of physiological disturbance in acute nephritis is the same as that of overtransfusion: the overexpansion of the circulation occurs because of the failure of the kidneys to balance water intake with output, and the appearances of heart failure are again belied by the performance of the heart.[3]

Failure to control the circulatory situation described above may stem from failure to realize the relatively large volume that must be lost rapidly from the circulation, which may be difficult if there is coincidental impairment of renal function. Treatment with morphine, aminophylline and digoxin, on the grounds that such a patient was suffering from heart failure, will not address the problem of the very large volume and has lead to death.

If the high atrial pressures are not reduced to well below the critical limit, ever worsening pulmonary oedema will produce, sometimes with surprising rapidity, a metabolic milieu of low oxygen tension, and ultimately hypercapnia in which the heart and all other organs fail. The work of breathing is greatly increased.[4] The condition is then infinitely

more difficult to treat, requiring positive pressure ventilation, inotropic support of the heart and the use of techniques such as haemofiltration to remove the fluid.

PULMONARY OEDEMA

There are many causes of pulmonary oedema (Table 3.1).

The interrelation of hydraulic and osmotic changes already described in the consideration of overtransfusion can cause pulmonary oedema. The albumin concentration in the oedema fluid in overtransfused patients appears to be proportional to the amount by which the critical value of pressure has been exceeded. Where the critical value has been grossly exceeded, the oedema fluid has the same protein concentration as the plasma, and

Table 3.1.   Classification of pulmonary oedema.

1 Physical forces:	Pulmonary capillary pressure
	Plasma oncotic pressure
	Negative pressure in chest
2 Membrane permeability:	Injections
	Aspirations of acid
	Toxins
	Disseminated intravascular coagulation
	Shock lung
	Immunological
3 Lymphatic insufficiency:	Lymphangitis carcinomatosis
	Fibrosis
4 Neurogenic	
5 Uncertain origin:	High altitude
	Poisoning
	Eclampsia

contains red cells and white cells. More modest excesses of pulmonary capillary pressure produce oedema fluid with albumin concentrations as low as half that of the plasma.

Neurogenic pulmonary oedema produced during the irritative phase of evolving cerebral medullary lesions is analogous to overtransfusion, except that the prime abnormality is an intense rise in both venous and arterial vascular tone, rather than a volume change.[5,6] Similarly, the enormous changes in vascular tone that occur in the often fatal pulmonary oedema seen in scuba divers appear to be triggered by an idiosyncratic reaction to cold.[7]

It is often suggested that the pulmonary oedema generated by high pulmonary capillary pressures ought to be amenable to treatment by raising the plasma albumin concentration. Salt-free albumin given in normal concentration raises the right atrial pressure, and, if given in high concentration with the intention of avoiding the circulatory volume load, still produces a rise in right and left atrial pressures by attracting fluid from the extracellular space. The possible benefits in the acute situation always seem to be offset by the attendant rise in atrial pressures.

Damage to the pulmonary capillary basement membrane will cause pulmonary oedema. Most commonly, this occurs in association with septicaemia, and sometimes following cardiopulmonary bypass procedures. Exposure to chlorine or formalin vapour, and paraquat poisoning are less common causes. Under these circumstances, the oedema appears at normal pulmonary capillary pressures, or even those that are lower than normal, and the albumin concentration approximates to that of the plasma.

Ligature of the thoracic duct or its right-sided homologue will produce pulmonary oedema. The distribution of the fluid is characteristic, being confined to the left upper lobe of the lung in the case of the thoracic duct, and involving the entire right lung and the lower lobe of the left in the case of the right-sided homologue. Again, the albumin concentration is similar to that of the plasma. The inadvertent tying of a pulmonary vein at operation is another cause of bizzarely localized pulmonary oedema.

It follows from what has been said that only a low albumin concentration in the oedema fluid relative to that of plasma is of diagnostic help, suggesting a hydraulic cause. If the albumin concentration is similar to that of plasma, any of the above causes are possible.

ACUTE MYOCARDIAL INFARCTION

Reduction of flow in the circulation can occur as a result of infarction of any part of the heart, but the events that predispose to pulmonary oedema are less common in inferior than in anterior and lateral infarction.[8,9] The question of paramount importance that has to be considered for each individual patient is what poses the greater threat to survival. Treatment likely to make pulmonary oedema better may further reduce peripheral perfusion and vice versa.

ACUTE ANTERIOR OR LATERAL MYOCARDIAL INFARCTION

Clinical features

Patients often have a short history of chest pain and extreme dyspnoea and orthopnoea. The venous pressure may not be raised. There is a productive cough and expectoration. The chest X-ray may show severe pulmonary oedema of a bat's wing distribution, and the electrocardiogram the changes of a developing anterolateral infarct.

Pathophysiology

The analysis of such a patient's circulatory state is presented in Fig. 3.2. The feature that presents the greatest threat to survival is uncontrolled pulmonary oedema, but here it occurs in the presence of a moderate reduction of peripheral perfusion.

The critical level of pulmonary capillary pressure above which pulmonary oedema will appear, approximates to 20 mmHg, the albumin concentration being 36 g/l. The equations of stroke volume show that a right atrial pressure of -2.5 mmHg corresponds to a pulmonary capillary pressure of 26 mmHg and a stroke volume of 40 ml, or a cardiac output of 4 l/min. At these pressures, oedema will continue to form at an appreciable rate.

As with the overtransfused patient, the key to the treatment of this situation lies in the venous compliance and the relative slopes of the stroke volume equations. These combine to make the patient prone to pulmonary oedema, and at the same time sensitive to treatment. The 7.5 : 1 ratio of the slopes and the figure of 110 ml/mmHg for the compliance of the capacity vessels infer that the removal of 250 ml from the circulation will reduce the right atrial pressure by 2.3 mmHg, and therefore the left atrial pressure by 17 mmHg, from 26 to 9 mmHg. This is

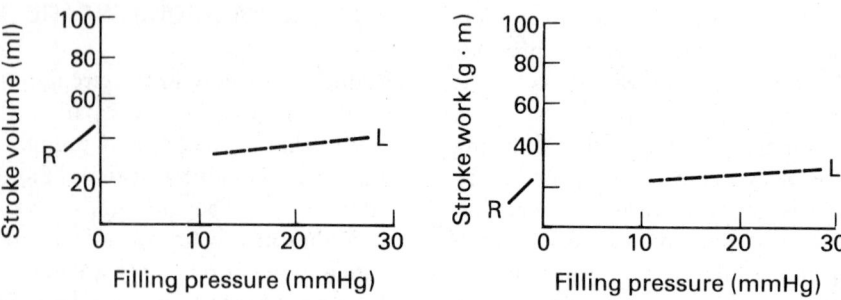

Fig. 3.2. Acute anterior myocardial infarction. Venous compliance = 110 ml/mmHg.

sufficient not only to prevent the generation of further oedema but to bring about its rapid reabsorption.

The ratio is such that sitting the patient upright or reduction of the venous tone with morphine are manoeuvres likely to effect the required reduction in right atrial pressure.

The loss of 250 ml from the circulation could be achieved with the passage of about 750 ml of urine, 250 ml of this coming directly from the circulation, and 500 ml coming through the circulation from the extracellular space. The amount of the contribution from the extracellular compartment would depend upon the partition coefficient for water between the two compartments. The treatment of pulmonary oedema due to acute myocardial infarction is morphine and diuretics; nitrates can be of value and, in an extreme situation, so can positive pressure ventilation.

Mechanism of destabilization

If attempts to reduce the atrial pressures fail, the patient will continue to generate pulmonary oedema and thereby enter a spiral of increasing lung stiffness, increasing respiratory workload,[4] diminishing efficiency of gas exchange, and increasing sympathetic activity, with rising venous tone and atrial pressures, from which there is no escape. Although it is essential to reduce the atrial pressures, this manoeuvre also reduces cardiac output. In normal clinical practice, minor changes of tissue perfusion are compatible with the continued function of all other organs, and only modest rises in urea and creatinine occur. Thus, there are no physical signs for the clinician to detect, but the patient experiences symptomatic deterioration, i.e. he or she is less capable of sustaining any activity, and the threshold at which exertion produces the small increase in right atrial pressure sufficient to

precipitate pulmonary oedema, would be lowered because of the increased venous tone.

Breathlessness

Patients experience the sensation of breathlessness before the atrial pressures reach the point at which oedema is produced in the lungs. Increments of right atrial pressure increase the stroke volume that the right heart delivers to the lungs. For a few beats, the stroke volume arriving in the pulmonary vessels exceeds that which the left heart is removing. This net transfer of blood from the systemic to the pulmonary circulation distends the pulmonary vessels, causing the lungs to become stiffer, and raises the filling pressure of the left heart so that its stroke output again matches that of the right heart. There is evidence that increasing stiffness of the lung is translated into the sensation of breathlessness by the alteration that it produces in the relation between tension and length in the respiratory muscles.[10] This is presumably sensed proprioceptively. Experimentally, abnormally high tension in the respiratory muscles in relation to the length to which they are stretched does produce the sensation of dyspnoea. Curarization abolishes muscular tension, which may account for the observation that it also abolishes the sensation of dyspnoea when it is used in patients being treated with intermittent positive pressure ventilation.

The factors that promote susceptibility to pulmonary oedema are depression of function of the left heart, and an increase in systemic vascular resistance, with preservation of the function of the right heart and a diminished pulmonary resistance. The last of these is an inevitable consequence of the volume shift into the pulmonary circulation. All of these changes are present in the example shown in Fig. 3.2.

ACUTE INFERIOR OR DIAPHRAGMATIC MYOCARDIAL INFARCTION

Clinical features

In most patients whose circulations are severely compromised as a result of this pattern of infarction, the patient is likely to complain of pain and tightness across the chest, radiating to the arms. There is restlessness, confusion, pallor, sweating, coldness of the limbs reaching above the elbows and knees, a tachycardia, and the venous pressure may be in excess of 10 cm, the blood pressure will probably be reduced, and the electrocardiogram shows changes of acute diaphragmatic myocardial infarction. The chest X-ray is usually normal.

Pathophysiology

The essential feature is poor tissue perfusion in the absence of pulmonary oedema; the findings are summarized in Fig. 3.3.

The compliance of the capacity vessels is small. Removal of only 56 ml from the circulation reduces the right atrial pressure by 1 mmHg, suggesting that the venous tone matches the very high systemic vascular resistance. These findings are in agreement with the clinical state described, and all suggest a high level of sympathetic activity.

Mechanism of destabilization

One of the commonest destabilizing influences in such a setting is treatment. The inordinately high right atrial pressure presents an almost irresistible temptation to treat the patient with diuretics. The

removal of < 0.5 l from the circulation reduces the right atrial pressure from 14 to 5 mmHg and the left atrial pressure from 17 to 9 mmHg. The results of diuretic therapy for the patient are disastrous because the cardiac output falls from 2.3 to 1.9 l/min, a level that leads to multiple organ failure. Inspection of the chest X-ray should make it clear that the patient is not at risk from pulmonary oedema, and treatment with diuretics can only make the flows worse.

THE FIVE POSSIBLE MEDICAL APPROACHES TO INADEQUATE TISSUE PERFUSION

MANIPULATION OF THE FILLING PRESSURES

Raising the filling pressures in order to increase the flows is likely to be most helpful in patients in whom there is some cardiac reserve and in whom both ventricles are affected. The aftermath of cardiopulmonary bypass operations,[11] and diaphragmatic myocardial infarction are most commonly associated with such an arrangement of function. In the former, optimal adjustment of the atrial pressures is an inevitable part of the postoperative management and, although much less commonly employed, is as advantageous in the presence of inferior infarction.

If monitoring of the pulmonary capillary pressure is possible, it is reasonable to raise this to 15 mmHg. If the pulmonary vascular resistance is normal, this level of pressure is commonly associated with the appearance of a right ventricular third sound, an observation offering some possibility of control by the use of physical signs. However, this device is of no value when the need is greatest, because there is no reserve of ventricular function.

THE USE OF INOTROPIC AGENTS

Inotropic agents cause the heart to produce more work at a given filling pressure, and by so doing will increase tissue perfusion. The major disadvantage of their use, especially in the context of ischaemic heart disease, is their impact on the internal metabolic economy of the heart.[12] They increase oxygen consumption, and if there is ischaemia they convert a lactate-consuming heart to lactate production. Also, the response they produce diminishes as the underlying state of the heart worsens. When the need for inotropy is greatest, the effect of such agents becomes difficult to measure.

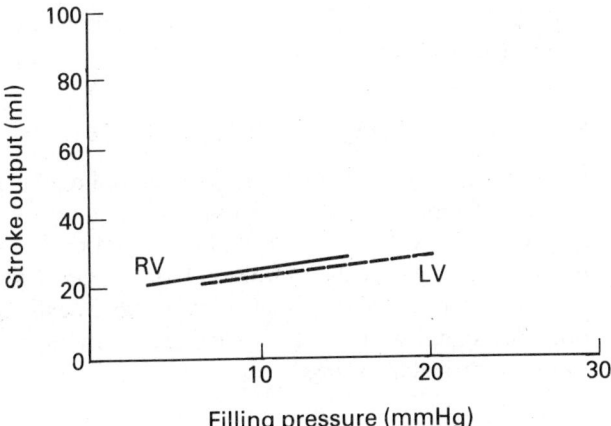

Fig. 3.3. Inferior or diaphragmatic myocardial infarction. Venous compliance = 56 ml/mmHg.

Despite these deficiencies, inotropic agents are used, often successfully, in what must be regarded as the limiting case of acute heart failure – cardiac arrest. Their undoubted value in this extreme situation deals summarily with the criticism that they should not be used in the presence of ischaemia. The heart has to generate its own blood supply and, used in conjunction with cardiac massage and metabolic correction, these agents offer the most rapid and effective method of restoring an adequate coronary perfusion pressure. The balance of effectiveness in terms of coronary perfusion versus cost of work should perhaps encourage the use of inotropic agents in that area of uncertainty between a heart that will not support life and one that will support renal function unaided.

In extreme situations, adrenaline and calcium are the inotropic agents of choice; they give rise to a modest improvement when the heart is beyond response to any of the other agents. In less severe circumstances, the choice will depend upon the ancillary properties of the inotropic agents, notably whether vasoconstrictor or vasodilator, and their effect on heart rate. The aim should be to tailor the effects to the individual pattern of circulatory disturbance (Table 3.2). Dopamine, in low dose, and dobutamine are dilators and can be used simultaneously for afterload reduction, and for their inotropic properties. Isoprenaline is both a dilator and a chronotrope.

AFTERLOAD REDUCTION

Afterload reduction has proved a most valuable manoeuvre. It depends upon a re-apportioning of the limited work of which the heart is capable. The useful work of the heart is consumed in generating both pressure and flow, and by reducing the resistance to ejection it is possible to achieve either greater flow at the same filling pressure or the same flow at a lower filling pressure.[13] If the latter is the object, because the problem is pulmonary oedema, the venodilatation that the agents employed inevitably produce is an added benefit. If an increase in flow is sought, it is important that the afterload reduction be accompanied by restoration of the filling pressures with a volume expander. The volume expansion dilates the vessels additionally, producing an even greater fall in vascular resistance.

The circulatory benefits are greater if the ventricle involved is abnormally dilated. As the resistance to ejection is reduced, the ventricular diameter also diminishes, and it follows from application of Laplace's Law[14,15] that the pressure generated is increased, at the same wall tension. The result is that afterload reduction in the presence of a dilated ventricle interferes less with the blood pressure than would be the case if the ventricle were small.

In the setting of acute infarction, vasodilatation carries an appreciable risk, probably because the accompanying hypotension reduces coronary perfusion. A trial of treatment of hypertension in acute infarction with sodium nitroprusside had to be abandoned because of the high mortality in the treated group.[16] If it were possible to select the group of patients whose acute infarction was the result of single-vessel disease, it is probable that they would benefit from afterload reduction.

Sodium nitroprusside or nitroglycerine, by intravenous infusion, are the most convenient drugs with which to test the effects of afterload reduction, because any change in dosage is effective within 3 min. The development in any individual of an undesirable degree of hypotension or oliguria can be reversed quickly.

PACING (PREFERABLY ATRIAL)

If the stroke volume is small and fixed, doubling the rate will double the output. This is effective up to paced rates between 90 and 100, but thereafter this manoeuvre ceases to be of value. Atrial or, in the presence of heart block, sequential pacing usually provides significantly better tissue perfusion than simple ventricular pacing.[17]

AORTIC COUNTERPULSATION

Balloon counterpulsation is physiologically ideal

Table 3.2. **Treatment of circulatory failure.**

LVEDP[a] (mmHg)	Blood pressure	Tissue perfusion	Treatment
> 18	Normal	Normal	Vasodilator
	Normal	Low	Vasodilator
	Low	Normal	Vasodilator/inotrope
	Low	Low	Inotrope and vasodilator
< 18	Normal	Normal	Observe
	Normal	Low	Vasodilator
	Low	Normal	Observe/inotrope
	Low	Low	Inotrope/?vasodilator
< 10	Low	Normal or low	Volume expansion
	Normal	Normal or low	Volume expansion

[a] LVEDP, Left ventricular end-diastolic pressure (often estimated from other measurements).

because it increases the cardiac output by about 0.5 l/min, increases coronary flow and diminishes the work of the heart and its oxygen consumption.[12] Unfortunately, published data show that the great majority of patients with acute infarction who cannot survive without counterpulsation will prove to be inseparable from the support. The few (<10%) who survive once separated from the pump have a very limited prognosis. In the aftermath of a cardiopulmonary bypass operation, where the function of the heart may improve considerably with the passage of time, counterpulsation is of established value.

ACUTE PULMONARY EMBOLISM

CLINICAL FEATURES

Patients develop sudden breathlessness and sometimes pain in the chest. The physical signs are those of heart failure: tachycardia, a raised venous pressure, cardiac enlargement, prominent third and fourth heart sounds, and expiratory ronchi, with a raised respiratory rate. Additionally, the extremities are cool and the blood pressure is normal or reduced. The electrocardiogram shows evidence of acute right ventricular overload. The chest X-ray is normal or shows areas of reduced perfusion.

The outstanding features are breathlessness and evidence from the arterial gases of considerable pulmonary shunting, without pulmonary oedema on the chest X-ray, in the presence of poor flows and a raised venous pressure. This is in contradistinction to left ventricular failure in which the arterial oxygen tension is little impaired until there is evident pulmonary oedema on the chest X-ray, and the flows are usually less reduced. The observation that sitting the patient up with legs dependent produces profound bradycardia and syncope, requiring cardiac massage, is highly relevant to the nature of the physiological disturbance.[1]

PATHOPHYSIOLOGY

The analysis of circulatory disturbance is presented in Fig. 3.4. The principal threat to the patient is impairment of the cardiac output due to obstruction of the circulation, the pulmonary resistance being very high. The secondary changes involve considerable constriction of the venous capacity vessels (53 ml volume change per mmHg change in right atrial pressure), and of the systemic arterial system (2960 dyne s/cm⁵).

The principal result of the above changes is that circulatory function is much better at high right atrial pressures, and is very sensitive to small volume changes. With a right atrial pressure of 3 mmHg, the patient is close to instability, the stroke volume being 21 ml, and the cardiac output only 1.9 l/min. The normal blood pressure, due to the high systemic resistance, should not be allowed to generate a false sense of security.

Infusion of only 0.5 l of plasma produces a most remarkable change. Because of the lack of compliance of the capacity bed, this small volume produces a large rise in the right atrial pressure from 3 to 12.5 mmHg, raising the right ventricular stroke work from 7 to 11 g·m. Briefly, as a result of this, the right heart pumps a larger volume into the pulmonary bed than the left heart removes. This volume change in the pulmonary circulation has the crucial effect of dilating all the pulmonary vessels, including those obstructed with emboli, reducing the measured pulmonary resistance (from 1120 to 560 dyne s/cm⁵). It is principally owing to this that the stroke output rises from 21 to 36 ml, and the cardiac output from 1.9 to 3.2 l/min.

MECHANISM OF DESTABILIZATION

Any change that lowers the right atrial pressure, either by diminishing venous tone or by removing volume from the circulation, is likely to prove lethal. The mechanism involves a fall in right ven-

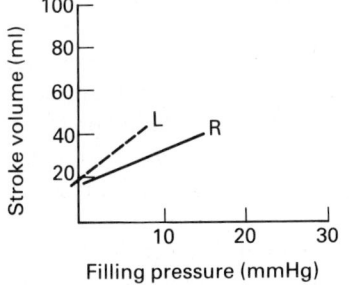

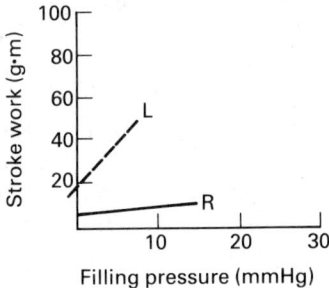

Fig. 3.4. Acute massive pulmonary embolism. Venous compliance = 53 ml/mmHg; systemic vascular resistance = 25–37 units (or 2000–2960 dyn·s/cm⁵); pulmonary vascular resistance = 7–14 units (or 560–1120 dyn·s/cm⁵).

tricular stroke volume, which is only balanced by an equal fall in left-sided stroke output, when volume has been lost from the pulmonary to the systemic circuit, allowing the left atrial pressure to fall. It is this net shift of volume from what little remains of the embolized pulmonary circuit that raises the pulmonary resistance to insupportable levels. In the context of acute as opposed to chronic pulmonary embolism, values of resistance > 15 times normal are likely to be fatal.

The interventions that commonly precipitate this unstable state are morphine administration, the induction of anaesthesia, the injection of contrast material (a venodilator) for angiography, inferior vena caval ligation, and the administration of diuretics in the mistaken belief that the patient has heart failure. Acute circulatory collapse triggered by venodilatation can be controlled with intravenous phenylephrine (1.5–4 ug/kg), which keeps the venous tone high.

There is a very considerable difference between the view that such patients have heart failure simply because of the physical signs and the understanding that in the earlier phases the problem is an obstructed circulation that can be manipulated, at least partially, by expansion of the obstructed vessels. Ultimately, the circulatory changes do involve failure of the heart which can to some extent be mitigated by infusion of adrenaline. Adrenaline is the inotropic agent of choice because it is also a venoconstrictor. Once the right atrial pressure is in excess of 15 mmHg (sternal angle as zero reference), the situation can be remedied only by open embolectomy and a period of supportive cardiopulmonary bypass to allow the right ventricle to recover.

Thrombolytic therapy has many attractions, provided that the patient has not recently undergone surgery. If such treatment is envisaged, it is important that invasive access to the circulation be kept to the absolute minimum because of bleeding at the access site. The best evidence of the efficacy of thrombolysis comes from a study involving the assessment of patency of the major pulmonary vessels obtained angiographically before and after treatment with streptokinase.[18] Thrombolysis has the disadvantage that it does not act as rapidly as may be required by the progress of events in acute pulmonary embolism. Volume expansion is effective within a few beats, and may account for many of the benefits that have been ascribed to thrombolytic therapy. These two forms of therapy are not exclusive but additive.

CHRONIC OBSTRUCTIVE AIRWAYS DISEASE

The term cor pulmonale is applied to the circulatory problems associated with both pulmonary embolism and chronic obstructive airways disease, albeit the first problem is acute and the second chronic. This suggests that the two may have common features; in truth, they differ in almost every respect.

The reason for considering the problems of obstructive airways in a section on acute circulatory disorder is that the circulatory sequelae appear as acute episodes.

CLINICAL FEATURES

The outstanding circulatory features of obstructive airways disease are gross limitation of exercise tolerance, a raised venous pressure, oedema, dilated warm extremities with full cutaneous veins, and a right ventricular third sound which although present may be obscured by the pulmonary signs of airways obstruction. Both the patient and the chest X-ray have appearances consistent with an enlarged functional residual capacity. The chest X-ray may also reveal the characteristic appearances of consolidation in overexpanded lung as an acute precipitating cause of decline in pulmonary function. The arterial blood gases always show evidence of carbon dioxide retention. In such a patient, a change from warm hyperdynamic extremities to those that are cold is a clinical warning of the onset of terminal instability.

PATHOPHYSIOLOGY

The circulatory findings typical of such a patient are detailed in Fig. 3.5. The principal threat is ventilatory rather than circulatory. The rise in pulmonary vascular resistance is moderate: 4 times normal in the case illustrated; it is most commonly within the range 2–6 times that of normal. Compensation for this change in resistance is achieved by the right heart doing more work than normal at any given filling pressure, the cardiac flows ranging between 5.5 and 7 l/min over the span of filling pressures illustrated. In as much as the left heart produces normal values of work in relation to filling pressure, and the right heart much more than normal thereby maintaining the cardiac output, neither the heart nor the circulation are failing.

Also, in contrast to the findings in acute pulmonary embolism, the systemic resistance is low, and

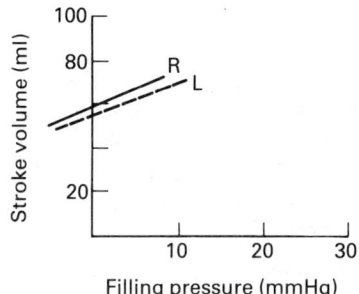 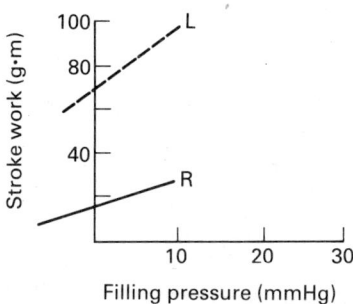

Fig. 3.5. Chronic obstructive airways disease. Venous compliance = 160 ml/mmHg; systemic vascular resistance = 15–16 units (or 1200–1280 dyn·s/cm⁵); pulmonary vascular resistance = 4 units (or 320 dyn·s/cm⁵).

the capacity vessels are dilated. A raised venous pressure in the presence of a low venous tone implies considerable salt and water retention, probably occurring in response to the ventilatory failure. In acute pulmonary embolism, there is not enough time for water–salt retention to occur, but in chronic packed pulmonary embolism, where the circulatory disturbance is of the same pattern, it is notable that the patients do not have systemic oedema, and the high venous pressure is generated by a high venous tone rather than by fluid retention.

The ultimate point of contrast is that patients with obstructive airways disease do not benefit from a high right atrial pressure. As has been pointed out, the raised venous pressure in this condition depends upon fluid retention rather than changes in venous tone, and any fluid retention increases the oedema of the chronically infected bronchial mucosa and therefore makes the airway obstruction worse.

It is common experience that the obstructed nasal airway associated with acute rhinitis is aggravated by the recumbent position and can often be cleared acutely by sitting upright. The mechanism relates to the gradient of pressure down the lymphatic system into the central venous system. The drainage of the chronically infected bronchial mucosa is into the same system, and lower values of right atrial pressure make such patients measurably easier to ventilate.

MECHANISM OF DESTABILIZATION

The circulatory state described above usually persists for several years, with modest fluctuations in pulmonary resistance occurring inversely with arterial oxygenation, and the adequacy of ventilation. Terminally, underventilation produces a metabolic milieu of gross hypoxia (with arterial oxygen tensions < 30 mmHg) and hypercapnic acidaemia in which the heart does fail, the pulmonary vascular resistance rises to values as high as 10 times that of normal and the hyperdynamic flows cease. As has

already been stated, an obvious change in peripheral perfusion is the clinical herald of this state lasting only a matter of hours, in which both sides of the heart fail to produce normal values of work and the pulmonary and systemic resistances both rise.

This unstable state can be reversed by artificial ventilation, which is an appropriate manoeuvre if it is thought possible that the patient's pulmonary function can be improved. The initiation of ventilation in such circumstances requires that the patient be oxygenated, given inotropic support, and deliberately underventilated, in that order. The reason for the initial underventilation is that the minute volume required to make a rapid inroad into the hypercapnia would increase the already very large functional residual capacity and raise the pulmonary vascular resistance to a level involving appreciable obstruction of the circulation.

SEPSIS AND THE CIRCULATION

Sepsis may cause either an increase or a decrease in the compliance of the capacity bed, and either an increase or decrease in the systemic or pulmonary vascular resistance. Moreover, any combination of these changes is possible, the tone of the various vascular beds altering in different directions and changing with time. In some patients, the function of the heart is diminished. Such enormous variability leads to complex circulatory adjustments. It also explains the failure of the relentless quest for a panacea that can be universally applied.

PATHOPHYSIOLOGY

The commonest combination of circulatory changes corresponds to those popularly associated with Gram-negative infection, although the nature of the infection is in no way predictive of the nature of the circulatory changes. The findings in a patient with a septicaemia are shown in Fig. 3.6. The venous

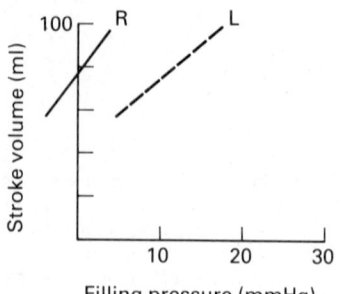

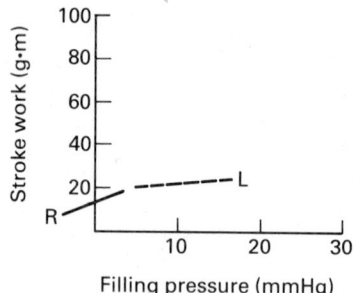

Fig. 3.6. Urethral dilatation – *Proteus* septicaemia. Venous compliance = 210 ml/mmHg; systemic vascular resistance = 2.8 units (*or* 224 dyn·s/cm⁵); pulmonary vascular resistance = 0.2 units (*or* 16 dyn·s/cm⁵).

system is relatively compliant, and both the systemic and pulmonary resistances are low. Over the range of right atrial pressures inspected, +2 to −3 mmHg, the stroke volume and cardiac output values are high, 90–70 ml and 10.8–8.4 l/min, respectively.

The clinical appearances of a hyperdynamic system with a normal venous pressure and no pulmonary oedema are not suggestive of heart failure, yet the ability of the heart to produce work in relation to its filling pressure can be grossly impaired. The patient detailed in Fig. 3.6 has a heart that is failing as a result of the infection.

The use of antibiotics alone to treat the sepsis may restore a heart which has failed for this reason, but not if the derangement is extreme. Frequently, it is obvious that the circulation cannot be maintained without support, because of gross hypotension and oliguria. If the resistances are low and the heart is failing, the drug that will tend to alter the circulation in the direction of normality is adrenaline because it is a constricting inotrope. The levels of dosage are regulated pragmatically by the result that each achieves. Dose levels as high as 50 µg/kg/ min may produce circulatory stability and an acceptable blood pressure. This is 10 times the dose rate required in any other condition, other than for very brief periods. Adrenaline, sometimes in combination with noradrenaline, will restore urine flow and peripheral perfusion when given to such patients; in a patient with a normal circulation, the opposite effect would occur.

Where sepsis produces a high systemic resistance and heart failure in the sense of diminished capacity to produce work, the treatment of choice is a dilating inotrope such as dopamine. Because dopamine has valuable effects on renal blood flow, but becomes a vasoconstrictor in doses > 5 µg/kg/min, it should be supplemented with dobutamine if greater dosage is required.

It has been claimed that steroids improve the distribution of blood flow and stabilize damaged capillary endothelia, reducing leakage of plasma from the vascular compartment. In a large multicentre, randomized double-blind trial,[19,20] high-dose steroids were found to be of no benefit and to be associated with a higher mortality in patients who had the syndrome of severe circulatory derangement associated with sepsis. The current balance of evidence suggests that they should not be used in this condition.

TAMPONADE

The important physiological disturbance that appears with tamponade is impairment of the cardiac output as a result of interference with the filling of the heart.

CLINICAL FEATURES

Restlessness, oliguria and hypotension stem from the diminished cardiac output. Breathlessness may be due to lung stiffness associated with the net transfer of blood from systemic to pulmonary vessels, which accompanies the rising left atrial pressure. The breathlessness may also be related to low cardiac output, because it certainly occurs with massive haemorrhage (air hunger breathing), in which all the intravascular pressures are low. The systolic descent in the venous pressure at the time of systole is due to a fall in pressure within the pericardial compartment at the time of ventricular ejection. When pulsus paradoxus (which is not pardoxical but an exaggeration of a normal phenomenon) appears in tamponade, it is principally due to failure of transmission of the intrathoracic pressure swings to the left atrium. During inspiration, the fall in intrathoracic pressure is transmitted to the pulmonary veins; if this fall is not also transmitted to the left atrium, it will produce a diminution in the effective filling pressure of the left heart, and a fall in the arterial pressure. The absence of pulsus paradoxus does not exclude the presence of tamponade, neither does the presence of a pericardial rub exclude a large pericardial effusion.

Confirmation of a pericardial effusion on echocardiography is usually correct although not always; a right atrial angiogram is the definitive investigation if the patient has a large enough effusion to produce tamponade.

PATHOPHYSIOLOGY

The venous tone is high. The volume of fluid within the pericardium, which may produce profound circulatory embarrassment, varies from about 300 ml, if the phenomenon occurs acutely, to as much as 2 l.

Until the effusion is drained, the cardiac output is best maintained with high right and left atrial pressures. If the heart is normal before the onset of tamponade, the right atrial pressure will rise from 0, and the left from 5 mmHg, as the effusion develops, until both pressures reach 15 mmHg. The safety of draining the pericardium has been much improved by not attempting to drain the effusion through the needle with which the puncture is made, but by replacing the needle with a soft catheter over a Seldinger guide-wire. The catheter should have multiple side-holes, and it is possible, by the use of dilators and sleeves in combination with the guidewire, to introduce a drain of appreciable size, if the fluid contains clot.

REFERENCES

1. Bradley, R.D. *Studies in Acute Heart Failure.* London: Edward Arnold, 1977.
2. Guyton, A.C. and Lindsey, A.W. Effect of elevated left atrial pressure and decreased plasma protein concentration on the development of pulmonary edema. *Circ. Res.* 1959; 7: 649–57.
3. Bradley, R.D., Jenkins, B.S. and Branthwaite, M.A. Myocardial function in acute glomerulonephritis. *Cardiovasc. Res.* 1971; 5: 223–5.
4. Aubier, M., Trippenbach, T. and Roussos, C. Respiratory muscle fatigue during cardiogenic shock. *J. Appl. Physiol. Respirat. Environ. Exercise Physiol.* 1981; 51: 499–508.
5. Sarnoff, S.J. and Bergelund, E. Neurohemodynamics of Pulmonary Edema. *Am. J. Physiol.* 1952; 170: 588.
6. Theodore, J. and Robin, E.D. Pathogenesis of neurogenic pulmonary oedema. *Lancet* 1975; ii: 749.
7. Wilmshurst, P.T., Nuri, M., Crowther, A., Betts, J.C. and Webb-Peploe, M.M. Recurrent Pulmonary Oedema in Scuba Divers; Prodrome of Hypertension: a new syndrome. *Underwater Physiol.* 1984; VIII: 327–39.
8. Cohn, J.N., Guiha, N.H., Broder, M.I. and Limas, C.J. Right ventricular infarction, clinical and hemodynamic features. *Am. J. Cardiol.* 1974; 33: 209–14.
9. Bradley, R.D., Jenkins, B.S. and Branthwaite, M.A. The influence of atrial pressure on cardiac performance following myocardial infarction complicated by shock. 1970; 42: 827–37.
10. Howell, J.B.L. and Campbell, E.J.M. *Breathlessness.* Oxford: Blackwell Scientific Publications, 1966.
11. Bradley, R.D., Jenkins, B.S. and Branthwaite, M.A. Cardiac function after open heart surgery. *Cardiovasc. Res.* 1973; 7: 297–305.
12. Mueller, H., Ayres, S.M., Gianelli, S., Conklin, E.F., Mazarra, J.T. and Grace, W.J. Effect of isoproterenol, L-norepinephrine and intra-aortic counterpulsation on haemodynamics and myocardial metabolism in shock following acute myocardial infarction. *Circulation* 1972; 45: 335–52.
13. Sarnoff, S.J., Mitchell, J.H., Gilmore, J.P. and Remensnyder, P. Homeometric autoregulation in the heart. *Circ. Res.* 1960; 8: 1077.
14. Woods, R.H. A few applications of a physical theorem to membrane in the human body in a state of tension. *J. Anat. Physiol.* 1892; 26: 302.
15. Burton, A.C. The importance of the shape and size of the heart. *Am. Heart J.* 1957; 54: 801.
16. Chatterjee, K., Parmley, W.W., Ganz, W., Forrester, J., Walkinsky, P., Crexells, C. and Swan, H.J.C. Hemodynamic and metabolic responses to vasodilator therapy in acute myocardial infarction. *Circulation* 1973; 28: 1183–93.
17. Chamberlain, D.A., Leinbach, R.C., Vassaux, C.E., Kastor, J.A., De Sanctis, R.W. and Sanders, C.A. Sequential atrioventricular pacing in heart block complicating acute myocardial infarction. *N. Engl. J. Med.* 1970; 282: 577–82.
18. Miller, G.A.H., Sutton, G.C., Kerr, I.H., Gibson, R.V. and Honey, M. Comparison of streptokinase and heparin in the treatment of isolated acute massive pulmonary embolism. *Br. Med. J.* 1971; ii: 681–4.
19. Bone, R.C., Fisher, C.J., Clemmer, T.P., Slotman, G.J., Metz, C.A. and Balk, R.A. A controlled clinical trial of high dose Methylprednisolone in the treatment of severe sepsis and septic shock. *N. Engl. J. Med.* 1987; 317: 653–8.
20. The Veterans Administration Sytemic Sepsis Study Group. Effect of high dose glucocorticoid therapy on mortality in patients with clinical signs of systemic sepsis. *N. Engl. J. Med.* 1987; 317: 659–65.

Chapter 4

Chronic Heart Failure: Causes, Pathophysiology, Prognosis, Clinical Manifestations, Investigations

P.A. Poole-Wilson

INTRODUCTION

The understanding, investigation and treatment of chronic heart failure have altered substantially in the last 20 years. These changes have resulted from advances in understanding the pathophysiology, new techniques for the investigation of patients, the availability of new drugs, and cardiac transplantation. Chronic heart failure has traditionally been treated with digoxin and diuretics. With modern diuretics, the elimination of oedema and the prevention of fluid overload are relatively simple. Other considerations are now of greater importance, such as the role of angiotensin converting enzyme inhibitors, positive inotropes or vasodilators in the treatment of heart failure, the origin of symptoms, delay in the progression of myocardial damage and reduction of mortality.

WORDS AND DEFINITIONS

A practical definition is that heart failure is a clinical syndrome (readily diagnosed by doctors) caused by an abnormality of the heart and recognized by a characteristic pattern of haemodynamic, renal, neural and hormonal responses.[1] This definition requires an abnormality of the heart to be present and states that much of the clinical picture is a consequence of the body's response to that abnormality. A briefer definition is ventricular dysfunction with symptoms.

The definition of heart failure has long been contentious. Some past definitions are shown in Table 4.1. Most of them are unsatisfactory because they emphasize one or other physiological or biochemical features of heart failure. As the symptoms of heart failure occur on exercise, definitions based on observations at rest are inevitably flawed.

With modern treatment, the classical physical signs of overt heart failure may be absent. Emphasis should not be placed on the ventricular filling pressure because this may be normal at rest, can be manipulated by diuretics, varies from moment to moment and in chronic heart failure is poorly related to symptoms.[2] The symptoms and clinical signs of treated heart failure are subtle. The phrases 'discharge its contents adequately', 'adequate circulation for the needs of the body' or 'requirements of the metabolizing tissues' do not have a precise meaning that can easily be tested. The limiting metabolic substrate of most tissues is oxygen and the oxygen content of blood in the femoral vein at peak exercise in heart failure is almost zero. The whole body oxygen consumption of patients with heart failure at rest or at low workloads is identical to that of normal persons and is only reduced towards the end of exercise when anaerobic metabolism is activated. Even then the reduction is small

Table 4.1. Some definitions of heart failure.

. . . a condition in which the heart fails to discharge its contents adequately
Thomas Lewis[26]

. . . a state in which the heart fails to maintain an adequate circulation for the needs of the body despite a satisfactory venous filling pressure
Paul Wood[27]

. . . a pathophysiological state in which an abnormality of cardiac function is responsible for the failure of the heart to pump blood at a rate commensurate with the requirements of the metabolizing tissues
Eugene Braunwald[28]

Practical definitions

A clinical syndrome caused by an abnormality of the heart and recognized by a characteristic pattern of haemodynamic, renal, neural and hormonal responses

Ventricular dysfunction with symptoms

because theoretical considerations and experimental data show that the ability of anaerobic metabolism to generate high-energy phosphates within the skeletal muscle cell is small in comparison to aerobic metabolism.

Many adjectives have been used to describe heart failure with particular features. These include high and low output cardiac failure, forward and backward failure, right and left heart failure, congestive heart failure, and acute and chronic heart failure. For practical purposes, it is necessary to consider only acute heart failure, which is a medical emergency closely allied to pulmonary oedema, and chronic heart failure. Chronic heart failure should be regarded as a dynamic rather than a steady-state condition since the function of the heart and the interaction of the heart and circulation vary with time. Many patients with chronic heart failure develop acute exacerbations which are often due to extraneous causes such as lung infection. The clinical entity whereby patients spontaneously recover and relapse with chronic heart failure might be called "undulating heart failure".

AETIOLOGY OF HEART FAILURE

Heart failure can be caused by arrhythmias, pericardial disease, extracardiac abnormalities, valve dysfunction or disease of the myocardium. Myocardial disease causes myocardial failure and has many causes (Table 4.2), the most common of which are atheromatous diseases of the coronary arteries or dilated cardiomyopathy.

Dilated cardiomyopathy is a term used to describe large hearts with reduced contractile function in the presence of normal coronary arteries. It is usually of unknown cause but when a cause is established the term may be preceded by an adjective, for example, myxoedematous or alcoholic dilated cardiomyopathy. Congestive cardiomyopathy is an older term used to describe the same condition. The use of the term ischaemic cardiomyopathy is often discouraged, but it has been used to describe the situation when global ventricular dysfunction occurs in the presence of coronary artery disease. It may be the consequence of 'stunned myocardium' or 'hibernating myocardium', or due to a reduction in the proportion of contractile proteins within a single myocardial cell.

Hypertension is a common cause of heart failure but the incidence of heart failure due to this cause has fallen as a result of improved detection and treatment of hypertension. The use of negative inotropic drugs (e.g. beta-adrenergic blockers, calcium antagonists, anti-arrhythmic agents) can precipitate heart failure and is a contributing cause which is easily remedied.

Traditionally, a distinction has been made between high and low output heart failure. So-called 'high output' heart failure can be caused by the conditions listed in Table 4.3. This entity does not strictly fall within the definition of heart failure given above because the primary abnormality is not in the heart; however, these conditions may present with physical signs similar to those of heart failure, such as fluid overload and neurohumoral abnormalities. I prefer to name these conditions according to their cause. I do not regard them as causes of heart failure.

Table 4.2. **Classification of heart failure due to myocardial disease (myocardial failure).**

1	Ischaemic heart disease:	Local dyskinesia
		Aneurysm
		'Hibernating'
		Diffuse
2	Dilated cardiomyopathy:	Alcohol
		Myocarditis
		Familial
		Unknown
3	Hypertension	
4	Drugs:	Beta-adrenergic blockers
		Calcium antagonists
		Anti-arrhythmic agents
5	Septicaemia, endocarditis, Chagas' disease, infections	
6	Some rarer diseases:	Hypertrophic cardiomyopathy
		Asymmetrical hypertrophy
		Amyloid
		Restrictive
		Thyroid
		Heavy metals

Table 4.3. **Causes of 'high output' failure.**

1	Anaemia
2	Nephritis
3	Arteriovenous fistula
4	Paget's disease
5	Beriberi
6	Thyrotoxicosis
7	Pregnancy

PATHOPHYSIOLOGY OF HEART FAILURE

METABOLIC CAUSES OF HEART FAILURE

Acute heart failure has many causes. The most common is myocardial ischaemia. The heart is critically dependent on a supply of oxygen from the coronary circulation. Occlusion of a coronary artery causes myocardial contraction to cease within 60 s. The loss of turgor in the coronary arteries occurs immediately and alters the end-diastolic shape of the heart. In man, this is a minor mechanism contributing to contractile failure. The major mechanisms are the development of intracellular acidosis from the breakdown of glucose and glycogen to lactate, the intracellular accumulation of phosphate from the breakdown of creatine phosphate and adenosine triphosphate (ATP), and eventually a lack of energy supply due to consumption of ATP and inhibition of production by acidosis and other retained metabolites. Hydrogen and phosphate ions interfere with the interaction between the cytosolic calcium and the shortening of the contractile proteins. Contractility is rapidly restored by the establishment of normal coronary flow. Some reduction of contractile function can persist for hours and even days after periods of ischaemia as short as 15 min. This condition has been called the 'stunned heart'.[3] If multiple episodes of ischaemia occurred continually, then normal function of the heart would never return. The term 'hibernating heart' has been applied to this condition, which is reminiscent of the older concept of 'chronic ischaemia'. Cell death occurs only if the ischaemic period exceeds 15 min.

Less is known about the mechanisms responsible for the reduced contractility of the myocardium in chronic heart failure. Minor and subtle changes in the make-up of the contractile proteins may result in a reduced sensitivity to the cytosolic calcium concentration or a reduced activity of myofibrillar ATPase, the enzyme determining the rate of energy consumption by the contractile proteins. The function of the sarcoplasmic reticulum may be abnormal during both the release of calcium in systole and the uptake of calcium during diastole. The cardiac myocyte may be overloaded with calcium, ATP synthesis may be inhibited or the heart may be limited in its contractile ability by extracellular fibrosis and collagen accumulation. Many other abnormalities have been described but these are probably the consequence of contractile failure rather than the cause. The role of the sympathetic nervous system is discussed below.

A distinction should be made between pump failure, myocardial failure and an abnormality of shortening of the myocyte. Pump failure can be caused by abnormalities of rhythm, the valves or pericardium, whereas myocardial failure is due to an abnormality of cardiac muscle. However, myocardial failure need not necessarily indicate malfunction of the myocyte, it can be the result of slippage of adjacent cells resulting in an enlarged and thinned heart, heterogeneous contraction of the myocardium (as in coronary heart disease), shape change of the ventricle and splinting of individual cells by fibrosis. A recent proposal is that some cardiomyopathies, for example, that associated with diabetes, are the result of multiple microscopic infarcts and subsequent fibrosis caused by vasospasm of small arterioles.[5] These mechanisms may cause myocardial failure in the absence of any abnormality of contraction of individual myocytes by the mechanisms outlined above.

The demonstration of a large heart with a low ejection fraction and minimal movement in systole does not necessarily mean that an abnormality of myocardial contractility is present. The reflexes in the body maintain the cardiac output at approximately 5 l/min. To achieve such a cardiac output, the ejection fraction of a large left ventricle and the movement of the ventricular wall must be greatly reduced. Thus, a low ejection fraction in the presence of a large ventricle is inevitable and does not necessarily indicate a poor exercise capacity or a diminished cardiac reserve.

SYSTOLIC OR DIASTOLIC ABNORMALITIES

The mechanism by which the cardiac output increases on exercise in heart failure varies according to the cause of the failure.[6] In dilated cardiomyopathy, the end-diastolic volume hardly changes and the stroke volume increases because of a smaller end-systolic volume, i.e. an increase of ejection fraction. By contrast, in patients with coronary artery disease, the end-diastolic volume tends to increase and the end-systolic volume is almost unaltered, i.e. a negligible change of ejection fraction. These volume changes are compatible with the idea that in dilated cardiomyopathy the end-diastolic volume is maximal, whereas in some patients with heart failure due to ischaemic heart disease the volume at end-diastole may be submaximal. Diastole can be divided into four periods (Table 4.4). Depending on the heart rate, abnorma-

Table 4.4. Components of diastole.

1 Isovolumic relaxation
2 Early rapid filling
3 Late filling
4 Atrial systole

lities of any diastolic event may influence the end-diastolic volume of the heart.

It is important that a distinction is made between systolic and diastolic heart failure.[7] In patients with diastolic heart failure, the stroke volume would be greater if filling during diastole were more complete. In some conditions, such as hypertrophic obstructive cardiomyopathy, following valve replacement for aortic stenosis, hypertensive heart disease with hypertrophy, and angina pectoris, relaxation may be incomplete at end-diastole particularly if a tachycardia is present. Even in these conditions a systolic abnormality may be evident on exercise. In the presence of ischaemic heart disease, the key abnormality may not be incomplete relaxation of myocytes (affecting primarily isovolumic relaxation and rapid filling during early diastole), but incoordinate relaxation of different regions of the ventricle (affecting the later passive phase of ventricular filling). The evidence that diastolic function is a major factor determining the function of dilated hearts is not compelling. Diastolic function should be considered in patients with heart failure and small hearts. The distinction has therapeutic implications. Patients with heart failure (especially those with small hearts and angina or breathlessness as a limiting symptom) due to myocardial ischaemia may benefit from nitrates or similar drugs because endocardial ischaemia is reduced, compliance increased and diastolic filling enhanced.

RESPONSES TO HEART FAILURE

There is a limited number of ways in which the body can respond to heart failure (Table 4.5). The most important and least understood is cardiac hypertrophy. Hypertrophy can vary substantially between patients with apparently equal stimuli to hypertrophy, such as high blood pressure or volume overload.

The second response is the increase of cardiac output resulting from an elevated ventricular filling pressure (Starling's law) associated with the retention of sodium and water.

The third response is activation of the neurohu-moral system.[8] This has received much emphasis in recent years. The sympathetic nervous system is stimulated in mild heart failure and the renin–angiotensin system to a lesser degree. The levels of plasma aldosterone, antidiuretic hormone (vasopressin), prostaglandins and atrial natriuretic peptide are all increased in severe heart failure. Numerous new peptides have been identified and many of these have powerful effects on sodium and water metabolism and on the systemic vascular resistance, but their role in heart failure has not been established as yet. The best known of these is atrial natriuretic peptide which is released from the atria in response to stretch and causes both natriuresis and vasodilatation. Atrial natriuretic peptide is increased in patients with heart failure, the increase being related to the magnitude of the left and right atrial pressures. Whether the increase of atrial natriuretic peptide in heart failure is a marker of a raised atrial pressure or an important pathological mechanism in heart failure is as yet unknown.

The sensor to activate this pattern of neurohumoral response is not known. In the absence of a response, the blood pressure would fall. Possible sensors are the baroreceptors in the heart and aorta, and low-pressure sensors in the ventricles and atria.

The hormonal changes described in the literature as being characteristic of heart failure have been measured in patients with treated heart failure. As diuretics are known to stimulate the renin–angiotensin system, at least part of the response to heart failure is a response to treatment. Measurements in untreated patients show that in mild heart failure the renin–angiotensin system is hardly activated, if at all, whereas the sympathetic system is

Table 4.5. Responses to heart failure.

1 Hypertrophy of the myocardium

2 Sodium retention and increase of the ventricular filling pressure (Starling's law)

3 Activation of the neurohumoral system:
    Sympathetic system
    Renin–angiotensin system
    Antidiuretic hormone (vasopressin)
    Atrial natiuretic peptide
    Prostaglandins
    Other hormones

4 Increased arteriolar resistance:
    Sodium retention in smooth muscle
    Extramural pressure on blood vessels from tissue oedema
    Endothelial cell swelling or dysfunction

5 Down-regulation of beta-adrenergic receptors in the myocardium

stimulated.[9] This may be partly due to suppression of initial activation of the renin–angiotensin system in heart failure by expansion of the circulating volume and sodium retention. Treatment with diuretics increases the plasma renin activity but reduces the plasma noradrenaline concentration. Activation of the sympathetic system is the earliest neuro-endocrine perturbation in heart failure.

The fourth response to heart failure is not well understood. Even in the presence of inhibitors of many of the neuro-endocrine systems, the systemic vascular resistance is still elevated at rest and blood flow to skeletal muscle on exercise is markedly reduced.[10] This suggests that in these vascular beds there are additional abnormalities limiting blood flow. The nature of such abnormalities is not clear. A popular and old hypothesis is that sodium is retained within smooth muscle causing vasoconstriction. An alternative explanation is endothelial cell swelling or an abnormality of endothelial cell function. Until the putative abnormality is corrected, the resistance to blood flow during exercise in the skeletal muscle bed remains high and exercise performance is diminished because maximal blood flow to exercising skeletal muscle is reduced. This mechanism may be the reason why most inotropic drugs, vasodilators and the angiotensin converting enzyme inhibitors do not bring about an increase in exercise capacity when given acutely, but can, particularly the angiotensin converting enzyme inhibitors, after treatment has been continued for several weeks.[11]

The fifth response to heart failure is molecular and affects the likely response to some therapeutic agents. The levels of plasma catecholamines are elevated in patients with heart failure. However, the response of the heart to beta-1 adrenoceptor stimulation is reduced (desensitization). This loss of sensitivity can be the result of internalization of receptors (a rapid and reversible mechanism) or, more usually, down-regulation (a loss of the proteins making up the receptor).

The responses of the body to heart failure are similar to the responses to exercise, stress and haemorrhage. It has been argued that the evolutionary origins of the response and the major factor initiating the response is the requirement to maintain a blood pressure sufficient to allow an immediate reaction to stress.[12,13]

THE KIDNEY IN HEART FAILURE

The clinical signs of heart failure are dominated by the renal response. In moderate heart failure, renal blood flow is reduced as a result of arterial vasoconstriction partly from the activation of the sympathetic and renin–angiotensin systems. Despite the fall in renal blood flow, the glomerular filtration rate is maintained as a result of greater constriction of the efferent arteries as opposed to the afferent arteries in the glomeruli. The filtration fraction is increased. One consequence is that the osmotic pressure of blood reaching the renal tubules is higher and will contribute to the retention of sodium in the distal tubule. An increased level of aldosterone and other hormonal changes will also stimulate tubular sodium reabsorption. In severe heart failure, renal blood flow is markedly reduced, the glomerular filtration rate falls and the levels of plasma urea and creatinine may increase. If the renin–angiotensin system is greatly activated by the use of high doses of diuretics in severe heart failure, the addition of angiotensin converting enzyme inhibitors can cause a further reduction of the glomerular filtration rate and an increase in the level of plasma urea despite an increase of blood flow. This occurs because angiotensin II has a greater effect on the efferent artery than on the afferent artery. A preferential reduction of resistance in the afferent artery will lead to a fall in the pressures determining the glomerular filtration rate. Under these circumstances, the filtration fraction will eventually fall.

The renal effects of mild heart failure are not well characterized.[14] The fall of total blood flow may be small, even negligible. Intrarenal redistribution of blood flow may contribute to the early retention of sodium. Alternatively, sodium retention may be explained by activation of neurohumoral systems.

THE SYMPATHETIC SYSTEM IN HEART FAILURE

The levels of plasma noradrenaline and adrenaline are increased at rest in patients with heart failure. At similar but low levels of physical activity, the sympathetic system is more activated in patients with heart failure than in normal subjects. At peak exercise, the converse is true. The level of plasma noradrenaline is higher in normal subjects than in patients. The sensitivity of most cardiovascular reflexes including the baroreflexes is blunted in heart failure.

The myocardial content of noradrenaline is reduced in severe heart failure, partly as a result of increased utilization. However, synthesis is also diminished as a consequence of reduced activity of tyrosine hydroxylase, the rate-limiting enzyme in the synthesis of catecholamines. Dopamine (the immediate precursor of noradrenaline) is increased because of a defect in the uptake mechanism into secretory vesicles in the nerve terminal. There is no close relation between plasma catecholamine concentrations and the content of cardiac tissue.

Studies on samples of heart muscle obtained from patients with severe heart failure undergoing heart transplantation have shown that beta-adrenergic receptors are reduced in number. Stimulation of myocardial adenylate cyclase by isoprenaline is diminished, and the contractile response of small strips of ventricular muscle to catecholamines may be lessened.[15] These findings have led to the idea that beta-adrenergic receptors in the heart are down-regulated. The human ventricle contains both beta-1 and beta-2 adrenergic receptors in the proportion of 70:30. Unlike many animal species, the beta-2 receptors are not localized solely to blood vessels but are also present on the cell membrane of myocytes. Beta-1 but not beta-2 receptors are down-regulated. The consequence is that the myocardium of patients with severe heart failure may be less responsive to adrenergic inotropic agents.

Beta-adrenergic blockers have been used to treat selected patients with heart failure. One possible mechanism is that the prevention of excessive beta-adrenergic stimulation of the myocardium allows up-regulation of beta-adrenergic receptors and a greater response of the myocardium to an increase of sympathetic stimulation on exercise. Alternative explanations are that tachycardia is avoided or that diastolic filling of the heart is improved.

CAUSE OF SYMPTOMS

The major symptoms of patients with heart failure are shortness of breath and fatigue. With the proper use of modern diuretics, shortness of breath can be minimized, the major symptom then being fatigue. The origin of these symptoms is poorly understood (Table 4.6).[2] In acute heart failure, shortness of breath is directly related to the left atrial pressure or the left ventricular end-diastolic pressure. Reduction of this pressure by therapeutic intervention brings immediate relief to the patient. In patients with chronic heart failure treated with diuretics, the origins of breathlessness are less clear and almost certainly more complex. There is no simple correla-

Table 4.6. **Origin of symptoms on exercise in chronic heart failure.**

1	Lungs:	Stiffness
		Left atrial pressure
		Physiological dead space
		Respiratory rate
2	Circulation:	Blood flow to skeletal muscle
		Production of metabolites
3	Skeletal muscle:	Rest atrophy
		? Specific abnormality

tion in this group of patients between peak oxygen consumption (a measure of exercise capacity) and estimates of left atrial pressure at peak exercise. Drugs which acutely reduce the left atrial pressure do not increase exercise capacity in such patients. Different types of exercise test give rise to different symptoms terminating exercise despite the values of left atrial pressure at peak exercise being identical. Changes of blood pH, and the level of plasma potassium and other metabolic signals almost certainly are contributory factors to shortness of breath in patients with chronic heart failure in addition to changes in the lungs, such as increased stiffness and an increased physiological dead space.

The cause of fatigue is more obscure. Patients with chronic heart failure have an increased resistance to blood flow in skeletal muscle at rest and on exercise.[10] Metabolic signals may arise from the leg muscles due to stimulation of anaerobic metabolism. In addition, skeletal muscle atrophies and the maximal strength of contraction is reduced. A metabolic defect in skeletal muscle has been postulated. Such abnormalities would result in the earlier onset of anaerobic metabolism in a particular muscle group for a given workload. In patients with chronic heart failure optimally treated with diuretics, improvement in symptoms will result only if blood flow to skeletal muscle on exercise is increased.

SPIRAL OF HEART FAILURE

In the 1970s, treatment with vasodilators was popular for patients with heart failure. The rationale was twofold: first, haemodynamics were altered in a manner considered to be beneficial (this assumption was unjustified, see below); and, second, the unloading of the left ventricle might alter the progression of heart disease within the myocardium.

The latter hypothesis has been tested in animal models in which it has been demonstrated that the progression of ventricular dysfunction after myocardial infarction,[16] or in response to hypertension, can be altered by vasodilators. The hypothesis is that in heart failure the increase in the systemic vascular resistance imposes a greater stress on the already damaged myocardium. This causes further damage to the heart muscle, worsening heart failure, activating neuro-endocrine systems and increasing the systemic vascular resistance. The sequence is a vicious spiral of heart failure. The clinical hope was and is that vasodilators in patients might delay the progression of heart disease. The extent to which the theory can be applied to humans is not known. The progression of heart disease in patients with coronary artery disease is probably dominated by the natural history of atheroma in the coronary arteries and subsequent ischaemic events. In some patients with cardiomyopathy, the prognosis is related to the continuing presence of the causal factor, for example, alcohol.

The anticipated benefit to patients from altered haemodynamics consequent upon the use of vasodilator drugs has not been demonstrated in controlled trials.[11] The reason is twofold: first, the assumption that left ventricular filling pressure was a major determinant of the symptom of shortness of breath has been shown to be erroneous; and, second, the increase of cardiac output observed at rest results in more blood being directed to previously constricted tissue beds, such as the skin and splanchnic circulations, but does not result in any substantial increase of skeletal muscle perfusion on exercise.

EPIDEMIOLOGY AND PROGNOSIS OF HEART FAILURE

PROGNOSIS

Epidemiological data on heart failure are sparse and most of that which is available originates in the USA.[17] The incidence of heart failure is 1%, the prevalence 4% and the admission rate to hospital 2% *per annum*. These figures may be confounded by the perennial problem of defining mild heart failure.

More precise information is available on prognosis. In the Framingham Study, the mortality for all grades of heart failure taken together was approximately 25% at 2 years. In mild heart failure, the 2-year mortality is 10–20% rising to 75% in severe heart failure. Wide variability exists in these figures. Patients with dilated cardiomyopathy may survive many years if the enlarged heart is a sign of a previous episode of cardiac damage that has not recurred. The prognosis in patients with coronary artery disease is related to the prognosis of atheromatous coronary artery disease as much as to the presence of heart failure. The prognosis is reported to be worse in patients with coronary artery disease when compared with that of patients with cardiomyopathy, but such a comparison is of doubtful validity because patients may not have been equally incapacitated by heart failure on entry into these studies.

PREDICTORS OF PROGNOSIS

Although many clinical features of patients with heart failure (symptoms, heart size, haemodynamics, plasma noradrenaline, arrhythmias) have been shown to have prognostic significance, such predictors show only that those who already have the features of heart failure will fare less well than an asymptomatic subject. Such predictors do not discriminate in terms of prognosis among a group of patients already classified as being in severe heart failure.

Information is becoming available on comparisons between the predictive power of many variables.[18] The two most powerful predictors are the ejection fraction at rest and the peak oxygen consumption on exercise. Other variables, such as heart size or the presence of arrhythmias, are of substantially less significance. The ejection fraction at rest reflects the extent of myocardial damage and the end-diastolic volume rather than ventricular function. The peak oxygen consumption is a measure of cardiac reserve. This information has important consequences for the investigation of patients, the classification of patients and methods for the assessment of the progression of disease and treatment.

SUDDEN DEATH AND ARRHYTHMIAS

The mode of death in heart failure has been studied extensively. A substantial proportion of patients (up to 50%) are said to die suddenly mostly from ventricular fibrillation. The remainder die from progression of heart disease. These two entities are not easy to distinguish and the definition of sudden death varies among studies. Sudden death is often defined as death within 6 h of the patient being known to be alive and well. Even if that time were to be reduced to 1 h, that is still sufficient time for the onset of acute pulmonary oedema or severe chest pain to precede death.

Arrhythmias (ventricular ectopic beats and non-sustained ventricular tachycardia) are common in patients with heart disease.[19] Treatment with anti-arrhythmic drugs is being evaluated in current trials and will provide compelling evidence as to whether instantaneous and opportunistic arrhythmias are an important cause of death. At present, it seems more probable that most arrhythmias are merely an indicator of the severity of heart disease and not an important independent determinant of prognosis.

CAUSE OF REDUCTION IN MORTALITY

Analysis of many small trials in heart failure has not provided any robust evidence that drug treatment in addition to the use of diuretics alters prognosis. By contrast, the results of two large trials have been able to demonstrate an effect on mortality. The first trial was from the Veterans Administration in the USA on patients with moderate heart failure,[20] in which a reduction in mortality over 2 years in patients treated with a combination of hydralazine and isosorbide dinitrate. The second trial was the CONSENSUS trial conducted in Scandinavia.[21] Enalapril (an angiotensin converting enzyme inhibitor) was added to conventional treatment in patients with severe heart failure; mortality was considerably reduced.

An important question is how these drugs brought about a reduction of mortality. None of these drugs are known to have direct anti-arrhythmic actions. Nitrates, but not enalapril, might influence the frequency and occurrence of coronary events. A direct effect on the myocardium has not been shown. A popular hypothesis is that the reduction of afterload on the heart reduced the progression of damage to the myocardium, the spiral of heart failure referred to above. An alternative possibility is that enalapril increased renal blood flow and improved sodium homeostasis so as to reduce the extent and occurrence of sodium overload. Clinical benefit in terms of exercise capacity could be accounted for if the improved sodium homeostasis resulted in reduced resistance in vascular beds and an increase of blood flow to skeletal muscle on exercise.

Heart transplantation leads to a dramatic reduction of mortality. Since the introduction of cyclosporin, the survival of patients who have undergone transplantation at 2 years is 80% contrasting with a mortality of > 75% which would be expected in such a group of patients treated medically. A control trial is not needed to demonstrate this obvious benefit.

CLINICAL HISTORY

The purpose of the clinical history is to establish the diagnosis, determine the cause of the heart failure, assess the severity of heart failure, predict the prognosis, and gain some indication of the most appropriate therapy.

The symptoms of patients with heart failure are easily established but are often a poor guide to the true disability of patients. Several gradings have been described, the best known being the New York Heart Association (NYHA) Classification of breathlessness (Table 4.7).[22] Although this classification is widely used, it has little advantage over a clinical assessment which uses the terms mild, moderate or severe heart failure. More sophisticated classifications have been devised. Some of these so-called 'instruments' are based on the response of the patient to a range of specific questions.

CLINICAL MANIFESTATIONS OF HEART FAILURE

The physical signs of heart failure are described in Chapter 7. The cause of heart failure is often evident from the presence of specific physical signs, such as rhythm, murmurs or indicators of coronary artery disease. The syndromes causing 'high output' failure must not be overlooked. Abnormalities of thyroid function are not always easy to discern.

Table 4.7. **New York Heart Association classification of breathlessness.**

Class I: No limitation. Ordinary physical activity does not cause undue fatigue, dyspnoea or palpitation

Class II: Slight limitation of physical activity. Such patients are comfortable at rest. Ordinary physical activity results in fatigue, palpitation, dyspnoea, or angina pectoris

Class III: Marked limitation of physical activity. Although patients are comfortable at rest, less than ordinary activity will lead to symptoms

Class IV: Inability to carry on any physical activity without discomfort. Symptoms of congestive failure are present even at rest. With any physical activity, increased discomfort is experienced

INVESTIGATIONS

The patient with heart failure should have an electrocardiogram, chest X-ray and echocardiogram taken. An exercise test is desirable. A blood sample should be obtained for a full blood count and the measurement of electrolytes, particularly the level of plasma or serum potassium and measures of renal function (such as urea and creatinine). Other blood tests may be necessary, for example, thyroid function tests.

Some patients will need further investigations, for example, a cardiac catheter or radionuclide study. Radionuclide studies provide an easy method for measuring the ejection faction and can be used to follow the progression of disease, but similar data can usually be obtained from the echocardiogram. A cardiac catheter study including coronary angiography is indicated if the diagnosis is uncertain or if a diagnosis which has a surgical remedy is entertained. Catheterization is not indicated merely to obtain the resting haemodynamics. Such information does not provide a reliable guide to different therapeutic regimes.

The indications for endomyocardial biopsy remain controversial.[23–25] Biopsy should be undertaken if rejection of a transplanted heart is suspected or when acute myocarditis, amyloid disease or endomyocardial fibrosis are possible diagnoses. The value of routine biopsy in patients with dilated cardiomyopathy is not established.

EXERCISE TESTING

In recent years, the exercise test has been widely advocated as a means of assessing the patient with heart failure. Exercise capacity confirms the severity of disability suspected from the clinical history, categorizes the severity of heart failure, predicts the prognosis and is useful in the subsequent assessment of therapy. The purpose of using an exercise test in patients with heart failure is different to that in patients with overt or suspected coronary artery disease in whom the presence or severity of coronary artery disease is being assessed.

Many uncertainties still exist with regard to exercise testing in patients with heart failure, including the most appropriate type of test (treadmill, erect or supine bicycle), the nature of the exercise protocol (fast or slow test, ramp or step increases in workload, fixed workload or patient-selected workload), reproducibility and sensitivity. A placebo effect of repeat exercise testing has been described, but of more significance is the increased confidence of patient and doctor as familiarity with the test increases. Contrary to often-stated opinion, exercise time is not an objective measurement and is influenced strongly by the doctor–patient relationship and by other factors such as anxiety and, in tests of long duration, boredom.

Sophisticated techniques exist for recording gas exchange during exercise. The measurement of peak oxygen consumption was introduced as an objective test for heart failure, which it is not. If patients can be persuaded to exercise beyond the point at which they believe they have achieved their maximum exercise capacity, oxygen consumption is increased. In contrast to athletes, patients with heart failure never achieve a plateau in their oxygen consumption. Nevertheless, the measurement of oxygen consumption is useful in that if changes of exercise time and peak oxygen consumption between two tests performed on different occasions are not similar then it is probable that one or both of the exercise tests has been influenced by factors other than heart failure, such as anxiety and the use of additional muscle groups during exercise to hold onto the frame of the exercise machine. Peak oxygen consumption is influenced by the muscle mass being used during exercise.

In an attempt to circumvent these problems, the concept of 'anaerobic threshold' has been applied to measurements of oxygen consumption and carbon dioxide production as an objective indicator of exercise performance in patients with heart failure. This concept is flawed because skeletal muscle contains mixed fibres with different metabolic pathways and anaerobic metabolism is not initiated in all muscle types at the same moment or to the same extent during exercise. The relationship between oxygen consumption and carbon dioxide production is affected by hyperventilation. Newer techniques are being developed which may allow a more objective assessment of patients during heart failure from measurements of gas exchange during exercise. The demonstration that the respiratory quotient is at least >1 and is increasing at the end of an exercise test does indicate that in the absence of lung disease or obstruction of peripheral arteries the patient has almost reached the limit of their exercise capability, and that the patient's exercise capacity is limited by the cardiovascular system.

The measurement of maximal exercise capacity is assumed to be an accurate indicator of the capacity of patients to lead a normal life; this may be an erroneous assumption. Some investigators are measuring the exercise time at submaximal workload. The six-minute walking test has been suggested as having a greater sensitivity for the effect of treatment in certain patients with heart failure. The six-minute walking test measures the maximum distance that a patient can walk in 6 min when invited to walk at their optimal speed.

REFERENCES

1. Poole-Wilson, P.A. Heart failure. *Med. Int.* 1985; **2**: 866–71.
2. Lipkin, D.P. and Poole-Wilson, P.A. Symptoms limiting exercise in chronic heart failure. *Br. Med. J.* 1986; **292**: 1030–1.
3. Braunwald, E. and Kloner, R.A. The stunned myocardium: prolonged, postischemic ventricular dysfunction. *Circulation* 1982; **66**: 1146–9.
4. Rahimtoola, S.H. A perspective on the three large multicenter randomized clinical trials of coronary bypass surgery for chronic stable angina. *Circulation* 1985; **72**(Suppl. 5): 123–35.
5. Factor, S.M. and Sonnenblick, E.H. The pathogenesis of clinical and experimental congestive cardiomyopathies: recent concepts. *Prog. Cardiovasc. Dis.* 1985; **XXVII**: 395–420.
6. Shen, W.E., Roubin, G.S., Hirasaw, K., Choong, C.Y.-P., Hutton, B.F., Harris, P.J., Fletcher, P.J. and Kelly, D.T. Left ventricular volume and ejection fraction response to exercise in chronic congestive heart failure: difference between dilated cardiomyopathy and previous myocardial infarction. *Am. J. Cardiol.* 1985; **55**: 1027–31.
7. Katz, A.M. Role of the basic sciences in the practice of cardiology. *J. Mol. Cell. Cardiol.* 1987; **19**: 3–17.
8. Francis, G.S. Neurohumoral mechanisms involved in congestive heart failure. *Am. J. Cardiol.* 1985; **55**: 15A–21A.
9. Bayliss, J., Norell, M., Canepa-Anson, R., Sutton, G. and Poole-Wilson, P. Untreated heart failure: clinical and neuroendocrine effects of introducing diuretics. *Br. Heart J.* 1987; **57**: 17–22.
10. Zelis, R. and Flaim, S.F. Alterations in vasomotor tone in congestive heart failure. *Prog. Cardiovasc. Dis.* 1982; **XXIV**: 437–59.
11. Lipkin, D.P. and Poole-Wilson, P.A. Treatment of chronic heart failure: a review of recent trials. *Br. Med. J.* 1985; **291**: 993–6.
12. Harris, P. Evolution and the cardiac patient. *Cardiovasc. Res.* 1983; **17**(6–8): 313–9; 373–8; 437–45.
13. Harris, P. Congestive cardiac failure: central role of the arterial blood pressure. *Br. Heart J.* 1987; **58**: 190–203.
14. Francis, G.S. Sodium and water excretion in heart failure: efficacy of treatment has surpassed knowledge of pathophysiology. *Ann. Intern. Med.* 1986; **105**: 272–4.
15. Fowler, M.B., Laser, J.A., Hopkins, G.L., Minobe, W. and Bristow, M.R. Assessment of the B-adrenergic receptor pathway in the intact failing heart: progressive receptor down-regulation and subsensitivity to agonist response. *Circulation* 1986; **74**: 1290–302.
16. Pfeffer, J., Pfeffer, M.A. and Braunwald, E. Influence of chronic captopril therapy on the infarcted left ventricle of the rat. *Circ. Res.* 1985; **57**: 84–95.
17. McFate Smith, W. Epidemiology of congestive heart failure. *Am. J. Cardiol.* 1985; **55**: 3A–8A.
18. Likoff, M.J., Chandler, S.L. and Kay, H.R. Clinical determinants of mortality in chronic congestive heart failure secondary to idiopathic dilated or to ischaemic cardiomyopathy. *Am. J. Cardiol.* 1987; **59**: 634–8.
19. Francis, G.S. Department of arrhythmias in the patient with congestive heart failure: pathophysiology, prevalence and prognosis. *Am. J. Cardiol.* 1986; **57**: 3B–7B.
20. Cohn, J.N., Archibald, D.G., Ziescah, S., Franciosa, J.A., Harston, W.E., Tristani, W.E., Dunkman, W.B., Jacobs, W., Francis, G.S., Flohr, K.H., Goldman, S., Cobb, F.R., Shah, P.M., Saunders, R., Fletcher, R.D., Loeb, H.S., Hughes, V.C. and Baker, B. Effect of vasodilator therapy on mortality in chronic congestive heart failure. Results of a Veterans Administration cooperative study. *N. Engl. J. Med.* 1986; **314**: 1547–52.
21. The CONSENSUS trial study group. Effects of enalapril on mortality in severe congestive heart failure. Results of the Cooperative North Scandinavian Enalapril Survival Study (CONSENSUS). *N. Engl. J. Med.* 1987; **316**: 1429–35.
22. The Criteria Committee of the New York Heart Association. *Diseases of the heart and blood vessels. Nomenclature and criteria for diagnosis.* 6th edn. Boston: Little-Brown, 1964.
23. Anonymous. Endomyocardial biopsy for the clinician (Editorial). *Lancet* 1984; **1**: 942–3.
24. Parillo, J.E., Aretz, H.T., Palacios, I., Fallon, J.T. and Block, P.C. The results of transvenous endomyocardial biopsy can frequently be used to diagnose myocardial diseases in patients with idiopathic heart failure. Endomyocardial biopsies in 100 consecutive patients. *Circulation* 1984; **69**: 93–101.
25. Shanes, J.G., Ghali, J., Billingham, M.E., Ferrans, V.J., Feroglio, J.J., Edwards, W.D., Tsai, C.C., Saffitz, J.E., Isner, J., Furrer, S. and Subramanian, R. Intraobserver variability in the pathologic interpretation of endomyocardial biopsy results. *Circulation* 1987; **75**: 401–5.
26. Lewis, T. *Diseases of the heart.* London and New York: Macmillan, 1933.
27. Wood, P. *Diseases of the heart and circulation.* Eyre and Spottiswoode, 1950.
28. Braunwald, E. *Heart disease. A textbook of cardiovascular medicine.* Philadelphia, London and Toronto: W.B. Saunders, 1980.

Chapter 5

Heart Failure, Management, Prevention and Drug Treatment

H.J. Dargie

INTRODUCTION

Heart failure is the common clinical expression of many diseases of the heart. However, neither the physical signs nor the symptoms are specific to the heart failure state; indeed, the clinical features of heart failure may not reflect the wide variety of cardiac pathologies that give rise to them. Pericardial, valvular, endocardial, vascular or myocardial abnormalities can all impair the cardiac output to the extent that they cause heart failure, emphasizing that heart failure is not a diagnosis in itself but a clinical syndrome. The improved safety and wider availability of definitive or palliative surgical techniques together with the increasing versatility of medical treatment require that a precise diagnosis be made before a rational therapeutic strategy can be adopted. Moreover, the development of an array of non-invasive cardiological techniques, including echocardiography and radionuclide ventriculography, has afforded not only improved diagnostic precision but also objective serial assessment of therapeutic response. Finally, it has become clear that the treatment of heart failure can reduce mortality[1,2] and thus it should be aimed not only at the alleviation of symptoms but also at retarding the progression of the underlying heart disease and improving patient survival.

PATHOPHYSIOLOGY OF HEART FAILURE RELEVANT TO MANAGEMENT

Sir Thomas Lewis deemed the heart to be failing when it was no longer able to supply sufficient oxygen for the needs of the metabolizing tissues.

But, as Harris has pointed out, the adequacy of the circulation is determined not by the degree of oxygenation of the tissues but by the blood pressure.[3] Thus, any fall in the arterial pressure, as a result of impaired cardiac function, activates several mechanisms designed to maintain it, including the sympathetic nervous system, the renin–angiotensin system and release of arginine vasopressin from the pituitary. Activation of the sympathetic nervous system increases the heart rate and redistributes blood flow from the splanchnic circulation and skin to the heart and skeletal muscles. Inadequate renal perfusion in turn stimulates renin release from the kidney. Ultimately, this results in the generation of angiotensin II, a powerful vasoconstrictor that stimulates the release of aldosterone from the adrenal glands which in turn leads to an increase in extracellular fluid volume.

Neuro-endocrine activation is not, however, omnipresent and it has been argued that it results, at least in part, from the treatment of heart failure, especially with diuretics and vasodilators. However, studies in early heart failure following myocardial infarction clearly demonstrate marked neuro-endocrine activation prior to diuretic therapy.[4]

These deleterious effects are to some extent counterbalanced by the actions of atrial natriuretic peptide which plays an important role in volume regulation (Fig. 5.1). Elevated levels of atrial natriuretic peptide occur in congestive heart failure;[5,6] these high levels are accompanied by depletion of the atrial storage granules, a finding that supports the concept of an activated system. Several studies have shown that infusion of atrial natriuretic peptide in patients with heart failure reduces arterial pressure and pulmonary capillary wedge

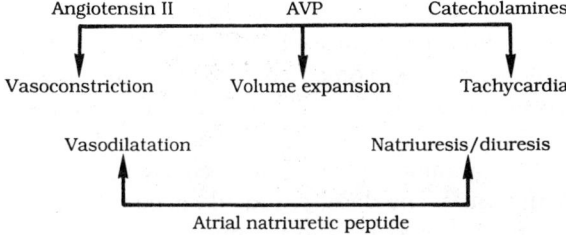

Fig. 5.1. Neuro-endocrine responses and effects in chronic heart failure.

pressure and increases urinary sodium excretion and cardiac output.[7,8]

Presumably, these so-called 'compensatory mechanisms' were designed to maintain arterial pressure, and thus perfusion, during short-lived periods of stress, particularly haemorrhage, dehydration, trauma and exercise. Their prolonged activation, however, as in severe heart failure, is potentially, disadvantageous to cardiac function. Vasoconstriction increases the afterload against which the heart must pump while the increase in intravascular volume also increases ventricular volume and myocardial oxygen consumption.

The aims of therapeutic intervention in heart failure, therefore, are to remove, where possible, the underlying or precipitating cause, to overcome the effects of the 'compensatory mechanisms' by preventing fluid retention, improve the loading conditions of the heart and, where appropriate, to enhance the contractility of the failing myocardium. Specific measures to achieve this include cardiac surgery, treatment with diuretics, conventional vasodilators, angiotensin converting enzyme inhibitors, calcium channel blockers, inotropes and beta-blockers. Other supportive pharmacological treatments include the use of anticoagulants and anti-arrhythmic agents; non-pharmacological measures include cessation of cigarette smoking and alcohol abuse, weight loss in the obese, appropriate decrease in activities and, in some cases, mild restriction of salt intake.

ACUTE RIGHT HEART FAILURE

Characteristic causes of acute right heart failure include massive pulmonary embolism and an acute deterioration of chronic right ventricular pressure overload, usually caused by chronic obstructive airways disease. These aspects are dealt with in Chapter 54.

The most important non-pulmonary cause of acute right heart failure in adults is that secondary to acute inferior or posterior myocardial infarction; about 50% of all inferior myocardial infarcts are associated with some degree of right ventricular infarction although isolated involvement of the right ventricle is much rarer.[9] Nonetheless, it is important to recognize this in view of the different management approach that has to be taken. It is one of the differential diagnoses of cardiogenic shock in acute myocardial infarction. The blood pressure will be low, the jugular venous pressure will be elevated, but the lung fields will be clear. Treatment is to increase the preload by intravenous fluids and not to decrease it with diuretics. This subject is discussed in more detail in the section on acute myocardial infarction.

ACUTE LEFT HEART FAILURE

The cause of this common medical emergency is usually easy to identify occurring, most commonly, as an early complication of acute myocardial infarction. Typically, the episode is managed using the simple clinical variables of heart rate, blood pressure, urine output and physical signs to monitor the outcome of a standard therapeutic strategy that includes opiates, diuretics and oxygen.

First, intravenous opiate, characteristically morphine or diamorphine, relieves the distressing dyspnoea and allays the patients anxiety; dosing varies from 2 to 5 mg according to the size of the patient and the clinical state. Second, intravenous diuretic is given, usually one or other of the rapidly acting powerful 'loop' diuretics, frusemide or bumetanide in initial doses of 40 mg or 1 mg, respectively. Third, oxygen is administered at up to 10 l/min via a facemask designed to deliver a high concentration of at least 60% oxygen.

A mild but occasionally moderate elevation of the blood pressure often accompanies left ventricular failure and may be regarded as being due to neuro-endocrine activation, but sustained hypertension may be contributing to the failure and require treatment in its own right.

Failure of the clinical situation to respond to these simple measures indicates that more intensive monitoring and other pharmacological or non-pharmacological interventions may be required.

More information about the underlying pathophysiology is required when there is, *de novo*, evidence of more severe haemodynamic disturbance including widespread crepitations beyond the mid-zone, peripheral circulatory failure, hypotension, mental obtundation or renal shutdown.

ADDITIONAL MONITORING

Additional monitoring is provided by Swan–Ganz cardiac catheterization which can be performed at the bedside.[10] A simple monitoring catheter provides information on pulmonary capillary 'wedge' pressure or indirect left atrial pressure, the pulmonary artery systolic and diastolic blood pressures and the right atrial pressure. If the pulmonary artery end-diastolic pressure and the 'wedge' coincide, the catheter may be more conveniently left in a main pulmonary artery leading to greater ease of monitoring.

More sophisticated monitoring catheters with associated computer systems allow cardiac output to be measured by thermodilution techniques; even more complex catheters incorporate a ventricular, atrial or atrioventricular sequential pacing facility. Intra-arterial monitoring of the blood pressure using a small radial artery cannula is also very useful especially when the pressure is low.

Such techniques clarify the nature and extent of the haemodynamic abnormality and establish a baseline from which the success or otherwise of a number of potential interventions can be judged. Importantly, it will reveal the occasional presence of a low filling pressure associated with right ventricular dysfunction or hypovolaemia caused by excessive diuresis.

Assuming an elevated left heart filling pressure, the initial interventions will be pharmacological and the choice of agents will depend largely on the systemic arterial pressure.

NORMOTENSION

When the blood pressure is >100 mmHg, a vasodilator may improve the stroke volume by reducing afterload, and lower the filling pressure and reduce pulmonary oedema by venodilatation.

Most commonly, the choice of intravenous agents is between nitroprusside and a nitrate. The arterial dilating effects of nitroprusside are greater than those of nitrates, and in the presence of a low cardiac output and high filling pressure this agent would seem to be the drug of choice. The drug has some disadvantages, however, which include the necessity to use silver foil to prevent loss of effect, the desirability of direct intra-arterial pressure recordings to facilitate dosing, the build-up of toxic metabolites in patients who have liver or renal dysfunction and a possible reduction in collateral blood flow, as compared with nitrate in experimental ischaemia.[11] Thus, intravenous nitrates are often used in the specific circumstance of left ventricular failure associated with acute myocardial infarction.[12] The dose is titrated against the systemic arterial pressure and the filling pressure: optimally, the latter should be reduced to the range 16–18 mmHg without lowering the former below the range 90–100 mmHg. If vasodilatation causes the blood pressure to fall below these limits, then, depending on the clinical state, inotropic therapy may be the best option (this is discussed below).

When the systemic arterial pressure is <100 mmHg, the immediate concern is that further reduction as a result of vasodilatation might compromise blood flow to the vital organs including the heart itself. Unfortunately, as coronary, cerebral or renal blood flow cannot be measured at the bedside, some arbitrary limits must be set which, in turn, may be influenced by clinical factors, such as the mental state, skin temperature, presence of peripheral vasoconstriction and the urine flow rate. Some patients respond to vasodilator therapy with a paradoxical rise in blood pressure as a result of the improvement in cardiac output. Thus, an important aspect of the management of these patients is adequate medical and nursing expertise backed up by accurate physiological measurement.

When the systolic blood pressure is <100 mmHg, the usual initial regimen is an intravenous inotrope, usually the beta$_1$-agonist dobutamine in a dose ranging from 5 μg/kg/min upwards.[13] Often, in the hope of increasing renal blood flow selectively and improving renal function, dopamine is given concurrently in its renal dose of <2.5 μg/kg/min.

Such treatment may stabilize the patient's condition but if a rise in the blood pressure is not accompanied by clinical improvement then vasodilatation can be instituted as previously described.

There is accumulating evidence that considerable neuro-endocrine activation occurs at an early stage in acute myocardial infarction, especially when it is complicated by left ventricular failure, and the treatment of such with diuretics, (Fig. 5.2) or by cardiogenic shock.[4] This has led to the cautious exploration of the place of angiotensin converting enzyme inhibitors in this situation (Fig. 5.3).[14,15] The haemodynamic effects are similar to those described in chronic heart failure and as the long-term effects of angiotensin converting enzyme inhibitors have been more encouraging than those

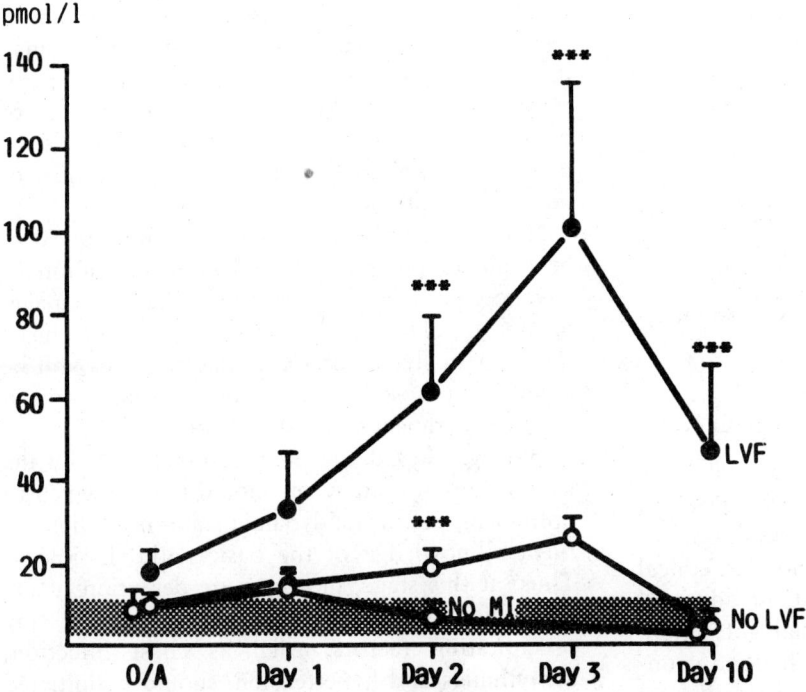

Fig. 5.2. Plasma concentrations of angiotensin II on admission (O/A) and following acute myocardial infarction in patients with left ventricular failure (LVF), no left ventricular failure (no LVF) compared with patients without myocardial infarction (no MI). Shaded area represents normal range for angiotensin II in pmol/l dose μp/l. ***$P < 0.001$.

of any other vasodilator, it seems likely that this approach will be used more widely in the near future. Recovery is usually heralded by the onset of a diuresis, whereupon gradual withdrawal of intravenous medications and replacement with oral drugs, principally diuretics and nitrates, should take place.

Despite these measures, some patients make only a modest improvement and enter a state of persistent left ventricular failure whose management becomes similar to that described below for patients who have chronic cardiac failure.

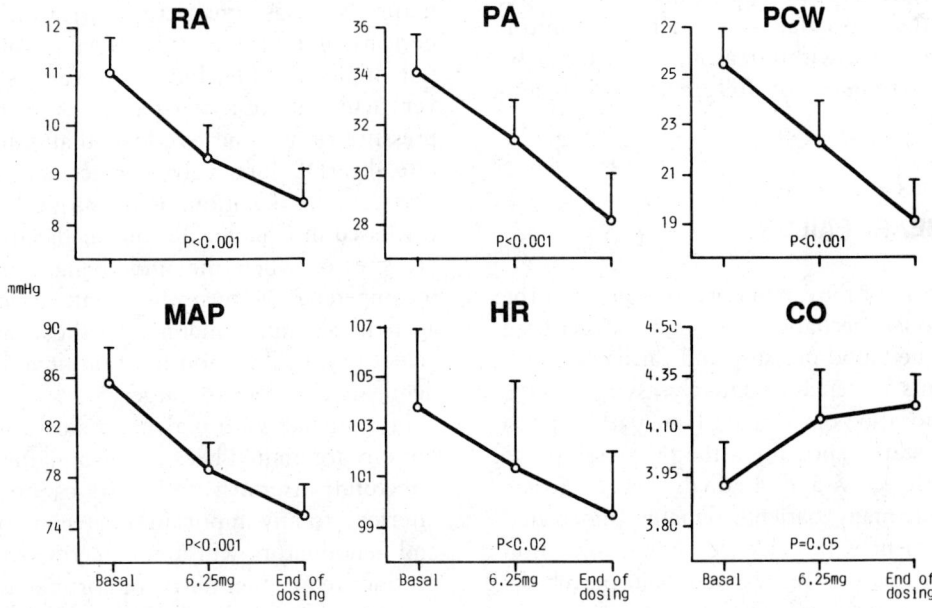

Fig. 5.3. Haemodynamic effects of a cumulative dose of captopril (6.25 mg or 12.5 mg orally) in 18 patients with left ventricular failure following acute myocardial infarction. RA, right atrial pressure; PA, pulmonary arterial pressure; PCW, pulmonary capillary wedge pressure; MAP, mean arterial pressure; HR, heart rate; CO, cardiac output.

ATRIAL FIBRILLATION

Atrial fibrillation is a characteristic precipitating or complicating factor in acute heart failure which usually responds to digoxin.[16]

Rapid digitalization is usually advised, digoxin being withdrawn on the restoration of sinus rhythm. Intravenous amiodarone may occasionally be required if the ventricular rate remains unacceptably high; it has the added advantage of being able to restore sinus rhythm sooner.[17] Occasionally, cardioversion will be necessary.

FAILURE TO RESOLVE ACUTE SITUATION

The persistence of pulmonary oedema and a low cardiac output despite these measures poses a difficult management problem the resolution of which involves an interplay among medical, ethical and logistic factors. In a young patient admitted soon after the onset of myocardial infarction, artificial ventilation and intra-aortic balloon counterpulsation, to improve and stabilize the clinical state, followed by cardiac catheterization, and, if technically feasible, coronary revascularization by angioplasty or coronary artery bypass surgery or even cardiac transplantation may be undertaken. However, these measures may not be available to or appropriate in many patients. Similarly, when non-invasive investigation has revealed a potentially reversible surgical cause for the acute heart failure, such as acute ventricular septal defect or mitral incompetence, then, within reason, age will not be the main determinant of full investigation and treatment.

CHRONIC HEART FAILURE

The very nature of the circulatory system, with the many and diverse mechanisms that may be recruited to maintain the blood pressure and cardiac output, allows patients to remain relatively asymptomatic despite deterioration of the underlying pathology to an advanced state, especially if the progression has been relatively slow and gradual. Thus, cardiac impairment in many patients remains undetected until they present with evidence of fluid retention giving rise to progressive dyspnoea and peripheral oedema. Very often on close questioning and in retrospect, a history of dyspnoea and tiredness attributed by the patient to advancing years can be elicited. At this stage, heart failure is a syndrome comprising cardiac, renal, neural and biochemical components. The nature of the cardiac disease may be obvious from the clinical features, the electrocardiogram and the chest X-ray; in most cases of doubt, the echocardiogram will usually provide the diagnosis as well as an indication of the severity of the cardiac pathology.

Not infrequently, the presentation may appear to be acute despite the subsequent identification of advanced pathology, whereupon the initial management is similar to that described for acute heart failure. Usually, the initial filling pressures will be higher than those in acute myocardial infarction so that the therapeutic aim will be different.

Having relieved the pulmonary oedema by the use of diuretics, attention should then be given to optimizing the haemodynamic state in the light of further knowledge of the basic pathophysiology. Thus, at this stage, more precise definition of the pathology is required and the treatment of any precipitating factors, such as chest infection, arrhythmias and hypertension, should be initiated or continued. Three broad categories of patients emerge, those with a potentially reversible aetiology, those with dilated poorly contracting ventricles and those with primarily diastolic dysfunction.

POTENTIALLY REVERSIBLE PATHOLOGY

Several pathologies of a physical or mechanical nature, such as constrictive pericarditis or chronic pericardial effusion, can present acutely and are potentially curable; but, in valvar disease, as it is ventricular dysfunction secondary to longstanding pressure or volume overload that usually precipitates heart failure, valve replacement will be only part of the solution. The surgical aspects are discussed in Chapter 35, but medically the options are greater when the underlying cause is valvar incompetence because these patients can be managed in a similar manner to those with primary ventricular dysfunction until full investigations can delineate the place of surgery.

In patients with valvar stenosis, the medical options are limited because vasodilators are usually unhelpful; arterial vasodilators cannot modify the afterload to any important degree in aortic stenosis and venodilators will almost certainly be counterproductive in either mitral or aortic stenosis. In such patients, the only hope for improvement lies with surgery; selected patients may obtain benefit from valvuloplasty.

It is essential to consider and exclude metabolic

and toxic causes, including alcohol abuse, haemochromatosis and thyroid disease.

DILATED POORLY CONTRACTING LEFT VENTRICLE (SYSTOLIC DYSFUNCTION)

This condition has been the focus of renewed interest in the subject of heart failure. Pivotal to that interest is that severe left ventricular dysfunction has been the substrate for most of the new therapeutic strategies in heart failure research.[18] Its management gives full expression to the increasing variety of those innovations aimed at improving symptoms, maintaining left ventricular function and improving the prognosis. (Fig. 5.4).

Management strategy (Table 5.1)

As this condition, by definition, presents at a fairly advanced stage in the disease, usually with evidence of fluid retention, treatment with diuretics remains the first stage in management. Typically, a potent diuretic in a modest dose clears the oedema and induces a marked clinical improvement, in which case diuretic therapy alone, or with the possible addition of a potassium-sparing diuretic or potassium supplement, may suffice at first.

However, if the dose of potent diuretics has to be increased to improve the clinical situation, the use of vasodilator therapy should be considered. For reasons that are discussed in detail later (p. 68), the treatment of choice at present is an angiotensin converting enzyme inhibitor, which usually obviates the need for potassium supplements, and, generally, is regarded as a contra-indication to potassium-sparing diuretics.

Conventional vasodilators, such as hydralazine and nitrates, often in combination, are indicated if

Table 5.1. Treatment of heart failure.

General treatment	Stop smoking
	Maintain optimum weight
	No added salt
	Treat hypertension
	Detect alcohol abuse

Specific treatment	
Mild heart failure:	Thiazide diuretic
Moderate heart failure:	Loop diuretic
	Digoxin
	Angiotensin converting enzyme inhibitor
	Other vasodilators
Severe heart failure:	Diuretic combinations
	Digoxin
	Angiotensin converting enzyme inhibitor
	Other inotropes
	Haemoperfusion
	Cardiac transplantation

angiotensin converting enzyme inhibitors have to be withdrawn or are contra-indicated for any reason.

Digoxin may be added to the diuretic–vasodilator regimen if the clinical situation has not satisfactorily resolved either during the initial management phase, which is often conducted in hospital, or, at a later stage, during outpatient management if symptoms are limiting or heart failure recurs. Atrial fibrillation is a specific indication for digoxin at any stage of management.

Failure to eradicate evidence of fluid retention and persistence of the heart failure state usually lead to the prescription of increasing doses of potent diuretics and the addition of a thiazide diuretic or metolazone to complement the effects of the more potent loop diuretics by blocking sodium reabsorption upstream and downstream from their site of action.

Intravenous inotropes or therapies, such as haemoperfusion, peritoneal dialysis or intra-aortic balloon counterpulsation, are probably preludes to cardiac transplantation or the ultimate expression of left ventricular dysfunction, death.

DIASTOLIC DYSFUNCTION

It is axiomatic that the cardiac output during systole is heavily dependent on the cardiac intake during diastole and, therefore, that a low cardiac output can result from diastolic dysfunction in the presence of normal systolic function.[19,20] The classic abnormality of diastolic cardiac dysfunction is mitral stenosis, in which the physical obstruction posed by

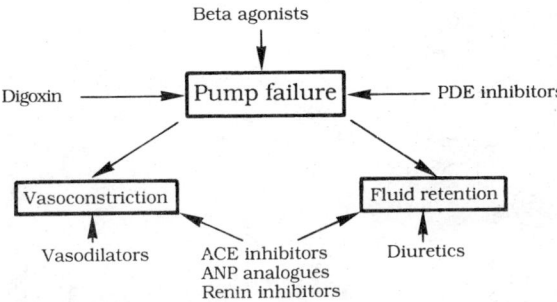

Fig. 5.4. Some of the new therapeutic strategies for heart failure secondary to left ventricular dysfunction. PDE, phosphodiasterase; ACE, angiotensin converting enzyme; ANP, atrial natriuretic peptide.

the narrowed mitral orifice impedes the ventricular filling. It is being increasingly recognized that functional impedance to ventricular filling is a feature of several myocardial disorders usually, but not specifically, affecting the left ventricle in which poor compliance is the principal pathophysiological expression of the intrinsic pathology.[21]

Restrictive cardiomyopathy falls into this group as does hypertrophic cardiomyopathy and hypertrophy secondary to left ventricular pressure overload. 'Little old lady's heart',[22] a syndrome comprising left ventricular hypertrophy and poor compliance in the elderly is an example of diastolic dysfunction that may result in heart failure (Fig. 5.5). Decreased compliance is also a recognized early feature of acute ischaemia.[23] Moreover, fibrosis adjacent to areas of hypertrophy may further complicate the pathophysiology.

Specific pathologies, such as restrictive cardiomyopathy, amyloid, sarcoidosis and severe concentric hypertrophy, give rise to diastolic dysfunction in the presence of systolic function that may be virtually normal and be severe enough to cause a reduced cardiac output and the features of heart failure. However, the contribution of diastolic dysfunction to the resultant haemodynamic abnormality in patients with severe systolic dysfunction as in dilated cardiomyopathy, for example, is difficult to assess at present.

Heart failure secondary to diastolic dysfunction is difficult to treat. As with mitral stenosis, venodilatation may be counterproductive leading to severe hypotension and a further fall in the cardiac output. Afterload reduction, however, seems a logical course, especially in the presence of abnormal vasoconstriction seen in the later stages of heart failure. This may be accomplished by treatment with hydralazine or a calcium antagonist.

The place of beta-blockers in the treatment of this condition remains controversial. Theoretically, an increase in the diastolic period due to the bradycardia should lead to a greater degree of filling and to an increased end-diastolic volume. This may be one mechanism for the benefit from beta-blockade claimed in other types of heart failure, notably that due to congestive cardiomyopathy.[24] It is speculation whether this points to an important diastolic component to the resultant cardiac dysfunction.

It has been claimed that calcium antagonists have a specific beneficial effect in hypertrophic cardiomyopathy, although the benefit would tend to be offset by tachycardia and shortening of the diastolic period resulting from peripheral vasodilatation.[25] The rate-modulating calcium antagonists, verapamil and diltiazem, may have an advantage in this situation.[26,27]

Apart from therapy with diuretics and arterial vasodilators, the results of medical treatment of this condition are disappointing. In a few suitable patients, cardiac transplantation is the only therapy

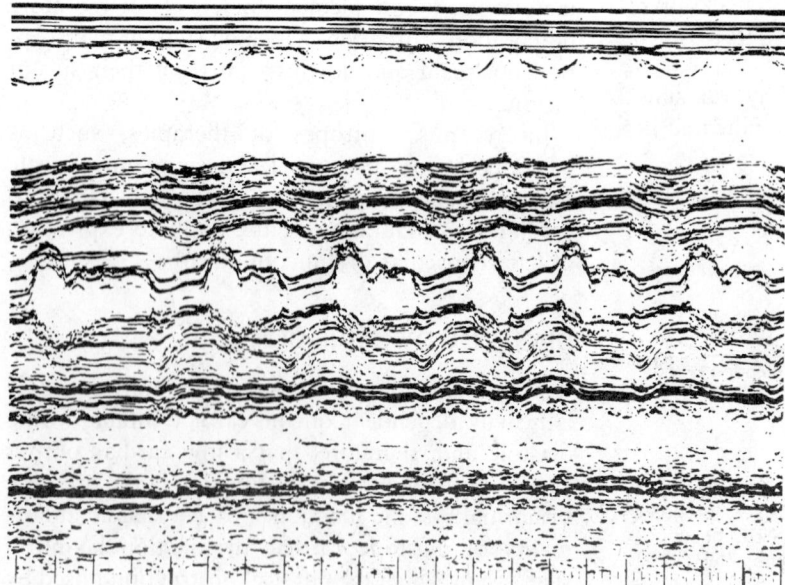

Fig. 5.5. Echocardiogram from a 75-year-old female patient with congestive cardiac failure and normal blood pressure showing hypertrophied and poorly compliant left ventricle with small left ventricular cavity.

to improve prognosis; conventional surgery on the inflow obstruction in hypertrophic cardiomyopathy or restrictive cardiomyopathy is only palliative at best.

CHRONIC STABLE HEART FAILURE

Patients rendered free of oedema by modern diuretic therapy may remain only mildly symptomatic for quite some time and with concomitant treatment with angiotensin converting enzyme inhibitors it may be possible to reduce substantially the dose of potent diuretics. Although the temptation exists to withdraw diuretic therapy, it has been shown that, in patients previously requiring diuretics, the cessation of such has led to a deterioration in clinical status.[28]

The availability of non-invasive techniques has heightened awareness of the prevalence and the spectrum of ventricular dysfunction. In many patients, cardiac haemodynamics may be entirely normal at rest, becoming abnormal only during exercise, with an insufficient rise in cardiac output coupled to a rise in left atrial pressure, and leading to the development of exertional fatigue and dyspnoea. In such patients, and according to the varying practices in different countries, digoxin or a diuretic might normally be prescribed. At present, considerable thought is being applied to identify the best management for such patients. The aims are, first, to ameliorate the symptoms and improve the quality of life, second, to preserve ventricular function by preventing or retarding the progress of further deterioration and, third, to prolong life of good or acceptable quality. Specific conditions such as amyloid or the cardiomyopathies presently elude effective specific treatment although in some cases of myocarditis and sarcoidosis benefit with steroids has been claimed.[29,30] In appropriate cases, revascularization offers the best hope of preventing further damage in patients with coronary heart disease.[31] Assuming that there is isolated ventricular dysfunction, could medical treatment significantly impede the progression of ventricular dysfunction? In the absence of specific treatment, the approach that seems most likely to have any impact is that of reducing the load on and the work of the heart.

Such effects could be provided by the angiotensin converting enzyme inhibitors in that they cause a persistent reduction in arterial pressure and specifically antagonize the compensatory neuro-endocrine and renal response to that fall in pressure thereby exposing the ventricle to a 'low pressure' circulatory system. This would lead to a long-term reduction in wall tension and stroke work both at rest and during exercise. Myocardial oxygen demands would be reduced thus ameliorating the effect of residual coronary stenosis. However, if the reduction in pressure in the presence of significant vascular obstruction in any organ system was too great, it could lead to a respective fall in organ blood flow. These aspects require further study.

NON-PHARMACOLOGICAL INTERVENTIONS

GENERAL

As physical exercise is the main factor in producing symptoms in patients with most types of chronic heart failure and it leads to stimulation of neuro-endocrine mechanisms, some restriction of activity is appropriate for many patients.

A careful explanation of the reasons for the symptoms is often useful in helping patients to reappraise their lives and make those adjustments necessitated by their change in circumstances. For some, this may mean abandoning previously precious more vigorous sporting exercise, whereas for others it may entail acceptance of a very severely limited exercise capacity. Rest periods during the day are particularly helpful in moderately severely affected patients; at a later stage, more prolonged periods of bed rest become increasingly necessary during episodes of frank decompensation.

Paradoxically, exercise training has been advocated for patients with poor left ventricular function but its role has yet to be fully evaluated.[32]

Other general methods include identification and correction of excess salt intake although strict salt restriction and the use of salt substitutes remain unpopular, unpalatable and probably impracticable additional detractions from an already impaired quality of life.

Ultimately, the care of patients with severe intractable heart failure becomes that of the terminally ill which entails the resolution of social, psychological and even psychiatric problems. These aspects of therapy must not be forgotten in the excitement generated by all the new therapeutic strategies now available for the management of subsequent patients.

DRUGS USED IN HEART FAILURE

DIURETICS

As fluid retention is the hallmark of heart failure, diuretics are the principal agents for treatment of this condition. In non-oedematous patients at an earlier stage of the disease, however, the logic of prescribing diuretics could be questioned.

Diuretics may be classified according to their potency which can be defined as the maximum percentage of the filtered load of sodium that the drug can cause to be excreted (Table 5.2). Although the list of compounds is extensive, in practice only three classes of diuretics are used: the moderately potent thiazides; the powerful 'loop' diuretics, of which only frusemide and bumetanide are used to any extent; and the weak diuretics that act in the distal tubule to inhibit the various sodium—potassium exchange mechanisms, amiloride triamterene and the aldosterone antagonist spironolactone.

The sites of action and clinical pharmacology of diuretics have been extensively reviewed elsewhere;[32,33] for practical purposes, it is important to appreciate their site of action in the nephron, their potency and that additive and beneficial effects, in terms of potency and potassium conservation, may be obtained by their combination.

Although the greatest percentage of the filtered load of sodium is reabsorbed in the proximal tubule, there are no powerful agents that act only at that site. Metolazone, a thiazide congener acting like other thiazides on the cortical diluting segment of the nephron, may owe part of its efficacy to a proximal action.[34] This may explain the widely held belief that its combination with a 'loop' diuretic is perhaps the most powerful natriuretic intervention available clinically (three sites of sodium reabsorption are inhibited).[35,36] Addition of a potassium-conserving diuretic, which acts in the distal tubule, completes what is in effect 'nephron blockade'. Few patients are resistant to such manipulation of modern diuretic therapy, the problems of which arise largely from volune depletion and electrolyte imbalances rather than from a lack of effect.

The spectrum of use and range of diuretic dosage in heart failure are wide, for example, from 5 mg of bendrofluazide on alternate days to 1 g/day of frusemide, according to individual practice or as part of a planned therapeutic strategy of increasing complexity. Many patients with mild symptoms can be managed with a thiazide diuretic, although eventually most patients will graduate to the more potent loop diuretics, frusemide or bumetanide. As a general rule, if monotherapy with frusemide (80 mg/day) is not effective, the use of vasodilator therapy should be considered. In refractory patients, increasing doses of potent diuretics may be complemented by the addition of a thiazide or metolazone. In the absence of an angiotensin converting enzyme inhibitor, the further addition of a potassium-conserving agent, such as amiloride, spironolactone or triamterene, completes the triple therapy approach to diuretic treatment. For clinical purposes, there is little to choose among the members of each diuretic class and individual usage varies widely. This subject has been extensively reviewed elsewhere.[37]

Adverse effects of diuretics

The main non-electrolyte metabolic complications of diuretic therapy, hyperuricaemia and hyperglycaemia, are not peculiar to heart failure and have been extensively reviewed elsewhere.[38]

The principal electrolyte abnormalities associated with diuretic therapy are hyponatraemia, hypokalaemia and hypomagnesaemia, all of which are important in the specific context of heart failure.

Table 5.2. **Site of action and potency of diuretics used in heart failure.**

Diuretic	Site of action	Potency (%filtered Na + excreted)
Frusemide/bumetanide	Ascending limb of Henle's loop	> 25%
Thiazides	Corticol diluting segment	10–15%
Potassium-sparing agents (amiloride, triamterene, spironolactone)	Distal tubule	<5%

The development of hyponatraemia usually indicates very severe heart failure and is an ominous prognostic sign;[39] hypokalaemia and hypomagnesaemia have been linked to ventricular arrhythmias which are also predictive of a poor prognosis.[40]

Hyponatraemia

In patients with untreated heart failure, total body sodium is increased although commonly the plasma sodium concentration is normal, thus implying equal retention of sodium and water by the kidney; hyponatraemia usually indicates increased body sodium but an even greater and inappropriate retention of water. Several mechanisms can be implicated including increased secretion of angiotensin II which, by reducing renal medullary blood flow and thereby increasing medullary osmolality, will provide the intrarenal conditions necessary for increased water reabsorption. This augmented water reabsorption may be facilitated by increased secretion of antidiuretic hormone, which has been reported in heart failure.[41,42] Angiotensin II may stimulate secretion of antidiuretic hormone directly and may also increase thirst, leading to further water intake and subsequent retention by the kidney. The resultant fall in plasma sodium concentration leads to further renin release, thus completing an unfavourable cycle of events. Although hyponatraemia can occur in the absence of diuretic therapy, it is most commonly seen in patients with severe heart failure who have been treated with high doses of diuretics. Hyponatraemia induced during diuretic therapy may occur for several reasons including urinary sodium loss, increased water intake caused by thirst and interference with maximal urinary dilution, leading to decreased free water clearance. As already noted, hyponatraemia may stimulate renin secretion thereby enhancing the angiotensin II-mediated mechanisms described above. It is not known to what extent hyponatraemia is a direct consequence of renal adaptations to declining cardiac function, to diuretic-induced stimulation of angiotensin II or to other unmeasured factors. Information is also lacking on the degree of activation of the renin–angiotensin system before treatment with diuretics or other drugs. Moreover, an inverse relationship between plasma renin and sodium concentrations has been described in several studies, indicating that hyponatraemia may be a marker for a high renin state in heart failure.[43]

Mild hyponatraemia is almost universal in patients with moderate or severe heart failure treated with diuretics. Clinically, the only way of managing hyponatraemia, or of preventing its development, is to institute some degree of fluid restriction, especially in patients with marked oedema receiving high doses of diuretics. Greater restriction (1–1.5 l/day) is essential when the plasma sodium concentration falls below 130 mmol/l; in the most severe cases of hyponatraemia, haemoperfusion or peritoneal dialysis may be required to correct this and other electrolyte abnormalities. As total body sodium is elevated in these patients, it seems illogical to correct a maldistribution of sodium and water with an infusion of sodium solutions.

Potassium

Like sodium, most of the potassium filtered at the glomerulus is reabsorbed in the proximal tubule; much of the potassium excreted results from secretion in the distal convoluted tubule in exchange for reabsorbed sodium. The extent of this exchange depends on several factors including acid–base status (hydrogen may also exchange with sodium), the distal delivery of sodium and potassium and plasma levels of aldosterone. Diuretic therapy may influence body potassium directly or through stimulation of the renin–angiotensin system, although there has been considerable controversy on the latter point. Low-dose diuretic therapy does not cause total body potassium depletion in patients who are eating a diet rich in potassium.[44–46] Although this may be the case in patients with mild heart failure, in several studies of patients with severe heart failure, these findings have not been confirmed.

In an unselected group of patients who were consecutively referred for investigation and management of severe heart failure, total body potassium (measured by whole-body counting of endogenous ^{40}K) was decreased.[47] This was not related to diuretic dose, duration of heart failure, functional class or decrease in lean body mass, but was closely and inversely related to plasma renin concentration. Although it is not surprising there is a close relationship between body potassium and the renin–angiotensin system in heart failure, it is surprising there is a good correlation between plasma potassium and total body potassium because, unlike sodium, most of the total body pool of potassium is intracellular. This is not the case in patients with essential hypertension receiving diuretics in whom hypokalaemia is common and depletion of total body potassium is rare.[46] Thus, plasma potassium concentration, like plasma sodium concentration, may be a useful clinical guide to the state of activation of the renin–angiotensin system in heart failure. Plasma potassium and total body potassium rise significantly during angiotensin converting enzyme inhibition leading to correction of the hypokalaemia and of the deficit in total body potassium.[48] Thus, angiotensin converting enzyme inhibitors have favourable effects on potassium status which are predictable from their known physiological effects. An important practical consideration is that concomitant therapy with potassium-sparing diuretics can aggravate any tendency to hyperkalaemia, especially in patients who have poor renal function.

In view of the propensity of patients with heart failure to develop potassium depletion, and since ventricular arrhythmias are relatively common in patients with severe heart failure, it should be routine to prescribe either potassium supplementation or, even better, a potassium-sparing diuretic to obviate the development of hypokalaemia.

VASODILATORS

The clinical application of those factors apart from contractility that regulate the stroke volume, together with a greater awareness of their interplay in the syndrome of heart failure, has led to the concept of unloading the heart, whereby an improvement in cardiac function can be obtained together with a reduction in cardiac work.[49,50]

Haemodynamic considerations relevant to vasodilation

Haemodynamically, cardiac function can be described in terms of the preload, afterload, myocardial contractility and compliance, and the heart rate.[49]

Preload, the extent of fibre stretch in diastole, is represented in the clinical setting by the end-diastolic volume which is determined by venous tone, the intravascular volume, ventricular compliance and the extent of ventricular systolic emptying. Although end-diastolic pressure and volume are not linearly related (pressure rising more steeply for any given increase in volume), the left ventricular end-diastolic pressure or filling pressure provides a useful indicator of preload. In the absence of any physical obstruction to blood flow from the lungs to the left ventricle, the left ventricular end-diastolic pressure correlates well with the pulmonary capillary wedge pressure and usually with the pulmonary artery end-diastolic pressure. In simple clinical terms, an increase in left ventricular preload may lead to pulmonary congestion and to the symptom of dyspnoea. Afterload, the left ventricular wall stress that must be overcome for the contents to be ejected, is determined by several factors including the radius of the ventricle, its thickness and its pressure, and by the arteriolar tone. As preload affects the volume and therefore the radius of the ventricle, it also influences the afterload. Systemic vascular resistance is the main contributor to and is used as a clinical approximation for the afterload. In heart failure, systemic vascular resistance increases in response to several of the vasoconstrictor stimuli that form part of the neuro-endocrine response.

Systolic and diastolic left ventricular dysfunction

In a ventricle with impaired contractility, increased peripheral resistance depresses the stroke volume to a greater extent than it does in a normal ventricle, emphasizing the importance of afterload not only in determining stroke volume but also as a mechanism worth modulating in efforts to increase it (Fig. 5.6). When contractility is impaired, stroke volume is maintained by an adaptive increase in end-diastolic volume which has been regarded, probably simplistically, as the recruitment of the Frank–Starling mechanism. Sodium and water retention by the kidney facilitates this by increasing intravascular volume, as does increased venous tone mediated mainly through the sympathetic nervous system. Both factors may be modulated by neuro-endocrine mechanisms, and the interaction of these and other factors has been well reviewed recently.[5,6] The left ventricular function curves relating filling pressure and cardiac output, together with the expected effects of vasodilatation (arterial or venous or both), are shown in Fig. 5.6.

When the left ventricle contracts well but relaxes poorly as in, for example, left ventricular hypertrophy, the acute effects of manipulation of preload and afterload are less predictable. Reduction of preload is likely to be counterproductive, leading to even poorer filling of the ventricle and, therefore, to falls in the cardiac output and systemic blood pressure. However, stroke volume can be increased by arteriolar vasodilators.

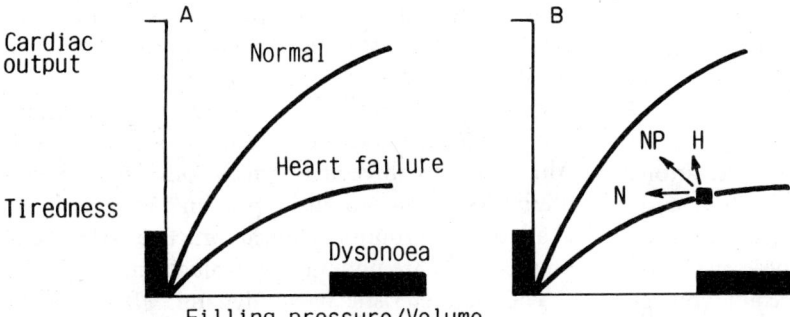

Fig. 5.6. (A) Normal and depressed left ventricular function curves relating cardiac output to failing pressure and end diastolic volume. The symptoms of tiredness and dyspnoea are notionally displayed to indicate the relationship to a low cardiac output and a high filling pressure, respectively. (B) Normal and abnormal left ventricular function curves displaying the responses to vasodilator therapy. N, nitrate; NP, nitroprusside; H, hydralazine.

Classification of vasodilators

As might be expected in a complex and intricately regulated system like the human circulation, the potential vasodilatory mechanisms or mediators identified thus far are many, including the sympathetic nervous system, slow calcium channels, histamine, prostaglandins, kinins, the renin–angiotensin system and the other ubiquitous peptides.[53] However, those vasodilators used in heart failure, by virtue of their specific arterial venous or mixed arterial and venous vasodilating effects, are relatively few. For clinical convenience, they may be divided into three groups: the 'conventional vasodilators' the angiotensin converting enzyme inhibitors and the calcium antagonists (Table 5.3). The conventional vasodilators are those that were originally and specifically applied as vasodilators, they have no other discernible pharmacological property and they have been used extensively in clinical practice. The angiotensin converting enzyme inhibitors have several other important properties that contribute to their observed clinical effects. The calcium antagonists are a heterogeneous group of compounds which have only recently been used in heart failure; they are discussed separately below.

In theory, the reduction of filling pressure or preload by a venodilator such as a nitrate may reduce pulmonary congestion and ameliorate dys-

ponea. Likewise, reduction of peripheral resistance and, therefore, afterload by an arteriolar dilator such as hydralazine can increase the stroke volume and cardiac output, thereby improving exercise capacity and tiredness. Thus, a 'balanced' vasodilator such as prazosin would be expected to reduce both preload and afterload and improve both dysponea and tiredness.

Place of conventional vasodilators in management

Although hydralazine, prazosin and the nitrates produce the acute haemodynamic effects predictable from their respective pharmacological profiles,[53] long-term oral therapy with these drugs has been disappointing because their favourable acute haemodynamic effects do not appear to be reflected in an improved exercise capacity even in the short term.[54] In long-term studies, neither hydralazine nor prazosin[55,56] has been shown to improve exercise capacity significantly. Part of the explanation for loss of the therapeutic effect during chronic dosing may be further activation of the compensatory mechanisms mentioned earlier.[57,58]

The results of studies of nitrate efficacy have also been conflicting, for which there are several reasons, including differing patient selection and study design, and the problem of nitrate tolerance.[59–61]

Although the results of long-term haemodynamic and clinical studies have not been universally encouraging, clinical interest in the conventional therapeutic approach of a vasodilator with nitrates and hydralazine was stimulated by the finding that patients with heart failure secondary to severe left ventricular dysfunction receiving this combination had improved survival. In contrast, prazosin had no impact on survival.[1]

Pharmacological innovation will ensure a continuing future for arterial and venous dilators. New generation calcium antagonists that have greater vascular selectivity, and hydralazine-like com-

Table 5.3. **Vasodilators used in long-term treatment.**

Drug	Mechanism	Arterial	Venous
Nitrates	Cyclic GMP	+	+
Hydralazine	Unknown	++	−
Prazosin	α–1–Antagonist	++	++
Angiotensin converting enzyme inhibitor	Angiotensin II	++	+
Calcium antagonists	calcium entry	++	−

pounds with greater potency and fewer long-term side-effects are already being investigated.[62,63]

Angiotensin converting enzyme inhibitors

The collective effects of neuro-endocrine activation seem to be unfavourable to cardiac function and could be responsible at least in part for the clinical syndrome of heart failure. Moreover, these mechanisms may be stimulated by and therefore antagonize the effects of conventional vasodilators such as hydralazine and prazosin, and therefore neuro-endocrine activation may be a factor in the decreased efficacy of these agents observed during chronic therapy.[57,58] Thus, there has been considerable interest in the development of agents that will antagonize the renin–angiotensin system at a number of sites. At present, the most interesting compounds are the angiotensin converting enzyme inhibitors. The first orally active compound to be developed was captopril; since then, enalapril and lisinopril have been introduced into clinical practice. A new group of compounds, the renin inhibitors, are of considerable experimental interest and of possible future clinical importance; they reduce the generation of angiotensin I by antagonizing the action of renin on its substrate.[64]

The major therapeutic effect of angiotensin converting enzyme inhibition in heart failure is vasodilatation associated with reduced plasma levels of angiotensin II. Thus, the angiotensin converting enzyme inhibitors can be regarded as vasodilators which have ancillary properties that block the activation of unwanted 'compensatory' mechanisms. It is not known whether inhibition of the degradation of bradykinin also contributes to the favourable haemodynamic effects of these drugs. Although only three angiotensin converting enzyme inhibitors, captopril, lisinopril and enalapril, are available for routine clinical practice at present, many others are undergoing evaluation.

The characteristic haemodynamic effects of the angiotensin converting enzyme inhibitors are those of a balanced vasodilator; they include falls in blood pressure, systemic vascular resistance and left ventricular filling pressure together with a small increase in stroke volume. Right atrial pressure also falls significantly, suggesting a venodilator effect.[65]

With long-term therapy, the reduction in angiotensin II concentration is accompanied by an improvement in several biochemical variables, including decreased plasma levels of aldosterone, vasopressin and noradrenaline. The levels of serum and total body potassium, which are often reduced in heart failure, may increase to a level within the normal range. These beneficial cardiac and biochemical effects are associated with a significant reduction in simple and complex ventricular arrhythmias (Fig. 5.7).[48]

Typically, the patient maintained on an angiotensin converting enzyme inhibitor and diuretic therapy for heart failure has a lower blood pressure than normal, which is usually well tolerated and which reduces left ventricular wall tension and

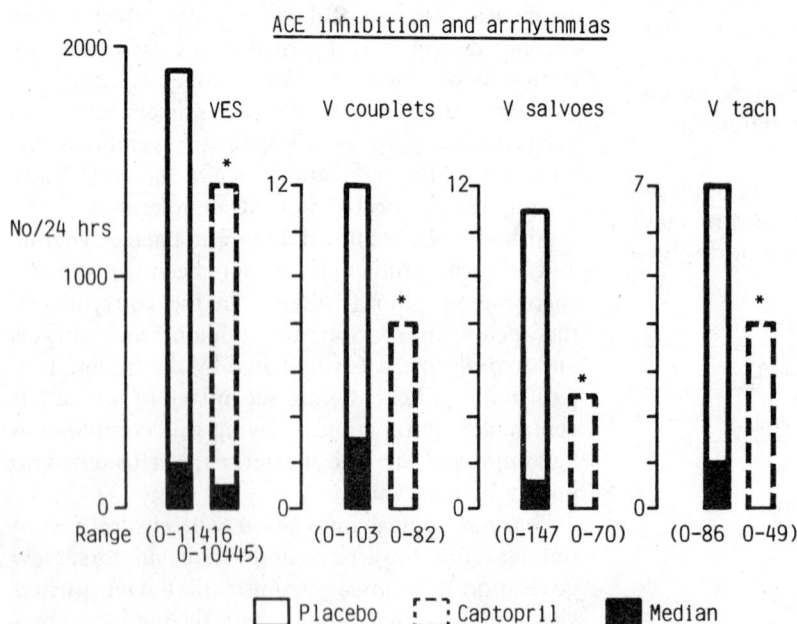

Fig. 5.7. The effect of chronic oral treatment with captopril on ventricular ectopic beats (VES), ventricular couplets (V couplets), ventricular salvoes (V salvoes) and ventricular tachycardia (V tach). Open columns represent mean frequency and closed area represents the median. Left-hand columns: placebo; right-hand columns, captopril. (From Cleland, J.G.F. *et al.* The effects of captopril on serum digoxin and urinary urea and digoxin clearances in patients with chronic heart failure. *Am. Heart J.* 1986; **112**: 130–5.)

myocardial work. The key to the long-term efficacy of angiotensin converting enzyme inhibitors may be the generation of a 'low pressure' state not accompanied by sodium retention and volume expansion. The reasons for this are complex and relate to the biochemical and renal effects of angiotensin converting enzyme inhibitors. Although renal perfusion pressure falls, effective renal plasma flow increases as a result of a fall in renal vascular resistance; despite this, the glomerular filtration rate falls. This apparent paradox arises because, in untreated heart failure, the glomerular filtration rate is initially preserved by preferential constriction of the efferent arteriole by angiotensin II which maintains glomerular hydrostatic pressure.[66] Thus, relaxation of the efferent arteriole by angiotensin converting enzyme inhibition reduces the glomerular filtration rate leading to a modest increase in serum urea and creatinine concentrations.[48,67] Despite the reduction in both renal perfusion and the glomerular filtration rate, sodium retention does not occur, presumably because renal tubular sodium excretion rises. It has yet to be determined whether this long-term reduction in blood pressure, which has an apparent benefit in terms of a reduction in myocardial work, will have favourable implications for the preservation of residual left ventricular function.

However, there is optimism that earlier treatment of heart failure with angiotensin converting enzyme inhibitors will alter the natural history of the condition. It is now apparent that marked stimulation of the renin–angiotensin and sympathetic nervous systems occurs during acute myocardial infarction, especially in patients who develop heart failure,[4] and it has recently been shown that captopril reduces infarct size in experimental acute myocardial infarction.[68] At present, studies of the effects of angiotensin converting enzyme inhibition on infarct expansion, preservation of left ventricular function the development of heart failure and mortality in humans are being undertaken.

Adverse effects of angiotensin converting enzyme inhibitors

Severe 'first dose' hypotension, a syndrome comprising hypotension, bradycardia, sweating and confusion,[69] is a form of vasomotor syncope. In a consecutive series of 100 first-dose administrations, 7 episodes of vasomotor syncope occurred which were unrelated to clinical state, aetiology of heart failure, pre-treatment blood pressure, serum sodium, plasma concentration of active renin or diuretic dose.[70] With captopril, hypotension occur-

red within 1 h of administration of a small oral dose (6.25 mg) and was abrupt in onset; following enalapril (5–10 mg), hypotension occurred approximately 2.5 h after dosing and was more prolonged.

Other side-effects of angiotensin converting enzyme inhibitors include rash, taste disturbance, neutropenia and proteinuria. It was hoped that enalapril would cause fewer side-effects than captopril; although this hope has not been fulfilled, both taste disturbance and skin rash appear to be less common with enalapril administration.[71] Recently, cough has been described as a side-effect of both captopril and enalapril.[72] This appears to be more common in women and is often severe enough to warrant drug withdrawal, which results in rapid recovery. The mechanism of action is unknown, although possible mediators include bradykinin and prostaglandins.

Place of angiotensin converting enzyme inhibitors in management

As there is now convincing evidence in favour of a sustained benefit on treatment with angiotensin converting enzyme inhibitors, they are the first choice of most physicians as the next step after diuretic therapy in the management of the patient with heart failure secondary to left ventricular dysfunction. As pointed out earlier, great care must be taken with their introduction because patients will already be receiving a variable dose of diuretics. One method is to omit the diuretic on the day the first dose of angiotensin converting enzyme inhibitor is given, but the patient should always be observed during the period of maximum effect of the particular preparation. For captopril, the period of maximum effect is short; if significant hypotension has not occurred during the first 2 h, it is unlikely to do so. The onset of hypotension with enalapril is delayed and can be prolonged. Patients should be given the lowest possible dose at first, i.e. 6.25 mg of captopril or 2.5 mg of enalapril. Thereafter, it is best to increase the dose according to changes in blood pressure and further by changes in renal function. At the bedside, it is difficult to predict the optimum dose which is generally taken to be that dose which does not result in either symptomatic hypotension (usually postural) or a serious rise in the blood urea.

The expected rise in serum potassium usually entails stopping any potassium supplements or potassium-sparing diuretics.

A further reason for the use of angiotensin converting enzyme inhibitors in patients with severe heart failure is the recent demonstration by the CONSENSUS study of a marked improvement in survival. This effect seems to have been due almost entirely to an improvement in heart failure since no effect on sudden death was demonstrated.

A proportion of patients cannot tolerate angiotensin converting enzyme inhibitors because of hypotension, a decrease in renal function or other side-effects; such patients are best managed with conventional vasodilators, often a combination of nitrates and hydralazine.

Calcium antagonists

Calcium antagonists are a heterogeneous group of compounds whose common principal action is relaxation of vascular smooth muscle in arteries and arterioles by inhibition of calcium entry through the slow calcium channels.[73] They have no detectable effect on venous tone, but, as calcium entry is important for myocardial contractility and the normal function of the sinus and atrioventricular nodes, potentially the calcium antagonists can have other effects.[74] Selectivity for different calcium channels has resulted in a range of effects. Verapamil is the most negatively inotropic and also slows the heart rate and atrioventricular conduction. Diltiazem possesses similar electrophysiological effects but has a less negative inotropic effect. As a group, the dihydropyridines, of which nifedipine was the first to be developed, are more selective for vascular calcium channels and therefore they are the most attractive of the calcium antagonists for use in heart failure.[73,74] Preliminary experience in heart failure has been conflicting.[75,76] Even the dihydropyridines, which do not have any direct electrophysiological effects on the sinus or atrioventricular nodes, have a spectrum of effects on the myocardium and smooth muscle. Agents such as nicardipine, nisoldipine and felodipine possess negligible negative inotropic effects and therefore hold promise for the future. At present, however, there is no reason to recommend these vascular selective agents in place of other arterial vasodilators or the angiotensin converting enzyme inhibitors in the management of heart failure.

In patients with diastolic dysfunction, the reflex tachycardia that might result from the dihydropyridines could be disadvantageous. Conversely, the rate-modulating effects of diltiazem and verapamil could be advantageous in this specific circumstance where any mild negative inotropic effect might not be important.[26,27]

INOTROPES

Failure to improve a patient's clinical state adequately by a combination of diuretic therapy and an angiotensin converting enzyme inhibitor or conventional vasodilator usually leads to additional therapy with an inotrope. At present and for practical clinical purposes, there are two main choices, intravenous dobutamine or oral digoxin.

Dobutamine

Intravenous therapy with the beta-agonist dobutamine is employed in very severe clinical situations when obvious features of a low cardiac output together with peripheral or pulmonary oedema persist, often in association with electrolyte imbalance and oliguria.[77] Initially, dobutamine can produce marked short-term diuresis and clearing of pulmonary and peripheral oedema. Some patients can then be weaned off this therapy and stabilized on oral treatment for a variable period. Others become inotrope dependent or even tolerant signalling the ultimate phase of the disease. A few will be suitable for cardiac transplantation and will survive until the operation can be carried out.

Although ambulatory therapy with dobutamine using micro-infusion pumps has been found to confer symptomatic improvement in patients awaiting transplantation, survival has been very poor in this group.[78]

Digoxin

The clinical pharmacology of digoxin has been extensively reviewed elsewhere.[79,80]

It must be appreciated that the inotropic effect of digoxin, so clearly demonstrated by the classic studies of McMichael and Sharpey Schafer,[81] is mild. Therefore, it has a role in chronic heart failure secondary to impairment of left ventricular function rather than in acute situations where more important inotropes such as dobutamine are the drugs of choice.

It is not known why only some patients derive long-term benefit from long-term digoxin therapy; in studies in which long-term digoxin therapy has been discontinued, congestive heart failure has recurred in some, but not all patients.[82,83] The nature of the underlying myocardial disease might determine the response to digoxin. The place of digoxin in the management of chronic heart failure is still a matter for debate. In the specific situation of a dilated poorly contracted ventricle, many clinicians are convinced of its short- and medium-term effects even in those patients in sinus rhythm. Atrial fibrillation is a specific indication; in such patients, digoxin should be continued long-term. The value of long-term digoxin-therapy in those patients in sinus rhythm does remain controversial. But, as novel agents continue to be developed for the treatment of heart failure, the results of several studies have shown that when digoxin is properly assessed in well-defined groups of patients it has significant beneficial effects.[84,85]

As the effect of digoxin is dose related, plasma concentrations should be monitored. Therapeutic drug monitoring is valuable and has been successful in several other areas of medicine.[86] Such practice will also help to reduce the possibility of toxicity from excessive plasma levels which might contribute to arrhythmia production.

Workers who favour the use of digoxin might concede that its role is as a supplement to primary treatment with a diuretic and a vasodilator.

It should be remembered that angiotensin converting enzyme inhibitors increase the plasma levels of digoxin.[87] Important drug interactions in the context of heart failure have been well reviewed recently.[88] Perhaps the most important drug interaction is that with diuretics. Long regarded as the standard treatment for congestive heart failure, any patient receiving this combination must be carefully monitored to obviate the development of hypokalaemia which might lead to the development of ventricular arrhythmia.

As will be discussed later (p. 75), the high frequency of asymptomatic ventricular arrhythmias in patients with left ventricular dysfunction is increasingly being recognized.[89,90] Recent studies have shown that the frequency of ventricular arrhythmia may be greater on long-term therapy with digoxin as compared with, for example, an angiotensin converting enzyme inhibitor.[85] Ultimately this may influence the future of long-term digoxin therapy in patients in sinus rhythm, especially if the presence of ventricular arrhythmias is shown conclusively to be an important predictor of subsequent mortality.

In contrast to the normal inotropes, which are more powerful but which tend to increase the heart rate, digoxin has a favourable bradycardic effect.

The peculiarities of digoxin assume a much lower profile when the drug is used properly.

Novel inotropes

Uncertainty about the continued beneficial effects of cardiac glycosides in conjunction with anxiety about their low therapeutic to toxic ratio has stimulated research into alternative inotropic agents. A better understanding of the several mechanisms of myocardial contraction has facilitated the development of several compounds which have differing effects.

Generally, it is believed the mechanism by which these drugs increase the force of myocardial contraction is by increasing the intracellular concentration of calcium, which is free to interact with the contractile proteins. Calcium enters the cell during the plateau phase of the action potential and triggers the release of further calcium from the cisternae of the sarcoplasmic reticulum, which then activates the contractile mechanism.[91] Relaxation occurs when calcium is taken up into the longitudinal part of the sarcoplasmic reticulum. The principal regulator of intracellular calcium kinetics is cyclic adenosine monophosphate, the production of which is stimulated by adenylate cyclase. Any intervention resulting in the stimulation of adenylate cyclase production or an increase in cyclic adenosine monophosphate by any other mechanism, such as inhibition of its degradation by phosphodiesterase, will lead to a greater rate of release of calcium from, and also enhancement of re-uptake into, the sarcoplasmic reticulum. Calcium transport out of the cell by sodium–calcium exchange is also an important part of the overall excitation–contraction, relaxation mechanism.

Beta-adrenoceptor agents

Although it has been claimed that cardiac function improves in patients with heart failure who are receiving either beta-agonists or beta-blockers, this is still an unresolved issue. The apparent success of beta-1-adrenoceptor stimulation in acute heart failure by intravenous agents such as dopamine and dobutamine has encouraged the development of orally active compounds. The chemistry of beta-adrenergic agents has been refined to the extent that, by appropriate substitution at various sites on a basic structure, the properties of the resulting compounds can be determined with considerable flexibility.[92] Thus, they may be cardioselective or non-cardioselective, pure beta-blockers or pure beta-agonists, or possess varying degrees of beta-agonistic and beta-blocking properties. Although it is possible to synthesize orally active pure agonist compounds, none has progressed far in clinical evaluation. However, beta partial agonists, have reached a more advanced stage of clinical evaluation.

Xamoterol (Corwin) Xamoterol is a selective beta-1-partial agonist that has a positive inotropic effect under resting conditions in man which is accompanied by only a slight increase in heart rate.[93] Systolic blood pressure rises, but diastolic blood pressure is unaffected. Although at higher doses in experimental animals, some beta-2-activity can be demonstrated, the compound is 13 times more active on beta-1-receptors. During these experimental studies, it was found that the increase in heart rate was 46% of that maximum produced by isoprenaline although, for equal degrees of chronotropic stimulation, similar increases in left ventricular contractility occurred. In normal subjects, xamoterol reduces maximum exercise-induced tachycardia, although the heart-rate response at lower workloads will be altered in proportion to the degree of sympathetic activity induced by the particular workload.[94] In patients who have left ventricular dysfunction, resting ejection fraction increases, as do the standard invasive indices of contractility, indicating a positive inotropic effect.[95] During exercise, the heart-rate response at low levels of exercise is unaffected, whereas maximum exercise-induced tachycardia is reduced. Presumably, when resting sympathetic activity is high, as in acute severe heart failure, partial agonists might not be advantageous. Similarly, in patients who have chronic impairment of left ventricular function but who may not be in frank heart failure, the beta-antagonistic effect, evident when sympathetic activity is high, such as during exercise, also does not appear to be beneficial. However, in placebo-controlled studies, exercise capacity was increased despite a lower heart rate, indicating that stroke volume must also have increased.[96] It has not been resolved whether this results from improved contraction or better filling, but findings such as these are partly responsible for renewed interest in diastolic dysfunction in heart failure. Double-blind placebo-controlled trials have shown that xamoterol has greater efficacy on exercise capacity and symptoms than digoxin.[97] More extensive trials with xamoterol are awaited with interest but the results of these phase 2 studies have been encouraging.

Ibopamine

Ibopamine is the di-isobutyryl ester of epinine, a naturally occurring catecholamine which has a pharmacological profile similar to that of dopamine. Thus, ibopamine is a pro-drug for epinine and is active after oral administration. In animal studies, it was found to increase cardiac output and reduce peripheral resistance; these haemodynamic effects were also observed in an acute double-blind placebo-controlled study of patients with severe heart failure.[98]

The bipyridines

The bipyridines possess both inotropic and vasodilatory properties, hence the use of the term 'inodilator'. Two compounds, amrinone and milrinone, have been studied in man,[99] both of which are phosphodiesterase inhibitors and increase the cyclic adenosine monophosphate content of cardiac muscle. Their effects are not blocked by alpha- or beta-adrenergic agents, H_1 or H_2 histamine-blocking agents or by inhibitors of prostaglandin synthesis; nor do the bipyridines inhibit Na^+/K^+-ATPase. Amrinone increases calcium uptake by the cells and increases the rate of calcium transport to the contractile proteins. Milrinone has a biphasic effect on canine myocardium suggesting a dual action: it is possible that it increases calcium uptake directly and also indirectly through increased formation of cyclic adenosine monophosphate.

In vascular smooth muscle, increased cyclic adenosine monophosphate causes relaxation so that peripheral vasodilatation may be an integral part of the action of these compounds.

In acute studies of patients who have congestive heart failure, intravenous and oral amrinone increased cardiac index and reduced the pulmonary capillary wedge and right atrial pressures with little change in heart rate or blood pressure. Qualitatively similar effects have been reported with milrinone, which is more potent than amrinone when compared on a weight basis.[100] In long-term open studies of both agents, it has been claimed that the beneficial acute effects persist in chronic dosing, but a recent randomized double-blind placebo-controlled study of amrinone produced less optimistic results.[101] Patients who had responded to oral amrinone with a significant increase in exercise capacity continued on amrinone or were changed to placebo in a double-blind fashion. No differences in a number of subjective and objective variables occurred suggesting that amrinone did not improve cardiac function in the long-term. The results of recent studies with milrinone have been more encouraging in terms of improving patients' symptoms and increasing their effort capacity.[102]

Enoximone

Several other novel inotropic agents are being evaluated in clinical trials. Of these, MDL 17043, enoximone, and its congener, MDL 19025, are imidazole derivatives which are also phosphodiesterase inhibitors.[103,104] Although structurally dissimilar to the bipyridines, their pharmacodynamic effects are similar being both inotropic and vasodilatory. In acute studies, both compounds increased cardiac index and stroke volume, reduced peripheral vascular resistance and caused minor increases in heart rate and minor decreases in blood pressure.

In a double-blind placebo-controlled study of enoximone, symptoms were improved significantly and exercise capacity and resting left ventricular ejection fraction increased in treated patients when compared with those receiving placebo.[105]

The problem that bedevils the use of all inotropes is that the inotropic effect seems inevitably to be accompanied by an increase in ventricular ectopy.[106] Further study of all the new inotropes is necessary to clarify this effect; the onus will be on the advocates of the use of inotropes to show that patient survival is not prejudiced in favour of a short-term improvement in their symptoms. Some workers might argue that in patients whose limitation of effort has imposed a miserable existence the quality and quantity of life should be viewed separately and dispassionately as equal but different goals.

Anti-arrhythmic therapy

Assuming that ventricular function can be preserved, the main factor favouring survival will be ventricular electrical stability. Although there is debate about the precise prevalence of sudden death in patients who have severe ventricular dysfunction, few workers would argue that it is an issue of no importance.[107,108] In several studies sudden or unexpected death has been identified as the most common mode of demise and frequent ventricular arrhythmias were found to be important predictors

of subsequent death (Fig. 5.8).[109] Ventricular arrhythmias are common in these patients and, often, asymptomatic. In patients with heart failure, the therapeutic options are limited by the negatively inotropic effects of most anti-arrhythmic drugs. To what extent this effect can be overcome by adjustment of the antifailure regimen is not clear at present. Amiodarone in the low dose of 200 mg/day has been shown to suppress effectively simple and complex ventricular arrhythmias without having any detectable effects on cardiac function when it is assessed subjectively and objectively.[110] When amiodarone is given in low doses, adverse reactions are few, and in this particular situation the risk to benefit ratio seems favourable. It has yet to be determined whether suppression of ventricular arrhythmia will prolong survival.

Another important question to be addressed is whether implantable defibrillators will be of use in the management of the patient with heart failure secondary to left ventricular dysfunction who has been found to have important ventricular arrhythmia during ambulatory monitoring.

ANTICOAGULANTS

The poorly contracting dilated ventricle may harbour thrombi which are a potential source of serious complications from embolization. Any manifestation of systemic embolization in such

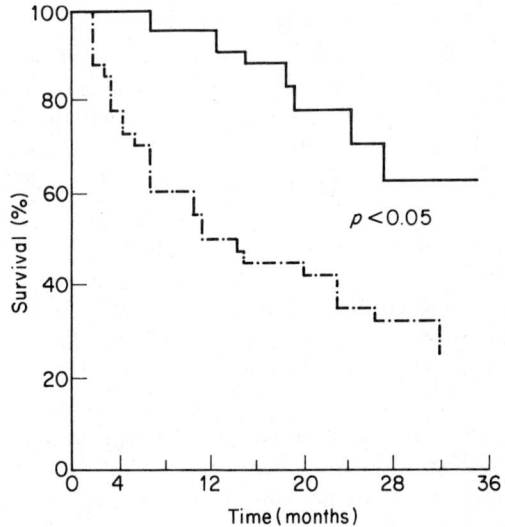

Fig. 5.8. Survival curves for patients with > 720 ventricular ectopic beats/24 h (○) and those with < 720 ventricular ectopic beats/24 h (●). (From Dargie, H.J. *et al*. Relation of arrhythmias and electrolyte abnormalities to survival in patients with severe chronic heart failure. *Circulation* 1987; **IV** (Suppl. 4): 98–107.)

patients is an immediate spur to consider treatment with anticoagulants as is the detection of left ventricular thrombi during echocardiography.

However, routine anticoagulation is not generally practised, but it is advocated in some patients with very dilated ventricles or aneurysm formation especially if atrial fibrillation also complicates their condition.

CONCLUSIONS

In common with many other areas of cardiovascular clinical pharmacology, the treatment of heart failure has entered an exciting period. Non-invasive cardiological investigation has provided information about cardiac function that previously was available only in the haemodynamic laboratory often under somewhat unphysiological conditions. Techniques such as echocardiography and radionuclide ventriculography yield qualitatively different but perhaps more relevant information about ventricular volume, contraction and relaxation, which can be used serially to assess the acute and long-term effects of new therapeutic interventions. Hence, the pre-occupation with acute haemodynamics has lessened and more attention is being given to aspects equally important to the patient's well-being and survival, such as the neuro-endocrine consequences of heart failure and its treatment, the body composition changes with which it is associated, and the frequency of arrhythmias and their relationship to prognosis.

Considerable activity in the pharmaceutical industry is being directed at the production of novel inotropic agents. It remains to be seen whether this is appropriate in the light of previous difficulties in demonstrating long-term efficacy, and of the potential of inotropes for arrhythmogenesis.

Vasodilators have highlighted the possibility of improving cardiac function while also reducing myocardial workload and, although long-term studies with conventional vasodilators have been less rewarding than would have been predicted from the acute effects, there is considerable promise that the beneficial effects of converting enzyme inhibitors will persist in the long-term. It is possible that their salutary effects are not simply due to vasodilatation in the conventional sense of unloading the heart; it is also possible that their important effects on the biochemistry of heart failure and on renal function are the reasons for their success. Further study of the renin inhibitors is awaited with interest; at least,

it should clarify whether the effects of converting enzyme inhibitors are solely related to the reduction in the levels of angiotensin II.

Agents that will simulate the effect or prolong the action of endogenous atrial natriuretic peptide are also being developed. Infusions of atrial natriuretic peptide cause natriuresis and diuresis without stimulating the renin–angiotensin system. If an orally active agent can be found that can produce these effects then further progress will have been made.

Cardiac transplantation is becoming a recognized clinical option for many patients; the scope for this form of management can only continue to expand.

The recognition and treatment of arrhythmias are likely to occupy more attention in the future as new pharmacological and non-pharmacological treatments continue to appear.

Although patients with severe and irreparable myocardial dysfunction cannot be expected to have a normal or near-normal survival after diagnosis, our understanding of the mechanisms involved in the heart failure syndrome and of the mode of action of new and potentially valuable drug treatments promises a brighter future.

The basic aim of treatment, to improve symptoms, has already been achieved; it is now possible to add to this achievement the 'prolongation of useful life'.

REFERENCES

1. Cohn, J.N., Archibald, D.G., Ziesches, et al. Effect of vasodilator therapy on mortality in chronic congestive heart failure N. Engl. J. Med. 1986; 314: 1547.
2. The Consensus Trial Group. Effect of enalapril on mortality in severe congestive heart failure: results of the cooperative North Scandinavian enalapril survival study. N. Engl. J. Med. 1987; 316: 1429.
3. Harris, P. Congestive cardiac failure: central role of the arterial blood pressure. Br. Heart J. 1987; 58: 190.
4. Dargie, H.J., McAlpine, H.M. and Morton, J.J. Neuroendocrine activation in acute myocardial infarction. J. Cardiovasc. Pharmacol. 1987; 9 (Suppl. 2): 21.
5. Burnett, J.C., Kao, P.C., Ju, B.E. et al. Atrial natriuretic peptide elevation in congestive heart failure in the human. Science 1986; 231: 1145.
6. Richards, A.M., Cleland, J.G., Tonolo, G. et al. Atrial natriuretic peptide in heart failure. Br. Med. J. 1986; 293: 409.
7. Riegger, A.J.C., Kramer, A.P. and Kochsiek, K. Human natriuretic peptide: plasma levels, haemodynamics, hormonal and renal effects in patients with severe congestive heart failure. J. Cardiovasc. Pharmacol. 1986; 8: 1107.
8. Crozier, R.G., Nicholls, M.G., Ikram, H., Espiner, E.A., Gomez, H.J. and Warner, J. Haemodynamic effects of atrial peptide infusion in heart failure. Lancet 1986; ii: 1242.
9. Tobinick, E., Schelbert, H.R., Henning, H. et al. Right ventricular ejection fraction in patients with acute anterior

and inferior myocardial infarction assessed by radionuclide angiography. *Circulation* 1978; 57: 1078.

10. Swan, H.J.C., Janz, W., Forrester, J.S., Marcus, H., Diamond, G. and Shonette, D. Catheterization of the heart in man with the use of a flow directed balloon tipped catheter. *N. Engl. J. Med.* 1970; **283**: 447.
11. Franciosa, J.A., Guiha, N.M., Limas, C.J., Rodriguera, E. and Cohn, J.N. Improved LV function during nitroprusside infusion in acute myocardial infarction. *Lancet* 1972; i: 650.
12. Rabinowitz, B., Timari, I., Elazar, E. and Neufeld, H.N. Intravenous isosorbide dinitrate in patients with refractory pump failure and acute myocardial infarction. *Circulation* 1982; **65**: 771.
13. Gillespie, J.A., Ambros, H.D., Sobel, B.E. and Roberts, R. Effects of dobutamine in acute myocardial infarction. *Am. J. Cardiol.* 1977; **39**: 588.
14. Lipkin, D.P., Fremeaux, M. and Maseri, A. Beneficial effect of captopril in cardiogenic shock. *Lancet* 1987; 2: 327.
15. McAlpine, H.M., Morton, J.G., Leckie, B. and Dargie, H.J. Haemodynamic effects of captopril in acute left ventricular failure complicated myocardial infarction. *J. Cardiovasc. Pharmacol.* 1987; 9 (Suppl. 2): 525.
16. Meigler, F.L. An 'account' of digitalis in atrial fibrillation. *J. Am. Coll. Cardiol.* 1985; 560A.
17. Cowan, J.C., Gardiner, P., Reid, D.S., et al. A comparison of amiodarone and digoxin in the treatment of atrial fibrillation, complicating acute myocardial infarction. *J. Cardiovasc. Pharmacol.* 1986; 8: 252.
18. Dargie, H.J. New therapeutic strategies in the management of heart failure in advanced medicine. In Brown, M.J., ed. Churchill Livingstone, Edinburgh and London 1986; 243.
19. Hamilton, A., Naccarelli, G.V., Gray, A.L. et al. Congestive heart failure with normal systolic function. *Am. J. Cardiol.* 1984; 54: 778.
20. Soufer, R., Wohltelerenter, D. and Vita, N.A. Intact systolic left ventricular function in clinical congestive heart failure. *Am. J. Cardiol.* 1985; 55: 1032.
21. Stewart, S., Mason, D.T. and Braunwald, D.E. Impaired rate of left ventricular filling in idiopathic hypertrophic subaortic stenosis and valvular aortic stenosis. *Circulation* 1968; 38: 8.
22. Topol, E.J., Traill, T.A. and Fortuin, N.J. Hypertensive hypertrophic cardiomyopathy in the elderly. *N. Engl. J. Med.* 1985; 312: 277–83.
23. Kumada, T., Karliner, J.S., Poulerur, H. et al. Effects of coronary occlusion on early ventricular diastolic events in unconscious dogs. *Am. J. Physiol.* 1979; 257: H542.
24. Waagstein, F., Hjalmarson, A., Varnauskas, E. and Wallentin, I. Effect of chronic beta adrenergic receptor blockade in congestive cardiomyopathy. *Br. Heart J.* 1975; 37: 1022.
25. Betocchi, S., Cannon, R.O., Watson, R.M. et al. Effect of sublingual nifedipine on hemodynamics and systolic and diastolic function in patients with hypertrophic cardiomyopathy. *Circulation* 1985; 72: 1001.
26. Bonow, R.O., Dilsizian, V., Rosing, D.R. et al. Verapamil induced improvement in left ventricular diastolic filling and increased exercise tolerance in patients with hypertrophic cardiomyopathy: short and long term effects. *Circulation* 1985; 72: 853.
27. Suwa, N., Hirota, Y. and Kalamura, K. Improvement in LV diastolic function during intravenous and oral diltiazem therapy in patients with hypertrophic obstructive cardiomyopathy: an echocardiographic study. *Am. J. Cardiol.* 1984; 54: 1047.
28. Richardson, A., Bayliss, J., Soriven, A.J., Parameshwar, J., Poole-Wilson, P.A. and Sutton, G.C. Double blind comparison of captopril alone against frusemide plus amiloride in mild heart failure. *Lancet* 1987; ii: 709–11.
29. Daly, K., Richardson, P.J., Olsen, E.G. et al. Acute myocarditis. Role of histological and virological examination in the diagnosis and assessment of immuno suppressive treatment. *Br. Heart J.* 1984; 51: 30.
30. Ishikawa, T., Condoh, H., Nakagawa, S., Koiwaya, Y. and Tanaka, K. Steroid therapy in cardiac sarcoidosis: increased left ventricular contractility concomitant with electrocardiographic improvement after prednisilone. *Chest* 1984; 85: 445.
31. Julian, D.G. The practical implications of the coronary artery surgery trials. *Br. Heart J.* 1985; 54: 343.
32. Lant, A. Diuretics; clinical pharmacology and therapeutic use (part 1). *Drugs* 1985; 29: 57.
33. Kokko, J.P. Site and mechanism of action of diuretics. *Am. J. Med.* 1984; 77: 11.
34. Dargie, H.J., Allison, M.E.M., Kennedy, A.C. and Gray, M.J.B. High dose metolazone in chronic renal failure. *Br. Med. J.* 1972; 4: 196.
35. Marone, C., Muggli, F., Lahn, W. and Frey, F.J. Pharmacokinetic and pharmacodynamic interaction between furosemide and metolazone in man. *Eur. J. Clin. Invest.* 1985; 15: 253.
36. Arnold, W.C. Efficacy of metolazone and furosemide in children with furosemide resistant oedema. *Pediatrics* 1984; 74: 872.
37. Davies, D.L. and Wilson, G.M. Diuretics: mechanism of action and clinical application. *Drugs* 1975; 9: 178–226.
38. Dargie, H.J. and Dollery, C.T. Adverse reactions to diuretics in Muiler's side effects of drugs. In: Dukes, M.N.G., ed. Amsterdam: Exerpta Medica, 1975, p. 483.
39. Lee, W.H. and Packer, M. Prognostic importance of serum sodium concentration and its modification by converting enzyme inhibition in patients with severe chronic heart failure. *Circulation* 1986; 73: 257.
40. Cleland, J.G.F., Dargie, H.J. and Ford, I. Mortality in heart failure: clinical variables of prognostic value. *Br. Heart J.* 1987; 58: 572–82.
41. Szatalowicz, B.L., Arnold, P.E., Chaimobitz, C., Bichet, D., Bart, T. and Schrier, R.W. Radioimmunassay of plasma arginine vasopressin in hyponatraemic patients with congestive heart failure. *N. Engl. J. Med.* 1981; 305: 263.
42. Goldsmith, S.R., Francis, G.S. and Cowley, A.W. Arginine vasopressin and the renal response to water loading in congestive heart failure. *Am. J. Cardiol.* 1986; 58: 295.
43. Schaer, G.L., Cobit, A.B., Laragh, J.H. and Cody, R.J. Association of hyponatraemia with increased renin activity in chronic congestive heart failure. Impact of diuretic therapy. *Am. J. Cardiol.* 1983; 51: 1635.
44. Lawson, D.H., Boddy, K., Gray, M.J.B., Mahaffey, M. and Mills, E. Potassium supplements in patients receiving longterm diuretics for oedema. *Q. J. Med.* 1986; 45: 469.
45. Morgan, D.B., Burkinshaw, L. and Davidson, C. Potassium depletion in heart failure and its relation to longterm treatment with diuretics: a review of the literature. *Postgrad. Med. J.* 1978; 54: 72.
46. Dargie, H.J., Boddy, K., Kennedy, A.C., King, P.C., Read, P.R. and Ward, D.M. Total body potassium on longterm frusemide therapy: is potassium supplementation necessary? *Br. Med. J.* 1974; 4: 316.
47. Cleland, J.G.F., Dargie, H.J., Robertson, I., Robertson, J.I.S. and East, B.W. Total body electrolyte composition in patients with heart failure: a comparison with normal subjects and patients with untreated hypertension. (Submitted for publication.)
48. Cleland, J.G.F., Dargie, H.J., Hodsman, G.P. et al. Captopril in heart failure: a double blind controlled trial. *Br. Heart J.* 1984; 52: 530.
49. Sonnenblick, E.H., Ross, J. Jr and Braunwald, E. Oxygen

consumption of the heart: new concepts of its multifactorial determination. *Am. J. Cardiol.* 1968; **22**: 328.

50. Schwartz, A.B. and Chatterjee, K. Vasodilator therapy in chronic congestive heart failure. *Drugs* 1983; **26**: 148.

51. Parmley, W.W. Pathophysiology of congestive heart failure. *Am. J. Cardiol.* 1985; **55**: 9A.

52. McCall, D. and O'Rourke, R.A. Congestive heart failure 1. Biochemistry, pathophysiology and neurohumeral mechanisms. *Mod. Conc. Cardiovasc. Dis.* 1985; **54**: 55.

53. Opie, L.H., Chatterjee, K. and Harrison, D.C. Vasodilating drugs. In: Opie, L.H., ed. *Drugs for the heart*. New York: Grune and Stratton, 1987, p. 131.

54. Dollery, C.T. and Corr, L. Drug treatment of heart failure. *Br. Heart J.* 1985; **29**: 57.

55. Chatterjee, K., Ports, T.A., Arnold, S. *et al.* Comparisons of haemodynamic effects of oral hydralazine and prazosin hydrochloride in patients with chronic congestive heart failure. *Br. Heart J.* 1979; **42**: 657.

56. Franciosa, J., Weber, K.T., Levine, T.B. *et al.* Hydralazine in the longterm treatment of chronic heart failure: lack of difference from placebo. *Am. Heart J.* 1982; **104**: 587.

57. Colucci, W.S., Williams, G. and Braunwald, E. Increased plasma norepinephrine during prazosin treatment for severe congestive heart failure. *Ann. Intern. Med.* 1980; **93**: 452.

58. Bayliss, J., Norell, M., Canepa-Ansen, R. *et al.* Neuroendocrine and haemodynamic interaction during exercise in chronic heart failure: double blind comparison of captopril and prazosin. *Br. Heart J.* 1985.

59. Franciosa, J.A. and Cohn, J.N. Sustained hemodynamic effects without tolerance during longterm isosorbide dinitrate treatment of chronic left ventricular failure. *Am. J. Cardiol.* 1980; **45**: 648.

60. Cohn, J.N. Nitrates for congestive heart failure. *Am. J. Cardiol.* 1985; **56**: 19A.

61. Jordan, R.A., Seth, L., Casebolt, P., Hayes, M.J., Wilen, M.M. and Franciosa, J. Rapidly developing tolerance to transdermal nitroglycerine in congestive heart failure. *Ann. Intern. Med.* 1986; **295**: 1–4.

62. Quyyumi, A.A., Wagstaff, D. and Evans, T.R. Acute haemodynamic effects of endralasine: a new vasodilator for chronic refractory congestive heart failure. *Am. J. Cardiol.* 1983; **51**: 1353.

63. Emanuelsson, H., Hjalmarson, A., Holmberg, S. and Waagstein, F. Acute haemodynamic effects of felodipine in congestive heart failure. *Eur. J. Clin. Pharmacol.* 1985; **28**: 489.

64. Haber, E. Renin inhibitors. *N. Engl. J. Med.* 1984; **311**: 1631.

65. Creager, M.A. Halperin, J.L., Bernard, D.B. *et al.* Acute regional circulatory and renal haemodynamic effects of converting enzyme inhibition in patients with congestive heart failure. *Circulation* 1981; **64**: 483.

66. Hadd, J.E., Deighton, A.C., Jackson, T.E. *et al.* Control of glomerular filtration rate by the renin angiotensin system. *Am. J. Physiol.* 1977; 366.

67. Cleland, J.G.F., Dargie, H.J., Hodsman, G.P. *et al.* Effects of enalapril in heart failure: a double blind study of effects on exercise performance, renal function, hormones and metabolic state. *Br. Heart J.* 1985; **54**: 305.

68. Ertl, G., Kloner, R.A., Alexander, R.W. and Braunwald, E. Limitation of experimental infarct size by an angiotensin-converting enzyme inhibitor. *Circulation* 1982; **65**: 40–8.

69. Cleland, J.G.F., Dargie, H.J., Semple, P.F. *et al.* Angiotensin II levels haemodynamics and sympathoadrenal function after low dose captopril in heart failure. *Am. J. Med.* 1984; **77**: 880.

70. Cleland, J.G.F., Dargie, H.J., McAlpine, H.M. *et al.* Severe hypotension after first dose of enalapril in heart failure. *Br. Med. J.* 1985; **291**: 1309.

71. Edwards, C.R.W. and Padfield, P.L. Angiotensin converting enzyme inhibitors: past, present and bright future. *Lancet* 1985; i: 30.

72. Semple, P.F. and Herd, G.W. Cough and wheeze caused by inhibitors of angiotensin converting enzyme. *N. Engl. J. Med.* 1986; **314**: 61.

73. Fleckenstein, A. Specific inhibitors in promoters of calcium action in the excitation contraction coupling of heart muscle and their role in the prevention or production of myocardial lesions. In: Harris, P. and Opie, L., eds. *Calcium and the Heart*. London and New York: Academic Press, 1970, p. 135.

74. Fleckenstein, A. Specific pharmacology of calcium in myocardium, cardiac pacemakers and vascular smooth muscle. *Ann. Ref. Pharmacol. Toxicol.* 1977; **17**: 149.

75. Elkayam, U., Waber, L., Torkin, B. *et al.* Acute haemodynamic effect of oral nifedipine in severe chronic congestive heart failure. *Am. J. Cardiol.* 1983; **53**: 1041.

76. Timmis, A.D. and Jewitt, D.E. Studies with felodipine in congestive heart failure. *Drugs* 1985; **29** (Suppl. 2): 66.

77. Francis, G.S., Sharma, B. and Hodges, M. *Am. Heart J.* 1983; **103**: 995.

78. Hodgson, J.M., Aja, M. and Sorkin, R.P. Intermittent ambulatory dobutamine infusions for patients awaiting cardiac transplantation. *Am. J. Cardiol.* 1984; **53**: 375.

79. Smith, T.W. and Haber, E. Digitalis. *N. Engl. J. Med.* 1973; **289**: 945–52; 1010–5; 1063–72; 1125–9.

80. Marsh, J.D. and Smith, T.W. Clinical use of cardiac glycoside in congestive heart failure. In: Smith, T.W., ed. *Digitalis Glycozides*. Orlando: Grune and Stratton, 1985, p. 83.

81. McMichael, J. and Sharpey-Schafer, E.P. *Q. J. Med.* 1944; **53**: 123.

82. Dal, G.L.C. *Br. Med. J.* 1972; 705.

83. Lee, D.C., Johnson, R.A., Bingham, J.B. *et al.* Heart failure in out patients: A randomized trial of digoxin versus placebo. *N. Engl. J. Med.* 1982; **306**: 699.

84. Di Banco, R., Shabetai, R., Kostuk, W., Moran, J., Schlant, R.C. and Wright, R. A comparison of oral milrinone, digoxin, and their combination in the treatment of patients with chronic heart failure. *N. Engl. J. Med.* 1989; **320**: 677–83.

85. The Captopril–Digoxin Multicenter Research Group. Comparative effects of therapy with Captopril and Digoxin in patients with mild to moderate heart failure. *JAMA* 1988; **259**: 539–44.

86. Duhme, D.W., Greenblatt, D.J. and Coch-Waser, J. Reduction of digoxin toxicity associated with measurement of serum levels. *Ann. Intern. Med.* 1974; **80**: 516.

87. Cleland, J.G.F., Dargie, H.J., Pettigrew, A., Gillen, G. and Robertson, J.L.S. The effects of captopril on serum digoxin and urinary urea and digoxin clearances in patients with chronic heart failure. *Am. Heart J.* 1986; **112**: 130–5.

88. Marcus, F.I. Pharmacokinetic interactions between digoxin and other drugs. *J. Am. Coll. Cardiol.* 1985; **5**: 82.

89. Meinertz, T., Hoffman, T., Casper, W. *et al.* The significance of ventricular arrhythmias in idiopathic dilated cardiomyopathy. *Am. J. Cardiol.* 1984; **53**: 902.

90. Unverfert, D.V., Majorian, R.D., Moeschberger, M.L., Baker, P.P. and Fetters, J.K. Factors influencing the one year mortality of dilated cardiomyopathy. *Am. J. Cardiol.* 1984; **54**: 147.

91. Blinks, J.R. Intracellular calcium measurements. In: Fozzard, D.H.A. Haber, E., Jennings, R.B., Katz, A.M. and Morgan, H.E. eds. *The Heart and Cardiovascular System*. New York: Raven Press, 1986, p. 671.

92. Main, B.G. Structure activity relation of beta adrenergic agents. *J. Chem. Tech. Biotech. Knowl.* 1982; **32**: 617.

93. Nuttall, A. and Snow, H.N. Cardiovascular effects of ICI 118 587, a beta I adrenoceptor partial agonist. *Br. J.*

Pharmacol. 1982; 77: 381.

94. Jennings, G., Bobik, A., Oddie, C. and Restall, R. Cardio selectivity kinetics, haemodynamics and metabolic effects of xamoterol. *Clin. Pharmacol. Ther.* 1984; 35: 594.

95. Rousseau, M.F., Pouleur, H. and Vincent, M.F. Effects of a cardioselective beta 1 partial agonist (Corwin) on left ventricular function and myocardial metabolism in patients with previous myocardial infarction. *Am. J. Cardiol.* 1983; 51: 1268.

96. Saltissi, S. *et al.* The effects of xamoterol (Corwin) on exercise tolerance and heart rate in patients with heart failure secondary to ischaemic heart disease. *Circulation* 1985; 72.

97. The German and Austrian Xamoterol Study Group. Double blind placebo controlled comparison of digoxin and xamoterol in chronic heart failure. *Lancet* 1988; i: 489–93.

98. Mengeot, P., Piette, S. and Mirgaux, M. Double blind haemodynamic study of a new dopamine derivative orally active in chronic congestive heart failure. *G. Ital. Cardiol.* 1981; 11: 1738.

99. Farah, A.E. and Alousi, A.A. New cardiotonic agents: a search for digitalis substitute. *Life Sci.* 1978; 22: 1139.

100. Benotti, J.R., Lesko, L.J., McCue, J.E. *et al.* Pharmacokinetics and pharmacodynamics of milrinone in chronic congestive heart failure. *Am. J. Cardiol.* 1985; 56: 685.

101. DiBianco, R., Shabetai, R. and Silverman, B.D. Oral amrinone for the treatment of chronic congestive heart failure: results of a multicentre randomised double blind and placebo controlled withdrawal study. *J. Am. Coll. Cardiol.* 1984; 4: 855.

102. Le Jemtel, T.H., Gumbardo, D., Chadwick, B., Rutman, H.I. and Sonnenblick, E.H. Milrinone for longterm therapy of severe heart failure: clinical experience with special reference to maximal exercise tolerance. *Circulation* 1986; 73 (Suppl. 3): 213.

103. Kereiakes, D. and Chatterjee, K. Intravenous and oral MDL 17043 (a new inotrope–vasodilator agent) in congestive heart failure; haemodynamic and clinical evaluation of 38 patients. *J. Am. Coll. Cardiol.* 1984; 4: 884.

104. Petain, M., Garberg, V., Carlyle, P. *et al.* Acute haemodynamic and neurohumeral effects of MDL 19205, a new inotropic agent in congestive heart failure. *J. Am. Coll. Cardiol.* 1983; 1675.

105. Choraria, S.K., Taylor, D. and Pilcher, J. Double blind crossover comparison of enoximone and placebo in patients with congestive heart failure. *Circulation* 1987; 76(6): 1307–11.

106. Holmes, J.R., Kubo, S.H., Cody, R.J. *et al.* Milrinone in congestive heart failure: observations on ambulatory ventricular arrhythmias. *Am. Heart J.* 1985; 110: 800.

107. Packer, M. Sudden unexpected death in patients with congestive heart failure: a second frontier. *Circulation* 1985; 72: 681.

108. Schultz, E.R.A. Jr., Strauss, H.W. and Pitt, B. Sudden death in the year following myocardial infarction: relation to ventricular premature contractions in the late hospital phase and left ventricular ejection fraction. *Am. J. Med.* 1977; 62: 192.

109. Cleland, J.G.F., Dargie, H.J., Ford, I. *et al.* Prognostic variables in heart failure. *Br. Heart J.* 1987.

110. Cleland, J.G.F., Dargie, H.J., Findlay, L.N. and Wilson, J.T. Clinical haemodynamic and antiarrhythmic effects of longterm treatment with amiodarone in patients with heart failure. *Br. Heart J.* 1987; 57: 436.

Chapter 6

Heart and Heart–Lung Transplantation

Christopher G.A. McGregor

CARDIAC TRANSPLANTATION

INTRODUCTION

It is now over twenty years since the first human cardiac transplant was performed by Barnard in December 1967 in Cape Town[1] and the first adult cardiac transplant in the USA by Shumway in January 1968. During this period, cardiac transplantation has evolved from a highly experimental procedure with a poor outcome to an accepted, validated form of surgical therapy for terminal heart disease with predictably good results in terms of patient survival and rehabilitation. This evolution has originated largely from surgical empiricism rather than from fundamental developments in immunology. Much credit is due to the group of workers at Stanford University, led by Dr Norman Shumway, who have pioneered several major advances in cardiac transplantation that have contributed significantly to the currently successful results.

These advances include the application of the endomyocardial biopsy technique[2] and the use of antithymocyte globulin[3] for the treatment of rejec-tion in the mid 1970s, and the introduction of cyclosporine for immunosuppression[4] in 1980. More gradual refinements have also occurred in recipient and donor selection, infectious disease management and improved organ preservation, resulting in increased survival, reduced morbidity and the concomitant reduction of hospital stay and cost.

The improvement in one-year survival at Stanford is illustrated in Fig. 6.1; this led to the widespread international application of cardiac transplantation in the 1980s (Fig. 6.2) such that the number of heart transplants performed in the UK and worldwide has risen from 3 and 62 in 1979 to 176 and 1415, respectively, in 1986. The groups at Stanford and Cape Town have recently reviewed their 20 years of experience with heart transplantation.[5,6]

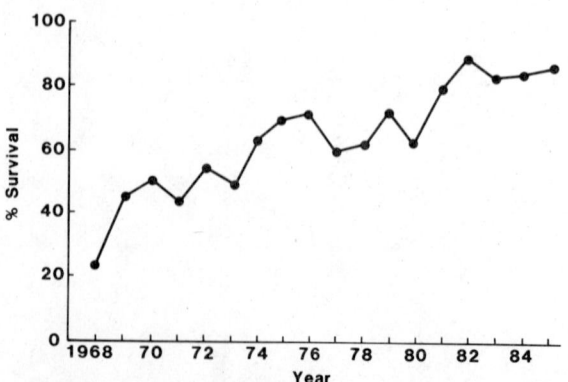

Fig. 6.1. Diagram illustrating the improvement in one-year survival following heart transplantation performed at Stanford University.

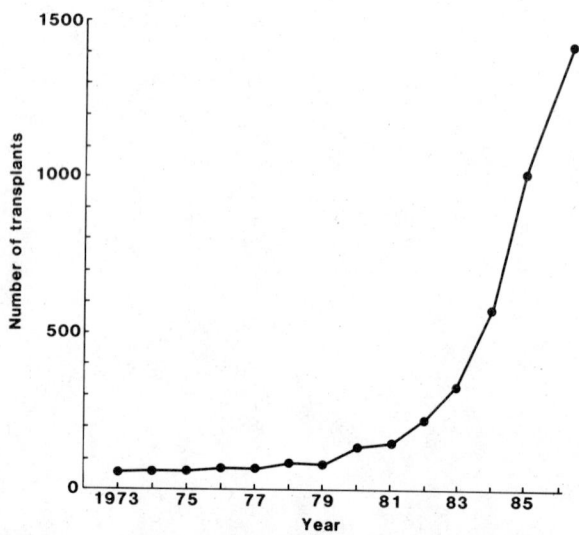

Fig. 6.2. Diagram illustrating the increase in the number of heart transplants performed worldwide during the 1980s. Data are taken from the Registry of the International Society for Heart Transplantation Fourth Official Report.

INDICATIONS FOR CARDIAC TRANSPLANTATION

The principal indication for cardiac transplantation is end-stage cardiac disease which is not amenable to more conventional medical or surgical therapy. Most patients will have New York Heart Association class III or IV symptoms of heart failure. The majority of patients suffer from either congestive cardiomyopathy or terminal ischaemic heart disease. Other less common indications include valvular or congenital heart disease, myocarditis unresponsive to therapy, cardiac tumour and other rarer entities.

Endomyocardial biopsy is indicated as part of transplant assessment to exclude the possibility of potentially controllable conditions, such as myocarditis or cardiac sarcoidosis.

Coronary artery bypass grafting, although a high-risk procedure, should be considered in some patients, especially in the presence of angina pectoris, even if the ejection fraction is low (< 25%). However, the results of mitral valve replacement for mitral regurgitation in the setting of cardiomyopathy have been disappointing.

The optimal timing of transplantation can be problematic, as the prognosis of end-stage cardiac disease is, at times, uncertain. Symptomatology, although important, is inadequate as the sole indicator of timing for transplantation. Stevenson has recently demonstrated a one-year survival of only 46% in 28 patients with known non-ischaemic dilated cardiomyopathy who were denied cardiac transplantation on the basis of lack of symptoms.[7] Low stroke volume or a history of ventricular arrhythmias were predictors of a poor outcome in this series.

Any condition that would limit patient prognosis or the likelihood of successful rehabilitation can be

Table 6.1. Possible contra-indications to cardiac transplantation.

Fixed elevated pulmonary vascular resistance (> 6 Wood units)
Serious irreversible organ disease, e.g. cirrhosis, emphysema, malignant neoplasm
Serious systemic diseases, e.g. peripheral vascular disease, collagen vascular disease
Severe hepatic or renal dysfunction (creatinine clearance < 30 ml/min)
Active infection
'Unstable' diabetes mellitus
Recent pulmonary infarction
Morbid obesity
Age > 60 years
History of alcohol or drug abuse
History of medical non-compliance

regarded as a possible contra-indication to transplantation (see Table 6.1). The introduction of cyclosporine has allowed some relaxation of selection criteria so that patients with 'stable' diabetes mellitus, recent pulmonary infarction (less than six weeks) or recently controlled infections can now be considered as heart transplant candidates. The upper age limit, formerly 50 years, has now been extended to 60 years, and paediatric cardiac transplantation has been successfully introduced. Irreversible pulmonary vascular hypertension remains a contra-indication to orthotopic cardiac transplantation, but the level of pulmonary vascular resistance above which it is unsafe to perform cardiac transplantation is unclear and will vary from patient to patient. Pulmonary vasodilator therapy should be employed at the time of cardiac catheterization in an attempt to assess reversibility of elevated pulmonary vascular resistance. In patients with long-standing heart failure, the presence of a significantly elevated pulmonary artery pressure with concomitant low cardiac output that does not respond to vasodilator therapy may preclude safe orthotopic cardiac transplantation.

The number of patients who would benefit from cardiac transplantation has been estimated at between 450 and 900 per annum in the UK, assuming more stringent selection criteria than are currently applicable.[8,9] These figures are probably a considerable underestimate; indeed, in the US, a working group in mechanical circulatory support reported to the National Institutes of Health that 15 000–35 000 patients per annum in the USA could be medically eligible for permanent circulatory support.[10]

DONOR SELECTION AND MANAGEMENT

The sera of potential cardiac transplant recipients are tested for cytotoxicity against a random panel of donor lymphocytes from around 50 patients who represent the major histocompatibility antigens in the community. If significant cytotoxicity is demonstrated, a prospective pre-operative cross-match is required between the specific donor and recipient.

The cardiac donor should have been pronounced 'brain dead' according to the relevant criteria, which in the UK have been designated by the Conference of the Medical Royal Colleges.[11] The cardiac donor and recipient are matched for ABO blood group compatibility, and donor weight should be within 20% of that of the intended recipient. Rhesus compatibility is not considered essential. In recipients with an elevated pulmonary vascular resistance, the use of a larger donor is indicated. Tissue-typing is performed retrospectively only, although it appears that close HLA matching is associated with improved long-term survival.[12] Logistically, it is not possible to match cardiac transplant patients for HLA prospectively. The upper limit for donor organ ischaemic time is around 4 h allowing travel distances of approximately 1000 miles using air transport. As travel time is a major part of the total ischaemic time, close co-ordination is required between the donor and recipient teams. Cardiac donors should be less than 35 years of age if male and less than 40 years of age if female with no history of heart disease. The use of older donors increases the risk of transplanting hearts which have undiagnosed coronary artery disease thus increasing the risk of the procedure. Donors should have no systemic infection, although many will have purulent sputum and lung infiltrates. Long periods of external cardiac massage or severe hypotension (systemic blood pressure < 60 mmHg) are contra-indications to cardiac donation. Brain death may result in severe cardiovascular changes and so careful clinical examination of potential donors is required with examination of the chest radiograph, electrocardiogram and, if necessary, cardiac enzymes and iso-enzymes and the echocardiogram. Central venous pressure measurement is helpful as a guide to fluid replacement for the optimization of cardiac output. If significant inotropic therapy is required in the presence of an adequate cardiac filling pressure in a non-vasodilated patient, the heart is not suitable for donation. Intermittent vasopressin administration may be required for control of diabetes insipidus and insulin therapy for control of hyperglycaemia. A heating blanket may be needed to maintain normothermia. Multi-organ donation is increasingly common with simultaneous removal of the heart, liver, kidneys and corneas.

Donor availability is likely to remain the principal limiting factor to the expansion of cardiac transplantation, both in the UK and the US.[13] There is clearly a discrepancy between the number of cardiac transplants needed and the number of organs available for donation. Up to one-third of patients on waiting lists in the UK have died while waiting for a suitable organ to become available.[14] In these circumstances, the use of an older donor or temporization with ventricular assist devices or artificial hearts may be an acceptable compromise.

SURGICAL TECHNIQUES

The cardiac donor operation does not require cardiopulmonary bypass and can be performed easily in any standard operating room. After systemic heparinization and cold cardioplegic arrest, the heart is excised and placed in cold saline or cardioplegic solution at 4°C for storage and transportation in a standard insulated container.[14]

Orthotopic cardiac transplantation is the technique of choice in most transplant centres and differs little from the original description by Lower and Shumway in 1960.[15] One additional modification introduced is that the right atriotomy incision is curved away from the donor sino-atrial node to avoid injury to that structure allowing for normal sinus rhythm in the transplanted heart. After the initiation of cardiopulmonary bypass, the recipient's own heart is excised at mid-atrial level leaving cuffs of right and left atrium with intervening interatrial septum. The aorta and pulmonary artery are divided at valvar levels. After preparation of the donor heart, the anastomoses are performed in the following order: left atrium, right atrium, aorta and pulmonary artery.

Heterotopic cardiac transplantation (piggy-back operation) is performed less frequently and probably should be reserved for circumstances in which the donor is of significantly smaller size than the recipient and where the donor heart could not be reasonably expected to maintain the recipient circulation. The operative technique has been described in detail elsewhere.[16] Advocates of this technique cite its usefulness in the presence of an elevated pulmonary vascular resistance, but this application remains to be adequately demonstrated. The ability of the recipient's own heart in rare circumstances to maintain the circulation at the time of severe donor heart rejection is another quoted advantage of the technique. The disadvantages of the method, however, are considerable and include thrombo-embolic complications from the poorly contractile remaining recipient heart, the need for anticoagulation, difficulty in performing endomyocardial biopsies, persistent angina in some patients and the danger of infection in the prosthetic graft material used to anastomose the donor and recipient pulmonary arteries.

POST-OPERATIVE MANAGEMENT

Circulatory management of cardiac transplant recipients is similar to that of general cardiac surgical patients apart from the need for an infusion of isoprenaline for 2–4 days post-operatively to act as a chonotropic agent and as a pulmonary vasodilator. Patients are generally reverse barrier-nursed in a single cubicle in the intensive care unit for up to one week. Early extubation and ambulation are encouraged. The average hospital stay is now around three weeks. Re-introduction of reverse barrier-nursing is indicated during periods of augmented immunosuppression, i.e. during treatment for severe rejection or when the white blood cell count is less than 3000/mm^3.

IMMUNOSUPPRESSION

Immunosuppressive methods have evolved over the last twenty years based on the empirical application by surgeons of different drugs and drug combinations. The introduction of cyclosporine for immunosuppression following cardiac transplantation in 1980 was a major landmark and although this drug remains the basis of nearly all immunosuppressive protocols, there is no agreement as to its optimal utilization. In recent years, there has been a clear trend to multiple drug therapy using lower doses of each drug in an attempt to minimize the side-effects of each. Prior to cyclosporine, 'conventional' therapy was employed consisting of azathioprine, corticosteroids and antithymocyte globulin (rabbit or equine) in high doses. Since the advent of cyclosporine, many drug protocols have been used and most current regimes consist of cyclosporine, azathioprine and corticosteroids, all in lower doses, sometimes supplemented by prophylactic antithymocyte globulin in the early post-operative period. The evolution of immunosuppressive therapy given at Stanford, based on the statistical analysis of defined patient groups, has been described by Oyer.[17]

More recently, OKT3 murine monoclonal antibody treatment has been introduced, and early experience with this agent used prophylactically after cardiac transplantation at the Universities of Utah[18] and Stanford has been very encouraging and may prove to be the most significant advance in immunosuppression since the introduction of cyclosporine. The level of immunosuppression needs to be greatest early after transplantation when the propensity to rejection is greatest, but, although the likelihood of rejection decreases with time, patients need to be on maintenance immunosuppressive therapy for life.

REJECTION

Prior to the introduction of cyclosporine, cardiac rejection could be detected by reduction in summated electrocardiographic voltages, the development of atrial dysrhythmias or the appearance of a gallop rhythm. Cardiac rejection associated with cyclosporine, however, cannot be detected reliably, clinically, and histological examination of endomyocardial biopsy specimens remains the 'gold standard' for the diagnosis of cardiac rejection. This technique, pioneered by Caves,[2] is performed under local anaesthesia using a percutaneous Seldinger technique under fluoroscopic control; it takes about 20 min. Three to five biopsies are taken, and the procedure can be performed on outpatients. Biopsies are performed each week for six weeks, every two weeks for a further six weeks, one each month for three months, and then every three months for life. There has been no mortality from over 5000 endomyocardial biopsies in the Stanford series (Billingham M.E., personal communication). Biopsies are graded according to severity with only moderate and severe changes considered to require augmented immunosuppression. The presence of a mild infiltrate alone is not an indication for additional therapy.

Much effort has been expended in searching for a reliable non-invasive method for the diagnosis of cardiac rejection, but nuclear medical techniques, echocardiography, cyto-immunological monitoring, nuclear magnetic resonance and more sophisticated electrocardiographic analysis have not yet proven to be of sufficient value to allow the discontinuation of cardiac biopsy.

MANAGEMENT OF INFECTION

Infection and rejection remain the two major causes of death following cardiac transplantation. The relative preponderance of one cause over another will reflect the balance of the immunosuppressive protocol used. If a particular immunosuppressive protocol tends to 'over' immunosuppression, the majority of deaths are likely to be due to infection rather than rejection; with 'under' immunosuppression, the reverse is true. It is interesting that the incidence of infection remains the same in patients treated with cyclosporine when compared with those treated in the pre-cyclosporine era, but the likelihood of a fatal outcome is much less. The majority of bacteriological infections occur in the lung, urinary tract and bloodstream, and, as with most immunosuppressed patients, the type of organism is highly variable.

Peri-operative prophylactic antibiotics are given until the intravenous lines and catheters are removed. In the presence of infection, 'blind' antibiotic therapy is contra-indicated unless life-threatening undiagnosed infection exists. Great efforts are put into the rapid investigation of any potential infection including the early use of invasive techniques, such as transthoracic needle biopsy and fibre-optic bronchoscopy for the diagnosis of pulmonary infection.

RESULTS OF CARDIAC TRANSPLANTATION

Actuarial survival (Cutler—Ederer life table method) for cardiac transplant recipients over three time-frames since the beginning of the clinical programme at Stanford are show in Fig. 6.3.

The calculated one- and five-year survival rates for patients receiving cyclosporine as the primary immunosuppressant (more than 100 patients beginning in December 1980) are 83% and 60%, respectively. The improvement in results of approximately 20% among patients in this most recent time-frame and those transplanted between January 1974 and December 1980 (99 patients) can largely be attributed to the introduction of cyclosporine. The improvement in results, again of approximately 20%, among patients transplanted between January 1974 and December 1980 (99 patients) and those receiving transplants between January 1968 and December 1973 (100 patients) is largely due to the application of the endomyocar-

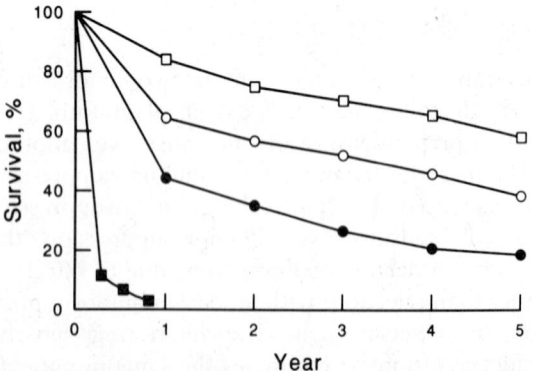

Fig. 6.3. Diagram illustrating the actuarial survival (Cutler–Ederer life table method) of cardiac transplant recipients operated upon at Stanford University over three time-frames. □, from December 1980 onwards; ○, from January 1974 to December 1980; ●, from January 1968 to December 1973; ■, not transplanted.

dial biopsy technique and the introduction of antithymocyte globulin for the prophylaxis and treatment of rejection.[2,3] These data are non-concurrent, but the introduction of cyclosporine does appear to have contributed significantly to improved results ($P < 0.005$, Gehan method). Patients depicted graphically in Fig. 6.3 as 'not transplanted' were accepted for cardiac transplantation, but no suitable donor heart became available. Their prognosis was extremely poor and, although this group is in no sense a 'control' group, these findings support the contention that cardiac transplantation provides improved survival in selected patients with terminal heart disease.

More than 80% of the one-year survivors of heart transplantation are considered to be well rehabilitated as judged by their ability to choose the life-style of their own choice.[5,19] The longest period of survival is now more than 18 years following heart transplantation.

LONG-TERM COMPLICATIONS

The major long-term complication of cardiac transplantation is the development of accelerated arteriosclerosis in the transplanted heart, and this is the major cause of death in patients who survive more than one year following heart transplantation. This disease is diffuse in distribution with intimal hyperplasia of both large, medium and small blood vessels. The vessel narrowing is concentric making angiographic diagnosis difficult. Accelerated arteriosclerosis occurs in almost half the patients examined angiographically five years after transplantation and appears to occur with equal frequency in patients whose pre-operative diagnosis was cardiomyopathy and in those with ischaemic heart disease. The cause of this process is unknown, but it has been attributed to immunologically mediated injury and labelled 'chronic rejection'. The incidence of this complication has not been reduced with the introduction of cyclosporine and no relationship has been demonstrated between its development and the frequency of biopsy-proven rejection episodes.

As the transplanted heart is denervated, patients are unaware of angina pectoris or the pain of myocardial infarction and so the diagnosis is frequently made following sudden death or unexplained cardiac failure. The nature of the disease process in most circumstances precludes treatment with angioplasty or coronary artery bypass grafting, and elective re-transplantation is indicated in selected patients. Many patients are treated with aspirin and dipyridamole prophylactically in an attempt to reduce the incidence of this complication, but the effectiveness of these measures is unknown.

COMPLICATIONS OF CYCLOSPORINE THERAPY

Nephrotoxicity following the use of cyclosporine was formerly considered to be transient and reversible. With further experience, it became clear that severe renal dysfunction with pathological changes in the kidney could occur in some patients.[20] The reduction of nephrotoxicity has been the main stimulus for reduction in the targeted serum levels of cyclosporine and in overall cyclosporine dosage. In patients with pre-operative renal dysfunction, many protocols allow for delay in initiating cyclosporine therapy until several days after transplantation to avoid compounding the nephrotoxic effects of cyclosporine and cardiopulmonary bypass.

Arterial hypertension requiring multiple medications was also seen early after the introduction of cyclosporine. This complication continues to occur although it has been lessened by reducing cyclosporine dosage.

The development of malignant disease, especially lymphoproliferative disorders, is a well-known complication of immunosuppressive therapy in general, and heart transplant recipients are no exception. Lymphoma, principally of the diffuse histiocytic type, often with central nervous system involvement was seen early in the cyclosporine era, but, with overall reduction in immunosuppression, the incidence of this complication is now much less. Many patients receive prophylactic therapy with acyclovir to obviate the risk of the Epstein–Barr virus-induced lymphoma.

The well-known long-term complications of high-dose corticosteroid therapy, such as cushingoid facies, skeletal demineralization and glucose intolerance, have been dramatically reduced by lowering overall steroid dosage.

Other complications such as hirsutism, tremor, convulsions, gum hypertrophy and hepatic dysfunction have not proved to be major management problems.

Constant awareness is required to detect drug interactions between cyclosporine and other medications used in transplant recipients.

COST OF CARDIAC TRANSPLANTATION

Since the introduction of cyclosporine, there has been a reduction in serious morbidity and hospital inpatient stay such that costs of cardiac transplantation have continued to fall. The DHSS Commission Brunel Report,[9] which analysed in detail the costs and benefits of cardiac transplantation in the UK, estimated a first-year cost of £17 000 and subsequent annual cost of £4500. The corresponding first-year cost of cardiac transplantation in the US is around $100 000.[5] These costs compare favourably with those for the treatment of other terminal diseases, such as dialysis for chronic renal failure, and home intravenous feeding.

FUTURE PROSPECTS

The major challenge in the coming years in the field of cardiac transplantation is the control of accelerated arteriosclerosis. It is unlikely that improved immunosuppression early after transplantation will result in dramatically better results than the 80–85% one-year survival now achieved. It is to be hoped that control of some of the long-term complications will allow significant improvement in the five-year survival of approximately 60%. Accelerated arteriosclerosis provides a great challenge in cardiac transplantation with possible implications for progress in arteriosclerosis research in general.

The possibility of improved immunosuppressive techniques allowing xenograftng may further expand the options for those with end-stage cardiac disease.

Paediatric cardiac transplantation is now being explored with early success, and this approach may become important in the future in the overall management of patients with severe congenital heart disease. There may be a 'window' of opportunity for transplanting infants without the need for steroid or azathioprine therapy, allowing for normal growth of these patients.

Whatever improvements are achieved in the management of cardiac transplant recipients, there are never going to be enough donor hearts to satisfy the demand. Inadequate supply of donor organs will continue to be a stimulus to the development of permanent left ventricular assist devices and artificial hearts to treat those patients who will be unable to receive biological cardiac replacement. The use of such devices as 'bridges' to cardiac transplantation has proved both successful and stimulating.[21]

CARDIOPULMONARY TRANSPLANTATION

INTRODUCTION

Early research into cardiopulmonary transplantation was carried out in the dog, with limited survival of a few days being achieved in the 1960s. The demonstration by Nakae[22] in 1967 that pulmonary denervation in the dog resulted in abnormal respiration secondary to absence of the Hering–Breuer reflex explained the death of these animals from respiratory failure. Further research was carried out in primates. Long-term survival after cardiopulmonary autotransplantation in primates was achieved by Castenada in 1972,[23] and extended survival was achieved by Reitz after allotransplantation using cyclosporine immunosuppression in 1980.[24] This laboratory programme provided the basis for the initiation of clinical heart and lung transplantation by Reitz and associates at Stanford University in March 1981.

The first successful heart–lung transplant recipient was a 45-year-old woman with primary pulmonary hypertension who was the first patient in the Stanford series who died of non-transplant-related pathology five years later. Prior to this time, there were three failed clinical attempts elsewhere. The number of heart–lung transplants performed in the UK was 51 and 71 in 1986 and 1987, respectively, with more than 350 having been performed worldwide by this time.

RECIPIENT SELECTION

In the early years of cardiopulmonary transplantation, most patients suffered from either pulmonary hypertension[25] or pulmonary hypertension secondary to Eisenmenger's syndrome,[26] but more recently heart–lung transplantation has been performed for patients with end-stage pulmonary disease.[27]

The place of combined heart–lung transplantation for end-stage respiratory disease remains to be defined. It appears that single-lung transplantation is an effective therapy for pulmonary fibrosis,[28] a relatively rare condition, but the efficacy of double-lung transplantation for emphysema and septic lung disease has yet to be determined.[29] If double-lung transplantation produces good results, then combined heart–lung transplantation may be reserved for patients with pulmonary hypertension. The disadvantage of combined heart–lung transplantation for primary lung disease is the removal of a healthy heart from the recipient and its replacement with a transplanted heart which will be subject to all the complications of transplantation of this organ such as accelerated arteriosclerosis.

Recipient selection criteria are similar to those for heart transplantation, but the average age tends to be younger than for the heart transplant population because priority is given to younger patients with end-stage disease and a deteriorating course. Previous intrathoracic surgery remains a relative contra-indication to combined heart–lung transplantation due to the likelihood of significant peri-operative haemorrhage contributing to serious morbidity and mortality. The number of patients who could benefit from combined heart–lung transplantation is unknown, but deaths from respiratory disease in England and Wales between the ages of 10 and 50 years, which could potentially be avoided with combined heart–lung transplantation, is around 180.[27]

DONOR MANAGEMENT

Until the last two years, it was necessary to move the body of the potential heart–lung donor to the recipient hospital, but more recently distant procurement of the heart and lungs has been achieved using several techniques. These include administration of cold crystalloid or colloid solutions into the pulmonary artery, the use of cardiopulmonary bypass to cool the whole body and the use of a ventilated perfused heart–lung preparation. Donor criteria for combined heart–lung transplantation are stricter than those for cardiac donation alone. Donors generally need to be obtained within five days of the initial injury and ventilation, as pulmonary complications, such as aspiration, pneumonitis or pulmonary oedema, often supervene in the brain-dead patient thereby contra-indicating heart–lung donation. A close thoracic cage size-match is important although the donor can be a little smaller than the recipient, but not vice versa as atelectasis and ventilation perfusion mismatch may develop post transplant. The chest radiograph and blood gases should be normal with normal pulmonary compliance. It is generally desirable to have a cardiac recipient of the same blood group held in reserve in the recipient hospital as often the heart–lung bloc cannot be used as expected due to deterioration of the donor lungs between the time of referral and harvest.

OPERATIVE FACTORS

The heart–lung donor operation does not require any special facilities and can be performed in any hospital operating room. Topical cooling of the heart and lungs is generally employed during transportation to supplement the initial technique of pulmonary preservation used.

The recipient operative technique has been described in detail.[30] Essential features of the procedure include preservation of the vagus phrenic, and recurrent laryngeal nerves, and meticulous haemostasis, as large bronchial collateral vessels are often present in the posterior mediastinum which become inaccessible after placement of the donor heart and lung bloc. This tendency to bleeding is accentuated by long cardiopulmonary bypass times and impaired coagulation secondary to chronic hepatic congestion.

The tracheal anastomosis is carried out first, followed by atrial and aortic anastomoses. Immunosuppressive techniques are similar to those for heart transplantation except that corticosteroids are not given for 14–21 days following heart–lung transplantation to avoid impairment of tracheal healing.

POST-OPERATIVE MANAGEMENT

Post-operative haemodynamic management is similar to that after cardiac transplantation. High inspired oxygen concentrations are avoided.

Currently, there is no reliable method of diagnosing pulmonary rejection after heart–lung transplantation, although the use of transbronchial biopsy appears encouraging.[31] It was previously accepted that cardiac and pulmonary rejection occurred concurrently and that pulmonary rejection could therefore be excluded by a normal cardiac biopsy, but this concept is now known to be flawed.[32] Apart from the use of transbronchial biopsy, the diagnosis of pulmonary rejection is largely made on clinical intuition and experience, and by the response to steroid therapy. The treatment of pulmonary rejection is by 'pulse' therapy with methylprednisolone, as used for cardiac rejection. The incidence of cardiac rejection following heart–lung transplantation appears significantly less than that after heart transplantation alone.[33]

RESULTS

One-year actuarial survival on a worldwide basis from the International Registry of Heart Transplantation for combined heart–lung transplantation is 55%.[34] One-year survival figures of around 70% have been achieved by the groups at Stanford University and Papworth hospital. The group at Pittsburgh have recently reviewed their experience.[35] The presence of previous intrathoracic surgery in the recipient, as mentioned above, has resulted in increased operative mortality in both the Pittsburgh and Stanford series.[35,36] The majority of early deaths are due to infection, principally cytomegalovirus infection or pneumocystis pneumonitis.

LONG-TERM COMPLICATIONS

Obliterative bronchiolitis has developed in half of the long-term survivors of the Stanford programme.[36] The onset of this complication has varied from months to years following transplantation. Symptoms include cough, often productive, and progressive shortness of breath. Chest radiography may demonstrate pulmonary infiltrates, with or without pleural thickening. Pulmonary function tests demonstrate a progressive obstructive physiology with superimposed restriction in a number of patients.[37] The cause of post-operative obliterative bronchiolitis is unknown, but it is believed to be due to chronic immunologically mediated lung injury.

Other complications including accelerated arteriosclerosis are shared with cardiac transplantation.

SUMMARY

Combined heart–lung transplantation remains an experimental procedure with a high one-year mortality (30–50%) and morbidity. Much further knowledge is needed in the fields of pulmonary preservation, the diagnosis of pulmonary rejection and the cause of obliterative bronchiolitis before widespread application of this operation is indicated. The early results, however, offer encouragement for future management of many hundreds of patients who would otherwise have no effective form of therapy.

REFERENCES

1. Barnard, C.N. The operation. *S. Afr. Med. J.* 1967; **41**: 1271–4.
2. Caves, P.K., Stinson, E.B., Billingham, M.E., Rider, A.K. and Shumway, N.E. Diagnosis of human cardiac allograft rejection by serial cardiac biopsy. *J. Thorac. Cardiovasc. Surg.* 1973; **66**: 461–6.
3. Bieber, C.P., Griepp, R.B., Oyer, P.E., Wong, J. and Stinson, E.B. Use of rabbit antithymocyte globulin in cardiac transplantation: Relationship of serum clearance rates to clinical outcome. *Transplantation* 1976; **22**: 478–88.
4. Oyer, P.E., Stinson, E.B., Jamieson, S.W., Hunt, S., Reitz, B.A., Bieber, C.P., Schroeder, J.S., Billingham, M.E. and Shumway, N.E. One year experience with cyclosporin-A in clinical heart transplantation. *Heart Transplantation* 1982; **1**: 285–95.
5. Schroeder, J.S. and Hunt, S. Cardiac transplantation, Update 1987. *JAMA* 1987; **258**: 3142–5.
6. Reichenspurner, M., Odell, J.A., Cooper, D.K.C., Novitzky, D., Human, P.A., Van Opell, U., Becerra, F., Boehm, D.H., Rose, A., Fasol, R., Zilla, P. and Reichart, B. Twenty years of heart transplantation at Groote Schuur Hospital. *J. Heart Transplantation* 1987; **66**: 317–23.
7. Stevenson, L.W., Fowler, M.B., Schroeder, J.S., Stevenson, W.G., Dracup, K.A. and Fond, V. Poor survival of patients with idiopathic cardiomyopathy considered too well for transplantation. *Am. J. Med.* 1987; **83**: 871–6.
8. British Cardiac Society. Report on cardiac transplantation in the United Kingdom. *Br. Heart J.* 1984; **52**: 679–82.
9. Buxton, M., Acheson, R.M., Caine, N., Gibson, S. and O'Brien, B. *Costs and benefits of heart transplant programmes at Harefield and Papworth Hospitals.* (The Brunel Report.) Research Report No. 12. London: HMSO, 1985.
10. The working group on mechanical circulatory support of the National Heart, Lung, and Blood Institutes. *Artificial heart and assist devices: Direction, needs, costs, societal, and ethical issues.* Bethesda, MD: NHLBI 1985.
11. Conference of the Medical Royal Colleges and their Faculties in the United Kingdom. Diagnosis of Brain Death. *Br. Med. J.* 1976; **2**: 1187–8.
12. Frist, W.H., Oyer, P.E., Baldwin, J.C., Stinson, E.B. and Shumway, N.E. HLA compatibility and cardiac transplant recipient survival. *Ann. Thorac. Surg.* 1987; **44**: 242–6.
13. Evans, R.W., Manningen, D.L., Garrison, L.P. and Maier, A.M. Donor availability as the primary determinant of the future of heart transplantation. *JAMA* 1986; **255**: 1892–8.
14. English, T.A.H., Spratt, P., Wallwork, J., Cory-Pearce, R. and Wheeldon, D. Selection and procurement of hearts for transplantation. *Br. Med. J.* 1984; **288**: 1889–91.
15. Lower, R.R. and Shumway, N.E. Studies on orthotopic transplantation of the canine heart. *Surg. Forum* 1960; **11**: 18–9.
16. Novitzky, B., Cooper, D.K.C. and Barnard, C.N. The surgical technique of heterotopic heart transplantation. *Ann. Thorac. Surg.* 1983; **36**: 476–82.
17. Oyer, P.E. Triple drug immunosuppressive therapy in cardiac transplantation. *Transpl. Immunol. Lett.* 1986; **3**: 3–11.
18. Bristow, M.R., Gilbert, G.M., Renlung, D.G., DeWitt, C.W., Burton, N.A. and O'Connell, J.B. Use of OKT3 monoclonal antibody in heart transplantation: Review of the initial experience. *Heart Transplantation* 1988; **7**: 1–11.
19. Baumgartner, W.A., Augustine, S., Borkon, A.M., Gardner, T.J. and Reitz, B.A. Present expectations in cardiac transplantation. *Ann. Thorac. Surg.* 1987; **43**: 585–90.
20. Myers, B.D., Ross, J., Newton, L., Luetscher, J. and Perlroth, M. Cyclosporine-associated chronic nephropathy. *N. Engl. J. Med.* 1984; **311**: 699–705.
21. Farrar, D.J., Hill, J.D., Gray, L.A., Pennington, D.G., McBride, C.R., Pierce, W.S., Pae, W.E., Glenville, B., Ross, D., Galbraith, T.A. and Zumbro, G.L. Heterotopic prosthetic ventricles as a bridge to cardiac transplantation. *N. Engl. J. Med.* 1988; **318**: 333–40.
22. Nakae, S., Webb, W.R., Theodorides, T. and Gregg, W.L. Respiratory function following cardiopulmonary denervation in dog, cat, and monkey. *Surg. Gynecol. Obstet.* 1967; **125**: 1285–92.
23. Castaneda, A., Zamora, R., Schmmidt-Habelman, P., Horung, J., Murphy, W., Ponto, D. and Moller, J.H. Cardiopulmonary autotransplantation in primates (baboons). Late functional results. *Surgery* 1972; **72**: 1064–70.
24. Reitz, B.A., Burton, N.A., Jamieson, S.W., Bieber, C.P., Pennock, J.L., Stinson, E.B. and Shumway, N.E. Heart and lung transplantation. Autotransplantation and allotransplantation in primates with extended survival. *J. Thorac. Cardiovasc. Surg.* 1980; **80**: 360–71.
25. Jamieson, S.W., Stinson, E.B., Oyer, P.E., Reitz, B.A., Baldwin, J., Modry, D., Dawkins, K., Theodore, J., Hunt, S. and Shumway, N.E. Heart–lung transplantation for irreversible pulmonary hypertension. *Ann. Thorac. Surg.* 1984; **38**: 554–62.
26. McGregor, C.G.A., Jamieson, S.W., Baldwin, J.C., Burke, C.M., Dawkins, K.D., Stinson, E.B., Oyer, P.E., Billingham, M.E., Zusman, D.R., Reitz, B.A., Morris, A., Yousem, S., Hunt, S.A. and Shumway, N.E. Combined heart and lung transplantation for end-stage Eisenmenger's syndrome. *J. Thorac. Cardiovasc. Surg.* 1986; **91**: 443–50.
27. Penketh, A., Higenbottam, T., Hakim, M. and Wallwork, J. Heart and lung transplantation in patients with end stage lung disease. *Br. Med. J.* 1987; **295**: 311–4.
28. The Toronto Lung Transplant Group. Lung Transplantation for Pulmonary Fibrosis. *N. Engl. J. Med.* 1986; **314**: 1140–5.
29. Patterson, G.A., Cooper, J.D., Dark, J.H., Jones, M.T. and the Toronto Lung Transplant Group. Experimental and clinical double lung transplantation. *J. Thorac. Cardiovasc. Surg.* 1988; **95**: 70–4.
30. Jamieson, S.W., Stinson, E.B., Oyer, P.E., Baldwin, J.C. and Shumway, N.E. Operative technique for heart–lung transplantation. *J. Thorac. Cardiovasc. Surg.* 1984; **87**: 930–5.
31. Penketh, A.R.L., Stewart, S., Zebro, T., Wallwork, J. and Higenbottam, T.W. Transbronchial biopsy in the diagnosis of pulmonary complications of heart–lung transplantation. Abstr. Eur. Soc. Organ Trans., Gothenburg, 1987.
32. McGregor, C.G.A., Baldwin, J.C., Jamieson, S.W., Billingham, M.E., Yousem, S.A., Burke, C.M., Oyer, P.E., Stinson, E.B. and Shumway, N.E. Isolated pulmonary rejection after combined heart–lung transplantation. *J. Thorac. Cardiovasc. Surg.* 1985; **90**: 623–6.
33. Baldwin, J.C., Oyer, P.E., Stinson, G.B., Starnes, V.A., Billingham, M.E. and Shumway, N.E. Comparison of cardiac rejection in heart and heart–lung transplantation. *J. Heart Transplantation* 1987; **6**: 352–6.
34. Kaye, M.P. The Registry of the International Society for Heart Transplantation: Fourth official report – 1987. *J. Heart Transplantation* 1987; **6**: 63–7.
35. Griffith, B.P., Hardesty, R.L., Trento, A., Paradis, I.L., Duquesnoy, R.J., Zeevi, A., Dauber, J.H., Dummer, J.S., Thompson, M.E., Gryzan, S. and Bahnson, H.T. Heart–Lung transplantation: lessons learned and future hopes. *Ann. Thorac. Surg.* 1987; **43**: 6–16.
36. Burke, C.M., Theodore, J., Baldwin, J.C. Tazelaar, H.D., Morris, A.J., McGregor, C.G.A., Shumway, N.E., Robin, E.D. and Jamieson, S.W. An evaluation of the results of human heart–lung transplantation. *Lancet* 1986; **1**: 517–9.
37. Burke, C.M., Theodore, J., Dawkins, K.D., Yousem, S.A., Blank, N., Billingham, M.E., Vankessel, A., Jamieson, S.W., Oyer, P.E., Baldwin, J.C., Stinson, E.B., Shumway, N.E. and Robin, E.D. Post-transplant obliterative bronchiolitis and other late lung sequelae in human heart–lung transplantation. *Chest* 1984; **86**: 824–9.

Chapter 7

Symptoms of Heart Disease

G.C. Sutton

It is generally acknowledged that more diagnostic information about both the patient and the disease is obtained by careful history-taking than any other aspect of physical examination or investigation. The assessment and interpretation of the history given by the patient must automatically lead to a logical sequence of steps in establishing the diagnosis with respect to the nature and severity of heart disease. Furthermore, the history will reveal fundamental aspects of the patient's character and their reaction to the symptoms, and will provide much of the necessary information that determines the need for therapeutic intervention.

In this section, the principal symptoms that might point to underlying heart disease will be discussed. In addition, the logical sequence of steps following on from the history will be described in order to discuss the differential diagnosis and to establish that a given symptom is indeed related to underlying cardiac pathology.

CHEST PAIN

Patients who have chest pain or discomfort are usually concerned that the pain arises from the heart and heralds or has something to do with a heart attack. Thus, the most common role for the clinician in the relationship with a patient is to establish whether chest pain is due to myocardial ischaemia.

MYOCARDIAL ISCHAEMIA

Myocardial ischaemia arises because the blood supply (via the coronary circulation) is inadequate to meet the demands of the myocardium thereby leading to myocardial hypoxia. The blood supply is inadequate because either the coronary flow is restricted (fixed narrowing or spasm in the coronary arteries) or the myocardial demand is so great (as in

hypertrophy of the myocardium) that a normal supply is insufficient, or both. If myocardial ischaemia is repetitively induced by the same provocative factor (for instance, physical exercise), the resulting chest pain or discomfort is known as *stable angina pectoris*. If myocardial ischaemia occurs apparently spontaneously (as in coronary artery spasm) or changes from a previous repetitively provoked pattern to one that is unpredictable, the resultant chest pain is called *unstable angina pectoris*.

The original description of angina pectoris was made by William Heberden in 1768. He described the four cardinal features of a patient's account of the pain which allow the clinician to make the diagnosis of angina based on the history and to infer that the underlying pathophysiological change is myocardial ischaemia.

1   The location of the pain is usually in the centre of the chest, but it may radiate to the left and into the left arm.
2   The pain is characteristically related to exertion.
3   The pain lasts a relatively short time (up to 5–10 min).
4   The quality of the pain is 'strangling', a pressure, heaviness or constriction in the chest, which causes the patient great anxiety.

Although such an account of stable angina is frequently given by the patient who develops myocardial ischaemia, many variations in these four features are possible. The location may vary to include the upper abdomen, the right side of the chest and right arm, the shoulders, back, neck, jaws and teeth. Sometimes these locations are part of the radiation of the pain, but sometimes they may be the sole location. Exertion does not necessarily mean only physical exertion: increased cardiac work associated with anxiety or nervous energy or digestion frequently gives rise to chest pain due to myocardial ischaemia (for instance, any source of excitement or following heavy meals with or without additional physical exercise). In some patients, myocardial ischaemia may result not in pain but in a tightness, a discomfort, or simply a sensation of breathlessness.

If myocardial ischaemia occurs without any obvious provocative factor (unstable angina), the patient will describe episodic chest pain or discomfort. The location, duration and quality of the pain resemble those for stable angina except there is no clear relation to exertion. A prolonged period of myocardial ischaemia may result in *myocardial infarction*. Thus, patients who describe chest pain lasting for more than 30 min and up to several hours may have acute myocardial infarction. The location of the pain is the same as in angina, but the severity is often dramatic and the sense of impending doom real. As in unstable angina, the pain of myocardial infarction is not related to exertion. Whereas the pain of myocardial ischaemia is relieved by nitroglycerine, the pain of myocardial infarction is not.

OTHER CAUSES OF CHEST PAIN

Pericarditis

Unlike the pain of myocardial ischaemia, inflammation of the parietal pericardium results in a chest pain which is sharp. The pain may be central or in the left chest but radiation to the neck and back, as well as the upper abdomen, may be described. The pain is exacerbated by inspiration and sometimes relieved by sitting upright and leaning forward. Twisting or swallowing may exacerbate the pain. The pain will usually last many hours or even days depending on the nature of the inflammatory process (viral, bacterial, neoplastic, following myocardial infarction, uraemic) and the development of pericardial effusion which tends to reduce the amount of pain.

Aortic dissection

The pain associated with acute dissection of the proximal aorta is usually even more severe than the pain of acute myocardial infarction. It is often present in the upper back and may not radiate elsewhere. Radiation of the pain into the neck and face is also a feature.

Oesophageal pain

The pain of oesophageal spasm closely resembles the pain of unstable angina. It is located in the centre of the chest and may radiate down the left arm. It usually lasts from 10 min up to 1 h and may have no obvious provocative factor. Nitroglycerine may relieve the pain of oesophageal spasm as quickly as it relieves transient myocardial ischaemia.

Prolonged vomiting from any cause may result in an oesophageal tear (the Mallory-Weiss syndrome) causing not only some vomiting of blood but also central chest pain.

The pain of gastro-oesophageal reflux (as in hiatus hernia) is usually located in the centre of the chest and epigastrium. It may be associated with an obvious regurgitation of acid into the mouth. It will be provoked by recumbency and relieved by adopting an upright posture and the taking of antacids.

Musculoskeletal pain

Musculoskeletal pain often follows sudden trauma, such as a rapid twisting movement or an injury to the chest and back. The pain is usually located on either side of the chest rather than the retrosternal area. It may persist for days or even weeks and is exacerbated by movements of the chest and arms. There may be a dull background ache with stabbing or sharp momentary exacerbations. Multiple locations of the pain or discomfort are common. Relief is usually obtained with the passage of time and the use of simple analgesics.

Emotional

Individuals who become tense as a result of anxiety often notice a tight sensation in the chest. Such a sensation will tend to persist until the situation provoking the anxiety no longer exists. Sometimes, as in some patients with stabbing musculoskeletal pain, the development of pain results in extreme anxiety with all the features of the hyperventilation syndrome.

Peptic ulceration and gall-bladder disease

Pathology in the stomach, duodenum or biliary system may result in chest pain although usually such pain is confined to the abdomen. The pain of peptic ulceration is typically related to meals, often burning in nature and usually relieved by antacids. Post-prandial pain of gastric ulceration may resemble the pain of myocardial ischaemia induced by the digestive process. Biliary pain is often colicky, sometimes related to certain foods and often right-sided in the upper abdomen and in the front and back of the chest.

Pleuritic pain

Inflammation of the pleura from any cause usually gives rise to chest pain. Such pain is usually sharp in nature and located to one side of the chest front or back. It is made worse by inspiration and in this respect resembles pericardial pain. The patient usually notices difficulty with breathing because it is restricted by the pain, or may become breathless (especially if there is underlying pulmonary disease or if a large pleural effusion develops).

FURTHER ASPECTS OF THE DIAGNOSIS OF MYOCARDIAL ISCHAEMIA

Stable angina

If the clinician interprets the patient's history as one of stable angina, the severity of the condition must be assessed as it will determine management; the clinician must also consider the nature of the pathological process that has resulted in myocardial ischaemia.

The assessment of severity is dependent on the extent that pain interferes with the patient's normal life. It would be possible to grade severity according to the level of exercise producing the pain: thus, extreme exertion, such as running, resulting in pain might be deemed 'mild' angina, whereas trivial emotion causing angina might be called 'severe' angina. But different levels of activity are important to different patients' lives and consequently each patient with angina needs to be assessed within his or her own life-style to determine the extent of interference in that life-style by angina.

Having established the patient's history is one of stable angina and having assessed its severity from the history, the basis of the pathophysiological process causing myocardial ischaemia needs to be considered. The causes of stable angina include coronary artery disease (usually atheroma but occasionally narrowing of the coronary ostia by an aortitis) or myocardial hypertrophy due to left ventricular outflow tract obstruction, such as aortic valve stenosis, sub-aortic stenosis or supravalvar aortic stenosis, coarctation of the aorta or systemic hypertension or idiopathic hypertrophic cardiomyopathy. Aortic regurgitation without involving the coronary ostia may occasionally also result

in stable angina. Thus, the basis of the physical examination of the patient who has stable angina is to look for physical signs of these conditions (see later). If the angina is due to coronary artery narrowing, the cardiovascular examination will be normal unless there has been significant damage to the myocardium (for instance, if the patient has had a myocardial infarct in the past); in the latter case, the physical signs will be those of left ventricular dysfunction.

There is an unusual group of middle-aged women who have normal coronary artery anatomy, and no other cause of myocardial ischaemia, and yet give a history sometimes of stable angina and sometimes of frequent episodic chest pain which sounds like myocardial ischaemia. The aetiology of this 'syndrome X' has not been established.

A variety of simple investigations needs to be carried out to confirm the diagnosis from the history and examination that the patient has stable angina due to myocardial ischaemia from coronary artery narrowing. The resting electrocardiogram and plain chest radiograph should be normal in the absence of myocardial damage. However, the electrocardiogram should show evidence of myocardial ischaemia during the kind of activity that the patient describes as resulting in pain. The demonstration of exercise-induced myocardial ischaemia may also be made by thallium myocardial scintigraphy.

If coronary artery narrowing alone is not the cause of myocardial ischaemia, investigations will be designed to establish other pathologies. Myocardial hypertrophy may be revealed by the resting electrocardiogram and particularly by echocardiography. Echocardiography may demonstrate different varieties of left ventricular outflow obstruction. Myocardial damage from coronary artery disease may be reflected in the resting electrocardiogram, in the plain chest radiograph, by echocardiography or radioisotope ventriculography. A number of factors may aggravate myocardial ischaemia and hence the extent of angina suffered by the patient. Anaemia can readily be investigated, as can hyper- and hypothyroidism. Hypertension may aggravate angina without causing myocardial hypertrophy.

Unstable angina

It is much more difficult to establish from the history that myocardial ischaemia is the cause of episodic chest pain than repetitively provoked chest pain is due to myocardial ischaemia. Some patients give an account of an episode of chest pain that might have occurred infrequently or over only a short period of time which has the features of myocardial ischaemic pain (location, duration and quality). If such an episode is part of a history that includes exertionally related pain, then unstable angina due to myocardial ischaemia is very likely. However, often there is no history of exercise-related pain. This diagnostic problem may be best resolved by recording the electrocardiogram during an episode of pain to determine whether there is evidence of myocardial ischaemia. Ambulatory monitoring of the electrocardiogram may also be useful. Although exercise-testing in such patients may reveal exercise-induced myocardial ischaemia, it does not prove that episodic chest pain is due to myocardial ischaemia.

The causes of episodic chest pain due to myocardial ischaemia include coronary artery spasm which may occur in association with fixed coronary artery narrowing (atheroma) or in normal coronary arteries. Another possibility for the development of episodic chest pain due to myocardial ischaemia in patients with fixed coronary artery narrowing is the occurrence of paroxysmal rhythm change. This may also be best detected by ambulatory monitoring of the electrocardiogram.

Occasionally, patients who have mitral valve prolapse complain of episodes of chest pain, the cause of which is uncertain, indistinguishable from the pain of myocardial ischaemia. Clinical examination or echocardiography should enable this diagnosis to be made.

Coronary arteriography and a history of chest pain

The demonstration of coronary artery narrowing by coronary arteriography (the 'gold standard' at present) is not a substitute for careful history-taking. There are many causes of chest pain apart from myocardial ischaemia due to coronary artery narrowing. As coronary artery narrowing due to atheroma is a common finding in individuals in the middle and elderly age-groups in most races, it does not follow that because a patient is shown to have coronary atheroma his symptoms are attributable to it. Only the history and the demonstration of myocardial ischaemia by the techniques indicated above enable the clinician to make a diagnosis of angina due to coronary artery disease.

DIFFICULTY WITH BREATHING

Many individuals notice difficulty with breathing, a symptom that is particularly difficult to assess as the reaction of different individuals varies depending on their psychological make-up. Furthermore, breathlessness is inevitable at a certain level of exercise for normal individuals, the level depending mainly on the degree of physical fitness. Thus, an elderly or physically disabled individual who lives a purely sedentary existence may notice breathlessness on climbing upstairs, whereas the trained athlete notices breathlessness at the termination of an athletic event: neither individual has heart or lung disease. An individual who has carried out normal sporting activities to the age of 40 years and who then stops those activities for a period of one year, for example, and then re-starts the old activities will notice breathlessness simply due to lack of fitness. A marked increase in weight is often associated with reduced fitness.

As such factors cause difficulty with breathing (dyspnoea), the clinician establishing the history of the individual needs to make a careful assessment of the normal or altered life-style of the individual in relation to the breathlessness. As in the patient with stable angina, it is necessary to establish the patient's normal exercise pattern.

The history-taking must also establish what the patient means by difficulty with breathing. Some individuals include 'sighing' or momentary catching of breath as a difficulty in breathing. Such a symptom may simply be an expression of a neurosis (for instance, claustrophobia) or may be due to an ectopic beat rather than a symptom revealing underlying heart or lung disease.

Anaemia often results in dyspnoea. The degree of anaemia is relevant as it is likely that only severe anaemia *per se* would cause breathlessness on exertion, whereas mild anaemia may be sufficient to cause breathlessness in the patient with pre-existing heart or lung disease.

DYSPNOEA ASSOCIATED WITH HEART DISEASE

The mechanisms by which heart disease cause dyspnoea are complex. They include increased lung stiffness due to fluid exuding into the alveoli because of high pulmonary venous pressures and hence increasing respiratory work, airways obstruction by fluid or spasm also increasing respiratory work, reduction in vital capacity due to pulmonary venous engorgement (sometimes with additional pleural effusions) and reflex hyperventilation due to hypoxia (as in pulmonary oedema) or from stretching of pulmonary receptors in congested lungs.

The patient may complain of breathlessness on exertion or present as an emergency with acute shortness of breath. The patient who has heart disease and notices exertional breathlessness needs careful assessment as this will determine management. As in the patient with angina, the symptom has to be appreciated within the patient's normal life-style and severity can then be assessed. Thus, a 45-year-old man, normally sedentary at work but walking one mile in each direction for the train that takes him to and from his work, may notice breathlessness at the end of the one-mile walk if he hurries ('mild' dyspnoea), has to stop after almost completing the walk at normal pace ('moderate' dyspnoea) or has to stop several times, struggling to complete the journey at a slow pace ('severe' dyspnoea). Other patients will become breathless on trivial exertion such as talking, which would be regarded as 'severe' if they are normally fit but less so if they normally carry out little exercise. It is reasonably common to hear patients with heart disease describing gradually diminishing exercise tolerance (able to walk less and less because of dyspnoea).

An objective assessment of a patient's limiting symptoms on exercise is to carry out an exercise test. In its simplest form, this involves going for a walk with the patient and observing their behaviour. More formal exercise testing using a 'heart failure' protocol and a treadmill may also be worthwhile, to compare different individuals and also to follow progress serially in the same individual.

Patients with heart disease notice breathlessness when lying flat and need to be propped upright when asleep. This symptom suggests a more precariously balanced circulation than that in patients with exertional dyspnoea alone. The increased venous return of recumbency increases the pulmonary venous pressure resulting in deterioration of dyspnoea. In addition, vital capacity may be critically reduced by the relatively high diaphragm in the recumbent position.

Sudden change in a patient's breathlessness and exercise tolerance always demands an explanation. The two most likely explanations are a change in cardiac rhythm and a change in medication. The patient may have noticed that the sudden deterioration in his breathing coincided with palpitation; the clinician will need to consider the possibility (perhaps carry out ambulatory monitoring of the electrocardiogram) as it may affect treatment. If breathlessness is due to myocardial disease, deterioration may be due to fresh damage to the myocardium (for instance, myocardial infarction). The presence of superadded pulmonary infection or embolism may result in deterioration of dyspnoea predominantly due to heart disease.

ACUTE BREATHLESSNESS (PULMONARY OEDEMA)

Patients with heart disease may wake at night fighting for breath (paroxysmal nocturnal dyspnoea). The mechanism may be similar to orthopnoea only the patient has failed to sit up. The attack may subside spontaneously on sitting up. A severe attack of breathlessness at night may be due to such striking elevation in pulmonary venous pressure that pulmonary oedema, the outpouring of fluid into the alveoli, results. The patient is usually too ill to give a detailed account. He has severe breathlessness, noisy breathing, cough, often productive of frothy blood-stained sputum, and is very ill. This condition may occur as the result of the remorseless progression of untreated heart disease, or as a result of a precipitating factor causing deterioration as described above. It is important to remember that not all cases of pulmonary oedema are due to heart disease. Severe renal impairment, fluid overloading and chemical alveolar damage can all result in pulmonary oedema.

BREATHLESSNESS DUE TO PULMONARY DISEASE

It is frequently impossible to distinguish whether breathlessness described by the patient is cardiac or respiratory in origin. Given either pathology, the patient will notice breathlessness on exertion or even acute episodes at rest. Exertional breathlessness in pulmonary disease usually reflects a long-standing process with important abnormalities of pulmonary function. On close questioning, the patient may reveal a long history of pulmonary disease or recurrent winter bronchitis, or the presence of chronic cough and sputum, sometimes infected. Pulmonary function tests at rest or on exercise may be necessary to demonstrate a pulmonary function abnormality sufficient to cause breathlessness, or unfitness, and to point to the nature of the pathological process causing the functional abnormality. The examination of the respiratory system, the plain chest radiograph, ventilation and perfusion isotope lung scanning, computed tomography scanning may all provide information confirming or suggesting that breathlessness is respiratory in origin in support of the clinician's assessment of the patient's history.

PULMONARY VASCULAR DISEASE

Pulmonary embolic disease is commonly associated with breathlessness. Chronic exertional dyspnoea is a feature of chronic thromboembolic pulmonary hypertension, as it is in pulmonary hypertension which may be idiopathic in origin, secondary to lung parenchymal disease, or in association with congenital heart disease and intracardiac shunts. The key diagnostic aspects are the detection of severe pulmonary hypertension by abnormal physical signs and plain chest radiograph and of consequent right ventricular hypertrophy on the electrocardiogram. Further specific evaluation of the cause may involve ventilation–perfusion lung scanning, computed tomography lung scanning or pulmonary function testing.

Acute severe breathlessness is a feature of acute massive pulmonary embolism. Such patients frequently develop acute circulatory collapse and on resuscitation they are observed to be tachypnoeic. The presence of predisposing factors for the development of thrombo-embolism and the features of acute reduction in cardiac output and right ventricular failure suggest the diagnosis, confirmed by demonstration of perfusion abnormality in the pulmonary vasculature. Acute minor pulmonary embolism, which may result in pulmonary infarction, may also cause acute breathlessness, but only if there is significant pre-existing cardiorespiratory disease. Difficulty in breathing results from the pleurisy caused by pulmonary infarction.

FURTHER ASPECTS OF THE DIAGNOSIS OF CARDIAC DYSPNOEA

It is apparent that it may be very difficult to determine with certainty whether a patient's difficulty in breathing is the result of heart disease. Initially, the clinician will need to establish there is significant cardiac pathology that might be associated with breathlessness. The possible cardiac pathology is most likely to be myocardial disease. This may be the consequence of damage to or ischaemia of the myocardium as a result of coron-

ary artery disease, or abnormalities of myocardial function for other reasons (pathophysiologically classified as dilated, hypertrophic or restrictive cardiomyopathy). If the cardiac pathology lies not in abnormalities of myocardial function, it may be due to valve disease, congenital heart disease or pericardial disease.

Thus, the physical examination of the patient suspected of having dyspnoea on a cardiac basis is directed to detecting abnormalities of myocardial function (double apical impulse, gallop rhythms, atrioventricular valvular regurgitation) or evidence of primary valvular abnormalities, such as mitral or aortic stenosis, congenital heart disease or pericardial constriction or tamponade. If myocardial dysfunction is the cause, the resting electrocardiogram is usually abnormal revealing evidence of prior myocardial infarction, left bundle branch block or left ventricular hypertrophy. If there are structural abnormalities, such as valvular disease, appropriate electrocardiographic features should be present. Non-invasive investigation of the heart (echocardiography, radioisotope ventriculography) should detect abnormalities of left ventricular function or other structural abnormalities. If these aspects of physical examination and investigation fail to demonstrate cardiac pathology, then breathlessness should not be attributed to the heart.

The importance of the plain chest radiograph in the assessment of breathlessness is crucial. If the patient presents with acute, severe breathlessness thought to be on a cardiac basis, the plain chest radiograph would be expected to show pulmonary oedema. There is little controversy that acute pulmonary oedema is related to acute elevations of pulmonary venous pressure whether due to myocardial disease or valve disease, such as mitral stenosis. Patients who describe exertional dyspnoea usually show less striking radiological features of pulmonary venous pressure elevation, such as pulmonary venous dilatation, upper lobe blood diversion, septal lines or additional pulmonary arterial dilatation. The clinician would expect such features to be present in patients whose dyspnoea has a cardiac basis. However, unlike acute pulmonary oedema, exertional breathlessness correlates less well with measured pulmonary venous pressure. Other features of the plain chest radiograph suggesting cardiac pathology in the patient with breathlessness is cardiac enlargement (due either to chamber dilatation, including the left atrium, or pericardial effusion), and specific features applicable to various types of congenital heart disease.

COMMENT

Many patients with known heart disease who develop breathlessness are automatically treated by clinicians as if they have 'heart failure' or breathlessness due to heart disease. This may result in unnecessary and inappropriate therapy being given. Unfortunately, at present, there is no certain method to determine that breathlessness is due to the heart disease, and only careful history-taking and assessment of all aspects of the patient will result in appropriate management. Furthermore, many patients are automatically treated with diuretics if they complain of dyspnoea without a proper attempt being made to establish whether the patient has heart disease. Such therapy may also be inappropriate.

FATIGUE AND WEAKNESS

These symptoms are frequently non-specific and extremely difficult to assess. However, it has to be recognized that they may relate to heart disease and particularly those patients who have heart failure. Fatigue seems to be related to low blood flows to exercising muscles. Tiredness, particularly on exertion, may be a side-effect of a cardiovascular drug, particularly a beta-adrenergic blocking agent. Weakness may be the result of hypokalaemia and hyponatraemia caused by excessive use of diuretics.

PALPITATION

When patients complain of palpitation, it usually means that they have become aware of the beating of the heart and find this sensation disturbing. The beating sensation may represent a normal heart beat, an irregular heart beat, a rapid heart beat or an increased intensity of the beat. Rarely, a patient will describe an unusually slow beating of the heart.

The two most common reasons for the patient to complain of palpitation are anxiety and the presence of ectopic beats. An anxious individual, particularly one who is thin and lying on the left side (thereby bringing the heart closer to the chest wall) in a quiet environment, may become aware of the normal beating of the heart. The more rapid beating of a sinus tachycardia induced by anxiety may be noticed. Such individuals also tend to notice the sinus tachycardia of exercise and particularly of emotional or stressful situations. The onset of such palpitation is gradual, lasts as long as the stimulus and is not a reflection of any underlying heart disease.

Cardiac conditions associated with an increased stroke volume (such as valvular regurgitation) or thyrotoxicosis and anaemia may result in patients becoming aware of the normal beating of their hearts or the sinus tachycardia of mild exertion. These diagnoses should become apparent from the examination and investigation of the patient. Occasionally, therapy, particularly vasodilator therapy, will induce sinus tachycardia noticed by the patient.

Other individuals, also often anxious and thin, notice ectopic beats. These usually do not indicate underlying heart disease. Most normal individuals will occasionally have an ectopic beat but it tends to be the anxious individual who notices it and describes it as palpitation. The description varies widely: sometimes the patient notices the compensatory pause following the ectopic and describes the heart missing a beat and the forceful beat following the pause; sometimes there is momentary faintness; sometimes the heart is said to jump; sometimes sensations occur in the abdomen or in the neck. In spite of the variety of descriptions, the sensation is always momentary, even though it may be repetitive, and it is this aspect that enables the clinician to make the diagnosis.

The symptom of palpitation may represent an awareness of the development of paroxysmal tachycardia. A patient with this kind of 'palpitation' often gives a clear and typical account of the sudden development of a tachycardia, usually without obvious provocative factors. The abrupt onset and often the abrupt cessation strongly suggests a diagnosis of paroxysmal tachycardia. It may be useful to ask the patient to beat out the nature of the tachycardia to attempt some assessment of its rate and whether it is regular; however, patients are less reliable at distinguishing the irregular beat of atrial fibrillation from the regular rapid rate of atrial tachycardia. Important aspects of such a history are the frequency and duration of attacks and associated features because they will determine the need for treatment. Patients who have underlying ischaemic heart disease will often develop angina during an episode of paroxysmal tachycardia. Other patients may notice breathlessness and faintness or dizziness. Occasionally, a patient with paroxysmal tachycardia will notice polyuria as a result of the attack. Paroxysmal tachycardia may indicate underlying cardiac pathology or may represent an electrical disturbance within the heart and conducting system without any disease process.

FURTHER ASPECTS OF THE DIAGNOSIS OF PALPITATION

The diagnosis of sinus tachycardia or ectopic beats due to anxiety in the presence of a normal heart may be certain on the basis of the history, complemented by the examination, resting electrocardiogram and plain chest radiograph of the patient. No further investigation should be carried out; reassurance is all that is required. If the diagnosis is not clear, and particularly if paroxysmal tachycardia is suspected, attempts need to be made to establish the nature of the palpitation by recording the electrocardiogram during an attack. If attacks are frequent, this may best be done by ambulatory recording of the electrocardiogram. If the attacks are infrequent, the patient may be loaned an 'event' ECG recorder to document the palpitation. If the episode is sufficiently long, rapid access to an ECG machine is all that is required. If the episode is related to exertion, an exercise test should reveal the nature of the symptoms. If there is a suspicion of underlying structural heart disease, this may be detected by investigations including echocardiography, radioisotope ventriculography or exercise testing.

SYNCOPE

A transient loss of consciousness due to inadequate cerebral perfusion results in the patient blacking out. Although the patient may describe such episodes to the clinician, it is frequently necessary to obtain another account of the episodes from a witness, such as a relative. Adequate cerebral perfusion depends on an adequate cardiac output, the maintenance of a constant cerebrovascular resistance and the maintenance of a systemic vascular resistance and blood pressure. Any factors that alter these variables may result in syncope.

The most frequent cause of syncope is the common faint (vasomotor or vasodepressor syncope). It is probably caused by a fall in systemic vascular resistance due to arterial dilatation in muscles with a resultant fall in blood pressure causing loss of consciousness. It is commonly a reaction to emotion or pain, but other factors, such as the sight of blood or physical debility, may be involved. It usually occurs when the individual is standing and is preceded by visual disturbance, yawning, weakness, sweating and nausea. Lying down aborts the episode as it restores cerebral perfusion. A witness may notice pallor in the individual, with a slow radial pulse, difficult to feel. If blood pressure falls excessively when a patient stands up, transient dizziness or blackout can occur. This may occur in patients receiving hypotensive therapy or it may occur in individuals with autonomic nervous system disease, such as diabetes mellitus. The pooling of blood in the legs on standing, prevented by arteriovenous constriction in normal individuals, is not prevented in some normal individuals and in those with an autonomic neuropathy.

Micturition syncope occurs in men who get up at night to pass urine. Syncope occurs immediately after passing urine. This is likely to be due to reflex vasodilatation from afferent vagal stimulation post-micturition in an individual already somewhat dilated from having been in bed. It may be accentuated by the valsalva manoeuvre induced by straining at micturition in the upright posture.

CARDIAC CAUSES OF SYNCOPE

Syncope can result from either very fast or very slow heart rates, which may significantly affect cardiac output and hence cerebral perfusion. Patients with paroxysmal tachycardia (either supraventricular or ventricular) may notice the sudden onset of palpitation before they black out, but often syncope occurs without any warning. Patients with slow heart rates or heart block are subject to episodes of cardiac arrest (Stokes–Adams attacks) due to either ventricular fibrillation or asystole. Such patients describe sudden loss of consciousness without warning, with recovery occurring after a collapse lasting 10–20 s. It is not uncommon for significant injury to occur when the patient blacks out as a result of the fall. The recovery is often accompanied by a hot flushing sensation spreading throughout the body. The frequency of such attacks varies in different individuals from several times a day to only once a year. Unlike epileptic attacks, an aura is not present, there are usually no convulsive movements or incontinence, and there is no post-ictal confusional state.

Exertional syncope occurs in a number of cardiac conditions including fixed left ventricular outflow tract obstruction (aortic valve stenosis or sub-aortic stenosis), hypertrophic obstructive cardiomyopathy and primary pulmonary hypertension. Inability of the heart to increase cardiac output on exercise is thought to be the mechanism, although exercise-induced arrhythmias may also occur, especially in aortic stenosis. A rare cause of unpredictable cardiac syncope is obstruction to the mitral valve orifice by either a left atrial myxoma or a ball-valve thrombus in the left atrium. An abnormally sensitive carotid sinus may also give rise to syncope from cardiac slowing or hypotension; it may be induced in such an individual by only light stimulation of the neck.

FURTHER ASPECTS OF THE DIAGNOSIS OF SYNCOPE

Obvious structural cardiac pathology, such as aortic valve stenosis, should be excluded by physical examination supported by investigation, such as echocardiography and Doppler examination. The resting electrocardiogram may indicate the presence of conducting tissue disease by showing abnormalities of the P–R interval, atrioventricular dissociation, with left or right bundle branch block, and abnormal axis deviation. Such an electrocardiogram strongly suggests the possibility of Stokes–Adams attacks as the cause of syncope. Abnormally slow heart rates or intermittent atrial arrhythmias may suggest the presence of a sick sinus. If the attacks are frequent, continuous monitoring of the electrocardiogram should establish whether any important rhythm abnormality is associated with the episode of syncope. Sometimes simultaneous electrocardiographic and electroencephalographic recording may be possible, particularly when there is doubt over whether the cause of syncope is a cardiac arrhythmia or epilepsy.

OEDEMA AND ASCITES

Unless swelling of the legs or abdomen is gross, it tends not to be noticed by the patient and is more likely to be elicited as an abnormal physical sign by the clinician. The accumulation of fluid in interstitial tissues is usually preceded by a substantial weight gain. The mechanism of the development of oedema in patients with heart disease is complex: reduced blood flow through the kidney as a consequence of an inadequate cardiac output leads to sodium retention and activation of the sympathetic and renin–angiotensin systems, which, in turn, stimulate the release of aldosterone and vasopressin; a high venous pressure increases the pressure at the venous end of a capillary as fluid fails to be re-absorbed and oedema results.

The patients who are most likely to develop oedema are those with tricuspid valve disease (and particularly tricuspid regurgitation), constrictive pericarditis and restrictive cardiomyopathy. Although many patients with left ventricular disease have abnormally activated neuro-endocrine systems which could produce oedema in their own right, it is particularly those with severe tricuspid regurgitation who seem to develop both oedema and ascites most readily. Patients with organic tricuspid valve abnormalities (such as those with rheumatic tricuspid stenosis, infective endocarditis or right atrial myxoma) and those with pericardial constriction or myocardial restriction are much less common than those with left heart disease and accompanying tricuspid regurgitation.

The localization of oedema is determined primarily by gravity. Thus, ambulant patients notice oedema in both feet, ankles and legs, whereas those who are bed-bound may have it mainly over the sacrum. If oedema is left untreated, it may spread over the genitalia and the abdominal and thoracic walls. Intraperitoneal fluid (ascites) often accompanies oedema in the periphery but is more obvious at a later stage.

Patients with high central venous pressures not only frequently develop oedema and ascites but, probably as a result of hepatic and mesenteric venous engorgement, also complain of anorexia, nausea and vomiting. Such patients may find themselves being investigated for abdominal conditions such as neoplasms if the high venous pressure is not noticed and attention is not paid to the heart. Alternatively, such symptoms may be thought to be due to digitalis intoxication, when in reality more 'aggressive' treatment for heart failure is required.

DIFFERENTIAL DIAGNOSIS OF CARDIAC OEDEMA AND ASCITES

Chronic venous insufficiency in the lower limbs is extremely common and gives rise to oedema. In this condition, the swelling may be unilateral, there may be obvious evidence of venous problems in the legs and the history is usually of longstanding swelling which is not present in the morning but develops during the day when the individual stands up. Increasing breathlessness is unlikely to be a feature of oedema from venous insufficiency whereas it usually, but not invariably, accompanies oedema from cardiac causes. In untreated oedema due to a cardiac cause, the jugular venous pressure is usually elevated; if the oedema is due to a venous problem in the legs, jugular venous pressure is not elevated.

Oedema around the face is a feature of angioneurotic oedema, acute glomerulonephritis, myxoedema and the nephrotic syndrome. Hypoproteinaemia from liver or renal disease may produce generalized oedema, but sometimes it is confined to the legs. When ascites is particularly marked, portal hypertension (hepatic cirrhosis) may be suspected.

Other causes of oedema include superior vena caval obstruction (for instance, from carcinoma of the bronchus), when the oedema is confined to the upper body, lymphatic obstruction (for instance, filariasis) and cyclical oedema (one aspect of the pre-menstrual syndrome).

CYANOSIS

Cyanosis is a bluish discoloration of the skin and mucous membranes caused by an increased amount of reduced haemoglobin (or, rarely, abnormal haemoglobin pigments) in the blood circulating through superficial capillaries and venules. Patients seldom complain of cyanosis but the bluish discolouration may be noticed by relatives if the patient is centrally cyanosed; however, an individual may complain of blue extremities (peripheral cyanosis). Central cyanosis is due to arterial oxygen desaturation from right-to-left shunting of blood bypassing the lungs or inadequate oxygenation of the blood by the lungs in certain lung diseases. Clubbing of the fingers or toes often accompanies longstanding central cyanosis.

Peripheral cyanosis is a consequence of peripheral vasoconstriction due to a cold extremity in normal individuals or low cardiac output in those with heart disease. Peripheral cyanosis can be abolished by warming the affected extremity, and mucous membranes (which are warm) will not be blue.

Central cyanosis due to lung disease may be diminished or abolished by breathing oxygen; this manoeuvre will have no effect if the cyanosis is due to an intracardiac shunt. Measurements of arterial oxygen saturation in centrally cyanosed individuals will be below about 85%, although arterial oxygen saturation will rise in polycythaemic individuals and fall in those who are anaemic.

COUGH AND HAEMOPTYSIS

Although cough and haemoptysis are usually features of pulmonary disease, they may be prominent symptoms in patients with heart disease. Cough is common in patients with pulmonary venous hypertension, either from left ventricular disease or from mitral valve disease, in whom it is usually a part of breathlessness as previously described. The cough may be unproductive, but if pulmonary oedema develops the cough may be associated with frothy sputum which can be pink. A persistent cough, especially that occurring at night, may be due to important left heart disease and be mistakenly treated as pulmonary disease, such as bronchitis.

There are many causes of haemoptysis, the coughing up of blood from the lungs. The rupture of a pulmonary or bronchial vein can occur in conditions associated with pulmonary venous hypertension and dilatation, such as mitral stenosis; the coughing up of pure blood will result. Patients with severe pulmonary hypertension (for instance, those with the Eisenmenger situation or primary pulmonary hypertension) often notice haemoptysis. Pulmonary infarction from minor pulmonary embolism is a fairly common complication of various cardiac conditions, including acute myocardial infarction and heart failure, mitral stenosis and pulmonary hypertension. If pulmonary infarction results in haemoptysis, it is usually accompanied by pleural pain but not invariably so. It may be difficult to differentiate between such pulmonary arterial infarction and pulmonary venous infarction associated with pulmonary venous hypertension causing haemoptysis in patients with acute myocardial infarction.

Hoarseness accompanying a cough usually suggests a neoplasm, such as a carcinoma of the bronchus. Rarely, however, there is a cardiological cause for compression of the recurrent laryngeal nerve and consequent hoarseness; an aortic aneurysm, a very large left atrium and even a dilated pulmonary artery can cause this symptom.

SYMPTOMATIC CLASSIFICATION OF CARDIAC FUNCTION

The New York Heart Association has produced a classification of functional capacity in heart disease based on patients' symptoms. Class I represents patients with known heart disease who do not have any limiting symptoms (pain, dyspnoea, fatigue or palpitation) in spite of ordinary activities. Class II includes patients with heart disease who have no symptoms at rest nor on mild exertion but who have some limiting symptoms on moderate or normal exertion. Class III encompasses patients with heart disease and marked limitation of physical ability due to the development of pain, dyspnoea, fatigue or palpitation on mild exertion. Class IV covers patients who have cardiac symptoms at rest, which are made worse by the slightest physical exertion. Other similar classifications (Canadian Cardiovascular Society Functional Classification, Specific Activity Scale) have subsequently been introduced to categorize an individual patient.

Such classifications have considerable limitations, notably that 'cardiac' symptoms in patients with known heart disease, however severe, may not be due to the heart disease but may be attributable to other factors (see above). However, classification is necessary to assess a change in a patient's condition over a period of time, with or without therapeutic intervention, and to compare groups of patients with different functional capacities.

Chapter 8

Examination of the Cardiovascular System

G.C. Sutton

The history obtained from the patient suggests the possibility or probability that disease of the heart and cardiovascular system is present. This focuses the attention of the clinician on examination of the cardiovascular system in order to obtain supportive evidence of cardiovascular abnormality. The findings of such a physical examination may provide information not only on the deranged anatomy (pathology) within the cardiovascular system but also on the haemodynamic consequences or physiological derangement resulting from the pathology.

A logical sequence of examination is necessary to extract maximum information. Such a sequence involves measurement of the blood pressure, an analysis of the arterial and venous pulses, palpation of the precordium, auscultation of the heart and a general inspection of the patient relevant to abnormalities in the cardiovascular system. At the end of such an examination, and in association with the knowledge gained from the history provided by the patient, the clinician is likely to have fairly precise knowledge of the anatomical and functional abnormalities present in the heart and circulation of many patients with cardiovascular disease. Appropriate investigations are then carried out to support such a clinical diagnosis and to elucidate it further.

In this section, the key physical signs in the examination of the cardiovascular system, and their modification by disease states, will be described.

THE BLOOD PRESSURE

Although precise measurement of arterial pressure requires intra-arterial catheterization, a close approximation is usually obtained by indirect blood pressure recording using a sphygmomanometer. The patient should rest comfortably propped up on a couch with the sphygmomanometer wrapped carefully around the bare upper arm 2–3 cm above the antecubital fossa. The size of the bag and cuff depends on the size of the arm; special small cuffs are used in children. The cuff is inflated until brachial artery pulsation is no longer felt; the cuff is then deflated slowly until pulsation reappears by palpation or sounds are heard by auscultating over the brachial artery. This moment represents the systolic blood pressure which can be read from the manometer attached to the inflatable bag. Gradual deflation of the bag results in the sounds changing in quality until they become muffled and, finally, extinct. The muffling of sounds is known as phase IV and extinction as phase V of the blood pressure. Historically, there has been disagreement over whether phase IV or phase V more accurately reflects the true diastolic blood pressure; both can be recorded. When making comparisons between different patients or the effect of interventions on the blood pressure, standardization is required among observers at either phase IV or phase V (phase V is used and accepted by most clinicians).

Blood pressure fluctuates considerably in individuals during a 24-h period and in response to innumerable stimuli. This variability causes difficulty in defining the pathological condition of hypertension, and also in assessing the response to treatment. Continuous ambulatory 24-h blood pressure recording may be valuable in resolving this problem. Arrhythmias also cause difficulty in blood pressure recording: a beat-to-beat variation will occur in atrial fibrillation and other arrhythmias. An average measurement over a number of beats needs to be obtained for both systolic and diastolic pressure.

Slight variations in blood pressure between the two arms are not uncommon but differences in systolic pressure of 15 mmHg between the right and left arm suggest obstructive lesions in the aorta or the origins of the innominate and subclavian arteries. Bruits over such blood vessels in combination with pressure differences would support the possibility of stenotic lesions. Measurement of blood pressure in the legs tends to be more difficult than in the arms, particularly in large adults. A large cuff is required, placed over the mid-thigh region, and the blood pressure auscultated in the popliteal fossa with the patient lying prone. The normal systolic pressure in the legs is up to 20 mmHg higher than that in the arms; however, the pressure will be lower than that in the arms in patients who have coarctation of the aorta.

THE ARTERIAL PULSE

The quality of the arterial pulse which is palpated by the clinician is determined by several factors, including the rate of ejection of blood from the left ventricle and the stroke volume of the ventricle, the capacity and stiffness of the arterial system into which blood has been ejected, and pressure waves along the arterial system from the left ventricle and reflected backwards from the peripheral circulation. Thus, many pathological conditions will alter the quality of the arterial pulse and, conversely, abnormal qualities of the arterial pulse will provide important clues to the presence of underlying abnormalities in the cardiovascular system.[1]

TECHNIQUE OF EXAMINATION

Of all the pulses that can be palpated, the carotid pulse most closely represents the pulse recorded by catheterization in the central aorta.[2] It can best be felt with the patient lying supine propped up at a 45° angle. The head needs to be resting comfortably with the neck slightly extended. In this position, the carotid pulsation may be visible, particularly in patients with large left ventricular stroke volumes and rapid rates of rise and fall of carotid pressure (Corrigan's sign).[3] Palpation of the carotid pulse may best be carried out using the thumb; palpation provides information not only on the quality of the pulse but also on the heart rate and rhythm. The carotid pulse provides the most accurate impression of the volume and rate at which blood leaves the left ventricle, least modified by the capacity and compliance of the arterial system. Examination of more peripheral pulses may reveal obstructive or stenotic lesions in the arterial system, and in conjunction with examination of the skin provides information on peripheral vasodilatation or vasoconstriction. Auscultation over central arteries such as the carotid or femoral may reveal bruits due to areas of stenosis.

NORMAL ARTERIAL PULSE

The normal carotid pulse shows an initial rapid rate of rise corresponding to the normal rapid ejection of blood from the left ventricle, followed by a more gradual rise to a peak. The downstroke of the pulse is more gradual as the rate of blood flow into the periphery exceeds the rate of left ventricular ejection. The downstroke is interrupted by the dicrotic notch corresponding to aortic valve closure. Indirect recording of the carotid pulse can be made using a pulse transducer placed over the carotid artery. The resultant recording can be made simultaneously with a phonocardiogram and electrocardiogram to allow analysis of the timing of various events (Fig. 8.1). Thus, the dicrotic notch can be seen to follow aortic valve closure by 0.02–0.05 s due to a delay in pulse transmission. The onset of the upstroke of the carotid pulse tracing is normally 0.12–0.15 s after the onset of the QRS complex.

The pulse recording often shows an initial wave called the 'percussion' wave corresponding with initial peak ejection from the left ventricle, and a second 'tidal' wave representing reflection of pulses from the periphery. A small third wave follows the dicrotic notch. Some would prefer to substitute 'early systolic' for 'percussion', attributing it to the arrival of the impulse generated by ventricular ejection, 'late systolic' for 'tidal', representing the echo of the wave from the upper part of the body, and 'diastolic' for 'dicrotic', representing the echo from the lower part of the body.[4]

As the pulse wave moves from the central aorta towards the periphery, a variety of factors alters the characteristics of the pulse contour: the initial upstroke becomes steeper and the systolic summit increases in magnitude. Thus, the peripheral pulse is less useful than the carotid pulse in revealing alterations in left ventricular ejection or aortic valve function. It follows, therefore, that the clinician should focus attention on examination of the carotid pulse to obtain information about left ventricular and aortic valve function; examination of the peripheral pulses should be reserved for detection of peripheral vascular abnormalities (e.g. obstructive lesions).

ABNORMALITIES OF THE ARTERIAL PULSE

Although the clinician may detect various qualita-

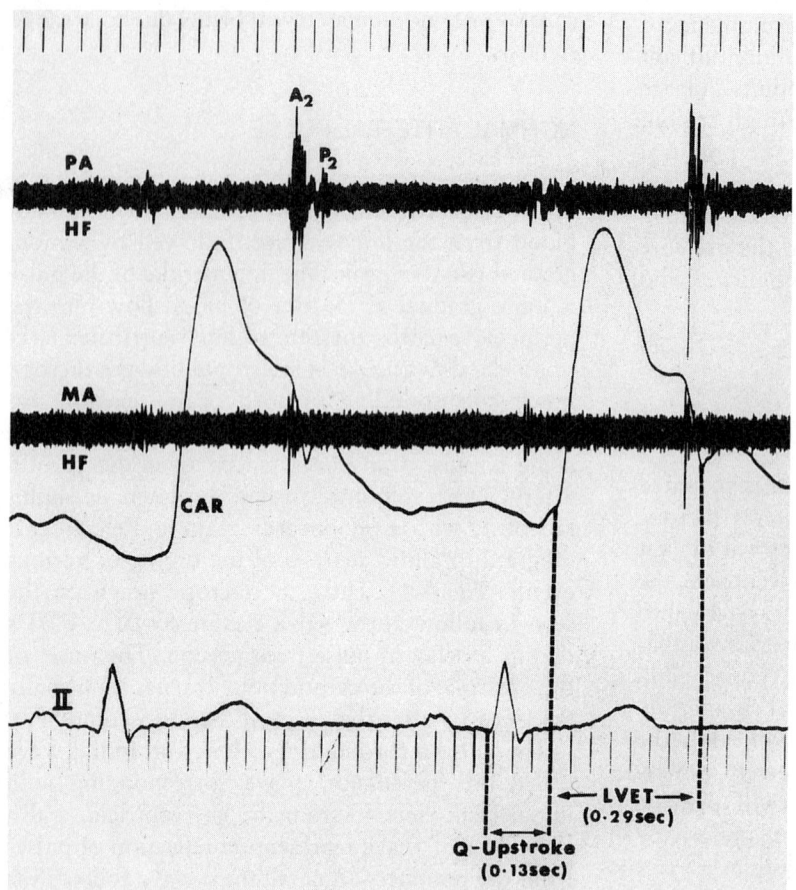

Fig. 8.1. Simultaneous phonocardiograms recorded in the pulmonary (PA) and mitral (MA) areas using high-frequency filters (HF) together with an indirect carotid artery recording and electrocardiogram in a normal individual. The onset of the carotid upstroke is 0.13 s after the Q wave on the electrocardiogram (lead II). The left ventricular ejection time (LVET) is 0.29 s. The dicrotic notch of the carotid tracing occurs slightly after the recorded aortic valve closure sound (A₂). Pulmonary valve closure (P₂) is also seen but only in the pulmonary area. Time-markers = 0.04 s.

tive abnormalities of the arterial pulse which provide information about underlying cardiovascular pathology, palpation of the pulse will not allow an estimate of the arterial pressure or left ventricular stroke volume to be made.

A slow upstroke to the carotid pulse indicates fixed obstruction to left ventricular emptying. This is the characteristic physical sign of significant aortic valve stenosis and the fibromuscular diaphragm of subaortic stenosis which is congenital in aetiology (Fig. 8.2). The slow upstroke distinguishes these patients from those with hypertrophic obstructive cardiomyopathy in which the carotid pulse is sharp in its upstroke (Fig. 8.3).[5] Fixed left ventricular outflow obstruction reduces the rate of rise of pressure in the aorta (although it is usually increased within the left ventricle) and prolongs the duration of left ventricular ejection. Indirect recordings of the carotid pulse enable the duration of left ventricular ejection to be measured (from the onset of arterial upstroke to the dicrotic notch—see Fig. 8.1) as well as the rate of rise of the pulse. Significant aortic stenosis is usually associated with

a measured slow rate of rise and prolongation of left ventricular ejection.[6,7] In some patients with severe aortic stenosis and reduced cardiac output, the carotid pulse may be impalpable or very difficult to feel.

A small, but not slow-rising, pulse which is difficult to feel (even though the upstroke is sharp) may be found in conditions associated with a reduced left ventricular stroke volume. Thus, it may occur in patients with acute heart failure due to myocardial infarction or in those with chronic heart failure due to dilated cardiomyopathy from any cause.

An abnormally sharp upstroke to the carotid pulse is observed in a variety of conditions associated with a hyperkinetic circulatory state (Fig. 8.4). In such conditions, left ventricular stroke volume is often increased with a reduction in peripheral vascular resistance and a wide pulse pressure. The pulse may be very obvious and bounding with a rapid upstroke to a high peak ('water-hammer pulse') and a rapid downstroke ('collapsing pulse'). Most patients will have both these characteristics

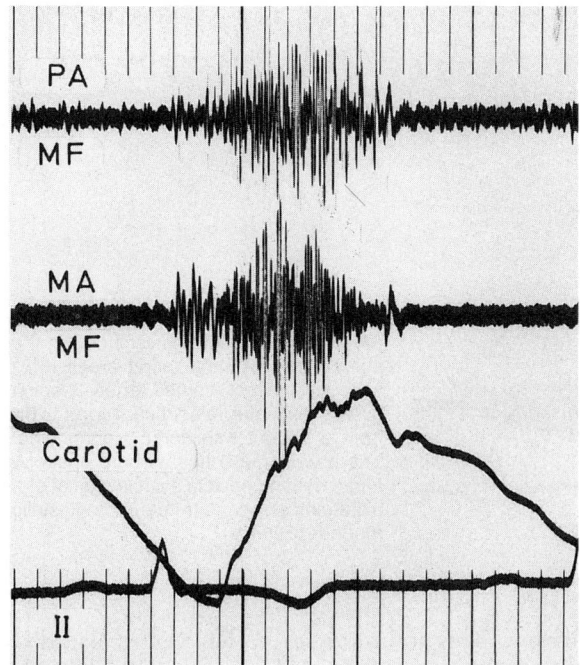

Fig. 8.2. Simultaneous phonocardiograms recorded in the pulmonary (PA) and mitral (MA) areas using medium-frequency filters (MF), indirect carotid artery recording and lead II of the electrocardiogram in a patient with aortic valve stenosis. The slow upstroke to the carotid pulse is seen (in contrast with Fig. 8.1) and the left ventricular ejection time is prolonged.

Peripheral vascular resistance is reduced when there is a run-off from the arterial system, as in aortic regurgitation, persistent ductus arteriosus, peripheral arteriovenous fistula or ruptured sinus of Valsalva. Conditions associated with hyperkinetic states and reduced peripheral resistance include pregnancy, anaemia, thyrotoxicosis, beriberi, cor pulmonale and fever. In all these conditions, the initial upstroke to the arterial pulse is sharp reflecting the rapid rate of ejection often of an increased left ventricular stroke volume. A subsequent decreased rate of ejection in systole together with a reduced peripheral resistance cause the systolic collapse of the pulse which may be further enhanced during diastole if there is a diastolic run-off from the arterial system as in aortic regurgitation.

Increased rate of initial emptying by the left ventricle without any significant alteration or even reduction in stroke volume may produce a sharp upstroke to the arterial pulse. This is a finding in hypertrophic obstructive cardiomyopathy and in 'left ventricular run-off' conditions such as mitral regurgitation and ventricular septal defect.[8] An increased stroke volume alone, as in slow heart rates, may also produce a sharp rise to the carotid pulse. The highest amplitudes of the sharp pulse will be found in conditions in which there is a large stroke volume, such as bradycardias and aortic regurgitation, whereas the lowest amplitudes will occur in conditions in which there is a small forward left ventricular stroke volume, such as mitral regurgitation.

which are exaggerated as the pulse wave is transmitted into the periphery. Thus, these abnormalities may be recognized more easily by palpating brachial or radial arteries rather than the carotids.

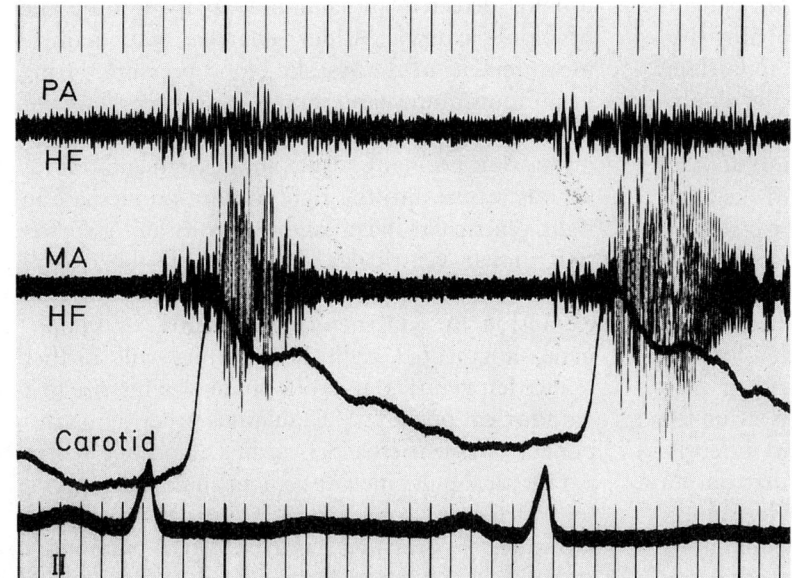

Fig. 8.3. Simultaneous high-frequency (HF) phonocardiograms from the pulmonary (PA) and mitral (MA) areas, indirect carotid artery recording and lead II of the electrocardiogram in a patient with hypertrophic obstructive cardiomyopathy. The rapid rate of rise of the carotid pulse (in contrast with Fig. 8.2) with a secondary 'hump' is seen.

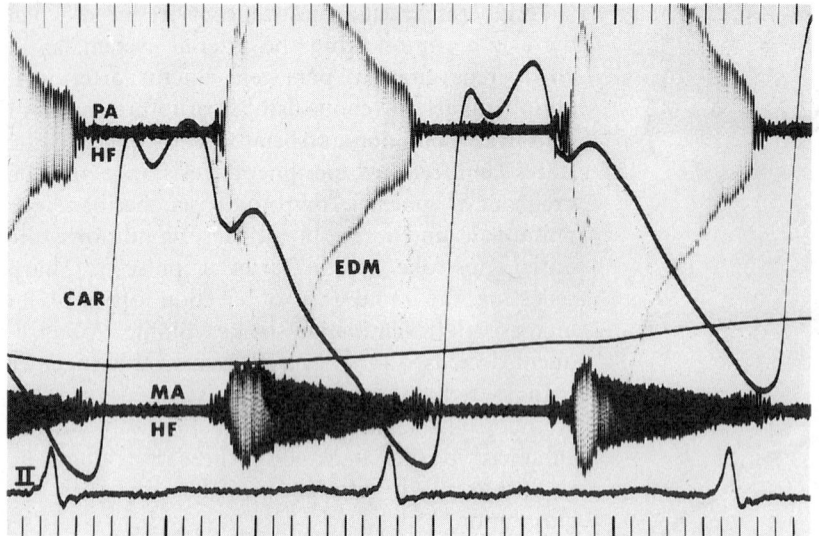

Fig. 8.4. Simultaneous high-frequency (HF) phonocardiograms recorded in the pulmonary (PA) and mitral areas (MA) with an indirect carotid artery tracing (CAR) and the electrocardiogram (II) from a patient with aortic regurgitation. The arterial pulse has a sharp upstroke and a second peak in systole typical of a bisferiens pulse. Note the early diastolic murmur (EDM).

OTHER ABNORMALITIES OF THE ARTERIAL PULSE

A bisferiens pulse is characterized by two systolic peaks best felt in the carotid pulse.[9,10] The first peak is due to a percussion (early systolic) wave of a large volume of blood rapidly ejected from the left ventricle; the second peak is due to a tidal (late systolic) wave as ventricular ejection is slowed and waves are reflected back from the periphery. The bisferiens pulse occurs in mixed aortic stenosis and regurgitation and in aortic regurgitation without stenosis (Fig. 8.4). A carotid pulse that has a sharp upstroke and a secondary wave or 'hump' preceding the dicrotic notch is sometimes recorded in patients with hypertrophic obstructive cardiomyopathy (Fig. 8.3), although in practice the clinician appreciates the initial sharp upstroke rather than the double beat.

A dicrotic pulse is a description given to another variety of pulse associated with two upstroke beats in each cardiac cycle.[11] It differs from the bisferiens pulse in that the second beat occurs in diastole after the dicrotic notch and not as two upstrokes in systole prior to the dicrotic notch. The dicrotic pulse may be seen in conditions in which a low left ventricular stroke volume is ejected into a high systemic vascular resistance: for example, acute left ventricular failure. It is said to occur also in febrile conditions associated with a normal cardiac output and presumably a low systemic vascular resistance.

Pulsus alternans is a description of alternating strong and weak pulses in a patient with sinus rhythm. This indicates severe left ventricular disease. Sometimes, alternate beats may not be felt at all. It needs to be distinguished from bigeminal rhythm in which alternate beats also vary in strength but the rhythm is not regular: each alternate beat is premature and weak with augmentation of the post-premature beat. Pulsus alternans is the result of alternation in left ventricular force of contraction in cardiac muscle probably reflecting disordered biochemistry.

A paradoxical pulse is an exaggeration of the normal (5–10 mmHg) fall in systolic blood pressure during inspiration (Fig. 8.5). If there is a marked fall in blood pressure during inspiration, it can be usually detected by a simple palpation of the brachial artery. Milder degrees may require measurement of the systolic blood pressure during inspiration and expiration. The mechanism of pulsus paradoxus is complex and controversial: inspiration normally results in an augmentation of venous return into the right atrium, an increase in right ventricular diastolic dimensions and a reduction in left ventricular dimension. If the overall capacity of the cardiac chambers is limited from expansion by constrictive pericarditis, or tamponade, augmented right heart filling will further reduce left ventricular stroke volume giving rise to a paradoxical pulse.[12–14] Conditions other than tamponade or constrictive pericarditis associated with a paradoxical pulse include asthma and emphysema[15] (in which there is marked respiratory fluctuation of intrapleural pressure) and massive pulmonary embolism.

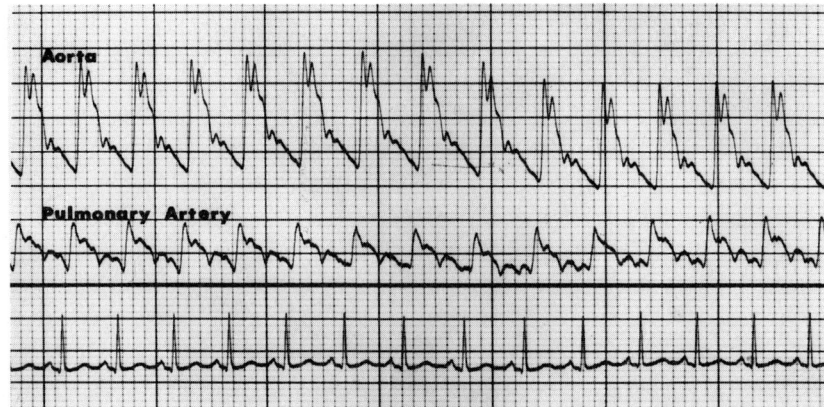

Fig. 8.5. Simultaneous aortic (upper) and pulmonary artery (lower) tracings together with the electrocardiogram in a patient with constrictive pericarditis. The fall in aortic pressure of about 20 mmHg occurs on inspiration as in pulsus paradoxus.

VARIATIONS IN PERIPHERAL PULSES

Palpation of carotid, brachial, radial, femoral, dorsalis pedis and posterior tibial pulses on both sides of the body may reveal abnormalities. Absence of a pulse indicates occlusion or severe narrowing of the artery or an anatomical variation. A pulse that is more difficult to feel (particularly by comparison with one on the other side) may indicate a proximal stenosis in the artery; there may be a bruit on auscultation over the artery to support this diagnosis. Narrowing or obstruction of an artery is usually due to atheroma but other pathologies such as aortic dissection involving proximal arterial compression will have the same effect.

A special reason for palpating peripheral pulses is to make the diagnosis of coarctation of the aorta.

Normally, the pulse wave arrives almost simultaneously at the radial and femoral arteries. In coarctation, the arrival of the pulse wave is delayed at the femoral artery and comparison of the radial and femoral pulses enables this delay in onset of upstroke to be readily appreciated (Fig. 8.6). Sometimes the femoral pulses may be impalpable or extremely difficult to feel in coarctation.

Supravalvular aortic stenosis is a lesion causing obstruction to left ventricular ejection, in which the pulses in the upper parts of the body may be asymmetric.[16] The localized supravalvular constriction may preferentially propagate a high-velocity jet into the innominate artery resulting in bounding pulses in the carotid and right arm. The left carotid and left arm pulses have a slow-rising upstroke and are more difficult to feel (Fig. 8.7). There may be a

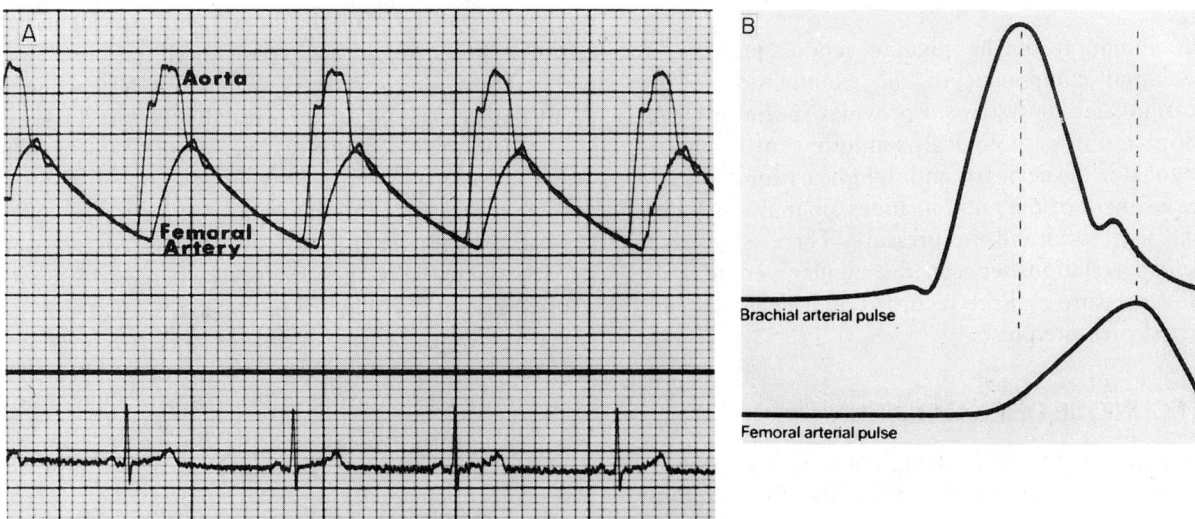

Fig. 8.6. (A) Pulses recorded in the aorta proximal to a coarctation and in the femoral artery together with the electrocardiogram. The systolic pressure difference is seen as well as the delay in onset of the upstroke of the femoral pulse. (B) Diagrammatic representation of simultaneous brachial and femoral arterial pulses in a patient with coarctation. The onset of the upstroke in the femoral pulse is delayed relative to the onset of the upstroke in the brachial pulse.

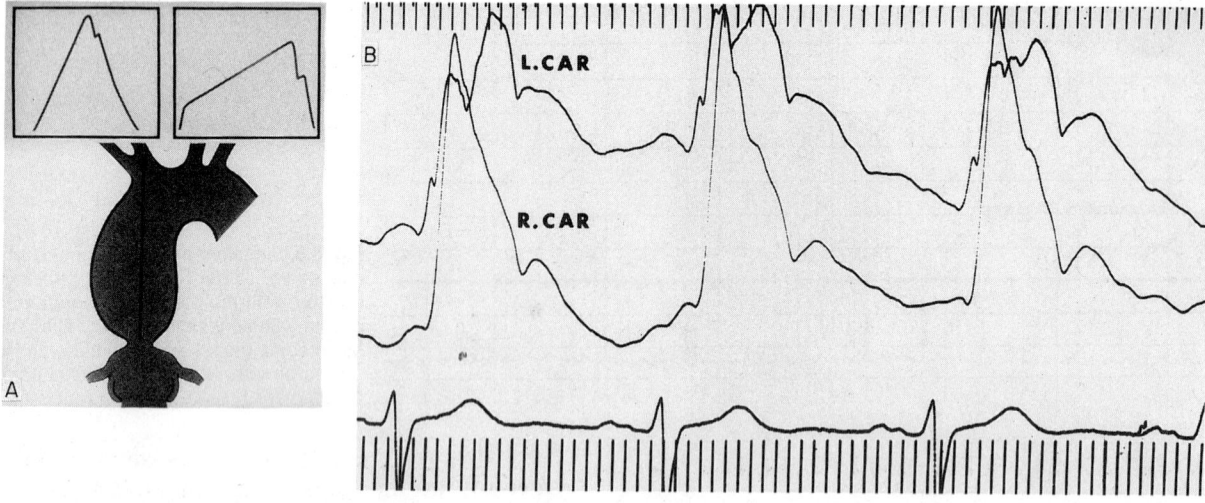

Fig. 8.7. (A) Diagrammatic representation of the right and left carotid pulses in supravalvular aortic stenosis. The right carotid pulse is sharp in upstroke, whereas the left is slow rising. (B) Superimposed indirect carotid artery recordings showing the left carotid artery (L.CAR) and right carotid artery (R.CAR) and the electrocardiogram from a patient with an aortic constriction between the innominate artery and the left carotid. The sharp upstroke on the right and the slower rise to a peak on the left can be seen.

higher systolic pressure in the right arm than in the left arm. Less frequently the anatomy of supravalvular aortic stenosis is such that the innominate orifice is bypassed by the jet stream so that the left carotid is sharp in its upstroke and bounding, while the right carotid is difficult to feel.

THE VENOUS PULSE

Examination of the jugular venous pulse is an essential component of the examination of the cardiovascular system; it provides special information about pathological conditions affecting the right side of the heart, and right heart function. The assessment of the pulse includes an analysis of both the waveform and the pressure. There is an excellent correlation between the jugular venous pulse and pressure and the recorded and measured right atrial pressure pulse.

TECHNIQUE OF EXAMINATION

The patient should be lying comfortably, propped up at an angle of 45° with the head slightly extended. Good illumination of the right side of the neck is essential. The internal jugular vein is examined because the pressure in the external jugular vein may not accurately reflect right atrial pressure. The right internal jugular vein is preferred

to the left as it is in a more direct line with the innominate vein and superior vena cava, whereas the left innominate vein may be kinked or compressed by normal structures, such as a dilated aorta. The right internal jugular vein is located deep in the neck behind the sternocleidomastoid muscle but the venous pulsation is transmitted readily to the skin surface where it is visible.

It may be difficult sometimes to distinguish venous pulsation in the neck from arterial pulsation. The normal points of distinction are:
1 venous pulsation is seen but not felt, whereas normal arterial pulsation is usually felt but not seen;
2 there are normally two peaks and two troughs within each cardiac cycle in the venous pulse whereas the arterial pulse has a single upstroke;
3 the venous pulse can be obliterated by compression at the root of the neck whereas this is not possible with visible arterial pulsation;
4 the jugular venous pressure may rise on abdominal compression and normally falls during inspiration, rising during expiration;
5 normal venous pulsation will disappear when the patient sits upright, whereas arterial pulsation remains unchanged.

It is normal to relate the height of the peak pressure in the venous pulse to the sternal angle. Thus, the upper limit of the normal height of the venous pressure is about 3–4 cm above the sternal angle (which is approximately a further 5 cm above

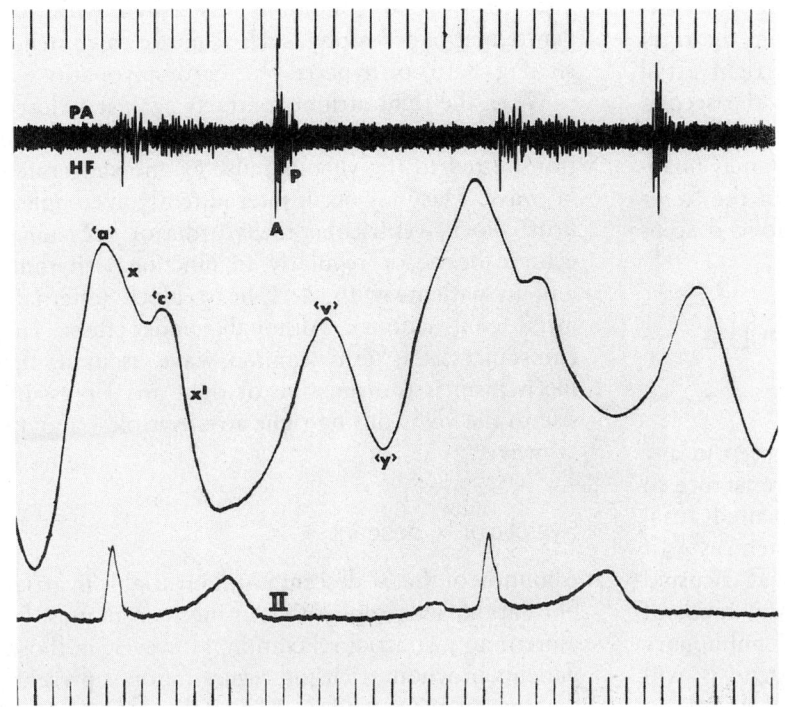

Fig. 8.8. Recording of the venous pulse in a normal individual simultaneously with a phonocardiogram and electrocardiogram. The 'a' wave follows the P wave of the electrocardiogram, the 'x' descent is interrupted by the 'c' wave with a following 'x¹' descent; the peak of the 'v' wave follows the second heart sound, while the 'y' descent would coincide with a third heart sound. PA–HF, Pulmonary area high-frequency phonocardiogram; A, aortic valve closure; P, pulmonary valve closure.

the mid-right atrium). Difficulty may be found in seeing the venous pulse if the pressure is very high or very low. If the patient is asked to sit upright instead of resting at 45°, a very high venous pressure pulse may become visible high in the neck, whereas if the patient lies supine or turns towards the left side when lying supine a low or normal venous pressure pulse may be seen more readily.

Graphic representation of the waveform of the venous pulse is made possible by the use of appropriate lightly held displacement transducers.[17] Such recording may complement visual inspection of the pulse, particularly when there is a tachycardia. Simultaneous recording of the electrocardiogram and phonocardiogram enables an accurate analysis of the waveform which relates excellently to the waveform recorded in the right atrial pressure pulse.

NORMAL WAVEFORM OF THE VENOUS PULSE

The normal visible waveform of the venous pulse consists of two peaks ('a' and 'v') and two troughs ('x' and 'y') with the first peak being normally dominant (Fig. 8.8). The normal initial venous upstroke is the 'a' wave. This is sharper in upstroke than the later 'v' wave and precedes the upstroke in the carotid pulse which can be palpated simul-

taneously on the left side of the neck as the venous pulse is observed on the right. The recorded 'a' wave follows the P wave of the electrocardiogram and precedes the QRS complex. The 'a' wave is due to venous distension during right atrial systole and is abolished in atrial fibrillation.

Following atrial systole, the venous pulse descends with atrial relaxation. Although usually not visible, the recorded 'systolic descent' following the 'a' wave is interrupted by a 'c' wave thought by some clinicians to be due to carotid artefact[18] and by others to be due to right ventricular contraction and forceful closure of the tricuspid valve.[17,19,20] The descent continues after the 'c' wave, probably as a result of downward displacement of the tricuspid valve ring as the right ventricle contracts. The relative contributions of atrial relaxation and downward movement of the tricuspid valve ring in producing the 'x' descent vary in different individuals and some authors have defined the descent as 'x' and 'x¹' according to the two different events.

The second venous upstroke is the 'v' wave resulting from increased distension of the veins and rise in right atrial pressure as the right atrium fills during ventricular systole. It tends to be later in systole in sinus rhythm than in atrial fibrillation when it occupies the whole of systole.

The second or 'y' descent of the venous pulse

begins as soon as the tricuspid valve opens. The descent continues as blood empties from the right atrium into the right ventricle and as right atrial pressure falls. The 'y' descent follows the second heart sound ('diastolic descent'). Simultaneous auscultation with venous pulse observation may facilitate the identification and distinction of the 'y' or diastolic descent from the 'x' or systolic descent which precedes the second heart sound.

ABNORMALITIES OF THE VENOUS PULSE

'a' Wave

An abnormally large 'a' wave may be seen in any condition in which there is increased resistance to right atrial emptying and hence augmented atrial systole. This may occur in tricuspid stenosis[21] (if sinus rhythm is present), or obstruction at tricuspid valve level by right atrial myxoma. Any cause of right ventricular hypertrophy, such as pulmonary hypertension (Fig. 8.9) or pulmonary stenosis, will also cause augmentation of right atrial systole in order to empty blood into the abnormally stiff right ventricle, and hence an increased 'a' wave in the venous pulse. However, in conditions with a coexisting ventricular septal defect (e.g. Fallot's tetralogy) the 'a' wave is not increased—an important distinguishing physical sign.[18] A large 'a' wave may

also be seen in conditions associated with left ventricular hypertrophy, such as aortic valve stenosis (Fig. 8.10) or hypertrophic cardiomyopathy.

When the right atrium contracts against a closed tricuspid valve, the increase in pressure will be transmitted to the venous pulse as an exaggerated 'a' wave. This may occur intermittently in complete heart block, ventricular tachycardia or occasional ectopic beats, or regularly in junctional rhythms and in patients with 2 : 1 heart block (alternate atrial contractions). Although, under these circumstances, the term 'cannon wave' is used, the mechanism is transmission of right atrial pressure rise to the veins during right atrial systole—a giant 'a' wave.

Systolic or 'x' descent

Abolition of the 'x' descent is not invariable in atrial fibrillation. This implies that its mechanism must be more than just atrial relaxation. However, in those patients in whom tricuspid regurgitation is present, the large 'v' wave tends to occupy the earlier part of ventricular systole and obliterates all of the systolic descent.

A dominant systolic descent of the venous pulse is an important physical sign in patients with cardiac

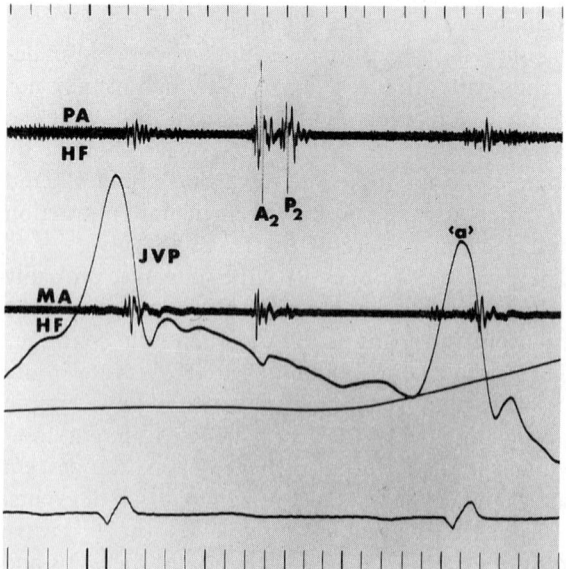

Fig. 8.9. Simultaneous high-frequency (HF) phonocardiograms in pulmonary (PA) and mitral (MA) areas, jugular venous pulse tracing (JVP) and electrocardiogram in a patient with primary pulmonary hypertension. The tall 'a' wave in the venous pulse is seen as well as wide splitting of the second heart sound. A_2, aortic valve closure; P_2, pulmonary valve closure.

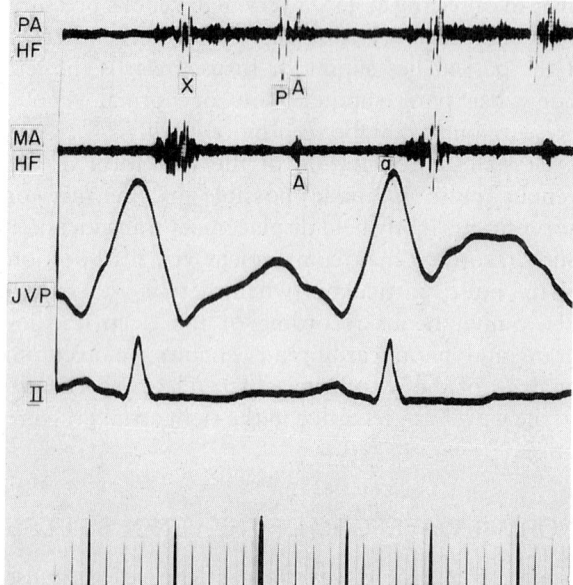

Fig. 8.10. Simultaneous high-frequency phonocardiograms in the pulmonary (PA–HF) and mitral (MA–HF) areas together with the jugular venous pulse (JVP) and lead II of the electrocardiogram in a patient with severe aortic stenosis. The large dominant 'a' wave is seen. (Note also reversed splitting of the second heart sound and an ejection sound.) X, ejection sound; P, pulmonary valve closure; A, aortic valve closure.

tamponade or in those cases of constrictive pericarditis where the myocardium is not significantly involved in the process.[22] In these situations, the descent is independent of atrial systole, dominating the venous pulse even in atrial flutter or fibrillation (Fig. 8.11). It may be explained by postulating that the moment in the cardiac cycle when the intrapericardial contents are at a minimum is during ventricular systole, and it is at this time that the veins can best empty into the right atrium.

'v' Wave

Exaggeration of the 'v' wave is the hallmark of tricuspid regurgitation (Fig. 8.12A). The more severe the regurgitation, the earlier the ascent of the 'v' wave during ventricular systole so that the venous pulse resembles the right ventricular systolic pressure pulse. In these circumstances, the 'v' wave may be aptly termed a 'systolic' wave in the venous pulse. Such a striking ascent of the venous pulse with a large excursion is readily visible in the neck and may cause movement of the earlobe. The wave may be palpable and cause confusion with arterial pulsation.

Diastolic or 'y' descent

A rapid 'y' descent is a feature of patients with tricuspid regurgitation (Fig. 8.12b). It represents the abnormally rapid inflow of blood from the right atrium into the right ventricle. If tricuspid stenosis is present the descent will be slow as right atrial emptying is obstructed: this physical sign in a patient with tricuspid regurgitation and mitral valve disease may provide a clue that there is organic (rheumatic) disease of the tricuspid valve as opposed to functional tricuspid regurgitation. In the absence of tricuspid stenosis, factors that influence the rate of right atrial emptying and right ventricular filling include the diastolic compliance of the myocardium and pericardium, the rate of ventricular relaxation and the end-systolic volume of the ventricle. Thus, a steep 'y' descent is seen in a variety of conditions (including coronary artery disease, and restrictive and dilated cardiomyopathy) in which there is myocardial dysfunction and an elevated venous pressure. In constrictive pericarditis with significant involvement of the myocardium, the 'y' descent is dominant (Fig. 8.13) in contrast to cardiac tamponade or pericardial constriction without significant myocardial involvement. The rapid diastolic collapse of the venous pulse is usually associated with an audible sound in early diastole coinciding with the nadir of the 'y' descent if simultaneous phonocardiograms and venous pulse tracings are recorded (Fig. 8.12A). If such a sound is clearly audible, it may be inferred that the dominant descent in the venous pulse is diastolic and not systolic. This finding has important therapeutic implications: if the 'y' descent is dominant and a diastolic sound present, pericardiectomy for con-

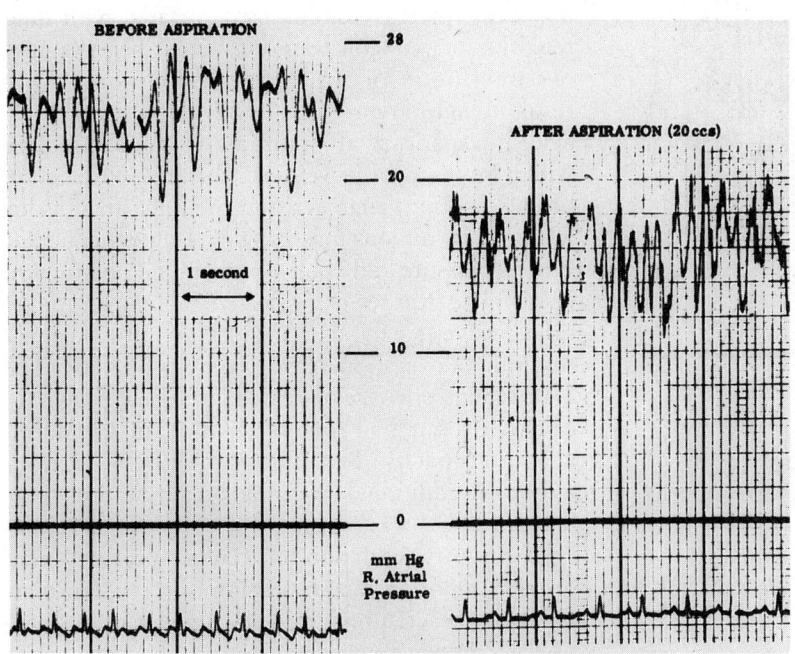

Fig. 8.11. Right atrial pressure recordings before and after aspiration of 20 ml of fluid in a patient with cardiac tamponade. Prior to aspiration, the patient is in atrial flutter, and the elevated right atrial pressure shows a dominant systolic descent. The relief of tamponade coincides with a reduction in right atrial pressure and a return to sinus rhythm.

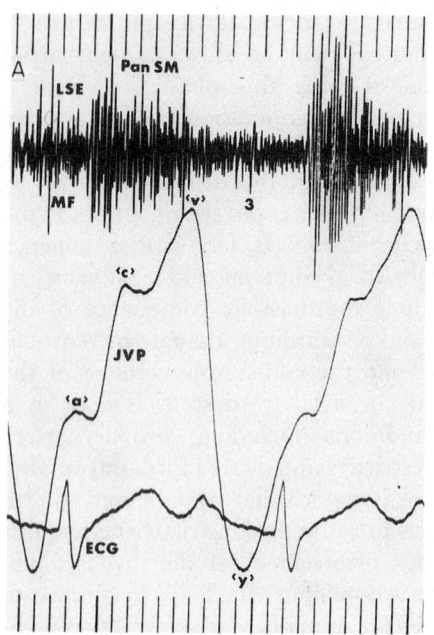

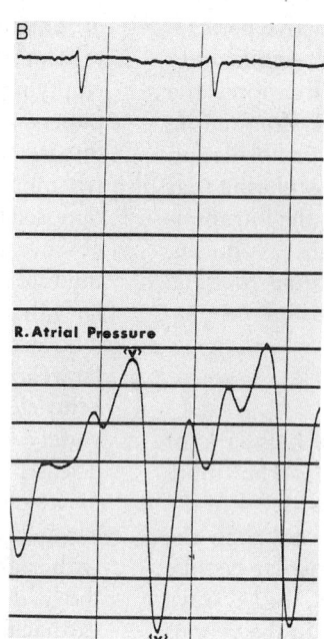

Fig. 8.12. (A) Simultaneous phonocardiogram at the left sternal edge (LSE) using medium-frequency filter (MF), jugular venous pulse recording (JVP) and electrocardiogram in a patient with tricuspid regurgitation. The dominance of the 'v' wave is seen as well as the nadir of the 'y' descent coinciding with a third heart sound (3). The 'a' and 'c' waves in the venous pulse are recorded; there is a pan-systolic murmur (Pan SM) in the phonocardiogram. (B) Right atrial pressure trace and electrocardiogram in a patient with severe tricuspid regurgitation. Note the deep 'y' descent as in (A).

strictive pericarditis is unlikely to be useful; if the venous pulse shows a dominant systolic descent and the diastolic sound is absent, the clinical diagnosis may be tamponade (requiring relief), or constrictive

pericarditis which may be usefully improved by pericardiectomy.

ABNORMALITIES OF THE VENOUS PRESSURE

Variations in the circulating blood volume or the capacity of the venous bed will cause variations in the height of the venous or right atrial pressure. Thus, conditions causing hypovolaemia or venodilatation, such as dehydration or excessive use of diuretics, will result in abnormally low venous pressure, whereas conditions associated with fluid retention or venoconstriction, such as heart failure, overtransfusion or acute glomerulonephritis, will result in high venous pressures. Increased intrathoracic, intrapericardial or intra-abdominal pressure will raise the jugular venous pressure. Obstruction of the superior vena cava and the right atrium (for instance, by tumour masses) will elevate the jugular venous pressure and abolish pulsation if obstruction is complete. Causes of a selective increase in the 'a' or 'v' wave, such as tricuspid valve disease, may result in an overall increase in venous pressure. The high venous pressure of heart failure may be mainly caused by salt and water retention in a reduced venous capacity bed due to vasoconstriction, although additional tricuspid regurgitation may play a part.

Respiratory variation in venous pressure may provide important diagnostic information. Normally, intrathoracic pressure decreases during inspiration, increasing venous return from the veins to the

Fig. 8.13. Right atrial pressure recording in a patient with constrictive pericarditis and extensive myocardial involvement in atrial fibrillation. The dominant 'y' descent is seen in the elevated right atrial pressure.

right atrium: thus, the venous pressure falls in inspiration and rises during expiration. Patients with constrictive pericarditis or with tamponade and some with severe myocardial failure show a rise in venous pressure during inspiration (Kussmaul's sign)[23]—the opposite of the normal response. (By contrast, the so-called paradoxical arterial pulse is an exaggeration of the normal arterial pressure response to inspiration.) The mechanism of Kussmaul's sign may be a rise in intrapericardial pressure obstructing venous return to the heart caused by the effect of inspiration distorting the pericardial 'box'.

PALPATION OF THE PRECORDIUM

Palpation of the precordium provides limited diagnostic information about underlying cardiac abnormalities. The location of the apical impulse or the point of maximal impulse provides less information than the quality of the impulse. Usually, the apical impulse represents activity by the left ventricle although this may be distorted and influenced by the right ventricle, particularly if it is dilated (as in an atrial septal defect). Pulsation may be felt in areas other than the apex; movement at the lower left sternal edge may represent abnormal right ventricular activity or systolic expansion of the left atrium as in chronic severe mitral regurgitation. Occasionally, abnormal right atrial activity may produce movement at the lower sternal edge. Rarely, abnormal pulsation of a dilated pulmonary artery may be felt in the region of the second left intercostal space.

TECHNIQUE OF PALPATING AND RECORDING THE APICAL IMPULSE

It is frequently impossible to feel the apical impulse in a normal individual lying supine, propped up at an angle of 45°, whereas the impulse can usually be felt if the individual turns to the left, 45° or more, and lies flat. In a normal individual lying in such a position, the apical impulse is felt as a fairly circumscribed movement of an intercostal space relative to the surrounding ribs. In most individuals, irrespective of their weight, a point of maximal impulse can be defined in this way. The limiting factor for feeling an impulse is rigidity of the intercostal space prohibiting the transmission of cardiac movement and vibration.

Recording of the apical impulse elucidates the findings of palpation. The graphic representation of apical movement is known as the apex cardiogram and is normally obtained by placing the centre of a transducer over the point of maximal impulse while the rim of the transducer rests on the adjoining ribs. Thus, movement of the intercostal space displaces the diaphragm of the transducer. Similar recordings can be made in other areas of the precordium where movement is apparent to the clinician.

THE NORMAL IMPULSE AND APEX CARDIOGRAM

The normal palpable apical impulse consists of a single brief brisk outward movement at the point of maximal impulse with each cardiac cycle. If such an impulse is recorded it will be seen to consist of several outward and inward movements, only one of which is obvious to palpation. It has to be recognized that the point of maximal impulse on the precordium is not the anatomical apex of the left ventricle but a point above the apex: this explains why the impulse moves outwards during isometric contraction at a time when the ventricle assumes a more spherical shape, with the anatomical apex rotating and moving away from the chest wall, but a point above it moving towards the chest wall.[24]

Following the P wave of a simultaneous electrocardiogram, there is a small outward movement reflecting the inflow of blood into the left ventricle during left atrial systole ('a' wave).[1,25] This movement is abolished in atrial fibrillation. Shortly after the Q wave of the electrocardiogram (about 0.02 s), there is a much larger and brisker outward movement which is the only aspect of the impulse that can normally be appreciated. The onset of upstroke of this systolic wave corresponds to the onset of the upstroke of the left ventricular pressure pulse.[26,27] The upstroke includes the period of isometric contraction and normally terminates at the 'E' point, which occurs approximately at the onset of left ventricular ejection. Subsequently, movement is mainly inward as ventricular volume diminishes. Much more rapid inward movement occurs around the time of the second heart sound reaching a nadir or 'O' point. The 'O' point coincides with the nadir of the left ventricular pressure pulse.[27] Following the 'O' point, outward movement re-commences and terminates at the end of the rapid filling wave: this moment (or 'F' point) coincides with the normal third heart sound. Finally, prior to atrial systole, there is a slow filling phase (Fig. 8.14).

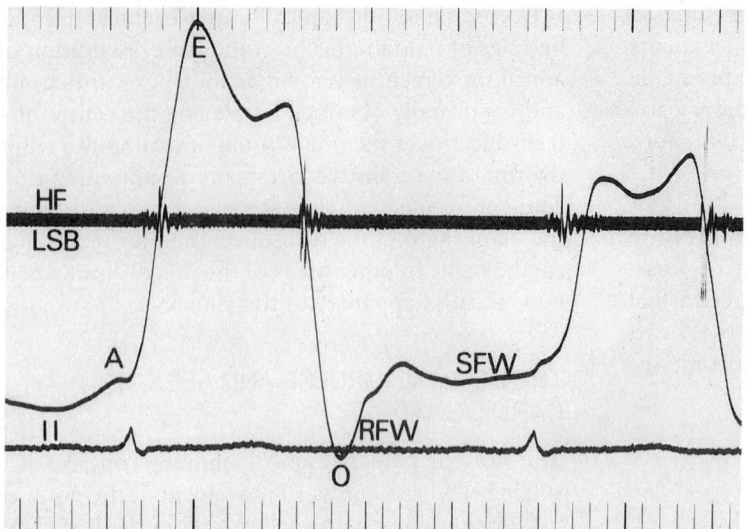

Fig. 8.14. Simultaneous apex cardiogram, high-frequency phonocardiogram, at the left sternal border (HF–LSB), and lead II of the electrocardiogram. The 'a' wave, 'E' point, 'O' point, rapid filling wave (RFW) and slow filling wave (SFW) are seen.

ABNORMALITIES OF THE APICAL IMPULSE

The 'a' wave

Augmentation of left atrial contraction results in an exaggeration, and often peaking, of the 'a' wave of the apex cardiogram. This may be felt as an additional separate outward movement from the normal single systolic outward movement. It is the most frequent explanation for feeling a 'double' apical impulse. This is a very valuable physical sign because it indicates that there is an underlying abnormality of the left ventricle which renders it abnormally stiff and results in augmentation of the force of left atrial contractions.[28–30] As patients with abnormalities of left ventricular function are very frequently seen in clinical practice, a 'double'

apical impulse may be the most commonly found abnormal physical sign in the examination of the cardiovascular system. The peak of the exaggerated 'a' wave of the apex cardiogram coincides with a fourth heart sound recorded by phonocardiography (Fig. 8.15). However, as the vibrations that produce these abnormalities occur at low frequencies, it may be easier to feel a 'double' impulse than it is to hear a fourth heart sound—the clinical implication is the same.

Because augmented atrial contraction is the mechanism, sinus rhythm is an essential requirement for a 'double' apical impulse. Although the sign indicates a stiff left ventricle, it cannot be used to distinguish between the causes of the stiffness, which include left ventricular hypertrophy from left ventricular outflow obstruction or systemic hyper-

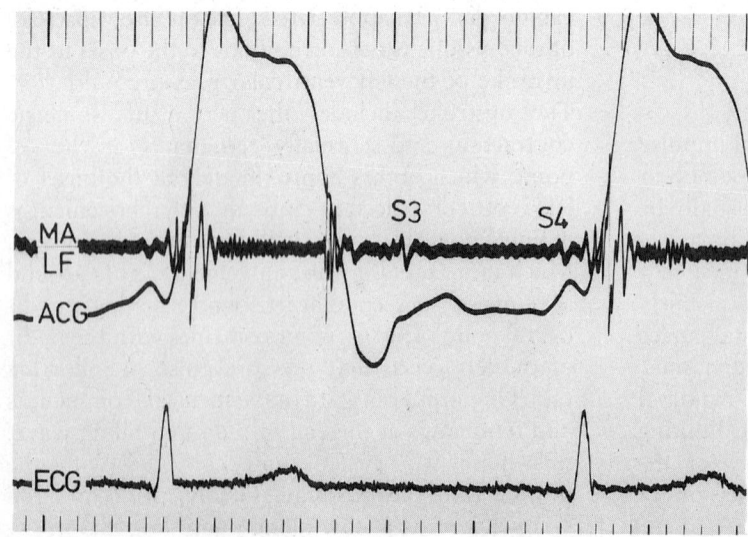

Fig. 8.15. Simultaneous apex cardiogram (ACG) and low-frequency mitral area (MA–LF) phonocardiogram and electrocardiogram. The peak of the 'a' wave in the ACG coincides with a fourth heart sound (S4), while the end of the rapid filling wave coincides with the third heart sound (S3).

tension, hypertrophic cardiomyopathy, left ventricular damage from ischaemic heart disease or dilated cardiomyopathy. Absence of the 'a' wave in the apex cardiogram is inevitable with atrial fibrillation, and the 'a' wave is diminished in mitral stenosis.

Systolic outward movement

Although the location of the apical impulse provides little useful information, the quality of the impulse gives some clues to the underlying pathophysiological disturbance affecting the left ventricle. The location of the impulse does not provide reliable information on heart size; this can be more readily obtained by plain chest radiography and echocardiography.

Three types of systolic outward movement can be palpated: normal, hyperdynamic and sustained (Fig. 8.16).[31] A normal outward movement implies

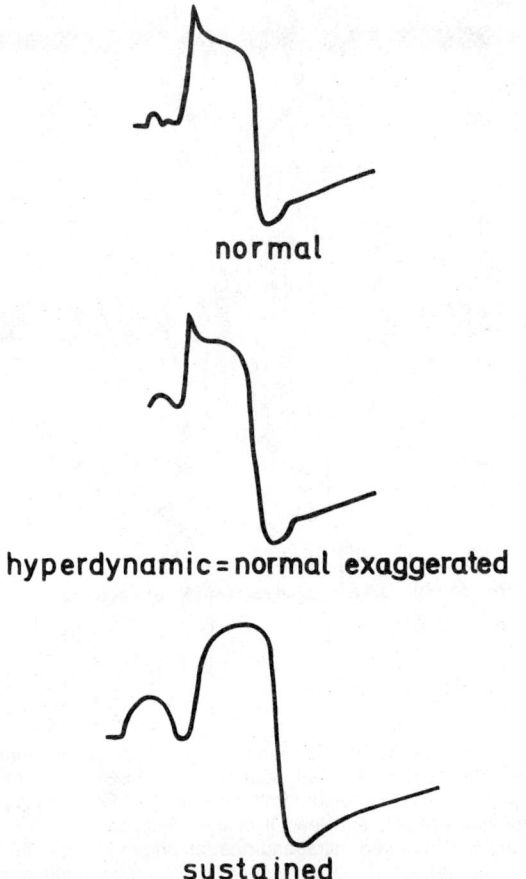

normal

hyperdynamic = normal exaggerated

sustained

Fig. 8.16. Diagrammatic representation of the three types of cardiac impulse: normal, hyperdynamic and sustained. Note the exaggerated 'a' wave which usually accompanies a sustained impulse.

no significant derangement with respect to pressure or volume characteristics of the left ventricle. A hyperdynamic impulse is characterized as an exaggerated normal impulse: the outward movement is brisker and larger than normal but it immediately falls away from the palpating finger after the 'E' point of the apex cardiogram, just as the normal impulse does. A hyperdynamic impulse implies that there is an increase in stroke volume of the left ventricle and the ejection fraction is preserved. Thus, a hyperdynamic impulse will be found in chronic severe mitral or aortic regurgitation or in hyperkinetic states such as hyperthyroidism.

A sustained outward movement is one in which the palpating finger does not fall inwards after the initial outward movement. The initial outward movement tends to be slower in reaching its outward limit by comparison with a normal or hyperdynamic impulse. The overall outward excursion tends to be less than that in a hyperdynamic impulse. Such an impulse is frequently accompanied by an exaggerated 'a' wave in the apex cardiogram, and consequently on palpation it is not only sustained but double. The apex cardiogram shows loss of the normal 'E' point (Fig. 8.17). The sustained outward movement is felt in conditions associated with a pressure-loaded left ventricle (e.g. aortic stenosis or hypertension) or hypertrophic cardiomyopathy and also in conditions in which the left ventricle is dilated, but has a reduced ejection fraction, such as dilated cardiomyopathy, or in which the ventricles are damaged by ischaemic heart disease.

The rapid filling wave

The rapid filling wave is rarely felt as a separate outward movement in early diastole. The apex cardiogram shows that it is abrupt cessation and immediate inward movement at the height of the rapid filling wave which is most frequently associated with an audible third heart sound (Fig. 8.18). Occasionally, in such circumstances, the peak of the rapid filling wave can be palpated; this is most likely to occur either in normal young individuals or in patients with chronic severe pure mitral regurgitation who have intact left ventricular systolic function. Unlike the fourth heart sound of left ventricular dysfunction which can be readily palpated as a 'double' impulse, the third heart sound associated with left ventricular disease and heart failure is virtually never felt as an abnormal rapid filling wave.

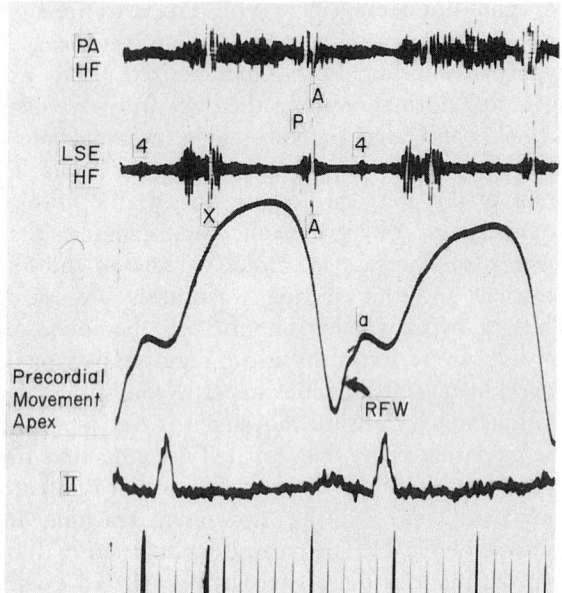

Fig. 8.17. Simultaneous high-frequency (HF) phonocardiograms in the pulmonary area (PA) and left sternal edge (LSE), apex cardiogram and lead II of the electrocardiogram in a patient with severe aortic stenosis. There is a peaked 'a' wave and sustained outward movement in the apex cardiogram with a preserved rapid filling wave (RFW). The 'E' point is absent. A fourth heart sound (4) coincides with the peak of the 'a' wave, and in addition an aortic ejection sound (X) and reversed splitting of the second heart sound [pulmonary valve closure (P) preceding aortic valve closure (A)] are seen.

Precordial movement at the left sternal edge

In normal adults, there is no appreciable movement of the precordium apart from that of the apex (described above). In children, however, movement can often be felt at the lower left sternal edge consisting of a brief outward non-sustained lift which has been thought to represent right ventricular activity.[32]

Abnormalities of right ventricular function are associated with movement at the left sternal edge in children and adults. Careful analysis of such movement, which can be either felt (with the patient supine) or recorded using identical equipment to that employed to record the apical impulse, provides diagnostic information regarding underlying right ventricular pathophysiology.[33] A marked exaggeration of outward movement, a hyperdynamic impulse, implies an increased stroke volume and a dilated right ventricle as in an atrial septal defect. A sustained outward movement is usually associated with right ventricular hypertrophy from pressure-loading such as pulmonary stenosis[34] or pulmonary hypertension. The lesion must be severe and long-standing for such changes to be present. In a way

analogous to the 'double' impulse of the stiff left ventricle, a separate outward thrust discrete from the sustained systolic outward movement can be felt at the left sternal edge in patients with right ventricular hypertrophy. The recording of precordial movement at the left sternal edge of such a patient will show a large 'a' wave due to the enhanced right atrial contraction.

Movement at the left sternal edge in Fallot's tetralogy is unlike that in pulmonary valve stenosis or pulmonary hypertension, even though right ventricular hypertrophy is present in all of these conditions. The movement is brief, not exaggerated, and not double. Just as the 'a' wave in the venous pulse is not exaggerated in Fallot's tetralogy when compared with that in pulmonary stenosis with

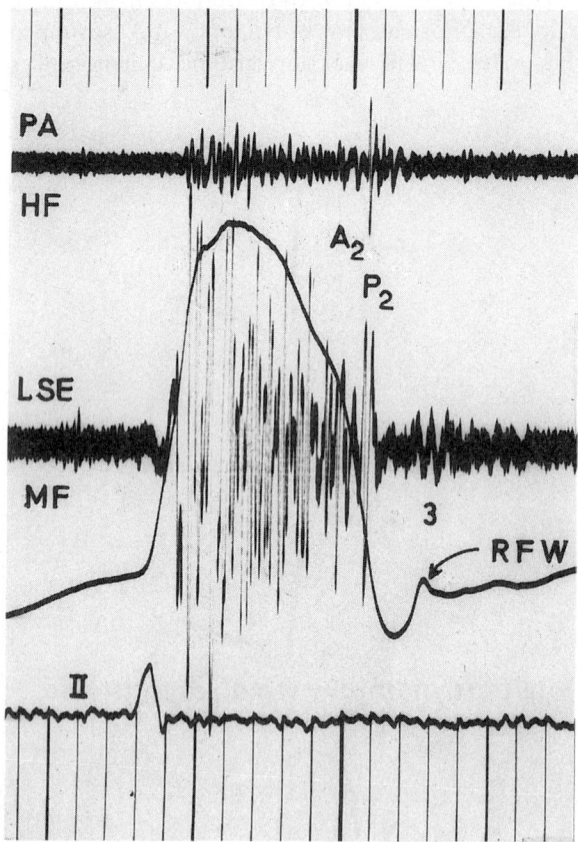

Fig. 8.18. Simultaneous phonocardiograms in the pulmonary area (PA) and at the left sternal edge (LSE) using high-frequency (HF) and medium-frequency (MF) filters with an apex cardiogram (ACG) and lead II of the electrocardiogram in a patient with ruptured mitral chordae tendineae in atrial fibrillation. The peaked rapid filling wave (RFW), coinciding with a third heart sound (3), is seen. There is an additional pansystolic murmur, and pulmonary valve closure (P_2) is louder than aortic valve closure (A_2) in the PA because of pulmonary hypertension. Note the absence of the 'a' wave in the ACG due to atrial fibrillation.

intact ventricular septum, the explanation for the difference is thought to be the run-off through the ventricular septal defect in Fallot's tetralogy.

Patients with severe, longstanding pulmonary hypertension may have striking dilatation of the central pulmonary arteries. Pulsation in such an artery may be felt high up the left sternal edge. The arterial nature of such pulsation can be determined by recordings that show a delay in the onset of the outward movement or upstroke in relation to the electrocardiographic Q wave by comparison with movement associated with a ventricle, which is much earlier.

In chronic severe mitral regurgitation, systolic outward movement may be felt or recorded at the left sternal edge representing the systolic expansion of dilated left atrium situated centrally and posteriorly moving the front of the chest wall. The systolic expansion peaks late in systole which if recorded will distinguish it from the sustained outward movement of right ventricular hypertrophy.

Left ventricular aneurysm

A ventricular aneurysm may sometimes be felt as a sustained outward bulge in different areas of the precordium depending on its location. An anterolateral or apical aneurysm may be felt best at the apex, but an anterior aneurysm may be felt several centimetres away from the apex. Some patients with dyskinetic left ventricles may have two distinct areas of rocking movement separated by several centimetres. As in other abnormalities of left ventricular function, patients with left ventricular aneurysm will have a palpable 'a' wave, and thus a double apical impulse.

Palpable sounds and murmurs

Heart sounds due to valve closure or, rarely, to valve opening, if sufficiently loud and having the appropriate frequency characteristics, may be palpated over the precordium. The 'tapping' apex of mitral stenosis represents a palpable mitral valve closure sound, whereas pulmonary valve closure in a dilated pulmonary artery with pulmonary hypertension may be felt in the second left intercostal space. Similarly, loud aortic valve closure sounds (A_2) may be felt and need to be distinguished from pulmonary valve closure (P_2) by recording the phonocardiogram and carotid pulse tracing; it is possible to identify A_2 and P_2 by their relationship to the dicrotic notch. Occasionally, a pulmonary ejection sound can be palpated in the second left intercostal space, or an aortic ejection sound at the apex.

If a murmur is sufficiently loud and contains certain low-frequency vibrations, it may be palpable as well as audible. A typical example is the systolic thrill in non-rheumatic primary mitral regurgitation. Little additional clinical diagnostic information can be derived from palpable thrills that cannot already be obtained from analysis of the murmur (see below).

AUSCULTATION OF THE HEART

A variety of vibrations throughout the cardiac cycle are generated by various structures within the heart and transmitted to the chest wall. These vibrations occur at various dominant frequencies which can be appreciated by the ear when transmitted through a stethoscope. The lowest frequency vibrations may be audible, but they are better appreciated as movement, whereas the highest frequencies are easier to hear. The stethoscope should fit the ears comfortably and the tubing should be thick walled and reasonably short. High-frequency sounds are best transmitted using a rigid diaphragm attachment applied to the chest; a gently applied bell attachment transmits low-frequency sounds (such as a third or fourth heart sound) best. Thus, the stethoscope should have both a bell and a diaphragm.

In order to appreciate all the possible auscultatory events within a cardiac cycle, the stethoscope has to be applied to several areas throughout the precordium. The low-frequency vibrations of a left-sided fourth or third heart sound or the mid-diastolic murmur of mitral stenosis can best be appreciated by using the bell and listening in the region of the cardiac apex ('mitral area'). The high-frequency aortic ejection sound or pan-systolic murmur of rheumatic mitral regurgitation will also be heard best in this area using the diaphragm. Murmurs originating from the tricuspid valve will be heard best at the lower sternal edge ('tricuspid area'), as will a right ventricular third or fourth heart sound. The two high-frequency components of the second heart sound are usually best heard using the diaphragm in the left second intercostal space ('pulmonary area'); the murmur of aortic stenosis may be best heard to the right of the sternum in the second intercostal space ('aortic area'). Although such traditional auscultatory areas exist, it cannot be assumed that because a murmur is heard best in the 'mitral' area it is necessarily of mitral origin. The same observation applies to all the other areas. The information derived from the location of murmurs is much less reliable in denoting the origin of the murmur than its timing. Thus, a pan-systolic murmur can be due to only mitral or tricuspid regurgitation or a ventricular septal defect, whereas an early diastolic murmur can be due only to aortic or pulmonary regurgitation, and a mid-diastolic murmur can be due to actual or relative mitral or tricuspid stenosis. Nevertheless, the entire precordial area may need to be scanned in order to hear individual heart sounds.

The optimum conditions for hearing the various auscultatory events are for the patient to be relaxed in a quiet room with a clinician practised at cardiac auscultation using a reliable stethoscope. The clinician should first auscultate with the patient supine, propped up at 45° and breathing quietly. Subsequently, the patient should be asked to turn towards the left in order to hear better the events audible at the cardiac apex. The experienced clinician will listen to each part of the cardiac cycle in turn, distinguishing brief events (heart sounds) from longer vibrations (a murmur). Events at the time of the first heart sound should be analysed first: there may be a single high-frequency sound (usually mitral valve closure), two high-frequency sounds (either separate mitral and tricuspid valve closure best heard at the left sternal edge, or mitral valve closure followed by an ejection sound) or a low-frequency sound as well as a high-frequency sound (a fourth sound followed by mitral valve closure). A high-frequency sound may be noticed in mid or late systole ('mid-systolic click'). The clinician should listen carefully in the pulmonary area to hear the two components of the second heart sound, both of high-frequency, and determine the relative intensities of the two components, and the variation of interval between them in relation to respiration ('splitting' of the second heart sound). Finally, an additional sound may be noticed after the second heart sound, which may be of high frequency (mitral or tricuspid opening snap) or low frequency (third heart sound) (Fig. 8.19).

The clinician should then listen for murmurs particularly noting their timing; first in systole (ejection, early, late or pan-systolic), then in diastole (early or mid-diastolic with pre-systolic accentuation) or, if the murmur appears to persist from

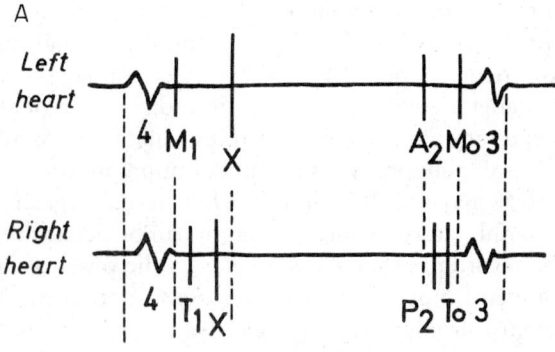

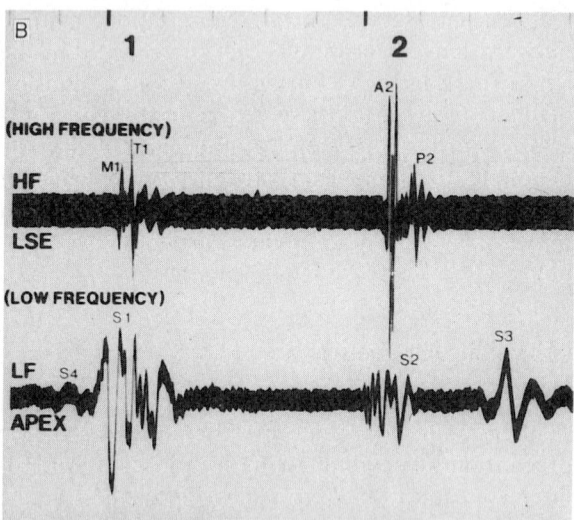

Fig. 8.19. (A) Diagrammatic representation of heart sounds originating from the left and right heart. Fourth (4) and third (3) heart sounds may originate from both sides as may ejection sounds (X). Mitral valve closure (M_1), tricuspid valve closure (T_1), aortic valve closure (A_2), pulmonary valve closure (P_2), tricuspid valve opening (To) and mitral valve opening (Mo) are shown in relation to each other with respect to normal timing. (B) Phonocardiograms recorded at the left sternal edge (LSE) using high-frequency filters (HF) and at the apex using low-frequency filters (LF) in a normal young individual. The components of the first heart sound (S1) are seen to contain an initial low frequency (S4) and two high frequencies—mitral (M1) and tricuspid (T1) valve closure. The second heart sound (S2) contains two high-frequency components—aortic (A2) and pulmonary (P2) valve closure. The low-frequency third heart sound (S3) is also seen.

systole into diastole passing through the second heart sound (continuous). At the end of such detailed auscultation, the experienced clinician may annotate what has been heard as part of the written clinical assessment of the patient with suspected heart disease. This sound and murmur notation can be added to a summary of the findings of the blood pressure, the quality and rhythm of the arterial pulse, the waveform and pressure of the venous pulse and a description of the cardiac impulse, together with any more distant observations to provide a clinical assessment of the cardiovascular system.

GRAPHIC REPRESENTATION OF HEART SOUNDS AND MURMURS (PHONOCARDIOGRAPHY)

Recordings of the arterial and venous pulses and of the cardiac impulse facilitate cardiac diagnosis and expand the information available from inspection and palpation. Phonocardiography is the graphic representation of auscultatory events.[35]. This technique, particularly when used in combination with carotid and venous pulse tracings, apex cardiograms and the electrocardiogram, elucidates the auscultatory findings.[36] The technique of echocardiography, unrelated to the recording of physical signs, complements the recording of physical signs to refine further the precise cardiac diagnosis.[37]

In phonocardiography, microphones applied to the chest (usually by suction) detect the various auscultatory events and, with appropriate amplification and filter systems, the sounds are recorded on paper. The filter can be used to emphasize high- or low-frequency sounds. Recording at fast paper speeds enables better separation of auscultatory events, and permits more accurate analysis of the time characteristics of sounds. The conditions for phonocardiography are the same as those for ideal auscultation: the room should be quiet and the microphones applied to the areas of maximum interest, as previously determined by auscultation. Phonocardiography is not a substitute for auscultation; there are high-frequency murmurs (for instance the murmur of aortic regurgitation), which are easier to hear than record. Only the clinician can know where the microphones should be placed to obtain the information required from the phonocardiogram. Ideally, one microphone should be used to record the area at which the two components of the second heart sound are best heard; the other microphone can be used to rove to other areas of interest. The recording should be made with a simultaneous electrocardiogram, an indirect carotid pulse tracing, sometimes a venous pulse tracing, and an apex cardiogram. All these other records facilitate the analysis of the phonocardiogram in addition to providing clinical information in their own right. The phases of respiration can also be recorded simultaneously, for instance, by using a nasal thermistor. The technique of

recording the M-mode echocardiogram when used simultaneously with phonocardiography is described in the section on echocardiography.

HEART SOUNDS

In a patient with heart disease, there is potential to hear at least 13 sounds in each cardiac cycle (Fig. 8.19): the mitral and tricuspid valve closure sounds forming the first heart sound, the aortic and pulmonary valve closure sounds forming the second heart sound, the opening or ejection sounds of an abnormal aortic or pulmonary valve or sounds generated from the aorta or pulmonary artery, the opening snap of an abnormal mitral or tricuspid valve, the left or right atrial fourth heart sounds, the left or right ventricular third heart sounds and the mid- or late systolic click of mitral valve prolapse. Each sound will be discussed in turn, as it is heard under normal circumstances (where appropriate) and its modification by deranged pathophysiology. The detection of abnormalities in a patient provides important clues to the underlying diagnosis.

First heart sound

Auscultatory analysis of the first heart sound provides considerably less diagnostic information than that of the second heart sound. There has been controversy over the genesis of the first heart sound; the argument centres on whether the main contributions to the sound come from atrioventricular valve closure.[38,39] The major factors responsible for its genesis are probably some initial low-frequency vibrations at the beginning of left ventricular contraction caused by muscular contraction together with abrupt deceleration of atrioventricular blood flow (these vibrations are normally inaudible), audible high-frequency vibrations caused by abrupt tension on the mitral valve as it completes closure, a second set of high-frequency vibrations at the time of tricuspid valve closure, and further inaudible low-frequency vibrations coinciding with acceleration of blood into the great vessels or completion of semilunar valve opening (which are normally inaudible but in pathological states they correspond to the ejection sound). Simultaneous catheter-tip micromanometric recording with phonocardiography shows that the rising left ventricular pressure crosses the left atrial pressure just before mitral valve closure is complete.[40,41] Similar right heart events occur in relation to tricuspid valve closure.[42] In practice, there is strong evidence that the major high-frequency components of the first heart sound are due to mitral valve closure (M_1) preceding tricuspid valve closure (T_1) in normal individuals by 0.02–0.03 s. M_1 is best heard and recorded phonocardiographically at the apex where T_1 is less audible and difficult to separate from M_1. T_1 is best heard and recorded separate from M_1 at the lower left sternal edge. Simultaneous phonocardiography and echocardiography[37] demonstrates mitral and tricuspid valve closure occurring at the time of the high-frequency components of the first heart sound (Fig. 8.20).

Abnormalities of splitting of the first heart sound (S_1)

Abnormal electrophysiological events may influence the relative timing of M_1 and T_1:[43] thus, abnormally wide splitting due to delay in T_1 will occur in right bundle branch block[44] or pacing from the left ventricle, both of which delay activation of the right heart. Delay in activation of the left ventricle may delay M_1, resulting either in a single S_1 (fused M_1–T_1, or reversed splitting (T_1 precedes M_1).[45] Reversed splitting is an echophonocardiographic diagnosis which it is not possible for the ear to appreciate. If left atrial pressure is raised M_1 will be delayed because the moment that left ventricular pressure exceeds left atrial pressure is later than normal. This situation occurs in mitral stenosis or left atrial myxoma, but it can be detected only by phonocardiography, and not by auscultation. The Q–M_1 interval has been used to make a rough assessment of the severity of mitral stenosis (based on the height of the left atrial pressure); it has also been combined with the interval from aortic valve closure to mitral opening snap[46] (which also depends partly on the height of the left atrial pressure) as another index of the severity of mitral stenosis.

Special diagnostic use of the first heart sound can be made in Ebstein's anomaly in which the combination of a large displaced tricuspid valve and right bundle branch block results in a loud late (up to 0.14 s after M_1) tricuspid closure sound. Simultaneous echocardiography of the mitral and tricuspid valves confirms the unusual asynchrony of valve closures.[47]

Intensity of S_1

Factors that influence the intensity of M_1 or T_1 include the mobility of the valves, the velocity of closure and the rate of rise of ventricular pressure at the moment of closure. If the mitral valve is calcified and immobile (as in some cases of rheumatic heart disease), M_1 is soft or absent. By contrast, the extremely mobile mitral valve in the floppy mitral valve syndrome may produce a loud M_1 even though mitral regurgitation is present.

The velocity of closure of M_1 contributes impor-

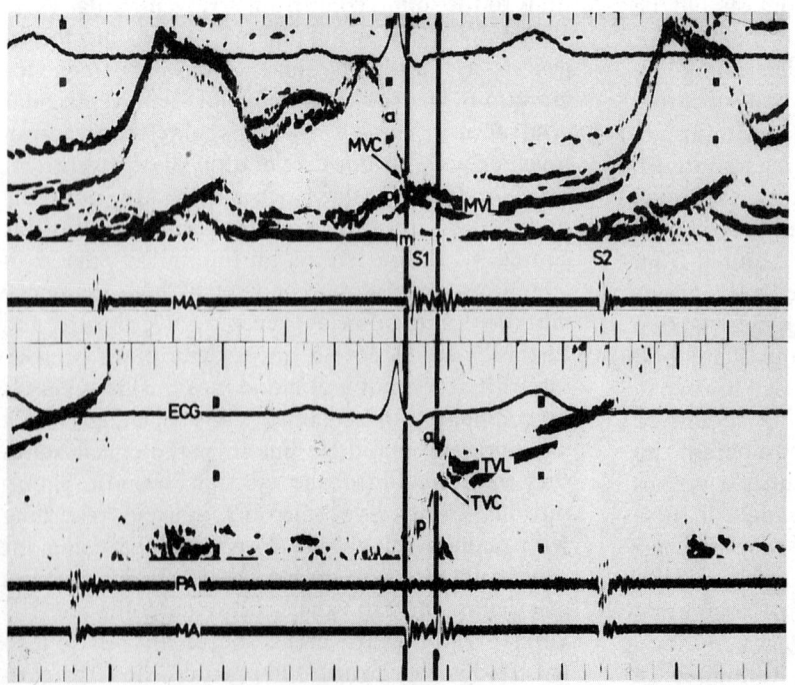

Fig. 8.20. Composite simultaneous M-mode echocardiography of the mitral valve (MVL) (upper) and tricuspid valve (TVL) (lower) with phonocardiograms in the mitral (MA) and pulmonary (PA) areas and electrocardiogram showing that the moment of mitral valve closure (MVC) of the anterior (a) and posterior (p) leaflets corresponds to the first high-frequency component (m) of the first heart sound (S1). The second high-frequency component (t) of S1 corresponds in timing to the moment when the anterior (a) and posterior (p) leaflets of the tricuspid valve close (TVC).

tantly to its intensity. If velocity is rapid, M_1 is loud. If the valve is completely closed at the onset of ventricular systole, as occurs in a long PR interval[48] or acute severe aortic regurgitation,[49] M_1 may be inaudible or seen (on echocardiography) to occur prior to the onset of ventricular depolarization (Q wave of the electrocardiogram). If the PR interval is short, the mitral leaflets are well down into the ventricular chamber as ventricular systole starts and rapidly closes the leaflets to produce a loud M_1. A similar mechanism can explain the loud T_1 in an atrial septal defect[50] because the tricuspid valve is held open by increased right atrial to right ventricular flow, to be finally closed abruptly by right ventricular systole.

Vigorous contraction of the left ventricle may be the main mechanism for a loud M_1 in states such as hyperthyroidism, exercise, increased sympathetic adrenergic activity and systemic hypertension. However, variations in the intensity of S_1 in atrial fibrillation, when a long diastolic pause would be expected to be associated with a loud S_1, are not invariable.[37]

The second heart sound (S_2)

All the evidence suggests that the genesis of the second heart sound (S_2) is the result of the closure and tensing of the aortic and pulmonary valves.[38] Echophonocardiographic studies show that the first high-frequency component of the second heart sound coincides with the moment of aortic valve closure seen on echocardiography,[37,51] while the second component coincides with pulmonary valve closure (Figs 8.21 and 8.22). Some workers, howev-

er, have shown a delay between the moment of aortic or pulmonary valve closure, as seen echocardiographically, and the moment of peak amplitude of A_2 or P_2 on a conventional phonocardiogram.[52] Phonocardiography with simultaneous indirect carotid pulse tracings shows that the aortic valve closure sound (A_2) precedes the dicrotic notch of the carotid by about 0.2 s and is normally audible and can be recorded throughout the precordium (Fig. 8.1). Pulmonary valve closure (P_2) is usually audible only high at the left sternal edge, although it may be heard more widely in young children or if P_2 is increased in intensity.

Much information about underlying cardiovascular abnormalities is provided by careful analysis of the second heart sound. It is essential to listen carefully to the second heart sound, noting the width of its splitting, the variation in splitting with respiration and the relative intensities of its two components, in every patient with suspected heart disease. As A_2 marks the end of left ventricular electromechanical systole and P_2 marks the end of right ventricular electromechanical systole, careful analysis of these two components provides comparative information from both sides of the heart. Although confirmation of the auscultatory findings may require more precise analysis by phonocardiography, the second heart sound remains the key to auscultation of the heart.

The normal second heart sound

In normal individuals, A_2 precedes P_2.[53] In expiration, the two components are usually fused and rarely separated by more than 0.02 s. The width of

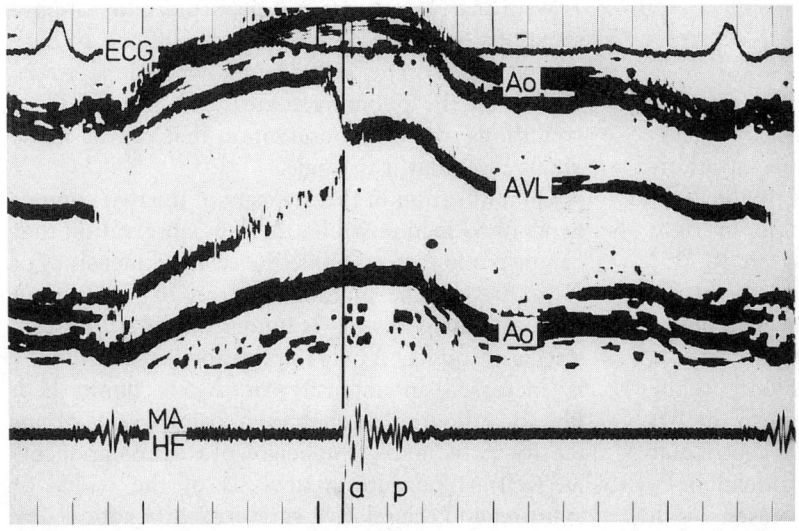

Fig. 8.21. Simultaneous M-mode echocardiogram of the aortic valve (AVL), phonocardiogram in the mitral area using high-frequency filters (MA–HF) and electrocardiogram. The closure of the aortic valve at the end of systole is seen to correspond in time with the first high-frequency component (a) of the second heart sound. P, pulmonary valve closure sound; Ao, aortic wall.

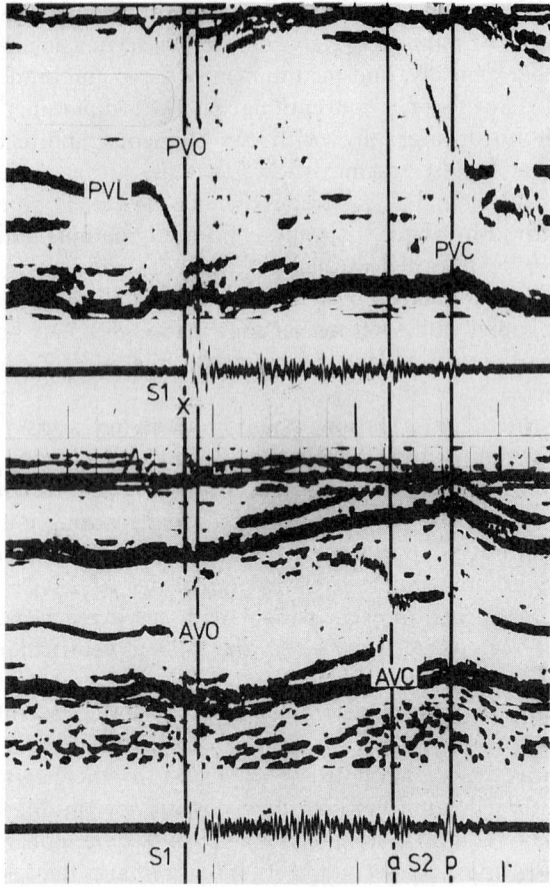

Fig. 8.22. Composite simultaneous M-mode echocardiograms of the pulmonary valve (upper) and aortic valve (lower) and phonocardiogram in the pulmonary area in a patient with pulmonary valve stenosis. The first high-frequency component (a) of the second heart sound (S2) coincides with aortic valve closure (AVC), while the second component (p) coincides with pulmonary valve closure (PVC). A pulmonary ejection sound (X) is seen to coincide with pulmonary valve opening (PVO) but not with aortic valve opening (AVO). PVL, pulmonary valve leaflets; S1, first heart sound.

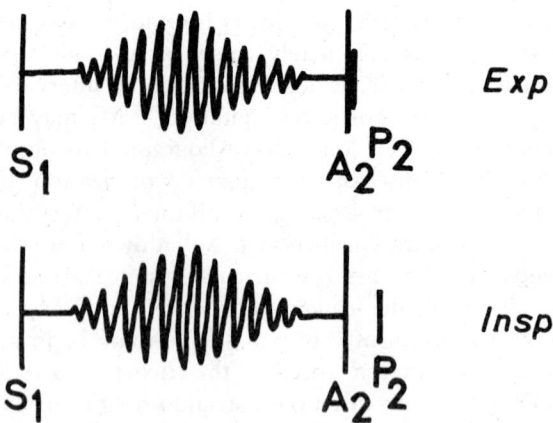

Fig. 8.23. Diagrammatic representation showing physiological splitting of the second heart sound in a patient with an innocent ejection systolic murmur. In expiration (Exp), aortic valve closure (A_2) and pulmonary valve closure (P_2) are almost fused, while in inspiration (Insp) A_2 and P_2 are obviously split mainly due to delay in P_2. S_1, first heart sound.

inspiratory splitting depends largely on the depth of inspiration, but it can be as great as 0.06 s (Fig. 8.23).[54] During inspiration, reduction in intrathoracic pressure allows increasing filling of the right ventricle and consequently prolongation of right ventricular systole and hence a delay in P_2.[38,55] (Inspiration may also increase the capacity of the pulmonary vascular bed which results in reduced vascular recoil to close the pulmonary valve—see below.) The inspiratory pooling of blood in the lungs causes a decrease in venous return to the left heart,[56] resulting in a shortened left ventricular systole and hence an earlier A_2. Thus, a delay in P_2 and an earlier A_2 contribute to the increased width

of splitting of S_2 during inspiration,[57] although the delay in P_2 is the more significant.

It has been shown that A_2 and P_2 coincide precisely with the dicrotic notches in the aorta and pulmonary artery, respectively. The dicrotic notch and A_2 closely follow the end of left ventricular ejection, but the low-resistance pulmonary vasculature produces a later recoil following right ventricular ejection, hence P_2 is later than A_2. The time between the end of ventricular ejection and the dicrotic notch in the appropriate great vessel is called the 'hangout' interval.[58] As pulmonary vascular resistance decreases in inspiration, the pulmonary 'hangout' interval lengthens and hence the width of splitting of A_2 and P_2 increases.

With increasing age, and particularly in emphysematous patients, P_2 may be very difficult to hear or to record. The only component of S_2 to be audible in the pulmonary area is A_2; under these conditions, the only observation that can be made about S_2 is that it is single.

Quantification of the intensity of the two components of S_2 is impossible; the only observation that can be made is to compare the relative intensities of A_2 and P_2 in the pulmonary area. In virtually all normal individuals, A_2 is louder than P_2;[54] indeed, if P_2 is as loud as A_2 the implication is that either P_2 is increased in intensity or A_2 is diminished. Phonocardiography enables a comparison of intensity to be made (the height of each component) as well as permitting analysis of the width of splitting and the relative variations of A_2 and P_2 by measurement of the Q–A_2 and Q–P_2 intervals during continuous respiration.

Abnormalities of splitting of S_2

Wide expiratory splitting

Wide expiratory splitting may be the result of delay in P_2 or a relatively early A_2. Electrical delay in P_2 causing wide expiratory splitting of S_2 occurs in right bundle branch block (Fig. 8.24) or in patients paced from the left ventricle; in both situations, activation of the right ventricle is delayed. A left ventricular ectopic beat would have the same effect. Haemodynamic factors causing prolongation in right ventricular systole and hence a delay in P_2 include right ventricular outflow obstruction (pulmonary valve stenosis or infundibular pulmonary stenosis) and increased right ventricular stroke volume (atrial septal defect or partial anomalous pulmonary venous drainage). With the exception of atrial septal defect, the width of splitting increases further, on inspiration, as it would normally.

The width of expiratory splitting is particularly valuable in assessing the severity of mild or moderate pulmonary valve stenosis (Fig. 8.25). It has been shown that there is a linear relationship between the width of expiratory splitting of S_2 and the right ventricular systolic pressure.[59] Similar findings apply to infundibular stenosis[60] with or without an associated ventricular septal defect.

In some cases of pulmonary embolism or primary or thrombo-embolic pulmonary hypertension, wide expiratory splitting of S_2 with further widening on inspiration occurs.[61–63] This may be due to pro-

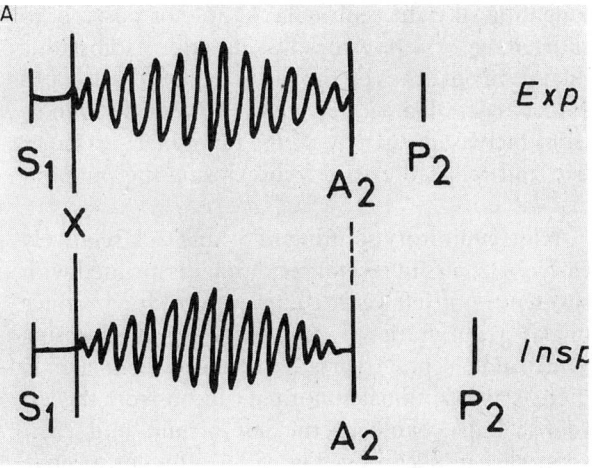

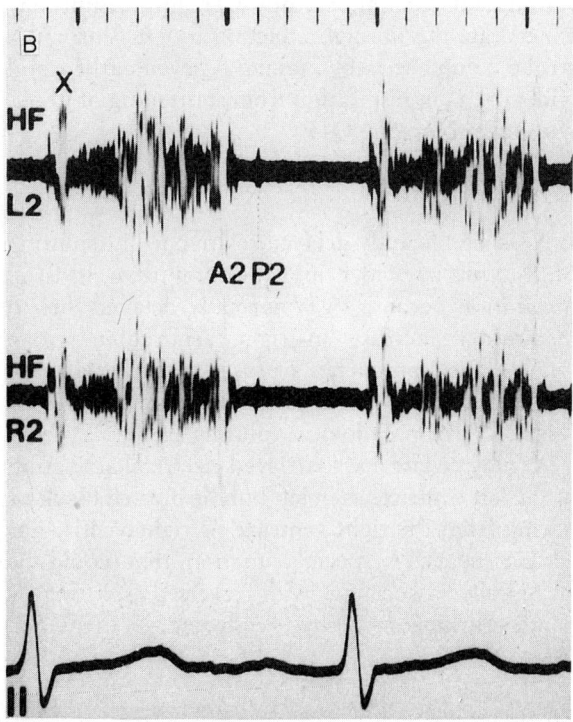

Fig. 8.25. (A) Diagrammatic representation showing wide, but physiological, splitting of the second heart sound in pulmonary valve stenosis. There is wide separation of aortic valve closure (A_2) and pulmonary valve closure (P_2) in expiration (Exp) widening further in inspiration (Insp) due to delay in P_2. A pulmonary ejection sound (X) and ejection systolic murmur are seen. S_1, first heart sound. (B) Simultaneous high-frequency phonocardiograms in the left second intercostal space (HF–L2) and right second space (HF–R2) together with lead II of the electrocardiogram in a patient with pulmonary valve stenosis. Wide separation (0.04 s) of aortic valve closure (A2) and pulmonary valve closure (P2) are seen as well as a pulmonary ejection sound (X).

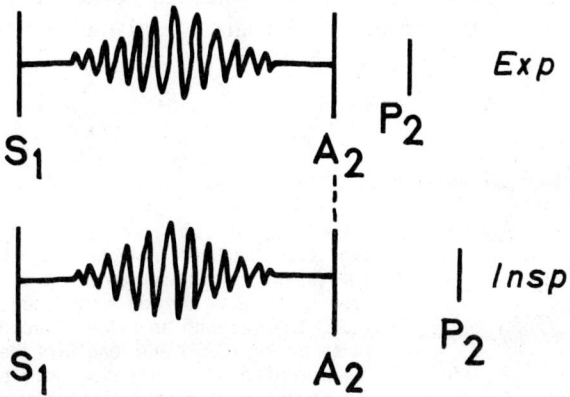

Fig. 8.24. Diagrammatic representation of wide, but physiological, splitting of the second heart sound as in right bundle branch block. Aortic valve closure (A_2) and pulmonary valve closure (P_2) are widely separated in expiration (Exp), but widen further on inspiration (Insp). S_1, first heart sound.

longation of right ventricular systole or possibly to shortening of left ventricular ejection. Idiopathic dilatation of the pulmonary artery[64,65] is also associated with a wide S_2 possibly due to delay in P_2 from increased capacity of the pulmonary vascular bed and reduced elastic recoil closing the pulmonary valve.

Wide expiratory splitting of S_2 due to a relatively early A_2 occurs in several conditions associated with shortening of left ventricular ejection, for instance mitral regurgitation[66] and left-to-right shunting ventricular septal defect,[67] conditions in which there is an additional abnormal run-off from the left ventricle in systole to the left atrium and right ventricle, respectively (Fig. 8.26). In constrictive pericarditis, right ventricular stroke volume is fixed and unaffected by inspiration (Q–P_2 constant throughout respiration); however, inspiration may exaggerate the normal reduction in left ventricular stroke volume thereby making A_2 even earlier, and widening S_2 in inspiration from shortening of Q–A_2 without prolonging Q–P_2.[68]

Reversed splitting of S_2

If A_2 is significantly delayed relative to P_2, splitting of S_2 will be wider in expiration than it is in inspiration because P_2 is normally delayed due to inspiratory increase in right ventricular stroke volume and approaches or fuses with the late A_2. This auscultatory observation is known as reversed (Fig. 8.27) or paradoxical splitting of S_2.[69]

A_2 may be late due to delayed electrical activation of the left ventricle as in left bundle branch block or pacing from the right ventricle or right ventricular ectopic beats. A special situation that could be electrically associated with reversed splitting is Wolff–Parkinson–White syndrome,[70] in which abnormally early activation of the right ventricle would result in a premature P_2.

Prolongation of left ventricular ejection, which thereby delays A_2, occurs in conditions associated with left ventricular outflow obstruction (aortic valve stenosis or hypertrophic obstructive cardiomyopathy), or where there is an increase in left ventricular stroke volume in a left-to-right shunting (persistent ductus arteriosus or aortic regurgitation). Reversed splitting may also be found in systemic hypertension and in patients with ischaemic heart disease[71] who have either chronic left ventricular dysfunction or acute myocardial infarction.

Single second heart sound

It is important to recognize that hearing a single component of S_2 in the pulmonary area does not mean that the sound is P_2 alone or A_2 alone, and, if it is loud, it should not be concluded that P_2 is loud and pulmonary hypertension is present.

A single S_2 may result from inaudibility or absence of P_2, inaudibility or absence of A_2, or fusion of A_2 with P_2 without the normal inspiratory separation of the two components. P_2 may be inaudible in normal individuals, particularly those who have emphysema. It may be inaudible because it is overshadowed by a murmur, as in aortic stenosis. The intensity of P_2 may be diminished, or P_2 may be absent, in pulmonary stenosis, Fallot's tetralogy or pulmonary atresia. Fusion of P_2 with A_2, thereby making the second heart sound appear to be single, occurs in an Eisenmenger ventricular septal defect.

Inaudibility or absence of A_2 may occur in aortic valve stenosis with a rigid calcified aortic valve: usually this results in total absence of the second

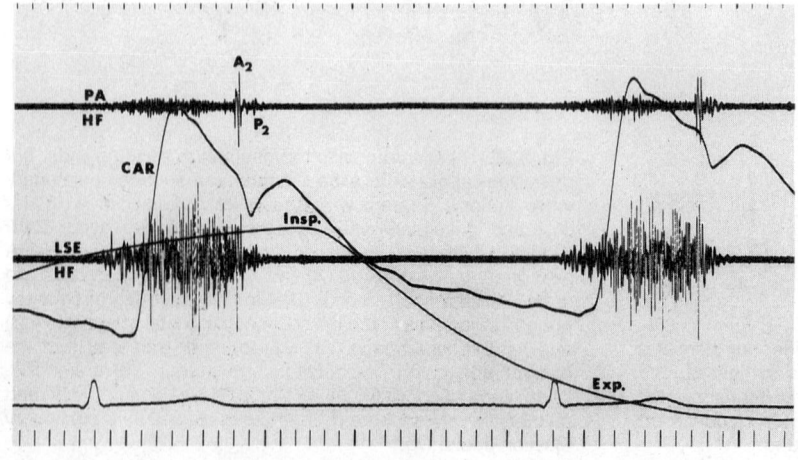

Fig. 8.26. Simultaneous high-frequency (HF) phonocardiograms in the pulmonary area (PA) and at the left sternal edge (LSE) together with an indirect carotid pulse tracing (CAR) and lead II of the electrocardiogram in a patient with a ventricular septal defect and left-to-right shunt. There is wide separation of aortic valve closure (A_2) and pulmonary valve closure (P_2) in both inspiration (Insp) and expiration (Exp). A pan-systolic murmur is seen.

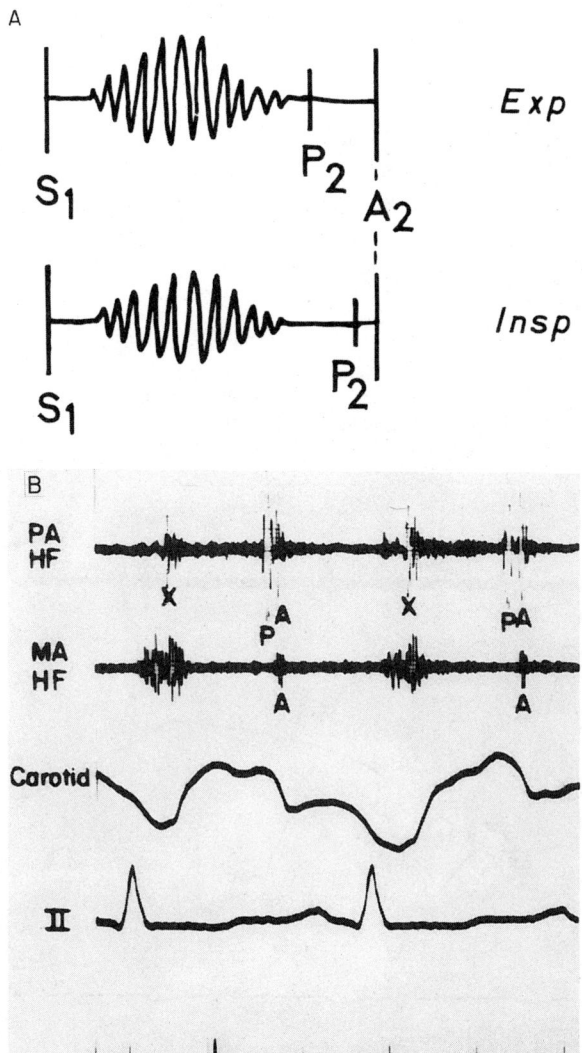

Fig. 8.27. (A) Diagrammatic representation of reversed splitting of the second heart sound. In expiration (Exp), the splitting of aortic valve closure (A_2) and pulmonary valve closure (P_2) is wider than in inspiration (Insp). P_2 precedes A_2 and delays normally in inspiration whereas A_2 remains unchanged in time during respiration. S_1, first heart sound. (B) Simultaneous high-frequency (HF) phonocardiograms in the pulmonary (PA) and mitral (MA) areas with an indirect carotid pulse tracing and lead II of the electrocardiogram in a patient with reversed splitting of the second heart sound. Note that both aortic valve closure (A) and pulmonary valve closure (P) precede the dicrotic notch of the carotid pulse with A identified by its close timing to the dicrotic notch and its presence in the MA. P is not seen or heard in the MA. The patient had aortic valve stenosis, and the ejection sound (X) and ejection systolic murmur can be seen.

heart sound (because P_2 is not audible either), but occasionally a single P_2 can be heard. A_2 can be rendered inaudible by a long systolic murmur passing through it (for instance, the pan-systolic

murmur of mitral regurgitation or a left-to-right shunting ventricular septal defect, or the long ejection systolic murmur of pulmonary valve stenosis). If a phonocardiogram is recorded simultaneously with a carotid pulse tracing, the moment of A_2 can be identified by the dicrotic notch.

Fixed splitting of S_2

Wide, fixed (no alteration in width throughout the respiratory cycle) splitting of the second heart sound (Fig. 8.28) is the hallmark of an atrial septal defect[50] irrespective of the level of pulmonary artery pressure and the presence or absence of pulmonary vascular disease.[61] The mechanism of this important clinical finding is the subject of controversy. It has been thought that the wide expiratory split represents prolongation of right ventricular mechanical systole from increased stroke volume, and possibly electrical delay from associated right bundle branch block. However, some workers have demonstrated normal right heart events but abnormally short left ventricular ejection[72] producing a relatively early A_2 rather than a delayed P_2. During inspiration, P_2 delays normally, while A_2, instead of moving earlier, also delays simultaneously with P_2, perhaps due to reduction in left-to-right atrial shunting or actual right-to-left atrial shunting.[55] Thus, phonocardiographically, $Q–A_2$ and $Q–P_2$ are seen to lengthen simultaneously during inspiration.[61]

Narrow or fused fixed splitting occurs in an Eisenmenger ventricular septal defect in which inspiration causes a simultaneous increase in right and left ventricular stroke volumes (through the ventricular septal defect) simultaneously delaying A_2 and P_2.

Intensity of S_2

Either component of the second heart sound may become accentuated or diminished in intensity by various factors. Factors that facilitate transmission of sound to the chest wall (e.g. when the heart assumes a position close to the chest wall) will alter the intensity of both components. The relative intensities of A_2 and P_2 (all that can be assessed by auscultation or phonocardiography) may be altered by selective increase or decrease in intensity of either component.

P_2 is increased in pulmonary hypertension, which results not only in P_2 being as loud or louder than A_2 in the pulmonary area but also in the possibility that P_2 may be heard away from the pulmonary

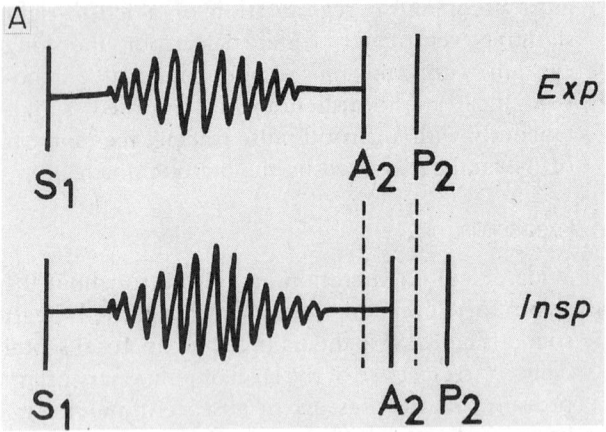

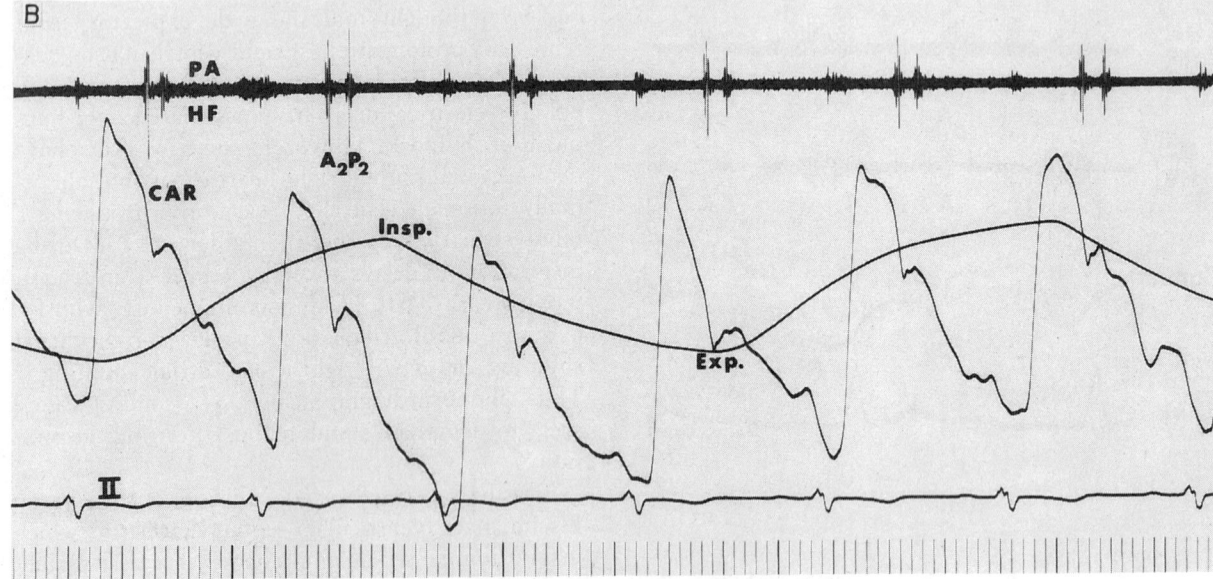

Fig. 8.28. (A) Diagrammatic representation of fixed wide splitting in an atrial septal defect. Aortic valve closure (A_2) and pulmonary valve closure (P_2) are widely split in expiration (Exp) and the split remains equally wide in inspiration (Insp) due to simultaneous delay in both A_2 and P_2. S_1, first heart sound. (B) High-frequency phonocardiogram in the pulmonary area (PA–HF) in a patient with an atrial septal defect. The carotid (CAR) pulse tracing and lead II of the electrocardiogram are shown. Wide (0.08 s) separation of aortic valve closure (A_2) and pulmonary valve closure (P_2) is present during inspiration (Insp) and expiration (Exp).

area, unlike the normal situation.[54,61] Irrespective of the cause of pulmonary hypertension (left ventricular disease, mitral valve disease, pulmonary vascular disease due to primary or thrombo-embolic pulmonary hypertension, the Eisenmenger situation, or respiratory disease, or left-to-right cardiac shunt), P_2 is accentuated. P_2 is also accentuated in atrial septal defect even when the pulmonary artery pressure is normal.

Although increase in P_2 relative to A_2 suggests pulmonary hypertension, it is the characteristics of

splitting that enable an assessment of the cause of pulmonary hypertension.[61] Thus, physiological splitting of S_2 with a loud P_2 suggests that either primary or thrombo-embolic pulmonary hypertension (Fig. 8.29), respiratory disease or Eisenmenger persistent ductus arteriosus is the cause. If the split is wide and fixed, atrial septal defect with either a left-to-right shunt (with or without pulmonary hypertension) or an Eisenmenger atrial septal defect is the cause. If A_2 and P_2 are fused, an Eisenmenger ventricular septal defect is the cause (Fig. 8.30). In

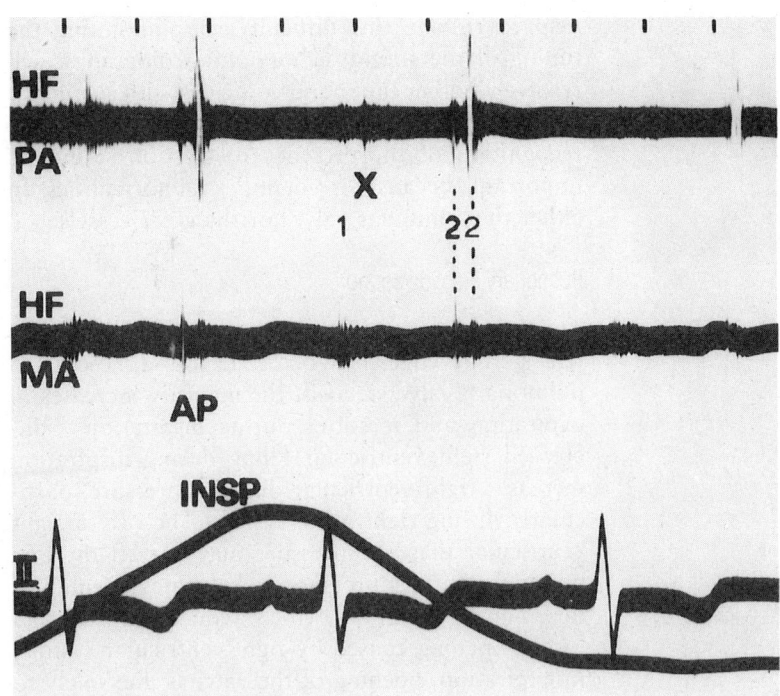

Fig. 8.29. Simultaneous high-frequency (HF) phonocardiograms in the pulmonary (PA) and mitral (MA) areas in a patient with primary pulmonary hypertension. There is a wide separation of aortic and pulmonary valve closure sounds in inspiration (INSP) and to a lesser extent in expiration with P louder than A and transmitted to the MA. A pulmonary ejection sound (X) is seen. 1, first heart sound; both aortic and pulmonary valve closure sounds are labelled as 2.

rheumatic mitral valve disease, P_2 may be accentuated by pulmonary hypertension and the splitting is physiological, but the opening snap may be mistaken for P_2 at the left sternal edge leading to the erroneous conclusion that P_2 is loud.

In severe pulmonary valve stenosis, P_2 is reduced (as well as delayed) in intensity or it may become totally inaudible. Complete absence of P_2 is a feature of pulmonary atresia or severe Fallot's tetralogy.

The intensity of A_2 may be increased when systemic arterial hypertension, aortic dilatation or coarctation of the aorta is present. The intensity will be reduced if the aortic valve is immobile and calcified (as in aortic valve stenosis) or there is a reduced rate of pressure change across the valve in early diastole (as in aortic regurgitation).[73] A reduced rate of left ventricular pressure fall also reduces pressure reversal and hence intensity of A_2 (as in left ventricular disease).

Ejection sounds

High-frequency sounds that occur early in systole closely following mitral and tricuspid closure at the time of maximum opening of the aortic and pulmonary valves are known as ejection sounds. These sounds are not heard in normal individuals but only in those patients who have abnormalities

of the semilunar valves[74,75] or dilatation of the aorta or pulmonary artery.[38]

The genesis of the ejection sound lies in the abrupt tensing at the moment of maximal opening of the semilunar valves. This has been demonstrated by simultaneous phonocardiography and echocardiography, showing the ejection sound coinciding with the opening of the semilunar valves (Figs 8.22 and 8.31). When the aortic or pulmonary valve is abnormal, the abrupt tensing and doming of the valve at the moment of complete, but limited, opening gives rise to the high-frequency sound. An abnormal valve provides a satisfactory explanation for such a 'valvular' origin of the ejection sound. However, ejection sounds can also be heard when there is no apparent abnormality of the semilunar valves and at the same time as a 'valvular' ejection sound.[76] Such sounds generally occur in conditions associated with dilatation of the great arteries. The ejection sound may then be termed 'vascular' in origin. As the timing of a 'vascular' ejection sound is identical to that of a 'valvular' sound, it suggests there is still vibration of the valve leaflets, perhaps distorted by the great vessel dilatation, which is responsible for the genesis of the sound.

The timing of a pulmonary ejection sound is about 0.09–0.11 s after the Q wave on the electrocardiogram, whereas the aortic ejection sound occurs 0.12–0.14 s after the Q wave. As these

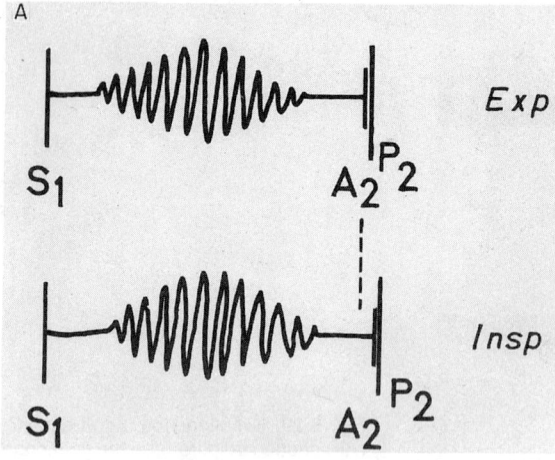

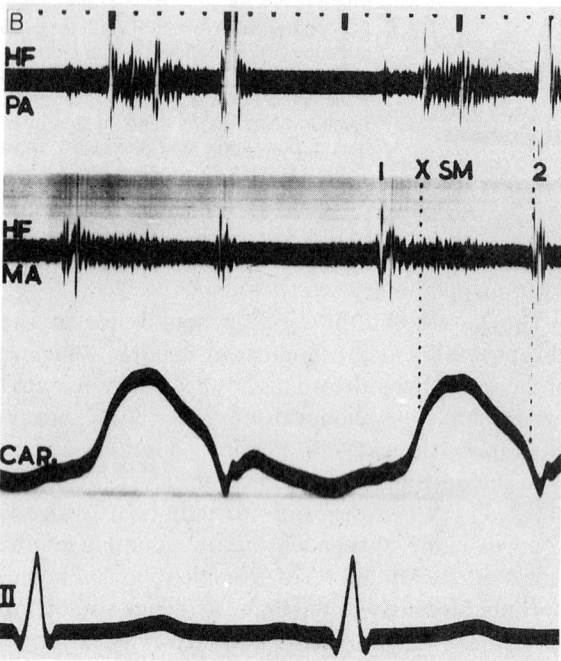

Fig. 8.30. (A) Diagrammatic representation of the fused second heart sound in an Eisenmenger ventricular septal defect. Aortic valve closure (A_2) and pulmonary valve closure (P_2) are scarcely separated and delay simultaneously on inspiration. P_2 is louder than A_2. S_1, first heart sound. (B) Simultaneous high-frequency (HF) phonocardiograms in the pulmonary (PA) and mitral (MA) areas in a patient with an Eisenmenger ventricular septal defect. Aortic and pulmonary valve closure sounds are fused and seen as a single broad sound (2). A pulmonary ejection sound (X) and systolic murmur (SM) can be seen. Indirect carotid pulse tracing (CAR) and lead II of the electrocardiogram are shown.

vibrations occur at high frequencies, it is apparent that auscultatory distinction between the two components of the first heart sound and an ejection sound may be difficult. Phonocardiography may help to resolve this difficulty by pinpointing the timing of the sound; echophonocardiography will resolve whether the sound coincides with semilunar valve opening or atrioventricular valve closure. The recognition of the presence of ejection sounds is important because it identifies abnormalities in either the semilunar valves or the great vessels.

Pulmonary ejection sound

The pulmonary ejection sound is best heard at the left sternal edge.[77] When the sound is due to pulmonary valve stenosis, the intensity increases in expiration and is softer during inspiration.[78] Increased right ventricular filling during inspiration increases right ventricular diastolic pressure, particularly during right atrial systole. The rise of right ventricular diastolic pressure may exceed the low pulmonary artery pressure and initiates opening of the pulmonary valve which reduces the normal forced opening caused by right ventricular systole. In expiration, opening of the valve is due solely to right ventricular systole allowing a fuller and more rapid excursion of the valve into its maximal opening position with a loud ejection sound. The more severe the stenosis, the earlier the pulmonary ejection sound.

Pulmonary ejection sounds occur in pulmonary valve stenosis (Fig. 8.22) but do not occur in right ventricular outflow tract obstruction without an abnormal pulmonary valve[60] (e.g. aberrant muscle bundle). The ejection sound will also be absent when the valve is severely dysplastic and immobile. Pulmonary ejection sounds also occur in some cases of pulmonary hypertension (particularly in those patients who have dilated central pulmonary arteries) and in idiopathic dilatation of the pulmonary artery. Under these circumstances, the later the ejection sound, the more severe the pulmonary hypertension[79] is likely to be, because the time taken for right ventricular systolic pressure to exceed pressure in the pulmonary artery and open the valve will increase with the level of pulmonary artery pressure.

Aortic ejection sound

Aortic ejection sounds are best heard at the cardiac apex. The intensity of the sound varies little with respiration. Unlike the pulmonary ejection sound, the timing of aortic ejection sounds has not been shown to relate to the severity of aortic valve stenosis.[80]

The sound occurs in a bicuspid aortic valve (Fig.

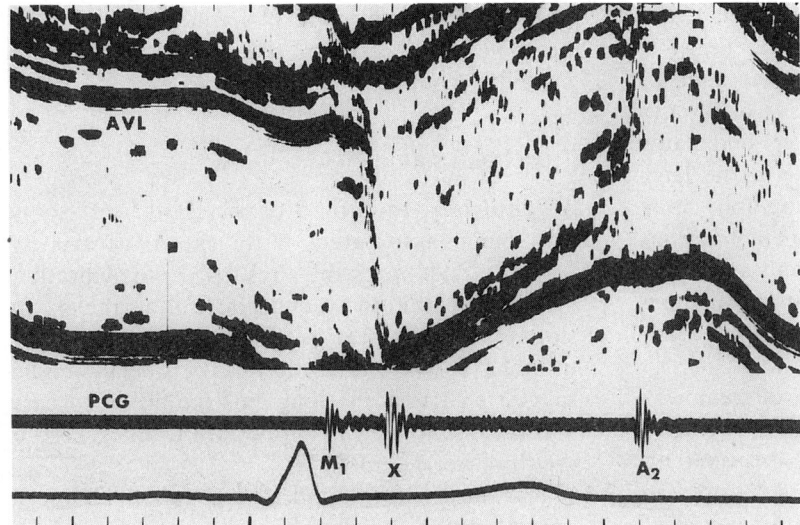

Fig. 8.31. Simultaneous aortic valve M-mode echocardiogram, phonocardiogram (PCG) and electrocardiogram in a patient with a bicuspid aortic valve. The moment of maximum opening of the aortic valve coincides with an aortic ejection sound (X). Note the eccentric diastolic closure line of the aortic valve (AVL). M₁, mitral valve closure; A₂, aortic valve closure.

8.31) or in aortic valve stenosis if the valve is not calcified and immobile.[81] Left ventricular outflow obstruction unassociated with aortic valve abnormality (subaortic stenosis, fixed or dynamic) does not result in an aortic ejection sound—an important clinical distinction. Aortic ejection sounds also occur in dilatation of the aorta and in systemic hypertension.

Opening snaps

The opening of the atrioventricular valves is analogous to the opening of the semilunar valves. Under normal circumstances, immediately after the left and right ventricular pressures fall below those in the left and right atria, the mitral and tricuspid valves open silently. However, when the valves are abnormal, the sudden halting at the maximum

opening of the valves is associated with high-frequency sounds known as opening snaps. In echophonocardiographic studies, the timing of these sounds has been shown to coincide with the moment of peak opening of the valves (Fig. 8.32). The normal tricuspid valve opens earlier than the normal mitral valve, but the timing of the opening snaps in diseased states varies considerably.

Mitral opening snap

The presence of an opening snap implies that the mitral valve is still pliable; the absence of the opening snap in rheumatic mitral valve disease is associated with a calcified immobile valve. The opening snap is best heard medial to the cardiac apex or at the left sternal edge with the patient turned halfway over to the left side. The opening

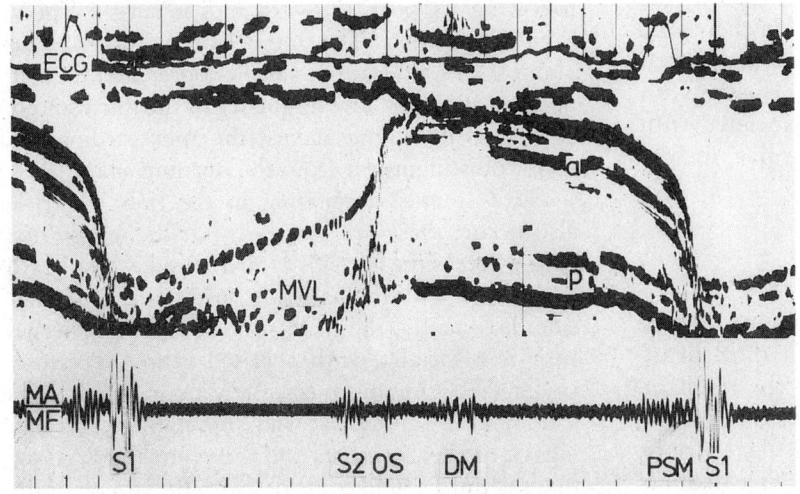

Fig. 8.32. Simultaneous mitral valve (MVL) M-mode echocardiogram and phonocardiogram in mitral area at medium-frequency (MA–MF) with electrocardiogram in a patient with mitral stenosis. The moment of maximum opening of the mitral valve coincides with the opening snap (OS). a, anterior leaflet mitral valve; p, posterior leaflet mitral valve; S1, first heart sound; S2, second heart sound; DM, diastolic murmur; PSM, pre-systolic murmur.

snap is frequently confused with P_2 (see above), and sometimes with a third heart sound. Features distinguishing between the opening snap and P_2 include variation in respiratory splitting of A_2 and P_2, whereas the A_2-opening snap interval remains constant, and the opening snap tends to be later than P_2 relative to A_2. Phonocardiography may permit recording of all three high-frequency components when the ear can distinguish only two. The third heart sound is later in timing than the opening snap and consists of low-frequency rather than high-frequency vibrations.

In the past, the A_2-opening snap interval was used to assess the severity of mitral stenosis (sometimes in conjunction with the Q–M_1 interval, see above). Although the timing of M_1 and the opening snap are partly dependent on the height of the left atrial pressure (the earlier the opening snap, the higher the left atrial pressure), several additional factors, such as left ventricular diastolic pressure, aortic pressure[82] and the presence of mitral regurgitation,[83] will influence the A_2-opening snap interval.

Although a mitral opening snap usually indicates rheumatic mitral valve disease, the snap can occur in conditions not associated with rheumatic heart disease. Abnormal mobility of the mitral valve when it is 'floppy' can cause an opening snap to be heard,[84] particularly when there is severe mitral regurgitation. In large left-to-right shunts, the increased flow through the normal mitral valve opening particularly quickly can also produce an opening snap.[85]

Tricuspid opening snap

The tricuspid opening snap is usually best heard at the lower left sternal edge. It is analogous to the mitral opening snap in that it is heard in rheumatic involvement of the tricuspid valve. The snap often increases in intensity with inspiration. The snap can sometimes be heard in conditions associated with high flow through a normal tricuspid valve, such as an atrial septal defect.[50,85]

Tumour plop

Occasionally, a right or left atrial tumour plop is confused with an opening snap or a third heart sound. The tumour plop is probably the result of the sudden halting of the atrial tumour on its stalk as it prolapses through the atrioventricular valve in early diastole.[86] The plop tends to be later than an opening snap and lower in frequency characteristics. The identification of this sound can readily be made by echophonocardiography.

Third heart sound

Traditionally, the origin of the third heart sound has been associated with rapid ventricular filling.[87,88] It probably results from vibrations generated within the ventricular wall as the expansion of the chamber is abruptly halted in early diastole. The results of recent experimental studies suggest that it is the long-axis limitation to early diastolic filling which is important to the genesis of the third heart sound.[89]

The third heart sound is a common finding in normal young individuals. It occurs in conditions associated with a high-output state such as hyperthyroidism or pregnancy. In non-rheumatic mitral regurgitation due to a floppy valve in which myocardial function is not impaired, a third heart sound occurs more frequently when the regurgitation is severe[84] than when it is mild. The third sound may also occur in conditions associated with left ventricular dysfunction. However, it is much more common in the dilated cardiomyopathies (whether due to ischaemic heart disease or without an obvious aetiology), than in the hypertrophic cardiomyopathies (as in aortic stenosis or hypertension); inability of the left ventricle to distend rapidly in early diastole may be the factor responsible for this distinction.

A constant feature of all left-sided third heart sounds is that they coincide with the peak of the rapid filling wave of the apex cardiogram (Fig. 8.33). The sounds best heard are usually associated with rapid retraction of the rapid filling wave following its peak outward movement—a 'spiky' rapid filling wave. The timing of the third sound is about 0.14 s after aortic valve closure, later than an opening snap; the low frequency of the third sound, as well as its timing against the apex cardiogram, help to distinguish it from the opening snap.

Third sounds originating in the right ventricle also occur; these are best heard at the left sternal edge whereas the left-sided third sound is best heard at the apex with the patient turned towards the left side. Frequently, the third sound at the left sternal edge is associated with a raised venous pressure. Under these circumstances, the venous pulse shows a dominant 'y' descent, and simultaneous recordings of the heart sounds and the venous pulse show that the third sound coincides with the trough of the

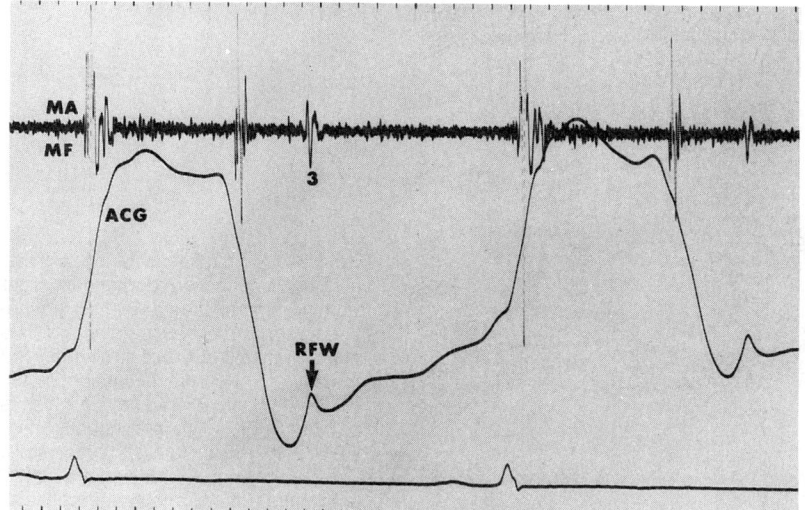

Fig. 8.33. Simultaneous medium-frequency mitral area (MA–MF), phonocardiogram, apex cardiogram (ACG) and electrocardiogram in a normal young individual. The third heart sound, 3, coincides with the peak of the rapid filling wave (RFW), which is 'spiky'.

'y' descent (Fig. 8.12).[17] The intensity of a right ventricular third heart sound increases during inspiration. It is likely that the pericardial 'knock' heard in cases of constrictive pericarditis[90] at the left sternal edge is little different from a right ventricular third sound. The sound is heard only in those patients with constrictive pericarditis in whom there is significant involvement and infiltration of the myocardium. It is not present when the constriction is 'pure' or when there is cardiac tamponade. The timing of the sound coincides with the nadir of the 'y' descent in the venous pulse; the 'y' descent is always dominant in such a case.

In those conditions associated with heart failure, the term diastolic (or S_3) gallop has been used, and should be distinguished from the physiological third heart sound, or that associated with high-output states or primary mitral regurgitation. There has been a tendency to overdiagnose this physical sign in studies connected with heart failure; often, it is more likely that a fourth heart sound (S_4) has been heard—it is particularly difficult to distinguish S_3 from S_4 at fast heart rates.

Fourth heart sound

In discussion of the genesis of the first heart sound (see above), it was observed that there were some initial inaudible low-frequency vibrations at the time of atrial contraction in normal individuals. When these vibrations become audible or palpable (since they occur at low frequencies),[28] they denote a pathological condition of the left ventricle which has rendered it abnormally stiff and resulted in an augmented atrial contraction to move blood into

the stiff ventricle.[30] The audible vibrations are known as the fourth heart sound. This phenomenon can occur on both the left and the right sides of the heart. If co-ordinated atrial contraction is absent (atrial fibrillation), the fourth heart sound cannot occur.

The left ventricle can have a reduced compliance during atrial systole from many causes; the most common cause is ischaemic heart disease,[25] but left ventricular hypertrophy from left ventricular outflow obstruction (aortic valve stenosis,[28] fixed subaortic stenosis, supravalvular aortic stenosis or hypertrophic obstructive cardiomyopathy[5]) or in isolation or associated with systemic hypertension are also frequent causes. Dilated cardiomyopathy from any cause is another condition in which fourth heart sounds are common.

A right-sided fourth heart sound is associated with conditions in which the right ventricle has a reduced compliance; right ventricular hypertrophy from pulmonary hypertension or right ventricular outflow obstruction (pulmonary valve stenosis or infundibular stenosis) are the most frequent causes.[33] Often, the presence of a right atrial sound is associated with unusual dominance of the 'a' wave in the jugular venous pulse.

Unlike the opening and closing sounds of the atrioventricular and semilunar valves, which originate as a result of vibration within the valves and supporting structures, the fourth heart sound, like the third sound, originates from the ventricular wall. It is sometimes known as an atrial or pre-systolic gallop to distinguish it from the diastolic gallop associated with the third sound. Patients with atrial gallops virtually always have elevated

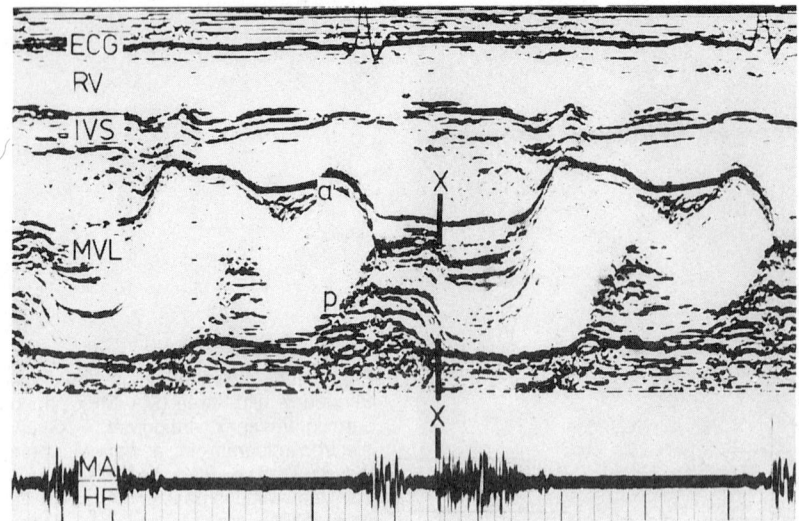

Fig. 8.34. Simultaneous M-mode mitral valve (MVL) echocardiogram with high-frequency mitral area (MA–HF) phonocardiogram and electrocardiogram in a patient with mitral valve prolapse. The moment of maximum excursion of the prolapsed posterior leaflet in systole coincides with a high-frequency mid-systolic click (X) initiating a late systolic murmur. RV, right ventricle; IVS, interventricular septum; a, anterior leaflet; p, posterior leaflet of the mitral valve.

ventricular diastolic pressures or obvious 'a' waves in the end-diastolic pressure. The timing of the atrial sound coincides with the peak of the 'a' wave of the apex cardiogram (Fig. 8.15).[91] If there is a sinus tachycardia resulting in a short diastole, the timing of the third and fourth heart sounds may be very close, thereby producing a 'summation' gallop. This can be identified on the apex cardiogram because the 'a' wave is superimposed on the rapid filling wave. The fourth sound generally occurs 0.10–0.16 s after the P wave on the electrocardiogram; it is thought that the earlier the sound, the stiffer the ventricle.[91]

Mid-systolic click

A characteristic finding associated with prolapse of the floppy mitral valve is a mid- or late systolic click with or without a late systolic murmur.[92] This high-frequency sound coincides with the abrupt halting of the floppy mitral valve leaflet as it prolapses into the left atrium at about the moment of peak left ventricular systolic pressure.[93] Simultaneous echophonocardiography demonstrates the relationship between the sound and the movement of the mitral valve leaflet very well (Fig. 8.34).

CARDIAC MURMURS

It is generally believed that turbulence of blood flow results in cardiac murmurs. Turbulence can be caused by any distortion of the normal passages through which blood flows; in particular, it will occur when there is a high rate of flow through either a normal or distorted orifice, a normal rate of flow through a distorted orifice or into a distorted chamber or vessel, and if there is abnormal backward flow into cardiac chambers. The higher the velocity of blood flow, the higher the frequency characteristic of the murmur. The turbulence occurs in the vessel or chamber beyond the area of distortion or high velocity, e.g. in the aorta in aortic stenosis or in the left ventricle in aortic regurgitation. Doppler studies will usually provide information on the source of a murmur because the technique is able to assess blood flow.

Murmurs are classified as systolic, diastolic or continuous. The timing of the murmur relative to the heart sounds provides the greatest information relating to its aetiology:[94] a pan-systolic murmur can be caused only by mitral regurgitation, tricuspid regurgitation or ventricular septal defect; a late systolic murmur denotes slight mitral regurgitation; a mid-diastolic murmur either mitral or tricuspid stenosis or increased flow through normal mitral or tricuspid valves; an early diastolic murmur aortic or pulmonary regurgitation. The relative timing of the first and second heart sounds having been established by auscultation the timing of the murmur relative to these sounds should also be determined. The phonocardiogram, which is *not* a substitute for careful auscultation, can elucidate further the timing of the murmur by identification of heart sounds or the moment of aortic valve closure from the dicrotic notch of the indirect carotid artery pulse. The radiation of a murmur depends on the direction of blood flow causing the murmur, the intensity of the murmur and, to a certain extent, its site of origin; however, radiation does not reveal the underlying pathophysiology in the way that the timing of a murmur does.

The main murmurs will be described indicating the deranged anatomy and haemodynamic state (pathophysiology) that give rise to each murmur.

Ejection (or mid-systolic) systolic murmurs

Ejection systolic mumurs start after the first heart sound (mitral and tricuspid valve closure) and have a crescendo–decrescendo characteristic terminating before the second heart sound (aortic and pulmonary valve closure). Classically, the murmur is caused by an abnormality of the semilunar valve resulting in turbulence as blood enters the distal great vessel. It follows, therefore, that the murmur cannot start until blood has been ejected into the great vessel. The mitral or tricuspid components of the first heart sound occur shortly after the left or right ventricular pressure exceeds the left or right atrial pressure, respectively. A murmur due to ejection into a great vessel cannot start until the left or right ventricular pressure has risen to exceed the diastolic pressure in the aorta or pulmonary artery, respectively. The murmur thus commences after the first heart sound, and after an aortic or pulmonary ejection sound if these are present (representing the opening of the aortic or pulmonary valve). The murmur has a crescendo and peaks at about the time of peak ventricular systolic pressure and flow, and then diminishes to terminate before the aortic or pulmonary valve closes (Fig. 8.35).

Causes of ejection systolic murmurs

Aortic valve stenosis Aortic stenosis is associated with several characteristic physical signs that enable it to be distinguished from other causes of ejection systolic murmur (Fig. 8.36): the arterial pulse is slow rising indicating fixed obstruction to left ventricular outflow; an ejection sound is present unless the valve is heavily calcified and immobile (in which case the calcification can be seen by cardiac screening or echocardiography); a double impulse or fourth heart sound is present because the left ventricle is hypertrophied and stiff; the left ventricular hypertrophy can be identified by echocardiography. In severe aortic stenosis associated with a low cardiac output and heart failure, the murmur may virtually disappear. The later the murmur peaks, the more severe the stenosis is likely to be, and the second heart sound is more likely to be reversed (as left ventricular ejection time is prolonged). The intensity of the murmur is not an index of severity, but prolongation of left ventricular ejection and left ventricular hypertrophy usually indicate severe obstruction to left ventricular outflow.

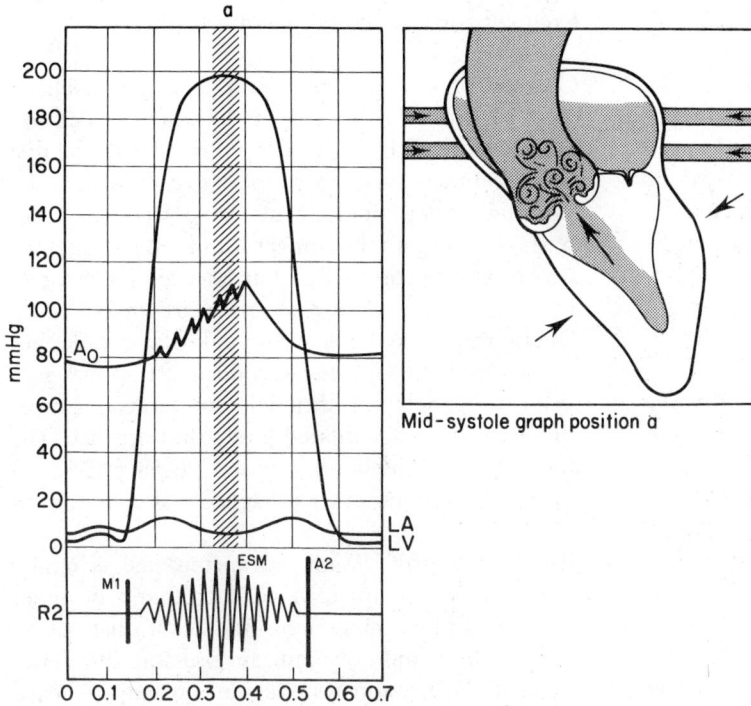

Mid-systole graph position a

Fig. 8.35. Diagrammatic representation of simultaneous pressure curves, phonocardiogram and blood flow from left ventricle to aorta in aortic valve stenosis. In mid-systole, most of the blood has left the left ventricle through the thickened distorted aortic valve to enter the aorta. The turbulent flow of blood has resulted in an ejection systolic murmur (ESM) initiated from the moment of aortic valve opening (after left ventricular (LV) pressure exceeds aortic (Ao) pressure) and terminating before aortic valve closure (A_2) (after left ventricular pressure falls below aortic pressure). LA, left atrial pressure; R2, right second intercostal space; M_1, mitral valve closure.

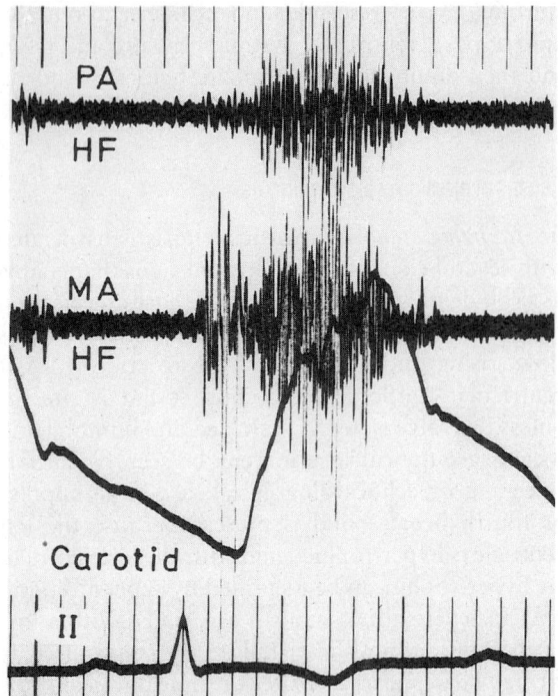

Fig. 8.36. Simultaneous high-frequency (HF) phonocardiograms in the pulmonary (PA) and mitral (MA) areas with the carotid pulse and lead II of the electrocardiogram in a patient with aortic valve stenosis. The ejection systolic murmur preceded by an ejection sound can be seen. Note the slow rise with shudder of the carotid pulse and the prolonged left ventricular ejection time.

Fixed subaortic stenosis (fibromuscular diaphragm) The physical findings are identical to those of aortic valve stenosis,[95,96] but, as the obstruction lies below the aortic valve, an aortic ejection sound will not be heard and an abnormal aortic valve will not be seen on screening or echocardiography. Early systolic closure of the aortic valve may be detected by M-mode echocardiography, but this is not a specific feature. Dilatation of the ascending aorta is not seen, unlike aortic valve stenosis. The diaphragm may be visualized directly by echocardiography.

Bicuspid (hydraulically imperfect) aortic valve The auscultatory features include an aortic ejection sound and an ejection systolic murmur (Fig. 8.37) but, because stenosis is absent, the carotid pulse is normal, the second heart sound is normal and there are no features of left ventricular hypertrophy. The biscuspid valve may be visualized directly by echocardiography.

Hypertrophic obstructive cardiomyopathy The ejection systolic murmur in this condition results from obstruction to blood leaving the left ventricular cavity as the anterior leaflet of the mitral valve meets the bulging hypertrophied septum thereby narrowing the outflow pathway.[97] Early in systole, ejection is rapid and unobstructed but, in mid-systole, the outflow pathway shuts down and the murmur is initiated. Thus, the murmur is delayed when compared with the murmur of aortic valve stenosis. Mitral regurgitation may also be a feature and contribute to the genesis of the murmur. The regurgitation does not occur until the anterior leaflet of the mitral valve moves forward. The distinguishing diagnostic features of this condition include a sharp upstroke to the carotid pulse (Fig. 8.3) and a double impulse due to the stiff left ventricle. Echocardiography demonstrates the hypertrophy (sometimes asymmetric) of the left ventricle and the systolic anterior motion of the mitral valve. In hypertrophic cardiomyopathy without obstruction, an ejection systolic murmur can also sometimes be heard.

Supravalvular aortic stenosis The murmur in this condition is indistinguishable from that of aortic valve or fixed subaortic stenosis. However, there is asymmetry of the right and left carotid and brachial pulses, those on the right being sharp in upstroke, whereas those on the left are slow rising (Fig. 8.7). An ejection sound is usually not heard,[98] and aortic regurgitation (often present in both aortic valve and fixed subaortic stenosis) is not a feature.

Coarctation of the aorta Although the murmur in coarctation of the aorta has a crescendo–decrescendo quality, it is delayed relative to the first heart sound more than aortic valve abnormalities (although a biscuspid aortic valve frequently co-exists) because it takes longer for blood to reach the area of constriction where turbulence is generated. Sometimes the murmur is best heard in the back. The murmur may be heard only during systole, but it may spill through the second heart sound as a result of the delay. Additional continuous murmurs may be heard over dilated intercostal arteries. The diminution and delay in femoral pulses relative to the radial pulse point to a diagnosis of coarctation.

'Aortic sclerosis' With advancing age, changes may occur in the aortic valve, such that it becomes distorted and yet there is no significant obstruction to blood flow and no significant pressure difference across it. An ejection systolic murmur may be heard as a result,[99] but without any of the other features

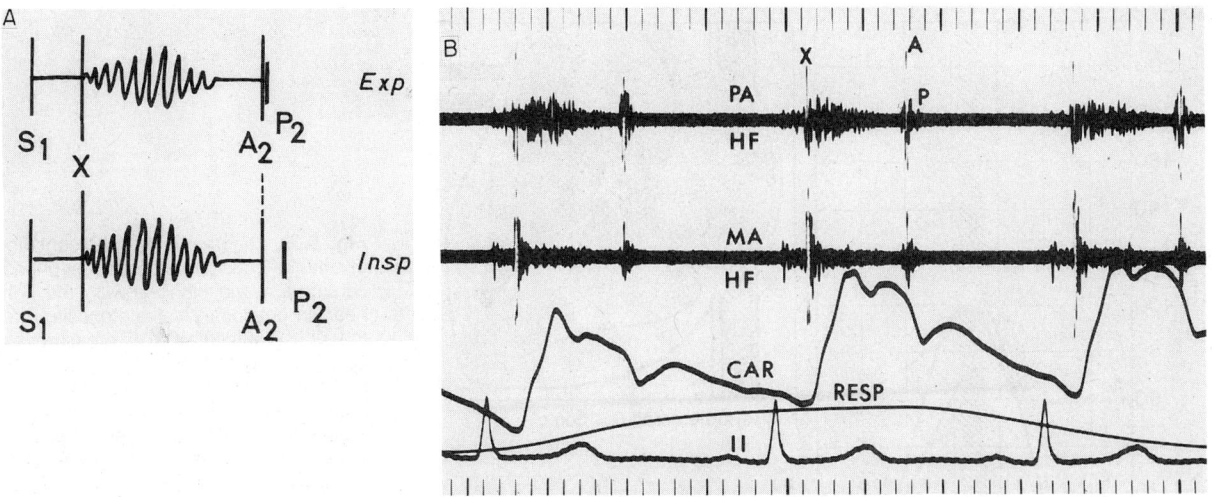

Fig. 8.37. (A) Diagrammatic representation of the sounds in a bicuspid aortic valve. The second heart sound is physiological, and there is an ejection sound (X) and ejection systolic murmur. A₂, aortic valve closure; P₂, pulmonary valve closure; S₁, first heart sound. (B) Simultaneous high-frequency (HF) phonocardiograms in the pulmonary (PA) and mitral (MA) areas with the indirect carotid pulse (CAR), lead II of the electrocardiogram and a respiratory (RESP) trace in a patient with a bicuspid aortic valve. The ejection sound (X) is well seen initiating an ejection systolic murmur. Physiological splitting of the second heart sound can be seen. A, aortic valve closure; P, pulmonary valve closure.

of obstruction (the pulse is normal, there are no features of left ventricular hypertrophy).

A similar murmur may be heard in conditions associated with distortion of the aortic root, such as atherosclerosis, aortic dilatation or aneurysm, with or without hypertension.

Hyperkinetic circulatory states Increased flow through a normal aortic valve may give rise to an ejection systolic murmur. Similarly, increased flow through a normal pulmonary valve may produce an ejection systolic murmur. Although it is fairly clear that the ejection systolic murmur of an atrial septal defect arises from the right ventricular outflow tract and pulmonary artery, or that the ejection murmur associated with pure aortic regurgitation arises from the left ventricular outflow tract in association with the increased left ventricular stroke volume, it is less certain whether the ejection systolic murmurs of hyperkinetic circulatory states, such as pregnancy, anaemia, fever or hyperthyroidism, arise in the left or right side of the heart.

In childhood, ejection systolic murmurs are common and in the absence of any other detectable abnormality on examination and investigation of the cardiovascular system, and particularly on auscultation (including physiological splitting of the second heart sound), these murmurs are called 'innocent'.[100] The murmurs sometimes have un-

usual frequency characteristics and are described as 'grunting' or 'musical'. The use of Doppler echocardiography should resolve the origin of these murmurs, which has previously been in dispute.

Pulmonary valve stenosis Pulmonary valve stenosis exemplifies the ejection systolic murmur that originates from the right ventricular outflow tract (Fig. 8.38). In systole, following tricuspid valve closure, the right ventricular pressure exceeds the pulmonary artery pressure and opens the pulmonary valve. In pulmonary valve stenosis, the valve is abnormal, halts abruptly at full opening and produces the pulmonary ejection sound. After the valve is open, turbulent blood flow is created as blood passes through the distorted valve; the murmur peaks at peak ejection, diminishing as the rate of blood flow falls. The murmur stops before pulmonary valve closure but, because P₂ is delayed in severe pulmonary stenosis,[59] the murmur may make A₂ inaudible as it passes through it, while remaining ejection with respect to P₂ (Fig. 8.25). The other features of pulmonary valve stenosis include right ventricular hypertrophy (diagnosed by electrocardiogram or palpation) and abnormal dominance of the 'a' wave in the venous pulse. The plain chest radiograph shows dilatation of the central and left pulmonary artery.

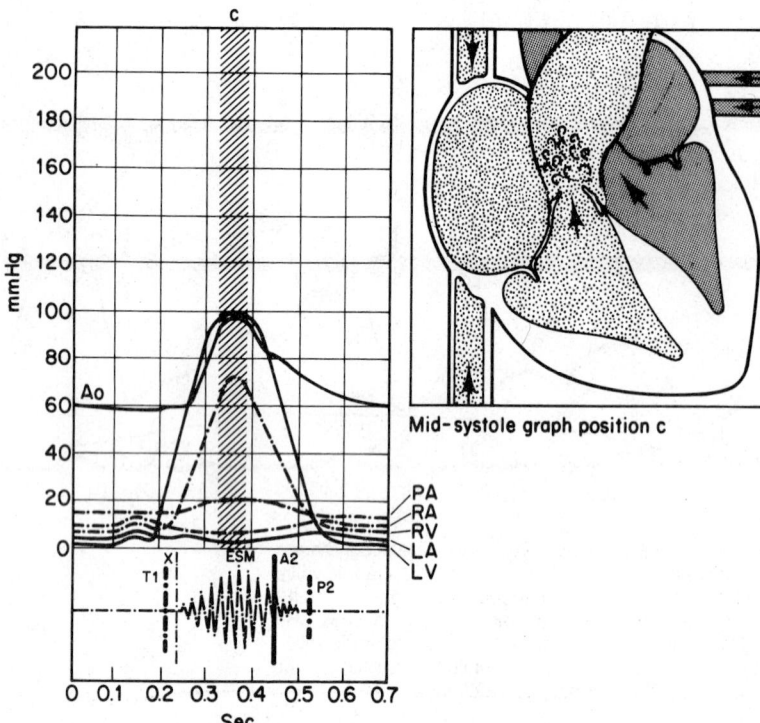

Fig. 8.38. Diagrammatic representation of simultaneous pressure curves, phono-cardiogram and blood flow in the right heart in pulmonary valve stenosis. After the right ventricular (RV) pressure exceeds the right atrial (RA) pressure, the tricuspid valve closes (T_1). After RV pressure exceeds pulmonary artery (PA) pressure, the abnormal thickened pulmonary valve opens with an ejection sound (X). Blood flows through the pulmonary valve in a turbulent way creating the systolic murmur which stops before the RV pressure falls below the PA pressure causing the pulmonary valve to close (P_2). Left heart events are also seen with aortic valve closure (A_2) occurring after left ventricular (LV) pressure has fallen below that in the aorta (Ao). There is wide splitting of A_2 and P_2. LA, left atrial pressure.

Infundibular pulmonary stenosis When infundibular pulmonary stenosis is present without a ventricular septal defect (e.g. aberrant right ventricular muscle bundles), the murmur is identical to that of pulmonary valve stenosis.[101] However, an ejection sound is not present and there is no dilatation of the pulmonary artery on the plain chest radiograph.

Fallot's tetralogy Obstruction to right ventricular outflow in this condition is at the infundibular level, but the pulmonary valve can also be abnormal. As the stenosis is usually severe, the shunt is from right-to-left through the septal defect. The ejection systolic murmur is usually well heard[102] although, if the outflow tract is severely narrowed or goes into spasm, the murmur may disappear completely. As the stroke volume of both ventricles is ejected mainly into the aorta, the aorta becomes dilated. The pulmonary valve closure sound becomes inaudible and a single loud A_2 is heard, often with an aortic ejection sound of 'vascular' origin. Right ventricular hypertrophy is less marked than in pulmonary valve stenosis and the 'a' wave in the venous pulse is not prominent.

Peripheral pulmonary artery stenosis This rare condition, which is usually associated with other congenital abnormalities, will give rise to a right-sided ejection systolic murmur.[103] The second heart sound may be abnormally widely split and sometimes the murmur spills through the second heart sound.

Idiopathic dilatation of the pulmonary artery Just as dilatation of the aorta may give rise to an ejection systolic murmur, dilatation of the pulmonary artery may cause a similar murmur in its own right or as a result of distortion of the pulmonary valve. The wide splitting of the second heart sound (see above) and an ejection sound are associated features.[64,65] The dilatation of the pulmonary artery can be visualized on plain chest radiography; the absence of obstruction at the level of the pulmonary valve may be demonstrated on Doppler.

Causes of pan-systolic (holosystolic) murmurs

A pan-systolic murmur is defined as starting immediately after the first heart sound and extending through systole until or just beyond the second heart sound. The haemodynamic explanation of the murmurs is that as soon as the mitral or tricuspid valve has closed after the ventricular pressure has risen to exceed atrial pressure, blood can exit from the ventricle to the atrium, if the atrioventricular valve is incompetent, or from the left to the right ventricle as soon as left ventricular pressure exceeds right ventricular pressure, if there is a ventricular septal defect.

The unusual escape of blood from the ventricle gives rise to turbulence and the onset of the murmur which will continue until the pressure in the ventricle falls below that in the atrium (Fig. 8.39) or equilibrates with right ventricular pressure in the case of a ventricular septal defect. This means that the murmur of mitral regurgitation does not finish until after A_2 or the murmur of tricuspid regurgitation until after P_2. Sometimes, the pan-systolic murmur of atrioventricular valve regurgitation has a late systolic accentuation, whereas the murmur of a left-to-right shunting ventricular septal defect has a crescendo–decrescendo characteristic. The origin of a pan-systolic murmur can be identified using the Doppler technique; the regurgitant flow can be readily detected when sampling in the left or right atrium or right ventricle.

Mitral regurgitation Mitral regurgitation may be rheumatic or non-rheumatic in aetiology. If mitral regurgitation is rheumatic, the pan-systolic murmur is usually associated with other evidence of rheumatic mitral valve disease, such as an opening snap or a mid-diastolic murmur. Pure rheumatic mitral regurgitation may occur in the acute phase of rheumatic fever. In mild rheumatic mitral regurgitation,

only the pan-systolic murmur will be heard and other physical signs are absent. In severe regurgitation, there will be an increase in left ventricular stroke volume resulting in a hyperdynamic apical impulse, and a third heart sound may be present if mitral stenosis is insignificant.[66,104] Echocardiography demonstrates the typical appearance of a rheumatic mitral valve.

Non-rheumatic mitral regurgitation may be due to either abnormalities of the leaflets and chordae tendineae ('primary' mitral regurgitation) or abnormalities of the left ventricular myocardium and papillary muscles ('secondary' mitral regurgitation). If regurgitation is trivial, the murmur may be confined to late systole (see below). If the lesion is moderate or severe, the murmur is usually pan-systolic but tends to have more low-frequency components than the pan-systolic murmur of rheumatic mitral regurgitation (Fig. 8.40). Sometimes the murmur is palpable. In primary chronic moderate-to-severe regurgitation, left ventricular stroke volume is increased so that the apical impulse is hyperdynamic and a third heart sound is heard.[84] Unlike rheumatic mitral valve disease, the rhythm remains sinus unless there has been severe regurgitation over a long period. Echocardiography will show the 'floppy' appearance of the mitral valve (redundant leaflets and enlongated chordae ten-

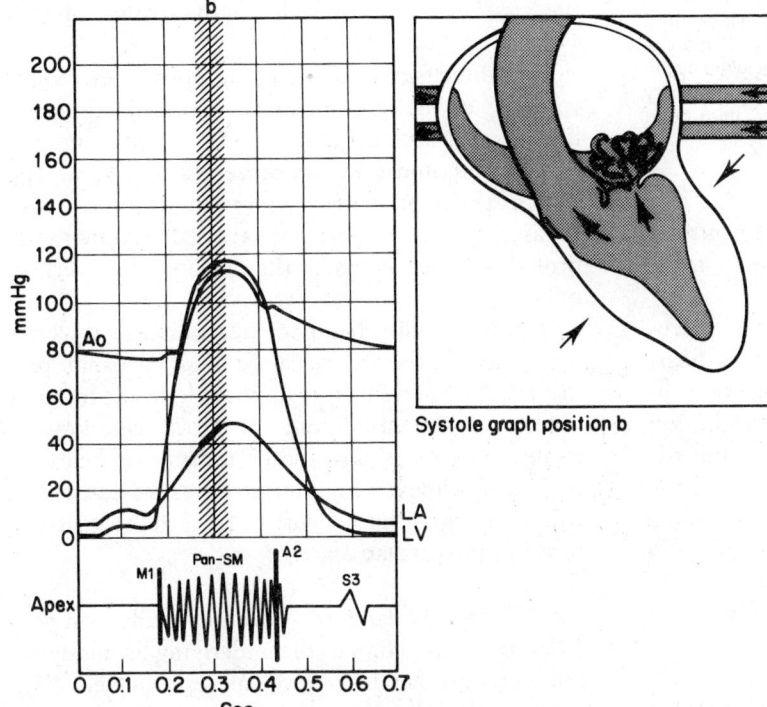

Systole graph position b

Fig. 8.39. Diagrammatic representation of simultaneous pressure curves, phonocardiogram at the apex and blood flow in mitral regurgitation. When left ventricular (LV) pressure exceeds left atrial (LA) pressure, the mitral valve closes (M_1). From this moment, because the valve is incompetent, blood flows from left ventricle to left atrium creating turbulence and hence a murmur. This flow can continue as long as there is a pressure difference from LV to LA and until LV pressure has fallen below aortic (Ao) pressure closing the aortic valve (A_2). The murmur is thus pan-systolic (Pan-SM). S_3, third heart sound.

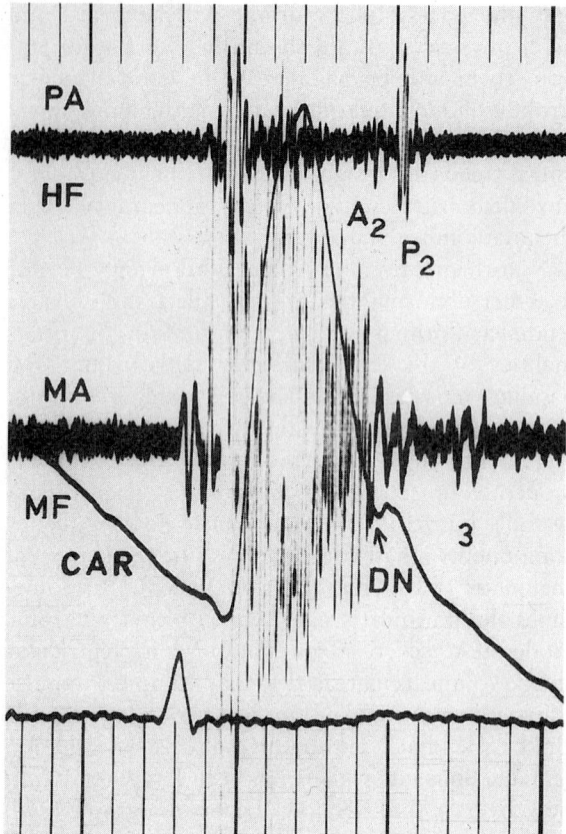

Fig. 8.40. Simultaneous phonocardiograms in the pulmonary area at high-frequency (PA–HF) and mitral area at medium-frequency (MA–MF) with the indirect carotid pulse (CAR) and electrocardiogram in a patient with non-rheumatic mitral regurgitation due to ruptured chordae tendineae. A pan-systolic murmur can be seen in the mitral area, with wide splitting of the second heart sound. Aortic valve closure (A_2) is identified by the dicrotic notch (DN) in the carotid pulse (CAR) and pulmonary valve closure (P_2) is louder than A_2 in the PA. A third heart sound (3) is seen in the mitral area.

dineae which may rupture), and intact left ventricular systolic function with an increased stroke volume.

In mitral regurgitation secondary to left ventricular disease (cardiomyopathy or ischaemic heart disease), the auscultatory features are indistinguishable from those of primary mitral regurgitation (although the murmur is seldom palpable), but the left ventricular stroke volume is decreased and the apical impulse tends to be sustained and double rather than hyperdynamic.[31] Echocardiography demonstrates impaired left ventricular systolic function with a normal or reduced stroke volume and a normal mitral valve.

Tricuspid regurgitation Tricuspid regurgitation

may be organic or functional. Organic tricuspid regurgitation is the result of abnormalities of the leaflets which are most frequently caused by rheumatism but can be caused by infective endocarditis, tumours of the right atrium interfering with tricuspid valve function or carcinoid disease. Functional tricuspid regurgitation is usually secondary to pulmonary hypertension although primary abnormalities of right ventricular function (e.g. right ventricular infarction) can cause tricuspid regurgitation.

Usually, the murmur is pan-systolic and best heard at the left sternal edge. The intensity of the murmur increases with inspiration. The diagnosis of tricuspid regurgitation is confirmed by the typically exaggerated 'v' or systolic wave in the jugular venous pulse (see above). If the aetiology is rheumatic, the additional findings of tricuspid stenosis (mid-diastolic murmur and opening snap at the left sternal edge) and a slow 'y' descent in the venous pulse may be helpful in the diagnosis. A right ventricular third heart sound often accompanies severe tricuspid regurgitation when the venous pressure is elevated, and expansile pulsation of the liver may be felt.

In some cases of tricuspid regurgitation due to non-rheumatic leaflet abnormalities, the murmur may be heard only in early systole[105] with a decrescendo rather than a pan-systolic quality. This may be explained by pressure equilibration between the right ventricle and the right atrium later in systole.

Two-dimensional echocardiography is extremely valuable in the assessment of tricuspid regurgitation. Leaflet abnormalities due to rheumatism may be detected, and tumours or vegetations seen. The sizes of the right ventricle and right atrium can also be assessed, although right ventricular function is probably better assessed using radionuclide techniques.

In patients with rheumatic heart disease in whom the venous pressure is raised and tricuspid regurgitation is present, it is impossible to diagnose at the bedside the co-existence of mitral regurgitation merely because a pan-systolic murmur is heard at the cardiac apex. This murmur may be caused by tricuspid regurgitation with a large right ventricle forming the cardiac apex.

Ventricular septal defect Careful auscultation provides important clues to the underlying haemodynamic derangement in ventricular septal defect (Fig. 8.41). A small left-to-right shunting ventricular

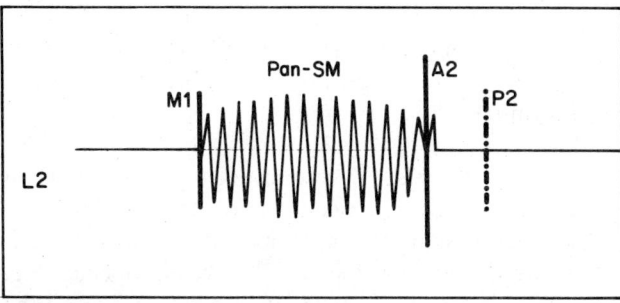

Small or moderate left-to-right shunt

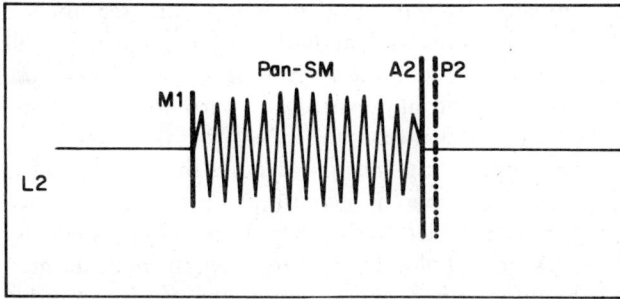

Large left-to-right shunt

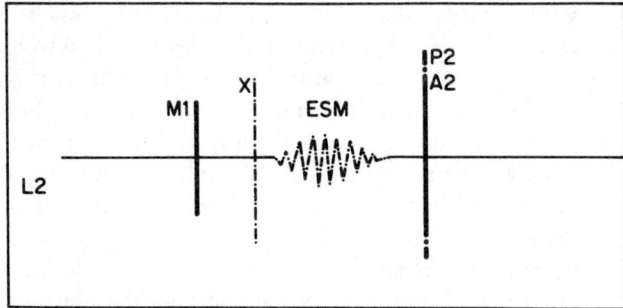

Eisenmenger's syndrome

Fig. 8.41. Diagrammatic representation of auscultatory findings in the second left intercostal space (L2) in ventricular septal defect. With a small or moderate left-to-right shunt, there is a pan-systolic murmur (Pan-SM) and wide splitting of the second heart sound, although the split is physiological and aortic valve closure (A_2) is louder than pulmonary valve closure (P_2). With a large left-to-right shunt, the second heart sound is normally split, but P_2 is accentuated. In the Eisenmenger syndrome, A_2 and P_2 are fused together, the murmur is ejection (ESM) and preceded by a pulmonary ejection sound (X). M_1, mitral valve closure.

septal defect with normal pulmonary artery pressure (maladie de Roger) (Fig. 8.26) has a pan-systolic murmur maximal at the left sternal edge with wide, but physiological, splitting of the second heart sound and A_2 louder than P_2.[67] With a large left-to-right shunting defect including an elevated pulmonary artery pressure (but not pulmonary vascular resistance), the murmur remains pan-systolic, but P_2 is accentuated and a mid-diastolic murmur, due to increased flow through a normal mitral valve, may be heard. When pulmonary vascular resistance is raised and the shunt is either right to left or bidirectional (Fig. 8.30), the pan-systolic murmur disappears; a pulmonary ejection sound and ejection systolic murmur may be heard, together with a 'fused' second heart sound in which

P_2 is accentuated.[61] The ventricular septal defect may be detected by Doppler and echocardiography.

Early systolic murmurs

Abbreviation of the pan-systolic murmur of mitral or tricuspid regurgitation or a ventricular septal defect can occur under certain unusual circumstances. In mitral or tricuspid regurgitation, equilibration of pressure between the ventricle and the atrium in mid-systole will prevent the continuation of regurgitation of blood; hence, the murmur will stop in mid-systole. This may occur in acute severe mitral regurgitation[106] when the regurgitant volume is met by a relatively non-compliant left atrium so that pressure rises very steeply as a 'v' or systolic wave. The same phenomenon may occur with tricuspid valve damage and although right ventricular systolic pressure remains normal the regurgitation causes a very high 'v' wave in the right atrium.

The cause of an early systolic murmur in a ventricular septal defect is different. If the defect lies in the muscular septum and is small, it may become closed during systole. Once the defect has closed, the murmur disappears.

Late systolic murmurs

A murmur that starts in mid- or late systole and then increases in intensity to reach the second heart sound is known as a late systolic murmur.[92] The murmur is often confused by the unpractised clinician with the pre-systolic murmur of mitral stenosis because it has a similar crescendo quality. The late systolic murmur is sometimes initiated by a mid- or late systolic click or clicks caused by the halting of a billowed mitral valve (Fig. 8.34). If the valve when stretched permits regurgitation to occur, a late systolic murmur will be heard. Occasionally, the murmur has musical or 'honking' characteristic. Although the murmur denotes slight mitral regurgitation, the underlying mitral valve abnormality can be secondary, not only to the floppy mitral valve but also to abnormalities of the left ventricular myocardium and papillary muscles, and even rheumatism affecting the leaflets. As the murmur occurs late in systole, the degree of regurgitation can never be severe.

Similar abnormalities causing late systolic murmurs arising from the tricuspid valve have also been described.

Diastolic murmurs

There are only two types of diastolic murmur: mid-diastolic and early diastolic.

Mid-diastolic murmurs

The mid-diastolic murmur has mainly low-frequency characteristics: it arises as a result of turbulence created in the ventricle due to distortion of blood flow through the atrioventricular valves as blood passes from atrium to ventricle. The distortion of blood flow may be the result of narrowing and pathological change of the atrioventricular valve (as in rheumatic mitral stenosis), increased blood flow through a normal atrioventricular valve (as in a left-to-right shunt) or normal blood flow

through a mitral valve that has been narrowed by partial premature closure caused by the regurgitant jet of aortic regurgitation (the Austin Flint murmur).[107]

Mitral stenosis The mid-diastolic murmur of rheumatic mitral stenosis cannot start until after the left ventricular pressure has fallen below the left atrial pressure and the mitral valve has opened (Fig. 8.42). There is therefore a gap between A_2 and the onset of the mid-diastolic murmur (Fig. 8.43). If the rheumatic mitral valve is pliable, the murmur is initiated by the mitral opening snap (see above). The duration and audibility of the murmur will depend partly on the severity of the stenosis and the rise in left atrial pressure, and partly on the volume of blood flow across the valve.[108] If flow is normal, the length of the murmur denotes the severity of the stenosis, as there is a continuing pressure difference between the left atrial and left ventricular diastolic pressures. If blood flow is reduced, the murmur may be difficult to hear, even if the stenosis is severe.[109] In mitral stenosis with sinus rhythm, a pre-systolic low-frequency murmur may be heard coinciding with atrial systole;[108] this represents the turbulence created by the increased blood flow of atrial systole across the abnormal mitral valve. Sometimes, this murmur accompanies a mid-diastolic murmur, but sometimes the stenosis is mild and only a pre-systolic murmur is heard. Although this murmur is attributed to atrial systole when sinus rhythm is present, a pre-systolic murmur is sometimes heard in mitral stenosis with atrial fibrillation. In this latter situation, it has been shown that the murmur occurs after the onset of ventricular systole and prior to the loud closing sound of the mitral valve: ventricular systole, by disturbing the abnormal valve, further narrows the left atrial to left ventricular pathway and produces the additional turbulence, even though atrial systole has not occurred.[110]

A left atrial myxoma or a ball valve thrombus within the left atrium may produce a mid-diastolic murmur indistinguishable from that of mitral stenosis. Changes of position may change the quality of the murmur.

Tricuspid stenosis The genesis of the mid-diastolic and pre-systolic murmurs of tricuspid stenosis is analogous to that in mitral stenosis although right heart haemodynamic events are concerned. Rheumatic tricuspid stenosis is much less common than rheumatic mitral stenosis, but when present

Pre–systolic murmur (PSM) and Mid–diastolic murmur (MDM)

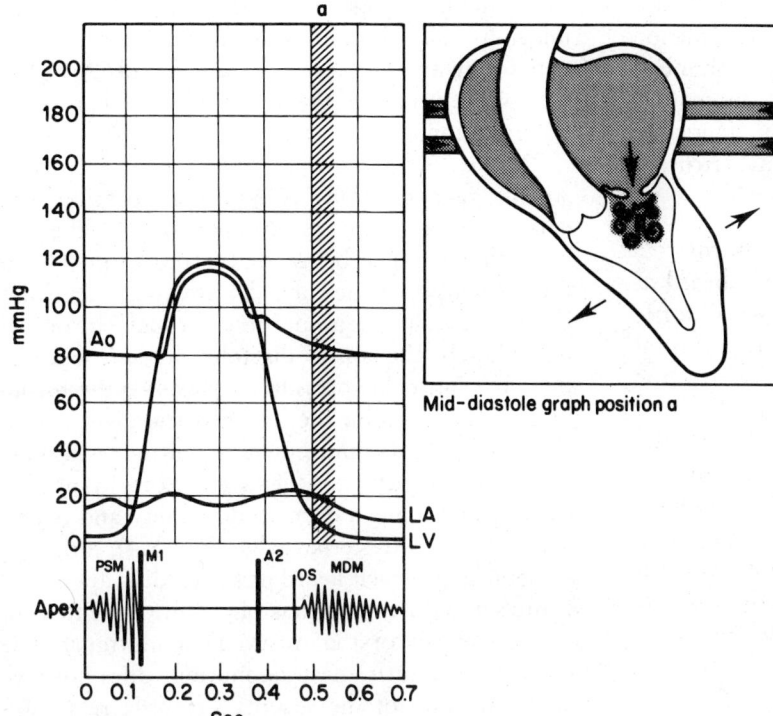

Mid-diastole graph position a

Fig. 8.42. Diagrammatic representation of simultaneous pressure curves, auscultatory findings at the apex, and blood flow in mitral stenosis. When left ventricular (LV) pressure exceeds left atrial (LA) pressure, the mitral valve closes (M_1). When LV pressure falls below aortic (A_0) diastolic pressure, the aortic valve closes (A_2). When LV pressure falls below LA pressure, the mitral valve opens and an opening snap (OS) is heard as the valve is abnormal. Blood flow through the abnormal mitral valve is turbulent generating a mid-diastolic murmur (MDM) and a pre-systolic murmur (PSM).

there is additional rheumatic mitral valve disease.[21] The venous pulse (see above) is an important marker of tricuspid valve disease; two-dimensional echocardiography will identify abnormalities at the level of the tricuspid valve and Doppler studies will provide confirmation. Inspiration, by increasing blood flow across the tricuspid valve, will intensify the murmurs of tricuspid stenosis.[111] A right atrial myxoma will mimic the physical signs of tricuspid valve disease, just as a left atrial myxoma mimics the physical signs of mitral valve disease.

Mid-diastolic murmurs due to increased blood flow If there is a large left-to-right shunt at the level of the ventricle or pulmonary artery (ventricular septal defect and persistent ductus arteriosus,

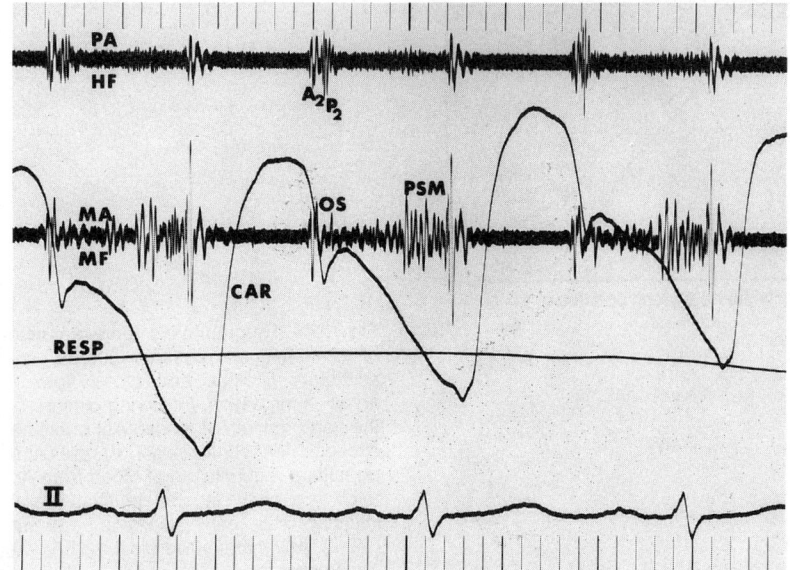

Fig. 8.43. Simultaneous high-frequency pulmonary area (PA–HF) and medium-frequency mitral area (MA–MF) phonocardiograms with an indirect carotid pulse (CAR), a respiratory trace (RESP) and lead II of the electrocardiogram in mitral stenosis. Physiological splitting of the second heart sound can be seen, but pulmonary valve closure (P_2) is louder than aortic valve closure (A_2) in the PA. An opening snap (OS) is seen in the MA, as well as a mid-diastolic and pre-systolic murmur (PSM).

respectively), the increased volume of blood passing through a normal mitral orifice results in a mid-diastolic murmur.[112,113] The same phenomenon occurs when there is a large left-to-right shunt at atrial level (atrial septal defect or anomalous pulmonary venous return), when an increased volume of blood passes through a normal tricuspid orifice.[50]

Austin Flint murmur   The Austin Flint murmur[107] is a mid-diastolic low-frequency murmur heard at the cardiac apex in some patients with aortic regurgitation who do not have rheumatic mitral valve disease. The murmur is *not* caused by the flutter of the anterior leaflet of the mitral valve that results from the aortic regurgitant jet; if it were, the murmur would occur early in diastole and not in mid-diastole. It has been shown that the regurgitant jet of aortic regurgitation moves the open anterior leaflet of the mitral valve to a position at which it impedes the flow of blood from left atrium to left ventricle, thereby causing a mid-diastolic murmur.[114]

Early diastolic murmurs

An early diastolic murmur is a high-frequency murmur that starts immediately after the aortic or pulmonary component of the second heart sound. This timing distinguishes it from the mid-diastolic murmur which does not start until there has been a gap following the second heart sound. An early diastolic murmur is the result of semilunar valve regurgitation.

Aortic regurgitation   Aortic regurgitation can commence as soon as the pressure in the left ventricle has fallen below that in the aorta. This is the moment of aortic valve closure and, if the valve is incompetent, regurgitation through it occurs immediately the aortic diastolic pressure exceeds the left ventricular pressure (Fig. 8.44): the turbulence created within the left ventricle gives rise to the early diastolic murmur. The murmur is usually of high frequency, is difficult to record by phonocardiography, has a decrescendo quality and is best heard at the left sternal edge (Fig. 8.4), although sometimes it is well heard at the cardiac apex (and confused with a mid-diastolic murmur either of mitral stenosis or the Austin Flint murmur). The length of the early diastolic murmur does not give any indication of the severity of aortic regurgitation, except in acute severe aortic regurgitation (see below).

In mild aortic regurgitation (whether due to

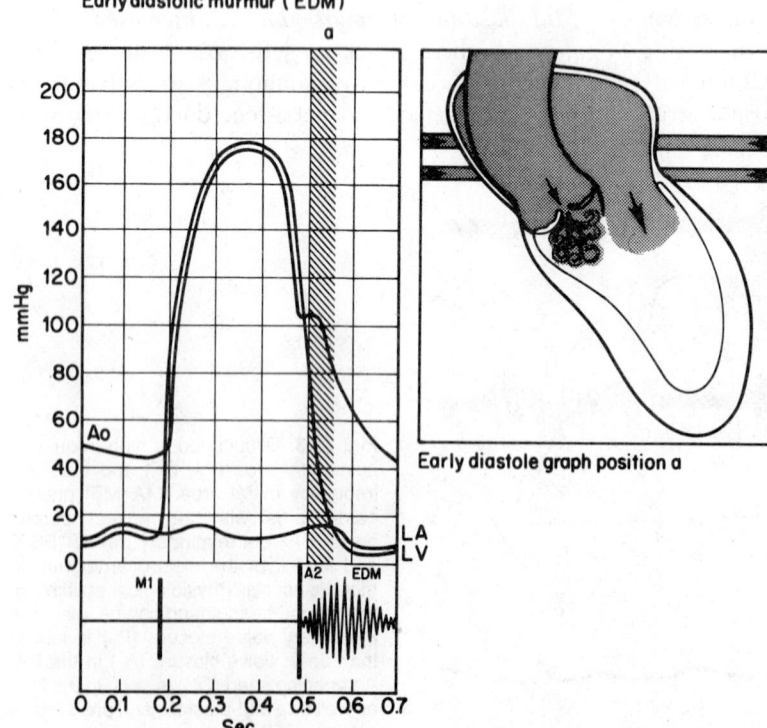

Fig. 8.44. Diagrammatic representation of simultaneous pressure curves, auscultatory findings and blood flow in aortic regurgitation. Following closure of the aortic valve (A$_2$), aortic (Ao) pressure exceeds left ventricular (LV) pressure permitting regurgitation of blood from Ao to LV through the incompetent valve, and initiating the early diastolic murmur (EDM). M$_1$, mitral valve closure; LA, left atrial pressure.

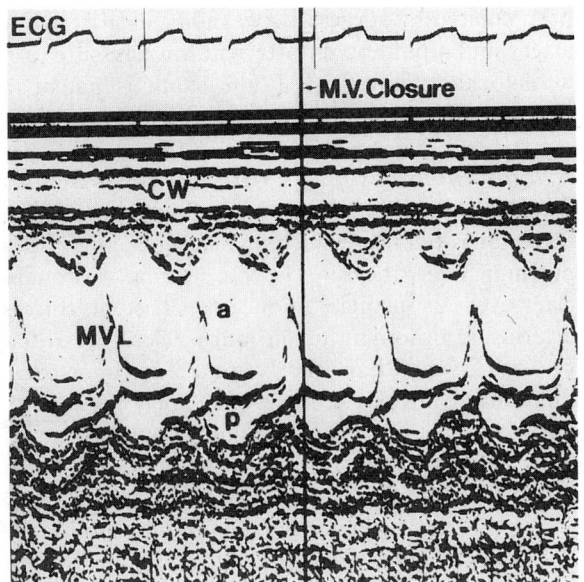

Fig. 8.45. M-mode echocardiogram and electrocardiogram in a patient with acute severe aortic regurgitation. The anterior (a) and posterior (p) leaflets of the mitral valve (MVL) are seen to close prior to the QRS complex on the electrocardiogram. Note the relatively normal left ventricular dimensions and excellent systolic function of the left ventricle. CW, chest wall.

leaflet abnormalities or aortic wall disease), the murmur may be the only abnormal finding. Flutter within the left ventricle on M-mode echocardiography provides confirmation of the existence of aortic regurgitation.

In chronic moderate or severe aortic regurgitation, the abnormal arterial pulse, wide pulse pressure and hyperdynamic apical impulse (see above) associated with the large left ventricular stroke volume provide important clues to severity; echocardiography shows the large left ventricular stroke volume and can be used to assess the aetiology in the aortic valve or aortic wall.

Acute severe aortic regurgitation (as in infective endocarditis with destruction of the valve leaflets) results in an unusual haemodynamic disturbance.[115] Severe regurgitation into the normal-sized and relatively non-compliant left ventricle causes extreme elevation of left ventricular diastolic pressure. The aortic and left ventricular diastolic pressures may be very similar and consequently an aortic early diastolic murmur may scarcely be heard. Left ventricular diastolic pressure rapidly rises to exceed left atrial pressure, resulting in the premature closure of the mitral valve.[49] Although this closure is inaudible, it may be identified by simultaneous M-mode echocardiography and electrocardiography (Fig. 8.45).

Pulmonary regurgitation The genesis of the high-frequency early diastolic murmur which immediately follows P_2 and is best heard at the left sternal edge is identical to that of aortic regurgitation. However, conditions resulting in pulmonary regurgitation are much less common than those causing aortic regurgitation.

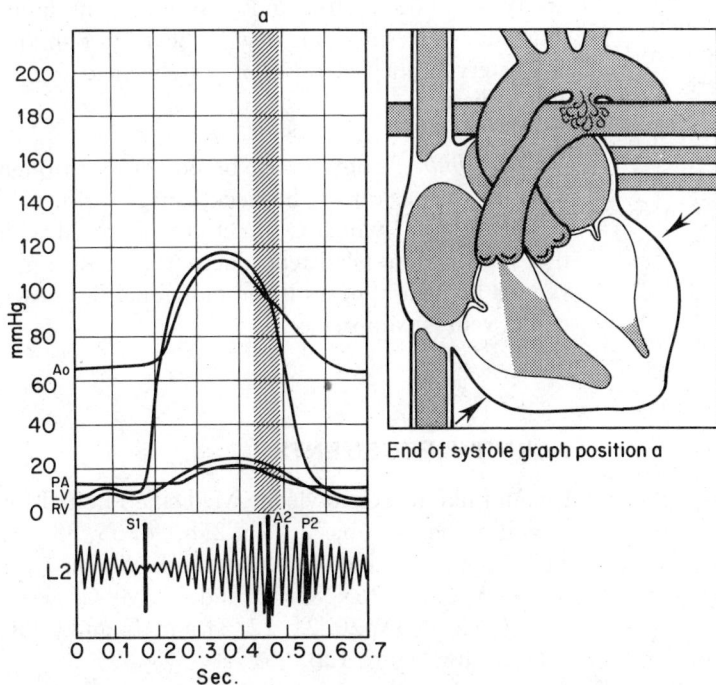

End of systole graph position a

Fig. 8.46. Diagrammatic representation of pressure curves, auscultatory findings in the left second space (L2) and blood flow in a persistent ductus arteriosus with a left-to-right shunt and normal pulmonary artery pressure. There is a pressure difference between aorta (Ao) and pulmonary artery (PA) throughout the cardiac cycle and hence a continuous murmur is heard. Blood flow from Ao to PA through the ductus is seen at the end of systole when the murmur peaks. (S_1, first heart sound; A_2, aortic valve closure; P_2, pulmonary valve closure; LV, left ventricular pressure; RV, right ventricular pressure.

The classical Graham Steell murmur of pulmonary regurgitation was described in patients with rheumatic mitral valve disease who had severe pulmonary hypertension.[116] Severe long standing pulmonary hypertension causes dilatation of the central pulmonary arteries and incompetence of the pulmonary valve by dilatation of the pulmonary valve ring.

Other causes of pulmonary hypertension may be associated with a similar phenomenon: the Eisenmenger situation, particularly with an Eisenmenger persistent ductus arteriosus; primary or chronic thrombo-embolic pulmonary hypertension; and, rarely, in chronic respiratory disease. Occasionally, pulmonary regurgitation occurs as a result of leaflet abnormalities, which may be seen following pulmonary valvotomy for pulmonary valve stenosis and in the absent pulmonary valve syndrome.

Continuous murmurs

Continuous murmurs start during systole and continue through the second heart sound (when they usually peak) into diastole. They are usually of high frequency and best heard over the abnormality responsible for their genesis. Any condition in which there is a pressure difference across a communication or a constriction in both systole and diastole and continuous blood flow may give rise to a continuous murmur.[117]

Persistent ductus arteriosus In a persistent ductus arteriosus with an aorta to pulmonary artery shunt and normal pulmonary artery pressure, there is a constant pressure difference in favour of the aorta. Blood can flow in both systole and diastole into the pulmonary artery through the ductus; a continuous murmur is the result (Fig. 8.46). The murmur is best heard in the second left interspace.

If pulmonary hypertension is present with a larger left-to-right shunt, the murmur usually becomes shorter and is confined to systole. The second heart sound is physiologically split, but P_2 is accentuated.[61] There may be a flow mid-diastolic murmur through the normal mitral valve.

When pulmonary vascular resistance is raised (Eisenmenger situation), the shunt is from the pulmonary artery to the aorta. The murmur is short in systole, P_2 remains accentuated and an early diastolic murmur due to pulmonary regurgitation may be heard.

An analogous situation occurs when a shunt has been created by surgery between a central systemic artery and a pulmonary artery at low pressure (e.g. a Blalock anastomosis). If the shunt is patent, a continuous murmur will be heard over it.

Arteriovenous fistulae Various arteriovenous fistulae, either congenital or acquired, exist. All of these can often be detected by hearing a continuous murmur over the site of the fistula. Coronary arteriovenous fistulae mimic a persistent ductus arteriosus, although the murmur is usually heard at a level lower than the second left interspace. Pulmonary arteriovenous fistulae may exist anywhere in the lungs, with continuous murmurs heard over the lung fields. In pulmonary atresia with ventricular septal defect, blood reaches the lungs through bronchopulmonary communications. Continuous murmurs over the lungs may be heard under these circumstances. A fistula may be created by trauma (e.g. bullet wounds) or deliberately created by surgery for the purpose of haemodialysis.

Ruptured aneurysm of the sinus of Valsalva This congenital lesion may rupture into any of the cardiac chambers but particularly into the right atrium or right ventricle. The continous murmur is best heard low down the sternal edge.

Arterial constriction A significant constriction in an artery creates a pressure difference from the proximal to distal end and, if flow through the artery is in both systole and diastole, a continuous murmur will result. This may be heard in pulmonary artery branch stenosis or, rarely, in coronary artery disease.

Venous hum Continuous blood flow through veins in the region of the neck can give rise to a venous hum,[118] which is sometimes confused with the sound of a persistent ductus arteriosus; the venous hum disappears if the individual lies down or the vein is compressed.

ACKNOWLEDGEMENTS

I would like to acknowledge Medicine Limited for providing figures 6b, 7a, 19b, 25b, 34, 35, 38, 39, 41, 42, 44, 45 and 46. Also Dr L. Shapiro for figures 5, 6a, 9, 26, 28b, 33 and 43, Mr G. Leech for figures 14, 15, 20, 21, 22, 31 and 32 and Dr R. Dawson for Figure 12b.

REFERENCES

1. Mackenzie, J. *The study of the pulse arterial venous and hepatic, and of the movements of the heart.* Edinburgh and London, 1902.
2. Van de Werf, F., Piessens, J. and Kesteloot, H. A comparison of systolic time intervals derived from the central aortic pressure and from the external carotid pulse tracing. *Circulation* 1975; **51**: 310.
3. Corrigan, D.J. On permanent patency of the mouth of the aorta, or inadequacy of the aortic valves. *Edin. Med. Surg. J.* 1832; **37**: 225.
4. O'Rourke, M.F. The arterial pulse in health and disease. *Am. Heart J.* 1971; **82**: 687.
5. Braunwald, E., Lambrew, C.T., Rockoff, S.D., Ross, J. and Morrow, A. Idiopathic subaortic stenosis: I. A description of the disease based upon an analysis of 64 patients. *Circulation* 1964; **30**(Suppl. IV): IV–3.
6. Robinson, B. The carotid pulse I. Diagnosis of aortic stenosis by external recordings. *Br. Heart J.* 1963; **25**: 51.
7. Epstein, E.J. and Coulshed, N. Assessment of aortic stenosis from the external carotid pulse wave. *Br. Heart J.* 1964; **26**: 84.
8. Elkins, R.C., Morrow, A.G., Vasko, J.S. and Braunwald, E. The effects of mitral regurgitation on the pattern of instantaneous aortic blood flow. Clinical and experimental observations. *Circulation* 1967; **36**: 45.
9. Fleming, P.R. The mechanism of pulsus bisferiens. *Br. Heart J.* 1957; **19**: 519.
10. Ikram, H., Nixon, P.G.F. and Fox, J.A. The haemodynamic implication of the bisferiens pulse. *Br. Heart J.* 1964; **26**: 452.
11. Ewy, G., Rios, J.C. and Marcus, F.I. The dicrotic arterial pulse. *Circulation* 1969; **39**: 655.
12. Dornhorst, A.C., Howard, P. and Leathart, G.L. Pulsus paradoxus. *Lancet* 1952; i: 746.
13. D'Cruz, I.A., Cohen, H.C., Prabhu, R. and Glick, G. Diagnosis of cardiac tamponade by echocardiography: changes in mitral valve motion and ventricular dimension, with special reference to paradoxical pulse. *Circulation* 1975; **52**: 460.
14. Settle, H.P., Adolph, R.J., Fowler, N.O., Engel, P., Agruss, N.S. and Levenson, N.I. Echocardiographic study of cardiac tamponade. *Circulation* 1977; **56**: 951.
15. Rebuck, A.S. and Pengelly, L.D. Development of pulsus paradox in the presence of airways obstruction. *N. Engl. J. Med.* 1973; **288**: 66.
16. Logan, W.F.W.E., Jones, E.W. and Walker, E. Familial supravalvar aortic stenosis. *Br. Heart J.* 1965; **27**: 547.
17. Hartman, H. The jugular venous tracing. *Am. Heart J.* 1960; **59**: 698.
18. Wood, P. *Diseases of the heart and circulation*, 2nd edition. London: Eyre & Spottiswoode, 1957.
19. Feder, W. and Cherry, R.A. External jugular phlebogram as reflecting venous and right atrial haemodynamics. *Am. J. Cardiol.* 1963; **12**: 383.
20. Rich, L.L. and Tavel, M.E. The origin of the jugular C wave. *Am. J. Cardiol.* 1970; **26**: 656.
21. Gibson, R. and Wood, P. The diagnosis of tricuspid stenosis. *Br. Heart J.* 1955; **17**: 552.
22. Gibson, R.V. Quoted in *Diseases of the heart and circulation* (Wood, P., ed.) 1957. London: Eyre & Spottiswoode.
23. Kussmaul, A. Ueber schwielige mediastino—pericarditis und der paradoxen Puls. *Klin. Wochenschr.* 1873; **10**: 433.
24. Coulshed, N. and Epstein, E.J. The apex cardiogram: its normal features explained by those found in heart disease. *Br. Heart J.* 1963; **25**: 697.
25. Benchimol, A. and Dimond, E.G. The apex cardiogram in ischaemic heart disease. *Br. Heart J.* 1962; **24**: 581.
26. Willems, J.L., De Geest, H. and Kesteloot, H. On the value of apex cardiography for timing intracardiac events. *Am. J. Cardiol.* 1971; **28**: 59.
27. Willems, J.L., Kesteloot, H. and De Geest, H. Influence of acute haemodynamic changes on the apex cardiogram in dogs. *Am. J. Cardiol.* 1972; **29**: 504.
28. Epstein, E.J., Coulshed, N., Brown, A.K. and Donkas, N.G. The 'a' wave of the apex cardiogram in aortic valve disease and cardiomyopathy. *Br. Heart J.* 1968; **30**: 591.
29. Fleming, J.S. The assessment of failure in aortic stenosis from the diastolic movements of the left ventricle. *Am. Heart J.* 1968; **76**: 235.
30. Gibson, T.C., Madry, R., Grossman, W., McLaurin, L.P. and Craige, E. The 'a' wave of the apex cardiogram and left ventricular diastolic stiffness. *Circulation* 1974; **49**: 441.
31. Sutton, G.C., Prewitt, T.A. and Craige, E. Relationship between quantitated precordial movement and left ventricular function. *Circulation* 1970; **41**: 179.
32. Craige, E. and Schmidt, R.E. Precordial movements over the right ventricle in normal children. *Circulation* 1965; **32**: 232.
33. Kesteloot, H. and Willems, J.L. Relationship between the right apex cardiogram and the right ventricular dynamics. *Acta Cardiol.* 1967; **22**: 64.
34. Schmidt, R.E. and Craige, E. Precordial movements over the right ventricle in children with pulmonary stenosis. *Circulation* 1965; **32**: 241.
35. Leatham, A. Phonocardiography. *Br. Med. Bull.* 1952; **8**: 333.
36. Tavel, M.E. *Clinical phonocardiography and external pulse recording*, 4th edition. Chicago: Year Book Medical Publishers, 1985.
37. Mills, P. and Craige, E. Echophonocardiography. *Prog. Cardiovasc. Dis.* 1978; **20**: 337.
38. Leatham, A. Splitting of the first and second heart sounds. *Lancet* 1954; ii: 607.
39. Di Bartolo, G., Nunez-Dey, D., Muiesan, G., MacCanon, D.M. and Luisada, A.A. Haemodynamic correlates of the first heart sound. *Am. J. Physiol.* 1961; **201**: 888.
40. Lariado, S., Yellin, E.L., Miller, H. and Frater, R.W.M. Temporal relation of the first heart sound to closure of the mitral valve. *Circulation* 1973; **47**: 1006.
41. Lakier, J.B., Fritz, V.U., Pocock, W.A. and Barlow, J.B. Mitral components of the first heart sound. *Br. Heart J.* 1972; **34**: 160.
42. Lakier, J.B., Bloom, K.R., Pocock, W.A. and Barlow, J.B. Tricuspid component of first heart sound. *Br. Heart J.* 1973; **35**: 1275.
43. Haber, E. and Leatham, A. Splitting of heart sounds from ventricular asynchrony in bundle branch block, ventricular ectopic beats and artificial pacing. *Br. Heart J.* 1965; **27**: 691.
44. Brooks, N., Leech, G. and Leatham, A. Complete right bundle branch block: echophonocardiography study of first heart sound and right ventricular contraction times. *Br. Heart J.* 1979; **41**: 637.
45. Burggraf, G.W. The first heart sound in left bundle branch block: an echophonocardiographic study. *Circulation* 1981; **63**: 429.
46. Craige, E. Phonocardiographic studies in mitral stenosis. *N. Engl. J. Med.* 1957; **257**: 650.
47. Crews, T.L., Pridie, R.B., Benham, R. and Leatham, A. Auscultatory and phonocardiographic findings in Ebstein's anomaly. Correlation of first heart sound with ultrasonic records of tricuspid valve movement. *Br. Heart J.* 1972; **34**: 681.
48. Leech, G., Brooks, N., Green-Wilkinson, A. and Leatham, A. Mechanism of influence of PR interval on loudness of

first heart sound. *Br. Heart J.* 1980; **43**: 138.

49. Meadows, W.R., Sharp, J.T. and Zachariudakis, S. Premature mitral valve closure: a haemodynamic explanation for absence of the first sound in aortic insufficiency. *Circulation* 1963; **28**: 251.

50. Leatham, A. and Gray, I. Auscultatory and phonocardiographic signs of atrial septal defect. *Br. Heart J.* 1956; **18**: 193.

51. Hirschfeld, S., Liebman, J., Borkat, G. and Bormuth, C. Intra-cardiac pressure-sound correlates of echocardiographic aortic valve closure. *Circulation* 1977; **55**: 602.

52. Chandraratna, P.A.N., Lopez, J.M. and Cohen, L.S. Echocardiographic observations on the mechanism of production of the second heart sound. *Circulation* 1975; **51**: 292.

53. Leatham, A. and Towers, M. Splitting of the second heart sound in health. *Br. Heart J.* 1951; **13**: 575.

54. Harris, A. and Sutton, G. Second heart sound in normal subjects. *Br. Heart J.* 1968; **30**: 739.

55. Aygen, M.M. and Braunwald, E. The splitting of the second heart sound in normal subjects and in patients with congenital heart disease. *Circulation* 1962; **25**: 328.

56. Shuler, R.H., Ensor, C., Gunning, R.E., Moss, W.G. and Johnson, V. The differential effects of respiration on the left and right ventricles. *Am. J. Physiol.* 1942; **137**: 620.

57. Boyer, S.H. and Chisholm, A.W. Physiologic splitting of the second heart sound. *Circulation* 1958; **18**: 1010.

58. Shaver, J.R., O'Toole, J.D., Curtis, E.I., Thompson, M.E., Reddy, P.S. and Leon, D.F. Second heart sound: the role of altered greater and lesser circulation. In: Leon, D.F. and Shaver, J.A., eds. *Physiologic Principles of Heart Sounds and Murmurs*, Monograph No. 46. New York: American Heart Association, 1975, p.58.

59. Leatham, A. and Weitzman, D.W. Auscultatory and phonocardiographic signs of pulmonary stenosis. *Br. Heart J.* 1957; **19**: 303.

60. Mills, P., Wolfe, C., Redwood, D., Leech, G., Craige, E. and Leatham, A. Non-invasive diagnosis of subpulmonary outflow tract obstruction. *Br. Heart J.* 1980; **43**: 276.

61. Sutton, G., Harris, A. and Leatham, A. Second heart sound in pulmonary hypertension. *Br. Heart J.* 1968; **30**: 743.

62. Cobbs, B.W., Logue, R.B. and Dorney, E.R. The second sound in pulmonary embolism and pulmonary hypertension. *Am. Heart J.* 1966; **71**: 843.

63. Sutton, G.C. Cardiovascular consequences of acute massive pulmonary embolism and the effect of treatment. MD Thesis, Cambridge, 1970.

64. Schrire, V. and Vogelpoel, L. The role of the dilated pulmonary artery in abnormal splitting of the second heart sound. *Am. Heart J.* 1962; **63**: 501.

65. Karnegis, J.N. and Wang, Y. The phonocardiogram in idiopathic dilatation of the pulmonary artery. *Am. J. Cardiol.* 1964; **14**: 75.

66. Brigden, W. and Leatham, A. Mitral incompetence. *Br. Heart J.* 1953; **15**: 55.

67. Leatham, A. and Segal, B. Auscultatory and phonocardiographic signs of ventricular septal defect with left-to-right shunt. *Circulation* 1962; **25**: 318.

68. Beck, W., Schrire, V. and Vogelpoel, L. Splitting of the second heart sound in constrictive pericarditis with observation of the mechanism of pulsus paradoxus. *Am. Heart J.* 1962; **64**: 765.

69. Gray, I.R. Paradoxical splitting of the second heart sound. *Br. Heart J.* 1956; **18**: 21.

70. March, H.W., Selzer, A. and Hultgren, H.N. The mechanical consequences of anomalous excitation (WPW syndrome). *Circulation* 1961; **23**: 582.

71. Yurchak, C.M. and Gorlin, R. Paradoxical splitting of the second heart sound in coronary heart disease. *N. Engl. J. Med.* 1963; **269**: 741.

72. Damore, S., Murgo, J.P., Bloom, K.R. and Rubal, B.J. Second heart sound dynamics in atrial septal defect. *Circulation* 1981; **64** (Suppl. 4): 28.

73. Sabbah, H.N., Khaja, F., Anbe, D.T. and Stein, P.D. The aortic closure sound in pure aortic insufficiency. *Circulation* 1977; **56**: 859.

74. Epstein, E.J., Criley, J.M., Raftery, E.B., Humphries, J.O. and Ross, R.S. Cineradiographic studies of the early systolic click in aortic valve stenosis. *Circulation* 1965; **31**: 842.

75. Leech, G., Mills, P. and Leatham, A. The diagnosis of a non-stenotic bicuspid aortic valve. *Br. Heart J.* 1978; **40**: 941.

76. Mills, P.G., Brodie, B., McLaurin, L.P., Schall, S. and Craige, E. Echocardiographic and hemodynamic relationships of ejection sounds. *Circulation* 1977; **56**: 430.

77. Leatham, A. and Vogelpoel, L. The early systolic sound in dilatation of the pulmonary artery. *Br. Heart J.* 1954; **16**: 21.

78. Hultgren, H.N., Reeve, R., Cohn, K. and McLeod, R. The ejection click of valvular pulmonary stenosis. *Circulation* 1969; **40**: 631.

79. Mills, P., Amara, I., McLaurin, L.P. and Craige, E. Non-invasive assessment of pulmonary hypertension from right ventricular isovolumic contraction time. *Am. J. Cardiol.* 1980; **46**: 272.

80. Gamboa, R., Hugenholtz, P.E. and Nadas, A.S. Accuracy of the phonocardiogram in assessing severity of aortic and pulmonic stenosis. *Circulation* 1964; **30**: 35.

81. Hancock, E.W. The ejection sound in aortic stenosis. *Am. J. Med.* 1966; **40**: 569.

82. Leo, T. and Hultgren, H. Phonocardiographic characteristics of tight mitral stenosis. *Medicine* 1959; **38**: 85.

83. Rich, C.B. The relation of heart sounds to left atrial pressure. *Can. Med. Assoc. J.* 1959; **81**: 800.

84. Sutton, G.C., Chatterjee, K. and Caves, P.K. Diagnosis of severe mitral regurgitation due to non-rheumatic chordal abnormalities. *Br. Heart J.* 1973; **35**: 877.

85. Milward, D.K., McLaurin, L.P. and Craige, E. Echocardiographic studies to explain opening snaps in presence of non-stenotic mitral valves. *Am. J. Cardiol.* 1973; **31**: 64.

86. Pitt, A., Pitt, B., Schaefer, J. and Criley, J.M. Myxoma of the left atrium: hemodynamic and phonocardiographic consequences of sudden tumor movement. *Circulation* 1967; **36**: 408.

87. Potain, C. Les bruits de galop. *La Sem. Med.* 1900; **20**: 175.

88. Kuo, P.T., Schnabel, T.G., Blakemore, W.S. and Whereat, A.F. Diastolic gallop sounds, the mechanism of production. *J. Clin. Invest.* 1957; **36**: 1035.

89. Ozawa, Y., Smith, D. and Craige, E. Origin of the third heart sound I. Studies in dogs. *Circulation* 1983; **67**: 393.

90. Tyberg, T.I., Goodyer, A.V.N. and Langrou, R.A. Genesis of pericardial knock in constrictive pericarditis. *Am. J. Cardiol.* 1980; **46**: 570.

91. Craige, E. The fourth heart sound. In: Leon, D.F. and Shaver, J.A. eds. *Physiologic principles of heart sounds and murmurs,* Monograph No. 46. New York: American Heart Association, 1975, p.74.

92. Barlow, J.B., Bosman, C.K., Pocock, W.A. and Marchand, P. Late systolic mumurs and non-ejection ('mid-late') systolic clicks. *Br. Heart J.* 1968; **30**: 203.

93. Criley, J.M., Lewis, K.B., Humphries, J.O. and Ross, R.S. Prolapse of the mitral valve: clinical and cineangiographic findings. *Br. Heart J.* 1966; **28**: 488.

94. Leatham, A. *Auscultation of the heart and phonocardiography.* London: J. & A. Churchill, 1970.

95. Hancock, E.W. Differentiation of valvar, subvalvar and supravalvar aortic stenosis. *Guy's Hosp. Rep.* 1961; **110**: 1.

96. Perloff, J.K. Clinical recognition of aortic stenosis; the physical signs and differential diagnosis of the various forms of obstruction to the left ventricular outflow. *Prog. Cardiovasc. Dis.* 1968; **10**: 323.

97. Shah, P.M., Gramik, R. and Kramer, D.H. Ultrasound localisation of left ventricular outflow tract obstruction in hypertrophic obstructive cardiomyopathy. *Circulation* 1969; **40**: 3.

98. Vogel, J.H.K. and Blount, S.G. Clinical evaluation in localising level of obstruction to outflow from left ventricle. Importance of early systolic ejection click. *Am. J. Cardiol.* 1965; **15**: 782.

99. Pomerance, A. Cardiac pathology and systolic murmurs in the elderly. *Br. Heart J.* 1968; **30**: 687.

100. Leatham, A., Segal, B. and Shafter, H. Auscultatory and phonocardiographic findings in healthy children with systolic murmurs. *Br. Heart J.* 1965; **25**: 451.

101. Vogelpoel, L. and Schrire, V. Auscultatory and phonocardiographic assessment of pulmonary stenosis with intact ventricular septum. *Circulation* 1960; **22**: 55.

102. Vogelpoel, L. and Schrire, V. Auscultatory and phonocardiographic assessment of Fallot's tetralogy. *Circulation* 1960; **22**: 73.

103. Perloff, J.K. and Lebauer, E.J. Auscultatory and phonocardiographic manifestation of isolated stenosis of the pulmonary artery and its branches. *Br. Heart J.* 1969; **31**: 314.

104. Nixon, P.G.F. The third heart sound in mitral regurgitation. *Br. Heart J.* 1961; **23**: 677.

105. Rios, J.C., Massumi, R.A., Breesman, W.T. and Sarin, R.K. Auscultatory features of acute tricuspid regurgitation. *Am. J. Cardiol.* 1969; **23**: 4.

106. Sutton, G.C. and Craige, E. Clinical signs of severe acute mitral regurgitation. *Am. J. Cardiol.* 1967; **20**: 141.

107. Flint, A. On cardiac mumurs. *Am. J. Med. Sci.* 1862; **44**: 29.

108. Wood, P. An appreciation of mitral stenosis. *Br. Med. J.* 1954; I: 1051 and 1113.

109. Heda, H., Sakamoto, T., Kawai, N., Watanabe, H., Vozumi, Z., Okada, R., Koboyasti, T. and Kaito, G. 'Silent' mitral stenosis. Pathoanatomical basis of the absence of the diastolic rumble. *Jap. Heart J.* 1965; **6**: 206.

110. Criley, J.M., Feldman, J.M. and Meredith, T. Mitral valve closure and the crescendo presystolic murmur. *Am. J. Med.* 1971; **51**: 456.

111. Perloff, J.K. and Harvey, W.P. Clinical recognition of tricuspid stenosis. *Circulation* 1960; **22**: 346.

112. Wood, P. Congenital heart disease. *Br. Med. J.* 1950; II: 639 and 653.

113. Ravin, A. and Darley, W. Apical diastolic mumurs in patent ductus arteriosus. *Ann. Intern. Med.* 1950; **33**: 903.

114. Fortuin, N.J. and Craige, E. On the mechanism of the Austin-Flint murmur. *Circulation* 1972; **45**: 558.

115. Rees, J.R., Epstein, E.J., Criley, J.M. and Ross, R.S. Hemodynamic effects of severe aortic regurgitation. *Br. Heart J.* 1964; **26**: 412.

116. Steell, G. The murmur of high pressure in the pulmonary artery. *Medical Chronicle, Manchester* 1888; **9**: 182.

117. Neill, C. and Mounsey, P. Auscultation in patent ductus arteriosus with a description of two fistulae simulating patent ductus. *Br. Heart J.* 1958; **20**: 61.

118. Potain, P.C.E. Des mouvements et des bruits qui se passent dans les veines jugularies. *Bull. et Mem. Soc. Med. Hop. de Paris* 1867; **4**: 3.

Chapter 9

The Resting Electrocardiogram

Derek J. Rowlands

Electrocardiography is concerned with the recording of electrical activity produced by the heart. No other investigative technique in cardiology has received such widespread and sustained acceptance and, despite the development of many additional investigative procedures, an electrocardiogram is an essential part of cardiovascular assessment.

HISTORICAL DEVELOPMENTS

In 1843, Carlow Matteucci noted that, in certain circumstances, electrical currents could be observed in strips of pigeon heart muscle. In 1856, Kollicker and Muller used a frog sciatic nerve–gastrocnemius preparation as a recording device (with the sciatic nerve draped across the myocardium of the exposed heart of another frog) and showed that a beating heart produced sufficient electrical activity to stimulate the sciatic nerve and induce contraction of the gastrocnemius. In 1878, John Sanderson and F.J.M. Page in England, using a capillary electrometer, recorded for the first time the current produced by the action of the heart. In 1887, Waller and Ludwig, also using a capillary electrometer, demonstrated that at the time of each cardiac contraction measurable current was detectable at the surface of the human body. Following the development of the string galvanometer by Willem Einthoven, the current from the human heart was first quantatively assessed in 1901. The term 'electrocardiogram' was coined by Einthoven. Between 1908 and 1926, a most fruitful liaison flourished between Einthoven (who occupied the chair of physiology at Lieden) and Sir Thomas Lewis from London. Einthoven's technical achievements were remarkable. He constructed the first reliable recording instrument (the string galvanometer) and he was instrumental in constructing a cable which connected his laboratory to the University Hospital approximately 1 mile away. To be able to obtain satisfactory readings of the body surface electrocardiogram with the 'electrodes' (actually bowls of saline) and the recorder separated by such a distance is nothing short of remarkable for the time. However, the enthusiasm of the local physicians was somewhat limited and the development of electrocardiography hinged predominantly on the relationship between Einthoven and Lewis. Sir Thomas Lewis was an excellent and indefatigable investigator who clearly demonstrated the usefulness of the electrocardiogram. Lewis's work was the first stage in the correlation of clinical data with electrical observation which has since formed the basis of the purely empirical discipline of electrocardiography. Correspondence and exchange visits between Lewis and Einthoven were frequent and productive. Einthoven labelled the deflections on the basic electrocardiographic waveform P, Q, R, S and T. The explanation for this choice of letters is not clear. One commentator suggests that he deliberately chose letters from the middle of the alphabet so as to leave room for extension but one must also presume that it is quite possible that in his earlier work (unrelated to the electrocardiogram) he had used labelling which had reached 'O'! Whatever the reason for the choice, this nomenclature has remained, as has his chosen arrangement of the connection of the limbs to give leads, I, II and III. The next major boost in the evolution of electrocardiography occurred as a result of the development by Frank Wilson in 1933 of the unipolar electrocardiogram. The recording technique has remained essentially unchanged since that time.

RHYTHM INFORMATION AND MORPHOLOGICAL INFORMATION

The 12-lead electrocardiogram contains both morphological information and rhythm information. Morphological information refers to information concerning the size and shape of the P waves, the QRS complexes and the ST segments and T waves (which provide information on, respectively, atrial myocardial depolarization, ventricular myocardial depolarization, and ventricular myocardial repolarization. Rhythm information refers to information concerning the frequency, regularity and timing of the P waves and of the QRS complexes, and the relationship between the two. There is some overlap between morphological and rhythm information (for example, during an ectopic ventricular tachycardia the QRS complexes will have abnormal morphology), but in most respects the two types of information remain discrete. In this chapter, I will deal with the 12-lead electrocardiogram during sinus rhythm. Arrhythmias will be described elsewhere. It is necessary first to describe the features of normal sinus rhythm.

ELECTROCARDIOGRAPHIC FEATURES OF NORMAL SINUS RHYTHM

The phrase 'the heart is in sinus rhythm' implies that the initiation of depolarization within the heart occurs at the sino-atrial node. Unless the term is qualified by some additional phrase (e.g. 'with first degree heart block', 'with right bundle branch block', 'with frequent ventricular ectopic beats' or 'with ventricular pre-excitation') this phrase may be held to imply also that the depolarization wave, once initiated at the sino-atrial node, then spreads through the atrial myocardium, through the normal atrioventricular conducting tissue and through the right and left bundle branches to the ventricles. The electrocardiographic appearances of sinus rhythm are shown in Fig. 9.1.

The normal rhythm of the heart is sinus rhythm with a regular rate of 60–100 beats/min. This definition is accepted by the Criteria Committee of the New York Heart Association. The term 'regular' is taken to mean that the cycle length (P to P

interval) does not vary by more than 10%. Note that a large number of criteria must be fulfilled before the simple statement 'the heart is in sinus rhythm' is a justifiable and sufficient description of the rhythm. These criteria are as follows:

1 there must be P waves;
2 the P waves must be morphologically usual for that subject;
3 all P waves must have the same morphology;
4 the P wave rate must be constant except for small changes due to sinus arrhythmia;
5 the P wave rate must not lie outside the limit 60–100 beats/min;
6 there must be QRS complexes;
7 the QRS complexes must have the morphology usual for that subject;
8 there must be one P wave to each QRS complex;
9 the P waves must be in front of the QRS complex;
10 the PR interval must be normal (i.e. within the limits 0.12–0.22 s);
11 the PR interval must be constant.

BASIC ASPECTS OF THE NORMAL 12-LEAD ELECTROCARDIOGRAM

THE 12-LEAD SYSTEM

The 12–lead electrocardiogram was not designed, it developed historically. This fact explains why it is such an unusual collection of leads: 3 bipolar leads in the frontal plane (I, II and III), 3 unipolar leads in the frontal plane (aVR, aVL and aVF) and 6 unipolar leads in the horizontal plane (V$_1$–V$_6$). The earliest electrocardiograms were 3-lead records (I, II and III) obtained using liquid electrodes into which the 4 limbs were immersed. (The right leg was, and still is, a simple 'ground' connection used for limiting noise.) These bipolar leads reflect the differences in voltage between the 2 electrodes and all voltage arrangements are difference values in any case. The 'unipolar' lead devised by Wilson con-

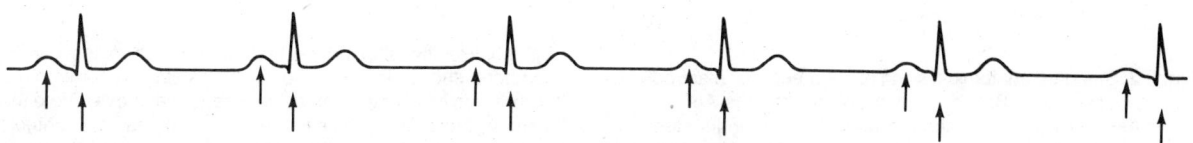

Fig. 9.1. The electrocardiographic appearance of sinus rhythm. The record is taken from a lead which shows well the P waves and QRS complexes. The P waves and QRS complexes are morphologically normal, the P waves are regular at 60 per minute, the P–R interval is both normal and constant. Since the P–R interval is constant and the P wave rate is constant, the QRS rate is also constant.

sisted of a system in which the *exploring electrode,* a'V' (i.e. voltage) lead, is attached to one terminal of the amplifier and a neutral lead, the *indifferent electrode* (consisting of simultaneous right arm, left arm and left leg connections) is attached to the other amplifier terminal. It can be proved that the sum of R, L and F (which is the voltage input to the indifferent terminal) is necessarily zero so that the V lead produces what is effectively a unipolar voltage recording. The 6 precordial leads, so produced, are therefore labelled V_1 to V_6 and the 3 unipolar leads are labelled VR, VL, and VF. In the early days of unipolar electrocardiography, the unipolar limb leads were amplified by omitting from the indifferent connection that limb to which the exploring electrode was attached, thus producing the *augmented unipolar limb leads,* aVR, aVL and aVF. The standard 12-lead electrocardiogram has come, by convention, to be as follows:

I, II, III	bipolar limb leads
aVR, aVL, aVF	unipolar limb leads
V_1–V_6	unipolar precordial leads

The limbs themselves act as linear conductors (i.e. they behave like wires) and the positioning of the electrode on the limb is therefore not critical. Anywhere between the periphery of the limb and the point of the limb's attachment to the torso will serve. However, the torso acts as a volume conductor and movement of the electrode position on the torso influences the recording produced. Standard positioning of the chest leads, therefore, had to be agreed, by international convention, and these are shown in Fig. 9.2.

An illustration of a horizontal cross-section through the heart showing the positioning of the precordial leads in relation to the ventricles is given in Fig. 9.3. It should be noted that the electrodes are not evenly spaced with respect to each other.

The precordial V leads are all situated close to the heart and each is powerfully influenced by electrical activity in underlying myocardium. The limb leads, however, are more remotely situated (Fig. 9.4) and give a general rather than a localized view.

THE BASIC WAVES OF THE ELECTROCARDIOGRAM

Most electrocardiograms contain three basic waves: *P waves* (indicative of atrial myocardial depolarization), *QRS complexes* (indicative of ventricular myocardial depolarization) and *T waves* (indicative of ventricular myocardial repolarization). Ventricular myocardial repolarization begins as the QRS ends and it follows that, although the ST segment is not strictly a 'wave', it is also part of the repolarization signal. A second repolarization wave (the *U wave*) is sometimes seen immediately after the T wave and this indicates the terminal part of the repolarization process. Atrial repolarization is indicated by the atrial T wave or *Ta wave,* which is a

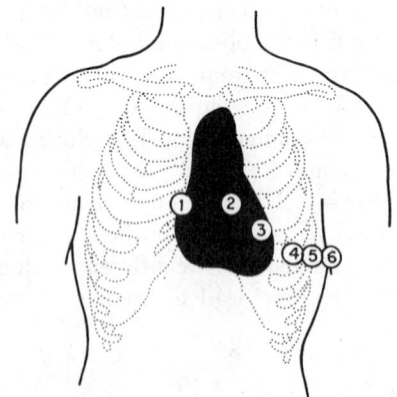

Fig. 9.2. Standard anatomical siting of the precordial electrodes agreed between the British Cardiac Society and the American Heart Association. The sitings are as follows: V_1, right sternal margin at fourth intercostal space; V_2, left sternal margin at fourth intercostal space; V_4, intersection of left mid-clavicular line and fifth intercostal space; V_3, midway between V_2 and V_4; V_5 intersection of left anterior axillary line with a horizontal line through V_4; V_6, intersection of mid-axillary line with a horizontal line through V_4 and V_5.

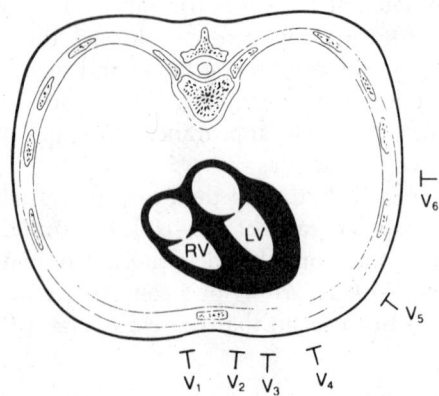

Fig. 9.3. Relationship of the precordial leads to the cardiac chambers shown in a horizontal cross-section through the thorax at the level of the ventricles (seen from above). Note that V_1 and V_2 face and lie close to the free wall of the right ventricle, V_3 and V_4 lie near to the interventricular septum and V_5 and V_6 face the free wall of the left ventricle but are separated from it by a substantial distance. V_4 is usually at the cardiac apex. Note, in particular, how far round the axilla is v_6. The novice electrocardiographer places V_5 and V_6 too anteriorly and does not get a true left ventricular recording.

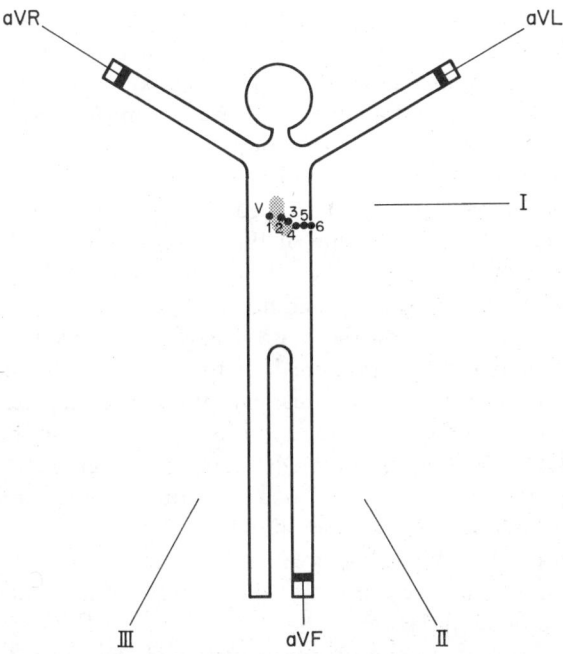

Fig. 9.4. The arrangement of the 6 frontal plane limb leads.

small asymmetric wave with a polarity opposite to that of the P wave. In most electrocardiograms, it is obscured by the QRS complexes and it usually becomes apparent only when there is atrioventricular dissociation (for example, in complete heart block), or where the Ta wave is increased in size, as during sinus tachycardia.

QRS WAVEFORM NOMENCLATURE

The deflections resulting from ventricular myocardial depolarization (QRS complexes) are usually large and they have the highest frequency components of the electrocardiographic recording. They may be uniphasic, biphasic or polyphasic, and a convention has been established to describe the main morphological features of any given QRS complex. The rules of this convention are as follows:

1 the first positive (upgoing) wave is labelled r or R;

2 any second positive wave is labelled r′ or R′;

3 a negative wave, i.e. one descending below the baseline, is labelled s or S wave if it follows an r or R wave;

4 a negative wave is labelled q or Q if it precedes an r or R (in which case it must inevitably also be the first wave to occur in the QRS);

5 any wave that is entirely negative is labelled qs or QS;

6 large deflections are given an upper case letter and small deflections a lower case letter.

Examples of the possible QRS waveforms together with the appropriate conventional abbreviated descriptions are shown in Fig. 9.5.

THE HEXAXIAL REFERENCE SYSTEM

The general disposition of the limb leads is shown in Fig. 9.4. The 6 frontal plane limb leads are shown also in Fig. 9.6. The arrangement of these 6 leads is such that, if each lead is produced through the origin, 6 lines are obtained which divide the full 360° of the frontal plane into 12 angles of 30° each. This is called the hexaxial reference system and it is

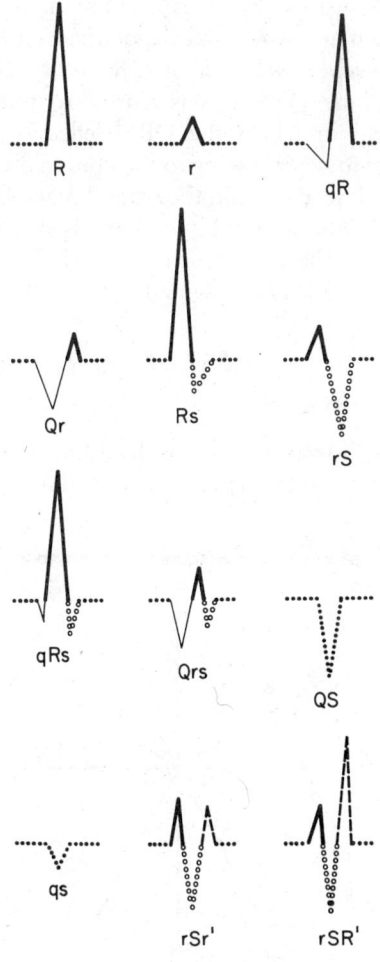

Fig. 9.5. Twelve of the possible variations in QRS waveform. Note that each is, in a generic sense, a QRS complex. r or R, first positive wave; r′ or R′, second positive wave; q or Q, negative wave before an r or R wave; s or S, negative wave following an r or R wave; qs or QS, entirely negative wave.

useful for describing positions within the frontal plane. Within this system (Fig. 9.6), lead I is arbitrarily assigned the value 0°, and the other points at the extremities of the lines are labelled as +30° to +180°, travelling clockwise from lead I, and as −30° to −180°, travelling counterclockwise from lead I. This bizarre, but universally accepted, convention results in the fact that the same point is described as either +180° or −180°.

THE FRONTAL PLANE QRS AXIS

Within a single QRS complex in any lead, the instantaneous direction of depolarization of ventricular myocardium is continuously varying. Nevertheless, for any given ventricular depolarization, there is usually a predominant direction of depolarization. That direction within the frontal plane which best describes the dominant direction of ventricular myocardial depolarization is known as the *mean frontal plane QRS axis*. The mean frontal plane QRS axis is closest to that frontal plane lead in which the QRS deflection is most positive. However, owing to the uneven distribution of the limb leads within the frontal plane (Fig. 9.6), the axis cannot reliably be assessed simply by looking for the position in the hexaxial reference system of the leads showing the tallest R wave.

DETERMINATION OF THE MEAN FRONTAL PLANE QRS AXIS

The axis, however, may be determined by inspection of the frontal plane leads as follows:

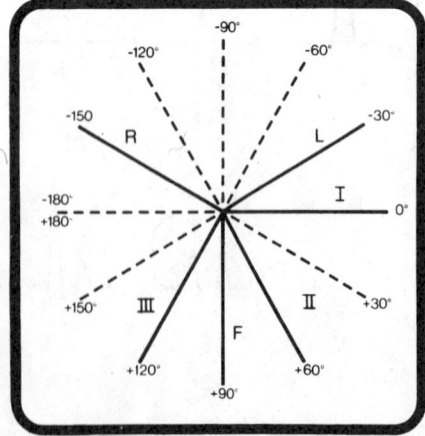

Fig. 9.6. The hexaxial reference system. The 12 subdividing lines of the system are constructed by producing each axial line through the origin.

1   Decide, by inspection, in which frontal plane lead the algebraic sum of QRS deflections most closely approximates to zero. The axis is approximately at right angles to this lead. It must lie, to a first order of approximation, in one of the two possible positions at right angles to this lead (these positions can be determined by reference to the hexaxial system). One of these two positions will inevitably lie on another of the 6 frontal plane leads within the hexaxial reference system.

2   The form of the QRS complex in this lead should now be examined. If there is a dominant positive deflection in this lead, the axis is approximately along this lead (and is at right angles to the lead first chosen). If the QRS complex is dominantly negative, the axis lies 180° away from this lead (and is still at 90° to the initial lead chosen). This procedure gives the axis to the nearest 30°. To improve the resolution to the nearest 15° a further step must be taken.

3   Return to the first lead chosen. It has already been decided that the algebraic sum of QRS deflections in this lead is close to zero. The question now to be asked is whether it is indistinguishable from zero, recognizably, but slightly, positive or recognizably, but slightly, negative. If it is indistinguishable from zero, the approximate axial position determined by the response to the first two questions is now seen to be accurate to ± 15°. If the QRS deflection in that lead in which the algebraic sum of deflections is closest to zero is actually slightly positive, the initial estimation of the axis (after answering the second question) has to be modified by adjusting it and bringing it 15° closer to that lead in which the algebraic sum approximates to zero. Conversely, if the algebraic sum, although close to zero, is actually slightly negative, the estimate of the axis which was made after answering the second question needs to be modified in such a way as to give an axis 15° further away from the lead in which the algebraic sum of QRS deflections was close to zero.

An example will help to clarify the technique. Consider the electrocardiogram shown in Fig. 9.7. The technique of calculating the axis is described in the caption to Fig. 9.7.

Several points should be noted about this technique for axis determination.

1   The plus and minus signs on the hexaxial reference system (Fig. 9.6) do not refer to the polarity of the QRS complexes in any lead. The signs are simply part of the arbitrary convention chosen to describe the position in the frontal plane.

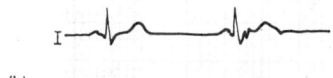

(b)

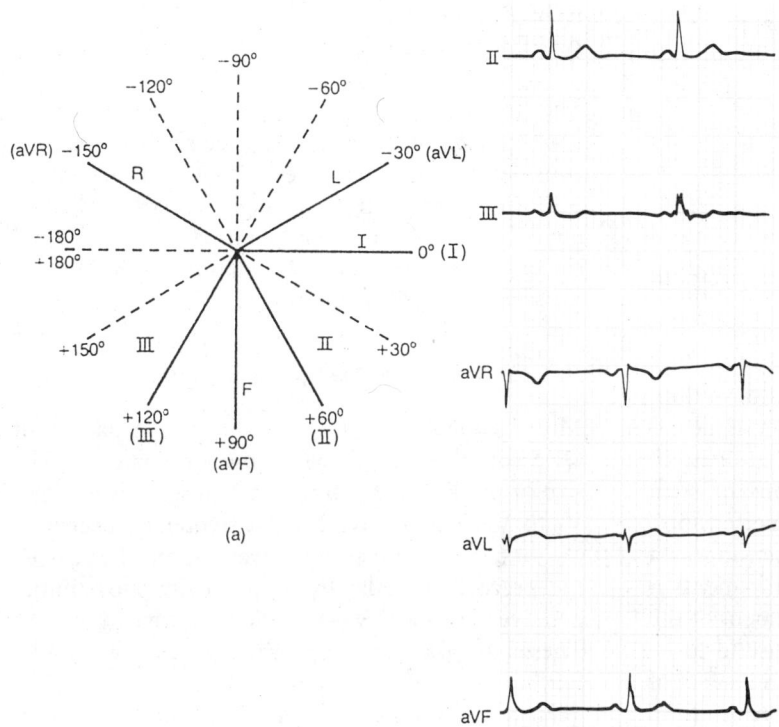

(a)

Fig. 9.7. The limb leads only are shown because the precordial leads are not relevant to the analysis of the frontal plane axis. Inspection of the 6 limb leads indicates that the algebraic sum of QRS deflections is most nearly equal to zero in aVL. The QRS axis therefore must be approximately at right angles to this lead. (a) two possible directions for the axis namely +60° and −120°, both of which are at right angles to lead aVL. One of these possible directions, +60°, lies on another lead (lead II). (b) Lead II shows a clearly positive dominant deflection of the QRS complex. Of the two possible directions, therefore, the axis must be along lead II, i.e. at +60°. This gives the axis to the nearest 30°. Further inspection of the QRS complex in lead aVL reveals that the algebraic sum of QRS complex deflections in this lead, although being closer to zero than in any other lead, is in fact slightly negative. It is therefore necessary to make an adjustment to the first estimate of the axis +60°) and to move the axis 15° further away from lead aVL (because the QRS is slightly negative in lead aVL). Thus, the final estimate of the axis is +75° and this is correct to the nearest 15°.

2   When there are two leads in which the algebraic sum of QRS complex deflections is close to zero, these leads will be either at 30° or at 150° to one another and the same answer for the axis to an accuracy of 15° will be given whichever lead is chosen first.

3   If all 6 frontal plane leads have QRS complexes with algebraic sums close to zero, the axis is indeterminate (by any technique) because the QRS complex vector is directed predominantly forwards or backwards and, in either case, subtends only a small angle at the frontal plane.

4   Slight variations in QRS complex morphology may occur with changes in the anatomical position of the heart such as those associated with respiration. A shift of 15° or occasionally of 30° in axis may occur spontaneously during the respiratory cycle.

THE SIGNIFICANCE OF THE ELECTRICAL AXIS

In the normal adult, the mean frontal plane QRS axis lies between −30° and +90° (Fig. 9.8). The axis is important for two independent reasons.

1   It has clinical significance in its own right.

2   The large potential normal range of the frontal plane axis explains the tremendous variation of normal appearances in the limb leads. Without an understanding of the normal variation in the frontal plane axis it is not easy to understand the range of normal and abnormal appearances in the frontal plane leads.

The descriptive terms *horizontal heart* and *vertical heart* can easily be understood from consideration of the cardiac axis. When the mean frontal plane QRS axis is in the region of +30° to −30° the heart is said to be horizontal. When the axis lies in the region of +60° to +90°, the heart is said to be vertical. The terms *right-axis deviation* and *left-axis deviation* can also be understood in relation to the axis and the hexaxial reference system. When the mean frontal plane QRS axis is more negative than −30° there is said to be left-axis deviation. When the mean frontal plane QRS axis is more positive

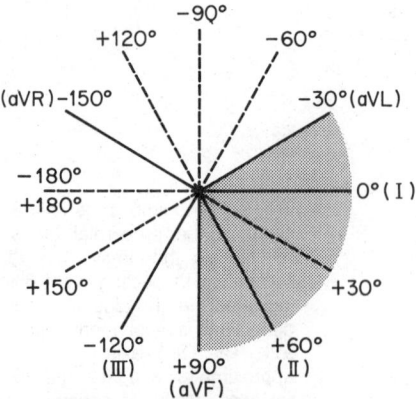

Fig. 9.8. The mean frontal plane QRS axis in the normal adult. The axis normally lies between −30° and +90°.

sive antero-lateral myocardial infarction, emphysema and a vertical heart in a tall thin subject.

NORMAL ELECTROCARDIOGRAPHIC APPEARANCES

The range of variation in the possible normal appearances of the 12-lead electrocardiogram is considerable and this presents one of the major obstacles to the initial learning of electrocardiography. The most consistent features of the normal electrocardiogram and the major variations on these features will be discussed below.

PRECORDIAL QRS MORPHOLOGY

Most frequently, lead V_1 will show an rS pattern of QRS complex and V_6 will show a qR pattern. The size of the R wave will increase progressively from V_1 to V_6. The S wave is most frequently deeper in V_2 than in V_1 and progressively diminishes across the precordial leads. V_1–V_3 typically show initial positive waves and V_4–V_6 initial negative (q) waves. These typical normal appearances are shown in Fig. 9.9.

However, numerous variations on this typical normal set of appearances are possible. These are illustrated in Fig. 9.10. Three important features should be noted:

1 The progressive increase in size of the r wave from V_1 to V_6 occurs because the myocardium underlying the electrodes becomes progressively thicker in the same sequence and because myocardial depolarization is always from endocardium to epicardium thus reflecting myocardial thickness.

2 However, as V_6, and to a lesser extent V_5, are further from the heart than the other precordial electrodes, the recorded R-wave voltage may be less in V_6 than it is in V_5. For the same reason, it may be less in V_5 than it is in V_4.

3 The tall positive waves in the left precordial leads are generated by depolarization on the left

than +90°, there is said to be right-axis deviation. The terms right-axis deviation and left-axis deviation are generic descriptive terms, the usefulness of which is confined to general discussions of such topics. They are similar to the word 'hypertension'. It is useful to be able to refer to hypertension as a generic term, but in respect of individual patients it is necessary to know the actual measurement of the blood pressure. In the same way, it is useful to be able to refer to 'left-axis deviation' but in respect of individual patients it is much more appropriate to be able to measure the axis. Quoting the actual axis rather than using the generic terms also precludes problems inherent in the fact that axes in the region of −180° to −150° could be called extreme right-axis deviation or extreme left-axis deviation. The commonest causes of abnormal left-axis deviation are block in the antero-superior division of the left bundle branch system (left anterior hemiblock), previous inferior myocardial infarction, ventricular pre-excitation, ostium primum atrial septal defect, artificial cardiac pacing from the apex of the right or left ventricle and hyperkalaemia. The important causes of abnormal right-axis deviation are block in the postero-inferior division of the left bundle branch system (left posterior hemiblock), right ventricular hypertrophy, atrial septal defect, exten-

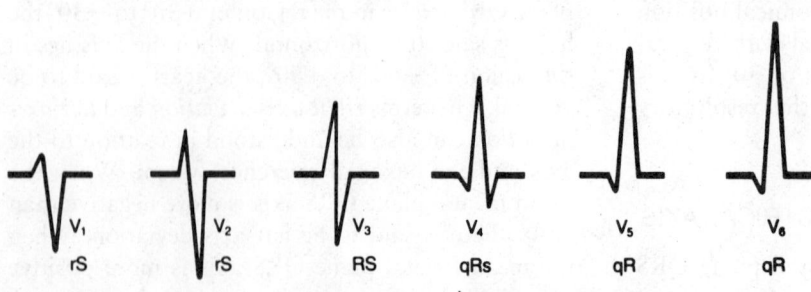

Fig. 9.9. Morphology of the QRS complexes in the precordial leads. Typical appearances.

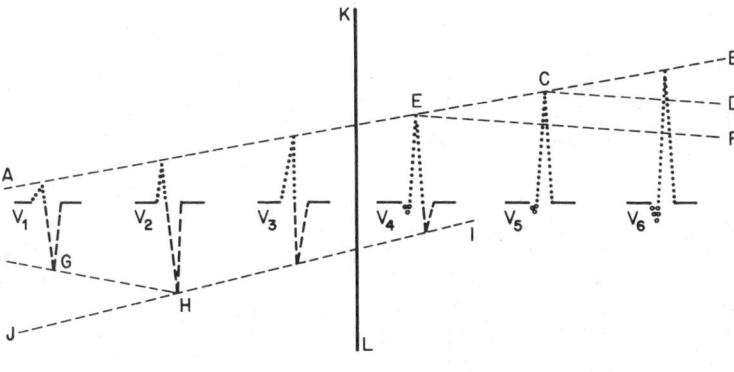

Fig. 9.10. Variations in the morphology of the QRS complexes in the precordial leads. Line AB illustrates that the R wave in each precordial lead is larger than that in the preceding lead in the series from V_1 to V_6. Line CD: it is quite normal for the R wave in V_6 to be smaller than that in V_5. Line EF: it is also normal for the R wave in V_5 to be smaller than that in V_4 provided that the R wave in V_6 is also smaller than that in V_5. Line JI: the size of the S wave diminishes progressively across the precordial leads and may ultimately disappear altogether. Line GH: the size of the S wave in V_2 is often greater than that in V_1. Leads before line KL have an initial deflection which is positive (an r wave). Leads after LK have an initial negative deflection (a q wave).

ventricular free wall. The same process gives rise to the deep S waves in the right precordial leads.

4   The initial part of each QRS deflection is produced by septal depolarization (the septum is the first part of the ventricular myocardium to depolarize). This is towards the right precordial leads and away from the left precordial leads. This explains why the initial part of the QRS defection is positive in the right precordial leads and negative in the left precordial leads.

Clockwise and counterclockwise cardiac rotation

The line KL in Fig. 9.10 indicates the electrocardiographic position of the interventricular septum. This conclusion is based on the fact that the interventricular septum, which normally depolarizes from left to right, gives negative waves in the left precordial leads and positive waves in the right precordial leads. This *transition zone* (indicated by KL) is most typically found between V_3 and V_4. However, when there is, electrically speaking, clockwise (seen from below) cardiac rotation, more of the electrical features of right ventricular activity come to underlie the recording electrodes and the transition zone moves to V_4/V_5 or V_5/V_6. Conversely, where there is counterclockwise electrical rotation (again observed from below), the transition zone moves between V_2/V_3 or V_1/V_2. Typical morphological appearances of the precordial leads in the usual intermediate position in clockwise cardiac rotation and in counterclockwise cardiac rotation are shown in Fig. 9.11.

When there is extreme clockwise cardiac rotation, there may not even be a q wave in V_6 and there

may be a QS complex in V_1; when there is extreme counterclockwise cardiac rotation, there may even be a q wave in V_1 (Fig. 9.12).

PRECORDIAL QRS DIMENSIONS

Within given QRS complexes, it is important to measure the depth and duration of any q waves present, the height of any r wave present, the S-wave depth, the total QRS duration and the ventricular activation time. The ventricular activation time is defined as the time-interval between the onset of a q wave and the peak of an R wave in any lead showing a left ventricular (qR) type of QRS complex. The way in which these important measurements are made are shown in Fig. 9.13.

The rules for normality of the QRS dimensions in the precordial leads are as follows.

1   Total QRS duration should not exceed 0.10 s (2.5 small squares)

2   At least one R wave should exceed 8 mm (assuming a standard electrocardiographic calibration)

3   The tallest R wave should not exceed 27 mm

4   The deepest S wave should not exceed 30 mm

5   The sum of the tallest r in the precordial leads and the deepest S in the precordial leads should not exceed 40 mm

6   The ventricular activation time should not exceed 0.04 s

7   Any Q wave seen should not have a depth exceeding one-quarter the height of the ensuing R wave

8   Any Q wave seen should not equal or exceed 0.04 s in duration.

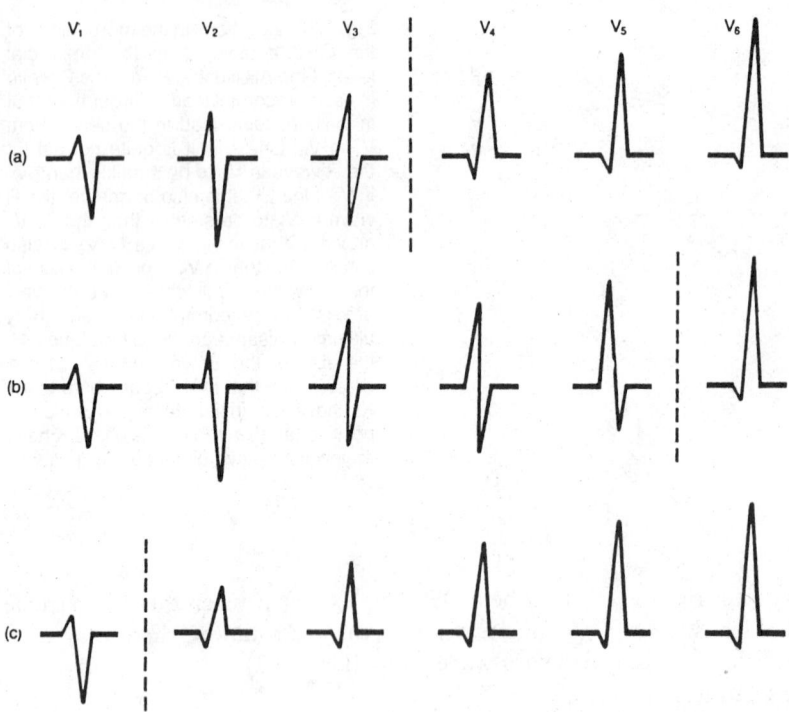

Fig. 9.11. The typical precordial QRS complexes of the intermediate position and of clockwise and counterclockwise rotation. (a) Intermediate position: transition zone between V_3 and V_4. (b) Clockwise rotation: transition zone between V_5 and V_6 (if appearance of q wave is taken as criterion) or between V_4 and V_5 (if dominant positive deflection is taken as criterion). (c) Counterclockwise rotation: transition zone between V_1 and V_2.

PRECORDIAL T-WAVE POLARITY AND SIZE

The rules for T waves are less precise than those for QRS complexes.

1   The T wave in V_1 may be upright, flat or inverted but if upright in earlier records it should still be upright.

2   The T wave in V_2 may be upright, flat or inverted but if upright in earlier records or simultaneously upright in V_1 it must be upright in V_2.

3   T waves from V_1 to V_6 must be upright.

In general, within any given lead, the taller the R wave the taller the T wave should be, but among leads the tallest T waves relative to the R-wave heights are to be seen in V_2 and V_3.

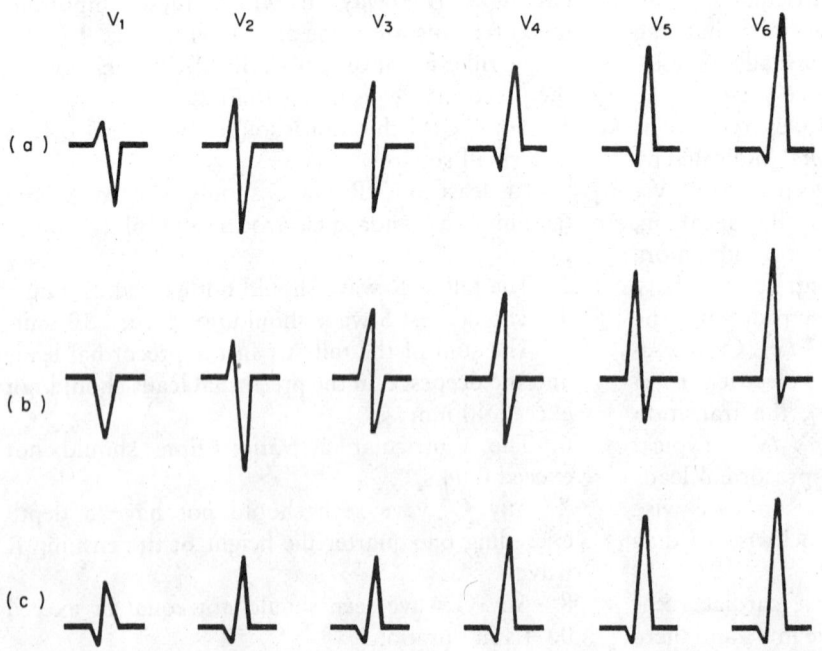

Fig. 9.12. Extreme rotation in which all leads record from one side of the interventricular septum only. (a) Intermediate position. (b) Extreme clockwise rotation: leads V_2–V_6 face the right ventricle. V_1 shows a QS complex because, like aVR (which is almost always looking into the cavity of the heart) it is looking into the cardiac cavity. (c) Extreme counterclockwise rotation: all leads show qR complexes, i.e. they face the left ventricle.

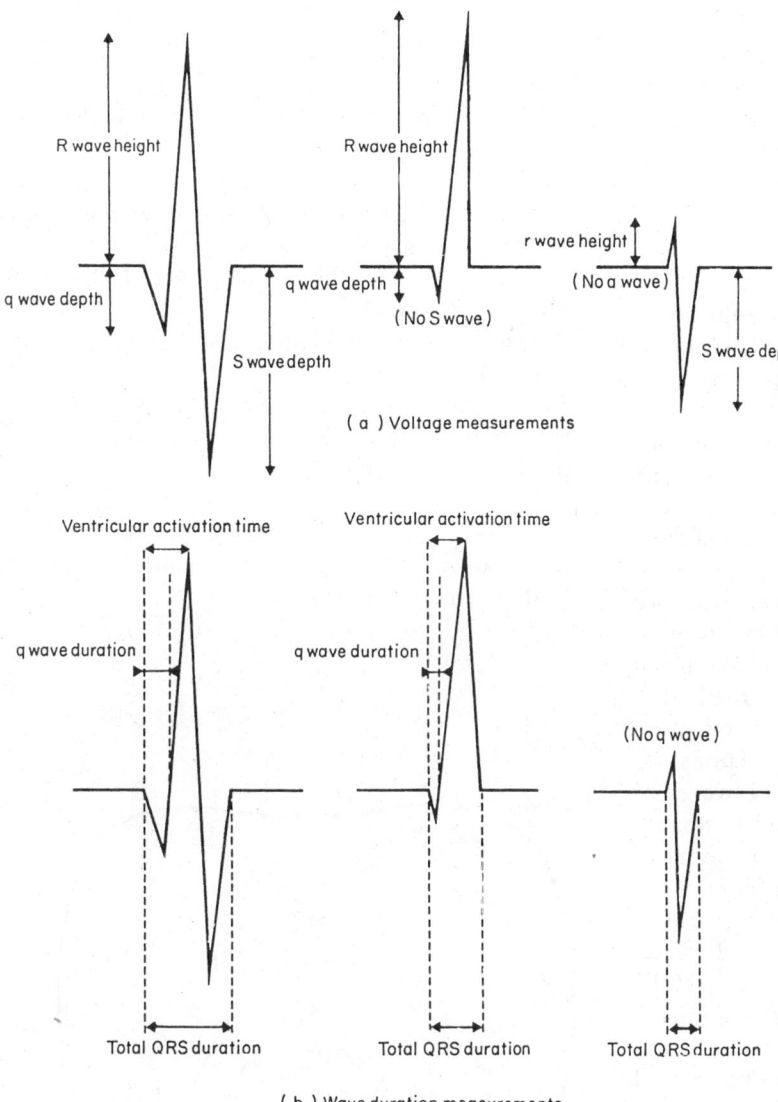

(a) Voltage measurements

(b) Wave duration measurements

Fig. 9.13. Diagram to illustrate the measurement of precordial QRS dimensions. (a) Voltage measurements. R-wave height: height in mm of the first positive wave above the baseline; Q-wave depth: depth in mm of any initial (i.e. preceding an R wave) negative wave below the baseline; S-wave depth: depth in mm below the baseline of any negative wave that follows an R wave. (b) Wave-duration measurements: q-wave duration: time in s from the onset of the q wave to the point where the upstroke of the R wave re-crosses the baseline; total QRS duration: time in s from the onset of the QRS complex (whether the initial wave be negative or positive) to the end of the QRS complex (whether the final wave be negative or positive); ventricular activation time: time in s from the beginning of the q wave to the peak of the R wave. It can be measured only in leads showing a qR type of QRS complex.

PRECORDIAL ST SEGMENTS

The ST segments of the precordial leads must not deviate from the iso-electric line by more than ± 1 mm. The iso-electric line is the time-interval between the end of the T wave and the beginning of the P wave. During sinus tachycardia, there may be little or no iso-electric line visible and assessment of minor degrees of ST-segment shift may therefore be difficult or impossible. The ST segment tends to be more discrete in V_5 and V_6 than it does in V_2 and V_3 and minor degrees of ST-segment elevation in V_2 and V_3 should be interpreted with great caution. It should be remembered that the ST segment *is* part of the repolarization process, as is the T wave; there is no intrinsic reason why it should always be recognizable as a discrete entity.

LIMB LEAD QRS COMPLEXES

The criteria required to assess normality or otherwise of the limb lead QRS complexes are relatively few.

1   A Q wave in aVL*, I, II or aVF should not equal or exceed 0.04 s in duration.

2   A Q wave in aVL*, I, II or aVF should not have a depth greater than one-quarter of the height of the ensuing R wave.

* Q waves > 0.04 s in duration or more than one-quarter the height of the ensuing R wave are permissible in lead aVL if the heart is vertical, i.e. has a mean frontal plane QRS axis of +60° or more positive.

3 The mean frontal plane QRS axis should not lie outside the range −30° to +90°.
4 The R wave in aVL should not exceed 13 mm and that in aVF should not exceed 20 mm.
Q waves visible only in aVR or lead III are of no significance.

LIMB LEAD T WAVES

In general, the T waves and the QRS complexes in the limb leads should be concordant. This means that when the QRS is recognized to be positive the T waves should be recognizably positive and when the QRS is clearly negative the T waves should be clearly negative. This rule allows an approximate general assessment of the T waves in the limb leads but it does not define the borderline cases and there are problems in deciding, for example, the significance of shallow T-wave inversion in the presence of a small positive QRS complex. One way of avoiding such difficulties is to work out the mean frontal plane T-wave axis using the same method as that for the calculation of the mean frontal plane QRS axis with the exception that all inspections and measurements are made in relation to T waves as opposed to QRS complexes. The rule for normality of the T waves in the limb leads is that the mean frontal plane T-wave axis should not differ from the mean frontal plane QRS axis by more than ± 45°. However, in the case of inferior myocardial infarction, when abnormal Q waves are present in II, III and aVF, T-wave inversion in these leads is said to be abnormal even though the angle between the frontal plane QRS and T-wave axes does not exceed the 45° limit.

LIMB LEAD ST SEGMENTS

The rule for the ST segment in the limb leads is exactly the same as for that in the precordial leads. A normal ST segment in the limb leads must not deviate from the iso-electric line by more than 1 mm (above or below).

THE P WAVES

During normal sinus rhythm, atrial myocardial depolarization is initiated from the sino-atrial node. In the frontal plane, atrial myocardial depolarization therefore travels predominantly from right to left and from above downwards and gives rise to positive deflections in lead II (and to a lesser extent in lead I and in the foot lead). Right atrial depolarization tends to give deflection towards the right precordial leads and left atrial depolarization deflection away from the right precordial leads (Fig. 9.14) and the resulting P wave in V_1 may therefore be biphasic (Fig. 9.15).

The P waves are most effectively assessed using leads II and V_1. The rules for normality or otherwise of the P waves are as follows.
1 The P waves should not exceed 0.12 s in duration in lead II.
2 The P waves should not exceed 2.5 mm in height in lead II.
3 Any negative component of the P wave in V_1 should not have a greater area than the initial positive component.

We are now in a position to consider the important morphological abnormalities of the 12-lead electrocardiogram.

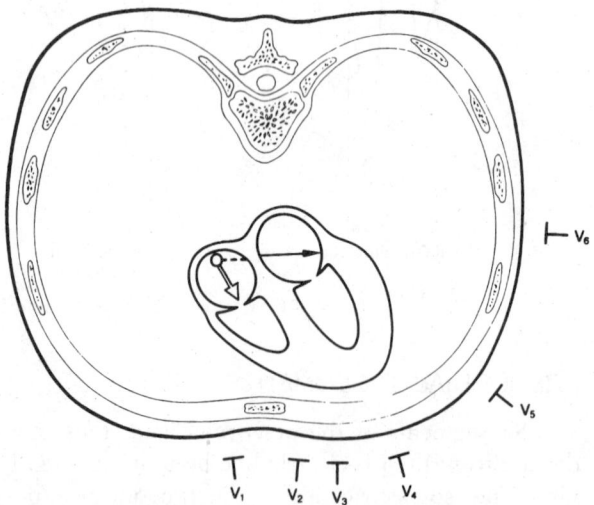

Fig. 9.14. The form of the P waves in the precordial leads. Atrial depolarization starts at the sino-atrial node and spreads simultaneously in all directions through the myocardium of the right atrium. That direction of spread of depolarization within the right atrium which produces the longest available pathway is the effective predominant direction of depolarization of the right atrium and this determines the direction of the right atrial P wave vector (arrow). The first part of the left atrium to be depolarized is that part lying on the shortest route from the sino-atrial node. From this point, depolarization spreads in all directions through the left atrial myocardium. That direction of spread of depolarization within the left atrium which provides the longest available pathway is the effective predominant direction of depolarization of the left atrium and this determines the direction of the left atrial P wave vector (arrow).

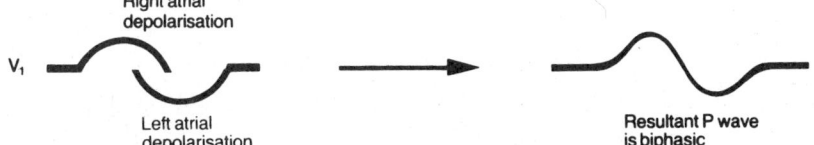

Fig. 9.15. Biphasic P wave in V_1.

INTRAVENTRICULAR CONDUCTION DISTURBANCES

When the normal sequence of conduction of a depolarization wave is disturbed after it has descended beyond the bifurcation of the bundle of His, an intraventricular conduction disturbance is said to have occurred. The following intraventricular disturbances are recognizable on the 12-lead electrocardiogram.

1 Right bundle branch block, partial or complete, permanent or intermittent.
2 Left bundle branch block, partial or complete, permanent or intermittent.
3 Left anterior hemiblock, also known as left superior interventricular block.
4 Left posterior hemiblock, also known as left inferior intraventricular block.
5 Right bundle branch block and left anterior hemiblock.
6 Right bundle branch block and left posterior hemiblock.
7 Diffuse intraventricular block.

RIGHT BUNDLE BRANCH BLOCK

When there is complete failure of conduction in the right bundle branch, the primary change induced is a delay in depolarization of the free wall of the right ventricle. There is no change in the timing or direction of depolarization in the interventricular septum or in the left ventricular free wall. The delay in depolarization of the free wall of the right ventricle gives rise to a late secondary R wave in the right precordial leads and a corresponding late secondary S wave in the left precordial leads. The R wave in the right precordial leads and the S wave in the left precordial leads are typically broad and slurred.

The criteria for the presence of right bundle branch block are (in relation to a supraventricularly initiated beat),
1 the total QRS duration is 0.12 s or more;
2 a secondary R wave (R′ wave) is seen in V_1.
Both criteria must be fulfilled before there is right bundle branch block. The QRS complex in V_1 may be rsr′, rSr′, rSR′, RSr′, RSR′, rSR′, or M shaped. Only these criteria are *necessary* for the diagnosis of right bundle branch block. Additional secondary changes frequently occur but are not part of the diagnostic requirement. If secondary changes are present, they should not lead to the conclusion that there is an additional abnormality. The secondary changes include the presence of deep slurred S waves in leads I, aVL and V_4–V_6 and ST-segment depression and/or T-wave inversion from V_1 to V_3. An example of right bundle branch block is shown in Fig. 9.16.

LEFT BUNDLE BRANCH BLOCK

Left bundle branch block produces more widespread and more impressive electrocardiographic changes than does right bundle branch block. Depolarization in the free wall of the left ventricle is delayed in left bundle branch block and this is a precise corollary of the delay in depolarization of the free wall of the right ventricle in right bundle branch block. However, in left bundle branch block, there is also reversal of the direction of septal depolarization. As the left bundle does not conduct, the septum cannot be depolarized from left to right as in the normal case and septal depolarization is therefore reversed. Since the first part of every QRS complex occurs as a result of septal depolarization, the direction of the initial part of each QRS is reversed and the electrocardiographic appearances are transformed.

The three diagnostic criteria for left bundle branch block, all of which must apply simultaneously, are as follows:
1 The total QRS duration is 0.12 s or more.
2 No initial Q wave is seen in V_5, V_6, lead I or aVL.
3 No secondary R wave is seen in V_1 to indicate the presence of right bundle branch block. (This last criterion is necessary to avoid confusion in cases in which there is simultaneously right bundle branch block and extreme clockwise cardiac rotation. The former feature would give rise to an RSr′− in V_1 and an increase in the total QRS duration and the

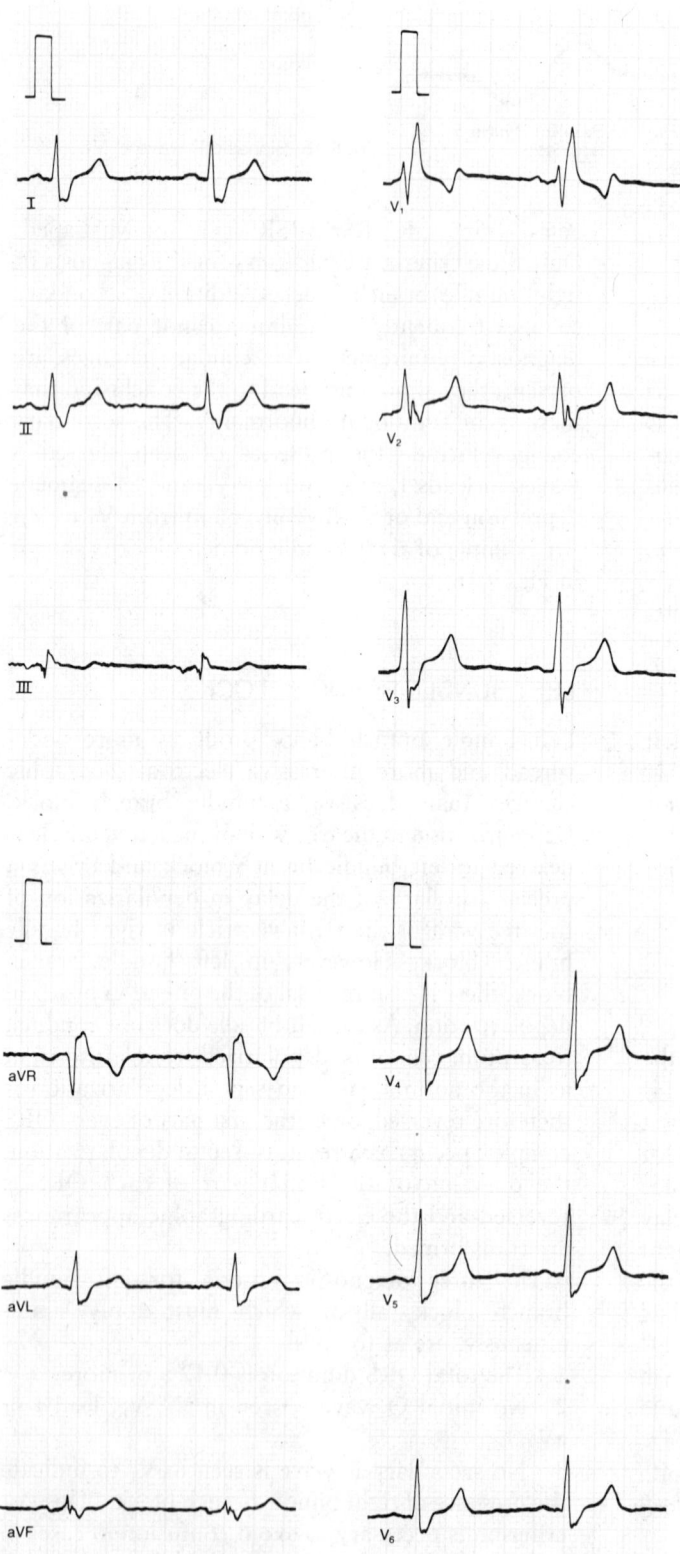

Fig. 9.16. The rhythm is sinus. The total QRS duration is abnormally long (0.16 s, most easily seen in the first QRS in V_1 or the second QRS in I). V_1 has a large secondary R wave (i.e. it has an rSR' complex). The combination of prolongation of the total QRS duration with a secondary R wave in V_1 is diagnostic of right bundle branch block. As is usually the case there is a broad, slurred S wave in V_6 (the equivalent of the broad, slurred R wave in V_1). The mean frontal plane QRS axis is indeterminate but, as is often the case, the QRS appearances in V_6 are transmitted to I and aVL. There is secondary S–T segment depression in V_1 (which often is present in V_2 and V_3 as well).

latter would give rise to absence of an initial q wave in V_5, V_6, lead I and aVL.)

As with right bundle branch block, secondary changes inevitably occur but they are not part of the diagnostic requirement. Such changes include secondary ST-segment depression and T-wave inversion most typically in leads I, aVL, V_4–V_6, broad QS complexes in V_1–V_3, notching of the R waves in the mid precordial leads to give M-shaped complexes and broad R waves in leads I, aVL and V_4–V_6. An example of left bundle branch block is shown in Fig. 9.17.

THE CONCEPT OF FASCICULAR BLOCK

That part of the atrioventricular conducting tissue from the bifurcation of the His bundle onwards was said earlier to consist of three fascicles, the right bundle branch, the anterior division of the left bundle branch and the posterior division of the left bundle branch. (The anatomical evidence suggests that there are four fascicles, there being three rather than two sub-divisions of the left bundle branch but from the point of view of the electrocardiographic changes it is convenient to consider two fascicles of the left bundle and therefore three fascicles in all.) Unifascicular block therefore means right bundle branch block, left anterior hemiblock or left posterior hemiblock, bifascicular block means right bundle branch block with left anterior hemiblock, right bundle branch block with left posterior hemiblock or left bundle branch block, and trifascicular block means complete heart block resulting from problems below the bifurcation of the His bundle. The features of right and of left bundle branch block have already been described. A description of left anterior hemiblock and of left posterior hemiblock follows. To understand left anterior and left posterior hemiblock it is necessary to recall that depolarization of the free wall of the left ventricle dominates all normal and most abnormal electrocardiograms, that the order of sequence of depolarization of the left ventricular myocardium is determined by the left bundle branch, its major divisions and the subsequent Purkinje network from these divisions, and that the anterior division of the left bundle branch (strictly speaking it is antero-superior) facilitates its preferential conduction towards the antero-superior part of the left ventricular myocardium and the posterior division of the left bundle branch facilitates preferential conduction towards the infero-posterior part of the left ventricular myocardium.

Left anterior hemiblock

If the anterior division is blocked, depolarization through the left ventricular myocardium begins initially inferiorly (orientated at about 90° in the frontal plane) and then the terminal part of left ventricular depolarization occurs as the activation wave passes superiorly into the left. This separation in the two parts of left ventricular depolarization produces a slight rightward shift of the initial part of the QRS complex and a dramatic leftward shift of the terminal part of the QRS complex resulting in an abnormal degree of left-axis deviation. The electrocardiographic diagnosis of left anterior hemiblock rests on the combination of an abnormal degree of left-axis deviation and absence of any other recognizable cause for such axis deviation. The commonest two causes of abnormal left-axis deviation are left anterior hemiblock and inferior myocardial infarction. The diagnosis of left anterior hemiblock therefore rests upon finding a mean frontal plane QRS axis more negative than −30° together with the presence of an initial r wave in aVF (which implies no evidence of previous inferior infarction). Obviously, these criteria cannot be applied if some alternative cause for left-axis deviation, e.g. ventricular pre-excitation, hyperkalaemia, and ostium primum atrial septal defect, is present.

Left posterior hemiblock

Just as left anterior hemiblock gives rise to abnormal left axis deviation so left posterior hemiblock gives rise to abnormal right axis deviation. Unfortunately, there are numerous causes of abnormal right-axis deviation (some of which are detailed above) and therefore it is never possible with confidence to make a diagnosis of left posterior hemiblock from the electrocardiogram alone. The finding of an abnormal degree of right-axis deviation without any obvious clinical cause raises the possibility that there is left posterior hemiblock. No statement stronger than this can be made.

BIFASCICULAR BLOCK

Left bundle branch block

The features of left bundle branch block have already been described. There are no means, from the electrocardiogram, of distinguishing left bundle branch block due to block in the two major

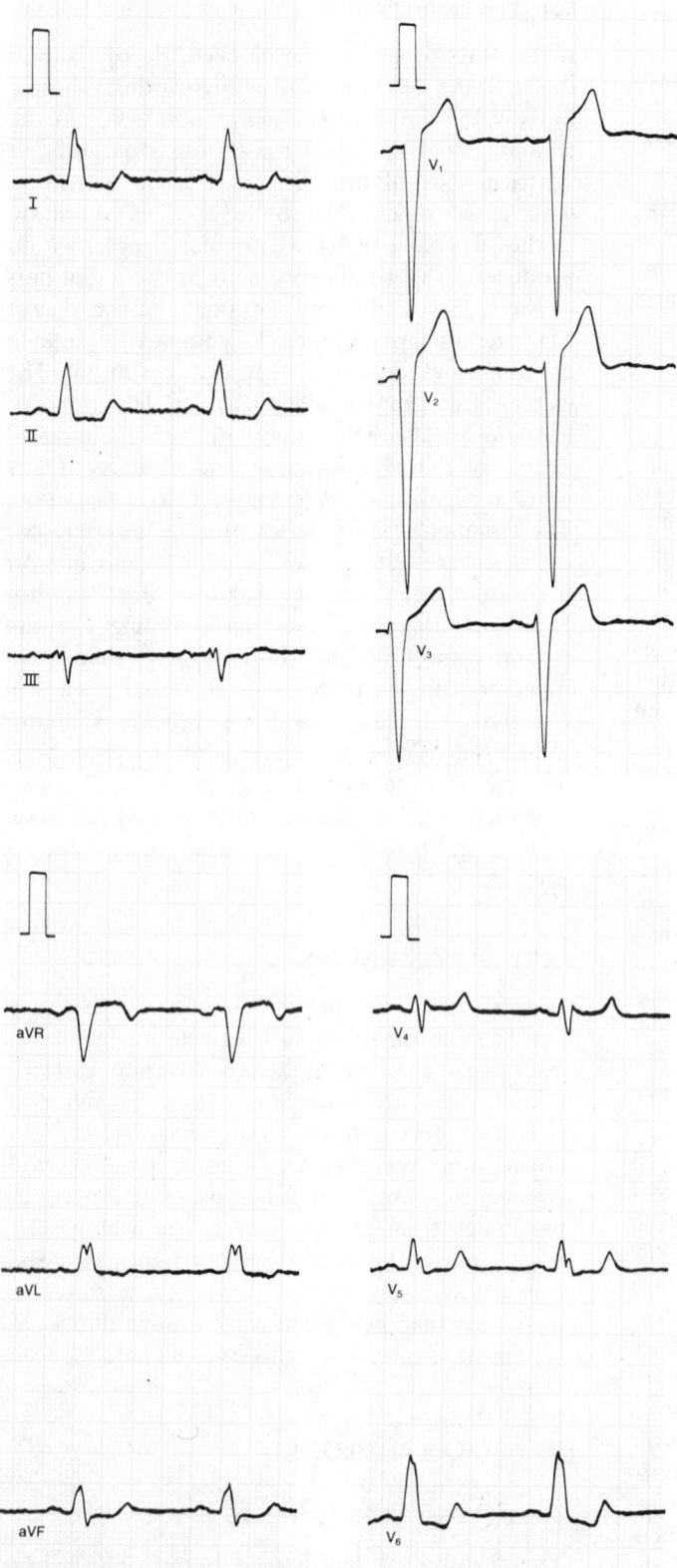

Fig. 9.17. The rhythm is sinus. The total QRS duration is abnormally long (0.14 s), most easily seen in the first QRS complex in V_6. No initial q waves are seen from V_4 to V_6 or in I or AVL. There is no secondary R wave in V_1 to indicate the presence of right bundle branch block. There is secondary ST-segment depression in V_6, leads I, II and aVL. The frontal plane QRS axis is within the normal range at $+15°$. This means that the heart is horizontal. The frontal plane QRS axis indicates the predominant direction of left ventricular depolarization. V_6 is a left ventricular surface lead. As regards the appearances in the limb leads in left bundle branch block, in general, it follows that appearances found in V_6 will also be found in those limb leads that are close to the position of the mean frontal plane QRS axis. In this case, therefore, lead I appears similar to V_6. Lead I will show appearances to V_6 whenever the heart is horizontal.

divisions of the left bundle from left bundle branch block due to a very proximal lesion occurring before the left bundle bifurcates.

Right bundle branch block with left anterior hemiblock

This is a common combination of bifascicular blocks. It can be recognized by the simultaneous presence of right bundle branch block with abnormal left-axis deviation, i.e. an axis more negative than $-30°$, in the absence of electrocardiographic evidence of previous inferior infarction.

Right bundle branch block with left posterior hemiblock

As left posterior hemiblock cannot be diagnosed with absolute confidence from the electrocardiogram, it follows that right bundle branch block with left posterior hemiblock cannot be diagnosed with absolute confidence from the electrocardiogram. The presence of this combination of lesions may be suspected when there is electrocardiographic evidence of right bundle branch block together with an abnormal degree of right-axis deviation, i.e. more positive than $+90°$; in the absence of any clinically adequate reason for right bundle branch block.

OTHER INTRAVENTRICULAR BLOCKS

Occasionally, abnormally wide QRS complexes may be seen in supraventricularly originated beats without the characteristic morphological appearances of either right bundle branch block or left bundle branch block. Such conduction delays are often referred to as 'non-specific intraventricular conduction defects' or as 'diffuse intraventricular conduction abnormalities'. They are thought to be due to diffuse disease in the Purkinje tissue or in the ventricular myocardium.

ATRIAL AND VENTRICULAR HYPERTROPHY

Appreciable hypertrophy of the right or of the left ventricle produces characteristic changes in the electrocardiogram; however, lesser degrees of hypertrophy may be present without any electrocardiographic changes being apparent or with only minor non-specific changes.

LEFT VENTRICULAR HYPERTROPHY

The increased bulk of the left ventricular myocardium in left ventricular hypertrophy increases the voltage induced during depolarization of the free wall of the left ventricle. This gives rise to taller R waves in the left precordial leads and deeper S waves in the right precordial leads. As the left ventricular free wall thickness is usually increased, the depolarization process takes longer to travel from endocardium to epicardium and this increased travel time is reflected in a prolongation of the ventricular activation time, i.e. the time-interval between the onset of the q wave and the peak of the R wave in any lead facing the left ventricle and showing a qR type of QRS complex. In addition to these primary changes in ventricular depolarization, secondary changes in repolarization occur with ST-segment depression and T-wave inversion. ST–T changes are always non-specific in appearance and their cause can be inferred only from any primary depolarization changes present or from the overall clinical picture. Left ventricular hypertrophy is not an 'all-or-none' diagnosis like left and right bundle branch block, but it is a graded diagnosis. The more criteria for the condition that are fulfilled the more likely it is that the condition exists. The recognized criteria for left ventricular hypertrophy are as follows.

1 R in V_4, V_5 or V_6 exceeds 27 mm.
2 S in V_1, V_2 or V_3 exceeds 30 mm.
3 R in V_4, V_5 or V_6 plus S in V_1, V_2 or V_3 exceeds 40 mm.
4 R in aVL exceeds 13 mm.
5 R in aVF exceeds 20 mm.
6 Ventricular activation time exceeds 0.04 s.
7 ST-Segment depression, T-wave flattening or T-wave inversion in leads facing the left ventricle (V_4, V_5 or V_6, leads I and aVL when the heart is horizontal and leads II and aVF when the heart is vertical).

An example of left ventricular hypertrophy is shown in Fig. 9.18.

SYSTOLIC AND DIASTOLIC LEFT VENTRICULAR OVERLOAD PATTERNS

The pattern produced by left ventricular hypertrophy caused by systolic overload of the left ventricle, as in systemic hypertension and aortic stenosis, is recognizably different in general from that produced by diastolic overload of the left ventricle, for example, by aortic incompetence or mitral incom-

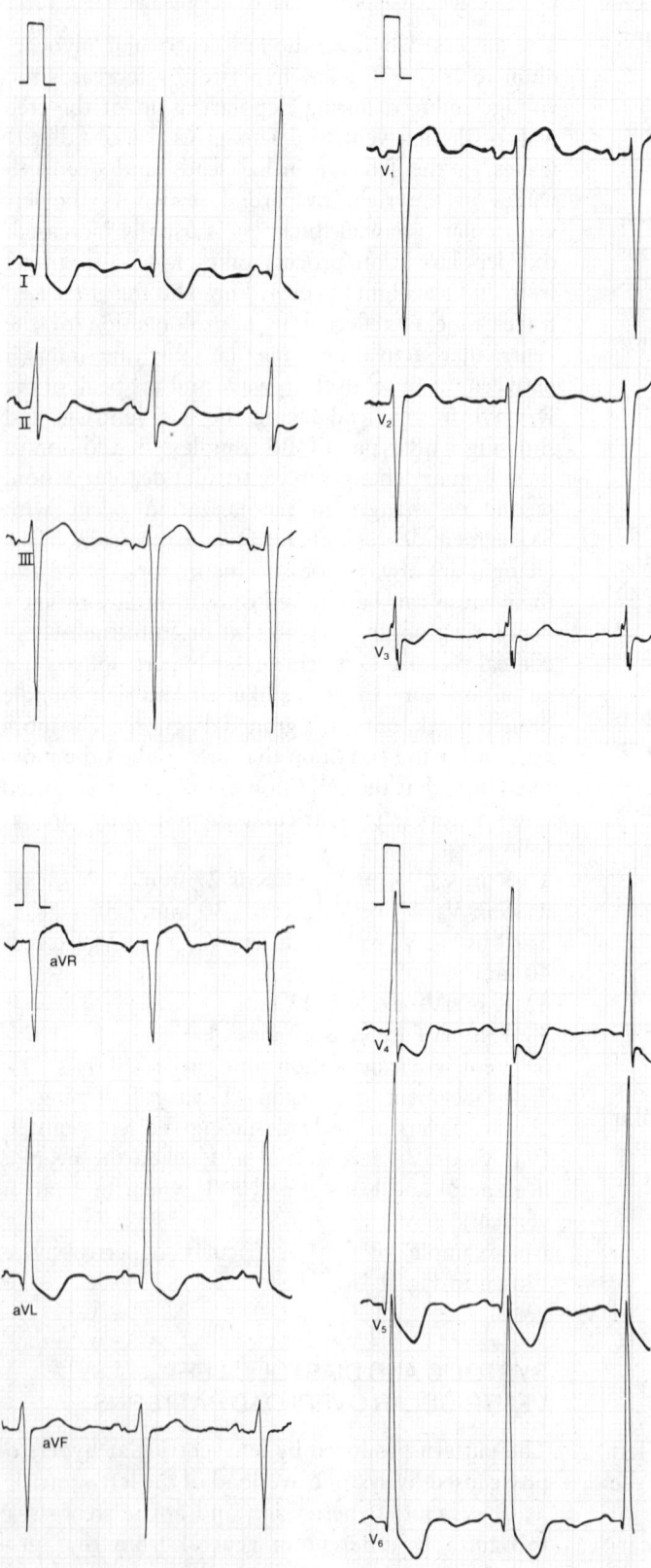

Fig. 9.18. The rhythm is sinus. The mean frontal plane QRS axis is −15°, i.e. the heart is horizontal. The R-wave height in V_5 and V_6 is abnormal (peak R-wave height in V_5 is 41 mm). The S-wave depth in V_1 is abnormal (31 mm). The ventricular activation time in V_5 and V_6 is prolonged (0.06 s). There is ST-segment depression and T-wave inversion in the left precordial leads. As the heart is horizontal, those changes that are seen in the left precordial leads are also reflected in I and aVL. In this case, there is also evidence of left atrial hypertrophy (see later).

petence. In the presence of systolic overload of the left ventricle, ST–T changes tend to be prominent whereas in situations of diastolic overload of the left ventricle ST–T changes tend to be minimal or absent and QRS-voltage changes are prominent. These distinctions, however, are not absolute or reliable. The term 'left ventricular strain' is sometimes used in association with changes of left ventricular hypertrophy in which the ST–T changes are particularly marked. The meaning of the term 'ventricular strain' is obscure and its use is unwise.

It should be noted that left ventricular hypertrophy does not usually give rise to left-axis deviation. The development of left ventricular hypertrophy is typically associated with a leftward shift of the axis of the order of 15° or, at most, 30°. If, before the development of left ventricular hypertrophy, the heart was horizontal, then borderline abnormal left-axis deviation can be anticipated. If, however, before the development of left ventricular hypertrophy, the heart was vertical, abnormal left-axis deviation does not develop. It should be realized that in normal individuals the axis moves progressively towards the left with advancing age, being typically of the order of +90° in subjects in their late teens and being in the region of 0° to −30° in subjects in their mid-60s. Counterclockwise cardiac rotation is often found when there is left ventricular hypertrophy simply because there is more left ventricle underlying the electrodes.

RIGHT VENTRICULAR HYPERTROPHY

The increased bulk of the right ventricle results in higher voltages being developed during right ventricular depolarization. This gives rise to an increase in the size of the positive deflection in the right precordial leads. In addition, the left ventricle no longer dominates the overall electrocardiographic appearances as obviously and the electrical axis of the heart moves towards the right. The diagnostic criteria for right ventricular hypertrophy are therefore an R wave in V_1 equal to or greater than the S wave, i.e. an R complex, an Rs, an RR′, a qR or a qRS, together with a mean frontal plane QRS axis more positive than +90°. Both these criteria must be present for a diagnosis of right ventricular hypertrophy. A dominant R wave in V_1 can also occur in true posterior infarction, in ventricular pre-excitation and in the Duchenne type of muscular dystrophy. As with left ventricular hypertrophy, secondary ST–T changes may be present with ST-segment depression and flattening or inversion of the T waves, but in the case of right ventricular hypertrophy these are seen in the right precordial leads. Examples of right ventricular hypertrophy are shown in Figs 9.19 and 9.20.

BIVENTRICULAR HYPERTROPHY

It may be difficult or impossible electrocardiographically to detect the simultaneous enlargement of right and left ventricles unless the degree of ventricular enlargement is more marked in one of the two ventricles. Theoretically, it is possible to have severe biventricular hypertrophy and to have a normal electrocardiogram, but in practice this is very unlikely because there would almost certainly at least be widespread non-specific ST–T changes. Biventricular hypertrophy should be suspected whenever there is clear electrocardiographic evidence of *left* ventricular hypertrophy together with *right*-axis deviation or clear electrocardiographic evidence of *right* ventricular hypertrophy together with *left*-axis deviation.

LEFT ATRIAL HYPERTROPHY

As indicated earlier, the P wave is best seen in lead II and in V_1. The normal P wave in lead II consists of a smooth rounded positive deflection. Something of the order of the initial fifth of the P wave consists exclusively of right atrial depolarization and something of the order of the terminal fifth of the P wave consists exclusively of left atrial depolarization. In the presence of left atrial enlargement, the terminal part of the P wave becomes taller and the P wave becomes broader. As the two parts of the P wave are no longer equal there is often a recognizable notch in the mid portion of the P wave and broad bifid P waves in lead II are characteristic of left atrial hypertrophy. As also indicated earlier, the P wave in V_1 consists of an initial positive and an initial negative component. The negative component is produced by left atrial depolarization and in the presence of left atrial hypertrophy this negative component increases in size.

The criteria for left atrial hypertrophy are as follows.

1 The P wave is notched and exceeds 0.12 s in duration in lead II (and possibly also in leads I, aVF and aVL).

2 The P wave in V_1 has a dominant negative component, i.e. the area of the negative component exceeds the area of the positive component which precedes it.

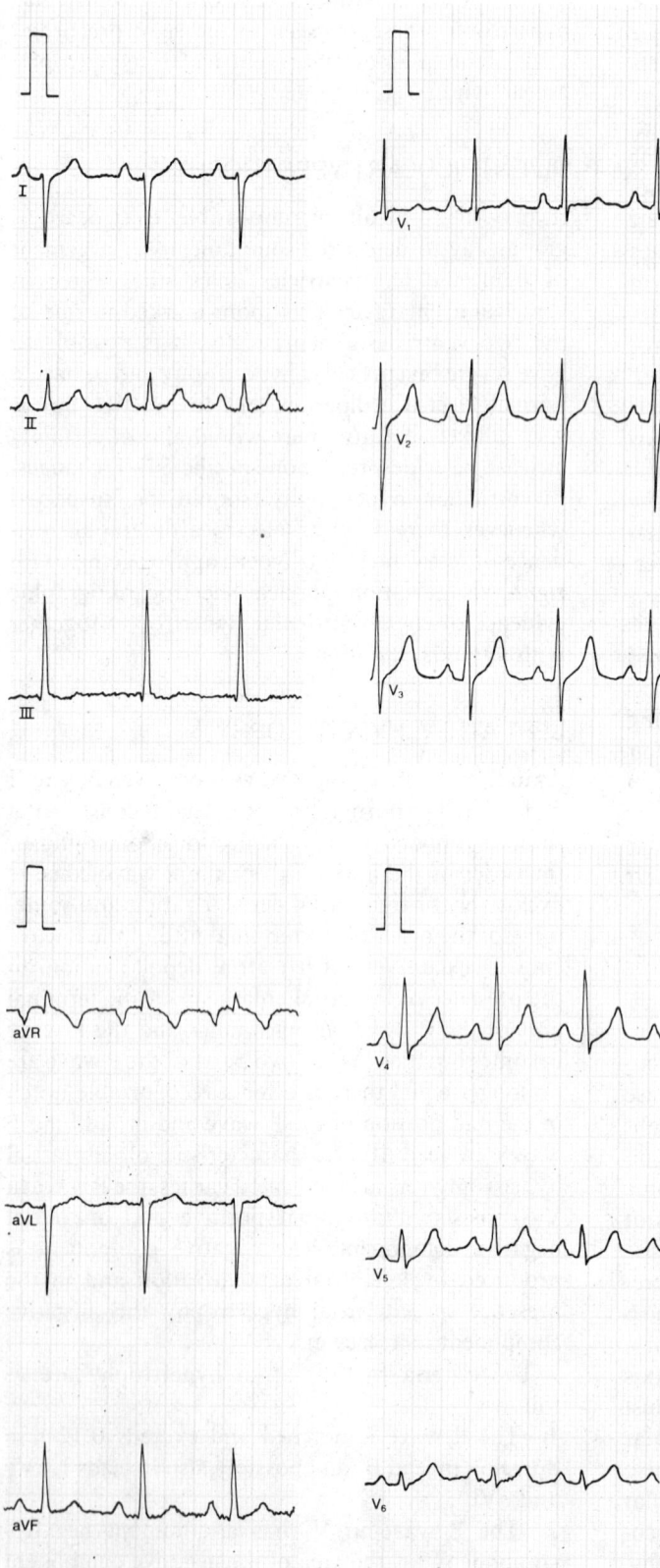

Fig. 9.19. There is an Rs complex in V₁ with the R wave clearly much larger than the S wave and there is an abnormal degree of right-axis deviation (+135°). These appearances are diagnostic of right ventricular hypertrophy. In this case, there are no secondary ST–T changes.

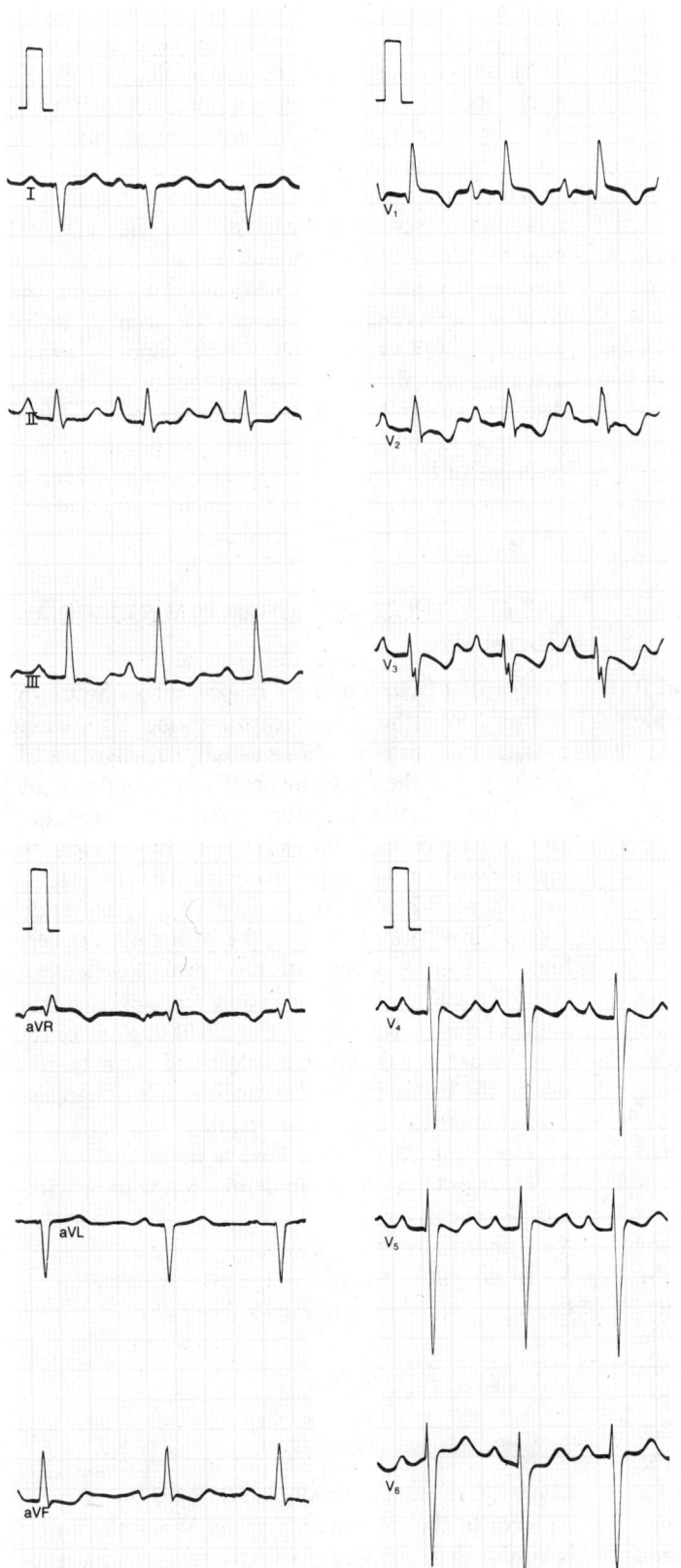

Fig. 9.20. There is a qR configuration in V_1, together with an abnormal degree of right-axis deviation (+135°). In addition, there are non-specific ST–T changes, from V_1 to V_4 and pronounced clockwise cardiac rotation. Clockwise cardiac rotation is common in right ventricular hypertrophy because there is more right ventricle underlying the electrodes.

It must be stressed that the second of these two independent criteria is far more sensitive than the first and that the first criterion is more specific than the second. An example of left atrial hypertrophy is shown in Fig. 9.21.

RIGHT ATRIAL HYPERTROPHY

Just as the left atrial component of the P wave increases in height and duration in left atrial hypertrophy, so the right atrial component of the P wave increases in height and in duration in association with right atrial hypertrophy. However, the increase in the duration of the right atrial component of the P wave is not sufficient to extend beyond the normal duration of the left atrial component so the width of the P wave is not increased in right atrial hypertrophy. The only obvious changes in right atrial hypertrophy are an increase in the P wave height in lead II and, occasionally, an increase in the positive component of the P wave in V_1.

The essential criterion for right atrial hypertrophy is a P-wave height of 3 mm or more in lead II and sometimes also in lead III and aVF. An example of right atrial hypertrophy is shown in Fig. 9.22.

ISCHAEMIC HEART DISEASE

The electrocardiogram is used more often in the detection and evaluation of ischaemic heart disease than in any other field of medicine. It has to be pointed out, however, that the electrocardiogram provides absolutely no information about the state of the coronary arteries except by inference. The electrocardiogram provides information concerning only depolarization and repolarization of myocardium. If, and only if, the degree of regional myocardial ischaemia induced by the presence of coronary atheroma is sufficient to induce recognizable alterations in myocardial depolarization or repolarization, will abnormalities be present on the electrocardiogram. A very significant number, which ranges between 25 and 75% depending on the series studied, of patients who present with unequivocal angina pectoris have, when first seen, absolutely normal resting 12-lead electrocardiograms. The commonest abnormality to find in the presence of ischaemic heart disease is evidence of a previous myocardial infarction. The second commonest abnormality to find is the presence of minor degrees of ST-segment depression or T-wave flattening or T-wave inversion. Although ST-segment depression and T-wave inversion are almost always non-specific, i.e. a recognizable cause cannot be assigned on the basis of the morphology of the ST segments and T waves alone, it must be emphasized that the term 'non-specific' does not in any sense imply 'non-significant'.

When electrocardiographic changes are seen in relation to ischaemic heart disease the range of possible changes is enormous. Since ischaemia can involve any part of the myocardium and or the conducting tissue, changes can be seen in the P waves, the QRS complexes, the ST segments or the T waves, and almost any arrhythmia or conduction disturbance can be induced. However, the majority of cases in which the electrocardiogram shows evidence of ischaemic heart disease can be classified as examples of myocardial ischaemia, myocardial injury or myocardial infarction.

THE ELECTROCARDIOGRAM IN MYOCARDIAL ISCHAEMIA

Myocardial ischaemia may be present without any changes on the electrocardiogram, but when changes are present these usually involve the T waves and or the ST segments. ST-segment changes and T-wave changes are almost always non-specific, and such changes may suggest, but never by themselves prove, the presence of underlying ischaemia. When there is deep and symmetrical T-wave inversion, however, the probability is very high that this is due to myocardial ischaemia. 'Symmetrical' T-wave inversion implies that the angle of downstroke and the angle of upslope of the T wave are equal. Myocardial ischaemia may give rise to the following electrocardiographic changes.
1   Symmetrical T-wave inversion.
2   Deep but asymmetric T-wave inversion.
3   Horizontal ST-segment depression with or without T-wave inversion.
4   Abnormally tall T waves.
5   Minor non-specific ST–T-wave changes.
Examples are shown in Figs 9.23–9.25.

MYOCARDIAL INJURY

Subendocardial ischaemia

Myocardial injury produces changes in the ST segment of the electrocardiogram. When the injury is confined to or predominantly involves the subendocardium, ST-segment depression is typically produced. The presence of horizontal, i.e. neither

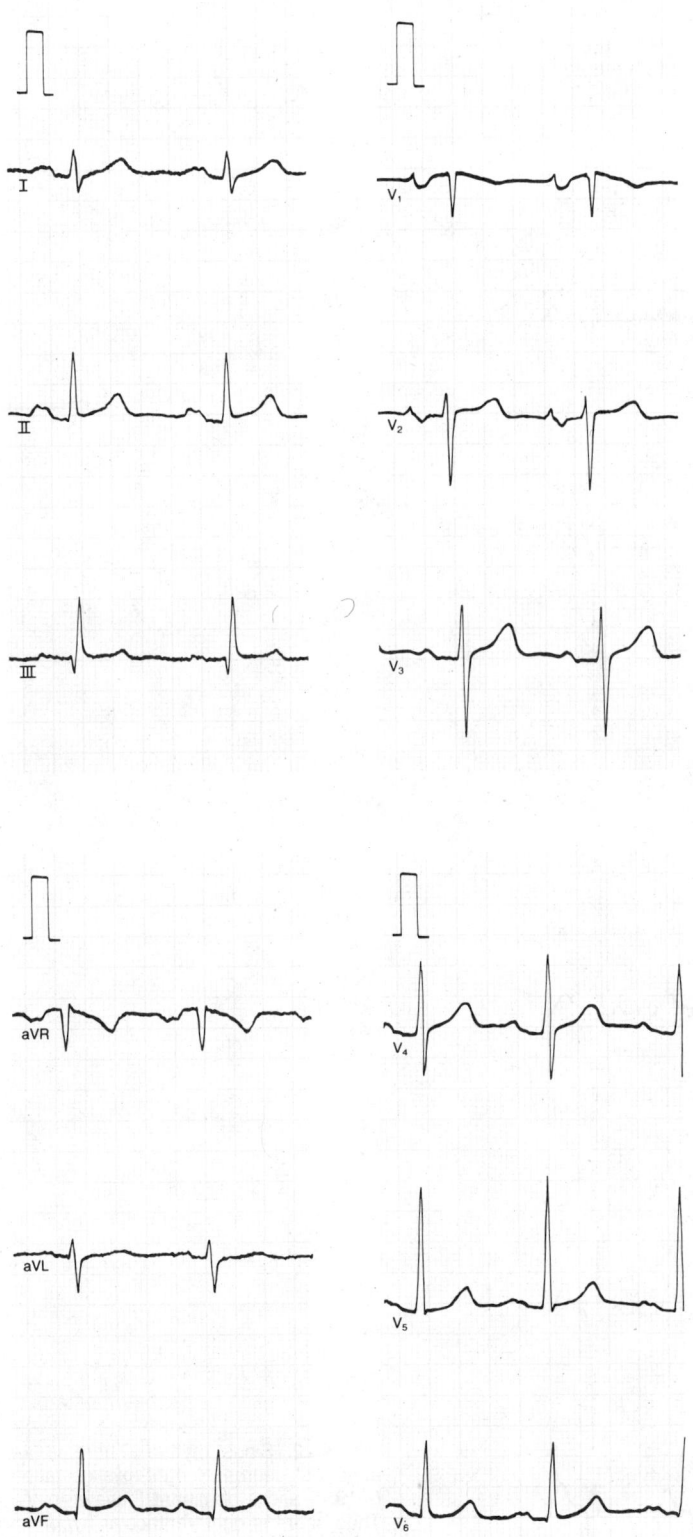

Fig. 9.21. The rhythm is sinus. The P waves are bifid in lead II. The P-wave duration in lead II is prolonged at 0.15 s. The P waves in V_1 are clearly biphasic. In this lead, there is a small, brief (and rather sharp-looking) initial positive component, followed by a deeper and very much broader negative component. The area of the negative component clearly exceeds that of the positive component.

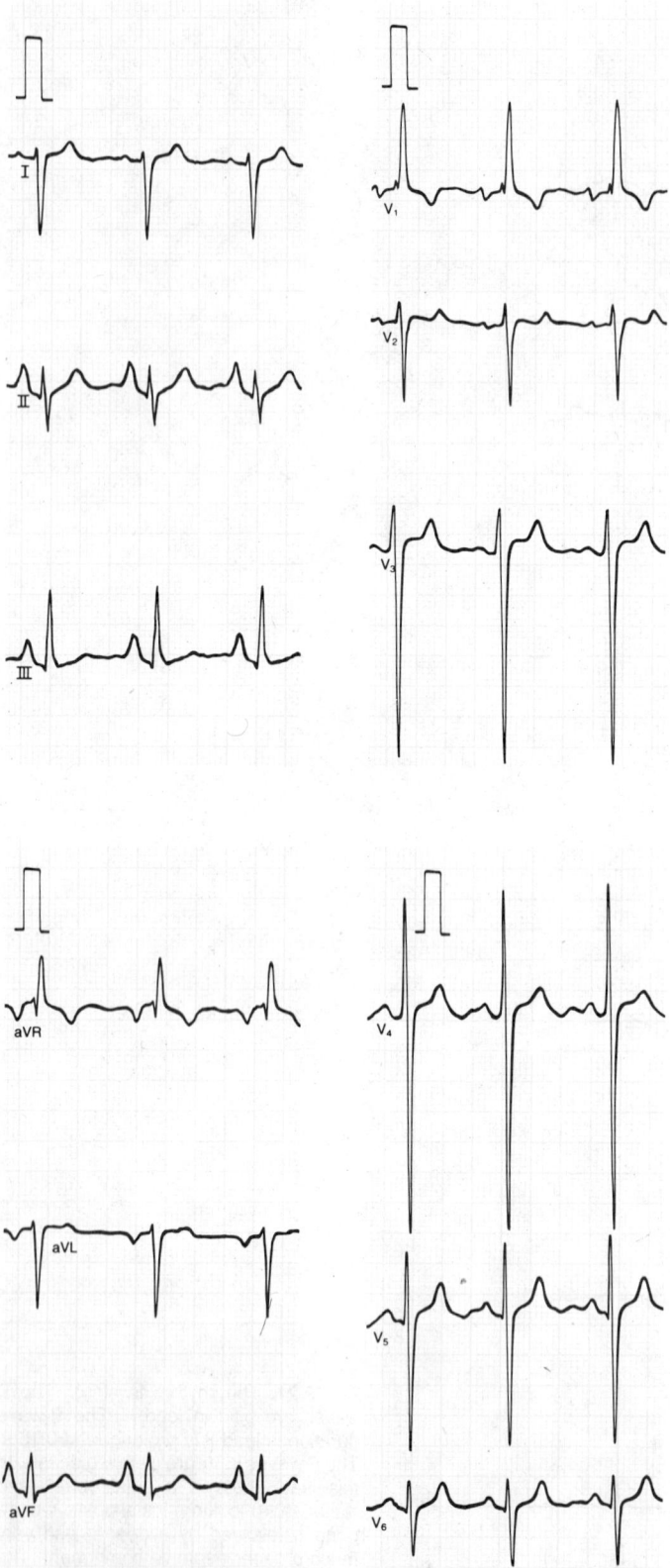

Fig. 9.22. Sinus rhythm. There is an abnormal degree of right-axis deviation (+165°) and a dominant R wave in V₁. Thus, there is right ventricular hypertrophy. The P waves are tall and pointed in lead II and are in excess of 3 mm. This provides unequivocal evidence of right atrial hypertrophy.

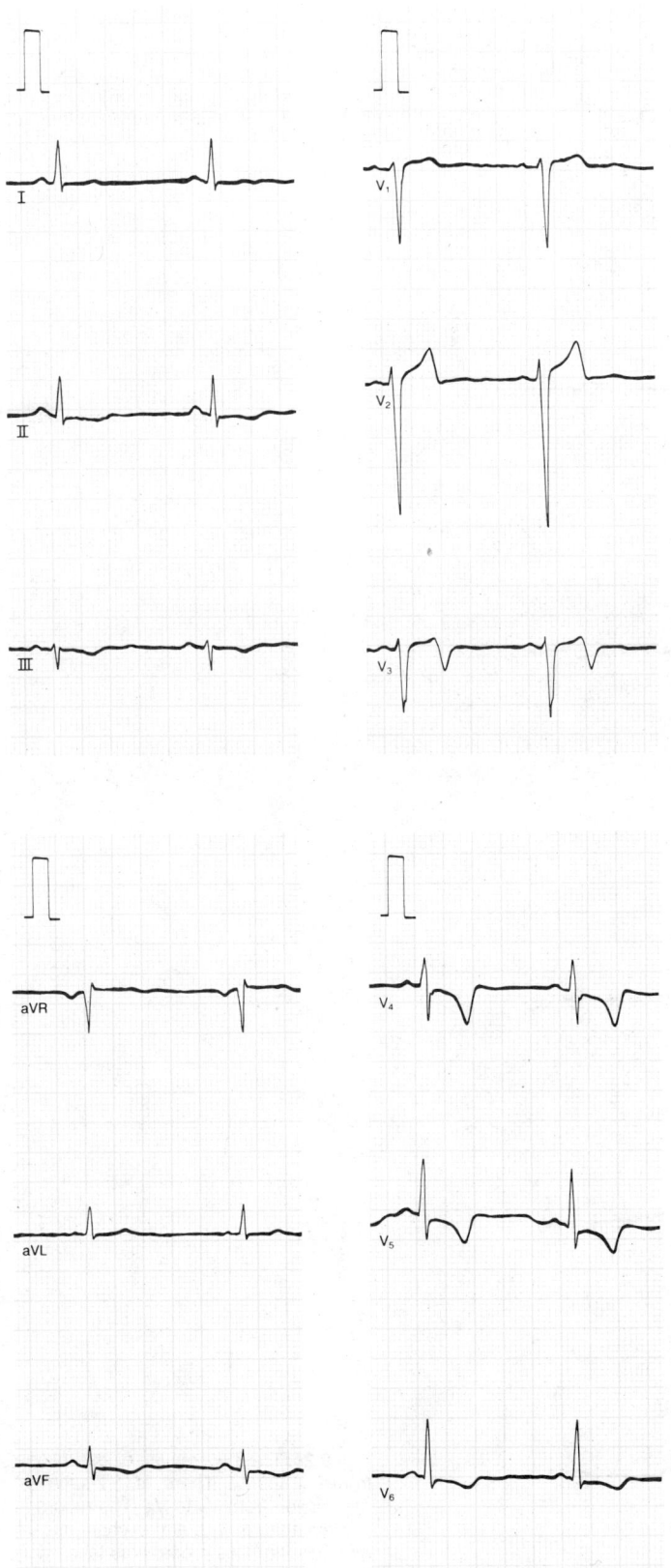

Fig. 9.23. There is T-wave inversion in V_3, V_4 and V_5. There is ST-segment depression with shallow T-wave inversion in V_6. These are non-specific but definitely abnormal changes. The deep symmetrical T-wave inversion in V_3 is very suggestive of an ischaemic origin. The T waves in the limb leads are also abnormal because the mean frontal plane QRS axis is highly determinate at $+15°$ whereas the frontal plane T-wave axis is indeterminate. Although, strictly speaking, all these changes are non-specific, the appearances are powerfully suggestive of myocardial ischaemia.

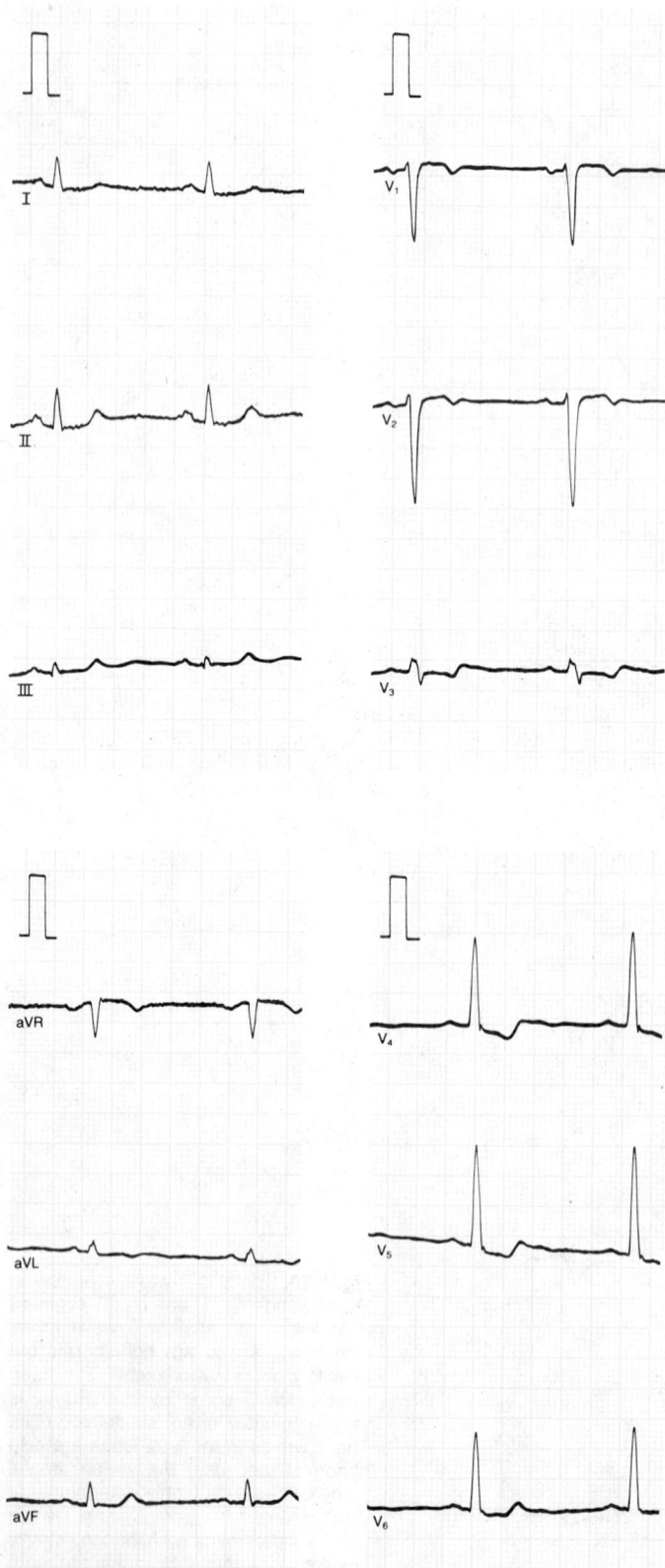

Fig. 9.24. The T waves are of low voltage from V_3 to V_6. There is ST-segment depression from V_3 to V_6 The record is frankly abnormal, but the changes are non-specific. This record was taken during a spontaneous attack of angina.

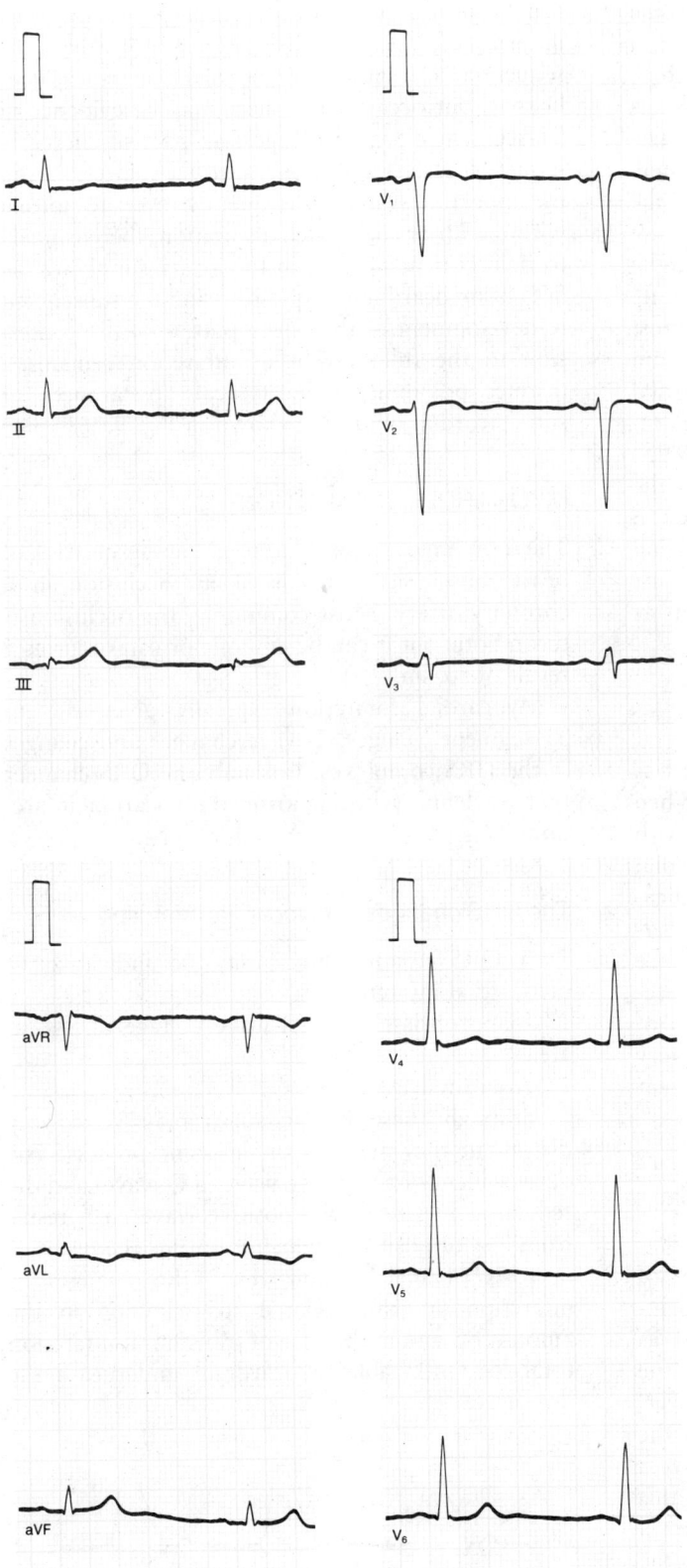

Fig. 9.25. This shows a record taken from the same subject as in Fig. 9.24 a few minutes later when the anginal pain had subsided. This record shows a substantial reduction in the non-specific ST–T changes noted in the earlier record (Fig. 9.24).

downsloping nor upsloping, ST-segment depression suggests sub-endocardial ischaemia or infarction. It is usually not possible to distinguish between these two possibilities but if the ST-segment depression is persistent, i.e. it does not clear within days, infarction is more likely than ischaemia as a cause; if there is clinical or enzyme evidence of infarction and the only electrocardiographic changes that occur are those of horizontal ST-segment depression, then the probability is that the latter changes indicate infarction rather than ischaemia. However, it must be made clear that an individual electrocardiogram alone cannot distinguish between sub-endocardial ischaemia and sub-endocardial infarction. Transient myocardial ischaemia (see Figs 9.24 and 9.25) is most commonly sub-endocardial because the sub-endocardium is that part of the myocardium most vulnerable to ischaemia. Transient myocardial ischaemia, whether occurring spontaneously or induced by exercise, is most frequently shown as ST-segment depression.

Sub-epicardial ischaemia

Transient sub-epicardial ischaemia is much less common than sub-endocardial ischaemia. When episodes of angina pectoris are associated with ST-segment elevation (indicative of sub-epicardial injury) rather than ST-segment depression (indicative of sub-endocardial injury), the terms *Prinzmetal's angina, atypical angina* or *variant angina* have been applied. Both spontaneous and exercise-induced sub-epicardial ischaemia, i.e. episodes of ischaemia with ST-segment elevation, are very much less common than angina with ST-segment depression (sub-endocardial ischaemia).

Myocardial injury in the early phase of myocardial infarction

During the electrocardiographic evolution of myocardial infarction, evidence of myocardial injury occurs early. This is usually manifested as ST-segment elevation. This may be because the dominant injury is in the sub-epicardium however, more often the injury is transmural and both the sub-epicardium and sub-endocardium are involved. Even if there is transmural myocardial injury in this way, the electrocardiographic appearances are, in effect, those of sub-epicardial injury because the electrical potential generated in the sub-epicardium is much greater than that in the sub-endocardium. When ST-segment elevation occurs as a result of an acute coronary occlusion, there is in the vast majority of cases a steady progression through the sequential changes of myocardial infarction (see below), but occasionally there may be evidence of ST-segment elevation suggesting part of the early sequence of changes of myocardial infarction and the appearances may subsequently revert to normal within 24 h or so. In such a situation, there is likely to be a critical stenosis in the artery supplying the area of myocardium in question and the subsequent re-development of the injury pattern with progression to the full pattern of infarction remains a distinct possibility. The typical appearances of sub-epicardial injury are shown in Fig. 9.26.

MYOCARDIAL INFARCTION

The term 'myocardial infarction' implies necrosis of heart muscle as a result of an occlusion in a coronary artery. Most commonly, the occlusion is thrombotic but it can be embolic or can occur as a result of spasm.

Myocardial infarction typically gives rise to ST-segment changes, T-wave changes and changes in the QRS complexes. It is only the QRS changes that are definitively diagnostic of myocardial infarction.

The QRS changes of myocardial infarction

Two QRS abnormalities may be indicative of myocardial infarction.
1 Inappropriately low R-wave voltage in a local area.
2 Abnormal Q waves.

Although these two changes may seem very dissimilar, they are part of the same process. The development of a negative wave (a Q wave) and the reduction in size of the positive wave each result from loss of positivity which in turn is the result of necrosis of myocardium. The QRS changes of infarction are thus related to reduction in the amount of, and in the case of transmural infarction total loss of, viable myocardium underneath the

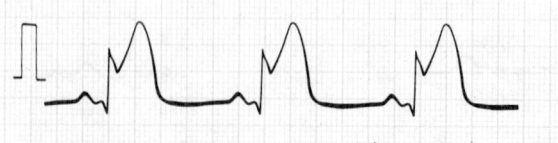

Fig. 9.26. Sinus bradycardia with marked ST-segment elevation typical of sub-epicardial injury.

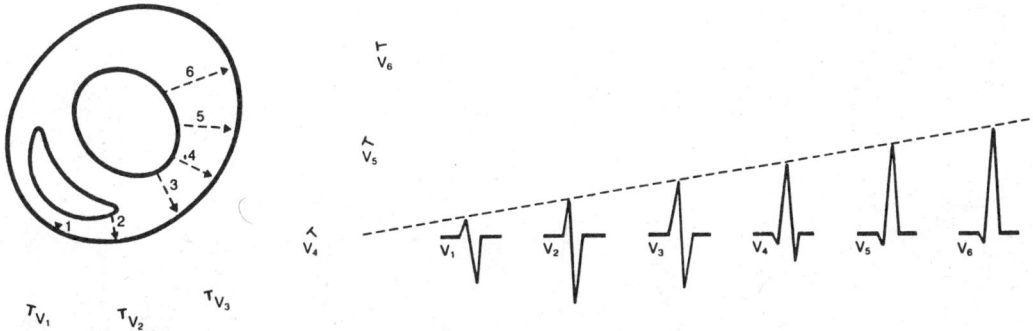

Fig. 9.27. The QRS complex in myocardial infarction. The progressive increase in R-wave height from right (V₁) to left (V₆) in the precordial series reflects the progressive increase in muscle depth (interrupted arrows) underlying the electrode because depolarization spreads from endocardium to epicardium.

exploring electrode. In the case of the precordial leads, the size of the positive wave in each lead is related to the thickness of viable myocardium underlying that electrode. In normal circumstances, this thickness increases progressively from right to left in the precordial series (Fig. 9.27).

Loss of R-wave voltage

If infarction occurs in a localized area of myocardium and if that infarction involves only part of the thickness of the myocardial wall, the QRS complexes recorded from the area of the infarction will show a reduction on R-wave voltage (Fig. 9.28).

Loss of R-wave height

Loss of R-wave height can be judged to be present only if either a previous record is available showing a significantly greater R-wave height in the appropriate leads before the infarction occurred or

the leads involved are two or more of the leads V₂–V₅ such that a normal R wave is seen on each side of the lead (V₁ and V₆) and interpolation between V₁ and V₆ permits estimation of the size of the anticipated normal R wave (see Fig. 9.28).

Abnormal Q waves and QS complexes

When infarction involves the full thickness of the myocardium ('transmural' infarction, i.e. from endocardium to epicardium), there will be *total* loss of R waves in leads overlying the infarcted zone (Fig. 9.29).

Total loss of R waves in the precordial leads gives rise to entirely negative waves. By definition, these waves are QS complexes. These negative waves are the result of depolarization of the posterior wall of the ventricle travelling from endocardium to epicardium (and therefore away from the precordial leads). These depolarization waves from the posterior wall of the heart are, in normal circumstances,

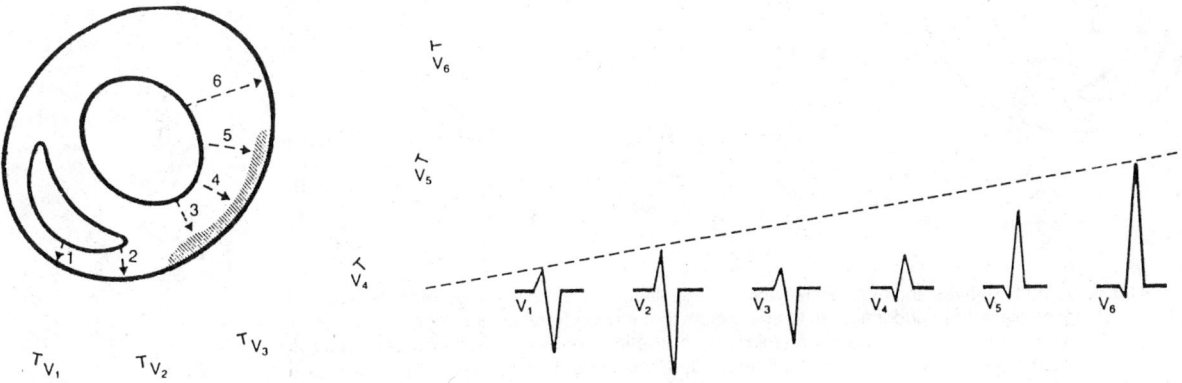

Fig. 9.28. Loss of R-wave voltage. The height of the R wave in each lead is related to the thickness of viable myocardium underlying the lead. With infarction of part of the wall thickness underlying leads V₃–V₅, there is loss of R-wave height in these leads.

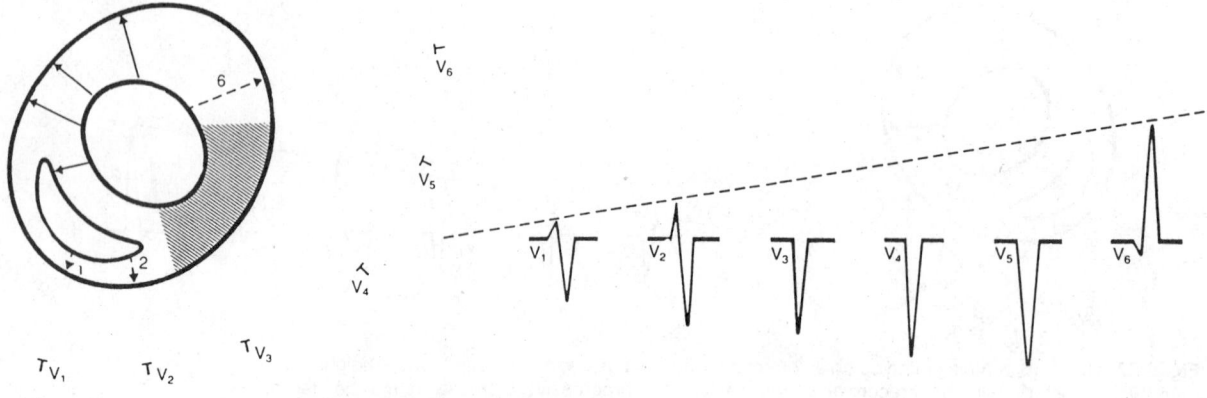

Fig. 9.29. Abnormal Q waves and QS complexes. When infarction involves the full thickness of the myocardium, i.e. from endocardium to epicardium ('transmural'), there will be total loss of the R waves. Depolarization of the normal free wall of the right and left ventricles takes place from endocardium to epicardium in areas underlying V_1, V_2 and V_6. However, leads V_3–V_5 are not influenced by the subjacent myocardium, which is electrically inert. These 3 leads reflect the depolarization of the interventricular septum and the posterior wall of the ventricle (continuous arrows). The depolarization also travels from endocardium to epicardium, but moves away from the precordial electrodes. The QRS complexes in V_3–V_5 show negative complexes, i.e QS complexes.

obscured by the dominant depolarization of the anterior wall of the ventricles which lie much closer to the precordial leads. When infarction involves less than the full thickness of the myocardium but still involves a major part of the wall thickness, less severe changes occur in which the R waves, although appreciably reduced in size, are still present and there are abnormal Q waves. The combination of abnormal Q waves (defined later)

and reduced R-wave voltage is the commonest electrocardiographic appearance in established infarction (Fig. 9.30).

The four possible QRS changes that may indicate the presence of myocardial infarction are as follows.
1   Reduced R-wave voltage where it can confidently be ascertained that this has occurred.
2   Abnormal Q waves without any conclusive evidence of R-wave reduction.

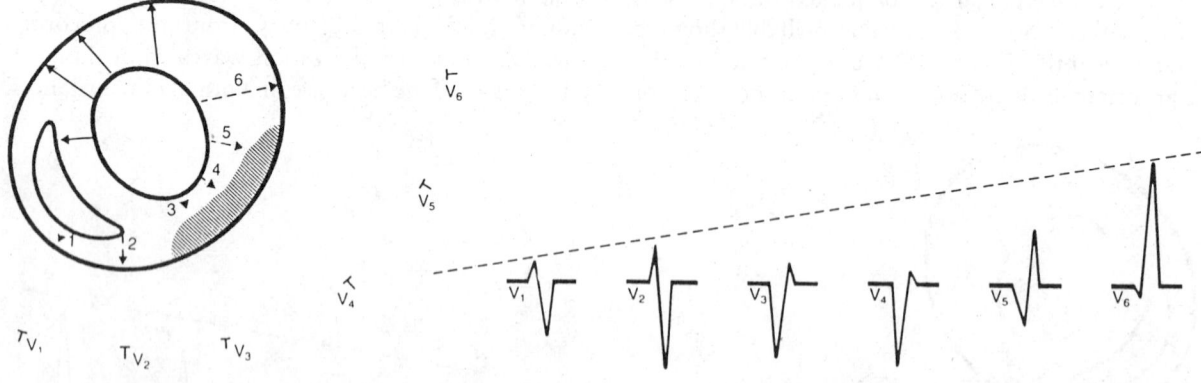

Fig. 9.30. Abnormal Q waves and reduced R-wave voltage. Depolarization of the normal free wall of the left ventricle takes place from endocardium to epicardium in areas underlying electrodes V_1, V_2 and V_6. However, infarction has occurred in a substantial part of the left ventricular wall in areas underlying V_3–V_5. As a result, the R-wave voltage is substantially diminished in these leads. The size of the residual R waves in V_3–V_5 is related to the thickness of remaining viable myocardium (interrupted arrows 3–5). This situation differs from that shown in Fig. 9.28 only by degree, i.e. the extent of wall thickness involved in the infarction. In this case, most of the wall thickness is involved and the thickness of the remaining viable myocardium is insufficient to overcome the effects of left ventricular wall depolarization passing away from the precordial leads giving rise to deep broad Q waves.

3 Abnormal Q waves with evidence of reduced R-wave voltage.

4 Abnormal QS complexes.

Normal and abnormal Q waves

The first part of each QRS complex is produced by depolarization of the upper part of the interventricular septum and all leads recording from the left side of the interventricular septum will necessarily, in normal circumstances, show normal q waves. Normal q waves will therefore be seen from V_4 to V_6 when the heart is intermediate in position but may be present from V_2 to V_6 if there is extreme counterclockwise cardiac rotation. In the limb leads, septal q waves will be seen in those leads that show a left ventricular configuration. The leads involved will depend upon the axis of the heart (Fig. 9.31).

When the heart is horizontal, normal qR complexes will be seen in leads I and aVL. When the heart is vertical, normal qR complexes will be seen in leads II and aVF.

A normal q wave is not more than one-quarter the height of the ensuing R wave and is also < 0.04 s in duration. Both criteria must be fulfilled for the q waves to be normal. Normal QS complexes occur in those leads that 'look' into the cavity of the myocardium. aVR is usually a cavity lead and therefore very frequently shows a QS complex (alternatively it may show an rS). Lead III is a cavity lead when the heart is horizontal, lead aVL is a cavity lead when the heart is vertical and lead V_1 is a cavity lead when there is pronounced clockwise cardiac rotation. QS complexes, therefore, may usually be found in aVR, will be found in lead III when the frontal plane QRS axis is in the region of $0°$ to $-30°$, will be found in aVL when the frontal plane QRS axis is in the region of $+60°$ to $+90°$ and will be found in V_1 when there is pronounced clockwise cardiac rotation. In all these situations, QS complexes are normal.

Abnormal Q waves are Q waves that are either abnormal in duration or abnormal in depth. A Q wave of 0.04 s or longer is abnormal in duration. A Q wave with a depth > 25% of the height of the ensuing R wave is abnormal.

The electrocardiographic criteria for the diagnosis of myocardial infarction from the QRS complexes

1 Reduction in R-wave height, from a normal level assessed either by a previous record ante-dating the infarction or by interpolation of the precordial leads.

2 The occurrence of QS complexes in V_1 (except in the presence of pronounced clockwise cardiac rotation), V_2, V_3, V_4, V_5, V_6, I, II, aVF and aVL (in the case of aVL, excepting those situations where the heart is vertical) or

3 Abnormally deep Q waves in V_1, V_2, V_3, V_4, V_5, V_6, lead I, lead II, aVF and aVL, except that abnormally deep Q waves (QS complexes) may be seen in V_1 in clockwise cardiac rotation and in aVL in vertical hearts.

4 Abnormally wide Q waves in V_1, V_2, V_3, V_4, V_5, V_6, lead I, lead II, aVF and aVL except that abnormally deep Q waves (QS complexes) may be seen in V_1 in clockwise cardiac rotation and in aVL in vertical hearts.

The ST-segment changes of infarction

As has already been indicated, it is only the QRS complexes that can provide definitive evidence of infarction. However, in the early stages of infarction, ST-segment elevation usually occurs and may occasionally be dramatic in degree. Such changes are indicative of injury rather than infarction, but the injury state is an unstable one and in the majority of cases evolutionary changes of infarction subsequently follow. Abnormal ST-segment elevation of this type usually occurs in leads facing the infarction in the case of both transmural infarction and sub-epicardial infarction. Leads looking at the heart from the opposite aspect will usually show 'reciprocal' ST-segment depression at a time when there is 'primary' ST-segment elevation in the leads related to the infarction. The precordial leads and lead I and aVL on the one hand and the inferior limb leads (II, III and aVF) on the other are mutually reciprocal in this respect.

The T-wave changes on infarction

A variety of T-wave changes may occur in association with myocardial infarction. These include flattening of the T waves, inversion of the T waves and abnormally tall T waves. None of these changes is specific. Sometimes, in the presence of sub-endocardial infarction, there may be widespread deep symmetrical T-wave inversion instead of the usual flat ST-segment depression. In such cases, sub-endocardial infarction can be inferred but cannot conclusively be diagnosed.

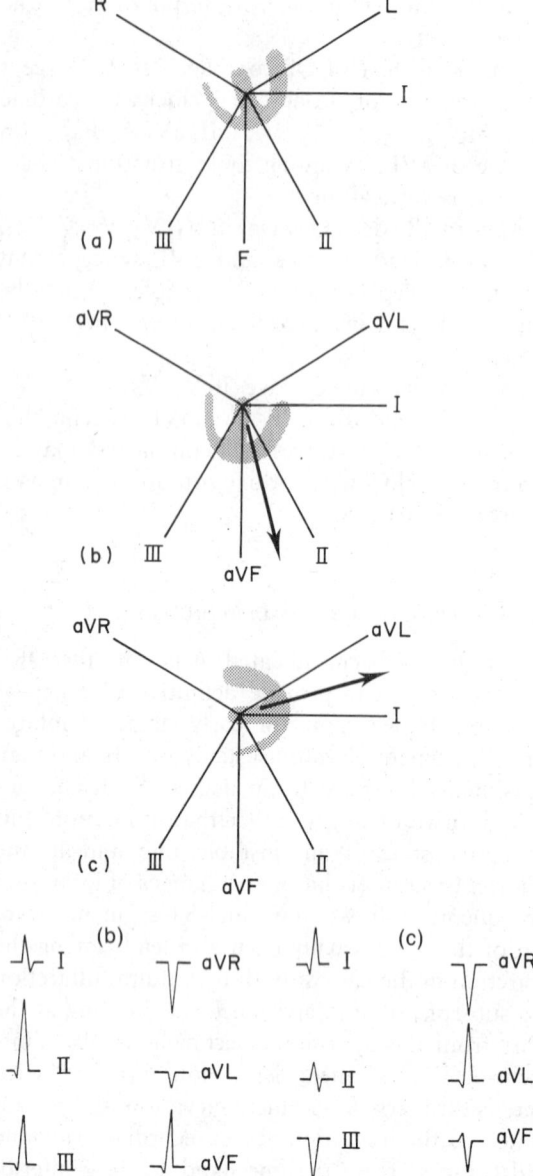

Fig. 9.31. (a) The orientation around the heart of the 6 limb leads. It should be noted that their distribution around the heart is uneven. Leads L and I 'look' at the antero-lateral aspect of the heart, leads II, F and III 'look' at the inferior aspect of the heart and lead R 'looks' into the cavity of the ventricles. **(b) and (c) Normal QS complexes** (the arrow indicates the direction of the mean frontal plane QRS axis in each case). (b) when the heart is vertical (in this case, the axis is +75°), aVL faces the cavity of the heart and shows a QS complex. Unless there is frankly abnormal right-axis deviation, i.e. an axis more positive than +90°, the resulting QS complex is usually relatively small. aVR has its usual QS configuration (this is normal unless there is extreme right-axis deviation, i.e. the axis is more positive than +120°, in which case aVR is no longer a cavity lead and may show a dominant positive deflection). (c) When the heart is horizontal (in this case, the axis is −15°), lead III faces the cavity of the heart and shows a QS complex. aVR also faces the cavity and shows its usual QS complex. *NB:* In this figure, the heart is shown to be *physically* vertical or horizontal. This is

The sequential changes of myocardial infarction

Although any or all of the changes described above may occur in myocardial infarction, a common typical *sequence* of changes is recognized. The more completely the described changes are present and the more closely the usual sequential patterns are followed, the more confident one can be of the diagnosis and the timing of infarction. The typical sequential changes of myocardial infarction occurring in a lead overlying the infarcted zone are shown in Fig. 9.32.

The location of changes in myocardial infarction

Primary electrocardiographic changes of the type described will occur in leads overlying the infarct.

Anterior infarction

The 'anterior' leads are the precordial leads (V_1–V_6) and lead I and aVL. If the infarction pattern involves V_1–V_3 the term 'antero-septal' is used. If the pattern involves V_4, V_5, V_6, I and aVL, the term 'antero-lateral' is used. If the pattern involves V_1–V_6 and I and aVL, the term 'extensive anterior' is used. If the pattern involves some of the group V_1–V_3 plus some of the group V_4–V_6, the term 'anterior' is used. If in the standard 12-lead electrocardiogram the pattern is seen only in aVL but is subsequently found also to be present in left-sided precordial leads taken one or more interspaces higher than the conventional positions, the term 'high lateral' is used.

Inferior infarction

Typically, inferior myocardial infarction shows primary changes in leads II, III and aVF. Not infrequently, the infarct also involves the apex of the ventricle in which case the term 'apical' or 'infero-lateral' is used and in this situation changes are expected in leads II, III, aVF, V_5 and V_6 (Fig. 9.33).

Less commonly, the infarct may be 'infero-septal', in which case changes may occur in leads II, III, aVF and V_1–V_3.

intended to facilitate understanding of what is an *electrical* rather than a physical concept. For example, the horizontal heart is one in which the main (left ventricular) electrical forces are directed horizontally and to the left.

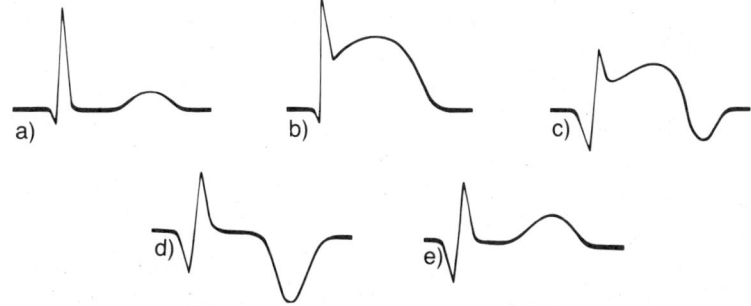

Fig. 9.32. The sequence of changes in acute myocardial infarction in a single lead. (a) The control normal appearances in a lead, which from the QRS morphology, clearly lies over the left ventricle. (b) Within hours of the clinical onset of infarction, there is ST-segment elevation. At this stage, no QRS-complex or T-wave changes have occurred. Although such a pattern is frequently referred to as showing 'acute infarction', no definitive evidence of infarction can be seen. There is evidence of myocardial damage. There is an unstable situation. In the vast majority of cases, evolutionary changes of infarction follow. Occasionally, the record returns to normal. (c) Within days, the R-wave voltage has fallen and abnormal Q waves (in this case, in both duration and depth relative to the R-wave height) have appeared. These changes are sufficient to prove the occurrence of infarction. In addition, T-wave inversion has appeared. The ST-segment elevation is less pronounced than it is in (b). (d) Within 1 or more weeks, the ST-segment changes revert to normal. The R-wave voltage remains reduced and the abnormal Q waves persist. Deep symmetrical T-wave inversion may develop at this stage. In some patients, this pattern remains permanently; in others, it progresses to the appearances shown in (e). (e) Months after the clinical infarction, the T waves may gradually return to normal. The abnormal Q waves and the reduced R-wave voltage persist.

Sub-endocardial infarction

Sub-endocardial infarction is diagnosed not so much by the location of the infarct pattern as by the fact that an atypical infarct pattern is produced (with horizontal ST-segment depression). Most commonly, this is shown in multiple leads.

Posterior infarction

Posterior infarction is a relatively uncommon infarct pattern in which changes that might be *anticipated* in true posterior leads can be estimated from changes that do *actually occur* in V_1 and V_2. Instead of having the primary infarct pattern of abnormally deep abnormally wide Q waves, loss of R-wave height and acute ST-segment elevation, there are abnormally tall abnormally broad R waves, loss of S-wave depth and ST-segment depression in V_1 and V_2 (Fig. 9.39), like Fig. 9.32(c) turned upside down.

Reciprocal changes of acute myocardial infarction

As indicated earlier, leads V_1–V_6, I and aVL on the one hand and leads II, III and aVF on the other hand are mutually reciprocal. Whenever primary ST-segment elevation is seen in one of these two groups of leads, there is a distinct possibility of the simultaneous occurrence of reciprocal ST-segment depression in the other group. When the primary ST-segment changes revert, the reciprocal ST-segment changes also clear. Thus, during acute inferior myocardial infarction, ST-segment elevation is to be anticipated in leads II, III and the foot lead and reciprocal ST-segment depression in some of the precordial leads. Likewise, in acute anterior myocardial infarction, primary ST-segment elevation is to be anticipated in the mid precordial leads and reciprocal ST-segment depression in the inferior limb leads.

Examples of the electrocardiogram in relation to myocardial infarction are shown in Figs 9.33–9.40.

Atrial infarction

There are no diagnostic changes of atrial infarction. Infarction of atrial myocardium is rare without simultaneous infarction of ventricular myocardium. The most specific electrocardiographic sign of atrial infarction is elevation or depression of the P–R segment. This is because the atrial repolarization wave (Ta wave or atrial T wave), which is the atrial equivalent of the ventricular T wave, tends to occur at the same time as the QRS complex. The PR interval corresponds in timing to the atrial equivalent of the ST segment. Elevation of the PR interval, therefore, can indicate acute atrial injury, and depression of the PR interval can indicate ischaemia of the atrium. A less specific but more sensitive indicator of atrial infarction is a bifid P wave in lead II or a biphasic P wave in V_1 with a dominant negative component. These P-wave changes cannot be distinguished from those of atrial hypertrophy.

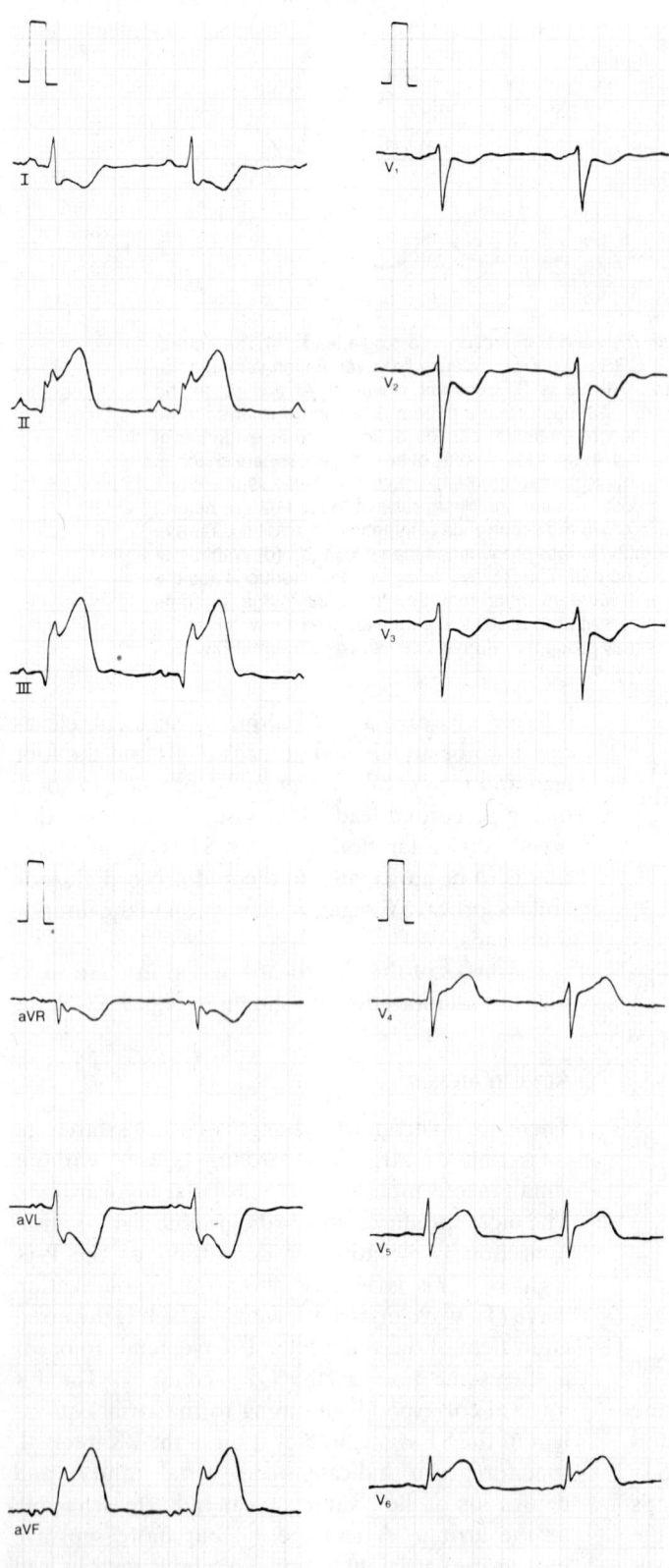

Fig. 9.33. There is ST-segment elevation in leads II, III, aVF, V_5 and V_6. These changes are indicative of infero-lateral myocardial damage. There is ST-segment depression in leads I, aVL, V_1 and V_2. These latter changes are reciprocal changes.

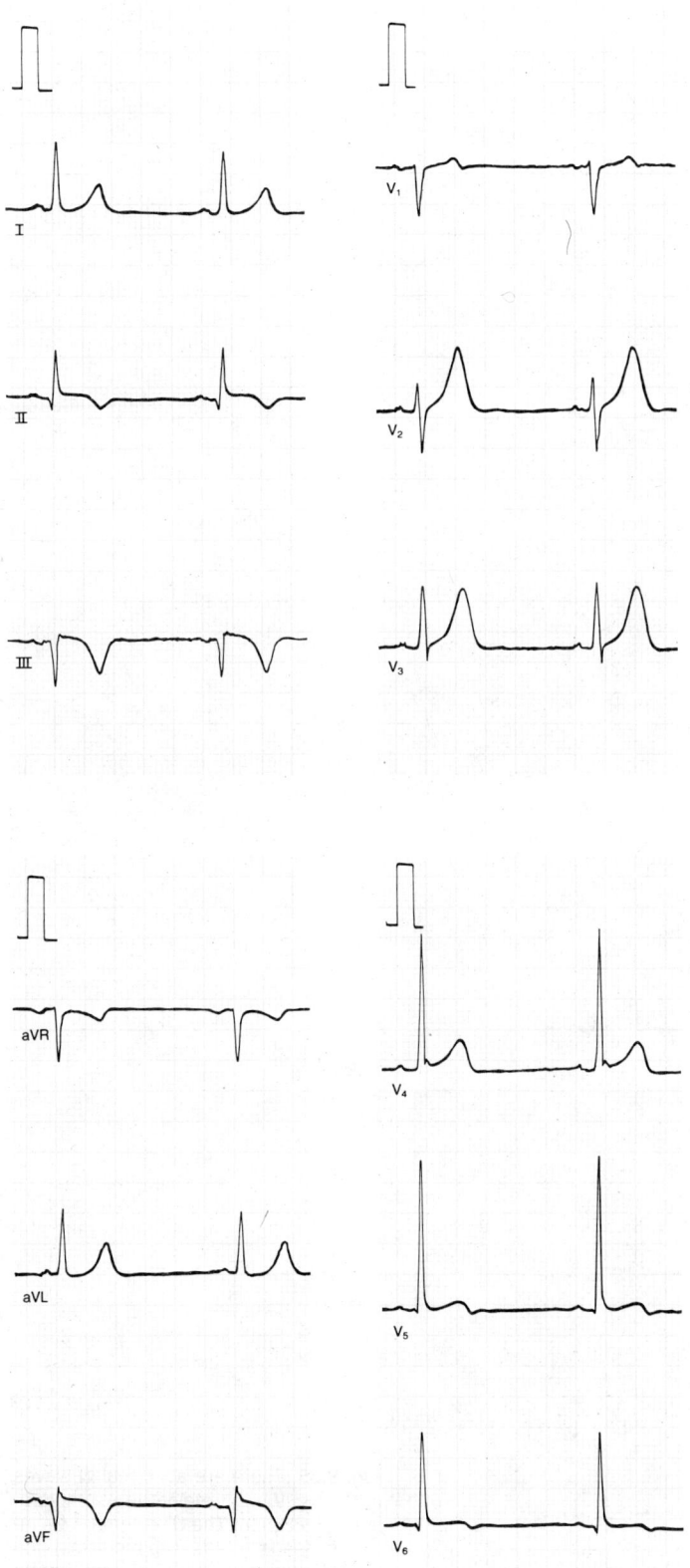

Fig. 9.34. There are abnormal Q waves in leads III and aVF, indicative of inferior myocardial infarction. There are minor ST–T changes in V_5 and V_6, suggesting antero-lateral ischaemic damage. The tall T waves in V_2 and V_3 raise the possibility of true posterior ischaemia.

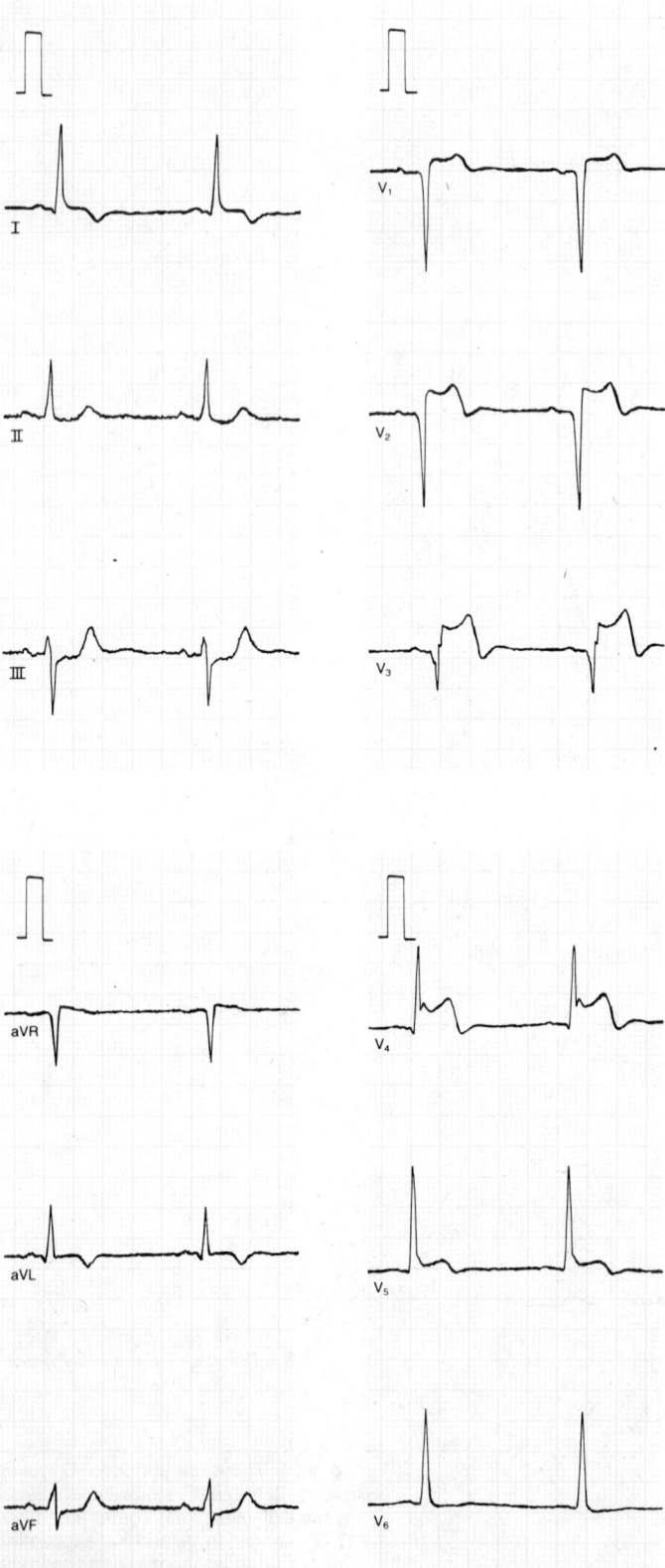

Fig. 9.35. There are abnormal Q waves in leads V_1–V_3, indicative of antero-septal infarction. The ST-segment elevation in leads V_1–V_5 suggests that the infarction is recent. The T-wave inversion in leads I and aVL suggests anterolateral ischaemia.

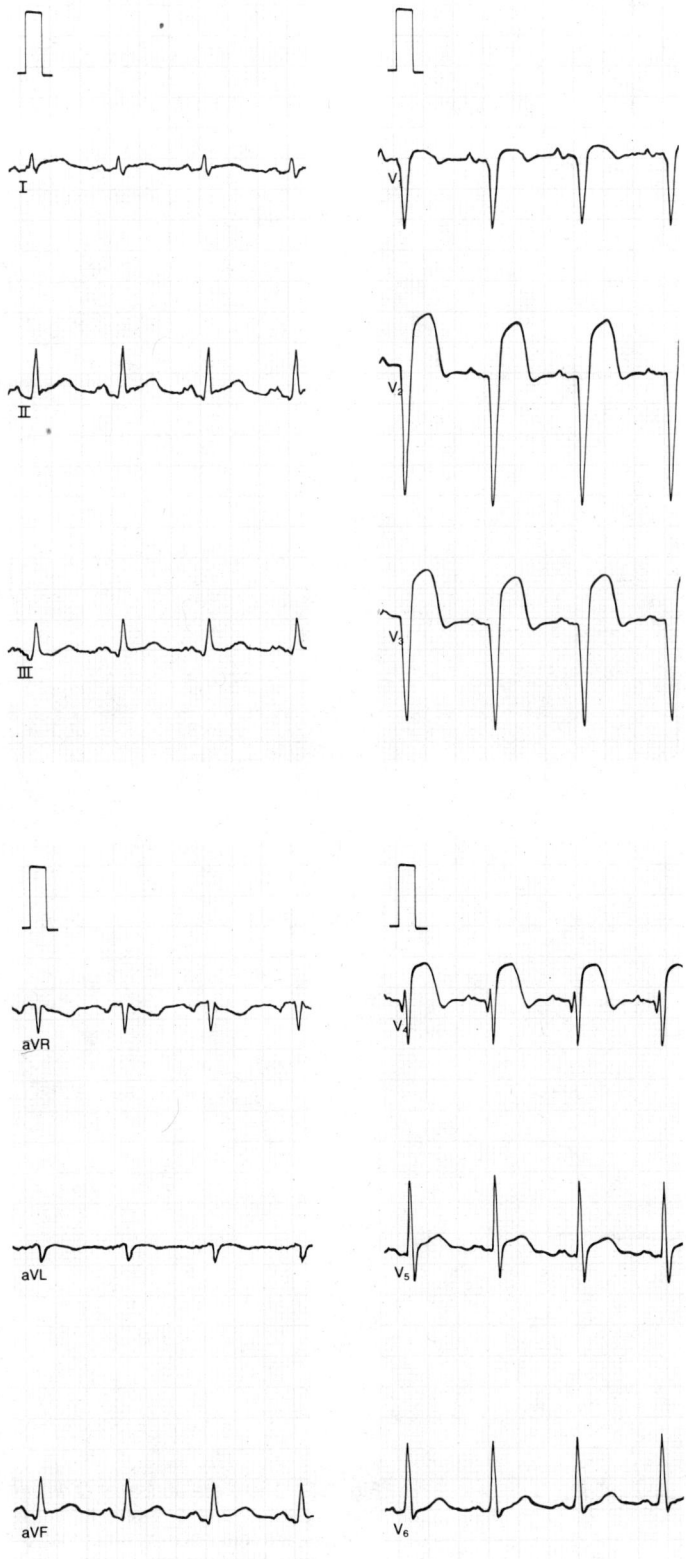

Fig. 9.36. There are abnormal Q waves from V$_1$ to V$_4$ indicating anteroseptal infarction and there is ST-segment elevation in these leads indicating that the infarction is recent.

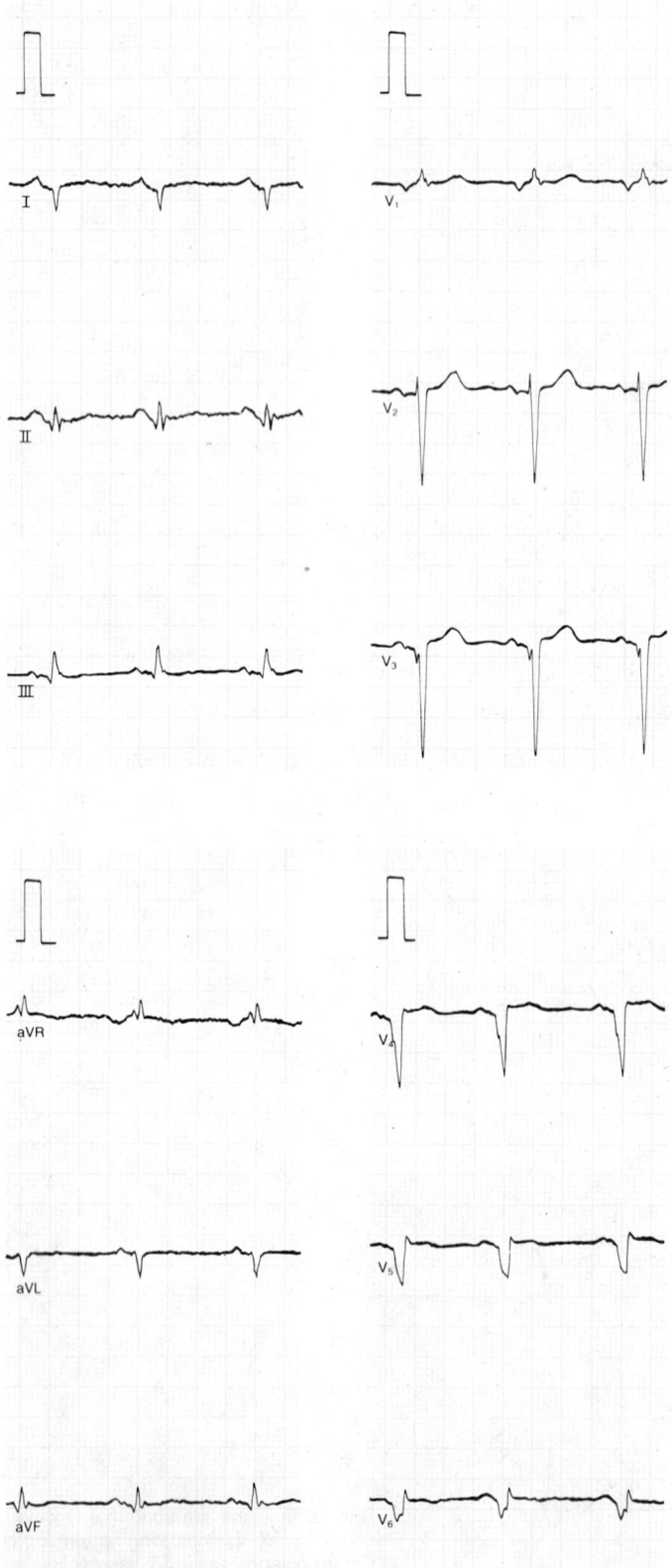

Fig. 9.37. There are abnormal Q waves from V_3 to V_6 and in I and II. These changes are indicative of antero-lateral infarction. The dominant r wave in V_1 suggests that there has probably also been true posterior infarction.

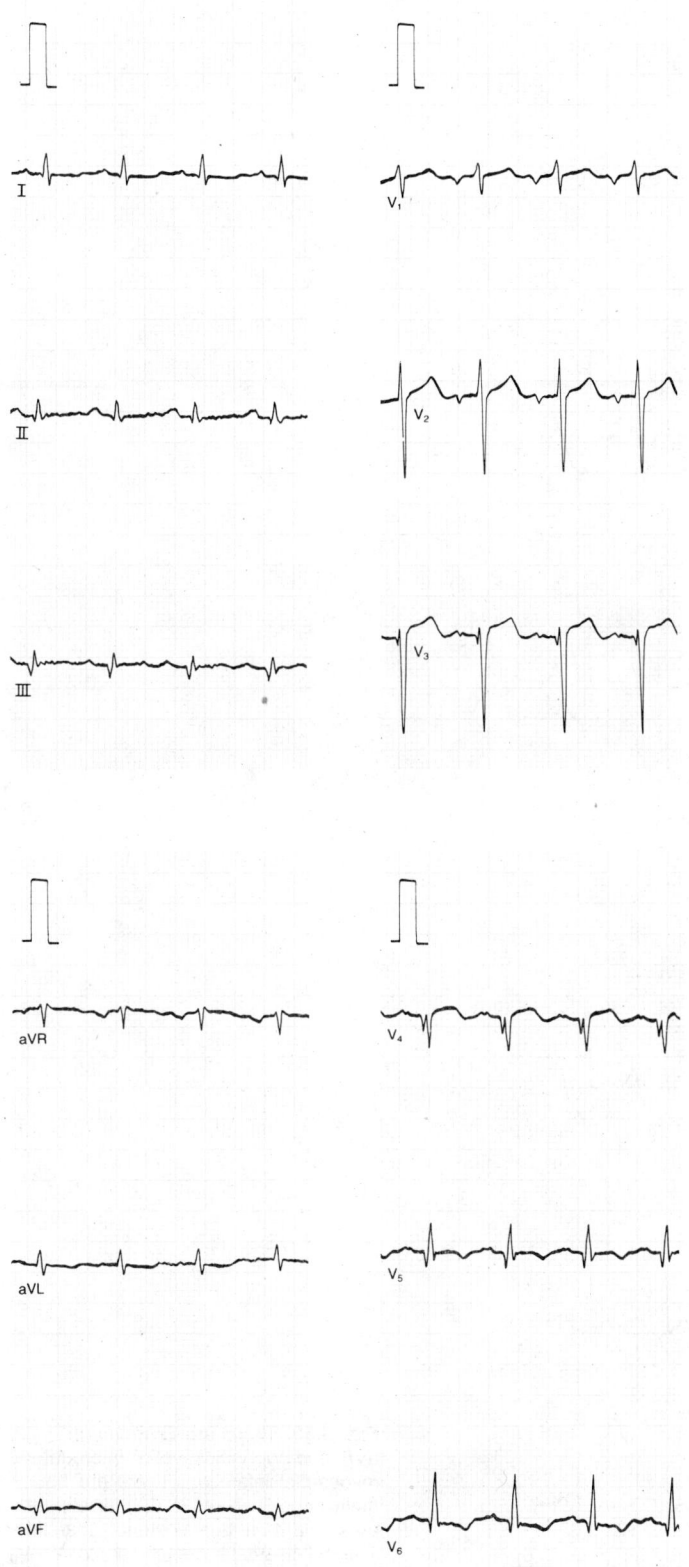

Fig. 9.38. There are abnormal q waves in V₄ and V₅, indicating a localized anterior infarction. There are widespread non-specific ST–T changes.

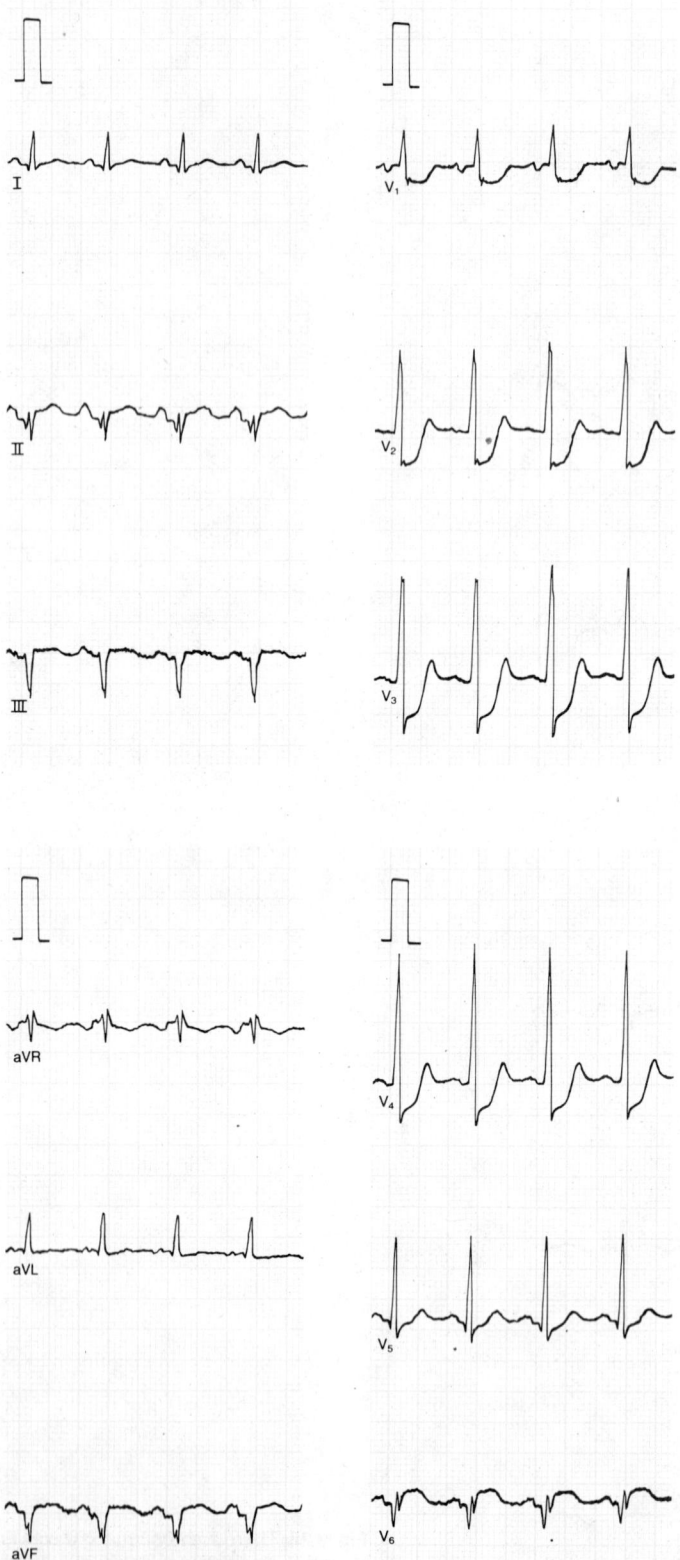

Fig. 9.39. There are Q waves in II, III, aVF and V_6, indicative of infero-lateral myocardial infarction. There are abnormally large R waves in V_1, indicating the presence of a true posterior infarction. The ST-segment depression in V_2–V_4 could indicate either anterior subendocardial ischaemia or (more probably) *recent* true posterior infarction.

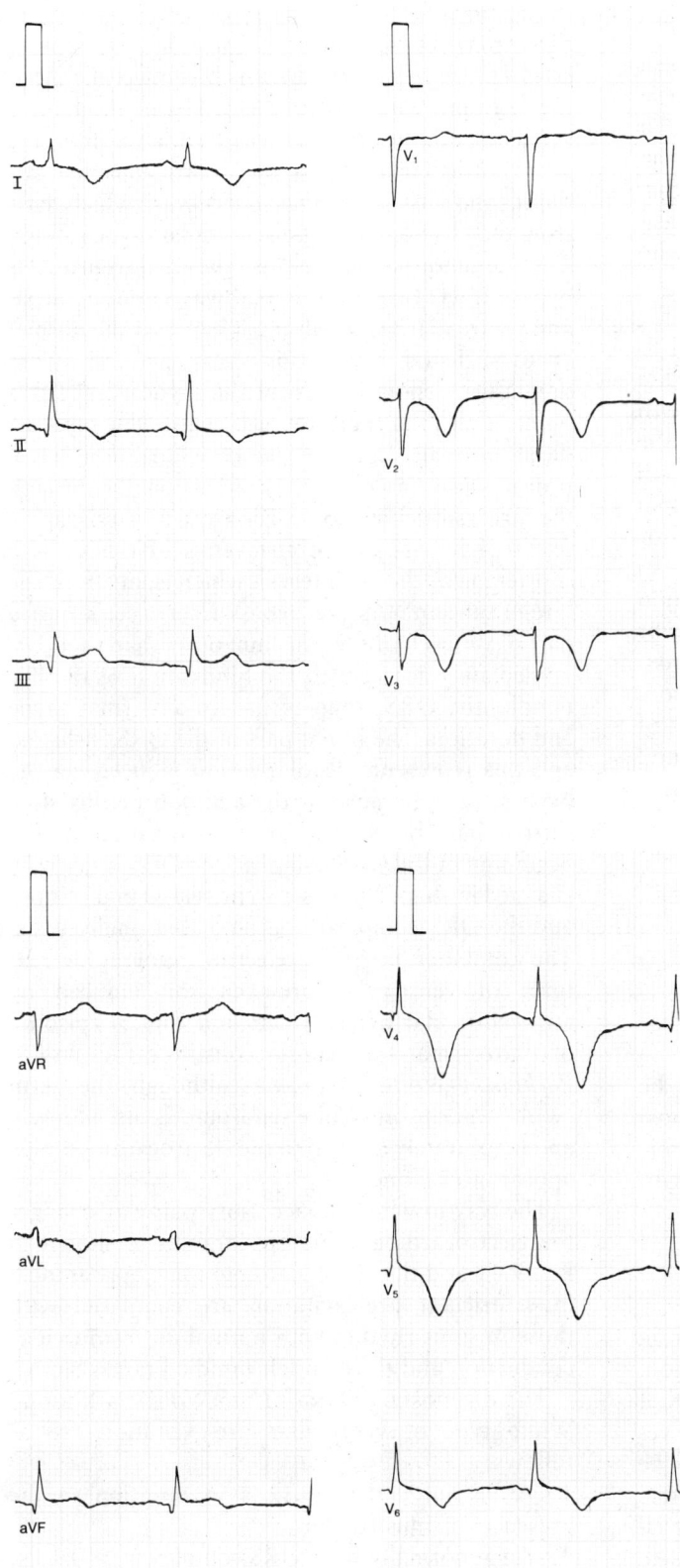

Fig. 9.40. The appearances in II, III and aVF suggest recent inferior infarction. The deep symmetrical T-wave inversion in V_2–V_6 and in I and aVL suggest sub-endocardial ischaemia or infarction.

VENTRICULAR ANEURYSM

It is widely believed that persistent ST-segment elevation occurring following acute infarction is indicative of a ventricular aneurysm. As 'ventricular aneurysm' is a haemodynamic concept rather than an anatomical one, it should not be expected that electrocardiography could provide a reliable basis for its diagnosis. The vast majority of patients who have ventricular aneurysms as a result of myocardial infarction have very large infarcts, and the persistent ST-segment elevation may be related to the presence of an extensive area of myocardial necrosis on the anterior wall of the ventricle (with loss of viable myocardium in this zone); the ST-segment elevation seen in the precordial leads in such cases may be a manifestation of additional sub-endocardial infarction on the true posterior wall, which would give ST-segment depression in true posterior leads and gives ST-segment elevation through the 'electrical window' of inert anterior wall myocardium. The mechanism of persistent ST-segment elevation is not completely understood. It certainly does occur in relation to some cases of ventricular aneurysm, but aneurysms can be found in the absence of this sign. When there is persistent and extensive ST-segment elevation, one can be reasonably confident that there is extensive myocardial infarction. In such situations, the finding of aneurysms is not uncommon.

MISCELLANEOUS ABNORMALITIES

Within this section, a variety of subjects will be covered which do not easily fit into major diagnostic categories; in addition, the electrocardiographic features of certain relatively common cardiac syndromes will be discussed.

VENTRICULAR PRE-EXCITATION

Ventricular pre-excitation is believed to occur in approximately 1 in 1000 of the normal population. The term 'ventricular pre-excitation' implies that some part of the ventricular myocardium receives the depolarization wave earlier than would be anticipated. This occurs as a resut of an abnormal (anomalous) 'accessory' pathway which links atrial and ventricular myocardium in such a way as to bypass the slowly conducting atrioventricular node. A variety of anatomical substrates permit ventricular pre-excitation. These include *atrioventricular*

connections (often referred to as Kent bundles and these may be left sided, right sided or septal), *atrio-Hisian bypass tracts,* which connect the atrial myocardium with the bundle of His or the bundle branches, *nodoventricular fibres,* which connect the atrioventricular node to the ventricular myocardium, and *fasciculoventricular fibres,* which pass from the His bundle to the ventricular myocardium. The commonest variety is the atrioventricular bypass tract. Because this pathway connects atrial and ventricular myocardium, it bypasses the normal atrioventricular conduction delay and results in premature depolarization of the myocardium at a point other than that at which ventricular myocardium normally initiates its depolarization when transmission has occurred conventionally through the atrioventricular node. The electrocardiographic result of bypass of the atrioventricular node is a shortening of the PR interval, which is, in effect, the 'pre-excitation'. As the bypass tract inserts into a part of ventricular myocardium other than that part immediately adjacent to the bifurcation of the His bundle, the QRS complex has an abnormal shape and duration. The initial part of the QRS is slurred and this represents depolarization induced via the bypass tract. Because of the addition of this slow slurred part of ventricular depolarization to the beginning of the QRS complex, the QRS is not only changed in shape but it is also increased in duration, and the QRS complexes become abnormally wide. The combination of the electrocardiographic features of ventricular pre-excitation induced by atrioventricular bypass tracts and clinical episodes of paroxysmal tachycardia constitute the *Wolff–Parkinson–White syndrome,* although the term 'Wolff–Parkinson–White syndrome' is often loosely and inaccurately applied to the electrocardiographic appearances alone.

The way in which an accessory pathway changes the electrocardiographic appearances is shown in Fig. 9.41 and the electrocardiographic appearances in ventricular pre-excitation are compared with those in sinus rhythm with normal atrioventricular conduction and those in left bundle branch block.

The diagnostic criteria of the Wolff–Parkinson–White type of ventricular pre-excitation are as follows.

1   A PR interval < 0.12 s in duration in the presence of sinus rhythm.

2   An abnormally wide QRS complex of > 0.10 s.

3   The presence of initial (first 0.03–0.05 s) slurring of the QRS complex.

All three criteria must be fulfilled for a diagnosis of

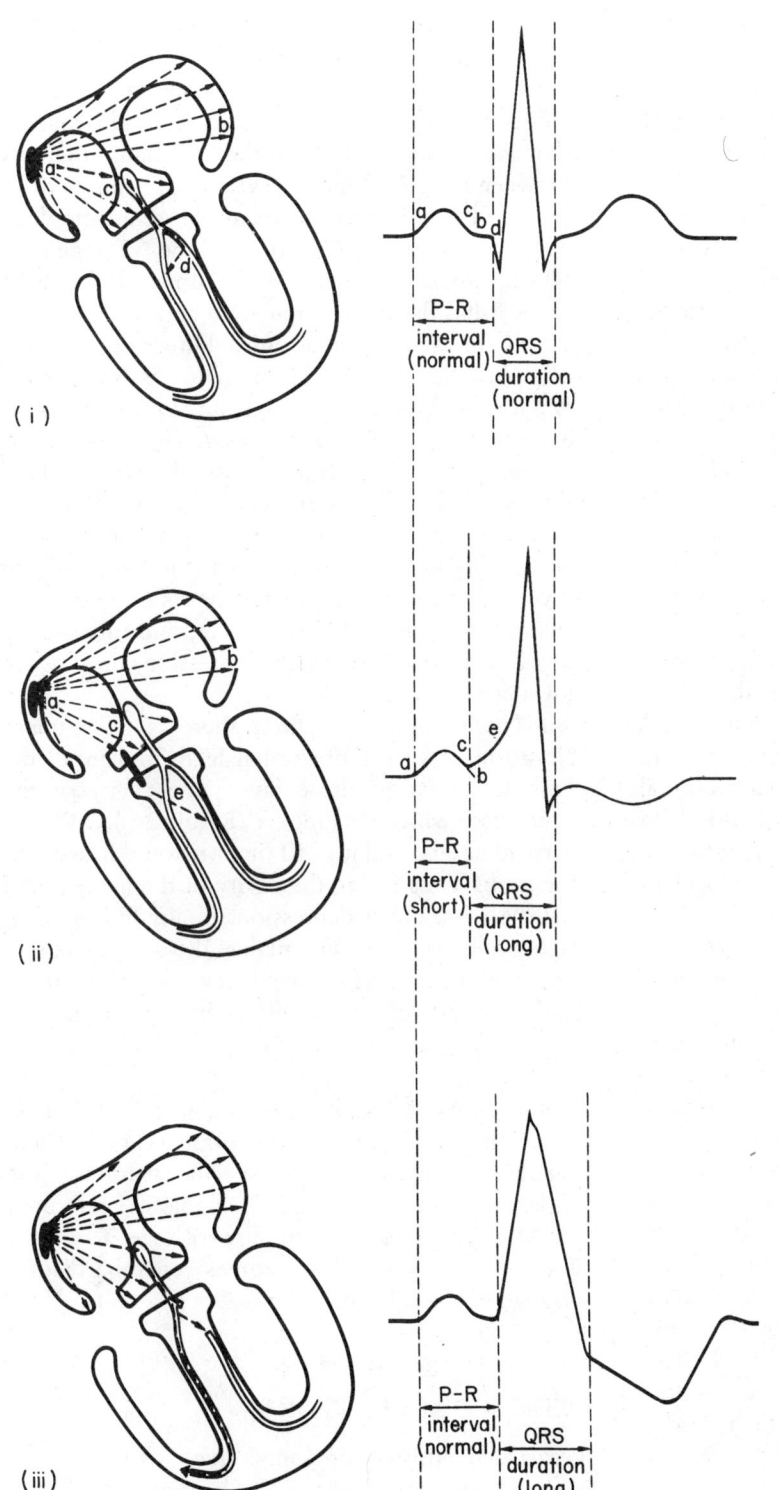

Fig. 9.41. The mechanism of accelerated atrioventricular conduction. (i) Normal atrioventricular conduction: the P wave is normal, the PR interval is normal, the QRS complex is normal, and the ST-segment and the T waves are normal. (ii) Ventricular pre-excitation: the P wave is normal, the PR interval is short, the QRS complex is abnormal in shape and duration and the ST-segment and the T waves are secondarily abnormal. (iii) Left bundle branch block: the P wave is normal, the PR interval is normal, the QRS complex is abnormal in shape and duration, and the ST-segment and T waves are secondarily abnormal.

pre-excitation of the Wolff–Parkinson–White type to be made.

The recognition of ventricular pre-excitation on the electrocardiogram is important for two practical reasons. The first is that subjects with such electrocardiographic appearances necessarily have some form of atrioventricular nodal bypass tract and are capable of having paroxysmal re-entrant atrioventricular tachycardia. The second is that the changes in the QRS complexes resulting from ventricular pre-excitation, if unrecognized, can easily be confused with right or left bundle branch block, right or left ventricular hypertrophy or myocardial infarction. As the initial part of each QRS complex may be changed radically by the presence of pre-excitation, the normal criteria for the QRS complexes cannot be applied once the presence of ventricular pre-excitation has been recognized.

An example of ventricular pre-excitation is shown in Fig. 9.42.

Compare Fig. 9.42 with Fig. 9.17. The form of the QRS complexes in these two records is very similar. The fundamental difference is that the PR interval is normal in Fig. 9.17 whereas in Fig. 9.42 the PR interval is short and there is a slurred initial delta wave. If the short PR interval and the delta wave are not recognized, this type of record can easily be mistaken for left bundle branch block.

A further example of ventricular pre-excitation is shown in Fig. 9.43. In this case, failure to recognize the presence of pre-excitation might give rise to a false diagnosis of myocardial infarction.

Another relatively common form of ventricular pre-excitation occurs when there are atrio-Hisian bypass tracts. In such a case, the atrioventricular node is bypassed but the ventricular myocardium receives the depolarization normally from the terminal part of the His bundle. The result of this combination is that the PR interval is abnormally short and there is no delta wave and no broadening of the QRS complexes. The electrocardiographic appearances again simply show a very short PR interval. An example is given in Fig. 9.44. The combination of this type of ventricular pre-excitation with episodes of paroxysmal tachycardia is called the *Lown–Ganong–Levine syndrome*.

PERICARDITIS

Acute pericarditis almost always gives rise to transient electrocardiographic changes of which by far the most typical and common is generalized ST-segment elevation. It is thought that this change is due to inflammation of the myocardium in the sub-epicardial region adjacent to the inflamed pericardium. The only other common cause of ST-segment elevation is acute myocardial ischaemic damage. It is widely taught that the main difference between the ST-segment elevation of acute pericarditis and that of acute myocardial ischaemic damage lies in the configuration of the ST segments, which are said to be convex upwards in acute myocardial ischaemic damage and concave upwards in acute pericarditis. However, a more obvious and reliable discriminator is ST-segment change: in ischaemic damage, it is *localized* whereas in pericarditis it is *generalized*. This is inevitable because acute pericarditis is usually a generalized inflammatory process involving the whole of the pericardium whereas myocardial ischaemic damage is typically localized to one area. The only form of myocardial ischaemic damage that is often generalized is sub-endocardial ischaemia, and this usually gives rise to ST-segment depression or T-wave inversion.

In pericarditis, therefore, there is ST-segment elevation in all the precordial leads and in all the limb leads except those facing the cavity of the ventricles, which includes aVR (always), aVL (in vertical hearts) and lead III (in horizontal hearts). In the limbs leads facing the cavity of the heart, there will be ST-segment depression. In any limb lead at right angles to the frontal plane QRS axis, there will be no significant ST-segment deviation since there will be only a very small QRS complex. An example of the changes of acute pericarditis is shown in Fig. 9.45.

Widespread ST-segment elevation is the hallmark of acute pericarditis. In the presence of chronic pericarditis, there are no specific features, just widespread non-specific ST–T changes. There may be ST-segment depression, low-voltage T waves, T-wave inversion and sometimes generalized low-voltage of the QRS complexes.

PERICARDIAL EFFUSION

Pericardial effusion does not give rise to specific electrocardiographic changes. There may be generalized reduction in the voltages of P waves, QRS complexes and T waves because of the interposition of pericardial fluid between the voltage generated in the myocardium and that recorded at the body surface. In addition, there may be non-specific ST–T changes.

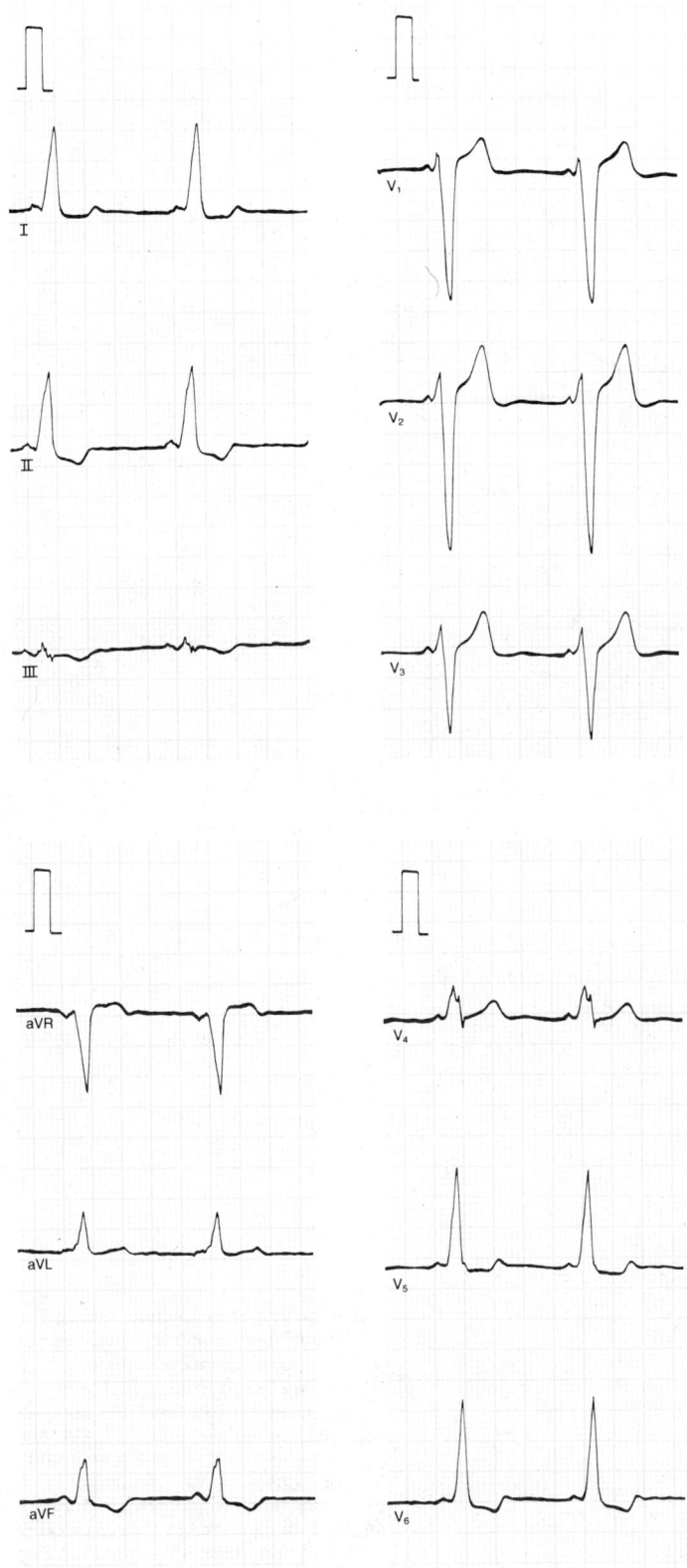

Fig. 9.42. The basic rhythm is sinus. The PR interval is abnormally short at 0.06 s (best seen in relation to the second complex in V_1). The total QRS duration is abnormally long at 0.18 s (well seen in both QRS complexes in V_2). The initial slurring of the QRS complex (the delta wave) is well seen in lead I, V_2, V_3 and V_4. The delta wave may not always be visible in all leads. It is always a small wave and leads that are approximately at right angles to the delta wave will hardly show it at all.

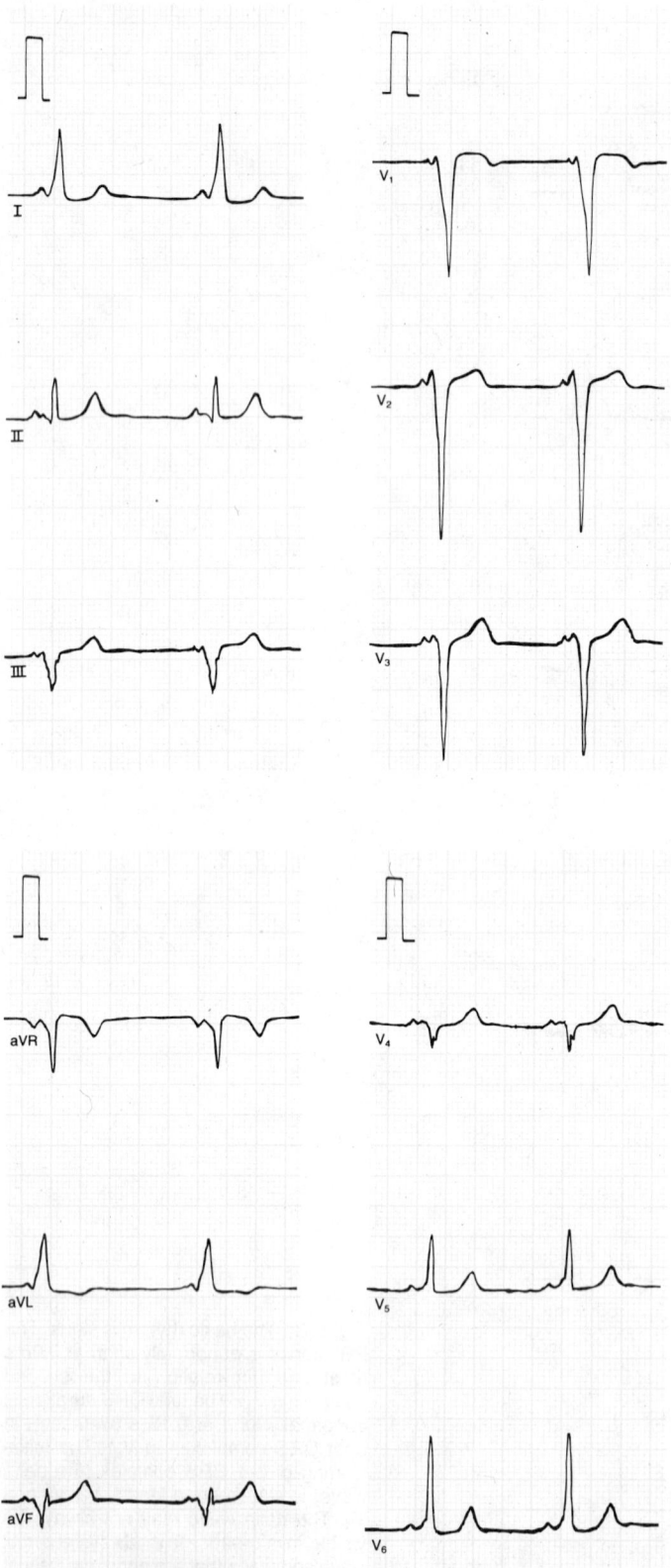

Fig. 9.43. The basic rhythm is sinus. The PR interval is short at 0.05 s (well seen in V₂). The QRS duration is prolonged at 0.14 s (well seen in lead I). There is a slurred initial part to the QRS complex (the delta wave) well seen in I, aVL and V₆. Abnormal Q waves are seen in aVF. In the absence of ventricular pre-excitation, these would indicate previous inferior infarction, but in the presence of ventricular pre-excitation no significance can be assigned to them other than the presence of ventricular pre-excitation.

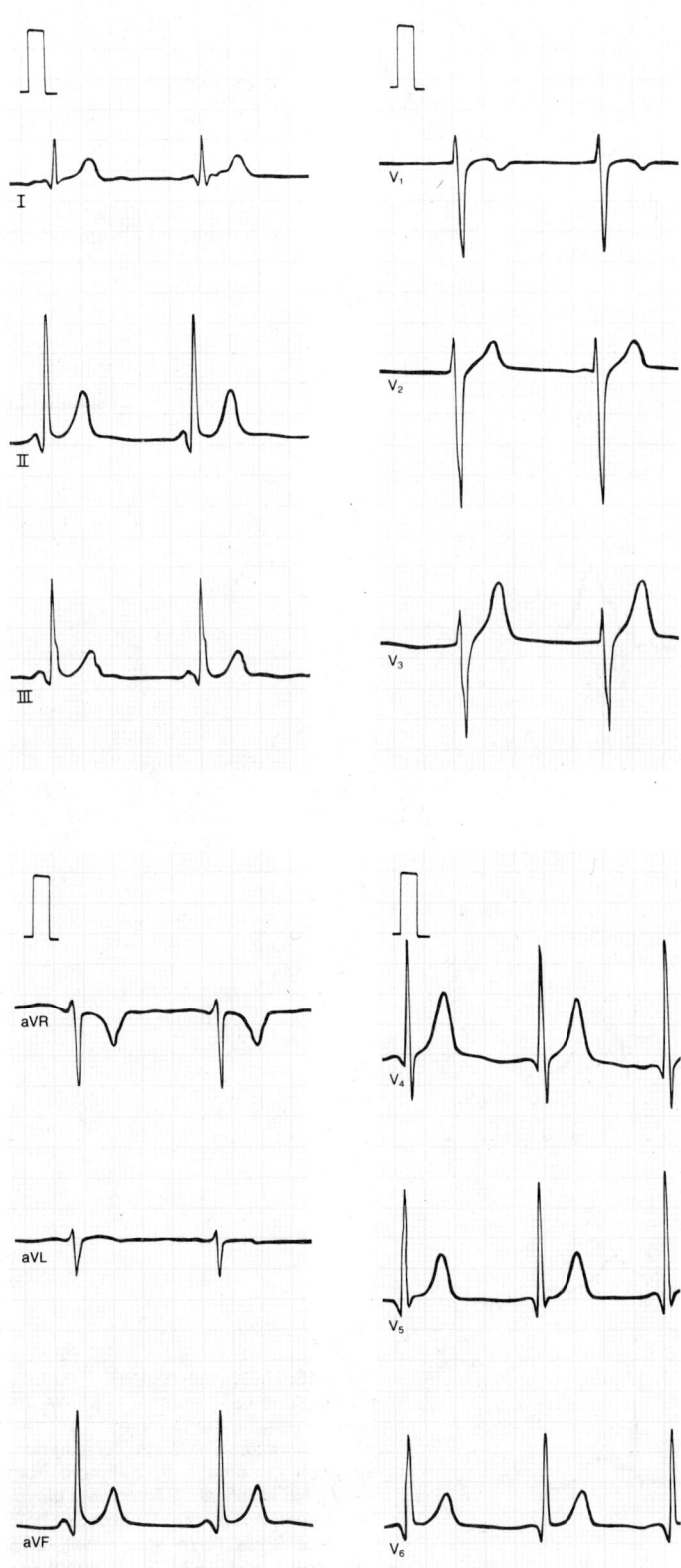

Fig. 9.44. The basic rhythm is sinus. The PR interval is abnormally short at 0.08 s. The QRS complexes are normal. The P waves are hardly visible in the precordial leads but can be seen clearly in leads III, aVR and aVF. This patient has episodes of paroxysmal tachycardia. The combination of such episodes with ECG evidence of a short P-R interval and no delta wave constitutes the Lown–Ganong–Levine syndrome.

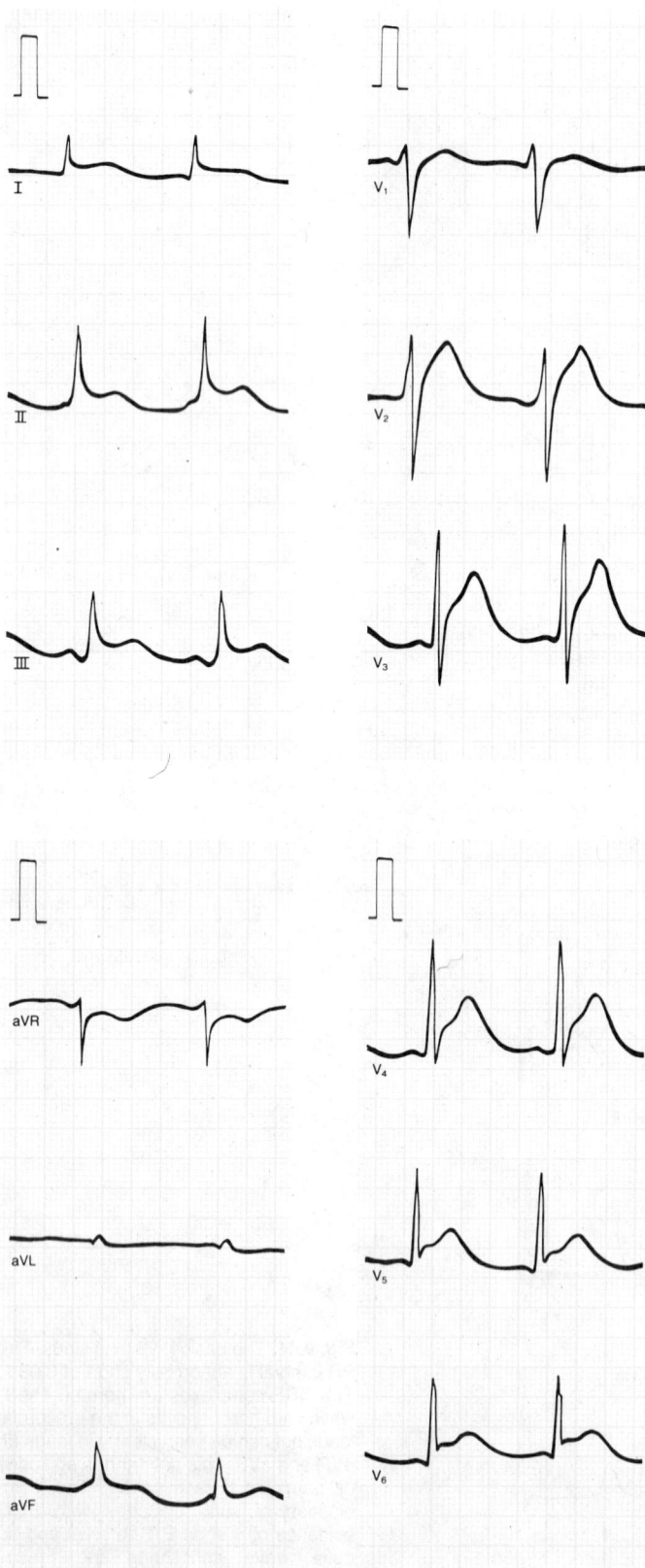

Fig. 9.45. The rhythm is sinus. The mean frontal plane QRS axis is +75°. As the heart is vertical, the Q waves in aVL are not abnormal. There is ST-segment elevation in leads I, II, aVF and from V₂–V₆. No significant ST-segment elevation is seen in aVL or in V₁ because both of these leads have very small QRS complexes, and slight ST-segment depression is seen in lead aVR as this is a cavity lead.

EFFECT OF DIGITALIS ON THE ELECTROCARDIOGRAM

As digitalis preparations are still relatively extensively used, it is important to be aware of the numerous changes that they may induce in the electrocardiogram. Digitalis preparations very frequently cause repolarization changes in the electrocardiogram (changes in the ST-segment, T wave and U wave) and these changes are known as *'digitalis effect'*. In addition, digitalis may cause a wide variety of cardiac arrhythmias, all of which are indicative of *digitalis toxicity*.

Digitalis effect

The most frequently recognized finding of digitalis effect is a downward sloping ST-segment depression; this is often associated with T-wave flattening and the combined appearance of a sloping ST segment and flattened T wave has been said to be similar to a reversed tick (or the tick made by a left-handed person). In addition, the QT interval may be shortened and the U-wave amplitude may be increased. The increase in U-wave amplitude is less impressive than that occurring in association with hypokalaemia or in response to quinidine therapy. The normal U wave is less than the height of the T wave that precedes it. In digitalis effect, the two tend to be of equal height or the U wave may be marginally greater than the T wave. Some shortening of the QT interval tends to occur in patients on digitalis. The shortening of the QT interval is not usually noticed on the 12-lead electrocardiogram and the changes are minor. It will be observed only if it is carefully looked for; it is not of major importance.

The morphology of the repolarization changes is shown in Fig. 9.46. An example of a 12-lead electrocardiogram showing appearances consistent with 'digitalis effect' is shown in Fig. 9.47.

It has to be emphasized that although the typical changes of ST-segment depression are those shown in Figs 9.46 and 9.47 these changes are in no way specific. Downsloping ST-segment depression can be caused by a variety of factors of which digitalis is only one. The recognition of digitalis effect does not imply the occurrence of digitalis toxicity.

Digitalis toxicity

The clinical syndrome of digitalis toxicity includes anorexia, nausea, vomiting and visual symptoms but the essential *electrocardiographic* manifestation of digitalis toxicity is the presence of digitalis-induced cardiac arrhythmias. A variety of cardiac arrhythmias may occur in digitalis toxicity. The commonest ones (in descending order of frequency of occurrence) are shown in Table 9.1. Examples of these various arrhythmias are shown in the section on cardiac arrhythmias.

EFFECT OF DRUGS OTHER THAN DIGITALIS ON THE ELECTROCARDIOGRAM

Numerous drugs produce relatively minor changes on the electrocardiogram. Some of the commoner and more important ones are listed below.

Quinidine

This drug produces reduction in the T-wave voltage or T-wave inversion, ST-segment depression, some prolongation of the QT interval, an increase in the height of the U wave and widening and notching of the P waves. In toxic doses, quinidine gives rise to widening of the QRS complexes and serious arrhythmias including heart block, ventricular tachycardia and ventricular fibrillation.

Beta-blocking drugs

The most obvious effect of beta-blocking drugs is the reduction of the heart rate. No significant

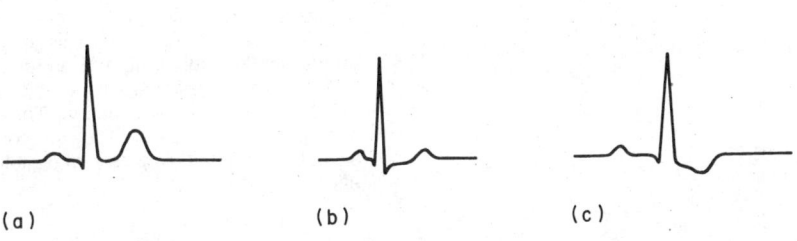

(a)   (b)   (c)

Fig. 9.46. The 'digitalis effect': ST-segment change. The electrocardiographic appearances in a left precordial lead in a normal subject (a) in the presence of mild (b) and more pronounced (c) changes of digitalis effect. (a) Normal QRS complexes, ST segment and T waves. (b) Non-specific ST-segment depression with a reduction in T-wave voltage. (c) Downward sloping ST-segment depression with flat T waves: highly typical but not diagnostic of digitalis effect.

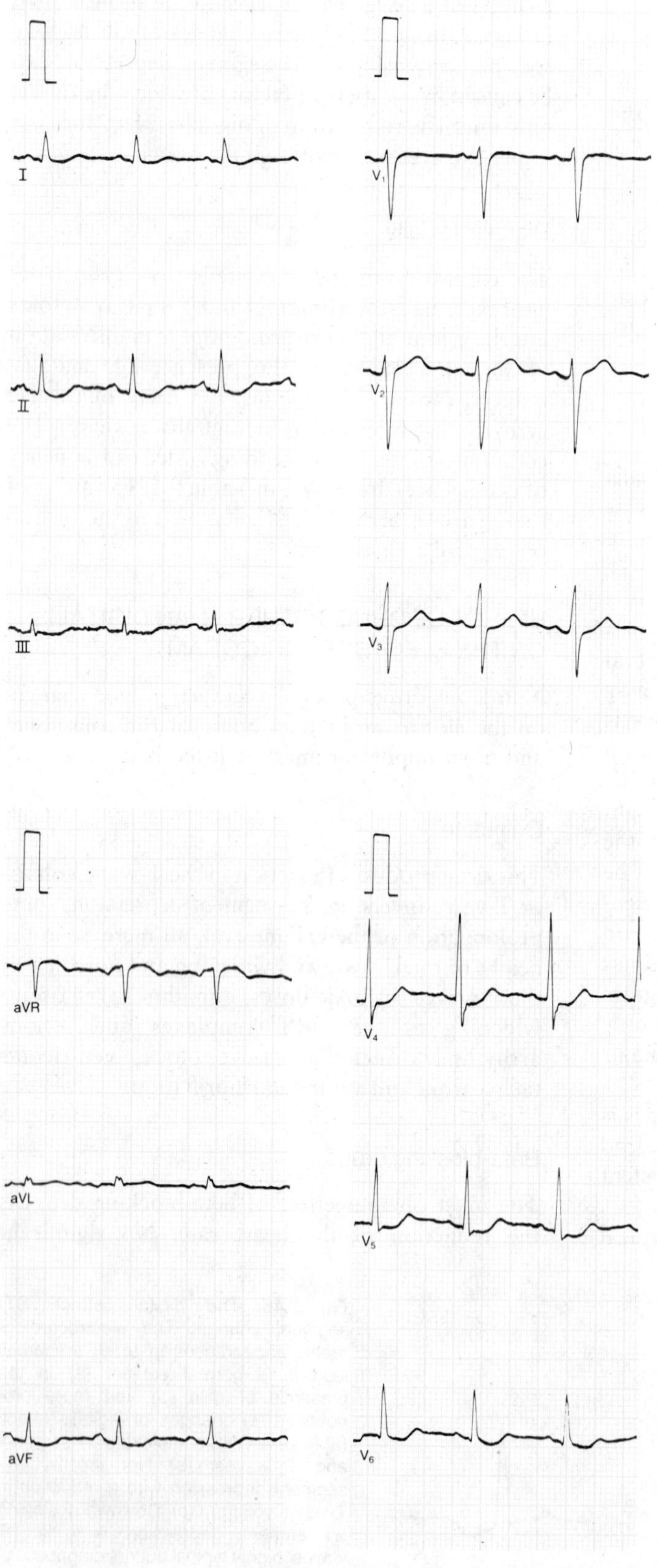

Fig. 9.47. The rhythm is sinus. The record is normal except for the presence of ST–T changes. There is ST-segment depression in leads II, III, aVF and from V_4 to V_6. The T waves are of low voltage in the limb leads and in V_5 and V_6. These changes are non-specific. They are consistent with but not diagnostic of digitalis effect.

Table 9.1. Digitalis-induced cardiac arrhythmias.

1 Non-paroxysmal atrioventricular junctional tachycardia
2 Ventricular coupling
3 Multiple premature ventricular ectopic beats
4 Sinus bradycardia
5 First degree heart block
6 Type I second degree heart block
7 Atrial tachycardia with varying atrioventricular block
8 Atrial or atrioventricular junctional premature ectopic beats with echo beats
9 Sino-atrial block or sinus arrest
10 Complete atrioventricular block
11 Atrioventricular junctional escape rhythm
12 Ventricular tachycardia
13 Multiform atrial tachycardia
14 Atrial fibrillation or atrial flutter
15 Ventricular asystole

---

changes in the QRS complexes, ST segments or T waves occur. Rarely, the degree of atrioventricular block may be increased in patients with atrioventricular conduction abnormalities. In patients with atrial fibrillation or atrial flutter, the ventricular rate is reduced.

Phenothiazine drugs and tricyclic antidepressants

These drugs produce changes similar to those of quinidine.

Lignocaine

In therapeutic doses, lignocaine has no recognizable effect on the electrocardiogram. In toxic doses, sinus tachycardia, sinus arrest or atrioventricular block may occur.

Mexiletine

The actions of mexiletine are similar to those of lignocaine.

Diphenylhydantoin

In normal doses, diphenylhydantoin produces no noticeable effect on the electrocardiogram. Occasionally, the PR interval may be increased and the QT interval diminished. In patients with extensive myocardial disease, the intravenous administration of this drug has occasionally been followed by bradycardia, atrioventricular block, asystole or ventricular fibrillation.

Procainamide

Therapeutic doses of procainamide produce only minimal changes. As the dose is increased, prolongation of the PR interval, QRS duration and QT interval occur. The T-wave voltage is reduced and the R-wave height increased. Toxic doses may give rise to gross widening of the QRS complexes, ventricular ectopic beats, ventricular tachycardia, ventricular fibrillation or asystole. These effects are more commonly seen after intravenous than after oral administration.

Disopyramide

In therapeutic doses, the effects of disopyramide are minimal. As the dose is increased, changes similar to those seen with quinidine occur.

Verapamil

Verapamil acts primarily by inhibiting the slow calcium channel in the myocardial cell membrane. It produces a slowing of the sinus rate and of conduction through the atrioventricular node. The latter effect gives rise ultimately to prolongation of the PR interval. There is no change in the QRS complex or in the QT interval. The effects of the drug on the sinoatrial and atrioventricular nodes are additive with those of beta-blocking drugs, and the simultaneous use of verapamil and beta-blocking drugs can occasionally give rise to profound and even catastrophic bradycardia, especially when one of the drugs is given intravenously.

Nifedipine

Although nifedipine is also a slow calcium channel blocker, its effect on the electrocardiogram is much less pronounced than that of verapamil. No significant changes in the P waves, PR interval or QS complexes occur, even at doses that produce profound haemodynamic effects.

Amiodarone

Amiodarone gives rise to prolongation of the QT interval and increase in the height of the U wave. This is in keeping with its characteristic electrophysiological effect of prolonging the actual potential duration.

HYPERKALAEMIA

Hyperkalaemia produces changes in the electrocardiogram which become increasingly more severe as the potassium ion concentration rises. There is, therefore, a direct correlation between the degree of increase in the serum potassium level and the resulting electrocardiographic change, but this correlation is neither precise nor totally consistent. There are no *diagnostic* changes of hyperkalaemia. All the changes are non-specific and may be seen in myocardial damage arising from other causes, e.g. infarction or the action of drugs. All parts of the electrocardiogram, P waves, QRS complexes, ST segments and T waves, may be affected in hyperkalaemia, and ultimately the cardiac rhythm becomes abnormal. The typical progressive changes of hyperkalaemia first involve the development of tall pointed narrow T waves, and then a reduction in the P-wave height and the R-wave height with widening of the QRS complexes and elevation or depression of the ST segments. At this stage, left anterior hemiblock and first degree heart block may develop. Subsequently, more advanced intraventricular block occur with very wide QRS complexes, bundle branch block or complete heart block. There may be multiple ectopic beats. Ultimately, the P waves disappear altogether and very broad bizarre QRS complexes occur. Finally, there may be ventricular tachycardia, ventricular fibrillation or ventricular asystole. The sequence of changes in hyperkalaemia are shown in Fig. 9.48.

HYPOKALAEMIA

Changes of hypokalaemia are much more frequently seen in clinical practice than those of hyperkalaemia but significant hypokalaemia can exist without recognizable changes necessarily being present on the electrocardiogram. Even when such changes are present, the correlation between the extent of the change and the degree of hypokalaemia is very poor.

The important changes of hypokalaemia (in descending order of frequency) are:
1 ST-segment depression, decreased amplitude of the T waves and increased U-wave height (all non-specific changes);
2 the development of cardiac arrhythmias; and
3 prolongation of the QRS duration and increase in P-wave amplitude and duration.
An example of the electrocardiographic changes of hypokalamia is shown in Fig. 9.49.

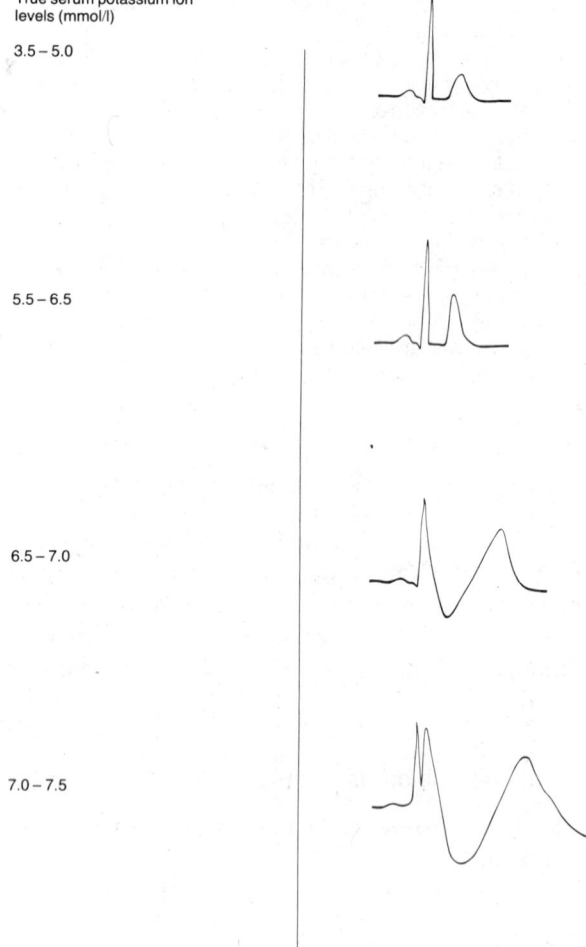

A few of the commoner, progressive changes of hyperkalaemia are illustrated.

True serum potassium ion levels (mmol/l)

3.5 – 5.0

5.5 – 6.5

6.5 – 7.0

7.0 – 7.5

Above 7.5

Fig. 9.48. Electrocardiographic changes in hyperkalaemia. Some of the commoner progressive changes of hyperkalaemia are shown. Serum potassium ion levels in mmol/l: 3.5–5.0, normal appearances (V_6); 5.5–6.5, T waves become abnormally tall and narrow; 6.5–7.0, P waves become broader and flatter, R-wave height decreases, QRS complexes become wider and ST-segment change (elevation in some leads, depression in others) occurs; 7.0–7.5, further widening and distortion of the QRS complex occurs, intraventricular block may develop, further ST-segment and T-wave changes develop with prolongation of the QT interval and ventricular ectopic beats may become frequent; > 7.5, ventricular fibrillation occurs.

HYPERCALCAEMIA

The main electrocardiographic change in hypercalcaemia is reduction in the QT interval. The T-wave duration appears to be unaffected, the reduction

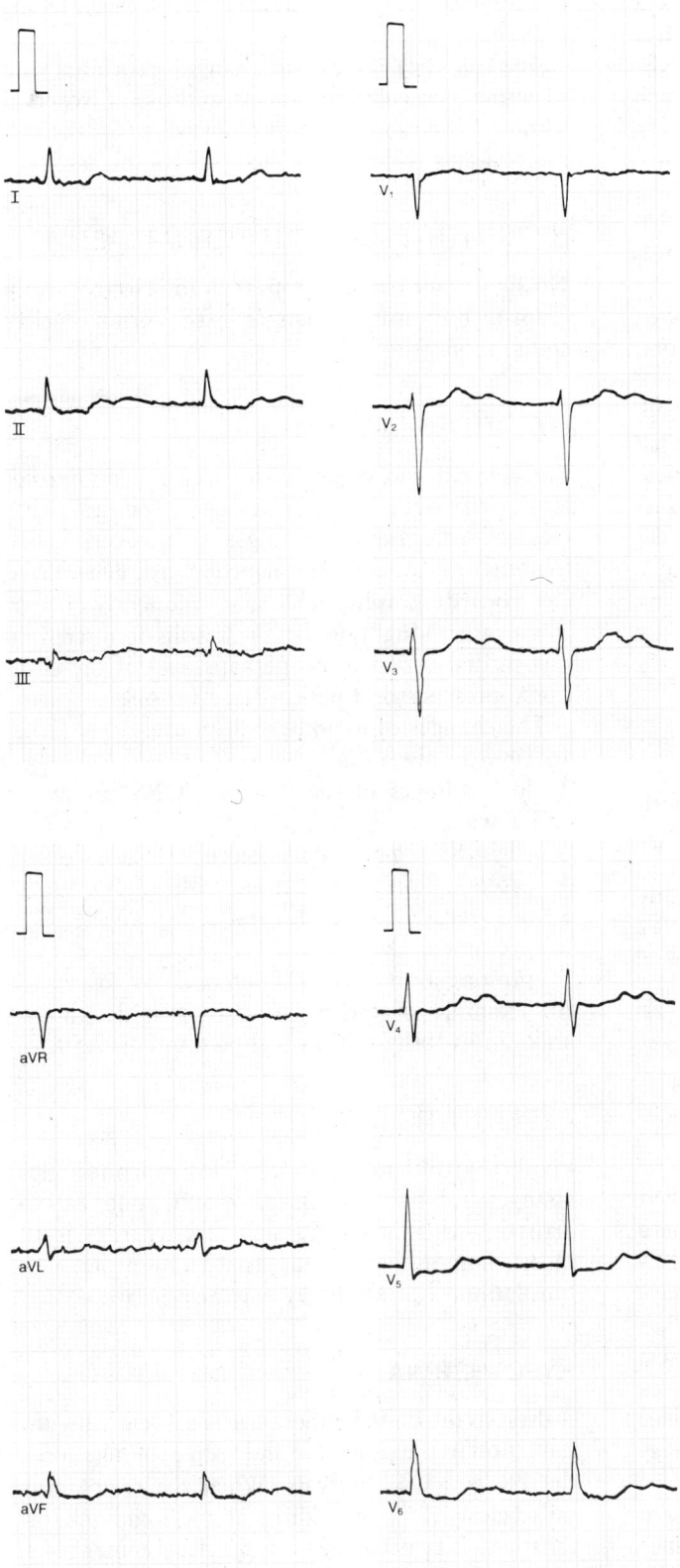

Fig. 9.49. The T waves are of low voltage, there is ST-segment depression in leads I, II, aVF and V4–V6. There are abnormally tall U waves in II, aVF and V4–V6. Although these changes are non-specific, they are powerfully suggestive of hypokalaemia.

being primarily in the duration of the ST segment itself. The degree of reduction in the QT interval is approximately proportional to the increase in the serum concentration of ionic calcium. At very high levels of serum calcium ions, this relationship breaks down because of progressive T-wave prolongation which offsets the effect of reducing ST-segment duration of the total QT interval. No appreciable changes occur in P, QRS or T morphology.

Significant cardiac arrhythmias do not often result from hypercalcaemia, but slight prolongation of the PR interval and occasionally second or third degree atrioventricular block have been described. Patients with hypercalcaemia have an increased sensitivity to digitalis; sinus arrest, sino-atrial block, atrioventricular ectopic beats, ventricular tachycardia and ventricular fibrillation have all been described in hypercalcaemia patients given digitalis. Occasional fatalities have been reported following the intravenous administration of calcium to a fully digitalized patient.

HYPOCALCAEMIA

The main electrocardiographic change in hypocalcaemia is prolongation of the QT interval due predominantly to an increase in the ST-segment duration. The T wave itself is not significantly changed. The electrocardiographic changes of hypocalcaemia appear to be of little or no clinical significance. Hypocalcaemia does not usually predispose to arrhythmias.

HYPOMAGNESAEMIA AND HYPERMAGNESAEMIA

Minor electrocardiographic changes are described in both of these electrolyte disturbances. As there are often simultaneous abnormalities of other electrolytes, their specificity is uncertain. In hypomagnesaemia, changes resembling those of hypokalaemia occur with flattening of the T waves, ST-segment depression, prominence of the U waves and occasionally prolongation of the PR interval. Like hypokalaemia and hypercalcaemia, hypomagnesaemia aggravates digitalis toxity. A variety of arrhythmias including ventricular fibrillation have been described in association with hypomagnesaemia, but it is difficult to know about the specificity of this relationship because frequently hypokalaemia is also present and many of the

patients in the recorded cases have been taking digitalis.

The electrocardiographic changes associated with hypermagnesaemia are similar to those of hyperkalaemia. There may be prolongation of the PR interval and widening of the QRS complexes.

HYPONATRAEMIA AND HYPERNATRAEMIA

No significant changes appear in the electrocardiogram in response to changes in the serum level of sodium ions.

HYPOTHYROIDISM

Biochemical and clinical evidence of hypothyroidism can occur without any recognizable electrocardiographic changes. However, when hypothyroidism is severe or prolonged, generalized electrocardiographic changes frequently occur. These are thought to be the result of interstitial myocardial oedema and perhaps also of the additional presence of a pericardial effusion.

The changes of hypothyroidism are:
1 sinus bradycardia;
2 low voltages of the P waves, QRS complexes and T waves;
3 slight ST-segment depression;
4 prolongation of the PR interval;
5 atrioventricular conduction disturbances;
6 prominent Q waves;
7 prolongation of the QT interval.
An example of the electrocardiographic appearances in hypothyroidism is shown in Fig. 9.50.

HYPERTHYROIDISM

Hyperthyroidism produces no morphological change in the electrocardiogram, but cardiac arrhythmias may occur. Sinus tachycardia is the most common finding, but atrial tachycardia, atrial fibrillation or atrial flutter may also occur.

HYPOTHERMIA

A drop in the body temperature is associated with a reduction in the sinus rate and with prolongation of the PR and QT intervals. When the temperature falls below 25°C, an additional and highly characteristic change occurs. This is the development of an extra deflection occurring at the end of the QRS complex and just overlapping the beginning of the ST segment. This deflection is called the 'J wave'. It

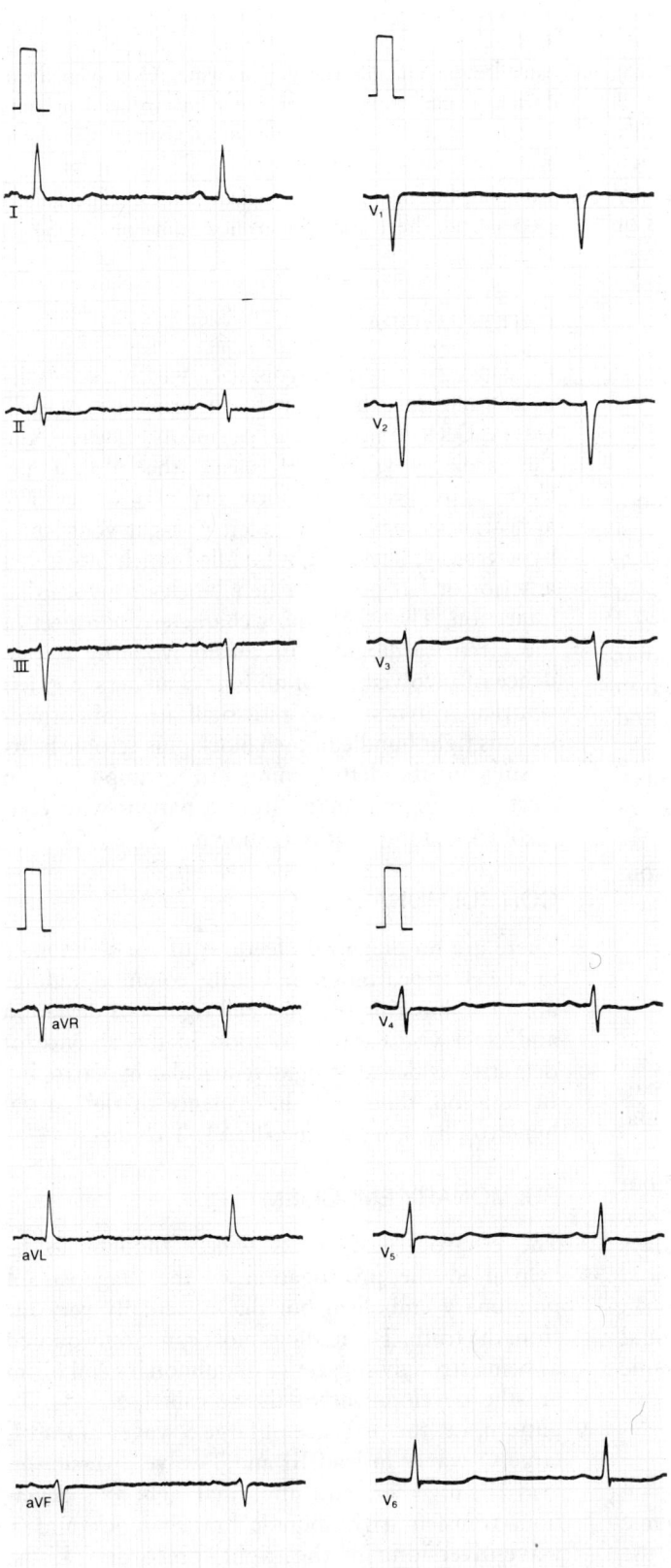

Fig. 9.50. *Hypothyroidism.* The cardiac rhythm is sinus bradycardia. The T waves are of low voltage in every lead. The P waves are of low voltage. The tallest R wave in the precordial leads is 8 mm (in V$_6$). This latter feature is an abnormality because at least one precordial R wave should exceed 8 mm in height. There is ST-segment depression in II and from V$_4$ to V$_6$. Prominent but not necessarily abnormal U waves are seen from V$_2$ to V$_6$.

is usually upright in the leads facing the left ventricle and increases in size as the temperature falls. It is often mistakenly interpreted as prolongation of the QRS duration. The broad second part of the QRS complex, which in V_1 may superficially resemble right bundle branch block, is also known as the 'camel hump sign' and it is accompanied by ST-segment depression and low-voltage T waves or T-wave inversion. Atrial fibrillation may develop. The QT interval may be prolonged. An example of hypothermia is shown in Fig. 9.51.

ELECTROCARDIOGRAPHIC CHANGES IN ACUTE DISORDERS OF THE CENTRAL NERVOUS SYSTEM

For reasons that are not adequately understood, several types of acute disturbance in the central nervous system give rise to electrocardiographic changes. Electrocardiographic changes can be seen in relation to infections or tumours in the central nervous system, following head injuries and after neurosurgery, but they are most commonly seen in association with subarachnoid haemorrhage and intracranial haemorrhage.

More than 50% of patients with subarachnoid or intracranial haemorrhage develop transient electrocardiographic changes. The most common changes in the electrocardiogram following central nervous system disease are:

1 deep T-wave inversion;
2 abnormally tall T waves;
3 prominent U waves;
4 ST-segment elevation or depression;
5 prolongation of the QT interval;
6 arrhythmias (sinus tachycardia, sinus bradycardia, nodal rhythm, atrial fibrillation and ventricular tachycardia).

The majority of the changes are non-specific but they can often be quite impressive. Records taken from the same patient within the first 8 days following admission for a proven subarachnoid haemorrhage are shown in Figs 9.52 and 9.53. In relation to Figs 9.52 and 9.53, the records could easily be misinterpreted as indicating ischaemic heart disease.

MYOCARDITIS

Transient myocarditis is very common in systemic virus infections and in acute rheumatic fever. In the majority of cases of viral myocarditis, the electrocardiogram shows non-specific flattening of the T waves, minimal ST-segment depression and the occurrence of frequent atrial or ventricular premature beats. Occasionally, abnormal Q waves simulating those found in myocardial infarction may occur. In acute rheumatic myocarditis, the commonest abnormality is prolongation of the PR interval, but second degree heart block (type I) may occur and there may be minor non-specific ST–T changes.

CARDIOMYOPATHY

In congestive cardiomyopathy, which is usually occult in origin, there may be abnormalities of the P waves, QRS complexes, ST segments, T waves and the cardiac rhythm. This means that almost any electrocardiographic abnormality may occur. The appearances may simulate left or right ventricular hypertrophy, left or right bundle branch block, left anterior or left posterior hemiblock or myocardial infarction. The single most characteristic aspect of the electrocardiogram in cardiomyopathy is evidence of involvement of all four chambers, e.g. left ventricular hypertrophy plus right atrial abnormality plus right bundle branch block plus ectopic beats arising in the left atrium. An example of an electrocardiogram taken from a patient with congestive cardiomyopathy is shown in Fig. 9.54.

COR PULMONALE

There are no diagnostic features of cor pulmonale on the electrocardiogram, but the common findings are a combination of abnormal right-axis deviation and clockwise cardiac rotation in the absence of definitive evidence of right ventricular hypertrophy. In addition, there may be evidence of right atrial hypertrophy and non-specific ST–T changes.

PULMONARY EMBOLISM

The electrocardiogram is widely thought to be helpful in the investigation of the diagnosis of pulmonary embolism but this is actually very far from the truth. The findings most commonly quoted as being strongly suggestive of pulmonary embolism are the development of the so-called, S_1, Q_3, T_3 pattern, i.e. the presence of large S waves in lead I, large Q waves in lead III and T-wave inversion in lead III, together with abnormal right-axis deviation, transient right bundle branch block and T wave-inversion in the right precordial leads. However, these appearances occur in only a minority of cases of pulmonary embolism (about 5%).

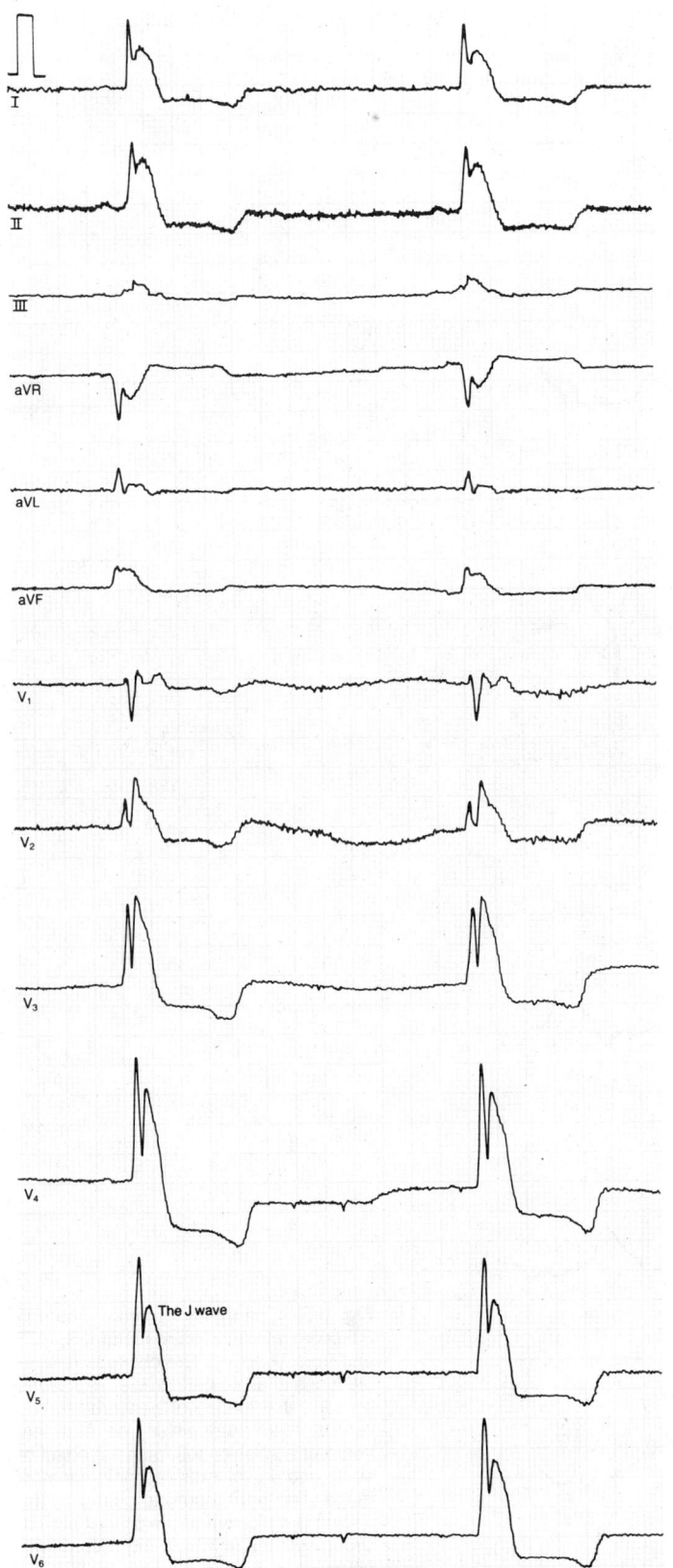

I

II

III

aVR

aVL

aVF

V₁

V₂

V₃

V₄

The J wave

V₅

V₆

Fig. 9.51. *Hypothermia.* The rhythm is sinus bradycardia. The rate is 28 per minute. The PR interval is 0.20 s. Broad slurred J waves are seen adjacent to the initial QRS deflection in all leads but they are most obvious in leads I, II and from V₄ to V₆. There is pronounced ST-segment depression and T-wave inversion.

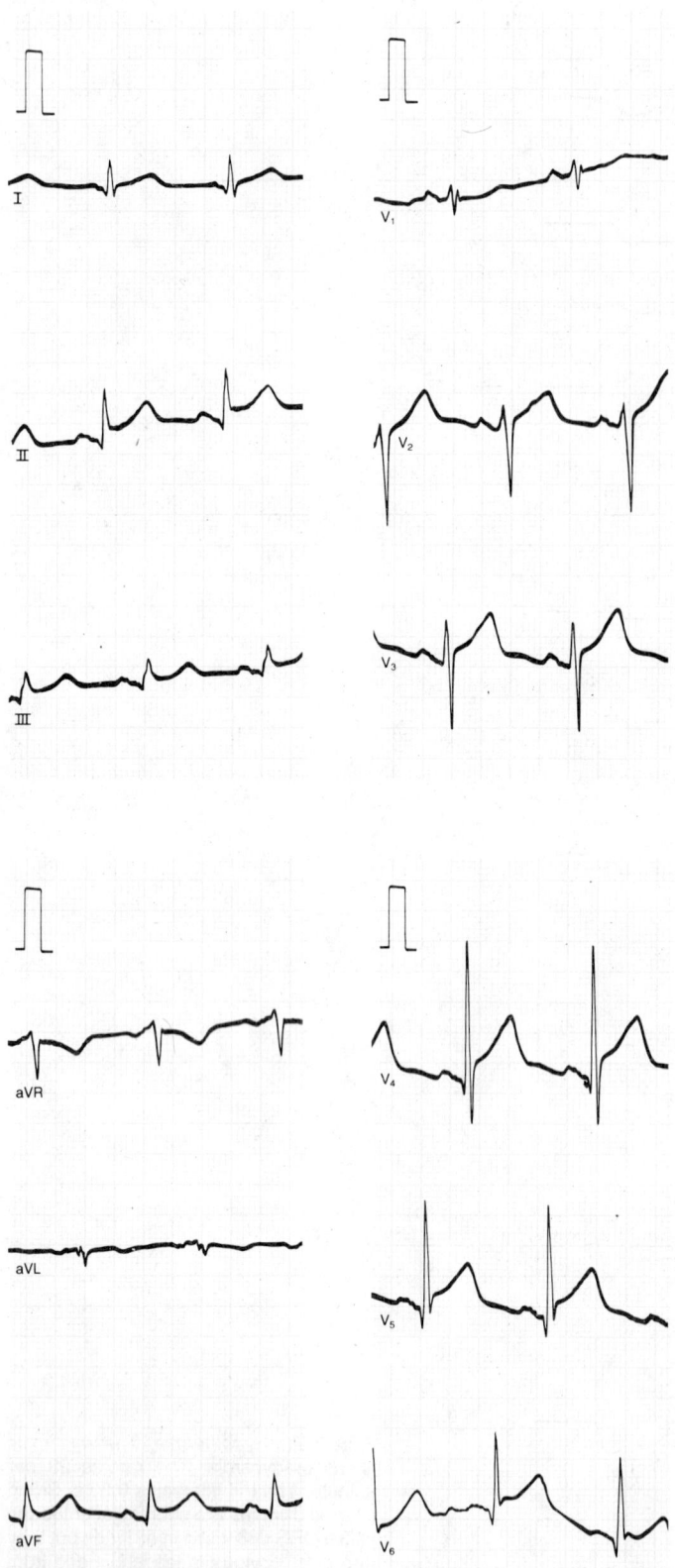

Fig. 9.52. The rhythm is sinus. There is ST-segment elevation in leads I, II, aVF and from V_2 to V_6. The changes resemble those of acute pericarditis. There was no clinical evidence of pericarditis. The record was taken within the first few hours of admission following the onset of acute and proven subarachnoid haemorrhage. The poor technical quality of the tracing is indicative of the difficult clinical circumstances in which the record was obtained.

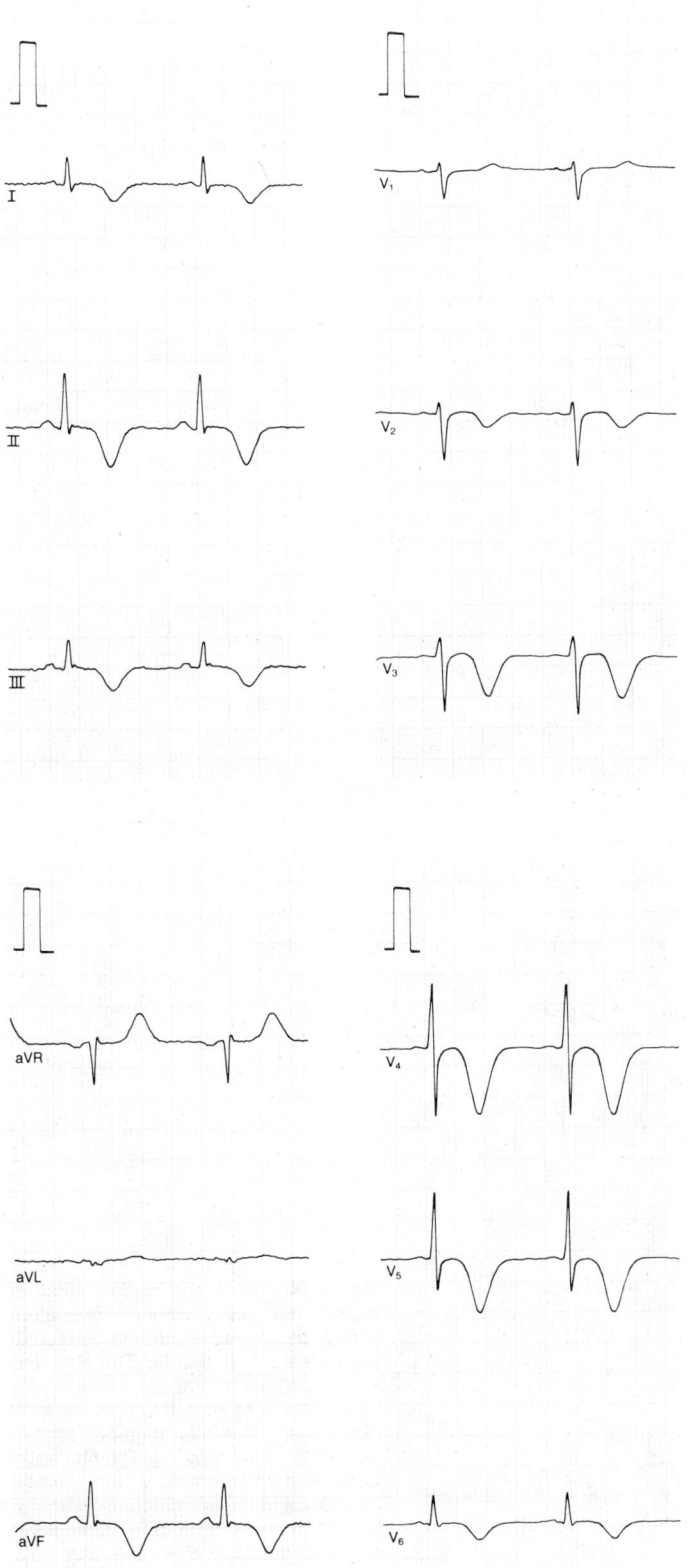

Fig. 9.53. The record is taken from the same subject as shown in Fig. 9.51, approximately 1 week later. There is deep symmetrical T-wave inversion involving all leads other than (a) cavity leads (in this case, aVR) and (b) leads positioned at right angles to the mean QRS vector (in this case, aVL).

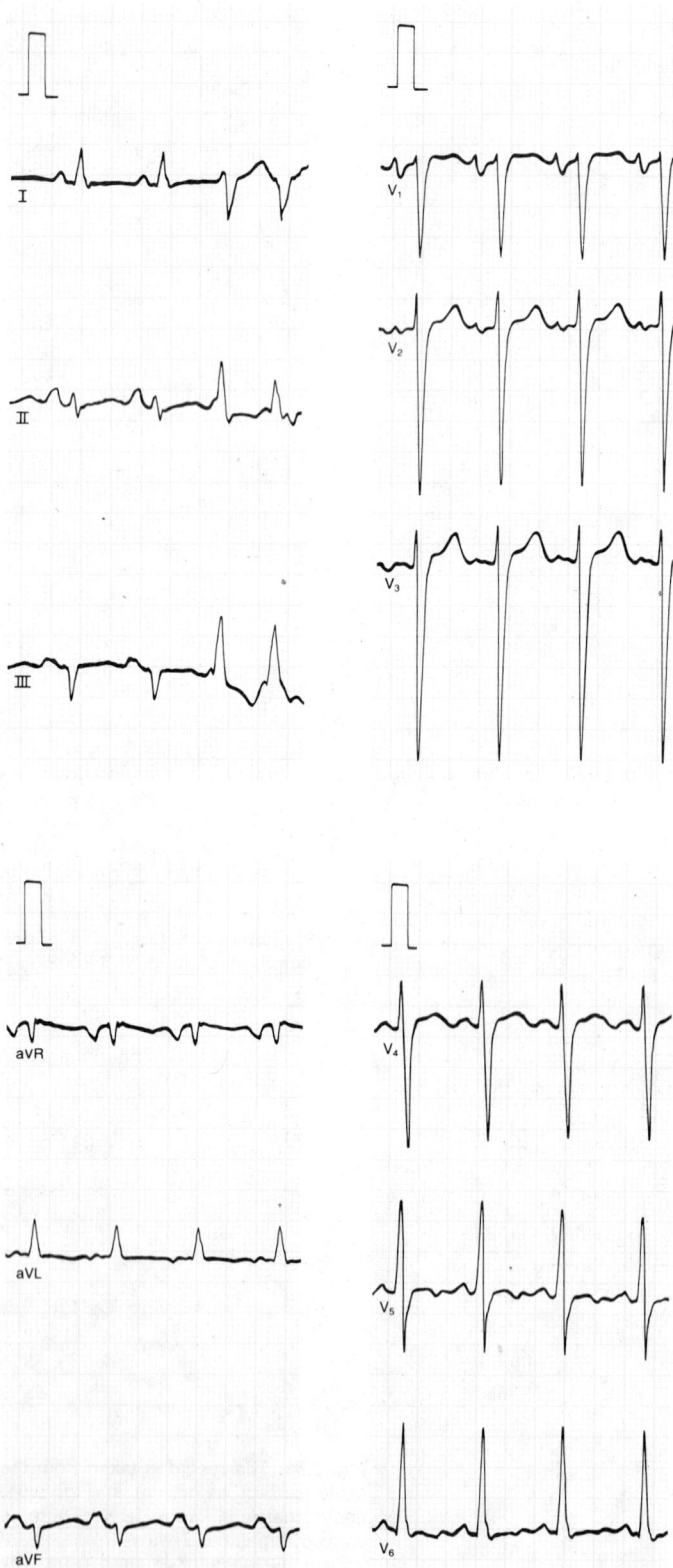

Fig. 9.54. The basic rhythm is sinus tachycardia but ventricular premature ectopic beats are seen during the recording of leads I, II and III. The P waves show evidence of right atrial abnormality (tall P waves in lead II) and of left atrial abnormality (dominant negative component to the P wave in V_1). The precordial QRS complexes satisfy the voltage criteria for left ventricular hypertrophy. There are non-specific ST–T changes in the limb leads and in the precordial leads. The mean frontal plane QRS axis is at the extreme left-hand end of the normal range at $-30°$.

Many cases of pulmonary embolism occur without any electrocardiographic changes at all and by far the most common electrocardiographic abnormality is non-specific T-wave changes which may be found in any of the precordial leads. Right-axis deviation occurs only in about 5–10% of patients with pulmonary embolism and the development of left-axis deviation is equally as common. ST–T changes of the left precordial leads are as common as those in the right precordial leads and only a minority of patients with pulmonary embolism develop atrial fibrillation or atrial tachycardia. The electrocardiogram thus contributes little or nothing to the diagnosis of pulmonary embolism.

MITRAL VALVE PROLAPSE

Mitral valve prolapse is an extremely common congenital abnormality, being present in about 10% of the female population. The electrocardiogram often shows non-specific abnormalities. The most common findings are flattening or inversion of the T waves in leads II, III and aVF. These changes are sometimes accompanied by slight ST-segment depression and they may wrongly be interpreted as evidence of inferior myocardial ischaemia. Occasionally, prominent U waves may be visible. The QT interval may be prolonged. Ventricular pre-excitation is found more commonly in subjects who have mitral valve prolapse than in those who do not. Supraventricular tachycardia, atrial fibrillation and atrial flutter may also occur.

HEREDOFAMILIAL NEUROMYOPATHIC DISORDERS

Three major hereditary and familial neuromyopathic disorders are often accompanied by electrocardiographic abnormalities: the progressive muscular dystrophies, dystrophia myotonica and Friedreich's ataxia.

Progressive muscular dystrophy

There are various different forms of progressive muscular dystrophy and any of them may show electrocardiographic changes. Many of them show sinus tachycardia, sometimes with an unusual degree of lability of the heart rate. They may also be associated with the sick sinus syndrome, atrial ectopic beats, ventricular ectopic beats, atrial flutter, atrial tachycardia, atrial fibrillation, paroxysmal ventricular tachycardia, right or left bundle branch block and various degrees of heart block. In addition, the Duchenne type of progressive muscular dystrophy frequently has an abnormal R/S ratio in V_1, i.e. the R wave is dominant in V_1. There may also be prominent Q waves in the limb leads or in the left precordial leads, and these may simulate infarction.

Dystrophia myotonica

In dystrophia myotonica, there may be a variety of cardiac arrhythmias, as listed above for progressive muscular dystrophy. The abnormal R/S ratio seen in the Duchenne type of muscular dystrophy does not seem to occur.

Friedreich's ataxia

In this condition inappropriate sinus tachycardia, arrhythmias as listed above for progressive muscular dystrophy and non-specific ST–T changes occur. Occasionally, the electrocardiogram satisfies the voltage criteria for left ventricular hypertrophy.

OBESITY

The most common electrocardiographic manifestation of obesity is a generalized reduction in the voltages of the P waves, QRS complexes and T waves. Sometimes, there is persistent sinus tachycardia.

PREGNANCY

Minor electrocardiographic changes may occur in relation to pregnancy. Sinus tachycardia is common. As pregnancy advances, there is usually a shift to the left of the mean frontal plane QRS axis (as the heart becomes physically more horizontal). Prominent Q waves may be seen in lead III, but their recognition should not be considered adequate grounds for the diagnosis of pregnancy!

DRESSLER'S SYNDROME (THE POST-MYOCARDIAL INFARCTION SYNDROME)

This is a syndrome in which pleuro-pericarditis occurs within the first 12 weeks following acute myocardial infarction. The electrocardiogram shows the typical diffuse ST-segment elevation as in pericarditis of any cause. In subsequent weeks, there may be flattening of the T waves and minor ST–T changes.

HAEMOCHROMATOSIS

In haemochromatosis, the electrocardiogram may show generalized low voltages of the QRS complexes and T waves and possibly also T-wave inversion. Ventricular and supraventricular ectopic beats and tachycardia may occur, and there may be right or left bundle branch block and first or third degree heart block.

AMYLOIDOSIS

Amyloidosis is not infrequently associated with cardiac involvement. There may be left-axis devia-

tion, left or right bundle branch block or complete heart block. A common finding is absence of the initial R wave from V_1 to V_3, simulating anteroseptal infarction.

DEXTROCARDIA

In dextrocardia, the electrocardiogram should be entirely normal apart from left–right inversion. The anatomical and electrocardiographic situations in dextrocardia are shown in Fig. 9.55. Interpretation of the electrocardiogram in case of true dextrocardia has the usual meaning only if the right and left

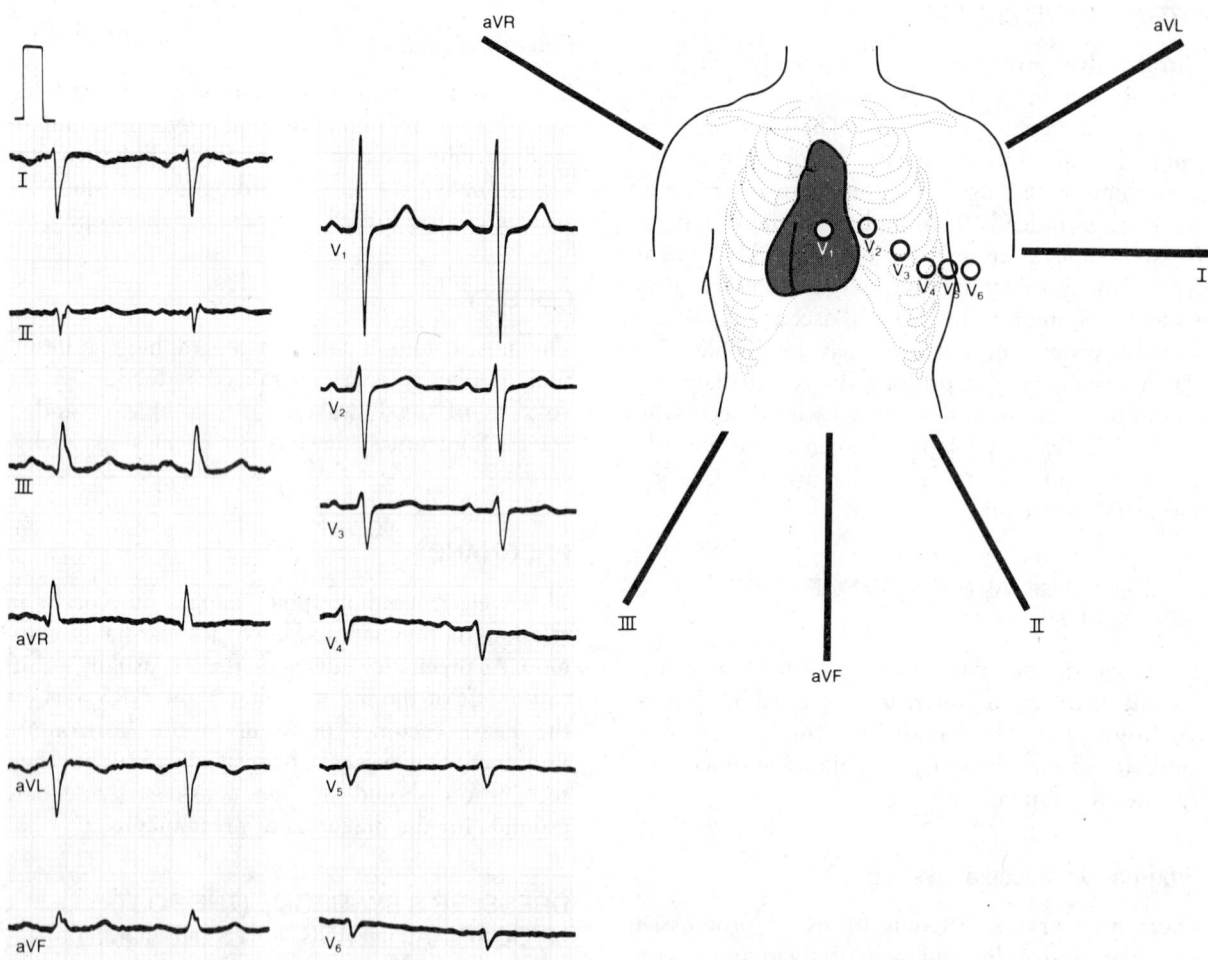

Fig. 9.55. As lead I equals +L −R, lead II equals +F −R and lead III equals +F −L, it follows that in dextrocardia lead I shows appearances similar to those normally found in lead I, but upside down, lead II shows appearances similar to those usually found in lead III and lead III shows appearances similar to those usually found in lead II. Similarly, aVR shows appearances similar to those usually found in aVL, and aVL shows appearances similar to those usually found in aVR. Lead aVF reveals the usual normal appearances. V_1–V_6 show completely abnormal appearances because they are being recorded at increasingly greater distances from the heart.

arm connections are reversed and the precordial leads are recorded on the right side of the chest instead of on the left (as in Fig. 9.56).

True dextrocardia is often associated with additional congenital abnormalities that may render the electrocardiogram abnormal.

TECHNICAL DEXTROCARDIA

This term implies the inadvertent interposition of the right and left arm connections during the recording. If the heart is actually located on the left side of the chest and the right and left arm leads are interposed, then the appearances produced in the limb leads resemble those seen in true dextrocardia whereas the appearances produced in the precordial leads are normal (assuming that the underlying electrocardiogram is normal). An example is shown in Fig. 9.57.

Interpretation of the electrocardiogram in case of true dextrocardia has the usual meaning only if the right and left arm connections are reversed and the precordial leads are recorded on the right side of the chest instead of on the left (as in Fig. 9.57). Technical dextrocardia is *much* commoner than true dextrocardia. It should be suspected whenever lead I shows inverted P and T waves and dominantly negative QRS complexes. Technical dextrocardia

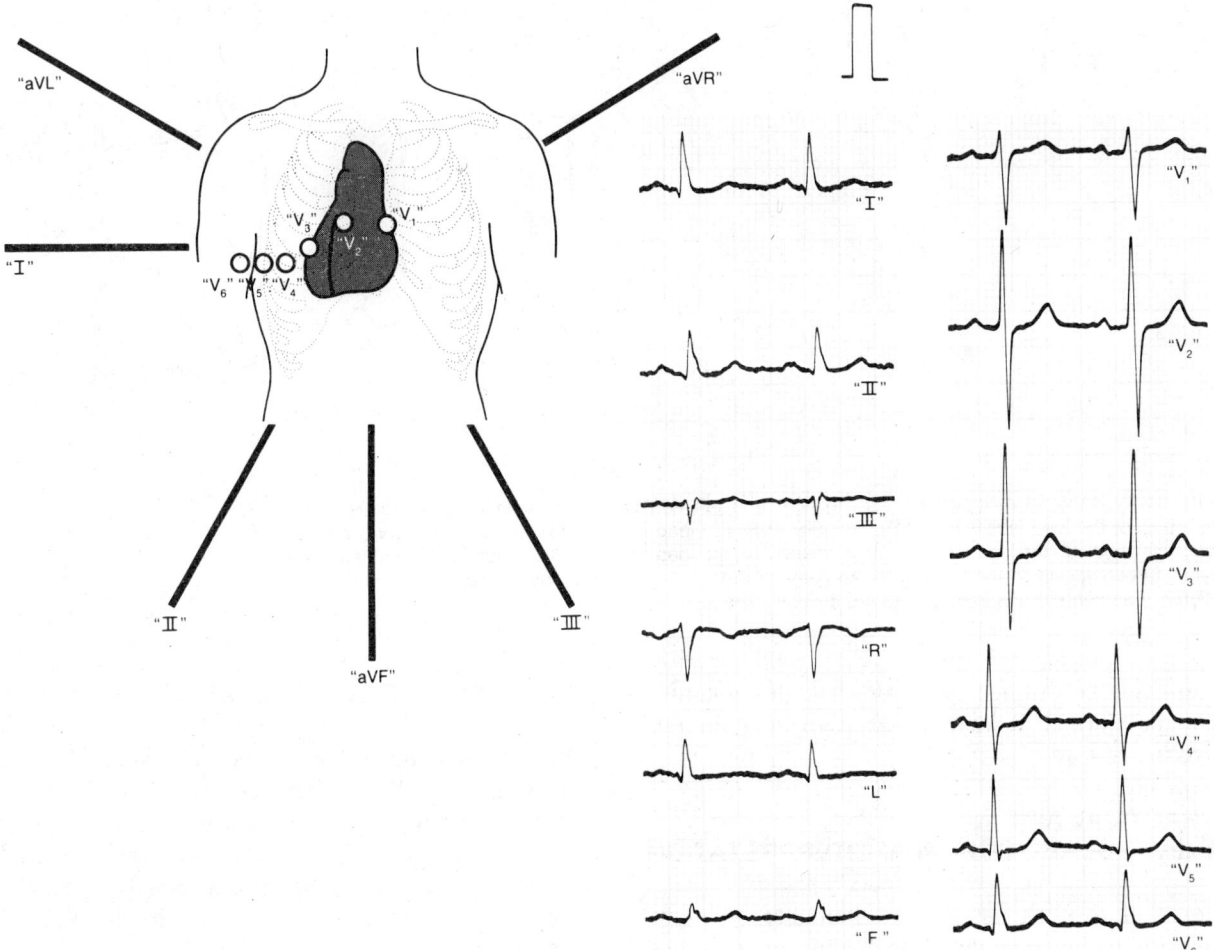

Fig. 9.56. In a patient with true dextrocardia, the electrocardiogram, recorded with the right and left arms interposed and with the precordial leads recorded from the right rather than the left side, shows appearances that allow of conventional electrocardiographic interpretation.

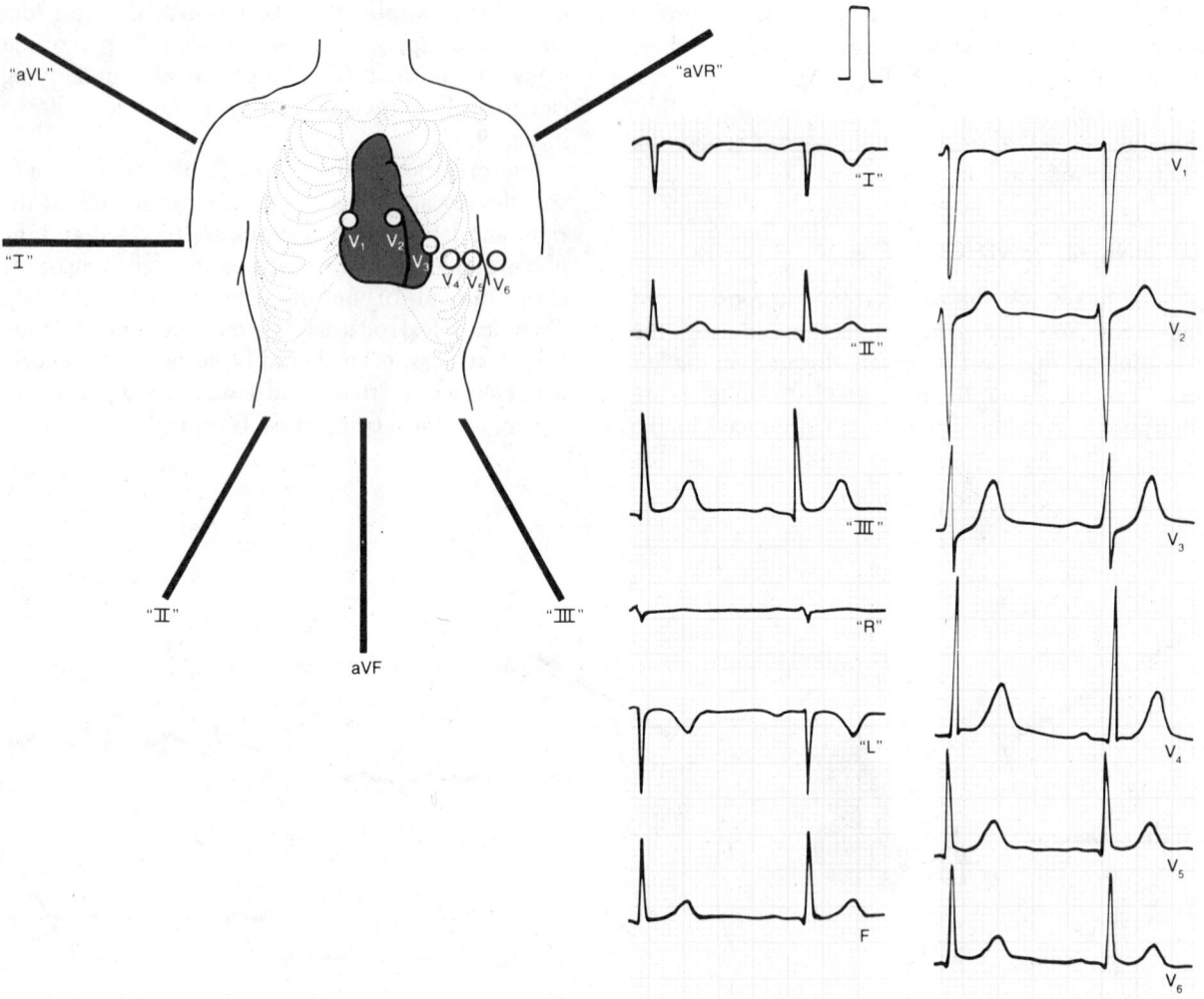

Fig. 9.57. Technical dextrocardia. As the right and left arm connections have been inadvertently interposed, the lead labelled "aVL" is actually aVR, the lead labelled "aVR" is actually aVL, aVF is correctly labelled, the lead labelled "II" is actually III, the lead labelled "III" is actually II, and lead "I", when turned upside down, shows the correct appearances. In this figure, inverted commas are used to signify lead connections that are (accidentally) incorrect.

can easily be distinguished from true dextrocardia by the normal R-wave progression seen in the precordial leads.

PRACTICAL AIDS IN ELECTROCARDIOGRAPHIC INTERPRETATION

Some of the criteria of the commoner or more important electrocardiographic abnormalities are shown in Table 9.2.

A scheme for the systemic interpretation of the electrocardiogram and the normal criteria for adults are shown in Table 9.3.

LIMITATIONS OF ELECTROCARDIOGRAPHY

The universal application of electrocardiography in the assessment of cardiac patients can easily lead to a completely mistaken view that the electrocardiogram is uniformly helpful in the diagnosis of heart disease. It must be emphasized that a normal electrocardiogram does not rule out significant organic disease and it is possible, for example, to have severe three-vessel coronary artery disease without any electrocardiographic abnormality. This simple but extremely important point is often neglected.

Table 9.2.   **Criteria for some of the commoner electrocardiographic abnormalities.**

Ventricular pre-excitation (Wolff–Parkinson–White type)	(a) PR interval of 0.11 s or less plus (b) QRS duration of 0.11 s or more plus (c) slurring of initial 0.03–0.05 s of QRS complex	In the presence of ventricular pre-excitation the normal criteria for QRS complexes, ST segments and T waves do not apply. **Take care not to make an incorrect diagnosis of left bundle branch block or myocardial infarction**
Left bundle branch block	(a) Total QRS duration of 0.12 s or more plus (b) absence of initial q wave in V_5, V_6, I and aVL plus (c) absence of secondary R wave in V_1 to indicate right bundle branch block	In the presence of left bundle branch block the normal criteria for QRS complexes, ST segments and T waves do not apply. The normal criterion for the frontal plane does apply. **Take care not to make an incorrect diagnosis of myocardial infarction or left ventricular hypertrophy**
Right bundle branch block	(a) Total QRS duration of 0.12 s or more plus (b) Secondary R wave in V_1	In the presence of right bundle branch block the normal criteria for the QRS complexes and for the frontal plane axis apply
Left anterior hemiblock	(a) Mean frontal plane QRS axis more negative than $-30°$ plus (b) absence of q-wave evidence of inferior infarction (i.e. initial r waves are visible in II and aVF)	Left anterior hemiblock and inferior infarction are the two commonest causes of left-axis deviation. The criteria for left anterior hemiblock are based on this. Other less common causes of left-axis deviation include ventricular pre-excitation, hyperkalaemia, tricuspid atresia, ostium primum atrial septal defect and artificial cardiac pacing
Left ventricular hypertrophy	One or more of:– (a) R in V_4, V_5 or V_6 exceeds 27 mm (b) S in V_1, V_2 or V_3 exceeds 30 mm (c) R in V_4, V_5 or V_6 plus S in V_1, V_2 or V_3 exceeds 40 mm (d) R in aVL exceeds 13 mm (e) R in aVF exceeds 20 mm (f) ventricular activation time exceeds 0.04 s (g) ST-segment depression, T-wave flattening, T-wave invasion in leads facing left ventricle	The reliability of the electrocardiographic diagnosis of left ventricular hypertrophy is directly related to the number of criteria fulfilled. Abnormal left axis deviation is not an expected finding in left ventricular hypertrophy
Right ventricular hypertrophy	(a) Dominant R in V_1 (i.e. R, Rs, RR′, qR or qRS) plus (b) frontal plane axis more positive than $+90°$	Dominant R in V_1 can occur in true posterior infarction, ventricular pre-excitation and Duchenne-type muscular dystrophy
Left atrial 'hypertrophy' (strictly 'abnormality')	(a) P duration longer than 0.12 s or P wave bifid in I, II, aVF and aVL or (b) P wave in V_1 has negative component with area greater than that of positive component	
Right atrial 'hypertrophy' (strictly 'abnormality')	(a) P-wave height 3.0 mm or more in II, III or aVF	
Myocardial infarction	(a) q waves 0.04 s or more in duration (excluding always leads aVR and III, and, when the frontal plane QRS axis $+75°$ or more positive, excluding also aVL). or (b) q waves more than ¼ the height of the ensuing R wave (excluding always leads aVR and III and, when the frontal plane QRS axis is $+75°$ or more positive, excluding also aVL).	The concomitant presence of significant ST-segment elevation suggests that the infarct is no more than days old. If the ST segments are normal but there is still T-wave inversion, it suggests that the infarct is not more than several weeks old. **It is always difficult, often impossible, and sometimes dangerous to diagnose infarction in the presence of left bundle branch block or ventricular pre-excitation**

Table 9.2. Continued.   **Criteria for some of the commoner electrocardiographic abnormalities.**

	or (c) qs or QS complexes (excluding always leads aVR and III and, when the frontal plane QRS axis is +75° or more positive excluding also aVL). or (d) Inappropriately low R-wave voltage in local area (when the facts can confidently be ascertained) NB The above 'diagnostic criteria' for myocardial infarction can occasionally be fulfilled in certain particular conditions which gives rise to 'pseudo-infarction' patterns. The most likely such condition is cardiomyopathy. The diagnosis of myocardial infarction is extremely unlikely to be incorrect if the full *sequence* of changes (ST-segment elevation, QRS changes, T-wave changes and restoration of normality to the ST segments) is seen	
Conditions in which 'normal' criteria do not apply	**In the presence of supraventricular arrhythmias, the normal criteria for P waves do not apply** In supraventricular arrhythmias, atrial depolarization begins from an abnormal site. The normal pathway for atrial myocardial depolarization cannot therefore be followed and the P waves are, in consequence, abnormal. Assuming there is normal intraventricular conduction, the normal criteria for QRS complexes, ST segments and T waves continue to apply	**In the presence of ventricular arrhythmias or of ventricular pre-excitation, the normal criteria for the QRS complexes do not apply** In ventricular arrhythmias, ventricular depolarization begins from an abnormal site and the normal pathway for ventricular myocardial depolarization cannot be followed. In consequence, the QRS complexes are abnormal. The ST segments and T waves are usually also abnormal in this situation for primary depolarization (QRS) abnormalities often result in secondary repolarization (ST segments and T wave) abnormalities.

Table 9.3.   **Systematic interpretation of the electrocardiogram and normal criteria for adults.**

1A	Determine cardiac rhythm	Criteria for normality of P waves only apply if rhythm is of sinus origin. Criteria for normality of QRS complexes, ST segments and T waves only apply if rhythm is of supraventricular origin
1B	Check PR interval	If 0.11 s or less, consider pre-excitation. If pre-excitation is present (defined by PR interval 0.11 s or less, plus total QRS duration 0.11 s or more, plus slurring of initial 0.03–0.05 s of QRS complex), normal criteria for QRS complexes, ST segments and T waves do not apply
2	Assess QRS morphology in precordial leads	(a) V_1 should have rS;

rS

V_6 should have qR but may have R, Rs or qRs.

qR   R   Rs   qRs

Table 9.3. Continued: **Systematic interpretation of the electrocardiogram and normal criteria for adults.**

	(In the presence of clockwise rotation, there may be no initial q in V_6 but a normal initial q may be seen in leads farther to left, i.e. I and aVL.) (b) r wave should progressively increase in size from V_1 to V_6. However, it is quite normal for the R wave in V_6 to be smaller than that in V_5 and it is also normal for the R wave in V_5 to be less than that in V_4 provided the R wave in V_6 is also less than that in V_5 (compare Figure 42). (c) Transition (from right ventricular to left ventricular complexes) zone in precordial leads marked either by change from initial r to initial q (e.g. V_3–V_4 below) or by development of dominant R wave (V_3 below)
	 V_1 V_2 V_3 V_4 V_5 V_6
3 Check QRS dimensions in precordial leads	(a) Total QRS duration should not exceed 0.10 s (2½ small squares). If QRS duration is 0.12 s or more and there is no initial q wave in V_6, I and aVL, and there is no secondary R wave in V_1 (and assuming the rhythm is supraventricular), there is left bundle branch block. In this situation, the normal criteria for the QRS complexes, ST segments and T waves do not apply. (b) At least one R wave should exceed 8 mm. (c) The tallest R wave should not exceed 27 mm (d) The deepest S wave should not exceed 30 mm (e) The sum of the tallest R and deepest S should not exceed 40 mm (f) The ventricular activation time should not exceed 0.04 s (g) Any q wave seen should not have a depth exceeding ¼ of the height of the ensuing R wave (h) Any q waves seen should not equal or exceed 0.04 s in duration
4A Assess precordial T waves	(a) The T wave in V_1 may be upright, flat or inverted. If upright in earlier records, it must be still upright (b) The T wave in V_2 may be upright, flat or inverted. If upright in earlier records of if upright in V_1, it must be upright (c) The T wave in V_3–V_5 must be upright. **In general**, the T wave should be more than ⅛ but less than ⅔ of the R wave height
4B Assess the U waves	The normal U wave is upright in all leads in which the T wave is upright. It should also be upright in the right precordial leads, even if the T waves are inverted here. Its average amplitude is < 0.5 mm. It tends to be largest in V_2 and V_3 where it may occasionally reach 2 mm in height. In general, it is less than 25% of the height of the preceding T wave. It is definitely abnormal when it is taller than the preceding T wave. Some authorities regard U waves taller than 1.5 mm as abnormal. U-wave inversion is abnormal

Table 9.3. Continued. Systematic interpretation of the electrocardiogram and normal criteria for adults.

5 Assess precordial ST segments	The ST segments must not deviate from the iso-electric line by more than ±1 mm. Note that this should not be rigidly applied in V_1 and V_2. Caution should also be exercised in the presence of a tachycardia which may render assessment of the iso-electric position difficult or impossible.
6 Assess QRS complexes in limb leads	(a) A q wave in aVL*, I, II or aVF should not equal or exceed 0.04 sec in duration (b) A q wave in aVL*, I, II or aVF should not have a depth greater than ¼ of the height of the ensuring R wave NB *q waves exceeding this criterion are acceptable in aVL if the frontal plane axis is more positive than +60° (i.e. +75° or more) (c) The R wave in aVL should not exceed 13 mm and that in aVF should not exceed 20 mm (d) The frontal plane axis should not lie outside the range −30° to +90°
7A Assess T waves in limb leads	(a) The mean frontal plane T-wave axis should not differ from the frontal plane QRS axis by more than ±45° (b) In the presence of abnormal q waves in II, III, and aVF, T-wave inversion in these leads is abnormal even if the above criterion is not fulfilled
7B Assess the U waves	The U waves should be upright where the T waves are upright. The criterion for U wave size is as given in 4B above
8 Assess ST segment in limb leads	These should not deviate by more than 1 mm above or below iso-electric line (see precautions under **5** above)
9 Assess P waves	(a) The P waves should not exceed 0.12 s in duration in II (b) The P waves should not exceed 2.5 mm in height in II (c) Any negative component to the P wave in V_1 should not have a greater area than the positive component
10 *Measure of QT interval	Make sure not to include a U wave. The number of 0.04 s intervals (i.e. small squares on the ECG graticule) between consecutive R waves should be counted and the normality or otherwise of the measured QT interval in relation to the observed RR interval determined. NB *Measurement of QT interval is difficult to make and is often unrewarding. An important exception is the patient with congenital Q-T prolongation. Abnormalities of QT duration are often discovered in retrospect when the primary abnormality (e.g. hypocalcaemia) is already apparent

ACKNOWLEDGEMENTS

All the illustrations in this chapter are reproduced, with permission from Rowlands, D.J. *Understanding the electrocardiogram*, Sections I–II, Gower Medical Publishers. The author acknowledges, with thanks, the help and generous co-operation of ICI PLC Pharmaceuticals Division in producing these illustrations.

FURTHER READING

Alboni, P. *Intraventricular Conduction Disturbances*. Martinus Nijhoff, 1981.

Armstrong, M.L. *Electrocardiograms*. Bristol: John Wright, I. 1985.

Barker, J.M. *The Unipolar Electrocardiogram*. Appleton-Century-Crofts, 1952.

Campbell, R.W.F. and Murray, A. *Dynamic Electrocardiography*. Churchill Livingstone, 1985.

Chou, T.-C. *Electrocardiography in Clinical Practice*, 2nd edn. Grune and Stratton, 1986.

Chung, E.K. *Electrocardiography: practical applications with vectorial principles*, 2nd edn. Harper and Row, 1980.

Constant, J. *Learning Electrocardiography*. Little, Brown and Co., 1981.

Conway, N. *An Atlas of Cardiology*. London: Wolffe Medical Publications, 1977.

Criteria Committee of the New York Heart Assocaition. *Nomenclature and Criteria for Diagnosis of Disease of the Heart and Great Vessels*. New York: Little, Brown and Co., 1973.

Marriott, H.J.L. *Practical Electrocardiography*, 7th edn. Baltimore: Williams and Wilkins, 1983.

Prineas, R.J. and Crow, R.S. *The Minnesota Code Manual of Electrocardiographic Findings*. John Wright, 1982.

Rowlands, D.J. *Understanding the Electrocardiogram, Section 1: The normal ECG*. London: Gower Medical Publishers, 1980.

Rowlands, D.J. *Understanding the Electrocardiogram, Section 2: Morphological Abnormalities*. London: Gower Medical Publishers, 1982.

Rowlands, D.J. *Understanding the Electrocardiogram, Section 3: Rhythm Abnormalities*. London: Gower Medical Publishers.

Schamroth, L. *The Electrocardiology of Coronary Artery Disease*, 2nd edn. Oxford: Blackwell Scientific Publications, 1984.

Summerall, C.P. III *EKG Interpretation*. Wiley Medical, 1982.

Wellens, H.J.J. and Kulbertus, H.E. *What's New in Electrocardiography*. Martinus Nijhoff, 1981.

Chapter 10

Ambulatory Monitoring of the Electrocardiogram

David E. Ward

The standard electrocardiogram (ECG) is recorded with the patient resting quietly, and a completed recording contains between 20 and 100 cycles in discontinuous strips. By its very nature, this type of ECG cannot provide much information about variations in the rhythm of the heart and is of very limited application in this area of cardiovascular investigation. The invention of real-time radio-telemetry[1] was an important step in the development of our understanding of arrhythmias in the hospitalized patient, but it was only with the perfection of ambulatory tape recording devices[2] that information about spontaneous arrhythmias during everyday life became available. The technique has become widely known as Holter monitoring, after its developer. It is preferable to use the following terms: ambulatory monitoring, long-term ECG monitoring and dynamic electrocardiography.

PRINCIPLES OF AMBULATORY MONITORING

Ambulatory tape recording is useful in a variety of circumstances (Table 10.1). In referring a patient for investigation of a particular symptom (for example, dizziness), it is hoped that such an episode will occur during the recording and will be accompanied by a change in heart rhythm appropriate to the severity of the symptom. Thus, if a patient being studied for the cause of recurrent black-outs has a syncopal episode accompanied by a period of asystole, such a recording would be judged as fully diagnostic and therefore clinically useful. Similarly, a recording showing no change in rhythm in a patient with recurrent palpitations will allow the physician to conclude that arrhythmias are not the cause of the symptoms. In analysing a continuous recording, therefore, it is necessary to establish the relationship between the symptom under investigation, spontaneous symptoms during the recording and rhythm changes.[3] With intermittent recording

techniques, the timing of the recordings is determined by fixed intervals, by the patient (when experiencing symptoms) or by automatic arrhythmia detection. At the time patients are fitted with a device and instructed in its use, they should be given a diary. It is imperative that patients should understand how important the diary is as a part of the investigation. For various reasons, some patients will not be able to complete the diary, thus limiting the value of the recording.

To some extent, the nature of the clinical problem determines the type of monitoring technique used. If the patient has symptoms very infrequently (for example, once a month), a single 24-hour recording cannot be expected to document an attack. In this case, the value of a single continuous tape recording might be to document electrocardiographic clues (for example, frequent ventricular premature beats in a patient with syncope due to ventricular tachycardia) or more frequent associated symptoms (for example, dizziness in a patient with infrequent syncope). Patient-activated recorders are of value only if patients can activate them at the appropriate moment. Thus, such a device is unsuitable for the investigation of disabling symptoms such as syncope.

Table 10.1. **Applications of ambulatory monitoring.**

1. Investigation of symptoms possibly referable to transient arrhythmias (syncope, breathlessness, etc.)
2. Establishment of an electrocardiographic diagnosis
3. Evaluation of anti-arrhythmic treatment (drugs, surgery, pacemaker function, etc.)
4. Evaluation of potential risk (after myocardial infarction)
5. Investigation of spontaneous myocardial ischaemia (pre-excitation syndromes, etc.)
6. Research studies

TECHNIQUES

CONTINUOUS TAPE RECORDING

The most commonly used method is that of continuous tape recording using a small portable cassette recorder. Cassettes of the C120 type are most often used. Modern machines allow continuous recording for 24–36 h. Recordings are either direct (amplitude modulated) or frequency modulated.[4] The frequency response of the recorders is generally 0.05–100 Hz. The upper band-pass of 0.05 Hz is designed to reduce the low-frequency interference caused by movement and low-frequency artefact. Frequency-modulated recordings reduce noise. In this as in all other systems, care should be taken to clean the skin and apply the electrodes correctly.

A single C120 cassette can be analysed in less than 30 min (60 times real time). Reel-to-reel recorders were in common use 10 years ago but they are no longer widely used. These systems allow faster analysis times because the tapes are more resilient.

Most systems provide at least two ECG channels. A time-signal channel is incorporated into most devices and this channel is often combined with a patient-activation signal generated by a push-button switch.

Data extracted from the recording can be presented in various ways.[5] The ECG can be presented as short strips containing automatically detected events or as a compressed full-disclosure of the entire recording period or selected parts (Fig. 10.1). Most analysers provide statistical data, such as total number of QRS complexes, number of wide QRS complexes, graphical trends (Fig. 10.2), histograms, etc. These facilities are useful for the assessment of drug effects.

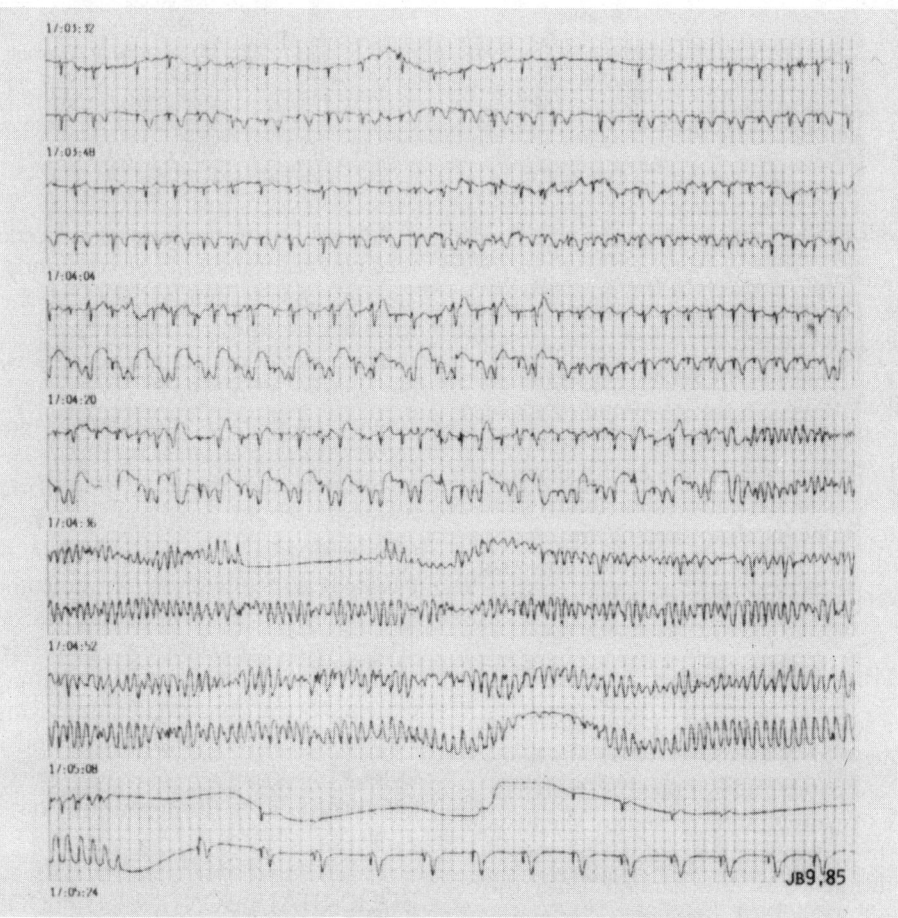

Fig. 10.1. Compressed display of the heart rhythm of an 8-year-old boy with recurrent syncope. After many recordings, this one finally and dramatically revealed the occurrence of ventricular fibrillation. During the minutes immediately preceding the syncopal event, there is a marked increase in the frequency of ventricular premature beats and at 4 min 20 s after 17 00 hours fibrillation is precipitated. Spontaneous termination occurred at 17:05:08 and was followed by bradycardia.

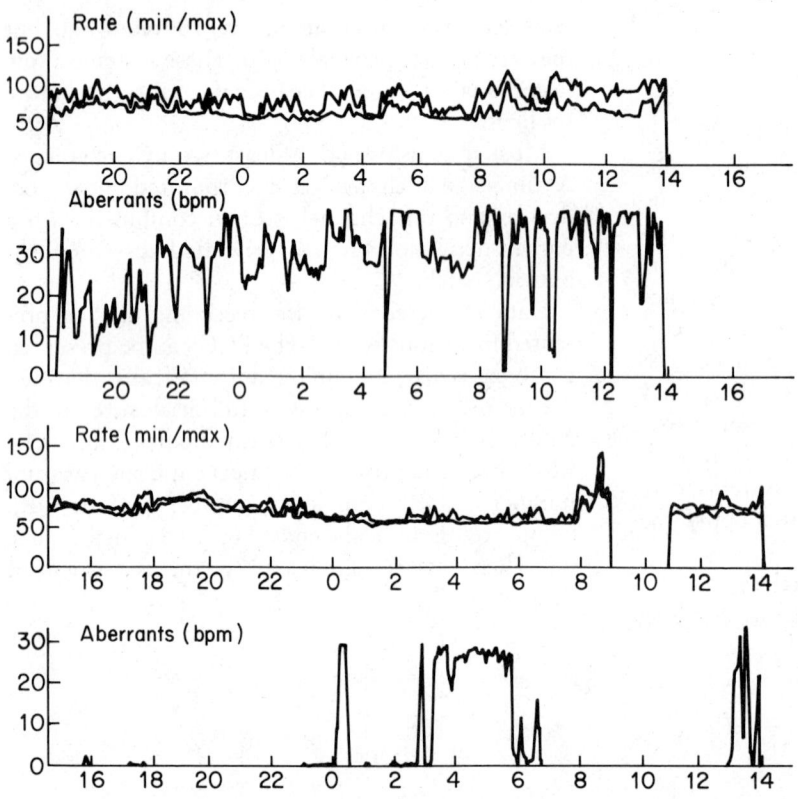

Fig. 10.2. Graphical representation (Reynolds Medical) of the maximum and minimum heart rates and the frequency of ventricular premature beats before (upper trace) and after (lower trace) treatment with sotalol. (The beginnings of the recordings were made at different times of day.)

EVENT RECORDERS

In this system, a tape recorder is activated by the patient when aware of symptoms or at any other time it is considered appropriate.[6] A major disadvantage of any intermittent recording device is that it is less likely to record the onset and offset of an event, especially if it is short-lived. The recording period is about 20–30 s and there is a built-in delay in some devices. This increases the chances of recording events immediately preceding the symptomatic arrhythmia and provides time for the patient to find and activate the push-button switch.

SOLID-STATE PORTABLE MEMORY DEVICE

More recently, solid-state devices have taken the place of the older type of recorder. These machines are carried by the patient and applied to the chest wall at the time of symptomatic episodes. The ECG is stored and can be transmitted down a telephone line at the convenience of the patient. Until the memory function was added, these portable monitors were difficult to use. It is not difficult to imagine the frustration of an unwell patient struggling with the device and desperately hoping to find a functioning telephone. For obvious reasons, a

dedicated line to the receiver is needed. Ideally, the receiving station should be constantly attended or in an area that is manned around the clock (e.g. a cardiac care unit).

These recorders are not easy to use especially by the elderly and infirmed. They are useless if patients cannot use them at the required moment. Patient-activated event monitoring systems provide little or no information about asymptomatic arrhythmias. Antman *et al.*[7] reported the results of transtelephonic ECG transmissions from 61 patients (51 patients with previously documented arrhythmias and 10 with infrequent symptoms suggestive of an arrhythmia). A clinically significant event was recorded in 11% of 650 transmissions. All 10 patients being investigated for symptoms had at least one positive transmission, and in 37% of the other 51 an event was detected. The number of calls per event in each group is, however, not stated.

SOLID-STATE CONTINUOUS LOOP RECORDERS

Technological advances have allowed the development of recorders with solid-state memories (see above). A recent development of this technology is the so-called SLOOP (solid state memory loop) developed by Davies in the early 1980s.[8] At any time 80 s of ECG are available for storage. The recording is stored in the memory if the patient activates the memory by pressing a button. The device is designed such that the 70 s prior to activation is stored together with 10 s following activation. In this way, electrocardiographic events immediately prior to and after patient-activation are available for inspection. In the currently available device, the length of the recording can be varied from one period of 160 s to 8 periods of 20 s. When the recorder is returned, it may be connected to a conventional electrocardiograph and the stored data are presented in the form of rhythm strips (Figs 10.3 and 10.4). This device can be used for long periods and is especially useful in the investigation of patients with infrequent symptoms. Brown et al.[8] detected 'clinically useful' information in 68% of patients. The lack of automatic recognition of asymptomatic or disabling arrhythmias (prohibiting patient-activation) is a disadvantage of this and other intermittent recording systems. Furthermore, long-term electrode contact is not reliable and patients must be taught to re-apply the electrodes at intervals or have to return to the clinic.

REAL-TIME ANALYSERS

The most recent development in ambulatory monitoring is the use of microprocessor-based devices which record and analyse the ECG.[9] Memory (usually solid state) storage limitations have so far prevented true full-disclosure of the 24-hour period and continuously monitored data are excerpted for storage according to predetermined software-encoded criteria (for example, wide complexes, runs of tachycardia, etc.). Some devices contain algorithms to prevent saturation of the memory with repeated similar sequences. One method of increasing storage capacity cuts out the iso-electric baseline and stores only the QRS complexes. The ECG is then reconstituted by the report-generating computer. Data is retrieved by plugging the recorder into a microcomputer which generates the report. Most devices have event markers. Clearly, the data collected is biased by the form of the detection algorithm and its reliability. The potential for automatic activation during disabling arrhythmias is an advantage over simpler patient-activated devices. At present, the precise application of this form of intermittent arrhythmia sampling is not clear and the technique must still be regarded as experimental.

IMPLANTED MONITORS

As yet, a purpose-built totally implantable monitoring device without stimulating facilities (Camm J., personal communication) is not available. However, some modern pacemakers have an inbuilt memory for recording events such as long pauses, tachycardias, number of paced events, etc. Thus, the utility of an implanted stimulating device may be

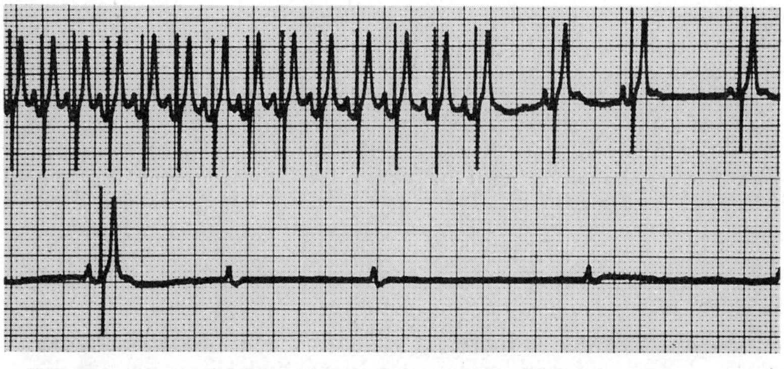

Fig. 10.3. Recordings from the SLOOP device. This 35-year-old patient had had occasional syncopal spells and despite numerous continuous 24-hour recordings no abnormality had been demonstrated. On this occasion, the patient was able to activate the device and the memory loop was activated showing the heart rhythm during a dizzy spell terminating in syncope. The recording shows sudden slowing of stable sinus rhythm with the emergence of complete atrioventricular block. The diagnosis was malignant vasovagal syncope. (Paper speed 10 mm/s.)

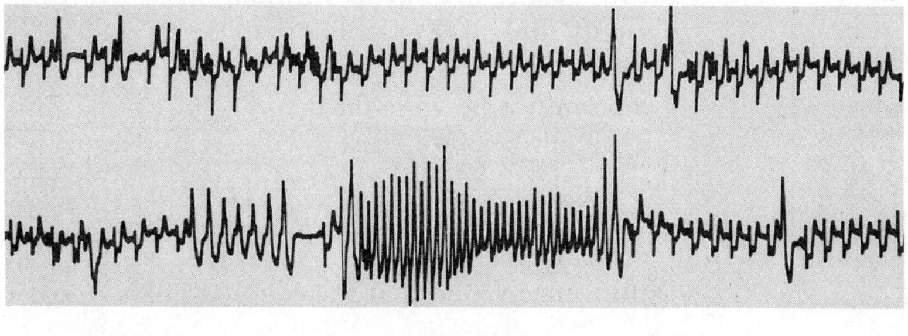

Fig. 10.4. Recordings from a 65-year-old man with recurrent dizzy spells and palpitations. Continuous recordings had shown only ventricular ectopic beats but no tachycardias. On this occasion, he had a brief episode of ventricular tachycardia causing dizziness and he activated the SLOOP. (Paper speed 100 mm/s.)

assessed in certain circumstances of bradycardia by storing the number of times stimulation was needed to terminate pauses of a certain duration[10] or terminate tachycardia in the case of tachycardia-terminating pacemakers.[11]

THE NORMAL AMBULATORY ELECTROCARDIOGRAM

Normal heart rates vary throughout the day. The highest rates occur in the morning after waking, and fall gradually throughout the day, falling more suddenly during sleep.[12] The range of rates varies with age as shown in Table 10.2.

Rates are on average about 5–10 beats/min faster in females than in males.[12] As the data in Table 10.2 indicates, the average minimum heart rates remain more or less unchanged with increasing age whereas upper heart rates decline. Heart-rate variability also decreases with age.[13]

The first important survey of the heart rhythm in normal individuals was reported by Hinkle et al. in 1969.[14] The results of this investigation of 301 normal telephone company employees challenged the view that in most healthy adults sinus rhythm is the single rhythm throughout the day. Ventricular ectopic activity was detected in 62% of subjects. Nineteen per cent of the total had between 1 and 10 ventricular premature beats per 1000 beats. Atrial premature beats were detected in 63%. So-called defects of conduction were detected in 7%. Similar findings have been reported by more recent studies.[12,15] Frequent or complex ventricular ectopic activity was further studied by Kennedy and Underhill.[16] In 25 healthy subjects with these findings on a resting ECG, ambulatory monitoring revealed a mean of 559 premature beats per hour and complex forms were present in all subjects. Montague et al. reported similar findings.[17] The natural history of ventricular ectopic activity in people apparently without heart disease is not known. There is no evidence that treatment mod-

ifies prognosis. Indeed, Kennedy and Underhill found that treatment was usually without effect.[16]

The prevalence of ventricular ectopic activity increases with age. Camm et al. detected it in 69% of subjects older than 75 years.[13] A higher prevalence of 80% was reported by Fleg and Kennedy.[18] High degrees of atrioventricular block and profound sinus bradycardia are unusual in the elderly but are not infrequent in younger healthier subjects. Brodsky et al. detected profound sinus bradycardia in 24% of male medical students and type I second degree atrioventricular block in 6%.[15] Junctional escapes were noted in 22%, presumably a reflection of the higher incidence of slow rates and brisker junctional escape mechanisms in this group. In 104 younger subjects between the ages of 7 and 11 years reported by Southall et al., 46% had junctional escapes at the slower rates.[19] Atrial premature beats were seen in 19% and ventricular premature beats in less than 1%. The results of this study also demonstrated that sinus pauses of up to 1.8 s must be regarded as normal in this age-group.

INVESTIGATION OF SYMPTOMS

The most important application of ambulatory monitoring is in the investigation of symptoms suspected to be of cardiac origin. The most common indications for monitoring are:

1 transient neurological symptoms, such as dizziness, faints, syncope, etc. (39%);
2 palpitations (19%);
3 assessment of treatment (including drugs, pacemakers, surgery etc.) (25%);
4 investigation of chest pain (7%);
5 other reasons (10%).[3]

The utility of ambulatory monitoring for the investigation of cardiac symptoms has not been widely studied. Ward et al. reported significant arrhythmias correlating with symptoms in 7.5% of a diverse group of 531 recordings.[3] Furthermore, many patients had symptoms other than that for which they were being investigated (21%) (e.g., breathlessness in patients with dizziness). Of these, about half had ECG abnormalities which were correlated with the 'other' symptoms. The indicated symptom was noted in the diary of 17% of patients but in only 76% of these was there an electrocardiographic abnormality at the time. Syncope during the recording occurred in only 3%, but this symptom was the reason for the test in 34%. Unfortunately, the diary was not available or the

Table 10.2. **Ranges of heart rates (beats/min) with age.**

Age	Heart rate		Reference
	Minimum	Maximum	
0–10 days	93 ± 12	175 ± 19	Southall et al.[98]
7–11 years	56 ± 6	164 ± 16	Southall et al.[19]
23–27 years	53 ± 6	141 ± 17	Brodsky et al.[15]
16–65 years	60	95	Clarke et al.[12]
> 60 years	53 ± 7	112 ± 18	Fleg and Kennedy[18]

indication not stated in the request in 21% of recordings! Thus, clinically useful information was obtained in the following categories.

1 Indicated symptoms with arrhythmia   7.5%
2 Indicated symptom with no arrhythmia 9.7%
3 Other symptom with arrhythmia   9.2%
          Total   26%

Whether the detection of asymptomatic arrhythmias (7.5%) can be regarded as clinically useful is debatable. Zeldis et al. documented symptomatic arrhythmias in only 13% of recordings.[20] In a further 34%, there were symptoms unrelated to ECG changes. It is probably not appropriate to infer that asymptomatic arrhythmias (for example, non-sustained tachycardia) during the recording may at other times cause the symptoms for which the patient is being studied. More than one type of arrhythmia is commonly recorded,[21] and interpretation of these findings is difficult. Clearly, however, clinical judgement is required. In a patient with syncope who had documented asymptomatic second degree atrioventricular block, it would not be unreasonable to consider a pacemaker. It is also likely that a single arrhythmia can cause more than one symptom (for example, paroxysmal sustained ventricular tachycardia may cause dizziness on one occasion and sudden dyspnoea on another).

The frequency with which symptoms occur is clearly a major factor in determining the outcome of a single study. Daily symptoms are likely to be documented, but those that occur monthly are less likely to be recorded. However, infrequent symptoms must not be regarded as a contra-indication to 24-hour continuous monitoring because other, possibly asymptomatic, arrhythmias may be recorded and provide clues to an underlying mechanism that may operate at times when the patient has symptoms (for example, intermittent pre-excitation in a patient with palpitations). Thus, at least one continuous recording should be performed before resorting to other techniques of monitoring (see above).

TRANSIENT NEUROLOGICAL EPISODES

Most patients who are referred to the cardiologist for investigation of these symptoms have been screened for neurological disorders beforehand or have given a history strongly suggestive of a cardiac cause. The commonest symptoms are dizziness, lightheadedness, near-syncope, syncope and unexplained falls in the elderly. Several studies have

addressed the utility of 24-hour tape monitoring in this group. Tzivoni and Stern reported on 110 patients with dizziness or syncope.[22] Only 11% had arrhythmias which were regarded as indications for the implantation of a pacemaker. Whether these arrhythmias were proven as the cause of the symptoms is not clear. Goldberg et al. found arrhythmias in 74% of 130 patients (including 48 with palpitations), but proof of a causal relationship with symptoms was not given.[21] In a larger series of 358 patients, Jonas et al. found symptomatic arrhythmias in only 3.9%, but in a further 5.1% they noted arrhythmias which were likely to cause symptoms but for some reason such symptoms were not indicated in the diary (for example, the patient had symptoms but did not or could not write in the diary, arrhythmias were asymptomatic, etc.).[23] De Bono et al. recorded symptomatic ECG abnormalities in only 3 of 89 patients attending neurology clinics for investigation of transient non-focal symptoms.[24] The precise nature of those abnormalities and the question of whether they were the cause of the symptoms for which the patient was being investigated are not clarified in the report. The results of ambulatory recording of 1512 patients referred for investigation of syncope were reported by Gibson and Heitzman.[25] An arrhythmia-related symptom was documented in 30 patients (1.9%). In the 7 patients with syncope, ventricular tachycardia was the commonest cause. Supraventricular tachycardia was the most frequent cause of pre-syncopal symptoms in 23 patients. Major arrhythmias without symptoms were very common. The difficulty in discovering the cause of non-focal transient neurological symptoms has led several investigators to use provocative electrophysiological testing (see Chapter 11). These symptoms can pose a particular problem in the elderly. Abdon and Nilsson found a high prevalence of cardiac arrhythmias in a group of patients suffering from frequent falls and fractures when compared with age-matched control subjects.[26]

Combined ambulatory monitoring of the ECG and the electroencephalogram has been made possible with purpose-built recorders.[27] This method of investigation may prove to be of especial value in carefully selected patients in whom the relationship between a possible neurological disorder and a cardiac arrhythmia is unclear.

PALPITATIONS

Few studies have been designed to address specifically the value of ambulatory monitoring for investigation of palpitations. Kunz *et al.* studied 319 recordings from 167 patients.[28] Symptomatic arrhythmias were recorded in 9.7%, whereas 39% had palpitations unrelated to arrhythmias. These results might be improved by careful history-taking before selecting patients for study.

CHEST PAIN

Early investigators of patients with chest pain failed to appreciate the inadequacy of the equipment when it was used for this purpose. The frequency-response characteristics of recorders removes low-frequency signals of the type contained in the ST segment and the T wave. The interpretation of early reports is confounded by this problem. More recently, technical modifications have made ST-segment monitoring more reliable. One such modification is frequency modulation of the signal.[29] Bragg-Remschel *et al.* formally compared several recorders of both the amplitude-modulated (AM) and frequency-modulated (FM) type and found none which conformed to the American Heart Association guidelines.[4] However, for crude ST-segment analysis, all but one type (an AM recorder) was satisfactory. In the study by Crawford *et al.* of 70 men with chest pain, ST-segment depression was recorded in 24 of 39 patients with coronary disease and in 12 of 31 without.[30] It would seem, therefore, that ambulatory monitoring is of limited value in excluding coronary disease. The results of a more recent study has shown that both ST-segment elevation and depression may occur in normal subjects.[31] It is now appreciated that in patients with coronary disease ischaemic episodes may not be associated with chest pain – so-called 'silent' ischaemia. This phenomenon and its significance are discussed in Chapter 47.

ESTABLISHMENT OF AN ELECTROCARDIOGRAPHIC DIAGNOSIS

TACHYCARDIAS

In patients suspected of having transient recurrent abnormalities of rhythm disturbance, the foremost consideration is documentation of the symptomatic episodes. In many instances, invasive electrophysiological studies have been valuable in that the arrhythmia can be initiated and its characteristics studied. From these tests, it is often possible to conclude that spontaneous occurrence of that arrhythmia is likely to account for the symptoms, especially so with junctional tachycardias of the re-entrant type and sustained monmorphic ventricular tachycardia (see Chapter 11). Most patients with these arrhythmias have relatively infrequent episodes (i.e. less than one a day). Ambulatory monitoring can be useful in providing information about the frequency of potential triggering events, such as premature stimuli or changes in heart rate, but the symptomatic tachycardia may not be recorded. Even if it is recorded, a precise mechanistic diagnosis (for example, atrioventricular versus intranodal re-entry) is often not possible. Wide complexes can be due to aberrancy or ventricular origin; distinction between these causes can be difficult with using only one or two channels. Lipkin *et al.* used intra-atrial electrograms to document atrioventricular dissociation in 8 or 9 patients confirming a ventricular origin.[32] The unusually low incidence of 1:1 retrograde conduction during tachycardia in this group no doubt favoured the success of the technique.

Investigation of intermittent symptomatic bradycardias is more difficult because such bradycardias cannot be reliably induced. Invasive studies have not proved especially useful in this respect because they usually provide only indirect evidence of an abnormality of impulse generation or conduction. Thus, intermittent sustained complete atrioventricular block or sinus pauses are not inducible whereas pacing-induced infraHis block or prolonged sinus recovery can be induced and provide circumstantial evidence for a more profound defect.

Ambulatory monitoring has been of complementary value in the study of sino-atrial disorders and atrioventricular block.

SINO-ATRIAL DISORDERS

The diagnosis of sino-atrial disorders is most reliably confirmed by ambulatory tape monitoring. Sinus pauses and sinus bradycardia are common in normal people[19,33] and must be distinguished from pathological states. Several criteria for the diagnosis of sino-atrial disorders from the ambulatory ECG have been proposed. Crook *et al.* were among the first to appreciate this problem.[34] They characterized the range of arrhythmias occurring in 27 patients with either second or 'third' degree sino-atrial block (NB third degree cannot reliably be diagnosed from surface recordings) or bradycardia of 56 beats/min or less. All patients were symp-

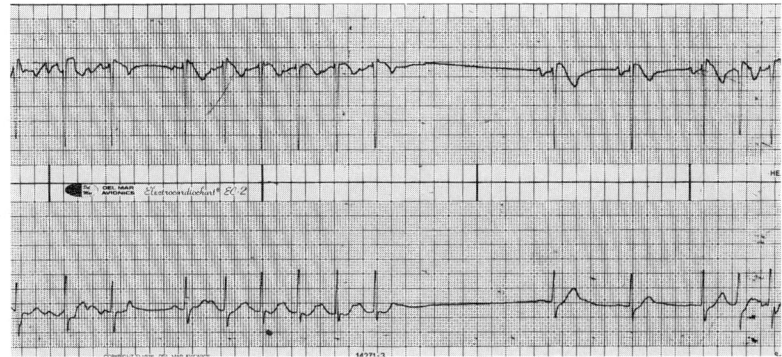

Fig. 10.5. This twin-channel segment from a continuous 24-hour recording (Avionics) shows intermittent atrial tachycardia interspersed with sinus pauses. The diagnosis was a sino-atrial disorder complicated with frequent atrial tachyarrhythmias (so-called 'tachy–brady' syndrome).

tomatic. Sinus pauses of up to 3.6 s, sinus bradycardia (36–56 beats/min), atrial fibrillation and other supraventricular tachycardias were recorded in the majority of patients. Many other studies have documented a similar variety of arrhythmias,[35] even in asymptomatic patients with resting bradycardia.[36]

The available evidence from normal subjects and those with known sino-atrial disorders would suggest that in adults rates below 40 beats/min and pauses of 2 s or greater must be considered as pathological,[37] unless there is a recognized physiological cause such as athletic training.

The presence of rapid atrial fibrillation or atrial tachycardias in addition to pauses is a variant of sino-atrial disorder known as the 'tachy-brady' syndrome (Fig. 10.5).

ATRIOVENTRICULAR BLOCK

Intermittent complete atrioventricular block during ambulatory ECG recording is very rare and usually short-lived. It is more commonly found in the elderly.[13,38] Even in symptomatic patients, numerous recordings are often needed to document the phenomenon.[39] If, in a symptomatic patient, there is a pre-existing intraventricular conduction defect,

it is often expeditious to pace rather than embark on a prolonged period of monitoring. Lesser degrees of block are more common. Brodsky et al.[15] and Clarke et al.[12] noted second degree atrioventricular block in 6% and 3.7% of subjects, respectively. In most instances, the pattern of block was type I, presumably reflecting variations in vagal tone (Fig. 10.6). Although this conduction abnormality is thought to be benign, Young et al. followed 16 young patients for 1–18 years and 7 developed complete atrioventricular block.[40] Two patients became symptomatic. These results suggest that young patients with second degree type I atrioventricular block should be followed closely. Intermittent first degree atrioventricular block has also been observed during monitoring. Rarely, this is due to the presence of dual atrioventricular nodal pathways (Fig. 10.7).

ASSESSMENT OF THERAPEUTIC INTERVENTIONS

DRUG STUDIES

Ventricular ectopic activity

Assessment of the effect of drugs on ventricular

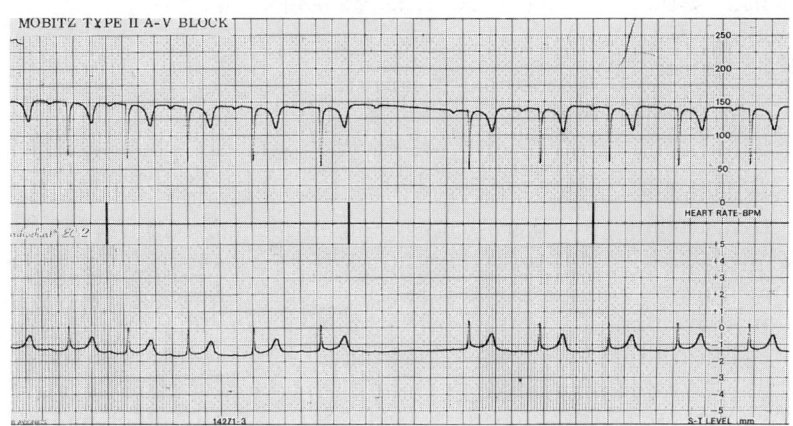

Fig. 10.6. Asymptomatic second degree type I atrioventricular block during a twin-channel 24-hour recording in a 25-year-old man with symptoms of dizziness. The number of cycles of PR lengthening prior to the dropped heart beat was often in excess of 6.

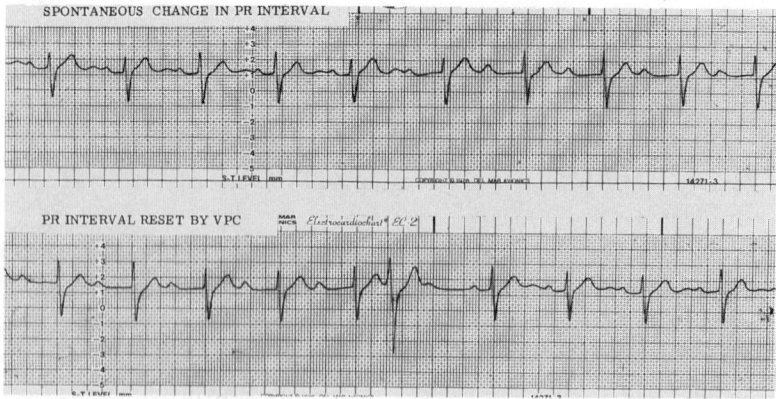

Fig. 10.7. Recordings from a patient with palpitations. None were documented during this recording but on several occasions there was a sudden increase in the PR interval (upper segment). The shorter PR interval was returned after a ventricular premature beat some minutes later. These phenomena are explained by the presence of dual atrioventricular nodal pathways. The transition from a short to a long interval reflects block in the faster pathway and sustained slow pathway conduction, although the precise mechanism of this transition is unclear. Sustained slow pathway conduction is presumably maintained by retrograde concealed conduction into the distal part of the fast pathway preventing anterograde expression. A ventricular premature beat results in early retrograde penetration of the faster pathway resetting its refractory period and allowing anterograde conduction on the next conducted beat. The cause of palpitations in this patient was conjectured to be the result of atrioventricular nodal re-entry.

ectopic activity is the most widely utilized application of ambulatory monitoring to assess treatment. It is outside the scope of this Chapter to review these studies in detail. However, several important principles have emerged. It has been known for some time that the frequency of ventricular ectopic beats may vary with time. In some circumstances, this natural variation may mimic the apparent effect suppressive of anti-arrhythmic therapy.[41] The half-hourly rate of ventricular ectopic beats varied from −99% to +1100%. Morganroth *et al.* suggested that a suppression of ventricular ectopic beats > 83% was required to be reliably attributable to a drug effect.[42] Michelson and Morganroth later suggested a 65% reduction for ventricular tachycardia (more than three ventricular ectopic beats consecutively) and 75% for couplets.[43] Although other authors have suggested different figures, the principle is widely accepted. The paradox is that, despite all these studies, there is very little evidence that treatment of ventricular ectopic activity influences survival; moreover, these studies are uncontrolled.[44]

It is now widely appreciated that anti-arrhythmic agents of all types may exacerbate ventricular arrhythmias. Therefore, similar considerations must be given to the definition of arrhythmogenicity. Morganroth *et al.* have proposed a simple algorithm which relates the supposed arrhythmogenic effect to the basal frequency of the ventricular premature beats;[42] for example, a 10-fold increase

in a control level of 1–50 premature beats per hour or a 5-fold increase over a control rate of 51–100 beats are regarded as pro-arrhythmic. Smaller increases are suggested for high basal frequencies.

Supraventricular tachycardias

Drug effects on supraventricular tachycardias assessed by ambulatory monitoring are less well defined. These arrhythmias occur less frequently and long periods of monitoring may be required. Therapy of junctional re-entrant tachycardias is much better assessed by invasive electrophysiological techniques which reliably initiate the tachycardia.[45] Control of recurrent paroxysmal atrial fibrillation using ambulatory recordings is unsatisfactory and possibly unnecessary because most episodes are symptomatic and a diary might suffice.[46]

Pacemaker function

Ambulatory monitoring is valuable in the investigation of patients with pacemakers. The main indications are as follows.
1 Persistent symptoms despite pacing. On examination such symptoms may be found to be due to other problems such as vertebrobasilar disease or postural hypotension, but pacemaker malfunction cannot be excluded unless ambulatory monitoring is performed during a symptomatic episode.[47] The results of monitoring

may reveal intermittent failure to capture with long pauses, transient spontaneous atrial or ventricular arrhythmias or those induced by inappropriate sensing of the pacemaker with consequent closely coupled stimulation.

2 New symptoms possibly related to the pacemaker. Some patients experience palpitations when the pacemaker cuts in. This can be distressing but it is difficult to treat. Retrograde conduction during long periods of ventricular pacing can cause breathlessness, dizziness and fatigue, the so-called pacemaker syndrome. In patients with dual chamber systems, palpitations can be caused by persistent retrograde conduction initiating pacemaker-mediated tachycardia (endless loop tachycardia). Myopotentials from movement can inhibit some pacemakers (e.g. VVI type) (Fig. 10.8) causing dizziness. Dual chamber systems may be falsely triggered resulting in pacemaker-mediated tachycardia. If pacing system malfunction is suspected, an attempt to elicit this in the clinic can be made using the programmer (for example, measuring threshold, myopotential inhibition (Fig. 10.7), initiating pacemaker-mediated tachycardia, etc.) before ambulatory monitoring is requested. Improved pacemaker programmability and flexibility have probably reduced the need for repeated ambulatory monitoring in symptomatic paced patients.

3 Assessment of pacemaker performance especially with dual chamber or rate-responsive systems for bradycardia or antitachycardia pacemakers. Complex pacing systems may need confirmation of normal function especially after adjustments have been made by programming. This applies especially to rate-responsive systems because the rate–response (the relationship between the input from the sensor and the final paced rate) is programmable in all types and fine-tuning for an optimal response is usually needed.

Many ambulatory tape systems incorporate an amplifier to detect and enhance the pacemaker stimulus artefact making failure to capture easier to detect.[48]

ASSESSMENT OF RISK

POST-MYOCARDIAL INFARCTION

Ambulatory monitoring has been used to acquire an enormous body of information about the frequency and pattern of ventricular ectopic activity following acute myocardial infarction. It is now appreciated that the presence of complex or frequent (> 10 per hour) ventricular premature beats is associated with a higher risk of death in the following year after infarction. After years of debate, it has now been shown that this risk is independent of the degree of left ventricular damage.[49] Thus, patients with both findings are at greater risk than those with either one or the other. However, it has not been shown that suppression of this ventricular ectopic activity improves prognosis. Several trials designed to answer this question are now underway.

A new approach to risk stratification using ambulatory ECG data is the analysis of heart–rate variability. Klieger et al. used the standard deviation of all normal cycles as an index of variability.[50] Multivariate analysis showed that heart-rate variability was most strongly correlated with mortality. The relative risk of death was over 5 times greater in patients with a variability of 50 ms or less compared with those in whom variability was 100 ms or more. Frequent and complex ventricular

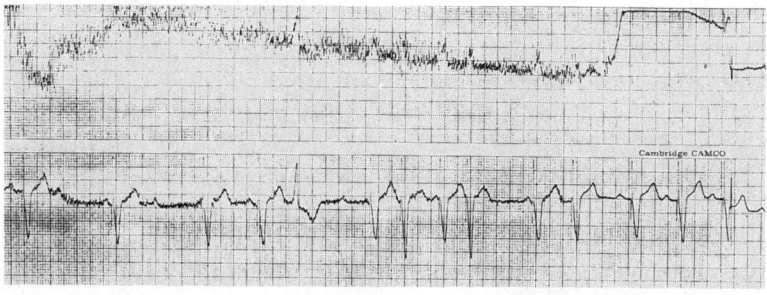

Fig. 10.8. Recordings during a twin-channel 24-hour continuous tape monitoring of a patient with a dual chamber pacemaker who complained of dizzy spells. Myopotential interference results in variable triggering of the atrial channel. At the onset of the trace, the atrial channel is inhibited and the pacemaker operates at its lower rate of 50 beats/min in the ventricular channel. Later in the recording, there is intermittent inappropriate triggering of the ventricular channel by myopotential sensed by the atrial channel. Normal function (VDD mode) resumes at the end of the segment of ECG.

premature beats were also strongly associated with heart-rate variability. Similar findings were reported by Martin et al.[51] This observation may indicate disturbed autonomic function after infarction.

OUT-OF-HOSPITAL CARDIAC ARREST

Over 90% of survivors of ventricular fibrillation occurring out of hospital manifest ventricular ectopic activity on a continuous tape recording,[52] and in about half complex forms are present. There is some evidence that suppression of this activity may improve survival,[53] but with such a high prevalence rate it is difficult to know how those at risk can be stratified.

AORTIC VALVE DISEASE

Sudden death is a recognized complication of patients with severe aortic stenosis, but information about the mechanism leading to death is scarce. Nikolic et al. reported on a patient who died whilst being monitored with a combined external pulse and ECG monitor.[54] This patient appeared to develop hypotension as a primary event in the absence of arrhythmias. Secondary asystole caused death. Olshausen et al. studied patients with aortic stenosis, aortic regurgitation and combined disease.[55] They found that the severity of ventricular arrhythmias on ambulatory monitoring correlated not with the type or severity of valve disease but with the extent of left ventricular impairment. In a later study, Klein found no correlation between frequency of arrhythmia and type of valve disease, severity of disease, presence or absence of coronary disease or left ventricular function.[56] Patients with greater degrees of hypertrophy and larger cavities had a greater tendency to develop complex arrhythmias. Thus, the factors contributing to ventricular ectopic activity in patients with aortic valve disease are far from being clarified.

MITRAL VALVE PROLAPSE

Patients with mitral valve prolapse are another group in whom ventricular arrhythmias may be a risk factor for sudden cardiac death.[57] This has been a subject of debate for some time. In the Framingham Study, the frequency of arrhythmias during 24-hour ambulatory monitoring in 61 patients with mitral valve prolapse was compared with that in 179 control subjects.[58] An excess of

supraventricular arrhythmias, complex or frequent ventricular premature beats and runs of ventricular tachycardia was found in the patients with mitral valve prolapse, but the difference between this group and the control subjects was not significant. Although in early reports it was suggested that the outlook for these subjects is good, there is increasing evidence that mitral valve prolapse (even in the absence of significant regurgitation) is not a harmless condition. Duren et al. reported the long-term follow-up of 300 patients with the condition.[59] Serious ventricular arrhythmias including fibrillation and tachycardia developed in 56 patients. Major complications other than arrhythmias occurred in another 57 patients. The value of ambulatory monitoring in the assessment of these risks in patients with mitral valve prolapse (of all degrees) remains to be determined.

LEFT VENTRICULAR HYPERTROPHY

That the risk of sudden cardiac death is increased in patients with left ventricular hypertrophy was shown in the Framingham Heart Study.[60] McLenachan et al. have shown that the severity and frequency of ventricular arrhythmias on ambulatory recordings are related to the extent of ventricular hypertrophy on echocardiography and the derived left ventricular mass.[61] Complex forms including non-sustained ventricular tachycardia were more common in patients with high left ventricular mass. Many patients, however, were receiving beta-blockade which may have had an independent effect. The performance of further studies may help to identify which patients are at risk of sudden death.

VENTRICULAR PRE-EXCITATION

Ambulatory monitoring is of little value in the study of supraventricular tachycardia associated with ventricular pre-excitation because they occur relatively infrequently (see above). Electrophysiological testing is superior (see Chapter 11). Ambulatory monitoring is useful in the detection of intermittency of ventricular pre-excitation (Fig. 10.9) Klein and Gulamhusein have reported that intermittent pre-excitation is correlated with a long refractory period of the anomalous pathway and therefore a decreased risk of a rapid response to atrial fibrillation.[62] Thus, ambulatory monitoring can be useful in the non-invasive assessment of risk in these patients.

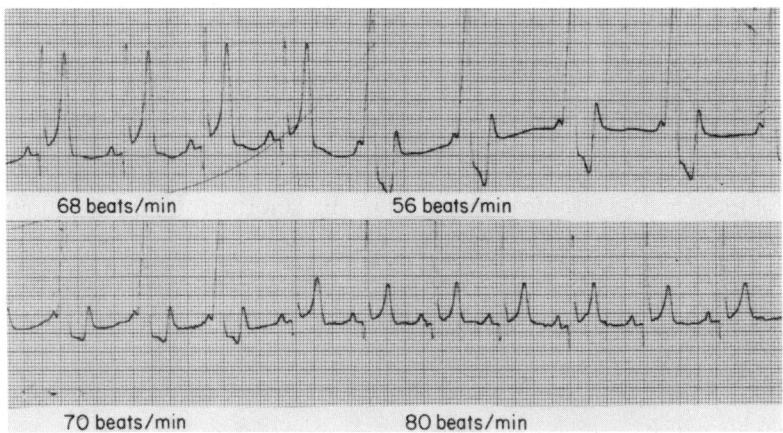

Fig. 10.9. A segment from a continuous 24-hour recording in a patient with the Wolff–Parkinson–White syndrome showing intermittent pre-excitation. As the heart rate slows from 68 to 56 beats/min the QRS complex changes with the appearance of a delta wave. When the rate increases again, pre-excitation disappears.

HYPERTROPHIC CARDIOMYOPATHY

Ambulatory monitoring has revealed ventricular arrhythmias in approximately 30% of patients with this disorder of heart muscle.[63] A high proportion of these have frequent and complex forms including ventricular tachycardia. Treatment of these arrhythmias with amiodarone has been shown to improve the survival rate.[64] Atrial arrhythmias are also common. Thus, prolonged ambulatory ECG monitoring should be considered a routine investigation in patients with hypertrophic cardiomyopathy. A significant number of patients with ventricular hypertrophy due to aortic valve stenosis or hypertension also have ventricular arrhythmias. The prognostic implications of these findings are not known (see above).

DILATED CARDIOMYOPATHY

Patients with dilated cardiomyopathy may die suddenly. The relationship between ventricular ectopic activity during ambulatory monitoring and the risk of sudden cardiac death has been investigated by several groups.[65] Despite intense study, no clear pattern has emerged. Olshausen et al. monitored 78 patients for 48 h and, although ventricular tachycardias during monitoring were a major indicator of risk, multivariate analysis failed to identify this variable as sufficiently powerful to distinguish between survivors and non-survivors.[66] Left ventricular function, on the other hand, was important in this respect.

CONGENITAL COMPLETE ATRIOVENTRICULAR BLOCK

Although the association of symptoms with complete congenital atrioventricular block is an undoubted indication for permanent pacing, the need for prophylactic pacing in patients who have this disorder but do not have symptoms has not been cleary defined.[67] Electrophysiological tests have helped to some extent, but a clear differentiation between those at risk of syncope and sudden death and those not at risk has not been demonstrated by the use of invasive tests as yet. Thus, there is still controversy about which patients with this potentially life-threatening disorder should receive a permanent pacemaker.[68]

In an important communication, Dewey et al. reported long-term follow-up data from ambulatory monitoring.[69] As a result of these studies, they concluded that patients with certain types of arrhythmia should be considered for prophylactic pacing: those with nocturnal exit block (Fig. 10.10) from the secondary junctional pacemaker (i.e.

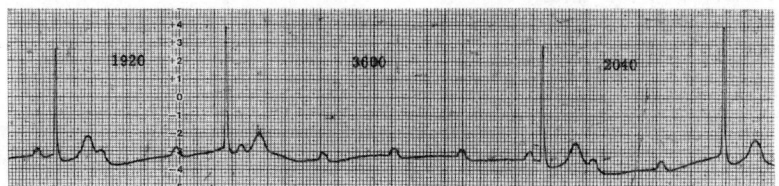

Fig. 10.10. Part of a continuous recording in a 36-year-old woman with 'congenital' complete atrioventricular block. At 05 30 hours she had several pauses which were approximately twice the base junctional escape interval. This is interpreted as junctional exit block and is regarded as an indication of unreliability of the subsidiary junctional pacemaker.

sudden pauses of approximately integer multiples of the basic junctional cycle length, described as junctional exit block); those with little or no change of the junctional escape rate on exertion; and those with associated tachycardias. Of the 8 patients who died suddenly or had syncopal spells or severe symptoms as a result of bradycardia, 6 of these had one or more of these ambulatory electrocardiographic findings. Many also had mean daytime junctional escape rates of 50 beats/min or less. The authors suggest that those patients with these manifestations of junctional instability or unreliability should undergo permanent pacemaker implantation. Although the optimal age at which permanent pacing should be undertaken has not yet been resolved, it is clear that ambulatory electrocardiographic monitoring is important in stratifying the risk of pacemaker candidates.

ARRHYTHMIAS FOLLOWING SURGICAL CORRECTION OF CONGENITAL DEFECTS

Damage to the atrioventricular conduction system following repair of congenital cardiac abnormalities is the most common indication for permanent pacing in children. Although early studies of this problem suggested that long-term prognosis was not adversely affected, more recent data have refuted this view.[67] Although ambulatory monitoring has not contributed in this area, it has brought to light the high incidence of atrial and ventricular arrhythmias in this population of patients. Two conditions have been extensively studied: palliative intra-atrial correction of *complete transposition* (ventriculo-arterial discordance) and *Fallot's tetralogy*.

Hayes and Gersony reported the results of monitoring patients for up to 13 years after atrial palliative surgery (Mustard's operation).[70] Atrial arrhythmias were noted in 20% of patients at discharge, but the prevalence increased to 75% at 6 years. There was also a high incidence of sinus pauses. Significant slow atrial or junctional escape rhythms were observed in 21% and 44% of patients, respectively. Six of 95 (6.3%) patients required permanent pacing. Post-operative ambulatory recordings therefore are of potential importance in such patients.

There are numerous studies of the prevalence of ventricular ectopic beats after repair of Fallot's tetralogy, and it is now recognized that ventricular tachycardia or fibrillation may be an important cause of mortality after this operation.[71] In the study by Garson *et al.*, ambulatory monitoring has revealed arrhythmias in about 12% of patients.[72] However, the study was uncontrolled and did not use actuarial techniques or multivariate analysis.[72] It wrongly claimed that treatment of these arrhythmias reduced the incidence of sudden death. This is improbable because the mortality rate[73] is about one-sixth of the prevalence of ectopic activity. Properly controlled prospective studies of the diagnostic, prognostic and therapeutic value of postoperative monitoring in this group of patients are needed.

SUDDEN INFANT DEATH

Sudden death in infancy has been the subject of debate and intensive research. It is clear from the many studies of this phenomenon that there is no single major cause.[74] Concern that cardiac arrhythmias are responsible for a proportion of deaths has been expressed by several investigators.[75] Apnoeic episodes accompanied by profound transient bradycardia have been demonstrated by combined ECG and respiratory monitoring.[76] The possibility of malignant ventricular arrhythmias has been suggested by the observation of an apparent lengthening of the QT interval.[77] However, the difficulties of defining and characterizing an abnormal QT interval have impeded the progress of this research.[78,79] Indeed, in a large prospective survey co-ordinated by Southall *et al.*, no such relationship between the QT interval during monitoring and later death was revealed.[80] A re-examination of this data, however, has shown that modulating effects of heart rate on the QT interval may be impaired in victims.[81] Whether this contributes to the generation of fatal ventricular arrhythmias remains to be demonstrated.

AMBULATORY ELECTROCARDIOGRAPHIC RECORDING DURING SUDDEN CARDIAC DEATH

In the last decade, there have been numerous reports of fortuitous ambulatory ECG recording during sudden cardiac death (Figs 10.11 and 10.12). Roelandt *et al.*, reviewing the literature in 1984, found reports of 20 cases and added 10 from their own experience.[82] In 23 patients, the terminal arrhythmia was ventricular fibrillation and in 7 patients bradycardias. In 10 of the patients with ventricular fibrillation, the terminal arrhythmia was

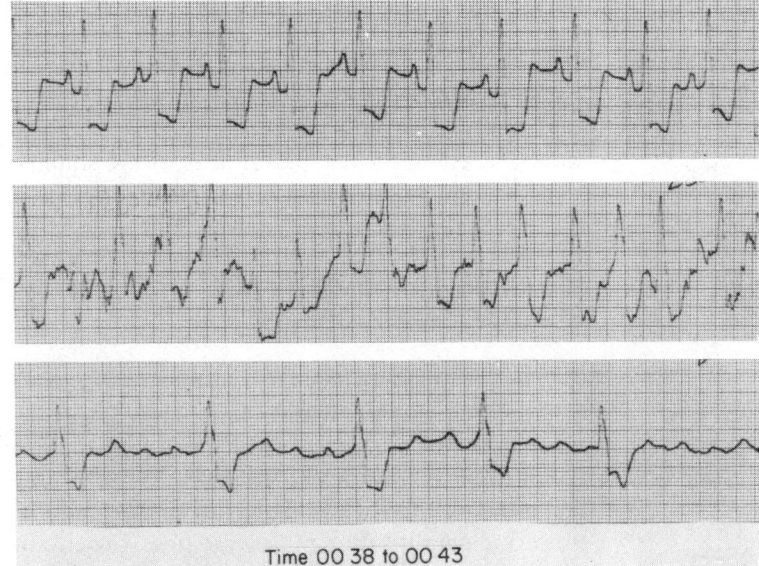

Time 00 38 to 00 43

Fig. 10.11. Ambulatory ECG recordings during the death of a patient with ischaemic heart disease. The harbinger of death is marked ST-segment depression (upper trace). This is followed several minutes later by a tachycardia possibly atrial or sinus in origin (middle trace). Minutes later (lower trace), the ECG shows atrial tachycardia with an irregular QRS complex rate indicating variable atrioventricular block (see also Fig. 10.12).

preceded by ventricular tachycardia. Panidis and Morganroth noted similar findings in 15 in-hospital deaths.[83] Bradycardias were seen in 3 patients and ventricular fibrillation in 12. In all 12 cases, fibrillation was preceded by tachycardia. Analysis of tapes showing spontaneous ventricular fibrillation confirms this phenomenon.[84] The relationship of these arrhythmias to ischaemia is not clear. The limitations of ambulatory ST-segment recording may be a contributory factor (see above). Pratt *et al.* did not detect any acute changes in the majority of patients.[84] In contrast, Savage *et al.* demonstrated marked ST-segment elevation or depression in 9 of

14 subjects who suffered sudden death, 10 of whom had ventricular fibrillation.[85] Furthermore, there was a distinct trend towards more marked changes in the hours preceding death. This was associated with an increasing frequency of ventricular ectopic activity including couplets and tachycardia. The most common time of death was in the early hours of the morning.

ELECTROCARDIOGRAPHIC ARTEFACTS

A wide range of electrocardiographic artefacts may

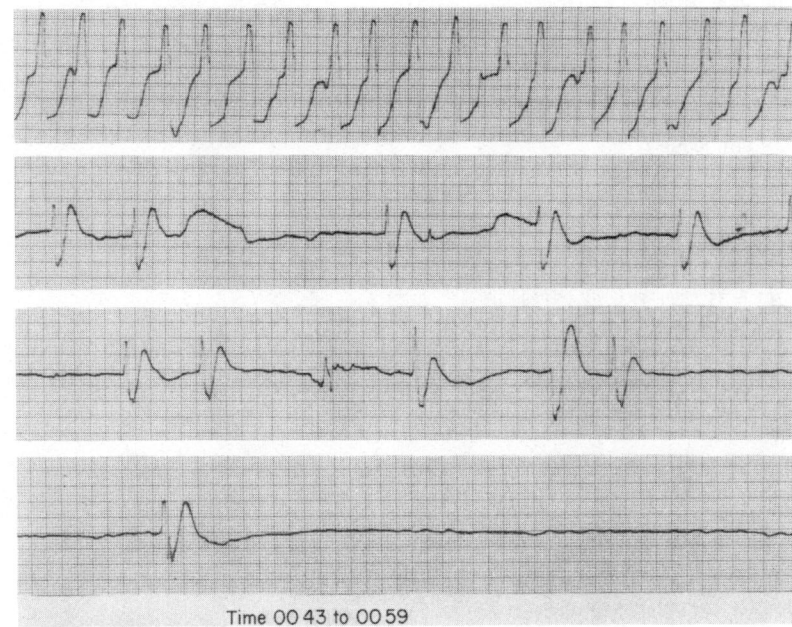

Time 00 43 to 00 59

Fig. 10.12. Continuation of the recording shown in Fig. 10.11. The tachycardia continues and the QRS complexes become wider. Minutes later, there is sinus and atrial arrest with erratic junctional and ventricular escape rhythms. Asystole is the terminal event.

Table 10.3. **The commonest types of artefacts on the electro-cardiogram.**

Problem	Possible ECG appearances
Variations of tape speed (Fig. 10.13)	Bradycardia with long PR, QT, wide QRS, tachycardia with narrow QRS, etc.
Disconnection of ECG (Fig. 10.14)	'Asystole'
Incomplete erasure (Fig. 10.15)	Atrioventricular dissociation
Interference (Fig. 10.16)	Tachycardia or fibrillation

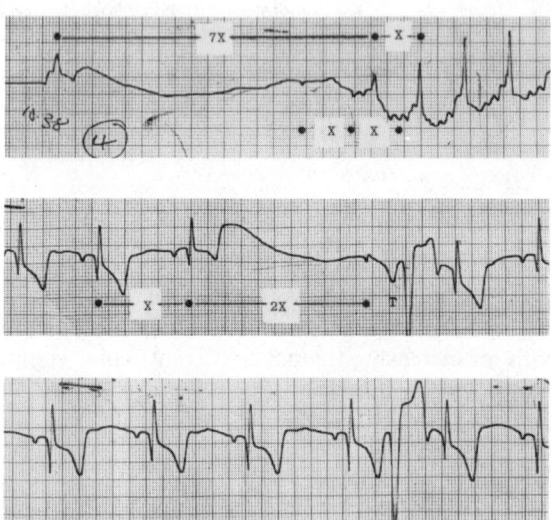

Fig. 10.13. Artefact during a 24-hour recording. The upper trace shows a pause terminated by a QRS complex and sinus tachycardia. The middle trace, several hours later, shows a similar event. This time the trace returns with a T wave followed by a ventricular ectopic beat. This provides the clue to the problem. Simple analysis of the pauses shows that the reappearance of the QRS is on-time, as is the T wave. The lower trace shows an interpolated ventricular premature beat during an intact recording. The cause is clear: intermittent electrode disconnection. This patient was referred for a permanent pacemaker because the pauses were erroneously interpreted as sinus pauses.

be observed during the analysis of ambulatory recordings.[86] It is important to recognize these and distinguish them from true electrocardiographic changes. Failure to recognize artefacts can lead to potentially inappropriate and dangerous intervention. The commonest types of artefact are summarized in Table 10.3 (see also Figs 10.13–10.16).

HIGH-RESOLUTION SURFACE ELECTROCARDIOGRAPHY

Recent advances in the technology of processing electrocardiographic signals has allowed the development of non-invasive methods of studying conduction in the heart. The most widely used technique is that of averaging to remove random noise and amplification in order to observe periodic events. The method has been used mainly to record His potentials[87] and to detect delayed potentials arising from areas of diseased myocardium.[88] Although there has been some clinical application of the non-invasive measurement of cardiac conduction intervals, most interest has centred on the application of high-resolution electrocardiography to detect late potentials (Fig. 10.17), especially in patients who have suffered from myocardial infarction.[89] The presence of these potentials is thought to indicate delayed activation and therefore the existence of slow conduction, which is known to be a prerequisite for the development of re-entrant ventricular tachycardia. There appears to be a significant association between late potentials and the propensity to spontaneous ventricular tachycardia.[90] The significance of late potentials as a risk factor after infarction was investigated by Denniss *et al.*[91] Late potentials were predictive of a sudden cardiac arrhythmic event (excluding those associated with re-infarction) with a sensitivity of

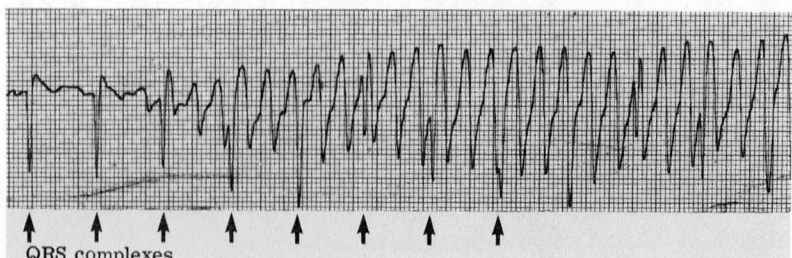

QRS complexes

Fig. 10.14. This recording alarmed the referring physician. Careful inspection revealed evidence of background sinus activity (arrows). Furthermore, the apparent arrhythmia persisted for several minutes and upon subsequent questioning the patient admitted no symptoms. This artefact is common and is often due to rapid body movements, such as hand-washing, or intermittent electrode contact. This patient was referred as an emergency for investigation of ventricular tachycardia.

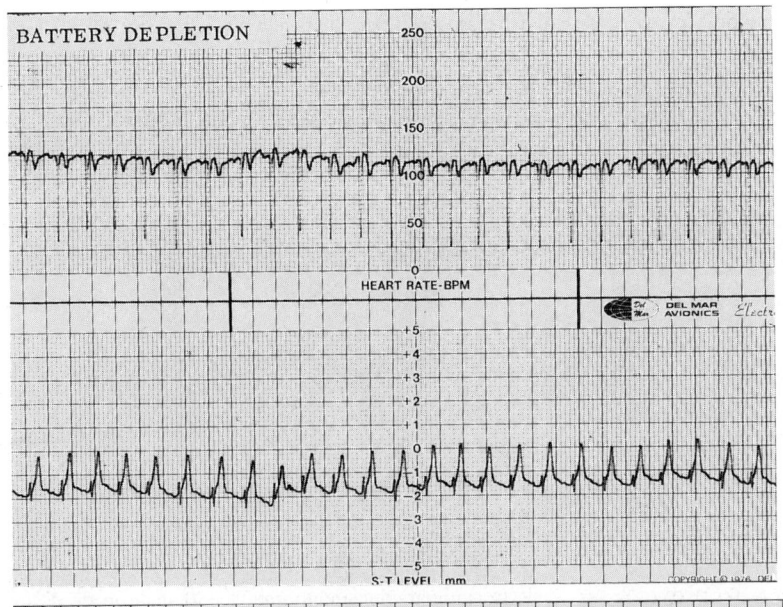

Fig. 10.15. Apparent atrial tachycardia. Further inspection shows that the PR interval, the QRS complex and the QT interval are all remarkably short. This is due to slowing of the tape as a result of battery depletion. Some modern devices have built-in timers which prevent this type of misleading display.

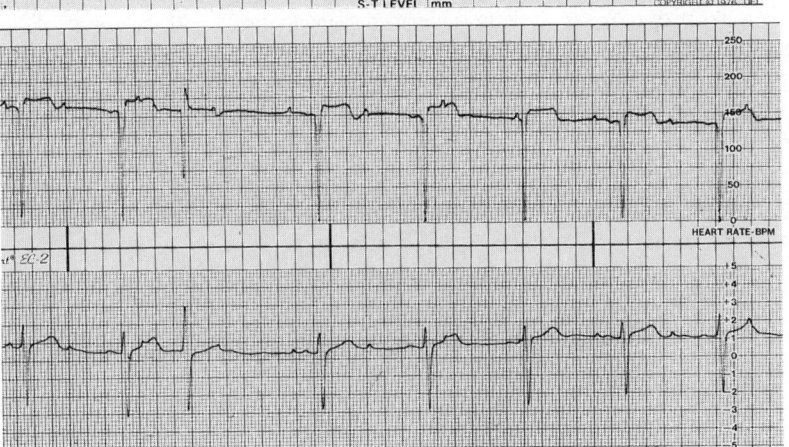

Fig. 10.16. The recording shows two dissociated rhythms. Upon casual inspection, this recording mimics atrioventricular dissociation, a diagnosis reinforced by the fortuitous occurrence of a premature QRS complex (possibly interpreted as a capture beat). Closer examination, however, reveals that all the QRS complexes are preceded by P waves. The smaller pseudo-P waves are the QRS complexes of a previous recording which has been incompletely erased.

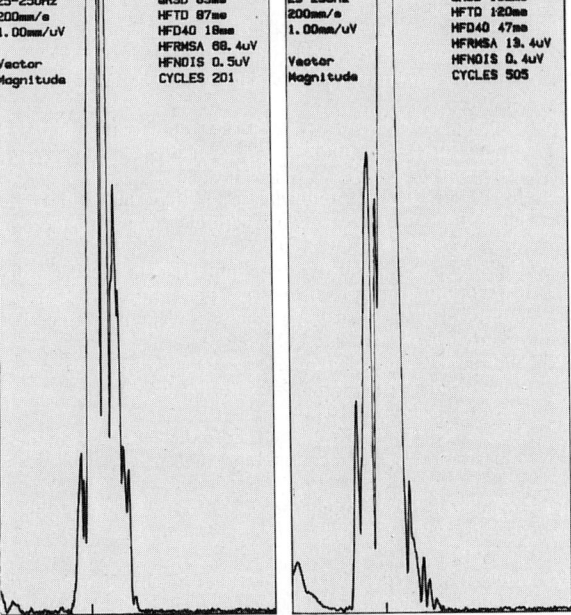

Fig. 10.17. Signal averaged electrocardiograms. The left recording shows a highly amplified (1 mm/μV) average 201 QRS complex of normal duration. The right recording (505 beats) was taken from a patient with recurrent ventricular tachycardias remote from acute anterior infarction. The tail-end of the recording shows low-amplitude activity for the last 47 ms of the complex at a root-mean-square amplitude of 13.4 μV. This reflects delayed myocardial activation and is abnormal. (Paper speed 200 mm/s.)

66%, a specificity of 78% and a predictive accuracy of 24%. When other factors such as ambulatory ECG data and left ventricular ejection fraction are taken into account these figures improve.[92] Thus, the combination of late potentials and an impaired ventricle (ejection fraction < 40%) gave a sensitivity of 80% with a specificity of 89%.

The technique has also been used in other settings in which ventricular tachycardia may be clinically important. Kuchar et al. found late potentials in 70% of patients with unexplained syncope and inducible ventricular tachycardia.[93] Poll et al. found that late potentials were more common in patients with dilated cardiomyopathy and sustained ventricular arrhythmias than in those without arrhythmias.[94]

Late potentials may also be analysed in the frequency domain (Fourier analysis).[95] Similar analysis of the entire QRS complex may also prove to be of clinical value. For example, rejection of transplanted hearts may be manifest by changes in the frequency content of the QRS complex.[96] Ambulatory recording of late potentials has to be obtained by averaging larger numbers of beats to reduce the high levels of noise during ambulation.[97]

The clinical utility of high-resolution electrocardiography remains to be determined. At present, it is useful in research studies but it is hoped that it may become important in the assessment of risk and the selection of patients for invasive electrophysiological studies.

REFERENCES

1. Holter, N.J. Radioelectrocardiography: a new technique for cardiovascular studies. Ann. N. Y. Acad. Sci. 1957; 65: 913–23.
2. Holter, N.J. New method for heart studies. Science 1961; 134: 1214–20.
3. Ward, D.E., Camm, A.J. and Darby, N. Assessment of the diagnostic value of ambulatory electrocardiographic monitoring. Biotelemetry and Patient Monitoring 1980; 7: 57–66.
4. Bragg-Remschel, D.A., Anderson, C.M. and Winkle, R.A. Frequency response characteristics of ambulatory monitoring systems and their implications for ST segment analysis. Am. Heart J. 1982; 103: 20–31.
5. Murray, A. Analysis techniques. In: Campbell, R.W.F. and Murray, A., eds. Dynamic Electrocardiography. London: Churchill Livingstone, 1985, pp. 1–13.
6. Kishida, H., Akazome, T., Kimura, E. and Rikli, A.E. A review of the pocket electrocardiograph (PECG) in a large general medical clinic. Circulation 1976; 53: 939–42.
7. Antman, E.M., Ludmer, P.L., McGowan, N., Bosak, M. and Friedman, P.L. Transtelephonic electrocardiographic transmission for management of cardiac arrhythmias. Am. J. Cardiol. 1986; 58: 1021–4.
8. Brown, A.P., Dawkins, K.D. and Davies, J.G. Detection of

arrhythmias: use of a patient activated ambulatory electrocardiogram device with a solidstate memory. Br. Heart J. 1987; 58: 251–3.
9. Kennedy, H.L. and Wiens, R.D. Ambulatory (Holter) electrocardiography using realtime analysis. Am. J. Cardiol. 1987; 59: 1190–5.
10. Shaw, D.B., Kekwick, C.A., Veale, D. and Whistance, T.W.T. Unexplained syncope—a diagnostic pacemaker? PACE 1983; 6: 720–5.
11. Scheunemeyer, T. A soft-ware based automatic pacemaker for the treatment of supraventricular tachycardia: a 12 month experience (Abstract). PACE 1986; 9: 303.
12. Clarke, J.M., Shelton, J.R., Hamer, J., Taylor, S. and Venning, G.R. The rhythm of the normal human heart. Lancet 1976; 2: 508–12.
13. Camm, A.J., Evans, K.E., Ward, D.E. and Martin, A. The rhythm of the heart in active elderly subjects. Am. Heart J. 1980; 99: 598–603.
14. Hinkle, L.E., Carver, S.T. and Stevens, M.S. The frequency of asymptomatic disturbances of cardiac rhythm and conduction in middle-aged men. Am. J. Cardiol. 1969; 24: 629–50.
15. Brodsky, M., Wu, D., Denes, P., Kanakis, C. and Rosen, K.M. Arrhythmias documented by 24 hour continuous electrocardiographic monitoring in 50 male medical students without apparent heart disease. Am. J. Cardiol. 1977; 39: 390–5.
16. Kennedy, H.L. and Underhill, S.J. Frequent or complex ventricular ectopy in apparently healthy subjects. A clinical study of 25 cases. Am. J. Cardiol. 1976; 38: 141–8.
17. Montague, T., McPherson, D.D., McKenzie, B.R., Spencer, C.A., Nanton, M. and Horacek, B.M. Frequent ventricular ectopic activity without underlying cardiac disease: analysis of 45 subjects. Am. J. Cardiol. 1983; 52: 980–4.
18. Fleg, J.L. and Kennedy, H.L. Cardiac arrhythmias in a healthy elderly population. Detection by 24-hour ambulatory electrocardiography. Chest 1982; 81: 302–7.
19. Southall, D.P., Johnston, F., Shinebourne, E.A. and Johnston, P.G.B. 24 hour electrocardiographic study of heart rates and rhythm patterns in a population of healthy children. Br. Heart J. 1981; 45: 281–91.
20. Zeldis, S.M., Levine, B.J., Michelson, E.L. and Morganroth, J. Cardiovascular complaints: correlation with cardiac arrhythmias on 24 hour electrocardiographic monitoring. Chest 1980; 78: 456–62.
21. Goldberg, A.D., Raftery, E.B. and Cashman, P.M.M. Ambulatory electrocardiographic records in patients with transient cerebral attacks or palpitation. Br. Med. J. 1975; 6: 569–71.
22. Tzivoni, D. and Stern, S. Pacemaker implantation based on ambulatory ECG monitoring on patients with cerebral symptoms. Chest 1975; 67: 274–8.
23. Jonas, S., Klein, I. and Dimant, J. Importance of Holter monitoring in patients with periodic cerebral symptoms. Ann. Neurol. 1977; 1: 470–4.
24. De Bono, D.P., Warlow, C.P. and Hyman, N.M. Cardiac rhythm abnormalities in patients presenting with transient non-focal neurological symptoms: a diagnostic grey area? Br. Med. J. 1982; 284: 1437–9.
25. Gibson, T.C. and Heitzman, M.R. Diagnostic efficacy of 24 hour electrocardiographic monitoring for syncope. Am. J. Cardiol. 1984; 53: 1013–7.
26. Abdon, N.J. and Nilsson, B.E. Episodic cardiac arrhythmia and femoral neck fracture. Acta Med. Scand. 1980; 208: 73–6.
27. Blumhardt, L.D. Ambulatory ECG and EEG monitoring of patients with blackouts. Br. J. Hosp. Med. 1986; 31: 354–60.
28. Kunz, G., Raeder, E. and Burckhardt, D. What does the symptom "palpitation" mean? Correlation between symp-

toms and the presence of cardiac arrhythmias in the ambulatory ECG. *Z. Kardiol.* 1977; **66**: 138–41.

29. Balasubramanian, B., Lahiri, A., Green, H.L., Stott, F.D. and Raftery, E.B. Ambulatory ST segment monitoring: problems, pitfalls, solutions and clinical application. *Br. Heart J.* 1980; **44**: 419–25.

30. Crawford, M.H., Mendoza, C.A, O'Rourke, R.A., White, D.H., Boucher, C.A. and Gorwit, J. Limitations of continuous ambulatory monitoring for detecting coronary artery disease. *Ann. Intern. Med.* 1978; **89**: 1–5.

31. Quyyumi, A.A., Wright, C. and Fox, K. Ambulatory electrocardiographic ST segment changes in healthy volunteers. *Br. Heart J.* 1983; **50**: 460–4.

32. Lipkin, D.P., Perrins, E.J., Shapiro, L.M., Ludgate, L. and Fox, K.M. Diagnosis of broad complex tachycardias with ambulatory monitoring of atrial electrography. *Br. Med. J.* 1984; **288**: 1713–4.

33. Camm, A.J., Ward, D.E. and Spurrell, R.A.J. Arrhythmias in ambulatory persons. A review and experience of 1000 consecutive recordings. *Biotelemetry and Patient Monitoring* 1978; **5**: 167–80.

34. Crook, B.R.M., Cashman, P.M.M., Stott, F.D. and Raftery, E.B. Tape monitoring of the electrocardiogram in ambulant patients with sinoatrial disease. *Br. Heart J.* 1973; **35**: 1009–13.

35. Lipski, J., Cohen, L., Espinoza, J., Motro, M., Dack, S. and Donoso, E. Value of Holter monitoring in assessing cardiac arrhythmias in symptomatic patients. *Am. J. Cardiol.* 1976; **37**: 102–7.

36. Reiffel, J.A., Bigger, J.T., Cramer, M. and Reid, D.S. Ability of Holter electrocardiographic recording and atrial stimulation to detect sinus nodal dysfunction in symptomatic and asymptomatic patients with sinus bradycardia. *Am. J. Cardiol.* 1977; **40**: 189–94.

37. Shaw, D.B. DCG in the investigation of bradyarrhythmias. In: Campbell, R.W.F. and Murray, A., eds. *Dynamic Electrocardiography*. London: Churchill Livingstone, 1985, pp. 58–73.

38. Shaw, D.B. and Kekwick, C.A. Potential candidates for pacemakers: survey of heart block and sinoatrial disorder (sick sinus syndrome). *Br. Heart J.* 1978; **40**: 99–105

39. McLeod, A.A. and Jewitt, D.E. Role of 24 hour ambulatory monitoring in a general hospital. *Br. Med. J.* 1978; **1**: 1197–9.

40. Young, D., Eisenberg, R., Fish, B. and Fisher, J.D. Wenckebach atrioventricular block (Mobitz I) in children and adolescents. *Am. J. Cardiol.* 1977; **40**: 393–9.

41. Winkle, R.A. Antiarrhythmic drug effect mimicked by spontaneous variability of ventricular ectopy. *Circulation* 1978; **57**: 1116–21.

42. Morganroth, J., Borland, M. and Chao, G. Application of a frequency definition of ventricular proarrhythmia. *Am. J. Cardiol.* 1987; **59**: 97–9.

43. Michelson, E.L. and Morganroth, J. Spontaneous variability of complex ventricular arrhythmias detected by long-term electrocardiographic recording. *Circulation* 1980; **61**: 690–5.

44. Graboys, T.B., Lown, B., Podrid, P.J. and DeSilva, R. Long-term survival of patients with malignant ventricular arrhythmia treated with antiarrhythmic drugs. *Am. J. Cardiol.* 1982; **50**: 437–43.

45. Ward, D.E. and Camm, A.J. Drug studies. In: *Clinical Electrophysiology of the Heart*. London: Edward Arnold, 1987, pp. 271–98.

46. Ward, D.E., Camm, A.J. and Spurrell, R.A.J. Clinical experience with disopyramide in paroxysmal atrial fibrillation. *Irish Med. J.* 1977; **70** (suppl.): 13–5.

47. Ward, D.E., Camm, A.J. and Spurrell, R.A.J. Ambulatory monitoring of the electrocardiogram. An important aspect of pacemaker surveillance. *Biotelemetry and Patient Monitoring* 1978; **4**: 109–14.

48. Murray, A. Pacemaker assessment in the ambulant patient. *Br. Heart J.* 1981; **46**: 531–8.

49. Bigger, J.T., Fleiss, J., Kleiger, R., Miller, J. and Rolnitzky, L. The relationships among ventricular arrhythmias, left ventricular dysfunction and mortality in the 2 years after myocardial infarction. *Circulation* 1984; **69**: 250–8.

50. Klieger, R.E., Miller, J.P., Bigger, J.T., Moss, A.J. and the Multicenter Post-Infarction Research Group. Decreased heart rate variability and its association with increased mortality after acute myocardial infarction. *Am. J. Cardiol.* 1987; **59**: 256–62.

51. Martin, G.J., Magid, N.M., Myers, G., Barnett, P.S., Schaad, J.W., Weiss, J.S., Lesch, M. and Singer, D.H. Heart rate variability and sudden death secondary to coronary artery disease during ambulatory electrocardiographic monitoring. *Am. J. Cardiol.* 1987; **60**: 86–9.

52. Weaver, W.D., Cobb, L.A. and Hallstrom, A.P. Ambulatory arrhythmias in resuscitated victims of cardiac arrest. *Circulation* 1982; **66**: 212–8.

53. Myerburg, R., Conde, C., Sheps, D.S., Appel, R.A., Kiem, M.S., Sung, R.J. and Castellanos, A. Antiarrhythmic drug therapy in survivors of prehospital cardiac arrest: comparison of effects on chronic ventricular arrhythmias and recurrent cardiac arrest. *Circulation* 1978; **59**: 855–63.

54. Nikolic, G., Haffty, B.G., Bishop, R.L., Singh, J.B., Flessass, A.P. and Spodick, D.H. Sudden death in aortic stenosis monitored by ear densitographic pulse and ECG. *Am. Heart J.* 1982; **104**: 311–2.

55. Olshausen, K., Schwarz, F., Apfelbach, J., Rohrig, N., Kramer, B. and Kubler, W. Determinants of the incidence and severity of ventricular arrhythmias in aortic valve disease. *Am. J. Cardiol.* 1983; **51**: 1103–9.

56. Klein, R.C. Ventricular arrhythmias in aortic valve disease: analysis of 102 patients. *Am. J. Cardiol.* 1984; **53**: 1079–83.

57. Campbell, R.W.F., Godman, M.G., Marquis, R.M. and Julian, D.G. Ventricular arrhythmias in syndrome of balloon deformity of mitral valve. *Br. Heart J.* 1976; **38**: 1053–7.

58. Savage, D.D., Levy, D., Garrison, R.J., Castelli, W.P., Kligfield, P., Devereux, R.B., Anderson, S.J., Kannel, W.B. and Feinleib, M. Mitral valve prolapse in the general population. 3. Dysrhythmias: The Framingham Study. *Am. Heart J.* 1983; **106**: 582–6.

59. Duren, D., Becker, A. and Dunning, A.J. Long-term follow-up of idiopathic mitral valve prolapse in 300 patients: a prospective study. *J. Am. Coll. Cardiol.* 1988; **11**: 42–7.

60. Kannel, W.B., Gordon, T. and Offutt, D. Left ventricular hypertrophy by electrocardiogram; prevalence, incidence and mortality in the Framingham study. *Ann. Intern. Med.* 1969; **71**: 89–105.

61. McLenachan, J.M., Henderson, E., Morris, K.I. and Dargie, H.J. Ventricular arrhythmias in patients with hypertensive left ventricular hypertrophy. *N. Engl. J. Med.* 1987; **317**: 787–92.

62. Klein, G.J. and Gulamhusien, S.S. Intermittent preexcitation in the Wolff–Parkinson–White syndrome. *Am. J. Cardiol.* 1983; **52**: 292–6.

63. McKenna, W.J. Arrhythmia and prognosis in hypertrophic cardiomyopathy. *Eur. Heart J.* 1983; **4** (Suppl. F): 225–34.

64. McKenna, W.J., Oakley, C.M., Krikler, D.M. and Goodwin, J.F. Improved survival with amiodarone in patients with hypertrophic cardiomyopathy and ventricular tachycardia. *Br. Heart J.* 1985; **53**: 412–6.

65. Packer, M. Sudden unexpected death in patients with congestive heart failure: a second frontier. *Circulation* 1985; **72**: 681–5.

66. Olshausen, K.V., Stienen, U., Schwarz, F., Kubler, W. and Meyer, J. Long-term prognostic significance of ventricular arrhythmias in idiopathic dilated cardiomyopathy. *Am. J. Cardiol.* 1988; **61**: 146–51.

67. Ward, D.E. The management of arrhythmias in children; are electrophysiological studies of value? *Int. J. Cardiol.* 1987; 11: 149–64.

68. Levy, A.M., Camm, A.J. and Keane, J.F. Multiple arrhythmias detected during nocturnal monitoring in patients with congenital complete heart block. *Circulation* 1977; 55: 247–53.

69. Dewey, R.C., Capeless, M.A. and Levy, A.M. Use of ambulatory electrocardiographic monitoring to identify high-risk patients with congenital complete heart block. *N. Engl. J. Med.* 1987; 316: 835–9.

70. Hayes, C.J. and Gersony, W.M. Arrhythmias after Mustard operation for transposition of the great arteries. *J. Am. Coll. Cardiol.* 1986; 7: 133–7.

71. Deanfield, J.E., McKenna, W.J. and Hallidie-Smith, K.A. Detection of late arrhythmia and conduction disturbance after correction of tetralogy of Fallot. *Br. Heart J.* 1980; 44: 248–53.

72. Garson, A., Randall, D.C., Gillette, P.C., Smith, R.T., Moak, J.P., McVey, P. and McNamara, D.G. Prevention of sudden death after repair of tetralogy of Fallot: Treatment of ventricular arrhythmias. *J. Am. Coll. Cardiol.* 1985; 6: 221–7.

73. Katz, N.M., Blackstone, E.H. Kirklin, J.W., Pacifico, A.D. and Bargeron, L.M. Late survival and symptoms after repair of tetralogy of Fallot. *Circulation* 1982; 65: 403–10.

74. Shannon, D.C. and Kelly, D.H. SIDS and near-SIDS. *N. Engl. J. Med.* 1982; 306: 959–65, 1022–8.

75. Schwartz, P.J. The quest for the mechanisms of the sudden infant death syndrome: doubts and progress. *Circulation* 1987; 75: 677–83.

76. Oren, J., Kelly, D. and Shannon, D.C. Identification of a high-risk group for sudden infant death syndrome among infants who were resuscitated for sleep apnoea. *Pediatrics* 1986; 77: 495–9.

77. Maron, B.J., Clarke, C.E., Goldstein, R.E. and Epstein, S.E. Potential role of QT interval prolongation in sudden infant death syndrome. *Circulation* 1976; 54: 423–30.

78. Gunteroth, W.G. The QT interval and sudden infant death syndrome. *Circulation* 1982; 66: 502–4.

79. Ward, D.E. Prolongation of the QT interval as an indicator of risk of a cardiac event. *Eur. Heart J.* 1988; 9: suppG. 139–44.

80. Southall, D.P. *et al.* Identification of infants destined to die unexpectedly during infancy: evaluation of predictive importance of prolonged apnoea and disorders of cardiac rhythm or conduction. *Br. Med. J.* 1983; 286: 1092–6.

81. Sadeh, D., Shannon, D., Abboud, S., Saul, J.P., Akselrod, S. and Cohen, R.J. Altered cardiac repolarization in some victims of sudden infant death syndrome. *N. Engl. J. Med.* 1987; 317: 1501–5.

82. Roelandt, J., Klootwijk, P., Lubsen, J. and Janse, M.J. Sudden death during longterm ambulatory monitoring. *Eur. Heart J.* 1984; 5: 7–20.

83. Panidis, I. and Morganroth, J. Sudden death in hospitalized patients: cardiac rhythm disturbances detected by ambulatory electrocardiographic monitoring. *J. Am. Coll. Cardiol.* 1983; 5: 798–805.

84. Pratt, C.M., Francis, M.J., Luck, J.C., Wyndham, C.R., Miller, R.R. and Quinones, M.A. Analysis of ambulatory electrocardiograms in 15 patients during spontaneous ventricular fibrillation with special reference to preceding arrhythmic events. *J. Am. Coll. Cardiol.* 1983; 5: 789–97.

85. Savage, H.R., Kissane, J.Q., Becher, E.L., Maddocks, W.Q., Murtaugh, J.T. and Dizadji, H. Analysis of ambulatory electrocardiograms in 14 patients who experienced sudden cardiac death during monitoring. *Clin. Cardiol.* 1987; 10: 621–32.

86. Krasnow, A.Z. and Bloomfield, D.K. Artifacts in portable electrocardiographic monitoring. *Am. Heart J.* 1976; 91: 349–57.

87. Hombach, V., Braun, V., Hopp, H.W., Gil-Sanchez, D., Scholl, H., Behrenbeck, D.W., Tauchert, M. and Hilger, H.H. The applicability of the signal averaging technique in clinical cardiology. *Clin. Cardiol.* 1982; 5: 107–24.

88. Simson, M.B. Use of signals in the terminal QRS complex to identify patients with ventricular tachycardia after myocardial infarction. *Circulation* 1981; 64: 235–42.

89. Breithardt, G., Becker, R., Seipel, L., Abendroth, R. and Ostermeyer, J. Non-invasive detection of late-potentials in man — a new marker for ventricular tachycardia. *Eur. Heart J.* 1981; 2: 1–11.

90. Breithardt, G. and Borggrefe, M. Pathophysiological mechanisms and clinical significance of ventricular potentials. *Eur. Heart J.* 1986; 7: 364–77.

91. Denniss, A.R., Richards, D.A., Cody, D.V., Russell, P.A., Young, A.A., Cooper, M., Ross, D.L. and Uther, J.B. Prognostic significance of ventricular tachycardia and fibrillation induced at programmed stimulation and delayed potentials detected on the signal averaged electrocardiograms of survivors of acute myocardial infarction. *Circulation* 1986; 74: 731–45.

92. Kuchar, D.L., Thorburn, C.W. and Sammel, N.L. Prediction of serious arrhythmic events after myocardial infarction: signal-averaged electrocardiogram, Holter monitoring and radionuclide ventriculography. *J. Am. Coll. Cardiol.* 1987; 9: 531–8.

93. Kuchar, D.L., Thorburn, C.W. and Sammel, N.L. Signal-averaged electrocardiogram for evaluation of recurrent syncope. *Am. J. Cardiol.* 1986; 58: 949–53.

94. Poll, D.S., Marchlinski, F.E., Falcone, R.A. and Josephson, M.E. Abnormal signal-averaged electrocardiograms in patients with nonischemic congestive cardiomyopathy: relationship to sustained ventricular tachyarrhythmias. *Circulation* 1985; 72: 1308–13.

95. Lindsay, B.D., Ambos, H.D., Schechtman, K.B. and Cain, M.E. Improved selection of patients for programmed ventricular stimulation by frequency analysis of signal-averaged electrocardiograms. *Circulation* 1986; 73: 675–83.

96. Haberl, R., Weber, M., Reichenspurner, H., Kemkes, B.M., Osterholzer, G., Anthuber, M. and Steinbeck, G. Frequency analysis of the surface electrocardiogram for recognition of acute rejection after orthotopic cardiac transplantation in man. *Circulation* 1987; 76: 101–8.

97. Kelen, G.J., Henken, R., Restivo, M., Zeiler, R.H., Caref, E.B. and El-Sherif, N. Signal averaging of high-gain Holter ECG recordings — validation of a new technique for detection of after-potentials. *J. Am. Coll. Cardiol.* 1986; 7: 104A.

98. Southall, D.P., Richards, J., Mitchell, P., Brown, D.J., Johnston, P.G.B. and Shinebourne, E.A. Study of cardiac rhythm in healthy newborn infants. *Br. Heart J.* 1980; 43: 14–20.

Chapter 11

Clinical Cardiac Electrophysiology

A. John Camm and Ghazwan S. Butrous

INTRODUCTION

The introduction of His bundle electrogram recording 30 years ago has refined the diagnosis and management of cardiac arrhythmias.[1-4] Stimulation of the heart can initiate and terminate the majority of paroxysmal arrhythmias.[3] Therefore, it is possible to study these tachycardias electively and record the cardiac activation sequence during the arrhythmia. Such studies, which were initiated in the late 1960s and early 1970s, form the basis of clinical cardiac electrophysiology which is now an important part of cardiology practice, providing useful clinical information for diagnosis and therapy.

INDICATIONS

The usual indications for clinical electrophysiology studies include elucidation of symptoms, evaluation of an abnormal electrocardiogram, assessment of risk and design of treatment.

SYMPTOMS

Palpitations, pre-syncope or syncope may be caused by transient cardiac arrhythmias which are difficult to capture on an electrocardiographic record.[5] The arrhythmia may be provoked at electrophysiology study; the relationship between the symptom and a precisely diagnosed arrhythmia can then be evaluated. Patients with undiagnosed recurrent sudden syncope merit electrophysiology study if neurological studies and non-invasive cardiac studies have been inconclusive. Recurrent paroxysmal rapid sustained palpitations should also be investigated if they are associated with features of cardiovascular insufficiency or distress.[6-8]

ABNORMAL ELECTROCARDIOGRAM

Sinus node pauses, conduction defects, such as bi-or tri-fascicular block, or undiagnosed tachycardia, such as broad complex tachycardia, merit further electrophysiology characterization.[7-9] In patients with symptoms suggestive of serious brachycardia, evaluation of sinus node function and atrioventricular conduction should be undertaken (in patients with symptoms suggestive of serious brady-cardia).[10-12] A broad complex tachycardia may originate from a supraventricular source (conducted with aberration) or from the ventricles. An electrophysiology study will help to make this important distinction. Narrow QRS complex tachycardias arise from a variety of substrates and successful therapy may depend on accurate information derived from electrophysiology study.[13,14]

RISK

Prognosis and the risk of morbidity can be clarified by electrophysiology study in patients who have survived an episode of cardiac arrest, have pre-excitation or have suffered myocardial infarction.[15-18]

THERAPY

The exact prescription of therapy for serious cardic arrhythmias is improved by using electrophysiology techniques. This is particularly useful for drug treatment of ventricular tachycardia, pacemaker/device treatment of tachyarrhythmia, operative or catheter ablation of tachycardia foci or conduction pathways, and pacemaker treatment of bradyarrhythmia (see below). The relative importance of conducting electrophysiology studies in a variety of situations is shown in Table 11.1.

METHODOLOGY

Clinical cardiac electrophysiology is an invasive technique which must be performed in a cardiac

Table 11.1. Indications for electrophysiology study.

Mandatory
Cardiac arrest survivors
Hypotensive ventricular tachycardia
Wolff–Parkinson–White with rapid atrial fibrillation

Usual
Syncope of unknown cause
Sustained ventricular tachycardia
Symptomatic Wolff–Parkinson–White syndrome

Useful
Symptomatic paroxysmal supraventricular tachycardia
Asymptomatic Wolff–Parkinson–White syndrome
Post myocardial infarction (high risk)
Undocumented paroxysmal tachycardia
Broad QRS tachycardia ? origin
Assessment of His–Purkinje conduction effects

catheterization laboratory where adequate fluoroscopy, electrocardiographic monitoring, resuscitation equipment, etc., are available. These studies should be performed by an appropriately trained cardiologist or, preferably, by two cardiologists working together. Additional personnel such as a nurse and a trained cardiac technician are also needed.[19]

EQUIPMENT

Equipment essential for electrophysiology studies is discussed below (Fig. 11.1).

Electrodes

Electrode catheters are used to record intracardiac signals and to stimulate the heart. The typical catheter is made of woven Dacron or polyurethane and has platinum ring electrodes. There are many types and shapes available which have been designed to perform specific functions. The basic electrode configuration is bipolar with 1 cm interelectrode spacing, but tripolar and quadripolar electrodes with different interelectrode spacing are also available.

Recording devices

The intracardiac signal is modulated by specially designed amplifiers, of which at least three must be available. The usual band width of these amplifiers is 50–500 Hz. The recording of monophasic action potentials requires a much lower high-pass setting, for example 0.05 Hz. Three or more intracardiac signals are recorded, together with at least three orthogonal, or approximately orthogonal surface electrocardiographic leads, for example, I, aVF and V_1. The physiological recorder must be a high-fidelity system (ink-jet, ultraviolet or electrostatic) capable of recording at paper speeds of at least 100 mm/s. The recorder is run almost continuously throughout the study, unless the signals are also being recorded on a high-fidelity tape recorder.

Monitoring devices

During the conduct of an electrophysiology study, cardiac arrhythmias will be provoked. Rapid correction of these arrhythmias may be required. The positioning of electrodes is assisted by electrographic confirmation. Real-time electrocardiographic monitoring is therefore essential. Multiple monitoring channels are needed to allow adequate arrhythmia diagnosis directly from the oscilloscope.

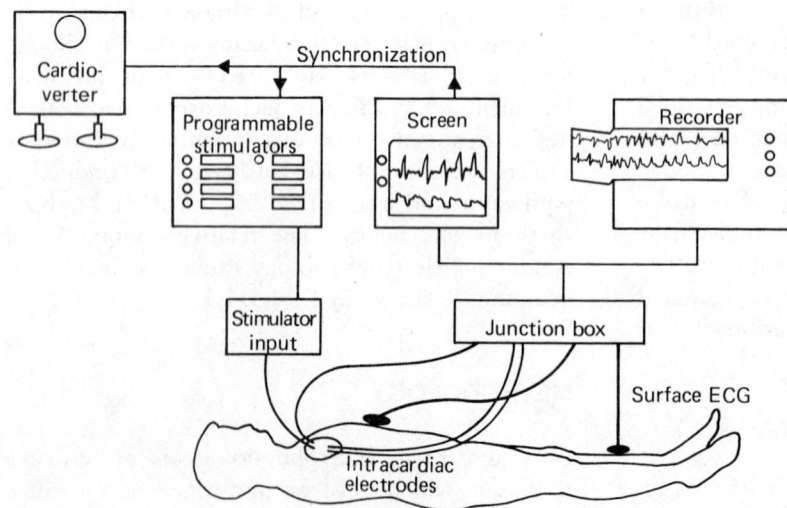

Fig. 11.1. The equipment necessary to perform an electrophysiology study comprises a programmable stimulator, multichannel physiological recorder, multichannel oscilloscope and isolated amplifiers. It is also essential that resuscitation equipment, including a defibrillator/cardioverter, is available.

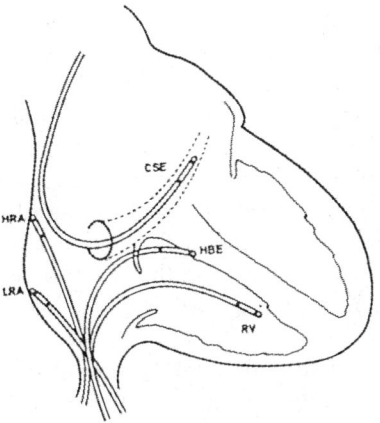

Fig. 11.2. Diagram demonstrating electrode disposition. HRA, high right atrium; LRA, low right atrium; CSE, coronary sinus electrodes; RV, right ventricle; HBE, His bundle electrodes.

In most laboratories, an 8-channel persistence monitor is chosen. In addition, a second monitor is used which usually has 3 or 4 channels and can be triggered by stimulation pulses to produce a frozen display.

Electrophysiology stimulators

Conventional pacemakers are inadequate for performing an electrophysiology study. The stimulator must be able to pace at a wide range (30–600 beats/min) of rates, for precise durations (or numbers of stimuli). It is necessary to introduce between 1 and 3 precisely timed extrastimuli during spontaneous or paced rhythms. The stimulus pulse width and amplitude must be independently variable.[20] Electrophysiology stimulators are commercially available and modern systems are microprocessor controlled.

Resuscitation equipment

As an electrophysiology study involves the placement of intracardiac electrode leads and the intentional provocation of potentially serious cardiac arrhythmias, it is essential to have resuscitation equipment, especially a defibrillator, immediately available. Direct current cardioversion of an arrhythmia, such as atrial fibrillation, that has been induced by the study is often necessary to allow successful completion of the study.

CLINICAL TECHNIQUE

Preparation

Prior to electrophysiology study, the patient is starved for about 12 h because of the possibility of inducing a cardiac arrest during the study. Heavy sedation is avoided because it may hamper the intended provocation of tachycardia and it may prevent the patient's active co-operation during the study. Light sedation with diazepam,[21] which does not affect the electrophysiological properties of the heart, may be necessary with nervous patients. Electrode leads are introduced under local anaesthetic, usually lignocaine (< 2.5 mg/kg).[22] Large amounts of lignocaine must not be given because it may suppress arrhythmia induction. General anaesthesia is occasionally necessary, particularly for young children. When the aim of the electrophysiology study is diagnosis and assessment of an arrhythmia, it is essential to discontinue anti-arrhythmic drugs 3–5 elimination half-lives prior to the study. It is often impracticable to discontinue amiodarone for 6 months or more but it should be stopped as long as possible prior to study. As contrast materials may disturb cardiac electrophysiology, it is unwise to combine coronary arteriography and electrophysiology study during the same procedure.

Catheterization

Electrode leads are introduced via the peripheral vascular system and negotiated under fluoroscopic and electrographic control into the appropriate intracardiac position (Fig. 11.2). Percutaneous puncture of the femoral or subclavian vein, or femoral artery, will allow the insertion of the leads. It is recommended that pressure recordings are made directly from the femoral or radial artery during study of ventricular tachycardia.

The number and location of intracardiac electrodes are determined by the purpose of the study (Table 11.2).

Useful information about the diagnosis of palpitations or the elucidation of an abnormal electrocardiogram can be obtained with a single atrial bipole. However, in most instances, it is necessary to record and stimulate in one or more cardiac chambers. A routine study for the evaluation of supraventricular tachycardia involves the placement of high right atrial, His bundle, coronary sinus and right ventricular electrodes (Fig. 11.2). A full study of ventricular tachycardia may require recording

Table 11.2. Types of electrophysiological study.

Type	Electrodes	Examples
Atrial	Single transvenous or oesophageal	Broad QRS tachycardia PSVT ? type WPW risk PSVT drug design
His	Single transvenous	AV/IV conduction
Ventricular	Single transvenous	Provocation of VT Drug design for VT
Pacemaker	Double transvenous	AV Wenckebach VA conduction time
Full	Four or more transvenous or arterial	Diagnostic PSVT study VT/WPW/AVNRT pre-surgery

Definitions: WPW, Wolff–Parkinson–White syndrome; AV, atrioventricular; IV, intraventricular; PSVT, paroxysmal supraventricular tachycardia; VT, ventricular tachycardia; AVNRT, atrioventricular nodal re-entrant tachycardia.

and stimulating in the left as well as the right ventricle.

The high right atrial electrodes are positioned as close as possible to the sinus node at the junction of the superior vena cava and right atrium. It is important to avoid right phrenic nerve stimulation. The His bundle electrode catheter is first inserted through the right atrium into the outflow tract of the right ventricle. As the lead is withdrawn, a clockwise torque is applied whilst recording signals from the electrodes. A stable electrode position which provides a consistent high-amplitude His bundle electrogram is selected.[23]

Catheterization of the coronary sinus may be difficult and is usually achieved in only about 90% of cases. Success is improved by the use of pre-shaped catheters inserted through the subclavian vein. Both the right ventricular apex and outflow tract should be stimulated when attempting to provoke ventricular tachycardia. Left ventricular stimulation and catheter mapping are often necessary for the complete evaluation of ventricular tachycardia. All catheters are positioned in order to obtain satisfactory pacing and sensing. Routine stimulation is performed with a 2-ms pulse set at twice the late diastolic threshold. Repeated threshold measurements are an essential part of each study protocol.[24]

ELECTROPHYSIOLOGY STUDY MEASUREMENTS

A typical example of a trace recorded at 100 mm/s

is illustrated in Fig. 11.3. The following measurements are usually made to an accuracy of 5 ms.

1 *PP interval* (sinus discharge interval): measured between adjacent high right atrial electrograms and averaged for 10 consecutive cycles.
2 *PA interval* (intra-atrial conduction time): from the earliest onset of atrial activity (on any lead) to the interinscoid deflection of the low right atrial electrogram (on the His bundle lead). The normal range of values in adults is 25–55 ms.[25,26]
3 *AH interval* (intra-atrioventricular nodal conduction time): from the interinscoid deflection of the low right atrial electrogram to the onset of the His bundle electrogram. The normal range is 60–120 ms.[25–27]

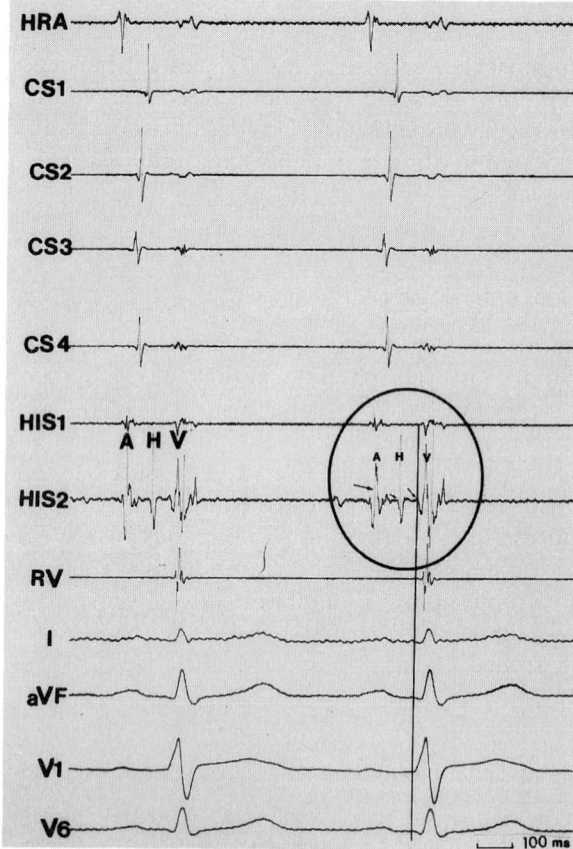

Fig. 11.3. Classic recordings derived during sinus rhythm. It is useful to record His bundle electrograms from two bipoles (HIS1 and HIS2) adjacent to the His bundle so that movement/displacement does not result in loss of the His bundle deflection. Multiple coronary sinus electrograms from electrodes situated proximally (CS4) and distally (CS1) should be recorded. These traces illustrate the method of measuring the AH and HV intervals (see text). HRA, high right atrium; RV, right ventricle.

4 *HV interval* (His-Purkinje conduction time): from the onset of the His bundle electrogram to the onset of the QRS complex (on any lead) (Fig. 11.3). Normally, this interval should be between 35 and 55 ms.[25,27]

5 *QRS duration* (ventricular activation time): earliest onset to latest offset on any and all surface leads (normally < 110 ms).

6 *QT interval* (an approximation of ventricular repolarization time): measured from the simultaneous surface ECG lead recordings.

These measurements are usually made during sinus rhythm and during atrial pacing at several cycle lengths, such as 600 and 400 ms. The ability of tissue to sustain conduction at high driving frequencies can be measured by slow acceleration to the point of conduction failure. An example of this technique is the determination of the *atrioventricular Wenckebach cycle length* by gradual increase of the atrial pacing rate until there is failure to conduct to the ventricles.[28,29]

Cardiac tissue refractoriness is assessed by pacing techniques which involve baseline stimulation at a fixed cycle length (usually 600 or 400 ms) for approximately 8 beats (S_1) followed by the introduction of an extrastimulus (S_2) coupled to the last basic drive beat by a progressively shorter interval (decrementation) (Fig. 11.4).[30,31] When the extrastimulus coupling interval is shorter than the *refractory period*, the extrastimulus will fail to excite tissue or to result in a propagated impulse. Examples of measures of refractoriness are given below.

1 *Atrial effective refractory period* (normal = 170–300 ms) is the longest atrial extrastimulus coupling interval (S_1–S_2) which fails to excite the atrium.

2 *Atrioventricular nodal effective refractory period* (normal = 230–430 ms) is the longest atrial depolarization coupling interval (A_1–A_2) measured from the His bundle electrode signal which fails to conduct through the atrioventricular node to the His bundle.

3 *Atrioventricular nodal functional refractory period* (normal = 330–500 ms) is the shortest His bundle depolarization interval (H_1–H_2) occurring as a result of atrial stimulation

4 *Ventricular effective refractory period* (normal = 180–280 ms) is the longest ventricular extrastimulus coupling interval (V_1–V_2) which fails to result in ventricular depolarization.

5 *Effective refractory period of an accessory pathway* is the longest atrial depolarization coupling interval (A_1–A_2), at a point near to the insertion of the accessory pathway, which fails to conduct through the pathway.

Cardiac tissue may conduct an impulse in a *decremental* or 'all or none' fashion. Atrioventricular nodal tissue usually responds decrementally and accessory pathways display 'all or none' conduction. Decremental conduction is characterized by progressive conduction delay in response to premature or faster stimulation. The functional refractory period of such tissue is longer than its effective refractory period. The difference between these types of conduction can be used to detect accessory pathway conduction.

Impulse generation or pacemaker behaviour can be tested by assessing the recovery of the pacemaker after a period of *overdrive suppression* or by testing the delay produced following the artificial insertion of a premature beat which conducts into the pacemaker and resets its cycle. These tests have been most widely applied to test sino-atrial node function but they have also been used to evaluate idio-junctional pacemakers.

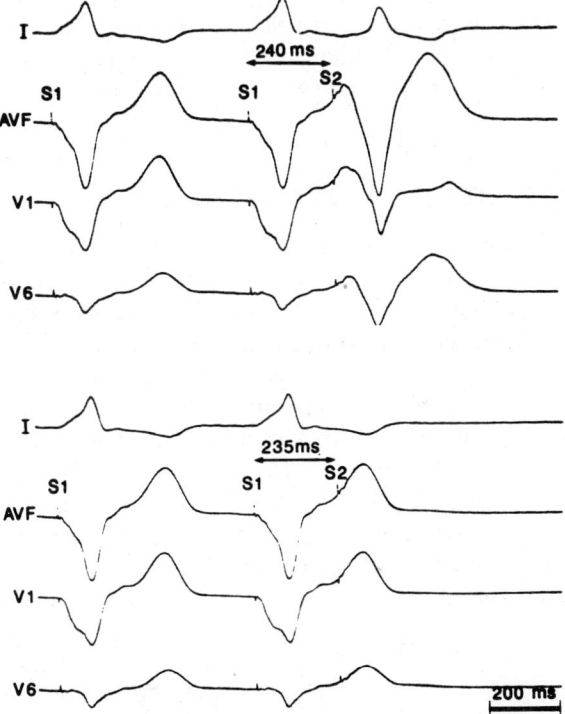

Fig. 11.4. The assessment of tissue refractoriness is illustrated in these two panels. After a period of constant rate ventricular pacing (S1 stimuli), a premature beat is introduced (S2). Ventricular depolarization results with an S1–S2 interval of 240 ms but not when the S1–S2 interval is reduced to 235 ms. In this case, the ventricular effective refractory period is 235 ms.

STIMULATION PROTOCOLS

The details of stimulation programmes depend on the purpose of the study. For example, the investigation of a patient with syncope and bundle branch block concentrates on the assessment of His–Purkinje conduction and attempted provocation of ventricular tachycardia. A patient with a history of syncope and Wolff–Parkinson–White pattern on the surface electrocardiogram is assessed by determining the refractory period of the accessory pathway, its conduction potential during induced atrial fibrillation and the location of the pathway. A baseline study, common to most investigations, includes measurement of anterograde (A to V) and retrograde (V to A) conduction intervals in response to atrial and ventricular stimulation, respectively, sinus node response to overdrive suppression (for example, by pacing for 1 min at a rate of 130 beats/min), atrioventricular and ventriculoatrial Wenckebach cycle lengths and atrial, atrioventricular nodal, ventricular and ventriculoatrial refractory periods.

USE OF ANTI-ARRHYTHMIC DRUGS IN ELECTROPHYSIOLOGY STUDIES

Drugs are used for 4 purposes: to identify tissue type by characteristic response to specific drugs, to provoke electrophysiological abnormalities, to evaluate therapeutic response and to assess risk.

Tissue electropharmacological characterization

An example is the differentation of atrioventricular nodal (decremental) tissue from accessory pathway tissue (all or none) by their response to class I (e.g. ajmaline) and class IV (e.g. verapamil) anti-arrhythmic drugs (Table 11.3).

Provocation of electrophysiological abnormalities

Disopyramide, flecainide and procainamide have been used to detect latent intraventricular conduction defects and sinus node dysfunction. Damaged or diseased tissue is markedly suppressed by these drugs but normal tissue is not much affected by them.

Assessment of therapeutic response

The inducibility and characteristics of tachyarrhythmias can be evaluated before and after treatment with anti-arrhythmic drugs. The prevention of tachycardia inducibility or a decrease in the rate of induced tachycardia following drug treatment suggests that the tachycardia will not occur spontaneously or will not cause serious symptoms, respectively, if the drug and/or drugs are prescribed for treatment.[32] Therapeutic testing may involve multiple drug trials. This may be achieved by repeat catheterization or by leaving one or more stable electrodes *in situ* whilst *serial drug testing* is carried out (Fig. 11.5).[33,34]

Assessment of risk

Conduction through accessory pathways with long effective refractory periods (> 270 ms) is more easily suppressed by some class I drugs (for example, procainamide) than is conduction through the more dangerous accessory pathways that recover more rapidly.

CATHETER MAPPING TECHNIQUES

If tachycardia can be induced, it is sometimes necessary to locate its origin or conduction pathway. When an accessory pathway is responsible for the expression or maintenance of tachycardia, its position should be accurately determined by recording electrograms from around the atrioventricular groove during the tachycardia. Bipoles with short interelectrode spacing (< 1 cm) record electrograms derived predominantly from local myocardium. The earliest electrogram recorded from the atrium, during atrioventricular re-entrant tachycardia, indicates the position of the accessory pathway.[35]

Table 11.3. **Electropharmacological tissue characterization.**

Tissue	Response to verapamil		Response to ajmaline	
	Conduction	Refractoriness	Conduction	Refractoriness
Atrioventricular node	Slowed	Increased	Not slowed	Not increased
Accessory pathway	Not slowed	Not increased	Slowed	Increased

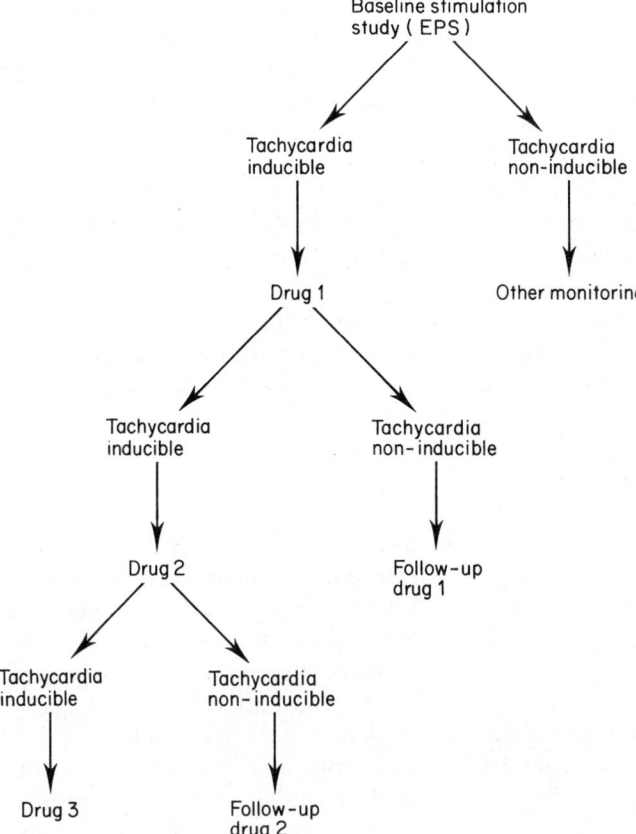

Fig. 11.5. Scheme to show serial drug testing.

Catheter mapping techniques are essential if it is proposed to ablate tissue by either catheter or surgical methods.

COMPLICATIONS

Most of the complications of an electrophysiology study[36,37] are similar to those of cardiac catheterization. As the procedure may take 2–3 h and sedation is not used, patient discomfort is common. The patient is exposed to more radiation than is usual with coronary angiography[36,37]. Bleeding (0.1–0.5%), thrombosis (0.5–0.6%), pulmonary embolus (< 0.3%) are no more frequent than is usual with cardiac catheterization. Pneumothorax may occur when percutaneous access to the subclavian vein is used. Arrhythmias are frequently provoked as an intentional part of the study. When unwanted arrhythmias are accidentally induced, they are treated conventionally. Drug treatment is avoided unless the study is otherwise complete. Catheter-induced trauma may cause transient right bundle branch block and, occasionally, accessory pathway conduction may be similarly blocked.

Death from this procedure is unusual, but occurs rarely in patients with severe left ventricular dysfunction, hypertrophic cardiomyopathy or left main coronary disease.[36,37]

ASSESSMENT OF SINUS NODE FUNCTION AND DISEASE

Sinus node dysfunction is most readily detected clinically and by long-term electrocardiographic recordings. However, electrophysiology tests of sinus node function, such as sinus node recovery time, sino-atrial conduction and sinus node refractoriness, are insensitive but specific.

SINUS NODE RECOVERY TIME

Sinus node recovery time is a measure of the automaticity of the atrioventricular node which is assessed by rapid atrial pacing at a rate of 100–160 beats/min for periods of 30 s to 2 min. Pacing-induced atrial beats repetitively depolarize the sinus node which takes time to recover when pacing is discontinued.[38,39] Sinus node dysfunction may be manifest as a prolongation of the recovery time which is measured from the high right atrial trace between the last paced atrial depolarization and the first spontaneous sinus depolarization. The result is usually expressed as the sinus node recovery time minus the spontaneous sinus cycle length. This *corrected sinus node recovery time* should be < 550 ms. The recovery time can also be corrected by expressing it as a percentage of the spontaneous sinus cycle length, which should be < 1.6 for patients with sinus cycle lengths > 800 ms and < 1.83 for faster sinus rates. Patients with sinus node dysfunction may also have secondary pauses which occur during the first 8–10 beats following the discontinuation of atrial pacing. This test has been estimated to have a sensitivity between 35 and 90%. This variable result is probably due to autonomic variation, age factors and the broad spectrum of sinus node disorders.[40,41]

SINO–ATRIAL CONDUCTION TIME

Sino-atrial conduction time is a measurement of the time taken for a depolarization to conduct from the atrium to the sinus node or vice versa. The *Strauss method*[42] for assessing this interval involves scanning the sinus cycle with a timed atrial premature beat. Late diastolic beats simply collide with the emerging spontaneous sinus beat but earlier beats depolarize the sinus node and reset its discharge cycle. The conduction time can be measured by subtracting the sinus cycle from the cycle following the atrial premature beat. The normal value is 50–150 ms. The *Narula method*[43] involves pacing the atrium for 8 beats at a rate 5–10 beats/min faster than the spontaneous sinus rate. The conduction time is measured by subtracting the average sinus cycle length from the first sinus cycle following the termination of pacing. Sinus node suppression induced by single or repeated atrial beats may artefactually lengthen the sino-atrial conduction time. *Direct recording*[44] of sinus node potentials through high-gain, low-frequency (0.1–20 Hz) amplifiers avoids this problem. The sino-atrial conduction time is measured from the start of the sinus potential to the beginning of the surface P wave. This method appears to be accurate but it has a low sensitivity because the potentials are difficult to record. Using this method the normal range of conduction times is 25–55 ms.

Changes in autonomic tone modulate sinus node activity and affect sinus node function tests. Much

of this variability can be removed by autonomic blockade with atropine 0.04 mg/kg and propranolol 0.2 mg/kg. Sick sinus syndrome can be differentiated from carotid sinus syndrome and other reflex forms of sinus node suppression by this technique.[45]

ASSESSMENT OF ATRIOVENTRICULAR CONDUCTION

In the normal heart, atrioventricular conduction involves transmission through the atrioventricular node, the His bundle and the Purkinje system. In conjunction with the surface electrocardiographic recording of low right atrial activity and the His bundle electrogram, conduction through the component parts can be individually assessed. The intervals recorded during normal sinus rhythm may demonstrate impaired conduction. For example, an HV interval > 55 ms suggests abnormal His-Purkinje conduction and an HV interval of 100 ms or more suggests such severely prolonged conduction that a pacemaker should be prophylactically implanted.[46,47] A split His bundle electrogram results from severe impairment of conduction within the His bundle itself. Delayed atrioventricular nodal conduction is manifest as a prolongation of the AH interval (Fig. 11.6).

Complete heart block can occur within the atrioventricular node (between the A and H deflections) or the His-Purkinje system (between the H and V electrograms). Congenital heart block, and other forms of heart block associated with narrow QRS escape rhythms, are due to block above the His bundle (block between the A and H electrograms). These conditions are relatively benign. The usual broad QRS complex forms of acquired heart block are due to conduction block below the His

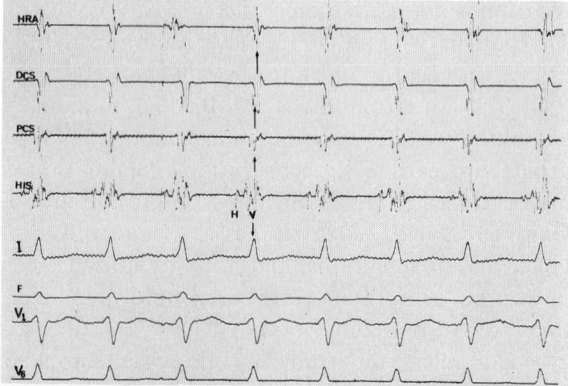

Fig. 11.6. These recordings demonstrate first degree atrioventricular block due to atrioventricular nodal conduction delay. The AH interval is prolonged. HB, His bundle recording.

bundle (between the H and V electrograms) (Fig. 11.7).[47,48]

Retrograde conduction intervals in response to ventricular pacing can also be measured. As the His depolarization is usually buried within the paced ventricular electrogram only the ventriculo-atrial interval can be routinely assessed. Retrograde conduction occurs in about 60% of patients with normal anterograde conduction.[49]

The atrioventricular conduction system can be 'stressed' by rapid atrial pacing or by the introduction of atrial premature beats. Rapid atrial pacing is used to provoke Wenckebach conduction block (Mobitz type I) within the atrioventricular node. This is characterized by progressive prolongation of the AH conduction time and subsequent conduction block within the atrioventricular node, between the A and H electrograms (Fig. 11.6).[28] The point at which block ensues is known as the *Wenckebach length*. Block within the His-Purkinje system occurs in Mobitz type II block. Suddenly, a His bundle depolarization is not followed by a ventricular electrocardiogram. This is usually associated with bundle branch block and suggests a need for pacemaker implantation. Careful measurement of HV intervals preceding the blocked beat often demonstrates slight progressive HV prolongation. More obvious Wenckebach cycles rarely occur at an infra-His level.

Anterograde conduction can be assessed by introducing a premature atrial beat after constant rate atrial pacing associated with stable conduction (basic drive). The intervals between the electrograms associated with the last beat of the basic drive

(A_1, H_1 and V_1) and the electrograms of the premature beat (A_2, H_2 and V_2) are used to construct an *anterograde conduction curve* (Fig. 11.8). The intervals between consecutive His bundle electrograms (H_1–H_2) and ventricular electrograms (V_1–V_2) are plotted against the atrial (A_1–A_2) intervals. The normal anterograde conduction curve is 'hockey stick' in shape because of the decremental conduction properties of the atrioventricular node. Bypass tracts conduct without decrement and modify the anterograde conduction curve depending on the proportion of the atrioventricular node (partial or total) that is bypassed. For example, a direct

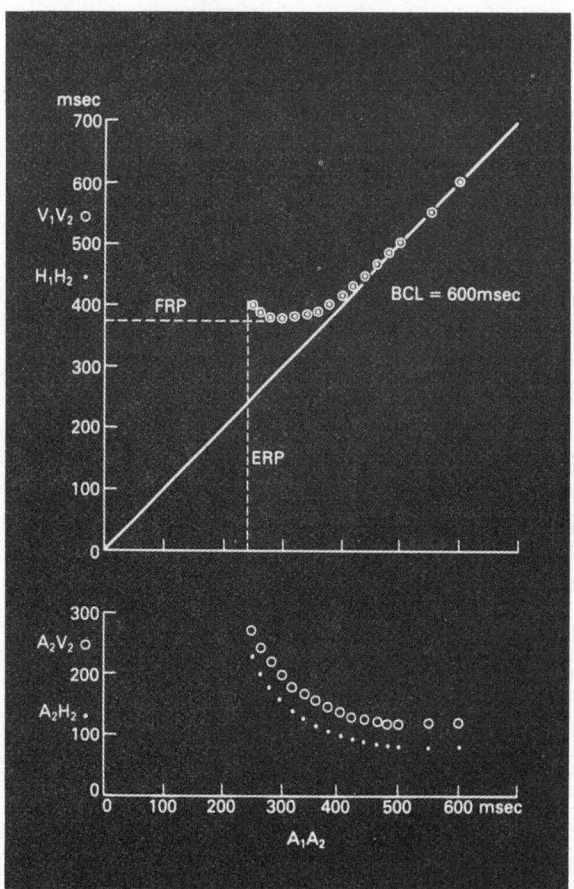

Fig. 11.8. An anterograde conduction curve is a plot of the response to a premature atrial extrastimulus. The resulting atrial beat (A_2) conducts to the His bundle (H_2) and the ventricle (V_2). The premature beat is delivered after a sequence of 8 beats delivered at a constant rate. The deflections associated with the normal beat are A_1, H_1 and V_1. The H_1–H_2 and V_1–V_2 intervals are plotted against the coupling interval of the atrial premature beat (A_1–A_2). The normal curve is continuous and 'hockey stick' in shape because of the additional atrioventricular nodal delay imposed by increasing prematurity of the atrial beat. ERP, effective refractory period of the atrioventricular node; FRP, functional refractory period of the atrioventricular node; BCL, basic cycle length of atrial pacing.

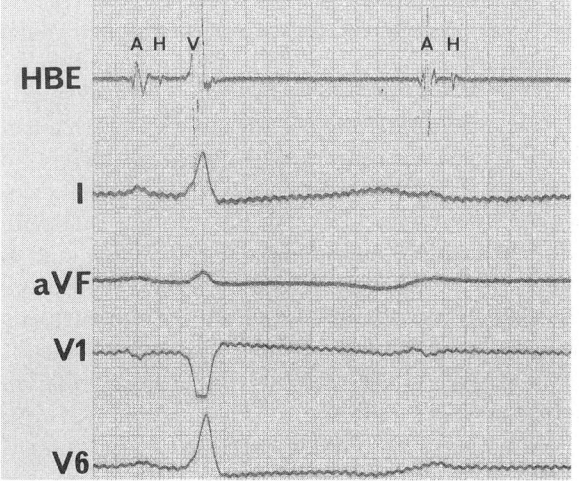

Fig. 11.7. Infra-Hisian block in patient with complete heart block. Notice that there is no conduction below His potential to the ventricles.

atrioventricular connection that totally bypasses the atrioventricular node results in a conduction curve that hugs the line of identity until the refractory period of the bypass is reached. Dual AH conduction can be recognized by a typical jump from slow to fast conduction in the anterograde conduction curve. The jump should be of at least a 50-ms increase in the H_1–H_2 interval for a 10-ms decrement in the A_1–A_2 interval.[28]

Retrograde conduction curves (A_1–A_2 against V_1–V_2) can also be constructed by introducing a ventricular premature beat after a short period of stable ventricular pacing. The shape of this curve is particularly useful in the diagnosis of retrograde conduction through a direct atrioventricular connection. In this case, the curve does not deviate from the line of identity.

ASSESSMENT OF SUPRAVENTRICULAR TACHYCARDIA

Supraventricular tachycardias that are paroxysmal in nature are usually re-entrant in origin (Fig. 11.9) and are amenable to electrophysiology study. The main indication for study is a tachycardia that has been difficult to contain with empiric treatment and which requires a more specific drug treatment, or a pacemaker/surgical solution. Other indications include differentiation between a ventricular and supraventricular origin if the tachycardia has a wide QRS complex, elucidation of recurrent palpitations not documented with an electrocardiogram and

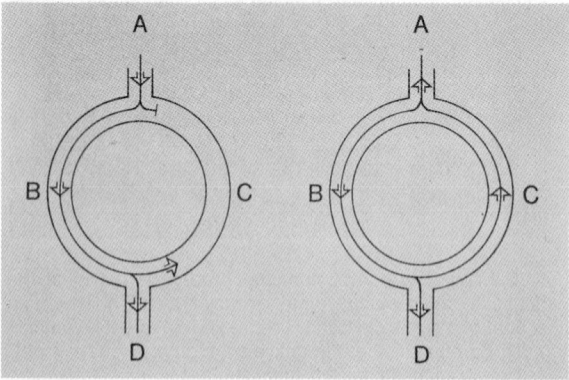

Fig. 11.9. This diagram illustrates the principle of re-entry. Conduction from A to D is possible through routes B or C. In this example, the conduction in pathway C is blocked. After travelling along pathway B, conduction may continue in the reverse direction (from D to A) along the previously blocked route C. If route B recovers in time, conduction may continue to circulate from A to D along that pathway.

ruling out the presence of an accessory pathway as the cause of tachycardia. The term supraventricular tachycardia includes all those regular tachycardias that arise from the atrial myocardium or the atrioventricular junction (which comprises the atrioventricular node, its atrial approaches and any accessory pathways that partially or completely bypass the atrioventricular node). Supraventricular tachycardias include those tachycardias that may arise from a large re-entrant circuit (macro circuit) involving atrial and ventricular myocardium. Most supraventricular tachycardias have narrow QRS complexes and normal HV intervals but aberrant His–Purkinje conduction (usually rate dependent) or pre-excitation (as in antidromic atrioventricular re-entrant tachycardia, see below) may result in wide QRS complex tachycardias. The major varieties of supraventricular tachycardia are sinus node re-entrant tachycardia, atrial re-entrant tachycardia, atrial flutter, atrioventricular nodal re-entrant tachycardia and atrioventricular re-entrant tachycardia. Atrial fibrillation is not usually regarded as a 'supraventricular tachycardia' although it is clearly a tachyarrhythmia arising from a supraventricular source.

Most supraventricular tachycardias can easily be initiated and terminated using atrial, and sometimes ventricular, stimulation. The manner of initiation and termination, the atrial activation sequence during tachycardia, the form of atrioventricular conduction and the atrioventricular relationship during tachycardia readily allow the differential diagnosis of these tachycardias. Their major electrophysiology characteristics are shown in Table 11.4.[50,51]

The most common types of supraventricular tachycardia are atrial flutter, atrioventricular nodal re-entrant tachycardia and atrioventricular tachycardia. *Atrial flutter* is easily induced, particularly by an atrial premature beat or rapid atrial pacing at a coupling interval or cycle length, respectively, of 200 ms. The flutter electrograms are usually sequenced from high to low and occur at a cycle length of 200 ms. The mechanism of this arrhythmia is probably large circuit re-entry through right atrial and septal myocardium. Induced flutter can easily be terminated by rapid atrial pacing at cycle lengths < 175 ms. However, transient atrial fibrillation often precedes reversion to sinus rhythm.[51,52,53]

Atrioventricular nodal re-entrant tachycardia is thought to be due to re-entry confined to the atrioventricular node or involving one intranodal and one immediately extranodal pathway.[54,55] This mechanism is suggested by the manner in which the

Table 11.4. Characteristics of supraventricular tachycardia.

	SNRT	AFL	ART	AVNRT	AVRT
Atrial activation sequence	Normal	Abnormal	Abnormal	Normal	Abnormal
AH interval	Normal	Normal	Normal	Normal	Normal
HV interval	Normal	Normal	Normal	Normal	Normal
Provocation	A	A	A	A or V	A or V
Termination	A	A	A	A or V	A or V
AV block	Possible	Usual	Possible	Possible	Impossible
Initiation with AH jump	Unlikely	Unlikely	Unlikely	Usual	Possible

Definitions: SNRT, sinus node re-entrant tachycardia; AFl, atrial flutter; ART, atrial re-entrant tachycardia; AVNRT, atrioventricular nodal re-entrant tachycardia; AVRT, atrioventricular re-entrant tachycardia; A, atrial pacing; V, ventricular pacing.

arrhythmia is initiated by atrial premature beats. At a critical coupling interval, an atrial premature beat conducts from atrium to His bundle with a sudden increase in the AH interval. This suggests that the anterograde effective refractory period of a relatively fast AH conduction pathway is reached and anterograde conduction continues in a slower AH conduction pathway. As tachycardia begins with this sequence, it is probable that the impulse returns towards the atrium through the fast pathway, thus completing a re-entrant circuit. This sequence is illustrated in Fig. 11.10. The atrial activation sequence during this arrhythmia is the normal retrograde sequence and, in the usual variety, atrial activation occurs almost simultaneously with the ventricular electrogram. This form of tachycardia is known as the *slow–fast variety* because of the sequence of atrioventricular nodal pathway

conduction.[56] An unusual form of atrioventricular nodal re-entry involves circulation in the reverse direction (fast pathway anterogradely and slow pathway retrogradely—*fast–slow variety*). In the fast–slow variety, atrial activation occurs at about mid-cycle. Rarely, atrioventricular block occurs during this arrhythmia. The arrhythmia can usually be initiated and terminated by both atrial and ventricular pacing techniques.

Atrioventricular re-entrant tachycardia is a form of large circuit re-entry dependent on the presence of an accessory pathway. Such tachycardias may be initiated by atrial or ventricular pacing sequences. As the re-entry involves circulation from atrium to ventricle through a slow pathway (atrioventricular node) and from ventricle to atrium through a fast pathway (the accessory connection), atrial electrograms closely follow ventricular electrograms. This tachycardia and its common variants are described in detail in the section below.

Atrial fibrillation is rarely amenable to electrophysiology study. However, it is possible to make an assessment of atrial 'vulnerability' to fibrillation by measuring the atrial refractory period, the duration of the atrial monophasic action potential and intra-atrial conduction times.[57] Failure of the atrial refractory period to shorten with an increase in the atrial drive rate also indicates vulnerability to atrial fibrillation. These measurements may be useful in the management of patients with paroxysmal atrial fibrillation.

Atrial fibrillation may complicate an electrophysiology study. It may revert spontaneously, often within a few minutes; if not, direct current cardioversion should be employed to allow the study to be completed. Atrial fibrillation is intentionally provoked during the assessment of the Wolff–Parkinson–White syndrome. In this situation, an

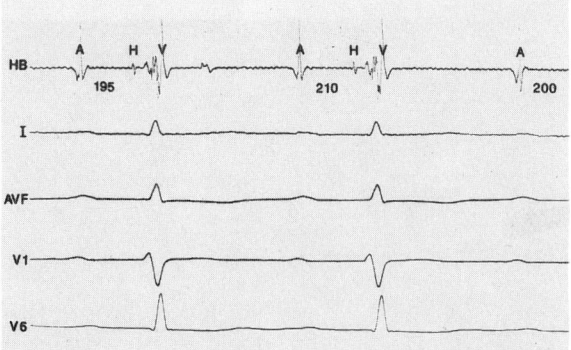

Fig. 11.10. In the usual variety of atrioventricular nodal re-entrant tachycardia, atrial and ventricular activation occurs simultaneously. The AH interval is longer than normal because of conduction in a 'slow' pathway. HRA, high right atrium; DCS, distal coronary sinus; PCS, proximal coronary sinus; HIS, His bundle.

appropriate anti-arrhythmic drug might be administered in order to assess its potential efficacy.

ASSESSMENT OF PRE-EXCITATION SYNDROMES

Fast non-decremental tissue (accessory pathway) that bypasses the decremental delaying properties of the atrioventricular node causes pre-excitation of the tissue into which it inserts. There are three major varieties of accessory pathway (Fig. 11.11).[58]

1 *Atrioventricular accessory connections* (or Kent pathways) link the atrial and ventricular myocardium directly across the atrioventricular groove. These pathways may be located in the anterior or posterior septum or along the right or left free wall. The pathway may conduct in both directions or in only one. Conduction in the atrioventricular direction produces a short PR interval and a broad QRS complex with a slurred start known as a 'delta wave' (the *Wolff–Parkinson–White* pattern)[59] because of early and eccentric activation of the ventricular myocardium (Fig. 11.12). Ventriculo-atrial conduction allows atrial re-entry of an impulse that has already conducted from atrium to ventricle over the normal atrioventricular node/His–Purkinje pathway. Repetition of this sequence results in *orthodromic* atrioventricular re-entrant tachycardia (Fig. 11.13). Occasionally, re-entrant tachycardia occurs in the reverse direction (*antidromic*). When the accessory pathway does not conduct in the atrioventricular direction, it is described as *concealed*.[60,61] Such a pathway does not produce the Wolff–Parkinson–White electrocardiographic pattern, but will sustain orthodromic (not antidromic) atrioventricular re-entrant tachycardia. Atrial fibrillation with potentially very rapid ventricular rates also occurs in this syndrome because atrial re-entry triggers the fibrillation, and atrioventricular conduction during atrial fibrillation is not controlled by the atrioventricular node.

2 *Nodo-(fasciculo-)ventricular connections* (or Mahaim fibres) connect the atrioventricular node or proximal His–Purkinje system directly to the ventricular myocardium. In this situation, atrioventricular conduction occurs over the atrioventricular node and the Mahaim fibre in series. The PR interval is usually normal, but the QRS is broad and begins with a delta wave because of early eccentric activation. Large circuit re-entry around the His–Purkinje system and the Mahaim fibres may occur.

3 *Atrionodal fibres* connect the atrial myocardium to the atrioventricular node or His bundle. As they bypass part or all of the atrioventricular node but insert into the normal conduction system, the surface electrocardiogram shows a short PR interval and a normal QRS complex. Associated tachycardias (the *Lown–Ganong–Levine* syndrome) may be due to re-entry involving the atrioventricular node and the accessory pathway.[62]

The electrophysiology evaluation of accessory pathways involves determining their origin and

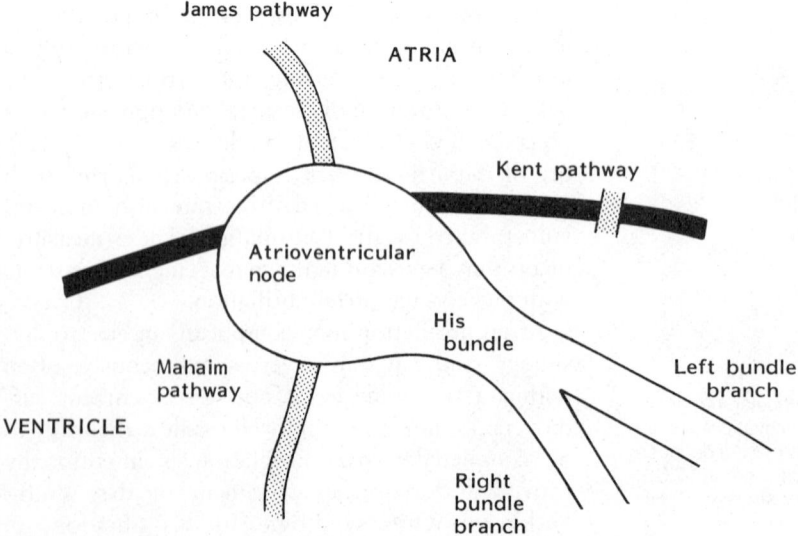

Fig. 11.11. The three major forms of accessory pathway are direct atrioventricular connection (Kent pathway), nodoventricular connection (Mahaim pathway) and atrionodal connection (James pathway).

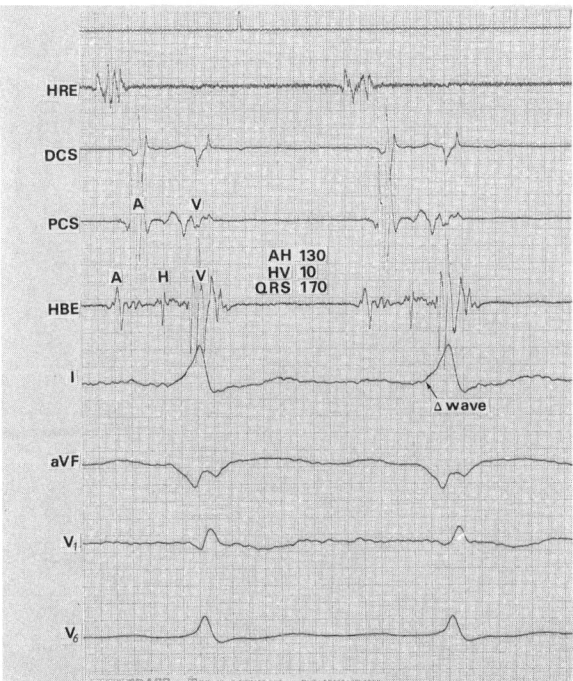

Fig. 11.12. In the Wolff–Parkinson–White syndrome, conduction from atrium to ventricle may occur over a direct atrioventricular accessory pathway. It is therefore possible for a beat that arises in the atrium to excite the ventricle before or just after the His bundle is depolarized via the atrioventricular node. The HV interval is short or negative. In this example, the His bundle is depolarized 10 ms before the onset of the delta wave.

insertion, elucidation of the tachycardias they support, and assessment of the risk they impose.[63] The location and functional properties (refractoriness, etc.) of the pathway(s) are demonstrated by pacing proximal and sensing distal to the pathway. For example, a left-sided atrioventricular connection may be located by pacing the ventricles and recording atrial electrograms with a series of electrodes placed along the length of the coronary sinus. Accessory pathway tissue is revealed by its non-decremental conduction properties and/or typical position. It cannot be assumed that the presence of an accessory pathway implies its participation in a re-entrant tachycardia circuit because many pathways are merely 'bystanders'. It may be difficult to establish that the accessory connection is a critical part of the re-entrant circuit, but there is a particularly elegant proof in the case of free wall direct atrioventricular connections. If the QRS complex associated with atrioventricular re-entrant tachycardia develops bundle branch block or delay on the same side as the accessory pathway which is part of

the tachycardia circuit, the ventriculo-atrial conduction time (and usually the cycle length) should be lengthened by the degree of delay imposed by the bundle branch block.

The risk associated with the Wolff–Parkinson–White syndrome is largely due to rapid atrial fibrillation.[16,64] An effective anterograde refractory period (Fig. 11.14) < 250 ms is regarded as unsafe. Another form of assessment requires initiation of atrial fibrillation (by atrial extrastimulation, rapid atrial pacing or alternating current) and measurement of the shortest interval between successive *pre-excited* QRS complexes. When this interval is < 215 ms, the pathway is capable of sustaining life-threatening ventricular rates.

The assessment of pre-excitation syndromes must include evaluation of the effect of potentially therapeutic drugs on the electrophysiological parameters of the bypass tract and the associated tachycardia(s). Thus, when a direct atrioventricular connection is present, an effective drug should prevent the inducibility of atrioventricular re-entrant tachycardia and slow the ventricular response to, or prevent the induction of, atrial fibrillation.[18,65]

The electrophysiological characteristics of the other forms of accessory pathway are compared with those of normal atrioventricular conduction in Table 11.5.

ELECTROPHYSIOLOGY STUDY PRIOR TO PACEMAKER IMPLANTATION

Implantable pacemakers are used to prevent bradycardia, ensure adequate rate response for metabolic requirements and restore the physiological sequence of cardiac activation. Three basic kinds of pacemaker are used: single chamber constant rate, single chamber rate modulated and dual chamber with or without additional rate modulation. The proper prescription of these devices requires clinical electrophysiology information; in particular, the status of atrioventricular conduction, the possibility and timing (ventriculo-atrial interval) of retrograde conduction, the reliability of sinus node function and the vulnerability of the atrial myocardium to atrial fibrillation can be assessed, especially when considering the implantation of an atrial or dual chamber device. Usually, the sinus node recovery time, the AH and HV intervals, the *atrioventricular Wenckebach cycle length* and the presence of ventriculo-atrial conduction in response to ventricular pacing are measured. An atrioventricular Wenc-

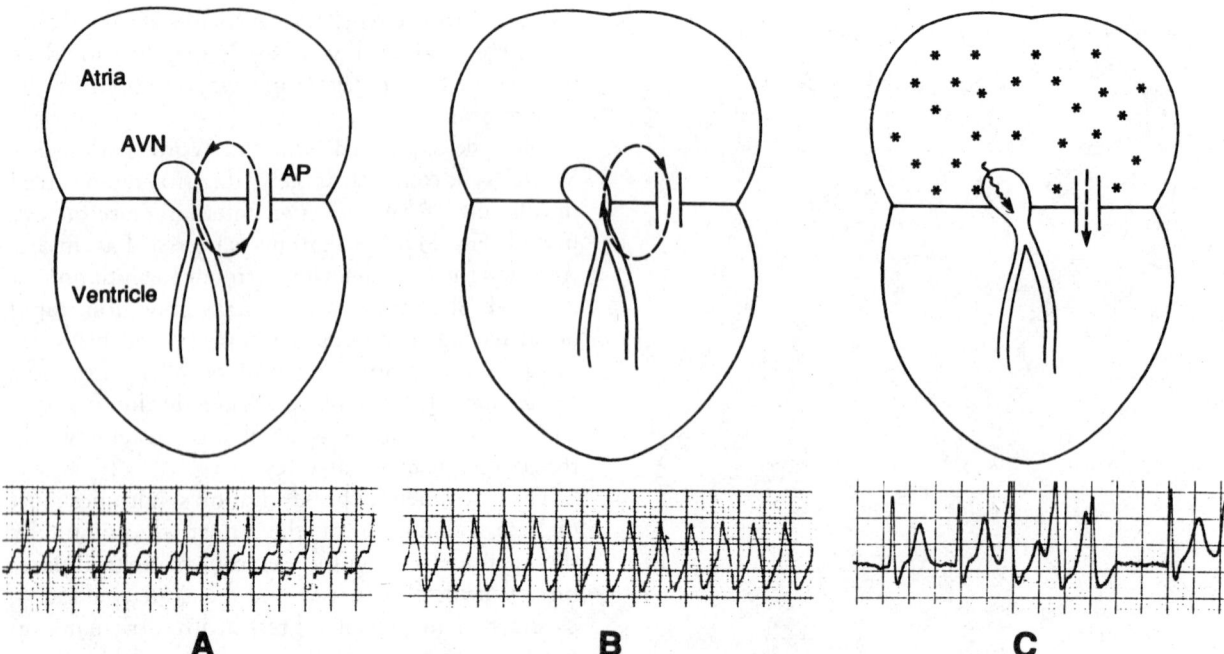

Fig. 11.13. The three arrhythmias associated with Wolff–Parkinson–White syndrome are: (A) orthodromic atrioventricular re-entrant tachycardia (regular narrow QRS complexes); (B) antidromic atrioventricular re-entrant tachycardia (regular pre-excited QRS complexes); and (C) atrial fibrillation (irregular narrow and pre-excited QRS complexes). AVN, atrioventricular node; AP, accessory pathway.

kebach rate < 120 beats/min excludes atrial pacing. The presence of retrograde conduction suggests that a dual chamber pacemaker is necessary and the *ventriculo-atrial interval* must then be measured in order to ensure that the device proposed for implantation can be programmed to a post-ventricular atrial refractory period (PVARP) that exceeds this interval. Unreliable sinus function, which should also be assessed by exercise testing, implies that additional rate modulation may be useful.[66]

ASSESSMENT OF VENTRICULAR TACHYCARDIA

Electrophysiology study of ventricular tachycardia (Table 11.6) is necessary to differentiate it from supraventricular tachycardias with aberrant or anomalous atrioventricular conduction, to determine the origin of the tachycardia, to assess its response to therapies, such as drugs and pacemakers, and to assess its possible role in producing symptoms, such as syncope or sudden death.

The electrophysiology *diagnosis* of ventricular tachycardia requires that the tachycardia is shown to be dissociated from atrial and, preferably, from His bundle activity. The broad QRS complexes of

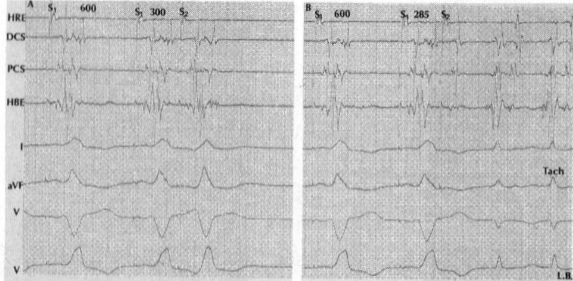

Fig. 11.14. The assessment of accessory pathway anterograde effective refractory period is demonstrated. An atrial premature beat coupled at 300 ms (a) conducts over the accessory pathway whereas the beat at 285 ms (b) finds the accessory pathway blocked and conducts to the ventricle over the normal His–Purkinje pathway.

Table 11.5. **Electrophysiological characteristics of accessory pathways.**

Accessory pathway	Sinus rhythm		Atrial premature beat	
	AH	HV	Delta AH	Delta HV
Normal	Normal	Normal	+++	0
Atrioventricular	Normal	Short or −ve	+++	−−
Nodoventricular	? Normal	Short	+++	−
Atrionodal	Short	Normal	+	0

Table 11.6. Aims of electrophysiology study for ventricular tachycardia.

1 To discover the cause of symptoms
2 To distinguish VT from SVT and AVRT
3 To localize origin of VT
4 To study mechanism of VT
5 To evaluate possible treatments:
   a) anti-arrhythmic drugs
   b) pacemaker
   c) internal cardioversion
   d) implantable defibrillator
   e) catheter ablation
6 To assess suitability for surgery

Definitions: VT, ventricular tachycardia; SVT, supraventricular tachycardia; AVRT, atrioventricular reentrant tachycardia.

supraventricular tachycardia should be preceded by His bundle deflections with normal HV times. In ventricular tachycardia, the His bundle deflection may be dissociated from, buried within, or just precede the ventricular electrogram. Atrioventricular dissociation, which occurs in about 75% of ventricular tachycardias,[67] can be established by atrial or oesophageal electrode catheterization, but an additional ventricular electrode pair is usually necessary to initiate the tachycardia. Depolarizations that affect the tachycardia without conducting to the His bundle or atria are useful additional proofs that the tachycardia arises from the ventricle. During the assessment, it is important to exclude the presence of an accessory pathway that conducts to produce QRS complexes identical to those recorded during tachycardia.

When it is proposed to eradicate the tachycardia using ablation techniques, it is essential to *map the origin* of tachycardia as precisely as possible.[68] This is achieved by moving a close electrode bipole within the cavities of the right and left ventricles and sampling local electrograms from each point during tachycardia. The tachycardia focus is located close to points from which mid-diastolic or pre-systolic activity is recorded during ongoing tachycardia. Alternatively, delayed, low-amplitude or fractionated electrograms during sinus rhythm can be used to identify possible substrate for tachycardia. This latter method is non-specific. Pace-mapping is a technique that can be used if tachycardia is not inducible at study, provided that a previously recorded 12-lead electrocardiogram of the tachycardia is available for comparison. The paced QRS complex should closely match the spontaneous QRS complex during tachycardia. Careful

biplane fluoroscopic localization of the electrode bipole is essential.

The 1-year mortality associated with newly diagnosed ventricular tachycardia approaches 40%. Careful prescription of effective *therapy* is therefore mandatory and serial drug testing is justified, (see above) even though it is a time-consuming and expensive procedure.[33,69] The order in which drugs are tested depends on the particular patient history but, in general, traditional class I drugs are tested before experimental compounds. Amiodarone is tested only as a last resort. Success with long-term treatment is likely if the tachycardia is rendered non-inducible following drug treatment. If tachycardia can still be provoked, a significant slowing of its rate following drug treatment indicates that the occurrence of sudden death will be unlikely although paroxysms of haemodynamically stable tachycardia may still occur. These outcomes seem to occur with the majority of class I drugs but not necessarily when using amiodarone or some class Ic drugs, such as propafenone.

Ventricular tachycardia may be the cause of recurrent syncope and out-of-hospital cardiac arrest. Electrophysiology studies may be used to *elucidate the cause of the symptoms*. Inducibility of ventricular tachycardia in patients who have suffered these symptoms suggest that this rhythm may be responsible for their symptoms. However, the protocol (Table 11.7) used to attempt to induce ventricular tachycardia determines the predictive accuracy of stimulation techniques.[70–73] Provided that stimulation is restricted to low energy (twice diastolic threshold) and no more than 2 ventricular extrastimuli, the test is highly specific (95%+) and moderately sensitive (65%). The sensitivity may be increased (up to 95%) by using more 'aggressive' protocols, such as 3 or 4 extrastimuli, additional isoprenaline and high-energy stimulation. However,

Table 11.7. Typical ventricular tachycardia stimulation protocol.

When ventricular tachycardia is only suspected:

Sinus rhythm	plus 1,
Ventricular pacing: 120 beats/min	then 2
Ventricular pacing: 140 beats/min	ventricular
Ventricular pacing: 160 beats/min	extrastimuli

When ventricular tachycardia has been recorded:

A third extrastimulus during sinus rhythm and ventricular pacing
High-energy pacing
Left ventricular pacing
Incremental ventricular burst pacing

this is justified only if a previous recording of a spontaneous ventricular tachycardia is available from which the clinical relevance of the induced tachycardia can be judged.

In clinical electrophysiology, definitions different to those in general use are employed (see below).

Repetitive ventricular response: 1–5 non-stimulated ventricular depolarizations.

Non-sustained ventricular tachycardia: tachycardia lasting more than 6 beats but < 30 s.

Sustained ventricular tachycardia: tachycardia lasting > 30 s or requiring emergency termination.

Polymorphic ventricular tachycardia: tachycardia with constantly varying QRS complexes.

Ventricular fibrillation: a sustained tachyarrhythmia with no clearly defined QRS complexes and no cardiac output.

Two specific forms of ventricular tachycardia with characteristic electrophysiological properties are fascicular tachycardia and His bundle tachycardia. *Fascicular tachycardia* has a re-entrant mechanism and may arise from a circuit within a single fascicle or involving several fascicles.[74] It may be provoked and terminated by atrial as well as ventricular stimulation. The QRS complexes, which are often relatively narrow, are usually 'preceded' by His spikes with negative HV intervals. Sometimes, the His electrograms are completely dissociated from the QRS complexes. *His bundle tachycardia* is usually ectopic in nature and arises from the main His bundle. The QRS complexes are narrow with a normal or short HV interval. Atrial activity is dissociated from His bundle and ventricular electrograms. These tachycardias cannot be provoked or terminated by electrostimulation.

PACEMAKER/IMPLANTABLE DEVICE PRESCRIPTION

Detailed electrophysiology study is necessary prior to the prescription or implantation of an electronic device designed to prevent or terminate tachycardia (Table 11.8).[75] Such studies aid the precise prescription of the device and the lead position, evaluate the potential success of the treatment and ensure that the device is not likely to provoke unwanted arrhythmias. Tachycardia is induced to allow a full diagnosis to be made. Potential pacing techniques for prevention and termination of tachycardia are assessed with various electrode locations. The rate and characteristics of induced tachycardia are com-

Table 11.8. Implantable devices for tachycardia control.

Pacing (about 25 µJ)	
Prevention:	overdrive
Termination	overdrive
	underdrive
	scanning
	burst
Cardioversion (about 2.5 J)	
Internal cardioverter	
Defibrillation (about 25 J)	
Implantable defibrillator	

pared with those of physiological (sinus) tachycardia in order to ensure that the tachycardias can be distinguished by the implantable device. Tachycardia termination by the proposed permanent technique is repeated many times at rest, on standing and during exercise. An external version of the implantable device should be used for this purpose.

If possible, prior to prescription of an *implantable defibrillator*, ventricular tachycardia is induced and mapped. During the implantation of the device, the energy required to revert the tachycardia (cardioversion threshold) and ventricular fibrillation (defibrillation threshold) are measured. Electrogram size and morphology adequate for tachycardia and fibrillation detection are ensured. During the convalescent phase after implantation, the success of the device in terminating ventricular tachycardia and ventricular fibrillation is assessed on provocation of these arrhythmias in the electrophysiology laboratory.[76,77]

OPERATIVE ELECTROPHYSIOLOGY

Surgical methods for ablation of foci of ectopic tachycardia and of conduction pathways responsible for the expression or continuation of tachycardia are now accepted techniques. All methods rely on accurate identification of the focus or pathway. Surgical *mapping techniques*, which involve point-by-point sampling of epicardial and/or endocardial signals, are the major electrophysiology investigation during the operation. Activation maps are derived by plotting the relative timing of signals collected during sinus rhythm and tachycardia. The endocardial surface is also mapped for fractionated or late activity during sinus rhythm. Recently, techniques have been devised for simultaneous mapping of the whole epicardial or endocardial surface. The arrhythmia usually arises close to the first point activated during tachycardia and from the areas of abnormal activation during sinus rhythm. Accessory pathways can be located by ascertaining the first point of atrial activation during atrioventricular tachycardia. *Cryothermal mapping*, which involves temporary freezing of the myocardium during the tachycardia, can also be used to identify its origin or critical conduction pathway because the reduction of temperature transiently abolishes myocardial conduction and automaticity.[78,79]

Electrophysiology techniques are used postoperatively to evaluate the success of surgery. Failure to elicit accessory pathway conduction or to initiate tachycardia indicates that the surgery has been successful.

CATHETER ABLATION TECHNIQUES

Clinical cardiac electrophysiology embraces several therapeutic techniques including transvascular catheter ablation. The method based upon the discharge of a *direct current cardioverter* through an electrode placed closely adjacent to the tissue to be ablated arose following a laboratory error. Accidental discharge through a His bundle catheter during attempted transcutaneous cardioversion resulted in permanent atrioventricular block. Extensive animal experimentation has now demonstrated that this effect probably results from very high current flow. Originally, a conventional defibrillator was used but various modifications have led to the development of modified current sources which do not cause explosive (*fulguration*) discharges. Conventional shocks give rise to. haemolysis, gas production and high intracardiac pressures. This may lead to ventricular dysfunction, myocardial perforation, cardiac arrhythmias and coronary disease. The newer techniques are probably much more safe. Electroshock ablation techniques require general anaesthesia.[80,81]

The *atrioventricular node/His bundle* may be ablated by placing an electrode in a position from which a high-amplitude atrial and His bundle deflection may be recorded. A pacing catheter is placed in the right ventricle to support the heart rate after the production of atrioventricular block. The technique is advised when rapid supraventricular arrhythmias are frequently recurrent and refractory to other therapies. Complete heart block is induced

in about 75% of cases and therapeutically effective but lesser degrees of block are produced in a further 15%. After the procedure the patient is dependent upon an artificial pacemaker and a rate-variable ventricular pacemaker is usually advised.

Accessory pathways can also be ablated.[82] The electrode is placed close to the pathway by positioning it against the right atrioventricular groove, within the proximal coronary sinus or against the left atrioventricular groove via a trans-septal puncture. Electrographic mapping, preferably during sustained atrioventricular re-entrant tachycardia, is used to locate the pathway. The results of these procedures have been variable (10–90%) but accessory pathways that have been ablated do not seem to recover. There is particular concern about direct current discharges delivered within the coronary sinus because there is a substantial risk of coronary sinus rupture.

The *focus of ventricular tachycardia* can be eradicated by this technique.[83] The focus is accurately located by detailed intraventricular mapping techniques searching for mid-diastolic and pre-systolic electrographic activity during induced ventricular tachycardia. Intracavitary discharge may ablate the focus or modify it sufficiently to render the tachycardia amenable to previously unsuccessful therapy. Results have been very variable. Some enthusiastic reports suggest virtually 100% success. The procedure is time consuming.

Successful and therapeutically satisfactory attempts to ablate other structures, such as the right bundle branch, atrial ectopic foci and the sinus node, have also been made.

In recent years, *radiofrequency energies* have been used for myocardial ablation. This technique has the advantages of allowing more carefully controlled energy discharge and avoiding general anaesthesia, because it is a painless procedure.[84] Transvenous delivery of laser energy is also being investigated as a potential method for myocardial ablation.[85]

ELECTROPHYSIOLOGY STUDY IN THE INVESTIGATION OF SYNCOPE

Recurrent undiagnosed syncope, sudden onset pallor during syncope and flushing following recovery suggest an arrhythmic aetiology and should be considered an indication for electrophysiology study. Symptoms derived from other causes, such as endocrine, metabolic or cardiovascular should be eliminated. It is appropriate to perform ambulatory electrocardiographic monitoring prior to electrophysiology testing because, although ambulatory recording is insensitive, it is non-invasive and relatively cheap. Electrophysiology study is warranted in about 50% of patients with recurrent syncope; in about half of these, a positive diagnosis is made which improves the outcome of treatment.[85–88]

The common diagnoses for syncope that may be made from an electrophysiology study are ventricular tachycardia, impaired His–Purkinje conduction, impaired atrioventricular nodal function, abnormal sinus node function, and rapid supraventricular tachycardias.

The diagnosis of 'vagotonia' can usually be made without resorting to expensive electrophysiology studies.

PROGRAMMED STIMULATION AFTER MYOCARDIAL INFARCTION

In the first year following myocardial infarction, 10–15% of survivors experience sudden unexpected death, in many cases due to ventricular tachycardia which rapidly degenerates to ventricular fibrillation.[89,90] Poor left ventricular function (ejection fraction < 35–40%), a high density of ventricular ectopy (> 10 ventricular premature beats per hour), a complicated acute course of infarction and persistent late potentials suggest the possibility of sudden death during follow-up. The value of programmed ventricular stimulation in stratifying risk after myocardial infarction is controversial.[91–95] Many of the initial studies were limited by non-specific definitions of a positive response (e.g. 4 unpaced beats and ventricular fibrillation) or by using insufficiently sensitive or specific stimulation protocols (e.g. only 1 or 2 extrastimuli or high-energy stimulation, respectively). Most of the early studies were too small or too short to detect sufficient events from which useful conclusions could be drawn. Recent studies[96] have proved sensitive (90–100%) in predicting arrhythmic events but the specificity of the studies has been variable (30–77%).[96] The stimulation protocol should include stimulation with up to 3 extrastimuli at 1 or 2 right ventricular sites. The only sensitive and specific response is the reproducible induction of a sustained monomorphic ventricular tachycardia.

Most patients who suffer arrhythmic events during convalescence from myocardial infarction have

several adverse risk indicators (see above). Ventricular stimulation after myocardial infarction should probably be reserved for those who have any one or several of these other risk factors.

ASSESSMENT OF SURVIVORS OF OUT-OF-HOSPITAL CARDIAC ARREST

Each year in the UK there are approximately 50 000 victims of sudden unexpected cardiac death. The provision of improved rescue services and the teaching of cardiopulmonary resuscitation to the lay public has led to the survival of increasing numbers of these patients. Although the majority of patients have extensive coronary artery disease, about two-thirds have not suffered an acute myocardial infarction. Subsequent mortality in the survivors is very high (35%+ in the first year).[97] Electrophysiology techniques may provoke ventricular tachyarrhythmias in as many as 80% of survivors,[98–100] and successful serial drug testing in this group leads to an apparently improved survival. Patients for whom no successful drug regimen can be identified should be considered for treatment with an *implantable defibrillator*. Electrophysiology tests have also demonstrated that sudden cardiac death may be due to inexpertly prescribed 'antiarrhythmic' treatment.[99–101]

CONCLUSION

Cardiac electrophysiology studies provide essential information on the mechanism and management of clinical arrhythmias. The ability to provoke and study paroxysmal arrhythmias allows their origin to be ascertained and potential treatments to be evaluated in a convenient clinical environment. Although clinical electrophysiology was initially a technique restricted to expert pioneers, it is now so useful that the basic method must be part of every cardiologist's approach to patients with arrhythmias. It requires very little expensive equipment additional to that found in ordinary catheter laboratories, but some experience in the practical performance of the studies is necessary. The technique can provide a satisfying, logical and effective approach to the investigation and treatment of cardiac arrhythmias.

REFERENCES

1. Alanis, J., Gonzales, H. and Lopez, E. Electrical activities of the bundle of His. *J. Physiol.* 1958; **142**: 127.

2. Castellanos, A., Castillo, C.A. and Agha, A.S. Contribution of His bundle recording to the understanding of clinical arrhythmias. *Am. J. Cardiol.* 1971; 28: 499.

3. Durrer, D., Schoo, L., Schuilenburg, R.M. and Wellens, H.J.J. The role of premature beats in the initiation and the termination of supraventricular tachycardia in the WPW syndrome. *Circulation* 1967; 36: 644.

4. Scherlag, B.J., Lau, S.H., Helfant, R.A., Berkowitz, W.D., Stein, E. and Damato, A.N. Catheter technique for recording His bundle activity in man. *Circulation* 1969; 39: 13.

5. Ezri, M., Lerman, B.B., Marchlinski, F.E., Buxton, A.E. and Josephson, M.E. Electrophysiologic evaluation of syncope in patients with bifascicular block. *Am. Heart J.* 1983; 106: 693.

6. Fisher, J.D. Role of electrophysiologic testing in the diagnosis and treatment of patients with known and suspected bradycardia and tachycardia. *Prog. Cardiovasc. Dis.* 1981; 24: 25.

7. Wellens, H.J.J. *Electrical stimulation of the heart in the study and treatment of tachycardias.* Leiden: H.E. Stenfert Kroese N.V. 1971.

8. Wellens, H.J.J. Value and limitations of programmed electrical stimulation of the heart in the study and treatment of tachycardias. *Circulation* 1978; 57: 845.

9. Dhingra, R.C., Denes, P., Wu, D., Wyndham, C., Amat-y-Leon, F., Town, W. and Rosen, K.M. Prospective observations in patients with chronic bundle branch block and marked HV prolongation. *Circulation* 1976; 53: 600.

10. Dhingra, R.C., Denes, P., Wu, D., Chuquimia, R. and Rosen, K.M. The significance of second degree atrioventricular block and bundle branch block: observations regarding site and type of block. *Circulation* 1974; 49: 638.

11. Gupta, P.K., Lichstein, E. and Chadda, K.D. Electrophysiological features of Mobitz type II A–V block occurring within the His bundle. *Br. Heart J.* 1972; 34: 1232.

12. Kelly, D.T., Brodsky, S.J., Mirowski, M., Krovetz, J. and Rowe, R.D. Bundle of His recordings in congenital heart block. *Circulation* 1972; 45: 277.

13. Wellens, H.J.J. Value and limitations of programmed electrical stimulation of the heart in the study and treatment of tachycardias. *Circulation* 1978; 57: 847.

14. Josephson, M.E. and Kastor, J.A. Supraventricular tachycardia: mechanisms and management. *Ann. Intern. Med.* 1977; 87: 346.

15. Bhandari, A.K. and Rahimtoola, S.H. Indications for intracardiac electrophysiologic testing in survivors of acute myocardial infarction: discussion. *Circulation* 1987; 75 (Suppl. III): 166.

16. Tonkin, A.M., Miller, H.C., Svenson, R.H., Wallace, A.G. and Gallagher, J.J. Refractory periods of the accessory pathway in the Wolff–Parkinson–White syndrome. *Circulation* 1975; 52: 563.

17. Denes, P., Dhingra, R.C., Wu, D., Wyndham, R.C., Amat-y-Leon, F. and Rosen, K.M. Sudden death in patients with bifascicular block. *Arch. Intern. Med.* 1977; 137: 1005.

18. Bashore, Th.M., Sellers, T.D., Gallagher, J.J. and Wallace, A.G. Ventricular fibrillation in the Wolff–Parkinson–White syndrome. *Circulation* 1976; 53 (Supp. II): II–187.

19. Gettes, L., Zipes, D.P., Gillette, P.C., Josephson, M.E., Laks, M.M., Mirvis, D.M., Scheinman, M., Sheffield, L.T. and Wu, D. Personnel and equipment required for electrophysiologic testing. Report of the Committee on Electrocardiography and cardiac Electrophysiology, council on clinical Cardiology, American Heart Association. *Circulation* 1984; 69: 1219A.

20. Sarma, J.S.M., Bhandari, A.K., Bilitch, M. and Sarma, R.J. Stimulators for cardiac electrophysiologic studies. A product review. *Clin. Prog. Pacing Electrophysiol.* 1984; 2: 373.

21. Ruskin, J.N., Caracta, A.R., Batsford, W.P. *et al.* Electrophysiologic effects of diazepam in man. *Clin. Res.* 1974; 22: 302A.

22. Nattel, S., Rinkenberger, R.L., Lehrman, L.L. and Zipes, D.P. Therapeutic blood lidocaine concentration, after local anaesthesia for cardiac electrophysiologic studies. *N. Engl. J. Med.* 1979; 301: 418.

23. Narula, O.S. Validation of His bundle electrograms: Limitations of the catheter technique. In: Narula, O.S., ed. *His Bundle Electrocardiography.* Philadelphia: F.A. Davis, 1975, p. 65.

24. Van Dam, R., Durrer, D., Strackee, J. and Van Der Tweel, L.H. The excitability of the dog's left ventricle, determined by anodal, cathodal and bipolar stimulation. *Circ. Res.* 1956; 4: 196.

25. Josephson, M.E. and Seides, S.F. *Clinical Cardiac Electrophysiology.* Philadelphia: Lea and Febiger, 1979.

26. Rosen, K.M. Evaluation of cardiac conduction in the cardiac catheterization laboratory. *Am. J. Cardiol.* 1972; 30: 701.

27. Narula, O.S., Scherlag, B.J. and Samet, P. Pervenous pacing of the specialized conduction system in man: His bundle and A-V node stimulation. *Circulation* 1970; 41: 77.

28. Ward, D.E. and Camm, A.J. Methodologic problems in the use of atrial pacing studies for the assessment of A-V conduction. *Clin. Cardiol.* 1980; 3: 155.

29. Denes, P., Levy, L., Pick, A. and Rosen, K.M. The incidence of typical and atypical A-V Wenckebach periodicity. *Am. Heart J.* 1975; 88: 26.

30. Denes, P., Wu, D., Dhingra, R., Pietras, R.J. and Rosen, K.M. The effect of cycle length on cardiac refractory periods in man. *Circulation* 1974; 49: 32.

31. Cagin, N.A., Kunstadt, D., Wolfish, P. and Levitt, B. Influence of heart rate on the refractory period of the atrium and A-V conducting system. *Am. Heart J.* 1973; 85: 358.

32. Prystowsky, E. Selection of Antiarrhythmic drugs based on electrophysiologic studies. In: Dreifus, L.S., ed. *Cardiac arrhythmias: Electrophysiologic techniques and management.* Philadelphia: F.A. Davis, 1985, p. 239–60.

33. Horowitz, L.N. Intracardiac electrophysiologic studies for drug selection in ventricular tachycardia. *Circulation* 1987; 75 (Suppl. III): 134.

34. Goren, C. and Denes, P. Role of electrophysiology in selection of antiarrhythmic therapy of ventricular tachycardia. In: Josephson, M.E., ed. *Ventricular tachycardia, mechanism and management.* New York: Futura Publications, 1982, p. 285–307.

35. Josephson, M.E., Scharf, D.L., Kastor, J.A. and Kitchen, J.G. III: Atrial endocardial activation in man. Electrode catheter technique for endocardial mapping. *Am. J. Cardiol.* 1977; 39: 972.

36. Ross, D.L., Farre, J., Bar, F.W. *et al.* Comprehensive clinical electrophysiologic studies in the investigation of documented tachycardias; time, staff problems and cost. *Circulation* 1980; 61: 1010.

37. DiMarco, J.P., Garan, H. and Ruskin, J.N. Complications in patients undergoing cardiac electrophysiologic procedures. *Ann. Intern. Med.* 1982; 97: 490.

38. Mandel, W.J., Hayakawa, H., Danzig, R. and Marcus, H.S. Evaluation of sino-atrial node function in man by overdrive suppression. *Circulation* 1971; 44: 59.

39. Jordan, J.L. and Mandel, W.J. Disorders of Sinus function. In: Mandel, W.J., ed. *Arrhythmias, their mechanisms, diagnosis and management.* Philadelphia: J.B. Lipponcott, 1987, pp. 143–85.

40. Narula, O.S., Samet, P. and Xavier, R.P. Significance of the sinus-node recovery time. *Circulation* 1972; 45: 140.

41. Benditt, D.G., Gornick, C.C., Dunbar, D., Almquist, A.

and Pool–Schneiden, S. Indications for electrophysiologic testing in the diagnosis and assessment of sinus-node dysfunction. *Circulation* 1987; 75: 93.

42. Strauss, H.C., Saroff, A.L., Bigger, J.T. Jr and Giardina, E.G.V. Premature atrial stimulation as a key to the understanding of sinoatrial conduction time in man: presentation of data and critical review of the literature. *Circulation* 1973; 47: 86.

43. Narula, O.S., Shantha, N., Vazquez, M., Towne, W.D. and Linhart, J.W. A new method for the measurement of sinoatrial conduction time. *Circulation* 1978; 58: 706.

44. Gomes, J.A.C., Hariman, R.I. and Chowdry, I.A. New application of direct sinus node recording in man: assessment of sinus node recovery time. *Circulation* 1984; 70: 663.

45. Kang, P.S., Gomes, J.A.C., Kelen, G. and El-Sherif, N. Role of autonomic regulatory mechanisms in sinoatrial conduction and sinus node automaticity in sick sinus syndrome. *Circulation* 1981; 64: 832.

46. Morady, F., Shen, E., Schwartz, A., Hess, D., Bhandari, A., Sung, R.J. and Scheinman, M.M. Long-term follow up of patient with recurrent unexplained syncope evaluated by electrophysiologic testing. *J. Am. Coll. Cardiol.* 1983; 2: 1309.

47. Scheinman, M., Peters, R., Sauve, M.J., Dasai, J., Abbott, J., Cogan, J., Wahl, B. and Williams, K. Value of the HQ interval in patients with bundle branch block and the role of prophylactic permanent pacing. *Am. J. Cardiol.* 1982; 50: 1316.

48. Denes, P., Dhingra, R.C., Wu, D. *et al.* Sudden death in patients with bifascicular block. *Arch. Intern. Med.* 1977; 137: 1005.

49. Akhtar, M. Retrograde conduction in man. *PACE* 1981; 4: 548.

50. Josephson, M.E. Paroxysmal supraventricular tachycardia: an electrophysiologic approach. *Am. J. Cardiol.* 1978; 41: 123.

51. Wu, D., Amat-y-Leon, F., Denes, P., Dhingra, R., Wyndham, C.R.C., Bauernfeind, R., Latif, P. and Rosen, K.M. Clinical, electrocardiographic and electrophysiologic observations in patients with paroxysmal supraventricular tachycardia. *Am. J. Cardiol.* 1978; 41: 1045.

52. Tenczer, J., Littman, L., Molner, F. *et al.* Atrial reentry in chronic repetitive supraventricular tachycardia. *Am. Heart J.* 1980; 99: 349.

53. Scheinman, M.M., Basu, D. and Hoolenberg, M. Electrophysiologic studies in patients with persistent atrial tachycardia. *Circulation* 1974; 50: 266.

54. Moe, G.K., Perston, J.B. and Burlington, H. Physiologic evidence for a dual A-V transmission system. *Circ. Res.* 1956; 4: 357.

55. Rosen, K.M., Mehta, A. and Miller, R.A. Demonstration of dual atrioventricular nodal pathways in man. *Am. J. Cardiol.* 1974; 33: 291.

56. Wu, D. and Denes, P. Mechanisms of paroxysmal supraventricular tachycardia. *Arch. Intern. Med.* 1975; 135: 437.

57. Debbas, N.M.G., Butrous, G.S., Mehta, D., Kingswell, S. and Camm, A.J. Assessment of atrial vulnerability using dynamic changes in endocardial monophasic action potential duration. *J. Am. Coll. Cardiol.* 1988; 11: 114A.

58. Anderson, R.H., Becker, A.E., Brechenmacher, C. *et al.* Ventricular preexcitation—a proposed nomenclature for its substrates. *Eur. J. Cardiol.* 1975; 3: 27.

59. Wolff, L., Parkinson, J. and White, P.D. Bundle branch block with short P-R interval in healthy young people prone to paroxysmal tachycardia. *Am. Heart J.* 1930; 5: 685.

60. Coumel, Ph. and Attuel, P. Reciprocating tachycardia in overt and latent pre-excitation. *Eur. J. Cardiol.* 1974; 1: 423.

61. Tonkin, A.M., Gallagher, J.J., Svenson, R.H. *et al.* Anterograde block in accessory pathways with retrograde conduction in reciprocating tachycardia. *Eur. J. Cardiol.* 1975; 3: 143.

62. Lown, B., Ganong, W.F. and Levine, S.A. The syndrome of short P-R interval, normal QRS complexes and paroxysmal rapid heart action. *Circulation* 1952; 5: 693.

63. Gallagher, J.J. and Sealy, W.C. The permanent form of junctional reciprocating tachycardia: further evaluation of the underlying mechanism. *Eur. J. Cardiol.* 1978; 8: 413.

64. Campbell, R.W.F., Smith, R.A., Gallagher, J.J. *et al.* Atrial fibrillation in the preexcitation syndrome. *Am. J. Cardiol.* 1977; 40: 514.

65. Wu, D., Amat-y-Leon, F., Simpson, R.J., Latif, P., Wyndham, C.R.C., Denes, P. and Rosen, K.M. Electrophysiological studies with multiple drugs in patients with atrioventricular reentrant tachycardia utilizing an extranodal pathway. *Circulation* 1977; 56: 727.

66. Greenspon, A.J. Electrophysiologic studies for pacemaker selection. In: Dreifus, L.S. ed., *Cardiac arrhythmias: electrophysiologic techniques and management.* Philadelphia: F.A. Davis, 1985, pp. 119–36.

67. Wellens, H.J.J., Brugada, P. and Stevenson, W. Programmed electrical stimulation of the heart in life threatening ventricular arrhythmias. What is the significance of induced arrhythmias and what is the correct stimulation protocol? *Circulation* 1985; 72: 1.

68. Josephson, M.E., Horowitz, L.N., Waxman, H.L., Spielman, S.R., Untereker, W.J. and Marchlinski, F.E. role of catheter mapping in evaluation of ventricular tachycardia. In: Josephson, M.E., ed. *Ventricular tachycardia. Mechanisms and Management.* New York: Futura Publications, 1982, pp. 305–30.

69. Horowitz, L.N., Josephson, M.E. and Kastor, J.A. Electrophysiologic studies as a method for the optimization of drug therapy in chronic ventricular arrhythmias. *Prog. Cardiovasc. Dis.* 1980; 23: 81.

70. Wellens, H.J.J., Duren, D.R. and Lie, K.I. Observations on mechanisms of ventricular tachycardia in man. *Circulation* 1976; 54: 237.

71. Echt, D., Swerdlow, C., Anderson, K., Mitchell, L., Mason, J. and Winkle, R. Value of adding extrastimuli vs. shortening drive cycle length in ventricular tachycardia induction. *PACE* 1983; 6: A–141.

72. Brugada, P. and Wellens, H.J.J. Comparison in the same patient of two programmed ventricular stimulation protocols to induce ventricular tachycardia. *Am. J. Cardiol.* 1985; 55: 380–3.

73. Prystowsky, E.N., Miles, W.M., Evans, J.J., Hubbard, J.E., Skale, B.T., Windel, J.R., Hegar, J.J. and Zipes, D.P. Induction of ventricular tachycardia during programmed electrical stimulation: analysis of pacing methods. *Circulation* 1986; 73: 32.

74. Ward, D.E., Nathan, A.N. and Camm, A.J. Fascicular tachycardia sensitive to calcium antagonists. *Eur. J. Cardiol.* 1984; 5: 896.

75. Camm, A.J. and Ward, D. *Pacing for tachycardia control.* Published by Telectronics, 1983.

76. Mirowski, M., Reid, P.R., Mower, M.M. *et al.* Termination of malignant ventricular arrhythmias with an implanted automatic defibrillator in human beings. *N. Engl. J. Med.* 1980; 303: 322.

77. Echt, D.S., Armstrong, K., Schmidt, P., Oyer, P.E., Stinson, E.B. and Winkle, R.A. Clinical experience: complications and survival in 70 patients with automatic implantable cardioverter-defibrillators. *Circulation* 1985; 71: 289.

78. Kupersmith, J. Electrophysiologic mapping during open heart surgery. *Prog. Cardiovasc. Dis.* 1976; 3: 167.

79. Fontaine, G., Guiraudon, G., Frank, R. *et al.* Intraopera-

tive mapping and surgery for the prevention of lethal arrhythmias after myocardial infarction. *Ann. N. Y. Acad. Sci.* 1982; **382**: 396.

80. Scheinman, M.M. The role of catheter ablation for patients with drug resistant cardiac arrhythmias. In: Mandel, W.J., ed. *Cardiac arrhythmias*. Philadelphia: J.B. Lippincott, 1987, pp. 754–63.

81. Scheinman, M.M., Evans-Bell, T. and the Executive Committee of the Percutaneous Mapping and Ablation Registry. Catheter ablation of the atrioventricular junction: a report of the percutaneous mapping and the ablation registry. *Circulation* 1984; **70**: 1024.

82. Camm, A.J. and Ward, D.E. Catheter ablation in the Wolff–Parkinson–White syndrome. In: Iwa, T. and Fontaine, G., eds. *Cardiac arrhythmias, recent progress in investigation and management*. Amsterdam: Elsevier, 1988, pp. 325–9.

83. Hartzler, G.O. Electrode catheter ablation of refractory focal ventricular tachycardia. *J. Am. Coll. Cardiol.* 1983; **2**: 1107.

84. Huang, S.K., Bharati, S., Graham, A. *et al.* Closed chest catheter Desiccation of the atrioventricular junction using radiofrequency energy—a new method of catheter ablation. *J. Am. Coll. Cardiol.* 1987; **9**: 349.

85. Akhtar, M., Shenasa, M., Denker, S. *et al.* Role of cardiac electrophysiologic studies in patients with unexplained recurrent syncope. *PACE* 1983; **6**: 192.

86. DiMarco, J.P., Garan, H., Harthorne, J.W. and Ruskin, J.N. Intracardiac electrophysiologic techniques in recurrent syncope of unknown cause. *Ann. Intern. Med.* 1981; **95**: 542.

87. Morady, F., Higgins, J., Peters, R.W., Schwartz, A.B., Shen, E.N., Bhandrai, A., Scheinman, M. and Sauve, M.J. Electrophysiologic testing in bundle branch block and unexplained syncope. *Am. J. Cardiol.* 1984; **54**: 587.

88. DiMarco, J.P. Electrophysiologic studies in patients with unexplained syncope. *Circulation* 1987; **75** (Suppl. III): 140.

89. Mulkarji, J., Rude, R.E., Poole, W.K. and the MILIS Study Group. Risk stratification and survival after acute myocardial infarction: two years follow up. *Am. J. Cardiol.* 1984; **54**: 31.

90. Kannel, W.B., Sorlie, P. and McNamara, P.M. Prognosis after initial myocardial infarction: the Framingham study. *Am. J. Cardiol.* 1979; **44**: 53.

91. Greene, H.L., Reid, P.R. and Schaeffer, A.H. The repetitive ventricular response in man: a predictor of sudden death.

N. Engl. J. Med. 1978; **299**: 729.

92. Hamer, A., Vohra, J., Hunt, D. and Sloman, G. Prediction of sudden death by electrophysiologic studies in high risk patients surviving acute myocardial infarction. *Am. J. Cardiol.* 1982; **50**: 223.

93. Richards, D.A., Cody, D.V., Denniss, A.R., Russell, P.A., Young, A.A. and Uther, J.B. Ventricular electrical instability: a predictor of death after myocardial infarction. *Am. J. Cardiol.* 1983; **51**: 75.

94. Richards, D., Taylor, A., Fahey, P., Irwing, L., Koo, C.C., Ross, D., Cooper, M., Kiat, H., Skinner, M. and Uther, J. Identification of patients at risk of sudden death after myocardial infarction: the continued Australian experience. In: Brugada, P. and Wellens, H.J.J., eds. *Cardiac arrhythmias, Where to go from here?* New York: Futura Publications, 1987, pp. 329–41.

95. Marchliniski, F.E., Buxton, A.E., Waxman, H.L. and Josephson, M.E. Identifying patients at risk of sudden death after myocardial infarction: Value of response to programmed stimulation, degree of ventricular ectopic activity, and the severity of left ventricular dysfunction. *Am. J. Cardiol.* 1983; **52**: 1190.

96. Uther, J.B., Richards, D.A.B., Denniss, A.R. and Ross, D.L. The prognostic significance of programmed ventricular stimulation after myocardial infarction: a review. *Circulation* 1987; **75** (Suppl. III): 161.

97. Schaffer, W.A. and Cobb, L.A. Recurrent ventricular fibrillation and modes of death in survivors of out-of-hospital ventricular fibrillation. *N. Engl. J. Med.* 1975; **193**: 259.

98. Ruskin, J.N., DiMarco, J.P. and Garan, H. Out of Hospital cardiac arrest: Electrophysiologic observations and selection of long-term antiarrhythmic therapy. *N. Engl. J. Med.* 1980; **303**: 607.

99. Skale, B.T., Miles, W.M., Heger, J.J., Zipes, D.P. and Prystowsky, E.N. Survivors of cardiac arrest: prevention of recurrence by drug therapy as predicted by electrophysiologic testing or electrocardiographic monitoring. *Am. J. Cardiol.* 1986; **57**: 113.

100. Wilber, D.J., Garan, H. and Ruskin, J.N. Electrophysiologic testing in survivors of cardiac arrest. *Circulation* 1987; **75** (Suppl. III): 146–8.

101. Roy, D., Waxman, H.L., Kienzle, M.G., Buxton, A.E., Marchlinski, F.E. and Josephson, M.E. Clinical characteristics and long term follow up in 119 survivors of cardiac arrest: relation to inducibility at electrophysiologic testing. *Am. J. Cardiol.* 1983; **52**: 969.

Chapter 12

Chest X-ray in Adult Heart Disease

Michael B. Rubens

During the last two decades, there have been remarkable advances in diagnostic imaging allowing detailed and accurate analysis of the heart and lungs. In most patients with acquired heart disease, the chest X-ray (CXR) is normal and infrequently provides a precise diagnosis. Nevertheless, a CXR remains part of the routine work-up of virtually all cardiac patients. The CXR is relatively inexpensive and non-invasive. It provides a record of heart size and shape, and may indicate specific chamber enlargement. Calcification of valves and other structures may be visible. Analysis of the pulmonary vascularity may indicate precise physiological disturbances. Analysis of the skeleton may provide information about systemic disease or previous surgery. Abnormalities of situs may be apparent. Finally, unsuspected non-cardiac abnormalities may be discovered.

TECHNIQUE[1]

A routine examination always includes a frontal view and usually a lateral view. Oblique views are now rarely performed. Ideally, the *frontal view* is postero-anterior (PA), with the patient upright and breath held in full inspiration. The ideal kilovoltage (kVp) for chest radiography is a matter of debate. Low-kVp films (60–80 kVp) are of high contrast and show the bones and calcification well and the lungs moderately well. The mediastinum, however, is poorly demonstrated, and a penetrated film with a grid (a filter comprising fine parallel lead strips that absorb scattered X-rays) may be necessary to show mediastinal anatomy and intracardiac calcification. High-kVp films (120–150 kVp) are of lower contrast; consequently the bones and calcification are less well visualized. However, the mediastinum is well penetrated, and the lungs are seen clearly (Fig. 12.1). For high-kVp films, a grid or air-gap is necessary to reduce scatter. The latter

may cause an apparent increase in heart size when compared with previous low-kVp CXRs.[2]

Patients too ill to be taken to the X-ray department may be examined with mobile equipment and an antero-posterior (AP) film is taken. Compared with a PA projection, the heart appears magnified because it is further from the film.

A lateral film, usually with the left side nearer the film, may be taken at a high or low kVp. It will give further information on heart size and shape, and cardiac calcification is often best seen in this view. Frontal and lateral films made with the patient having swallowed barium may provide data on left atrial size and the presence of aberrant branches of the great vessels.

Currently, the usual routine cardiac series comprises a high-kVp PA film and a lateral film.

THE NORMAL CHEST X-RAY[3]

Four levels of radiographic contrast are seen on a normal conventional CXR. Air appears black, and calcium (in cortical bone) appears white. Soft tissues, blood vessels and fluid appear white, but not as densely white as calcium; fat appears grey. The structures that make up the cardiovascular silhouette can be identified only where they form a 'border' and abut air-filled lung.

THE CARDIOVASCULAR SILHOUETTE

On the *frontal CXR* (Fig. 12.2), the right border of the cardiovascular silhouette comprises, from above inferiorly, the superior vena cava, the body of right atrium and the inferior vena cava. The normal superior vena cava may be difficult to identify. If visible, it is a low-density vertical shadow, just lateral to the spine. On a supine film, it enlarges and becomes visible (Fig. 12.3). The azygos vein may be visible just above the origin of the right bronchus,

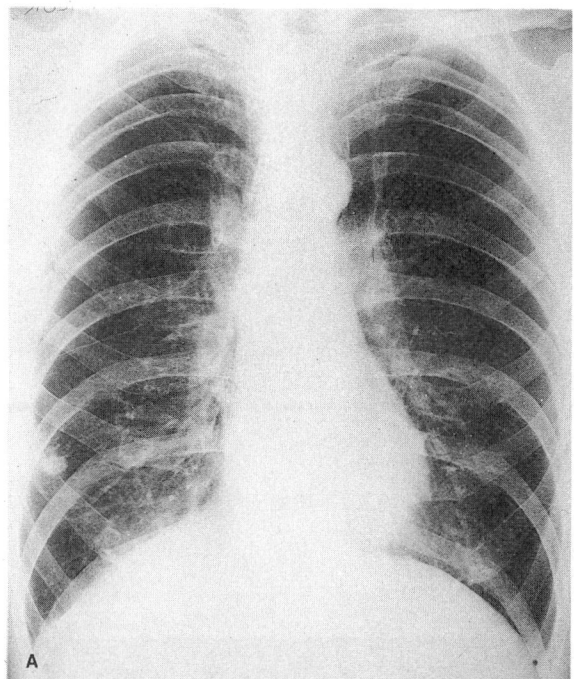 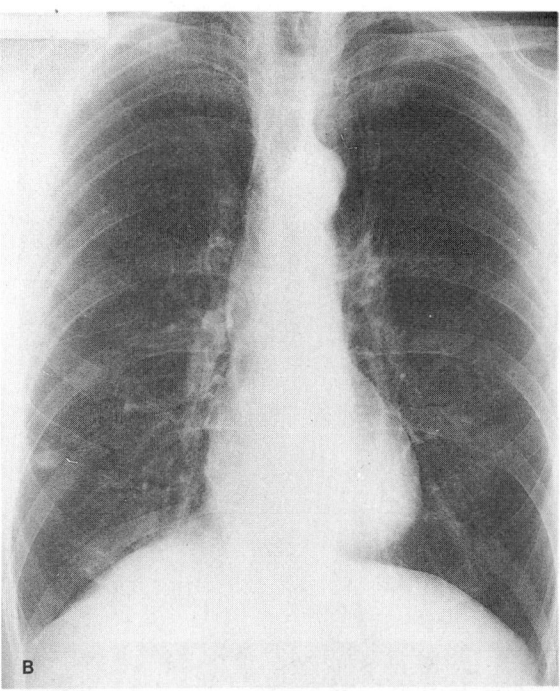

Fig. 12.1. (A) Low-kVp film: high contrast, showing ribs and calcified right lower zone granuloma well. The mediastinum is poorly penetrated. (B) High-kVp film of same patient: lower contrast with better demonstration of mediastinum and pulmonary vasculature, especially behind the heart. The ribs and granuloma appear less dense.

where it arches anteriorly to drain into the superior vena cava. The lower half of the right side of the cardiovascular silhouette is convex and produced by the body of the right atrium. Occasionally, the inferior vena cava is visible as a short vertical shadow in the right cardiophrenic angle.

The left border of the cardiovascular silhouette comprises, from above inferiorly, the aortic knuckle, the pulmonary trunk, the left atrial appendage and the left ventricle. The aortic arch is usually left sided, arching posteriorly over the left bronchus. The aortic knuckle is produced by the posterior part of the arch; the proximal part of the descending aorta may be visible as a vertical shadow, continuous with the knuckle and eventually merging with the left paraspinal shadow. The pulmonary trunk is projected below the aortic knuckle, and below this is a short segment produced by the left atrial appendage. The left ventricle forms the bulk of the left heart border. Frequently, the left cardiophrenic angle is filled in by a low-density shadow representing an apical pericardial fat pad (Fig. 12.4). Less commonly, a fat pad is visible in the right cardiophrenic angle.

On the *lateral film* (Fig. 12.5), the heart is seen anteriorly, in contact with the lower half of the sternum. The anterior border of the heart shadow is formed almost entirely by the right ventricle, although in atrial diastole the right atrial appendage may touch the sternum. The right ventricular outflow tract is continuous with the main pulmonary artery, which arches posteriorly and continues into the left pulmonary artery. The branches of the right pulmonary artery, where they emerge from the pericardium, cast an ovoid shadow anterior to the right bronchus. The distal part of the ascending aorta may be visible above the pulmonary trunk, and the aortic arch is seen passing posteriorly and then descending for a variable distance. The aortic arch is separated from the left pulmonary artery by the aortico-pulmonary window. The upper part of the posterior aspect of the cardiac silhouette is formed by the body of left atrium and the pulmonary veins and the lower part by the left ventricle. The inferior vena cava may be visible as a short straight vertical shadow extending from diaphragm and overlapping the posterior heart border.

The shape of the cardiovascular silhouette changes with age. In infancy, the thymus occupies a large part of the anterior mediastinum and may obscure the aorta, the pulmonary trunk and the right ventricular outflow tract. By early adolesc-

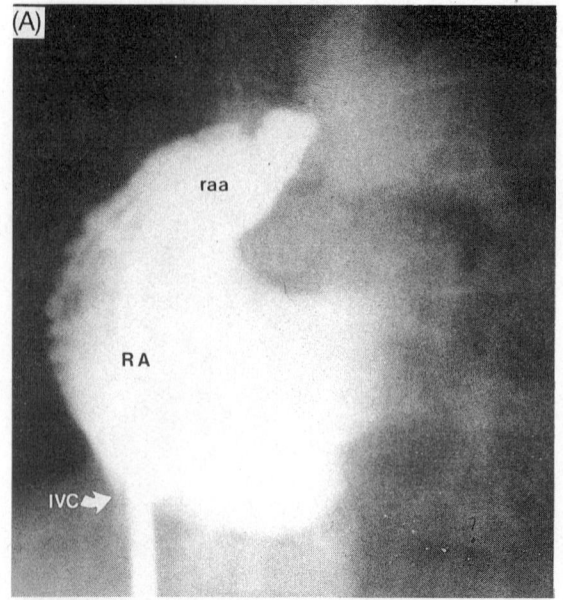

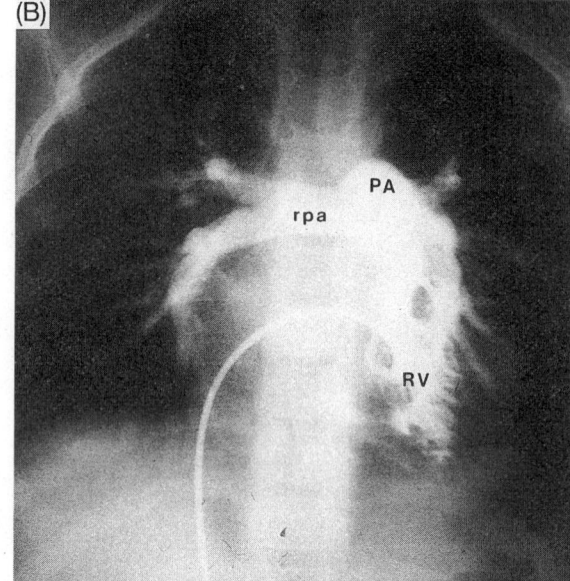

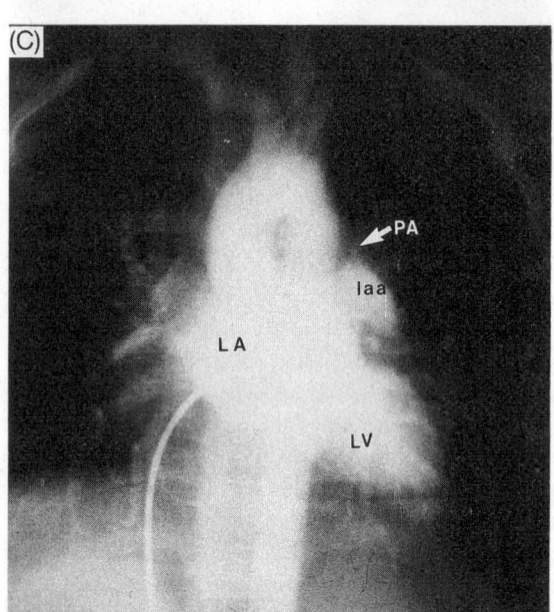

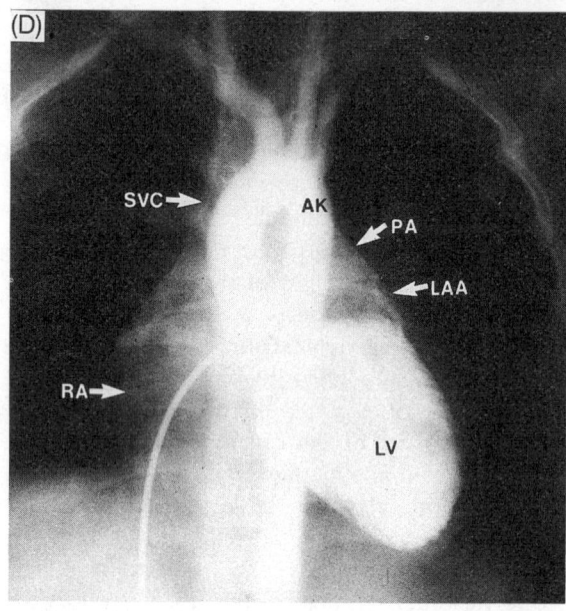

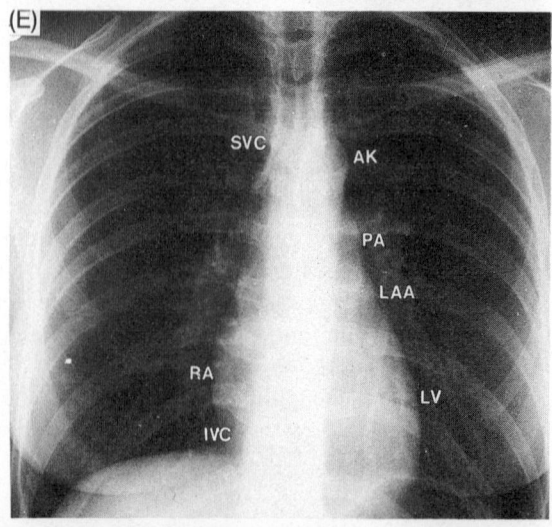

Fig. 12.2. Frontal CXR anatomy—the cardiovascular silhouette. (A) Right atriogram. Catheter in inferior vena cava (IVC). Body of right atrium (RA) forms right heart border. The right atrial appendage (raa) is well demonstrated. (B) Right ventriculogram. The right ventricle (RV) is not a border-forming structure. The pulmonary trunk (PA) forms a short segment of the left cardiovascular silhouette. The right pulmonary artery (rpa) is intrapericardial. (C) Same injection as (B)—laevophase. The body of the left atrium (LA) is not a border-forming structure, but its appendage (laa) is. The left ventricle (LV) forms the bulk of the left heart border; PA, pulmonary trunk. (D) Left ventriculogram. The ascending aorta is not a border-forming structure, being medial to the superior vena cava (SVC). The aortic knuckle (AK) lies above the pulmonary artery (PA). LAA, left atrial appendage; RA, right atrium; LV, left ventricle. (E) The normal frontal cardiovascular silhouette (labels as previously).

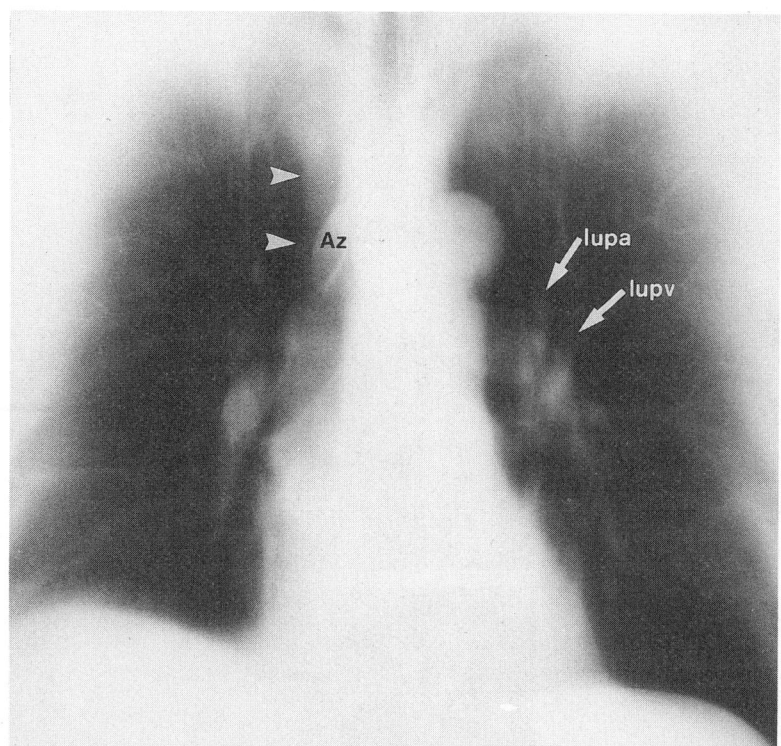

Fig. 12.3. Normal antero-posterior tomogram. Patient supine. The superior vena cava (arrowheads) and azygos vein (Az) are well demonstrated. The left upper lobe pulmonary vein (lupv) is lateral to the left upper lobe pulmonary artery (lupa).

ence, the thymus is not visible on the CXR, and the normal pulmonary trunk is often prominent. In adulthood, the pulmonary trunk becomes less

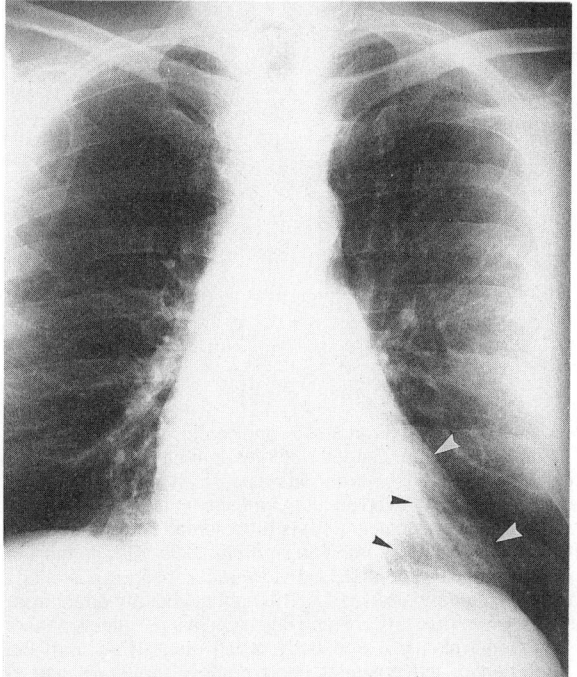

Fig. 12.4. Pericardial fat pads. A large apical fat pad (white arrowheads) is situated over the cardiac apex (black arrowheads). A smaller fat pad is present in the right cardiophrenic angle.

prominent, and with advancing years the left ventricular contour becomes more convex. In old age, the ascending aorta may become tortuous and project lateral to the superior vena cava, and the aortic knuckle and descending aorta may be increasingly prominent.

THE PULMONARY VASCULATURE

As described above, the pulmonary trunk usually forms a short segment of the left heart border. In adults, it is usually straight, but in normal children and young women it may be slightly convex. The pulmonary arteries are not visible until they emerge from the pericardium and are surrounded by lung. The right pulmonary artery lies anterior to the right bronchus and usually divides into upper lobe and descending branches just before emerging from the pericardium. The descending branch passes inferiorly and is usually clearly seen lateral to the right heart border, forming the bulk of the right hilum. Its diameter should not exceed 15 mm in females and 16 mm in males. The left pulmonary artery arches posteriorly over its bronchus, and, therefore, the left hilum is higher than the right. The branching pattern of the pulmonary arteries is similar to that of the bronchi. As the pulmonary arteries pass peripherally, they taper smoothly and are not

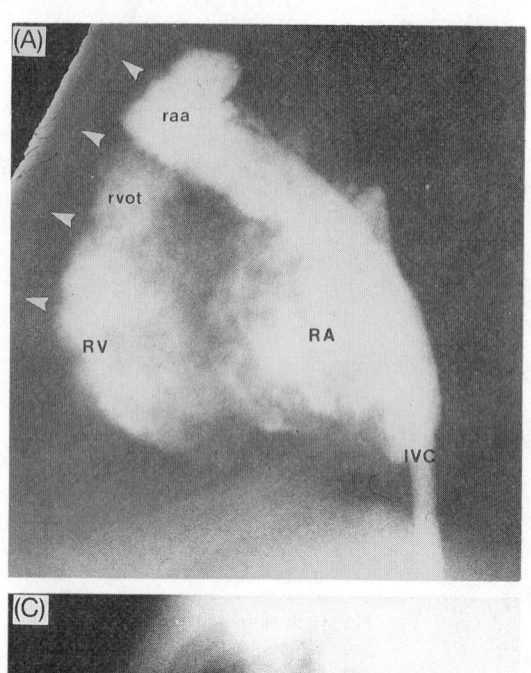

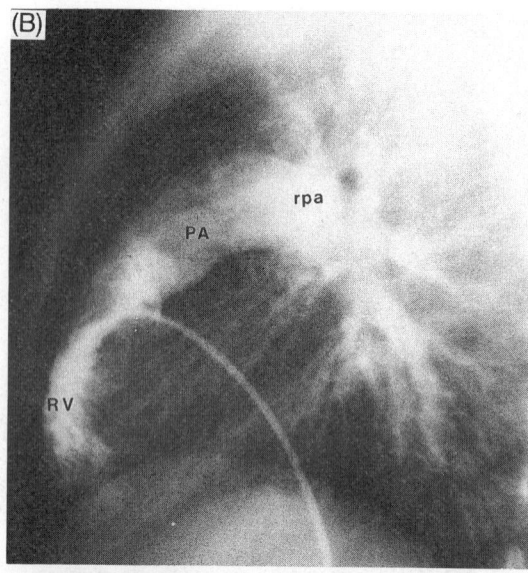

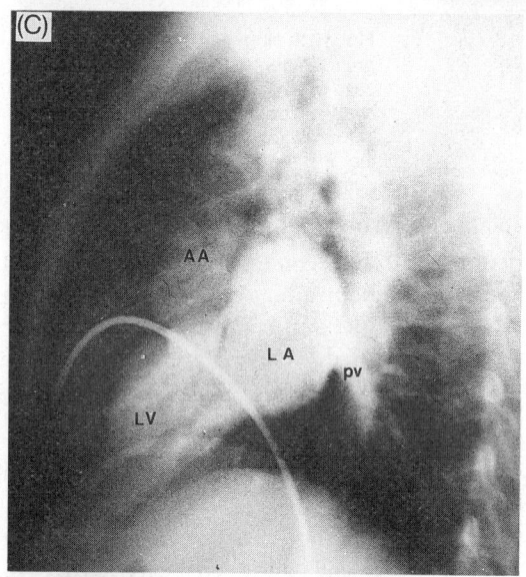

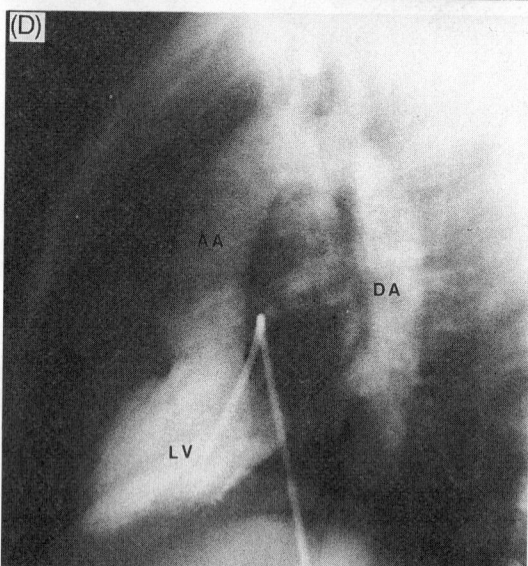

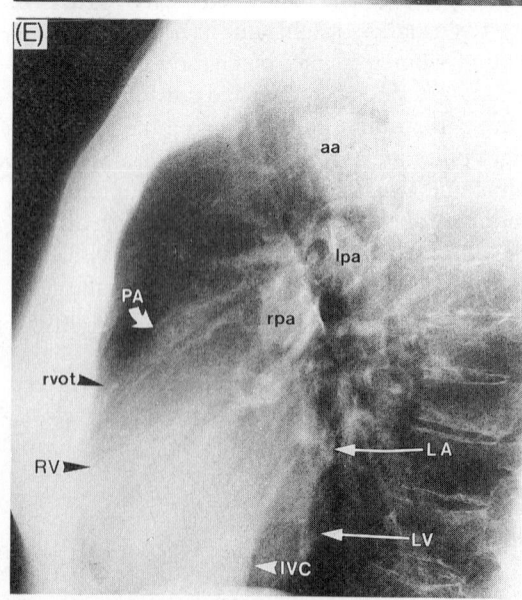

Fig. 12.5. Lateral CXR anatomy—the cardiovascular silhouette. (A) Right atriogram. Catheter in inferior vena cava (IVC). The right atrial appendage (raa) lies close to the sternum (white arrowheads) and overlies the right ventricular outflow tract (rvot). The right ventricle (RV) is retrosternal. RA, right atrium. (B) Right ventriculogram. The right ventricle (RV) forms the anterior heart border, and its outflow tract continues posteriorly as the pulmonary artery (PA). The right pulmonary artery (rpa) is seen 'en face'. (C) Same injection as (B)—laevophase. Pulmonary veins (pv) and body of left atrium (LA) form the upper part of the posterior heart border. The lower part is formed by left ventricle (LV). The ascending aorta (AA) after emerging from pericardium may be seen above the pulmonary artery. (D) Left ventriculogram. The left ventricle (LV), ascending aorta (AA) and descending aorta (DA) are well demonstrated. (E) The normal lateral cardiovascular silhouette. The aortic arch (aa) and left pulmonary artery (lpa) are well shown on this film. (Other labels as previously.)

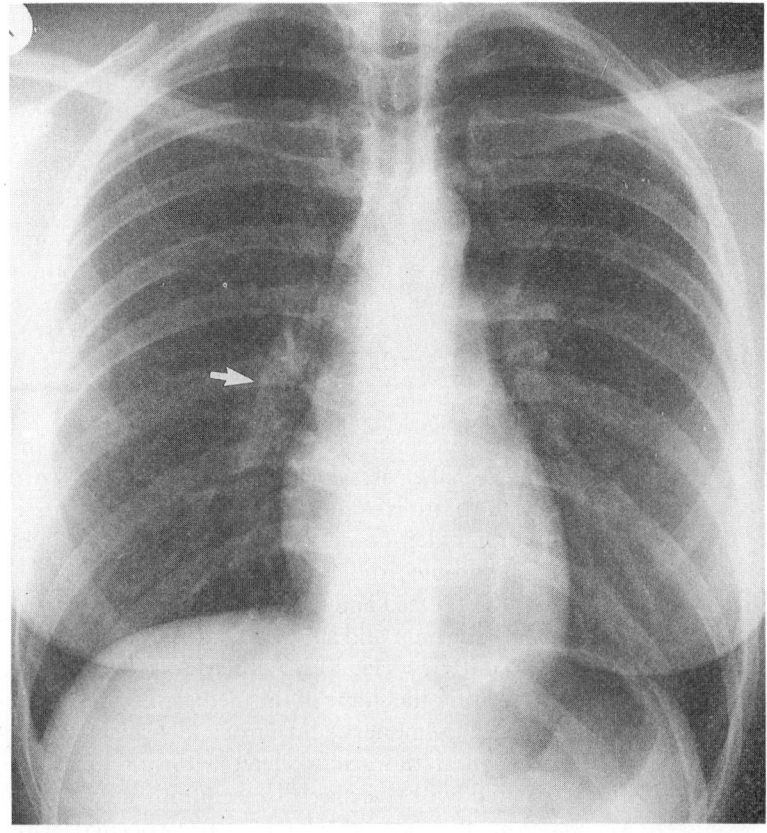

Fig. 12.6. Normal pulmonary vascular pattern. The descending branch of the right pulmonary artery is arrowed.

normally visible in the outer third of the lung (Fig. 12.6).

The pulmonary venous anatomy is somewhat variable. The upper lobe veins run lateral to the corresponding pulmonary arteries and may be identified crossing the pulmonary arteries at the hilum (Fig. 12.3) before entering the left atrium. The lower lobe veins run more horizontally and medially than the accompanying arteries. Radiographically, the hilum is the area where the upper lobe vein crosses the basal artery.

On the frontal CXR of a normal subject, the peripheral pulmonary vessels should be clearly visible and are larger in the lower zones than in the upper zones. The upper zone veins in the first anterior intercostal space should not exceed 3 mm in diameter. On a supine film, the upper zone and lower zone vessels are similar in size.

HEART SIZE

The commonest methods of assessment of cardiac size using the CXR are the measurement of the transverse cardiac diameter and the measurement of cardiothoracic ratio.

The transverse cardiac diameter is measured on a PA film by adding the maximum distance of the right heart border from the mid-line to the maximum distance of the left heart border from the mid-line (Fig. 12.7). The upper limit of normal is 16 cm for men and 15 cm for women. A change of 1.5 cm in cardiac diameter is significant. Apparent increase in heart size may be due to a poor inspiration (Fig. 12.8). When using air-gap techniques and AP films, geometric magnification of the heart shadow occurs.

The cardiothoracic ratio is the ratio of transverse cardiac diameter to maximum internal diameter of the thorax (Fig. 12.7). There are racial differences in the normal ratio. The ratio should not exceed 50% in white subjects or 55% in black subjects.

The cardiac volume may be calculated using PA and lateral films and assuming the heart shape to be between a paraboloid and an ellipsoid (Fig. 12.9).[4] Long and broad diameters are measured on the PA film and the depth is measured on the lateral film. The product of these 3 diameters, a geometric

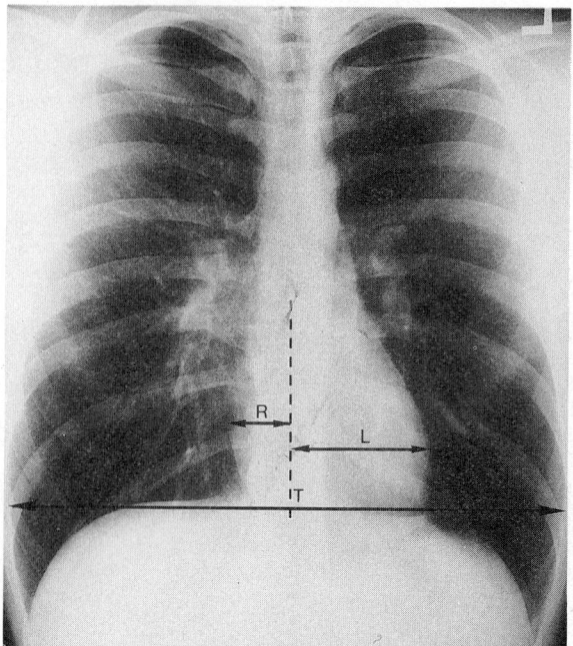

Fig. 12.7. Measurement of heart size—see text.

Transverse cardiac diameter = R + L

Cardiothoracic ratio = $\dfrac{(R + L)}{T}$

constant (0.63) and a magnification factor, which depends upon the X-ray technique, gives the cardiac volume, which may then be related to the patient's surface area. Measurement of cardiac volume is not a routine clinical procedure.

ANALYSIS OF THE CHEST X-RAY

As in other areas of clinical examination, the CXR should be analysed in a strict systematic manner. Poor radiographic technique may produce spurious appearances. The cardiovascular silhouette is such an obvious focus of attention that the bones, soft tissues and upper abdomen may be overlooked. The heart shadow may provide information about anatomy, but the lungs provide information about haemodynamics. A proposed order of analysis is as follows: technical factors, the bones, the upper abdomen, the lungs and, finally, the heart.

THE ABNORMAL CHEST X-RAY

TECHNICAL CONSIDERATIONS

The lungs on an over-exposed CXR are blacker than usual and may suggest oligaemia. Conversely, an under-exposed film may accentuate the pulmonary vascular pattern, or even suggest diffuse lung disease. A film made on expiration may show increased basal shadowing and suggest pulmonary oedema or other interstitial lung disease, and the heart and other mediastinal structures may appear enlarged (Fig. 12.8). A rotated film may make some structures appear unusually prominent and others unusually small.

THE BONES

Thoracic deformity may alter the appearance of the heart. Sternal depression usually causes a leftward shift and rotation of the heart giving a characteristically straight left border (Fig. 12.10). In the 'straight back syndrome', the antero-posterior thoracic diameter is decreased and the heart may be compressed between sternum and spine and appear enlarged on the frontal view (Fig. 12.11). Severe scoliosis may not only alter the shape of the mediastinum but may also cause pulmonary and cardiac disease.

Congenital thoracic skeletal deformity may be associated with cardiac disease. Both sternal depression and 'straight back' are associated with mitral valve prolapse. Many systemic diseases and congenital syndromes affecting the heart may have skeletal manifestations e.g. in Down's syndrome there may be an endocardial cushion defect and only 11 pairs of ribs.

Rib notching[5] is usually associated with coarctation of the aorta (Fig. 12.12), but it may be seen following a Blalock–Taussig shunt and in pulmonary atresia and vena caval obstruction. Evidence of previous surgery, such as rib deformity, sternal sutures and prosthetic valves, is easily seen on the CXR (see Fig. 12.24B).

THE UPPER ABDOMEN

Occasionally, patients presenting to the cardiologist with chest pain have a hiatus hernia or gallstones which may be visible on the CXR. In patients with congenital heart disease, information about situs may be visible on the CXR. In these cases, it is worth noting on which side the stomach and liver lie, and also whether the spleen is visible and its location. However, the best indication of abdominal situs is given by the tracheobronchial anatomy, and the interested reader should refer to Chapter 25.

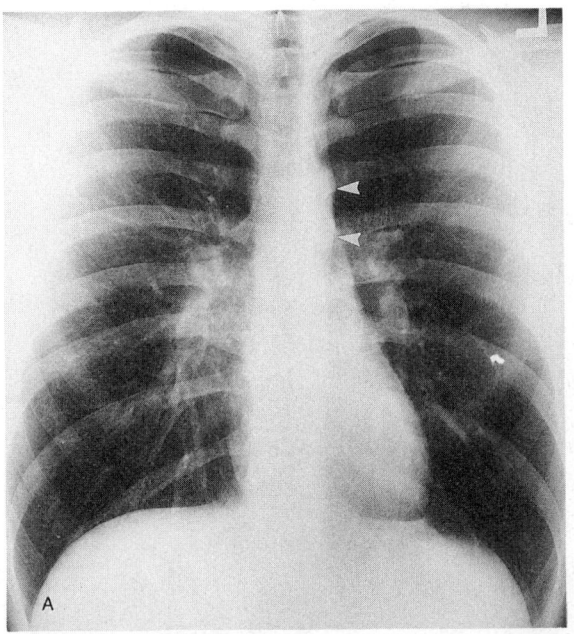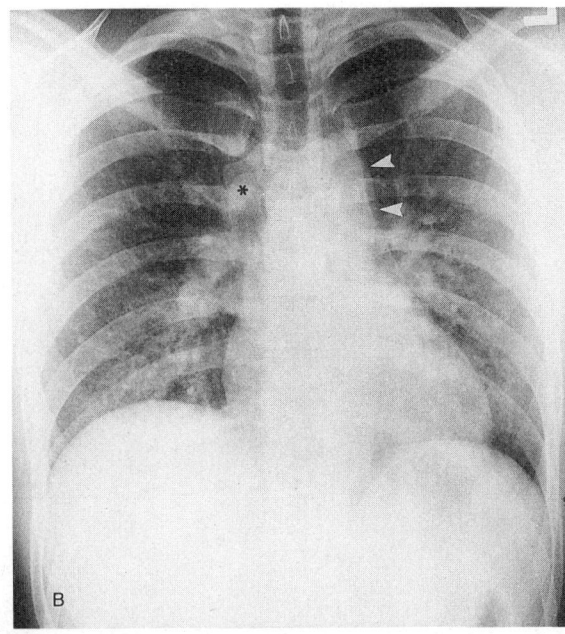

Fig. 12.8. (A) Normal CXR on inspiration. Descending aorta is arrowed. (B) Same patient: CXR on expiration. The heart size has increased, the lower zone vessels are less distinct, the descending aorta is more prominent (arrowheads) and the azygos vein (asterisk) has enlarged.

THE LUNGS

Pulmonary vascularity may be normal, increased, decreased or uneven. A normal pulmonary vascular pattern does not exclude significant myocardial disease, mild valvular disease or a small intracardiac shunt.

The normal radiographic appearance of the lung is produced by pulmonary vessels outlined by air-filled alveoli. Any opacity that is not a vessel should be carefully considered. As smoking is an important aetiological factor in both heart and lung disease, it is not surprising that the routine CXR in a cardiac patient may uncover previously unsuspected lung disease (Fig. 12.13).

There are four distinct patterns of increased pulmonary vascularity:
1 pulmonary venous hypertension;
2 pulmonary arterial hypertension;
3 pulmonary over-circulation;
4 systemic supply to the lungs.
Any of these patterns may co-exist.

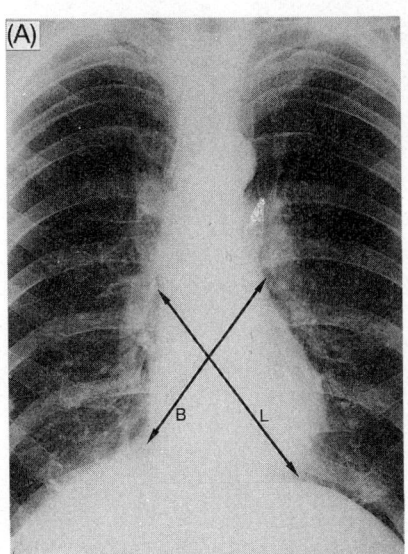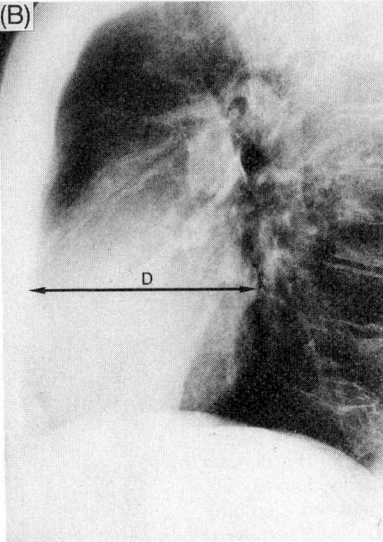

Fig. 12.9. Measurement of cardiac volume—see text.

Cardiac volume = B × L × D × 0.63 × magnification factor.

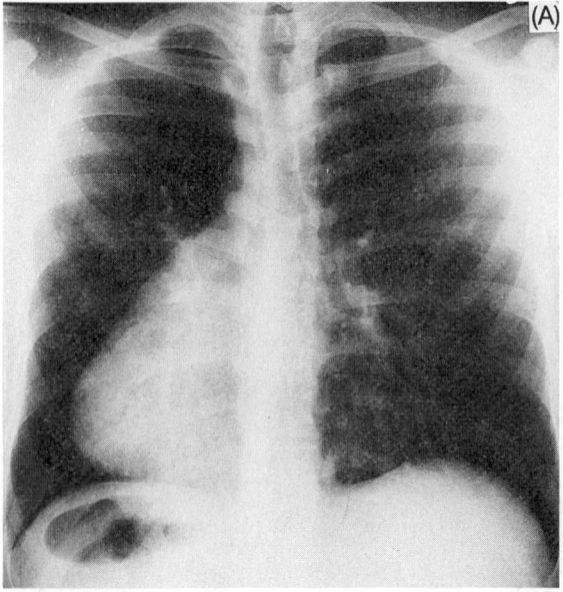

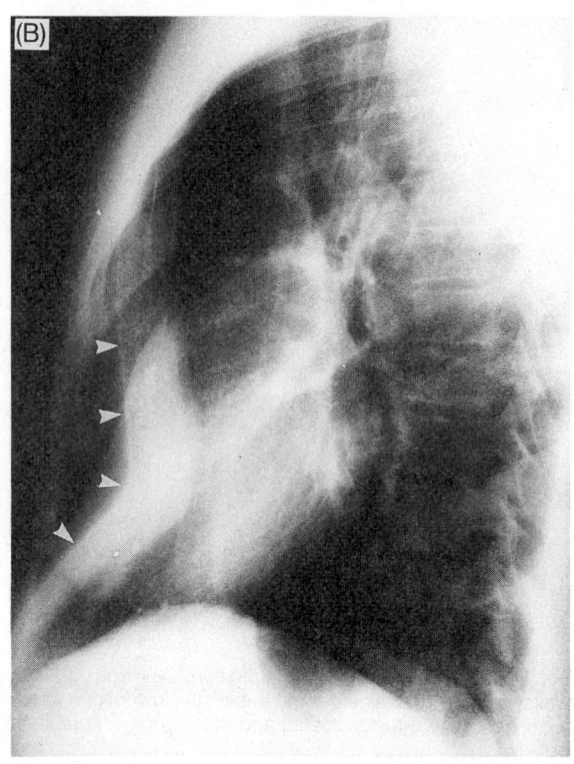

Fig. 12.10. Sternal depression. (A) on the frontal film, the heart is shifted to the left and the left heart border appears straightened. (B) The lateral film clearly shows that this is due to the depressed sternum (arrowheads).

Pulmonary venous hypertension

The commonest causes of pulmonary venous hypertension are left ventricular failure, mitral valve disease and aortic valve disease. Rarely, it is due to

pulmonary venous obstruction. As pulmonary venous pressure rises, the upper lobe veins distend and become similar in size to the lower lobe veins; eventually, they become larger. This phenomenon

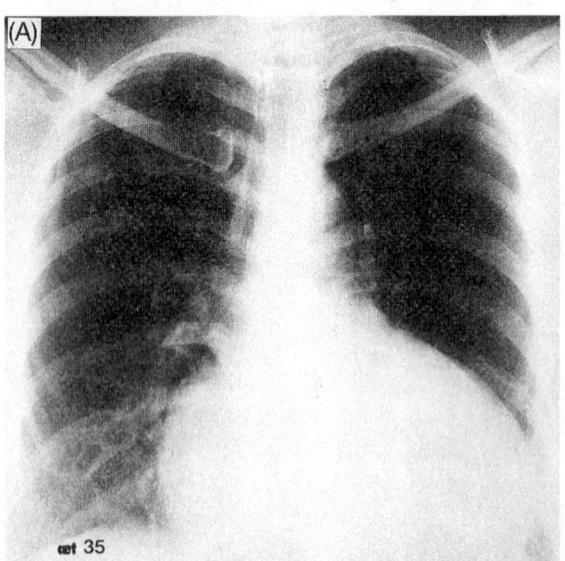

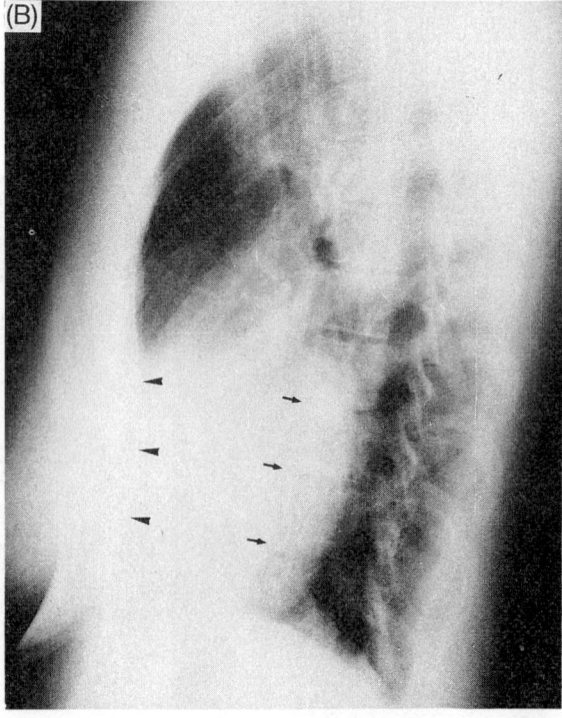

Fig. 12.11. Straight back. On the frontal film (A), the heart appears enlarged. The lateral film (B) shows that the dorsal spine is straightened, the thoracic antero-posterior diameter is decreased, and the heart is compressed between sternum (arrowheads) and spine (arrows).

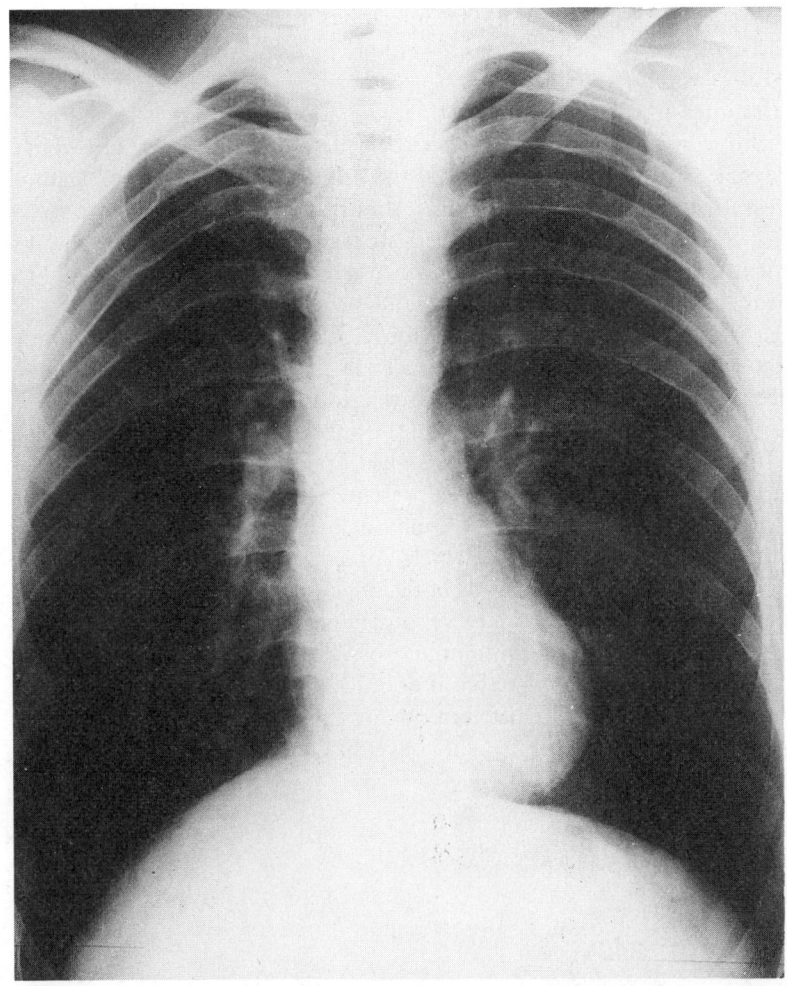

Fig. 12.12. Rib notching due to coarctation of aorta. The inferior surfaces of the 4th–9th ribs show well-defined indentations with sclerotic margins, due to pressure from enlarged intercostal arteries. The contour of the aortic knuckle is abnormally flattened.

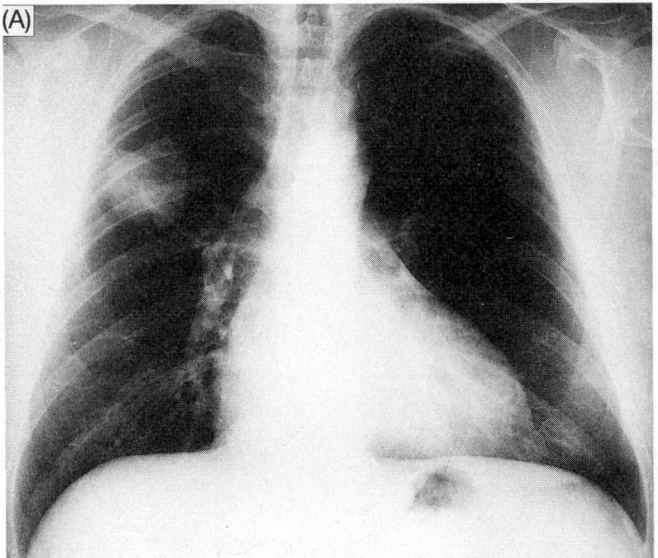
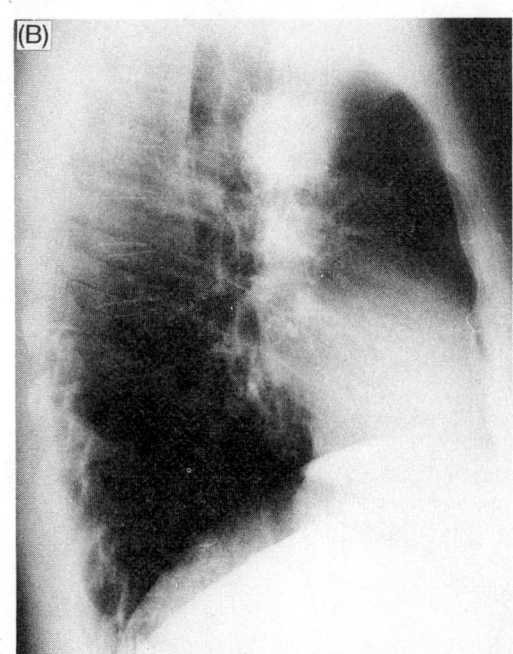

Fig. 12.13. (A) and (B) Lung cancer in a 53-year-old asymptomatic smoker, 6 years after coronary artery bypass surgery. Right upper lobe carcinoma discovered on routine CXR.

may be described as 'redistribution of blood flow' or 'upper lobe blood diversion' (Fig. 12.14). If the pulmonary venous pressure exceeds the plasma osmotic pressure, fluid accumulates in the interstitial spaces of the lung. Radiographically, this appears as interstitial pulmonary oedema (Fig. 12.15). The lower zone and hilar vessels may become indistinct (perihilar haze) and interstitial lines may appear. Kerley B lines are caused by fluid-filled interlobular septa and appear as fine non-branching horizontal lines in the periphery of the lower zones. Kerley A lines are less common and are longer, fine-line shadows that radiate from the hila into the mid and upper zones. They also represent distended interlobular septa. Interstitial fluid around bronchi may appear as peribronchial cuffing (Fig. 12.16C). A further increase in pulmonary venous pressure leads to accumulation of fluid in the alveolar spaces (Fig. 12.16). Alveolar pulmonary oedema may be indistinguishable from other causes of pulmonary consolidation. Classically, alveolar oedema is perihilar, but it may be patchy and asymmetric, even nodular. Pleural effusions are common in pulmonary venous hyper-

tension. The interlobar fissures may appear thickened due to either pleural fluid or sub-pleural oedema.

In the untreated patient, there is a fairly close correlation between the pulmonary capillary wedge pressure and the signs of pulmonary venous hypertension.[6] A normal vascular pattern corresponds to a wedge pressure of < 12 mmHg, that of redistribution of blood flow corresponds to 12–18 mmHg, interstitial oedema corresponds to 18–22 mmHg, and above 22 mmHg, there is usually alveolar oedema. If a patient has received diuretic therapy, this correlation is less reliable.

In patients with longstanding pulmonary venous hypertension, signs of pulmonary arterial hypertension may be present. Chronic pulmonary venous hypertension may also be associated with haemosiderosis, which appears as a fine nodular pattern throughout both lungs (Fig. 12.17). Severe chronic pulmonary venous hypertension may be associated with pulmonary ossicles (Fig. 12.18). These are calcified basal nodules, up to 1 cm in diameter.

Redistribution of blood flow may occur in patients who have basal emphysema and no evi-

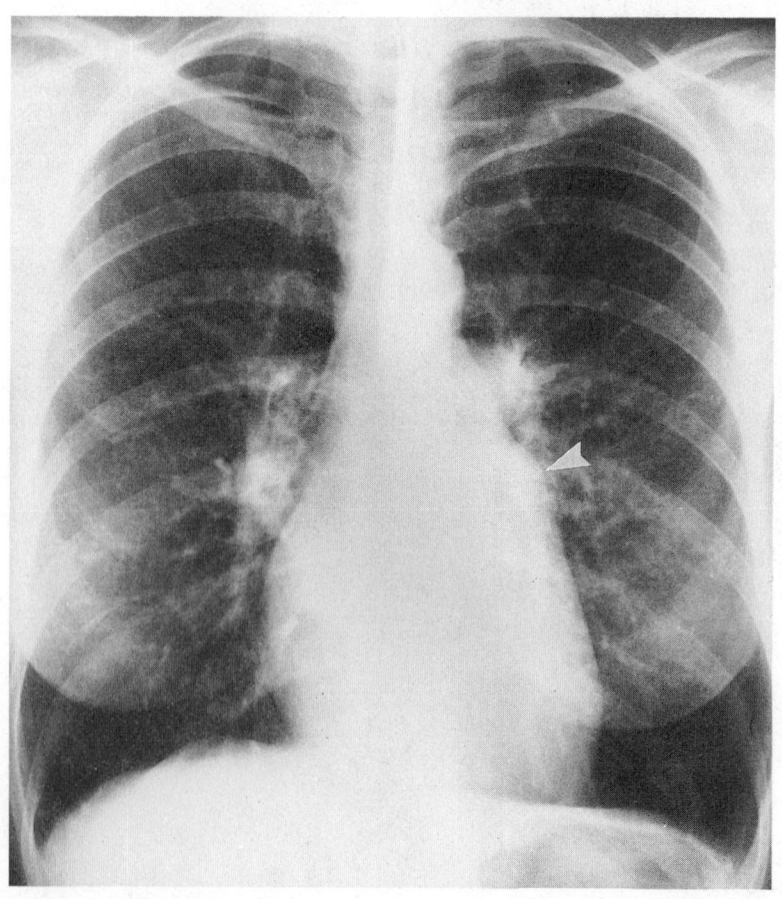

Fig. 12.14. Redistribution of blood flow. Mitral stenosis. The upper zone vessels are larger than the lower zone vessels. The left atrial appendage is enlarged (arrowhead).

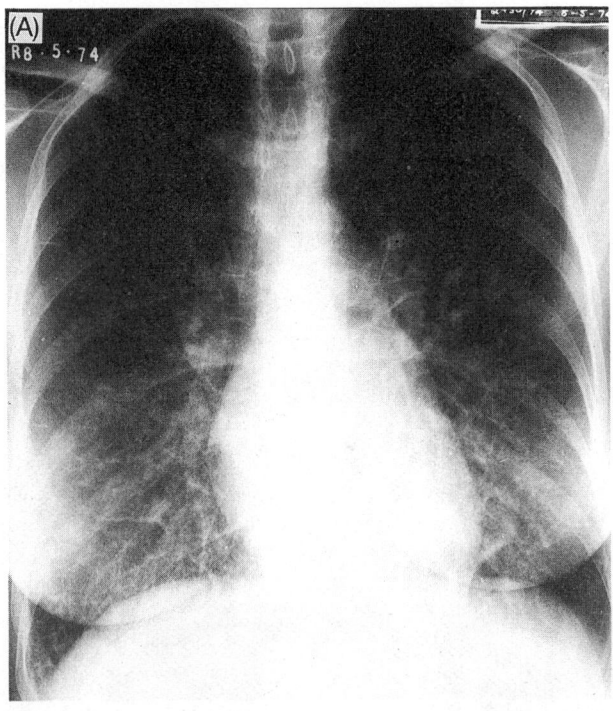

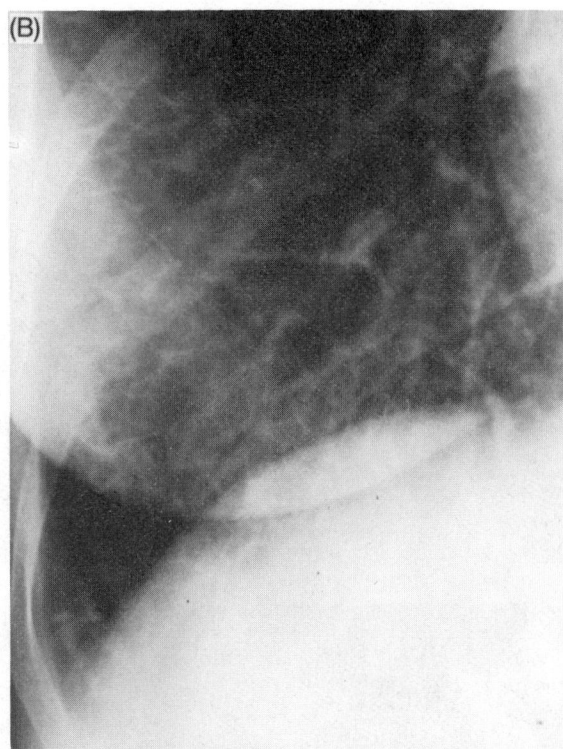

Fig. 12.15. Interstitial pulmonary oedema in mitral stenosis. (A) The lower zone and hilar vessels are indistinct. Kerley B lines are present in the periphery of both lower zones. (B) An enlargement of (A). Increased interstitial shadows are present. Kerley B lines are present adjacent to the lateral chest wall.

dence of pulmonary venous hypertension (Fig. 12.19). Septal lines may be seen in non-cardiogenic pulmonary oedema (Fig. 12.20), lymphangitis carcinomatosa, sarcoidosis and silicosis.

Pulmonary arterial hypertension

Pulmonary arterial hypertension exists when the pulmonary artery systolic pressure is > 30 mmHg. The main causes of this condition are chronic lung disease, pulmonary emboli, pulmonary venous hypertension, shunts and idiopathic. The essential radiographic appearances are enlargement of the central pulmonary arteries and pruning of the peripheral arteries (Fig. 12.21). In severe longstanding pulmonary arterial hypertension, calcification may be seen in the central pulmonary arteries.

Clues to the basic cause may be present on the CXR, for example, there may be signs of chronic obstructive airways disease or pulmonary embolism (Fig. 12.22). Bilateral hilar lymph node enlargement may mimic enlarged central pulmonary arteries, but usually lymphadenopathy is lobulated, whereas enlarged arteries have a smooth outline.

Pulmonary over-circulation

Pulmonary over-circulation or plethora implies increased blood flow through the lungs. It is usually due to a left-to-right shunt, less commonly due to bidirectional shunting and rarely due to increased cardiac output. Small shunts may not be perceptible on the CXR, but shunts with a pulmonary-to-systemic flow ratio of 2:1 or greater should be apparent unless there is co-existing heart failure. The central pulmonary arteries are larger than normal and peripheral pulmonary vessels are visible in the outer third of the lung (Fig. 12.23). Pulmonary plethora in a non-cyanosed patient indicates a left-to-right shunt, whereas in the presence of central cyanosis it indicates bidirectional shunting.

Systemic supply to the lungs

Systemic supply to the lungs, which is often known as bronchial circulation, develops in patients with severe right ventricular outflow obstruction. The pulmonary trunk is either small or absent, and the peripheral vessels are disorganized and may pro-

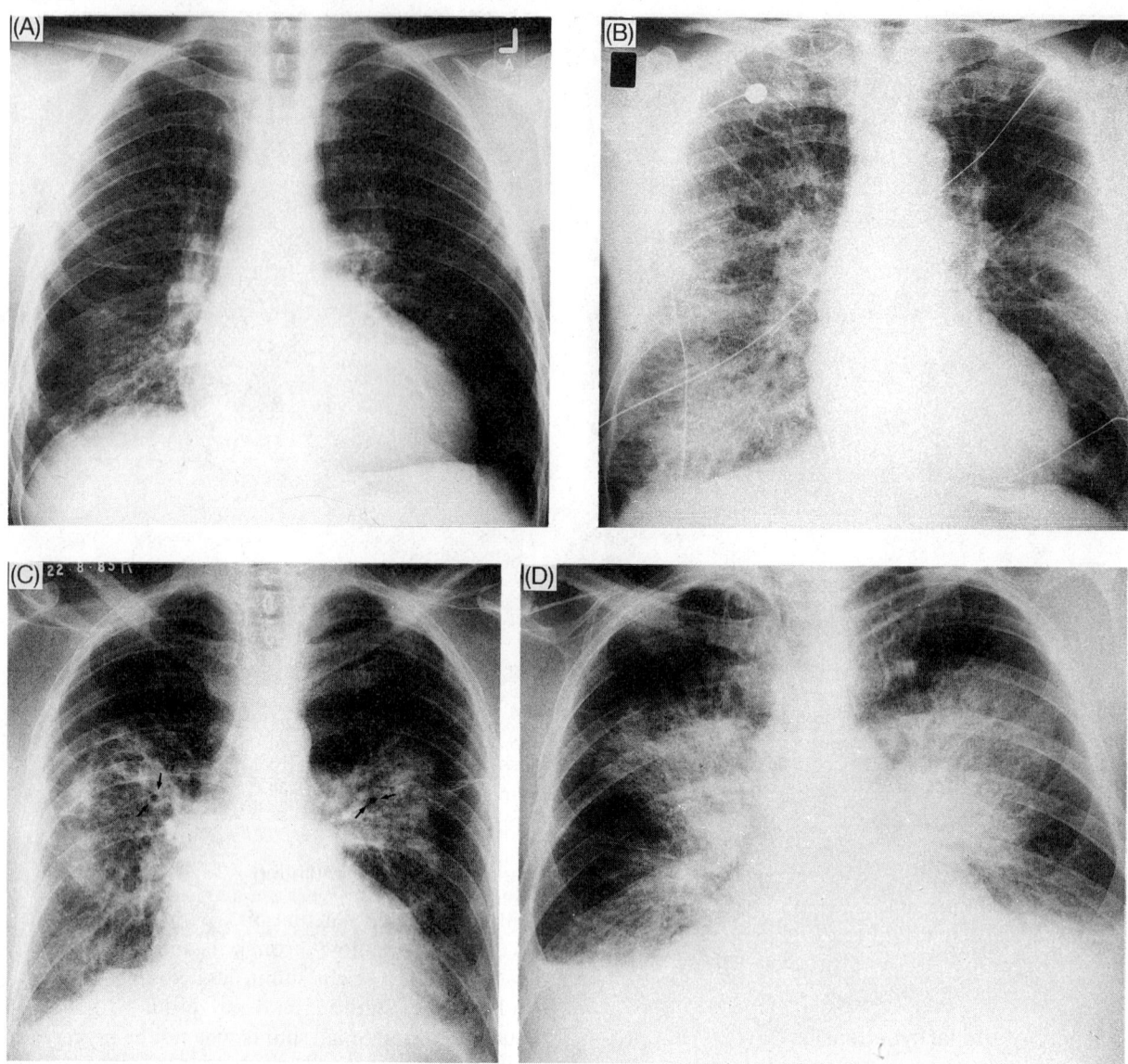

Fig. 12.16. Alveolar pulmonary oedema. (A) Coarctation of aorta and bicuspid aortic valve. Localized consolidation is present in the right lower zone. Lamellar pleural effusions are present and the horizontal fissure is thickened. Note rib notching, left ventricular enlargement and flattened aortic knuckle. (B) Myocardial infarction. Consolidation is present in both mid-zones and the right lower zone. There is perihilar haze, and Kerley B lines are visible at the right base. (C) Congestive cardiomyopathy. Bilateral perihilar consolidation is present. Peribronchial cuffing is well shown (arrows). Note left ventricular enlargement. (D) Acute myocardial infarction. Bilateral perihilar consolidation and moderate pleural effusions are present.

duce a reticular or nodular pattern similar to that of interstitial lung disease. There may be areas of oligaemia (Fig. 12.24).

Pulmonary oligaemia

Pulmonary oligaemia implies decreased blood flow through the lungs. It is usually due to right ventricular outflow obstruction in association with a right-to-left shunt. It may also occur with restricted filling of the right heart, such as occurs in cardiac tamponade, but such oligaemia is rarely perceptible on the CXR. The lungs appear to have fewer and smaller vessels than usual, and the pulmonary trunk may be small or inapparent (Fig. 12.25).

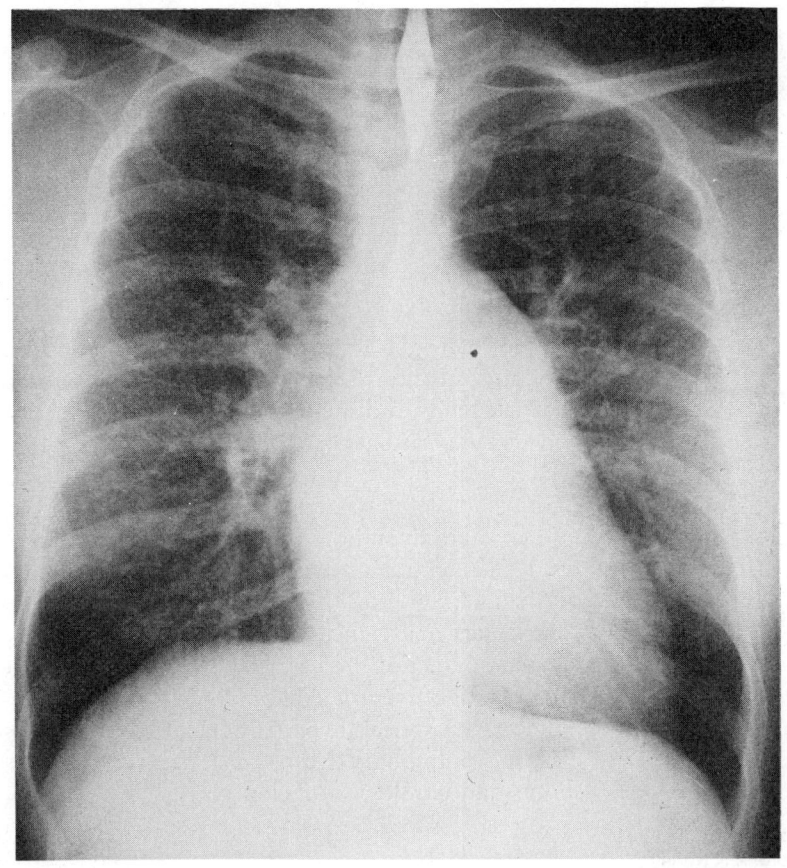

Fig. 12.17. Haemosiderosis. Longstanding rheumatic mitral valve disease. Small nodular shadows are present throughout both lungs. The pulmonary trunk is enlarged consistent with pulmonary arterial hypertension.

Uneven vascularity

Minor degrees of rotation of the patient or thoracic skeletal deformity may make one lung appear darker than the other. Uneven vascularity is most commonly due to pulmonary disease, for example, fibrosis, segmental or lobar collapse or emphysema. A previous lung resection will obviously alter the vascular pattern. Apart from pulmonary thrombo-embolism, cardiovascular causes of uneven vascularity are uncommon, but include previous shunt operations for congenital heart disease, pulmonary artery stenoses and pulmonary arteriovenous fistulae.

ABNORMALITIES OF THE HEART AND GREAT VESSELS

The systemic veins

The superior vena cava may be enlarged by either increased flow or increased pressure. Increased flow occurs in anomalous pulmonary venous return. Increased pressure occurs in right heart failure,

tricuspid valve disease (see Fig. 12.29), cardiac tamponade (see Fig. 12.45B) and constrictive pericarditis. The superior vena cava may also be obstructed by mediastinitis and mediastinal tumours. A tortuous or dilated ascending aorta or right-sided aortic arch may displace the superior vena cava laterally (Fig. 12.25). A persistent left superior vena cava is present in 0.5% of the normal population and in a higher proportion of patients with congenital heart disease. It may produce a low-density shadow in the left upper mediastinum.

The azygos may be enlarged for the same reasons as those that apply to enlargement of the superior vena cava; an enlarged azygos is also seen in superior vena caval obstruction (Fig. 12.26), portal vein obstruction and absence of the hepatic portion of the inferior vena cava in polysplenia.

The inferior vena cava may become enlarged in right heart failure (Fig. 12.27).

The right atrium

Right atrial enlargement rarely occurs in isolation, and is usually associated with right ventricular

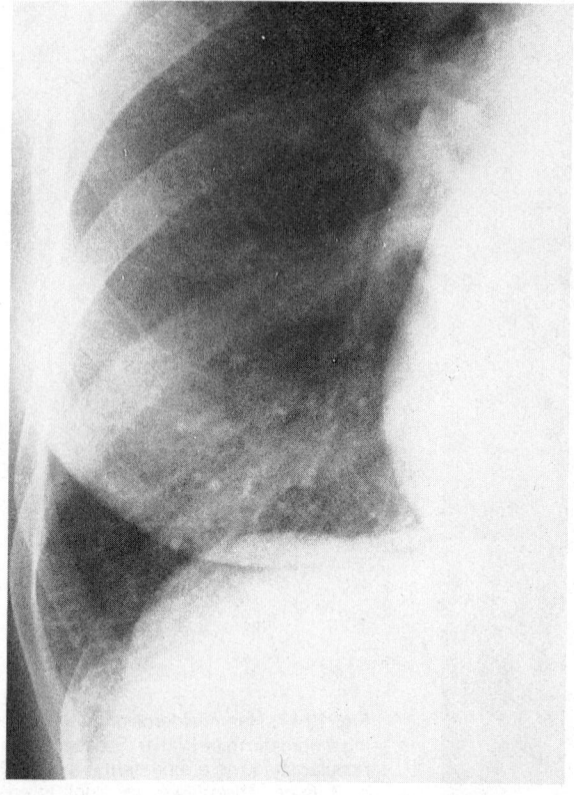

Fig. 12.18. Pulmonary ossicles. Longstanding rheumatic mitral valve disease. Small calcified basal nodules are present. Kerley B lines are also visible.

enlargement. Classically, right atrial enlargement produces increased prominence of the lower half of the right side of the cardiac shadow (Figs. 12.28 and 12.29). Right atrial enlargement occurs in right heart failure, tricuspid valve disease and in atrial septal defect and other shunts that enter the right atrium.

The right ventricle

The normal right ventricle is not a border-forming structure on the frontal CXR. An enlarging right ventricle tends to displace the left ventricle laterally and so the cardiac apex becomes elevated (Fig. 12.23A). In gross right ventricular enlargement, the right ventricle may actually form the left heart border, and dilatation of its outflow tract may produce an extra convexity just below the pulmonary trunk (Fig. 12.28). On the lateral view, right ventricular enlargement is made manifest by increased contact of the heart with the sternum (Fig. 12.30). Right ventricular enlargement occurs in pulmonary arterial hypertension, tricuspid valve disease, pulmonary valve disease, left-to-right shunts and tetralogy of Fallot.

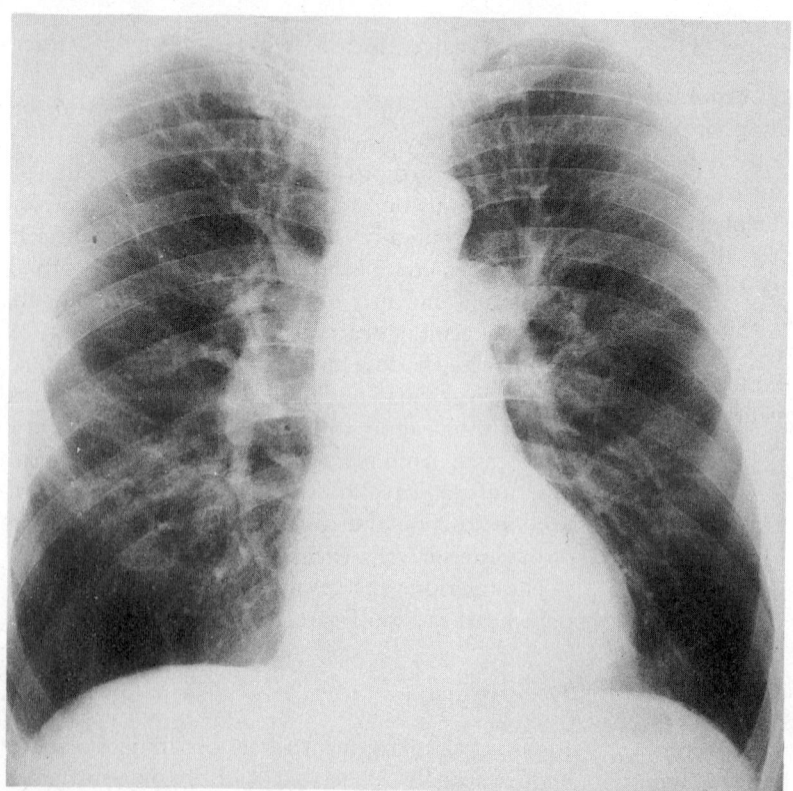

Fig. 12.19. Redistribution of blood flow due to basal emphysema in patient with alpha-1-anti-trypsin deficiency. Enlargement of the central pulmonary arteries indicates pulmonary arterial hypertension.

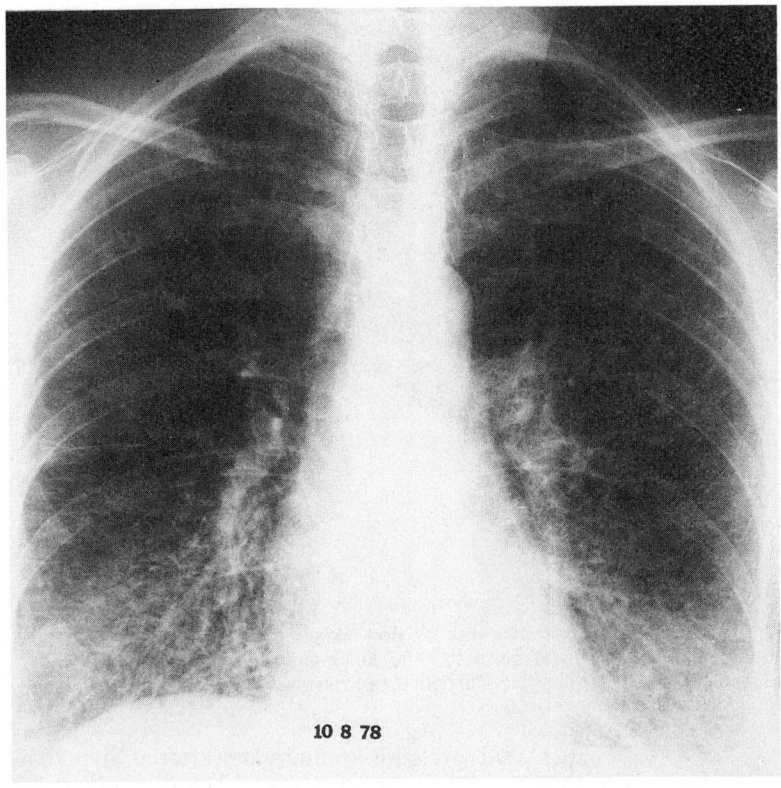

Fig. 12.20. Non-cardiogenic pulmonary oedema due to heroin overdose. Multiple Kerley B lines are present in addition to extensive lower zone interstitial shadowing and generalized nodular shadows.

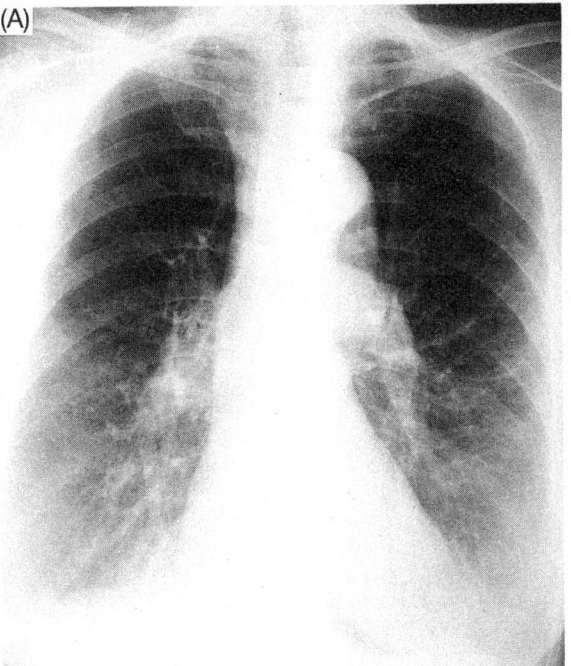

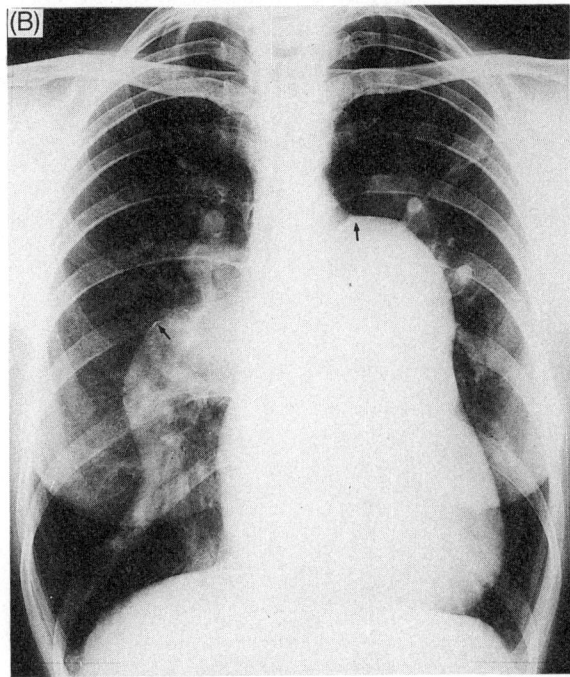

Fig. 12.21. Pulmonary arterial hypertension. (A) Chronic obstructive airways disease. The central pulmonary arteries are markedly enlarged. The lungs are hyper-inflated. (B) Eisenmenger atrial septal defect. The central pulmonary arteries are enormously dilated and there is dramatic peripheral pruning. Pulmonary arterial calcification (arrows) indicates severe chronic pulmonary arterial hypertension.

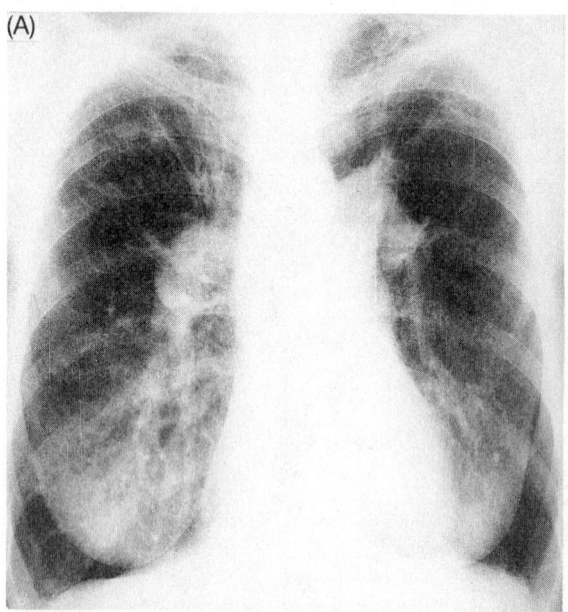

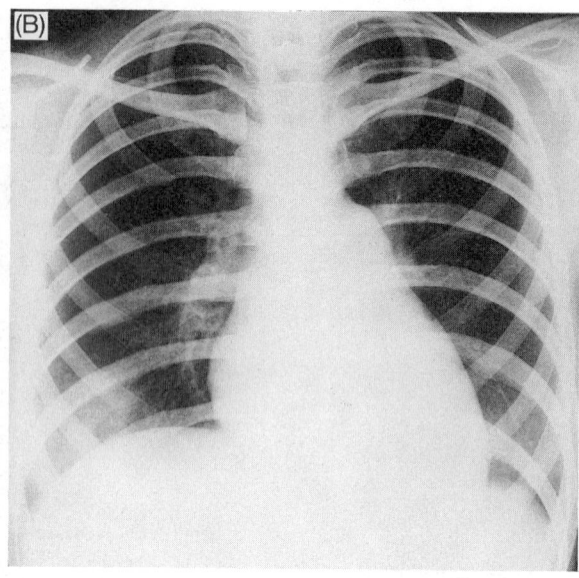

Fig. 12.22. Pulmonary arterial hypertension. (A) Chronic obstructive airways disease and bilateral upper lobe fibrosis. The central pulmonary arteries are enlarged and elevated. The lungs are hyper-inflated. (B) Multiple pulmonary emboli. The pulmonary trunk is enlarged. The right upper zone is oligaemic. Right basal consolidation represents pulmonary infarction.

The pulmonary trunk

Enlargement of the pulmonary trunk is due to increased pressure, increased flow, post-stenotic dilatation or idiopathic dilatation. In conditions of increased pressure (pulmonary arterial hypertension), it is associated with enlargement of the central pulmonary arteries and peripheral pruning (Figs 12.21 and 12.22). In situations of increased flow, it is associated with pulmonary plethora (Fig.

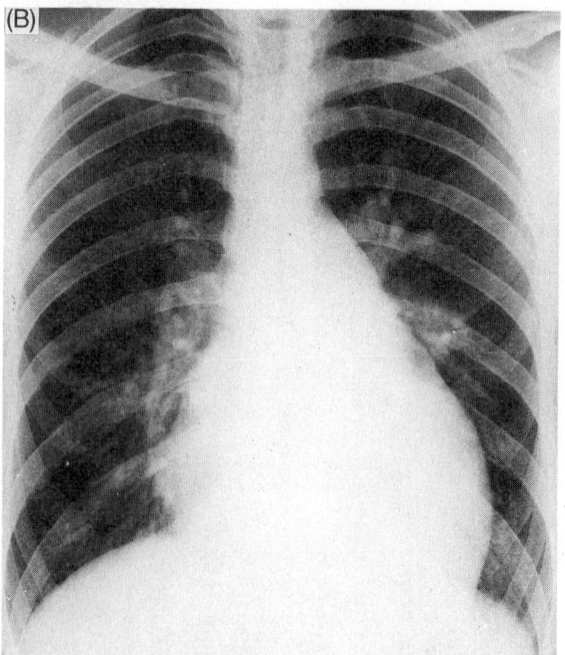

Fig. 12.23. Pulmonary plethora. (A) Atrial septal defect. The pulmonary trunk is prominent and the normal peripheral vascular pattern is accentuated. The cardiac apex is elevated. (B) Ventricular septal defect.

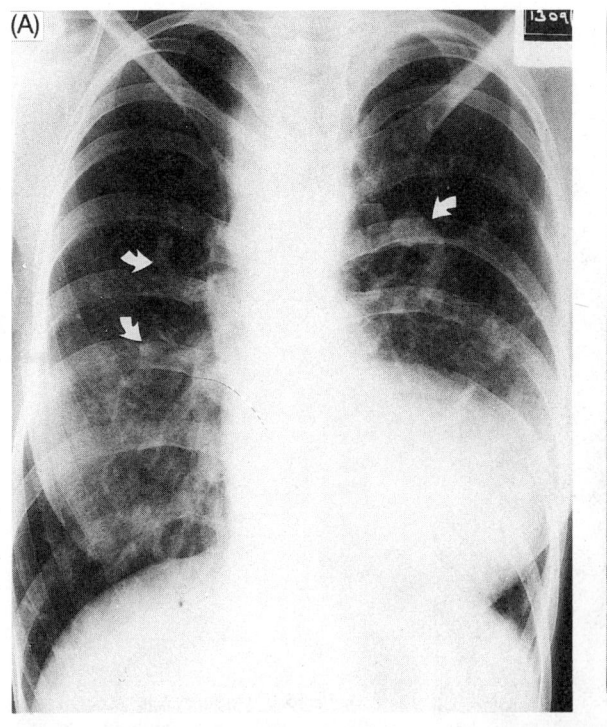 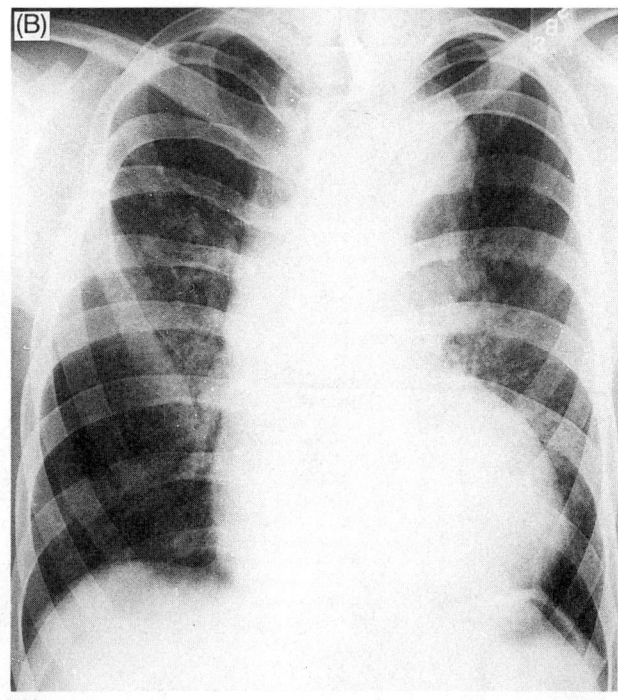

Fig. 12.24. Systemic supply to the lungs. (A) Pulmonary atresia. A pulmonary bay is present. Large systemic collateral arteries (arrows) supply the lungs. The aortic arch is right-sided and the cardiac apex is elevated. (B) Pulmonary atresia with right Blalock–Taussig shunt. A pulmonary bay is present. A fine nodular pattern is present in both mid-zones. The aorta is large. Surgical changes are present in the right 4th rib.

12.23). In cases of post-stenotic and idiopathic dilatation, it is usually associated with enlargement of the left pulmonary artery and normal peripheral vascularity (Fig. 12.31).

In corrected transposition of the great arteries, the pulmonary trunk is not visible on the CXR. In tetralogy of Fallot and pulmonary atresia, the pulmonary trunk is small, producing an obvious pulmonary bay (Figs 12.24 and 12.25).

The left atrium

The body of the left atrium is situated beneath the carina and in front of the oesophagus. Enlargement superiorly may increase the angle between the left and right bronchi by elevating the left bronchus and displacing it posteriorly (Fig. 12.32). Posterior enlargement may displace the oesophagus posteriorly (Fig. 12.33). Enlargement to the right may produce an extra density over the right heart border (Fig. 12.34), and in gross enlargement the left atrium may form the right heart border (Fig. 12.35). Enlargement of the left atrial appendage causes straightening or convex bulging of the upper left heart border (Fig. 12.14). Left atrial enlargement

occurs most obviously in mitral valve disease, but is seen in other forms of left heart failure, in shunts at ventricular and great vessel level and in association with left atrial tumours.

The left ventricle

Left ventricular hypertrophy produces increased convexity of the left heart border (Fig. 12.36), but not cardiac enlargement unless heart failure develops. Left ventricular dilatation causes displacement of the cardiac apex downward and to the left (Fig. 12.37). On the lateral view, the heart shadow extends more posteriorly than usual (Fig. 12.38). Left ventricular hypertrophy results from systolic overload, and dilatation from diastolic overload.

In left ventricular aneurysm, a discrete bulge may develop on the left heart border (Fig. 12.39).

The aorta

Selective enlargement of the ascending aorta is seen in post-stenotic dilatation due to aortic valvar stenosis (Fig. 12.36) and in association with aneurysms (Fig. 12.40). The aortic knuckle may be

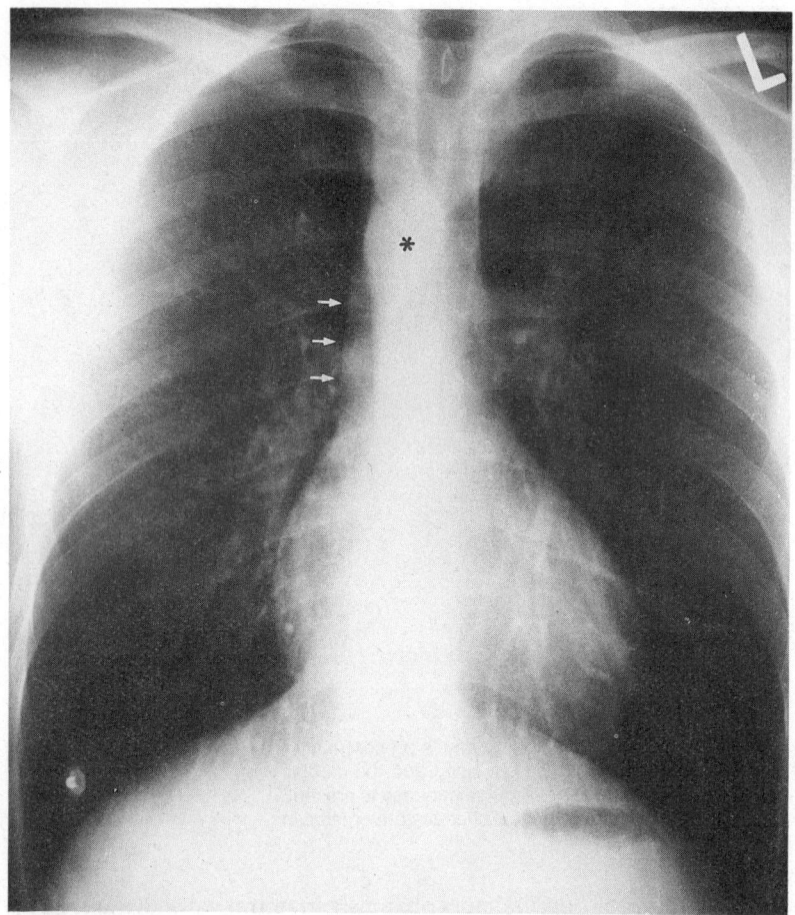

Fig. 12.25. Pulmonary oligaemia. Tetralogy of Fallot. The peripheral vascular pattern is attenuated and a pulmonary bay is present. The left pulmonary artery is enlarged due to post-stenotic dilatation, the pulmonary valve being stenosed. The aortic arch is right-sided (asterisk) displacing the superior vena cava (arrows), and indenting the right side of the trachea.

prominent due to aneurysm (Fig. 12.41), patent ductus arteriosus, tetralogy of Fallot and pulmonary atresia (Fig. 12.24B). In coarctation of the aorta, the knuckle always appears abnormal—it may be prominent, flat, high, low or have an abnormal contour (Figs 12.12 and 12.16A). In non-obstructing coarctation or pseudocoarctation, the arch appears elongated and kinked (Fig. 12.42).

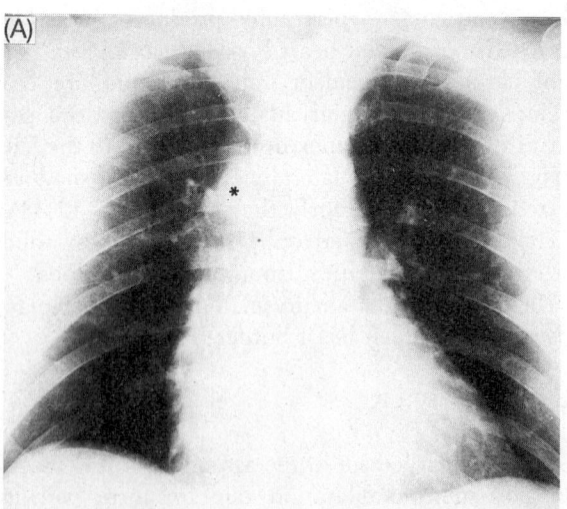

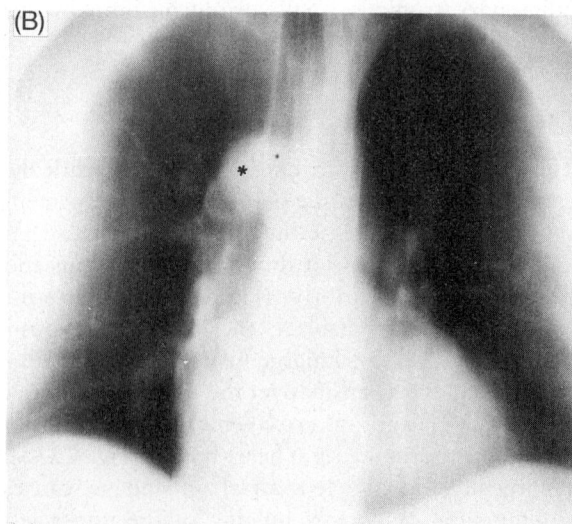

Fig. 12.26. Dilatation of azygos vein (asterisk) in superior vena caval occlusion. (A) CXR. (B) Tomogram.

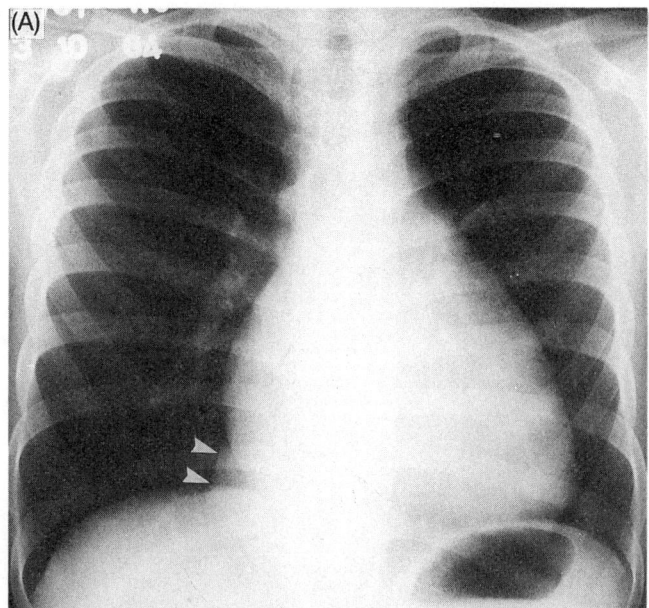

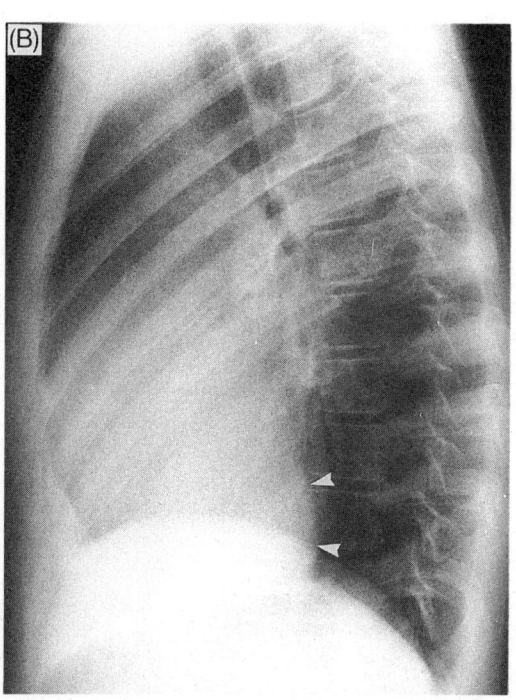

Fig. 12.27. Dilatation of inferior vena cava (arrowheads) in Ebstein's anomaly. (A) Postero-anterior. (B) Lateral. Note enlarged right atrium and ventricle.

Selective enlargement of the descending aorta may be due to aneurysm (Fig. 12.43). Generalized prominence of the thoracic aorta may be part of the ageing process but is also seen in systemic hypertension and aortic regurgitation.

Occasionally, the aorta arches over the right bronchus (Fig. 12.25). In such cases, the knuckle is

seen indenting the right side of the trachea, and the usual shadow of the left arch is absent. It may displace the superior vena cava laterally. A right arch with an aberrant left subclavian artery is not usually associated with heart disease, but if its branches are the mirror image of normal there is a high incidence of congenital heart disease. Tetralo-

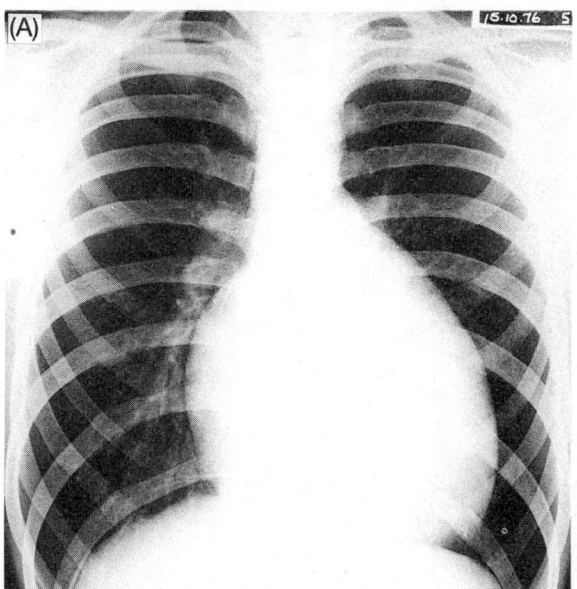

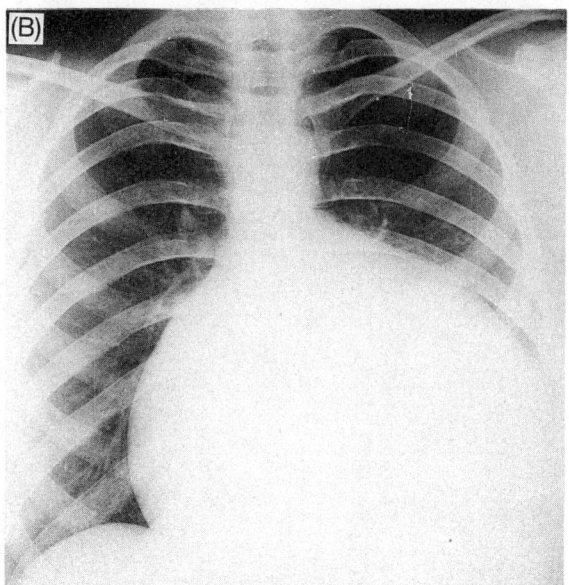

Fig. 12.28. Right heart enlargement. (A) Ebstein's anomaly. The convexity of the right heart border is greater than normal, indicating right atrial enlargement. Increased convexity of the upper left heart border is due to dilatation of the right ventricular outflow tract. (B) Ebstein's anomaly. Severe dilatation of right atrium and ventricle.

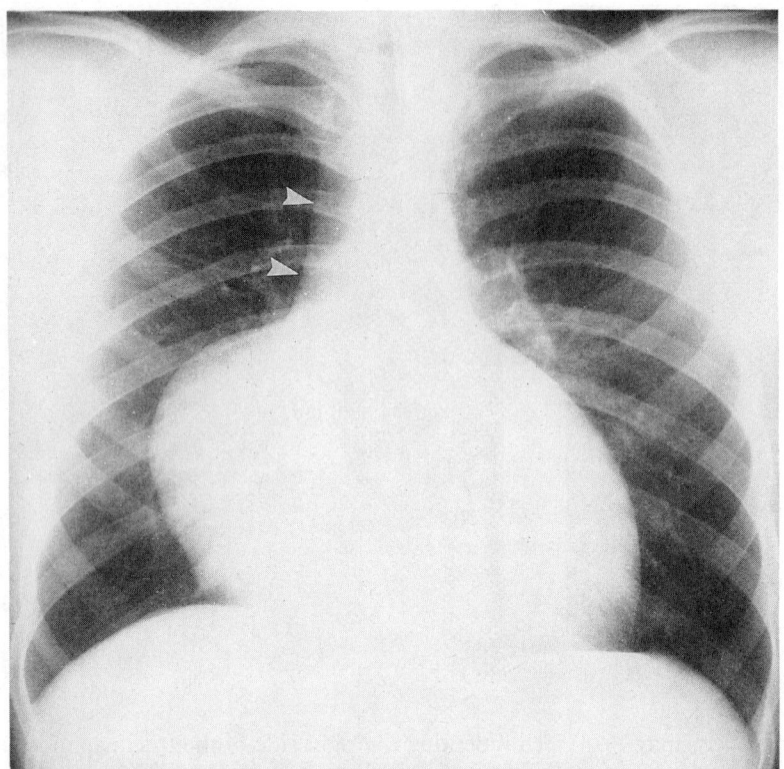

Fig. 12.29. Right atrial enlargement. Congenital tricuspid stenosis. The right heart border is prominent; the superior vena cava is dilated (arrowheads).

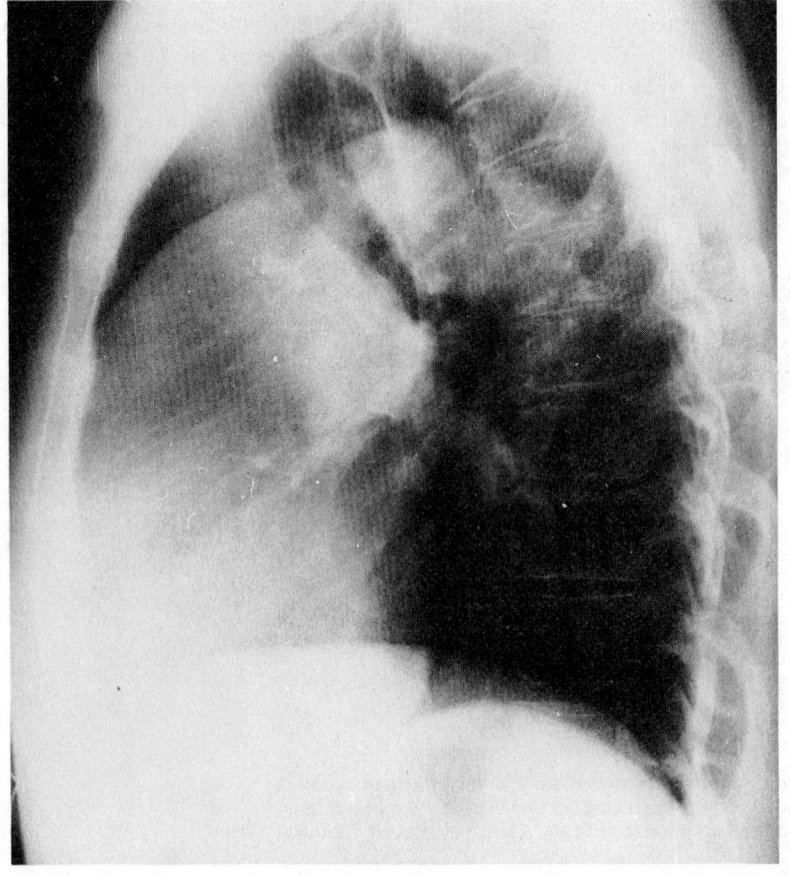

Fig. 12.30. Right ventricular enlargement. Primary pulmonary hypertension. There is increased contact of the anterior aspect of the heart with the sternum. The right ventricular outflow tract is prominent.

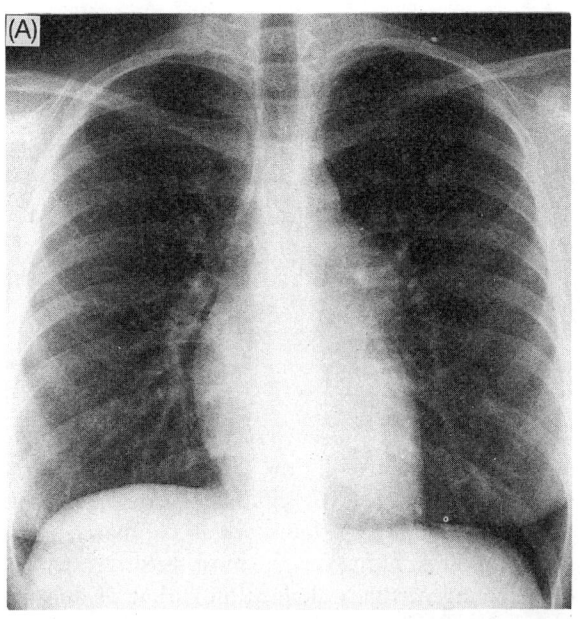
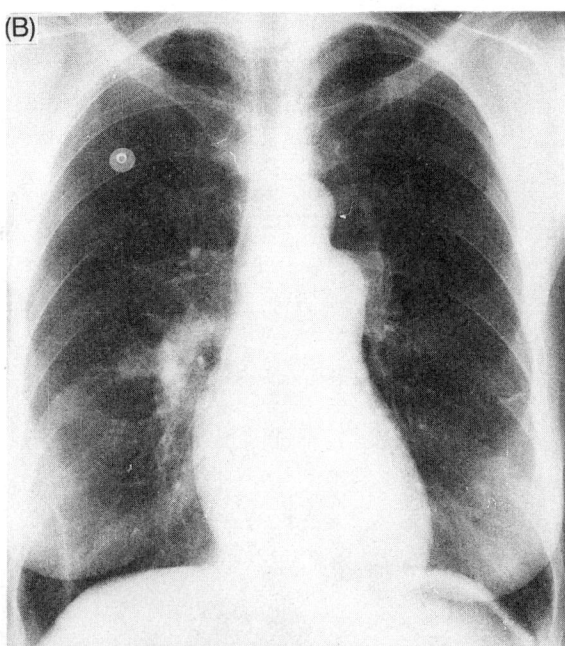

Fig. 12.31. (A) Pulmonary valvar stenosis. The pulmonary trunk and left pulmonary artery are prominent. The peripheral vessels are normal. (B) Idiopathic dilatation of the pulmonary artery. The pulmonary trunk and left pulmonary artery are enlarged. The right pulmonary artery is mildly enlarged. The peripheral vessels are normal.

gy of Fallot, pulmonary atresia, truncus arteriosus and ventricular septal defect may be associated with a right arch. An aberrant subclavian artery can be identified on a barium swallow (Fig. 12.44).

The pericardium

Pericardial effusion may produce non-specific globular enlargement of the heart shadow (Fig.

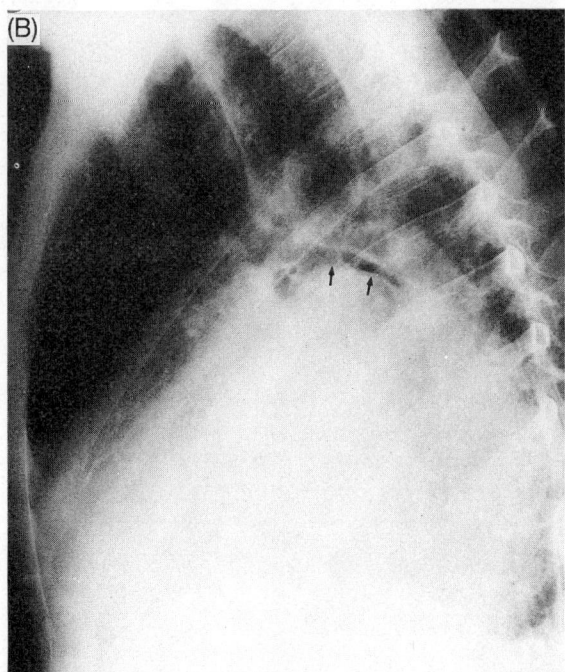

Fig. 12.32. (A) and (B) Left atrial enlargement. Mitral valve disease. The body of the left atrium is grossly enlarged displacing the left bronchus (arrows) superiorly and posteriorly. A double density is visible over the right heart (arrowheads).

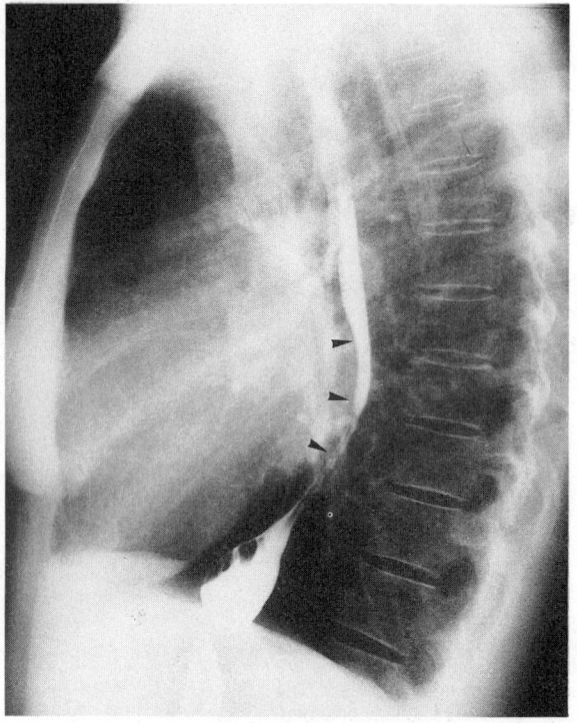

Fig. 12.33. Left atrial enlargement. Mitral stenosis—same patient as in Fig. 12.14. The body of the left atrium is displacing the barium-filled oesophagus posteriorly (arrowheads).

12.45). The pulmonary vascularity is usually normal. Rapid increase in heart size on serial films is suggestive of pericardial effusion. A pericardial cyst may appear as a well-circumscribed rounded opacity adjacent to the heart (Fig. 12.46). Partial pericardial defects may allow herniation of the left atrial appendage causing a prominent bulge on the left heart border. Congenital absence of the pericardium is made manifest by the displacement of the heart to the left.

Cardiac calcification

Calcification may occur in any cardiovascular structure, and is usually the result of inflammatory disease or infarction. Calcification is more difficult to see on high-kVp films when compared with low-kVp films. However, the most sensitive method of detecting cardiac calcification is that of fluoroscopy, in which movement of an abnormally calcified structure aids its detection, in contrast to the CXR where movement causes blurring.

Myocardial and endocardial calcification most commonly occur in the left ventricle as a consequence of coronary artery disease. Curvilinear calcification may occur in the wall of left ventricular

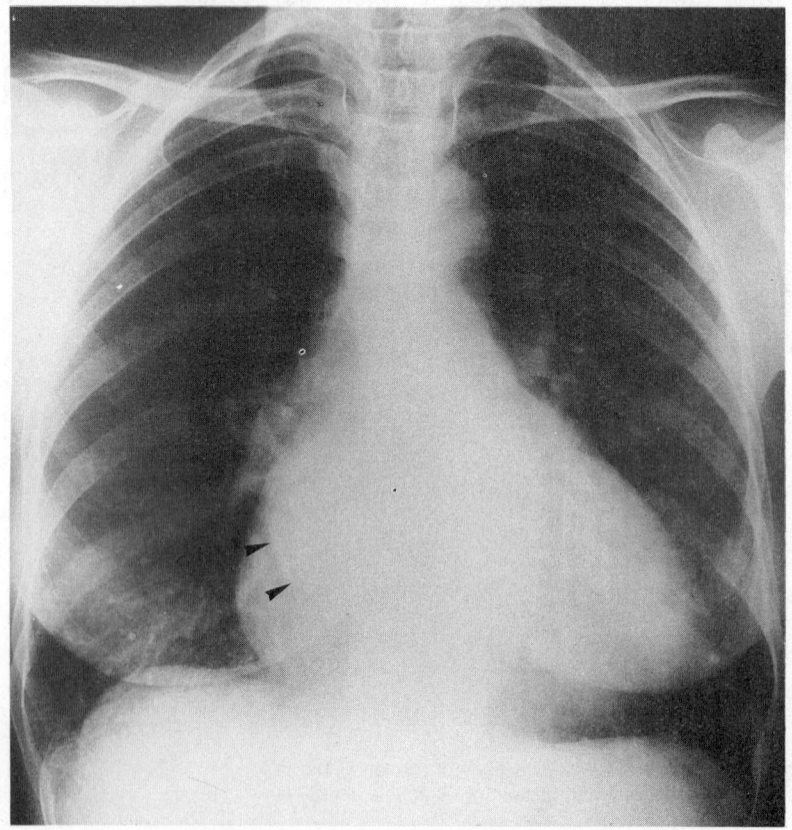

Fig. 12.34. Left atrial enlargement. Mitral valve disease—same patient as in Fig. 12.18. The enlarged left atrium is producing an extra density (arrowheads) over the right atrial shadow.

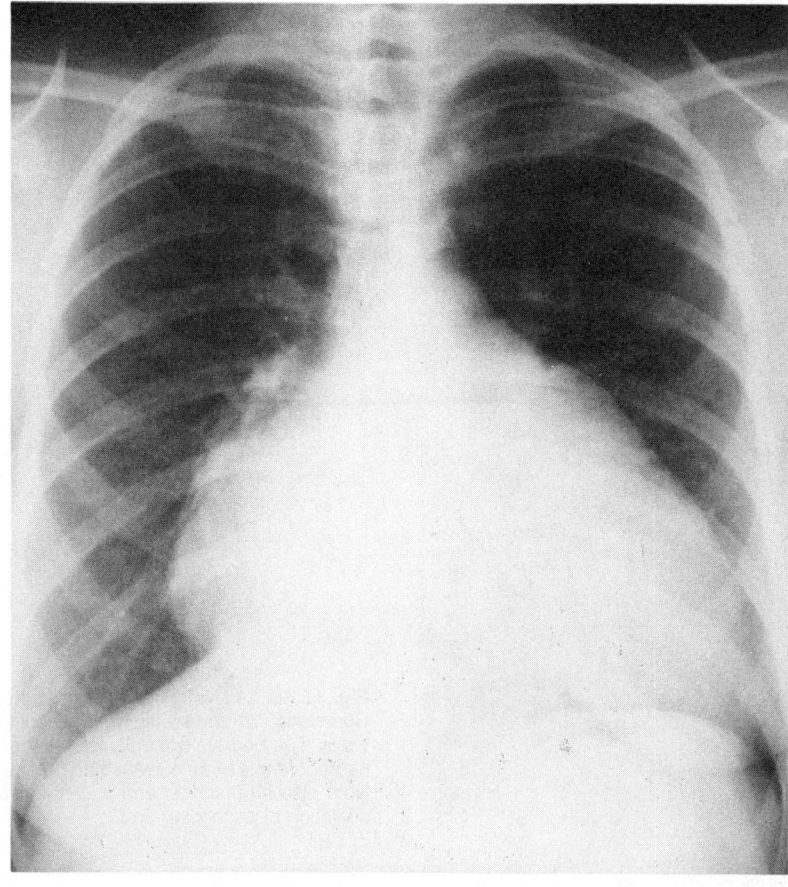

Fig. 12.35. Gross left atrial enlargement. Mitral valve disease. The left atrium is forming the right heart border. The left atrial appendage is prominent, and the left ventricle is enlarged.

aneurysms (Fig. 12.47), in thrombus and in infarcted areas. Left atrial wall calcification may be seen as a result of rheumatic myocarditis, and left atrial thrombi may calcify.

Aortic valve calcification usually lies over the spine on the frontal CXR and is obscured. It is well seen on the lateral view, and tends to lie mostly above a line drawn from the carina to the anterior costophrenic angle (Fig. 12.48). Mitral valve calcificiation usually lies to the left of the spine, and on a lateral view it lies below the line drawn from carina to the anterior costophrenic angle (Fig. 12.49). Calcification is rarely seen in the tricuspid and pulmonary valves, but commonly occurs in right ventricular outflow tract homografts.

Calcification is frequently seen in the aortic arch of older patients as part of the normal ageing process. Extensive aortic calcification is most likely to be due to atheroma (Fig. 12.40), but may be seen in syphilis (Fig. 12.41), which characteristically involves the ascending aorta, and in arteritis. Calcification in a healed dissecting aneurysm (Fig. 12.43) may be seen in any part of the aorta. Chronic traumatic aneurysms in the region of the aortic

isthmus may calcify (Fig. 12.50).

Coronary artery calcification (Fig. 12.51) indicates atheroma, but does not necessarily correspond to significant coronary artery narrowing.[7] A patent ductus arteriosus may calcify (Fig. 12.52), and calcification may develop in the central pulmonary arteries in longstanding, severe pulmonary arterial hypertension (Figs 12.21B and 12.52).

Pericardial calcification may be a sequel to pericarditis and haemopericardium, and is densest in the atrioventricular grooves (Fig. 12.53). It may be associated with pericardial constriction.

Rare causes of cardiac calcification include tumours, hydatid disease and coronary artery fistulae.

FURTHER READING

Elliott, L.P. and Schiebler, G.L. *X-Ray Diagnosis of Congenital Cardiac Disease*, 2nd edition. Springfield: Charles C. Thomas, 1979.

Jefferson K. and Rees S. *Clinical Cardiac Radiology*, 2nd edition. London, Boston: Butterworths, 1980.

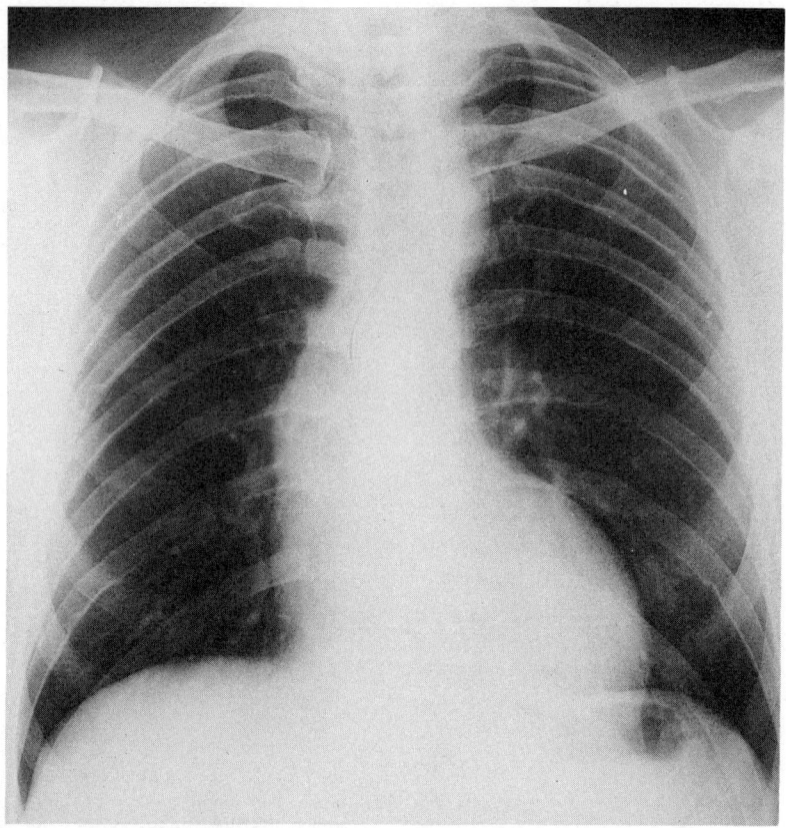

Fig. 12.36. Left ventricular hypertrophy. Coarctation of aorta with bicuspid aortic valve. The heart is not enlarged; the left heart border is more convex than normal. Note also rib notching and post-stenotic dilatation of ascending aorta.

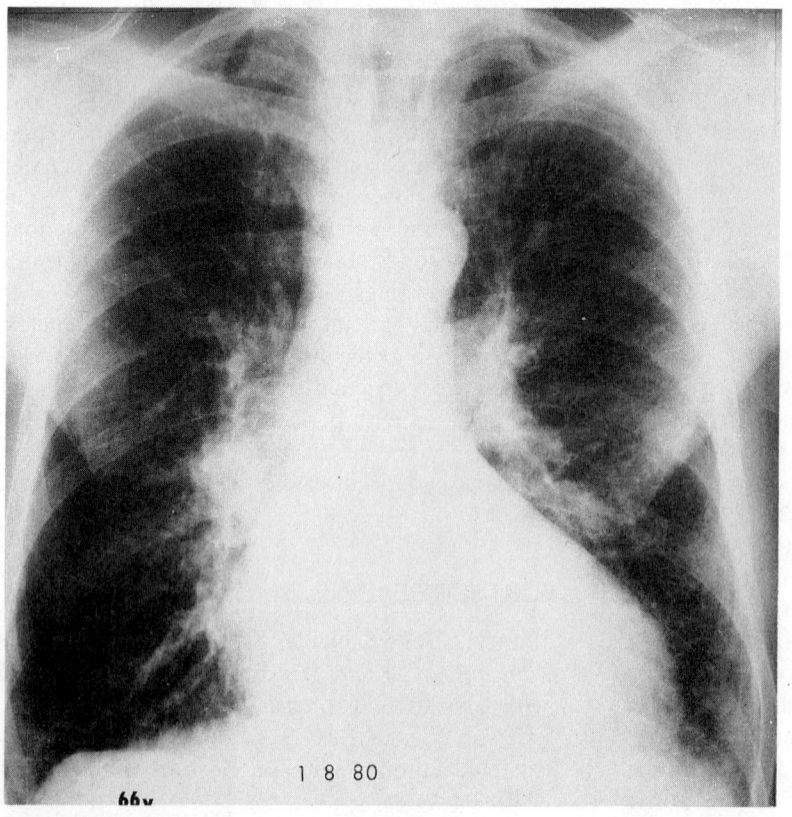

Fig. 12.37. Left ventricular enlargement. Aortic stenosis. The heart is enlarged and the apex is displaced downward. Note redistribution of blood flow and bilateral Kerley B Lines.

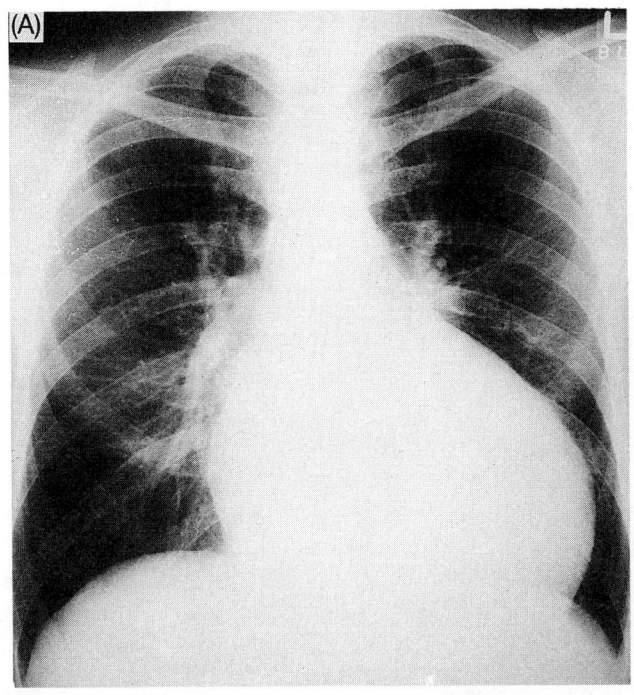

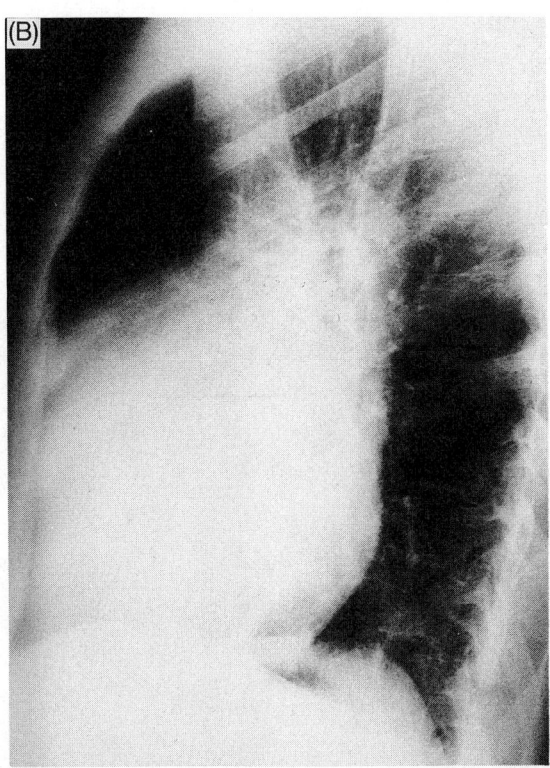

Fig. 12.38. Left ventricular enlargement. Congestive cardiomyopathy. Gross cardiac enlargement. (A) Frontal film shows convex left heart border with downwardly displaced apex. Note redistribution of blood flow and bilateral basal interstitial lines. (B) Lateral film shows left ventricle extending posteriorly and almost overlapping spine.

REFERENCES

1. Jacobson, G., Bohlig, H. and Kiviluoto, R. Essentials of chest radiography. *Radiology* 1970; **95**: 445.
2. Perry, N.M., Irfan, S.P., Simmons, S.P., Thomas, J.M. and Rees, R.S.O. Heart size in high kilovoltage chest radiography *Clin. Radiol.* 1985; **36**: 335.
3. Simon, G. The anterior chest radiograph—criteria for normality derived from a basic analysis of the shadows. *Clin. Radiol.* 1975; **26**: 429.
4. Jonsell, S. Method for the determination of heart size by teleroentgenography (heart volume index) *Acta Radiol.* 1939; **20**: 325.
5. Boone, M.L., Swenson, B.E. and Felson, B. Rib notching: its many causes. *Am. J. Roentgenol.* 1964; **91**: 1075.
6. McHugh, T.J., Forrester, J.S. and Adler, L. Pulmonary vascular congestion in acute myocardial infarction; hemodynamic and radiologic correlations. *Ann. Intern. Med.* 1972; **76**: 29.
7. McCarthy, J.H. and Palmer, F.J. Incidence and significance of coronary artery calcification. *Br. Heart J.* 1974; **36**: 499.

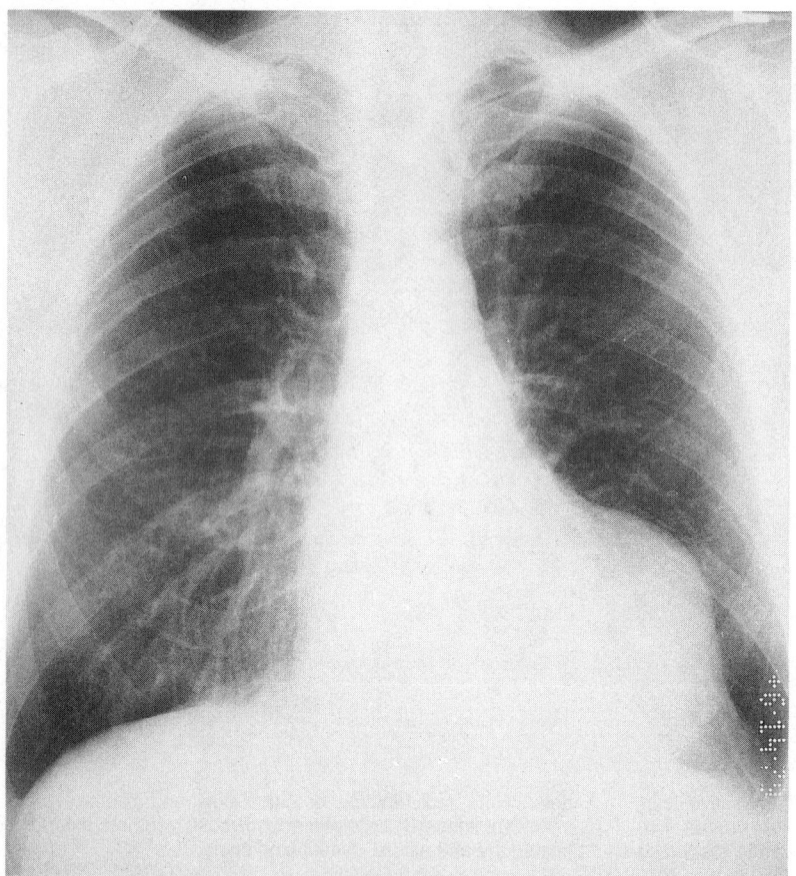

Fig. 12.39. Left ventricular aneurysm. There is a localized bulge on the left heart border.

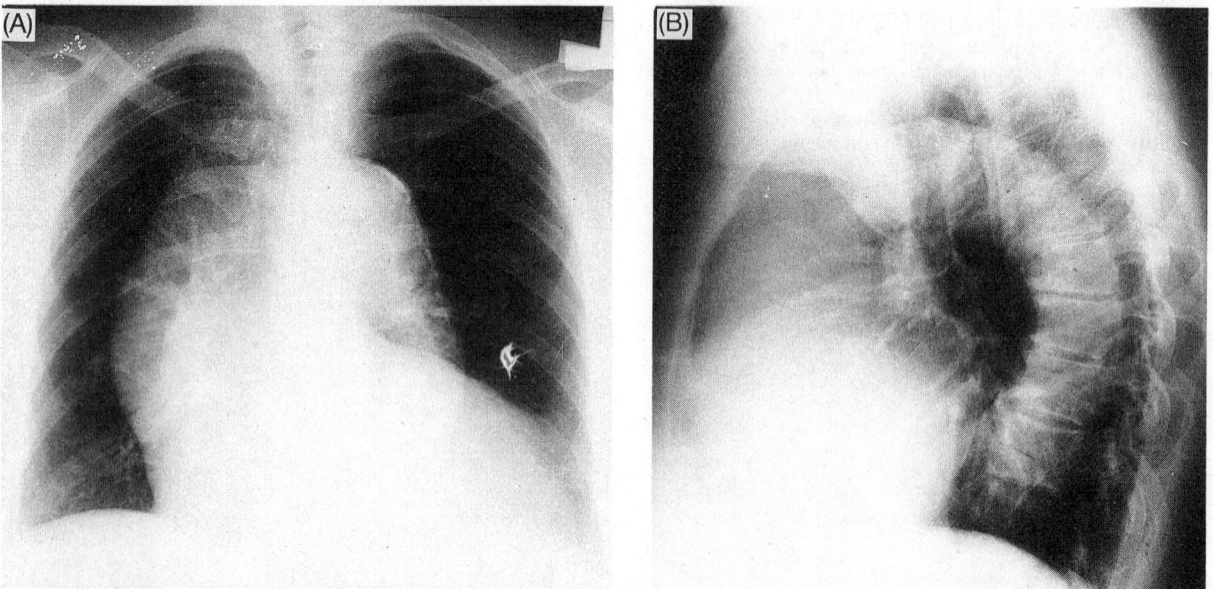

Fig. 12.40. (A) and (B) Large aneurysm of ascending aorta in an elderly 'arteriopath'. The descending aorta is diffusely calcified and mildly dilated.

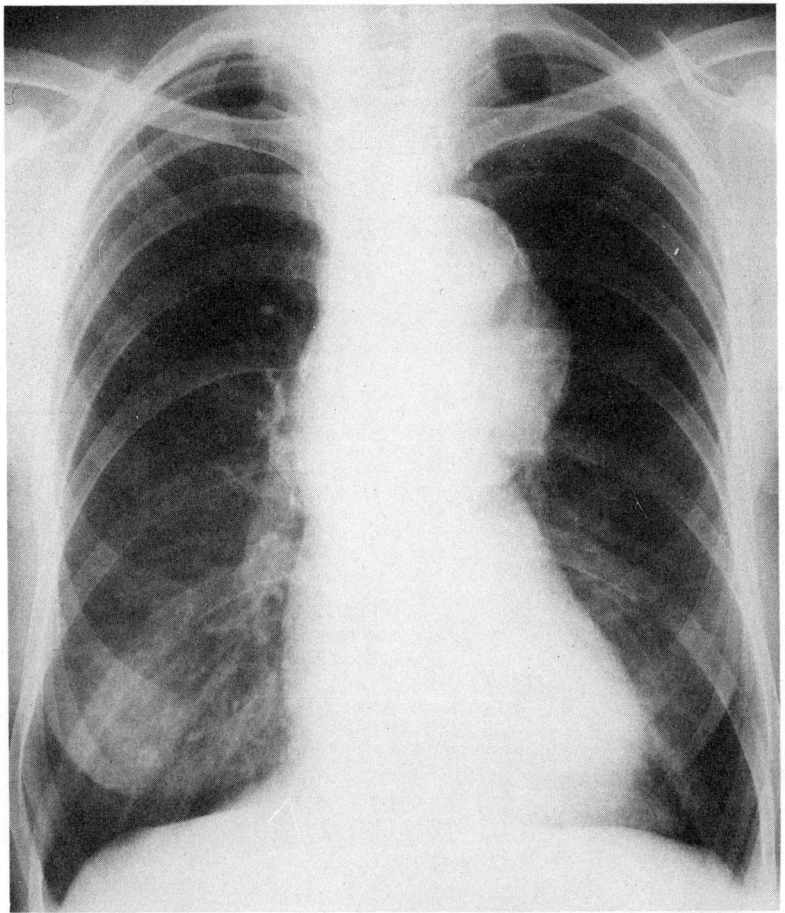

Fig. 12.41. Aneurysm of aortic arch. Syphilitic aortitis. Calcification is seen in the ascending aorta, the aortic knuckle and descending aorta.

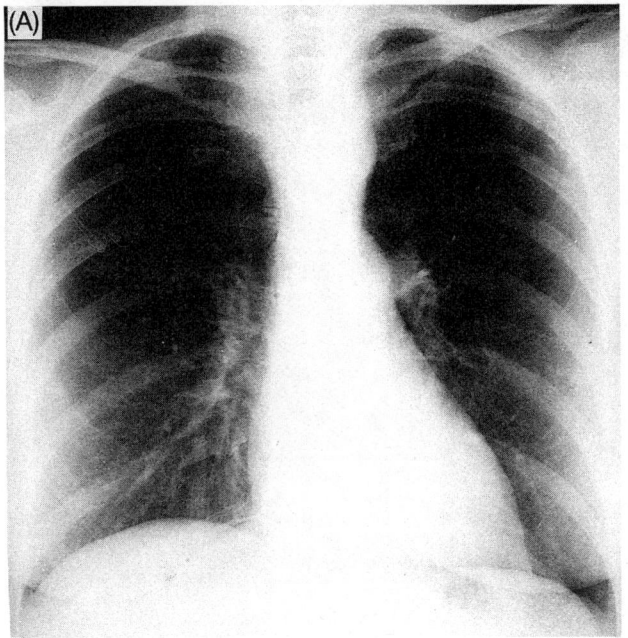

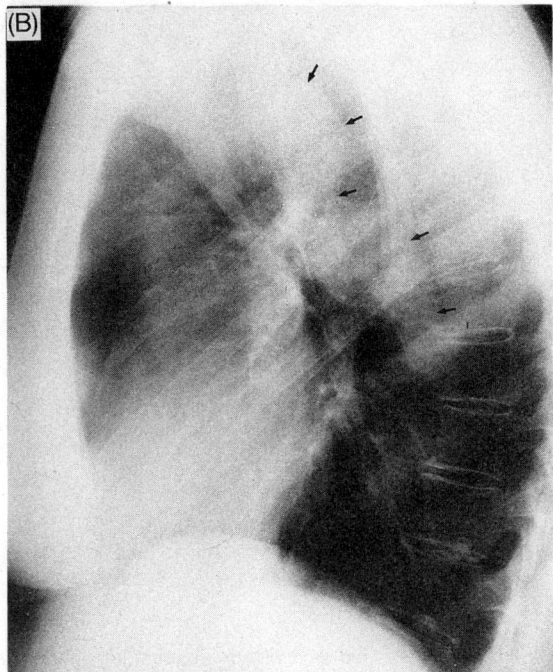

Fig. 12.42. Non-obstructing coarctation of aorta. (A) On the frontal film, the aortic arch is unusually high and has an abnormal contour. (B) The lateral view shows the aorta to be kinked (arrows).

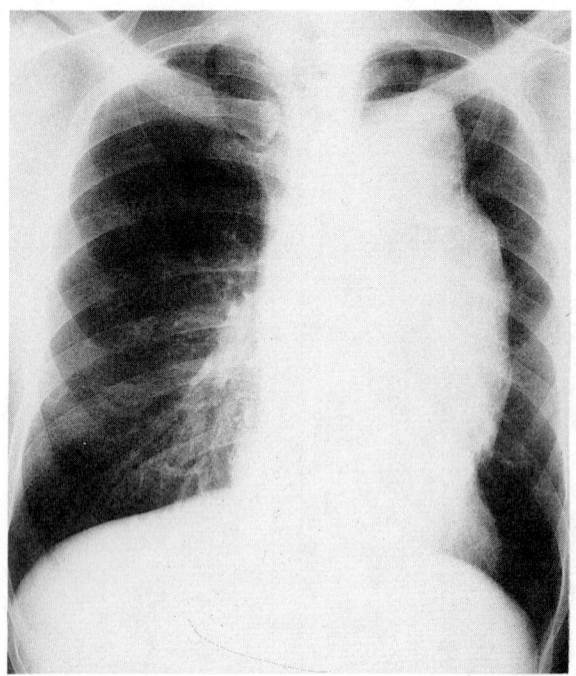

Fig. 12.43. Type III dissecting aneurysm of aorta. The descending aorta is dilated and calcified.

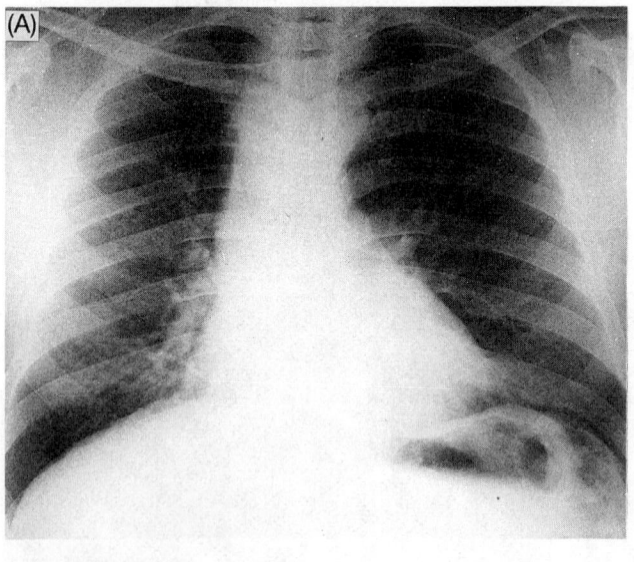

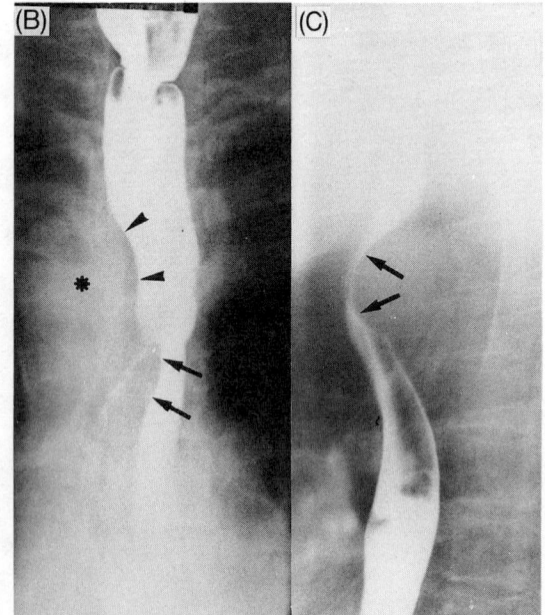

Fig. 12.44. Right-sided arch with an aberrant left subclavian artery. (A) The right arch displaces the superior vena cava (arrowheads) laterally. (B) and (C) Barium swallow shows the right aortic arch (asterisk) indenting the right side of the oesophagus (arrowheads) and the aberrant subclavian artery causes an oblique posterior impression on the oesophagus (arrows).

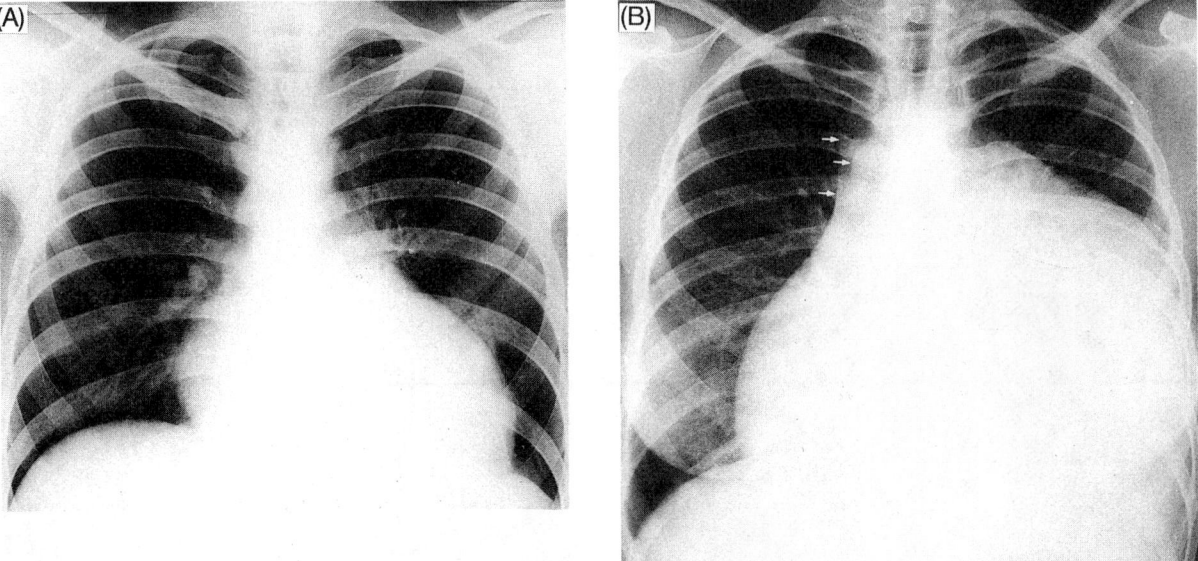

Fig. 12.45. Pericardial effusion. (A) Tuberculous pericarditis. Moderate globular enlargement of heart shadow. The pulmonary vascularity is normal. (B) Large pericardial effusion. The lungs are clear. The superior vena cava and azygos vein are prominent (arrows).

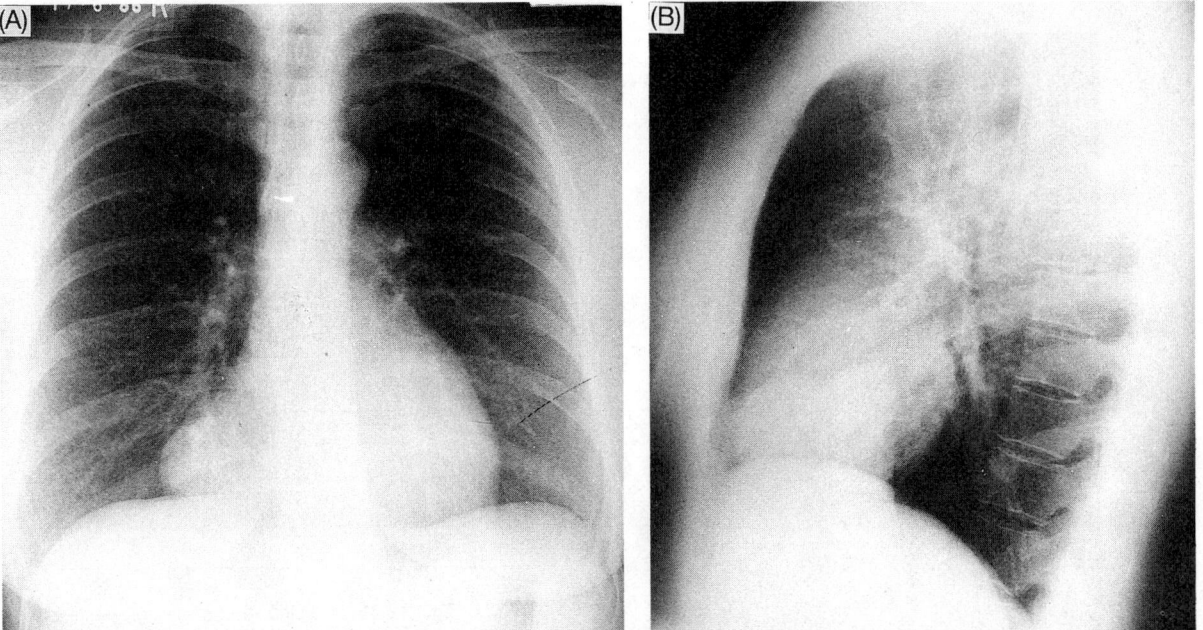

Fig. 12.46. (A) and (B) Pericardial cyst. A well-defined rounded opacity is contiguous with the right heart border.

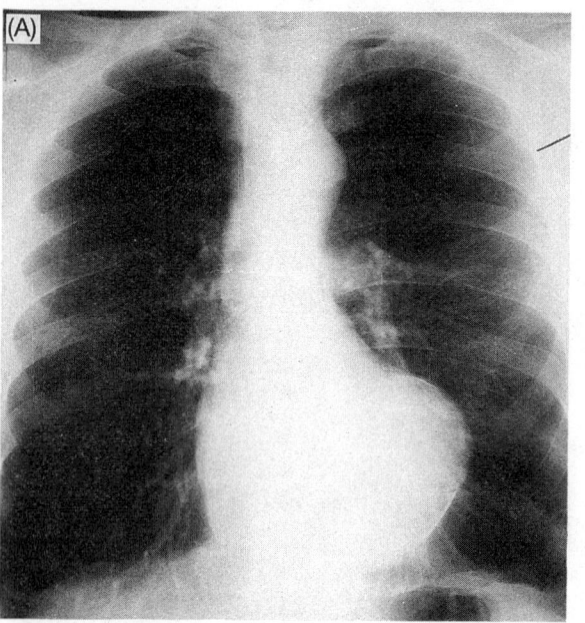
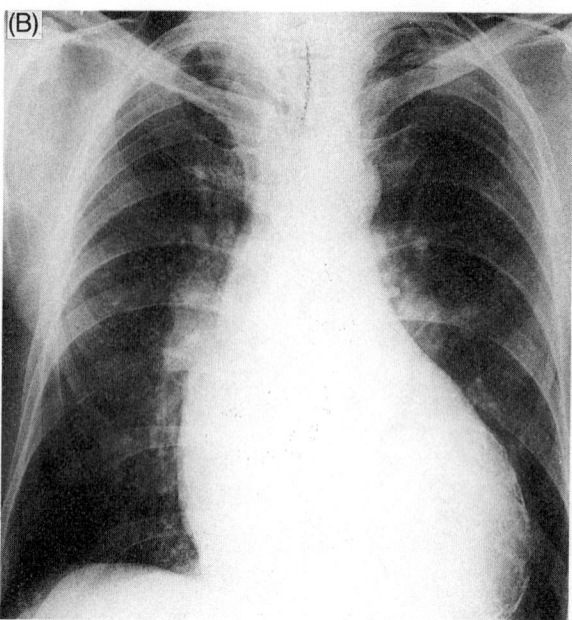

Fig. 12.47. Calcified left ventricular aneurysms. (A) Normal size heart with discrete calcified bulge at apex. (B) Left ventricular enlargement and calcification over apex.

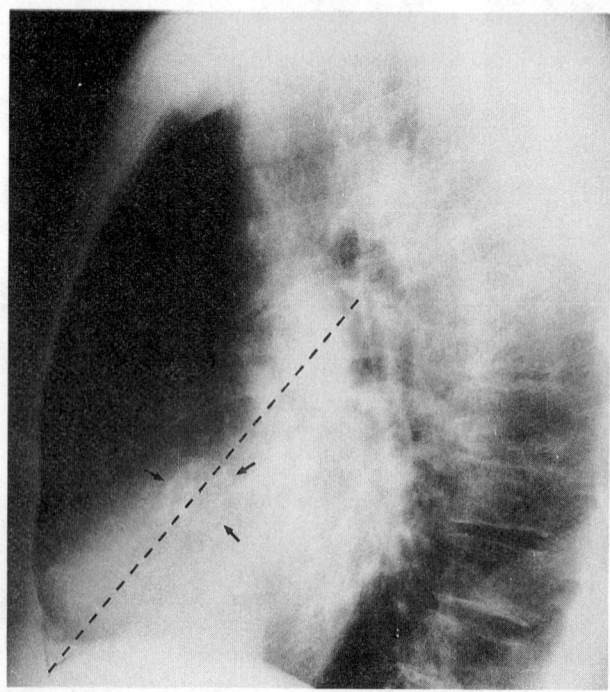

Fig. 12.48. Calcific aortic stenosis—same patient as in Fig. 12.37. The calcified aortic valve (arrows) straddles a line drawn from the carina to the anterior costophrenic angle.

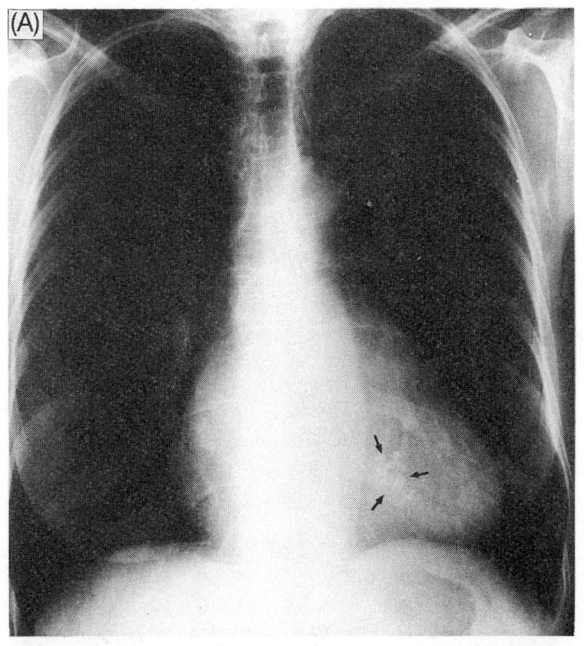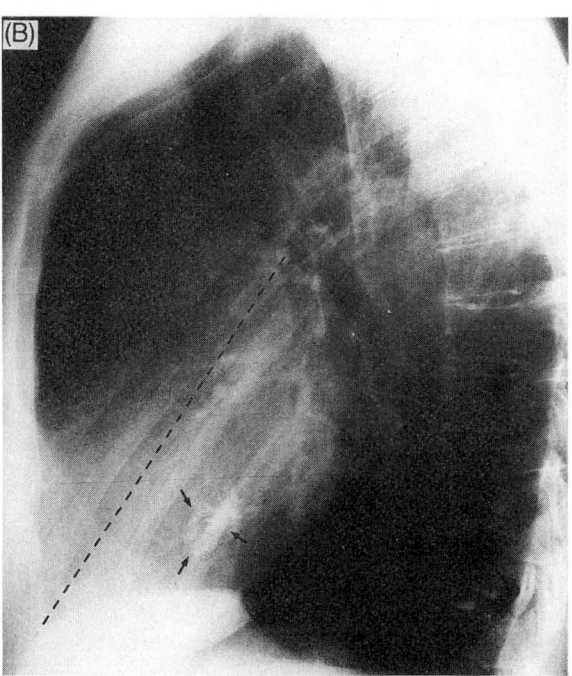

Fig. 12.49. Mitral valve calcification. (A) On the frontal view, the calcified valve (arrows) is lateral to the spine. (B) On the lateral view, the calcification (arrows) is posterior to a line drawn from the carina to the anterior costophrenic angle.

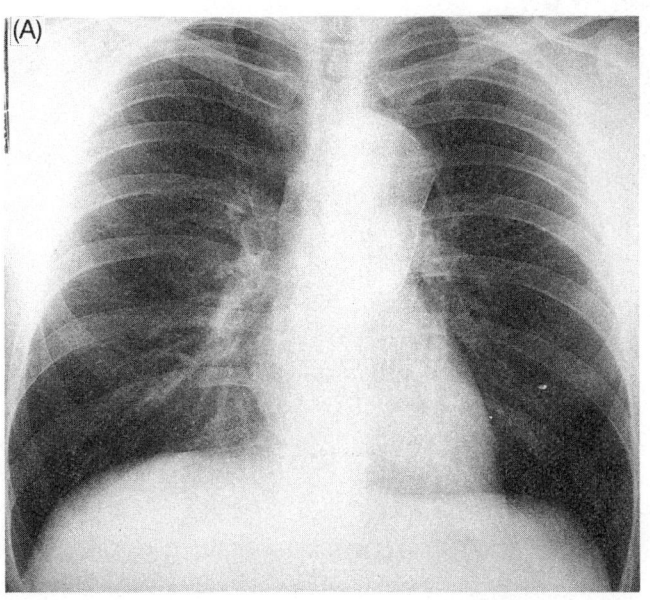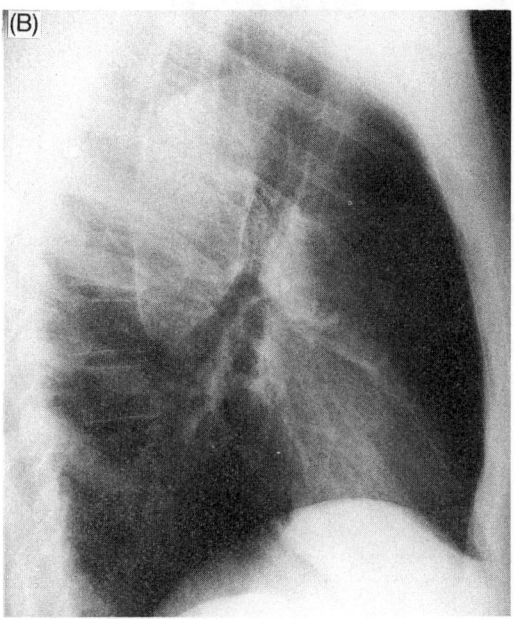

Fig. 12.50. (A) and (B) Calcified traumatic aortic aneurysm. Road-traffic accident 7 years earlier. A calcified aneurysm in the region of the aortic isthmus was found on routine CXR.

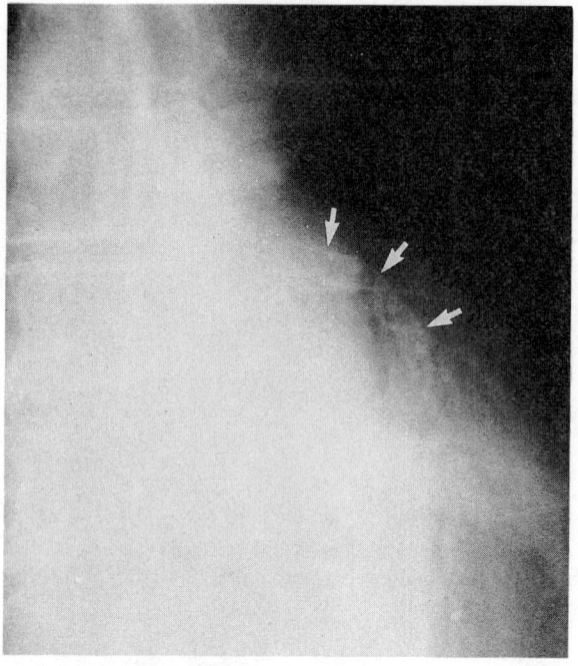

Fig. 12.51. Calcification (arrows) in left anterior descending artery.

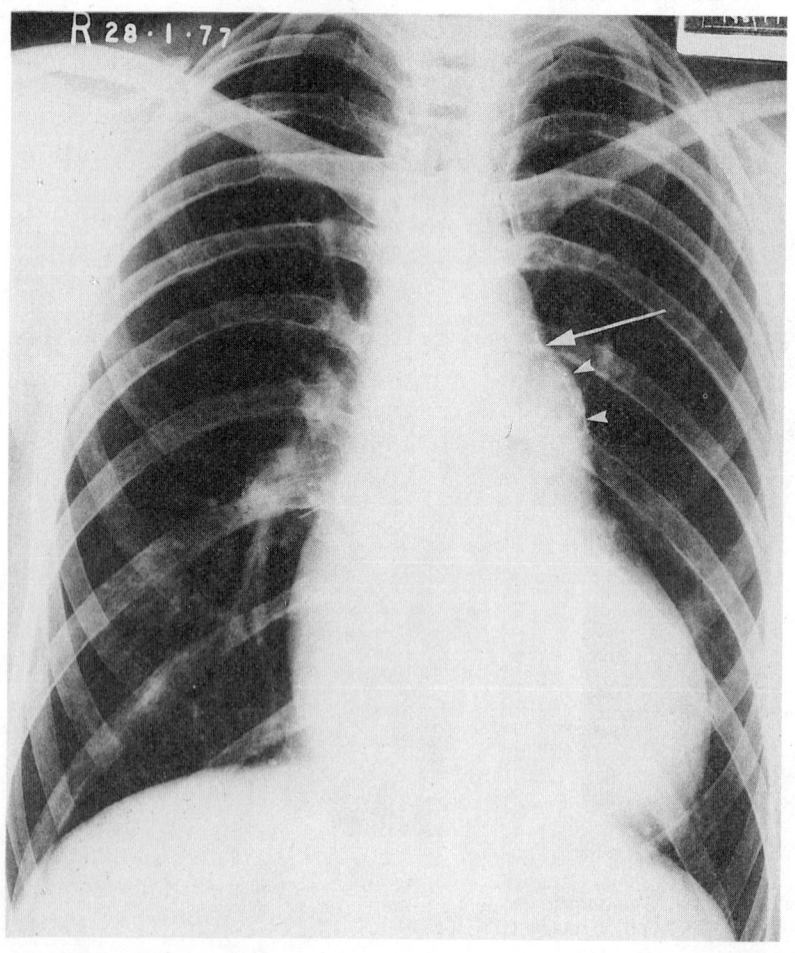

Fig. 12.52. Eisenmenger patent ductus arteriosus. The duct is calcified (arrow) and calcification is also present in the pulmonary trunk (arrowheads).

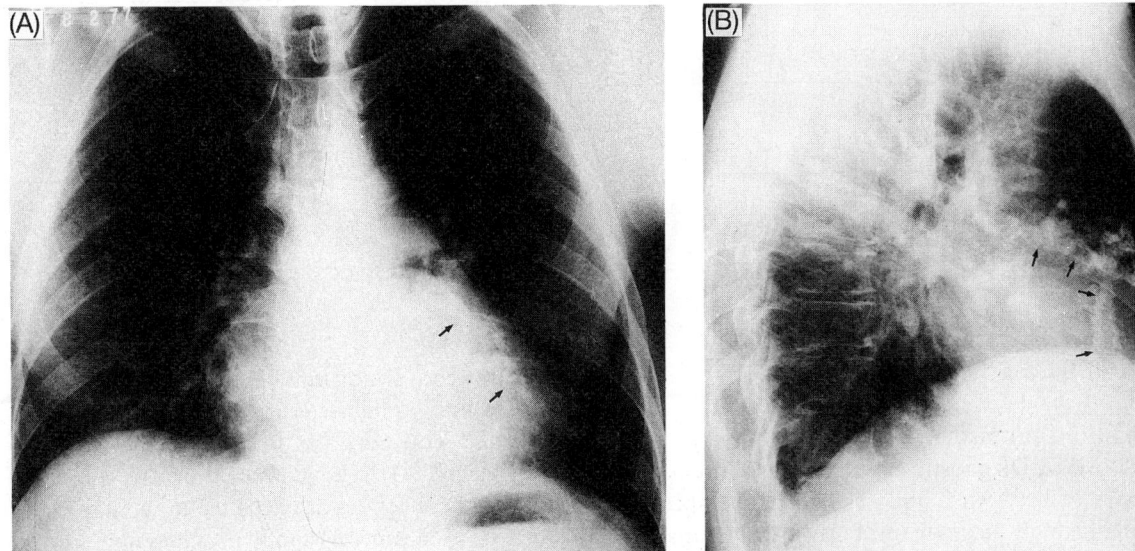

Fig. 12.53. (A) and (B) Pericardial calcification. Constrictive pericarditis. Dense calcification is present in the atrioventricular and interventricular grooves (arrows).

Chapter 13

Echocardiography

Stewart Hunter and Roger Hall

PRINCIPLES OF ECHOCARDIOGRAPHY

By definition, ultrasound has a frequency of > 20 000 MHz. Diagnostic cardiac ultrasound uses frequencies of between 2 and 7.5 MHz. The speed of sound through most of the body tissues, apart from bone, does not vary greatly and it is therefore possible to compute distance by measuring the time elapsed from emission of the ultrasound until it returns to the crystal having been reflected by cardiac structures. Fortuitously, there are small but detectable differences in ultrasonic reflectivity between the various tissues of the body making it possible to differentiate, for instance, between pericardium and myocardium or between valve cusps and papillary muscles. Provided workers adhere to well-established limits of power output, ultrasound produced by the current devices is innocuous; there is no evidence in any of the published work to prove that ultrasound damages tissue when used to investigate human subjects.

Three types of cardiac ultrasound are available on existing echocardiograph machines and all have their particular place in cardiac investigation. M-mode echocardiography (the oldest modality) is derived from a single crystal which produces a very thin slice through the heart in one dimension, the second dimension of the technique being time. Echoes returning from the insonated cardiac struc-

tures are converted into instantaneous dots of energy falling on light-sensitive paper which is then drawn at a constant and known speed across the display (Fig. 13.1). The parts of the heart that have produced these echoes are depicted moving in space against elapsed time. M-mode provides a great deal of accurate information every second from a very localized segment of the heart. The thickness of the heart walls and the movement of cardiac structures can be studied elegantly and in great detail. However, the technique is 'blind' and very dependent on operator skill. The echocardiographer cannot be certain of the angle of insonation and this can lead to inaccuracy of measurement. In addition, the simultaneous visualization of all cardiac chambers is impossible.

Cross-sectional echocardiography was developed initially using mechanical scanners or linear arrays (Fig. 13.2a,b). Although the *linear array* was popular for non-cardiac imaging, it was never satisfactory for cardiac work because the transducer was too big to slip between the ribs and consequently rib echoes interfered with the picture. However, *mechanical scanners* had smaller transducers that could be placed between the ribs or in the subcostal or suprasternal position without difficulty. Some very sophisticated echo machines still use mechanical scanning to this day. One or more crystals rotate or wobble so that they sweep through a pre-set but

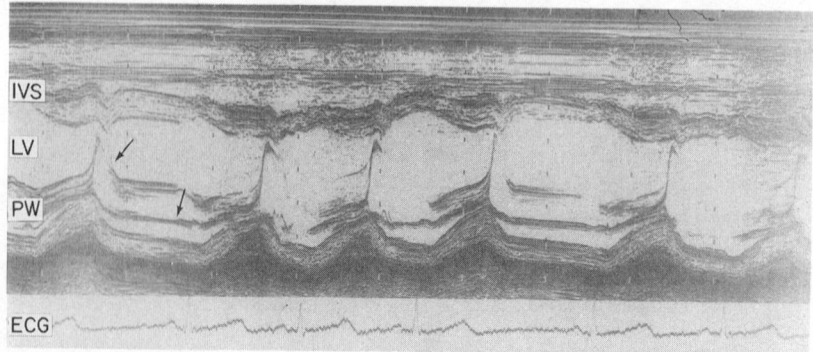

Fig. 13.1. A normal M-mode echocardiogram of a left ventricle. The septum and posterior left ventricular wall either side of the left ventricular cavity are seen moving towards each other in systole and away from each other in diastole. There is also an overall movement of the cavity of the left ventricle posteriorly and then anteriorly with respiration. This echocardiogram is recorded at the mid mitral valve level—part of the mitral valve cusps and some chordal echoes are seen (arrows). IVS = interventricular septum, LV = left ventricle, PW = posterior wall of left ventricle.

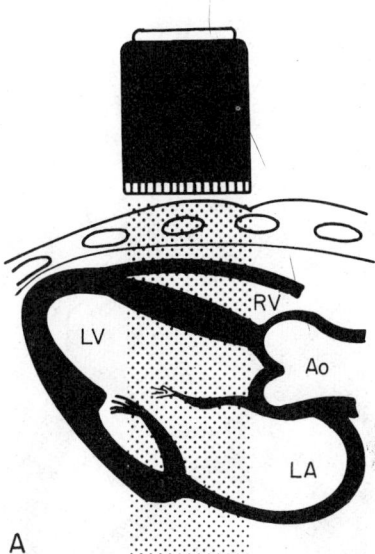

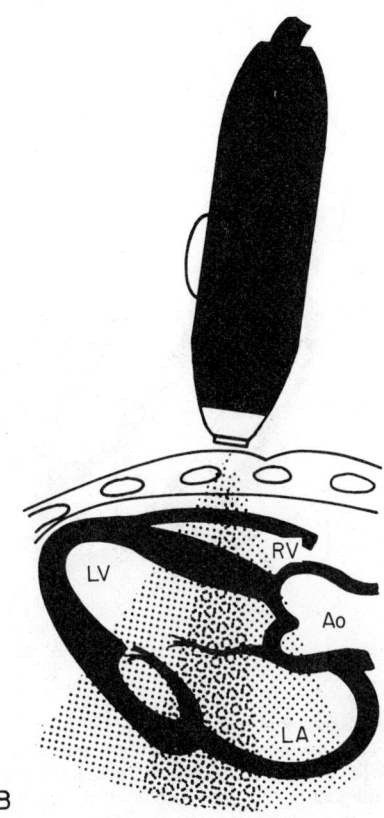

Fig. 13.2. (A) Linear array scanner. This device utilizes a linear multi-element transducer in which the sound beam is transmitted and received by the elements along the array and the entire array is scanned at a high rate thus presenting a real-time two-dimensional picture. (B) Sector scanner. A single transducer is mechanically angled rapidly from a fixed spot on the patient's chest. The information from the transducer position and the returned echoes produce a real-time dynamic image on the monitor. Ao = aorta, LV and LA = left ventricle and atrium, RV = right ventricle.

variable sector which is triangular in shape. The crystal(s) fire between 16 and 30 times per second as they scan across the heart and a compilation of the resulting scans gives a real-time picture. In recent years, the *phased array* has become the transducer of choice. Multiple (up to 64) small fixed crystals within the head of the scanner are focused and electronically fired in sequence. The head and the crystals remain static but the beam is electronically swept and focused so that the resulting sector is the same as that for the mechanical transducer. Mechanical scanners are cheap to manufacture and can produce much higher frequencies than phased arrays which do not exceed 5 MHz and are very expensive to manufacture. Both systems can produce first class image quality.

There are a series of standard views of the heart using cross-sectional imaging. It is possible to examine the length of the left ventricle, aorta and the left atrium in the *long-axis* view which can be recorded from the left parasternal window and from the apex (Fig. 13.3). From the parasternal window, a *short-axis* view of the left ventricle and the proximal parts of the great arteries is achieved by turning the transducer through 90° from the long-axis view (Fig. 13.4). The anatomical details of

papillary muscles, the orifice of the mitral valve, the orifice of the aortic valve and the main and branch pulmonary arteries can all be well visualized in these views. From the apex, both the *four-chamber* and the *four-chamber plus aortic root* views can be recorded (Fig. 13.5). Although the remaining ultrasound windows for the heart are valuable, they are less frequently obtained in adults. Subcostal short-axis views, four-chamber views and four-chamber plus aortic root views can be obtained in many patients, but it may be impossible to image the heart from its window particularly in the obese subject. The suprasternal notch gives access to the arch of the aorta and its tributaries in a series of transverse sagittal views. From this position, in many adult patients, it is difficult to see either the aortic valve or the aorta much beyond the left subclavian origin.

In middle-aged and older patients, obesity and lung disease frequently preclude satisfactory ultrasonic imaging in all the views mentioned above. These factors have significantly limited the usefulness of cardiac ultrasound in the elderly, in patients in the intensive care unit and in those in the coronary care unit. The recent development of a small phased array transducer attached to the end of a gastroscope may eliminate these practical

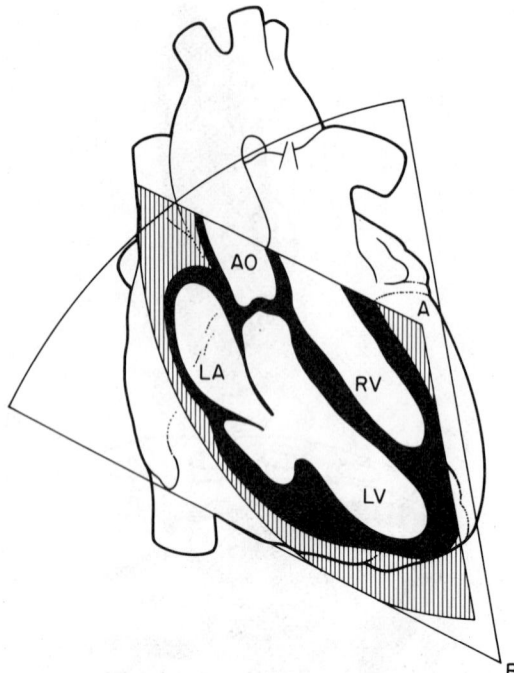

Fig. 13.3. Cross-sectional echocardiography: long-axis parasternal view. The view obtained from the transducer at the left sternal border (A) and the echo sector directed in the long axis of the heart (almost in the sagittal plane). A similar picture, showing the same structures, is obtained by placing the transducer at the cardiac apex with the sector in the same plane (B). This echo plane is at 90° to the apical four-chamber view (see Fig. 13.5). AO, aorta; LA, left atrium; RV, right ventricle; LV, left ventricle.

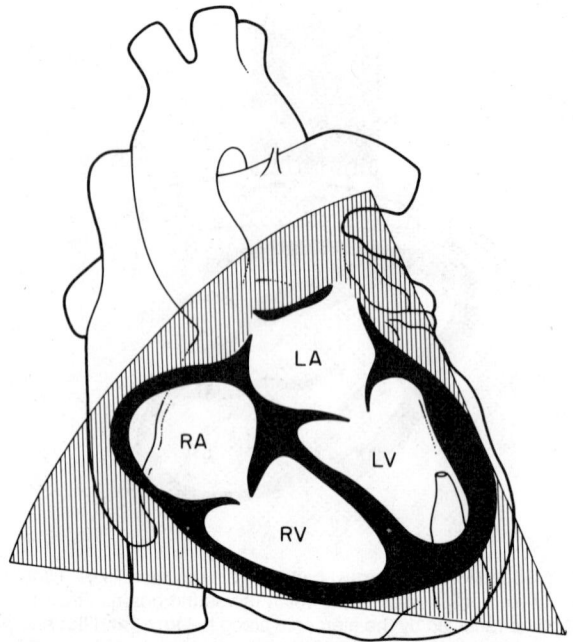

Fig. 13.5. Cross-sectional echocardiography: apical four-chamber view. This view from the cardiac apex shows all 4 cardiac chambers and demonstrates the atrioventricular junction particularly well. The view obtained from this site by rotating the plane of the echo by 90° (the apical two-chamber or long-axis view) is shown in Fig. 13.3B.

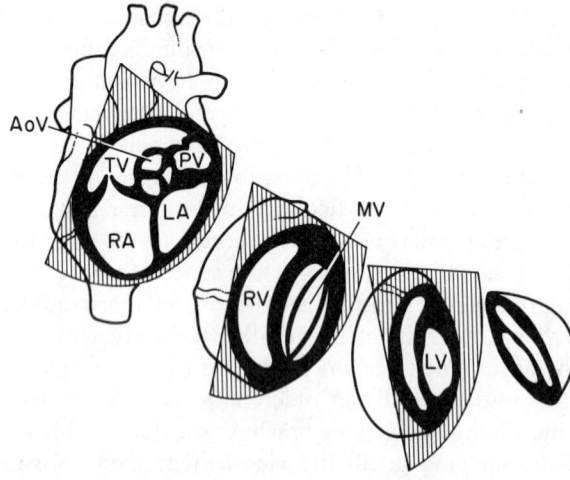

Fig. 13.4. Cross-sectional echocardiography: short-axis parasternal view. Multiple cuts along the short axis of the heart obtained from the left parasternal area. This view shows the aortic (AoV) and mitral (MV) valve orifices in cross-section. PV, pulmonary valve; TV, tricuspid valve; LA, left atrium; RA, right atrium; RV, right ventricle; LV, left ventricle.

difficulties by allowing imaging of the heart from the fundus of the stomach. Trans-oesophageal echocardiography is recommended as a safe technique. Its value in clinical practice has yet to be fully evaluated, but the initial results are very encouraging.

With the advent of high-resolution cross-sectional devices, echocardiographers began to appreciate changes in shape and size of the cardiac cavities and to identify with certainty anomalies of arterial and venous connections. The measurement of cavity size and of rates of wall movement from the sector scan is open to many inaccuracies. Measurements made within axial resolution are usually reproducible and reliable, but those lying outside in lateral resolution cannot be relied upon. However, the sector enables the operator to angle the M-mode beam with great reliability thereby improving its potential for accuracy and reproducibility (Fig. 13.6).

The most important property of M-mode echocardiography is its ability to define precisely the timing of movement of intracardiac structures and to measure accurately the dimension of the cardiac chambers and walls. Analysing echocardiograms using a digitizing tablet linked to a small computer

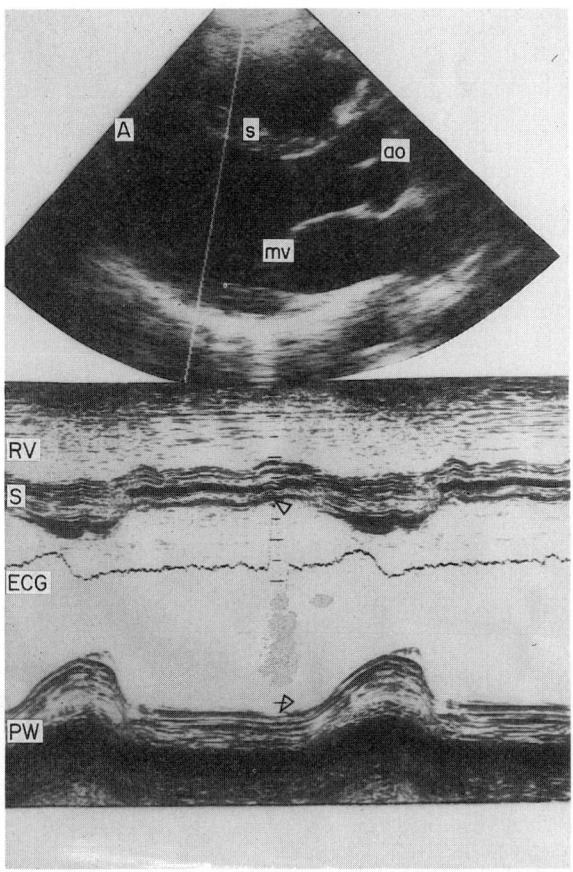

Fig. 13.6. The relationship between cross-sectional echocardiography and M-mode. Upper panel: a cross-sectional echo parasternal long-axis view of the left ventricle, aorta, mitral valve and left atrium. Across it runs a cursor which can be manipulated within the sector. Lower panel: the M-mode derived from the cross-sectional echo at the level of the cursor. A, apex; s, ventricular septum; mv, mitral valve; ao, aorta; RV = right ventricle, LV = left ventricle, PW = posterior wall.

allows these properties of M-mode echocardiography to be used to their full potential; the movement and changes in dimension of intracardiac structures can be quantified as can their timing and rate of change.[1]

Digitization of M-mode echocardiograms has provided a large amount of basic information about cardiac function. It has helped advance the concept that left ventricular contraction is a co-ordinated event and that this co-ordination is often severely disturbed in heart disease even when overall motion is normal. It has given insight into the mechanism of left ventricular filling and the ways in which it may be deranged in ischaemic heart disease, valve disease and hypertrophy.[1-3]

In addition to elucidating physiological mechanisms, this technique provides a small amount of

practical help in some clinical situations. In the past, this technique proved useful in assessing the severity of mitral stenosis.[4] As the left ventricular inflow obstruction slows the rate of left ventricular filling in early diastole, there is no longer a definite early rapid filling period and left ventricular filling continues at about the same rate throughout diastole (Fig. 13.7). This filling rate is reflected by the rate of increase of left ventricular dimension in diastole which is reduced in proportion to the area of the mitral valve. Although this proved to be the most accurate M-mode method of predicting the severity of mitral stenosis, it is time-consuming and requires perfect echocardiograms which can be obtained in only 60–70% of patients. Consequently, it has been abandoned because both cross-sectional echocardiography and the Doppler technique allow mitral stenosis to be assessed more rapidly and accurately.

Digitized echocardiograms may be of some use in the assessment of prosthetic mitral valves[5] because this can be difficult using either M-mode or cross-sectional echocardiography due to the highly reflective nature of the mechanical prostheses (Fig. 13.8A) or of the supporting structures to which bioprostheses are sewn. All prosthetic valves in the mitral position are at least mildly obstructive and therefore digitized M-mode echocardiograms reveal a slow rate of increase in left diastolic ventricular dimension similar to that seen in mild mitral stenosis. If the valve begins to leak, there is an increase in the rate of left ventricular filling to normal or increased levels which can be detected easily by the digitized echocardiogram (Fig. 13.8B). However, digitization is not particularly successful in the detection of obstructed valves since there is a considerable overlap in rate of dimension change between normally functioning and obstructed prosthetic valves. Doppler ultrasound has improved the assessment of prosthetic valves considerably and is now replacing the use of digitized M-mode echocardiograms in this area.

Digitizing M-mode echocardiography therefore has a reduced role in clinical cardiology not only because the information is difficult to obtain but also because the same information can often be provided more easily by the cross-sectional and Doppler techniques. It remains a valuable technique for research, particularly when studying left ventricular function.

Most modern echo machines have the capability of using the Doppler effect first described in the nineteenth century by J.C. Doppler. Ultrasound

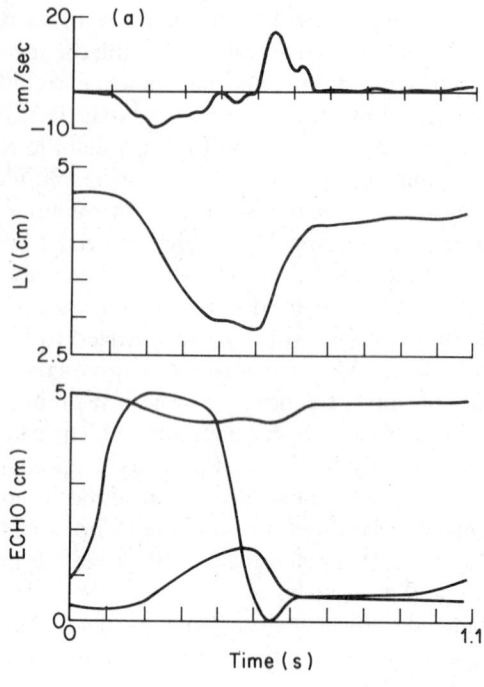
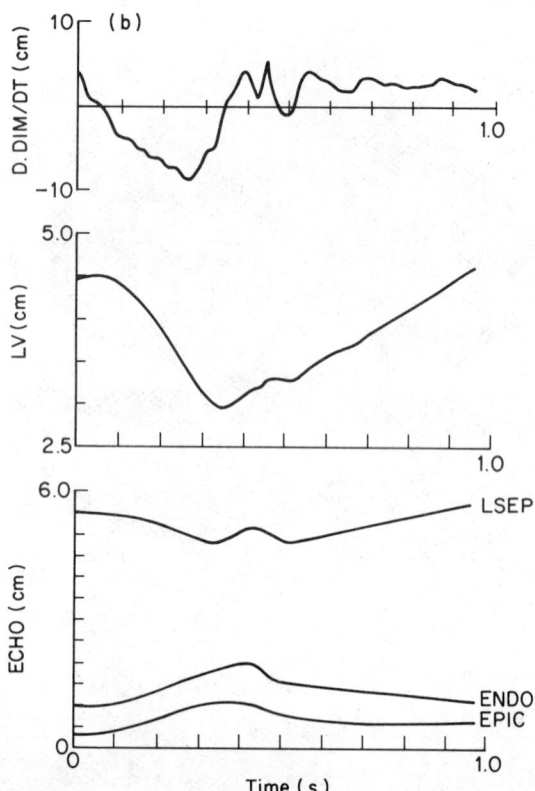

Fig. 13.7. Digitized M-mode echocardiograms from a normal subject and a patient with mitral stenosis. In (A) and (B), the lower tracing represents the original echocardiogram, the middle tracing the left ventricular dimension change with time and the upper tracing the rate of change of left ventricular dimension (cm/s). In (A) (normal subject), the left ventricular dimension increases rapidly in early diastole; following this, there is little further change in dimension during diastole. The peak rate of left ventricular diastolic dimension change is approximately 17 cm/s. By contrast, in (B) (mitral stenosis), left ventricular dimension is seen to increase slowly throughout diastole with a peak rate of change (upper trace) of approximately 4 cm/s. There is an apex cardiogram on the lower tracing of (A).

emitted from a fixed source is reflected from a moving structure. The reflected frequency recorded at the transducer is different from the transmitted frequency and this difference, known as the 'frequency shift', which occurs as a result of the motion of the target, is directly proportional to the velocity of the moving object. The change in frequency is measured; when this change is inserted into the Doppler equation, the velocity of blood flow can be calculated.[6]

The Doppler technique is used in three different ways.

1   *Continuous wave*. A continuous beam of ultrasound is emitted by one crystal and after reflection by moving red cells is received by a separate crystal within the same transducer. The beam is manoeuvred blindly and all the velocities encountered along the length of the ultrasonic beam are registered through a spectral analyser without selection or range-gating for depth. This technique is capable of measuring very high velocities but requires considerable operator skill.

2.   *Pulsed Doppler*. A range-gating system is applied to a source of ultrasound to recover flow information from a particular point in the circulation. This point is indicated by the position of a sample volume accurately located using a cross-sectional image and a cursor. Owing to the physics of ultrasound, the velocities measured by this mode are low, i.e. they are seldom above 1.5–2 m/s in the normal adult. Even mild mitral stenosis can give rise to velocities in excess of this value; in aortic stenosis, a velocity of 5–6 m/s is not uncommon. If the velocity is too high, *aliasing* occurs and the velocities disappear from the recording device and reappear in the opposite part of the picture. 'High-pulsed repetition frequency' Doppler ultrasound was introduced to combine a directed beam with high-velocity measurement. This technique has not proved particularly successful except in small chil-

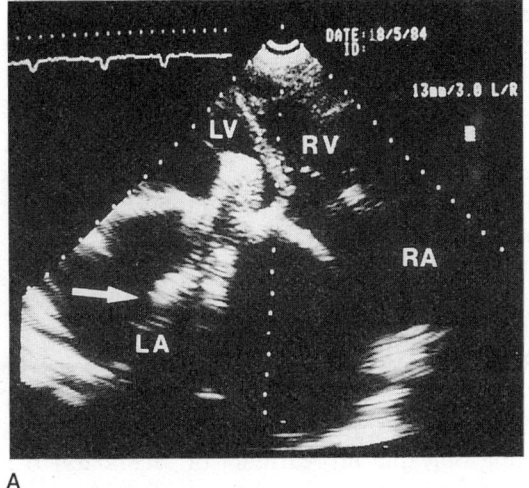

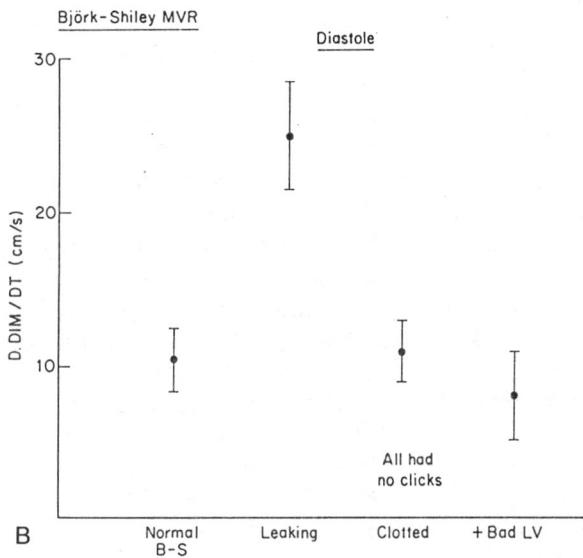

Fig. 13.8. (A) Cross-sectional echocardiogram from a patient with Starr–Edwards mitral prosthesis (apical four-chamber view). The strong reflection from the mitral prosthesis does not allow any detail of the valve to be seen and there are multiple spurious echoes (arrow) in the left atrium (LA) due to reverberation. RA, right atrium; RV, right ventricle; LV, left ventricle. (B) The peak rate of change of left ventricular dimension in diastole from a series of patients with Björk–Shiley (B-S) mechanical mitral valve prosthesis. The most striking feature is the high rate of diastolic dimension change in patients with a paraprosthetic leak. In patients with normally functioning and clotted valves, there is no significant difference in the peak rate of left ventricular dimension change in diastole. Similarly, patients with deterioration due to poor left ventricular function (BAD LV) cannot be distinguished from those with thrombosed valves by this parameter. (Data for this figure derived from Dawkins *et al., Br. Heart J.* 1984; **51**: 168–74.)

dren in whom velocities of a slightly higher order can be measured by pulsed Doppler.

However, it is possible to quantify valvar stenosis with considerable accuracy using continuous wave Doppler. The increase in velocity of blood flow across a stenotic valve or orifice is related to the pressure drop across the orifice. This relation has been described in the Bernoulli equation, of which a simplified version was shown by Hatle *et al.*[7] to allow pressure drop to be inferred with sufficient accuracy to make good clinical decisions.

The newest and most intriguing of the Doppler formats is colour flow mapping. This technique uses pulsed Doppler to select multiple sites of interrogation within the heart. The direction of flow at these sites is coded using colour so that blood flowing away from the transducer is shown as blue and that flowing towards the transducer as red. Although this format is still at an early stage of development, it has already made the diagnosis of regurgitation, shunts and stenosis easier.

In summary, cardiac ultrasound is a major

diagnostic advance; its immediacy, relative cheapness and lack of side-effects have made it invaluable to the clinician. By utilizing all modalities, it is now possible to make accurate diagnoses in valvular heart disease, congenital heart disease and myocardial disease. At present, it lacks the ability to interrogate the coronary arteries to any useful extent but the developing fields of intra-operative and trans-oesophageal ultrasound may make this practicable. It has been demonstrated that ultrasound eliminates the need for invasive investigation in many instances.[8] To gain the maximum information the operator must be familiar with and use all three modalities of ultrasound—M-mode echocardiography, cross-sectional echocardiography and the Doppler technique.

REPRODUCIBILITY OF CARDIAC ULTRASOUND

A knowledge of its reproducibility is essential to the

development of any clinical technique. The assessment of reproducibility is time-consuming, frequently difficult and therefore often not performed. Reproducibility should not be confused with accuracy. The precision of a technique such as M-mode or cross-sectional echocardiography is mediated by many factors. For practical purposes, it is assumed that the speed of sound through the different body tissues does not change but this is not strictly accurate. Nonetheless, this assumption is used to estimate distance based on recorded time-delay. This source of error is not large and can be disregarded for most clinical situations.

It is essential to know whether cardiac studies carried out by two investigators on one patient are comparable or whether a repeat investigation performed on a different day can be compared with the first. Several authors have found echocardiography to be reproducible in both contrasts. Martin[9] identified the areas of variability in the M-mode echocardiogram. There are similar studies for cross-sectional echo[10] and Doppler ultrasound.[11]

In repeated investigations of the same patient, a standardized patient position is essential. Intracardiac structures can be used as markers to allow the operator to duplicate previous positions. Variation with respiration can make a difference of as much as 3 mm in ventricular dimension[12] between peak inspiration and expiration.

There is also variability in the measurement of the echo tracings. For instance, end-diastole has been measured at the onset of the Q wave, on the peak of the R wave or at the maximum diastolic dimensions. Such variability should not cause problems provided the clinician always uses the same convention when interpreting the tracings. Digitization of M-modes has been used in the assessment of rates of change of wall thickness or cavity size. However, Bullock et al.[13] demonstrated that the variability of this method was much more than that of direct echo measurement. They suggested that the replicated component of variance (i.e. the difference between measurements made from a single recording) was the largest source of variability and this could be halved by repeating the digitization on 4 occasions.

There is also considerable variability during the recording and assessment of a cross-sectional echocardiogram. In a study of segmental wall movements in ischaemic heart disease, Peart and his colleagues[10] investigated reproducibility in this difficult group of patients. Choosing a simple segmental scheme of the left ventricle, they showed that the echocardiographer contributed little to variability when looking at segmental wall movement and that the greatest source of variability was in analysis of the recording. There were large within and between analyser components of variability. The results of this study suggested that care and circumspection was necessary in the use of this technique and the echocardiographer should be aware of where the variability may lie.

ECHOCARDIOGRAPHY OF THE CARDIOMYOPATHIES

Cardiomyopathy can be a primary disease process affecting only the myocardium or secondary to a systemic disorder. The primary cardiomyopathies are divided into dilated, hypertrophic and restrictive cardiomyopathy. In most centres, echocardiography has replaced the use of invasive investigations in these conditions.

DILATED CARDIOMYOPATHY

The echo features of dilated cardiomyopathy are similar, whether it is idiopathic or secondary to myocarditis or ischaemic heart disease. The left ventricular end-diastolic cavity is greatly enlarged on both M-mode and cross-sectional echo (Fig. 13.9). End-systolic dimension is also much greater than normal so that the change between diastole and systole is small. The left ventricular cavity loses its ellipsoidal shape and tends toward a spheroid. The left ventricular outflow tract is widely open and the duration of rapid filling of the left ventricle is short. Within the dilated left ventricle, the mitral valve remains close to the posterior wall, at a greater distance than usual from the posterior aortic wall and the interventricular septum. The morphology of the mitral valve is not intrinsically abnormal although chordal echoes frequently superimpose on the valve cusps. The amplitudes of movement of anterior and posterior mitral leaflets are equally reduced. The left atrium is usually enlarged; at a late stage in the disease, the right ventricle may also be dilated. Doppler studies may often demonstrate the presence of functional mitral regurgitation which may not be audible clinically.

Differentiation between dilated cardiomyopathies secondary to ischaemic heart disease or viral myocarditis and the idiopathic form is not always possible, although ischaemic patients tend to have more obvious incoordination of contraction. Thrombus is frequently seen within the left ventri-

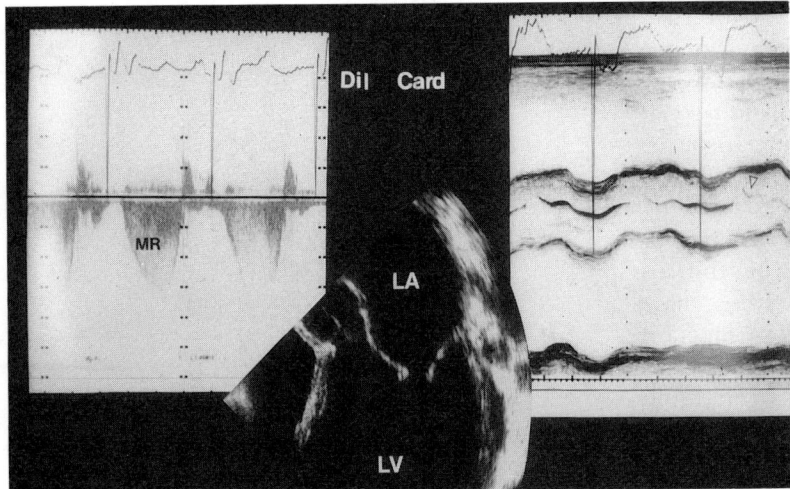

Fig. 13.9. Dilated cardiomyopathy. The three modalities of ultrasound used to investigate a patient with dilated cardiomyopathy. The gross left ventricular enlargement can be appreciated from the cross-sectional echo in the centre. Left atrial enlargement and failure to maintain opening of the aortic valve during ejection are shown on the right-sided M-mode and on the left the mitral regurgitant jet can be used to deduce a high left atrial pressure. LA, left atrium; LV, left ventricle.

cles of ischaemic patients, either as a layered structure, usually at the apex, or less commonly as a pedunculated clot higher up in the ventricle. When the cavity is very large, the blood flow is disordered and swirls around the chamber causing a haze of fine echoes within the ultrasound beam and in the centre of the cavity. The origin of these echoes is not known but it is thought that they represent gas forced out of solution for a brief period due to disorganized flow.

HYPERTROPHIC CARDIOMYOPATHY

The most specific feature of hypertrophic cardiomyopathy is asymmetric septal hypertrophy, although up to 20% of affected hearts also have hypertrophy of the left ventricular free wall (Fig. 13.10). The classic asymmetric hypertrophy is found mid way between the apex and the aortic valve ring but it may also be found in the upper or lower thirds of the septum.[13] The results of family studies suggest that septal hypertrophy may be genetically transmitted as an autosomal dominant. Asymmetric hypertrophy used to be diagnosed on M-mode when the ratio of septal to posterior wall thickness was found to be above the normal range. This ratio could be modified artefactually to a very significant degree if the M-mode did not cut the posterior wall of the ventricle and the interventricular septum at right angles. More recently, cross-sectional echocardiography has been shown to improve the accuracy of the diagnosis. Although asymmetric septal hypertrophy is sensitive for the diagnosis of hypertrophic cardiomyopathy, it is not specific because it is found in several other conditions that cause left ventricular hypertrophy, includ-

ing aortic valve stenosis, discrete subvalvar aortic stenosis and coarctation. An abnormal septal to

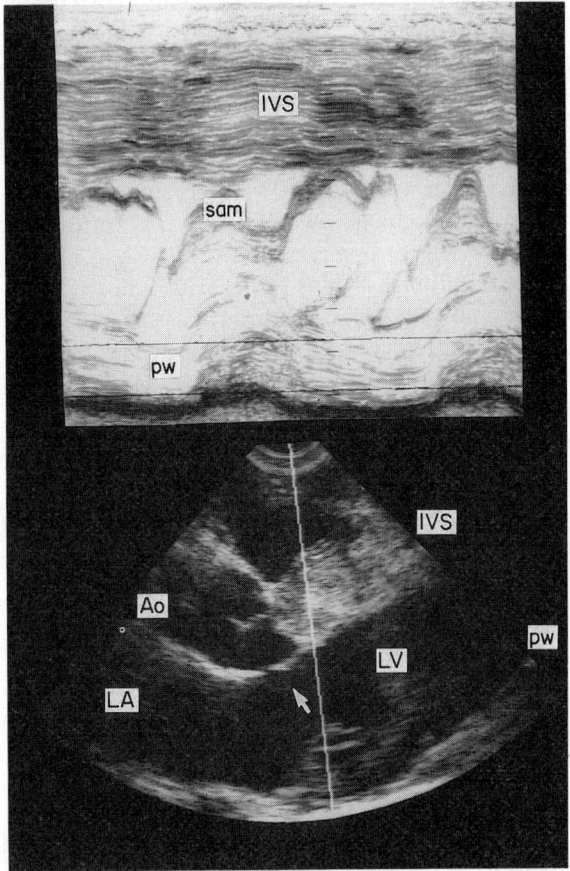

Fig. 13.10. Cross-sectional echocardiogram and M-mode derived from it in a case of hypertrophic obstructive cardiomyopathy. The cross-sectional echo and the M-mode both may demonstrate gross asymmetric septal hypertrophy. The M-mode demonstrates systolic anterior movement (sam) with the anterior mitral leaflet touching the septum. IVS, interventricular septum; pw, posterior wall.

posterior wall ratio may be found in myocardial infarction when scarring leads to thinning of the posterior wall of the left ventricle. Finally, the septum increases in thickness with age and normal age-related values must be used for comparison.

Systolic function in hypertrophic cardiomyopathy is usually normal, as measured by fractional shortening, peak rates of thickening of the septum and peak rates of shortening of ventricular dimension. In very severe end-stage cases, these indices may be abnormally low. Diastolic function of the left ventricle is more frequently abnormal. The left ventricular filling rate is significantly reduced in many patients as judged by assessment from the screen or digitization of septal and posterior left ventricular walls during diastole.[15]

The left ventricular outflow tract in hypertrophic cardiomyopathy is characteristically narrowed, and a systolic pressure difference exists when the condition is obstructive. There is not a close correlation between ventricular septal thickness and narrowness of the outflow. However, outflow tract obstruction correlates fairly well with the presence or absence of systolic anterior movement of the anterior mitral leaflet (Fig. 13.11). There is controversy over what causes systolic anterior movement. Although it is an important feature of hypertrophic cardiomyopathy, it is also found in other conditions, such as transposition of the great arteries. It is almost certainly associated with changes in left ventricular shape when the left ventricular cavity becomes small or partly obliterated. This change in shape probably contributes also to mitral regurgitation which is a frequent occurrence in hypertrophic cardiomyopathy. Partial mid-systolic closure of the aortic valve is a characteristic feature of hypertrophic obstructive cardiomyopathy which correlates with left ventricular outflow tract obstruction and mirrors the haemodynamic events during systole (Fig. 13.12), but must be distinguished from the disturbances of aortic valve motion seen in other situations, e.g. subaortic stenosis, mitral valve prostheses, etc. These conditions often cause partial closure of the aortic valve *earlier* in systole.

Doppler ultrasound in hypertrophic cardiomyopathy can demonstrate the degree of outflow obstruction and the presence of mitral regurgitation. Dynamic outflow tract obstruction has a characteristic Doppler pattern. The gradually increasing obstruction during early systole produces a classic 'scimitar' appearance (Fig. 13.13). Doppler will also detect a high-velocity jet if mitral reg-

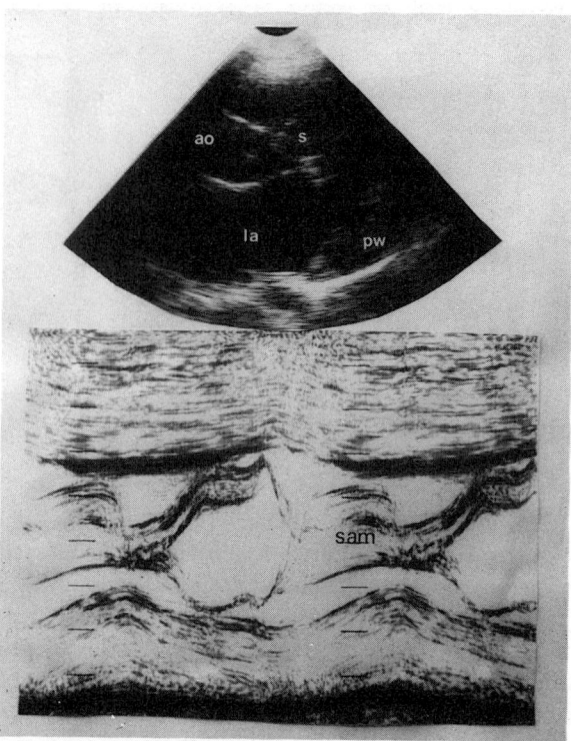

Fig. 13.11. Systolic anterior movement and left ventricular outflow tract narrowing. Cross-sectional echo at the top shows extreme narrowing of the left ventricular outflow tract as the anterior mitral leaflet touches the septum in systole—systolic anterior movement. ao, aorta; la, left atrium; s, ventricular septum; pw, posterior wall; sam, systolic anterior movement.

urgitation is present.

The echocardiographer must therefore endeavour to demonstrate asymmetric septal hypertrophy, narrowing of the left ventricular outflow tract, systolic anterior movement of the mitral valve and partial systolic closure of the aortic valve cusps to make the diagnosis of hypertrophic obstructive cardiomyopathy. However, hypertrophic car-

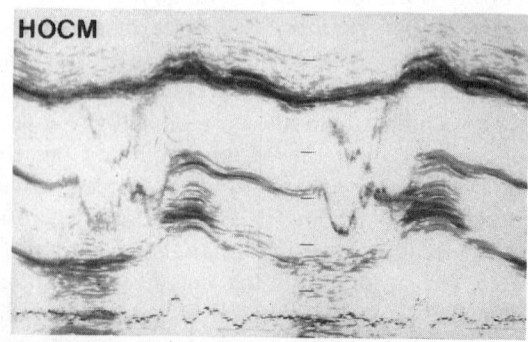

Fig. 13.12. The aortic valve in hypertrophic obstructive cardiomyopathy. This M-mode shows mid-systolic collapse of the right coronary and non-coronary cusps of the aortic valve.

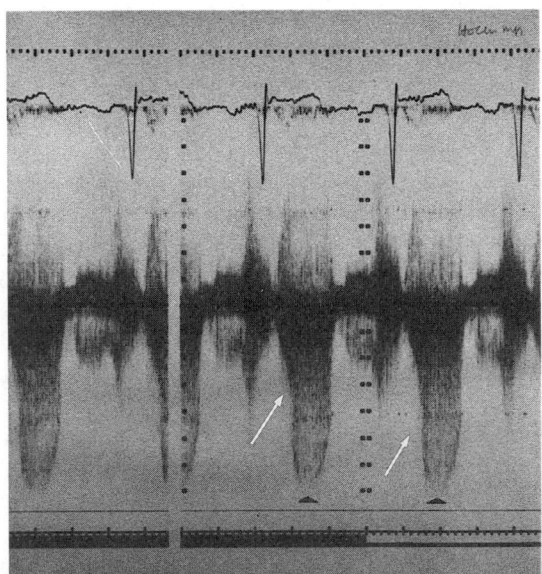

Fig. 13.13. Ventricular outflow tract Doppler in a severely obstructed case of hypertrophic cardiomyopathy. This patient had extreme left ventricular outflow tract obstruction and there was the characteristic slow upstroke to be seen on the left ventricular outflow tract Doppler envelope (arrows). This was recorded from the apex of the left ventricle.

diomyopathy can be diagnosed in some patients from the presence of only one of the above features.

RESTRICTIVE CARDIOMYOPATHY

Restrictive cardiomyopathy is a poorly understood entity. It is the least common of the cardiomyopathies. The primary restrictive car-

diomyopathy is a rare lesion of the left ventricle with reduced ventricular compliance but often with well-preserved systolic function.[16] The echocardiogram (Fig. 13.14) frequently reveals enlargement of the atria, and normal or only slightly depressed global systolic function with normal myocardial thickness. More commonly, restrictive cardiomyopathy is part of a disease process affecting other systems. It is usually associated with amyloidosis, but it can also occur with glycogenosis, haemochromatosis and neoplasia. In any of these entities, the myocardium appears more thickened and is hyper-refractile, particularly in patients with cardiac amyloid,[17] which sometimes causes a bright 'scintillating' appearance of the myocardium on cross-sectional echocardiography. In the secondary forms, the infiltrative processes gradually become more severe, limiting the ability of the myocardium to thicken or thin during the cardiac cycle. Constrictive pericarditis which may give a similar clinical picture to restrictive cardiomyopathy can usually be distinguished because of normal wall thickness, normal posterior left ventricular wall movement and the characteristic abnormal septal movements.

THE ATHLETE'S HEART

Cross-sectional and M-mode echocardiography demonstrate the presence of ventricular hypertrophy with clarity and accuracy. Athletes in training may develop cardiac chamber enlargement, left ventricular hypertrophy and frequently bradycardia, features very similar to those of hypertrophic car-

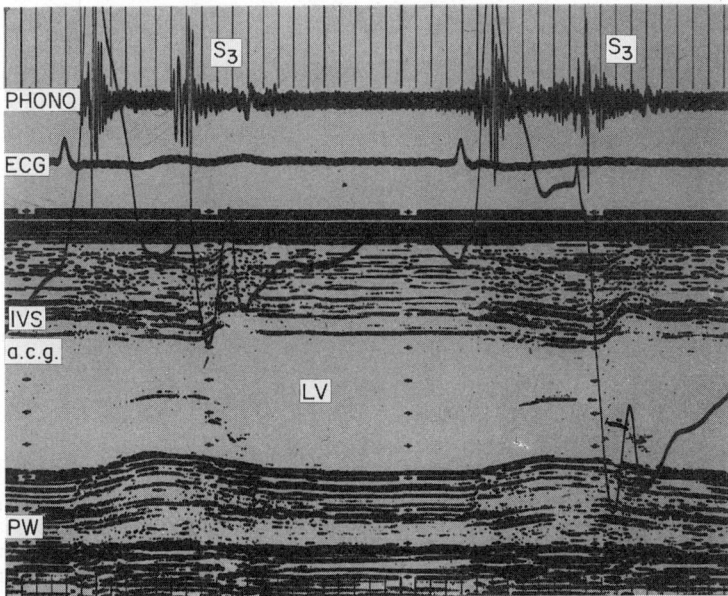

Fig. 13.14. Restrictive cardiomyopathy. This echocardiogram is from a patient with a restrictive cardiomyopathy showing ventricular wall hypertrophy and poor movement of ventricular walls between systole and diastole. There is also a phonocardiogram (phono) which shows a loud third heart sound (S_3) and an apexcardiogram (a.c.g.). IVS = interventricular septum, LV = left ventricle, PW = posterior wall.

diomyopathy and therefore a cause of concern to the clinician.[18,19] As many more people now take part in physical exercise, the differentiation between physiological and pathological hypertrophy is of considerable importance. In athletes in training, left ventricular mass increases in a similar way and to a similar degree as it does in hypertensive patients and in patients with left ventricular outflow tract obstruction and cardiomyopathy. The type of exercise is important. Athletes may be divided into anaerobic exercisers, e.g. wrestlers and shot putters, and aerobic exercisers, e.g. distance runners and swimmers. When wall thickness and cavity size are corrected for body mass, there is probably little difference between the normal heart and that of the anaerobic exerciser. However, the aerobic exerciser frequently has asymmetric septal hypertrophy and an increase in diastolic cavity dimension of the left ventricle. This increase, which may be as much as 10%, occurs rapidly after vigorous training and regresses equally quickly after cessation of training.[20] Changes in cavity size can be attributed to the bradycardia apart from the genuine increase in posterior left ventricular and septal wall thickness. After very prolonged periods of training, top-class athletes show cavity dimensions greatly increased beyond the level seen in non-aortic subjects and there is probably a direct relationship between the amount of exercise and the increase in left ventricular size, the highest grade of athletes having the largest increase. Shapiro[20] has summarized the features that differentiate the athlete's heart from pathological hypertrophy (see also Chapter 63). No athlete's heart should have a free wall thicker than 2 cm. Although asymmetric septal hypertrophy can occur in athletes, systolic anterior movement does not. Athletes never have reduced cavity size but this is not uncommon in patients with hypertrophic cardiomyopathy. Indices of diastolic performance are frequently abnormal in those with hypertrophic cardiomyopathy, but athletes usually have normal systolic and diastolic function.

ECHOCARDIOGRAPHY OF CARDIAC TUMOURS

Most cardiac tumours are secondary to disseminated malignant disease elsewhere in the body and are associated with pericardial involvement and fluid. Primary heart tumours are rare. In adults, most of the primary tumours are myxomas; in childhood, the common tumour is the rhabdomyoma.

The classic intracardiac tumour is the left atrial myxoma first recognized by echocardiography in 1959 by Effert and Domanig.[21] The diagnosis can be made quite reliably with M-mode echocardiography. The mitral valve is similar in appearance to calcific mitral stenosis with a slow diastolic closure rate and dense echoes from the tumour filling in the space behind the anterior mitral leaflet (Fig. 13.15). In most patients, the M-mode pattern is sufficiently specific for surgery to be undertaken without further investigation. Cross-sectional echocardiography makes the diagnosis easier. It also allows an appreciation of the tumour size and of its site of attachment, which is nearly always on the interatrial septum (Fig. 13.16). Calcification or cyst formation may occur in myxomas and can be demonstrated by cross-sectional echocardiography. The main differential diagnosis is between myxomas and large vegetations attached to the atrioventricular valves. Vegetations are usually more shaggy and irregular and interfere with the movement of the valve leaflets. Some intracavity tumours are sarcomas rather than myxomas and it is not possible to differentiate between the two on the echocardiogram.

Intramural tumours are extremely rare and occur more often in childhood than in later life. Many patients are asymptomatic. The echo appreciation of such tumours is often difficult and depends on recognizing a difference in the intensity of the echoes reflected from the tumour and the rest of the heart wall.

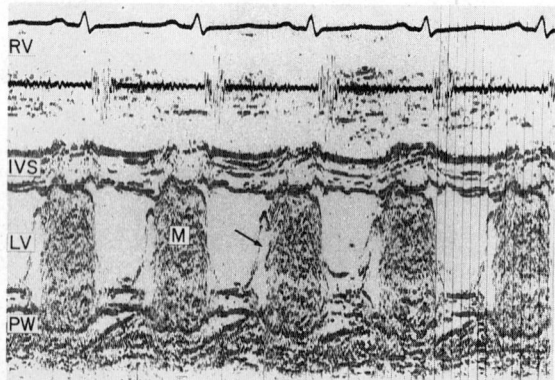

Fig. 13.15. M-mode echocardiogram showing a left atrial myxoma (M). The tumour is seen filling the mitral valve orifice in diastole. There is a small echo–free space in early diastole just before the tumour moves from the left atrium into the open mitral valve (arrow). IVS; interventricular septum, LV; left ventricle, PW; posterior wall, RV; right ventricle.

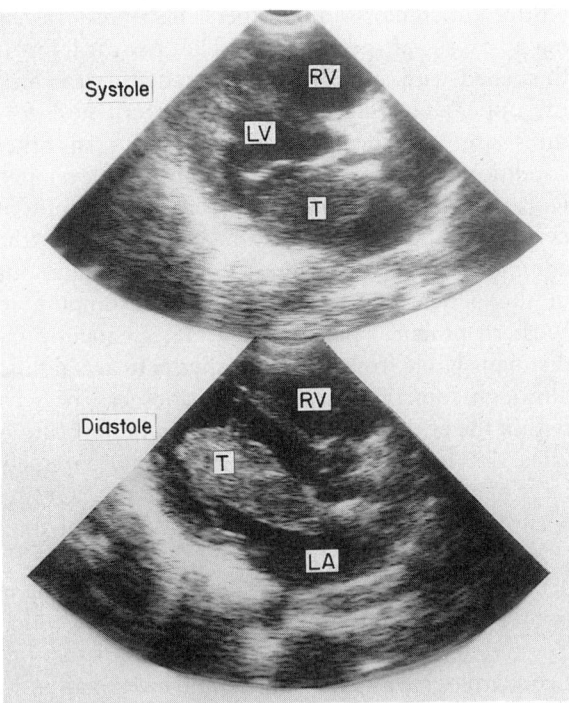

Fig. 13.16. Cross-sectional echocardiogram of left atrial myxoma. A large atrial myxoma attached to the inter-atrial septum is seen prolapsing through the mitral valve in diastole in the lower figure. This is a long axis, parasternal view. T = myxoma, RV = right ventricle, LA = left atrium.

Metastases from disseminated malignancy regularly affect the pericardium. The pericardium is frequently thickened, and a pericardial effusion is almost invariable. The features will be described in the section on pericardial effusions.

ECHOCARDIOGRAPHY OF INTRACARDIAC THROMBI

Intracardiac thrombi could never be reliably identified by M-mode echocardiography although they were frequently suspected when multiple echoes were seen along the posterior left atrial wall or in the left ventricular apex. Although cross-sectional echocardiography can identify intracardiac thrombi, it is sometimes misleading. New thrombi usually appear as a mass of echoes, which are frequently quite faint and seem to be filamentous and shaggy. As the thrombus ages, its appearance becomes more circumscribed and dense (Fig. 13.17). Differentiation between a clot and a vegetation can be very difficult; the clinical picture and the cavity in which the mass is seen aid in the differentiation. For

example, following a myocardial infarction, the presence of a mass in the apex of the left ventricle is likely to suggest thrombus rather than vegetation. There is considerable argument over the size of thrombus that can be detected by echocardiography. Mobile or pedunculated thrombi are much more easily recognized than the static cessile thrombus lining the wall of a chamber. Although clot in the left atrium and left atrial appendage can be missed on cross-sectional or M-mode echocardiography, the use of trans-oesophageal echocardiography may solve this diagnostic problem.

ECHOCARDIOGRAPHY OF PERICARDIAL DISEASE

Echocardiography is undoubtedly the method of choice for demonstrating pericardial fluid. Normally the potential space between the visceral and parietal pericardium is invisible to the echocardiographer. When disease processes produce increased pericardial fluid, these layers separate and the space is immediately apparent on M-mode or cross-sectional echocardiography (Fig. 13.18). Cross-sectional echocardiography is superior to the M-mode in that it gives a better impression of the extent and depth of the fluid. Accurate quantification of pericardial fluid is difficult and most operators confine themselves to reporting small, medium or large accumulations and commenting on the presence or absence of haemodynamic effects.

Cardiac tamponade occurs when the accumulation of fluid within the pericardial space interferes

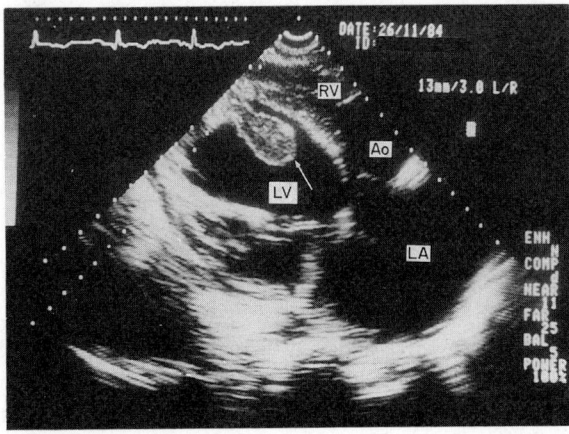

Fig. 13.17. Thrombus in left ventricle (arrow). This penduculate clot is attached to the left ventricular wall near the apex (arrow). Ao; aorta, LA; left atrium, LV; left ventricle, RV; right ventricle.

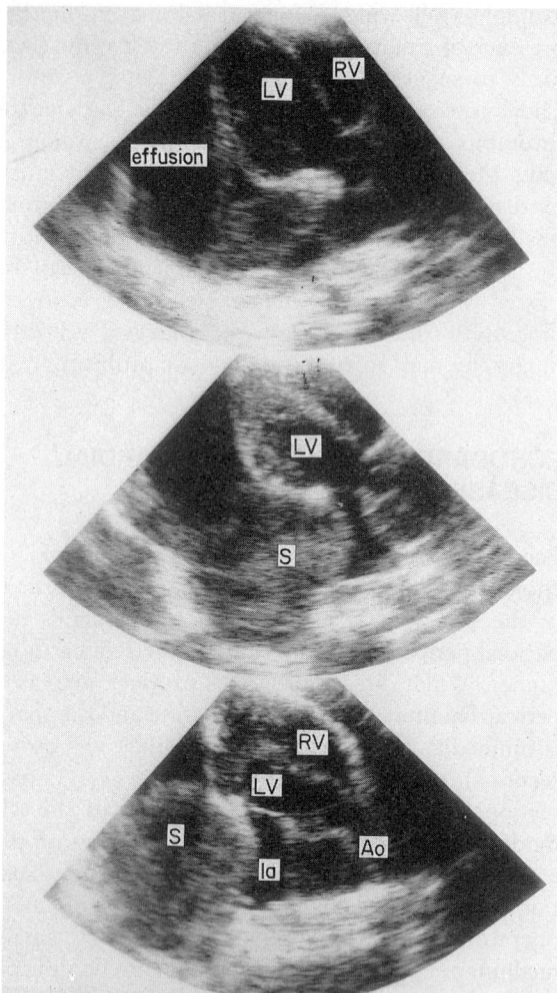

Fig. 13.18. A very large pericardial effusion in a patient with sarcoma(s) involving the left atrial walls which in the lower 2 pictures can be seen to be thickened. RV, right ventricle; LV, left ventricle; la, left atrium; ao, aorta. These pictures are a series of slices obtained from positions between a long axis parasternal and a four-chamber apical view.

with the function of the heart. Martin *et al.*[22] demonstrated that the right ventricular free wall collapsed during diastole in tamponade (Fig. 13.19). This effect was also noted on the right atrial wall in diastole. These abnormal appearances disappeared after aspiration of pericardial fluid. Experimental work suggests that these abnormal wall movements can be detected before major changes in systemic blood pressure occur, indicating that 'echocardiographic tamponade' is a relatively early finding preceding overt clinical tamponade.

Pericardial fluid accumulation generally follows infection or malignant disease. In many parts of the world, tuberculosis and other infections are the main cause of pericarditis. The pericardium is thickened with strands of fibrin radiating towards the upper epicardial surface. However, these features are not specific and may occur in other conditions including malignancy. In the developed world, malignant disease is the commonest cause of pericardial fluid accumulation and probably the commonest cause of tamponade. Surprisingly, pus in the pericardium (not particularly common in Western practice) produces features frequently indistinguishable from those of other pericardial fluid although sometimes fibrinous strands can be seen within the effusion. When pericardial fluid accumulates slowly, the effusion may become extremely large before tamponade develops. By contrast, acute accumulation of relatively small amounts of fluid (often blood) caused by trauma (e.g. road traffic accidents, wounding, etc.) may cause tamponade because the pericardium has not had time in which to stretch as it does in the chronic situation. Echocardiography is an important investigation in the patient with trauma who shows an unexpected degree of cardiovascular collapse.

The diagnosis of constrictive pericarditis can present a problem for the echocardiographer. In established cases, there is probably a characteristic echo appearance. The cavities are of normal size and particularly when visualized in the four-chamber view, the free walls hardly move or at most they demonstrate a sudden cessation of expansion in early diastole. In the centre of the heart, the septum moves briskly backwards and forwards appearing to provide most of the systolic movement of the ventricle. Using ultrasound, it is not possible to assess pericardial thickness accurately, particularly in the presence of calcification. Only when there is an adjacent and simultaneous pleural effusion is it possible to see both sides of the pericardium and to make some estimate of the true thickness. The new imaging techniques, such as magnetic resonance and computer tomography, may become valuable in assessing pericardial thickening, and they are likely to be superior to echocardiography.[23]

ECHOCARDIOGRAPHY OF THE AORTA

In infancy, the entire aorta, from the aortic valve to the bifurcation, can be visualized using several echo windows. In the middle-aged and elderly, it may be possible to see no more than a few centimetres of

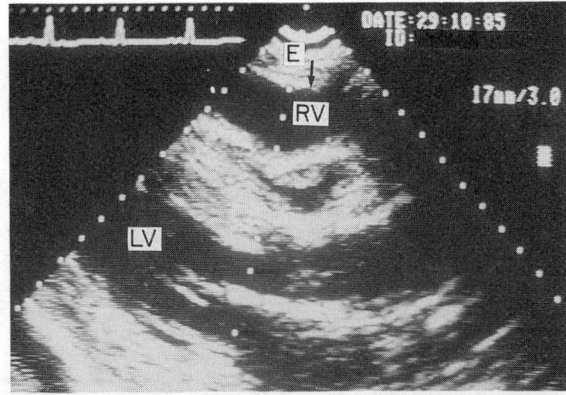

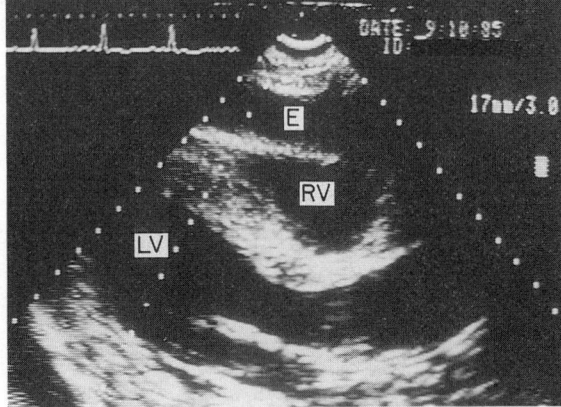

A

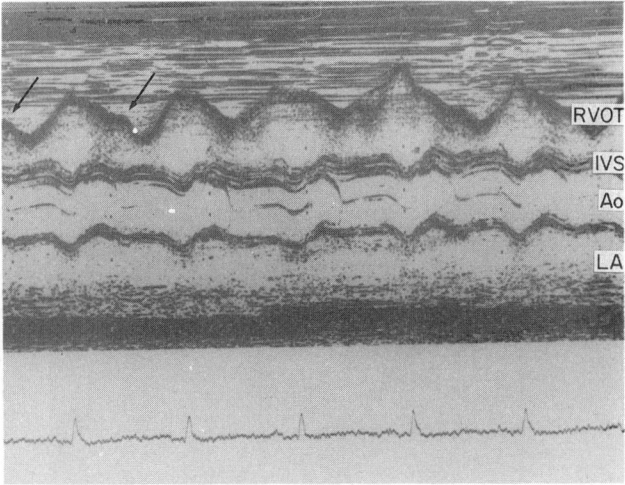

B

Fig. 13.19. (A) Parasternal cross-sectional echocardiograms from a patient with tamponade. The RV collapses in early diastole (arrow) and expands again later in diastole. E = pericardial effusion, LV and RV = left and right ventricle. (B) M-mode echocardiogram from another patient showing the same phenomenon. This recording is obtained (RVOT) slightly oblique across RV outflow (RVOT), which is seen to collapse in diastole (arrow), septum (IVS), aorta (Ao) and left atrium (LA).

the root of the aorta and a few more centimetres in mid arch. When examining patients who have aortic lesions, all possible views must be recorded in an attempt to define aortic structure. The ascending aorta should be studied from the third and fourth left intercostal space in the parasternal long axis. The suprasternal notch should be used to examine the transverse arch and the origin of the main head and neck vessels. Part of the abdominal aorta can be visualized in a subcostal approach in most patients. With the advent of trans-oesophageal echocardiography, it may be possible to obtain high-quality images of all parts of the aorta with ultrasound.

Aneurysms of the aorta can affect any part of the structure and be secondary to trauma, dissection, Marfan's syndrome or degeneration of the vessel wall. They are recognized by dilatation of certain segments of the aorta in conjunction with the occurrence of normal dimensions elsewhere. Angiocardiography, computer tomographic scanning and nuclear magnetic resonance give superior pictures and are better suited to examination of the whole aorta than standard transthoracic and sternal notch echocardiography. Nonetheless, the cheapness and mobility of cross-sectional echocardiogra-

phy makes it valuable in the diagnosis of aneurysms and in the follow-up of patients (Fig. 13.20).

In aortic dissection, duplication of echoes from the aortic wall associated with root dilatation or dilatation of other parts of the aorta are commonly seen (Fig. 13.21). In such a view, the inner echoes

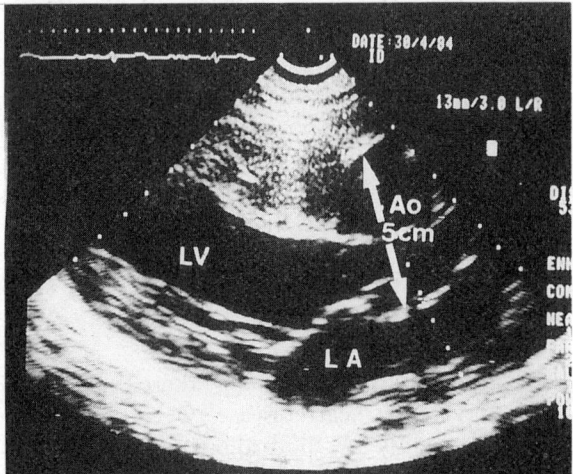

Fig. 13.20. Cross-sectional echo of aortic dilatation in Marfan's syndrome. The parasternal long-axis view in this patient shows gross enlargement of the aortic root just above the valve cusps. LA, left atrium; LV, left ventricle; Ao, aorta.

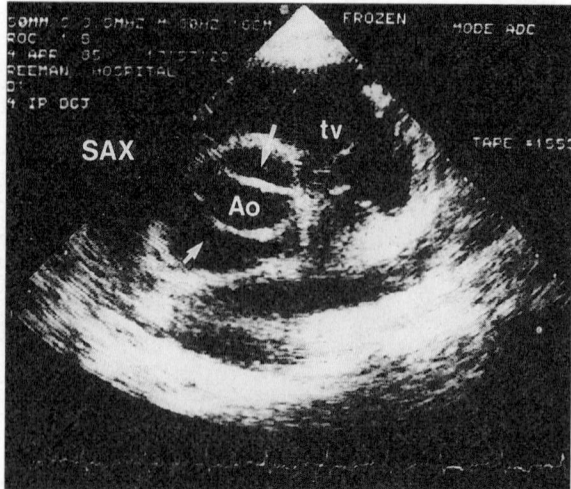
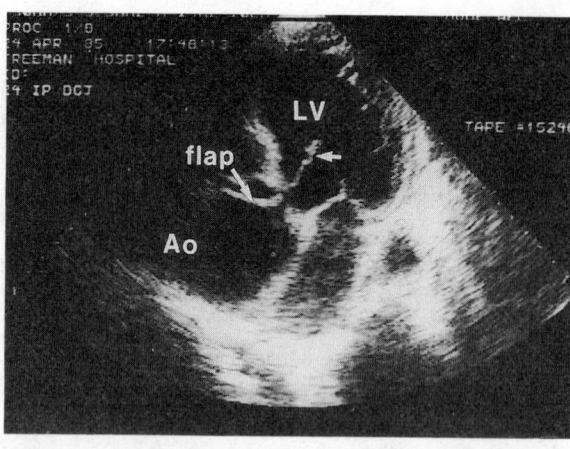

Fig. 13.21. (A) Short-axis view of a patient with dissection of the aorta. The false lumen is arrowed and the area marked Ao is the true lumen. tv, tricuspid valve. (B) The same patient in a slightly oblique view which is close to a parasternal long-axis view. The flap caused by the dissection is arrowed as is a piece of aortic endothelium which prolapses into the LV. LV, left ventricle; Ao, aorta.

usually represent the limits of the true lumen and the outer echoes the false lumen. Aortic dissection can be mimicked by abscesses of the ventricular septum or dilatation of the sinuses of Valsalva. Aortic regurgitation and pericardial effusion which both frequently result from dissection can be detected by ultrasound and may indicate the true diagnosis.

Coarctation of the aorta is rare in adults; in neonates it is the most common cause of heart failure. The echocardiogram can visualize aortic narrowing in the classic post-ductal position, and a combination of imaging in the suprasternal approach and gradient assessment using continuous wave Doppler is usually sufficient to obviate the need for angiography (Fig. 13.22). In older adult patients, the area of the coarctation is not always visible using cross-sectional echocardiography and it is necessary to perform other techniques. Associated lesions must be sought, in particular, a bicuspid aortic valve or a ventricular septal defect, defects commonly associated with coarctation.

VALVE DISEASE

Echocardiography has gradually altered the assessment of valvular heart disease. Over the last 10 years, the quality of echocardiographic images has improved, more information about the significance of changes seen on echocardiography has been accumulated and the pitfalls of the technique have been recognized. The information provided by echocardiography frequently allows the clinician to diagnose the valve lesions with enough accuracy to obviate the need for cardiac catheterization before surgery.[8] Direct inspection of the cardiac valves with echocardiography gives anatomical information about their involvement in the disease process. Echocardiography may also indicate the degree of stenosis or regurgitation, but this information is achieved more directly from the Doppler technique. The echocardiogram also gives information about left ventricular function, which is important not only in the assessment of this parameter itself but also because abnormalities of wall motion may indicate the severity of valve lesions, particularly those causing regurgitation.

Although the pre-operative assessment of patients with valve disease has been revolutionzed by echocardiography, the problem of assessing coronary artery disease remains. Small ultrasound probes can be run directly over the coronary artery at operation to detect narrowings within them, but at present their use is experimental.[24]

The next major object in the echocardiographic investigation of valve disease is to improve the assessment of patients before operation so that irreversible deterioration of left ventricular function is prevented, particularly in valvar regurgitation. M-mode echocardiography is already being used to follow the course of left ventricular enlargement with these lesions, but there is considerable dispute, and a lack of knowledge, about the appropriate timing of therapeutic intervention.

The use of echocardiography in valve lesions can

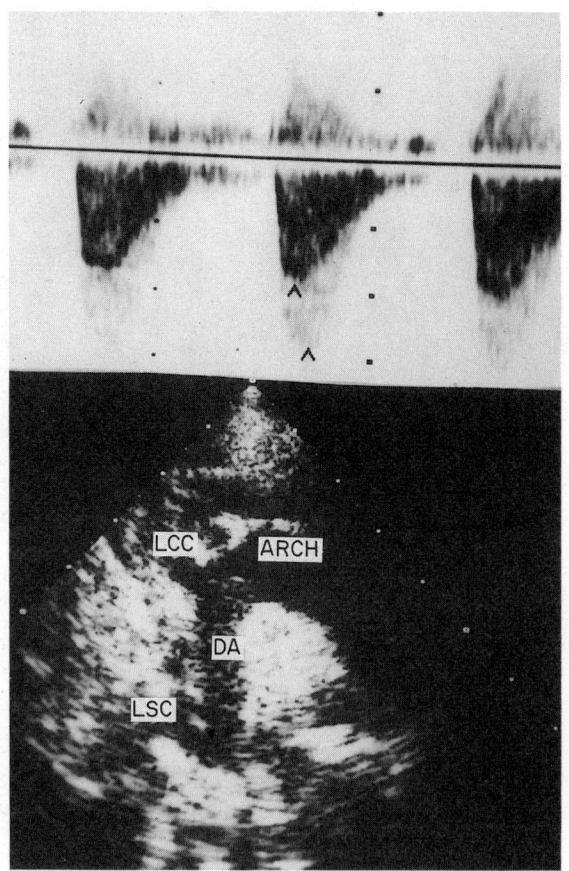

Fig. 13.22. Doppler and cross-sectional echocardiography in a case of coarctation. The continuous wave Doppler above shows a double Doppler envelope (see arrows) suggesting the presence of both aortic valve stenosis and coarctation of the aorta. A cross-sectional echo below taken from the suprasternal approach demonstrates the difficulties in obtaining good echo images at the site of coarctation which in this case is just distal to the origin of the left subclavian artery. DA, descending aorta; LCC, left common carotid artery; LSC, left subclavian artery.

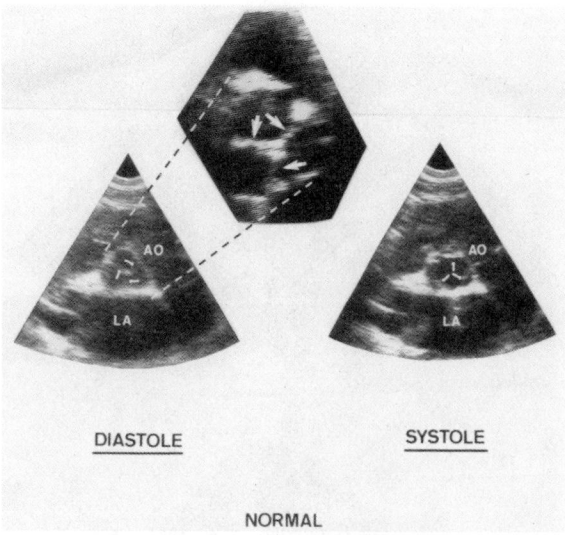

Fig. 13.23. Cross-sectional echocardiogram of a normal aortic valve in systole and diastole in the parasternal short-axis view. The three aortic valve cusps were seen to be closed in diastole and to open widely in systole. LA, left atrium; AO, aorta.

be discussed under two main headings: direct inspection of the valve and assessment of the effect of the valve lesion on left and/or right ventricular function.

AORTIC VALVE DISEASE

Aortic stenosis

In most adults, the diagnosis of significant aortic stenosis is excluded if a thin freely mobile aortic valve, opening fully with each systole, is seen on either M-mode or cross-sectional echocardiography (Fig. 13.23). Occasionally, young adults (usually below the age of 30 years) show full valve opening on the M-mode echocardiogram but have significant aortic stenosis. This deceptive appearance is the result of the thin M-mode echobeam transecting the wide proximal portion of the doming aortic valve leaflets. This doming can usually be detected on a good quality cross-sectional echocardiogram, but it is occasionally missed (Fig. 13.24).

If echocardiography shows the aortic valve cusps to be abnormally thickened and to have reduced mobility, a diagnosis of significant aortic stenosis is possible but not certain. When the valve is grossly thickened and immobile (Fig. 13.25) or simply appears as a mass of immobile echoes filling the aortic root, stenosis is nearly always severe. When thickening and immobility are less marked, an assessment of the severity of stenosis by echocardiography is more difficult. Some valves which show moderate thickening and reduction of mobility of the valve cusps are severely stenotic, whereas others that have similar echocardiographic appearance may produce little or no stenosis.[8] Similarly, heavily calcified valves that are not particularly stenotic reflect ultrasound strongly and produce artefacts due to reverberation of the echoes striking the valve, which appear to fill the aortic root and give the impression of severe stenosis. Attempts have been made to correlate the degree of stenosis with the amount of valve-cusp separation seen on the cross-sectional echocardiogram. Cusp separa-

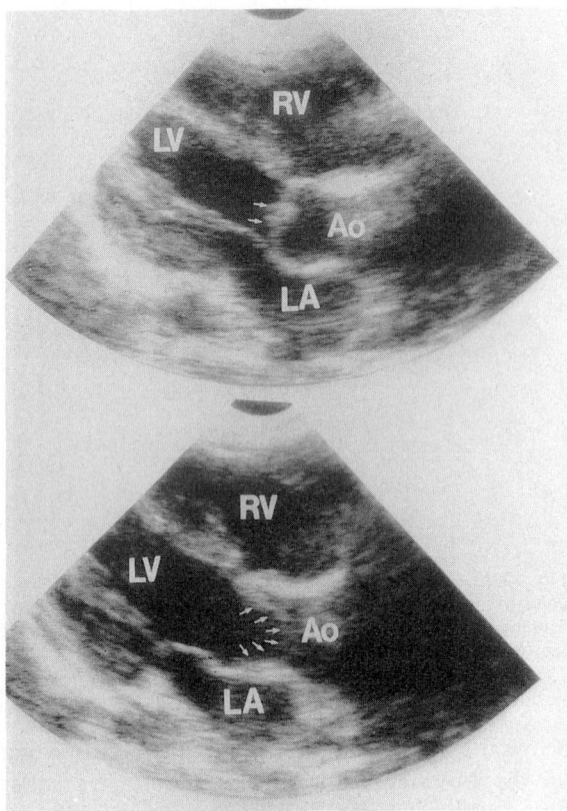

Fig. 13.24. Cross-sectional echocardiogram in the long-axis parasternal view of a domed bicuspid aortic valve. Upper panel: the thickened aortic valve is seen coapted in diastole (arrows); lower panel: the bicuspid valve is seen to dome in systole into the aortic root (arrows). LA, left atrium; LV, left ventricle; RV, right ventricle; Ao, aorta.

tion > 12 mm excludes severe stenosis whereas cusp separation < 6 mm suggests that stenosis is severe. Up to 40% of patients with suspected stenosis have between 7 and 12 mm of detectable valve opening, consequently it is not possible to use this technique to assess the severity of stenosis in this group of patients.[25] Assessment of the degree of aortic stenosis from the echocardiogram alone is frequently unreliable unless the lesion is very severe or very mild. The introduction of the Doppler technique has overcome many of these problems. Using the modified Bernoulli equation, as described by Hatle,[7] the peak pressure difference across the valve is calculated from the maximum velocity of flow recorded across the valve by continuous wave Doppler. This is not the same as the 'peak to peak' pressure difference recorded at catheterization; the peak pressure difference is usually higher and occurs earlier. This method is reliable and it is used widely to make decisions about the need for surgery or balloon valvuloplasty.

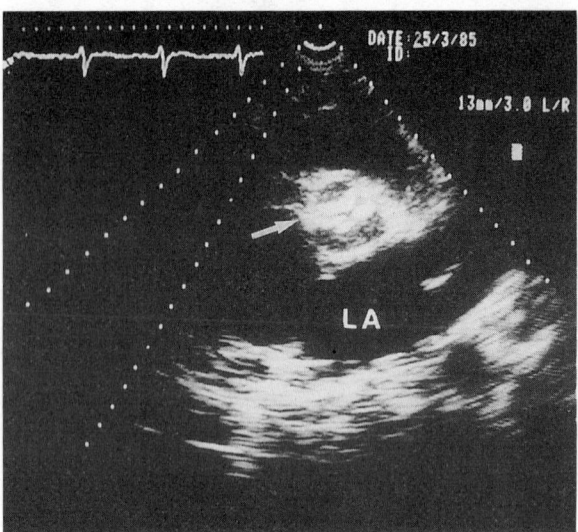

Fig. 13.25. Cross-sectional echocardiogram from a patient with severe aortic stenosis in the parasternal short-axis view. The calcified thickened aortic cusps are seen and there is a thin crack-like opening between the three valve cusps (arrow). This is the widest extent of opening seen in systole. LA, left atrium.

Echocardiography can usually distinguish between tricuspid and bicuspid aortic valves. In 70% of patients with a bicuspid aortic valve, the diagnosis is suggested on the M-mode echocardiogram by either an extremely eccentric closure line, or multiple closure lines in diastole.[26] The cross-sectional technique is more reliable in the detection of bicuspid valves, particularly when the valve can be visualized in the parasternal short-axis view (Fig. 13.26).[27] Although this distinction between bicuspid and tricuspid valves has no importance in the assessment of the severity of stenosis, it has some relevance as far as follow up is concerned. A normal tricuspid aortic valve at echocardiography is unlikely to cause problems in the future. A bicuspid valve, even if it is not stenotic at the time of investigation, may in future become stenotic or act as a focus for infective endocarditis.

Although non-valvar aortic stenosis, or the sub- or supravalvar variety, is rare in adults, echocardiography may provide useful diagnostic information. In neither type can M-mode echocardiography reliably show the obstruction itself, although in subvalvar stenosis there is often a characteristic abnormality of aortic valve motion (Fig. 13.27). The obstruction proximal to the aortic valve causes a disturbance in the flow through it and early partial closure of the cusps. Although this appearance is characteristic, it is not specific because other conditions that disturb flow below the valve, such as a

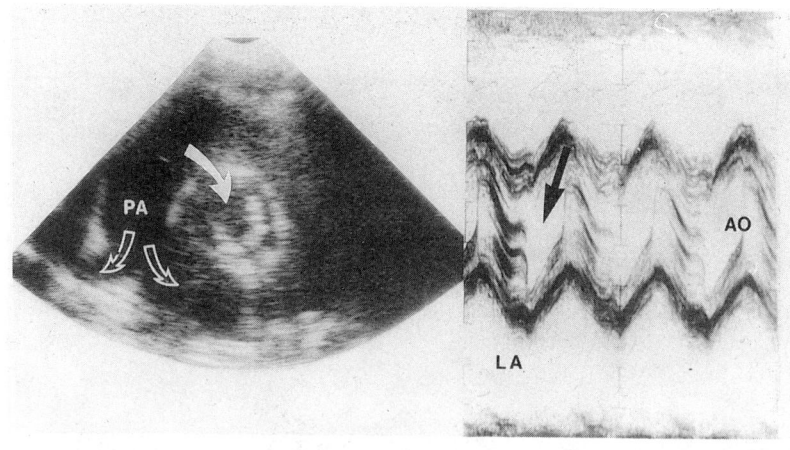

Fig. 13.26. Cross-sectional echocardiogram in the short-axis parasternal view on the left and an M-mode derived from this view on the right. The patient has a bicuspid aortic valve with vertical leaflets. In some patients who have a bicuspid aortic valve, the cusps lie in a horizontal position. Although this valve is stenotic the M-mode shows apparently wide opening of the cusps due to doming (black arrow). The M-mode also shows multiple echoes from the aortic valve, a feature suggesting that it is abnormal and bicuspid. AO, aorta; LA, left atrium; PA, pulmonary artery.

mitral prosthetic valve projecting into the left ventricular outflow, an aneurysmal aortic root, dissecting aneurysm and hypertrophic cardiomyopathy, produce similar abnormalities. Although there are subtle distinguishing features between the types of movement seen in subvalvar aortic stenosis and those of these other conditions, all possibilities should be considered if abnormal early closure of the aortic valve is seen. Occasionally, the subvalvar obstructing membrane is well seen on M-mode echocardiography and it may be mistaken for vegetation (Fig. 13.28).

The cross-sectional echocardiogram is more useful in the assessment of non-valvar aortic stenosis. It can usually define the site of obstruction (Figs 13.29 and 13.30), although this is achieved more easily in subvalvar than supravalvar stenosis because the obstructing bar of tissue or membrane below the aortic valve is usually seen in conventional echo views.[28] Supravalvar narrowings may be seen from the parasternal approach, but more frequently a suprasternal transducer position is necessary. These views can usually be obtained in children but in

adults this may prove difficult and is often impossible.[29] The severity of supra- or subvalvar aortic stenosis can be assessed reliably using continuous wave Doppler. As supravalvar stenosis is often associated with William's syndrome, the echocardiographer should also scan as much of the pulmonary arterial tree as possible, searching for associated pulmonary artery branch stenosis.

As aortic stenosis becomes more severe, it causes increasing degrees of left ventricular hypertrophy. This hypertrophy is usually concentric with the thickness of the interventricular septum and posterior wall increasing to the same extent. Occasionally, hypertrophy is markedly asymmetric, the septal thickness being far in excess of that of the posterior wall.[3] Left ventricular cavity size remains normal except in severe longstanding aortic stenosis, in which it begins to increase progressively and systolic function, as judged by fractional shortening, falls (Fig. 13.31). The dilated ventricle of end-stage aortic stenosis shows increased wall thickness and this feature helps distinguish aortic stenosis from dilated cardiomyopathy.[30] Cross-

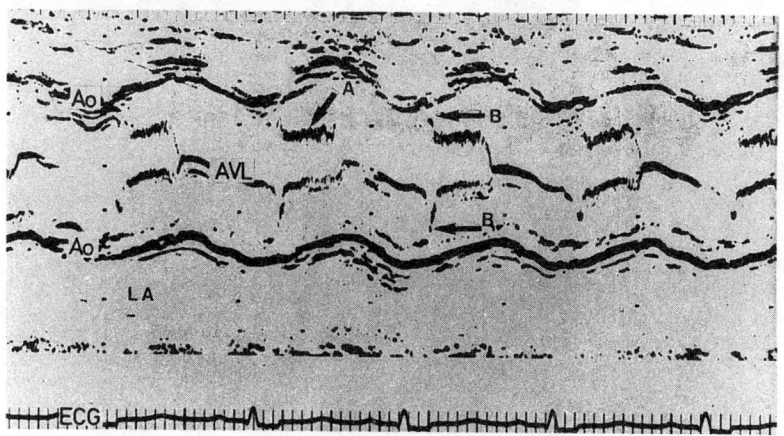

Fig. 13.27. M-mode echocardiogram of the aortic valve in a patient with subaortic stenosis. The valve is seen to open widely in early systole (arrow B) but quickly regains a mid-position (arrow A) for the rest of systole. LA, left atrium; Ao, aorta; AVL, aortic valve leaflet.

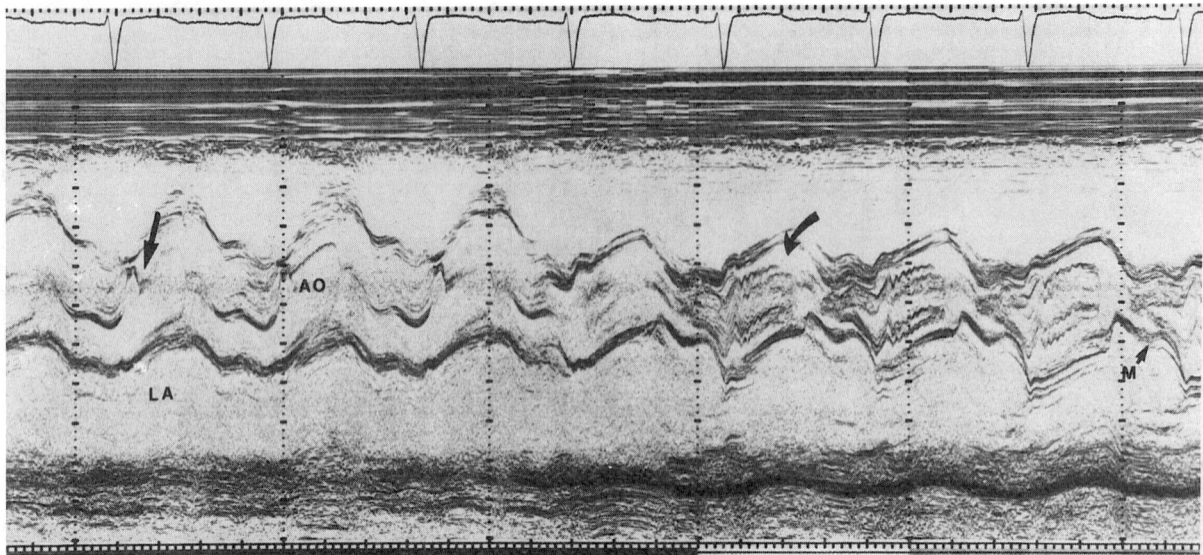

Fig. 13.28. M-mode echocardiographic sweep from the left ventricular outflow (left) to the aorta (right). A vibrating mass of echoes (curved arrow) is seen anterior to the mitral valve (M) and is present until the sweep reaches the aortic valve. These appearances were due to a membrane-producing subaortic stenosis. There is early systolic partial closure of the aortic valves (straight arrow, left) characteristic of this condition. LA, left atrium; AO, aorta.

sectional echocardiography gives an overall impression of left ventricular cavity size and wall motion and thickness, but more precise measurements of wall thickness can be made using the M-mode technique.

The degree of hypertrophy detected by M-mode echocardiography usually correlates with the degree of stenosis because hypertrophy tends to continue to increase until wall stress has been normalized. In young people with aortic stenosis, this correlation is close enough to make fairly accurate predictions of aortic valve gradients in groups of patients;[31,32] in some individuals, this technique produces inaccurate results and in practical terms it is not reliable enough for clinical decision-making.

The assessment of left ventricular systolic function using simple echocardiographic parameters, such as fractional shortening or the velocity of circumferential fibre shortening, can be extremely misleading. If these parameters are normal, it is certain that left ventricular function is normal. However, if they are reduced, left ventricular function may still be normal; the parameters may be depressed because of the extremely high afterload

Fig. 13.29. Cross-sectional parasternal long-axis view of a patient with subaortic stenosis. The subvalvar membrane is seen below the aortic valve (ao.v.) and is marked by small arrows. lv, left ventricle; m, mitral valve; la, left atrium; rv, right ventricle.

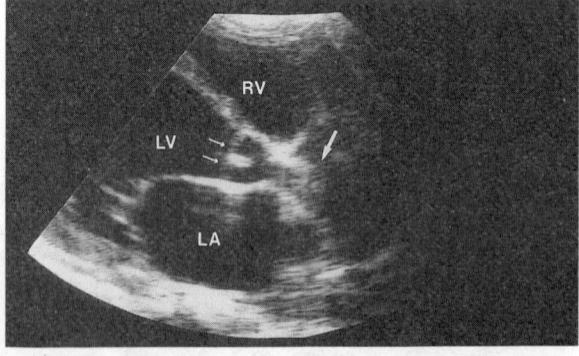

Fig. 13.30. Parasternal long-axis view of a patient with supravalve aortic stenosis. The thickened cusps of the aortic valve are shown closed in diastole (small arrows) and the narrowing is seen just above that level (large arrow). The left ventricle is enlarged and in this case left ventricular function was significantly impaired by the severe outflow obstruction. LV = left ventricle, LA = left atrium, RV = right ventricle.

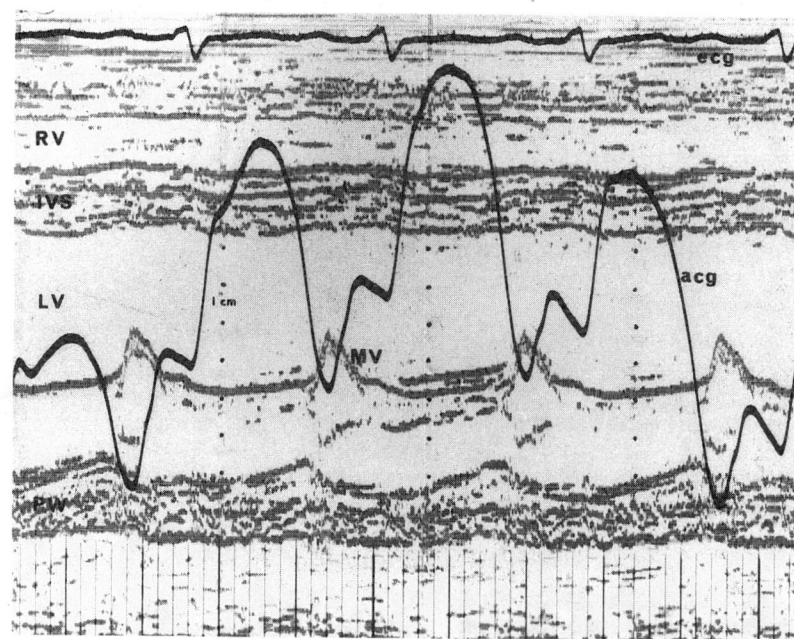

Fig. 13.31. M-mode echocardiogram of the left ventricle in a patient with end-stage aortic stenosis. The left ventricular dimensions are moderately increased, the left ventricular wall motion is extremely poor, there is thickening of both the interventricular septum (IVS) and posterior wall (PW) of the left ventricle. There is also an apex cardiogram (acg) on this tracing. RV, right ventricle; LV, left ventricle; MV, mitral valve; ecg, electrocardiogram.

on the left ventricle. Changes in diastolic function, of which prolonged isovolumic relaxation and slow left ventricular filling are the most prominent, can be detected by digitized echocardiograms.[3] These abnormalities of diastolic function probably result from a combination of hypertrophy, interstitial fibrosis, and sub-endocardial ischaemia caused by the high intraventricular pressure, and do not influence clinical decision-making. However, they may complicate the assessment of the severity of associated mitral stenosis using digitized M-mode echocardiography, with implications concerning the symptomatic relief expected and obtained from surgery.

Aortic regurgitation

Echocardiographic imaging of the aortic valve itself in patients with aortic regurgitation is of limited value. Severe aortic regurgitation can occur through an aortic valve that appears normal echocardiographically. If the cause of regurgitation is rheumatic, the leaflets are usually thickened and have some restriction of movement. More rarely, vegetations on the valve due to infective endocarditis or a flail aortic valve cusp can be identified (Fig. 13.32).[33] Vegetations and a fluttering flail cusp can produce very similar echocardiographic appearances when they prolapse into the left ventricular outflow tract in diastole. Defects of the membranous part of the interventricular septum often lead to prolapse of an

aortic valve leaflet and aortic regurgitation. This prolapse can often be detected echocardiographically; occasionally, the valve cusp prolapses through the ventricular septal defect and is seen as a vibrating structure in the right ventricular outflow in diastole.[34] The clinical significance of the aortic valve prolapse which occurs alone or in association with mitral prolapse has yet to be properly defined, as have the echocardiographic criteria for its diagnosis.

The shape and size of the aortic root sometimes suggests the cause of aortic regurgitation. Conditions that cause aortic root dilatation (e.g. Marfan's syndrome, hypertension and inflammatory diseases such as ankylosing spondylitis) lead to aortic regurgitation. The echocardiogram will show the increased aortic root dimensions in such patients. Occasionally, echocardiography shows a dissecting aneurysm of the aortic root as the cause of aortic regurgitation,[35] but the diagnosis may be missed when using conventional echocardiography. Preliminary results with trans-oesophageal echocardiography suggest that it can detect this condition with considerable reliability.

The indirect effects of aortic regurgitation on the movement of the mitral valve sometimes provide useful information. The best known but least useful finding is high-frequency diastolic fluttering of the anterior cusp of the mitral valve (Fig. 13.33),[36] which must be distinguished from lower frequency fluttering that can occur in normal subjects, parti-

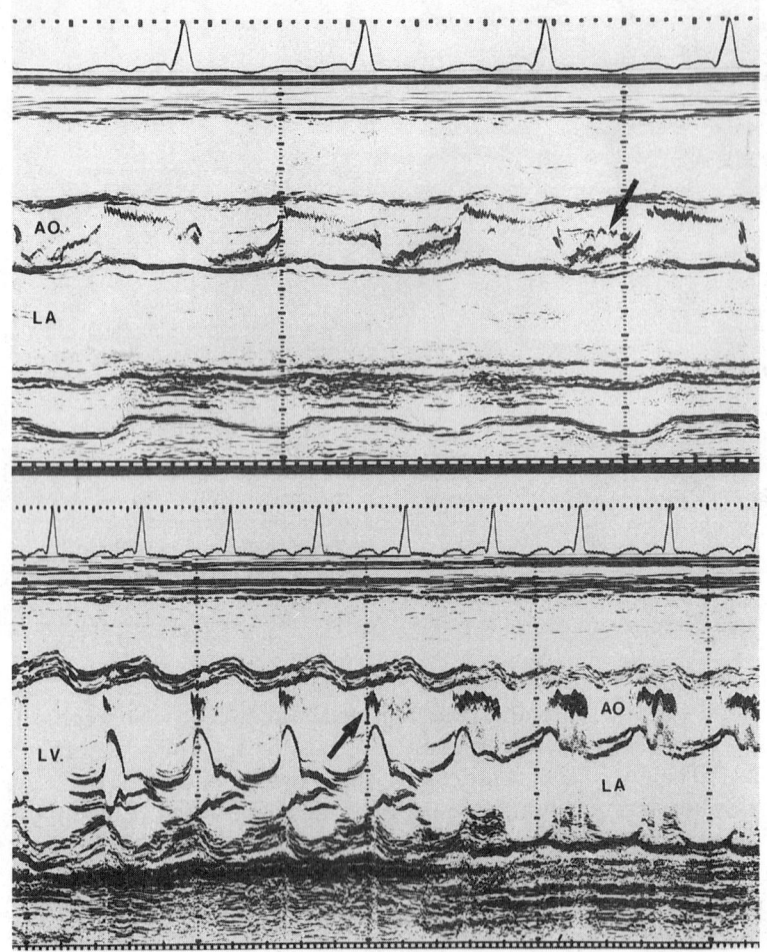

Fig. 13.32. M-mode echocardiogram from a patient with a flail aortic valve cusp. Upper panel: M-mode echocardiogram of the aortic valve shows multiple vibrating echoes in the aortic root due to the flail cusp (arrow). Lower tracing: a sweep from the aortic root (left) to the left ventricle (right), showing a vibrating structure in the aortic root which can also be detected in the left ventricle anterior to the mitral valve (arrow). This is the flail aortic valve leaflet. AO, aorta; LA, left atrium; LV, left ventricle.

cularly in the presence of atrial fibrillation. High-frequency diastolic fluttering can be detected reliably only by M-mode echocardiography, because it is too rapid to be detected by the slow frame rate of cross-sectional echocardiography. It is usually present when aortic regurgitation is clinically significant, but its intensity does not correlate with the severity of regurgitation and it is quite often absent when aortic regurgitation is trivial. If the mitral valve is thickened due to mitral stenosis, it may not be able to vibrate; in such patients, careful inspection of the echocardiogram may reveal similar high-frequency diastolic vibration of the interventricular septum and posterior left ventricular wall. The only diagnostic value of diastolic mitral valve vibration is that occasionally it helps to establish whether an early diastolic murmur is due to aortic or pulmonary regurgitation. Today this distinction is best made using Doppler.

Early mitral valve closure is an important finding

in severe aortic regurgitation (Fig. 13.34). It is seen in acute aortic regurgitation or following a sudden and marked increase in the severity of chronic aortic regurgitation.[37,38] As the left ventricle has not had time in which to dilate sufficiently to deal with the enormous volume load imposed on it, a sudden and rapid rise in intraventricular pressure is incurred during early diastole causing the mitral valve to close prematurely. This rise in pressure as blood regurgitates from the aorta into the left ventricle exceeds left atrial pressure in early diastole and closes the mitral valve. This abnormality can be detected reliably only by M-mode echocardiography with a simultaneous echocardiogram. The mitral valve closes well before the next QRS complex and often before the next P wave rather than at or just after the next QRS complex. Measurement of the time during which the mitral valve remains open has been suggested as a means of confirming that premature mitral valve closure is

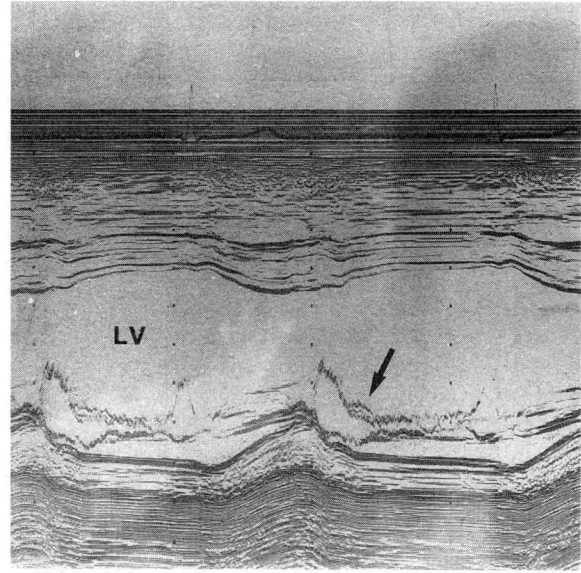

Fig. 13.33. M-mode echocardiogram from a patient with severe aortic regurgitation. High-frequency vibration of the mitral valve in diastole is clearly seen (arrow). LV, left ventricle.

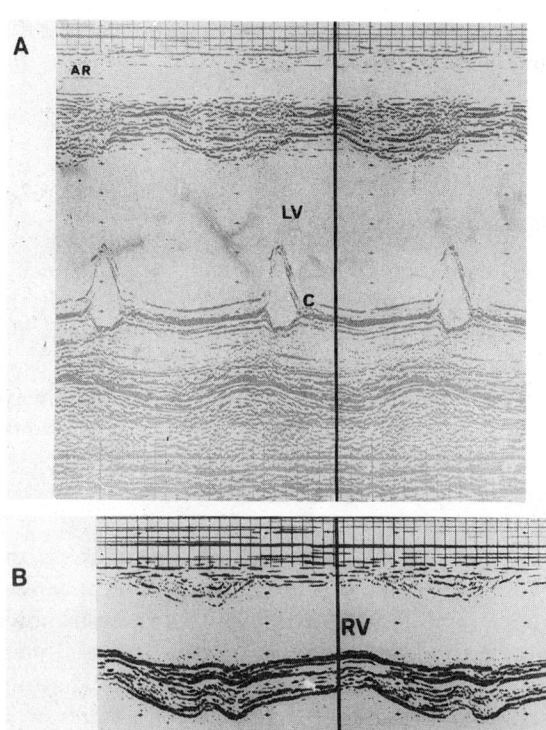

Fig. 13.34. (A) M-mode echocardiogram showing premature closure of the mitral valve in the presence of acute aortic regurgitation due to infective endocarditis. The mitral valve is seen to close (c) *well before* the next QRS complex which is marked with a vertical line. LV, left ventricle. (B) Echocardiogram obtained from a patient with chronic aortic regurgitation. The QRS complex is marked with a vertical line and it can be seen that mitral valve closure occurs *well after* this point (C). LV, left ventricle; RV, right ventricle.

present. If the valve remains open for < 0.04 s (normal = 0.05–0.07 s), mitral valve closure is likely to be premature. The main disadvantage of using this method is that sinus tachycardia, present in most patients who are haemodynamically compromised for whatever reason, also reduces the time during which the mitral valve remains open.

In acute aortic regurgitation, left ventricular dimensions are normal or slightly increased; fractional shortening is usually in the lower part of the normal range, but it may be reduced.

The left ventricle dilates and hypertrophies as a result of the volume load imposed on it by chronic aortic regurgitation. As the ventricle dilates, end-diastolic and end-systolic dimensions increase. Initially, the former increases more than the latter and simple measures of left ventricular ejection, such as fractional shortening, remain normal. Later in the course of the illness, the increase in end-systolic dimension exceeds that of end-diastolic dimension and fractional shortening decreases. Left ventricular wall thickness is usually normal or slightly increased because the increased muscle mass is spread out to surround the enlarged ventricle, i.e. there is an increased amount of ventricular wall of normal or slightly increased thickness. Changes in left ventricular dimension and fractional shortening usually occur gradually, often over many years. Serial M-mode echocardiograms are a convenient way of following this

protracted clinical evolution. Changes in left ventricular function may alert the clinician to the need for aortic valve replacement. At present, there is no agreement over which parameters of left ventricular function are the most reliable when assessing the need for valve replacement.[39] The most commonly used are a fall in fractional shortening below normal or an increase in end-systolic dimension to > 5.5 or 6 cm.[40] When comparing the results of various studies, it should be remembered that a change in left ventricular dimension must be of the order of 5 mm if it is to be regarded as valid;[9] the serial echocardiograms must be of high quality and recorded from the same rib interspace at the same level in the ventricle.

MITRAL VALVE DISEASE

Mitral stenosis

The stenotic mitral valve has a characteristic echocardiographic appearance (Fig. 13.35). Both the M-mode and cross-sectional techniques show the thickening and restricted motion of the valve cusps. Extremely thick and immobile valves are always severely stenotic, but they do retain some mobility. When the echoes returning from the valve cusps are particularly bright and thick, it is likely that they are calcified.

In the past, attempts were made to assess the severity of stenosis from the M-mode echocardiographic appearances of the valve. The best known parameter of the severity of mitral stenosis, measured directly from the mitral valve, is the diastolic closure rate.[41] Although the initial studies were encouraging, later work suggested that the diastolic closure rate does not give an accurate assessment of the severity of stenosis, particularly in patients who have undergone a previous mitral valvotomy. A similar but more complicated parameter, depending upon the movement of both the anterior and posterior mitral valve cusps (the mitral valve closure index), was also proposed but it has similar shortcomings.[42] Using the M-mode echocardiogram to measure the extent to which the mitral valve cusps separate is unreliable, mainly because it is not possible to know which part of the funnel-shaped mitral valve is traversed by the M-mode beam and because the valve orifice is often elongated and irregular. As direct inspection of the mitral valve using M-mode echocardiography was an unsatisfactory way of assessing the severity of stenosis, other techniques using digitized M-mode echocardiography were developed.[1,4,30] Although these techniques provide an improved assessment of the severity of stenosis, their use is limited to those patients in whom a high-quality echocardiogram can be obtained; thus they are tedious to perform and may be rendered inaccurate by other factors that influence left ventricular filling, such as hypertrophy due to co-existent aortic stenosis (see above). Consequently, this technique is no longer widely used.

Although M-mode echocardiography is useful as a way of detecting rheumatic mitral stenosis, it has been abandoned as a technique for assessing severity because cross-sectional echocardiography is superior (Figs 13.36 and 13.37). Long-axis parasternal views demonstrate the limitation of cusp motion and the extent to which valve cusps and subvalvar apparatus are thickened and shortened. The short-axis parasternal view delineates the mitral valve orifice in cross-section and allows its size to be measured,[43] but considerable care is required in interpretation. The echo sector has to be scanned up and down the long axis of the mitral valve to find the true orifice. Inappropriate gain settings may cause the mitral valve orifice area to be underestimated, because reverberations from the anterior leaflet, particularly if calcified, tend to fill in the orifice. Some patients with low output states who do not have stenosis appear to have reduced mitral valve areas because the low flow through the mitral valve fails to open it completely. Differentiation between this state and mitral stenosis is easy using the M-mode echocardiogram which shows thin normal valve cusps that move at a normal speed but over a smaller distance than usual.

Left ventricular dimensions and wall thickness are normal in mitral stenosis. The characteristic slow filling of the left ventricle, discussed in the section on digitized echocardiograms, can often be appreciated by inspecting either the M-mode or the

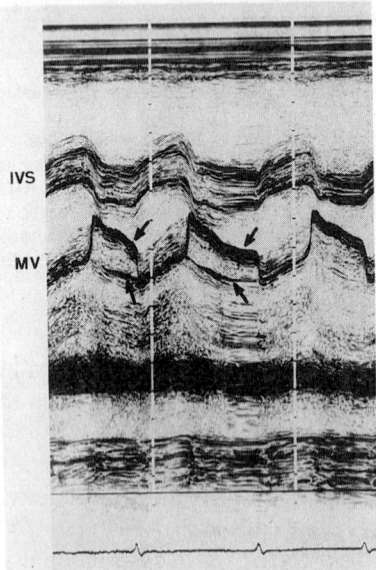

Fig. 13.35. M-mode echocardiogram showing the mitral valve in a patient with mitral stenosis. The characteristic appearance of the mitral valve cusp (MV) is seen with some thickening and a slow diastolic closure rate. The anterior and posterior cusps are marked with arrows. The posterior cusp is seen to move the anterior cusp during diastole. IVS, interventricular septum.

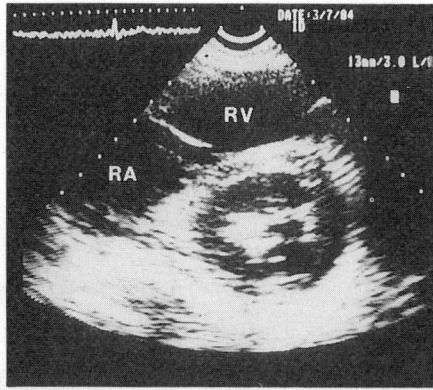

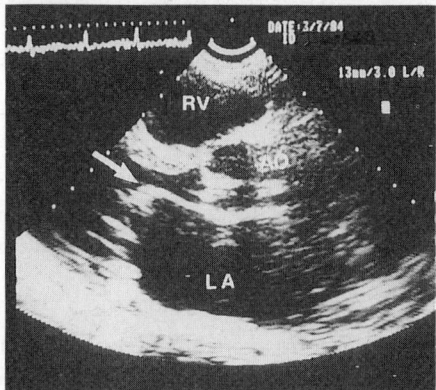

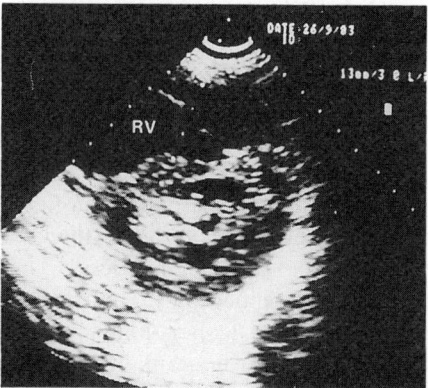

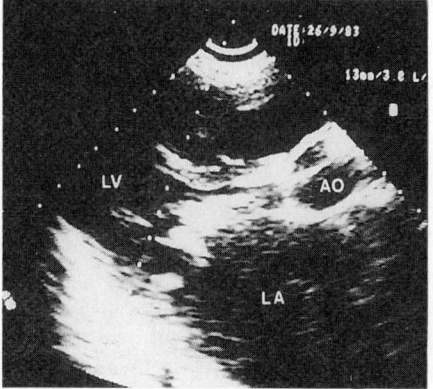

Fig. 13.36. Cross-sectional echocardiograms from a patient with severe mitral stenosis in the parasternal short-axis view (above) and in the parasternal long-axis view (below). Upper panel: the mitral valve orifice is seen in cross-section during diastole and is narrowed. There is considerable thickening of one of the commissures on the left side; lower panel: the long-axis view in which the valve is open, the anterior cusp bowing anteriorly (arrow). This is the so-called 'hockeystick' appearance when the valve cusp retains some mobility but is tethered to the posterior cusp at its margins. LA, left atrium; RA, right atrium; LV, right ventricle; AO, aorta.

Fig. 13.37. Cross-sectional echocardiogram presented in the same manner as Fig. 13.36. This patient had severe mitral stenosis with calcification and severe thickening of the valve. In the parasternal short-axis view (above), the orifice is slit like and irregular. In the long-axis view (below), a considerable thickening of the anterior cusp of the mitral valve can be seen and the left atrium is also grossly enlarged. AO, aorta; LA, left atrium; LV, left ventricle; RV, right ventricle.

cross-sectional echocardiogram. In early diastole, the M-mode echocardiogram shows posterior movement of the intraventricular septum in most patients who have significant mitral stenosis.[42]

At present, Doppler ultrasound is a valuable alternative method of assessing mitral valve stenosis.[7] The greater the obstruction, the longer it takes for the pressures to equalize. The time taken for the pressure to drop by 50% (the pressure half-time) gives a good estimation of severity of obstruction regardless of the presence or absence of mitral regurgitation.

Rheumatic mitral regurgitation and mixed stenosis and regurgitation

It is unusual to encounter pure rheumatic mitral

regurgitation in Western cardiological practice. If pure rheumatic mitral regurgitation does occur, the mitral valve appears thickened on both the M-mode and the cross-sectional echocardiogram. Valve cusp motion is limited but much less than that in patients with mitral stenosis. The cross-sectional echocardiogram shows that the mitral valve area is normal or slightly reduced. Direct measurement of the valve orifice or cusp motion gives no indication of the severity of regurgitation. Information about severity derived from the echocardiogram is indirect and imprecise. Increased left ventricular end-diastolic dimension combined with vigorous wall motion seen either on the M-mode or the cross-sectional echocardiogram suggests volume overload and hence significant regurgitation. Rapid left ventricular filling, as assessed by the digitized M-mode echocardiogram (often in excess of 20 cm/s), strongly suggests that regurgitation is severe.[44]

Neither echo evidence of volume overload nor increased filling rate gives an accurate assessment of severity.

More commonly, rheumatic mitral regurgitation is combined with some degree of mitral stenosis. The echocardiographic appearances vary with the relative degrees of stenosis and regurgitation and the extent to which the valve is thickened and immobilized by the rheumatic process. The degree of stenosis can be defined by the mitral valve area seen in the parasternal short-axis view with the cross-sectional echocardiogram. The appearances are often identical to those described for mitral stenosis. Left ventricular dimensions and wall motion indicate how much regurgitation there is. Left ventricular filling rates will be in the normal range, because the effects of stenosis and regurgitation offset each other. If there is significant regurgitation, the early diastolic posterior motion of the interventricular septum, seen on the M-mode echocardiogram in mitral stenosis, is not usually present.

Echocardiographic evidence of left ventricular hypertrophy in the form of increased wall thickness is unusual in patients with mitral regurgitation, because the hypertrophy is evenly distributed around the enlarged left ventricular cavity in a similar manner to that in aortic regurgitation (see above).

Non-rheumatic mitral regurgitation

Most severe mitral regurgitation seen in Western cardiological practice is non-rheumatic. The echocardiographic appearances of the left ventricle are similar to those described for rheumatic mitral regurgitation. As severe mitral regurgitation is often well tolerated by the patient for long periods, the left ventricular enlargement may be considerable, although wall motion, as measured by fractional shortening, remains normal (Fig. 13.38) until the disease is very advanced. This well-maintained wall motion may mislead the clinician over the true state of left ventricular function and, therefore, over the appropriate timing of mitral valve replacement.[45] If valve replacement is deferred until left ventricular wall motion is reduced, the operative results are likely to be poor: while mitral regurgitation is present, left ventricular afterload is low because impedance to the run-off into the left atrium is low, therefore systolic wall motion of normal amplitude can occur even after left ventricular function has begun to deteriorate. Once regurgitation is corrected, the ventricle has to eject against a consider-

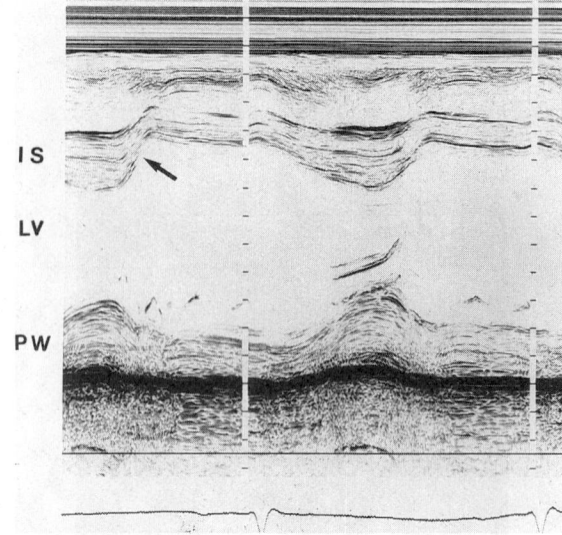

Fig. 13.38. M-mode echocardiogram for left ventricle (LV) from a patient with severe mitral regurgitation. Note the vigorous wall movement and the rapid outward anterior movement of the interventricular septum (IS) in early diastole that is often seen in this situation (arrow). PW, posterior wall.

ably increased afterload—thus surgery may unmask hitherto undetected deterioration of left ventricular function that occurred before surgery.[46] Changes in left ventricular function in mitral regurgitation are discussed in more detail in Chapter 29.

Although echocardiography is a poor method of assessing the severity of mitral regurgitation, it may reveal the underlying cause (Fig. 13.39), the most important of which are summarized in Table 13.1. It must be remembered that significant mitral regurgitation can occur through an echocardiographically normal mitral valve.

Calcification of the mitral valve annulus

Calcification on the mitral valve annulus is commonly seen in the elderly, particularly females.[47] It can be identified on the M-mode echocardiogram as a thick bright echo moving parallel to the posterior left ventricular wall just behind the mitral valve cusps. On the cross-sectional echocardiogram, it is best seen in the long-axis parasternal view as a bright echo posterior to the mitral valve at or just on the ventricular side of the atrioventricular junction.

Mitral valve prolapse

The echocardiographic diagnosis of mitral valve prolapse can be difficult (see the section on mitral

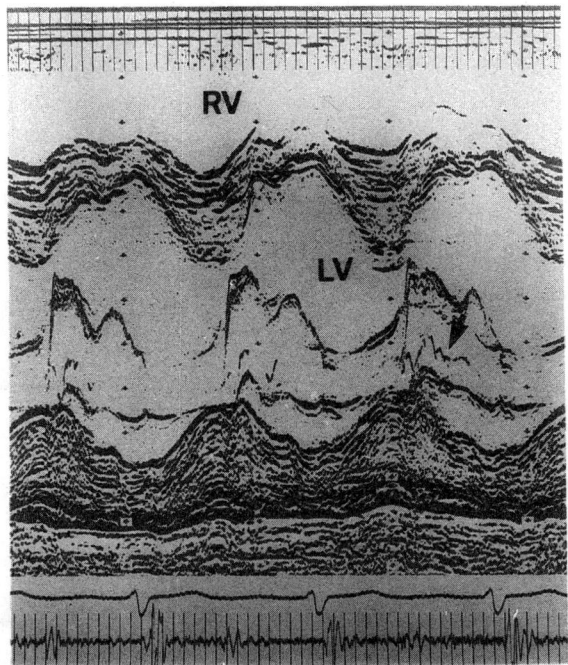

Fig. 13.39. M-mode echocardiogram of the left ventricle and mitral valve from a patient with severe mitral regurgitation due to chordal rupture. The left ventricle is not enlarged but there is vigorous wall movement denoting volume overload. Within the mitral valve, fine rapidly oscillating echoes originating from the ruptured chordae and the unsupported edges of the valve cusps are seen (arrow). RV, right ventricle; LV, left ventricle.

valve prolapse, Chapter 29).[48] There is no consensus over what constitutes mitral valve prolapse. Different authors have used different criteria for the diagnosis, and series of patients are not necessarily comparable in their age, sex or ethnic background.[49,50] Moreover, the high incidence of echocardiographic abnormalities often thought to represent mitral valve prolapse occur frequently in normal subjects.[51] About 15% of patients in whom prolapse can be definitely identified on echocardiography have no clinical signs of the syndrome; conversely, between 10 and 20% of patients with characteristic clinical signs have no echocardiographic abnormality.[52,53]

Despite these problems, some echocardiographic appearances are considered to be characteristic (Fig. 13.40). Approximately 40% of patients show 'buckling', a sharp posterior dip of the mitral valve in mid or late systole which exceeds the systolic mitral closure line by 2 mm. This finding is very specific. The remaining 40% of patients show 'hammocking', a posterior motion of the mitral valve throughout systole. As mild backward movement of this type is common in normal subjects, strict criteria of definition are necessary. Various authors have suggested that between 2 and 5 mm of

Table 13.1. **Echocardiographic detection of the principal causes of mitral regurgitation.**

Cause	Main echo features
Rheumatic	1. Cusp thickening ± calcification 2. Restricted cusp motion 3. Shortening and thickening of subvalvar apparatus
Mitral valve prolapse	1. Late or pan-systolic posterior motion (> 3 mm)—M-mode 2. Bowing of cusps beyond the mitral valve annulus (towards left atrium) in late systole—CSE[a] four-chamber view 3. Apparent thickening and excessive motion of redundant cusp 4. Associated chordal rupture
Chordal rupture	1. Chaotic fluttering and multiple echoes in systole and diastole from unsupported cusp and its chordae 2. Prolapse of unsupported cusp
Papillary muscle rupture (in acute myocardial infarction)	1. Features of chordal rupture 2. The head of ruptured papillary muscle attached to chordae moves rapidly towards left atrium in systole and may move chaotically
Infective endocarditis	1. Vegetations 2. Features of chordal rupture (holes valve cusps not usually seen)
Calcified mitral annulus	1. Strong echoes seen behind normally moving thin mitral leaflets

NB Significant mitral regurgitation can occur through an echocardiographically normal mitral valve.
[a] CSE, cross-sectional echocardiography.

displacement are required before the diagnosis can be made; 3 mm can be regarded as a reasonable compromise.[54] In addition to these specific abnormalities, other non-specific changes have been described, including thickening of the mitral valve, multiple echoes probably due to redundant valve cusp tissue and wide excursion of the mitral valve leaflets (Fig. 13.40). When using M-mode echocardiography to diagnose mitral valve prolapse, attention to detail is necessary. High-quality echoes are needed and incorrect positioning of the transducer can produce false-positive or false-negative results. The former usually occur when the transducer is placed too high on the chest wall and the latter if it is placed too low. Ideally, the mitral valve echo should be identified with the transducer perpendicular to the chest wall. Although there is no close correlation between the auscultatory findings and the presence of 'buckling' or 'hammocking', the latter tends to be more commonly associated with a pan-systolic murmur.

Cross-sectional echocardiography allows the anterior and the posterior mitral valve leaflets to be inspected in several planes. When definite prolapse is present, it affects the anterior and the posterior cusps in 80% of cases.[55] Prolapse can be identified in all long-axis views of the heart (Fig. 13.41), but it is usually best seen on the apical four-chamber view.[56] This view shows the mitral valve leaflets and also the mitral valve annulus, which can be used as a fixed point against which the position of the valve leaflets can be compared. Prolapse is judged to be present if the valve cusps move or bow towards the left atrium beyond this fixed point. However, this criterion for mitral valve prolapse may be too sensitive in some patient groups; some systolic motion of the mitral valve towards the left atrial side of the mitral valve annulus has been observed in 35% of normal subjects between the ages of 10 and 18 years.[57] If an 'abnormality' occurs in such a large number of normal subjects, it should be regarded as a normal variant rather than as an abnormality.

When the condition is severe and there is considerable stretching of the valve cusps and supporting chordae, leading to the true floppy valve, the echocardiographic appearances are usually unequivocal. The voluminous cusps prolapse well beyond the mitral valve annulus and often have a thickened appearance because of the large amount of redundant tissue.

In practice, the echocardiographic diagnosis of mitral valve prolapse divides patients into three groups: those who definitely have prolapse, those who definitely do not have prolapse and those in whom it is impossible to be sure. In all patient groups, the echocardiogram should be regarded simply as a confirmation of the clinical situation rather than creating a disease in its own right. The difficulties of diagnosis are emphasized by the results of a recent study which showed that the reproducibility of the echocardiographic diagnosis of mitral valve prolapse is poor.[58]

Chordal rupture frequently occurs in association

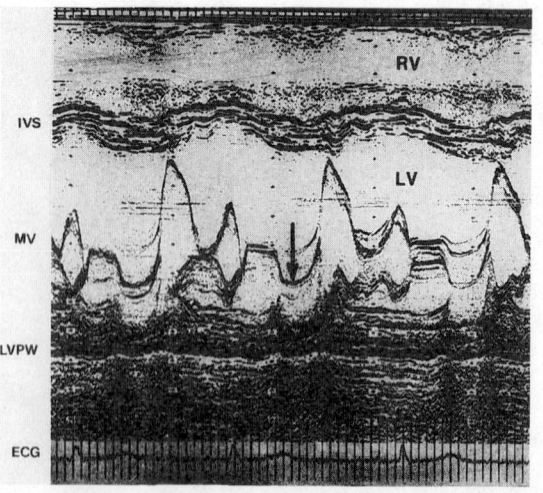
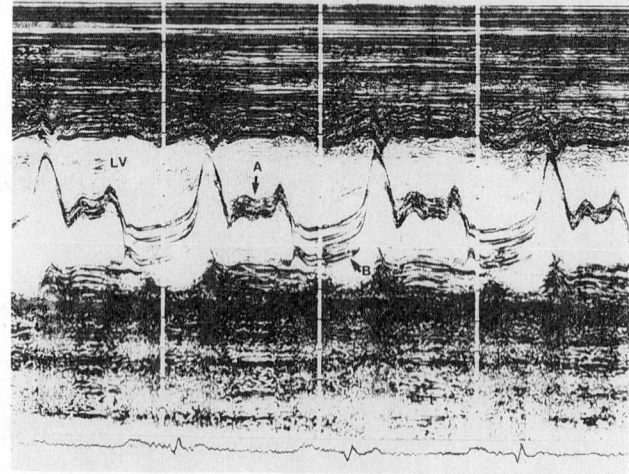

Fig. 13.40. M-mode echocardiograms from the left ventricle (LV) and mitral valve (MV) from two patients with mitral valve prolapse. In (A) there is characteristic late systolic prolapse of the valve and in (B) there is pan-systolic 'hammocking' of the valve (arrow, B). This recording also shows the thickened appearance of the valve (arrow, A) due to its redundant nature and also the wide excursion over the valve with the anterior cusp coming into contact with the interventricular septum (IVS) in early diastole. LVPW, left ventricular posterior wall; RV, right ventricle.

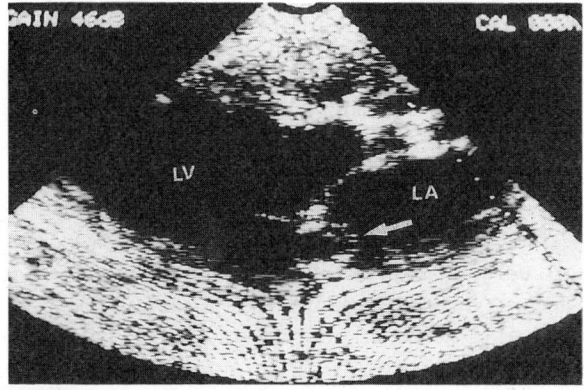

Fig. 13.41. Cross-sectional long-axis parasternal view of a patient with mitral valve prolapse. The posterior cusp of the mitral valve can be seen prolapsing towards the left atrium (LA) in systole (arrow). LV, left ventricle.

with mitral valve prolapse and can be identified echocardiographically. Rupture is much more common than was previously thought and is often present in a clinically stable situation.[59] The M-mode echocardiogram is often useful, showing multiple thin rapidly moving echoes between the two leaflets of the mitral valve during diastole, and along their closure line and prolapsing towards the left atrium during systole. (Fig. 13.42). The cross-sectional echocardiogram will also show fluttering and excessive movement of the unsupported part of the mitral valve as it prolapses into the left atrium during systole. In some patients with chordal rupture, an important artefact can be seen; a mass appears to be attached to the mitral valve and may be mistaken for a vegetation. This artefact

is caused by the bunching together of the ruptured chordae and the unsupported redundant valve tissue.

TRICUSPID VALVE DISEASE

The tricuspid valve is difficult to image by M-mode echocardiography; the cross-sectional technique gives a better assessment of the valve, usually from the apical or subcostal approach. In these views, it is often possible to see the anterior and the septal cusps of the valve. Thickening of the tricuspid valve detected on echocardiography may be caused by rheumatic tricuspid valve disease, carcinoid heart disease,[60] and tricuspid valve prolapse; it is also seen in cardiac infiltrative conditions, such as cardiac amyloid and eosinophilic endomyocardial disease. Although thickening is non-specific, the associated valve motion may help make the diagnosis. In rheumatic tricuspid valve disease, the restricted motion and doming of the valve towards the right ventricle in diastole are characteristic (Fig. 13.43). Many other conditions causing valve thickening are associated with normal free valve motion, for example, tricuspid valve prolapse, Ebstein's anomaly and cardiac amyloid. Valve motion can be abnormal but the abnormalities are different from those in rheumatic disease. For example, in carcinoid heart disease, the valve leaflets appear to be stuck in a mid position (Fig 13.44),[60] rather than showing the characteristic doming of rheumatic tricuspid valve disease. Echocardiography cannot assess the severity of tricuspid stenosis accurately,

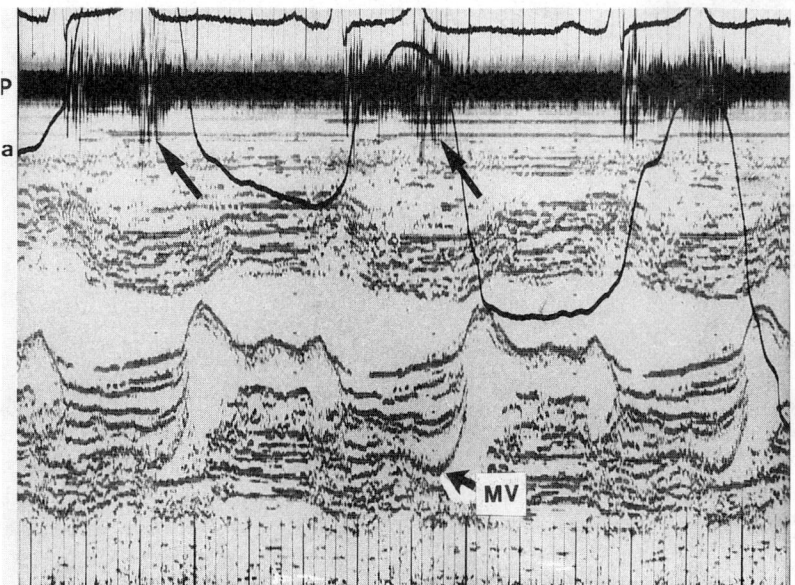

Fig. 13.42. M-mode echocardiogram and phonocardiogram (P) from a patient with a floppy mitral valve and chordal rupture. There are multiple echoes from the mitral valve (MV) because it is redundant and is also partially unsupported due to chordal rupture. The valve cusps prolapse further at the end of systole and this coincides with an increase in the intensity of the murmur arrowed on the phonocardiogram (P). There is also an apex cardiogram (a) on this recording.

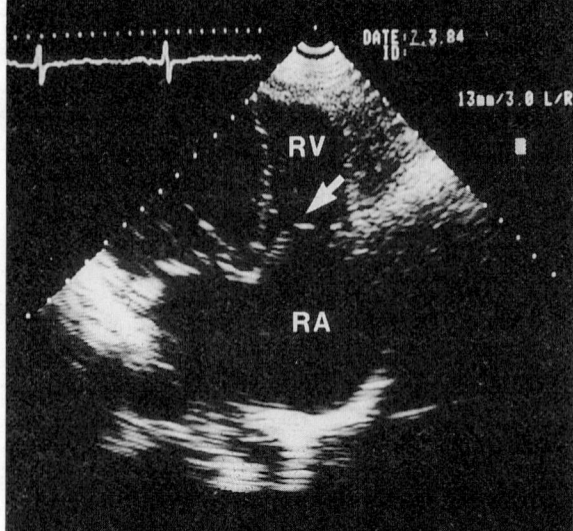

Fig. 13.43. Cross-sectional echocardiogram apical four-chamber view from a patient with rheumatic tricuspid stenosis. The tricuspid valve (arrow) can be seen doming towards the right ventricle (RV) in diastole. RA, right atrium.

but this can be achieved using Doppler ultrasound. Most other lesions of the tricuspid valve result predominantly in tricuspid regurgitation if they achieve haemodynamic significance. Echocardiography can detect vegetations on the tricuspid valve in patients who have right-sided infective endocarditis, but is much less successful than it is in detecting vegetations on the mitral and aortic valves.[61] Among patients with rheumatic heart disease in whom echocardiographic thickening of

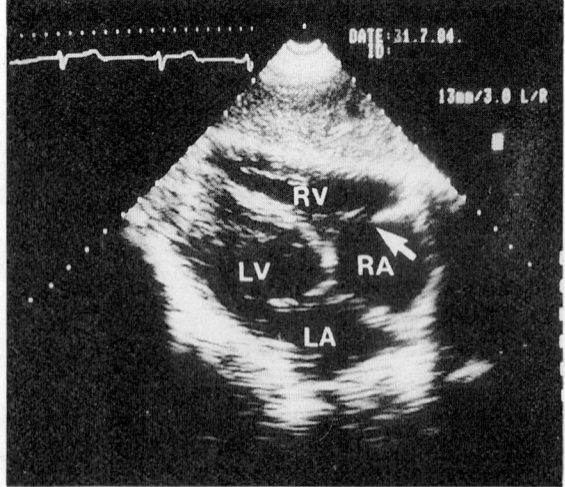

Fig. 13.44. Cross-sectional echocardiogram subcostal four-chamber view from a patient with carcinoid involvement of the tricuspid valve which is thickened and stuck in-mid position throughout the cardiac cycle (arrow). RV, right ventricle; RA, right atrium; LV, left ventricle; LA, left atrium.

the tricuspid valve is detected, about 75% have tricuspid regurgitation alone, whereas 20% have significant tricuspid stenosis.[62] Tricuspid valve prolapse has been reported, usually in patients who have mitral valve prolapse. Tricuspid valve prolapse is rare and the criteria for diagnosis are less well defined than those for mitral valve prolapse.[63]

When tricuspid regurgitation is significant, echocardiography detects dilatation of the right ventricle due to volume overload. This is usually associated with reversed septal motion, the explanations of which are complex.[64] Tricuspid regurgitation is more frequently *functional* than organic in origin, i.e. secondary to right ventricular dilatation, and the valve leaflets usually appear to be normal. As the conventional echocardiographic features of tricuspid regurgitation and those of other conditions that cause right ventricular overload are non-specific, other techniques using ultrasound have been sought to improve diagnosis and aid in the assessment of severity. Contrast echocardiography has been used widely.[65] This technique depends on an injection of echocardiographic contrast, usually in the form of 5% dextrose into an upper limb vein. Echocardiographic imaging of the inferior vena cava just below its entrance into the right atrium reveals whether tricuspid regurgitation is present. Contrast enters the right ventricle first and then if there is tricuspid regurgitation it refluxes in systole to the inferior vena cava via the right atrium. This method of investigation has significant shortcomings; false-positive and false-negative results are common.[66] The Doppler technique provides a reliable method of detecting tricuspid regurgitation. Unfortunately, the assessment of severity with all techniques described, including that of Doppler, is at best approximate.

ACQUIRED PULMONARY VALVE DISEASE

Acquired pulmonary stenosis is a rare lesion in adults. The pulmonary valve is spared by rheumatic heart disease, and the valve itself becomes narrowed only as a consequence of the carcinoid syndrome.[60] If the pulmonary valve can be imaged, the cross-sectional echocardiogram shows thickening and immobility of the pulmonary valve cusps.[60,67] Most commonly acquired pulmonary regurgitation is the result of pulmonary valve ring dilatation secondary to pulmonary hypertension.[68] The M-mode and cross-sectional echocardiograms show an increase in pulmonary artery dimensions. If the regurgitation is severe, right ventricular volume overload may also be detected. Occasionally, diastolic fluttering of the anterior leaflet of the tricuspid valve is seen, but this is much less common than the fluttering of the mitral valve in aortic regurgitation, because the anatomy of the right ventricle directs the regurgitant jet away from the tricuspid valve. Congenital lesions of the pulmonary valve are discussed below.

DIAGNOSTIC PROBLEMS IN VALVE DISEASE

Echocardiography is valuable in resolving many of the common problems encountered when assessing valvular heart disease. These are summarized in Table 13.2. Occult mitral and aortic stenosis are both reliably revealed. The much rarer occult regurgitant lesions, of which mitral regurgitation is the most common, may be suggested by the presence of left ventricular volume overload on echocardiography. Fortunately, the Doppler technique can detect regurgitant lesions with a high degree of sensitivity, although invasive investigation, such as cardiac catheterization, may sometimes be necessary to assess the severity of the lesion.

INFECTIVE ENDOCARDITIS

Echocardiography is a valuable technique for the assessment of patients who have suspected infective endocarditis. It can be used to help diagnose infective endocarditis and to identify and assess complications. The echocardiographic diagnosis of infective endocarditis is based on the detection of vegetations (Figs 13.45A,B). Vegetations must be > 2 mm in diameter to be visualized although occasionally smaller vegetations can be seen if they are calcified.[69] Large vegetations (> 5 mm in diameter) are nearly always detected. Vegetations are usually attached to the surface of the valve; in this position, they can be detected by both M-mode and cross-sectional echocardiography. Occasionally, they are attached to the endocardium near the valve or its subvalvar apparatus. M-mode echocardiography is rarely able to detect these vegetations but sometimes they can be seen on cross-sectional echocardiography. On M-mode echocardiography, vegetations often have a characteristic appearance which is fuzzy or shaggy due to rapid oscillation.

Table 13.2.   Use of ultrasound for resolving problems in valve disease diagnosis.

Condition	Clinical problem	Ultrasound imaging			Comments
		M-Mode	CSE[a]	Doppler	
Atrial myxoma	? MVD (or TVD)	++	++	−	Imaging = best
HCM	? MR ? AS	+	++	(+)	
ASD	? MVD	(+)[see 2]	++[see 1]	(+)	1 Beware artefactual drop out of echoes in four-chamber view 2 Evidence of RV overload (non-specific)
VSD or MR post MI	Collapse with murmur post MI	(+)	+	++	M-Mode may show chaotic MV motion with ruptured papillary muscle. CSE shows VSD. Pulsed Doppler can differentiate
Occult valve disease (a) AS	CF ? cause	+	+	++	Best estimate of severity is by Doppler
(b) MS	CF ? cause, or COAD	+	+	++	Best estimate of severity by Doppler
(c) AR (acute infective endocarditis)	Collapse during infective endocarditis	++[see comment]	+	+	Early mitral valve closure (only detected by M-mode)
(d) MR	CF ? cause	(+)	(+)	++	Rarely occult. Imaging (M-mode and CSE) are non-specific. Doppler very helpful

HCM, hypertrophic cardiomyopathy; ASD, atrial septal defect; VSD, ventricular septal defect; MR, mitral regurgitation; AR, aortic regurgitation; CSE, cross-sectional echo; AS, aortic stenosis; MS, mitral stenosis; CF, cardiac failure; COAD, chronic obstructive airways disease; MVD, mitral valve disease; TVD, tricuspid valve disease; MI, myocardial infarction.
(+), occasionally helpful but non-specific; +, helpful and sometimes diagnostic; ++, very useful—method of choice.

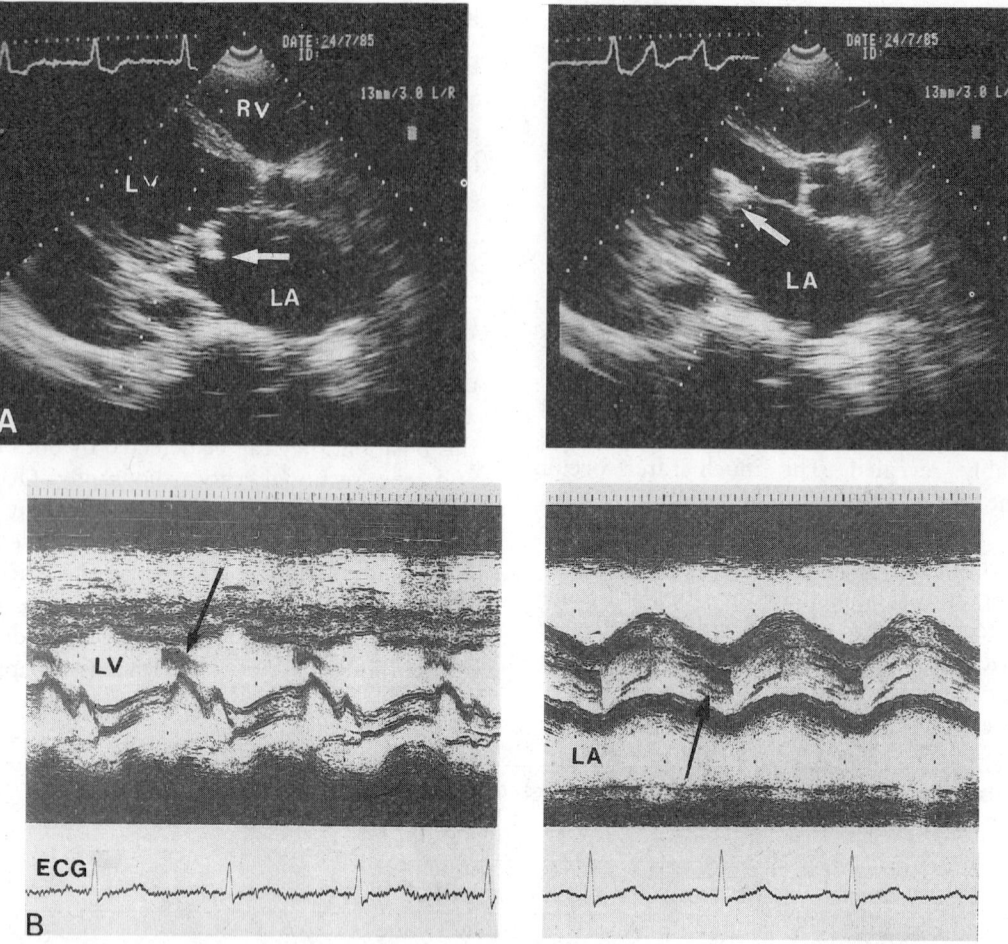

Fig. 13.45. (A) Cross-sectional echocardiograms: parasternal long-axis view recorded in systole on the left and diastole on the right from a patient with a large vegetation attached to the anterior cusp of the mitral valve (arrows). This can be seen to prolapse into the left atrium in systole on the left. LV, left ventricle; LA, left atrium; RV, right ventricle.
(B) M-mode echocardiograms from a patient with infective endocarditis and a vegetation on the aortic valve. The view of the aortic valve from the right shows the vegetation attached to the aortic valve (arrow) and when the echo beam is tilted towards the left ventricle (left) the vegetation prolapses into the left ventricular outflow tract anterior to the mitral valve (arrow). LA, left atrium; LV, left ventricle.

This shagginess cannot be appreciated on the cross-sectional echocardiogram which does not have the ability to resolve rapid motion. However, the cross-sectional echocardiogram gives better definition of the site, size and mobility of the vegetation.

The frequency with which vegetations are detected in infective endocarditis varies from 55 to 80%.[70,71] Cross-sectional echocardiography is more sensitive than M-mode echocardiography, detecting vegetations in at least 20% of patients in whom they are not seen when using the M-mode technique.[71] Vegetations are particularly difficult to detect by echocardiography in certain situations, of which endocarditis on a prosthetic valve and

right-sided heart lesions are the most important.[61] Prosthetic valves generate strong echoes from the prosthetic valve structure which tend to mask the weaker echoes produced by vegetations, and valve lesions on the right side of the heart cannot be imaged as well as those on the left. In both instances, cross-sectional echocardiography can detect some vegetations whereas the M-mode technique can detect only a few. The frequency with which vegetations are detected depends on the skill of the echocardiographer and on the patient population studied. A higher incidence of vegetations is found in series reported from teaching centres, because patients seen at these centres often tend to have been referred for surgery and have a more advanced and aggressive form of disease. Vegetations tend to increase in size as the disease progresses and are very rarely detected during the first 2 weeks of infection.

Although vegetations often have a characteristic appearance, occasionally intracardiac masses generated by other disease processes are mistaken for vegetations. The conditions most commonly confused with vegetations are summarized in Table 13.3. Frequently, doubt about whether a mass is a vegetation can be resolved using a combination of cross-sectional and M-mode echocardiography. The cross-sectional echocardiogram is used to locate the mass and guide the M-mode on which there may be the characteristic appearance of a vegetation; if not, doubt over the diagnosis remains. It must be remembered that the detection of a vegetation on echocardiography does not necessarily indicate that the patient has active endocarditis. Even when endocarditis has been cured by antibiotic therapy, vegetations may persist for many months or even years in up to 60% of patients.[71,72] Occasionally, echocardiography helps make the diagnosis in patients with *culture-negative* endocarditis.[73]

Complications of endocarditis

Cross-sectional echocardiography is the best technique available for diagnosing extension of infection from the involved valve into the surrounding myocardium which produces a valve ring or intracardiac abscess (Fig. 13.46).[74] Occasionally, this complication can also be detected on M-mode echocardiography. More rarely, echocardiography

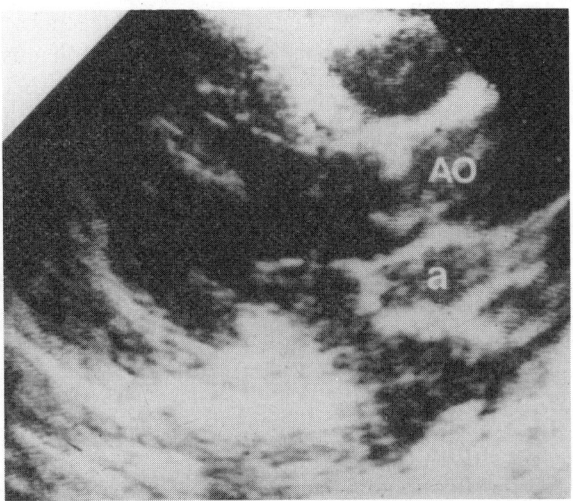

Fig. 13.46. Cross-sectional echocardiogram parasternal long-axis view from a patient with infective endocarditis involving the aortic valve. There is a large abscess cavity (a) posterior to the aortic root (AO).

will reveal a large mass of vegetations obstructing the aortic or mitral valve orifice,[75] or demonstrate chordal rupture or a flail cusp caused by infection eroding the valves and their surrounding tissue.[34] Perforations of valve cusps, which are common in this condition, cannot usually be detected on echocardiography.

Echocardiography is also useful in following the clinical course of patients with infective endocarditis. Serial echocardiograms will show whether left ventricular enlargement is due to increasing regurgitation caused by the endocarditis. In addition, M-mode echocardiograms are helpful in assessing patients who have acute severe aortic regurgitation. Often, these patients do not have many signs of acute aortic insufficiency and they present with heart failure. Patients with endocarditis in whom vegetations are detected on echocardiography have a much higher incidence of haemodynamic deterioration, unresolved infection or embolization than patients in whom vegetations are not detected.[67] Although the results of some studies have suggested that 90–100% of patients with vegetations need surgical intervention, those of a prospective study have shown that 70% of such patients will do well on medical treatment.[72] The most likely explanation for the worse clinical course of patients with vegetations is that they have more severe and advanced disease.

Recently, a new technique, known as transoesophageal cross-sectional echocardiography, has provided promising results in patients with

---

Table 13.3. Conditions that may produce echocardiographic findings that are confused with vegetations.

1   Intracardiac tumours, particularly small atrial myxomas

2   Flail valve leaflets:
   a chordal rupture
   b papillary muscle rupture
   c ruptured aortic valve cusp

3   Chordae tendineae may bunch together when ruptured

4   Head of ruptured papillary muscle attached to mitral chordae

5   Intracardiac thrombus. Most commonly mobile thrombi are seen in right atrium, but mobile thrombi in other cardiac chambers may cause confusion.

6   Partially detached patch, particularly on a ventricular septal defect

7   A mobile subaortic membrane in subaortic stenosis

8   A mobile intimal flap due to a dissecting aneurysm of the ascending aorta

endocarditis.[76] When the cross-sectional echocardiographic transducer is placed in the oesophagus, it is much closer to the heart valves and their surrounding structures than it is when used from the chest wall, therefore definition is better because the structures are imaged in the near field of the transducer. Preliminary results suggest a much higher rate of detection of vegetations and of the complications of endocarditis, such as valve ring abscesses.

ECHOCARDIOGRAPHY OF CONGENITAL HEART DISEASE

The most common form of congenital heart disease seen in adult cardiological practice is aortic stenosis. Discrete subvalvar and supravalvar aortic stenosis are relatively uncommon lesions.

PULMONARY VALVE STENOSIS

Pulmonary valve stenosis in adult practice is usually mild because most severe cases have been dealt with in childhood. The changes seen on cross-sectional imaging of the pulmonary valve may be minimal. Patients who have pulmonary stenosis are usually asymptomatic and referred because of basal murmurs. If mild thickening and doming are recognizable on the parasternal short axis, the diagnosis can be made. However, other causes of basal murmurs, such as atrial septal defects and aortic stenosis, should be excluded. When pulmonary stenosis is present, Doppler ultrasound will demonstrate an increased velocity of flow across the pulmonary valve and turbulent flow in the main pulmonary artery. The peak velocity reliably predicts the severity of the stenosis. Other features detected by echocardiography are post-stenotic dilatation of the pulmonary artery and right ventricular hypertrophy (Fig. 13.47).

ATRIAL SEPTAL DEFECTS

There are three kinds of atrial septal defect. The most common is the secundum atrial septal defect lying in the central part of the interatrial septum in the region of the oval fossa (Fig. 13.48). The so-called 'primum' and 'sinus venosus' are less common. It is arguable that these are not solely defects of the atrial septum. The sinus venosus defect is frequently associated with anomalous drainage of the right upper pulmonary vein into the right atrium.

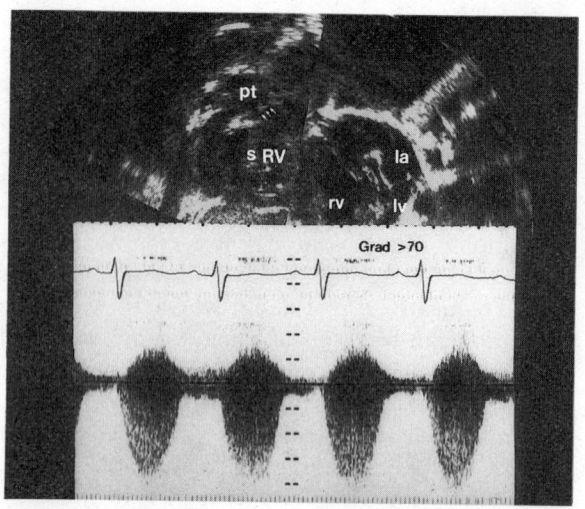

Fig. 13.47. Composite echo and Doppler picture of pulmonary valve stenosis. In the cross-sectional echo, combined short-axis and four-chamber views show extreme right ventricular hypertrophy and a thickened bar-like pulmonary valve. **Lower panel:** continuous wave Doppler picture from the parasternal approach shows significant pulmonary stenosis with a gradient > 70 mmHg predicted using the Bernoulli equation. RV = right ventricle, la = left atrium, s = septum, lv = left ventricle, pt = pulmonary trunk.

The 'primum atrial septal defect' is considered to be part of a spectrum of anomalies of the atrioventricular septum, the structure that lies between the left ventricle and the right atrium.[77] The structure involved in most atrioventricular septal defects is the atrioventricular muscular septum. Normally, the tricuspid valve inserts onto the ventricular septum at a lower level than the mitral valve. The space between the two insertions is the atrioventricular septum (Fig. 13.49). When the atrioventricular septum is partly or wholly deficient, the atrioventricular valve structures are continuous with each other and lie at a common level echocardiographically (Fig. 13.50). In the partial defect, there are usually two atrioventricular rings although the structure of the atrioventricular valve is common and continuous from the right to the left border of the heart. The complete atrioventricular septal defect (once called a 'canal defect') extends below the atrioventricular valve structures to produce a ventricular septal defect (13.51). In the complete defect, there is usually a single atrioventricular valve ring with anterior and posterior bridging leaflets crossing the cavities of the left and right ventricles. Atrioventricular septal defects, whether complete or partial, are suited to diagnosis by cross-sectional echocardiography. The diagnosis can be made using the four-chamber view with

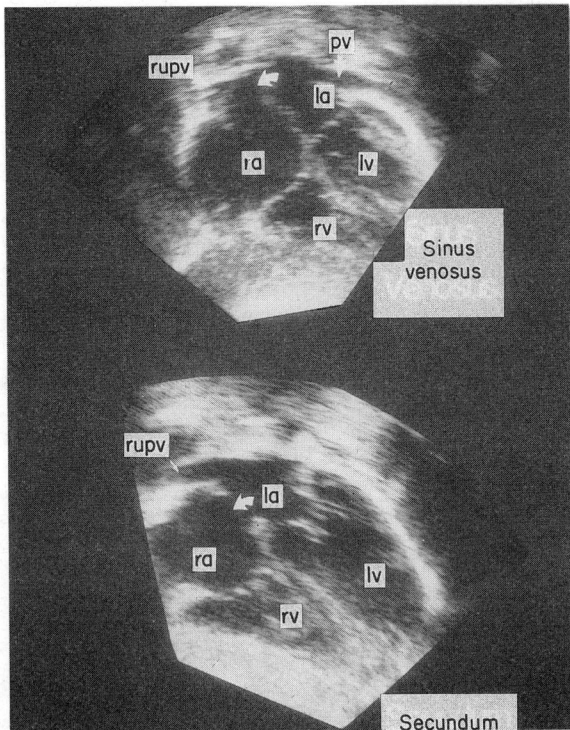

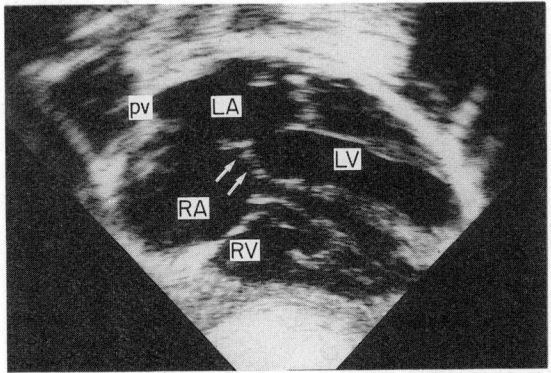

Fig. 13.48. Atrial septal defects on cross-sectional echocardiography. **Upper panel:** a high posterior atrial septal defect in a four-chamber view from the subcostal approach. The right upper pulmonary vein (rupv) is seen to drain into the top of the right atrium and the arrow demonstrates the typical sinus venosus defect. **Lower panel:** a classic central or secundum atrial septal defect (arrow). This picture also demonstrates the atrioventricular septum lying between the insertion of the mitral and tricuspid valves. la, left atrium; pv, pulmonary vein; ra, right atrium; rv, right ventricle; lv, left ventricle.

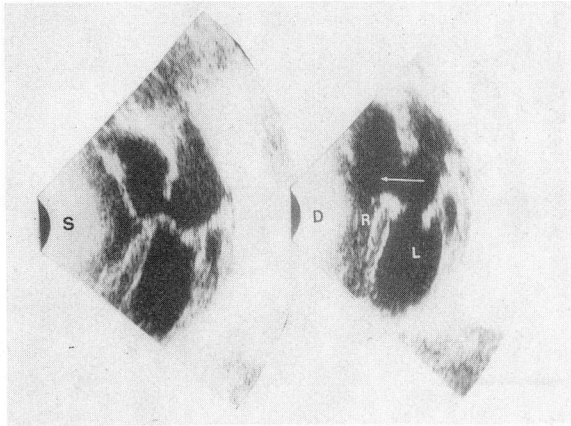

Fig. 13.50. Systolic and diastolic frames for cross-sectional echocardiogram in a patient with partial atrioventricular septal defect. The arrow in the picture on the right shows the low or primum atrial septal defect. Both figures show the common insertion of the atrioventricular valve structures onto the crest of the ventricular septum. R, right ventricle; L, left ventricle; S, systole; D, diastole.

Fig. 13.49. Four-chamber subcostal view. This patient has a secundum atrial septal defect. The mitral valve inserts into the free wall via a papillary muscle and the tricuspid valve inserts into the right side of the ventricular septum. There is obvious offsetting of the septal leaflet insertion—the mitral valve being inserted superiorly to the tricuspid valve. The area of the septum between these two insertions is the atrioventricular septum (arrows). pv, pulmonary vein; LA, left atrium; RA, right atrium; RV, right ventricle; LV, left ventricle.

either an apical or subcostal approach; the detail of the atrioventricular valve leaflets and the attachment are well seen.

All intra-atrial communications should be capable of resolution by cross-sectional echocardiography, particularly when it is used in combination with pulsed Doppler or colour flow mapping. Enlargement of the right ventricle and right atrium associated with paradoxical septal movement (Fig. 13.52) indicates the presence of right ventricle volume overload, which is seen in secundum atrial septal defects and also in anomalous pulmonary venous drainage, tricuspid regurgitation and pulmonary regurgitation. In atrioventricular septal defects, right ventricular volume overload can be demonstrated, but it is often masked by pulmonary hypertension (which normalizes the direction of the septal movement).

All intra-atrial communications should be examined echocardiographically by both the apical *and* subcostal routes in the four-chamber view. From the apex, the sector runs parallel to the intra-atrial septum. At its mid-point, this structure is very thin and a drop out of echoes may produce an artefact which suggests a central or secundum atrial septal defect. Subcostally, the sector cuts the atrial septum *en face*. Only in this view can the echocardiographic diagnosis of an atrial septal defect be made with certainty (Fig. 13.49).

VENTRICULAR SEPTAL DEFECTS

Ventricular septal defects are among the com-

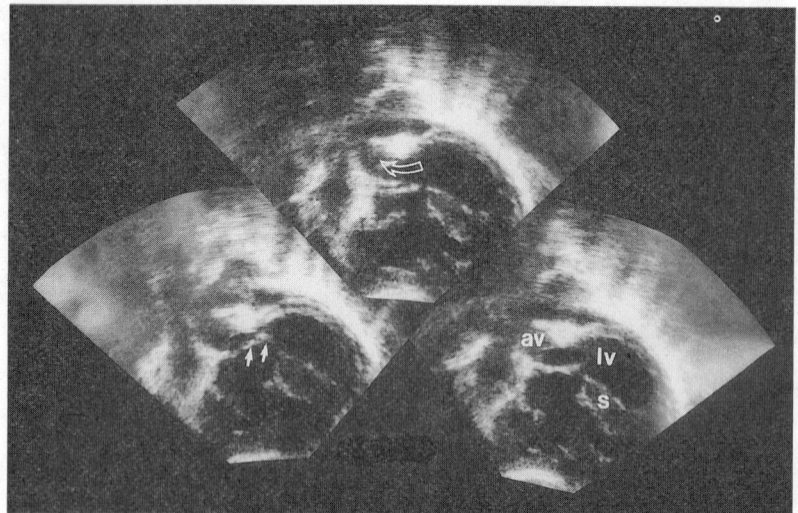

Fig. 13.51. Cross-sectional montage of three views of a patient with complete atrioventricular septal defect. The pictures are in four-chamber plus aortic root views and show the bending of the left ventricular outflow tract (large arrow) which was described by angiocardiographers as the 'goose-neck' deformity. In the lower two pictures, the bridging leaflets of the atrioventricular valve structure can be seen passing across the crest of the ventricular septum into the left ventricular cavity. Underneath this leaflet is the ventricular component of the defect. av, aortic valve; lv, left ventricle; s, septum.

monest congenital anomalies at all ages. As a high percentage of them close spontaneously, the defect is less common in adults. This lesion is suited to echocardiographic diagnosis. All echocardiographic views both parasternally and apically should be used because different parts of the septum are preferentially profiled by particular views.[78] The parasternal long-axis view demonstrates defects of the outlet septum, such as seen in the tetralogy of Fallot (Fig. 13.53). Muscular trabecular ventricular septal defects are better seen in short-axis views (Fig. 13.54). Perimembranous defects are best seen in four-chamber plus great artery views (Fig. 13.55). The approximate size of a defect can be assessed by comparing it with the aortic root dimension. Doppler ultrasound can provide further haemodynamic information in patients with ven-

tricular septal defects. Using continuous wave ultrasound and the modified Bernouilli equation, the peak velocity and the derived pressure drop across the ventricular septal defect can be determined.[79] If the pressure drop between left and right ventricles is subtracted from the systolic blood pressure, the right ventricular systolic pressure can be predicted accurately.

EBSTEIN'S ANOMALY

Echocardiography can demonstrate congenital atrioventricular valve anomalies such as Ebstein's abnormality of the tricuspid valve. The tricuspid valve ring in this condition is sited normally but the septal leaflet is attached to the septum at a level much lower than usual and the anterior leaflet is

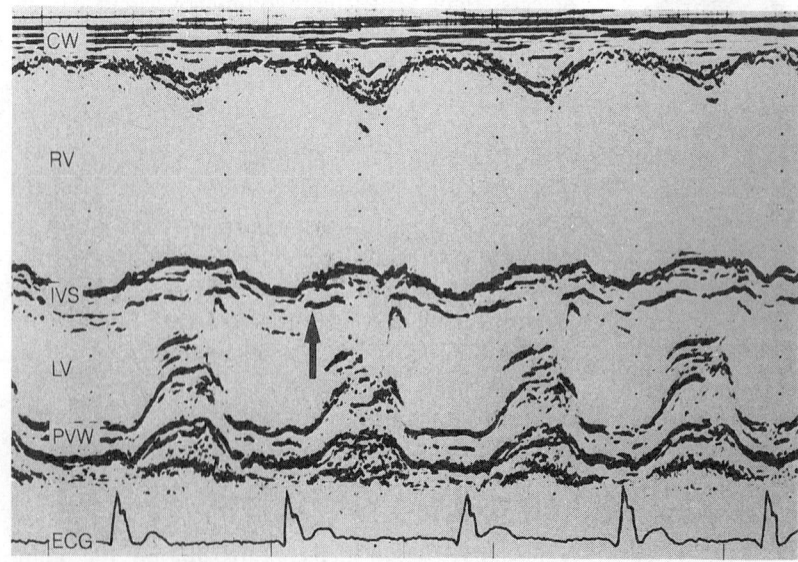

Fig. 13.52. M-mode echocardiogram showing right ventricular volume overload. The right ventricle (RV) is grossly enlarged and the interventricular septum (IVS) shows reversed or paradoxical movement (arrow). LV, left ventricle; PVW, posterior ventricular wall. CW, chest wall.

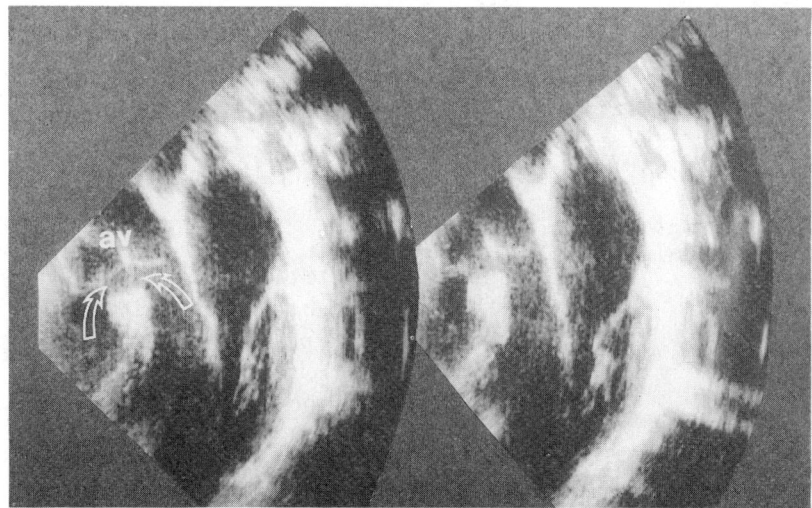

Fig. 13.53. A subarterial ventricular septal defect seen in a case of tetralogy of Fallot by parasternal long-axis views. The arrows demonstrate where the ventricular septal defect lies directly under the closed aortic valve (av). If the interventricular septum and the closed aortic valve cusp echo are compared it would be seen that the aorta overrides the interventricular septum by at least 50%.

frequently large and sail like (Fig. 13.56). There is tricuspid regurgitation, which can be demonstrated by Doppler.

ASSESSMENT OF PULMONARY HYPERTENSION BY ECHOCARDIOGRAPHY AND DOPPLER

The non-invasive evaluation of pulmonary artery pressure is one of the most significant contributions made by cardiac ultrasound. Prior to the advent of Doppler and echo, systolic time-intervals were the only non-invasive method for assessing right heart pressures[80] These have been shown to be insuf-

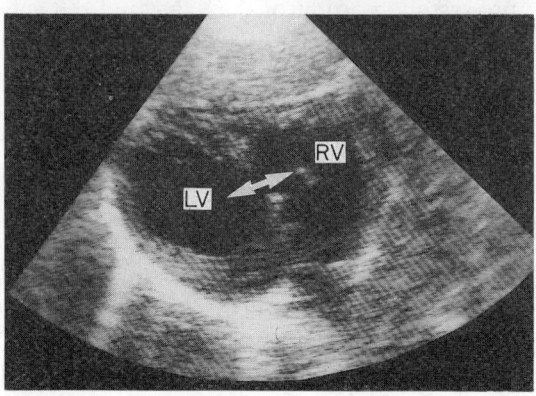

Fig. 13.54. Short-axis subcostal view of the left and right ventricles demonstrating a sizeable trabecular ventricular septal defect. LV, left ventricle; RV, right ventricle.

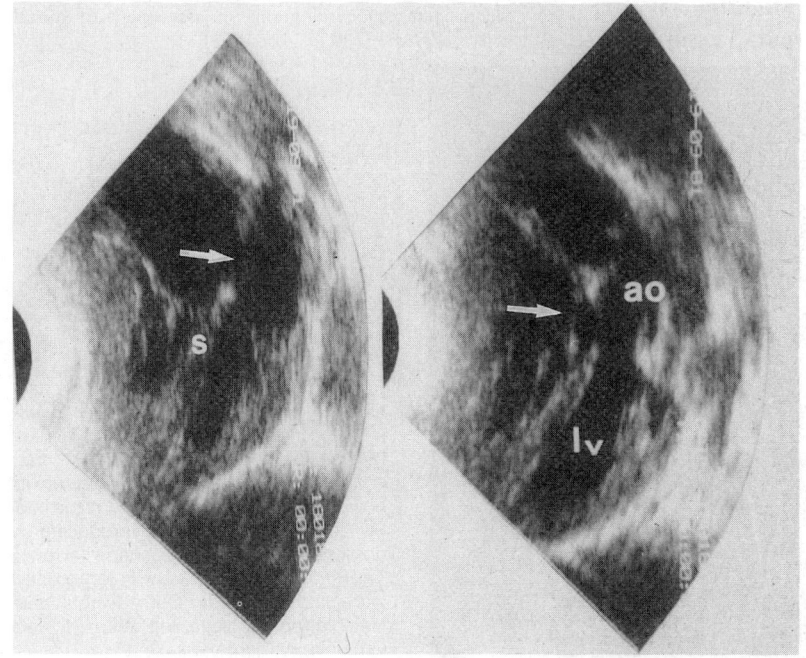

Fig. 13.55. Perimembranous ventricular septal defect shown by cross-sectional echocardiography in two views from the apical four-chamber and apical four-chamber plus aortic root positions. The patient also has a secundum atrial septal defect (arrowed in the left echo). The right echo shows a ventricular septal defect immediately below the aortic valve in the characteristic position for a perimembranous defect. ao, aorta; lv, left ventricle; s, septum.

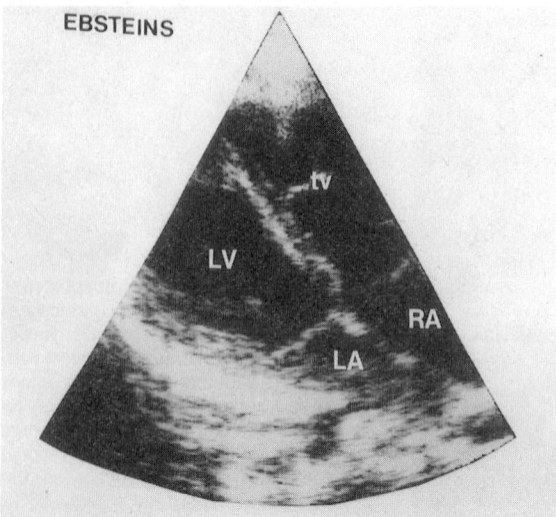

Fig. 13.56. Apical four-chamber view with the apex uppermost. The tricuspid valve septal leaflet (tv) is shown inserted far down on the ventricular septum and in a characteristic position for this lesion. LV, left ventricle; LA, left atrium; RA, right atrium.

ficiently sensitive for clinical use, particularly for the assessment of pulmonary hypertension.[81]

Most patients with pulmonary hypertension have tricuspid regurgitation which can be detected by Doppler. By measuring the peak velocity in the regurgitant jet and substituting this value within the modified Bernouilli equation, the pressure drop in systole across the tricuspid valve can be assessed. Good agreement with catheterization data has been reported.[82] If an approximation of right atrial pressure is added to the trans-tricuspid pressure drop, pulmonary artery systolic pressure can be estimated. If the patient also has a ventricular septal defect, the pulmonary artery pressure can be confirmed.[79]

Elevated right ventricular pressure whether primary or secondary results in typical changes in the cross-sectional echocardiogram (Fig. 13.57). The right ventricle becomes hypertrophied and the cavity is increased in size during both diastole and systole. This change in shape is readily apparent in the right ventricle and it pushes the interventricular septum across into the left ventricular cavity causing an alteration in the configuration of that structure also.

The systolic opening of the pulmonary valve is large in amplitude, there is an absence of 'a' dip on the pre-systolic portion of the valve and the valve lies within an enlarged pulmonary artery. During systole, the valve cusps vibrate and may gradually approximate to each other, but this feature is not specific for pulmonary hypertension.

REFERENCES

1. Upton, M.T. and Gibson, D.G. Study of left ventricular function from digitised echocardiograms. *Prog. Cardiovasc. Dis.* 1978; **20:** 359–84.
2. Upton, M.T., Gibson, D.G. and Brown, D.J. Echocardiographic assessment of abnormal left ventricular relaxation in man. *Br. Heart J.* 1976; **38:** 1001–9.
3. Gibson, D.G., Traill, T.A., Hall, R.J.C. and Brown, D.J. Echocardiographic features of secondary left ventricular hypertrophy. *Br. Heart J.* 1979; **41:** 54–9.
4. Furukawa, K., Matsuura, T., Endo, N. *et al.* Use of digitised left ventricular echocardiograms in assessment of mitral stenosis. *Br. Heart J.* 1979; **42:** 176–81.

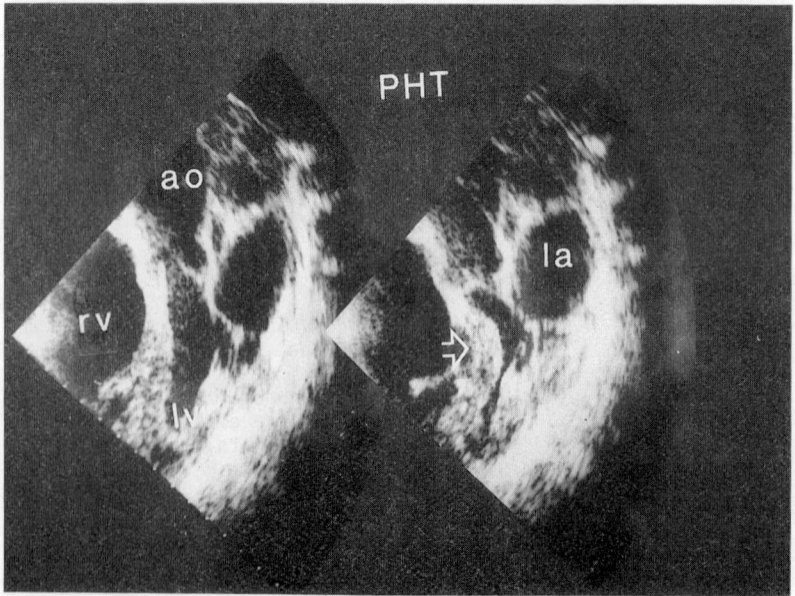

Fig. 13.57. Two cross-sectional echocardiographic pictures in long-axis view showing the effect of pulmonary hypertension on the shape of the cardiac chambers. The interventricular septum is bowed by the enlarged right ventricle into the left ventricular cavity producing a deformed left ventricular shape (arrow). The right ventricular cavity is greatly increased in size in both systole and diastole. ao, aorta; la, left atrium; lv, left ventricle; rv, right ventricle.

5. Dawkins, K.D., Cotter, L. and Gibson, D.G. Assessment of mitral Björk–Shiley prosthetic dysfunction using digitised M mode echocardiography. *Br. Heart J.* 1984; **51**: 168–74.

6. Doppler, J.C. Ueber das farbige Licht der Doppelsterne und einiger anderer Gesterne des Himmels. *Abhandl d Konigl Bohemischen Gesellschaft der Wissenschaften* 1843; **Sers 2**: 465–82.

7. Hatle, L., Brubakk, A., Tromsdal, A. and Angelsen, B. Non-invasive assessment of pressure drop in mitral stenosis by Doppler ultrasound. *Br. Heart J.* 1978; **40**: 131–40.

8. Hall, R.J.C., Kaduski, O.A. and Evemy, K. Need for cardiac catheterisation in assessment of patients for valve surgery. *Br. Heart J.* 1983; **49**: 268–75.

9. Martin, M.A. Reproducibility of M mode echocardiography. In: Hunter, S. and Hall, R.J.C., eds. *Clinical Echocardiography*. Tunbridge Wells: Castle House Publications, 1986, pp. 1–7.

10. Peart, I., Austin, A., Appleton, D., Hall, R.J.C. Reproducibility in cross sectional echocardiography. In: Hunter, S. and Hall, R.J.C., eds. *Clinical Echocardiography*. Tunbridge Wells: Castle House Publications, 1986, pp. 8–18.

11. Gardin, J.M., Burn, C., Hughes, C. and Henry, W.L. Are Doppler aortic flow velocity measurements reproducible? *Circulation* 1981; **62**(Suppl. IV): 205.

12. Lewis, B.S., Lewis, N. and Gotsman, M.S. Effect of respiration on echocardiographic ventricular dimensions and relationship to the second heart sound. *Eur. J. Cardiol.* 1979; **10**: 89–99.

13. Bullock R.E., Appleton, D., Griffiths, C., Albers, C.J., Amer, H. and Hall, R.J.C. Precision of digitised M mode echocardiograms for clinical practice. *Eur. Heart J.* 1984; **5**: 941–7.

14. van Dorp, W.G., ten Cate, F.J., Vletter, W.B., Dohmen, H. and Roelandt, J. Familial prevelance of asymmetric hypertrophy. *Eur. J. Cardiol.* 1976; **4**: 439.

15. St John Sutton, M.G., Tajik, A.J., Gibson, D.G., Seward, J.B. and Guiliani, E.R. Echocardiographic assessment of left ventricular filling and septal and posterior wall dynamics in idiopathic hypertrophic subaortic stenosis. *Circulation* 1977; **57**: 512–20.

16. Seward, J.B. and Tajik, A.J. Primary cardiomyopathies: classification, pathophysiology, clinical recognition and management. *Cardiovasc. Clin.* 1980; **10**: 199–230.

17. Siqueira-Filho, A., Cunha C.L.P., Tajik, A.J. *et al.* M mode and two dimensional echocardiographic features in cardiac amyloidosis. *Circulation* 1981; **63**: 188–96.

18. Bullock, R.E., Albers, C.J. and Hall, R.J.C. The athlete's heart. In: Hunter, S. and Hall, R.J.C., eds. *Clinical Echocardiography*. Tunbridge Wells: Castle House Publications, 1986, pp. 19–24.

19. Shapiro, L.M. The differentiation of physiological from pathological left ventricular hypertrophy. In: Hunter, S. and Hall, R.J.C., eds. *Clinical Echocardiography*. Tunbridge Wells: Castle House Publications, 1986, pp. 25–32.

20. Shapiro, L.M. and Smith, R.J. The effect of training on left ventricular structure and function: an echocardiographic study. *Br. Heart J.* 1983; **50**: 534–9.

21. Effert, S. and Domanig, E. Diagnostik intraaurikularer Tumoren und grober Thromben mit dem Ultraschall Echoverfahren. *D. Med. Wochenschr.* 1959; **84**: 6–8.

22. Martin, R.P., Rakowski, H., French, J. and Popp, R.L. Localization of pericardial effusion with wide angled phased array echocardiography. *Am. J. Cardiol.* 1978; **42**: 904–12.

23. Soulen, R.L., Stark, D.D. and Higgins, C.B. Magnetic resonance imaging of constrictive pericardial disease. *Am. J. Cardiol* 1985; **55**: 480–4.

24. Sahn, D.J., Barratt-Boyes, B.G., Graham, K. *et al.* Ultrasonic imaging of the coronary arteries in open chest humans; evaluation of coronary atherosclerotic lesions during cardiac surgery. *Circulation* 1982; **66**: 1043–44.

25. Motro, M., Vered, Z., Rath, S. *et al.* Correlation between echocardiography and cardiac catheterisation in assessing the severity of aortic stenosis. *Eur. Heart J.* 1983; **4**: 117–20.

26. Johnson, M.L., Warren, S.G., Waugh, R.A. *et al.* Echocardiography of the aortic valve in non-rheumatic left ventricular outflow tract lesions. *Radiology* 1974; **112**: 677.

27. Fowles, R.E., Martin, R.P., Abrams, J.M. *et al.* Two dimensional echocardiographic features of bicuspid aortic valve. *Chest* 1979; **75**: 434–40.

28. Ten Cate, F.J., Van Dorp, W.G., Hugenholtz, P.G. and Roelandt, J. Fixed subaortic stenosis: value of echocardiography for diagnosis and differentiation between different types. *Br. Heart J.* 1979; **41**: 159–66.

29. Weyman, A.E., Caldwell, R.L., Hurwitz, R.A. *et al.* Cross sectional echocardiographic characteristics of aortic obstruction. I. Supravalvularaortic stenosis and aortic hypoplasia. *Circulation* 1978; **57**: 491–7.

30. Morgan, D.J. and Hall, R.J.C. Occult aortic stenosis as a cause of intractable heart failure. *Br. Med. J.* 1979; **1**: 784–7.

31. Bennett, D.W., Evans, D.W. and Raj, M.V.J. Echocardiographic left ventricular dimensions in pressure and volume overload. Their use in assessing aortic stenosis. *Br. Heart J.* 1975; **37**: 971–7.

32. Aziz, K.U., van Grondelle, A., Paul, M.H. and Muster, A.J. Echocardiographic assessment of the relation between left ventricular wall and cavity dimensions and peak systolic pressure in children with aortic stenosis. *Am. J. Cardiol.* 1977; **40**: 775–80.

33. Krivokapich, J., Child, J.S. and Skorton, D.J. Flail aortic valve leaflet: M mode and two dimensional echocardiographic manifestations. *Am. Heart J.* 1980; **99**: 425–37.

34. Aziz, K.U., Cole, R.B. and Paul, M.H. Echocardiographic features of supracristal ventricular septal defect with prolapsed aortic valve leaflet. *Am. J. Cardiol.* 1979; **43**: 854–9.

35. Victor, M., Mintz, G., Kotler, M. *et al.* Two dimensional echocardiographic diagnosis of aortic dissection. *Am. J. Cardiol.* 1981; **48**: 1155.

36. D'Cruz, I., Cohen, H.C., Prabhu, R. *et al.* Flutter of left ventricular structures in patients with aortic regurgitation, with special reference to patients with associated mitral stenosis. *Am. Heart J.* 1976; **92**: 684.

37. Botvinick, E.H., Schiller, N.B. *et al.* Echocardiographic demonstration of early mitral valve closure in severe aortic insufficiency. Its clinical implications. *Circulation* 1975; **52**: 836.

38. Mann, T., McLaurin, L., Grossman, W. and Craige, E. Assessing the haemodynamic severity of acute aortic regurgitation due to infective endocarditis. *N. Engl. J. Med.* 1975; **293**: 108.

39. Fioretti, P., Roelandt, J., Bos, R.J. *et al.* Echocardiography in chronic aortic unsufficiency; is valve replacement too late when left ventricular systolic volume reaches 55 mm? *Circulation* 1983; **67**: 216.

40. Henry, W.L., Bonow, R.O., Roing, D.R. and Epstein, S.E. Observations on the optimum time for operative intervention for aortic regurgitation. *Circulation* 1980; **61**: 484.

41. Elder, I. Ultrasound cardiography in mitral valve stenosis. *Am. J. Cardiol.* 1967; **19**: 18–31.

42. Hall, R.J.C., Austin, A. and Hunter, S. M mode echogram as a means of distinguishing between mild and severe mitral stenosis. *Br. Heart J.* 1980; **46**: 486–91.

43 Martin, R.P., Rakowski, H., Kleinman, J.H. *et al.* Reliability and reproducibility of two dimensional echocardiographic measurement of the stenotic mitral valve orifice area. *Am. J. Cardiol.* 1979; **43**: 560–8.

44. Hall, R.J.C. Place of M mode echocardiography in the clinical decision. *Herz* 1983; **5**: 199–212.

45. Carabello, B.A., Nolan, S.P. and McGuire, L.B. Assessment of pre-operative left ventricular function in patients with

mitral regurgitation: value of the end systolic wall stress end systolic volume ratio. *Circulation* 1981; **64**: 1212–7.

46. Wong, C.Y.H. and Spotnitz, H.M. Systolic and diastolic properties of the human left ventricle during valve replacement for chronic mitral regurgitation. *Am. J. Cardiol.* 1981; **47**: 40.

47. Osterberger, L.E., Goldstein, S., Khaja, F. and Lakier, J.B. Functional mitral stenosis in patients with massive mitral annular calcification. *Circulation* 1981; **64**: 472–6.

48. Barlow, J.B. and Pocock, W.A. Billowing, floppy, prolapsed or flail mitral valves. *Am. J. Cardiol.* 1985; **55**: 501–2.

49. Procacci, P.M., Savran, S.V., Schreiter, S.L. *et al.* Prevalance of clinical mitral valve prolapse in 1169 young women. *N. Engl. J. Med.* 1976; **294**: 1086–8.

50. Markiewicz, W., Stoner J., London, E. *et al.* Mitral valve prolapse in one hundred presumably healthy young females. *Circulation* 1976; **53**: 464–73.

51. Perloff, J.K. Evolving concepts of mitral valve prolapse. *N. Engl. J. Med.* 1982; **307**: 369–70.

52. DeMaria, A.N., Neumann, A., Lee, G. *et al.* Echocardiographic identification of the mitral valve prolapse syndrome. *Am. J. Med.* 1977; **62**: 819–29.

53. Malcolm, A.D., Bonghaner, D.R., Kostuk, W.J. *et al.* Clinical features and investigative findings in presence of mitral leaflet prolapse. Study of 85 consecutive patients. *Br. Heart J.* 1976; **38**: 244–56.

54. Jerasaty, R.M. *Mitral valve prolapse.* New York: Raven Press, 1979.

55. Gilbert, B.W., Schatz, R.A., VonRamm, O.T. *et al.* Mitral valve prolapse. Two dimensional echocardiographic and angiographic correlation. *Circulation* 1976; **54**: 716–23.

56. Naito, M., Morganroth, J., Mardelli, T.J. and Chen, C.C. Apical cross sectional echocardiography: The standard for diagnosis of mitral valve prolapse (Abstract). *Circulation* 1979; **59,60** (Suppl. II): II–154.

57. Warth, D.C., King, M.E. *et al.* Prevalence of mitral valve prolapse in normal children. *J. Am. Coll. Cardiol.* 1985; **5**: 1173–7.

58. Wan, L.S., Gross, C.M., Wakefield, R.J. and Kalbfleisch, J.H. Diagnostic precision of echocardiography in mitral valve prolapse. *Am. Heart J.* 1985; **109**: 803–8.

59. Grenadier, E., Keidar, S., Sahn, D.J. *et al.* Ruptured mitral chordae tendinae may be a frequent and insignificant complication in the mitral valve prolapse syndrome. *Eur. Heart J.* 1985; **6**: 1006–15.

60. Callahan, J.A., Wroblewski, E.M., Reeder, G.S. *et al.* Echocardiographic features of carcinoid heart disease. *Am. J. Cardiol.* 1982; **50**: 762–8.

61. Smith, M.D., Kwan, O.L. and DeMaria, A.N. The role of echocardiography in the diagnosis and management of infective endocarditis. *Prac. Cardiol.* 1984; **10**: 78.

62. Daniels, S.J., Mintz, G.S. and Kotler, M.N. Rheumatic tricuspid valve disease. Two dimensional echocardiographic hemodynamic and angiographic correlations. *Am. J. Cardiol.* 1983; **51**: 492.

63. Brown, A.K. and Anderson, V. Two dimensional echocardiography and the tricuspid valve. Leaflet definition and prolapse. *Br. Heart J.* 1983; **49**: 495–500.

64. Feneley, M. and Gavaghan, T. Paradoxical and pseudoparadoxical interventricular septal motion in patients with right ventricular volume overload. *Circulation* 1986; **74**: 230–8.

65. Meltzer, R.S., van Hoogenhuyze, D., Serruys, P.W. *et al.* Diagnosis of tricuspid regurgitation by contrast echocardiography. *Circulation* 1981; **63**: 1093–9.

66. Skjaerpe, T. and Hatle, L. Diagnosis of tricuspid regurgitation. Sensitivity and Doppler ultrasound compared with contrast echocardiography. *Eur. Heart J.* 1985; **6**: 429–36.

67. Nanda, N.C. Echocardiography of tricuspid and pulmonary valves. *Cardiovasc. Clin.* 1978; **9**: 97.

68. Weyman, A.E., Dillon, J.C., Feigenbaum, H. and Chang, S. Pulmonary valve echo motion in pulmonary regurgitation. *Br. Heart J.* 1975; **37**: 1184–90.

69. Thompson, K.R., Nanda, N. and Bramika, R. The reliability of echocardiography in the diagnosis of infective endocarditis. *Radiology* 1975; **125**: 473.

70. Kisslo, J., Guadalajara, J.F., Stewart, J.A. and Stack, R.S. Echocardiography in infective endocarditis. *Herz* 1983; **8**: 271.

71. Smith, M.D., Kwan, O.L. and DeMaria, A.N. The role of echocardiography in the diagnosis and management of infective endocarditis. *Prac. Cardiol.* 1984; **10**: 78.

72. Stewart, J.A., Slimperi, D., Harris, P. *et al.* Echocardiographic documentation of vegetative lesions in infective endocarditis: clinical implications. *Circulation* 1980; **61**: 374.

73. Rubenson, D.S., Tucker, C.R., Stinson, E.B. *et al.* The use of echocardiography in diagnosing culture negative endocarditis. *Circulation* 1981; **64**: 641.

74. Scanlan, J.G., Seward, J.B. and Tajick, A.J. Valve ring abscesses in infective endocarditis: visualization with wide angle two dimensional echocardiography. *Am. J. Cardiol.* 1982; **49**: 1794.

75. Ghosh, P.K., Miller, H.I. and Vidne, B. Mitral obstruction in bacterial endocarditis. *Br. Heart J.* 1983; **53**: 341.

76. Erbel, R., Rohmann, S. *et al.* Diagnostic value of transoesophageal echocardiography in infective endocarditis (Abstract). *Circulation.* 1986; **74**(Suppl. II): 55.

77. Becker, A.E. and Anderson, R.H. Atrioventricular septal defects. What's in a name? *J. Thorac Cardiovasc. Surg.* 1982; **83**: 461–86.

78. Sutherland, G.R., Goodman, M.J., Smallhorn, J.F., Guiterras, P., Anderson, R.H. and Hunter, S. Ventricular septal defects. Two dimensional echocardiographic and morphological correlations. *Br. Heart J.* 1982; **47**: 316–28.

79. Hatle, L. and Rokseth, R. Non-invasive diagnosis and assessment of ventricular septal defect by Doppler ultrasound. *Acta Med. Scand.* 1981; Suppl. **645**: 47–56.

80. Burstin, L. Determination of pressure in the pulmonary artery by external graphic recordings. *Br. Heart J.* 1967; **29**: 396–404.

81. Marin-Garcia, J., Moller, J.H. and Mirvis, D.M. The pulmonic valve echogram in the assessment of pulmonary hypertension in children. *Paediatr. Cardiol.* 1983; **4**: 209–14.

82. Yock, P.G., Popp, R.L. Non-invasive estimation of ventricular pressures by Doppler ultrasound in patients with tricuspid regurgitation (Abstract). *Circulation* 1983; **68**: 111–230.

Chapter 14

Doppler Ultrasound

G. Sutherland

INTRODUCTION

With the development of ultrasound in cardiac imaging from the early M-mode machines to the modern high-resolution two-dimensional images, the cardiologist now has a technique at his or her disposal that allows accurate morphological and (to a lesser degree) functional assessment of the heart and great vessels. Although some haemodynamic information concerning both flows and pressures can be inferred from echocardiographic images, in many cases such information can be misleading. With the development of the Doppler modalities (pulsed, continuous and colour flow imaging) over the past 10 years, and their appropriate integration into two-dimensional imaging systems, a comprehensive range of non-invasive ultrasound techniques has become available to the cardiologist.

WHAT IS DOPPLER? HISTORICAL PERSPECTIVE

In 1842, Johann Christian Doppler, an Austrian physicist and mathematician, first presented his paper 'On the coloured light of stars and some other heavenly bodies'.[1] In this paper, he related changes in the wavelength of light emitted from stars to the relative motion of the observer and the light source. It is interesting to note that in this description of what is now known as the 'Doppler principle' Johann Doppler did not relate his findings to sound waves. Subsequent proof of the 'Doppler principle' in relation to sound waves was obtained by Buys Ballot in 1844 in his famous experiment on the Dutch railway which compared the changing pitch of a note from a trumpet player mounted on a moving train with the same note emitted by two stationary trumpet players standing beside the railway track.

Interestingly, the Doppler principle as applied to the colour shift of light from stars has subsequently been shown to be incorrect, whereas that applied to sound by Ballot has stood the test of time and is the basis of all cardiac Doppler investigations. The initial application of the Doppler principle to cardiology was first reported in 1956 when Satomura[2] described its use in the measurement of blood flow velocity. Little appeared in the cardiology literature until the mid 1960s when Lindstrom and Edler demonstrated the frequency spectrum for mitral flow.[3] A further decade passed until the first machine integrated pulsed Doppler into an M-mode system with spectral analysis of the Doppler signal performed by time-interval histography. The first clinically effective cardiac Doppler systems only became available when fast Fourier transform was applied to spectral display to allow the accurate linear analysis of velocity curve profiles. The subsequent development and application of continuous wave Doppler, the integration of both pulsed and continuous wave Doppler into two-dimensional imaging systems to create Duplex scanning systems and finally the addition of the pulsed Doppler-based colour flow imaging systems have all taken place within the last 10 years.

THE DOPPLER PRINCIPLE[4]

The Doppler principle, as defined by Johann Christian Doppler, states that any apparent shift in transmitted frequency occurs as a result of motion of either the source or the target. In cardiology, the source is the ultrasound transducer and the target is the red blood cells moving in the heart and great vessels. The frequency shift detected by the Doppler mode (be it pulsed, high pulsed repetition frequency or continuous wave—see below) is directly related to the velocity at which the red blood cells are travelling within the ultrasound beam and to the cosine of the angle (θ) at which the red cells are insonated by the stationary transducer, i.e.

$$V = \frac{C \times F}{2 \text{ (transmitted frequency)} \times \text{cosine } \theta}$$

where V is the velocity of blood cells, C is the speed of ultrasound in the medium and F is the frequency shift in KHz. Modern ultrasound machines directly compute velocity from frequency shift. When Doppler is used in clinical cardiology, the precise intercept angle (θ) between the ultrasound beam and the direction of blood flow is usually unknown. As the velocity measured depends on the cosine of this angle, and cosines of angles $< 20°$ are $\simeq 1$, it is important to attempt to align the ultrasound beam as near parallel to blood flow as possible. The error in underestimation of velocity increases exponentially once the angle to flow increases above 30° (Fig. 14.1).

From the above, it will be obvious that it is essential to align to the direction of flow as best as possible in any Doppler examination. This may involve trying many transducer positions and varying the angle of the sound beam to derive the clearest velocity envelope with the high velocities arranged around the outside of the envelope. Conventionally, all Doppler-derived information is displayed in a standard manner around a zero velocity line. Flow that is directed towards the transducer is displayed above the zero velocity line and flow directed away from the transducer is displayed below the zero velocity line.

The two major uses of Doppler in cardiac ultrasound are in the assessment of the pressure drop across any obstruction within the heart and great vessels and in the measurement of volume flow across a known cross-sectional area. The former measurement can be used to calculate intracardiac pressures and evaluate valvar obstruction; the latter can be used to estimate cardiac output and the degree of intracardiac shunting.

THE PRINCIPLES OF EVALUATING A PRESSURE DROP[4]

Any isolated pressure drop within a fluid-filled system can be evaluated from the Doppler information obtained by using a modification of the classical Bernoulli equation. In its full form, the Bernoulli equation states that in a steady haemodynamic state the pressure drop across an obstruction within a fluid-filled vessel is proportional to both the flow rate and the resistance encountered in the system.

$$_1 - P_2 = \tfrac{1}{2}\,\rho\,(V_2^2 - V_1^2) + \int_1^2 dv/dt \times ds + R(v)$$
$$\qquad\qquad (A) \qquad\qquad\qquad (B) \qquad\quad (C)$$

where P_1 and P_2 represent the pressures before and after the stenosis, V_1 and V_2 are the peak velocities at the same sites, ρ is the density of blood, dv/dt = rate of change of velocity and ds the distance over which it occurs and $R(v)$ is the viscous resistance × the local velocity. Term (A) represents the convective acceleration, Term (B) flow acceleration and Term (C) viscous friction. In practical terms, in the human circulation, both flow acceleration and viscous friction have little effect on the pressure-drop calculation and can be omitted from the equation. The equation thus modified by Holen and Hatle and referred to as the modified (or simplified) Bernoulli equation is thus:

$$P_1 - P_2 = 4V^2$$

where P_1 is the peak distal pressure, P_2 is the proximal peak pressure and V is the velocity gain over the obstruction. The equation should more correctly be written as:

$$P_1 - P_2 = 4\,(V_2^2 - V_1^2)$$

where V_2 = the distal peak velocity and V_1 = the proximal (or pre-obstruction) peak velocity, but where V_1 is less than unity the proximal velocity can be ignored. However, when the volume of forward flow is increased above normal parameters (such as in patients with raised cardiac output or valve incompetence—see below), V_1 can be increased significantly (i.e. to 2 m/s) and must be incorporated

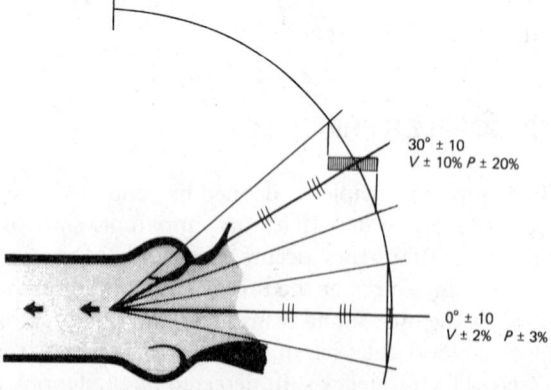

Fig. 14.1. The effect of changing angle of alignment of the ultrasound beam to the direction of bloodflow. Note that the error increases almost exponentially as the angle of incidence increases above 30 degrees (figure reproduced with permission of Houston and Simpson, taken from Cardiac Doppler Ultrasound, published by Wright).

into the modified Bernoulli equation in order that a correct evaluation of the stenotic element of the valve can be made.

THE PRINCIPLES OF EVALUATING VOLUME FLOW[4]

DOPPLER MODES

Three different Doppler modes, each with unique advantages and disadvantages, are used in clinical practice: pulsed Doppler, continuous wave Doppler and colour flow imaging. A fourth mode, high pulsed repetition frequency (PRF) Doppler, is incorporated into some machines but it is essentially a variation on the pulsed technique and is not dealt with in detail here. A short description of the way in which each mode derives its information is required so that the advantages and disadvantages inherent in each technique and their application to the analysis of the range of normal and abnormal flows encountered in cardiology can be understood.

Continuous wave[5]

Continuous wave Doppler is perhaps the simplest of the three modes to understand. Two ultrasound crystals are mounted on the same transducer, one continuously transmits the ultrasound beam and one continuously receives reflected sound waves (Fig. 14.2). The great advantage of this arrangement

is that, with appropriate crystal frequency selection, very high velocities can be recorded from within the heart and accurately displayed on a monitor. Continuous wave Doppler can record any high velocity encountered even in the most severe case of valvar obstruction. Although continuous wave Doppler can record high velocities it is not capable, because of the manner in which the information is obtained, of determining where the signal originated because all the frequency shifts detected along the path of the Doppler beam will be incorporated in the final signal display. Thus, continuous wave Doppler has *range ambiguity* as its main drawback.

Pulsed mode

Pulsed doppler is almost the direct opposite of continuous wave in both its advantages and disadvantages. In a pulsed Doppler system, only one crystal is used which transmits and receives information (Table 14.1 and Plate 14.1). Clearly, this single crystal cannot transmit and receive information continuously. In effect, the ultrasound signal is transmitted at a given frequency for a specific length of time; as the speed of sound is relatively constant in fluid and tissue, the transmitting crystal can be electronically switched to a 'listening mode' at a given time-interval after the transmission of the initial signal and the Doppler information received at that time-interval will represent Doppler information derived at a known depth (i.e. the sample

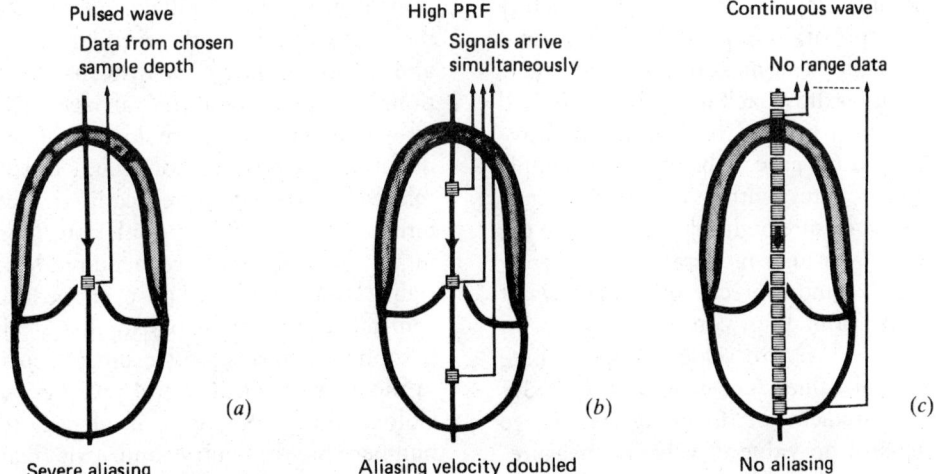

Pulsed wave
Data from chosen sample depth

High PRF
Signals arrive simultaneously

Continuous wave
No range data

(a)   (b)   (c)

Severe aliasing   Aliasing velocity doubled   No aliasing

Fig. 14.2. The three Doppler modalities used in interrogation of trans mitral flow. Note that in Fig. 2A the sample volume is placed at the tip of the mitral leaflets. Fig. 2B illustrates the use of high PRF Doppler. The maximum velocity prior to the onset of aliasing is doubled by the use of multiple sample volumes. In Fig. 2C continuous wave Doppler is demonstrated. This system continuously transmits and receives ultrasound information and thus no range data is obtainable (reproduced by permission of Houston and Simpson, Clinical Doppler Ultrasound, published by Wright).

Table 14.1. **Maximal velocities recorded noninvasively with Doppler ultrasound in normal individuals.**

	Children	Adults
	(m/s)	(m/s)
Mitral flow	1.00 (0.8–1.3)	0.90 (0.6–1.3)
Tricuspid flow	0.60 (0.5–0.8)	0.50 (0.3–0.7)
Pulmonary artery	0.90 (0.7–1.1)	0.75 (0.6–0.9)
Left ventricle	1.00 (0.7–1.2)	0.90 (0.7–1.1)
Aorta	1.50 (1.2–1.8)	1.35 (1.0–1.7)

Reproduced by permission of Hatle and Angelsen, *Doppler Ultrasound in Cardiology*, second edition, Published by Lea & Febiger.

volume). By increasing the time-interval over which the receiving crystal listens to the reflected information, the sample volume can be made larger (i.e. less depth specific) or conversely by reducing the listening interval a greater specificity of sampling site is achieved. In any pulsed Doppler system, the maximum frequency shift that can be measured unambiguously is related to both the frequency of the crystal used and the depth being interrogated. The maximum frequency that may be measured at a specific depth is half the pulse repetition frequency of the crystal; this value is known as the Nyquist frequency. Converted to velocity, this value is known as the Nyquist limit and can be calculated at depth R using the following equation:

$$V_\mathrm{m} = c2/ (8F'R)$$

where V_m is the maximum velocity, F' is the transducer frequency and c is the acoustic velocity. When the Nyquist limit is exceeded, ambiguity occurs in the interpretation of any velocity information displayed. This phenomenon is termed 'aliasing' and is the major drawback in the use of pulsed Doppler. Thus, in contrast to continuous wave Doppler, pulsed Doppler can be used to sample velocity at specific sites within the heart but it cannot be used to measure high velocities, e.g. in the range encountered through moderately or severely stenosed valves. It is more precise in its analysis of low-velocity waveforms than continuous wave. In practical terms, it can record velocities up to three times physiological values (i.e. peak velocities 3.5 m/s equivalent to gradients of 50 mmHg), but above these values it is of no value in velocity measurement. The importance of pulsed Doppler as a diagnostic modality has now been largely supplanted by colour flow imaging but it remains an essential requirement for an accurate analysis of low-velocity waveforms.

Colour flow imaging[6]

Colour flow imaging is essentially a multigate pulsed Doppler technique. Multiple pulsed sample volumes are interrogated across the two-dimensional image. From the Doppler information derived from these multiple sampling sites, a colour display representing a number of facets of blood flow is overlain on the black and white cross-sectional image. Various colours are either varied in intensity or mixed to produce patterns that represent blood flow direction, mean velocity and turbulence. Traditionally, laminar flow towards the transducer is illustrated as red and laminar flow away from the transducer as blue. Turbulence is normally encoded as green which produces a colour mosaic when added to the normal red and blue colour display. The greater the degree of turbulence the more green is added to the display. The colour information is processed separately from the imaging information within the ultrasound system and is overlain on the black and white cross-sectional structural information when processing is complete. The overall effect produced is that of ultrasonic angiography. The information derived is at best semi-quantitative but used appropriately can impart unique flow information that cannot be obtained from any other Doppler modality. At its present state of development, colour flow imaging has virtually replaced conventional pulsed Doppler in its diagnostic role (but has had no impact on the quantifying roles of pulsed and continuous wave Doppler). It allows a rapid evaluation and distinction of abnormal from normal flow and provides the relative novice with a rapid means of identifying and understanding flow disturbances that conventional Doppler modalities can never achieve. Colour flow imaging has its main role in complex flow disturbances both in congenital heart disease and relatively rare complex acquired lesions encountered in the adult population, such as post-infarction septal rupture, acquired left ventricular–right atrial shunting post endocarditis and left ventricular pseudoaneurysm. Its use in the trans-oesophageal ultrasound examination is invaluable in the assessment of mitral prosthesis malfunction. Colour flow imaging can identify the site and number of the entry and exit tears in aortic dissection as well as demonstrating the abnormal and diagnostic flow patterns in both the aortic true and false lumens; it is superior to conventional angiography in this respect. The value of colour flow imaging in individual lesions will be discussed

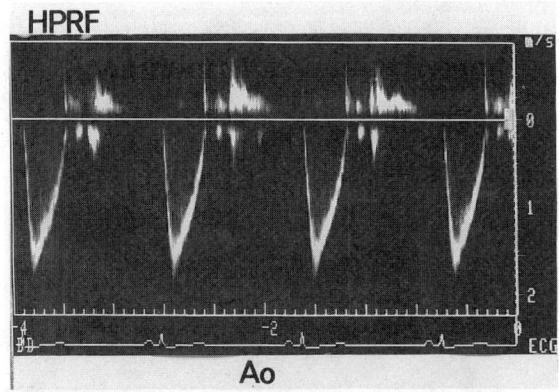

Fig. 14.3. Normal ascending aortic flow—peak velocity 1.7 m/s. High pulse repetition Doppler (HPRF). Apical transducer position. Note the early transient diastolic flow reversal in the ascending aorta (Ao). This is a normal finding.

subsequently under the heading of each lesion to which it makes a significant diagnostic contribution.

AORTIC VALVE DISEASE

NORMAL AORTIC FLOW

Flow across the aortic valve can be recorded from a number of transducer positions: subcostal, apical, left precordial, high right parasternal and suprasternal. Normal flow is only systolic. Neither transthoracic nor oesophageal echocardiography have suggested there is any significant incidence of 'physiological' aortic incompetence (cf. the mitral, pulmonary and tricuspid valves). The range of velocities recorded across the normal aortic valve is 1.0–1.7 m/s (Fig. 14.3).

VALVAR AORTIC STENOSIS[7-22]

Perhaps the most important aspect of the introduction of Doppler into cardiology has been the use of continuous wave Doppler to assess the peak instantaneous gradient in valvar aortic stenosis. Symptoms and physical signs in this lesion may all be confusing, especially when essential hypertension co-exists. In addition, it has become a lesion more frequently encountered as the percentage of elderly in the population increases. With the correct use of the continuous wave Doppler investigation, an accurate assessment of the transvalve pressure gradient across the aortic valve can be achieved in virtually every case.[7] Cardiac catheterization provides little additional information in this respect. The main problem that remains is what clinical management decision is made based on the combination of the clinical information and the derived Doppler pressure gradient. Valvar aortic stenosis is a fixed obstructive lesion. With mild-to-moderate obstruction, continuous wave Doppler will identify a pressure gradient which rises to a peak almost immediately (Figs 14.4 and 14.5). With aortic stenosis of increasing severity, the peak pressure gradient is increasingly delayed.[4] Initial correlative catheter and continuous wave Doppler studies of the estimation of pressure gradient in valvar aortic stenosis produced disappointing results. In these studies (the majority of which were non-simultaneous), the pressure gradient derived by continuous wave Doppler was compared with the left 'peak to peak' ventricular–aortic withdrawal gradient as measured by a fluid-filled catheter. It was only when it was understood that the two techniques were measuring differing entities that the

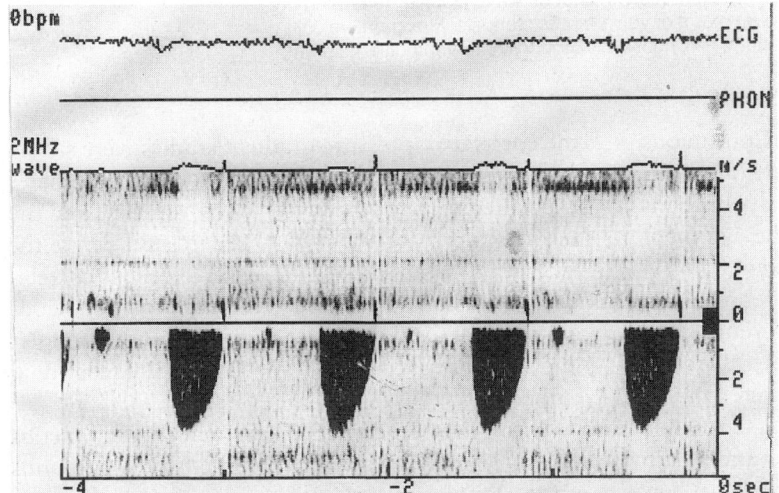

Fig. 14.4. Valvar aortic stenosis (moderate). Continuous wave Doppler. Apical transducer position. This example demonstrates the characteristic 'fixed obstruction' velocity profile associated with valvar aortic stenosis. There is a rapid rise in the pressure gradient in systole to a peak velocity of 4 m/s. As the peak velocity of the pre-valve flow was negligible, the modified Bernoulli equation ($P = 4V^2$) can be used to derive a maximal instantaneous gradient of 64 mmHg. No co-existing aortic incompetence was recorded in this patient.

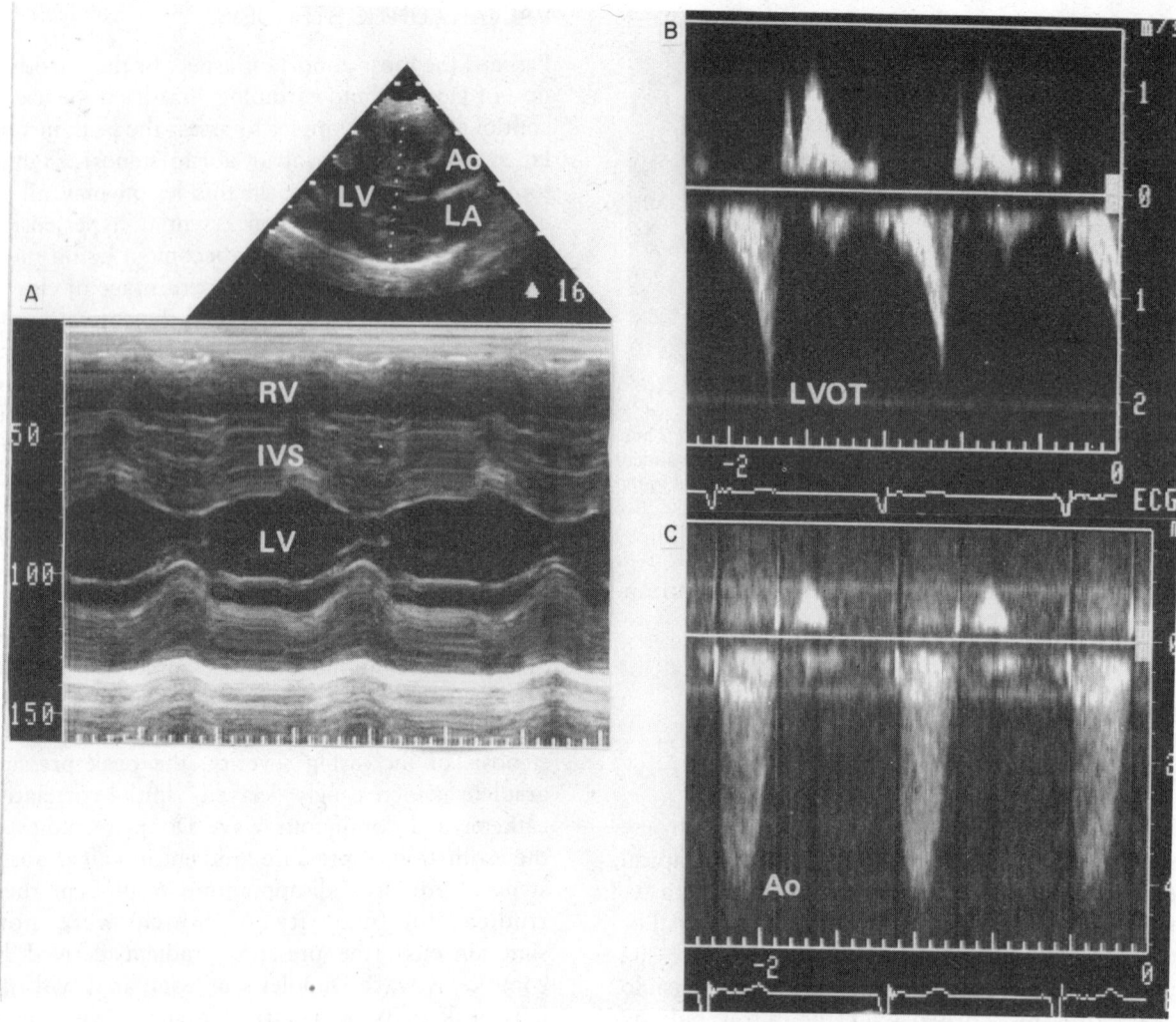

Fig. 14.5. Valvar aortic stenosis (severe). Co-existing fixed (valvar) and dynamic (subvalvar) velocity waveforms. These two waveforms frequently co-exist if severe ventricular hypertrophy is present. (A) M-Mode echocardiogram demonstrating severe concentric left ventricular hypertrophy and a relatively small left ventricular cavity. (B) Pulsed Doppler interrogation of the left ventricular outflow tract identifies a dynamic obstruction waveform below the aortic valve. Peak velocity = 1.8 m/s. This is secondary to hypertrophy caused by the distal severe valvar obstruction. (C) Continuous wave Doppler recording of transaortic valve flow. Note the fixed obstruction waveform of valvar aortic stenosis. Maximum velocity = 4.6 m/s. Ao, aorta; LV, left ventricle; LA, left atrium; RV, right ventricle; IVS, interventricular septum; LVOT, left ventricular outflow tract.

discordant results were understood. Continuous wave Doppler, because it samples velocity (and thus the gradient) across the valve continuously throughout the cardiac cycle, can measure the maximal instantaneous transaortic pressure gradient. This is a true physiological gradient which does exist in real time and which is created by left ventricular contraction. The 'peak to peak' gradient, traditionally evaluated in the cardiac catheterization laboratory, is an artificial gradient that does not exist in real time since the left ventricular and aortic pressures reach their peaks at different times. When the correlative pressure gradient studies were subsequently repeated using two high-fidelity manometer tip catheters (one placed in the left ventricle and the second in the aortic root), to record and derive the true peak instantaneous gradient, excellent correlation was confirmed between the peak instantaneous gradient derived from continuous wave Doppler and that derived simultaneously from the dual catheters.[13,15]

With experience, the maximal instantaneous pressure gradient can be recorded by continuous wave Doppler in over 95% of patients with aortic stenosis. It is relatively easy to record in children and young adults, but it may present problems in the elderly. Signals from multiple transducer positions should be recorded in every case to attempt to record the maximal velocity envelope as the jet may be extremely eccentric in origin and direction. Such an examination technique should allow the continuous wave beam to be directed approximately parallel to flow thus eliminating the need to perform angle correction calculations. Colour flow imaging can be of value in the estimation of pressure gradient by defining the jet direction and thus allowing a rapid alignment of the continuous wave beam to flow. Measurement inaccuracies may occur at both ends of the pressure gradient spectrum. Normally, both flow acceleration and viscous friction are negligible and are omitted from the Bernoulli equation to give the modified Bernoulli equation used in everyday clinical ultrasound practice. This is justifiable in the vast majority of cases but both these entities become significant at peak instantaneous gradients > 150 mmHg. Failure to include them into the pressure gradient calculation will lead to an increasing underestimation of the pressure gradient as the gradient itself increases. Similarly, inaccuracies may occur in gradient estimation between 0 and 40 mmHg with a degree of gradient overestimation taking place. This is normally due to failure to take the pre-valve flow velocity into account and simply deriving the pressure gradient from the post-valve peak flow velocity and assuming that pre-valve flow was less than unity. Thus, for clinical practice, the Doppler-derived peak instantaneous gradient for aortic stenosis is at its most accurate in the range of 40–150 mmHg. This is precisely the range over which it is of most value in clinical decision-making. A false-positive diagnostic error can be made by mistaking the high-velocity jet of mitral incompetence for the jet of aortic stenosis. The timing of the commencement of the abnormal jet, the direction of flow and the transducer angulation will allow accurate differentiation between the two entities. In inexperienced hands, this differentiation can be a problem. Where colour flow imaging is available, the differentiation of the two entities is readily effected by the identification and location of turbulent flow in either the ascending aorta or the left atrium.

The peak systolic gradient across the aortic valve is determined by the valve area and the systolic flow across the valve. Thus, this gradient may differ considerably among patients with the same degree of valve narrowing as a result of many variables including:

1 heart rhythm;
2 heart rate;
3 left ventricular function;
4 the presence of co-existing aortic incompetence;
5 co-existing mitral valve disease.

The effect of atrial fibrillation with widely varying R–R intervals on the peak instantaneous gradient is shown in Fig. 14.6. In such cases, the gradient should be calculated over a large number of beats with an R–R interval approximating to a normal heart rate. Left ventricular function should be evaluated in every patient undergoing assessment of aortic stenosis. With severe impairment of left ventricular failure (either acute or chronic), the left ventricle may fail to produce a significant gradient despite critical aortic valve narrowing. Where such a case is suspected, the judicious use of an inotropic agent during the Doppler examination may provoke a significant gradient as left ventricular contractility improves. Although poor left ventricular function may cause underestimation of the severity of the aortic valve lesion, co-existing severe aortic incompetence will lead to an overestimation of the stenotic component if only the peak velocity in the ascending aorta is used to estimate the transvalve gradient. This problem, created by the large left ventricular stroke volume, may be circumvented by measuring the pre-valve peak velocity using pulsed Doppler and using the full modified Bernoulli equation $P_1 - P_2 = 4 (V_2^2 - V_1^2)$ which takes the pre-valve velocity into account. This will increase diagnostic accuracy. It should be remembered

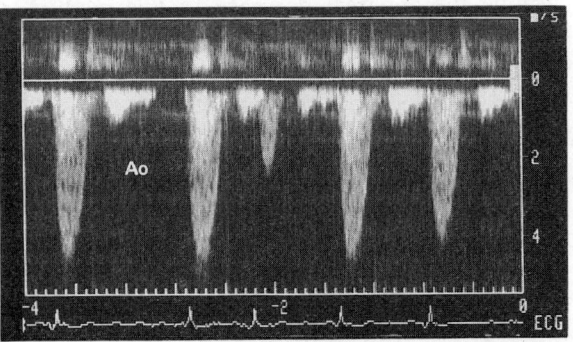

Fig. 14.6. Valvar aortic stenosis. The effect of cardiac rhythm on the instantaneous pressure gradient. In this patient with atrial fibrillation, note the variation in peak velocity and hence pressure gradient with changing R–R interval. Clearly, a mean pressure gradient should be calculated over many beats to derive a meaningful estimation of the severity of the obstruction. Ao, aorta.

however that the increased systolic transvalve flow, as the blood regurgitated in the previous diastole plus the forward cardiac output enters the aorta, truly produces an increased systolic gradient for a particular degree of stenosis. Another method of circumventing the problems inherent in the evaluation of valve stenosis in patients with either severe aortic incompetence or poor left ventricular function may be to use the continuity equation to assess the *aortic valve area*.[16-22] The continuity equation states that the net forward flow at any cross-sectional area within the heart must be equal to the net forward flow at any other cross-section. Thus, for a patient with mixed aortic valve disease, the net forward flow in the left ventricular outflow tract must equal the net forward flow over the stenotic orifice of the aortic valve. As net forward flow at a particular point is the product of the cross-sectional area at that point and the mean spatial velocity of flow across the vessel lumen at that point, then for the aortic valve

$$V.\text{LVOT} \times A.\text{LVOT} = V.\text{AoV} \times A.\text{AoV}.$$

Both *V*.LVOT and *A*.LVOT can be measured; the former using pulsed Doppler with the sample volume placed in the LVOT and the latter by measuring the LVOT dimension at the point of Doppler sampling from the cross-sectional image. *V* AoV is taken as the peak velocity of flow across the stenotic aortic orifice and is assumed to be the main spatial velocity at that point. Thus, the only unknown in the equation is the aortic valve area and this can easily be calculated from the three measurements (*V*.LVOT, *A*.LVOT and *V*.AoV) derived above. Several correlative catheter/Doppler studies have now appeared in the literature confirming the apparent accuracy of this method of deriving aortic valve area. A simplified form of the continuity equation has been suggested in which the peak velocities are substituted for the mean spatial velocities and this would appear to be equally effective in determining the area of the aortic valve orifice in clinical practice.[16]

AORTIC INCOMPETENCE[23-27]

The jet of aortic incompetence is normally easily detected by continuous wave Doppler (Fig. 14.7A, B). As all normal native aortic valves appear competent to a precordial Doppler study, any aortic incompetence recorded must be pathological. Since continuous wave Doppler is such a sensitive technique, the problem immediately arises of how to

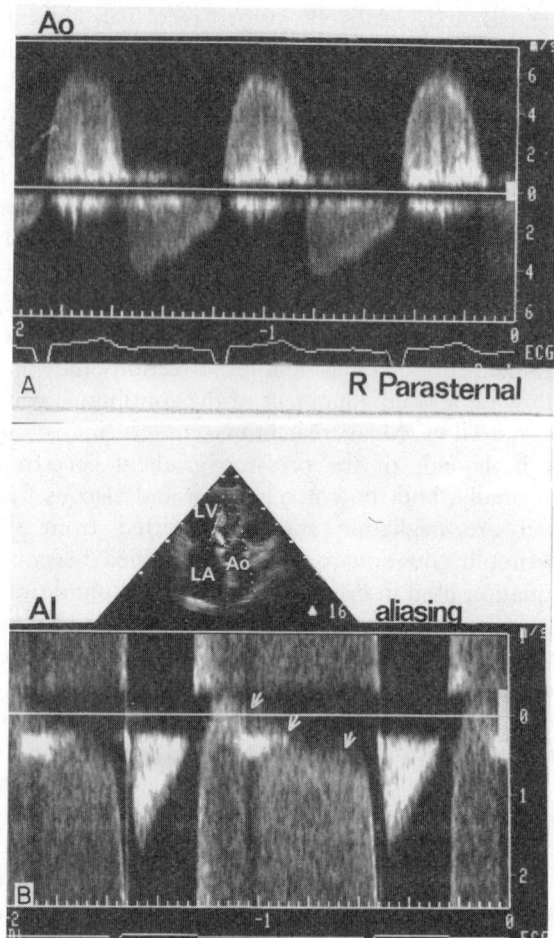

Fig. 14.7. (A) Mixed aortic valve disease (severe). Continuous wave Doppler. High right parasternal transducer position. Frequently, the highest velocity in the ascending aorta (Ao) will be recorded from this transducer position in patients with aortic stenosis. Note that the stenotic jet velocity envelope now appears above the zero velocity line as the jet is directed towards this transducer position (c.f. the apical transducer position—Figs 14.4–14.6). Maximal jet velocity = 6 m/s. Note also the aortic incompetence diastolic waveform below the zero line. (B) Aortic incompetence (mild). The upper panel is a black and white reproduction of cross-sectional image with colour flow imaging showing the regurgitant jet on the left ventricular side of the aortic valve. The lower panel shows the continuous wave recording of this jet. Waveform aliasing of continuous wave Doppler occurs. Apical transducer position. With inappropriate use of both the velocity range and zero-line positioning as in this example, aliasing can be created when using continuous wave Doppler (aliasing is normally the feature of pulsed Doppler). In this example, the diastolic waveform of aortic incompetence 'wraps itself' around the zero velocity line one time. The waveform, however, remains entirely interpretable and the maximum velocity envelope (arrowed) can still be analysed. LV, left ventricle; LA, left atrium; Ao, aorta.

assess the severity of any valve incompetence recorded. Usually the jet of aortic incompetence originates from the centre of the valve and is directed downwards and posteriorly to strike the anterior mitral valve leaflet as it opens, and is then directed down the anterior mitral leaflet to mix with mitral inflow. In severe incompetence, the turbulent jet may extend as far down as the left ventricular apex. Previous haemodynamic and angiographic studies have linked the severity of aortic incompetence to jet width and jet length, both of which reflect jet volume to some extent. In Doppler studies assessing the severity of aortic regurgitation, an attempt has been made to measure jet length and jet width and correlate these with 'non-Doppler' indices of severity; in addition, several other Doppler-derived parameters have been analysed. Initial reports on 'flow mapping' of the aortic incompetence jet used single-gate pulsed Doppler to track the 'aliased' area of flow disturbance caused by aortic incompetence within the left ventricle. This

method was accurate in experienced hands but the results were only semi-quantitative, grading aortic incompetence as mild, moderate or severe. Despite the apparent crudity of the technique and the numerous inherent pitfalls, a series of studies correlating the technique with angiography suggested that pulsed Doppler flow mapping was as accurate as cinéangiography in the assessment of aortic incompetence. The rather cumbersome flow mapping technique has now been wholly supplanted by colour flow imaging. This multigate pulsed Doppler system derives essentially the same information as 'flow mapping' in a very short time and at present it would appear to be the Doppler technique of choice in analysing aortic incompetence.[6]

Where colour flow imaging is not available, a further series of indices can be used in addition to 'flow mapping' in an attempt to determine the severity of the incompetence. Where a clear maximum velocity envelope of aortic incompetence is obtained, the 'pressure half-time' of the incompetence jet can be calculated. Clearly, the more rapid the rate of fall of the diastolic pressure gradient between aorta and left ventricle the more severe is the incompetence. In the most severe cases, equalization of pressures on either side of the aortic valve will occur during late diastole and there is no late diastolic pressure gradient. Analysis of the rate of decay of the pressure gradient (the pressure half-time) will allow a broad differentiation into mild, moderate and severe incompetence (Fig. 14.8). An aortic incompetence pressure half-time of < 250 ms with a normal heart rate is always indicative of severe incompetence. Other parameters that can provide useful additional information include:

1 the increase in forward flow velocity in the left ventricular outflow in systole due to the left ventricular volume overload;
2 the duration of diastolic flow reversal in the descending aorta (Fig. 14.9);
3 the Doppler evaluation of regurgitant fraction;
4 the signal strength of the incompetence jet (the higher the signal strength the more the incompetence).

With this spectrum of parameters to measure, it should be clear that their use in combination should and does lead to a reproducible and clinically valuable semi-quantitative estimation of aortic incompetence which at worst is equal to angiography. However, no more than subdivision into mild,

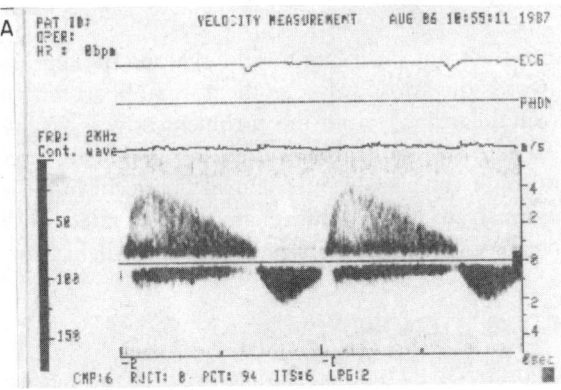

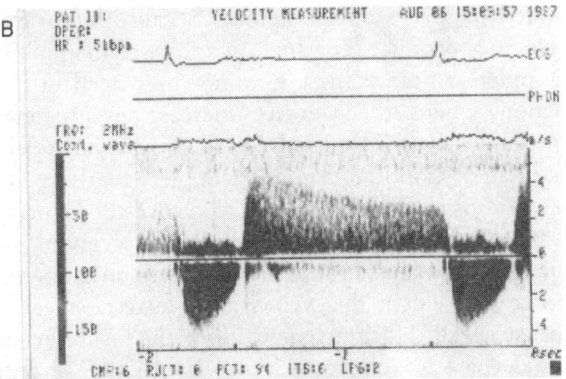

Fig. 14.8. Aortic incompetence. The value of the waveform in determining the severity of the lesion. Continuous wave Doppler. Apical transducer positions. (A) severe aortic incompetence. Note the rapid diastolic fall in the aorta/left ventricular pressure gradient to near zero by end-diastole. This is in marked contrast to the persistence of the pressure gradient during the whole of diastole (B) which is the hallmark of mild aortic incompetence.

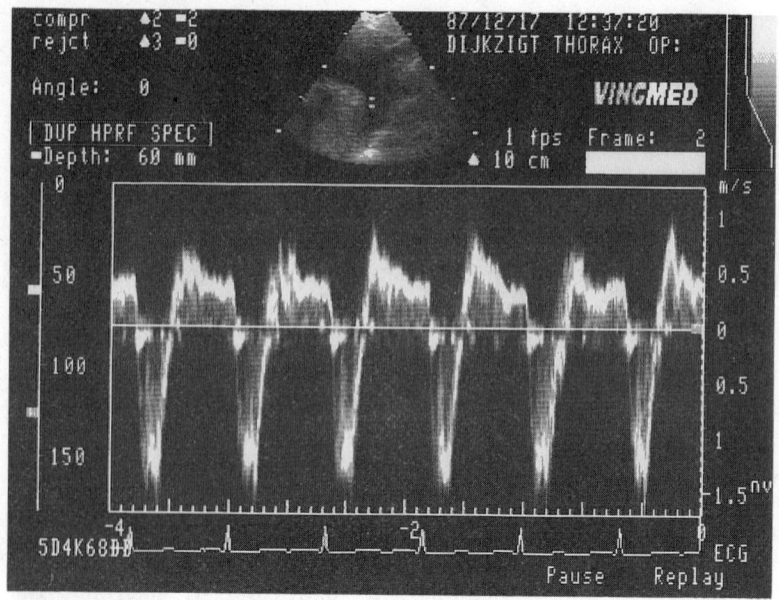

Fig. 14.9. Severe aortic incompetence. Descending aortic flow characteristics. High pulse repetition frequency mode. Suprasternal transducer position. In the normal patient, diastolic flow reversal in the descending aorta is confined to the first third of diastole. With increasing severity of aortic incompetence, this becomes a pan-diastolic event. The above flow pattern is diagnostic of severe 'run-off' from the descending aorta and in the context of aortic valve disease represents severe incompetence. The lower panel shows the high pulse repetition frequency recording; the upper panel shows the position of the sample volume in the descending aorta as seen from the suprasternal view.

moderate or severe incompetence should be attempted.

MITRAL VALVE DISEASE

NORMAL MITRAL FLOW

Both pulsed and continuous wave Doppler can be used to record normal mitral flow. Alignment to flow is best achieved by using the apical transducer position. Normal mitral flow is biphasic with an initial passive filling component occurring with left ventricular relaxation and a later active component occurring as a result of atrial contraction. The initial passive filling phase is termed the E wave and the atrial filling phase is termed the A wave. In the normal situation, the peak velocity of the E wave is always higher than that of the A wave. The normal peak velocity of flow across the mitral valve is between 0.6 and 1.3 m/s. A similar flow pattern is seen across the tricuspid valve but the mitral peak velocity is invariably higher than tricuspid velocity in the normal heaart and shows much less respiratory variation. Colour flow imaging of normal mitral flow from the apical transducer position demonstrates the red (laminar flow towards the transducer) transatrial flow entering the mitral orifice and passing down the mitral funnel to exit along the lateral wall of the left ventricular cavity and then progress downwards towards the cardiac apex. Mitral inflow then turns around in the cardiac apex and passes upwards (seen as blue, i.e. away

from the transducer laminar flow) along the septum towards the aortic valve. In the normal heart with a normal cardiac output, no turbulent flow is visualized across the mitral inflow. With rapid heart rates and high cardiac outputs, mitral flow will initially demonstrate the colour changes associated with aliasing prior to demonstrating any turbulent flow.

MITRAL STENOSIS[6,28–34]

Theoretically, Doppler should provide the perfect technique to evaluate mitral stenosis. Pulsed Doppler can record the increased flow velocities over moderately stenotic valves but it cannot be interpreted in severe mitral stenosis because high flow velocities produce 'aliasing'. In addition, the pulsed Doppler sample volume may not be placed in the region where the velocity increase is greatest; consequently, the transvalve gradient will be underestimated. Continuous wave Doppler clearly is the method of choice with which to record the velocity waveforms in mitral stenosis because it is capable of measuring the fastest velocities and will not miss the point at which the velocity is fastest since it measures all velocity changes along the beam. From the derived waveforms (Figs 14.10–14.14), several indices can be calculated using the modified Bernoulli equation. The peak diastolic gradient and the end-diastolic gradient can be measured. Both are dependent on a number of variables (i.e. heart rate, heart rhythm, transmitral volume flow, atrial compliance and left ventricular compliance). The mean diastolic gradient can be calculated by sampling at

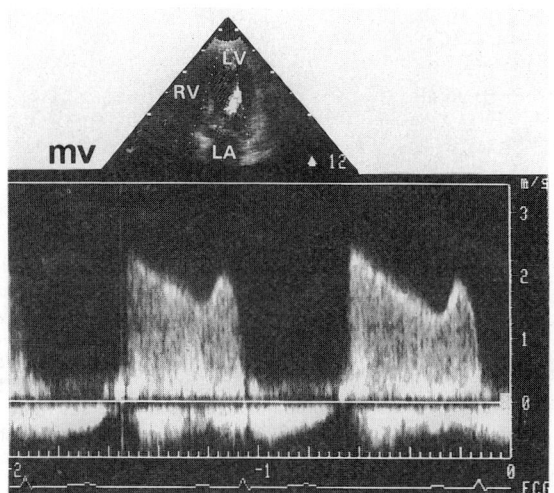

Fig. 14.10. Moderate mitral stenosis. Sinus rhythm. Continuous wave Doppler. Apical transducer position. This is the characteristic velocity waveform of mitral stenosis with the patient in sinus rhythm. Note the significant contribution that atrial contraction plays in mitral flow in late diastole, which produces a second peak in the velocity tracing. The upper panel is a black and white reproduction of a colour flow image in the same patient which shows the characteristic pattern of a mitral stenosis yet on the left ventricular side of the mitral valve (MV).

several equidistant points along the mitral diastolic flow velocity curve. The mean diastolic gradient is similarly altered by changing transmitral flow, heart rate, etc. In an attempt to minimize the effect of changing flow over the valve another measurement has been developed, that of the pressure half-time (PHT). In essence, the pressure half-time can be recorded for any transvalvar flow and represents the time taken for the initial peak pressure grdient across the valve to decrease to half its initial value. The normal range of the pressure half-time for the mitral valve is 20–60 ms. With mild mitral obstruc-

tion, the pressure half-time increases to between 80 and 180 ms; in moderate obstruction, it lies between 180 and 300 ms and with severe obstruction to > 300 ms. The pressure half-time is relatively accurate where transmitral flow is normal or only moderately increased, but it becomes increasingly prone to measurement inaccuracies as the severity of mitral stenosis increases. It is, however, less altered by flow or heart rate than either the peak or mean gradient. It will give a more accurate assessment of the stenotic component of a mitral valve abnormality in the presence of co-existing mitral regurgitation than any other index of diastolic flow. From correlative invasive catheter data, Hatle *et al.* demonstrated that the mitral valve orifice area can be derived from the pressure half-time by dividing a constant value of 220 by the derived pressure half-time (i.e. mitral valve area = 220/PHT). Correlation of valve area derived from two-dimensional imaging and Doppler with that from surgical findings suggests that Doppler-derived indices are at least as accurate as indices derived by cross-sectional imaging. Cardiac rhythm clearly has an effect on the transmitral pressure gradient. In sinus rhythm, the velocity waveform is relatively unchanging from beat to beat and representative indices for the transvalvar flow can be calculated from as few as 3–5 sequential beats. However, in the presence of atrial fibrillation or multiple atrial premature beats, the transmitral flow velocity curve will vary considerably with changing R–R interval; flow indices must be calculated as mean values derived from 10 or more consecutive beats.

Abnormal haemodynamic events other than mitral stenosis will prolong the pressure half-time.

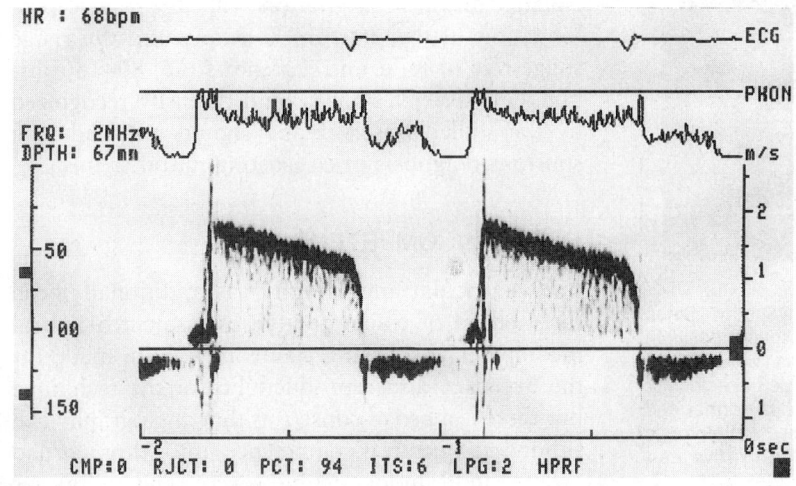

Fig. 14.11. Severe mitral stenosis. Atrial fibrillation. Pulsed Doppler. Apical transducer position. Note that in this patient there is no late diastolic velocity increase as the active atrial filling phase has been lost because of the onset of atrial fibrillation.

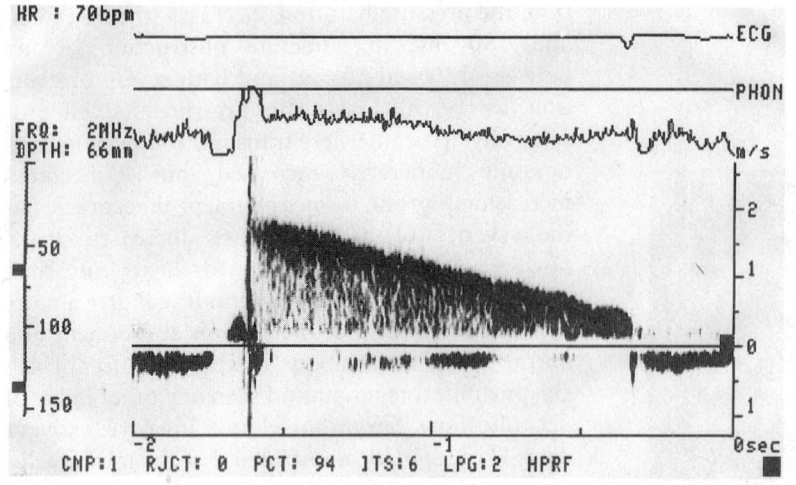

Fig. 14.12. Very severe mitral stenosis. Atrial fibrillation. Continuous wave. Apical transducer position. Note the very prolonged pressure half-time indicative of very severe mitral stenosis. The mean diastolic gradient does not appear elevated in this patient but this is due to underestimation of the maximal velocity envelope because of poor alignment of the continuous wave beam to transmitral flow.

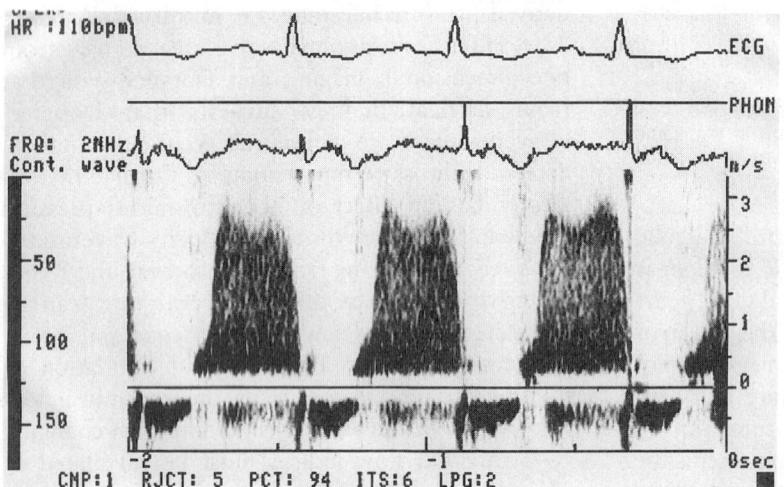

Fig. 14.13. Severe mitral stenosis. Sinus rhythm. Continuous wave Doppler. Apical transducer position. Note the very high mean diastolic gradient in this patient. This may be caused by isolated stenosis but may in part be caused by significant co-existing mitral incompetence. Calculation of the pressure half-time will normally allow a more accurate assessment of the stenotic component, than simply calculating the pressure gradient.

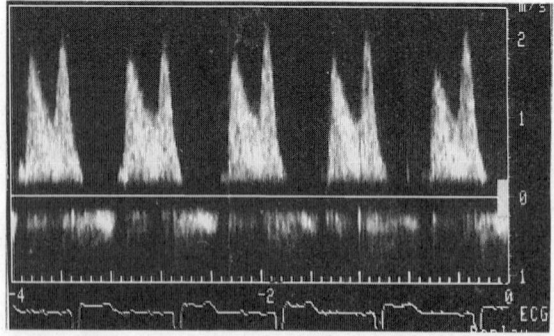

Fig. 14.14. Mitral inflow—restrictive cardiomyopathy. Sinus rhythm. Continuous wave Doppler. Apical transducer position. Note the dominant atrial active filling phase with a high end-diastolic velocity indicative of a high left ventricular end-diastolic pressure. The pressure half-time is normal and thus mitral stenosis is excluded. This velocity waveform is associated with either primary or secondary restrictive cardiomyopathy.

Severe aortic regurgitation, conditions causing abnormal left ventricular filling and significant isolated mitral regurgitation will all produce prolongation of the pressure half-time into the range suggestive of mild mitral stenosis (i.e. 80–180 ms) but these other lesions should be easily recognized by the skilled observer and should not lead to a spurious diagnosis of co-existing mitral stenosis.

MITRAL INCOMPETENCE[4,6,35]

Left ventricular angiography has traditionally been the method of choice for the assessment of mitral incompetence. Varying claims have been made for the accuracy and reproducibility of the technique but there is a broad consensus that angiography can subdivide mitral incompetence into three broad groups: mild, moderate and severe. The limitations

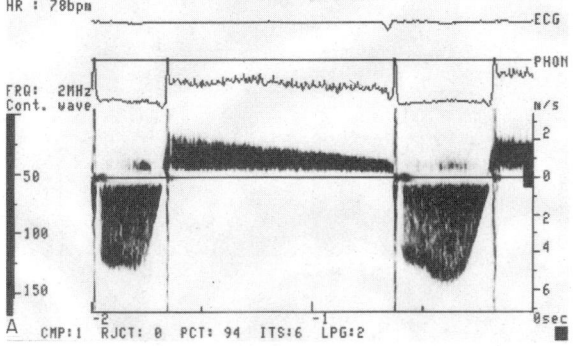

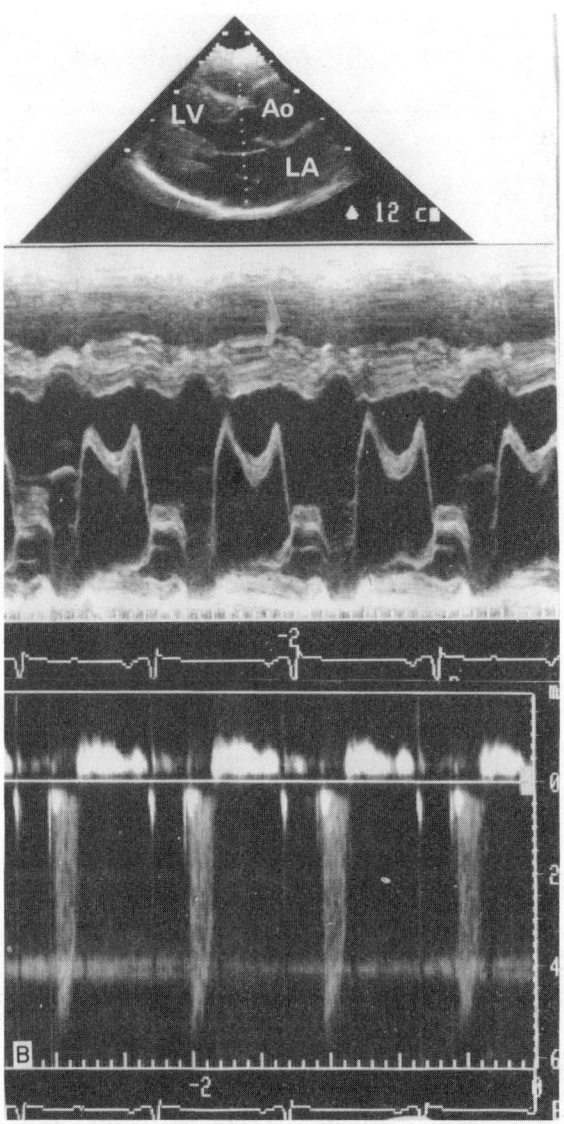

of the angiographic technique are that it is invasive, it is an assessment taken at one moment in time often with preload and afterload conditions which differ from those present in everyday life, it is significantly affected by heart rate and the presence of ectopic beats and the interpretation of the images is extremely subjective. Intra- and interobserver error variation has been demonstrated to be highly significant. What role does Doppler evaluation have in the assessment of mitral incompetence?

Continuous wave Doppler is an extremely sensitive technique for the detection of a mitral incompetence jet. Transthoracic continuous wave studies have failed to record any 'physiological' incompetence of the normal mitral valve but the results of transoesophageal continous wave studies have suggested that very small amounts of 'physiological' mitral incompetence, which is of no clinical significance, may be present in approximately 20% of apparently normal individuals selected at random. This physiological mitral incompetence recorded by transoesophageal studies in the normal individual and the mitral incompetence associated with rheumatic, ischaemic and myopathic heart disease is a holosystolic event. This contrasts markedly with the mid-to-late systolic onset of the mitral incompetence associated with mitral valve prolapse. Continuous wave Doppler will clearly demonstrate these timing differences (Fig. 14.15A, B).

The results of studies *in vitro* have suggested that continuous wave Doppler is sufficiently sensitive to detect a mitral incompetence jet of about 5–10 ml and these appear to be confirmed in clinical practice. The derived velocity waveform and peak velocity of the mitral incompetence jet reflect the changing instantaneous pressure gradient between the left ventricle and the left atrium. The waveform is constant in appearance over the range of mild-to-moderate/severe mitral incompetence, only showing a late-systolic rapid equalization of pressures when regurgitation is severe and left atrial pressure rises very rapidly. In theory, left atrial pressure should be calculable from the mitral incompetence waveform

Fig. 14.15. (A) Mixed mitral valve disease. Atrial fibrillation. Continuous wave Doppler. Apical transducer position. Severe mitral stenosis co-exists in this patient with mitral incompetence. The systolic mitral incompetence waveform is visualized below the zero velocity line. Little can be said about the severity of the mitral incompetence from this tracing. However the pan-systolic nature of the incompetence waveform is characteristic of a rheumatic or myopathic aetiology. Upper panel: cross-sectional image. Middle panel: M-mode recording at the mitral valve level shows the late systolic prolapse of the mitral valve. (B) Posterior mitral leaflet prolapse (Marfan's syndrome). Sinus rhythm. Continuous wave Doppler. Apical transducer position. Upper panel: derived M-mode. Lower panel: late systole onset of mitral regurgitation (below zero line) characteristic of mitral valve prolapse. Note the different timing and waveform of the incompetence jet compared to (A).

but in practice alignment to the jet to reduce cosine θ to zero is the major source of the significant inaccuracy in this Doppler measurement.

Although waveform changes (see above) and the signal strength of the incompetence jet can give valuable information on the severity of the lesion, the information obtained can be very misleading. Pulsed Doppler evaluation using the 'jet area mapping' technique to track the turbulent margins of the defect and thus estimate jet area increases the accuracy of the assessment but it still has major inherent limitations and potential sources of error. This rather cumbersome technique has now been totally superseded by colour flow imaging.

Colour flow imaging rivals continuous wave Doppler in its sensitivity and specificity for mitral incompetence. Moreover, it is specific for jet direction, jet width and jet length allowing a more accurate evaluation of jet area. It can demonstrate the differing jet direction associated with the different forms of mitral prolapse. In anterior leaflet prolapse, the jet can be demonstrated to be directed laterally and posteriorly whereas in posterior leaflet prolapse the jet is directed medially towards the atrial septum. These jet directions can be readily distinguished from mitral incompetence due to other causes in which the central orifice jet is normally directed superiorly and posteriorly towards the pulmonary veins.

Colour flow imaging used from the oesophageal approach gives an even more accurate assessment of the number and morphology of the regurgitant jet(s). This approach circumvents the problems inherent in the trans-thoracic approach in patients with heavily calcified native valves, or prosthetic valves which form a physical obstruction between the regurgitant flow and the transducer and thus often prevent accurate detection of such a jet.

In summary, the combined use of the different Doppler modalities can provide a non-invasive assessment of the severity of mitral incompetence equal to, or better than, left ventricular angiography. It can subdivide mitral incompetence into the same three broad groups: mild, moderate and severe; at present, precise quantification of jet volume cannot be achieved. This may become possible with future developments in estimation of jet kinetic energy derived from the colour flow images. Thus, with the appropriate use of Doppler to assess left heart valve stenosis and regurgitation a very accurate haemodynamic profile can be built up (Fig. 14.16) in multivalve disease.

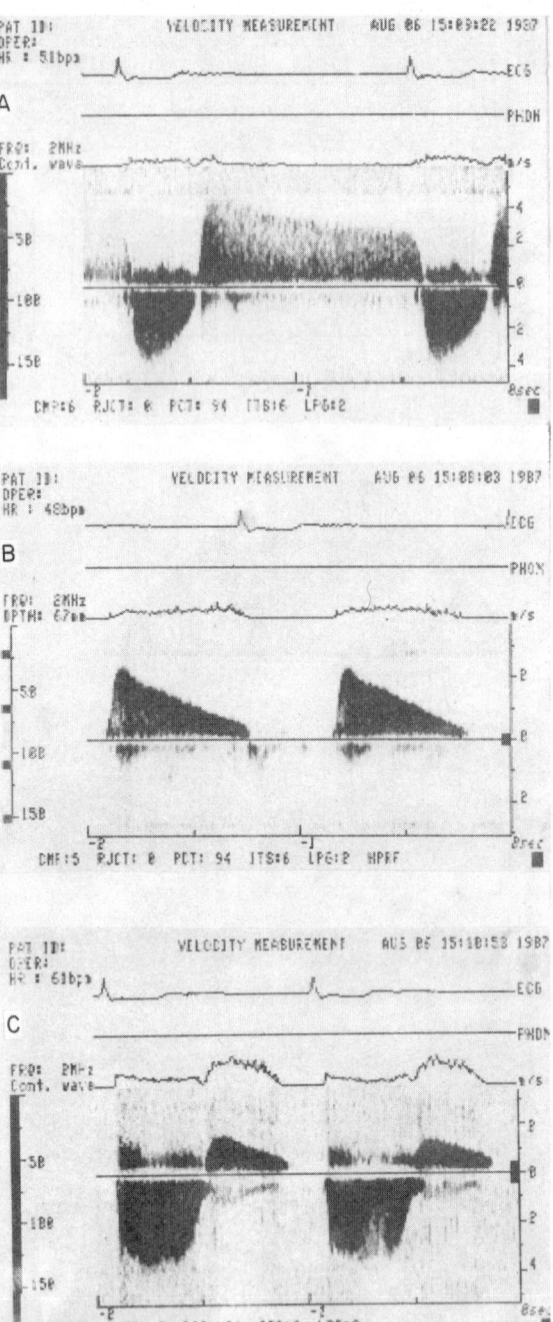

Fig. 14.16. Rheumatic heart disease. Atrial fibrillation. Continuous wave Doppler registrations of aortic (A), mitral (B) and tricuspid (C) valve velocity profile. Significant aortic stenosis is present—peak systolic velocity = 4 m/s. The aortic incompetence waveform is suggestive of mild/moderate incompetence. Moderate/severe mitral stenosis is present. The tricuspid incompetence peak jet velocity is 4 m/s. This will give a derived right ventricular peak systolic pressure of approximately 64 mmHg ($4V^2$) plus the right atrial pressure assessed clinically. This is presumed to be raised as a consequence of the severity of the left heart disease. Cardiac catheterization has little further to offer in the evaluation of the valvar lesions in this instance.

LEFT VENTRICULAR OUTFLOW TRACT OBSTRUCTION

HYPERTROPHIC OBSTRUCTIVE CARDIOMYOPATHY[36-38]

Hypertrophic obstructive cardiomyopathy is normally either an M-mode or (more reliably) a cross-sectional imaging diagnosis. The request for the ultrasound examination is commonly based on clinical suspicion but the lesion is not infrequently identified for the first time at the initial ultrasound study. The abnormal septal hypertrophy, the abnormal relationship of the anterior mitral valve leaflet and its subvalve apparatus to the left ventricular outflow tract and the abnormal appearance of the outflow tract itself are readily apparent on imaging. Involvement of the right ventricular outflow tract (frequently present in children and adolescents) in this condition is not well assessed by cross-sectional imaging. Despite the wealth of morphological detail that can be obtained by imaging, it imparts little haemodynamic information. The appearances on imaging can be identical in a patient with only a small resting left ventricular outflow tract gradient and in a patient who has a high resting gradient (e.g. in excess of 100 mmHg). Pulsed Doppler, continuous wave and colour flow imaging studies have all contributed to our understanding of the multiplicity of haemodynamic abnormalities encountered in the left ventricular inflow and outflow tracts in this complex spectrum of abnormalities. In addition, they have allowed therapeutic interventions to be assessed in a physiologic setting rather than in the artificial invasive environment of the catheter laboratory.

The Doppler hallmark of the obstructive form of this lesion is the dynamic pressure gradient present in the left ventricular outflow tract. This systolic pressure gradient differs from those found in other forms of left ventricular outflow obstruction (i.e. aortic valve stenosis, fibromuscular membranes, supravalvar stenosis) in that it is dynamic rather than fixed. The intraventricular or outflow tract pressure gardient may occur at many levels from the ventricular apex to the site of the apposition of the mitral valve anterior leaflet with the septum. It most commonly occurs at a single level but can occasionally occur at several different points. The pressure gradient across the site of obstruction characteristically increases gradually throughout systole to reach its late systole peak (Fig. 14.17). This velocity waveform is readily distinguished

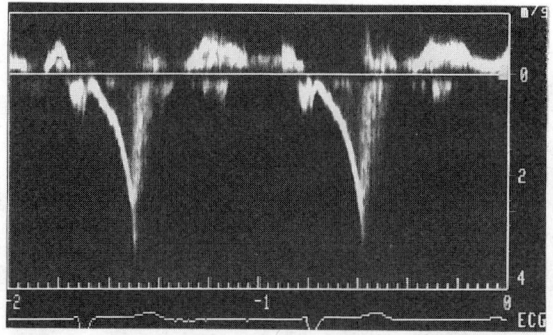

Fig. 14.17. Hypertrophic obstructive cardiomyopathy. Sinus rhythm. High pulse repetition frequency. Apical transducer position. This left ventricular outflow tract obstruction waveform (peak velocity = 3.8 m/s) is a characteristic finding in the obstructive form of this lesion. Note the gradual increase in the peak pressure drop until it achieves its late systolic peak.

from the characteristic velocity waveform of fixed left ventricular outflow obstruction (for example, Figs 14.4–14.6 and 14.18). The dynamic obstructive velocity waveform is the hallmark of a muscular obstruction which actively narrows during systole as opposed to the fixed obstructive velocity waveform which is associated with a rigid fibrous or calcified obstruction that presents an unchanging resistance to flow throughout systole. In various studies *in vivo*, which have involved correlating the dual catheter measurement of peak instantaneous dynamic pressure gradients with simultaneously recorded Doppler maximum velocity envelopes, it has been demonstrated how accurately continuous wave Doppler can measure the dynamic gradient both at rest and during exercise or during inotropic or chronotropic stimulation. Although measuring the peak instantaneous gradient, continuous wave Doppler cannot demonstrate the site of maximal obstruction because of the range ambiguity inherent in the technique. Single-gate pulsed Doppler can be used to demonstrate the low-velocity flows within the left ventricle but it will demonstrate 'aliasing' some distance before the region of maximal dynamic obstruction is approached and also for some distance after the obstruction as 'velocity shedding' takes place. Thus, pulsed Doppler is of restricted value in determining the precise site of obstruction in hypertrophic cardiomyopathy. It is in this complex analysis problem that high pulsed repetition frequency Doppler (HRPF) has its major role in cardiology. Using the inherent 'controlled' range ambiguity of this system, it is possible to scan the whole of the left and right ventricles (if the latter chamber is involved) to determine the site (or sites)

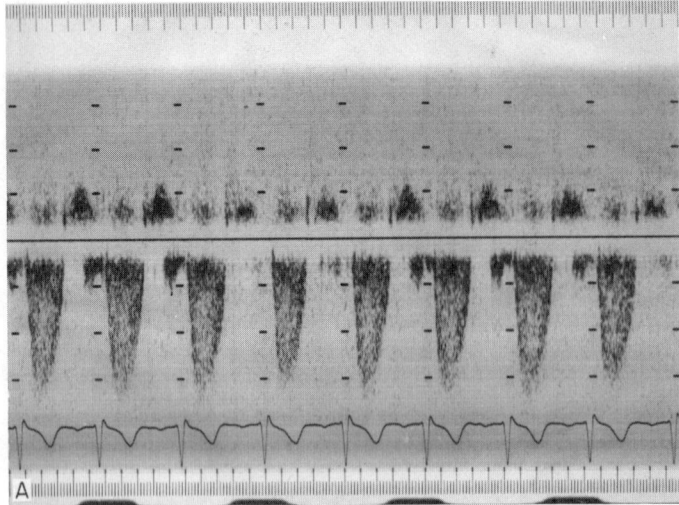
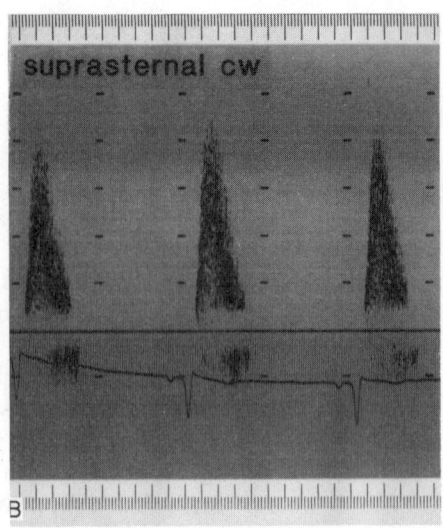

Fig. 14.18. (A) Subaortic membrane. Sinus rhythm. Continuous wave Doppler. Apical transducer position. A fixed obstruction waveform (peak velocity = 3.5 m/s). The invariably co-existing aortic incompetence is not visualised on this tracing. (B) Supravalvar aortic stenosis. Suprasternal transducer position. Continuous wave Doppler. Sinus rhythm. In this case of William's syndrome, HPRF Doppler confirmed that the peak velocity of aortic valve systolic flow was normal. Mild aortic regurgitation was present. It was only when the ascending aorta was interrogated from the suprasternal position that a high velocity jet (peak velocity = 4.5 m/s) suggestive of a severe supravalve stenosis was recorded. Subsequent aortography confirmed the diagnosis.

of obstruction and to determine the precise intracavitary gradient at each site interrogated. Colour flow imaging has added much to the investigation of these patients by clearly demonstrating the site(s) of turbulence (i.e. the sites of obstruction) within the left ventricle. It also demonstrates the direction of the jet originating from these obstructions and thus allows accurate alignment of the continuous wave beam to the obstructive jet so that a more accurate measurement of the pressure gradient can be obtained. Where combined continuous wave and colour flow imaging studies demonstrate no flow disturbance within the left ventricle, it is safe to assume that the patient has no resting gradient.

Many other inherent associated complex flow abnormalities can be demonstrated using pulsed Doppler. Mitral inflow is frequently abnormal due to the abnormal relaxation of the hypertrophied left ventricular myocardium. The pressure half-time of the mitral valve flow is frequently prolonged to values between 60 and 120 ms (normal < 60 ms), the increase in pressure half-time being directly related to the degree to which left ventricular function is impaired. In addition, in patients in sinus rhythm, there is frequently an abnormally marked increase in late diastolic flow velocity through the mitral valve resulting from atrial contraction. These changes are non-specific and are encountered across the spectrum of patients with hypertrophied ventri-

cles. Pulsed Doppler can similarly demonstrate the abnormalities of ascending aortic flow present in the obstructive forms of this lesion. The peak velocity of flow is frequently elevated to 1.5–2.0 m/s and the velocity curve is abnormal with flow occurring predominatly in early systole. With increasing intraventricular obstruction, late systolic aortic flow is progressively reduced. A major problem in the measurement of the intracavitary gradient in this lesion is the misinterpretation of the mitral regurgitant jet (almost invariably present) for the dynamic obstructive velocity waveform. These two jets are normally very closely aligned to the apical or low parasternal interrogating continuous wave beam and are frequently superimposed upon one another. Colour flow imaging allied to a steerable continuous wave beam will normally circumvent this difficult problem by allowing accurate alignment of the continuous wave Doppler and thus separate interrogation of each discrete flow disturbance.

OTHER FORMS OF LEFT VENTRICULAR OUTFLOW TRACT OBSTRUCTION

Cross-sectional imaging remains the diagnostic technique in defining the morphology of left ventricular outflow obstruction. With good image quality, it will normally readily distinguish valvar from subvalvar obstruction. It is only in the context of supravalvar aortic obstruction that transthoracic ultrasound may fail to define the exact morphology of the obstruction. Transoesophageal studies will now provide all the morphological information required for diagnosis in such patients.

Left ventricular outflow tract obstruction can exist in three main forms: hypertrophic cardiomyopathy, a discrete subaortic fibrous membrane and a fibromuscular tunnel. Cross-sectional imaging will define which of these entities is present but rarely gives any indication of the severity of the obstruction present. Continuous wave Doppler can accurately measure the peak instantaneous gradient over the obstruction caused by either a subaortic membrane or a tunnel. High pulsed repetition frequency Doppler can be used to determine the site of the maximal subvalvar obstruction and to exclude any co-existing valve obstruction (mild-to-moderate co-existing aortic incompetence is invariably present in patients with subaortic membranes but it is less common in patients with fibromuscular tunnels). Both a subaortic membrane and a fibromuscular tunnel give rise to a fixed obstruction waveform (Fig. 14.18A) but the time of onset to peak obstruction is delayed when compared with an obstruction of similar severity at aortic valve level. These lesions thus lie in the middle of a spectrum between a fixed and a dynamic obstruction. Colour flow imaging can be of great help in defining a subvalvar obstruction in patients in whom cross-sectional imaging is non-diagnostic by demonstrating the location of the subvalvar area of turbulent flow. Where supravalvar aortic stenosis is present, this may be missed on imaging because of poor visualization of the ascending aorta. Continuous wave Doppler from the precordial approach can fail to record the high-velocity jet associated with the supravalvar obstruction and will record only normal transaortic valve systolic velocities. The suprasternal position should be used to align the continuous wave beam to the ascending aortic jet, and the peak velocity recorded will normally accurately reflect the severity of the obstruction (Fig. 14.18B). Mild-to-moderate co-existing aortic valve incompetence is an almost invariable finding in this lesion.

PULMONARY VALVE ABNORMALITIES

PULMONARY STENOSIS[39]

Valvar pulmonary stenosis is a common lesion in

paediatric cardiology but is more rarely encountered in adult practice. It may exist as an isolated lesion or be part of a more complex right ventricular outflow tract obstructive lesion such as that seen in tetralogy of Fallot. Continuous wave Doppler is equally as effective in assessing isolated pulmonary valve stenosis as it is in assessing valvar aortic stenosis. The main difference lies in the examination technique. In young children, a subcostal transducer position is frequently the most effective in recording the highest velocities but in every case the pulmonary valve should be studied from multiple precordial and suprasternal positions to ensure that the maximal velocity envelope has been recorded. A similar examination technique will normally accurately record the gradient across a surgically placed pulmonary artery band. In virtually all cases of pulmonary valve stenosis or pulmonary artery banding, a co-existing diastolic jet of pulmonary incompetence will be recorded using continuous wave Doppler (Fig. 14.19). Colour flow imaging will normally confirm that this is a trivial lesion by identifying short jet width and short jet length. Care must be taken when assessing pulmonary valve flow

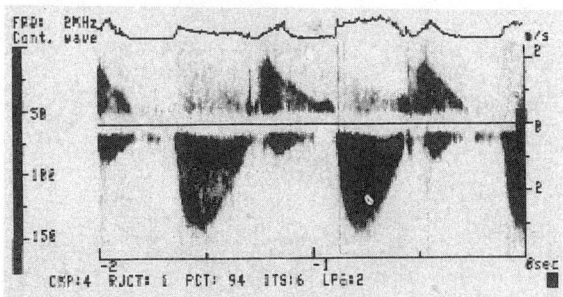

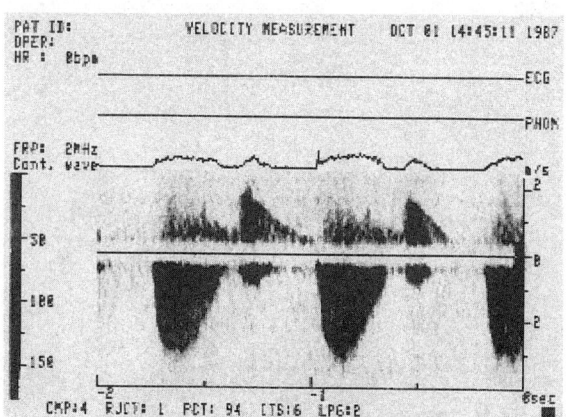

Fig. 14.19. Combined mild valvar pulmonary stenosis and incompetence (top and bottom tracings). Sinus rhythm. Continuous wave Doppler. Mild left parasternal position. These two lesions virtually always co-exist. The pulmonary incompetence is invariably mild.

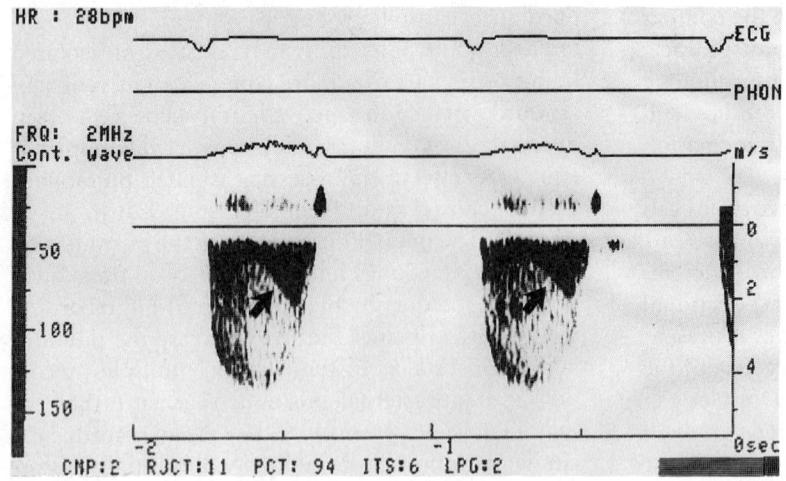

Fig. 14.20. Dominant valvar pulmonary stenosis with secondary infundibular obstruction. Continuous wave. Subcostal transducer position. Note the fixed obstruction waveform (peak velocity = 4.6 m/s) of valvar pulmonary stenosis. Within this velocity envelope (arrow) a second velocity waveform has been recorded (peak velocity = 2 m/s) which has the characteristic dynamic obstructive waveform. This represents the secondary infundibular dynamic obstruction which is almost invariably present in the right ventricular outflow tract in patients with severe valvar pulmonary stenosis or tetralogy of Fallot.

in a patient with a large left-to-right intracardiac shunt. In such cases, pulmonary stenosis is normally more apparent than real and is caused by the abnormally large amount of flow crossing the normal pulmonary valve. Where such an intracardiac shunt is suspected, it is essential to determine the pre-valve peak flow velocity. This is frequently elevated and must be taken into consideration when using the modified Bernoulli equation to calculate the transpulmonary pressure gradient. Frequently dynamic subpulmonary obstruction is present in cases of pulmonary stenosis (Fig. 14.20). This may be either an intrinsic part of an associated cardiac lesion (as in tetralogy of Fallot) or a secondary acquired lesion due to the severity of the more distal valve obstruction. Every study of the right ventricular outflow tract should include a careful search for dynamic subpulmonary obstruction. The relative severity of multilevel obstruction can be assessed by using high pulsed repetition frequency Doppler. Colour flow imaging is of value in aiding the correct alignment of continuous wave Doppler to flow.

PULMONARY INCOMPETENCE[40–42]

Trivial pulmonary incompetence is a normal physiological finding in more than 40% of the normal healthy population. This has been clearly demonstrated in both continuous wave and colour flow imaging studies. The onset of regurgitation is early diastolic and persists to the end of diastole. Physiological pulmonary incompetence is of low velocity (i.e. peak velocity 2 m/s reflecting the normal low diastolic pressure drop that exists between the pulmonary artery and the right ventricle. The waveform changes with respiration (Fig. 14.21). Colour flow imaging will identify a narrow nonturbulent high-velocity 'flame-like' jet which originates at the point of diastolic valve leaflet coaptation and is directed downwards about 1–2 cm towards the ventriculo-infundibular fold. This physiological jet never extends to the apex of the right ventricle.

The differentiation of physiological incompetence from mild pathological incompetence is difficult. However, where right ventricular pressure is nor-

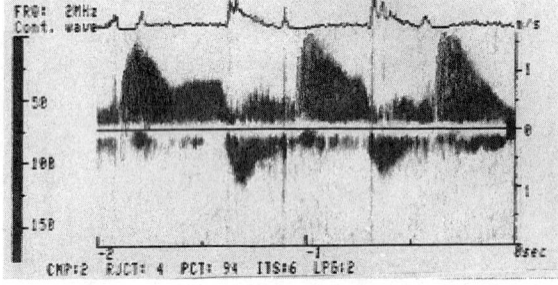

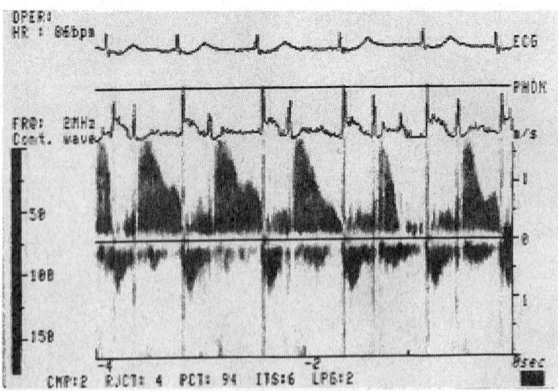

Fig. 14.21. Physiological pulmonary incompetence. Vary diastolic waveforms. Continuous wave Doppler. Mid-left parasternal position. This demonstrates normal physiological pulmonary incompetence (above the zero line). Note the low peak velocity (< 2 m/s) and the respiratory variation in the diastolic waveform which is characteristic of normal pulmonary haemodynamics.

mal, a mid-diastolic equalization of the pulmonary artery and right ventricular pressures on the continuous wave tracing with cessation of the regurgitant signal is suggestive of at least moderate incompetence. Colour flow imaging gives the most accurate assessment of the severity of pulmonary incompetence by visualizing both the breadth and extension of the incompetence jet.

The peak velocity, the end-diastolic velocity and the pulmonary incompetence waveform potentially can give useful information on pulmonary artery pressure and pulmonary vascular resistance. The peak pulmonary artery–right ventricular pressure difference occurs at the onset of diastole. At this point, right ventricular pressure is almost zero and therefore the pressure difference measured will approximate to the early diastolic pressure in the pulmonary artery. The end-diastolic pressure in the pulmonary artery can be estimated in a similar way. Where pulmonary artery pressure is very elevated and pulmonary resistance is irreversibly high, the velocity of the pulmonary incompetence jet is high throughout diastole with no end-diastolic fall. Although the pulmonary incompetence waveform is of value in the detection of both raised pulmonary artery pressure and pulmonary vascular resistance, it is not sufficiently accurate to replace precise evaluation of pulmonary vascular resistance by cardiac catheterization.

TRICUSPID VALVE

NORMAL TRICUSPID VALVE

Doppler signals from diastolic flow across the tricuspid valve are best recorded with the transducer positioned either apically or between the apex and the lower left sternal edge (the subcostal transducer position rarely allows the transducer beam to be aligned to flow and should not be used unless the precordial approach is unsatisfactory).

The normal tricuspid diastolic flow pattern, like the normal mitral diastolic flow pattern, is biphasic; the initial peak occurs immediately after tricuspid valve opening and the second peak occurs as a result of atrial systole. In either the pre-term or term infant with persistence of the fetal vascular resistance or with parenchymal lung disease, the second peak caused by atrial contraction is dominant and may achieve a peak velocity about 2–3 times that of initial peak velocity as a result of the increased atrial contractility required to drive blood into the hyper-

trophied and non-compliant right ventricle. This dominance of atrial filling rapidly disappears with the reduction in right ventricular pressure as pulmonary vascular resistance falls. By 1 year of age, the initial peak velocity is the higher of the two and this situation then holds true for the diastolic flow profile throughout the rest of normal life. Another characteristic of normal tricuspid flow (and one that differentiates it from mitral flow) is the marked variation in flow velocity and flow profile with normal respiration. Inspiration increases tricuspid flow velocities throughout diastole whereas expiration decreases them. It should be noted that maximal tricuspid diastolic velocity recorded in the normal heart will always be less than the maximal diastolic velocity recorded across the mitral valve because the tricuspid orifice is invariably greater in size than the mitral orifice while mean flow across both is the same. Tricuspid peak velocity is normally some two-thirds of mitral peak velocity. The normal range of tricuspid flow velocities is 0.5–0.8 m/s in children and 0.3–0.7 m/s in adults (tricuspid velocities either should be measured midway through the respiratory cycle or should be averaged over 3–5 complete respiratory cycles).

PHYSIOLOGICAL TRICUSPID INCOMPETENCE[40,43–50]

Prior to the introduction of Doppler studies, clinical examination and right ventricular angiography suggested that the normal tricuspid valve is a competent structure. However, with the use of increasingly sophisticated spectral analysis, continuous wave Doppler has demonstrated the tricuspid valve to be 'physiologically' incompetent in between 35 and 46% of normal individuals. What then is meant by 'physiologically incompetent'? First, it should be stressed that this is a normal finding and does not indicate any intrinsic tricuspid valve dysfunction. Physiological tricuspid incompetence is most easily recorded by continuous wave Doppler. The less sensitive pulsed Doppler mode fails to record the tricuspid waveforms in a significant number of patients in whom continuous wave succeeds. It is probably best for the inexperienced operator to record the systolic waveform representative of tricuspid incompetence using Duplex continuous wave Doppler because the jet of physiological tricuspid incompetence is constant in both its site of origin from the tricuspid valve and the direction of its extension into the right atrium. To record tricuspid incompetence, the inlet of the heart should be imaged and the tricuspid orifice, right atrium and interatrial septum identified. In this position, the jet of 'physiological incompetence' will commencce at the central point of systolic tricuspid leaflet coaptation and will be directed 1–3 cm posteriorly into the right atrium towards the lower third of the atrial septum (the jet extension or 'jet length' can be confirmed by tracking it back into the atrium using pulsed Doppler or by visualizing its extension using colour flow imaging). The normal physiological tricuspid incompetence waveform is pan-systolic with the peak velocity recorded between one-third and halfway through systole. The complete velocity envelope with a clear maximal velocity should be obtained prior to any assessment of the trans-tricuspid pressure drop being attempted.

'Physiological' tricuspid incompetence is difficult to record in the pré-term and newborn infant. The incidence with which 'physiological' tricuspid incompetence can be recorded increases to a peak in adolescence and thereafter remains unchanged. The peak velocity of the tricuspid incompetence jet can be used to estimate the peak systolic pressure in the right ventricle in every case in which it is clearly recorded. Many authors have confirmed this finding by simultaneous Doppler/catheter studies. With normal right ventricular pressure (i.e. a systolic pressure < 30 mmHg), the peak velocity of the tricuspid incompetence jet will be between 1.7 and 2.5 m/s. It is frequently of great practical value in the assessment of cardiac or respiratory disease to record a tricuspid incompetence peak velocity in the normal range and, hence, be certain that the right heart pressures are normal.[44–47]

PHYSIOLOGICAL VERSUS PATHOLOGICAL TRICUSPID INCOMPETENCE

To determine whether tricuspid incompetence is physiological or mildly pathological using Doppler is a problem. Less difficulty is encountered when distinguishing physiological from moderately severe pathological tricuspid incompetence. However, although well-defined problem areas do exist, the Doppler modalities may be used to assess the severity of tricuspid incompetence with reasonable accuracy. Several methods may be of value in assessing its severity:

1   the systolic velocity waveform;
2   the signal strength of the regurgitant jet;
3   the extension of the tricuspid incompetence jet into the right atrium, inferior vena cava and hepatic veins;
4   the jet width;
5   the volume of the jet estimated by colour flow imaging;
6   the diastolic tricuspid flow velocity waveform.

If tricuspid incompetence (either pathological or physiological) is present in an adolescent or adult, the skilled examiner should be able to identify systolic backflow from right ventricle to right atrium in virtually every case using continuous wave Doppler. Where tricuspid incompetence is physiological, the peak velocity of the incompetence jet will be < 2.5 m/s (i.e. right ventricular peak systolic pressure will be normal). However, in up to 40% of cases where a tricuspid incompetence signal is recorded, a complete velocity envelope may not be obtained and uncertainty may exist as to the precise peak systolic velocity. With an increase in tricuspid incompetence from a mild to a moderate degree, the systolic waveform will remain the same but the signal strength will normally increase. Where tricuspid incompetence is physiological, the incompetence jet can normally be 'tracked back' only about 2–3 cm into the right atrium using pulsed Doppler. The physiological incompetence jet never extends to the superior atrial wall. No abnormal flow disturbance will be noted in the hepatic veins or inferior vena cava. Finally, colour flow mapping can readily determine the origin, length and width of the physiological incompetence jet, thereby clearly distinguishing this from significant pathological tricuspid incompetence.

PATHOLOGICAL TRICUSPID INCOMPETENCE (FIGS. 14.22 AND 14.23)

Pathological tricuspid incompetence has many causes. It may occur as a result of organic tricuspid valve disease, such as Ebstein's anomaly or rheumatic carditis, or secondary to endocarditis. It is commonly found in patients with complete heart block. It is frequently present following right ventricular infarction (this latter group may either have normal or elevated right heart systolic pressures). Finally, tricuspid incompetence may be secondary to either acute or chronic elevation of the right ventricular systolic pressure. In a study of 416 patients with a broad spectrum of left heart disease, the incidence of moderate-to-severe tricuspid incompetence increased with the severity of the left heart disease, being present in 96% of those with

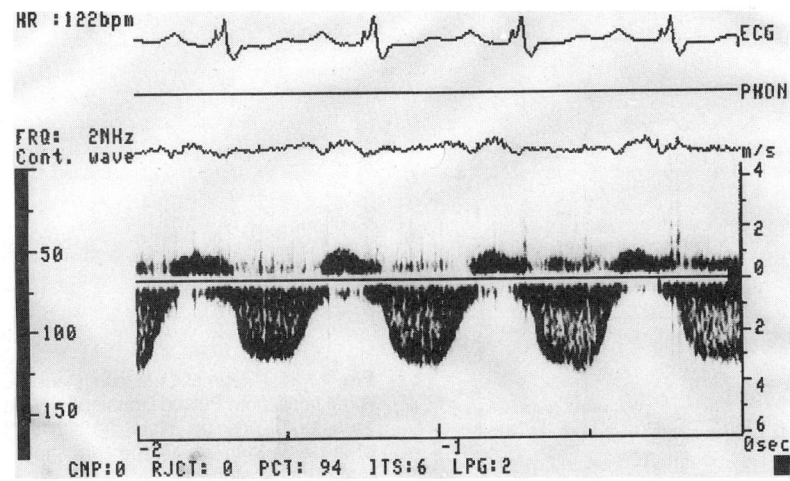

Fig. 14.22. Tricuspid incompetence. Sinus rhythm. Continuous wave Doppler. Low parasternal position. This represents mild pathological tricuspid incompetence secondary to raised right heart pressure. The waveform is normal but the signal intensity is increased. The peak systolic velocity is increased at 3.4 m/s which gives a calculated right ventricular/right atrium peak systolic pressure difference in excess of 45 mmHg. Assuming a mean right atrial pressure of 5 mmHg, the peak right ventricular systolic pressure will be in excess of 50 mmHg. If Doppler confirms normal pulmonary flow with no right ventricular outflow tract pressure gradient, 50 mmHg can be assumed to be the peak systolic pulmonary artery pressure.

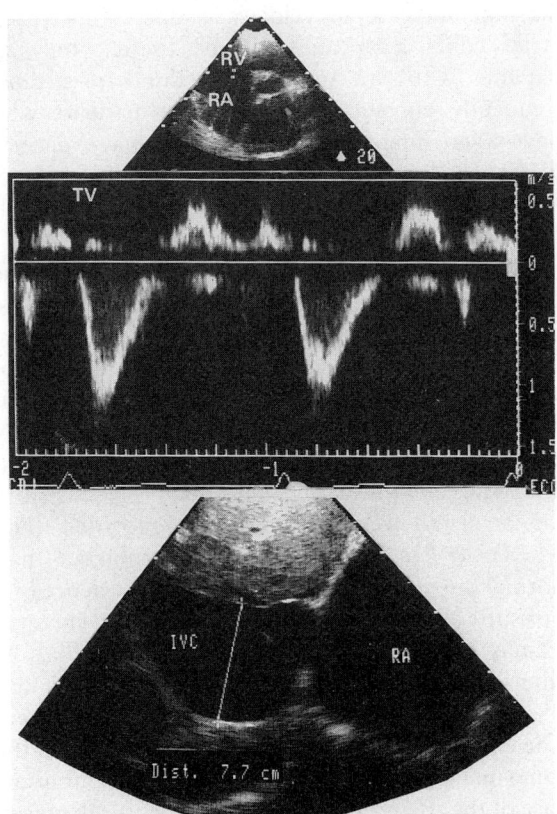

Fig. 14.23. Severe tricuspid incompetence due to an intrinsic abnormality of the tricuspid valve. HPRF Doppler. Low left parasternal position. Upper panel: in contrast to Fig. 14.22, the tricuspid incompetence waveform here demonstrates a rapid late systolic equalization of atrial and ventricular pressure indicative of free tricuspid regurgitation. Note the low peak velocity of the waveform (< 1.5 m/s) indicative of normal right ventricular pressure. Lower panel: note the extremely dilated inferior vena cava which has resulted from prolonged severe tricuspid regurgitation. RV, right ventricle; RA, right atrium; TV, tricuspid valve; IVC, inferior vena cava.

severe ischaemic or valvar left heart disease irrespective of the lesion. It should be emphasized that severe tricuspid incompetence may occur in the setting of a normal or an elevated right ventricular pressure; the latter is the more common finding.

Which Doppler findings are of most value in distinguishing physiological from pathological tricuspid incompetence? Pathological incompetence will normally be associated with an increase in signal strength of the incompetence jet thus making it easier to record. However, this is not an invariable finding and in cases where right atrial and right ventricular pressures are virtually equal (e.g. in severe Ebstein's anomaly) and where cardiac output is low, the tricuspid incompetence signal may be difficult to record despite the severity of the incompetence. Pathological incompetence is frequently, but not invariably, associated with an elevation in the peak systolic jet velocity to values > 2.6 m/s (indicating an elevated right ventricular systolic pressure). Where incompetence is severe and there is an early equalization of right ventricular and right atrial pressures, a characteristic late systolic change in the incompetence waveform occurs (Fig. 14.23). This invariably indicates severe tricuspid incompetence. Another change in the tricuspid incompetence waveform may co-exist if severe right ventricular dysfunction is the direct cause of the pathological incompetence. In this situation, the initial rate of rise in the velocity waveform may be reduced when compared with that in the patient with normal ventricular function. The incompetence waveform may be similarly altered when caused by ventricular premature beats. Although peak velocity, systolic waveform and

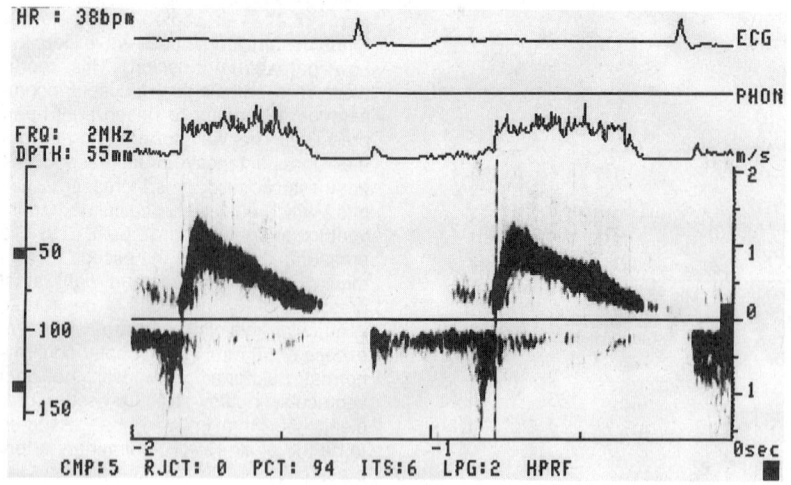

Fig. 14.24. Rheumatic tricuspid stenosis. Atrial fibrillation. Pulsed Doppler. Low left parasternal position. Note the similarity of the waveform (above the zero line) to that of mitral stenosis.

signal strength are of value in assessing the severity and cause of the tricuspid incompetence, all may be misleading. The experienced echocardiographer can often derive more clinically useful information from determining jet length and jet width within the right atrium and jet extension into the inferior vena cava and hepatic veins. A tricuspid incompetence jet tracked back to the superior atrial wall or into the hepatic veins using pulsed Doppler invariably indicates severe tricuspid incompetence. Colour flow imaging has greatly assisted this evaluation.

ABNORMAL TRICUSPID DIASTOLIC FLOW VELOCITIES AND WAVEFORMS

The peak velocity of diastolic flow across the tricuspid valve may be increased to abnormal values by several factors. The most common of these is the increased flow across a structurally normal valve, best exemplified by the pan-diastolic velocity increase associated with the left-to-right atrial shunt of an atrial septal defect. Such high tricuspid flows increase velocity throughout diastole, but they have their major effect on early diastolic velocities, with the peak velocity in some cases reaching twice normal values. Such flows do not alter the calculated pressure half-time. In addition, high-flow situations tend to eliminate the respiratory variation in the tricuspid waveform that occurs with normal flow. An abnormally increased tricuspid velocity in early diastole, higher than that of the mitral valve at the corresponding point in diastole, is strong evidence of a significant atrial shunt. Tricuspid peak velocity may also be abnormally increased in late diastole in patients who have either severe tricuspid stenosis (a very rare lesion) or non-compliant

usually hypertrophic right ventricles. This late-diastolic increase in velocity is due to increased atrial contraction and will be present only in patients who are in sinus rhythm. It is most frequently encountered in younger patients who have severe lung disease, severe pulmonary vascular disease or severe right ventricular outflow tract obstruction. It is less commonly found in adult patients.

Doppler is probably the most sensitive technique available with which to diagnose tricuspid stenosis. Cross-sectional imaging is unreliable in diagnosing this entity, and frequently dual high-fidelity manometer tip catheter studies are misleading. Continuous wave and pulsed Doppler are equally effective in ascertaining the diagnosis. When tricuspid stenosis is present, it is normally obvious from the tricuspid velocity waveform recorded (Fig. 14.24). Tricuspid diastolic velocities higher than normal are recorded with abnormal persistence of a pressure gradient throughout diastole. There is usually a slow decrease in velocity during diastole similar to that encountered in mitral stenosis and the pressure half-time is significantly prolonged. The calculated mean pressure drop is derived in the same manner as that for the mitral valve, but in the case of the tricuspid valve lower values for the mean pressure drop (i.e. > 3 mmHg) can be taken to represent severe obstruction. Increases in the mean pressure drop are normally particularly noticeable during inspiration and fall with expiration. It is probably best to estimate the mean pressure drop and pressure half-time in mid respiratory cycle, taking the average of 5 such beats. Isolated tricuspid incompetence may increase the mean pressure drop in patients with tricuspid valve disease, but neither the velocity waveform nor the pressure half-time will suggest tricuspid stenosis.

TRICUSPID VALVE PROSTHESES

All tricuspid prostheses, whether mechanical or bioprosthetic, are mildly stenotic. Each will have its own flow characteristics including velocity profile, normal mean pressure drop and pressure half-time. In each case, these should be recorded following operation; prosthetic function should then be monitored at appropriate time-intervals in the postoperative period. The criteria used for the diagnosis of tricuspid prosthetic stenosis are similar to those assessed when evaluating native tricuspid valve stenosis and are clearly defined above.

VENTRICULAR SEPTAL DEFECTS[51–58]

Ventricular septal defects should be subdivided into two distinct haemodynamic groups when considering the information derived by Doppler.

1 Restrictive defects in which a pressure gradient exists across the ventricular septum in systole;
2 Non-restrictive defects in which peak systolic pressure is equal in the two ventricles.

Single or multiple ventricular septal defects may occur in either haemodynamic group.

RESTRICTIVE DEFECTS

Continuous wave Doppler will invariably record a high-velocity trans-septal jet in such lesions (Fig. 14.25). The derived peak velocity may vary from 2 to 5 m/s and when the interrogating Doppler beam is correctly aligned to flow this peak velocity is directly related to the trans-septal pressure gradient. The results of many studies have now confirmed the accuracy with which continuous wave Doppler can estimate the right ventricular peak systolic pressure in patients with these lesions in the absence of any left ventricular outflow tract obstruction (Fig. 14.26). This parameter can be derived in the following manner. If the systolic blood pressure is known (normally recorded from the right arm using a sphygmomanometer cuff) and continuous wave Doppler confirms normal left ventricular outflow and trans-aortic flow, the left ventricular peak systolic pressure can be assumed to equal the systolic blood pressure. The modified Bernoulli equation can then be used to derive the trans-septal

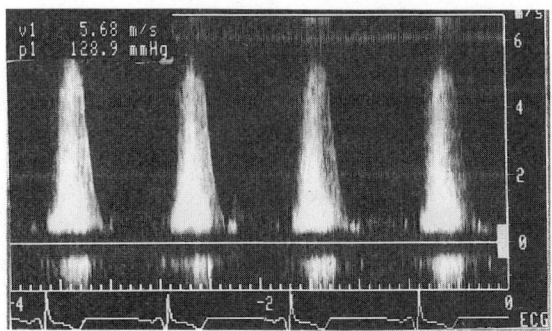

Fig. 14.25. The characteristic systolic jet of a small restrictive ventricular septal defect. Continuous wave Doppler. Mid-left parasternal position. Peak jet velocity = 5.1 m/s. Derived interventricular pressure gradient = 129 mmHg. As the right arm systolic blood pressure was 140 mmHg at the time of the recording (= left ventricular systolic pressure), the right ventricular peak systolic pressure will be approximately 11 mmHg (140–129 mmHg). No diastolic shunting has been recorded in this instance (in the majority of restrictive ventricular septal defects diastolic left to right shunting will be recorded).

gradient. Subtraction of the trans-septal gradient from the left ventricular peak systolic pressure (= right arm systolic pressure as Doppler has confirmed no left ventricular outflow obstruction exists) will derive the right ventricular peak systolic pressure. Once this has been derived, Doppler analysis of the flow over the right ventricular outflow tract will allow peak systolic pulmonary artery pressure to be calculated. A useful check on the reliability of the estimation of the right ventricular peak systolic pressure would be to evaluate right ventricular pressure using the peak velocity of the normally co-existing tricuspid incompetence. Unfortunately, this is not possible because the interrogating continuous wave beam must cross the disturbed flow in the right ventricular flow resulting from the ventricular septal defect jet. This leads to ambiguity in the interpretation of any co-existing tricuspid incompetence signal.

Many authors have suggested that Doppler can accurately evaluate the Qp:Qs ratio where a significant left-to-right intracardiac shunt exists. For a ventricular septal defect, this is dependent on accurate Doppler measurement of the volume flow in both the aorta (or left ventricular outflow tract) and the main pulmonary artery. For any vessel, pulsed Doppler in theory can derive the mean spatial flow velocity whereas cross-sectional imaging can measure its dimension at the site where the mean velocity was sampled. From these indices, volume flow in the pulmonary and systemic circuit can be calculated. Despite many theoretical and

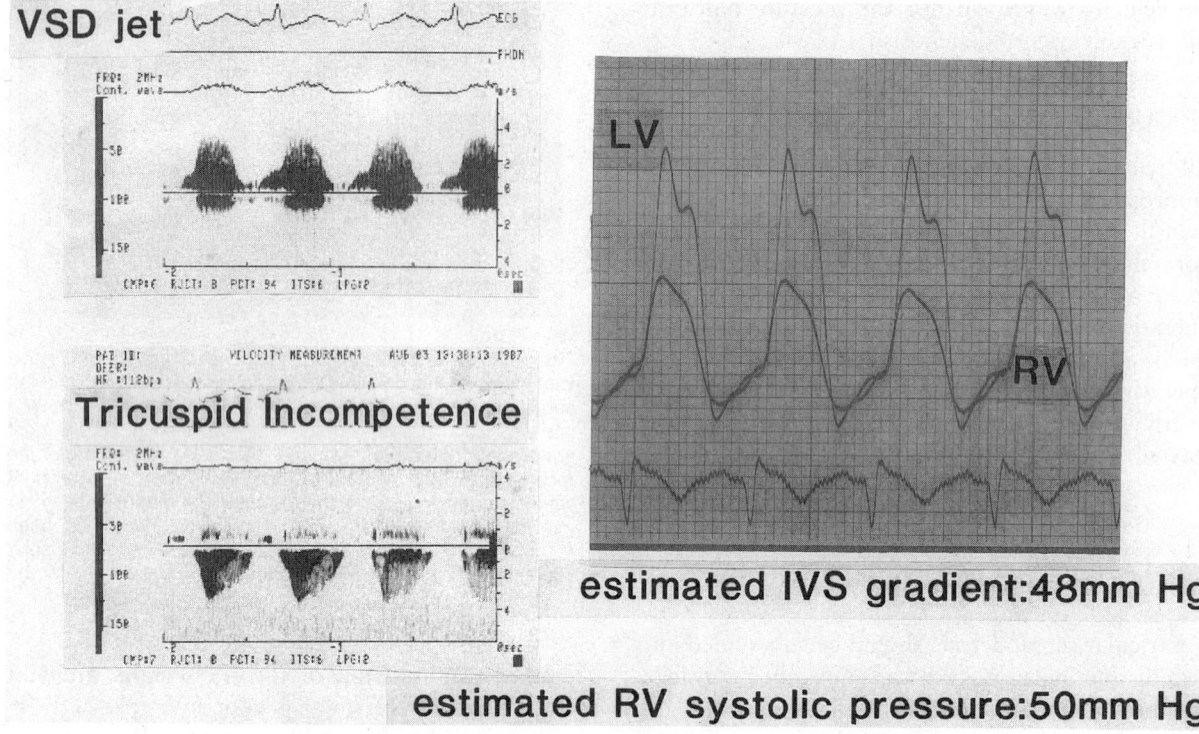

Fig. 14.26. The haemodynamic evaluation of a post-infarction ventricular septal defect. Continuous wave Doppler. Upper left panel: the characteristic ventricular septal defect jet. Peak velocity = 3.6 m/s. This gives an estimated interventricular pressure gradient of 48 mmHg. This is confirmed by the simultaneous peak instantaneous interventricular pressure gradient derived at cardiac catheterization (right panel). Lower left panel: the tricuspid incompetence waveform demonstrates rapid late diastolic equalization of right ventricular and atrial pressures and is diagnostic of severe tricuspid incompetence. In the setting of a recent infarct, this finding is diagnostic of significant right ventricular damage. The peak jet velocity (= 3.5 m/s) indicates that right ventricular pressure is significantly raised. LV, left ventricle; RV, right ventricle; IVS, interventricular septum.

practical problems inherent in such measurements, surprisingly few workers have cast doubts on the ability of Doppler to evaluate $Qp:Qs$ ratio in children and adults with isolated ventricular and atrial septal defects,[67–72] but in clinical decision-making such data should be regarded as no more than a rough guide to the size of the shunt.

NON-RESTRICTIVE DEFECTS

As the peak systolic ventricular pressures are equal in these defects, no high velocity trans-septal jet will be present and, thus, low-velocity (i.e. < 1.5 m/s) laminar flow will occur across such defects. Thus, continuous wave interrogation of the septum will reveal no apparent abnormality. However, positioning a pulsed Doppler sample volume within the ventricular septal defect will frequently reveal low-velocity multiphasic 'to and fro' flow across the septum (this is more frequently recorded if there is co-existing bundle branch block). As there is no turbulent flow disturbance within the right ventricle (cf. restrictive defects), continuous wave Doppler will normally record the velocity envelope of any co-existing tricuspid incompetence and thus allow accurate confirmation of the raised right ventricular systolic pressure (Fig. 14.27). In contrast to the characteristic diagnostic trans-septal high-velocity jet of restrictive defects, the diagnosis of an isolated non-restrictive ventricular septal defect remains a cross-sectional imaging diagnosis. The Doppler modalities (including colour flow imaging) have little positive diagnostic contribution to make in this haemodynamic situation. However, where a significantly sized defect is visualized within the ventricular septum and continuous wave Doppler, used appropriately, fails to record a high-velocity trans-septal jet, it may be presumed that the ventricular systolic pressures are equal, and further evidence of this situation is obtained if the systolic blood pressure (in the absence of left ventricular outflow obstruction) and right ventricular systolic

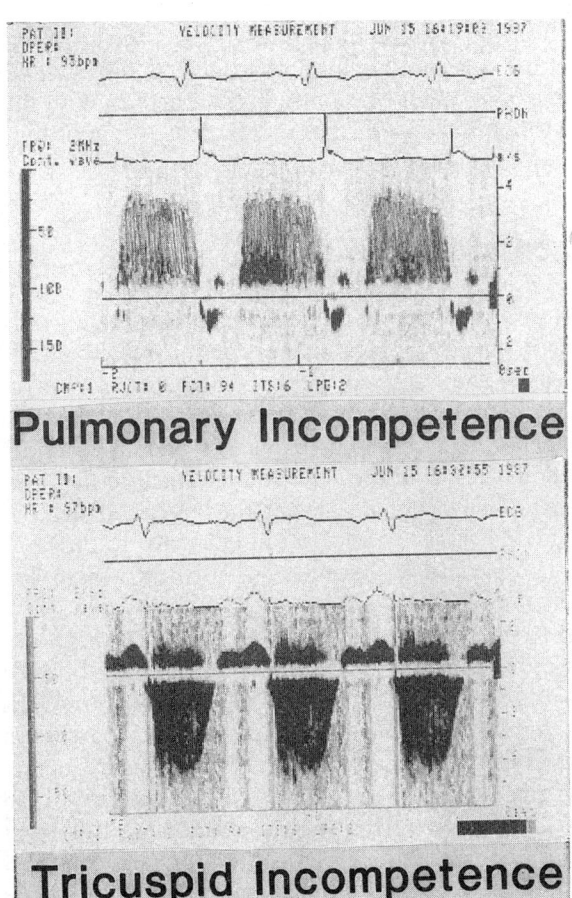

Pulmonary Incompetence

Tricuspid Incompetence

Fig. 14.27. The diagnostic findings in an Eisenmenger ventricular septal defect. Continuous wave Doppler. In this patient, a large perimembranous defect was seen on cross-sectional imaging. No high-velocity ventricular septal jet could be found on continuous wave Doppler study since left and right ventricular pressures are the same. Pulsed Doppler confirmed low-velocity flow within the defect. Continuous wave Doppler analysis of pulmonary flow (upper panel) identified high-velocity pulmonary incompetence (= 4 m/s) with a high end-diastolic pressure gradient. The tricuspid incompetence jet peak velocity (5 m/s) confirms the very high right heart pressure. The combined findings are characteristic of irreversible pulmonary vascular disease secondary to an Eisenmenger ventricular septal defect.

pressure calculated from any tricuspid incompetence jet are the same or similar.

SINGLE VS MULTIPLE VENTRICULAR SEPTAL DEFECTS

In theory, pulsed Doppler interrogation of the right ventricular aspect of the ventricular septum should identify the turbulence associated with the exit of the high-velocity jet of any restrictive defect. Where a single defect exists this is frequently possible. Thus, the position in the septum of small defects,

not visualized by cross-sectional imaging, can be found by identifying their exit site by pulsed Doppler scanning. In theory, multiple exit points could be identified and distinguished from each other, thereby allowing multiple restrictive defects to be diagnosed. Although a theoretical possibility, this method produces too many false-positive and false-negative results to be clinically reliable.

Colour flow imaging is a rapid and sensitive method for use in identifying the turbulent transseptal flow and right ventricular flow disturbance associated with a restrictive defect. Where a defect is non-restrictive, an initial systolic non-turbulent flow acceleration may be visualized across the area of septal drop-out or in the adjacent right ventricular cavity as flow commences across the defect. No turbulence will be encoded. In some instances, no flow may be visualized within the defect. From the above, it will be clear that colour flow imaging is a useful adjunct in the diagnosis of multiple restrictive ventricular septal defects but it is of only limited diagnostic value in multiple non-restrictive defects in which no turbulent flow occurs. Thus, all Doppler techniques may fail to identify multiple ventricular septal defects.

ATRIAL SEPTAL DEFECTS[59]

Defects in the atrial septum may be of four basic types:

1 sinus venosus;
2 secundum;
3 coronary sinus;
4 partial atrioventricular defect.

Partial atrioventricular defect is one of the complex series of abnormal hearts that are classified as atrioventricular defects, and shunting at atrial level is only one aspect of the multiple haemodynamic abnormalities present.

The assessment of atrial septal defect morphology is normally a cross-sectional imaging diagnosis. Where adequate images are obtained, the four types of defect are readily identified and classified. The main diagnostic problem areas are poor image quality and false-positive areas of echo drop-out in the atrial septum image. In theory, the use of Doppler should have significantly improved diagnostic accuracy by identifying flow through an atrial septal defect. Pulsed Doppler can be used to confirm such flow (Fig. 14.28). This flow is laminar in the great majority of defects but it can be

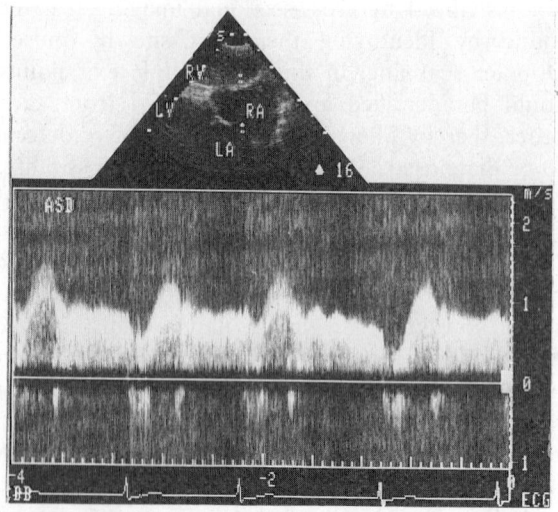

Fig. 14.28. The characteristic continuous flow profile of a non-restrictive secundum atrial septal defect. A HPRF Doppler study with the sample volume placed within the area of septal 'drop-out' on the cross-sectional image (above). This is diagnostic of defect flow.

turbulent where a secundum defect is restrictive and left atrial pressure is high. Transatrial septal flow is essentially continuous throughout the cardiac cycle with a peak velocity in diastole and variable systolic flow reversal. Pulsed Doppler, however, can be misleading in the diagnosis of transatrial septal flow because both superior vena caval flow and coronary sinus flow can be misinterpreted as transatrial septal flow. The use of colour flow imaging has significantly improved diagnostic accuracy over the spectrum of atrial septal defects. Trans-septal flow can readily be visualized and distinguished from caval and coronary sinus flow. Flow due to abnormalities (left superior vena cava in coronary sinus defects and anomalous right upper pulmonary vein drainage in sinus venosus defects) are also readily visualized. Colour jet width may accurately reflect the defect dimensions. Assessment of jet volume by analysis of the colour flow map can potentially facilitate $Qp:Qs$ estimation. The degree of intracardiac shunting present can be assessed with reasonable accuracy by standard pulsed Doppler evaluation and comparison of the volume flows in the main pulmonary artery and the left ventricular outflow tract. Pulmonary artery and right ventricular peak systolic pressures are estimated in the standard Doppler manner using continuous wave Doppler to record both the tricuspid incompetence waveform (almost invariably present) and the pulmonary systolic flow. Thus, combined and judicious use of

all the ultrasound modalities can provide an exceptionally accurate morphological and haemodynamic assessment of an atrial septal defect. With this level of diagnostic accuracy, cardiac catheterization should seldom be required.

AORTIC COARCTATION

A proximal stenosis in the descending aorta would at first sight appear to be a lesion which should readily be assessed by a combination of cross-sectional imaging and continuous wave Doppler. The aortic arch and proximal descending aorta can be imaged from the suprasternal notch in the great majority of patients. From this position, the continuous wave transducer can be angled to direct its beam parallel to descending aortic flow irrespective of the position of the descending aorta. It is therefore surprising that although diagnostic Doppler information can frequently be obtained on the site and severity of a coarctation, major problems still exist. In the neonate, an aortic coarctation rarely exists as an isolated lesion but it is frequently associated with a patent ductus arteriosus. In addition, there is a high incidence of associated intracardiac lesions, many of which are complex, and these add to the diagnostic problems. The neonatal coarctation should be thought of as part of a coarctation syndrome rather than as a discrete entity. The coarctation site is most commonly around the origin of the left subclavian artery from the descending aorta and is opposite the entry point of the ductus into the descending aorta. When the neonatal pulmonary resistance is high and the ductus is widely patent, pulmonary artery and systemic pressures will be equal. Pressure above the coarctation will be maintained by the left ventricle and pressure below the coarctation (if severe) by the right heart circulation via the ductus. Thus, although a severe coarctation is present, no significant pressure gradient will exist across it and no high-velocity signal will be recorded by continuous wave Doppler. As the ductus closes spontaneously, a pressure gradient will evolve over the coarctation. This normally occurs by 3–4 weeks of neonatal life. Before this time, the confirmation of the site and severity of a coarctation remains a cross-sectional imaging (and, if that fails, angiographic) diagnosis. With the evolution of a gradient across the coarctation, an obstructive velocity waveform will be recorded by continuous wave Doppler. The precise nature of the velocity waveform will vary with the

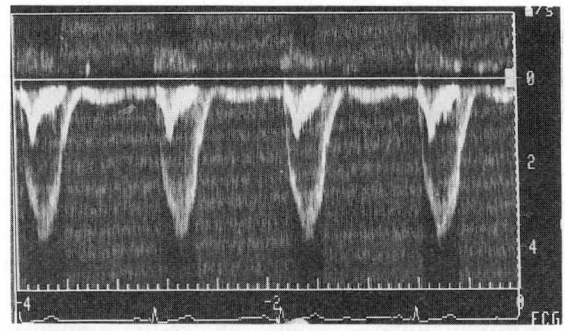

Fig. 14.29. The descending aortic flow profile in an adolescent with a mild 'ring form' aortic coarctation. HPRF Doppler has been used. One sample volume has been placed proximal to the coarctation and one distal. The calculated pressure drop is about 46 mmHg. Note that high-velocity flow is restricted to systole. This is typical of a mild lesion.

severity of the obstruction and the precise morphology of the lesion.

In infants, the descending aortic coarctation may be a complex multilevel lesion with further discrete or long segment narrowings in both the aortic arch and the descending aorta. Such complex lesions may have to be analysed as lesions in 'series' and the pressure drop may have to be calculated for individual lesions to determine which components are the most significant. Discrete lesions separated by > 1.5 cm must be analysed individually. It is not possible to make satisfactory estimations of long segment aortic lesions with Doppler and long segment aortic arch obstruction cannot be assessed accurately by suprasternal continuous wave interrogation, even using the angle correction technique. The common form of coarctation encountered in the older child or adult is the 'ring' form found in

the juxtaductal position in the descending aorta. The severity of this lesion may range from a 'pinhole' orifice with multiple collateral vessels bypassing the obstruction to a mild concentric aortic narrowing with no associated collateral vessels. The waveforms recorded by continuous wave Doppler may vary similarly. Where the coarctation is mild or moderate, the abnormal high-velocity jet in the descending aorta is normally easily recorded. In severe coarctations, the jet may be extremely difficult to record or may be missed. The velocity waveform also varies. In patients with mild obstructions and no collaterals, the high-velocity jet is restricted to systole (Fig. 14.29). With increasing severity of coarctation, the high-velocity jet spills over into diastole. With a very severe coarctation, flow is continuous with an incomplete pressure equalization even in late diastole (Fig. 14.30). The origin of the pan-diastolic velocity waveform is not known. Some authors suggest that it originates from collateral flow and others suggest that it represents flow across the severely coarcted region. Both mechanisms in isolation have been demonstrated to produce an identical flow pattern. With a good-quality signal and trans-coarctation flow restricted to systole, an accurate assessment of the pressure drop will normally be obtained. When flow is prolonged into diastole, the accuracy of the technique diminishes and increasingly gradient underestimation is a problem. Similar problem areas are encountered when using continuous wave Doppler to assess the surgical results of coarctation repair. Colour flow imaging has added little to diagnostic accuracy in this lesion.

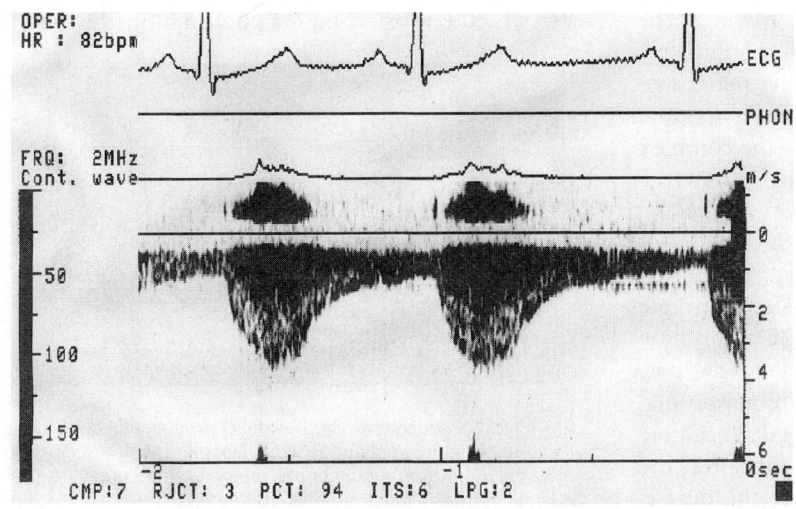

Fig. 14.30. The descending aortic flow profile in a patient with a severe coarctation with multiple collateral vessel formation. Although the peak velocity is approximately the same as that in Fig. 14.29 (*NB*: the scales are different), the waveform now indicates that high-velocity flow now takes place over the coarctation or the collateral vessels in diastole as well. This is always associated with a severe coarctation.

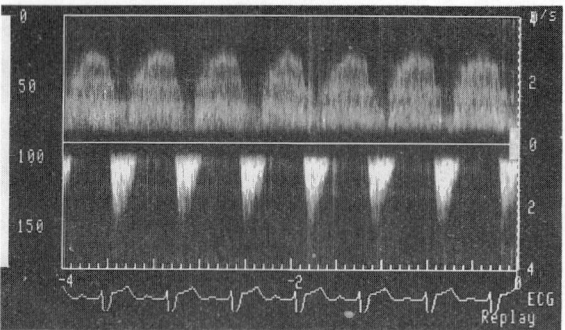

Fig. 14.31. Patent ductus arteriosus. Pulmonary artery flow. Continuous wave Doppler. Upper left parasternal position.

PATENT DUCTUS ARTERIOSUS AND OTHER FORMS OF HIGH-VELOCITY CONTINUOUS SHUNTING[60-66]

Continuous high-velocity shunting of blood within the heart and great vessels is a rare finding in adult patients but a relatively common occurrence in children. The commonest cause is the presence of a patent ductus arteriosus. In the neonate, the ductus is frequently of large diameter and thus non-restrictive to both flow and pressure. With the rapidly varying parameters of pulmonary and systemic resistance and of duct diameter in the perinatal period, a spectrum of complex flow abnormalities across the ductus may be encountered. However, when the ductus constricts to become restrictive to flow and the pulmonary resistance falls, the shunting of blood across the duct becomes left to right and is continuous throughout the cardiac cycle with a peak velocity occurring in early systole. Unless an Eisenmenger reaction occurs later, this flow pattern persists through adult life. Continuous wave Doppler will normally record this flow pattern with ease (Fig. 14.31) with the beam directed towards the pulmonary artery from the precordial or suprasternal transducer positions. Pulsed Doppler may be of less value due to the inherent insensitivity of the technique (cf. continuous wave) and to the complex flow patterns produced by the ductus within the pulmonary artery. Ideally, the flow should be recorded from within the duct itself, but this cannot always be imaged to allow positioning of the pulsed wave sample volume. It is therefore easier to sample flow in the main pulmonary artery. Colour flow imaging has indicated that the complex flow patterns within this vessel could lead to an inappropriate use of pulsed Doppler giving false-negative results. Colour flow imaging demonstrates that the high-velocity turbulent jet exiting from the duct is directed downwards along the lateral wall of the main pulmonary artery to hit the lateral pulmonary valve cusp. The duct flow is then deflected onto the medial wall of the pulmonary artery and passes up this wall mixing with flow entering the pulmonary artery from the ventricle. Much of the initial jet velocity has now been shed. Thus, sampling with pulsed Doppler in the medial portion of the main pulmonary artery may not give a characteristic duct signal.

Aortopulmonary shunts (Waterston, modified Blalock) will give rise to an identical continuous flow pattern on continuous wave interrogation (Fig. 14.32). In theory, the maximal pressure drop recorded across the shunt should allow an accurate calculation of the peak pressure drop from the systolic blood pressure. However, in several studies, inherent errors in this approach have been demonstrated due in the main to underestimation of the peak pressure drop across the shunt because of poor alignment to flow. If an aortopulmonary shunt is patent and there is a pressure drop across it, the careful use of continuous wave Doppler should always allow the flow profile to be recorded. Failure to record this by an experienced observer is strongly suggestive of shunt closure. Other abnormal communications from the aorta to a low-pressure chamber (either congenital or acquired) will also give rise to continuous intracardiac shunting (Figs 14.33 and 14.34). Examples of this are aorto-right ventricular and aorto-atrial fistulae, such as those arising from a ruptured aneurysm of a sinus of Valsalva.

DOPPLER EVALUATION OF PROSTHETIC VALVE FUNCTION[73]

Perhaps the most complex challenge in the use of

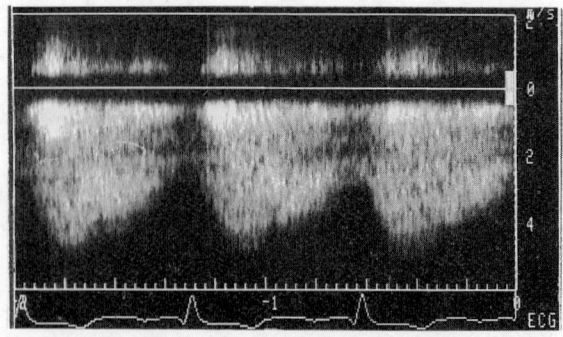

Fig. 14.32. Waterston shunt—the characteristic continuous flow, recorded by continuous wave Doppler (peak velocity = 5 m/s, the peak aorto–pulmonary artery systolic pressure gradient is in this instance at least 100 mmHg).

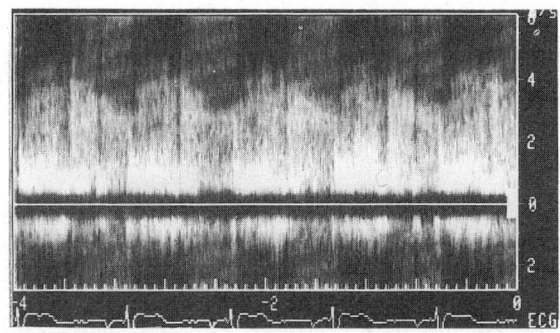

Fig. 14.33. The continuous wave Doppler waveform of an aorto–right ventricular fistula (acquired following aortic valve endocarditis). This is identical to the flow pattern obtained from a ductus arteriosus or aortopulmonary shunt. It is only by using pulsed Doppler to map the origin and extension of the jet or better by using colour flow imaging that such complex abnormalities can be accurately defined.

Doppler to evaluate normal and abnormal function is in the assessment of prosthetic values. Prosthetic values may be divided into three main types categorized by their generic design.

1 Tissue valves (homograft or autograft);
2 Bioprostheses (constructed from both biological and synthetic materials);
3 Mechanical valves. There are a number of very different mechanical valve types:
  a tilting disc;
  b ball and cage;
  c disc and cage.

All types of mechanical valve pose differing problems to the cardiologist attempting to evaluate their function.

Clinical evaluation can often be misleading, but clear clinical signs of valve malfunction do exist. Catheterization is frequently difficult and the results are unsatisfactory. Both M-mode and cross-sectional imaging have proved to be of limited value in their assessment of prosthesis malfunction. Any ultrasound assessment of prosthetic function is severely limited by the effect prosthetic material has on the normal propagation of ultrasound within the heart. Ultrasound will not penetrate through metal or many of the other materials used in prosthesis construction. In addition, many artefactual lateral reverberant echoes will also be created which cause very significant analysis problems; such reverberations often make it impossible to detect significant thrombus or vegetations on or around the prosthesis. Thus, precordial imaging of a prosthetic valve containing metal or plastic material to derive information on possible valve dehiscence, valve

thrombus or vegetations is of very limited value. Although positive diagnostic information can on rare occasions be obtained by such a study, e.g. grossly exaggerated prosthetic motion when there is major dehiscence sometimes with a hingeing appearance about the remaining point of attachment, an apparently normal prosthetic valve

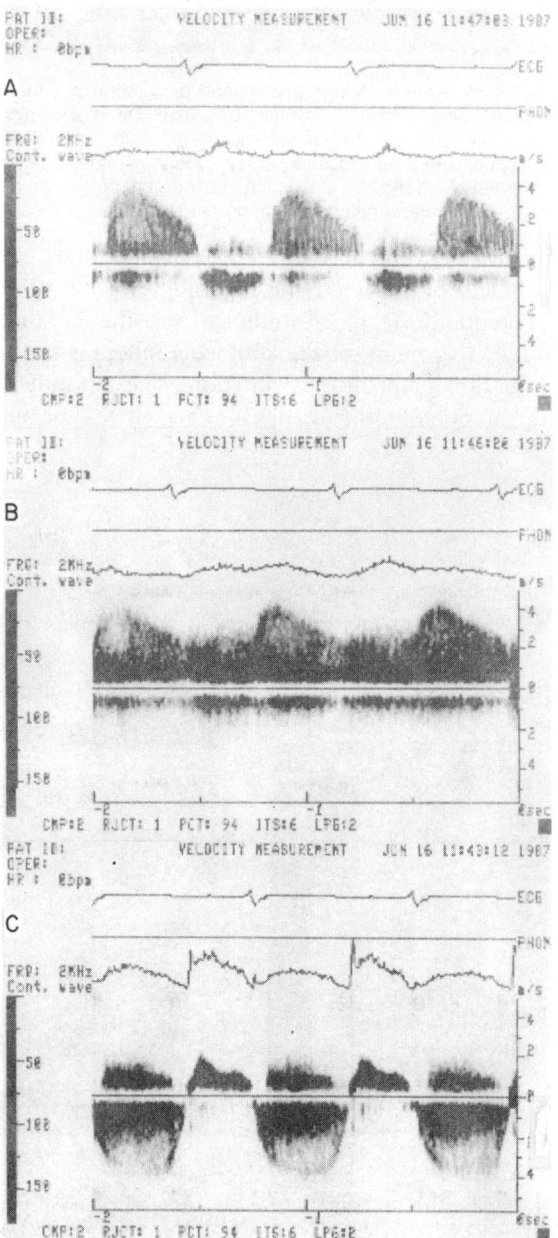

Fig. 14.34. Sinus of Valsalva fistula. The multiple abnormal intracardiac high velocity waveforms that may co-exist with a complex anatomic lesion. (A) The associated severe aortic incompetence. (B) The high-velocity continuous flow of the sinus of Valsalva fistula. (C) Co-existing functional mitral incompetence due to left ventricular dilatation.

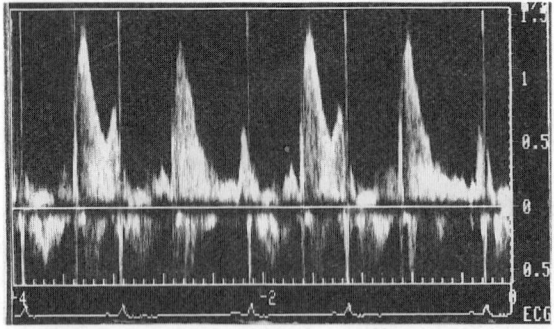

Fig. 14.35. Normal Björk (mechanical) disc mitral prosthetic function. Sinus rhythm. Continuous wave Doppler. Apical transducer position. The prosthetic valve clicks are readily visualized. The peak diastolic velocity, mean diastolic velocity and pressure half-time are within the normal range for the prosthesis size and orientation in the mitral position.

appearance on cross-sectional imaging does not exclude serious underlying pathology.

Potentially, Doppler studies of prosthetic valves could solve many of the problems inherent in the evaluation of prosthesis function. The amount of information obtained varies for each valve type and

analysis of function may be difficult as similar penetration problems exist for the continuous wave ultrasound beam as for the cross-sectional beam.

MITRAL PROSTHETIC FUNCTION

From a precordial position, diastolic inflow into the left ventricle across a mitral prosthesis can readily be recorded with no intervening prosthetic materials to cause problems (Fig. 14.35). By contrast, 'flow masking' of much of the left atrial cavity occurs directly behind a mitral prosthesis. Each type of mitral prosthesis has its own unique ultrasound shadow that is cast directly behind it. It is only around the prosthetic sewing ring that the ultrasound beam can penetrate into the left atrium; some Doppler information on prosthetic regurgitation can be obtained from interrogation of these areas (Fig. 14.36). However, from the above, it will be obvious that major problems exist in the Doppler evaluation of mitral prosthetic valvar and paravalvar leakage using the precordial approach. The

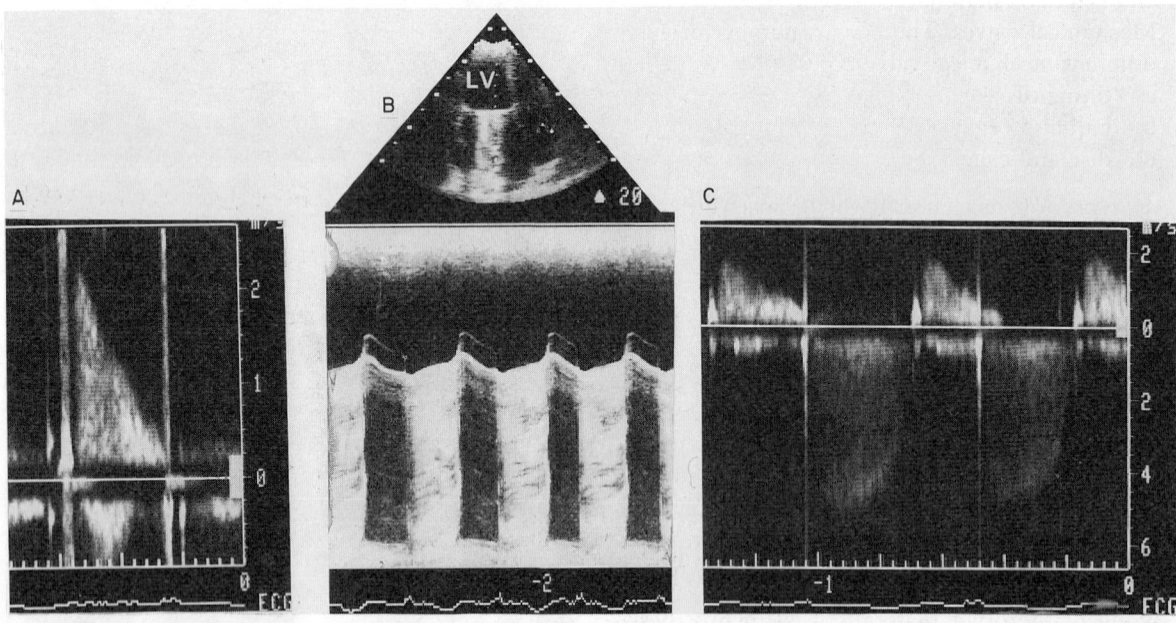

Fig. 14.36. The problems inherent in assessing mitral prosthesis regurgitation. (A) The normal continuous wave diastolic flow profile for the valve type size and orientation in the mitral position. (B) The cross-sectional image and derived M-mode recorded from the apical transducer position. Note the dense abnormal echoes representing the area of ultrasound 'shadowing' behind the mitral prosthesis in the left atrium. No meaningful ultrasound information can be obtained from this area using a transthoracic transducer position. (C) Continuous wave Doppler—mitral valve flow in the same patient. By angulation of the continuous wave beam lateral to the prosthesis, the lateral aspect of the left atrium can be interrogated. In this patient, a mitral incompetence waveform has been recorded. This indicates that a lateral paravalvar leak is present. LV, left ventricle; LA, left atrium; RA, right atrium.

flow-masking problems within the left atrium can be overcome by using the transoesophageal approach. From within the oesophagus, the ultrasound beam can carry out complete imaging, colour flow and continuous wave studies of the left atrium and atrial aspect of the mitral prosthesis to evaluate prosthetic function without any intervening artefact occurring within the atrial cavity. Therefore, transoesophageal imaging and Doppler studies have enormous advantages over all other non-invasive techniques in this situation.

All prosthetic mitral valves are designed to have a small amount of incompetence to effect valve closure. The pattern and degree of incompetence vary with the valve design. Transoesophageal colour flow imaging can readily distinguish these 'normal' regurgitant flow patterns from the large turbulent incompetence jets associated with either central orifice or paravalvar leakage. Multiple paravalvar leaks can readily be detected and accurately located using this technique. Each type of mitral prosthetic valve has its own range of normal values for peak diastolic gradient, mean gradient and pressure half-time (Fig. 14.37). These should be known for the specific valve being studied. It should be appreciated that the indices of mitral prosthetic function are sensitive to change of cardiac output, heart rate and atrial and ventricular compliance when compared with a native valve. In essence, all mitral prostheses are stenotic to some degree; they become increasingly stenotic on mild-to-moderate exercise. However, an abnormal or changing diastolic flow profile over a mitral prosthesis should alert the cardiologist to a possible deterioration in valve function, e.g. a greatly increased but rapidly declining diastolic flow pattern suggests regurgitation even when a systolic jet is not detected from the precordial approach while an increased or normal diastolic flow velocity that is abnormally persistent throughout diastole suggest prosthetic stenosis.

AORTIC PROSTHETIC FUNCTION

In contrast to the mitral valve, it is possible to obtain ultrasound information from both sides of an aortic prosthesis using a combination of precordial, high right parasternal and suprasternal transducer positions (Fig. 14.38). Information on valvar or paravalvar leakage can be obtained by recording continuous wave or colour flow imaging information from an apical or precordial transducer position. Colour flow imaging is the technique of choice because it has the ability to identify and locate multiple incompetence jets. Transvalvar systolic flow is best evaluated from above the valve using continuous wave Doppler to estimate the peak systolic velocity. As virtually all aortic prostheses are smaller in diameter than the native left ventricular outflow into which they are inserted, some flow acceleration always occurs before flow enters the valve orifice. Thus, it is essential in every case to incorporate the maximal pre-valve systolic velocity into the modified Bernoulli equation when estimating the true transvalve gradient. If this is not incorporated into the equation, an overestimation of the degree of prosthetic stenosis will result. As with prosthetic mitral valves, each aortic prosthesis has its own range of normal Doppler parameters and any change in these parameters should be viewed as suggestive of changing valve function which requires an explanation. Doppler evaluation would appear to be an extremely sensitive method of monitoring aortic prosthetic function (Fig. 14.39).

PULMONARY PROSTHETIC FUNCTION

Pulmonary valve replacement is an extremely rare occurrence. Little is known of the function of prostheses in this position. The assessment of prosthetic valve function is much more complex when such a valve is placed in a right ventricular–pulmonary artery conduit. Within such conduits, multilevel obstructions may occur, of which the potential valve obstruction may be only one component. Very skilled examinations using all the available Doppler modalities are required to derive a

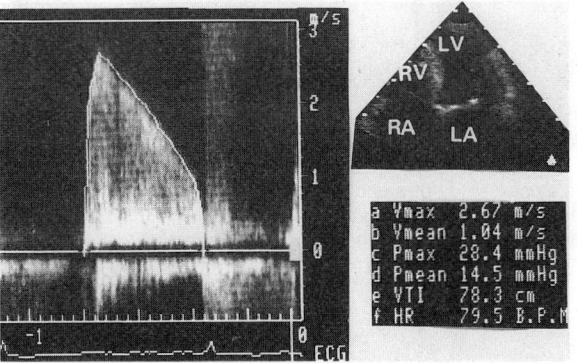

Fig. 14.37. A continuous wave Doppler study of a Hancock (porcine) tissue prosthesis in the mitral position demonstrating the indices of mitral prosthesis which can be measured. Vmax = maximal diastolic velocity; Vmean = mean diastolic velocity; Pmax = maximal diastolic pressure drop; Pmean = mean diastolic pressure drop.

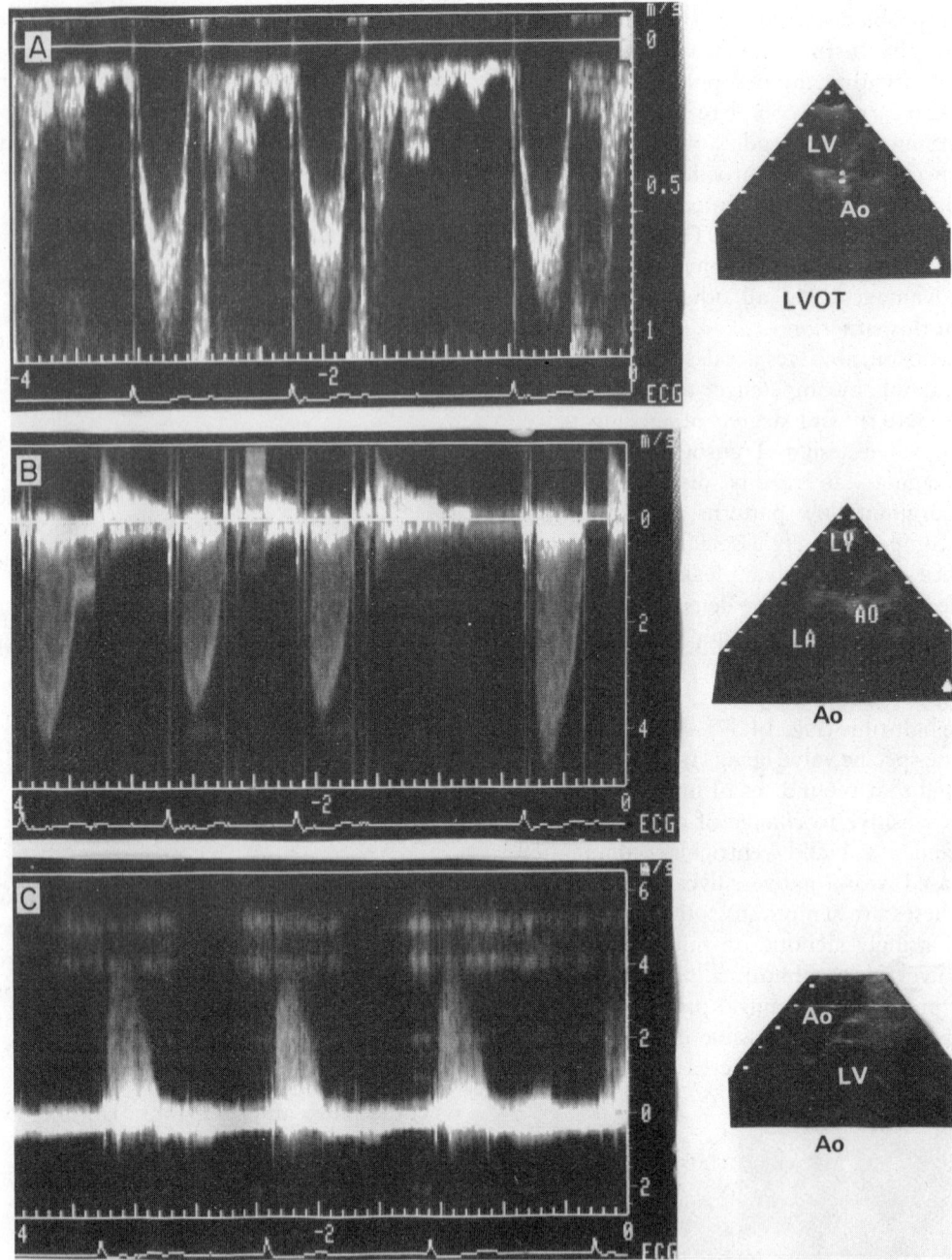

Fig. 14.38. A pulsed (A) and continuous wave (B and C) Doppler study of aortic prosthetic (size 21 Björk) function. Both the pre-valve left ventricular outflow tract maximal systolic velocity (A) and the post valve ascending aortic peak systolic velocity must be recorded to accurately assess prosthetic gradient. (B) A continuous wave recording from the apex. (C) A suprasternal recording. LV, left ventricle; LA, left atrium; LVOT, left ventricular outflow tract; Ao, aorta.

correct evaluation of valved conduit function (Fig. 14.40).

TRICUSPID PROSTHETIC FUNCTION

See section on tricuspid valve disease above (p. 345).

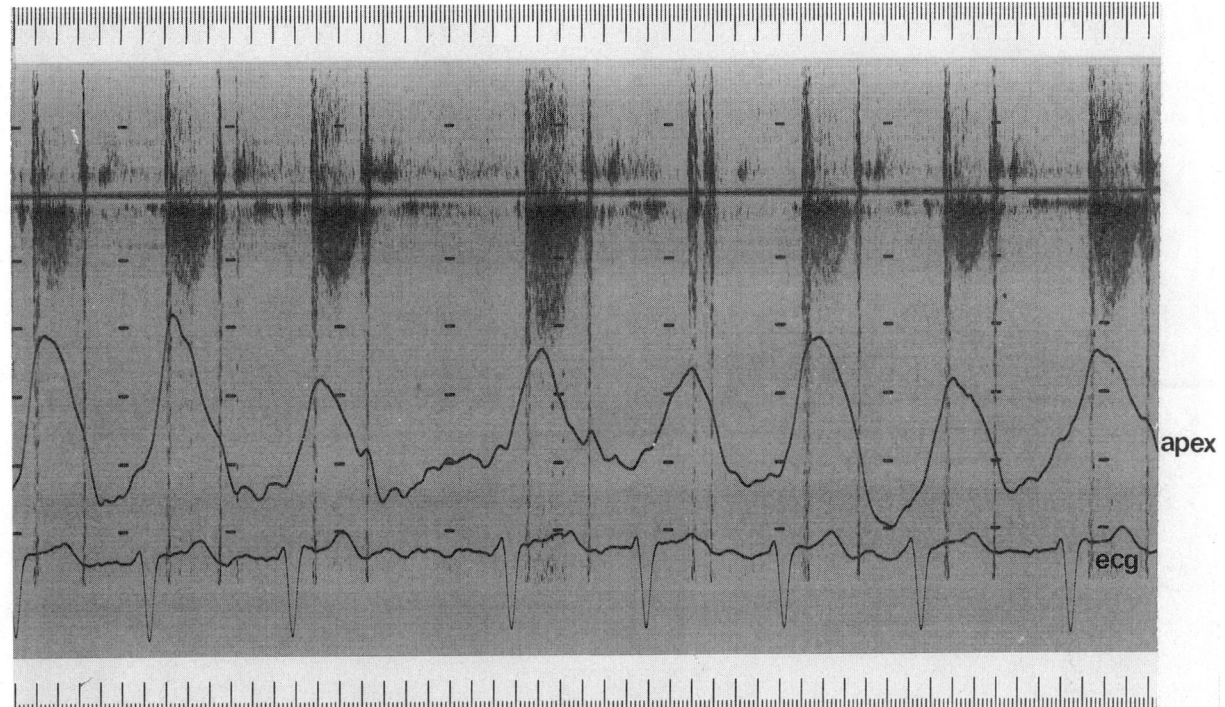

Fig. 14.39. Aortic prosthesis malfunction. A continuous wave study. Apical transducer position. A simultaneous apex cardiogram has been recorded to monitor left ventricular function. With an appropriate R–R interval, neither valve opening nor valve flow is recorded in the fifth beat. This is despite the apparently normal apex cardiogram. The conclusion must be that the prosthetic valve is intermittently 'sticking' and that valve malfunction is present.

REFERENCES

1. Doppler, C.J. Ueber das farbige Licht der Doppelsterne. Abhandlungen der Koniglichen Bohmischen Gesellschaft der Wissenschaften 1842; II: 465.
2. Satomura, S. A study on examining the heart with ultrasonics. I. Principles. II. Instrument. *Japanese Circulation* 1956; 20: 227.
3. Edler, I. and Lindstrom, K. Ultrasonic Doppler technique used in heart disease. I. An experimental study.
4. Hatle, L. and Angelsen, B. *Doppler ultrasound in Cardiology: Physical principles and clinical applications.* Philadelphia: Lea & Febiger: 1982.
5. Hatle, L., Brubakk, A., Tromsdal, A. and Angelsen, B. Noninvasive assessment of pressure drop in mitral stenosis by Doppler ultrasound. *Br. Heart J.* 1978; 40: 131–40.
6. Kisslo, J., Adams, D.B. and Belkin, R.N. *Doppler flow color imaging.* New York: Churchill Livingstone, 1988.
7. Hatle, L., Angelsen, B.A. and Tromsdal, A. Noninvasive assessment of aortic stenosis by Doppler ultrasound. *Br. Heart J.* 1980; 43: 284–92.
8. Hatle, L. Noninvasive assessment and differentiation of left ventricular outflow obstruction by Doppler ultrasound. *Circulation* 1981; 64: 381–7.
9. Berger, M., Berdoff, R.L., Gallerstein, P.E. and Goldberg, E. Evaluation of aortic stenosis by continuous wave ultrasound. *J. Am. Coll. Cardiol.* 1984; 3: 150–6.
10. Lima, C.O., Sahn, D.J., Valdes-Cruz, L.M., Allen, H.D., Goldberg, S.J., Grenadier, E. and Vargas-Barron, J. Prediction of the severity of left ventricular outflow tract obstruction by quantitative two-dimensional echocardiographic Doppler studies. *Circulation* 1983; 68: 348–54.
11. Callahan, M.J., Tajik, A.J., Su-Fan, Q. and Bove, A.A. Validation of instantaneous pressure gradients measured by continuous-wave Doppler in experimentally induced aortic stenosis. *Am. J. Cardiol.* 1985; 56: 989–93.
12. Smith, M.D., Dawson, P.L., Elion, J.L., *et al.* Correlation of continuous wave Doppler velocities with cardiac catheterization gradients: an experimental model of aortic stenosis. *J. Am. Coll. Cardiol.* 1985; 6: 1306–14.
13. Currie, P.J., Seward, J.B., Reeder, G.S., *et al.* Continuous-wave Doppler echocardiographic assessment of severity of calcific aortic stenosis: a simultaneous Doppler-catheter correlative study in 100 adult patients. *Circulation* 1985; 71: 1162–9.
14. Hegrenaes, L. and Hatle, L. Aortic stenosis in adults: non-invasive estimation of pressure differences by continuous wave Doppler echocardiography. *Br. Heart. J.* 1985; 54: 396–404.
15. Currie, P.J., Hagler, D.J., Seward, J.B. *et al.* Instantaneous pressure gradient: a simultaneous Doppler and dual catheter correlative study. *J. Am. Coll. Cardiol.* 1986; 7: 800–6.
16. Otto, C.M., Pearlman, A.S., Comes, K.A., Reamer, R.P., Janko, C.L. and Huntsman, L.L. Determination of the stenotic aortic valve area in adults using Doppler echocardiography. *J. Am. Coll. Cardiol.* 1986; 7: 509–17.
17. Skjaerpe, T., Hegrenaes, L. and Hatle, L. Noninvasive estimation of valve area in patients with aortic stenosis by Doppler ultrasound and 'two-dimensional echocardiography. *Circulation* 1985; 72: 810–18.
18. Zoghbi, W.A., Farmer, K.L., Soto, J.G., Nelson, J.G. and Quinones, M.A. Accurate noninvasive quantification of stenotic aortic valve area by Doppler echocardiography. *Circulation* 1986; 73: 452–9.

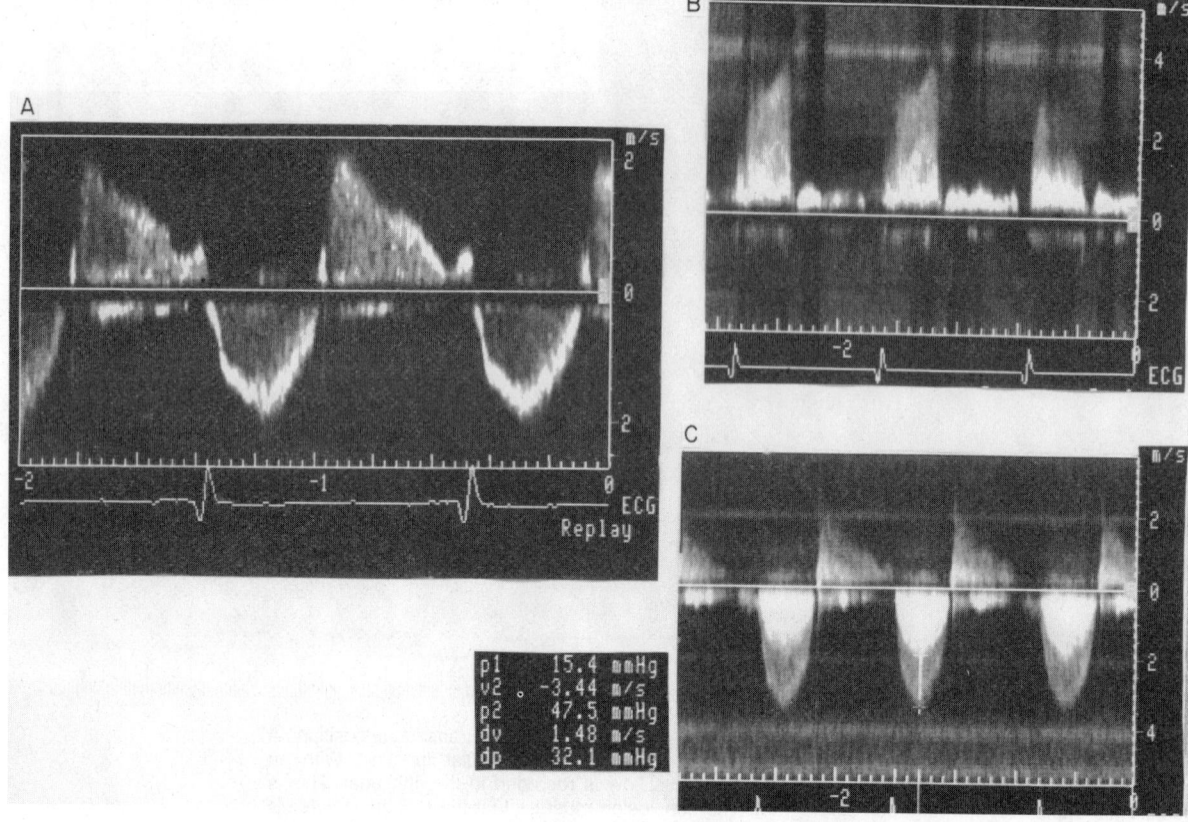

Fig. 14.40. A post-operative Doppler study from a young adult 4 years post correction of a double outlet right ventricle. A right ventricular–pulmonary artery conduit containing a homograft valve was used in the repair. (A) Pre-homograft conduit flow. HPRF Doppler. This demonstrates normal velocity systolic flow with a diastolic waveform suggestive of moderate conduit valve incompetence. (B) The high-velocity jet of a small residual restrictive ventricular septal defect demonstrated by continuous wave Doppler. The trans-septal pressure gradient is 64 mmHg (derived from the ventricular septal defect maximal jet velocity) and thus right ventricular pressure is mildly elevated. (C) Continuous wave Doppler confirms that mild conduit homograft stenosis is present with a peak pressure drop of 32 mmHg. This study demonstrates the very detailed haemodynamic information which a complete Doppler study can derive in patients who have residual lesions following complex cardiac surgery.

19. Teirstein, P., Yeager, M., Yock, P.G. and Popp, R.L. Doppler echocardiographic measurement of aortic valve area in aortic stenosis: a noninvasive application of the Gorlin formula. *J. Am. Coll. Cardiol.* 1986; 8: 1059–65.
20. Nishimura, R.A. and Jamil Tajik, A. Determination of left-sided pressure gradients by utilizing Doppler aortic and mitral regurgitant signals: validation by simultaneous dual catheter and Doppler studies. *J. Am. Coll. Cardiol.* 1988; 11: 317–21.
21. Richards, K.L., Cannon, R.S., Miller, J.F. and Crawford, M.H. Calculation of aortic valve area by Doppler echocardiography: a direct application of the continuity equation. *Circulation* 1986; 73; 5: 964–9.
22. Rijsterborgh, H. and Roelandt, J. Doppler assessment of aortic stenosis: Bernoulli revisited. *Ultrasound in Med. & Biol.* 1987; 13; 5: 241–8.
23. Ward, J.M., Baker, D.W., Rubenstein, S.A. and Johnson, S.L. Detection of aortic insufficiency by pulsed Doppler echocardiography. *J. Clin. Ultrasound* 1977; 5: 5–10.
24. Quinones, M.A., Young, J.B., Waggoner, A.D., Ostojic, M.C., Ribeiro, L.G.T. and Miller, R.R. Assessment of pulsed Doppler echocardiography in detection and quantification

of aortic and mitral regurgitation. *Br. Heart. J.* 1980; 44: 612–20.
25. Diebold, B., Peronneau, P., Blanchard, D., Colonna, G., Guermonprez, J.L., Forman, J., Sellier, P. and Maurice, P. Non-invasive quantification of aortic regurgitation by Doppler echocardiography. *Br. Heart J.* 1983; 49: 167–73.
26. Segadal, L., Engedal, H., Folling, M. and Matre, K. Measurement of aortic regurgitation fraction by pulsed ultrasonic Doppler technique. In: Peronneau, P. and Diebold, B. (Eds), *Cardiovascular Applications of Doppler Echocardiography* Paris: Inserm, 1983; p. 358.
27. Smith, M.D., Grayburn, P.A., Spain, M.G., DeMaria, A.N., Ling Kwan, O. and Banks Moffett, C. Observer variability in the quantification of Doppler color flow jet areas for mitral and aortic regurgitation. *J. Am. Coll. Cardiol.* 1988; 11: 579–84.
28. Holen, J., Aaslid, R., Landmark, K. and Simonsen, S. Determination of pressure gradient in mitral stenosis with a noninvasive ultrasound Doppler technique. *Acta Med. Scand.* 1976; 199: 455–60.
29. Hatle, L., Angelsen, B. and Tromsdal, A. Noninvasive assessment of atrioventricular pressure half-time by Doppler

ultrasound. *Circulation* 1979; **60**: 1096–104.

30. Holen, J. and Simonsen, S. Determination of pressure gradient in mitral stenosis with Doppler echocardiography. *Br. Heart J.* 1979; **41**: 529–35.

31. Holen, J., Aaslid, R., Landmark, K., Simonsen, S. and Ostrem, T. Determination of effective orifice area in mitral stenosis from noninvasive ultrasound Doppler data and mitral flow rate. *Acta Med. Scand.* 1977; **201**: 83–8.

32. Holen, J., Hoie, J. and Froysaker, T. Determination of pre- and postoperative flow obstruction in patients undergoing closed mitral commissurotomoy from noninvasive ultrasound Doppler data and cardiac output. *Am. Heart J.* 1979; **97**: 499–504.

33. Kalmanson, D., Veyrat, C., Bouchareine, F. and Degroote, A. Noninvasive recording of mitral valve flow velocity patterns using pulsed Doppler echocardiography. *Br. Heart J.* 1977; **39**: 517–28.

34. Stamm, B.R. and Martin, R.P. Quantification of pressure gradients across stenotic valves by Doppler ultrasound. *J. Am. Coll. Cardiol.* 1974; **2**: 707–18.

35. Kalmanson, D., Veyrat, C., Abitbol, G. and Farjon, M. Doppler echocardiography and valvular regurgitation with special emphasis on mitral insufficiency. Advantages of two-dimensional echocardiography with real-time spectral analysis. In: *Echocardiology.* Rijsterborgh, H. Ed. The Hague, Martinus Nijhoff. 1981; pp. 279–290.

36. Shah, P.M., Gramiak, R., Adelman, A.G. and Wigle, E.D. Role of echocardiography in diagnostic and hemodynamic assessment of hypertrophic subaortic stenosis. *Circulation* 1971; **44**: 891–8.

37. Henry, W.L., Clark, C.E., Glancy, D.L. and Epstein, S.E. Echocardiographic measurement of the left ventricular outflow gradient in idiopathic subaortic stenosis. *N. Engl. J. Med.* 1973; **288**: 989–93.

38. Joyner, C.R., Harrison, F.S. and Gruber, J.W. Diagnosis of hypertrophic subaortic stenosis with a Doppler velocity flow detector. *Ann. Intern. Med.* 1971; **74**: 692–6.

39. Oliveira Lima, C., Sahn, D.J., Valdes-Cruz, L.M., Goldberg, S.J., Vargas Barron, J., Allen, H.D. and Grenadier, E. Noninvasive prediction of transvalvular pressure gradient in patients with pulmonary stenosis by quantitative two-dimensional echo Doppler studies. *Circulation* 1983; **67**: 866–871.

40. Waggoner, A.D., Quinones, M.A., Young, J.B., Brandon, T.A., Shah, A.A., Verani, M.S. and Miller, R.R. Pulsed Doppler echocardiographic detection of right-side valve regurgitation. *Am. J. Cardiol.* 1981; **47**: 279–86.

41. Miyatake, K., Okamoto, M., Kinoshita, N., Matsuhisa, M., Nagata, S., Beppu, S., Park, Y., Sakakibara, H. and Nimura, Y. Pulmonary regurgitation studied with the ultrasonic pulsed Doppler technique. *Circulation* 1982; **65**: 969–76.

42. Patel, A.K., Rowe, G.G., Dhanani, S.P., Kosolcharoen, P., Lyle, L.E.W. and Thomsen, J.H. Pulsed Doppler echocardiography in diagnosis of pulmonary regurgitation: its value and limitations. *Am. J. Cardiol.* 1982; **49**: 1801–5.

43. Veyrat, C., Kalmanson, D., Farjou, M., Manin, J.P. and Abitbol, G. Non-invasive diagnosis and assessment of tricuspid regurgitation and stenosis using one and two-dimensional echopulsed Doppler. *Br. Heart J.* 1982; **47**: 596–605.

44. Hatle, L. Non-invasive methods of measuring pulmonary artery pressure and flow velocity. Cardiology, an international perspective. 1984. New York: Plenum Press, p. 783–90.

45. Skjaerpe, T. and Hatle, L. Diagnosis and assessment of tricuspid regurgitation with Doppler ultrasound. In: *Echocardiology* Rijsterborgh, H. (Ed), The Hague; Martinus Nijhoff, 1981; pp. 299–304.

46. Yock, P.G., Popp, R.L. Noninvasive estimation of ventricular pressures by Doppler ultrasound in patients with tricuspid or aortic regurgitation. *Circulation* 1983; **68** (suppl. III): 230 (abstract).

47. Skjaerpe, T. and Hatle, L. Noninvasive estimation of pulmonary artery pressure by Doppler ultrasound. Cardiac Doppler Diagnosis (Ed. Spencer, M.), The Hague; Martinus Nijhoff. 1983; pp. 247–54.

48. Lieppe, W., Behas, V.S., Scallion, R. and Kisslo, J.A. Detection of tricuspid regurgitation with two-dimensional echocardiography and peripheral vein injection. *Circulation* 1978; **57**: 128.

49. Meltzer, R.S., van Hoogenhuyze, D., Serruys, P.W., Haalebos, M.M.P., Hugenholtz, P.G. and Roelandt, J. Diagnosis of tricuspid regurgitation by contrast echocardiography. *Circulation* 1981; **63**: 1093–9.

50. Hatle, L., Angelsen, B.A.J. and Tromsdal, A. Noninvasive estimation of pulmonary artery systolic pressure with Doppler ultrasound. *Br. Heart J.* 1981; **45**: 157–165.

51. Stevenson, J.G. Echo Doppler analysis of septal defects. Cardiovascular Applications of Doppler Echocardiography. (Eds. Peronneau, P., Diebold, B.), Inserm, Paris. 1983; **111**: 515–40.

52. Stevenson, J.G., Kawabori, I., Dooley, T. and Guntheroth, W.G. Diagnosis of ventricular septal defect by pulsed Doppler echocardiography—sensitivity, specificity and limitations. *Circulation* 1978; **58**: 322–6.

53. Hatle, L. and Rokseth, R. Noninvasive diagnosis and assessment of ventricular septal defect by Doppler ultrasound. *Acta Med. Scand.* 1981; suppl. **645**: 47–56.

54. Skjaerpe, T., Hegrenaes, L. and Hatle, L. Noninvasive estimation of right ventricular pressure by Doppler ultrasound in VSD. *Fifth Symposium on Echocardiology*, Rotterdam, *Ultrasonar. Bull.* 1983; **92** (abstract).

55. Stevenson, J.G., Kawabori, I. and Guntheroth, W.G. Differentiation of ventricular septal defects from mitral regurgitation by pulsed Doppler echocardiography. *Circulation* 1977; **56**: 14–8.

56. Daniels, O., Kapusta, L. and Hopman, J.C.W. The advantage of two-dimensional Doppler flow imaging in the diagnosis: small ventricular septal defect with left to right shunt (abstr) *Int. Cong. Card. Doppler* 1986; **113**.

57. Ortiz, E., Robinson, P.J., Deanfield, J.E. *et al.* Localization of ventricular septal defects by simultaneous display of superimposed colour Doppler and cross sectional echocardiographic images. *Br. Heart J.* 1985; **54**: 53.

58. Ludomirsky, A., Huhta, J.C., Vick, G.W. *et al.* Color Doppler detection of multiple septal defects. *Circulation* 1986; **74**; 6: 1317–22.

59. Dittmann, H., Jacksch, R., Voelker, W., Karsch, K.R. and Seipel, L. Accuracy of Doppler echocardiography in quantification of left to right shunts in adult patients with atrial septal defect. *J. Am. Coll. Cardiol.* 1988; **11**: 338–42.

60. Daniels, O., Hopman, J.C.W., Stelinga, G.B.A., Busch, H.J. and Peer, P.G.M. Doppler flow characteristics in the main pulmonary artery and A/Ao ratio before and after ductral closure in healthy newborns. *Pediatr. Cardiol.* 1982; **3**: 99–104.

61. Stevenson, J.G., Kawabori, I. and Guntheroth, W.G. Pulsed Doppler echocardiographic diagnosis of patent ductus arteriosus: sensitivity, specificity, limitations and technical features. *Cathet. Cardiovasc. Diagn.* 1980; **6**: 255–63.

62. Stevenson, J.G., Kawabori, I. and Guntheroth, W.G. Noninvasive detection of pulmonary hypertension in patent ductus arteriosus by pulsed Doppler echocardiography. *Circulation* 1979; **60**: 355–9.

63. Swenssen, R.E., Valdes-Cruz, L.M., Sahn, D.J. *et al.* Real time Doppler color flow mapping for detection of patent ductus arteriosus. *J. Am. Coll. Cardiol.* 1986; **8**: 1059–65.

64. Allen, H.D., Sahn, D.J., Lange, L. and Goldberg, S.J. Noninvasive assessment of surgical systemic to pulmonary artery shunts by range-gated pulsed Doppler echocardiogra-

phy. *J. Pediatr.* 1979; **94**: 395–402.

65. Stevenson, J.G., Kawabori, I. and Bailey, W.W. Noninvasive evaluation of Blalock-Taussig shunts: determination of patency and differentiation from patent ductus arteriosus by Doppler echocardiography. *Am. Heart J.* 1983; **106**: 1121–32.

66. Marx, G.R., Allen, H.D. and Goldberg, S.J. Doppler echocardiographic estimation of systolic pulmonary artery pressure in patients with aortic-pulmonary shunts. *J. Am. Coll. Cardiol.* 1986; 7; 4: 880–5.

67. Goldberg, S.J., Sahn, D.J., Allen, H.D., Valdes-Cruz, L.M., Hoenecke, H. and Carnahan, Y. Evaluation of pulmonary and systemic blood flow by two-dimensional Doppler echocardiography using fast Fourier transform spectral analysis. *Am. J. Cardiol.* 1982; 50: 1394–1400.

68. Sanders, S.P., Yeager, S. and Williams, R. Measurement of systemic and pulmonary blood flow and QP:QS ratio using Doppler and two-dimensional echocardiography. *Am. J. Cardiol.* 1983; 51: 952–6.

69. Stevenson, J.G. and Kawabori, I. Noninvasive determination of pulmonic to systemic flow ratio by pulsed Doppler echo.

Circulation 1982; **66** (suppl. II): 232 (abstract).

70. Meyer, R.A., Kalavathy, A., Korfhagen, J.C. and Kaplan, S. Comparison of left to right shunt ratios determined by pulsed Doppler/2D-echo and Fick method. *Circulation* 1982; **66** (suppl. II): 232 (abstract).

71. Valdes-Cruz, L.M., Mesel, E., Horowitz, S., Sahn, D.J., Fischer, D.C., Larson, D., Goldberg, S.J. and Allen, H.D. Validation of two-dimensional echo Doppler for measuring pulmonary and systemic flows in atrial and ventricular septal defects: a canine study. *Circulation* 1982; **66** (suppl. II): 231 (abstract).

72. Vargas Barron, J., Sahn, D.J., Valdes-Cruz, L.M., Oliveira Lima, C., Grenadier, E., Allen, H.D. and Goldberg, S.J. Quantification of the ratio of pulmonary: systemic blood flow (QP:QS) in patients with ventricular septal defect by two-dimensional range gated Doppler echocardiography. *Circulation* 1982; **66** (suppl. II): 318 (abstract).

73. Jones, M., McMillan, S.T., Eidbo, E.E., Ren Woo, Y. and Yoganathan, A.P. Evaluation of prosthetic heart valves by Doppler flow imaging. *Echocardiography* 1986; 3; 6: 513–25.

Chapter 15

Cardiac Catheterization and Angiography

Roger Hall

INTRODUCTION

The first recorded use of catheterization in man was when Forssman introduced a catheter into his own right atrium in the 1920s. During the 1930s, various investigators used this technique to gain new and interesting information about patients with a variety of heart disease. The widespread use of cardiac catheterization did not occur however until the 1950s and 1960s when cardiac surgery began to develop and accurate pre-operative assessment of patients with cardiac disease was required. As surgery became more sophisticated, cardiac catheterization developed and found many applications, some of which have been superseded in the last decade with the rapid improvement in non-invasive techniques, of which ultrasound has been by far the most important.

Cardiac catheterization is most useful as an investigative technique when it is carried out by an operator who possesses all the clinical facts about a patient and understands the important questions to be answered. Unfortunately, in some centres, the erroneous notion that an investigation can be a "complete" investigation grew up; in some places, this notion still persists. The correct use of cardiac catheterization demands a targeted approach; the primary object of the investigator is to answer questions that have not yet been satisfactorily resolved by non-invasive investigation prior to catheterization. This leads to shorter procedures, which involve less discomfort and risk to the patient; this is particularly important when the patient is severely ill and unlikely to be able to withstand a prolonged investigation. Another misunderstanding slowly being corrected is that cardiac catheterization provides, in all circumstances, a "gold standard" for other investigations. In some circumstances, better anatomical and haemodynamic information is provided by echocardiography and Doppler ultrasound. Finally, it is extremely impor-

tant to remember that the technique is valueless unless it is carried out with meticulous attention to detail.

PRACTICAL CONSIDERATIONS

Cardiac catheterization consists of techniques designed to introduce catheters into the arterial and venous systems, and the chambers of the left and right side of the heart so that pressures can be recorded and angiographic contrast injected in appropriate positions to gain the desired information. The catheters used in adult work are usually between 6 and 8F. There are many different designs of catheter for different procedures, which will not be described in detail here. Frequently, catheters used for pressure measurement have a single end-hole (Fig. 15.1); these catheters are inappropriate for power injections of large quantities of contrast material as there is a risk of intramyocardial injection of large quantities of contrast which can have serious effects on cardiac performance and rhythm. For this reason, the catheters used for this type of angiography either do not have an end-hole and instead have several small holes near their tip (Fig. 15.1) (e.g. the NIH catheter) or have both end- and side-holes (e.g. the pigtail and Gensini catheters). When angiography is performed by hand injection of contrast, for example when visualizing the coronary arteries, end-hole catheters are used (Fig. 15.1).

Generally, cardiac catheterization is carried out as an inpatient procedure, although in certain units patients of moderate or low risk are investigated as day cases quite safely.[1] The patient is fasted before the procedure. This is particularly important because patients occasionally develop extreme nausea after the injection of contrast material and this has obvious dangers (the inspiration of vomit) when the patient is lying on his or her back under X-ray equipment. Premedication for the procedure varies

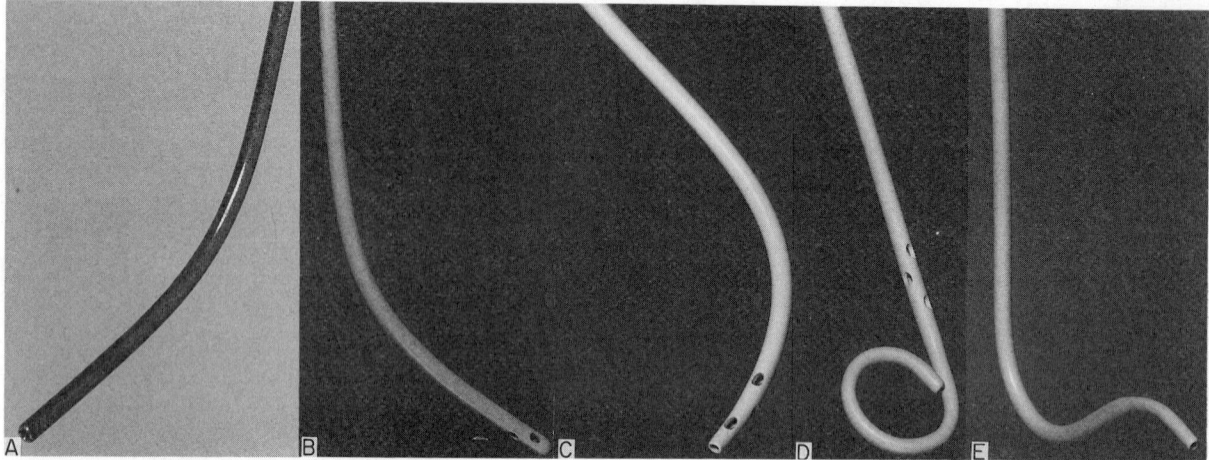

Fig. 15.1. Various types of cardiac catheters in common use. (A) *Cournand*. This has a single end-hole and is used for pressure measurement mainly in the right side of the circulation. (B) *NIH*. This has a closed end and several side-holes near the tip. It is used for angiography. (C) *Gensini*. This has an end-hole but, like the NIH, it has side-holes near the tip. It is used for angiography and has the advantage that because of the presence of an end-hole a guidewire can be passed through it. (D) *Pigtail* catheter. The reason for the name is obvious. It is an excellent angiographic catheter and will also take a guidewire because it has both end- and side-holes. The curled end enables it to 'roll' past obstacles and rendering it relatively atraumatic when compared with catheters which have a straight tip. (E) *Amplatz*. This catheter is for coronary angiography from the femoral approach. It has been designed to enter the left coronary artery. It is often used in patients in whom there is difficulty engaging the left coronary orifice with a Judkins' catheter. Similar shaped but shorter catheters are available for use from the brachial approach (Castillo catheter).

considerably among centres. A small amount of anxiolytic drug (usually an opiate or benzodiazepine) probably reduces apprehension and is helpful. Many operators use atropine routinely, administered either during the procedure or with the premedication. This can prove an extremely useful precaution because vagal reactions are not uncommon, as a result of fear, pain or manipulation of the catheter within the vascular system. Prophylactic administration of atropine, however, should be avoided in patients who are in atrial fibrillation because it often causes an excessive tachycardia. The use of anticoagulation with systemic heparinization during the procedure varies considerably from centre to centre. It reduces the incidence of thrombus formation at the end of the catheter and possible embolization and thrombosis at the site of arterial access. These advantages, however, are obtained at the expense of a higher incidence of haematomas after the procedure. Although the use of heparin when catheterization is carried out percutaneously from the femoral artery (see below) is not universal, nearly all operators would regard heparinization either systemically or locally as mandatory when the brachial artery approach is used. When trans-septal catheterization is likely to be attempted, it should be omitted because of the risk

of perforation of the heart with the trans-septal needle.

The procedure is normally carried out under local anaesthetic, but very occasionally an extremely nervous patient may need general anaesthesia. Venous access can be obtained from any large vein. Usually either a percutaneous puncture of the femoral vein or a percutaneous puncture or cut-down on an arm vein is used to introduce the venous catheter, which is then manipulated to the right atrium, right ventricle and pulmonary artery. The catheter can then be advanced further to wedge in a small branch of the pulmonary artery to give an indirect measurement of left atrial pressure (pulmonary artery wedge pressure). Occasionally, the venous catheter passes from the right atrium through an atrial septal defect or patent foramen ovale (present in about 5% of the adult population) to enter the left atrium. From here, it can be manipulated either into the pulmonary veins or onward into the left ventricle through the mitral valve. Generally, catheterization has to be performed from the femoral vein to give the catheter the right angle of approach to the atrial septum so that it can pass through to the left atrium. Ventricular septal defects are rarely crossed by cardiac catheterization from the venous side except in patients with other abnormalities of anatomy (for example, Fallot's tetralogy).

Arterial access is usually obtained either by percutaneous puncture of the femoral artery using the Seldinger technique or via the brachial artery usually using an arteriotomy (although small catheters may be introduced percutaneously into this artery). The use of arteriotomy requires a considerable degree of training before it can be done safely.

All chambers of the heart, except the left atrium, can be easily reached in most patients using a combination of venous catheterization and retrograde arterial catheterization. Indirect left atrial pressure can be measured using the pulmonary artery wedge pressure and, if a direct atrial pressure is required, this can be obtained by trans-septal puncture using a Brockenbrough needle with a Teflon catheter over it. The needle ensheathed by the catheter is advanced from the right femoral vein into the right atrium and, after appropriate manoeuvres, puncture of the interatrial septum is performed with the needle, and the catheter is then advanced over the needle into the left atrium. Further manipulation may allow the catheter to be introduced into the left ventricle via the mitral valve. This technique has advantages in the occasional patient in whom the left ventricle cannot be entered retrogradely, for example, when there is severe aortic stenosis or a mechanical aortic valve prosthesis. An alternative technique for entering the left ventricle under these circumstances is to use direct needle puncture of the left ventricle through the chest wall. Although this technique sounds horrific, it has a very low complication rate in experienced hands. Angiography by this route, however, is extremely difficult or impossible. When difficulties are experienced in manipulating standard catheters through the right heart and into the pulmonary artery, Swan–Ganz balloon catheters can be helpful.

One of the most common applications of cardiac catheterization is coronary arteriography. This can be performed from either the femoral or the brachial route and is described in more detail below.

The radiation received by the patient during the average cardiac catheterization is in the order of 0.3 mGy (30 mrad). The operator receives about half this dose.[2] Some modern procedures, particularly coronary angioplasty, require more radiation. It is important that all catheter laboratory staff are carefully monitored for radiation exposure and that all possible precautions are taken to reduce this exposure.

INFORMATION DERIVED FROM CARDIAC CATHETERIZATION

Cardiac catheterization provides information about intracardiac pressure and flow, and, combined with angiography, gives information about both function and anatomy. Information of these different types can be combined: for example, measurements of pressure and flow can be used to calculate vascular resistance, and valve areas (see below). Occasionally, further information is derived from cardiac biopsies and metabolic studies obtained during catheterization.

PRESSURE MEASUREMENTS

Pressure measurements are meaningless unless they are accurate. Accuracy demands high-quality tracings and well-maintained and calibrated equipment which has a suitable frequency response.[3] For practical purposes, fluid-filled systems produce pressure measurements that are suitable for clinical decision-making. These pressure measurements, however, are often delayed and distorted, although this probably is kept to a minimum by keeping the length of tubing between the end of the catheter and the transducer as short as possible. If accurate and undistorted pressure tracings are required, specialized equipment such as catheter tip manometers are required.

Assuming that suitable equipment is available, there are certain situations in which measurements may be misleading. Excessive mobility and whip of the catheter caused by cardiac motion may sometimes artificially raise pressures by as much as 10–15 mmHg. This is usually easily recognizable because the pressure tracing has a spiky nature. Perhaps the pressure measurement most prone to error is the pulmonary artery wedge measurement. In ideal conditions, the waveform of the pulmonary artery wedge pressure corresponds to that of the left atrial pressure tracing. There is a small delay due to the time taken for the pressure pulse to spread back to the wedged catheter via the pulmonary venous and capillary system (Fig. 15.2). This delay is usually of no practical importance and, if a simultaneous measurement of left ventricular and left atrial tracings is required, for example, in the assessment of mitral stenosis, the pulmonary artery wedge pressure has to be moved back. This can be done if the patient is in sinus rhythm by ensuring that the 'a' wave present in both the pulmonary wedge pressure and left ventricular pressure occurs

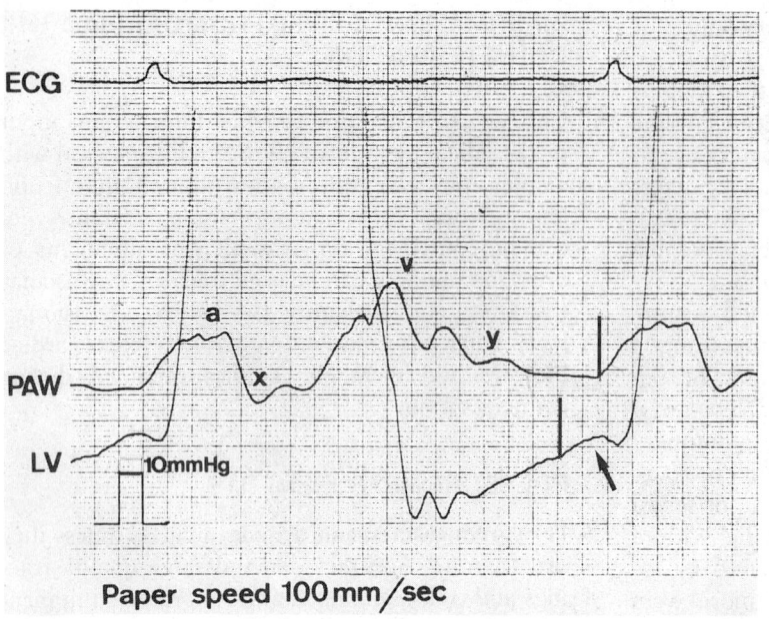

ECG

PAW

LV

10mmHg

Paper speed 100 mm/sec

Fig. 15.2. Simultaneous left ventricular (LV) and pulmonary artery wedge (PAW) pressures from a patient with mitral stenosis. There is a pressure gradient between them throughout diastole indicating that there is significant mitral stenosis. This patient is in sinus rhythm and the 'a' wave is seen in both traces. The beginning of the 'a' wave is marked on both and allows the delay in the PAW trace to be appreciated (arrow).

synchronously. In patients with atrial fibrillation, such a correction is more difficult. Delay in the wedge pressure, however, is not the main problem with this pressure measurement. The main errors occur because the pulmonary artery wedge pressure, although phasic and obtained from a properly wedged position, often overestimate left atrial pressure.[4,5] Accurate wedge pressures are particularly difficult to obtain in patients with chronically raised pulmonary artery pressure, because either the tracing is distorted by pulmonary vascular disease or it is impossible to wedge the catheter satisfactorily.

A further common error is an assumption that peripheral arterial tracings correspond in pressure to those obtained from the aorta. This is not usually the case and the peripheral pulse often gives a systolic pressure which is as much as 10–15 mmHg *higher* than that derived from the aortic pressure trace (Fig. 15.3). Consequently, if a peripheral arterial tracing is recorded simultaneously with the left ventricular pressure to assess the gradient across the aortic valve, such a gradient is underestimated.[6]

Pressure tracings are used in several different ways to derive information about the patient's clinical state. Elevation of pressures above normal may suggest the presence of an abnormality; the extent to which the pressure is elevated may give some idea of severity. Normal values are given in Table 2 of the appendix. However, when interpret-

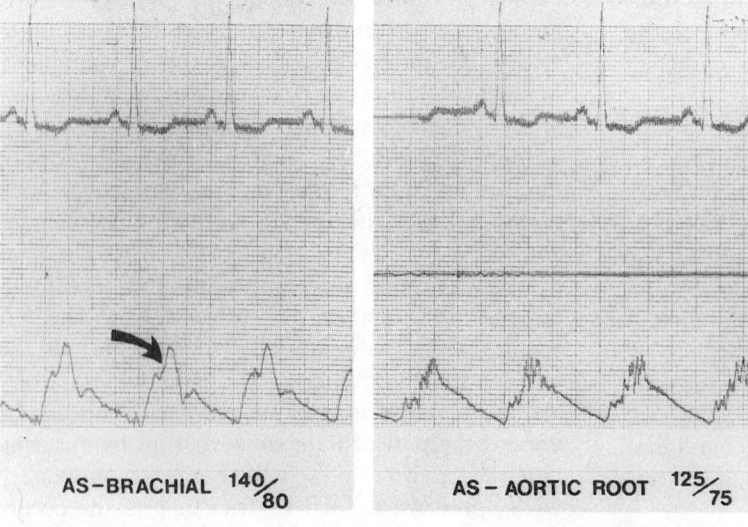

AS–BRACHIAL 140/80   AS – AORTIC ROOT 125/75

Fig. 15.3. Pressure tracings from the brachial artery (left) and aorta (right) in a patient with aortic stenosis (AS). There is a considerable difference in both the amplitude of the pulse (greater in the brachial) and the pressure waveform. This shows that the pulse changes as it goes towards the periphery. The arrow shows the anacrotic notch in the brachial recording. This is not seen as clearly in the aortic trace which has a more obvious shudder on its upstroke.

ing intracardiac pressures, it should be remembered that they may be altered by factors other than cardiac disease. First, the patient going to the cardiac catheterization laboratory may be on medication that alters the intracardiac pressures. For example, diuretics, powerful premedication or vasodilators may all lower intracardiac pressures. Beta-blockade tends to produce an elevation of left ventricular end-diastolic pressure and left atrial pressure. Second, the volume load produced by angiography may alter intracardiac pressures during the procedure, as will the occurrence of ischaemia which may lead to increases, particularly in left ventricular end-diastolic and left atrial pressures. Third, anxiety may elevate intracardiac pressures and in particular the arterial pressure.

In addition to alterations in intracardiac pressures that may suggest disease, specific patterns of pressure tracings may prove useful. The presence of prominent 'v' waves in the left atrial or pulmonary wedge pressure suggests the presence of mitral regurgitation (Fig. 15.4). If these are particularly sharp and high, significant mitral regurgitation is almost certainly present, but significantly increased 'v' waves of a lesser degree may occur in patients without mitral regurgitation. Similarly, large 'v' waves in the right atrial pressure trace strongly suggest the presence of tricuspid regurgitation (Fig. 15.5). Perhaps the most characteristic change in intracardiac pressures occurs in patients with pericardial constriction, in whom the ventricular pressure tracings have a particularly characteristic appearance. In early diastole, the pressure rises sharply to an abnormally high level and then remains at this plateau until the end of diastole. This appearance has been compared to the square root

sign (Fig. 15.6). In addition to this characteristic distortion of ventricular diastolic pressures, which usually occurs to the same extent in both left and right ventricles (Fig. 15.7), the mean right atrial pressure and the mean pulmonary artery pressure are also, usually, similar or identical to the ventricular end-diastolic pressures. Confusion can occur however in the rare patient with restrictive cardiomyopathy. Although various techniques have been described, including volume loading, to distinguish between these two situations, in practice this is often very difficult. The presence of severe pulmonary hypertension, however, is uncommon in constrictive pericarditis but relatively common in severe restrictive cardiomyopathy.

Pressure tracings are the main way in which a distinction can be made between functional and organic tricuspid regurgitation. This distinction is not absolute, but the following rules are useful. If severe tricuspid regurgitation is present with a normal or slightly elevated right ventricular systolic pressure, regurgitation is almost certainly organic. If there is significant pulmonary hypertension with a raised right ventricular systolic pressure, it is likely that tricuspid regurgitation is functional although this finding does not exclude the possibility of organic disease. Sometimes, echocardiography may be helpful by showing structural abnormalities of the tricuspid valve, but often the final diagnosis has to be left to the cardiac surgeon.[7]

Cardiac catheterization allows pressure gradients across all the cardiac valves to be measured (Figs 15.8 and 15.9). Commonly, these gradients are used in isolation to assess the severity of stenotic lesions. This approach has one major problem—it assumes that cardiac output is normal. The gradient across a

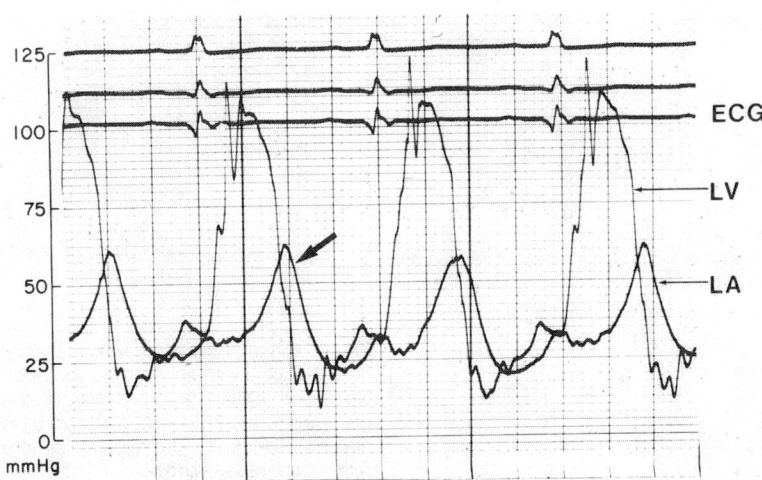

Fig. 15.4. Simultaneous left ventricular (LV) and left atrial (LA) pressures from a patient with severe mitral regurgitation. The left atrial pressure trace shows a prominent 'v' wave of about 60 mmHg (arrow) and the left ventricular end-diastolic pressure is elevated being about 30 mmHg.

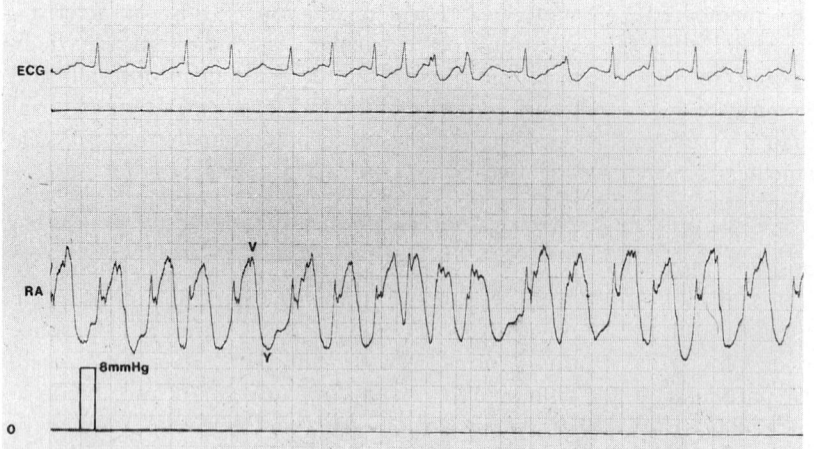

Fig. 15.5. Right atrial (RA) pressure trace from a patient with severe tricuspid regurgitation. There is a very prominent 'v' wave of 22 mmHg and a sharp 'y' descent.

cardiac valve is determined by the valve area and the flow across the valve. If the flow is increased, a mildly stenotic valve may have a high pressure gradient across it; conversely, and often more importantly, a severely stenotic valve may only produce a small pressure gradient when the cardiac output is low.[8] For these reasons, simultaneous measurement of transvalvar flow and gradient with calculation of the valve area (see below) is necessary in difficult cases.

As many cardiac symptoms occur on exercise, the finding of normal haemodynamics at rest may lead to a false impression of the true clinical situation.

For this reason, on occasions, exercise is used in conjunction with cardiac catheterization. Using either leg raising or a bicycle suspended over the catheter table, the patient is exercised while intracardiac pressures are measured. For example, this may lead to a sudden rise in end-diastolic pressure in a patient with compromised left ventricular function, for whatever reason, whereas the normal reaction is for this pressure to remain normal or near normal during exercise. Similarly, the increase in flow produced by exercise increases transvalvar pressure gradients, particularly in the assessment of patients with mitral stenosis. Those with moderate

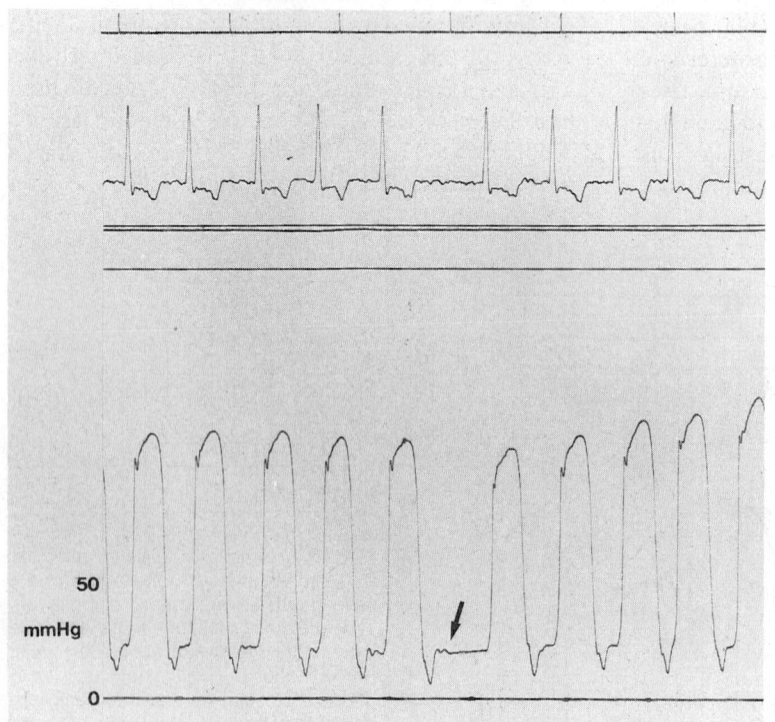

Fig. 15.6. Left ventricular pressure trace from a patient with constrictive pericarditis, which shows a rapid rise in the pressure in early diastole followed by a plateau leading to the typical 'square root' appearance (arrow).

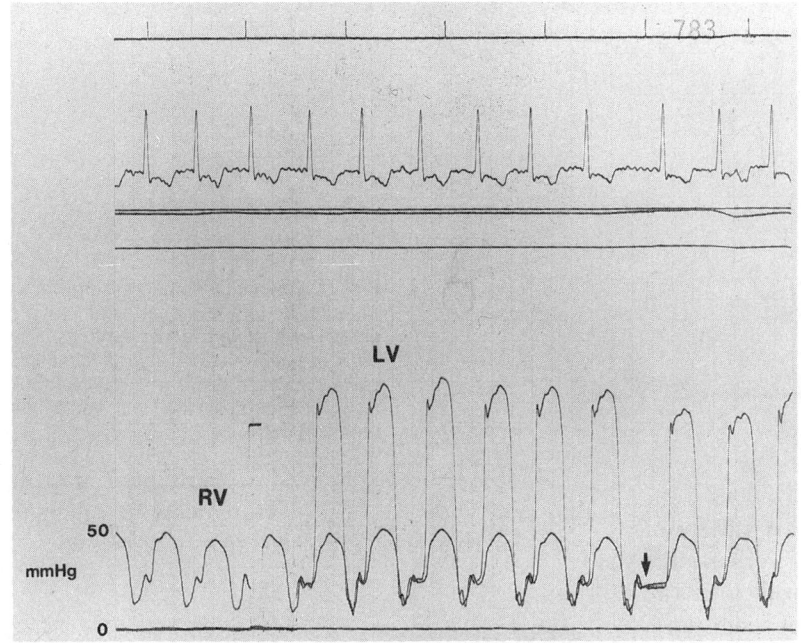

Fig. 15.7. Left ventricular (LV) and right ventricular (RV) pressure traces from the same patient as in Fig.15.6. The RV shows an identical pattern of pressure change in diastole.

stenosis may have a normal left atrial pressure at rest and this will rise sharply with the increase in cardiac output produced by exercise. This gives the clinician some idea of the level to which left atrial pressure rises during exercise in such patients and it may help to account for the symptoms, although recent studies of patients with heart failure have revealed imprecise correlations between left atrial pressure and the sensation of breathlessness.

Finally, pressure monitoring is helpful when manipulating catheters. Any loss or change in pressure suggests that the catheter has impinged on the wall of a vessel or cardiac chamber and therefore should be withdrawn slightly and re-manipulated. In addition, simultaneous pressure measurements, particularly when performing coronary angiography, ensure that the catheter is not obstructing the coronary orifice.

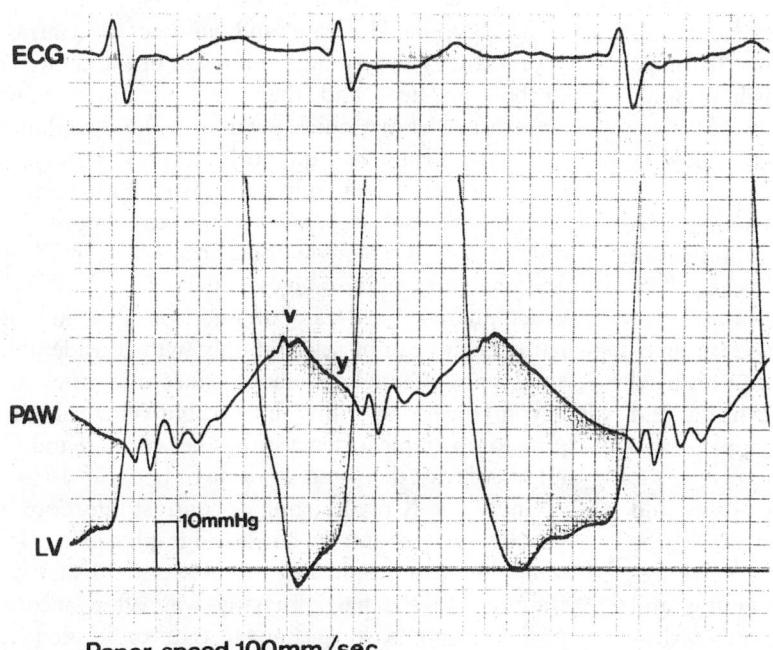

Fig. 15.8. Left ventricular (LV) and pulmonary artery wedge (PAW) pressure tracings from a patient with severe mitral stenosis and atrial fibrillation. There is a large pressure gradient throughout diastole indicating severe mitral stenosis. The end-diastolic gradient is greater when the cycle length is short (left) being about 30 mmHg. When it is longer (right), the gradient falls to 20 mmHg.

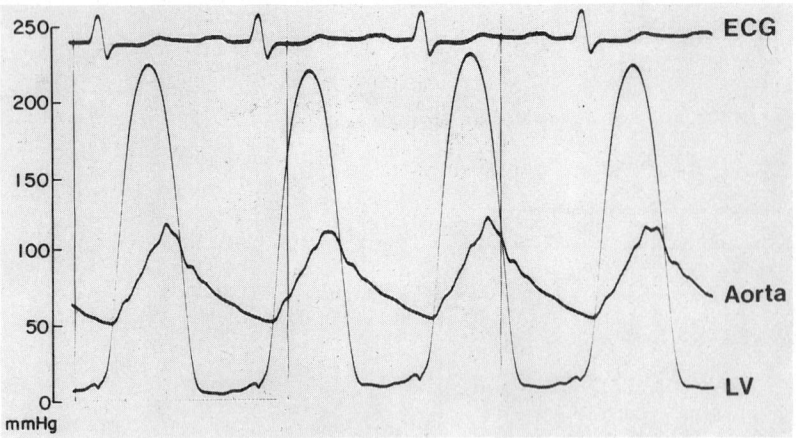

Fig. 15.9. Simultaneous pressure traces from the aorta and the left ventricle in a patient with severe aortic stenosis. The peak-to-peak gradient across the aortic valve in systole is 110 mmHg. Note the slow upstroke of the left ventricular pressure trace.

FLOW MEASUREMENT

Intracardiac flow can be measured in a variety of ways during cardiac catheterization. Perhaps the commonest method is to use the Fick principle. The Fick principle states that the amount of a substance taken up or released by an organ is the product of its blood flow and the difference in concentration of the substance in its arterial and venous blood. Using the lungs' capacity to take up oxygen, the sampling of the oxygen concentration of blood entering and leaving the lungs allows cardiac output to be calculated if oxygen consumption is known. Either oxygen consumption can be measured during cardiac catheterization, or sometimes it is simply derived by tables constructed for patients of varying age and sex[9] (Table 1, Appendix p. 385). The latter method is far less accurate. If there is no intracardiac shunt, the values for oxygen saturation taken from pulmonary artery and aorta are satisfactory to make this measurement. If there is an intracardiac shunt, both pulmonary and systemic flows can be calculated. The use of the Fick principle is described in the appendix to this chapter (p. 385).

The second most frequently used technique is based on the dilution of a known amount of indicator introduced into the vascular system.[10,11] The most commonly used indicators are Indocyanine Green or a bolus of cold saline (thermodilution) where heat, or rather the lack of it, is used as the indicator. The principles of dye dilution and thermodilution are also discussed in the appendix to this chapter.

In addition to estimating total cardiac output and the extent of shunts, these techniques can also be used to assess valvular regurgitation[12,13] (see below). These techniques are time-consuming and infrequently used in modern cardiac catheterization.

Flow measurements are frequently used in combination with pressure measurements to calculate vascular resistance and valve areas (see below).

ANGIOGRAPHY

Angiograms are produced by injecting radiopaque iodine-containing contrast agents at the appropriate place in the circulation via cardiac catheters. When small quantities of contrast are required to produce an angiogram, for example, when a vessel is selectively cannulated, between 5 and 10 ml of contrast material can be injected by hand via the catheter. When larger quantities of contrast have to be delivered, for example, to opacify the left ventricle, it is impossible to inject sufficiently quickly by hand and a power injection delivered by special equipment is used. The rate and volume of contrast required vary depending on the size of the chamber to be opacified, and the speed of blood flow. Contrast must mix quickly with the blood so that it is present in sufficient quantities to produce a good image. If insufficient contrast is injected too slowly, it will be washed away by the circulation too quickly for an adequate concentration to build up and therefore poor images will be obtained. The exact quantity and rate of injection vary among patients and can be selected only with considerable experience. Guidelines about exact quantities are beyond the scope of this chapter, but ventriculography, for example, often requires between 30 and 60 ml of contrast delivered at a rate of between 10 and 20 ml/s. The X-ray imaging of contrast injections is usually carried out by cinéangiography using 35-mm film at a frame rate of between 30 and 50 frames/s. In the past, imaging was often accomplished using a film changer that took pictures about the size of an average chest X-ray several times a second. This technique is still used for pulmonary angiography, does not produce the definition of movement obtained by cinéangiography and is very expensive because of the amount of X-ray film used, but it does allow a large field to be imaged. In the future, it is likely that techniques of digital subtraction angiography (see Chapter 17) will become more popular, allowing angiographic information to be stored in a computer and the images to be reconstructed when required, and videotape will take over from ciné film, particularly when video discs become more widely available. These will allow cheap storage of large numbers of angiograms which will be easy to access quickly.

Contrast agents for angiography

All contrast agents used for angiography contain iodine in high concentrations, which makes them radiopaque. Conventional contrast agents, such as Urografin (meglumine/sodium diatrizoate) and Cardioconray (meglumine/sodium iothalamate) are extremely hyperosmolar. Their molar concentration is between 5 and 8 times physiological level, and many of their adverse effects are related to this hyperosmolarity. They expand intravascular volume by attracting fluid into the circulation, reduce peripheral vascular resistance and may also alter intracardiac pressures and cardiac output. Intracardiac pressures often rise, and cardiac output may rise or fall depending on the individual patient. Although serious complications from the contrast material injected at angiography are rare, many patients develop minor unpleasant side-effects, of which flushing, nausea and the feeling that they may have been incontinent are perhaps the most common. Major side-effects including cardiovascular collapse, pulmonary and cerebral oedema, bronchospasm and anaphylaxis can sometimes occur. The precise mechanism of action of many of these adverse effects is poorly understood but many of the effects have been reduced by the recent introduction into clinical practice of new imaging agents that have considerably lower osmolarity. As these new agents seem to produce a lower incidence of major and minor side-effects,[14,15] they are rapidly gaining in popularity. The low incidence of serious problems with conventional agents in low-risk patients means that the use of the new agents is not obligatory in such cases, and, in some centres, because of the considerably higher cost of the new agents, they may be restricted to high-risk patients. Ideally, they should be used for all cases because patients find them much less unpleasant.

The reduced osmolarity but equal radiopacity of these new agents has been achieved by halving the number of particles in solution while maintaining the same concentration of iodine. This can be achieved in two ways. Some agents are non-ionic, and thus produce half as many particles in solution as the conventional ionic agents. Examples of this type of contrast medium are metrizamide (Amipaque) and iopamidol (Niopam). An alternative approach is to produce a compound that has twice as many iodine atoms for the number of particles in solution but which still ionizes. An example of this type of agent is ioxaglate (Hexabrix). Halving the number of particles in solution theoretically reduces osmolarity to 50%, but, in reality, these agents have only 30% osmolarity of conventional agents because some aggregation also occurs in solution which further reduces the number of particles.

Types of angiography

Coronary angiography

Visualization of the coronary arteries is the most commonly used form of angiography in cardiology (Fig. 15.10). High-quality angiograms can be produced only by selectively intubating the coronary orifices. Injections of contrast into the coronary sinuses rarely produce angiograms of sufficiently high quality for diagnostic use. Selective intubation of the coronary orifices can be achieved using several standard techniques. The most common is the Judkins' technqiue using preformed catheters introduced via the femoral route (Fig. 15.11). The catheters for right and left coronary arteries are of different shapes. The coronary arteries can also be intubated by the femoral route using catheters of alternative design, for example, the Amplatz catheter (Fig. 15.1E), but these are usually reserved for patients in whom difficulty is experienced using the Judkins' technique. Occasionally, Judkins' catheters are used from the left arm because with this approach they traverse the aortic arch in a similar direction to catheters introduced from the leg. More commonly, when coronary angiography is carried out from the arm, access is gained by the right brachial artery and the Sones' technique is used. The Sones' catheters have a long tapering tip and are flexible so that the operator can form loops and manipulate the end of the catheter into either the right or left coronary artery. This technique needs more training and expertise but in skilled hands the

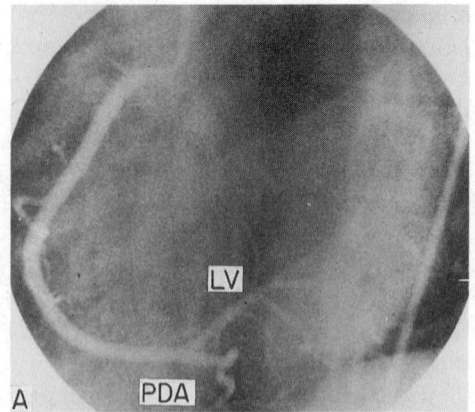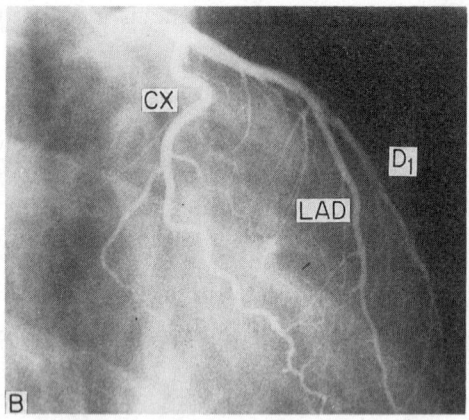

Fig. 15.10. Normal coronary arteries. The right coronary (A) is shown in the left anterior oblique (LAO) projection and the left coronary (B) in the right anterior oblique (RAO) projection. PDA, posterior descending artery; LV, left ventricular branch; CX, circumflex; LAD, left anterior descending; D₁, first diagonal. (Orientation is similar to that in Fig. 15.13.).

results are as good as with the Judkins' technique (Fig. 15.12).

Preformed catheters, similar in shape to the Amplatz catheter, are available for use from the arm. The choice of approach depends on many factors. In some patients with peripheral vascular disease, an arm approach has to be used. In other patients, the choice of technique depends on individual practice and training. In skilled hands, the results obtained from the arm and the leg are equally good and the risks similar. However, the Judkins' technique is more popular and requires less training.

Regardless of the technique used, careful attention to detail is essential. It is particularly important that the system is free of air and thrombus so that embolism into the coronary arteries does not occur at the time of angiography. It is equally important that the catheter is not allowed to occlude the vessel being imaged. This is avoided by continuous press-

ure monitoring from the tip of the catheter. As long as the catheter is free with flow around it occurring into the coronary arteries, a normal aortic pressure will be recorded. If the pressure recorded falls suddenly or shows a distorted waveform, occlusion of the coronary orifice should be suspected and the catheter withdrawn. Continuous electrocardiographic monitoring also helps to detect the occurrence of complications. If progressive ischaemic changes begin to occur, the catheter should be withdrawn to allow full flow into the coronary artery, although transient ischaemic changes, sometimes accompanied by angina, are not uncommon during or just after injection of contrast. Occasionally, rhythm disturbances occur while coronary angiography is being performed, usually just after the injection of contrast. The most common is sinus bradycardia which may be very severe and occurs most often with injection into the right coronary

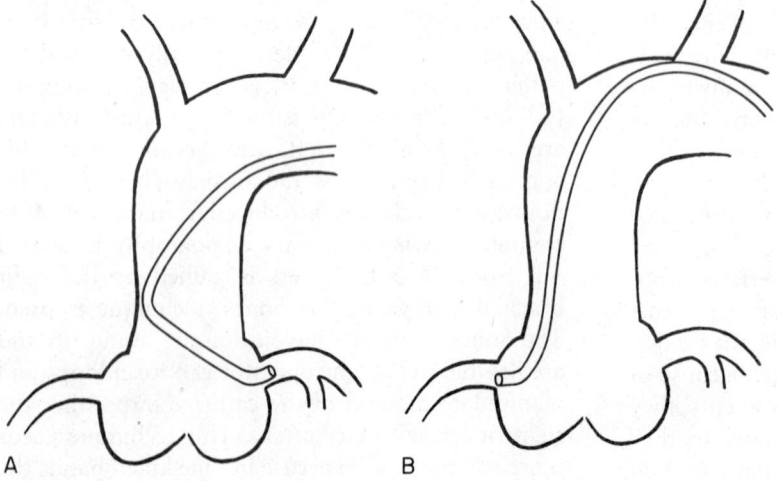

Fig. 15.11. Drawings showing the coronary arteries selectively intubated using the Judkins' technique from the femoral approach. The catheters for the left (A) and right (B) coronary arteries are of different shapes and each comes in a range of different sized curves to suit the individual patient.

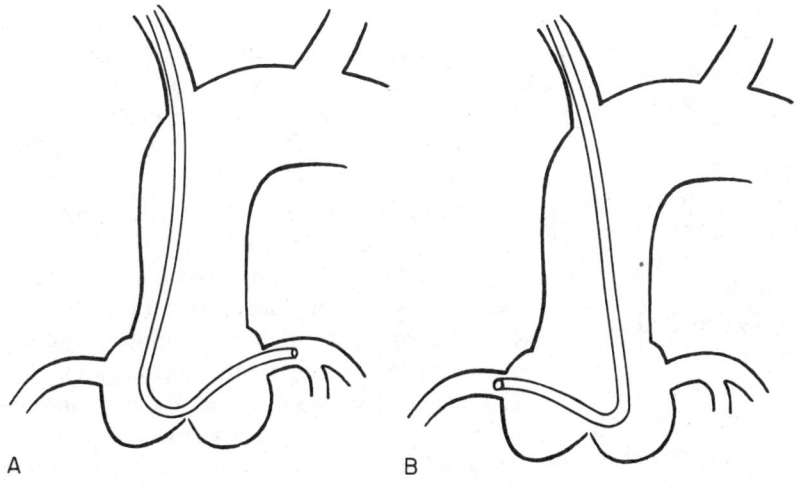

Fig. 15.12. Drawings showing the coronary arteries selectively intubated using a Sones' catheter from the brachial approach. The same tapering catheter is used to enter both coronary arteries: (A) left coronary artery; (B) right coronary artery.

artery. Acutely, this can usually be treated by asking the patient to cough because this reflexly reduces the vagal tone. If bradycardia is prominent, occurring with every injection and persisting between injections, atropine should be given. Far less often, ventricular fibrillation may occur during or immediately after a coronary injection. For this reason, a defibrillator should be available in the catheterization laboratory. Usually, a single shock is sufficient to restore the patient to sinus rhythm without any long- or short-term sequelae. A single episode of ventricular fibrillation does not usually necessitate termination of the procedure, although many operators would give the patient an anti-arrhythmic agent, such as lignocaine, and wait for a few minutes before continuing angiography.

Angiograms are obtained by hand injection of contrast into the coronary orifices. Usually 5–10 ml are required for adequate opacification. The rate and quantity of injections are regulated by the operator who watches the images as they appear and alters the rate of injection to obtain good images. While the contrast material is being injected by hand, ciné film is recorded and is allowed to run after the end of the hand injection to image any collateral flow that may appear late.

The quality of coronary angiograms depends on a variety of factors. To obtain both high-quality angiograms and useful diagnostic information, the equipment used must be of high quality, the vessel must be selectively intubated and sufficient contrast must be injected at an adequate rate. In addition, it is essential that the operator analyses the changes as they are found during the procedure so that adequate views can be taken to define any suspected pathology.

Angiographic projections used in coronary angiography

The aim of coronary angiography is to visualize the entire coronary artery system and to show any suspected lesion in at least two orthogonal projections (at right angles to each other). This is required because coronary angiography produces a silhouette of the structure being visualized. The X-ray equipment used for coronary angiography usually allows the image intensifier and X-ray tube to be rotated around the patient to almost any angle and also to be tilted in either a cranial or caudal direction.

Left coronary artery The left coronary artery is usually imaged in right anterior oblique, postero-anterior, left anterior oblique and lateral views. Addition of cranial or caudal tilt to the oblique views frequently allows vessels to be separated and lesions to be defined more precisely. A particularly important use of this tilting is to view the proximal part of the left anterior descending coronary artery by applying cranial tilt to a left anterior oblique projection. In most centres, this would be regarded as a standard view. In addition to these standard views, any combination of obliquity and tilt may be needed to define a particular lesion.

Right coronary artery The right coronary system is simpler, with fewer branches than the left coronary system. As a result, a smaller number of views is normally used and a combination of right and left anterior oblique projections is usually sufficient. Cranial or caudal tilt in the individual patient may help to define lesions more clearly, particularly at the bifurcation into the posterior descending and left ventricular branches (Fig. 15.13B).

Coronary anatomy

The anatomy of the coronary artery system has been described in detail elsewhere but is shown in Fig. 15.13. There is considerable variation in coronary anatomy among individuals. The most prominent and common variation is the dominance of the coronary arteries. The right or left coronary artery is referred to as being dominant if it supplies the posterior descending artery. In the majority of patients, the posterior descending artery is supplied by the right coronary artery, but in about 10% of patients the right coronary artery is very small and the circumflex coronary artery supplies the posterior descending artery. Although, in most patients, the left anterior descending and circumflex coronary arteries are formed by the division of the left main coronary artery, this is not always so. The left main coronary artery varies in length considerably and on occasions becomes so short that it disappears and the circumflex and left anterior descending coronary arteries originate from a common orifice or even separate orifices in the left coronary sinus. This variation is relatively common and may make coronary angiography technically difficult if the coronary catheter will enter only one or other of the two branches, or occludes the origin of one while entering the other. Very occasionally, more extreme variations in coronary anatomy occur,[16] in which a coronary artery arises from an unusual situation and then may run in an aberrant direction for at least part of its course. The most common aberrant vessel is the circumflex, which may arise either as a separate vessel from the right coronary sinus or as a branch of the right coronary artery (Fig. 15.14). Under these circumstances, it runs posterior to the aorta before reaching its normal territory. This situation may be missed during coronary angiography but can usually be recognized because of the dearth of vessels in the circumflex territory when the left coronary artery is injected (Fig. 15.14B). Re-inspection of the left ventriculogram will usually show the aberrant circumflex end-on running behind the aortic root (Fig. 15.15) (the so-called 'aortic root' sign).[17] It is important that this situation is recognized because there may be significant disease within the aberrant vessels giving rise to the patient's symptoms. Other less common aberrations of the coronary circulation can occur, of which probably the most important is origin of the left anterior descending coronary artery from the right coronary sinus. In young subjects, this anomaly, which is fairly rare, has been found to be associated with ischaemic symptoms and sudden death on exertion. Occasionally, coronary arteries may arise from the pulmonary artery, but these are always associated with ischaemic problems during early childhood.

At present, coronary angiography requires selective injection of the coronary arteries. In future, techniques such as digital subtraction angiography may produce satisfactory images of the coronary arteries with non-selective injections into the aortic root, but to date these hopes have not been fulfilled (see Chapter 17).

Uses of coronary angiography

Coronary artery disease

The most common use of coronary arteriography is in the investigation of coronary artery disease where it has many applications.

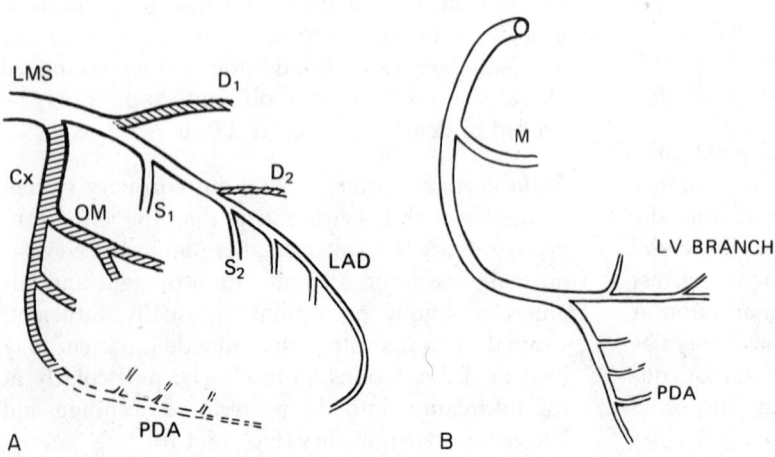

Fig. 15.13. Diagrams of the left (A) and right (B) coronary arteries; (A) is drawn from the right anterior oblique position and (B) from the left anterior oblique with cranial tilt. The posterior descending coronary artery (PDA) is usually a branch of the right coronary (the right dominant system), but in about 10% of patients it arises as a branch of the circumflex (Cx) and this is known as a left dominant system (dotted lines on the diagram of the left coronary artery). The shaded branches on the diagram of the left coronary vessel are those that run on the back of the heart. M, marginal; LMS, left main stem; LAD, left anterior descending; D_1 and D_2, first and second diagonals; S_1 and S_2, first and second septals; OM, obtuse marginal; LV branch, left ventricular branch.

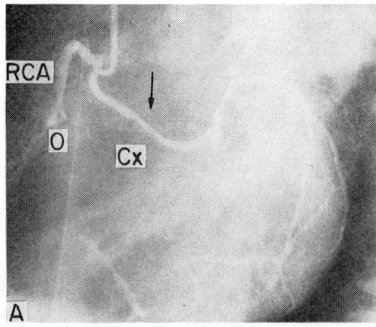
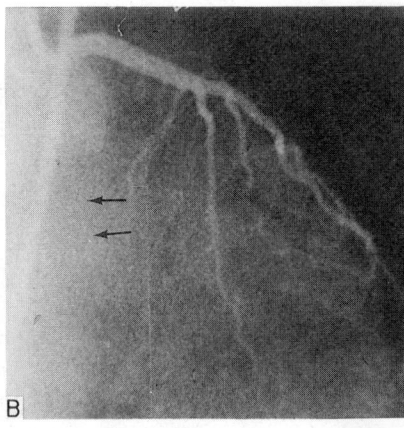
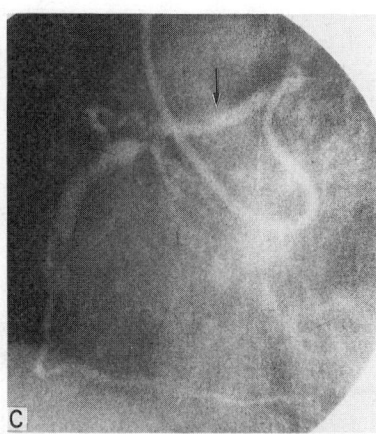

Fig. 15.14. (A) An aberrant circumflex vessel (LAO) arising from the right coronary artery and passing to the left behind the aorta to gain its usual territory (arrow). The distal right coronary artery is occluded (O). (B) The left coronary artery in a patient who has an aberrant circumflex vessel as in (A). Note the complete absence of any branches from this vessel to the circumflex territory (arrows). (C) Significant disease in a *right* coronary artery (LAO) that arises aberrantly from the *left* coronary sinus and runs around the aortic root to the right coronary territory.

Coronary arteriography is used to define the position and severity of obstructive lesions within the coronary artery tree.[18] As the results of experimental studies in animals and *in vitro* indicate that a 70% reduction in cross-sectional areas of the coronary artery, which is equivalent to a 50% reduction in diameter, is sufficient to produce a reduction of regional flow and myocardial ischaemia at peak exercise,[19] lesions of this severity are usually regarded as being significant. Confusion often occurs because it is not clear whether the information in the angiographer's report refers to a reduction in the diameter of the vessel or in the area of the vessel. Usually, reduction in diameter is quoted because this information is directly available from the angiogram. Problems also arise because the angiogram merely demonstrates the effect of arterial wall disease on the contour of the arterial lumen in one particular projection, therefore any lesion must reduce diameter by at least 50% in two views at right angles to each other before significance is reached. Although this appears to be straightforward, in practice the situation is much more complicated. The coronary angiogram can reliably identify a normal coronary artery and there is little doubt about the presence of coronary disease when lesions are either very severe or vessels are occluded. Further evidence about the haemodynamic effects of lesions is obtained if retrograde filling of portions of coronary arteries beyond lesions is seen via collaterals. The conventional grading of lesions in coronary arteries by 'eyeballing' them and then assigning an arbitrary figure to their degree of severity is notoriously inaccurate.[18] Some experts have suggested that it is more sensible to grade coronary lesions as mild, moderate or severe.[18] In addition to the severity and morphology of the stenosis, i.e. whether that stenosis is eccentric or concentric, variations also occur in the length of stenotic lesions. More severe obstruction to flow is caused by long coronary stenoses and, although stenoses occurring in series may have an additive effect, little is known or understood about this problem and it is certainly not taken into account in cardiological practice.[19] As the grading of coronary stenoses by eye is inaccurate, various attempts have been made to use advanced imaging technology assisted by computers to assess the severity of coronary artery lesions.[20] These techniques, often relying on edge detection performed by computer, are rudimentary, and at present they are time-consuming and not universally available.

Despite the problems of grading coronary lesions into percentage severity without measurement, this technique is in common usage. Patients with coronary disease are then usually classified into having disease of one, two or three coronary arteries. Some patients with coronary lesions in all three coronary arteries may have considerably less coronary disease than other patients. The severity of stenosis within the individual vessel, the number of large diseased or undiseased branches and the extent of collaterals will all contribute to disease severity. Despite these shortcomings, in most of the large studies designed to examine the relationship between the severity of coronary artery disease and the effects of coronary

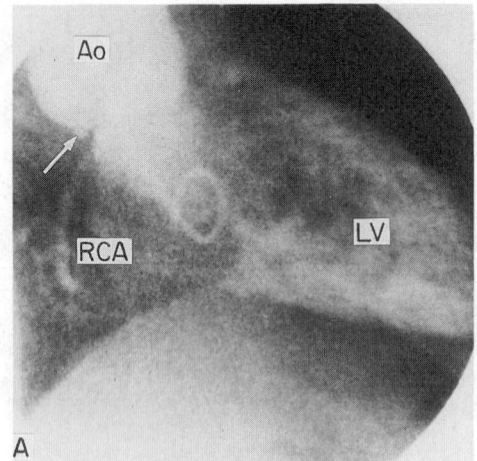

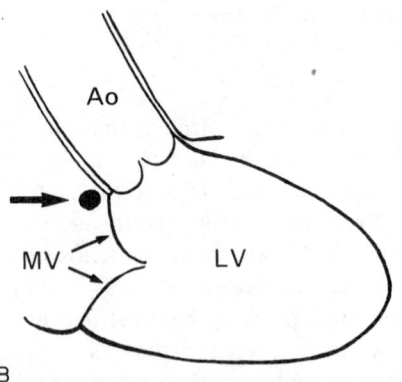

Fig. 15.15. The aortic root sign' seen in the right anterior oblique (RAO) left ventriculogram in patients in whom the circumflex coronary artery arises from the right and passes behind the aorta. In this projection, the aberrant vessel is seen end-on as a dot behind the aorta (arrow). (A) Angiogram; (B) drawing to illustrate angiogram. Ao, aorta; LV, left ventricle; RCA, right coronary artery

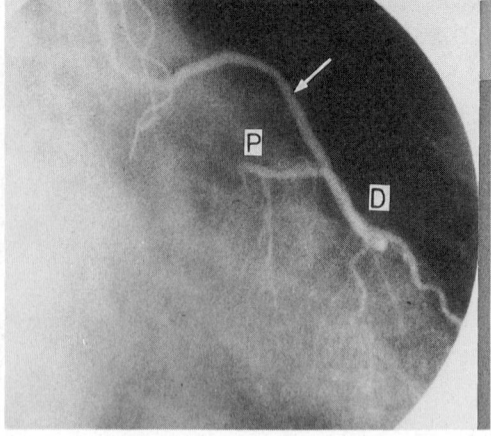

Fig. 15.16. Selective injection of contrast into a coronary artery bypass graft (arrow) to the left anterior descending. This arises from the anterior wall of the aorta and in this case the surgeon has marked the graft with a wire loop. The distal vessel (D) fills well and there is some retrograde flow in the native vessel to show part of the proximal left anterior descending artery (P) and a septal branch.

artery surgery on prognosis and symptoms, this classification has been used[21] and it forms the basis upon which many clinical decisions are made in such patients. It is likely that this method of classification will persist into the foreseeable future.

The identification of *graft patency* usually requires selective intubation of the individual grafts so that patency and any stenosis in the grafts or at the point at which they enter the coronary arteries can be defined. These grafts usually have their proximal end placed on the anterior surface of the aorta (Fig. 15.16). They can usually be entered using conventional Judkins' catheter designed for the right coronary artery or specially adapted catheters for graft intubation. Grafts can also be entered using the Sones' technique. Graft angiography can be time-consuming and difficult, but it is usually suc-

cessfully achieved. Special catheters are available for entering internal mammary arteries in patients in whom this artery has been used to bypass lesions. Non-selective techniques using digital subtraction angiography can identify the patency of coronary grafts but they usually fail to delineate them with sufficient clarity to allow stenoses to be defined.

Other uses of coronary angiography

Occasionally, coronary angiography is used to identify rare conditions, such as coronary artery fistulae and aneurysms, abnormalities of coronary artery anatomy associated with congenital heart disease, which may prove important to the surgeon when correcting the congenital defect, and coronary anomalies, which may occasionally be the cause of symptoms, for example, an aberrant left anterior descending coronary artery. Occasionally, spasm is detected during a coronary arteriogram. If spasm occurs at the origin of the coronary artery, usually the right, during angiography, it is nearly always due to mechanical stimulation caused by the catheter and is of no clinical significance (Fig. 15.17). More rarely, spasm producing ischaemic pain and occurring more distally in the artery often originating at a coronary lesion is of clinical significance. This type of spasm can be revealed by the administration of vasoconstrictors, such as ergometrine, during the procedure. This technique is now used far less frequently because it may produce severe

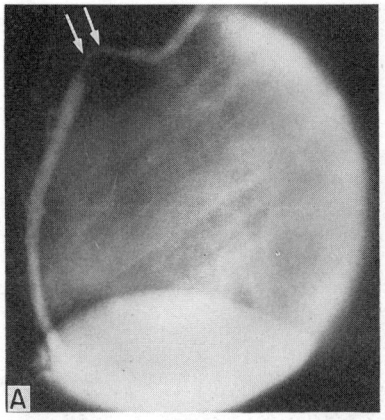 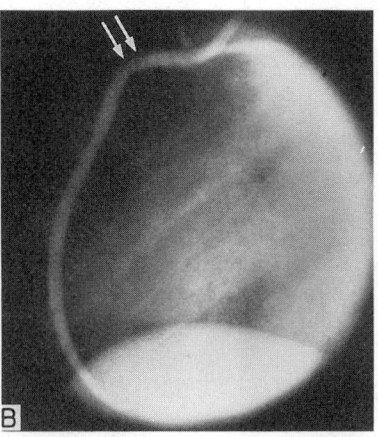

Fig. 15.17. (A) Spasm near the orifice of the right coronary artery of the type that is occasionally induced by the angiographic catheter. (B) The same vessel a few minutes later following the administration of intracoronary nitroglycerine.

and irreversible spasm with serious consequences for the patient.[22] Generally, in a patient in whom coronary artery spasm is suspected, a safer approach is to make strenuous attempts to record an electrocardiogram, or even a thallium perfusion image, during spontaneously occurring episodes of pain. This is considerably safer than giving ergometrine during coronary angiography. Failing this, a therapeutic trial of calcium antagonists is preferable.

Intubation of the coronary arteries to carry out therapeutic manoeuvres such as angioplasty and thrombolysis are important applications of the technique.

Ventriculography

Ventricular function and regurgitation Angiograms of the ventricles are carried out for two main reasons: first, to assess ventricular function; and second to detect regurgitation through the atrioventricular valves. The left ventricle lends itself to angiographic study much better than the right. Its shape allows wall motion to be analysed and ventricular volume to be calculated using methods such as those of Sandler and Dodge or by Simpson's rule (see Appendix to this chapter).[23-25] It is easily imaged in two planes, of which the most commonly used are the right anterior oblique projection and a left anterior oblique or lateral projection. Addition of the second plane adds to the accuracy of the calculations of volume. Left ventricular angiograms are usually carried out via catheters that enter the ventricle retrogradely through the aortic valve. This catheter position does not interfere with atrioventricular valve function and thus regurgitation through the mitral valve can be assessed (Fig. 15.18). In contrast, the right ventricle has a more

complicated crescentic shape with a trabeculated wall; these factors make measurement of volume difficult or impossible. Similarly, the assessment of wall motion is likely to be inaccurate because of this complicated shape. Assessment of tricuspid regurgitation by right ventriculography is sometimes rendered inaccurate by the fact that the catheter used for injecting contrast into the ventricle passes into it anterogradely via the tricuspid valve and may thereby interfere with its function and result in spurious tricuspid regurgitation.

In clinical practice, assessment of left ventricular function by ventriculography is usually carried out by a subjective assessment of the extent of wall motion and ventricular size. Although this type of analysis is fraught with error, it is sufficiently accurate to distinguish very poor from normal ventricular function. Similarly, assessment of regurgitation is usually performed by a simple subjective grading of the regurgitation observed into slight, mild, moderate or severe. This grading of severity is inaccurate with wide interobserver variation.[26,27] Despite these difficulties, this method of assessing left ventricular function and regurgitation is often taken as the 'gold standard' against which other cardiac measurements are compared. In addition to the problems of measurement suggested above, both ventricular function and regurgitation are highly dependent on ventricular loading, which may vary widely with time in the same patient, consequently measurements such as the degree of regurgitation or the extent of wall motion may be very different from day to day. Although this aspect cannot be eliminated by attention to detail, measurement of left ventricular wall motion can be improved using modern computer-assisted techniques. However, these require a considerable amount of time to perform and analyse and are

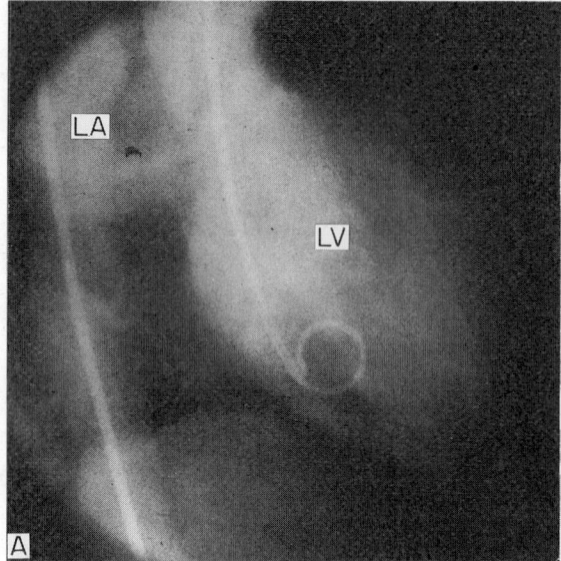 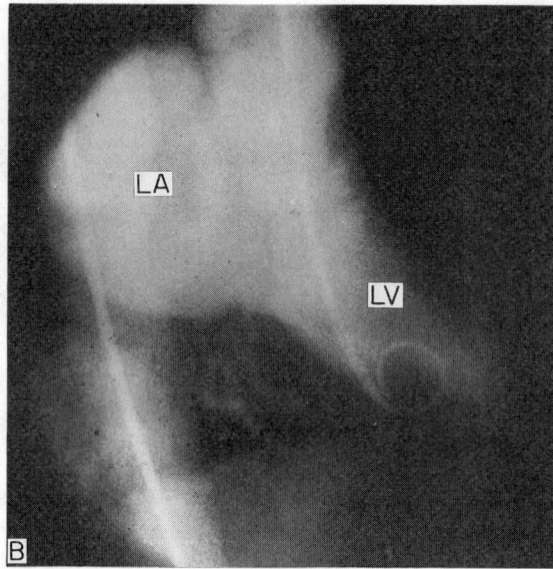

Fig. 15.18. Diastolic (A) and systolic (B) frames from a left ventriculogram in a patient with severe mitral regurgitation. Note that the left atrium in (B) is completely opacified by the contrast; this is the first systolic frame and therefore the mitral regurgitation is very severe. The large difference between the left ventricular dimensions in systole and diastole shows that the ejection fraction is high. LV, left ventricle; LA, left atrium.

probably not cost-effective in everyday clinical practice.

Other uses of ventriculography Ventriculograms have many other uses, all of which are relatively uncommon. They may identify particular abnormalities within the ventricle, such as left ventricular aneurysm or an interventricular filling defect due to clot or tumour. Defects in the interventricular septum will be shown by the passage of dye through the defect and valve cusps (aortic, pulmonary, tricuspid or mitral depending on the site of injection) may be seen in silhouette. It may also allow thickening or abnormal motion of the aortic and mitral valves to be identified (Fig. 15.19).

Aortography

The main use of aortography is to identify the shape and size of the aortic root and the presence or absence of aortic regurgitation (Fig. 15.20). This may be useful in a patient with a suspected aneurysm (Fig. 15.21) or abnormality such as Marfan's syndrome or aortic dissection. Injection of contrast (30–50 ml) into the aortic root has to be carried out rapidly (20–30 ml/s) so that the aorta is filled before the dye is washed away. The catheter is

positioned above the aortic valve in such a way that it does not interfere with the aortic valve itself, and the amount of aortic regurgitation can be assessed from the degree to which the left ventricle opacifies. This type of assessment has the same shortcomings as grading mitral regurgitation by eye. Gross aortic regurgitation or its absence are easy to identify but the accurate assessment of moderate degrees of aortic regurgitation is difficult.[27] Aortography will also reveal other abnormalities such as coarctation (Fig. 15.22).

Other angiography

Occasionally, angiography in other intracardiac sites is required. Pulmonary arteriography is used mainly to assess diseases of the pulmonary circulation but can also be used to assess left ventricular function; contrast injection into the pulmonary artery usually reaches the left ventricle rapidly and with modern cinéangiographic equipment good imaging of the left ventricle is easily obtained. This method has the advantage that arrhythmias and ectopic beats are usually avoided; however, as the left atrium is also opacified this technique cannot be used to assess mitral regurgitation.

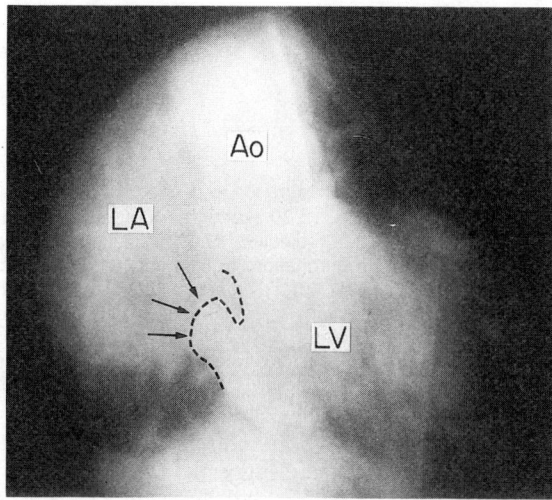 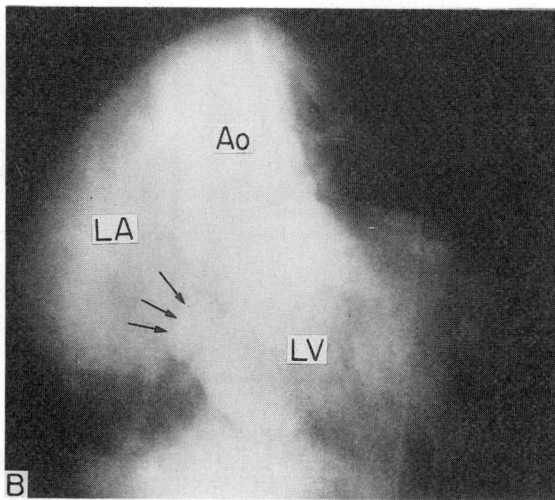

Fig. 15.19. Left ventriculogram (right anterior oblique projection) from a patient with a prolapsing floppy mitral valve. These are identical systolic frames and the prolapsing scallops of the posterior mitral valve cusp can be seen in addition to opacification of the left atrium due to mitral regurgitation. In (A), the prolapsing portion of the valve (arrows in A and B) has been traced with a dotted line. Ao, aorta; LV, left ventricle; LA, left atrium.

COMBINED USE OF DIFFERENT TYPES OF VARIABLES DURING CARDIAC CATHETERIZATION

Measurements of pressure and flow are combined to calculate various important haemodynamic variables.

Vascular resistance

If the blood flow and pressure drop across a vascular bed are known, its resistance can be calculated. The formulae for calculating pulmonary and systemic vascular resistance are given in Table 3 of the Appendix to this chapter. Calculation of systemic vascular resistance has little practical application but is often used when experimentally assessing vasodilator drugs. Pulmonary vascular resistance is calculated more often. It is frequently raised in patients with chronic mitral valve lesions and occasionally when there is severe left ventricular dysfunction. This measurement is particularly important in patients being assessed for cardiac transplantation. If the pulmonary vascular resistance is high, usually as a result of chronic left ventricular disease, the patient may be *unsuitable for cardiac transplantation* because the normal thin-walled right ventricle of the donor heart is unable to cope with the resistance offered by the recipient's lungs. High levels of pulmonary vascular resistance used

to be regarded as a contra-indication to mitral valve surgery but nowadays with improved surgical and anaesthetic technique patients are rarely rejected for surgery because of a high pulmonary resistance. Despite this, it is useful to know the level of pulmonary vascular resistance before surgery because this may indicate whether potential problems will arise during the operative course. A raised pulmonary vascular resistance is also a feature of some patients with longstanding left-to-right shunt. If the pulmonary vascular resistance is sufficiently high to cause the shunt to reverse and become a right-to-left shunt, such patients are unlikely to benefit from surgery to close the defect causing the shunt. Finally, a raised pulmonary vascular resistance is a feature of intrinsic disease of the pulmonary circulation, such as primary pulmonary hypertension, and of patients with severe chronic lung disease. If patients with chronic lung disease have co-existent cardiac lesions, it is difficult to distinguish how much of the raised pulmonary vascular resistance is due to the pulmonary lesion and how much is due to the cardiac lesion.

Calculation of valve areas

The need for assessing valve stenosis by calculating valve areas rather than relying on pressure gradients alone has been discussed above. Formulae for esti-

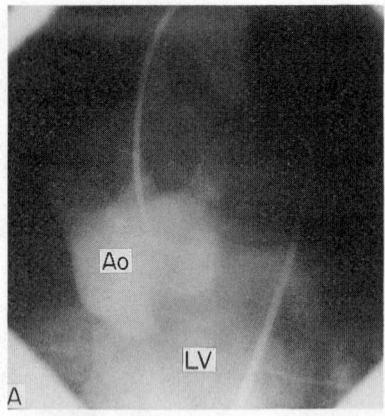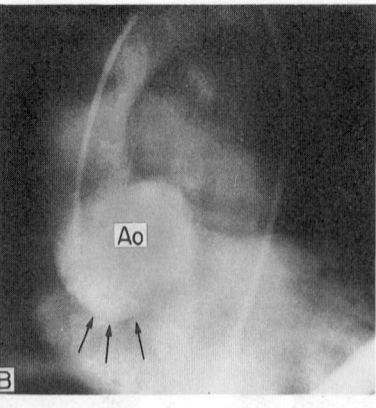

Fig. 15.20. Aortogram (left anterior oblique projection) from a patient with aortic regurgitation due a prolapsing aortic valve cusp as the result of a high ventricular septal defect (VSD). (A) The prolapsing cusp (arrows); a later frame (B), demonstrates that the left ventricle is opacified by contrast that has regurgitated through the incompetent valve.

mating mitral and aortic valve areas were first proposed by Gorlin and Gorlin in 1951.[28] These equations were further modified in 1972.[29] Although the Gorlin formulae are often used as a value against which all other methods for assessing stenosis are compared, they have many shortcomings. They are derived by assuming that flow across the valves is non-pulsatile. Although it is reasonable to make this assumption about the mitral valve, it does not apply to the aortic valve. Furthermore, the formulae require the use of constants originally derived from a small number of patients in whom the degree of stenosis was validated at surgery.

Further experiments have suggested that these 'constants' probably vary with the size of gradient and the cardiac output. The Gorlin formulae seem to be least satisfactory when applied to valves with an area of < 1.5 cm^2, the range in which valvar stenosis becomes clinically important. Owing to the shortcomings of the Gorlin formulae, various alternative formulae have been suggested in recent years but many require further validation.[30] Finally, any calculation of valve area depends on accurate pressure and flow measurement both of which can prove difficult.

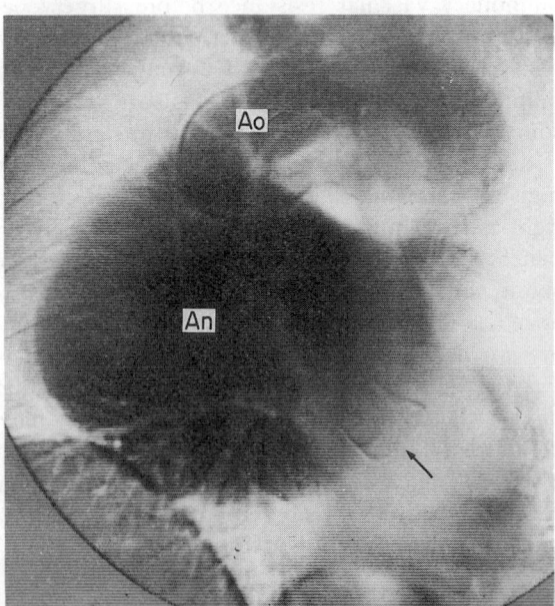

Fig. 15.21. Aortogram (left anterior oblique projection) obtained by digital subtraction angiography. This patient who has an aortic valve bioprosthesis (arrow) has an enormous aneurysmal dilatation of the aortic root (An). The aorta beyond the aneurysm is of normal size (Ao).

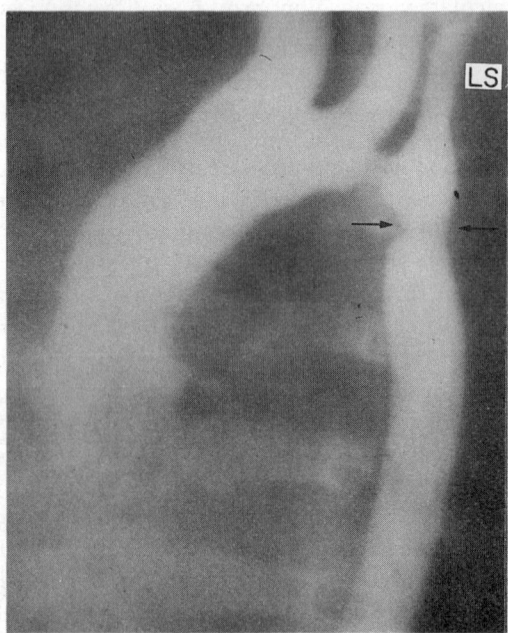

Fig. 15.22. Aortogram (left anterior oblique projection) from a child with coarctation of the aorta. The coarctation is seen (arrows) at the usual site just beyond the left subclavian artery (LS). There is also a more minor narrowing of the aorta just before the left subclavian artery.

Assessment of regurgitation

The assessment of regurgitation by inspection of angiograms can be inaccurate. For this reason, methods have been introduced for calculating regurgitant fraction, i.e. the percentage of the stroke volume that regurgitates with each beat (see Appendix p. 387). These methods depend on calculating the forward flow with each beat, using assessments of cardiac output and heart rate, and the total amount ejected by the ventricle with each beat, using an angiographic technique. The difference between these two measurements gives the amount of the total stroke volume that regurgitates with each beat. Regurgitation at two valves will invalidate these techniques. Such measurements are difficult when the heart rate is irregular, for example, in atrial fibrillation. Under these circumstances, the values derived from 5 or 10 beats have to be averaged to calculate regurgitant fraction. If either cardiac output measurement or ventriculographic technique is imprecise, the results will be inaccurate.

An alternative approach, rarely used nowadays because of practical problems and doubtful accuracy, is the use of indicator curves to assess the severity of regurgitant lesions.[12,13] It is possible to obtain an idea of the severity of regurgitation by studying the shape of an indicator curve seen peripherally after a single injection downstream from the regurgitant lesion. The assessment will be more accurate if two dilution curves are obtained, one proximal to the regurgitant valve to estimate the volume of blood regurgitated and one distal to the point of regurgitation (usually from the descending aorta) to estimate the degree of forward flow.

Complex measurements of left ventricular function

The combined use of pressure information, derived from catheters within the heart, and measurements of left ventricular volume, obtained by angiography, can be used for the assessment of left ventricular pressure–volume relationships. These relationships, which are complicated, give information about ventricular performance (usually the left ventricle). Although these techniques are too complicated for clinical practice, they do provide important pathophysiological information about ventricular performance and are of considerable value in research.[31]

MYOCARDIAL BIOPSY

Biopsy of the myocardium was first introduced in the 1950s by Weisberg. His technique involved a limited thoracotomy and drill biopsy of the ventricle which was a major undertaking. In 1962, Konno and co-workers in Japan managed to introduce biopsy forceps pervenously into the right ventricle to obtain fragments of myocardium.[32] Since then, biopsy forceps have been further refined and can now be introduced into either the right or left ventricle without difficulty.[33] There are two main techniques. Most commonly, the right ventricle is biopsied pervenously from the right internal jugular vein using a Caves' bioptome. This instrument is slightly curved and its handles face in the same direction as the curve. This allows an experienced operator to introduce the forceps directly and quickly into the right ventricle and point them towards the interventricular septum. The ease with which this procedure can be accomplished by an experienced operator means that it can be used repeatedly in patients after cardiac transplantation to obtain samples to assess whether rejection is occurring, now the major use of cardiac biopsy.

Alternatively, the left ventricle can be biopsied using the King's bioptome. This is similar to the instrument originally introduced by Konno but smaller. The easiest method is to introduce an 8F sheath via the right femoral artery, which is long enough to cross the aortic valve into the left ventricle, and through which the biopsy forceps are introduced.

Satisfactory specimens of cardiac muscle, for both techniques, can be obtained in over 90% of patients with very little risk. The main problems that can occur are those associated with any form of cardiac catheterization (see below); in addition, there is a small risk of perforation of the heart at the biopsy site; even when perforation does occur, it is often minor with only a small leak of blood into the pericardium, sometimes accompanied by pain. Occasionally, tamponade may occur and require pericardial aspiration or even operative intervention. The risk of perforation is greater if the right ventricular free wall is biopsied rather than the interventricular septum or when repeated biopsies of the left ventricle are taken from the same point. Although the operator usually tries to avoid this, the long sheath sometimes tends to direct the biopsy forceps repeatedly to the same place in the ventricle.

Although initially it was hoped that biopsy would be useful in the management of patients with congestive cardiomyopathy, this has not proved to be the case except in special circumstances. Occasionally, it may allow the differentiation of myocarditis from dilated cardiomyopathy. If biopsy shows active inflammatory changes, the use of steroids and immunosuppressive drugs may sometimes give benefit to the patient. Occasionally, endomyocardial biopsy is useful in diagnosing rare conditions, such as cardiac amyloidosis, primary or secondary tumours of the heart or endomyocardial fibrosis. Very rarely, vasculitis or a sarcoid granuloma may be detected; however, the small size of the biopsy and the scattered nature of granulomata or vasculitic lesions means that they will not usually be found.

CARDIAC CATHETERIZATION: COMPLICATIONS

Cardiac catheterization and angiography can occasionally result in serious complications and death.[34] The occurrence of complications can sometimes be predicted before the investigation from the clinical condition of the patient. Severe angina, poor left ventricular function, low cardiac output and uncontrolled heart failure are all factors that predict a higher than normal risk; advanced age acts as an additional risk factor both independently and because elderly patients have, in general, more advanced disease.

The incidence of complications has been reported in several large series, of which the most important are the Coronary Artery Surgery Study (CASS)[35] and the Registry of the Society for Cardiac Angiography[36] which give the complication rates of invasive cardiac investigations in 7553 and 53 581 patients, respectively. The vast majority of patients in these studies underwent coronary angiography alone, but both studies included patients with valve disease. Investigations for valve disease tend to be more prolonged and complicated and carry an increased risk of all complications when compared with coronary angiography alone.

MORTALITY

The mortality of cardiac catheterization for coronary artery disease is between 0.1 and 0.2%;[35,36] it is higher in patients with valve disease (possibly double). In certain groups of patients with valve disease, catheter-related mortality can be very high. McHenry found a 7% mortality in patients with aortic stenosis severe enough to compromise left ventricu-

lar function sufficiently to lead to pulmonary hypertension.[37] When death does complicate cardiac catheterization, it usually occurs because of a considerable worsening of the haemodynamic state of the patient during the investigation. Occasionally, however, it is due to either myocardial or cerebral embolization or intractable rhythm disturbances. Death may occur during the first 24–48 h after an apparently uneventful investigation.[37] This late collapse is most commonly seen in patients with severe aortic stenosis and severe pulmonary hypertension.

The potential for death during or after cardiac catheterization should never be forgotten. The shorter and less traumatic the investigation and the smaller the amount of contrast used, the lower will be the complication rate. If cardiac catheterization must be carried out in patients with pre-existing haemodynamic compromise, then all of the non-invasive data should be assessed and the primary objectives of the invasive investigation decided beforehand. Once these objectives are achieved, the procedure should be terminated. There is no virtue in a so-called 'complete' investigation which is both time-consuming and dangerous. A targeted approach to cardiac catheterization is particularly important in an emergency, and has been made possible by advances in echocardiography and Doppler ultrasound.

SYSTEMIC COMPLICATIONS

The most important complications are embolization, adverse effects of contrast material, arrhythmias and trauma caused by the catheter.

Emboli

Emboli usually originate from the catheter tip, but occasionally clot or friable calcium which is already present in the heart and great vessels or the cardiac valves is dislodged by the catheter. Such material when dislodged can embolize to any site. Emboli occur in approximately 1% of cardiac catheterization and, fortunately, the consequences are usually minor and transient. Routine use of heparin during catheterization reduces the risk (see above). Occasionally, minor pulmonary embolism occurs during or soon after catheterization because of clot originating on the right heart catheter, or from the invaded vein or occurring in other veins due to the immobility associated with the procedure. The results of one study showed a 12% incidence of new perfusion lung scan defects after catheterization.[38] These small pulmonary emboli are usually asymptomatic.

Adverse effects of contrast material

Minor problems are frequent. Nausea and vomiting may cause problems during catheterization because vomiting produces powerful vagal effects with cardiovascular depression. This problem is reduced by the use of atropine before the procedure. The occurrence of severe nausea and vomiting also shakes the patient's confidence, which it is extremely important to maintain to ensure a trouble-free investigation. Flushing and transient hypotension do not usually cause any problems; in patients with a lesion that prevents a compensatory rise in cardiac output (for example, those with severely increased pulmonary vascular resistance or a tightly stenosed aortic valve), the vasodilatation that occurs can produce serious hypotension and sometimes cardiovascular collapse.

Mild sensitivity with urticaria is common and of no significance. Occasionally, major anaphylactic reactions occur which may be fatal (1 in 40 000 catheterizations).[39] The treatment of such reactions is empirical because they occur too infrequently for treatment to have been established scientifically. The general principles are to give adrenaline, to maintain blood pressure and counteract bronchospasm, in combination with antihistamines and intravenous steroids in large doses. Patients often become extremely hypotensive because they leak fluid into the tissues and require fluid replacement (with careful monitoring of left atrial pressure) and artificial ventilation.

The volume effects of contrast material are particularly important in the sick and frail patient; care should be taken to confine the volume used to the lowest possible level without sacrificing angiographic quality. The prophylactic use of intravenous diuretics or even venesection at the end of the procedure may forestall problems in the susceptible patient.

Angiographic contrast material can be nephrotoxic and may cause either a transient deterioration of renal function or renal failure.[39,40] Diabetics and dehydrated patients are at particular risk.

Arrhythmias

Acute arrhythmias may occur during cardiac catheterization but they are usually easily treated. Ventricular fibrillation occurs in between 0.3 and 0.6% of patients,[35,36] is usually precipitated by coronary angiography and is easily reversed by direct current cardioversion. Atrial fibrillation and supraventricular tachycardia may be triggered by catheter manipulation in the right heart; episodes often last for only a few minutes and will usually revert spontaneously. Transient heart block is rare but can occur as the catheter is manipulated across the tricuspid valve and comes into contact with the atrioventricular node and the bundle of His. Severe bradycardia with hypotension secondary to high vagal tone is probably the most serious and common problem encountered during catheterization. It is frequently the result of a combination of pain and fear and can often be avoided by the timely use of sufficient premedication, atropine and anaesthesia.

Trauma by catheter

Trauma by catheter is rare, but occasionally the catheter tip dissects the origin of a coronary artery or the wall of the aorta, the trans-septal needle punctures the aorta from the right atrium or the pericardium, rather than the left atrium, or a catheter will penetrate the right ventricular wall and enter the pericardium. Many of these problems can be avoided by careful and gentle manipulation of the cardiac catheter; occasionally, despite all precautions, trauma occurs. In these circumstances, conservative management with careful observation for tamponade is sufficient and the consequences are often minor. The main exception is dissection of the coronary artery which may lead to extensive myocardial infarction and death. Urgent surgical intervention to graft the vessel should be considered. Localized dissections in the aorta, which are not uncommon, rarely cause trouble and should be treated conservatively, with careful observation of the pulses distal to the site of injury.

LOCAL COMPLICATIONS

The overall mortality of catheterization from the femoral and brachial route is probably similar in experienced hands.[34] Regardless of the site of access, thrombosis or dissection occurs in the artery used in between 0.5 and 0.6% of patients. A rare complication at the access site, more likely when the femoral artery is used, is the creation of an arteriovenous fistula.[41] If arterial complications occur, they must be handled promptly and surgical advice requested as soon as possible. Early intervention is best if there is any doubt about limb perfusion distal to the entry site. A rare late complication, usually involving the femoral artery, is the development of a pseudo-aneurysm which may require surgical treatment.

The complication rate of cardiac catheterization can be reduced by attention to detail, adequate premedication and operator expertise; however, even in the most skilful hands, it cannot be abolished. As the result of cardiac catheterization can be death, the procedure should not be undertaken lightly or in centres where surgical help with full cardiopulmonary bypass facilities is not immediately available. These strictures do not apply to procedures involving only venous catheterization, for example, pulmonary angiography and the insertion of Swan–Ganz catheters.

REFERENCES

1. Rogers, W.F. and Noothart, R.W. Outpatient arteriography and cardiac catheterization: Effective alternatives to inpatient procedures. *Am. J. Radiol.* 1985; **144**: 233–4.
2. Reuter, F.G. Physician and patient exposure during cardiac catheterization. *Circulation* 1978; **58**: 134.
3. Bertrand, M.E. and Widimsky, J. Pressures. *Eur. Heart J.* 1985; **6** (Suppl. C): 5–9.
4. Hosenpud, J., McAnulty, J. and Morton, M. Overestimation of mitral valve gradients obtained by phasic pulmonary capillary wedge pressure. *Cathet. Cardiovasc. Diag.* 1983; **9**: 283–90.
5. Schoenfeld, M.H., Palacios, I.F. *et al.* Underestimation of prosthetic mitral valve areas: role of transseptal catheterization in avoiding unnecessary repeat mitral valve surgery. *J. Am. Coll. Cardiol.* 1985; **5**: 1387–92.
6. Folland, E.D., Parisi, A.F. and Carbone, C. Is peripheral arterial pressure a satisfactory substitute for ascending aortic pressure when measuring aortic valve gradients? *J. Am. Coll. Cardiol.* 1984; **4**: 1207–12.
7. Hall, R.J.C., Kadushi, O.A. and Evemy, K. Need for cardiac catheterisation in assessment of patients for valve surgery. *Br. Heart J.* 1983; **49**: 268–75.
8. Morgan, D.J.R. and Hall, R.J.C. Occult aortic stenosis as cause of intractable heart failure. *Br. Med. J.* 1979; **1**: 784.
9. Robertson, J. and Reid, D. Standards for the basal metabolism of normal people in Britain. *Lancet* 1952; **i**: 940–3.
10. Kinsman, J., Moore, J. and Hamilton, N. Studies in Circulation. I. Injection method: Physical and Mathematical Considerations. *Am. J. Physiol.* 1929; **89**: 322–30.
11. Yang, S., Bentivoglio, L., Maranhao, V. and Goldberg, H. In: *From Cardiac Catheterisation Data to Haemodynamic Parameters.* 2nd Edn. F.A. Davis, pp. 64–75 and 77–9.
12. Jose, A., McGaff, C. and Milnor, W. The value of injection of dye into the left heart in the study of mitral and aortic valve disease by catheterization of the left heart. *Am. Heart J.* 1960; **60**: 408–16.
13. Lopez, J.F., Hanson, S., Orchard, R.C. and Tann, L. Quantification of mitral valvular incompetence. *Cathet. Cardiovasc. Diag.* 1985; **11**: 139–52.
14. Fraser, A.G., Culling, W., Singh, H. *et al.* The haemodynamic effects of left ventriculography in coronary artery disease and mitral valve disease: A comparison of high and low osmolality contrast media. *Eur. Heart J.* 1984; **5**: 727–34.
15. Dawson, P., Graigner, R.G. and Pitfield, J. The new low-osmolar contrast media: A simple guide. *Clin. Radiol.* 1983; **34**: 221–6.
16. Chaitman, B.R., Lesperance, J., Saltiel, J. and Bourassa, M.G. Clinical, angiographic and hemodynamic findings in patients with anomalous origin of the coronary arteries. *Circulation* 1976; **53**: 122–31.
17. Page, H.L., Engel, H.J., Campbell, W.B. and Thomas, C.S. Anomalous origin of the left circumflex coronary artery. *Circulation* 1974; **50**: 768–73.
18. Paulin, S. Assessing the severity of coronary lesions with angiography. *N. Engl. J. Med.* 1987; **316**: 1405–7.
19. Robbins, S.L. and Bentov, I. The kinetics of viscous flow in a model 1 vessel: effect of stenoses of varying size, shape and length. *Lab. Invest.* 1967; **16**: 864–74.
20. Sandor, T., Als, A.V. and Paulin, S. Cine-densitometric measurement of coronary artery stenoses. *Cathet. Cardiovasc. Diag.* 1979; **5**: 229–45.
21. European Coronary Surgery Study Group. Long term results of prospective randomised trial for coronary bypass surgery: survival data. *Lancet* 1982; **ii**: 1173–80.
22. Crevey, B.J., Owen, S.F. and Pite, B. Irreversible coronary occlusion related to administration of ergonovine. *Circulation* 1981; **64**: 853–6.
23. Dodge, H.T., Sandler, H., Ballew, D.W. and Lord, J.D. The use of biplane angiocardiography for the measurement of left ventricular volume in man. *Am. Heart J.* 1960; **60**: 762–6.
24. Rackley, C.E. Quantitative evaluation on left ventricular function by radiographic techniques. *Circulation* 1976; **54**: 862–79.
25. Froehlicher, V. Angiographic assessment of ventricular volume mass and wall motion. *Eur. Heart J.* 1986; **6** (Suppl. C): 29–31.
26. Chaitman, B.R., DeMott, S., Bristow, J.D. *et al.* Objective and subjective analysis of left ventricular angiograms. *Circulation* 1975; **52**: 420.
27. Croft, C.H., Lipscomb, K., Mathis, K. *et al.* Limitations of qualitative angiographic grading in aortic or mitral regurgitation. *Am. J. Cardiol.* 1984; **53**: 1593–8.
28. Gorlin, R. and Gorlin, S.G. Hydraulic formula for calculation of the area of the stenotic mitral valve, other cardiac valves and central circulatory shunts. *Am. Heart J.* 1951; **41**: 1–28.
29. Cohen, N. and Gorlin, R. Modified orifice equation for the calculation of mitral valve area. *Am. Heart J.* 1972; **84**: 839.
30. Odemuyiwa, O. and Hall, R.J.C. Assessing the severity of valve stenosis. *Br. Heart J.* 1986; **55**: 117–9.
31. Fifer, M.A. and Braunwald, E. End-systolic pressure–volume and stress–length relations in the assessment of ventricular function in man. *Adv. Cardiol.* 1985; **32**: 36–55.
32. Sakakibara, S. and Konno, S. Endomyocardial biopsy. *Jpn Heart J.* 1962; **3**: 537.
33. Laser, J.A., Fowles, R.E. and Mason, J.W. Endomyocardial Biopsy. *Cardiovasc. Clin.* 1985; **15**: 141–63.
34. Kron, J. The case for continued scrutiny of catheterization—related complications. *Chest* 1985; **87**: 707–8.
35. Davis, K., Kennedy, J.W., Kemp, H.G. *et al.* Complications of Coronary Arteriography from the Collaborative Study of Coronary Artery Surgery. *Circulation* 1979; **59**: 1105–11.
36. Kennedy, J.W. and the Registry Committee of the Society for Cardiac Angiography. Complications associated with cardiac catheterization and angiography. *Cathet. Cardiovasc. Diag.* 1982; **8**: 5–11.
37. McHenry, M.M., Rice, J., Matlof, H.J. and Flamm, M.D. Jr. Pulmonary hypertension and sudden death in aortic stenosis. *Br. Heart J.* 1979; **41**: 463–7.
38. Primm, R.K., Segall, P.H., Alison, H.W. *et al.* Incidence of

new pulmonary perfusion defects after routine cardiac catheterization. *Am. J. Cardiol.* 1979; **43**: 529–32.

39. D'Elia, J.A., Gleason, R.E., Alday, M. *et al.* Nephrotoxicity from angiographic contrast material. A prospective study. *Am. J. Med.* 1982; **72**: 719–25.

40. Eisenberg, R.L., Bank, W.O., Hedgecock, M.W. Renal failure after major angiography. *Am. J. Med.* 1980; **68**: 43–6.

41. Picus, O. and Tolly, W.G. Iatrogenic femoral arteriovenous fistulae: Evaluation by digital vascular imaging. *Am. J. Radiol.* 1984; **142**: 566–70.

42. Hillis, L., Firth, B. and Winniford, M. Analysing of factors affecting the variability of Fick versus Indicator-Dilution measurements of Cardiac Output. *Am. J. Cardiol.* 1985; **56**: 764–8.

43. Rahimtoola, S. and Swan, H. Calculation of cardiac output from Indicator dilution curves in the presence of mitral regurgitation. *Circulation* 1965; **311**: 711–8.

44. Hyman, A.L. *et al.* A comparative study of the detection of cardiovascular shunts by oxygen analysis and indicator dilution methods. *Ann. Intern. Med.* 1962; **56**: 535.

45. Grossman, W. (ed.) *Cardiac catheterisation and angiography*, 3rd ed. Philadelphia: Lea & Febiger, 1986.

46. Sandler, H. and Dodge, H. The use of single plane angiocardiograms for the calculation of left ventricular volume in man. *Br. Heart J.* 1965; **75**: 325–34.

47. Chapman, C., Baker, O., Reynolds, J. and Bonte, F. Use of biplane cineflurography for measurement of ventricular volume. *Circulation* 1958; **18**: 1105–17.

48. Bloomfield, D., Battersby, E. and Sinclair Smith, B. Use of Indicator Dilution techniques in measuring combined aortic and mitral insufficiency. *Circ. Res.* 1966; **18**: 97–100.

49. Cannon, S.R., Richards, K.L. and Crawford, N. Hydraulic estimation of stenotic orifice area: A correction of the Gorlin formula. *Circulation* 1985; **71**: 1176–8.

50. Bach, R.J., Wang, Y. and Jorgensen, C.R. Haemodynamic effects of exercise on isolated valvular aortic stenosis. *Circulation* 1971; **44**: 1003.

51. Seitz, W., Marino, T., Zanolla, L. *et al.* Cardiac valve orifice equation independent of valvular flow intervals: application to mitral valve area computation in mitral stenosis and comparison with the Gorlin formula and direct anatomical measurements. *Cardiovasc. Res.* 1984; **18**: 669–74.

52. Hakki, A.H., Iskrandian, A.S., Bermis, C.E. *et al.* A simplified valve formula for the calculation of stenotic cardiac valve areas. *Circulation* 1981; **63**: 1050–5.

APPENDIX

CALCULATION OF CARDIAC OUTPUT

Direct Fick (oxygen uptake) method

The Fick principle states that the amount of a substance taken up or released by an organ is the product of that organ's blood flow and the concentration of the substance in the organ's arterial and venous blood.

As the lung takes up oxygen and the pulmonary blood flow can be considered as equivalent to cardiac output, provided there is no intracardiac shunting, the Fick principle can be applied to pulmonary blood flow to calculate cardiac output. Although the bronchial supply to the lungs upsets this assumption slightly, it is nearly always insufficient to be of importance. Therefore:

$$\text{Cardiac output (l/min)} = \frac{O_2 \text{ uptake (l/min)}}{\text{a-v } O_2 \text{ difference (vol. \%)}}$$

Oxygen uptake is measured from the concentration of oxygen in a timed (usually 3 min) collection of expired air (the inspired oxygen concentration must be known and is usually room air). The arterial oxygen concentration is measured in a specimen from any systemic artery, and the mixed venous specimen is obtained from the pulmonary artery. These specimens are taken at the mid-point of the gas collection for oxygen uptake. Measurement of oxygen uptake can be technically difficult and it is time-consuming; many workers resort to assumed values for oxygen uptake (Table A15.1).[9] Measurements of cardiac output must be made while the patient is in a steady state.

The oxygen content of the blood is calculated using the fact that each gram of haemoglobin binds 1.36 ml of oxygen at 100% saturation.

Table A15.1. Assumed values for oxygen consumption (ml O_2/m^2 body surface area/min)[1].

Age (years)	Male	Female
3	208	188
4	200	186
5	195	183
6	187	179
7	180	173
8	173	167
9	166	160
10	161	153
11	156	146
12	152	140
13	148	135
14	145	131
15	142	127
16	139	124
17	137	122
18	136	121
19	134	119
20	133	118
25	128	118
30	126	118
35	124	116
40	123	113
45	118	111
50	117	110
55	115	109
60	114	108
65	113	107
70	112	106

Oxygen bound to haemoglobin (vol %)

$$Hb.(G) \times 1.36 \times \% \text{ saturation.}$$

Dissolved oxygen

In addition to haemoglobin-bound oxygen, a small amount is dissolved in the plasma, and this can be calculated since 0.003026 ml O_2 dissolved in 100 ml of blood per mmHg partial pressure of O_2 in the blood and added to the Hb-bound O_2.

$$Po_2 \times 0.003026 \text{ ml/100 ml.}$$

Unless the patient has a high inspired Po_2 the dissolved portion can be ignored with only a small overestimate of cardiac output.

Indicator methods

Indicator methods are employed less often than the much simpler direct Fick (O_2) method. They depend on the use of the Hamilton equation[10] which states:

$$\text{Cardiac output} = \frac{1 \times 60}{\text{Cm} \times t}$$

where I is the amount of indicator injected, t the total duration of the concentration curve (S), Cm the mean indicator concentration/l, and 60 is 60 s/min. I and Cm must be in the same units.

The principles of the indicator methods are straightforward, but the measurements and calculations can be time-consuming. The indicator is injected, mixes with the blood completely and then its concentration curve is measured downstream. In practice, the agent used most commonly is Indocyanine Green. This is injected into the right atrium and blood is withdrawn at a steady rate from the aorta as the injected bolus reaches this point, and its concentration curve is obtained by passing the blood through a suitably calibrated densitometer. There are a variety of methods for measuring the mean concentration of the indicator from the concentration curve and as the end of the descending limb of this curve also detects re-circulation of a small amount of dye this has to be allowed for by extrapolation of the primary curve (Fig. A15.1). These methods of calculation are beyond the scope of this appendix but are described in detail elsewhere.[11]

The dye dilution technique can be applied to the calculation of total forward cardiac output by injecting in the right atrium and sampling in the aorta, but it can also be applied to the calculation of flow in restricted areas of the circulation by using other

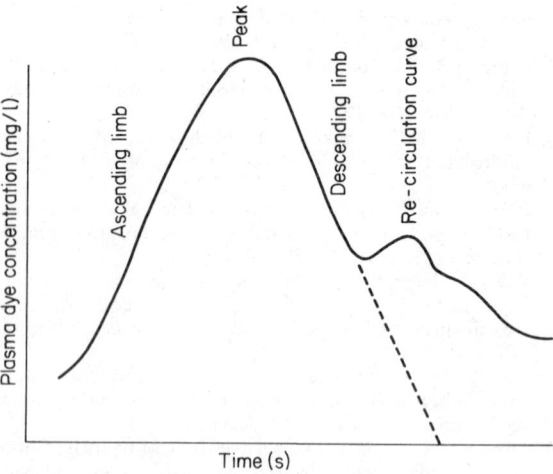

Fig. A15.1. Indicator curve recorded in a systemic artery after injection of the indicator in the right atrium of a normal patient. The dotted line is the extrapolation of the descending limb just before re-circulation begins.

injecting and sampling sites. All applications are dependent on complete mixing of the indicator with the blood and constant blood volume and flow during the measurements. An example of a measurement other than total cardiac output is the use of indicator curves for assessing regurgitant fraction, e.g. in mitral regurgitation.[13] The backward flow from the left ventricle to the left atrium can be measured by injecting in the left ventricle and sampling in the left atrium, whereas total left ventricular forward flow is obtained by conventional use of the technique to measure cardiac output or by sampling in the aorta simultaneously with the left atrium. Using such a short distance between the injection site (LV) and sampling site (LA) introduces inaccuracies due to inadequate mixing.

Thermodilution

Measurement of blood flow by thermodilution employs temperature (or rather lack of it) as the indicator and depends on the same principles as dye dilution.[11] It has the advantages that there is virtually no re-circulation and, usually, no lengthy calculation is involved because the thermistors that detect the 'dilution curve' are connected to a dedicated computer which performs all the necessary calculations. For cardiac output measurement, cold (or room temperature) 5% dextrose is injected into the right atrium and mixes with blood in the right ventricle; this indicator is then detected in the main pulmonary artery by a thermistor mounted on the end of the catheter. The calculation of cardiac output depends on the Hamilton equation in a modified form.[11]

Comparison of methods

In general, all methods produce an acceptable level of agreement; however, when there are significant left-sided regurgitant lesions or the cardiac output is low, there may be important differences. Both situations may result in primary dye dilution curves that are so prolonged that re-circulation occurs before the downslope of the primary curve.[42] Furthermore, re-circulation of dye within the coronary vascular bed may produce similar problems when the primary curve is prolonged.[43] This will either vitiate the measurement or, if re-circulation is not recognized, it will lead to underestimation of the cardiac output by enlarging the primary curve and thus increasing the value of the denominator in the Hamilton equation.

CALCULATION OF SHUNTS

Direct Fick (oxygen uptake) method

Intracardiac shunts are expressed as the ratio between systemic flow (Qs) and pulmonary flow (Qp) which can be calculated as follows:

$$Qs = \frac{\text{Oxygen consumption}}{O_2 \text{ content systemic artery} - O_2 \text{ content mixed venous}}$$

$$Qp = \frac{\text{Oxygen consumption}}{O_2 \text{ content pulmonary vein} - O_2 \text{ content pulmonary artery}}$$

A left-to right shunt is then calculated as $Qp-Qs$ and a right-to-left shunt as $Qs-Qp$.

Bidirectional shunts

Bidirectional shunts can be calculated using the formulae below:[44,45]

$$\text{Right to left} = Qs \times \frac{O_2 \text{ PV} - O_2 \text{ content systemic artery}}{O_2 \text{ content PV} - O_2 \text{ content mixed venous}}$$

$$\text{Left to right} = Qp \times \frac{O_2 \text{ content PA} - O_2 \text{ content mixed venous}}{O_2 \text{ content PV} - O_2 \text{ content mixed venous}}$$

where PA stands for pulmonary artery and PV pulmonary vein.

Sources of error

1 If the sampling of blood for measurement of oxygen saturation for a variety of sites takes some time to accomplish, changes in cardiac output and shunting may occur while this is being done.
2 It is difficult to establish the true mixed venous saturation when a shunt is at atrial level. Usually a mean of inferior vena cava (IVC) and superior vena cava (SVC) concentration is used. The IVC sample is particularly variable because there may be streaming of hepatic (low O_2 content) and renal (high O_2 content) blood in the IVC just below the right atrium. To minimize this, the mean value of two SVC samples and one IVC sample is often used.
3 When the lesion is a high ventricular septal defect, blood in the pulmonary artery may not be completely mixed; when the lesion is a patent ductus arteriosus it is usually impossible to obtain a true estimate of pulmonary artery oxygen content.
4 A sample from the pulmonary vein often cannot be obtained; if there is no lung disease, pulmonary vein saturation is usually regarded as being 97%.

Indicator dilution

The calculation of shunts using indicators is extremely complicated and beyond the scope of this Appendix. Full accounts can be found elsewhere.[11,44,45]

QUANTIFICATION OF VALVAR REGURGITATION

Regurgitation is usually measured as the regurgitant fraction (RF). This is calculated from the effective stroke volume (Sef), which is the volume of blood ejected into the systemic circulation with each heart beat, and the regurgitant stroke volume (Sr), which is the amount of blood regurgitating with each heart beat.

$$RF = \frac{Sr}{Sr + Sef}$$

A variety of methods have been used to calculate RF. Both Sr and Sef can be obtained using dye dilution (see above), or Sef may be calculated by dividing total cardiac output obtained by any method by the heart rate and obtaining total stroke volume (Sef + Sr) by measuring the left ventricular volumes at end-systole and end-diastole from a left ventriculogram (e.g. with the area–length method[23,46] or Simpson's rule[47]).

These techniques become difficult or impossible to perform when more than one valve is regurgitant, because most methods assess only the total regurgitant volume,[48] or when the heart rate is irregular.

Radionuclide methods are also available for calculating regurgitant volume but they cannot be applied when there are two regurgitant valves.

NORMAL INTRACARDIAC PRESSURES

Normal intracardiac pressures are shown in Table A15.2.

VASCULAR RESISTANCE

Resistance is defined as the ratio of the driving pressure to the mean flow and thus its measurement requires knowledge of the pressure drop and flow across a vascular bed. In cardiological practice, hybrid resistance units (HRU) (mmHg/l/min) are usually used for convenience because this involves dividing the pressure difference (mmHg) by flow (l/min). Absolute resistance units (ARU) are used less often. An ARU is resistance to flow of 1 ml/s under a driving pressure of 1 dyne/cm². HRUs can be converted to ARUs by multiplying by 80.

This simple concept of resistance is clinically useful but contains several sources of inaccuracy: it ignores the contributions of viscosity and pulsatile flow; and resistance may vary with pressure, e.g. some vascular beds may open up with increased driving pressure or increased pressure may produce vasoconstriction.

The most commonly used measurements of vascular resistance are summarized in Table A15.3.

VALVE AREAS

Another important application of pressure and flow information in combination is the measurement of valve areas. Most methods are based on the formulae published by Gorlin and Gorlin[28] and subsequently modified.[29] These were derived from two simple formulae that describe laminar and steady-state flow. As flow across cardiac valves is probably never laminar and is often pulsatile (particularly in the case of the aortic valve), these formulae must by their nature be inaccurate. The two formulae are:

$$\text{i}\quad F = A \times V$$
$$\text{ii}\quad V = c\sqrt{g} \times \sqrt{\bar{\Delta} p}$$

and are combined to produce the Gorlin formula:

$$A = \frac{F}{K\sqrt{\bar{\Delta} p}}$$

where A is the valve area in cm², F the flow across the valve in ml/s, V the volume, c a constant primarily describing that part of the pressure gradient that creates flow rather than overcomes friction, $\bar{\Delta} p$ the mean pressure gradient in mmHg, g the gravitational constant and K a constant. The constant (K) for the mitral valve was obtained from pressure and flow data obtained at catheterization and measurement of mitral valve area at surgery; it is usually taken to be 38. A similar constant for the aortic valve of 44.3 seems to have no experimental basis. The two non-constant components ($\bar{\Delta} p$ and F) are obtained as follows:

Table A15.2.   Normal intracardiac pressures.

Site	Systole (mmHg)	Diastole (mmHg)	Mean (mmHg)
Right atrium	'a' up to 7 'v' up to 5	'x' up to 3 'y' up to 3	< 5
Right ventricle	Up to 25	End pressure before 'a' up to 3. End pressure at 'a' up to 7	Not applicable
Pulmonary artery	Up to 25	Up to 15	Up to 20
Left atrium or pulmonary artery wedge	'a' up to 12 'v' up to 10	'x' up to 7 'y' up to 7	Up to 12
Left ventricle	120	End pressure before 'a' up to 7. End pressure at 'a' up to 12	Not applicable

Table A15.3.   Formulae for vascular resistance.

Variable	Formula	
TPR	$\dfrac{\text{PAm}}{\text{CO}}$	TPR = total pulmonary (vascular) resistance PAm = mean pulmonary arterial pressure
PAR	$\dfrac{\text{PAm}-\text{LAm}}{\text{CO}}$	PAR = pulmonary arteriolar (vascular) resistance LAm = mean left atrial pressure
SVR	$\dfrac{\text{SAm}-\text{RAm}}{\text{CO}}$	SVR = systemic vascular resistance SAm = mean systemic arterial pressure RAm = mean right atrial pressure
TSR	$\dfrac{\text{SAm}}{\text{CO}}$	TSR = total systemic resistance CO = cardiac output

1 **Flow (*F*)**: this is the *mean* rate of flow across the valve when it is open. This requires a measurement of cardiac output and the number of seconds per minute that the valve is open, obtained from simultaneous pressure traces across the valve in question.

$$F \text{ (ml/s)} = \frac{\text{Cardiac output (ml/min)}}{\text{Relevant flow period (s/min)}}$$

2 **Mean pressure gradient ($\bar{\Delta}p$)**: this is obtained by planimetering the area between the simultaneous pressure tracing obtained on either side of the valve. Both F and $\bar{\Delta}p$ must be assessed over at least 10 beats in atrial fibrillation.

The problems with assessment of valve area using the Gorlin method are well known and have been reviewed.[30,49] The main problems are that flow through cardiac valves is neither laminar nor steady, and the 'constants' may not be constant and vary with flow rate,[50] and that the presence of regurgitation disturbs these calculations severely because the true transvalvar flow is much higher than that calculated from the cardiac output. The Gorlin formula performs badly when the valve area is moderately or severely reduced, the situation in which such a calculation is most often required.

For these reasons, there have been many attempts to modify the original Gorlin formula or to derive new formulae.[49,51,52] Although these formulae have theoretical advantages, many require further clinical validation before they supersede the Gorlin method.

A final caution: it is unreasonable to validate new techniques (e.g. echo and Doppler assessment of valve area) against the Gorlin method alone.

The references to this appendix appear in the reference section to the chapter.

Chapter 16

Interventional Cardiac Catheterization: Transluminal Angioplasty

M.F. Shiu

INTRODUCTION

Percutaneous transluminal coronary angioplasty (PTCA) was first performed by Grüntzig in 1977. Within a year, he published his experience of the first 50 cases, in 60% of which he achieved a successful dilatation.[1] Although at the time balloon dilatation of peripheral arteries was an established technique, its application in the coronary circulation was met with surprise and incredulity. For some years, workers at only a few centres in Europe and the USA were prepared to adopt the technique. With justifiable caution, a registry was set up by the National Heart Lung and Blood Institute, Bethesda, MD, in 1979 to monitor the success and complication rates of coronary angioplasty for single-vessel disease. By the time the registry was closed in 1982, 3567 procedures had been entered, and the conclusion was that the procedure is safe and appropriate for single-vessel disease.[2] Nevertheless, doubts remained about the long-term effectiveness of coronary angioplasty and its safety in comparison with coronary artery bypass grafting. Despite such reservations, the next 5 years saw a rapid expansion of the application of PTCA in the Western world. Indications were extended from stable angina to unstable angina and acute myocardial infarction, and from single-vessel disease to multivessel disease and even to palliative treatment of inoperable triple-vessel disease. The number of procedures performed has virtually doubled every year with little sign of slowing down. The reason for such growth is largely the continued improvement in equipment and operator experience, resulting in better success rates and fewer complications.[3] As the technique is still evolving, it will be some years before its full role is clearly defined. Meanwhile, coronary angioplasty has become established as an alternative therapeutic option to surgical treatment of angina pectoris in an increasing proportion of patients.

MECHANISM OF PTCA

Balloon dilatation of diseased arterial segments was originally thought to have been brought about by compression of the atheromatous plaque. This simplistic mechanism has not been substantiated by the results of pathological studies,[4] which have suggested there is a complex combination of disruption of the plaque and of the arterial wall. The extent of such disruption depends on the pathological condition of the vessel and the region of balloon dilatation. Following an effective dilatation, there is at the very least desquamation of the endothelium and splitting of the atherosclerotic plaque. In most cases, there is also injury to the medial layer of the arterial wall with tears in the medial smooth muscle. Very occasionally, the tear extends to the tunica externa leading to a localized false aneurysm. These observations have helped to explain the angiographic appearances following angioplasty, as well as some of the common acute and late complications. Disruption of the normal endothelial layer and exposure of collagenous tissue to the bloodstream leads to platelet deposition and aggregation.[5,6] In the absence of antiplatelet drugs and anticoagulant agents, this would lead to acute occlusion of the vessel. Even with such agents, acute occlusion occasionally occurs and is the major early drawback of balloon angioplasty. Both inadequate dilatation and excessive dilatation may predispose to acute occlusion. Insufficient platelet antagonism with superimposed spasm are also important contributory factors. Clearly, the optimal dilatation is one that would restore full patency without excessive medial dissection but this may not be possible in severely stenosed segments.

The repair process is not fully understood, but the following sequence of events probably occurs: first, the endothelial layer regenerates over the denuded surfaces; and, second, macrophages move into the area and remove debris, resulting in remodelling of the vessel. Such re-modelling can be documented by repeated coronary angiography showing continued improvement following angioplasty. Restenosis, however, occurs in up to one-third of cases. An excessive fibrocellular response to the initial injury rather than regeneration of the atheromatous plaque has been shown to be responsible for recurrence of stenosis at the dilatation site.[7] Factors predisposing to restenosis will be discussed in a later section.

CLINICAL INDICATIONS

Indications for coronary angioplasty are widening as the technique develops. At present, the procedure is performed for various manifestations of coronary artery disease, such as stable angina, unstable angina, acute myocardial infarction and post-infarction angina. However, the main indication is undoubtedly that of severe angina resistant to medical therapy. This would represent the bulk of patients investigated with a view to coronary artery bypass grafting although only some will be suitable according to angiographic criteria. The possibility of non-operative revascularization by coronary angioplasty has led to a lower threshold for coronary angiography in patients with angina, some of whom may not otherwise be considered as candidates for surgery. Certainly, in patients in whom coronary artery bypass grafting is relatively contra-indicated, such as the elderly and patients with serious associated medical conditions, coronary angioplasty has become a substitute for coronary artery surgery.

Unstable angina, post-infarction angina and acute myocardial infarction are all clinical situations in which surgery is possible but associated with an increased risk. Early experience has shown that coronary angioplasty in these conditions is highly effective in restoring normal coronary flow and abolishing symptoms. However, acute complications and late restenosis are more common following PTCA for these conditions when compared with PTCA for stable angina. A growing number of patients are undergoing PTCA following coronary artery bypass surgery. Dilatation of stenosed coronary artery bypass grafts has a high initial success rate, although repeat dilatations frequently have to be performed as restenosis is more common in vein grafts than it is in native vessels.

ANGIOGRAPHIC SELECTION

The coronary angiogram is ultimately the main determinant of a patient's suitability for coronary angioplasty. Angiographic criteria, like clinical criteria, are evolving and many previous contra-indications have been removed or modified. Much depends on the experience of the angioplasty operator. The need for high-quality diagnostic coronary arteriograms cannot be overemphasized. Apart from assessment of the severity of lesions and the run-off beyond, additional information, such as morphology of the lesion, its relationship to side branches and the presence or absence of collaterals, is crucial to decision-making in coronary angioplasty. Mild lesions of < 60% diameter reduction are generally not suitable for dilatation, partly because the haemodynamic significance of such lesions is doubtful, and partly because the incidence of acute complications and late restenosis is no less than for those of severe lesions. Similarly, dilatation of isolated distal lesions is rarely justified. The majority of lesions selected are proximal lesions not involving any major side branches. Although cases of single, discrete lesions are ideal, more complex multilesion and multivessel angioplasty is becoming common in experienced centres. Increasingly, long, eccentric lesions, total occlusions and branch lesions are being tackled with high success rates. Diffuse distal disease and chronic total occlusions of over 3 months' duration are generally not considered suitable for coronary angioplasty because of the low success rate.

It should be emphasized that decision for coronary angioplasty should not be on angiographic evaluation alone. Evaluation involves both an estimate of the chance of a successful dilatation and the risks of a serious complication. Mild and technically easy lesions may be haemodynamically important. Total occlusions, although technically more demanding, are associated with fewer complications. The severity of major complications can be estimated from the anatomical situation of the 'target' lesion. For example, dilatation of a right coronary artery that supplies a significant amount of collateral flow to either the circumflex or left anterior descending territory or vice versa would place a large amount of myocardium in jeopardy should occlusion of the target vessel occur. Similarly, stenosis involving the left main branch or combined stenosis of both proximal circumflex and left anterior descending branches carries substantial risk. Single-vessel angioplasty in patients with multivessel disease implies incomplete revascularization. Such procedures carry a higher incidence of residual angina.

Angiographic selection for multivessel angioplasty is complicated and depends on operator experience and clinical indications. In general, the more dilatations required the higher the risk, as each lesion dilated increases the risk of an acute occlusion. Currently, most operators would consider routine triple-vessel angioplasty unwarranted. The presence of severe left ventricular dysfunction has also been shown to increase morbidity and mortality. Such cases are tackled only if the risks of coronary angioplasty are deemed to be less than those of bypass surgery.

THE PTCA SYSTEM

The dilatation system consists of the guiding catheter, balloon catheters (Fig. 16.1) and steerable wires. Ancillary equipment includes such items as arterial and venous sheaths, Y junctions, adjustable 'O' rings, wire introducers and inflation devices. Several firms manufacture these products, many of which are interchangeable. It is possible, but not advisable, to use one line of products exclusively. Detailed understanding of all the components of the system is necessary for the performance of PTCA to be safe and successful. The so-called 'learning curve' of operators can partly be ascribed to the time required to become familiar with all aspects of the equipment.

THE GUIDING CATHETER

The guiding catheter serves several functions: it provides a stable base from which the balloon catheter is advanced into the coronary artery and it allows selective contrast injection and pressure monitoring at the coronary ostium. Manoeuvres of the guiding catheter may cause damage to the ostium, consequently, 'soft tip' guides have been introduced which are probably a significant improvement. Early catheters were all 9F, but 8F

catheters with larger lumens are now available, allowing less trauma to the arterial access point. Each size has particular merits. The 8F catheter, apart from reducing the size of arterial puncture, allows easier manipulation of the catheter. This is more important when dilating the right coronary artery because more manipulation is necessary to enter the ostium of the right when compared with the left coronary artery. The smaller size also makes the catheter less likely to occlude the vessel completely. The advantage of the 9F guiding catheter is its stability once it is engaged in the vessel, thus providing firmer 'back-up' when crossing lesions with the balloon catheter.

The Judkins-type of guiding catheters are in common use and their shape and sizing systems are equivalent to diagnostic catheters. In the right coronary and circumflex arteries, the Amplatz shape guides often provide much better support for the passage of the balloon through severely stenotic lesions, although these should be considered as second-line catheters. Manipulation of catheters other than the Judkins-type demands greater operator skill and there is an increased risk of damaging the coronary ostium.

BALLOON CATHETERS

With few exceptions, balloon catheters in current use are of the steerable type (Fig. 16.2). These have a through lumen which enables a steerable wire to pass and move freely beyond the balloon. In this way, trauma to the vessel by the sharp-tipped balloon catheters is avoided. This distal lumen also allows the measurement of pressure before, during and after balloon dilatation, thus providing a means of assessing the progress of the procedure (Fig. 16.3). Important differences exist in the material and the construction of balloon catheters by different manufacturers. Material used may be polyvinyl chloride or polyethylene, both of which have a very high tensile strength allowing high inflation pressures. The former is more compliant and this property can be used to increase the effective balloon size beyond the nominal diameter by overinflation. The internal construction also varies among models, and users should be familiar with the different venting systems for balloon inflation and deflation (Fig. 16.3). Balloon sizes are a standard 2.0 cm in length (though some short ones are now available for lesions on curves) and range from 1.5 to 4.2 mm in diameter. In general, the larger balloons have a larger collapsed profile than

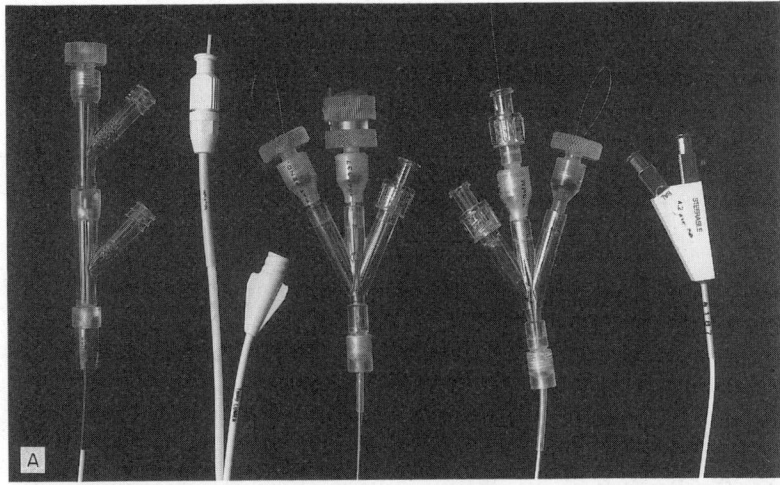

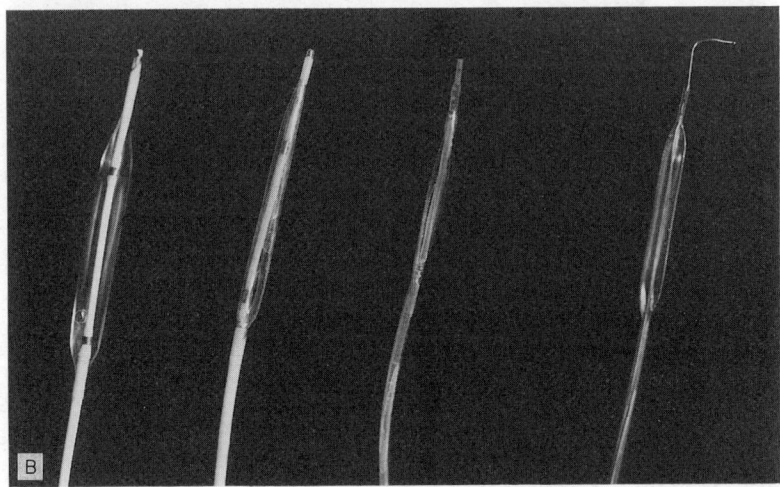

Fig. 16.1. The proximal (A) and distal (B) ends of some of the coronary angioplasty balloon catheters in common use. A detailed knowledge of their design and physical characteristics is important in their preparation and proper use.

the smaller ones. Although balloons have been constructed to withstand higher pressure, balloon rupture is a risk at pressures above 8 atm (1 atm ≈ 100 kPa).

There are several important features which it is desirable that a balloon catheter possess: the collapsed profile needs to be small for passage through tight lesions; the shaft of the catheter should be sufficiently flexible to negotiate curves in the vessel and yet stiff enough to transmit the longitudinal force needed to cross tight lesions. As some of these features are incompatible with one another, there is no single make of balloon ideal for the dilatation of all lesions and a range of balloons should be stocked. Operators should become familiar with two to three models that have different handling characters and select them accordingly.

THE STEERABLE WIRE

The freely movable guidewire is responsible for a dramatic improvement in the success rate and safety of PTCA.[3] It is used to enter sub-selectively the target vessel, cross the stenosis and assist passage of the balloon without the risk of creating a false channel. Also, after balloon dilatation, the balloon can be removed from the vessel with the wire still across the lesion, thus allowing full antegrade perfusion and contrast imaging. If necessary, further balloon dilatation is possible without any further re-exploration. Most wires are constructed to give a high amount of torque which allows accurate steering inside the coronary artery. The tips are radiopaque for full visualization and 'floppy' to avoid damage to the vessel wall. Wire sizes vary

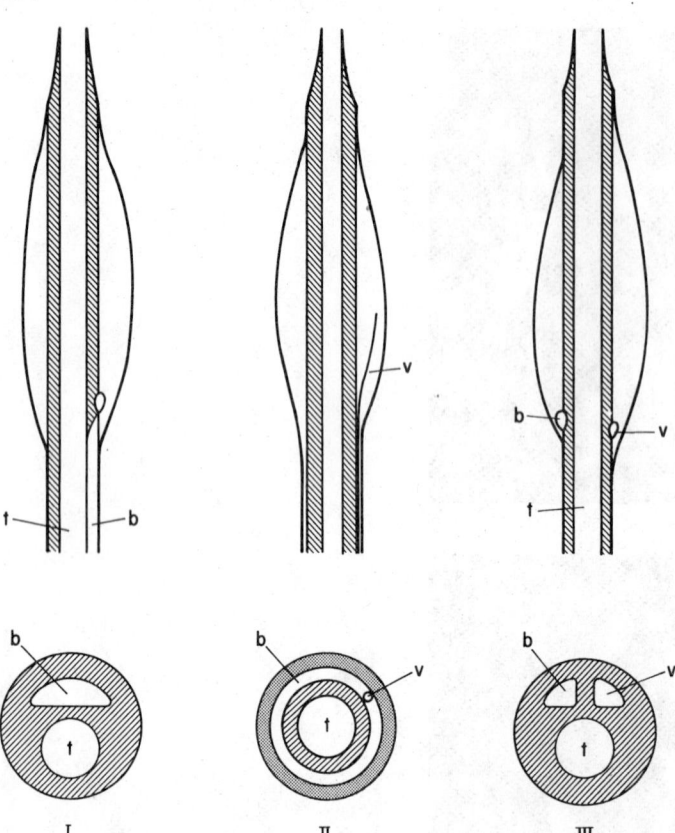

Fig. 16.2. Schematic diagram showing the internal construction of three commonly used steerable balloon catheters. T, through lumen for wire passage; V, vent for expelling air during balloon preparation; B, balloon inflation channel.

from 0.010 to 0.018″ to suit various situations and balloon sizes. A small wire can be used in a larger balloon but some of the smaller low-profile balloons will only accept wires up to a certain size. Too close a fit between wire and balloon also leads to loss of distal pressure recordings. By using a double length wire, it is also possible to exchange balloons for one of a larger or smaller size without losing access to the vessel.

THE ANGIOPLASTY PROCEDURE

PREPARATION OF THE PATIENT

The patient should be prepared as for cardiac catheterization, i.e. fasted and premedicated. Written consent should be obtained after full explanation of the nature and risks of balloon angioplasty. Aspirin 300 mg orally should be given daily from the time of admission. Except in those patients with unstable symptoms, beta-blocking agents should be stopped and a calcium antagonist started if not already taken. Nitrates may be administered in various ways, but a convenient and effective method is to give isosorbide dinitrate by a venous

infusion pump at a rate of 3–5 mg/h starting 1 h before the procedure.

The procedure is usually performed via a femoral artery puncture. It is not necessary to insert a temporary pacing wire electively, but a short sheath should be placed in the femoral vein in case the need should arise. As soon as all lines are in place, 10 000 units intravenous heparin are given and the time noted. If the procedure lasts longer than 1 h, 5000 units are administered and 2000 units hourly thereafter.

If there has been any significant time-lapse since the last diagnostic study, a full set of angiograms should be repeated to exclude appearance of new diseased segments. This will also provide another chance to choose the best view to use for the dilatation procedure. The correct size of balloon is chosen and prepared. The guiding catheter should be placed into the femoral artery and advanced to the aortic root. Once the guiding catheter is properly engaged in the coronary ostium, the balloon is advanced with the guidewire leading.

CROSSING THE LESION

Using small injections of contrast medium into the

guiding catheter, the target lesion is visualized and displayed in the most favourable view. If at all possible, the balloon should be kept back in the guiding catheter until the guidewire is placed across and well distal to the target lesion. Failure to cross the lesion with the wire is rare except in cases of total or sub-total occlusion. Very occasionally, the wire can be 'splinted' by having the balloon placed very close to the lesion.[8] This manoeuvre increases the risk of trauma to the vessel and should be used only when initial wire passage fails.

The correct position of the wire should be checked by contrast injection in at least two views before balloon passage is attempted. The wire should be in the main vessel rather than in any side branch including those distal to the lesion. Balloon crossing is best performed with one operator adjusting the guiding catheter while advancing the balloon and the other constantly adjusting the position of the wire. Careful attention should be paid to the position of the guiding catheter during balloon passage. The proximal pressure should also be monitored; a fall in this pressure indicates over-engagement of the guide catheter. More commonly, the guide catheter is pushed out of the ostium by the force required for crossing the lesion, and constant minor adjustment of its position is critical to the success of the procedure. Failure to cross the lesion with the balloon may be due to a lack of firm guiding catheter support or a balloon profile that is too large. Recognition of which is the contributory factor is important. Once the balloon is across the lesion, its position is again checked angiographically with a hand injection of contrast via the guiding catheter (Fig. 16.3). The initial pressure gradient is recorded and balloon dilatation can begin.

BALLOON DILATATION

There are no rules regarding the duration and number of inflations. Between 2 and 4 dilatations lasting up to 60 s each are usually made. Angina accompanied by ST-segment changes often occurs during inflation of the balloon but it should resolve with the cessation of each inflation. Adequacy of balloon distension can be seen by the absence of any indentation in the inflated balloon; progress in the procedure can be checked by a reduction in the pressure gradient across the lesion (Fig. 16.4) and by further contrast injection with the balloon pulled back into the guiding catheter while the wire remains across the lesion. It is recommended that after the last inflation the wire is left across the lesion for several minutes to ensure that antegrade flow is well maintained and that dissection or spasm is not causing sufficient residual stenosis to require further dilatation.

ANGIOPLASTY OF THE RIGHT CORONARY ARTERY

Problems with PTCA of the right coronary artery often relate to the guiding catheter. The Judkins-type size 4 or 5 guiding catheter has a tendency to jam in the first part of the vessel with partial or total occlusion affecting pressure and flow. Attempts to withdraw the catheter may result in the catheter flipping out of the artery. Use of an 8F catheter or a catheter with side-holes may allow engagement without compromising flow. Even so, the problem is often one of support, in allowing either intricate manoeuvring of the guidewire across a lesion, or later passage of the balloon. The proximal portion of the right coronary artery sometimes forms a sharp curve, not unlike the top of a shepherd's crook, making both guide catheter engagement and balloon passage difficult (Fig. 16.5). The options are to change to an Amplatz guide (Fig. 16.6) or to use a small-sized balloon catheter at the start of the procedure.

The Amplatz catheter is less easy to control than the Judkins-type catheter. The main advantage of the Amplatz catheter is allowing firm support when the tip of the catheter is advanced well into the vessel. Control of the depth of engagement may be difficult; if engagement is too deep, there may be impairment of forward flow. The catheter is usually selected only after the safer Judkins-type catheter fails to give adequate support.

ANGIOPLASTY OF THE LEFT ANTERIOR DESCENDING CORONARY ARTERY

The left anterior descending coronary artery is the most common vessel for PTCA and has the highest success rate. Part of the reason is the ease of use of the guiding catheter. The Judkins-type guide catheter is of the same configuration as the diagnostic catheters, but it has greater rigidity. The increased stiffness is intended to provide support for balloon passage. The correct choice of size is in the range from 3.5 to 6; the size of the diagnostic catheter can be used as a guide. Apart from the aortic root size, attention should be given to the orientation of the left main artery and the first portion of the left

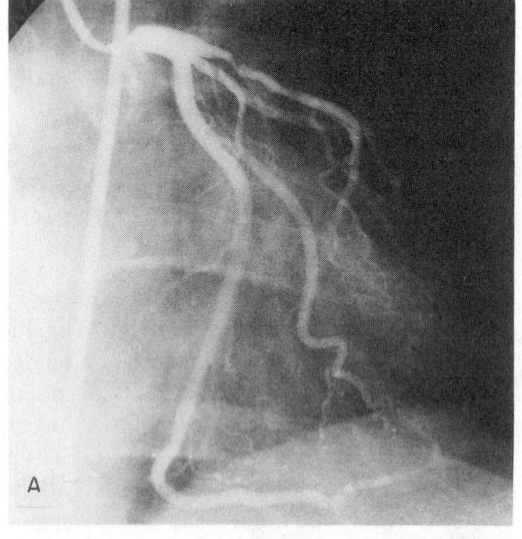
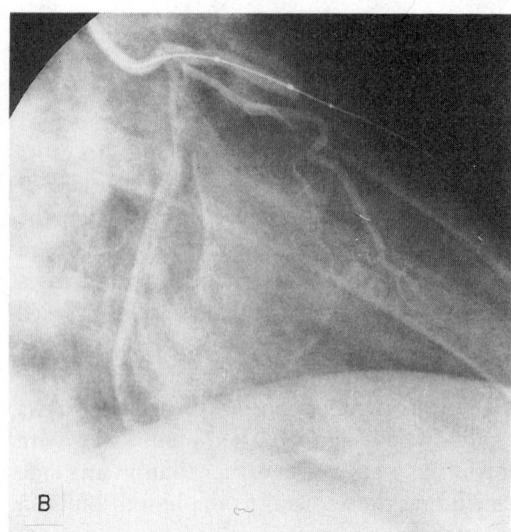
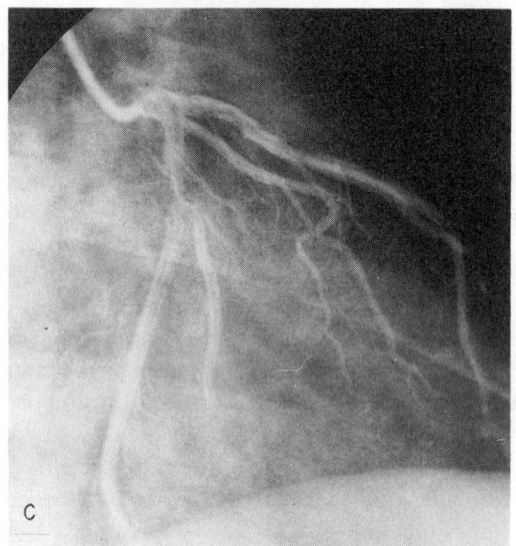

Fig. 16.3. Single-vessel angioplasty of a discrete left anterior descending lesion. (A) Left coronary angiogram showing a severe stenosis of the proximal left anterior descending branch. (B) After sub-selective entry of the left anterior descending artery with the steerable wire, the balloon was placed across the lesion and inflated for 40 s. (C) After repeated dilatations, a final repeat angiogram was taken to demonstrate successful dilatation of the narrowed segment and patency of all branches.

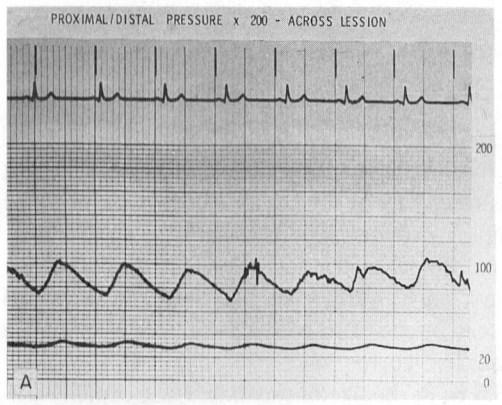
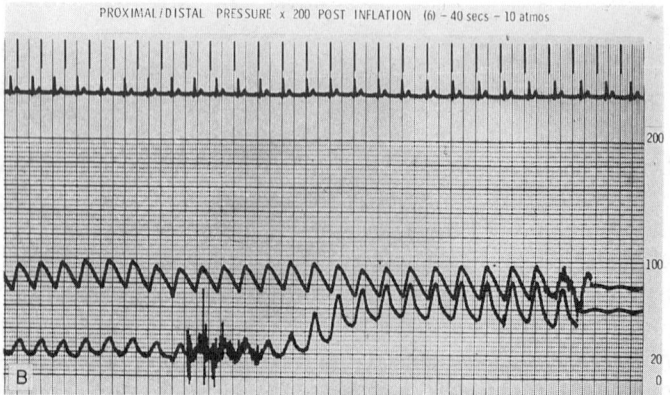

Fig. 16.4. (A) Simultaneous pressure recordings taken with the balloon catheter across the stenosis prior to balloon dilatation. This showed an initial pressure gradient of about 60 mmHg. (B) Pressure recording following repeated dilatation resulting in a final trans-stenotic pressure gradient of 20 mmHg.

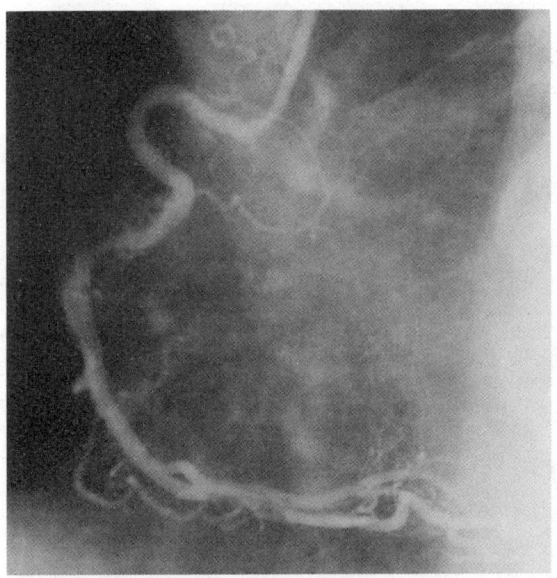

Fig. 16.5. A right coronary artery angiogram in the left anterior oblique view showing a stenosis in the mid-portion. The tortuosity of the proximal portion giving the 'snepherd's crook' appearance often causes difficulties in balloon passage.

anterior descending artery. Under-sizing of the catheter causes the tip to point upwards and over-sizing downwards. After correct engagement of the guide, the balloon catheter should be advanced with the steerable wire leading. The system can be moved as a whole, or the wire can be moved independently, as desired, as long as the balloon catheter is kept well out of the coronary vessel at this stage. Selective passage of the vessel

avoiding septal and diagonal branches is usually best done in the left anterior oblique view, although confirmation by a second plane is mandatory before balloon passage.

Close attention should be given to the seating of the guiding catheter any resistance at the lesion is likely to result in 'back-off' of the guide from the ostium with the loss of further support. In experienced hands, the guiding catheter can be cautiously advanced well into the left anterior descending branch for further support (Fig. 16.7). The manoeuvre may require lowering of the secondary curve of the guide into the aortic root thereby forming a 'swan neck'. Some of the stiffer makes of guiding catheters cannot be made to curve in this way, but they provide firmer support because of their pre-configured shape.

ANGIOPLASTY OF THE CIRCUMFLEX ARTERY

The circumflex artery poses a problem because the first part of the artery usually forms a 'Z' bend (Fig. 16.8), which explains the low success rate of dilating this vessel during the earlier years of coronary angioplasty. With the advent of steerable systems, results now approximate those of other vessels. Even so, distal circumflex lesions are often in the marginal branch adding more curvature to the eventual path of the balloon. As in the 'shepherd's crook' of the right coronary artery, such curvature reduces the axial force required to cross severe stenoses. In addition, the Judkins-type guid-

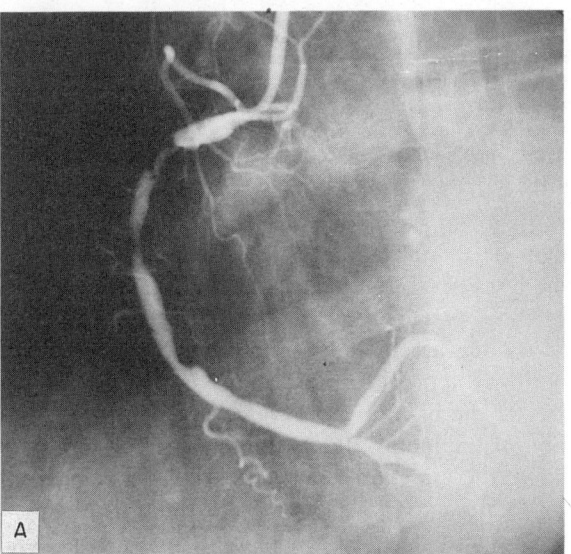
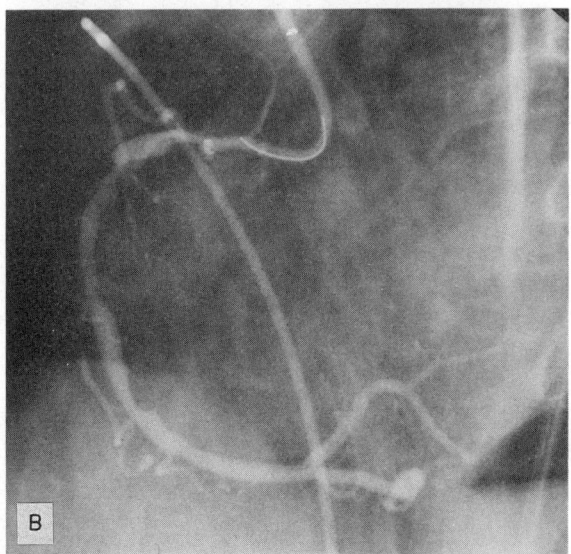

Fig. 16.6. (A) Angiogram taken before dilatation of a right coronary artery showing a series of stenotic lesions in the proximal and middle portions of the vessel. (B) Angiogram taken after dilatation using an Amplatz-type guiding catheter. The dilating balloon and wire have been withdrawn into the guide.

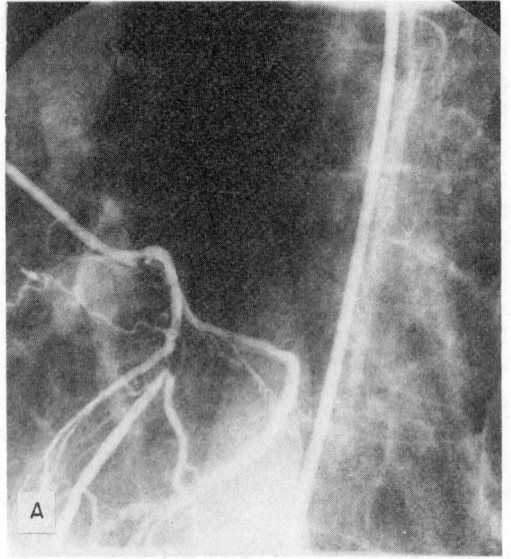

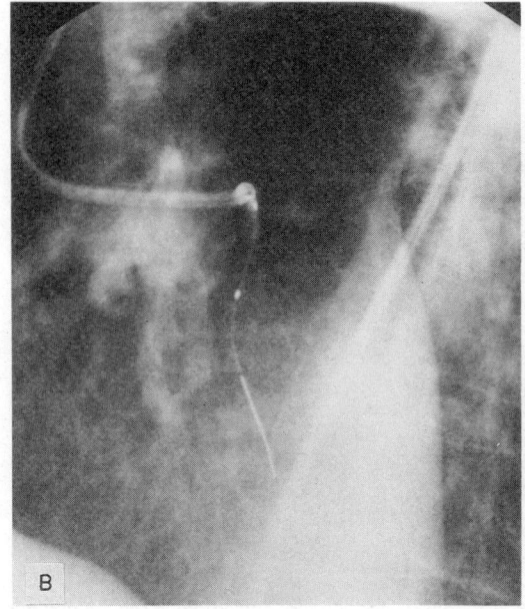

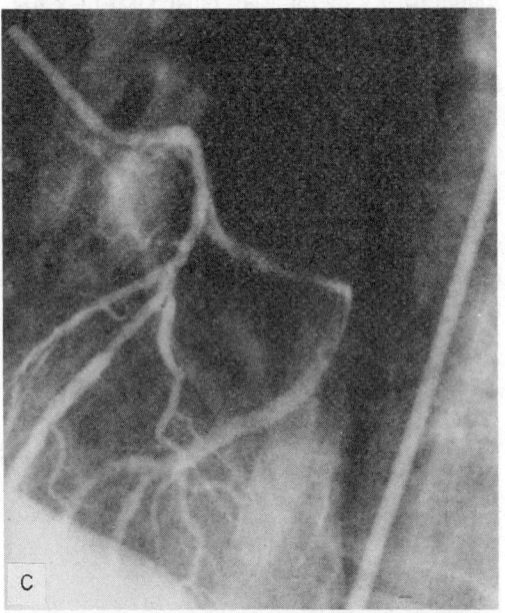

Fig. 16.7. A case in which deep engagement of the guide was necessary to facilitate balloon passage. Before (A), during (B) and after (C) balloon dilatation. Note the characteristic horizontal lie of the tip of the Judkins-type guiding catheter needed to enter sub-selectively the left anterior descending branch. All three angiograms were taken in the same left anterior oblique and cranial tilt projection.

ing catheter cannot be advanced into the circumflex as it can into the left anterior descending. It is sometimes necessary to use an Amplatz-type guiding catheter, which, when advanced into the vessel, effectively eliminates the proximal curve and provides excellent support.

MULTIPLE LESION CORONARY ANGIOPLASTY

Multiple lesion PTCA requires careful additional planning beforehand. Where all the lesions involve a single vessel, the wire should be placed across all the lesions in the first instance. The lesions should

then be dilated sequentially, usually starting with the most severe one, regardless of its position (Fig. 16.9). This will allow early establishment of a good flow rate, thereby improving visibility and reducing occlusive complications. It is not necessary to retract the balloon from the vessel between dilatation of the lesions unless there is doubt about flow down the vessel, in which case it would be prudent to obtain a good view with only the wire left in.

Coronary angioplasty of more than one vessel should be undertaken with a clear plan of the order of procedure (Figs 16.10 and 16.11). In general, the lesion that would be expected to cause the least

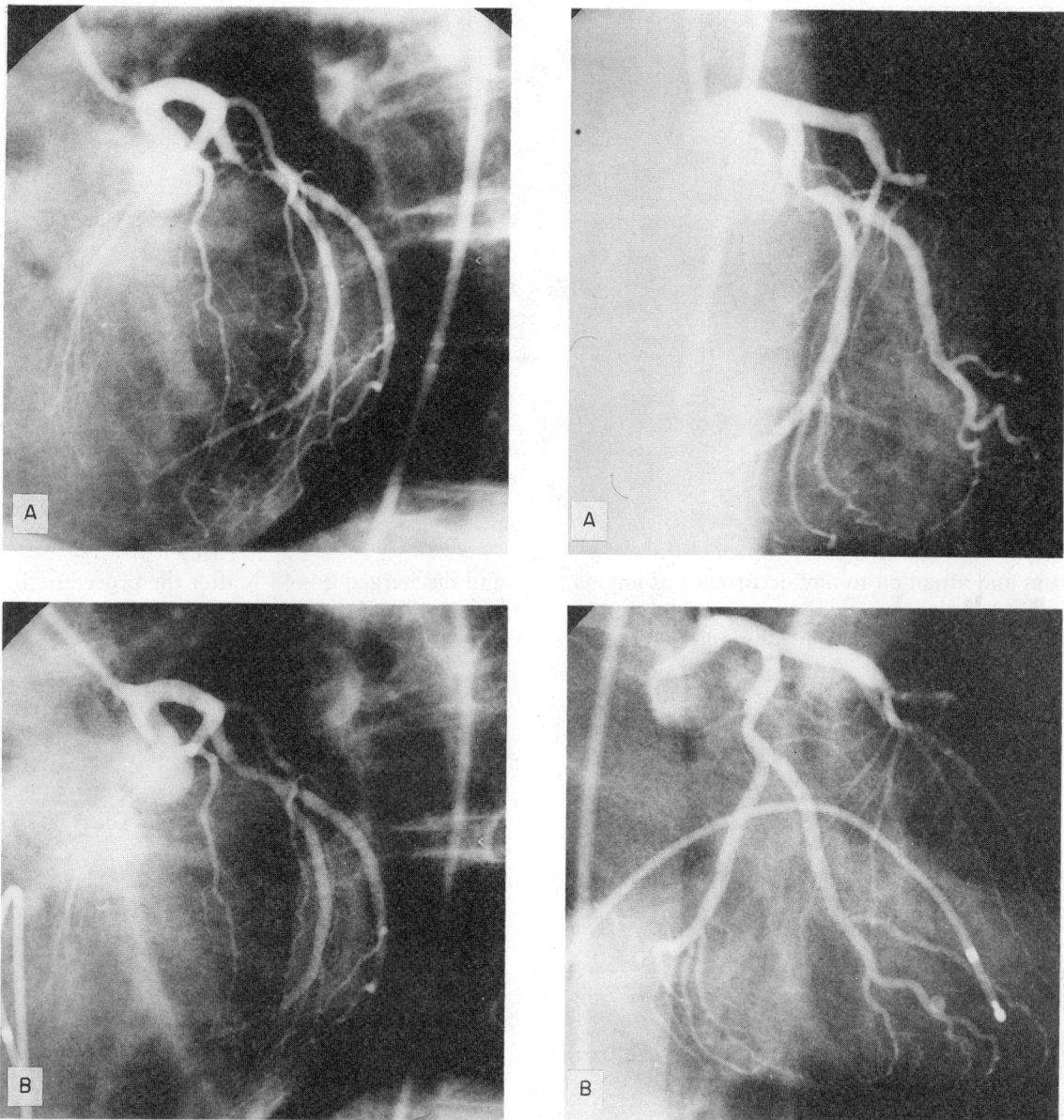

Fig. 16.8. Angiograms of the left coronary artery showing circumflex stenosis before (A) and after (B) angioplasty. Both the left anterior oblique (left) and right anterior oblique (right) views show the 'Z' bend of the main circumflex vessel which commonly causes difficulties in balloon passage.

myocardial damage, should acute occlusion occur, should be tackled first. For this reason, total occlusion, if deemed suitable, should be recannulated and dilated first. As a general rule, if the most severe lesion cannot be successfully dilated, other lesions should not be attempted. Each lesion should be carefully assessed after dilatation with respect to the adequacy of dilatation and presence and extent of medial dissection. If there is some doubt about the stability of the lesion, it would be best to 'stage'

the procedure and do further dilatations a few days later.

PATIENT MANAGEMENT IMMEDIATELY AFTER CORONARY ANGIOPLASTY

After the procedure, the patient should be observed in the Coronary Care Unit or an equivalent high dependency area with close monitoring of cardiac

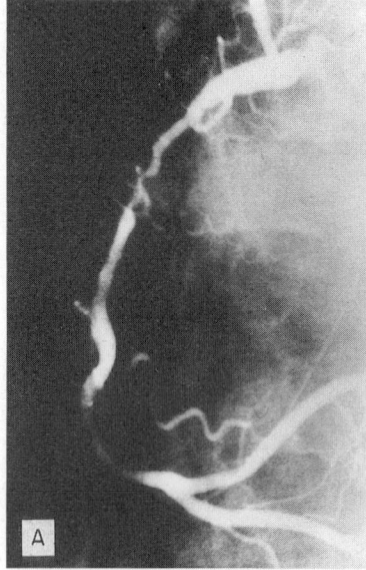
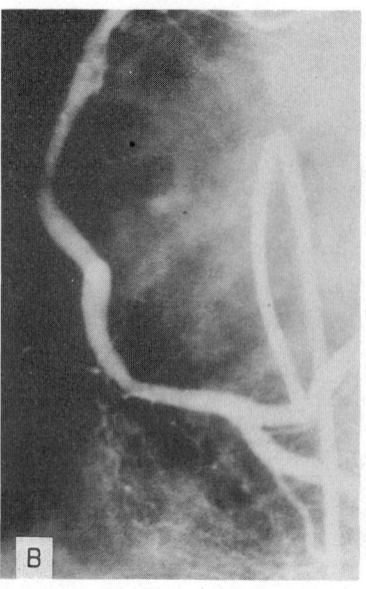

Fig. 16.9. Angiograms taken before (A) and after (B) dilatation of a right coronary artery in the left anterior oblique view. Four sequential lesions were all dilated with the same balloon catheter. The proximal two 'tandem' lesions were dilated first as these were the most severe.

rhythm and attention to any occurrence of angina. A full 12-lead electrocardiogram should be recorded for reference and only fluids allowed for the first hour. It is standard practice not to reverse the effect of heparin with protamine sulphate and to leave the femoral sheaths in place for 4–5 h in case repeat angiography is required. Sufficient analgesia, for example, 10 mg Omnopon intramuscularly should be given prior to removal of the sheaths. Atropine 0.3–0.6 mg intramuscularly is also recommended because reflex bradycardia is common due to pain. The patient can be mobilized the next day

and discharged 24–48 h after the procedure if free of angina. Estimation of the level of cardiac enzymes should be made the day after the procedure to detect the presence of any myocardial damage. An electrocardiogram should be done after the procedure and before discharge.

DEFINITION OF A SUCCESSFUL DILATATION

Successful angioplasty is a procedure in which the target lesion or lesions are dilated satisfactorily

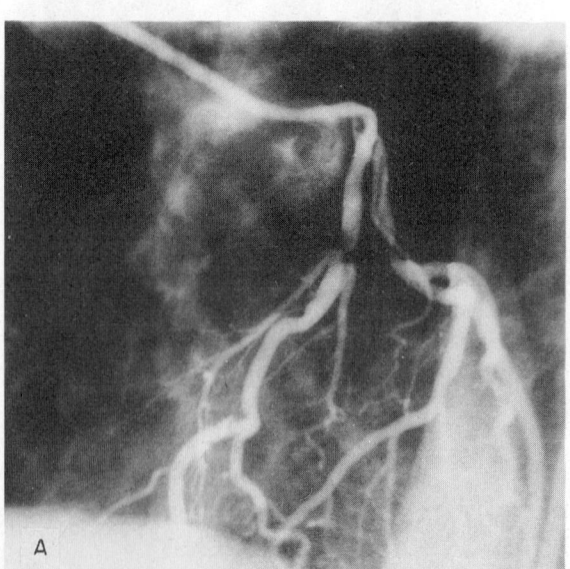
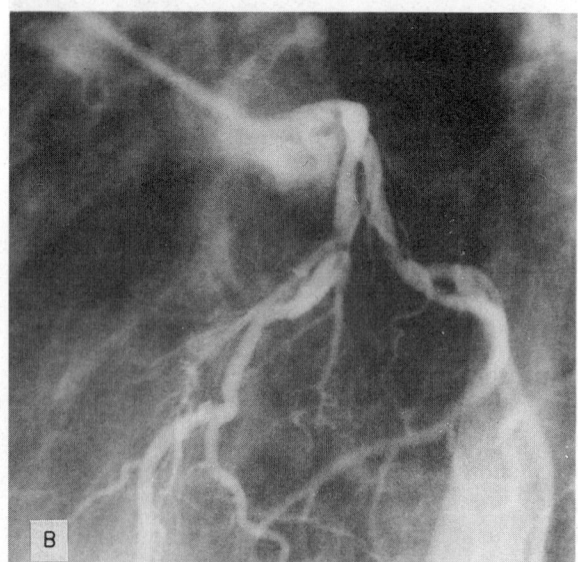

Fig. 16.10. Multivessel angioplasty in a case of left anterior descending and circumflex branch stenosis. Both lesions were proximal and discrete (A). The left anterior descending branch lesion was dilated first and the circumflex lesion was approached only after the LAD was seen to be successfully dealt with. Both were satisfactory at the end (B).

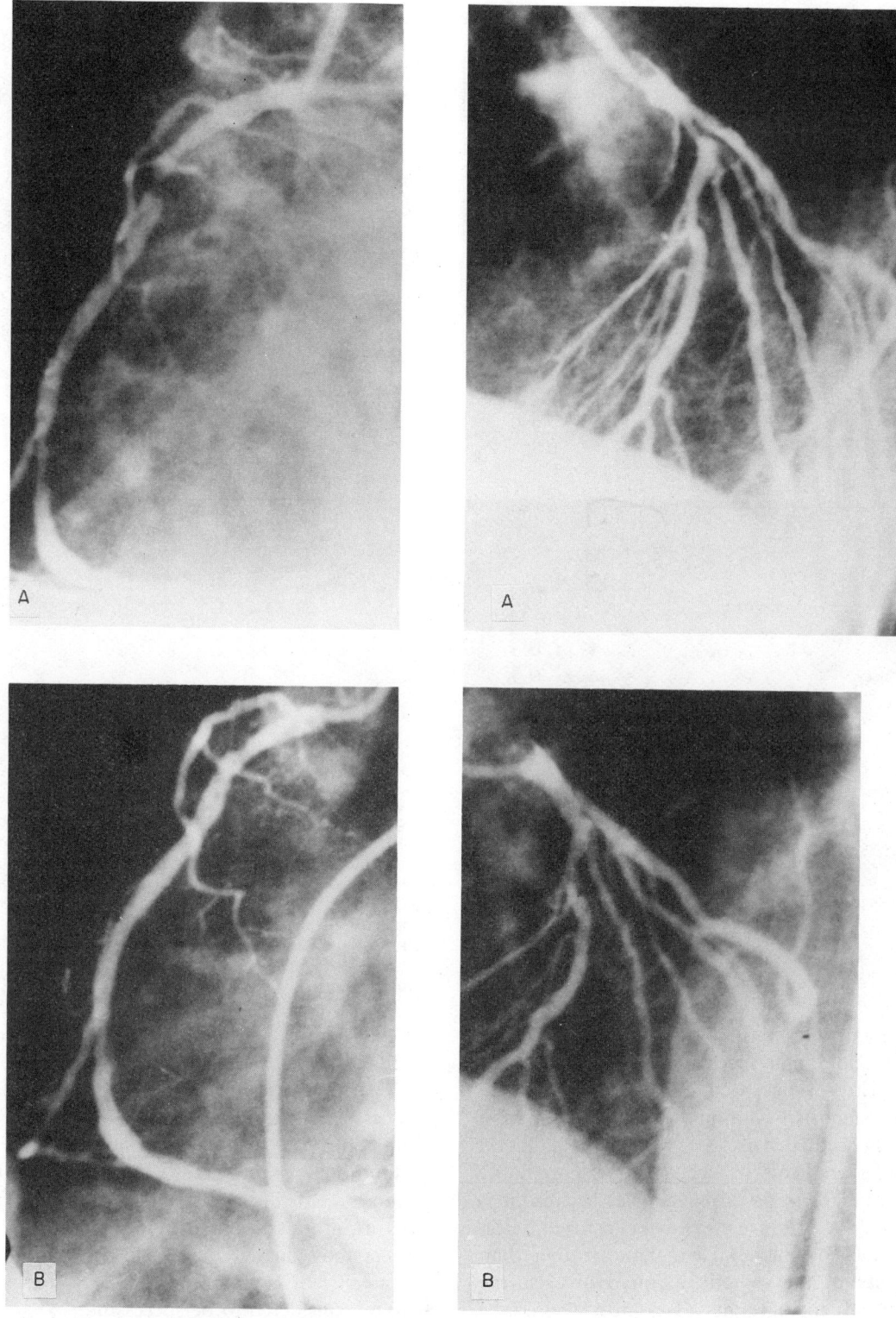

Fig. 16.11. Multivessel angioplasty in a case of right coronary artery (A left) and left anterior descending artery stenosis (A right). Both lesions were severe (A) but as the right coronary artery was almost totally occluded this was dilated and seen to be uncomplicated before (B left) the other vessel was attempted. (B) shows the successful results in both lesions.

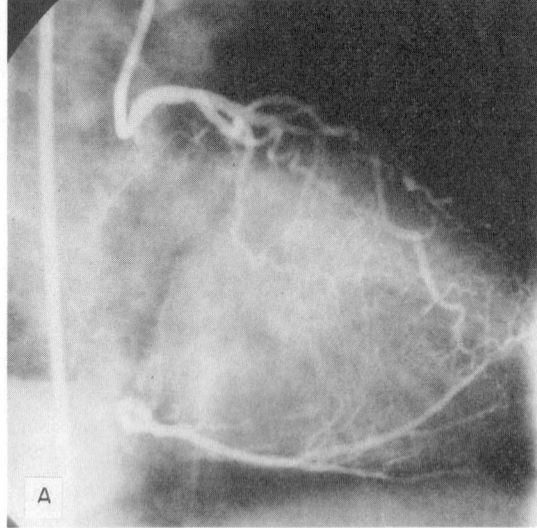

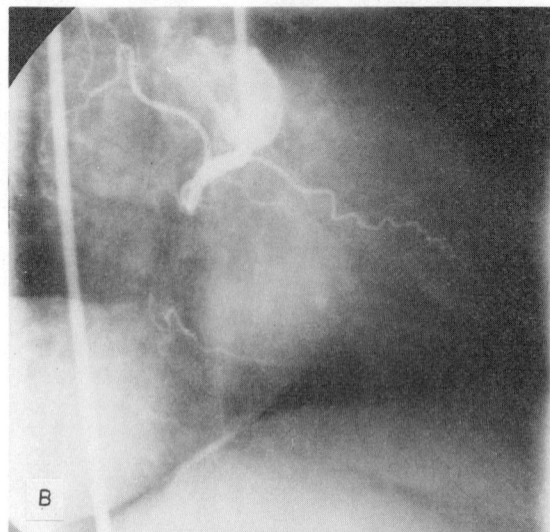

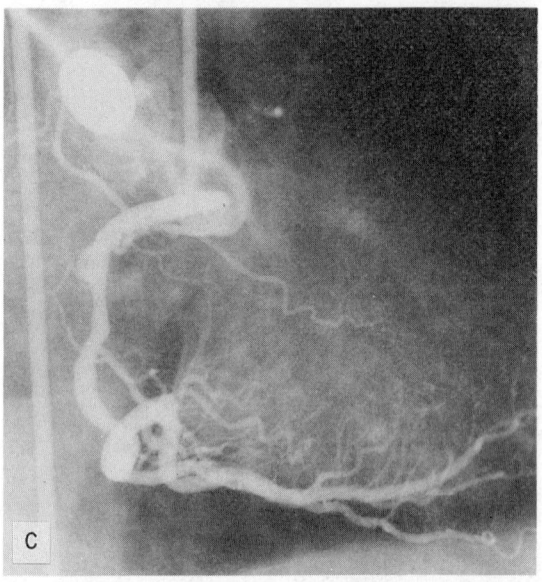

Fig. 16.12. Multivessel angioplasty in left anterior descending stenosis and right coronary total occlusion. The patient had had a recent (10 days) sub-endocardial inferior infarction followed by persistent angina pectoris at rest. (A) shows a mid left anterior descending stenosis and filling of the distal right coronary artery which was occluded near the origin (B). After successful dilatation of the right coronary artery (C), the left anterior descending lesion was dilated 1 week later with no complications.

without incurring any major complication. Definitions of angiographic success vary. One commonly used in early series was a 20% reduction in diameter stenosis. Currently, a more common criterion is residual stenosis of < 50%.[9] Reduction of pressure gradients has become less commonly used as a means of assessing stenosis because it is clear that distal pressure measurements often reflect the adequacy of collateral circulation rather than the severity of the stenotic lesion. However, the limitation of angiographic assessment should be recognized.[10] The presence of quite extensive intimal dissection does not negate a successful dilatation as long as antegrade flow is not compromised, but it does make assessment of a stenosis virtually impossible. Acute occlusion, often dealt with im-

mediately by repeat dilatation, is also compatible with a good long-term result if there is no evidence of a peri-operative infarction.[11,12] The evaluation of success in multivessel angioplasty is more complicated and no general agreement exists. A rigid definition would be the absence of a residual stenosis > 50%, but workers at most centres adopt the attitude that if the most severe lesion is successfully dilated there is often clinical success with relief of angina, and therefore the procedure can be considered to be successful.

PROCEDURAL FAILURE

Despite advances in angioplasty technique and

equipment technology, dilatation is unsuccessful in over 5% of cases in most reported series. This may be due to failure to cross the lesion either with the steerable wire or the balloon catheter. Occasionally, despite repeated dilatation with a balloon catheter of suitable size, the stenosis is not relieved or complications occur which result in a myocardial infarction or require emergency bypass grafting. The primary success rate is influenced by many factors, both clinical and angiographic. Earlier differences in success rates in different vessels have all but disappeared and, in most instances of single-vessel coronary angioplasty for chronic stable angina, the success rate can be expected to be well over 90%.[3,9] The success rate for more complicated coronary angioplasty is necessarily lower.[13] Chronic total occlusions and lesions affecting major junctions or multiple lesions along the same vessel all increase the complexity of the procedure and therefore decrease the primary success rate.

COMPLICATIONS OF CORONARY ANGIOPLASTY

Minor complications include reversible rhythm disturbances, chest pain or local complications at the access site. The most important complications of coronary angioplasty are myocardial infarction, emergency bypass grafting and death.[14] Most of these occur as a result of vessel occlusion at or around the site of balloon dilatation. Failure to cross a lesion or to dilate it satisfactorily poses significant risk of vessel occlusion. However, even with an apparently straightforward initial dilatation, acute occlusions can occur. The mechanism of such occlusions is not always obvious but it may be secondary to vessel dissection, spasm, thrombus formation or a combination of these factors.[4-6] The onset of such occlusion is usually within the first 1–2 h of the procedure and rarely occurs after 6 h.

DISSECTION

Dissection accounts for more than half the cases of vessel occlusion. Dissection may occur as a result of wire or balloon manipulation but more often as a direct result of balloon dilatation. It occurs more often in women than in men and in vessels with lesions that are eccentric or situated at sharp curves. It should be emphasized that small areas of dissection at the site of the lesion commonly occur in straightforward procedures without any comprom-

ise of flow (Fig. 16.13). It is likely that for severe stenoses adequate dilatation is not possible without dissecting both the plaque and the vessel.[15] On the other hand, it has been shown that the presence of a sizeable dissection greatly increases the chances of acute occlusion.[16] The dissection may be discovered during the course of the procedure or after removal of the balloon catheter (Fig. 16.14). It may be necessary to examine the angiogram in several planes before the typical appearance of the intimal flap is seen. If forward flow appears satisfactory, no action is required other than careful observation for 10–20 min to ensure that the dissection does not encroach into the true lumen. If this happens and forward flow is reduced, the lesion should be re-crossed and re-dilated with the balloon catheter. If this occurs after the steerable wire has been removed, re-crossing is possible but careful exploration with the wire is important to avoid increasing the extent of the dissection. In the majority of cases, repeat dilatation results in enlargement of the true lumen and maintenance of forward flow (Fig. 16.15).

SPASM

Coronary artery spasm leading to total occlusion of the artery may occur at any time during coronary angioplasty. In critically severe lesions, it is not uncommon to observe transient episodes of occlusion from spasm prior to balloon crossing. Spasm probably plays a significant role in vessel occlusion secondary to extensive dissection, because vasoactive substances are released as a result of interaction between platelets and the exposed medial smooth muscle. Intracoronary nitroglycerine should be given in doses of 200–300 μg. Nifedipine may also be given, either sublingually (by piercing a 10-mg capsule with a needle and asking the patient to chew it) or by intracoronary injection of 200 μg. Repeat dilatation is sometimes necessary to prevent further occlusive episodes.

THROMBO-EMBOLIC OCCLUSION

Thrombo-embolic occlusion usually results from under-heparinization or incorrect PTCA procedures. Inadequate flushing of the guiding catheter, especially when using long exchange wires without a balloon catheter, has caused problems. Adherence to the regime of additional heparinization for procedures lasting longer than 1 h is therefore important; dosage adjustment with tests of partial

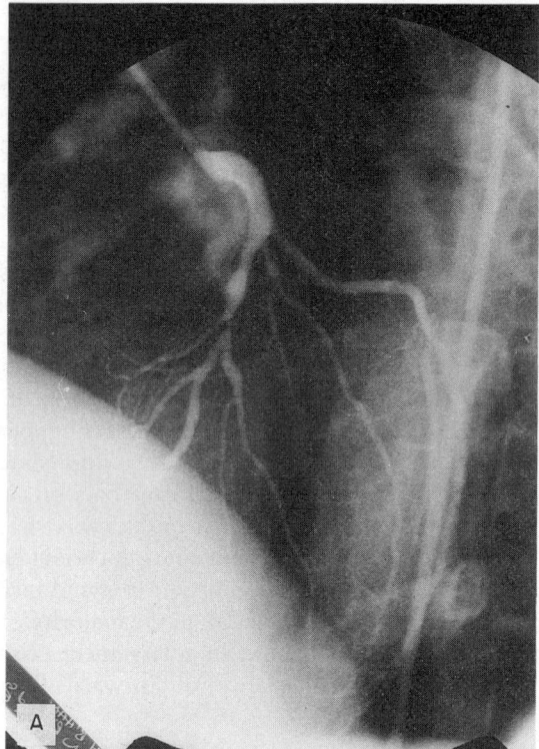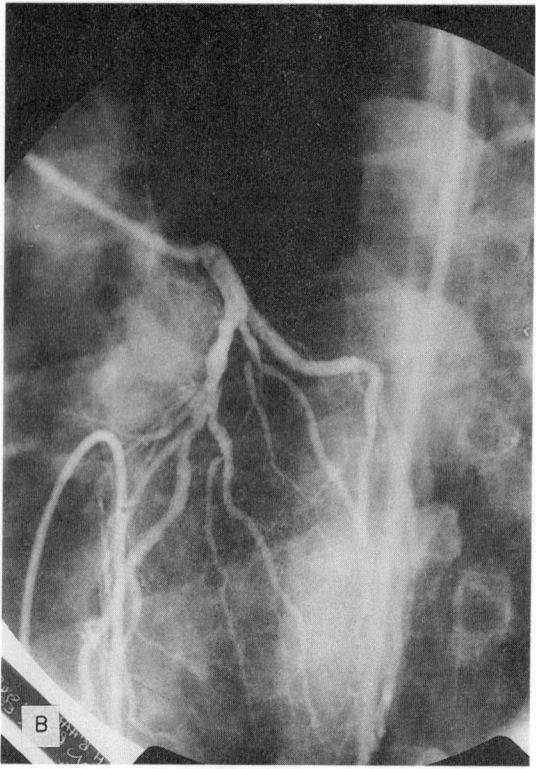

Fig. 16.13. Angiograms taken before (A) and after (B) dilatation in a patient with left anterior descending stenosis showing significant dissection without any compromise of forward flow. The patient had a good immediate and long-term result.

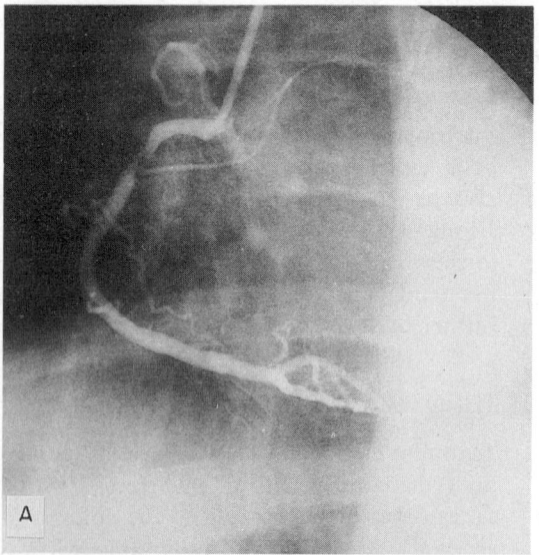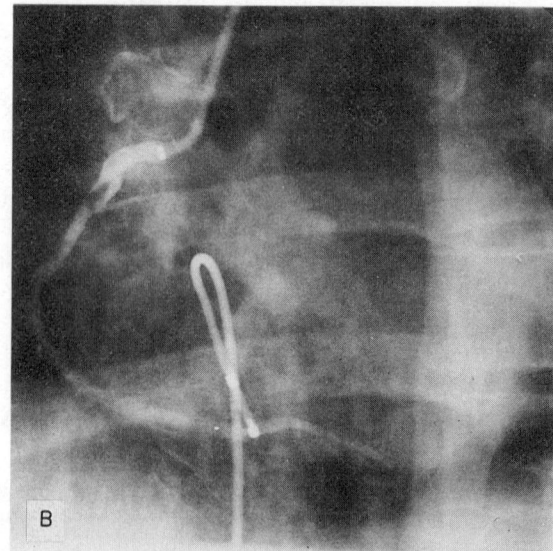

Fig. 16.14. Occlusive dissection complicating coronary angioplasty of a right coronary artery lesion (A). The dissection was observed during the course of the dilatation. Despite repeated balloon inflation, the lumen was not sufficiently wide to maintain adequate forward flow (B) and emergency coronary bypass grafting was undertaken for an evolving infarction.

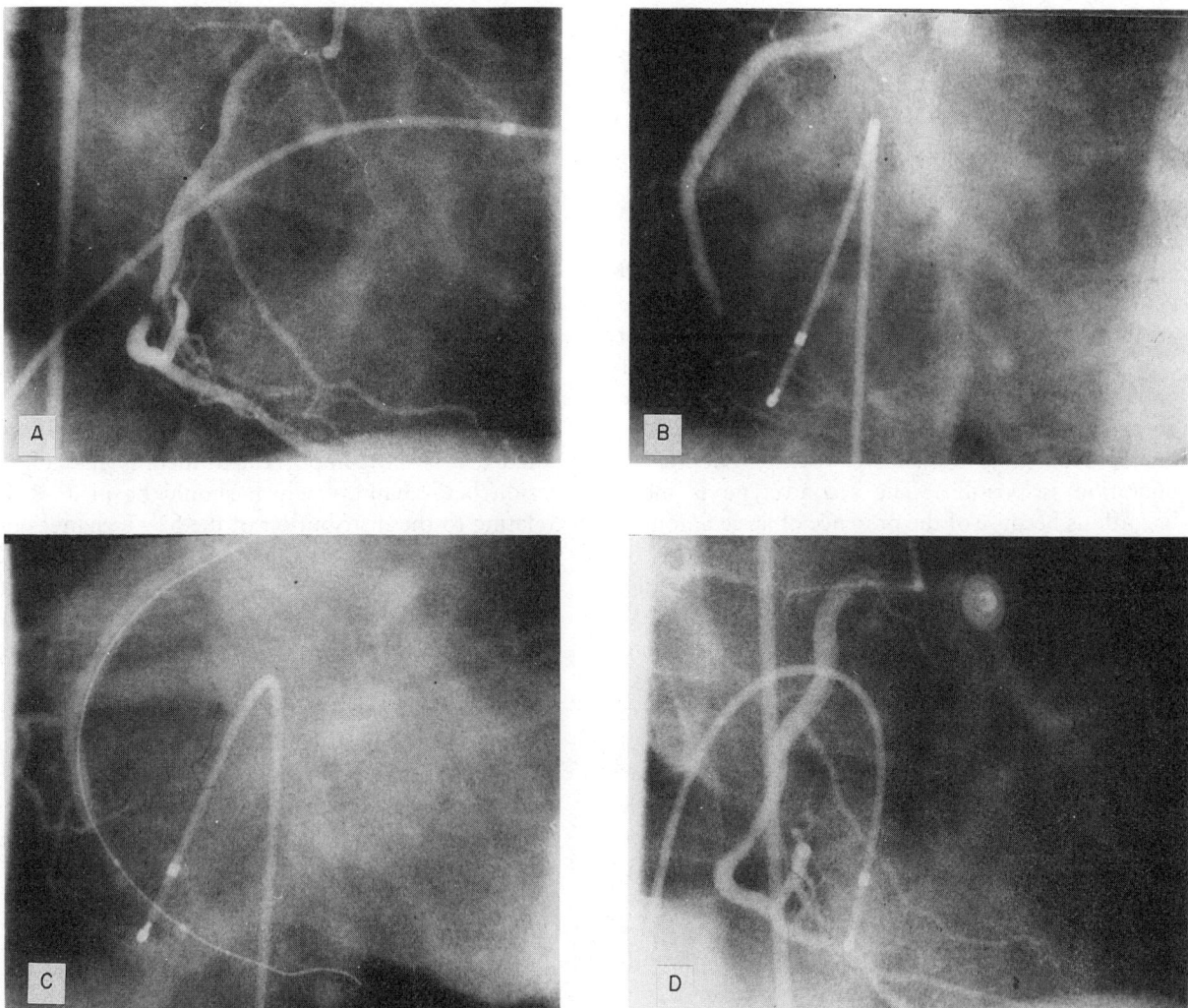

Fig. 16.15. Occluding dissection resolved by immediate repeat angioplasty. (A) A severe distal right coronary artery lesion. Following an apparently uneventful dilatation, acute occlusion occurred (B) around a small area of dissection at the dilatation site. The occlusion was re-opened with the steerable wire and dilated (C) with good results (D).

thromboplastin time has been suggested. In occlusions due to any cause, undue delay in re-establishing forward flow can result in secondary thrombotic occlusion of the vessel and its distal branches. Therefore, it is probably prudent to give additional heparin immediately acute occlusion is observed.[11,12] Extensive intracoronary thrombus formation cannot be dealt with by repeat balloon dilatation, and emergency bypass grafting is needed.

MEDICATION AFTER CORONARY ANGIOPLASTY

Following successful PTCA, anti-anginal medication, such as beta-blocker and oral nitrates is

usually withdrawn. Aspirin, started prior to PTCA, should be continued for some months in an attempt to reduce restenosis. Research into pharmacological agents that will prevent restenosis continues. There is no evidence that either oral anticoagulation or calcium antagonists have a protective role, although the latter are often prescribed to reduce the possible occurrence or coronary artery spasm early after PTCA.[17,18]

ANGIOPLASTY OF CORONARY ARTERY BYPASS GRAFTS

Several mechanisms are responsible for the development of stenosis in aortocoronary saphenous vein bypass grafts.[21] Proximal or ostial stenosis and stenoses at the distal anastomotic site are often caused by the technical problems of inserting a graft. Angioplasty of such lesions may be attempted, but the success rate is slightly lower than that for mid-graft lesions, which may be of two types: discrete, often concentric lesions affecting grafts in the first few years after surgery which have been ascribed to intimal proliferation and eccentric, and extensive lesions due to the development of large atheromatous plaques, which tend to be found in older grafts. The first type of lesion is ideal for balloon dilatation and has a high initial success rate with few complications. Recurrence of stenosis is higher than that for native vessels, but repeat dilatation is possible. The second type is more hazardous because of the presence of large amounts of loose atheromatous material. Embolization of such material into the native circulation leading to a myocardial infarction has been reported.

The technique of coronary angioplasty in coronary artery bypass grafts is similar to those of angioplasty in native vessels. The proper selection of a guiding catheter is important as the anatomy of grafts varies greatly. Although angiographic visualization is often possible with the Judkins-type right coronary type catheter, the Amplatz-type guide is better suited for secure seating in the graft. Coronary angioplasty in patients who have undergone previous coronary artery bypass grafting poses a problem in the instituting of emergency cardiopulmonary bypass in such patients. However, in experienced hands, the occurrence of complications is rare and symptomatic relief common. Considering the higher operative mortality of repeat surgery, PTCA should be the treatment of choice for recurrent angina after coronary artery bypass surgery if technically dilatable lesions are present in the grafts or native vessels.

NON-ELECTIVE CORONARY ANGIOPLASTY

There are several clinical situations in which PTCA is carried out either as an emergency or at least as a semi-urgent procedure. Ad-hoc angioplasty is the performance of PTCA at the same sitting as the diagnostic investigation.[21] This approach has been justified on various clinical and economical grounds but its widespread use is not appropriate. Lack of proper prior discussion of the nature and risk of the procedure with the patient is an obvious drawback. Careful review of the cinéangiogram is a prere-

quisite of safe coronary angioplasty and this may be difficult on a non-elective basis. Nevertheless, recent expansion in the application of PTCA to the treatment of unstable angina and acute myocardial infarction will result in more angioplasty procedures being done immediately after the diagnostic angiogram. Indeed, angioplasty is increasingly becoming the preferred procedure in the treatment of unstable angina and of myocardial infarction; the initial results are very promising.[22]

UNSTABLE ANGINA

In contrast to chronic stable angina, in unstable angina, it is most important to identify the culprit lesion beforehand,[23] which should be in a vessel relating to the distribution of the ST–T changes on the electrocardiogram observed during periods of chest pain. The lesion is often severe (85% to sub-total occlusion) or shows features of recent plaque rupture with overhanging edges or intraluminal clot in or just distal to the stenosis (Fig. 16.16). Such lesions are usually easy to cross with the balloon catheter and successful dilatation results in rapid control of anginal symptoms. However, acute occlusion is more common and in most series a higher incidence of procedural related myocardial infarction as compared with stable angina has been reported.[24]

ACUTE MYOCARDIAL INFARCTION

Mechanical disobliteration of the thrombus in acute myocardial infarction was introduced at around the same time that treatment with intracoronary streptokinase was advocated. The technique of percutaneous transluminal coronary recanalization (PTCR) is the use of a soft-tipped guidewire to probe open the vessel after the infusion of nitrate and before that of streptokinase. Later, it was shown that once the vessel was patent, balloon dilatation could be carried out, with or without concomitant use of thrombolytic therapy. Advocates of PTCA argue that full recanalization is more rapid with this method than by thrombolysis, thereby resulting in better myocardial salvage.[25] However, considering the manpower and resources required for such procedures, emergency PTCA is unlikely to be feasible in the majority of centres. A more important emerging role for PTCA is dilatation after thrombolytic therapy. It has been shown that up to two-thirds of patients have severe residual stenosis at the site of previous thrombosis;

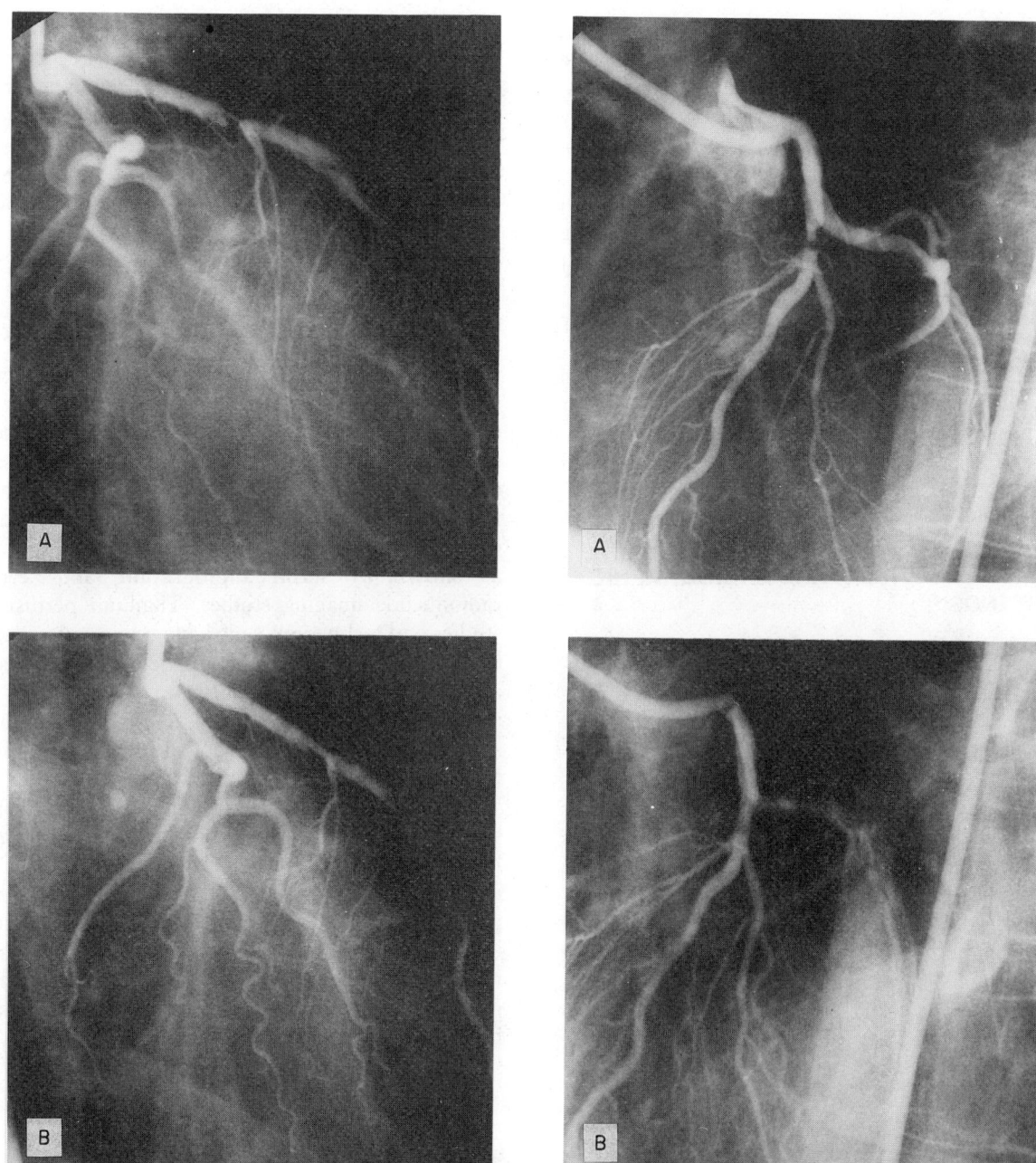

Fig. 16.16. Coronary angioplasty in a patient with unstable angina. This case illustrates the common angiographic finding of a sub-totally occluded vessel with 'fuzziness' around the lesion, suggestive of recent plaque eruption or adherent thrombi. (A) After dilatation, the angiographic appearance was unremarkable.

coronary angioplasty appears to be an appropriate therapy, although the timing and long-term benefit of such an intervention need to be defined by future trials.[26]

SURGICAL STANDBY FOR CORONARY ANGIOPLASTY

Since the initial clinical use of coronary angioplasty, the need for surgical standby for emergency bypass grafting has been repeatedly stressed. Although there are rare occasions when prompt surgical intervention may salvage a substantial amount of myocardium and improve survival, emergency bypass grafting is generally performed in the context of an evolving or even completed myocardial infarction. The morbidity and mortality of such emergency operations are substantially higher than those for elective operations. The advent of the steerable system has greatly facilitated recanalization of acute occlusions complicating coronary angioplasty, and the recent development of a perfusion catheter allows sufficient antegrade flow through occlusions to provide enough time in which to conduct a less hurried bypass operation.[27] Owing to these developments, it is becoming acceptable not to have surgical standby that is immediately available. However, the establishment of coronary angioplasty in centres without surgical facilities is controversial. Where possible, arrangements should be made for emergency transportation of the patient to a nearby surgical centre, but the angioplasty team at each centre should develop a philosophy and protocol for the management of acute events.

RECURRENT ANGINA AND ANGIOGRAPHIC RESTENOSIS

Reports documenting medium- to long-term follow-up of patients after successful PTCA are accumulating, and they provide a consistent picture of the incidence and pattern of recurrent stenosis.[28,29] Despite pharmacological and procedural modifications, restenosis remains the 'Achilles heel' of coronary angioplasty (Figs 16.17–16.19). Figures for the rate of restenosis vary, partly due to differences in definition and partly due to incompleteness of follow-up angiography. The NHLBI registry report in 1985 documented a recurrence rate of 36.2% for men and 22.5% for women followed for a mean period of 18 months.[28] In a large series of 998 patients with single-vessel disease treated at Emory University, there was a similar rate of recurrence of 30.2% using 50% stenosis at follow-up angiography as a criterion.[29] Although other series have lower restenosis rates, it is generally agreed that the true rate is likely to be about 30%; however, not all episodes of restenosis are associated with symptomatic relapse or require further dilatation. Restenosis nearly always occurs within the first 6 months of the initial procedure and very rarely after 1 year. There are small but significant differences in restenosis rates in different coronary arteries, the left anterior descending artery being most prone and the circumflex least prone to restenosis. Total occlusion prior to dilatation and stenosis of coronary artery bypass grafts are associated with a higher restenosis rate of approximately 50%. Patients with unstable angina, especially those with demonstrable artery spasm, have a higher incidence of restenosis.[30] There is less information available about restenosis in patients following multivessel PTCA. So far, some reports indicate that the rate of restenosis is only slightly increased, a finding which suggests that restenosis may be patient-dependent and not directly related to the number of sites dilated.

DIAGNOSIS AND MANAGEMENT OF RECURRENT STENOSIS

Restenosis may be suspected because of recurrent symptoms, positive stress tests or routine repeat coronary arteriography. Symptomatic recurrence strongly suggests angiographic restenosis, whereas routine angiography in asymptomatic patients showed a restenosis rate of only 4%.[31] The process of restenosis probably starts a few days after PTCA, as shown by serial angiographic and serial radionuclide imaging studies. Thallium perfusion studies and technetium ventriculograms at 1 month have been shown to be 75% predictive of restenosis at 6 months.[32] Pre-discharge exercise testing is sometimes advocated. If the result is positive at this state, it suggests inadequacy of the dilatation rather than the occurrence of restenosis.

Although the majority of patients with recurrent stenosis can be successfully treated by repeat PTCA, it has been shown that the risk of further recurrence is similar to, and possibly higher than, that of the primary procedure. It should be stressed that with longer periods of follow-up recurrent symptoms may not be due to restenosis; beyond 1 year, the recurrence of angina is increasingly more likely to be caused by the development of new lesions.

LONG-TERM RESULTS OF CORONARY ANGIOPLASTY

In several series, long-term follow-up after coronary angioplasty has shown very favourable outcomes for patients up to 8 years after the procedure. Late restenosis is rare, and the incidence of myocardial infarction and death is very low. Although these results may reflect the selection of low-risk patients in the early series, they do highlight that the initial benefit of PTCA is not lost with time, as is the case for coronary artery bypass grafting. Patients with multivessel disease suffered most of the cardiovascular events during follow-up, confirming

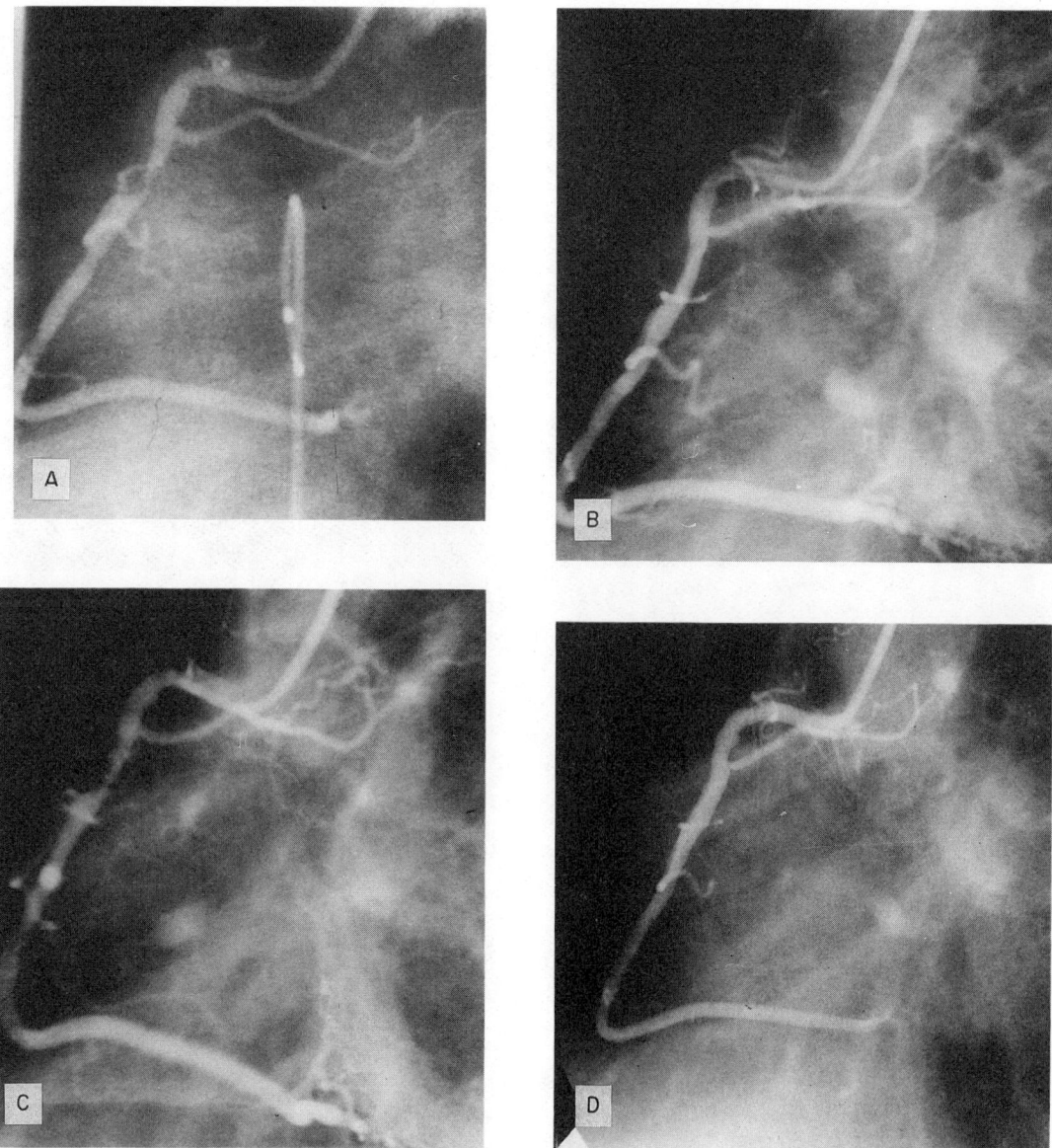

Fig. 16.17. Recurrent stenosis in a young man with single-vessel disease affecting the right coronary artery (A). Despite full dilatation (B), the stenosis recurred at 6 months (C). After repeat dilatation, the vessel remained normal up to 1 year later (D).

that progressive disease rather than restenosis is the main determinant of long-term prognosis.

ECONOMIC CONSIDERATIONS

PTCA has been estimated to be one-third to one-quarter of the cost of coronary artery bypass grafting. In the UK, the cost of a PTCA procedure is approximately £1400, which includes a 4-day stay in hospital and use of disposable PTCA equipment, drugs and radiographic material. Even when the cost of repeat procedures is taken into account, the cost of PTCA compares very favourably with that of bypass grafting. With an increased volume of sales, PTCA equipment should become less costly; however, the largest impact on resources would be the need for dedicated intervention laboratories and specially trained medical and ancillary staff. The growth in the use of PTCA has been spectacular in the USA and all Western European countries. The rate of growth depends on the health economics of the country and, in the UK, it is likely to be restricted by considerations of both manpower and

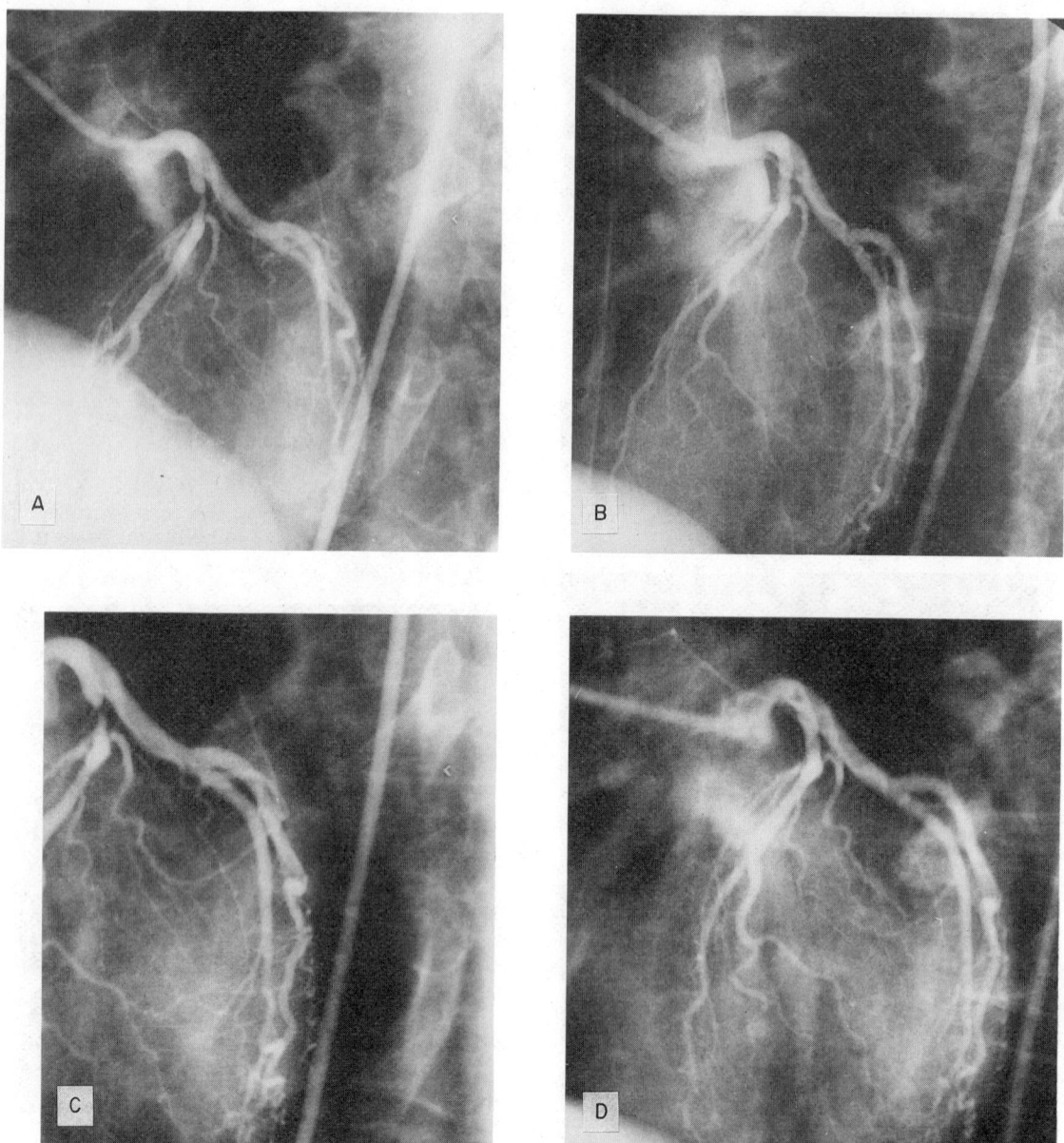

Fig. 16.18. Recurrent stenosis in a young woman with exercise-induced angina and ventricular tachycardia. A severe proximal left anterior descending stenosis (A) was fully dilated (B) but recurred 2 months later (C) at the same site, accompanied by recurrent angina pectoris and arrhythmia. She had repeat dilatation at 2 months, and again at 6 months following which restenosis did not occur (D).

resources. It is not possible to make projections too far into the future, but it is becoming increasingly clear that many patients with disabling chronic stable angina and unstable angina can be treated by PTCA instead of by coronary artery bypass grafting. As the adoption of thrombolysis for the treatment of acute myocardial infarction becomes more widespread, many more patients will have subsequent therapy by coronary angioplasty.

CONCLUSION

In the short time-span of 10 years since the beginning of coronary angioplasty, the procedure has become a standard form of treatment for many patients with various manifestations of coronary artery disease. Future developments will not be restricted to balloon dilatation. Percutaneous coronary angioscopy already provides direct

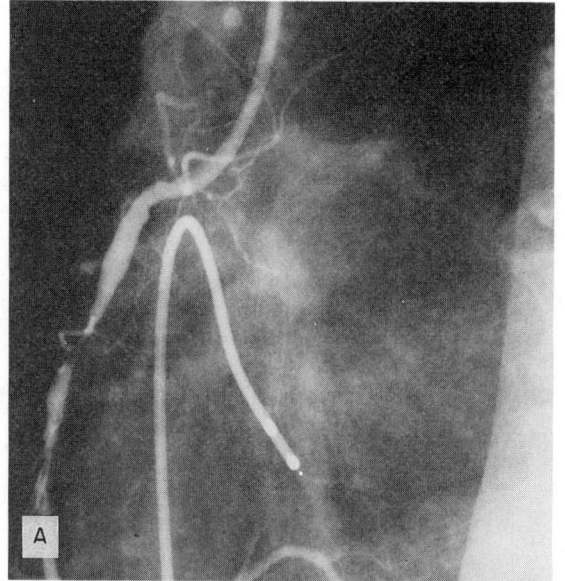

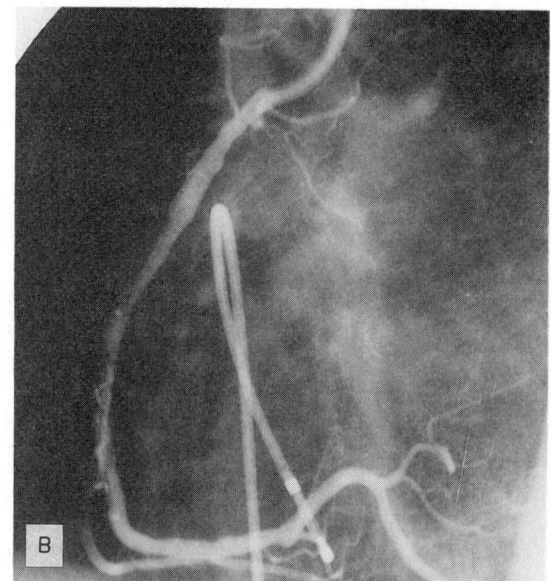

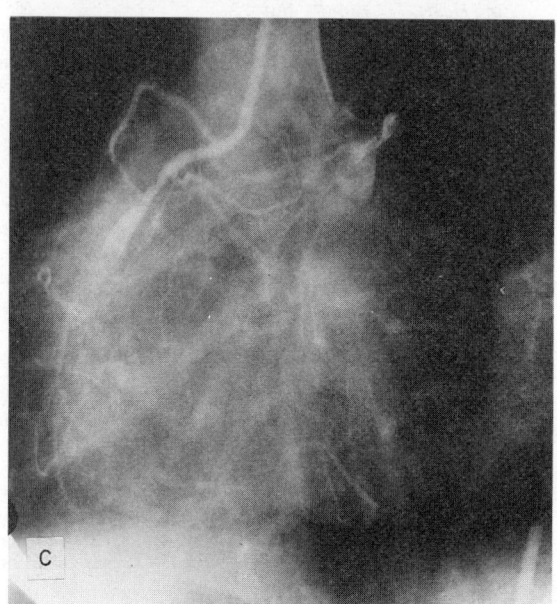

Fig. 16.19. Angiograms in a patient with severe angina pectoris and critical stenosis of the mid right coronary artery (A). After an uneventful and successful dilatation (B), angina returned at 1 month due to total occlusion of the vessel. Repeat dilatation was not attempted and the patient underwent elective coronary artery bypass grafting.

observation of acute and chronic atheromatous lesions *in vivo*. Various mechanical, thermal, electrical and laser devices are currently being evaluated for use in the 'plastic' reconstruction of obstructed coronary arteries. All these exciting developments sprang from the late Dr Andreas Grüntzig's first inspired and brave step of inflating a balloon catheter inside the coronary circulation.

REFERENCES

1. Grüntzig, A.R. Transluminal dilatation of coronary artery stenosis. *Lancet* 1978; i: 263.
2. Kent, K.M., Bentivoglio, L.G., Block, P.C. *et al.* Percutaneous transluminal coronary angioplasty. Report from the Registry of the National Heart, Lung and Blood Institute. *Am. J. Cardiol.* 1982; **49**: 2011–20.
3. Harston, W.E., Tilley, S., Rodeheffer, R., Forman, M.B. and Perry, J.M. Safety and success of the beginning percutaneous

transluminal coronary angioplasty program using the steerable guidewire system. *Am. J. Cardiol.* 1986; 57: 717–20.

4. Sanborn, T.A., Faxon, D.P., Haidenscheld, C., Gottsma, S.B. and Rayan, T.J. The mechanism of transluminal angioplasty: evidence of formation of aneurysms in experimental atherosclerosis. *Circulation* 1983; 68: 1136–40.

5. Essed, C.E., Van den Brand, M. and Becker, A.E. Transluminal coronary angioplasty and early re-stenosis. Fibrocellular occlusion after wall laceration. *Br. Heart J.* 1983; 49: 393–6.

6. Block, P.C. Mechanism of transluminal angioplasty. *Am. J. Cardiol.* 1984; 53: 69C–71C.

7. Austin, G.C., Ratliff, N.B., Hollman, J., Tabei, S. and Phillips, D.F. Intimal proliferation of smooth muscle cells as an explanation for recurrent coronary artery stenosis after percutaneous transluminal coronary angioplasty. *J. Am. Coll. Cardiol.* 1985; 6: 369–75.

8. Seth, A., Perry, R.A., Hunt, A. and Shiu, M.F. Angioplasty of total coronary occlusion. Improved success rates with the use of a wire splinting technique. *Br. Heart J.* 1988; 59: 603(P).

9. Holmes, D. Jr, Vlietstra, R.E., Smith, H.C., Vetrovec, G.W., Kent, K.M., Cowley, M.J., Faxon, D.P., Gruentzig, A.R., Kelsey, S.F., Detre, K.M. *et al.* Restenosis after percutaneous transluminal coronary angioplasty (PTCA): a report from the PTCA Registry of the National Heart, Lung, and Blood Institute. *Am. J. Cardiol.* 1984; 53: 77C–81C.

10. Bourdillon, P.D. Assessing the success of percutaneous transluminal coronary angioplasty. *Br. Heart J.* 1987; 58: 185–9.

11. Hollman, J., Gruentzig, A.R., Douglas, J.S., King, S.B., Ischinger, T., Meier, B. Acute occlusion after percutaneous transluminal coronary angioplasty—a new approach. *Circulation* 1983; 68: 725–32.

12. Marquis, J.E., Schwartz, L., Aldridge, H., Majid, P., Henderson, M. and Matushinsky, E. Acute coronary artery occlusion during percutaneous transluminal coronary angioplasty treated by redilation of the occluded segment. *J. Am. Coll. Cardiol.* 1984; 6: 1268–71.

13. Cowley, M.J., Vetrovec, G.W., DiSciascio, G., Lewis, S.A., Hirsh, P.D. and Wolfgang, T.C. Coronary angioplasty of multiple vessels: short-term outcome and long-term results. *Circulation* 1985; 72: 1314–20.

14. Reul, G.J., Cooley, D.A., Hallman, G.L., Duncan, J.M., Liversay, J.J., Frazier, O.H., Ott, D.A., Angelini, P., Massumi, A. and Mathur, V.S. Coronary artery bypass for unsuccessful percutaneous transluminal coronary angioplasty. *J. Thorac. Cardiovasc. Surg.* 1984; 88: 685–94.

15. Hoshino, T., Yoshida, H., Takayama, S., Iwase, T., Sakata, K., Shingu, T., Yokoyama, S., Mori, N. and Kaburagi, T. Significance of intimal tears in the mechanism of luminal enlargement in percutaneous transluminal coronary angioplasty: correlation of histologic and angiographic findings in postmortem human hearts. *Am. Heart J.* 1987; 114: 503–10.

16. Leimgruber, P.P., Roubin, G.S., Anderson, H.V., Bredlau, C.E., Whitworth, H.B., Douglas, J.S. Jr, King, S.B. and Greuntzig, A.R. Influence of intimal dissection on restenosis after successful coronary angioplasty. *Circulation* 1985; 72: 530–5.

17. Thorton, M.A., Gruentzig,A.R., Hollman, J., King, S.B. and Douglas, J.S. Coumadin and aspirin in the prevention of recurrence after transluminal coronary angioplasty: a randomized study. *Circulation* 1984; 69: 721–7.

18. Whitworth, H.B., Roubin, G.S., Hollman, J., Meier, B., Leimgruber, P.P., Douglas, J.S. Jr, King, S.B. and Gruentzig, A.R. Effect of nifedipine on recurrent stenosis after percutaneous transluminal coronary angioplasty. *J. Am. Coll. Cardiol.* 1986; 8: 1271–6.

19. Waller, B.F., Gorfinkel, H.J., Dillon, J.C., Girod, D.A. and Rothbaum, D.A. Morphologic observations in coronary arteries, aortocoronary saphenous vein bypass grafts, and infant aortea following balloon angioplasty procedures. *Cardiol. Clin.* 1984; 2: 593–619.

20. El Gamal, M.E., Bonnier, J.J., Michels, H.R. and van Gelder, L.M. Improved success rate of percutaneous transluminal graft and coronary angioplasty with the El Gamal guiding catheter. *Cathet. Cardiovasc. Diag.* 1985; 11: 89–96.

21. Feldman, R.L., Macdonald, R.G., Hill, J.A., Conti, R., Pepine, C.J., Carmichael, M.J., Knauff, D.G. and Alexander, J.A. Coronary angioplasty at the time of initial cardiac catheterization. *Cathet. Cardiovasc. Diag.* 1986; 12: 219–22.

22. Safian, R.D., Snyder, L.D., Snyder, B.A., McKay, R.G., Lorell, B.H., Aroesty, J.M., Pasternak, R.C., Bradley, A.B., Monrad, E.S. and Baim, D.S. Usefulness of percutaneous transluminal coronary angioplasty for unstable angina pectoris after non-Q-wave acute myocardial infarction. *Am. J. Cardiol.* 1987; 59: 263–6.

23. de Feyter, P.J., Serruys, P.W., Arnold, A., Simoons, M.L., Wijns, W., Geuskens, R., Soward, A., van den Brand, M. and Hugenholtz, P.G. Coronary angioplasty of the unstable angina related vessel in patients with multivessel disease. *Eur. Heart. J.* 1986; 7: 460–7.

24. de Feyter, P.J., Serruys, P.W., van den Brand, M., Balakumaran, K., Mochtar, B., Soward, A.L., Arnold, A.E. and Hugenholtz, P.G. Emergency coronary angioplasty in refractory unstable angina. *N. Engl. J. Med.* 1985; 313: 342–6.

25. Prida, X.E., Holland, J.P., Feldman, R.L., Hill, J.A., MacDonald, R.G., Conti, C.R. and Pepin, C.J. Percutaneous transluminal coronary angioplasty in evolving acute myocardial infarction. *Am. J. Cardiol.* 1986; 57: 1069–74.

26. Satler, L.F., Pallas, R.S., Bond, O.B., Green, C.E., Pearle, D.L., Schaer, G.L., Kent, K.M. and Rackley, C.E. Assessment of residual coronary arterial stenosis after thrombolytic therapy during acute myocardial infarction. *Am. J. Cardiol.* 1987; 56: 1231–3.

27. Hinohara, T., Simpson, J.B., Phillips, H.R., Behar, V.S., Peter, R.H., Kong, Y., Carlson, E.B. and Stack, R.S. Transluminal catheter reperfusion: a new technique to reestablish blood flow after coronary occlusion during percutaneous transluminal coronary angioplasty. *Am. J. Cardiol.* 1986; 57: 684–6.

28. Cowley, M.J., Mullin, S.M., Kelsey, S.F., Kent, K.M., Gruentzig, A.R., Detre, K.M. and Passaman, E.R. Sex differences in early and long-term results of coronary angioplasty in the NHLBI PTCA Registry. *Circulation* 1985; 71: 90–7.

29. Leimgruber, P.P., Roubin, G.S., Hollman, J. *et al.* Restenosis after successful coronary angioplasty in patients with single vessel disease. *Circulation* 1986 73: 710–7.

30. Bertrand, M.E., La Blanche, J.M., Thieule, F.A., Fourrier, J.L., Traismel, G. and Asseman, P. Comparative results of percutaneous transluminal coronary angioplasty in patients with dynamic versus fixed coronary stenosis. *J. Am. Coll. Cardiol.* 1986; 8: 504–8.

31. Ernst, S.M., Hillebrand, F.A., Klein, B., Ascoop, C.A., van Tellingen, C. and Plokker, H.W. The value of exercise tests in the follow-up of patients who underwent transluminal coronary angioplasty. *Int. J. Cardiol.* 1985; 7: 267–79.

32. Wijns, W., Serruys, P.W., Reiben, J.H.C. *et al.* Early detection of restenosis after successful percutaneous transluminal coronary angioplasty by exercise redistribution Thallium scintigraphy. *Am. J. Cardiol.* 1985; 55: 357–61.

Chapter 17

Digital Subtraction Angiography

M.J. Raphael

Radiologists were soon disabused of the idea that computers could produce high-quality arteriograms from a small injection of contrast made into a peripheral vein; however, many of our clinical colleagues still give some credence to it.

INTRODUCTION

What is digital subtraction angiography (DSA) and what can it do? A photographic subtraction technique was suggested by Ziedses des Plantes in 1935.[1] In this technique, an X-ray exposure of the part to be studied by angiography is made before any contrast arrives. Another film is then exposed after the contrast has arrived. The non-contrast-bearing film is reversed by contact printing onto film so that the dark areas become light and the light areas dark. This reversed film is known as the mask. It is superimposed on the contrast-bearing film. If the density and contrast range of the mask are correct, an image of uniform grey is produced, i.e. black areas in the contrast film being cancelled out by white areas in the mask and vice versa, so that only the contrast medium in the vessels stands out because it has not been subtracted. A contact print is made leaving the subtracted background as light grey and the contrast-bearing vessels in high contrast. In DSA, all these manoeuvres are performed at high speed and with a wide adjustability by a digital computer.

TECHNICAL ASPECTS[2,3]

After passage through the patient, X-rays produce an image on the input phosphor of an image intensifier. A light amplified version of this image is produced on the outlet phosphor and photographed by a TV camera which scans the image converting it into an electrical signal. The electrical signal, after amplification, produces the image on the TV monitor. For DSA, the electrical signal is passed t an analogue to digital (A–D) converter. This converts the continuously variable analogue signal from the TV camera into a series of discrete digital signals, the values of which are stored in the memory of the computer in the form of a square matrix of points called pixels (picture elements). The computer stores the non-contrast bearing frame (Fig. 17.1A) and can reverse its polarity to give the negative mask (Fig. 17.1B), equivalent to the photographic mask, instantaneously. The computer stores the contrast-bearing image in a similar matrix form (Fig. 17.1C) and can subtract the corresponding pixel values of the mask from those of the contrast image leaving only the electrical signal due to the contrast, which can then be amplified and processed by the computer (Fig. 17.1D). Both brightness and contrast can be adjusted by the computer (Fig. 17.2) and a variety of masks can be chosen, even moved, to obtain correct superimposition (registration) after the study (post-processing).

Two types of subtraction process may be utilized. The most common is temporal subtraction in which the contrast image is exposed at a different time from the mask image. The other form, energy subtraction, is based on the differential absorption by tissue of X-rays of different energies and requires a high- and a low-energy X-ray exposure which are made as close together as possible. Combined temporal and energy subtraction is known as hybrid subtraction.[4] What follows applies primarily to temporal subtraction, although the physical limitations of the apparatus tend to be similar for both techniques.

IMAGE FORMATION[5]

The modern image intensifier has a very high resolution and is unlikely to be the significant factor in influencing image quality in DSA.

The TV camera must have high dynamic range

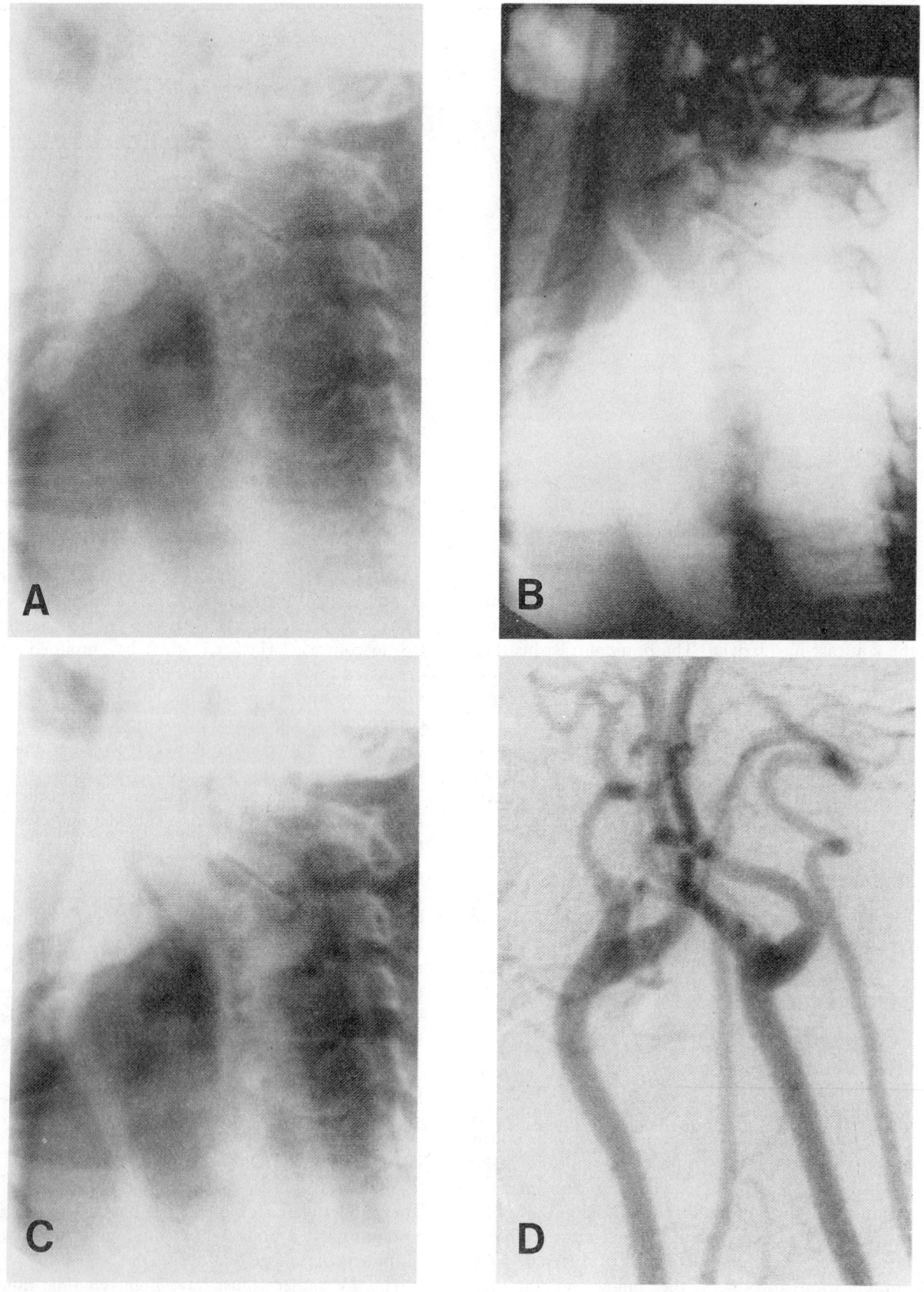

coupled with low noise, as it is the main source of electronic noise. This is a problem only when contrast medium is of too low a concentration and great amplification is necessary.

The speed of the A–D converter is a major limitation in the image formation chain. In electronic terms, this is the slowest part of the system and imposes one of two possible limitations: either imaging rates must be reduced if imaging is taking place in a high-resolution matrix (512 × 512), or resolution must be reduced at high imaging rates by using a smaller matrix (256 × 256 or 128 × 128) (Fig. 17.3). Once the image has been digitized, no further electronic degradation occurs.

The computer limits the quality of the image only in so far as its memory capacity is limited. It will be able to study only a limited number of large matrix images.

In summary, DSA has the following limitations, in apparatus terms, as compared with conventional angiography. The limitations of X-ray generation are shared by both:

1 Digital subtraction angiography is severely limited by the field size of the image intensifier. Currently, most are 9″ or 10″ fields, although a few 14″ image intensifiers are becoming available. For most applications, DSA is limited to a 6″ square field. In conventional angiography, a rapid film changer using 14″ square films gives a full 14″ square field of coverage.

2 The spatial resolution of DSA, as compared with conventional angiography, is currently limited by the size of matrix in the computer. The current largest matrix, 512 × 512, will, in optimized apparatus, produce spatial resolution of up to 2 line-pairs/mm (lp/mm). A comparable conventional film angiogram should achieve a spatial resolution of 6 lp/mm. Whether the gain in resolution by increasing the matrix size to 1024 × 1024 would be worth the enormous expense of increasing computer memories and slowing image acquisition rates is as yet unclear.[6]

3 Contrast resolution in DSA is limited by the noise of the system but is currently taken to be at least four times as high as it is in conventional angiography. The advantage of this much higher contrast resolution is that acceptable images may be obtained with far lower concentrations of contrast than in conventional angiography, allowing either the intravenous injection of contrast to obtain arteriograms or the use of much lower doses of contrast for intra-arterial work.

FEATURES OF THE EXAMINATION

Compared with a conventional cut-film angiogram, DSA shows the following features.

1 The field size is usually less than the 14″ × 14″ of the conventional angiogram.
2 Spatial resolution is only one-third as good as that of the conventional angiogram.
3 Contrast resolution is 4–8 times better than that of the conventional angiogram.
4 Radiation dose per exposure is similar.
5 The dynamic range is greater in DSA enabling detail to be seen within a well-opacified vessel.
6 There is no delay while films are being developed.
7 Hard copy is cheap: many frames may be printed on one sheet of film.

PATIENT FACTORS

Three factors that relate to the patient are crucial to the quality of the subtracted image.

REGISTRATION

Registration is the ability to select a mask that will exactly subtract from the contrast frame. In temporal subtraction, it actually means the ability of the patient to keep absolutely still while holding their breath between exposure of mask and angiogram. Poor registration of the mask and contrast images

Fig. 17.1. Stages in the subtraction process. (A) The mask frame is exposed before the arrival of the contrast. In DSA, this is simply stored in the computer. Here, it has been recalled from the computer memory merely to illustrate the process of subtraction. (B) The mask has been electronically reversed. Structures which appear previously black are now white and vice versa. Again, this process has been performed within the computer memory but is reproduced here for illustrative purposes. (C) The contrast-bearing frame. This has been stored in another part of the computer memory and is reproduced for illustrative purposes. It is part of a venous study of the carotid arteries in the neck and hence there is low density of opacification of the vessels and difficulty in identifying them in the presence of obscuring background structures. (D) The background, stored in one part of the computer memory, has been subtracted from the contrast-bearing frame, stored elsewhere, leaving only the electrical signal due to the contrast itself. This has been amplified so that it appears dense and conspicuous. In this example, registration is particularly good and no misregistration artefacts have been created.

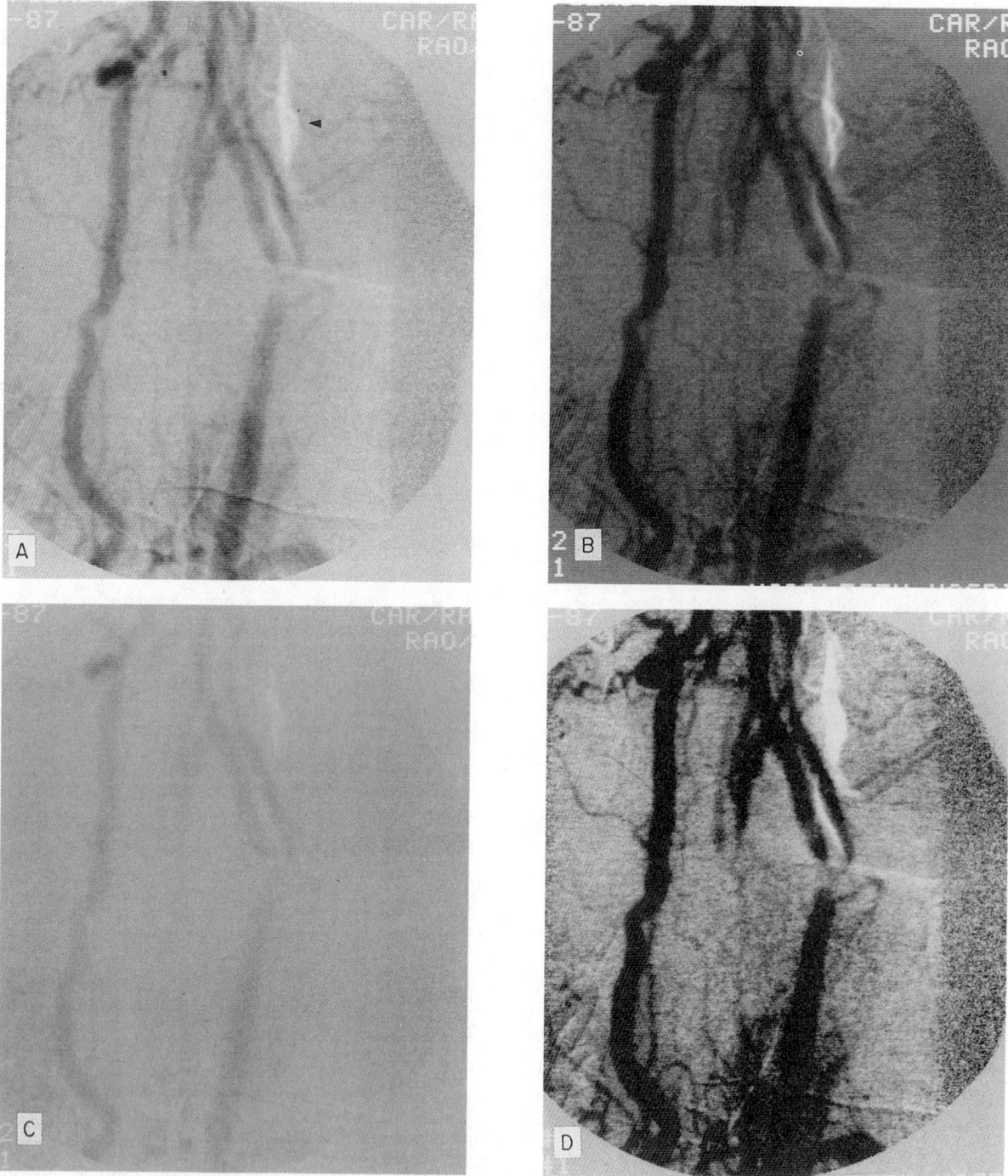

Fig. 17.2. Some of the effects of electronic image processing. (A) Correct settings for image reproduction. The vessels in this IV DSA study are moderately well seen. A misregistration subtraction artefact (arrow) has been produced. (B) The contrast settings are unchanged, but density has been increased. The result is a darker image, although most of the information is still present. (C) The overall density setting is unchanged, but contrast has been reduced. A flat picture with reduced information content results. (D) Overall density setting is unchanged, but contrast has been exaggerated. The result is a conspicuous display of the vessels, but resolution has not been improved because 'noise' has also been increased. In addition, detail within opacified vessels has been lost.

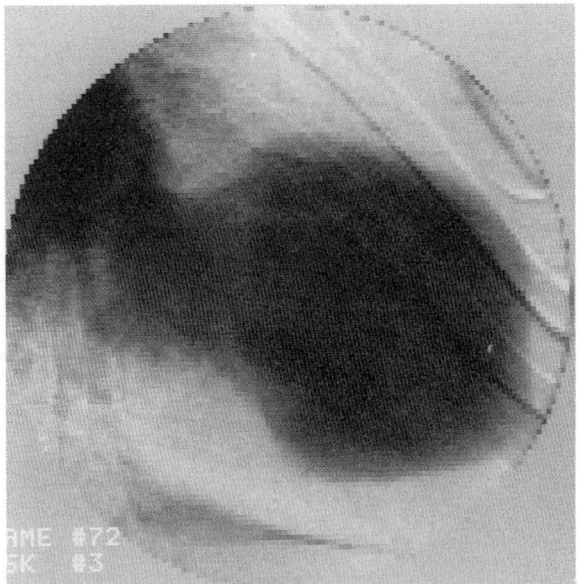

Fig. 17.3. 128 × 128 matrix image. Note the coarseness of the pixels making up the picture and the consequent loss of resolution.

not only removes any advantages there might be in the subtraction technique, but it can also introduce confusing artefacts. It is particularly difficult to obtain good subtraction images in areas like the lungs where both respiratory movements and vessel pulsations cause registration problems: even with perfect registration it is usually impossible to subtract very high (or low) density structures satisfactorily. Thus, opaque metal fragments or gas shadows (in the abdomen) will not subtract fully and, in the latter case, lead to difficulties in interpretation.

COMPACTION

The quality of a digital angiogram varies with the contrast medium concentration. Concentration of the contrast medium may be increased by giving more contrast more quickly and also by giving it more centrally so that the bolus remains compact and not dispersed. In patients with poor cardiac output and valvular heart disease, particularly valvular incompetence, the bolus will be slurred and compaction reduced, leading to a low concentration of contrast medium and a poor angiogram.

RADIATION

Contrast resolution varies with the square root of the radiation doses of the exposure. Hence, the image quality may be improved by increasing the radiation dose for each exposure, although the potential for improvement in this way is limited.

VENOUS DIGITAL SUBTRACTION ANGIOGRAPHY

It is important to remember that venous DSA (IV DSA) requires the passage of a 4F or 5F catheter from a peripheral vein to the central circulation (either to the venae cavae or preferably the right atrium itself). Contrast, in a bolus of 40 ml, is delivered at 18–20 ml/s during suspended respiration. Non-ionic contrast is preferred because it produces less of a sensation of heat and the patients tend to move less. Each study is viewed immediately and supplementary examinations made. Venous DSA can be performed as an outpatient procedure. The patient needs no premedication, should not eat or drink during the 2 h preceding the study, and is able to leave immediately after.

Venous DSA is particularly useful in the following situations.

1 When the vessels to be imaged are large and imaging is not markedly restricted by the limited spatial resolution and low contrast concentration.

2 If a localized segment of the arterial system is to be imaged, IV DSA, because of the limited field covered by the image intensifier, is best used when the suspected site of vascular pathology can be covered by a single position of the intensifier. Lesions at multiple sites require multiple large injections of contrast which are time-consuming. Consequently, extensive pathology is better imaged using conventional angiography.

3 When direct access to the arterial system is difficult.

CLINICAL INDICATIONS FOR VENOUS DIGITAL SUBTRACTION ANGIOGRAPHY

Extracranial cerebrovascular disease

The extracranial blood supply to the brain can be visualized to diagnostic quality in over 70% of patients by IV DSA,[7] showing both atheromatous strictures and ulcers without narrowing (Fig. 17.4). The study is performed on an outpatient basis and requires a pair of angulated oblique views of the carotid bifurcations, usually a frontal view of the intracranial circulation, and, if there is clinical indication, a view of the arch of the aorta in the

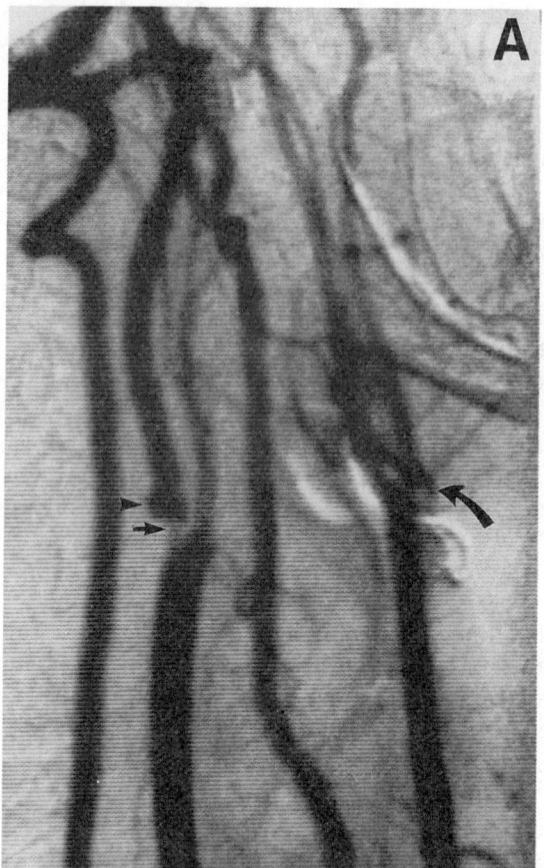

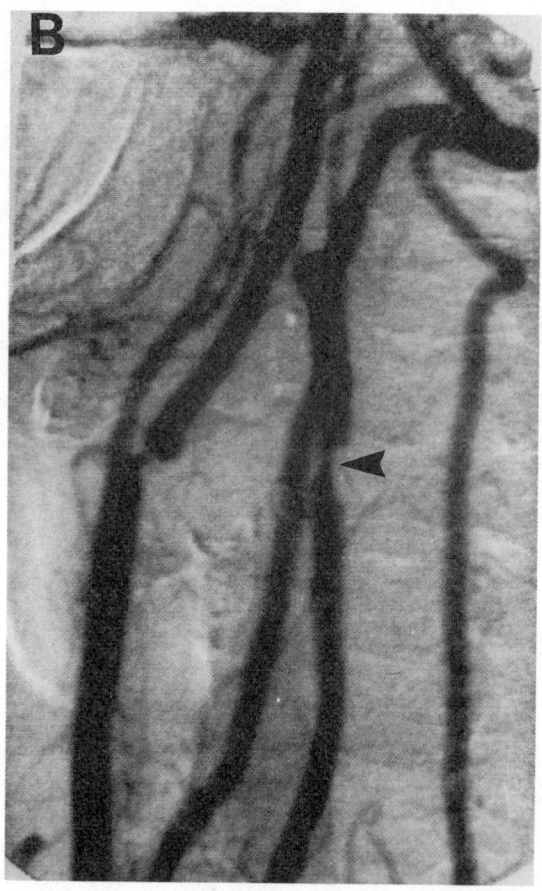

Fig. 17.4. Venous DSA of the extracranial cerebral vessels. (A) Left anterior oblique view. The right vertebral artery and right carotid bifurcation are well seen and a right internal carotid stenosis (arrow) is demonstrated with a possible atheromatous ulcer (arrowhead) beyond it. The left bifurcation (curved arrow) is obscured by vessel overlap and a misregistration artefact from gas in the larynx caused by the patient swallowing at the arrival of the contrast medium. (B) Right anterior oblique projection. The right internal carotid stricture is still well seen. The right vertebral artery now overlaps the upper left carotid branches but a left internal carotid stricture (arrowhead) has been revealed. The left vertebral artery, previously coiled on itself, is now well seen.

right posterior oblique views (LAO equivalent). The ease of performance of IV DSA and its very low morbidity allow the indications for investigation to be extended widely so that patients with apparently trivial or infrequent symptoms, or even relatively asymptomatic patients with physical signs indicating carotid disease, may be investigated.

Studies of the neck vessels reveal the difficulties attached to IV DSA as well as its advantages. Numerous errors of interpretation may occur, even in apparently adequate diagnostic studies.[8] Very short web-like strictures may not be resolved using this system. Strictures may appear worse than they are when misregistration of wall calcium in the vessel leads to subtraction artefacts. Lesions may not be identified if misregistration occurs from movement due to swallowing. Unfortunately, even the arrival of non-ionic contrast medium in the neck produces an urge to swallow in some patients. Lesions may be obscured by overlap of vessels. All vessels in the area are opacified because IV DSA is a non-selective procedure. An additional problem when imaging the neck is that plaque development begins posteriorly and is preferably imaged by a very steep oblique or true lateral view which cannot be obtained with IV DSA because overlap will always be produced. By close attention to the details of radiography and by exercising care in the interpretation of the images, these potential errors can be reduced. It is now usual for the physician to accept a good-quality negative study as correct, and for a surgeon to operate on the basis of a good-quality study showing carotid stenoses. Only when IV DSA is indeterminate will a small proportion of patients need to proceed to hospital admission to undergo the potentially hazardous arch aortogram and selective carotid arteriogram.

As a screening and diagnostic procedure, IV DSA of the carotid arteries must be compared with the totally non-invasive evaluation of the carotid bifurcation by Doppler ultrasound. With the technical improvements in Doppler interrogation systems now combined with imaging of the carotid bifurcations, atheroma in the wall of the carotid can be identified, strictures can be seen and the haemodynamic disturbance to flow that they produce identified.[9] At this moment, the technique is still under evaluation and its accuracy, when compared with that of IV DSA, may be as good or better.

Arch aortography

The aorta, being a large and relatively immobile vascular structure in the thorax and close to the heart, is a reasonably good object for investigation by IV DSA, although the simultaneous opacification of the pulmonary veins degrades the image quality (Fig. 17.5). Coarctation (Fig. 17.5) is usually well visualized in co-operative subjects. All that is required is the visualization of the site of the

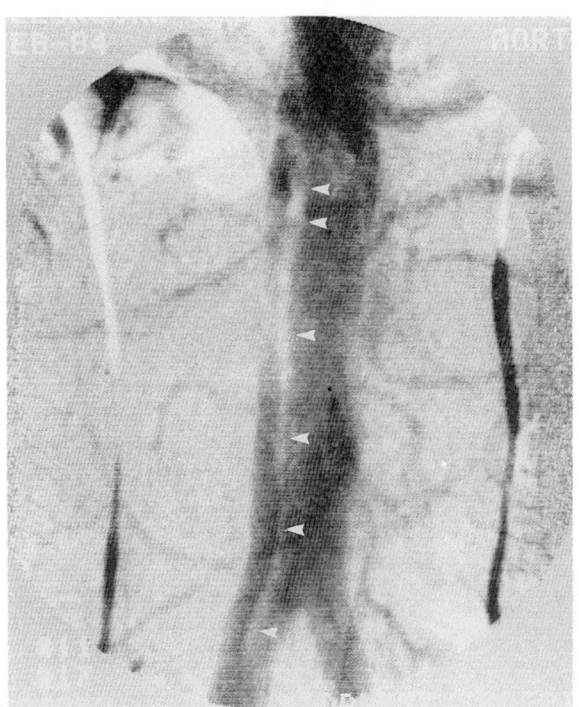

Fig. 17.6. Aortic dissection. This patient suffered a traumatic dissection of his abdominal aorta at cardiac catheterization two months previously. Venous DSA demonstrates that the elevated intimal flap (arrowheads) is still present and has not healed. This patient was clinically well, without valvular heart disease and with a good cardiac output, allowing good subtraction. Few workers have found IV DSA of great value in spontaneous acute dissection of the aortic arch when these factors are absent.

coarctation and the length of affected aorta. As no haemodynamic data are required, IV DSA is usually perfectly adequate as the only investigation for isolated coarctation. Other congenital anomalies of the aorta, provided there is no associated heart disease, may also be visualized adequately by IV DSA. Aneurysms of the aorta may be demonstrated, although modern computed tomography will also show them and requires only a slow infusion of contrast into a peripheral vein. Dissections of the aorta have been demonstrated by IV DSA (Fig. 17.6), but detail is poor and modern computed tomography is the investigation of choice.

Renal arteriography[11]

Venous DSA has been used as a screening test for renal artery stenosis in hypertensive patients (Fig. 17.7). Providing the circulation is normal, the bolus remains compact and density of opacification of the aorta and renal arteries is usually adequate.

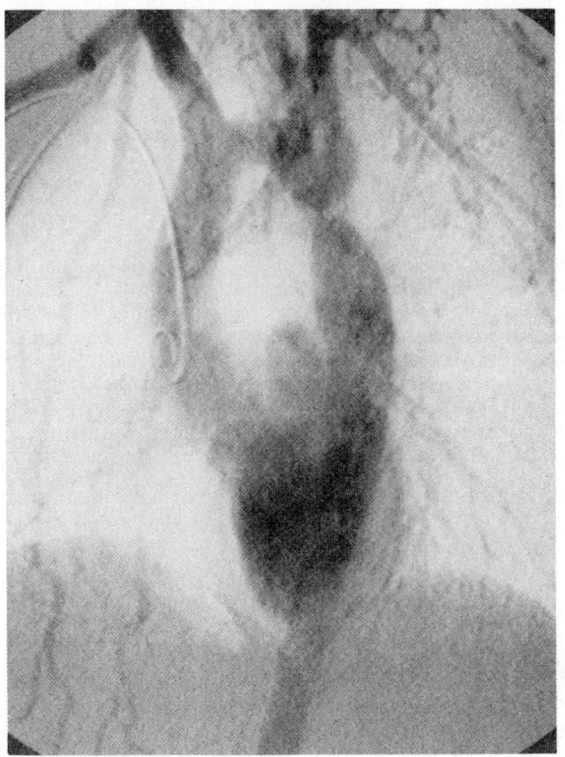

Fig. 17.5. Arch aortography. This patient had clinically severe coarctation as an isolated lesion. Venous DSA demonstrates that the lesion is in the typical site and suitable for reconstruction.

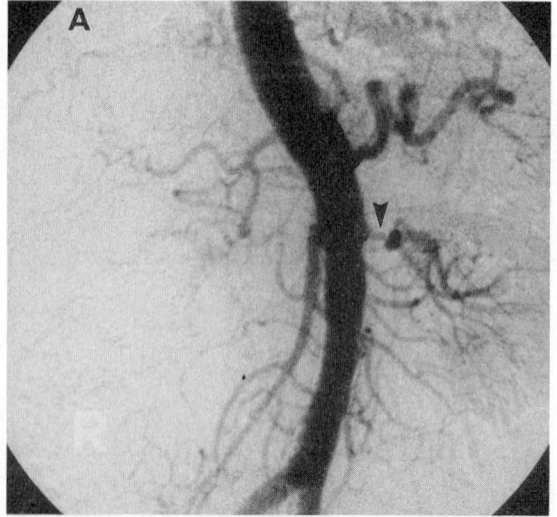

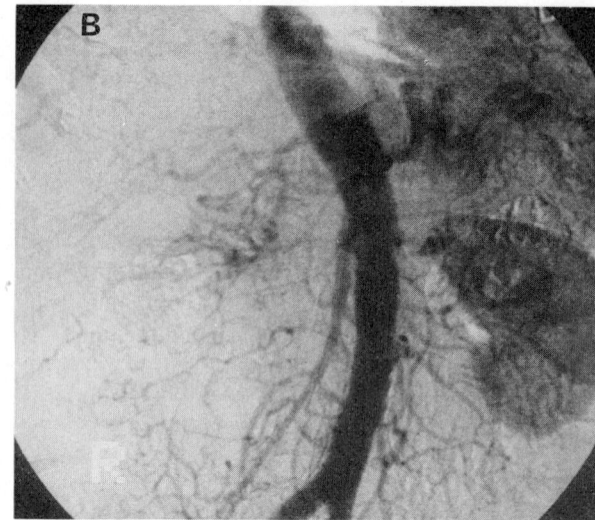

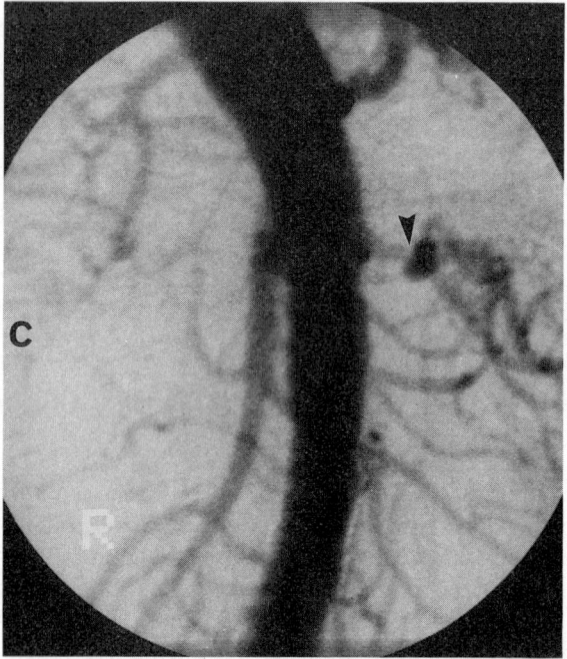

Fig. 17.7. Venous DSA in renal arteriography. A patient with worsening hypertension. (A) Large field view in the arterial phase. Only the left renal artery (arrowhead) is identified. (B) Nephrogram phase. Only a left nephrogram has developed. (C) Magnified view of (A) reveals a stenosis (arrowed) at the left renal artery.

Peripheral vascular disease

With the a 9″ image intensifier, a complete study of the vessels of the lower limb involves radiography in 9 positions, each requiring its own bolus of contrast medium. In addition, bowel gas in the sigmoid colon very frequently obscures the iliac arteries, it being immediately over the area of interest. In the legs, however, registration and hence subtraction are usually very satisfactory. Because of the large volumes of contrast medium involved and the time taken to set up and expose each position, even with the larger image intensifiers becoming available, IV DSA is not currently used to investigate peripheral vascular disease of the lower limbs. It is valuable, however, when the site of a suspected pathology is known, for example, when checking the results of an angioplasty or the appearance of a surgical graft (Fig. 17.8).

Pulmonary angiography

Venous DSA can satisfactorily image the main pulmonary artery and its first two or three divisions. Beyond this, the vessels are small and misregistration artefacts seriously degrade the detail. Thus, although it may have a limited use in identifying large and central pulmonary emboli, resolution is usually inadequate to identify an embolus in the

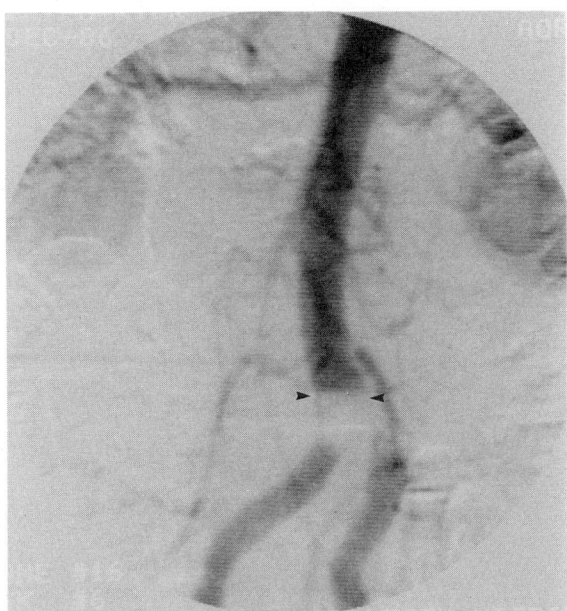

Fig. 17.8. Venous DSA in peripheral vascular disease. Following cardiac surgery, this patient developed what was thought clinically to be a saddle embolus. Venous DSA avoids arterial catheterization in a patient receiving anticoagulation, confirms the diagnosis and demonstrates the embolus (arrowheads) at the lower end of the abdominal aorta.

segmental vessels and beyond. In general, it gives little information in patients with pulmonary embolus that cannot be obtained by isotope studies. It can however occasionally show rarer abnormalities of the pulmonary arteries, such as congenital absence, hypoplasia or proximal stenosis and involvement of the pulmonary arteries and more generalized arteriopathic conditions.

INTRA-ARTERIAL DIGITAL SUBTRACTION ANGIOGRAPHY

Intra-arterial contrast injection, combined with DSA, has a number of advantages over film radiography. Small catheters, 5F or even 4F, may be used enabling patients to be studied on a day-case basis. Small volumes of dilute contrast may be injected relatively slowly and high-quality pictures may be produced. A low cardiac output or valvular heart disease are not contra-indications to intra-arterial DSA (IA DSA). The disadvantages are that patient co-operation with breath-holding and immobility are still required, the field size of the image intensifier is small and all vessels fill, and an unwanted vessel may overlap the area of interest. The advantages of IA DSA mean that there has been a trend toward its increased use, particularly

because contrast volume and delivery rate may be reduced and flush injections may provide a diagnosis without the necessity of proceeding to selective arteriography. It may be the technique of choice where its contrast-enhancing advantages outweigh its lack of spatial resolution.[14] The smaller amounts of contrast save money and reduce patient discomfort and risk if heart failure or renal failure is present. Film costs are dramatically reduced. In areas where subtraction technique is valuable in its own right, such as neuroradiology investigations, IA DSA has found particular favour. The technique of 'road mapping' is of great value to radiologists during interventional procedures: the subtracted angiogram may be frozen on the monitor and catheter manipulation, visualized by fluoroscopy, can be superimposed on the image to aid selective catheterization.

CARDIAC DIGITAL SUBTRACTION ANGIOGRAPHY[15–17]

Venous DSA is able to opacify all the cardiac chambers quite well, even in cases with poor ventricular function, provided that there is no gross valvular heart disease. Two variations of the subtraction technique may be used within the heart. The commonest is the technique previously described in which a single mask is subtracted from each contrast-bearing image in turn. In more sophisticated apparatus, the mask itself may be prepared by a composite from a number of different mask frames. In the technique uniquely applied to the heart, each frame becomes the mask being subtracted from the following frame which in turn becomes the mask and is subtracted from the next frame. This continuous subtraction process is known as ciné subtraction.

Venous DSA may be used for studying left ventricular function in two ways. The volume of the left ventricle may be measured directly by opacifying the chamber. Measurement of the systolic and diastolic volumes makes it possible to calculate the stroke volume and hence the ejection fraction. In addition, if rapid sequence exposures (up to 30 frames/s or fps) are taken, regional wall movement abnormalities may be seen (Fig. 17.9). Ventricular volumes and regional wall movement abnormalities observed by IV DSA have been compared with those in the same patient studied by the technique of standard ciné left ventriculography with good correlation.[18]

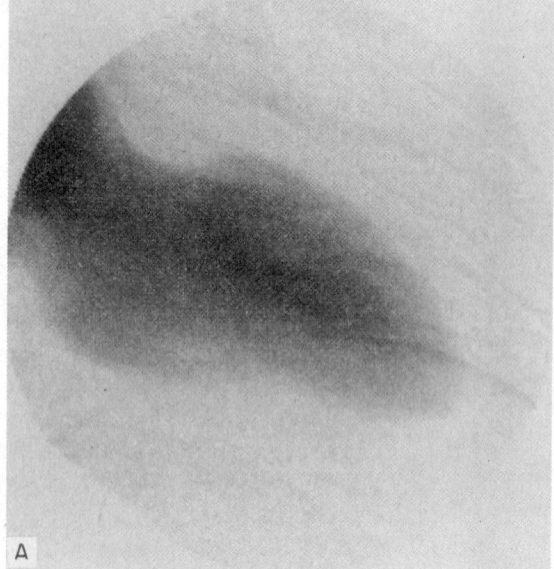 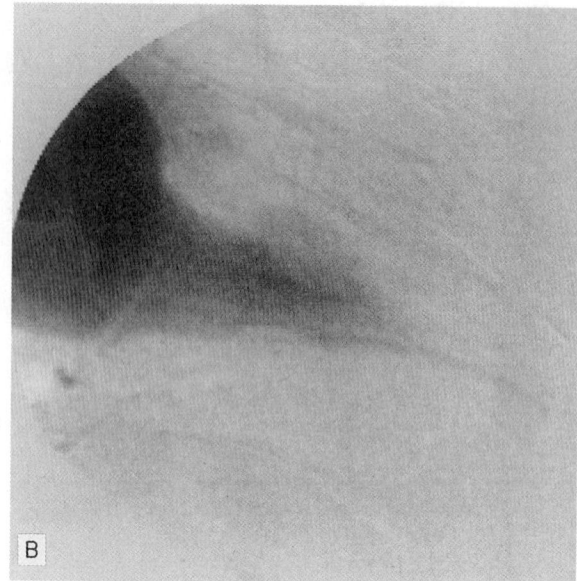

Fig. 17.9. Venous DSA in left ventriculography. (A) Diastole; (B) systole. The ventricle is well opacified and resolution is superior to that obtained by nuclear techniques. In this case, ventricular contraction can be clearly identified as being concentric and normal.

As computer technology extends, it has become possible to record very rapidly (up to 40 frames/s) large numbers of high-resolution digital images, and digital ventriculography (with or without subtraction) may replace direct ciné ventriculography. This will allow very low doses of contrast to be used and saves on expensive ciné film, its processing and storage. In addition, the direct recording of the image in digital format will allow further computer processing. The ventricle in each frame may be outlined by an edge-detection programme, ventricular volume calculated in systole and diastole and from these the ejection fraction. More advanced programmes enable localized abnormalities of ventricular wall movement to be directly assessed by the computer. All this should allow a safer, cheaper and more detailed evaluation of left ventricular function.[19]

Venous DSA can also be used to study left ventricular function using a totally different principle. The internal computer allows a region of interest (ROI) to be designated by the user within the outline of the left ventricle. The computer then directly calculates the intensity of the transmitted X-rays at the ROI, and from this the quantity of iodine in the beam at that point. By measuring the transmission and its difference between diastole and systole, the proportion of iodine ejected from the ventricle with each beat can be calculated and hence the ejection fraction determined. This method does not depend on any geometric assumptions about the shape of the ventricle. However, it does systematically underestimate the ejection fraction as compared with the ventricular volume measurements. This type of computer analysis of the DSA images of the left ventricle closely follows those used in nuclear cardiology. Nuclear studies are less invasive and more flexible, they require only an injection into a peripheral vein and they can be easily repeated and performed during exercise. Using multiple gated acquisition (MUGA) techniques, repeated studies may be made. Venous DSA of the left ventricle can be repeated far fewer times because of the radiation and contrast load, but it does have significantly more spatial resolution than the nuclear image.

Other chambers within the heart may be studied by IV DSA. Tumours and other pathological processes have been demonstrated, but the technique has little advantage over cross-sectional echocardiography, unless ultrasound access is impossible.

CORONARY ARTERIES

Occasionally, the proximal parts of the coronary arteries are visualized in high-quality IV DSA. The pictures are never diagnostic. Intra-arterial DSA with injections into the aortic root provides too capricious a filling of the coronary arteries for systematic diagnosis. Up to now, ungated selective intracoronary injections have lacked sufficient re-solution due to poor registration. However, expo-sure of the images in a designated part of the cardiac cycle, usually diastole, by gating the exposure to the electrocardiogram, significantly improves image quality (Fig. 17.10).

Again, the advantage of direct recording of the image into digital format, either in place of the ciné coronary arteriogram or simultaneously with it, is that computer processing of the image becomes possible. Programmes are commercially available to quantify the degree of narrowing demonstrated on selective coronary arteriograms using edge-detection techniques. However, the value is not clear in view of the well-known eccentricity of narrowings that develop in the coronary arteries. Evaluation of the degree of stenosis and, it is claimed, the pressure gradient may also be made by measuring the reduction in X-ray transmission, and hence the iodine content, in the coronary artery and its stenosed area. These techniques still require operator intervention to supervise the correct func-tioning of the computer, and they need to undergo extensive clinical evaluation.

Coronary flow and myocardial perfusion may be assessed by digital subtraction techniques. Coron-ary flow (indeed, flow in any vessel) may be calculated by measuring the diameter of the vessel (hence, its cross-sectional area) and the distance the

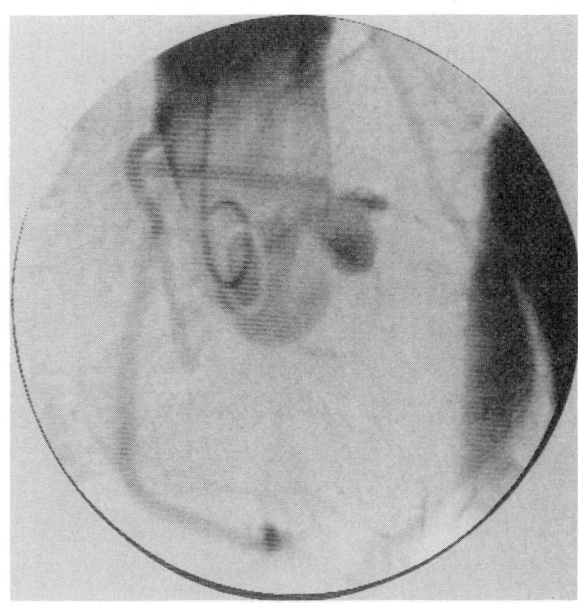

Fig. 17.11. Intra-arterial DSA of the aortic root in a patient with coronary artery bypass grafts. Note the two images of the pigtail catheter tip. It has moved its position between the mask and the contrast-bearing frame. The grafts themselves are particularly well visualized in this study and appear to be widely patent. Even here, no detail of the native coronary circulation can be seen.

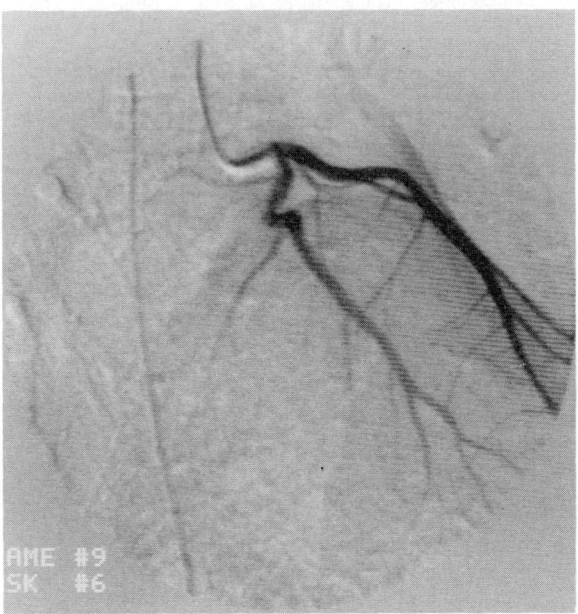

Fig. 17.10. Intra-arterial gated DSA of a selective left coronary artery injection. Although resolution is good, it is no better than that of high-quality ciné-radiography which has numerous other advantages.

blood, and contrast, move along the vessel in a known time. Myocardial perfusion may be mea-sured, with some limitations, by centring an ROI over a segment of myocardium and using the technique to measure an iodine washout curve by the change in X-ray transmission after the end of the selective intracoronary contrast injection. Whereas absolute measurements may as yet not be very reliable comparisons of flow or perfusion in the same patient, they may be possible after interven-tions such as intra-coronary papaverine to access coronary flow reserve.

Venous DSA has also been investigated as a method for studying coronary artery saphenous vein bypass grafts. It did not prove satisfactory due to poor contrast density and poor registration. However, intra-arterial DSA has proven significant-ly more successful (Fig. 17.11). A 5F or even 4F pigtail may be introduced percutaneously from the femoral artery and positioned above the aortic valve. A power injection of a bolus of 30–40 ml over 2 s usually gives excellent opacification of the aorta and adequate opacification of grafts. Almost all patent grafts can be identified from a single injection in the LAO projection.[20] This technique, however, is limited because it produces images of such poor detail it is possible to determine only graft patency; strictures may be missed and the state of the native circulation cannot be determined. It seems likely that high-speed high-resolution computed tomography scanning will demonstrate the patency of coronary artery bypass grafts as accurately as intra-arterial DSA and much less invasively.

CONCLUSION

Digital subtraction angiography does not have a unique role in any sphere of routine cardiac investigation. It has a useful but limited role in demonstrating the patency of coronary artery bypass grafts. It seems unlikely that IV DSA in any form will visualize the coronary arteries satisfactorily; it is more likely that an intra-arterial aortic root injection, combined with gating, may act as a screening test for coronary artery disease in the future. Stenosis measurement, coronary blood flow and myocardial perfusion studies will become routinely possible during selective coronary arteriography in future, and the use of digital techniques to evaluate function as well as anatomy will become widespread.

Lesions of the thoracic aorta are usually well demonstrated, but IV DSA is probably not good for imaging dissections. Venous DSA demonstrates only the proximal pulmonary arteries satisfactorily. In other arteries, IV DSA is indicated usually only when intra-arterial injections are inappropriate, perhaps due to lack of arterial access or a bleeding diasthesis, and the resolution difficulties of DSA are acceptable. In the investigation of the carotid arteries, DSA has become established as the investigation of first choice, although the introduction of duplex Doppler ultrasound scanning may change this. As image intensifiers become larger, and their fields of coverage larger, the indications for DSA will be extended because fewer injections will cover larger areas, which will lead to the substitution of DSA for conventional film angiography because it is cheaper and quicker.

REFERENCES

1. Ziedses des Plantes, B.G. Subtraction. *Fortschr. Rontgenstr.* 1935; 52: 67–79.
2. Brody, W.R., Enzmann, D.R., Miller, D.C. *et al.* Intravenous arteriography using digital subtraction techniques. *JAMA* 1982; 248: 671–4.
3. Mistretta, C.A., Crummy, A.B. and Strother, C.M. Digital angiography: A perspective. *Radiology* 1981; 139: 273–6.
4. Foley, W.D., Benes, J., Smith, D.F. *et al.* Intravenous and intra-arterial hybrid digital subtraction angiography: Clinical evaluation. *Am. J. Roentgenol.* 1986; 147: 613–20.
5. Verhoeven, L.A.J. DSA imaging: some physical and technical aspects. *Medicamundi* 1985; 30: 46–55.
6. Gomes, A., Papin, P.J., Markovich, N.I. *et al.* Digital subtraction angiography: A comparison of 512 × 512 and 1024 × 1024 imaging. *Am. J. Roentgenol.* 1986; 146: 835–8.
7. Foley, D.W., Smith, D.F., Mieke, M.W. *et al.* Intravenous DSA, examination of patients with suspected cerebral ischaemia. *Radiology* 1984; 151: 651–9.
8. Turski, P.A., Zwiebel, W.I., Strother, C.M., Crummy, A.B., Celesia, G.G. and Sackett, J.F. Limitations of intravenous digital subtraction angiography. *AJNR* 1983; 4: 271–3.
9. Sumner, D.S., Russell, J.B. and Miles, R.D. Are non-evasive tests sufficiently accurate to identify patients in need of carotid arteriography? *Surgery* 1982; 91: 700–6.
10. Grossman, L.B., Buonocore, E., Modic, M.T. *et al.* Digital subtraction angiography of the thoracic aorta. *Radiology* 1984; 150: 323.
11. Wilms, G.E., Baert, A.L. and Stuessen, J.A. Renal artery stenosis: Evaluation with intravenous digital subtraction angiography. *Radiology* 1986; 160: 713–5.
12. Ferris, F.J., Holder, J.C., Lim, W.N. *et al.* Angiography of pulmonary emboli: Digital studies and balloon occlusion cine angiography. *Am. J. Roentgenol.* 1984; 142: 369–73.
13. Kaufman, S.L., Chang, R., Kadir, S. *et al.* Intra-arterial digital subtraction angiography in diagnostic arteriography. *Radiology* 1984; 151: 323–7.
14. Hemmingway, A.P., Virjee, N. and Allison, D.J. Digital subtraction angiography in gastrointestinal disease. *Medicamundi* 1986; 31: 91–5.
15. Struyven, J.L., Delcour, C., Brion, J.P. *et al.* Digital subtraction angiography of the heart and coronary arteries. *Medicamundi* 1986; 31: 16–22.
16. Myerowitz, P.D., Shaw, C.G., Swann, D.K. *et al.* Computerised fluoroscopy: New technique for the non-invasive evaluation of the aorta, coronary artery bypass grafts, and left ventricular function. *J. Thorac. Cardiovasc. Surg.* 1982; 83: 65–73.
17. Detrano, R., Yiannikis, J., Simpfendorfer, R.E. *et al.* Exercise digital subtraction ventriculography for the detection of ischaemic wall motion abnormalities in patients without myocardial infarction. *Br. Heart J.* 1986; 56: 131.
18. Nissen, S.E., Booth, D., Waters, J. *et al.* Evaluation of left ventricular contractile pattern by intravenous digital subtraction ventriculography: Comparison with cine angiography and assessment of inter-observer variability. *Am. J. Cardiol.* 1983; 52: 1293–1298.
19. Hunter, G.J.S., Hunter, J.V. and Brown, N.J.G. Parametric imaging using digital subtraction angiography. *Br. J. Radiol.* 1986; 59: 7–11.
20. Guthaner, D.F., Wexler, I. and Bradlel, B. Digital subtraction angiography of coronary grafts: Optimisation of technique. *Am. J. Roentgenol.* 1985; 145: 1185–1190.

Chapter 18

Magnetic Resonance Imaging and Computed Tomography

Martin Been

INTRODUCTION

The development of nuclear magnetic resonance imaging has excited considerable interest and much speculation about its future potential in cardiology. Despite the enthusiasm often associated with new technology, the initial high expectations are not always fulfilled. Although developments and refinements in magnetic resonance imaging (MRI) are continuing, it is now possible to assess critically what has been achieved and what advances may realistically be expected in the medium term.

Computed tomography (CT) has been available for about 10 years longer than MRI, but it has found only a limited application in the investigation of cardiac disease. Recent technical innovations, such as the introduction of ultrafast cine-CT scanners designed for cardiac imaging, have expanded the potential role of computed tomography. However, the advent, success and relative cost-effectiveness of cross-sectional echocardiography are important in determining the limited role of CT scanning in cardiology and these factors will continue to operate with respect to MRI.

At first sight, the transverse images obtained with CT scanning resemble MR images but the underlying physical principles and nature of the biological information they provide are very different and the two techniques will be considered separately.

MAGNETIC RESONANCE IMAGING

Currently available imaging systems selectively 'tune in' to the resonant frequency of single protons (^{1}H). The images are therefore constructed from signals derived from the hydrogen nucleus (^{1}H), thus giving rise to the term 'proton nuclear magnetic resonance imaging'.

Magnetic resonance imaging can be performed on other atoms if the nucleus contains an odd number of protons or neutrons, such as ^{13}C, ^{23}Na and ^{31}P. The relatively low abundance of these atoms in biological systems means that the detected signal is correspondingly small. Despite the low signal-to-noise ratio, it has been possible to obtain sodium images from myocardium *in vivo*, but only if prolonged imaging times are used; as yet these images have not been obtained in man.

PRINCIPLES OF MAGNETIC RESONANCE IMAGING

Physical principles

Protons are most suited for MRI because hydrogen is by far the most abundant atom in living systems. Most tissues consist mainly of water, and each molecule of water has two protons capable of contributing to the MR signal. Hydrogen is also a significant constituent in other tissue components such as lipids.

The creation of magnetic resonance images can be considered in three stages (see 1–3 below) but also depends on naturally occurring nuclear magnetism. Protons are electrically charged and have an inherent spin which produces a tiny magnetic field around each proton (Fig. 18.1Ai). In the normal state, the direction of these individual magnetic fields is random (Fig. 18.1Aii) and results in no net magnetization.

1 Creation of a uniform *magnetic* field (Fig. 18.1B). When a person enters a strong uniform magnetic field, the direction of the atomic spins of all electrically charged atoms, including protons, will tend to align themselves parallel to the external magnetic field in either direction (Fig. 18.1Bi,ii). In fact, there will be a slightly

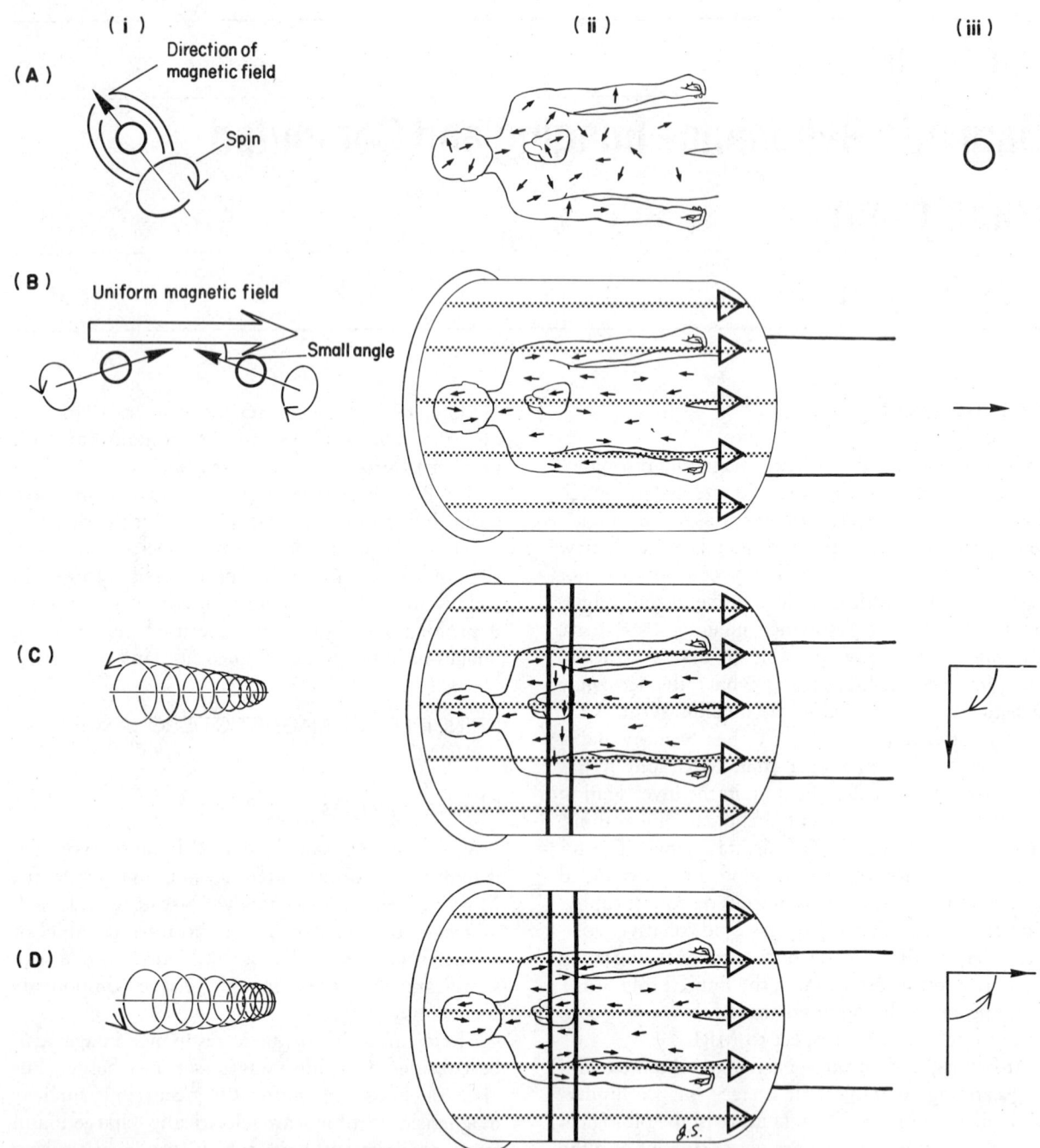

Fig. 18.1. (A)(i) Single proton indicating spin and (random) direction of the tiny magnetic field so induced. (ii) Random orientation of protons before entering magnetic field. (iii) Direction of net magnetization — zero. (B)(i) Protons aligned along the direction of the uniform magnetic field. (ii) Alignment with magnetic field but with slight excess in one direction. (iii) Direction of net magnetization. (C)(i) Precession. (ii) Tilting of the magnetic moment in the imaging section. (iii) Direction of net magnetization. (D)(i) Precession (in reverse direction). (ii) Return of magnetic moment to alignment with uniform field. (iii) Direction of net magnetization.

greater number of protons in the direction of the external magnetic field and this difference results in a net magnetization or magnetic moment in the direction of the uniform magnetic field.

2   Radiofrequency pulse (*resonance*) (Fig. 18.1C).

A smaller oscillating magnetic field (radiofrequency pulse) is then applied perpendicular to the uniform magnetic field at the correct frequency for a particular nucleus (the Larmor frequency) and the additional force results in the radiofrequency pulse is applied the angle of the proton spins relative to the uniform magnetic field direction increase, and the spins also rotate about this direction at the Larmor frequency. The net effect of this is to tilt the magnetic moment (Fig. 18.1Cii). The angle of tilt, often referred to as the flip angle, is dependent on the magnitude and duration of the radiofrequency pulse. In practice, the pulse sequences used usually result in alteration of direction of net magnetization by 90 or 180°. A gradient is applied that selects the imaging section, which is usually of between 5 and 15 mm (Fig. 18.1Ciii).

3   Signal detection (*imaging*) (Fig. 18.1D). When the radiofrequency pulse is turned off, the nuclei precess back, so that they are once again aligned along the direction of the uniform magnetic field (Fig. 18.1Di–iii). During this precession, the protons in turn emit a radiofrequency signal which is detected by the same transmitting coil or by a separate receiving coil. This signal is composed of a range of different frequencies, close to the Larmor frequency, which provide coding for spatial information. By using a complex mathematical technique, known as a two-dimensional Fourier transform, the frequency components can be determined thus allowing an image to be reconstructed from 128 or 256 different signals.

One advantage of MRI is its ability to obtain images in different planes. Transverse images are most commonly used in practice, but sagittal and coronal views can provide useful additional information. The ability to obtain oblique slices is of particular value in cardiac imaging because it allows optimal orientation along the desired cardiac axis. Furthermore, as the position of signals obtained from multiple slices is known, the three-dimensional reconstruction of images is possible, although time-consuming.

More detailed descriptions of the techniques employed are available elsewhere.[1,2]

Parameters that make up magnetic resonance images

In their simplest form, images can be constructed from information about the density of protons. These are essentially proton density maps in which image intensity is a direct reflection of the density of protons in each pixel (individual picture element).

parameters, T_1 and T_2. These parameters are a measure of the efficiency of relaxation in the longitudinal (T_1) or transverse (T_2) plane (see below). Magnetic relaxation times differ among and sometimes within tissues because individual nuclei are not only subjected to the uniform and oscillating magnetic fields but are also constrained by the surrounding environment.

In practice, images are usually constructed from signals which contain proton density information as well as a weighting of T_1 or T_2 information. To understand the importance of these parameters for medical imaging, it is necessary to consider the biophysical principles of magnetic resonance imaging.[3]

Biophysical principles

Proton density (displays structure)

The proton signal is derived primarily from water; intracellular and extracellular water comprises around 80% of most biological systems. Many tissues have a high water content: ventricular myocardium, lung tissue and liver, for example, all consist of about 80% water. Therefore, using proton density alone, it would be difficult to differentiate among tissues and particularly between pathological and normal tissue in the same organ.

Cardiac structures, however, can be well demonstrated because of the natural contrast provided by flowing blood and by air in the lungs (Fig. 18.2). Blood flow provides contrast because many protons that precess in response to the radiofrequency pulse will have left the imaging field before transmitting their signal. Similarly, air in the lungs greatly reduces the density of protons resulting in a minimal signal.

The limitations of proton density imaging are that subtle differences within the myocardium cannot be seen and, in cases in whom blood is static or flow is slow, the intracavitary signal may increase greatly making it impossible to distinguish from myocardium.

Relaxation parameters and tissue characterization

The relaxation parameters T_1 and T_2 are measurements in milliseconds, related to the exponential decay of the signal produced by precession. T_1

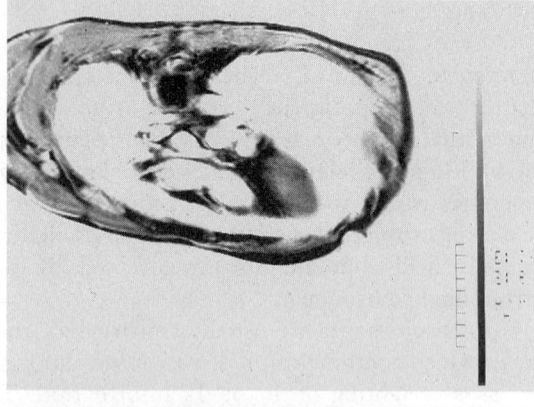

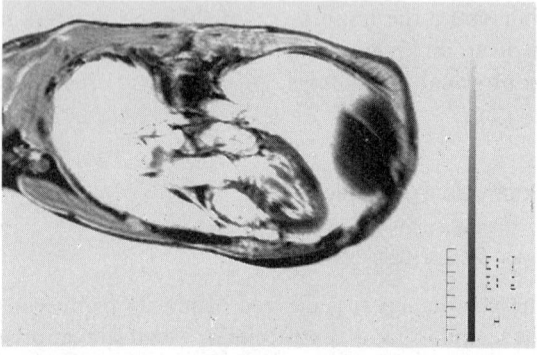

Fig. 18.2. Transverse section through the left ventricle showing high-quality anatomical detail of both ventricles and the papillary muscles. (Courtesy of Dr M.A. Smith.)

measures longitudinal and T_2 transverse relaxation times.

Tissue characterization is possible because precession of individual protons is influenced by their surrounding environment. Water in living systems exists to a varying degree as 'bound' or 'free' water, and the state of water is thought to be an important influence on the relaxation parameters. Three types of water have been postulated.[4]

1 Bound water, i.e. water that is an integral part of macromolecular structures (primary hydration layer).
2 Surface bound, i.e. water bound to the surface of macromolecules (secondary hydration layer).
3 Free water, i.e. unbound water.

The relationship between molecular size, the binding of water and the magnetic resonance parameters T_1 and T_2 is complex. Although T_1 (influenced by macromolecular size) and T_2 (affected by interactions with other resonating nuclei) are both prolonged as the ratio of free to bound water increases, they provide complementary information. T_1 measurements are affected by the field strength, and so quoted values from different systems cannot be compared directly.

In practice, the ability to estimate T_1 and T_2 depends on the particular radiofrequency pulse sequences used. Thus, images may be constructed primarily from proton density information or have a varying degree of T_1 or T_2 'weighting'.

Discrimination between tissues

There are large differences between both T_1 and T_2 values of tissue constituents. Fat always gives a low T_1 with progressively higher values for fibrous tissue, myocardium and static fluid. The differences in T_1 values are readily appreciated when the values are colour coded (Plates 18.1–18.3). Fat, liver and myocardium are seen to have progressively higher values. This ability for tissue characterization is also illustrated by examining the pericardial region in Plates 18.1–18.3. At echocardiography, such patients would have an echo-free space in the region of the pericardium, but on MRI there is clear differentiation between fluid fat and pericardium. It may even be possible to differentiate between a bloody and serous pericardial effusion.

Discrimination between normal and pathological tissue

Some pathological processes alter the ratio of bound to free water within tissues, thereby altering T_1 and T_2 in the affected region (Pl. 18.1). Diseases that produce myocardial oedema are particularly likely to alter relaxation parameters, but other factors are also involved.[3] An increase (or decrease) in T_1 or T_2 is not specific to any one disease but the magnitude, timing and distribution of changes may differentiate among various disease processes, and serial studies should allow assessment of the myocardial response to therapeutic interventions. The current status of tissue characterization is considered in more detail below.

Factors specifically related to cardiac imaging

Cardiac gating

The natural contrast provided by flowing blood in MRI is an important advantage but associated cardiac motion causes difficulties. Cardiac gating is usually employed to obtain fine anatomical detail and is important for the precise measurement of magnetic relaxation parameters; however the techniques required for gated T_1 and T_2 images are complex.[5] Most commonly, the electrocardiogram is used to trigger the pulse sequence, although a mechanical trigger detecting a peripheral arterial pulse can be used.

Further improvements in image quality are possible with respiratory gating, but for routine cardiac imaging the technical difficulties and consequent lengthening of imaging time do not justify the relatively modest improvement obtained. New techniques that compensate for respiratory motion may prove to be of value.

Phase imaging (or flow imaging)

Phase imaging refers to an imaging system that specifically examines protons moving in a selected direction such that only flowing blood produces a signal. This signal is related to flow because there is a delay between the radiofrequency stimulating pulse and signal detection. There are several methods of quantifying blood flow. With phase encoding, the image is composed of maps of flow rates in a selected plane. The direction and magnitude of flow can be displayed alongside or superimposed upon a structural image.

Using gating techniques, flow at any point in the cardiac cycle can be measured. By imaging at several points through the cardiac cycle, and with flow colour coded to indicate direction and velocity (similar to colour Doppler), a moving display can be obtained, but at the cost of increased imaging time.

Flow imaging has undoubted potential but also some drawbacks. Although the problem of aliasing which may occur with very high velocities can be resolved, the signal loss caused by turbulent flow appears to be a more fundamental difficulty.

Echo-planar imaging (or real-time imaging)

Rather than building up an image over many cardiac cycles, echo-planar imaging displays the signal obtained following each radiofrequency pulse, giving a real-time, moving image[6] similar to that obtained with cross-sectional echocardiography. However, image definition is reduced using this technique.

Cine images

Because of the inherent problems of real-time imaging, moving images of the heart are usually constructed from a series of images gated to different times through the cardiac cycle. These are then replayed as a continuous loop displaying wall motion, wall thickness and blood flow.

Spectroscopy

The hope that simultaneous biochemical and anatomical information might be obtained[7] by using very high-field magnets has not been realized. However, spectroscopy using small-bore magnets with the aid of surface coils has been used to study peripheral (skeletal) muscle in patients with heart failure[8,9] and has demonstrated metabolic abnormalities. The nuclear magnetic resonance spectrum for ^{31}P has separate peaks for inorganic phosphate, phosphocreatine and each of the three forms of ATP and it allows pH to be calculated. The findings from a single case of cardiomyopathy in an 8-month-old girl showed an abnormal ratio of phosphocreatine to inorganic phosphate. Furthermore, selective improvement in this ratio was obtained by intravenous administration of glucose and by a high glucose–medium chain triglyceride meal.[10]

Technical limitations have not yet allowed metabolic studies in adult hearts, but innovations such as passing intravascular receiver coils have allowed high resolution spectra to be obtained from canine hearts.[11]

Spectroscopic studies in animals may also shed light on metabolic changes after mechanical or therapeutic interventions. In a rabbit model of acute myocardial infarction, phosphocreatine fell rapidly and recovered quickly after reperfusion. ATP fell later, but did not recover after reperfusion.[12] Future studies may provide important information leading to improved methods of myocardial salvage.

CHOICE BETWEEN COMMERCIALLY AVAILABLE SYSTEMS

A wide range of machines is available, the differences between machines being primarily related to the magnetic field strength and pulse sequences used. The cost of installing and running a system is generally proportional to field strength. As image definition tends to improve with increasing field strength, there has been a trend towards favouring higher field systems. However, adequate images can be obtained using low-field systems, particularly when body surface coils are used. Furthermore, the capacity for tissue characterization by measuring T_1 and T_2 seems to be better at lower field strengths.[13]

Thus, MRI systems must compete against each other as well as against alternative technologies.[14]

Low-field imagers (resistive and permanent magnets)

Magnetic field strength is measured in Tesla. Most low-field imagers use a *resistive* magnet with field strengths in the region of 0.012–0.2 Tesla. For comparison, the strength of the earth's magnetic field is about 0.00005 T.

Resistive magnets produce their magnetic field when current passes through their core. Heat generated by flowing current is dissipated by a water cooling system. Because of the limited radius of significant magnetic fields with resistive (and permanent) magnets, they require less screening from their surroundings and so less space. Installation within existing buildings is therefore easier and less expensive.[15]

The capital cost of low-field systems is currently in the region of £500 000; the running costs are about 10% of this figure per annum.

High-field imagers (superconducting magnets)

A higher magnetic field can be obtained by reducing the electrical resistance to zero. The very low temperatures required are achieved by cooling the system with liquid helium or nitrogen. Such systems typically operate at about 0.5 T but much higher field strengths are available. Although a better signal-to-noise ratio is obtained, resulting in greater stability of the magnetic field, there are several negative consequences of using higher field strengths.

1 Increased capital cost.
2 Increased installation cost.
3 Increased running cost.
4 Greater working area required.
5 Loss of tissue characterization?
6 Greater potential hazards.

SAFETY OF MAGNETIC RESONANCE IMAGING

Apart from its use in a small number of specific clinical situations, the technique of magnetic resonance imaging appears to be remarkably safe. The uniform (and oscillating) magnetic fields, even with superconducting magnets, involve very low energies which do not disrupt chemical bonds or result in any tissue damage.[16] The oscillating field used for magnetic resonance is in the radiofrequency band and is generally safe. However, at high power levels, radiofrequency radiation is thermogenic; increases in body temperature have been shown using a high-field imaging system.[17] There is understandable concern about the safety of imaging in patients with metallic implants. The two commonest situations in which MRI might be considered in cardiac patients with metallic implants are in patients with prosthetic valves and in those with a pacemaker. Fortunately, most modern implants are not ferromagnetic and so movement will not occur. Where ferromagnetic material is present, high-field systems may be more dangerous.

Prosthetic valves

Experimental work[18] and clinical experience have shown that magnetic resonance imaging in patients with prosthetic valves in currently available imagers is safe. Although some image distortion may occur, it is usually localized and does not interfere with the interpretation of the remainder of the image.

Pacemakers

The radiofrequency field appears to pose a greater problem than the uniform field with respect to cardiac pacemakers and may result in rapid pacemaker discharge. In general, it has been considered to be a contra-indication to performing MRI, but recent work suggests that in some circumstances it may be safe.[19] As there may be differences in the response to radiofrequency fields among various types of pacemaker and different manufacturers more information is required before firm guidelines can be given. Furthermore, pacemakers implanted in the usual pre-pectoral position will result in a large area of signal loss with image distortion because of the metal generator casing.

The safety of MRI must be considered against that of alternative techniques. Despite the problems discussed above, the lack of ionizing radiation (or the need for contrast agents) with MRI is a major advantage when compared with CT scanning or angiography.

Paramagnetic contrast agents

Additional contrast can be obtained by administering paramagnetic material, such as manganese or gadolinium,[19] but there are reservations about the use of such agents in man. By careful selection of appropriate pulse sequences, surface coils and magnetic fields, the inherent ability of MRI should be powerful enough to provide tissue discrimination without resort to potentially hazardous agents.

Safer paramagnetic contrast agents are being investigated.

ADVANTAGES AND DISADVANTAGES OF MAGNETIC RESONANCE IMAGING

The main advantages of MRI are as follows.
1 No contrast media are required.
2 Ionizing radiation is not used.
3 Imaging can be performed in any plane.
4 Serial studies are possible.
5 The technique is versatile.

The main disadvantages are:
1 the high cost;
2 the relatively long (but reducing) imaging times required;
3 the difficulty in imaging sick patients, particularly those with breathlessness; and
4 the claustrophobic effect induced in some patients.

MAGNETIC RESONANCE IMAGING OF THE HEART

The current state of MRI with regard to the demonstration of cardiac structure, function and tissue characterization will now be reviewed.

Demonstration of anatomy

Although the accuracy of measurements varies between different imaging systems, the following general conclusions can be drawn.
1 Measurement of chamber volumes *in vitro* and *in vivo* and wall thickness can be performed with a high degree of accuracy.[20–22] Cardiac gating is essential for accurate measurements.
2 Measurement of myocardial thickness yields values similar to those obtained with echocardiography.[23] With multiple-slice imaging, the calculation of total myocardial mass is possible and accurate.[24,25] Such measurements do have limitations and the following factors are important:
  i Careful attention to the timing of end-systole and end-diastole is required for accurate measurements and this is difficult with MR imaging.[23]
  ii The allied problems of partial volume effects and difficulties with border definition will introduce small inaccuracies.
  iii The alteration of the imaging plane by rotation of the axis of imaging gives superior images and more precise measurements by allowing optimal short-axis slices to be obtained.[26–28] This alteration will minimize the problems outlined under ii.

3 Imaging of normal and abnormal myocardium can provide high-quality anatomical definition. Owing to its cost, its use for structural imaging is likely to be restricted. For most patients, echocardiography will remain the investigation of choice, particularly for those with valvular heart disease. Magnetic resonance imaging should be used in those patients who are poor candidates for echocardiography. Magnetic resonance imaging of cardiac structure has been reported in the following conditions.
  i Chronic ischaemic heart disease. The geometry of the left ventricle is readily seen, as is regional wall thinning[29] and aneurysm formation[30] in areas of previous myocardial infarction (Pls 18.1 and 18.2). Intracardiac thrombus can also be detected, but care in the timing of the image and use of particular pulse sequences may be required. In patients with heart failure, pleural effusions are frequently found and quantification is possible (Pl. 18.3).
  ii Myocardial hypertrophy. The distribution and extent of hypertrophy can be readily appreciated in both hypertrophic cardiomyopathy and hypertrophy secondary to increased afterload.[31]
  iii Congenital heart disease in adults. Complex anomalies, particularly those involving the great vessels, can be defined with MRI.[32] Ventricular septal defects are generally easily seen, but, as with echocardiography, false positive atrial septal defects are not uncommon.[33] Combined anatomical and flow imaging to provide functional assessment of shunts will be valuable in the investigation of congenital heart disease.
  iv Tumours. Intracardiac tumours, such as atrial myxomas,[34] are well shown and magnetic resonance imaging is of value in defining the site of attachment and extent of infiltration into surrounding structures.[35]
  v Pericardial disease. Magnetic resonance imaging is ideally suited to the investigation of pericardial disease: the entire pericardium can be imaged, its thickness assessed (Pl. 18.3) and MRI is of value in the diagnosis of pericardial constriction.[36]

Assessment of myocardial function

Function derived from structural imaging and measurements

Comparison of systolic and diastolic images allows accurate assessment of regional wall motion[29] and, as total intracardiac volume can be measured, cardiac output can be derived. Such calculations accord well with values obtained by other techniques.[21] Highly accurate measurements are obtained by using multiple sections which allow for complex geometrical shapes. This may be of particular value in the assessment of the right ventricle.

Function derived from flow information

Flow in the heart. Colour-coded ciné sequences of blood flow are very sensitive at detecting valvular regurgitation and flow through atrial or ventricular septal defects.[38] At present, only semi-quantitative assessment of valvular regurgitation is possible using these techniques because apparent severity is influenced by technical factors.

Flow in arteries and veins. The ascending and descending aorta are ideally suited to magnetic resonance phase imaging (Pl. 18.4) because they are large and lie in a convenient plane. The sensitivity of this technique is illustrated by its ability to demonstrate differential velocity of blood flow in the normal aorta.[39] Increased velocity is seen in aortic stenosis, but the accuracy of velocity measurement is severely hampered by signal loss due to turbulence.

Two important areas in which magnetic resonance phase imaging appears likely to play a significant role are the assessment of coronary artery vein graft patency and flow and the assessment of carotid artery disease. Coronary artery vein grafts lie along the plane of the aorta for most of their course and initial reports indicate that phase imaging is useful for assessing graft patency and measuring graft flow.[40] Coronary arteries are often seen incidentally on magnetic resonance images, but clinically useful coronary flow imaging has yet to be achieved. The difficulties to be overcome relate not only to the small size of the coronary arteries, but more importantly to their constantly changing direction as they run along the epicardial surface. Magnetic resonance imaging will not replace coronary angiography in the foreseeable future.

Flow in shunts. Patency and flow in palliative systemic to pulmonary artery shunts can be assessed,[41] but these measurements may require imaging of multiple sections and considerable skill in obtaining the correct imaging plane.

Tissue characterization

Tissue characterization is potentially important, but it has been less widely studied because the cardiac gating of T_1 and T_2 images is difficult. The relationship of relaxation parameter changes (see above) to histopathological findings is poorly understood, but 'free water' plays an important part in the prolongation of relaxation times. Thus, conditions resulting in myocardial oedema or inflammation cause T_1 and T_2 to increase. There are several areas, detailed below, in which the unique ability of magnetic resonance imaging for tissue characterization shows particular promise.

Myocardial infarction

Animal studies in vitro. Experimental work using animal models *in vitro* has shown an increase in T_1 within 30 min of coronary occlusion. T_1 prolongation tends to increase progressively with occlusion times of 1 and 2 h.[42] In some animal experiments in which coronary occlusion is followed by reperfusion, T_1 and T_2 are further increased.[43,44] The relevance of this finding is unclear as occlusion and reperfusion times are arbitrary and measurements have been performed on excised hearts.

Animal studies in vivo. Imaging *in vivo* has also shown increasing signal intensity (related to magnetic resonance relaxation times) during the first 4 h after coronary occlusion.[45] However, the percentage increase in the early stages is small and the area of infarction may not be visible during the first few hours. It has been shown that signal intensity increases over several days following coronary occlusion, reaching a peak around the end of the first to second week.[46]

Recently, a new paramagnetic contrast agent, Fe-pyrophosphate, was shown to localize in the border zone around the infarct.[47]

Studies in man in vivo. Increases in T_1[48] and T_2[49] following myocardial infarction in man have been reported. The increase is confined to the area of infarction and there may be associated wall thinning (Fig. 18.2 and Pls 18.1 and 18.5). Several hours or even days may be required before the increase is noticeable, consequently the technique is unable to differentiate between reversible and irreversible ischaemia. During the second week after infarction, the highest T_1 values are found and the largest area is affected.[50] By performing complete images of the heart at this time, it may be possible to obtain an index of infarct size.

Thus far, no differences between patients with and without coronary reperfusion have been noted, but the technique shows great promise for the assessment of changes *within the myocardium* during the healing stage of myocardial infarction.

Myocardial inflammation

Systemic lupus erythematosus. Increases in myocardial T_1 in some patients with systemic lupus erythematosus have been seen, even when the results of other cardiac investigations have been negative. This reflects the limited ability of other non-invasive techniques to provide useful information about changes within the myocardium. As T_1 changes probably reflect the activity of inflammation they may prove to be useful indications in the assessment of the efficacy of treatment in this and other inflammatory diseases. In contrast to the localized findings in acute myocardial infarction, there is a diffuse but generally less intense increase in T_1 in patients with systemic lupus erythematosus (Pl. 18.6).

Cardiac allograft transplantation and rejection. Magnetic resonance imaging may provide useful anatomical information following cardiac transplantation (Pl. 18.3), and be of value in assessing cardiac rejection. After heterotopic transplantation, rejection is characterized by an increase in T_1 and T_2 in rats[51] and in dogs.[52] In man, cardiac transplantation results in an increase in T_1 and T_2 suggesting that there is scope for improvement in methods of preservation. Magnetic relaxation parameters fall towards normal by about three weeks after transplantation. Increases in T_1 and T_2 after 25 days have been shown to be sensitive indicators of late graft rejection.[53]

Myocarditis. The diagnosis of myocarditis is often difficult to make and our understanding of the processes involved is limited. Tissue characteristics may be altered in the acute phase of myocarditis.

COMPARISON WITH OTHER TECHNIQUES

The power of MRI is illustrated by the fact that it can be favourably compared to chest radiography, echocardiography, Doppler ultrasound, CT (+ ultrafast CT), radionuclide angiography, aortography and left ventriculography. Nevertheless, the costs involved are considerable and, unless MRI can provide useful information that cannot be obtained using other less expensive techniques, its role will be limited. For this reason, it is likely that its major impact in the investigation of adult cardiac disease will be its ability to characterize tissue and quantify blood flow.

X-RAY COMPUTED TOMOGRAPY

TECHNICAL ASPECTS

Images are obtained by projecting and rotating a narrow beam of conventional X-rays through 360°. The non-absorbed photons are detected, so providing the information by which tomographic sections can be reconstructed by computer. High-resolution images are obtained by measuring absorption values from each pixel. The imaging plane can be adjusted by patient angulation to allow optimal orientation. With newer systems, images can be reconstructed in any plane by computer after the collection of several adjacent transverse sections.

The absorption values are displayed as a greyscale and measurements expressed in Hounsfield units. As there is considerable overlap in the absorption values of various tissues, the degree of tissue discrimination provided by measuring the relative radiological density of tissues is limited. (The values obtained are *not* related to the relaxation parameters measured in MRI.)

With modern conventional whole-body scanners, image acquisition takes several seconds which is too slow to prevent motional blurring of cardiac images. Recently, two different approaches have been used to solve this problem: cardiac gating, performed either prospectively or by retrospective analysis of the acquired data, or ultrafast scanning, in which images are acquired in 30–50 ms. These systems have been specifically designed for cardiac imaging; however, they are expensive and experience with them is limited.

Computed tomography scanning relies on the use of ionizing radiation and, for many cardiological investigations, radiopaque contrast material (injected into a peripheral vein) is required.

IMAGING WITH CONVENTIONAL COMPUTED TOMOGRAPHY SCANNERS

Computed tomography has a useful role in the investigation of conditions in which echocardiographic examination has limitations.

The size and position of thoracic aortic aneurysms can be defined and, where dissection has taken place, contrast medium enhancement confirms the diagnosis by demonstrating a double lumen. Aortography is often required for demonstration of the intimal flap, because it may not be seen on CT;[54] conversely, aortography may give falsely negative results, even when the diagnosis is clear on computed tomographic images.[55]

Patency and flow in coronary artery bypass grafts can be accurately assessed.[56] Pericardial content, thickness and consistency may be of help in the diagnosis of pericardial constriction.

Intracardiac tumours are well visualized on echocardiography, but CT scanning is usually superior when the lesion involves the myocardium or is extracardiac.

There have been a few reports of CT tissue characterization being of value, but, in patients with cardiac amyloidosis, tissue density measured in Hounsfield units is significantly lower than that of normal myocardium.[57]

After bolus injection of contrast media, myocardial perfusion can be assessed: there is lack of early uptake in regions of acute infarction, giving the appearance of a filling defect, followed by late enhancement in the infarct region.[58]

ULTRAFAST (CINE) COMPUTED TOMOGRAPHY

This provides very rapid imaging while maintaining high resolution. Its ability to define clearly myocardial wall thickness and cavity size sequentially throughout the cardiac cycle gives it similar capabilities to MRI with respect to anatomical information and functional derivatives, although contrast injections are still required.

It is too soon to be certain of the eventual place of ultrafast CT scanning. In terms of cost, cine cannot compete with echocardiography and Doppler studies, although the speed of imaging should allow a large throughput of patients. Cine CT is faster than MRI, the associated expenses are similar and cine CT appears to be potentially useful in many of the same clinical settings. The versatility and truly non-invasive nature of MRI suggest that it will become the more widely used of the two techniques for cardiac investigation.

REFERENCES

1. Pykett, I.L. NMR imaging in medicine. *Sci. Am.* 1982; **246**: 78–88.
2. Kean, D.M. and Smith, M.A. *Magnetic Resonance Imaging: Principles and Applications*. London: William Heinemann Medical Books, 1986.
3. Mathur-De Vre, R. Biomedical implications of the relaxation behaviour of water related to NMR imaging. *Br. J. Radiol.* 1984; **57**: 955–76.
4. Franks, F. Solvation interactions of proteins in solution. *Phil. Trans. R. Soc. Lond. B* 1977; **278**: 89–96.
5. Smith, M.A., Ridgway, J.P., Brydon, J.W.E. *et al.* ECG gated T1 images of the heart. *Phys. Med. Biol.* 1986; **31**: 771.
6. Ordridge, R.J., Mansfield, P., Coupland, R.E. Rapid biomedical imaging by NMR. *Br. J. Radiol.* 1981; **54**: 850–5.
7. Berger, H.J. and Pettigrew, R.I. Cardiovascular imaging and evaluation of myocardial metabolism. *J. Am. Coll. Cardiol.* 1985; **5**: 750–3.
8. Massie, B., Conway, M., Yonge, R., Frostick, S., Rajagopalan, B. and Radda, G.K. P nuclear magnetic resonance evaluation of skeletal muscle metabolism during exercise in congestive heart failure (abstract). *Br. Heart J.* 1986; **55**: 527.
9. Wilson, J.R., Fink, L., Maris, J., Ferraro, N., Power-Vanwart, J., Eleff, S. and Chance, B. Evaluation of energy metabolism in skeletal muscle of patients with heart failure with gated phosphorus-31 nuclear magnetic resonance. *Circulation* 1985; **71**: 57–62.
10. Whitman, G.J.R., Chance, B., Bode, H. *et al.* Diagnosis and therapeutic evaluation of a pediatric case of cardiomyopathy using phosphorus-31 nuclear magnetic resonance spectroscopy. *J. Am. Coll. Cardiol.* 1985; **5**: 745–9.
11. Kantor, H.L., Briggs, R.W. and Balaban, R.S. In vivo P nuclear magnetic resonance measurements in canine heart using a catheter-coil. *Circ. Res.* 1984; **55**: 261–6.
12. Rajagopalan, B., Ramsey, J., Harmsen, E., Bore, P. and Radda, G.K. Biochemical changes during repeated occlusion and reperfusion of a coronary artery in the rabbit: a 31P magnetic resonance spectroscopy study (abstract). *Br. Heart J.* 1986; **55**: 527–8.
13. Richards, M.A., Webb, J.A.W., Reznek, R.H. *et al.* Detection of spread of malignant lymphoma to the liver by low field strength magnetic resonance imaging (abstract). *Br. Med. J.* 1986; **293**: 1126–8.
14. Petitti, D. Competing Technologies: Implications for the costs and complexity of medical care. *N. Engl. J. Med.* 1986; **315**: 1480–3.
15. Smith, M.A., Best, J.J.K., Douglas, R.H.B. and Kean, D.M. The installation of a commercial resistive NMR imager. *Br. J. Radiol.* 1984; **57**: 1145–8.
16. Budinger, T.F. Potential medical effects and hazards of human NMR studies. In: Kaufman L., Crooks, L.E. and Margulis, A.R., eds, *NMR imaging in medicine*. New York: Igaku-Shoin, 1981, Chapter 10.
17. Shellock, F.G. and Crus, J.V. Temperature, heart rate, and blood pressure changes associated with clinical MR imaging at 1.5T. *Radiology* 1987; **163**: 259–62.
18. Soulen, R.L., Budinger, T.F. and Higgins, C.R. Magnetic resonance imaging of prosthetic heart valves. *Radiology* 1985; **154**: 705–7.
19. Fetter, J., Aram, G., Holmes, D.R., Gray, J.E. and Hayes, D.L. The effects of nuclear magnetic resonance imagers on external and implantable pulse generators. *PACE* 1984; **7**: 720–7.

20. Rehr, R.B., Malloy, C.R., Filipchuk, N.G. and Peshock, R.M. Left ventricular volumes measured by MR imaging. *Radiology* 1985; **156**: 717–9.

21. Mogelvang, J., Thomsen, C., Mehlsen, J., Brackle, G., Stubgaard, M. and Henriksen, O. Evaluation of left ventricular volumes measured by magnetic resonance imaging. *Eur. Heart J.* 1986; **7**: 1016–21.

22. Longmore, D.B., Underwood, S.R., Hounsfield, G.N. *et al.* Dimensional accuracy of magnetic resonance in studies of the heart. *Lancet* 1985; **1**: 1360–2.

23. Friedman, B.J., Waters, J., Ling Kwan, O. and DeMaria, A.N. Comparison of magnetic resonance imaging and echocardiography in determination of cardiac dimensions in normal subjects. *J. Am. Coll. Cardiol.* 1985; **5**: 1369–76.

24. Florentine, M.S., Grosskreutz, C.L., Chang, W. *et al.* Measurement of left ventricular mass in vivo using gated nuclear magnetic resonance imaging. *J. Am. Coll. Cardiol.* 1986; **8**: 107–12.

25. Keller, A.M., Peshock, R.M., Malloy, C.R., Buja, L.M., Nunnally, R., Parkey, R.W. and Willerson, J.T. In vivo measurement of myocardial mass using nuclear magnetic resonance imaging. *J. Am. Coll. Cardiol.* 1986; **8**: 113–7.

26. Feiglin, D.H., George, C.R., MacIntyre, W.J., O'Donnell, J.K., Go, R.T., Pavlicek, W. and Meaney, T.F. Gated cardiac magnetic resonance structural imaging: Optimization by electronic axial rotation. *Radiology* 1985; **154**: 129–32.

27. Murphy, W.A., Gutierrez, F.R., Levitt, R.G., Glazer, H.S. and Lee, J.K.T. Oblique views of the heart by magnetic resonance imaging. *Radiology* 1985; **154**: 225–6.

28. Akins, E.W., Hill, J.A., Fitzsimmons, J.R., Pepine, C.J. and Williams, C.M. Importance of imaging plane for magnetic resonance: Imaging of the normal left ventricle. *Am. J. Cardiol.* 1985; **56**: 366–72.

29. Underwood, S.R., Rees, R.S.O., Savage, P.E. *et al.* Assessment of regional left ventricular function by magnetic resonance. *Br. Heart J.* 1986; **56**: 334–40.

30. Higgins, C.B., Lanzer, P., Stark, O. *et al.* Imaging by nuclear magnetic resonance in patients with chronic ischemic heart disease. *Circulation* 1984; **69**: 523–31.

31. Been, M., Kean, D., Smith, M.A., Douglas, R.H.B., Best, J.J.K. and Muir, A.L. Nuclear magnetic resonance in hypertrophic cardiomyopathy. *Br. Heart J.* 1985; **54**: 48–52.

32. Higgins, C.B., Byrd, B.J., Farmer, D.W., Osaki, L., Silverman, N.H. and Cheitlin, M.D. Magnetic resonance imaging in patients with congenital heart disease. *Circulation* 1984; **70**: 851–60.

33. Dinsmore, R.E., Wismer, G.L., Guyer, D. *et al.* Magnetic resonance imaging of the interatrial septum and atrial septal defects. *AJR* 1985; **145**: 697–703.

34. Go, R.T., O'Donnell, J.K., Feiglin, D.H. *et al.* Comparison of gated cardiac MR1 and 2D echocardiography of intracardiac neoplasms. *AJR* 1985; **145**: 21–5.

35. Freedberg, R.S., Kronzon, I., Rumancik, W.M. and Liebeskind, D. The contribution of magnetic resonance imaging to the evaluation of intracardiac tumours diagnosed by echocardiography. *Circulation* 1988; **77**: 96–103.

36. Soulen, R.L., Stark, D.D. and Higgins, C.B. Magnetic resonance imaging of constrictive pericardial disease. *Am. J. Cardiol.* 1985; **55**: 480–4.

37. Markiewicz, W., Sechtem, U. and Higgins, C.B. Evaluation of the right ventricle by magnetic resonance imaging. *Am. Heart J.* 1987; **113**: 8–15.

38. Underwood, S.R., Firmin, D.N., Klipstein, R.H. Rees, R.S.O. and Longmore, D.B. Magnetic resonance velocity mapping: clinical application of a new technique. *Br. Heart J.* 1987; **57**: 404–12.

39. Klipstein, R.H., Firmin, D.N., Underwood, S.R, Rees, R.S.O. and Longmore, D.B. Magnetic resonance blood flow patterns in the human aorta studied by magnetic resonance.

Br. Heart J. 1987; **58**: 316–23.

40. Underwood, S.R., Firmin, D.N., Klipstein, R.H., Rees, R.S.O. and Longmore, D.B. The assessment of coronary artery bypass grafts by magnetic resonance imaging with velocity mapping: Clinical application of a new technique. *Br. Heart J.* 1987; **57**: 404–12.

41. Jacobstein, M.R., Fletcher, B.D., Nelson, A.D. *et al.* Magnetic resonance imaging: evaluation of palliative systemic–pulmonary artery shunts. *Circulation* 1984; **70**: 650–6.

42. Williams, E.S., Kaplan, J.L., Thatcher, F., Zimmerman, G. and Knoebel, S.B. Prolongation of proton spin-lattice relaxation times in regionally ischaemic tissue from dog hearts. *J. Nucl. Med.* 1980; **21**: 449–53.

43. Ratner, A.V., Okada, R.D., Newell, J.B. and Pohost, G.M. The relationship between proton nuclear magnetic resonance relaxation parameters and myocardial perfusion with acute coronary arterial occlusion and reperfusion. *Circulation* 1985; **71**: 823.

44. Johnston, D.L., Brady, T.J., Ratner, A.V. *et al.* Assessment of myocardial ischemia with proton magnetic resonance: effects of a three hour coronary occlusion with and without reperfusion. *Circulation* 1985; **71**: 595.

45. Pflugfelder, P.W., Wisenberg, G., Prato, F.S., Carroll, S.E. and Turner, K.L. Early detection of canine myocardial infarction by magnetic resonance imaging *in vivo*. *Circulation* 1985; **71**: 587–94.

46. Pflugfelder, P.W., Wisenberg, G., Prato, F.S., Turner, K.L. and Carroll, S.E. Serial imaging of canine myocardial infarction by in vivo nuclear magnetic resonance. *J. Am. Coll. Cardiol.* 1986; **7**: 843–69

47. Maurer, A.H., Knight, L.C., Siegel, J.A., Adler, P.I. and Elfenbein, I.B. Magnetic resonance contrast enhancement of acute myocardial infarction with paramagnetic pyrophosphate (Abstract). *Circulation* 1987; **76** (Suppl. IV): 159.

48. Been, M., Ridgeway, J.P., Douglas, R.H.B. *et al.* Characterisation of acute myocardial infarction by gated magnetic resonance imaging. *Lancet* 1985; **2**: 348–50.

49. McNamara, M.T., Higgins, C.B., Schechtman, N. *et al.* Detection and characterization of acute myocardial infarction in man with use of gated magnetic resonance. *Circulation* 1985; **71**: 717.

50. Been, M., Smith, M.A., Ridgeway, J.P., Best, J.J.K., de Bono, D.P. and Muir, A.L. Serial changes in the T_1 magnetic relaxation parameter after myocardial infarction in man. *Br. Heart J.* 1988; **59**: 1–8.

51. Sasaguri, S., Laraia, P.J., Fabri, B.M. *et al.* Early detection of cardiac allograft rejection with proton nuclear magnetic resonance. *Circulation* 1985; **72** (Suppl. I): 231–6.

52. Aherne, T., Tscholakoff, D., Finkbeiner, W., Sechtem, U., Derugin, N., Yee, E. and Higgins, C.B. Magnetic resonance imaging of cardiac transplants: the evaluation of rejection of cardiac allografts with and without immuno-suppression. *Circulation* 1986; **74**: 145–56.

53. Wisenberg, G., Pflugfelder, P.W., Kostuk, W.J. *et al.* Diagnostic applicability of magnetic resonance imaging in assessing human cardiac allograft rejection. *Am. J. Cardiol.* 1987; **60**: 130–6

54. Iliceto, S., Ettorre, G., Francisoso, G., Antonelli, G., Biasco, G. and Rizzon, P. Diagnosis of aneurysm of the thoracic aorta. Comparison between two non-invasive techniques: two-dimensional echocardiography and computer tomography. *Eur. Heart J.* 1984; **5**: 545–55.

55. Singh, H., Fitzgerald, E. and Ruttley, M.S.T. Computed tomography: the investigation of choice for aortic dissection? *Br. Heart J.* 1986; **56**: 171–5.

56. Foster, C.J., Sekiya, T., Brownlee, W.C. and Isherwood, I. Computed tomographic assessment of coronary artery bypass grafts. *Br. Heart J.* 1984; **52**: 24–9.

57. Sekiya, T., Foster, C.J., Isherwood, I., Lucas, S.B., Kahn,

M.K. and Miller, J.P. Computed tomographic appearances of cardiac amyloidosis. *Br. Heart J.* 1984; 51: 519–22.

58. Masuda, Y., Yoshida, H., Morooka, N., Watanabe, S. and Inagaki, Y. The usefulness of x-ray computed tomography for the diagnosis of myocardial infarction. *Circulation* 1984; 70: 217–25.

Chapter 19

Radionuclide Investigations in Adult Heart Disease

A.L. Muir

Many aspects of cardiac function in health and disease can be assessed using radionuclides, but their principal use is in the investigation of ischaemic heart disease to provide information that is not as easily obtained by other techniques. They are used mainly to document ventricular function at rest and during physiological or pharmacological stress, to provide information about pulmonary or myocardial blood flow and myocardial metabolism and to detect and localize myocardial necrosis and thrombus (Table 19.1). Their rational use depends on a knowledge of the disordered pathophysiology, the radiopharmaceuticals and necessary instrumentation.

RADIOPHARMACEUTICALS

A radionuclide is unstable and seeks stability through a process of decay, i.e. by emitting particles or photons. Radionuclides used diagnostically decay through beta or gamma decay (Table 19.2). Beta particles deposit their energy within very short distances. As they do not escape from the body, they cannot be detected; moreover they lose energy when colliding with atoms or molecules and so contribute to radiobiological damage. In contrast, gamma rays are widely used in imaging; they are a form of electromagnetic radiation produced when an excited nucleus decays to a lower energy by the emission of a photon. This is indistinguishable from an X-ray, which is created by the interaction of electrons with the orbital electrons of an atom. These photons may escape from the body and can be detected by external counting equipment.

The commonest radionuclide in clinical use is the gamma-emitting technetium-99m (^{99}Tc^m) (Table 19.3). It has several useful properties. Its single photon energy of 140 keV is high enough for a high proportion of the photons to escape from the body (about 50% of the photons pass through 4 cm of average tissue), but not too high for efficient detection by modern gamma cameras. ^{99}Tc^m (half-life 6 h) is the product of the decay of molybdenum-99 (^{99}Mo) (half-life 66 h); the two may be separated by washing isotonic saline over an ion-exchange column of ^{99}Mo. This combination of a long half-life, required to enable distribution of the radionuclide to hospitals, with a short half-life, which is desirable in patient studies, makes ^{99}Tc^m ideal for clinical use. It is readily available in a form (ionic pertechnetate) that may be used to label many organic and inorganic compounds. Thus, technetium can be used to label the blood pool when bound to either albumin or the patient's erythrocytes, to detect myocardial necrosis when bound to pyrophosphate, to deter-

Table 19.1. Common cardiac problems referred for radionuclide investigation.

1 Is the chest pain angina pectoris?
2 Can the prognostic significance of the angina be estimated?
3 Can the coronary artery involved be deduced?
4 Has there been a recent myocardial infarction?
5 If so, what is the prognosis?
6 Is this an ischaemic or an idiopathic cardiomyopathy?
7 Is there any evidence of an intracardiac shunt?
8 The pre-operative assessment of ventricular function.
9 The assessment of right ventricular function in pulmonary heart disease and inferior myocardial infarction.
10 Has there been a pulmonary embolism?

Table 19.2. Radionuclides used in the investigation of heart disease.

	Half-life		Principal photons (keV)	Abundance (%)
^{99}Tc^m	6.0 h		140	90
^{201}Tl	73.0 h		73–81	94
^{133}Xe	5.2 days		81	37
^{113}In^m	100 min		392	64
^{111}In	67.2 h		171, 245	90, 94
^{11}C	20.4 min	($\beta+$)	511	200
^{15}O	2.0 min	($\beta+$)	511	200

Tc: technetium, Tl: thallium, Xe: xenon, In: indium, C: carbon, O: oxygen

Table 19.3. **Radiopharmaceuticals commonly used for the investigation of heart disease.**

Radiopharmaceutical	Investigation	Max. usual activity	Effective dose-equivalent (mSv)	Approximate cost (£)
		MBq		
^{99}Tc^m-Human albumin complex	Blood pool imaging &	800	5	10
^{99}Tc^m-Red blood cells	Ventriculography	800	6	10
^{99}Tc^m-Human albumin macro-aggregates or microspheres	Perfusion lung scanning	80	1	4
^{99}Tc^m-pyrophosphate	Myocardial infarction detection	600	4	12
^{201}Tl	Myocardial perfusion imaging	80	7	35

mine the distribution of blood flow when bound to microspheres or macro-aggregates of albumin, most commonly in the detection of pulmonary emboli. The half-life of ^{99}Tc^m (6 h) is a useful length of time for most types of study, but a major disadvantage when rapid serial studies have to be undertaken. If cardiac function is being examined repeatedly, ^{99}Tc^m labelled to diethylenetriaminepentaacetic acid (DPTA) has been used because the technetium can be rapidly cleared by renal excretion.

More recently, several investigators have used ultra short-lived radionuclides, such as gold-195m which has a half-life of 30 s and a gamma energy of 262 keV, to perform repeat studies examining ventricular function in multiple projections. However, the high-energy photons of ^{195}Au^m result in scattered radiation. This and the high cost of the generator have limited the widespread application of ^{195}Au^m. The use of other ultra short-lived isotopes, such as tantalum-178 and iridium-191m, is being investigated.

DETECTION DEVICES

The absorption of a gamma photon by a sodium iodide crystal, impregnated with thallium impurities, causes a flash of light. As the amount of light is small, the signal has to be amplified by a photomultiplier.

A cardiac probe is a specialized form of a simple scintillation detector connected to a dedicated microcomputer to detect counts over the precordium and display ventricular time–activity curves. Smaller probes using cadmium telluride crystals have been described which have portability advantages for cardiac imaging.

The single-Crystal (Anger) gamma camera consists of a single large sodium iodide crystal, about 25–50 cm in diameter and 0.5–1 cm thick with a bank of photomultiplier tubes in an hexagonal array. When a photon strikes the crystal, its position is noted electronically and the energy pulse is analysed to select events within a specified energy range for display on a cathode ray tube or storage in a computer for subsequent analysis. The percentage of the observed counts to the incident photons is termed the detection efficiency which is greater for low-energy photons. Although a thicker crystal is more efficient, the spatial resolution (sharpness) of the image is reduced. Two other characteristics are important in defining the performance of a gamma camera: the field uniformity, or ability to respond uniformly to an identical source of radioactivity, and the temporal resolution (or dead time), which is the time taken to process an event before another pulse can be processed.

Multicrystal cameras have a special role in cardiovascular investigation; they have a high count-rate capability but a poorer spatial resolution. The detector head consists of 294 separate sodium iodide crystals arranged in a 14/21 elements. Each crystal is optically connected to two photomultiplier tubes to allow location of X and Y axes. The information is then processed in a similar way to that obtained using the more conventional single-crystal gamma camera.

Multiwire proportional counter gamma cameras are being developed. They are highly compact and lightweight and have count-rate capabilities superior to those of conventional gamma cameras. They are particularly suited to cardiac investigation using low-energy short half-life isotopes, such as tantalum (^{178}Ta). Although they are not yet commercially available, the simplicity of the electronics and detector suggests production costs should be significantly lower.[1]

The *collimation* or focusing of photons is necessary so that only photons travelling in the appropriate direction are allowed to strike the crystal. Collimators are usually made of lead and the thickness of the lead and the size and the length of the holes will alter the number of photons allowed onto the crystal. High count rates can be achieved by large holes and thin lead, but the accuracy of determining the position of recorded events is decreased. In most systems, there is a compromise between the need for adequate count rates and spatial accuracy. Converging, diverging and slant hole are examples of specialized collimators, but for most work a low-energy parallel collimator will suffice.

Attenuation: Only a small fraction of the photons emitted from the body will travel in a straight optical path to the detector. In addition, other photons are lost by interactions with matter. The first of these interactions is called photo-electric absorption in which a photon is absorbed by an atom with the release of an electron; this is the predominant interaction of lower energy photons in heavy elements. In Compton scattering, the photon collides with an electron and loses energy; in contrast to photo-electric absorption, the photon still has sufficient energy to escape and it can be detected although at a different energy and from a different direction. Compton scatter is the major cause of attenuation and image degradation in radionuclide cardiovascular investigations.

TOMOGRAPHY

Early attempts to obtain three-dimensional information used specialized slant-hole or seven-pinhole collimators to produce longitudinal tomographic reconstructions; transaxial tomography, however, produces images of better quality. The image plane is perpendicular to the long axis of the body and in *single photon emission computed tomography* (SPECT) single- or double-headed cameras rotate around the thorax detecting the gamma emission. Reconstruction of the images is carried out in a similar manner to that of X-ray computed tomography.

POSITRON EMISSION TOMOGRAPHY (PET)

Positrons are particles with the mass of an electron but an opposite charge. As the positron loses kinetic energy, it interacts with an electron and both particles are annihilated and their mass converted in two 511-keV photons that leave the site of the interaction in exactly opposite directions. Detection of this interaction allows precise spatial location, which is not possible with gamma-emitting nuclides. Detectors are placed at opposite sides of the thorax to note annihilation by coincidence-counting of the pairs of 511-keV photons. To date, isotopes that are positron emitters are largely produced as short-lived isotopes from a cyclotron, principally oxygen-15, nitrogen-13, carbon-11, and fluorine-81. However, it is also possible to use a generator similar to that for the production of $^{99}Tc^m$ and several positron emitters, such as rubidium-82, gallium-68 and copper-62, have been produced. These compounds can be used to label the blood pool, to indicate blood flow or to study cardiac metabolism. ^{11}C-palmitate and ^{18}F-2-deoxyglucose have been of particular importance for the study of myocardial metabolism.

CARDIAC FUNCTION

FIRST PASS TECHNIQUES

Cardiac output

When a bolus of radionuclide (typically 700 MBq of $^{99}Tc^m$ labelled to red blood cells or albumin) is injected intravenously, its passage through the heart can be recorded by a gamma camera–computer system. (For units of measurement used in nuclear medicine see Appendix 1.) In analysis, regions of interest (ROIs) are placed around the right or left ventricle and activity–time curves obtained. If the discrete time-intervals during which counts are collected are relatively long (0.5 s), a standard indicator dilution curve is produced (Fig. 19.1). Cardiac output may then be assessed using the Stewart–Hamilton principle in which

$$\text{cardiac output} = i/(c.t)$$

where i is the quantity injected, c the average concentration of the indicator during its first pass and t the total duration of the curve. Interpretation of the area under the curve (A) and the duration of the curve can be improved by using mathematical functions such as the 'gamma variate' fit. As external sampling is used the quantity of radionuclide injected (i in counts per minute) can be assessed only by assuming that this equals the equilibrium

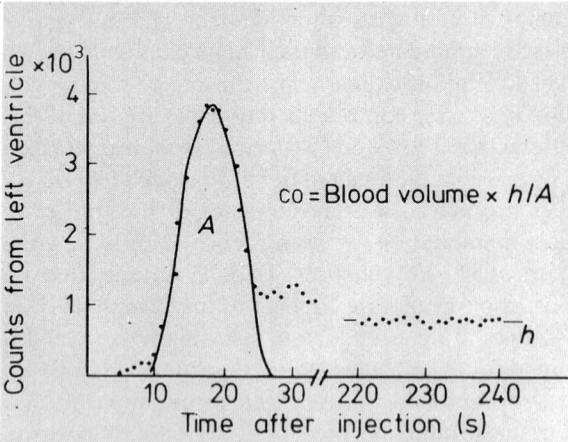

Fig. 19.1. A radionuclide indicator dilution curve. Counts from the left ventricle are recorded as a bolus of $^{99}Tc^m$-labelled red blood cells passes through the heart. The cardiac output is derived from the area under the curve (A), the height at equilibrium (h) and the blood volume. The blood volume is calculated from the total distribution of the blood pool marker by measuring its dilution in serial plasma samples. (Reproduced, by permission, from Hannan, W.J. et al. Clin. Phys. Physiol. Meas. 1980; **1**: 125–34.[2])

concentration or counts (C_{eq} in counts per minute per ml) multiplied by the blood volume (BV in ml).[2]

$$i = C_{eq} . BV$$

Thus, for the radionuclide method:

$$\text{Cardiac output} = (BV.h)/A$$

where h is the height of the curve at equilibrium. This assumption limits the accuracy of radionuclide-determined cardiac output because the lung and chest wall contain more activity during equilibrium than during the first pass and Compton scatter is greater at equilibrium. Various solutions have been proposed but none has found universal favour. Radionuclide methods tend to overestimate cardiac output.

Pulmonary blood volume

By determining the difference in transit times (t) of the indicator curves from the right and left ventricles, the *pulmonary blood volume* (V) may be calculated:

$$V = Ft$$

where F is flow or cardiac output. The precise value is dependent on the accuracy of the cardiac output but differences in transit time are seen clearly in different patient groups.[3]

Shunt detection

In patients with left-to-right shunt, when a bolus of radionuclide is injected, some passes back from the left side of the heart to the right side resulting in early recirculation of tracer. The ratio of pulmonary to systemic flow can be calculated from the indicator dilution curves recorded from the right lung where the portion due to systemic circulation is separated from the portion due to recirculation by mathematical techniques involving gamma variate fitting of the curve or deconvolution analysis. The pulmonary dilution time–activity curve prior to recirculation is subtracted from the total pulmonary curve and the resultant curve represents recirculation. The area under the first curve represents the flow through the lungs (Q_P), whereas the area under the second curve represents pulmonary less systemic flow ($Q_P - Q_S$). Shunt determination by this technique may be superior to conventional oximetric analysis of pulmonary to systemic flow ratio.[4]

Right-to-left shunting can be assessed by injecting intravenously an inert gas in solution, such as xenon-133. Normally, this gas would be extracted on passing through the lung, but it will appear in the systemic circulation if there is a significant right-to-left shunt. The same principle also holds for the intravenous injection of $^{99}Tc^m$-macro-aggregates which would normally be arrested in the pulmonary circulation. An estimate of the magnitude of the shunt can be made by counting the activity from the lungs and from the rest of the body, but the total number of particles injected must be small or there is a risk of embolization in the brain and other organs.

Valvular regurgitation

Observation of the passage of the bolus of radionuclide through the cardiac chambers can give some indication of chamber size or delay in emptying, and a number of quantitative methods based on distortion of the indicator dilution curves have been advocated for quantifying regurgitation.[5] Gated ventriculography can also be used to compute the amount of regurgitation using the stroke count output of left and right ventricles. The left to right ventricular stroke index should be close to unity but in regurgitation of the mitral or aortic valves the ratio is greater than 1.35.[6] Tricuspid regurgitation may be assessed by observing an increase in liver blood volume in systole. These techniques are of limited value and become difficult or impossible to interpret if more than one valve is leaking.

First pass ejection fraction

If the passage of the bolus is examined in much smaller time-frames (30 ms), clear oscillations caused by the contribution of each beat can be seen (Fig. 19.2). The count rate at the peak of each beat is proportional to the end-diastolic volume and the trough to the end-systolic volume. The ejection fraction is obtained from:

$$\text{Ejection fraction} = \frac{\text{Diastolic counts} - \text{Systolic counts}}{\text{Diastolic counts} - \text{Background counts}}$$

For statistical reliability, 3–5 cardiac cycles should be averaged. Background correction is made by counting from a rim of tissue around the free margin of the left ventricle or from the region of the left ventricle immediately prior to the arrival of the bolus. Similar methods are used to determine right ventricular ejection fraction with background correction from the inferior margin of the right ventricle. This method of calculating ejection fraction requires a good bolus injection and has the disadvantage of needing repeated injections of a radionuclide if more than one estimate is made, but it minimizes the problem of chamber overlap and different chamber views can be obtained. It is best used with multicrystal cameras which have high count-rate capabilities.[7] Summing several cardiac

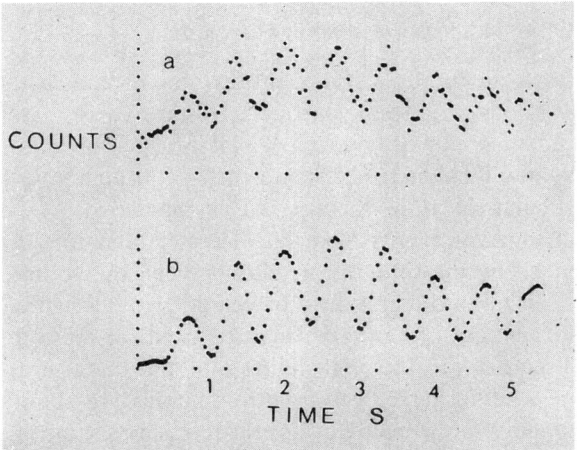

Fig. 19.2. Time–activity curve recorded from the left ventricular region during the passage of a bolus of intravenously administered $^{99}Tc^m$-red blood cells. The top panel shows the recorded count rate and the bottom panel shows the same data after a mathematical filter. Each peak represents end-diastole and each trough end-systole.

cycles increases the counts in each picture frame and improves the quality of the displayed images which can be shown in apparent 'movie' sequence or as systolic and diastolic images so that cardiac wall motion can be studied (Fig. 19.3).

Gated ventriculography

Workers in most departments opt for a general purpose single-crystal camera because it is more versatile, having many applications within a nuclear medicine department. However, as these cameras do not usually have the high count-rate capabilities of multicrystal cameras, ventricular function is better assessed using the gated blood pool method rather than the first pass method. A radionuclide that remains in the blood pool (i.e. $^{99}Tc^m$-red blood cells) is injected and imaging is carried out over a large number of cardiac cycles, usually between 300 and 500 beats. The counts from the heart, detected by the gamma camera, are stored in a computer using the R wave of the electrocardiogram as a marker of the start of each cardiac cycle. Frames of 20–40 ms are accumulated to produce an average activity in each specified phase of the cardiac cycle of the number of beats acquired. The images are then displayed in rapid or 'movie' sequence. This method achieves good counting statistics and images. It is possible to view the heart in different projections and many repeat studies can be obtained from a single radionuclide injection, but quantitative information about the left ventricle can be obtained only in the left anterior oblique projection which optimizes separation of the left and right ventricles. The ejection fraction is calculated in the same manner as in the first pass method, but background subtraction is more critical because up to 50% of the counts coming from the region of the left ventricle are due to background. Various methods of accounting for background activity have been proposed, but most use the free border of the left ventricle and many now use a region that follows the rim of the ventricle as it contracts. As the counting statistics of the equilibrium technique are better, it provides a more accurate representation of the ventricular volume curve (Fig. 19.4) than first pass studies.

Although there are theoretical advantages and disadvantages associated with these two methods of radionuclide ventriculography, the technique chosen is usually determined by the equipment available. Both methods have been shown to provide measurements of ejection fraction that are

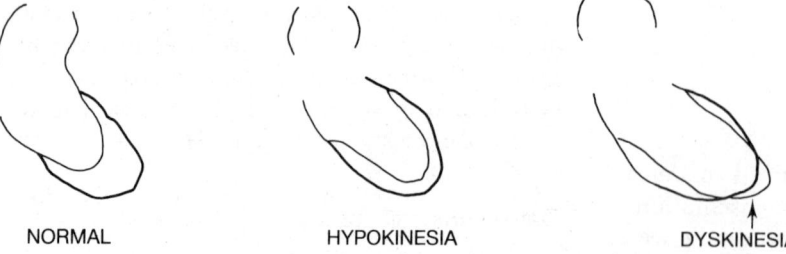

NORMAL   HYPOKINESIA   DYSKINESIA

Fig. 19.3. End-systolic and end-diastolic outlines in the right anterior oblique view from a normal subject, a patient with a hypokinetic ventricle and a patient with a dyskinetic segment taken from their respective 'first-pass' radionuclide ventriculograms.

comparable to those measured using contrast angiography.[8–10]

As both methods use counts as a measure of volume, they are free from the errors of any geometrical assumptions; moreover, being semi-automated, they show little inter- and intra-observer variability. However, photon attenuation may lead to some errors when imaging very large hearts because there is greater attenuation of events from the posterior wall of the ventricle than from the anterior wall.[11] Edge detection is not as precise as with contrast angiography and minor degrees of abnormal wall motion may go undetected.

Functional images

A variety of computational methods are used to improve visual appreciation of normal and abnormal wall movement. These are termed functional images because each derived image represents a function of the ventricle. The 'stroke volume' image

is made by dividing the background subtracted end-systolic image from the end-diastolic image. This can be further divided by the end-diastolic image to produce an 'ejection fraction' image which gives a representation of regional ejection fractions. If the end-diastolic frame is subtracted from the end-systolic frame, the image will show parts of the ventricle that exhibit paradoxical wall motion.[12] Regional asynchrony can be best assessed by 'phase' imaging. In this technique, the activity curve from each picture-cell element (pixel) is fitted to a sine wave by Fourier analysis and a phase angle determined. Each phase angle is given a colour and displayed (Pl. 19.1) If the ventricle is contracting synchronously, it will be represented by a uniform colour, whereas asynchrony is shown by a variation in the colour code. Even in normal ventricles, there is some variation in ventricular activation and the earliest phase angle is at the base of the interventricular septum. In patients with left bundle branch block, it begins in the right ventricle. Myocardial segments with delayed phase or amplitude can be easily identified and can aid the detection of regional ventricular disease.[13]

Other indices of ventricular function

Both first pass and equilibrium radionuclide methods produce a ventricular volume curve, parts of which may provide additional information about ventricular function. The normalized mean left ventricular ejection fraction rate is calculated as the changes in counts from diastole to end-systole divided by the time taken; alternatively, the volume expelled in the first third of systole or the weighted mean time of emptying may be used. In diastole, alterations in the peak filling rate and the time to peak filling have been used to demonstrate abnormalities in the behaviour of the left ventricle during diastole. Most of these measurements and those of the rate of change of volume are influenced by the curve-fitting procedures and filtering required to make the measurements and caution is required to avoid over-interpretation of such data.[14,15]

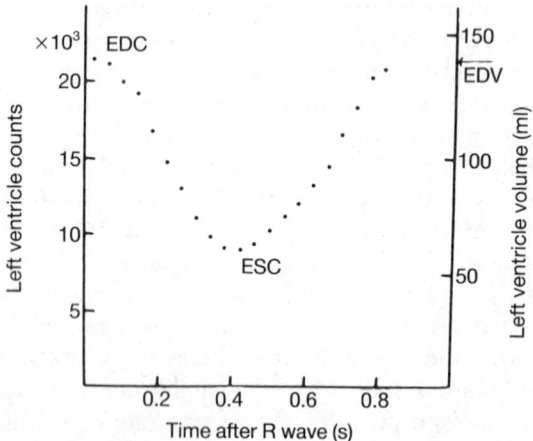

Fig. 19.4. A ventricular volume curve from gated blood pool imaging. The background corrected counts for each time-interval from the onset of the R wave of the electrocardiogram from the left ventricle for the total acquisition period are displayed. End-diastole and end-systole are indicated. An absolute calibration can be achieved by using stroke volume calculated from the initial indicator dilution curve: SV = EDC − ESC. (Reproduced, by permission, from Hannan, W.J. *et al. Clin. Phys. Physiol. Meas.* 1980; **1**: 125–34).[2]

STRESS TESTING

Ventricular function may become abnormal only when stressed. *Supine* bicycle exercise is the most frequently used stress for radionuclide ventriculography because a good position for imaging can be maintained easily. After resting measurements have been taken, the exercise load is increased in 25-W increments at 3-min intervals until the patient experiences angina, dyspnoea, undue fatigue, hypotension, ST-segment changes on the electrocardiogram or arrhythmias. Imaging takes place in the last 2 min of each exercise stage. In some laboratories, *upright* bicycle exercise is preferred as a more normal stress. Most responses in the two positions are similar, although differences in end-diastolic volumes have been noted.[16]

Other forms of stress, including isometric exercise (handgrip),[17] the cold pressor test,[18] atrial pacing[19] and pharmacological interventions, e.g. intravenous dipyridamide[20] have all been used, although less widely than dynamic exercise, and they are usually reserved for patients who cannot use a bicycle ergometer.

RADIONUCLIDE VENTRICULOGRAPHY: CLINICAL APPLICATIONS

Radionuclide ventriculography is of particular use in clinical problems that can be resolved by a knowledge of ventricular performance at rest or during appropriate stress. Its major use has been in the assessment of ischaemic heart disease and in the evaluation of congestive heart failure. It is also used to document ventricular function in valvular heart disease and the cardiovascular response to drugs.

ISCHAEMIC HEART DISEASE

The normal response to exercise is for the ejection fraction to increase by at least 5% (Fig. 19.5). Patients with ischaemic heart disease usually show a deterioration in left ventricular performance during exercise, manifest as abnormalities in regional wall motion and increases in pulmonary blood volume. Left ventricular ejection fraction fails to increase during exercise and may even decrease.[21] In patients with coronary artery disease and normal resting left ventricular function, this response is usually easy to elicit. In patients with abnormal resting left ventricular function, exercise performance depends on the extent of scar tissue and on the presence and extent of exercise-induced ischaemia; changes in ejection fraction may be small and inconsistent.

In the literature, it has been suggested that analysis of the ejection fraction and regional wall motion response to exercise gives a sensitivity and specificity of around 95% for the detection of coronary artery disease, although the selection of the study population must influence the precise values.[22] Patients with other forms of heart disease will often have an abnormal response to exercise. Older subjects and some women may show a reduced response to exercise, but often this is because the

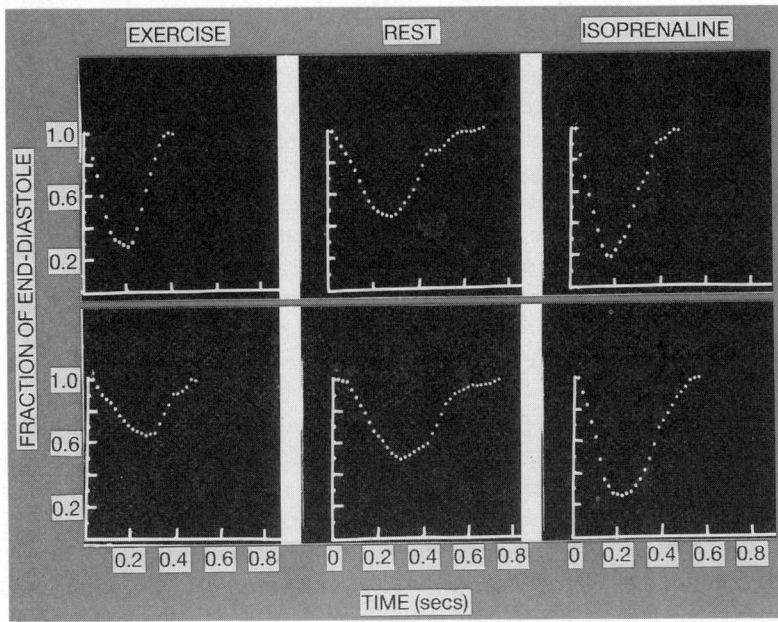

Fig. 19.5. Ventricular volume curves constructed from gated blood pool ventriculography in a normal subject (top panels) and a patient with coronary artery disease (bottom panels). Both have normal resting left ventricular function at rest and respond to isoprenaline by increasing their ejection fractions. The normal subject also increased ejection fraction on exercise, but ejection fraction decreases in the patient with coronary artery disease. (Reproduced, by permission, from Sapru, *et al. Cardiology* 1982; **69**: 91–7[19]).

exercise may have been inadequate, terminated by general fatigue, an inability to manage the leg co-ordination necessary for cycling or lack of motivation. To avoid this, it is important to ensure that there is an adequate heart-rate response to the exercise. Drug therapy may also influence the response: beta-blockade may blunt the rise in ejection fraction in normal subjects, conversely, it may improve ventricular function in patients with coronary artery disease;[23] vasodilators may also improve ventricular performance in patients with angina.[24] Therefore, if clinically appropriate, patients should be studied either off drugs or whilst receiving only short-acting nitrates.

Prediction of the vessel stenosed can be attempted on the basis of local regional dysfunction; in the standard left anterior oblique view, septal motion abnormalities indicate disease in the left anterior descending coronary artery, and postero-lateral abnormalities disease of the circumflex coronary artery. A decrease in right ventricular function may indicate disease in the right coronary artery.[25] Interpretation of these changes is not always simple, and it is often subjective. It is particularly difficult if there has been a previous infarction or if multivessel disease is present. A decrease in ejection fraction is more likely to be seen in patients who have multivessel coronary artery disease,[26] but some may have a near-normal response, other patients with single-vessel disease show a profound impairment of the ventricular response to exercise. A closer correlation is found between the ventricular response to exercise and an assessment of coronary artery disease severity when a scoring system that accounts for the site and severity of the lesion, the dominance of the vessel and the presence or absence of collaterals is used.[27] The extent of the abnormal response to exercise is a function of the total amount of ischaemic myocardium. Exercise left ventricular ejection fraction appears to be the most important predictor of both cardiac events and death; exercise heart rate and exercise duration are significant, but weaker, predictors in patients with suspected coronary artery disease.[28] It remains to be shown that this test can be used reliably to predict patients with angina at high risk of infarction or death or those who require coronary artery surgery or angioplasty.

MYOCARDIAL INFARCTION

After myocardial infarction, the ejection fraction is often reduced; the reduction is usually greatest in those who have sustained an anterior transmural myocardial infarction, intermediate in those with inferior transmural myocardial infarction and least in those with non-Q wave infarction.[29] In those with anterior infarction, there is a close correlation with the total enzyme release, but this is not as close in patients who have inferior infarction.[30] The immediate and long-term prognosis after infarction is determined mainly by the extent of muscle damage and this is reflected by the reduction in ejection fraction. A reduction in global ejection fraction in the first 24 h has been shown to be the best predictor of risk when combined with the Killip clinical score. Patients with left ventricular ejection fraction (< 30% in Killip class II had a mortality of 39% at 30 days and of 47% at 90 days, whereas patients in Killip class II with left ventricular ejection fraction > 30% had a 30-day mortality of 13%.[31] In some patients, there may be a partial recovery in ejection fraction over the first 48 h, but in the majority there is little improvement. There is very little change in left ventricular ejection fraction from 3 days onwards; the left ventricular ejection fraction at around 10 days is often used as an assessment of infarct size in patients who have sustained their first infarction.[32] The long-term prognosis after infarction can also be assessed, and a resting and submaximal exercise ventriculogram can be used to stratify risk after infarction. Patients with a resting ejection fraction < 30% have a high risk of heart failure, sudden death, ventricular tachycardia and fibrillation.[30] A decrease in ejection fraction during a submaximal exercise test can predict those at risk of developing angina in the year after infarction. About half of the patients surviving the hospital phase of acute infarction will have moderately preserved ventricular function and a near-normal response to exercise. Such patients have a very good prognosis.

As the reduction in ejection fraction after a first myocardial infarction can be closely related to infarct size, ventriculography has been used to assess the effects of thrombolytic therapy in acute infarction. The underlying assumption is that the better preserved the ejection fraction, the less myocardial damage has occurred. Patients with anterior infarction who have undergone thrombolysis have higher ejection fractions than similar patients who have been treated with placebo,[33] suggesting some myocardial salvage. Such an effect was not seen in patients with inferior infarction, but it may be difficult to demonstrate significant change in this group of patients irrespective of treatment.

because they have better preserved resting ejection fractions. However, radionuclide techniques may also underestimate changes in the posterior portion of the ventricle due to tissue attenuation of the counts,[11] such that small differences between treatment groups may be masked.

Radionuclide assessment of right ventricular function is also of value in managing hypotension complicating acute myocardial infarction.[34] Although the treatment of cardiogenic shock in patients with poor left ventricular function has disappointing results, patients with impaired right ventricular function often respond well to increasing the blood volume. Gated radionuclide ventriculography quickly identifies those patients who have poor right ventricular function but relatively well preserved left ventricular function who should respond well to volume loading.

Right ventricular performance is often impaired in patients with inferior infarction, in some of whom the long-term prognosis relates as much to damage to the right as to the left ventricle. An assessment of right ventricular function should be incorporated into any risk stratification or prognostic index for this group of patients.

OTHER HEART DISEASE

Radionuclide ventriculography can help in the assessment of congestive cardiomyopathy. Regional dyskinesia implies coronary artery disease as the underlying pathology, whereas a globally poorly functioning ventricle is more likely to indicate a generalized cardiomyopathic process. Ventriculography is also of value in identifying isolated right ventricular cardiomyopathy, particularly in young patients with tachyarrhythmias. Patients with hypertrophic cardiomyopathy usually have supernormal ejection fractions, with near obliteration of the ventricle during systole, but prolonged isovolumic relaxation.[35]

Ventricular performance may also be used to assess prognosis in aortic regurgitation, and it has been suggested, but not proven (see p. 747) that a fall in resting left ventricular ejection fraction to < 50% in serial studies or impairment of functional reserve with an abnormal response to exercise are indications for surgical correction.[36] The technique can be used to document abnormal cardiac function in many diseases. Diabetic patients have abnormal systolic and diastolic function suggestive of a specific cardiomyopathy.[37] There is altered function in hyperthyroidism which is independent of beta-

adrenoceptor activity.[38] Patients with obstructive lung disease have impaired right ventricular function which may precede the development of the clinical syndrome of cor pulmonale; once it has developed, there is a reduction of both right and left ventricular function which can be partially corrected by therapy with vasodilators or oxygen.[39]

A decrease in ventricular performance is an indicator of drug cardiotoxicity and is used to monitor the response to chemotherapeutic drugs, such as doxorubicin.[40] Ventriculography may also be used to determine the effectiveness of a drug in an individual patient or to investigate the action of a new agent. Although the equilibrium blood pool method is particularly suited to the assessment of the effects of drug therapy on cardiovascular function because serial determinations of the acute response can be made without further radiation burden, such assessment is complicated by the fact that ejection fraction and other ejection phase indices will be influenced by changes in loading conditions caused by the particular drug.

A vasodilating drug will almost invariably cause an increase in ejection fraction although it may have no effect on contractile state. Some account of preload changes can be made by examining alterations in end-diastolic volume counts after administration of a drug. To discriminate between changes in contractile state and afterload is more difficult; however, the volume of the left ventricle at end-systole is independent of preload but dependent on afterload. When left ventricular end-systolic pressure and volume are determined at different levels of afterload, the slope of the end-systolic pressure–volume relation may be calculated and used as an index of contractility. Afterload is determined by a number of factors, but in clinical practice it is often assumed to be the end-systolic pressure with the further simplification of equating this to the sphygmomanometer-determined systolic blood pressure. This pressure is then related to end-systolic volume as determined from the ventricular volume curve.[38]

There are theoretical and practical objections to this approach. As calibration of the ventricular volume curve and hence the calculation of end-systolic volume is achieved either by determining the cardiac output and hence the stroke volume from the initial passage of the bolus of isotope or by attenuation correction methods, there is imprecision in the volume measurements. Recently, single photon emission computed tomography has been used in an attempt to establish more precise values for ventricular volumes,[41] but the procedure becomes more complicated. Systolic pressure measured by sphygmomanometry is only an approximation of the end-systolic pressure. Even when using micromanometer/tipped catheters, the end-systolic pressure may not reflect true afterload because ventricular wall thickness is necessary to calculate the left ventricular end-systolic stress. Patients may not always tolerate the changes in afterload needed to produce the slope of the pressure to volume ratios. Finally, the changes in afterload induced by physiological or pharmacological means may induce reflex changes in contractility. Attempts to inhibit the reflex changes may further alter contractility. Provided these strictures are understood, the method does help to expose the action of drugs on the circulation.

An additional advantage of the equilibrium method when used to examine drug action on the cardiovascular system is that the blood pool is already labelled, and changes in regional counts from a limb or organ will largely reflect changes in venous volume because approximately 80% of the blood volume is contained within the venous as opposed to the arterial system. For example, hydrallazine, known to act mainly on the arterial bed, produces marked arterial vasodilatation without any changes in venous volume. In contrast, venoactive drugs, such as glyceryl trinitrate, cause less impressive changes in systemic arterial pressure but a 12% increase in venous volume. As many cardioactive drugs act on venous tone, an assessment of changes in venous volume provide a more complete understanding of the drugs' mechanisms of action.[42]

THALLIUM-201 FOR MYOCARDIAL PERFUSION IMAGING

A variety of radionuclides have been used for myocardial perfusion studies. The first of these was potassium-43 and since then several potassium analogues have been used including caesium-129, rubidium-81 and thallium-201. Thallium-201 is now the most widely used in the clinical evaluation of perfusion defects in ischaemic heart disease. It has biological properties similar, but not identical, to potassium and is probably transported into the cell by the sodium pump. Thallium-201 has a physical half-life of 73.1 h and it decays by electron capture to mercury-201, emitting X-rays of 69–83 keV and gamma rays mainly of 167 keV. Owing to

the greater abundance of X-rays, imaging is carried out at the 69–83-keV mercury X-ray photo peak.

The initial distribution of ^{201}Tl to the heart, following intravenous administration, is proportional to that fraction of the cardiac output perfusing the myocardium and the percentage of thallium extracted by the myocardium during the first pass through the heart.[43] The uptake of thallium into a myocardial cell depends on the integrity of the Na^+–K^+ ATPase on its surface membrane which maintains the transmembrane gradients of sodium and potassium.[44] Inhibition of oxidative phosphorylation or the glycolytic pathways reduces cellular uptake of thallium.[45] A large carbohydrate meal may decrease, and fasting increase, the diagnostic yield of thallium imaging.[46] Drug therapy may also alter thallium kinetics.[47]

MYOCARDIAL INFARCTION

Areas of myocardium that are either ischaemic or infarcted do not take up thallium and will be seen as a 'cold spot' on the image. However, only about 55% of patients with a previous myocardial infarction have a positive thallium scintigram. When the infarct has been small or is inferiorly located, the thallium image may be normal.[48] The main application of thallium imaging is in the assessment of effort angina.

STRESS TESTING WITH THALLIUM

The patient undergoes a graded exercise test to try to achieve target heart-rate response either on a treadmill or a bicycle. At target heart rate, or when there is electrocardiographic change or chest pain sufficient to warrant early cessation of exercise, 80 MBq of ^{201}Tl is injected via an indwelling venous cannula. The patient should be exercised for a further 30–60 s to maintain ischaemia during the uptake of thallium. In patients in whom exercise is not possible, a pharmacological stress test is performed in which 400 mg of dipyridamole is used as an alternative stress.[49] Stress testing combining exercise and dipyridamole has also been used.[50] Imaging is commenced within 5 min of the injection of the isotope, first using the 45° left anterior oblique projection followed by anterior and left lateral projections. It is important these views are obtained as soon as possible after the injection and before there is significant redistribution of tracer. If a cold spot is identified the patient returns to the laboratory 2–3 h later by which time redistribution of tracer should have occurred. Control images are then recorded in the same projections. In a few cases in whom there is uncertainty about the adequacy of reperfusion and there appears to be a non-reversible defect, without clinical evidence of myocardial infarction, a repeat testing image may be obtained 1 week later following a second ^{201}Tl injection. Images can be recorded on Polaroid or X-ray film or better inspected using a computer to display exercise and recovery images simultaneously. Similar background subtraction is applied to both images. More elaborate computerized analysis of ^{201}Tl imaging, with analysis of washouts, has been extensively reported and, in some series, improved the sensitivity and specificity of the technique,[51] but it is not widely used in clinical practice. Some workers have gated the thallium images to take account of cardiac motion and suggest this procedure enhances image interpretation. In addition, some assessment of ventricular function can also be obtained. Transaxial computed tomography can also be performed (Pl. 19.2) and high-quality images with much greater definition obtained.[52] Undoubtedly, tomography improves the contrast between the myocardium and surrounding structures, but there is some concern that redistribution of thallium may take place during imaging if the time taken to acquire the two-dimensional data is longer than 20–30 min. With this stricture, ^{201}Tl rotational tomography does appear to provide a highly accurate technique for determining the presence and location of coronary artery disease.[53]

Lung uptake

An increased concentration of thallium in the lung is frequently noted in patients with myocardial ischaemia or left ventricular dysfunction.[54] Greater uptake in the lung correlates with a prolonged transit through the lungs and the severity of heart disease.[55] The increased thallium uptake in the lungs probably reflects the increased pulmonary capillary hydrostatic pressure that occurs in these patients during exercise.

DETECTING CORONARY ARTERY DISEASE

Perfusion scintigraphy with thallium provides a greater overall sensitivity and specificity for diagnosing coronary artery disease than the exercise electrocardiogram.[56] However, thallium is not cheap, neither is the radiation burden negligible and imaging should be carried out only when the exercise electrocardiogram is not diagnostic or is abnormal in an asymptomatic patient in whom there is a moderate probability of coronary artery disease.

Exercise thallium imaging provides an objective guide to the severity of the patient's coronary artery disease, but because of the limitations of planar imaging it has not proved particularly useful in determining the number of stenotic coronary arteries or in identifying which vessels are diseased. It provides reasonable sensitivity for diagnosing disease in the left anterior descending artery which usually supplies the septum, anterior wall and apex of the left ventricle, the best visualized portions of the myocardium. The right coronary artery perfuses the inferior left ventricle wall and this can be identified on the anterior or left lateral views with reasonable sensitivity and specificity, but these same segments may also be perfused to the circumflex artery. This artery most commonly supplies the left ventricular posterior wall and is best visualized in a 45° left anterior oblique view, but partly because it supplies that part of the myocardium which is most poorly visualized and partly because of anatomical variation sensitivity and specificity for disease in this artery is poor.[57] Some improvement in detecting individual arterial involvement can be expected with the wider use of SPECT imaging of ^{201}Tl uptake by the myocardium.[53]

The presence of a 75% or greater stenosis in the left main coronary artery can produce exercise-induced ischaemia in anterior septal and posterolateral left ventricular portions of the myocardium, but the findings are not highly specific.[58] The technique is also useful for detecting graft patency.

Other conditions causing myocardial ischaemia will also cause abnormal thallium scans: muscular myocardial bridges and aortic stenosis in the presence of normal coronary arteries. Transient defects in thallium images are also seen when coronary artery spasm occurs at rest.[59] Right ventricular uptake is often seen on exercise scans, but when seen on a resting thallium image it usually indicates right ventricular hypertrophy.

Thallium scanning has also been used to detect the presence of co-existing coronary artery disease in patients with valvular heart disease. As noted above, patients with aortic stenosis may have an abnormal stress image without having coronary artery disease and similar findings have been reported in patients with aortic regurgitation[60] who have apical defects which may be related to volume overload. In patients with mitral valve prolapse, fixed and reversible defects have been described, although the presence of an exercise-induced defect usually indicates associated coronary artery disease.[61] A recent report[62] has suggested that the technique is valuable in the detection of coronary artery disease in patients with mitral stenosis and regurgitation and, provided apical defects are ignored, it can be used in patients with aortic valve disease. Until the completion of studies in which larger numbers of patients are investigated the value of thallium stress imaging in the detection of coronary artery disease in patients with aortic valve disease cannot be ascertained.

There are still several technical limitations to thallium imaging. In particular, the energy is too low for conventional gamma cameras and thus image quality and resolution are poor. As tech-

netium is an almost ideal isotope for imaging, several compounds that can be labelled with technetium have been developed.[63] Of these, the newer isonitriles, such as $^{99}Tc^m$-butylisonitrile or $^{99}Tc^m$-methoxymethylpropylisonitrile, appear to be the most promising agents for myocardial perfusion imaging (Fig. 19.6). The kinetics governing the uptake of the isonitriles in myocytes are poorly understood, but the isonitriles do appear to bind to myocytes in a manner proportional to the delivery of the complex to the extracellular spaces.[64]

COMPARISON OF STRESS IMAGING USING THALLIUM OR VENTRICULOGRAPHY IN THE DETECTION OF CORONARY ARTERY DISEASE

As the assessment of myocardial perfusion is being considered, the advantages should lie with thallium scintigraphy, the technique that measures myocardial blood flow. Multiple views can be obtained from a single injection and the more familiar treadmill exercise can be used as the stress. Reperfusion can be examined after recovery to give an assessment of the reversible defect. However, despite extensive work to extract the maximum information from the images, the technique itself is limited by the physical characteristics of ^{201}Tl. The superior imaging characteristics of technetium give a technical advantage to ventriculography. Perfusion is then assessed indirectly from the adequacy of the ventricular response to exercise. Thallium imaging, although improved by computer enhancement, does not require quantification; ventriculography requires computer facilities and is probably more demanding technically than planar imaging. However, advanced computer facilities are required for rotational tomographic imaging with thallium and the subsequent complex analysis that is now possible to perform.[65] Some patients with multivessel disease may have a general but balanced reduction in ^{201}Tl uptake such that the images may not be grossly abnormal, but the ventriculogram will show impaired function. Moreover, ventriculography may be easier to interpret in patients with previous infarction. Ventriculography is probably more sensitive but less specific in detecting coronary artery disease because other forms of heart disease also cause impaired ventricular function. Finally, it is less expensive. Ultimately, the test chosen will depend on the equipment available and local experience.

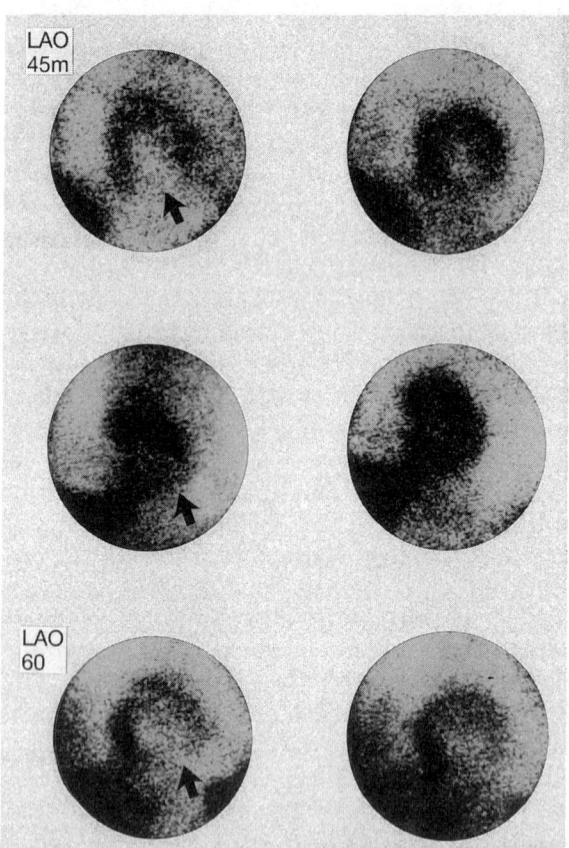

Fig. 19.6. Technetium-99m-butylisonitrile perfusion images taken immediately after exercise (left-hand panels) and after redistribution (right-hand panels). The perfusion defect indicated in the post-exercise sequence is shown to be reversible indicating an ischaemic but not infarcted segment of myocardium. The patient had a stenosis in the right coronary artery. (By courtesy of Dr M. Khalil.)

ALTERNATIVE METHODS OF MEASURING MYOCARDIAL PERFUSION

Myocardial perfusion can also be assessed by a variety of invasive techniques using radionuclides. These include the injection of microspheres into the left atrium or the coronary arteries,[66] injection of the positron emitter rubidium-82 directly into the coronary arteries and inert gas washout methods.[67] Owing to their complexity, these methods are not in clinical use. However, the quantification it is possible to perform when using these techniques gives them important applications in research.

MYOCARDIAL METABOLISM

Ischaemic myocardium is unable to metabolize fats and several techniques have been adopted to utilize this fact and try to measure biochemical changes in the heart in man. The most attractive have involved the use of positron emission tomography because it has the spatial resolution to differentiate between regions of abnormal and those of preserved myocardial metabolism. Carbohydrate metabolism can be analysed using 2-fluoro-2-deoxyglucose, which becomes trapped in the cell and is not used as a substrate for futher glycolysis. The clearance half-time of ^{11}C-palmitate indicates the rate of oxidation of free fatty acids while blood flow may be studied using ^{13}N-ammonia.[68] These methods, or developments from them, may provide a greater understanding of the viability of ischaemic tissue and improve the selection of patients for revascularization. However, the expense of positron cameras for imaging and of the cyclotrons necessary to produce the radionuclides makes it unlikely that these techniques will be used beyond specialized research centres.

Several gamma-emitting metabolic tracers have been used, the most common being iodine-123-labelled fatty acids. The patterns of uptake and washout give some indication of fatty acid turnover, but doubt over the significance of the clearance half-times and concern about the diffusion of free iodide have limited the wider application of this method.[69]

INFARCT AVID SCANNING

Early attempts to identify myocardial infarction used fluorescein or tetracycline because they were known to concentrate in infarcted muscle. Bonte and colleagues,[70] stimulated by the observations of Shen and Jennings[71] indicating that calcium is deposited in crystalline or sub-crystalline form in irreversibly damaged myocardial cells, investigated technetium-99m pyrophosphate (PYP) as an infarct-imaging agent. Although there is still uncertainty about the precise mechanisms of PYP uptake, this is now the most widely used hot-spot infarct-imaging agent. Infarcted myocardium accumulates $^{99}Tc^m$ PYP within 6 h of coronary occlusion and there is a progressive uptake for the next 24–72 h. Uptake remains abnormal for up to 6 days after infarction and then diminishes.

Scanning procedure

The optimal time for clinical scanning is usually between 24 and 48 h after infarction.[72] A negative scintigram performed within 24 h of suspected acute myocardial infarction does not exclude such an event. Good-quality imaging can be obtained after the intravenous injection of 500 MBq of $^{99}Tc^m$ PYP. Scintigrams are taken after the blood pool has cleared and before there is intense uptake by bone. The optimal time is about 2 h after the injection of PYP but if there is a diffuse pattern the patient should be re-scanned 2 h later to determine whether further clearance of the radioisotope has taken place. Imaging is performed with a low-energy all-purpose parallel-hole collimator coupled to the gamma camera, and views in the anterior 45° left anterior oblique and left lateral are taken (Fig. 19.7). In certain circumstances, a gated ventriculogram can also be constructed in the first 5 min after the injection of $^{99}Tc^m$ PYP before there is significant loss from the blood pool, although the image quality tends to be poorer than when ventriculograms are constructed after the injection of blood pool labels.

Scintigraphic abnormalities are classified first as localized or diffuse and then the intensity of the pattern is compared with that of the ribs[69] (greater intensity than bone 4+; equal intensity to bone 3+; moderate intensity but less than that of bone 2+; slight 1+; none 0). When the activity in the myocardium is equal to or greater than that in bone, the result is unequivocally positive, i.e. 3+ and 4+. Focal uptake graded at 2+ also represents infarcted tissue, but diffuse uptake at this level of intensity is more difficult to interpret. Berman *et al.*[73] suggested this should be graded as 'equivocal' because such a grading conveys the necessary degree of uncertainty to other clinicians. Scans graded at 0–1+ are consi-

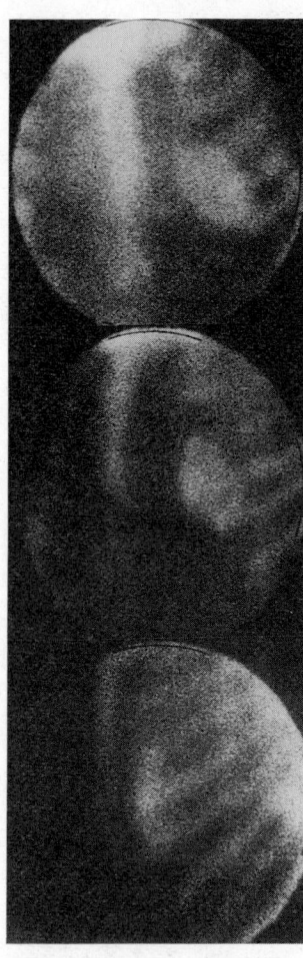

Fig. 19.7. Anterior (top) left anterior oblique and lateral views of a $^{99}Tc^m$ PYP image in a patient who had sustained an anterior myocardial infarction.

dered to show no evidence of infarction. Localized uptake is more likely to indicate transmural infarction, and diffuse uptake sub-endocardial or non-Q-wave infarction, but this is not always so. The descriptive term 'doughnut' pattern is applied to a large circular uptake of $^{99}Tc^m$ PYP which is always associated with a large transmural myocardial infarction.

Sensitivity and specificity

Localization of infarction is easiest in patients with anterior infarction and poorest in those who have non-Q-wave infarction. False-positive results are recorded in those patients with chest wall trauma, breast cancer, left ventricular aneurysms and myocarditis. After cardioversion, a positive scan could indicate myocardial damage or chest wall injury. Increased anatomical accuracy can be achieved using tomographic techniques (Pl. 19.3).[74] Values for specificity and sensitivity will depend on patient selection, but the results of most studies suggest the rates of false-positive and false-negative tests are between 10 and 15%.

PRACTICAL USE OF PYROPHOSPHATE SCINTIGRAPHY

Late diagnosis of myocardial infarction

The diagnosis of myocardial infarction is usually easily confirmed by electrocardiographic and enzyme changes so that in general $^{99}Tc^m$ PYP scintigrams are reserved for those patients in whom interpretation of these criteria is difficult. When an infarct is suspected to have occurred some days before hospital admission or outpatient consultation, evolutionary changes are unlikely to be seen on the electrocardiogram, and even changes in late rising enzymes, such as lactic dehydrogenase, may be missed. In contrast, because a positive $^{99}Tc^m$ PYP scan can be obtained 6 days or longer after infarction, this technique may prove helpful in the diagnosis of late suspected infarction. A positive pyrophosphate scan that is negative 2–3 weeks later strongly supports the diagnosis of recent infarction. In patients in whom the electrocardiogram can be misleading, such as in those with left bundle branch block or in those who have had previous infarctions, the diagnosis of further infarction is difficult. Even if there is a rise in cardiac enzymes, localization of the site of infarction may be impossible. As the site of infarction has considerable influence on prognosis, $^{99}Tc^m$ PYP scintigraphy should be carried out to locate the site of infarction.

Myocardial contusion

Blunt chest trauma can produce myocardial contusion with non-specific electrocardiographic findings and enzymic abnormalities that may or may not be due to skeletal muscle trauma. Damage to the myocardium can be demonstrated by $^{99}Tc^m$ PYP scintigraphy[75] and can alert clinicians to the possibility of life-threatening arrhythmias.

Unstable angina

Patients who have anginal pain at rest that responds poorly to therapy (unstable angina) pose a particular clinical problem. By definition, these patients do not have electrocardiographic or enzymic evidence of myocardial infarction, but about one-third of them have a low-grade positive $^{99}Tc^m$ PYP myocardial scintigram. The uptake seems to be associated with multifocal irreversible myocardial damage, consisting of myocytolysis, coagulation necrosis and/or fibrosis.[76] In these patients with unstable angina, small areas of necrosis may have developed over a period of days, such that the total enzyme released into the bloodstream is small; however, as the uptake of PYP continues for 6–7 days after infarction the scan may detect the accumulated damage over that period. Patients with unstable angina and abnormal images have a poorer prognosis than those with normal PYP images.

Peri-operative infarction

The myocardium is particularly vulnerable at the time of circulatory arrest during cardiac surgery, but the diagnosis of myocardial damage following cardiac surgery is difficult. Non-specific electrocardiographic abnormalities frequently occur, and increases in serum enzymes are often noted in the absence of myocardial infarction. In contrast a positive $^{99}Tc^m$ PYP scan is indicative of acute infarction,[77] provided the pre-operative scan was negative and the operative procedure did not involve the excision of myocardial tissue.

Other infarct-avid imaging agents

As the localization of isotope in bone is minimized by tomographic imaging, more accurate localization and sizing of damage to the myocardium can be accomplished by SPECT. However, the uptake of $^{99}Tc^m$ PYP relates too closely to myocardial blood flow and the half-life of $^{99}Tc^m$ is still too long to allow frequent repeated observations in the acute phase. Other infarct-avid imaging agents are being investigated and antimyosin antibodies show particular promise because they localize in proportion to the amount of muscle cell injury.[78] However, labelling of these antibodies with isotopes possessing a short half-life has not yet been accomplished.. Another approach has been to label the patient's neutrophils with indium-111. Provided the labelling and re-injection of the autologous cells is performed early in the course of infarction, uptake of neutrophils in the infarcted myocardium can be seen.[79] Although the technique should be of value when examining the role of the neutrophil in reperfusion injury or infarction, it is not intended to have a diagnostic role.

PERFUSION AND VENTILATION IMAGING OF THE LUNG

PERFUSION IMAGING

Pulmonary perfusion is usually assessed by the intravenous injection of macro-aggregates or microspheres of albumin labelled with $^{99}Tc^m$.[80] The particles are between 15 and 40 μm in diameter and lodge in pulmonary capillaries in proportion to the blood flow. The particles disintegrate slowly and the half-life in the capillaries is about 6 h. There is earlier loss of technetium from the particles and imaging is best carried out as soon as is practical after injection, the recorded counts being a direct representation of blood flow. The technique rarely causes any complications. It has been estimated that the injection of 500 000 particles will occlude < 0.1% of the capillaries, and the injection does not change the pulmonary diffusing capacity;[81] however, fatal reactions have been reported in patients with severe pulmonary hypertension.[82] Images are acquired in the anterior, posterior, left lateral, right lateral and left and right posterior oblique views. Good-quality images require at least 400 000 counts per image. As the distribution of perfusion to the lung is dependent upon posture, it is best to inject the particles when the patient is supine. As clumping of the particles will cause abnormal images, it is important to mix the particles before injection and that the injection is clean and not contaminated with blood drawn back into the syringe. Patient breath-holding must also be avoided. A normal perfusion scan shows a uniform distribution of counts in both lung fields. Inhomogeneity can be produced by abnormalities of the pulmonary circulation due to congenital or acquired disease or to extraluminal compression, as seen in some patients with bronchial tumours. Intraluminal obstruction is usually due to thromboembolism, but it may also be caused by tumour embolism, parasites, amniotic fluid or air. Parenchymal disease of the lung, in which there is distortion of the lung architecture, will also cause an abnormal perfusion scan making interpretation difficult, particularly in patients who have obstructive lung disease. In patients in whom interpretation is difficult, ventilation scanning may help.

VENTILATION IMAGING

Various methods are used to document the distribution of ventilation; the existence of so many approaches suggests that none is optimal. The best images are obtained using krypton-81m derived from a rubidium-81 generator. With a photon energy of 190 keV, it provides high-resolution images and imaging can be carried out once an abnormality has been noted on the perfusion scan because the energy levels of the $^{99}Tc^m$ perfusion scan will not cross into the higher energy window. Multiple images can be made because the half-life of $^{81}Kr^m$ is only 13 s. However, as the generator has a half-life of only 4 h, $^{81}Kr^m$ is not readily available for routine imaging.

Patients can inhale microspheres labelled with $^{99}Tc^m$ and good-quality images are obtained, but the imaging cannot be carried out simultaneously with technetium perfusion images and there is considerable concern that the distribution of the particles may not properly reflect the distribution of ventilation in patients with parenchymal lung disease.[83] The intrapulmonary distribution of ^{133}Xe gas is used in many centres. This radionuclide is readily available and accurately mirrors ventilatory patterns, but it has a low energy and, as there is

substantial scattering of $^{99}Tc^m$ into the ^{133}Xe window, imaging has to be carried out before the results of the perfusion scanning are known. Xenon-127 is being increasingly used because it has a higher photon energy. Initially, expense limited its use, but its long half-life (32 days) gives it the advantage of a long shelf-life, and increasing use has reduced its cost. It can be administered after an abnormal perfusion scan has been identified and ventilation imaging can be carried out in the same view as the most abnormal perfusion image. Respiratory gating can be used to enhance image appearance and permit calculation of regional tidal volume in a manner analogous to that of equilibrium blood pool imaging.[84]

PULMONARY EMBOLISM

The main clinical use of perfusion and ventilation imaging is in the identification of pulmonary embolism. A normal perfusion scan virtually excludes a pulmonary embolism within the previous 48 h. Acute pulmonary embolism usually produces sharply delineated segmental or lobar defects and most patients have multiple defects. The perfusion scan must be interpreted in conjunction with the chest X-ray because any parenchymal lung defect will also produce an abnormal defect on the perfusion scan. Defects in remote areas from the radiological abnormality are suggestive of an embolism, but further help can be obtained from the ventilation scan. Although patients with obstructive lung disease may have a normal chest X-ray, emphysematous bullae will usually produce abnormal perfusion images with a matched ventilation defect.

The detection of pulmonary embolism is not absolute and it should be recognized that imaging presents the clinician with a diagnostic probability,[85] although the diagnosis of recent embolism is excluded by a normal perfusion scan. Sub-segmental defects are unlikely to indicate pulmonary embolism and the diagnosis is unlikely unless there are other supporting clinical or investigative features.[86] Patients with a single segmental or lobar defect and a normal chest X-ray and a normal ventilation scan are likely to have sustained a pulmonary embolism, but if there is doubt about the clinical features or the scanning interpretation a pulmonary angiogram should be carried out. In patients with multiple defects and a normal chest X-ray and ventilation scan (Fig. 19.8), there is a very high probability of pulmonary embolism. The most difficult patients to assess are those with

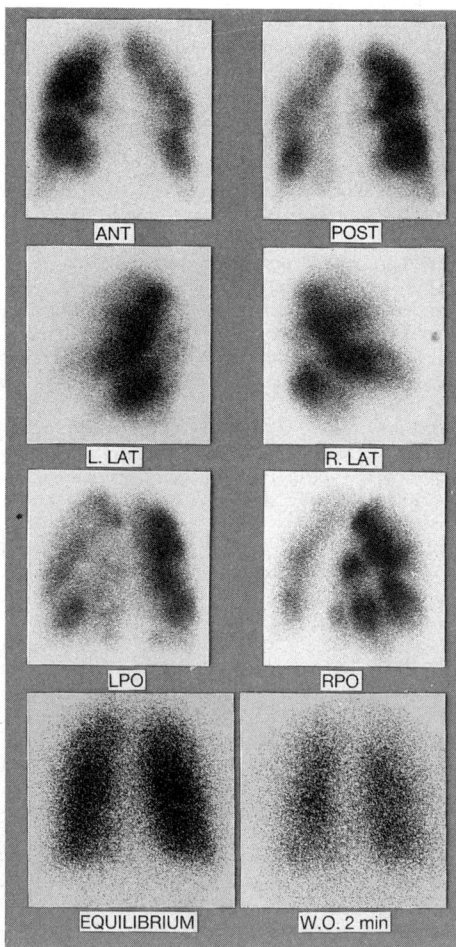

Fig. 19.8. Ventilation/perfusion images of a patient with pulmonary embolism. The perfusion scan (top 3 panels) shows multiple filling defects but the ventilation scan (posterior view) shows a normal distribution of ventilation and a normal washout of the inhaled ^{127}Xe.

obstructive airways disease in whom pulmonary angiography may be required to confirm or refute the diagnosis; unfortunately, in these patients, interpretation of the angiogram may also be difficult and treatment may have to be based on clinical suspicion.

FURTHER READING

Berman, D.S. and Mason, D.T. eds. *Clinical Nuclear Cardiology*. New York: Grune & Stratton, 1981.

Iskandrian, A.S. *Nuclear Cardiac Imaging: Principles and Applications*. Philadelphia: F.A. Davis & Co., 1986.

Gerson, M.C. *Cardiac Nuclear Medicine*. New York: McGraw-Hill, 1987.

REFERENCES

1. Lacy, J.L., Verani, M.S., Ball, M.E., Boyce, T.M., Gibson, R.W. and Roberts, R. First-pass radionuclide angiography using a multi-wire gamma camera and tantalum-178. *J. Nucl. Med.* 1988; **29**: 293–301.
2. Hannan, W.J., Vojacek, J., Dewhurst, N.J. and Muir, A.L. The sequential measurement of ventricular volumes and cardiac output by radionuclides. *Clin. Phys. Physiol. Meas.* 1980; **1**: 125–34.
3. Hannan, W.J., Vojacek, J., Connell, H.M., Dewhurst, N.G. and Muir, A.J. Radionuclide determined pulmonary blood volume in ischaemic heart disease. *Thorax* 1982; **36**: 922–7.
4. Baker, E.J., Ellam, S.V., Lorber, A., Jones, O.D.H., Tynan, M.J. and Maisey, M.N. Superiority of radionuclide over oximetric measurement of left to right shunts. *Br. Heart J.* 1985; **53**: 535–40.
5. Hannan, W.J., Vojacek, J., Dewhurst, N.G. and Muir, A.L. An index of valvular regurgitation from a radionuclide bolus. *Clin. Phys. Physiol. Meas.* 1981; **2**: 27–33.
6. Nicod, P., Corbett, J.R., Firth, B.G., Demmer, G.J., Markham, R.V., Hillis, L.D., Willerson, J.T. and Lewis, S.E. Radionuclide techniques for valvular regurgitant index: comparison in patients with normal and depressed ventricular function. *J. Nucl. Med.* 1982; **23**: 763–9.
7. Hecht, H.S., Mirrel, S.G., Rollett, E.L. and Blahd, W.H. Left ventricular ejection fraction and segmental wall motion by peripheral first-pass radionuclide angiography. *J. Nucl. Med.* 1978; **19**: 17–23.
8. Kaul, S., Boucher, C.A., Okada, R.D., Newell, J.B., Strauss, H.W. and Pohost, G.M. Source of variability in the radionuclide angiographic assessment of ejection fraction; a comparison of first pass and gated equilibrium techniques. *Am. J. Cardiol.* 1984; **53**: 823–8.
9. Burow, R.D., Strauss, H.W., Singleton, R., Pond, M., Rehn, T., Bailey, I.K., Griffith, L.C., Nickoloff, E. and Pitt, B. Analysis of left ventricular function from multiple gated acquisition cardiac blood pool imaging: comparison to contrast angiography. *Circulation* 1977; **56**: 1024–8.
10. Dymond, D.S., Elliott, A., Stone, D., Hendrix, G. and Spurrell, R. Factors that affect reproducibility of measurements of left ventricular function from first-pass radionuclide ventriculograms. *Circulation* 1982; **65**: 311–22.
11. Yeh, E.L. and Yeh, Y.S. Theoretical error in radionuclide ejection fraction study due to photon attenuation. *Eur. J. Nucl. Med.* 1981; **6**: 69–71.
12. Dewhurst, N.G., Hannan, W.J., Brash, H.M., Wraith, P.K. and Muir, A.L. The prevalence and prognosis of ventricular dyskinesis after myocardial infarction using radionuclide ventriculography. *Eur. Heart. J.* 1981; **2**: 409–17.
13. Ormerod, O.J.M., Barber, R.W., Stone, D.L., Taylor, N.C., Wraight, E.P. and Petch, M.C. Improved selection of patients for aneurysmectomy by combined phase and amplitude analysis of gated cardiac scintigraphy. *Eur. Heart J.* 1985; **6**: 921–9.
14. Muir, A.L., Hannan, W.J., Sapru, R.P., Boardman, A.K., Wraith, P.K. and Brash, H.M. The effects of isoprenaline, atropine & dobutamine on ventricular volume curves obtained by radionuclide ventriculography. *Clin. Sci.* 1980; **58**: 357–64.
15. Bacharach, S.L., Green, M.V., Vitale, D., White, G., Douglas, M.A., Bonow, R.V. and Larson, S.M. Optimal filtering of cardiac data: a minimum-error method. *J. Nucl. Med.* 1983; **24**: 1176–84.
16. Manyari, D.E. and Kostuk, W.J. Left and right ventricular function at rest and during bicycle exercise in the supine and sitting positions in normal subjects and patients with coronary artery disease. *Am. J. Cardiol.* 1983; **51**: 36–42.
17. Bodenheimer, M.M., Banka, V.S., Fooshee, C.M., Gillespie, J.A. and Helfant, R.H. Detection of coronary heart disease

using radionuclide determined regional ejection fraction at rest and during handgrip exercise; comparison with coronary arteriography. *Circulation* 1978; 58: 640–8.

18. Vojacek, J., Hannan, W.J. and Muir, A.L. Ventricular response to dynamic exercise and the cold pressor test. *Eur. Heart. J.* 1982; 3: 211–22.

19. Stone, D., Dymond, D., Elliott, A.T., Britton, K.E., Spurrel, R.A.J. and Banim, S.O. Use of first-pass radionuclide ventriculography in assessment of wall motion abnormalities induced by incremental atrial pacing in patients with coronary artery disease. *Br. Heart J.* 1980; 43: 369–75.

20. Sapru, R.P., Muir, A.L., Hannan, W.J., Smith, H.J., Brash, H.M. and Wraith, P.K. Effect of exercise and isoprenaline on left ventricular ejection fraction in patients with angina pectoris as assessed by radionuclide angiography. *Cardiology* 1982; 69: 91–7.

21. Borer, J.S., Kent, K.M., Bacharach, S.L., Green, M.V., Rosing, D.R., Seides, S.F., Epstein, S.E. and Johnston, G.S. Sensitivity, specificity and predictive accuracy of radionuclide cineangiography during exercise in patients with coronary artery disease: comparison with exercise electrocardiography. *Circulation* 1979; 60: 572–80.

22. Berman, D.S., Maddahi, J., Garcia, E.V., Freeman, M.R., Shah, P.K. Assessment of left and right ventricular function with multiple gated equilibrium cardiac blood pool scintigraphy. In: *Clinical Nuclear Cardiology*. Berman, D.S. and Mason, D.R., eds. New York: Grune & Stratton, 1981, p. 248.

23. Dehmer, G.D., Falkoff, M., Lewis, S.E., Hillis, L.D., Parkey, R.W. and Willerson, J.T. Effect of oral propranolol on rest and exercise, left ventricular ejection fraction, volumes and segmental wall motion in patients with angina pectoris: assessment with equilibrium blood pool. *Br. Heart J.* 1981; 45: 656–66.

24. Steele, P.P., Rainwater, J. and Jensen, D. Isosorbide dinitrate-induced improvement in left ventricular ejection fraction during exercise in coronary artery disease. *Chest* 1978; 74: 526–30.

25. Johnson, L.L., McCarthy, D.M., Sciacca, R.R. and Cannon, P.J. Right ventricular ejection fraction during exercise in patients with coronary artery disease. *Circulation* 1979; 60: 1284–300.

26. De Pace, N.L., Hakki, A.H., Wenreich, D.J. and Iskandrian, A.S. Non-invasive assessment of extent of coronary artery disease. *Am. J. Cardiol.* 1983; 52: 714–20.

27. Iskandrian, A.S., Hakki, A.H., Goel, I.P., Mundth, E.D., Kane-Marsch, S.A. and Schenk, C.L. The use of rest and exercise radionuclide ventriculography in risk stratification in patients with suspected coronary artery disease. *Am. Heart J.* 1985; 110: 865–72.

28. Iskandrian, A.S. and Hakki, A.H. Radionuclide evaluation of exercise left ventricular performance in patients with coronary artery disease. *Am. Heart J.* 1985; 110: 851–6.

29. Reduto, L.A., Berger, H.J., Cohen, L.S., Gottchalk, A. and Zaret, B.L. Sequential radionuclide assessment of left and right ventricular performance after acute myocardial infarction. *Ann. Intern. Med.* 1978; 89: 441–7.

30. Dewhurst, N.G. and Muir, A.L. Comparative prognostic value of radionuclide ventriculography at rest and during exercise in 100 patients after first myocardial infarction. *Br. Heart J.* 1983; 49: 111–21.

31. Ong, L., Green, S., Reiser, P. and Morrison, J. Early prediction of mortality in patients with acute myocardial infarction: a prospective study of clinical and radionuclide risk factors. *Am. J. Cardiol.* 1986; 57: 33–8.

32. Buda, A.J. Dubbin, J.D., Meindok, H. Radionuclide assessment of regional left ventricular function in acute myocardial infarction. *Am. Heart J.* 1986; 111: 36–41.

33. Res, J.C., Simoons, M.L., Van der Wall, E.E., Eenige, M.J., Vermeer, F., Verheugt, F.W.A., Wijns, W., Braar, S., Remme, W.J., Surruys, P.W. and Roos, J.P. Long term improvement in global left ventricular function after early thrombolytic therapy in acute myocardial infarction. *Br. Heart J.* 1986; 56: 414–21.

34. Rodrigues, E.A., Dewhurst, N.G., Smart, L.M., Hannan, W.J. and Muir, A.L. Diagnosis and prognosis of right ventricular infarction. *Br. Heart J.* 1986; 56: 19–26.

35. Betocchi, S., Bonow, R.V., Bacharach, S.K., Rosing, D.R., Maron, B.J. and Green, M.V. Isovolumic relaxation period in hypertrophic cardiomyopathy: assessment by radionuclide angiography. *J. Am. Coll. Cardiol.* 1986; 7: 74–81.

36. Lumia, F.J., MacMillan, R.M., Germon, P.A., Kornberg, B., Fernandez, J. and Maranhao, V. Rest-exercise radionuclide angiographic assessment of left ventricular function in chronic aortic regurgitation: significance of serial studies in medically versus surgically treated groups. *Clin. Cardiol.* 1985; 465–76.

37. Fisher, B.M., Gillen, G., Lindop, G.B.M., Dargie, H.J. and Frier, B.M. Cardiac function and coronary arteriography in asymptomatic Type 1 (insulin-dependent) diabetic patients: evidence for a specific diabetic heart disease. *Diabetologia* 1986; 29: 706–12.

38. Forfar, J.C., Muir, A.L., Sawers, S.A. and Toft, A.D. Abnormal left ventricular ejection fraction in hyperthyroidism: evidence for a possible reversible cardiomyopathy. *N. Engl. J. Med.* 1982; 307: 1165–70.

39. MacNee, W., Morgan, A.D., Wathen, C.G., Muir, A.L. and Flenley, D.C. Right ventricular performance during exercise in chronic obstructive pulmonary disease: the effects of oxygen. *Respiration* 1985; 48: 206–15.

40. Alexander, J., Daniak, N., Berger, H.J., Goldman, L., Johnstone, D., Reduto, L., Duffy, T., Schwarz, P., Gottschalk, A. and Zaret, B.L. Serial assessment of duxorubicin cardiotoxicity with quantitative radionuclide angiography. *N. Engl. J. Med.* 1979; 300: 278–83.

41. Underwood, S.R., Walton, S., Laming, P.J., Jarritt, P.H., Ell, P.J., Emanuel, R.W. and Swanton, R.H. Left ventricular volume and ejection fraction determined by gated blood pool emission tomography. *Br. Heart J.* 1985; 53: 216–22.

42. Wathen, C.G., Hannan, W.J., Adie, C.J. and Muir, A.J. A radionuclide method for the simultaneous study of the effects of drugs on central and peripheral haemodynamics. *Br. J. Clin. Pharmacol.* 1983; 16: 45–50.

43. Pohost, G.M., Alpert, N.A., Ingwall, J.S. and Strauss, H.W. Thallium-201 redistribution: mechanisms and clinical utility. *Semin. Nucl. Med.* 1980; 10: 70–93.

44. Gehring, P.J. and Hammond, P.B. The interrelationship between thallium and potassium in animals. *J. Pharmacol. Exp. Ther.* 1967; 55: 187.

45. Weich, H.F., Strauss, H.W. and Pitt, B. The extraction of thallium-201 by the myocardium. *Circulation* 1977; 56: 188–91.

46. Wilson, R.A., Sullivan, P.J., Okada, R.D., Boucher, C.A., Morris, C., Pohost, G.M. and Strauss, H.W. The effect of eating on thallium myocardial imaging. *Chest* 1986; 89: 195–8.

47. Tono-oka, I., Satoh, S., Kanaya, T., Komatani, A., Takahashi, K., Tsuiki, K. and Yasui, S. Alterations in myocardial perfusion during exercise after isosorbide dinitrate infusion in patients with coronary disease: assessment by thallium-201 scintigraphy. *Am. Heart J.* 1986; 111: 525–32.

48. Uthurralt, N., Parodi, O., Severi, S., Davies, G.J. and Maseri, A. Thallium-201 scintigraphy for diagnosis of old myocardial infarction: comparison with electrocardiographic, ventriculographic and coronary arteriographic findings. *Br. Heart J.* 1980; 43: 527–34.

49. Leppo, J., Boucher, C.A., Okada, R.D., Newell, J.B., Strauss, H.W. and Pohost, G.M. Serial thallium-201 myocardial imaging after dipyridamole infusion: diagnostic utility in detecting coronary stenoses and relation to regional

wall motion. *Circulation* 1982; **66**: 649–57.

50. Walker, P.R., James, M.A., Wilde, R.P.H., Wood, C.H. and Rees, J.R. Dipyridamole combined with exercise for thallium-201 myocardial imaging. *Br. Heart J.* 1986; **55**: 321–9.

51. Vantrain, K.P., Berman, D.S., Garcia, E.V., Berger, H.J., Sands, M.J., Friedman, J.D., Freeman, M.R., Pryzlak, M., Ashburn, W.L., Norris, S.L., Green, A.M. and Maddahi, J. Quantitative analysis of stress thallium-201 myocardial scintigrams: a multicenter trial. *J. Nucl. Med.* 1986; **27**: 17–25.

52. Wolfe, C.L., Jansen, D.E., Corbett, J.R., Lipscomb, K., Gabliani, G., Filipchuk, N., Redish, G., Lewis, S.E. and Willerson, J.T. Determination of left ventricular mass using single photon emission computed tomography. *Am. J. Cardiol.* 1985; **56**: 761–4.

53. DePasquale, E.E., Nody, A.C., DePuey, E.G., Garcia, E.V., Pilcher, G., Bredlau, C., Roubin, G., Gober, A., Gruentzig, A., d'Amato, P. and Berger, H.J. Quantitative rotational thallium-201 tomography for identifying and localizing coronary artery disease. *Circulation* 1988; **77**: 316–27.

54. Liu, P., Kiess, M., Okada, R.D., Strauss, H.W., Block, P.C., Pohost, G.M. and Boucher, C.A. Increased thallium lung uptake after exercise in isolated left anterior descending coronary artery disease. *Am. J. Cardiol.* 1985; **55**: 1469–73.

55. Bingham, J.B., McKusik, M.A., Strauss, H.W., Boucher, C.A. and Pohost, G.M. Influence of coronary artery disease on pulmonary uptake of thallium-201. *Am. J. Cardiol.* 1980; **46**: 821–6.

56. Kaul, S., Boucher, C.A., Newell, J.B., Chesler, D.A., Greenberg, J.M., Okada, R.D., Strauss, H.W., Dinsmore, R.E. and Pohost, G.M. Determination of the quantitative thallium imaging variables that optimize detection of coronary artery disease. *J. Am. Coll. Cardiol.* 1986; **7**: 527–37.

57. Berman, D.S., Garcia, E.V. and Maddahi, J. Thallium 201 myocardial scintigraphy in the detection and evaluation of coronary artery disease. In: Berman, D.S. and Mason, D.T., eds *Clinical Nuclear Cardiology*. New York: Grune & Stratton, 1981, p. 87.

58. Dash, H., Massie, B.M., Botvinick, E.H. and Brundage, B.H. The non-invasive identification of left main and three vessel coronary artery disease by myocardial stress perfusion scintigraphy and treadmill exercise electro-cardiography. *Circulation* 1979; **60**: 276–84.

59. Maseri, A., Parodi, O. and Severi, S. Transient transmural reduction of myocardial blood flow, demonstrated by thallium-201 scintigraphy, as a cause of variant angina. *Circulation* 1976; **54**: 280–8.

60. Pfisterer, M., Muller-Brand, J., Brundler, H. and Cueri, T. Prevalence and significance of reversible radionuclide ischaemic perfusion defects in symptomatic patients with or without concomitant coronary disease. *Am. Heart J.* 1982; **103**: 92–6.

61. Gaffney, F.A., Wohl, A.J., Blomqvist, C.G., Parkey, R.W. and Willerson, J.T. Thallium-201 myocardial perfusion studies in patients with mitral valve prolapse syndrome. *Am. J. Med.* 1978; **64**: 21–26.

62. Huikuri, H., Korkonen, U.R., Heikhila, J. and Takhunen, J.T. Detection of coronary artery disease by thallium scintigraphy in patients with valvular heart disease. *Br. Heart J.* 1986; **56**: 146–51.

63. Khalil, M.N., Thornback, J., Early, M.Y., Morton, D.B., Berry, J.M. and Hubner, P.J.B. Technetium-99m isonitrile complex as a potential myocardial imaging agent. *Nucl. Med. Commun.* 1985; **6**: 615–22.

64. Piwnica-Worms, D., Kronauge, J.F., Holman, B.L., Lister-James, J., Davison, A. and Jones, A.G. Hexakis (Carbomethoxyisopropylisonitrile) technetium (I), a new myocardial perfusion imaging agent: binding characteristics in cultured chick heart cells. *J. Nucl. Med.* 1988; **29**: 55–61.

65. Botvincik, E.H., O'Connell, W.J., Dae, M.W., Hattner, R.S. and Schechtmann, N.M. Analysis of thallium-201 'washout' from parametric colour coded images. *J. Nucl. Med.* 1988; **29**: 302–10.

66. Ashburn, W.L., Braunwald, E., Simon, A.L., Peterson, K.L. and Gault, J.H. Myocardial perfusion imaging with radionuclide labelled particles injected directly into the coronary circulation of patients with coronary artery disease. *Circulation* 1971; **44**: 851–65.

67. Cannon, P.J., Dell, R.B. and Dwyer, E.M. Measurement of regional myocardial perfusion in man with 133 xenon and a scintillation camera. *J. Clin. Invest.* 1972; **51**: 964–77.

68. Bergmann, S.R., Fox, K.A.A., Geltman, E.M. and Sobel, B.G. Positron emission tomography of the heart. *Prog. Cardiovasc. Dis.* 1985; **28**: 165–94.

69. Styles, C.B., Noujaim, A.A., Jugdutt, B.I., Sykes, T.R. and Turner, C. Omega-iodo fatty acid scintigraphy: what are we measuring. *Eur. Heart J.* 1985; **6**(suppl B): 103–4.

70. Bonte, F.J., Parkey, R.W., Graham, K.D., Moore, J. and Stokely, E.M. A new method of radionuclide imaging of myocardial infarcts. *Radiology* 1974; **110**: 473–4.

71. Shen, A.C. and Jennings, R.B. Myocardial calcium and magnesium in acute ischaemic injury. *Am. J. Pathol.* 1972; **67**: 412–40.

72. Willerson, J.T., Parkey, R.W., Buja, M.L., Lewis, S.E. and Bonte, F.J. Detection of acute myocardial infarcts using myocardial scintigraphy techniques. In: Parkey, R.W., Bonte, J.F., Buja, M.L. and Willerson, J.T., eds, *Clinical Nuclear Cardiology*. New York: Appleton, 1979, p. 141.

73. Berman, D.S., Amsterdam, E.A., Hines, H.H., Selel, A.F., Bailey, G.J., Denardo, G.L. and Mason, D.T. New approach to interpretation of technetium pyrophosphate scintigraphy in detection of acute myocardial infarction. *Am. J. Cardiol.* 1977; **39**: 341–6.

74. Tamaki, S., Kadota, K., Kambara, H., Suzuki, Y., Nohara, R., Murakami, T., Kawai, C., Tamaki, N. and Torizuka, K. Emission computed tomography with technetium-99m pyrophosphate for delineating location and size of acute myocardial infarction in man. *Br. Heart J.* 1984; **52**: 30–7.

75. Go, R.T., Doty, D.B., Chiu, C.L. and Christie, J. A new method of diagnosing myocardial contusion in man by radionuclide imaging. *Radiology* 1975; **116**: 107–10.

76. Donsky, M.S., Curry, G.C., Parkey, R.W., Meyer, S.L., Bonte, F.J., Willerson, J.T. and Platt, M.R. Unstable angina pectoris. Clinical, angiographic and myocardial scintigraphic observations. *Br. Heart J.* 1976; **38**: 257–63.

77. McGregor, C.G.A., Muir, A.L., Smith, A.F., Miller, H.C., Hannan, W.J. and Cameron, E.W.J. Myocardial infarction related to coronary artery by pass graft surgery. *Br. Heart J.* 1984; **51**: 399–406.

78. Khaw, B.A., Strauss, H.W., Pohost, G.M., Fallon, J.T., Katus, H.A. and Haber, E. Relations of immediate and delayed thallium-201 distribution to localization of ^{125}I-antimyosin antibody in acute experimental myocardial infarction. *Am. J. Cardiol.* 1983; **51**: 1428–32.

79. Bell, D., Jackson, M., Millar, A.M., Nicoll, J.J., Connell, M. and Muir, A.L. The acute inflammatory response to myocardial infarction: imaging with indium-111 labelled autologous neutrophils. *Br. Heart J.* 1987; **57**: 23–7.

80. Neumann, R.D., Sostman, H.D. and Gottschalk, A. Current status of ventilation–perfusion imaging. *Semin. Nucl. Med.* 1980; **10**: 198–217.

81. Rootwelt, K. and Vale, J.R. Pulmonary gas exchange after intravenous injection of ^{99m}Tc-sulphur-colloid albumin macroaggregates for lung perfusion scintigraphy. *Scand. J. Clin. Lab. Invest.* 1972; **30**: 14–21.

82. Vincent, W.R., Goldberg, S.J. and Desilets, D. Fatality immediately following rapid infusion of macroaggregates of ^{99m}Tc-albumin (MAA) for lung scan. *Radiology* 1968; **91**: 1181–4.

83. Hannan, W.J., Emmett, P.C., Aitken, R.J., Love, R.G., Millar, A.M. and Muir, A.L. Effective penetration of lung periphery using radioactive aerosols. *J. Nucl. Med.* 1982; **23**: 872–7.

84. Muir, A.L., Adie, C.J., Kirby, T.P., Bell, D., Brash, H.M. and Hannan, W.J. Regional tidal volume assessed by gated lung imaging. *Nucl. Med. Commun.* 1985; **6**: 127–39.

85. McNeil, B.J. A diagnostic strategy using ventilation–perfusion studies in patients suspect for pulmonary embolism. *J. Nucl. Med.* 1976; **17**: 613–6.

86. Biello, D.R., Mattar, A.G., Osei-Wusu, A., Alderson, P.O., McNeil, B.J. and Siegel, B.A. Interpretation of indeterminate lung scintigrams. *Radiology* 1979; **133**: 189–94.

APPENDIX
Units used in nuclear medicine.

The unit of activity is one disintegration per second – the becquerel (1 Bq = 1 s^{-1})

The obsolete unit of activity is the curie (Ci)

$$1 \text{ Ci} = 3.7 \times 10^{10} \text{ Bq}$$
$$1 \text{ Bq} = 2.7 \times 10^{-11} \text{ Ci}$$

The dose-equivalent is the sievert (Sv)

This replaces the rem (rem)

$$1 \text{ Sv} = 100 \text{ rem}$$

Chapter 20

Exercise Testing

O. Odemuyiwa and R.J.C. Hall

In this chapter, the normal cardiovascular response to upright exercise, the methods available for exercise testing and the interpretation of exercise tests in patients with cardiovascular disease are addressed.

PHYSIOLOGY

The energy for muscular contraction comes directly from the breakdown of ATP but there are only 5 mmol of ATP stored in each kg of muscle,[1] enough to maintain intense exercise for only a few seconds. It follows that if exercise is to be sustained the ATP sources in muscle have to be continually replenished. The rise in intracellular ADP when ATP is broken down stimulates oxidative phosphorylation during which nutrients are oxidized in the mitochondria. The electrons released are passed down the respiratory chain, more ATP is formed, and the electrons finally combine with hydrogen to form water. The function of the cardiorespiratory system is to maintain the supply of oxygen and nutrients to contracting muscle and to remove carbon dioxide, heat and metabolites from the immediate vicinity for detoxification, recycling or excretion. Only 50% of respiratory capacity is necessary to respond to light or moderately heavy workloads[2] so normal respiratory function ordinarily places no limitations on exercise tolerance. Therefore, we shall concentrate on the cardiovascular response to exercise.

THE NEUROVASCULAR RESPONSE TO EXERCISE

During exercise, unmyelinated endings in the mechanical and chemical receptors situated in skeletal muscle are activated and the afferent signals are received in the medulla (by the vasomotor centre) and in the hypothalamus.[3,4] This results in an increase in efferent sympathetic traffic to the cell bodies of the preganglionic neurons in proportion to the speed and force of muscle contraction.[5] Accompanying this reflex outflow is an anticipatory sympathetic response which probably starts in the higher centres and ends directly, or via the medulla, on the preganglionic neurons. Postganglionic neurons release noradrenaline at the target organ whose response depends on the particular combination of specialized adrenergic receptors which it possesses. The stimulation of cardiac beta-1 adrenergic receptors increases heart rate and cardiac contractility; the latter is reflected in a smaller left ventricular end-systolic volume and an increased stroke volume. The greatest increase in stroke volume occurs at the transition from mild to moderate exertion but, as exercise becomes more intense, so increases in heart rate become a more important mechanism for increasing cardiac output. Cardiac output (which is usually around 5 l/min at rest) may reach 40 l/min during exercise and is sustained because arterial baroreceptors are reset at a higher level.[6] Moreover, the stretch on special cardiac and pulmonary mechanoreceptors is reduced during exercise. Their normal inhibitory input to the vasomotor centre is reduced, thereby further reinforcing the sympathetic outflow.

Unlike the heart, the cell walls of vascular smooth muscle are rich in alpha-1 adrenergic receptors. Unopposed stimulation of these receptors by noradrenaline results in vasoconstriction, but during exercise vasoconstriction is most marked in the relatively inactive splanchnic and renal beds whereas in the muscles other competing influences lead to a marked vasodilatation. Only about 3% of muscle capillaries are open at rest,[7] but at the onset of exercise other capillaries open up in proportion to the force of muscular contraction. This vasodilation (exercise hyperaemia) is in part mediated by the action of adrenaline on the beta-2 adrenergic receptors in the vessel wall. Adrenaline is released by the postganglionic stimulation of the adrenal medulla and it in turn releases more noradrenaline from terminal sympathetic neurons. Adrenaline also increases venous return by increasing the tone of the capacitance vessels.[8] Exercise hyperaemia may also be mediated via sympathetic vasodilator fibres which originate in the higher centres, bypass the vasomotor centre and travel with adrenergic fibres to the target organs.[9] An increase in local temperature, and a rise in the concentration of substances such as histamine, prostaglandins, H^+ ions and metabolites[10-12] also help to maintain exercise hyperaemia. The onset and duration of exercise hyperaemia may also depend on the type, duration and intensity of exercise and probably on the predominant type of muscle involved in the exercise. Vessel wall tone and stiffness may also be important in conditions such as chronic heart failure in which oedema and the content of sodium and calcium ions in the vessel wall could interfere with vasodilation. Exercise hyperaemia increases the exchange of nutrients between blood and tissue whereas the vasoconstriction in other tissues serves to redistribute blood to the active muscles. Redistribution alone has been estimated to direct an extra 2 l of blood per minute to the skeletal muscles, equivalent to about 500 ml of oxygen per minute.[13] Overall, muscle blood flow can increase from 4–7 ml/100 g at rest (15% of cardiac output) to as much as 75 ml/100 g during severe exercise (80% of cardiac output). Conversely, renal blood flow falls from 1100 ml/min at rest (20% of cardiac output) to 250 ml/min during intense exercise (about 1% of cardiac output). Skin blood flow also falls during severe exertion.

About 200 ml of oxygen are carried in every 1000 ml of blood; 50 ml of which is extracted at rest but nearly all of which is extracted during very severe exertion. Therefore, there is a potential threefold increase in aerobic work capacity simply by increasing oxygen extraction. An increase in muscle myoglobin content, capillary density, the size and number of mitochondria and anaerobic enzyme activity have been found in trained subjects,[14] but Saltin and Gollnick estimated that the potential capacity of the aerobic enzyme systems far outstrips the maximum oxygen consumed during exercise.[15] It is therefore unlikely that the extraction of oxygen by the tissues is an important limitation to exertion, at least not during normal daily activity.

At the cellular and molecular level, the local increases in temperature, Pco_2 and acidity result in a shift of the oxygen dissociation curve to the right (Bohr effect) reducing the affinity of haemoglobin for oxygen and helping the extraction of oxygen by the tissues. The affinity of haemoglobin for oxygen is also reduced by the attachment of 2,3-diphosphoglyceric acid, formed during red cell glycolysis, to sub-units of the haemoglobin molecule. Myoglobin, the iron-containing pigment protein, surrenders oxygen at a much lower Po_2 (around 5 mmHg) then haemoglobin and so serves as a reservoir of oxygen for use during prolonged exertion.

METABOLIC CHANGES IN EXERCISE

Most of the fuel oxidized by skeletal muscle for energy at rest is free fatty acid. In steady, moderately severe exercise, such as jogging, the replacement of ATP is met by glycogenolysis—the full combustion of the carbohydrates provided from the breakdown of muscle glycogen stores. A small amount of lactate is formed during these reactions, but it does not accumulate because its rate of disposal remains faster than its rate of production. As exercise progresses, fatty acids become more important sources of energy. During severe exercise, as the requirements for oxygen outstrip its supply or utilization, glycolysis becomes the main and most rapid means of replacing ATP. Glycolysis provides only 5% of the ATP produced by the complete mitochondrial oxidation of carbohydrates, but this is compensated for by the high concentration and activity of the cytoplasmic enzymes. The H^+ ions produced are transferred to pyruvate to form lactate. This reaction, without which glycolysis will stop, is catalysed by lactate dehydrogenase and frees NADH for the oxidation of phosphoglyceraldehyde earlier in the glycolytic chain. The point at which lactate begins to accumulate reflects predominantly anaerobic work. Lactate has a low dissociation constant readily releasing H^+ ions which are then buffered by HCO_3^-. The detection of the extra carbon dioxide formed from this buffering over and above the normal respiratory production of carbon dioxide forms the basis for the determination of the *anaerobic threshold*.[16,17]

The onset and degree of lactic acidaemia during exercise is multifactorial, and will vary with the blood supply to the working muscles, the size of glycogen stores, the intensity of exercise and, to a lesser extent, oxygen utilization. The type of muscle involved in a particular form of exercise may also affect lactic acidaemia. The fast twitch (type II) muscle fibres perform phasic contractions, are rich in glycolytic enzymes and therefore generate more lactic acid than the slow twitch (type I) muscle fibres which perform tonic postural reactions and are rich in oxidative enzymes. In fast vigorous exercise, lactate levels are higher than in slow gentle exertion.[18] The accumulation of lactate may be partly responsible for fatigue by altering intracellular pH and enzyme activity and slowing down the production of ATP.

CARDIAC METABOLISM DURING EXERCISE

The heart is unique because it has a limited capacity for anaerobic metabolism, its main sources of ATP being glucose, fatty acids and lactate. During exercise, the utilization of lactate increases by about three times as much as does the use of glucose and fatty acids, but fatty acids still supply up to 70% of the energy requirement. This is because one molecule of fatty acid yields 463 molecules of ATP compared with the 36 molecules of ATP formed from one molecule of glucose. The coronary blood flow at rest is 60 ml/100 g/min or 200–250 ml/min (5% of cardiac output) with an arteriovenous oxygen extraction ratio of between 70 and 80%. As heart rate and contractility increase, so does the myocardial oxygen demand. The myocardial oxygen consumption is also increased in direct proportion to chamber diameter, wall tension and speed of circumferential fibre shortening.

The basal myocardial oxygen extraction is very high, but cardiac muscle, unlike skeletal muscle, cannot increase oxygen extraction much more and, therefore, increases in oxygen requirement during exercise have to be met by an increase in coronary blood flow. Coronary flow is proportional to the fourth power of the radius of the coronary arteries and to the pressure difference between the aorta and the left ventricular cavity in diastole during which most coronary flow occurs. Coronary vasodilatation results from an increase in the concentration of metabolites, such as adenosine,[19] and from the activation of cholinergic sympathetic nerves. Coronary blood flow is also increased by the rise in aortic pressure. Together these adaptations can increase coronary blood flow 300% to 240 ml/100 g/min. Sympathetic-mediated vasoconstriction of the coronary arteries also occurs during exercise; this is more marked during isometric than during isotonic exercise,[20] and the extent to which it limits the magnitude of coronary vasodilatation during exercise is unknown.

As there is a linear relationship between myocar-dial oxygen consumption and the product of systolic blood pressure and heart rate (the rate–pressure product or 'double product') this is often used as a non-invasive estimate of myocardial oxygen consumption.[21,22] When coronary artery stenoses limit coronary reserve, cardiac ischaemia can occur during exercise. This may be manifested as angina pectoris, ST-segment depression or elevation, hypotension or by the abnormal release of lactate, potassium, adrenaline and other myocardial constituents.

CLINICAL

INDICATIONS FOR EXERCISE TESTING[23,24]

This section outlines the role of exercise tests. Aspects of exercise testing unique to particular clinical situations are discussed under appropriate sections elsewhere.

In patients with suspected angina, exercise testing may confirm the diagnosis of ischaemic heart disease and indicate the severity and prognostic importance of coronary artery lesions. In patients with definite ischaemic heart disease, the exercise test may be used to follow the progression of disease and the effect of therapy including drugs, angioplasty or coronary artery surgery. Following myocardial infarction, exercise testing is performed to allow risk stratification; patients identified as being at low risk for death or re-infarction can be reassured and those at high risk can be managed appropriately.

In specific groups, such as pilots, the exercise test is sometimes used to screen for asymptomatic coronary artery disease. This approach, however, is not considered appropriate for screening large numbers of asymptomatic subjects because of the high proportion of false-positive tests obtained from such a population (see below). Exercise tests are also used to establish the functional capacity of subjects who wish to participate in strenuous sport or take up regular exercise after a long period of inactivity.

The functional capacity of patients in chronic heart failure can be assessed by exercise testing and, occasionally, may be extended to patients with valve disease, especially mitral, particularly when there is a discrepancy between the patient's symptoms and the clinical and laboratory findings. Patients whose hypertension is well controlled at rest but who are likely to engage in vigorous sport are sometimes exercised formally to see whether there is a dangerous rise in blood pressure. Similarly, after surgery for coarctation of the aorta, an exaggerated rise in blood pressure in exercise may identify patients who will require antihypertensive therapy.

Occasionally, exercise testing may be clinically helpful as a means of provoking arrhythmias and in assessing sino-atrial function and may even assist in the choice of pacemaker for the individual patient.

CONTRA-INDICATIONS TO EXERCISE TESTING

Exercise testing is absolutely contra-indicated in the presence of any acute illness, for example, myocarditis, pericarditis or pneumonia, nor should exercise testing be performed in patients with severe aortic stenosis, untreated life-threatening arrhythmias, severe congestive cardiac failure or unstable angina.

Relative contra-indications to exercise testing include moderate aortic stenosis and severe hypertension. Certain features of the resting electrocardiogram may render the test uninterpretable, e.g. digoxin effects, left bundle branch block, frequent ventricular ectopic beats, hypokalaemia and Wolff–Parkinson–White syndrome (see Table 20.2), and as such may make exercise testing pointless.

METHOD

In patients with coronary heart disease, cardiac ischaemia often limits exercise before the maximum potential is reached.

In the past, exercise tests were carried out using Master's two-step protocol.[25] This had the advantage of needing little or no special equipment but was not stressful enough for diagnostic use in many patients. The bicycle ergometer and the motorized treadmill are now the most widely used means for exercise testing. The former is cheap, small and the ECG recordings are of high quality because there is minimal motion artefact. The patient's energy output can be predicted more accurately and is less dependent on bodyweight than treadmill exercise. The work rate can be pre-selected but the oxygen uptake varies with pedal speed. In some bicycles, the product of pedal speed and resistance is kept constant but should the subject tire and slow down there is a disconcerting rise in pedal resistance which may force a premature end to the test. The maximum rate–pressure products achieved with the bicycle are in a similar range to those achieved with the treadmill but the highest rate–pressure products

are seen with the latter.[26] Many patients find bicycle exercise awkward and unfamiliar, and pain and fatigue in the quadriceps muscle may precede the onset of cardiac symptoms. The motorized treadmill involves activity which is similar to that which usually produces the patient's symptoms, i.e. walking, and the workload can easily be regulated. In clinical practice, using either the bicycle ergometer or treadmill, uninterrupted exercise is performed under steadily increasing workloads until a particular endpoint is reached. In a maximal test, this endpoint is the patient's maximal ability to exercise until stopped usually by fatigue, shortness of breath or chest pain. The test may be stopped earlier in the interest of the patient's safety. A submaximal test is stopped when the subject reaches a pre-defined target, such as 85% of maximum predicted heart rate or a particular duration of exercise (Table 20.1). Submaximal tests are usually performed in the elderly, unfit or early after myocardial infarction.

Exercise tests in patients with suspected cardiac disease should be supervised by a doctor and an assistant, both of whom should be familiar with cardiopulmonary resuscitation and remain in attendance until the end of the recovery phase.

The room should be large enough for adequate resuscitation and must be equipped with a defibrillator. A properly maintained cardiac resuscitation trolley must be available. Patients can walk barefoot or in comfortable low-heeled shoes. They should be sensibly clothed so that they are neither shivering nor too hot. No smoking is allowed on the day of the test and no meals or sublingual glyceryl trinitrate should be taken within 2 h of the test, but routine medication can be taken unless stated otherwise.

Some clinicians stop anti-anginal medication before the exercise test to reduce the chance of a false-negative result, but in some patients this may

Table 20.1. Table of approximate age-predicted maximal heart rate (220 beats/min – age in years) Figures in parentheses represent 85% of the maximum heart rate.

Age (years)	Male	Female
20–29	200 (170)	195 (166)
30–39	190 (162)	186 (158)
40–49	180 (153)	178 (150)
50–59	170 (145)	166 (141)
60–69	160 (136)	157 (134)
70–79	150 (128)	148 (126)
80–	140 (120)	138 (117)

result in unstable angina or even myocardial infarction, especially when beta-blockers are stopped abruptly.[27,28] This is more likely to occur in patients whose angina was severe before treatment was started. The safer alternative is to exercise the patient while taking medication and then, if the results on therapy are equivocal, repeat the exercise test off medication. The patient should arrive at least 15 min before the test is scheduled to start to allow for a rest, explanation and a quick history and examination. A few questions will help to relax the patient and corroborate the medical history, including events such as recent myocardial infarction or unstable angina which may modify or contra-indicate exercise testing. This interview also provides some idea of the patient's usual physical activity and probable exercise tolerance.

An examination should exclude severe aortic valve disease, an absolute contra-indication to exercise testing. The patient is asked to exercise to the best of his ability with the reassurance that the test will be stopped as soon as the request is made to do so.

The patient is stripped to the waist. The areas of electrode placement are shaved if necessary and then rubbed with fine grounded sandpaper to remove the upper horny layer of the epidermis so that better contact is made between the electrolyte

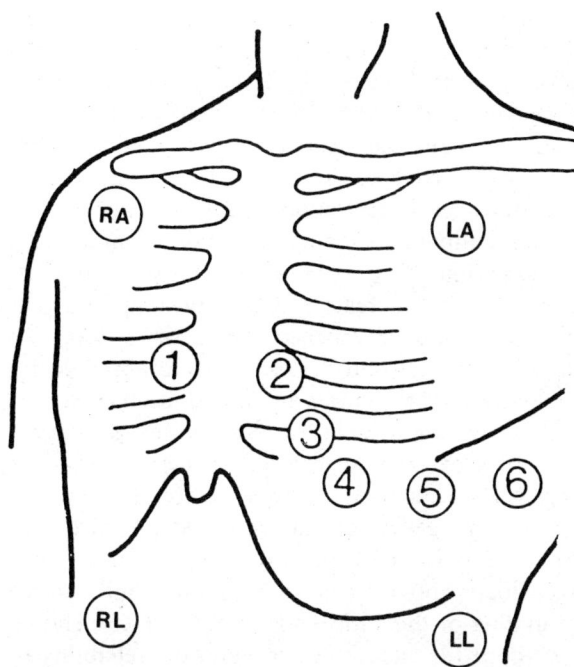

Fig. 20.2. The modified Mason and Liker 12-lead system. The limb leads can be placed on either the front or the back of the chest.

paste in the electrodes and the better conducting lower layers of the skin. Skin adhesiveness is increased by rubbing the same areas with light gauze soaked in isopropyl alcohol. Lightweight silver electrodes are then attached to the skin as dictated by the particular lead system employed (Figs 20.1 and 20.2). The electrodes can be further secured by applying sticky tape and a tube of elastic net bandage can be pulled down over them to reduce the motion artefact.

A variety of lead systems are in use. The most popular bipolar lead placement with a single-channel recorder is lead CM_5 with the positive electrode in position V_5 and the negative electrode on the manubrium (Fig. 20.1). Leads II and CM_5 are used with a two-channel recording system and leads II, aVF and V_5 when a three-channel system is available. A modification of the Mason and Likar 12-lead system is now widely used (Fig. 20.2).[29] In this system, the precordial leads are placed in their standard locations but the limb electrodes are placed on the chest (Fig. 20.2). Although pathological Q waves in the inferior leads may be missed by this lead system, most of the recent information on exercise testing has been obtained using it; however, the resting tracing should never be used as a substitute for a standard 12-lead electrocardiogram in the routine assessment of a patient. The patient's

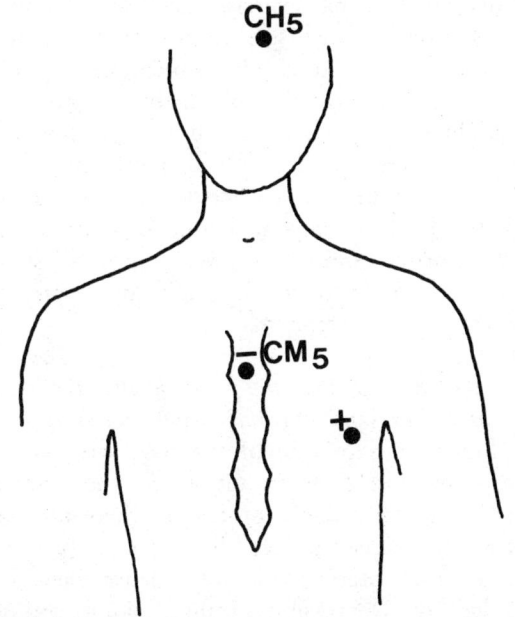

Fig. 20.1. The lead placings for bipolar systems. The positive lead is attached to the 5th intercostal space anterior axillary line and the negative electrode is placed on the manubrium (CM_5), 5th left intercostal space (CC_5), the forehead (CH_5) or the back (CA_5).

blood pressure and a 12-lead electrocardiogram should be recorded at rest, and an oscilloscopic display of at least one lead should be maintained throughout the test. When exercise starts, the patient should walk as naturally as possible, keeping to the front of the treadmill and holding the handrails gently for support while looking straight ahead. Pulling or gripping the handrail can increase exercise times and, because it is a form of isometric exercise, also increase oxygen consumption. The patient should be watched for pallor, cyanosis or signs of distress and the oscilloscope observed for arrhythmias or changes in the ST segments. The blood pressure is recorded at least once during the last 30 s of each stage of exercise but should be repeated or taken more frequently if there is a drop of 10 mmHg or more in the blood pressure. The brachial pulse may be difficult to hear at high workloads above the noise of the treadmill and the pounding of the patient's feet, and exercise should be stopped if there is doubt about the reliability or accuracy of the blood-pressure readings. In the occasional anxious patient, the blood pressure may be high at rest but shows an initial drop when exercise starts; such patients are usually recognizable from the history, increased resting heart rate and the sudden increase in heart rate that occurs as soon as exercise starts. The onset and detailed description of any chest pains should be noted, but the onset of symptoms need not necessarily mean the end of the test unless the patient asks to stop. The reason for stopping should be recorded since this may help in management. The test should be stopped immediately if the patient looks unsteady, pale, cyanosed or is distressed in any way; if the blood pressure falls by 10 mmHg or more; if there are three or more consecutive ventricular ectopic beats or frequent ventricular ectopic beats or if there is 3 mm or more of horizontal or downsloping ST-segment depression measured 0.08 s after the J point of the QRS complex. The blood pressure and a 12-lead electrocardiogram are recorded immediately after exercise, 3 min into recovery and at subsequent 2-min intervals until the electrocardiogram returns to normal and the patient is comfortable.

Auscultation of the heart is necessary if the test has been complicated by arrhythmias or hypotension and if exercise-induced left ventricular dysfunction or mitral regurgitation is being sought through the appearance of abnormal precordial bulge, third or fourth heart sounds or characteristic murmurs. Spirometry should be performed before and after exercise if exercise induced asthma is suspected.

INTERPRETATION

In interpreting an exercise test, two important questions must be answered.
1 *Is the test adequate?*
   The adequacy of the test depends on the patient's performance and the quality of recordings obtained. Exercise must be continued until it is stopped by: symptoms, such as angina or fatigue in a maximal test; the achievement of a pre-defined target in a submaximal test; or the development of diagnostic ischaemic changes. The workload is considered to place an adequate stress on the cardiovascular system if the heart rate reaches 85% of the maximum predicted heart rate and the blood pressure rises by at least 20 mmHg. The workload can be expressed as multiples of resting metabolic rate (METS) measured as oxygen consumption in ml/kg/min. One MET is equal to 3.6 ml/kg/min. Normal sedentary adults usually achieve up to 10–11 METS on exercise but 8 METS is usually enough to provoke angina in patients with important coronary artery disease.[30,31] If an exercise test does not satisfy the criteria for a positive test and the peak workload is not high enough, then that exercise test should be interpreted as inconclusive rather than negative. Until recently, exercise ECG recordings were of poor quality because of the distortion caused by baseline drift and noise from respiration and muscle tremor and electrical interference from the wire and the skin–electrode interface. Computer signal analysis, better electrodes and monitoring equipment have improved signal quality and removed a significant source of intra-observer error.[32,33]

2 *Is the test positive and what is the likelihood that it represents coronary artery disease?*
   This is perhaps one of the most contentious aspects of test interpretation. As there are as many exercise test protocols as there are patterns of exercise-induced ST-segment abnormalities, the criteria for a positive test vary considerably. Depression of the J point without significant ST-segment depression (Fig. 20.3) is a normal response to exercise and occurs most commonly in young adults. The first common pattern of abnormal ST-segment depression is

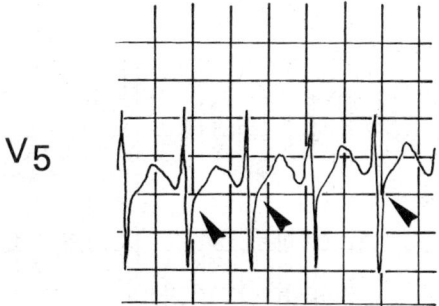

Fig. 20.3. Example of depression of the J point without significant ST-segment depression.

horizontal or downsloping whereas in the second pattern, the ST segments are upsloping (Fig. 20.4a, b). When a 12-lead system is used, the most widely accepted definition of a positive exercise test is the development of at least 1 mm of horizontal or downsloping ST-segment depression measured 0.08 s after the J point of the QRS complex. The signal amplitude is higher when lead CM_5 is used and at least 2 mm of depression is required for a positive test when using this system. The distinction between a positive test *per se* and the likelihood of coronary artery disease in the patient tested will be discussed later. Most workers accept that a 70% reduction in the cross-sectional area of a major epicardial artery (about 50% reduction in diameter) is sufficient to cause cardiac ischaemia during maximal exercise. Exercise test criteria are defined in relation to their ability to identify this degree of coronary artery stenosis.

Test characteristics

The ability of an exercise test to detect coronary artery disease, i.e. its sensitivity, is calculated from:

$$\text{Sensitivity} = \frac{TP}{TP + FN}$$

where TP stands for true positives, i.e. the number of patients with a positive test who have coronary artery disease, and FN stands for false negatives, the number of patients with a negative test but who have coronary artery disease. TP + FN is total number of patients in the sample who have coronary artery disease.

Sensitivity depends on many factors. It is higher with maximal tests than submaximal or fixed workload tests because maximal tests are more strenuous and by definition last longer. The early

Master's two-step test resulted in too many false-negative tests because often it was not stressful enough to elicit cardiac ischaemia. Single-lead systems are less sensitive than 12-lead systems.[34] Lead CM_5 was found to detect 89% of the abnormalities detected by the 12-lead system.[35] The sensitivity increases with the severity of coronary artery disease.[34] The site of disease is also important. The circumflex vessel supplies a region which is relatively electrically silent compared with the left anterior descending and right coronary arteries and there are more false negative tests in patients with isolated disease in this artery. Anti-anginal therapy, such as beta-blockade lowers sensitivity by reducing the number of positive tests.[24] Sensitivity also depends on the accuracy with which important variables are measured. For example, a consistent overestimation of the severity of coronary artery stenosis will result in an apparent increase in the number of patients with coronary artery disease and a false reduction in the sensitivity of the test.

As we shall see, the number of false-positive tests is influenced by the prevalence of coronary artery disease in the population tested, but other factors are important. Digoxin therapy is a common cause of false-positive tests and should be stopped 10–14 days before the exercise test. False-positive tests are also common in patients with mitral valve prolapse, left bundle branch block, Wolff–Parkinson–White syndrome or left ventricular hypertrophy (Table 20.2). When the diagnosis of ischaemic heart disease is uncertain in the presence of any of these conditions, a thallium exercise test is a useful alternative method because it does not depend on exercise-induced ST-segment changes.

The ability of an exercise test to identify patients without coronary artery disease, its specificity, or the probability that a patient with a negative test does not have the disease, is expressed as

$$\text{Specificity} = \frac{TN}{TN + FP}$$

Table 20.2. Common causes of false-positive exercise tests.

Digitalis
Wolff–Parkinson–White syndrome
Mitral valve prolapse
Left bundle branch block
Left ventricular hypertrophy
Right ventricular hypertrophy
Resting ST–T wave abnormalities
Hypokalaemia
Hyperventilation
Antidepressants, e.g. amitriptyline

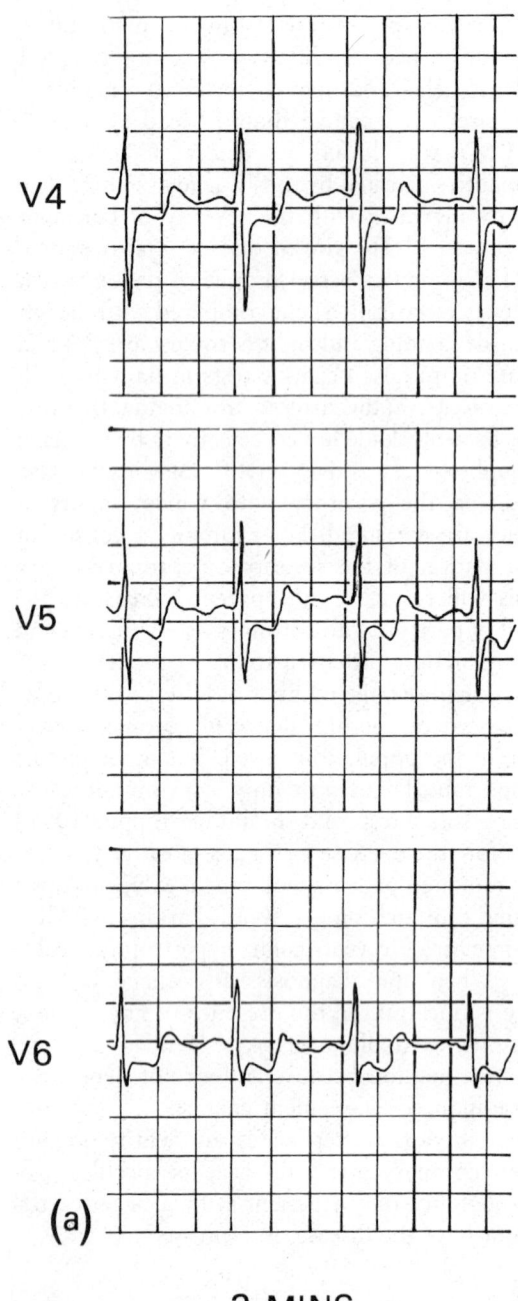

V4

V5

V6

(a)

3 MINS

V4

V5

(b)

Fig. 20.4. (a) Example of downsloping ST-segment depression 3 min into exercise. (b) Example of upsloping ST-segment depression.

where TN stands for true negative, i.e. the number of patients tested who have a negative test who do not have coronary artery disease, and FP stands for false positive, i.e. the number of patients tested who have a positive test but who do not have coronary artery disease. TN + FP is total number of patients who do not have coronary artery disease.

When the definition of a positive test is relaxed, e.g. from 1.0 to 0.5 mm of ST-segment depression, the sensitivity of the test will improve because there will be an increase in the number of true-positive tests but the number of false-positive tests will also rise so that specificity is reduced. The reverse occurs when the criteria are stricter, i.e. specificity increases and there is a fall in sensitivity. Therefore, the criterion for a positive test is a compromise between sensitivity and specificity, i.e. the test must correctly identify patients who have coronary artery disease (true positive) without an unacceptably high number of false positives. The sensitivity and specificity are unique characteristics of the test and are not influenced by the prevalence of coronary artery disease.

The predictive value of a *positive* test is the likelihood that the individual has coronary artery disease, and is calculated from the following ratio:

$$\text{Predictive value} = \frac{TP}{TP + FP}$$

Bayes *theorem of conditional probability* formally combines the sensitivity, specificity and prevalence of disease in the population tested to obtain the predictive value:[36]

$$\frac{\text{prevalence of coronary artery disease} \times \text{sensitivity}}{\text{sensitivity} \times \text{prevalence} + (1-\text{specificity}).(1-\text{prevalence})} \quad \text{(equation 20.1)}$$

If we assume that the prevalence of coronary artery disease in a group of middle-aged hypertensive cigarette-smoking diabetic males is 90% and the sensitivity of an exercise test is 70% with a specificity of 90%, then, substituting in equation 20.1, the predictive value of a positive test will be:

$$\frac{= 0.9 \times 0.7}{0.9 \times 0.7 + (1 - 0.9).(1 - 0.9)} = 98\%$$

Therefore, in a population in which the prevalence of coronary artery disease is high, the predictive value of a positive test is also very high.

Similarly, in a second hypothetical population of non-smoking young women with a disease prevalence of 2%, the predictive value of a positive test will be 12.5%. Therefore, there is a 7:1 chance that any positive test will be a false-positive test in this latter group.

In the first example, the probability that a patient with a negative test does not have coronary artery disease can also be calculated. The prevalence of negative disease is $100 - 90 = 10\%$, the test sensitivity is 90% and specificity is 70% (the reverse of a positive test). Substituting in equation 20.1 again, the predictive value is 25%, i.e. the probability that a patient with a negative exercise test in this group does not have coronary artery disease is only 25%. In the female patients, the negative predictive value of a negative test is 99%. So a negative test in this group of patients means that they almost certainly do not have coronary artery disease.

In summary, the post-test likelihood of disease (predictive value) depends on the pre-test likelihood (prevalence) of disease in the population tested or from which the patient is taken.

Exercise test analysis

The analysis of ST-segment depression alone results in unacceptably high numbers of false-positive and false-negative results especially in asymptomatic subjects.[37,38] Several attempts have been made to tackle this problem. For example, McHenry and co-workers[39] calculated an ST index by adding the mean values for the ST slope and the ST-segment depression derived from the 25 most abnormal complexes. When this sum was negative, it indicated ischaemia.

A more detailed analysis by Elamin and co-workers[40] was based on the assumption that when ST-segment depression occurs at a lower heart rate, i.e. a lower myocardial oxygen demand, it represents more severe coronary stenoses than the same degree of ST-segment depression at a higher heart rate. The steepest slope of their plot of ST-segment depression against heart rate (ST/HR slope) separated, without overlap, patients with no, single-, two- and three-vessel coronary artery disease. These results have been disputed and difficult to reproduce.[41–43] The main criticism has been the precision of their results despite the influence of such factors as the severity and location of coronary stenoses, the transmural perfusion pressure and the abundance of collateral vessels on myocardial oxygen consumption and the onset of cardiac ischaemia in the individual patient.

On a similar basis, Hollenberg et al.[44] derived a treadmill exercise score (TES) by dividing the total area of ST-segment depression in leads aVF and V_5 by the percentage of maximum predicted heart rate achieved. Detrano et al.[45] derived the heart rate-adjusted ST-segment depression by a similar approach.

In normal subjects, the degree of ST-segment depression is directly proportional to the height of the R wave,[46] but the routine correction of ST-segment depression for R-wave dimensions is unnecessary. Measuring the height of the R wave during exercise is also unnecessary, especially in patients who have no history of a myocardial infarction.[47,48] It had been suggested that an increase in the height of the R wave would reflect the increase[49] in left ventricular volume during cardiac ischaemia.

Post-infarction exercise testing

Exercise testing in patients who have had a myocardial infarction is aimed at defining patients who are at high risk of death or re-infarction. The interpretation of such tests extends beyond whether the test is 'positive' or 'negative'. About 60% of survivors of myocardial infarction will be able to perform this test; the remainder will be precluded by severe angina or heart failure or by the presence of orthopaedic, neurological or other non-cardiac disease. Some clinicians employ a submaximal exercise test 10 days after infarction or just before discharge from hospital whereas others prefer a maximal or symptom-limited exercise test 4–6 weeks after infarction. The initial stages of the test protocol are normally less strenuous than in routine outpatient exercise tests (see later). Submaximal tests are usually stopped at a heart rate of 130 beats/min (120 beats/min if the patient is taking beta-blockers) or at about 70% of predicted maximum heart rate. Alternatively, an endpoint of about 5 METS is often used. Both types of test are safe and provide useful prognostic information, but a maximal test may detect evidence of ischaemia that could have been missed on a submaximal test. A maximal test may be more reassuring because the patients can see how well they perform rather than being stopped at an arbitrarily pre-defined point. High-risk patients are probably identified equally well by both types of exercise test.

Again, when interpreting the test, the characteristics of the population tested must be considered. For example, the prognosis in young survivors of myocardial infarction is better than that in older, otherwise comparable, patients and therefore exercise test variables such as ST-segment depression may not have the same discriminatory value in young patients.[50,51] These and other aspects are discussed in detail in Chapter 50.

Other parameters

The exercise duration, heart rate and blood-pressure response, the rate–pressure product, the duration and morphology of abnormalities of the ST–T wave complex after exercise and the development of angina or ventricular arrhythmias are variables used in exercise test interpretation.[52] Thus, up to 28% of patients with an early positive exercise test, i.e. within Stage I or II of the Bruce protocol, had significant stenosis of the left main stem or severe multivessel disease.[53,54] A similar pattern of disease has been found in 90% of patients whose ST-segment depression worsened after exercise.[55] An inadequate rise (< 20 mmHg) or a fall in blood pressure during exercise in patients who are not on beta-blockers indicates poor left ventricular function due to severe ischaemia or previous myocardial damage.[56–58] Kansal et al.[59] showed a peak heart rate < 80% of the maximum predicted heart rate to be most significantly related to the presence of coronary artery disease.

During 4 years follow-up, Ellestad and Wan[60] found that patients who show evidence of ischaemia after < 3 min of exercise experience four times the incidence of cardiovascular death or events than patients who exercise for 7 min or more without ischaemia. In the study by Dagenais et al.[61] of medically treated patients with angina who had 2 mm of ST-segment depression on Bruce protocol exercise testing, the 5-year survival rate was only 50% in those whose exercise duration was < 3 min. Survival improved with increasing exercise duration; it was 86% in patients who completed the third stage of the Bruce protocol (i.e. 9 minutes of exercise).

Heart failure

Exercise testing is sometimes used in the assessment of patients in chronic heart failure because there is often very little correlation between the severity of the patient's symptoms and the indices of left ventricular function measured at rest.[62,63] As there are no objective or physical markers for dyspnoea or fatigue as endpoints, the duration of exercise depends not only on the patient's cardiovascular disabilities but also on subjective influences, such as patient motivation, previous training and the bias of the supervisor. The use of visual analogue score systems can increase the reproducibility of endpoints, such as shortness of breath and fatigue, but a more objective measure of aerobic capacity is still necessary. The oxygen consumption, Vo_2, during exercise is the product of cardiac output and peripheral oxygen extraction. The latter is near maximal, even at rest, in patients with heart failure. Therefore, the maximum oxygen consumption, $Vo_{2\,max}$, during exercise is an indirect but useful measure of maximum cardiac output and hence of cardiovascular reserve. The anaerobic threshold[16,17] (see above) can also be identified. It occurs at approximately 60% of maximal aerobic capacity in healthy subjects. The more severe the heart failure and the more vigorous the exercise, the earlier the anaerobic threshold is reached.[18]

Exercise test protocols (Tables 20.3–20.5)

Treadmill exercise test protocols are based on the

Table 20.3. The Bruce protocol for exercise testing.

Stage	Speed (mph)	Grade (%)	Duration (min)	METS (units)
0[a]	1.7	0	—	—
½[a]	1.7	5	—	—
1[b]	1.7	10	3	4
2	2.5	12	3	6–7
3	3.4	14	3	8–9
4	4.2	16	3	15–16
5	5.0	18	3	21
6	5.5	20	3	—
7	6.0	22	3	—

[a] Stages in the 'modified' Bruce protocol.
[b] The starting point of the full Bruce protocol.

Table 20.4. The Naughton protocol for exercise testing.

Stage	2.0 mph Grade (%)	3.0 mph Grade (%)	3.4 mph Grade (%)	Duration (min)	METS (units)	Total time elapsed (min)
1	—	—	—	2	1	2
2	0.0	—	—	2	2	4
3	3.5	0.0	—	2	3	6
4	7.0	2.5	2.0	2	4	8
5	10.5	5.0	4.0	2	5	10
6	14.0	7.5	6.0	2	6	12
7	17.5	10.0	8.0	2	7	14
8	—	12.5	10.0	2	8	16
9	—	15.0	12.0	2	9	18
10	—	17.5	14.0	2	10	20
11	—	20.0	16.0	2	11	22
12	—	22.5	18.0	2	12	24
13	—	25.0	20.0	2	13	26
14	—	27.5	22.0	2	14	28
15	—	30.0	24.0	2	15	30
16	—	32.5	26.0	2	16	32

Table 20.5. The Ellestad protocol for treadmill exercise testing.

Stage	Speed (mph)	Grade (%)	Duration (min)	Total time elapsed (min)	METS (units)
1	1.7	10	3	3	4
2	3.0	10	2	5	6–7
3	4.0	10	2	7	8–9
4	5.0	10	3	10	10–12
5	5.0	15	2	12	13–15
6	6.0	15	3	15	16–20

resting oxygen consumption. The workload is increased at intervals, usually of 3 min, to allow a near steady state of oxygen consumption between increments.

The protocol selected must be suited to the clinical situation and the subject's anticipated exercise capacity. A vigorous exercise protocol may be used in younger relatively healthy subjects, whereas a more sedate protocol, e.g. the Naughton, will be required in patients with known cardiorespiratory limitations. The Bruce protocol is probably the most popular and is especially useful in the assessment of patients with known or suspected coronary artery disease because the test is often positive in under 9 min of exercise. The protocol is also used in the evaluation of anti-anginal therapy and coronary artery surgery or angioplasty, but is considered too vigorous for pre-discharge post-myocardial infarction exercise testing. Some patients, particularly those of small stature, have to run during or after Stage III and this produces motion artefact on the electrocardiogram which may render it uninterpretable. Running, even at a low speed, requires more energy than walking and this may make comparisons between patients difficult unless oxygen consumption is measured. A modified Bruce protocol with two extra less strenuous stages preceding the standard first stage is often used in patients, after infarction, in chronic heart failure or in other situations where exercise capacity is limited. The Naughton protocol is less stressful than the Bruce because its initial workload and its increments are lower than those in the Bruce protocol, and it can therefore be used in submaximal post-myocardial infarction tests. Familiarity with two protocols will suffice in most laboratories.

With proper supervision, adequate facilities and close adherence to the measures discussed earlier, the risk of exercise testing is very small. A survey of 170 000 tests carried out in 73 medical centres showed a mortality of 0.01%; only 0.02% of the patients had complications requiring admission to hospital.[67] In another study of 15 000 maximal exercise tests, there were no deaths reported.[68] Exercise testing, properly performed, provides information that is useful in planning patient management and it is now a routine part of cardiological investigation.

REFERENCES

1. Hultman, E. Studies in muscle metabolism of glycogen and active phosphate in man with special reference to exercise

early work of Bruce[64,65] and Astrand[66] and are designed so that exercise ends within 6–15 min, an interval that allows the patient to warm up but is not long enough for fatigue and boredom to become important endpoints. The initial workload is within the subject's capability and each increase in workload usually approximates to a multiple of the and diet. *Scand. J. Clin. Lab. Invest. Suppl.* 1967: 94.

2. Jones, N.L., Campbell, E.J., Edwards, R.H. and Robertson, D.G. In: *Clinical Exercise Testing.* W.B. Saunders, 1975, pp. 25–9.

3. Alam, M. and Smirk, F.M. Observations in man upon a blood pressure raising reflex arising from voluntary muscles. *J. Physiol. Lond.* 1972; **271**: 589–600.

4. Tallarida, G., Baldoni, F., Perruzi, G., Raimondi, G., Massaro, M., Sangiorgi, M. Cardiovascular and respiratory reflexes from muscles during dynamic and static exercise. *J. Appl. Respirat. Environ. Exercise Physiol.* 1981; **50**: 786–91.

5. Shepherd, J.T. In: *Handbook of Physiology. The Cardiovascular System.* Bethesda, M.D.: American Physiological Society, 1983, pp. 349–58.

6. Robinson, B.F., Epstein, S.E., Beiser, G.D. and Braunwald, E. Control of heart rate by the autonomic nervous system. Studies in man on the inter-relation between baroreceptor mechanisms and exercise. *Circ. Res.* 1966; **19**: 400–11.

7. Zweifach, B.J. The microcirculation of the blood. *Sci. Am.* 1959; **January**: 954.

8. Shepherd, J.T. Behaviour of resistance and capacity vessels in human limbs during exercise. *Circ. Res.* 1967; **20–21** (Suppl. I): 70–82.

9. Folkow, B. and Neil, E. In: *Circulation.* London: Oxford University Press, 1971.

10. Barcroft, H. An inquiry into the nature of the mediator of vasodilatation in skeletal muscle in exercise and during circulatory arrest (Abstract). *J. Physiol. Lond.* 1972; **222**: 99–118.

11. Hilton, S.M., Hudlicka, O. and Marshall, J. Possible mediators of functional hyperaemia in skeletal muscle. *J. Physiol. Lond.* 1978; **282**: 131–47.

12. Sparks, H.V. Jr and Belloni, F.L. The peripheral circulation: local regulation. *Ann. Rev. Physiol.* 1978; **40**: 67–92.

13. Rowell, B. Human Cardiovascular Adjustments to Exercise and Thermal Stress. *Physiol. Rev.* 1974; **54**: 75.

14. Holloszy, J.O. and Booth, F.W. Biochemical adaptations to endurance in muscle. *Ann. Rev. Physiol.* 1976; **38**: 273–91.

15. Saltin, B. and Gollnick, P. Skeletal muscle adaptability. Significance for metabolism and performance. In: *Handbook of Physiology; Skeletal Muscle*, Section 10. Bethesda, MD: American Physiological Society, 1983, p. 555.

16. Wasserman, K. and McIlroy, M.B. Detecting the threshold of anaerobic metabolism in cardiac patients during exercise. *Am. J. Cardiol.* 1964; **14**: 844–8.

17. Matsumura, N., Nishijima, H., Kojima, S., Hashimoto, F., Minani, M. and Yasuda, H. Determination of anaerobic threshold for assessment of functional state in patients with chronic heart failure. *Circulation* 1983; **68**: 360–7.

18. Lipkin, D., Canepa Anson R., Stephens, M. and Poole-Wilson, P. Factors determining symptoms in heart failure: comparison of fast and slow exercise tests. *Br. Heart J.* 1986; **55**: 439–45.

19. Knabb, R., Ely, S., Bacchus, A., Rubio, R. and Berne, R. Consistent parallel relationships among myocardial oxygen consumption, coronary blood flow and pericardial infusate adenosine concentration with various interventions and beta blockade in the dog. *Circ. Res.* 1983; **53**: 33–41.

20. Shepherd, J.T., Blomqvist, C.G., Lind, A.R., Mitchell, J.H. and Saltin, B. Isometric exercise. Retrospection and Introspection. *Circ. Res.* 1981; **48**: 1179–88.

21. Nelson, R.R., Gobel, R.L., Jorgenson, C.R., Wang, K., Wang, Y. and Taylor, H.L. Haemodynamic predictors of myocardial oxygen consumption during static and dynamic exercise. *Circulation* 1974; **50**: 1179–89.

22. Gobel, F.L., Nordstrom, L.A., Nelson, R.R., Jorgenson, C.R. and Wang, Y. The rate pressure product as an index of myocardial oxygen consumption during angina in patients with angina pectoris. *Circulation* 1978; **57**: 549–56.

23. Council on Scientific Affairs, American Medical Association: Indications and contraindications for exercise testing. *JAMA* 1981; **246**: 1015.

24. Schlant, R., Blomquist, G., Brandenburg, R. *et al.* Guidelines for exercise testing. A report of the Joint American College of Cardiology/American Heart Association Task Force on assessment of cardiovascular procedures (Sub-committee on Exercise Testing). *Circulation* 1986; **74**: 653(A)–667(A).

25. Master, A.M. The two-step test of myocardial function. *Am. Heart J.* 1935; **10**: 495.

26. Wicks, J.R., Sutton, J.R., Oldridge, N.B. and Jones, N.L. Comparison of the electrocardiographic changes induced by maximum exercise testing with treadmill and cycle ergometer. *Circulation* 1978; **6**: 1066–70.

27. Miller, R., Olson, H., Amsterdam, E. and Mason, D. Propranolol—withdrawal rebound phenomenon. Exacerbation of coronary events after abrupt cessation of antianginal therapy. *N. Engl. J. Med.* 1975; **293**: 416–8.

28. Mizgala, H. and Coumell, J. Acute coronary syndromes following abrupt cessation of oral propranolol therapy. *CMA Journal* 1976; **114**: 1123–6.

29. Mason, R.E. and Likar, I. A new system of multiple lead exercise electrocardiography. *Am. Heart J.* 1966; **71**: 196.

30. Kleiner, J.P., Nelson, W.P. and Boland, M.J. The 12 lead electrocardiogram in exercise testing. *Arch. Intern. Med.* 1978; **138**: 1572–3.

31. Chung, E.K. In: *Manual of exercise ECG testing.* Yorke Medical Books, 1986, p. 4.

32. Sheffield, T.L. and Roitman, D. Stress Testing Methodology. *Prog. Cardiovasc. Dis.* 1976; **19**: 33–49.

33. Watanabe, K., Bhargava, V. and Froelicher, V. Computer analysis of the exercise ECG: A review. *Prog. Cardiovasc. Dis.* 1980; **22**: 423–46.

34. Fortuin, N.J. and Weiss, J.L. Exercise stress testing. *Circulation* 1978; **56**: 699–712.

35. Chaitman, B.R. and Hanson, J.S. Comparative sensitivity and specificity of exercise electrocardiographic lead systems. *Am. J. Cardiol.* 1981; **47**: 1335–49.

36. Diamond, G.A. and Forrester, J.S. Analysis of probability as an aid in the clinical diagnosis of coronary artery disease. *N. Engl. J. Med.* 1979; **300**: 1350–8.

37. Borer, J., Brensike, J., Redwood, D. *et al.* Limitations of the electrocardiographic response to exercise in predicting coronary artery disease. *N. Engl. J. Med.* 1975; **283**: 367–71.

38. Redwood, D.R., Borer, J.S. and Epstein, E.S. Whither the ST segment during exercise? *Circulation* 1976; **54**: 703–6.

39. McHenry, P.L., Phillips, J.F. and Knoebel, S.B. Correlation of computer quantitated treadmill exercise electrocardiogram with arteriographic location of coronary artery disease. *Am. J. Cardiol.* 1972; **30**: 747–52.

40. Elamin, M.S., Boyle, R., Kardash, M. *et al.* Accurate detection of coronary artery disease by new exercise test. *Br. Heart J.* 1982; **48**: 311–20.

41. Fox, K.M. Exercise heart rate/ST segment relation. Perfect predictor of coronary disease? *Br. Heart J.* 1982; **48**: 309–10.

42. Quyyumi, A., Raphael, M., Wright, C., Bealing, L. and Fox, K. Inability of the ST segment/heart rate slope to predict accurately the severity of coronary artery disease. *Br. Heart J.* 1984; **51**: 395–8.

43. Balcon, R., Brooks, M. and Layton, C. Correlation of heart rate/ST slope and coronary angiographic findings. *Br. Heart J.* 1984; **52**: 304–7.

44. Hollenberg, M., Budge, R., Widneski, J. and Gertz, E. Treadmill score quantifies electrocardiographic response to exercise and improves test accuracy and reproducibility. *Circulation* 1980; **2**; 276–85.

45. Detrano, R., Salcedo, E., Passalacqua, M. and Friis, R. Exercise electrocardiographic variables: A Critical Apprais-

al. *J. Am. Coll. Cardiol.* 1986; **8**: 836–47.

46. Geson, M., Morris, S. and McHenry, P. Relation of exercise-induced physiologic S-T segment depression to R-wave amplitude in normal subjects. *Am. J. Cardiol.* 1980; **46**: 778–82.

47. Alijarde-Guimera, M., Evangelista, A., Galve, E., Olive, S., Anivar, I. and Soler-Soler, J. Useless diagnostic value of exercise induced R-wave changes in coronary artery disease. *Eur. Heart J.* 1983; **4**: 614–21.

48. Hopkirk, J., Uhl, G., Hickman, J. and Fischer, J. Limitation of exercise induced R-wave amplitude changes in detecting coronary artery disease in asymptomatic men. *J. Am. Coll. Cardiol.* 1984; **3**: 821–6.

49. Brody, D.A. A theoretical analysis of intracavitary blood mass on the heart–lead relationship. *Circ. Res.* 1956; **4**: 731.

50. Peart, I., Seth, L., Albers, C., Odemuyiwa, O. and Hall, R.J.C. Post infarction exercise testing in patients under 55 years. Relation between ischaemic abnormalities and the extent of coronary artery disease. *Br. Heart J.* 1986; **55**: 67–74.

51. Roubin, G.S., Harris, P.J., Bernstein, L. and Kelly, D.T. Coronary anatomy and prognosis after myocardial infarction in patients 60 years of age or younger. *Circulation* 1983; **67**: 743–9.

52. McNeer, F.J., Margolic, J.R., Leek, L. *et al.* The role of the exercise test in the evaluation of patients for ischaemic heart disease. *Circulation* 1978; **57**: 64–70.

53. Schneider, R.M., Seaworth, J.F., Dohrmann, M.L. *et al.* Anatomic and prognostic implications of an early positive treadmill exercise test. *Am. J. Cardiol.* 1982; **50**: 682–8.

54. Goldschlager, N., Selzer, A. and Cohn, K. Treadmill stress tests as indicators of presence and severity of coronary disease. *Ann. Intern. Med.* 1976; **85**: 277–86.

55. Weiner, D.A., McCabe, C.H. and Ryan, T.J. Identification of patients with left main and three vessel coronary artery disease with clinical and exercise test variables. *Am. J. Cardiol.* 1980; **46**: 21–7.

56. Thomson, P.D. and Kelemen, M.H. Hypotension accompanying the onset of exertional angina. A sign of severe compromise of left ventricular blood supply. *Circulation* 1975; **52**: 28–32.

57. Morris, S.N., Phillips, J.F., Jordan, J. and McHenry, P.L. Incidence and significance of decreases in systolic blood pressure during graded treadmill exercise testing. *Am. J. Cardiol.* 1978; **41**: 221–6.

58. Hakki, A., Munley, B.M., Hadjimiltiades, S., Meissner, S. and Iskrandian, A. Determinants of abnormal blood pressure response to exercise in coronary artery disease. *Am. J. Cardiol.* 1986; **57**: 71–5.

59. Kansal, S., Roitman, D., Bradley, E. and Sheffield, T. Enhanced evaluation of treadmill tests by means of scoring based on multivariate analysis and its clinical application. A study of 608 patients. *Am. J. Cardiol.* 1983; **52**: 1155–60.

60. Ellestad, M.H. and Wan, M.K. Predictive implications of stress testing. Follow-up of 2700 subjects after maximum treadmill stress testing. *Circulation* 1975; **51**: 363–9.

61. Dagenais, G., Jacques, R., Christen, A. and Fabia, J. Survival of patients with strongly positive electrocardiogram. *Circulation* 1982; **65**: 452–6.

62. Weber, K.T. and Janicki, J.S. Cardiopulmonary exercise testing for evaluation of chronic cardiac failure. *Am. J. Cardiol.* 1985; **55**: 22A–31A.

63. Franciosa, J., Park, M. and Levine, T. Lack of correlation between exercise capacity and indices of resting left ventricular performance in heart failure. *Am. J. Cardiol.* 1981; **47**: 33–9.

64. Bruce, R.A. and Hornsten, T.R. Exercise stress testing in evaluation of patients with ischaemic heart disease. *Prog. Cardiovasc. Dis.* 1969; **11**: 371–390.

65. Bruce, R.A., Blackman, J.R., Jones, J.W. and Strait, G. Exercise testing in adult normal subjects and cardiac patients. *Paediatrics* 1963; **32**: 742.

66. Astrand, P.O. Quantification of exercise capability and evaluation of physical capacity in man. *Prog. Cardiovasc. Dis.* 1976; **19**: 51–67.

67. Rochmis, P. and Blackburn, H. Exercise tests: A survey of procedures, safety and litigation experience in approximately 170,000 tests. *JAMA* 1971; **217**: 1061.

68. Bruce, R.A. In: Yu, P. and Goodwin, J.F., eds, *Progress in Cardiology*, Vol. 3. Philadelphia: Lea and Febiger, 1974, pp. 113–72.

Chapter 21

Left Ventricular Function

Derek Gibson

Left ventricular disease is a very important cause of disability and death, and even its presence has a profound effect on prognosis. It may manifest itself as structural or functional abnormalities. Structural abnormalities may be macroscopic, such as an abnormal increase in the size of the cavity or of the thickness of its wall, or as a localized or generalized change within the myocardium itself. Although such changes are often associated with disturbances in function, this is not always the case. Functional abnormalities are recognized as a disturbance to the normal processes of energy transfer from the myocardium to the circulation. They may be apparent at rest, or, in less severe cases, can be demonstrated only with a physiological stress such as exercise. In man, myocardial performance is very sensitive to the conditions under which the heart is called upon to function. It is greatly affected by reflex activity, for example, sympathetic stimulation causes an increase in heart rate and the force of myocardial contraction. It also depends on mechanisms within the myocardium itself. The increased force of contraction occurring with increased end-diastolic fibre length referred to as Starling's Law of the Heart is a well-recognized example. Finally, the overall performance of the heart depends on the demands made upon it by the circulation, particularly on venous return and on the properties of the arterial bed into which it is ejecting, factors often called 'loading conditions'. Even in the normal subject, therefore, the problem of dissociating intrinsic cardiac performance from the possible effects of these external factors is a very complex one, and difficulties are compounded in disease.

NORMAL VENTRICULAR FUNCTION

Normal changes in left ventricular volume and pressure during ejection and filling are very characteristic and are shown in Fig. 21.1. Resting end-

diastolic volume is in the range 100–150 ml, and stroke volume between 75–100 ml. The ratio of stroke volume to end-diastolic volume is referred to as the ejection fraction, and in normal subjects this is in the range 55–70%. A low ejection fraction is good evidence of left ventricular disease and usually appears before any fall in resting stroke volume or cardiac output. Cavity volume can be determined by a number of techniques including contrast angiography, cross-sectional echocardiography,

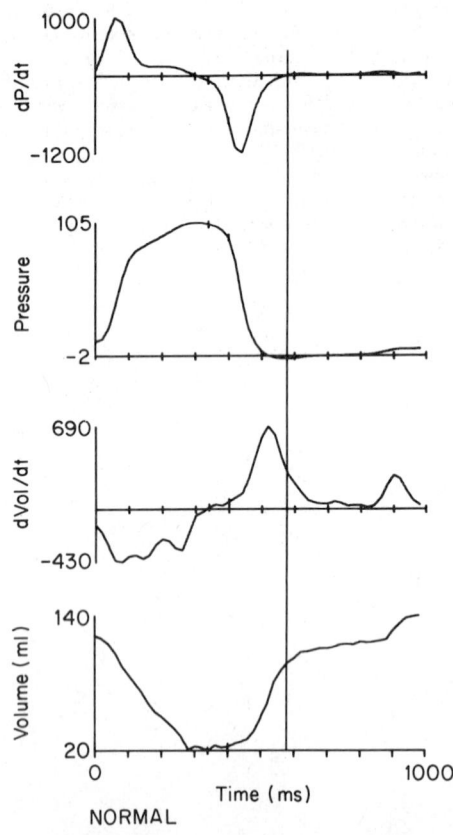

Fig. 21.1. Normal left ventricular pressure and volume changes throughout the cardiac cycle. Ventricular volume is measured by contrast angiography, and simultaneous pressure with a micromanometer. Absolute values and their rates of change are shown.

and magnetic resonance imaging. Radionuclide angiography can be used to measure ejection fraction as the ratio of the fall in counts during systole to end-diastolic counts without having to determine absolute ventricular volumes. The way in which wall motion in different parts of the ventricle contributes to the fall in cavity volume is apparent from Fig. 21.2, which shows the superimposed endocardial outlines from successive ciné frames at 20-ms intervals during systole from a normal subject. As cavity size falls, the relative shortening of the transverse axis is greater than that of the long, or base to apex, axis so that the shape of the cavity changes during ejection to become longer and thinner. The extent of minor axis shortening is quantified as the shortening fraction or (Dd − Ds)/Dd expressed as a percentage, where Dd and Ds are the end-diastolic and end-systolic dimensions, respectively.[1] Normal values are in the range 25–40% and can readily be measured by M-mode echocardiography. The degree of this minor axis shortening is remarkable when it is considered that, under normal loading conditions, a sarcomere shortens by only 10%, and when unloaded by only 15%.[2] With normal myocardium arranged circumferentially around a spherical cavity, sarcomere shortening of 10% would lead to an ejection fraction of only 30%.[3] A normal ejection fraction becomes possible only when the cavity is elongated, for example, when it is an ellipsoid, and when the muscle fibres are arranged spirally.

Although the extent of left ventricular wall motion varies with position, the timing of its inward motion is almost synchronous. It starts within an interval of only 60 ms, the latest portion to start moving inwards is that towards the apex on the free wall. Peak inward movement in all regions coincides with aortic valve closure to within 40 ms.[4] Synchronous wall motion is very characteristic of normal. It is unaffected by loading conditions or reflex changes, a property that makes its loss a valuable indicator of disease. The timing of wall motion can be displayed from radionuclide or digital subtraction angiograms, and displayed as phase shifts.[5] Changes in cavity outline can be mapped in considerable detail from successive frames of a contrast angiogram;[6] unfortunately, subjective analysis of ventriculographic images is not a satisfactory way of appreciating these subtle disturbances of function.

RATE OF EJECTION

The characteristics of blood flow into the aorta during ejection make a sensitive index of left ventricular systolic function. Peak ejection rate is of the order of 500–700 ml s^{-1} at rest, increasing to approximately double this value on exercise severe enough to raise the heart rate to 140 beats/min. It can be measured from angiograms as the rate of fall of ventricular volume,[7] or much more simply from Doppler records of flow velocity in the ascending aorta, and converted to flow, knowing the cross-section of the outflow tract.[8] Normal peak flow velocities are in the range 1–1.5 m s^{-1}, with peak acceleration at the onset of ejection around 2–3 g. An increase in peak flow velocity and particularly in peak acceleration have proved very sensitive in detecting positive inotropic stimuli.[9] Peak acceleration is little affected by aortic pressure suggesting that early in ejection blood flow into the aorta is determined mainly by cardiac factors rather than loading conditions. Later in ejection, as flow decelerates, exactly the opposite applies: aortic pressure is now characteristically higher than that in the left ventricle, indicating that blood flow is largely inertial and no longer depends directly on left ventricular wall stress.[10] It is not surprising, therefore, that, in contrast to peak acceleration, measurements of peak blood flow velocity or flow rate as well as of stroke volume and ejection time are all very sensitive to arterial loading conditions. This sensitivity greatly limits their use in detecting the possible inotropic effects of drugs, but may account for much of the benefit of vasodilator treatment in disease.

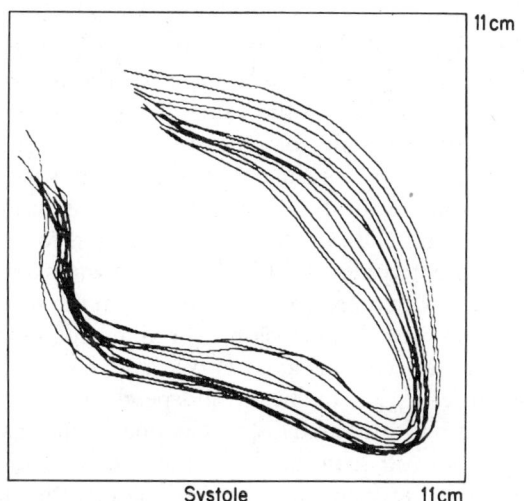

Fig. 21.2. Normal left ventricular cavity outlines during systole from successive frames of a contrast angiogram. The time-interval between frames is 20 ms.

Some indication of the speed of ejection can also be gained from measuring the rate of change of dimension during systole. The dimension most commonly chosen is the minor transverse axis of the ventricle, which can be measured by M-mode echocardiography or contrast angiography. The results are usually presented as an entity termed velocity of circumferential fibre shortening (VCF),[1] which is calculated as:

$$(Dd - Ds)/Dd. ET$$

where Dd and Ds are the end-diastolic and end-systolic dimensions, respectively, and ET is left ventricular ejection time measured from an indirect carotid pulse or an aortic valve echogram. Circumferential fibre shortening is thus a normalized velocity with the dimensions of s^{-1}, and is simply shortening fraction divided by ejection time. Normal values are in the range $0.8 - 1.2 \ s^{-1}$. Although it may be regarded as an index of the rate of change of minor dimension, for the reasons described above, its behaviour should not be equated with those of any circumferential muscle fibre.

LEFT VENTRICULAR PRESSURE

Left ventricular pressure directly reflects changes in myocardial tension. The onset of pressure rise is the earliest mechanical event detectable within the left ventricular cavity after the QRS complex. Peak rate of rise of pressure (peak dP/dt) occurs during isovolumic contraction.[11] Normal values are within the range $1500–2500 \ mmHgs^{-1}$ at rest, increasing with exercise and positive inotropic stimuli. The timing of peak dP/dt usually corresponds with aortic valve opening. Thus, the peak value is reduced if the valve opens early or increased if it opens late as may occur, in aortic regurgitation or aortic stenosis, respectively. Peak dP/dt thus depends on arterial pressure as well as on the rate of tension development and its value as a measure of systolic myocardial function is limited.

Pressure and volume changes can be displayed as a pressure-volume loop (Fig.21.3). The area of the loop represents work done on the circulation by the ventricle. These loops form the basis of another approach to assessing ventricular systolic function, potentially independent of the effects of loading conditions.[12] It arises from the observation that the end-systolic tension of isolated cardiac muscle depends only on end-systolic length and contractile state, and not on end-diastolic length or the mode of contraction, whether isotonic or isometric. At any

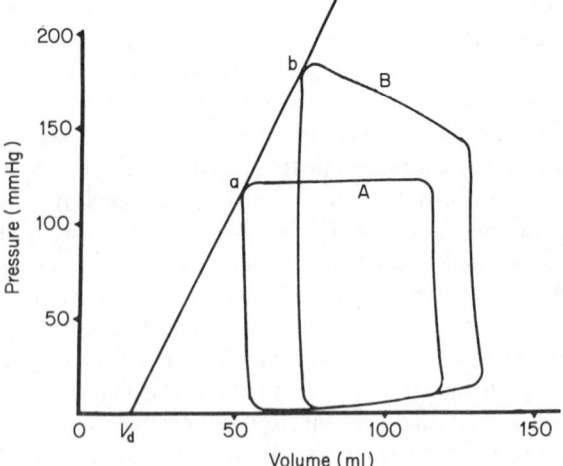

Fig. 21.3. Left ventricular pressure-volume loops under control conditions (A) and after administration of a pressor agent (B). The end-systolic points, a and b, respectively, lie on a line that intercepts the volume axis at V_d. The slope of this line represents E_{max}. A postitive inotropic stimulus is associated with an increase in E_{max}.

time during the cardiac cycle, left ventricular elasticity can be defined as:

$$E = P/(V - V_d),$$

where E is elastance, P and V ventricular pressure and volume, and V_d an intercept corresponding to volume at zero pressure. On this basis, increased systolic wall tension can be taken as reflecting the effect of reduced elastance, so that elastance itself can be thought of as changing continuously throughout the cardiac cycle. The idea is thus referred to as 'time-varying elastance'. The highest value of cavity elastance (E_{max}) in the normal left ventricle occurs at end-systole, just before the onset of pressure fall (Fig. 21.3). This maximum value cannot be determined from a single pressure-volume loop because the value of V_d is unknown. However, if a series of pressure-volume loops are constructed by infusing a vasopressor, such as methoxamine, or by a sudden change in venous return, their end-systolic points are found to move approximately along a straight line, upwards and to the right with a pressor stimulus, and in the reverse direction with hypotension. The intercept of this line on the volume axis, is V_d, and its slope is therefore E_{max}. In being independent of both preload and afterload, E_{max} has one of the major properties of 'contractility', the entity held to represent intrinsic systolic ventricular function, independent of any external factor. Contractility was originally defined as peak shortening velocity of the contractile elements at extrapolated zero afterload.[13] It is now considered doubtful whether these measurements were ever valid;[14] unfortunately, the term contractility has never been rigorously defined, although it is still widely invoked in cardiological literature. E_{max} is, from its derivation, a measure of elasticity and not of velocity, so it cannot possibly be identical with an entity whose definition depends on a velocity. Nevertheless, E_{max} does increase with administration of a drug with a positive inotropic action, and at the same time the end-systolic pressure-volume line moves to the left.[15] Normal values of E_{max} in adults are in the range 4–6 mmHgml^{-1}. Higher slopes are found in children, because end-systolic volume changes more than pressure with age.

In practice, E_{max} has usually been determined from contrast angiography with a simultaneous high-fidelity pressure which has made the method cumbersome to perform. It is thus more convenient to measure left ventricular volume by radionuclide angiography, so that multiple points can be determined. If end-systolic dimension, measured by echocardiography, is substituted for volume, and end-ejection pressure determined sphygmomanometrically for that at end-systole, the resulting related but not identical measurement becomes completely non-invasive.[16] An impedance catheter capable of measuring ventricular volume continuously has been constructed, and, if validated, will make these measurements much simpler to perform in man.[17]

Relations between cavity size, wall thickness and pressure during systole can also be considered in terms of wall stress.[18] A stress is a force per unit area within the wall. Stresses have direction as well as magnitude, and, within the ventricle, can be directed circumferentially, i.e. around the minor dimension, or longitudinally. In addition, shear stress can develop across the wall. Wall stress cannot be measured directly, but, if it is assumed that it is in equilibrium with pressure in the cavity, it can be calculated from Laplace's relation:

$$F - Pr/t$$

where F is wall stress, P cavity pressure, r cavity radius and t wall thickness.

This formulation makes a number of assumptions. Although apparently taking wall thickness into account, it is strictly valid only when thickness is less than one-tenth of the cavity radius. It also assumes that the wall is homogeneous and isotropic, whereas myocardium is arranged as fibres with a definite local architecture. The assumption that pressure and wall stress are in equilibrium applies rigorously only in the arrested heart, and major departures may occur in the beating heart, particularly at times of rapid pressure or volume change. Even more fundamental, the simple Laplace approach implicitly assumes that the tension in the wall is the direct result of pressure in the cavity, rather as with the boiler of a steam engine. In the ventricle, of course, the reverse applies: the pressure is secondary to the tension in the wall. This inverted computation has proved surprisingly difficult to undertake with any rigour, particularly when the complex left ventricular anatomy is taken into account, and indeed the problem has not been completely solved. Using the Laplace approach, peak mid-systolic wall stress is of the order of 200–400 gcm^{-2} (Fig 21.4). Unlike ventricular elastance, peak wall stress is registered early in systole; values decrease later in ejection as cavity size falls and wall thickness increases. Stress varies across the left ventricular wall, being much higher in the sub-endocardial than the sub-epicardial region. It

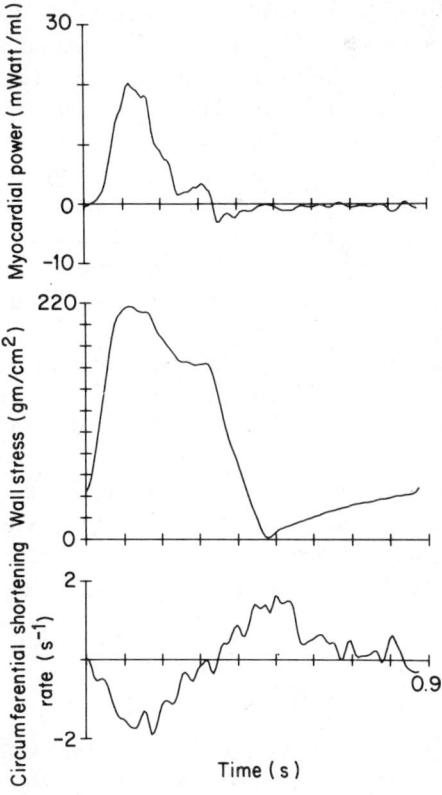

Fig 21.4. Normal myocardial mid-wall stress, derived from simultaneous M-mode echocardiogram and high-fidelity pressure. Pressure, wall stress and shortening rate are shown. Peak wall stress is reached early in systole and falls off as ejection proceeds. Myocardial power, the product of wall stress and shortening rate, is also displayed.

may also vary around the left ventricular cavity, being greater in regions such as the mid portion of the free wall where curvature (the reciprocal of radius of curvature) is low. Curvature of the ventricle is frequently reversed along the normal inferior wall, which is convex rather than concave towards the cavity.[19] The Laplace relation would predict a negative wall stress during systole, an unlikely conclusion, which illustrates how limited this approach is even in the normal heart.

SYSTOLIC VENTRICULAR DISEASE

Abnormal left ventricular systolic function is common in disease. It is still often attributed to impaired contractility, which, from its definition,[20] would imply that the primary disturbance is a reduction in the peak rate of tension development (V_{max}). This approach has proved very disappointing in providing any understanding of the nature of clinical systolic left ventricular disease. It has not been possible to dissociate the effect of loading conditions from estimates of V_{max} made in the beating heart. Values for V_{max} have been reported in the literature, but their normal range is very wide, and there is considerable overlap between normal subjects and patients with severe and obvious disease, which has been confirmed, for example, by strikingly reduced ejection fraction.[21,22] The idea of depressed contractility, defined in terms of reduced V_{max} and implying slow contraction, being the dominant or even a significant mechanism of clinical disease has been generally abandoned. Alternative criteria of disease that have been found useful include cavity enlargement with reduction in ejection fraction, localized disturbances in the amplitude of wall motion and loss of the normal pattern of synchrony. At a more general level, it has become apparent that there is no single mechanism underlying ventricular disease, but that many, potentially separable, disturbances exist in individual patients.

CAVITY DILATATION

Cavity dilatation is a common feature of ventricular disease. End-diastolic cavity size may be increased from the upper limit of normal of around 150–180 ml to 500 ml or more. If stroke volume remains normal, ejection fraction must be strikingly reduced, sometimes to 20% or below. Wall thickness is usually normal, but left ventricular mass is

nevertheless increased. These findings are present in a number of conditions including dilated cardiomyopathy, coronary artery disease, the late stages of valvular heart disease and heart muscle disease due to toxic compounds, such as alcohol or daunorubicin. They are confirmed in man by demonstrating reduced ejection and shortening fractions to below the lower limits of normal of 50% and 25%, respectively. Associated low values of mean VCF to < 0.8 s^{-1} might be taken as evidence that contraction velocity is also reduced. However, ejection time is either normal or short in ventricular disease, so, from its derivation, a low VCF directly reflects reduced shortening fraction and is not evidence of a primary reduction in contraction velocity.

When the cavity is dilated and ejection fraction low, the myocardium in its wall is placed at a considerable mechanical disadvantage. If wall thickness is normal, wall stress must be increased to maintain a physiological ventricular pressure. In addition, the reduction in cavity dimension and the increase in wall thickness normally occurring during ejection are both reduced; wall stress therefore falls less as the ventricle ejects. Thus, high values of wall stress must be generated throughout systole, with a corresponding requirement for oxygen. The highest values of wall stress occur in the subendocardium. In combination with an elevated end-diastolic pressure, which effectively reduces coronary perfusion pressure, this may lead to local ischaemia. A high wall stress increases the afterload of myocardial fibres in the wall even when cavity pressure is normal; their shortening rate is further reduced, mimicking a reduction in contractility. In practice, this fall in velocity proves to be proportionately greater than the increase in wall stress, so that power production (Fig. 21.4), the product of force and velocity, also falls. The relation between a power source and operating resistance is referred to as matching. Optimal matching allows maximum power transfer. Significant mismatch between the heart and circulation contributes to the disturbed energy transfer when cavity size is increased.[25]

Although it is clear that the function of myocardium in the wall of a dilated cavity is greatly impaired, it is much less certain whether the dilatation itself is always the direct result of primary myocardial disease. It is often assumed that dilatation reflects the workings of Starling's law; impaired myocardial function invokes increased preload to compensate so that end-diastolic fibre length becomes increased.[20] This mechanism would predict that average sarcomere length in myocardium from a dilated ventricle is greater than normal. Experimentally, overall sarcomere length, measured as the distance from one Z line to another, has been shown to be normal in such ventricles, suggesting that a dilated ventricle is not simply a small one stretched, but that a fundamental alteration in myocardial architecture has occurred.[26] This process is referred to as slippage, and dissection has demonstrated a large increase in the number of circumferentially arranged fibres. The exact relation between these anatomical abnormalities and impaired sarcomere function remains to be determined. Certainly, non-specific biochemical disturbances can be demonstrated, but it is not known whether these are the result of the increased and prolonged wall stress associated with subendocardial ischaemia or they represent primary metabolic disturbances. Even if they do, the mechanism of slippage has yet to be established. No clear causal mechanism between reduced sarcomere function and changes in cardiac anatomy is apparent, neither is there any evidence of any other way in which a primary disturbance of fibre arrangement might occur. Nevertheless, its result is loss of those anatomical features which are the basis of a normal ejection fraction: oblique fibre angle and an elongated cavity shape. Once they have been lost, a normal ejection fraction is not possible despite normal sarcomere shortening. Thus, it could be argued that ejection fraction is more an index of the integrity of myocardial architecture than it is of contractile function. The mechanical disadvantages of myocardium in the wall of a dilated cavity provides instructive insight into the biological advantages of a normal ejection fraction and, by inference, of intact myocardial anatomy.

Cavity dilatation may also develop in association with volume overload. If the overload is severe, stroke volume will be correspondingly increased. This increase is accommodated in part by a larger end-diastolic volume and in part by a reduction in end-systolic volume, particularly if the resistance to ejection is low. The former is usually more prominent in patients with aortic regurgitation, and the latter in those with uncomplicated mitral regurgitation or a ventricular septal defect. In contrast to the cavity dilatation occurring in patients with myocardial disease, therefore, ejection fraction is normal or even increased when the resistance to ejection is low. The ventricular enlargement of uncomplicated volume overload frequently differs from that seen in dilated cardiomyopathy in that wall thickness (t) is

also increased, so that the ratio between it and cavity radius (r) (the r/t ratio) usually remains within the normal range. This ratio remains virtually constant during growth,[27] and indeed throughout a wide range of mammalian hearts because peak systolic wall stress is similarly constant regardless of cavity size. If the cavity enlarges without a corresponding increase in wall thickness, Laplace's law predicts that systolic wall tension will rise. One way of looking at hypertrophy is thus to consider it a homeostatic mechanism maintaining peak systolic wall tension approximately constant. In these terms, an increase in r/t implies that the increase in wall thickness has been inadequate to prevent systolic wall tension rising.[28] Such failure to maintain the r/t ratio is seen late in the natural history of valvular heart disease, either stenotic or regurgitant, and adversely affects survival independent of ejection fraction. The ratio between cavity volume and ventricular mass, measurements that can conveniently be made at contrast angiography, gives similar information.

END-SYSTOLIC PRESSURE-VOLUME RELATIONS

When the left ventricle is enlarged, and its ejection fraction low, end-systolic cavity volume is likely to be increased. Not surprisingly, therefore, end-systolic pressure-volume relations are abnormal. The characteristic findings are a reduction in the slope of the end-systolic pressure-volume points, i.e. in E_{max} from normal values of 4–6 to 1 mmHgml^{-1} or less, and displacement of the curve to the right due to the increase in cavity volume.[15,29] Values of the intercept V_d in disease are variable, ranging from small and positive to large and negative, the physical significance of the latter not being clear. This change in end-systolic pressure-volume relations is exactly the opposite of that occurring with a positive inotropic stimulus. In patients with disease, E_{max} is closely related to ejection fraction, not only in the abnormal range but throughout the normal range. This relation is not surprising as both E_{max} and ejection fraction are calculated from end-systolic volume. The way in which end-systolic pressure-volume relations are affected by non-uniform ventricular function has yet to be determined. Definite evidence that measurements of E_{max} can detect subclinical ventricular disease as distinct from acute changes in inotropic state is still not available.

NON-UNIFORM CONTRACTION

Non-uniform ventricular wall motion is well recognized in patients with coronary artery disease, but, if specifically sought, it can be demonstrated in dilated or hypertrophic cardiomyopathy and valvular heart disease. As predictable differences in the extent and timing of regional wall motion occur in normal subjects, their presence alone has no pathological significance.[30] In disease, it is the amplitude of wall motion that has received most attention. Reduced amplitude is referred to as hypokinesis, the absence of wall motion as akinesis, reversed motion as dyskinesis, and an abnormal increase in amplitude as hyperkinesis. Although it is straightforward to document these disturbances when they are severe, the lower 95% confidence limit of normal amplitude for the region in question must be known, and such limits are wide.[31] Wall motion abnormalities must be distinguished from overall movement of the heart within the thorax; a variety of schemes for correcting for this possibility have been described, but none is completely satisfactory.

ASYNCHRONOUS WALL MOTION

In spite of being very common in disease, abnormalities in the timing as distinct from the overall amplitude of wall motion have received little attention. From their nature, they are harder to detect and display. A number of patterns may occur. At the start of systole, the onset of inward motion may be delayed or even reversed because tension develops late or is inadequate to cause inward movement until late in ejection.[6,32] Asynchronous wall motion during early diastole causes striking changes in cavity shape during isovolumic relaxation, because tension persists in abnormal regions while relaxation, has already started elsewhere. Finally, wall motion is often incoordinate when the ventricular filling rate is low.[33,34]

Although the detailed study of asynchrony may seem an esoteric activity, its presence profoundly modifies the results of simpler tests of left ventricular function. When the onset of tension development is asynchronous, the peak rate of rise of ventricular pressure (peak dP/dt) is reduced;[35] incoordination thus mimics slow contraction, and peak dP/dt or quantities derived from it cannot be used to assess the isotropic state. Also, this asynchronous wall motion, rather than a generalized reduction in inotropic state, is the main reason for the prolongation of the pre-ejection period in patients with ventricular disease.[36] The possibility of incoordination was never considered in the original studies which attempted to explain the behaviour of a diseased ventricle on the basis of an isolated papillary muscle.[20] Asynchrony also affects the apparent pattern of regional wall motion demonstrated by the standard method of superimposing end-diastolic and end-systolic frames.[37] Incoordinate relaxation implies that the timing of the onset of diastole, and thus the timing of end-systole, differs in different parts of the ventricle. This spread in time may be wide, stretching from aortic valve closure to mitral valve opening. There is thus no single frame that can be identified as 'end-systolic' on a left ventriculogram. The consequences of altering the timing of end-systole from that of aortic closure to mitral opening on the apparent pattern of wall motion is shown in Fig. 21.5. In the former case, the picture is of inferior akinesis with normal wall motion on the anterior wall, whereas in the latter generalized hypokinesis is present. In patients with coronary artery disease and regional wall motion abnormalities, this two-frame method of display gives ambiguous results in nearly half the

AVC

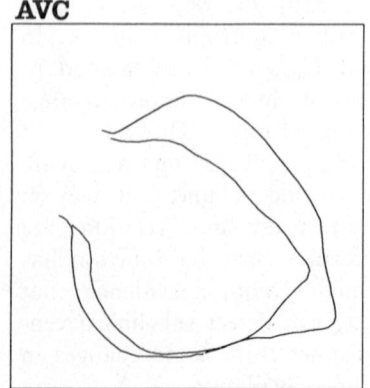

MVO

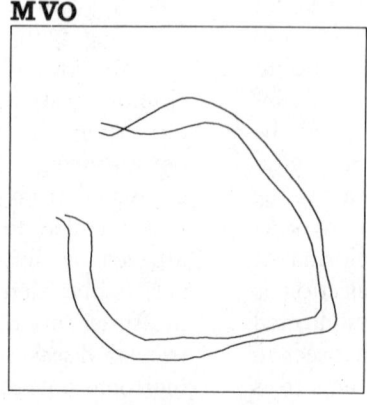

Fig 21.5. Effect of ventricular asynchrony on the apparent pattern of wall motion displayed by the two-frame method. Both displays come from the same beat. In that on the left, 'end-systole' is taken as the time of aortic valve closure (AVC), and on the right as mitral valve opening (MVO). Note the difference in the pattern of wall motion between the two.

cases, arising from this lack of definition in the timing of end-systole.

Incoordination has major effects on energy transfer from the myocardium to the circulation, changes in cavity shape resulting in a striking loss of mechanical efficiency and dissociation of local myocardial function from that of the ventricle as a whole. Its presence is a useful sign of potentially reversible left ventricular disease. In the first few hours after coronary artery occlusion in man, the predominant disturbance of wall motion is asynchrony rather than simple akinesis or dyskinesis.[38] The onset of inward wall motion is delayed in the territory of the affected artery. This delay continues into the period of isovolumic relaxation. Despite this asynchrony, the overall amplitude of inward motion during systole is frequently normal in such patients, although that during ejection is often strikingly reduced. Incoordinate relaxation may cause changes in cavity shape during isovolumic relaxation and thus impair function in otherwise unaffected parts of the ventricle. Finally, a return to normal wall motion after thrombolysis or revascularization is much commoner in regions showing asynchronous motion in comparison with those where it is akinetic.[39] More widespread study of asynchrony will probably not be undertaken until the problems of collection, analysis and display of data have been improved thereby making the results available for patient management.[40]

DIASTOLIC FUNCTION

Diastolic function is as important as systolic in maintaining normal stroke volume, particularly on exercise when the time available for filling is considerably less than that for ejection. Normal diastolic function differs from normal systolic function in that many aspects change progressively with age.

Diastole is normally taken as starting with aortic valve closure, which marks the onset of the period of isovolumic relaxation.[41] This lasts until mitral valve opening and the start of ventricular filling. Isovolumic relaxation time is most conveniently determined by echo-phonocardiography.[42] Aortic closure is identified either from cusp apposition on the aortic echogram, or from A2, the onset of the first high-frequency vibration of the aortic component of the second heart sound. Mitral opening is taken as the time of cusp separation on a mitral echogram or the onset of diastolic flow by Doppler,

the two methods agreeing closely. The normal isovolumic relaxation time is 60 ± 10 ms, with shorter times in children and longer ones in the elderly. In disease, isovolumic relaxation time is determined by both loading factors and ventricular disease.[43,44] It is short when end-diastolic pressure is high, and may be zero when the end-diastolic pressure is >30 mmHg. Isovolumic relaxation time is prolonged when aortic pressure is raised. Superimposed on this simple relation is prolongation by ventricular disease, sometimes to values of >150 ms (Fig. 21.6). A long isovolumic relaxation time with normal filling pressures is seen in patients with left ventricular hypertrophy, coronary artery disease or diabetes mellitus with evidence of microangiopathy. The duration of isovolumic relaxation time is thus an excellent example of interactions that may occur between a primary cardiac abnormality and loading conditions. Although isovolumic relaxation time can readily be defined, the same cannot be said of the term 'relaxation'. 'Relaxation' has been taken as referring to the termination of systolic tension development, i.e. 'deactivation',[45] implying that it has a biochemical basis. It has also been defined as any process leading to the ventricle returning to its end-diastolic configuration,[46] and thus would include passive elastic restoring forces. Other authors include events during filling, such as the peak rate of dimension increase,[47] and the compliance of the ventricle;[48] even events during left atrial systole have been held to reflect abnorma-

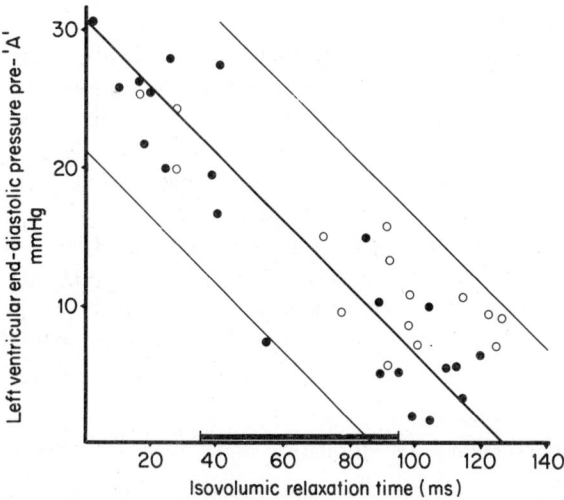

Fig. 21.6. Relation between the duration of isovolumic relaxation and left ventricular end-diastolic pressure in patients with coronary artery disease. Note the inverse relation between the two. ●, Patients not receiving beta-blockers; ○, patients receiving propranolol.

lities of relaxation. As there is such chaos in the use of words, it is not surprising that misunderstanding occurs. Until terminology has been standardized, context must be used to establish the meaning that individual authors give to the term.

Left ventricular pressure starts to fall during late ejection, marking the onset of the period termed 'protodiastole' by Wiggers.[41] Peak rate of fall of pressure occurs just after A2. The absolute magnitude of the rate of fall is load dependent, being closely related to peak systolic pressure. It is also modified in disease, being reduced, for example, in acute ischaemia.[49] Less dependent on loading conditions is the time-constant of left ventricular pressure fall (often referred to as the time-constant of 'relaxation').[50] In order to derive a time-constant, it must be assumed that the left ventricular pressure curve is exponential, and that the zero pressure to which it is tending (the asymptote) is known. Time-constant is calculated for the portion of the curve between peak negative dP/dt and mitral valve opening. The time-constant changes little with arterial pressure, heart rate or end-systolic volume. It is prolonged in ventricular disease, particularly hypertrophy and coronary artery disease.[51] The time-course of pressure fall may correlate with ventricular filling rate later in diastole[52] once the mitral valve has opened. When relaxation is incoordinate, as in hypertrophic cardiomyopathy, the pressure curve may depart so significantly from an exponential that the calculation cannot be made. In some patients with coronary artery disease, two exponentials have been recognized, one during the first 40 ms of exponential fall and the other for the remainder, but two exponentials can also be recognized in normal subjects, which revert to one when the value of the asymptote is varied from zero to a value, usually significantly below zero, which gives the best fit.[51] When left atrial pressure is high, isovolumic relaxation time may be very short,[43] such that the time-constant cannot be calculated at all. Subject to these limitations, an abnormal time-course of left ventricular pressure fall can be used to detect the presence of abnormalities early in diastole, but it gives no indication of their nature.

VENTRICULAR FILLING

Ventricular filling is obviously as important as ventricular ejection in maintaining stroke volume. At rest, the time available for filling, which can be estimated as the interval that the mitral valve cusps are separated during diastole, is much longer than that required for ejection. As heart rate increases, however, this disparity is reversed. Towards peak exercise, when heart rate is around 160 beats/min, left ventricular filling time drops to 100 ms or less, at a time when ejection time is maintained at 150 ms. In normal subjects, therefore, mean left ventricular filling rate, at rest must be of the order of 1 ls^{-1}.

The normal pattern of ventricular filling is apparent on the volume curve (Fig. 21.1). Its three phases were recognized in the early years of the twentieth century. There is an early period of rapid filling when approximately 70% of the stroke volume enters.[54] When heart rate is slow, this is followed by a mid-diastolic period of diastasis, when volume changes little. The remaining 25–30% of the normal stroke volume enters during left atrial systole. As heart rate increases, the duration of rapid filling and atrial systole remain unaltered, so that the period of diastasis is encroached upon, and at moderate heart rates rapid filling and atrial systole become continuous.

Rapid filling

Rapid filling is a complex process. Ventricular pressure continues to fall after the mitral valve opens, as volume rises, so that minimum left ventricular pressure does not occur until after the time of peak filling rate.[55–57] The mechanism underlying this apparently paradoxical relation between pressure and volume has not been established. It may represent continuing decay of the active state within the myocardium after mitral valve opening, so that throughout the greater part of the rapid filling period myocardial tension is falling.[58] Thus, the driving pressure leading to ventricular filling would be developed solely in the left atrium and opposed by the effects of tension persisting in the ventricular myocardium. Alternatively, forces may be present in the left ventricular wall at end-systole restoring its cavity towards its end-diastolic configuration.[59,60] These forces, energized during systole, are unrelated to decay of the active state within the myocardium and probably reside in connective tissue elements. It follows from simple physical principles that acceleration of blood flow during filling cannot occur without a positive pressure difference between left atrium and left ventricle, which is reversed at the time of peak filling rate. The question, therefore, is whether this pressure difference results solely from a driving pressure in the left atrium or there is an additional negative pressure difference across the ventricular wall during early diastole resulting from restoring forces and leading to 'ventricular suction'.[61] Whatever the exact mechanism of generation of the atrioventricular pressure gradient, ventricular filling in normal subjects and in patients with heart disease is very sensitive to an increase in left atrial pressure.[62,63] This load dependency may underline at least part of the predictable increase in filling rate that occurs with exercise.

Filling rate can be determined directly from rate of change of ventricular volume measured by contrast angiography. Radionuclide angiography is often used to give relative filling rates, in terms of end-diastolic volume per second; a low value therefore may result from a low transmitral blood flow rate or an increase in ventricular cavity size,[64,65] two different entities. Doppler measurements of blood velocity across the mitral valve can be combined with estimates of mitral ring area to give blood flow.[66]

Peak left ventricular filling rate falls normally with age. It is also commonly modified in disease. It is low in patients with mitral stenosis, the direct result of obstruction.[67] Low values are also seen in patients with left ventricular disease of a variety of types, including ventricular hypertrophy[68] and coronary artery disease,[69] and also in a number of less common conditions, such as with microvascular diabetes, or in association with skeletal muscular dystrophies.[70] Slow filling does not invariably accompany left ventricular disease. In left ventricular hypertrophy, the filling rate may be normal, or increased, suggesting restriction. Similarly, disturbed filling is a poor marker for ventricular involvement in coronary artery disease;[64] when present, it is often associated with reduced ejection fraction and with abnormal wall motion during isovolumic relaxation.[33] Reduced filling rate is probably more significant during exercise than at rest, when the filling period is long. The failure of ventricular filling period to shorten normally during exercise in patients with left ventricular hypertrophy is shown is Fig. 21.7. The additional 100 ms required for filling must be gained from elsewhere in the cardiac cycle; it comes mainly from the shortening of isovolumic relaxation time, probably by elevation of left atrial pressure, and to a lesser extent from the shortening of ejection time.

Passive ventricular filling

Passive ventricular filling may be said to start when pressure and volume increase together. Its onset is

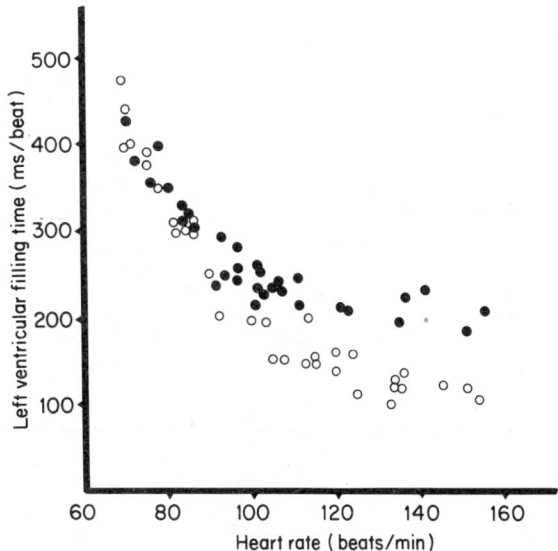

Fig. 21.7. Relation between left ventricular filling time (the total period of mitral valve opening during diastole) and heart rate in normal subjects (○) and those with left ventricular hypertrophy (●). Note that at a heart rate of 160 beats/min, filling time falls to 100 ms or less in normal subjects, but does not drop below 200 ms in patients with left ventricular hypertrophy.

thus toward the end of the period of rapid filling, and it includes the period of diastasis. It is during this period that ventricular stiffness can be measured. Assessing the passive diastolic properties of the ventricle has proved to be remarkably complicated.[71] A ventricular pressure-volume curve is shown diagrammatically in Fig. 21.8 as AB. It is curvilinear, the slope increasing as filling proceeds.[72] The compliance of the ventricle at any point is given by the relation dV/dP, where dV and dP represent small increments of volume and pressure, respectively, and their ratio the slope of the curve. The shape of the pressure-volume curve shows that compliance falls, i.e. the ventricle becomes stiffer as it gets larger. The curve AC represents a ventricle with a steeper pressure-volume relation than that for which AB applies. Its slope at a volume of 110 ml is greater than that of AB, although early in diastole the slopes of the two are the same. If the blood volume of the patient represented by AB is increased, however, such that the end-diastolic volume rises to 150 ml, then compliance becomes the same as that at end-diastole on curve AC. Thus, manipulation of volume can lead to identical values of compliance being measured even if the underlying pressure-volume curves are widely different, and, conversely, that different values of compliance can occur on the same pressure-volume curve. Ideally, therefore, the

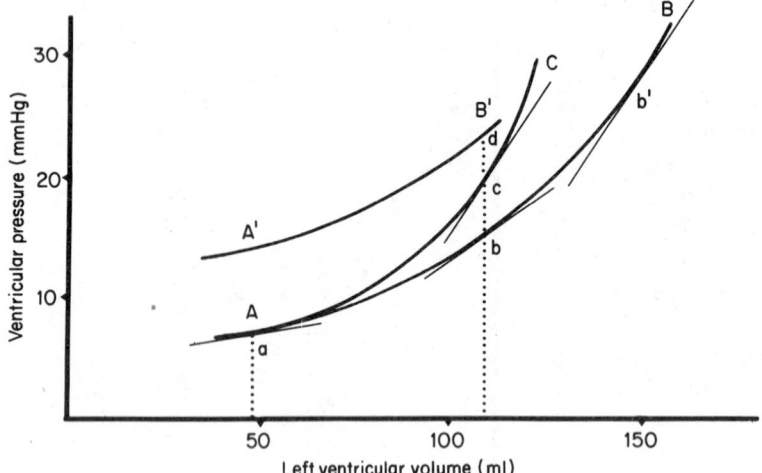

Fig. 21.8. Schematic diagram to illustrate features of left ventricular pressure-volume relations during passive filling. For discussion, see text.

absolute extent of filling at which the measurement is made should be specified. To do this, the unstressed volume, i.e. the volume in equilibrium with zero pressure must be known. Unfortunately, this cannot be determined in the beating heart. Another difficulty is that, in certain circumstances, the pressure-volume curve as a whole can be displaced upwards or downwards.[73] Upward displacement to A′B′ may occur during an attack of angina, and downward displacement with the administration of vasodilators or beta-blocking drugs. Although end-diastolic pressure has increased at constant end-diastolic volume, when AB has been displaced to A′B′, there has been no increase in cavity compliance because the slope of the curve at B′ is unaltered. It is thus not possible to infer anything about cavity stiffness from single pairs of measurements of end-diastolic pressure and volume, still less from end-diastolic pressure alone.

Despite these difficulties, end-diastolic values for ventricular compliance in disease are reduced in patients with hypertrophy or cavity dilatation.[74] The mechanism of this reduction in compliance is not clear. In some cases, particularly those with hypertrophy, it may be due to increased myocardial collagen. In others, particularly those with cavity dilatation, it seems to be related more to cavity shape. In intact man, measurements of diastolic pressure and volume can be made only as the ventricle is filling; thus, they might be affected by some aspect of the filling process itself and so differ from the values that would have been obtained had pressure and volume been allowed to reach equilibrium. The dynamic factor most likely to affect apparent cavity stiffness is viscosity, which is directly related to the rate of filling. Viscous forces

lead to an increase in measured stiffness above equilibrium values, proportional to filling velocity and the coefficient of viscosity.[75] Conversely, inertial forces, which vary with rate of change of filling velocity, lead to the measured stiffness being lower than that in equilibrium.[76] Whether either of these two effects are of clinical importance is uncertain in spite of extensive investigation. Finally, the left ventricle cannot be considered to be independent of surrounding structures. It is well established that diastolic disease of either ventricle alters the apparent passive stiffness of the other. In part, this may arise from distortion of the cavity shape, and in part from their sharing common muscle fibres. An accentuated 'a' wave in the right atrial pulse, for example, is often seen in patients with left ventricular hypertrophy. This was originally described by Bernheim and attributed to the septum bulging into the right ventricular cavity. A second possible factor is restraint by the pericardium. This may be caused by an increase in pericardial pressure, making transmyocardial pressure gradients throughout diastole less than those measured with respect to an external reference point.[77,78] Alternatively, the pericardium may restrain the outward movement of myocardium only at end-diastole, as does the net around the bulb of a sigmoidoscope. In man, the contribution of the pericardium is not known. It is obviously important in the syndromes of pericardial constriction or tamponade, and possibly in many patients after open-heart surgery irrespective of whether the pericardium is closed (Fig. 21.9). However, its contribution to a raised end-diastolic pressure in disease, or its effect on measured ventricular compliance or displacement of the pressure-volume curve, remains uncertain.

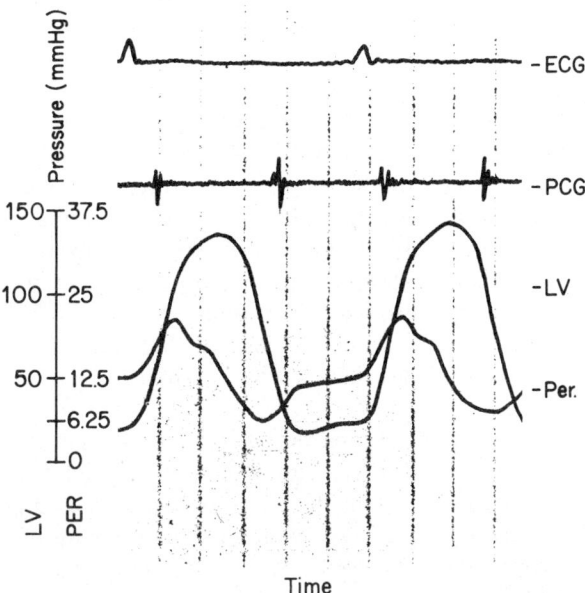

4/11/74 15.50 hrs. LV = 25:1. PER = 6.25:1.

Fig. 21.9. Simultaneous left ventricular (LV) and pericardial (PER) pressures measured early after open-heart surgery in man. Pericardial pressure was measured with a solid-state transducer applied to the epicardium. Note that part of the elevation of left ventricular diastolic pressure during ventricular filling is due to corresponding elevation of pericardial pressure, with a consequent reduction in the trans-myocardial pressure difference.

An alternative approach to studying ventricular diastolic properties is to estimate myocardial stress–strain relations in order to assess the physical properties of the myocardium itself in terms of its elastic modulus.[18] To do this realistically involves complicated calculations, making it a procedure of research interest with, as yet, limited clinical application.

From these considerations, it is clear that the stiffness of a ventricle cannot be measured in the same way as, for example, its ejection fraction. As pointed out, unstressed length cannot easily be measured in the beating heart, therefore it is not possible to compare measurements between patients, as there is no way of identifying equivalent volumes between them. A volume of, for example, 150 ml may occur during rapid filling in one patient, during diastasis in a second, and not be registered at all in a third. Measurements are frequently presented in terms of an exponential relation between pressure and volume, but there is no compelling reason why such a relation should apply; inspection of original data often shows that

wide departures have not prevented authors analysing their results in this way. How the pressure–volume curve becomes displaced with ischaemia or drugs is poorly understood.[79] It is often implied that a reduction in peak left ventricular filling rate is evidence of reduced cavity compliance, although there is no direct evidence to support this contention. Filling rate is a rate of change of volume with time, and compliance a rate of change of volume with pressure. Peak filling rate occurs at a time when compliance cannot be measured, because pressure and volume are moving in opposing directions;[56,57] no study has examined the relation between peak filling rate and compliance later in diastole using well-validated methods. Finally, it seems unlikely that disturbed cavity compliance is a major cause of symptoms. It can show itself only during diastasis and thus when the heart rate is low. At the limits of exercise tolerance, heart rate is likely to be increased so that early rapid filling becomes continuous with atrial systole and diastasis is lost.

Left atrial systole

At rest, approximately one-third of the stroke volume at rest normally enters the left ventricle during atrial systole. In patients with diastolic left ventricular disease, this proportion may be increased to 50% or more. In an individual patient, evidence of increased left atrial activity may be useful evidence of abnormal ventricular diastolic function. This evidence may take several forms. An increase in the height of the 'a' wave may be apparent on the left ventricular pressure trace itself. Events on the apexcardiogram during diastole are closely related in timing to those of the ventricular pressure, such that this technique can also give evidence of an abnormal rise in cavity pressure during atrial systole. At the same time, there may be an abnormal increase in ventricular volume during atrial systole, which can be detected using an imaging method such as contrast or radionuclide angiography (Fig. 21.10). Finally, Doppler may show transmitral flow velocity to be increased during atrial systole (A).[80,81] This may be expressed in absolute terms, or related to the early diastolic peak (E), so that the ratio A/E becomes greater than one. Clearly, these measurements are not identical. The increase in ventricular pressure depends on the increase in volume during atrial systole as well as on some function of the stiffness of the cavity. The increase in blood velocity is likely to depend on atrial systolic as well as on ventricular diastolic

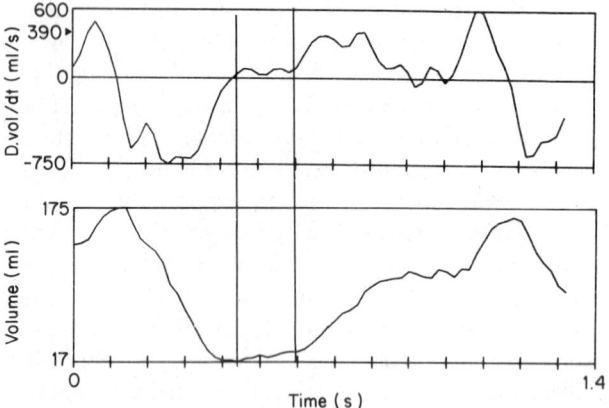

Fig. 21.10. Left ventricular filling curve from a patient with systemic hypertension, measured from a contrast angiogram. Note that filling rate is reduced during early diastole, and that peak filling rate occurs during left atrial systole. Compare this figure with Fig. 21.1.

function, and there is no reason to suppose that an invariable relation exists between the two in all forms of heart disease. In many cases of severe left ventricular hypertrophy, for example, an 'a' wave is readily apparent on the apexcardiogram but not on the Doppler flow velocity trace. Conversely, in early hypertension, the height of the Doppler 'a' wave is increased in the absence of evidence of left ventricular hypertrophy.

CLINICAL ASSESSMENT OF LEFT VENTRICULAR FUNCTION

The extent of the literature on left ventricular function and the number of 'indices' described make if difficult to determine what measurements should be made in an individual patient. It has become clear that there is no single index of left ventricular function and there are many aspects of both systolic and diastolic performance that can vary independently of one another. It would seem reasonable therefore to adopt an analytical approach, and try to identify the disturbances present in an individual patient, rather than thinking only in terms of ill-defined entities such as 'contractility' or 'relaxation'.

Among the most fundamental aspects of left ventricular function are cavity size and shape at end-systole and end-diastole, and hence ejection fraction along with the presence or distribution of any increase in wall thickness. Cavity size and shape determine the relation between muscle and pump function, reflecting the integrity of myocardial fibre

architecture. Myocardial cells function at a mechanical disadvantage in a dilated ventricle, their reduced shortening velocity mimicking depressed contractility.

A second characteristic feature of the normal ventricle is the synchrony of its movement in systole and diastole. Loss of this normal co-ordination can mimic more generalized disturbances of function. In systole, for example, its presence is directly associated with prolongation of the pre-ejection period or reduced peak dP/dt and its derivatives, abnormalities previously ascribed to impaired contractility. Similarly, in diastole, the slow filling seen in patients with coronary artery disease or left ventricular hypertrophy is associated with strikingly incoordinate wall motion.

Some aspect of contraction velocity should also be measured. The velocity of circumferential fibre shortening can easily be measured by almost any imaging technique. Low values in disease are nearly always associated with increased cavity size of which it is the direct geometrical consequence, whereas acute changes in individual patients are more likely to be load dependent rather than reflect any change in inotropic state. Alternatively, peak left ventricular ejection rate can be assessed, either from rate of fall of ventricular volume or from flow velocities measured in the ascending aorta by the Doppler technique. Although E_{max} is largely independent of preload and afterload, there are indications that it may be sensitive to stroke volume. Nevertheless, it appears to be useful in giving an overall index of left ventricular systolic function, closely related to ejection fraction. Its units are those of elastance, and so it is conceptually independent of contraction velocity; it is a measure of overall function, and thus gives no indication of regional disturbances.

Wherever possible, measurements of ventricular systolic function undertaken at rest should be supplemented by those taken during physiological stress. Several methods have been used, including isometric exercise or the cold pressor test, whose main effect is to increase arterial pressure, or isotonic exercise which increases cardiac output. Their influence on any aspect of ventricular function can be studied, but ejection fraction or the relation between stroke volume and filling pressure have proved the most popular. Again, the overall response is determined by the complicated interactions between ventricular function itself and the loading conditions.

Diastolic performance must also be assessed. The

time-constant of ventricular pressure fall has been widely used, although its rate-limiting step is not known. Simple prolongation of isovolumic relaxation time or incoordinate wall motion during the isovolumic period are evidence of early diastolic abnormality, and both have been correlated with peak filling rate once the mitral valve has opened. The characteristics of the rapid filling period are probably crucial for determining stroke volume. Measurements of cavity stiffness must be undertaken during diastasis, and, therefore, it is possible to perform them only when the heart rate is slow. They are complicated to perform, their significance is not well understood and no relation to exercise tolerance or prognosis has been established. Finally, evidence of increased left atrial activity may suggest abnormal diastolic function. This increase may be seen in the pressure curve, in cavity size or in blood velocity. The way in which these various manifestations interact with one another, and how they depend on atrial systolic function remain to be determined, as does the exact diastolic disturbance or disturbances that they reflect. Measurements based on Doppler methods are relatively simple to perform, and have attracted much recent popularity, but when these different aspects of diastolic function are compared in patients with uncomplicated left ventricular hypertrophy, there is evidence of at least four, apparently independent underlying mechanisms;[81] it would seem unwise, therefore, to restrict measurements to one technique.

The approach to the study of left ventricular disease suggested here is an analytical one. It avoids assuming that myocardial function is uniform, and allows disturbances in individual patients to be defined. Although terms such as 'heart failure' or 'decompensation' are convenient and attractive, they cover a variety of different physiological abnormalities. Only when these are analysed in detail will it be possible for their individual contribution to symptoms or prognosis to be determined and optimum treatment established.

REFERENCES

1. Paraskos, J.A., Grossman, W., Soltz, S., Dalen, J.E. and Dexter, L. A noninvasive technique for the determination of the velocity of circumferential fiber shortening in man. *Circ. Res.* 1971; **29**: 610.
2. Ross, Jr J., Sonnenblick, E.H., Covell, J.W., Kaiser, G.A. and Spiro, D. Architecture of the heart in systole and diastole. Technique of rapid fixation and analysis of left ventricular geometry. *Circ. Res.* 1967; **21**: 409–21.
3. Carew, T.E. and Covell, J.W. Fiber orientation in hypertrophied canine left ventricle. *Am. J. Physiol.* 1979; **236**: H487–H493.
4. Hammermeister, K.E., Brooks, R.C. and Warbasse, J.R. The rate of change of left ventricular volume in man. I. Validation and peak systolic ejection rate in health and disease. *Circ. Res.* 1974; **49**: 729–38.
5. Ratib, O. and Rutishauser, W. Recent developments in cardiac digital radiography. *Int. J. Cardiac. Imag.* 1985; **1**: 29–48.
6. Gibson, D.G., Prewitt, T.A. and Brown, D.J. Analysis of left ventricular wall movement during isovolumic relaxation and its relation to coronary artery disease. *Br. Heart J.* 1976; **38**: 1010–9.
7. Hammermeister, K., Gibson, D.G. and Hughes, D. Regional variation in the timing and extent of left ventricular wall motion in normal subjects. *Br. Heart J.* 1986; **56**: 226–35.
8. Huntsman, L.L., Stewart, D.K., Barnes, S.R., Franklin, S.B., Colocousis, J.C. and Hessel, E.A. Noninvasive Doppler determination of cardiac output in man. *Circulation* 1983; **67**: 593–602.
9. Noble, M.I.M., Trenchard, D. and Guz, A. Left ventricular ejection in conscious dogs. I. Measurement and significance of the maximum acceleration of blood from the left ventricle. *Circ. Res.* 1966; **19**: 139–47.
10. Spencer, M.P. and Greiss, F.C. Dynamics of ventricular ejection. *Circ. Res.* 1962; **10**: 274–9.
11. Gleason, W.L and Braunwald, E. Studies on the first derivative of the ventricular pressure pulse in man. *J. Clin. Invest.* 1962; **41**: 80.
12. Sagawa, K. The end-systolic pressure–volume relation of the ventricle: definition, modifications and clinical use (Editorial). *Circulation* 1981; **63**: 1223–7.
13. Braunwald, E., Sonnenblick, E.H., Ross, J. and Gault, J.H, Insights into cardiovascular physiology derived from muscle mechanics. *Am. J. Cardiol.* 1967; **20**: 705.
14. Noble, M.I.M. Problems concerning the application of muscle mechanics to the determination of the contractile state of the heart (Editorial). *Circulation* 1972; **45**: 252.
15. Mehmel, H.C., Stockins, B., Ruffmann, K., von Olshausen, K., Schuler, G. and Kubler, W. The linearity of the end-systolic pressure–volume relationship in man and its sensitivity for assessment of left ventricular function. *Circulation* 1981; **63**: 1216–22.
16. Colan, S.D., Borow, K.M., Gamble, W.J. and Sanders, S.P. Effects of enhanced afterload (methoxamine) and contractile state (dobutamine) on left ventricular late-systolic wall stress-dimension ratio. *Am. J. Cardiol.* 1983; **52**: 1304–9.
17. Baan, J., Jong, T.T.A., Kerkhof, P.L.M., Moene, R.J., van Dijk, A.D., ven der Velde, E.T. and Koops, J. Continuous stroke volume and cardiac output from intra-ventricular dimensions obtained with impedance catheter. *Cardiovasc. Res.* 1981; **1**: 328–34.
18. Yin, F.C.P. Ventricular wall stress. *Circ. Res.* 1981; **49**: 829–42.
19. Greenbaum, R.A. and Gibson, D.G. Regional non-uniformity of left ventricular wall movement in man. *Br. Heart J.* 1981; **45**: 29–34.
20. Braunwald, E., Ross, J. and Sonnenblick, E.H. Mechanisms of contraction in the normal and failing heart. *N. Engl. J. Med.* 1967; **227**: 1012.
21. Peterson, K.L., Skloven, D., Ludbrook, P., Uther, J.B. and Ross, Jr J. Comparison of isovolumic and ejection phase indices of myocardial performance in man. *Circulation* 1974; **39**: 1088–101.
22. Kreulen, T.H., Bove, A.A., McDonough, M.T., Sands, M.J. and Spann, J.F. The evaluation of left ventricular function in man. A comparison of methods. *Circulation* 1975; **51**: 677–88.
23. Burton, A.C. The importance of the size and shape of the heart. *Am. Heart J.* 1957; **54**: 801.

24. Falsetti, H.L., Mates, R.E., Greene, D.G. and Bunnell, I.L. Left ventricular wall stress calculated from one-plane cineangiography. An approach to force–velocity analysis in man. *Circ. Res.* 1970; **26**: 71–83.

25. Ross, J. Afterload mismatch and preload reserve: a conceptual framework for analysis of ventricular function. *Prog. Cardiovasc. Dis.* 1976; **18**: 255.

26. Linzbach, A.J. Heart failure from the point of view of quantitative anatomy. *Am. J. Cardiol.* 1960; **5**: 370–82.

27. Ford, L.E. Heart size. *Circ. Res.* 1976; **39**: 297–303.

28. Gaasch, W.H. Left ventricular wall thickness ratio. *Am. J. Cardiol.* 1979; **43**: 1189–93.

29. Grossman, W., Braunwald, E., Mann, T., McLaurin, L.P. and Green, L.H. Contractile state of the left ventricle in man as evaluated from end-systolic pressure–volume relations. *Circulation* 1977; **56**: 845–52.

30. Herman, M.V. and Gorlin, R. Implications of left ventricular asynergy. *Am. J. Cardiol.* 1969; **23**: 538–47.

31. Chaitman, B.R., Bristow, J.D. and Rahimtoola, S.H. Left ventricular wall motion assessed by using fixed external reference systems. *Circulation* 1973; **48**: 1043–50.

32. Gibson, D.G., Doran, J.H., Traill, T.A. and Brown, D.J. Abnormal left ventricular wall movement during early systole in patients with angina pectoris. *Br. Heart J.* 1978; **40**: 758–66.

33. Hui, W.K.K. and Gibson, D.G. Mechanisms of reduced left ventricular filling rate in coronary artery disease. *Br. Heart J.* 1983; **50**: 362–71.

34. Yamagishi, T., Ozaki T., Kumada, T., Ikezono, T., Shimizu, T., Furutani, Y., Yamaoka, H., Ogawa, H., Matsuzaki, M. and Matsuda, Y. Asynchronous left ventricular diastolic filling in patients with isolated disease of the left anterior descending coronary artery: assessment with radionuclide ventriculography. *Circulation* 1984; **69**: 933–42.

35. Gibson, D.G. and Brown, D.J. Assessment of left ventricular systolic function in man from simultaneous echocardiographic and pressure measurements. *Br. Heart J.* 1976; **38**: 8–17.

36. Chen, W. and Gibson, D. Mechanisms of prolongation of the pre-ejection period in patients with left ventricular disease. *Br. Heart J.* 1979; **42**: 304–10.

37. Marier, D.L. and Gibson, D.G. Limitations of two frame method for displaying regional left ventricular wall motion in man. *Br. Heart J.* 1980; **44**: 555–9.

38. Gibson, D., Mehmel, H., Schwarz, F., Li, K. and Kubler, W. Asynchronous left ventricular wall motion early after coronary thrombosis. *Br. Heart J.* 1986; **55**: 4–13.

39. Gibson, D., Mehmel, H., Schwarz, F., Li, K. and Kubler, W. Changes in left ventricular regional asynchrony after intracoronary thrombolysis in patients with impending myocardial infarction. *Br. Heart J.* 1986; **56**: 121–30.

40. Brunt, J.N.H., Love, H.G. and Rowlands, D.J. Objective analysis of left ventricular cine-angiograms. In: Rowlands D.J. ed. *Recent Advances in Cardiology*, No. 9. Edinburgh: Churchill Livingstone, 1984, pp. 321–42.

41. Wiggers, C.J. Studies on the duration of the consecutive phases of the cardiac cycle. I. The duration of the consecutive phases of the cardiac cycle and criteria for their precise determination. *Am. J. Physiol.* 1921; **56**: 415–38.

42. Chen, W. and Gibson, D.G. Relation of isovolumic relaxation to left ventricular wall movement in man. *Br. Heart J.* 1979; **42**: 51–6.

43. Mattheos, M., Shapiro, E., Oldershaw, P.J., Sacchetti, R. and Gibson, D.G. Non-invasive assessment of changes in left ventricular relaxation by combined phono-, echo-, and mechanography. *Br. Heart J.* 1982; **47**: 253–60.

44. Gamble, W.H., Salerni, R. and Shaver, J.A. The noninvasive assessment of pulmonary capillary pressure in mitral regurgitation. *Am. Heart J.* 1984; **107**: 950–8.

45. Weisfeldt, M.L., Weiss, J.L., Frederiksen, J.T. and Yin,

F.C.P. Quantification of incomplete left ventricular relaxation: relationship to the time constant for isovolumic pressure fall. *Eur. Heart J.* 1980; **1**: A119–29.

46. Brutsaert, D.L., Rademakers, F.E., Sys, S.U., Gillebert, T.C. and Housmans, P.R. Analysis of relaxation in the evaluation of ventricular function of the heart. *Prog. Cardiovasc. Dis.* 1985; **28**: 143–63.

47. Goldberg, S.J., Feldman, L., Reinecke, C., Stern, L.Z., Sahn, D.J and Allen, H.D. Echocadiographic determination of contraction and relaxation measurements of the left ventricular wall in normal subjects and patients with muscular dystrophy. *Circulation* 1980; **62**: 1061–9.

48. Danford, D.A., Huhta, J.C. and Murphy, D.J. Doppler echocardiographic approaches to ventricular diastolic function. *Echocardiography* 1986; **3**: 33–40.

49. Frederiksen, J.W., Weiss, J.L. and Weisfeldt, M.L. Time constant of isovolumic pressure fall: determinants in the working left ventricle. *Am. J. Physiol.* 1978; **235**: H701–H706.

50. Weiss, J.L., Frederiksen, J.W and Weisfeldt, M.L. Hemodynamic determinants of the time-course of fall in canine left ventricular pressure. *J. Clin. Invest.* 1976; **58**: 751–60.

51. Thompson, D.S., Waldron, C.B., Coltart, D.J., Jenkins, B.S. and Webb-Peploe, M.M. Estimation of time constant of left ventricular relaxation. *Br. Heart J.* 1983; **49**: 250–8.

52. Thompson, D.S., Waldron, C.B., Juul, S.M., Naqvi, N., Swanton, R.H., Coltart, D.J., Jenkins, B.S. and Webb-Peploe, M.M. Analysis of left ventricular pressure during isovolumic relaxation in coronary artery disease. *Circulation* 1982; **65**: 690–7.

53. Rousseau, M.F., Veriter, C., Detry, J.-M., Brasseur, L. and Pouleur, H. Impaired early left ventricular relaxation in coronary artery disease; effects of nifedipine. *Circulation* 1980; **62**: 764–72.

54. Henderson, Y., Scarbrough, M.M. and Chillingworth, F.P. The volume curve of the ventricles of the mammalian heart, and the significance of this curve in respect to the mechanics of the heart-beat and the filling of the ventricles. *Am. J. Physiol.* 1906; **16**: 325–67.

55. Katz, L.N. The role played by the relaxation in filling of the ventricle. *Am. J. Physiol.* 1930; **95**: 542.

56. Gibson, D.G. and Brown, D.J. Relation between diastolic left ventricular wall stress and strain in man. *Br. Heart J.* 1974; **36**: 1066–77.

57. Fioretti, P., Brower, R.W., Meester, G.T. and Serruys, P.W. Interaction of left ventricular relaxation and filling during early diastole in human subjects. *Am. J. Cardiol.* 1980; **46**: 197–203.

58. Ishida, Y., Meisner, J.S., Tsujioka, K., Gallo, J.I., Yoran, C., Frater, R.M.W. and Yellin, E.L. Left ventricular filling dynamics : influence of left ventricular relaxation and left atrial pressure. *Circulation* 1986; **74**: 187–96.

59. Winegrad, S., Weisber, A. and McClennan, G. Are restoring forces important to relaxation. *Eur. Heart J.* 1980 (Suppl. A); **1**: 59–66.

60. Sonnenblick, E.H. The structural basis and importance of restoring forced and elastic recoil for the filling of the heart. *Eur. Heart J.* 1980 (Suppl. A); **1**: 107–110.

61. Brecher, G.A. Critical review of recent work on ventricular diastolic suction. *Circ. Res.* 1958; **6**: 554–66.

62. Carroll, J.D., Hess, O.M., Hirzel, H.O. and Krayenbuehl, H.P. Dynamics of left ventricular filling at rest and during exercise. *Circulation* 1983; **68**: 59–67.

63. Carroll, J.D., Hess, O.M., Hirzel, H.O. and Krayenbuehl, H.P. Exercise-induced ischemia: the influence of altered relaxation on early diastolic pressures. *Circulation* 1983; **67**: 521–8.

64. Bonow, R.O., Bacharach, S.L., Green, M.V., Kent, K.M., Rosing, D.R., Lipson, L.C., Leon, M.B. and Epstein, S.E. Impaired left ventricular diastolic filling in patients with

coronary artery disease: assessment with radionuclide angiography. *Circulation* 1981; **64**: 315–23.

65. Reduto, L.A., Wickemeyer, W.J., Young, J.B., Del Ventura, L.A., Reid, J.W., Glaeser, D.H., Quinones, M.A. and Miller, R.R. Left ventricular diastolic performance at rest and during exercise in patients with coronary artery disease. Assessment with first pass radionuclide angiography. *Circulation* 1981; **63**: 1228–37.

66. Rokey, R., Kuo, L.C., Zoghbi, W.A. *et al*. Determination of parameters of left ventricular diastolic filling with pulsed Doppler echocardiography: comparison with angiography. *Circulation* 1985; **71**: 543–51.

67. Hui, W.K.K., Lee, P.K., Chow, J.S.F. and Gibson, D.G. Analysis of regional left ventricular wall motion during diastole in mitral stenosis. *Br. Heart J.* 1983; **50**: 231–9.

68. Gibson, D.G., Traill, T.A., Hall, R.J.C. and Brown, D.J. Echocardiographic features of secondary left ventricular hypertrophy. *Br. Heart J.* 1979; **41**: 54–9.

69. Shapiro, L.M., Leatherdale, B.A., Mackinnon, J. and Fletcher, R.F. Left ventricular function in diabetes millitus. II: Relation between clinical features and left ventricular function. *Br. Heart J.* 1981; **45**: 129–32.

70. Venco, A., Saviotti, M., Besana, D., Finardi, G. and Lanzi, G. Noninvasive assessment of left ventricular function in myotonic muscular dystrophy. *Br. Heart J.* 1978; **40**: 1262–6.

71. Mirsky, I. Assessment of passive elastic stiffness of cardiac muscle: Mathematical concepts, physiologic and clinical considerations, direction of future research. *Prog. Cardiovasc. Dis.* 1976; **18**: 277–308.

72. Grossman, W. and McLaurin, L.P. Diastolic properties of the left ventricle. *Ann. Intern. Med.* 1976; **84**: 316–26.

73. Alderman, E.L. and Glantz, S.A. Acute hemodynamic interventions shift the diastolic pressure–volume curve in man. *Circulation* 1976; **54**: 662.

74. Fester, A. and Samet, P. Passive elasticity of the human left ventricle. The "parallel elastic element". *Circulation* 1974; **50**: 609–18.

75. Hess, O.M., Grimm, J. and Krayenbuehl, H.P. Diastolic simple elastic and viscoelastic properties of the left ventricle in man. *Circulation* 1979; **59**: 1178–87.

76. Tallarida, R.J., Rusy, B.F. and Loughnane, M.H. Left ventricular wall acceleration and the law of Laplace. *Cardiovasc. Res.* 1970; **4**: 217–23.

77. Tyberg, J.V., Misbach, G.A., Galnyz, S.A., Moores, W.Y. and Parmely, W.W. A mechanism for shifts in the diastolic, left ventricular, pressure–volume curve: the role of the pericardium. *Eur. J. Cardiol.* 1978; **7** (suppl.) 163–75.

78. Smiseth, O.A., Frais, M.A., Kingma, I., Smith, E.R. and Tyberg, J.V. Assessment of pericardial constraint in dogs. *Circulation* 1985; **71**: 158–64.

79. Glantz, S.A. and Parmley, W.W. Factors which affect the diastolic pressure – volume curve. *Circ. Res.* 1978; **42**: 171–80.

80. Ohkushi, H., Asai, M., Ishito, T. *et al*. Left ventricular diastolic filling patterns in hypertrophic cardiomyopathy and myocardial infarction: studies by pulsed Doppler echocardiography and multigate blood pool scans. *J. Cardiogr.* 1984; **14**: 95–114.

81. Shapiro, L.M. and Gibson, D.G. Patterns of diastolic dysfunction in left ventricular hypertrophy. *Br. Heart J.* 1988; **9**: 438–45.

Chapter 22

The Pathology of Arrhythmias, Conduction Disturbances and Sudden Death

M.J. Davies and David E. Ward

SINO-ATRIAL DISEASE AND ATRIAL ARRHYTHMIAS

STRUCTURE OF SINUS NODE

In the 80 years that have elapsed since Keith and Flack described the sino-atrial node as the origin of sinus rhythm in the mammalian heart, histological, ultrastructural and electrophysiological data have been integrated to delineate the best understood component of the conduction system.[1]

In man, the sino-atrial node is tiny with a length of 5.2–8.5 mm and a maximal thickness of 1.5 mm. The sinus node of the rabbit is larger than that of man, indicating that nodal size and heart size are not related. In mammalian hearts, including the human heart, three types of myocyte can be identified within the node by ultrastructural studies. The myocytes in the centre of the node are interwoven, interspersed with connective tissue, and contain very few myofilaments, thus they appear to have empty cytoplasm. Animal studies suggest these myocytes (P cells) are the dominant pacemaking foci; in the rabbit node, the number of these cells is estimated at a maximum of 5000. External to the deep portion of the node is a transitional layer of myocytes, which contain more myofilaments, and a final layer of cells, which are virtually indistinguishable from ordinary atrial myocytes, containing specific atrial granules and with over 50% of the cell cytoplasm occupied by myofilaments. In the rabbit heart, only the deepest nodal myocytes behave as the primary pacemakers; there is no reason to believe the human heart is different in this respect. Abundant nerve tissue ramifies in the nodal connective tissue and ganglia are present in the adjacent atrial tissue.

In man, age-related changes in the sinus node are very striking. In young individuals, the node is made up of approximately equal proportions of connective tissue and nodal myocytes (Fig. 22.1). By 70 years of age, many normal subjects have only 10% of the node made up of myocytes (Fig. 22.2), as measured by the proportion of the volume they occupy relative to connective tissue.[2] The node does not increase in size with age and the data indicate an overall fall in the number of nodal myocytes, but the quantitative methods employed are too crude to allow an assessment of whether there is a differential effect on the deepest nodal cells. Many elderly subjects with otherwise normal hearts, however, will have very few sino-atrial nodal cells. As the fall in the proportion of myocytes to collagen in the human node is linear with respect to age, it can be predicted that if many members of the population became centenarians very few would be in sinus rhythm.

In man, the node often has a small central artery around which the deep nodal fibres are arranged, a

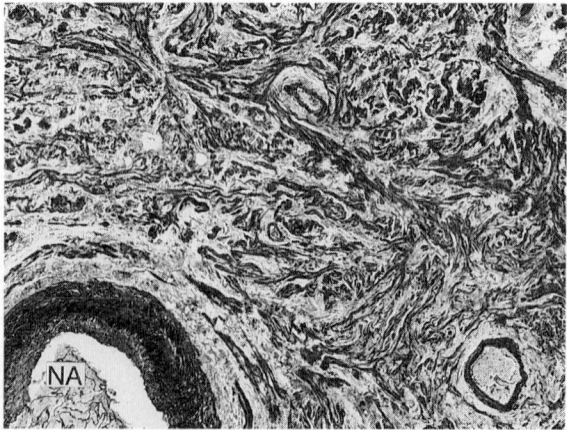

Fig. 22.1. The normal sinus node consists of a mass of small darkly stained interweaving myocytes embedded in a connective tissue framework. The whole structure closely surrounds the nodal artery (NA).

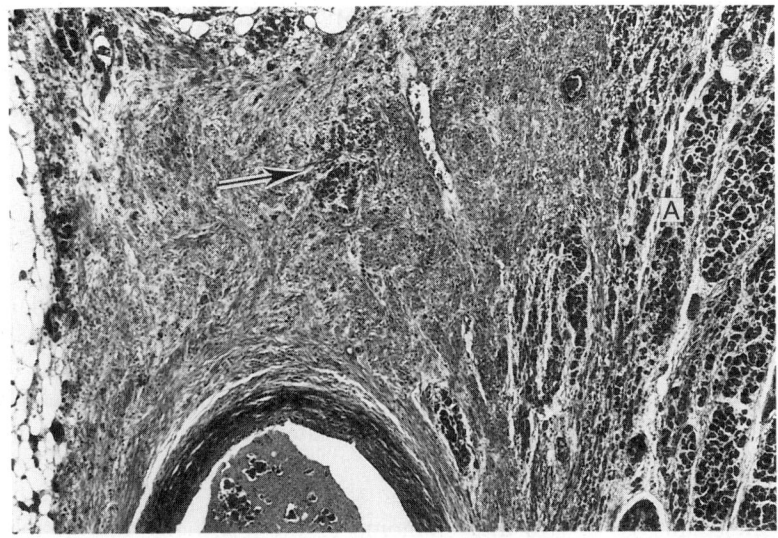

Fig. 22.2. A sinus node with non-specific reduction of myocyte numbers. Within the node, there is a single clump of myocytes (arrow). The perinodal myocytes are more numerous (A).

pattern that has led to suggestions that arterial pulsation can influence the rate of sinus discharge.[3] This hypothesis seems negated by the occurrence of cases in whom the artery is absent or alongside, rather than within, the node. The age-related loss of nodal myocytes is independent of the degree of arteriosclerosis present.[4]

MORPHOLOGICAL STUDIES IN CHRONIC SINO-ATRIAL DISEASE

Pathological studies of the heart in chronic sino-atrial disease are rare, reflecting the relatively benign course of the disease, but a consistent pattern can be perceived.[4–7] Amyloid deposition within the node and adjacent atrial myocardium is one cause of sino-atrial block. A second cause is associated with a marked loss of nodal myocytes beyond that normal for the age of the patient. This means the virtual absence of myocytes in a node that is recognizable as being of normal size by its collagenous outline. The reason for the accentuated loss of nodal myocytes is obscure; in epidemiological studies, previous diphtheria, myocarditis, autoimmunity or rheumatic disease have all been postulated as the cause for this loss.[8] Some morphological and clinical evidence suggests that there is a concomitant loss of conduction fibres in the more distal conduction system.[5] The third morphological pattern responsible for sino-atrial block is an aplastic or hypoplastic node in which even the basic collagenous structure is absent or small. This form has been found in sino-atrial block in children[9] and may be responsible for familial cases.[10] Finally, cases of idiopathic sino-atrial disease are described

in whom no morphological abnormality, using conventional light microscopy, can be found and the explanation must lie in abnormal physiology or abnormal neural influences. None of these morphological patterns can be linked with atheroma affecting the epicardial coronary arteries. Seventeen patients with ischaemic heart disease who had obstruction to the right coronary artery, proximal to or at the origin of the sinus node artery, showed no electrophysiological evidence of abnormal function of the node.[11] Six patients with the sick sinus syndrome and ischaemic heart disease had normal sinus node arteries.[11] The Devon Regional Survey found that only 11 of 106 patients wth chronic sino-atrial disease had had previous myocardial infarction.[8] An angiographic study of 25 cases of chronic sino-atrial disease at autopsy[12] has shown complete block of the sinus node artery in two and poor filling in a further three; these results indicate that coronary atheroma is not the principal cause of chronic sino-atrial block. Detailed morphometry shows no association between arteriosclerosis of the smaller intramyocardial arteries and nodal myocyte loss.[4]

MORPHOLOGICAL STUDIES IN ATRIAL FIBRILLATION

Chronic atrial fibrillation is associated with a very wide range of clinical conditions but it is also related to age; up to 15% of elderly patients without overt evidence of heart disease are not in sinus rhythm.[13] Studies of the node itself[14] show that an accentuated, or even total, loss of nodal myocytes is almost universal in established atrial fibrillation, suggesting that generation of a sub-threshold sinus impulse may be an important mechanism. There is also an almost constant association of chronic atrial fibrillation with intersection of the atrial septal muscle by fibrous and/or adipose tissue providing a substrate for multiple re-entry circuits.[14] Atrial fibrillation is also accompanied by atrial dilatation which may be largely secondary but will, in itself, potentiate any tendency to fibrillation.

ATRIAL TACHYCARDIAS

In most instances, atrial tachycardias arise in micro re-entry circuits close to the sinus node or elsewhere in the atrial septum. The anatomical abnormality probably lies in fibrosis isolating islands and strands of atrial muscle; this view is supported by the occurrence of such tachycardias after operations involving patching or suturing of the atrial septum. In one case, excision of a small localized atrial aneurysm abolished the tachycardia.[15] Paroxysmal atrial tachycardia is also associated with focal tumour deposits within atrial muscle. Atrial tachycardia due to a focus of abnormal automaticity is usually associated with cardiac disease, but no pathological studies of an excised focus initiating the arrhythmias are known.

JUNCTIONAL TACHYCARDIAS

Junctional tachycardias arise in the atrioventricular junctional tissue or depend on these tissues for their continuation.[16] The junctional tissues comprise the atrioventricular node and the penetrating atrioventricular bundle as well as accessory or anomalous atrioventricular connections. The term junctional tachycardia thus includes:

1 re-entry tachycardias involving atrioventricular anomalous pathways in the septum or lateral atrioventricular rings;
2 intranodal re-entrant tachycardias;
3 tachycardias associated with nodoventricular pathways;
4 focal His bundle tachycardia.

An understanding of the micro-anatomy of the atrioventricular node and the atrioventricular rings is central to an understanding of these arrhythmias.

The atrioventricular node lies just beneath the endocardium of the right atrium within the triangle of Koch; this triangle is bounded by the coronary sinus, the continuation of the Eustachian valve as the tendon of Todaro and the insertion of the septal cusp of the tricuspid valve (Fig. 22.3). At the apex of the triangle is the central fibrous body. The node lies closer to the apex of the triangle than to the base which is formed by the ostium of the coronary sinus. The sub-epicardial fat invaginates into the

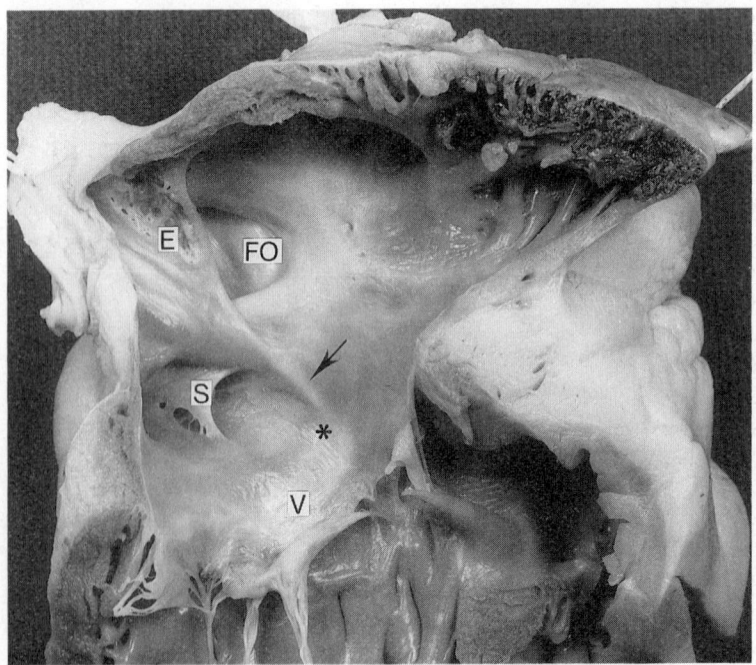

Fig. 22.3. The interatrial septum viewed from the right side. The triangle of Koch is formed by the coronary sinus (S), the tendon of Todaro (arrow) and the septal cusp of the tricuspid valve (V). The node (*) lies at the apex of the triangle. E, Eustachian valve; FO, foramen ovale.

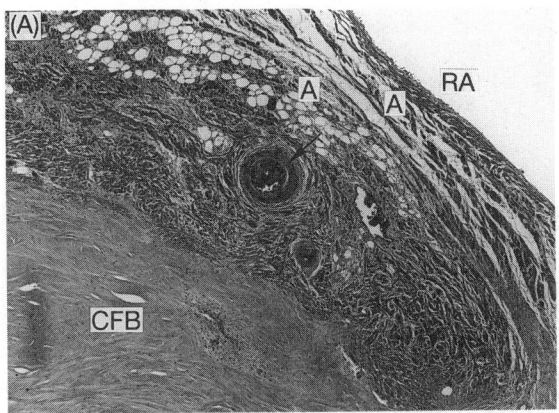
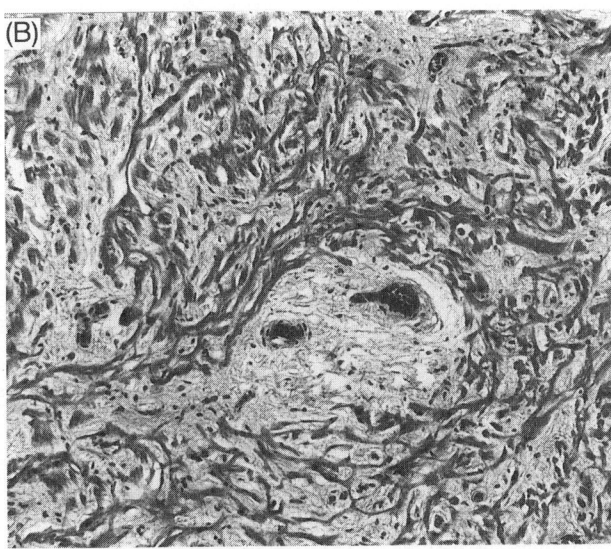

Fig. 22.4. (A) The atrioventricular node consists of an oval mass of small myocytes surrounding the nodal artery (arrow). The node is applied to the central fibrous body (CFB) and lies beneath the endocardium of the right atrium (RA). Layers of atrial myocytes (A) separate the endocardium from the node. (B) The myocytes of the deep inner portion of the node are small and arranged in an interwoven pattern. Such an arrangement is associated with very slow conduction.

posterior aspect of the atrial septum in the floor of the coronary sinus, almost reaching the node, and contains the nodal artery as it runs in from the origin of the posterior descending coronary artery in the interventricular sulcus. The morphology of the node is best appreciated in histological sections taken in the long axis of the atrial septum (Fig. 22.4). The compact or deep portion of the atrioventricular node is made up of an interweaving mass of small muscle cells embedded in a fibrous stroma closely resembling the sino-atrial node in appearance. This portion of the node is half-oval in shape and applied closely to the central fibrous body (Fig. 22.5). Anteriorly, the deep node begins to sink into the central fibrous body, finally becoming encased in a fibrous tunnel, to form the penetrating atrioventricular bundle (Fig. 22.6). The deep portion of the node is covered by a superficial layer of transitional myocytes which make contact with the atrial myocardium (Fig. 22.5). Another more superficial layer of atrial muscle sweeps down over the node just beneath the endocardium to end in the base of the septal cusp of the tricuspid valve, but no contact is made with the node itself in the majority of hearts. There may not be concordance between the anatomical and electrophysiological definition of what is nodal or atrial. The nodal complex comprises a deep and a superficial layer; only the former contains small interweaving nodal myocytes. When using the term nodal, the elec-

trophysiologist may mean these deep cells but the morphologist will include the whole complex, deep and superficial, within the term.

Ultrastructural studies of the human atrioventricular node confirm that a high proportion of the myocytes do not have transverse tubules, and possess scanty myofibrils,[17] but there is a far greater mixture of the types of myocyte found throughout the atrioventricular node as compared with that found within different layers of the sino-atrial node.

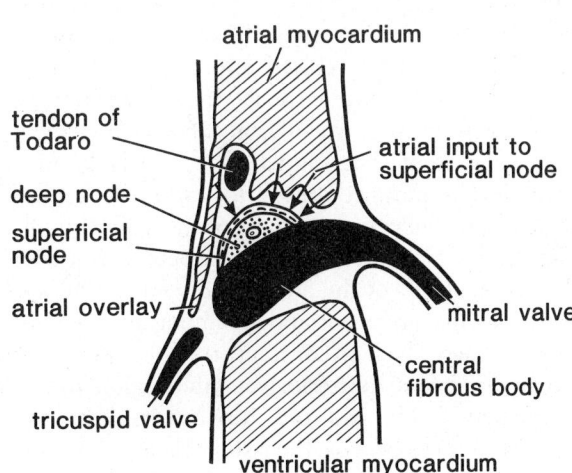

Fig. 22.5. Diagrammatic representation of the relation of the atrioventricular node and its atrial connections to the central fibrous body.

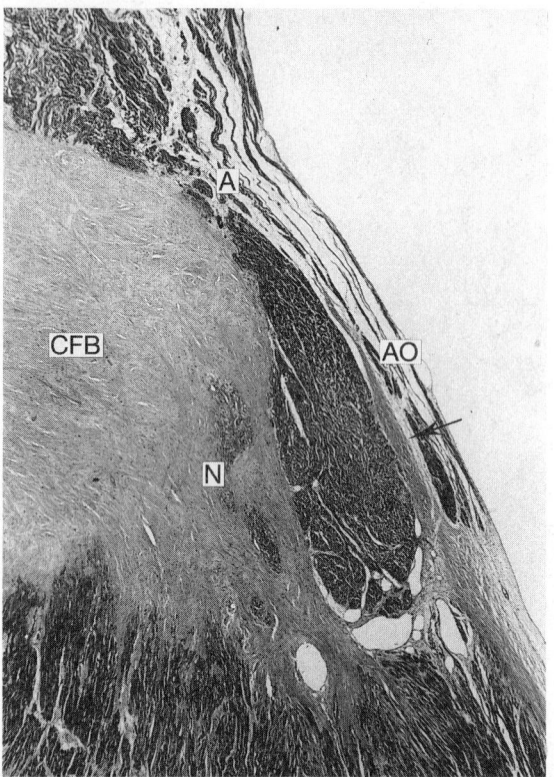

Fig. 22.6. The atrioventricular node is beginning to penetrate the central fibrous body (CFB) and becoming partially enclosed by a layer of fibrous tissue (arrow). The last atrial connection (A) is made from myocytes in the middle of the septum. The atrial overlay (AO) myocytes do not connect with the penetrating atrioventricular bundle. Buried within the central fibrous body are some separate islands of nodal tissue (N).

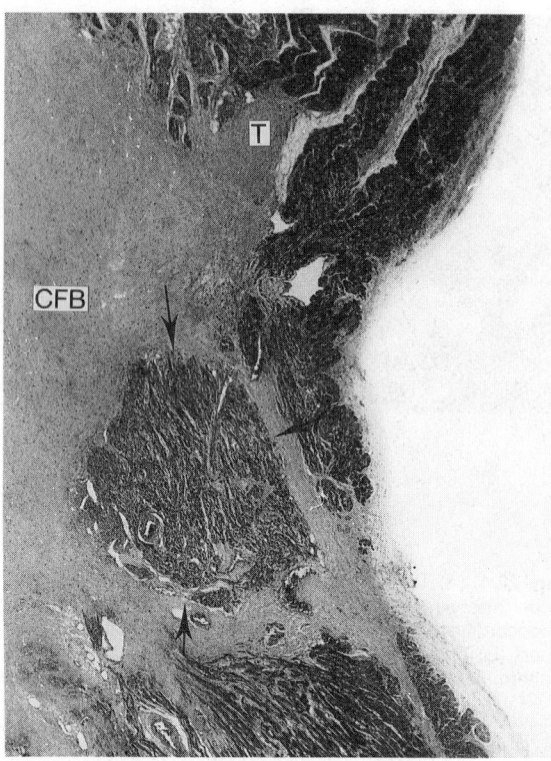

Fig. 22.7. The penetrating atrioventricular bundle (arrows) is now fully encased by the central fibrous body (CFB) to which the tendon of Todaro is attached (T).

This fact further confuses the definition of a nodal cell. The point at which the atrioventricular node ends and the penetrating bundle begins is best regarded as occurring when the roof of the fibrous tunnel is completely closed and thus there is no possibility of a further atrial input. Within the tunnel, a nodal-type irregular myocyte arrangement may be present, but ultimately the cells become arranged in parallel arrays to form the typical structure of the penetrating atrioventricular bundle (Fig. 22.7). Considerable disagreement exists over the arrangement of the atrial inputs into the node, reflecting the great variability among individuals. James[18] described a constant tract of myocytes which originated posteriorly in the region of the Eustachian valve and ran forward beneath the endocardium to become the last input into the node. This tract would bypass much of the delay-producing deep nodal area, but its existence in normal hearts has not been confirmed by other workers. The last nodal input is variable but it is usually derived from either the superficial transitional fibres or atrial muscle in the mid part of the septum.[19]

The nodal artery passes through the centre of the deep portion of the node and enters the central fibrous body, separate from the penetrating atrioventricular bundle, to reach the upper ventricular septum; a series of parallel arterioles continue within the penetrating atrioventricular bundle. The central fibrous body is also penetrated by one or more venous sinusoids. The deep node is closely applied to the edge of the central fibrous body, but in many normal young subjects isolated islands of nodal-type tissue are embedded within the fibrous tissue (Fig. 22.8). Strands of myocardial cells also accompany the vessels entering the central fibrous body. It is not known whether these archipelagos of nodal tissue interconnect with each other to form loops with the deep node. It is well established that some otherwise normal hearts contain tracts that penetrate the fibrous body to reach the ventricular septum establishing nodoventricular or fasciculoventricular contact independent of the normal conduction axis (Mahaim fibres) (Fig. 22.9).

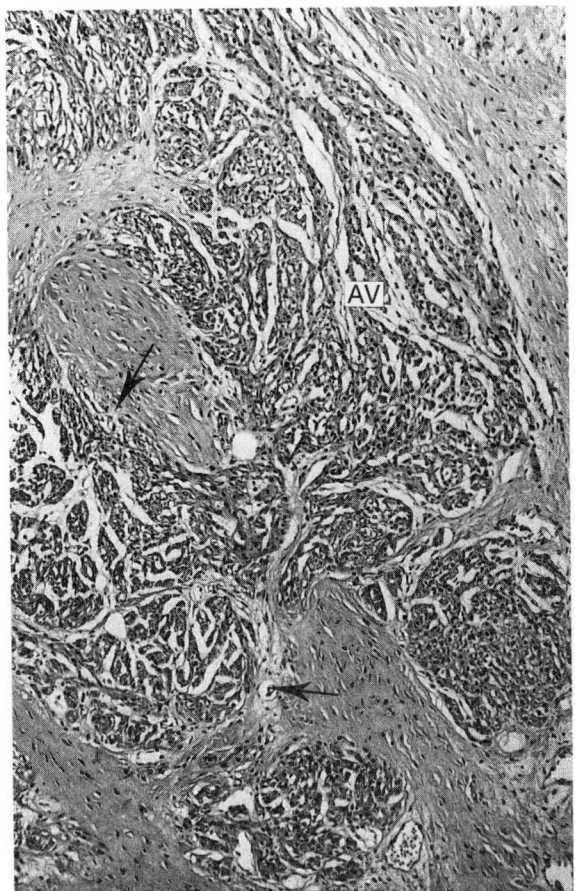

Fig. 22.8. The atrioventricular node (AV) in this infant heart connects with separate islands of nodal tissue (arrows) embedded within the central fibrous body.

The central fibrous body separates the atrial and ventricular myocardium within the septum. Exceptions are points where the penetrating bundle of Mahaim fibres establish continuity. In addition, in up to 50% of normal hearts, the central fibrous body posterior to the node is deficient where there is a pad of fat in the floor of the ostium of the coronary sinus. The gap is normally filled by adipose tissue but it may contain strands of atrial muscle which thereby come into contiguity with ventricular myocardium. Bundles of atrial muscle, however, do not normally enter and ramify in the ventricular septum to establish atrioventricular continuity. A similar defect occurs in many hearts at the point where the base of the septal cusp of the tricuspid valve meets the central fibrous body allowing the superficial atrial atrioventricular nodal overlay fibres to lie directly alongside ventricular myocardium.

In the ventricular free walls, atrial and ventricular myocardium are often regarded as being totally separated by the collagen of the valve rings. The tricuspid valve ring, however, is partially formed in most hearts and a pad of fat separates atrial and ventricular myocardium, the valve cusp being inserted into the endocardium. In addition, a node-like mass of tissue exists as a remnant of the fetal atrioventricular ring conduction tissue in up to 30% of normal adult hearts.[20] This tissue, identified by Kent, does not create a potential for pre-excitation because, although atrial and ventricular muscle may abut, no muscle bundles actually cross the atrioventricular junction to establish continuity in normal hearts.

ACCESSORY CONDUCTION PATHWAYS

Accessory paths can be divided[19] into those that lie in the left or right atrioventricular valve rings (parietal) and those that lie within the septum (Fig. 22.10). Posterior septal pathways may activate

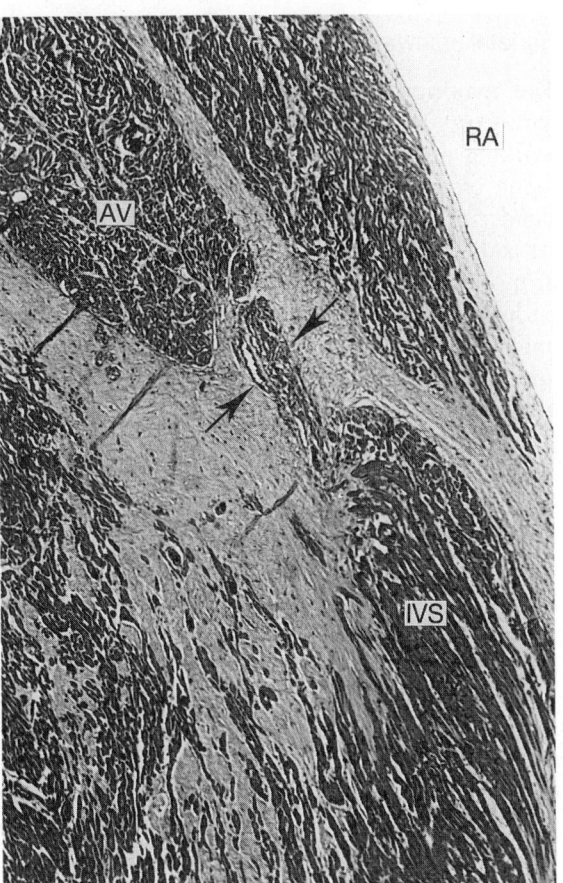

Fig. 22.9. Mahaim fasciculoventricular tract (arrows) joining the penetrating bundle (AV) to the right side of the upper interventricular septum (IVS). RA, right atrium.

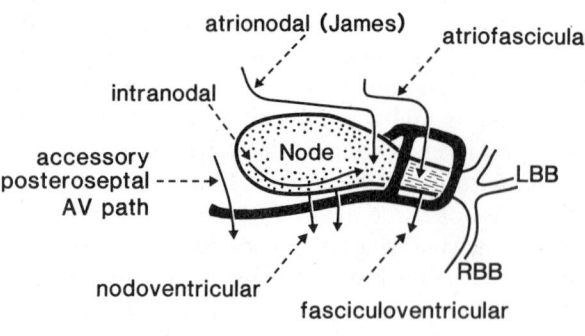

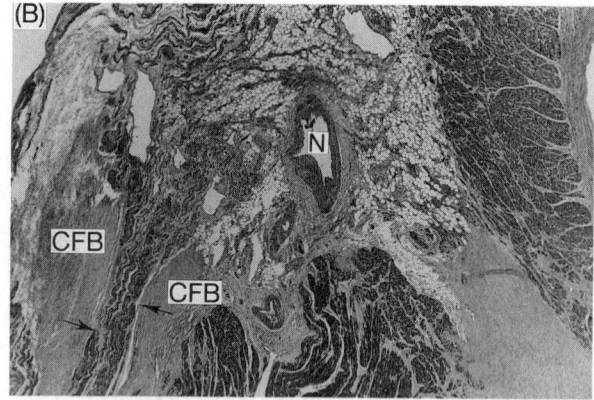

Fig. 22.10. (A) Diagrammatic representation of the accessory conduction pathways and anomalous connections in the region of the atrioventricular node. (B) Postero-septal anomalous atrioventricular connection (arrows) consisting of a bundle of longitudinally arranged atrial myocytes which penetrate the central fibrous body (CFB). The nodal artery is shown (N) just as it is beginning to enter the region of the node. The central fibrous body is seldom complete at this point and in this case is made up of three separate fibrous masses.

either the right or the left side and are difficult to distinguish from posterior parietal pathways by electrocardiographic criteria.

Parietal pathways

The majority of parietal anomalous conduction pathways consist of slender strands of normal working atrial myocytes embedded in connective tissue crossing the atrioventricular ring. Multiple slender strands and an arborization of the ventricular end of the pathway over an area of a centimetre or more are common.[19] There are rare examples of paths that arise in persistent nodal-type tissue in the anterior tricuspid ring area, which should be appropriately regarded as Kent bundles,[19] but in general there is no morphological evidence of a delay-producing area in the vast majority of parietal accessory paths. On the left side, parietal anomalous bundles run in epicardial fat closely applied to the fibrous annulus of the mitral valve (Fig. 22.11). On the right side, pathways simply run through the fat pad separating atrial and ventricular muscle.

Septal pathways

In the area immediately posterior to the atrioventricular node in the floor of the ostium of the coronary sinus, strands of normal atrial muscle may pass through the defect which commonly exists in the central fibrous body at this site. Access to this area can be achieved surgically by burrowing into the fat from the posterior interventricular sulcus because the pericardium is invaginated almost as far anteriorly as the atrioventricular node.[21]

Connections may also be present between the superficial atrial overlay myocytes beneath the endocardium of the right atrium and the ventricular septum through defects between the base of the septal cusp of the tricuspid valve and the central fibrous body. These paths are composed of normal atrial myocytes.

FUNCTIONAL CORRELATES IN JUNCTIONAL TACHYCARDIAS

To have any validity, morphological studies in this field must involve a large number of serial histological sections. Even when the serial sectioning is adequate, different levels of correlation exist. The simplest level is the demonstration of an abnormally arranged conduction system in a patient who has

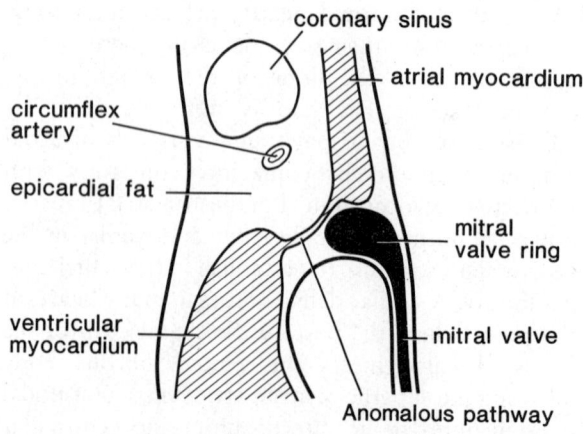

Fig. 22.11. Diagrammatic representation of the anatomical relations of a left atrioventricular anomalous connection.

died suddenly but in whom there are no electrocardiographic or electrophysiological data. The next level is the demonstration of an anomalous connection in a patient known to have pre-excitation. The most sophisticated level is when electrophysiological studies have shown the involvement of an anomalous pathway, which is confirmed to be present at autopsy, in maintaining tachycardia. The number of reported cases in the third category remains very small.

PRE-EXCITATION AND RE-ENTRANT TACHYCARDIA INVOLVING ANOMALOUS ATRIOVENTRICULAR PATHWAYS

Anomalous atrioventricular pathways lead to the early activation of a segment of ventricular myocardium due to avoidance of the delay normally imposed by the deep portion of the atrioventricular node. The anomalous pathways may conduct in either one or both directions and can act as the afferent or the efferent limb of a re-entry circuit using the conventional conduction system as the other limb. In pathological studies, all types of anomalous parietal and septal pathways have been shown to be associated with pre-excitation and tachycardia. Evidence of the function of these pathways is best shown by the success of surgical division and ablation in abolishing both pre-excitation and tachycardia. All these pathways are thought to represent persistence of atrioventricular connections that exist in all developing mammalian hearts. There is a significant familial trend, with an autosomal dominant inheritance for persistence of these pathways.[22] Multiple accessory pathways have been reported[23] in up to 13% of patients with pre-excitation and are more common in the right parietal and postero-septal position.

Virtually all the anomalous pathways described either have a higher content of connective tissue than ordinary working myocardium or run within tunnels in collagenous tissue. In general, fibrosis increases with time and if the same applies to conduction paths their electrophysiological properties either might alter with age or their function might cease. Fibrous proliferation is particularly striking around the central fibrous body and the concept that active re-modelling of the margins of the node might contribute to sudden death or arrhythmias in infants has been put forward.[24] The prevalence of nodoventricular and fasciculoventricular Mahaim pathways does fall with age, being lower in adult than in infant hearts. Small strands of nerve tissue often accompany anomalous pathways and might be responsible for alterations in electrophysiological behaviour.

CONDITIONS ASSOCIATED WITH PRE-EXCITATION

Patients with anomalous conduction paths are not immune to other diseases and cases of ischaemic heart disease or cardiomyopathy with pre-excitation probably reflect no more than coincidence. The myocardium of patients with uncomplicated pre-excitation is not morphologically abnormal. A pre-excitation pattern is found in a high proportion of patients with Ebstein's anomaly,[25] and the anomalous connections are usually septal and/or right parietal. Two factors militate for the presence of anomalous pathways: the downward displacement of the septal cusp, increasing the chance of the atrial overlay fibres connecting with the septum, and connections via the dysplastic valve cusps often extensively covered by a layer of atrial muscle. In one case, the anomalous pathway originated in persistent nodal tissue in the anterior tricuspid ring.[26] Multiple pathways are common in Ebstein's anomaly.[23]

Hypertrophic cardiomyopathy has been shown to have an undue association with pre-excitation and in some families the two conditions are inherited together.[27] The pathways present have been both parietal and septal, and usually they are inserted into areas of abnormally arranged ventricular muscle. It is not known whether there is a chance association with anomalous pathways or whether the abnormal growth of the ventricular myocardium actually establishes atrioventricular connections through areas where deficits in the fibrous body or annuli existed. Other abnormal myocyte configurations, such as the rhabdomyomatous transformation of tuberous sclerosis[28] and infantile histiocytoid cardiomyopathy,[29,30] are also associated with pre-excitation in infancy and may have an analogous mechanism. In infantile histiocytoid cardiomyopathy, nodules of lipid containing clear vacuolated cells develop within both the atrial and the ventricular myocardium. The condition has been given many names reflecting a belief that either these cells are of histiocytic origin or they represent transformed myocytes. The latter belief is more in accord with the consistent association of the condition with pre-excitation[29] and atrial and ventricular tachycardia.[30] The current view is that these nodules are myocardial hamartomas which possibly have a Purkinje cell element. The mortality of the condition is very high; the excision of nodules producing symptoms has now been reported.[30]

Pre-excitation has also been linked to mitral valve prolapse. There is no inherent reason why myxomatous changes in the floppy mitral cusp should invoke anomalous conduction because the paths are alongside the annulus rather than passing through it. An alternative view[31] is that the anomalous pathway itself causes asynchronous contraction of the posterior wall of the left ventricle leading to prolapse of a cusp which is anatomically normal.

There is also a rare association of posterior left parietal paths with aneurysmal dilatation of the coronary sinus regarded as abnormal persistence of a cuff of atrial muscle associated with the sinus venosus.[32]

INTRANODAL RE-ENTRY TACHYCARDIA

Atrioventricular nodal re-entrant tachycardias are common and arise from dual conduction pathways within or close to the atrioventricular nodal area itself. Electrophysiological studies have shown a slowly conducting anterograde and a rapidly conducting retrograde limb within the node, beginning and ending in nodal tissue.[33] In contrast, dissection around the nodal area has been described as highly successful in abolishing atrioventricular nodal re-entry tachycardia[34] a result that indicates one limb of the circuit is paranodal. Such conflicting views pre-suppose that the limits of the atrioventricular node are being defined in an identical manner. The node contains a deep central portion, easily recognizable by its interweaving small myocytes, but the superficial node is made up of successive layers of myocytes which become more like those of atrial muscle. The complexity of these layers makes histological demonstration of two conduction pathways and the limits of the node difficult. Arguments, however, are likely to continue over whether the intranodal tachycardias use atrial muscle immediately adjacent to the node as one pathway. In one autopsy study in which intranodal tachycardia had been demonstrated prior to death, no atrial connections to the node were found suggesting a pure intranodal origin for the re-entry pathways.[35] A further possibility is that dual pathways are associated with the interconnecting islands of nodal tissue interspersed in the central fibrous body. This appearance, often known as fetal dispersion of the node, is found in a proportion of normal adult hearts. Incessant tachycardia associated with

atrioventricular nodal re-entry and a long RP' interval have also been postulated to represent accessory atrioventricular nodal tissue close to the normal conduction axis,[36] a role for which nodal tissue in the central fibrous body is an obvious candidate. However, one autopsy study revealed a long and tortuous septal anomalous connection between atrial and ventricular muscle made up of normal atrial myocytes.[37]

TACHYCARDIA ASSOCIATED WITH NODO- AND FASCICULOVENTRICULAR PATHWAYS

The nodo- and fasciculoventricular pathways described by Mahaim have been associated with both pre-excitation and tachycardia in several clinico-pathological studies.[38,39] However, there is continuing clinical debate over whether the anomalous connection plays a part in maintaining tachycardia or whether it is merely a bystander phenomenon. Ward and Camm[16] have reviewed evidence showing that this group of connections may co-exist with intranodal re-entry which may be the main cause of tachycardia. It is becoming increasingly clear to morphologists working in this field that nodoventricular and fasciculoventricular connections are very common in otherwise normal hearts taken from subjects not known to have any arrhythmias. If these pathways are important in initiating tachycardias, the question is why they become functional in a minority of subjects who possess such paths.

FOCAL HIS BUNDLE TACHYCARDIA

Focal His bundle tachycardia is thought to be due to an abnormal autonomous focus within the distal atrioventricular node or atrioventricular bundle with normal ventricular conduction and is found almost exclusively in children. The findings of one pathological study support there being a focal lesion in the atrioventricular bundle.[40]

THE SHORT PR INTERVAL/NORMAL QRS COMPLEX

The Lown–Ganong–Levine syndrome with its short PR interval and normal QRS complex is, as yet, not firmly based on an anatomical substrate. James[41] and Brechenmacher[42] have described paths that join the atria either to the distal atrioventricular node or to the penetrating atrioventricular bundle itself but these reports lack electrophysiological data which would exclude the presence of fast intranodal pathway. Another postulated mechanism is hypoplasia of the node itself.

ATRIOVENTRICULAR CONDUCTION DEFECTS

One aspect of any histopathological study of the conduction system is confirmation of the anatomical site at which atrioventricular block has occurred. In this respect, excellent correlations with electrophysiological studies can be found and confirm that the site of chronic atrioventricular block is, most frequently, distal to the atrioventricular node.

A second aspect lies in determining the nature of the destructive process. In this respect, distinction must be made between patients in whom heart block is the sole manifestation and patients who may have any of the known systemic or cardiac diseases which can be complicated by atrioventricular block. The relative proportions of the causes of chronic atrioventricular block in any clinical series will be influenced by the selection of patients.

In large series of patients referred for long-term pacing who did not have other overt systemic disease, the commonest cause of chronic atrioventricular block was found to be the entity known as idiopathic bilateral bundle branch fibrosis. Although this term is clumsy, it is an accurate description of a process in which conduction fibres vanish from the bifurcating atrioventricular bundle and proximal bundle branches. The disease was known to the pathologists who made the first morphological studies of atrioventricular block in the late nineteenth century but two somewhat different forms of the disease have been stressed subsequently by Lev[43] and Lenegre.[44] Both authors emphasize that the disease is most common in subjects over 65 years of age and is the culmination of a process which may evolve over 10 years or more. Lev stresses a form of the disease in which the initial loss of conduction fibres takes place in the proximal left bundle branch. The left bundle branch has numerous fine fascicles arising independently from the bifurcating bundle, each runs between the endocardium of the ventricular outflow and the connective tissue of the upper ventricular septum (Fig. 22.12). Lev postulates that the fascicles are hammered between the two masses of collagen each time the ventricle contracts. The conduction fibres ultimately vanish leaving open spaces which still outline the original site of the bundle branch in the connective tissue (Fig. 22.13). The process is ubi-

quitous in old age and appears to be accelerated by hypertension; it is only in extreme cases that the loss of conduction tissue extends into the bifurcating bundle and atrioventricular block develops, usually after a long period of left bundle branch block. Lev envisages the process as a combination of age and 'wear and tear'. In many cases, there is some associated fibrosis and microscopic foci of calcification in the upper interventricular septum. In a proportion of cases, there is also hyaline thickening of the small arterial vessels within the penetrating atrioventricular bundle, a process that could be either a primary or a secondary change. There is no evidence to suggest that atheroma of epicardial coronary arteries is implicated directly in Lev's disease. The age of the patients and the association with left ventricular hypertrophy means that some patients with Lev's disease have concomitant coronary atheroma.

Lenegre described cases of idiopathic bundle branch fibrosis in whom either diffuse or focal

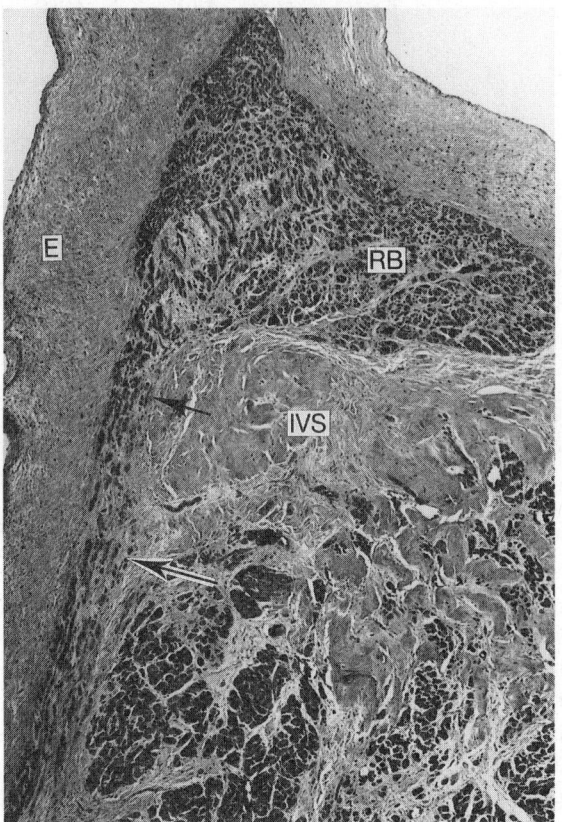

Fig. 22.12. Micro-anatomy of the bifurcating atrioventricular bundle. The right branch (RB) is a single large bundle of darkly staining myocytes. The left branch consists of multiple slender fascicles (arrows) each of which runs in a narrow pass between the endocardium (E) of the left ventricular outflow and the collagenous apex of the interventricular septum (IVS).

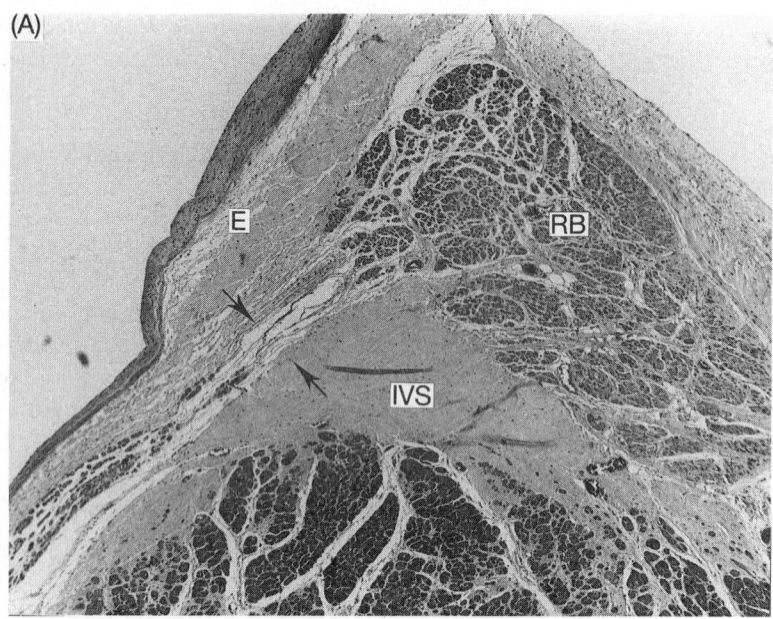

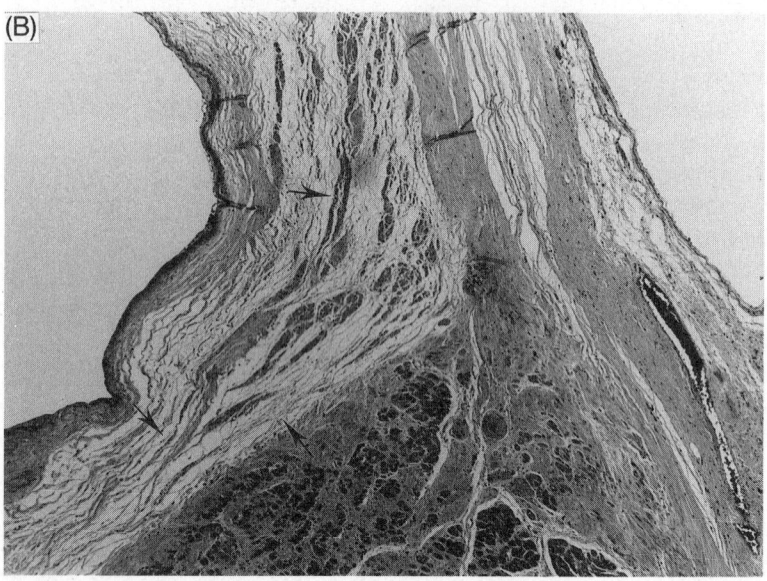

Fig. 22.13. (A) Mild loss of conduction fibres (arrows) in the proximal left bundle branch in aging and hypertrophied hearts. (B) Severe Lev-type bundle branch fibrosis with open spaces (arrows) in the atrioventricular bundle and left bundle branch with a marked loss in conduction fibres. E, endocardium; RB, right branch; IVS, interventricular septum.

segments of both the right and left bundle branches showed a progressive loss of conduction fibres with replacement fibrosis, but the spaces so characteristic of Lev's disease were absent (Fig. 22.14). In these areas of fibrosis, occasional degenerate conduction cells survive associated with small foci of chronic inflammatory cells, but in general there is no evidence of an acute myocarditis (Fig. 22.15). The myocardium immediately adjacent to the bundle branches is normal. Loss of conduction fibres also extends into the more distal portions of the right and left branches. In extreme cases, conduction fibres are lost throughout the Purkinje network of the left ventricle.

Speculation with regard to the aetiology of Lenegre's disease includes previous acute myocarditis and a 'myopathic' process selective for conduction fibres. The latter is supported by the similarity of the morphological changes to those found in the conduction system in patients with familial conduction disturbances or dilated cardiomyopathies, the association of Lenegre's disease with an increase in left ventricular mass with mild diffuse interstitial fibrosis and the occasional occurrence of the disease

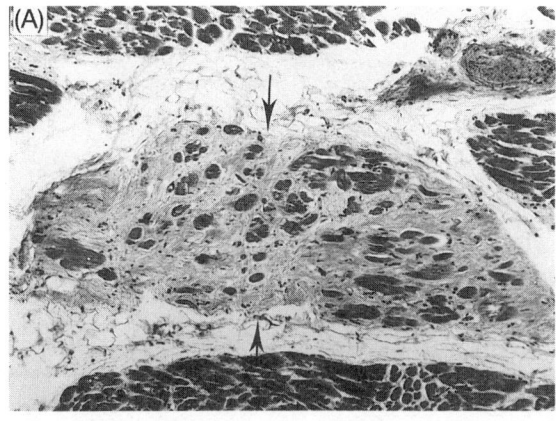

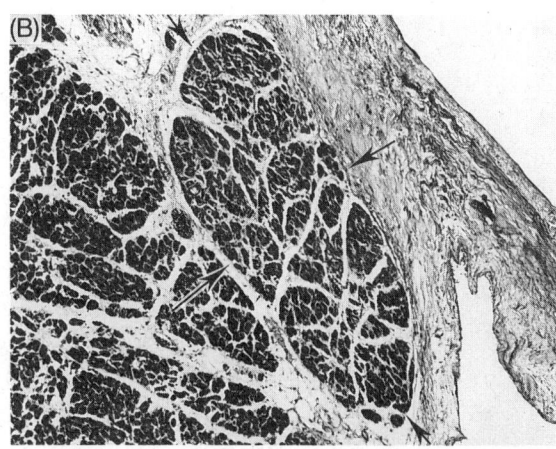

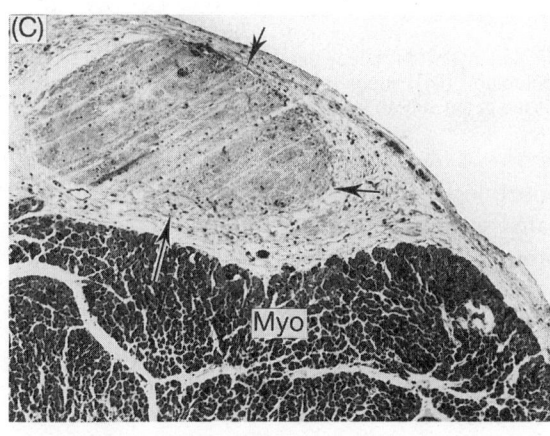

Fig. 22.14. (A) Normal right branch (arrows). (B) Lenegre-type bundle branch fibrosis with the right branch (arrows) containing about 50% of the normal number of conduction fibres. (C) Lenegre-type bundle branch fibrosis with total loss of conduction myocytes in the right branch (arrows). The adjacent myocardium (Myo) is normal.

in relatively young individuals. Although auto-antibodies specific for Purkinje cells have been demonstrated,[45] immune-based destruction of the conduction system has not been established as a contributory factor in bundle branch fibrosis.

Within the spectrum of idiopathic bundle branch fibrosis, overall, more cases conform to the Lev than the Lenegre type, but many cases have features of both diseases. It is, therefore, impossible to determine from a morphological study of autopsy cases whether idiopathic bundle branch fibrosis represents the end-stage of one, two or several disease processes.

ISCHAEMIC HEART DISEASE AND CHRONIC ATRIOVENTRICULAR BLOCK

Coronary atheroma is responsible for chronic atrioventricular block when acute infarction destroys totally a segment of the conduction system and the patient survives. The most common pattern encountered is destruction of both bundle branches

within one or more episodes of septal infarction due to occlusion of the left anterior descending artery. An occlusion of the right coronary artery that has extended into the nodal artery itself with subsequent destruction of the node is more rare. In one study of 13 patients with ischaemic chronic atrioventricular block, 10 were found to have infraHisian block with left anterior descending disease and 3 to have nodal block with right coronary artery disease.[46]

CALCIFIC ATRIOVENTRICULAR BLOCK

The term calcific atrioventricular block is usually applied to transection of the conduction system by a mass of calcium large enough to be visible on X-ray or echocardiography in life and by naked eye examination at autopsy.[47] The penetrating atrioventricular bundle is anatomically very close to the medial aspect of the mitral valve ring, to the membranous interventricular septum and to the aortic valve. Nodular calcification at any of these

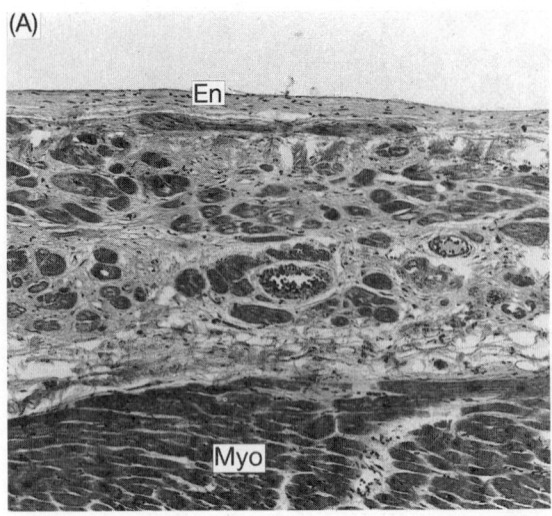
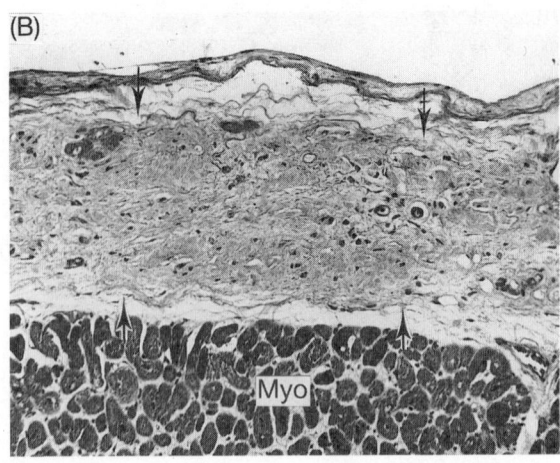

Fig. 22.15. (A) Normal left bundle branch in the mid-septal area. The conduction myocytes occupy the sub-endocardial zone (arrows). En, endocardium; Myo, contractile myocardium. (B) Lenegre-type bundle branch fibrosis. Conduction myocytes are absent from the fibrous tissue in the sub-endocardial zone (arrows). The contractile myocardium (M) is normal.

sites, due to any cause, may extend outward sufficiently to disrupt the conduction system. Extension of calcium from the valve into the upper septum may complicate any form of aortic stenosis whether in a tricuspid or bicuspid valve. The clinical association of atrioventricular block with massive mitral ring calcification in old age is often known as Rytand's syndrome.[48,49] Accelerated soft-tissue calcification in Paget's disease of bone or renal failure may lead to similar mitral ring calcification and atrioventricular block.

CARDIOMYOPATHY AND ATRIOVENTRICULAR BLOCK

Patients with idiopathic dilated cardiomyopathy have diffuse loss of conduction fibres with replacement fibrosis, particularly in the distal bundle branches, which is manifest clinically as a high incidence of left bundle branch block. Complete atrioventricular block is rare due to the short clinical course. In comparison, subjects with familial cardiomyopathies have a tenfold incidence of atrioventricular block and those with inherited neuromyopathies have an even higher incidence of cardiac involvement characterized by conduction rather than contraction abnormalities. Conduction abnormalities may precede any manifestation of skeletal muscle disease.[50,51] In dystrophia myotonica, conduction fibres are replaced by fat rather than fibrous tissue; the results of electrophysiological studies suggest that the loss is at all levels in the

conduction system. Detailed pathological studies of isolated examples of many of the rarer forms of neuromyopathies indicate a non-specific loss of conduction tissue at all levels. The results of clinical studies of patients with progressive external ophthalmoplegia suggest that the Purkinje cells of the more distal bundle branches are involved selectively.[52]

Familial conduction defects are heterogeneous.[53–55] The simplest form is absence of a segment of a bundle branch, usually the right, not associated with progression of the conduction defect. Another form is a slowly progressive loss of conduction fibres throughout both bundle branches and both nodes culminating in complete atrioventricular block late in life. In all affected families, sudden death seems to be more common than would be anticipated from the severity of the conduction defect.

CONGENITAL COMPLETE ATRIOVENTRICULAR BLOCK

Congenital heart block which is not associated with other complex congenital cardiac malformations has been shown to have two morphological varieties.[56] In the most common form, the inferior limbus of the atrial septum inferior to the foramen ovale is deficient in atrial myocytes and is formed predominantly of adipose tissue. Buried within the central fibrous body is tissue representing the deep portion of the atrioventricular node but, in the absence of an atrial nodal component, no connection is established between atrial muscle in the upper septum and the atrioventricular conduction axis. The more distal penetrating and bifurcating atrioventricular bundles are normal. This form of atrioventricular block has been specifically linked with maternal connective tissue disorders, predominantly systemic lupus erythematosus but also rheumatoid arthritis and dermatomysitis.[57,58] The mothers are characterized by possession of anti-RO(SS-A) antibodies to soluble tissue ribonucleoprotein antigens. These antibodies cross the placenta and will bind fetal cardiac tissue, but specificity for conduction tissue has not been well established. Subclinical maternal lupus is one cause of several siblings having congenital atrioventricular block and may be confused with an inherited familial conduction tissue defect.

The second form of congenital heart block has a well-formed node with a deep and a superficial portion but no continuity is made with the ventricular conduction axis (nodoventricular dissociation). This rarer form of congenital block is not related to maternal connective tissue disorder. It may be related to some of the familial bundle branch defects. The rare primary 'tumour' of the atrioventricular node (mesothelioma) is due to growth of rests of pericardial tissue persisting within the node and reflecting its original histogenesis on the posterior interventricular sulcus. Atrioventricular block is usually present in early life simulating clinically true 'congenital' block.[59]

THE CONDUCTION SYSTEM IN CONNECTIVE TISSUE DISEASES

An inflammatory aortitis is found in association with the HLA-B24-related diseases including ankylosing spondylitis and Reiter's syndrome.[60] The distortion of the aortic root leads to aortic regurgitation while extension of the inflammatory process outside the aorta may involve the immediately adjacent atrioventricular node.[61] Conduction disturbances and aortic regurgitation are therefore closely linked. Heart block is predominantly supraHisian in HLA-B24-related disease.[62] A different mechanism is responsible for complete atrioventricular block in rheumatoid arthritis where a granuloma in the upper septum or mitral/aortic rings transects the conduction system usually at the level of the bifurcating atrioventricular bundle.[63] In systemic sclerosis, connective tissue within the atrioventricular node proliferates and, in associa-

tion with small vessel obliteration, leads to nodal destruction.[64-66] Bundle branch destruction also occurs in association with the widespread myocardial scarring. In adult systemic lupus, focal necrosis and fibrosis associated with an arteritis in the node have been described.[67] Similar changes occur in polyarteritis.[68] About 70% of cases of dermatomyositis have evidence of cardiac involvement with conduction defects being common and one of the leading causes of death.[69] The cardiac damage which principally affects the bundle branches[70] has been linked to antibodies to ribonucleoproteins,[58] although it is not known why there are similar antibodies in systemic lupus erythematosus that affect only the fetus and not the mother.

MYOCARDITIS AND ATRIOVENTRICULAR BLOCK

All forms of myocarditis may develop conduction system involvement with the bundle branches being particularly vulnerable. Mild cases are usually detected by electrocardiography in patients with systemic viral infections.[71,72] Complete atrioventricular block identifies the rare examples of more severe involvement, but even so reversion to sinus rhythm is usual. In one series of 10 patients with myocarditis and complete atrioventricular block, only 2 had permanent conduction defects.[73] Histological confirmation of an inflammatory infiltrate in the conduction system exists only in case-reports.[74] Although most cases of atrioventricular block with myocarditis are assumed to be caused by a Coxsackie infection, virtually every virus has been implicated in individual case-reports, with mumps being the most common.[75] Idiopathic giant cell (granulomatous) myocarditis also involves the conduction system.[76] In patients with acute rheumatic fever, vasculitis and inflammatory infiltration of the connective tissue around the node may lead to conduction disturbances, but there seems to be no significant risk of long-term sequelae.[77] Diphtheria has a very high incidence of atrioventricular block in the acute phase due to the direct effect of the exotoxin on conduction myocytes. Long-term conduction defects are an appreciable risk.[78] Chagas' disease (South American trypanosomiasis) carries a high risk of bundle branch block and atrioventricular block in the initial acute myocarditic phase and in the later chronic stage. In the latter, bundle branch destruction occurs as part of a generalized myocardial scarring; arrhythmias may be enhanced by the neuronal damage that occurs within the heart in Chagas' disease.[79] Worldwide, Chagas' disease may be the commonest cause of chronic atrioventricular block. Septal gummata in syphilis used to be a classic cause of complete atrioventricular block and they are still reported sporadically,[80] as are tuberculomas destroying the conduction system.[81] Sarcoidosis, when involving the heart, may produce a large granulomatous mass most frequently occurring in the upper interventricular septum and the atrial muscle in the vicinity of the aortic root. Destruction of the conduction system leads to sudden death and atrioventricular block.[82] Sudden death may reflect either conduction defects or the high frequency of ventricular arrhythmias associated with myocardial scarring and aneurysm formation. Involvement of the sinus node by giant cell granulomas in sarcoid is also recorded.[83]

THE MORPHOLOGICAL BASIS OF BUNDLE BRANCH BLOCK

Many myocardial diseases are associated with bundle branch block; conversely, mass electrocardiographic surveys have revealed that many apparently healthy individuals have the same patterns. The prognosis of bundle branch block reflects that of the underlying myocardial disease and is therefore very variable.

LEFT BUNDLE BRANCH

Common to all descriptions of the anatomy of the left bundle branch is that a series of slender fascicles arise from a considerable length of the bifurcating atrioventricular bundle as it lies at the crest of the muscular interventricular septum.[84] Some individuals possess anterior and posterior streams of fascicles of equal size, some have a preponderance of one and others have an additional middle stream in the upper third of the septum. In all individuals, however, by the time the fascicles reach the lower third of the septum, there is a contiguous sheet of conduction tissue in the sub-endocardium.[84] There is general agreement that complete left bundle branch block is associated with severe loss of conduction tissue. This may be proximal and focal, as in old age, hypertension, aortic valve disease and some patients with ischaemic heart disease, or diffuse and distal, as in the myopathies and severe ischaemic damage. The electrocardiographic patterns described as indicating partial bundle branch block, hemiblock or left-axis deviation are now

agreed to be due to lesser degrees of fascicular loss than that of complete bundle branch block.[84] Left anterior hemiblock has not been found to be specifically associated with damage confined to the anterior portion of the bundle branch but to more diffuse loss.[85] In contrast, left posterior hemiblock, particularly in association with inferior infarction, is associated with damage concentrated on the posterior division of the left branch.[86] The age-related sclerosis of the upper interventricular septum potentiated by any disease causing left ventricular hypertrophy[87] is the non-specific factor unifying the many causes of left bundle branch block.

RIGHT BUNDLE BRANCH

The right bundle branch is the continuation of the penetrating atrioventricular bundle and runs as a single discrete bundle beneath the endocardium of the ventricular septum to reach the base of the anterior papillary muscle; from here, it runs in the moderator band to form a rich anastomosing network of conduction fibres throughout the right ventricle.

The discrete nature and sub-endocardial position of the bundle branch at the rim of the right ventricular outflow make it liable to mechanical trauma from catheters (a situation that has no analogue on the left side of the heart). The main stem of the right branch is very variable in size and in the number of myocytes it contains as viewed in cross-section. Focal hypoplasia is one cause of congenital right bundle branch block. The discrete nature of the right bundle branch also means that destruction within an area of infarction, particularly anteroseptal in distribution, is common.[88] Severe right ventricular hypertrophy is associated with diffuse sub-endocardial fibrosis within the outflow tract, a process that may also involve the right bundle branch.[88]

VENTRICULAR TACHYCARDIA

The results of electrophysiological studies suggest that ventricular arrhythmias reflect non-homogeneous intramyocardial conduction leading to re-entry. As an acute phenomenon, this may be due to focal areas containing damaged, but viable, myocytes with abnormal transmembrane potentials and it is typical of acute ischaemic damage or acute myocarditis. Common to the many chronic conditions causing ventricular arrhythmias is disruption of the homogeneity of the myocardial mass of myocytes into cords or islands by fibrous tissue or infiltration by amyloid.

ISCHAEMIC HEART DISEASE

The margins of the fibrous scars that result from myocardial infarction are never sharply defined and, at the lateral borders, clumps and strands of surviving myocardium are embedded in collagen. In the great majority of infarcts, a thin layer of myocardium survives just beneath the endocardium forming ribbon-like anastomosing strands of muscle (Fig. 22.16). This sheet of muscle, up to 1 mm and 10 cells in thickness,[89] owes its survival to diffusion of oxygen across the endocardium from the cavity of the left ventricle and contains inevitably a number of conduction myocytes (Purkinje cells). This muscle sheet joins with more normal myocardium at the lateral margins of the infarct. Complete transmural infarction is rare and a thin sheet of sub-pericardial surviving muscle is also common in ischaemic scars. Therefore, a potential substrate for a re-entry circuit, either around the complete circumference of the infarct or confined to the sub-endocardial zone, exists in many ischaemic scars.[89] It is clear, however, that only a minority of patients who have ischaemic scars are troubled by ventricular arrhythmias; the results of autopsy studies and examination of the material resected during successful eradication of tachycardia have shown the importance of several additional factors.

Clinical studies in which the origin of the tachycardia is mapped show that, over the ischaemic scar, potentials are fractionated and early endocardial activation relative to the epicardium occurs.[90,91] The area of endocardium over which a re-entry circuit can be located is recorded[92] as being from small (2–3 cm^2) to very large (10–12 cm^2) in size. Resection particularly of the margins of an aneurysmal scar is often successful in abolishing tachycardia. Histological examination of resected material from successful ablations (93–95) shows the endocardium to be thickened by elastic tissue and collagen, beneath which there is a layer of collagenous tissue in which there are embedded strands of myocardial muscle cells comprising 10–50% of the tissue (Fig. 22.17). Ultrastructural studies[93] show that the myocytes comprise both contractile and conduction (Purkinje) cells. The contractile myocytes show marked myocytolysis, that is, a loss of myofibrillary content thought to represent a chronic hypoxic state, whereas the Purkinje cells are normal in structure. Following a successful sub-endocardial resection, the endocardium once again undergoes fibro-elastic thickening but the arrhythmia does not recur in the absence of surviving sub-endocardial myocytes. It is not possible in morphological studies to establish the mechanism by which the tachycardia is initiated but such studies do indicate the importance of a particular geometric configuration of anastomosing ribbons of sub-endocardial myocytes embedded in collagen. An important additional factor is chronic hypoxia perhaps related to increasing endocardial

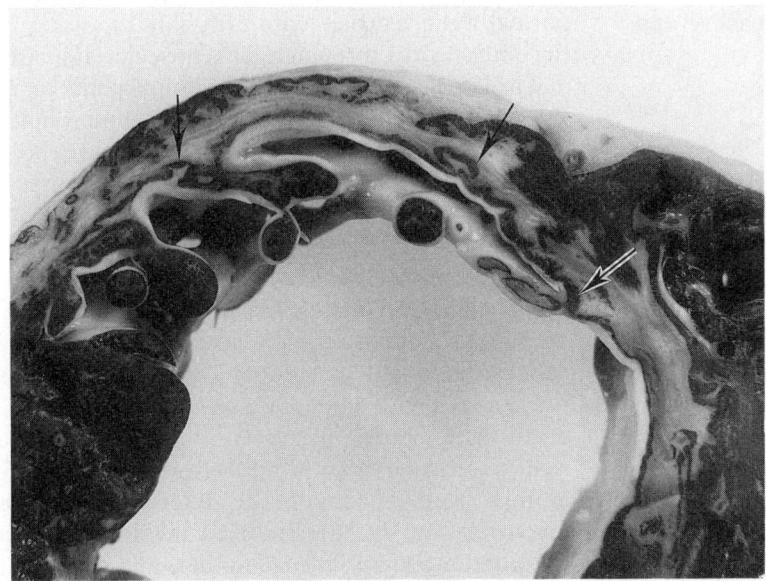

Fig. 22.16. Old myocardial infarct associated with ventricular arrhythmias. The endocardium is thick and white. Immediately beneath the endocardium is a thin ribbon of surviving myocytes (arrows).

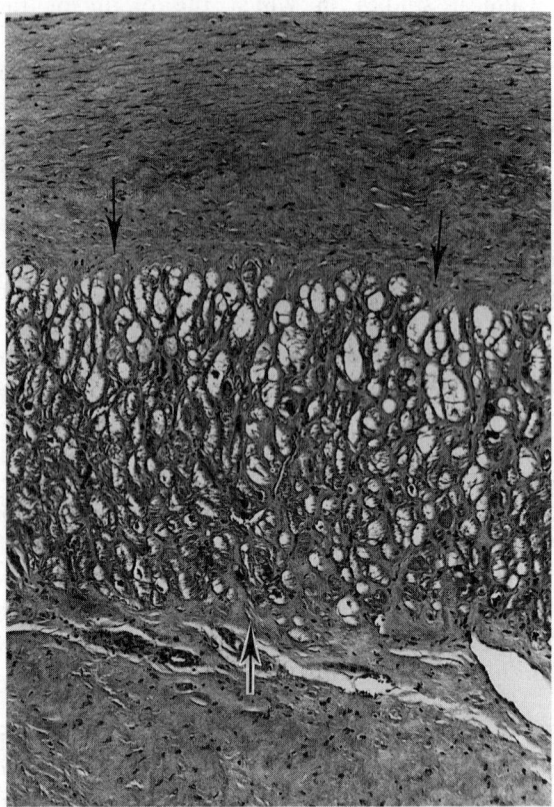

Fig. 22.17. Histology of the ribbons of myocytes (arrows) in Fig. 22.16. The myocytes are embedded in collagen and are very vacuolated (myocytolysis).

fibro-elastosis. It is not known whether it is essential for Purkinje cells to be present among the myocytes, but they would inevitably be present in an area of sub-endocardial myocardium as large as several square centimetres.

NON-ISCHAEMIC ARRHYTHMOGENIC VENTRICULAR DISEASE

The concept of fibrosis breaking the mass of myocardial cells into smaller interconnecting units thereby providing a basis for re-entry, with or without acute myocyte damage, is also relevant to non-ischaemic disease. Hypertrophic cardiomyopathy is associated with a high incidence of ventricular tachycardia[96,97] and the configuration of whorls of myocytes arranged around foci of connective tissue seems an ideal substrate for re-entry. The presence of foci of acute myocyte necrosis is a further common factor potentiating the risk. The end-stage of a dilated cardiomyopathy is also associated with considerable interstitial fibrosis and evidence of acute myocyte damage.[98] Ventricular arrhythmias are also strongly associated with myocardial sarcoidosis in both the acute phase, when granulomas are present, and the burnt-out phase, when granulomas are absent. The scars resulting from healed sarcoidosis are irregular in outline and often become aneurysmal suggesting that similar mechanisms to those in ischaemic scars will operate.

Any ventricle in which there is severe hypertrophy will undergo a marked increase in interstitial fibrosis and focal myocyte damage thereby providing a substrate for arrhythmias and, as would be anticipated, the incidence rises as ventricular function fails.[99] Gross right ventricular hypertrophy is associated with course fibrous trabeculae subdividing the myocardium, particularly the infundibular portion.

Ventricular arrhythmias arising in the right ventricle

Gross right ventricular hypertrophy is associated with considerable interstitial fibrosis which occurs in a coarser pattern than that found in left ventricular hypertrophy. The formation of trabeculae of muscle divided by broad bands of connective tissue is particularly characteristic of the outflow tract in Fallot's tetralogy and may explain the occurrence of arrhythmias even after surgical correction.[100,101]

There is a spectrum of morphological changes in non-hypertrophied right ventricles associated with recurrent ventricular tachycardia. These changes range, at one extreme, from what is an apparently normal right ventricle with arrhythmias arising in the outflow tract through right ventricular dysplasia and isolated right ventricular cardiomyopathy to, at the other extreme, Uhl's anomaly. The morphological features to which these names have been applied merge and overlap to such an extent that it is not certain whether they do represent different conditions.

In Uhl's anomaly, the whole of the right ventricle is paper-thin and dilated. Histology shows virtually no myocardial muscle, with close apposition of the endocardium and epicardium; islands of fibrous tissue mixed with adipose tissue are present however. In right ventricle dysplasia,[102] a segment of the right ventricular wall is thinned and replaced by adipose and fibrous tissue intermingled with myocytes (Fig. 22.18). The area involved is often the anterior free wall related to the outflow tract but

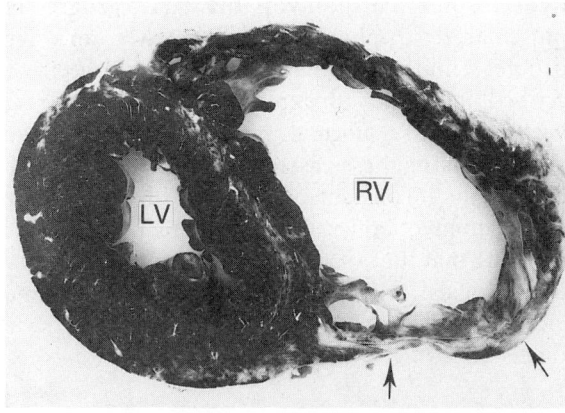

Fig. 22.18. Right ventricular dysplasia. The heart is shown in a short-axis view. The right ventricle (RV) is dilated and thin-walled with obvious fibrous scarring (arrows) on the posterior wall. Taken from a male of 19 years with no coronary atheroma and sudden death. LV, left ventricle.

it may also be lateral or posterior. In what is described as right ventricular isolated cardiomyopathy, the changes are similar but more diffuse in distribution.[103,104] Adipose tissue is normally present in the right ventricular free wall and therefore its presence in an abnormal ventricle cannot be regarded as specific for any condition in which myocytes are replaced by fibrous tissue. The name applied to any individual ventricular arrhythmia in which there is a demonstrable contraction abnormality reflects whether the worker applying the name believes the condition is a familial dysplasia,[105,106] i.e. maldevelopment of a segment of the ventricle, or an acquired condition, possibly representing a healed myocarditis in which the right

ventricle was selectively involved. Patients with right ventricular tachycardia but without clinical evidence of any contractile abnormality are often regarded as idiopathic or 'innocent'. A high incidence of morphological abnormality detected by biopsy is reported.[107-110] A small proportion of patients do have an occult myocarditis, the majority of the remainder show a mild increase in the amount of interstitial fibrosis, and overall about one-third of patients have a normal biopsy. As yet, no relation has been found between a mild increase in interstitial fibrosis and right ventricular dysplasia.

SUDDEN DEATH AND THE CONDUCTION SYSTEM

Autopsies on victims of sudden natural death will always define the major groups as those in whom there is a clear non-cardiac cause, such as dissection of the aorta, or a clear cardiac cause, such as ischaemic heart disease, myocarditis or cardiomyopathy. In up to 5% of sudden natural deaths, however, no clear cause of death is found, no coronary atheroma is present and the possibility of an abnormality of the conduction system is raised. This possibility is not unreasonable given the known risk of sudden death in conditions such as pre-excitation, the long QT interval and atrioventricular block. A large catalogue of morphological abnormalities of the conduction system found to be present at autopsy in sudden death without cause exists, mainly in the form of individual case-reports.

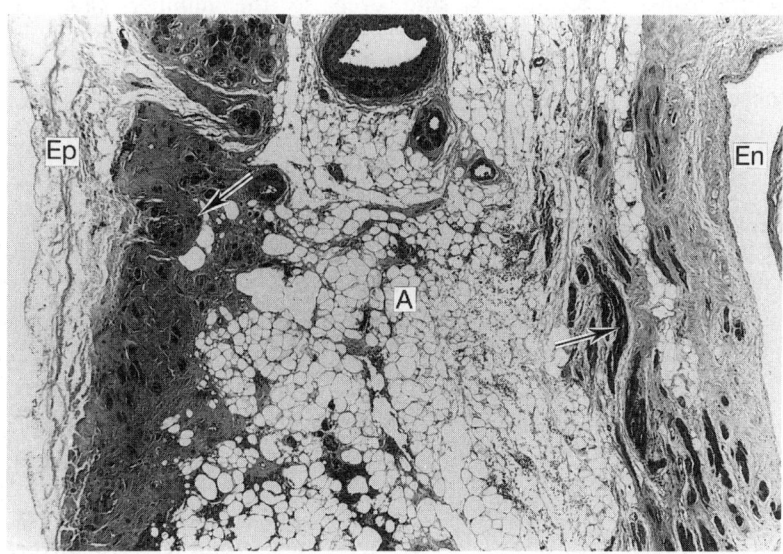

Fig. 22.19. Histology of right ventricular dysplasia. The right ventricular wall shows strands and islands of dark-staining myocytes (arrows) embedded in paler connective tissue. There is abundant adipose tissue present (A). En, endocardium; Ep, epicardium.

POST-NATAL MORPHOGENESIS OF THE ATRIOVENTRICULAR NODAL AREA

James[111] has suggested that the margin of the atrioventricular node with the central fibrous body undergoes active remodelling from the first week of life for up to months or years later. In this process, the margin of the node is smoothed with obliteration of the archipelagos of nodal tissue within the fibrous body and severing of Mahaim fibres. It has been postulated that abnormal re-modelling allows loops of nodal tissue that have a potential for microreentry to survive or nodoventricular connections that have a macroreentry potential. Excess fibrous proliferations in the central fibrous body may obliterate or even narrow the penetrating bundle. All these processes have been implicated as contributing to the sudden death syndrome in infants and in adults,[111,112] but they are not consistently found.

SMALL VESSEL DISEASE

In the context of the conduction system, the term small artery includes vessels up to 1 mm in diameter which are branches of the atrial arteries. Arteries of this size are not involved primarily by atheroma. The sinus node artery is the termination of a major atrial artery arising from the proximal portion of the right coronary (60%), the proximal left circumflex (30%) or more distally. Within the sinus node, the artery is often, but not always, centrally placed and supplies the node via smaller vessels. The atrioventricular node artery is the termination of a vessel running in the atrial septum and arising from the origin of the posterior descending coronary artery. It also supplies smaller vessels to the node itself.

Pathological processes that have been observed in the nodal arteries[68] include arteritis and fibrinoid necrosis in polyarteritis nodosa and systemic lupus and inflammation and concentric intimal thickening in scleroderma, dermatomyositis and ankylosing spondylitis. In these cases, nodal damage can be clearly shown and linked to nodal artery occlusion and thus to conduction disturbances. Embolic occlusion of the nodal arteries may occur in ischaemic heart disease; it also occurs in thrombotic thrombocytopenic purpura.

Fibrous proliferation of the intima and disorderly fibromuscular proliferation of the media of the nodal arteries have also been described in a range of cardiomyopathies including Friedreich's ataxia,[113] hypertrophic cardiomyopathy and progressive muscular dystrophy as well as in Marfan's syndrome. Similar vascular changes have been described in sudden unexplained death in subjects with otherwise normal hearts. Major evidence against linking these vascular changes with arrhythmias is the inconstant presence of such changes in the cardiomyopathies, the lack of angiographic data showing that the vessels are narrowed when filled at physiological pressures and the lack of morphological evidence for damage to the nodal myocytes themselves.

PROLONGED QT INTERVAL AND SUDDEN DEATH

Prolongation of the vulnerable period of ventricular repolarization is associated with a high risk of ventricular arrhythmias and sudden death, particularly when inherited, and with or without associated nerve deafness. Experimental imbalance of sympathetic stimulation may prolong the QT interval; this finding has focused attention on the cardiac neurones in human cases, supported by the clinical benefit obtained from left stellate ganglionectomy in man. A focal 'neuritis', i.e. degeneration of axons and an infiltration by lymphocytes of nerves and ganglia, was described consistently in humans.[114] Similar findings in ganglia were reported in cases of sudden unexpected death without previous electrocardiographic study.[115] Other workers[116] have failed to confirm these findings in the long QT interval syndrome. Histological examination of peripheral neural tissue is difficult because axons are not easily identified, unless stained by silver techniques, and even so the number and the thickness of axons have to be quantified rather than assessed subjectively. Supporting glial cells are almost impossible to distinguish from lymphocytes using routine staining methods. The confirmation of neural changes in the long QT syndrome requires the performance of studies in which specific neural markers with monoclonal antibodies are used.

A different view of the pathology of the long QT syndrome describes fatty infiltration of the approaches to the atrioventricular node in four of six cases and a 'chronic' mild myocarditis in all.[117] Although the authors state that morphological changes cannot be ignored because they do not fit the electrophysiological theories, morphological changes must be quantified and compared with those found in control subjects before any credence can be placed in the findings. Another view of the long QT syndrome[118] comes from a case in which ultrastructural study was carried out showing mitochrondrial deposits of calcium suggesting a possible defect in intracellular calcium metabolism. As yet, the morphological basis of the long QT syndrome is undefined.

STRUCTURAL ABNORMALITIES OF THE CONDUCTION SYSTEM IN SUDDEN UNEXPLAINED DEATH

Numerous case-reports suggest that examination of the conduction system for structural abnormalities may elucidate the cause of sudden unexplained death, particularly in young subjects. Numerous abnormalities are described including persistent fetal dispersion of the atrioventricular node,[119] nodoventricular and fasciculoventricular connections,[120] an intramyocardial course for the right bundle branch[121] and undue sclerosis or fatty infiltration of the conduction system for the age of the subject.[122] Sudden death has been documented in patients with pre-excitation who have not had previous episodes of significant tachycardia and no other abnormality at autopsy apart from an anomalous conduction pathway.[123]

In a study of the conduction system in 18 cases of unexplained sudden death in South East Asian immigrants,[120] it was found that 14 had fetal dispersion of the atrioventricular node and 13 had accessory conduction pathways, of which 3 were atriofascicular, 8 nodoventricular and 5 fasciculoventricular. In a control group of 124 hearts taken from subjects in whom death was accidental, 35 were found to have similar perinodal anatomical abnormalities. It seems that anatomical abnormalities of the conduction system are not uncommon in normal hearts but they may be more common in the hearts of subjects suffering sudden unexpected death. However, it is important to bear in mind that the vast majority of reports linking sudden unexplained death to morphological abnormalities of the conduction system are case-reports and therefore uncontrolled.

REFERENCES

1. Bouman, L.N. and Jongsma, H.J. Structure and function of the SA node: a review. Eur. Heart J. 1986; 7: 94.
2. Davies, M.J. Pathology of atrial arrhythmias. In: Davies, M.J., Anderson, R.H. and Becker, A.E., eds. The Conduction System of the Heart. London: Butterworths, 1983, p. 203.
3. James, T.N. The sinus node. Am. J. Cardiol. 1977; 40: 965.
4. Thery, C., Gosselin, B., Lekieffre, J. and Warembourg, H. Pathology of sinoatrial node. Correlation with electrocardiographic findings in 111 patients. Am. Heart J. 1977; 93: 735.
5. Evans, R. and Shaw, D.B. Pathological studies in sinoatrial disorder (Sick Sinus Syndrome). Br. Heart J. 1977; 39: 778.
6. Demoulin, J.C. and Kulbertus, H.E. Histopathological correlations of sinoatrial disease. Br. Heart J. 1978; 40: 1384.
7. Sugiura, A. and Ohkawa, S. A clinicopathologic study on sick sinus syndrome with histologic approach to the sinoatrial node. Jap. Circ. J. 1980; 44: 497.
8. Shaw, D.B. and Kekwick, C.A. Potential candidates for pacemakers. Br. Heart J. 1978; 40: 99.
9. Bharati, S., Nordenberg, A., Bauerfiend, R. et al. The anatomic substrate for the sick sinus syndrome in adolescence. Am. J. Cardiol. 1980; 46: 163.
10. Lorber, A., Maisuls, E. and Palant, A. Autosomal dominant inheritance of sinus node disease. Int. J. Cardiol. 1987; 15: 252.
11. Engel, T.R., Meister, S.G., Feitosa, G.S., Fischer, H.A. and Frankl, W.S. Appraisal of sinus node artery disease. Circulation 1975; 52: 86.
12. Shaw, D.B., Linker, N.J., Heaver, P.A. and Evans, R. Ischaemia and chronic sinoatrial disease (Sick Sinus Syndrome). Br. Heart J. 1988; 58: 598.
13. Camm, A.J. and Ward, D.E. Clinical electrocardiography. In: Martin, A. and Camm, A.J., eds. Heart disease in the elderly. Chichester: John Wiley and Sons, 1984, p. 149.
14. Davies, M.J. and Pomerance, A. Pathology of atrial fibrillation in man. Br. Heart J. 1972; 34: 520.
15. Perulman, M.S. and Krikler, D.M. Termination of focal atrial tachycardia by adenosine triphosphate. Br. Heart J. 1987; 58: 528.
16. Ward, D.E. and Camm, A.J. Clinical Electrophysiology of the Heart. London: Edward Arnold, 1987, p. 173.
17. Vassal-Adams, P.R. Ultrastructure of the human AV conduction tissues. Eur. Heart J. 1983; 4: 449.
18. James, T.N. Anatomy of the human A–V node with remarks pertinent to its electrophysiology. Am. Heart J. 1961; 62: 756.
19. Becker, A.E. Morphological basis of pre-excitation. In: Davies, M.J., Anderson, R.H. and Becker, A.E., eds. London: Butterworths, 1983, p. 183.
20. Anderson, R.H., Davies, M.J. and Becker, A.E. Atrioventricular ring specialised tissue in the normal heart. Eur. J. Cardiol. 1974; 2: 219.
21. Sealy, W.C. and Gallagher, J.J. The surgical approach to the septal area of the heart based on experience with 45 patients with Kent bundles. J. Thorac. Cardiovasc. Surg. 1980; 79: 542.
22. Vidaillet, H.J., Presley, J.C., Henke, E., Harrell, F.E. and Ferman, L.D. Familial occurrence of accessory atrioventricular pathways (pre-excitation syndrome). N. Engl. J. Med. 1987; 317: 65.
23. Colavita, P.G., Packer, D.L., Presley, J.C. et al. Frequency, diagnosis and clinical characteristics of patients with multiple accessory atrioventricular pathways. Am. J. Cardiol. 1987; 59: 601.
24. Marino, T.A. and Kane, B.M. Cardiac atrioventricular junctional tissues in hearts from infants who died suddenly. J. Am. Coll. Cardiol. 1985; 5: 1178.
25. Smith, W.M., Gallagher, J.J. et al. The electrophysiological basis and management of symptomatic recurrent tachycardia in patients with Ebstein's anomaly of the tricuspid valve. Am. J. Cardiol. 1982; 49: 1223.
26. Becker, A.E. Morphological basis of pre-excitation. In:

Davis, M.J., Anderson, R.H. and Becker, A.E., eds. *The Conduction System of the Heart*. London: Butterworths, 1983, p. 195.

27. Hauser, A.M., Gordon, S. and Timmis, G.C. Familial hypertrophic cardiomyopathy and pre-excitation. *Am. Heart J.* 1984; 107: 176.

28. Jayakar, P.B., Stanwick, R.S. and Seshia, S.S. Tuberous scelerosis of Wolff–Parkinson–White Syndrome. *J. Pediatr.* 1986; 108: 259.

29. Gottlieb, A.V., Chan, M., Palmer, W.H. and Huang, S.N. Ventricular pre-excitation syndrome. Accessory left atrioventricular connection and rhabdomyomatous myocardial fibres. *Arch. Pathol. Lab. Med.* 1977; 101: 486.

30. Kearney, D.L., Titus, J.L., Hawkins, E.P., Ott, D.A. and Garson, A. Pathologic features of myocardial hamartomas causing childhood tachycardia. *Circulation* 1987; 75: 705.

31. Drake, C.E., Hodsden, J.E., Sridharan, M.R. and Flowers, N.C. Evaluation of the association of mitral valve prolapse in patients with WPW type electrocardiogram and its relation to ventricular activation pattern. *Am. Heart J.* 1985; 109: 83.

32. Gerlis, L.M., Davies, M.J., Boyle, R., Williams, G. and Scott, H. Pre-excitation due to accessory sinuoventricular connections associated with coronary sinus aneurysms. A report of two cases. *Br. Heart J.* 1985; 53: 314.

33. Miller, J.M., Rosenthal, M.E., Vassallo, J.A. and Josephson, M.E. Atrioventricular nodal reentry tachycardia: Studies on upper and lower "common pathways". *Circulation* 1987; 75: 930.

34. Ross, D.L., Johnson, D.C., Denniss, A.R., Cooper, M.J., Richards, D.A. and Uther, J.B. Curative surgery for atrioventricular junctional ("AV Nodal") reentrant tachycardia. *J. Am. Coll. Cardiol.* 1985; 6: 1383.

35. Scheinman, M.M., Gonzalez, R., Thomas, A., Ullyot, D., Bjarati, S. and Lev, M. Re-entry confined to the AV node: electrophysiology and anatomic findings. *Am. J. Cardiol.* 1983; 49: 1814.

36. Ward, D.E. and Camm, A.J. Ventriculo-atrial conduction over accessory pathways exhibiting decremental properties. *Eur. Heart J.* 1982; 3: 267.

37. Critelli, G., Gallagher, J.J., Monda, V., Coltorti, F., Scherillo, M. and Rossi, L. Anatomic and electrophysiologic substrate of the permanent form of junctional reciprocating tachycardia. *J. Am. Coll. Cardiol.* 1984; 4: 601.

38. Lev, M., Fox, S.M., Bharati, S., Rosen, K.M., Langendorf, R. and Pick, A. Mahaim fibres as a basis for a unique variety of pre-excitation. *Am. J. Cardiol.* 1975; 35: 152.

39. Gmenier, R., Ng, C.K., Hammer, I. and Becker, A.E. Tachycardia caused by an accessory nodo-ventricular tract: a clinico-pathological correlation. *Eur. Heart J.* 1984; 3: 233.

40. Brechenmucher, C., Coumel, P. and James, T.N. Intractable tachycardia in infancy. *Circulation* 1976; 53: 377.

41. James, T.N. The Wolff–Parkinson–White syndrome: evolving concepts of its pathogenesis. *Prog. Cardiovasc. Dis.* 1970; 50: 159.

42. Brechenmacher, C. Atrio-His bundle tracts. *Br. Heart J.* 1975; 37: 853.

43. Lev, M. The pathology of complete atrioventricular block. *Prog. Cardiovasc. Dis.* 1964; 6: 317.

44. Lenegre, J. Aetiology and pathology of bilateral bundle branch fibrosis in relation to complete heart block. *Prog. Cardiovasc. Dis.* 1964; 6: 409.

45. Fairfax, A.J. and Doniach, D. Autoantibodies to cardiac conduction tissue and their characterisation by immunofluoresence. *Clin. Exp. Immunol.* 1976; 23: 1.

46. Ginks, W., Sutton, R., Siddons, H. and Leatham, A. Unsuspected coronary artery disease as a cause of chronic atrioventricular block in middle age. *Br. Heart J.* 1980; 44: 699.

47. Fulkerson, P.K., Beaver, B.M. Auseon, J.C. and Graber, H.L. Calcification of the mitral annulus. Aetiology, clinical associations, complications and therapy. *Am. J. Med.* 1979; 66: 967.

48. Paulsen, S. and Vetner, M. Rytand–Lipsitch syndrome. *Arch. Pathol.* 1975; 99: 246.

49. Takamoto, T. and Popp, R.L. Conduction disturbances related to the site and severity of mitral annular calcification. A 2 dimensional echo and electrocardiographic correlative study. *Am. J. Cardiol.* 1983; 51: 1644.

50. Davies, M.J. Conduction tissues in systemic disease. In: Davies, M.J., Anderson, R.H. and Becker, A.E., eds. *The Conduction System of the Heart*. London: Butterworths, 1983, p. 204.

51. Dunnigan, A., Pierpont, M.E., Smith, S.A. et al. Cardiac and skeletal myopathy associated with cardiac dysrhythmias. *Am. J. Cardiol.* 1984; 53: 731.

52. Roberts, N.K., Perloff, J.K. and Kark, R.A. Cardiac Conduction in the Kearns–Sayre Syndrome. *Am. J. Cardiol.* 1979; 44: 1396.

53. Gault, J.H., Cantwell, J. and Lev, M. Fatal familial cardiac arrhythmias. Histological observations on the cardiac conduction system. *Am. J. Cardiol.* 1972; 29: 548.

54. Lynch, H.T., Mohiuddin, S., Moran, J., Kaplan, A., Sketch, M., Zencka, A. and Rurco, V. Hereditary progressive atrioventricular conduction defect. *Am. J. Cardiol.* 1975; 36: 297.

55. Barak, M., Herschkowitz, S., Shapiro, I. and Roguin, N. Familial combined sinus node with atrioventricular conduction dysfunctions. *Int. J. Cardiol.* 1987; 15: 231.

56. Ho, S.Y., Esscher, E., Anderson, R.H. and Michaelsson, M. Anatomy of congenital complete heart block and relation to maternal RO antibodies. *Am. J. Cardiol.* 1986; 58: 291.

57. Taylor, P.V., Scott, J.S., Gerlis, L.M., Esscher, E. and Scott, O. Maternal antibodies against foetal cardiac antigens in congenital complete heart block. *N. Engl. J. Med.* 1986; 315: 667.

58. Behan, W.M.H., Behan, B.O. and Gairns, J. Cardiac damage in polymyositis associated with antibodies to tissue ribonucleoproteins. *Br. Heart J.* 1987; 57: 176.

59. Evans, D.W. and Stoven, P.G.I. Fatal heart block due to Mesothelioma of the AV node. *Br. Heart J.* 1986; 56: 572.

60. Hassel, D., Heinsimer, J., Califf, R.M. et al. Complete heart block in Reiter's syndrome. *Am. J. Cardiol.* 1984; 53: 967.

61. Davies, M.J. Disorders of the conduction system. In: Ansell, B.M. and Simkin, P.A., eds. *The Heart and Rheumatic Disease*. London: Butterworths, 1984, p. 65.

62. Bergfeldt, L., Vallin, H. and Edhag, O. Complete heart block in HLAB27 associated disease–electrophysiological and clinical characters. *Br. Heart J.* 1984; 51: 184.

63. Ahern, M., Lever, J. and Cosh, J. Complete heart block in rheumatoid arthritis. *Ann. Rheum. Dis.* 1983; 42: 389.

64. Roberts, N.K. and Cabeen, W.R. Atrioventricular nodal function in progressive systemic sclerosis. Electrophysiological and morphological findings. *Br. Heart J.* 1980; 44: 529.

65. Bulkley, B.H., Ridolfi, R.L., Salyer, W.R. and Hutchins, G.M. Myocardial lesions of progressive systemic sclerosis—a cause of cardiac dysfunction. *Circulation* 1976; 53: 483.

66. Roberts, N.K. The prevalence of conduction defects and cardiac arrhythmias in progressive systemic sclerosis. *Ann. Intern. Med.* 1981; 94: 38.

67. Bharati, S., Fuente, J., Kallen, R.J., Freij, Y. and Lev, M. Conduction system in systemic lupus with AV block. *Am. J. Cardiol.* 1975; 35: 299.

68. James, T.N. Small arteries of the heart. *Circulation* 1977; 56: 2.

69. Askari, A.D. and Huettner, T.L. Cardiac abnormalities in polymyositis and dermatomyositis. *Semin. Arthritis Rheum.* 1982; **12**: 208.

70. Lightfoot, P.R., Bharati, S. and Lev, M. Chronic dermatomyositis with intermittent trifascicular block—an electrophysiological conduction system correlation. *Chest* 1977; **71**: 413.

71. Levander-Lindgren, M. Studies in myocarditis. *Cardiologia* 1965; **47**: L139.

72. Karjalainen, J., Viitasalo, M., Kala, R. and Keikkila, J. 24-hour electrocardiographic recordings in mild acute infectious myocarditis. *Ann. Clin. Res.* 1984; **16**: 34.

73. Lim, C.H., Toh, C.C., Chia, B.L. and Low, L. Stokes–Adams attacks due to acute non-specific myocarditis. *Am. Heart J.* 1975; **90**: 172.

74. Fujiwara, T., Akiyama, Y., Narita, H. *et al.* Idiopathic acute myocarditis with complete AV block in a baby. Clinicopathological study of the AV conduction system. *Jap. Heart J.* 1981; **22**: 275.

75. Arita, M., Ueno, Y. and Masuyama, Y. Complete heart block in mumps myocarditis. *Br. Heart J.* 1981; **16**: 342.

76. Lindvall, K., Edhag, O., Erhardt, O., Erhardt, L.T., Sjogren, A. and Swahn, A. Complete heart block due to granulomatous giant cell myocarditis. Report of 3 cases. *Eur. J. Cardiol.* 1978; **8**: 349.

77. Clarke, M. and Keith, J.D. AV conduction in acute rheumatic fever. *Br. Heart J.* 1972; **34**: 472.

78. Moffat, R.C. Diphtheritic heart block. A case report demonstrating the progressive development of complete heart block. *Angiography* 1972; **23**: 609.

79. Andrade, Z.E., Andrade, S.G., Oliviera, G.B. and Alonso, B.R. Histopathology of the cardiac conduction system in Chagas myocarditis. *Am. Heart J.* 1978; **95**: 316.

80. Nicholas, G., Leborgne, P., Meneut, J.C., Bouhour, J.B., Pony, J.C. and Godin, J.F. A case of complete AV block caused by syphilitic gumma of the IV septum. *Arch. Mal. Coeur* 1973; **66**: 295.

81. Stovin, P.G. Isolated interventricular septal tuberculoma causing complete heart block. *Thorax* 1982; **45**: 49.

82. Fleming, H.A. Sarcoid heart disease. *Br. Med. J.* 1986; **292**: 1095.

83. Silverman, K.J., Hutchins, G.M. and Bulkley, B.H. Cardiac sarcoid: a clinicopathological study of 84 unselected patients with systemic sarcoidosis. *Circulation* 1978; **58**: 1204.

84. Kulbertus, H.E. *The Hemiblocks—Ten Years' Experience.* Boehringer-Ingelheim, 1979.

85. Demoulin, J.C., Simar, L.J. and Kulbertus, H.E. Quantitative study of left bundle branch fibrosis in left anterior hemiblock. A stereological approach. *Am. J. Cardiol.* 1975; **36**: 751.

86. Rizzon, P., Rossi, L., Baissus, C., Demoulin, J.C. and Dibaise, M. Left posterior hemiblock in acute myocardial infarction. *Br. Heart J.* 1975; **37**: 711.

87. Lev, M., Unger, P.N., Rosen, K.M. and Bharati, S. The anatomic base of the ECG abnormality of left bundle branch block. *Adv. Cardiol.* 1975; **14**: 16.

88. Lev, M., Unger, P.N., Lesser, M.E. and Pick, A. Pathology of the conduction system in acquired heart disease; complete right bundle branch block. *Am. Heart J.* 1961; **61**: 593.

89. Bolik, D.R., Hackel, D.B., Reimer, K.A. and Ideker, R.E. Quantitative analysis of myocardial infarct structure in patients with ventricular tachycardia. *Circulation* 1986; **74**: 1266.

90. Cox, J.L. Anatomic–electrophysiologic basis for the surgical treatment of refractory ischaemic ventricular tachycardia. *Ann. Surg.* 1983; **198**: 119.

91. Josephson, M.E., Horowitz, L.N. and Spielman, S.R. Comparison of endocardial catheter mapping with intraoperative mapping of ventricular tachycardia. *Circulation* 1980; **61**: 395.

92. Horowitz, L.N., Josephson, M.E. and Harken, A.H. Epicardial and endocardial activation during sustained ventricular tachycardia in man. *Circulation* 1980; **61**: 1227.

93. Fenoglio, J.J., Pham, T.D., Harken, A.H., Horowitz, L.N., Josephson, M.E. and Wit, A.L. Recurrent sustained ventricular tachycardia: structure and ultrastructure of subendocardial regions in which tachycardia originates. *Circulation* 1983; **68**: 518.

94. Silver, M.A., Cohen, A.I., and Katz, N.M.L. Cardiac morphological findings late after partial left ventricular endomyocardial resection for recurrent ventricular tachycardia. *Am. J. Cardiol.* 1984; **54**: 233.

95. Silver, M.A. Morphologic substrates of ventricular arrhythmias. *Clin. Prog. Electrophys. Pacing* 1986; **4**: 1.

96. McKenna, W.J., England, D., Doi, Y.L., Deanfield, J.E., Oakley, C. and Goodwin, J. Arrhythmia in hypertrophic cardiomyopathy. Influence on prognosis. *Br. Heart J.* 1981; **46**: 168.

97. Bjarnason, I., Hardarson, T. and Jonsson, S. Cardiac arrhythmias in hypertrophy cardiomyopathy. *Br. Heart J.* 1982; **48**: 198.

98. Huang, S.K., Messer, J.V. and Denes, P. Significance of Ventricular Tachycardia in Idiopathic Dilated Cardiomyopathy: Observations in 35 patients. *Am. J. Cardiol.* 1983; **51**: 507.

99. Olshausen, K., Amann, E., Hofmann, M., Schwartz, F., Mehmel, H.C. and Kubler, W. Ventricular arrhythmias before and late after aortic valve replacement. *Am. J. Cardiol.* 1984; **54**: 142.

100. Karey, R.E.W., Blackman, M.S. and Sondheimer, H. Incidence and severity of chronic ventricular dysrhythmia after repair of Tetralogy of Fallot. *Am. Heart J.* 1982; **103**: 342.

101. Sullivan, I.D., Presbitero, P., Gooch, V.M., Aruta, E. and Deanfield, J.E. Is ventricular arrhythmia in repaired tetralogy of Fallot an effect of the operation or a consequence of the course of the disease? A prospective study. *Br. Heart J.* 1987; **58**: 40.

102. Marcus, F.I., Fontaine, G.H., Guiraudon, G., Frank, R., Laurenceau, J.L., Malergue, C. and Grosgogeat, Y. Right ventricular dysplasia: a report of 24 adult cases. *Circulation* 1982; **65**: 384.

103. Fitchett, D.H., Sugrue, D.D., Macarthur, C.G. and Oakley, C.M. Right ventricular dilated cardiomyopathy. *Br. Heart J.* 1984; **51**: 25.

104. Ibsen, H.H.W. Baandrup, U. and Simonsen, E.E. Familial right ventricular dilated cardiomyopathy. *Br. Heart J.* 1985; **54**: 156.

105. Laurent, M., Descaves, C., Biron, Y., Deplace, C., Almange, C. and Daubert, J.C. Familial form of arrhythmogenic right ventricular dysplasia. *Am. Heart J.* 1987; **113**: 827.

106. Rakovec, P., Rossi, L., Fontaine, G., Sasel, B., Markez, J. and Voncina, D. Familial arrhythmogenic right ventricular disease. *Am. J. Cardiol.* 1986; **58**: 377.

107. Morgera, T., Salvi, A.E., Silvestri, F. and Camerini, F. Morphological findings in apparently idiopathic ventricular tachycardia. An echocardiographic haemodynamic and histologic study. *Eur. Heart J.* 1985; **6**: 323.

108. Sugrue, D.D., Holmes, D.R., Gersh, B.J., Edwards, W.D., McLaran, C., Wood, D.L., Osborn, M.J. and Hammill, S.C. Cardiac histological findings in patients with life threatening ventricular arrhythmias of unknown origin. *J. Am. Coll. Cardiol.* 1984; **4**: 952.

109. Strain, J.E., Grose, R.M., Factor, S.M. and Fisher, J.D. Results of endomyocardial biopsy in patients with spontaneous ventricular tachycardia but without apparent

structural heart disease. *Circulation* 1983; **68**: 1171.

110. Hosenpud, J.D., McAnulty, J.H. and Niles, N.R. Unexpected myocardial disease in patients with life threatening arrhythmias. *Br. Heart J.* 1986; **56**: 55.

111. James, T.N. Normal variations and pathologic changes in structure of the cardiac conduction system and their functional significance. *J. Am. Coll. Cardiol.* 1985; **5**: 71B.

112. Marino, T.A. and Kane, B.M. Cardiac atrioventricular junctional tissues in hearts from infants who died suddenly. *J. Am. Coll. Cardiol.* 1985; **5**: 1178.

113. James, T.N., Cobbs, B.W., Coghlan, H.C., McCoy, W.C. and Fisch, C. Coronary disease, cardioneuropathy and conduction system abnormalities in the cardiomyopathy of Friedreich's ataxia. *Br. Heart J.* 1987; **57**: 446.

114. James, T.N., Froggatt, P., Atkinson, W.J. *et al*. Observations on the pathophysiology of the long QT syndromes with special reference to the neuropathology of the heart. *Circulation* 1978; **57**: 1221.

115. James, T.N., Pearce, W.N. and Givhan, E.G. Sudden death while driving—role of sinus perinodal degeneration and cardiac neural degeneration and ganglionitis. *Am. J. Cardiol.* 1980; **45**: 1095.

116. Pellegrino, A., Ho, S., Anderson, R.H., Hegerty, A., Godman, M.J. and Michaelsson, M. Prolonged QT interval and the cardiac conduction tissues. *Am. J. Cardiol.*

1986; **58**: 1113.

117. Bharati, S., Dreifus, L., Bucheleres, G. *et al*. The conduction system in patients with a prolonged QT interval. *J. Am. Coll. Cardiol.* 1985; **6**: 1110.

118. Moothart, R.W., Pryor, R., Hawley, R.L., Clifford, N.J. and Blount, S.G. The heritable syndrome of prolonged QT interval syncope and sudden death—electron microscopic observations. *Chest* 1976; **70**: 263.

119. James, T.N. and Marshall, T.K. Persistent foetal dispersion of the AV node and His bundle within the central fibrous body. *Circulation* 1976; **53**: 1026.

120. Kirschner, R.H., Echner, F.A.O. and Baron, R.C. The cardiac pathology of sudden unexplained nocturnal death in SE Asian refugees. *JAMA* 1987; **256**: 2700.

121. Bharati, S. and Lev, M. Congenital abnormalities of the conduction system in sudden death in young adults. *J. Am. Coll. Cardiol.* 1986; **8**: 1096.

122. Bharati, S., Baverfeind, R., Miller, L.B., Strasbourg, D. and Lev, M. Sudden death in three teenagers: conduction system studies. *J. Am. Coll. Cardiol.* 1983; **1**: 879.

123. Weidermann, C.J., Becker, A.E., Hopferwieser, T., Muhlberger, V. and Knappe, E. Sudden death in a young competative athelete with WPW syndrome. *Eur. Heart J.* 1987; **8**: 651.

Chapter 23

The Recognition and Management of Tachyarrhythmias

A. John Camm

This chapter concerns the care of patients who suffer from tachyarrhythmias. It is divided into two sections: individual arrhythmias and specific modalities of treatment.

INDIVIDUAL ARRHYTHMIAS

PREMATURE BEATS

The mechanisms that cause premature beats are not known for certain but various responsible factors such as hypoxia, acidosis, application of chemicals, physical contact and stretch of the myocardium are well appreciated. A wide range of diseases and disorders therefore may provoke premature beats (Table 23.1).[1] Judging by a routine 12-lead electrocardiogram, ventricular premature beats are more common (< 1%) than atrial premature beats (< 0.5%) and junctional premature beats are uncommon in the apparently normal population.[2] However, 24-hour electrocardiography reveals that premature beats occur in the majority of adults[3] and in practically every old person.[4] These arrhythmias tend to become more frequent as age advances[5] and are generally noted more frequently in men.[6] Ventricular premature beats are more common during exercise.[6]

Electrocardiographic appearance

Atrial premature beats

An atrial premature beat is characterized by an abnormally shaped atrial depolarization wave (P' wave) which occurs prior to the next anticipated sinus beat. Several electrocardiographic leads may be needed to distinguish the different P'-wave shape and in the rare case of sinus node premature beats

the P' wave will be identical. The interval following the premature P wave is usually similar to the basic sinus interval or a little longer due to penetration and reset of the sinus node by the premature beat.

Table 23.1. Common causes and provocations of premature beats.

Structrual heart disease:
Myocardial infarction
Hypertension
Stable coronary disease
Post-myocardial infarct
Cardiomyopathy
Heart failure
Myocarditis
Mitral valve prolapse

Endocrine disorder:
Thyrotoxicosis[a]

Neurogenic causes:
Sleep
Exercise
Anxiety
Vagal stimulation

Intoxication:
Digitalis
Alcohol
Caffeine
Catecholamines
Tobacco
Anti-arrhythmic drugs
Anaesthetic agents

Electrolyte disturbance:
Hypokalaemia
Hypomagnesaemia

Other diseases:
Pneumonia[a]
Bronchial carcinoma[a]
Hypoxia

[a] Particularly atrial premature beats.

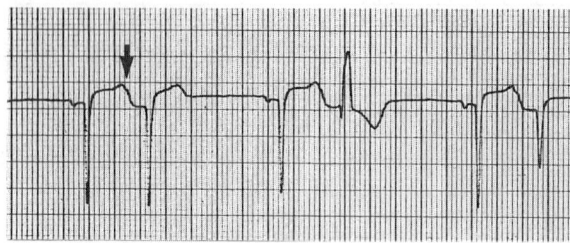

Fig. 23.1. Atrial premature beats with and without (arrow) aberration. The beat that does not aberrate has a very slightly longer coupling interval (450 ms) than those that do (440 ms).

Occasionally, the post-ectopic interval may be longer due to suppression of sinus node automaticity. The premature beat may conduct normally, encounter some degree of intraventricular block (aberration) (Fig. 23.1) or block completely (blocked atrial premature beat) (Fig. 23.2). When conducted to the ventricles, an atrial premature beat usually enounters slight atrioventricular delay and the P'R interval is therefore marginally longer than that of normal sinus beats. Aberrant conduction is discussed below with reference to the distinction between supraventricular and ventricular tachycardia. Blocked atrial premature beats may masquerade as pauses or bradycardias when P waves are not seen. The T wave of those beats that precede a pause should be carefully inspected to detect any 'hidden' premature P' wave.

Junctional premature beats

The atrioventricular junction comprises the atrioventricular node, the bundle of His, the atrium immediately adjacent to the atrioventricular node and any closely applied bypass tract. Most junctional premature beats probably arise from the proximal His bundle[7] or the atrium—the term 'atrioventricular nodal premature beat' is therefore inappropriate. The premature beat usually conducts antegradely to the ventricles (with or without aberration) and retrogradely to the atria. The timing of the retrograde P wave (inverted in II, III and aVF, and upright in aVR) relative to the QRS complex depends on the site of origin of the beat and the conduction times from there to the atria and to the ventricles. The retrograde P wave, therefore, may occur immediately before, during or following the QRS complex. The length of the post-ectopic interval depends on whether the retrograde P wave resets the sinus node.

Ventricular premature beats

The morphology of a ventricular premature beat depends on its site of origin. Beats that arise close to the intraventricular conduction system tend to be narrow and more similar to supraventricular beats because they conduct rapidly after accessing the proximal part of the specialized conduction system. These premature beats are known as *fascicular* beats.[8] However, most ventricular premature beats are wide (> 120 ms) and bizarre in shape. Beats arising in the left ventricle tend to be right bundle branch block-like in appearance (positive in lead V_1) whereas a right ventricular origin shows as a left bundle branch block-like appearance (negative in lead V_1). In chronic ischaemic heart disease, ectopic beats arising from the interventricular septum may have either morphology. Ventricular premature beats arising from a 'normal' heart usually have a right ventricular shape.[9] If the premature beat conducts back to the atria, a retrograde P wave may be seen in the ST segment/T wave.[10] More often, sinus P waves are not affected by the ventricular premature beat, which may however prevent the

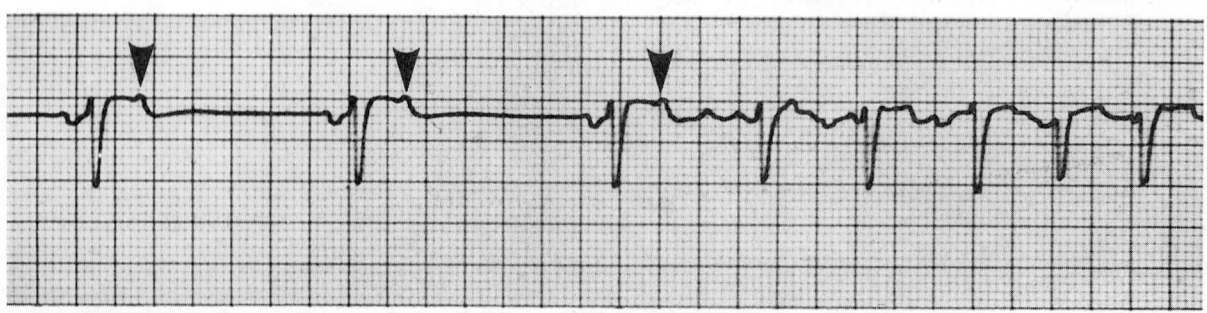

Fig. 23.2. An example of non-conducted atrial premature beats (arrows) occurring in a bigeminal pattern. This results in a slow ventricular rate. The third atrial premature beat provokes atrial fibrillation.

sinus beat from conducting to the ventricles, thus producing the so-called 'complete compensatory pause'.

Various forms of *complexity* are described.

1 **Multiform (pleomorphic)**: two or more distinctly different shapes (note that the term *multifocal* is not appropriate because beats from the same origin may be conducted differently and give rise to different shapes).
2 **Bigeminy, trigeminy and quadrigeminy**: recurring premature beats separated by one (bigeminy), two (trigeminy), or three (quadrigeminy) normal beats.
3 **Couplets and salvos**: pairs or multiples (3 or more with variable coupling intervals) of premature beats.

Significance of premature beats

Symptoms

Premature beats may not give rise to any symptoms especially when they conduct normally through the His–Purkinje system (atrial and junctional origins). Palpitation is the most common symptom and usually consists of an awareness of the premature beat itself, of the following pause, usually described as a 'missed beat', or of the more forceful 'post-extrasystolic beat'. These palpitations are most often felt at night, especially when the patient lies on the left side, whilst sitting quietly, and during exercise or immediately afterwards. Uncomfortable neck pulsations, due to venous cannon waves, sometimes occur. In some patients, the palpitations induce anxiety and associated dyspnoea and hyperventilation. Occasionally, stabbing or searing chest pain may be caused by premature beats but this usually occurs in the setting of 'effort (Da Costa's) syndrome'. Frequent premature beats, especially when interpolated within a normal sinus interval, may produce relative tachycardia, hypotension and classical angina pectoris.

Triggers of sustained arrhythmia

Premature beats may provoke sustained tachyarrhythmias because the majority of these clinical arrhythmias seem to be due to the mechanisms of re-entry or triggered automaticity. Atrial premature beats induce atrial tachycardia, flutter and fibrillation, junctional tachycardias and occasionally ventricular tachycardia.[11] Ventricular premature beats may provoke ventricular or junctional tachyar-

rhythmias. Atrial fibrillation may be triggered by ventricular premature beats when retrograde conduction is present, especially when this conduction occurs through an accessory pathway. These arrhythmias are generally initiated by premature beats occurring at critical coupling intervals. Ventricular fibrillation may be induced by closely coupled (R-on-T) ventricular premature beats and also by relatively late coupled premature beats.[12] Torsade de pointes is usually initiated by a specific 'short–long–short' sequence seen with ventricular bigeminy or when ventricular premature beats are associated with sinus bradycardia.[13]

Markers of prognosis

Atrial and junctional premature beats seem to have no prognostic significance. The prognostic importance of ventricular premature beats in otherwise normal individuals is controversial.[14] It may be that the premature beat signals otherwise latent disease but in many patients no such disease comes to light. Although there is an excess mortality in such patients, this has usually been ascribed to co-existing risk factors.[15] Recently, it has been claimed that some of the risk for sudden cardiac death is due to the premature beat.[16] However, it should be emphasized that this risk is small. Ventricular premature beats carry an adverse prognosis in patients convalescing from myocardial infarction, in patients with otherwise stable coronary disease, in patients with heart failure and in patients with cardiomyopathy, especially the hypertrophic variety. In patients followed-up after myocardial infarction, the reduction in lifespan associated with frequent premature beats (> 10/h) is additional to that predicted by poor ventricular function.

Treatment

Neither atrial nor junctional premature beats usually need treatment because they are rarely symptomatic and they do not have prognostic significance. Symptomatic premature beats should be managed by eliminating provoking factors, such as caffeine or alcohol and by treating any underlying condition, such as pneumonia or thyrotoxicosis. Ventricular premature beats should be treated for symptomatic purposes by similar measures but often anti-arrhythmic drugs are needed. Because the application of such drugs may aggravate rather than ameliorate the arrhythmia, their use should be carefully monitored using 24-h electrocardiography, exercise testing and blood levels as appropriate.

When significant structural heart disease or left ventricular dysfunction is present, frequent or complex ventricular premature beats should probably be treated on prognostic grounds. Routine treatment of premature beats, even when frequent, following myocardial infarction is not justified because it has not been proved in formal trials that such treatment is valuable. Patients at great risk of sudden cardiac death or hypotensive ventricular tachycardia should receive carefully prescribed and monitored treatment to suppress premature beats.

ATRIAL ARRHYTHMIAS

Atrial flutter

Atrial flutter is one of the most common causes of regular supraventricular tachycardias encountered clinically, but, unlike paroxysmal re-entrant atrioventricular tachycardia, atrial flutter usually occurs in association with atrial disease. Atrial distension and intra-atrial delay are predisposing factors,[17] and atrial flutter is a re-entrant arrhythmia.

Atrial flutter is rarely seen in normal subjects. It was found only once among 67 000 United States Air Force personnel.[18] It may occur at all ages, even in infancy, and it is more common than atrial fibrillation in the first few years of life.[19] However, flutter is most commonly encountered in patients with ischaemic heart disease over the age of 40 years, and paroxysms complicate 2–5% of cases of acute myocardial infarction.[20]

Atrial flutter may be paroxysmal or chronic: paroxysmal atrial flutter may occur in patients without organic heart disease, whereas chronic persistent atrial flutter is usually associated with underlying organic heart disease. The causes of atrial flutter include atrial dilatation from septal defect, pulmonary emboli, mitral and tricuspid valve disease, ventricular failure, thyrotoxicosis, alcoholism, pericarditis and digitalis toxicity. Occasionally, atrial flutter may be congenital[21] or even occur *in utero*.[22] In children, continued episodes of atrial flutter are associated with an increased possibility of sudden cardiac death.[23]

Clinical features

Patients with atrial flutter usually present with rapid palpitations. The arrhythmia usually responds to carotid sinus massage with a decrease in ventricular rate. Very rarely, sinus rhythm results from carotid sinus massage. Exercise by enhancing the sympathetic or by lessening the parasympathetic tone, may improve atrioventricular conduction and produce a doubling of the ventricular rate.

Rapid flutter waves may be observed in the jugular venous pulse. If the relationship of flutter waves to conducted QRS complexes remains constant, the first heart sound will have a constant intensity. Occasionally, sounds caused by atrial contraction may be heard with the stethoscope.

Diagnosis

The flutter waves in the electrocardiogram are called F waves. Their pattern is variable, but the most common is typical sawtooth waves in leads II, III and aVF (Fig. 23.3) and more discrete waves separated by iso-electric intervals in V_1 and other precordial leads. When the rate is slow, a definite iso-electric 'shelf' appears in the limb leads. Rarely, the F waves may be notched or undulating, rather than serrated.[20] The flutter waves are commonly inverted (negative) in leads II, III and aVF and less often they are upright (positive).

The atrial rate during classical or type I atrial flutter is usually 250–350 beats/min[24] but antiarrhythmic drugs such as quinidine and amiodarone may reduce the rate to the range of 200 beats/min. The rate in type II atrial flutter is 350–450 beats/min.[24]

The commonest atrioventricular conduction ratio is 2:1 and alternate F waves are often hidden by the QRS complex, so that the underlying mechanism may be overlooked. When tachycardia presents with a ventricular rate of about 150 beats/min, electrocardiography should be performed in an attempt to reveal underlying atrial flutter waves. A 4:1 ratio is common especially after therapy with digitalis or propranolol. Atrial flutter with 1:1 atrioventricular conduction should always be suspected when a tachycardia with a rate of about 300 beats/min is seen.[20]

Treatment

The aims of treatment are to control the ventricular rate and to restore and maintain sinus rhythm. When urgent treatment for arrhythmias is required, direct current cardioversion using low energies (25 J) is appropriate. Intravenous verapamil,[25] diltiazem[26] or propranolol[27] are effective in slowing the ventricular rate by increasing atrioventricular

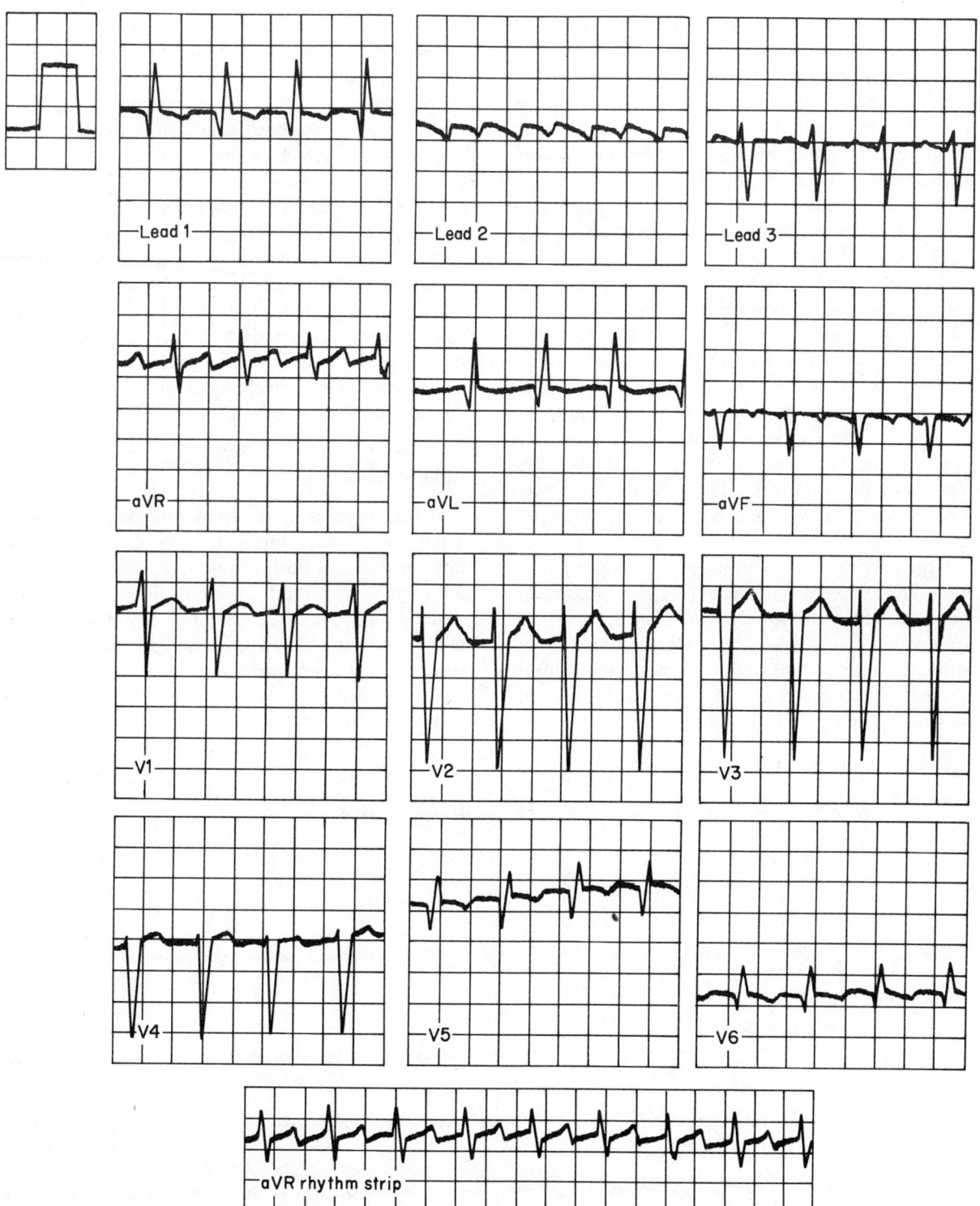

Fig. 23.3. This 12-lead electrocardiogram was recorded from a patient with atrial flutter and 2:1 atrioventricular conduction. The ventricular rate is 130 beats/min. The flutter waves (F waves) are not immediately obvious because of the QRST complexes. However, careful inspection of lead II shows the typical sawtooth F waves of atrial flutter.

block. Verapamil is given as an initial intravenous bolus of 5–10 mg, followed by a constant infusion at a rate of 5 μg/kg/min.[28]

If the flutter cannot be cardioverted or if it recurs at frequent intervals, digitalis may be administered to induce atrial fibrillation. Sinus rhythm may then be restored on withdrawing the digitalis. If atrial flutter persists, quinidine (disopyramide, procainamide or amiodarone) may restore sinus rhythm (Fig. 23.4). Any underlying disorders such as thyrotoxicosis must be effectively treated in order to achieve conversion to sinus rhythm.

It is important to emphasize that quinidine, procainamide, disopyramide and similar drugs should not be used unless atrioventricular block has been achieved with digitalis, verapamil or propranolol. Quinidine and disopyramide have a vagolytic effect on the atrioventricular node and all these drugs slow the atrial rate. These combined effects may result in a 1:1 ventricular response to the atrial flutter.

In the post-operative cardiac patient, termination of flutter by rapid atrial pacing (Fig. 23.5) has been very successful.[29] In other circumstances, reversion is more difficult.[30] Rapid atrial pacing effectively terminates type I atrial flutter but not type II atrial flutter.[29] A pacing rate 20–25 beats/min faster than the atrial flutter rate is usually required, and after atrial entrainment has been achieved and the tachycardia broken pacing may be stopped to reveal sinus rhythm.[31,32]

For chronic prophylaxis, quinidine and disopyramide remain standard drugs, although amiodarone may be effective for otherwise refractory cases. If recurrences cannot be prevented, therapy is directed towards controlling the ventricular rate with digitalis alone or combined with propranolol or verapamil. If recurrent or sustained atrial flutter or atrial fibrillation occurs and the ventricular rate cannot be adequately controlled by drugs, ablation of atrioventricular conduction and permanent pacemaker implantation may be useful. Specific atrial surgery or ablation techniques may also be considered.

Atrial fibrillation

Atrial fibrillation is more common than the other atrial tachyarrhythmias. It may be chronic or intermittent and both forms may occur in patients who have apparently normal hearts. However, underlying heart disease is more usual in patients with atrial flutter than in those with atrial fibrillation. The causes of atrial fibrillation are similar to those of atrial flutter. Rheumatic heart disease, especially mitral valve disease, atrial septal defect,[33]

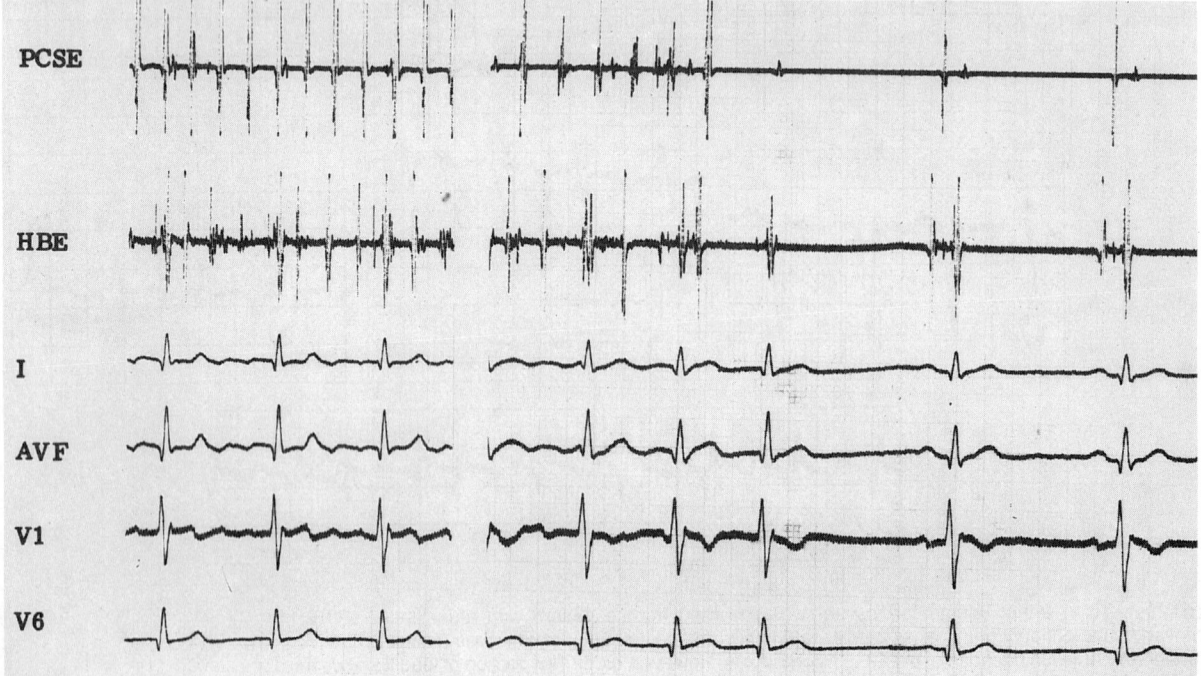

Fig. 23.4. Recordings before (left) and after (right) treatment of atrial flutter with intravenous disopyramide. Atrial flutter slows from 290 to 198 beats/min and then terminates.

3

6/92 — Day o Thorp bulletin.

A. FL push less with of thanks embolia

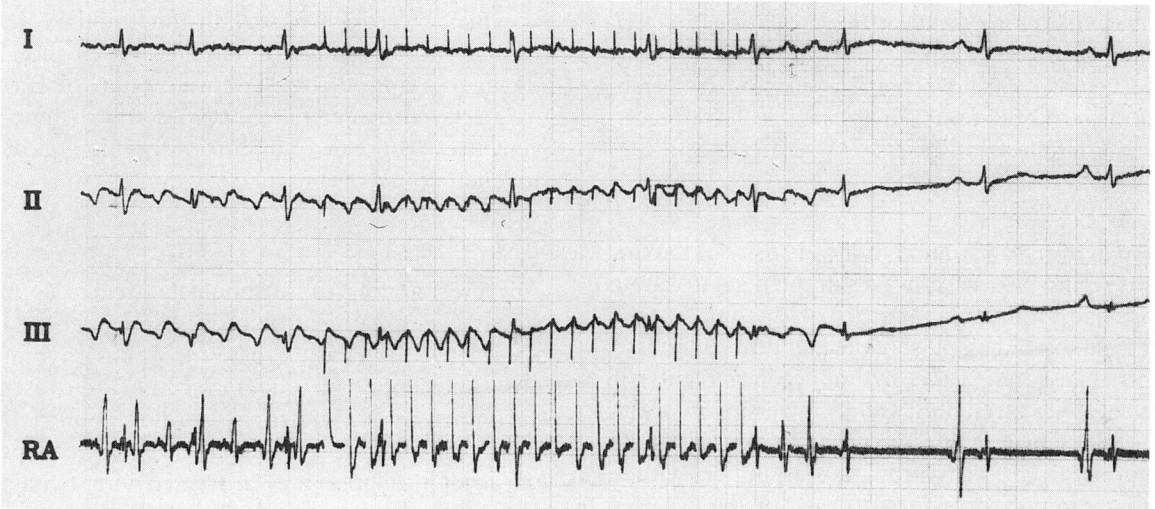

Fig. 23.5. Atrial flutter converts to sinus rhythm following a short burst of atrial pacing (400 beats/min) at a rate faster than the spontaneous flutter frequency (275 beats/min). Note (particularly, in leads II and III) that before the pacing is stopped atrial entrainment occurs (increase in the rate but no change in shape). Entrainment implies that the pacemaker-induced depolarization enters the re-entrant circuit. When tachycardia circulation breaks, the entrained rhythm changes in rate and in shape. When the pacing burst concludes, there is a very short run of atrial fibrillation before sinus rhythm resumes.

cardiomyopathy, pulmonary emboli, coronary heart disease, and post cardiac surgery[34] are common causes of atrial fibrillation; however, hypertensive cardiovascular disease is the most common cause. Pericarditis may be important although the results of a recent report suggests that pericarditis alone does not cause arrhythmias.[35] Occult or manifest thyrotoxicosis should always be considered in a patient with atrial fibrillation of recent onset.[36] In susceptible persons with otherwise apparently normal hearts, the arrhythmia is occasionally precipitated by alcohol ingestion (holiday heart).[37] The duration of a single paroxysm or intermittent atrial fibrillation may range from seconds to weeks. Atrial fibrillation may become permanent in 25% of these patients observed for more than 1 year.[38] Mortality is unchanged or only slightly increased in patients who have paroxysmal atrial fibrillation with no other cardiovascular impairment. However, paroxysmal atrial fibrillation with associated mitral stenosis or coronary artery disease incurs a significantly increased mortality. The development of chronic atrial fibrillation is associated with a doubling of the overall mortality and of the mortality from cardiovascular disease.[39] Mortality is highest in patients with mitral stenosis.[40] Occasionally, patients with longstanding atrial fibrillation may develop spontaneous reversion to sinus rhythm.[41] Patients with chronic

atrial fibrillation are at greatly increased risk of embolic stroke, particularly at the onset and termination of the atrial fibrillation. Chronic atrial fibrillation is associated with a fivefold increase in the incidence of stroke which rises to seventeenfold in patients with rheumatic heart disease. The occurrence of stroke increases directly with the duration of atrial fibrillation.[42] Approximately 30% of patients with longstanding chronic atrial fibrillation experience at least one embolic episode during the course of the fibrillation.

Subjects with 'lone' atrial fibrillation (atrial fibrillation in the absence of recognizable structural heart disease) have no increased risk of coronary heart disease and congestive heart failure, but they have a greater incidence of strokes.[43]

Atrial fibrillation is reported in 7–16% of continuously monitored patients with myocardial infarction.[20] Patients who develop atrial fibrillation within 1 year after acute myocardial infarction have higher total mortality and a greater frequency of ventricular tachyarrhythmias than do patients who do not develop atrial fibrillation.[44] Those who develop atrial fibrillation at the time of their acute myocardial infarction have a higher pulmonary wedge pressure and are usually older.[45]

The presence of atrial fibrillation appears to be related to the type of underlying heart disease and to left atrial size. The left atrial diameter as measured by echocardiography is smaller in patients with paroxysmal atrial fibrillation that terminates spontaneously than in those who require direct current cardioversion, those who have persistent atrial fibrillation[46] or those who have recurrences after electrical reversion.[47]

Clinical features

There is a slight variation in the intensity of the first heart sound, absent 'a' waves in the jugular venous pulse and an irregular ventricular rhythm. A significant apex–radial pulse deficit appears with fast ventricular rates. If the rhythm becomes regular in patients with atrial fibrillation, conversion to one of the following rhythms may be suspected: sinus rhythm, atrial tachycardia, atrial flutter with a constant ratio of conducted beats, or the development of junctional or ventricular tachycardia.

Diagnosis

Atrial fibrillation is characterized by totally disorganized atrial depolarization without effective atrial contraction. Electrical activity of the atrium may be detected electrocardiographically as small irregular baseline undulations of variable amplitude and morphology, known as f waves, at a rate of 350–600 beats/min. The f-wave amplitude does not correlate with left atrial size, the type of heart disease[48] or the chronicity of the atrial fibrillation. In uncomplicated atrial fibrillation, the QRS complexes are usually of normal configuration. Atrial fibrillation with aberrantly conducted beats may be mistaken for ectopic ventricular activity. Aberration is particularly likely to occur if a long ventricular cycle is immediately followed by a short cycle when the beat ending the short cycle shows aberrant conduction (Ashman phenomenon) (Fig. 23.6).[49] The ventricular response is grossly irregular and, in the untreated patient with normal atrioventricular conduction, it is usually between 100 and 160 beats/min. In patients with Wolff–Parkinson–White syndrome, the ventricular rate during atrial fibrillation may exceed 300 beats/min and lead to ventricular fibrillation. Many atrial impulses are concealed, owing to a collision of wavefronts, or are blocked in the atrioventricular junction without reaching the ventricles (concealed conduction), which accounts for the irregular ventricular rhythm.

Treatment

Any precipitating cause should be treated appropriately. The treatment objectives are either to slow the ventricular rate or to restore sinus rhythm. If atrial fibrillation results in acute cardiovascular decompensation, electrical cardioversion is the treatment of choice. If the patient is not collapsed, the atrial fibrillation may be treated with digitalis to maintain a resting apical rate of 60–80 beats/min that does not exceed 100 beats/min after exercise. The speed, route, dosage and type of digitalis preparation administered are determined by the status of the patient. The use of digitalis in combination with a beta-blocker or calcium antagonist[25] may be useful in slowing the ventricular rate. Reversion to sinus rhythm may occur with digoxin treatment and is most likely to occur after 4–8 h of treatment. Quinidine must often be given with digitalis to achieve conversion to sinus rhythm.

Prior to possible direct current cardioversion, quinidine sulphate should be administered for a few days and normal sinus rhythm will resume in 10–15% of patients. In 90% of the remainder, direct current cardioversion successfully establishes normal sinus rhythm. However, sinus rhythm persists for 12 months or more in only 30–50% of patients. Patients with atrial fibrillation of < 12 months' duration have a greater chance of maintaining sinus rhythm after cardioversion. Disopyramide or procainamide may be tried instead of quinidine.[50] Propafenone and flecainide are both effective for conversion of short-lived atrial fibrillation.[6] Long-term prevention of recurrences is

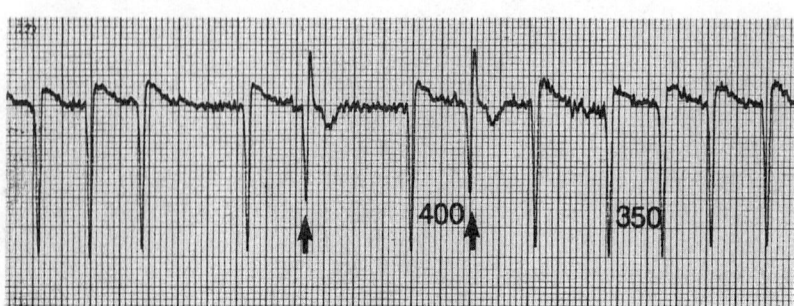

Fig. 23.6. The Ashman phenomenon describes aberration of beats (arrowed) following long–short cycles. The short cycle immediately preceding the aberrant beat is longer (400 ms) than cycles that do not result in aberration. The explanation is that the long penultimate cycle leads to increased His–Purkinje refractoriness which thus results in delayed intraventricular conduction in response to the following short cycle.

best achieved by treatment with drugs that stabilize the atrial myocardium, such as quinidine, disopyramıde (Fig. 23.7), procainamide and sotalol. Amiodarone is very effective but, because of its serious side-effects, it should not be used routinely to treat this relatively benign arrhythmia.

Atrial tachycardia

There are several varieties of atrial tachycardia, some of which are re-entrant and others of which are automatic. The electrocardiographic characteristic of atrial tachycardias is a P'R interval less than the RP' interval. The shape of the P' wave largely depends on the origin of the tachycardia.

Sino-atrial re-entry tachycardia

This is a rare type of re-entrant tachycardia. Diagnosis is suggested by a sudden increase in the atrial rate with no change in the morphology of the P wave. Usually the rate of tachycardia is relatively slow in the range of 100–140 beats/min. At electrophysiology study, the atrial activation sequence during tachycardia is indistinguishable from that during sinus rhythm. Atrial conduction times (PA) are also similar. It is difficult to differentiate sino-atrial re-entry from atrial tachycardia arising from in the upper part of the atrium. Treatment with beta-blockade is usually successful.

Atrial re-entrant tachycardia

Atrial re-entrant tachycardia presents in a paroxy-

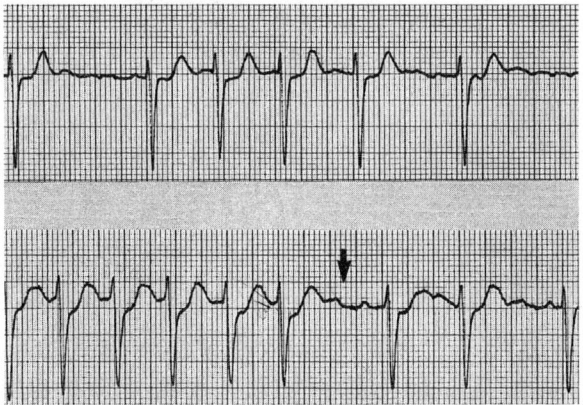

Fig. 23.7. These traces show the effect of disopyramide (2 mg/kg i.v.) on acute onset atrial fibrillation. The pre-treatment trace is shown on the top panel. In the lower panel, there is a trace recorded 14 min after the start of a 10-min infusion. The ventricular rate during atrial fibrillation is noticeably faster and more regular just before the atrial fibrillation gives way to sinus rhythm (arrow).

smal form. The PR interval depends on the rate of tachycardia and is longer than in sinus rhythm at the same rate. The tachycardia is usually rather slow (125–150 beats/min) and it can be initiated and terminated by atrial premature beats. Vagotonic manoeuvres rarely slow the tachycardia. Quinidine, disopyramide and beta-blockers may be successful treatments.

Automatic atrial tachycardia

Automatic atrial tachycardia accelerates or 'warms up' before reaching rates between 125 and 200 beats/min. The P'-wave morphology is different to that seen during sinus rhythm and the PR interval is longer. Importantly, the initial P' wave is usually the same as the subsequent tachycardia P' waves. This arrhythmia is not started or terminated by atrial premature beats. Automatic atrial tachycardia is usually due to digitalis toxicity, chronic pulmonary disease, ischaemic heart disease and alcohol. Treatment consists of potassium replacement, digoxin withdrawal where appropriate, and atrial membrane stabilizing drugs, such as quinidine, disopyramide and procainamide.

Atrial tachycardia with block

Atrial tachycardia with block occurs most commonly in patients with significant organic heart disease, such as coronary artery disease, with or without myocardial infarction, cor pulmonale, or digitalis intoxication. Digitalis toxicity accounts for 50–75% of cases. The signs, symptoms and prognosis are usually related to the underlying cardiovascular status. Because this arrhythmia occurs primarily in patients suffering from serious heart disease, clinical deterioration may result from the arrhythmia.

The rhythm depends on the varying degree of atrioventricular block (Fig. 23.8) and the first heart sound has variable intensity depending on the variability of the P'R interval. A wave may be seen in the jugular venous pulse and carotid sinus massage increases the degree of atrioventricular block by slowing the ventricular rate in a stepwise fashion. However, carotid sinus massage should be performed cautiously in patients with digitalis toxicity because serious ventricular arrhythmias may result.

The atrial rate is generally 150–200 beats/min. When the tachycardia is due to excess digitalis, the atrial rate may increase gradually as the digitalis is administered. As the atrial rate increases and atrioventricular conduction becomes impaired,

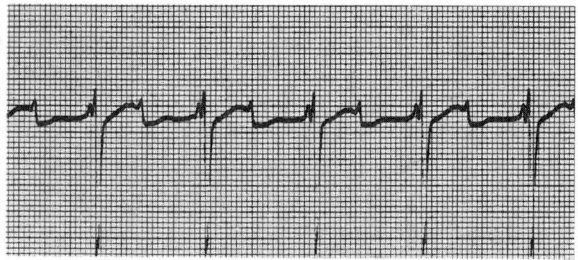

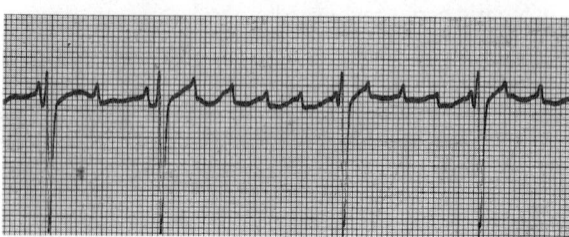

Fig. 23.8. These two short electrocardiographic strips are recorded from the same patient who was suffering from digitalis toxicity. Both traces show atrial tachycardia with block. Note the abnormal and rapid P waves, a proportion of which do not conduct to the ventricles. The lower strip demonstrates another feature of this rhythm: the P wave rate suddenly accelerates from 140 to 230 beats/min.

second degree atrioventricular block develops. Characteristic iso-electric intervals between P waves are usually present in all leads. At rapid atrial rates, it may be difficult to differentiate between atrial tachycardia with block and atrial flutter.

If atrial tachycardia with block occurs in a patient receiving digitalis, treatment requires stopping digitalis and giving potassium replacement if serum potassium is not abnormally elevated. Often the ventricular response is not excessively fast, and simply withholding digitalis is all that is necessary. Atrial tachycardia occurring in a patient not receiving digitalis is treated in a similar way to other atrial tachyarrhythmias.

Multifocal atrial tachycardia

Multifocal atrial tachycardia is characterized by rapid, irregular, discrete P waves of three or more different morphologies. It is a rare arrhythmia, but it is seen in childhood, in association with lung disease, digitalis toxicity and diabetes. Potassium replacement and the treatment of the underlying causes are the most effective therapies.

JUNCTIONAL TACHYCARDIA INCLUDING WOLFF–PARKINSON–WHITE SYNDROME

All narrow complex regular tachycardias were previously loosely grouped together as paroxysmal atrial tachycardia. Further understanding of surface electrocardiograms and advances in intracardiac electrophysiology techniques have permitted clinically relevant subgrouping of narrow complex regular tachycardias. Using such techniques, it has been established that the majority of such tachycardias are due to the mechanism of re-entry (circus movement) and only a small proportion are due to ectopic impulse information in the atrium, the atrioventricular node or His bundle.

Re-entrant junctional tachycardia

Re-entrant tachycardia is due to the circulation of a wave of depolarization (Fig. 23.9). This may be over a relatively well-defined pathway as in Wolff–Parkinson–White syndrome or through functionally distinct parts of otherwise homogeneous tissue such as the atrioventricular node or the atrial myocardium. Re-entry is initiated when:

1   two functionally distinct conduction pathways are present;

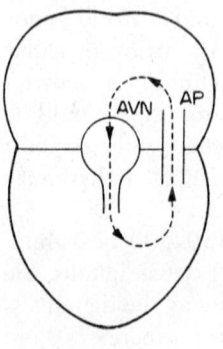

Orthodromic AVRT

Antidromic AVRT

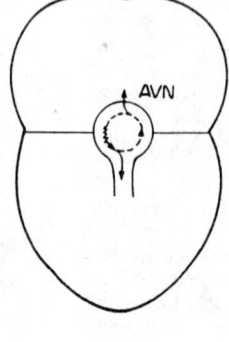

AVNRT

Fig. 23.9. Three varieties of junctional re-entrant tachycardia. AVN, atrioventricular node; AP, accessory pathway; AVRT, atrioventricular re-entrant tachycardia; AVNRT, atrioventricular nodal tachycardia. (Reproduced from Macfarlane, P. and Lawrie, V. (eds) *Comprehensive Electrocardiology. Theory and Practice in Health and Disease.* New York: Pergamon, 1988).

2 unidirectional block is induced in one pathway for example by a premature stimulus or by a physiological tachycardia;

3 sufficiently slow conduction exists to allow recovery of excitability in the blocked pathway and permit retrograde conduction over that pathway and completion of the circuit.

Electrophysiological features suggestive of re-entry in supraventricular tachycardias include:

1 initiation and termination by a 'precisely timed' premature beat;

2 an initial ectopic P wave different in shape from the subsequent P' (tachycardia) waves;

3 absence of tachycardia acceleration after initiation (no warm-up period).

Approximately one half of re-entrant supraventricular tachycardias (Fig. 23.9) are due to re-entry within the atrioventricular node (and closely adjacent atrial myocardium) and the other third are due to re-entry over a route that includes an accessory pathway.[51-54] A small number result from re-entry within the sinus node[55-57] or atrial myocardium.[58,59] In the absence of pre-excitation during sinus rhythm, the most frequent cause of supraventricular tachycardia is re-entry within the atrioventricular node (Table 23.2).

Clinical features

Re-entrant supraventricular tachycardias tend to appear first in youth and the attacks recur throughout life. Occasionally, certain events such as emotional upset, nervousness, fatigue, indigestion or alcohol ingestion precipitate attacks. Polyuria is often present during or after a prolonged attack. Usually no other cardiac abnormality is found (besides Wolff–Parkinson–White syndrome) but supraventricular tachycardias has been reported in 6–10% of patients with mitral valve prolapse.[61,62] Wolff–Parkinson–White syndrome is associated with Ebstein's anomaly. In the absence of an

underlying cardiac abnormality, supraventricular tachycardia should be considered benign unless the rate is very rapid (> 250 beats/min) or the episodes very prolonged. Extremely rapid rates (300–400 beats/min), more frequently seen in infants, might cause the normal heart to fail. In the presence of intraventricular conduction disturbances, supraventricular tachycardias may resemble ventricular tachycardia, and the differentiation may be difficult. Transoesophageal or transvenous atrial recordings may be required to demonstrate the sequence of cardiac activation and suggest the correct diagnosis. The relationship between the P' and the R waves provides important diagnostic information (Fig. 23.10).

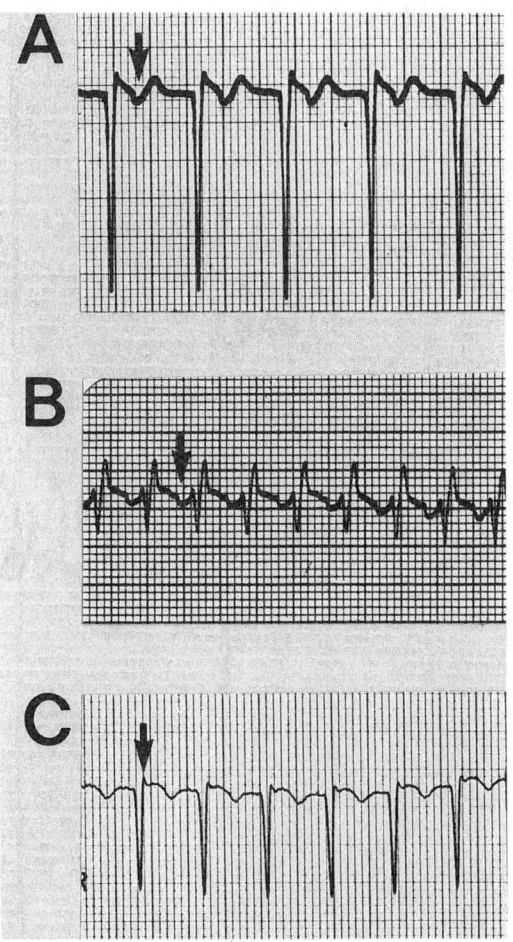

Fig. 23.10. Electrocardiograms of three varieties of paroxysmal supraventricular tachycardia. (A) Atrioventricular re-entry—notice the P' wave (arrow) in the ST segment following the QRS. The RP' is shorter than the P'R. (B) Atrial re-entry—the P' wave (arrow) is seen before each QRS complex. The RP' is longer than the PR'. (C) Atrioventricular nodal re-entry—the P wave is either masked by the QRS complex or seen as a small terminal r' wave.

Table 23.2. Incidence of various types of supraventricular tachycardia[52,53,60] (excluding atrial flutter and atrial fibrillation).

Supraventricular tachycardia	Incidence (%)
Atrioventricular nodal re-entry	50
Re-entry via accessory pathway (concealed)	30
Intra-atrial re-entry	8
Atrial automaticity	5
Miscellaneous	7

Atrioventricular nodal re-entrant tachycardia

This tachycardia is not usually associated with structural disease of the heart. The electrocardiogram during sinus rhythm in patients with atrioventricular nodal re-entrant tachycardia is usually normal. Precisely timed atrial and ventricular premature beats can initiate and terminate the tachycardia, and re-entry is the underlying mechanism for the arrhythmia. Patients with this form of tachycardia may have two functionally distinct intranodal pathways with different conduction velocities and refractory period properties which are described as slow and fast, or alpha and beta, pathways, respectively.[63–65] During sinus rhythm, an atrial premature beat may block in the fast pathway if it has a longer refractory period than the slower pathway. The His bundle is therefore activated via the slow pathway. However, by the time the impulse has conducted through the slow pathway, it stimulates the distal end of the fast pathway, which by now has recovered, to conduct retrogradely. Circus movement is initiated in this way. Thus, initiation of the tachycardia is associated with delayed atrioventricular conduction (slow pathway) and sudden prolongation of the AH interval at the initiation of tachycardia. In typical atrioventricular nodal re-entry tachycardia, the AH interval measured on the His bundle recording is prolonged (antegrade conduction down the slow pathway) and the HA interval is short. Much less often, the slow pathway has a long refractory period, the premature atrial impulse blocks antegradely in the slow pathway but conducts over the fast pathway and returns over the slow pathway ('fast–slow' tachycardia/atypical atrioventricular nodal re-entry tachycardia.[66,67] Thus, during tachycardia, the AH interval is short but the HA' is long (correspondingly a long RP' interval on the surface electrocardiogram). Although the functional basis of atrioventricular nodal re-entry tachycardia seems to be duality of atrioventricular nodal conductive tissue, the anatomical basis for this is not known and dual atrioventricular nodal pathways have not been demonstrated histologically.

Atrioventricular nodal re-entrant tachycardias respond to treatment with beta-blockers, calcium antagonists (Fig. 23.11) or digitalis glycosides. Acute termination of the attack is possible with vagal manoeuvres, adenosine, etc.

Diagnosis   Onset of tachycardia is associated with a prolonged PR interval. In classic atrioventricular

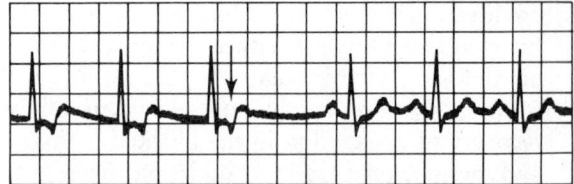

Fig. 23.11. The termination of a rather slow (100 beats/min) atrioventricular re-entrant tachycardia by an intravenous bolus of verapamil (0.1 mg/kg in 2 min). Note the retrograde P wave (arrow) in the ST segment after each tachycardia QRS complex. During sinus rhythm, only the sinus P wave is seen. Tachycardia terminates in the atrioventricular limb of the circuit.

nodal re-entrant tachycardia (slow–fast) the P' is either lost inside the QRS complex because of rapid retrograde conduction, or is barely visible at the end of the QRS complex (Fig. 23.12). Atypical atrioventricular nodal re-entrant tachycardia is characterized by a long RP' interval such that the P' waves can be seen in the latter half of the RR interval. However, when the RP' is greater than the P'R interval, the tachycardia is more likely to be due to atrial re-entry or re-entry over a slowly conducting accessory pathway[68,69] situated in the posterior septal region. Such tachycardias are rare.[70]

Atrioventricular re-entrant tachycardia

The anatomical basis for atrioventricular re-entrant tachycardia is an abnormal muscle connection between atrial and ventricular myocardium. This arrhythmia occurs in approximately 30% of patients with 'paroxysmal atrial tachycardia' who have no ventricular pre-excitation during sinus rhythm. In the majority of patients with the Wolff–Parkinson–White syndrome, narrow QRS complex tachycardia is due to atrioventricular re-entry.[53,71] In this tachycardia, one limb of the re-entrant circuit is the normal atrioventricular pathway and the other is the anomalous connection. In the majority of cases, antegrade conduction

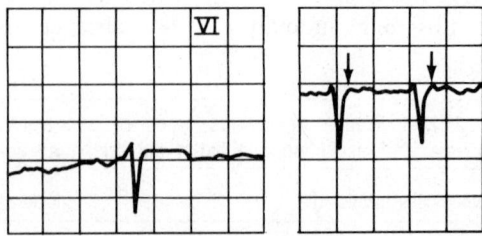

Fig. 23.12. Lead V₁ during sinus rhythm (left panel) and atrioventricular nodal re-entrant tachycardia (right panel). The retrograde P wave during tachycardia is seen as a small positive deflection at the end of the QRS complex (arrow). This deflection is not present during sinus rhythm.

during tachycardia is over normal atrioventricular nodal tissue and the abnormal connection forms the retrograde limb of the circuit pathway. The QRS complexes are usually similar to those seen during sinus rhythm but they may show rate-dependent aberration. The electrocardiogram during sinus rhythm may show pre-excitation if the accessory pathway is capable of conduction in the antegrade direction, but it is normal if the pathway conducts only in the retrograde direction, so-called concealed accessory pathway.[71–73]

Diagnosis   During the arrhythmia, the retrograde P′ wave may be seen in the ST segment and this alone should suggest the diagnosis, with or without overt pre-excitation during sinus rhythm. Retrograde P waves occur later in atrioventricular re-entrant tachycardia than in atrioventricular nodal re-entrant tachycardia because atrial activation follows ventricular activation in the former. In atrioventricular nodal re-entrant tachycardia, the atria and ventricles are activated simultaneously. The importance of making the diagnosis of atrioventricular re-entrant tachycardia in the absence of pre-excitation during sinus rhythm is twofold.

1   'Latent' pre-excitation may be present. In this situation, pre-excitation may be revealed by vagal manoeuvres or by other means of delaying atrioventricular nodal conduction (such as intravenous adenosine) and allowing conduction to occur through the accessory connection in an antegrade direction. These patients require electrophysiological evaluation in order to assess risk of rapid pre-excited tachycardias.[74]
2   Surgical treatment for these tachycardias is highly successful and may be preferable to anti-arrhythmic drug therapy in some patients.

Treatment

Acute termination of re-entrant paroxysmal supraventricular tachycardia may be achieved by applying vagotonic physical manoeuvres or by the intravenous injection of verapamil, beta-blockers or adenosine. Long-term control can be established by anti-arrhythmic drug treatment designed to suppress premature beats or to modify the characteristics of the re-entrant circuit such that it cannot support continued circulation. Prolongation of the refractoriness of the atrioventricular node (with beta-blockers or calcium antagonists) or of an accessory pathway (with disopyramide, procaina-

mide, quinidine or flecainide) is usually successful. Resistant cases may be considered for pacemaker, surgical or catheter ablation therapies.

Pre-excitation syndromes

This term refers to activation of the ventricular muscle, by an impulse arising in the atrium, earlier than would be expected if conduction occurred via the normal atrioventricular conduction pathway. The term was first used to describe electrocardiographic abnormalities in patients with typical Wolff–Parkinson–White syndrome.[75] However, three major types of pre-excitation are recognized.

1   Anomalous atrioventricular conduction over a pathway directly connecting atrial and ventricular myocardium (accessory atrioventricular connection, previously known as a bundle of Kent). The resulting syndrome of short PR interval (< 0.12 s) with a prolonged QRS complex (≥ 0.12 s) with an initial delta wave and paroxysmal tachycardias is known as the Wolff–Parkinson–White syndrome (Fig. 23.13).
2   Anomalous conduction over accessory nodoventricular or fasciculoventricular connections previously known as Mahaim fibres. This also presents as Wolff–Parkinson–White syndrome but the PR interval tends to be normal (only part of the normal atrioventricular conduction system is bypassed).
3   Anomalous conduction via intranodal or atriofascicular bypass tracts (previously known as James fibres) causing pre-excitation of the atrioventricular node or of the His bundle. The syndrome of short PR interval associated with a normal QRS complex and paroxysmal tachycardia is called the Lown–Ganong–Levine syndrome.

The clinical significance of pre-excitation is related to the common association with arrhythmias and the bizarre and misleading electrocardiographic patterns produced by the pre-excitation. The most important supraventricular arrhythmias to complicate the syndrome are atrioventricular re-entrant tachycardia and atrial fibrillation. In patients with the Wolff–Parkinson–White syndrome and tachyarrhythmias, most have atrioventricular re-entrant tachycardia and about one-third have atrial fibrillation.

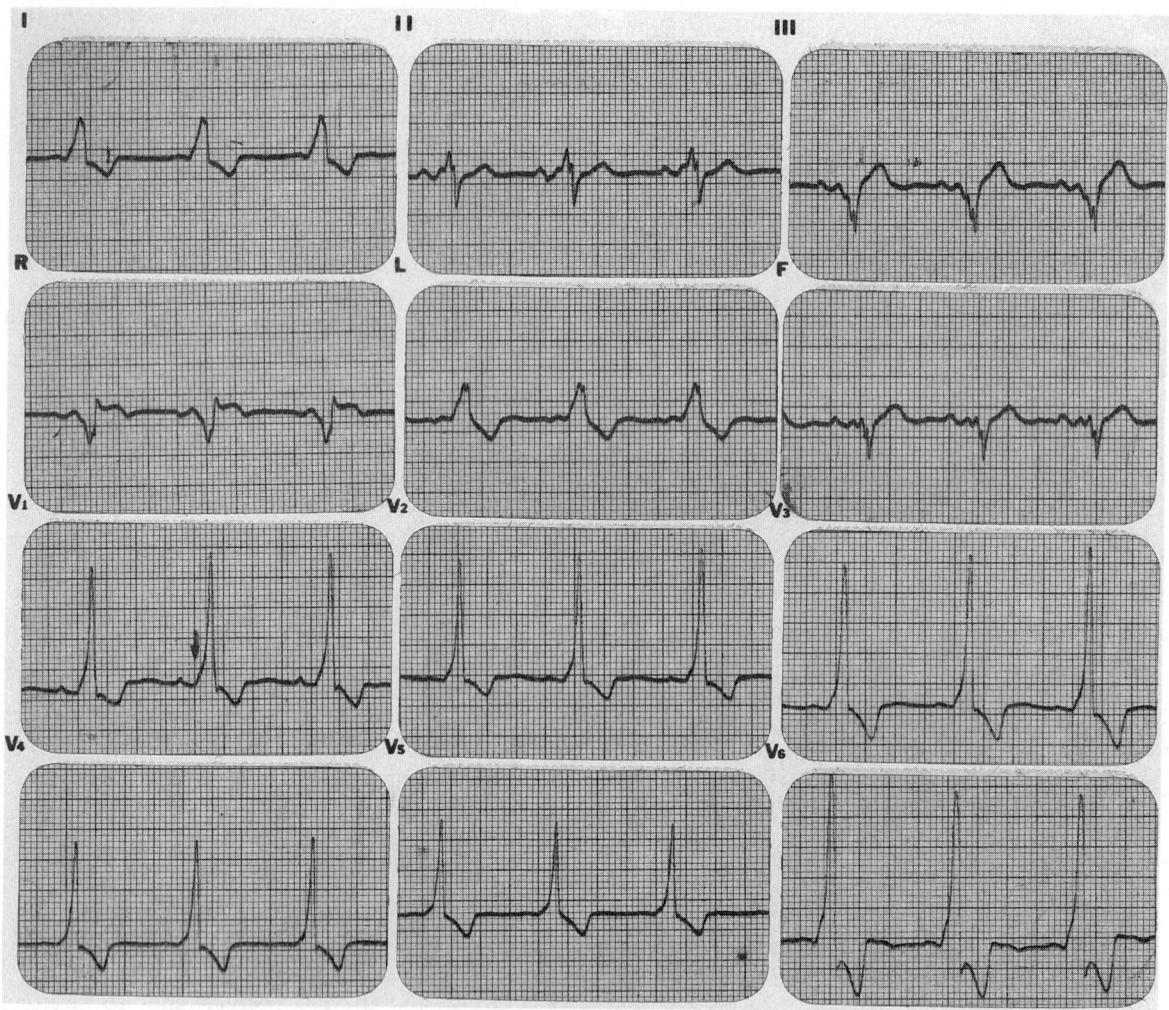

Fig. 23.13. 12-Lead electrocardiogram demonstrating the Wolff–Parkinson–White pattern (short PR interval and wide QRS with an initial slurred component (delta wave—arrow)). This particular example is typical of a posterior free wall left atrial-to-left ventricular connection. The pattern is described as 'type A', i.e. the delta wave is positive in V_1.

Wolff–Parkinson–White syndrome

Atrioventricular pathways that conduct antegradely produce a disturbed QRS complex beginning with a delta wave, the axis of which depends upon the location of the pathway. The Wolff–Parkinson–White syndrome is classified as type A (positive delta wave in V_1) and type B (negative delta wave in V_1) varieties which are associated with left- and right-sided pre-excitation, respectively.[76,77] Pathways can be more precisely localized using the initial polarity of the delta wave.[77] Pathways not conducting antegradely produce normal electrocardiograms during sinus rhythm. However, these latent pathways may be revealed by vagal stimulation or by the infusion of isoprenaline.[78] In approximately 10–20% of cases of Wolff–Parkinson–White syndrome, more than one accessory pathway is present.

Atrial fibrillation associated with the Wolff–Parkinson–White syndrome During atrial fibrillation, antegrade conduction over the accessory pathway results in a wide QRS complex tachyarrhythmia which may be mistaken for ventricular tachycardia (Fig. 23.14). Atrial fibrillation associated with the Wolff–Parkinson–White syndrome may be life-threatening if the accessory pathway has a short refractory period allowing a very rapid ventricular rate. Ventricular fibrillation may result if the antegrade impulse reaches the ventricles

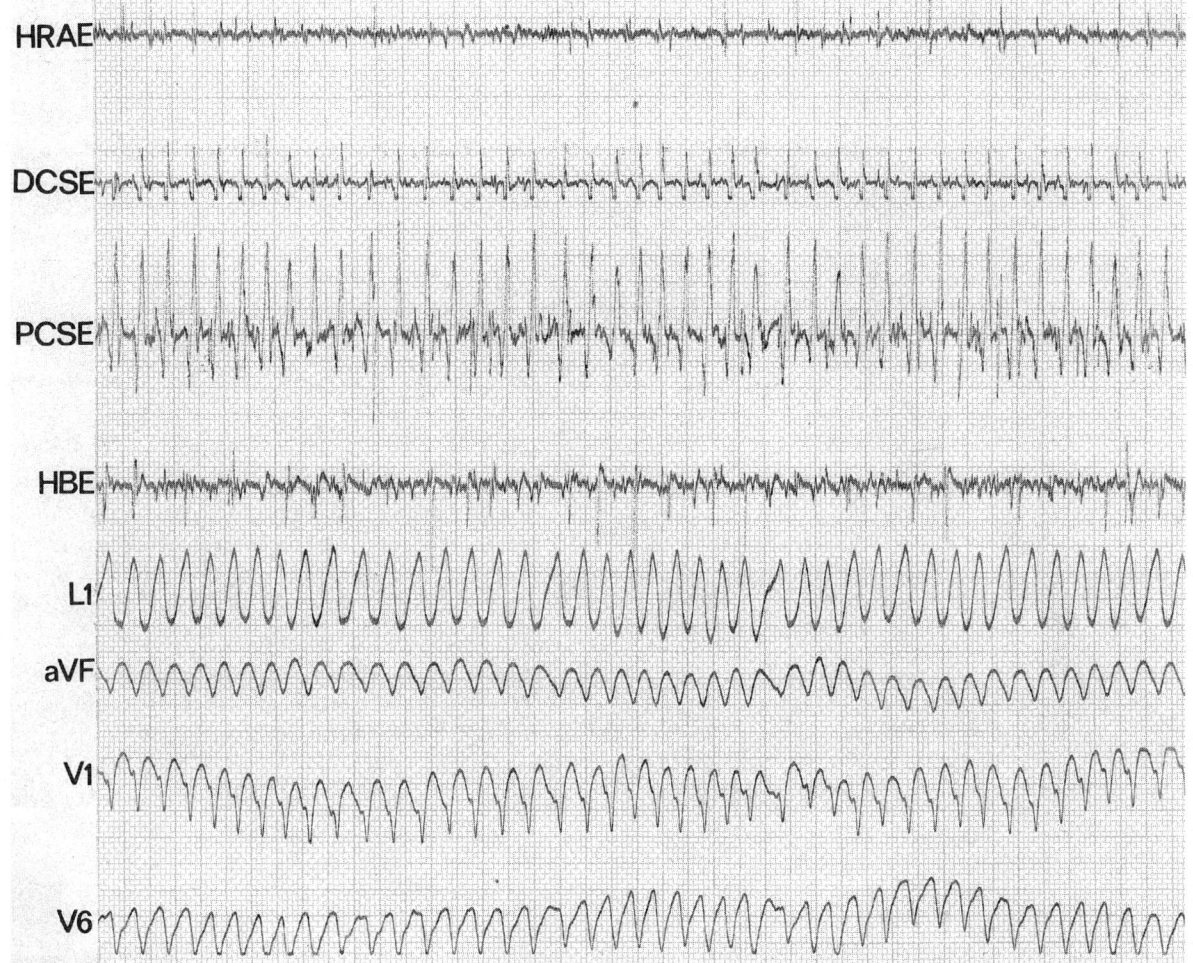

Fig. 23.14. Tracings from a clinical electrophysiology study demonstrating the response to atrial fibrillation of a patient with Wolff–Parkinson–White syndrome. Note the very rapid ventricular rate (at times > 300 beats/min) with pre-excited QRS complexes. HRAE, high right atrial electrogram; DCSE, distal coronary sinus electrogram; PCSE, proximal coronary sinus electrogram; HBE, His bundle electrogram. Lead I, aVF, V1 and V6 are simultaneously recorded surface ECG leads. Paper speed is 25 mm/s.

during the 'vulnerable period'. The pathways with the shortest refractory period are associated with the highest risk. An RR interval between consecutive pre-excited complexes of 250 ms or less is associated with rapid ventricular rates which are particularly dangerous.[74,79,80] On the other hand, a larger and safer refractory period is suggested, but not certain, when pre-excitation is intermittent or disappears on exercise.[81]

Surgical therapy is advised for life-threatening Wolff–Parkinson–White syndrome. Medical therapy with drugs that prolong the recovery of accessory pathways and stabilize the atrial myocardium may be used to reduce the occurrence of atrial fibrillation and decrease the ventricular rate during attacks. Paroxysmal supraventricular tachycardias are treated by conventional techniques (see above).

Lown–Ganong–Levine syndrome

The Lown–Ganong–Levine syndrome consists of a short PR interval and a normal QRS complex (Fig. 23.15) associated with supraventricular tachycardia.[82] A short PR interval (< 0.12 s) by itself could be due to small size, excessive adrenergic tone or atrioventricular conduction via an intranodal or extranodal anomalous AH pathway. Paroxysmal tachycardia occurs in approximately 10% of patients with a short PR interval and normal QRS complex compared with 0.5% patients who have a

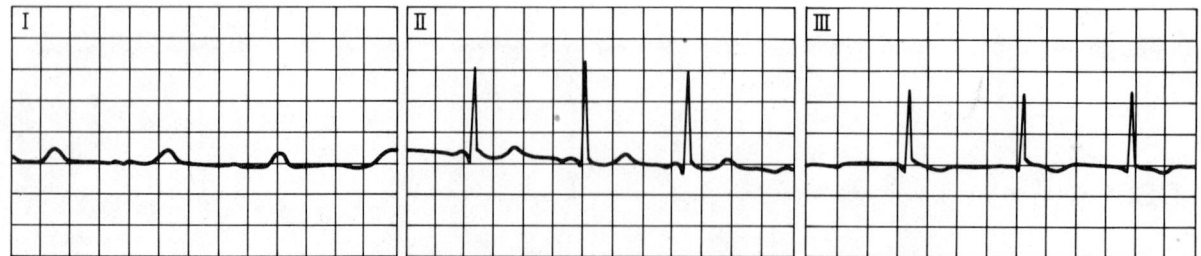

Fig. 23.15. These three ECG leads are recorded from a young woman with the Lown–Ganong–Levine syndrome. Notice the short PR interval (0.09 s) and narrow QRS complex (0.07 s) without any evidence of a delta wave.

normal PR interval and normal QRS complex durations.[82] Although supraventricular tachycardias, atrial flutter and atrial fibrillation can be associated, most tachycardias in the Lown–Ganong–Levine syndrome have atrioventricular nodal or atrioventricular re-entrant mechanisms.[83]

VENTRICULAR TACHYARRHYTHMIAS

Ventricular tachycardia

Ventricular tachycardia and ventricular fibrillation are the major causes of sudden unexpected cardiac death. Interest in their treatment has grown since the introduction of direct current cardioversion and the use of clinical electrophysiology techniques. They remain difficult to treat because there is no medical therapy which is broadly effective. However, surgical and transvenous catheter ablation techniques have provided alternative treatments and the recent development of the implantable automatic defibrillator offers a most effective therapy.

The principal mechanism of ventricular tachycardia is re-entry or circus movement. This mechanism requires an area of slow conduction, preferably with unidirectional block. Other important mechanisms of ventricular tachycardia are reflection, which is a form of microre-entry involving electrotonic conduction, triggered or abnormal automaticity and macrore-entry around the His–Purkinje system (bundle branch re-entry).[84] Triggered automaticity is due to delayed afterdepolarizations and is mediated by calcium channels and induced by intracellular calcium overload. This may be produced by metabolic disturbances including digoxin inactivation of the sodium/potassium pump or catecholamine activation of adenyl cyclase. Abnormal automaticity is chara-

cterized by rapid phase–4 depolarization of the ventricular myocardium, probably because of abnormal potassium or sodium conductance.[85]

An indication of the mechanism may be obtained on electrophysiology testing. Abnormal automaticity cannot be induced with extrastimulation, although it can be terminated by overdrive pacing, or occasionally by using extrastimuli. Both re-entry and triggered automaticity can be stimulated and terminated by extrastimulation. With triggered automaticity, the length of the first cycle of tachycardia is directly related to the prematurity of the extrastimulus, whereas with a re-entrant mechanism there is an inverse relationship.[86] Reset or entrainment of the tachycardia by pacing techniques favours a re-entrant mechanism, but to be sure of this electrograms from the tachycardia circuit must be entrained and slow conduction must be demonstrated.[87]

Most ventricular tachycardias are related to ischaemic heart disease, and they are seen as an early consequence of myocardial infarction. The mechanism is probably abnormal automaticity or re-entry. In this setting, ventricular tachycardia frequently degenerates to ventricular fibrillation and it is responsible for a significant proportion of sudden cardiac death in the community. Chronic recurrent ventricular tachycardia is less common, and it is most commonly related to a healed myocardial infarction, often with aneurysm formation. The areas of slow conduction are located within the endocardium often close to an aneurysm. Histologically, these areas are a patchwork of viable myocardium and scar tissue. During mapping of these tachycardias, the earliest activation is on the endocardial surface in a region of slow conduction. Activation of the unscarred ventricle is rapid, and the activation pattern usually has a 'figure-of-eight' appearance with the cross of the eight situated in the area of slow conduction.[88] In patients with non-ischaemic cardiomyopathy, the areas of slow conduction and the origin of the ventricular tachycardia are often intramyocardial. Other causes of ventricular tachycardia include congestive and hypertrophic cardiomyopathies, right ventricular dysplasia, repolarization abnormalities, such as the long QT syndrome, and some relatively rare idiopathic ventricular tachycardia syndromes, such as the right ventricular outflow tachycardias and the fascicular tachycardias.

Definitions

Ventricular tachycardia is defined as 5 or more consecutive beats arising below the atrioventricular node with an RR interval of < 500 ms (120 beats/min). *Sustained* ventricular tachycardia lasts > 30 s or requires termination because of haemodynamic collapse; *non-sustained* tachycardia terminates spontaneously in < 30 s.

Monomorphic tachycardia has only one morphology during each episode; *multiple monomorphic* (or *pleomorphic*) ventricular tachycardia has more than one morphology at different times. *Polymorphic* ventricular tachycardia describes an arrhythmia with morphology that changes during a single paroxysm. *Bidirectional* ventricular tachycardia[89] is a rare form of tachycardia with two alternating morphologies, usually right bundle branch block-like with alternating left- and right-axis deviation (Fig. 23.16). Rapid irregular, polymorphic ventricular tachycardia cannot easily be distinguished from ventricular fibrillation

Ventricular tachycardia may occur in paroxysmal, repetitive or incessant forms. Repetitive monomorphic ventricular tachycardia is a specific syndrome characterized by short runs of tachycardia, separated by brief spells of sinus rhythm (Fig. 23.17). It occurs in young patients with apparently normal hearts.[90]

Clinical features

The clinical presentation of ventricular tachycardia depends on the haemodynamic disturbance it produces. Rapid tachycardias, long-lasting tachycardias, poor left ventricular function and atrioventricular dissociation tend to contribute to haemodynamic collapse which may present as pre-syncope, syncope or sudden death. When cardiac output and blood pressure are maintained, and when the tachycardias are short-lived, the arrhythmia may present as recurrent palpitations, breathlessness or chest pain. Acute ischaemia may be the cause rather than the consequence of ventricular tachycardia. Occasionally, patients are completely asymptomatic during tachycardia. A history of ischaemic heart disease or congestive heart failure in men older than 35 years suggests that tachycardia will be ventricular in origin, but the absence of this history does not make the diagnosis one of supraventricular tachycardia.[91]

Physical examination in a patient with ventricular tachycardia may give evidence of haemodynamic distress, such as low blood pressure, heart failure and cardiogenic shock. If retrograde ventriculo-atrial block is present, atrioventricular dissociation may be apparent by a changeable pulse pressure, irregular cannon waves in the jugular venous pulse and a variable first heart sound. However, none of these signs will be present if there is retrograde ventriculo-atrial conduction which is present in 20–30% of cases. In this situation, atrial systole coincident with ventricular systole will produce regular cannon waves.

Investigations

The initial presentation of ventricular tachycardia is often a medical emergency. The differential diagnosis is between supraventricular tachycardia with aberrant (for example, bundle branch block) or eccentric (pre-excited) conduction. This is an important distinction because it has important immediate and long-term implications for management and prognosis.[92–95].

If the haemodynamic situation will allow, a 12-lead electrocardiogram should be recorded before definitive treatment is undertaken. This may

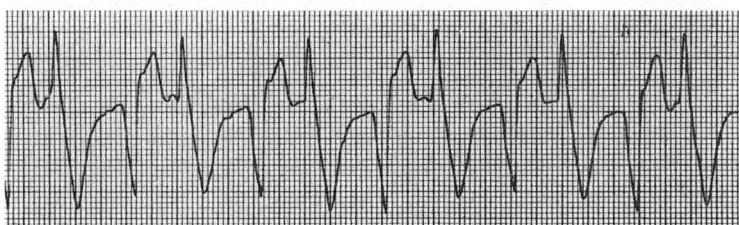

Fig. 23.16. This lead I of the electrocardiogram demonstrates an example of bidirectional ventricular tachycardia in a patient with digitalis toxicity. Both QRS complexes are 'right bundle branch block-like' but the frontal plane axis alternates between inferior and superior axes.

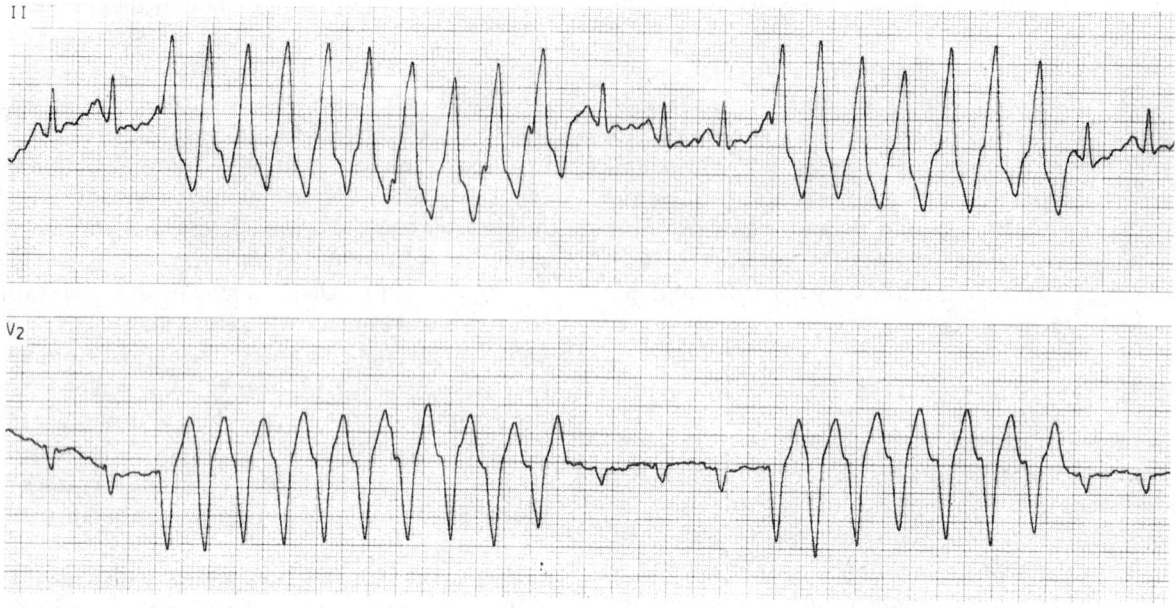

Fig. 23.17. An example of repetitive monomorphic ventricular tachycardia in a man with an apparently normal heart. Note that the brief paroxysms of tachycardia are separated by even shorter runs of sinus rhythm. The electrocardiogram (leads II and V₂) suggests that this tachycardia arises from the right ventricular outflow tract (left bundle branch block-like with right-axis deviation). (By courtesy of Dr D. Ward.)

provide an accurate diagnosis if the following features are considered.[96]

1   Ventricular tachycardia presents with a QRS complex wider than 110 ms and the RR intervals are usually regular (< 40 ms beat-to-beat variation).

2   *Atrioventricular dissociation* may be seen as independent atrial activity especially in lead II or as 2:1 or 3:1 retrograde block with a P wave following every second or third QRS complex. Intermittent capture of the ventricles by conduction from the independent atrial activity will produce *fusion beats* (slightly premature or on-time beats with a shape intermediate between sinus and tachycardia morphologies) due to a depolarization of the ventricles partially by the tachycardia beat (Fig. 23.18) and partially by the sinus beat, or *capture beats* (premature beats with the morphology of conducted beats) due to complete depolarization of the ventricles by the sinus beat. Because ventricular tachycardia may conduct retrogradely to the atrium, atrioventricular dissociation is not always present.

3   Abnormally wide QRS complexes produced by supraventricular tachycardias usually have a typical bundle branch block or pre-excited pattern. QRS shapes produced from ectopic ventricular foci are usually unlike these typical conducted beats. However, when severe myocardial disease is present, very abnormally shaped conducted QRS complexes may be produced.

When the QRS is predominately *positive in lead V₁* (right bundle branch block-like pattern) the following electrocardiographic features suggest a ventricular origin to the tachycardia:

a   left-axis deviation;
b   QS or R/S ratio of < 1 in lead V₆,
c   purely positive QRS deflections in leads V₁–V₆ (positive concordance);
d   monophasic (R) or biphasic complex (QR or RS) in lead V₁, or where the complex is triphasic the initial R wave is taller than the R′ wave.

When the QRS complex is predominantly *negative in lead V₁* (left bundle branch block-like pattern), the distinction between ventricular and supraventricular tachycardia is more difficult. The typical morphology in lead V₁ comprises:

a   a wide initial r wave (> 30 ms);

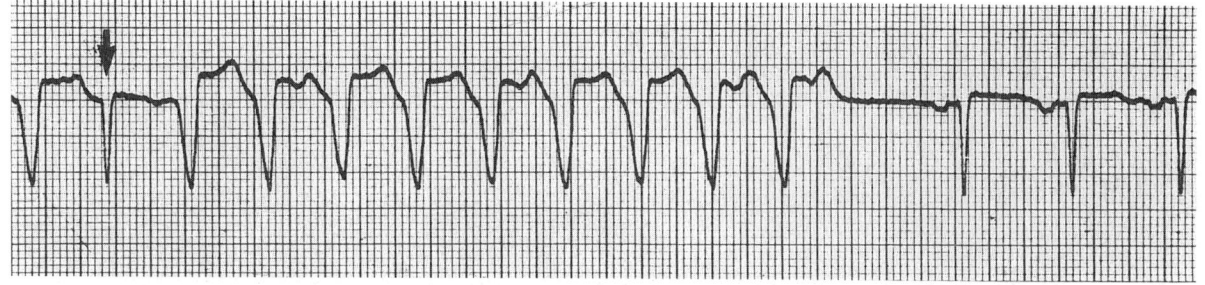

Fig. 23.18. Paroxysmal ventricular tachycardia with a capture beat (arrow) and independent P-wave activity. The capture beat has the same morphology as the QRS complex seen during sinus rhythm.

b a delayed nadir to the subsequent S wave (> 60 ms);

c a notch on the downstroke of the S wave (Fig. 23.19).

These characteristics probably hold only for ventricular tachycardia of ischaemic origin. The following characteristic morphologies also suggest the diagnosis of ventricular tachycardia:

a QS or predominantly negative deflection in lead V_6;

b purely negative deflections in leads V_1–V_6 (negative concordance).

When the tachycardia has been terminated further information may be gained from the 12-lead electrocardiogram in sinus rhythm. If bundle branch block is present but with a different morphology or axis to that during tachycardia, the tachycardia is ventricular in origin. If delta waves are present and they have the same initial polarity as the QRS complexes of tachycardia, the diagnosis is likely to be that of the Wolff–Parkinson–White syndrome with either an atrial or antidromic tachycardia. Using solely information from the electrocardiogram, up to 90% of broad complex tachycardias may be diagnosed correctly.

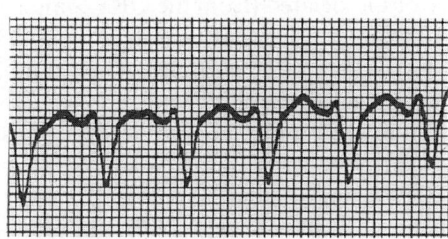

Fig. 23.19. This V_1 rhythm strip records ventricular tachycardia with a left bundle branch block-like morphology. Notice the characteristic features: a broad initial r wave (> 30 ms), a delayed nadir of the subsequent S wave (> 60 ms), and a notch on the downstroke of the S wave.

If definite electrocardiographic diagnosis is not possible, transvenous (Fig. 23.20) or transoesophageal electrograms, echocardiography or Doppler sonography can be performed.[97] Echocardiographic visualization of the atrial wall gives direct information,[98] and the irregularity of mitral valve opening time[99,100] or Doppler ascending aorta flow[97] gives indirect evidence of independent atrial activity.

Recently, it has been shown that adenosine, a naturally occurring nucleoside with a powerful but short-lived negative dromotropic effect on the atrioventricular node, will terminate or reveal most supraventricular tachycardias[101–103] and will not affect most ventricular tachycardias. It can therefore be given intravenously in doses up to 0.25 mg/kg as a diagnostic agent.[104] Verapamil should not be used in this way because when given during ventricular tachycardia it frequently causes life-threatening hypotension.[93–95]

Long-term electrocardiographic monitoring is used to document spontaneous ventricular tachycardia, and the effectiveness of the technique is directly related to the frequency of the attacks of tachycardia. A negative result does not exclude the diagnosis. This method is also used to monitor drug treatment of ventricular tachycardia, usually on the basis of ventricular premature beat counts over 24-h periods. The rationale behind the technique is that suppression of premature beats abolishes the trigger to the tachycardia. Holter monitoring can be used only if there are frequent premature beats on the baseline recording and its predictive power is poor because of the high degree of spontaneous variation of premature beats.[105]

Exercise testing should be used in the assessment of patients with ventricular tachycardia in order to document the likelihood of underlying coronary artery disease, the possibility of exercise inducing the tachycardia and the relationship between

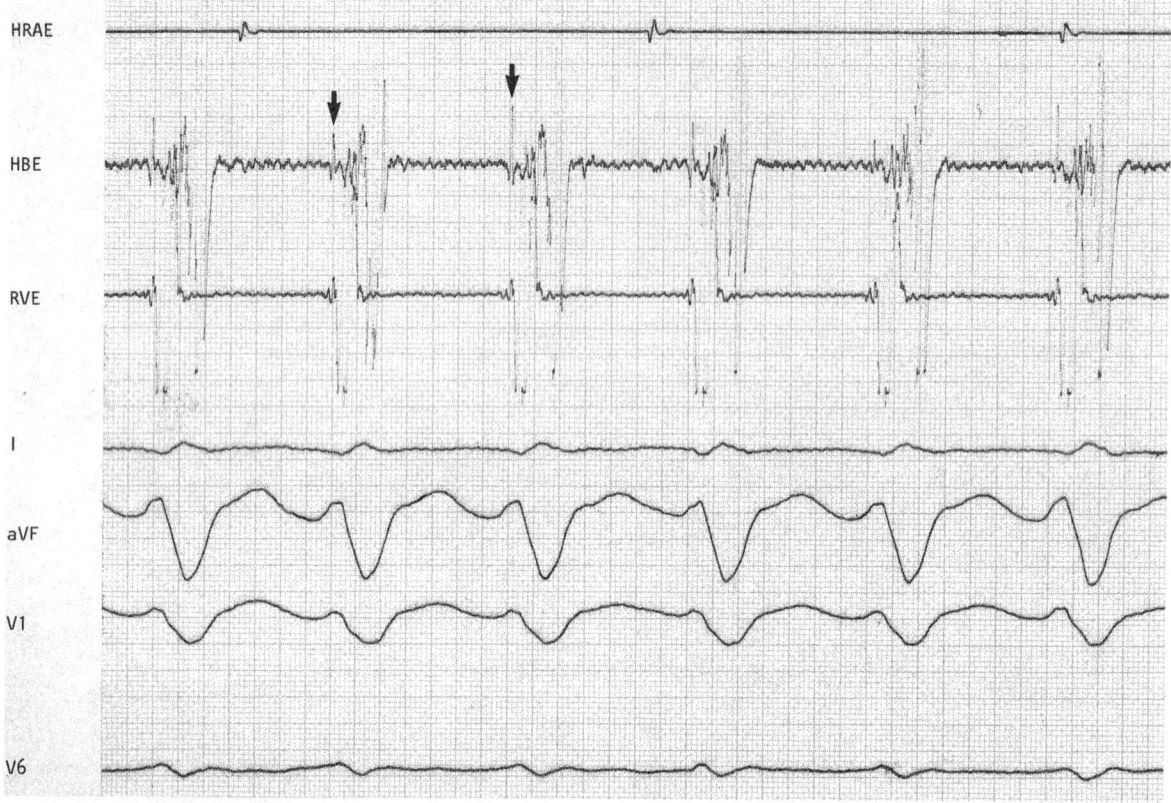

Fig. 23.20. An electrophysiology study is sometimes necessary to distinguish the origin of broad complex tachycardia. In this case, there was no obvious independent atrial activity on the surface electrocardiogram but intracardiac recordings (HRAE, high right atrial electrogram) clearly demonstrated independent atrial activity. In this example, a His-bundle deflection (arrow) is seen in association with each QRS complex but the His bundle is activated after the onset of the QRS complex on the surface electrocardiogram, further confirming the ventricular origin of tachycardia. HBE, His bundle electrogram; RVE, right ventricular electrogram.

ischaemia and the tachycardia. Stress testing is particularly relevant in patients with a history of exercise-induced palpitations or syncope. In patients with ischaemic heart disease, the development of ventricular tachycardia during exercise in association with chest pain or ST-segment depression strongly suggests that the tachycardia is induced by ischaemia. In such cases, revascularization alone will usually prevent further episodes of ventricular tachycardia.[106] However, ventricular tachycardia is more often seen during recovery from exercise and is not usually related to active ischaemia. Beta-blockers or calcium antagonists may be effective therapy in these patients. Use of exercise testing to monitor the treatment of ventricular tachycardia is complicated by the large spontaneous variation in the response to exercise. However, the method is useful in demonstrating a potential arrhythmogenic response to anti-arrhythmic drug treatment.

Programmed electrical stimulation should be performed in patients with suspected ventricular tachycardia to confirm the diagnosis and evaluate possible therapies. Electrophysiology recordings allow the diagnosis of ventricular tachycardia to be made with certainty by demonstrating a short, negative or dissociated (from the QRS complex) His depolarization during tachycardia (Fig. 23.20), provided that there is no evidence of any anomalous pathway bypassing the His bundle.

Programmed stimulation is the technique used to provoke tachycardia. One or two closely coupled paced extrastimuli are delivered to the right ventricular apex during sinus rhythm and after short runs (8 beats) of ventricular pacing at rates of 100, 120 and 140 beats/min. This protocol is 83% sensitive for provoking tachycardia and it is highly specific (near to 100%).[107,108] It is usual to stimulate with pacing pulses of 2-ms duration and an

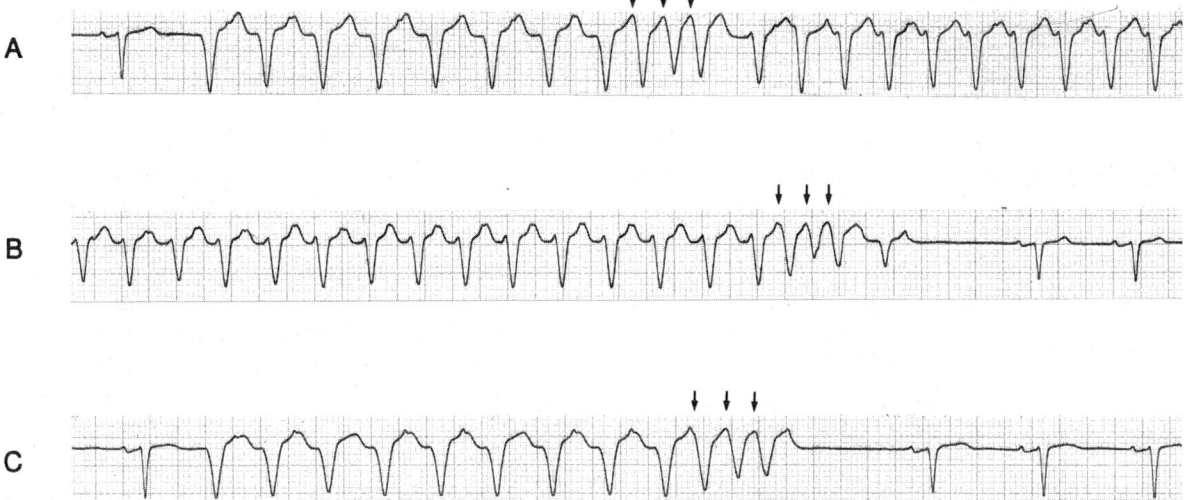

Fig. 23.21. Electrocardiographic traces (lead aVF) demonstrating a ventricular stimulation study. Trace A shows the initiation of ventricular tachycardia by regular right ventricular apical pacing followed by 3 ventricular paced beats. Trace B illustrates that the ventricular tachycardia can also be terminated by stimulated ventricular premature beats. Trace C was recorded after the patient had been treated with flecainide. Ventricular stimulation did not initiate tachycardia. (These traces were kindly provided by Dr M.J. Griffith.)

amplitude of twice the diastolic threshold. A third extrastimulus increases the sensitivity to over 90% but reduces specificity such that the clinical relevance of the induced arrhythmia is less certain. Pacing from more sites (the right ventricular outflow or the left ventricle) does not increase sensitivity much.[109,110] High-frequency burst pacing, the use of higher stimulation energies or pre-treatment with isoprenaline does increase sensitivity but results in a higher yield of non-clinical tachycardias. These latter manoeuvres should be restricted to those patients in whom tachycardia has been previously documented. Any tachycardia identical in rate and morphology to the clinical tachycardia should be regarded as significant. Monomorphic ventricular tachycardia induced with one or two extrastimuli is significant even when that morphology has not yet been recorded clinically.[111] Even if no spontaneous ventricular tachycardia has been recorded previously, any sustained monomorphic ventricular tachycardia induced with one or two extrastimuli is likely to be significant.[112] Induced polymorphic ventricular tachycardia or ventricular fibrillation is probably not significant, especially if an 'aggressive' protocol has been used[107,113] unless a spontaneous and similar arrhythmia has been previously recorded.

It is possible to terminate induced ventricular tachycardia in over 80% of patients. Single, then double ventricular extrastimuli are tried first. If this method fails, burst ventricular pacing, usually at a rate 50 beats/min faster than the tachycardia, is used. Obvious and full capture of the ventricles is essential for termination unless pacing occurs very close to the area of slow conduction, the depolarization of which may not be apparent from the surface electrocardiogram.

The ease of induction of clinical ventricular tachycardia can be used to guide treatment. The more extrastimuli required to induce ventricular tachycardia the more likely a drug will be found to suppress re-induction.[114] If ventricular tachycardia is induced only when isoprenaline has been given, beta-blockade will probably be effective therapy, especially if the clinical tachycardia is exercise induced.[115] The attempt to induce ventricular tachycardia is repeated after oral loading with an anti-arrhythmic drug (Fig. 23.21). If tachycardia induction is suppressed by the drug, it is likely that the tachycardia will not occur clinically.[116] If tachycardia induction is made more difficult or the induced tachycardia is slower and better tolerated, spontaneous tachycardia may still occur but the incidence of sudden death is reduced.[117] However, if tachycardia is induced just as easily or is faster, less well tolerated or degenerates more readily, the drug is less likely to be beneficial.[118] Repeat testing after several drugs tried in succession is known as *serial drug testing* (Fig. 23.22).

These generalities hold true for most drugs except possibly amiodarone[119] and propafenone.[120] With these drugs, complete suppression predicts a good response but failure to suppress re-induction does not predict a poor response. In the case of amiodarone, this may be because of the drug's complicated pharmacokinetic profile and, therefore, it is recommended that repeat testing should not take place until the drug has been given for at least 2 weeks. Programmed stimulation is also used to induce tachycardia in order to locate its origin by catheter mapping prior to surgical or transvenous ablation.

When a patient has both inducible ventricular tachycardia and frequent and complex ventricular ectopic beats, both Holter monitoring and programmed stimulation can be used to guide therapy. If used alone, programmed stimulation is more effective than Holter monitoring and exercise testing.[121,122] However, the combination of both techniques can be advantageous. If ventricular tachycardia induction is suppressed, the clinical response will be good, whatever the Holter demonstrates. If ventricular tachycardia induction is not suppressed but the Holter shows a significant reduction of spontaneous ventricular ectopic activity, a good clinical response will occur.[123] On the other hand, failure to demonstrate suppression by Holter monitoring predicts a poor outcome.

Electrocardiographic signal averaging is a technique designed to reveal low-voltage, high-frequency signals at the end of the QRS complex (Fig. 23.23). Such signals are thought to emanate from areas of fibrosis and disease that conduct slowly and provide a substrate for ventricular tachycardia. They have been detected in up to 90% of patients with ischaemic ventricular tachycardia.[124] The method involves averaging up to 100–400 consecutive normal sinus beats, usually using the sum of orthogonal leads, to reduce noise. The presence of late potentials is defined as a filtered QRS duration of > 120 ms (in the absence of bundle branch block) or a root-mean-square voltage of the last 40 ms of the QRS < 25 µV (Fig. 23.21). The discovery of late potentials may indicate that ventricular tachycardia is the cause of previously unexplained syncope,[125] and the potentials are useful in risk stratification after myocardial infarction.[126] When late potentials are present, it may be worth performing an electrophysiology study on patients with non-sustained ventricular tachycardia.

In most patients with ventricular tachycardia, it is important to document the state of the coronary arteries. Left and right ventricular angiography may be indicated to exclude cardiomyopathy, and endomyocardial biopsy is necessary if sarcoid heart disease, active myocarditis or occult cardiomyopathy is suspected. Left and right ventricular function can also be assessed using echocardiography and nuclear angiography.

Specific conditions

Ischaemic heart disease

Acute arrhythmias In the 48 h after myocardial infarction, ventricular tachycardia and ventricular fibrillation are relatively common. The aetiology of these rhythms is thought to be altered automaticity,

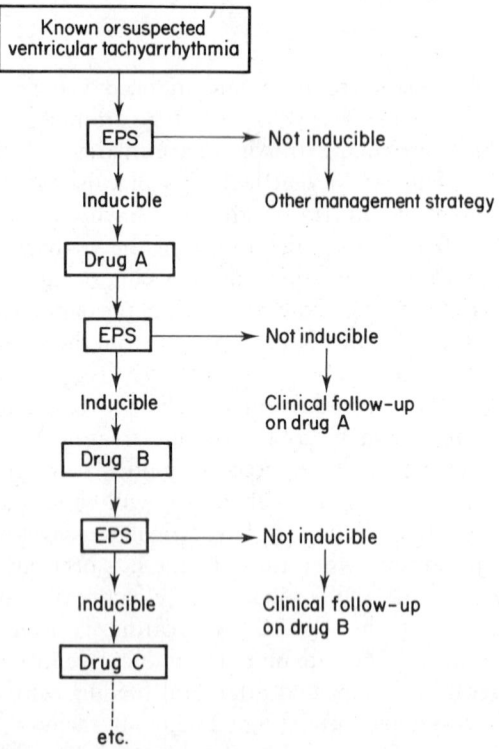

Fig. 23.22. Schematic for serial drug testing. This protocol can be applied to therapy monitored by electrophysiology study (EPS) or 24 h electrocardiogram and exercise testing. F.U., follow up. (Reproduced from: Ward, D.E. and Camm, A.J. *Clinical Electrophysiology of the Heart*. London: Edward Arnold, 1987).

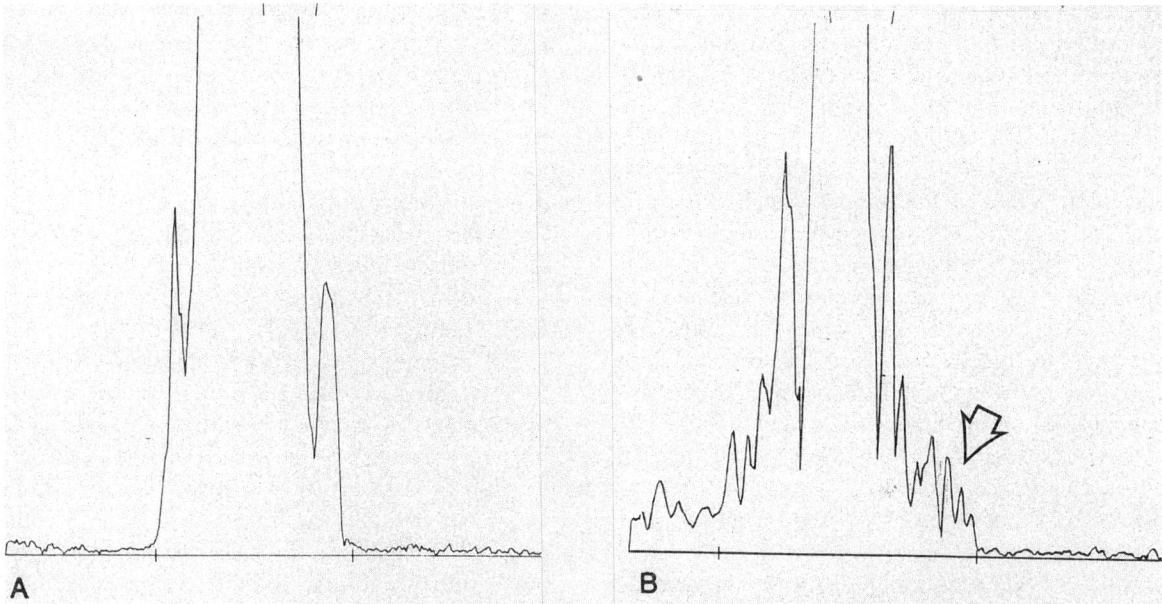

Fig. 23.23. Signal-averaged electrocardiograms. (A) Normal subject: the filtered QRS duration is 90 ms and there is no delayed activity (late potential). (B) Post-infarction patient with ventricular tachycardia. The filtered QRS duration is 131 ms with a distinct late potential (open arrow).

although re-entry may also play a part. As the substrate of these tachycardias is self-limiting, the management is usually direct-current cardioversion and short-term prophylaxis, usually with lignocaine over 24 h. There is controversy over the significance of ventricular tachycardia or ventricular fibrillation in the immediate post-infarction period but they probably do not indicate independently a poor prognosis.[127]

Chronic arrhythmias The substrate of these tachycardias is thought to be focal slow conduction in the endocardium allowing re-entry. Presentation may be with sudden death, syncope or palpitations. Atypical presentations with chest pain or breathlessness are due to the associated haemodynamic effects. Nearly all patients have late potentials and the ventricular tachycardia is inducible with programmed stimulation. After a single episode, the patient should be offered prophylactic therapy, guided if possible by programmed stimulation together with Holter and exercise testing. Surgery should be reserved for those patients in whom medical therapy fails.

Dilated cardiomyopathy Ventricular tachycardia occurs in association with dilated cardiomyopathy,[128] probably due to slowed conduction pro-

ducing intramyocardial re-entry. The development of ventricular tachycardia in a patient with dilated cardiomyopathy and a reduced ejection fraction places the patient at high risk for sudden cardiac death.[129] The tachycardias are rarely inducible by exercise but they can often be stimulated by pacing techniques. Late potentials are usually detectable,[130] especially when there is marked cardiomegaly.[131] Multiple morphologies are common such that surgical resection is unlikely to be successful. In patients with complex ventricular premature beats, multiform, pairs or ventricular tachycardia, amiodarone has been shown to improve survival.[132]

Hypertrophic cardiomyopathy Sustained ventricular tachycardia is unusual,[133] but frequent or polymorphic ventricular premature beats and nonsustained ventricular tachycardia are poor prognostic markers.[134] Treatment of these patients with amiodarone has been shown to improve survival.[135] Electrophysiology testing in these patients can be dangerous.

Arrhythmogenic right ventricular cardiomyopathy Arrhythmogenic right ventricular cardiomyopathy may be a less extreme form of *Uhl's anomaly* (parchment right ventricle) and is characterized by focal disease of the right ventricle with a histopathological appearance of fatty infiltration and fibrosis. Usually there is echocardiographic or angiographic evidence of right ventricular dilatation.[136] The tachycardias arise from the right ventricle and their typical electrocardiographic appearance is that of 'left bundle branch block with right axis deviation'.[137] During sinus rhythm, there is often right bundle branch block and large-amplitude late potentials (epsilon waves) may be seen.[138] The tachycardias, which are probably re-entrant in mechanism, can be provoked by pacing methods but not usually by exercise. Patients, who are more often males, may present with recurrent tachycardia or with right ventricular failure. The disease may progress to involve the left ventricle and there is an associated mortality.[139]

Tetralogy of Fallot   Sudden death and ventricular tachycardia may occur several years after repair of tetralogy of Fallot.[140] The arrhythmias are probably due to re-entry around the ventriculotomy scar, related to the repair of the ventricular septal defect or due to disturbed right ventricular depolarization.[141] The tachycardias often respond to medical treatment and long-term therapy may be necessary. Surgical resection of the scar has also proved valuable.[142] Routine prophylactic administration of anti-arrhythmic drugs post repair has been undertaken[143] but it is probably not justified.

Mitral valve prolapse   The ventricular arrhythmias that occur in this condition are probably due to the distorted geometry of the left ventricle and abnormally stretched papillary muscles. Ventricular tachycardia can sometimes be provoked by pacing techniques.[144,145] The prognosis is generally good, but sudden death has been reported.

Ventricular tachycardia with a 'normal' heart   Approximately 10% of patients with ventricular tachycardia do not have clinically obvious heart disease to account for the arrhythmia. The tachycardias in these patients is often called idiopathic, primary or even 'benign'. The diagnosis is made when all known cardiac and systemic causes of cardiac arrhythmias, such as ischaemic heart disease, dilated and hypertrophic cardiomyopathy, mitral valve prolapse, congenital heart disease, arrhythmogenic dysplasia, metabolic and electrolyte abnormalities, drug intoxications and long QT syndrome, have been excluded.

These tachycardias may be early manifestations of cardiac disease which is otherwise clinically latent or may be due to a primary electrical abnormality of the ventricular muscle. Recent investigations of these patients by echocardiography, angiography and endomyocardial biopsies have shown a proportion (45–92%) to have evidence of underlying heart disease.[146–149] The presence of underlying heart disease is associated with adverse electrophysiological features of the arrhythmias and worsened prognosis.[146,147] As the majority of the patients with 'idopathic' ventricular tachycardia have tachycardia of right ventricular origin (left bundle branch block morphology), close assessment of the right ventricle is particularly important, more so as subclinical right ventricular cardiomyopathy is increasingly recognized as a cause of sudden arrhythmic death in young people.[146,150–152] Apart from the patients who on evaluation are found to have ventricular disease such as cardiomyopathy, the following two subgroups are presently identified.

(i) Repetitive monomorphic ventricular tachycardia   This arrhythmia is usually due to *right ventricular outflow tract tachycardia* which presents with a left bundle branch block-like morphology and an inferior axis (Fig. 23.24) with a relatively slow ventricular rate (110–150 beats/min).[153–155] The origin of the tachycardia is in the right ventricular outflow tract.[153] The tachycardias are usually non-sustained, and they present as sinus rhythm interrupted by repetitive monomorphic ventricular extrasystoles or salvos of ventricular tachycardia. Exercise can precipitate or suppress ventricular tachycardia.[155] Because the arrhythmia is not induced by programmed electrical stimulation, its mechanism is thought to be abnormal automaticity or triggered activity.[153] These tachycardias may respond to verapamil, beta-blockade or class I anti-arrhythmic agents.

(ii) Sustained ventricular tachycardia with right bundle branch block pattern and left axis   This form of tachycardia is known as *fascicular tachycardia* (Figure 23.25) and is usually seen in young patients who have otherwise normal hearts.[156,157] The QRS complex is relatively narrow (90–110 ms) and ventricular tachycardia can be induced by atrial or ventricular stimulation; thus, it is often misdiagnosed as being supraventricular in origin.

The earliest ventricular activation is in the region of the left ventricle supplied by the posterior division of the left fascicle.[157] His bundle activity

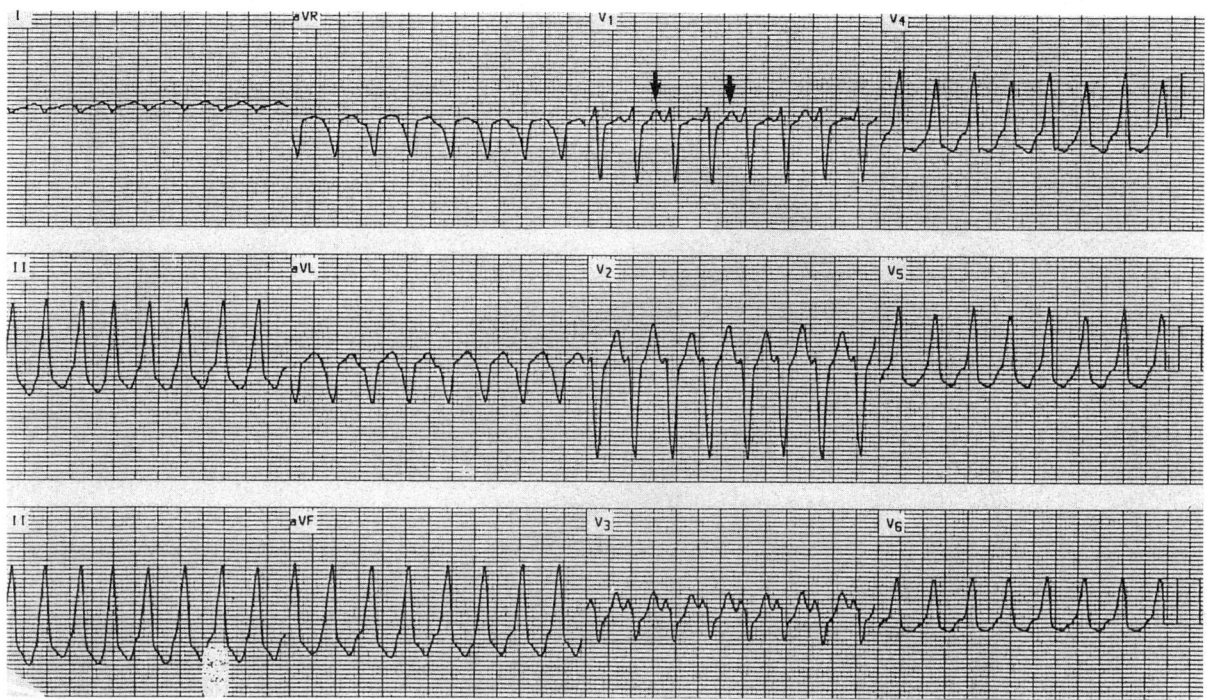

Fig. 23.24. 12-Lead electrocardiogram of right ventricular outflow tract tachycardia in a young man with an 'apparently' normal heart. The QRS complexes are broad with the appearance of left bundle branch block and right-axis deviation but independent P-wave activity is also apparent. (By courtesy of Dr D. Mehta.)

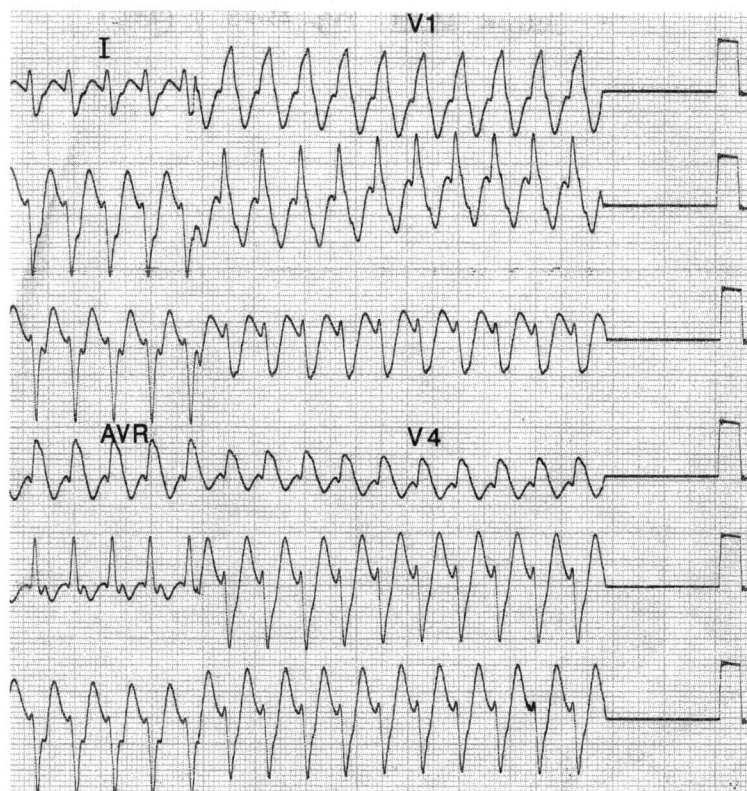

Fig. 23.25. 12-Lead electrocardiogram showing an example of a fascicular tachycardia in a middle-aged woman. The QRS complexes are wider than is usual with fascicular tachycardia, but the morphology is otherwise typical—right bundle branch block-like with left-axis deviation. (By courtesy of Dr D. Mehta.)

has a 1:1 relationship with the ventricular electrogram and either a short or negative HV interval, suggesting early retrograde conduction to the His bundle. Re-entry located within the proximal part of the left posterior fascicle seems the more likely cause for the relatively narrow QRS complexes, early retrograde His deflection during ventricular tachycardia, and possible induction by atrial beats. These tachycardias respond best to verapamil.[157]

In the small proportion of patients with 'idiopathic' ventricular tachycardia, the tachycardia is the manifestation of cardiomyopathy. These patients tend to have sustained tachycardias, usually of right ventricular origin. As they originate in the inflow tract or the body, the tachycardias have a superior frontal plane axis. Signal-averaged electrocardiograms are frequently abnormal and show late potentials.[158] Underlying myocardial disease, although not clinically identifiable, is often detected by detailed echocardiographic examination and confirmed by endomyocardial biopsies.[159] The histology invariably shows features of non-specific cardiomyopathy.[148,149] At programmed electrical stimulation, the tachycardias are usually inducible which makes therapeutic assessment easy and more specific.

Thus, what is commonly referred to as 'idiopathic' ventricular tachycardia, has protean clinical manifestations (Table 23.3) and several potential causes, which to some extent can be identified by the morphology of the arrhythmia, clinical evaluation and routine investigations, such as echocardiography and ventricular biopsy. If correctly identified, these conditions can be specifically treated.

Management

Emergency management

All patients with ventricular tachycardia should be admitted to hospital, and therapy should be administered with continuous electrocardiographic monitoring. The method of terminating the tachycardia is principally determined by the haemodynamic status of the patient. The collapsed unconscious patient should be immediately cardioverted by direct current shock and full cardiopulmonary resuscitation should be instigated. If the patient is collapsed but conscious, sedation or light anaesthesia should be provided before attempting cardioversion. If the patient is well, the following options are available.

1. Elective direct current cardioversion with general anaesthesia.
2. Medical cardioversion with anti-arrhythmic drugs.
3. Conversion using pacing techniques.

Drug cardioversion should first be attempted with intravenous lignocaine 1.5 mg/kg. If this fails, a second drug such as disopyramide 2 mg/kg or procainamide 50 mg/min up to a total dose of 500–2000 mg may be given. It is not wise to use more drugs because their additional effects and their interactions are unpredictable.

Pacing termination using a transvenous temporary pacing wire will terminate up to 80% of episodes of ventricular tachycardia. A burst of 20–50 paced beats introduced at a rate of 50 beats/min faster than the tachycardia is usually effective. Pacing may be more successful after the administration of an anti-arrhythmic drug which slows the tachycardia.[160] Direct current cardioversion should be tried if the tachycardia is rapid, polymorphic, associated with pulmonary oedema, cardiogenic shock or hypotension, or refractory to pacing and drug treatment. Direct current cardioversion may also be necessary if the former techniques result in tachycardia acceleration.

The patient should not be discharged from

Table 23.3. Characteristics of idiopathic ventricular tachycardia.

Characteristic	Right ventricular outflow tract	Fascicular	Cardiomyopathy
Morphology	Left bundle branch block	Right bundle branch block	Usually left bundle branch block
Frontal axis	Right-axis deviation	Usually left-axis deviation	Usually left-axis deviation
Sustained/non-sustained	Non-sustained	Sustained	Sustained/non-sustained
Exercise test	+	−	−/+
Late potentials	−	−	+ (unless mild)
Echocardiogram	Usually normal	Always normal	Always abnormal
Inducibility	−	+	+
Beta-blockade	+	−/+	+/−
Verapamil	+/−	+	−

hospital until the mechanism, aetiology and long-term effective therapy of the tachycardia have been established.

Long-term management

All patients with recurrent sustained ventricular tachycardia are at risk of sudden cardiac death, as high as 40% in the first year after initial presentation. Therefore, effective therapy must be sought. First, any cause for ventricular tachycardia should be reversed when possible;[161] in particular, electrolyte abnormality (hypokalaemia and hypomagnesaemia), acute ischaemia, acute infarction, drug toxicity, underlying bradycardias and structural cardiac abnormalities should be allowed to recover or should be corrected. Thereafter, treatment with anti-arrhythmic drugs is considered.

Anti-arrhythmic drugs   The choice of which drug to assess first for the treatment of ventricular tachycardia is largely empirical, and it is often based on the expected effectiveness balanced against the expected side-effects in individual patients. These effects are detailed in the Appendix. It is usual to try first a Vaughan Williams class IA drug, and follow with classes IB, IC and finally class III. Beta-blockade is often prescribed concurrently.

Class I drugs are the mainstay of medical treatment for ventricular tachycardia. All these drugs suppress sodium influx at the onset of the action potential. However, there are three subgroups, IA, IB and IC, based on the effects on repolarization. Class IA drugs delay both conduction and repolarization, so widening the QRS complex and prolonging the QT interval. It has been suggested that the response to procainamide will predict the efficacy of other drugs.[162] Class IB drugs slow conduction and possibly shorten the QT interval. Lignocaine is widely used in the acute management of ventricular arrhythmias, particularly when associated with acute infarction. Response to lignocaine does not accurately predict the long-term efficacy of oral analogues (other class IB drugs) such as tocainide and mexiletine. Drugs in class IC are the most powerful sodium channel blockers and have little effect on repolarization. All class IC anti-arrhythmic drugs are potent suppressants of ventricular tachyarrhythmias, but all are difficult to use in patients with significant heart disease because they are negatively inotropic (for example, disopyramide) and tend to aggravate arrhythmias especially in those with low ejection fractions (for example,

flecainide). Flecainide should be used with particular care when given intravenously because it may produce an incessant form of ventricular tachycardia that is difficult to control.[163] Encainide has at least two cardio-active metabolites and its full electrophysiological effect is not achieved for several weeks. Newer drugs in this class, such as propafenone, diprafenone, indecainide and recainam, are currently under investigation.

Antisympathetic drugs constitute class II. Various forms of exercise—or isoprenaline-induced ventricular tachycardia respond to beta-blockade. This is the only form of 'anti-arrhythmic therapy' that has been shown to reduce the incidence of sudden death. Nadolol is often recommended for chronic use because of its long half-life. Esmolol with a half life of < 10 min may have a role in the emergency situation. In some cases, permanent pacing must be instituted to overcome the bradycardia that beta-blockade may produce.

Class III drugs prolong repolarization. Amiodarone has additional class I and class II properties and is probably the most effective empirical therapy available. However, its long half-life (30–60 days), the presence of a cardio-active metabolite (desethyl amiodarone), the difficulty in assessing efficacy and the serious side-effects associated with long-term administration (in up to 80% of patients[164] mean that it should be reserved for patients with persistent sustained ventricular tachycardia despite otherwise optimal therapy. Amiodarone improves prognosis in patients with cardiomyopathies.[132,135] Sotalol is highly effective in suppressing the inducibility of ventricular tachycardia. At low doses, the racemic compound acts principally as a beta-blocker,[165] but at higher doses the class III effect of the dextro-isomer becomes more apparent. The actions of bretylium are complex; it must be given intravenously and it produces profound postural hypotension. It is useful in the emergency situation, particularly since it is not negatively inotropic. Bethanidine is a ganglion-blocker, which should be given with protriptyline to counter peripheral vasodilatation effects; it is sometimes effective as long-term therapy.

Class IV drugs, calcium antagonists, are generally contra-indicated for use in the treatment of ventricular tachyarrhythmias because of the negative inotropic and peripheral vasodilatation effects. However, verapamil is effective for the treatment of fascicular tachycardia[166] and triggered (cyclic AMP dependent) ventricular tachycardia.[167]

Treatment with drug combinations is attractive

because a unique electropharmacological effect can be achieved by combining drugs of different classes, or a more powerful single effect without side-effects can be obtained by combining drugs with similar therapeutic actions and different adverse effects. Probably the most effective combinations have been amiodarone with class I or class II agents. Combinations of class I agents (for example, IA with IB) have been described.[168]

Failure to respond to drug treatment prompts consideration of surgical or transcutaneous ablation therapy or pacing and cardioverter/defibrillator treatment.

Surgery Surgery is usually reserved for patients with recurrent sustained ventricular tachycardia unresponsive to medical therapy, primarily when there is an ischaemic aetiology. Most surgery is carried out in patients with discrete aneurysms and carries a hospital mortality of about 10% and an efficacy in up to 85% of cases.[169] For surgical success, the tachycardia should be inducible, monomorphic and associated with a structural problem such as an aneurysm.

Transvenous catheter ablation After very careful endocardial catheter mapping, a high-energy shock can be delivered against that part of the endocardium from which the tachycardia arises. Using the tip of the electrode of the transvenous catheter as a cathode, about 50% of tachycardias can be ablated.[170]

Automatic implantable cardioverter/defibrillator These devices are indicated for patients with recurrent ventricular tachycardia unresponsive to drug therapy, especially when the tachycardias occur relatively infrequently and are associated with haemodynamic collapse and syncope.[171,172] New devices with more sophisticated sensing systems and more flexible therapy (combined pacing, cardioversion—low-energy synchronized shocks—and defibrillation) will allow the indications for the device to be expanded.

Anti-tachycardia pacing Although pacing techniques using a variety of protocols have been shown to be effective in terminating ventricular tachycardia in up to 80% of cases, there is also a significant incidence (10%) of tachycardia acceleration or degeneration into ventricular fibrillation. Automatic devices should not be implanted without defibrillator back-up.[173]

Prognosis

Sustained ventricular tachycardia in the setting of ischaemic heart disease or dilated cardiomyopathy marks out a poor prognosis, with as many as 40% of patients dying in the first year after presentation. If effective suppression with drugs is achieved, mortality from sudden death falls to around 5% per annum. However, as many as 40% of patients will need further therapy, such as surgery or an implantable defibrillator, particularly if there is poor left ventricular function. In patients with ventricular tachycardia and an apparently normal heart, the prognosis is much better.

Torsade de pointes and the long QT syndromes

This form of non-sustained ventricular tachycardia is often repetitive and may trigger ventricular fibrillation. Torsade de pointes means 'a twist of points' and refers to the electrocardiographic appearance of spikey QRS complexes which rotate irregularly around the iso-electric line.[174] Between attacks, there is usually a long QT (Fig. 23.26) (or QT/U) interval (when the QT is 'corrected' using Bazett's formula ($QT_c = QT/[R-R]^{-2}$) it should not exceed 440 ms). Often a significant bradycardia, such as complete heart block, sinus bradycardia or ventricular premature beats with long post-ectopic pauses, is present. The U wave may be unduly prominent. The arrhythmia frequently initiates with a short–long–short sequence (Fig. 23.27).[175]

The arrhythmia may be due to the phenomenon of reflection, in this case, the reactivation of recovered myocardium by adjacent tissue which is still depolarized because of the dispersion of recovery which is present.[176] Early after-depolarizations on the downslope of the action potential have been noted in experimental tissue preparations[177] and also in clinical electrophysiology studies using monophasic action potential recording techniques.[178] The arrhythmia may also be caused by the continued discharge of 2 or more ventricular ectopic foci with different and variable discharge rates.[179]

The combination of torsade de pointes and a long QT interval is known as the *long QT syndrome*. There are two forms: congenital and acquired. The causes of long QT syndrome are shown in Table 23.4.

Patients with the congenital variety of the long QT syndrome have a strong family history of sudden death, often in infancy, and present with

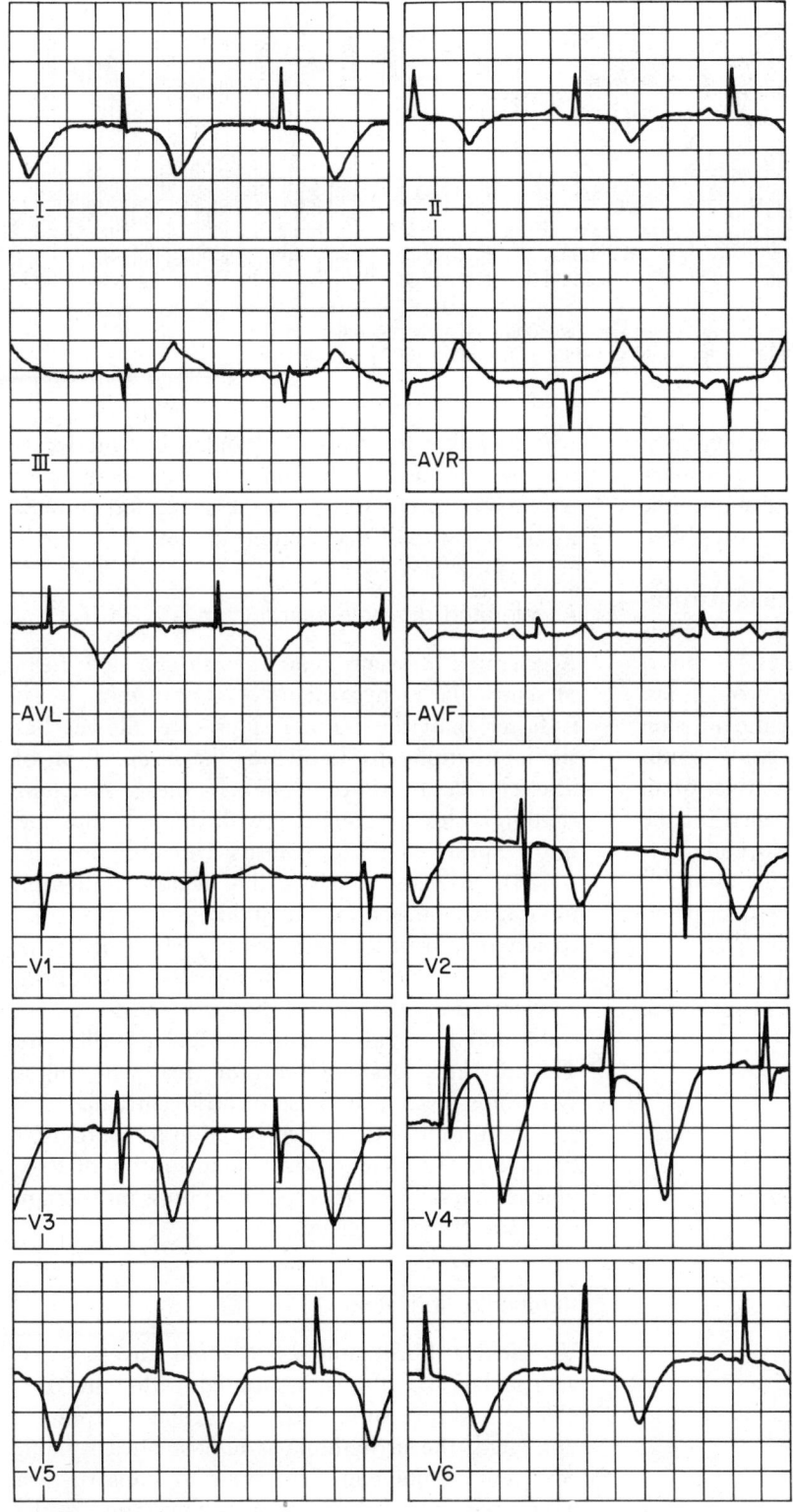

Fig. 23.26. 12-Lead electrocardiogram of a case of acquired long QT syndrome. In this middle-aged man the syndrome was due to severe left main stem coronary stenosis. The QT interval dramatically shortened after surgical revascularization. (By courtesy of Dr D. Ward.)

dizzy spells, syncope or sudden death.[180] When congenital deafness co-exists, the syndrome is called *Jervell–Lange–Nielsen syndrome*[181] and is inherited in an autosomal recessive manner. Without deaf-

ness, the *Romano–Ward syndrome*[182,183] is inherited as an autosomal dominant condition. The QT interval is often grossly prolonged (500 ms or more), the QT interval may vary with time, and

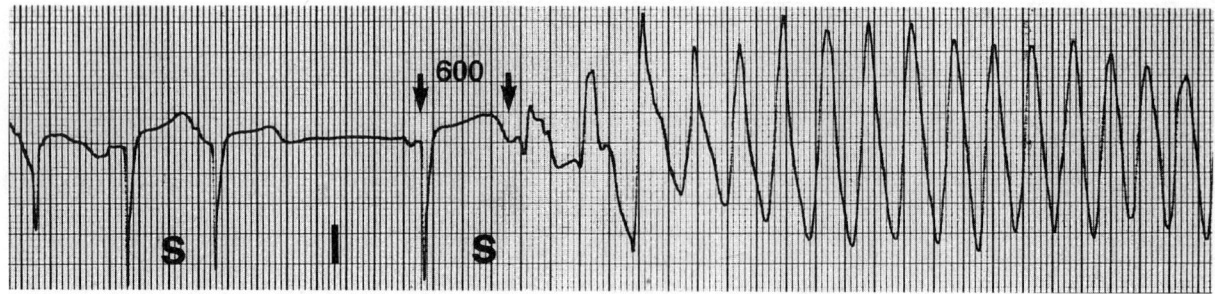

Fig. 23.27. In this electrocardiogram, a short–long–short (s–l–s) sequence immediately precedes the onset of torsade de pointes (atypical ventricular tachycardia). Note the long QT interval (600 ms) of the sinus beat before the onset of torsades.

there may be deep symmetrical T-wave inversion in association. The condition may be due to a primary myocardial abnormality, but disturbed autonomic innervation (dominant left sympathetic supply to the heart) may also play a role.[180]

Attacks usually occur without warning, particularly in the early morning or when the patient is suddenly alarmed. Between attacks, the QT abnormality may not be obvious but it can be brought out by exercise, the Valsalva manoeuvre or the infusion of catecholamines. Electrophysiology study is not usually rewarding.[184] All first degree relatives of an affected family member should be screened for the condition. Treatment relies on beta-blockade, left stellate ganglionectomy or the combination.[185] Sometimes, cardiac pacing can be successful, particularly if there is associated bradycardia.[186]

The acquired forms of long QT syndrome should be treated by restitution of depleted electrolytes,

---

Table 23.4. Causes of the long QT syndrome

Congenital:
Jervell and Lange–Nielson
Romano–Ward

Drugs:
Classes I and III anti-arrhythmics
Tricyclic antidepressants
Phenothiazines
Erythromycin

Metabolic abnormality:
Hypokalaemia
Hypomagnesaemia
Liquid protein diet

Central nervous system abnormality:
Subarachnoid haemorrhage

Cardiac abnormality:
Myocardial infarction
Mitral valve prolapse
Significant bradycardia

---

withdrawal of toxic causes, avoidance of bradycardia by the use of a temporary or permanent pacemaker (preferably at atrial level), and perhaps by the infusion of magnesium sulphate.

Accelerated idioventricular rhythm

Accelerated idioventricular rhythm is a slow form of ventricular tachycardia (< 120 beats/min), but it is faster than the normal sinus rate. Slower but similar rhythms are known as the *escape* form of idioventricular rhythm. When the ventricular rhythm is slow, it competes with sinus rhythm and both capture and fusion beats are common (Fig. 23.28). It characteristically occurs following myocardial infarction, but unlike the paroxysmal variety of ventricular tachycardia, which occurs in association with acute myocardial infarction, accelerated idioventricular rhythms tend to remain stable and do not give rise to ventricular fibrillation. This rhythm does not warrant treatment unless symptoms develop because of atrioventricular dissociation, rapid rate or degeneration to ventricular fibrillation. The intravenous administration of atropine is generally sufficient, but suppressant therapy must sometimes be given.

Ventricular fibrillation

Ventricular fibrillation is a rapid disorganized ventricular arrhythmia associated with unrecordable blood pressure and no cardiac output. If untreated, the arrhythmia is almost always fatal; very few spontaneous reversions to sinus rhythm have been recorded. Ventricular fibrillation is the most common cause of out-of-hospital cardiac arrest, accounting for approximately three-quarters of cases. Although the majority of victims have demonstrable coronary disease, less than half seem

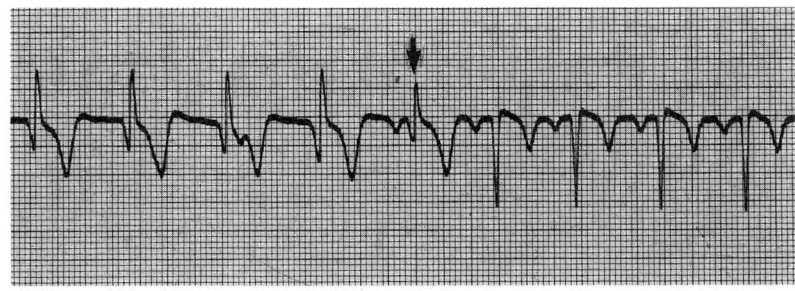

Fig. 23.28. Accelerated idioventricular rhythm (91 beats/min) fusing (arrow) and competing with sinus rhythm (100 beats/min).

to have suffered an acute myocardial infarction just prior to the attack. Almost any cardiac insult may give rise to ventricular fibrillation (Table 23.5).

During ventricular fibrillation, the electrocardiogram shows rapid (150–400 beats/min), irregular, shapeless QRST undulations of variable amplitude. Some examples of apparent asystole may be low-amplitude or *fine* ventricular fibrillation.[187] Ventricular flutter is a 'sinusoidal' waveform at a rate of 150–300 beats/min which is also associated with haemodynamic embarrassment (Fig. 23.29). During an acute myocardial infarction, ventricular fibrillation may be initiated by a ventricular premature beat falling in the vulnerable period (R-on-T) (Fig. 23.30), but, in patients who have not recently sustained an infarction, the arrhythmia more often results from degeneration of ventricular tachycardia (Fig. 23.31). More uncommon modes of initiation include 'escape' from asystole, degeneration from torsade de pointes, degeneration from rapid supraventricular arrhythmia (particularly atrial fibrillation), and pacing (Fig. 23.32) or electrical stimulation in the vulnerable period. The treatment for witnessed ventricular fibrillation is immediate direct current shock (200 J), followed by full resuscitation measures if necessary.

ARRHYTHMIAS IN CHILDHOOD

The mechanisms of many arrhythmias in childhood are similar to those in later life but their effect on the circulation may be more serious. In small infants and neonates, systolic function is reduced because the ventricle is less compliant and greater force is required to distend it during diastole. The neonatal ventricle is working at near peak performance even at rest and there is little reserve to enable the young child to adapt to the insult of a tachyarrhythmia.[188] During the first year of life, therefore, an attack of supraventricular tachycardia may present as severe cardiac failure or cardiovascular collapse.[189] Children who have undergone cardiac surgery may be subject to late arrhythmias, and in a circulation already compromised these may result in sudden late death.[190]

Supraventricular tachycardia

Supraventricular tachycardias are the commonest arrhythmias seen during childhood. In the first year of life, 90% of these are atrioventricular re-entry tachycardias involving an accessory pathway. In older children, atrioventricular nodal re-entry tachycardia is a common mechanism of supraventricular tachycardia. Optimum management of these more common tachycardias during childhood differs in some respect from management in adult patients. Vagal manoeuvres are similarly useful for termination of an acute attack, and a cold cloth or bag of ice placed on the face or immersion

---

Table 23.5. **Causes of ventricular fibrillation.**

Acute myocardial infarction, ischaemia, hypoxia and acidosis

Chronic ischaemic heart disease and any other cause of ventricular tachycardia

Competitive ventricular pacing

Electrocution, lightning strike, unsynchronized direct current shock.

Overdose of cardio-active drugs, for example quinidine, tricyclic drugs and other causes of long QT syndrome and torsade de pointes

Rapid atrial fibrillation, for example, with Wolff–Parkinson–White or Lown–Ganong–Levine syndromes

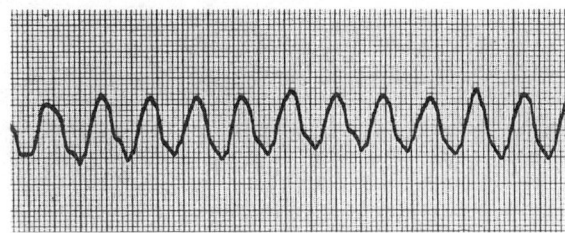

Fig. 23.29. Electrocardiographic trace of ventricular flutter—a 'sinusoidal' ventricular tachycardia. In this case, the rate is 165 beats/min. A similar appearance was seen in all 12 leads of the electrocardiogram.

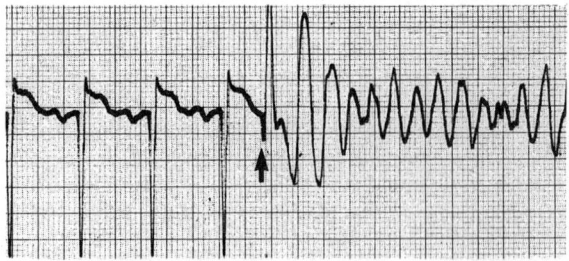

Fig. 23.30. Ventricular fibrillation initiated by an R-on-T ventricular premature beat (arrow). This patient had sustained an acute myocardial infarction several hours previously.

of the child's face in cold water are very often effective. Older children are quick to adapt and will learn to interrupt recurrent attacks with such tricks as eating a cold ice-cream or standing on their head.

Direct current cardioversion is effective and rapid, and a shock of 1 J/kg is recommended. Elegant techniques for overdrive pacing supraventricular tachycardia utilizing an oesophageal electrode[191,192] have been described in children as well as adults.

The rapid occurrence of congestive cardiac failure influences the choice of drug therapy for the acute termination of an attack of supraventricular tachycardia in a child. For this reason, digoxin has remained a popular drug in paediatric practice. Although it is not negatively inotropic, it does have disadvantages. It is often slow to work. It may enhance countershock arrhythmias and if mistakenly given to a child with ventricular tachycardia digoxin may precipitate ventricular fibrillation[193] Verapamil is highly effective in the paediatric age-group and works rapidly,[194,195] but there have been reports of profound and irreversible circulatory collapse in children following its intravenous use.[196] One of the newer drugs currently being evaluated is adenosine. This endogenous purine nucleoside with a short half-life (10–15 s) offers a rapid action and, when given as a bolus dose in a conscious child, it appears to be safe even in the presence of severe cardiac failure with no persisting detrimental effects on blood pressure.[103,197] Efficacy in re-entry arrhythmias involving the atrioventriuclar node as one limb of the circuit is high,

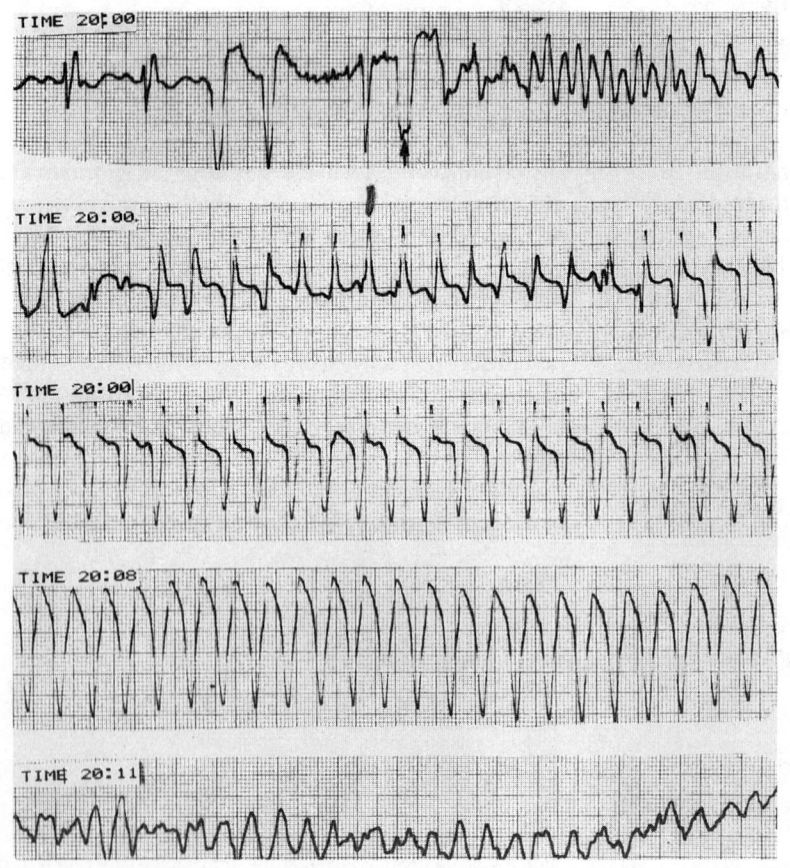

Fig. 23.31. This series of electrocardiographic traces show the electrocardiographic events, recorded on an ambulatory recorder, as a patient with long-standing coronary disease dies suddenly. At 20 00 hours, the electrocardiogram shows the development of ventricular tachycardia which continues and accelerates for a little more than 8 min. By 20 11 hours, the tachycardia has degenerated to ventricular fibrillation.

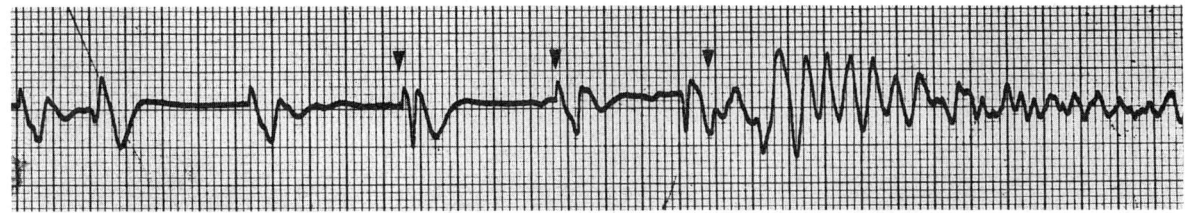

Fig. 23.32. This trace shows the provocation of ventricular fibrillation due to competitive ventricular pacing. The bipolar pacing stimuli, which are not clear on the tracing, are indicated by the arrows. Ventricular fibrillation is provoked when the stimulus falls in the T wave of a spontaneous beat.

usually interrupting the circuit in the atrioventricular node.[197] Anti-arrhythmic drugs which are commonly used in children are listed in Table. 23.6.

Few arrhythmias of childhood, if recognized and treated promptly, are life-threatening, but one such arrhythmias that is is His bundle tachycardia.[198] This is seen in the immediate post-operative period following cardiac surgery and occasionally it is congenital. The diagnosis is made from the surface electrocardiogram by demonstrating atrioventricular dissociation and a narrow QRS complex. These electrocardiographic features represent an automatic tachycardia arising from an ectopic focus situated in the His bundle above the bifurcation (Fig. 23.33). The aetiology remains unknown; trauma to this region during surgery or catheterization has been suggested.[199] The arrhythmia is resistant to standard forms of therapy: direct current cardioversion, vagal manoeuvres, overdrive pacing and conventional anti-arrhythmic agents. Tachycardia is usually incessant and heart failure rapidly develops. In the post-operative patient in whom myocardial

function is already compromised following cardiopulmonary bypass, a rapid tachycardia rate and loss of atrioventricular synchrony severely reduces cardiac output and this arrhythmia is associated with a high mortality and morbidity. His bundle ablation may be useful in the congenital form of His bundle tachycardia.[200] In the post-operative form, if cardiac output can be supported, the arrhythmia usually resolves spontaneously 3–4 days following surgery.

The long R–P tachycardia (Coumel's tachycardia) is another arrhythmia more commonly seen in childhood (Fig. 23.34). Tachycardia characteristically commences when the sinus rate accelerates and therefore it tends to be persistent, stopping and starting throughout the day following short episodes of sinus rhythm. This tachycardia is usually refractory to conventional medical therapy, but surgical division of the accessory pathway can be performed if the tachycardia is sufficiently symptomatic.[462]

A similar persistent arrhythmia of childhood is

Table 23.6. Doses of anti-arrhythmic drugs in children.

Drug	Intravenous	Oral
Adenosine	0.05–0.3 mg/kg (bolus)	—
Amiodarone	5 mg/kg (30 min)	LD: 350 mg/m^2/day (7–10 days) MD: 200 mg/m^2/day
Atropine	20–40 µg/kg	
Bretylium	5–10 mg/kg	
Digoxin	LD: 25–30 µg/kg/day 3 divided doses	LD: 40 µg/kg/day MD: 10 µg/kg/day 2 divided doses
Disopyramide	2 mg/kg (bolus 1–10 mg/kg/h (infusion)	—
Flecainide	2 mg/kg (10–15 min)	6 mg/kg/day 3 divided doses
Lignocaine	1 mg/kg (bolus) 1–3 mg/kg/h (infusion)	—
Propranolol	0.05–0.1 mg/kg (bolus)	3 mg/kg/day 3 divided doses
Verapamil	0.15 mg/kg (bolus) 1–10 mg/kg/h (infusion)	2.5–7 mg/kg/day 3 divided doses

LD, loading dose; MD, maintenance dose.

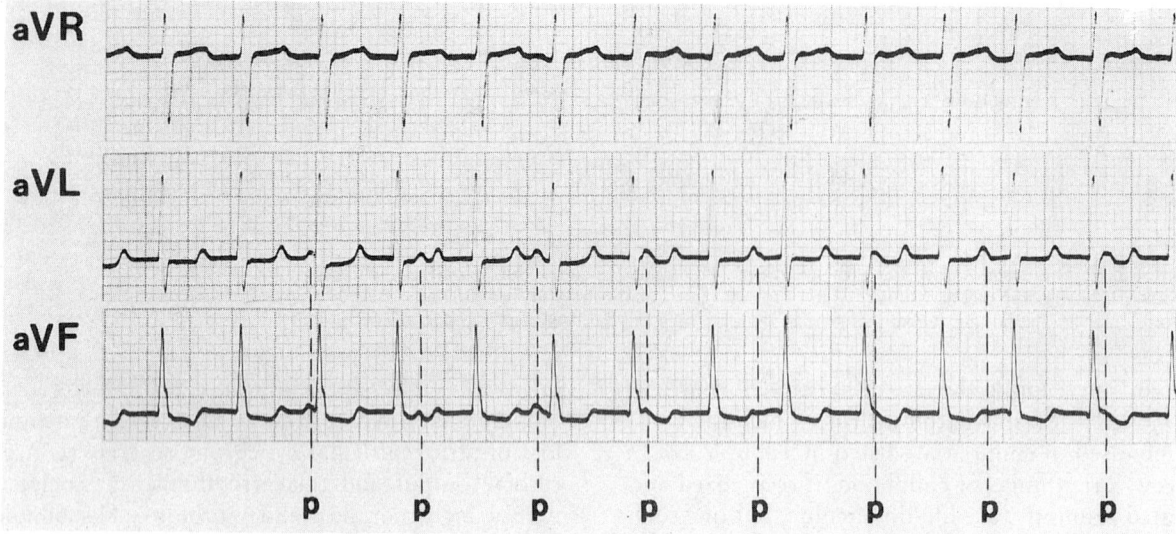

Fig. 23.33. His bundle tachycardia in a young child following cardiac surgery. The electrocardiogram trace shows narrow complex tachycardia at a rate of 165 beats/min and independent sinus P waves at a rate of 110 beats/min. (By courtesy of Dr J. Till.)

ectopic atrial tachycardia. This is estimated to account for 10% of supraventricular tachycardia in children.[201] This is an automatic tachycardia and recognition relies on many of the features of automaticity, i.e. there is a warm-up phase, the

arrhythmia will not terminate with vagal manoeuvres, it is responsive to changes in autonomic tone and, thus, significant variability in rate during tachycardia occurs, and it fails to terminate in response to overdrive pacing. As ectopic foci are

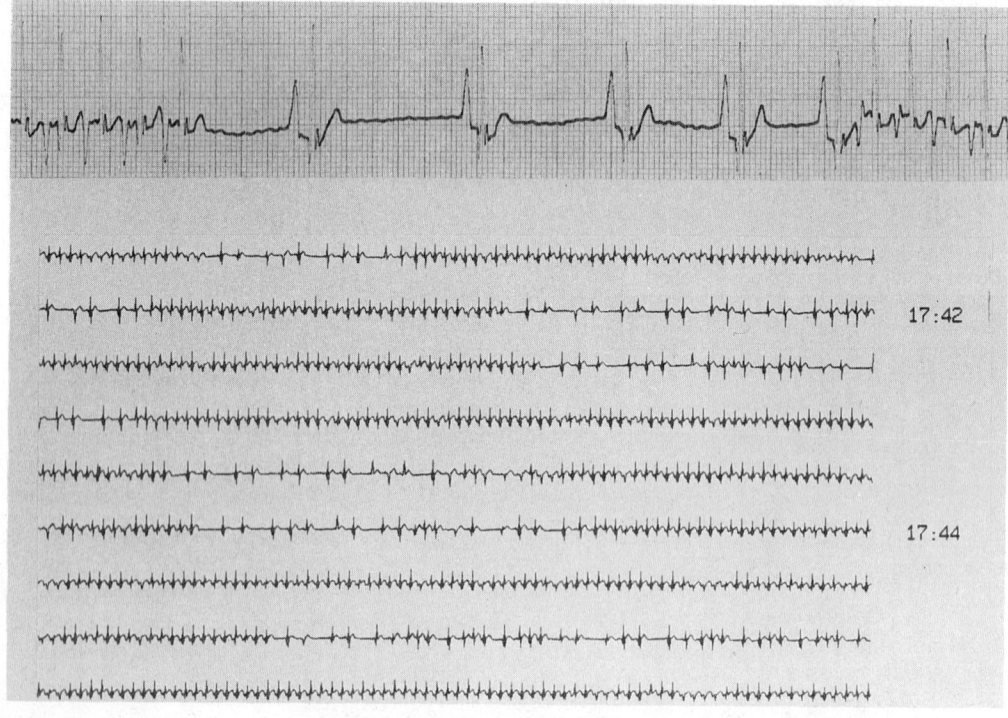

Fig. 23.34. Electrocardiographic strip (upper panel) and long recording (lower panel) demonstrating the incessant long RP′ tachycardia and intermittent sinus rhythm. (By courtesy of Dr J. Till.)

more commonly found in the right rather than the left atrium, differentiation from sinus rhythm may be difficult. This arrhythmia may continue for months, and some authors have suggested that chronicity may result in myocardial dysfunction. Certainly, children have presented with ectopic atrial tachycardia and cardiomyopathy which, on control of tachycardia, has resolved.[202,203] The arrhythmia is generally refractory to conventional anti-arrhythmic agents but digoxin has been reported to decrease tachycardia. Propranolol similarly has been reported to decrease the tachycardia rate in approximately 50% of cases. Amiodarone may be effective,[204] but long-term control with amiodarone may produce unacceptable side-effects. A successful combination of surgical excision and cryo-ablation has been described.[202]

Atrial flutter is unusual in children who have a normal heart, and atrial fibrillation is rare. A small number of children present with atrial flutter in association with secundum atrial septal defect, cardiomyopathy or occasionally with Wolff–Parkinson–White syndrome, but the largest group at risk are those children who have undergone atrial surgery for correction of complete transposition of the great arteries.[205–207] Therapy of atrial tachycardias in this situation is difficult and some authors have recommended that no drug other than digoxin should be used without insertion of a permanent pacemaker.[208]

Ventricular tachycardia

Ventricular tachycardia is unusual in childhood but supraventricular tachycardia with aberrancy is even less common.[209] Therefore, wide complex supraventricular tachycardia should be assumed to be ventricular tachycardia and treated as such, unless a positive diagnosis to the contrary can be confidently made. Failure to manage the child in this way may lead to the inappropriate treatment of ventricular arrhythmias with drugs such as verapamil or digoxin which can prove dangerous in such a situation because they may induce ventricular fibrillation. The aetiology of ventricular tachycardia in children is varied and prognosis depends on the underlying cause.

Incessant ventricular tachycardia may present in infancy. The rate is rapid and the tachycardia is refractory to conventional medical therapy. At surgery, tumour tissue (largely Purkinje-like cells) is evident, which when resected abolishes the tachycardia.

Ventricular arrhythmias associated with the long QT syndrome (Fig. 23.35) should be identified early because treatment is specific and the mortality high. There are two forms of the congenital long QT syndrome: one associated with bilateral sensorineural deafness, which is inherited as an autosomal recessive (Jervell–Lange-Nielsen syndrome), and one unassociated with deafness and inherited as an autosomal dominant (Romano–Ward syndrome).[181] Children with these syndromes suffer from a variety of atypical ventricular tachycardia known as torsade de pointes (Fig. 23.36). Treatment with beta-blockers reduces the mortality of these conditions from 71 to 7%.[180] The optimum treatment of those children who remain refractory to beta-blockade is controversial. Left stellate ganglionectomy or cardiac pacing may be necessary.[210]

The concept that ventricular tachycardia in a child is benign if the heart is 'normal' has long been debated and one of the difficulties is which criteria should be used to judge normality.[211] If aggressive investigation is performed, including both echocardiography and angiography, entities such as right ventricular dysplasia may be excluded, and it does appear that most children have a good prognosis.[209] However, catecholamine-sensitive ventricular tachycardia is a disorder that is certainly not benign even though children with this disorder may have an ostensibly normal heart.[212,213] This condition is found in a small number of older children and adolescents. These children have an atypical history of collapse on exercise or excitement and are difficult to distinguish from children who have the long QT syndrome. Some of them may indeed represent a variant of long QT syndrome with a normal QT interval on the surface electrocardiogram.

A further group of children to consider are those who have undergone repair of congenital cardiac disease and are left with a ventriculotomy scar. There is a small incidence of late sudden death in all children who have had a ventriculotomy,[214] particularly following repair of tetralogy of Fallot. The incidence of late sudden death in this group has been estimated to be as high as 5%.[215] Originally, this was thought to result from late onset of complete atrioventricular block, but it has since been realised that ventricular arrhythmia represents a greater risk.[140] In some series, up to 10% of children are thought to have premature ventricular ectopic beats on the routine electrocardiogram, 30% ventricular arrhythmias on exercise, and 50% ventricular arrhythmias on Holter monitoring.

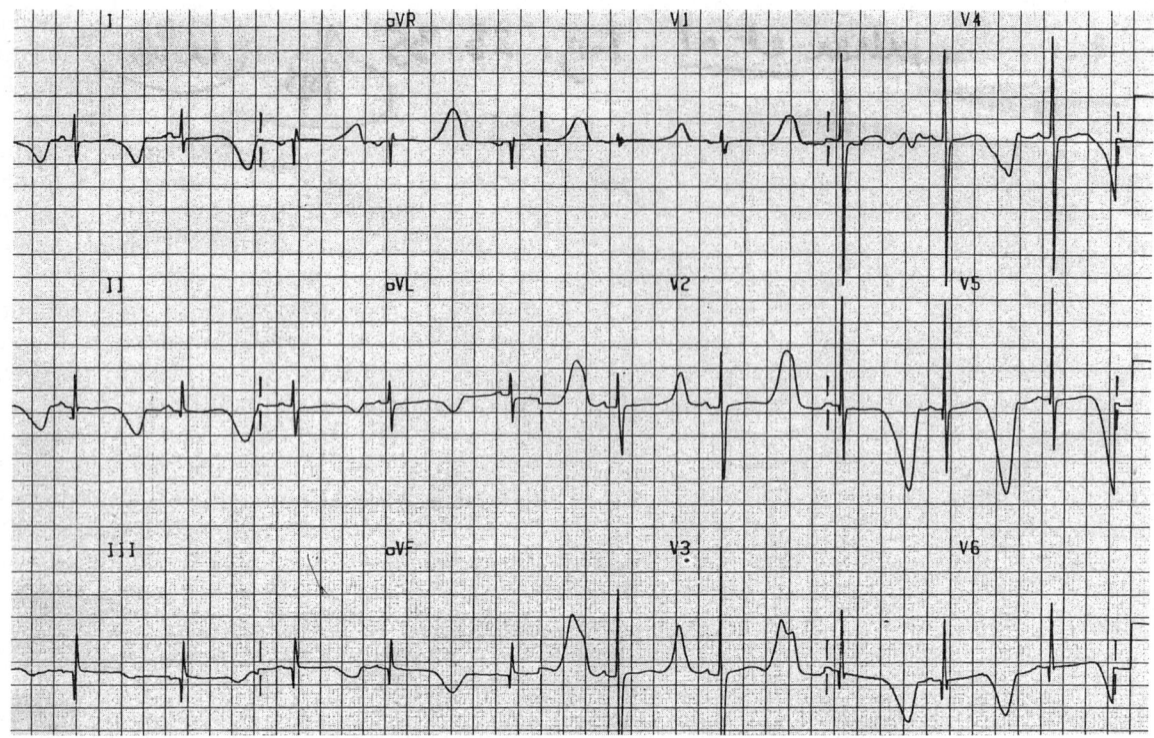

Fig. 23.35. This electrocardiogram was recorded from a young boy with the Jervell and Lange-Neilsen syndrome. It shows marked QT prolongation (> 650 ms) even after correction using Bazett's formula (QTc = 680 ms). Note the variation/alteration in the morphology of the T wave, for example, in leads V_1 and V_2.

Those children with the worst haemodynamic result seem to be at greater risk, as are those who undergo repair at an older age.[216]

SPECIFIC MODES OF TREATMENT

STRATEGIES AND MODES OF TREATMENT

A wide range of treatments is available for cardiac arrhythmias (Table 23.7) because they present in such a diverse manner, the mechanisms are so variable and the prognoses range from totally benign to extremely dangerous. Occasionally, an arrhythmia may be cured, for example, by excising the focus of an arrhythmia or by dividing an anomalous pathway, but usually the arrhythmia can only be controlled by terminating an acute

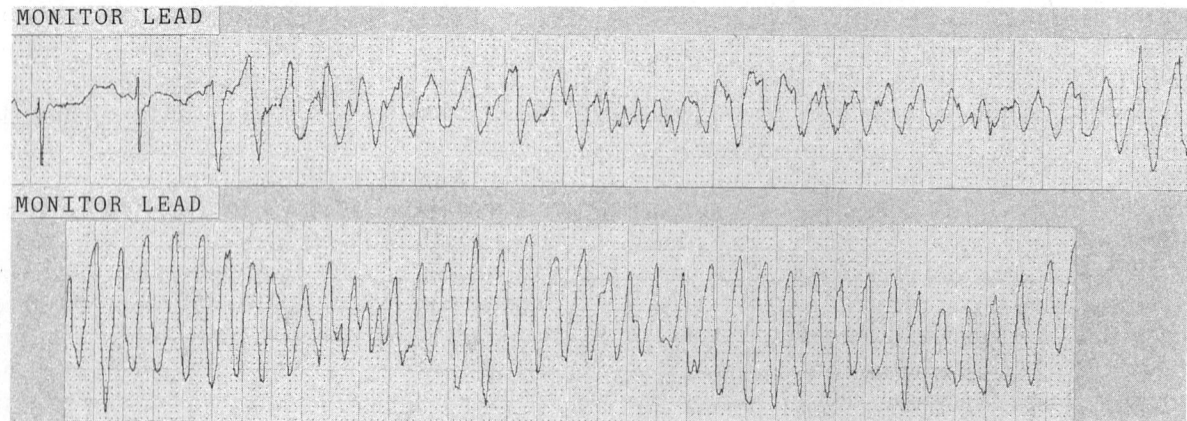

Fig. 23.36. An example of torsades de pointes in a 5-year-old boy with the Jervell–Lange-Nielsen syndrome. (By courtesy of Dr N.J. Linker.)

Table 23.7. Strategies and modes of treatment.

Strategies:
Terminate arrhythmia
Slow the heart rate
Improve haemodynamic results
Prevent recurrence
Cure

Modes:
Reassurance
Physical manoeuvres
Pacing and implantable devices
Anti-arrhythmic drugs
Ablation methods

attack, slowing the rate or improving the haemodynamic situation during the continuing arrhythmia. Most therapeutic effort is directed towards preventing the recurrence of arrhythmia, usually by the use of suppressant anti-arrhythmic drug therapy.

The modes of treatment available for cardiac arrhythmias are equally diverse ranging from simple reassurance to cardiac surgery. The choice of treatment depends on prognosis, symptoms, underlying disease, treatment efficacy and the patient's wishes. For example, a patient with mildy symptomatic Wolff–Parkinson–White syndrome may prefer surgical correction, or the physician may press a patient to accept this therapy when the associated arrhythmia is potentially dangerous. The specific indications for the treatment of individual arrhythmias have already been discussed, and the methods of treatment are described in detail below.

PHYSICAL MANOEUVRES

Patients often volunteer that a particular action may initiate or terminate their arrhythmia. Most of these actions result in vagal efferent stimultion to the heart which produces sinus node slowing, increased refractoriness and slowed conduction in the atrioventricular node, and shortened atrial refractoriness. The ventricles are only sparsely innervated by the vagus. The likely response of various arrhythmias to these manoeuvres can be deduced from the distribution and the effect of vagal activity on the heart (Table 23.8). Because transient atrioventricular block is the predominant effect of vagal stimulation, atrial arrhythmias may be revealed during the atrioventricular block, and atrioventricular junctional arrhythmias in which conduction within the atrioventricular node is essential for their continuation will terminate. Vagal manoeuvres are generally more effective in younger patients who have reactive autonomic nervous systems.

Carotid sinus massage

Rotatory pressure over the carotid sinus stimulates afferent responses in the nerve of Hering (a radical of the glossopharyngeal nerve). In turn, this results in vagal stimulation of the heart which may slow or terminate tachycardia (see Table 23.8). The result may depend on which (left or right) carotid sinus is chosen but this is inconsistent. Firm, and often uncomfortable, pressure must be applied. Carotid sinus stimulation may be associated with reduced cerebral blood flow, hemiparesis and hypotension. As with other vagal manoeuvres, carotid sinus stimulation may induce ventricular arrhythmias.[217,218] It is best performed with the patient recumbent after checking that there are no carotid bruits.

Ocular pressure, by a similar reflex (oculocardiac), can also be used to terminate tachycardia. However, it is painful to apply and no more effective than other less uncomfortable manoeuvres.

Valsalva manoeuvre

During the strain phase of the manoeuvre, raised intrathoracic pressure results in decreased venous

Table 23.8. Effect of vagal manoeuvres on cardiac arrhythmias.

Arrhythmia	Effect
Sinus tachycardia	Transient slowing
Atrial tachycardia	Slowing or termination
Atrial flutter	Increased atrioventricular block
Atrial fibrillation	Increased atrioventricular block
Atrioventricular nodal re-entrant tachycardia	Occasional termination
Atrioventricular re-entrant	Frequent termination
Ventricular tachycardia	Rare termination*

* Right ventricular outflow tract tachycardia.

return and reduced cardiac output. A sympathetically activated pressor and tachycardic response occurs. In the relaxation phase (Fig. 23.37), the sudden increase of venous return boosts cardiac output and blood pressure, reflexly activating a parasympathetic response.

Supraventricular arrhythmias often terminate in the vagal predominant relaxation phase, although occasionally a tachycardia may terminate during strain, presumably due to an increase in the rate of tachycardia which exceeds the decrease in circuit refractoriness. The Valsalva manoeuvre is easily taught to patients and is the most effective of the physical manoeuvres. It is best performed in the recumbent position in order to reduce coincident sympathetic stimulation. Some ventricular tachycardias will terminate in response to the Valsalva manoeuvre, especially those arising from the right ventricular outflow tract.[219]

Diving reflex

Apnoeic facial immersion results in trigeminal afferent stimulation and then vagal efferent traffic to the heart and a pressor response. The intensity of the stimulation depends inversely on the temperature of the water.[220] This reflex is effective in terminating junctional tachycardias, especially in children and neonates.[221]

The mechanism is less clear in a variety of other manoeuvres, such as sudden changes in posture, deep inspiration, coughing, drinking ice-cold water and isometric exercise, which are often developed spontaneously by patients to effect termination of their tachycardias.

DEFIBRILLATION AND CARDIOVERSION

Early devices successfully utilized alternating current to defibrillate the heart,[222,223] but safe and effective cardioversion, the conversion of rhythms other than ventricular fibrillation to sinus rhythm, requires the synchronized delivery of direct current.[224] Re-entrant arrhythmias may be successfully cardioverted when the excitable tissue between the advancing head of the re-entrant wave and its receding refractory tail is depolarized by the shock. The mechanism of the rare termination of an automatic rhythm is unknown, but it is probably related to stimulation of the cardiac nerves by the discharge.[225]

Indications

Re-entrant arrhythmias readily respond to cardioversion, but automatic arrhythmias, such as parasystole, accelerated idioventricular rhythms and some atrial tachycardias, are less amenable.

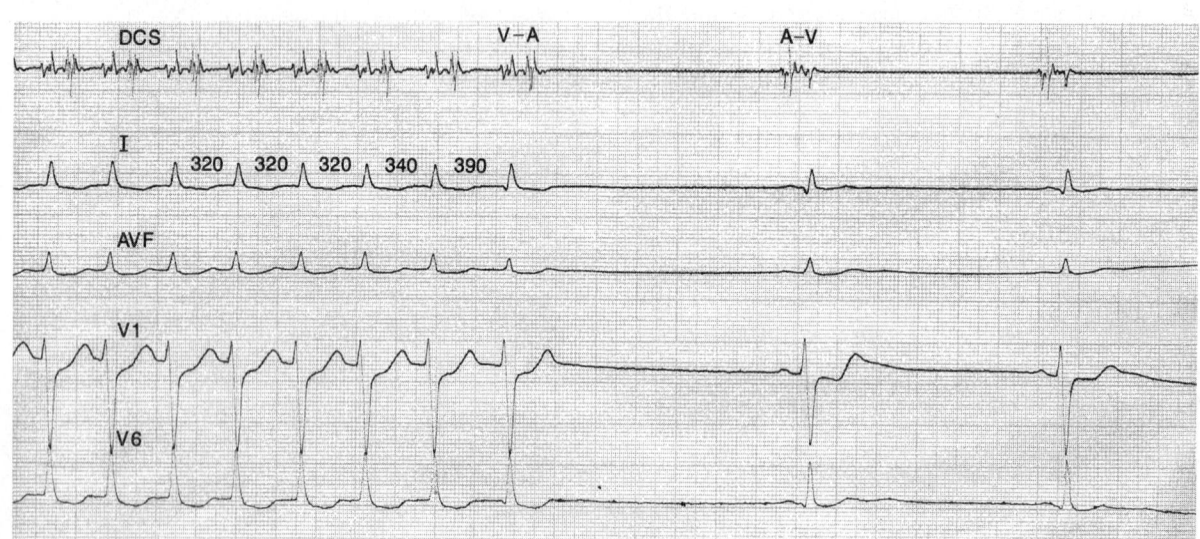

Fig. 23.37. These traces demonstrate the termination of atrioventricular re-entrant tachycardia during the release phase (phase IV) of the Valsalva manoeuvre. The increased vagal tone at this stage of the manoeuvre causes slowing and termination within the atrioventricular node. The last event during tachycardia is atrial activation (A). V, ventricular electrogram; A, atrial electrogram; DCS, distal coronary sinus; I, aVF, V₁ and V₆ are surface ECG leads. Recording speed is 50 mm/s. (By courtesy of Dr C. Garratt.)

Although it may be possible to convert an incessant or frequently repetitive tachycardia to sinus rhythm, the arrhythmia will re-initiate spontaneously within a short time rendering the procedure useless. Toxic rhythm disturbances, including those due to digoxin, anti-arrhythmic drugs, hypokalaemia and thyrotoxicosis, will generally not respond well and may degenerate. Torsade de pointes, induced by electrolyte disturbance, drug toxicity or congential causes, is generally a self-limiting arrhythmia and does not justify cardioversion unless it has degenerated to sustained ventricular tachycardia. Although re-entrant junctional arrhythmias will cardiovert readily, they are also easily treated with simple vagal manoeuvres or anti-arrhythmic drugs, and cardioversion is rarely needed. The emergency presentation of ventricular fibrillation, hypotensive ventricular tachycardia and atrial fibrillation with a rapid response demands urgent treatment with defibrillation/cardioversion. Some other rhythm disturbances such as 'controlled' atrial fibrillation, atrial flutter and stable ventricular tachycardia merit elective treatment (Table 23.9).

Ventricular tachycardia

When the onset of tachycardia is witnessed, a chest thump[226] can be administered in an attempt to terminate it ('thumpversion'). If established ventricular tachycardia is haemodynamically unstable or proves resistant to intravenous lignocaine, and possibly one other intravenous anti-arrhythmic such as disopyramide, electrical cardioversion is the treatment of choice. Intravenous lignocaine should be given if tachycardia fails to respond to this therapy. Full cardiopulmonary resuscitation (*see* Chapter 72) may be needed if hypotensive ventricular tachycardia does not convert.

Atrial fibrillation

In chronic cases, medical conversion with oral quinidine or intravenous disopyramide or flecainide should be considered prior to electrical cardioversion. Atrial fibrillation should be cardioverted if it is symptomatic and capable of conversion. The points in favour and against attempting cardioversion are given in Table 23.10. Particular caution should be applied to those patients who have a history of bradycardia (bradycardia/tachycardia syndrome) or those with slow ventricular rates during the atrial fibrillation suggesting the possibility of high-grade atrioventricular block.

Atrial flutter

Cardioversion is the treatment of choice for paroxysmal atrial flutter that does not respond to conventional medical therapy such as combined digoxin and quinidine.

Procedure

Cardioversion is applied in two circumstances: urgently and electively. In an emergency, there may be little opportunity for preparation but, when possible, all should be done to ensure that the patient is ready to receive a brief anaesthetic or neuroleptic. In the case of atrial fibrillation of > 1 week's duration, anticoagulants should be administered for 1–2 weeks prior to attempted cardioversion. If there is a history of sinus node disease or atrioventricular block, a pliable temporary pacing wire should be inserted. A modern defibrillator utilizes capacitor discharge through an inductor to damp the oscillations of the waveform. Typically, a capacitor of 30–40 μF and an inductor of 30–

Table 23.9. Indications for cardioversion and defibrillation.

Urgently indicated:
Ventricular fibrillation
Hypotensive ventricular tachycardia
Atrial fibrillation with a rapid ventricular rate

Electively indicated:
Atrial flutter
Ventricular tachycardia unresponsive to drugs
Atrial fibrillation of short duration (< 1 year)

Not indicated:
Incessant arrhythmia
Automatic rhythms
Toxic arrhythmias
Torsade de pointes

Table 23.10. Favourable and unfavourable factors for the cardioversion of atrial fibrillation.

Favourable:
Symptoms (angina, dyspnoea, palpitations)
Rapid ventricular rate
Refractory to drug conversion
Refractory to rate control
No structural heart disease
No continuing toxic cause

Unfavourable:
Frequently repetitive
Large left atrium
Slow ventricular rate
Bradycardia–tachycardia syndrome
Longstanding atrial fibrillation (> 1 year)

50 mH produces a critically damped (1 oscillation only) sinusoidal discharge with a duration of 2–3 ms and an amplitude of 4–5000 V. The energy chosen for cardioversion in adults depends more on the arrhythmia than on the size of the patient.[227] Neonates and infants require a low-energy shock between 1 and 5 J/kg bodyweight. The usual energy requirements for cardioversion and defibrillation are given in Table 23.11.

The paddles, about 12 cm in diameter,[228] should be centred over the right second intercostal space just to the right of the sternum and over the apex (*apex–anterior position*) or below the left scalpula and over the apex (*apex–posterior position*). Polarity seems to make little difference to the success of the technique. Good electrical contact is best achieved by placing gel pads impregnated with electrolyte between the paddle and the chest wall. In patients who have frequently recurrent arrhythmias, adhesive gel pads/disposable paddles can be stuck to the patient's chest until the arrhythmia is successfully controlled. Except for ventricular fibrillation, it is advisable to use a shock synchronized to the R wave of the electrocardiogram in order to avoid the discharge falling in the vulnerable period (on the T wave). It is sometimes difficult to synchronize to the sinusoidal waveforms of fast or drug-induced ventricular tachycardia. In these circumstances, the ventricular tachycardia may be converted into ventricular fibrillation in which case a second shock should be given immediately.

Complications

Minor complications occur in as many as half of the patients undergoing cardioversion, but significant complications are uncommon.[229] Transient arrhythmias need no treatment but sustained bradycardias or tachycardias may occur which warrant treatment. Sinus node arrest, sinus bradycardia or atrioventricular block should be treated with atropine initially, but temporary pacing may be needed. Ventricular tachyarrhythmias usually occur if the discharge is not delivered synchronously (Fig. 23.38) with the R wave, but occasionally properly synchronized shocks provoke ventricular arrhythmias.[228] Atrial fibrillation may result, particularly when attempting to cardiovert atrial flutter, because there is no attempt to synchronize to atrial depolarization.

Patients with digoxin toxicity are vulnerable to the provocation of arrhythmias,[230] but digoxin treatment need not be stopped before cardioversion, provided that there is no suggestion of toxicity.[231] Hypokalaemia and quinidine toxicity may also favour the development of post-shock arrhythmias. Embolic complications can be largely prevented by elective anticoagulation[232] of patients who have atrial fibrillation and mitral valve disease, a large left atrium or a prosthetic mitral valve. Although tissue injury can occur in cell cultures,[233] in animals given high-energy shocks[234] and in patients receiving intracardiac discharges, it is unusual with therapeutic transthoracic cardioversion. The rise in CK enzyme is largely due to injury to skeletal muscle[235] and the ST/T-wave changes on the electrocardiogram may be due to autonomic nervous consequences of the shock.[225] Pulmonary oedema and hypotension have occasionally occurred after cardioversion. Pacemakers may be damaged by cardioversion,[236] particularly if the shock is given along the axis of the pacemaker can/electrode tip. Energy from the discharge may be picked up by the electrode acting as an aerial, and myocardium at the electrode tip may be burnt. Zener diodes largely protect the pacemaker, but re-programming of the device may occur. Pacemakers should be carefully checked following cardioversion or defibrillation.

Automatic and advisory defibrillators

These devices have been developed for use by lay and paramedical personnel in order to improve cardiac resuscitation outside the hospital.[237] The devices automatically recognize ventricular fibrillation and then deliver a shock through previously applied paddles (automatic defibrillator) or instruct the operator to deliver a shock (advisory defibrillator).

In order to ensure that ventricular fibrillation is correctly distinguished from artefact, the impedance between the paddles is continuously measured.

Table 23.11. **Energy levels (stored) for cardioversion and defibrillation.**

Arrhythmia	Energy level (J)	
	Elective procedure	Emergency procedure
Ventricular fibrillation		200, 200, 400
Ventricular tachycardia	50	200, 200, 400
Atrial fibrillation	200	400
Atrial flutter	25	100, 200, 400

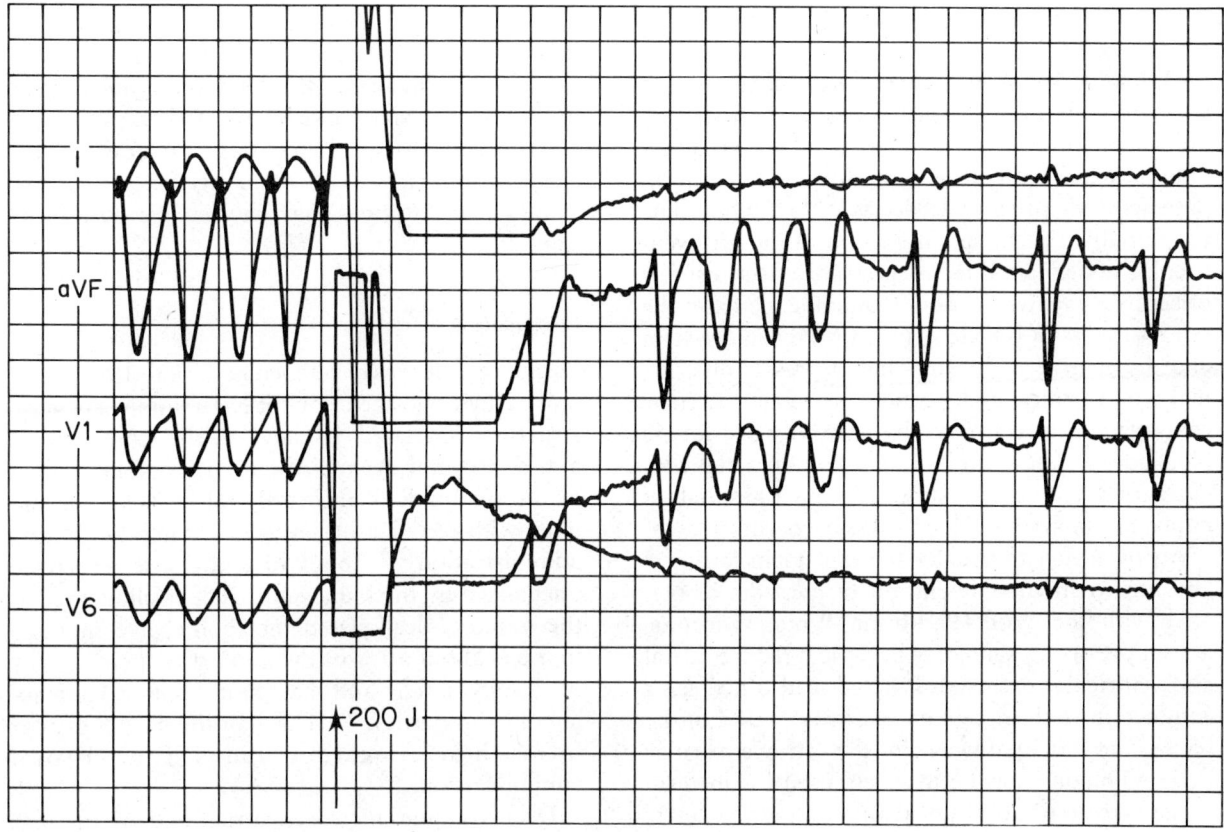

Fig. 23.38. These simultaneous recordings demonstrate cardioversion from ventricular tachycardia (left) to sinus rhythm (right) following a shock of 200 J. Note the irregular and rapid ventricular arrhythmia which immediately follows the discharge. Such arrhythmias are more common when the shock is inadequately synchronized, which may have been so in this case. However, when the tachycardia is sinusoidal, it is difficult to know to which part of the QRS to synchronize.

ANTI-ARRHYTHMIC DRUGS

The number of anti-arrhythmic agents available has greatly increased in recent years. There is no universally accepted classification of anti-arrhythmic drugs; however, the most widely used format (Vaughan Williams) classifies drugs mainly by their cellular electrophysiological effects (Table 23.12).[238,239] A second classification is based on clinical electrophysiological effects and is less commonly used.[240]

Class IA drugs

Quinidine

Quinidine is an alkaloid which was introduced about 300 years ago. Quinidine sulphate is rapidly absorbed after oral administration with a bioavailability of 60–80%, although the gluconate salt is more slowly absorbed with a systemic availability of only 70%.[241,242] Peak plasma levels occur 1.5–2 h after ingestion of the sulphate and 4 h after ingestion of the gluconate.[243] Quinidine is partly excreted unchanged and partly metabolized by the liver, with the 3-hydroxy metabolite having some

Table 23.12. Vaughan Williams' classification of anti-arrhythmic drugs.

Class I: Membrane-stabilizing agents (fast sodium channel blockers)
a Delayed repolarization, widening of action potential duration, e.g. quinidine
b Accelerated repolarization, shortening of action potential duration, e.g. lignocaine
c Action potential duration unchanged, *powerful* membrane stabilizing effect, e.g. flecainide

Class II: Beta-adrenergic blocking agents, e.g. propranolol

Class III: Agents delaying action potential repolarization, e.g. amiodarone

Class IV: Agents inhibiting slow calcium channel, e.g. verapamil anti-arrhythmic activity.[241] The elimination half-life is 5–9 h.

Quinidine has a direct depressant effect on the sinus node, but this is usually masked by vagolytic influences and tachycardic reflexes, although quinidine may markedly depress sinus node function in patients with sinus node disease.[244,245] Quinidine has variable effects on conduction in the atrioventricular node.[241] a direct depressant effect, usually offset by a vagolytic action. Quinidine increases the refractoriness of the atria, the His–Purkinje system and the ventricles.[246] Quinidine depresses myocardial contractility and reduces systemic vascular resistance, primarily by alpha-adrenergic blockade.[244] These effects can be counteracted with glucagon,[247] and with slow infusion rates only a minor fall in systolic blood pressure occurs.

Atrioventricular nodal re-entrant tachycardia[248] and atrioventricular re-entrant tachycardia associated with the Wolff–Parkinson–White syndrome are suppressed by quinidine because it reduces atrial and ventricular extrasystoles, and it also decreases conduction in the accessory pathway[241] and in the retrograde fast pathway in the atrioventricular node. Quinidine has been widely used for medical cardioversion of atrial fibrillation and atrial flutter with success rates of 65–85%, and it is successful in maintaining sinus rhythm after cardioversion. It has been reported in several studies that quinidine suppresses ventricular extrasystoles; in general, approximately 50% of patients will have 65% suppression of extrasystoles, and 11% will have 99–100% suppression.[249] Quinidine has also been used for the treatment of sustained ventricular tachycardia, and it has been shown to suppress inducibility in about 20% of patients when given either intravenously or orally.[250]

Because of its vagolytic effect, quinidine can increase the ventricular response to atrial fibrillation. The most important side-effect of the drug is torsade de pointes.[251,252] This is an idiosyncratic response and it is usually associated with marked prolongation of the QT interval. It can be exacerbated by a low level of serum potassium.[252] Prolongation of the QT interval and widening of the QRS complex are not useful signs for predicting arrhythmogenesis, but the association of bradycardia with QT prolongation is ominous and often heralds torsade de pointes.[252]

Gastro-intestinal side-effects, particularly diarrhoea are common, often requiring withdrawal of treatment. Large doses may cause cinchonism, consisting of tinnitus, headache, blurred vision and other visual disturbances, loss of hearing and confusion, in addition to the cardiotoxic effects.[253]

Quinidine increases the level of serum digoxin and can potentiate anticoagulant therapy.[254] The anti-adrenergic effects can potentiate the hypotension caused by other agents. Drugs that induce liver enzymes may shorten the half-life of quinidine.

Disopyramide

Disopyramide was developed in the late 1960s as an anti-arrhythmic agent; and it has a unique chemical structure unrelated to any of the conventional anti-arrhythmic agents. About 90% of an oral dose of disopyramide is absorbed and 80% is bioavailable, with peak serum levels occurring 2–3 h after administration.[255] About 50% of a dose is excreted unchanged by the kidney and 20% is eliminated as the mono-N-dealkylated metabolite, a compound that has about 50% of the anti-arrhythmic activity of disopyramide and has more potent anticholinergic properties.[256] The half-life is 4.5 h after intravenous injection and 7 h after oral administration.[257]

Disopyramide increases atrial and ventricular refractoriness, slows the sinus rate and increases the refractory period of the atrioventricular node.[258,259] However, owing to the strong anticholinergic effect of the drug, there may be an increase in sinus rate and enhanced atrioventricular nodal conduction (Fig. 23.39).[259] Dose-dependent widening of the QRS interval and prolongation of the QT interval may be seen, especially in patients with pre-existing abnormalities in these parameters.[256] Intravenous disopyramide decreases contractility of the normal ventricle, but this effect is much more marked when there is left ventricular dysfunction.[260,261] Patient selection is important because cardiac failure occurs in 55% of patients who have a history of congestive cardiac failure.[262]

Disopyramide will terminate approximately 40% of atrioventricular nodal re-entrant tachycardias with an intravenous dose of up to 2 mg/kg;[263] it is effective in prolonging refractoriness in accessory pathways,[264] although, unlike class IC agents, the increase in accessory pathway refractoriness is dependent on the refractory period before drug administration.[265] Oral disopyramide in doses of 400–800 mg daily has been shown to be effective in suppressing ventricular extrasystoles.[266] The drug has a 50% success rate for conversion of ventricular tachycardia, although it may cause hypotension

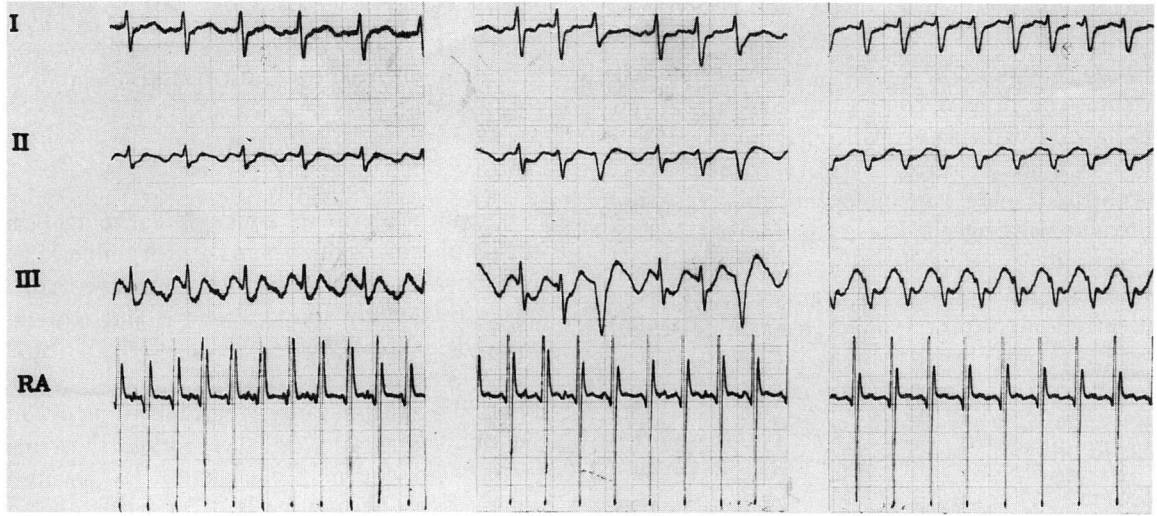

Fig. 23.39. The effect of intravenous disopyramide on atrial flutter is demonstrated on this series of electrocardiograms. On the baseline trace (left panel), the atrial rate is 270 beats/min but because of 2:1 atrioventricular conduction the ventricular rate is 135 beats/min. After disopyramide (2 mg/kg i.v.), the atrial rate has slowed to 200 beats/min but 1:1 atrioventricular conduction is present. The ventricular rate, therefore, has increased to 200 beats/min. In the middle trace, 4:3 atrioventricular Wenckebach is seen (note the aberrant conduction of the final QRS in each Wenckebach period).

particularly in patients with impaired left ventricular function.[267]

Anticholinergic side-effects of disopyramide are very common. However, they can be avoided by the concomitant use of pyridostigmine without any loss of anti-arrhythmic activity.[268] Marked changes in intraventricular repolarization may be produced by the drug, often in an idiosyncratic manner, causing prolongation of the QT interval and torsade de pointes.[269,270] The drug should be avoided in any patients with atrioventricular block, sinus node disease, severe bradycardia, glaucoma or myasthenia gravis.[256]

Procainamide

Procainamide was introduced in 1951 having been developed from the agent procaine hydrochloride in the 1940s. Absorption is between 75 and 95% in most subjects, with peak plasma concentrations occurring about 1 h after administration.[271] The drug is extensively tissue bound and nearly 50% of the drug is excreted unchanged in the urine. About 10–23% of the drug is converted to the active metabolite, N-acetyl procainamide. The biological half-life of the drug is 3.1 h with a range of 2.2–4.0 h.[256]

There is minimal prolongation of atrioventricular nodal conduction, and prolongation of His–Purkinje conduction, with an increase in the refractory periods of the atria. His–Purkinje system and ventricles.[227] The PR and QT intervals are often prolonged. Intravenous procainamide decreases myocardial contractility and may cause hypotension via peripheral vasodilatation, probably as a result of ganglionic blockade.[244] This effect is less marked with oral administration but care should be exerted in patients who have cardiac failure.

Procainamide is effective in a wide range of ventricular and supraventricular arrhythmias, but it should be avoided in the treatment of digitalis-induced ventricular arrhythmias, where its action is unpredictable. Procainamide is effective in controlling up to 50% of atrioventricular nodal re-entrant tachycardias and atrioventricular re-entrant tachycardias. Procainamide may be used to convert atrial fibrillation to sinus rhythm,[278] but an acceleration of the ventricular response has been reported.

Procainamide is relatively effective in controlling ventricular extrasystoles. In published series, 65% suppression was achieved in 57% of patients and 99–100% suppression in 9%.[249] Response rates for suppression of sustained ventricular tachycardia range from 35 to 75% which may be due in part to differences in patient selection.[279]

Torsade de pointes has been reported, although it is not as common as with quinidine. Gastro-intestinal side-effects occur and long-term therapy is associated with a high incidence (50–70%) of the development of high anti-nuclear antibody titres.[256] In 20% of cases, a 'lupus-like' syndrome will develop. The drug is contra-indicated in patients who have myasthenia or glaucoma and in patients with a significant degree of atrioventricular block. Procainamide may potentiate anticholinergic and antihypertensive agents. It has an additive effect on the neurological side-effects of other local anaesthetic agents, such as lignocaine. Plasma concentrations of procainamide may be decreased by warfarin and phenytoin.

Class IB drugs

Lignocaine

Lignocaine is a local anaesthetic agent, synthesized in 1946 and first used successfully as an anti-arrhythmic drug in 1950. It must be administered parenterally because of extensive first-pass hepatic metabolism. Increased plasma levels and toxicity may occur in patients with liver disease or if there is reduced hepatic blood flow, as in cardiac failure.[280] Following intravenous injection, plasma levels fall rapidly. The drug has a metabolic half-life of about 100 min, although the duration of the anti-arrhythmic effect is only 20 min.[281]

Therapeutic doses of lignocaine produce minimal effects on heart rate, atrioventricular and intraventricular conduction. The drug has no consistent effect on the effective refractory period of the atria or atrioventricular node.[282] In patients with impaired atrioventricular conduction, lignocaine has precipitated complete heart block, at an infra-Hisian level.[283] Therapeutic doses of lignocaine cause little haemodynamic effect, although transient depression of myocardial function has been noted in patients with pre-existing cardiac failure.[284]

Lignocaine is an effective agent for the emergency treatment of ventricular arrhythmias. It is ineffective in the control of atrial arrhythmias and should be avoided in atrial flutter where enhanced atrioventricular nodal conduction may occur with 1:1 atrioventricular conduction.[285] Intravenous lignocaine is a very effective agent against life-threatening ventricular arrhythmias, and it is widely used in patients with acute myocardial infarction resuscitated from ventricular fibrillation.[280] Recent evidence suggests that lignocaine may be effective in preventing the first episode of ventricular fibrillation during the early phase of myocardial infarction.[286]

Adverse reactions are very uncommon, but with overdosage central nervous system symptoms occur including drowsiness, disorientation and convulsions.[287]

Mexiletine

Mexiletine is a primary amine similar to lignocaine, but its pharmacokinetics make it suitable for oral use. It was initially developed as an anorectic but was subsequently found to have anti-arrhythmic properties. Mexiletine is well absorbed from the gastro-intestinal tract with a systemic bioavailability of 90%. The majority of its absorption occurs in the duodenum and, as such, drugs that inhibit gastric emptying may markedly delay its absorption.[281] Peak plasma levels occur within 2–4 h of ingestion. The drug is approximately 70% protein bound and is extensively metabolized in the liver to inactive products.[288] Ten per cent of the drug is excreted unchanged in the urine. The elimination half-life is 10–12 h, which may be prolonged if hepatic blood flow is reduced or if there is renal impairment.

Mexiletine has little effect on sinus node automaticity and on the refractory periods of the atria, atrioventricular node and ventricles. Mexiletine has been shown to have little effect on left ventricular ejection fraction even in patients with pre-existing left ventricular dysfunction.[289,290]

Mexiletine has been shown to be effective in suppressing ventricular extrasystoles. Overall it suppresses 65% of extrasystoles in 55% of patients and in 7% of patients it suppresses 99–100%.[249] In patients with sustained ventricular tachycardia, mexiletine suppressed the arrhythmia in about 30% of cases as assessed by invasive or non-invasive methods.[291]

Gastro-intestinal side-effects of nausea and vomiting tend to limit the usefulness of the drug as these occur in 25–50% of patients.[292] Up to one-third of patients develop central nervous system side-effects of dizziness, blurred vision, paraesthesiae and fatigue. Mexiletine interacts with a variety of drugs because of its intensive hepatic metabolism. In particular, phenytoin and rifampicin increase the clearance of mexiletine by inducing drug-metabolizing enzymes in the liver.[293]

Class IC drugs

Flecainide

Flecainide is a recently introduced fluorinated derivative of procainamide developed in the late 1970s as a potent anti-arrhythmic agent. It is well absorbed orally, with a bioavailability of 90% or greater.[294] Peak plasma levels are obtained in 3–4 h, with a terminal elimination half-life of 13–16 h, compatible with twice daily administration.[295] Approximately 85% of the drug is excreted in the urine as parent compound and metabolites, which are produced in the liver. Flecainide may accumulate in renal failure and is not removed by dialysis.

Flecainide does not have a significant effect on normal sinus node function;[296] however, in patients with sinus node disease, flecainide has been shown to produce marked depression of sinus node activity.[297] The drug produes a significant lengthening of intra-atrial, atrioventricular and intraventricular conduction (Fig. 23.40).[296,298,299] An analysis of multiple studies[299] showed that flecainide increased the PR interval by between 17 and 29% and the duration of the QRS complex by between 11 and 29%. Although prolongation of the QT interval by 4–13% was observed, this was found to be due mainly to QRS widening, there being no significant effect on the JT interval (JT = QT − QRS).

In patients with dual atrioventricular nodal pathways, flecainide selectively affects retrograde conduction via the 'fast' pathway.[300] Flecainide increases the pacing threshold by more than 100%.[301] Intravenous flecainide increases right atrial, pulmonary artery and pulmonary wedge pressures.[302–304] Oral flecainide has a mild negative inotropic effect, producing congestive cardiac failure in 4%.[303]

Intravenous flecainide terminates over 85% of atrioventricular nodal re-entrant tachycardias.[300,305,306] Following termination, tachycardia can be re-induced in 31–44% of patients.[305,306] In atrioventricular tachycardia involving an accessory pathway, flecainide increases the tachycardia cycle length by 30% and terminates the tachycardia in 50% of patients.[300,305,307,308] The increase in cycle length and termination are invariably due to retrograde block in the accessory pathway. Flecainide is also effective in pre-excited atrial fibrillation, terminating the arrhythmia in 24–50% of patients and significantly shortening the minimum pre-excited RR interval in the remainder.[309]

In patients with sustained ventricular tachycardia, flecainide will suppress the arrhythmia in the majority of patients, but incessant tachycardia and cardiac arrest may occur.[295] In 89% of patients, flecainide achieves 65% suppression of all ectopics, in 75% it achieves 80% suppression and, in 50%, 100% suppression.

The main cardiovascular side-effect of flecainide is its arrhythmogenicity which occurs in 5-10% of patients and should limit its use for termination of ventricular tachycardia to coronary care units where temporary pacing is available. The most

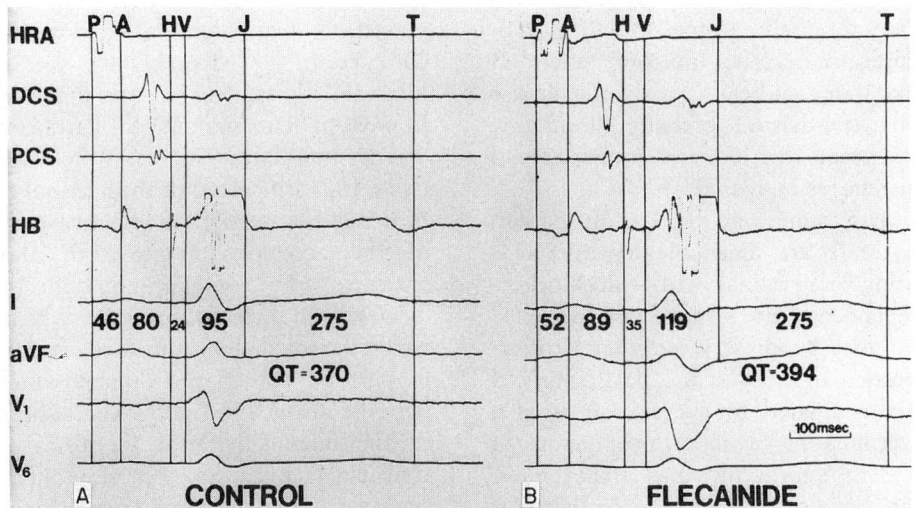

Fig. 23.40. Recordings of sinus rhythm from an electrophysiology study before and after the administration of flecainide acetate (2 mg/kg bodyweight). All conduction intervals are prolonged following flecainide. HRA, high right atrium; DCS, distal coronary sinus; PCS, proximal coronary sinus; HB, His bundle region; lead I, aVF, V₁ and V₆ are surface ECG leads. Paper speed is 100 mm/s.

frequent non-cardiovascular side-effects are dizziness and visual disturbances, which occur in approximately 30% of patients and appear to diminish during long-term therapy.[310] Digoxin levels are increased by 13–25% when flecainide treatment is initiated.[311] Addition of flecainide therapy to patients on amiodarone results in increased pharmacological effects from flecainide.[312]

Class II drugs

There are many beta-blocking agents available at present, all of which have a similar spectrum of anti-arrhythmic efficacy with the exception of sotalol. Propranolol will be discussed here as a representative agent for the group.

Propranolol

Propranolol is well absorbed from the gastrointestinal tract but has a bioavailability of < 30% due to extensive first-pass metabolism.[313] Peak plasma levels occur 1–2 h after an oral dose and the half-life of a single dose is 2–4 h, although this is increased to 4–6 h in patients taking the drug long-term due to saturation of the excretion pathway.

Propranolol exerts its main effect by inhibiting beta-adrenoceptors in the heart, removing the arrhythmogenic effect of excessive sympathetic drive. Propranolol slows the sinus rate, increases the AH interval and prolongs the refractory period of the atrioventricular node. It does not affect ventricular conduction or refractoriness.[314] Propranolol has a significant negative inotropic effect. It decreases stroke index and causes a significant rise in left ventricular end-diastolic pressure. Blood flow to all tissues except the brain is reduced, and peripheral resistance is increased.

No specific arrhythmia and no specific patient with an arrhythmia are amenable to any beta-blocker. Treating arrhythmias with beta-blockers assumes a dependence on sympathetic drive.[315] Such treatment may suppress ventricular extrasystoles and ventricular tachycardia, particularly if the arrhythmia is related to exercise. It is also effective in terminating a large proportion of regular paroxysmal supraventricular arrhythmias. The ventricular response during atrial fibrillation is reduced by beta-blockade.

Left ventricular failure may be precipitated by propranolol, and asthma is exacerbated. Other side-effects include excessive bradycardia, hypoglycaemia (which may be unrecognized in diabetic subjects due to the masking effect of the drug on the manifestations), and disturbed sleep. Worsening of symptoms in patients with intermittent claudication or Raynaud's phenomenon may occur.

Class III drugs

Amiodarone

Amiodarone is a benzofuran derivative initially investigated in the early 1960s in the field of the management of angina pectoris. It was not until 1974 that the clinical anti-arrhythmic properties of the drug were reported.[316]

The pharmacokinetics of amiodarone have not been completely evaluated in man. Oral absorption after a single dose is protracted (peak concentration is reached in a mean time of 8 h) with a low mean bioavailability of 35%.[317] The drug has a very large volume of distribution and a very long terminal elimination half-life (1–2 months).[318] Monitoring of plasma levels of amiodarone and its principal metabolite, desethyl amiodarone, following cessation of chronic oral therapy indicates an exceptionally long half-life for the elimination of both compounds.[319] Following intravenous injection, the onset of anti-arrhythmic effect is almost immediate and lasts from 20 min to 4 h.[320]

The electrophysioligical effects of amiodarone include depression of sino-atrial node automaticity,[321] prolongation of intra-atrial conduction time and atrial effective refractory period,[322] depression of atrioventricular nodal conduction,[323] lengthening of the HV interval[324,325] and an increase in the QT interval.[326] In most patients with Wolff–Parkinson–White syndrome, amiodarone increases the anterograde effective refractory period of the accessory pathway and prolongs the retrograde effective refractory period of the accessory pathway in about 50% of patients.[327] Following a rapid bolus injection, there is a fall in arterial pressure which produces a baroreflex-mediated sinus tachycardia.[328] This may in part be due to the diluent which consists of benzylic alcohol and polysorbate, because injection of the diluent without the drug also causes a transient tachycardia.[329] A slow intravenous injection in patients with good left ventricular function presents no danger: heart rate either falls or remains unchanged despite a decrease in arterial pressure.[330] Cardiac output increases significantly due to a decrease in systemic vascular resistance.[330]

Table 23.13. Indications for amiodarone treatment.

Definitely indicated:
Wolff–Parkinson–White syndrome with rapid atrial fibrillation when surgery is inappropriate or unacceptable

Probably indicated:
Life-threatening ventricular arrhythmias in:
    hypertrophic cardiomyopathy,
    dilated cardiomyopathy,
    congestive cardiac failure.
Highly symptomatic paroxysmal atrial fibrillation arrhythmias, such as atrial flutter or atrioventricular nodal re-entry tachycardia, not controlled by other treatment

Not indicated:
Non-life-threatening arrhythmias with the exceptions noted above
Arrhythmias likely to be controlled by other drugs
Pregnancy
Breast feeding
Thyroid dysfunction

Amiodarone is a very powerful anti-arrhythmic agent but unfortunately its use is restricted by potentially dangerous side-effects; however, it does have an important role in many arrhythmias (Table 23.13).[330]

Corneal microdeposits (Pl. 23.1) develop in nearly all adult patients receiving long-term amiodarone treatment. They are rarely associated with symptoms or impairment of visual acuity. Photosensitivity is frequently seen and in patients taking high maintenance dosages a slate-grey pigmentation of exposed areas may develop (Fig. 23.41). This regresses only slowly after cessation of therapy. As amiodarone contains 2 iodine molecules and bears a structural resemblance to the iodothyronines, it interferes with assays of thyroid hormones and makes all biochemical assessment of thyroid function unreliable. Overt hypothyroidism or hyperthyroidism develops in 2–16% of patients and may even occur several months after discontinuing the drug.[331] Proximal muscle weakness, peripheral neuropathy and neural symptoms (tremor, impaired memory, insomnia) rarely occur. Impaired liver function tests may occur in 10–20%.[332] Prolonged high-dose therapy may also induce an interstitial pneumonitis which may lead to irreversible pulmonary fibrosis, although if the complication is recognized early enough withdrawal of amiodarone and treatment with corticosteroids may produce regression.[333]

Amiodarone potentiates the anticoagulant effect of warfarin and the maintenance dose of the latter should be reduced by about one-third. Amiodarone increases the plasma digoxin concentration predisposing to digitalis toxicity.[334] Serum concentrations of quinidine, procainamide and flecainide are increased when amiodarone is given concomitantly. In addition, combining amiodarone with a class IA agent may predispose to the development of torsade

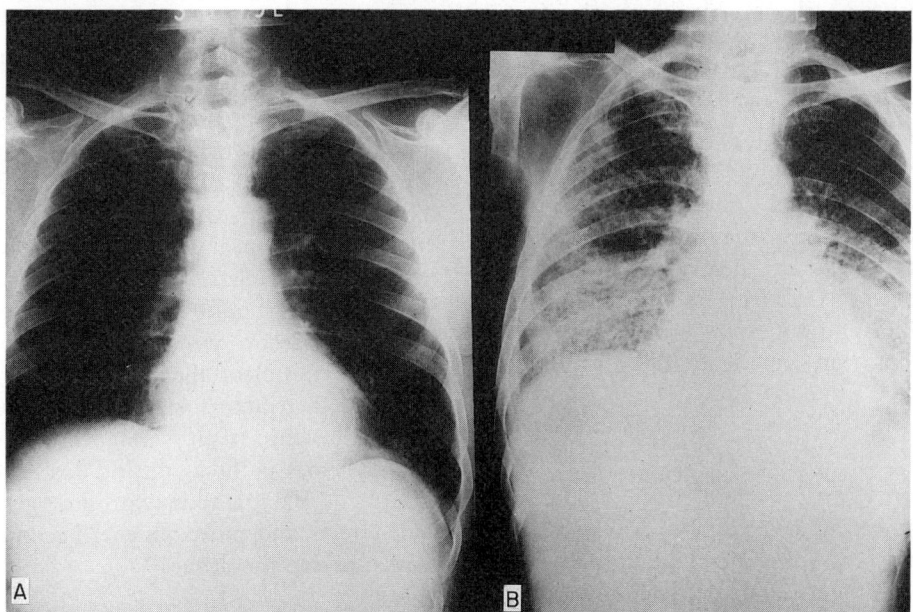

Fig. 23.41. Chest X-rays of a patient with a thinly calcified ventricular aneurysm before (left) and after (right) treatment with amiodarone 400 mg daily for a few weeks. The development of interstitial pulmonary fibrosis (amiodarone lung) is obvious.

de pointes. Finally, amiodarone may potentiate the depressant effects of calcium antagonists and beta-blockers on the conducting system.[335]

Bretylium

Bretylium was originally introduced as an anti-hypertensive agent in 1959 and was subsequently found to have anti-arrhythmic properties.[336] Because oral absorption is unreliable and tends to produce unacceptable hypotension, the drug is usually given intravenously, as a bolus dose in an emergency or as a continuous infusion. It is excreted without metabolic alteration and the average half-life is 9.8 h.

The release of catecholamines on administration of bretylium is accompanied by a reduction in both the action potential duration and myocardial refrac-toriness, often causing transient worsening of the cardiac rhythm.[337–339] Following the acute effects, bretylium then exhibits a direct class III action and may have an antifibrillatory action.[340] Bretylium has little effect on sustained tachycardia/fibrillation.[341,342] However, in selected cases, brety-lium can be a useful second-line agent in refractory ventricular arrhythmias.

Sotalol

Sotalol has combined class II and class III actions. The class III action is due to the effects of the *d*-isomer, which has little beta-blocking activity and is an effective anti-arrhythmic agent in its own right.[343] Sotalol has fewer side-effects than amiodarone but it may not be as effective. Furth-ermore, torsade de pointes has been reported secondary to sotalol therapy,[344] especially when it is combined with potassium-losing diuretic therapy. However, the drug has useful advantages over ordinary beta-blockers when an added anti-arrhythmic element is required, and it is effective in controlling supraventricular and ventricular tachy-cardia in a proportion of patients.[345,346]

Class IV drugs

Verapamil

Verapamil was introduced initially as a coronary vasodilator and was subsequently found to have anti-arrhythmic properties.[347] Systemic absorption is complete, but verapamil undergoes extensive first pass metabolism in the liver so that it has only 10–22% bio-availability. The drug has a half-life of 3–7 h, with 70% being excreted in the urine.[348]

Verapamil predominantly affects nodal tissue. It suppresses the sino-atrial and atrioventricular nodes and increases atrioventricular nodal re-fractoriness.[349] The depressant effect on the sino-atrial node is usually more than compensated for by a reflex tachycardia, secondary to peripheral vasodilatation. Verapamil has no appreciable effect on myocardial refractoriness.[348] Verapamil exerts a negative inotropic effect, particularly when given intravenously.[350] With oral administration, there is a lesser but still significant effect, seen most commonly in patients with underlying left ventricu-lar dysfunction.[25]

Intravenous verapamil is a useful agent for terminating supraventricular arrhythmias. It has been used to terminate and prevent sinus node re-entrant tachycardia.[351] Verapamil is widely used to terminate re-entrant tachycardias involving the atrioventricular node (Fig. 23.42). It is effective in terminating 90% of these arrhythmias irrespective of whether they involve an accessory pathway. The usual intravenous dose is 10 mg (or 0.145/mg/kg), given as a slow bolus injection. Intravenous verapa-mil should be avoided in patients taking beta-blockers because this combination produces signi-ficant negative inotropic and chronotropic effects.[352] Unfortunately, oral verapamil is not as effective in the long-term prevention of these arrhythmias, being effective in only 5–10% of cases[351] and often requiring high doses (360–720 mg daily).

Verapamil is rarely effective in terminating ven-tricular tachycardia, with the exception of tachycar-dias arising from the posterior fascicle of the left bundle branch, which have a characteristic electro-cardiographic appearance of right bundle branch block with left-axis deviation. These unusual arrhythmias appear to be particularly sensitive to calcium antagonists.[108]

Verapamil should be avoided in patients with Wolff–Parkinson–White syndrome who have atrial fibrillation, unless the electrophysiological prop-erties of their accessory pathway have been deter-mined, because it may enhance conduction down the accessory pathway during this arrhythmia (Fig. 23.43).[353] Verapamil may produce gastro-intestinal side-effects and most patients become constipated whilst taking the drug.

Unclassified anti-arrhythmic agents

Adenosine

Adenosine, an endogenous purine nucleotide, is a

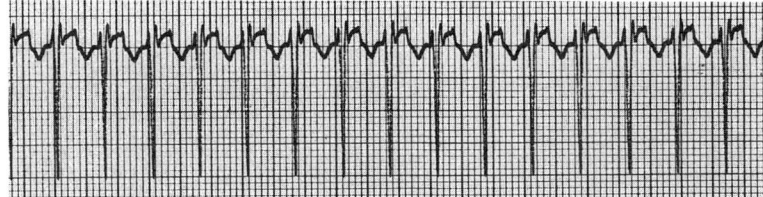

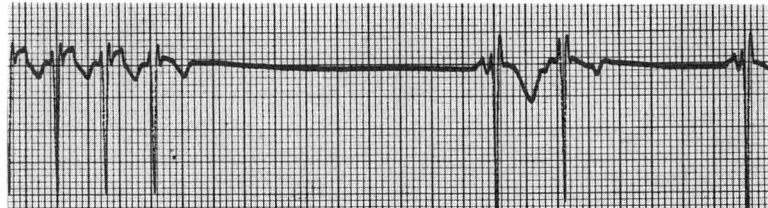

Fig. 23.42. Intravenous verapamil is given to rapid atrioventricular re-entrant tachycardia (195 beats/min) (top panel). When the tachycardia stops, there is sinus node arrest (bottom panel). This patient had sinus node disease in addition to atrioventricular re-entry.

potent atrioventricular nodal blocking agent, producing prolongation of the AH interval and increasing the atrioventricular nodal effective refractory period.[101] It increases the sinus cycle length but has no effect on the HV interval. It has interesting pharmacokinetics, in that it can be given only by intravenous injection, and has a half-life of 10–30 s. The results of studies performed to date have shown that given in doses of 0.05–0.25/mg/kg it is effective in terminating 80–100% of atrioventricular re-entrant tachycardias and atrioventricular nodal re-entrant tachycardias (Fig. 23.44).[101–103] It is ineffective in most cases of ventricular tachycardia, but unlike verapamil it has not been shown to cause any deleterious effects and it is safe to give in cases of broad complex tachycardia in which the diagnosis is uncertain.[104]

Digoxin

Digoxin is still one of the most widely used anti-arrhythmic agents (see recent review by Smith[354]). In particular, it is one of the most useful agents for the control of the ventricular rate in atrial fibrillation. It exerts its effect predominantly by increasing vagal tone which increases the refractoriness and decreases condution in the atrioventricular node. As vagal tone is reduced during exercise, digoxin is less effective in controlling the ventricular rate in these circumstances. The drug is of little use in controlling other arrhythmias and should be particularly avoided in Wolff–Parkinson–White syndrome where it can enhance conduction through the accessory pathway and result in an increased ventricular response to atrial fibrillation, often with disastrous consequences.

The wide range and variety of anti-arrhythmic agents at present available attest to the fact that no one agent is vastly superior to the others. Certain drugs are more potent, e.g. amiodarone, but potency must be weighed against side-effects. The search continues for the ideal anti-arrhythmic agent but because of the diversity of mechanism for arrhythmias it is unlikely that such a drug will be found in the near future.

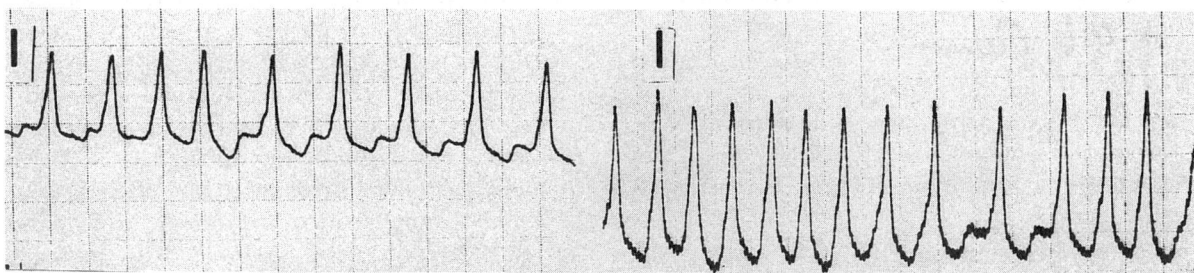

Fig. 23.43. Pre-excited atrial fibrillation in a patient with Wolff–Parkinson–White syndrome before (left) and after (right) administration of intravenous verapamil. Note that the ventricular rate greatly accelerates following the verapamil. Paper speed is 25 mm/s.

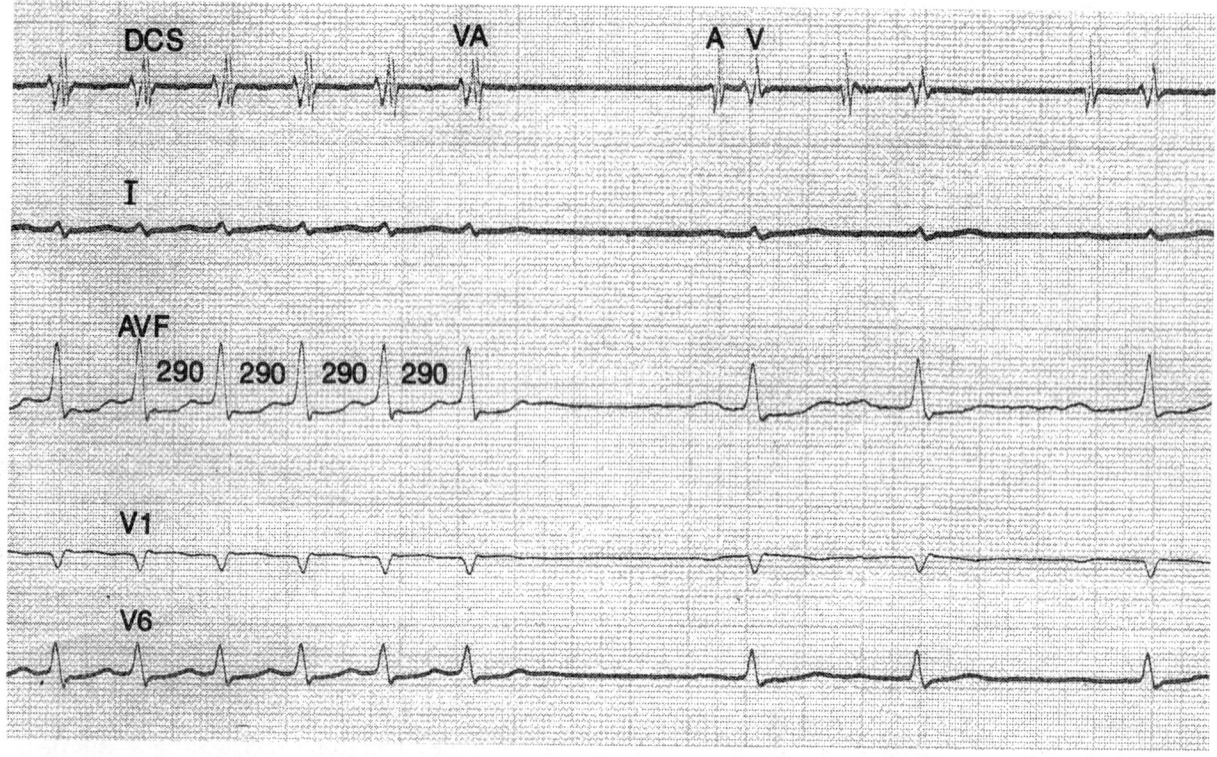

Fig. 23.44. Termination of paroxysmal atrioventricular nodal re-entrant tachycardia by the intravenous administration of adenosine. The tachycardia stops suddenly without first slowing. V, ventricular electrogram; A, atrial electrogram; DCS, distal coronary sinus; I, aVF, V$_1$ and V$_6$ are surface ECG leads. Recording speed is 50 mm/s. (By courtesy of Dr C. Garratt.)

Arrhythmogenic effects of anti-arrhythmic drugs

Most, if not all, anti-arrhythmic drugs have the potential to aggravate rather than relieve cardiac arrhythmias. Digitalis toxicity is well known to produce cardiac arrhythmias, even in patients who do not have a history of cardiac arrhythmia.[355] Of the remaining anti-arrhythmic compounds, beta-blockers are probably the least arrhythmogenic but even they may aggravate sinus bradycardia or worsen atrioventricular block. The serious import of these arrhythmogenic effects was first suggested when quinidine syncope was described,[251] but it has taken many years for this problem to be fully appreciated. Anti-arrhythmic compounds exert powerful electrophysiological effects which on occasion will be helpful but in other circumstances may be harmful.

New arrhythmias may develop or existing arrhythmias may be 'aggravated' by becoming more numerous, more prolonged or more haemodynamically unstable. These effects are described as *pro-arrhythmic* or *arrhythmogenic*.

Types of pro-arrhythmic event

Premature beats, bradycardias and tachycardias may occur. Sinus node function and atrioventricular nodal and intraventricular conduction are impaired by flecainide, disopyramide and other Vaughan Williams class I drugs, particularly in patients with pre-existing disorders of impulse generation and conduction.[356,357] Improved atrioventricular conduction may be a problem when there is an atrial tachyarrhythmia with some degree of atrioventricular block. In such circumstances, drugs that slow the atrial tachyarrhythmia without effecting termination, or improve atrioventricular nodal or accessory pathway conduction, may lead to acceleration of the ventricular response rate to the atrial arrhythmia. This potential arrhythmogenic effect is common with quinidine or disopyramide which slow atrial tachycardia and improve atrioventricular nodal conduction. Drugs such as verapamil, lignocaine and digitalis increase the anterograde conduction frequency through accessory pathways, and therefore they are contra-indicated for the treatment of atrial fibrillation complicating Wolff–Parkinson–White syndrome.

An increase in the frequency of ventricular premature beats may be an arrhythmogenic effect, but it is difficult to differentiate such an effect from normal variation.[358] However, from a statistical viewpoint, it has been suggested that the increase in frequency should be related to the baseline incidence of the arrhythmia. Therefore, if the baseline recording reveals 50 or less premature beats per hour, a tenfold increase in frequency is necessary to define an arrhythmogenic effect whereas an increase of only four-fold is needed if the baseline incidence is more than 100 per hour.[359]

Two major varieties of ventricular tachycardia are provoked by drugs. Class IA drugs,[360] which slow conduction and lengthen the action potential of myocardial cells and therefore prolong the QT interval (both the QRS and JT portions), and to a lesser extent class III drugs,[361] which prolong only the JT part of the QT interval, may induce a type of polymorphic ventricular tachycardia known as *torsade de pointes* (Fig. 23.45) because the QRS complexes appear to 'twist' around the iso-electric line. These arrhythmias may be due to early after-depolarizations induced by the drugs[362] and they often occur in patients who have no history of ventricular tachycardia. There does not seem to be a relationship between dose or serum level of the drug and the provocation of the arrhythmia. However, co-existing hypokalaemia[362] or ischaemia[363] may be important in the genesis of the arrhythmia. The second form of ventricular tachycardia is a sustained monomorphic variety, often with shapeless or 'sinusoidal' QRS complexes (Fig. 23.46). This complication occurs particularly with class IC compounds such as encainide,[364] flecainide[359] and propafenone.[365] In this case, the arrhythmias are more common in those patients with left ventricular dysfunction and a history of ventricular tachycardia,[336] the QRS complex is widened but the JT section of the QT interval is not prolonged and the serum level of the drug is often raised. It is likely that class IC drugs, which are powerful membrane depressants, slow conduction in a potential re-entrant circuit sufficiently to allow emergence of tachycardia.

Incidence of arrhythmogenic events

Anti-arrhythmic drug-induced arrhythmias occur in between 5 and 10% of patients,[358,367] but not all are serious or significant.[368] Such arrhythmias can be subdivided according to their clinical effects (Table 23.14).

With the most arrhythmogenic agents, for exam-

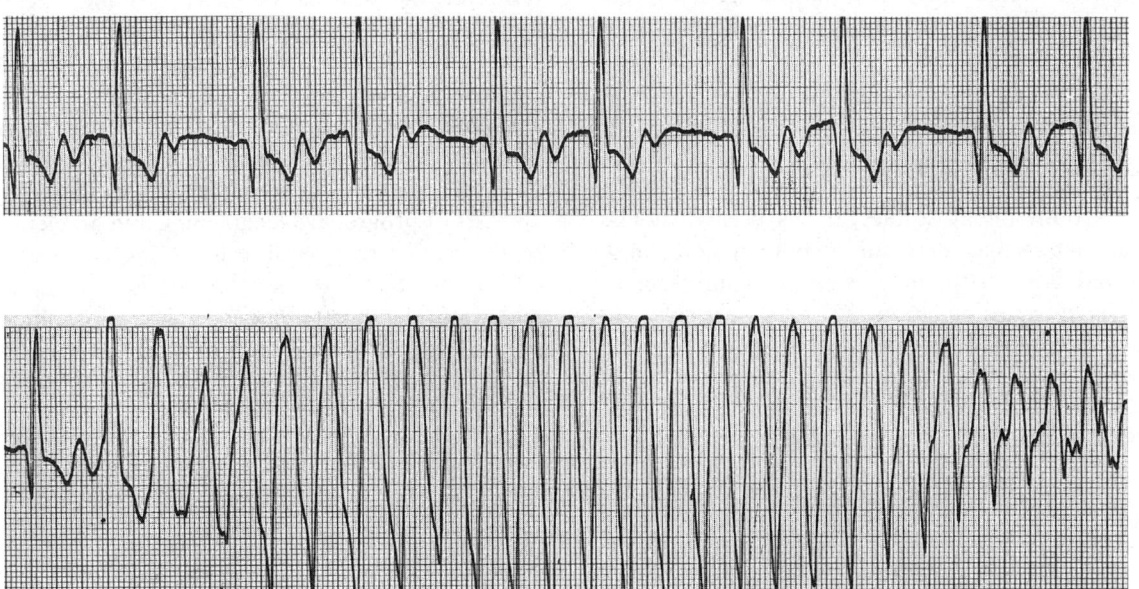

Fig. 23.45. An example of atypical ventricular tachycardia (torsades de pointes) developing in a patient who was treated with disopyramide (lower trace) because of symptomatic atrial premature beats (upper trace).

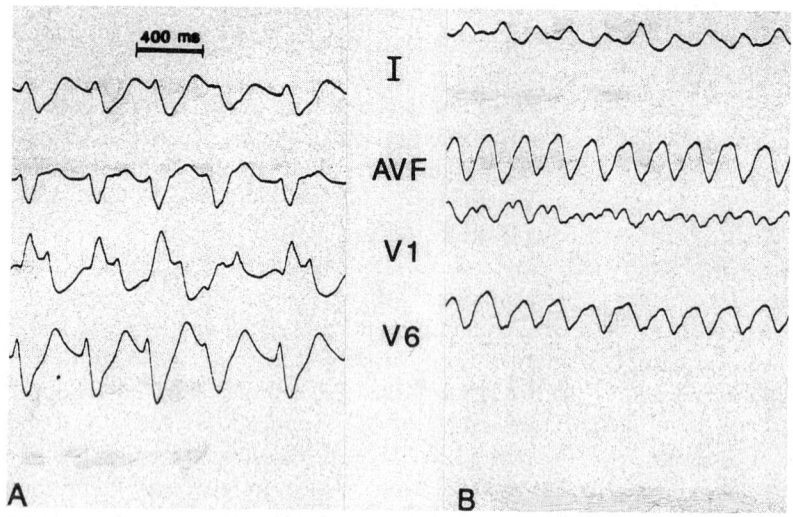

Fig. 23.46. Ventricular tachycardia before (A) and after (B) treatment with intravenous flecainide acetate. Note the acceleration of tachycardia and the change of morphology to a more sinusoidal' pattern.

ple, flecainide and encainide, serious pro-arrhythmic effects occur in < 10% of cases and deaths are unusual (1–3%) in patients treated for lethal ventricular arrhythmias.[359] In patients treated for less serious arrhythmias, deaths are very rare (< 0.1%) and other aggravated arrhythmias are correspondingly less. The pro-arrhythmic problem therefore is small but significant. An important confirmation of its significance is the report that a proportion of the victims resuscitated from out-of-hospital sudden cardiac arrest may have the potentially fatal arrhythmia reproduced in the electrophysiology laboratory only when they have been given the anti-arrhythmic medication they were taking at the time of their arrest.[369]

PACING AND IMPLANTABLE DEFIBRILLATORS

In electrophysiology studies, it has been demonstrated that tachycardias due to both re-entry and triggered automaticity may be initiated and terminated by electrostimulation.[370,371] In particular, a high percentage of sustained monomorphic ven-

tricular tachycardia,[372] atrial flutter[373] and all forms of junctional re-entrant tachycardias[374] may be successfully treated in this way.

The ability of an artificially induced depolarization to reach and influence tachycardia depends on the distance between the pacing site and the focus of tachycardia. When the rate of tachycardia is rapid, stimulation close to the origin or circuit of tachycardia is essential. Between the receding refractory tail and the advancing head of a re-entrant tachycardia wavefront is tissue that has fully recovered. This is known as the excitable 'gap' and in order to terminate tachycardia the pacemaker must depolarize this tissue by using critically timed stimulation. This can be achieved by scanning the tachycardia cycle with 1 or more extrastimuli or by using a sustained burst, possibly with a variable pacing rate. The single most successful modality of pacing has been called the 'universal' pacing mode.[375,376] It consists of progressive lengthening and acceleration of the pacing rate because following every unsuccessful burst an additional faster pacing cycle is added to the burst. The techniques of ultrafast pacing have not proved clinically valuable.

Table 23.14. **Classification of arrhythmogenic effects of anti-arrhythmic drugs.**

1 Deaths: sudden death within a few days of starting therapy or increasing dose

2 Clinically serious: new sustained ventricular tachycardia requiring urgent intervention

3 Clinically relevant: new ventricular tachycardia requiring reduction of dose or cessation of treatment

4 Clinically unimportant: increased frequency of ventricular premature beats or tachycardia without
the need to adjust therapy

Pacing techniques for the management of tachycardia

A wide range of pacing methods (Table 23.15) have been devised in order to improve the efficacy and safety of the tachycardia termination techniques.[377] In general, atrial pacing is preferred to ventricular pacing and long slower bursts are better than one or more closely coupled premature beats. Pacing techniques may induce or aggravate arrhythmias[378] when high-stimulation energy or fast pacing rates are used, and when there is co-existing drug toxicity (for example, digitalis), electrolyte disturbance or metabolic upset.

Automatic tachycardia recognition is essential to the proper working of these pacemakers.[379] All current systems rely on heart rate or a derivative of heart rate (for example, rate of change of heart rate, heart rate variability or the duration of high rate) to identify tachycardia. Proposed systems will use other biosensors and techniques of electrogram analysis to determine whether tachycardia is pathological and to provide a more specific diagnosis.

Permanent pacing

Permanent pacing techniques may be used to relieve the bradycardic background from which tachycardias may emerge, or to prevent the specific patterns such as the 'short–long–short' sequence which may initiate *torsade de pointes*. Permanent pacemakers have been used to treat successfully such arrhythmias when associated with either the congenital or acquired forms of the long QT syndrome.[186]

Several manufacturers produce implantable devices specifically intended for the termination of paroxysmal tachycardia. These devices can be considered as those that need patient activation, usually with a magnet or an external control box, and those that respond automatically. Automatic activation is preferred because patient co-operation is not required, no external apparatus is needed and tachycardia can be recognized and terminated before significant symptoms develop. Automatic pacemakers are usually used for termination of sporadic attacks of medically refractory re-entrant supraventricular tachycardia. Burst atrial pacing is the most commonly employed technique (Fig. 23.47). Despite the ready availability of these devices, they are not widely employed because there is concern about the provocation of unwanted arrhythmias or aggravation of the arrhythmia being treated, and the long-term efficacy of these pacemakers is not well known.[380–382]

The indications for the treatment of tachycardia with an implantable pacemaker are set out in Table 23.16. Prior to implantation, the patient must undergo a complete cardiac electrophysiology investigation during which the origin and mechanism of the tachycardia are established and its susceptibility to termination using pacemaker techniques is evaluated. Multiple trials of pacemaker therapy are then undertaken to confirm the efficacy and safety of the technique.

The implantation of a tachycardia-terminating pacemaker system involves the induction of the arrhythmia at the time of the implant so that it can be ascertained whether the pacemaker can recognize and terminate the tachycardia. Following

---

Table 23.15. Pacing methods for tachycardia control.

Tachycardia prevention:
1 Prevention of bradycardia and 'escape' tachycardias
2 Physiological overdrive pacing at a rate higher than normal sinus rhythm
3 Pre-excitation pacing (two sites, e.g. atrium and ventricle in Wolff–Parkinson–White syndrome)
4 Pre-emptive pacing (pacing ahead of the first return beat)

Tachycardia termination:
1 Single (or several) beat:
    underdrive (pacing rate < tachycardia rate)
    scanning extrastimulus

2 Multiple beat:
    asynchronous versus synchronous burst
    constant rate versus accelerating or decelerating burst
    single rate or 'concertina' (next attempt faster or slower rate) burst
    adaptive (adjusted to tachycardia rate) burst
    fixed duration or expanding burst
    very high-frequency burst

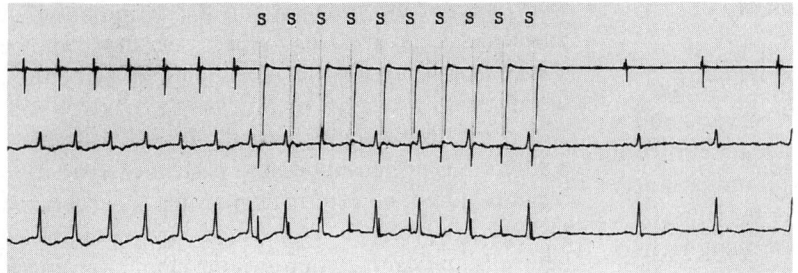

Fig. 23.47. These traces (top, atrial electrogram; middle, lead I; bottom, lead aVF) demonstrate the successful conversion from atrioventricular re-entrant tachycardia (left) to sinus rhythm (right) by overdrive atrial pacing with a burst of 10 stimulations (S).

discharge of the patient from hospital, careful follow-up is essential because re-programming is often necessary to ensure continued efficacy of the device. However, with careful patient selection, the techniques are safe and effectively reduce hospital admissions and the need for the patients to consult doctors.

Implantable cardioverter/defibrillator

Devices of this sort were first suggested in the early 1970s and first released for the treatment of human arrhythmias in 1980.[383] Essentially, they are miniaturized defibrillators comprising a small lithium power supply, capacitors capable of storing and discharging up to 35 J, and the electronic circuitry necessary to recognize automatically ventricular tachyarrhythmias and initiate a sequence of shock therapies. The present generation of devices have the theoretical capacity for several hundred shocks and a projected lifespan of about 3 years.[384] The arrhythmias are sensed predominantly by the recognition of a fast heart rate although more sophisticated sensing systems (such as the probability–density function—an assessment of how much of the time the signal spends on the iso-electric baseline) are available.

These devices should be considered for those at high risk of sudden unexpected cardiac death. The indications for device implantation are set out in Table 23.17. Patients with poor left ventricular function must be considered because they have the poorest long-term survival if treated with anti-arrhythmic drugs. Implantable cardioverter/defibrillator therapy considerably reduces mortality even in this high-risk group.[385–387] In the USA and Continental Europe, implantable cardioverter/defibrillator implantation rates are increasing dramatically. Cost considerations limit the availability of the device in some countries, including the UK.

Prior to the implantation of a cardioverter/defibrillator, the patient should undergo an electrophysiology study to assess the rate, origin and relevance of any inducible ventricular tachyarrhyth-

---

Table 23.16. **Indications for treatment of tachycardia by implanted pacemakers.**

Definite:
1 Atrial or junctional tachycardia which terminates readily when simple forms of atrial pacing are used and which does not degenerate to atrial fibrillation in response to atrial pacing, provided that other forms of therapy are unsuitable or ineffective, or the patient prefers pacing over other treatments
2 Bradycardia-tachycardia syndrome in which both elements of the syndrome may be treated with the implanted pacemaker

Probable:
1 Supraventricular tachycardia (including atrial flutter) which is usually terminated by atrial pacing and which does not provoke unwanted arrhythmias provided that anti-arrhythmic drugs are used concurrently
2 Ventricular tachycardia which terminates in response to atrial pacing
3 Ventricular tachycardia which responds readily to ventricular pacing but is not otherwise treatable (physician activation usually essential)
4 Ventricular tachycardia when pacing is used in combination with an implanted defibrillator.

Not indicated:
1 Ventricular tachycardia with a few exceptions as noted above
2 Tachycardia which degenerates in response to pacing
3 Wolff–Parkinson–White syndrome with a short accessory pathway effective refractory period

Table 23.17. **Indications for the implantation of a cardioverter/defibrillator.**

Definite:
1 Survivors of documented out-of-hospital sudden unexpected cardiac death not due to transient or correctable cause (for example, acute myocardial infarction, hypokalaemia, trauma)
2 Sufferers from recurrent inducible but non-suppressible hypotensive or syncopal ventricular tachyarrhythmias

Probable:
1 Survivors of undocumented out-of-hospital sudden unexpected cardiac death
2 Sufferers from recurrent documented but non-inducible ventricular tachycardia
3 Patients who have undergone potentially effective but uncertain therapy for ventricular tachyarrhythmias (for example, following surgery for ventricular tachycardia)
4 Patients for whom ventricular pacing therapy is used to terminate paroxysms of ventricular tachycardia

Not indicated:
1 Patients who are not expected to survive for 6 months because of another co-existing disease
2 Patients who suffer from ventricular tachyarrhythmias too frequently
3 Patients with frequent non-sustained tachycardias sufficient to trigger the device
4 Patients with incessant ventricular tachycardia

mia and to study the patient's vulnerability to atrial arrhythmias. Exercise testing and Holter monitoring are also carried out to evaluate spontaneous arrhythmias and to determine the maximum sinus rate (to ensure that the device will be able to distinguish between sinus tachycardia and the ventricular tachyarrhythmias).

The device is usually implanted in the anterior abdominal wall in the pararectal position. It is connected to the heart via a number of electrodes: patch electrodes (for example, on the anterior and posterior surfaces of the heart) are used to deliver the cardioversion/defibrillation shock and a trans-venous bipolar electrode catheter[388] (or 2 epicardial screw-in electrodes) are used to sense the arrhythmia. Access to the heart may be gained via the sternotomy, thoracotomy or sub-xiphoid approaches.[389] Cardiopulmonary bypass is not usually required although about one-third of patients also undergo additional cardiac surgery, such as coronary artery bypass grafting, aneurysmectomy and endocardial resection.

There is now some successful experience with the use of a new electrode system which comprises a right ventricular apical cathodal electrode set against a right atrial anode combined with a subcutaneous anode plate electrode positioned over the left ventricular apex (Fig. 23.48). This technique will provide a less traumatic and non-thoracotomy method of implantation.

Following surgery, the device is not activated until post-operative arrhythmias have settled down. The patient usually undergoes further electrophy-

siology testing to ascertain that the device works correctly prior to discharge from hospital. Complications from the surgery (Table 23.18) include those expected from any thoracic operation, those related to the implantation of a device and those specific to the current generation of device.[390] Some complications are inevitable with the use of such a treatment method, in particular, psychological reactions are not uncommon. These complications can, however, be reduced by careful peri-operative counselling.

Patient survival following cardioverter/defibrillator implantation testifies to the remarkable success of this form of therapy.[390,391] Survival from sudden death at 1 year is 98% and at 5 years 94%. Total survival at 1 year is 92% and at 5 years 76%.[392] These results compare very favourably with the dismal results from anti-arrhythmic drug treatment or arrhythmia surgery. Furthermore, the therapy has been shown to be remarkably cost-effective. Over 8000 units have now been implanted, largely from one manufacturer, and mostly in the USA. More than half of the patients who have received the device have coronary artery disease and about a third suffer from cardiomyopathy. A few patients have the long QT syndrome, mitral valve prolapse, clinically normal hearts or congenital heart disease. On average, the ejection fraction of patients in most series has averaged between 30 and 35%. There are already devices available from several manufacturers and in the near future others will be released. These newer systems will combine high-energy defibrillation therapy with pacing tech-

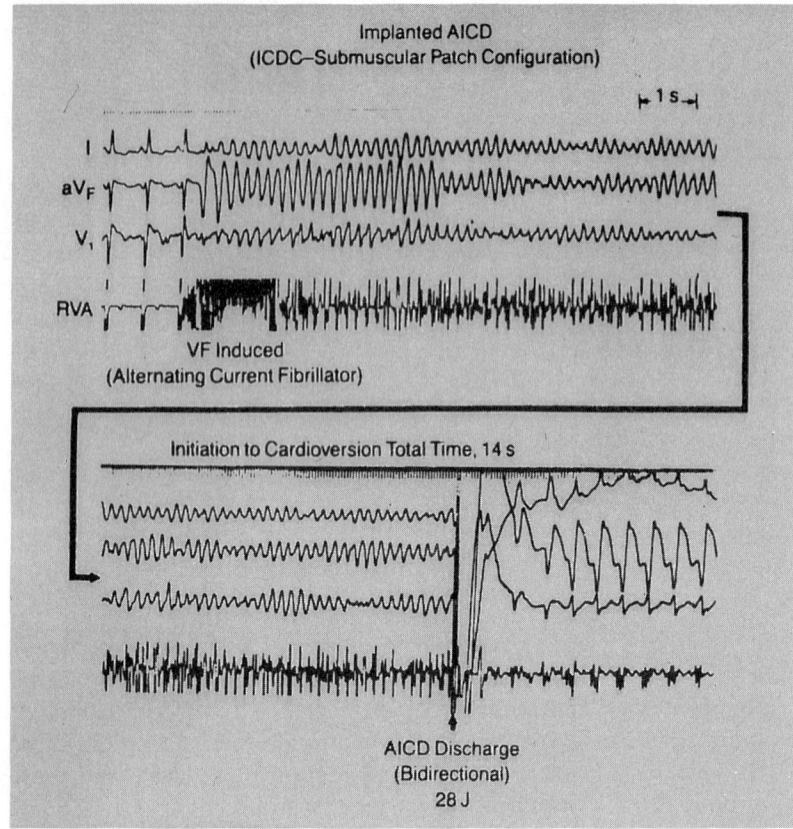

Fig. 23.48. The top panel shows the provocation of ventricular fibrillation by the application of alternating current. Reversion occurs following a 28J discharged between a single cathode in the apex of the right ventricle and two anodes, in the right atrium and subcutaneously over the left ventricle. The discharge results in the restoration of sinus rhythm. This system can be implanted transvenously (except for the subcutaneous patch electrode). AICD, automatic implantable cardioverter/defibrillator. (Reproduced from Saxena, S. and Parsonett, Implantation of a cardiovascular/defibrillator without thoracotomy using a simple electrode system. *J.A.M.A.* **259**: 69, 1988).

niques and low-energy cardioversion, and will incorporate more sophisticated and reliable sensing and Holter functions. However, this form of therapy is essentially designed to terminate the arrhythmia once it has started. It is, therefore, unsatisfactory for a fully effective form of therapy.

ABLATION

Catheter techniques

The first example of His bundle ablation occurred when a patient with supraventricular tachycardia received a transthoracic defibrillation shock during

---

Table 23.18.   **Complications of therapy with implantable cardioverter/defibrillator.**

Common to all implants:
Lead fracture and/or disconnection
Lead dislodgement
Infection of wound or pocket
Erosion of device or leads
Superior vena caval thrombosis

Surgical complications:
Operative and peri-operative deaths
Pericarditis
Pneumothorax and haemothorax
Bleeding (needing transfusion)
Post-operative arrhythmias

Complications common to current devices:
Mis-triggering, undersensing (shock not delivered), oversensing (unnecessary shock given)
Interaction with implanted pacemakers

Unavoidable complications:
Psychological reactions (fear, anxiety, insecurity)
Persistent arrhythmia despite maximum shocks

---

the course of an electrophysiology study.[393] The discharge accidentally shorted through the His bundle recording catheter and the patient developed heart block. Initial animal investigations[394] were soon followed by results of His bundle ablation in patients with supraventicular tachycardia,[395,396] especially atrial fibrillation. From these early results, it seemed that the technique was both effective and safe and it was soon widely used. However, the realization that the technique was potentially dangerous lead to detailed investigation of its mechanism which in turn lead to modifications of the technique to improve its safety.

Biophysical effects

When high energy is discharged through a small electrode, the fluid in contact with the electrode vaporizes producing insulation around the electrode. However, if the energy is sufficiently high, the insulation breaks down and arcing occurs. A fireball, consisting of gas bubbles and a flash of light, a pressure wave and explosive sounds are formed. The temperature may rise to more than 1700°C (the melting point of platinum) and a pressure of several atmospheres is produced. Such physical effects may be sufficient to disrupt the myocardium or the coronary sinus.[397]

The gas bubbles formed in blood contain principally hydrogen and nitrogen; the volume of gas is greater for anodal discharge. Similarly, blood haemolysis is greater with anodal shocks.[398]

The immediate effect of fulgurative discharge on cardiac tissue is to produce contraction band necrosis and loss of cell nuclei.[399] This is followed acutely by a local inflammatory response. Finally, the myocardium becomes thin and is replaced by adipose and fibrous tissue. Presumably, the integrity of the myocyte membrane is sufficiently damaged by the shock to prevent polarization. The cause of this damage is likely to be the high voltage and current,[400] whereas the more gross damage, especially myocardial perforation, must be due to barotrauma.

Techniques, equipment and indications

Most clinicians use a conventional defibrillator energy source and deliver the discharge to the myocardium via a standard woven Dacron catheter with a platinum electrode. Usually the myocardial electrode is connected to the cathodal output of the defibrillator whereas the anode is formed by a large electrode placed against the back of the patient (Fig. 23.49). Anodal shocks and bipolar shocks have also been used. Irrespective of where the shock is delivered, arrhythmias may be provoked and transient atrioventricular block may occur. It is therefore mandatory to pass a soft (to prevent myocardial perforation when the shock is given) temporary pacing wire into the apex of the right ventricle and to provide comprehensive resuscitation equipment. High-energy capacitor discharges are painful and a general anaesthetic must be used.

For His bundle (atrioventricular nodal) ablation, a bipolar electrode catheter is placed against the His

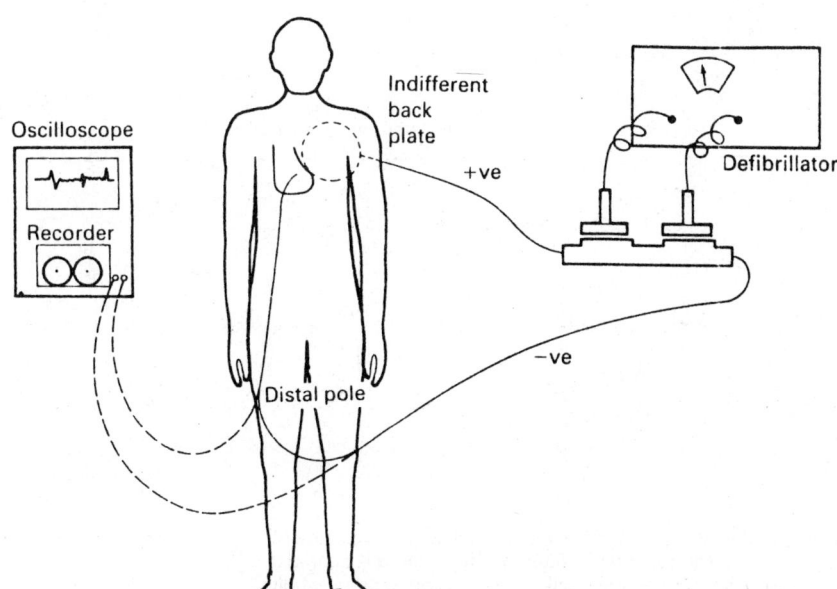

Fig. 23.49. Diagram of the set-up of equipment for His bundle ablation. In this case, the standard defibrillator was used. (Reproduced from: Ward, D.E. and Camm, A.J. *Clinical Electrophysiology of the Heart*. London: Edward Arnold, 1987).

bundle so that both atrial and His bundle potentials can be recorded through the electrode intended for the ablation. Between 50 and 350 J is then delivered. A second shock may be necessary to achieve atrioventricular block (Fig. 23.50) and the procedure may have to be repeated on a subsequent occasion if conduction resumes. Anomalous pathways may be ablated by placing the catheter as close as possible to the bypass tract, perhaps using Kent potentials or the earliest atrial activation during orthodromic re-entrant tachycardia. The catheters may be placed within the coronary sinus or across its ostium, against the right atrioventricular groove, or on the left atrial side of the atrioventricular groove using a trans-septal puncture. Obviously, shocks delivered into a thin-walled coronary sinus may rupture the vessel. It is suggested that this technique be either avoided or restricted to very low energy (< 50 J). For the ablation of foci of ventricular tachycardia, it is crucial to locate the origin of tachycardia or the area of critically slowed conduction that supports the circus movement causing tachycardia. Detailed catheter mapping is necessary. For ventricular tachycardias of septal origin, trans-septal shocks have been advocated. Other cardiac structures such as the right bundle branch and atrial ectopic foci have also been ablated successfully.

Anomalous pathway ablation remains experimental and its further use should be restricted to the experimental setting. Ventricular tachycardia can be successfully ablated but the procedure is time consuming and potentially dangerous. It should be offered to those with ventricular tachycardia of a single or perhaps two morphologies which are refractory to drug treatment and unsuitable for surgery or therapy with an implantable cardioverter/defibrillator. His bundle ablation is now commonplace and should be considered in the following circumstances.

1 Bradycardia–tachycardia syndrome when a pacemaker is necessary and the tachycardia is refractory to other therapy.
2 Paroxysmal atrial arrhythmias (particularly atrial flutter and atrial fibrillation) that remain uncontrolled despite optimal drug treatment.
3 Chronic (established) atrial arrhythmias when it is impossible to control atrioventricular conduction (through the atrioventricular node).
4 Incessant or frequently recurrent atrioventricular re-entrant tachycardia for which drug treatment fails and surgery is not appropriate or acceptable.
5 Seriously symptomatic atrioventricular nodal re-entrant tachycardia when drugs are ineffective.

Destruction of the normal atrioventricular conduction system renders the patient dependent on an idioventricular escape rhythm which may not be reliable. For this reason, permanent pacemaker implantation is always advised following an

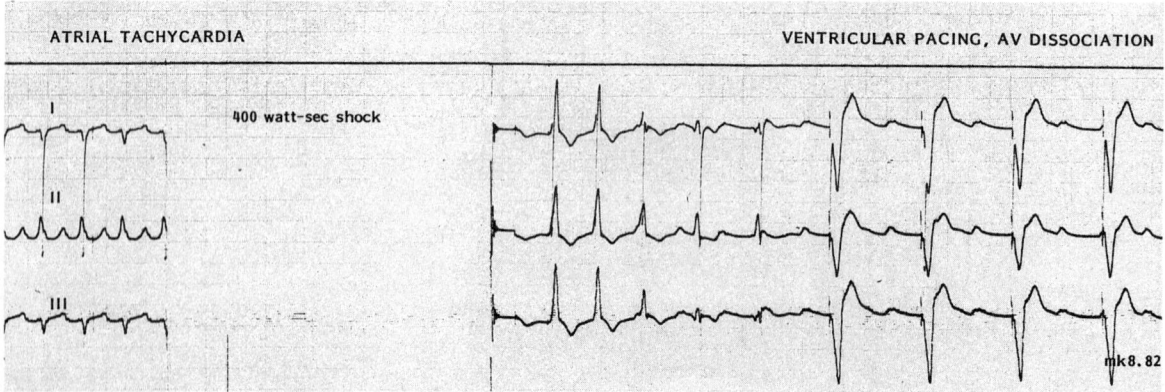

Fig. 23.50. These electrocardiograms were recorded at the time of His bundle ablation. The treatment was advised because of incessant atrial tachycardia with block (left). After the shock there is sporadic polymorphic ventricular activity until a demand ventricular pacemaker takes over control when ventricular bradycardia develops. (This trace was kindly provided by Dr D. Ward.)

atrioventricular node/His bundle ablation procedure. As atrioventricular block may develop later, a pacemaker should be fitted even if the attempted ablation has apparently failed. Rate-responsive ventricular pacing is preferred. The use of dual chamber devices may be complicated by pacemaker-related tachycardias.

Results of ablation procedures

His bundle ablation In about 70% of patients, complete atrioventricular block is permanently established and in a further 20% conduction resumes but the arrhythmia is greatly improved. However, half of these patients need to take anti-arrhythmic drugs which were previously unsuccessful. In the remaining 10%, the procedure is a failure.[401] The normal atrioventricular conduction system is more easily interrupted using catheter techniques than resorting to open heart surgery.

Anomalous pathway ablation Some results suggest that it is possible to ablate postero-septal pathways with certainty and safety.[402–404] This has been achieved by the delivery of high-energy shocks at the orifice of the coronary sinus. Other reports are not so optimistic and coronary sinus rupture has occurred with this technique.[405] Left free wall pathways are very difficult to localize and ablate. Effective techniques involve the delivery of shocks to the endocardial surface of the left atrium, or between poles sited in the coronary sinus and the left ventricle. Right atrioventricular pathways are easily accessible but difficult to localize closely. Results have sometimes been good with this sort of pathway.

Ventricular tachycardia focus ablation The role of catheter ablation techniques for the management of ventricular tachycardia is still uncertain. Although the tenor of initial reports was optimistic,[406,407] later results have not been as good. According to the International Ablation Registry, about 50% of ventricular tachycardias respond to this therapy.[408] However, many need continued anti-arrhythmic drug treatment, and recurrences are common.

Complications

Transient hypotension and short-lived arrhythmias occur commonly. More serious complications, such as pulmonary oedema, myocardial perforation, coronary sinus rupture and thrombosis, electromechanical dissociation and cardiac tamponade,

are very uncommon. There has been a small incidence of sudden cardiac death during the follow-up of patients who had undergone atrioventricular nodal/His bundle ablation. Most of these patients did have significant underlying heart disease but some did not. Furthermore, inducible and clinical forms of chronic ventricular tachycardia have been reported following ablation and there is concern that the technique may occasionally be *arrhythmogenic*. Chronic chest pain, dyspnoea, impaired ventricular function and reduced exercise tolerance[409] have also been reported. Implanted pacemakers may be re-programmed by the discharge and should be thoroughly checked before the patient is allowed to go home. A transient increase in pacing threshold may occur.

Future development of the ablation procedure

The present ablation technique is rather crude and although it has proved to be a valuable clinical tool it will shortly be improved. Special energy sources,[410] designed to provide very high voltages without arcing, will reduce damage due to barotrauma whilst retaining the effectiveness of the technique. Lower energies are effective if an active fixation electrode is used to ensure that the energy is delivered directly to the myocardium.[411,412] Purpose-built catheters will also feature improved electrode geometry and better insulation. It would be better not to produce atrioventricular block but to modify conduction properties in such a way as to prevent tachycardia.[413] Lower energy, better electrode placement and controlled targeted discharges may allow this. Other forms of energy may have advantages. Radiofrequency (for example, 300–700 MHz) and pulsed argon lasers are being evaluated.[414,415]

Surgical techniques

Surgery offers a cure or amelioration of symptoms to some patients with tachycardias resistant to drug treatment. Both supraventricular and ventricular tachycardias are amenable to this form of therapy but each tachycardia requires a different surgical approach.[416] The most important indication for surgery is the failure of medical therapy to control the arrhythmia. However, surgery may be the treatment of first choice for the Wolff–Parkinson–White syndrome and for concealed accessory pathways in young fit patients.[416] Intolerance or unsuitability of anti-arrhythmic drugs are also important indications for surgery.

Pre-operative evaluation

All patients undergoing anti-tachycardia surgery require pre-operative electrophysiological assessment to establish the electrophysiological diagnosis, to locate the substrate and to evaluate conduction from the substrate to the remainder of the heart. The presence, location and involvement in clinical arrhythmias of possible accessory pathways must be determined. Their electrophysiological properties, such as the ventricular response to induced atrial fibrillation, must also be assessed. The site of origin of atrial or ventricular tachycardia should be determined by catheter mapping[417] in order to reduce the time spent in mapping during the operation and to allow surgery to proceed if the tachycardia cannot be induced on the day of surgery. However, catheter mapping provides only an approximate resolution and it is not an adequate substitute for intra-operative mapping.[418]

Surgical treatment of specific tachycardias

Atrial tachycardia, atrial flutter and atrial fibrillation Pathological sinus tachycardia has been treated by subtotal excision and surgical exclusion of the right atrium[419,420] but atrial fibrillation developed in all patients. Atrial tachycardias have been successfully managed by excising the atrial focus.[421–424] The results of electrophysiologically guided cryoablation of left and right atrial foci in young patients is encouraging, 11 out of 12 patients were cured in a recent series.[425] Atrial fibrillation and atrial flutter may be treated by creating artificial atrioventricular block by exposure, dissection and cryoablation of the atrioventricular node and insertion of a permanent pacemaker,[426] but surgery is now being largely replaced by catheter ablation. This procedure is acceptable in the elderly, but it may cause a significant fall in cardiac output in young patients despite the use of dual chamber pacemakers. Recently, it has proved possible to isolate a substantial proportion of both atria whilst preserving normal atrioventricular conduction by leaving a strip or *corridor* of intact non-fibrillating myocardium between the sinus and atrioventricular nodes.[427] Preliminary experience suggests that atrial flutter may be successfully abolished by an incision carefully placed in the low right atrium.[428]

Atrioventricular nodal re-entrant tachycardias Surgery for atrioventricular nodal tachycardia is warranted when the arrhythmia is refractory to medical therapy. The recognition that atrioventricu-

lar nodal re-entry pathways may be separate from the atrioventricular node itself has lead to the development of a curative operation preserving normal atrioventricular conduction.[429] Two types of extranodal pathway have been identified: an antero-medial pathway with a short (< 40 ms) retrograde conduction time (type A) and a posterior pathway with a longer retrograde conduction time (type B). After identification with intra-operative electrogram and cryothermal mapping of the type of pathway involved in the tachycardia, the antero-medial or posterior space is dissected in order to disconnect the atrioventricular node from the atrium at that point. In a large series from one centre, it has been shown that post-operatively tachycardia cannot be induced but atrioventricular conduction is preserved.[429] An alternative approach, with excellent results, is to make a grid of cryothermal lesions in the triangle of Koch while monitoring atrioventricular conduction.[430]

Atrioventricular re-entrant tachycardias and Wolff–Parkinson–White syndrome Surgical division of direct atrioventricular pathways is now established as safe and effective and should no longer be considered as experimental.[431] There are 4 main locations of direct accessory pathways in the Wolff–Parkinson–White syndrome: left free wall, right free wall, postero-septal and antero-septal.[432] With the exception of the antero-septal location, these pathways may be divided by an epicardial approach which allows the operation to be performed on a normothermic beating heart.[433,434] The division of antero-septal pathways requires an endocardial approach on cardiopulmonary bypass; some workers prefer this approach for all pathways. The location of the accessory pathway is determined by careful intra-operative mapping and may be confirmed by cryomapping, i.e. inactivating the pathway by cooling (Fig. 23.51). The atrial insertion is best demonstrated by timing electrograms recorded from the endocardial or epicardial surface during orthodromic tachycardia. This avoids confusion with retrograde atrioventricular nodal conduction which occurs in response to ventricular pacing unless reduced or abolished by atrioventricular nodal blocking drugs. The ventricular end of the pathway can be located by epicardial mapping during atrial pacing at a rate sufficient to expose pre-excitation. Between 10 and 20% of patients with the Wolff–Parkinson–White syndrome have multiple pathways,[431,435] and it is, therefore, important to repeat the intra-operative electrophysio-

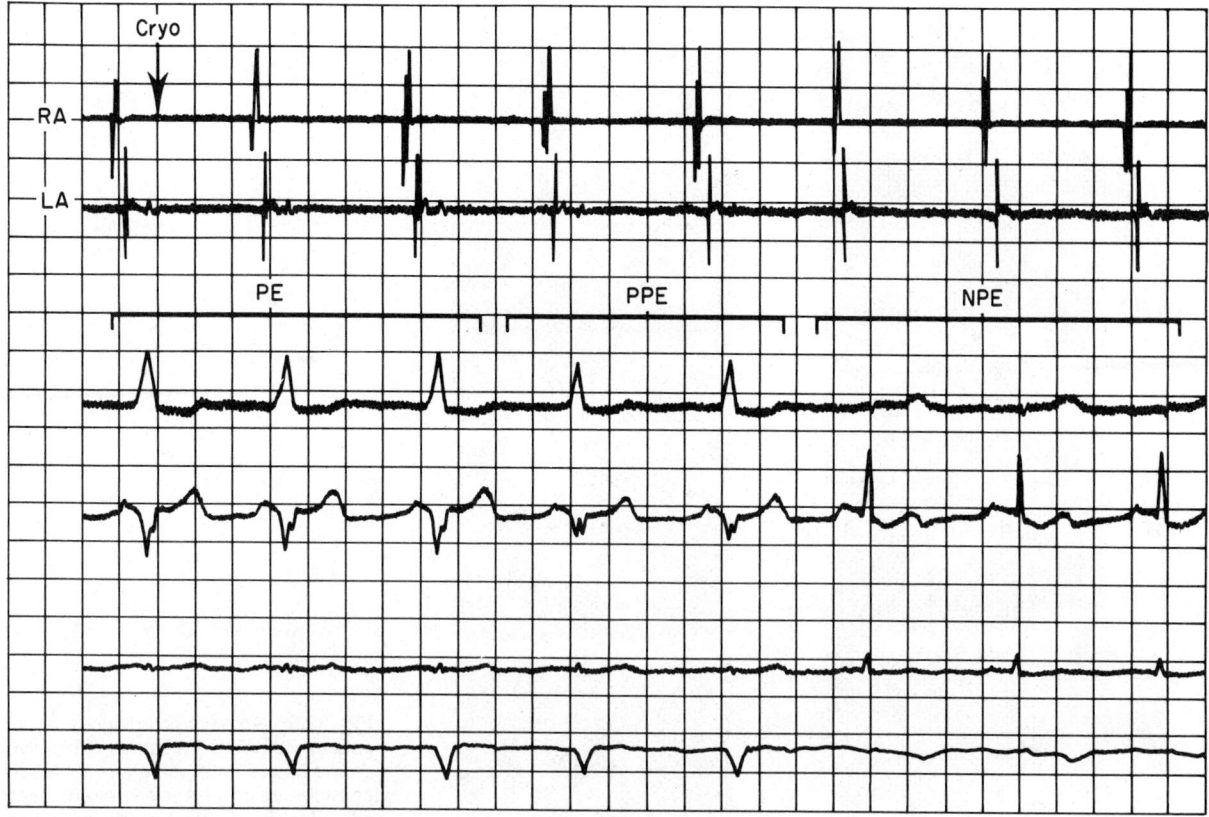

Fig. 23.51. At operation for Wolff–Parkinson–White syndrome, cryosurgical 'mapping' is often performed after electrographic mapping has suggested the approximate location of the pathway. In this case, the application of the cryoprobe achieved block of anterograde anomalous pathway conduction within a few seconds indicating that the probe was positioned very close to the pathway. The traces are from the right atrium (RA), left atrium (LA) and 4 surface ECG leads. PE, pre-excited complexes; PPE, partially pre-excited complexes; NPE, non-pre-excited complexes.

logical assessment of atrioventricular conduction before concluding surgery. In experienced centres, the cure rate of surgery for Wolff–Parkinson–White syndrome is now about 95% (Fig. 23.52) and the peri-operative mortality is < 1%. Patients who have undergone surgery for the Wolff–Parkinson–White syndrome should have a post-operative electrophysiology study (using implanted epicardial electrodes) to confirm the lack of pre-excitation.

Ventricular tachycardia Patients with ventricular tachycardia unresponsive to medical therapy should be considered for surgical treatment, especially when the tachycardia is of a single morphology, due to ischaemic heart disease, related to a distinct aneurysm, and/or situated on the anterior surface of the left ventricle.[436] In each case, careful mapping to locate the origin or path of the tachycardia is essential to the success of the treatment. Activation mapping is preferred,[437,438] but identification of

fragmented or fractionated electrograms during sinus rhythm (*fragmentation mapping*)[439,440] or simulating the tachycardia complex by ventricular pacing (*pace mapping*)[441] may be employed if tachycardia cannot be induced at the time of surgery (Fig. 23.53). About 10% of ventricular tachycardias involve identifiable macrore-entrant circuits, whereas the rest appear to arise from an area of myocardium between 3 and 6 cm wide[442] in which the present mapping methods are inadequate to delineate the detailed excitation pattern. Mapping of well-sustained tachycardia can be performed with a hand-held probe but multi-electrode arrays with computerized data analysis[88] are necessary for mapping short runs of tachycardia. Most ischaemic ventricular tachyarrhythmias seem to arise in the endocardium and mapping is therefore often performed through a ventriculotomy. Electrophysiological mapping improves the results: only 11% of patients developed ventricular tachycardia

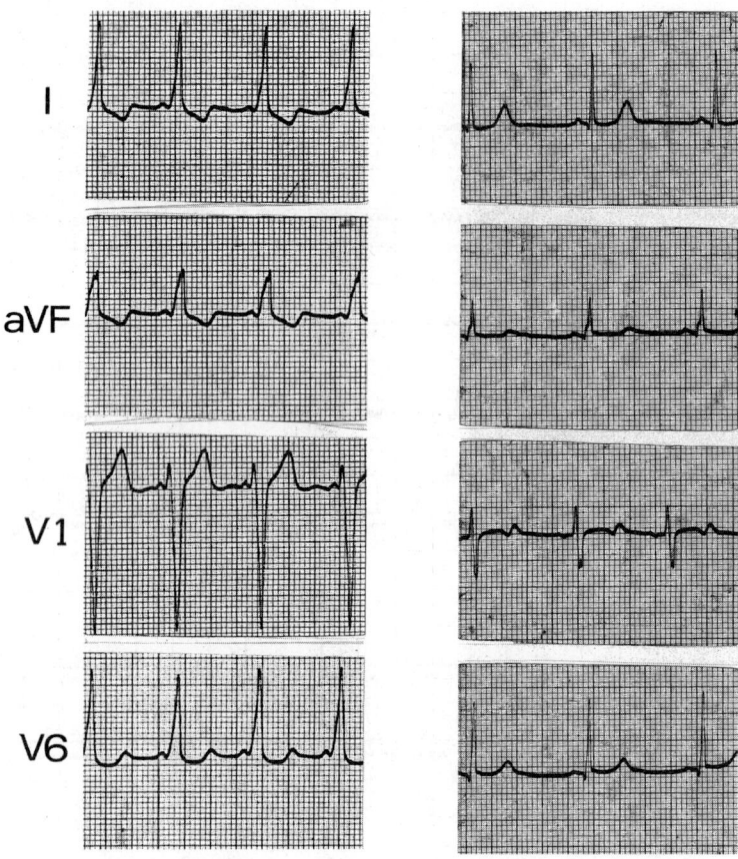

Fig. 23.52. An electrocardiogram from a patient with Wolff–Parkinson–White syndrome before (left) and after (right) successful division of a left free wall direct left atrial-to-left ventricular accessory pathway.

post-operatively as opposed to 50% of patients in whom the arrhythmia was not mapped.[443] There are four basic approaches: resection, ablation, interruption and isolation.

(i) Resection Aneurysmectomy with or without revascularization is usually performed when a distinct aneurysm is present, but the mortality is 20–50%.[444] In patients with ischaemic heart disease but no discrete aneurysm, a limited endocardial resection can be undertaken, provided that the origin of the tachycardia or site of re-entry can be identified. However, in a proportion of patients, the tachycardia cannot be mapped and more extensive resection must be undertaken without map guidance.[445] The mortality for these procedures ranges from 6 to 17%[446,447] and the technique is successful in approximately 65% of cases.[447] Cardiac tumours[448] and ventriculotomy scars (for example, following surgery for tetralogy of Fallot)[449] can also be resected

(ii) Ablation Cryotherapy[450] or laser (pulsed argon or Nd-YAG)[451,452] may be used to ablate

tissue that supports tachycardia. These techniques are employed intra-operatively under direct vision. Cryotherapy is particularly valuable for the ablation of tachycardia foci that cannot be resected, for example, within the papillary muscles.[453]

(iii) Interruption A simple ventriculotomy may be used for interrupting macrore-entrant ventricular tachycardias, such as those related to arrhythmogenic right ventricular dysplasia,[454] bundle branch re-entry[455] or other forms of right ventricular cardiomyopathy.

(iv) Isolation A ventriculotomy may be used to encircle and isolate any focus of tachycardia,[456] but when this was performed on the left ventricle it led to an unacceptable incidence of ventricular failure probably by compromising myocardial blood flow.[457] However, an encircling cryosurgical lesion[458] may successfully isolate the arrhythmia without depressing myocardial function. The right ventricle can be disconnected from the septum such that free wall right ventricular tachycardia cannot conduct to the left ventricle,[459] but this operation

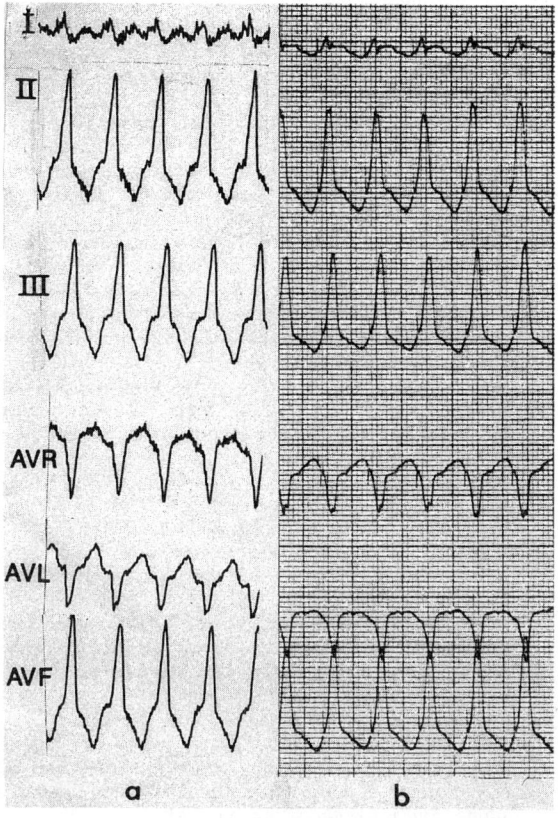
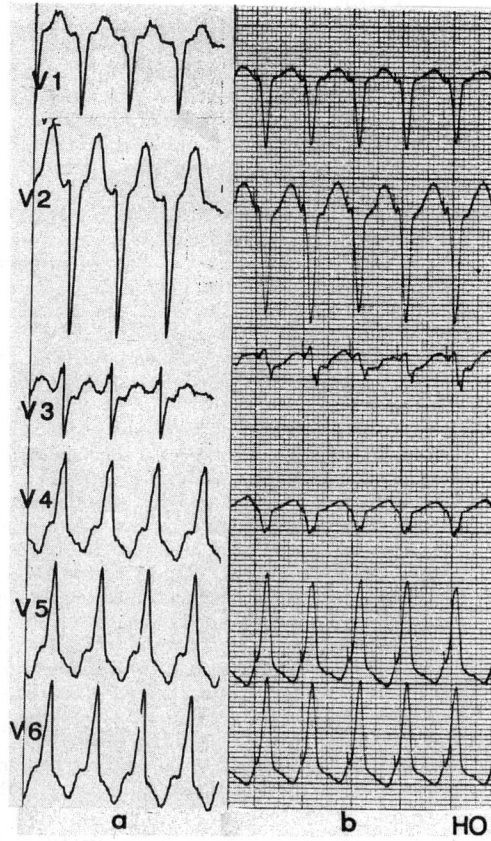

Fig. 23.53. An example of ventricular 'pace-mapping'. Traces from the spontaneous ventricular tachycardia (right of each panel), which arises from the right ventricular outflow tract, are compared with traces produced by pacing from the right ventricular outflow tract (left). (By courtesy of Dr D. Mehta.)

has been associated with post-operative dilatation of the right ventricle.[460] Following surgery for ventricular tachycardia, 24-h electrocardiography and electrophysiology study is undertaken. The failure to induce or record clinical tachycardia following surgery implies a good prognosis.[461]

CONCLUSIONS

Of the many therapies available for the manage-

ment of cardiac arrhythmias, some can be applied by the patient but others need medical intervention. Medical treatments range from those that can be applied in the consulting room to those that need the facilities of a cardiac surgical unit (Table 23.19).

It is possible to manage successfully the vast majority of cardiac arrhythmias. However, there remain those arrhythmias that are simply an expression of a dying heart for which no treatment is necessary or possible.

Table 23.19. **The use of anti-arrhythmic treatments.**

Treatment	Primary care	Secondary care	Tertiary care
Reassurance	++++	+	+
Physical manoeuvres	+++	++	+
Anti-arrhythmic drugs	++	++++	+++
Defibrillation	+	+	+
Cardioversion	0	++	+
Implantable devices	0	0	+
Catheter ablation	0	0	+
Surgical ablation	0	0	+

REFERENCES

1. Scherf, D. and Schott, A. *Extrasystoles and Allied Arrhythmias.* London: William Heinemann, 1973.
2. Hiss, R.G. and Lamb, L.E. Electrocardiographic findings in 67, 375 asymptomatic subjects. X. Normal values. *Am. J. Cardiol.* 1960; **6**: 200.
3. Hinkle, L.E., Carver, S.T. and Stevens, M. The frequency of asymptomatic disturbances of cardiac rhythm and conduction in middle aged men. *Am. J. Cardiol.* 1969; **24**: 629.
4. Fleg, J.L. and Kennedy, H.L. Cardiac arrhythmias in a healthy elderly population. Detection by 24-hour ambulatory electrocardiography. *Chest* 1982; **81**: 302.

5. Moss, A.L. Clinical significance of ventricular arrhythmias in patients with and without coronary artery disease. *Prog. Cardiovasc. Dis.* 1980; 23: 33–52.

6. Ekblom, B., Hartley, L.H. and Day, W.C. Occurrence and reproducibility of exercise-induced ventricular ectopy in normal subjects. *Am. J. Cardiol.* 1979; 43: 35–40

7. Scherlag, B.J., Lazzara, R. and Helfant, R.H. Differentiation of "A–V junctional rhythms". *Circulation* 1973; 48: 304.

8. Rosenbaum, M.B., Halpern, M.S., Nau, G.J. Elizari, M.V. and Lazzari, J.O. The mechanism of narrow ventricular ectopic beats. In: *Symposium of Cardiac Arrhythmias.* Sodertalje, Sweden: AB Astra, 1970, p. 223.

9. Montague, T.J., McPherson, D.D., Mackenzie, B.R., Spencer, C.A., Nanton, M.A. and Horacek, B.M. Frequent ventricular ectopic activity without underlying cardiac disease: Analysis of 45 subjects. *Am. J. Cardiol.* 1983; 52: 980.

10. Kistin, A. and Landowne, M. Retrograde conduction from premature ventricular contractions, a common occurrence in the human heart. *Circulation* 1951; 3: 738.

11. Zipes, D.P., Foster, P.R., Troup, P.J. and Pedersen, D.H. Atrial induction of ventricular tachycardia. Re-entry or triggered automaticity? *Am. J. Cardiol.* 1979; 44: 1.

12. Roberts, R., Ambos, H.D., Loh, C.W. and Sobel, B.E. Initiations of repetitive ventricular depolarizations by relatively late premature complexes in patients with acute myocardial infarction. *Am. J. Cardiol.* 1978; 41: 678.

13. Cranfield, P.F. and Aronson, R.S. Torsade de pointes and other pause-induced ventricular tachycardias: the short–long–short sequence and early after depolarizations. *Pacing Clin. Electrophysiol.* 1988; 11: 670–78.

14. Campbell, R.W.F. Ventricular ectopic activity and its relevance to aircrew licensing. *Eur. Heart J.* 1984; 5 (Suppl. A): 95–98.

15. Hinkle, L.E., Carver, S.T. and Argyros, D.C. The prognostic significance of ventricular premature contractions, in healthy people and in people with coronary heart disease. *Acta. Cardiol. Suppl.* 1974; 18: 5–32.

16. Cullen, K., Wearne, K.L., Stenhouse, N.S. and Gumpston, G.N. Q waves and ventricular extrasystoles in resting electrocardiograms. A 16-year follow-up in Busselton study. *Br. Heart J.* 1982; 47: 209.

17. Leier, C.V., Meacham, J.A. and Schaal, S.F. Prolonged atrial conduction; a major predisposing factor for the development of atrial flutter. *Circulation* 1978; 57: 213.

18. Fosmoe, R.J., Averill, K.H. and Lamb, L.E. Electrocardiographic findings in 67,375 asymptomatic subjects: II. Supraventricular arrhythmias. *Am. J. Cardiol.* 1960; 6: 84.

19. Langendorf, R. and Pick, A. Cardiac arrhythmias in infants and children. In: Gasul, B.M., Arcilla, R.A. and Lev, M, eds. *Heart Disease in Children*, Philadelphia: J.B. Lippincott, 1966, p. 121.

20. Marriott, H.J.L. and Myerburg, R.J. Recognition of arrhythmias and conduction abnormalities. In: Hurst, J.W., ed. *The Heart, Arteries and Veins*. New York: McGraw Hill, 1986, p. 443.

21. Silverman, N.H., Enderlein, M.A., Stanger, P., Teitel, D.F., Heyman, M.A. and Golbus, M.S. Recognition of foetal arrhythmias by echocardiography. *J. Clin. Ultrasound* 1985; 13: 225.

22. Garson, A. Jr., Bink-Boelkens, M., Hesslein, P.S., Hordof, A.J., Keane, J.F., Neches, W.J. and Porter, C.J. Atrial flutter in the young: A collaborative study of 380 cases. *J. Am. Coll. Cardiol.* 1985; 6: 871.

23. Wells, J.L. Jr., Maclean, W.A.H., James, T.M. and Waldo, A.L. Characterisation of atrial flutter. Studies in man after open heart surgery using fixed atrial electrodes. *Circulation* 1979; 60: 665.

24. Robertson, C.E. and Miller, H.C. Extreme tachycardia complicating the use of disopyramide in atrial flutter. *Br. Heart J.* 1980; 44: 602.

25. Singh, B.N., Ellrodt, G. and Peter, C.T. Verapamil: A review of its pharmacological properties and therapeutic use. *Drugs* 1978; 15: 169.

26. Betriu, A., Chaitman, B.R., Bourassa, M.G., Brevers, G., Scholl, J.M., Bourassa, P., Gagne, P. and Chabot, M. Beneficial effects of intravenous Diltiazem in acute management of paroxysmal supraventricular tachyarrhythmias. *Circulation* 1983; 67: 88.

27. Singh, B.N. and Jewitt, D.E. β-adrenergic receptor blocking drugs in cardiac arrhythmias. *Drugs* 1974; 7: 426.

28. Waxman, H.L., Myeburg, R.J., Appel, R. and Sung, R.J. Verapamil for control of ventricular rate in paroxysmal supraventricular tachycardia and atrial fribrillation or flutter: A double blind randomized cross over study. *Ann. Intern. Med.* 1981; 94: 1.

29. Waldo, A.L., Maclean, W.A.H., Karp, R.B., Kouchoukos, N.T. and James, T.N. Entrainment and interruption of atrial flutter with rapid atrial pacing: Studies in man following open heart surgery. *Circulation* 1977; 56: 737.

30. Batchelder, J.E. and Zipes, D.P. Treatment of tachyarrhythmias by pacing. *Arch. Intern. Med.* 1975; 135: 1115.

31. Campbell, R.M., Dick, M., Jenkins, J.M. *et al.* Atrial overdrive pacing for conversion of atrial flutter in children. *Pediatrics* 1985; 75: 730.

32. Graboys, T.B., Podrid and Lown, B. Efficacy of atrial flutter and fibrillation and the termination of atrial flutter by esophageal pacing. *Pacing Clin. Electrophysiol.* 1983; 6, 60.

33. Brandenburg, R.O. Jr., Holmes, D.R. Jr., Brandenburg, R.O. and McGoon, D.C. Clinical follow up study of paroxysmal supraventricular tachyarrhythmias after operative repair of a secundum type atrial septal defect in adults. *Am. J. Cardiol.* 1983; 51: 273.

34. Ormerod, O.J., McGregor, C.G., Stone, D.L., Wisbey, C. and Petch, M.D. Arrhythmias after coronary artery bypass surgery. *Br. Heart J.* 1984; 51: 618.

35. Spodick, D.H. Frequency of arrhythmias in acute pericarditis determined by Holter monitoring. *Am. J. Cardiol.* 1984; 53: 852.

36. Porfan, J.C., Miller, H.C. and Toff, A.D. Occult thyrotoxicosis: A correctable cause of idiopathic atrial fibrillation. *Am. J. Cardiol.* 1979; 44: 9.

37. Engel, T.R. and Luck, J.C. Effect of whisky on atria vulnerability and holiday heart. *J. Am. Coll. Cardiol.* 1983; 1: 816.

38. Takahashi, N., Seki, A., Imataka, K. and Fujii, J. Clinical features of paroxysmal atrial fibrillation: An observation of 94 patients. *Jpn. Heart J.* 1981; 22: 143.

39. Kannel, W.B., Abbot, R.D., Savage, D.D. and McNamara, P.M. Epidemiological features of chronic atrial fibrillation: The Framingham study. *N. Engl. J. Med.* 1982; 306: 1018.

40. Gajewski, J. and Singer, R.B. Mortality in an insured population with atrial fibrillation. *JAMA* 1981; 245: 1540.

41. Olsson, S.B., Orndahl, G., Ernestrom, S., Eskielson, J., Persson, S., Grennert, M.L. and Johanson, B.W. Spontaneous reversion from longstanding atrial fibrillation to sinus rhythm. *Acta Med. Scand.* 1980; 207: 5.

42. Wolf, P.A., Kannel, W.B., McGee, D.L., Meeks, S.L., Bharucha, N.E. and McNamara, P.M. Duration of atrial fibrillation and imminence of stroke: The Framingham study. *Stroke* 1983; 14: 664.

43. Brand, F.N., Abbot, R.D., Kannel, W.B. and Wolf, P.F. Characteristics and prognosis of lone atrial fibrillation. 30 year follow up in the Framingon study. *JAMA* 1985; 254: 3449.

44. Hunt, D., Sloman, G. and Penington, C. Effects of atrial fibrillation on prognosis of acute myocardial infarction.

Br. Heart J. 1978; **40**: 303.

45. Sugiura, T., Iwasaka, T., Ogawa, A., Shiroyama, Y., Tsuji, H., Onoyama, H. and Inada, M. Atrial fibrillation in acute myocardial infarction. *Am. J. Cardiol.* 1985; **56**: 27.

46. Ewy, G.A., Ulfers, L., Hager, W.D., Rosenfeld, A.R., Roeske, W.R. and Goldman, S. Response of atrial fibrillation to therapy: Role of etiology and left atrial diameter. *J. Electrocardiol.* 1980; **13**: 119.

47. Hoglund, C. and Rosenhamer, G. Echocardiographic left atrial dimension as a predictor of maintaining sinus rhythm after conversion of atrial fibrillation. *Acta Med. Scand.* 1985; **217**: 411.

48. Morganroth, J., Horowitz, L.N., Josephson, M.E. and Kastor, J.A. Relationship of atrial fibrillatory wave amplitude to left atrial size and etiology of heart disease. An old generalisation reexamined. *Am. Heart. J.* 1979; **97**: 194.

49. Gouaux, J.L. and Ashman, R. Auricular fibrillation with aberration simulating ventricular paroxysmal tachycardia. *Am. Heart J.* 1947; **34**: 366.

50. Halpern, S.W., Ellrodt, G., Singh, B.N. and Mandel, W.J. Efficacy of intravenous procainamide infusion in converting atrial fibrillation to sinus rhythm. Relation to left atrial size. *Br. Heart J.* 1980; **44**: 589.

51. Josephson, M.E. and Seides, S.F. Clinical cardiac electrophysiology: Techniques and interpretation. Philadelphia: Lea and Febiger, 1979, pp. 148–176.

52. Wu, D., Denes, P. and Amat-Y-Leon, F. Clinical electrocardiographic and electrophysiological observations in patients with paroxysmal supraventricular tachycardia. *Am. J. Cardiol.* 1978; **41**: 1045.

53. Josephson, M.E. Paroxysmal supraventricular tachycardia: An electrophysiological approach. *Am. J. Cardiol.* 1978; **41**: 1123.

54. Benditt, D.G., Pritchett, E.L.C., Smith, W.M. *et al.* Ventriculo-atrial intervals: Diagnostic use in paroxysmal supraventricular tachycardias. *Ann. Intern. Med.* 1979; **91**: 161.

55. Weisfogel, G.M., Batsford, W.P., Paulay, K.L. *et al.* Sinus node re-entrant tachycardia in man. *Am. Heart J.* 1975; **90**: 295.

56. Wu, D., Amat-Y-Leon, F., Denes, D. *et al.* Demonstration of sustained sinus and atrial reentry as a mechanism of paroxysmal supraventricular tachycardia. *Circulation* 1975; **51**: 234.

57. Gomes, J.A., Hariman, R.J., Kang, P.S. *et al.* Sustained symptomatic sinoatrial reentrant tachycardia: Incidence, clinical significance, electrophysiologic observations and the effects of antiarrhythmic agents. *J. Am. Coll. Cardiol.* 1985; **5**: 45.

58. Coumel, P., Flammang, D., Attuel, P. *et al.* Sustained intra-atrial reentry tachycardia, electrophysiological study of 20 cases. *Clin. Cardiol.* 1979; **2**: 167.

59. Tenczer, J., Littman, L., Molnar, F. *et al.* Atrial reentry in chronic repetitive supraventricular tachycardia. *Am. Heart J.* 1980; **99**: 349.

60. Farshidi, A., Josephson, M.E. and Horowitz, L.N. Electrocardiographic characteristics of concealed bypass tracts: Clinical and electrocardiographic correlates. *Am. J. Cardiol.* 1978; **41**: 1052.

61. DeMaria, A.N., Vismara, L.A., Neumann, A. *et al.* Arrhythmias in mitral valve prolapse syndrome: Prevalence, nature and frequency. *Ann. Intern. Med.* 1976; **84**: 656.

62. Josephson, M.E., Horowitz, L.N. and Kastor, J.A. Paroxysmal supraventricular tachycardia in patients with mitral valve prolapse. *Circulation* 1978; **57**: 111.

63. Mendez, C. and Moe, G.K. Demonstration of a dual A–V nodal conduction system in an isolated rabbit heart. *Circ. Res.* 1966; **19**: 378.

64. Denes, P., Dhingra, R.C., Chuquimia, R. *et al.* Demonstration of dual A–V nodal pathways in patients with paroxysmal supraventricular tachycardia. *Circulation* 1973; **43**: 549.

65. Ahktar, M., Damato, A.N., Ruskin, J.N. *et al.* Anterograde and retrograde conduction characteristics in 3 patterns of paroxysmal atrioventricular junctional tachycardia. *Am. Heart J.* 1978; **95**: 22.

66. Brugada, P., Farre, J., Green, M. *et al.* Observations in patients with supraventricular tachycardia having a P-R interval shorter than the R-P interval; Differentiation between atrial tachycardia and reciprocating atrioventricular tachycardia using an accessory pathway with a long conduction time. *Am. Heart J.* 1984; **107**: 556.

67. Gallagher, J.J. and Sealy, W.C. A permanent form of junctional reciprocating tachycardia: further elucidation of the underlying mechanism. *Eur. J. Cardiol.* 1978; **8**: 413.

68. Guarnieri, T., Sealy, W.C., Kassell, J. *et al.* The non-pharmacological management of the permanent form of junctional reciprocating tachycardia. *Circulation* 1984; **69**: 269.

69. Guarnieri, T., German, L.D. and Gallagher, J.J. Long RP' tachycardias. *Pacing Clin. Electrophysiol.* 1987; **10**: 103.

70. Gallagher, J.J., Gilbert, M., Svenson, R.H. *et al.* Wolff–Parkinson–White syndrome: The problem evaluation, and surgical correction. *Circulation* 1975; **51**: 1975.

71. Zipes, D.P., DeJoseph, R.L. and Rothbaum, D. Unusual properties of accessory pathways. *Circulation* 1974; **49**: 1200.

72. Pritchett, E.L.C., Gallagher, J.J. and Sealy, W.C. Supraventricular tachycardia dependence upon the accessory pathway in the absence of preexcitation. *Am. J. Med.* 1978; **64**: 214.

73. Barold, S.S. and Coumel, P. Mechanism of atrioventricular tachycardia. Role of reentry and concealed accessory bypass tracts. *Am. J. Cardiol.* 1977; **39**: 97.

74. Wellens, H.J.J. Wolff–Parkinson–White syndrome. Part 1. Diagnosis, arrhythmias and identification of the high risk patient. *Mod. Conc. Cardiovasc. Dis.* 1983; **52**: 53.

75. Ohnell, R.F. Preexcitation: a cardiac abnormality. *Acta Med. Scand.* 1944; **152** (Suppl.): 1.

76. Rosenbaum, F.F., Hecht, H.H., Wilson, F.N. *et al.* The potential variations of the thorax and the esophagus in anomalous atrioventricular (Wolff–Parkinson–White syndromes). *Am. Heart J.* 1945; **29**: 281.

77. Tonkin, A.M., Wagner, G.S., Gallagher, J.J. *et al.* Initial forces of ventricular depolarization in the Wolff–Parkinson–White syndrome. *Circulation* 1975; **52**: 1030.

78. Pryzbylski, J., Chiale, P.A., Halpern, *et al.* Unmasking the ventricular preexcitation by vagal stimulation or isoproterenol administration. *Circulation* 1980; **61**: 1030.

79. Bauernfiend, R.A., Wyndham, C.R., Swiryn, S.P. *et al.* Paroxysmal atrial fibrillation in the Wolff–Parkinson–White syndrome. *Am. J. Cardiol.* 1981; **47**: 562.

80. Wellens, H.J.J. and Durrer, D. Wolff–Parkinson–White syndrome and atrial fibrillation. Relation between refractory period of the accessory pathway and the ventricular rate during atrial fibrillation. *Am. J. Cardiol.* 1974; **34**: 777.

81. Klein, G.J. and Gulamhusien, S.S. Intermittent preexcitation in the Wolff–Parkinson–White syndrome. *Am. J. Cardiol.* 1983; **52**: 292.

82. Lown, B., Ganong, W.F. and Levine, S.A. The syndrome of short PR interval, normal QRS complex and paroxysmal rapid heart rate. *Circulation* 1952; **5**: 693.

83. Benditt, D.G., Pritchett, E.L.C., Smith, W.M. *et al.* Characteristics of atrioventricular conduction and the spectrum of arrhythmias in LGL syndromes. *Circulation* 1978; **57**: 454.

84. Welch, W.J., Strasberg, B., Coelho, A. and Rosen, K.M. Sustained macroreentrant ventricular tachycardia. *Am.*

Heart J. 1982; **104**: 166.

85. Bigger, J.T. Electrophysiology for the clinician. *Eur. Heart J.* 1984; **5**: 1.

86. Brugada, P. and Wellens, H.J.J. The role of triggered activity in clinical ventricular arrhythmias. *Pacing Clin. Electrophysiol.* 1984; **7**: 260.

87. Okumura, K., Olshansky, Henthorn, R.W., Epstein, A.E., Plumb, V.J. and Waldo, A.L. Demonstration of the presence of slow conduction during sustained ventricular tachycardia in man:use of transient entrainment of the tachycardia. *Circulation* 1987; **75**: 369.

88. Harris, L., Downar, E., Mickleborough, I., Shaikh, N. and Parson, I. Activation sequence of ventricular tachycardia: Endocardial and epicardial mapping studies in the left ventricle. *J. Am. Coll. Cardiol.* 1987; **10**: 1040.

89. Levy, S., Hilaire, J., Clementy, J. *et al.* Bidirectional tachycardia. Mechanism derived from intracardiac recordings and programmed electrical stimulation. *Pacing Clin. Electrophysiol.* 1982; **5**: 633.

90. Buxton, A.E., Marchlinski, F.E., Doherty, J.U. *et al.* Repetitive, monomorphic ventricular tachycardia: Clinical and electrophysiologic characteristics in patients with and without organic heart disease. *Am. J. Cardiol.* 1984; **54**: 997.

91. Baerman, J.F., Morady, F., DiCarlo, L.A. and de Buitler, M. Differentiation of ventricular from supraventricular tachycardia with aberration: Value of the clinical history. *Ann. Emerg. Med.* 1987; **16**: 40.

92. Anonymous. Looks like SVT (Editorial). *Lancet* 1986; **ii**: 612.

93. Rankin, A.C., Rae, A.P. and Cobbe, S.M. Misuse of intravenous verapamil in patients with ventricular tachycardia. *Lancet* 1987; **ii**: 472.

94. Dancy, M., Camm, A.J. and Ward, D. Misdiagnosis of chronic recurrent ventricular tachycardia. *Lancet* 1985; **ii**: 320.

95. Stewart, R.B., Bardy, G.H. and Greene, H.L. Wide complex tachycardia: Misdiagnosis and outcome after emergent therapy. *Ann. Intern. Med.* 1986; **104**: 766.

96. Wellens, H.J., Bar, F.W.H.M. and Lei, K.I. The value of the electrocardiogram in the differential diagnosis of a tachycardia with a widened QRS complex. *Am. J. Med.* 1978; **64**: 27.

97. Griffith, M.J., Mehta, D., Ward, D.E. and Camm, A.J. Ascending aorta Doppler echocardiography to identify atrioventricular dissociation during broad complex tachycardias. *Am. Heart J.* 1988; **116**: 555.

98. Drinkovic, N. Subcostal M-mode echocardiography of the right atrial wall for differentiation of supraventricular tachyarrhythmias with aberration. *Am. Heart J.* 1984; **107**: 326.

99. Wren, C., Cambell, R.W.F. and Hunter, S. Role of echocardiography in the differential diagnosis of broad complex tachycardia. *Br. Heart J.* 1985; **54**: 166.

100. Manyari, D.E., Ko, P., Gulamhusein, S., Boughner, D.R., Kostuk, W.J. and Klein, G.J. A simple echocardiographic method to detect atrioventricular dissociation. *Chest* 1982; **81**: 67.

101. DiMarco, J.P., Sellers, T.D., Lerman, B.B., Greenberg, M.L., Berne, R.M. and Belardinelli, L. Diagnostic and therapeutic use of adenosine in patients with supraventricular tachyarrhythmias. *J. Am. Coll. Cardiol.* 1985; **6**: 417.

102. Munoz, A., Leenhardt, A., Sassine, A., Galley, P. and Puech, P. Therapeutic use of adenosine for terminating spontaneous paroxysmal supraventricular tachycardia. *Eur. Heart J.* 1984; **5**: 735.

103. Clarke, B., Till, J., Rowland, E., Ward, D.E., Barnes, P.J. and Shinebourne, E.A. Rapid and safe termination of supraventricular tachycardia in children by adenosine.

Lancet 1987; **i**: 299.

104. Griffith, M.J., Linker, N., Ward, D.E. and Camm, A.J. Adenosine in the diagnosis of broad complex tachycardias. *Lancet* 1988; **i**: 672.

105. Winkle, R.A. Antiarrhythmic drug effect mimicked by spontaneous variability of ventricular ectopy. *Circulation* 1978; **57**: 1116.

106. Rasmussen, K., Lunde, P.I. and Lie, M. Coronary bypass surgery in exercise induced ventricular tachycardia. *Eur. Heart J.* 1987; **8**: 44.

107. Wellens, H.J.J., Brugada, P. and Stevenson, W.G. Programmed electrical stimulation of the heart in patients with life threatening arrhythmias: What is the significance of induced arrhythmias and what is the correct stimulation protocol. *Circulation* 1985; **72**: 1.

108. Ward, D.E. Can the technicalities of electrophysiological testing for ventricular tachycardia be simplified. *Br. Heart J.* 1987; **58**: 437.

109. Kudenchuk, J., Kron, J., Walance, C. and McAnulty, J. The limited value of programmed electrical stimulation from 2 right ventricular sites in patients with clinical sustained ventricular tachyarrhythmias. *Pacing Clin. Electrophysiol.* 1987; **10**: 448 (abst.).

110. Huang, L., Mann, D.E. Luck, C. *et al.* Prospective comparison of right and left ventricular stimulation for induction of sustained ventricular tachycardia. *Am. J. Cardiol.* 1987; **59**: 559.

111. Henthorn, R.W., Moreira, D.A.R., Olshansky, B., Epstein, A.E. and Waldo, A.L. Does induced "non-clinical" monomorphic ventricular tachycardia become manifest clinically? *J. Am. Coll. Cardiol.* 1987; **9**: 109.

112. Morady, F., Shapiro, W., Shen, E., Sung, R.J. and Scheinman, M.M. Programmed ventricular stimulation in patients without spontaneous ventricular tachycardia. *Am. Heart J.* 1984; **10**: 875.

113. Brugada, P., Green, M., Abdollah, H. and Wellens, H.J.J. Significance of ventricular arrhythmias initiated by programmed ventricular stimulation: the importance of the type of ventricular arrhythmia induced and the number of extrastimuli required. *Circulation* 1984; **69**: 87.

114. Amann, F.W., Blatt, C.M., Podrid, P.J. and Lown, B. Relationship between ease of inducibility of arrhythmia with electrophysiologic testing and response to antiarrhythmic therapy. *Am. Heart J.* 1986; **111**: 625.

115. Olshansky, B. and Martins, J.B. Usefulness of isoproterenol facilitation of ventricular tachycardia induction during extrastimulus testing in predicting effective chronic therapy with beta-adrenergic blockade. *Am. J. Cardiol.* 1987; **59**: 573.

116. Mason, J.W. and Winkle, R. Accuracy of the ventricular tachycardia induction study for predicting long-term efficacy of antiarrhythmic drugs. *N. Engl. J. Med.* 1980; **303**: 1073.

117. Waller, T.J., Kay, H.R., Spielman, S.R, Kutalek, S.P. and Greenspan, A.M. Reduction in sudden death and total mortality by antiarrhythmic drug testing: Criteria of efficacy in patients with sustained ventricular tachyarrhythmia. *J. Am. Coll. Cardiol.* 1987; **10**: 83.

118. Swerdlow, C.D., Winkle, R.A. and Mason, J.W. Determinants of survival in patients with ventricular tachyarrhythmias. *N. Engl. J. Med.* 1983; **308**: 1436.

119. Brugada, P. Should electrophysiological studies be performed to assess drug efficacy in patients receiving amiodarone. *Am. J. Cardiol.* 1987; **51**: 1415.

120. Kim, S.G., Seiden, S.W., Felder, S.D., Waspe, L.E. and Fisher, J.D. Is programmed stimulation of value predicting the long term success of antiarrhythmic drug therapy for ventricular tachycardias? *N. Engl. J. Med.* 1986; **315**: 356.

121. Mitchell, L.B., Duff, H.J., Manyari, D.E. and Wyse, D.G.

A randomized clinical trial of the noninvasive and invasive approaches to drug therapy of ventricular tachycardia. *N. Engl. J. Med.* 1987; **317**: 1681.

122. Platia, E.V. and Reid, P.R. Comparison of programmed electrical stimulation and ambulatory (Holter) monitoring in the management of ventricular tachycardia and ventricular fibrillation. *J. Am. Coll. Cardiol.* 1984; **3**: 493.

123. Kim, S.G. The management of patients with life threatening ventricular arrhythmias: programmed electrical stimulation or Holter monitoring (either or both). *Circulation* 1987; **76**: 1.

124. Simson, M.B. Clinical application of signal averaging. *Clin. Cardiol.* 1983; **1**: 109.

125. Gang, E.S., Peter, T., Rosenthal, M.E., Mandel, W.J. and Lass Y. Detection of late potentials on the surface of electrocardiogram in patients with unexplained syncope. *Am. J. Cardiol.* 1986; **58**: 1014.

126. Kuchar, D.L., Thorburn, C.W. and Sammel, N. Prediction of serious effects after myocardial infarction: Signal averaged electrocardiogram, Holter monitoring and radionuclide ventriculography. *J. Am. Coll. Cardiol.* 1987; **9**: 531.

127. Tofler, G.H. and the MILIS study group. Prognosis after cardiac arrest due to ventricular tachycardia or ventricular fibrillation associated with acute myocardial infarction (the MILIS study). *Am. J. Cardiol.* 1987; **60**: 755.

128. Von Olshausen, K., Schafer, A., Mehmel, H.C., Schwartz, F., Senges, J. and Kubler, W. Ventricular arrhythmias in idiopathic dilated cardiomyopathy. *Br. Heart J.* 1984; **51**: 195.

129. Meinertz, T., Hofmann, T., Kasper, W., *et al.* Significance of ventricular arrhythmias in idiopathic dilated cardiomyopathy. *Am. J. Cardiol.* 1984; **53**: 902.

130. Poll, D.S., Marchlinski, F.E., Falcone, R.A. and Simson, M.B. Abnormal signal averaged ECG in non ischemic congestive cardiomyopathy: Relationship to sustained ventricular arrhythmias. *Circulation* 1984; **70**: 253.

131. Coto, H., Maldonado, C., Palakurthy, P. and Flowers, N.C. Late potentials in normal subjects and in patients with ventricular tachycardia unrelated to myocardial infarction. *Am. J. Cardiol.* 1984; **55**: 384.

132. Neri, R., Mestroni, L., Salvi, A., Pandullo, C., Camerini, F. Ventricular arrhythmias in dilated cardiomyopathy: Efficacy of amiodarone. *Am. J. Cardiol.* 1987; **113**: 707.

133. Kowey, P.R., Eisenberg, R. and Engel, T.R. Sustained arrhythmias in hypertrophic cardiomyopathy. *N. Engl. J. Med.* 1984; **315**: 1566.

134. Borggrefe, M., Kuhn, H., Koniger, H.H., *et al.* Arrhythmias in hypertrophic obstructive and non-obstructive cardiomyopathy. *Eur. Heart J.* 1983; **4** (Suppl. F): 245.

135. McKenna, W.J., Oakley, C.M., Krikler, D.M. and Goodwin, J.F. Improved survival with amiodarone in patients with hypertrophic cardiomyopathy and ventricular tachycardia. *Br. Heart J.* 1985; **53**: 412.

136. Robertson, J.H., Bardy, G.H., German, L.D., Gallagher, J.J. and Kisslo, J. Comparison of two-dimensional echocardiographic and angiographic findings in arrhythmogenic right ventricular dysplasia. *Am. J. Cardiol.* 1985; **55**: 1506.

137. Fontaine, G., Frank, R., Tonet, J.L., *et al.* Arrhythmogenic right ventricular dysplasia: a clinical model for the study of chronic ventricular tachycardia. *Jpn. Circ. J.* 1984; **48**: 515.

138. Fontaine, G., Frank, R. and Gallais, Hammono, F. Electrocardiographie des potentials tardifs du syndrome de post-excitation. *Arch. Mal. Coeur* 1978; **78**: 854.

139. Blomstrom-Lundquist, C., Sabel, K. and Olsson, S.B. A long term follow up of 15 patients with arrhythmogenic right ventricular dysplasia. *Br. Heart J.* 1987; **58**: 477.

140. Gillette, P., Yeoman, M., Mullins, C. and McNamara, D. Sudden death after repair of tetralogy of Fallot. Electrocardiographic and electrophysiologic abnormalities. *Circulation* 1977; **56**: 566.

141. Deanfield, J., McKenna, W. and Rowland, E. Local abnormalities of right ventricualr depolarisation after repair of tetralogy of Fallot: A basis for ventricular arrhythmia. *Am. J. Cardiol.* 1985; **55**: 552.

142. Horowitz, L., Vetter, V., Harken, A. and Josephson, M. Electrophysiologic characteristics of sustained ventricular tachycardia occurring after repair of tetralogy of Fallot. *Am. J. Cardiol.* 1980; **46**: 446.

143. Garson, A., Randall, D., Gillette, P., Smith, R., Moak, J., Mcvey, P. and McNamara, D. Prevention of sudden death after repair of tetralogy of Fallot: Treatment of ventricular arrhythmias. *J. Am. Coll. Cardiol.* 1985; **6**: 221.

144. Morady, F., Shen, E., Bhandari, A., Schwartz, A. and Scheinman, M.M. Programmed ventricular stimulation in mitral valve prolapse: Analysis of 36 patients *Am. J. Cardiol.* 1984; **53**: 135.

145. Rosenthal, M.E., Hamer, A., Gang, E.S., Oseran, D.S., Mandel, W.J. and Peter, T. The yield of programmed ventricular stimulation in mitral valve prolapse patients with ventricular arrhythmias. *Am. Heart J.* **110**: 970, 1985.

146. Deal, B.J., Miller, S.M., Scagliotti, D., Prechel, D., Gallastegui, J.L. and Hariman, R.J. Ventricular tachycardia in a young population without overt heart disease. *Circulation* 1986; **73**: 1111.

147. Foale, R.A., Nihoyannopoulos, P., Ribeiro, P., McKenna, W.J., Oakley, C.M., Krikler, D.M. and Rowland, E. Right ventricular abnormalities in ventricular tachycardias of right ventricular origin: Relation to electrophysiologic abnormalities. *Br. Heart J.* 1986; **56**: 45.

148. Mogera, T., Salvi, A., Alberti, E., Silvestri, F. and Camerini, F. Morphological findings in apparently idiopathic ventricular tachycardia. An echocardiographic haemodynamic and histologic study. *Eur. Heart J.* 1985; **6**: 323.

149. Strain, J.E., Grose, R.M., Factor, S.M. and Fisher, J.D. Results of endomyocardial biopsy in patients with spontaneous ventricular tachycardia but without apparent heart disease. *Circulation* 1983; **68**: 1171.

150. James, T.N., Forggatt, P. and Marshall, T.K. Sudden death in young athletes. *Ann. Intern. Med.* 1967; **67**: 1013.

151. Maron, B.J. Right ventricular cardiomyopathy: Another cause of sudden death in the young. *N. Engl. J. Med.* 1988; **318**: 178.

152. Thiene, G., Nava, A., Corrado, D., Rossi, L. and Pennelli, N. Right ventricular cardiomyopathy and sudden death in young people. *N. Engl. J. Med.* 1988; **318**: 129.

153. Buxton, A.E., Marchlinski, F.E., Doherty, J.U. *et al.* Repetitive, monomorphic ventricular tachycardia: clinical and electrophysiologic characteristics in patients with and patients without heart disease. *Am. J. Cardiol.* 1984; **54**: 997.

154. Gallavardin, L. Extrasystolie ventriculaire à paroxysmes tachycardiques prolongés. *Arch. Mal. Coeur* 1922; **15**: 298,

155. Zimmerman, M., Maisonblanche, P., Cauchemez, B., Leclercq, J. and Coumel, P. Determinants of the spontaneous ectopic activity in repetitive monomorphic idiopathic ventricular tachycardia. *J. Am. Coll. Cardiol.* 1986; **7**: 1219.

156. Belhassen, B., Shapira, I., Pelleg, A., Copperman, I., Kauli, N. and Laniado, S. Idiopathic recurrent sustained ventricular tachycardia responsive to verapamil: An ECG electrophysiologic entity. *Am. Heart J.* 1984; **108**: 1034.

157. Ohe, T., Shimomura, K., Aihara, N. *et al.* Idiopathic sustained ventricular tachycardia: Clinical and electrophysiologic characteristics. *Circulation* 1988; **77**: 560.

158. Mehta, D., Ward, D.E., Davies, M.J. and Camm, A.J. Value of signal averaged electrocardiograms and myocardial biopsies in ventricular tachycardia associated with 'normal heart'. *Circulation* 1988; 78:II–301.

159. Mehta, D., Odawara, H., McKenna, W.J., Davies, M.J. and Camm, A.J. Echocardiographic and histologic evaluation of the right ventricle in ventricular tachycardias of left bundle branch morpology without overt cardiac abnormality. *Am. J. Cardiol.* 1989 (in press).

160. Naccarelli, G.V., Zipes, D.P., Rahilly, G.T., Heger, J.J. and Prystowsky, E.N. Influence of tachycardia cycle length and antiarrhythmic drugs on pacing termination and acceleration of ventricular tachycardia. *Am. Heart J.* 1983; 105: 1.

161. Rubin, D.A., Nieminski, K.E., Monteferrante, J.C. Magee, T., Reed, G.E. and Herman, M.V. Ventricular arrhythmias after bypass graft surgery: Incidence, risk factors and long-term prognosis. *J. Am. Coll. Cardiol.* 1985; 6: 307.

162. Waxman, H.L., Buxton, A.E., Sadowski and Josephson, M.E. The response to procainamide during electrophysiological study for sustained ventricular tachyarrhythmias predicts the response to other medications. *Circulation* 1983; 67: 30.

163. Reid, P.R., Griffiths, L.S.C., Platia, E.V. and Ord, S. Evaluation of flecainide acetate in the management of patients at high risk of sudden cardiac death. *Am. J. Cardiol.* 1984; 53: 108B.

164. Bauman, J.L., Berk, S.I., Hariman, R.J. *et al.* Amiodarone for sustained ventricular tachycardia: Efficacy, safety and factors influencing long-term outcome. *Am. Heart J.* 1987; 114: 1436.

165. Anastasiou-Nana, M.I., Anderson, J.L., Askins, J.C., Gilbert, E.M., Nanas, J.N. and Menlove, R.L. Long term experience with sotalol in the treatment of complex ventricular arrhythmias. *Am. Heart J.* 1987; 114: 288.

166. Ward, D.E., Nathan, A.W. and Camm, A.J. Fascicular tachycardia sensitive to calcium antagonists. *Eur. Heart J.* 1984; 5: 896.

167. Lerman, B.B., Belardinelli, L., West, A., Berne, R.M. and DiMarco, J. Adensosine-sensitive ventricular tachycardia: Evidence suggesting cyclic AMP-mediated triggered activity. *Circulation* 1986; 74: 270.

168. Duff, H.J., Mitchell, L.B., Manyari, D. and Wyse, D.G. Mexiletine-Quinidine combination: electrophysiological correlates of a favourable antiarrhythmic interaction in humans. *J. Am. Coll. Cardiol.* 1987; 10: 1149.

169. Haines, D.E., Lerman, B.B., Kron, I.L. and DiMarco, J.P. Surgical ablation of ventricular tachycardia with sequential map-guided subendocardial resection: Electrophysiological assessment and long-term follow-up. *Circulation* 1988; 77: 131.

170. Morady, F., Scheinman, M.M., DiCarlo, L.A. *et al.* Catheter ablation of ventricular tachycardia with intracardiac shocks: results in 33 patients. *Circulation* 1987; 75: 1037.

171. Mirowsky, M. The automatic implantable cardioverter-defibrillator: An overview. *J. Am. Coll. Cardiol.* 1985; 6: 461.

172. Gabry, M.D., Brodman, R., Johnston, D. *et al.* Automatic implantable defibrillator experience. *J. Am. Coll. Cardiol.* 1987; 9: 1349.

173. Fisher, J.D., Johnston, D.R., Furman, S., Mercando, A.D. and Kim, S.G. Long-term efficacy of antitachycardia pacing for supraventricular and ventricular tachycardias. *Am. J. Cardiol.* 1987; 60: 1133.

174. Fontaine, G., Frank, R. and Grosgogeat, Y. Torsades de pointes. Definition and management. *Mod. Conc. Cardiovasc. Dis.* 1982; 51: 103.

175. Kay, G.N., Plumb, V.J., Arciniegas, J.G., Henthorn, R.W. and Waldo, A.L. Torsade de pointes: The long-short initiation sequence and other clinical features. Observa-

tions on 32 patients. *J. Am. Coll. Cardiol.* 1983; 2: 806.

176. Surawicz, B. and Knoebel, S.B. Long QT: Good, bad or indifferent? *J. Am. Coll. Cardiol.* 1984; 4: 398.

177. Schecter, E., Freeman, C.C. and Lazzara, R. Afterdepolarizations as a mechanism for the long QT syndrome: Electrophysiologic studies of a case. *J. Am. Coll. Cardiol.* 1984; 3: 1556.

178. Bonatti, V., Rolli, A. and Botti, G. Monophasic action potential studies in human subjects with prolonged repolarization and long QT syndromes. *Eur. Heart J.* 1985; 6 (Suppl. D): 131.

179. Baroy, J.H., Ungerleider, R.M., Smith, W.M. and Ideker, R.E. A mechanism of torsades de pointes in a canine model. *Circulation* 1983; 67: 52.

180. Schwarts, P.J. Idiopathic long QT Syndrome: Progress and questions. *Am. Heart J.* 1985; 109: 405.

181. Jervell, A. and Lange-Nielsen, F. Congenital deaf-mutism, functional heart disease with prolongation of the QT interval and sudden death. *Am. Heart J.* 1957; 54: 59.

182. Romano, C., Gemme, G. and Pongiglione, R. Aritmie cardiache rare dell'eta pediatrica. II Accessi sincopali per fibrillazione ventricolare parossitica. *La Clinic Paed* 1963; 45: 656.

183. Ward, O.C. New familial cardiac syndrome in children. *J. Irish Med. Assoc.* 1964; 54: 103.

184. Bhandari, A.K., Shapiro, W.A., Morady, F., Shen, E.N., Mason, J. and Scheinman, M.M. Electrophysiologic testing in patients with the long QT syndrome. *J. Am. Coll. Cardiol.* 1985; 6: 1110.

185. Moss, A.J., Schwartz, P.J., Crampton, R.S., Locati, E. and Carleen, E. The long QT syndrome: A prospective international study. *Circulation* 1985; 71: 17.

186. Wilmer, C.I., Stein, B. and Morris, D.C. Atrioventricular pacemaker placement in Romano–Ward syndrome and recurrent torsades de pointes. *Am. J. Cardiol.* 1987; 59: 171.

187. Ewy, G.A. Ventricular fibrillation masquerading as asystole. *Ann. Emerg. Med.* 1984; 13: 811.

188. Friedman, W.F. Physiological properties of the developing heart. In: *Paediatric Cardiology* 6th edn. Marcelletti, Anderson, Becker, Corno, di Coalo, Mazzeru, eds. Churchill Livingstone: 1986.

189. Gikonyo, B., Dunnigan, A. and Woodrow Benson, D. Cardiovascular collapse in infants: Association with paroxysmal atrial tachycardia. *Paediatrics* 1985; 76: 922.

190. Garson, A., Smith, R., Moak, J., Ross, B. and McNamara, D. Ventricular arrhythmias and sudden death in children. *J. Am. Coll. Cardiol.* 1985; 5: 130B.

191. Woodrow Benson, D., Dunugan, A., Stoba, R. and Benditt, D.G. Atrial pacing from the esophagus in the diagnosis and management of tachycardia and palpitations. *J. Pediatr.* 1983; 102: 40.

192. Gallagher, J.J., Smith, W.M., Kerr, C.R. *et al.* Esophageal pacing: a diagnostic and therapeutic tool. *Circulation* 1982; 65: 336.

193. Garson, A., Smith, R.T., Moak, J.P. *et al.* Incessant ventricular tachycardia in infants: myocardial hamartomas and surgical cure. *J. Am. Coll. Cardiol.* 1987; 10: 619.

194. Shahar, E., Barzilay, Z. and Frand, M. Verapamil in the treatment of paroxysmal supraventricular tachycardia in infants and children. *J. Pediatr.* 1981; 98: 323.

195. Soler-Soler, J., Sagrista-Sauleda, J., Cabrera, A. *et al.* Effect of verapamil in infants with paroxysmal supraventricular tachycardia. *Circulation* 1979; 59: 876.

196. Epstein, M.L., Kiel, E.A. and Victoria, B.E. Cardiac decompensation following verapamil therapy in infants with supraventricular tachycardia. *Paediatrics* 1985; 75: 737.

197. Overholt, E.D., Rheuban, K.S., Gutgesell, H.P., Lerman, B.B. and Di Marco, J.P. Usefulness of adenosine for

arrhythmias in infants and children. *Am. J. Cardiol.* 1988; **61**: 336.

198. Garson, A. and Gillette, P.C. Functional ectopic tachycardia in children: Electrocardiography, electrophysiology and pharmacologic response. *Am. J. Cardiol.* 1979; **44**: 298.

199. Kerr, C. and Mason, M. Incidence and clincial significance of accelerated junctional rhythm following open heart surgery. *Am. Heart J.* 1985; **110**: 966.

200. Gillette, P., Garson, A., Porter, C. *et al.* Junctional automatic ectopic tachycardia: new proposed treatment by transcatheter His bundle ablation. *Am. Heart J.* 1983; **106**: 619.

201. Gillette, P. and Garson, A. *Paediatric Cardiac Dysrhythmias* London: Grune and Stratton, 1981.

202. Gillette, P., Smith, R., Mullins, C. *et al.* Chronic supraventricular tachycardia. A curable cause of congestive cardiomyopathy. *J. Am. Med. Assoc.* 1985; **253**: 391.

203. Kugler, J., Baisch, S., Cheatham, J. *et al.* Improvement of left ventricular dysfunction after control of persistent tachycardia. *J. Pediatr.* 1984; **105**: 543.

204. Mehta, A.V., Sanchez, G.R., Sacks, E.J., Casta, A., Dunn, J.M. and Donner, R.M. Ectopic automatic atrial tachycardia in children: clinical characteristics, management and follow-up. *J. Am. Coll. Cardiol.* 1985; **11**: 379.

205. Duster, M., Bink-Boelkens, M., Wampler, D., Gillette, P., McNamara, D. and Cooley, D. Long term follow-up of dysrhythmias following the Mustard procedure. *J. Am. Coll. Cardiol.* 1985; **109**: 1323.

206. Hayes, C.J. and Gersony, W.M. Arrhythmias after the Mustard operation for transposition of the great arteries: a long-term study. *J. Am. Coll. Cardiol.* 1986; **7**: 133.

207. Garson, A., Bink-Boelkens, M., Hesslein, S.P. *et al.* Atrial flutter in the young: A collaborative study of 380 cases. *Paediatr. Cardiol.* 1985; **6**: 871.

208. Gillette, P.C., Wampler, D.G., Shannon, C. and Ott, D. Use of cardiac pacing after the Mustard operation for transposition of the great arteries. *J. Am. Coll. Cardiol.* 1986; **7**: 138.

209. Garson, A. Ventricular arrhythmias in the young: differences and similarities to adults. *Clin. Prog. Electrophysiol Pacing* 1986; **4**: 175.

210. Eldar, M., Griffin, J.C., Abbott, J.A. *et al.* Permanent cardiac pacing in patients with the long QT syndrome. *J. Am. Coll. Cardiol.* 1987; **10**: 600.

211. Fulton, D.R., Chung, K.J., Tabakin, B.S. and Keane, J.F. Ventricular tachycardia in children without heart disease. *Am. J. Cardiol.* 1985; **55**: 1328.

212. Coumel, P., Fidelle, J., Lucet, V., Attuel, P. and Bouvrain, Y. Catecholamine-induced severe ventricular arrhythmias with Adams–Stokes syndrome in children: Report of four cases. *Br. Heart J.* 1978; **40** (Suppl.): 28.

213. Deal, B.J., Scagliotti, D., Miller, S.M., Gallastegni, J.L., Hariman, R.J. and Levitsky, S. Electrophysiologic drug testing in symptomatic ventricular arrhythmias after repair of tetralogy of Fallot. *Am. J. Cardiol.* 1987; **59**: 1380.

214. Garson, A. Medicolegal problems in the management of cardiac arrhythmias in children. *Pediatrics* 1987; **79**: 84.

215. James, F., Kaplan, S. and Chou, T. Unexpected cardiac arrest in patients after surgical correction of tetralogy of Fallot. *Circulation* 1975; **52**: 691.

216. Chen, D. and Moller, J. Comparison of late clinical status between patients with different haemodynamic findings after repair of tetralogy of Fallot. *Am. Heart J.* 1987; **113**: 767.

217. Lamb, L.E., Dermksian, G. and Sarnoff, C.A. Significant cardiac arrhythmias induced by common respiratory manoeuvers. *Am. J. Cardiol.* 1958; **2**: 563.

218. Cohen, M.V. Ventricular fibrillation precipitated by carotid sinus pressure: Case report and review of the literature.

Am. Heart J. 1972; **84**: 681.

219. Waxman, M.B., Wald, R.W., Finley, J.P., Bonet, J.F., Downar, E. and Sharma, A.D. Valsalva termination of ventricular tachycardia. *Circulation* 1980; **62**: 843.

220. Hunt, H.G., Whitaker, D.K. and Wilmott, N.J. Water temperature and diving reflex (letter). *Lancet* 1975; **i**: 572.

221. Wildenthal, K., Leshin, S.J., Atkins, J.M. and Skelton, C.L. The diving reflex used to treat paroxysmal atrial tachycardia. *Lancet* 1975; **i**: 12.

222. Beck C.S. Resuscitation for cardiac standstill and ventricular fibrillation occurring during operation. *Am. J. Surg.* 1941; **54**: 273.

223. Zoll, P.M., Linenthal, A.J., Gibson, W., Paul, M.H. and Norman, L.R. Termination of ventricular fibrillation in man by externally applied electric countershock. *N. Engl. J. Med.* 1956; **254**: 727.

224. Lown, B., Amarsingham, R. and Neuman, J. New method for terminating cardiac arrhythmias—use of synchronized capacitor discharge. *J. Am. Med. Assoc.* 1962; **182**: 548.

225. Cobb, F.R., Wallace, A.G. and Wagner, G.S. Cardiac inotropic and coronary vascular responses to countershock: evidence for excitation of intracardiac nerves. *Circ. Res.* 1968; **23**: 731.

226. Cotoi, S. Precordial thump and termination of cardiac reentrant tachyarrhythmias. *Am. Heart J.* 1981; **101**: 675.

227. Crampton, R. Accepted, controversial and speculative aspects of ventricular defibrillation. *Prog. Cardiovasc. Dis.* 1980; **3**: 167.

228. Kerber, R.E., Jensen, S.R. Grayzel, J., Kennedy, J. and Hoyt, R. Elective cardioversion: Influence of paddle electrode location and size on success rates and energy requirements. *N. Engl. J. Med.* 1981; **305**: 658.

229. Resnekov, J. and McDonald, L. Complications in 220 patients with cardiac dysrhythmias treated by phased direct current shock, and indications for electroversion. *Br. Heart J.* 1967; **29**: 926.

230. Rabbino, M.D., Likoff, W. and Dreifus, L.S. Complications and limitations of direct current countershock. *J. Am. Med. Assoc.* 1964; **190**: 417.

231. Mann, D.L., Maisel, A.S., Atwood, J.E., Engler, R.L. and Le Winter, M.M. Absence of cardioversion-induced ventricular arrhythmias in patients with therapeutic digoxin levels. *J. Am. Coll. Cardiol.* 1985; **5**: 882.

232. Bjerkelund, C.K. and Orning, O.M. The efficacy of anticoagulant therapy in preventing embolism related to DC electrical conversion of atrial fibrillation. *Am. J. Cardiol.* 1969; **23**: 208.

233. Jones, J.L. and Jones, R.E. Decreased defibrillator-induced dysfunction with biphasic rectangular waveforms. *Am. J. Physiol.* 1983; **245**: H60.

234. Babbs, C.F., Tacker, W.A., Van Fleet, J.F., Bourland, J.D. and Geddes, L.A. Therapeutic indices for transchest defibrillator shocks: effective, damaging and lethal electrical doses. *Am. Heart J.* 1980; **99**: 734.

235. Ehsani, A., Ewy, G.A. and Sobel, B.E. Effects of electrical countershock on serum creatinine phosphokinase (CPK) isoenzyme activity. *Am. J. Cardiol.* 1976; **37**: 12.

236. Levine, P.A., Barold, S.S., Fletcher, R.D. *et al.* Adverse acute and chronic effects of electrical defibrillation and cardioversion on implanted unipolar cardiac pacing systems. *J. Am. Coll. Cardiol.* 1983; **1**: 1413.

237. Cummins, R.O., Eisenberg, M.S., Litwin, P. *et al.* Automatic external defibrillators used by emergency medical technicians. *J. Am. Med. Assoc.* 1987; **257**: 1605.

238. Vaughan Williams, E.M. A classification of antiarrhythmic actions reassessed after a decade of new drugs. *J. Clin. Pharmacol.* 1984; **24**: 129.

239. Cobbe, S.M. Clinical usefulness of the Vaughan Williams classification system. *Eur. Heart J.* 1987; **8** (Suppl. A.): 65.

240. Touboul, P., Attalah, G., Gressard, A., Michelon, G.,

Chatelain, M.T. and Delahaye, J.P. Effets electrophysiologiques des agents antiarythmiques chez l'homme. *Arch. Mal. Coeur* 1979; **72**: 72.

241. Cosin-Aguilar, J. and Hernandez-Martinez, A. The clinical usefulness of the antiarrhythmic drug quinidine. *Eur. Heart J.* 1987; **8** (Suppl. A): 1.

242. Greenblatt, D.J., Pfeifer, H.J., Ochs, H.R. *et al.* Pharmacokinetics of quinidine after intravenous, intramuscular, and oral administration. *J. Pharmacol. Exp. Ther.* 1977; **202**: 365.

243. Kessler, K.M., Lowenthal, D.T., Warner, H., Gibson, T., Briggs, W. and Reidenberg, M.M. Quinidine elimination in patients with congestive heart failure or poor renal function. *N. Engl. J. Med.* 1974; **290**: 706.

244. Hoffman, B.F., Rosen, M.R. and Wit, A.L. Electrophysiology and pharmacology of cardiac arrhythmias. VII. Cardiac effects of quinidine and procain amide. B. *Am. Heart J.* 1975; **90**: 117.

245. Mason, J.W., Winkle, R.A., Rider, A.K., Stinson, E.B. and Harrison, D.C. The electrophysiologic effects of quinidine in the transplanted human heart. *J. Clin. Invest.* 1977; **59**: 481.

246. Josephson, M.E., Seides, S.F., Batsford, W.P. *et al.* The electrophysiologic effects of intramuscular quinidine on the atrioventricular conducting system in man. *Am. Heart J.* 1974; **87**: 55.

247. Prasad, K. Use of glucagon in the treatment of quinidine toxicity in the heart. *Cardiovasc. Res.* 1977; **11**: 55.

248. Wu, D., Hung, J.S., Kuo, C.T., Hsu, K.S. and Sheih, W.B. Effects of quinidine on atrioventricular nodal reentrant paroxysmal tachycardia. *Circulation* 1981; **64**: 823.

249. Salerno, D.M. Review: Antiarrhythmic drugs: 1987. Part II: Class IA and IB antiarrhythmic drugs: a review of their pharmacokinetics, electrophysiology, efficacy, and toxicity. *J. Electrophysiol.* 1987; **1**: 300.

250. Di Marco, J.P., Garan, H. and Ruskin, J.N. Quinidine for ventricular arrhythmias: value of electrophysiologic testing. *Am. J. Cardiol.* 1983; **51**: 90.

251. Selzer, A. and Wray, H.W. Quinidine syncope. Paroxysmal ventricular fibrillation during treatment of chronic atrial arrhythmias. *Circulation* 1964; **30**: 17.

252. Roden, D.M., Woosley, R.L., Bostick, D., Bernard, I. and Primm, R.K. Quinidine-induced long QT syndrome: Incidence and presenting features. *Circulation* 1983; **68** (Suppl. III): III.

253. Cohen, I.S., Hershel, J. and Cohen, S.I. Adverse reactions to quinidine in hospitalized patients: findings based on data from the Boston Collaborative Drug Surveillance Program. *Prog. Cardiovasc. Dis.* 1977; **20**: 151.

254. Schenck-Gustafsson, K., Jogestrand, T., Nordlander, R. and Dahlquist, R. Quinidine-induced changes of digoxin in serum and skeletal muscle. *Eur. Heart J.* 1984; **5** (Abstr. Suppl. 1): 204.

255. Hinderling, P.H. and Garret, E.R. Pharmacokinetics of the antiarrhythmic disopyramide in healthy humans. *J. Pharmacokinet Biopharm* 1976; **4**: 199.

256. Ribeiro, C. and Longo, A. Procainamide and disopyramide. *Eur. Heart J.* 1987; **8** (Suppl. A): 11.

257. Harrison, D.C., Meffin, P.J. and Winkle, R.A. Clinical pharmacokinetics of antiarrhythmic drugs. *Prog. Cardiovasc. Dis.* 1977; **20**: 217.

258. Danilo, P. Jr. and Rosen, M.R. Cardiac effects of disophyramide. *Am. Heart J.* 1976; **92**: 532.

259. Birkhead, J.S. and Vaughan Williams, E.M. Dual effects of disopyramide on atrial and atrioventricular conduction and refractory periods. *Br. Heart J.* 1977; **390**: 657.

260. Jensen, G., Sigurd, B. and Uhrenholt, A. Circulatory effects of intravenous disopyramide in heart failure. *J. Intern. Med. Res.* 1976; **4**: (Suppl. I): 42.

261. Vismara, L.A., DeMaria, A.N. Amsterdam, E.A. and

Mason, D.T. Hemodynamic assessment of intravenous disopyramide phosphate effects on ventricular function and peripheral circulation in coronary heart disease. *Pharmacologist* 1975; **17**: 282.

262. Podrid, P.J., Schoenberger, A. and Lown, B. Congestive heart failure caused by oral disopyramide. *N. Engl. J. Med.* 1980; **302**: 614.

263. Brugada, P. and Wellens, H.J.J. Effects of intravenous and oral disopyramide on paroxysmal atrioventricular nodal tachycardia. *Am. J. Cardiol.* 1984; **53**: 88.

264. Spurrell, R.A.J., Thorburn, C.W., Camm, A.J., Sowton, E. and Deuchar, D.C. Effects of disopyramide on elecrophysiologic properties of specialized conduction system in man and on accessory atrioventricular pathway in Wolff–Parkinson–White syndrome. *Br. Heart J.* 1975; **37**: 861.

265. Wellens, H.J.J., Bar, F.W., Dassen, W.R.M., Vanagt, E.J. and Farre, J. Effect of drugs in the Wolff–Parkinson–White syndrome. Importance of initial length of effective refractory period of accessory pathway. *Am. J. Cardiol.* 1980; **46**: 665.

266. Smith, W.S., Vismara, L.A. and Kalmansohm, R.B. Clinical studies of Norpace. Part I. *Angiology* 1975; **26** (Suppl. I): 124.

267. Mizgala, H.F. and Huvelle, P.R. Acute termination of cardiac arrhythmias with intravenous disopyramide. *J. Intern. Med. Res.* 1976; **4** (Suppl. I): 82.

268. Teichman, S.L., Ferrick, A., Kim, S.S., Matos, J.A., Waspe, L.W. and Fisher, J.D. Disopyramide-pyridostigmine interaction: Selective reversal of anticholinergic symptoms with preservation of antiarrhythmic effect. *J. Am. Coll. Cardiol.* 1987; **10**: 633.

269. Meltzer, R.S., Robert, E.W., Mcmorrow, M. and Martin, R.P. Atypical ventricular tachycardia as a manifestation of disopyramide toxicity. *Am. J. Cardiol.* 1978; **42**: 1049.

270. Tzivoni, D., Keven, D. and Stern, S. Disopyramide-induced torsade de pointes. *Arch. Intern. Med.* 1980; **140**: 413.

271. Koch-Weser, J. and Klein, S.W. Procainamide dosage schedules, plasma concentrations and clinical effects. *J. Am. Med. Assoc.* 1971; **215**: 1454.

277. Josephson, M.E., Caracta, A.R., Ricauti, M.A., Lau, S.H. and Damato, A.N. Electrophysiologic properties of procainamide in man. *Am. J. Cardiol.* 1974; **33**: 596.

278. Kayden, H.J., Brodie, B.B. and Steele, J.M. Procaine amide—a review. *Circulation* 1957; **15**:118.

279. Marchlinski, F.E., Buxton, A.E., Vassallo, J.A. *et al.* Comparative electrophysiologic effects of intravenous and oral procainamide in patients with sustained ventricular arrhythmias. *J. Am. Coll. Cardiol.* 1984; **6**: 1247.

280. Branch, R.A., Shand, D.G., Wilkinson, G.R. and Nies, A.S. The reduction of lidocaine clearance by DL-propranolol—an example of a hemodynamic drug interaction. *J. Pharmacol. Exp. Ther.* 1973; **184**: 515.

281. Rizzon, P., Di Biase, M., Favale, S. and Visani, L. Class IB agents lidocaine, mexiletine, tocainide, phenytoin. *Eur. Heart J.* 1987; **8** (Suppl. A): 21.

282. Rosen, K.M., Lau, S.H., Weiss, M.B. and Damato, A.N. The effect of lidocaine on atrioventricular and intraventricular conduction in man. *Am. J. Cardiol.* 1970; **25**: 1.

283. Roos, J.C. and Dunning, A.J. Effects of lidocaine on impulse formation and conduction defects in man. *Am. Heart J.* 1975; **89**: 686.

284. Schumaker, R.R., Lieberson, A.D., Childress, R.H. and Williams, J.F. Jr. Hemodynamic effects of lidocaine in patients with heart disease. *Circulation* 1968; **37**: 965.

285. Marriott, H.J.L. and Bieza, C.F. Alarming ventricular acceleration after lidocaine administration. *Chest* 1972; **61**: 682.

286. Koster, R.W. and Dunning, A.J. Intramuscular lidocaine for prevention of lethal arrhythmias in the prehospitaliza-

tion phase of acute myocardial infarction. *N. Engl. J. Med.* 1985; **313**: 1105.

287. Bigger, J.T. Jr. and Heissenbuttel, R.H. The use of procaine amide and lidocaine in the treatment of cardiac arrhythmias. *Prog. Cardiovasc. Dis.* 1969; **11**: 515.

288. Danilo, P. Jr. Mexiletine. *Am. Heart J.* 1979; **97**: 399.

289. Stein, J., Podrid, P.J. and Lown, B. Effects of oral mexiletine on left and right ventricular function. *Am. J. Cardiol.* 1984; **54**: 575.

290. Chew, C.Y.C., Collett, J. and Singh, B.N. Mexiletine: a review of its pharmacological properties and therapeutic efficacy in arrhythmias. *Drugs* 1979; **17**: 161.

291. Schoenfeld, M.H., Whitford, E., McGovern, B., Garan, H. and Ruskin, J.N. Oral mexiletine in the treatment of refractory ventricular arrhythmias: the role of electrophysiologic techniques. *Am. Heart J.* 1984; **107**: 1071.

292. Rutledge, J.C., Harris, F. and Amsterdam, E.A. Clinical evaluation of oral mexiletine therapy in the treatment of ventricular arrhythmias. *J. Am. Coll. Cardiol.* 1985; **6**: 780.

293. Pentikainen, P.J., Koivula, I.H. and Hitunen, H.A. Effect of rifampicin treatment on the kinetics of mexiletine. *Eur. J. Clin. Pharmacol.* 1982; **23**: 261.

294. Conard, G.J. and Ober, R.E. Metabolism of flecainide. *Am. J. Cardiol.* 1984; **53**: 41B.

295. Salerno, D.M. Review: antiarrhythmic drugs: 1987. Part III: Class IC antiarrhythmic drugs—a review of their pharmacokinetics, electrophysiology, efficacy, and toxicity. *J. Electrophysiol.* 1987; **1**: 435.

296. Camm, A.J. Cardiac electrophysiology of four new antiarrhythmic drugs—encainide, flecainide, lorcainide and tocainide. *Eur. Heart J.* 1984; **5** (Suppl. B): 75.

297. Vik-Mo, H., Ohm, O.-J. and Lund-Johansen, P. Electrophysiologic effects of flecainide acetate in patients with sinus nodal dysfunction. *Am. J. Cardiol.* 1982; **50**: 1090.

298. Hellestrand, J.J., Bexton, R.S., Nathan, A.W., Spurrell, R.A.J. and Camm, A.J. Acute electrophysiological effects of flecainide acetate on cardiac conduction and refractoriness in man. *Br. Heart J.* 1982; **48**, 140.

299. Este, N.A.M., Garan, H. and Ruskin, J.N. Electrophysiologic properties of flecainide acetate. *Am. J. Cardiol.* 1984; **53**: 26B.

300. Hellestrand, K.J., Nathan, A.W., Bexton, R.S., Spurrell, R.A.J. and Camm, A.J. Cardiac electrophysiologic effects of flecainide acetate for paroxysmal reentrant junctional tachycardia. *Am. J. Cardiol.* 1983; **51**: 770.

301. Hellestrand, K.J., Nathan, A.W., Bexton, R.S. and Camm, A.J. Electrophysiologic effects of flecainide acetate on sinus node function, anomalous atrioventricular connections, and pacemaker thresholds. *Am. J. Cardiol.* 1984; **53**: 30B.

302. Cohen, A.A., Daru, V., Covelli, G., Gonzalez, M., Villamayor, R. and Tronge, J.E. Hemodynamic effects of intravenous flecainide in acute noncomplicated myocardial infarction. *Am. Heart J.* 1985; **110**: 1193.

303. Josephson, MA., Ikeda, N. and Singh, B.N. Effects of flecainide on ventricular function: clinical and experimental correlations. *Am. J. Cardiol.* 1984; **53**: 95B.

304. Serruys, P.W., Vanhaleweyk, G., Van Den Brand, M., Verdouw, P., Lubsen, J. and Hugenholtz, P.G. The hemodynamic effect of intravenous flecainide acetate in patients with coronary artery disease. *Br. J. Clin. Pharmacol.* 1983; **16**: 51.

305. Bexton, R.S., Hellestrand, K.J., Nathan, A.W., Spurrell, R.A.J. and Camm, A.J. A comparison of the antiarrhythmic effects on AV junctional re-entrant tachycardia of oral and intravenous flecainide acetate. *Eur. Heart J.* 1983; **4**: 92.

306. Neuss, H., Golling, F.R., Weismuller, P., Schlepper, M. and Thormann, J. Effects of flecainide (F) in atrioventricular nodal (AVN) reentrant tachycardia. *Eur. Heart J.*

1984; **5** (Abstr. Suppl. 1): Abstr. 1155.

307. Neuss, H., Buss, J., Schlepper, M. *et al.* Effects of flecainide on electrophysiological properties of accessory pathways in the Wolff–Parkinson–White syndrome. *Eur. Heart J.* 1983; **4**: 347.

308. Orning, O.M. The use of tocainide, encainide, lorcainide and flecainide for supraventricular arrhythmias. *Eur. Heart J.* 1984; **5** (Suppl. B): 81.

309. Kim, S.S., Lal, R. and Ruffy, R. Treatment of paroxysmal supraventricular tachycardia with flecainide acetate. *Am. J. Cardiol.* 1986; **58**: 80.

310. Gentzkow, G.D. and Sullivan, J.Y. Extracardiac adverse effects on flecainide. *Am. J. Cardiol.* 1984; **53**: 101B.

311. Lewis, G.P. and Holtzman, J.L. Interaction of flecainide with digoxin and propranolol. *Am. J. Cardiol.* 1984; **53**: 52B.

312. Shea, P., Lal, R., Kim, S.S., Schechtman, K. and Ruffy, R. Flecainide and amiodarone interaction. *J. Am. Coll. Cardiol.* 1986; **7**: 1127.

313. Conolly, M.E., Kesting, F. and Dollery, C.T. The clinical pharmacology of beta-adrenoreceptor-blocking drugs. *Prog. Cardiovasc. Dis.* 1976; **19**: 203.

314. Wit, A.L., Hoffman, B.F. and Rosen, M.R. Electrophysiology and pharmacology of cardiac arrhythmias. IX. Cardiac electrophysiologic effects of beta adrenergic receptor stimulation and blockade. Part C. *Am. Heart J.* 1975; **90**: 795.

315. Coumel, P., Leclerq, J.-F. and Escoubet, B. Beta-blockers: use for arrhythmias. *Eur. Heart J.* 1987; **8** (Suppl. A): 41.

316. Rosenbaum, M.B., Chiale, PA., Ryba, D. and Elizari, U.M. Control of tachyarrhythmias associated with Wolff–Parkinson–White syndrome by amiodarone hydrochloride. *Am. J. Cardiol.* 1974; **34**: 215.

317. Holt, D.W., Tucker, G.T., Jackson, P.R. and Storey, G.C.A. Amiodarone pharmacokinetics. *Am. Heart J.* 1983; **106**: 840.

318. Storey, G.C. and Holt, D.W. High performance liquid chromotographic measurements of amiodarone and desethyl amiodarone in plasma or serum at the concentrations obtained following a single 400 mg dose. *J. Chromatogr.* 1982; **245**: 377.

319. Wilkinson, P.R., Rees, J.R., Storey, G.C. and Holt, D.W. Amiodarone prolonged elimination following cessation of chronic therapy. *Am. Heart J.* 1984; **107**: 787.

320. Benaim, R., Denizeau, J.P., Melon, J. *et al.* Les effets antiarythmiques de l'amiodarone injectable. A propos de 100 cas. *Arch. Mal. Coeur* 1976; **69**: 513.

321. Touboul, P., Atallah, G., Gressard, A. and Kirkorian, G. Effects of amiodarone on sinus node in man. *Br. Heart J.* 1979; **42**: 573.

322. Waleffe, A., Bruninx, P. and Kulbertus, H.E. Effects of amiodarone studied by programmed electrical stimulation of the heart in patients with paroxysmal reentrant supraventricular tachycardia. *J. Electrocardiol.* 1981; **11**: 253.

323. Marcus, F.I., Fontaine, G.H., Frank, R. and Grosgogeat, Y. Clinical pharmacology and therapeutic applications of the antiarrhythmic agent, amiodarone. *Am. Heart J.* 1981; **101**: 480.

324. Reddy, C.P. and Kuo, C.S. Effect of amiodarone on retrograde conduction and refractoriness of the His–Purkinje system in man. *Br. Heart J.* 1984; **51**: 648.

325. Shanasa, M., Denker, S.T., Mahmud, R., Lehmann, M., Estrada, A. and Akhtar, M. Effect of amiodarone on conduction and refractoriness of the Purkinje system in the human heart. *J. Am. Coll. Cardiol.* 1984; **4**: 105.

326. Pritchard, D.A., Singh, B.N. and Hurley, P.J. Effects of amiodarone on thyroid function in patients with ischaemic heart disease. *Br. Heart J.* 1975; **37**: 856.

327. Wellens, H.J.J., Lie, K.I., Bar, F.W. *et al.* Effect of

amiodarone in the Wolff–Parkinson–White syndrome. *Am. J. Cardiol.* 1976; 38: 189.

328. Cote, P., Bourassa, M.G., Delaye, J., Janin, A., Froment, R. and David, P. Effects of amiodarone on cardiac and coronary hemodynamics and on myocardial metabolism in patients with coronary artery disease. *Circulation* 1979; 59: 1165.

329. Sicart, M., Besse, P., Choussat, A. and Bricaud, H. Action hemodynamique de l'amiodarone intra-veineuse chez l'homme. *Arch. Mal. Coeur* 1977; 70: 219.

330. Schwartz, P., Shen, E., Morady, F., Gillespie, K., Scheinman, M. and Chatterjee, K. Hemodynamic effects of intravenous amiodarone in patients with depressed left ventricular function and recurrent ventricular tachycardia. *Am. Heart. J.* 1983; 106: 843.

331. Liechti, B., Burger, A. and Ferrero, C. Amiodarone et fonction thyroidienne. *Therap. Umschl.* 1980; 37: 105.

332. Salerno, J.A., Bressan, M.A., Vigano, M. *et al.* Medical and surgical treatment of sustained and recurrent post-infarction ventricular tachycardia. *Eur. Heart J.* 1985; 6: 1054.

333. Rotmensch, H.H., Liron, M., Tupilski, M. and Laniado, S. Possible association of pneumonitis with amiodarone therapy (letter). *Am. Heart J.* 1980; 100: 412.

334. Nademanee, K., Kannan, R., Hendrickson, J., Ookhtens, M., Kay I. and Singh, B.N. Amiodarone-digoxin interaction: clinical significance, time course and development, potential pharmacokinetic mechanisms and therapeutic implications. *J. Am. Coll. Cardiol.* 1984; 4: 111.

335. Marcus, F. Drug interactions with amiodarone. *Am. Heart J.* 1983; 106: 924.

336. Bacaner, M.B. Treatment of ventricular fibrillation and other acute arrhythmias with bretylium tosylate. *Am. J. Cardiol.* 1986; 21: 530.

337. Cardinal, R. and Sasyniuk, B.I. Electrophysiological effects of bretylium tosylate on subendocardial Purkinje fibers from infarcted canine hearts. *J. Pharmacol. Exp. Ther.* 1978; 204: 159.

338. Patterson, E. and Gibson, J.K. Prevention of chronic canine ventricular tachyarrhythmias with bretylium tosylate. *Circulation* 1981; 64: 1045.

339. Patterson, E., Gibson, J.K. and Lucchesi, B.R. Postmyocardial infarction re-entrant ventricular arrhythmias in conscious dogs: suppression by bretylium tosylate. *J. Pharmacol. Exp. Ther.* 1981; 216: 453.

340. Wenger, T.L., Lederman, S., Startmer, F., Brown, T. and Strauss, H.C. A method for quantitating antifibrillatory effects of drugs after coronary reperfusion in dogs: improved outcome with bretylium. *Circulation* 1984; 69: 142.

341. Bauernfeind, R.A., Hoff, J.V., Swiryn, S. *et al.* Electrophysiologic testing of bretylium tosylate in sustained ventricular tachycardia. *Am. Heart J.* 1983; 105: 973.

342. Greene, H.L., Werner, J.A., Gross, B.W. and Sears, G.K. Failure of bretylium to suppress inducible ventricular tachycardia. *Am. Heart J.* 1983; 105: 717.

343. Taggart, P., Sutton, P. and Donaldson, R. D-Sotalol: a new potent class III anti-arrhythmic agent. *Clin. Sci.* 1985; 69: 631.

344. McKibbin, J.K., Pocock, W.A., Barlow, J.B., Millar, R.N. and Obel, I.W. Sotalol, hypokalaemia, syncope and torsade de pointes. *Br. Heart J.* 1984; 51: 157.

345. Rizos, I., Senges, J., Jauernig, R. *et al.* Differential effects of sotalol and metoprolol on induction of paroxysmal supraventricular tachycardia. *Am. J. Cardiol.* 1984; 53: 1022.

346. Nademanee, K., Feld, G., Hendrickson, J., Singh, P.N. and Singh, B.N. Electrophysiologic and antiarrhythmic effects of sotalol in patients with life-threatening ventricular tachyarrhythmias. *Circulation* 1985; 72: 555.

347. Schamroth, L., Krikler, D.M. and Garrett, C. Immediate effects of intravenous verapamil in cardiac arrhythmias. *Br. Med. J.* 1972; i: 660.

348. Schomerus, M., Spiegelhalder, B., Stieren, B. and Eichelbaum, M. Physiological disposition of verapamil in man. *Cardiovasc. Res.* 1976; 10: 605.

349. Roy, P.R., Spurrell, R.A.J. and Sowton, E. The effect of verapamil on the cardiac conduction system in man. *Postgrad. Med. J.* 1974; 50: 270.

350. Singh, B.N. and Roche, A.H.G. Effects of intravenous verapamil on hemodynamics in patients with heart disease. *Am. Heart J.* 1977; 94: 593.

351. Rowland, E. Antiarrhythmic drugs—class IV. *Eur. Heart J.* 1987; 8 (Suppl. A): 61.

352. Packer, M., Meller, J., Medina, N. *et al.* Hemodynamic consequences of combined beta-adrenergic and slow calcium channel blockade in man. *Circulation* 1982; 65: 660.

353. Gulamhusein, S., Ko, P., Carruthers, S.G., and Klein, G.J. Acceleration of the ventricular response during atrial fibrillation in the Wolff–Parkinson–White syndrome after verapamil. *Circulation* 1982; 65: 348.

354. Smith, T.W. Digitalis: mechanisms of action and clinical use. *N. Engl. J. Med.* 1988; 318: 358.

355. Bigger, J.T. Digitalis toxicity. *J. Clin. Pharmacol.* 1985; 25: 514.

356. Hellestrand, K., Nathan, A.W., Bexton, R.S. and Camm, A.J. Response of an abnormal sinus node to intravenous flecainide acetate. *Pacing Clin. Electrophysiol.* 1984; 7: 436.

357. Goldberg, D., Reiffel, J.A., Davis, J.D., Gang, E.S. and Livelli, F.D. Electrophysiologic effects of procainamide on sinus node function in patients with and without sinus node disease. *Am. Heart J.* 1982; 103: 75.

358. Velebit, V., Podrid, P., Lown, B., Cohen, B.H. and Grayboys, T.B. Aggravation and provocation of ventricular arrhythmias by antiarrhythmic drugs. *Circulation* 1982; 65: 886.

359. Morganroth, J. and Horowitz, L.N. Flecainide: Its proarrhythmic effect and expected changes on the surface electrocardiogram. *Am. J. Cardiol.* 1984; 53: 89B.

360. Bauman, J.L., Bauernfeind, R.A., Hoff, J.V., Strasberg, B., Swiryn, S. and Rosen, K.M. Torsades de pointes due to quinidine: observations in 31 patients. *Am. Heart J.* 1984; 107: 425.

361. McKibbin, J.K., Pocock, W.A., Barlow, J.B., Miller, R.N.S. and Obel, I.W.P. Sotalol, hypokalaemia, syncope and torsade de pointes. *Br. Heart J.* 1984; 51: 157.

362. Roden, D.M. and Hoffman, B.F. Action potential prolongation and induction of abnormal automaticity by low quinidine concentrations in canine Purkinje fibers. Relationship to potassium and cycle length. *Circ. Res.* 1985; 56: 857.

363. Bardy, G., Ungerleider, R., Smith, W. and Ideker, R. A mechanism of torsades de pointes in a canine model. *Circulation* 1983; 67: 52.

364. Winkle, R.A., Mason, J.W., Griffin, J.C. and Ross, D. Malignant ventricular tachyarrhythmias associated with the use of encainide. *Am. Heart J.* 1981; 102: 857.

365. Stavens, C.S., McGovern, B., Garan, H. and Ruskin, J.N. Aggravation of electrically provoked ventricular tachycardia during treatment with propafenone. *Am. Heart J.* 1985; 110: 24.

366. Morganroth, J., Anderson, J.L. and Gentzkow, G.D. Classification by type of ventricular arrhythmia predicts frequency of adverse cardiac events from flecainide. *J. Am. Coll. Cardiol.* 1986; 8: 607.

367. Podrid, P.J., Lampert, S., Grayboys, T.B., Blatt, C.M. and Lown, B. Aggravation of arrhythmia by antiarrhythmic drugs—incidence and predictors. *Am. J. Cardiol.* 1987; 59: 38E.

368. Morganroth, J. Risk factors for the development of

proarrhythmic events. *Am. J. Cardiol.* 1987; **59**: 32E.

369. Ruskin, J.N., Mcgovern, B., Garan, H., DiMarco, J.P. and Kelly, E. Antiarrhythmic drugs: a possible cause of out-of-hospital cardiac arrest. *N. Engl. J. Med.* 1983; **309**: 1302.

370. Barold, S.S., Linhart, J.W., Samet, P. and Lister, J.W. Supraventricular tachycardia initiated and terminated by a single electrical stimulus. *Am. J. Cardiol.* 1969; **24**: 37.

371. Bertholet, M., Demoulin, J.C., Waleffe, A., Kulbertus, H. Programmable extrastimulus pacing for long-term management of supraventricular and ventricular tachycardias: clinical experience in 16 patients. *Am. Heart J.* 1985; **110**: 582.

372. Fisher, J.D., Mehra, R., Furman, S. Termination of ventricular tachycardia with bursts of rapid ventricular pacing. *Am. J. Cardiol.* 1978; **41**: 94.

373. Hunt, N.C., Cobb, F.R., Waxman, M.B., Zeft, H.J., Peter, R.H. and Morris, J.J. Conversion of supraventricular tachycardias with atrial stimulation. Evidence for reentry mechanisms. *Circulation* 1968; **38**: 1060.

374. Den Dulk, K., Brugada, P., Waldecker, B., Begemann, M., van der Schatte, Oliver T. and Wellens, H.J.J. Automatic pacemaker termination of two different types of supraventricular tachycardia. *J. Am. Coll. Cardiol.* 1985; **8**: 201.

375. Den Dulk, K., Brugada, P., Karsschot, I., Dassen, W., Wellens, H.J.J. Is there a universal anti-tachycardia pacemaker mode? *Pacing Clin. Electrophysiol.* 1986; **9**: 902.

376. Den Dulk, K., Richards, D., Wellens, H. *et al.* A versatile pacemaker system for termination of tachycardias with a programmable patient activator. *Circulation* 1982; **66**: Supp. II: II-217, 1982.

377. **Camm, A.J. and Ward, D.E.** *Pacing for Tachycardia Control.* Sydney, Australia: Telectronics.

378. Fisher, J.D., Lawrence, K.A., Waspe, L.E. and Matos, J.A. Mechanisms for success and failure of pacing for termination of ventricular tachycardia: clinical and hypothetical considerations. *Pacing Clin. Electrophysiol.* 1983; **6**: 1094.

379. Spurrell, R.A.J., Nathan, A.W., Bexton, R.S., Hellestrand, K.J., Nappholz, T. and Camm, A.J. Implantable automatic scanning pacemaker for termination of supraventricular tachycardia. *Am. J. Cardiol.* 1982; **49**: 753.

380. Peters, R.W., Shafton, E., Frank, S., Thomas, A.N. and Scheinman, M.M. Radiofrequency triggered pacemakers: Uses and limitations. *Ann. Intern. Med.* 1978; **88**: 17–22.

381. Fisher, J.D., Johnston, D.R., Furman, S., Waspe, L.E. and Kim, S.G. Long-term efficacy of antitachycardia pacing for supraventricular and ventricular tachycardias. *Am. J. Cardiol.* 1987; **60**: 1311.

382. Lau, C.P., Cornu, E. and Camm, A.J. Fatal and non fatal cardiac arrest in patients with an implanted antitachycardia device for the treatment of supraventricular tachycardia. *Am. J. Cardiol.* 1988; **61**: 919.

383. Mirowski, M., Reid, P.R., Mower, M.M. *et al.* Termination of malignant ventricular arrhythmias with an implanted automatic defibrillator in human beings. *N. Engl. J. Med.* 1980; **303**: 322.

384. Mirowski, M., Reid, P.R., Mower, M.M., Watkins, L. and Platia, E.W. Clinical performance of the implantable cardioverter-defibrillator. *Pacing Clin. Electrophysiol* 1984; **7**: 1345.

385. Winkle, R.A., Stinson, E.B., Echt, D.S., Mead, R.H. and Schmidt, P. Practical aspects of automatic cardioverter/ defibrillator implantation. *Am. Heart J.* 1984; **108**: 1335.

386. Marchlinski, F.E., Flores, B.T. and Buxton, R.E. The automatic implantable cardioverter–defibrillator: efficacy, complications, and device failures. *Ann. Intern. Med.* 1986; **104**: 481.

387. Echt, D.S., Armstrong, K., Schmidt, P., Oyer, P., Stinson,

E.B. and Winkle, R.A. Clinical experience, complications, and survival in 70 patients with the automatic cardioverter–defibrillator. *Circulation* 1985; **71**: 289.

388. Winkle, R.A., Bach, S.M. and Echt, D.S. The AICD local ventricular bipolar sensing to detect ventricular tachycardia and fibrillation. *Am. J. Cardiol.* 1983; **52**: 256.

389. Watkins, L., Mirowski, M. and Mower, M.M. Implantations of the automatic defibrillator: the subxiphoid approach. *Ann. Thorac. Surg.* 1982; **34**: 515.

390. Veltri, E.P., Mower, M.M., Guarnieri, T. and Mirowski, M. Clinical efficacy of the automatic implantable defibrillator: 6 year cumulative experience. *Circulation* 1986; **74**: II, 109.

391. Gabry, M.D., Brodman, R., Johnston, D., Frame, R., Fisher, J.D. and Furman, S. AICD longevity, shock delivery, patient survival. *Cardiac Pacing Electrophysiol* 1986; **4**: 29.

392. Wilber, D.J., Garan, H., Finkelstein, D. *et al.* Out-of-hospital cardiac arrest: use of electrophysiologic testing in the prediction of longterm outcome. *N. Engl. J. Med.* 1988; **318**: 19.

393. Vedel, J., Frank, R., Fontaine, G. *et al.* Bloc auriculo-ventriculaire infrahisien definitif induit au cours d'une exploration endoventriculaire droite. *Arch. Mal. Coeur* 1979; **72**: 107.

394. Gonzales, R., Scheinman, M.M., Margaretten, W. and Rubenstein, M. Closed-chest electrode-catheter technique for His bundle ablation in dogs. *Am. J. Physiol.* 1981; **241**: B283.

395. Gallagher, J.J., Svenson, R.B., Kassell, J.P. *et al.* Catheter technique for closed chest ablation of the atrioventriuclar conduction system. *N. Engl. J. Med.* 1982; **306**: 194.

396. Scheinman, M.M., Morady, F., Hess, D.S. and Gonzales, B. Catheter-induced ablation of the atrioventricular junction to control refractory supraventricular arrhythmias. *J. Am. Med. Assoc.* 1982; **248**: 851.

397. Boyd, E.G.C.A. and Holt, P. An investigation into the electrical ablation technique and a method of electrode assessment. *Pacing Clin. Electrophysiol* 1985; **8**: 815.

398. Holt, P. and Boyd, E.G.C.A. Haematological effects of the high energy endocardial ablation technique. *Circulation* 1986; **73**: 1029.

399. Holt, P. and Boyd, E. The high energy catheter ablation technique in the management of tachyarrhythmias. In: Camm, A.J. and Ward, D.E., eds. *Clinical Aspects of Cardiac Arrhythmias.* Lancaster: MTP Press, 1988, pp. 359–73.

400. Jones, J.L., Proskauer, C.C., Paull, W.K., Lepeschkin, E. and Jones, R.G. Ultrastructural injury to chick myocardial cells in vitro following 'electrical countershock'. *Circ. Res.* 1980; **46**: 387.

401. Scheinman, M.M. and Evans-Bell, T. and the Executive Committee of the Percutaneous Mapping and Ablation Registry. Catheter ablation of the atrioventricular conduction system: a report of the Percutaneous Mapping and Ablation Registry. *Circulation* 1984; **70**: 1024.

402. Morady, F., Scheinman, M.M., Winston, S.A. *et al.* Efficacy and safety of transcatheter ablation of posteroseptal accessory pathways. *Circulation* 1985; **72**: 70.

403. Morady, F. and Scheinman, M.M. Transvenous catheter ablation of an accessory pathway in a patient with Wolff–Parkinson–White syndrome. *N. Engl. J. Med.* 1984; **310**: 705.

404. Ward, D., Drysdale, M. and Redwood, D. Interruption of anomalous atroventriular conduction using a transvenous electrode catheter to deliver shocks in the coronary sinus. *Br. Heart J.* 1984; **51**: 686.

405. Fisher, J.D., Brodman, R., Kim, S.C. *et al.* Attempted non-surgical electrical ablation of accessory pathways via the coronary sinus in the Wolff–Parkinson–White syn-

drome. *J. Am. Coll. Cardiol.* 1984; **4**: 685.

406. Hartzler, G.O. Electrode catheter ablation of refractory focal ventricular tachycardia. *J. Am. Coll. Cardiol.* 1983; **2**: 1107.

407. Tonet, J.L., Fontaine, G., Frank, R. and Grosgogeat, Y. Treatment of refractory ventricular tachycardias by endocardial fulguration. *Circulation* 1985; **72**: III 388.

408. Evans, T.G., Scheinman, M.M. and the Executive Committee of the Percutaneous Cardiac Mapping and Ablation Registry. *Catheter ablation for control of cardiac arrhythmias: A report of the Percutaneous and Cadiac Mapping and Ablation Registry in Nonpharmacological Therapy of Tachyarrhythmias.* Breithardt, G., Borggrefe, M. and Zipes, D.P. New York: Futura Publishing Co., 1987, pp. 243–256.

409. Schofield, P.M., Bowes, R.J., Brooks, N. and Bennett, D.H. Exercise capacity and spontaneous heart rhythm after transvenous fulguration of atrioventricular conduction. *Br. Heart J.* 1986; **56**: 358.

410. Cunningham, A.D., Rowland, E. and Rickards, A.F. A low energy power source for ablation and a new index for ablating devices. *Clin. Prog. Electrophysiol Pacing* 1986; **4**: 125.

411. Holt, P., Boyd, E.C.G.A., Crick, J.C.P. and Sowton, E. Low energies and Helifix electrodes in the successful ablation of atrioventricular conduction. *Pacing Clin. Electrophysiol* 1985; **8**: 639.

412. Polgar, P., Bolnar, K., Worum, B., Bekassy, S., Kovacs, P. and Lorinerz, I. Closed chest ablation of the His Bundle: A new technique using suction electrode catheter and DC shock. In: Steinbach, K., ed. *Cardiac Pacing* Steinkopff Verlag, Darmstadt, pp. 883–90.

413. McComb, J.M., McGovern, B.A., Garan, H. and Ruskin, J.W. Management of refractory supraventricular tachyarrhythmias using low energy transcatheter shocks. *Am. J. Cardiol.* 1986; **58**: 959–63.

414. Borggrefe, M., Budde, T.H., Podczeck, A. and Breithardt, G. High-frequency alternating current ablation of an accessory pathway in man. *J. Am. Coll. Cardiol.* 1987; **10**: 576.

415. Lee, G., Ikeda, R.M., Theis, J. *et al.* Effects of laser irradiation delivered by a flexible fiberoptic system on the left ventricular internal myocardium. *Am. Heart J.* 1983; **106**: 587.

416. Cox, J.L. The status of surgery for cardiac arrhythmias. *Circulation* 1985; **71**: 413.

417. Josephson, M.E., Horowitz, L.N., Speilman, S.R., Waxman, H.L. and Greenspan, A.M. Role of catheter mapping in the preoperative assessment of ventricular tachycardia. *Am. J. Cardiol.* 1982; **49**: 207.

418. Hauer, R.N.W., Heethaar, R.M., deZwart, M.T.W. *et al.* Endocardial catheter mapping validation of a cineagiographic method for accurate localization of left ventricular sites. *Circulation* 1986; **74**: 862.

419. Yee, R., Guiraudon, G.M., Gardener, M.J. *et al.* Refractory paroxysmal sinus tachycardia: Management by subtotal right atrial exclusion. *J. Am. Coll. Cardiol.* 1984; **3**: 400.

420. Guiraudon, G.M., Klein, G.J., Sharma, A.D. *et al.* Surgical treatment of supraventricular tachycardias. A five year experience. *Pacing Clin. Elecrophysiol* 1986; **9**: 1376.

421. Gillette, P.C., Garson, A., Hesslein, P.S. *et al.* Successful surgical treatment of atrial, junctional and ventricular tachycardia unassociated with accessory connections in infants and children. *Am. Heart J.* 1981; **102**: 984.

422. Iwa, T., Ichihashi, T., Hashizume, Y., Ishida, K. and Okada, R. Successful surgical treatment of left atrial tachycardia. *Am. Heart J.* 1985; **109**: 160.

423. Olsson, S.B., Blomstrom, P., Sabel, K.G. and William-Olsson, G. Incessant ectopic atrial tachycardia: Successful surgical treatment with regression of dilated cardio-myopathy. *Am. J. Cardiol.* 1984; **53**: 1465.

424. Josephson, M.E., Spear, J.F., Harken, A.H. *et al.* Surgical excision of automatic atrial tachycardia: Anatomic and electrophysiologic correlates. *Am. Heart J.* 1982; **104**: 1076.

425. Ott, D.A., Garson, A., Cool, D. *et al.* Cryoablation techniques in the treatment of cardiac arrhythmias. *Ann. Thorac Cardiovasc. Surg.* 1987; **43**: 138.

426. Sealy, W.C., Anderson, R.W. and Gallagher, J.J. Surgical treatment of supraventricular tachycardias. *J. Thorac Cardiovasc. Surg.* 1977; **73**: 511.

427. Guiraudon, G.M., Campbell, C.S., Jones, D.L. *et al.* Combined sinoatrial node and atrioventricular isolation: A surgical alternative to His bundle ablation in patients with atrial fibrillation. *Circulation* 1985; **72**: III–220.

428. Klein, G.J., Guiraudon, G.M., Sharma, A.D. and Milstein, S. Demonstration of macro-reentry and feasibility of operative therapy in the common type of atrial flutter. *Am. J. Cardiol.* 1986; **57**: 587.

429. Ross, D.L., Johnson, D.C., Dennis, A.R., Cooper, M.J., Richards, D.A. and Uther, J.B. Curative surgery for atroventricular junctional ("AV nodal") reentrant tachycardia. *J. Am. Coll. Cardiol.* 1985; **6**: 1383.

430. Cox, J.L. and Cain, M.E. Discrete cryosurgical ablation of AV node reentry tachycardia in patients. *J. Am. Coll. Cardiol.* 1987; **9**: 249.

431. Cox, J.L., Gallagher, J.J. and Cain, M.E. Experience with 118 consecutive patients undergoing operation for the Wolff–Parkinson–White syndrome. *J. Thorac Cardiovasc. Surg.* 1985; **90**: 490.

432. Selle, J.G., Sealy, W.C., Gallagher, J.J. *et al.* Technical considerations in the surgical approach in multiple accessory pathways in the Wolff–Parkinson–White syndrome. *Ann. Thorac Surg.* 1987; **43**: 579.

433. Guiraudon, G.M., Klein, G.J., Sharma, A.D. *et al.* Closed heart technique in WPW syndrome: further experience and potential limitations. *Ann. Thorac Surg.* 1986; **42**: 651.

434. Bredikis, J., Bukauskas, F., Zebrausas, R. *et al.* Cryosurgical ablation of right parietal and septal accessory without use of extracorporeal circulation. *J. Thorac Cardiovasc. Surg.* 1985; **90**: 206.

435. Uther, J.B., Johnson, D.C., Baird, D.K. et al. Surgical section of AV electrical connections in 108 patients. *Am. Heart J.* 1982; **49**: 995.

436. Miller, J.M., Lienzle, M.G., Harken, A.H. and Josephson, M.E. Subendocardial resection for ventricular tachycardia: Predictors of surgical success. *Circulation* 1984; **70**: 624.

437. Gallagher, J.J., Kassell, J.H. *et al.* Techniques for intraoperative electrophysiologic mapping. *Am. J. Cardiol.* 1982; **49**: 221.

438. Josephson, M.E., Horowitz, L.N., Speilman, S.R. *et al.* Comparison of endocardial catheter mapping with intraoperative mapping of ventricular tachycardia. *Circulation* 1980; **61**: 395.

439. Wiener, I., Mindich, B. and Pitchon, R. Fragmented endocardial electrical activity in patients with VT: a new guide to surgical therapy. *Am. Heart J.* 1984; **107**: 86.

440. Kienzle, M.G., Falcone, R.A., Kenpf, F.C. *et al.* Intraoperative endocardial mapping: relation of fractionated electrograms in sinus rhythm to endocardial activation in ventricular tachycardia. *J. Am. Coll. Cardiol.* 1983; **1**: 582.

441. O'Keeffe, D.B., Curry, P.V.L., Prior, A.L. *et al.* Surgery for ventricular tachycardia using operative paced mapping. *Br. Heart J.* 1980; **43**: 116.

442. Miller, J.M., Harken, A.H., Hargreve, W.C. *et al.* Pattern of endocardial activation during sustained ventricular tachycardia. *J. Am. Coll. Cardiol.* 1985; **6**: 1280.

443. Mason, J.W., Stinson, E.B., Winkle, R.A *et al.* Relative

efficacy of blind left ventricular aneurysm resection for the treatment of recurrent ventricular tachycardia. *Am. J. Cardiol.* 1982; **49**: 241.

444. Buda, A.J., Stinson, E.B. and Harrison, D.C. Surgery for life threatening tachyarrhythmias. *Am. J. Cardiol.* 1979; **44**: 1171.

445. Kron, I.L., Lerman, B.B. and DiMarco, J.P. Extended subendocardial resection. A surgical approach to ventricular tachyarrhythmias that cannot be mapped intraoperatively. *J. Thorac Cardiovasc. Surg.* 1985; **90**: 586.

446. Garan, H., Nguyen, K., McGovern, B. *et al.* Perioperative and longterm results after electrophysiologically guided ventricular surgery for recurrent ventricular tachycardia. *J. Am. Coll. Cardiol.* 1986; **8**: 201.

447. Borggrefe, M., Podczek, A., Ostermeyer, J. and Breithardt, G. Long-term results of electrophysiologically guided antitachycardia surgery in ventricular tachyarrhythmias: A collaborative report on 665 patients. In: Breithardt, G., Borggrefe, M., Zipes, D.P., eds. *Non-Pharmacological Therapy of Tachyarrhythmias.* New York: Futura, 1988, pp. 109–132.

448. Garson, A., Gillette, P.C., Titus, J.L. *et al.* Surgical treatment of ventricular tachycardia in infants. *N. Engl. J. Med.* 1984; **310**: 1443.

449. Garson, A., Porter, C.B., Gillette, P.C. and McNamara, D.G. Induction of ventricular tachycardia during electrophysiologic study after repair of Tetralogy of Fallot. *J. Am. Coll. Cardiol.* 1983; **1**: 1493.

450. Camm, J., Ward, D., Cory-Pearce, R., Rees, G.M. and Spurrell, R.A.J. The successful cryosurgical treatment of paroxysmal ventricular tachycardia. *Chest* 1979; **75**: 621.

451. Svenson, R.H., Gallagher, J.J., Selle, J.G. *et al.* Successful intraoperative Nd-YAG laser ablation of ventricular tachycardia. *J. Am. Coll. Cardiol.* 1986; **7**: 237A.

452. Saksena, S. and Gadhoke, A. Laser therapy for tachyarrhythmias: a new frontier. *Pacing Clin. Electrophysiol* 1986; **9**: 531.

453. Kron, I.L., DiMarco, J.P., Nolan, S.P. and Lerman, B.B. Resection of scarred papillary muscles improves outcome after surgery for ventricular tachycardia. *Ann. Surg.* 1986; **203**: 685.

454. Fontaine, G., Guiraudon, G., Frank, R., Fillette, F.,

Cabrol, C. and Grosgogeat, Y. Surgical management of ventricular tachycardia unrelated to myocardial ischemia or infarction. *Am. J. Cardiol.* 1982; **49**: 397.

455. Spurrell, R.A.J., Sowton, E. and Deuchar, D.C. Ventricular tachycardia in 4 patients evaluated by programmed electrical stimulation of heart and treated in 2 patients by surgical division of the anterior radiation of the left bundle branch. *Br. Heart J.* 1973; **35**: 1014.

456. Guiraudon, G., Fontaine, G., Frank, R., Escande, G., Etievant, P. and Cabrol, C. Encircling endocardial ventriculotomy: a new surgical treatment for life-threatening ventricular tachycardias resistant to medical treatment following myocardial infarction. *Ann. Thorac Surg.* 1978; **26**: 438.

457. Boineau, J.P. and Cox, J.L. Rationale for a direct surgical approach to control ventricular arrhythmias. Relation of specific intraoperative techniques to mechanism and location of arrhythmic circuit. *Am. J. Cardiol.* 1982; **49**: 381.

458. Guiraudon, G.M., Klein, G.J., Vermeulen, F.E., Yee, R. and Van Hemel, N.M. Encircling endocardial cryoablation: a technique for surgical treatment of ventricular tachycardia after myocardial infarction. *Circulation* 1983; **68**: III–176.

459. Guiraudon, G.M., Klein, G.J., Gulamhusein, S.S. *et al.* Total disconnection of the right ventricular free wall: Surgical treatment of right ventricular tachycardia associated with right ventricular dysplasia. *Circulation* 1983; **67**: 463.

460. Cox, J.L., Bardy, G.H., Damiano, R.J. *et al.* Right ventricular isolation procedures for nonischemic ventricular tachycardia. *J. Thorac Cardiovasc. Surg.* 1985; **90**: 212.

461. Borggrefe, M., Podczek, A., Ostermeyer, J., Schwartmaier, J. and Breithardt, G. Induction of non-clinical ventricular tachycardia after map-guided surgery for refractory ventricular tachyarrhythmias: incidence and clinical significance. *J. Am. Coll. Cardiol.* 1987; **9**: 108A.

462. Guarnieri, T., Sealy, W.C., Kasell, J.H., German, L.D. and Gallagher, J.J. The nonpharmacologic management of the permanent form of junctional reciprocating tachycardia. *Circulation* 1984; **69**: 269.

Chapter 24

The Management of Bradycardias

David H. Bennett

Bradycardia due to impaired function of either the sinus node or atrioventricular junction can cause syncope, near-syncope, exertional dyspnoea, heart failure, tachyarrhythmia or it may be asymptomatic. Management will be influenced by the presence or absence of symptoms and by whether treatment is likely to improve prognosis. Usually, treatment consists of temporary or long-term artificial cardiac pacing, but occasionally drug therapy is indicated.

CARDIAC PACING FOR BRADYCARDIAS

An artificial cardiac pacemaker generates electrical stimuli which can initiate myocardial contraction. The stimuli are usually delivered to the heart by transvenous leads or less commonly via epicardial, oesophageal or transthoracic electrodes. For temporary treatment, an external pulse generator is used, whereas an implanted system is used for long-term pacing.

Experiments involving electrical stimulation of the heart were reported in the eighteenth and nineteenth centuries. Temporary cardiac pacing for Adams–Stokes attacks was first described in 1952.[1] Subsequent important advances include the implantation of a long-term rechargeable pacemaker with myocardial electrodes in 1958[2] and the implantation of a transvenous pacing system in 1962.[3] Over the following 25 years, rapid progress in technology and an increasing awareness of the benefits of pacing have led to pacemakers being widely used. Patients of all ages, from the newborn to those over 100 years, have been paced; the average age at first implantation is 72 years.

In the UK, the results of surveys have suggested that the annual rate of new pacemaker implantation should be at least 174–198 patients per million of the population.[4,5] The annual implantation rate has increased over the years and is currently 180 per million per year,[6] although there are some health districts with very low implantation rates. In 1986, implantation rates for the USA, France, Belgium and Germany were much higher than that in the UK, approximately 400 per million per year. In North America, in 1981, the implantation rate was 518 per million of the population.[7]

INDICATIONS FOR LONG-TERM CARDIAC PACING

The main considerations in deciding whether to implant a pacemaker are as to whether relief of symptoms and/or improvement in prognosis will be achieved. In some patients with asymptomatic impairment of the specialized cardiac conducting system, other factors may also be pertinent, such as the need for medication which may cause unwanted bradycardia or concern in a motor vehicle driver that an accident might result should syncope occur.

Long-term pacing is not indicated if bradycardia is unlikely to recur, e.g. if caused by drug toxicity or acute myocardial ischaemia. Atrioventricular dissociation, in which the ventricular rate exceeds the atrial rate, and non-conducted atrial extrasystoles are sometimes erroneously diagnosed as heart block; clearly, there is no need for pacing.

Complete atrioventricular block

The most common reason for pacemaker implantation is syncope or near-syncope caused by complete atrioventricular block. The occurrence of a single episode is a sufficient indication and, as the next blackout may cause injury or be fatal, delay in implantation should be minimal. Even patients who have a short life-expectancy, should be considered for pacing if by preventing syncope, independence may be preserved and serious injury, which may lead to greater demands on medical resources than pacing, may be avoided.

Complete heart block can reduce cardiac output

and thereby lead to exertional dyspnoea and sometimes to cardiac failure. Pacing usually, but not invariably, improves these problems. Mental impairment is sometimes attributed to heart block but it does not always improve with pacing; if there is doubt, it is best to undertake a trial of temporary pacing.

Without pacing, the prognosis in patients with complete heart block is poor.[8] With an artificial pacemaker, life-expectancy approaches that of the general population although those with overt coronary heart disease or heart failure do not have such a good prognosis.[9] Pacemaker implantation should be considered in asymptomatic patients with complete atrioventricular block, particularly when the ventricular rate is 40 beats/min or less, on purely prognostic grounds.[10]

The occurrence of narrow ventricular complexes during complete atrioventricular block suggests that the interruption in conduction is at the atrioventricular nodal level and that, in contrast to infranodal block, a subsidiary pacemaker placed within the His bundle will discharge reliably at a relatively rapid ventricular rate. However, in practice, patients with narrow ventricular complexes during complete heart block may experience syncope and impaired exercise tolerance. In the UK, one-third of patients who receive pacemakers for complete atrioventricular block have narrow QRS complexes.[6]

Congenital heart block

Congenital heart block, i.e. complete atrioventricular block discovered in a neonate or child which is not caused by acquired disease, is widely regarded as benign.[11] However, some patients do develop symptoms or die suddenly. In a series of 44 patients followed for 12 years, two died suddenly and nine required a pacemaker.[12] Broad ventricular complexes, a ventricular rate < 50 beats per minute, QT-interval prolongation and ventricular ectopy suggest a poor prognosis, but these factors are not sufficiently specific to be reliable in the individual patient. In asymptomatic patients, the risks of not implanting a pacemaker have to be weighed against the possibility of complications associated with several decades of pacing. Unpaced patients should undergo ambulatory and exercise electrocardiography at regular intervals.

Second degree atrioventricular block

The management approach to second degree atrioventricular block is similar to that for complete atrioventricular block.

Mobitz type II atrioventricular block often progresses to complete atrioventricular block.[10] The results of a recent study showed that symptoms were commonly associated with Mobitz type II atrioventricular block and that although the prognosis was poor in unpaced patients it was similar to that of the general population in paced patients.[13] The findings of this study also refuted the previously held view that Mobitz type I atrioventricular block is benign;[14] the incidence of symptoms, prognosis and influence of pacing were the same as those for patients with Mobitz type II block. This poor outlook, however, does not apply to young people with transient and often nocturnal Wenkebach block which is due to high vagal tone and is benign.

First degree atrioventricular block

First degree atrioventricular block is not itself an indication for cardiac pacing. If a patient presents with first degree block and syncope or near-syncope it is possible that the symptoms are due to transient second or third degree atrioventricular block, but a pacemaker should not be implanted without proof of this, e.g. from ambulatory electrocardiography.

Bundle branch and fascicular blocks

The risk of high degree atrioventricular block developing in an asymptomatic patient with either left or right bundle branch block is extremely small[15] and pacing is not indicated. In patients who present with syncope or near-syncope, the management approach should be the same as that for first degree atrioventricular block.

In bifascicular block, it is possible that the remaining functioning fascicle may fail to conduct, intermittently or persistently, and cause high degree atrioventricular block. In patients with a good history of Adams–Stokes attacks, pacemaker implantation is indicated to prevent syncope without further investigation. With atypical symptoms, high degree atrioventricular block must be documented first.

In asymptomatic bifascicular block, the chance of progression to complete atrioventricular block is in the order of 2% per year, and the major determinants of prognosis are the presence of coronary artery or myocardial disease; prophylactic pacing is generally not indicated.[16] Additional first degree atrioventricular block or His bundle electrographic evidence of prolonged infranodal conduction suggest that conduction in the functioning fascicle is also impaired. However, there is no evidence of a higher risk.

Atrioventricular and bundle branch block after myocardial infarction

Atrioventricular block due to inferior myocardial infarction usually resolves within a few days and almost always by three weeks. When anterior infarction is complicated by high degree atrioventricular block, there is usually extensive myocardial damage and hence the prognosis is poor; although block may persist it is prudent to ensure that the patient is going to survive before implanting a pacemaker. Pacemaker implantation should not be considered unless second or third degree atrioventricular block is present 3 weeks after myocardial infarction.

Bifascicular block persisting after acute anterior infarction complicated by atrioventricular block raises the possibility that complete atrioventricular block might recur. Although transient bradycardia has been demonstrated to occur in some patients with post-infarction bifascicular block,[17] prophylactic pacing does not reduce mortality.[18]

Sick sinus syndrome

Sick sinus syndrome accounts for one-quarter of pacemaker implantations.[6] Pacing is indicated when syncope or near-syncope are caused. It should be borne in mind that sinus bradycardia and pauses in sinus node activity for up to 2.0 s, particularly if nocturnal, can be physiological.

In patients with the bradycardia–tachycardia syndrome, pacing may be required to avoid severe bradycardia caused by anti-arrhythmic drugs. Sometimes, tachyarrhythmias that start during bradycardia will be prevented by atrial pacing.

Pacing for sick sinus syndrome does not improve prognosis[19] and is not usually indicated in asymptomatic patients. However, pauses in cardiac activity for several seconds might be considered an indication for pacing in those who operate machinery, including a motor car, to guard against the possibility of an accident should syncope occur.

Hypersensitive carotid sinus syndrome

Hypersensitive carotid sinus syndrome is applied to patients who suffer from near-syncope or syncope without evidence of impaired function of the sinus node or atrioventricular junction in whom unilateral carotid sinus massage for 5 s causes sinus arrest or complete atrioventricular block for at least 3 s; pacing is indicated.[20] Pacing is not indicated in asymptomatic patients with hypersensitive carotid sinus reflexes.

PACEMAKER MODES

The first generation of pacemakers functioned in a fixed-rate mode: the pacemaker stimulated the ventricles regularly, usually at 70 beats/min, irrespective of any spontaneous cardiac activity (Fig. 24.1). Competition with a spontaneous rhythm could cause irregular palpitation, and stimulation during ventricular repolarization could possibly initiate ventricular fibrillation.[21]

Subsequent developments enabled sensing of spontaneous activity via the stimulating lead to facilitate demand pacing:[22] a sensed event resets the timing of delivery of the next pacemaker stimulus to avoid competition with spontaneous activity (Fig. 24.2). With the advent of reliable transvenous atrial pacing leads, it became straightforward to pace and sense in the atrium as well as in the ventricle,[23] thus allowing both atrial and ventricular 'single chamber' pacing and also 'dual chamber' pacing, whereby stimulation and/or sensing can take place at both atrial and ventricular levels. These developments have permitted a more physiological approach to cardiac stimulation.

Pacing system code

A five-letter code is widely used to describe the

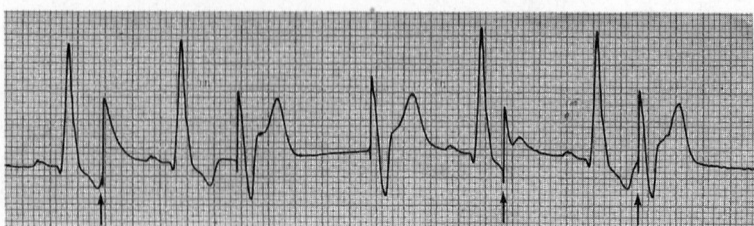

Fig. 24.1. Fixed rate ventricular pacing during sinus rhythm. Three stimuli fall on or close to a T wave.

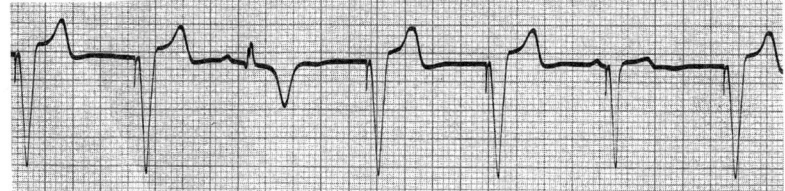

Fig. 24.2. Ventricular demand pacing. Beats of sinus node origin inhibit pacemaker output (third complex) and result in a fusion beat due to simultaneous pacemaker output (sixth complex).

various pacing modes; the first three characters are the most important.[24]

The first character identifies the chamber(s) paced: 'A' for atrium, 'V' for ventricle and 'D' for double if both atrium and ventricle can be stimulated.

The second character indicates the chamber or chambers whose activity is sensed: in addition to the use of A, V and D, 'O' indicates that the pacemaker is insensitive.

The third character denotes the response to the sensed information: 'I' indicates that pacemaker output is inhibited by a sensed event, 'T' that stimulation is triggered by a sensed event and 'D' that ventricular sensed events inhibit pacemaker output whereas atrial sensed events trigger ventricular stimulation; 'O' indicates that there is no response to sensed events.

The fourth character denotes whether the generator is programmable: 'O' indicates that it is not; 'P' that it is a simple programmable unit (for one or two parameters e.g. rate and output); and 'M' that it is multiprogrammable. 'C' indicates that, in addition, the pacemaker has facilities for telemetry. The facility for rate modulation in response to a sensed variable (see below) is denoted by 'R'.

The fifth character relates to anti-tachycardia functions: 'O', none; 'P', anti-tachycardia pacing (low-energy stimulation); 'S', shock (i.e. cardioversion or defibrillation); and 'D', both anti-tachycardia pacing and shock.

Single-chamber pacing

Atrial demand pacing

In the absence of spontaneous atrial activity, an atrial demand pacemaker, like a fixed-rate unit, delivers stimuli at a regular rate (Fig. 24.3).

However, if spontaneous activity is sensed via the atrial lead, the timing of delivery of the next pacemaker output is reset to avoid competition.

In atrial inhibited (AAI) pacemakers, a sensed event terminates the current stimulation cycle, thus inhibiting pacemaker output, and starts a new cycle. In contrast, a sensed event during atrial triggered (AAT) pacing immediately triggers delivery of a pacing stimulus which will consequently fall during the myocardial refractory period and will thus be ineffective; the subsequent cycle will then start from delivery of the triggered impulse.

The pacemaker is rendered insensitive immediately after a paced or sensed event for an interval that approximates the duration of myocardial depolarization and repolarization in order to prevent sensing the atrial electrogram which is produced by the event; this interval is referred to as the refractory period. In all pacemakers, the refractory period is at least 250–300 ms. With atrial pacing, it is usually somewhat longer to avoid sensing the 'far field' ventricular electrogram which may be sensed via the atrial lead and inappropriately inhibit the pacemaker.

Atrial pacing is indicated for treatment of the sick sinus syndrome unless atrioventricular conduction is impaired. By stimulating the atria rather than the ventricles, the normal sequence of cardiac chamber activation is maintained, loss of which can reduce cardiac output by up to one-third. Sick sinus syndrome can be associated with impaired atrioventricular conduction.[25] However, the risk of impaired atrioventricular conduction developing if there is no evidence of it at the time of atrial pacemaker implantation is low.[26]

Ventricular demand pacing

The timing cycles of ventricular inhibited (VVI) and the less commonly used ventricular triggered (VVT)

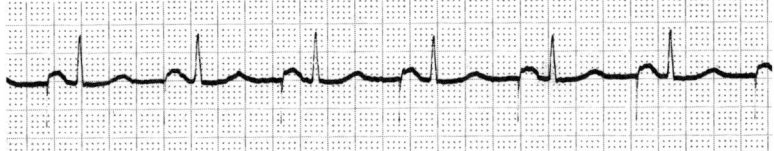

Fig. 24.3. Atrial pacing. Each stimulus initiates a P wave which is followed by a QRS complex.

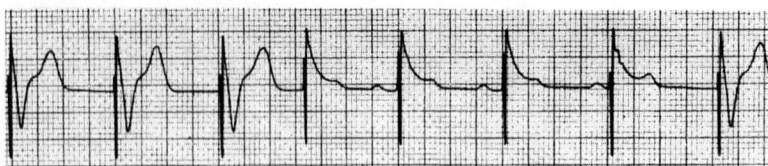

Fig. 24.4. Ventricular triggered (VVT) pacing. After the first three paced beats, there is sinus rhythm. A stimulus is delivered after the onset of the next four spontaneous QRS complex.

modes (Figs. 24.2 and 24.4) are the same as for atrial demand pacing, as described above.

Ventricular demand pacing is the most commonly employed mode, but its use is diminishing as its disadvantages—the inabilities to facilitate the normal sequence of cardiac chamber activation and to provide a chronotropic response to exercise—become more widely appreciated (see below).

Unequivocal indications for ventricular demand pacing include bradycardia associated with persistent atrial fibrillation, second and third degree atrioventricular block in patients who are limited by impaired cerebral or locomotor function and patients with infrequent bradycardia in whom the pacemaker is mainly on 'standby'.

Dual chamber pacing

Atrioventricular sequential pacing

In atrioventricular sequential (DVI) pacing the atria are stimulated first and then, after a delay that approximates the normal PR interval, the ventricles are stimulated (Fig. 24.5). As with other dual chamber modes, both atrial and ventricular electrodes are required. The pacemaker is inhibited by spontaneous ventricular activity but no sensing occurs in the atrium.

There are non-committed and committed versions of atrioventricular sequential pacing. In the former, a sensed ventricular event during the interval between atrial and ventricular stimulation will inhibit delivery of the ventricular stimulus. In the latter, ventricular stimulation will always follow the atrial stimulus.

Fusion beats are commonly seen during DVI pacing and are sometimes misinterpreted as pacemaker malfunction: whereas the pacemaker is inhibited by an event sensed in the ventricles, the

first chamber to be stimulated is the atrium; it is therefore possible for pacemaker output to occur at the same time as spontaneous atrial depolarization because the resultant ventricular depolarization has not yet occurred.

The main indication for atrioventricular sequential pacing is sick sinus syndrome associated with impaired atrioventricular conduction.

Atrial synchronized ventricular pacing

In atrial synchronized ventricular pacing, ventricular stimulation is triggered by a sensed atrial event after an interval similar to the normal PR interval (Fig. 24.6). It thereby maintains the normal sequence of cardiac chamber activation and permits a chronotropic response to exercise provided sinus node function is normal.

If an atrial event is not sensed, ventricular stimulation continues at a fixed and usually fairly long cycle length, otherwise atrial standstill might lead to ventricular asystole. To avoid atrial tachycardia or fibrillation triggering inappropriately fast ventricular pacing rates, there is an atrial refractory interval: the atrial channel is rendered insensitive during the atrioventricular delay and for a period after ventricular stimulation. Sensed atrial activity at a cycle length shorter than this period will not trigger ventricular stimulation. The upper rate at which atrial activity will trigger ventricular output is determined by the 'total atrial refractory period' which consists of the atrioventricular delay plus the post-ventricular stimulus atrial refractory period. For example, if the atrioventricular delay is 125 ms and the atrial refractory period is 250 ms, the upper rate limit will be 60 000/375 = 160 beats/min.

In earlier years, sensing took place only in the atrium and pacing occurred only in the ventricle (VAT). Thus, ventricular ectopic beats or rhythms

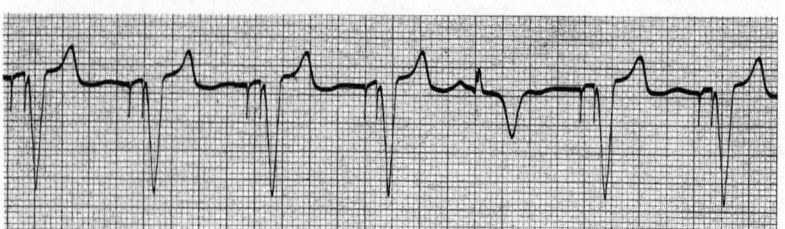

Fig. 24.5. Atrioventricular sequential (DVI) pacing: pacing stimuli precede both atrial and ventricular complexes. After four paced beats, a spontaneous beat inhibits the pacemaker.

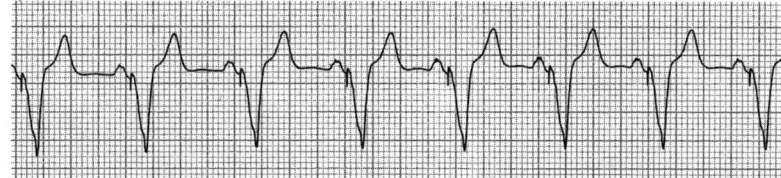

Fig. 24.6. Atrial synchronized (VAT) pacing; each P wave triggers ventricular stimulation.

faster than the sinus node rate would not inhibit ventricular output. More recently, VDD pacing has been introduced whereby sensing also takes place in the ventricles, such that spontaneous ventricular activity will inhibit the pacemaker.

Atrial synchronized ventricular pacing is indicated in second and third degree atrioventricular block when sinus node function is normal. It is contra-indicated in sick sinus syndrome or when atrial tachyarrhythmias are present.

'Endless loop tachycardia' If a ventricular stimulus is conducted retrogradely to the atria via either the atrioventricular junction or, if present, an accessory atrioventricular pathway, and the timing of the resultant atrial activation is outside the pacemaker's atrial refractory period, it will trigger ventricular stimulation and hence initiate an 'endless loop tachycardia' (Fig. 24.7). Ventriculo-atrial conduction has been demonstrated in approximately two-thirds of patients with sick sinus syndrome and one-fifth of those with atrioventricular block. Endless loop tachycardia can usually be prevented by prolongation of the atrial refractory period but at the expense of a reduction in the upper rate limit for ventricular stimulation.[27]

Recently, several measures to prevent or interrupt quickly endless loop tachycardia have been devised. These include:

1 automatic extension of the atrial refractory period after ventricular extrasystoles;
2 immediate atrial stimulation on sensing a ventricular extrasystole making the atria refractory to retrograde atrial activation;
3 recognition of re-entrant tachycardia by a regular cycle length—atrial tracking is prevented for one cycle thereby interrupting the re-entry circuit;

4 setting the atrial sensing threshold so that anterograde atrial activity is sensed but the usually lower amplitude retrograde activity is rejected;[28]
5 distinguishing atrial tachycardia due to sinus node activity from that due to re-entry on the basis of whether the atrial cycle length has gradually or suddenly increased.[29]

The facility discussed in 5 also helps to deal with another problem. Atrial synchronized pacemakers have an upper rate limit above which ventricular pacing is no longer synchronized to atrial activity. In some patients, sinus node rates during exercise may exceed the upper rate limit at which point many pacemakers simply track alternate atrial waves.[30] The resultant abrupt drop in ventricular rate can be disabling. An algorithm has been developed so that the pacemaker responds by a gentle reduction in rate in a Wenckebach fashion when the pacemaker recognizes a physiological increase in atrial rate.[29]

Atrioventricular universal pacing

In this mode (DDD), both sensing and pacing can take place at atrial and ventricular levels. It allows the pacemaker to function in atrial demand (AAI), atrioventricular sequential (DVI) or atrial synchronized (VDD) modes depending on the spontaneous heart rhythm (Fig. 24.8). If there is sinus bradycardia, it functions as an atrial demand pacemaker; if there is impaired atrioventricular conduction, ventricular pacing is triggered by either spontaneous atrial activity or delivery of an atrial stimulus. When sinus node function is normal, it functions in the atrial synchronized mode thus providing a chronotropic response to exercise. The pacemaker is inhibited by both atrial and ventricular ectopic

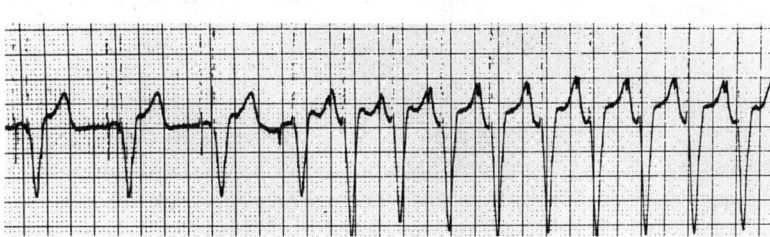

Fig. 24.7. Pacemaker-mediated or endless loop tachycardia starts after four cycles of dual chamber' pacing.

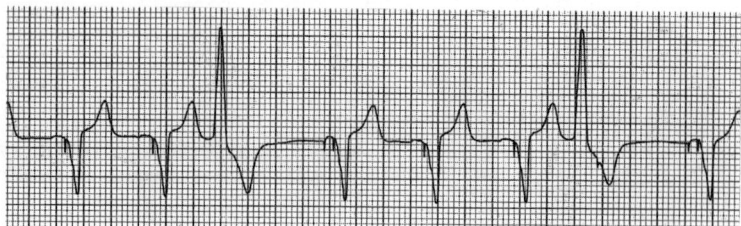

Fig. 24.8. Universal (DDD) pacing. Spontaneous P waves trigger ventricular stimulation. After the second and fifth paced beats, ventricular extrasystoles inhibit the pacemaker and depress sinus node function so they are followed by atrioventricular paced beats.

beats. Endless loop tachycardia may occur if there is retrograde atrioventricular conduction.

DDD pacing is indicated in second and third degree atrioventricular block and in sinus node dysfunction. Atrial tachyarrhythmias are a contraindication.

'PHYSIOLOGICAL PACING'

Ventricular demand pacing presents the least technical challenge and continues to be the most commonly employed pacing mode. However, important disadvantages of this mode are its inabilities to maintain the normal sequence of cardiac chamber activation and to provide a chronotropic response to exercise.

Atrial synchronized ventricular pacing

Atrial synchronized ventricular pacing maintains atrioventricular synchronization and facilitates a chronotropic response; it has been shown to increase cardiac output at rest and during exercise when compared with ventricular pacing at 70 beats/min.[31] Exercise capacity is of greater practical importance than haemodynamic measurements, and has been measured in a double-blind manner[32–34] during ventricular pacing at 70 beats/min and during atrial synchronized ventricular pacing. The latter mode was shown to increase maximal exercise capacity by about 30%. However, individual patients varied in the degree to which they benefited: in a few patients, there was little improvement in exercise capacity, whereas in a significant proportion there was a dramatic increase. Neither age nor cause of heart block predicted the amount of benefit gained. Previously, it was thought that 'physiological' pacing was of greatest value to patients with poor ventricular function, but this is not the case; patients with high venous pressures may not benefit.[35,36]

Atrial synchronized pacing also improves other parameters: shortness of breath, dizziness and palpitation are less frequent; whereas constant rate pacing tends to impair the normal blood-pressure response to exercise and leads to higher levels of arterial lactate, respiratory rate and perceived exertion during submaximal exercise.[32,34,36] The advantages of atrial synchronized pacing have been shown to be maintained in the long term.[36]

There are limitations to atrial synchronized ventricular pacing. First, normal or at least near-normal sinus node activity is required. Second, the current generation of pacemakers cannot distinguish between a rise in atrial rate caused by a physiological increase in sinus node activity and that due to an atrial tachyarrhythmia. Third, an atrial as well as a ventricular pacing lead is required.

Rate-responsive systems

In terms of exercise capacity, the ability to increase heart rate is far more important than maintaining atrioventricular synchronization.[31] This has been demonstrated by measuring exercise tolerance during three pacing modes: fixed rate, atrial synchronized and ventricular pacing at a rate commensurate with but not synchronized to atrial activity. The latter two forms of chronotropic pacing increased exercise performance to a similar degree when compared with fixed rate pacing.[37] Loss of atrioventricular synchronization has been shown to be compensated for by an increase in ventricular ejection fraction.[38]

Several pacing systems are available or are being developed that can facilitate a chronotropic response independent of atrial activity: a change in stimulation rate is achieved in response to a parameter that alters with exercise. These have the advantages of requiring only one pacing lead, of not necessitating normal sinus node activity and of not causing endless loop tachycardia.

Evoked QT response

Although it has been known for many years that the QT interval decreases with increasing heart rate, it has only recently been appreciated that sympathetic nervous system activity is a major independent determinant of the duration of the QT interval; the QT interval shortens during exercise even during fixed rate pacing.[39,40] The 'TX' pacemaker senses, via a conventional ventricular pacing electrode, the interval between pacing stimulus and the evoked T wave; a decrease in the interval leads to an increase in stimulation rate.[41]

Problems relating to inadequate T-wave sensing have occurred particularly with the first generation of TX pacemakers and with older types of pacing lead.[42] The sensitivity of the system to changes in the QT interval and the period during which T-wave sensing occurs have to be programmed for each individual. Not infrequently, fine adjustments to these functions have to be made to ensure a progressive chronotropic response to exercise and to avoid inappropriate acceleration of the pacemaker at rest.[43]

Muscle vibration

A system that senses vibration resulting from muscle activity, using a piezo-electric crystal attached to the inner surface of the pacemaker can, has been shown to provide a satisfactory chronotropic response to exercise.[44] It can be used for atrial as well as ventricular pacing.

Respiratory rate

There is a close relation between respiratory and heart rates.[45] An implantable system is available, the discharge of which is governed by the respiratory rate; the respiratory rate is monitored by means of an electrode implanted subcutaneously in the chest wall using the impedance principle. A system using changes in intravascular impedance as a measure of respiration has also been developed.[46]

Blood temperature

Skeletal muscle activity generates heat which is transferred to the blood. There is a useful relation between the level of exercise and right ventricular blood temperature. One problem, however, is that there is a latency in the system due to the delay of 1 or 2 min before blood temperature rises after the start of exercise.[47,48]

Mixed venous oxygen saturation

Mixed venous oxygen saturation is an index of cardiac output and can be measured by means of an optical detector in the right ventricle. A fall in oxygen saturation would trigger an increase in pacing rate.[49]

Other sensors

Blood pH, P_{CO_2}, P_{O_2}, the integral of the intracardiac ventricular complex and right ventricular stroke volume are parameters being investigated for use in rate-responsive pacing. Information on long-term reliability of sensors is not yet available.

'Multisensor pacing'

Dual chamber pacemakers have now been developed that, in addition to sensing atrial activity, respond to parameters related to exercise, such as vibration.

'Pacemaker syndrome'

It is at rest that the disadvantage of the loss of atrioventricular synchrony caused by ventricular pacing may become apparent. When normal atrioventricular synchronization is lost, atrial contraction may occur against closed mitral and tricuspid valves. Atrial pressure will rise and impede venous return so that during the next diastolic period the ventricles will be underfilled with a resultant reduction in stroke volume. The loss of properly timed atrial systole results in a reduction in cardiac output of up to one-third[50] this fall in cardiac output may cause hypotension (Fig. 24.9); near-syncope and syncope can result.[51] Ventriculo-atrial conduction causes even greater haemodynamic upset: the resultant atrial distension may actually initiate a reflex vasodepressor effect.[52]

Hypotension is likely to be more marked whilst standing. It is most severe during the first few seconds of ventricular pacing, before vasoconstrictor compensatory mechanisms can come into play, so ventricular pacing is particularly unsuitable for patients who are mainly in sinus rhythm but who often develop bradycardia at a rate less than the cycle length of the ventricular pacemaker, i.e. those with sick sinus or carotid sinus syndrome. Atrioventricular sequential pacing or, when atrioventricular conduction is not impaired, atrial pacing will avoid this problem. This has been demonstrated by recording ambulatory blood pressure in patients with ventricular demand pacemakers. The onset of ventricular pacing was followed by hypotension which was greater in those who had complained of syncope and near-syncope. Atrioventricular sequential pacing prevented hypotension and syncope.[53]

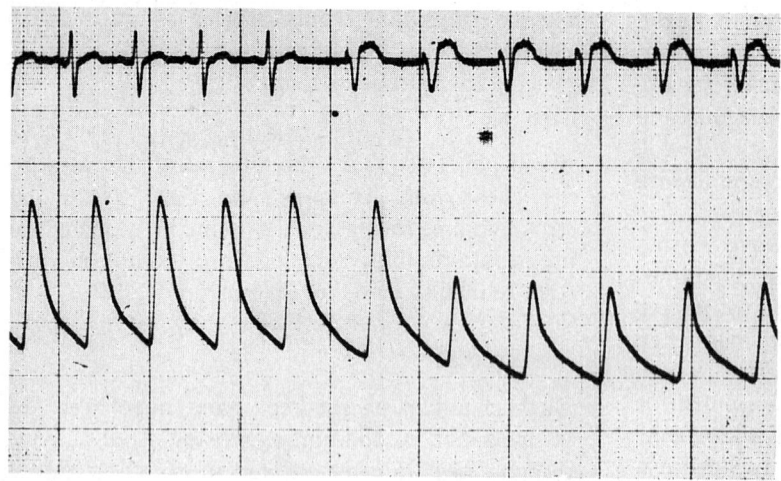

Fig. 24.9. Marked reduction in arterial systolic and pulse pressure after the second paced ventricular beat. (The first paced beat is preceded by a P wave.)

PACEMAKER HARDWARE

Pulse generator

A pulse generator consists of a power source and electronic circuits to control the timing and characteristics of the impulses which the power source generates.

In the past, several sources have been used including mercury–zinc cells, rechargeable nickel–cadmium cells and nuclear energy. Now, lithium iodide and lithium copper sulphide cells are used almost exclusively. They have replaced the other widely used power source, the mercury–zinc cell, the lifetime of which was limited to 24–48 months and which produced hydrogen, making it impractical to seal the pacemaker hermetically. Lithium pacemakers have a lifespan of 4–15 years and a predictable progressive discharge behaviour. They are contained in a hermetically sealed titanium can, weigh 35–50 g and generally have a maximum diameter of no more than 50 mm and a thickness of as little as 6 mm.

Pacemaker leads

Stimuli produced by the pulse generator are conducted to the heart via a lead consisting of an insulated wire with an electrode at its tip which is attached to the heart.

Leads that are sewn on to the epicardium or screwed into the myocardium necessitate thoracotomy; with the advent of reliable transvenous leads, they are rarely used now unless pacemaker implantation is undertaken at the time of open heart surgery, or venous thrombosis or tricuspid valve

prosthesis preclude a transvenous approach. There is doubt about the long-term reliability of epimyocardial leads.

Transvenous leads are used in over 95% of pacemaker implantations. A modern lead consists of a multifilar, helically coiled wire which is insulated by a material that does not cause tissue reaction or thrombosis—silicone rubber or polyurethane. Polyurethanes have a higher tensile strength so that the insulation and hence the lead itself can be thinner. Furthermore, they have a low coefficient of friction enabling both atrial and ventricular leads to be manipulated within the same vein. One manufacturer's polyurethane was associated with a high incidence of failure but other polyurethanes have performed well.

At the lead tip is the cathode which is composed of an inert material such as platinum–iridium, elgiloy, steel or vitreous carbon. For effective stimulation, the cathode must be securely and closely attached to the endocardium. If fibrous tissue, which is non-excitable, develops between cathode and endocardium the amount of energy required to stimulate the heart will increase and may exceed the output capability of the pacemaker.

In order to achieve a low threshold for stimulation and a secure endocardial attachment, several 'fixation devices' have been employed. 'Passive' fixation devices include tines, flanges or fins position proximal to the lead tip which can become entrapped in the trabeculae. 'Active' devices include an electrode in the shape of a helix which, by rotation of the lead, can be wound around a trabeculum, and a retractable metal screw which can be screwed into the endomyocardium. Recently, 'porous' metal or carbon electrodes have been introduced: the surface of the cathode consists of many microscopic pores which promote rapid tissue ingrowth and hence very secure fixation. Movement between electrode and endocardium, and thus generation of fibrous tissue, is minimized. One new electrode even elutes dexamethasone to minimize local tissue reaction and, hence, stimulation threshold. Attachment of atrial leads was impracticable until the advent of fixation devices. The distal portion of atrial leads are often 'J'-shaped to facilitate positioning in the right atrial appendage.

The amount of energy required to stimulate the heart is related to the surface area of the cathode. Nowadays, electrodes of small surface area are used, in the order of 6–12 mm^2. Porous-surfaced leads provide a large surface area for sensing whilst maintaining a small area (high current density) for stimulation.

Unipolar versus bipolar pacing

In unipolar pacing, the anode is remote from the heart, usually it is the metal can containing the pulse generator. In bipolar pacing, which is less widely used, both anode and cathode are within the cardiac chamber to be paced, the anode being positioned along the lead near to its cathodal tip. A commonly held view is that an electrogram sensed by a unipolar lead is larger than that from a bipolar lead. In most cases, there is little difference between bipolar and unipolar electrograms or stimulation thresholds.[54] Bipolar pacing has the advantage that inappropriate sensing of electromagnetic interference and skeletal muscle electromyograms is much less likely, as is extracardiac stimulation. Reasons for favouring unipolar pacing are that there is greater experience with unipolar leads, the leads have in the past been thinner and surface electrocardiographic unipolar pacemaker spikes are larger. Furthermore, until the recent introduction of 'in-line' connectors to the pulse generator, it was necessary with bipolar pacing to utilize two bulky connectors.

Costs

In the UK, the current approximate costs of a pulse generator plus leads for single chamber, programmable single chamber and dual chambered pacing systems are £500, £850 and £1600, respectively.

High costs have led to the increasing use of explanted re-sterilized generators. Anticipated problems have been hypothetical rather than practical. The main difficulties have been medicolegal.[55]

PACEMAKER IMPLANTATION

Facilities for fluoroscopy, electrocardiographic monitoring and cardiopulmonary resuscitation are required. The procedure is usually carried out under local anaesthesia and takes 15–45 min.

Subclavian approach

The subclavian approach is now widely used and is especially useful if more than one lead is to be inserted.[56] The pacemaker lead(s) is/are introduced via infraclavicular subclavian vein puncture and are connected to the pulse generator which is implanted in a subcutaneous pocket fashioned over the pectoralis major.

An incision is made 2 cm below the junction of the middle and inner thirds of the clavicle and is extended in a lateral and usually inferior direction for approximately 7 cm. A subcutaneous pocket large enough to accommodate the pulse generator is created by blunt dissection.

Puncture of the subclavian vein is easier if the vein is distended; a slight head-down position will help. A needle is introduced just below the inferior border of the clavicle at the junction of its middle and inner thirds and directed towards the sternoclavicular joint so that it passes behind the posterior surface of the clavicle. As the needle punctures the vein, venous blood will be aspirated easily; if only a trickle occurs, it suggests that the needle is not in the vein. Aspiration of air or bright pulsatile blood indicates puncture of the pleura or subclavian artery, respectively. If the patient has a 'deep' chest, and particularly if the clavicle bows anteriorly, it may be necessary to introduce the needle a little more laterally and to point it slightly posteriorly.

Cannulation of the vein is then achieved by introducing a flexible guidewire, preferably with a J-shaped tip, through the needle. Resistance to its passage indicates that the wire is not in the vein. The wire is passed into the superior vena cava and its position checked by fluoroscopy. The needle is then withdrawn and a sheath, within which is a vessel dilator, is passed over the wire into the vein. The guidewire and dilator are then removed and the pacing lead inserted into the sheath. If it is planned to introduce a second pacing lead, the guidewire can be left in place to permit introduction of a second introducer and sheath. 'Peel-away' sheaths are used so that their removal is not prevented by the connector at the proximal end of the lead.

Cephalic vein approach

An alternative to subclavian vein puncture is to cut down onto the cephalic vein in the deltopectoral groove. Although this approach avoids the risks of subclavian vein puncture, it has its own disadvantages. The vein may not be big enough to accommodate two leads and sometimes it is too small for one lead. It is sometimes difficult to manipulate the lead from the cephalic vein into the superior vena cava.

Occasionally, a cut-down technique is used with the jugular, axillary or pectoral vein.

Positioning of a ventricular lead

To facilitate manipulation of long-term pacing leads, which are very flexible, a wire stylet is passed down the centre of the lead. Bending the distal part of the stylet or its partial withdrawal will often aid positioning.

The lead is passed into the right atrium. Sometimes, the lead can then be directly advanced through the tricuspid valve to the right ventricular apex. More often, it is necessary to form a loop in the atrium by impinging the lead tip on the atrial wall and then advancing the lead a little further. By rotating the lead, its tip can then be positioned near the tricuspid valve. Slight withdrawal of the lead will allow it to 'flick' through the valve into the ventricle. Ventricular ectopic beats are usually provoked as the valve is crossed. If these do not occur, it is possible that the coronary sinus has been entered. Entry into the ventricle can be confirmed by advancing the lead into the pulmonary artery. Once in the right ventricle, the lead tip is positioned in or near the ventricular apex by a process of lead rotation, advancement and withdrawal (Fig. 24.10). A stable position should be ensured by checking for continuous pacing and for absence of excessive lead tip movement during deep inspiration and coughing. Once a satisfactory position has been achieved in terms of stability and measurements (see below), it is very important that the lead is secured by placing a short length of rubber sleeve around it near its point of entry into the vein and fixing it to the underlying muscle with a non-adsorbable suture.

Positioning of an atrial lead

The right atrial appendage is the usual site for atrial pacing. If necessary, it is possible to carry out atrial pacing from the coronary sinus or by using a 'screw-in' lead to pace from the septal or free right atrial walls.

For pacing the right atrial appendage, a lead with a J-shaped terminal portion is usually used. First, using a straight stylet, the lead tip is straightened and advanced to the mid-right atrium. The lead is then rotated so that its tip is near the triscuspid valve. Partial withdrawal of the stylet causes the lead to assume its J shape and slight withdrawal of the lead itself allows the lead tip to enter the appendage. It is possible to position a straight lead in the appendage by use of a stylet, the terminal 5–7.5 cm of which have been shaped into a tight 'J'.

Correct positioning will be demonstrated by the lead tip moving from side to side with atrial systole. Lateral screening should demonstrate that the lead is pointing anteriorly. Lead stability should be confirmed by twisting the lead 45° in either direc-

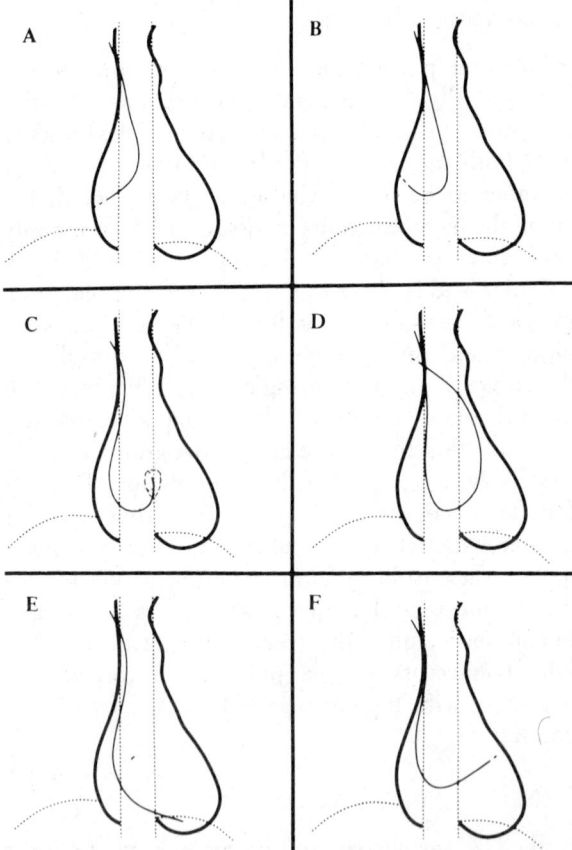

Fig. 24.10. Diagram illustrating the positioning of the ventricular lead. A loop is formed in the right atrium (A and B) which is then positioned near the tricuspid valve, indicated by the oval of dashes(C). Entry into the right ventricle can be confirmed by passing the lead into the pulmonary artery (D). The lead is then positioned in the right ventricular apex (E). (F) The characteristic appearance of a lead in the coronary sinus. (From Bennett, D.H. *Cardiac Arrhythmias.* Bristol: John Wright & Sons, by permission.)

tion: the lead tip should not turn. It is important that there is the correct amount of slack in the lead: during inspiration, the angle between the two limbs of the J should not exceed 80°.

Measurement of stimulation and sensing thresholds

Achievement of low stimulation and sensing thresholds is essential for satisfactory long-term pacing. High thresholds suggest that the cathode is not in close apposition to excitable tissue. Thresholds rise after pacemaker implantation, usually peaking 3 weeks to 3 months after surgery (Fig. 24.11). If they become high, they may exceed the stimulation and sensing capabilities of the pulse generator.

Thresholds are usually measured with a commercially produced pacing systems analyser. It is preferable to match the analyser with the generator to be implanted so that they have similar impulse-generating and impulse-sensing circuits. The same unipolar or bipolar electrode configuration should be used as that which it is planned to use with the implanted system.

Stimulation threshold

The stimulation threshold is the smallest electrical stimulus (delivered by the cathode outside the ventricular effective and relative refractory periods) that will consistently depolarize the myocardium and thereby pace the heart.

To measure the stimulation threshold, the analyser is set to deliver impulses at 70 beats/min (or if there is no bradycardia at the time, 10 beats/min in excess of the spontaneous rate) with an impulse duration commensurate with that which the implanted pulse generator will deliver (often 0.5 ms) and a voltage output of 5 V. The threshold is then established by progressively reducing the output until failure of capture occurs; it should be noted that if the patient has no spontaneous rhythm, pacemaker output will have to be promptly increased to avoid asystole. At a pulse duration of 0.5 ms, a voltage threshold of < 1.0 V is satisfactory; usually, the threshold will be in the region of 0.5 V.

Strength–duration curve

The longer the duration of the pacing stimulus the more energy is delivered and hence the lower is the stimulation threshold. However, the relationship is not linear: the range of efficient impulse duration, in terms of energy consumption, is 0.25–1.0 ms.[57] A strength–duration curve can be created by measuring the threshold, in terms of voltage, current (mA) or energy (μJ) at several different pulse durations (Fig. 24.12). If the stimulation threshold is mea-

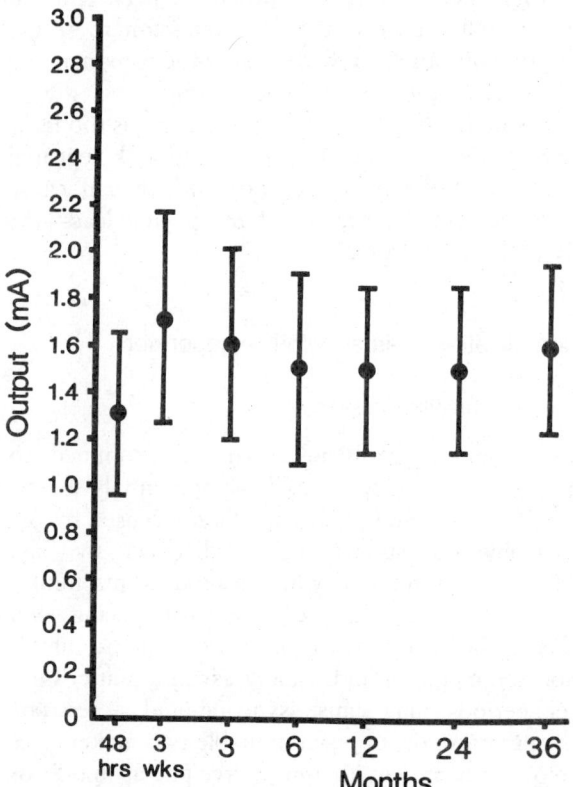

Fig. 24.11. Stimulation thresholds (mean and standard deviation) measured at intervals over three years from 400 patients with porous-surfaced pacing electrodes.

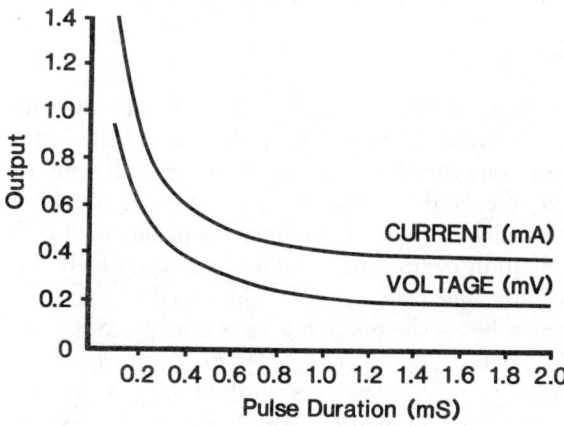

Fig. 24.12. Typical strength–duration curves measured at pacemaker implantation; there is no significant reduction in stimulation threshold when the pulse duration is increased above 1.0 ms.

sured by progressively increasing the output from a subthreshold level, it will be found to be slightly higher—the Wedensky phenomenon.

Sensing threshold

For satisfactory sensing, it is important to ensure that the intracardiac electrogram resulting from spontaneous activity in the cardiac chamber to be paced is of sufficient amplitude. This is usually done using a pacing systems analyser. Ventricular and atrial electrograms should be > 4 and > 2 mV, respectively. In 'borderline' cases, the slew rate, i.e. the rate of change of signal voltage, is also important; low slew rates may result in failure to sense.

Lead impedance

The pacing systems analyser can also be used to measure lead impedance which is a measure of resistance to flow of current in the lead. It varies with lead type but is usually in the order of 400–800 Ω. A low impedance suggests a break in insulation and hence a leakage of current whereas a high impedance indicates lead fracture.

COMPLICATIONS OF PACEMAKER IMPLANTATION

Surgical complications

Haematoma

Mild bruising is not uncommon but, occasionally, poor haemostasis will result in a haematoma which should be evacuated if tense.

Infection

Infection should occur in < 1% of implantations and is virtually always staphyloccocal. Unless it is only superficial explantation will usually be required even if antibiotics appear to help initially. It is usually not possible to remove a pacing lead with a fixation device safely without resorting to thoracotomy. The lead should be shortened so that it no longer lies in the infected area and its proximal end should be capped and fixed with a suture. Occasionally, infection persists on the lead and causes a bacteraemia in which case thoracotomy may be necessary.

Prophylactic antibiotics are widely used but there is no evidence that they are of value.[58]

Erosion

Although erosion is a late complication, it is often a consequence of implantation technique. Factors that predispose to erosion include creation of a pacemaker pocket which is too tight or too superficial, a very thin patient and use of a generator with sharp corners. The skin will be found to be thinned around the site of erosion. Infection is often present but it is secondary to erosion. If 'threatened' erosion is detected, it may be possible to re-site the generator; if the skin is broken, explantation will be necessary.

Lead displacement

Lead displacement was once a common problem but with modern leads it occurs in less than 1% of implantations;[59] it necessitates re-operation.

Other surgical complications

Complications of attempted subclavian vein puncture are infrequent; they include pneumothorax, haemothorax, air embolism, brachial plexus damage and puncture of the subclavian artery.

Very occasionally, intermittent or persistent failure to pace may result from omission to secure tightly with a set screw the pin at the proximal end of the pacing lead into the generator.

Fashioning of a generator pocket that is too large may allow spontaneous or intentional repeated rotation of the pulse generator which can cause dislodgement or fracture of the pacing lead—the 'twiddler's syndrome'.

Complications related to pulse generator

Electromyographic interference

This common problem is virtually confined to unipolar pacing systems.[60] Myopotentials generated from the underlying muscle are sensed by the pacemaker as spontaneous cardiac activity (Fig. 24.13). In systems in which sensed events inhibit output, inappropriate cessation of pacing will occur. Short periods of electromyographic inhibition are common and usually asymptomatic. Longer periods may cause syncope and necessitate re-operation, or, in programmable pacemakers (see below) adjustment to sensitivity, pacing mode or polarity.

Susceptibility to electromyographic inhibition can be demonstrated by asking the patient to extend

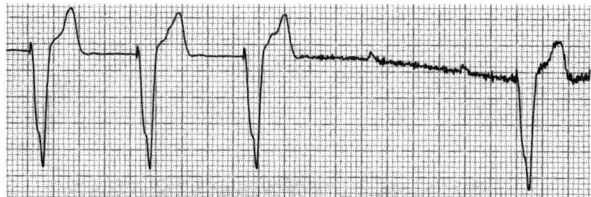

Fig. 24.13. Electromyographic inhibition. After three paced beats, pectoral muscle activity inappropriately inhibits pacemaker output.

his/her arms and then press his/her hands firmly together. It is only significant if pacemaker inhibition lasts for several seconds and particularly if the patient's symptoms are reproduced.

Muscle stimulation

Muscle stimulation is also related to unipolar pacing. It is a consequence of the pacemaker can being the anode; stimulation of the underlying pectoral muscle occurs and can be very troublesome. Most unipolar pacemakers now have an insulating covering applied to the back and sides of the pacemaker such that the only anodal contact is with the subcutaneous tissues.

Generator failure

Premature generator failure does occur occasionally, even at the time of implantation.

Complications related to pacing lead

Exit block

The development of excessive fibrous tissue, which is non-excitable, around the cathode may increase the stimulation threshold to a level higher than the pacemaker's output. The result will be intermittent or persistent failure to pace without evidence of lead displacement (Fig. 24.14). Exit block is most likely to occur in the first 3 weeks to 3 months after implantation when a stimulation threshold is at its highest. Sometimes, exit block is transient, otherwise lead re-positioning will be required unless

generator output can be increased by reprogramming (see below). Modern leads with poroussurfaced electrodes of small surface area and positive fixation devices rarely give rise to this complication.

Lead fracture

With the advent of modern leads, lead fracture is rare. If it does occur, it is usually at the point at which the lead enters the venous system, at the site of a fixation suture or wherever there is excessive angulation of the lead. Lead fracture will cause intermittent or persistent failure to pace and sense. Lead fracture can often be detected radiographically but it should not be confused with 'pseudofracture'—the pressure of a tight ligature directly applied to the lead may compress the insulation and spread the coils of wire inside without interfering with lead function.

Insulation breakdown

Insulation breakdown will allow leakage of current, which may cause stimulation of adjacent muscles and, hence, premature battery depletion. A tight ligature anchoring the lead without use of a rubber sleeve is the commonest cause.

Phrenic nerve and diaphragmatic stimulation

The phrenic nerve or diaphragm can sometimes be stimulated through the intervening thin myocardial walls by atrial and ventricular leads, respectively. Lead re-positioning will be required unless, in programmable pacemakers, cessation of extracardiac stimulation can be achieved by output reduction.

Venous thrombosis

Clinically apparent subclavian vein thrombosis is rare and pulmonary embolism even rarer. Anticoagulant therapy is indicated. In angiographic studies, the occurrence of asymptomatic venous thrombosis was not infrequent.

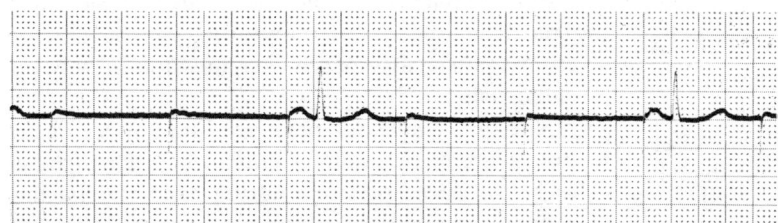

Fig. 24.14. Intermittent exit block during atrial pacing; only the third and sixth stimuli capture the atria.

PACEMAKER PROGRAMMABILITY

A programmable pacemaker can be non-invasively adjusted in one or more of its functions by radiofrequency signals emitted from an external programming device. Programmability enables achievement of optimal pacemaker function for the individual patient and can also be used in the diagnosis and treatment of certain pacemaker complications: it reduces the need for re-operation by one-fifth. Some authorities regard their use as mandatory.[61]

Simple programmable pacemakers permit alteration to rate and output. In multiprogrammable pacemakers, a wide variety of parameters can be adjusted. These are listed below together with typical options.

1 Lower rate limit (30–150 beats/min)
2 Output (2.5–5.0 V or 1–12 mA)
3 Sensitivity (0.5–8 mV)
4 Pacing mode (e.g. inhibited, triggered or fixed rate)
5 Refractory period (200–500 ms)
6 Pacing polarity (uni- or bipolar)
7 Atrioventricular delay (0–250 ms)*
8 Upper rate limits (100–180 beats/min)*

Recently, software-based pacemakers have been introduced. Many functions are controlled by a microcomputer within the pacemaker which can be externally programmed; functions can be modified and new developments incorporated that had not been anticipated at the time of implantation.

Some examples of the advantages of programmability are discussed below.

In patients who are mainly in sinus rhythm, reduction of the standby rate will allow sinus rhythm to be maintained for longer periods and therefore will help to avoid the haemodynamic disadvantages of ventricular pacing.[62] Reduction of stimulation rate may occasionally help in the management of angina. Temporary rate reduction will enable study of the patient's intrinsic rhythm. Sometimes, an increase in rate is of help in the treatment of cardiac failure or arrhythmias.

Usually, the stimulation threshold is a lot lower than the maximum output of a pacemaker; a reduction in output will prolong battery life. At regular intervals, the threshold can be measured by progressive reduction in output and then the output programmed to the threshold value plus a safety margin. Extracardiac stimulation can often be

* For dual chamber pacemakers.

stopped by reduction in output without approaching the threshold level. Some pacemakers have a high output facility (e.g. ability to increase output from 5 to 10 V); use of this may avoid the need for re-operation should exit block, which may be a temporary problem, occur.

Increase in sensitivity of the amplifier circuits may help with undersensing whereas inappropriate sensing of T waves or afterpotentials may be dealt with by reduction in sensitivity or prolongation of refractory period.

Reduction in sensitivity may prevent electromyographic inhibition. Alternatively, re-programming from inhibited to triggered mode will at least prevent bradycardia even if the electromyographic potentials reset the stimulation cycle. Another solution, which may also help with extracardiac stimulation, is to change from unipolar to bipolar pacing in systems that have this facility.

Atrial pacemakers require a higher sensitivity, because the atrial electrogram is usually of lower amplitude than its ventricular counterpart, and a longer refractory period to avoid sensing the far-field ventricular electrogram. A multiprogrammable generator can be adjusted for use as either an atrial or ventricular pacemaker.

In dual chamber pacing systems, adjustments to atrioventricular delay, atrial refractory period and/or sensitivity may prevent endless loop tachycardia (see above). In patients with sick sinus syndrome, re-programming from DDD to DVI or AAI mode will prevent this problem. Alteration from the DDD to VVI mode may be required should atrial fibrillation develop.

Pacemaker clinic

Patients with implanted pacemakers should regularly attend a follow-up clinic. The main purposes of this clinic are to check that the pacemaker is working satisfactorily, to ensure that there are no pacing complications, to detect impending battery depletion, so that generator replacement can be carried out before the patient is at risk, and to maintain a record of patients' locations should a recall of a particular generator or lead be necessary. Transtelephonic ECG monitoring can be used to ensure satisfactory pacemaker function in between clinic visits.

The main indicator of impending battery depletion is a reduction in the stimulation rate which has to be measured precisely during fixed rate pacing, usually initiated by placing a magnet over the pacemaker. Each type of pacemaker has its own characteristic 'end-of-life rate', which is usually of the order of a 5–10% reduction of the 'beginning-of-life' rate.

Some pulse generators have the facility to transmit data to the programmer, i.e. telemetry. Information about how the pacemaker has been programmed, battery status, the stimulation and sensing thresholds, lead impedance, patient details and even intracardiac electrograms can be obtained.[63] A rise in lead impedance suggests lead fracture.

Electromagnetic interference

External electromagnetic interference may be sensed by demand pacemakers and cause either inhibition or reversion to the fixed rate mode, but the pacemaker will not be damaged. The many sources include electric motors in household devices, internal combustion engines, microwave ovens, radio transmitters, theft and weapon detection systems, arc welding apparatus and radar. In practice, however, very few problems are encountered and patients should be reassured that the risks are minimal.[64] Clearly, if a patient feels dizzy near electrical equipment, they should quickly walk away from it. If a job of work brings the patient into close proximity with strong sources of electromagnetic interference, a bipolar or triggered pacemaker should be implanted.

Cardioversion may cause pacemaker damage, but this should be prevented if the paddles are at least 15 cm from the generator and preferably positioned such that they are at right angles to the pacing system. Pacemaker function should be checked after the procedure.

Diathermy may damage a pacemaker, cause inappropriate inhibition or possibly precipitate ventricular fibrillation. These risks can be avoided if the active electrode is kept at least 15 cm from the generator and the indifferent electrode sited as far away as possible so that its dipole is perpendicular to the pacing system. The pulse should be monitored so that diathermy could be interrupted if prolonged inhibition occurred.

Radiation for diagnostic purposes will not affect a pacemaker, but therapeutic levels may cause damage. The pacemaker should be shielded and, if this is not possible, re-siting of the generator should be considered.

Limited experience with magnetic resonance imaging indicates that all pacemakers will revert to fixed rate mode and some will pace at a dangerously fast rate.[65]

Short-wave diathermy can cause pacemaker inhibition.

Advice on practical matters

Patients should be encouraged to lead a normal life. It may be prudent to avoid contact sports because of the risk of damage to the pacemaker or pacemaker site.

In the UK, the presence of complete heart block should be notified to the Driving and Vehicle Licensing Centre and driving should not be permitted. Patients may resume driving 1 month after implantation of a pacemaker provided its function is checked regularly. However, patients are generally not allowed to hold a public or heavy goods vehicle licence although exceptional cases may be considered by the Honorary Medical Advisory Panel.[66]

Although air travel does not cause any problems for patients with pacemakers, patients should carry details about their pacemakers in case the pacemaker activates an airport metal detector and/or a pacing problem occurs whilst they are abroad.

A pacemaker must be explanted before cremation to avoid explosion.

TEMPORARY CARDIAC PACING

The transvenous route is usually used for temporary pacing but, in emergencies, transcutaneous and oesophageal approaches are possible short-term alternatives.

Temporary transvenous pacing

Ventricular, atrial or dual chamber pacing can be carried out by means of pacing leads introduced percutaneously or by cut-down, and connected to an external pulse generator.

Indications

The various indications include symptoms due to a bradycardia which is likely to be a short-term problem and symptomatic bradycardia in patients awaiting implantation of a long-term pacemaker.

Temporary pacing is often necessary in acute myocardial infarction which has caused a high degree of atrioventricular block. In inferior infarction, however, because interruption of conduction is at the atrioventricular nodal level, the ventricular rate is rarely very slow and pacing is necessary only if the rate is below 40 beats/min or if there is shock or ventricular arrhythmia. In anterior infarction, temporary pacing is also indicated when sinus rhythm is complicated by bifascicular block which has not hitherto been documented.

Insertion of temporary transvenous pacemaker

Atrial and/or ventricular leads are usually introduced via percutaneous subclavian vein puncture which, together with methods of lead placement, has been described above. Alternative routes of access include cut-down on a medially sited antecubital vein, internal jugular vein puncture and, for brief periods, femoral vein puncture.

Ventricular pacing is the usual mode, but, in patients with a critically low cardiac output, atrial or dual chamber pacing will be of further benefit. A J-shaped lead for temporary use in the atrium is available.

The stimulation threshold should be checked daily and the pacemaker output adjusted accordingly. If necessary, a temporary lead can be left *in situ* for several weeks provided it is not infected. Pyrexia without other obvious cause suggests lead infection; an infected lead must be removed.

Temporary transcutaneous pacing

Transcutaneous cardiac pacing was first attempted many years ago but it was usually unsuccessful and caused severe discomfort due to skeletal muscle stimulation. Recently, considerable success with less discomfort has been achieved by using skin electrodes of large surface area and stimuli of much longer duration than are used for endocardial stimulation (20–40 ms). The latest generation of transcutaneous pacemakers function in the demand mode and have a maximum output in the region of 150 mA. One electrode is applied to the front of the chest and the other to the back over the right scapula. Pacing is likely to stimulate the atria at the same time as the ventricles. It is not always possible to ascertain from the electrocardiogram that the heart is being stimulated; monitoring of an arterial pulse may be necessary. As with transvenous pacing, transcutaneous pacing is unlikely to be successful after a prolonged period of cardiac arrest.[67]

Temporary oesophageal pacing

A long impulse duration is necessary (10 ms). Success is more often encountered when stimulating the atria than the ventricles.[68]

DRUGS FOR TREATMENT OF BRADYCARDIA

Drugs have a limited role in the treatment of bradycardias. In patients with symptomatic sinus or junctional bradycardia, particularly when due to acute myocardial infarction or vagal hyperactivity, the anticholinergic action of atropine can be effective. The dose is 0.3–1.0 mg given intravenously. Atropine may be useful when atrioventricular block is due to impaired conduction in the atrioventricular junction rather than in the bundle branches. In the latter case, intravenous isoprenaline or adrenaline can sometimes be useful as a 'first-aid' measure, but pacing is safer and more effective. Before the advent of reliable pacemakers, slow-release isoprenaline tablets were widely used for the treatment of chronic heart block, but they are no longer indicated.

Xamoterol, a partial beta$_1$-adrenoceptor agonist, has been reported as having a beneficial effect in a small number of patients with the sick sinus syndrome.[69]

REFERENCES

1. Zoll, P.M. Resuscitation of the heart in ventricular standstill by external electrical stimulation. *N. Engl. J. Med.* 1952; 247: 768.
2. Elmquist, R. and Senning, A. Implantable pacemaker for the heart. In: Smyth, C.N., ed. *Medical Electronics*. Proceedings of the Second International Conference on Medical Electronics. Paris, June 1959. London: Iliffe and Sons, 1960.
3. Parsonnet, V. Permanent transvenous pacing in 1962. *PACE* 1978; 1: 265.
4. Shaw, D.B. and Kekwick, A. Potential candidates for pacemakers. *Br. Heart J.* 1978; 40: 99.
5. Malcolm, A.D. and Menon, D.K. Analysis of pacing policy and outcome in single district pacing service with high implant rate: overenthusiasm or responsible practice? *Br. Heart J.* 1985; 53: 680.
6. Data collected by British Pacing and Electrophysiology Group.
7. Parsonnet, V., Furman, S., Smythe, N.P.D. and Bilitich, M. Optimal resources for implantable pacemakers. *Circulation* 1983; 68 (Suppl. 1): 1–227–44A.
8. Edhag, O. and Swahn, A. Prognosis of patients with complete heart block or arrhythmic syncope who were not treated with artificial pacemakers: A long-term follow-up study of 101 patients. *Acta Med. Scand.* 1976; 200: 457.
9. Fitzgerald, W.R., Graham, I.M., Cole, T. and Evans, D.W. Age, sex, and ischaemic heart disease as prognostic indicators in long-term pacing. *Br. Heart J.* 1979; 42: 57.
10. Frye, R.L., Collins, J.J., DeSanctis, R.W. *et al.* Guidelines for permanent pacemaker implantation, May 1984. A report of

the Joint American College of Cardiology/American Heart Association Task Force on Assessment of Cardiovascular Procedures. *Circulation* 1984; 70: 331A.

11. Campbell, M. and Emmanuel, R. Six cases of congenital heart block followed for 34–40 years. *Br. Heart J.* 1967; 97: 577.

12. Esscher, E.B. Congenital complete heart block in adolescence and adult life. A follow up study. *Eur. Heart J.* 1981; 2: 281.

13. Shaw, D.B., Kekwick, C.A., Veale, D., Gowers, J. and Whistance, T. Survival in second degree atrioventricular block. *Br. Heart J.* 1985; 53: 587.

14. Strasberg, B., Amat-Y-Leon, F., Dhingra, R.C. *et al.* Natural History of Chronic Second-degree Atrioventricular Nodal block. *Circulation* 1981; 63: 1043.

15. Rowlands, D.J. Left and right bundle branch block, left anterior and posterior hemiblock. *Eur. Heart J.* 1984; 5A: 99.

16. McAnulty, J.H., Rahimtoola, S.H., Murphy, E.S. *et al.* Natural history of "high risk" bundle-branch block: Final report of a prospective study. *N. Engl. J. Med.* 1982; 307: 137.

17. Edhag, O., Bergfeldt, L., Edvardsson, N., Holmberg, S., Rosenqvist, M. and Vallin, H. Pacemaker dependence in patients with bifascicular block during acute anterior myocardial infarction. *Br. Heart J.* 1984; 42: 408.

18. Watson, R.D.S., Glover, D.R., Page, A.J.F. *et al.* The Birmingham trial of permanent pacing in patients with intraventricular conduction disorders after acute myocardial infarction. *Am. Heart J.* 1984; 108: 496.

19. Shaw, D.B., Holmann, R.R. and Gowers, J.I. Survival in sinoatrial disease (sick-sinus syndrome). *Br. Med. J.* 1980; 280: 139.

20. Morley, C.A., Perrins, E.J., Grant, P., Chan, S.L., McBrien, D.J. and Sutton, R. Carotid sinus syncope treated by pacing. Analysis of persistent symptoms and role of atrioventricular sequential pacing. *Br. Heart J.* 1982; 47: 411.

21. Bilitch, M., Cosby, R.S. and Cafferky, E.A. Ventricular fibrillation and competitive pacing. *N. Engl. J. Med.* 1967; 276: 598.

22. Lemberg, L., Castellanos, A. and Berkovits, B. Pacing on demand in AV block. *JAMA* 1965; 191: 12.

23. Parsonnet, V. and Bernstein, A.D. Cardiac Pacing in the 1980s: Treatment and techniques in transition. *J. Am. Coll. Cardiol.* 1983; 1: 339.

24. Berstein, A.D., Camm, A.J., Fletcher, R.D., Gold, R.D., Rickards, A.F., Smyth, N.P.D., Spielman, S.R. and Sutton, R. The NASPE/BPEG Generic code for Antibradyarrhythmia and Adaptive-Rate Pacing and Antitachyarrhythmia Devices. *PACE* 1987; 10: 794.

25. Narula, O.S. Atrioventricular conduction defects in patients with sinus bradycardia. *Circulation* 1971; 44: 1096.

26. Hayes, D.L. and Furman, S. Stability of AV conduction in patients with implanted atrial pacemakers. *Am. Heart J.* 1983; 107: 644.

27. Den Dulk, K., Lindemans, F.W. and Wellens, H.J.J. Merits of various antipacemaker circus movement tachycardia features. *PACE* 1986; 9: 1055.

28. Klementowicz, P.T. and Furman, S. Selective atrial sensing in dual chamber pacemakers eliminates endless loop tachycardia. *J. Am. Coll. Cardiol.* 1986; 7: 590.

29. Gascon, D., Errazquin, F., Nieto, J., Burgos, J., Diaz, A., Candelon, B. and Castillon, L. Preliminary Clinical Evaluation of a new DDDM pacemaker (Quintech DDD 931). *PACE* 1985; 8: A78.

30. Furman, S. Dual Chamber Pacemakers: Upper Rate Behaviour. *PACE* 1985; 8: 187–214.

31. Karlof, I. Haemodynamic effect of atrial triggered versus fixed rate pacing at rest and during exercise in complete block. *Acta Med. Scand.* 1975; 197: 195.

32. Fananapazir, L.F., Srinivas, V. and Bennett, D.H. Comparison of Resting Haemodynamic Indices and Exercise Performance During Atrial Synchronised and Asynchronous Ventricular Pacing. *PACE* 1983; 6: 202.

33. Perrins, E.J., Morley, C.A., Chan, S.L. and Sutton, R. Randomised controlled trial of physiological and ventricular pacing. *Br. Heart J.* 1983; 50;: 112.

34. Kristensson, B., Arnman, K., Smedgard, P. and Ryden, L. Physiological Versus Single-Rate Ventricular Pacing: A Double-Blind Cross-Over Study. *PACE* 1985; 8: 73.

35. Greenberg, B., Chattergee, K., Parmley, W.W., Werner, J.A. and Holly, A.N. The influence of left ventricular filling pressure on atrial contribution to cardiac output. *Am. Heart J.* 1979; 98: 742.

36. Kruse, I., Arnman, K., Conradson, T.B. and Ryden, L. A comparison of acute and longterm hemodynamic effects of ventricular inhibited and atrial synchronous ventricular inhibited pacing. *Circulation* 1982; 65: 846.

37. Fananapazir, L.F., Bennett, D.H. and Monks, P. Atrial synchronised Ventricular Pacing: Contribution of the Chronotropic Response to Improved Exercise Performance. *PACE* 1983; 6: 601.

38. Ausubel, K., Steingart, R.M., Shimshi, M., Klementowicz, P. and Furman, S. Maintenance of exercise stroke volume during ventricular versus atrial synchronous pacing: role of contractility. *Circulation* 1985; 72: 1037.

39. Rickards, A.F. and Norman, J. Relations between QT interval and heart rate. New design of physiological adaptive pacemaker. *Br. Heart J.* 1981; 45: 56.

40. Fananapazir, L.F., Bennett, D.H. and Faragher, E.B. Contribution of heart rate to QT interval shortening during exercise. *Eur. Heart J.* 1983; 4: 265.

41. Donaldson, R.M., Fox, K. and Rickards, A.F. Initial Experience with a physiological, rate responsive pacemaker. *Br. Med. J.* 1983; 286: 667–71.

42. Boute, W., Derrien, Y. and Wittkampf, F.H.M. Reliability of evoked endocardial T-wave sensing in 1500 pacemaker patients. *PACE* 1986; 9: 948.

43. Fananapazir, L.F., Rademaker, M. and Bennett, D.H. Reliability of the Evoked Response in Determining the Paced Ventricular Rate and Performance of the QT or Rate Responsive (TX) Pacemaker. *PACE* 1985; 8: 701.

44. Benditt, D.L., Mianulli, M., Fetter, T. *et al.* Single Chamber cardiac pacing with activity-initiated chronotropic response: evaluation by cardiopulmonary exercise testing. *Circulation* 1987; 75: 184.

45. Rossi, P., Aina, F., Rognoni, G., Occhetta, E., Plichhi, G. and Prando, M.D. Increasing Cardiac Rate by Tracking the Respiratory Rate. *PACE* 1984; 7: 1246.

46. Nappholtz, T., Valenta, H., Maloney, J. and Simmons, T. Electrode configurations for a respiratory impedance measurement suitable for rate responsive pacing. *PACE* 1986; 9: 960.

47. Laczkovics, A. The Central Venous Blood Temperature as a Guide for Rate Control in Pacemaker Therapy. *PACE* 1984; 7: 822.

48. Jolgren, D., Fearnot, N. and Geddes, L. A Rate-responsive Pacemaker Controlled by right Ventricular Blood Temperature. *PACE* 1984; 7: 794.

49. Wirtzfeld, A., Heinze, R., Stanzl, K., Hoekstein, K., Alt, E. and Liess, H.D. Regulation of Pacing Rate by Variations of Mixed Venous Oxygen Saturation. *PACE* 1984; 7: 1257.

50. Samet, P, Bernstein, W.H., Nathan, D.A. and Lopez, A. Atrial contribution to cardiac output in complete heart block. *Am. J. Cardiol.* 1965; 16: 1.

51. Nishimura, R.A., Gersch, B.J., Vliestra, R.E., Osborn, M.J., Ilstrup, D. and Holmes, D.R. Haemodynamic and Symptomatic Consequences of Ventricular Pacing. *PACE* 1982; 5: 903.

52. Erlebacher, J.A., Danner, R.L. and Stelzer, P.E. Hypotension

with ventricular pacing. An atrial vasopressor reflex in human beings. *J. Am. Coll. Cardiol.* 1984; **4**: 550.

53. Jones, R.I., Cashman, P.M.M., Hornung, R.S., Prince, H., Bassein, L. and Raftery, E.B. Ambulatory blood pressure and assessment of pacemaker function. *Br. Heart J.* 1986; **55**: 462.

54. DeCaprio, V., Hurzeler, P. and Furman, S. A comparison of unipolar and bipolar electrograms for cardiac pacemaker sensing. *Circulation* 1977; **56**: 750.

55. Boal, B.H. Report of the policy conference on pacemaker re-use sponsored by the North American Society of Pacing and Electrophysiology. *PACE* 1985; **8**: 161.

56. Parsonnet, V., Werres, P.V., Atherley, T. and Littleford, P.O. Transvenous insertion of double sets of permanent electrodes. Atraumatic technique for atrial synchronous and atrioventricular sequential pacemakers. *JAMA* 1980; **243**: 62.

57. Furman, S., Hurezeler, P. and Mehra, R. Cardiac pacing and pacemakers. IV. Threshold of Cardiac stimulation. *Am. Heart J.* 1977; **94**: 115.

58. Ramsdale, D.R., Charles, R.G., Rowlands, D.B., Singh, S.S., Gautam, P.C. and Faragher, E.B. Antibiotic prophylaxis for pacemaker implantation: a prospective randomised trial. *PACE* 1984; **7**: 844.

59. Fananapazir, L., Martin, T.S., Martin, V. *et al.* Experience with 407 transvenous, finned pacing leads with a sintered porous-surfaced electrode. *PACE* 1984; **7**: 132.

60. Ohm, O.J., Bruland, H., Pedersen, O.M. and Waerness, E. Interference effect of myopotentials on function of unipolar demand pacemakers. *Br. Heart J.* 1974; **36**: 77.

61. Levine, P.A., Belott, P.H., Bilitch, M. *et al.* Recommendations of the NASPE policy conference on pacemaker programmability and follow-up. *PACE* 1983; **6**: 1221.

62. Rosenqvist, M., Vallin, H.O. and Edhag, K.O. Rate hysteresis pacing: how valuable is it? A comparison of the stimulation rates of 70 and 50 beats per minute and rate hysteresis in patients with sinus node disease. *PACE* 1984; **7**: 332.

63. Levine, P.A., Sholder, J. and Duncan, J.L. Clinical Benefits of Telemetered Electrograms in Assessment of DDD function. *PACE* 1984; **7**: 1170.

64. Gold, R.G. Interference to cardiac pacemakers—how often is it a problem? *Prescribers' J.* 1984; **24**: 115.

65. Holmes, D.R., Hayes, D.L., Gray, J.E. and Meredith, J. The effects of magnetic resonance imaging on implantable pulse generators. *PACE* 1986; **9**: 360.

66. *Medical Aspects of Fitness to Drive,* 4th edn. London: Her Majesty's Stationery Office, 1985.

67. Noe, R., Cockrell, W., Moses, H.W., Dove, J.T. and Batchelder, J.E. Transcutaneous pacemaker use in a large hospital. *PACE* 1986; **9**: 101.

68. Touberg, P., Anderson, H.R. and Pless, P. Low-current bedside emergency atrial and ventricular cardiac pacing from the oesophagus. *Lancet* 1982; **1**: 166.

69. Tsen, F.L., Morley, C.A. and Macintosh, A.F. Oral xamoterol in patients with sinoatrial disease. *Br. Heart J.* 1986; **56**: 469.

Chapter 25

Congenital Heart Disease

Michael Tynan and Robert H. Anderson

INCIDENCE

The incidence of congenital cardiac abnormalities is still uncertain and varies in different age-groups.[1,2] It is probable that congenital cardiac anomalies are found in at least 0.75% of livebirths. Nowadays, it is rare for patients with any of these lesions to present in adult life. Technical improvements in treatment, however, are producing an ever increasing pool of adult survivors requiring care. Furthermore, among school children with cardiac ailments, the incidence of congenital malformations has been increasing in relation to that of rheumatic heart disease. In Western countries, congenital defects are responsible for the vast majority of heart disease in childhood.

The simpler cardiac malformations are the most common.[3] Isolated ventricular septal defect alone accounts for 25–30% of all congenital heart disease. Persistence of the arterial duct (ductus arteriosus) is next most common, making up a further 10% of the total. These two anomalies, together with pulmonary stenosis, atrial septal defect, coarctation of the aorta, aortic stenosis and the tetralogy of Fallot constitute two-thirds of the organic heart disease seen by paediatric cardiologists. Of the more complex malformations, the commonest are complete transposition, atrioventricular septal defect and the hypoplastic left heart syndrome, each accounting for 4 or 5% of cases.

Congenital heart disease is the fourth most important cause of childhood death in developed countries. In pre-school age-groups, it causes at the most 1 death in every 20 000 living children.[4] In infancy (i.e. from birth to 1 year of age), the picture is different. Approximately 2 of every 1000 liveborn infants die as a result of congenital heart defects.[5] As approximately one-quarter of all those born with congenital heart disease die in the first year of life, early diagnosis is of supreme importance.

AETIOLOGY

Several aetiological factors can be identified in congenital heart disease.[6] A small proportion of affected individuals have intrinsic defects in the developing embryo including chromosomal anomalies and mutant gene syndromes. Environmental insults to the fetus account directly for a further small proportion, but the majority of cases appear to occur sporadically. Evidence suggests that sporadic occurrence is not a chance phenomenon; rather it is due to the combination of environmental and genetic interactions known as multifactorial inheritance.

The available information on the aetiology of congenital heart defects gives little indication of the basic cause or mechanism of their production. Its importance lies in counselling parents of an affected child and adults with congenital heart defects on the risks of recurrence in the family. When the defect is part of a syndrome with Mendelian inheritance, the risks can be accurately stated. Hence, the importance of recognizing these syndromes. The risk of recurrence in the family of sporadic cases with multifactorial inheritance can be estimated only by analysis of the family history and the frequency with which a given lesion occurs in the general population. The existence of an affected first degree relative (sibling or parent) demonstrates a family predisposition to congenital heart defects. Subsequent pregnancies then carry a risk for the same lesion which can be roughly stated as the square root of its natural occurrence rate when expressed as a decimal. As an example, the frequency of ventricular septal defect is approximately 25 per 10 000 livebirths or 0.0025. The square root of this is 0.05 or 5%. Calculated risk rates compare well with those observed in family studies. The observed risk rates are trebled when 2 first degree relatives are affected. With 3 or more affected relatives,

subsequent pregnancies may be expected to carry a
risk of up to or exceeding 50%; these families have
a genetic predisposition that requires little or no
environmental insult to precipitate the defect. Two
people with congenital heart disease should be
aware that the risk to their children will be about
3–15% depending on the type of lesions from
which the parents suffer. When families with more
than one first degree relative affected are counselled,
the expert services of a clinical geneticist are
invaluable. Known environmental triggers should
be avoided, particularly in families with an already
demonstrated predisposition to congenital heart
defects. Immunization against rubella is indicated in
all girls, not already immune, before they reach
child-bearing age. If possible, teratogenic drugs
should be substituted by non-teratogenic ones.
Prospective mothers should be encouraged to abstain from alcohol or at least to limit their intake
severely. Should there be a family history of
congenital heart disease (or should there have been
exposure to a known teratogen) then fetal echocardiography should be recommended.

DESCRIPTION OF AND APPROACH TO CONGENITALLY MALFORMED HEARTS

The majority of congenital cardiac lesions exist in
hearts which are otherwise normal. These can be
considered as 'simple' anomalies and described in a
few words such as 'ventricular septal defect'. Other
lesions seem to be more complicated because they
are either abnormalities of connexion of the cardiac
segments or else due to abnormal structure of the
cardiac components. Considerable danger of confusion ensues if these malformations are described
with brief titles such as 'asplenia' or 'single ventricle' (Table 25.1).

Confusion can be eliminated by simple sequential
segmental analysis of the cardiac structures.[7] The
basis of this approach is that there are limited
morphological variations in the make-up of the
three cardiac segments. Thus, there are only morphologically right or left atriums (the chambers
with morphological characteristics of the right-
sided and left-sided atrial chambers seen in the
normal individual[8]—see Chapter 1). Ventricles can
only be morphologically right, left or indeterminate; the arterial trunks can be aortic, pulmonary or
common. Within these limited basic morphological
options, however, there are innumerable permutations of connexions and relations. Description of

Table 25.1. Descriptions of congenitally malformed hearts.

Confusing term	Better description
Asplenia	Right atrial isomerism
Polysplenia	Left atrial isomerism
Single ventricle	Double-inlet ventricle
Dextrocardia	Right-sided heart
Corrected transposition	Discordant atrioventricular and ventriculo-arterial connexions
Complete transposition	Concordant atrioventricular and discordant ventriculo-arterial connexions
Truncus arteriosus	Common arterial trunk
Endocardial cushion defect	Atrioventricular septal defect
Atrioventricular canal	
Ductus arteriosus	Arterial duct
Ductus venosus	Venous duct
Situs solitus	Usual atrial arrangement
Situs inversus	Mirror-image atrial arrangement

these possibilities starts with atrial arrangement.
This is the most difficult step for the clinician since
the atrial appendages, which are the most characteristic feature of the atriums, do not lend themselves
to clinical identification. Almost always, therefore,
the clinician takes advantage of the fact that atrial
arrangement, with very few exceptions, reflects the
arrangement of the abdominal and thoracic organs.
This gives two basic patterns: the usual arrangement (so-called 'solitus') and its mirror-image
variant (so-called 'inversus'). The greater majority
of patients with congenitally malformed hearts have
usual arrangement of their organs whereas a very
small minority have mirror-image arrangement
(Fig. 25.1). These two patterns do not cater for all
hearts. There is a significant minority which have a
jumbled-up arrangement of the abdominal
organs—so-called visceral heterotaxy. In terms of
the thorax, such patients are often said to have an
ambiguous arrangement of the lungs and atriums.
Careful analysis shows that they have an isomeric
arrangement, with bilateral manifestations of either
morphologically right or left characteristics. The
minority of cases that are neither usual nor mirror-
image can be described as right or left isomerism
(Fig. 25.1). In rare cases, atrial arrangement will be
disharmonious with either thoracic or abdominal
arrangement. In these circumstances, analysis of
each body segment should be done separately and
recorded, but cardiac analysis should be based upon
the determined arrangement of the atriums. This
will rarely be necessary. In practical terms, therefore, atrial arrangement can be inferred from

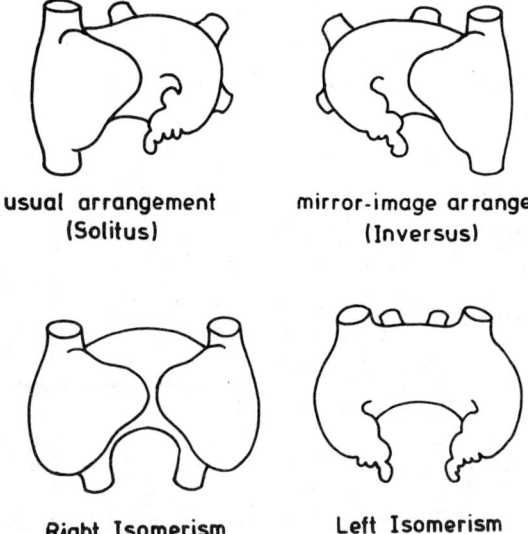

Fig. 25.1. Diagram showing the four possible combinations of morphologically right and left atriums. These underscore the atrial arrangement or so-called 'situs'.

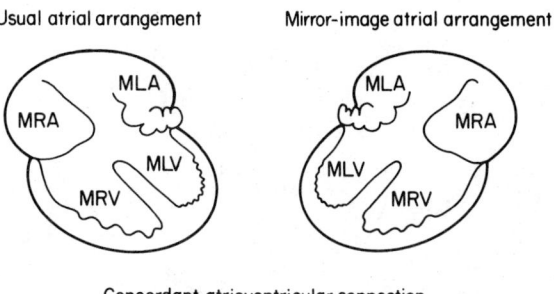

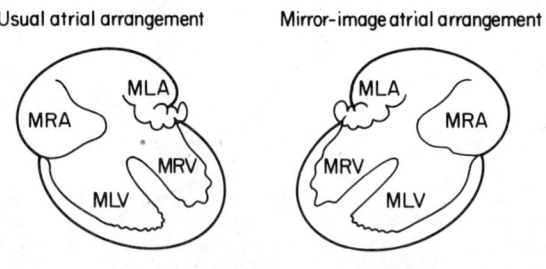

Fig. 25.2. The connexions of atriums and ventricles producing concordant and discordant arrangements.

clinical identification of bronchial morphology by means of penetrated chest radiography or analysis of the relationship of the abdominal great vessels to the spine by ultrasonography.

Having determined atrial arrangement, the next step in sequential segmental analysis is to decide how the atriums are connected to the ventricles. This is conditioned by both atrial arrangement and ventricular morphology. Usually arranged or mirror-image atriums can connect to either appropriate or inappropriate ventricles. This produces concordant or discordant atrioventricular connexions (Fig. 25.2). Isomeric atriums can themselves be connected to paired ventricles arranged in usual or mirror-image pattern (Fig. 25.3). The ventricular topology is itself described in terms of right-handedness or left-handedness of the ventricular mass. The combination of a biventricular connexion of isomeric atriums is called an ambiguous connexion. The three connexions described above all produce a biventricular atrioventricular connexion. There are then three further patterns of connexion which are not accounted for by these variants. These further options are unified because the atrial chambers (of usual, mirror-image or isomeric arrangement) connect to only one ventricle (univentricular atrioventricular connexion). They are double-inlet, absent right and absent left connexion. All three can exist when the ventricle connected to the atriums is of left morphology (the right ventricle being incomplete and rudimentary),

of right morphology (with an incomplete and rudimentary left ventricle), or solitary and of indeterminate morphology (Fig. 25.4). Equally sig-

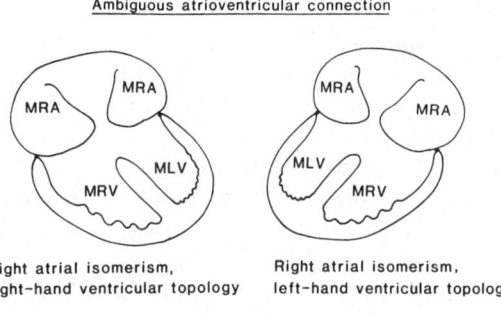

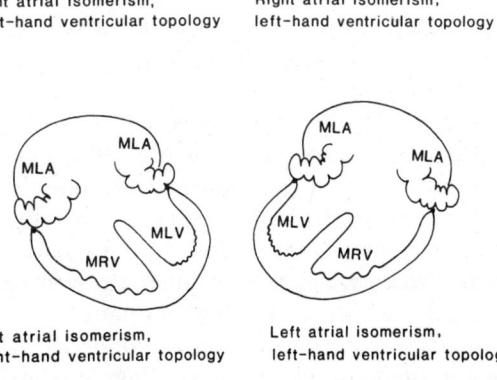

Fig. 25.3. When each of two isomeric atriums is connected to its own ventricle, the atrioventricular connexion must be ambiguous (neither concordant nor discordant) irrespective of the ventricular topology (architecture of the ventricular mass).

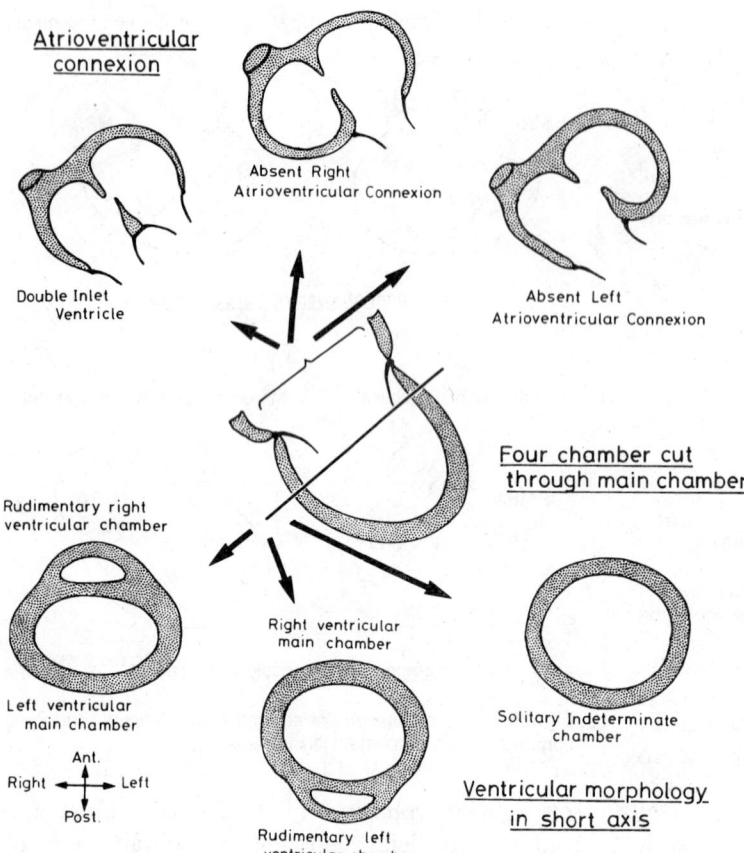

Atrioventricular connexion

Absent Right Atrioventricular Connexion

Double Inlet Ventricle

Absent Left Atrioventricular Connexion

Four chamber cut through main chamber

Rudimentary right ventricular chamber

Left ventricular main chamber

Right ventricular main chamber

Solitary Indeterminate chamber

Ant.

Right ← → Left

Post.

Rudimentary left ventricular chamber

Ventricular morphology in short axis

Fig. 25.4. The combinations underscoring a univentricular atrioventricular connexion. The central panel shows the idealized situation of the atriums joined to only one ventricle. The upper three panels show the specific arrangements underscoring this situation. The lower panels show the ventricular morphologies that can co-exist. Note that in only one (solitary and indeterminate chamber) is there only one ventricle present.

nificant at the atrioventricular junction is the morphology of the atrioventricular valves, a feature we call the mode of connexion. When both atriums are connected to the ventricular mass (concordant, discordant, ambiguous and double-inlet connexions), the junction can be guarded by separate right and left valves or by a common valve (Fig. 25.5). These valves have the options of straddle (tension apparatus astride the ventricular septum) and/or override (the junction shared between two ventricles). The precise degree of override will condition the precise connexion (the 50% law—Fig. 25.6). Either a right or left valve can be imperforate, producing valve atresia in the setting of concordant, discordant, ambiguous or double-inlet connexions. When there is absence of one atrioventricular connexion, which gives a different pattern of valve atresia, the solitary valve can be connected exclusively to one ventricle or can straddle or override.

Analysis of type and mode of connexions is then repeated at ventriculo-arterial level. Here the options are governed by the nature of the ventricular mass (two ventricles or a solitary ventricle) and the pattern of the arterial trunks (aortic, pulmonary or common). When there are two ventricles, the connexions may be concordant, discordant or double or single outlet from the right or left venticles, be they normal, dominant or incomplete. With only one ventricle, the connexions must be either double or single outlet. The modes of connexion are limited at ventriculo-arterial level. Only a common trunk can be guarded by a common valve. Aortic or pulmonary valves can be imperforate or can override, as can (and usually does) a common valve.

Relationships throughout the heart are accounted for with the detail required to provide clear and unambiguous description using simple terms like right, left, anterior, posterior, and so on. Associated lesions are tabulated going through the heart from venous to arterial poles. Finally, cardiac position is described according to the position of the heart within the chest and, when accurately identified, the orientation of its apex.

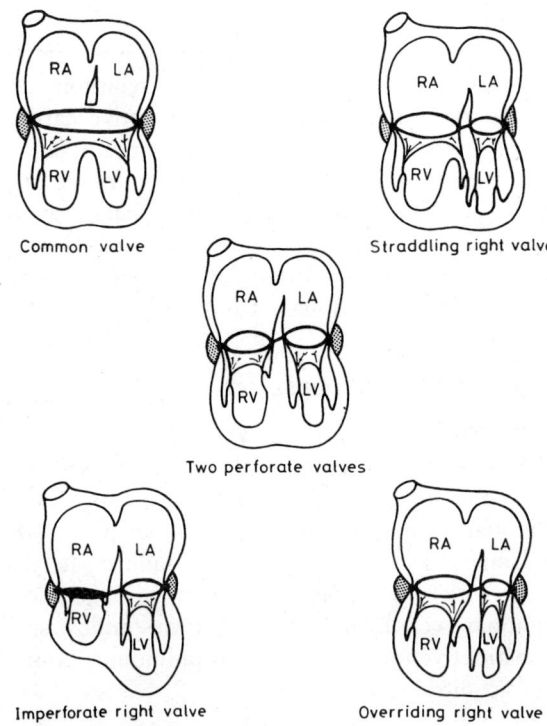

Fig. 25.5. These diagrams show the variable morphologies of the valves that guard the atrioventricular junction when two atriums connect with the ventricles. Straddling, overriding and imperforateness can affect the left as well as the right valve. RA, right atrium; LA, left atrium; RV, right ventricle; LV, left ventricle.

THE DEVELOPMENT OF THE HEART

Most textbooks concerned with congenital heart disease carry a section devoted to cardiac development. This is often used subsequently to provide explanations, and names, for lesions which are presumed to represent an arrest of normal development. Such assumptions are speculative and often wrong. They add little to the understanding of the anatomy of the malformations and have a potential for confusion. It is the anatomy which underscores the understanding and diagnosis of congenital heart defects. For this reason, we will avoid any embryological speculations; instead, we will concentrate on descriptions of the anatomy as it is observed.

GENERAL PATHOLOGY AND SYMPTOMATOLOGY

The presentation and management of infants with congenital heart disease are influenced by the changes that occur with the transition from the fetal to the mature extra-uterine circulation.[9,10] The placenta dominates the fetal circulation (Fig. 25.7). As the placenta is the organ of gas exchanges, blood flow is directed towards it and away from the lungs.

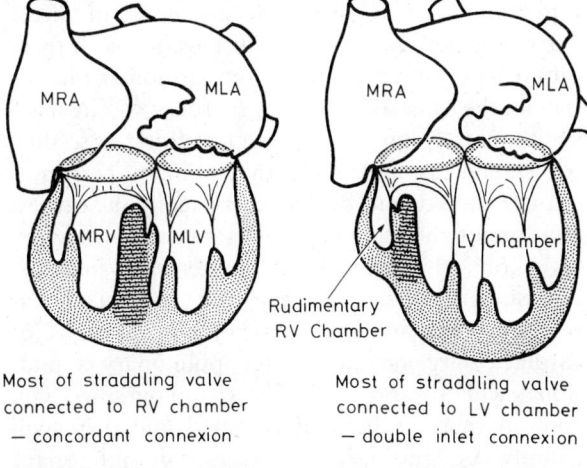

Fig. 25.6. Diagrams showing how the extent of override of the straddling right valve can change a concordant into a double-inlet atrioventricular connexion. M, morphologically. Other abbreviations as for Fig. 25.5.

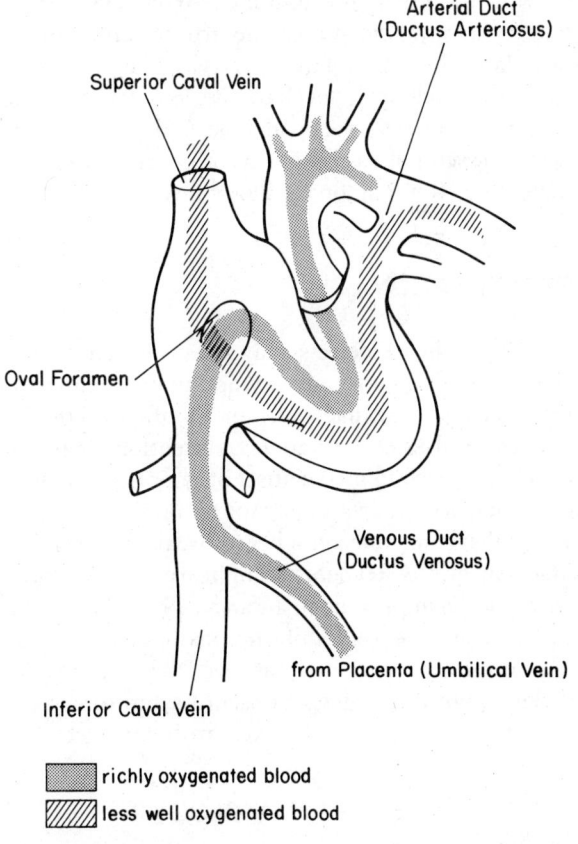

Fig. 25.7. The course of the fetal circulation.

This circulatory pattern is achieved by the maintenance of a high pulmonary vascular resistance. Thus, blood arriving in the pulmonary trunk is diverted to the descending aorta through the arterial duct (ductus arteriosus) whose patency is maintained throughout fetal life. Richly oxygenated blood returning to the heart from the placenta to the inferior caval vein is directed to the left atrium through the oval hole (foramen ovalis). The basic route of fetal circulation, therefore, is that superior caval venous return passes from right atrium to right ventricle and pulmonary trunk. A major part then passes through the arterial duct to the lower body and the placenta via the two umbilical arteries. Blood returning from the lower body and from the placenta to the umbilical vein then passes from the inferior caval vein via the right atrium and oval hole to the left atrium and ventricle and then to the ascending aorta. In this way, the richly oxygenated blood is directed to the developing brain. The deoxygenated blood returning from the brain passes through the right atrium, right ventricle, pulmonary trunk and arterial duct before returning to the placenta (Fig. 25.7). The active events that dominate transition from this to the free-living circulatory pattern are the closure of the arterial and venous ducts and the fall in pulmonary vascular resistance from the high fetal level to the low level of the infant. Closure of the oval hole, although important, is essentially a passive event dependent on the increase in the pulmonary blood flow after birth.

PRESENTATION

Congenital heart defects may be suspected at any age by the finding of any asymptomatic abnormality, such as a cardiac murmur or absence of the femoral pulses. Alternatively, attention may be drawn to the child by the onset of symptoms such as breathlessness or cyanosis. Approximately 70% of all deaths from congenital heart disease occur in the first year of life. Recognition of heart disease is thus particularly important in infancy. Not only is the early recognition of manifestations of heart disease important in order to improve the chances of survival, but the timing of onset of symptoms gives clues to the type of lesion likely to be present.

PRESENTING SYMPTOMATOLOGY IN INFANCY

In the case of infants, the word 'symptom' refers to abnormalities noted by the parents or medical or lay attendants. Broadly speaking, presentation in infancy is due to the appearance of symptoms of pulmonary venous congestion, congestive cardiac failure, cyanosis or to circulatory collapse. It is rare that other symptoms bring the infant to the attention of the cardiologist. These include 'spells' in the tetralogy of Fallot and paroxysmal distress seen with anomalous origin of the left coronary artery from the pulmonary trunk.

Pulmonary venous congestion

The earliest symptom is tachypnoea due to interstitial pulmonary oedema. With increasing severity, dyspnoea and frank pulmonary oedema may occur. Pulmonary venous congestion is seen as part of the syndrome of congestive cardiac failure. It also occurs when the lesion is a primary obstruction to pulmonary venous return or left atrial outflow such as obstructive totally anomalous pulmonary connexion or mitral atresia.

Congestive cardiac failure

The syndrome of congestive cardiac failure in infants is different from that seen in adults and older children. Pitting peripheral oedema is rarely a feature of the syndrome in infancy. Oedema is undoubtedly present, as evidenced by the excessive weight gain seen in such infants, but they are rarely obviously oedematous. An exception is heart failure occurring in fetal life (hydrops fetalis). Another difference is the evidence of increased systemic venous pressure. In infancy, this is manifested by rapid increase in liver size rather than easily detectable peripheral venous distension. With these differences, the principles of recognition in infancy remain the same as in older age-groups.[11] The main symptom is dyspnoea at rest or on effort. As feeding is the main sustained effort that an infant performs, poor feeding due to dyspnoea is usually the earliest abnormality noticed. Clinical examination will then reveal objective signs of dyspnoea, such as intercostal, subcostal, suprasternal and supraclavicular recession. Hepatic enlargement, clinical signs of cardiac enlargement and, often, pulmonary crepitations will be present. Chest radiography will confirm that the heart is enlarged and there will usually be radiographic signs of pulmonary plethora or congestion.

The commonest cause of congestive cardiac failure in infancy is a large left-to-right shunt due most frequently to a large ventricular septal defect or a large persistent arterial duct and less frequently to other lesions allowing a systemic to pulmonary communication with an unrestricted pulmonary blood flow. The time of onset of symptoms will depend, to a great extent, on the state of the pulmonary vascular resistance.[12] At birth, the resistance is high and little shunt will occur. As the pulmonary resistance falls, blood flow to the lungs will be progressively less restricted, the left atrial and ventricular filling and output will have to increase, and finally cardiac enlargement, cardiac decompensation and pulmonary venous congestion will become evident. In these situations, the congestive cardiac failure is dependent on the fall in pulmonary vascular resistance and occurs later than is the case when, for instance, mitral regurgitation, primary myocardial disease or a peripheral arteriovenous fistula is the cause. The time of onset of congestive cardiac failure due to these latter lesions will be determined mainly by their severity. The earliest presenting lesions causing pulmonary venous congestion and/or congestive cardiac failure will be those with severe obstruction to pulmonary venous drainage or left atrial emptying. The classic examples are totally anomalous pulmonary venous connexion to the portal vein on the one hand and mitral atresia on the other. These conditions cause severe illness in the first days of life. Non-dependent cardiac failure, as seen in atrioventricular septal defect with incompetence of the left-sided component of the common valve or endocardial fibroelastosis, tends to cause symptoms in the early weeks of life. In dependent cardiac failure (for instance, with a large ventricular septal defect), the onset of symptoms may be delayed to the second or third month of life.

Cyanosis

When caused by heart disease, blue coloration of the skin and mucous membrane indicates that there is admixture of systemic venous return with the systemic arterial output. It is most evident when the aorta is connected to the ventricle receiving the systemic venous return as exemplified in complete transposition. It also occurs when systemic venous blood is denied access to the pulmonary arterial tree by pulmonary or tricuspid atresia. In all these instances, cyanosis is usually noticed at or shortly after birth. When obstruction to pulmonary flow is not total, as in the tetralogy of Fallot, the appearance of cyanosis is dependent on the severity of the

pulmonary stenosis. This is often progressive, such that cyanosis may not be present at birth but is usually evident by 1 year of age. Cyanosis can be present but difficult to detect when venous admixture to the systemic circulation is not accompanied by a restricted pulmonary blood flow (as in the case of common arterial trunk and other common mixing situations). When suspected, the effect of breathing 100% oxygen should be assessed (the nitrogen wash-out test). If the arterial Po_2 does not rise above 160 Torr after 5 min of breathing 100% oxygen, venous admixture to the systemic arterial blood is present. If it does rise above this level, cyanosis, if present, is unlikely to be due to a cardiac cause. A case can be made for re-defining cyanotic congenital heart disease as those conditions failing to give a normal response to the nitrogen wash-out test. In complex congenital heart malformations (such as complete transposition), pulmonary venous congestion, congestive cardiac failure and cyanosis may co-exist.

Collapse

Sudden circulatory collapse in the neonatal period is usually the result of closure of the arterial duct when part of the circulation is dependent for its perfusion on ductal patency as, for example, in aortic atresia.

PRESENTATION OF HEART DISEASE IN CHILDHOOD

Health surveillance of children in Western countries by well-baby clinics, pre-school examinations and, in some instances, examinations to assess fitness for leisure activities frequently leads to the discovery of congenital heart defects before the onset of symptoms. Congestive cardiac failure, although a rare presenting syndrome in childhood, does occur. It is usually heralded by shortness of breath on effort. Cyanosis is occasionally the first sign of heart disease in childhood. Rare instances of tetralogy of Fallot present during the second year of life, but when cyanosis is seen in older children with no previous history of heart disease it often indicates an increase in pulmonary vascular resistance due to pulmonary vascular disease established from infancy. The basic cardiac lesion, such as a ventricular septal defect, will have remained undetected because shunt flow was limited by the high pulmonary resistance. Syncope should alert the physician to the possibility of aortic stenosis or of an arrhythmia, whereas it is well known that the first symptom of aortic coarctation can be a subarachnoid haemorrhage.

SYSTEMIC MANIFESTATIONS OF CONGENITAL HEART DISEASE

GROWTH RETARDATION

Congenital heart disease is included as one of the causes of 'failure to thrive' in childhood. Although growth retardation is a feature of all severe congenital cardiac malformations,[13] it is rarely a presenting feature. Failure to gain weight is most evident in infants with congestive cardiac failure. It is also seen in severe cyanotic heart disease, such as tetralogy of Fallot. The cause of growth failure in infants and children with congenital heart disease is not clear. It appears that hypoxia in cyanotic conditions can of itself cause slowing of physical growth but, in acyanotic conditions, inadequate caloric intake is probably the major factor. In either case, palliative or corrective surgery can cause a growth spurt even to the extent of ensuring normal stature.

INTELLECTUAL DEVELOPMENT

There is some evidence to suggest that prolonged severe cyanosis results not in mental retardation but in a lower intelligence quotient than would normally be attained by the patient. Palliative and corrective surgery can result in an improvement in intelligence quotient whilst corrective surgery can be performed in infancy with preservation of normal intellectual function.[14,15]

RESPIRATORY INFECTIONS

Infants and children with large left-to-right shunts are subject to recurrent respiratory infections. It is often during one of these infections that the congenital heart defect is discovered. A respiratory infection may precipitate the patient into congestive cardiac failure. The altered lung mechanics secondary to high pulmonary blood flow and pulmonary venous congestion probably account for the increased susceptibility of these infants and children to respiratory infections.

CEREBRAL COMPLICATIONS OF CONGENITAL HEART DISEASE

Cerebrovascular accidents and cerebral abscess are mainly complications of cyanotic congenital heart defects. They can occur with acyanotic conditions, such as atrial septal defect (the paradoxical embolus), but are rare. Cerebrovascular accidents (usually cerebral venous thromboses but often a mixture of venous and arterial occlusions) generally occur in infancy and are rare after 3 years of age. In contrast, cerebral abscesses are rare before 3 years of age but they are the most frequently encountered cerebral complications after this age. Both forms of cerebral complication appear to be more related to arterial hypoxaemia and relative anaemia than to polycythaemia.[16,17] Increased blood viscosity plays a part in the causation of these complications, particularly when they are exacerbated by dehydration due to an intercurrent illness. The much more important role of hypoxaemia, however, should lead to consideration of the possibility of surgical improvement of arterial oxygenation rather than venesection to lower the hematocrit.

PULMONARY VASCULAR DISEASE

An elevation of pulmonary vascular resistance may be found in many forms of congenital heart disease. When such an elevation persists (or recurs after the usual age of involution of the fetal pulmonary vascular pattern), it is known as pulmonary vascular disease. It exists in a continuum of clinical and pathological severity. When associated with a simple anomaly, such as ventricular septal defect, it may be severe enough to cause a right-to-left shunt. This clinical situation, with cyanosis appearing in a previously pink patient, has been called the Eisenmenger syndrome. It represents one end of the clinical spectrum of pulmonary vascular disease.

Factors that predispose to the development of pulmonary vascular disease are a high-pressure communication between pulmonary and systemic circulations (such as found with a large enough ventricular septal defect to permit equalization of ventricular pressures), a high pulmonary blood flow (as with any large left-to-right shunt), a high pulmonary venous pressure (which may also accompany a large left-to-right shunt) and systemic arterial hypoxaemia, such as found in complete transposition. The most important factors are a high-pressure communication and systemic arterial hypoxaemia. When occurring together, as in complete transposition with a large ventricular septal defect, pulmonary vascular disease is almost inevitable.[18]

The natural history of pulmonary vascular disease in congenital heart disease is that it becomes established by the age of 1–2 years and then steadily progresses through childhood.[12] The best chance of prevention is to make operative interventions during infancy. Any patient with pulmonary hypertension should have either corrective surgery or banding of the pulmonary trunk. This is even more important in those subjects with cyanosis (other than that due to a high pulmonary resistance) or pulmonary venous hypertension. Although this account of pulmonary vascular disease is a good working clinical model, the many exceptions to this pattern demonstrate that there is much that we do not yet understand.

HISTORY AND PHYSICAL EXAMINATION

Nowadays, early detection of congenital heart disease is the rule. A definitive diagnosis is arrived at by 1 month of age in 70% of patients. Indeed, this stage is reached in nearly half the patients by the age of 1 week.[4] Thus, in many instances, it is the medical and paramedical support personnel who notice something amiss, rather than the parents seeking medical advice for problems they have encountered. This means that the burden of recognition of affected infants is on the professionals. The signs that direct attention towards the heart include tachypnoea, dyspnoea, poor feeding, abnormalities of weight gain and cyanosis. Although all of these can be manifestations of diseases other than those of the cardiovascular system, the possibility of heart disease must always be entertained. Although signs noted by professionals are of great importance, complaints by the parents of poor feeding, cyanosis or 'funny turns' must never be ignored.

In many instances, advice is sought because a murmur has been detected at a routine medical examination. The history serves to assist in the assessment of the significance of the murmur to the presence of structural or functional heart disease. It also helps in ascertaining the functional status of the patient who has heart disease, in the uncovering of any aetiological factors and in establishing any genetic predisposition that might influence counselling and management.

As many children have few (if any) symptoms, history-taking frequently comes to resemble an interrogation rather than a medical interview; this must be guarded against. Parents and children must be given time and encouraged to ask questions and voice their concerns no matter how distant they may appear from the purely technical decisions that have to be made. Although a checklist of questions has to be worked through, this must be done with sympathy and interested attention on the part of the physician.

As far as possible, examination should be carried out in a warm, quiet and congenial environment. The temptation immediately to reach for the stethoscope must be resisted. Inspection, particularly in the case of young infants and newborns, is of paramount importance for diagnosis. Infants are usually examined as they lie flat; older children should be sitting at 45°. This is to facilitate inspection of the jugular venous pressure and pulse.

An overall impression of the general health of the child must be obtained. Is the state of nutrition good? The presence or absence of cyanosis is often best assessed by examining the finger- and toenail beds. At the same time, finger and toe clubbing is looked for. Tachypnoea and dyspnoea, although obvious, must consciously be sought since they are often missed or more probably disregarded. Subcostal, intercostal and supraclavicular recession are present and indicate dyspnoea. The accessory muscles of respiration may be in use.

Apart from features bearing directly on the cardiovascular system, attention must be given to appearances that indicate recognizable syndromes of malformation known to be associated with cardiac lesions.[6] In many instances, it will be recognition of such a syndrome that has brought the heart under suspicion. Chromosomal anomalies like Down's syndrome, or those genetically determined like the Ulrich-Noonan syndrome, will be obvious. William's syndrome and the asymmetric cry or cardiofacial syndromes are less obvious and, unless careful examination is made, they may be missed. Intermittent 'cannon waves' will be seen with heart block. With congestive cardiac failure, the overall jugular venous pressure will be elevated; restricted filling of the heart (as in constrictive pericarditis) and overall high venous pressure are accompanied by deep and jerky 'x' and 'y' descents. Cardiac tamponade is evidenced by increasing venous pressure on inspiration (Kussmaul's sign). Hepatojugular reflux is of little significance except where caval venous obstruction is suspected, for example, after venous redirection operations for complete transposition. Here, presence of the hepatojugular reflux is reassuring.

Although the information obtained from palpation (or auscultation) must be systematized and complete, the approach to the child and strategies used to achieve this information are varied.[19] They depend on the personality of the child (and the family) and that of the clinician. The experienced physician may at times be able to examine the child while talking to his or her parents. This can be almost before the child has realized an examination is taking place. To this end, distraction is always better than coercion. The pulses should be examined in the upper and the lower limbs. The carotids or superficial temporals should also be palpated. Important signs include absent or weak femoral pulses with normal or increased upper limb pulses. These indicate coarctation of the aorta.

Qualitative abnormalities in the pulses are more difficult to assess. High-volume pulses are found with persistent patency of the arterial duct. In the premature baby, they are the major diagnostic sign of this condition. Pulses of similar character, even amounting to collapsing pulses, are seen with other causes of rapid aortic run-off, for example, aortic regurgitation or ruptured aneurysm of the sinus of Valsalva. As the arterial duct closes, weak pulses become evident in newborns with aortic atresia. In infants with severe aortic stenosis, weak or absent pulses, rather than the classical slow-rising pulse, are of diagnostic importance. Palpation of the carotid pulse (and also the suprasternal notch) will reveal a systolic thrill with aortic stenosis or with bicuspid aortic valve. In the latter case, the thrill is very delicate and can be obliterated by finger pressure. Irregularities of the pulse will be noticed during arrhythmias. Analysis of the arterial and venous pulses can give assistance in the elucidation of arrhythmias but the electrocardiogram is better.

The apex beat should be localized. Its recognition provides a clinical impression of cardiac size, although this is more reliably determined from the chest radiograph. The character of the cardiac impulse gives further information. A parasternal heave indicates right ventricular hypertrophy. Especially in infants, such palpation is superior to the radiograph in differentiating between left, right, and combined ventricular hypertrophy. Thrills during the cardiac cycle are detected by palpation with the flat hand using the metacarpal heads as low-frequency sensors. Accurate timing should be by the apex beat and is rarely a problem. Further information includes palpation of a loud (pulmonary) component to the second heart sound in the presence of severe pulmonary vascular disease. A palpable second heart sound (aortic) may also be found in any malformation with an anteriorly placed aorta.

Measurements of the blood pressure should be part of the physical examination of patients of all ages. Technical difficulties in performing this test have been largely overcome by the introduction of Doppler shift detection of either arterial flow or wall motion. In this simple form, an ultrasound Doppler probe is placed over the radial or posterior tibial artery whilst a cuff of appropriate size is deflated.[20]

Auscultation must be carried out in a quiet warm room with a warm stethoscope of a size appropriate to the child. Owing to the small radius of curvature of the infant chest, a stethoscope with a small diaphragm is essential to ensure even application. The bell size is less critical. Low-pitched sounds are best heard with the lightly applied bell; high-pitched sounds are ideally auscultated with the diaphragm. An early diastolic murmur may be audible only with the diaphragm. The best overall performance, if a compromise is necessary, is obtained using the bell and varying the pressure of application. Such a compromise may be necessary with a restless or uncooperative child when auscultation is needed urgently. If a child is uncooperative, it is best not to fight, but perhaps to accept a limited examination to gain his or her confidence. In certain circumstances, particularly if the electrocardiogram and chest radiograph are normal, a return visit at a later date may be the only answer.

Systematic examination of the cardiovascular system together with careful history-taking will frequently lead to the correct diagnosis. It is certainly the most important aspect of the differentiation of innocent from pathological murmurs. At the very least, such a careful approach will make the choice of investigations logical and economic. However, attention must not be focused solely on the heart. Careful enquiry and examination should be made to exclude associated congenital malformations. When appropriate, the signs of intercurrent illness (such as pneumonia, urinary tract infection or infective endocarditis) must be sought. Systemic diseases with cardiac involvement must be borne in mind. These aspects are discussed in Chapter 60.

SPECIAL INVESTIGATIONS

CHEST RADIOGRAPHY

General features to be noted in the examination of the chest radiograph include bone abnormalities (such as hemi-vertebrae in the Klippel-File syndrome, which is often associated with congenital heart defects) and rib notching seen in older children with aortic coarctation. Hyperinflation of the lungs due to airways obstruction is found in patients with left-to-right shunts and associated respiratory infections, whereas pulmonary arteriovenous fistulas present discrete opacities in the lung fields.

Thymic shadow

In infants and small children, the upper mediastinum will appear wide in the frontal projection and the retrosternal area opaque in the lateral projection. This shadow, often sail-like, is due to the normal thymus (Fig. 25.8). It is particularly evident in healthy children but it is decreased in size in the sick, particularly those with cyanotic heart disease.

Cardiac position and atrial arrangement

The cardiac shadow may be predominantly located in the left chest (laevocardia), in the right chest (dextrocardia) or may be centrally located (sometimes called mesocardia). The disposition of the

heart within the thorax does not predict or deny intracardiac abnormalities. A mid-line or right-sided heart is not of itself a sinister finding; isomerism of the atriums is. Consequently, determination of the atrial arrangement is of far more significance than the position of the heart. The importance of recognizing abnormalities of cardiac position is that they are easy to detect and should always prompt a thorough examination of visceral (and therefore atrial) arrangement. Satisfactory chest radiographs invariably include the upper abdomen and allow a judgement to be made concerning the arrangement of the abdominal organs. In the usual abdominal arrangement, the stomach bubble is to the left; it is to the right with the mirror-image arrangement. When the position of the heart and of the abdominal organs are as anticipated and appropriate to one another (left-sided heart with usual or right-sided heart with mirror-image arrangement), the plain chest film will almost always suffice for identification of atrial arrangement. In contrast, when cardiac position and abdominal arrangement are not appropriate, or when either is indeterminate, atrial arrangement must be determined from the bronchial anatomy. The main bronchus of the morphologically left

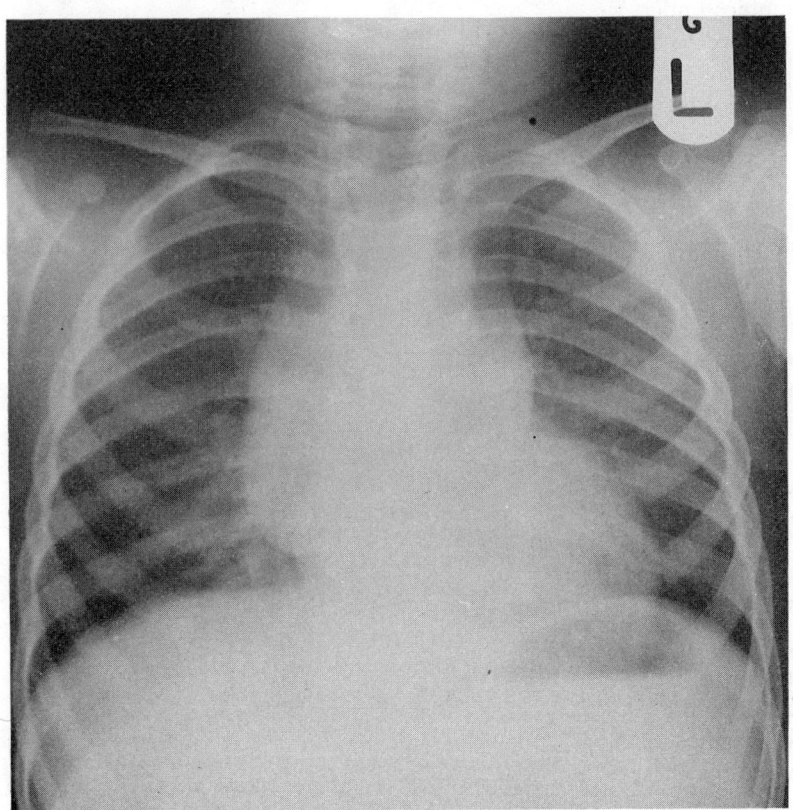

Fig. 25.8. Normal chest radiograph of an infant. The lobulated shadow widening the mediastinal shallow is the normal thymus.

(two-lobed) lung is longer from the carina to its first branch than that of the main bronchus to the morphologically right (three-lobed) lung. Thus, in usual atrial arrangement, the longer bronchus is on the left; in mirror-image arrangement, it is on the right. When both bronchi are more or less the same length, atrial isomerism is almost invariably present. Severe cardiac abnormalities can be predicted in the presence of atrial isomerism (see p. 626).

Cardiac size and silhouette

The principles of recognition of the components of the cardiac silhouette are similar in adults and children. In infants and small children, however, it is almost impossible to differentiate left from right ventricular enlargement on the basis of the chest radiograph alone. Usually, the only judgement that can be made is that the heart is enlarged. In general, cardiac enlargement is considered to be present when, on a standardized postero-anterior radiograph with a tube-to-film distance of 2 m, the cardiothoracic ratio is greater than 50%. This judgement is complicated in the neonatal period because the cardiothoracic ratio may normally approach 60% on the first day of life. This is particularly true when films are taken (as they often are at this age) with the baby supine under non-standard conditions. Even with standard techniques, the cardiothoracic ratio diminishes over the first few days of life. Thus, at birth, a ratio of 60% or over is abnormal but, by the age of 1 week, a ratio of over 50% is abnormal.

Specific abnormalities of the cardiac silhouette

A prominent pulmonary knob is seen in patients with large left-to-right shunts or pulmonary hypertension. When stenosis is present at valvar levels, it is due to post-stenotic dilatation of the pulmonary trunk. Mild but definite degrees of prominence of the pulmonary knob are sometimes detected in children without heart disease. Concavity at the usual site of the pulmonary knob is seen in pulmonary arterial hypoplasia in the tetralogy of Fallot and pulmonary atresia. A narrow upper mediastinum is seen in these latter conditions but, when associated with cardiomegaly, it strongly suggests complete transposition. Absence of a left-sided aortic knob with a right-sided descending aortic shadow (a right aortic arch) is seen with the tetralogy of Fallot, pulmonary atresia with ventricular septal defect and common arterial trunk. A wide

upper mediastinum with enlargement of the superior caval vein and a somewhat fainter shadow of a left-sided ascending pulmonary vein (snowman, cottage loaf or W.C. Fields heart) is strongly suggestive of totally anomalous supracardiac pulmonary venous connexion. The diagnostic shadow associated with anomalously connected right-sided pulmonary veins is the 'scimitar' shadow which accompanies the syndrome of that name.

Pulmonary vascularity

Apart from evidence of lung disease, examination of the lung fields provides useful information regarding the state of the pulmonary circulation. Several patterns are discernible. Pulmonary plethora indicates a high pulmonary blood flow (Fig. 25.9). All the pulmonary arteries are enlarged from the hilum to the periphery. When doubt exists, it is useful to examine the arterial shadows accompanying the bronchi. The bronchial and arterial shadows are normally of similar diameter but, when pulmonary plethora is present, the arterial shadows have a greater diameter than those of the bronchi.

Pulmonary venous congestion in infants and small children rarely shows the regional distribution seen in the adult. A generalized 'fluffy' or reticular

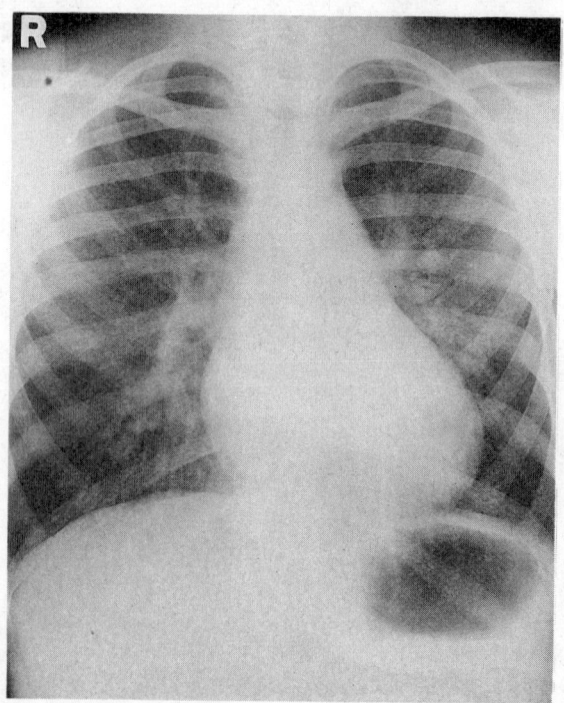

Fig. 25.9. Increased pulmonary vascular markings of pulmonary plethora. This patient had an atrial septal defect.

pattern is seen, together with septal lines (often seen best in the lateral film). The appearances suggest severe pulmonary venous hypertension as occurs with obstructed totally anomalous pulmonary venous connexion.

Enlarged central pulmonary arteries with diminished peripheral vascular shadowing is the classic picture of established severe pulmonary vascular disease. This sign is of limited diagnostic value, because it is not seen in early stages of the condition when diagnosis is imperative if treatment is to be effective.

Pulmonary oligaemia (Fig. 25.10) is found when pulmonary blood flow is diminished and pulmonary perfusion pressure is low as, for example, in the tetralogy of Fallot. The lungs have a generally translucent appearance with vascular shadows being smaller in diameter than the bronchi. In pulmonary atresia, the origin of the pulmonary blood supply from large tortuous systemic to pulmonary collateral arteries can sometimes be discerned.

Asymmetrical perfusion of the lungs

When one pulmonary artery is atretic, the lung it

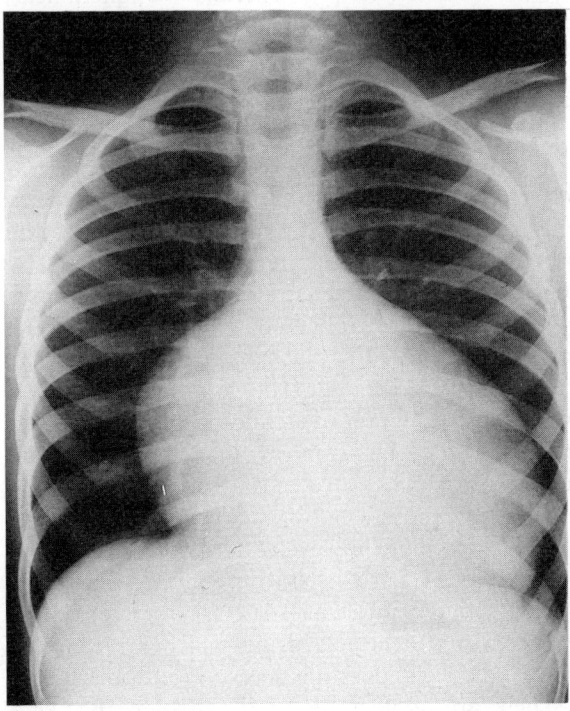

Fig. 25.10. The decreased pulmonary vascular markings of pulmonary oligaemia. The heart is enlarged. This radiograph is typical of Ebstein's malformation.

originally supplied will be oligaemic compared with the other. When the blood supply to one lung arises directly from the aorta, that lung will be plethoric when compared with the other. Asymmetrical vascularity is seen in complete transposition even though both lungs are perfused via the pulmonary arteries.

ELECTROCARDIOGRAPHY

The principles of electrocardiography are the same in infants and children as they are in adults. Minor differences in technique include the use of small chest electrodes to obtain adequate separation of the chest lead position, together with the recording of at least one additional right-sided chest lead, usually lead V_4R. The proximity of the heart to the anterior chest wall in childhood often leads to large QRS deflections in the anterior chest leads, particularly V_2–V_5. Abnormalities of QRS voltages are best detected in the leads most distant from the ventricular mass, i.e. V_6 and V_1 and V_4R. Lead V_4R is useful in confirming that abnormally high R-wave voltages detected in lead V_1 are not solely due to the proximity of this lead to the right ventricle. In addition, V_4R often reveals abnormalities of initial ventricular depolorization (such as those seen with discordant or univentricular atrioventricular connexions). Apart from these technical differences, the normal electrocardiogram in infancy and childhood differs from that of the adult as a consequence of the changes that occur in the circulation with the transition from intra- to extra-uterine life. At full term, the fetal right and left ventricles eject against more or less the same resistance. The fetal and newborn right ventricle is thus relatively more massive than that in the mature subject. The electrocardiogram of the full-term neonate, therefore, shows right ventricular dominance with the mean frontal QRS vector being directed inferiorly and to the right.

Changes in the frontal QRS axis

The mean frontal QRS axis normally changes during infancy from a prevalent direction of $+135°$ to one of $+65°$, the major changes occurring during the first 3 months of life. There is, however, a wide distribution in the normal population.

Changes in QRS voltages

As with the mean frontal QRS axis, there is a

change from right to left ventricular dominance during childhood. The general tendency is decreases in voltage of the R wave in leads V_4R and V_1 and of the S wave in V_6 with a reciprocal increase in voltage of the S wave in leads V_4R and V_1 and of the R wave in V_6. As there is a wide variation of normality, the diagnosis of ventricular hypertrophy on voltage criteria is only secure when it is marked. Minor degrees of hypertrophy can be suggested but not definitely diagnosed on the basis of an isolated electrocardiogram. In general, the direction of initial activation in the horizontal plane (septal activation) is to the right in infants as in adults. In a small number of newborns, it may be to the left. A Q wave is then seen in lead V_4R with at most a small Q wave in V_6. In these subjects, the initial activation becomes directed to the right with increasing age. The QR pattern in lead V_4R rarely persists after the first few weeks of age.

Changes in the T wave

The T waves may be upright in lead V_1 and inverted in lead V_6 at birth and for the first 8 hours of life. After 8 hours of age, the T waves in the right chest leads become inverted. By 24 hours, the usual infant pattern is established of an upright T wave in lead V_6 and inverted T waves in V_4R–V_4. The T waves become upright across the chest from left to right during childhood and adolescence, that in V_4 being upright by 5 years of age, V_3 by 10 years of age, V_2 by 12 years of age and V_1 by 16 years of age.

Heart rate and rhythm

Heart rate is generally faster in infancy than in older children, but observed heart rates depend on the time of recording and on the method used. Isolated electrocardiograms show average heart rates of 120–160 beats/min during the first year of life reducing to 70–80 beats/min by the age of 12 years. Recordings taken over a 24-h period show that there are extreme variations in heart rate throughout the day. Rates as high as 220 beats/min and as low as 59 beats/min may be observed in young infants and children. Similarly, although sinus rhythm dominates in normal children, tape monitoring over long periods has revealed that atrial ectopic beats, multiple ventricular ectopic beats, sinu-atrial block and sinus arrest occur in a significant number of normal children.

Interpretation of the electrocardiogram in childhood

Criteria for the diagnosis of disturbances of heart rhythm, atrioventricular conduction, intraventricular conduction and atrial hypertrophy are little different in infants and children than in adults. Differences occur in the assessment of ventricular hypertrophy and of deviations of the mean frontal QRS axis from normal.[21] A useful electrocardiographic sign is a superiorly directed axis. This is seen in atrioventricular septal defects and in tricuspid atresia. It is also seen with an inlet ventricular septal defect whether this occurs alone or in association with other abnormalities, such as double-outlet right ventricle or complete transposition. Patients with the Ullrich-Noonan syndrome are the only group known to have a naturally occurring superior QRS frontal axis without an abnormality of the inlet portion of the septum. It is not understood why the axis is directed superiorly in many of these conditions, but this does not diminish the usefulness of this sign. The combination of a superior axis and right bundle branch block occurring after closure of a ventricular septal defect strongly suggests proximal damage to the conduction tissues, and is associated with the development of late post-operative complete heart block.

ECHOCARDIOGRAPHY

The introduction of cross-sectional echocardiography has revolutionized the recognition of congenitally malformed hearts. Details of cardiac anatomy previously seen only by the morphologist are now routinely observed and used for diagnostic purposes by the echocardiographer. A detailed account of the techniques used are given in Chapter 13. The approach used in adults, however, is not always pertinent in infants and children. This is not to imply that the heart is more difficult to interrogate in younger patients. Access is easier in the neonate, and through more windows. In those with congenital malformations, however, the cardiac structures, or even the heart itself, may not be in their anticipated location. Each structure, therefore, must be positively identified, using whichever echocardiographic view gives the necessary information.

There are no features of the atriums that lend themselves to direct echocardiographic recognition. It is the appendages that are the most reliable anatomical marker, but they cannot be consistently identified. The venous connexions can be recognized, but these can themselves be anomalous. Because of this, the echocardiographer must infer atrial arrangement from the relationships of the abdominal great vessels relative to the spine (Fig. 25.11). When the aorta and the inferior caval vein are on opposite sides of the spine, there is either usual or mirror-image atrial arrangement and the morphologically right atrium is on the side of the caval vein. When the vessels are to the same side of the spine, there is atrial isomerism. In almost all cases, an anterior venous channel is indicative of right isomerism whereas an anterior aorta suggests left isomerism.[22]

It is much easier to recognize the ventricles directly. The morphologically right ventricle has its atrioventricular valve tethered to the inlet septum whereas the left ventricle does not (Fig. 25.12). If seen, off-setting of the septal attachments of the atrioventricular valves is also a marker of the morphology of the ventricles. The tricuspid valve is always inserted more towards the apex than is the mitral valve, differentiating in this way the right from the left ventricle. When there is a univentricular atrioventricular connexion, the rudimentary right ventricle is always located antero-superiorly whereas rudimentary left ventricles are found in postero-inferior position (Fig. 25.13). The great arteries are readily recognized from their branching pattern (Fig. 25.14). By these means, therefore, it is possible to determine accurately the sequential segmented connexions of the heart and, subsequent-

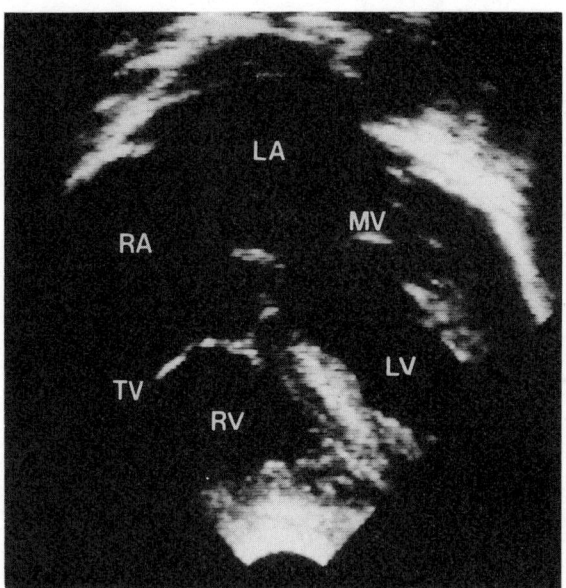

Fig. 25.12. Standard parasternal four-chamber echocardiographic section demonstrating the right and left atriums (RA and LA) and right and left ventricles (RV and LV). There is normal offsetting of the septal attachments of the tricuspid valve (TV) and mitral valve (MV). The membranous and muscular parts of the atrioventricular septum are demonstrated. (Figure courtesy of Dr M.L. Rigby).

ly, to identify almost all of the associated lesions.[23] The diagnostic criteria of the individual lesions will be described in the subsequent section.

Doppler echocardiography

In congenital as in other forms of heart disease, Doppler estimates of blood flow velocity enable the detection of valvar regurgitation and the quantification of valvar stenosis.[24] They permit unequivocal identification of persistence of the arterial duct. It is also possible to estimate pulmonary arterial pressure by this means. However, as the estimation of pulmonary arterial pressure in infants is often of critical importance, it should be measured properly. Useful information can be obtained from the flow velocity across a ventricular septal defect. This information has been made easier to obtain by the introduction of colour coding of the direction of flow.

The anatomical and functional information that can be obtained from ultrasonography have rendered it the major and indispensable diagnostic method for congenital heart disease.

NUCLEAR ANGIOGRAPHY

Using technetium-99 as the basic isotope, three

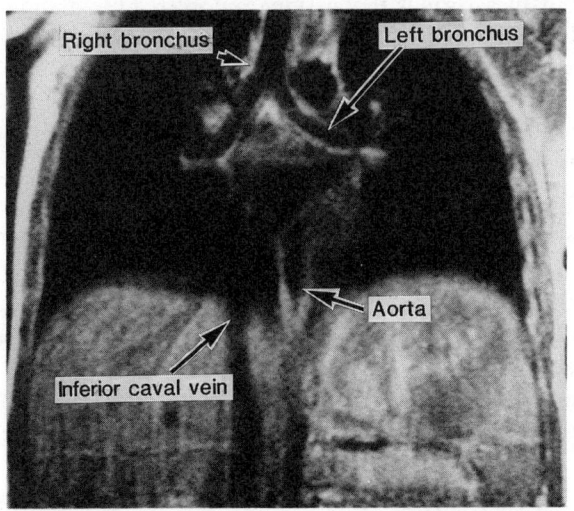

Fig. 25.11. Sagittal plane magnetic resonance image showing the features of usual atrial arrangement. The left bronchus is longer than the right, the inferior caval vein is to the right and the aorta is to the left. (Figure courtesy of Dr E.J. Baker).

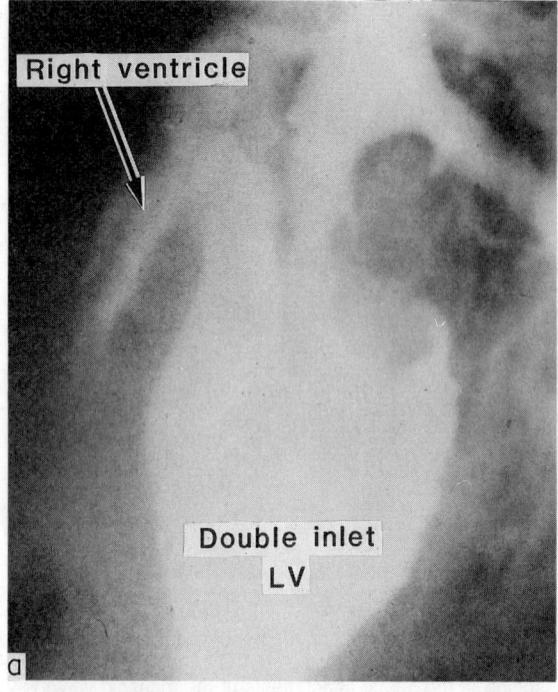

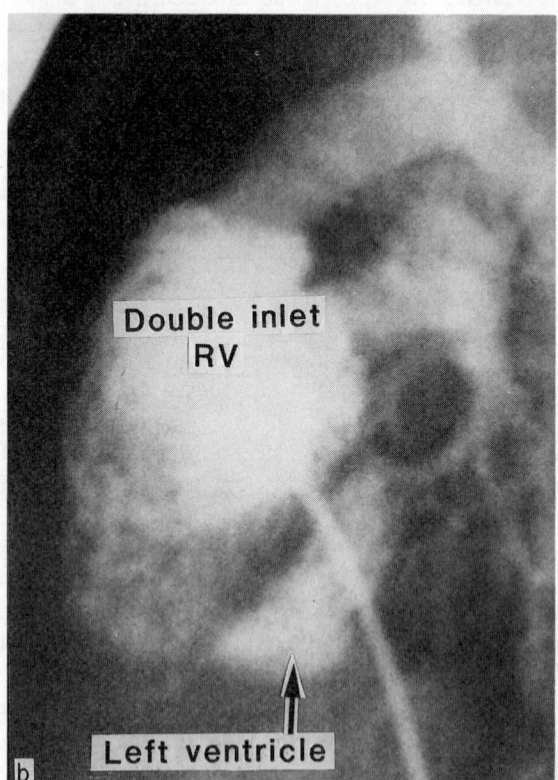

Fig. 25.13. (a) Left ventricular angiogram showing double-inlet left ventricle with an antero-superior rudimentary ventricle. (b) Right ventricular angiogram in double-inlet right ventricle showing the rudimentary left ventricle in postero-inferior location.

types of study can be of use in congenital heart disease. The first passage of the isotope through the heart gives information regarding the sequence of filling of the chambers and vessels. Thus, if the aorta fills at the same as or before the pulmonary trunk, a right-to-left shunt can be diagnosed. Similarly, if there is prolonged activity in the pulmonary arteries, a left-to-right shunt can be recognized and quantified.[25] When red cells are labelled with technetium-99, it is possible to obtain multiple acquisition blood pool images of the heart. Left ventricular performance can be estimated.[26] If labelled microspheres or albumin is used, it is possible to ascertain the distribution of pulmonary blood flow.[27] In practice, the main clinical uses of nuclear angiography in children are the quantification of left-to-right shunts and recordings for the sequential assessment of cardiac performance.

MAGNETIC RESONANCE IMAGING

Magnetic resonance imaging is as yet unproven as an accurate diagnostic technique in congenital heart disease. It has the potential to make accessible those parts of the circulation that cannot be visualized on echocardiography. Thus, the distal aortic arch and the major branches of the pulmonary arteries can now be demonstrated non-invasively (Fig. 25.15). Furthermore, recent advances enabling the heart and great arteries to be studied in its own axes, even in infancy, allow the anatomy to be displayed in a fashion comparable to that on echocardiography but in a format that is much more readily assimilated (Fig. 25.16).

CARDIAC CATHETERIZATION AND ANGIOCARDIOGRAPHY

The principles of cardiac catheterization and angiocardiography in children are similar to those in adults. Normal cardiac connexions cannot be assumed and an unusual course of the catheter will need an anatomical explanation. Fortunately, the efficacy of echocardiography in anatomical diagnosis has eradicated some of the surprises and the operator can now undertake diagnostic catheterization with more calm. Usually, cardiac catheterization is performed to resolve a specific haemodynamic question (for example, to estimate the pulmonary vascular resistance), to obtain a specific angiocardiogram or to enable a catheter intervention to be performed.

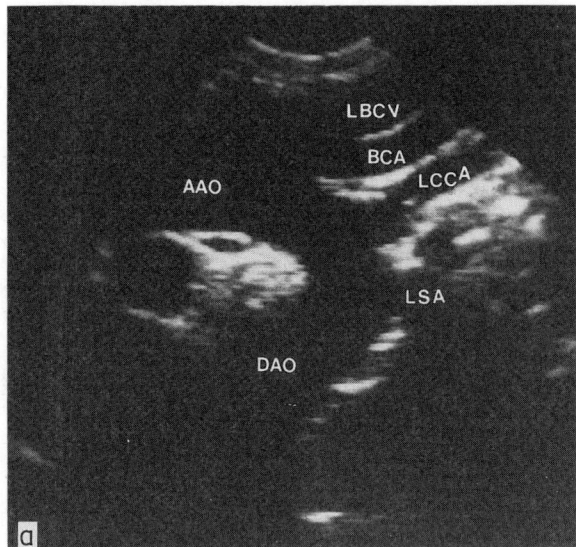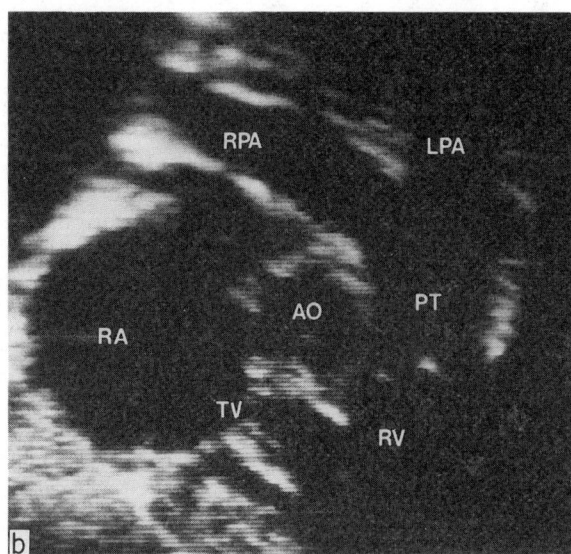

Fig. 25.14. (a) Normal branching pattern of the aorta obtained from a suprasternal parasagittal echocardiographic section. AAO, ascending aorta; DAO, descending aorta; BCA, brachiocephalic artery; LCCA, left common carotid artery; LSA, left subclavian artery; LBCV, left brachiocephalic vein. (b) Subcostal right oblique echocardiographic section demonstrating the normal branching pattern of the pulmonary trunk. RA, right atrium; TV, tricuspid valve; RV, right ventricle; AO, aortic root; PT, pulmonary trunk; RPA, right pulmonary artery; LPA, left pulmonary artery. (Figure courtesy of Dr M.L. Rigby).

PRINCIPLES OF MANAGEMENT

The majority of deaths from congenital heart disease occur in the early months of life. The management of infants and newborns with symptomatic heart disease depends in the first instance on the type and complexity of the abnormality present. In many instances, surgical treatment is imperative, for example, in totally anomalous pulmonary venous connexion. In others, surgery is indicated only when medical treatment fails to control the situation as, for example, with an isolated ventricular septal defect. Decisions about how long to pursue a conservative course can only be made with full knowledge of the anatomy and physiology of the congenital anomaly. Thus, when investigating infants, special techniques including echocardiography, cardiac catheterization and angiocardiography are frequently performed as a

Fig. 25.15. Transverse plane magnetic resonance image showing hypoplastic pulmonary arteries. The pulmonary trunk is much smaller than the ascending aorta. (Figure courtesy of Dr E.J. Baker).

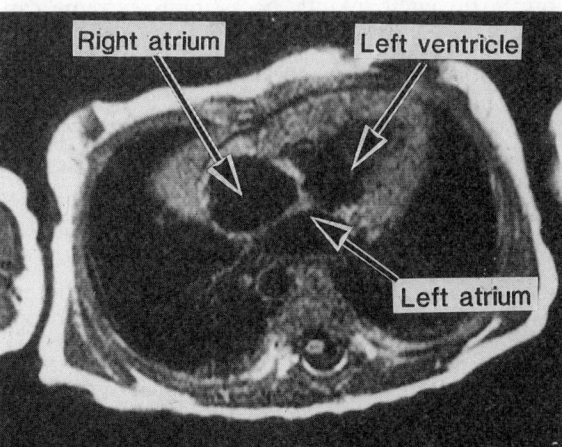

Fig. 25.16. Transverse plane magnetic resonance image showing both atriums connected to ventricle of left ventricular morphology. This is a double-inlet connexion. (Figure courtesy of Dr E.J. Baker).

matter of urgency or even emergency. Echocardiography provides adequate information for the planning of treatment in the majority of young infants. If any doubt exists as to the necessity for cardiac catheterization, it is best to perform it because, if a condition demanding surgery is present, waiting can lead only to deterioration. An early comprehensive diagnosis is required in all infants presenting in heart failure, in all cyanosed infants and in all infants suspected of having severe obstructive lesions such as aortic stenosis or coarctation of the aorta.

MEDICAL MANAGEMENT

Congenital heart disease in infants

Even before the full diagnosis is established, it is reasonable to start medical treatment. Rest is an important aspect of treatment. All dyspnoeic infants, therefore, should be rested by giving feeds through a nasogastric tube. Humidified oxygen should be administered if a pulmonary contribution to cyanosis is suspected. Blood gas analysis should be performed if ventilatory insufficiency is suspected. Mechanical ventilation is started if this is confirmed. The ambient temperature must be adjusted to restore and maintain a normal body temperature. Heart failure is treated with diuretics initially and with digoxin traditionally. The role of digoxin in the chronic treatment of congestive cardiac failure is a matter of debate although in both adults and children it appears to have some beneficial effect on left ventricular performance.[28] The incidence of toxicity, however, particularly in low birthweight infants, necessitates extreme caution in its use.[29] It is our practice to commence the treatment of congestive cardiac failure with frusemide and to introduce digoxin only if diuretics do not effect control. This approach is particularly applicable in cases where congestive cardiac failure continues or occurs after surgical treatment. When digoxin is used, it must be controlled by frequent estimations of its levels in the blood. In resistant heart failure, the introduction of vasodilators should not be delayed. The progress of an infant in congestive cardiac failure is assessed by daily weighing. Excessive weight gain indicates the accumulation of oedema; subnormal weight gain indicates inadequate oral intake of calories. If an infant in heart failure cannot maintain a steady (even if slow) weight gain on oral feeding, and then requires tube feeding, the heart failure is uncontrolled.

Co-existent infections are often suspected in symptomatic newborns with heart disease. Frequently, a respiratory infection precipitates an infant into heart failure. Confirmation of the presence of infections usually awaits the bacteriological cultures of sputum, blood, urine or cerebrospinal fluid. Antibiotics, therefore, are often indicated before an infection is confirmed. These should be administered only after the appropriate samples have been taken for culture. It is reasonable in neonates who present collapsed or severely cyanosed to consider the administration of E type prostaglandins,[30] even without a firm diagnosis. This is because the systemic or pulmonary circulation may be compromised by closure of the arterial duct. The basic plan of management of an infant presenting with heart disease is the institution of general resuscitative measures and the commencement of treatment of heart failure and infections if these are present. Early complete diagnosis is necessary; the younger the infant, the more urgent this is. When achieved, the decisions regarding surgical or medical treatment can be made with full knowledge of the anatomy and physiology of the cardiac malformation.

Congenital heart disease in older children

With certain exceptions, all congenital heart defects that are amenable to surgical correction should be corrected before the child starts full-time schooling. The exceptions include aortic valvar stenosis (where the timing of surgery depends entirely on the severity of the obstruction) and those conditions requiring prosthetic conduits or valves; in these instances, surgery should be delayed, if possible, until the child has grown enough to have a prosthesis of adequate size for an adult. In children awaiting the optimal age for surgery, in those unsuitable for surgery and those in whom surgery is not necessary, the doctor must give advice on lifestyle. Two factors should be borne in mind. First, most psychological problems encountered in long-term survivors of surgery for congenital heart disease probably stem from overprotection of the child before and after surgery.[31] Second, sudden death in children with congenital heart disease is rarely related to physical activity. It is, therefore, the responsibility of the physician to encourage the patient to lead an active life. The parents and school authorities should similarly be encouraged to allow the child to take part in all activities, including competitive sports, up to the child's tolerance for these activities. Even when the child has a low exercise tolerance, as much participation as possible should be encouraged. It is not possible for a cyanosed boy with tricuspid atresia to be an effective sprinter, but he may be able to play soccer as a goalkeeper. When exercise limitation is indicated, as in severe aortic stenosis, it should be enforced only until surgical relief has been obtained.

Congenital heart disease in the adolescent and adult

Several categories of patients survive into adolescence and adulthood. The first category are those with trivial heart defects that do not deteriorate in adult life. Examples are small ventricular septal defects and mild pulmonary stenosis. These people should be encouraged to lead a normal life, the only precaution necessary being the usual prophylactic measures against infective endocarditis. It is advisable for them to continue to be followed-up, because crisis points in their lives will occur and then the opinion of a cardiologist will be sought. These occasions include impending marriage, pregnancy and career decisions. In our opinion, the long-term care of these patients should involve the paediatric cardiologist irrespective of the age of the patient. Continuity of care is ensured in this way and unnecessary invasive investigations are avoided. The second category are the survivors of the surgery. In this group, the intensity of follow-up will depend on the severity of the lesion and the presence or absence of post-operative complications. As some complications may appear late after surgery, and as the long-term outcome in many conditions is still not known, regular assessment of functional capacity, cardiac rhythm and cardiac performance is needed in most patients. Advice will be required at the crisis points of their lives. The cardiologist's opinion will additionally be sought concerning the patient's suitability for life insurance or to hold a driving licence. The third category are those surviving with inoperable heart disease. Advice on all the above matters will be needed, but a major consideration in these patients is the possibility of heart or heart–lung transplantation. It is our experience that this possibility should be discussed sooner rather than later because many of these patients have adjusted their outlook to the perceived hopeless nature of their condition. They need time and the opportunity for discussion in order to readjust their outlook. Similar considerations apply in those who have had a poor outcome from surgery or who have deteriorated following an apparently successful operation.

INTERVENTIONAL CATHETERIZATION

In recent years, the possibilities of balloon angioplasty and catheter embolization have been, and are being, explored in congenital heart disease. Progress has been so rapid that balloon valvoplasty has already supplanted surgery as the treatment of first choice in most cases of valvar pulmonary stenosis irrespective of the age of the patient. The principal considerations involved in deciding which lesions to approach in this way are the effectiveness and the safety of the technique in each individual anomaly. At present, an unqualified recommendation for balloon angioplasty or valvoplasty can be given only for pulmonary valve stenosis. Support is growing for its use in aortic valve stenosis and post-operative re-coarctation. Use of the technique remains controversial in the primary treatment of aortic coarctation, of peripheral pulmonary stenosis, of subvalvar aortic stenosis and of the palliative dilatation of subvalvar pulmonary stenosis in conditions such as tetralogy of Fallot.[32] Catheter embolization using detachable balloons or coils has an established place as the primary treatment of many arteriovenous malformations, for example, those in the lungs. These methods are also gaining acceptance for closure of aortopulmonary collateral arteries.[32] New devices are being investigated in clinical trials for the catheter closure of persistent patency of the arterial duct; others are under development for closure of atrial septal defect. The field of interventional catheterization is in a rapid state of development.

PRINCIPLES OF SURGICAL MANAGEMENT

There are four basic approaches to the surgical treatment of congenital heart disease: palliation, anatomical correction, radical palliation and transplantation. Radical palliation implies that the overall route of circulation is 'corrected', but the anatomical derangement is left unaltered. This is the case in venous redirection for complete transposition of the great arteries and the Fontan operation for tricuspid atresia. The choice of approach will be determined by the anatomy of the malformation. For aortic coarctation, anatomical correction is the treatment of choice at any age. The age at which surgery is necessary may influence the decision. In the tetralogy of Fallot with unfavourable anatomy, when hypoxia necessitates operation in the first year of life, a palliative aortopulmonary shunt may be used as a temporizing procedure. Thus, palliative operations may permit corrective surgery to be delayed until that surgery entails a low risk. In very complex malformations, however, such as some that are encountered in association with atrial isomerism, palliation may be the only treatment available. Transplantation, its indications and feasibility, in congenital heart disease is at present an experimental procedure. When deciding on the particular approach to be applied in a particular patient, the anatomy, the age and the risk–benefit equation must be assessed. To do this, the cumulative risk of alternative operative strategies must be taken into account, bearing in mind the surgical skills of the unit involved.

SPECIFIC ANOMALIES

Up to this point, congenital heart disease has been discussed in general terms. Knowledge of the normal and abnormal physiological events that occur in childhood is useful for the initial recognition that a child has a heart defect. Once identified, broad groupings can be made on the basis of the physiological derangements. For accurate prognos-

tication and treatment, however, detailed anatomical and physiological diagnosis is essential. In the subsequent pages, the features of the major specific congenital heart defects are described. As far as is possible, these have been arranged in segmental fashion, starting with venous anomalies and progressing through to malformations of the arteries.

ANOMALOUS SYSTEMIC VENOUS CONNEXION

Anomalous connexion of a systemic vein is rarely an anomaly of consequence in its own right. Most frequently, it is found as an associated malformation with more complex defects. It rarely causes a significant haemodynamic disturbance. On most occasions, although the morphology of a systemic vein may be found to be abnormal, it drains to the systemic venous atrium. This is seen with the commonest systemic venous malformation, drainage of the left superior caval vein to the coronary sinus (Fig. 25.17).[33] Drainage of a systemic vein to the pulmonary venous atrium can occur, and is a more serious anomaly. It is a very rare cause of cyanosis. The most severe systemic venous anomalies are found in the presence of atrial isomerism when they are the rule (see p. 626). The diagnosis of anomalous systemic venous connexion is usually

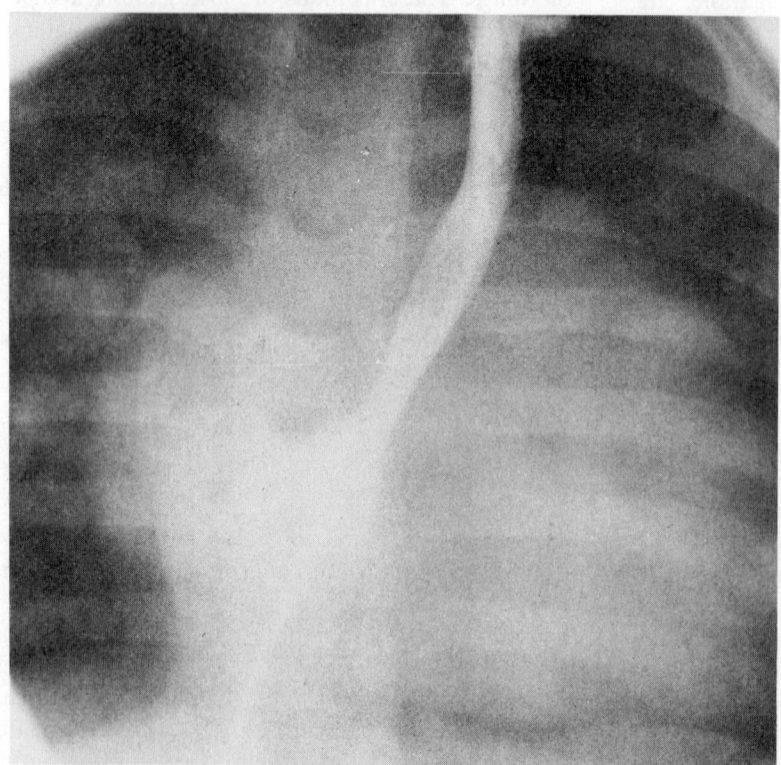

Fig. 25.17. Angiogram demonstrating a left superior caval vein draining to the coronary sinus. There is no connexion to the right superior caval vein.

made echocardiographically or at cardiac catheterization when the catheter course is observed to be abnormal.

ANOMALOUS PULMONARY VENOUS CONNEXION

Some or all of the pulmonary veins may connect to anatomical sites other than the left atrium. In other words, anomalous pulmonary venous connexion may be partial or total. The partial form usually involves part or the whole of the return from one lung and, when it is an isolated lesion, rarely requires surgical treatment. In totally anomalous pulmonary venous connexion, the haemodynamic disturbance is more severe and is always associated with systemic venous admixture to the systemic arterial circulation. The condition exists when none of the pulmonary veins drain to the left atrium. The anomalously connected veins may all terminate in the same systemic site or different veins may drain separately to different systemic sites. The latter arrangement is called mixed anomalous connexion. The site of connexion may be supracardiac, cardiac or infradiaphragmatic (Fig. 25.18).[34] In the supracardiac form, the anomalous veins connect to either the right or left superior caval veins, directly or via the azygos venous system. In the cardiac pattern, the veins connect most frequently to the coronary sinus but can join directly to the right atrium. The infracardiac or infradiaphragmatic type of connexion is characterized by the anomalous channel descending through the diaphragm to terminate almost always in the portal venous system but very rarely in the inferior caval vein. An atrial septal defect co-exists, usually within the oval depression.

Totally anomalous pulmonary venous connexion results in a high pulmonary blood flow, unless the pulmonary venous return is obstructed or there is pulmonary vascular disease. As all of the pulmonary venous return is directed to the right side of the heart, the high pulmonary flow is associated with right ventricular volume overload. Systemic blood flow is derived from that portion of the mixed pulmonary and systemic venous return which crosses the atrial septum to reach the left atrium and left ventricle. Some degree of systemic arterial desaturation is present but, with a high pulmonary blood flow, this may be difficult to detect clinically. In some cases, a restrictive interatrial communication may limit the flow from right to left atrium and thus limit the systemic cardiac output.[35]

When unrestricted pulmonary flow accompanies totally anomalous connexion, tachypnoea is usually present during the first month of life. This will often progress to dyspnoea on feeding and poor weight gain during the first 3 months of life. Frank cardiac failure may supervene during this period but some patients may survive through infancy and early childhood without heart failure. Cyanosis may be difficult to detect. The nitrogen washout test may be necessary to reveal its presence. The first heart sound is usually loud but the most impressive sign is the ease with which splitting of the second sound is detected.[35] In contrast, when there is obstruction to a totally anomalous connexion, presentation is usually in the first week of life, often on the first day. Pulmonary venous congestion causes early

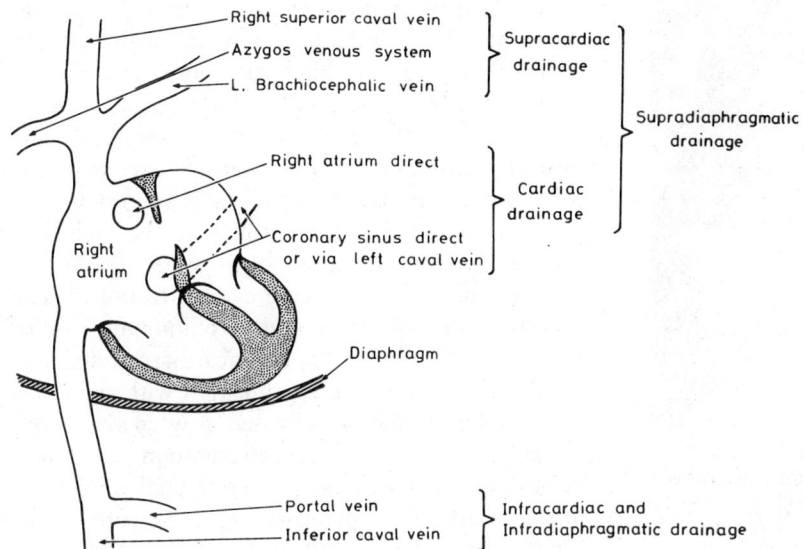

Fig. 25.18. Diagram showing the potential sites of drainage of anomalously connected pulmonary veins.

tachypnoea. With the rapid onset of pulmonary oedema, dyspnoea and profound cyanosis become apparent. Hepatic enlargement is early and marked. The pulmonary arterial pressure is always elevated and thus the second heart sound is invariably loud.

The chest radiograph with unrestricted pulmonary blood flow reveals cardiac enlargement with a prominent pulmonary knob. A typical cardiac silhouette (the snowman, cottage loaf or W.C. Fields) is seen when the anomalous connexion is to the left brachiocephalic vein (Fig. 25.19). With an obstructed connexion, the heart is of normal size with a prominent pulmonary knob, the lung fields showing all the features of pulmonary oedema. There is little in the electrocardiogram in infancy that gives clues to the diagnosis of the condition itself whether the anomalously connected veins are obstructed or non-obstructed connexions.

Cross-sectional echocardiography is diagnostic when the pulmonary vein can be traced to a confluence which does not then connect to the left

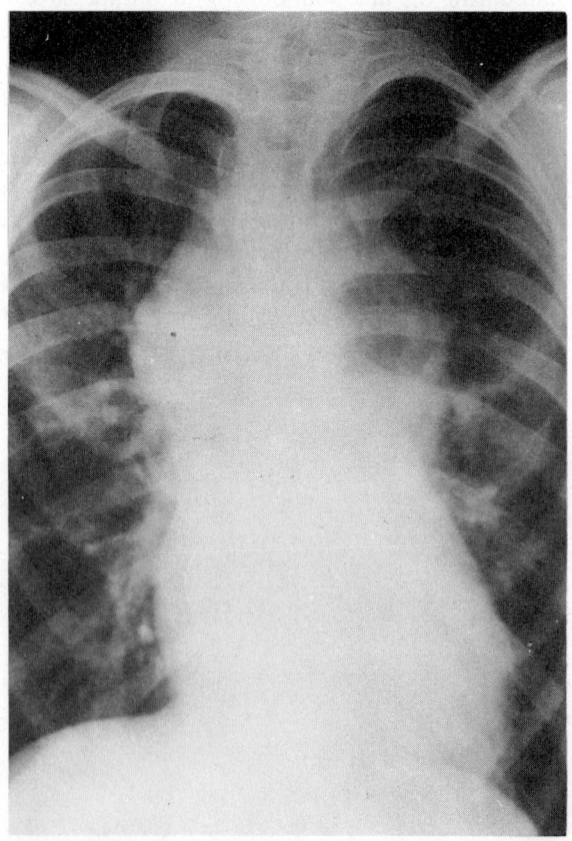

Fig. 25.19. Classic chest radiograph of total anomalous pulmonary venous connexion to the ascending vein—the snowman, cottage loaf or W.C. Fields heart. The ascending vein is in the semilucent shadow in the left mediastinum.

atrium.[36] In skilled hands, the site of anomalous connexion can reliably be identified (Fig. 25.20), Doppler flows demonstrating well an infra-diaphragmatic connexion. However, there may be difficulties in distinguishing partially anomalous connexions. Catheterization will demonstrate a left-to-right shunt in the right atrium when totally anomalous connexion is to that atrium or the coronary sinus. Alternatively, highly saturated blood will first be encountered in the superior caval or left innominate vein when the connexion is supracardiac or within the inferior caval vein when it is infradiaphragmatic. Desaturated blood is found in the left atrium, left ventricle and in the systemic arteries. The pulmonary arterial pressure is usually mildly elevated in early infancy but becomes severely elevated if pulmonary vascular disease has supervened in older children. The left atrium is easily reached but no pulmonary veins can be entered from it. It is always possible to enter the anomalously connected pulmonary veins themselves by careful catheter exploration when the connexion is cardiac or supracardiac. Direct injection is the best method of demonstrating angiographically the connexion of the anomalous vein or veins, particularly when there are multiple sites of entry. Alternatively, angiocardiography in the pulmonary trunk with prolonged recording of the image can be used to obtain diagnostic pictures.

Totally anomalous connexion usually gives problems in the first days or weeks of life, and the majority of patients with this lesion die soon after presentation unless they are surgically corrected. When no obstruction is present, life may be prolonged. Medical treatment can be only a temporizing measure. It has an important role to play in those infants who may present to the cardiac unit in critical condition, usually with pulmonary venous obstruction or when pulmonary blood flow is unrestricted but heart failure is severe. These critically ill infants require intensive care from the time of presentation. At some stage, surgery will be required; it is better if this can be achieved immediately after diagnosis by cross-sectional echocardiography, thus avoiding catheterization.[37] The objective is to join the common pulmonary vein to the left atrium. In the supracardiac and infra-diaphragmatic types, the connexion with the systemic venous circulation is ligated. A wide anastomosis is then created between the common pulmonary venous channel and the posterior wall of the left atrium. The final operative step is closure of the atrial septal defect. When the pulmonary veins

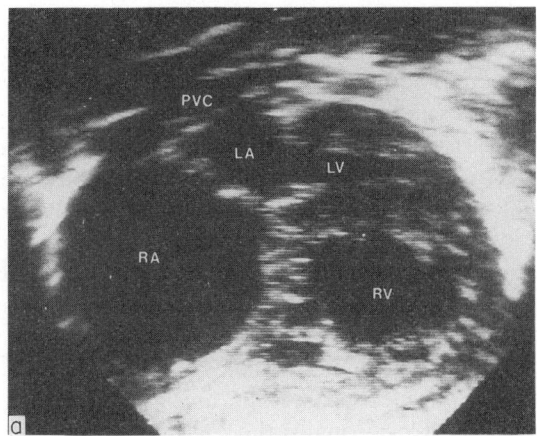

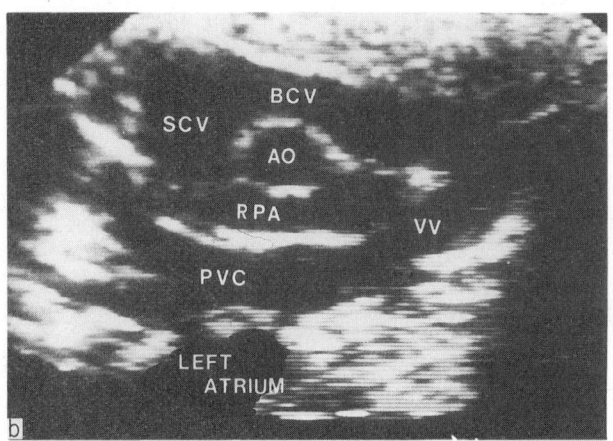

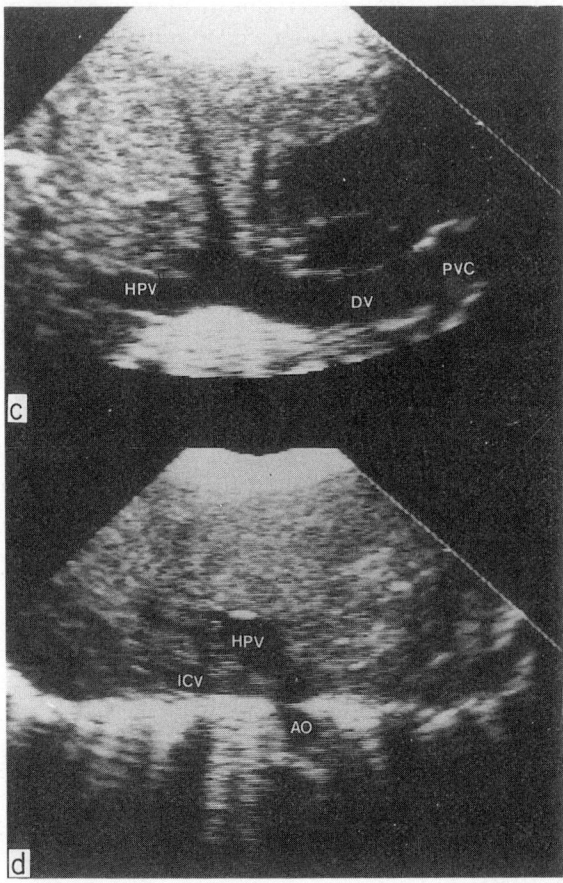

Fig. 25.20. (a) Subcostal four-chamber echocardiographic section illustrating totally anomalous pulmonary venous connexion. The right atrium (RA) and right ventricle (RV) are relatively large when compared with the left atrium (LA) and left ventricle (LV). The pulmonary venous confluence (PVC) can be seen superior to the left atrium and four pulmonary veins can be seen entering the confluence. (b) Suprasternal paracoronal echocardiographic section demonstrating supracardiac total anomalous pulmonary venous connexion. The pulmonary venous confluence (PVC) connects via a vertical vein (VV) to the left brachiocephalic vein (BCV) and right superior caval vein (SCV). AO, aortic arch; RPA, right pulmonary artery. (c) Subcostal parasagittal echocardiographic section demonstrating infracardiac total anomalous pulmonary venous connexion. The pulmonary venous confluence (PVC) connects to the hepatic portal vein (HPV) via the descending vein (DV) which passes behind the heart and through the diaphram. (d) Subcostal short-axis section demonstrating the dilated hepatic portal vein (HPV). ICV, inferior caval vein; AO, aorta. (Figure courtesy of Dr M.L. Rigby).

drain into the right atrium or coronary sinus, the interatrial communication is enlarged and a patch inserted to redirect the pulmonary veins into the left atrium.

The 'scimitar' syndrome is a rare form of partially anomalous pulmonary venous connexion, recognized by the presence of a broad crescentic shadow close to the border of the right atrium descending to the right diaphragm.[38] This shadow represents the course of the anomalous pulmonary venous connexion from the right lung to the inferior caval vein. The syndrome also includes anomalous arterial supply directly from the aorta to the right lung. In addition, the right lung is frequently hypoplastic. The diagnosis is usually made on the chance finding of the 'scimitar' shadow. The majority of patients are asymptomatic until late adult life, but the syndrome has been associated with heart failure in infancy. Partially anomalous connexion in general rarely presents in infancy, being consistent with survival well into adult life. It may never cause symptoms; if symptoms are produced, they usually appear in middle life.

DIVIDED ATRIAL CHAMBERS ('COR TRIATRIATUM')

There are several anatomical arrangements that give the impression of the existence of three atrial chambers. The right atrial chamber can be divided because of persistence of the valves of the embryonic sinus venosus. Generally, however, the term 'cor triatriatum', when used without qualification, refers to division of the morphologically left atrium. One of the compartments receives part or all of the pulmonary venous return, whereas the other communicates with the mitral valve and the left atrial appendage. The orifice between the two divided components is variable in size, but it is frequently small enough to produce pulmonary venous obstruction (Fig. 25.21).[39]

Presentation depends on the severity and timing of obstruction to pulmonary venous return. As most cases appear normal at birth, it is probable that the obstruction is progressive. Dyspnoea, tachypnoea and persistent cough are noted most frequently in the first months of life. These features, together with poor feeding and failure to thrive, frequently draw attention to the illness. Haemoptysis and anaemia

can occur; occasionally, the presenting feature may be severe pulmonary oedema. Later presentation in childhood or adult life is the consequence of a larger orifice between the left atrial chambers. The anomaly has rarely been observed in asymptomatic subjects. On examination, the signs of dyspnoea are usually obvious. Fine crepitations will be heard over the lung fields in the presence of pulmonary oedema. Auscultation of the heart reveals a loud second sound due to pulmonary hypertension, this in turn being secondary to the pulmonary venous obstruction. Murmurs are undiagnostic but there is frequently an ejection systolic murmur at the left sternal edge. Occasionally, there is an early diastolic murmur due to pulmonary regurgitation. Chest radiography shows either a heart of normal size or cardiac enlargement due to dilatation of the right ventricle. The lung fields are congested with variable signs of pulmonary oedema depending on the severity of the obstruction. The electrocardiogram is non-specific, showing right-axis deviation and right ventricular hypertrophy, dependent upon the degree of obstruction. Cross-sectional echocardiography is diagnostic (Fig. 25.22) and, nowadays, catheterization and angiography are unnecessary.[40] Once diagnosed, the treatment involves surgical excision of the obstructive membrane.

ATRIAL ISOMERISM

It has long been known that the syndromes which include asplenia and polysplenia are usually associated with congenital heart defects. The splenic

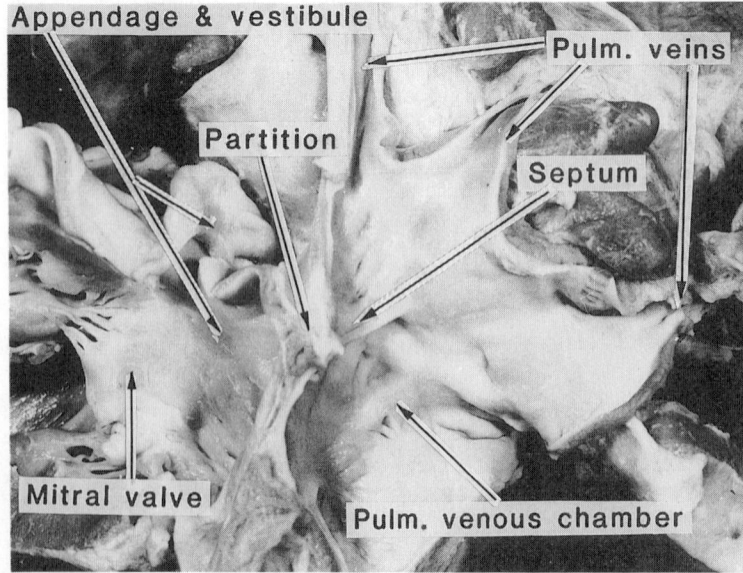

Fig. 25.21. Lateral view of the left-sided chambers in a case with divided left atrium ('cor triatriatum').

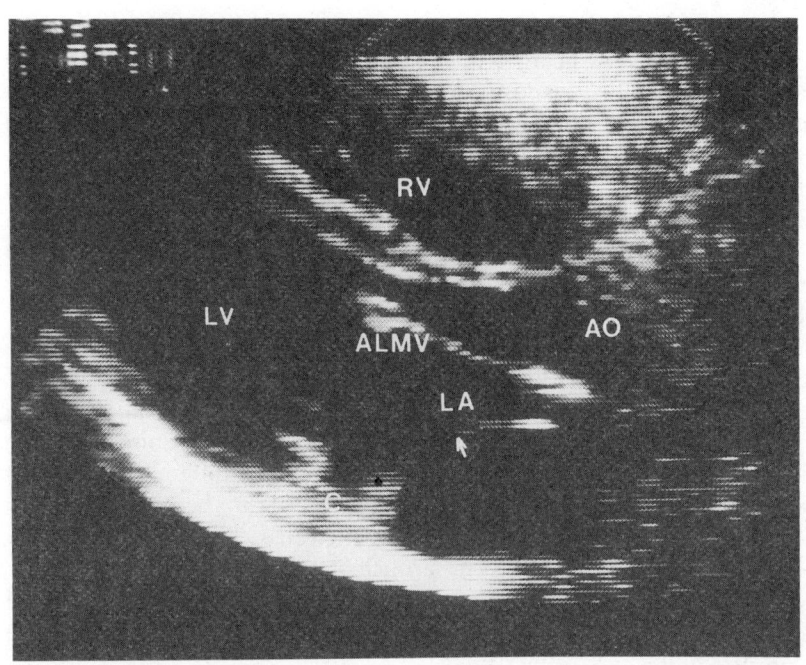

Fig. 25.22. Parasternal long-axis section demonstrating divided left atrium ('cor triatriatum'). The arrow demonstrates the membrane within the left atrium (LA). The anterior leaflet of the mitral valve (ALMV) is clearly visualized. LV, left ventricle; RV, right ventricle; AO, ascending aorta. (Figure courtesy of Dr M.L. Rigby).

abnormalities are merely reflexions of the overall visceral abnormalities which result from the lack of the laterilization that characterizes normality. Instead, the paired organs have similar morphology and unpaired organs are either absent or centrally placed. This results in isomerism. There are two variants (Fig. 25.23), one with bilateral paired organs having 'right' morphology (right isomerism), and the other with bilateral paired organs of 'left' morphology (left isomerism). Isomerism of the lungs is reflected in isomerism of the bronchial pattern and this can be determined by chest radiography. The key to diagnosis lies in the atrial anatomy. Patients with right isomerism have bilateral right atrial appendages and bilateral terminal crests. Bilateral superior caval veins are usually found opening directly into the atriums, each in relation to its terminal crest. The coronary sinus is absent and cardiac veins drain directly to the atriums by several separate orifices. As the primary pulmonary vein is a left atrial structure, anomalous pulmonary venous connexion is invariable. The

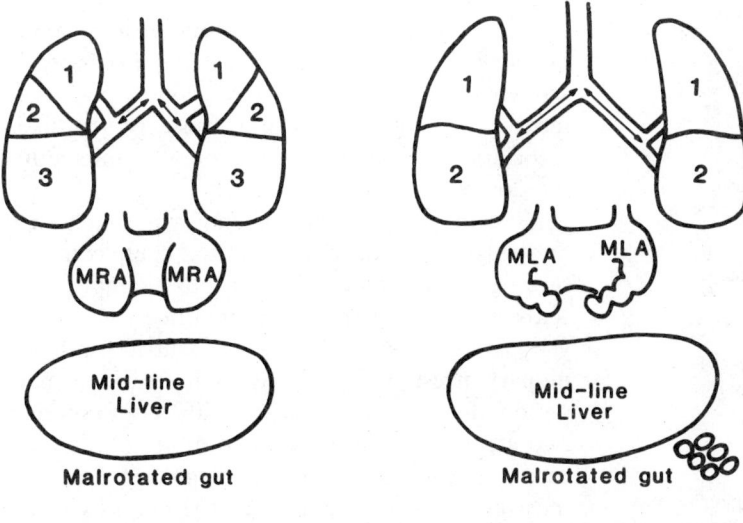

Right Isomerism   **Left Isomerism**

Fig. 25.23. Diagrams showing the basic arrangements of the organs in the setting of isomerism as opposed to lateralization.

atrial chambers themselves are either unseptated or minimally septated, a muscle bar frequently spanning the atrial chamber in mid-line position. A common atrioventricular valve is almost invariably present, but ventricular morphology and ventriculo-arterial connexions are variable. Pulmonary stenosis or atresia is frequent enough to be considered as part of the syndrome.

In left isomerism, the atrial chambers show evidence bilaterally of morphologically left features. Atrial septal structures are better formed; because of this, there may be two atrioventricular valves, although a common valve is still a frequent finding. Bilateral superior caval veins may drain directly to the atrial chambers, but more usually only one is present. Pulmonary venous connexion tends to be bilaterally symmetrical. The most frequent systemic venous anomaly is that of continuation of the inferior caval vein via the azygos system of veins (Fig. 25.24), presumably because the right vitelline vein is a right-sided structure and that portion of the inferior vena cava from which it is formed is therefore absent. As with right isomerism, atrioventricular connexions, ventricular morphology and arterial connexions are variable. Pulmonary stenosis or atresia are less frequent in left than right isomerism, but in contrast coarctation or obstructive lesions of the aortic arch are more frequent.[41]

There are no specific clinical features of atrial isomerism. The symptoms will reflect the complexity of the cardiac anatomy. Thus, single outlet of the heart with pulmonary atresia will present with cyanosis, but double-outlet ventricle without restriction of pulmonary blood flow can present in congestive cardiac failure. It is important to recognize the possibility that failure of lateralization is present. Clues to this are a centrally placed liver on examination, a heart of indeterminate position on chest radiography and an abnormal P-wave vector on the electrocardiogram.

Once the diagnosis is suspected, the most accurate way of establishing the presence or absence of isomerism is by radiographic visualization of the main bronchi,[42] remembering that, sometimes, the bronchial arrangement will be different from atrial arrangement. The feature can be determined by examination of a penetrated chest radiograph (Fig. 25.25), but bronchial tomography may be necessary. The finding of left and right main bronchi of unequal length in the ratio > 1.6 : 1 will exclude isomerism.

Despite the complexity of the visceral and cardiac malformations, many patients with atrial isomerism are surgically treatable. For this reason, all such patients should have full echocardiography and, if necessary, cardiac catheterization and angiographic diagnosis. Nowadays, the diagnosis of the condition and recognition of most associated lesions will be achieved using cross-sectional echocardiography or magnetic resonance imaging (Fig. 25.26). Catheterization will hardly ever be performed in ignorance of the existence of isomerism. If needed, the invasive study can be properly planned. In right isomerism, a major task will be to confirm the site of connexion of all the pulmonary veins. When left isomerism is present, the systemic venous connexions will be the target. When left isomerism is known to exist, the catheterization is performed most easily from the arm because of the likely association of azygos continuation of an interrupted inferior caval vein.

As with the presentation and symptomatology, the prognosis is dependent on the complexity and severity of the lesions present. For example, cases with right isomerism, anomalous pulmonary venous connexion, double-inlet ventricle and pulmonary atresia will be likely to die in the neonatal period. In contrast, patients with left isomerism, two atrioventricular valves and more simple intracardiac lesions may remain undiagnosed. Each case must be treated on its merits. The majority can at least be palliated, either by shunting where pulmonary flow is limited or by banding the pulmonary

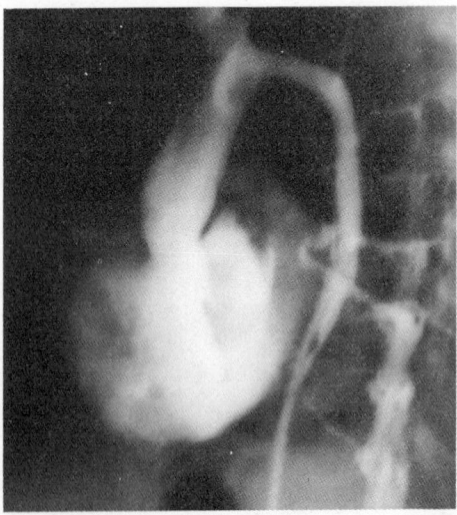

Fig. 25.24. Lateral projection of an angiogram with injection into the azygous vein from a catheter introduced into the femoral vein. This angiogram shows azygous continuation of the inferior caval vein.

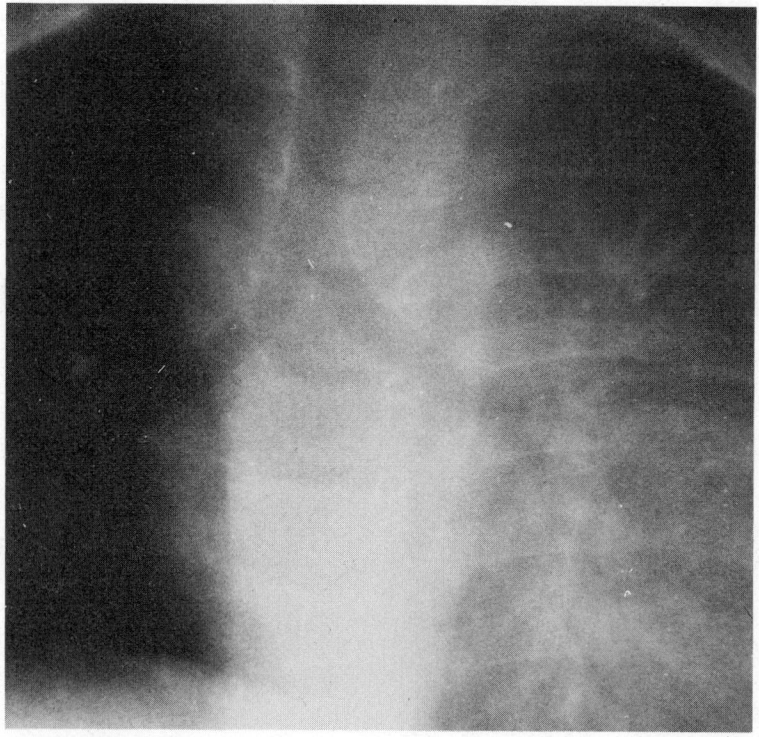

Fig. 25.25. Filtered chest radiograph demonstrating bilaterally long bronchi in a patient with left atrial isomerism. (Figure courtesy of Dr M.L. Rigby).

trunk where an intraventricular communication results in unrestricted pulmonary flow and leads to congestive heart failure. In a proportion of cases, corrective surgery will be possible, even with complicated malformations. Success will be dictated by the combination of lesions present.[43]

ATRIAL SEPTAL DEFECT

Atrial septal defect is one of the commonest congenital cardiac malformations. It is of particular importance because long-term survival is usual and presentation in adult life is not infrequent. Atrial septal defects of all forms account for 10–15% of congenital cardiac malformations. The commonest variety is found within the oval fossa (so-called 'secundum' defects). The other defects permitting an interatrial communication are not within the atrial septum and not, therefore, strictly 'septal defects' (Fig. 25.27). Ostium primum defects are due to a deficiency of the atrioventricular septum and are discussed in the section devoted to atrioven-

tricular septal defects. Sinus venosus and coronary sinus defects will be discussed in this section. Taken together, atrial septal defects occur twice as frequently in women than men.[44] The aetiology of the majority of cases can best be considered under the heading of multifactorial inheritance. An autosomal dominant mode of inheritance is seen in a minority of cases as in the Holt–Oram syndrome and in the syndrome of oval fossa defects associated with a prolonged atrioventricular conduction time.[45]

Understanding of the morphology of interatrial communications demands knowledge that the extent of the atrial septum is confined to the oval fossa and its immediate surrounds. The true atrial septal defects, therefore, can exist only within the confines of the fossa. They are due to perforation or deficiency of the floor of the fossa. The so-called patent oval foramen is only an interatrial communication when right atrial pressure is higher than left. In circumstances of normal physiology, the higher left atrial pressure closes the septum and prevents any shunt. The sinus venosus variety of

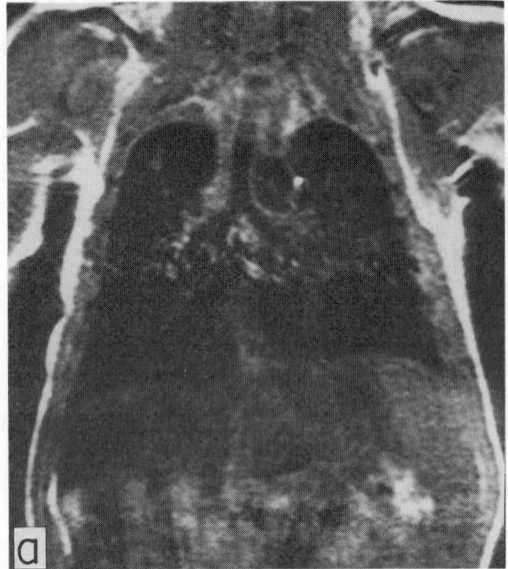
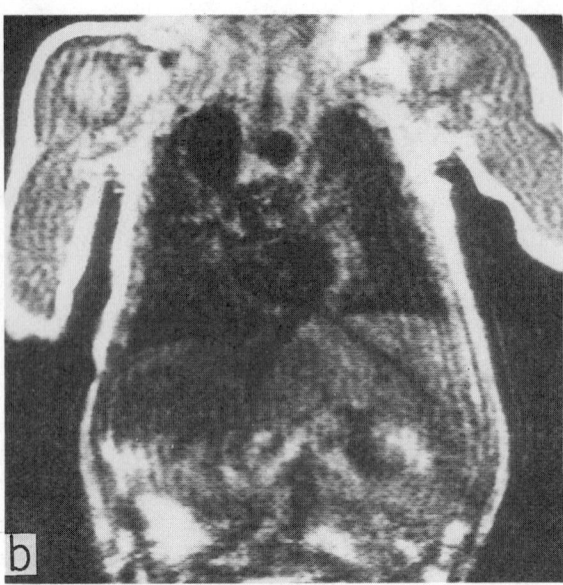

Fig. 25.26. (a) Magnetic resonance scan showing bilaterally short bronchi in right atrial isomerism. (b) Magnetic resonance scan showing central liver and hepatic veins draining directly to the atrium in atrial isomerism.

interatrial communication is related to the orifice of either the superior or inferior caval veins. It exists when either the caval veins themselves or anomalously connected pulmonary veins provide an interatrial conduit outside the confines of the atrial septum (Fig. 25.28). The coronary sinus defect exists at the orifice of the coronary sinus when the 'party wall' between the sinus and left atrium is effaced. The sinus is then in free communication with the left atrium. Usually, it co-exists with a

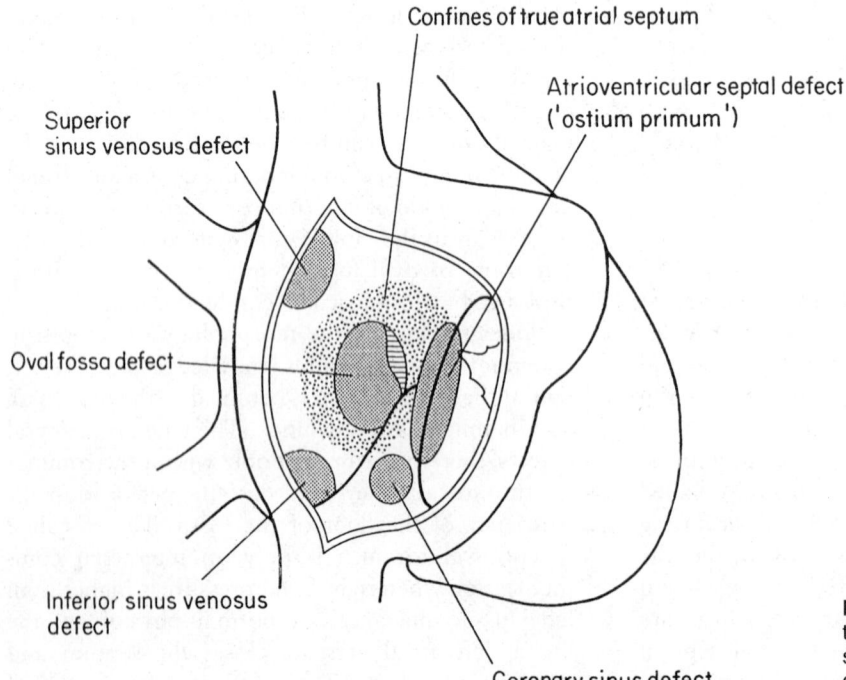

Confines of true atrial septum

Atrioventricular septal defect ('ostium primum')

Superior sinus venosus defect

Oval fossa defect

Inferior sinus venosus defect

Coronary sinus defect

Fig. 25.27. Diagram showing the holes that produce the potential for interatrial shunting of blood. Only those within the oval fossa are true atrial septal defects.

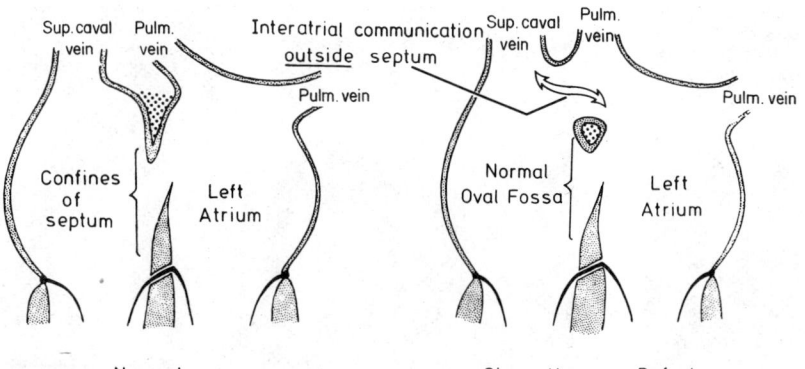

Sup. caval vein — Pulm. vein — Interatrial communication outside septum — Sup. caval vein — Pulm. vein — Pulm. vein — Confines of septum — Left Atrium — Pulm. vein — Normal Oval Fossa — Left Atrium — Normal — Sinus Venosus Defect

Fig. 25.28. Diagrams showing the usual anatomical mechanism underscoring the existence of a so-called 'sinus venosus' atrial septal defect (right) as compared with the normal heart.

persistent left superior caval vein draining to the atrial roof of the left atrium, hence the alternative term of 'unroofed coronary sinus'.

Atrial septal defects are usually large enough to provide little obstruction to flow. The magnitude and direction of flow through them is determined by the resistances to filling of the two ventricles and the relative pressures in and flows into the two atriums. In the early weeks of life, when the right ventricle is relatively more massive than in adult life, resistance to filling is also relatively higher, and little flow may occur across the defect. As the resistance to filling of the right ventricle falls relative to that of the left ventricle, a left-to-right shunt occurs. The pulmonary blood flow is often more than three times the systemic blood flow, but pulmonary hypertension is rare in childhood. Although a predominant left-to-right shunt is the rule in atrial septal defect, small right-to-left shunts can occur in early atrial systole.[46] These are rarely reflected in detectable systemic arterial desaturation. When the defect is adjacent to the inferior caval vein (and in cases of unroofed coronary sinus), a large right-to-left shunt may occur in addition to the left-to-right shunt. As both of these malformations are rare, obstructive lesions such as tricuspid valve disease (for example, Ebstein's malformation) must be excluded before streaming is evoked as the cause of a right-to-left shunt.

Symptoms are rare in childhood. The usual presenting feature is an incidentally discovered heart murmur. In the majority of patients, growth is normal. Exercise tolerance is usually considered to be normal, and most patients lead a normal life as children and young adults. By contrast, parents often remark on an improvement in physical performance in their children after closure of the defect, suggesting that children with atrial septal defect frequently suffer a mild limitation of exercise ability. Severe symptoms, such as cyanosis or those associated with the onset of congestive cardiac failure, are rare in childhood. Their presence must alert the cardiologist to the possibility that the malformation is more complex. In adult life, cyanosis is associated with the development of severe pulmonary vascular disease. Congestive cardiac failure, rare in childhood, increases in frequency in the fourth, fifth and sixth decades. Its onset is often precipitated by supraventricular arrhythmias. Arrhythmias can occur in childhood but are more common in middle life.

The fully developed picture of an uncomplicated atrial septal defect consists of clinical evidence of right ventricle hypertrophy with an active cardiac impulse of right ventricular type. The first heart sound is normal, the second heart sound is widely split and the split does not vary with the phases of respiration. This feature was first remarked on by Mr W. W. Dicks, Senior Cardiac Technician at the London Hospital.[47] An ejection systolic murmur is present at the upper left sternal edge. The murmur is usually of grade 2–3 in intensity. A thrill is rarely present. When the shunt is large, a mid-diastolic murmur can be heard at the lower left sternal edge indicating high flow through the tricuspid valve. Other added sounds are rare, but a mid-systolic click and an apical systolic murmur can be heard with the frequent association of prolapse of the mitral valve.

As judged radiographically, the heart is usually at the upper limit of normal for size or mildly enlarged in infants and young children. Cardiac enlargement, predominantly involving the right ventricle, is usual in older children and adults. At all ages, a significant shunt is associated with enlargement of the pulmonary knob and pulmonary plethora.

The electrocardiogram is characterized by an rsR pattern in the right chest leads. This is sometimes

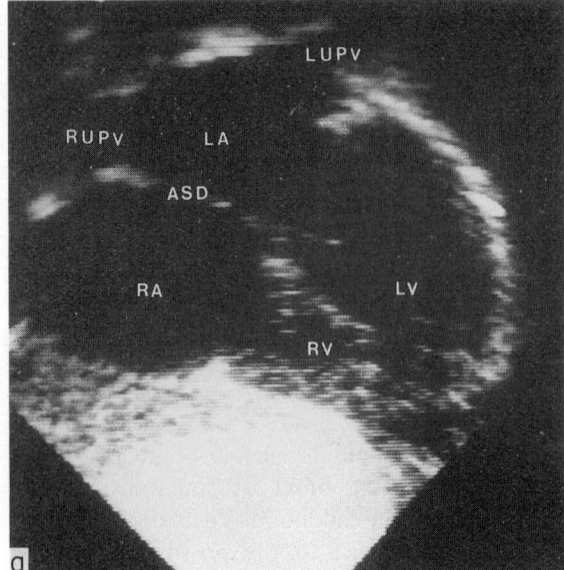
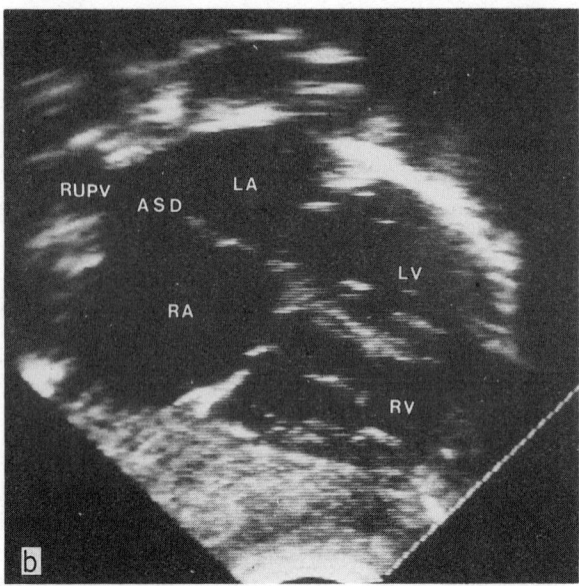

Fig. 25.29. (a) Subcostal four-chamber section demonstrating an oval fossa atrial septal defect. The right upper and left upper pulmonary veins (RUPV and LUPV) are seen entering the left atrium (LA). RA, right atrium; RV, right ventricle; LV, left ventricle. (b) Parasternal four-chamber section demonstrating a sinus venosus atrial septal defect. The right upper pulmonary vein (RUPV) overrides the atrial septum at the site of the atrial septal defect (ASD). LA, left atrium; RA, right atrium; LV, left ventricle; RV, right ventricle. (Figures courtesy of Dr M.L. Rigby).

referred to as 'incomplete right bundle branch block'. The QRS pattern probably indicates right ventricle cavity enlargement rather than discrete delay in the right bundle branch. Voltages suggestive of right ventricular hypertrophy are common in older children and adults. The QRS frontal axis usually ranges from +90° to +180°. In a minority (about 2%), the axis is superiorly orientated and resembles the tracing of an atrioventricular septal defect. Atrioventricular conduction is delayed in one-third of patients. This is manifested by prolongation of the PR interval. Electrocardiographic evidence of right atrial hypertrophy is present in about one-quarter of children with defects within the oval fossa.

Cross-sectional echocardiography using the four-chamber view can differentiate the various forms of interatrial communication from one another and also from the 'primum' variety of atrioventricular septal defect (Fig. 25.29).[48]

If catheterization is deemed necessary, it is usually easy to cross the defect from right to left atrium. This is facilitated using the saphenous venous approach but can be accomplished with little difficulty from the arm. A left-to-right shunt is detected. Pulmonary arterial pressure is normal, except when pulmonary vascular disease is present.

Even when the pulmonary arterial pressure is normal, however, the right ventricular systolic pressure is frequently elevated to 40 or 50 mmHg because of the increased pulmonary blood flow resulting in a small systolic gradient from right ventricle to pulmonary artery. Right and left atrial pressures are quantitatively similar, although the waveforms may be different. It is hazardous to diagnose a simple defect within the oval fossa when left and right atrial pressure are quantitatively different. In sinus venosus defects, it is frequently possible to enter a right pulmonary vein close to the junction of the superior caval vein with the right atrium.

A four-chamber angiocardiogram with injection into the left atrium at the origin of the right pulmonary veins will differentiate a high (usually sinus venosus) defect, a defect with the oval fossa and a primum (atrioventricular septal) defect (Fig. 25.30). Left ventricular angiography will demonstrate the integrity of the mitral valve; pulmonary venous angiography is indicated when anomalous pulmonary venous connexion is suspected.

Death is extremely rare in infancy and childhood. Symptoms are more frequently encountered in adult life and increase in frequency and severity with age. The commonest manifestation of an isolated atrial

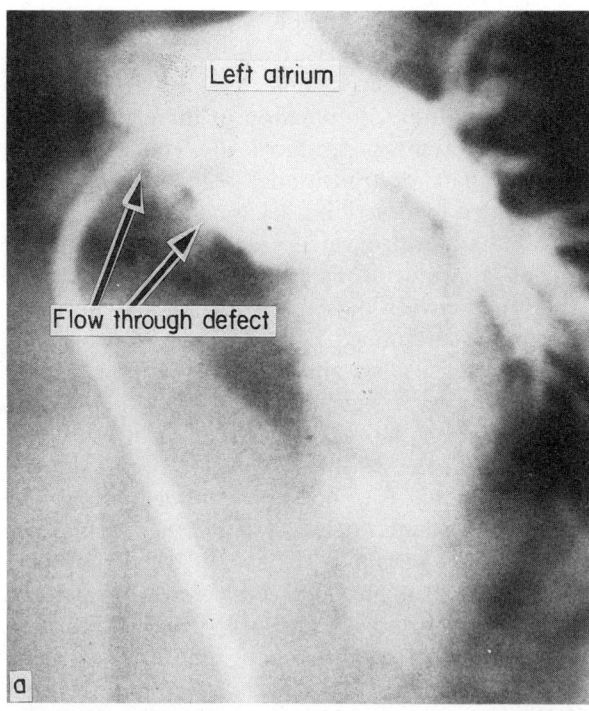
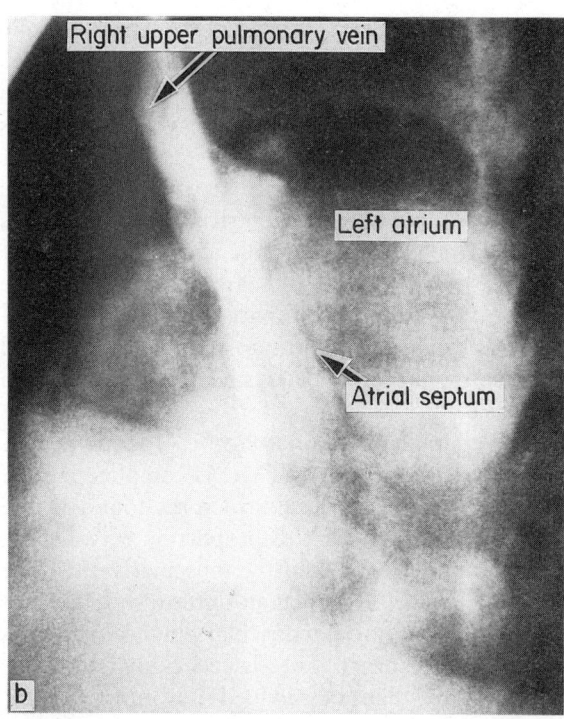

Fig. 25.30. Angiocardiograms in the four-chamber projection. (a) Contrast passing from the left to the right atrium in the region of the oval foramen. (b) Contrast passing from the superior caval vein to either side of the atrial septum; a sinus venosus defect.

septal defect in adult life is congestive cardiac failure. This can occur when the patient is in sinus rhythm, but atrial fibrillation is also a frequent occurrence in the older patient. Nowadays, the average length of life with an untreated atrial septal defect within the oval fossa is probably about 50 years. As heart failure in this condition is slowly progressive, this does not mean 50 asymptomatic years. Apart from heart failure with or without an atrial arrhythmia, causes of death include embolism and pulmonary vascular disease. Mitral stenosis was a frequent accompaniment of atrial septal defect in previous years (Lutembacher's syndrome). With the fall in the incidence of rheumatic heart disease in Western countries, this is now rare.

Pulmonary vascular disease in association with atrial septal defect is also rare. Pulmonary hypertension is unusual in infancy and early childhood, but after the age of 20 years some elevation of pulmonary arterial pressure is seen in approximately one-fifth of patients. Prolapse of the mitral valve occurs frequently. It may be the substrate for those very rare cases of subacute infectious endocarditis. Its known association with arrhythmias may account for at least some of the rhythm problems seen in untreated and surgically corrected patients.

Except in those cases with severe pulmonary vascular disease, all atrial septal defects should be surgically corrected. Ideally, this should be performed as soon after diagnosis as possible. If the diagnosis is made in infancy, closure is indicated at some time before the child starts schooling. When isolated atrial septal defect presents with classic clinical and non-invasive investigatory findings, it should be possible to recommend surgery without prior cardiac catheterization. Elective repair of an uncomplicated atrial septal defect is now possible with < 1% operative mortality. Major complications are unusual, and the post-operative course is usually uncomplicated.[49] Although surgery is at present the treatment of choice, prostheses now exist which can be introduced at catheterization. These devices are at an experimental stage but promise a new era in the treatment of, at least, those defects in the oval fossa.[50]

ATRIOVENTRICULAR SEPTAL DEFECTS

Atrioventricular septal defects ('atrioventricular canal malformations' or 'endocardial cushion defects') are a group of malformations unified because of the complete absence of normal atrioventricular septal structures (Fig. 25.31). The defects usually occur in patients with concordantly connected hearts; they can be observed with some frequency in patients with atrial isomerism and ambiguous atrioventricular connexions and rarely in patients with discordant atrioventricular connexion. In the normal population, atrioventricular septal defects are rare, the group as a whole accounting for only about 4% of congenital heart disease. They are frequently encountered in patients with trisomy 21 (Down's syndrome), approximately one-third of all atrioventricular septal defects being associated with this syndrome.

The characteristic anatomy is found at the atrioventricular junction. There is complete lack of the atrioventricular septal structures found in the normal heart along with disproportion between the inlet and outlet lengths of the muscular ventricular septum. The left ventricular outflow tract is not 'wedged' into the atrioventricular junction as occurs in the normal heart. The defects united by these features can then be divided according to the anatomy of the valve mechanism which guards the common atrioventricular junction. There may be a common valve or separate right and left atrioventricular valves (Fig. 25.32). Five leaflets can be distinguished in the common valve: left parietal, right parietal, superior and inferior bridging, and right antero-superior leaflets, respectively. Separate valve orifices are found when the facing edges of the bridging leaflets are fused to one another by a connecting tongue of leaflet tissue.

Atrioventricular septal defects are often described as 'complete' or 'partial' depending on the presence or absence of a common atrioventricular valve. Other workers use the presence or absence of an interventricular communication as the distinguishing feature. Combination of these two criteria by some authors produces the concept of the 'intermediate' or 'transitional' lesion. All of this can be avoided by describing separately the presence of a common orifice versus separate right and left valves along with the anatomical potential for shunting between the cardiac chambers. This latter feature is determined by the relationship between the bridging leaflets and the atrial and ventricular septal structures (Fig. 25.33).

In practice, the defect most frequently encountered will be the so-called 'complete' form. This has a common valve orifice and confluent atrial and ventricular septal defects. The other commonly encountered variant is the so-called 'partial' form (or 'ostium primum' atrial septal defect), which has separate right and left atrioventricular orifices and the anatomical potential only for atrial shunting. Atrioventricular septal defects with separate right and left atrioventricular valves, however, may have ventricular septal defects. Malformations may also rarely exist with the potential for shunting exclusively at ventricular level. Irrespective of these variations, the left atrioventricular valve in all atrioventricular septal defects has a characteristic three-leaflet arrangement. The left ventricular outflow tract is always narrow and is particularly susceptible to obstruction. Other associated malformations include additional muscular ventricular septal defects, valvar pulmonary stenosis or more complex lesions like Fallot's tetralogy or double

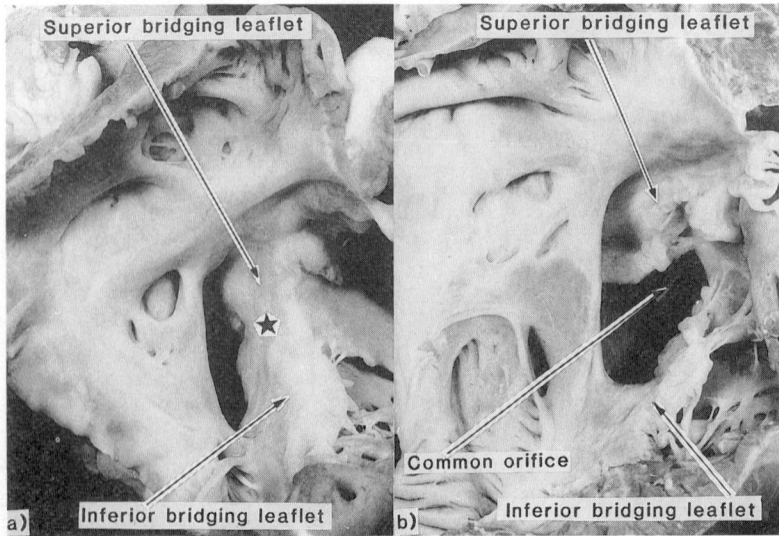

Fig. 25.31. These hearts both have deficient atrioventricular septation in the setting of separate right and left atrioventricular valves (a) and a common valve (b). The difference between the two is the presence of a tongue of leaflet tissue connecting the bridging leaflets (starred) in (a).

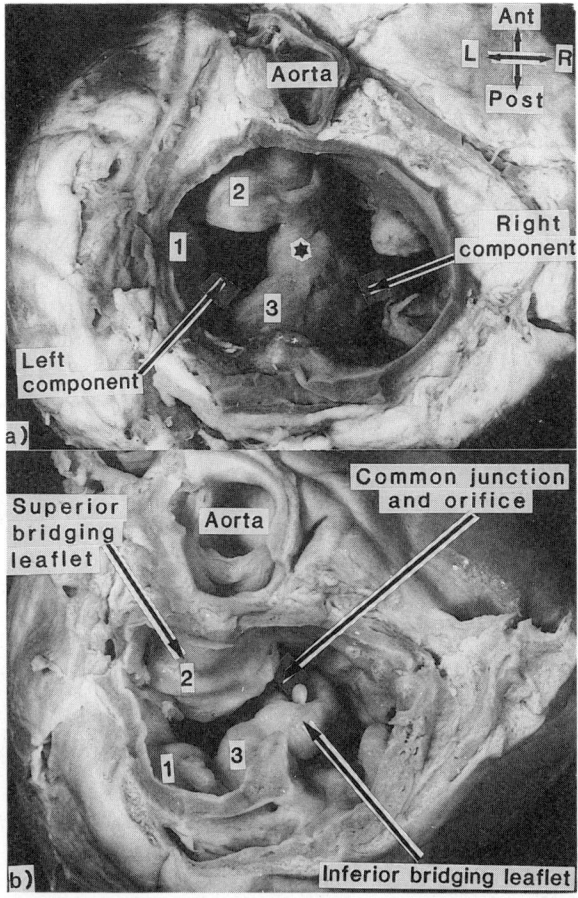

Fig. 25.32. The arrangement of the common atrioventricular junction in hearts with atrioventricular septal defect and (a) separate right and left valves as opposed to (b) a common valve. The compass shows orientation (L, left; R, right). Note the tongue (starred) connecting the bridging leaflets in (a) and the three-leaflet arrangement of the left valve (#1, mural leaflet; #2 and 3 left ventricular components of bridging leaflets) in both hearts.

outlet right ventricle.

The severity of the haemodynamic disturbance is related to the severity of the basic anatomical lesion

and the presence or absence of atrioventricular valvar regurgitation. A left-to-right shunt occurs at atrial level in those who have an 'ostium primum' defect but who do not have regurgitation through the left valve. Such defects are indistinguishable haemodynamically from atrial septal defects. Most defects are a common atrioventricular orifice (complete defect), and a few of those with separate valve orifices, add a left-to-right ventricular shunt to that occurring at atrial level. Elevation of pulmonary arterial pressure in childhood is mainly determined by the size of this ventricular component. Regurgitation through the left atrioventricular valve (when present) leads to additional left ventricular volume overload. The development of pulmonary vascular disease in those subjects with an 'ostium primum' defect is similar to the progression in those with atrial septal defect. In those with the potential for ventricular shunting, pulmonary disease develops more rapidly than in those with 'isolated' ventricular septal defect.[51] Once developed, the majority of patients with pulmonary hypertension have a fixed elevation of pulmonary vascular resistance by the age of 1 or 2 years. In some cases, this may occur by as early as 6 months of age.

The age and mode of presentation depend on the severity of the haemodynamic disturbance. Early onset of congestive cardiac failure is seen in patients with a common atrioventricular orifice, dyspnoea and poor feeding becoming evident during the first months of life. Symptoms occurring in the first 1 or 2 weeks of life suggest severe incompetence of the atrioventricular valve. Subjects with an 'ostium primum' defect and little or no regurgitation through the left valve are usually asymptomatic. They often present with cardiac murmurs discovered at routine medical checks. When atrioventricular septal defects are associated with more complex lesions (such as tetralogy of Fallot), the

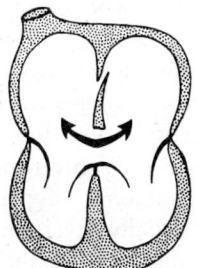

Bridging leaflets attached to Interventricular septum — Interatrial communication ('Ostium primum ASD')

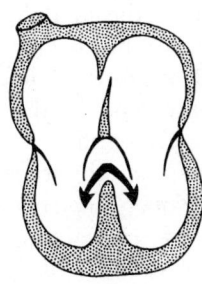

Bridging leaflets attached to Interatrial septum Interventricular communication ('Isolated VSD')

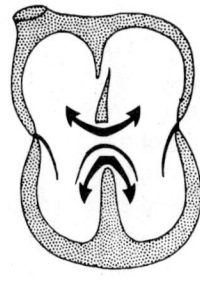

Floating bridging leaflet(s) Interatrial and interventricular communications (Usually common orifice)

Fig. 25.33. Diagrams in four-chamber projection showing how the potential for shunting is determined by the relationship of the bridging leaflets to the atrial and ventricular septal structures. ASD, atrial septal defect; VSD, ventricular septal defect.

clinical features will be dominated by the more complex defect. In these cases, the discovery of the atrioventricular septal defect may be an unwelcome surprise.

The physical signs, like the symptoms, depend on the severity of the lesion. Those subjects with no ventricular shunting and competent atrioventricular valves will have the signs of an atrial septal defect. An interventricular communication will be accompanied by a pan-systolic murmur. When regurgitation through the left atrioventricular valve is present, a pan-systolic murmur may radiate to the right of the sternum as well as being audible at the left sternal edge and the apex. Pulmonary hypertension will be associated with a loud pulmonary component of the second heart sound. Fixed splitting, heard in ostium primum defects, is not a feature of those with a common valve orifice.

The characteristic electrocardiographic abnormality is a superiorly orientated mean QRS vector axis.[52] The axis in the majority is between $-30°$ and $-120°$. Right ventricular hypertrophy is usual when shunting is confined at the atrial level; biventricular hypertrophy is found with common orifice and/or regurgitation through the left valve. Conduction defects, usually a prolonged PR interval, are frequently present.

There are no diagnostic features on the chest radiograph. Those subjects with shunting confined at atrial level have the appearances of atrial septal defects; patients with a common valve orifice have appearances similar to those of ventricular septal defects. When significant left atrial enlargement is seen, it suggests that regurgitation through the left atrioventricular valve is associated with a restrictive interatrial communication.

Cross-sectional echocardiography has revolutionized the diagnosis of atrioventricular septal defects and the differentiation of the specific forms.[53] The four-chamber views are the most useful, from either apical or subcostal windows (Fig. 25.34). Two atrioventricular valve orifices are seen in the 'ostium primum' defect, the bridging leaflets being attached to the ventricular septum. In the variants with common orifice, it is possible to judge the potential for interventricular shunting beneath both bridging leaflets. In all defects, the three-leaflet arrangement of the left valve is readily visualized together with an abnormal disposition of the left ventricular papillary muscles (Fig. 25.35). Doppler techniques permit detection and quantification of regurgitation through the left atrioventricular valve.

At catheterization, the left atrium is easily entered in the majority of patients. Wayward behaviour of the catheter, which enters all chambers easily and moves from one to another with little manipulation, is a clue to the presence of a common valve orifice. A left-to-right shunt is usually detected first at atrial level, but subsequent rises in oxygen saturation in the right ventricle or pulmonary trunk do not differentiate the various forms. More important is the presence or absence of pulmonary hypertension. The pulmonary arterial pressure is usually normal when shunting is only at atrial level but high in those with common valves. The left atrial pressure provides little indication concerning the presence or severity of regurgitation through the left atrioventricular valve. It will be elevated only if the interatrial communication is restrictive.

The classic angiographic features reflect the basic unifying anatomical features.[54] The 'sprung' position of the aorta elongates the outlet dimension of the left ventricle as seen in the antero-posterior projection; the deficient inlet portion of the ventricle gives rise to the 'goose neck' deformity (Fig. 25.36a). Valuable as this sign is, the 'four-chamber' view is the most informative projection for visualization of the anatomy (Fig. 25.36b). A left atrial injection demonstrates the interatrial communication. Left ventricular injections visualize the common valve when present. Passage of contrast under the superior bridging leaflet is easily seen. Similar shunting is sometimes seen under the inferior leaflet.

Three factors have a major effect on longevity:

1 the presence and severity of regurgitation through the left atrioventricular valve;
2 the development of pulmonary vascular disease (which is usually related to the presence and size of any interventricular communication);
3 the integrity of the conduction tissues.

Patients with shunting at atrial level but without regurgitation through the left valve who do not develop heart block carry a prognosis similar to those with atrial septal defects within the oval fossa. At the other end of the spectrum, patients with common valve orifice, valvar regurgitation and a large ventricular shunt frequently succumb during the first year of life. Those with pulmonary hypertension who survive infancy have usually developed pulmonary vascular disease. Because of this, they have a limited life-expectancy. Infective endocarditis can occur in any patient, even those who have apparently uncomplicated defects.

Treatment of the lesion is surgical, almost always

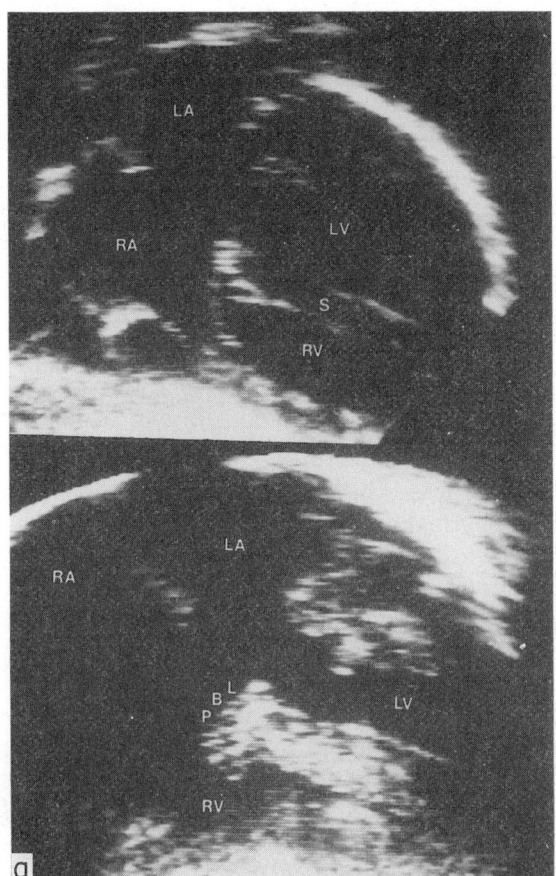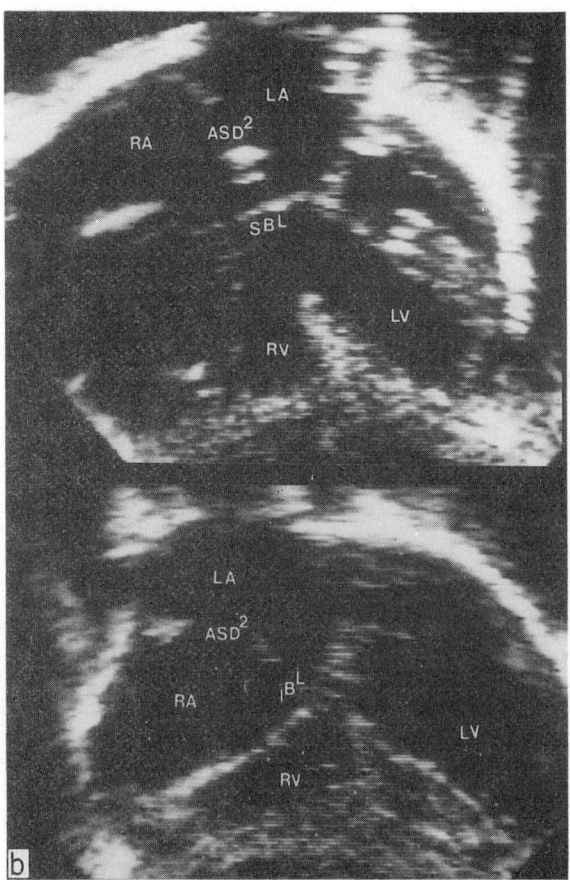

Fig. 25.34. (a) Four-chamber echocardiographic sections demonstrating an atrioventricular septal defect with two separate valves. The lower illustration is a subcostal four-chamber view which demonstrates the primum atrial septal defect and shows the posterior bridging leaflet (PBL) bound to the crest of the interventricular septum. The upper frame is a parasternal four-chamber section showing the two separate valves and the primum atrial septal defect. LA, left atrium; RA, right atrium; LV, left ventricle; RV, right ventricle; S, ventricular septum. (b) Four-chamber echocardiographic sections demonstrating an atrioventricular septal defect with common orifice. The lower illustration is a subcostal four-chamber section demonstrating the inferior bridging leaflet of the common orifice bound down to the crest of the ventricular septum. Immediately above the inferior bridging leaflet is a primum atrial septal defect. There is also an oval fossa atrial septal defect (ASD2). The upper illustration is a parasternal four-chamber section which demonstrates the superior bridging leaflet (SBL) of the common orifice. Immediately above the superior bridging leaflet is the primum atrial septal defect and immediately below the interventricular component. RA, right atrium; LA, left atrium; RV, right ventricle; LV, left ventricle. (Figures courtesy of Dr M.L. Rigby).

by complete repair, although some infants with common atrioventricular valves do benefit from initial banding of the pulmonary trunk. Patients with shunting exclusively at atrial level rarely, if ever, require surgery in infancy. Should surgery be required at this time, it must be corrective because palliation of a defect with only interatrial shunting is of little value. Elective surgery for asymptomatic children should be performed prior to school age. Mortality for repair of defects with only atrial shunting performed at specialized centres is now < 5%.

The surgery of those defects with a common orifice is complicated by the need to reconstruct separate valve orifices from the common valve and to close the interatrial and interventricular communications. Experience with primary correction now permits this to be the operation of choice in all but the extremely ill infant seen in the first month of life. When possible, the operation should be performed within the first year of life because of the risk of development of pulmonary hypertension. In the best series, the risk is no greater in this period than in later life. Mortality from primary repair,

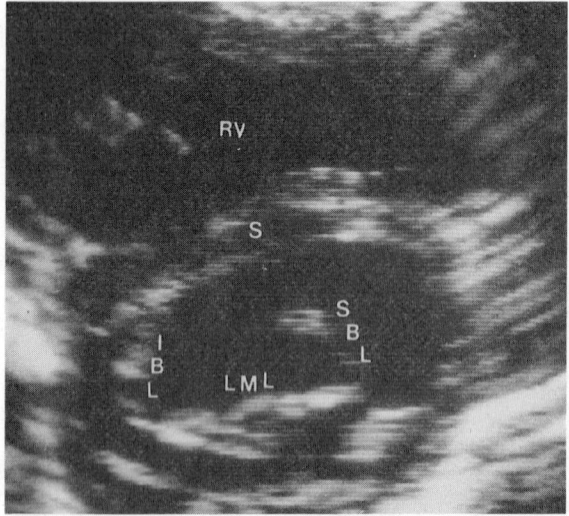

Fig. 25.35. Parasternal short-axis echocardiographic section demonstrating a three-leaflet left atrioventricular valve in an atrioventricular septal defect. The so-called 'cleft' is the commissure between the inferior bridging leaflet (IBL) and superior bridging leaflet (SBL). The left mural leaflet (LML) is also demonstrated clearly. S, interventricular system; RV, right ventricle. (Figure courtesy of Dr M.L. Rigby).

even in patients < 2 years of age, has decreased dramatically in recent years but it is higher than that for correction of patients with ostium primum defects.[55]

The influence of associated non-cardiac anomalies on the management of patients with congenital heart disease must be judged in each individual case. No surgery would be recommended for a patient with trisomy 13 disease; these babies never survive the first year or two. In Down's syndrome, however, surgery is indicated to relieve symptoms such as spells in the tetralogy of Fallot. However, more radical surgery, such as correction of complete atrioventricular septal defects, may not be advisable because there is evidence to suggest that such surgery does not confer a better chance of long-term survival when compared with conservative management.

VENTRICULAR SEPTAL DEFECTS

Interventricular communications are the most frequently encountered congenital cardiac anomaly. They can occur in isolation or as an integral part of more complex pathological entities such as tetralogy of Fallot, common arterial trunk and double-outlet ventricles. They also exist in association with other abnormalities such as complete or congenitally corrected transposition, pulmonary atresia or univentricular atrioventricular connection. When occurring in these more complex settings, the pathology and clinical picture are overshadowed by the associated anomalies (see appropriate sections). Consideration in this section will be confined to ventricular septal defect as an 'isolated' lesion.

Defects of the ventricular septum can be divided morphologically into holes bordered by the central fibrous body or tissue of the cardiac valves and those with entirely muscular rims (Fig. 25.37).[56] The defects with fibrous rims are of two types. The commonest is found in the region of the membranous septum. Such defects result from deficiency of the muscular components of the septum and are more properly termed perimembranous (Fig 25.38a). They may extend to open predominantly into the inlet or outlet components of the right

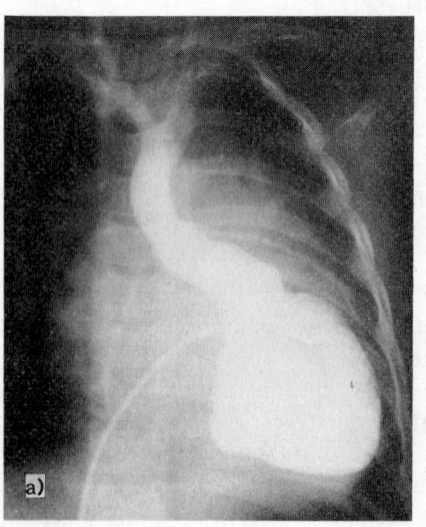

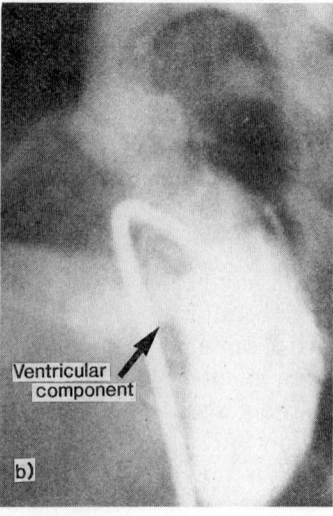

Ventricular component

a)

b)

Fig. 25.36. (a) A left ventricular angiogram in the frontal projection in an atrioventricular septal defect. The gooseneck deformity is well seen. (b) A four-chamber projection left ventricular angiogram in complete atrioventricular septal defect. Contrast is passing to the right ventricle via the ventricular component of the defect. This is taking place beneath the inferior bridging leaflet of the common atrioventricular valve.

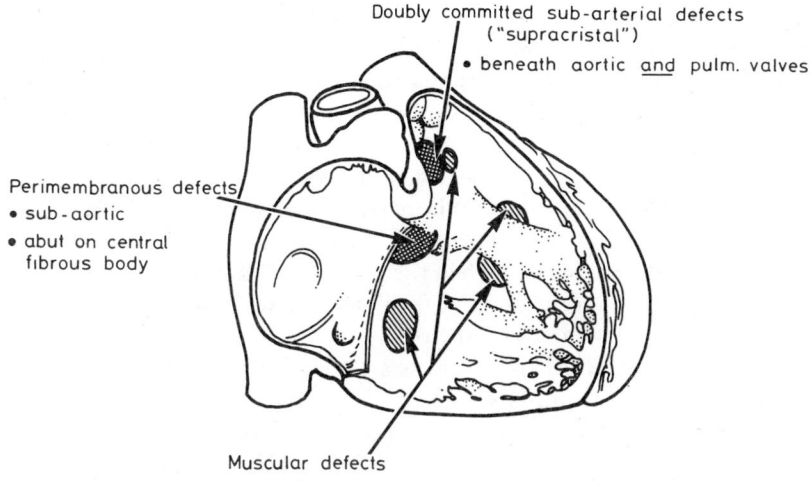

Doubly committed sub-arterial defects
("supracristal")
• beneath aortic and pulm. valves

Perimembranous defects
• sub-aortic
• abut on central fibrous body

Muscular defects
• entirely enclosed in muscular septum

Fig. 25.37. Diagram showing the typical anatomical positions of the three basic types of ventricular septal defect.

ventricle or may be confluent. All perimembranous defects have in common the feature that the atrioventricular bundle lies in their postero-inferior rim. The other defect with a fibrous rim is that known as the doubly committed and subarterial ('supracristal'). The upper border of this defect is the fused leaflets of the aortic and pulmonary valves (Fig. 25.38c). It results from absence or deficiency of the outlet septum together with the 'septal' component of the sub-pulmonary infundibulum. Because of this, the leaflets of the aortic valve may prolapse into the right ventricle. Muscular defects may be found in all parts of the septum. Muscular defects of the inlet septum must be distinguished from those that are perimembranous, because the

atrioventricular conduction axis will be superior to the muscular defect. Defects within the apical trabecular septum may be single or multiple, the latter being termed 'Swiss cheese' defects (Fig. 25.38b). Muscular outlet defects are rare. Muscular defects of any type may co-exist with a perimembranous septal defect.

The direction of the flow of blood through a ventricular septal defect depends on the relative resistances in the pulmonary and systemic circuits. When, as is usual, pulmonary resistance is less than systemic, flow will be from left to right. When pulmonary resistance exceeds the systemic, flow will be from right to left (a reversed shunt). Increasing resistance to flow in the lungs is seen

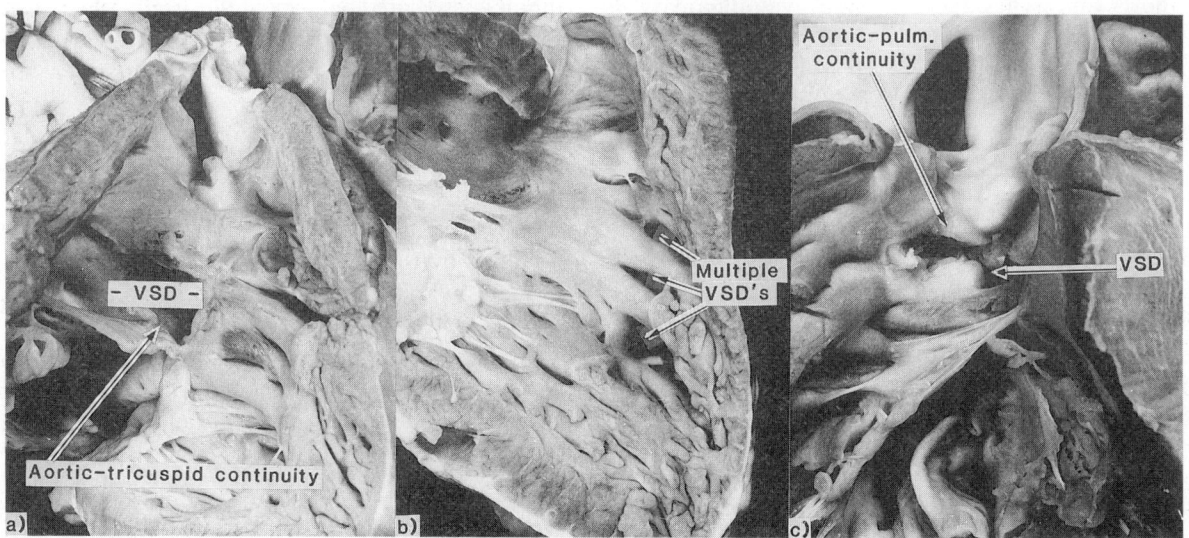

a) — VSD —
Aortic-tricuspid continuity
b) Multiple VSD's
c) Aortic-pulm. continuity   VSD

Fig. 25.38. The right ventricle showing the salient anatomical features of (a) perimembranous, (b) muscular and (c) doubly committed and subarterial ventricular septal defects.

with pulmonary vascular disease (so-called Eisenmenger reaction) or with muscular subvalvar pulmonary obstruction. If the ventricular septal defect is small enough to restrict flow, its size will be the major determinant of the magnitude of the shunt. With restrictive defects, the left ventricular pressure will exceed that in the right ventricle and pulmonary trunk. In contrast, the ventricular pressures will be equal with unrestrictive defects, and pulmonary arterial systolic pressure will be similar to that in the aorta. When pulmonary resistance is not much elevated and a high pulmonary flow exists, the pulmonary arterial diastolic pressure is less than aortic diastolic pressure. This situation is known as hyperdynamic pulmonary hypertension.

In fetal life, the pulmonary resistance is high enough to limit blood flow into the lungs. Pulmonary resistance begins to fall at birth with the onset of breathing. The fall to normal adults levels is not instantaneous and takes some days or weeks to be completed. In the early days of life of a patient with ventricular septal defect, therefore, there will be little shunting across the defect such that the lesion may be clinically undetectable. As pulmonary resistance falls, the shunt will increase and the defect may be detected. Its severity cannot be established until the fall in pulmonary resistance is complete. The age of completion is extremely variable. Some babies develop cardiac failure at 1 week; in others, this may be delayed until 2 or 3 months. In a small proportion of patients with ventricular septal defect, pulmonary resistance never falls. Then, the defect is detected only in later childhood when cyanosis supervenes due to progressive pulmonary vascular disease.

Patients with small shunts are asymptomatic and acyanotic and have a very favourable prognosis. Patients with large ventricular septal defects and large shunts show evidence of underdevelopment, recurrent pulmonary infections and early congestive heart failure. Death may rarely occur as a direct consequence of the septal defect. Cyanosis may be present in patients with marked pulmonary vascular disease when there is intermittent or continuous reversal of the shunt (the so-called Eisenmenger complex). It may also occur in some patients only during exercise, pulmonary infections or with the development of heart failure. Although congestive heart failure appears early, it tends to disappear after the first 1 or 2 years of life and may recur in later childhood or adult life.

The characteristic physical sign in patients with a small ventricular septal defect is a distinctive, usually loud and harsh pan-systolic murmur with maximal intensity in the third or fourth left interspaces near the sternum. It frequently extends beyond closure of the aortic valve. In small muscular septal defects (which may be closed during cardiac contraction), there may be only a short murmur in the early part of systole. A murmur that does not extend throughout systole may also be present when there is increased pulmonary vascular resistance. A thrill accompanies the murmur in the majority of cases.

The second heart sound is normally split or the split is widened. Unlike the wide split of an atrial septal defect, it varies normally with respiration. With normal or only slightly elevated pulmonary pressure, the sound of pulmonary closure is normal. With very large left-to-right shunts, a third sound is regularly audible and followed by a rumbling mid-diastolic murmur at the apex due to high flow through the mitral valve. There is also a pulmonary ejection systolic murmur which is usually obscured by the systolic murmur of the defect.

When there is severe pulmonary hypertension due to increased pulmonary vascular resistance, the systolic murmur does not last throughout systole. When dilatation of the pulmonary trunk is present, it is associated with an ejection systolic murmur and an ejection click. There is no systolic thrill. There is an increased intensity of the pulmonary element of the second sound and there may be an early high-pitched decrescendo murmur of pulmonary regurgitation. A third heart sound is not audible and there is no low-pitched mid-diastolic apical rumble. Associated patency of the arterial duct gives rise not to a continuous murmur but to an early diastolic murmur resembling that of pulmonary or aortic regurgitation.

The greater majority of patients with ventricular septal defect can survive to the age of 40 years without surgical treatment.[57] The relative infrequency of ventricular septal defect in adult life is explained by the high rate of spontaneous closure. Estimates vary, but in some series spontaneous closure is reported in up to 50% of patients. Spontaneous closure occurs most frequently up to the first 5 years, but occasionally it happens later and even in adult life. Perimembranous defects are closed by growth of tissue tags from the leaflets of the tricuspid valve or by adhesion of leaflet tissue across the defect. Muscular defects close by myocardial hypertrophy.

The small minority of infants in whom the ventricular septal defect itself is life-threatening are usually symptomatic by the age of 1 or 2 months. In these, the pulmonary resistance will have fallen sufficiently to allow a large left-to-right shunt which causes congestive cardiac failure. If untreated, these infants may die. In asymptomatic subjects, a normal life may be threatened by intercurrent disease. Respiratory infections may be life-threatening in infants and young children. Infective endocarditis and aortic regurgitation are life-threatening complications in older children, adolescents and adults. Infective endocarditis occurs with greater frequency in adults than in children: longevity predisposes to its occurrence. Surgical closure of a defect, although lowering the risk of bacterial endocarditis, does not completely eliminate it. Similarly, endocarditis may occur in a patient in whom a defect has closed spontaneously. Aortic regurgitation occurs most frequently with subaortic defects and is due to prolapse of the aortic leaflets bordering the defect. Simple closure of the defect may not cure this complication. These facts mean that patients with ventricular septal defects must be followed up carefully even after surgery or spontaneous closure. A small number of patients with isolated ventricular septal defect will develop sub-pulmonary infundibular obstruction. This may lead to an amelioration of their clinical condition by limiting the left-to-right shunt.

There is usually no distinctive cardiac silhouette on the chest X-ray. Moderate increases in pulmonary blood flow may be indicated by dilatation of the pulmonary vessels without any increase in heart size. With large defects, the left ventricular load is increased and the left ventricle becomes enlarged, the pulmonary trunk prominent and its smaller branches dilated. The left atrium is likewise enlarged. Both ventricles may be enlarged when a large shunt is associated with both high pulmonary blood flow and right ventricular systolic hypertension. The aortic knob is small. When pulmonary hypertension is marked, there is a right-to-left shunt through the ventricular septal defect. The findings are then those of the Eisenmenger complex with prominence of the pulmonary knob and engorgement of the central pulmonary arteries.

There is no significant electrocardiographic change when defects are small. With larger defects, the right chest leads often show an rSr complex. The typical pattern is left ventricular hypertrophy. The degree of hypertrophy depends on the size of the left-to-right shunt and the response of the left ventricle to the additional load. A qR is usually present in leads V_5 and V_6. In cases with high pulmonary arterial pressure, the electrocardiogram usually shows evidence of biventricular hypertrophy. With severe pulmonary hypertension due to increased pulmonary vascular resistance, the electrocardiogram shows only right ventricular hypertrophy. The mean frontal QRS vector axis is usually normal, but a superior axis is sometimes seen and suggests that the defect involves the inlet septum.

Cross-sectional echocardiography permits distinction of the type of defect and its position within the ventricular septum.[58] Perimembranous defects are distinguished by the finding of aortic-tricuspid valvar continuity in the roof of the defect. Those extending to open into the inlet of the right ventricle have the mitral and tricuspid valves in continuity at the same level in the roof of the defect (Fig. 25.39a). Muscular defects have the muscle of the septum separating all their borders from the attachments of both atrioventricular and arterial valves (Fig. 25.39b). Doubly committed subarterial defects exhibit the characteristic feature of fibrous continuity between the aortic and pulmonary valves (Fig. 25.39c). Malalignment of septal structures is readily seen. Doppler echocardiography can confirm the presence of small muscular defects while, in skilled hands, it can permit an estimate to be made of right ventricular pressure. Radionuclide angiograms can be used as a minimally invasive way of demonstrating and quantifying localizing shunts. Magnetic resonance imaging also demonstrates well the morphology (Fig. 25.40) but offers little information over and above that provided by the skilled echocardiographer.

At catheterization, the catheter usually follows the normal course from the right atrium to the right ventricle and then to the pulmonary trunk. The defect may be crossed by the catheter and the left ventricle and aorta may be entered from the right ventricle. This is not always the case. Failure to cross the defect has no implications regarding its presence or size. The oxygen saturation in the right ventricle usually exceeds that in the right atrium. Caution must be exercised when inferring the anatomical site of the defect from the level at which the step-up in oxygen saturation is detected. In the absence of an interatrial communication, detection of the step-up in the right atrium does suggest that the shunt is from left ventricle to right atrium. The left ventricular, aortic and right atrial pressures are usually normal. Elevation of left atrial pressure is often present in infants with a large shunt and a high pulmonary blood flow. Right ventricular and pulmonary arterial systolic pressures depend on the

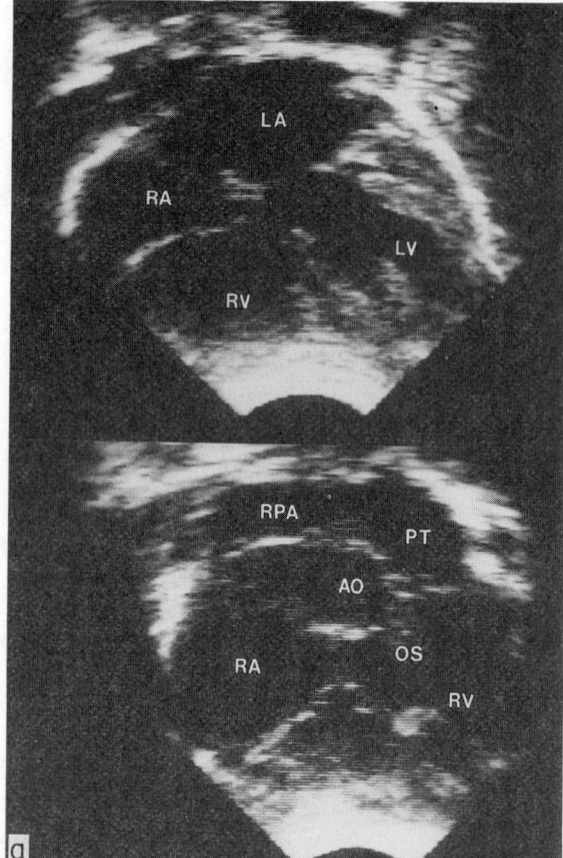

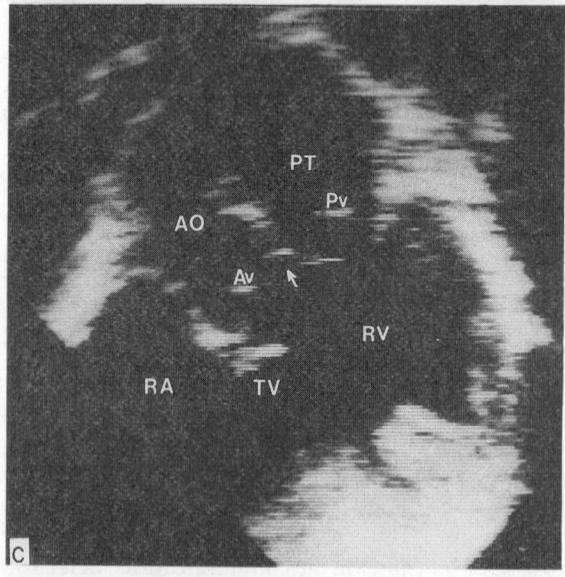

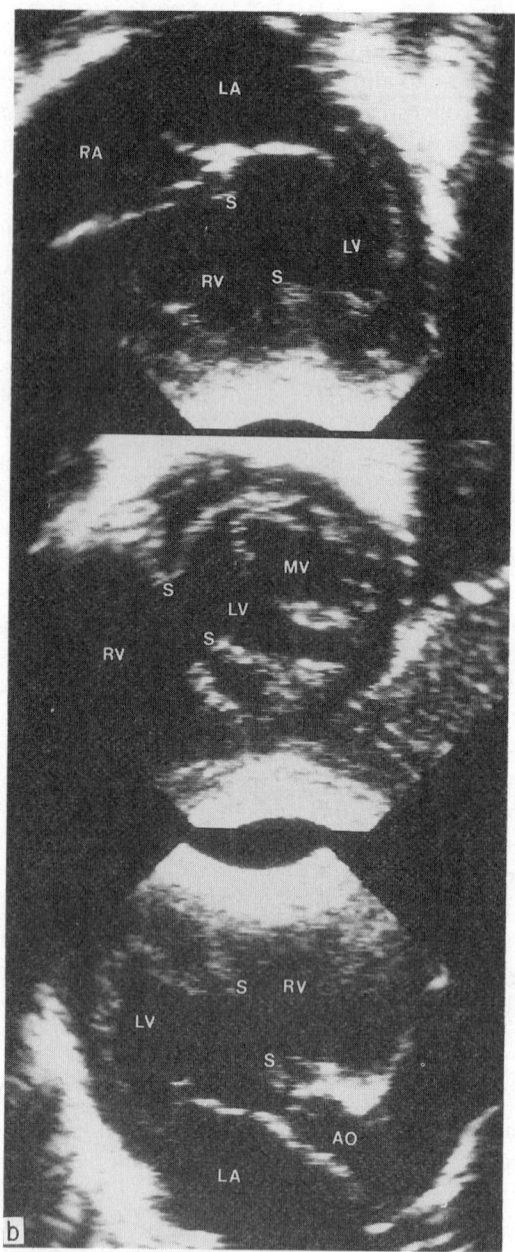

Fig. 25.39. (a) Echocardiographic sections from a heart with a perimembranous confluent ventricular septal defect. The upper illustration is a conventional parasternal four-chamber section demonstrating a perimembranous ventricular septal defect roofed superiorly by the mitral and tricuspid valves in fibrous continuity. The lower illustration is a subcostal right oblique section in which the outlet septum (OS) is profiled within the morphologically right ventricle (RV). RPA, right pulmonary artery; PT, pulmonary trunk; AO, aortic root; RA, right atrium,

LA, left atrium; RV, right ventricle; LV, left ventricle. (b) Echocardiographic sections demonstrating a large confluent muscular ventricular septal defect. The upper illustration is a parasternal four-chamber section showing normal offsetting of the atrioventricular valves and a supero-posterior muscular rim to the ventricular septal defect. The middle illustration is a subcostal short-axis view with the ventricular septal defect shown at the level of the mitral valve. The lower illustration is parasternal long-axis section also showing the large ventricular septal defect. RA, right atrium; LA, left atrium; S, interventricular septum; RV, right ventricle; LV, left ventricle; MV, mitral valve; AO, ascending aorta. (c) Subcostal right oblique echocardiographic section demonstrating fibrous continuity (arrow) between the aortic valve (AV) and pulmonary valve (PV) in the presence of a doubly committed subarterial ventricular septal defect. RA, right atrium; TV, tricuspid valve; RV, right ventricle; AO, aorta; PT, pulmonary trunk. (Figure courtesy of Dr M.L. Rigby).

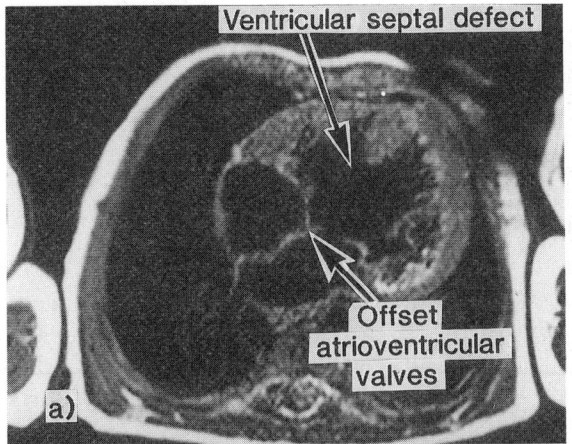
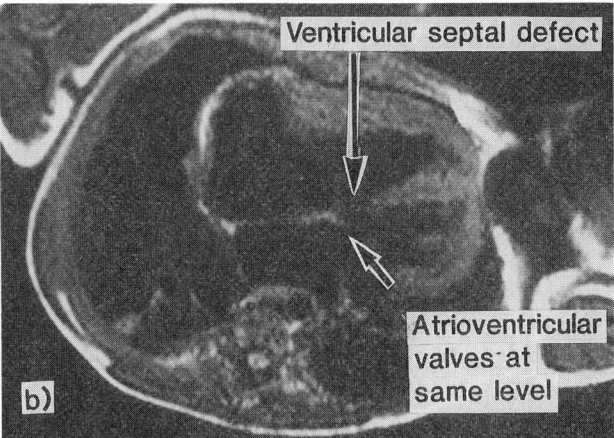

Fig. 25.40. Transverse plane magnetic resonance scans in ventricular septal defect. (a) A large perimembranous defect. The normal offset of the atrioventricular valves is contrasted with the lack of offset in (b) where the defect is in the inlet portion of the septum. (Figure courtesy of Dr E.J. Baker).

size of the defect and the pulmonary vascular resistance.

The precise localization of ventricular septal defects is possible using left ventricular contrast injections in long-axis and four-chamber projections (Fig. 25.41).[56] Outlet defects are best seen in the long axis view whereas defects opening to the right ventricular inlet are best seen in the four-chamber projection. Both views may be needed to assess accurately the position and number of defects in the apical trabecular septum.

The majority of patients with ventricular septal defect require no specific treatment. They all need prophylaxis against bacterial endocarditis but, apart from this, should lead entirely normal lives. Patients presenting in heart failure in infancy

require intensive medical therapy including digoxin and diuretics and afterload reduction. Where severe congestive failure is present, tube feeding is necessary. Inability of the infant to suck is the prime symptom of congestive cardiac failure. Its persistence despite medical therapy is the major indication that the cardiac failure is intractable. This is the major indication for surgery. In addition to the specific treatment for cardiac failure, antibiotics may be necessary because respiratory infection is frequently a precipitating factor. If the medical treatment is successful, and the infant is able to feed normally, urgent surgery is not required. The patient should be followed and cardiac catheterization performed or repeated at 6–9 months of age when in the presence of pulmonary hypertension,

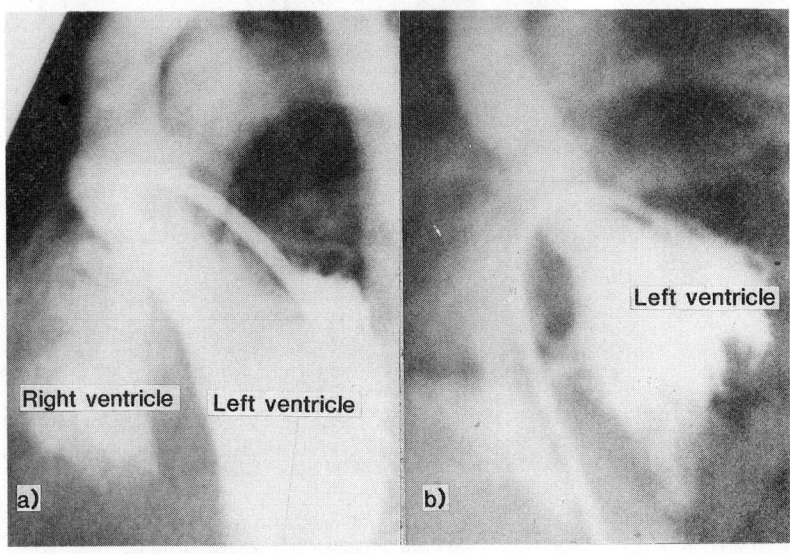

Fig. 25.41. Left ventricular angiograms in ventricular septal defect. (a) A long-axial oblique projection showing a perimembranous defect adjacent to the aortic valve. (b) A four-chamber projection showing a muscular inlet defect.

surgery may be necessary to prevent pulmonary vascular disease. Surgery can then be performed as an elective procedure before the age of 1 year. If surgery is not indicated in early infancy, either as a life-saving procedure or in order to prevent pulmonary vascular disease, there is usually steady clinical improvement with medical treatment.

Formerly indications for surgery depended on cardiac catheterization findings. However now catheterization is no longer needed for diagnosis and is therefore only indicated prior to corrective surgery when multiple defects cannot be excluded by non-invasive investigations. A further indication is in infants who have responded to treatment for heart failure but in whom a Doppler echocardiogram at six to nine months of age does not exclude pulmonary hypertension. Any patient in whom the clinical picture, electrocardiogram or echocardiogram suggests pulmonary hypertension also requires catheterization, as do patients who, for one reason or another, have not been diagnosed in infancy but present when older with signs of high pulmonary flow, cardiomegaly or congestive cardiac failure.

Surgery should be performed in all infants with heart failure resistant to medical treatment and in all patients with pulmonary hypertension but a pulmonary resistance < 5 units. If the resistance is > 5 units, closure carries a high risk and may not necessarily prevent progression of the pulmonary disease. In most specialized units, the risks of surgery are now < 5% for uncomplicated closure even if it is performed during infancy.[59]

ABNORMALITIES OF THE RIGHT ATRIOVENTRICULAR JUNCTION

Abnormalities of the right atrioventricular junction include tricuspid atresia, tricuspid stenosis and tricuspid regurgitation. The last two named anomalies are rare in the setting of a normally positioned valve in the absence of other lesions, but occur as part of the expression of Ebstein's malformation, probably the most notable of the lesions of the morphologically tricuspid valve.

Tricuspid atresia

When considered haemodynamically, tricuspid atresia is the condition in which systemic venous return must pass across the atrial septum from a blind-ending right atrium in order to enter the ventricular mass and reach the great arteries. In morphological terms, this clinical picture can be produced by several chamber combinations. One particular arrangement is by far the most frequent. It is often thought that this variant, which can be considered as 'classic' tricuspid atresia, is due to an imperforate tricuspid valve interposed between right atrium and ventricle. Such hearts do exist, but they are rare. When seen, they tend to exist in the setting of imperforate Ebstein's malformation. In fact, the 'classic' lesion is due to complete absence of the right atrioventricular connexion, with the left atrium connected to a dominant left ventricle, the right ventricle being rudimentary and incomplete (Fig. 25.42). In the setting of this 'classic' tricuspid atresia, there is still further variability in the downstream anatomy, particularly with different ventriculo-arterial connexions which modify markedly the physiological derangement.

Tricuspid atresia is a rare anomaly. Although estimates of its frequency vary from 0.3 to 5% of all congenital cardiac malformations, the estimates cluster around 1–2.5% in autopsy and in clinical series. This results in an incidence of tricuspid atresia of 1 in every 10 000–20 000 births. There is little sex difference in the incidence (a minimally

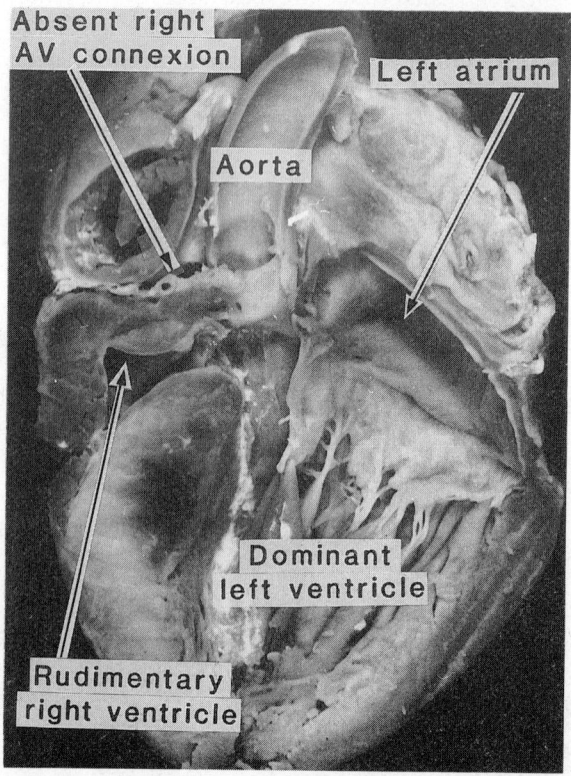

Fig. 25.42. Section in oblique long-axis projection shows the anatomical features of classical tricuspid atresia.

higher incidence in boys). Tricuspid atresia with a discordant ventriculo-arterial connexion ('transposition') definitely occurs more frequently in boys. No specific aetiological factor can be demonstrated in the majority of cases, but the condition has been reported following thalidomide ingestion and is known to be part of the 'cat eye' syndrome.

The outstanding morphological feature of the classic variant is that, on opening the morphologically right atrium, there is no sign whatsoever of the right atrioventricular connexion. The atrium has a complete muscular 'floor', which in reality is the lateral wall of the appendage. Sometimes, a muscular 'dimple' may be seen anterior to the orifice of the coronary sinus which is often presumed to be the site of the right atrioventricular orifice. Sectioning through this dimple shows that it 'points' to the outflow tract of the morphologically left ventricle. The right atrial blood must perforce exit to the left atrium through an atrial septal defect, usually within the oval depression. The left atrium drains to a dominant left ventricle which communicates in turn with a rudimentary right ventricle lacking any inlet component. The septum separating the two ventricles has only apical trabecular and outlet components. It extends to the acute point of the atrioventricular junction, not reaching the crux as in a heart with a biventricular atrioventricular connexion. The rudimentary right ventricle is therefore carried on the antero-superior shoulder of the ventricular mass. The anatomy described thus far is relatively constant for almost all examples of classic tricuspid atresia.[60] Variability is mostly related to the ventriculo-arterial connexion and to the presence of outflow tract stenosis. The subgrouping most frequently used depends upon these features. Thus, the lesion is usually considered in terms of subgroups with concordant ('normally related', Type I) or discordant ('transposed', Type II) great arteries. Each of these subgroups is described with totally obstructed (Type A), decreased (Type B) or increased (Type C) pulmonary blood flow.[61] This alphanumeric approach, although useful in many cases, is not universally applicable. We prefer a descriptive approach to categorization.

Most usually, tricuspid atresia is found with a concordant ventriculo-arterial connexion and with the aorta posterior and to the right of the pulmonary trunk ('normal relations'). The volume of pulmonary blood flow is then dependent on the size of the ventricular septal defect which also conditions the size of the rudimentary right ventricle. The second most frequent ventriculo-arterial connexion

is a discordant one. If stenotic, the ventricular septal defect then produces subaortic obstruction, almost always with concomitant coarctation and isthmal hypoplasia. Subpulmonary obstruction is less frequent. When found, it is due to deviation of the outlet septum into the left ventricle or to 'tissue tags'. Other ventriculo-arterial connexions are rare. A double outlet connexion can be found, usually from the dominant left ventricle but rarely from the rudimentary right ventricle. Single outlet due to a common arterial trunk also exists but is exceedingly rare, as is solitary pulmonary trunk with aortic atresia. Pulmonary atresia with a solitary aortic trunk is commoner. With pulmonary atresia, almost always the pulmonary blood flow is duct dependent. Most of the associated malformations that complicate classic tricuspid atresia have already been referred to, notably the atrial septal defect, the ventricular septal defect and the substrates of outflow tract obstruction. Any malformation however, must be anticipated to exist. Anomalies of systemic venous return are frequent, particularly a persistent left superior caval vein draining to the coronary sinus.

Whatever the morphological nature of tricuspid atresia, the basic route of circulation is the same. Systemic venous return must exist from the right to the left atrium via an interatrial communication. In the left atrium, it is joined by the pulmonary venous return and thence the mixed systemic and pulmonary venous returns enter the dominant left ventricle via the left atrioventricular valve. The mixed venous return is then ejected to both the aorta and the pulmonary trunk. Thus, in all cases of tricuspid atresia, there is complete systemic and pulmonary venous admixture. Of necessity, there is always systemic arterial desaturation. The degree depends upon the rate of pulmonary blood flow. When this is low, cyanosis is difficult to detect. Determinants of pulmonary blood flow include the type of ventriculo-arterial connexion and the presence or absence of pulmonary outflow obstruction, as discussed above. The presence or absence of pulmonary vascular disease is also important. In the majority of cases with a concordant ventriculo-arterial connexion, pulmonary blood flow is restricted. The site of obstruction is usually the ventricular septal defect. With discordant ventriculo-arterial connexions, there is usually unrestricted pulmonary blood flow. Such patients are not initially deeply cyanosed. Pulmonary stenosis, usually subvalvar, leads to restricted pulmonary blood in a minority of cases. When both great arteries arise from either the right or the left ventricle, the level of pulmonary blood flow (and therefore the degree of cyanosis) will depend on the presence or absence of pulmonary outflow obstruction. In any infant with obstruction to pulmonary blood flow, persistent patency of the duct will, by increasing pulmonary flow, ameliorate the systemic arterial desaturation. Those cases with initially unrestricted pulmonary blood flow also have pulmonary hypertension. They are at risk for the development of pulmonary vascular disease, which is usually established by the age of 1 year. Its progression, with progressive decrease in pulmonary blood flow, will lead to deepening cyanosis. Until this time, the effect of unrestricted pulmonary blood flow is to produce volume overload of the left ventricle. This leads in many cases to congestive cardiac failure.

Rarely, there may be obstruction to flow into the aorta. This is usually seen in cases with a discordant ventriculo-arterial connexion when the ventricular septal defect is restrictive. There is usually associated coarctation of the aorta. The combination of unrestricted pulmonary blood flow and restricted systemic arterial flow leads to early presentation in heart failure with metabolic acidosis. The rarity of this combination of defects suggests that it may be lethal in fetal life.

Obstruction to pulmonary or systemic blood flow in tricuspid atresia is not a static phenomenon. There is progressive decrease in size of the ventricular septal defect which may progress to complete closure.[62] Such changes are seen with both concordant and discordant ventriculo-arterial connexions. If obstruction to pulmonary blood flow becomes total, either persistent patency of the duct or, rarely, systemic-to-pulmonary collateral arteries are necessary to maintain life. Patients with tricuspid atresia are usually of normal size at birth but, by the end of their first year of life, significant growth retardation is often evident. Although no comprehensive data are available, patients with tricuspid atresia and cyanosis presumably exhibit similar limitation of intelligence to that seen in other forms of cyanotic heart disease.

The route of circulation in tricuspid atresia results in all patients having some degree of systemic arterial desaturation. Those with obstruction to pulmonary blood flow (the majority of cases) present with cyanosis. Those with unrestricted blood flow (about one-fifth) will not be clinically blue. Desaturation may be revealed only by failure of the systemic arterial Po_2 to rise while the patient is breathing 100% oxygen. Thus, the extremes of the spectrum of patients with tricuspid atresia are those with cyanosis and those who are clinically pink. Many who present with little or no cyanosis will, with the passage of time, become blue. Some of those who are mildly cyanosed will become grossly cyanosed. It must be excessively rare in the absence of surgical treatment for patients to become less cyanosed with age.

Half of all patients present on the first day of life. Two-thirds have presented by the age of 1 week and four-fifths by the age of 1 month. It is cyanosis that brings the majority to the physician. In those not cyanosed, a systolic murmur may lead to referral. Tachypnoea and dyspnoea may be the presenting features in those with high pulmonary blood flow. Although the clinical features are dominated by systemic arterial hypoxaemia, hypercyanotic spells are not seen nearly as frequently as in patients with tetralogy of Fallot.

On examination, patients will generally be small for their age. Those with a low pulmonary blood flow will be cyanosed. Towards the end of the first year of life, they may exhibit clubbing of the fingers and toes. Systemic venous congestion with raised jugular venous pressure may be seen in older patients, but this is rare in infancy. When pulmonary blood flow is severely limited by a restrictive ventricular septal defect (or similar lesion), only a single second heart sound is heard. Otherwise the heart sounds are of little significance. With subpulmonary obstruction, an ejection murmur will be heard which is propagated into the lung fields. This is not usually associated with a thrill. Tachypnoea and dyspnoea are seen in the minority of patients with a high pulmonary blood flow when the liver may be enlarged.

There are no pathognomonic features in the chest radiograph. As with most other congenital cardiac malformations, the picture reflects the haemodynamics. With diminished pulmonary blood flow, the heart is of normal size with little or no pulmonary knob and the lung fields are oligaemic. When pulmonary blood flow is increased, the heart is enlarged with plethoric lung fields.

The classic electrocardiographic features are right atrial hypertrophy, a mean frontal QRS axis of 0°–90° and diminished right ventricular forces. A superior QRS axis is seen in almost all the patients in whom the ventriculo-arterial connexion is concordant and in approximately half of those with discordant ventriculo-arterial connexions. One-sixth of the patients have a prolonged PR interval on the standard electrocardiogram.

The cross-sectional echocardiographic examination reflects the anatomy in considerable detail.[63] Subcostal four-chamber, paracoronal and apical four-chamber views (Fig. 25.43) show that there is only one atrioventricular valve. In the majority of cases, this valve enters a dominant left ventricle. Those rare variants with a dominant right ventricle should immediately be demonstrable. The diagnosis of absent right atrioventricular connexion is a positive one. It depends on demonstrating that, at the echocardiographic crux of the heart, the 'dimple' of the atrioventricular membranous septum is bounded by the left ventricular outflow and the thick echogenic sulcus tissue. No aspect of the rudimentary right ventricle or a right atrioventricular valve is present in this view. When more anterior projections are examined, the relationship of the right atrial floor to the rudimentary right ventricle varies with the position and size of that ventricle. If present, an imperforate valve will be seen as a thin membrane at the crux of the heart. Complete echocardiographic examination demonstrates the ventricular septal defect, the ventriculo-arterial connexion and the associated malformations. The information seen on cross-sectional echocardiography is also readily obtainable from magnetic resonance imaging.

First pass nuclear angiography demonstrates the route of circulation, a right-to-left atrial shunt being visualized. In older patients, in whom isotope dose levels provide adequate counts, the first pass study allows estimation of left ventricular performance.

The most obvious finding on cardiac catheterization is the failure to enter the right ventricle from the right atrium. The catheter route is from the right atrium to the left atrium and thence to the left ventricle. From the left ventricle it is usually possible to enter a great artery. This is the aorta when the ventriculo-arterial connexion is concordant or the pulmonary trunk when it is discordant. When the ventricular septal defect is large, both great arteries may be entered. When small, as is often the case with a concordant ventriculo-arterial connexion, it may be impossible to enter the artery that arises from the rudimentary right ventricle. Oximetry demonstrates a right-to-left shunt. Oximetric evidence of complete mixing will be obtained when both the aorta and pulmonary trunk are entered. With discordant ventriculo-arterial connexions, there will generally be a high pulmonary arterial pressure and blood flow. With concordant connexions, the pulmonary blood pressure and flow will be low.

Angiocardiography is now rarely required for the diagnosis of tricuspid atresia, but it is still indicated prior to definitive surgery (Fig. 25.44). Right atrial angiocardiography demonstrates the separation of the right atrium from the ventricular mass, the 'incisura' at the expected site of the right atrioventricular connexion being visualized. Left ventricular angiocardiography in the long-axial oblique projection demonstrates the rudimentary right ventricle,

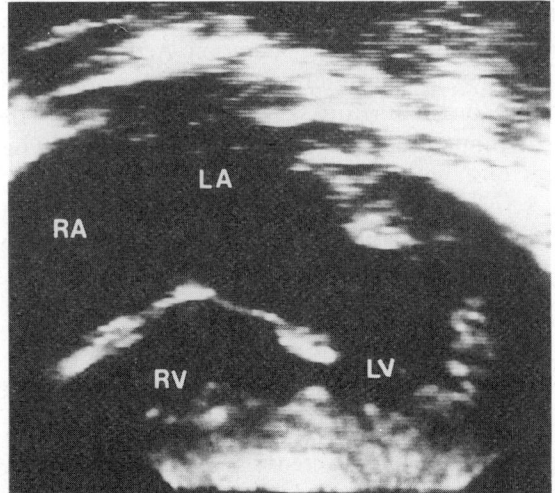

Fig. 25.43. Parasternal four-chamber echocardiographic section demonstrating absence of the right atrioventricular connexion in classic tricuspid atresia. Sulcus tissue interposes between the floor of the right atrium (RA) and the ventricular mass. The left atrium (LA) connects to the morphologically left ventricle (LV). There is a large ventricular septal defect. RV, right ventricle. (Figure courtesy of Dr M.L. Rigby).

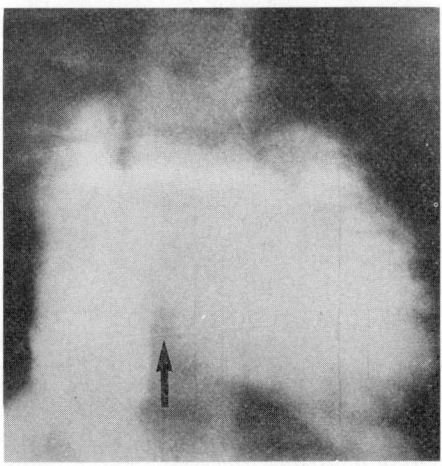

Fig. 25.44. Right atrial angiogram, in the frontal projection, of classic tricuspid atresia. The arrow indicates the incisure of the absent right atrioventricular connexion.

the ventriculo-arterial connexion and the site and size of the ventricular septal defect. Additional malformations (such as valvar pulmonary stenosis, coarctation of the aorta and aortic arch hypoplasia) are seen on appropriate angiocardiography.

The overall prognosis without treatment for patients with tricuspid atresia is poor. Only rare cases survive into middle life without surgical treatment. Even into the era of palliative surgery, two-fifths of patients died under the age of 6 months, half by 1 year and only one-tenth survived for 10 years. Increasing hypoxaemia is to be expected in patients with concordant ventriculo-arterial connexions. If untreated, it has a profound adverse effect on survival. It is related to closure of the duct or to diminution in size of the ventricular septal defect. As with other cyanotic conditions, cerebrovascular accidents occur in a small percentage of children. Deterioration in patients with tricuspid atresia and discordant ventriculo-arterial connexions is usually manifested by congestive cardiac failure. Although the major determinant of this is the high pulmonary blood flow, the common association of aortic arch anomalies (including aortic coarctation) is an exacerbating factor in affected infants. Diminution in size of the ventricular septal defect with resulting aortic outflow obstruction is a potentially lethal complication. For this reason, those surviving the early months of life, either because of the development of pulmonary vascular disease or as a result of banding of the pulmonary trunk, are at risk for sudden death. The tendency for the ventricular septal defect to close is a hazard for patients with either concordant or discordant ventriculo-arterial connexions.

Palliative treatment in patients with diminished pulmonary blood flow and consequent severe cyanosis is directed at augmenting the pulmonary flow. Maintenance or establishment of patency of the duct by the use of prostaglandin E_1 and E_2 should be attempted in critically ill neonates. Once the diagnosis is established, palliative surgery is usually essential. Palliation for those with diminished blood flow consists of construction of the modified Blalock shunt using a Gore-Tex or similar prosthetic graft from the subclavian artery to the pulmonary artery. In patients over 6–12 months of age, however, the Glenn operation may be performed. The superior caval vein is anastomosed to the right pulmonary artery, the right pulmonary artery is ligated proximal to the anastomosis and the superior caval vein ligated on the atrial side of the anastomosis. In those with excessive blood flow,

the pulmonary trunk is banded.

Although the results of palliative surgery are continually improving, a normal lifespan cannot be assured by these manoeuvres and a definitive operation is necessary. This is offered at present by modifications of the Fontan procedure. This operation achieves separation of the pulmonary from systemic circuits by establishing continuity between the right atrium and the pulmonary arteries. With discordant ventriculo-arterial connexions, the right atrium is directly connected to the pulmonary trunk either using a valved conduit or by direct anastomosis. When the ventriculo-arterial connexion is concordant, the Fontan operation may be modified in that the right atrium is connected to the rudimentary right ventricle and the ventricular septal defect closed. This also can be done with a conduit or by direct anastomosis. More usually, however, an atriopulmonary anastomosis is preferred in this setting. Success of the procedure is heavily dependent upon the haemodynamics, and rigid selection criteria are needed to obtain optimal results. When patients are chosen carefully, the Fontan operation produces acceptable operative mortality. Nowadays, less than one-tenth of patients will die. Statistically significant higher mortality, however, is seen in patients under 4 and over 16 years of age. The trend in mortality is upwards from the age of 7 years onwards.[64]

Complications in the intermediate and longer term include residual interatrial and interventricular shunts and conduit obstruction. These complications may necessitate re-operation. Arrhythmias are a further complication, causing deterioration in about one-tenth of survivors. Control of the arrhythmia usually restores the patient to his or her previous clinical state.

Actuarial analysis following surgery is encouraging and nine-tenths of the survivors are in New York Heart Association (NYHA) functional class I or II.

Tricuspid stenosis

Apart from its presence in association with Ebstein's malformation, stenosis is rare as an isolated lesion. It can occur with greater frequency associated with pulmonary atresia and intact ventricular septum or with Uhl's anomaly. In these cases, it is frequently miniaturization of the valve that leads it to be stenotic. Straddling of the right atrioventricular valve may also result in functional stenosis. In those rare cases of isolated stenosis, the valve is usually dysplastic. The physical signs include a large 'a' wave in the venous pulse, a pre-systolic murmur, which is louder on inspiration, and, rarely, an opening snap. The electrocardiogram shows right atrial hypertrophy. The chest radiograph gives little diagnostic information. Echocardiography shows limitation of the diastolic closure slope of the valve and reveals dysplasia of the valve leaflets. Cardiac catheterization is diagnostic, there being a high right atrial pressure with an end-diastolic gradient across the valve. Treatment is rarely required until adult life. Commissurotomy may be attempted, although the valve may be so dysplastic that replacement is required. It is important to recognize the rarity of this anomaly and to exclude more complex cardiac lesions, particularly Ebstein's malformation.

Tricuspid regurgitation

As an isolated lesion in the absence of Ebstein's malformation, tricuspid regurgitation is extremely rare. It does occur in the setting of a normal valve as a transient phenomenon in the newborn period.[65] When persistent, there is usually significant dysplasia, particularly of the medial (septal) leaflet. It may be the least severe lesion of the spectrum of Ebstein's malformation. There is also a well-recognized anomaly in which the leaflets of the valve are totally lacking so that the tricuspid orifice is unguarded. Usually, however, this lesion co-exists with some form of pulmonary atresia, which is then the dominant malformation. Recently tricuspid regurgitation due to tricuspid dysplasia has become recognized as a cause of fetal cardiac dysfunction leading to fetal or neonatal death.

Whatever the cause, tricuspid regurgitation may result in neonatal cyanosis, due to right-to-left shunting through the oval foramen, accompanied by a systolic murmur and thrill at the lower left sternal edge. The electrocardiogram shows right ventricular and right atrial hypertrophy. The chest radiograph may show gross cardiomegaly with pulmonary oligaemia. The diagnosis is made by Doppler echocardiography or by cardiac catheterization and angiography. A prominent 'V' wave with an elevated right atrial pressure are suggestive, whereas Doppler and right ventricular angiography will demonstrate the regurgitation. When occurring as an isolated lesion, the best treatment is conservative. As the name indicates transient ischaemia of the newborn usually regresses spontaneously. Surgery may on rare occasions

be indicated in older children. As with tricuspid stenosis, it is important to exclude more complex cardiac malformations before accepting the diagnosis of isolated regurgitation.

Ebstein's malformation

The hallmark of this lesion is displacement of the proximal attachment of the tricuspid valve leaflets into the cavity of the right ventricle (Fig. 25.45). Thus, although the right atrioventricular 'annulus' remains in its normal position, the displaced attachment effectively transforms part of the right ventricle into part of the right atrium. The degree of downward displacement varies. In its mildest form, only the adjacent parts of the septal and inferior leaflets are plastered down onto the walls of the ventricular inlet portion, the antero-superior leaflet being normally formed and positioned. In the severe form, the inferior and septal leaflets are displaced to the inlet–trabecular junction of the right ventricle, and the free edge of the antero-superior leaflet becomes anomalously attached to a muscular ridge formed apically at the inlet–trabecular junction. This latter arrangement produces severe tricuspid stenosis, the blood being able to pass to the distal parts of the right ventricle only through the slit-like antero-septal and inferior commissures of the valve (Fig. 25.46). In intermediate forms of the anomaly, the degree of displacement can vary, as can the degree of linear apical attachment of the antero-superior leaflet. All the leaflets of the valve can show dysplastic features which may render them stenotic, incompetent or both. It is possible for the malformation to be even more severe with the commis-

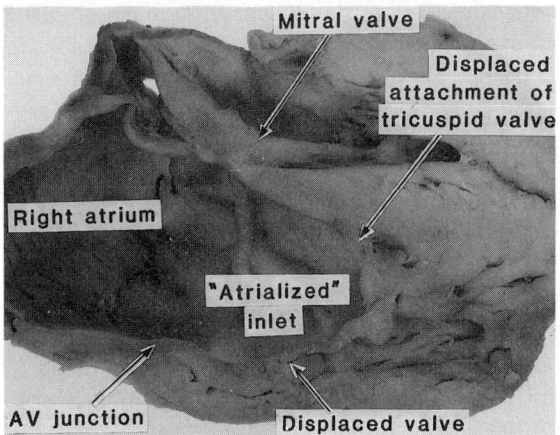

Fig. 25.45. A four-chamber section showing downward displacement of the attachments of the septal and mural leaflets of the tricuspid valve. This is pathognomonic of Ebstein's malformation.

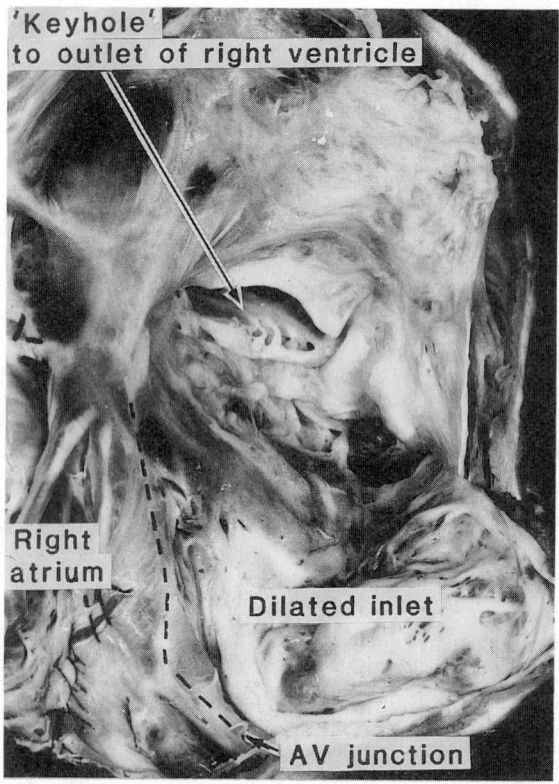

'Keyhole' to outlet of right ventricle

Right atrium

Dilated inlet

AV junction

Fig. 25.46. Photograph of the opened right atrioventricular junction showing the features of severe Ebstein's malformation. AV, atrioventricular.

sures being fused, producing an imperforate shelf and, hence, tricuspid atresia.[66]

Ebstein's malformation can exist as an isolated anomaly. In its mildest form, it is frequently a chance finding at autopsy. More often, it is associated with other lesions such as atrial septal defect, ventricular septal defect or pulmonary stenosis. When associated with pulmonary atresia and intact ventricular septum, the malformation of the tricuspid valve is usually of secondary importance. There is an important association between Ebstein's anomaly and the Wolff–Parkinson–White syndrome, with right-sided accessory pathways being found.[67]

With mild forms, the diagnosis may be indicated by the chance finding of abnormal physical signs. In contrast, three-quarters of the sufferers are cyanosed, indicating more severe forms with an associated atrial septal defect or persistent oval foramen. The cyanosis is characteristically variable in severity at its onset which may be as early as the first week of life. Dyspnoea is frequent in association with cyanosis but may occur alone. It is always present when congestive cardiac failure occurs. The

age at presentation is variable, but the most severely affected patients are the earliest to present. The frequent association of pre-excitation syndromes leads to tachyarrhythmias which may be the presenting feature. On physical examination, a systolic thrill may be felt at the left sternal edge. The cardiac impulse may appear weak in the anterior precordium. A systolic murmur, frequently described as scratchy, is characteristic and is heard over the lower sternal border and may on occasion be pan-systolic. A mid-diastolic or pre-systolic murmur is usually also present in this area. The first heart sound is widely split because of the delayed closure of the sail-like antero-superior leaflet. A third heart sound is frequently heard. When tricuspid regurgitation is marked, a prominent systolic wave may be seen in the jugular venous pulse. The characteristic murmurs and multiple heart sounds are strongly suggestive of the diagnosis.

Clinical course is as variable as the different grades of severity of the lesion. Mild degrees are consistent with a normal lifespan whereas with the most severe forms death can occur in infancy. Those patients who survive the first year of life rarely die in childhood. The onset of congestive cardiac failure is a grave prognostic sign. Following the onset of cyanosis, prolonged survival is unusual, but not unknown. Death in childhood or adult life may be the result of a tachyarrhythmia.[68]

Although the heart size may be normal on the chest radiograph, the majority of patients have generalized cardiac enlargement. There is usually right atrial dilatation, and the left cardiac border is convex, although the heart shadow may appear globular. The pulmonary vascular markings are normal or decreased (Fig. 25.10). The electrocardiogram usually shows right bundle branch block with small R and S waves in the right chest leads. The PR interval is frequently prolonged. The major exception to this is when the Wolff–Parkinson–White syndrome is present. This is found in one-tenth of patients and is usually of type B.

Echocardiography is diagnostic. The M-mode technique reveals delayed closure of the antero-superior leaflet with asynchronous septal motion. Cross-sectional investigation reveals the exaggerated off-setting of the septal attachments of the atrioventricular valves (Fig. 25.47). It also shows the extent of apical tethering of the antero-superior leaflet.[69]

It used to be held that cardiac catheterization carried a high risk in patients with Ebstein's

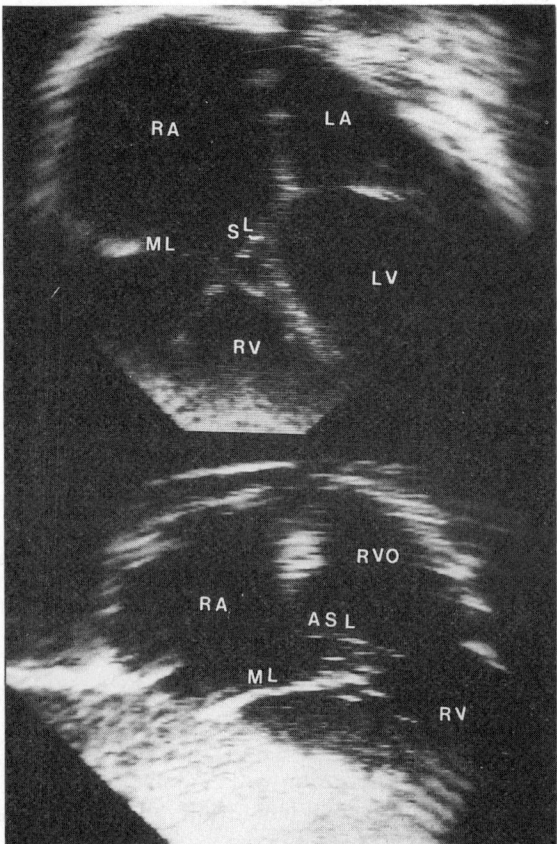

Fig. 25.47. Echocardiographic sections from a patient with Ebstein's anomaly of the tricuspid valve. The upper illustration is a parasternal four-chamber section. The right atrium (RA) is large. The septal leaflet (SL) of the tricuspid valve is displaced into the body of the right ventricle and is short with rolled edges. In this projection, the mural leaflet of the tricuspid valve (ML) is not displaced but also has rolled edges. The lower illustration is a subcostal right oblique projection which shows some displacement of the mural leaflet into the morphologically right ventricle (RV). The antero-superior leaflet of the tricuspid valve (ASL) is seen and the right ventricular outflow tract (RVO). (Figure courtesy of Dr M.L. Rigby).

malformation. With appropriate care, this is no longer the case. When catheterization is performed, the first clue to diagnosis may be the difficulty with which the catheter is manipulated from the large right atrium through the tricuspid valve to the right ventricle and pulmonary trunk. When the atrial septum is patent, a right-to-left shunt may be detected across it. This may occur without there being obvious obstruction to inflow to or outflow from the ventricular portion of the right ventricle. Injection into the right ventricle shows the portion distal to the tricuspid valve to be small. There is frequently angiographic evidence of tricuspid regurgitation and, with this or with an atrial injection,

the deformed valve can be seen and distinguished from the more proximal true atrioventricular junction. The valve is displaced to the junction of the inlet and trabecular portions of the right ventricle, frequently with a prominent shelf at this site (Fig. 25.48).

Many patients survive with a normal life span having received little medical attention; some will require treatment for arrhythmias, whereas others have severe enough haemodynamic disturbances to need surgery. Severe cyanosis and congestive cardiac failure are the chief indications for operation. The options are either reconstruction of the valve or its replacement by a prosthesis. Owing to the varied morphology, each case must be treated on its merits. Whether reconstruction or replacement is performed, it is usually necessary to plicate the atrialized inlet portion of the right ventricle. If the valve is replaced, care must be taken to avoid the atrioventricular node and penetrating bundle, particularly as the displacement of the septal leaflet may distort the usual atrial landmarks. If an atrial septal defect is present, it is closed. Results vary, being acceptable in adult life but poor when surgery is required in infancy. No palliative approach has been successful. If pre-excitation is present, the accessory atrioventricular connexion, usually right-sided, should be identified and divided. This may be done as an operation in its own right, but it should always be performed if surgical correction of the valvar lesion is necessary.[70]

ABNORMALITIES OF THE LEFT ATRIOVENTRICULAR JUNCTION

Congenital malformations of the left atrioventricular junction include mitral stenosis, mitral regurgitation, absence of the left atrioventricular connexion and imperforate left atrioventricular valve.

Congenital mitral stenosis

This is a rare problem and may be due to several pathological processes. The valve leaflets may be dysplastic and the commissures fuse to form a stenotic orifice somewhat like that of rheumatic stenosis. The tendinous cords may be short, thickened and fused. They may be attached to one major papillary muscle, producing the so-called 'parachute' mitral valve. A combination of dysplastic and fused leaflets and anomalies of the tension apparatus may be present.[71] Congenital mitral stenosis

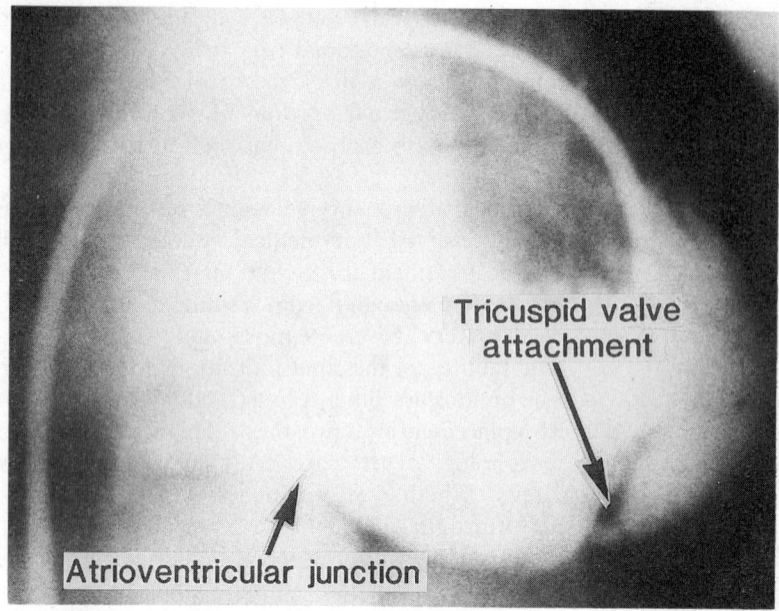

Tricuspid valve attachment

Atrioventricular junction

Fig. 25.48. A frontal projection of a right ventricular angiogram in Ebstein's anomaly. The insertion of the tricuspid valve is more apical than the normal atrioventricular junction. The right ventricle distal to the tricuspid valve is small.

can occur as an isolated malformation, but it is more frequently associated with other conditions such as aortic coarctation, complete transposition or double-outlet right ventricle.

The effect of congenital mitral stenosis is to obstruct left atrial emptying. The left atrial and pulmonary venous pressures are thus elevated causing tachypnoea and, if the obstruction is severe, pulmonary oedema. Reflex elevation of the pulmonary vascular resistance leads to pulmonary hypertension.

Presentation can be at any age and depends on the severity of the stenosis and of the associated anomalies. Tachypnoea and dyspnoea are usually the first symptoms, and when stenosis is very severe they may occur in the first week of life.

The signs found on auscultation are similar to those of mitral stenosis in adult life, but with the rapid heart rates encountered in infancy pre-systolic accentuation of the mid-diastolic murmur is difficult to appreciate. As the leaflets and cords are frequently dysplastic and stiff, the first heart sound is often soft and an opening snap may not be heard.

The chest radiograph frequently shows cardiomegaly due to right ventricular enlargement secondary to pulmonary hypertension. The lung fields are usually congested with septal lines as evidence of chronic pulmonary oedema. There is right-axis deviation on the electrocardiogram together with right and left atrial and right ventricular hypertrophy. Echocardiography demonstrates slow diastolic closure of the mitral valve. Although

the mural leaflet usually moves anteriorly, in some instances of congenital mitral stenosis its direction of motion may be normal.

Cardiac catheterization will demonstrate a pressure gradient from the left atrium (or pulmonary arterial wedge pressure) to the left ventricular end-diastolic pressure. Pulmonary hypertension will be either demonstrated or excluded. Left ventricular angiography frequently shows the type of lesion involved, for example, a parachute deformity. The major indication for catheterization, however, is the exclusion or delineation of associated anomalies.

Initial management, particularly in infancy, is supportive with the use of diuretics and digitalis. Surgical treatment includes valvotomy or valve replacement. Either approach has a better chance of success in the older child than in the infant. Any surgical treatment is only palliative.

The prognosis of congenital mitral stenosis depends on the severity of the lesion and the presence of associated cardiac malformations. Survival is rare when the disease is severe enough to present in the first year of life. The older the patient, the better the prognosis. Even with surgery, the long-term outlook is not known.

Congenital mitral regurgitation

Mitral regurgitation is a not uncommon accompaniment of other congenital cardiac anomalies. It is a frequent problem in endocardial fibro-elastosis and coarctation of the aorta, and as a result of ischaemic damage to papillary muscles. It can also occur as an isolated lesion due to intrinsic pathology of the valve or its tension apparatus. Prolapse with an intact tension apparatus can result in regurgitation. A cleft aortic (anterior) leaflet is another cause of regurgitation, together with parachute deformity, double-orifice valve and anomalous arcade.[72] Regurgitation may also result from or be exacerbated by dilatation of the left ventricle.

The symptoms, age at presentation and prognosis are a function of the severity of the regurgitation. Dyspnoea on effort, poor weight gain and frequent respiratory infections are common. When regurgitation is severe, congestive cardiac failure is common. The initial physical examination may suggest that the patient has a ventricular septal defect. Careful auscultation reveals that the pan-systolic murmur and thrill are maximal over the apex rather than at the left sternal border.

The electrocardiogram shows left ventricular, and frequently left atrial, hypertrophy. There is cardiac enlargement and frequently pulmonary congestion on the chest radiograph. Enlargement of the left atrium may be detected on the lateral projection, but it is more frequently identified in older children than in infants. Echocardiography can demonstrate the nature of the lesion responsible for regurgitation.

Cardiac catheterization may show elevation of the left atrial or pulmonary artery wedge pressure with a prominent 'v' or systolic wave. The pulmonary arterial pressure may be elevated. The diagnosis is confirmed and the severity assessed by retrograde left ventricular angiography, which may also reveal the anatomy of the valve lesion, for example, a parachute deformity.

Many cases can be maintained in good health by medical treatment. If congestive cardiac failure cannot be controlled or if there is severe pulmonary hypertension, surgery must be performed. Valve replacement is a feasible operation even in small children, but at present there is no suitable prosthetic valve. The complications of anticoagulant therapy and the realization that replacement in small children is only palliative make conservative treatment more attractive. In some centres, reconstructive operations show promise of offering a surgical alternative to valve replacement.

Hypoplastic left ventricle

The association of mitral stenosis or atresia with hypoplasia of the morphologically left ventricle and atresia of the aortic orifice is usually characterized as the hypoplastic left heart syndrome (Fig. 25.49). It is the commonest cause of heart failure on the first

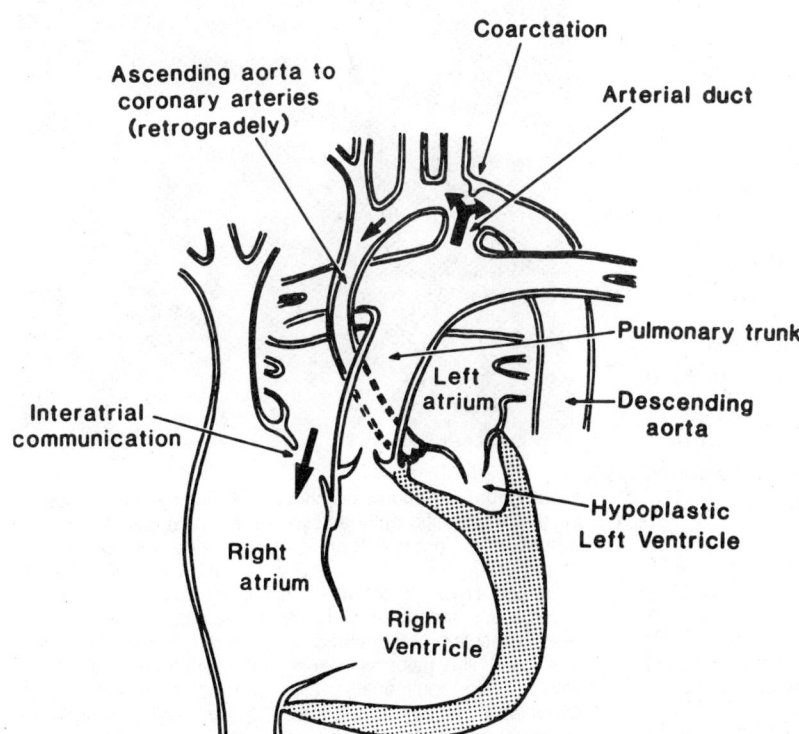

Fig. 25.49. Diagram illustrating the typical features of so-called hypoplastic left heart syndrome.

day of life and of death from congenital heart disease in the neonatal period.

There are two discrete anatomical variants. In one, the hypoplastic left ventricle contains a miniature and dysplastic but perforate mitral valve. It gives rise to a hypoplastic ascending aorta with atresia of its outflow. The left ventricular endocardium is thickened by fibro-elastosis, which also involves the mitral valve and its tension apparatus.[73] In the second type, aortic atresia and hypoplasia of the morphologically left ventricle are associated with atresia of the left atrioventricular valve. In the majority of cases, no mitral valve can be detected, these hearts having absence of the left atrioventricular connexion.[74] The left ventricle is then rudimentary in that it lacks an inlet portion. Such a ventricle may be so small that careful sectioning of the heart may be needed to demonstrate its presence.

In both varieties, the aorta has no patent connexion with the ventricular mass and all the systemic blood flow must leave the heart via the pulmonary trunk and the arterial duct. The brachiocephalic and coronary arteries are perfused in retrograde fashion through the aortic isthmus. The ascending aorta is narrow because it is solely a conduit for coronary flow. The systemic circulation is dependent on the maintenance of patency of the arterial duct. Ductal closure, therefore, produces a sudden deterioration in the condition of the patient. Even with a patent duct, coronary perfusion (and that of the upper limbs and head) may be compromised by the frequently associated aortic coarctation. Similarly, the only outlet for blood entering the left heart via the pulmonary veins is through the oval hole to the right atrium. This is against the direction of flow allowed by the flap valve of the hole so that left atrial and pulmonary venous hypertension are usually present.

Affected patients present during the first few days of life with tachypnoea and dyspnoea due to pulmonary venous hypertension. This rapidly progresses to pulmonary oedema and congestive cardiac failure with rapid enlargement of the liver. Sudden collapse with cyanosis and shock occur with closure of the duct.

The electrocardiogram shows severe right ventricular hypertrophy. The chest radiograph reveals gross cardiomegaly with congested lung fields. Cross-sectional echocardiography is diagnostic and shows a large right ventricle, a small or unidentifiable left ventricle and a very small aortic root (Fig. 25.50). Further studies are not usually indicated. If cardiac catheterization is performed, the pulmonary arterial pressure is found to be elevated, the aorta is entered via the duct and frequently the aortic pressure is lower than that in the pulmonary artery. This indicates ductal constriction. The left atrial pressure is found to be elevated, and often a left-to-right shunt is present at atrial level. Pulmonary arterial angiography leads to retrograde opacification of the aortic arch and visualizes the hypoplastic ascending aorta and the coronary arteries. When the mitral valve is perforate, it is possible to demonstrate angiographically the hypoplastic left ventricle. More usually, the left ventricle is not entered and left atrial angiography shows no evidence of left ventricular filling, contrast leaving the left atrium via the foramen ovale.

Death usually occurs within the first week of life.

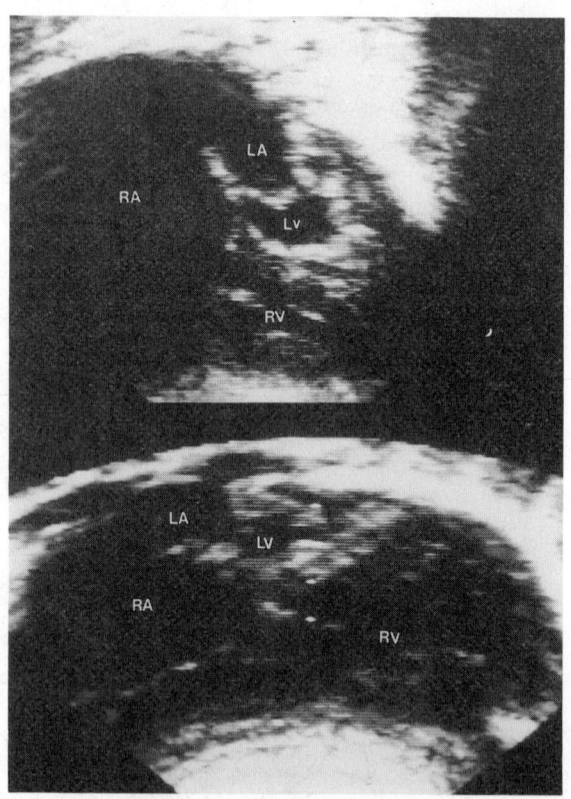

Fig. 25.50. Four-chamber echocardiographic sections illustrating the hypoplastic left heart syndrome. The upper illustration is a parasternal four-chamber section showing a hypoplastic left atrium (LA), a thickened and dysplastic miniaturized mitral valve and a hypoplastic left ventricle (LV). The right atrium (RA) is large and septal attachments of the tricuspid valve to the interventricular septum can be seen in the right ventricle (RV). The lower illustration is a subcostal four-chamber section in which dilated pulmonary veins can be seen entering the hypoplastic left atrium and the relatively small size of the left ventricle can be seen when it is compared with the right ventricle. (Figure courtesy of Dr M.L. Rigby).

Longer survival may occur if, for instance, there is an atrial septal defect rather than a patent oval foramen. Left atrial hypertension and pulmonary oedema do not then occur. In addition, if the duct remains patent, systemic perfusion may be maintained by the right ventricle. Even then, survival is not prolonged beyond a few months. Treatment is possible. Atrial septostomy may prevent pulmonary oedema and prostaglandin therapy may maintain ductal patency long enough for a palliative operation to be performed. These operations consist of bilateral banding or isolation of the pulmonary arteries and creation of a pulmonary to aortic shunt. They are not corrective and have a high mortality. In some cases, however, they prepare the patient for subsequent correction using a modification of the Fontan procedure.[75] As this carries an equally high, or higher, mortality, the success of operative intervention so far has not been great. A more promising alternative may be cardiac transplantation, either during the neonatal period or after initial palliation. However the condition is detectable in fetal life by echocardiography and thus termination of pregnancy is a realistic alternative.

'Mitral atresia' with patent aortic root

In contrast to the hypoplastic left heart syndrome, atresia of the left atrioventricular orifice can rarely occur with a patent aortic outflow. Atresia of the left atrioventricular valve results in all the pulmonary venous return having to exit from the left atrium across the atrial septum, against the direction of opening of the flap valve. As with aortic atresia, unless there is a large atrial septal defect, left atrial and pulmonary venous hypertension are the main pathophysiological effects and lead to pulmonary oedema. Additional anomalies such as aortic coarctation are common and further complicate the anatomy and physiology.

Infants usually present early, during the first week of life, with tachypnoea or dyspnoea. Congestive cardiac failure frequently occurs. Although prolonged survival is possible with medical treatment, death usually occurs within the first weeks or months of life.

The electrocardiogram is non-specific. Occasionally, when survival is prolonged, left atrial hypertrophy may be apparent. The ventricular electrical forces reflect the anatomy. The chest radiograph in general shows globular cardiac enlargement with plethoric lung fields or even obvious pulmonary oedema. The echocardiogram will de-monstrate the anatomy present which, if necessary, can be confirmed by cardiac catheterization and angiocardiography.

The treatment of left atrioventricular valve atresia with patent aortic root, like that of the hypoplastic left heart syndrome, is subject to debate. Atrial septostomy or septectomy is indicated in patients surviving the early days of life. Once free communication between the atria has been created, congestive cardiac failure due to high pulmonary blood flow may ensue. This usually requires medical treatment, but banding of the pulmonary trunk may be needed.[76] The options for 'corrective' treatment are as for the hypoplastic left heart syndrome.

TETRALOGY OF FALLOT

The tetralogy of Fallot is a combination of ventricular septal defect, infundibular pulmonary stenosis, overriding of the ventricular septum by the aorta and right ventricular hypertrophy. With respect to both symptomatology and pathophysiology, the ventricular septal defect and pulmonary stenosis are the essential defects. The degree of aortic override varies considerably but this is of less functional significance. Some patients have the aorta predominantly in connexion with the left ventricle; in other patients with similar basic morphology, the aorta arises in its greater part from the right ventricle. In other words, the anatomical complex which is the tetralogy of Fallot can exist with concordant or double-outlet ventriculo-arterial connexions. The right ventricular hypertrophy is a secondary development. Probably the greatest morphological variation of functional note is in the degree of right ventricular outflow tract obstruction. When minimal, the patient may be acyanotic, but complete obstruction may result in one of the varieties of pulmonary atresia with ventricular septal defect.

Tetralogy of Fallot is the commonest clinical form of cyanotic congenital heart disease permitting survival to adult life. It accounts for at least 15% of all children > 2 years of age who have congenital heart disease. If a person unversed in paediatric cardiology made a diagnosis of tetralogy in every cyanotic child seen who was more than 2 years old, the diagnosis would be right in about three-quarters of the patients.

The essential feature of morphology is the abnormal insertion of the septal extension of the outlet septum cephalad and anterior to the septomarginal trabeculation (Fig. 25.51). This abnormal position results in subpulmonary infundibular stenosis and

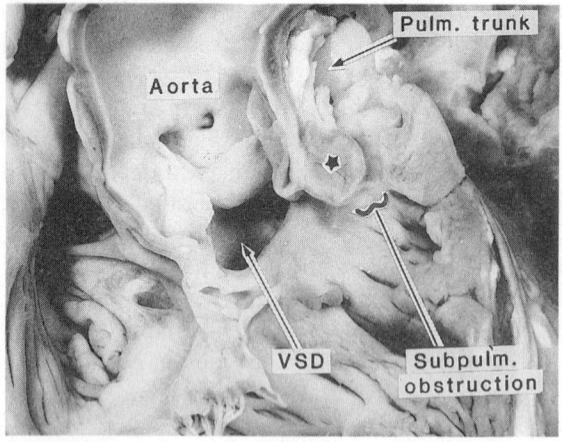

Fig. 25.51. This section, simulating the oblique subcostal paracoronal echocardiographic plane, illustrates the salient anatomical features of tetralogy of Fallot. The hallmark of the anomaly is malalignment of the outlet septum (starred) relative to the rest of the ventricular septum. VSD, ventricular septal defect; pulm, pulmonary.

ensures the presence of a large subaortic ventricular septal defect.[77] The degree of aortic override correlates with the position of the parietal insertion of the outlet septum. The malalignment ventricular septal defect thus formed is usually perimembranous but, in a proportion of cases, it has a muscular postero-inferior rim. In some hearts, the outlet septum is absent so that there is aortic–pulmonary valvar continuity. Such hearts are often considered as variants of tetralogy. As they lack muscular subpulmonary obstruction, they are better placed in a separate group. Valvar pulmonary stenosis, although in itself not part of the tetralogy, often co-exists with infundibular stenosis. The stenotic valve is almost always bicuspid. Absence of the leaflets of the pulmonary valve is also a significant association, being found with dilated pulmonary arteries. Stenosis in the pulmonary tree may be found at the level of the trunk, at the bifurcation, in the right or left pulmonary arteries or at the origin of more peripheral branches. One pulmonary artery may be absent or may arise directly from the aorta. Systemic–pulmonary collateral arteries are found in some cases but are more usual when there is associated congenital pulmonary atresia. Tetralogy of Fallot can co-exist with an atrial septal defect, an atrioventricular septal defect or with an additional ventricular septal defect, particularly in the muscular inlet septum. Coronary arterial anomalies may have considerable surgical significance, notably origin of the anterior descending artery from the right coronary artery. In about three-quarters of the

cases of tetralogy, the aortic arch is on the left; in one-quarter, it is on the right.

The age of onset of symptoms varies considerably and depends on the severity of the right ventricular outflow obstruction. In the severest cases, the parents or medical attendants may notice cyanosis in the first month of life. More usually, cyanosis occurs (and is noted) later during the first year. The first symptom may be severe spells occurring in a child thought to be acyanotic.[78] The initiating factor of these attacks is unknown. Whatever the trigger, hyperventilation, a decreasing arterial oxygen saturation and increasing metabolic acidosis are the result. These in turn perpetuate the attack. Usually, the attacks are terminated by loss of consciousness. Death may occur rarely during a spell. More importantly, cerebrovascular accidents sometimes result. Spells *may* be terminated by morphine or general anaesthesia. When they are severe or recurrent, surgery is indicated.

Growth is usually normal early in infancy but, in later childhood, growth retardation becomes evident. Intellectual development may appear normal in any individual case but severe cyanosis does appear to result in some intellectual retardation. Cyanosis and clubbing of the fingers and toes are usual after the first year of life. There may be large 'a' waves in the jugular venous pulse but this sign is difficult to elicit in small children. A right parasternal heave, sometimes visible, indicates the presence of right ventricular hypertrophy. The first heart sound is normal; the pulmonary component of the second sound is usually diminished or even inaudible. The aortic component may be loud as a consequence of the more anterior position of the aorta. An ejection systolic murmur is usually heard in the second and third intercostal spaces at the left sternal edge. The murmur may radiate into the lung fields and the neck vessels. Its intensity is not consistently related to the severity of the stenosis. With extreme stenosis, the murmur may be soft and short because less blood is flowing across the right ventricular outflow tract.

The chest X-ray typically shows a heart of normal size associated with diminished pulmonary vascularity. The pulmonary trunk is never prominent and the portion of the left heart border it usually occupies may be concave. With the exception of infants presenting with a high pulmonary flow, when the heart will be enlarged and the lung fields plethoric, these features are present at all ages. The classic configuration of the 'coeur en sabot' (like a wooden clog) is seen when right ventricular hypertrophy elevates the apex of the heart. This sign is generally seen in older patients. When a right-sided aortic arch is present, the aortic knob will not be in its usual left-sided position but may be recognized on the right cardiac border.

Electrocardiography usually reveals pronounced right-axis deviation. There may be ST-segment depression and an inverted T in leads II and III. Evidence of right ventricular hypertrophy is virtually always present except in patients with mild pulmonary stenosis and substantial left-to-right shunt. These may show an incomplete right bundle branch block pattern.

Cross-sectional echocardiography is diagnostic,[79] particularly using the sub-costal window to obtain oblique views of the right ventricular outflow tracts. This approach demonstrates the degree of subpulmonary obstruction and the precise nature of the ventricular septal defect (Fig. 25.52). Interrogation of the ventricular inlets will reveal an atrioventricular septal defect, a second muscular inlet ventricular septal defect or straddling of the tricuspid valve should any of these lesions co-exist. These features are all demonstrated by magnetic resonance imaging. When cyanosis is clinically difficult to detect, the effect of breathing 100% oxygen will reveal the presence of a right-to-left shunt. This can be confirmed by a first pass nuclear angiocardiogram.

Catheterization is still needed for full documentation of the pulmonary arterial pathways. The right

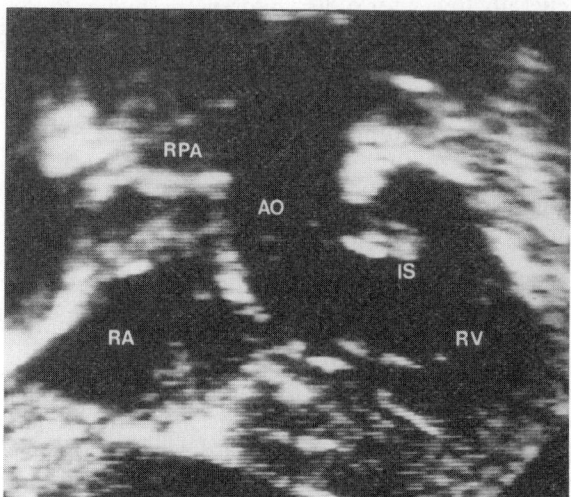

Fig. 25.52. Subcostal right oblique echocardiogram in a patient with tetralogy of Fallot. There is anterior and cephalad deviation of the infundibular (outlet) septum (IS) giving rise to muscular subpulmonary stenosis. (RA, right atrium; RV, right ventricle; AO, ascending aorta; RPA, right pulmonary artery). (Figure courtesy of Dr M. Rigby).

ventricle is usually entered from the right atrium. From the right ventricle, it is almost always possible to enter the aorta across the ventricular septal defect. Indeed, it is usually easier to enter the aorta than the pulmonary trunk. The left heart chambers are often entered via a patent oval hole or a septal defect. Such a patent atrial septum does not usually cause any haemodynamic disturbance but must be sought and commented upon because, if present, it must be closed at the time of corrective surgery. The right and left ventricular pressures are usually similar. Pulmonary arterial systolic pressure is low as a result of the right ventricular outflow tract obstruction. The site or sites of obstruction can usually be identified by recording pressures on withdrawal from the peripheral pulmonary arteries to the right ventricle. Classically, there is a right-to-left shunt with desaturation detectable in the aorta and frequently in the left ventricle. The extent of the right-to-left shunt depends on the severity of the pulmonary stenosis.

Angiocardiography demonstrates the characteristic anatomy of tetralogy of Fallot,[80] even in those young infants who have not yet developed cyanosis (Fig. 25.53). The right ventricular angiocardiogram shows the anterior and leftward deviation of the outlet septum narrowing the outflow tract of the right ventricle. The antero-posterior projection taken at 45° head-up visualizes the entire outflow tract, the pulmonary trunk and its branching pattern, facilitating the diagnosis of valvar and arterial stenoses. The overriding of the aorta is best demonstrated by a left ventricular angiogram profiled in long-axis projection. This latter view will also show any additional ventricular septal defects. When an atrioventricular septal defect is suspected, the four-chamber projection of the left ventricular angiogram should be recorded.

The course of patients presenting in infancy is variable.[81] Those with severe outflow tract obstruction and pulmonary arterial hypoplasia at birth present at this time with severe cyanosis and rarely survive the first 2 years without surgical treatment. Those with more favourable outflow tract anatomy gradually become cyanosed over the first year, but at any time may have 'spells' requiring urgent surgery. An unusual presentation is seen in infants with minimal pulmonary stenosis at birth. Initially, they have a left-to-right shunt through the ventricular septal defect in early infancy. By 2–4 months of age they may be in congestive cardiac failure only to become cyanosed with increasing subvalvar pulmonary stenosis.

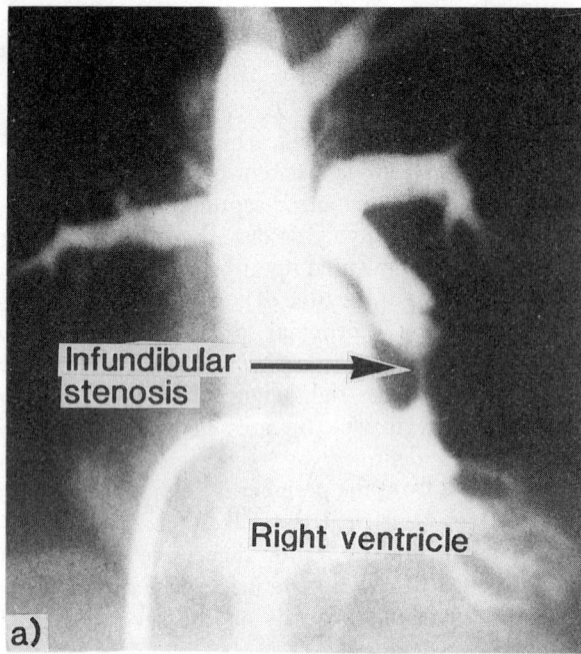
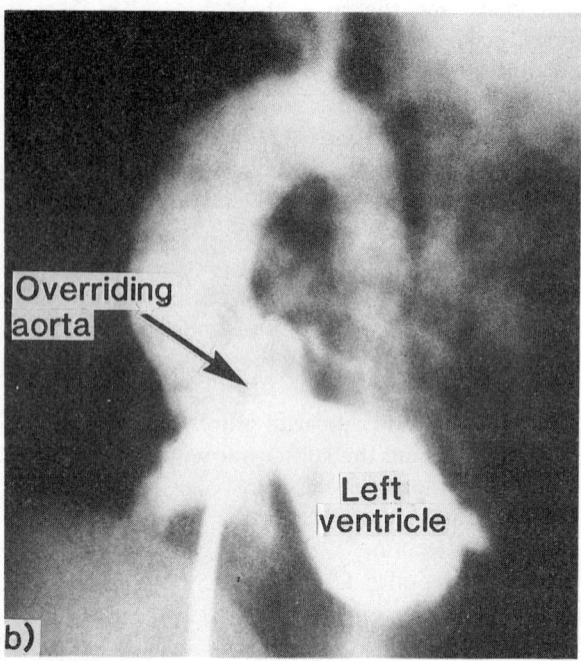

Fig. 25.53. Angiocardiograms in the tetralogy of Fallot. (a) Right ventricular injection in the frontal projection with 45° head-up tilt. The aorta, which is right sided, and the pulmonary artery fill. There is typical infundibular and valvar stenosis with moderate hypoplasia of the pulmonary arteries. (b) Left ventriculogram in the long-axis projection demonstrating overriding of the aorta.

All patients with the tetralogy should have a totally corrective operation. The timing of this operation is a matter of debate.[82] Prolonged cyanosis has a deleterious effect on both physical growth and intellectual development. The longer a patient awaits corrective surgery, the greater is the risk of cerebral complications. Palliative surgery in the form of a shunt operation will ameliorate the growth and intellectual retardation but it will not prevent strokes or brain abscess. The decision regarding the type of surgery to be performed must depend on the relative risks of primary correction. In most centres, results of palliative surgery are now so good that the best overall treatment is provided by palliating symptomatic infants and delaying the definitive operation. At some centres, excellent results are obtained when performing primary correction in all but those with the most severely hypoplastic pulmonary arteries. In any event, the corrective procedure should be performed prior to school age, as should primary correction in patients with less severe disease. Medical treatment of patients with spells includes sedation with morphine and the administration of oxygen. More prolonged treatment with beta-adrenergic blocking drugs has been suggested. In our experience, it rarely has a dramatic effect whereas successful

surgery is entirely reliable in preventing these episodes. The long-term surgical results for tetralogy of Fallot are excellent, and the operative mortality has continuously diminished, now ranging between 3 and 10%. The operative risk is generally lower for older children and higher in the infant group. In most patients, the clinical and physiological status is greatly improved and, in long-term evaluations, excellent results have been reported in up to nine-tenths.[83]

DOUBLE-OUTLET VENTRICLE

Double-outlet ventricle does not describe a heart, but only a small part of the heart, namely a ventriculo-arterial connexion. We define this connexion as the one in which more than half of both great arteries take origin from the same ventricle. That ventricle may be a right ventricle, a left ventricle or the solitary chamber of a univentricular heart. Double outlet must always be qualified by stating the nature of the ventricle supporting the arteries, and then the segmental arrangement of the heart itself.[84] By far the commonest variety is double outlet from a morphologically right ventricle. Much rarer is double outlet from the left ventricle, which will be considered briefly. Double outlet from a solitary and indeterminate ventricle is exceedingly rare and will not be considered.

Double-outlet right ventricle

There is still considerable scope for morphological variability when both great arteries arise for their greater parts from the right ventricle. The major subdivision of this anomaly is into hearts with concordant, discordant or ambiguous atrioventricular connections. Variability in presentation in all situations depends upon the position of the ventricular septal defect, which forms the only outlet from the left ventricle. Also significant are the presence or absence of arterial stenosis and the morphology of any other associated lesions. The ventricular septal defect is usually large and may be situated beneath the aorta (Fig. 25.54a), beneath the pulmonary trunk (Fig. 25.54b), beneath both great arteries or beneath neither. The position of the defect is itself related to the positions of the great arteries. Usually, the aorta is right sided and somewhat posterior. In these circumstances, the defect is usually subaortic. When the aorta is anterior and to the right of the pulmonary trunk, the defect tends to be subpulmonary, giving one variant of the so-called Taussig-Bing malformation. Rarely, the aorta is anterior and to the left and then the defect is usually subaortic. Considerable emphasis has been laid on the infundibular morphology of double-outlet right ventricle, some authorities demanding the presence of a bilateral infundibulum before making the diagnosis. This criterion ignores the fact that presence or absence of muscle between

the arterial and atrioventricular valves in no way affects the connexion between ventricles and arteries. Usually, hearts with double outlet from the right ventricle do exhibit a bilateral infundibulum, but this is not a prerequisite for the ventriculo-arterial connexion. The remainder of the discussion in this section will be devoted to double-outlet right ventricle in the setting of usual atrial arrangement with a concordant atrioventricular connexion.

When the defect is subaortic, pulmonary infundibular stenosis is a frequent finding, and the hearts resemble tetralogy of Fallot. When the defect is subpulmonary, it is more usual to find aortic infundibular stenosis, frequently associated with coarctation and tubular hypoplasia of the aortic arch. When the defect is beneath both great arteries, both tend to override the septum and it is often difficult to determine if the connexion is double inlet from the right or left ventricle. Of the important associated anomalies, mitral atresia occurs with some frequency, while juxtaposition of the atrial appendages is frequently found with a left-sided and anterior aorta.[85]

When both great arteries arise from the right ventricle, there will be mixing of the systemic and pulmonary venous returns. Some degree of systemic arterial desaturation is therefore to be expected. The presence of detectable cyanosis and its severity depend on the site of the ventricular septal defect and the presence or absence of restriction of pulmonary blood flow. When the defect is subaortic, pulmonary venous blood will be preferentially directed into the aorta. If pulmonary blood flow is not restricted, systemic arterial desaturation may be

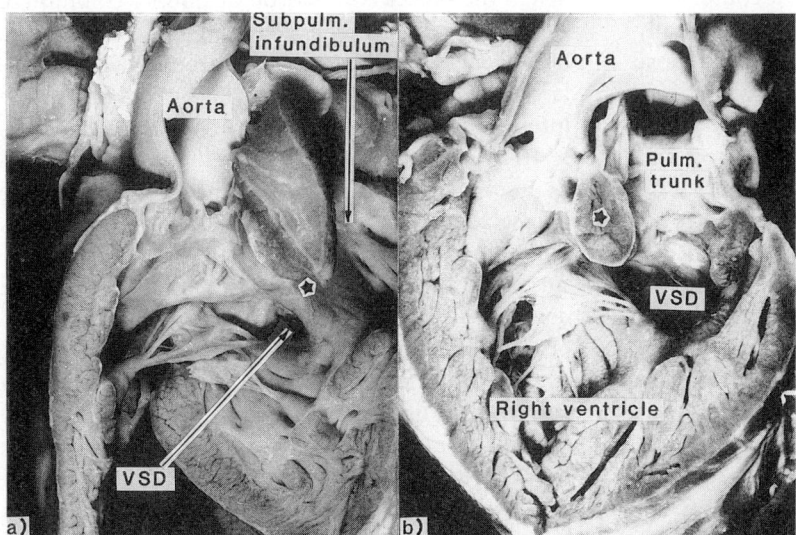

Fig. 25.54. Photographs of the right ventricle showing the features of double-outlet right ventricle with (a) a subaortic and (b) a subpulmonary (pulm.) ventricular septal defect (VSD). The outlet septum is starred.

clinically undetectable. Conversely, when the defect is subpulmonary, the pulmonary venous return will be preferentially directed to the pulmonary trunk resulting in less oxygenated blood being ejected into the aorta. When the pulmonary blood flow is restricted by pulmonary stenosis or pulmonary vascular disease, cyanosis will be more obvious whatever the site of the ventricular septal defect. The degree of cyanosis will depend entirely on the magnitude of the pulmonary blood flow.[86]

When pulmonary blood flow is unrestricted, the clinical presentation is similar to that seen in patients with isolated ventricular septal defect and a high pulmonary blood flow. Such patients usually present in infancy with heart failure, with a pan-systolic murmur at the left sternal edge, an apical mid-diastolic murmur and a loud pulmonary component of the second heart sound. Suspicion that this is not a simple ventricular septal defect is aroused by a poor response to breathing 100% oxygen (the nitrogen wash-out test). Patients with a subpulmonary ventricular defect and unrestricted pulmonary blood flow present in a similar fashion. In the presence of subaortic stenosis and coarctation of the aorta, however, the key feature will be absence of the femoral pulses, or the fact that they are felt only intermittently. With a non-committed or doubly committed ventricular septal defect, the degree of arterial desaturation depends upon the magnitude of the pulmonary blood flow. In all cases with double-outlet right ventricle, cyanosis will become more obvious and severe with the development of pulmonary vascular disease.

The clinical course is as variable as are the anatomical features. The combination with subaortic outflow obstruction with or without coarctation of the aorta, unless treated surgically, is usually fatal in early infancy. Survival is more likely in those with a subaortic defect than in those in whom it is below the pulmonary trunk. The most favourable prognosis is in patients with a subaortic defect and pulmonary stenosis. There are no specific radiographic features, the chest film reflecting the haemodyamic state. The heart is usually of normal size in the presence of pulmonary stenosis while the lung fields are oligaemic. When pulmonary blood flow is unrestricted, the heart is usually enlarged and the lung fields are plethoric. Similarly, there are no diagnostic electrocardiographic features, but right-axis deviation and right ventricular hypertrophy are typical findings as is right atrial enlargement. When pulmonary blood flow is high (or when there is aortic outflow obstruction), left ventricular forces will be prominent and there will be evidence of biventricular hypertrophy.

Cross-sectional echocardiography is diagnostic in 'classic' cases showing the precise ventriculo-arterial connexion and the site and morphology of the ventricular septal defect (Fig. 25.55). Assessment of the degree of overriding of arterial valves in equivocal cases may be difficult. The technique also demonstrates the nature of the associated lesions.

Catheterization is usually needed to confirm the diagnosis. The aorta and pulmonary trunk are both entered from the right ventricle. There is usually some degree of desaturation of the aortic blood, this being marked when streaming is disadvantageous. Desaturation is most evident when pulmonary blood flow is limited by pulmonary stenosis or pulmonary vascular disease. Pressures recorded on withdrawal from the aorta and the pulmonary trunk to the right ventricle will demonstrate aortic or pulmonary outflow obstruction if present. A pressure in the left ventricle higher than that in the right ventricle will be found when the ventricular septal defect is small and restrictive. Angiocardiography with injections into both ventricles is the ideal technique. Angled views should be taken in order to profile the ventricular septum and the origins of the great arteries. Good details can then be obtained of the outflow tract morphology and of the relationship of the ventricular septal defect to the great arteries.

The indications for surgical treatment and operative technique depend upon the location and size of the ventricular septal defect, the relationship of the atrioventricular conduction axis and the presence or absence of subpulmonary or subaortic stenosis.[88] When the defect is subaortic or doubly committed, surgical repair can be achieved by directing the blood leaving the left ventricle through the ventricular septal defect to the aorta by means of an interventricular patch. If the septal defect is restrictive, it may need to be enlarged. If subpulmonary obstruction is present, the obstructive tissue is resected or bypassed. When the septal defect is non-committed, there are usually two options for surgical 'correction'. The aortic valve and septal defect may both be closed and a conduit placed between the left ventricular apex and the aorta. Alternatively, the pulmonary trunk may be closed, a valved conduit be placed between the left ventricle and the pulmonary arteries and an atrial redirection procedure performed. In exceptional circumstances, the anatomy may permit construction of a patch between the non-committed defect and the aorta.

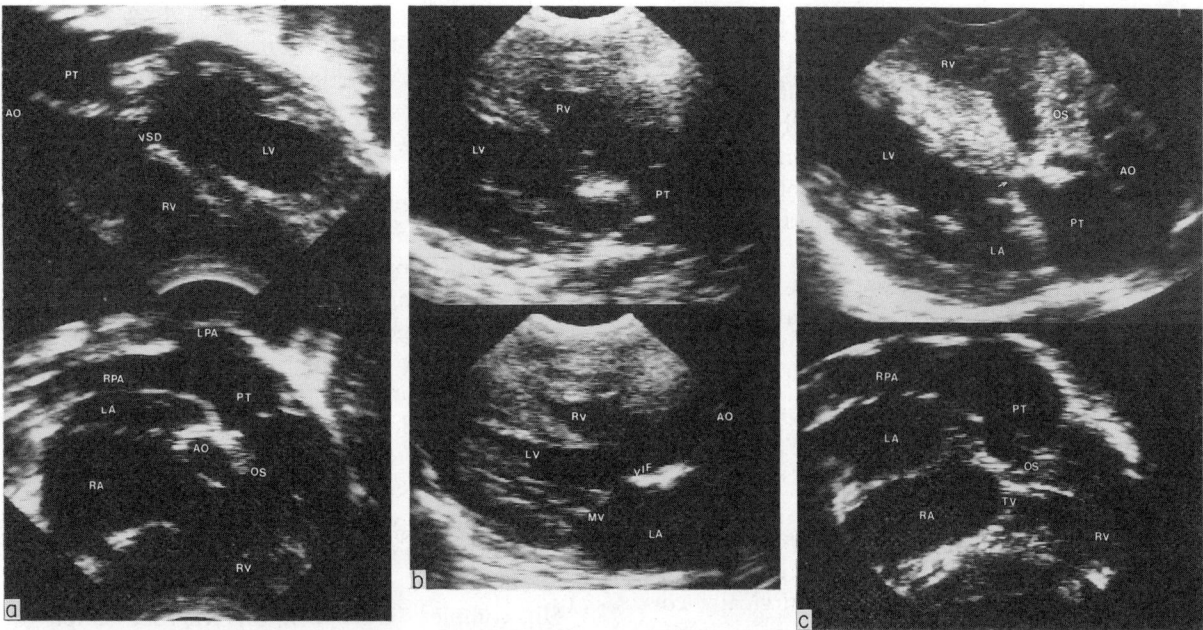

Fig. 25.55. (a) Subcostal echocardiographic sections illustrating double-outlet right ventricle with a subaortic ventricular septal defect. The upper illustration demonstrates the ascending aorta (AO) arising from the morphologically right ventricle and shows the ventricular septal defect (VSD). LV, left ventricle. The lower illustration is a subcostal right oblique projection showing the outlet septum (OS) within the right ventricle (RV). LA, left atrium; RA, right ventricle; AO, ascending aorta; RPA, right pulmonary artery; LPA, left pulmonary artery. (b) Parasternal long-axis echocardiographic sections from the same patient illustrated in (a) with double-outlet right ventricle and a subaortic ventricular septal defect. The upper illustration demonstrates the pulmonary trunk (PT) arising from the morphologically right ventricle (RV). The lower illustration shows the aorta (AO) overriding the ventricular septum and arising predominantly from the right ventricle. The left ventriculo-infundibular fold (VIF) interposes between the posterior wall of the aorta and the anterior leaflet of the mitral valve (MV). LA, left atrium; LV, left ventricle. (c) Echocardiographic sections from a patient with double-outlet right ventricle and a small restrictive subpulmonary ventricular septal defect. Bilateral infundibula are present and there is both subaortic and subpulmonary stenosis. The upper illustration demonstrates an anterior aorta (AO) and posterior pulmonary trunk (PT) arising from the right ventricle (RV). There is gross hypertrophy of the outlet septum (OS) giving rise to subaortic and subpulmonary stenosis. The left ventricle (LV) communicates with the pulmonary trunk through a small and restrictive ventricular septal defect (arrow). The lower illustration is a subcostal right oblique projection from the same patient which shows the extreme hypertrophy of the outlet septum and the muscular subpulmonary obstruction. The right pulmonary artery (RPA) is well visualized and the tricuspid valve (TV) is seen between the right atrium and right ventricle. (Figure courtesy of Dr M.L. Rigby).

When the ventricular septal defect is subpulmonary, it is usually necessary to place a patch in order to connect the ventricular septal defect and the subpulmonary outflow tract. This then necessitates correction of the circulation, at either the atrial or the arterial level. Increasingly, the trend is to resort to correction at arterial level (the arterial switch procedure—see below). The results of corrective surgery depend largely upon the complexity of the intracardiac anatomy. When the ventricular septal defect is subaortic, success is now achieved in most cases (up to 90% or more). The late results depend upon the status of the pulmonary vascular bed. Similar success can now be obtained in specialized centres for correction of patients with a subpulmon-

ary ventricular septal defect (the Taussig–Bing malformation[89]) using the arterial switch procedure. In the less common and more complex types of double-outlet right ventricle, the risks of corrective surgery are considerably higher. Despite this high operative risk, however, corrective operation offers the only prospect for a near-normal life. When obstructive pulmonary vascular disease is not present, most survivors of corrective surgery lead essentially normal lives. In some patients, however, the anatomy is such that definitive palliation offers the best chance of success. This can be achieved with shunt procedures or with modification of the Fontan approach.

Double-outlet left ventricle

As with double-outlet right ventricle, this diagnosis implies only that more than half of both great arteries arise from the morphologically left ventricle. Although rare, it has already been reported as existing with various segmental combinations. Exactly the same variability in arterial interrelationship, septal defect position and infundibular morphology must be anticipated as is found in double-outlet right ventricle. Similar associated anomalies may be found.

The pathophysiological and clinical features are extremely variable. All patients demonstrate some degree, from mild to profound, of cyanosis, or at least a failure to manifest a normal response to the nitrogen wash-out test. The diagnosis must always be considered when investigating patients known to have complex defects. Although some patients with double-outlet left ventricle can be surgically corrected, many cannot. The frequent association of a hypoplastic right ventricle is of particular importance.[90] Surgical treatment must never be attempted unless every aspect of the anatomy has been fully demonstrated.

COMPLETE TRANSPOSITION

Complete transposition is the combination of concordant atrioventricular and discordant ventriculo-arterial connexions (Fig. 25.56). The aorta arises from the morphologically right ventricle which is connected to the right atrium while the pulmonary trunk takes origin from the morphologically left ventricle which is connected to the left atrium. The use of the term 'complete' does not imply that there are 'partial' forms of transposition. It is merely used to differentiate this variety of discordant ventriculo-arterial connexion from the congenitally corrected and other forms. Complete transposition is the commonest life-threatening form of cyanotic congenital heart disease in the first year of life. It occurs once in every 2000–4000 livebirths and is twice as common in boys as in girls.[91]

The chamber combinations defined as complete transposition can exist with either usually arranged or mirror-image atrial arrangement but not with atrial isomerism. Complete transposition, signifying the presence of a discordant ventriculo-arterial connexion, cannot co-exist with a double-outlet connexion. It is usually the presence of an atrial septal defect or persistent patency of the oval hole that permits survival through the early days or weeks of life. In absence of other anomalies, this combination is frequently termed simple complete transposition. Complex complete transposition is the term used when other anomalies, typically a ventricular septal defect or pulmonary stenosis, are present.

In complete transposition, whether simple or complex, the aortic valve is most frequently to the right of the pulmonary valve in individuals with usual atrial arrangement (or to the left in those with mirror-image arrangement); however, in approximately one-third of cases with usual atrial arrangement, the aorta is not to the right,[92] being either directly anterior, to the left or even posterior. Similarly, although usually the aorta has a muscular infundibulum and the pulmonary valve lacks a complete infundibulum, this is not always the case. There may be a bilateral infundibulum or a sub-pulmonary infundibulum with aortic–atrioventricular valvar continuity. The morphology of a ventricular septal defect, if present, can be analysed in similar fashion for the 'isolated' lesion. Most frequently, it is a malalignment defect between the outlet component and the rest of the muscular septum. It may extend to become perimembranous but more usually it has a completely muscular postero-inferior rim. The defect is frequently crossed by tension apparatus of the tricuspid valve arising from the outlet septum. Defects in other parts of the septum may occur alone or in combination with the malalignment defect. Malalignment of the septal structures is also of importance in the setting of pulmonary stenosis. Usually the septum is to the right of the rest of the muscular septum. If the outlet septum inserts into the left ventricle, it narrows the sub-pulmonary outflow tract. Pure valvar pulmonary stenosis is rare, but stenosis may be produced by aneurysm of the membranous septum or anomalous attachment of the tension apparatus of the atrioven-

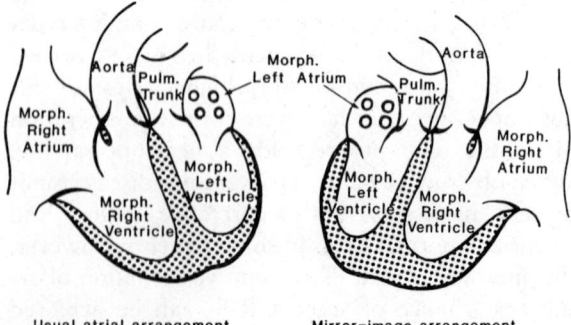

Usual atrial arrangement   Mirror-image arrangement

Fig. 25.56. Diagram showing the segmental combinations underscoring the lesion best termed complete transposition.

tricular valves within the left ventricular outflow tract. These lesions produce obstruction most frequently in association with ventricular septal defect. When the septum is intact, a fibromuscular tunnel or shelf is the most usual cause of discrete pulmonary stenosis.

Other anomalies frequently co-exist with complete transposition, persistent patency of the arterial duct and aortic coarctation being of greatest importance and frequency. Complete transposition can rarely exist with a common atrioventricular valve or, more frequently, with straddling and overriding of either the tricuspid or mitral valve. These, as with the combination of coarctation and arterial duct, are lethal malformations, particularly if unrecognized prior to surgical intervention. Abnormalities in the epicardial course of the coronary arteries are frequent and have been well documented. Their major significance is their potential effect on any proposed arterial 'switch' operation. In this context, the important point is that almost always the coronary arteries arise from the aortic sinuses which 'face' the pulmonary trunk, so that relocation of the arteries is unlikely to pose problems.[93]

The basic abnormal pathophysiological mechanism is that systemic venous blood is re-circulated to the aorta whereas the pulmonary venous return is re-circulated to the pulmonary trunk. The pulmonary and systemic circulations are separate and not arranged in series as is the case in hearts with concordant chamber connections. This circulatory separation is exemplified in the simplest anatomical variant, complete transposition with no other abnormalities other than an interatrial communication. The re-circulation of systemic venous blood to the aorta results in profound systemic arterial hypoxaemia which in turn leads to a high cardiac output (high systemic blood flow). The re-circulation of pulmonary venous blood to the left atrium via the low-resistance pulmonary circuit results in a high left atrial pressure and a high left ventricular preload. This combination predisposes to a high pulmonary blood flow. Separation of the two circulations can never be absolutely complete and still allow even limited survival. Some cross-flows between the circuits must occur. In the simplest variant (complete transposition with a patent oval hole), these cross-flows are minimal. It is the objective of palliative treatment to improve them. The classic physiological situation (of extreme systemic arterial hypoxaemia, high cardiac output and high pulmonary blood flow all leading

to congestive cardiac failure) is seen only when the pulmonary vascular resistance has fallen significantly from the high fetal levels towards the levels of normal extra-uterine life.[94] Pulmonary blood flow does not exceed systemic in the first few days of life. Although profound cyanosis is present, cardiac enlargement and congestive cardiac failure are not usually evident. Life therefore, is maintained by the amount of cross-flows that occur between the two circulations (Fig.25.57). Some systemic venous blood must cross to the left atrium and ventricle to take up oxygen in the lungs—the 'effective pulmonary flow'. Similarly, some pulmonary venous blood must cross to the right atrium and ventricle to supply oxygenated blood to the body—the 'effective systemic flow'. Although beat-to-beat variations occur in these cross-flows, they must equalize over time. The higher these 'effective flows' are, the higher the systemic arterial oxygen saturation will tend to be. The prime requirement for adequate effective flows is a communication or communications of unrestrictive size between the two circuits. In general, this is provided by palliative treatment, but, even with unrestrictive intercirculatory communications, cross-flows vary in magnitude. A high systemic flow with the resultant large volume of desaturated blood entering the aorta predisposes to a low arterial oxygen saturation for any given level of effective flow. A high pulmonary flow in itself appears to predispose to a high effective flow and, therefore, to a higher arterial oxygen saturation for any given level of systemic flow. The most beneficial state is that of a pulmonary blood flow in excess of the systemic flow. Although oxygen delivery to the tissues is a grave problem, carbon dioxide elimination appears to be adequately dealt with even when effective flows are small.

Associated malformations are, initially, beneficial in the setting of complete transposition. Persistence of the arterial duct or a ventricular septal defect, by providing an additional intercirculatory communication and by their tendency to increase the pulmonary blood flow, will predispose to a higher systemic arterial oxygen saturation. When they are large enough to cause pulmonary hypertension, however, they impart a high risk of developing pulmonary vascular disease. This is usually established by the age of 1 year.[95] When the pulmonary resistance has reached sufficiently high levels to reduce pulmonary blood flow, the effect of such a communication is to decrease systemic arterial oxygen saturation. Pulmonary vascular disease occurs less frequently when there is no high-

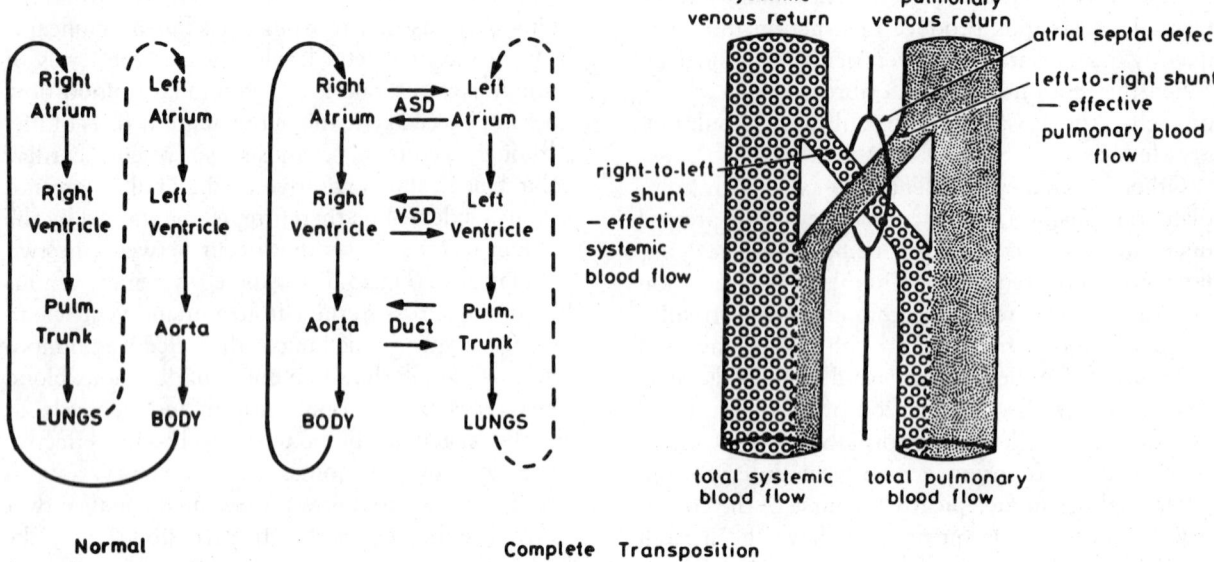

Fig. 25.57. Diagram showing the pattern of circulation in complete transposition as compared with the normal heart. Shunts are necessary at either atrial (ASD), ventricular (VSD) or ductal level to permit mixing between the parallel systemic and pulmonary circuits.

pressure communication between the two circuits. When it does occur, as with an atrial defect, for example, the time-course is similar to that seen with a ventricular septal defect or a patent duct. Obstruction of the left ventricular outflow can occur with or without a ventricular septal defect. It is often a progressive lesion when it occurs with an intact ventricular septum. In either case, it decreases pulmonary blood flow and leads to increasing cyanosis.

Cyanosis, usually noted at or shortly after birth, is the most obvious clinical feature of complete transposition. The infant is not usually distressed. Dyspnoea, fluid retention and the full picture of congestive cardiac failure develop only if treatment is delayed. Cyanosis may be difficult to detect in presence of a large duct or ventricular septal defect. The effect of breathing 100% oxygen is then helpful in differentiating between cyanosis of cardiac and cyanosis of respiratory origin.

The pulses are usually normal, although, as expected, the femoral pulses are diminished or absent when aortic coarctation co-exists. The first and second heart sounds are loud and often palpable. Cardiac murmurs, when present, usually indicate an associated malformation such as a ventricular septal defect, persistent arterial duct or pulmonary stenosis. The infants are of normal size at birth, but growth retardation becomes evident by the age of 1 year unless corrective surgery is

performed. Severe cyanosis over this period will be associated with polycythaemia, clubbing and the development of varices on the fingers and toes.

The supposedly classic radiographic appearance of an enlarged heart with a narrow upper mediastinum (egg on its side) and pulmonary plethora is rarely seen in the first weeks of life. Instead, the heart is of normal size or only slightly enlarged and the lung fields are normal or mildly plethoric. The right lung tends to be more plethoric; plethora is more obvious in association with a ventricular septal defect or an arterial duct. The lung fields may be oligaemic with left ventricular outflow obstruction. In this setting, the radiographic appearance may be indistinguishable from that seen in the tetralogy of Fallot.

The electrocardiogram may also be normal in the first days of life. Evidence of right ventricular hypertrophy is usually seen by 1 week and right-axis deviation is then usually persistent. The presence of a superiorly orientated mean frontal QRS axis suggests the presence of an atrioventricular septal defect or an inlet ventricular septal defect with or without a straddling atrioventricular valve. Isolated left ventricular hypertrophy is rarely seen even in the presence of pulmonary stenosis. Biventricular hypertrophy suggests the presence of a ventricular septal defect with or without pulmonary stenosis.

Cross-sectional echocardiography is diagnostic,[96]

demonstrating the combination of concordant atrioventricular and discordant ventricular arterial connexions (Fig. 25.58). Associated malformations should all be demonstrated and distinguished.

Nuclear angiography is also diagnostic. The first pass study demonstrates early filling of the aorta; the multiple acquisition blood pool study shows the discordant ventriculo-arterial connexion. This anatomy is seen with greater facility using magnetic resonance imaging (Fig. 25.59).

Despite advances in non-invasive diagnosis, catheterization is still indicated in many cases. The classic findings are seen in patients whose only intercirculatory communication is at atrial level. The catheter is advanced from the right atrium to the right ventricle, where the pressure is at the systemic level, and thence to the aorta. Right atrial pressure is usually within the normal range. The atrial septum is usually crossed, and pressures in the left atrium are found to be similar or in excess of

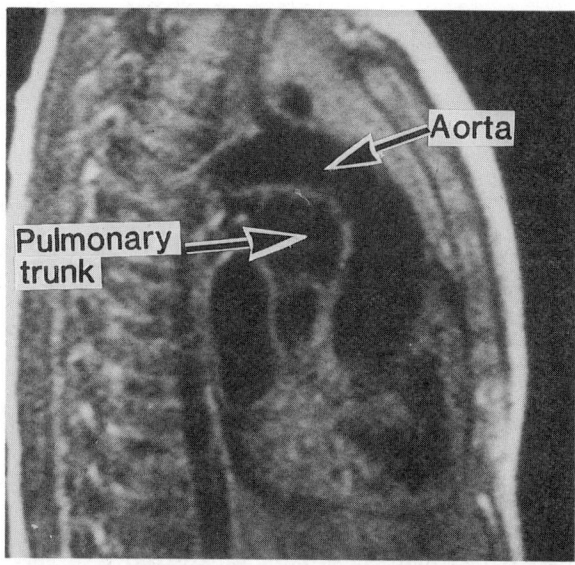

Fig. 25.59. In this magnetic resonance image in a sagittal section, the relationships of the great arteries typical of transposition is seen. The aorta is anterior to the pulmonary artery. (Figure courtesy of Dr E.J. Baker).

those in the right atrium. From the left atrium, the catheter can usually be manoeuvred from the left ventricle to the pulmonary trunk. Pulmonary arterial pressure is usually normal and a small pressure gradient (10–20 mmHg) across the pulmonary valve is the rule. Oximetry reveals severe desaturation in the aorta and right ventricle with high saturations in the pulmonary trunk, left atrium and left ventricle. A bidirectional shunt is usually detected at atrial level. The findings are modified early in the first month of life by persistence of the high fetal pulmonary vascular resistance. When seen on the first day of life, therefore, the pulmonary arterial and left ventricular pressures are usually elevated. With time, the left-sided pressures fall and are usually low by the age of 1–6 weeks.

When present, a large duct or ventricular septal defect will cause pulmonary hypertension, usually with a high pulmonary flow. Such pulmonary hypertension, if it persists after the first 6–8 weeks of life, predisposes to the development of pulmonary vascular disease. These associated lesions, therefore, are an indication for early surgical treatment. Pulmonary stenosis produces a high pressure gradient between the left ventricle and the pulmonary trunk. When found in the setting of an intact ventricular septum, pressure in the left ventricle may exceed that in the right ventricle. Pulmonary stenosis in the presence of a ventricular septal defect will manifest similar pressures in right and left

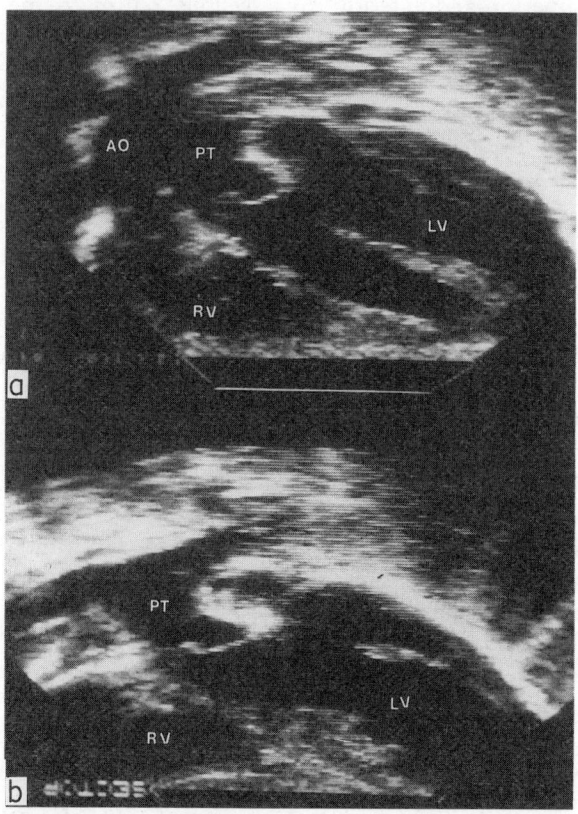

Fig. 25.58. (a) Subcostal echocardiographic section illustrating complete transposition of the great arteries with the right ventricle (RV) giving rise to the aorta (AO). (b) Subcostal long-axis section from the same patient showing the pulmonary trunk (PT) bifurcating into right and left pulmonary arteries and arising from the morphologically left ventricle (LV). (Figure courtesy of Dr M.L. Rigby).

ventricles with normal or low pulmonary arterial pressures.

Angiography confirms the existence of concordant atrioventricular and discordant ventriculo-arterial connexions. Injections should be made in both ventricles, particularly when associated defects are suspected.

If untreated, 90% of infants with complete transposition will die during their first year of life. Prior to the advent of balloon atrial septostomy,[97] the best prognosis was provided by association with ventricular septal defect and pulmonary stenosis. The worst prognosis was in those infants with no additional defects apart from an interatrial communication. Nowadays, the presence of a ventricular septal defect is associated with the more rapid development of pulmonary vascular disease which may render many unsuitable for corrective surgery. It is the advent of medical palliation that has revolutionized prognosis. This is achieved by balloon atrial septostomy performed at the diagnostic study. All patients should have this procedure irrespective of associated abnormalities unless they are to undergo immediate surgical correction. Balloon septostomy is achieved via the long saphenous or femoral vein, the catheter being passed across the oval hole into the left atrium. The catheter position within the left atrium is now best confirmed using cross-sectional echocardiography. The entire procedure can be performed in the neonatal nursery using echocardiographic control.[98] When it is confirmed that the catheter is in the left atrium, the balloon is inflated. With a quick jerk, it is then pulled through the oval pit, taking care to prevent impaction in the inferior caval vein. The procedure is repeated until no resistance is felt to withdrawal across the atrial septum. There should be some rise in arterial saturation after the procedure, ideally to 50–60%, and only a minimal residual interatrial pressure gradient should be found.

Sometimes balloon septostomy is not successful. The patient may be too old, in which case the atrial septum is too tough for it to be ruptured by the balloon. Balloon septostomy rarely works in infants older than 3 months. More frequently, oxygen saturation falls after the procedure because of adverse haemodynamics despite the production of a defect of adequate size. Two courses of action are possible after failed septostomy. The septum may be removed at surgery or, better, the patient may be sent immediately for surgical correction. Nowadays, surgical septectomy is rarely indicated. Surgical palliation is usually limited to those patients in whom correction cannot be achieved because of irreversible pulmonary vascular disease or those in whom 'preparation' of the left ventricle is needed prior to an arterial switch procedure.[99]

In most centres, corrective surgery is now performed within the first year of life, although patients with the combination of a ventricular septal defect and left ventricular outflow tract obstruction are best deferred to the age of 5 years. Correction is most frequently achieved at atrial level although there is a worldwide trend towards the arterial switch procedure. Those patients with the combination of a ventricular septal defect and pulmonary stenosis are usually treated with the Rastelli procedure.

For the past 20 years, the mainstay of surgery has been atrial redirection, initially with the Mustard procedure,[100] but lately with the Senning operation.[101] The essence of the Mustard operation is removal of the major portion of the atrial septum and insertion of an interatrial patch which directs superior and inferior caval venous return to the mitral valve and the pulmonary venous return to the tricuspid valve. The procedure was initially plagued with post-operative complications such as pulmonary and systemic venous obstructions and arrhythmias. Modifications in the operative procedure have largely succeeded in eradicating these problems. Mustard's operation performed in the best centres now carries an operative mortality of < 5%. Follow-up extends to over 20 years, the majority of patients living normal lives but with abnormal haemodynamics revealed by careful testing. The question remains whether the Mustard operation will allow a normal life-span.

The Senning procedure redirects venous return in a similar way to the Mustard operation, the major difference being that no atrial tissue is excised. Instead, the atrial septum is re-positioned to form a major part of the interatrial baffle, thus permitting more normal atrial growth and function. Like the Mustard procedure, it can be performed with excellent short-term results. Whether it has any long-term advantages has yet to be proven.

The more obvious approach to 'correction' of complete transposition is transection of both arterial trunks, re-suturing each to its appropriate ventricle with transplantation of the coronary arteries to the 'new' aorta. The major problem with the arterial 'switch' procedure is that the left ventricle of complete transposition, functioning at low pressure, has suddenly to subserve a systemic function. The procedure is most suitable, therefore, in cases where the left ventricle is already at systemic or near systemic levels. This is usually because of associated defects. In such cases, particularly those with ventricular septal defects, the arterial switch is now the operation of choice and can be performed with a mortality of < 10%.[102] The problem remains of how best to utilize the approach in the more common situation of an intact ventricular septum. Some surgeons have chosen to 'prepare' the left ventricle in the neonatal period by banding the pulmonary trunk and creating an aortopulmonary shunt.[99] Although good results have been achieved, a better alternative is to perform the arterial switch itself in the neonatal period. If the operation is performed prior to the fall in pulmonary vascular resistance, experience has shown that the left ventricle is able to assume a systemic role. Surgeons in selected centres using this approach have achieved successes comparable to those obtained with atrial redirection procedures. There is, however, a well-recognized learning curve for the arterial option. It remains to be seen if surgeons throughout the world can adapt to the technique.[103]

Those patients with the combination of a large ventricular septal defect and pulmonary stenosis can be corrected by connecting the aorta to the left ventricle via the septal defect, closing the pulmonary trunk and placing a valved conduit between the right ventricle and the pulmonary arteries (the Rastelli procedure). Success demands a ventricular septal defect of sufficient size and in the appropriate position to allow the connection to be made between the left ventricle and the aorta. Like the arterial switch procedure, it has the advantage of using the left ventricle in its 'correct' systemic role. It has yet to be employed with acceptably low

mortality until the patient has reached the age of 4–5 years.

CONGENITALLY CORRECTED TRANSPOSITION

Congenitally corrected transposition is the commonest condition characterized by a discordant atrioventricular connexion, the additional feature being a discordant connexion also at ventriculo-arterial level (Fig. 25.60). The particular combination of connexions is usually associated with abnormalities of the spatial arrangement of both the ventricles and the great arteries. Thus, in the individual with usual atrial arrangement, the morphologically right ventricle is usually to the left of the morphologically left ventricle ('ventricular inversion') and the aorta is usually to the left of the pulmonary trunk. This abnormal relationship of the great arteries has lead to the introduction of the term 'l-transposition' as a synonym. This is inadvisable, because not all hearts with corrected transposition have a left-sided aorta whereas many patients without corrected transposition do. Congenitally corrected transposition is the best brief term for the combination of discordant atrioventricular and ventriculo-arterial connexions, but the term defines only one particular ventriculo-arterial connexion in the setting of hearts with a discordant atrioventricular connexion. Other ventriculo-arterial connexions are possible and have been described. The commonest of these is double-outlet right ventricle. As all hearts with a discordant atrioventricular connexion have anatomical similarities despite differences of ventriculo-arterial connexion, they will be described here as related conditions.

Taken together, congenitally corrected transposi-

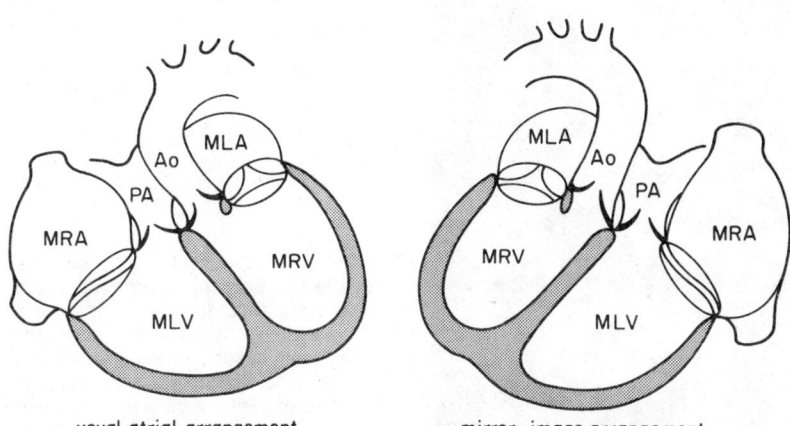

usual atrial arrangement   mirror-image arrangement

Discordant atrioventricular connection and discordant ventriculo-arterial connection

Fig. 25.60. The segmental combinations underscoring the existence of the lesion best termed congenitally corrected transposition.

tion and its related anomalies are extremely rare, accounting for only about 1% of congenital heart defects.

The anatomical hallmark of congenitally corrected transposition is that the right atrium connects to the morphologically left ventricle via a mitral valve whereas the left atrium connects to the morphologically right ventricle via a tricuspid valve. The morphologically left ventricle gives rise to the pulmonary trunk and the morphologically right ventricle to the aorta (Fig. 25.61).[104] This chamber arrangement is found in patients with usual and patients with mirror-image atrial arrangement. Although abnormal connexions can occur without additional abnormalities, it is rare. The most frequent associated abnormality is a perimembranous ventricular septal defect. Pulmonary stenosis is common as are abnormalities of the morphologically tricuspid valve. A consequence of the discordant atrioventricular connexion is malalignment of the atrial and ventricular septal structures. This malalignment prevents the regular atrioventricular node from making contact with the ventricular conduction tissues. Instead, an anomalous anterior atrioventricular node effects connexion with the atrioventricular bundle which then encircles the pulmonary outflow tract on its anterior and lateral quadrants.[105] There tends to be better alignment of the septal structures when corrected transposition occurs in the mirror-image arrangement. Normal conduction systems have been described in such hearts.

Clinical presentation with a discordant atrioventricular connexion is governed by the associated lesions. Patients without associated abnormalities can and do lead normal lives. When a ventricular septal defect is present without restriction of pulmonary flow, the presentation will be with dyspnoea and subsequent congestive cardiac failure as in 'isolated' ventricular septal defect. Similarly, a ventricular septal defect associated with pulmonary stenosis will present similar clinical features to those encountered in patients with tetralogy of Fallot. Severe regurgitation through the morphologically tricuspid valve will lead to pulmonary venous congestion and pulmonary venous hypertension. Unless the discordant connexion is recognized, the combination will seem to be typical of mitral regurgitation.

Children with congenitally corrected transposition frequently present with an asymptomatic heart murmur, such murmurs being due to small and restrictive ventricular septal defects or to mild tricuspid regurgitation. The symptoms and clinical signs give no indication of the abnormal chamber connexions. These clues must be found in the special investigations.

The prognosis is extremely varied, depending to a great extent on the associated malformations. Approximately three-quarters of patients present during the first year of life due to the effects of an unrestrictive ventricular septal defect or to cyanosis when pulmonary stenosis accompanies such a defect. Approximately one-third of deaths without treatment occur during the first year of life. Those with a large ventricular septal defect and pulmonary hypertension who survive the first year have a high risk of developing pulmonary vascular disease. A

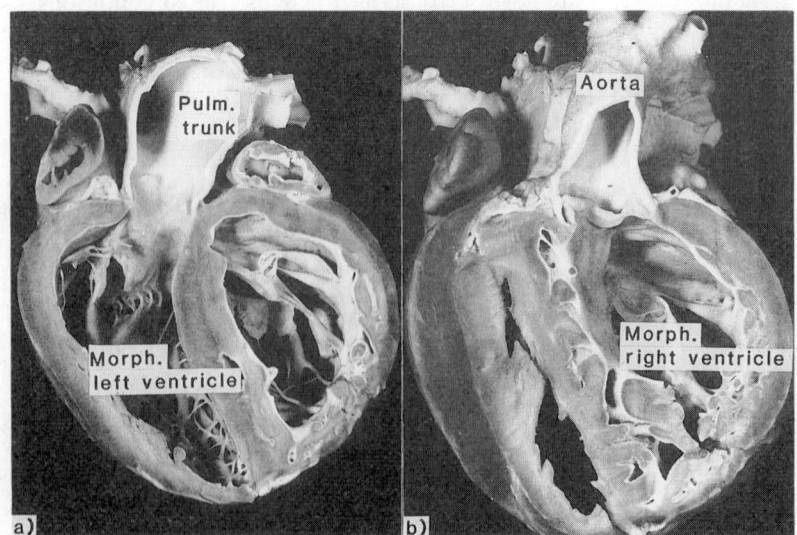

Fig. 25.61. Sections in coronal plane showing the discordant ventriculo-arterial connexions in a heart with congenitally corrected transposition and usual atrial arrangement. Note that the morphologically (morph) left ventricle is right sided (a) in comparison to the right ventricle (b). The aorta is to the left of the pulmonary trunk.

normal life-span with normal health is rare, because, even in the absence of other associated defects, tricuspid regurgitation and spontaneously occurring complete heart block frequently complicate the course in adult life.

The abnormal relationships of the ventricles leads to the classic and characteristic electrocardiographic findings. There is loss of the normal septal q waves in leads V_6 and V_7 and presence of an initial q wave in leads V_4R and V_1.[106] The voltages of the precordial leads reflect, to some extent, the haemodynamic situation. Increased left-sided forces are present when a ventricular septal defect is associated with a high pulmonary flow. Increased right-sided forces are present when there is pulmonary stenosis. Conduction disturbances are frequent, a long PR interval being the most common. More severe degrees of atrioventricular block also occur. Ventricular pre-excitation is seen in several cases.

As with the electrocardiogram, the radiographic features are suspicious rather than diagnostic. The origin of the aorta from the left-sided morphologically right ventricle will often lead to a prominent straight left cardiac border. This feature is also seen in some patients with univentricular connexion to a dominant left ventricle and also in some normal subjects. Cardiac enlargement with increased pul-

monary vascular markings indicates a large ventricular septal defect whereas pulmonary oedema suggests severe incompetence of the tricuspid valve. Oligaemic lung fields suggest the presence of pulmonary stenosis and a ventricular septal defect.

Cross-sectional echocardiography is diagnostic.[107] In addition, it is possible to identify and characterize the nature of all associated anomalies (Fig. 25.62). Doppler techniques are useful in quantifying the competence of the morphologically tricuspid valve. Magnetic resonance imaging will also identify all features with precision. Although the condition can be diagnosed non-invasively, catheterization will be performed in most instances. The intracardiac pressures and oximetry will reflect the haemodynamics of the associated lesions. No definite indication of a discordant atrioventricular connexion is obtained from this information. Clues are obtained from the course of the catheter. An unusually medial position of the pulmonary trunk when entered via venous catheterization and an unusually lateral position of the aorta entered retrogradely or via a ventricular septal defect should alert the operator to the possibility of a discordant atrioventricular connexion. Angiography confirms the diagnosis (Fig. 25.63).[108] Injection of contrast into the systemic venous ventricle shows the pul-

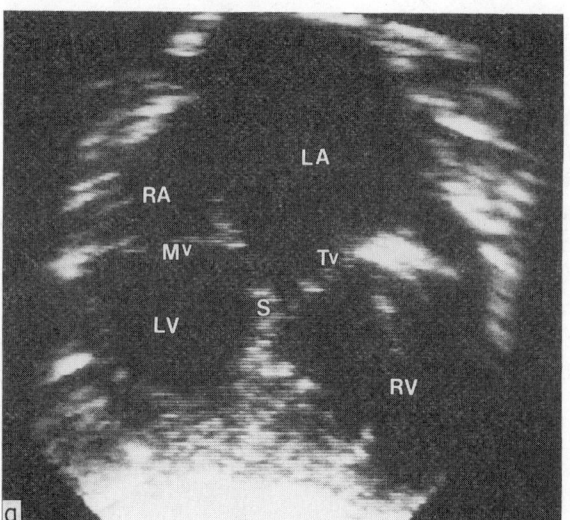
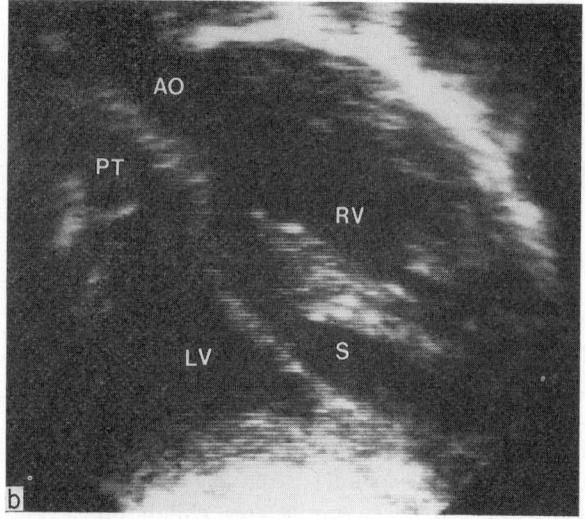

Fig. 25.62. (a) Parasternal four-chamber echocardiographic section illustrating usual atrial arrangement with a discordant atrioventricular connexion and Ebstein's anomaly of the tricuspid valve (TV). The septal leaflet of the tricuspid valve is displaced into the body of the right ventricle and there is marked and reversed offsetting from the septal leaflet of the mitral valve (MV). RA, right atrium; LA, left atrium; LV, left ventricle; S, interventricular septum. (b) Subcostal long-axis sections from a patient with usual atrial arrangement, discordant atrioventricular connexion and discordant ventriculo-arterial connexion showing the pulmonary trunk (PT) arising from the left ventricle (LV) and aorta (AO) arising from the right ventricle (RV). The right ventricle is to the left of the left ventricle and the interventricular septum (S) is hypertrophied. (Figure courtesy of Dr M.L. Rigby).

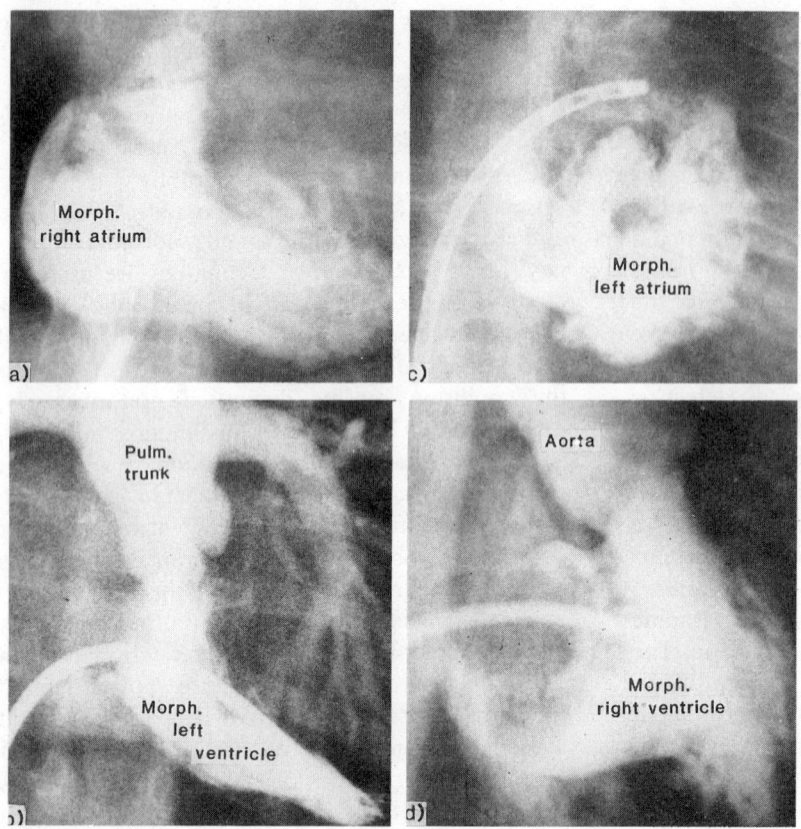

Fig. 25.63. Angiograms showing the chamber arrangements in congenitally corrected transposition.

monary trunk arising from the morphologically left ventricle. Follow-through demonstrates the aorta arising from the morphologically right ventricle. Selective injection into the ventricle giving rise to the aorta demonstrates more distinctly its right ventricular morphology. Injection into this ventricle also delineates with more accuracy the presence or absence of a ventricular septal defect.

Patients without additional abnormalities require treatment only when complications arise. Careful follow-up, even when asymptomatic, is indicated to chart the onset of severity of tricuspid regurgitation and conduction disturbances. Patients with additional malformations may require treatment for these. Corrective surgery may be deferred until school age or even until later childhood. Even nowadays, in the infant with pulmonary stenosis and ventricular septal defect, severe cyanosis should probably be treated initially by a systemic-to-pulmonary arterial shunt. Heart failure due to an unrestrictive ventricular septal defect should be treated initially by medical means, surgery in infancy being reserved for those with intractable heart failure and those with pulmonary hyperten-

sion.

Corrective surgery is complicated by the course of the conduction tissue. Knowledge of its position now permits it to be avoided during closure of a ventricular septal defect. Damage to the conduction system is extremely likely to occur if a direct attempt is made to relieve the pulmonary stenosis. Placement of a conduit from the morphologically left ventricle to the pulmonary trunk should therefore be employed. All the procedures required to minimize surgical induction of atrioventricular block are more easily accomplished in older children than in infants. Hence the conservative approach to treatment suggested in this age-group.[109,110]

DOUBLE-INLET VENTRICLE

The diagnosis and appropriate surgical treatment of patients with a double-inlet atrioventricular connexion has been hampered over the past 20 years by lack of a unifying nomenclature or definition for the morphology involved. Thus, although classic 'single ventricle with outlet chamber' has been generally recognized as being the same entity as double-inlet left ventricle, there has been no agreement over whether hearts with double-inlet right ventricle should be analysed in the same group, or whether it is appropriate to include other patients who simply have a huge ventricular septal defect. Confusion has been compounded by the fact that the commonest type of 'single ventricle' has two ventricular chambers, namely a double-inlet left ventricle and a rudimentary right ventricle. In recent years, terminology has changed; the terms 'single ventricle' or 'univentricular heart' no longer need to be used because hearts can be described in terms of atrioventricular connexion and the ventricular morphology. Thus, 'single ventricle with outlet chamber' becomes double-inlet left ventricle with rudimentary right ventricle.[111]

The majority of patients with double inlet have both atria connected to a dominant left ventricle in the presence of a rudimentary right ventricle. The rudimentary right ventricle is always found in basically antero-superior position. The major subdivision depends on the ventriculo-arterial connexion. Most frequently, this is discordant ('transposition'). Stenosis or atresia of the ventricular septal defect in this setting leads to subaortic obstruction and is often associated with coarctation and/or aortic arch hypoplasia or interruption. Less common is a concordant ventriculo-arterial connexion. Hearts with this connexion are often termed the 'Holmes' heart'. Stenosis or obstruction of the ventricular septal defect in this setting results in subpulmonary stenosis. Double outlet from the rudimentary right ventricle can occur but it is infrequent. More frequent is double outlet from the dominant left ventricle. Single outlet can also occur. Most frequently, the trunk is the aorta with pulmonary atresia, but either a common trunk or a solitary pulmonary trunk with aortic stenosis are possible ventriculo-arterial connexions.

Hearts with double-inlet right ventricle are almost always found with a rudimentary left ventricle located in postero-inferior position, usually to the left, but rarely to the right. Two separate atrioventricular valves are encountered but most frequently the connexion is via a common valve committed exclusively or predominantly to the right ventricle. The ventriculo-arterial connexion is most freqently double outlet from the dominant right ventricle or single outlet with pulmonary atresia, the aorta arising from the right ventricle. Hearts are found rarely with double inlet to a solitary ventricle

of indeterminate morphology. Usually the ventricle is coarsely trabeculated and is criss-crossed by prominent freestanding muscle bundles which support the atrioventricular valve tension apparatus. Sometimes it is difficult to differentiate an indeterminate left ventricle from a right ventricle solely on the basis of its trabecular pattern. Ventriculo-arterial connexions are limited (because of the solitary ventricle) to the possibilities of double outlet or single outlet of the heart. Hearts also exist in which most of the ventricle septum is absent, but an apical rim persists dividing the predominantly common ventricle into right ventricular and left ventricular components. We prefer to categorize these as large ventricular septal defects, while recognizing they have some affinity with the other hearts described within this section.

Double-inlet ventricle is said to make up about 1.5% of clinical cases of congenital heart disease. Difficulties in diagnosis, particularly before the advent of cross-sectional echocardiography, cast some doubt on the reliability of this figure. In our experience, the incidence is closer to 5% of symptomatic infants seen with heart disease in clinical series.

The major consequence of the double-inlet atrioventricular connexion is obligatory mixing of the atrial streams in the dominant ventricle, irrespective of its morphology. In most patients, mixing is incomplete and streaming within the ventricle usually leads to differences in pulmonary arterial and aortic oxygen saturations, with that in the aorta being the higher. Usually, such streaming plays a minor role in determining arterial oxygen saturation. The major determinant is the magnitude of pulmonary blood flow: when it is low, cyanosis is severe; when it is high, the patient may appear pink. The higher arterial saturation is achieved, however, at the cost of a considerable volume overload to the ventricle.

When present, a ventricular septal defect has a tendency to become smaller with increasing age. If the aorta originates from the rudimentary right ventricle in patients with double-inlet left ventricle, this will result in increase of subaortic obstruction. This tendency appears to be increased by banding of the pulmonary trunk. If the pulmonary trunk arises from the rudimentary right ventricle, progressive reduction in the size of the ventricular septal defect causes subpulmonary obstruction with increasing cyanosis. When no pulmonary obstruction is present the pulmonary arterial systolic pressure is similar to that of the aorta. Long-term survival, without surgery, is accompanied by early development of pulmonary vascular disease.

Presentation and symptoms are independent of ventricular morphology but strongly related to associated lesions. Thus, patients with stenosis of the left atrioventricular valve tend to present in infancy with congestive heart failure and pulmonary congestion. Apart from this, the mode of presentation is almost entirely dependent on the degree of pulmonary stenosis. At one extreme are patients with pulmonary atresia who present with severe cyanosis without heart failure on the first day of life. If no pulmonary stenosis is present, infants present in the first month or two of life with severe heart failure, often without clinically evident cyanosis. The heart failure is exacerbated by the co-existence of interruption of the aortic arch or coarctation. Between the extremes of severe cyanosis and flooded lungs are those patients who have a degree of pulmonary stenosis sufficient to prevent heart failure but not to cause cyanosis. Patients in this category may present as asymptomatic children, or rarely, as adults with murmurs detected at routine physical examination.

Just over half the patients are clinically cyanosed from birth, four-fifths become so by the end of the first year of life and about 5% are never cyanosed. One-third present with signs of heart failure and, in these, cyanosis tends to be mild or absent. The first heart sound is usually normal, but the second heart sound is single in half of the patients. In the remainder, physiological splitting is present. Pulmonary closure may be accentuated in patients with pulmonary hypertension. A long ejection systolic murmer is present in almost all patients, being particularly loud in those with moderate pulmonary stenosis. Those with severe pulmonary vascular obstructive disease may develop high-pitched early diastolic murmurs of pulmonary regurgitation together with ejection clicks due to pulmonary arterial dilatation. If the second heart sound is split with accentuation of pulmonary closure, this indicates pulmonary hypertension. A loud single second heart sound can indicate pulmonary vascular disease, proximity of the aortic valve to the chest wall with a posterior pulmonary valve or subvalvar or valvar pulmonary stenosis.

Chest radiography will often reflect an abnormally located heart, particularly when double-inlet ventricle exists with atrial isomerism. An unusual relationship of the great arteries may be suggested by a straight upper left border of the heart shadow. Otherwise the radiograph reflects the haemodynamic picture with cardiomegaly in the presence of heart failure, plethora with unobstructive flow and oligaemia with restricted pulmonary flow. With balanced flow, the chest X-ray may be normal.

The electrocardiogram is more readily interpreted when it is known that the patient has double-inlet ventricle. Making the diagnosis prospectively from the electrocardiogram is much less secure. Double-inlet ventricle should be considered whenever q waves are seen in V_1 but not in V_6 or when a child appears to have a uncomplicated condition yet the electrocardiogram is atypical.

Cross-sectional echocardiography is the most reliable method of diagnosing double-inlet ventricle.[112] Not infrequently, angiocardiographic diagnoses have to be revised in the light of cross-sectional echocardiographic findings. The key to the diagnosis lies in the demonstration of two atrioventricular valves (one of which may be imperforate) or a common valve opening into one ventricle. This is best achieved from the subcostal or apical windows. In hearts with two ventricles, the displaced septum separating the dominant from the rudimentary ventricle will be readily identified. If not, it should be searched for assiduously.

If no rudimentary ventricle is identified, the ventricular morphology can be presumed to be indeterminate. If the septum is anterior to the atrioventricular valves, the diagnosis is double-inlet left ventricle. If it is posterior, double-inlet right ventricle is present. Once the existence and morphology of any rudimentary ventricle has been determined, the ventriculo-arterial connexion can be established in the usual way. Echocardiography also demonstrates the nature of any obstruction beneath the arterial valves. All this information can be seen with magnetic resonance imaging but radionuclide angiography is of no value in diagnosis. Palliative surgery, either banding of the pulmonary trunk or a systemic-to-pulmonary arterial shunt, can be performed on the basis of the echocardiogram. Cardiac catheterization is indicated prior to definitive surgery. The main objective is to measure pulmonary arterial pressure and to obtain an estimate of pulmonary vascular resistance. The pulmonary arteries must be entered. When this is difficult from the venous approach, retrograde arterial catheterization of the ventricle will usually allow manipulation of the catheter into the pulmonary trunk.

Angiocardiography will demonstrate the ventricular morphology and ventriculo-arterial connexions, but it requires the use of carefully angled projections.

If untreated surgically, half of the patients with double-inlet ventricle will be dead within the first month of life, and three-quarters will be dead within the first 6 months. Consequently, most patients will need palliative surgery in the neonatal period or early infancy.

Cyanosed newborns with severe restriction to pulmonary blood flow will benefit from maintenance of patency of the arterial duct by the administration of prostaglandin E_1 or E_2. Exceptions are those with pulmonary atresia and obstructed pulmonary venous drainage. This combination with double-inlet ventricle is frequently encountered in right atrial isomerism. Knowing that the possibility exists should not lead to withholding prostaglandin treatment from a sick cyanosed baby, but, prostaglandins should be withdrawn if deterioration rather than improvement occurs.

Palliative surgery is aimed at optimizing pulmonary blood flow and pressure. Patients who have pulmonary hypertension in infancy should undergo immediate banding of the pulmonary trunk if they are in intractable failure. They probably should undergo banding in any case in order to protect them against pulmonary vascular obstructive disease. Although banding may carry the risk of inducing subaortic obstruction in those patients with a discordant venticulo-arterial connexion, this risk is smaller than the risk of death or of pulmonary vascular obstructive disease. Relief of inadequate pulmonary blood flow is usually achieved by construction of systemic-to-pulmonary arterial shunts. This is now usually done with the modified Blalock approach using a prosthetic graft. In older infants and children in whom the intention eventually is to perform the Fontan procedure, the Glenn operation has the theoretical advantage of increasing pulmonary blood flow without overloading the dominant ventricle.

When considering more corrective surgery, septation of the dominant ventricle is the most logical approach to repair. Septation, however, carries a high mortality and is difficult to perform. In selected patients, it can produce excellent results, but such patients are in a minority. The alternative to septating the dominant ventricle is to use the ventricle to supply the systemic circulation and leave the right atrium to supply the pulmonary circulation. The use of this, the Fontan approach, in patients with double-inlet ventricle necessitates closing the right atrioventricular valve or inserting an atrial patch in order to prevent passage of

systemic venous blood through a common atrioventricular valve. The right atrial blood is usually directed to the pulmonary circulation by direct anastomosis to the pulmonary arteries. Results of using the Fontan procedure are now approaching those obtained for tricuspid atresia. It has become established as the operation of choice. Nine-tenths of patients should now be expected to survive the procedure when it is performed in centres experienced in its use. The intermediate results are excellent although sophisticated exercise testing shows reduced capacity and some evidence of ventricular dysfunction. The long-term prognosis, therefore, remains in some doubt.[113]

COMMON ARTERIAL TRUNK

This rare anomaly accounts for < 1% of congenital heart defects. It is the condition in which a single arterial trunk leaves the base of the heart through a common arterial valve to supply directly the coronary arteries, at least one pulmonary artery and the majority of the systemic circulation (Fig 25.64).

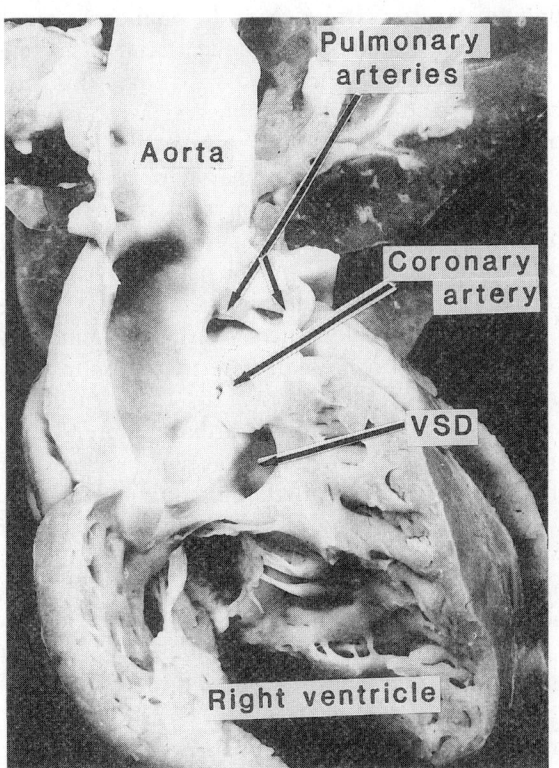

Fig. 25.64. Heart opened through the right ventricle showing a common arterial trunk. The trunk overrides a subarterial ventricular septal defect (VSD) and gives rise directly to the aorta, pulmonary and coronary arteries.

Variation occurs in the setting of common trunk according to the origin of the pulmonary arterial supply from the ascending trunk. A confluent segment may branch from the common trunk to form the right and left pulmonary arteries or else the common trunk itself gives rise directly to the ascending aorta and separate right and left pulmonary arteries. The variety of solitary arterial trunk in which the pulmonary supply is exclusively via systemic–pulmonary collateral arteries is better classified as a single trunk with pulmonary atresia. Usually, the common trunk arises astride the ventricular septal defect which is almost invariably present and is committed in approximately equal amounts to left and right ventricles. Less frequently, the trunk may arise exclusively from either right or left ventricle or be committed in its greater part to one or other ventricle. The truncal valve most frequently has three leaflets, but it may have four or, less frequently, two or five. The valve usually shows some evidence of dysplasia. Aortic arch malformations are a frequent association, particularly interruption of the aortic arch, the descending aorta then being supplied via an arterial duct. The aortic arch itself may be right sided. The anomaly in which one pulmonary artery arises from the pulmonary trunk whereas the other arises from the ascending aorta is sometimes called 'Hemitruncus'. We find this term confusing and classify such hearts as anomalous origin of one pulmonary artery from the aorta.

The origin of the pulmonary arteries together with the aorta from a common trunk means that the pulmonary vascular bed is perfused at the same pressure as the systemic. As the pulmonary vascular resistance falls from the high fetal levels, so the pulmonary blood flow increases. If the pulmonary resistance falls to normal, unrestricted pulmonary blood flow will be sufficient to cause early left ventricular and congestive cardiac failure. If the pulmonary vascular resistance remains high, or increases after an initial fall, pulmonary blood flow will be diminished and heart failure will not occur or will be less severe. Because the pulmonary arterial pressure remains at systemic level, there is always a high risk of developing pulmonary vascular disease in those who survive the early months of life.

Symptoms tend to occur very early. Approximately one-third of afflicted patients reach a centre of paediatric cardiology during the first week of life; nine-tenths present by the age of 3 months. Patients with a low pulmonary vascular resistance are tachypnoeic, dyspnoeic, feed poorly and fail to gain weight. Heart failure develops early. Because of the high pulmonary blood flow, cyanosis may not be clinically evident. Breathing 100% oxygen may be required to demonstrate the occurrence of systemic venous admixture to the arterial circulation. By contrast, when the pulmonary vascular resistance is high, tachypnoea and dyspnoea are usually not present at rest but the patient is markedly cyanosed.

On physical examination, the baby is usually obviously dyspnoeic, often poorly nourished but rarely obviously cyanosed. The heart is usually palpably enlarged with a systolic thrill at the left sternal border. The pulses are of high volume when pulmonary flow is increased or when truncal valve regurgitation is present and severe. The first heart sound is normal, the second is loud and should be single. Singularity is often more apparent retrospectively, many cases being reported as having split second heart sounds. A systolic murmur is usually found, frequently pan-systolic, and is indistinguishable from that of a ventricular septal defect. An apical mid-diastolic murmur indicates a high pulmonary blood flow; an early diastolic murmur is heard when the truncal valve is incompetent. An ejection click may be heard even in those infants with no audible murmurs. In those patients surviving into childhood, the development of pulmonary vascular disease is usual. This results in the onset of cyanosis and diminution in intensity of the systolic murmur. If left untreated, the majority of patients die within the first 3 months of life, usually due to intractable heart failure. Truncal valve incompetence is one of the factors contributing to early demise. Survival without surgery is usually accompanied by the development of pulmonary vascular disease, which is usually established by the age of 1 year. Surviving patients tend to grow poorly and to be limited in their activity by cyanosis.

When the pulmonary blood flow is high, the heart is enlarged on the chest radiograph and the lung fields are plethoric. There is no typical cardiac silhouette but a sharp angulation is sometimes seen below the pulmonary bay. The shadows from the pulmonary arteries are frequently higher in the chest than normal. The heart shadow may be normal in size when the pulmonary vascular resistance is elevated but there is no enlargement of the pulmonary knob. Electrocardiographically, the mean frontal QRS axis is generally normal or directed to the right. Left ventricular or biventricular hypertrophy are the usual findings. Cross-sectional echocardiography or magnetic resonance imaging are diagnostic.[114] Should catheterization be deemed necessary, the trunk is usually entered from the right ventricle. When the pulmonary arteries are entered, this is always from the trunk or else retrogradely from the aorta. Aortic oxygen saturation is usually below normal but ranges from 80–90%, as does the oxygen saturation in the pulmonary arteries. Similar systolic pressures are found in common trunk, aorta, pulmonary arteries and both ventricles. Left ventricular angiography demonstrates the ventricular septal defect and suggests the presence of a common trunk. An aortic or truncal injection is usually needed to confirm the diagnosis, although this is often more difficult than echo diagnosis.

Medical treatment is usually of little avail in those infants presenting early. Surgery, either palliative or corrective, offers the only hope. Banding of the pulmonary arteries offers some prospect of controlling the heart failure but the mortality is high, usually at least 50%. Corrective surgery consists of closing the ventricular septal defect so that the left ventricle ejects into the common trunk. Disconnection of the pulmonary artery or arteries from the trunk is then performed with closure of the defects thus created. A conduit is then anastomosed proximally to the right ventricle and distally to the pulmonary artery or arteries. If the atrial septum is patent, it is closed.

Immediate operative results in older children are good with reported operative mortalities as low as 10%. Many children reaching the age of 5–7 years, however, already have established pulmonary vascular disease,[115] consequently the long-term outlook is poor. Some workers, therefore, have performed primary reconstruction during infancy with excellent results.[116] This has yet to be uniformly achieved. Surgical treatment of common arterial trunk remains a considerable challenge.

PULMONARY ATRESIA

Pulmonary atresia simply means a blockage of the pulmonary trunk. Its classification depends upon the ventricular origin of the atretic pulmonary trunk, the ventricular origin of the aorta and the connexions of the cardiac segments. Irrespective of this consideration, the primary subclassification of pulmonary atresia depends upon whether the ventricular septum is intact or not, because this affects not only the morphology but the clinical presentation and progress.

When found with an intact ventricular septum, almost always the connexion is concordant and the aorta arises from the left ventricle. Rarely, it may exist as a variant of complete or corrected transposition. In almost all instances, the pulmonary trunk can be traced to the infundibulum of the right ventricle, but two patterns are observed at the ventriculo-arterial junction. In one, the pulmonary valve is formed but imperforate; the right ventricular chamber is usually hypoplastic but of reasonable size and the tricuspid orifice reasonably formed although its leaflets are dysplastic. In the other variety, there is no evidence of formation of a pulmonary valve, the right ventricle and tricuspid annulus are small and there is infundibular atresia. Even in this group, there is wide variation in ventricular size. When considering all variants, the right ventricle is usually small even though the spectrum of ventricular size includes some that may be normal or dilated. Whatever the ventricular size, the diameter of the tricuspid annulus is a good indicator of its dimensions.[117] No matter how small the right ventricle, it is rare for there to be atresia of the entire pulmonary trunk and its main branches, which is in contrast to the situation often encountered when pulmonary atresia is associated with a ventricular septal defect. With intact septum, the pulmonary arteries are usually of good dimension and are fed by an arterial duct. A complicating feature is the frequent finding of sinusoids connecting the right ventricular cavity to the coronary arteries. The small hypertrophied right ventricle frequently shows endocardial fibro-elastosis.

The absence of any outlet from the right ventricle in the presence of an intact ventricular septum necessitates a right-to-left shunt at atrial level. Tricuspid regurgitation is common, being particularly obvious in cases with a dilated right ventricle. The right ventricular pressure is frequently higher than the left. The pulmonary circulation is maintained via the arterial duct and its closure precipitates profound hypoxia and shock. If present, the sinusoids connecting the right ventricle to the coronary arterial circulation are a striking anatomical and angiocardiographic feature. The precise mechanics of the sinusoidal circulations is unclear, but they are deleterious.

Cyanosis noted during the first days of life is the usual presenting feature. The cyanosis becomes profound with narrowing of the arterial duct, closure leading to collapse of the infant. Congestive cardiac failure is common when tricuspid regurgitation is severe. Approximately one-quarter of the infants have no audible murmurs but the remainder have systolic or continuous murmurs originating at the tricuspid valve or the arterial duct.

There is a wide variation in cardiac contour as seen in the chest radiograph. The heart may be normal in size in cases with a diminutive right ventricle; in those with large right ventricles and gross tricuspid regurgitation, the right atrial and ventricular enlargement can lead to gross cardiomegaly. It is usual for the lung fields to be grossly oligaemic.

Although the p waves of the electrocardiogram may be normal in the first week of life, after this time right atrial hypertrophy is the rule. The frontal QRS vector axis is usually normal or deviated to the right. Right ventricular hypertrophy is found in approximately one-third of patients and left ventricular hypertrophy is seen in about one-half. In the remaining one-sixth, combined ventricular hypertrophy is found, although rare cases may have a normal electrocardiogram. The electrocardiogram correlates poorly with the size of the right ventricle except at the extremes of ventricular size.

Cross-sectional echocardiography demonstrates the presence of pulmonary atresia and reveals the size of the right ventricle and pulmonary arteries. Doppler interrogation distinguishes atresia from critical pulmonary stenosis.

Catheterization reveals severe systemic arterial hypoxaemia with a right-to-left shunt at atrial level. It is frequently difficult to enter the right ventricle, and the pulmonary trunk is never entered in anterograde fashion. The pressure in the right ventricle is usually elevated and often exceeds that in the left ventricle. The right and left atrial pressures are usually similar, although the right atrial pressure will be higher if the interatrial communication is restrictive in size.

Right ventricular angiography is essential; it will confirm the diagnosis of atresia and define its level (Fig. 25.65). It will exclude even pinhole pulmonary valvar stenosis and will define the size of the right ventricle and the presence or absence of tricuspid regurgitation. In addition, the size and ramification of any myocardial sinusoids can be visualized.[118] Left ventricular angiocardiograms demonstrate the arterial duct and show the size of the pulmonary arteries.

The majority of untreated patients die in the first year of life. Approximately one-third are dead before they reach 2 weeks of age. Survival into childhood without treatment is very rare and survival into adult life is even rarer. Sudden deterioration is usually related to closure of the

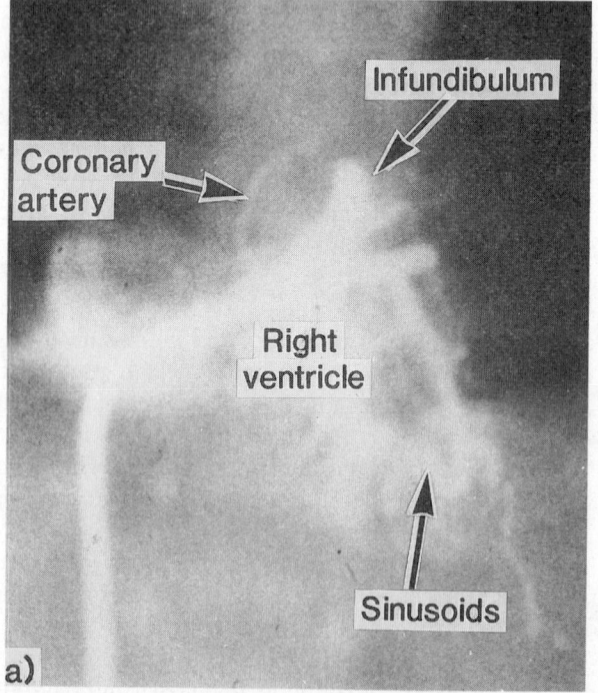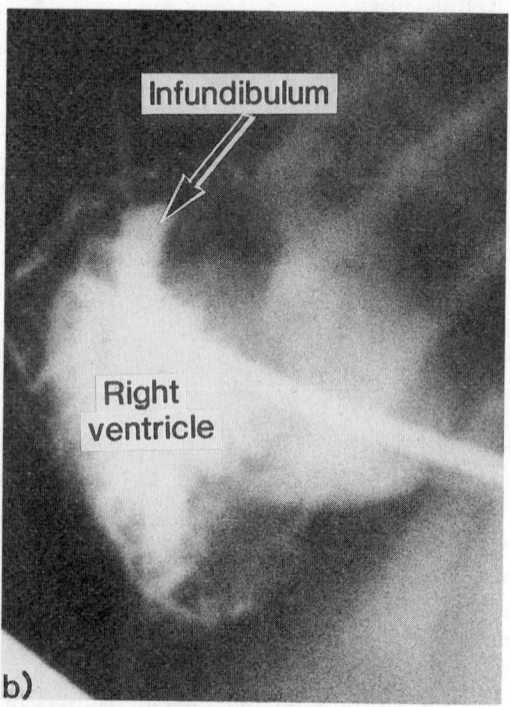

Fig. 25.65. A right ventricular angiogram in frontal (a) and lateral (b) projections. The blind-ending infundibulum and diminutive right ventricle are seen. Also, sinusoidal connection of the right ventricular cavity to the coronary arterial circulation are demonstrated.

duct, survival being contingent upon its patency. Most infants die hypoxic deaths.

Even with surgical treatment, the outlook is relatively poor. The surgical approach depends on the anatomy. When pulmonary infundibular or truncal atresia is present, direct attack on the atretic segment is precluded. When the atresia is solely valvar, the approach is determined by the size of the right ventricle. When it is close to normal, pulmonary valvotomy is the most usual approach. If the right ventricle is small, a systemic-to-pulmonary arterial shunt is the treatment of choice. This usually follows a balloon atrial septostomy performed at the diagnostic catheterization. The decision regarding the surgical approach must be made at the diagnostic catheterization because atrial septostomy is contra-indicated if a direct attack on the pulmonary valve is intended. This underlines the close co-operation necessary between cardiologist and surgeon when dealing with infants who have heart disease.

Having decided on the surgical approach, the patient must be maintained in the best possible condition prior to operation. In this regard, the most important factor is the patency of the arterial duct, which can be maintained by intravenous administration of prostaglandin E_1 or E_2.

The presence of a defect in the ventricular septum has a profound effect on the immediate prognosis of patients with pulmonary atresia. As when the septum is intact, various patterns can exist depending upon the atrioventricular and ventriculo-arterial connexions. The commonest form is that with concordant connexions, in which the atretic pulmonary trunk can usually be traced to the right ventricular infundibulum whilst the aorta overrides the ventricular septum. The anterior position of the remnant of the outlet septum indicates that, in essence, the anomaly is tetralogy of Fallot with pulmonary atresia (Fig. 25.66). Within the basic intracardiac anatomy, considerable variation is encountered in the anatomy of the pulmonary arteries and in the route of pulmonary blood supply. The right and left pulmonary arteries may be confluent or either left or right or both pulmonary arteries may be absent. The central pulmonary arteries may be supplied from the aorta, via a left- or right-sided arterial duct, rarely via bilateral ducts or, in many instances, from major aortopulmonary collateral arteries[119] arising from the aorta, the head or upper limb arteries, the intercostal arteries or rarely from the coronary arteries.

There being no direct connexion between the

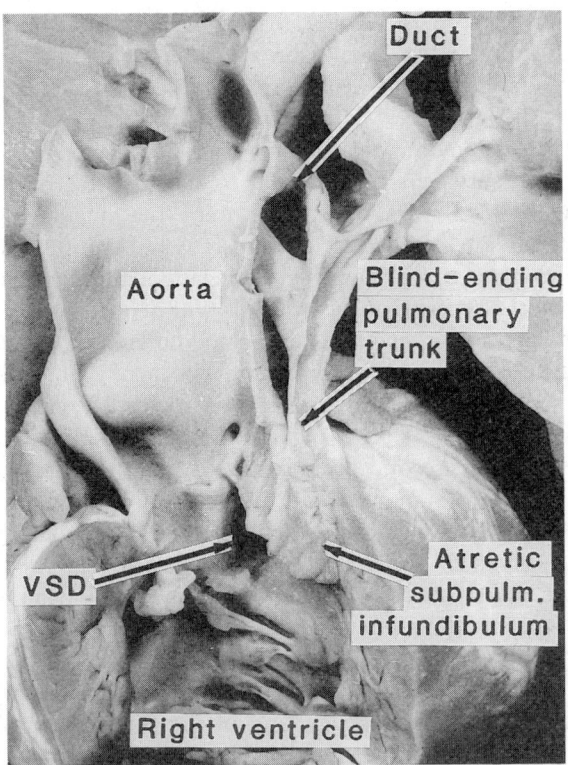

Fig. 25.66. Heart dissected to show the right ventricle, exhibits pulmonary atresia due to an atretic subpulmonary (pulm.) infundibulum in the setting of tetralogy of Fallot. VSD, ventricular septal defect. The pulmonary arterial supply is derived through the arterial duct.

heart and the pulmonary arterial system, all the systemic venous return is diverted via the ventricular septal defect to the aorta. The pulmonary blood flow is then supplied according to the anatomical pathways. There is always systemic arterial desaturation but its severity depends on the magnitude of the pulmonary blood flow. This is usually low but it may be increased, especially in the presence of large systemic–pulmonary collateral arteries. The ventricular septal defect is rarely restrictive and so the pressures in the right and left ventricles are usually similar. Confluent pulmonary arteries are usually supplied by a solitary arterial duct. They may also be found in the presence of one or more major collateral arteries. In these circumstances, the role of the confluent pulmonary arteries in lung perfusion is not known, nor is the extent of the distribution of their branches to the lung segments. Major aortopulmonary collateral arteries usually communicate with the segmental branches of the intrapulmonary arteries close to the hilum of the lung. The junction is frequently the site of stenosis. It cannot be assumed that the perfusion pressure in the lungs is the same as that in the aorta. The pressures must be measured in the confluent pulmonary arteries when an arterial duct is present or in the peripheral intrapulmonary arteries entered via as many major collateral arteries as possible.

Patients usually present at or shortly after birth with severe cyanosis. Closure of the duct may precipitate increased cyanosis. When supply is through major systemic–pulmonary collateral arteries, the severity of the cyanosis will depend on the magnitude of the pulmonary blood flow. Even when cyanosis is minimal, breathing 100% oxygen will demonstrate the existence of a right-to-left shunt. Other physical signs include a single unsplit and often loud second heart sound. Freqently, there is also an ejection click. Murmurs will depend on the collateral circulation. When the pulmonary blood supply is via confluent pulmonary arteries supplied via a duct, a classic ductal murmur is usually heard. When the pulmonary perfusion is via major aorto-pulmonary collateral arteries, murmurs will be localized and continuous, particularly when stenosis is present at the junction of the collateral and intrapulmonary portions of the artery.

The heart is usually of normal size on the chest radiograph, but the pulmonary knob is absent and the cardiac contour often resembles that seen in tetralogy. This resemblance is reinforced when the aortic arch is right sided. The lung fields are oligaemic early in life but, later in childhood, a 'spotty' picture of collateral arterial supply may be seen. The lungs (or segments of the lungs) may appear plethoric when the pulmonary circulation is through major aortopulmonary collateral arteries.

There are no characteristic electrocardiographic features, but right ventricular hypertrophy is usual. Right atrial hypertrophy is also frequently seen.

Cross-sectional echocardiography shows the large aorta straddling the ventricular septum. The pulmonary trunk is not usually identified, but confluent pulmonary arteries may be demonstrated when supplied by an arterial duct. It may also be possible to identify collateral arteries at their aortic origin, but this is better seen with magnetic resonance imaging.

At catheterization, the aorta is usually entered from the right ventricle via the ventricular septal defect. A right-to-left shunt is found at ventricular level or in the aorta. The pulmonary arteries are never entered directly from the heart and very rarely entered, even via arterial duct. The right ventricular, left ventricular and aortic systolic pressures are similar. The atrial septum may or may not be patent

Angiocardiograms in the right and left ventricles demonstrate that only one great artery, the aorta, takes origin from the heart. Crucial to the treatment, and therefore to the complete diagnosis, is the pattern of pulmonary arterial blood supply. This is best demonstrated angiographically. When confluent pulmonary arteries are supplied by an arterial duct, this can be shown by aortography. When this is not the case, it may be necessary to search very hard before concluding that there are no confluent pulmonary arteries. Injection of contrast into major aortopulmonary collateral arteries may visualize the central pulmonary arteries, as may aortography performed with the patient sitting head-up at 45° (Fig. 25.67). Probably the most reliable way of

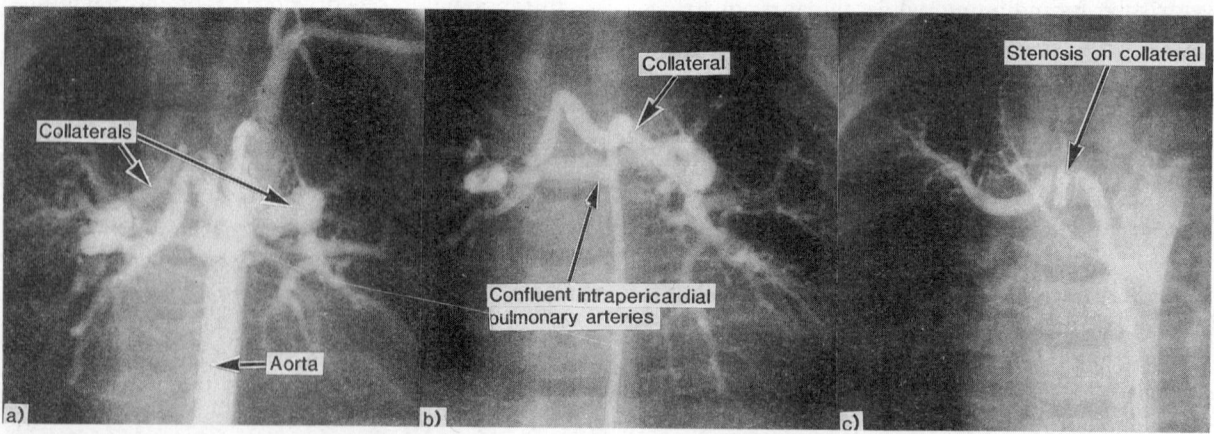

Fig. 25.67. Major aortopulmonary collateral arteries in pulmonary atresia shown by an aortogram (a). On selective injections, a collateral is shown anastomosing with the confluent pulmonary arteries (b) and as the sole blood supply to a pulmonary segment (c). This artery is stenosed as it enters the lung.

showing or excluding central confluent pulmonary arteries is by pulmonary venous wedge angiography,[120] which should always be performed before a patient is declared inoperable.

Without treatment, the majority of patients do not survive the first year of life; a small minority survive into older childhood and adult life. Early death is most likely in those patients whose pulmonary circulation is dependent on the arterial duct. As with pulmonary atresia and intact ventricular septum, sudden deterioration during early infancy may be due to its closure. Untreated survivors are at risk for the complications of cyanotic congenital heart disease, such as cerebrovascular accidents and cerebral abscess.

Action may need to be taken in the neonatal period to establish a secure route of pulmonary circulation in those infants whose pulmonary blood flow depends on their arterial duct. As a temporary measure, a prostaglandin E_2 infusion is instituted and maintained up to the time of surgery. A palliative shunt operation can then be done with the patient in good condition.

Palliative surgery is aimed at ensuring survival to an age when corrective surgery can be safely performed. At present, this is best delayed until the patient is between 5 and 7 years old. Corrective surgery is aimed at establishing continuity between the right ventricle and the pulmonary arteries by means of a conduit, preferably an aortic homograft. The ventricular septal defect is closed so that the left ventricle ejects into the aorta. The operative risks are high even at the best centres.[121] The risk factors include pulmonary arteries that are too small to form an adequate conduit for transmitting the whole cardiac output to the lungs and the arrangement in which central pulmonary arteries do not perfuse the entire pulmonary tree. It is essential to determine accurately the distribution of the branches of the central pulmonary arteries. When identified, major aortopulmonary collateral arteries can be subjected to temporary blockage with a balloon catheter to assess the effects of their permanent occlusion at surgery or by transcatheter embolization after intracardiac reconstruction.

When it has been determined that the pulmonary arteries are too small or inadequately distributed to permit a corrective operation, a two-stage approach is advocated. The first stage is the establishment of right ventricle to pulmonary arterial continuity with a valve conduit or by an onlay gusset. Alternatively, a shunt may be constructed combined with unilocalization (if necessary) of the pulmonary arteries. The second stage is delayed until there is evidence that the pulmonary arteries have increased in size sufficiently to allow closure of the ventricular septal defect with diversion of all the systemic venous return to the lungs. This may never prove feasible. The short- and intermediate-term results of conduit reconstruction are encouraging but there are, as yet, few long-term survivors.

PULMONARY STENOSIS

Obstruction to the right ventricular outflow tract can occur as an isolated lesion or in combination with many cardiac malformations. In its complex forms, the morphological setting and the anatomy of the pulmonary stenosis are closely related. For instance, the pulmonary stenosis in the tetralogy of Fallot is always basically infundibular. In this section, we will concentrate only on pulmonary stenosis without complex additional anomalies.

Pulmonary stenosis with concordant atrioventricular and ventriculo-arterial connexions and an intact ventricular septum is a common anomaly, accounting for 8–10% of congenital heart defects. Stenosis at the level of the valve leaflets is the most common form, isolated subvalvar and supravalvar lesions being much rarer. As with other congenital heart defects that apparently occur sporadically, valvar pulmonary stenosis conforms to the multifactorial model of inheritance with a recurrence rate in first degree relatives of between 2 and 3%. Exceptions to this mode of inheritance include the Ullrich–Noonan syndrome and the multiple lentigines syndrome, both of which are Mendelian dominants and have pulmonary valvar stenosis as part of the syndrome. Peripheral pulmonary arterial stenosis is much rarer than valvar stenosis, but it is a frequent concomitant of the idiopathic hypercalcaemia (or elfin face) syndrome in which supravalvar aortic stenosis is also found.

In the normally connected heart with an intact ventricular septum, stenosis of the right ventricular outflow tract can occur within the trabecular portion of the ventricle, at infundibular level, at valvar level or above the level of the pulmonary valve. Stenosis within the trabecular component of the ventricle is frequently termed 'two-chambered right ventricle'. The obstructing lesion is muscular, and represents hypertrophy of the muscular ring normally present between the inlet and outlet portions of the ventricle. Infundibular stenosis occurs at the junction of the trabecular and outlet components of the ventricle. It can be either in the form of a fibromuscular diaphragm, or the infundibulum may be concentrically thickened up to the level of the valve, the latter frequently occurring in association with valve stenosis. Valve stenosis itself is usually due to doming of a three-leaflet valve, the leaflets fusing at the commissures and leaving a circular opening at the crest of the dome. This is associated with post-stenotic dilatation of the pulmonary arteries. Rarely, a two-leaflet pulmonary valve may be stenotic. Stenosis of a dysplastic pulmonary valve is found particularly in the Ullrich–Noonan syndrome, when post-stenotic dilatation may not be present.[122] Supravalvar stenosis can affect the pulmonary trunk, one or both pulmonary arteries or the peripheral pulmonary arteries. In the latter case, multiple stenoses are usually present. In any form of pulmonary stenosis, it is usual to find hypertrophy of the trabecular part of the right ventricle. In all forms, the degree of hypertrophy is related to the degree and duration of obstruction. Atrial septal defects may also be present with any variety of pulmonary stenosis.

Obstruction to pulmonary flow results in pressure overload of the right ventricle with consequent right ventricular hypertrophy. This in turn tends to result in decreased right ventricular compliance with an increased filling pressure of the ventricle. These effects are directly related to the severity of the stenosis, mild stenosis causing little ventricular hypertrophy whereas severe stenosis can result in a massive increase in the right ventricular muscle mass. Prolonged severe right ventricular hypertrophy leads to degenerative changes in the myocardium. When stenosis is severe, and right ventricular filling pressure is increased, the resulting increase in right atrial pressure can cause a right-to-left atrial shunt if there is a patency of the atrial septum, whether an atrial septal defect or a patent oval pit. On occasions, such a right-to-left shunt becomes evident only after surgical relief of the stenosis.

Severe pulmonary stenosis with a patent atrial septum usually presents as cyanotic heart disease in infancy. Sometimes right ventricular failure with tricuspid regurgitation is present, but frequently this is not the case. In the absence of right ventricular failure, it is difficult clinically to differentiate this variant from the tetralogy of Fallot. When there is no interatrial shunt, presentation is usually due to the discovery of a murmur in an asymptomatic child. Heart failure can occur but high right ventricular pressures can be sustained for many years without symptoms. Severe stenosis with marked right ventricular hypertrophy can rarely be associated with angina pectoris.

The physical signs of valvar pulmonary stenosis are dependent on its severity. When it is severe, the jugular venous pulse will show a prominent 'a' wave and the precordium may exhibit a visible right ventricular impulse. Even if not visible, a right ventricular heave is usually palpable together with a systolic thrill at the upper left sternal edge. The first heart sound is normal, but splitting of the second sound is increased. Unlike the situation in atrial septal defect, the widely split second sound has a normal respiratory variation. A loud long ejection systolic murmur is audible at the upper left sternal edge and is propagated into the lung fields or the carotids. With severe valvar stenosis and in all cases of infundibular or supravalvar stenosis, an ejection click is not heard. An ejection click is the rule in mild-to-moderate valvar stenosis. It is present unchanged throughout the respiratory cycle in mild stenosis, but disappears on inspiration in moderately severe cases. The presence of the ejection click suggests that right atrial systolic pressure is low and that right ventricular hypertrophy is not severe.[123]

The abnormality of cardiac contour seen most frequently on the radiograph is enlargement of the pulmonary knob due to post-stenotic dilatation of the pulmonary trunk. This dilatation is frequently continued into the left pulmonary artery. Post-stenotic dilatation is not seen in cases with predominantly subvalvar stenosis and when valvar stenosis occurs in the setting of the Ullrich–Noonan syndrome. The heart size is frequently normal. Cardiac enlargement is most often seen in infancy when severe stenosis is present.

The electrocardiogram is usually normal with mild-to-moderately severe stenosis. Severe stenosis is associated with right ventricular hypertrophy. Right-axis deviation is present with prominent R waves in the right chest leads, often being in excess of 30 mm. The presence of a q wave in V_4R and V_1 and of T-wave inversion in lead V_4 indicate severe right ventricular hypertrophy and suggest right ventricular pressures in excess of 100 mmHg. More complex correlations between the electrocardiographic and clinical features and the right ventricular pressures have been made but these have a wide standard error. The QRS axis is usually superiorly orientated in patients with the Ullrich–Noonan syndrome such that right ventricular hypertrophy with left-axis deviation are the typical findings.

Cross-sectional echocardiography reveals the levels of stenosis and, if present, shows dysplasia of the valve leaflets. Doppler interrogation, by use of the Bernoulli equation, can give a good indication of the transvalvar gradient. The echocardiogram is also useful in the Ullrich–Noonan syndrome in demonstrating the presence or absence of associated hypertrophic cardiomyopathy.

The diagnosis is confirmed at catheterization by demonstrating a systolic pressure gradient from the right ventricle to the peripheral pulmonary arteries. Caution must be employed in small infants when interpreting small pressure gradients from main to branch pulmonary arteries because the catheter itself is of a size sufficient to cause partial obstruction. In these circumstances, pressure gradients of 10–15 mmHg are normal findings. Nowadays, the major purpose of catheterization will be to perform balloon valvoplasty.

Selection of patients with pulmonary stenosis for treatment demands as accurate as possible an assessment of the severity of the lesion. The longstanding approach in asymptomatic children has been a combination of measurement of the peak systolic gradient across the obstruction together with the angiographic appearances. This is now often achieved using Doppler echocardiography. However measured, a peak systolic gradient of > 80 mmHg is generally considered to indicate severe stenosis. A gradient of < 40 mmHg is generally considered to be trivial. Between these values, clinical findings will have a role in determining the place of treatment.

In general, the clinical course is determined by the severity of the obstruction. Prior to the introduction of open heart surgery, deaths due to severe pulmonary stenosis occurred throughout childhood and early adult life. The highest mortality was under the age of 1 year. Today, the worst prognosis is still in those infants presenting in congestive cardiac failure, few of whom survive their first birthday without valvotomy. The most favourable group are those over the age of 12 years with mild-to-moderately severe obstruction. Increase in severity is rare in this group and can be excluded with confidence. No such confident prediction can be made in children under the age of 4 years. In this age-group, increase in severity is quite frequent.[124]

In addition to infants presenting in heart failure, infants and children with pulmonary stenosis and a right-to-left atrial shunt comprise a high-risk group. Although at high risk, these patients more frequently survive into childhood. In children over the age of 1 year, cyanosis is usually associated with very severe stenosis such that they are exposed to the double risk of cyanotic heart disease and of right ventricular failure. Once the diagnosis is made, valvotomy is a matter of urgency. Paradoxically, a right-to-left shunt can occur in infancy with less severe degrees of pulmonary stenosis. Unless the right ventricular outflow pressure gradient is trivial, these patients should also undergo valvotomy. When a right-to-left atrial shunt is associated with trivial pulmonary stenosis, an alternative explanation (for example, Ebstein's malformation) should be sought. The clinical course of pulmonary stenosis may be complicated by infective endocarditis which, although rare, does occur. As the risk is not eliminated by valvotomy, all children managed medically or surgically should have routine prophylaxis. When stenosis is severe, the onset of congestive cardiac failure or of hypoxic spells at any age has grave prognostic implications. Sudden death occurs occasionally in patients with severe stenosis and its possibility provides a further impetus for early treatment.

The assessment of severity of pulmonary stenosis and changes in severity with increasing age are the major aspects of medical management, coupled nowadays with valvotomy at catheterization.[125] When stenosis is clinically severe, or when doubt exists about the degree of severity, cardiac catheterization is indicated for both assessment and valvotomy. As stated above, increasing severity of obstruction is not uncommon under the age of 12 years. Therefore, all children with pulmonary stenosis initially assessed as mild or moderate should be carefully followed. The onset of symptoms of congestive cardiac failure, of hypoxic spells, of angina or syncope indicates that the period of non-intervention has been too long. Similarly, the development of cardiomegaly suggests that there has been an unjustified delay in definitive treatment. The presence or appearance of significant right ventricular hypertrophy on the electrocardiogram is probably the most sensitive indication that severity is increasing. Thus regular follow-up with electrocardiographic and radiological control are mandatory. The only indication for medical management of severe pulmonary stenosis is inoperability. This is usually confined to patients with multiple peripheral pulmonary artery stenoses. In such cases, supportive treatment is all that can be offered.

Most patients can now have definitive treatment by balloon valvotomy (Fig 25.68). Infundibular obstruction often regresses after this procedure. Surgical relief is now confined to cases where balloon valvoplasty has failed to relieve severe right ventricular outflow tract obstruction or those with

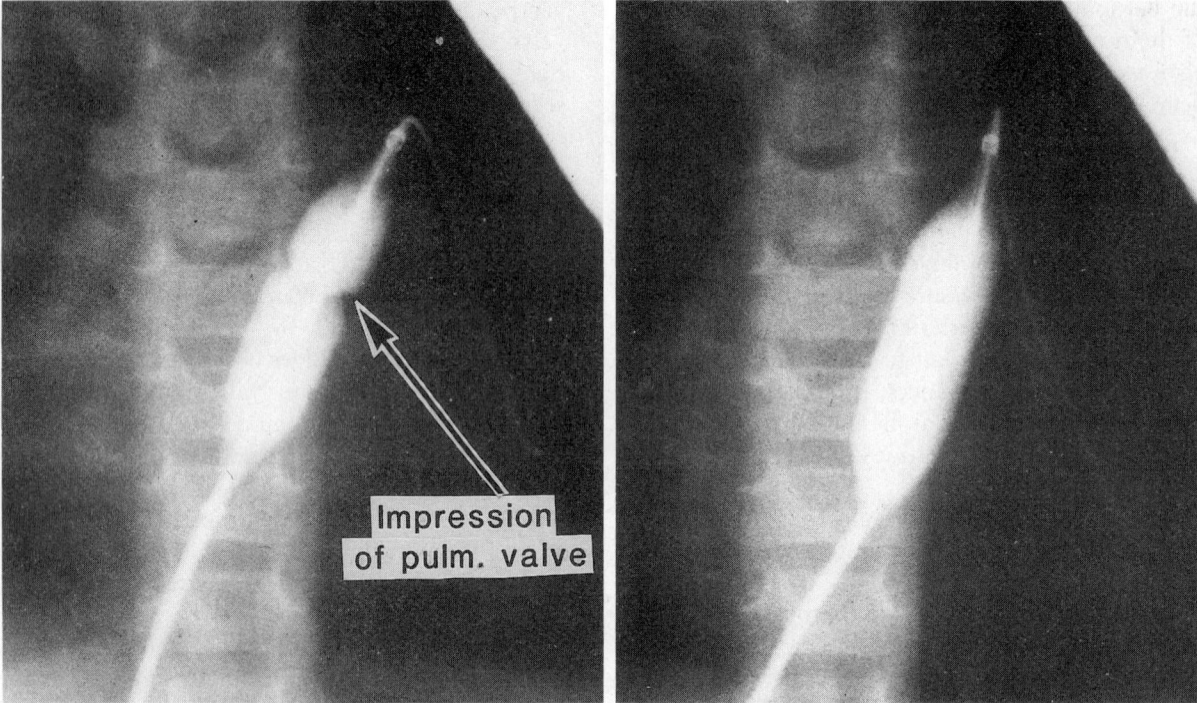

Fig. 25.68. Balloon pulmonary valvoplasty. There is an indentation on the balloon produced by the stenosed valve (a) which is eliminated when the stenosis is relieved. Note the position of the guidewire with its tip in the periphery of the left pulmonary artery.

associated shunts, particularly interatrial defects, requiring closure. The operative mortality is 1–3%. Long-term follow-up demonstrates that 75–85% of the patients have a result that is good to excellent without evidence of recurrence of the obstruction.[126]

AORTIC STENOSIS

Congenital aortic stenosis accounts for 5–8% of all congenital cardiac anomalies. In approximately 85%, the stenosis is at valve level. The remainder have either subvalvar stenosis (5–10%) or, somewhat less frequently, supravalvar stenosis.[127] With valvar aortic stenosis, boys are affected four times more frequently than girls; in the subvalvar variety, the ratio is 2:1, but in the supravalvar form there is no sex predilection.

'Supravalvar' stenosis is conventionally considered to be a narrowing above the level of the aortic sinuses. The aortic valve itself is involved in about one-third of cases, the leaflets being thickened, but valves with two leaflets are encountered no more frequently than in the general population. The coronary arteries may be normal, but most fre-

quently they are large, dilated and tortuous. Left ventricular hypertrophy is usual, particularly in the presence of severe stenosis.

There are several forms of congenital valvar stenosis. In the so-called unicuspid form, there may be either a domed valve with a central perforation but no obvious commissures or an eccentric keyhole opening in a valve with a single commissure. Most frequently, the stenotic valve has two leaflets, in which case a raphe is frequently found in one of them. When a three-leaflet valve is stenotic, it is usual for the leaflets to show marked disparity in size. Four-leaflet valves rarely exhibit stenosis. Unicuspid valves are stenotic from birth, and are the usual finding in infants with critical aortic stenosis, although occasionally gross thickening and dysplasia of a three-leaflet valve may be encountered. A two-leaflet valve although a congenital abnormality rarely presents problems at birth. It generally becomes obstructive with the onset of acquired disease processes in later life. Aortic valve stenosis is accompanied by left ventricular hypertrophy in proportion to the degree of stenosis and by post-stenotic dilatation of the ascending aorta. Left ventricular hypoplasia and endocardial fibro-elastosis may be encountered in infants.

Subvalvar stenosis also results from several pathological lesions. These can be divided into fixed and dynamic forms. Fixed stenosis itself is of two major patterns. In the most common, a fibrous thickening is found on the smooth septal surface of the left ventricular outflow tract extending onto the outflow aspect of the aortic leaflet of the mitral valve and continuing onto the parietal wall of the ventricle to form a ring-like obstruction. In the second form, the area of thickening is more widespread so that a fibromuscular tunnel is formed between the septum and the mitral valve. The dynamic type of subaortic stenosis is the consequence of hypertrophy of the muscular part of the ventricular septum. This lesion enjoys a multiplicity of synonyms, but it is basically hypertrophic cardiomyopathy. Frequently, the facing surface of the mitral valve shows 'kiss' lesions. The leaflets of the aortic valve and the ascending aorta are fairly normal, whereas the left ventricular walls may be hypertrophied, and cavity size of the left ventricle together with that of the right ventricle, is characteristically reduced.

Obstruction to the left ventricular outflow, whether valvar, supravalvar or subvalvar, leads to the development of left ventricular hypertrophy. The extent of hypertrophy relates to the severity of the obstruction and to its duration. The muscular hypertrophy is usually concentric and involves the free wall and septal portions of the ventricle in similar degree. With severe hypertrophy, left ventricular end-diastolic pressure rises. It is rarely grossly elevated in childhood, and cavity dilatation is rarely seen. This contrasts with aortic stenosis in middle life and critical aortic stenosis presenting in infancy. In both these situations, dilatation of the left ventricular cavity is an important feature.

The diastolic pressure in the aorta is not elevated in either valvar or subvalvar stenosis, nor is diastole prolonged. Thus, the increased oxygen demand due to ventricular hypertrophy may not be matched by increased oxygen supply. Under these conditions, the sub-endocardial layers of the left ventricle may become ischaemic, particularly on exercise. T-Wave inversion is seen over the left chest leads when sub-endocardial ischaemia occurs. This gives a so-called 'left ventricular strain pattern' on the electrocardiogram.

Severe stenosis of the aortic valve presenting in infancy, which is rare, has its own symptomatology and clinical features (see below). In childhood and adolescence, the usual presenting feature is a murmur discovered incidentally. Symptoms are rare, but may include diminished exercise tolerance, dyspnoea on exertion and anginal pain. Generally, symptoms are unreliable indicators of the severity of stenosis. An exception is the occurrence of syncope at rest or on effort. Syncope suggests that the aortic obstruction is severe enough to limit cardiac output in response to increased systemic oxygen demand. When the obstruction is severe, a left ventricular apex beat may be discernible and will have the typical left ventricular lift. The pulse tends to be slow rising, a sign difficult to appreciate in small children. Cardiac enlargement is not usual in children and adolescence, but occurs when cardiac failure supervenes. A thrill is usually palpable in the second right intercostal space at the right sternal edge, in the suprasternal notch and over both carotid arteries. A systolic ejection murmur heard maximally in the second right intercostal space radiates into the carotid arteries. An early diastolic murmur of aortic regurgitation may be heard in the setting of a valve with two leaflets, when there is gross inequality of leaflet size in a valve with three leaflets or following an attack of subacute infective endocarditis. The murmur heard in children and adolescents is preceded by an ejection click which is best heard at the left sternal edge or even the apex. This is important, because it differentiates valvar from other forms of aortic stenosis. The second heart sound usually shows close splitting with normal respiratory variation. In very severe cases, the splitting is heard on expiration and not inspiration. A third sound is common but this is a normal finding in childhood. A fourth heart sound usually indicates severe obstruction.

As discussed above, aortic stenosis rarely causes symptoms in infancy; when it does, they are usually so severe that the condition is life-threatening. Critical stenosis is usually present with a small outflow tract and a grossly deformed valve. Endocardial fibro-elastosis is a frequent finding; myocardial infarction with papillary muscle involvement often leads to associated mitral regurgitation. Patients may present as early as the first day of life with signs of pulmonary venous congestion. They have a poor peripheral circulation, hypotension and generally weak peripheral pulses. Congestive cardiac failure rapidly develops and is usually severe. The murmur is often not characteristic of aortic stenosis. In the most severe cases, there may be no murmur at all. Diagnosis is helped by the electrocardiographic findings which usually show left ventricular hypertrophy and ST-segment changes of sub-endocardial ischaemia. When right ventricular and right atrial hypertrophy co-exist, they cause confusion. As with all critically ill infants with heart disease, rapid diagnosis and interventional therapy is essential because any response to medical treatment is rarely prolonged. Once the diagnosis is established, emergency valvotomy should be performed either surgically or at catheterization.[128] The results are disappointing. In particular, associated endocardial fibro-elastosis or mitral regurgitation presages a poor prognosis.

Supravalvar aortic stenosis is often an expression of a generalized abnormality of conducting arteries. There is also an association between supravalve aortic stenosis, elfin face and mental retardation (Williams' syndrome). This suggests that, in a number of cases, there is a generalized embryopathy. In cases not exhibiting this syndrome, occurrence may be sporadic but sometimes there is a familial incidence inherited as an autosomal dominant. The cardiac signs are those of aortic stenosis but without an ejection click. When the pulmonary arteries are involved, a murmur, whose intensity will depend on the severity of the lesion, will be heard conducted into the lungs. When associated with Williams syndrome, mild skeletal abnormalities, strabismus and an extrovert personality will be present.[129]

Presentation and general clinical features in discrete subaortic stenosis are similar to those seen in valvar stenosis. Clinical differentiation of the two conditions is difficult; an ejection click is rarely heard in subaortic stenosis whereas an early diastolic murmur is more frequent. Asymmetry and thickening of the valve with consequent poor apposition of the leaflets may cause aortic regurgitation.

The electrocardiogram in aortic stenosis usually shows left ventricular hypertrophy for age, but, in rare instances, significant obstruction can be seen with a normal pattern. Abnormalities of left ventricular ST segments, flattening of the T wave and inversion of the T wave with ST-segment depression all indicate severe stenosis even if their absence does not exclude it.

The cross-sectional echocardiogram demonstrates the nature of aortic stenosis and reveals the associated lesions when present. Doppler echocardiography permits an assessment to be made of the transvalvar gradient. Other non-invasive techniques, such as the use of systolic time-intervals and pulse-wave tracings, have proved of little value in the diagnosis or assessment of severity of aortic stenosis in childhood.

Diagnosis can now be made non-invasively, but cardiac catheterization and angiocardiography are usually performed. Retrograde catheterization of the left ventricle is the most valuable technique because not only can it be used to assess severity but also to detect the level of the stenosis. In valvar stenosis, an abrupt gradient is seen at the transition from left ventricular to aortic pressure. In subvalvar stenosis, the systolic pressure falls to the level of aortic pressure, but the end-diastolic pressure is that of the left ventricle. In supravalvar stenosis, the transition from ventricular to aortic pressure shows no fall in systolic pressure, the gradient being demonstrated after further withdrawal into the ascending aorta. Catheterization of the right heart should always be performed to exclude intracardiac shunts, along with pulmonary arterial and subvalvar stenosis. Associated obstruction to right ventricular outflow is seen in Williams syndrome, but it can occur in the absence of this syndrome.

Left ventricular angiography and aortography should be performed in the left anterior oblique projection. This allows precise identification of the site and type of stenosis, assessment of the structure and function of the mitral valve, detection of aortic regurgitation and assessment of left ventricular function. Valvar aortic stenosis is characterized by thickened immobile leaflets, subvalvar stenosis by a discrete or tunnel lesion in the left ventricle and discrete or diffuse supravalvar stenosis by lesions distal to the aortic sinuses.

Most children with aortic stenosis survive into adult life. Deaths are most frequent in those presenting with critical stenosis in infancy. Congestive cardiac failure is seen in infancy and later adult life, but it is rare in childhood. Death in childhood and adolescence occurs suddenly in about 2% of cases, but controversy exists about its frequency. Sudden death is usually associated with severe obstruction, but it has been known to occur in patients with normal electrocardiograms.[130] Syncope also occurs mainly in those with severe stenosis, but it is not clear whether it is a prodromal symptom for sudden death. Nevertheless, it should be treated as such. Another cause of death in childhood is subacute infective endocarditis, which occurs in at least 2% of cases. Aortic regurgitation following endocarditis may lead to an unfavourable outcome. Aortic stenosis is frequently a progressive disease in childhood, as in adult life. Thus, a small gradient measured on one occasion does not mean that severe stenosis will not subsequently occur.

Medical treatment plays little part in the management of children with aortic stenosis. It is used in the resuscitation of infants, but, at all ages, if treatment is required, it must be by interventional catheterization or surgical. Valvotomy (or, if regurgitation is present or created, valve replacement) is indicated when the peak systolic pressure gradient is > 75 mmHg or the orificial area of the aortic valve is < 0.5cm^2/m^2 body surface area. Although this value is arbitrary, it serves in the absence of objective criteria, erring, as it does, on the side of safety. The crux of the management of aortic stenosis is choosing the appropriate time to perform a cardiac catheterization. Absolute indications can be given by symptoms (syncope, dyspnoea or chest pain), signs (such as fourth heart sound) and investigatory findings (such as radiographic cardiomegaly, ST-segment changes suggesting subendocardial ischaemia or electrocardiographic evidence of left ventricular hypertrophy).

Echocardiographic indices suggesting severe stenosis will influence the decision with respect to asymptomatic subjects. It is also difficult to ignore vaguer symptoms, such as diminished exercise tolerance. It must be borne in mind that the patient with aortic stenosis will require repeated cardiac catheterizations because the disease is often progressive even after aortic valvotomy. Recent developments in interventional techniques have also posed the dilemma as to whether valvotomy should be attempted during catheterization or whether the patient should be referred for surgical relief.

The operative results depend upon the age of the patient, the type of valvar obstructive lesion, and the experience of the surgical team. The operative mortality is low in children and young adults (0–2%) but remains much higher in infants, despite improvements in cardiopulmonary bypass and postoperative care. The majority of operative survivors are asymptomatic following operation, although the long-term results of valvotomy are still not known. The procedure is often palliative, because the valve leaflets remain deformed. Some patients require re-operation due to residual stenosis, calcification, or aortic regurgitation.[131] It is against this background that the results of balloon valvotomy must be assessed. Initial reports are favourable and compare well with results of surgery.[132] Worse results are obtained in those who do least well when treated surgically and have the highest mortality, namely those with critical stenosis in infancy. It may be that, as with pulmonary stenosis, increasing experience will demonstrate balloon valvotomy to be the treament of choice for aortic stenosis.

Hypertrophic cardiomyopathy is a particularly discrete form of subaortic stenosis. About one-third of cases are familial, the mode of inheritance being a Mendelian dominant. The remaining two-thirds occur sporadically. The condition rarely manifests itself in childhood, but symptomatic cases have been reported from the newborn period onwards. It can occur as a manifestation of other systemic diseases, such as the multiple lentigenes syndrome, Pompe's disease, Friedreich's ataxia, and it is seen in infants of diabetic mothers, when it may be a transient phenomenon. Hypertrophic cardiomyopathy has also been reported in association with congenital heart defects which themselves affect mainly the right heart, for example, pulmonary stenosis and atrial septal defect. The clinical profile, diagnosis and treatment of obstructive cardiomyopathy in adults are discussed in Chapter 39. They differ little in childhood. It should be recognized, however, that the condition occurs in childhood. When present, this type of left ventricular outflow obstruction must be differentiated from the other types.

PERSISTENT PATENCY OF THE ARTERIAL DUCT

The arterial duct (ductus arteriosus) is an essential part of the fetal circulation (Fig. 25.7). Failure of closure shortly after birth is abnormal. As an isolated lesion, persistent patency occurs once in every 1500 livebirths and accounts for approximately 10% of congenital heart defects. The overall incidence is greater than this because it can occur in combination with almost any other congenital malformation. In the majority of cases, the aetiology is not known. Maternal rubella with consequent fetal infection is known to cause the anomaly. The model of multifactorial inheritance applies to those in whom there is no identifiable environmental trigger and it is supported by the well-established risk rate of 2% for the offspring of one affected parent.

The normal arterial duct is a left-sided structure extending from the pulmonary trunk to the descending aorta (Fig. 25.69). It forms a major pathway in the fetal circulation. In this context, much has been made of the supposed disproportion in size between the duct and the aortic isthmus; the results of recent morphological and echocardiographic studies of the fetal pathways have shown

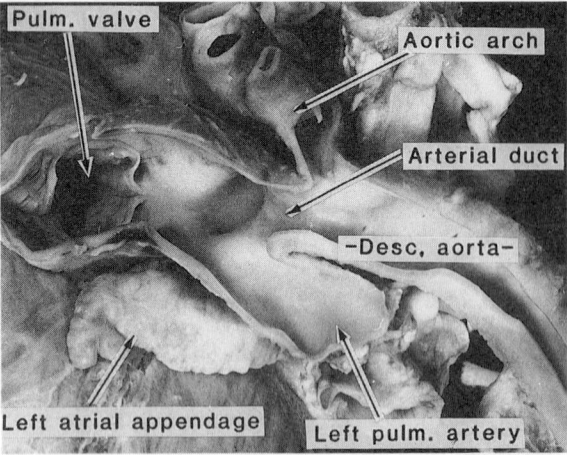

Fig. 25.69. This dissection in simulated echocardiographic plane across the aortic arch shows persistent patency of the arterial duct.

the structures to be comparable in size. Unlike the elastic aorta and pulmonary arteries, the arterial duct has muscular walls and can be distinguished very easily by its histology. This make-up is important in normal closure, but muscular constriction is not the only factor involved. Towards term, structural changes occur which are of equal importance. These are disruptions of the internal elastic lamella and the development of intimal mounds together with mucoid lakes within the muscle. These closely related phenomena produce irregular luminal narrowing and facilitate complete obliteration of the duct. The intimal mounds are particularly well seen in the closing duct. They are much less obvious in the lumen of the persistently patent duct, which also has an intact internal elastic lamella. These observations allow the histological differentiation of the persistently patent duct from one undergoing delayed closure, for example, as a consequence of prematurity.[133] Functional closure normally occurs within the first day of life. Anatomical closure is effected in most cases within the first week but in a minority it may take 2–8 weeks. The obliterated arterial channel is usually converted to a fibrous chord (the arterial ligament) within the first 3 months of life.

When a persistent duct is an isolated lesion, it is a thin, smooth-walled and usually wide channel. In contrast, the arterial duct associated with complex lesions is usually a narrower channel with thicker walls. In this setting, the duct frequently contains intimal mounds, thus giving it the appearance of a closing duct which, in fact, it may be. This is

significant because frequently such a duct may be the only channel supplying either the aortic or pulmonary circulation (see hypoplastic left heart, pulmonary atresia, coarctation and interruption of the aortic arch). Closure often occurs in these circumstances and precipitates an immediate crisis.

Usually, the arterial duct is a left-sided structure, but, particularly in the presence of pulmonary atresia, it may be right sided. This tends to occur when the arch system as a whole is right sided. More rarely, the right pulmonary artery may be supplied by a right duct in the presence of a left arch, the duct then arising from the brachiocephalic artery. In rare circumstances, a right- and a left-sided duct may co-exist. When suspected, it is important to distinguish bilateral ducts from systemic–pulmonary collateral arterial channels.

As discussed, patency of the arterial duct after birth can be due to failure of structural maturation leading to the truly persistent duct. Alternatively, there may be delayed closure in the presence of normal structural maturation, as seen in many infants born prematurely. These two variants can be distinguished histologically and their behaviour in response to pharmacological interventions is probably also different. Attempts to close the duct by prostaglandin synthetase inhibition with indomethacin[134] and attempts to maintain patency by the administration of prostaglandins[135] produce unpredictable results. It is probable that these methods are successful in cases where structural maturation is normal and are less successful when the histology is that of persistent patency. The definitive clinical differentiation between persistence and delayed closure is retrospective, depending on the occurrence of spontaneous closure or of a positive response to indomethacin or prostaglandins. As life-threatening patency can occur in either setting, it must be treated similarly in both. When the duct causes no symptoms, or when symptoms can be controlled by decongestive treatment, it is reasonable to wait for some months to elapse after birth to allow for the possibility of spontaneous closure.

In terms of pathophysiology, the arterial duct provides a channel of communication between the aorta and the pulmonary arteries. The direction of flow through an isolated duct is determined by the pulmonary vascular resistance. A left-to-right shunt occurs when this is low, as is usually found in children after evolution of the pulmonary vasculature. A right-to-left shunt occurs in isolated patency when, as a result of pulmonary vascular disease, the pulmonary resistance exceeds the systemic. The pulmonary vascular resistance is also one of the determinants of the magnitude of blood flow through the duct, the other being its size. Thus, little ductal blood flow occurs in the early days of life before normal extra-uterine levels of resistance have been achieved. Later, the flow may increase to levels sufficient to cause congestive cardiac failure. When the duct is small, the left-to-right shunt will also be small, even though the pulmonary resistance is normal.

The pulmonary arterial systolic pressure depends entirely on the size of the duct. When a large duct causes pulmonary arterial systolic hypertension, the diastolic pressure is dependent on the pulmonary vascular resistance. In the classic form of isolated persistent duct with normal pulmonary resistance, blood flow occurs throughout the cardiac cycle because aortic pressure is always greater than pulmonary. Blood flow is maximal at the end of systole. With elevation of the pulmonary resistance, blood flow is limited during diastole. Further elevation results in systolic blood flow from the aorta to the pulmonary arteries being diminished. Ultimately, when pulmonary resistance exceeds systemic resistance, blood flow is reversed so that it occurs from the pulmonary arteries to the aorta.

A persistent arterial duct rarely causes symptoms in older children, and the commonest mode of presentation is an incidentally discovered murmur. Detailed enquiry often reveals that the children have suffered an excess of respiratory infections and thus have not been entirely asymptomatic. In infants and premature babies, the left-to-right shunt through the duct may be sufficient to cause congestive cardiac failure with all its symptoms. Should pulmonary vascular disease be established, cyanosis may occur as a result of right-to-left ductal flow.

When presenting without symptoms in childhood, the patients appear normal and the physical signs are confined to the cardiovascular system. The pulse is of high volume and may be collapsing. A thrill may be palpable in the second and third left interspaces and it is usually limited to systole. The pulse pressure is usually in excess of 40 mmHg. The classic murmur is also typical. As described by Gibson,[136]

"the murmur is rough and thrilling. It begins softly and increases in intensity so as to reach its acme just about, or immediately after, the incidence of the second sound and from that point gradually wanes until its termination."

In younger children the rough, thrilling or machinery quality may not be as striking as it is in older patients. Despite this, the cadence of the murmur is unmistakable. The first heart sound is normal but the second sound may be loud even without severe pulmonary hypertension.

When heart failure has occurred (as is the case in approximately one-third of patients), growth retardation is usually evident, even after successful medical treatment of the heart failure. In infants presenting in congestive cardiac failure, the murmur may be abbreviated to systole while heart failure is uncontrolled but becomes continuous when control is achieved by medical therapy. These cases are atypical. A clinical diagnosis can usually be made from the combination of high-volume 'bouncy' pulses and a murmur which, if not absolutely classic, does accentuate towards the second sound and exhibits some diastolic component. A mid-diastolic murmur may be heard at the apex when pulmonary blood flow is high.

The heart size as seen radiographically is usually normal in the absence of congestive cardiac failure. Some enlargement of the pulmonary knob is usually seen in older children, and there is also some pulmonary plethora. Overall, there are no specific radiological features for patency of the arterial duct.

An abnormal electrocardiogram is found in two-thirds of patients, being particularly frequent in those under 2 years of age. The usual abnormalities are voltage criteria for left ventricular hypertrophy and prominent Q waves in the left chest leads. Biventricular hypertrophy may be encountered in infants, but right ventricular hypertrophy alone is exceedingly rare at all ages. Its presence suggests a more complex lesion. The correlation of electrocardiographic changes with ductal size is poor, but patients with high pulmonary blood flow and cardiomegaly usually have more evidence of left ventricular hypertrophy.

Patency of the duct is readily distinguished using cross-sectional echocardiography, particularly when infants are scanned from the suprasternal window (Fig. 25.70). Echocardiography, particularly Doppler techniques, is most useful in the diagnosis and monitoring of treatment in pre-term infants because the mere demonstration of patency of the duct does not indicate flow through it. The presence of ductal patency can also be shown with magnetic resonance imaging, but it is most unlikely that this expensive technique will ever be used as a first-line study; the technique may prove valuable in demonstrating ductal patency in the setting of more

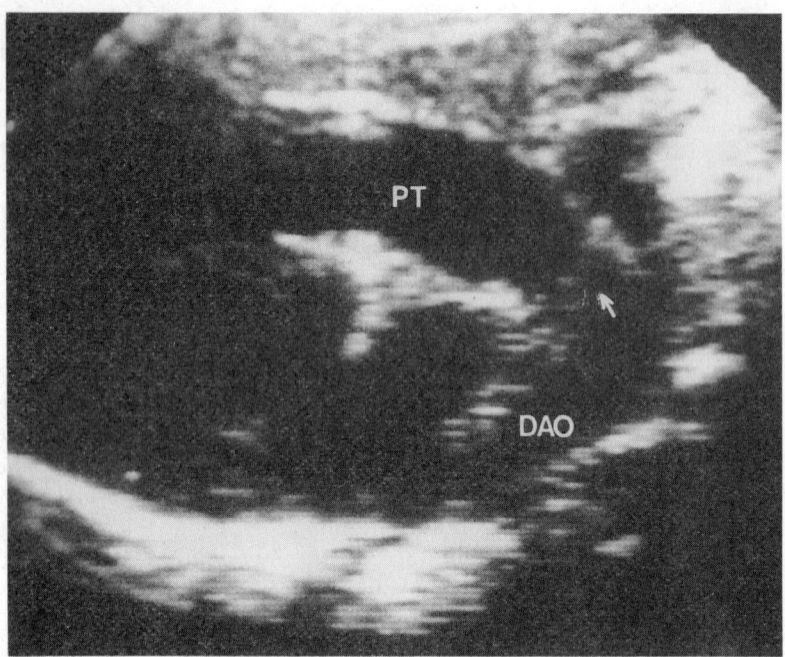

Fig. 25.70. Subclavicular parasagittal section showing an arterial duct (arrow). The duct connects the pulmonary trunk (PT) with the descending aorta (DAO). (Figure courtesy of Dr M.L. Rigby).

complex malformations.

It is also unlikely nowadays that catheterization will be used for the diagnosis of ductal patency. Should it be performed, the venous catheter in many cases passes from the pulmonary trunk to the descending aorta via the duct. Failure to traverse the duct, however, does not exclude its presence. In the majority of cases, the pulmonary arterial pressure is normal and a pressure gradient from the aorta to the pulmonary arteries is easily demonstrated. A left-to-right shunt is usually detected at pulmonary arterial level. As the arterial blood has not passed through a mixing chamber, calculation of the pulmonary blood flow is extremely inaccurate. This is important in the presence of pulmonary hypertension because it makes calculation of the pulmonary vascular resistance equally inaccurate. Angiography is no longer indicated in the setting of an isolated duct. When the diagnosis is less clear, or when a duct is suspected as a complicating lesion in other conditions, aortography (like magnetic resonance imaging) may be helpful in elucidating the full anatomical picture.

Special problems are produced by delayed closure of the duct in infants born prematurely. The proportion of such infants who are affected is unknown. In most cases, delayed closure may be expected because of either structural immaturity of the duct or neonatal hypoxia, for instance, the respiratory distress syndrome. Ductal patency during fetal life is maintained by continuous produc-

tion of prostaglandins which prevent contraction of the muscular walls.[137] Sensitivity to prostaglandins is highest in the young fetus and declines towards term. Sensitivity is also increased by hypoxaemia, which exists normally in the fetus. A third factor is therefore introduced in delayed closure after birth, namely sensitivity to prostaglandins. This will be greatest in the most premature. It is in this age-group that hypoxia due to the respiratory distress syndrome is most likely and most severe. Now that mechanical ventilation has improved the survival of these immature and hypoxic babies, delayed ductal closure becomes a life-threatening situation. In these surviving neonates, the patent duct leads to high pulmonary blood flow, pulmonary venous congestion and congestive cardiac failure. All of these may be further exacerbated by high fluid intake regimes. The clinical picture in these infants is usually that of dependence on mechanical ventilation, accompanied by high-volume pulses and a cardiac murmur which is usually abbreviated with only a short diastolic component. Cardiomegaly is seen on the chest radiograph while echocardiography confirms the presence of ductal flow. Closure of the duct can lead to a rapid amelioration of symptoms with early cessation of mechanical ventilation. Ligation of the duct can be performed in premature infants with an acceptable mortality, but nowadays it is more usual to achieve closure pharmacologically, using indomethacin to inhibit the prostaglandin mechanisms that prevent ductal constriction.[138] The majority of patients treated in this way show evidence of constriction or closure with improvement in their clinical state. Re-opening of the duct is, however, a frequent occurrence. A repeat course of the drug will usually effect permanent closure. Although medical therapy is attractive, it is not universally applicable. Indomethacin administration is contra-indicated in babies with active infections, those with necrotizing enterocolitis and when there is evidence suggesting a bleeding tendency or diminished renal function. When indomethacin can be used, the dose is 0.2 mg/kg repeated every 24 h up to a total of 0.6 mg/kg. The drug is administered orally but, when available, an intravenous preparation can be used.

The contra-indications to the use of indomethacin discussed above, together with its failure to close the duct in a small number of infants, mean that surgical ligation cannot be abandoned. It is still preferred as the primary course of action at some centres. Whichever method is used, ductal closure should not be delayed if the complications of prolonged ventilation and oxygen administration are to be avoided. An initial trial of diuretics to control the heart failure is reasonable, but pre-term infants with symptomatic patency of the arterial duct should not be allowed to remain dependent on mechanical ventilation for more than 7–10 days before closure is attempted by one or other method.

In those patients with persistent patency of the duct (as opposed to delayed closure), attempted pharmacological closure is ineffective. In all but the premature infant, therefore, surgical treatment is still needed for closure of the isolated duct. Nowadays, surgical closure in uncomplicated cases should not result in death.

The risk of surgery is greater in the adult or in the patient with pulmonary hypertension. Indeed, in patients with pulmonary hypertension it is questionable whether operative closure should be performed. A trial occlusion may then be indicated, ultimate ligation being carried out only if a decrease in pulmonary arterial pressure is accompanied by simultaneous increase in systemic pressure. A further alternative to surgery is now provided by the design and development by Rashkind of a safe technique for closure by catheterization. The technique involves insertion of polyurethane sponge discs carried on collapsible umbrellas. Results have been reported of an extensive clinical experience in several American centres;[139] we have used the device in a smaller number of patients in the UK (Fig. 25.71). Closure can be achieved safely and with reasonable consistency although, as yet, it is not achieved uniformly. Problems do occur in a minority of cases with embolization of the device, but this complication has not yet caused serious morbidity. The major drawback is that the closure attempt is unsuccessful and the patient has to be submitted for surgical closure. Catheter closure of the arterial duct, therefore, is feasible and safe. Its role in infants has yet to be established. This system has advantages over previous approaches[140] in that it is compact and employs a venous approach. In our opinion, it will become the treatment of choice, certainly in older children and adults.

An arterial duct is often found complicating other lesions. Treatment of this contingency is considered in the sections dealing with those lesions. However, the possibility of maintaining ductal patency by pharmacological means is mentioned here. In conditions such as pulmonary atresia, the duct may form the only route of pulmonary blood supply. Frequently, the duct closes or narrows with rapid

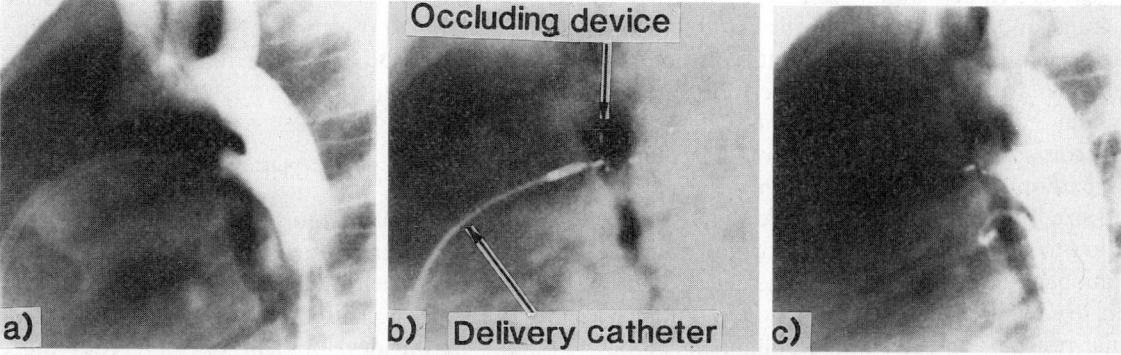

Fig. 25.71. (a) The arterial duct with a catheter traversing it. The pulmonary end of the duct is at the anterior border of the trachea. (b) The occluding device positioned prior to release. The post-release aortogram (c) shows successful occlusion of the device.

deterioration in clinical condition. Surgical treatment with creation of a systemic to pulmonary anastomosis then becomes extremely hazardous. Administration of intravenous prostaglandin E$_1$ can maintain patency of the duct and can cause a closing duct to re-open. The patient usually improves dramatically allowing surgical intervention to be more safely performed.

It should also be remembered that, as with ventricular septal defect, pulmonary vascular disease can develop in patients with persistent patency of the arterial duct. There is a small number of patients in whom an elevation in pulmonary vascular resistance has been documented to occur in later life and who thus might be prevented from developing this complication by ligation in childhood. In the majority of instances of pulmonary vascular disease, the vascular lesions are established in the first year of life. They may develop so early that they prevent manifestation of a left-to-right shunt. Any infant with isolated persistent patency of the arterial duct and a systolic pressure in the pulmonary artery equal to the aortic pressure should undergo closure during the first 6 months of life if the occurrence of pulmonary vascular disease is to be prevented.

AORTOPULMONARY WINDOW

Hearts with aortopulmonary window have some features comparable with a common arterial trunk, but they are characterized by each arterial trunk having its own arterial valve. The characteristic morphology is a communication between the ascending portions of the aorta and pulmonary trunk. The size of the communication varies from a small hole between the ascending trunks to the trunks themselves being coalesced into a common ascending channel above the sinuses of the arterial valves. Such windows can exist with other cardiovascular anomalies such as aortic or pulmonary atresia. Usually, however, the ventriculo-arterial connexions are concordant in the presence of aortopulmonary window. Discordant ventriculo-arterial connexions have been observed.

The pathophysiological effects depend primarily on the size of the defect. Small defects give rise to small left-to-right shunts with little or no elevation of pulmonary arterial pressure. Large defects cause pulmonary hypertension and, when the pulmonary vascular resistance is low, a high pulmonary blood flow. In some infants, the pulmonary vascular resistance never appears to fall to normal levels and, in these, pulmonary hypertension is not accompanied by a high pulmonary blood flow. As with other high-pressure communications between the systemic and pulmonary circuits, survival into childhood is invariably associated with the development of pulmonary vascular disease.

When a high pulmonary blood flow is present, tachypnoea, dyspnoea and frank congestive cardiac failure are frequently encountered during early infancy. In contrast, some patients are asymptomatic, particularly when the defect is small or when the pulmonary vascular resistance is high. A continuous murmur is heard when there is a significant left to right shunt. It is frequently localized to the second left intercostal space and may be extremely difficult to differentiate from that due to persistent patency of the arterial duct.

There are no specific radiological or electrocardiographic features. The diagnosis is made by cross-sectional echocardiography,[141] and can be confirmed by the other techniques such as magnetic resonance imaging. Should catheterization be deemed necessary, it will frequently be found that the catheter passes from the pulmonary trunk into the aorta and the head and neck arteries. Aortography demonstrates the communication between the ascending aorta and the pulmonary trunk, but the picture may be more difficult to interpret than the cross-sectional echocardiographic findings. It should be remembered that an arterial duct may co-exist with an aortopulmonary window.

Surgical closure should be performed in all patients with a low pulmonary vascular resistance.[142] Those with small defects can be operated upon electively in childhood but, when the defect is large, closure in infancy is necessary. In the pre-operative assessment, special attention should be paid to the origin of the coronary arteries because the left coronary artery may arise on the pulmonary arterial side of the defect. In selected cases, it may prove possible to occlude the window using an umbrella device inserted during cardiac catheterization.

COARCTATION OF THE AORTA

Coarctation of the aorta has been recognized as a pathological entity for some 200 years. Its clinical profile has been understood for a century and its successful surgical correction in 1945 was a milestone in the development of surgery of the cardiovascular system.[143]

Coarctation is one of the most frequently occurring congenital heart lesions, accounting for approximately 5% of congenital heart defects; it will be seen in approximately 1 in every 4000 children. It is found at routine examination in approximately 1 in 10 000 otherwise healthy subjects. There is a higher frequency in males than females. It is the most frequently seen congenital malformation in Turner's syndrome, but it is not uncommon in girls with normal chromosomes.

The word 'coarctation' means a narrowing or a 'drawing together'. In pathological terms, it describes an obstructive lesion of the aortic arch. There have been numerous attempts to classify the condition. The classic concept was that it could be divided into infant and adult forms. Realizing this to be an oversimplification, subsequent investigators have concentrated upon the haemodynamic or surgical aspects of classification. In anatomical terms, there are two distinct types of narrowing (Fig. 25.72). The first is a discrete shelf-like lesion almost always found at the junction of the aortic isthmus with the arterial duct (or its ligamental remnant) and the descending aorta. The second is tubular hypoplasia, normally present maximally at the isthmus but sometimes spreading more pro-

ximally into the transverse arch. The arterial duct itself may be closed or be a small non-conducting channel. The coarctation lesion is then usually discrete and shelf-like and found in the posterior wall of the aortic arch. In contrast, when the duct is a widely patent channel, the lesion tends to be more complicated and a shelf-like lesion continuous with the ductal wall usually co-exists with tubular hypoplasia of the arch of varying degree.

The simple form of coarctation with a closed duct is most usually seen as an isolated malformation, although it can occur in association with lesions such as bifoliate aortic valve or anomalous origin of one subclavian artery. The more complex form of coarctation, in which the patent arterial duct is an integral part of the malformation, is frequently associated with other malformations, particularly ventricular septal defect, complete transposition, obstructive lesion of the left side of the heart or hearts with univentricular atrioventricular connexion which produce obstruction to aortic flow. Coarctation of either sort is a most unexpected finding in the cyanotic group of congenital anomalies where the cyanosis is related to obstruction of

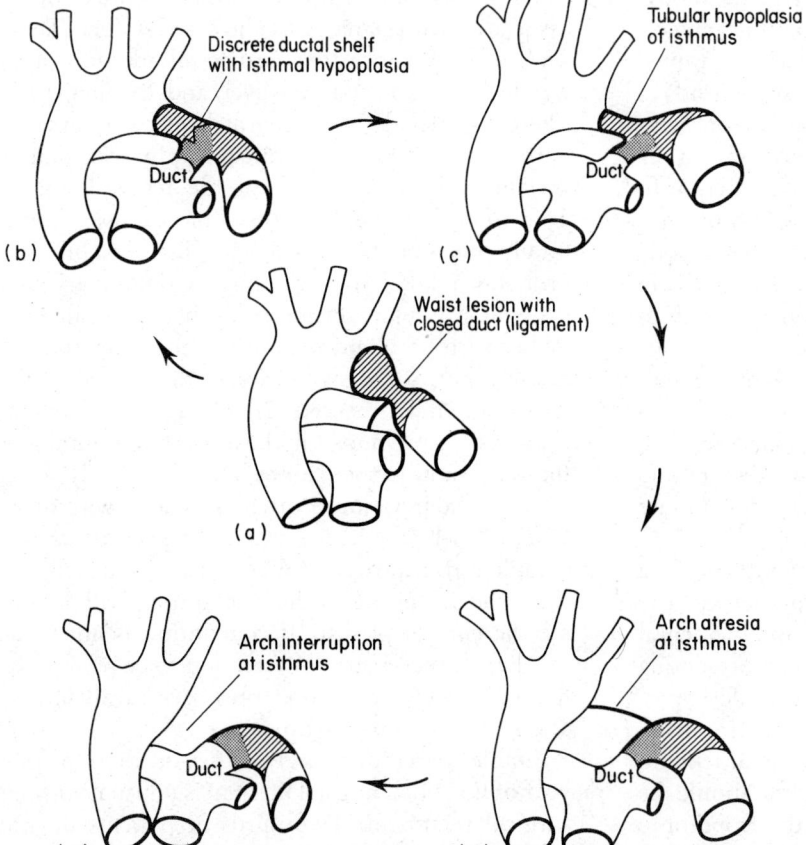

Fig. 25.72. Diagrams showing the spectrum of obstructive lesions of the aortic arch from various types of coarctation (a–c) through arch atresia to interruption of the arch at the isthmus.

pulmonary blood flow. Left ventricular hypertrophy occurs as a consequence of the hypertension, as does development of premature atherosclerotic changes in the ascending aorta and coronary arteries. Collateral arterial channels are present from an early age in all forms of coarctation, developing from the internal mammary, intercostal and scapular arteries to bypass the obstruction.

In terms of pathophysiology, simple coarctation of the aorta is associated with upper limb hypertension and a decreased pulse volume below the obstruction. There is controversy concerning the cause of the hypertension; one view is that the mechanical obstruction to the left ventricular outflow is causative; alternatively, renal mechanisms have been invoked. The rapid fall of blood pressure which usually follows resection of coarctation is adduced as evidence for the mechanical thesis. But persistent hypertension is seen after resection of the coarctation. This suggests that the mechanical lesion is not the sole aetiological agent of hypertension in coarctation and that renal mechanisms are involved in at least a proportion of children with coarctation.

Coarctation with isthmal or tubular hypoplasia (complex coarctation) presents different haemodynamic problems. Some degree of upper limb hypertension is usually present, but it is rarely the most obvious abnormality. The condition usually leads to congestive cardiac failure in early infancy. Persistent patency of the arterial duct is an integral part of the complex and the presence of severe obstruction to flow from the ascending to descending aorta means that perfusion to the lungs and to the lower body depends mainly on the right ventricle. Early in systole, blood flows from the pulmonary artery to the aorta. Late in systole, because the systemic vascular resistance is usually higher than the pulmonary resistance, blood flow is reversed and occurs from the aorta to the pulmonary arteries. This combination of right ventricular pressure and volume overload leads to congestive cardiac failure in early infancy.

Children with isolated coarctation in the setting of a closed duct are rarely symptomatic. The majority are discovered because of incidental findings at a routine examination. The presenting findings are often a heart murmur, systolic hypertension or impalpability of the femoral pulses. Rarely, patients may present with subarachnoid haemorrhage. Coarctation of the aorta should be excluded in all young people with this condition. Some patients are not identified during routine health surveillance; any patient with hypertension (even an adult) should be examined to exclude coarctation. Upper limb hypertension, although present, may not be marked in childhood. Blood pressures of 120 and 140 mmHg are not infrequent even in the presence of severe aortic narrowing. Lower limb blood pressures are usually lower, being in the region of 60-100 mmHg. Delay in the femoral pulses, when compared with those in the upper limbs, is rarely appreciated in childhood, but it is an important sign in adult life. Often there is a prominent suprasternal pulsation. When an associated bifoliate aortic valve is present (approximately 10-20%), a thrill will be felt in the aortic area, in the suprasternal notch and over the carotids. The heart sounds are usually unremarkable. An ejection systolic murmur is heard in the majority along the left sternal border. This murmur radiates to the back in older children. The left ventricular nature of the apex suggests hypertrophy in severe and longstanding cases. When collateral circulation is marked, usually in older children or adults, arterial pulsation may be visible over the scapular anastomoses. A continuous bruit is then also audible in this region.

Tachypnoea, dyspnoea and poor feeding are the usual presenting symptoms when coarctation is associated with patency of the arterial duct. These lead to frank congestive cardiac failure with rapid weight gain, an enlarged liver and cardiomegaly. There is usually a precordial ejection systolic murmur, but the most valuable physical sign is variability of the volume of the femoral pulses. These may be palpable on some occasions, but totally impalpable on others. This variability is probably related to variations in pulmonary and systemic vascular resistances. There is usually a higher systolic blood pressure in the arms than in the legs but, to be significant in the newborn, the difference must exceed 20 mmHg. Differential cyanosis, with cyanosis in the lower limbs but not in the face and upper limbs, is exceedingly rare. Complex coarctation is often associated with other lesions such as a ventricular septal defect or complete transposition. When thus associated, the signs and symptoms of these conditions will dominate the clinical picture. If coarctation is not to be missed, it is necessary for attention to be paid to the femoral pulses and blood pressures in all infants and children with heart disease.

Simple coarctation rarely causes death in the first year of life, but a normal lifespan is unusual without surgical treatment. Two-thirds of patients do not survive the age of 40 years, approximately half being dead by the age of 30 years. Death may be due to cerebrovascular accidents, rupture of the aorta, infective endocarditis of the aortic valve or bacterial infection of the arterial wall near the site of the coarctation. All are more common after the age of 10 years. Sudden unexpected death can also occur. The course of complex coarctation is more predictable, patients rarely surviving the first year of life without treatment.[144]

When survival does occur without treatment, the infants have usually developed severe pulmonary vascular disease, thus rendering them inoperable. Death is usually in congestive cardiac failure. Even when the failure is apparently well controlled, sudden death can still occur. Consequently, there is no place for long-term medical treatment of complex coarctation.

The chest radiograph reveals a heart of normal size when the duct is closed although the ascending aorta is often dilated. The cardiac silhouette often suggests left ventricular hypertrophy in older children and adults. The most obvious sign is the rib-notching due to a marked collateral circulation through the intercostal arteries. Interestingly, although collateral circulation is present at all ages, the physical and radiological signs of it are rarely apparent before the age of 3 years. Occasionally, the site of coarctation can be seen as an indentation of the descending aortic shadow, the so-called '3' sign. No specific radiological features exist. When the duct is patent, cardiomegaly and pulmonary plethora are usually present, but they are non-specific.

After the first year of life, the electrocardiogram reveals signs of left ventricular hypertrophy. In contrast, combined ventricular or right ventricular hypertrophy are commoner in infants and young children. In either event, a normal electrocardiogram is rare.

Cross-sectional echocardiography reveals the nature of the coarctation lesion, the state of the arterial duct and the existence of associated malformations.[145] The site of coarctation can also be shown with exquisite detail using magnetic resonance imaging, even in neonates (Fig. 25.73).

Invasive investigation is now unnecessary in older children because the rib-notching identifies the site of coarctation as thoracic. Invasive investigation may be required if doubt exists about the location of the coarctation or when interruption of the aortic arch has not been ruled out by echocardiographic investigation. Magnetic resonance imaging is particularly effective in this lesion.

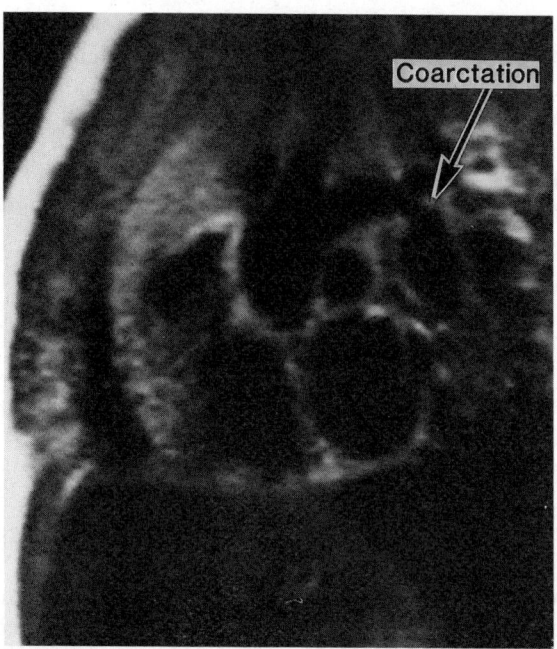

Fig. 25.73. Magnetic resonance image showing coarctation of the aorta with post-stenotic dilatation of the aorta. (Figure courtesy of Dr E.J. Baker).

The haemodynamic findings in the presence of a closed duct are left ventricular and ascending aortic hypertension with a lower pressure and lower pulse volume in the descending aorta. Aortography shows the site of the coarctation and the collateral circulation. When the duct is patent, cardiac catheterization reveals pulmonary arterial and right ventricular pressures at systemic level. Usually the catheter passes easily through the duct into the descending aorta. The left ventricular and ascending aortic pressures are often higher than those in the pulmonary artery and descending aorta, but this is not invariably so. A right-to-left shunt is detected through the duct. Angiography reveals the site of the coarctation and the degree of isthmal hypoplasia in addition to delineating or excluding more complex cardiac malformations.

There is no effective medical treatment for coarctation. Surgical correction[146] should be performed as soon after diagnosis as is technically possible. Surgery is usually a matter of urgency when the duct is patent or when the lesion is associated with other cardiac malformations. Treatment of the coarctation is usually the initial step in management. When the duct is closed, it is usually possible to resect the coarcted segment of the aorta and achieve end-to-end anastomosis. In complex coarctation, where the arch and isthmus are usually hypoplastic, end-to-end anastomosis rarely produces adequate surgical relief although some surgeons espouse this technique. More usually, the left subclavian artery is used as on onlay either by means of the flap procedure, having divided the arteries, or by its removal from the arch with re-anastomosis across the coarcted segment. In either event, it is crucial to resect the shelf lesion composed of ductal wall. Incorporation of prosthetic patches is an alternative procedure, but this is becoming less popular because of the observed frequency of aneurysm formation. Whatever the operation performed, there is a small risk of causing spinal cord injury during the period of aortic occlusion. Associated anomalies can either be corrected at the same time as the coarctation is relieved, or be deferred for staged repair. Staged repair is often possible when the associated lesion is a ventricular septal defect, complete transposition or mitral valve malformations. When the associated anomaly is itself life-threatening, for example obstructed totally anomalous pulmonary venous connexion, total correction is unavoidable. If staged repair is considered, the principles of treatment of the associated lesion are followed. The operative risk of simple coarctation should be < 5% in children, but it may be slightly higher in adults. The risks of repair in infancy are higher chiefly because of the associated lesions. In most patients, satisfactory relief of hypertension follows surgery. Increased hypertension in the immediate postoperative period is a well-recognized complication and can be controlled with sodium nitroprusside and propranolol. Some patients require antihypertensive agents for a variable period of time following surgery and a few remain hypertensive even with appropriate medication. When postoperative hypertension lasts for more than a few days, it is frequently accompanied by abdominal pain. This usually responds to symptomatic and antihypertensive treatment. Rarely, the pain is severe and may be accompanied by abdominal rigidity. Laparotomy in these cases has revealed necrotizing arteritis sometimes requiring bowel resection. Irrespective of the type of surgery performed, re-coarctation is a problem in a minority of cases. It may require re-operation but, more recently, it has been shown that balloon dilatation of the narrowed segment provides relief.[147] Fibrosis around the initial site of operation contains the necessary rupture of the aortic wall. Some workers have also advocated balloon dilatation of native coarctation lesions. In this setting, however, there is nothing to support the ruptured wall and a proportion of cases have been noted to develop aneurysmal expansion at the site of dilatation.[148] Clinicians at most centres, therefore, are reserving judgement concerning the role of balloon dilatation of native coarctation.

INTERRUPTION OF THE AORTIC ARCH

An interrupted arch is the extreme form of tubular hypoplasia. It occurs in three sites (Fig. 25.74). The first is at the isthmus between the left subclavian artery and the descending aorta, the arterial duct then supplying blood to the lower body. Alternatively, the arch may be interrupted between the left common carotid and the left subclavian arteries. The duct then supplies the left arm as well as the lower body. These two varieties are found with approximately equal frequency. The third site, which is much rarer, is between the brachiocephalic and left common carotid arteries. Any type of interruption can co-exist with retro-oesophageal origin of the right subclavian artery, in which case the right arm is fed through the duct. Many infants have other cardiovascular malformations in addition to the patent arterial duct. The commonest are ventricular septal defect or subaortic stenosis due to

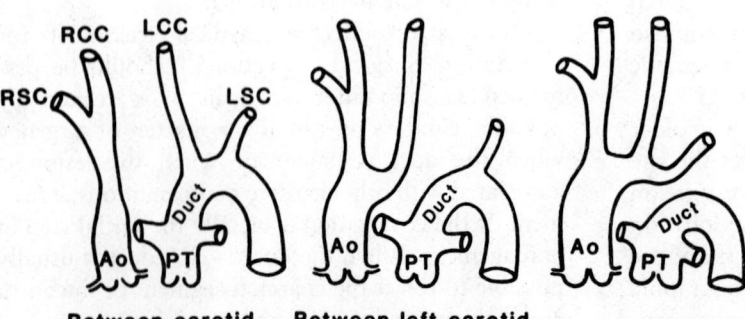

Between carotid arteries   **Between left carotid and left subclavian arteries**   **At isthmus**

Fig. 25.74. Diagrams showing the three possible variants for interruption of the aortic arch.

any cause. In rare circumstances, ducts may be closed at the time of diagnosis and the distal aortic segment is then fed through collateral arteries.

The pathophysiology of the condition is similar to that of severe coarctation of the aorta in the setting of a patent duct. The presentation and clinical course of the two conditions are also similar. Affected children rarely survive the first year of life, although infants with interruption usually present somewhat earlier than those with coarctation. Only in those rare cases where the interruption is between the brachiocephalic and the left common carotid arteries (or else there is retro-oesophageal origin of the right subclavian artery) do physical signs help. In such cases, inequality of the arm and neck pulses may provide a clue to the presence of interruption of the aortic arch. In general, the diagnosis is made by cross-sectional echocardiography,[149] or angiocardiography when absence of an aortic segment is either positively identified or else inferred from the course and distribution of the head and neck arteries. Until recently, surgical correction has been successful only in those rare cases surviving into older childhood. Results in recent reports suggest that correction in early infancy is possible,[150] but the determining factor in survival is often the presence and severity of subaortic stenosis.

CONGENITAL MALFORMATIONS OF THE CORONARY ARTERIES

Congenitally malformed coronary arteries can be found as isolated lesions in otherwise anatomically normal hearts. These lesions are rare. More frequently, the coronary arteries may be malformed in a heart which is itself abnormal. Where the deformed coronary arterial pattern is part of a more major lesion, the abnormality is described in the appropriate section. In this section, we consider only anomalies of the coronary arteries in otherwise normal hearts. These in themselves may be abnormalities in the origin of the arteries, either from the pulmonary trunk or from the aorta itself, abnormalities in their epicardial course, occlusive inflammatory arterial disease or arteriovenous fistulas.

Usually, the coronary arteries arise one from each of two aortic sinuses that 'face' the pulmonary trunk. They arise from the sinus well below the junction with the tubular aorta. Variations in the normal anatomy include one artery arising above the aortic bar and both arteries arising from the same sinus or from a single coronary ostium.

Another variation is the origin of the left circumflex or infundibular coronary arteries directly from the aortic sinuses in addition to the usual right and left coronary arteries. Presence of additional ostia is of no clinical significance, but abnormal origin may produce symptoms. When a coronary artery does not arise within a sinus, its course through the aortic wall is more oblique than usual and this may produce stenosis. Although, in most cases, these variations are symptomless, it has recently been suggested that anomalous origin may produce angina pectoris or be a cause of sudden death.[151]

The rare finding of anomalous origin of a coronary artery from the pulmonary trunk accounts for < 1% of congenital cardiac malformations. The most frequently encountered variant is that in which the left coronary artery, supplying the entire left system, arises from the left sinus of the pulmonary trunk, usually called the Bland–White–Garland syndrome. The effect of the anomalous origin is to produce ischaemia of the left ventricle. When seen at autopsy, there is usually marked ventricular dilatation with little hypertrophy (Fig. 25.75). Patchy fibrosis is evident, and endocardial fibro-elastosis is frequently encountered. Patchy myocardial calcification is also found in many affected hearts. The anomalous origin has no deleterious effect during fetal life. After birth, however, the fall in pulmonary arterial pressure results in a fall in the perfusion pressure of the artery with ectopic origin. Its territory is perfused at low pressure with blood that has mixed venous oxygen saturation. These factors predispose to myocardial ischaemia. The major factor is the low coronary arterial perfusion pressure. Patients with ectopic origin of the right coronary artery may survive a normal lifespan whilst those with severe cyanosis but a normal perfusion pressure, as encountered in the tetralogy of Fallot, do not have acute ischaemic episodes. If present collateral communications between the right and left coronary systems can mitigate to a certain extent the effect of the ectopic origin.[152] Although the presence of a good collateral circulation produces a higher oxygen saturation in the territory of the ectopic artery, the perfusion pressure will still be related to the pulmonary arterial pressure. Once the pulmonary resistance has fallen to normal, an effective steal is established from the ectopic coronary artery to the pulmonary trunk.

Symptoms occur after the fall of pulmonary vascular resistance has been accomplished. The infants appear normal at birth, but deteriorate rapidly by the second or third month of life. Babies usually show evidence of paroxysmal discomfort often accompanied by pallor and sweating. Their anxious look suggests that they are experiencing anginal pain. These intermittent attacks progress to symptoms of congestive cardiac failure. The ensuing dyspnoea and tachycardia, accompanied by crepitations heard throughout the lung fields, frequently suggest a diagnosis of pneumonia or bronchiolitis. Clinical cardiac enlargement and hepatomegaly suggest a cardiac aetiology. Rarely are any murmurs heard.

The chest radiograph establishes the presence of cardiac enlargement. The electrocardiogram shows evidence of myocardial ischaemia. In ectopic origin of the left coronary artery, this will indicate anterior ischaemia. Cross-sectional echocardiography in skilled hands will reveal the anomalous origin of the coronary artery.[153] Thallium scintigraphy demonstrates anterior perfusion defects. The diagnosis can be confirmed by aortography with either selective aortic sinus injections or, where feasible, selective coronary arteriography.

Very few affected infants survive the first year of life. If they survive this year, such patients may live into adult life. When questioned, they have usually manifested no symptoms or signs in infancy and have a well-developed coronary collateral circulation. Infants presenting in heart failure should be given decongestive treatment, which improves their general condition and may also improve myocardial perfusion. Re-implantation of the aberrant artery is the surgical treatment of choice and can be accomplished in infants under 3 months of age. Saphenous vein grafting or re-implantation of the ectopic artery appear to be equally applicable in older patients.[154]

It is becoming increasingly common (although still exceedingly rare in the overall context of paediatric heart disease) to encounter aneurysms of the coronary arteries. These may be discovered in infants presenting with severe heart failure or as isolated lesions in older children. Although seen infrequently in Western centres, these lesions are much more common in the Far East where they have been recognized as part of the mucocutaneous lymph node syndrome. The cardiac part of this syndrome is now widely referred to as Kawasaki's disease.[155] Sporadic cases with identical morphology have been well known for many years in Western countries and described as infantile polyarteritis nodosa. The anatomical lesions in the two are the same: massive aneurysms of the main stems and branches of both the right and left coronary arterial systems (Fig. 25.76), with similar aneurysm being found in the worst affected cases in the renal, cerebral and abdominal arteries. Those patients who are severely affected frequently die in the acute phase of the febrile illness, but if they recover they may then present with symptoms of their aneurysms during adolescence or rupture may be a cause of sudden death.

Fistulous connexions between the coronary arteries and the right heart chambers, either directly or via the coronary sinus, are rare malformations. Usually, they present in adult life but exceedingly rarely they may be encountered in infancy.

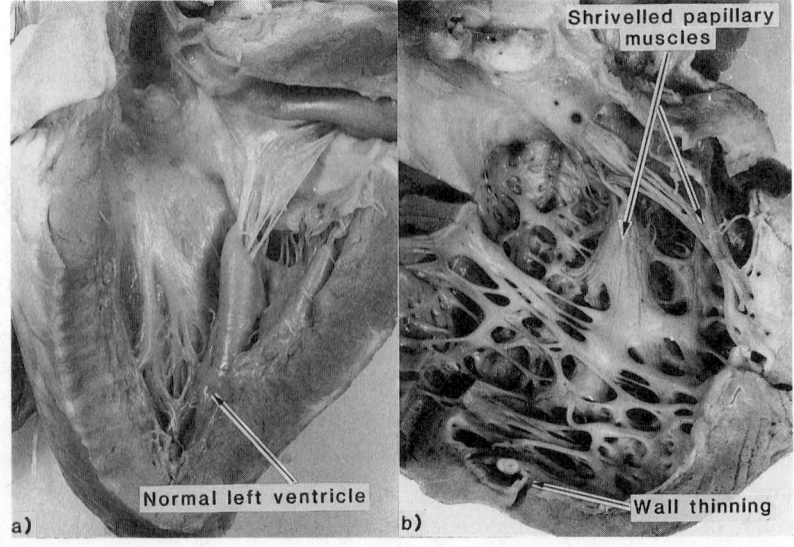

Fig. 25.75. Photographs showing a normal left ventricle (a) compared with an ischaemic ventricle (b) in the setting of anomalous origin of the left coronary artery from the pulmonary trunk.

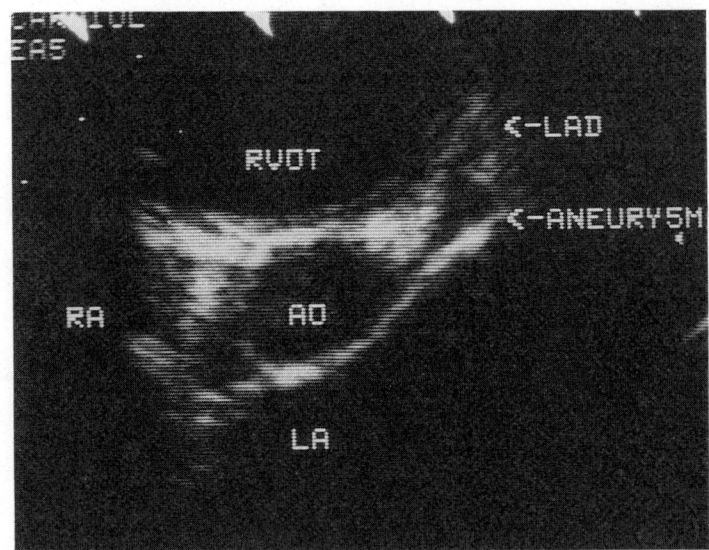

Fig. 25.76. Parasternal short axis section of the aortic root (AO) in a patient with Kawasaki's disease showing an aneurysm of the left coronary artery at its bifurcation into left anterior descending (LAD) and circumflex branches. (RA, right atrium; LA, left atrium; RVOT, right ventricular outflow tract).

ANOMALIES OF THE PULMONARY ARTERIES

The major anomalies of the pulmonary arterial tree are the absence of one pulmonary artery, idiopathic dilatation of the pulmonary trunk, origin of the left pulmonary artery from the right pulmonary artery (vascular sling) and pulmonary arteriovenous malformations.

Although one of these lesions is often decribed as 'absence' of one pulmonary artery, it is very rare for there to be no pulmonary arterial supply to one of the lungs. More usually, there is discontinuity between one lung and the pulmonary trunk which supplies only the other lung. The vascular supply to the disconnected lung may come from various sources, either directly from the ascending aorta, via an arterial duct, or by collateral arteries from the descending aorta or the head and neck arteries. 'Absence' of a pulmonary artery is usually associated with intracardiac anomalies such as the tetralogy of Fallot. In these instances, the signs and symptoms are usually those of the associated cardiac malformation. In its isolated form, symptoms depend on the magnitude of blood flow to the disconnected lung. When the blood supply is via an anomalous artery from the ascending aorta, there is usually a high pulmonary blood flow. This results in early development of congestive heart failure and often in death in infancy. Other sources of arterial supply usually have a low flow and patients may be asymptomatic through childhood. Mild exertional dyspnoea and occasionally haemoptysis may then be experienced. There are few physical signs in the absence of congestive heart failure. The discon-

nected lung tends to be hypoplastic and there is asymmetry of the chest. Chest radiography will demonstrate asymetric pulmonary blood flow. The affected lung will be plethoric when flow is excessive and oligaemic when it is diminished. Nuclear angiography may be of value in demonstrating the abnormal delayed filling of the affected lung. The diagnosis is established by contrast angiocardiography, cross-sectional echocardiography or magnetic resonance imaging. Asymptomatic patients require no treatment. When one large artery arises from the ascending aorta, continuity between this artery and the pulmonary trunk should be surgically re-established.

Idiopathic dilatation of the pulmonary trunk is rare and, usually, asymptomatic. It tends to be discovered through the observation of an enlarged knob on the chest radiograph performed for no cardiac reasons. The diagnosis is confirmed by angiocardiography or cross-sectional echocardiography. As affected individuals have a normal lifespan, invasive studies should be performed only when other cardiac problems are suspected.

Anomalous origin of the left pulmonary artery from the right pulmonary artery, passing to the left hilum between the trachea and the oesophagus, is termed a 'vascular sling'.[156] The course of the aberrant artery tends to compress the trachea and right main bronchus giving rise to respiratory symptoms which are usually present from birth. Affected infants sustain recurrent respiratory infections. Symptoms are usually severe and, unless treated, death usually occurs in the first 6 months of life. The changes will be evident on the chest radiograph. An oesophagogram often shows an anterior identation but may be normal. Pulmonary arterial angiography should be performed when the condition is suspected, or the anatomy should be demonstrated with magnetic resonance imaging. The treatment is surgical. The left pulmonary artery is divided at its anomalous origin and re-attached appropriately to the pulmonary trunk.

Pulmonary arteriovenous malformations are exceedingly rare, being seen in approximately 1 per 5000 autopsies. They vary greatly in size but may be up to 5 cm in diameter. They are frequently multiple and may be widespread. Haemangiomata of the skin and mucous membranes are present in one-third of the patients. Flow through the malformation is often of sufficient magnitude to cause systemic arterial desaturation. Affected individuals may be asymptomatic, but exertional dyspnoea, haemoptysis and chest pain are frequently experienced. Physical examination reveals a fit and well-nourished but cyanosed patient. Systolic or continuous murmurs are usually heard, which increase in intensity during inspiration. The chest radiograph shows some evidence of the malformation in almost every case. The classic picture is of a rounded or nodular opacity with dilated vessels connecting it to the hilum of the lung. Contrast echocardiography and nuclear angiography have been suggested as useful screening techniques. Pulmonary angiography or magnetic resonance imaging delineates the lesions accurately, although multiple and small lesions may be difficult to detect. Surgery, with excision of the malformation by lobectomy or segmental resection, has been the mainstay of treatment; now transcatheter embolization has been shown to be effective.[157] This is performed using detachable balloons or coils and is particularly applicable to multiple lesions.

AORTIC ARCH ANOMALIES AND VASCULAR RINGS

Anomalies of the aortic arches and their major branches are legion.[156] Many are entirely asymptomatic and some, although giving rise to no symptoms, are important from the surgical point of view when associated with other defects. In this category is the anomalous left subclavian artery arising below a complex aortic coarctation. This type of origin complicates surgical correction. There are, however, varieties which do cause symptoms or

confusion and it is with these that we concern ourselves here.

All the varied aortic arch malformations are well explained on the basis of an hypothetical double aortic arch with bilateral arterial ducts (Fig. 25.77). The hypothetical double arch can be divided at various points in its circle to explain the different lesions. Following such division, one or more of the head and arm arteries become isolated from the major arch, and may be supplied either via an arterial duct or from the contralateral persisting segment of the descending aorta. The hypothetical double-arch system accounts well for the morphology seen with an anomalous origin of the right subclavian artery from a left aortic arch (Fig. 25.78). The system can be used in similar fashion to explain all known malformations of the aortic arch. We shall restrict ourselves to the most common examples.

The major anomalies occurring with a left aortic arch are:

1 anomalies of the brachiocephalic arteries (with or without tracheal compression);
2 aberrant origin of the right subclavian artery;
3 a left arch with a right-sided proximal descending aorta.

The commonest of these lesions is aberrant origin of the right subclavian artery (Fig. 25.79). Reported as being found in approximately 0.5% of autopsies, this may be an isolated defect but it is frequently

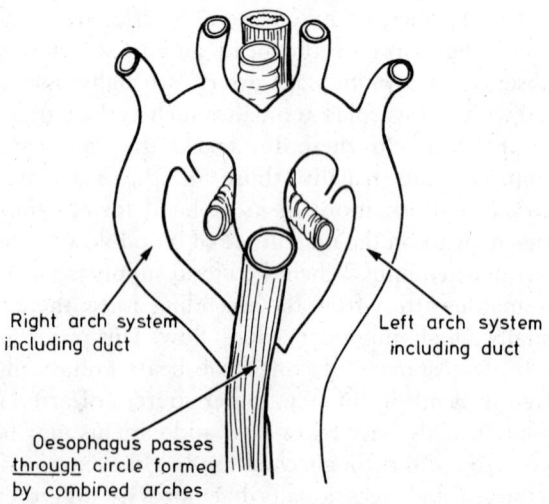

Head, neck and arm arteries have potential to connect to whichever arch system is present

Right arch system including duct

Left arch system including duct

Oesophagus passes through circle formed by combined arches

Fig. 25.77. Diagram showing the hypothetical arrangement of a perfect double aortic arch.

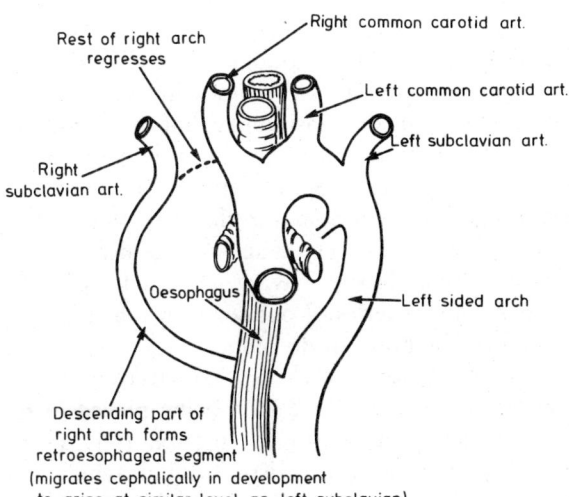

Fig. 25.78. Diagram showing how retro-oesophageal origin of the right subclavian artery is explained on the basis of interruption of a double aortic arch system.

found associated with other congenital malformations. The association with coarctation is an important one, because, if the aberrant and normally connected subclavian arteries are on either side of the coarcted segment, the blood pressure will differ in the two arms and there may be unilateral rib-notching.

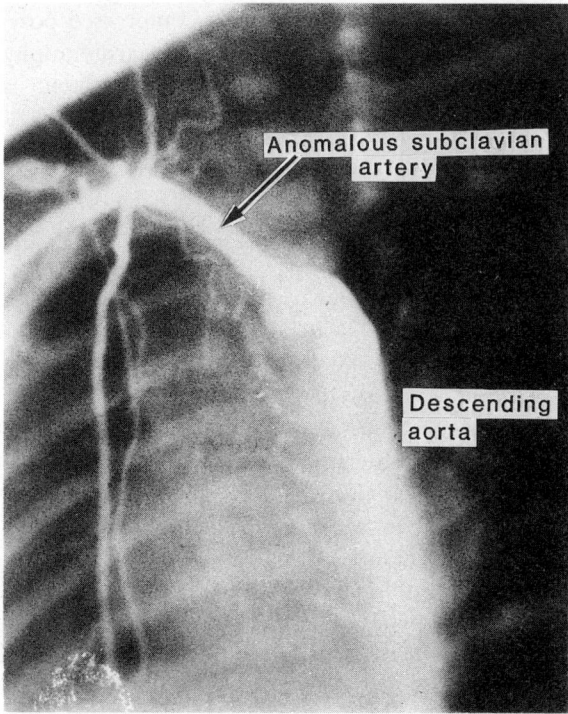

Fig. 25.79. A countercurrent aortogram from a right brachial artery injection showing anomalous origin of the right subclavian artery from the descending aorta.

Aberrant right subclavian artery usually presents with dysphagia, this being the classic cause of 'dysphagia lusoria'. Far more frequently, the condition is asymptomatic, being discovered during gastro-intestinal radiological examination or incidentally at post-mortem. It is possible although uncommon for respiratory distress to be the presenting feature in infants and children. An oesophagogram is the most important diagnostic test. A wedge-shaped impression is seen in lateral projection on the posterior oesophageal wall just at or below the level of the aortic arch. Confirmation by angiography is rarely warranted unless symptoms exist. When symptoms are present, treatment should first be medical using a soft diet. If this is unsuccessful, or if respiratory obstruction is present, surgical division of the aberrant artery should be performed.

A right aortic arch in itself is not uncommon and it is frequently observed with such lesions as tetralogy of Fallot, pulmonary atresia and common arterial trunk. The head and neck arteries are formed in mirror-image pattern, but an arterial duct, when present, is usually a left-sided structure. No vascular ring is produced when there is simply mirror-image branching with a right arch. The symptomatology in such cases is entirely dependent upon the associated congenital malformations. All the aberrant arterial patterns as described above can be found with a right arch or with a left arch. Thus, the most frequently encountered lesions are an aberrant left subclavian artery, an aberrant left brachiocephalic artery and isolation of the left subclavian artery from the aorta.

When the left subclavian artery arises aberrantly from a right arch, the order of arterial branching is left common carotid, right common carotid and then right and left subclavian arteries. As with aberrant right artery, the left subclavian passes behind the oesophagus during its anomalous course forming a partial vascular ring. Persistence of a left-sided arterial duct will connect the aberrant left subclavian to the left pulmonary artery and produce a complete vascular ring. The complete ring frequently causes symptoms. These are mild, and surgery is required in only a small minority. The appearances of oesophagography are the mirror image of those found with aberrant right subclavian artery.

An aberrant left brachiocephalic artery with a right arch is a rare anomaly that is similar to aberrant left subclavian. In the rare cases described, there has always been a left-sided duct and thus a complete vascular ring. Treatment is surgical. Isolation of the left subclavian artery is also a rare condition. The subclavian artery has no attachment to the aortic arch, being fed instead by a patent left-sided duct. It exists in various patterns, all of which can be explained on the basis of the 'hypothetical double arch'.

The most extreme form of vascular ring, of necessity complete, is when both right and left arches persist to encircle the trachea and oesophagus (Fig 25.80). It is a rare malformation. The relative size of the lumens of each arch, the patency of each arch and the side of an arterial duct (if present) are all variable. Usually, the right arch is dominant. A double arch tends to be an isolated anomaly, only one-fifth of patients having associated cardiac lesions. Ventricular septal defect and tetralogy of Fallot are the most frequent. Presence or absence of symptoms depends on the tightness of the compressing ring. Presentation under the age of 2 years is usually due to severe symptoms. Over this age, symptoms are milder or the condition may be discovered by chance. Symptoms, usually occurring shortly after birth, range from mild stridor with wheezing to severe respiratory obstruction, dysp-

noea and cyanosis. Recognition of a double arch from the plain chest radiograph is difficult and oesophagography gives the best results. Aortography confirms the diagnosis and delineates the size of the arches, the arterial pattern and the presence of any atretic segments. Some patients can be treated medically but symptomatic children will almost certainly require surgery. This involves dividing the ring at a suitable site, having identified the major segments and arteries. If one segment is atretic, this should be the point of division.

A cervical aortic arch is characterized by the transverse portion of the arch being placed in the neck rather than within the thorax. It is a rare anomaly that usually is isolated but which can occur with other congenital cardiac lesions. Of the cases described, over half were associated with a descending right aorta. There is variation in anatomy among the few cases described, but all cases have similar presentation and symptomatology. There is a pulsatile supraclavicular mass and symptoms of tracheoesophageal compression have occurred in several cases. There is a thrill and systolic murmur over the mass, compression of which obliterates the femoral pulse. The chest radiograph shows widening of the superior mediastinum on the side of the arch. The trachea may be displaced laterally and is usually compressed posteriorly by the descending aorta. Angiocardiography or aortography defines the lesion. Treatment is necessary only for symptomatic cases. If there is a complete vascular ring, it should be divided.

MISCELLANEOUS CONDITIONS

Endocardial fibro-elastosis is characterized by diffuse thickening of the endocardium. It most frequently affects the left ventricle, but the left atrium, right ventricle and right atrium may be involved.[158] It is found in approximately 1 per 6000 livebirths and in some instances has a familial incidence. The aetiology is unknown but, when a familial incidence is not found, it has been suggested that fetal infection with Coxsackie B virus may be the cause. The affected chamber, usually the left ventricle, is often grossly enlarged with diffuse thickening of the endocardium. The valves are also thickened and, when involved, the tension apparatus is short and deformed. The myocardium is somewhat, but not grossly, thickened and may show evidence of necrosis, calcification or fibrosis. Endocardial fibroelastosis is frequently associated with severe obstructive lesions such as aortic stenosis, aortic

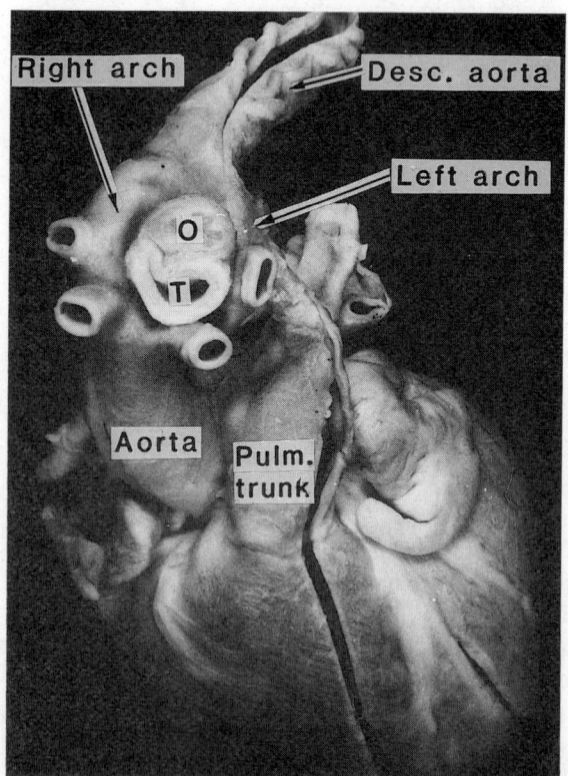

Fig. 25.80. A double aortic arch encircling the tracheo-oesophageal (T,O) pedicle in a patient with tetralogy of Fallot.

atresia or rarely pulmonary stenosis. In this section, we are concerned with the picture of isolated (or primary) fibro-elastosis. In the majority of cases, the onset is during the first 9 months of life. Rarely are symptoms first noted after the age of 1 year. Dyspnoea and poor feeding may be the features noticed first but, more frequently, infants present with the rapid onset of congestive cardiac failure. There is usually clinical evidence of cardiac enlargement but, unless valvar lesions are present, murmurs are absent or unimpressive. A third heart sound and gallop rhythm are usually noted. The chest radiograph shows generalized cardiac enlargement and, when mitral regurgitation is severe, signs of pulmonary venous congestion. Left ventricular hypertrophy is evident on the electrocardiogram. The patients are usually in sinus rhythm, but partial or complete heart block are not infrequently encountered. There may be T-wave inversion or flattened T waves in all the chest leads in the early months of life. Echocardiography demonstrates dilatation of the left ventricle with poor left ventricular function. The thickened endocardium is seen and its tissue character differs markedly from normal. Cardiac catheterization adds little to the diagnosis apart from excluding severe obstructive lesions. Angiocardiography confirms the global left ventricular dysfunction and demonstrates the presence or absence of valvar lesions and other congenital cardiac malformations. Most affected children die in the first year of life. Patients have occasionally died in adult life at which time autopsy confirmation of the diagnosis was obtained. Of these patients diagnosed as endocardial fibro-elastosis by exclusion, a number continue to survive and, in our experience, some appear to improve with age. Supportive treatment of the congestive cardiac failure and prompt treatment of infections are all that can be offered. Approximately half the patients now survive childhood.

ARTERIOVENOUS MALFORMATIONS

Arteriovenous malformations can occur in the systemic or pulmonary circulations. The latter form cause cyanosis and have been dealt with already. Systemic arteriovenous malformations may be single or multiple. They may be located in the brain, neck, limbs, the thoracic wall, the heart or the liver. The most common are those occurring in the brain, which account for approximately one-third of the total. Heart failure may ensue when the arteriovenous communication is large. When located outside the brain or liver, malformations are usually easy to detect by inspection and by hearing a continuous murmur over their site. Those in the brain and liver are more difficult to detect but should be suspected when an infant is in heart failure which has no obvious cardiac cause. The circulation appears hyperkinetic as evidenced by a high-volume or collapsing pulse.[159] Inspection of the neck may reveal prominent pulsation when the lesion is in the brain; hepatomegaly may be present when the liver is the site. As with more superficial arteriovenous malformations, a continuous murmur may be heard over the head or the liver. The diagnosis should be suspected when heart failure is associated with a structurally normal heart on the echocardiograms and when no other cause can be found. Confirmation can be obtained angiographically, but cerebral or abdominal ultrasonography and magnetic resonance imaging should give the diagnosis. Most patients with large malformations, particularly those in the brain, die in infancy. Ligation or clipping or embolization of the feeding arteries is the usual treatment. Little can be done when the malformation is in the liver. In general, results of treatment are disappointing.

ACKNOWLEDGEMENTS

We would like to thank Dr M.L. Rigby for supplying the echocardiograms and Dr E.J. Baker for supplying the magnetic reasonance images. We are also grateful for Dr J.R. Zuberbuhrer for providing the facilities of Childrens Hospital of Pittsburg for photographing many of the specimens.

REFERENCES

1. Carlgren, L.E. The incidence of congenital heart disease in Gothenberg. The Third Edgar Mannheimer Memorial Lecture. *Proc. Ass. Eur. Paed. Card.* 1969; **5**: 2–8.
2. Hoffheinz, H.Z., Glaser, E. and Rodewald, G. Uber die Haufigheit angeborener im Hamburger Sektionsgut. *Zentralbl. Chir.* 1964; **89**: 326–40.
3. Hoffman, J.I.E. and Christianson, R. Congenital heart disease in a cohort of 19,502 births with long-term follow-up. *Am. J. Cardiol.* 1978; **42**: 641–7.
4. Dickinson, D.F., Arnold, R. and Wilkinson, J.L. Congenital heart disease among 160,480 liveborn children in Liverpool 1960 to 1969. Implications for surgical treatment. *Br. Heart J.* 1981; **46**: 55–62.
5. Fyler, D.C., Buckley, L.P., Hellenbrand, W.E. and Cohn, H.E. Report of the New England Regional Infant Cardiac Program. *Pediatrics* 1980; **65** (Suppl.): 375–461.
6. Burn, J. Aetiology of congenital heart disease. In: Anderson, R.H., Macartney, F.J., Shinebourne, E.A. and Tynan, M., eds. *Paediatric Cardiology*, Vol. 1. Edinburgh: Chur-

chill Livingstone, 1987, pp. 15–63.

7. Anderson, R.H., Becker, A.E., Lucchese, F.E., Meier, M.A., Rigby, M.L. and Soto, B. Sequential segmental analysis. *Morphology of Congenital Heart Disease. Angiocardiographic, echocardiographic and surgical correlates.* Tunbridge Wells: Castle House Publications, 1983, pp. 1–22.

8. Anderson, R.H. and Becker, A.E. *Cardiac Anatomy—An Integrated Text and Colour Atlas.* London and Edinburgh: Gower–Churchill Livingstone, 1980.

9. Olley, P.M. and Coceani F. Prostaglandins and the ductus arteriosus. *Ann. Rev. Med.* 1981; 32: 375–85.

10. Dawes, G.S. *Fetal and neonatal physiology.* Chicago: Year Book Medical Publishers, 1968.

11. Rudolph, A. *Congenital Diseases of the Heart.* Chicago: Year Book Medical Publishers, 1974.

12. Haworth, S.G. Pulmonary vasculature. In: Anderson, R.H. Macartney, F.J., Shinebourne, E.A., and Tynan, M., eds. *Paediatric Cardiology*, Vol. 1. Edinburgh: Churchill Livingstone, 1987, pp. 123–58.

13. Feldt, R.H., Strickler, G.B. and Weidman W.H. Growth of children with congenital heart disease. *Am. J. Dis. Child,* 1969; 117: 573–77.

14. Messmer, B.J., Schallberger, U., Gattiker, R. and Senning, A. Psychomotor and intellectual development after deep hypothermia and circulatory arrest in early infancy. *J. Thor. Card. Surg.* 1976; 72: 495–502.

15. Haka-Ikse K, Blackwood, M.J.A. and Steward, D.J. Psychomotor development of infants and children after profound hypothermia during surgery for congenital heart disease. *Dev. Med. Child. Neurol.* 1978; 20: 62–70.

16. Phornphutkul, C., Rosenthal, A., Madas, A.S. and Berenberg, W. Cerebrovascular accidents in infants and children with cyanotic congenital heart disease. *Am. J. Cardiol.* 1973; 32: 329–34.

17. Fishbein, C.A., Rosenthal, A., Fischer, E.G., Madas, A.S. and Welch, K. Risk factors for brain abscess in patients with congenital heart disease. *Am. J. Cardiol.* 1974; 34: 97–102.

18. Newfeld, E.A., Paul, M.H., Muster, A.J. and Idriss, F.S. Pulmonary vascular disease in complete transposition of the great arteries. A study of 200 cases. *Am. J. Cardiol.* 1974; 34: 75–80.

19. Anderson, R.H., Macartney, F.J., Shinebourne, E.A. and Tynan, M. History and physical examination. In: *Paediatric Cardiology* Vol. 1. Edinburgh: Churchill Livingstone, 1987, pp. 183–90.

20. Elseed, A.M., Shinebourne, E.A. and Joseph, M.C. Assessment of techniques for measurement of blood pressure in infants and children. *Arch. Dis. Child.* 1973; 48: 932–36.

21. Garson, A. Electrocardiography. In: Anderson, R.H., Macartney, F.J., Shinebourne, E.A. and Tynan, M., eds. *Paediatric Cardiology*, Vol. 1. Edinburgh: Churchill Livingstone, 1987, pp. 235–318.

22. Huhta, J.C., Smallhorn, J.F. and Macartney, F.J. Two dimensional echocardiographic diagnosis of situs. *Br. Heart J.* 1982; 48: 97–108.

23. Silverman, N.H., Hunter, S., Anderson, R.H., Ho S.Y., Sutherland, G.R. and Davies, M.J. Anatomical basis of cross sectional echocardiography. *Br. Heart J.* 1983; 50: 421–30.

24. Hatle, L., Angelsen, B. and Tromsdal, A. Non invasive assessment of aortic stenosis by Doppler ultrasound. *Br. Heart J.* 1980; 43: 284–93.

25. Baker, E.J., Ellam, S.V., Lorber, A., Jones, O.D.H., Tynan, M.J. and Maisey, M.N. Superiority of radionuclide over oximetry measurement of left to right shunts. *Br. Heart J.* 1985; 53: 535–40.

26. Parrish, M.D., Graham, J.P.Jr, Born, M.L. and Jones, J. Radionuclide evaluation of right and left ventricular

function in children: validation of methodology. *Am. J. Cardiol.* 49; 1241–47.

27. Baker, E.J., Malamitsi, J., Jones, O.D.H., Maisey, M.N. and Tynan, M.J. Use of radionuclide labelled microspheres to show the distribution of the pulmonary perfusion with multifocal pulmonary blood supply. *Br. Heart J.* 1984; 52: 72–6.

28. Hofstetter, R., Land, E. and Von Bernuth, G. Effect of digoxin on left ventricular contractility in newborns and infants estimated by echocardiography. *Eur. J. Cardiol.* 1979; 9: 1–11.

29. Myberg, L. and Wettrell, G. Digoxin dosage schedules for neonates and infants based on pharmacokinetic considerations. *Clinical Pharmacokinetics*, 1978; 3: 453–61.

30. Heymann, M.A. and Rudolph, A.M. Ductus arteriosus dilatation by prostaglandin E in infants with pulmonary atresia. *Paediatrics*, 1977; 59: 325–9.

31. Garson, A.Jr, Williams, R.B.Jr. and Reckless, J. Long-term follow-up of patients with tetralogy of Fallot: physical health and psychopathology. *J. Pediatr.* 1974; 85: 429–33.

32. Baker, E.J. Valvoplasty, angioplasty and embolotherapy in congenital heart disease. (Editorial review). *Int. J. Cardiol.* 1986; 12: 139–45.

33. Winter, F.S. Persistent left superior vena cava: a survey of world literature and report of 30 additional cases. *Angiology*, 1954; 5: 90–132.

34. DeLisle, G. Ando, M., Calder, A.L., Zuberbuhler, J.R., Rochenmacher, S., Alday L.E., Mangino, O., Van Praagh, S. and Van Praagh, R. Total anomalous pulmonary venous connection: report of 93 autopsied cases with emphasis on diagnostic and surgical considerations. *Am. Heart J.* 1976; 91: 99–122.

35. Gathman, G.E. and Nadas, A.S. Total anomalous pulmonary venous connection. Clinical and physiological observations of 75 pediatric patients. *Circulation* 1970; 42: 143–54.

36. Huhta, J.C., Gutgesell, H.P. and Nihill, M.R. Cross sectional echocardiographic diagnosis of total anomalous pulmonary venous connection. *Br. Heart J.* 1985; 53: 525–34.

37. Stark, J., Smallhorn, J., Huhta, J., de Leval M., Macartney F.J., Rees, P.G. and Taylor, J.F.M. Surgery for congenital heart defects diagnosed with cross-sectional echocardiography. *Circulation*, 1983; 68: II:129–38.

38. Neill, C.A., Ferencz, C., Sabiston, D.C. and Sheldon, H. The familial occurrence of hypoplastic right lung with systemic arterial supply and venous drainage "scimitar syndrome". *Johns Hopkins Med. J.* 1960; 107: 1–15.

39. Gasul, B.M., Arcilla, R.A. and Lev, M. Cor triatriatum. In: *Heart Disease in Children*. Philadelphia: J.B. Lippincott Company, 1966, pp. 869–81.

40. Ostman-Smith, I., Silverman, M.H., Oldershaw, P., Lincoln, C. and Shinebourne, E.A. Cor triatriatum sinistrum. Diagnostic features on cross-sectional echocardiography. *Br. Heart J.* 1984; 51: 211–19.

41. Anderson, R.H., Macartney, F.J., Shinebourne, E.A. and Tynan, M. Atrial isomerism. In: *Paediatric Cardiology*, Vol. I. Edinburgh: Churchill Livingstone, 1987, pp. 473–95.

42. Partridge, J.B., Scott, O., Deverall, P.B. and Macartney, F.J. Visualization and measurement of the main bronchi by tomography as an objective indicator of thoracic situs in congenital heart disease. *Circulation*, 1975; 51: 188–96.

43. Kirklin, J.W. and Barratt-Boyes, B.G. Atrial isomerism. In: *iac Surgery. Morphology, Diagnostic Criteria, Natural History, Techniques, Results, and Indications.* New York: John Wiley & Sons, 1986, pp. 1333–46.

44. Weidman, W.H., Swan, H.J.C., DuShane, J.W. and Wood, E.H. A hemodynamic study of atrial septal defect and associated anomalies involving the atrial septum. *J. Lab.*

Clin. Med. 1957; **50**: 165–85.

45. Bizarro, R.O., Callaghan, J.A., Feldt R.H., Kurland, L.T., Gordon, H. and Brandenburg, R.O. Familial atrial septal defect with prolonged atrioventricular conduction: a syndrome showing the autosomal dominant pattern of inheritance. *Circulation,* 1970; **41**: 677–83.

46. Seward, J.B., Tajik, A.J., Spangler, J.G. and Ritter, D.G. Echocardiographic contrast studies: initial experience. *Mayo Clin. Proc.* 1975; **50**: 163–69.

47. Wood, P. *Diseases of the Heart and Circulation.* London: Eyre and Spottiswood, 1956, pp. 362.

48. Bierman, F.Z. and Williams, R.G. Subxyphoid two-dimensional imaging of the interatrial septum in infants and neonates with congenital heart disease. *Circulation,* 1979; **60**: 80–90.

49. Kirklin, J.W. and Barratt-Boyes, B.G. Atrial septal defect and partial anomalous pulmonary venous connection. In: *Cardiac Surgery, Morphology, Diagnostic Criteria, Natural History, Techniques, Results, and Indications.* New York: John Wiley & Sons, 1986, pp. 463–98.

50. Rashkind, W.J. Interventional cardiac catheterization in congenital heart disease. *Int. J. Cardiol.* 1985, 7: 1–11.

51. Haworth, S.G. Pulmonary vascular disease in different types of congenital heart disease: implications for interpretation of lung biopsy findings in early childhood. *Br. Heart J.* 1984; **52**: 557–71.

52. Toscano-Barbosa, E., Brandenburg, R.U. and Burchell, H.B. Electrocardiographic studies of cases with intracardiac malformations of the atrioventricular canal. *Proc. Staff Meet. Mayo Clin.* 1956; **31**: 513–23.

53. Anderson, R.H., Becker, A.E., Lucchese, F.A., Meier, M.A., Rigby, M.L. and Soto, B. *Morphology of Congenital Heart Disease. Angiocardiographic, echocardiographic and surgical correlates.* Tunbridge Wells: Castle House Publications Ltd, 1983, 65–83.

54. Soto, B., Bargeron, L.M.Jr, Pacifico, A.D., Vanini, V. and Kirklin, J.W. Angiography of atrioventricular canal defects. *Am. J. Cardiol.* 1981; **48**: 492–9.

55. Mavroudis, C., Weinstein, G., Turley, K. and Ebert, P.A. Surgical management of complete atrioventricular canal. *J. Thorac. Cardiovasc. Surg.* 1982; **83**: 670–9.

56. Soto, B., Becker, A.E., Moulaert, A.J., Lie, J.T. and Anderson, R.H. Classification of ventricular septal defects. *Br. Heart J.* 1980; **43**: 332–43.

57. Corone, P., Doyen, F., Gaudeau, S., Guerin, F., Vernant, P., Ducam, H., Rumeau-Rouquette, C. and Gaudeul, P. Natural history of ventricular septal defect. A study involving 790 cases. *Circulation,* 1977; **55**: 908–15.

58. Baker, E., Leung, M.P., Anderson, R.H., Fischer, D.R. and Zuberbuhler, J.R. The cross-sectional anatomy of ventricular septal defects: a reappraisal. *Br. Heart J.* 1988; **59**: 339–51.

59. Macartney, F.J., Taylor, J.F.N., Graham, G.R., de Leval, M. and Stark, J. The fate of survivors in cardiac surgery in infancy. *Circulation,* 1980; **62**: 80–91.

60. Anderson, R.H., Wilkinson, J.L., Gerlis, L.M., Smith, A. and Becker, A.E. Atresia of the right atrioventricular orifice. *Br. Heart J.* 1977; **39**: 414–28.

61. Vlad, P. Tricuspid atresia. In: Keith, J.D., Rowe, R.D. and Vlad, P., eds. *Heart Disease in Infancy and Childhood.* 3rd. Edition. New York: Macmillan Publishing Co. Inc., 1978, pp. 518–41.

62. Rao, P.S. The natural history of ventricular septal defect in tricuspid atresia. In: Rao, P.S., ed. *Tricuspid Atresia.* Mount Kisco, New York: Futura Publishing Company, 1982, pp. 201–29.

63. Sutherland, G.R., Godman, M.J., Anderson, R.H. and Hunter S. The spectrum of atrioventricular valve atresia: A two-dimensional echocardiographic/pathological correlation. In: Rijsterborgh, H., ed. *Echocardiology.* The Hague,

Boston, London: Martinus Nijhoff Publishers, 1981, pp. 345–53.

64. Fontan, F., Deville, C., Quaegebeur, J., Ottenkamp, J., Sourdille, N., Choussat, A. and Brom, G.A. Repair of tricuspid atresia in 100 patients. *J. Thorac. Cardiovasc. Surg.* 1983; **85**: 647–60.

65. Finley, J.P., Howman-Giles, R.B., Gilday, D.L. and Rowe R.D. Transient myocardial ischaemia of the newborn infant demonstrated by thallium myocardial imaging. *J. Pediatr.* 1979; **94**: 263–70.

66. Zuberbuhler, J.R., Allwork, S.P. and Anderson, R.H. The spectrum of Ebstein's anomaly of the tricuspid valve. *J. Thorac. Cardiovasc. Surg.* 1979; **77**: 202–11

67. Becker, A.E., Anderson, R.H., Durrer, D. and Wellens, H.J.J. The anatomical substrates of Wolff-Parkinson-White Syndrome: a clinico-pathologic correlation in seven patients. *Circulation,* 1978: 57: 870–79

68. Fischer Hansen, J., Leth, A., Dorph, S. and Wennevold, A. The prognosis in Ebstein's disease of the heart. Long-term follow-up of 22 patients. *Acta Med. Scand.* 1977; **201**: 331–35.

69. Silverman, N.H. and Birk, E. Ebstein's malformation of the tricuspid valve: cross sectional echocardiography and Doppler. In: Anderson, R.H., Neches, W.H., Park, S.C. and Zuberbuhler, J.R., eds. *Perspectives in Pediatric Cardiology,* Vol. I. Mount Kisco, New York: Futura Publishing Company Inc., 1988, pp. 113–25

70. Kirkin, J.W. and Barratt-Boyes, B.G., Ebstein's malformation. In: *Cardiac Surgery. Morphology, Diagnostic criteria, Natural History, Techniques, Results, and Indications.* New York: John Wiley & Sons, 1986, pp. 889–910.

71. Becker, A.E. Valve pathology in the paediatric age group. In: Anderson, R.H., Macartney, F.J., Shinebourne, E.A. and Rynan, M., eds. *Paediatric Cardiology,* Vol. 5. Edinburgh: Churchill Livingstone Edinburgh, 1983, pp. 345–60.

72. Carpentier, A., Branchini, B., Cour, J.C., Asfaou, E., Villani, M., Deloche, A., Relland, J., D'Allaines, C.L., Blondeau, P. and Piwnica, A. Congenital malformations of the mitral valve in children. Pathology and surgical treatment. *J. Thorac. Cardiovasc. Surg.* 1976; **72**: 854–66.

73. Mickell, J.J., Mathews, R.A., Anderson, R.H., Zuberbuhler, J.R., Lenox, C.C., Neches, W.H., Park, S.C. and Fricker, J.J. The anatomical heterogeneity of hearts lacking a patent communication between the left atrium and the ventricular mass ('mistral atresia') in presence of a patent aortic valve. *Eur. Heart J.* 1983; **4**: 477–86. F.J., Neches, W.H. and Zuberbuhler, J.R. Left atrioventricular valve atresia: clinical management. *Circulation,* 1980; **61**: 123–27

74. Gittenberger-de-Groot, A.C. and Wenink, A.C.G. Mitral atresia: morphological details. *Br. Heart. J.* 1984; **51**: 252–8.

75. Norwood, W.I., Lang, P. and Hansen, D.D. Physiologic repair of the aortic atresia-hypoplastic left heart syndrome. *New Engl. J. Med.* 1983; **308**: 23–6.

76. Mickell, J.J., Mathews, R.A., Park, S.C., Lenox, C.C., Fricker, F.J., Neches, W.H. and Zuberbuhler, J.R. Left atrioventricular valve atresia: clinical management. *Circulation,* 1980; **61**: 123–7.

77. Becker, A.E., Connor, M. and Anderson, R.H. Tetralogy of Fallot: a morphometric and geometric study. *Am. J. Cardiol.* 1975; **35**: 402–12.

78. Wood, P. Attacks of deeper cyanosis and loss of consciousness (syncope) in Fallot's tetralogy. *Br. Heart. J.* 1958; **20**: 282–6.

79. Anderson, R.H., Macartney, F.J., Shinebourne, E.A. and Tynan, M. Fallot's tetralogy. In: *Paediatric Cardiology,* Vol. 2. Edinburgh: Churchill Livingstone, 1987, pp. 765–98.

80. Soto, B., Pacifico, A.D., Ceballos, R. and Bargeron, L.M.Jr. Tetralogy of Fallot: an angiographic-pathologic correlative study. *Circulation*, 1981; **64**: 558–66.

81. Shinebourne, E.A., Anderson, R.H. and Bowyer, J.J. Variations in clinical presentation of Fallot's tetralogy. Angiographic and pathogenetic implications. *Br. Heart J.* 1975; **37**: 946–55.

82. Kirklin, J.W. and Barratt-Boyes, G.C. Ventricular septal defect and pulmonary stenosis or atresia. In: *Cardiac Surgery. Morphology, Diagnostic Criteria, Natural History, Techniques, Results, and Indications*. New York: John Wiley & Sons, 1986, pp. 699–820.

83. Vogt, J., Wesselhoeft, H., Luig, H., Schmitz, L., De Vivie, E.R., Weber, H. and Beuren, A.J. The preoperative and postoperative findings in 627 patients with tetralogy of Fallot. *Thorac. Cardiovasc. Surgeon*, 1984; **32**: 234–43.

84. Wilkinson, J.L. Double outlet ventricle. In: Anderson R.H., Macartney, F.J., Shinebourne, E.A. and Tynan, M., eds. *Paediatric Cardiology*, Vol. 2. Edinburgh: Churchill Livingstone, 1987, pp. 889–911.

85. Wilkinson, J.L., Wilcox, B.R. and Anderson, R.H. Anatomy of double outlet right ventricle. In: Anderson, F.J., Macartney, F.J., Shinebourne, E.A. and Tynan, M., eds. *Paediatric Cardiology*, Vol. 5. Edinburgh: Churchill Livingstone, 1983, pp. 397–407.

86. Sridaromont, S., Feldt, R.H., Ritter, D.G., Davis, G.D. and Edwards, J.E. Double outlet right ventricle. Hemodynamic and anatomic correlations. *Am. J. Cardiol.* 1976; **38**: 85–94.

87. Anderson, R.H., Becker, A.E., Lucchese, F.E., Meier, M.A., Rigby, M.L. and Soto, B. Double outlet right ventricle. In: *Morphology of Congenital Heart Disease. Angiocardiographic, echocardiographic and surgical correlates*. Tunbridge Wells: Castle House Publications Ltd., 1983, pp. 51-64.

88. Kirklin, J.W. and Barratt-Boyes, B.G. Double outlet right ventricle. In: *Cardiac Surgery. Morphology, Diagnostic Criteria, Natural History, Techniques, Results and Indications*. New York: John Wiley & Sons, 1986, pp. 1219–50.

89. Taussig, H.B. and Bing, R.J. Complete transposition of the aorta and a Levoposition of the pulmonary artery. Clinical, physiological and pathological findings. *Am. Heart J.* 1949; **37**: 551–59.

90. Sharratt, G.P., Sbokos, C.G., Johnson, A.M., Anderson, R.H. and Monro, J.L. Surgical "correction" of solitus-concordant, double-outlet left ventricle with l-malposition of tricuspid stenosis with hypoplastic right ventricle. *J. Thor. Card. Surg.* 1976; **71**: 853–8.

91. Liebman, J., Cullum, L. and Belloc, N. Natural history of transposition of the great arteries. Anatomy, birth history and death characteristics. *Circulation* 1969; **40**: 237–62.

92. Carr, I., Tynan, M.J., Aberdeen, E., Bonham-Carter, R.E., Graham, G., Waterstone, D.J. Predictive accuracy of the loop-hole in 109 children with classic complete transposition of the great arteries (Abstract). *Circulation* 1968; **38** (Suppl. I), 52.

93. Anderson, R.H., Macartney, F.J., Shinebourne, E.A. and Tynan, M. Complete Transposition. In: *Paediatric Cardiology*, Vol. 2. Edinburgh: Churchill Livingstone, 1987, pp. 829–65.

94. Tynan, M.J. Transposition of the great arteries: changes in the circulation after birth. *Circulation*, 1972; **46**: 809–15.

95. Rabinovitch, M., Haworth, S.G., Castaneda, A.R., Nadas, A.S. and Reid, L.M. Lung biopsy in congenital heart disease: a morphometric approach to pulmonary vascular disease. *Circulation*, 1978; **58**: 1107–21.

96. Daskalopoulos, D.A., Edwards, W.D., Driscoll, D.J., Seward, J.B., Tajik, A.J. and Hagler, D.J. Correlation of two-dimensional echocardiographic and autopsy findings in complete transposition of the great arteries. *J. Am. Coll. Cardiol.* 1983; **2**: 1151–7.

97. Rashkind, W.J. and Miller, W.W. Creation of an atrial septal defect without thoracotomy. A palliative approach to complete transposition of great arteries. *JAMA*, 1966; **196**: 991–2.

98. Baker, E.J., Allan, L.D., Tynan, M.J., Jones, O.D.H., Joseph, M.C. and Deverall, P.B. Balloon atrial septostomy in the neonatal intensive care unit. *Br. Heart J.* 1984; **51**: 377–8.

99. Yacoub, M., Keck, E. and Radley-Smith, R. An evaluation of one and two stage anatomic correction of simple transposition of the great arteries. (Abstract). *Circulation*, 1983; **68**: III–48.

100. Mustard, W.T., Keith, J.D., Trusler, G.A., Fowler, R. and Kidd, L. The surgical management of transposition of the great vessels. *J. Thorac. Cardiovasc. Surg.* 1964; **48**: 953–8.

101. Senning, A. Surgical correction of transposition of the great arteries. *Surgery*, 1959; **45**: 966–80.

102. Quaegebeur, J.M., Rohmer, J., Ottenkamp, J., Buis, T., Kirklin, J.W., Blackstone, E.H. and Brom, A.G. The arterial switch operation: An eight-year experience. *J. Thorac. Cardiovasc. Surg.* 1986; **92**: 361–84.

103. Kirklin, J.W. and Blackstone, E.H. Current management of patients with complete transposition. In: Anderson, R.H., Neches, W.H., Park, S.C. and Zuberbuhler, J.R., eds. *Perspectives in Pediatric Cardiology*, Vol. I. Mount Kisco, New York: Futura Publishing Company Inc., 1988, pp. 281–95.

104. Losekoot, T.G., Anderson, R.H., Becker, A.E., Danielson, G.K. and Soto, B. *Congenitally Corrected Transposition*. Edinburgh: Churchill Livingstone, 1983.

105. Becker, A.E. and Anderson, R.H. The atrioventricular conduction tissues in congenitally corrected transposition. In: Van Mierop, L.H.S., Oppenheimer-Dekker, A. and Ch Bruins, C.L.D., eds. *Embryology and Teratology of the Heart and the Great Arteries*. (Boerhaave Course 13). The Hague: Leiden University Press, 1978, pp. 79–87.

106. Anderson, R.C., Lillehei, C.W. and Lester, R.G. Corrected transposition of the great vessels of the heart, a review of 17 cases. *Paediatrics*, 1957; **20**: 626-46.

107. Sutherland, G.R., Smallhorn, J.F., Anderson, R.H., Rigby, M.L. and Hunter, S. Atrioventricular discordance. Cross-sectional echocardiographic-morphological correlative study. *Br. Heart J.* 1983; **50**: 8–20.

108. Soto, B, Bargeron, L.M.Jr, Bream, P.R. and Elliott, L.P. Conditions with atrioventricular discordance—angiographic study. In: Anderson, E.H. and Shinebourne, E.A., eds. *Paediatric Cardiology*, 1977. Edinburgh: Churchill Livingstone, 1978, pp. 207–21.

109. Danielson, G.K. Surgical treatment of atrioventricular discordance. In: Losekoot, T.G., Anderson, R.H., Becker, A.E., Soto, B. and Danielson, G.K., eds. *Congenitally Corrected Transposition*. Edinburgh: Churchill Livingstone, 1983, pp. 177–90.

110. De Leval, M., Bastos, P., Stark, J., Taylor, J.F.N., Macartney, F.J. and Anderson, R.H. Surgical technique to reduce the risks of heart block following closure of ventricular septal defect in atrioventricular discordance. *J. Thor. Card. Surg.* 1979; **78**: 515–26.

111. Anderson, R.H., Macartney, F.J., Tynan, M., Becker, A.E., Freeman, R.M., Godman, M.J. and Hunter, S. *et al.* Univentricular atrioventricular connection: the single ventricle trap unsprung. *Ped. Cardiol.* 1983; **4**: 272–80.

112. Rigby, M.L., Anderson, R.H., Gibson, D., Jones, O.D.H., Joseph, M.C. and Shinebourne, E.A. Two-dimensional echocardiographic categorisation of the univentricular heart. Ventricular morphology, type, and mode of atrioventricular connection. *Br. Heart. J.* 1981; **46**: 603–12.

113. Anderson, R.H., Crupi, G. and Parenzan, L. Double Inlet Ventricle. *Anatomy, Diagnosis and Surgical Management*. Tunbridge Wells: Castle House Publications Ltd., 1987.

114. Hagler, D.J., Tajik, A.J. Seward, J.B., Mair, D.D. and Ritter, D.G. Wide-angle two-dimensional echocardiographic profiles of conotruncal abnormalities. *Mayo Clin. Proc.* 1980; 55: 73–82.

115. Marcelletti, C., McGoon, D.C., Danielson, G.K., Wallace, R.B. and Mair, D.D. Early and late results of surgical repair of truncus arteriosus. *Circulation*, 1977; 55: 636–41.

116. Parenzan, L., Crupi, G., Alfieri, O., Bianchi, T., Vanini, V., Locatelli, G., Tiraboschi, R., Di Benedetto, G., Villani, M. et al. Surgical repair of persistent truncus arteriosus in infancy. *Thorac. Cardiovasc. Surgeon.* 1980; 28: 18–20.

117. Zuberbuhler, J.R., Fricker, F.J., Park, S.C., Anderson, R.H., Lenox, C.C., Neches, W.H. and Mathews, R.A. Pulmonary atresia with intact ventricular septum: morbid anatomy. In: Goodman, M.J. and Marquis, R.M., eds. *Paediatric Cardiology*, Vol. 2. *Heart Disease in the Newborn*. Edinburgh: Churchill Livingstone, 1979, pp. 285–96.

118. Freedom, R.M. and Harrington, D.P. Contribution of intramyocardial sinusoids in pulmonary atresia and intact ventricular septum to a right sided circular shunt. *Br. Heart J.* 1974; 36: 1061–5.

119. Macartney, F.J., Deverall, P.B. and Scott, O. Haemodynamic characteristics of systemic arterial blood supply to the lungs. *Br. Heart J.* 1973; 35: 28–37.

120. Singh, S.P., Rigby, M.L. and Astley, R. Demonstrations of pulmonary arteries by contrast injection into pulmonary vein. *Br. Heart J.* 1978; 40: 7.

121. Alfieri, O., Blackstone, E.H., Kirklin, J.W., Pacifico, A.D. and Bargeron, L.M.Jr. Surgical treatment of tetralogy of Fallot with pulmonary atresia. *J. Thorac. Cardiovasc. Surg.* 1978; 76: 321–35.

122. Koretzky, E.D., Moller, J.H., Korns, M.E., Schwartz, C.J. and Edwards, J.E. Congenital pulmonary stenosis resulting from dysplasia of valve. *Circulation*, 1969; 40: 43–53.

123. Weyman, A.E., Dillon, J.C., Feigenbaum, H. and Chang, S. Echocardiographic patterns of pulmonary valve motion in valvular pulmonary stenosis. *Am. J. Cardiol.* 1974; 34: 644–51.

124. Nugent, E.W., Freedom, R.M., Nora, J.J., Ellison, R.C., Rowe, R.D. and Nadas, A.S. Clinical course in pulmonary stenosis. *Circulation*, 1977; 56: I.38–46.

125. Kan, J.S., White, R.I., Mitchell, S.E. and Gardner, T.J. Percutaneous balloon valvuloplasty: a new method for treating congenital pulmonary-valve stenosis. *New Engl. J. Med.* 1982; 307: 540–2.

126. Tynan, M., Baker, E.J., Rohmer, J., Jones, O.D.H., Reidy, J.F., Joseph, M.C. and Ottenkamp, J. Percutaneous balloon pulmonary valvuloplasty. *Br. Heart J.* 1985; 53: 520–4.

127. Somerville, J. Aortic stenosis and incompetence. In: Anderson, R.H., Macartney, F.J., Shinebourne, E.A. and Tynan, M., eds. *Paediatric Cardiology*, Vol. 2. Edinburgh: Churchill Livingstone, 1987, pp. 977–99.

128. Rupprath, G. and Neuhaus, K.L. Percutaneous balloon valvuloplasty for aortic stenosis in infancy. *Am. J. Cardiol.* 1985; 55: 1655–6.

129. Williams, J.C.P., Barratt-Boyes, B.G. and Lowe, J.B. Supravalvular aortic stenosis. *Circulation*, 1961; 24: 1311–8.

130. Hossack, K.F., Neutze, J.M., Lowe, J.B. and Barratt-Boyes, B.G. Congenital valvar aortic stenosis. Natural history and assessment for operation. *Br. Heart J.* 1980; 43: 561–5.

131. Kirklin, J.W. and Barratt-Bóyes, B.G. Congenital aortic stenosis. In: *Cardiac Surgery. Morphology, Diagnostic*

Criteria, Natural History, Techniques, Results, and Indications. New York: John Wiley & Sons, 1987, 971–1012.

132. Lababidi, Z., Wu, J. and Walls, J.T. Percutaneous aortic valvuloplasty: results in 23 patients. *Am. J. Cardiol.* 1984; 53: 194–7.

133. Gittenberger-de-Groot, A.C., Moulaert, A.J., Harinck E. and Becker, A.E. Histopathology of the ductus arteriosus after prostaglandin E1 administration in ductus dependent cardiac anomalies. *Br. Heart J.* 1978; 40: 215–20.

134. Heymann, M.A., Rudolph, A.M. and Silverman, N.H. Closure of the ductus arteriosus in premature infants by inhibition of prostaglandin synthesis. *N. Engl. J. Med.* 1976; 295: 530–3.

135. Olley, P.M. Coceani, F. and Bodach, E. E-type prostaglandins. A new emergency therapy for certain cyanotic congenital heart malformations. *Circulation*, 1976; 53: 728–31.

136. Gibson, G.A. *Diseases of the Heart and Aorta*. Edinburgh: Pentland, 1898, pp. 61, 303, 310–12.

137. Heymann, M.A. and Rudolph, A.M. Control of the ductus arteriosus. *Physiol Rev.* 1975; 55: 62–77.

138. Gersony, W.M., Peckham, G.S., Ellison, R.C., Meittenen, O.S. and Nadas, A.S. Effects of indomethacin in premature infants with patent ductus arteriosus: results of a national collaborative study. *J. Pediatr.* 1983; 102: 895–906.

139. Rashkind, W.J., Mullins, C.E., Hellenbrand, W.E. and Tait, M.A. Non-surgical closure of patent ductus arteriosus: clinical application of the rashkind P.D.A. occluder system. *Circulation*, 1987; 75: 583-92.

140. Porstmann, W., Wierny, L., Warnke, H., Gerstberger, G. and Romaniuk, P.A. Catheter closure of patent ductus arteriosus. 62 cases treated without thoracotomy. *Rad. Clinics Nth. America* 1971; 9: 203–18.

141. Smallhorn, J.F., Anderson, R.H. and Macartney, F.J. Two dimensional echocardiographic assessment of communications between ascending aorta and pulmonary trunk or individual pulmonary arteries. *Br. Heart J.* 1982; 47: 563-72.

142. Deverall, P.B., Aberdeen, E., Bonham-Carter, R.E. and Waterston, D.J. Aorticopulmonary window. *J. Thorac. Cardiovasc. Surg.* 1969; 57: 479–86.

143. Crafoord, C. and Nylin, G. Congenital coarctation of the aorta and its surgical treatment. *J. Thorac. Cardiovasc. Surg.* 1945; 14: 347–50.

144. Sinha, S.N., Kardatzke, M.L., Cole, R.B., Muster, A.J., Wessel, H.U. and Paul, M.J. Coarctation of the aorta in infancy. *Circulation*, 1969; 40: 385–98.

145. Huhta, J.C., Gutgesell, H.P., Latson, L.A. and Huffines, F.D. Two-dimensional echocardiographic assessment of aorta in infants and children with congenital heart disease. *Circulation*, 1984; 70: 417–24.

146. Kirklin, J.W. and Barratt-Boyes, B.G. Coarctation of the aorta and aortic arch interruptions. In: *Cardiac Surgery. Morphology, Diagnostic Criteria, Natural History, Techniques, Results, and Indications*. New York: John Wiley & Sons, 1986, pp. 1035–80.

147. Tynan, M. Balloon angioplasty in congenital heart disease. *Herz* 1988; 13: 59–70.

148. Morrow, W.R., Vick, G.W., Nihill, M.R., Rokey, B., Johnston, D.L., Hedrick, T. and Mullins, C.E. Balloon dilation of unoperated coarctation of the aorta: short and intermediate term results. *J. Am. Coll. Cardiol.* 1988; 11: 133–8.

149. Smallhorn, J.F., Anderson, R.H. and Macartney, F.J. Cross-sectional echocardiographic recognition of interruption of aortic arch between left carotid and subclavian arteries. *Br. Heart J.* 1982; 48: 229–35.

150. Norwood, W.I., Lang, P., Castaneda, A.R. and Hougen, T.J. Reparative operations for interrupted aortic arch with ventricular septal defect. *J. Thorac. Cardiovasc. Surg.*

1983; **86**: 832–7.

151. Becker, A.E. Congenital malformations of the coronary arteries. In: Anderson, R.H., Neches, W.H., Park, S.C. and Zuberbuhler, J.R., eds. *Perspectives in Pediatric Cardiology*, Vol. 1. Mount Kisco, New York: Futura Publishing Company, Inc., 1988, pp. 369–77.

152. Perry, L.W. and Scott, L.P. Anomalous left coronary artery from pulmonary artery: report of 11 cases, review of indication for and results of surgery. *Circulation* 1970; **41**: 1043–50.

153. King, D.H., Danford, D.A., Huhta, J.C. and Gutgesell, H.P. Noninvasive detection of anomalous origin of the left main coronary artery from the pulmonary trunk by pulsed Doppler echocardiography. *Am. J. Cardiol.* 1985; **55**: 608–9.

154. Siewers, R.D. Origin of the left coronary artery from the pulmonary trunk: clinical spectrum and operative management. In: Anderson, R.H., Neches, W.H., Park, S.C. and Zuberbuhler, J.R., eds. *Perspectives in Pediatric Cardiology*, Vol. 1. Mount Kisco, New York: Futura Publishing Company Inc. 1988, pp. 405–10.

155. Neches, W.H. Kawasaki syndrome. In: Anderson, R.H., Neches, W.H., Park, S.C. and Zuberbuhler, J.R., eds. *Perspectives in Pediatric Cardiology*, Vol. 1. Mount Kisco, New York: Futura Publishing Company Inc., 1988, pp. 411–24.

156. Park, S.C. and Zuberbuhler, J.R. Vascular ring and pulmonary sling. In: Anderson R.H., Macartney F.J., Shinebourne E.A., Tynan M., eds. *Paediatric Cardiology*, Vol. 2. Edinburgh: Churchill Livingstone, 1987, pp. 1123–36.

157. White, R.I. Jr, Ursic, T.A., Kaufman, S.L, Barth, K.H., Kim, W. and Gross, G.S. Therapeutic embolisation with detachable balloons: physical factors influencing permanent occlusion. *Radiology*, 1978; **126**: 521–3.

158. Losekoot, T.G. and Becker, A.E. Primary endocardial fibroelastosis. In: Anderson, R.H., Macartney, F.J., Shinebourne, E.A. and Tynan, M., eds. *Paediatric Cardiology*, Vol. 2. Edinburgh: Churchill Livingstone, 1987, pp. 1223–8.

159. Rowe, G.G., Castillo, C.A., Alfonso, S. and Crumpton, C.W. The systemic and coronary hemodynamic effect of arteriovenous fistulas. *Am. Heart. J.* 1962; **64**: 44–9.

Chapter 26

Aortic Stenosis

Roger Hall

INTRODUCTION

There have been dramatic changes in the incidence of individual valve lesions during the last few decades. The decline of rheumatic fever has led to a steady reduction of mitral stenosis. In contrast, the improved survival of the general population has led to an increase in the number of cases of aortic stenosis because most of these are degenerative rather than rheumatic in origin. Valvar aortic stenosis is now the commonest valve lesion seen in adult cardiological practice in the Western world.

Aortic stenosis may involve the valve cusps themselves or be located in the supravalvar or subvalvar positions. The main causes are congenital, calcific and rheumatic. Regardless of aetiology, calcification of the aortic valve and its annulus occurs in most longstanding valvar cases. The vast majority of cases are valvular; supravalvar stenosis is a very rare congenital disorder; subvalvar stenosis occurs more often but nevertheless is uncommon.

AETIOLOGY

VALVAR AORTIC STENOSIS

Early pathological studies revealed that virtually all cases of adult aortic stenosis were rheumatic in origin.[1,2] Nowadays, the majority of cases of aortic stenosis seen in Western countries occur in individuals with congenitally bicuspid aortic valves that have become calcified (Table 26.1).[3]

The effects of congenital malformations of the aortic valve are variable.[4] When there is stenosis at birth or soon after, the condition is referred to as *congenital aortic stenosis*. This definition excludes congenitally abnormal (usually bicuspid) aortic valves that function quite satisfactorily until they calcify in later life (see below). The most common abnormality causing congenital aortic stenosis is a bicuspid valve with fusion of the edges of the cusp

and a central orifice. Perhaps the most severely abnormal valve is one with a single cusp, a single commissure and a small eccentric aperture. This type of valve is usually composed of soft bulky tissue and is not particularly amenable to valvuloplasty or valvotomy and often leads to fatal aortic stenosis in infancy. Finally, a dome-shaped valve, formed by fusion of three cusps or composed of a homogeneous membrane, can occur. The very severely abnormal valves (e.g. unicuspid) cause severe stenosis at birth. Other patients with anatomically abnormal and fused valves develop significant stenosis in early childhood, adolescence or early adult life, the timing depending on the severity of the initial malformation and the degree of further thickening and fusion of the cusps.

Congenital aortic stenosis is quite separate from aortic stenosis resulting from degeneration of a congenitally bicuspid aortic valve that initially has no significant commissural fusion. This type of valve occurs in 1–2% of the population, is more common in males than females and usually produces no problems until it calcifies in later life. Some congenitally malformed valves are tricuspid, but the cusps themselves are of unequal size with variable degrees of commissural fusion. Fenoglio *et al.*,[5] studying the natural history of bicuspid aortic valves, predicted that one-third will have normal function throughout life, one-third will eventually calcify and cause aortic stenosis while the remaining third will cause aortic regurgitation.

Table 26.1. **Relative frequency of causes of aortic stenosis.**

Calcified valve:		
Bicuspid	56%	} 68%
Tricuspid	12%	
Rheumatic:		
Isolated aortic lesion	2%	} 17%
Mitral disease	15%	
Other or aetiology unknown		15%

Congenital abnormalities of the aortic valve may be associated with other cardiac lesions of which the most important and frequent are coarctation of the aorta and persistent ductus arteriosus.

Calcific valvar aortic stenosis

In its broadest sense, calcific valvar aortic stenosis refers to all cases of aortic stenosis in adults because all varieties calcify if longstanding. As rheumatic aortic stenosis is usually considered separately, in clinical practice this term is reserved for calcification affecting either bicuspid or tricuspid valves, in which the rheumatic process is not involved.[6–9]

The exact cause of calcification is unclear, but it seems likely that the tension in the abnormally shaped valve cusps and the trauma imposed by turbulence of flow over the valve for long periods of time are responsible. It is possible that repetitive deposition and organization of micro-thrombi may be important. The calcification, which is not usually associated with commissural fusion (cf. congenital aortic stenosis and rheumatic aortic stenosis), causes the valve cusps to become immobile and narrowed (Figs 26.1 and 26.2). The calcification itself is often exuberant and causes considerable lumpy thickening of the valve cusps.

The calcification may also involve structures adjacent to the cusp. The most important are the bundle of His in the interventricular septum, calcification of which may result in conduction abnormalities, and the anterior mitral valve leaflet. There is an association between calcification of the aortic valve and calcification of the mitral valve annulus.

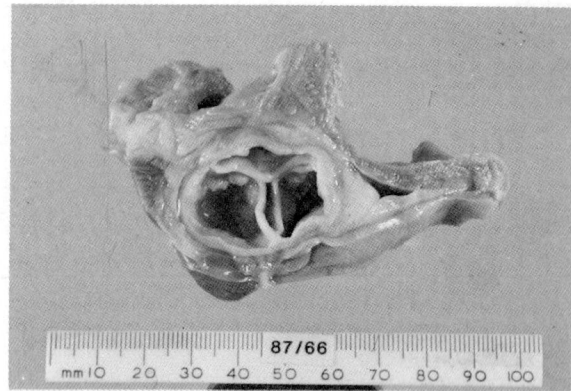

Fig. 26.2. A calcified tricuspid aortic valve which was the cause of severe aortic stenosis. Note that the cusps are irregular and calcified, but there is no significant commissural fusion.

Fortunately, calcification rarely involves the coronary ostia. However, calcific emboli may be occasionally released into the coronary arteries causing ischaemia or infarction.[10]

Rheumatic aortic stenosis

The rheumatic process affects the free edges of the valve cusps, with thrombotic deposits eventually leading to early commissural fusion.[11] This fusion usually affects all three commissures and produces a small triangular central aperture to the valve. There is often some retraction and shortening of the cusps with the disease process, leading to inability of the valve to close properly and some regurgitation. In some cases, fusion occurs less evenly and may cause two of the three valve cusps to stick together producing an apparent 'acquired bicuspid valve'. Calcification is nearly always present in patients over the age of 40 years.

In most cases of rheumatic aortic stenosis, there is also associated mitral valve disease (see Table 26.1).[4] Rheumatic aortic stenosis appears to take longer to develop than mitral stenosis. This leads to a characteristic clinical pattern.[4] A patient with mitral valve disease comes to surgery for their mitral valve lesion and at pre-operative assessment is found to have mild aortic valve disease. Subsequently, after mitral valve surgery has been successful, the patient again develops symptoms some years later as the aortic valve disease progresses.

Other causes of aortic stenosis. Very occasionally aortic stenosis may be caused by atherosclerotic involvement of the aortic valve, particularly in patients with severe hypercholesterolaemia (Types II and III). Onchronosis and rheumatoid disease can

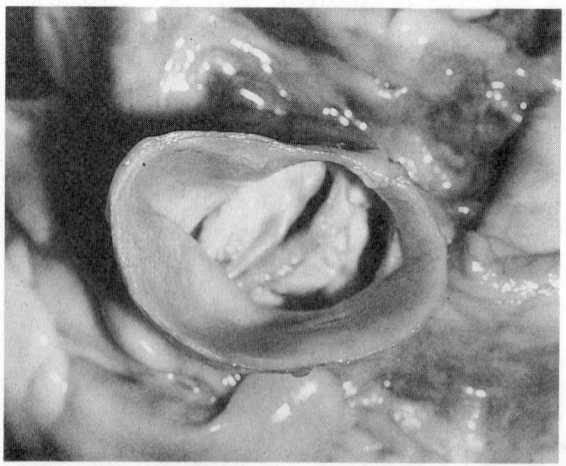

Fig. 26.1. A calcified bicuspid aortic valve seen from the aortic root. Note the nodular irregularity of the cusps due to calcification, and the lack of commissural fusion.

occasionally affect the aortic valve to produce stenotic lesions, although rheumatoid involvement usually leads to aortic regurgitation.

SUPRAVALVAR AORTIC STENOSIS

This rare congenital anomaly is most often a component of a syndrome (Williams' syndrome)[12] characterized by 'elfin facies', mental retardation, multiple branch stenoses in the pulmonary arteries, inguinal hernia, squint, dental abnormalities and hypocalcaemia. Occasionally, cases of supravalvar aortic stenosis are seen without these accompanying abnormalities.

There are three anatomical varieties: an hour-glass type, in which there is an annular constriction at the superior margin of the sinus of Valsalva, a membranous type, with a fibrous or fibromuscular diaphragm that has a small central opening, and a hypoplastic type, in which part of the ascending aorta is underdeveloped. The coronary arteries which arise below the stenosis are subjected to a high pressure and are often dilated and tortuous.

SUBAORTIC STENOSIS

Discrete subaortic stenosis (subvalvar) accounts for about 10% of all cases of congenital aortic stenosis and is twice as common in males as it is in females. There are two main types: the membranous variety in which a fibrous diaphragm encircles the left ventricular outflow tract extending from just below the non-coronary aortic cusp to the anterior cusp of the mitral valve with which it fuses (Fig. 26.3), and,

more rarely, the type in which there is a tunnel of fibrous tissue extending from the mitral to the aortic valve. The latter is often associated with hypoplasia of the aortic valve ring and thickening of the aortic valve cusps. The aortic valve is nearly always mildly regurgitant in cases of subaortic stenosis.

PATHOLOGY

The pathological abnormalities occurring in the aortic valve have been described above.

The left ventricle hypertrophies; in general, the extent of this hypertrophy is proportionate to the severity of the stenosis (Fig. 26.4). Occasionally, however, gross hypertrophy is seen in the presence of only moderate stenosis, whereas in other patients who have very severe stenosis the degree of hypertrophy is less than expected. Left ventricular cavity dimensions remain normal except in patients in whom the stenosis is severe and longstanding and in whom heart failure has begun to develop. In these patients, a moderate degree of left ventricular dilatation occurs. If this late stage is reached and, as as a consequence, heart failure develops, right ventricular hypertrophy may ensue and there may be enlargement of both atria.

The ascending aorta is frequently abnormal in aortic stenosis. In patients in whom the stenosis is at valvar level, the ascending aorta is usually dilated and occasionally this dilatation may become so gross that a saccular post-stenotic aneurysm may develop.[13] The systolic jet through the aortic valve seems to be responsible for the dilatation of the

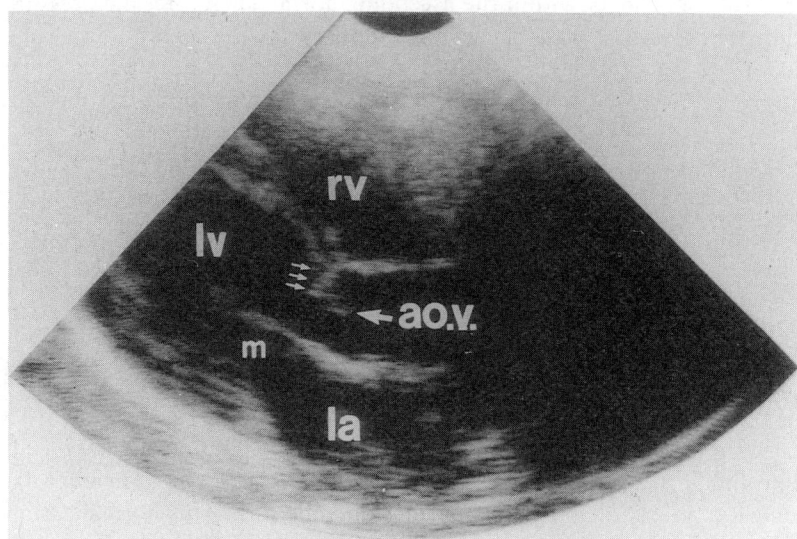

Fig. 26.3. Cross-sectional echocardiogram from a patient with subaortic stenosis (parasternal long-axis view). There is a membrane (small arrows) just below the aortic valve (Ao. v.). lv, left ventricle; rv, right ventricle; m, mitral valve; la, left atrium.

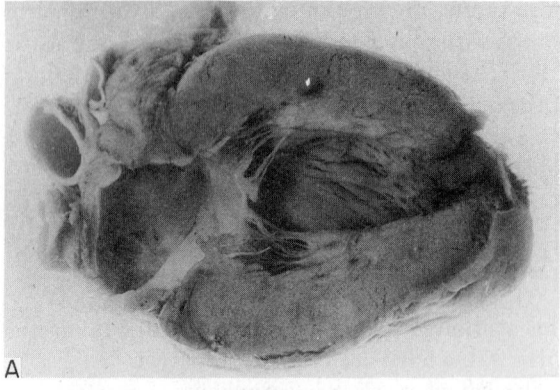

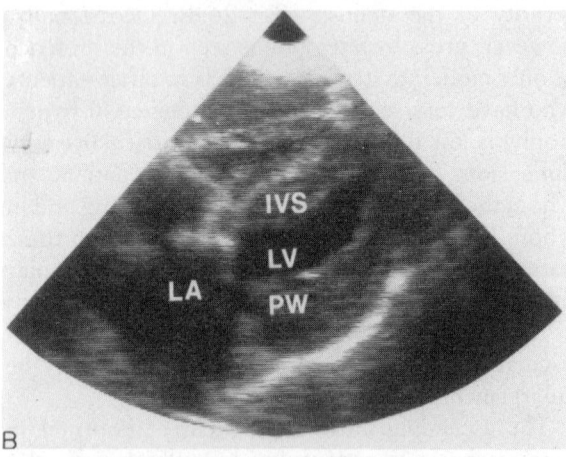

Fig. 26.4. (A) Long-axis section of the heart of a patient with aortic stenosis. There is severe left ventricular hypertrophy which is concentric (i.e. it affects the posterior wall and septum to a similar extent). (B) Cross-sectional echocardiogram demonstrating the same features as in (A). This is a sub-xiphoid long-axis view. LA, left atrium; LV, left ventricle; IVS, interventricular septum; PW, posterior wall.

ascending aorta. Post-stenotic dilatation is rare in subaortic stenosis.

PATHOPHYSIOLOGY

In normal adults, the aortic valve orifice is between 2.6 and 3.5 cm^2.[14] A reduction of this area to 1 cm^2 is required before a pressure gradient develops across the aortic valve. Generally, aortic stenosis is considered to be critical when the peak systolic pressure gradient across the aortic valve exceeds 50 mmHg (in the presence of a normal cardiac output) or if the effective aortic valve orifice is 0.4 cm^2/m^2 body surface area.[15] Although moderate degrees of stenosis may be associated with significant aortic regurgitation, when the stenosis becomes very severe, the size of the orifice, which tends to be fixed,

does not permit a significant degree of aortic regurgitation. The pressure gradient is related to the flow across the aortic valve orifice. The relationship is not linear: the flow is related to the square root of the pressure gradient and a constant. Therefore, small changes in flow across the aortic valve can produce large changes in pressure gradients. Furthermore, when stenosis is severe but cardiac output is low, the pressure gradient across the valve may be of the order of only 20–30 mmHg.[16] As the aortic pressure is maintained and regulated by the normal baroreceptor mechanisms, it tends to remain constant and the pressure gradient is produced by an increase in left ventricular pressure; however, if the aortic stenotic lesion is very severe, the aortic pressure tends to be in the low normal range. Exceptions to this occur and, very occasionally, patients who have hypertensive levels of aortic pressure may also have significant valvar aortic stenosis. This is because the left ventricular pressure gradient can reach levels in excess of 300 mmHg. The relationship between cardiac output, valve area and pressure gradient is complex and varies depending on the type of obstruction to left ventricular outflow. When the cusps are fused with a small central orifice, the valve area tends to be fixed. If, however, the patient has stiffened cusps without commissural fusion (Fig. 26.1) (the normal situation in an elderly patient with a calcified non-rheumatic valve), then increased force on these cusps may increase the valve area. Under these circumstances, an increase in cardiac output may produce slightly wider opening of the stiffened cusps and therefore a larger valve area.[4]

In supravalvar stenosis the pressure drop occurs within the ascending aorta. Therefore, the pressure just above the aortic valve has a systolic value similar to that of the left ventricle and a diastolic valve similar to that in the aorta above the obstruction. In discrete subvalvar aortic stenosis, the pressure drop occurs before the aortic valve and therefore the systolic pressure in the subvalvar chamber is similar to that in the aorta whereas the diastolic pressure is similar to that in the left ventricle.

The left ventricular hypertrophy that occurs in aortic stenosis has two main beneficial results. First, the increased muscle bulk allows more forceful ejection which can maintain normal cardiac output despite outflow obstruction. Second if the increase in wall thickness is sufficient, it normalizes wall stress, which is a major determinant of myocardial oxygen consumption and work. This normalization occurs because of the relationship between wall stress, pressure, dimension and wall thickness, which is most simply stated by the Laplace relationship for a sphere:

$$\text{Wall stress} = \frac{\text{Pressure} \times \text{Dimension}}{4 \text{ (Wall thickness)}}$$

This equation has been modified for the left ventricle by Mirsky.[17–19] Consequently, wall stress will remain constant when intraventricular pressure rises if dimension does not increase and wall thickness increases by the necessary amount. This is usually the situation in 'compensated' aortic stenosis. When the ventricle begins to fail, it usually dilates; this has the opposite effect because it produces an increase in left ventricular dimension and a fall in wall thickness, both of which increase left ventricular wall stress with a resulting increase in oxygen consumption and a deterioration of left ventricular function. If left ventricular hypertrophy is longstanding, interstitial fibrosis may occur in the myocardium,[20] this may play an important part in altering left ventricular function.

LEFT VENTRICULAR FUNCTION

Systolic function

Patients with well-compensated aortic stenosis have adequate hypertrophy to maintain normal left ventricular wall stress and in general have normal indices of contractility,[21] although some authors have postulated subtle changes in function[22] related to an intrinsic abnormality of the contractile function of hypertrophied muscle.

In severe disease, when left ventricular function can no longer be regarded as 'compensated' because of evidence of either clinical symptoms and signs of heart failure or evidence of left ventricular dilatation (for example, on echocardiography), several factors may operate. First, if hypertrophy is not adequate for the level of intraventricular pressure, wall stress will rise. Despite normal contractility, this will cause variables of left ventricular function, which are dependent on afterload (for example, ejection fraction and the velocity of circumferential fibre shortening), to diminish.[23] Some workers have suggested that, in patients who develop heart failure, afterload mismatch is only partly responsible and an abnormality of contractility is also common[24,25] and that may be one of the factors leading to cardiac failure.

The mechanisms underlying any reduction in contractility are unclear. Pressure overload itself may produce some deleterious effects on myocardial contractility: hypertrophied muscle may not function as efficiently as normal muscle and longstanding high intraventricular pressure may produce sub-endocardial ischaemia and fibrosis in the chronically hypertrophied myocardium which may also impair contractility.

In the clinical setting, it is usually impossible to differentiate between the relative importance of impaired contractility and afterload mismatch in the individual patient. As afterload mismatch alone without impaired contractility can produce very low ejection fractions (as low as 19%),[23] and since the prognosis of aortic stenosis with poor left ventricular function is so appalling unless surgery is undertaken, no patient with significant aortic stenosis should be regarded as having left ventricular function too poor to preclude surgery (Fig. 26.5). If further research discloses parameters that will reliably identify patients in whom heart failure has occurred but who have low wall stress and mild aortic stenosis, it may be possible to isolate a group of patients in whom surgery is not appropriate because the main effect of surgery is to lower wall stress, an unnecessary exercise in those in whom it is already low.[25]

Diastolic function

Although attention is usually focused on systolic function in aortic stenosis because the primary problem is systolic outflow obstruction, marked abnormalities of left ventricular diastolic function are common. In patients with moderate or even severe but well-compensated aortic stenosis in whom heart failure has not occurred, the most prominent abnormality is slow left ventricular filling, particularly in early diastole.[26] This abnormality is also seen in left ventricular hypertrophy of any other cause (Fig. 26.6).[26] Once cardiac failure occurs and left ventricular diastolic pressure increases, filling rates will return towards normal presumably because of the higher filling pressure.[27,28]

The changes in left ventricular filling that occur in aortic stenosis are not fully understood. Most are due to complex changes in left ventricular geometry, but altered left ventricular *chamber* stiffness and compliance may also be important.[29,30] Such changes in the properties of the whole left ventricular chamber do not necessarily imply changes in the properties of the muscle itself. Indeed, hyper-

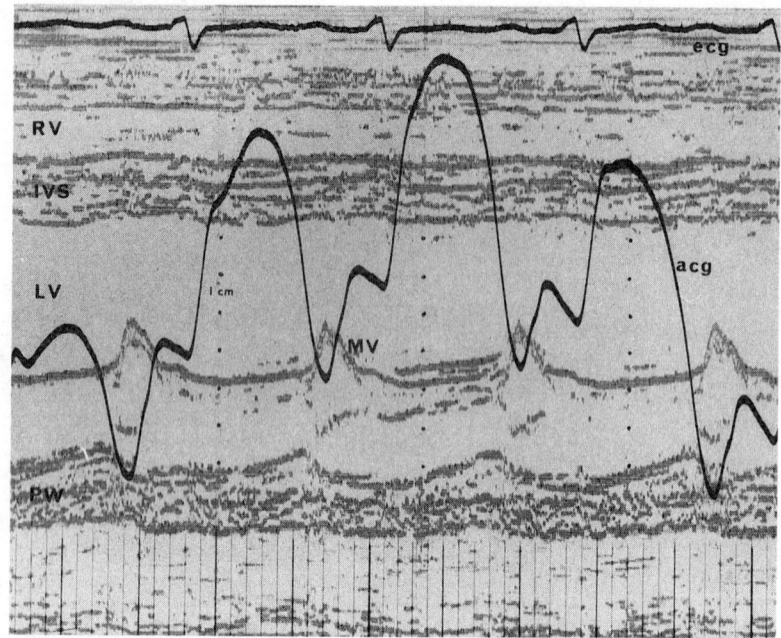

Fig. 26.5. M-Mode echocardiogram from a patient with severe end-stage aortic stenosis and congestive heart failure. The left ventricle is considerably dilated and wall motion is poor, although there is evidence of left ventricular hypertrophy. This patient underwent a successful aortic valve replacement and returned to a completely normal life. RV, right ventricle; IVS, interventricular septum; LV, left ventricle; PW, posterior wall. There is also an apex cardiogram (acg) on this tracing which shows a prominent 'a' wave. MV, mitral valve.

trophied muscle probably has normal stiffness;[31] only when fibrosis occurs in longstanding hypertrophy, do the *intrinsic* properties of the muscle change.

Regardless of the mechanisms leading to the diastolic abnormalities of left ventricular function, this impairment of filling confers increased importance on the atrial component of left ventricular filling. For this reason, a large 'a' wave is a characteristic feature of left atrial and left ventricular pressure traces, and loss of atrial contraction, if atrial fibrillation occurs, has an adverse effect on cardiac function. The importance of atrial contraction can also be seen non-invasively. The echocardiogram often shows that an increased proportion of left ventricular filling occurs as a result of atrial contraction, and on the Doppler echocardiogram the late diastolic velocity of left ventricular inflow

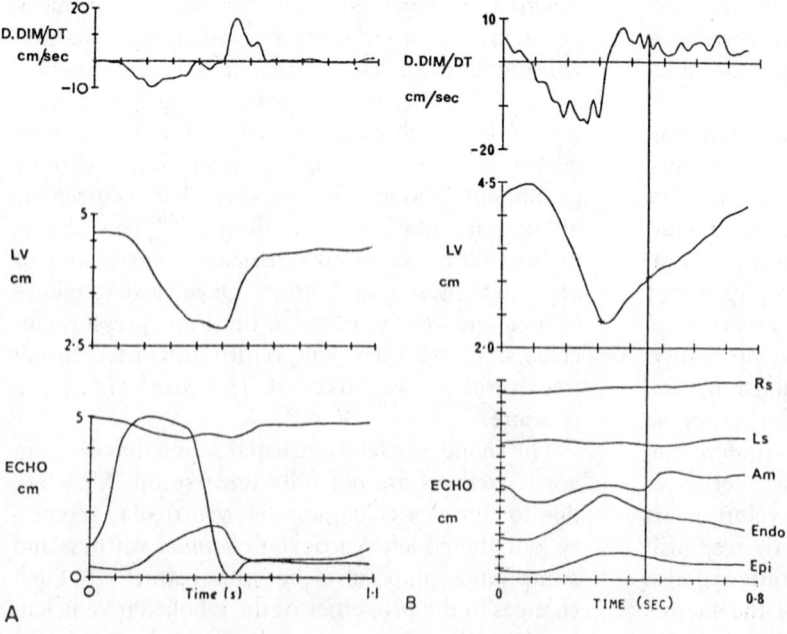

Fig. 26.6. Digitized M-mode echocardiograms from a normal subject (A) and a patient with severe aortic stenosis (B). In both (A) and (B), the lower trace is of the original echocardiogram, the middle trace is a representation of the change in left ventricular dimension with time and the upper trace is the rate of change of left ventricular dimension. Note that, in the normal subject (A), left ventricular filling occurs rapidly in early diastole and that the peak rate of change of dimension (upper trace) is approximately 17 cm/s. In the patient with aortic stenosis (B), left ventricular filling occurs slowly throughout diastole and there is no rapid filling period in early diastole. The peak rate of change of dimension (upper tracing) is approximately 7 cm/s. On the normal trace (A), there is also an apex cardiogram and on the trace from the patient with aortic stenosis the vertical line represents the point at which the mitral valve opens, which is considerably delayed compared with normal due to abnormal diastolic left ventricular function. Rs, right side of septum; Ls, left side of septum, Am, anterior mitral valve leaflet; Endo, endocardium; Epi, epicardium.

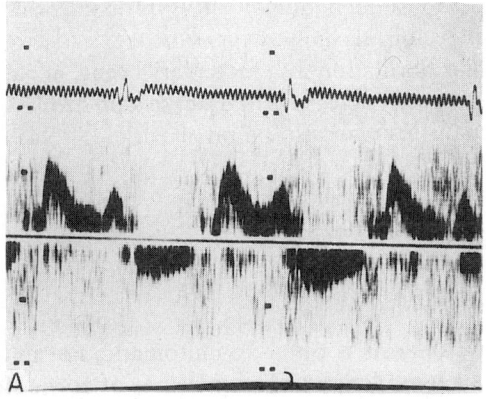

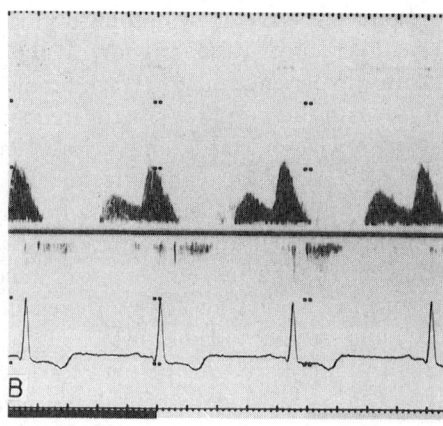

Fig. 26.7. Doppler recordings from the left ventricular inflow (mitral valve) in a normal subject (A) and a patient with aortic stenosis (B). Note that in the normal subject early diastolic inflow occurs at a higher velocity than the late inflow due to atrial contraction. The situation is reversed in the patient with aortic stenosis (B) and the velocity of flow generated by atrial contraction is considerably faster than early diastolic flow. Both recordings were obtained from the cardiac apex. The scale is 1 m/s between the vertical dots.

due to atrial contraction is often much more marked than that in normal subjects (Fig. 26.7).

Disturbances in the co-ordination of relaxation may also occur in aortic stenosis.[32] In the normal heart, the sequence of relaxation and outward wall movement during diastole is highly organized occurring almost synchronously throughout the ventricle. This synchronization has been shown to be disturbed in hypertrophied vessels such that, although outward wall motion occurs at a normal or near-normal rate in individual areas, these areas are not co-cordinated. This robs the ventricle of the explosive, co-ordinated, early diastolic outward wall motion that aids left ventricular filling in the normal ventricle.

OTHER HAEMODYNAMIC CHANGES IN AORTIC STENOSIS

In the compensated state, the mean left atrial pressure remains normal, although the 'a' wave becomes more prominent. When left ventricular failure ensues, the left atrial pressure begins to rise and consequently there is an elevation in pulmonary capillary pressure and pulmonary arterial pressure. The pulmonary artery pressure is usually only modestly raised even when cardiac failure occurs, but occasionally a patient develops very severe pulmonary hypertension, secondary to an unusual degree of pulmonary vasoconstriction. The right ventricular systolic pressure reflects that in the pulmonary artery, but right ventricular end-diastolic pressure does not usually rise until a late stage of the disease when congestive cardiac failure has occurred.

Cardiac output is usually within normal limits at rest, even in the presence of severe stenosis, although, in the most advanced cases or when there is concomitant mitral valve disease, it may be low. When this occurs, the peak gradient across the aortic valve is frequently <50 mmHg despite extreme narrowing,[16] which emphasizes the importance of measuring cardiac output and calculating valve area whenever the severity of aortic stenosis is in doubt.

Coronary blood flow is usually increased in aortic stenosis. This is appreciated at coronary angiography when the angiographer has difficulty in injecting contrast rapidly enough to fill the enormous coronary arteries. Despite this, the coronary blood flow is normal or even subnormal when corrected for myocardial mass.[33] In the most severe and advanced cases of aortic stenosis, there is clearly a mismatch between coronary supply and demand. Oxygen has to diffuse over a longer distance than normal from the capillaries to the centre of hypertrophied fibres, and the raised left ventricular systolic pressure, prolonged ejection and the high intramyocardial pressure impede coronary blood flow during systole while diastolic flow is limited by the raised left ventricular end-diastolic pressure.[4] Sub-endocardial ischaemia may result.

A further factor that may impair coronary blood flow in aortic stenosis is the possible occurrence of a Venturi phenomenon (a fall in pressure due to the rapid rate of flow through a constricted orifice) in the aortic root which will impair inflow into the coronary orifices.[34]

EFFECTS OF EXERCISE IN AORTIC STENOSIS

In normal exercising subjects, cardiac output increases as a result of both an increased heart rate and an increased stroke volume. The increase in stroke volume is achieved mainly by a fall in end-systolic volume although the end-diastolic volume may increase slightly.[35] In aortic stenosis, the response of the left ventricle depends on the severity of the lesion. When stenosis is mild, this may be normal but generally it is highly abnormal. Stroke volume and the end-systolic and the end-diastolic volumes do not change,[35,36] and any increase in cardiac output with exercise occurs simply from an increase in heart rate. Furthermore, abnormalities of filling due to disturbed diastolic function have their maximum impact and may become the main factor limiting an increase in cardiac output during exercise because the time available for ventricular filling is reduced by an increasing heart rate.[37]

MECHANISMS OF SYNCOPE AND SUDDEN DEATH IN AORTIC STENOSIS

Three main mechanisms have been suggested for the occurrence of syncope in aortic stenosis: cardiac arrhythmias, sudden failure of an overloaded left ventricle during the stress of exercise and peripheral vasodilatation occurring suddenly and inappropriately in the face of a fixed cardiac output. There is little or no evidence to support the existence of the first two mechanisms.[4] Any arrhythmias that occur seem to be secondary events following an abrupt fall in blood pressure.[38] The possibility of a sudden failure of the left ventricle as a result of the demands of exercise is difficult to prove or disprove. It seems unlikely because syncope often occurs prior to any other suggestion of left ventricular dysfunction. Most evidence supports inappropriate vasodilatation usually during or just after exercise as the cause of syncope.[39–41] This probably arises via reflexes originating in the left ventricle; patients with syncope have been found to have higher left ventricular systolic pressures than those in patients without syncope.[42] The sudden and severe rise of left ventricular intraventricular pressure during exercise produces reflex peripheral vasodilatation. As the cardiac output cannot increase to compensate for this, severe hypotension results.

The mechanism of sudden death is not known but it is probably related to the mechanism of syncope because patients prone to syncope are also those prone to sudden death.[4] It is probable that the hypotension accompanying syncope leads to ventricular fibrillation as a secondary event. In patients with severe left ventricular dysfunction, other mechanisms may also be involved.[4]

CLINICAL FEATURES

SYMPTOMS

Aortic stenosis is often asymptomatic; not uncommonly, a moderate or severe degree of aortic stenosis is discovered as an accidental finding at necropsy. Patients with the congenital forms of aortic stenosis frequently develop symptoms during childhood or adolescence. Patients with calcific aortic stenosis often experience their first symptoms in the fifth to seventh decades, although frequently a murmur has been detected long before. Patients with rheumatic aortic stenosis frequently have associated mitral valve disease, which often reaches clinical significance before the aortic valve lesion.[4]

The classic triad of symptoms in aortic stenosis is one of syncope, angina pectoris on exertion and dyspnoea, but fatigue and dizziness may be early symptoms. Angina and syncope tend to occur before dyspnoea at a stage when left ventricular function is normal or near normal. Only when left ventricular function begins to deteriorate does the dyspnoea become a prominent symptom. Some patients never experience either angina or syncope and present with dyspnoea alone once left ventricular function begins to deteriorate.

Sudden death can be the first evidence of serious heart disease, but fortunately it is usually preceded by other symptoms albeit often for a short time.

Angina pectoris

Angina pectoris is much more common in aortic stenosis than in any other valve lesion. It occurs in about two-thirds of adult patients with severe lesions, approximately half of whom will have significant coronary disease.[43] If angina is not a symptom, coronary artery disease is less common than in other valve lesions but it may occur.[4] The precise incidence of angina varies according to the population studied; it occurs more often with increasing age but may be prominent in children or young adults. The characteristics of angina caused by aortic stenosis do not differ essentially from those of angina due to ischaemic heart diesase.

Myocardial infarction is a relatively rare complication, although occasionally it occurs due to coronary embolization of calcific or thrombotic material from the diseased valve or vegetations during an attack of infective endocarditis.

Syncope

About 25% of symptomatic patients with aortic stenosis experience syncope. It usually occurs during or immediately after the completion of exertion and is often, but by no means invariably, associated with angina pectoris.

Dyspnoea

Although mild dyspnoea may be the first symptom of aortic stenosis, severe breathlessness and in particular symptoms that suggest left ventricular failure, such as paroxysmal nocturnal dyspnoea, are usually relatively late manifestations of the illness and are associated with a sinister prognosis.

Other symptoms

Arrhythmias, particularly of ventricular origin, may occur but they are not particularly common in aortic stenosis[42] and rarely cause symptoms. Occasionally, patients present with the features of infective endocarditis. Even more rarely, aortic stenosis presents with peripheral embolization of calcific deposits from the aortic valve. The symptoms experienced depend on the site of embolism.

PHYSICAL SIGNS

Pulse and blood pressure

In mild cases of aortic stenosis, the pulse is normal. Once the lesion becomes severe, the pulse is of small amplitude and rises slowly. Its slow-rising nature gives it the form of a plateau and it is sometimes possible to feel a notch on the upstroke (Fig. 26.8). When this is present, the pulse is described as anacrotic. In addition to a notch on the upstroke, systolic vibrations may be present and appreciated by palpation as the pulse rises slowly to its peak (Fig. 26.9). If there is associated aortic regurgitation, the pulse may feel double (pulsus bisferiens). These abnormalities of the pulse are usually best appreciated by palpating the carotid pulse, although they are also often present in the brachial pulse. The radial pulse is generally small in volume but, be-

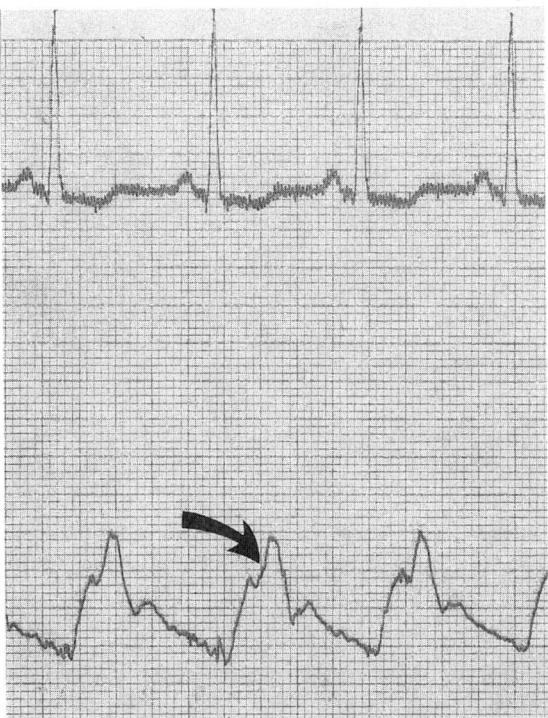

Fig. 26.8. Pulse recording from the brachial artery in a patient with severe aortic stenosis. Note the notch (arrow) on the upstroke of the arterial pulse.

cause of its distance from the heart, does not usually show the characteristic waveform.

The jugular venous pressure is usually normal except when right ventricular failure supervenes secondary to left ventricular failure. There may sometimes be a prominent 'a' wave if the right ventricular cavity is distorted by a hypertrophied ventricular septum (Bernheim's syndrome).

As mentioned above, the blood pressure frequently remains normal until the disease is very advanced. The aortic valve gradient is achieved by a rise in left ventricular pressure. Indeed, patients with hypertension may remain hypertensive despite the development of significant aortic stenosis. When the stenosis is very severe, the systolic pressure is diminished and the pulse pressure small.

In elderly patients, who are being seen with increasing frequency, the characteristic abnormalities of the carotid pulse and the somewhat reduced blood pressure may be absent. The sclerotic vessels of the elderly distort the pressure trace in such a way as to eliminate these characteristic findings.

Cardiac signs

There is usually no abnormality on inspection ex-

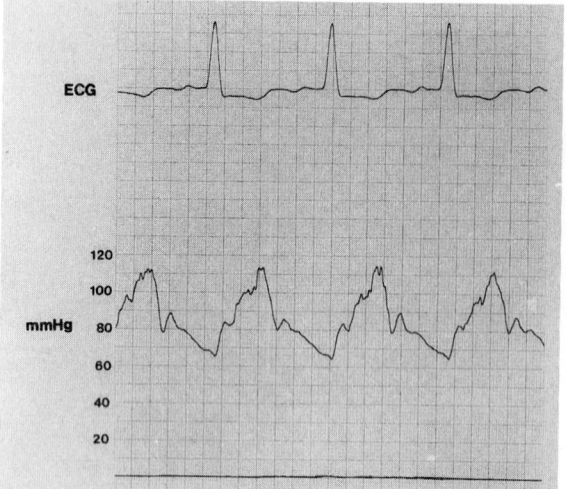

Fig. 26.9. Pulse tracing from the carotid artery in a patient with severe aortic stenosis. Note the slow-rising and shuddering nature of the upstroke of the pressure pulse.

cept in very thin individuals in whom a thrusting cardiac apex due to the hypertrophied left ventricle can be seen. Unless the disease is very advanced and left ventricular dilatation has occurred, the apical impulse is not usually displaced to the left, but on palpation a definite left ventricular lift or thrust can be appreciated and often a pre-systolic pulsation, leading to a double apical impulse and resulting from atrial contraction, can be felt. If this cannot be detected with the patient lying supine, turning the patient into the left lateral position brings the heart against the chest wall and allows this abnormality to be appreciated.

There is often a systolic thrill at the base of the heart to the right of the sternum, which is frequently best felt with the patient sitting up or leaning forward in full expiration. This thrill is often conducted into the vessels of the neck and the suprasternal notch. Occasionally, a thrill may also be felt at the cardiac apex (see 'Systolic Murmur' below).

The first heart sound is normal and when the valve is mobile it is frequently followed by an ejection click 0.04–0.08 later. This click is often loudest at the cardiac apex. It disappears when calcification renders the valve immobile and is absent if the site of aortic stenosis is either sub- or supravalvar. The ejection click is synchronous with the early systolic halting of the diaphragm-like valve (Fig. 26.10).

Characteristic changes may occur in the second heart sound. When aortic stenosis is mild, the second heart sound is normally split. As it becomes more severe, the duration of left ventricular ejection is increased and the aortic component of the second heart sound becomes increasingly later in the cardiac cycle. Initially, it becomes superimposed on the pulmonary component and therefore the second heart sound becomes single. Later, it may occur after the pulmonary component of the second heart sound. Since inspiration moves the pulmonary component of the second heart sound later in the cardiac cycle, reverse splitting occurs with inspiration (i.e. the pulmonary and aortic components of the second heart sound move closer). These abnormalities of the second heart sound depend on a mobile aortic valve. Once thickening and calcifica-

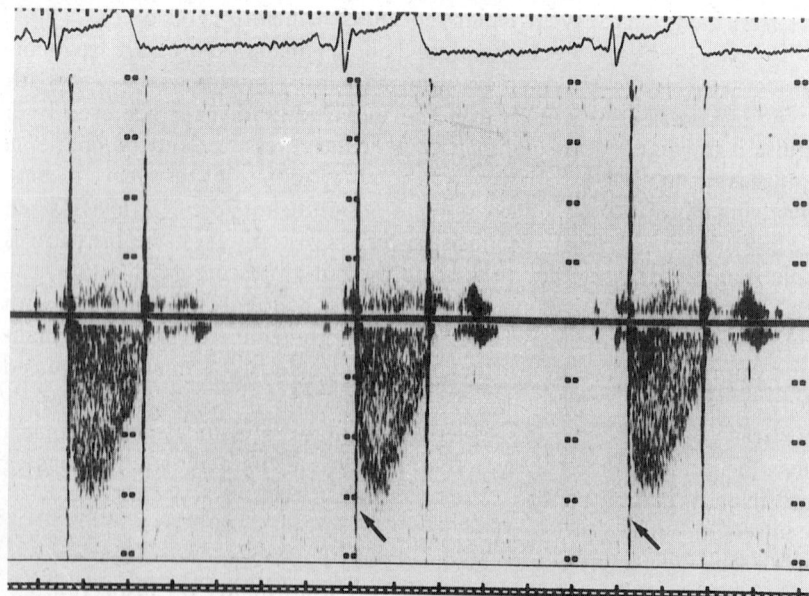

Fig. 26.10. Continuous wave Doppler trace from a patient with mild aortic stenosis due to a bicuspid aortic valve. The recording is obtained from the cardiac apex and therefore the deflection is away from the transducer. The peak gradient across the valve is < 40 mmHg. The peak velocity occurs early in systole and this corresponds with the early peaking murmur in this type of patient with mild stenosis. The aortic velocity trace is preceded by a sharp deflection due to the opening click of the valve (arrows).

tion of the aortic valve cusps occur the aortic component of the second heart sound disappears completely and the second heart sound is single in character.

A fourth heart sound leading to an atrial (pre-systolic) gallop is audible in many cases of severe aortic stenosis. Its presence usually suggests a high pressure gradient across the aortic valve, marked left ventricular hypertrophy and left atrial hypertrophy. A third heart sound is heard only in the late stages of the disease once left heart failure has developed.

The murmur of aortic stenosis is mid-systolic in timing and usually rough, rasping or squeaky in character. Although traditional teaching states that it is usually heard best at the second or third right intercostal space, it is frequently heard best at the left sternal border or even at the cardiac apex, particularly in the elderly. This leads to problems because apical murmurs due to aortic stenosis are often mistakenly attributed to mitral regurgitation. This is further complicated in advanced aortic stenosis because, once left ventricular dilatation begins to occur, mitral regurgitation is also frequently present. In young patients, the murmur is often best heard at the lower left sternal edge and this may be confused with the murmur of ventricular septal defect. Regardless of where the murmur is best heard over the precordium, it nearly always radiates into the neck. As aortic stenosis becomes increasingly severe, the murmur tends to become louder and

to peak later in systole. Once the lesion becomes very severe the murmur may start to become softer again because the flow across the valve producing the murmur is diminished as cardiac output falls. In its most extreme form aortic stenosis may occur with little or no audible systolic murmur.[16] The murmur of aortic stenosis is increased by squatting or lying flat or by the inhalation of amylnitrite, whereas it is decreased during the strain phase of the Valsalva manoeuvre. In atrial fibrillation, it varies in intensity from beat to beat.

A diastolic murmur due to associated aortic regurgitation is quite frequently present even when the haemodynamic lesion is almost exclusively aortic stenosis. This is usually the case in patients with calcific and rheumatic stenosis but less common in patients with the congenital forms of aortic stenosis occurring in childhood. When aortic stenosis is of the discrete subaortic variety, aortic regurgitation, which is usually mild, is almost invariable.

INVESTIGATION

THE ELECTROCARDIOGRAM

The electrocardiogram usually shows left ventricular hypertrophy which becomes increasingly pronounced as the lesion becomes more severe (Fig. 26.11). Despite this, a few patients with severe aortic stenosis have normal electrocardio-

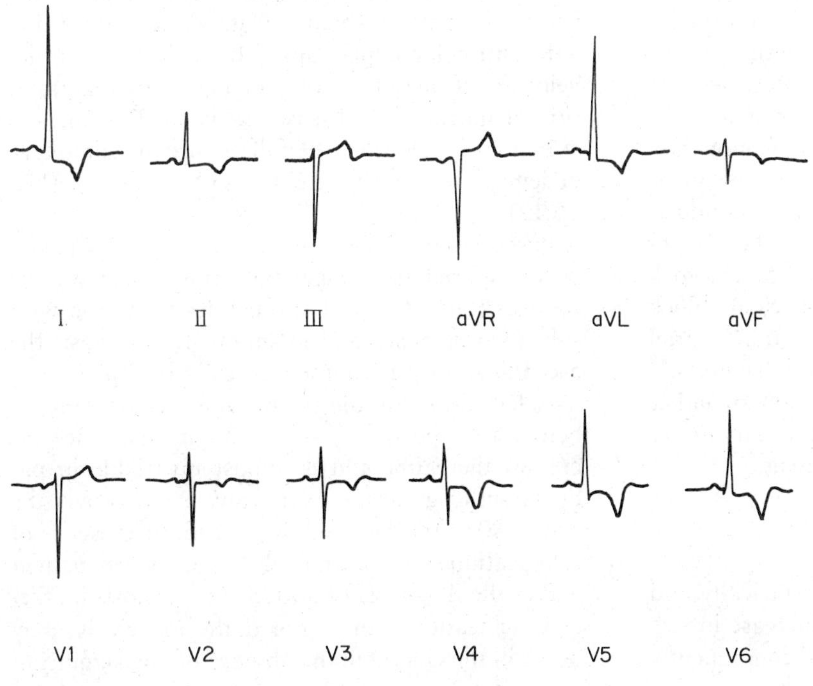

I   II   III   aVR   aVL   aVF

V1   V2   V3   V4   V5   V6

Fig. 26.11. Electrocardiogram from a patient with severe aortic stenosis showing marked left ventricular hypertrophy, which is most obvious in the standard leads (1 and aVL). The relative lack of height of the R wave in the left chest leads is due to the mild degree of left axis deviation present. (Standardization 10 mm = 1 mV.)

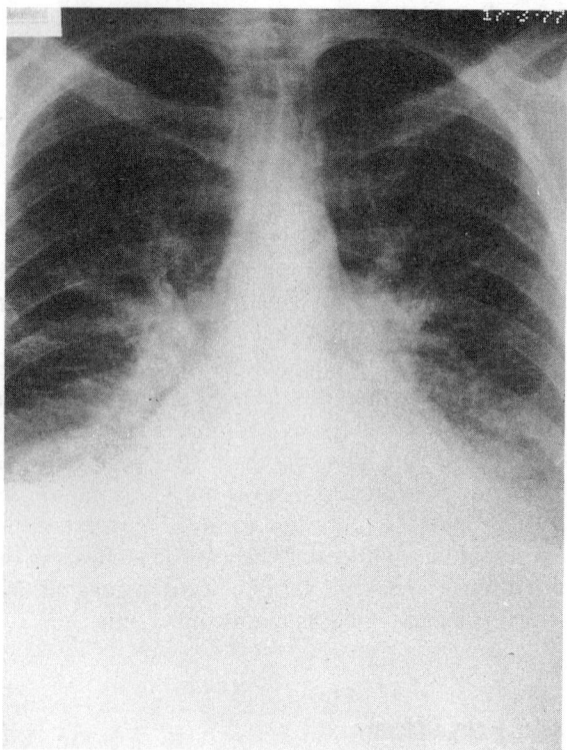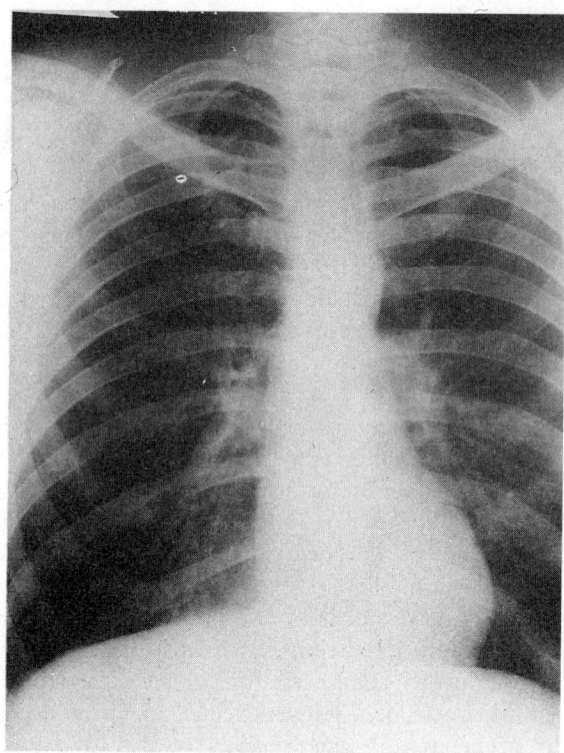

Fig. 26.12. Chest X-ray from a patient with severe aortic stenosis leading to pulmonary oedema (left). One year later, following successful aortic valve replacement, there was no significant abnormality on the chest X-ray (right).

grams.[45–47] Left-axis deviation may occur and cause the R waves to disappear from the right precordial leads (V_1–V_3) sometimes giving the impression of antero-septal myocardial infarction. As left ventricular function begins to deteriorate, the features of left atrial hypertrophy, of which the most common is a large negative component to the P wave in lead V_1, become evident. Conduction abnormalities are a characteristic feature of aortic stenosis and occur as calcium invades the conducting tissue. First degree heart block may be present and left-axis deviation and left bundle branch block are common.[42] Complete atrioventricular block occurs as a late manifestation but is rare.[48] Atrial fibrillation is uncommon in pure aortic stenosis.[42] Its presence should lead to a suspicion of either concomitant mitral valve disease or coronary artery disease, although neither may be present.

CHEST X-RAY

The left ventricle hypertrophies concentrically and the left ventricular cavity does not increase in size until the late stages of the disease, and consequently the cardiac shadow on the chest X-ray is usually of normal size. However, there may be a blunting or rounding of the left lower cardiac contour and some protrusion posteriorly in the lateral view suggesting left ventricular hypertrophy. If cardiac failure develops or if there is accompanying aortic regurgitation or mitral valve disease, cardiac enlargement is common. In addition, the full picture of pulmonary oedema is seen in the late stages of the disease (Fig. 26.12).

Post-stenotic dilatation of the aorta is usual in both acquired and congenital forms of aortic valve stenosis (Fig. 26.13). It is much less common with subvalvar stenosis, and in supravalvar stenosis the ascending aorta is characteristically hypoplastic.

Calcification of the aortic valve is uncommon before the age of 20 years, but its incidence increases thereafter and is almost invariable in patients with significant aortic valve stenosis over the age of 40 years (Fig. 26.14). Indeed, the absence of calcification of the aortic valve in an elderly patient makes the diagnosis of aortic valve stenosis unlikely. Calcification in the region of the aortic valve may occur in the elderly in the absence of any significant

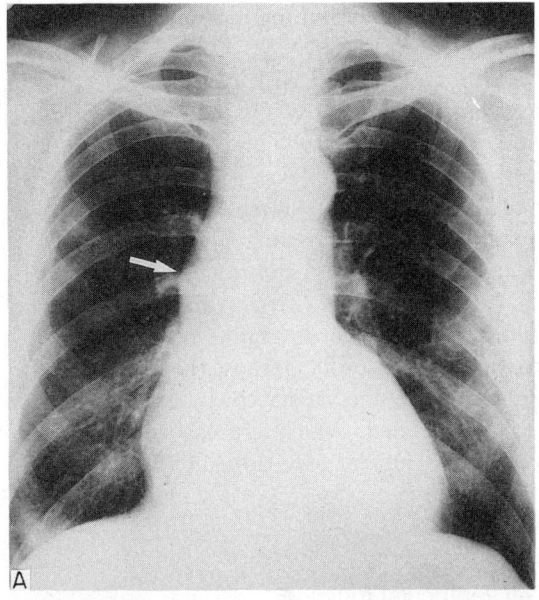

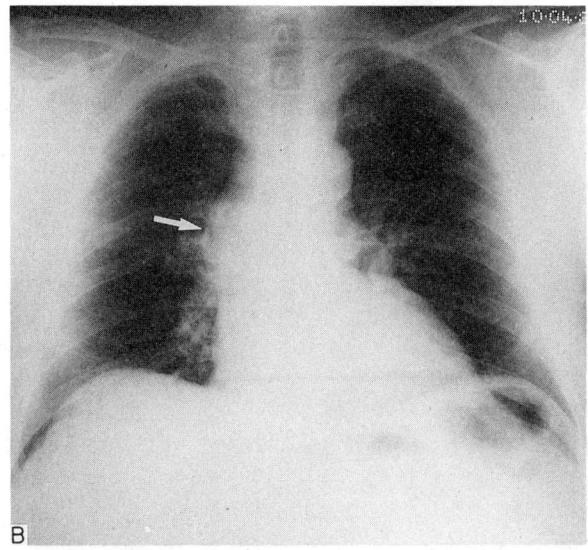

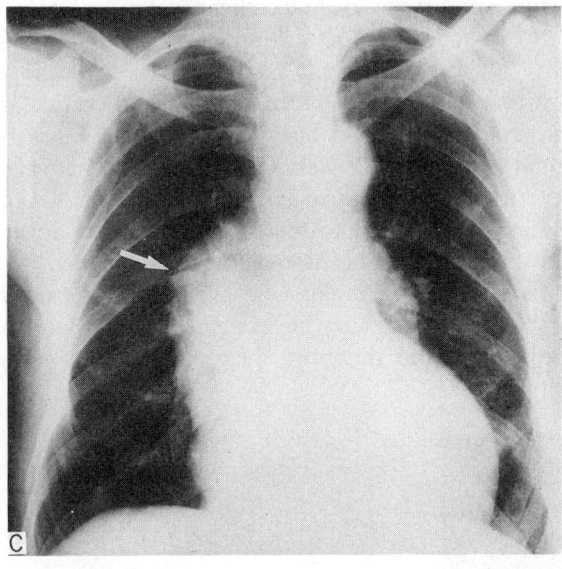

Fig. 26.13. Chest x-ray appearances in three patients with aortic stenosis. In all three, there is post-stenotic dilatation of the aorta (arrow). The degree of post-stenotic dilatation increases from (A) to (C). In (C) it has reached the proportions at which the dilatation of the aortic root has become aneurysmal.

aortic valve narrowing. Aortic valve calcium can be detected on the lateral chest X-ray but is best detected by fluoroscopy.

ECHOCARDIOGRAPHY

The echocardiographic features of aortic stenosis are discussed in detail in Chapter 13. The most important features are summarized below.

Assessment of site and degree of stenosis

Echocardiographic imaging of the aortic valve may give an idea of the severity of the stenosis and may identify the number of cusps (Fig. 26.15). If the valve is normal with freely mobile cusps, this excludes significant aortic stenosis in the adult. Occasionally, in children, a doming valve may appear to open fully, particularly on M-mode examination (Fig. 26.16), because the narrowed and fused part of the mitral valve is not in the echo plane.[49] This is rare, however, in adults. If a moderate degree of thickening and immobility of aortic valve is seen with the valve opening between 7 and 12 mm in systole, it is usually impossible to define, from valve movement and appearance, whether haemodynami-

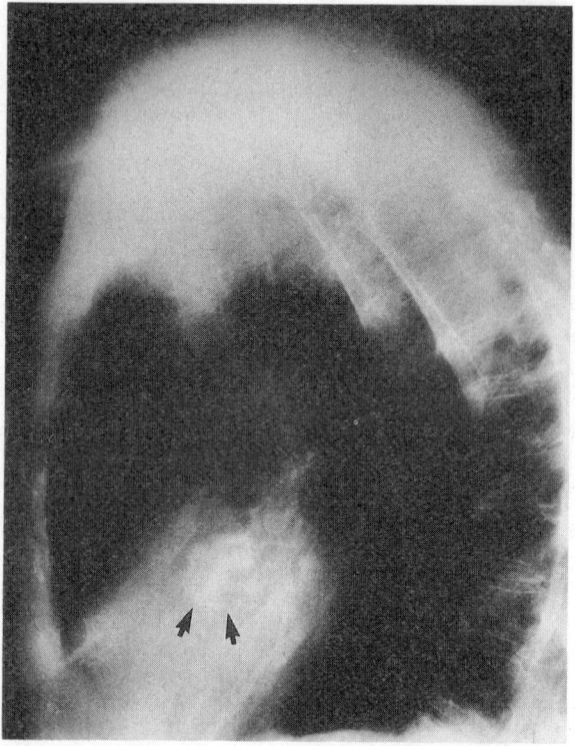

Fig. 26.14. Lateral chest X-ray from a patient with calcific aortic stenosis showing gross calcification of the aortic valve (arrows).

cusps artefactually filling in the aortic valve orifice on echocardiography.

Echocardiography will usually define the site of left ventricular outflow obstruction. Valvar obstruction, if present, is nearly always identified. Obstruction at a subvalvar level is usually easily seen by echocardiography with either a tunnel or membrane-like narrowing below the aortic valve being identified best in the parasternal long-axis view (Fig. 26.3).[53,54] Supravalvar stenosis may be detected on echocardiography but it can be missed, particularly in adults, because the ascending aorta is difficult to image satisfactorily. Suprasternal views may be needed, which are easy to obtain in the young but much more difficult to obtain in older patients.[55]

Left ventricular function

Echocardiography is an excellent method of assessing left ventricular size, contraction and hypertrophy. In aortic stenosis, as the degree of outflow obstruction becomes more severe, left ventricular hypertrophy increases but the left ventricle remains small and contracts well. The relationship between severity and left ventricular hypertrophy has led to the construction of formulae which predict aortic valve gradients from the extent of hypertrophy.[56,57] Although these formulae work well for large groups of patients, they can be extremely inaccurate in individuals and therefore they are of little or no clinical use.

cally significant aortic stenosis is present.[50,51] When the valve is extremely immobile and thickened, the patient nearly always has severe aortic stenosis; very occasionally, there are exceptions[52] due to reverberating echoes from heavily calcified valve

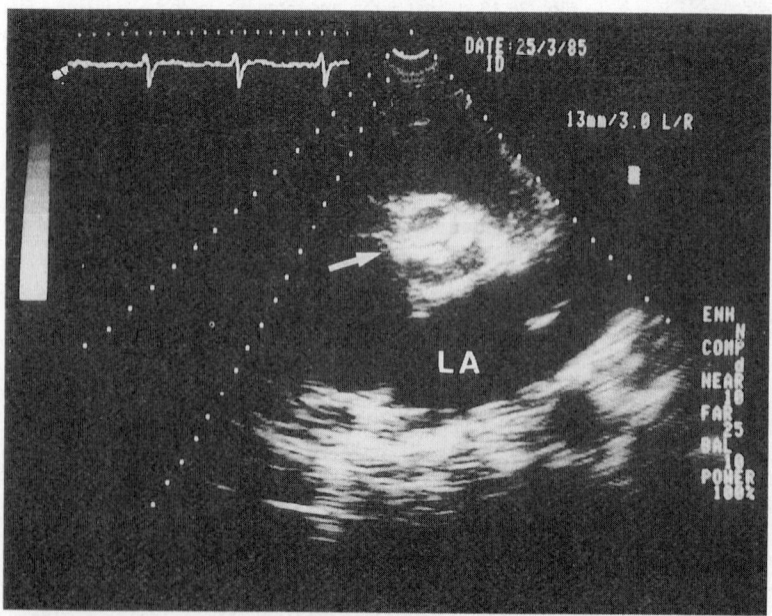

Fig. 26.15. Cross-sectional echocardiogram (parasternal short-axis view) from a patient with severe aortic stenosis. This echocardiogram was obtained in systole, and the slit-like opening of the three heavily thickened and calcified aortic valve cusps can be seen (arrow). LA, left atrium.

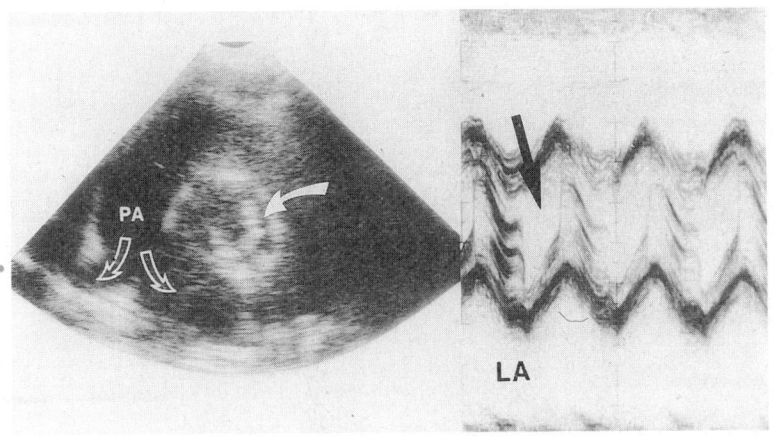

Fig. 26.16. Cross-sectional echocardiogram and M-mode echocardiogram from a patient with a bicuspid aortic valve which was significantly stenotic and domed in systole. The cross-sectional echocardiogram on the left (parasternal short-axis view) shows that the valve is bicuspid (solid arrow). Despite the significant stenosis, the M-mode echocardiogram on the right shows apparently normal opening of the aortic valve (arrow) since the doming valve has been transected below its stenotic orifice. LA, left atrium.

When aortic stenosis is very advanced and heart failure develops, left ventricular wall motion is decreased; and this is easily assessed as a reduction in fractional shortening. In some patients, considerable left ventricular dilatation occurs at this stage, although left ventricular wall thickness remains increased.[16] In other patients, there is only a slight increase in left ventricular dimensions, but wall movement is poor (Fig. 26.17).

Conditions that masquerade as aortic stenosis

Echocardiography can identify the two conditions most likely to masquerade as aortic stenosis—hypertrophic cardiomyopathy and subvalvar mitral regurgitation. However, it is worth remembering that the left ventricular hypertrophy produced by aortic stenosis may be sufficiently asymmetric on occasions to cause confusion with hypertrophic cardiomyopathy (Fig. 26.18).

DOPPLER

The introduction of the Doppler technique has resolved many of the problems in the assessment of aortic stenosis (see Chapter 14); the main features

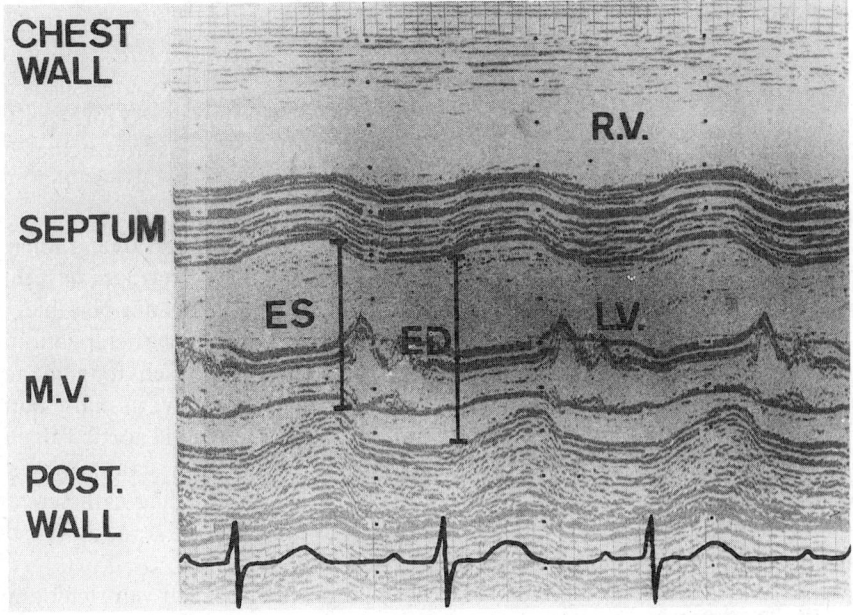

Fig. 26.17. M-Mode echocardiogram from a patient with severe aortic stenosis and very poor left ventricular function. The left ventricle has not dilated but is grossly hypertrophied. Wall motion is extremely poor; this is shown by the very small difference in end-systolic and end-diastolic (ES and ED) left ventricular dimensions. LV, left ventricle; RV, right ventricle; MV, mitral valve.

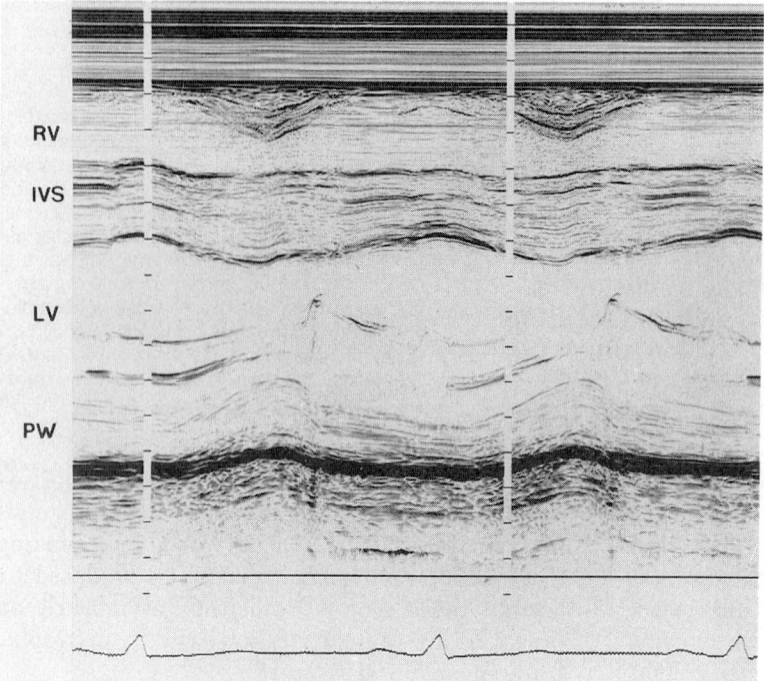

Fig. 26.18. M-Mode echocardiogram from a patient with severe aortic stenosis. Note that the interventricular septum (IVS) has, in this case, hypertrophied far more than the posterior wall (PW). This can occasionally lead to confusion with hypertrophic cardiomyopathy. RV, right ventricle; LV, left ventricle.

are summarized below. The site of outflow obstruction can be defined by using the sample volume of the pulsed Doppler to detect the site at which blood flow velocity is increased. However, this increase in velocity is so great when stenosis is significant that the pulsed Doppler technique, although capable of its detection, is unable to measure it because of aliasing. For this reason, continuous wave Doppler has to be used to assess the degree of stenosis.[58] The best sites for obtaining continuous wave Doppler signals are the cardiac apex, the suprasternal notch or the right parasternal area. Using these approaches, good signals can be obtained from at least one of these sites in most (90%) patients (Fig. 26.19). The highest success rate is achieved with the apical approach. The Doppler technique is usually used to measure velocity through the valve; this information can be used to calculate the pressure gradient using the modified Bernoulli equation (Chapter 14). It is important to remember that the gradient measured by Doppler is the *peak gradient*, whereas that measured by catheter is usually the *peak-to-peak gradient*. The former is usually greater than the latter, often by 10–15 mmHg (Fig. 26.20). Other more complicated techniques have been introduced recently that can be used to assess aortic valve area.[59] This may be valuable when cardiac output is low and as a consequence the pressure gradient and hence velocity of flow has fallen.

CARDIAC CATHETERIZATION AND ANGIOGRAPHY

Previously it was nearly always necessary to perform cardiac catheterization to assess the severity of aortic stenosis. In general, gradients > 50 mmHg indicate significant aortic stenosis if cardiac output is normal. If there is any suspicion that cardiac output is not normal, the aortic valve area should be calculated from pressure tracings and cardiac output measurements using the Gorlin formula (p. 388).

Usually, the aortic valve gradient is obtained by passing a catheter retrogradely through the valve (Fig. 26.21). If this is not possible, other techniques such as trans-septal catheterization or left ventricular puncture, are used to gain access to the left ventricle. Fortunately, in many patients, such good information about the aortic valve gradient and left ventricular function can now be obtained non-invasively; that cardiac catheterization is unnecessary or needed only to assess the state of the coronary arteries.

Traditionally, a left ventriculogram has been used to assess left ventricular function but if the aortic valve is not crossed echocardiography can often supply this information. A left ventriculogram would also reveal whether there is mitral regurgitation and show the movement of the aortic valve

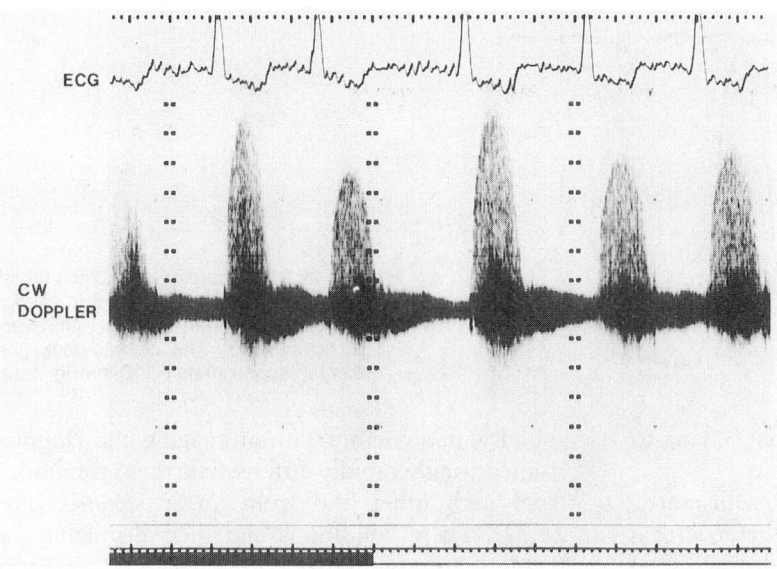

Fig. 26.19. Continuous wave Doppler recording from a patient with severe aortic stenosis and atrial fibrillation. The peak velocity across the valve varies considerably from beat to beat. The lowest peak velocity on this trace is 4.7 m/s, corresponding to a transvalvar gradient of 88 mmHg. The highest recorded is 6.8 m/s, corresponding to a gradient of 185 mmHg. Each division on the vertical scale is 1 m/s. As this recording was obtained from the suprasternal notch, the aortic jet is towards the transducer.

cusps and the extent of their thickening. Aortography allows concomitant aortic regurgitation to be assessed.

DIAGNOSIS

A diagnosis of aortic stenosis is often first suspected

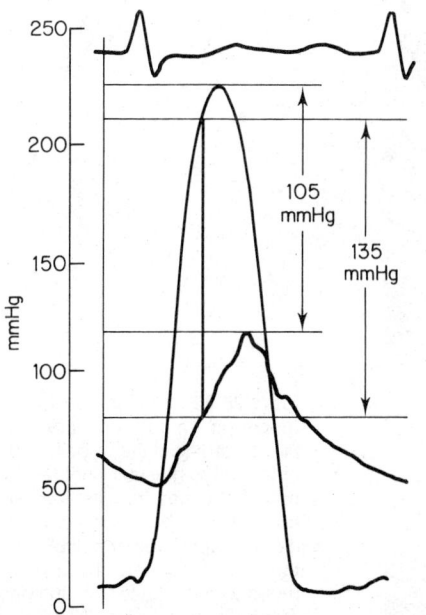

Fig. 26.20. Simultaneous pressure traces of the aorta and left ventricle in a patient with severe aortic stenosis. The *maximum pressure gradient* during systole is 135 mmHg and corresponds to the gradient that is obtained from the peak velocity derived from the continuous wave Doppler. The *peak-to-peak* gradient is 105 mmHg, and is the gradient measured conventionally at cardiac catheterization.

when a murmur is heard on routine physical examination. Adults who develop significant aortic stenosis in later life are often aware that they have had a murmur detected during childhood or adolescence.

The diagnosis should always be suspected in a patient who presents with one or more of the classic triad of symptoms of angina pectoris, syncope and breathlessness. It is particularly important that patients presenting with angina are carefully examined before treatment is started and any patient with a significant heart murmur is assessed by a cardiologist to determine whether significant aortic stenosis is present. The most important diagnostic features are the murmur and the quality of the carotid pulse. Abnormalities of the pulse are not always reliable however. Patients who are elderly and have sclerotic vessels may not demonstrate the classic slow-rising pulse despite having severe aortic stenosis, and patients with small or abnormal carotid pulsations and bruits in the neck may have these because of carotid disease. The differentiation of carotid bruits and murmurs radiating into the neck from the aortic valve can be very difficult. Generally, carotid bruits do not radiate into the chest and may be associated with unequal pulses in the neck, with the vessel demonstrating the bruit having a reduced pulsation when compared with the pulse in the other side of the neck. This is not always the case, however, and often the differentiation is difficult or impossible without resorting to further tests. The recent introduction of Duplex scanning of the carotid arteries (Doppler and echo) and the Doppler assessment of aortic valve gradients have made this

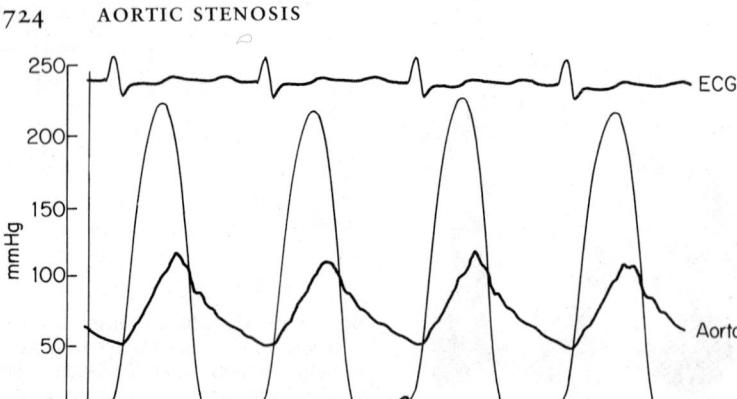

Fig. 26.21. Recordings of aortic and left ventricular pressure obtained at cardiac catheterization from a patient with severe aortic stenosis. The peak-to-peak gradient is approximately 110 mmHg.

differentiation very much easier without having to perform catheterization and angiography.

Conditions likely to be confused with aortic stenosis are all characterized by the presence of a systolic murmur. They can usually be distinguished from aortic stenosis by the character of the murmur, the absence of the characteristic carotid pulse of aortic stenosis and changes in the splitting on the second heart sound. Fortunately, cardiac ultra-

sound with a combination of imaging and Doppler studies usually rapidly differentiate these conditions from each other and from aortic stenosis (Fig. 26.22). These conditions and their distinguishing features are summarized in Table 26.2. Patients with ejection systolic murmurs are often diagnosed as having 'aortic sclerosis'. As patients become elderly, their aortic valves become stiff but they may not necessarily be significantly stenosed. Such valves

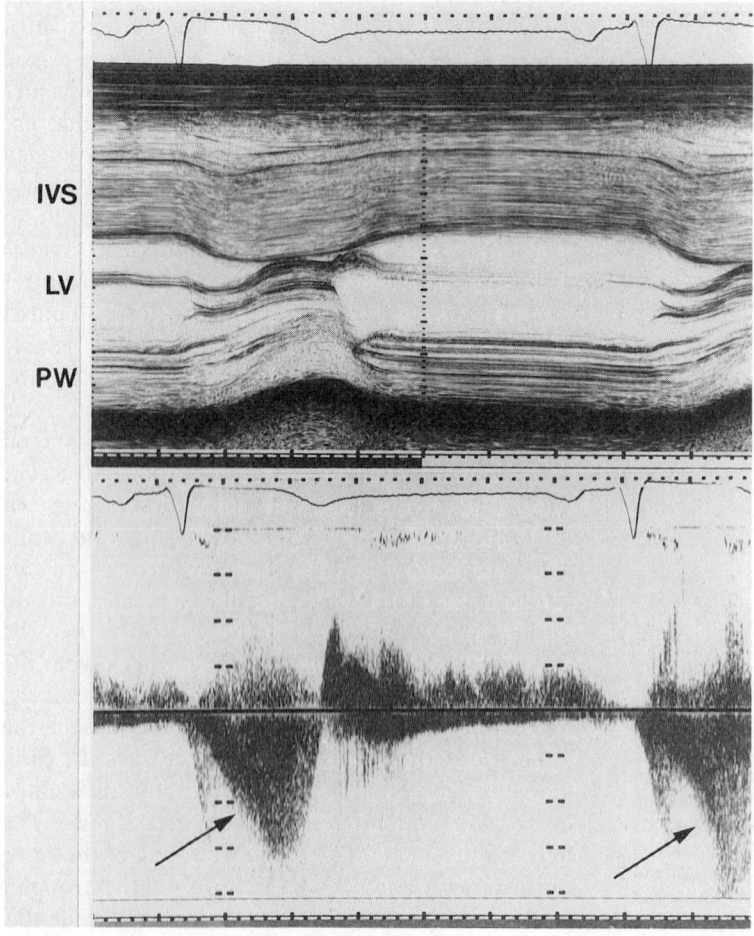

Fig. 26.22. M-Mode echocardiogram (upper panel) and continuous wave Doppler recording of the velocity of blood flow in the left ventricular outflow tract (lower panel) obtained from the cardiac apex in a patient with hypertrophic cardiomyopathy. Note the different shape to the velocity signal (arrows) when compared with the trace from the patient with aortic stenosis in Fig. 26.19. In patients with hypertrophic cardiomyopathy, the upstroke of the velocity trace is slower and often slightly curved due to the steady increase in gradient occurring as left ventricular contraction progresses. This is a 'dynamic' gradient. IVS, interventricular septum; LV, left ventricle; PW, posterior wall.

Table 26.2. Aortic stenosis—differential diagnosis.

Diagnosis	Important points	Carotid pulse	Radiation of murmur to neck	Echo	Doppler
Aortic sclerosis	Elderly	N	+	Normal	No gradient at aortic valve
Flow murmur (e.g. pregnancy, anaemia and thyrotoxicosis)	Murmur musical, heard at left sternal border and may radiate to apex and neck. No thrill	Large volume	+	Normal (vigorous left ventricle)	No gradient
Bicuspid valve without stenosis	Ejection sound ± early peaking ejection systolic murmur. S_2 normal	N	+	70% detected	No gradient
Mitral regurgitation	(a) Rheumatic not usually confused (pan-systolic murmur of even intensity throughout systole)	Sharp or normal	—	Rheumatic mitral valve seen	Detects mitral regurgitation and absence of an aortic valve gradient
	(b) Subvalvar, e.g. chordal rupture. Murmur may be harsh, crescendo or even ejection type. Loudest at apex but radiates widely (can go to neck). Third sound plus mid-diastolic murmur if severe	Sharp	+/−	Underlying mitral valve abnormality often detected, e.g. prolapse or chordal rupture	"
Hypertrophic cardiomyopathy	Murmur usually either late systolic or pan-systolic, increasing towards S_2. May be harsh and heard at left sternal border and apex	Sharp 'jerky' pulse	+/−	Left ventricular hypertrophy +/− asymmetric septal hypertrophy +/− systolic anterior motion of mitral valve	May show *dynamic* outflow gradient +/− mitral regurgitation (Fig. 26.22)
Ventricular septal defect	Usually loud at sternal border with thrill	Normal	+/−	Normal if defect small, defect seen if moderate or large	Jet across defect detected by Doppler

give rise to murmurs, which are not usually associated with any pulse abnormality although the valve may be thickened or even calcified. Doppler shows that there is no significant gradient across the aortic valve and the echocardiogram shows that the aortic valve cusps open well (Fig. 26.23). Aortic sclerosis is a diagnosis made too frequently by non-cardiologists in patients who really have significant aortic stenosis. This is therefore a diagnosis of exclusion which can be made only when non-invasive investigations have shown that there is no significant gradient across the aortic valve.

Certain clinical features help to distinguish the various sites of left ventricular outflow obstruction. Valvar aortic stenosis is many times more common than the sub- or the supravalvar varieties. When the

aortic valve retains its mobility, cases of valvar aortic stenosis usually demonstrate an ejection sound which is loud and snapping, best heard at the cardiac apex preceding the murmur. This type of ejection sound is not heard in the sub- or supravalvar varieties. Abnormalities and alterations of the second heart sound tend to be similar in all types of aortic stenosis and depend on the extent of left ventricular outflow obstruction. The possibility of the diagnosis of supravalvar aortic stenosis may be suggested by the characteristic facies and other associated abnormalities.[12] In addition, these patients may have a continuous murmur heard anywhere in the thorax due to associated multiple pulmonary branch stenoses which are sometimes present. Finally, the unequal pulses and blood press-

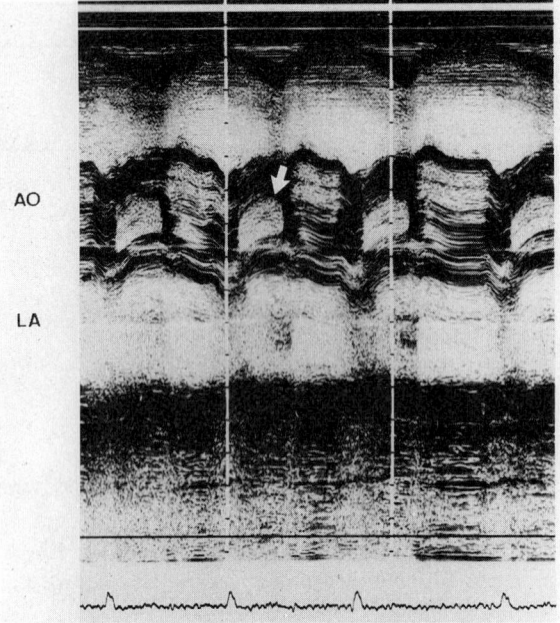

Fig. 26.23. M-Mode echocardiogram from a patient with a thickened aortic valve but no significant stenosis who was 80 years old. Note the heavy echoes (arrow) from the aortic valve but its wide opening. Ao, aorta; LA, left atrium.

ures in the upper extremities may suggest the diagnosis. Subvalvar stenosis is not associated with any particular syndrome and is simply suggested by the absence of an ejection sound in a relatively young patient and confirmed by the characteristic non-invasive findings.

It should be remembered that aortic stenosis can occasionally occur without murmurs, and cause intractable cardiac failure.[16] Such apparently moribund patients derive enormous benefit from aortic valve replacement and it is therefore extremely important to suspect the diagnosis in patients with cardiac failure of unknown aetiology.

COMPLICATIONS

Sudden death is an important complication and occurs in about 10–20% of all patients with significant aortic stenosis[60] and probably in about 1% of children with congenital aortic stenosis.[4] The evidence strongly suggests that patients who die suddenly have severe disease and have nearly always been symptomatic prior to death,[4] although, in one series reported by Glew *et al.*, 4 of 33 patients who died suddenly had had no symptoms before death.[61]

Another important complication of aortic steno-

sis is the onset of cardiac failure which usually leads to death unless surgical intervention is undertaken.

Arrhythmias and conduction abnormalities may occur (see above).

Another important complication of calcific aortic stenosis is the embolization of calcium deposits from the aortic valve. These are usually small and cause little trouble except when they embolize into a coronary artery.

Infective endocarditis is an important complication and should always be suspected in patients with aortic stenosis who have an unexplained illness however vague and difficult it is to define.

NATURAL HISTORY AND PROGNOSIS

PROGRESSION OF AORTIC STENOSIS

The progression of aortic stenosis depends to some extent on its underlying cause. Broadly speaking, congenital cases with a fixed orifice tend to remain static during childhood as long as the growth of the aortic valve is the same as that of the aorta. Occasionally, patients show an increase or a decrease in the level of stenosis.[4]

Studies of the haemodynamic progression of aortic stenosis in adults have been reported; these show that the natural history is very variable.[62–66] In some patients, the stenosis remains static for many years, whereas in others it progresses slowly; in others, it progresses quite rapidly. Wagner and Selzer[62] have shown that progression tends to be most rapid in patients with calcific aortic stenosis; it is particularly marked in the more elderly patient. In rheumatic cases, stenosis due to commissural fusion is usually not very severe initially, and there is often associated regurgitation. Later, calcification causes the lesion to increase in severity.

Aortic stenosis has a poor prognosis irrespective of the age at which it is detected. When significant aortic stenosis develops in infancy, those who survive early childhood often continue in apparently good health until their third decade; 10–20% of patients detected in infancy will die during childhood. Although some of these deaths are sudden, the majority occur due to progressive heart failure.

Similarly, in adults, aortic stenosis carries a poor prognosis. The mortality rate is approximately 50% at 3 years, 60% at 5 years and 90% at 10 years.[67,68] The prognosis tends to vary depending on the presenting symptom. Of the three major components of the symptom triad, left ventricular failure and breathlessness carry the worst prognosis with a life-expectancy of considerably less than 2 years from the onset of this symptom. Syncope is said to be associated with a life-expectancy of around 3 years and angina of about 5 years.[44,69]

TREATMENT

MEDICAL TREATMENT

Medical treatment has little or no part to play in the management of aortic stenosis. Careful supervision is necessary however, and particular attention should be paid to the prevention of infective endocarditis. Furthermore, patients in whom surgery is contra-indicated may derive some benefit from the treatment of cardiac failure and arrhythmias when they occur. Patients with a moderate degree of aortic stenosis in whom surgery is planned for the future should avoid very strenuous exertion. This is often a difficult aspect of treatment particularly in the young asymptomatic patient with a moderate degree of aortic stenosis who is keen on sport. The risks in this situation are not known and the advice given to patients tends to vary considerably from physician to physician. However, there have been very few reports of young adults with unsuspected aortic stenosis dying suddenly during athletic events. This is in sharp contrast to hypertrophic cardiomyopathy and congenital abnormalities of the coronary arteries, conditions frequently found in the young patient dying suddenly during exercise. This suggests that aortic stenosis in asymptomatic young adults may not be as dangerous as is often thought. Nonetheless, advice should err on the conservative side if there is any doubt. The recent introduction of balloon valvuloplasty may mean that earlier treatment can be undertaken in such patients to allow them to participate in normal sporting activities while postponing the hazards of aortic valve replacement and cardiopulmonary bypass.

SURGICAL TREATMENT

Indications for surgical treatment are also discussed in Chapter 35. In general, surgery is advisable whenever patients have symptoms that are attributable to aortic stenosis. Problems arise in two circumstances: first, when patients are asymptomatic but have evidence of severe aortic stenosis and, second, when patients have symptoms that could be due to aortic stenosis but objective measurements of the severity of their stenosis suggest that it is only mild to moderate.

Opinions vary widely as to the correct management for asymptomatic patients. The advantage of operating early is that the patient may return to a normal and active life without the risk of sudden death on exertion; the disadvantage of surgical intervention is that all prosthetic valves have considerable problems. Tissue valves degenerate and require re-replacement, particularly in young patients, and re-operation is technically more demanding; all mechanical valves carry a small but significant risk of systemic embolism and the oral anticoagulation required with these valves also has associated risks. Bearing these facts in mind and that patients who die suddenly are rarely if ever asymptomatic prior to this event, careful supervision and postponement is often the most sensible course of action. The decision made in the individual patient depends considerably on the patient's lifestyle; for instance, a professional athlete may require early correction of aortic stenosis whereas a sedentary middle-aged patient could be managed conservatively for longer with the same degree of stenosis.

If the valve gradient seems inadequate to account for the symptoms, it is important to calculate the valve area, in case the valve gradient is underestimating the severity of stenosis due to a reduction in cardiac output, and to consider the possibility of other causes for the symptoms. For example, syncope may have an arrhythmogenic basis and angina pectoris may be due to coronary artery disease. Replacement of an aortic valve that is only mildly stenotic is unlikely to be of benefit to a patient and should not generally be undertaken.

Nowadays, age is not normally a contra-indication to surgical therapy and many patients can be successfully treated by surgery in their eighth or ninth decade with excellent results. The indications for surgical treatment of non-valvar aortic stenosis are similar to those of valvar aortic stenosis.

BALLOON VALVULOPLASTY

Balloon valvuloplasty was initially introduced for the treatment of pulmonary valve stenosis.[70-72] Recently, it has been applied to aortic stenosis Fig. 26.24). Its use varies depending on the type of aortic stenosis. In infants with severe aortic stenosis, the results of surgery are poor since surgical valvotomy

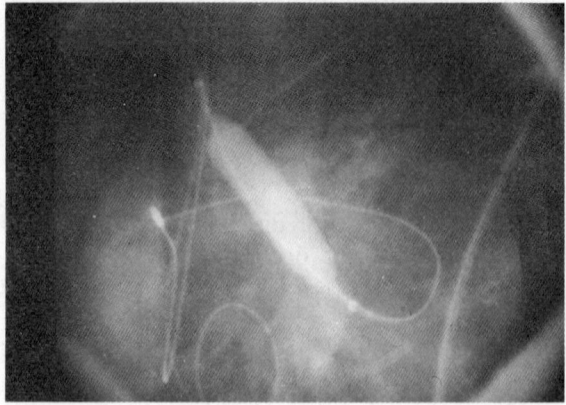

Fig. 26.24. A balloon full of radiographic contrast inflated in the aortic valve in a patient with severe aortic stenosis. The aortic valve is at the mid-point of this balloon and has been completely dilated, hence the absence of any constriction at this point. There is a guidewire beyond the balloon in the left ventricle. There are also two pacing wires in place because this patient had a dual chamber pacemaker.

is difficult and the valve cannot be replaced. In some of these patients, very good results are obtained by balloon valvuloplasty. In children and young adults in whom the valve remains pliable and the gradient is high, excellent results can often be obtained by splitting the valve using balloon valvuloplasty. Under these circumstances, this technique may be used to postpone the need for aortic valve surgery until later in adult life.

Although originally introduced for patients with flexible valves, balloon valvuloplasty is being used increasingly in elderly patients with calcific aortic stenosis. In the short term, this can produce moderately good haemodynamic results, often with the gradient being halved, and excellent symptomatic results. The safety and long-term effectiveness of this procedure have yet to be established. In elderly patients, it seems to increase valve mobility by fracturing the calcified tissue in the aortic valve. It seems likely that these plaques re-form with the passage of time. To establish the place of balloon valvuloplasty in the treatment of calcific aortic stenosis, it must be shown that it can produce better results than those for aortic valve replacement which are excellent in both the short and long term. The role of valvuloplasty and the choice of patients for the procedure remain controversial at present, and aortic valve replacement remains the treatment of choice for most patients.

REFERENCES

1. Clawson, B.J., Noble, J.F. and Lufkin, N.H. The calcified nodular deformity of the aortic valve. *Am. Heart J.* 1938; **15**: 58.
2. Karsner, H.T. and Koletsky, S. *Calcific disease of the aortic valve.* Philadelphia: J.B. Lippincot, 1947.
3. Davies, M.J. *Pathology of cardiac valves.* London: Butterworths, 1980.
4. Selzer, A. Changing aspects of the natural history of valvular aortic stenosis. *N. Engl. J. Med.* 1987; **317**: 91–8.
5. Fengolio, J.J. Jr, McAllister, H.A. Jr, DeCastro, C.M. *et al.* Congenital bicuspid aortic valve after age 20. *Am. J. Cardiol.* 1977; **39**: 164–9.
6. Pomerance, A. Pathogenesis of aortic stenosis and its relation to age. *Br. Heart J.* 1972; **34**: 569–74.
7. Hultgren, H.N. Calcific disease of the aortic valve. *Arch. Pathol.* 1948; **45**: 694–706.
8. Koletsky, S. Congenital bicuspid aortic valves. *Arch. Intern. Med.* 1941; **67**: 129–56.
9. Campbell, M. Calcific aortic stenosis and congenital bicuspid aortic valves. *Br. Heart J.* 1968; **30**: 606–16.
10. Holley, K.E., Bahn, R.C., McGoon, D.C. and Mankin, H.T. Spontaneous calcific embolization associated with calcific aortic stenosis. *Circulation* 1963; **27**: 197–202.
11. Tweedy, P.S. The pathogenesis of valvular thickening in rheumatic heart disease. *Br. Heart J.* 1956; **18**: 173–85.
12. Williams, J.C.P., Barratt-Boyes, B.G. and Lowe, J.B. Supravalvular aortic stenosis. *Circulation* 1961; **24**: 1311.
13. Ditchek, T. and Bookstein, J.J. Saccular aortic aneurysm due to aortic valve stenosis. *Circulation* 1965; **31**: 127.
14. McMillan, I.K.R. Aortic stenosis: A postmortem cinephotographic study of valve action. *Br. Heart J.* 1955; **17**: 56.
15. Morrow, A.G., Roberts, W.C., Ross, J. Jr *et al.* Clinical staff conference. Obstruction to left ventricular outflow. Current concepts of management and operative treatment. *Ann. Intern. Med.* 1968; **69**: 1255.
16. Morgan, D.J. and Hall, R.J.C. Occult aortic stenosis as a cause of intractable heart failure. *Br. Med. J.* 1979; **1**: 784–7.
17. Mirsky, I. Left ventricular stress in the intact human heart. *Biophys. J.* 1969; **9**: 189.
18. Grossman, W., Jones, D. and McLaurin, L.P. Wall stress and patterns of hypertrophy in the human left ventricle. *J. Clin. Invest.* 1975; **56**: 56–65.
19. Hood, W.P., Rackley, C.E. and Rolett, E. Wall stress in the normal and hypertrophied left ventricle. *Am. J. Cardiol.* 1968; **22**: 550–8.
20. Hess, O.M., Schneider, J., Koch, R. *et al.* Diastolic function and myocardial structure in patients with myocardial hypertrophy: special reference to normalized visco-elastic data. *Circulation* 1981; **63**: 360–71.
21. Levine, H.J., McIntyre, K.M., Lipana, J.G. and Bing, O.H.L. Force of velocity relationships in failing and non-failing heart in subjects with aortic stenosis. *Am. J. Med. Sci.* 1970; **259**: 79.
22. Mason, D.T. Regulation of cardiac performance in clinical heart disease. Interactions between contractile state, mechanical abnormalities and ventricular compensatory mechanisms. *Am. J. Cardiol.* 1973; **32**: 437.
23. Gunther, S. and Grossman, W. Determinants of ventricular function in pressure overload hypertrophy in man. *Circulation* 1979; **59**: 679–88.
24. Huber, D., Grimm, J., Koch, R. and Krayenbuehl, H.P. Determinants of ejection performance in aortic stenosis. *Circulation* 1981; **64**: 126–34.
25. Carabello, B.A., Green, L.H., Grossman, W. *et al.* Hemodynamic determinants of prognosis of aortic valve replacement in critical aortic stenosis and advanced congestive heart failure. *Circulation* 1980; **62**: 42–8.

26. Gibson, D.G., Traill, T.A., Hall, R.J.C. and Brown, D.J. Echocardiographic features of secondary left ventricular hypertrophy. *Br. Heart J.* 1979; **41**: 54–9.

27. Murakami, T., Hess, O.H., Gage, J.E. *et al.* Diastolic filling dynamics in patients with aortic stenosis. *Circulation* 1986; **73**: 1162–74.

28. Lavine, S.J., Follanbee, W.P., Shreiner, P.P. and Amioi, H. Left ventricular diastolic filling in valvular aortic stenosis. *Am. J. Cardiol.* 1986; **57**: 1349–55.

29. Krayenbuehl, H.P., Hess, O. and Hirzel, H. Pathophysiology of the hypertrophied heart in man. *Eur. Heart J.* 1982; **3** (Suppl. A): 125–31.

30. Paulus, W.J. and Brutsaert, D.L. Relaxation abnormalities in cardiac hypertrophy. *Eur. Heart J.* 1982; **3** (Suppl. A): 133–7.

31. Hess, O.M., Grimm, J. and Krayenbuehl, H.P. Diastolic simple elastic and viscoelastic properties of the left ventricle. *Circulation* 1979; **59**: 1178–87.

32. Hui, W.K.K. and Gibson, D.G. The dynamics of rapid left ventricular filling in man. In: *Advances in Cardiology*, Vol. 32. Basle: Karger, 1985, p. 735.

33. Bertrand, M.E., LaBlanche, J.M., Tilmant, P.Y. *et al.* Coronary sinus blood flow at rest and during isometric exercise in patients with aortic valve disease. Mechanisms of angina pectoris in presence of normal coronary arteries. *Am. J. Cardiol.* 1981; **47**: 199.

34. Bellhouse, B. and Bellhouse, F. Fluid mechanics of model normal and stenotic aortic valves. *Circ. Res.* 1969; **25**: 693–704.

35. Dancy, M., Leech, G. and Leatham, A. Changes in echocardiographic left ventricular minor axis dimensions during exercise in patients with aortic stenosis. *Br. Heart J.* 1984; **52**: 446–50.

36. Gorlin, R., McMillan, I.K.R., Medd, W.E. *et al.* Dynamics of the circulation in aortic valve disease. *Am. J. Med.* 1955; **18**: 855–70.

37. Oldershaw, P.J., Dawkins, K.D. and Gibson, D.G. The effect of exercise on left ventricular filling in left ventricular hypertrophy. *Br. Heart J.* 1983; **49**: 568–73.

38. Schwartz, L.S., Goldfischer, J., Sprague, G.J. and Schwartz, S.P. Syncope and sudden death in aortic stenosis. *Am. J. Cardiol.* 1969; **23**: 647–58.

39. Johnson, A.M. Aortic stenosis, sudden death and left ventricular baroreceptors. *Br. Heart J.* 1971; **33**: 1–5.

40. Mark, A.L., Kioschos, J.M., Abboud, E.M. *et al.* Abnormal responses to exercise in patients with aortic stenosis. *J. Clin. Invest.* 1973; **52**: 1138–46.

41. Richards, A.M., Nicholls, M.G., Ikram, H. *et al.* Syncope in aortic valvular stenosis. *Lancet* 1984; **ii**: 1113–6.

42. Lombard, J.T. and Seltzer, A. Valvular aortic stenosis: clinical and hemodynamic profile of patients. *Ann. Intern. Med.* 1987; **106**: 292–8.

43. Hakki, A.H., Kimbiris, D., Iskandrian, A.S. *et al.* Angina pectoris and coronary artery disease in patients with severe aortic valvular disease. *Am. J. Cardiol.* 1980; **100**: 441.

44. Ross, J. Jr and Braunwald, E. Aortic stenosis. *Circulation* 1968; **38** (Suppl. V): V-61–V-67.

45. Jones, R.C., Walker, W.J., Jahnke, E.J. and Winn, D.F. Congenital aortic stenosis. Correlation of clinical severity with hemodynamic and surgical findings in forty-three cases. *Ann. Intern. Med.* 1963; **58**: 486.

46. Romhilt, D.W., Bove, K.R. and Norris, R.J. A critical appraisal of the electrocardiographic criteria for the diagnosis of left ventricular hypertrophy. *Circulation* 1969; **40**: 185.

47. Sanders, C.A. and Freidlich, A.L. Misleading electrocardiographic findings in severe aortic stenosis. *Medicine* 1964; **43**: 393–9.

48. Pluth, J.R., Connolly, D.C. and Kirklin, J.W. Calcific aortic stenosis and complete heart block: incidence and manage-

ment (Abstract). *Circulation* 1964; **29–30** (Suppl. 3): III–141.

49. Chang, S., Clements, S. and Chang, J. Aortic stenosis: echocardiographic cusp separation and surgical description of aortic valve in 22 patients. *Am. J. Cardiol.* 1977; **39**: 499.

50. Yeh, H., Winsberg, F. and Mercer, E.N. Echographic aortic valve orifice dimension: its use in evaluating aortic stenosis and cardiac output. *J. Clin. Ultrasound* 1973; **1**: 182.

51. Motro, M., Vered, Z., Rath, S. *et al.* Correlation between echocardiography and cardiac catheterisation in assessing the severity of aortic stenosis. *Eur. Heart J.* 1983; **4**: 117–20.

52. Hall, R.J.C., Kadushi, O.A. and Evemy, K. Need for cardiac catheterisation in assessment of patients for valve surgery. *Br. Heart J.* 1983; **49**: 268–75.

53. Ten Cate, F.J., Van Dorp, W.G., Hugenholtz, P.G. and Roelandt, J. Fixed subaortic stenosis: value of echocardiography for diagnosis and differentiation between various types. *Br. Heart J.* 1979; **41**: 159.

54. Wilcox, W.D., Seward, J.B., Hagler, D.J. *et al.* Discrete subaortic stenosis: two-dimensional echocardiographic features with angiographic and surgical correlation. *Mayo Clin. Proc.* 1980; **55**: 425.

55. Weyman, A.E., Caldwell, R.L., Hurwitz, R.A. *et al.* Cross-sectional echocardiographic characteristics of aortic obstruction. I. Supravalvular aortic stenosis and aortic hypoplasia. *Circulation* 1978; **57**: 491.

56. Bennett, D.W., Evans, D.W. and Raj, M.V.J. Echocardiographic left ventricular dimensions in pressure and volume overload. Their use in assessing the aortic stenosis. *Br. Heart J.* 1975; **37**: 971–7.

57. Aziz, K.U., van Grondelle, A., Paul, M.H. and Muster, A.J. Echocardiographic assessment of the relation between left ventricular wall and cavity dimensions and peak systolic pressure in children with aortic stenosis. *Am. J. Cardiol.* 1977; **40**: 775–80.

58. Stamm, B.R. and Martin, R.P. Quantification of pressure gradients across stenotic valves by Doppler ultrasound. *J. Am. Coll. Cardiol.* 1984; **2**: 707–18.

59. Zhang, Y., Myhre, E. and Nitter-Hauge, S. Non-invasive quantifications of the aortic valve area in aortic stenosis by Doppler echocardiography. *Eur. Heart J.* 1985; **6**: 998.

60. Hohn, A.R., van Praagh, S., Moore, A.A.D. *et al.* Aortic stenosis. *Circulation* 1965; **32** (Suppl. 3): III–4.

61. Glew, R.H., Varghese, P.J., Krovetz, L.J. *et al.* Sudden death in congenital aortic stenosis: a review of eight cases with an evaluation of premonitory clinical features. *Am. Heart J.* 1969; **78**: 615–25.

62. Wagner, S. and Selzer, A. Patterns of progression of aortic stenosis: a longitudinal hemodynamic study. *Circulation* 1982; **65**: 709–12.

63. Bogart, D.B., Murphy, B.L., Wong, B.Y.S. *et al.* Progression of aortic stenosis. *Chest* 1979; **76**: 391–6.

64. Cheitlin, M.D., Gertz, E.W., Brundage, B.H. *et al.* Rate of progression of severity of aortic stenosis. *Am. Heart J.* 1979; **98**: 689–700.

65. Jonasson, R., Jonasson, B., Nordlander, R. *et al.* Rate of progression of severity of aortic stenosis. *Acta Med. Scand.* 1983; **213**: 51–4.

66. Nestico, P.F., DePace, N.L., Kimbiris, D. *et al.* Progression of isolated aortic stenosis: analysis of 29 patients having more than 1 cardiac catheterization. *Am. J. Cardiol.* 1983; **52**: 1054–8.

67. Frank, S., Johnson, A. and Ross, J. Jr. Natural history of valvular aortic stenosis. *Br. Heart J.* 1973; **35**: 41.

68. Rapaport, E. Natural history of aortic and mitral valve disease. *Am. J. Cardiol.* 1975 **35**: 221.

69. Olesen, K.H. and Warburg, E. Isolated aortic stenosis—the late prognosis. *Acta Med. Scand.* 1957; **160**: 437–46.

70. McKay, R.G., Safian, R.D., Lock, J.E. *et al.* Balloon dilata-

tion of calcific aortic stenosis in elderly patients: postmortem, intraoperative, and percutaneous valvuloplasty studies. *Circulation* 1986; 74: 119–25.

71. Lababidi, Z., Wu, J. and Walls, J.T. Percutaneous balloon valvuloplasty: results in 23 patients. *Am. J. Cardiol.* 1984; 53: 194–7.

72. Cribier, A., Savin, T., Saoudi, I. *et al.* Percutaneous transluminal valvuloplasty of acquired aortic stenosis in elderly patients: an alternative view to valve replacement? *Lancet* 1986; i: 63–7.

Chapter 27

Aortic Regurgitation

Roger Hall

AETIOLOGY AND PATHOLOGY

Aortic regurgitation is one of the commonest valvular lesions and has many causes. As with other valve lesions, there has been a change in the relative frequency of the pathologies causing it over the last 50 years. In 1932, Campbell reported that 67% of cases of aortic regurgitation were rheumatic in origin while 19% were caused by syphilis.[1] Nowadays, rheumatic fever is far less common; in a recent report of 100 cases, Davis considered that only 26% of cases were rheumatic and he did not find a single example of syphilitic aortic regurgitation.[2] A cause being reported increasingly in recent years is idiopathic dilatation of the aortic root. In Davis' series, this comprised approximately 40% of cases; further work from the USA has confirmed these findings.[3,4] The relative frequencies of the various underlying causes of aortic regurgitation are reviewed in Table 27.1.

SPECIFIC CAUSES

Rheumatic aortic regurgitation

When an aortic valve is involved by the acute rheumatic process, it becomes inflamed and thickened by oedema. If commissural fusion occurs, either aortic stenosis or combined aortic stenosis and regurgitation results. If the cusps do not fuse but fibrose and retract, the valve becomes incompetent with stiff, thickened and deformed valve cusps. Aortic regurgitation is seldom found as an isolated lesion in chronic rheumatic heart disease; it is nearly always associated with some mitral involvement. Similarly, it is rarely a pure lesion; there is often some stenosis due to a degree of commissural fusion. In addition to deformity of the aortic valve, some aortic valve annulus dilatation may occur and add to the degree of regurgitation.

Syphilitic aortic regurgitation

The cause of regurgitation is aortic root dilatation particularly affecting the first few centimetres. Syphilis virtually never attacks the valve cusps directly. Occasionally, a localized aneurysm or gumma may form in the aortic root. When the process is chronic, there is often quite extensive calcification of the ascending aorta which has a characteristic thin plate-like appearance, that can often be detected by chest X-ray.

Other forms of inflammatory aortitis

In ankylosing spondylitis, there is irregular fibrosis

Table 27.1. The main causes of aortic regurgitation.

Cause	Incidence (%) in series of 100 patients (Davies, 1980[2])*
Rheumatic	26
Inflammatory:	8
Rheumatoid	
Reiter's syndrome	
Ankylosing spondylitis	
Aortic root dilatation:	23
Idiopathic	
Connective tissue disorder	
Dissecting aneurysm	
Bicuspid aortic valve	16
Endocarditis	21†
Others:	4
Aortic valve prolapse[20]	
Trauma[81,82]	
Syphilitic	
Spontaneous tears	
Associated with congenital heart disease	
(e.g. ventricular septal defect)[21]	
No obvious cause	2

* Several of the rarer causes of aortic regurgitation were not seen in this particular review.
† 11 on a tricuspid valve, 10 on a bicuspid valve.

which distorts the aortic root extending into the base of the aortic valve, sometimes reaching as far as the mitral valve[5] This inflammatory process may also involve the conducting tissue, consequently varying degrees of heart block are a common complication.[6] Similar appearances are seen in association with rheumatoid arthritis,[7] psoriasis and Reiter's syndrome.[8] The aortic regurgitation associated with these inflammatory diseases can sometimes be quite acute in onset, in which case the valve is found to be somewhat oedematous and inflamed at surgery. A few cases are the result of a non-specific aortitis,[9] in some of which there may be evidence of a giant cell aortitis or involvement of the aorta in a more generalized giant cell arteritis.[10]

Aortic regurgitation due to non-inflammatory aortic root dilatation

In many cases of aortic regurgitation, dilatation of the aortic root of unknown aetiology appears to be the underlying cause. There is no evidence of inflammation but the media of the aorta shows varying degrees of destruction of its elastic tissue and smooth muscle. These degenerative lesions are often localized as discrete round areas. This condition has been given various names, including idiopathic aortic root dilatation,[11] aortic annulus ectasia[12] and idiopathic medial aortopathy.[13] In some cases, the aortic root dilatation is concentric leading to a central defect whereby the three cusps fail to meet. The valve cusps are not normal, showing some rolling and thickening of their edges. Occasionally, dilatation is eccentric leading to prolapse of a valve cusp. Idiopathic aortic root dilatation rarely causes problems until middle age and is often seen in the elderly.

Although most cases of aortic root dilatation are idiopathic, in a few there are associated syndromes which cause more widespread defects. The most important of these is Marfan's syndrome (Fig. 27.1).[14,15] Aortic root dilatation also occurs in the Ehlers–Danlos syndrome[16] and osteogenesis imperfecta.[17]

Bicuspid aortic valve

Bicuspid valves are common (occurring in about 1% of the population); if such a valve causes a haemodynamic problem, it is usually one of stenosis but occasionally it can lead to a mainly regurgitant lesion,[18] which is usually mild unless occurring secondary to infective endocarditis.

Dissecting aneurysm

Dissecting aneurysm is a serious condition; it frequently produces aortic regurgitation as one of its features (Fig. 27.2).[19] The intimal tear, which is followed by blood tracking into the wall of the aorta to produce the dissection, often occurs only a few centimetres above the aortic valve. When the dissection tracks down towards the supra-aortic ridge, the integrity of the aortic valve is disturbed and aortic regurgitation occurs. The presence of aortic regurgitation in dissecting aneurysm indicates that urgent surgical repair of the aneurysm is required. The right coronary cusp and intimal flaps may prolapse into the left ventricle (Fig. 27.3).

Infective endocarditis

Infective endocarditis is an important cause of aortic regurgitation. Infection may occur on a valve previously affected by the aortic stenosis or regurgitation or on one upon which there is a minor abnormality, for example, a congenitally bicuspid aortic valve. Regurgitation is due to rupture or perforation of valve cusps (Fig. 27.4) and can occur suddenly. Sometimes infective endocarditis may attack a normal aortic valve, particularly if the infecting organism is *Staphylococcus aureus*, which can produce a disease that develops over a few days or even hours and may lead to a rapid deterioration and death in a short period of time.

Other important causes of aortic regurgitation

Other important causes of aortic regurgitation are summarized in Table 27.1. Aortic valve prolapse is

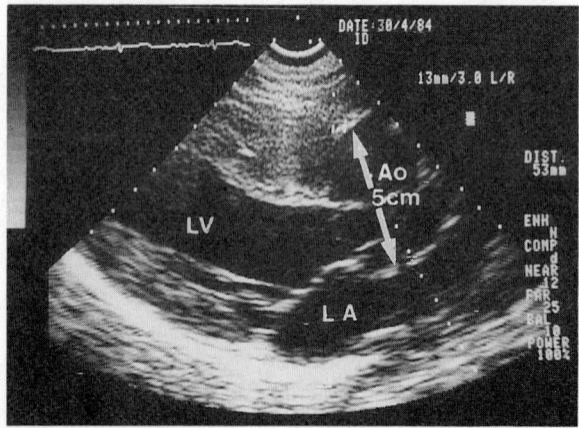

Fig. 27.1. Cross-sectional echocardiogram from a patient with Marfan's syndrome. The aortic root is grossly dilated. LV, left ventricle; LA, left atrium; Ao, aorta.

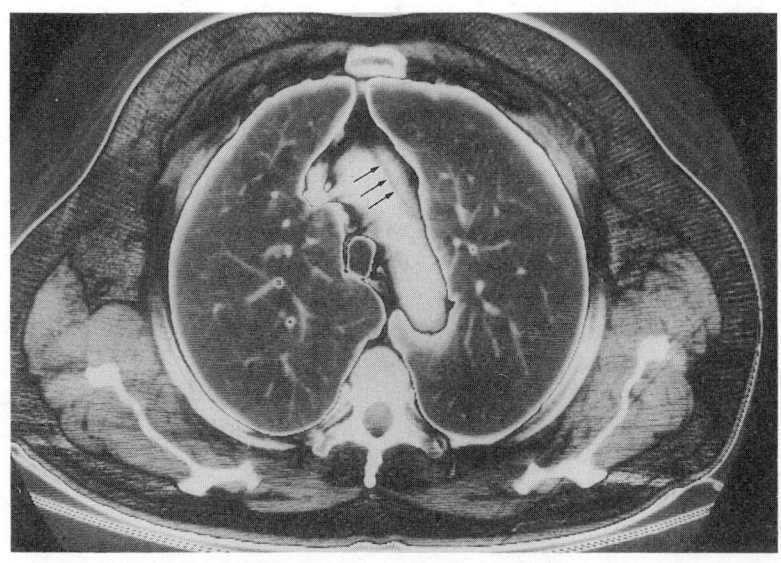

Fig. 27.2. Computed tomographic scan from a patient with a dissecting aneurysm of the aorta. The dissection flap is clearly seen (arrows) at the level of the aortic arch.

a poorly understood condition which is identified by echocardiography.[20] It rarely causes significant aortic regurgitation. The most important cause of aortic regurgitation in congenital heart disease is the prolapse of an aortic valve cusp into a ventricular septal defect just below the valve.[21] Although the ventricular septal defects that lead to this type of aortic regurgitation are often small and cause no significant haemodynamic problems themselves, the aortic regurgitation they produce may become increasingly severe and often requires surgical intervention in adolescence or adult life. The combination of a ventricular septal defect and aortic regurgitation may simulate a continuous

murmur because the harsh murmur of ventricular septal defect tends to merge into that of early diastole caused by aortic regurgitation.

PATHOPHYSIOLOGY

The adverse effects of aortic regurgitation result from the load imposed on the left ventricle by the regurgitation of substantial volumes of blood from the aorta to the left ventricle during diastole. Occasionally, as much as 80% of the ejected stroke volume may leak back into the left ventricle during the next diastole. The severity of regurgitation

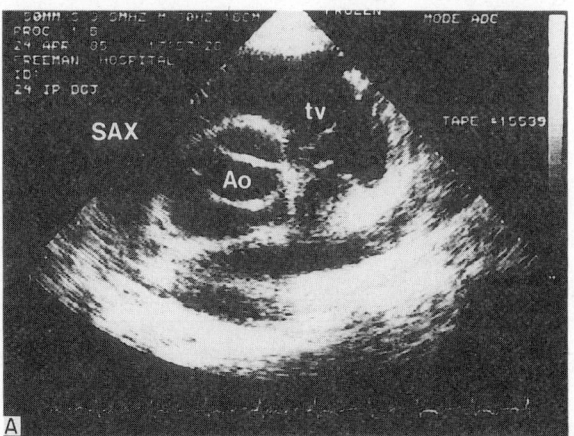

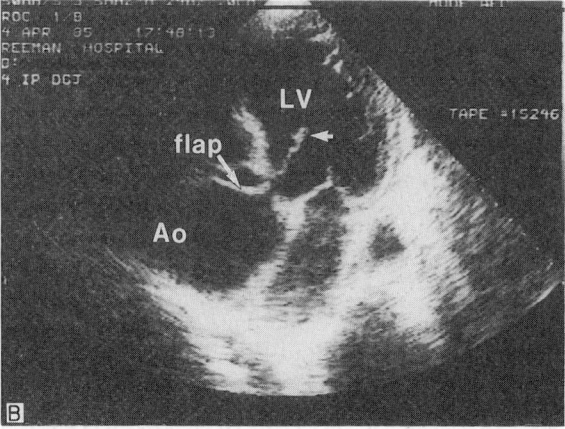

Fig. 27.3. Cross-sectional echocardiograms from a patient with an extensive dissecting aneurysm of the aortic root. (A) Parasternal short-axis view (SAX). The false lumen can be seen both in front of and behind the true lumen (marked Ao). (B) Long-axis view of the heart obtained from the cardiac apex and tilted to include the aortic root. The dissection flap (flap) can be seen in the aortic root and within the left ventricle there is a strip of intima (arrow) which has prolapsed from the aorta into the left ventricular outflow. tv, tricuspid valve; LV, left ventricle. In (B) the orientation is a mirror image of the normal orientation i.e. in this picture the aorta is presented to the left and the LV to the right.

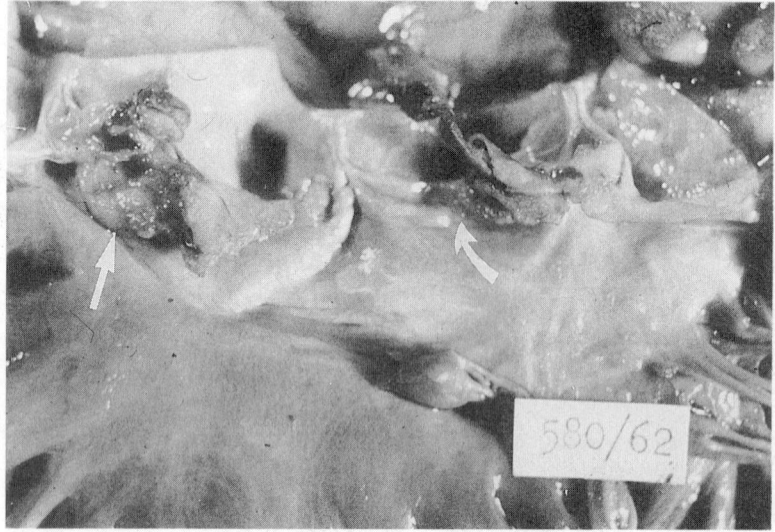

Fig. 27.4. Pathological specimen of the aortic valve from a patient who died of infective endocarditis. There is a large vegetation on one of the aortic valve cusps (left-hand arrow) and one of the valve cusps is perforated (right-hand arrow).

depends on four main factors.

1 *The size of the aortic valve orifice in diastole.* Severe regurgitation occurs through diastolic apertures of 0.3–0.7 cm^2.[22,23]

2 *Systemic vascular resistance.* A high systemic vascular resistance encourages aortic regurgitation while a low systemic vascular resistance will reduce it. This has therapeutic implications, since vasodilating drugs can be used to reduce the severity of regurgitation.

3 *The heart rate.* The amount of time available for regurgitation per minute is decreased by a rapid heart rate; as the heart rate rises, systole remains relatively constant in duration but diastole becomes very much shorter. Conversely, bradycardia increases the amount of diastole per unit time available for regurgitation.

4 *The diastolic properties of the left ventricle.* In chronic aortic regurgitation, the left ventricle is usually compliant and easily accommodates the regurgitated volume.[24] In acute aortic regurgitation, the unprepared left ventricle has a relatively low compliance and therefore limits the amount of regurgitation that can occur at the expense of a gross rise in left ventricular diastolic pressure which leads to pulmonary oedema (Fig. 27.5). This subject is discussed in more detail below.

LEFT VENTRICULAR FUNCTION IN AORTIC REGURGITATION

The volume load imposed on the left ventricle in chronic aortic regurgitation eventually leads to considerable left ventricular dilatation and hypertrophy. Although wall thickness does not approach

that seen in severe aortic stenosis, moderate increases in wall thickness combined with dilatation lead to some of the largest and heaviest hearts encountered by the pathologist. The left ventricle is able to accommodate the large regurgitant volume by dilatation and thereby maintain a normal cardiac output until the late stages of the disease. Consequently, patients often tolerate severe aortic regurgitation for a long time without developing symptoms; 75% of asymptomatic patients with significant aortic regurgitation and initially normal left ventricular function will still be asymptomatic 7 years after diagnosis.[25] The ability of the left ventricle to accommodate severe aortic regurgitation without developing symptoms is at the centre

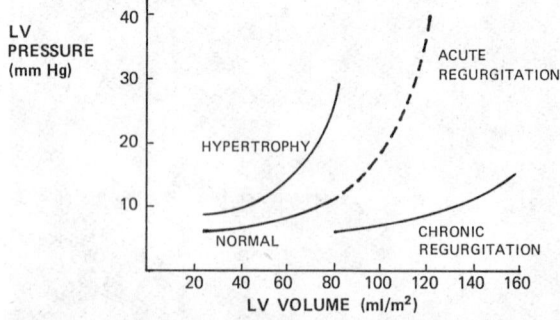

Fig. 27.5. The pressure–volume relationships of the left ventricle in normal subjects, patients with hypertrophy and those with acute and chronic regurgitation. It can be seen that hypertrophy produces a small change from normal, that patients with acute regurgitation behave as if they are on the extreme right-hand side of the normal relationship, and that the relationship is completely altered in patients with chronic regurgitation, when large volumes of blood are accommodated with only a small rise in the left ventricular pressure.

of the common dilemma of the timing of aortic valve replacement. The main concern is that, while the ventricle dilates and the patient remains asymptomatic, irreversible damage to the left ventricle may be occurring that will ultimately affect the symptomatic result and possibly the mortality of subsequent aortic valve replacement. As information about the natural history and reversibility by surgery of abnormalities of left ventricular function is incomplete, this clinical dilemma persists.

Systolic function

Mild degrees of aortic regurgitation cause little disturbance of left ventricular function; a small increase in ejection fraction compensates for the abnormality. When regurgitation is more severe, the increase in end-systolic and end-diastolic dimensions allows a larger than normal stroke volume to be produced without any appreciable increase in ejection fraction. Generally, when aortic regurgitation is severe, there is a moderate increase in heart rate which tends to limit the degree of regurgitation (see above). Interpretation of 'ejection phase' indices of left ventricular performance (for example, ejection fraction) and left ventricular dimensions, is difficult because both are dependent on afterload and preload.[26-28] A fall in ejection fraction or a change in left ventricular dimension may be due to either a deterioration of left ventricular function or an increase in the severity of regurgitation. Despite these problems, many workers have found a rough correlation of both falling ejection fraction and increasing left ventricular dimension with surgical outcome.[29,30] The results of early studies showed a relationship between surgical mortality and a dilated poorly contracting ventricle. Recent improvements in surgical and anaesthetic techniques have decreased surgical mortality in these patients who were at high risk. Altered operative mortality is no longer a useful way of assessing the impact of pre-operative left ventricular function; it is now more valid to examine the symptomatic results and late survival following surgery.[31] It has been shown that simple ejection phase parameters of left ventricular function may help to predict long-term survival.[32] For patients in whom the pre-operative ejection fraction was < 45% survival at 5 years after valve replacement was 52%, whereas patients who had a pre-operative ejection fraction > 45% had a 5-year survival rate of 96%. The prognostic significance of this reduction in ejection fraction was stronger if it had been present for more than 18

months before surgery or was combined with poor exercise tolerance as assessed by treadmill testing. Other workers have not been able to show a clear predictive value for these simple measurements.[33-35]

As ejection phase indices, recorded at rest, are difficult to interpret, attempts have been made to derive other variables of left ventricular function that may help to determine the optimal time for surgery. The use of end-systolic pressure–volume or stress–strain indices has the advantage of being virtually independent of loading, and such indices have been applied to this situation.[36] Scognamiglio et al. used this approach in patients with aortic regurgitation.[37] The ratio between peak arterial pressure and end-systolic volume (derived from echocardiography) was related to the ejection fraction. In patients in whom this relationship was normal, surgery gave excellent short- and long-term results. In contrast, patients in whom this relationship was similar to that in patients with cardiomyopathy fared much worse: 25% died in the post-operative phase and a further 33% developed cardiac failure in the year after operation.

As in patients with aortic stenosis, the development of an appropriate degree of left ventricular hypertrophy normalizes the increase in wall stress which would otherwise be produced by an increase in cavity dimension and intraventricular pressure. Information about the effectiveness of this adaptation in aortic regurgitation is conflicting, possibly due to differences in patient selection between studies. In general, however, it appears that appropriate hypertrophy has a beneficial effect on left ventricular function,[38] before and after operation; in these patients, the hypertrophy tends to regress following surgery. Both inadequate and excess hypertrophy (of an inappropriate degree) may have deleterious effects on both pre- and post-operative myocardial function.[39,40]

Diastolic function

Although abnormalities of left ventricular diastolic function are common in aortic regurgitation, their clinical significance is poorly understood.

Since aortic regurgitation begins as soon as systole has finished, a true isovolumic relaxation period does not exist. Information about the pattern of left ventricular filling in aortic regurgitation is conflicting. Osbakken and Bove[41] have described normal left ventricular filling patterns in patients with symptomatic aortic regurgitation but found that left ventricular filling was later and slower once patients developed heart failure. Lavine *et al.*[42] who studied a larger group of patients found abnormalities of diastolic function to be more widespread even in the absence of heart failure. The explanations of these changes in diastolic function are largely unsatisfactory; hypertrophy, fibrosis, ischaemia and altered loading conditions have all been incriminated. Surgery has not been found to reverse these abnormalities of diastolic function.

As well as the alterations in the filling patterns of the ventricle during diastole, there are also changes in its diastolic pressure–volume relationships when regurgitation is chronic. The stiffness of the left ventricle is reduced so that a large left ventricular volume can be managed at relatively low diastolic pressures.[43] This adaptation (Fig. 27.5) has obvious advantages and it is probably the most important factor underlying the ability of patients with severe aortic regurgitation to remain asymptomatic for a long time, but its mechanism is poorly understood. Slippage of muscle fibres and the formation of additional sarcomeres during hypertrophy such that sarcomere length remains normal, combined with increased wall thickness, which reduces wall stress, may all contribute. Finally, the pericardium, which normally limits ventricular filling to some extent, may stretch and thereby cause less restriction than it does in the heart that has not adapted.

ACUTE AORTIC REGURGITATION

The pathophysiology of acute aortic regurgitation is different to that of chronic aortic regurgitation. Sudden and severe regurgitation into the unprepared ventricle which is neither dilated or hypertrophied causes a rapid rise in left ventricular diastolic pressure which may be as high as 60–70 mmHg.[44] This pressure is transmitted back into the lungs and leads to acute pulmonary oedema. As the pressure equalizes between the aorta and the ventricle early in diastole, the time during which aortic regurgitation can occur is limited, consequently the early diastolic murmur is sometimes inconspicuous or absent. The early rise in left ventricular diastolic pressure caused by the torrential regurgitation into the unprepared and thus non-compliant left ventricle quickly exceeds left atrial pressure and therefore the mitral valve closes early in diastole (Fig. 27.6).[45] The clinical features and diagnosis of acute aortic regurgitation are discussed further below.

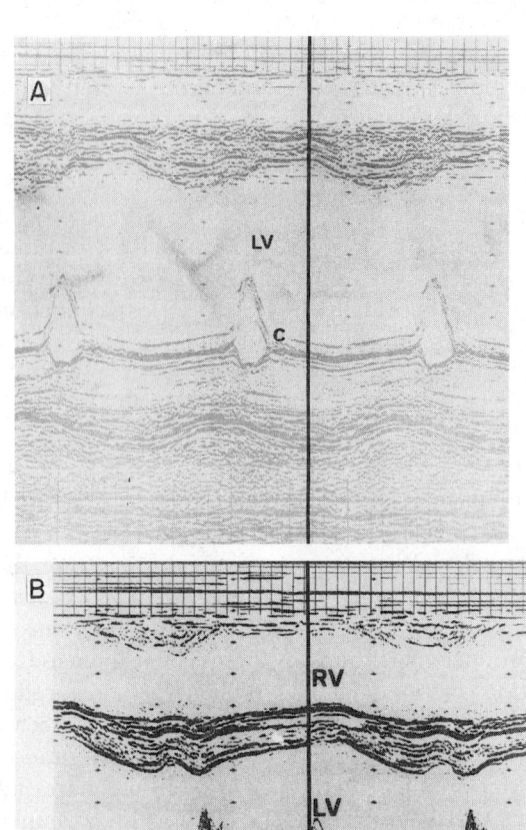

Fig. 27.6. M-Mode echocardiograms from a patient with acute aortic regurgitation due to infective endocarditis (A) and a patient with chronic stable aortic regurgitation (B). The vertical lines mark the onset of the QRS complex which is not easy to see in A. The closure of the mitral valve is marked (C). It can be seen that in acute aortic regurgitation the mitral valve closes well *before* the onset of the next QRS complex despite the fast heart rate. In the patient with chronic stable aortic regurgitation, mitral valve closure occurs well *after* the QRS complex. RV, right ventricle; LV, left ventricle.

CORONARY BLOOD FLOW

Coronary blood flow is largely dependent on aortic diastolic pressure. When this falls to low levels, coronary blood flow is compromised particularly when there is a raised left ventricular end-diastolic pressure.

EFFECT OF EXERCISE IN AORTIC REGURGITATION

In general, the proportion of cardiac output that

regurgitates into the left ventricle, the regurgitant fraction, is reduced by exercise. At peak exercise, this reduction is usually about 20%[46] and occurs regardless of the state of left ventricular function at rest or on exercise. The most important factor in the reduction of the regurgitant fraction is the increase in heart rate which reduces the duration of diastole per unit time.

In addition to the reduction in regurgitant fraction, other changes in left ventricular function occur. Generally, patients who have severe aortic regurgitation and normal resting left ventricular function show a normal increase in ejection fraction and stroke volume. Unlike normal subjects in whom the increase in stroke volume on exercise is achieved almost exclusively by an increase in end-diastolic volume, patients with significant aortic regurgitation show a reduction in both systolic and end-diastolic left ventricular volume.[46,47] The reduction in end-diastolic volume is explained, at least in part, by the reduction in regurgitant fraction but the encroachment on end-systolic volume, which is similar to that seen in trained athletes, suggests 'a higher inotropic state' of the myocardium.[46] The reduction in ventricular volume on exercise has the advantage of lowering wall stress which, combined with the increase in mean aortic pressure, favours coronary flow while limiting myocardial oxygen consumption which is highly dependent on wall stress (and heart rate).

In contrast, patients who have impaired resting left ventricular function show a progressive fall in ejection fraction and an increase in both systolic and diastolic left ventricular volumes on exercise.[48] These volume changes occur despite the fall in regurgitant fraction and serve to increase wall stress and myocardial oxygen consumption. Exceptions to these patterns may occur. Occasionally, patients with apparently normal resting left ventricular function show a fall in ejection fraction during exercise whereas others in whom resting left ventricular function appears abnormal do not show any further deterioration with exercise.

The marked fall in regurgitant fraction with exercise is probably very important in determining the long asymptomatic periods seen in many patients with this condition.

Recently, exercise and stress have been investigated as means of unmasking early abnormalities of left ventricular function in patients with aortic regurgitation.[48,49] These techniques, which commonly use non-invasive assessment of ejection fraction by radionuclide angiography, can show differences in the reaction to exercise between patients with apparently identical resting left ventricular function. The clinical significance of these changes is not yet known but in future they may prove useful in determining the correct time for aortic valve replacement.

CLINICAL FEATURES

Patients with aortic regurgitation often remain asymptomatic for many years. Although the onset of the valve lesion may occur at an early age, for example, during an attack of rheumatic fever, it rarely gives rise to symptoms until the middle or late years. Occasionally, individuals with marked aortic regurgitation, although unrestricted in their physical activity, may be aware of unusually vigorous action of the heart or prominent peripheral arterial pulsation, particularly during exercise. In contrast to this slowly progressive form of chronic aortic regurgitation, acute aortic regurgitation is nearly always associated with an immediate onset of severe symptoms, of which breathlessness is the most prominent.

SYMPTOMS

The main symptoms of aortic regurgitation are dyspnoea, tiredness and angina pectoris. Dyspnoea occurs as a result of an increase in left ventricular end-diastolic pressure, particularly on exercise; tiredness is probably related to an impairment of cardiac output mainly during exertion. As the disease progresses further, the left ventricle is no longer able to accommodate the large volume of regurgitation, and left heart failure ensues. This increases exertional dyspnoea; orthopnoea sometimes associated with episodes of paroxysmal nocturnal dyspnoea may develop. At a late stage of the illness, congestive heart failure ensues producing ankle swelling and hepatic engorgement.

Angina pectoris occurs in pure aortic regurgitation but is considerably rarer than in either a combined aortic stenosis and regurgitation or pure aortic stenosis. It has the features of exertional angina that occur in any other clinical setting. Its occurrence in a patient with pure aortic regurgitation should raise the possibility that it is the result of concomitant coronary artery disease. In syphilitic aortic regurgitation, angina is likely to be due to stenosis of the coronary ostia.

Other symptoms

Several curious symptom complexes may occur. Carotid sheath pain experienced as episodes of bilateral throbbing pain of sudden onset in the region of the carotid arteries, associated with tenderness over these arteries, is considered to be a rare but distinctive feature of severe aortic regurgitation.[50] Episodes of abdominal pain often with angina or heart failure, and nocturnal paroxysms of angina during which there is a sudden rise in blood pressure with an increase in pulse and respiratory rates associated with vasomotor disturbance such as flushing and sweating, have been described.[50,51]

PHYSICAL SIGNS

When aortic regurgitation is mild, the only abnormal feature is the early diastolic murmur; with moderate to severe lesions, the peripheral signs are usually well marked.

Peripheral signs

Arterial pulse

The arterial pulse in chronic aortic regurgitation is large in volume (Fig. 27.7), rises and falls abnormally quickly and is usually described as collapsing. This abnormality is appreciated in all peripheral pulses but it is often most striking in the carotid arteries. Occasionally, the pulse has a bisferiens (two peaks) character, which usually implies associated aortic stenosis but it can occur in pure regurgitation. The pulse rate is normal except when the lesion becomes severe in which case a slight or moderate resting tachycardia occurs. This tachycar-

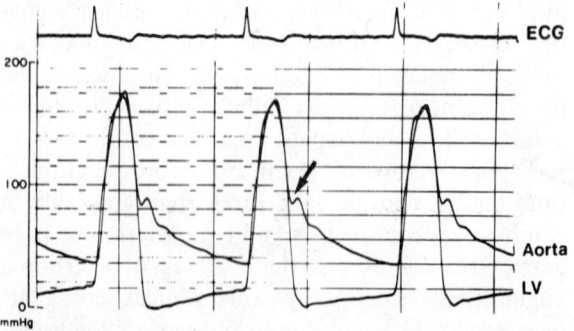

Fig. 27.7. Simultaneous recording of left ventricular and aortic pressures in a patient with severe aortic regurgitation. Note the large sharply rising aortic pressure pulse, the low diastolic pressure (< 40 mmHg) and the low dicrotic notch (arrow). The dicrotic notch is synchronous with aortic valve closure.

dia is beneficial because it limits the degree of aortic regurgitation. The rhythm is usually sinus; atrial fibrillation develops only very rarely in pure aortic regurgitation. If it does occur, associated mitral valve disease is often found.

The sudden forceful ejection of large volumes of blood into the aorta in systole and rapid leak of blood back into the left ventricle during diastole give rise to several unusual physical signs which are summarized in Table 27.2.

Blood pressure

Typically, when aortic regurgitation is more than mild, the diastolic blood pressure is low and the systolic blood pressure slightly raised, causing the

Table 27.2. Abnormalities of the pulse in aortic regurgitation.

Name	Physical sign	Comment
Water-hammer pulse	Vigorous tapping felt when forearm or wrist grasped	Increased by raising arm vertically
Corrigan's pulse	Collapsing pulse plus visible pulsation in neck, temporal arteries and elsewhere	—
De Musset's sign	Head nodding in time with the pulse	Named after French poet with syphilitic aortic regurgitation
Quincke's pulse	Capillary pulsation, seen best in fingertips by transillumination	May be accentuated by gentle pressure on nail, may also be seen in lips and earlobes. Can occur in vasodilated normal subjects
Hill's sign	Excess of femoral systolic pressure compared with brachial	Femoral systolic pressure exceeds brachial by as much as 60–100 mmHg. Normal difference is 10–20 mmHg
Duroziez's sign	Auscultation of slightly compressed femoral artery produces to-and-fro systolic and diastolic murmur	May occur in vasodilated normal subjects
'Pistol shot' femorals	Booming sound synchronous with the pulse, heard by auscultation over femoral artery	—

pulse pressure to be wider than normal (Fig. 27.7). In severe cases, the diastolic blood pressure is usually < 50 mmHg and frequently the pressure in the sphygmomanometer can be lowered to zero without the sound disappearing. In such cases, muffling rather than disappearance should be taken as being closer to the true diastolic pressure. Elevation of systolic blood pressure is usually moderate; systolic blood pressures of 150–160 mmHg are typical. Whereas in normal subjects the pulse pressure is usually in the region of 30–50 mmHg, in aortic regurgitation it often exceeds 80 mmHg and sometimes reaches 100 mmHg. The pulse pressure tends to be particularly wide in elderly subjects with sclerotic arteries. If cardiac failure develops, the systolic blood pressure may fall and the diastolic blood pressure rise.[52] In patients with underlying hypertension, the diastolic blood pressure may not reflect the severity of regurgitation as accurately as it does in patients who are not hypertensive.

Cardiac signs

Inspection and palpation

When regurgitation is minor, inspection and palpation are normal. Once regurgitation becomes more severe, a vigorous but diffuse apex beat, displaced downwards and outwards, can be seen and on palpation this is found to be 'heaving' in characer. In the most severe cases, the apex beat is displaced into the mid-axillary region. Precordial thrills are not usually felt unless a valve cusp has been ruptured or perforated.

Auscultation

The characteristic murmur of aortic regurgitation is an immediate or early diastolic murmur. It is nearly always of high frequency and decrescendo. Occasionally, there is a slight increase in intensity before the decrescendo begins. The murmur starts immediately after the aortic component of the second heart sound but occasionally there is a short pause. Although its intensity is a poor guide to the severity of regurgitation, the murmur is usually soft in milder cases. The duration of the murmur is the key to the severity of regurgitation, although this is not a completely reliable sign.[51,53]

The murmur is usually best heard along the left side of the sternum in the third or fourth left interspace. Occasionally, particularly when the ascending aorta is dilated, it is loudest in the second right intercostal space; less frequently, it is best heard in the pulmonary area or at the cardiac apex. The chances of hearing the murmur, which may be soft and high pitched, are improved by auscultation with the patient leaning forward in held expiration. When aortic regurgitation is the result of rupture of an aortic valve cusp, it may be extremely loud and either musical or harsh. It has been likened to the cooing of a dove or the cry of a seagull (seagull murmur). A precordial diastolic thrill is most likely to be felt in these cases.

Two other murmurs are frequently heard in aortic regurgitation. Nearly all patients with significant aortic regurgitation have an ejection systolic murmur, usually heard in the same area as the early diastolic murmur, caused by the high forward flow across the aortic valve in systole as the regurgitated blood is pumped back into the aorta. It can be difficult to differentiate this systolic component from the murmur of concomitant aortic stenosis. The second murmur is named after Austin Flint who, in 1862, described a pre-systolic murmur in two cases of aortic regurgitation.[54] Today, the term Austin Flint murmur is used to describe a low-frequency mid-diastolic murmur best heard at the cardiac apex which may show pre-systolic accentuation. The murmur is virtually indistinguishable from that of mitral stenosis, but it is not preceded by an opening snap. There is no close correlation between the presence of this murmur and the severity of the aortic regurgitation. The exact mechanism causing this murmur is not yet known. As vibration of the anterior leaflet of the mitral valve is frequently seen echocardiographically in patients with aortic regurgitation, this has been considered as a possible mechanism but studies by Fortuin and Craige[55] suggest that this is not the case. They found that the vibrations of the anterior leaflet of the mitral valve (Fig. 27.8) were related to the timing of the early diastolic murmur and not the low-frequency Austin Flint murmur, which they regard as due to vibrations set up by anterograde flow of blood across a closing mitral valve orifice. Other authors have suggested that late diastolic accentuation of this murmur could be the result of diastolic mitral regurgitation caused by a raised end-diastolic pressure,[56,57] but Fortuin and Craige[55] point out that when a high diastolic pressure causes premature closure of the mitral valve the late diastolic phase of the Austin Flint murmur is usually eliminated. It is hazardous to regard a mid-diastolic murmur heard in a patient

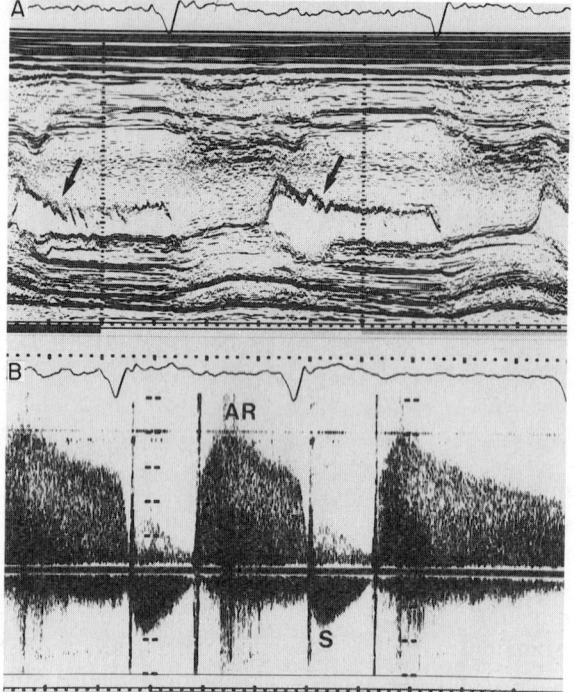

Fig. 27.8. M-Mode echocardiogram (A) and continuous wave Doppler recording (B) from a patient with severe aortic regurgitation. Although the mitral valve shows slight thickening and is probably rheumatic, it still demonstrates vigorous vibration during diastole (arrows). The continuous wave Doppler signal, obtained from the cardiac apex, depicts regurgitation above the zero line because it is coming towards the transducer. There is a strong regurgitant signal (AR). The systolic signal (S) is of normal velocity (cf. Fig. 27.12).

with aortic regurgitation as being of the Austin Flint variety, particularly if the aetiology of the valve disease is rheumatic, because such an assumption would lead to mitral valve disease being overlooked. Echocardiography provides the most reliable means of determining whether a mid-diastolic murmur is due to mitral stenosis or is an Austin Flint murmur.

A pan-systolic murmur is sometimes present at the cardiac apex in patients with advanced aortic regurgitation in whom left ventricular dilatation led to functional mitral regurgitation. It is particularly likely to occur with the sudden onset of aortic regurgitation in infective endocarditis.

The first heart sound is often normal, but in severe acute cases (see below) when there is premature close of the mitral valve it may be virtually absent.[58] Following the first heart sound, an early systolic ejection click may be present particularly when the underlying cause of aortic regurgitation is a bicuspid valve. The second heart

sound is also normal in most cases, although the aortic component is absent if the valve cusps are calcified and immobile. Once heart failure is advanced and pulmonary hypertension has occurred, the pulmonary component of the second heart sound may be accentuated. A third heart sound develops when left ventricular failure is imminent or has occurred, but it may be masked by the Austin Flint murmur at the apex or when the early diastolic murmur radiates to the cardiac apex and is loud.

CLINICAL FEATURES OF ACUTE AORTIC REGURGITATION

Acute aortic regurgitation nearly always results from the perforation and/or rupture of a valve cusp due to infective endocarditis, although it can result from other mechanisms such as dissecting aneurysm or cardiac trauma. Its clinical picture is different to that of chronic aortic regurgitation. *Chronic* aortic regurgitation has a long asymptomatic period, whereas *acute* aortic regurgitation of any severity subjects the unprepared left ventricle to a sudden volume load and therefore there is an immediate and marked rise in left ventricular end-diastolic pressure (Fig. 27.5)[44,45] Almost immediately, this leads to the symptoms of left heart failure, of which dyspnoea, orthopnoea and paroxysmal noctural dyspnoea are the most striking.

The physical signs are also different. In *chronic* aortic regurgitation, many of the characteristic signs are due to the enormous volume of blood ejected with each systole by the hypertrophied and dilated left ventricle. In the *acute* situation the previously normal left ventricle suddenly subjected to aortic regurgitation is incapable of producing a large stroke volume and therefore the characteristic abnormalities of the pulse are not seen. The physical signs are those of a low output state associated with left ventricular failure. There is usually obvious dyspnoea at rest. The patient may be cyanosed with a cold periphery and coughing due to the presence of pulmonary oedema which may be expectorated. There is a sinus tachycardia and the pulse is sharp in character and of low volume. The blood pressure is low and the pulse pressure is not increased. On auscultation, the early diastolic murmur due to aortic regurgitation is short, frequently soft and may be inaudible because the duration of regurgitation is short (see above) and the total volume of blood regurgitated is low. The most prominent auscultatory feature is usually a loud third and occasionally a fourth heart sound leading to a marked gallop rhythm. Sometimes an apical systolic murmur due to functional mitral regurgitation is also heard.

This clinical picture is confined to patients with no pre-existing aortic regurgitation. Sometimes acute aortic regurgitation occurs in patients who already have a significant degree of chronic aortic regurgitation and subsequently develop infective endocarditis. This leads to a mixed picture in which some of the signs of chronic regurgitation persist but tachycardia, pulmonary oedema and heart failure with a shortening of the early diastolic murmur and a decrease in the pulse pressure are superimposed upon them. Under these circumstances, the diagnosis of aortic regurgitation is usually not difficult, but in the patient with a previously normal aortic valve and left ventricle it may be very difficult, unless it is suspected and appropriate tests, of which echocardiography is the most important, are used (Fig. 27.6).

INVESTIGATIONS

CHEST X–RAY

When aortic regurgitation is mild, the chest X-ray is normal. As the condition advances, progressive cardiomegaly occurs, mainly due to an increase in the size of the left ventricle. This causes the lower left cardiac border to extend laterally downwards on the postero-anterior chest film, and posterior bulging of the left ventricle towards the spine may be seen on the lateral film. In many cases, the ascending aorta is dilated and becomes prominent on the postero-anterior film. Some degree of valvular calcification may be detected on the lateral chest film; in syphilitic regurgitation, linear calcification in the wall of the ascending aorta is a characteristic feature. Once left ventricular failure develops, pulmonary congestion and oedema are seen; eventually, enlargement of the left atrium and main pulmonary arteries may also be detected, but this is unusual and a very late feature.

ELECTROCARDIOGRAM

Aortic regurgitation causes left ventricular and left atrial hypertrophy. Left ventricular hypertrophy is initially shown by a considerable increase in the voltage of the electrocardiogram, particularly in the precordial leads. Later, the ST-segment and T-wave changes of hypertrophy develop. The characteristic changes of left atrial hypertrophy with broadening of the P wave in lead II and a large negative component in lead V_1 are commonly seen when aortic regurgitation is severe. The PR interval may also be prolonged in severe cases.[51]

Twenty-four hour electrocardiographic recording rarely reveals atrial arrhythmias of significance but ventricular arrhythmias are quite common. These are particularly prominent when left ventricular function deteriorates as the disease enters its advanced stages.

ULTRASOUND

Both echocardiography and Doppler are extremely helpful in the detection and assessment of patients with aortic regurgitation. Although the main features have been described in Chapters 13 and 14, they are reviewed below.

Detection of aortic regurgitation by echocardiography is indirect and it should be remembered that severe aortic regurgitation can occur through a valve which appears, echocardiographically, to be normal. The most common echocardiographic clue to the presence of aortic regurgitation is the characteristic high-frequency fluttering of the anterior cusp of the mitral valve during diastole (Fig. 27.8). This fluttering is also seen on other intracardiac structures including the posterior cusp of the mitral valve, the interventricular septum and, less commonly, the posterior wall of the left ventricle. In patients with concomitant rheumatic mitral stenosis, the mitral valve is frequently too thick to flutter but vibration of these other structures is usually detected if high-quality echocardiograms are obtained.[59] Diastolic fluttering is detected reliably only by M-mode echocardiography. Its presence and severity are not closely correlated with the severity of aortic regurgitation.[59] Although it may be absent in patients with significant aortic regurgitation, it is so common that its absence should raise the possibility that the physical signs ascribed to aortic regurgitation are due to some other cause. The rapid diastolic vibration of the mitral valve seen in aortic regurgitation must be distinguished from the coarser fluttering of the mitral valve commonly occurring in patients with atrial fibrillation (Fig. 27.9).

The Doppler technique is the best method for detecting aortic regurgitation (Fig. 27.8). It is extremely sensitive and can demonstrate even minor degrees of regurgitation which are not detectable

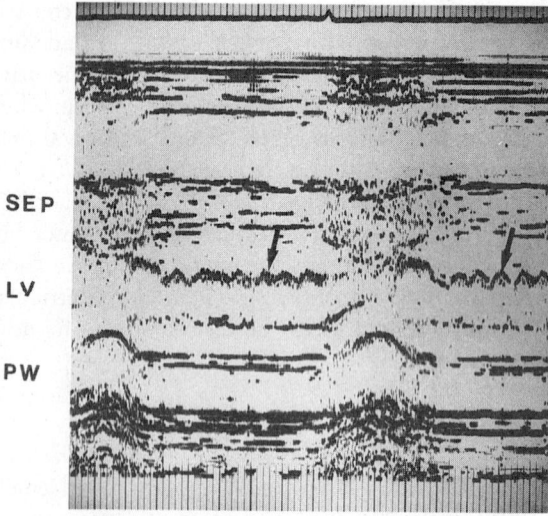

Fig. 27.9. M-Mode echocardiogram from a patient with atrial fibrillation. There is coarse fluttering of the anterior leaflet of the mitral valve (arrows). This must be distinguished from the finer vibrations seen in aortic regurgitation (see Fig. 27.8). SEP, septum; LV, left ventricle; PW, posterior wall.

clinically. It is also an excellent method for distinguishing aortic regurgitation from conditions that may be confused with it. The most important is pulmonary regurgitation but occasionally patients with a ruptured sinus of Valsalva or a persistent ductus arteriosus may be misdiagnosed clinically as having aortic regurgitation.

Echocardiography and Doppler ultrasound used in combination will always distinguish whether a mid-diastolic murmur heard in a patient with aortic regurgitation is due to concomitant mitral stenosis or is an Austin Flint murmur.

Echocardiography may establish the cause of aortic regurgitation (see Chapter 13). Direct visualization of the aortic valve will reveal the thickened leaflets of a rheumatic valve, vegetations

due to aortic regurgitation or a flail aortic valve leaflet caused by disruption usually during the course of the infective endocarditis. Echocardiography has also been used to identify aortic valve prolapse,[20] a condition for which the criteria are at present inadequately defined and the clinical significance not known. Patients with a high ventricular septal defect in the membranous part of the septum frequently develop aortic regurgitation due to prolapse of the right coronary cusp of the aortic valve into the left ventricular outflow tract during diastole. Occasionally, this cusp prolapses through the ventricular septal defect and can be seen as a vibrating structure in the right ventricular outflow tract.[60]

The echocardiographic appearance of the aortic root sometimes gives some information about the cause of aortic regurgitation. When aortic regurgitation is due to aortic root dilatation (for example, Marfan's syndrome, hypertension, some inflammatory conditions of the aortic root and idiopathic dilatation of the aortic root), the echocardiogram shows increased aortic root dimensions (Figs 27.1 and 27.10). This increase is usually only moderate (a few centimetres), but occasionally the diameter of the aortic root may double or even treble. Dissecting aneurysm as a cause of aortic regurgitation can often (Fig. 27.3), but not always, be detected by echocardiography. In general, the overall anatomy of the aortic root is seen by the cross-sectional technique and the dimension in various parts can be measured by using the cross-sectional technique to guide the M-mode beam to the appropriate place. Although the presence of dissecting aneurysm can be suspected from M-mode echocardiography (Fig. 27.11)[61] the cross-sectional technique is nearly always needed to make this diagnosis[62] but it is not completely reliable. Similarly, although the M-mode technique may give more

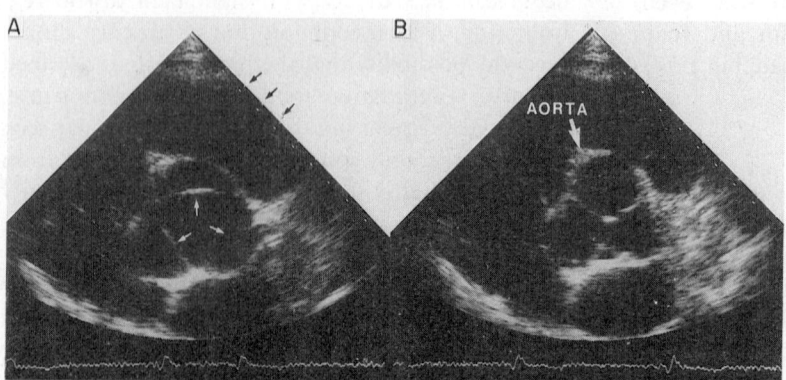

Fig. 27.10. Cross-sectional echocardiogram from a patient with Marfan's syndrome (parasternal short-axis view). The enormously dilated aortic root containing three valve cusps can be seen. The valve cusps are open in systole (A) (arrows) and closed in diastole (B). There is definite dilatation of each sinus of Valsalva to give a trefoil appearance to the aortic root. The normal aortic root usually appears almost circular at this level. The calibrations (1 cm apart) are highlighted by small black arrows. The aortic root is > 5 cm in diameter (normal < 3 cm).

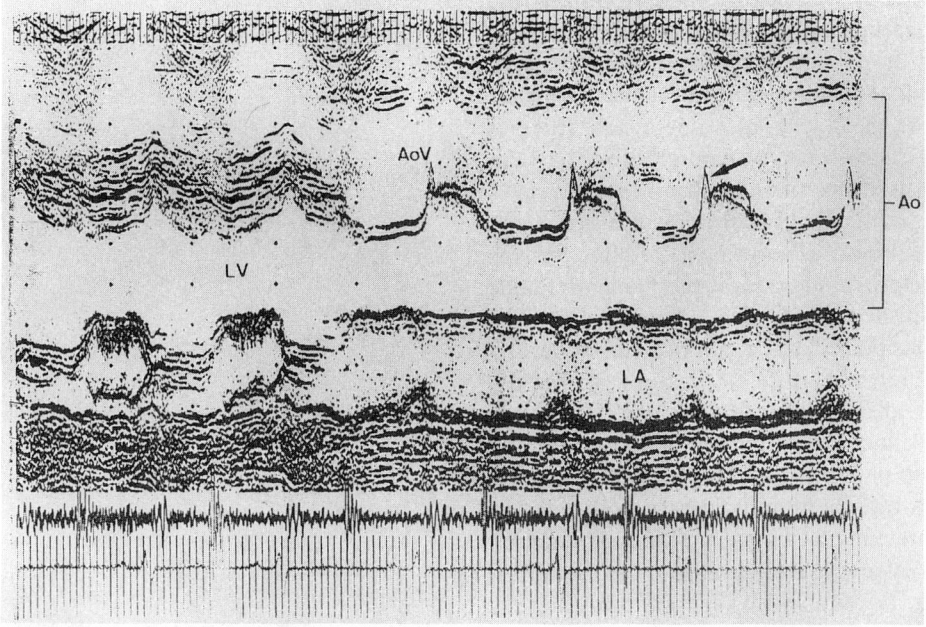

Fig. 27.11. M-Mode echocardiogram from a patient with a dissecting aneurysm of the aorta. The echo beam has been swept from the left ventricle (left) to the aorta (right). There is gross dilatation of the aortic root (approximately 5 cm) and very abnormal movement of the aortic valve (arrow). The mitral valve shows coarse vibration of its anterior leaflet due to aortic regurgitation. Although these findings suggest a dissecting aneurysm, they are non-specific. LV, left ventricle; Aov, aortic valve; LA, left atrium.

information about the fine structure and movement of aortic valve cusps, the cross-sectional technique is far superior in defining valve prolapse, flail leaflets or vegetations. The new technique of trans-oesophageal echocardiography is superior in the detection of both dissecting aneurysm and vegetations and computed tomographic scanning is a useful technique for diagnosing dissecting aneurysm (Fig. 27.2).

Serial studies of left ventricular dimension and wall movement are important in the follow-up of patients with aortic regurgitation. Although the exact role of echocardiographic criteria in the decision to recommend surgery remains uncertain, changes in left ventricular dimensions and function, detected by echocardiography, may signal that the time for surgery is approaching. The frequency with which serial echocardiograms need to be carried out depends on the clinical situation; studies every year in stable patients are probably sufficient whereas studies at 3–6-month intervals are necessary if the patient's state begins to change either clinically or echocardiographically. When using serial studies, a change of at least 5 mm is needed before it can be regarded as reflecting a true alteration in left ventricular dimension.

Echocardiography is particularly useful in pa-

tients with severe acute aortic regurgitation. The most important feature, reflected by the echocardiographic findings, is the rapid rise in diastolic pressure as severe regurgitation occurs into the unprepared left ventricle. This causes the mitral valve to close early in diastole (Fig. 27.6),[63,64] an abnormality which is best detected by the M-mode technique. Using the M-mode technique and the electrocardiogram simultaneously, valve closure occurring well before the next QRS complex (and often before the next P wave), rather than at or just after the next QRS complex, is deemed premature. It has also been suggested that if the mitral valve stays open for < 400 ms (normal range 500–700 ms), mitral valve closure is likely to be premature. The main disadvantage of assessing premature mitral valve closure by measuring the time during which the valve remains open is that the period of mitral valve opening is curtailed by sinus tachycardia. The assessment of mitral valve movement in relation to the electrocardiogram is generally more reliable.

CARDIAC CATHETERIZATION

As the diagnosis of severe aortic regurgitation and the assessment of its effect on left ventricular function is usually well documented by clinical and ultrasound features, full cardiac catheterization is not required. In patients with angina, it is essential to carry out coronary arteriography. Cardiac catheterization is chiefly of value when there is doubt about the severity of regurgitation, particularly if there is concomitant mitral echocardiography which may mask physical signs of a significant aortic valve lesion. Pressure recordings during cardiac catheterization confirm the haemodynamic changes suspected by clinical examination. The aortic pressure pulse has a rapid rise and fall and a low dicrotic notch (Fig. 27.7). Pressures within the left ventricle are usually normal during the early stages of the illness but later a raised end-diastolic pressure is common. In advanced cases, the diastolic pressure rises rapidly in mid-diastole to exceed left atrial pressure in late diastole. This may lead to early mitral valve closure and also *diastolic* mitral regurgitation. In pure aortic regurgitation, there is no systolic gradient across the aortic valve but when there is even a minor degree of concomitant aortic stenosis the very high systolic flow due to the blood regurgitated during the previous diastole returning to the aorta across the slightly narrowed valve produces an exaggerated gradient (Fig. 27.12).

An aortogram, performed by injecting contrast into the ascending aorta, has two main purposes. It allows assessment of the degree of aortic regurgitation from the amount of contrast material seen entering the left ventricle, which is usually quantified by eye and is only moderately accurate.[65] More accurate assessment of the degree of regurgitation can be derived from calculating the regurgitant fraction. Incorrect positioning of the angiographic catheter may lead to spurious aortic regurgitation if the catheter interferes with the aortic valve.

Aortography also outlines the anatomy of the aortic root. Usually, a mild-to-moderate degree of dilatation of the aortic root is seen. Sometimes this is extreme, particularly in patients who have a connective tissue abnormality, for example, Marfan's syndrome. The dilated aortic root, which is particularly bulbous just above the aortic valve ring, is said to resemble a Chianti bottle. Aortography usually but not always detects dissecting aneurysm with its characteristic appearances of a double lumen. The point of entry of dissection into the media may be detected and the dissection flap itself often has a characteristic 'wave' movement. Aortography will also detect other rare causes of regurgitation such as prolapse of a cusp associated

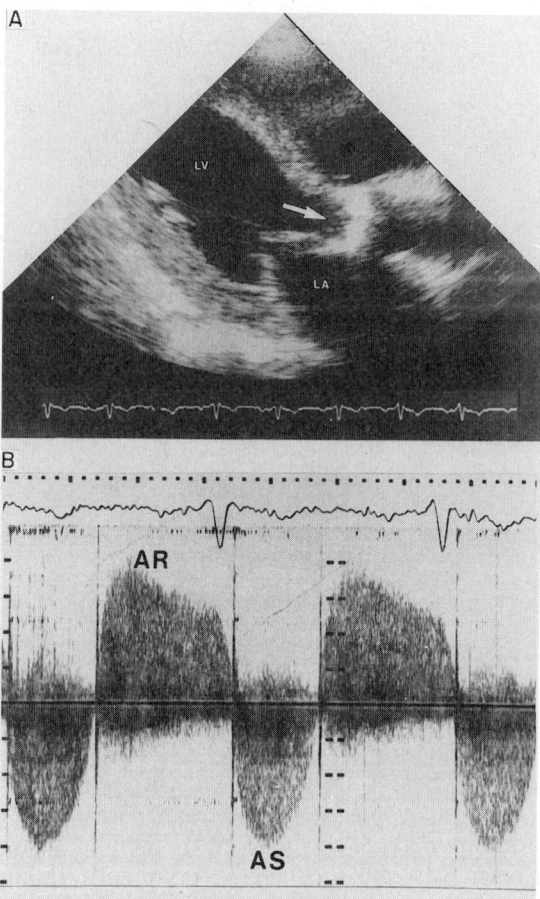

Fig. 27.12. Cross-sectional echocardiogram (A) and continuous wave Doppler recording (B) from a patient with severe mixed aortic valve disease. There is a strong regurgitant signal (AR) (above the zero line) in the Doppler tracing. The systolic peak velocity (AS) is approximately 4 m/s giving a peak gradient across the aortic valve in systole of 64 mmHg. This gradient exaggerates the severity of the aortic stenosis which is only mild, and results from the very high flow across the aortic valve in systole as the blood regurgitated in the previous diastole plus the forward cardiac output returns to the aorta. The aortic valve is thickened and had reduced mobility (arrow). LV, left ventricle; LA, left atrium.

with a ventricular septal defect (Fig. 27.13). It may outline paravalvular abscesses (Fig. 27.14) in patients with infective endocarditis but generally invasive procedures are avoided in such patients and the diagnosis is made using echocardiography.

The left ventriculogram shows the extent to which the left ventricle is dilated and its wall motion impaired. Impairment is usually global rather than regional. The coronary arteries, which take a very high flow of blood to the hypertrophied ventricle, are often extremely large and difficult to fill during

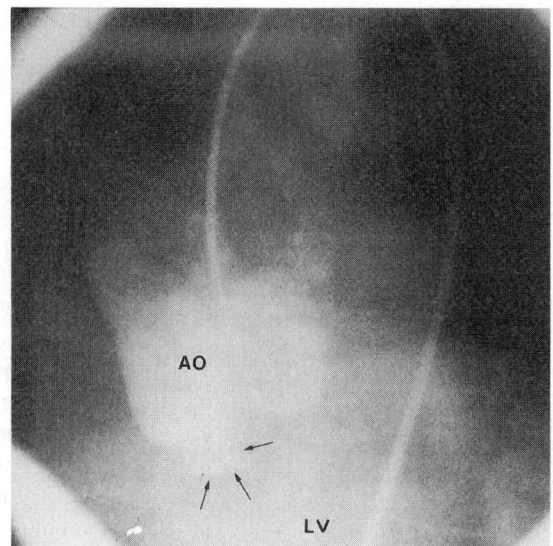

Fig. 27.13. Aortogram obtained from a patient with aortic regurgitation due to the prolapse of an aortic valve cusp into a high ventricular septal defect. The prolapsing cusp is shown by arrows. Ao, aorta; LV, left ventricle.

coronary angiography; sometimes the dilatation of the aortic root may make it difficult to engage the coronary ostia to perform selective coronary angiography.

DIAGNOSIS AND DIFFERENTIAL DIAGNOSIS

When aortic regurgitation is moderately severe its characteristic physical signs make it unmistakeable. Mild aortic regurgitation may be missed because the murmur is not detected and peripheral signs have not yet developed.

The most important condition to distinguish from aortic regurgitation is pulmonary regurgitation. It should be borne in mind that some patients with aortic and mitral disease of rheumatic origin may also have pulmonary and aortic regurgitation. Most often, pulmonary regurgitation is secondary to pulmonary hypertension which causes dilatation of the pulmonary valve ring. Occasionally, pulmonary regurgitation occurs in the absence of pulmonary hypertension, particularly when there has been previous surgery on the pulmonary valve. Although the presence of physical signs suggestive of pulmonary hypertension are in favour of a diagnosis of pulmonary regurgitation, this does not exclude the possibility that the murmur is due to aortic regurgitation or that both aortic and pulmonary regurgitation are present in the same patient. The

The only way to make this distinction with certainty is using Doppler ultrasound which can accurately detect both conditions and distinguish them from each other.

Occasionally, confusion arises in patients with persistent ductus arteriosus because the systolic and diastolic murmurs of aortic regurgitation may resemble a continuous murmur. Usually, these two conditions can be distinguished on the basis of the character of the murmur and its site. In persistent ductus arteriosus, the maximal murmur is usually heard well to the left of the sternum and even under the middle of the clavicle, whereas in aortic regurgitation the murmur is usually loudest at the sternal border. The distinction of the murmurs caused by these two conditions depends on the experience of the auscultator. The Doppler technique allows accurate distinction of these two conditions. A further unusual situation which must be distinguished from pure aortic regurgitation is the combination of a ventricular septal defect and aortic regurgitation. As mentioned above a high membranous ventricular septal defect causes the prolapse of one of the aortic valve cusps leading to aortic regurgitation. In such patients, the auscultatory findings are of a loud harsh systolic murmur best heard at the left sternal border followed by an

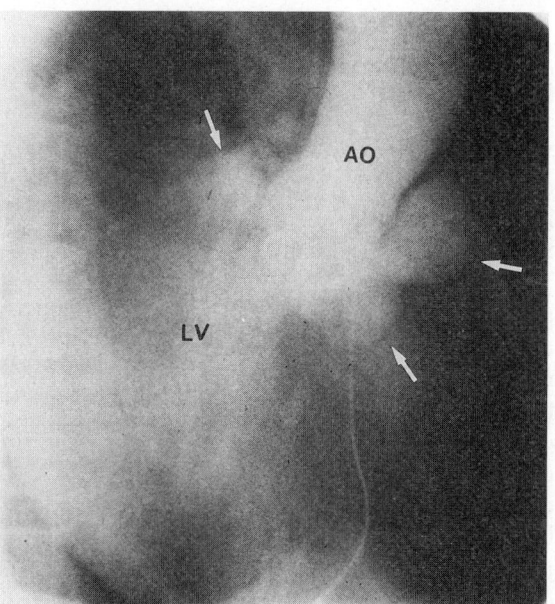

Fig. 27.14. Aortogram (right lateral projection) from a patient who had undergone re-operation (aortic valve replacement) for infective endocarditis involving a previous mechanical aortic valve prosthesis. There are enormous paravalvular abscess cavities (arrows) which were debrided by the surgeon at the time of re-replacment, fortunately with favourable results. Ao, aorta; LV, left ventricle.

early diastolic murmur. The systolic component usually extends for longer than the systolic murmur heard in aortic regurgitation alone but sometimes this distinction can be difficult. Again, echocardiography and Doppler ultrasound immediately resolve this problem. More rarely, other causes of a continuous heart murmur such as a ruptured sinus of Valsalva have to be distinguished from aortic regurgitation. Generally, the physical signs do not appear to be exactly those of aortic regurgitation and characteristic ultrasound findings confirm or refute the diagnosis. Diagnosis of unusual conditions such as a VSD and associated regurgitation at a ruptured sinus of Valsalva has been greatly facilitated by the advent of colour flow Doppler.

Although syphilitic aortic regurgitation is now rare, it is important to exclude this condition in patients with aortic regurgitation by carrying out the necessary serological tests. General clinical examination will reveal evidence of associated disorders such as ankylosing spondylitis, rheumatoid arthritis or connective tissue disorders such as Marfan's syndrome. The unexpected finding of aortic regurgitation should always prompt a thorough search for other evidence of infective endocarditis.

COMPLICATIONS

When aortic regurgitation leads to disability and death, it nearly always does so through deteriorating left ventricular function leading to left ventricular failure and eventually right ventricular failure. The time-course of these events is usually extremely protracted. Infective endocarditis is an important and dangerous complication. Death may occur as a result of the infective consequences of the condition; more often, it is caused by the sudden and catastrophic increase in the amount of regurgitation caused by valve perforation or rupture. Atrial arrhythmias are not common, although occasionally atrial fibrillation develops. Ventricular arrhythmias occur much more commonly; ventricular ectopic beats and runs of ventricular tachycardia are detected frequently, particularly when left ventricular function has begun to deteriorate. There is no evidence that treatment of these arrhythmias has any effect on prognosis, nor is it known whether they are corrected by satisfactory aortic valve replacement.

NATURAL HISTORY AND PROGNOSIS

The prognosis and natural history of aortic regurgitation depend to a great extent on the underlying cause. If it is rheumatic in origin and detected at the time of acute rheumatic fever, it frequently remains unchanged over the next 2–3 decades. Friedberg[66] emphasized that the majority of patients with rheumatic aortic regurgitation have a favourable outlook, particularly when the diastolic blood pressure is normal, when there are no peripheral manifestations and cardiac enlargement is slight. If deterioration occurs in early adult life in a patient with rheumatic aortic regurgitation, the possibility of another valve lesion, usually mitral, or infective endocarditis should be suspected.[67] In contrast, aortic regurgitation of acute or subacute onset has a poor prognosis unless corrected surgically, for example, in patients with aortic regurgitation due to infective endocarditis in whom early surgery is needed, in those with a dissecting aneurysm, in whom involvement of the aortic valve ring implies extensive dissection, and in some patients with inflammatory lesions of the aortic root, for example rheumatoid arthritis, in whom progression of aortic regurgitation can be rapid. Similarly, patients in whom there is a severe abnormality of collagen, for example, those with Marfan's syndrome, often show progressive deterioration over only a few years.

Once patients become symptomatic, deterioration is relatively rapid therefore surgery should be considered without undue delay. The prognosis tends to be worse in patients with large hearts.[68] Spagnuolo et al.[69] reported that 87% of patients with a triad of left ventricular enlargement judged radiologically, electrocardiographic evidence of left ventricular hypertrophy and a wide pulse pressure (a systolic pressure > 140 mmHg and a diastolic pressure < 40 mmHg) developed heart failure or died within 6 years. An elevated left ventricular end-diastolic pressure at cardiac catheterization is another feature indicative of a poor prognosis.[67]

TREATMENT

MEDICAL TREATMENT

Asymptomatic patients do not require any therapy except for appropriate antibiotic prophylaxis to prevent infective endocarditis. If aortic regurgitation is thought to be syphilitic, a full course of anti-syphilitic therapy should be given. When patients develop minor symptoms, relief is often gained for some time using a small dose of diuretics (and possibly digoxin). Vasodilators, including hydralazine,[70] nifedipine[71] and angiotensin converting enzyme inhibitors[72] may be valuable in reducing chronic regurgitation and alleviating symptoms. Although such measures may produce symptomatic improvement, the occurrence of symptoms means that surgery should not be delayed for long. If angina occurs, beta-blockade is inappropriate because by slowing the heart rate it lengthens diastole and increases regurgitation. More appropriate therapy, which may be successful, is the use of either calcium antagonists, which are principally vasodilating agents, or nitrates.

Medical treatment should be regarded only as a temporary substitute for patients who are suitable for surgical treatment.

SURGICAL TREATMENT

Surgical treatment is required for patients with aortic regurgitation except for those who have the most minor symptoms. The surgery of aortic regurgitation is discussed in detail in Chapter 35. Surgery is undertaken for two purposes: to abolish symptoms and to improve prognosis. In a patient who is symptomatic and has not already sustained severe damage to left ventricular function, surgery will relieve symptoms and probably improve prognosis. However, in the symptomatic patient in whom there is marked impairment of left ventricular function the decision to perform surgery is more difficult. Although improvements in anaesthetic and surgical skills have reduced operative mortality in such patients,[31,32] the effects on prognosis and the late symptomatic results of surgery may be disappointing;[32] it is arguable whether surgery or energetic medical therapy produces the best results. For the individual patient it is better to undertake surgery because some patients will experience a dramatic and unexpected improvement; for those who fail to improve, medical treatment is still available.

The most difficult clinical problem is presented by the patient who has no cardiac symptoms, severe aortic regurgitation and evidence that left ventricular function is beginning to deteriorate. This complex situation arises mainly for the following reasons. The true predictive value of the parameters of left ventricular function used to assess aortic regurgitation are unknown and are dependent on ventricular loading. They may change either because left ventricular function has deteriorated or because regurgitation has become more severe. The simplest and most widely used parameter is a left ventricular end-systolic dimension > 55 mm on M-mode echocardiography. Some workers reported a worse progress after aortic valve replacement once this dimension is exceeded,[73] but others have obtained convincing evidence that this is not a reliable detector of a poor prognosis.[33,34] Others have used haemodynamic variables such as an ejection fraction < 50%[74] or an elevation of end-diastolic pressure,[75] but the reliability of these criteria has not been established.[75] Despite these reservations, there would be no dilemma if aortic valve replacement was a procedure free of complications. In some centres, immediate mortality may be between 5 and 10%, and up to 60% of patients with prosthetic valves (either mechanical or tissue) will experience some complication within 7 years of operation. For these reasons, although the ultimate objective is to replace the aortic valve before severe and irreversible left ventricular damage occurs,[76] the case for carrying out aortic valve replacement in asymptomatic patients simply to preserve left ventricular function cannot be regarded as proven. Although some authors[77,78] recommend surgery if the ejection fraction falls below 55% or the end-systolic left ventricular volume rises above 70 ml/m^2, others regard the problems of prosthetic valves as being highly significant and recommend that aortic valve replacement should not be undertaken until the onset of symptoms.[79] However, the onset of symptoms may not be easy to define: patients may deny symptoms, some may lead such inactive lives that they do not experience symptoms and others may exaggerate their symptoms. Consequently, some workers have added an objective assessment of exercise tolerance using treadmill testing to their assessment of aortic valve disease; the detection of impaired exercise tolerance has been shown to be additional and possibly independent predictor of a poor prognosis.[32]

COMBINED AORTIC STENOSIS AND REGURGITATION

All the conditions that lead to aortic stenosis may also cause aortic regurgitation or a combination of the two lesions (Figure 27.12).[80] By comparison, many of the conditions leading to aortic regurgitation do this indirectly by causing enlargement of the aortic root and never lead to aortic stenosis.

Mixed stenosis and regurgitation produce clinical features that are a combination of those of the two lesions and tend to reflect the predominant one. Dyspnoea and tiredness are symptoms common to both lesions and therefore they occur most frequently. The presence of angina pectoris and syncope without much change in heart size suggests that aortic stenosis is the predominant lesion. If the pulse is of large volume, with a wide pulse pressure, and cardiac enlargement is prominent, aortic regurgitation is likely to be the main lesion.

As combined aortic stenosis and regurgitation and aortic regurgitation alone produce systolic and early diastolic murmurs, auscultation may not be helpful. Generally, the systolic murmur in aortic regurgitation is not as harsh as that heard when there is also significant aortic stenosis. The most useful physical sign when trying to decide the relative degrees of stenosis and regurgitation is the carotid pulse. A small-volume plateau pulse indicates that aortic stenosis is the most prominent lesion. When the lesion is evenly balanced, the pulse is often bisferious. When aortic stenosis is more marked than regurgitation, the pulse may still be of large volume but have an upstroke that is slower than normal, often with a shudder. This pulse may have either a single or a double peak.

As aortic stenosis carries the risk of sudden death, patients in whom stenosis is judged to be an important component should be treated as patients who have pure aortic stenosis; surgery should be undertaken without delay as soon as symptoms appear.

REFERENCES

1. Campbell, M. Aortic valvular disease. *Br. Med. J.* 1932; 1: 328.
2. Davies, M.J. *Pathology of Cardiac Valves.* London: Butterworths, 1980.
3. Lakier, J.B., Copans, H., Rosman, H.S. *et al.* Idiopathic degeneration of the aortic valve. A common cause of isolated aortic regurgitation. *J. Am. Coll. Cardiol.* 1985; 5: 347.
4. Olsen, L.J., Subramanian, R. and Edwards, W.D. Surgical pathology of pure aortic insufficiency: A study of 225 cases. *Proc. Mayo Clin.* 1984; 59: 835–41.
5. Bulkley, B.H. and Roberts, W.C. Ankylosing spondylitis in aortic regurgitation. Description of the characteristic cardiovascular lesion from study of 8 necroscopy patients. *Circulation* 1973; 68: 1014.
6. Liu, S.M. and Alexander, C.S. Complete heart block and aortic insufficiency in rheumatoid spondylitis. *Am. J. Cardiol.* 1969; 23: 888.
7. Roberts W.C., Kehoe, J.A., Carpenter, D.F. and Golden, A.

Cardiac valvular lesions in rheumatoid arthritis. *Arch. Intern. Med.* 1968; 122: 141.
8. Paulus, H.E., Pearson, C.M. and Pitts, W. Aortic insufficiency in 5 patients with the Reiter's syndrome. A detailed clinical and pathological study. *Am. J. Med.* 1972; 53: 564.
9. Gula, G., Pomerance, A., Bennet, M. and Yacoub, M.H. Homograft replacement of aortic valve and ascending aorta in a patient with nonspecific giant cell aortitis. *Br. Heart J.* 1977; 39: 581.
10. Howe, J. and Strachan, B.W. Case Reports. Aortic regurgitation as a manifestation of giant cell arteritis. *Br. Heart J.* 1978; 40: 1052.
11. Olsen, E.G.J. Cardiovascular system. In *Recent Advances in Pathology*, 9. Edinburgh: Churchill Livingstone, 1975.
12. Lemon, D.K. and White, C.W. Annular aortic ectasia; angiographic, haemodynamic and clinical comparison with aortic valve insufficiency. *Am. J. Cardiol.* 1978; 41: 482.
13. Marquis, Y., Richardson, J.B., Richie, A.C. and Wigle, E.C. Idiopathic medial aortopathy and arteriopathy. *Am. J. Med.* 1968; 4: 939.
14. Sinclair, R.J.G., Kitchin, A.H. and Turner, R.W.D. The Marfan syndrome. *Q. J. Med.* 1960; 29: 19.
15. Lewis, M.G. Idiopathic medionecrosis causing aortic incompetence. *Br. Med. J.* 1965; 1: 1478.
16. Leier, C.V. *et al.* The spectrum of cardiac defects in the Ehlers-Danlos syndrome, Types I and III. *Am. Intern. Med.* 1980; 92: 171.
17. Criscitiello, M.G., Ronan, J.A., Besterman, E.M.M. and Schoenwitter, W. Cardiovascular abnormalities in osteogenesis imperfecta. *Circulation* 1965; 31: 255.
18. Mills, P., Leed, G., Davies, M. and Leatham, A. The natural history of non-stenotic bicuspid aortic valve. *Br. Heart J.* 1978; 40: 951–7.
19. Roberts, W.C. and Honig, H.S. The spectrum of cardiovascular disease in the Marfan syndrome. A clinico-morphologic study of 18 necropsy patients and comparison to 151 previously reported necropsy patients. *Am. Heart J.* 1982; 104: 115.
20. Shapiro, L.M., Thwaites, B., Westgate, C. and Donaldson, R. Prevalence and significance of aortic valve prolapse. *Br. Heart J.* 1985; 54: 179.
21. Halloran, K.H., Talmer, N.S. and Browne, M.J. A study of ventricular septal defect associated with aortic insufficiency. *Am. Heart J.* 1965; 69: 320.
22. Wiggers, C.J. and Maltby, A.B. Further observations of experimental aortic insufficiency. *Am. J. Physiol.* 1931; 97: 689.
23. Morrow, A.G., Brawley, R.K. and Braunwald, E. Effects of aortic regurgitation on left ventricular performance. *Circulation* 1965; 31 (Suppl. I): 1–80.
24. Sonnenblick, E.H., Spiro, D. and Sponitz, I. The ultrastructural basis of Starling's law of the heart. *Am. Heart J.* 1964; 69: 336.
25. Bonnow, R.O., Rosing, D.R., McIntosh, C.L. *et al.* The natural history of asymptomatic patients with aortic regurgitation and a normal left ventricular function. *Circulation* 1983; 68: 509–17.
26. Fifer, M.A. and Braunwald, E. End-systolic pressure–volume and stress–length relations in the assessment of left ventricular function in man. *Adv. Cardiol.* 1985; 32: 36–55.
27. Quinones, M.A., Gaasch, W.H. and Alexander, J.K. Influence of acute changes in pre-load, after-load, contractile state and heart rate on ejection phase and isovolumetric indices of myocardial contractility in man. *Circulation* 1976; 53: 293.
28. Grossman, W., Braunwald, E., Mann, P. *et al.* Contractile state of the left ventricle in man as evaluated from end-systolic pressure–volume relations. *Circulation* 1977; 56: 845–52.
29. Cohn, P.F., Gorlin, R., Cohn, L.H. and Collins, Jr. J.J. Left

ventricular ejection fraction as a prognostic guide in surgical treatment of coronary and valvular heart disease. *Am. J. Cardiol.* 1974; **34**: 136.

30. Henry, W.L., Bonnow, R.O., Borer, J.S. *et al*. Observations on the optimum time for operative intervention in aortic regurgitation. I. Evaluation of the results of aortic valve replacement in symptomatic patients. *Circulation* 1980; **61**: 471.

31. Turina, J., Turina, M., Rothlin, M. and Krayenbuehl, H.P. Improved late survival in patients with chronic aortic regurgitation by earlier operation. *Circulation* 1984; **70** (Suppl. I): 1–147.

32. Bonow, R.O., Picone, A.L., McIntosh, C.L. *et al*. Survival and functional results after valve replacement for aortic regurgitation from 1976–1983: impact of pre-operative left ventricular function. *Circulation* 1985; **72**: 1244–56.

33. Fioretti, P., Roelandt, J., Bos, R.J. *et al*. Echocardiography in chronic aortic insufficiency: is valve replacement too late when left ventricular systolic dimension reaches 55mm? *Circulation* 1983; **67**: 216.

34. Fioretti, P., Roelandt, J., Sclavo, M. *et al*. Post-operative regression of left ventricular dimensions in chronic aortic insufficiency: a long-term echocardiographic study. *J. Am. Coll. Cardiol.* 1985; **5**: 856.

35. Daniel, W.G., Hood, W.P., Siart, A. *et al*. Chronic aortic regurgitation: the assessment of the prognostic value of pre-operative left ventricular end-systolic dimension and fractional shortening *Circulation* 1985; **71**: 669.

36. Osbakken, M., Bove, A.A. and Spann, J.F. Left ventricular function in chronic aortic regurgitation with reference to end-systolic pressure, volume and stress relations. *Am. J. Cardiol.* 1981; **47**: 193.

37. Scognamiglio, R., Roelandt, J., Fasoli, G. *et al*. Relation between myocardial contractility, hypertrophy and pump performance in patients with chronic aortic regurgitation: An echocardiographic study. *Int. J. Cardiol.* 1984; **6**: 473–84.

38. Gaasch, W.H., Carroll, J.D., Levine, H.J. and Criscitiello, M.G. Chronic aortic regurgitation: Prognostic value of left ventricular end-systolic dimension and end-systolic radius/thickness ratio. *J. Am. Coll. Cardiol.* 1983; **1**: 775–9.

39. Wisenbaugh, T., Booth, D., DeMaria, A. *et al*. Relationship of contractile state to ejection performance in patients with chronic aortic valve disease. *Circulation* 1986; **73**: 47–53.

40. Almeida, P., Cordoba, M., Goicolea, J. *et al*. Relation of mid-wall circumferential systolic stress to equitorial mid-wall fibre shortening in chronic aortic regurgitation. Value as a predictor of post-operative outcome. *Br. Heart J.* 1984; **52**: 284–91.

41. Osbakken, M.D. and Bove, A.A. Use of left ventricular filling and ejection patterns in assessing severity of chronic mitral and aortic regurgitation. *Am. J. Cardiol.* 1984; **53**: 1054–60.

42. Lavine, S.J., Follansbee, W.P., Shreiner, D.P. *et al*. Pattern of left ventricular diastolic filling in chronic aortic regurgitation: a gated blood pool assessment. *Am. J. Cardiol.* 1985; **55**: 127–32.

43. Lewis, B.S. and Gotsman, M.S. Current concepts of left ventricular relaxation and compliance. *Am. Heart J.* 1980; **99**: 101–12.

44. Rees, J.R., Epstein, E.J., Criley, J.M. and Ross, R.S. Haemodynamic effects of severe aortic regurgitation. *Br. Heart J.* 1964; **26**: 412.

45. Wright, J.L., Tojscano-Barboza, E. and Brandenburg, R.O. Left ventricular and aortic pressure pulses in aortic valve disease. *Proc. Mayo Clin.* 1956; **31**: 120.

46. Thompson, R., Ross, I., Leslie, P. and Easthope, R. Haemodynamic adaptation to exercise in asymptomatic patients with severe aortic regurgitation. *Cardiovasc. Res.* 1985; **19**: 212–8.

47. Iskandrian, A.S., Hakki, A.H., Amenta, A. *et al*. Regulation of cardiac output during upright exercise in patients with aortic regurgitation. *Cardiovasc. Cathet. Diag.* 1984; **10**: 573–82.

48. Greenberg, B., Massie, D., Thomas, D. *et al*. Association between the exercise ejection fraction response and systolic wall stress in patients with chronic aortic insufficiency. *Circulation* 1985; **71**: 458–65.

49. Weiss, R.J., Buda, A.J., LeMire, M.S. and Pitt, B. Assessment of dysfunction in aortic regurgitation by stress–shortening relationship. *Int. J. Cardiol.* 1985; **8**: 475–86.

50. Harvey, W.P., Segal, J.P. and Hufnagel, C.A. Unusual clinical features associated with severe aortic insufficiency. *Ann. Intern. Med.* 1957; **47**: 27.

51. Engloff, E. Aortic incompetence: Clinical, haemodynamic and angiocardiographic evaluation. *Acta Med. Scand.* 1972; **193** (Suppl. 538): 3.

52. Gorlin, R. and Goodale, W.T. Changing blood pressures in aortic insufficiency. *N. Engl. J. Med.* 1956; **255**: 77.

53. Reichek, N., Shelbourne, J.C. and Perloff, J.K. Clinical aspects of rheumatic valvular disease. *Prog. Cardiovasc. Dis.* 1973; **15**: 49.

54. Flint, A. On cardiac murmurs. *Am. J. Med. Sci.* 1982; **44**: 29.

55. Fortuin, N.J. and Craige, E. On the mechanism of the Austin Flint murmur. *Circulation* 1972; **45**: 558.

56. Aldridge, H.E., Lansdown, E.L. and Wigle, E.D. Diastolic mitral insufficiency. *Circulation* 1966; Suppl. 33–34: III–42.

57. Lochaya, S., Igarashi, M. and Schaffer, A.B. Late diastolic regurgitation secondary to aortic regurgitation: Its relationship to the Austin Flint Murmur. *Am. Heart J.* 1967; **74**: 161.

58. Meadows, W.R., Van Praagh, S., Indreika, M. and Sharp, J.T. Premature mitral valve closure. A hemodynamic explanation for absence of the first sound in aortic insufficiency. *Circulation* 1963; **28**: 251.

59. D'Cruz, I., Cohen, H.C., Prabhu, R. *et al*. Flutter of left ventricular structures in patients with aortic regurgitation, with special reference to patients with associated mitral stenosis. *Am. Heart J.* 1976; **92**: 684.

60. Aziz, K.U., Cole, R.B. and Paul, M.H. Echocardiographic features of supracristal ventricular septal defect with prolapsed aortic valve leaflet. *Am. J. Cardiol.* 1979; **43**: 854.

61. McLeod, A.A., Monaghan, M.J., Richardson, P.J. *et al*. Diagnosis of acute aortic dissection by M-mode and cross-sectional echocardiography. A five year experience. *Eur. Heart J.* 1983; **4**: 196.

62. Victor, M., Mintz, G., Kotler, M. *et al*. Two-dimensional echocardiographic diagnosis of aortic dissection. *Am. J. Cardiol.* 1981; **48**: 1155.

63. Botvinick, E.H., Schiller, N.B. *et al*. Echocardiographic demonstration of early mitral valve closure in severe aortic insufficiency. Its clinical implications. *Circulation* 1975; **51**: 836.

64. Mann, T., McLaurin, L., Grossman, W. and Craige, E. Assessing the hemodynamic severity of acute aortic regurgitation due to infective endocarditis. *N. Engl. J. Med.* 1975; **293**: 108.

65. Croft, C.H., Lipscomb, K., Mathis, K. *et al*. Limitations of qualitative angiographic grading in aortic and mitral regurgitation. *Am. J. Cardiol.* 1984; **53**: 1593–8.

66. Friedberg, C.K. *Diseases of the Heart*, 3rd edn. Philadelphia: W.B. Saunders Co., 1966.

67. Goldschlager, N., Pfeifer, J., Cohn, K. *et al*. The natural history of aortic regurgitation: A clinical and hemodynamic study. *Am. J. Med.* 1973; **54**: 577.

68. Smith, H.J., Neutze, Roche, A.H.G. *et al*. The natural history of rheumatic aortic regurgitation and the indications for surgery. *Br. Heart J.* 1976; **38**: 147.

69. Spagnuolo, M., Kloth, H., Taranta, A. *et al*. Natural history

of rheumatic aortic regurgitation: Criteria predictive of death, congestive heart failure and angina in young patients. *Circulation* 1971; **44**: 368.

70. Greenberg, B.H., DeMots, H., Murphy, E. and Rahimtoola, S. Beneficial effect of hydralazine on rest and exercise hemodynamics in patients with chronic severe aortic insufficiency. *Circulation* 1980; **62**: 49.

71. Fioretti, P. *et al.* Afterload reduction with nifedipine in aortic insufficiency. *Am. J. Cardiol.* 1982; **49** 1728.

72. Heck, I., Schmidt, J., Mattern, H. *et al.* Reduktion der regurgitation bei aorten—und mitralinsuffizienz durch captopril im akut—und langzeitversuch. *Schweiz. Med. Wschr.* 1985; **115**: 1618.

73. Henry, W.L., Bonow, R.O., Rosing, D.R. and Epstein, SE. Observations on the optimum time for operative intervention for aortic regurgitation. *Circulation* 1980; **61**: 484.

74. Fischl, S.J., Gorlin, R. and Herman, M.W. Cardiac shape and function in aortic valve disease: Physiologic and clinical implications. *Am. J. Cardiol.* 1977; **39**: 170.

75. Pine, M., Hahn, G., Paton, B. *et al.* Homograft and prosthetic aortic valve replacement. A comparative study. *Circulation* 1976; Suppl. 54: III–84.

76. Roberts, D.L., DeWeese, J.A., Mahomey, E.G. and Yu, P.N. Long-term survival following aortic valve replacement. *Am. Heart J.* 1976; **91**: 311.

77. Rubin, J.W., Moore, H.W., Hillson, R.F. and Ellison, R.G. Thirteen year experience with aortic valve replacement. *Am. J. Cardiol.* 1977; **40**: 345.

78. Thompson, R. Aortic regurgitation—how do we judge optimal timing for surgery? *Aust. N.Z. J. Med.* 1984; **14**: 514.

79. Rahimtoola, S.H. Early valve replacement for preservation of ventricular function? *Am. J. Cardiol.* 1977; **40**: 472.

80. Subramanian, R., Olson, L.J. and Edwards, W.D. Surgical pathology of combined aortic stenosis and insufficiency: A study of 213 cases. *Proc. Mayo Clin.* 1985; **60**: 247–54.

Chapter 28

Rheumatic Mitral Valve Disease

Roger Hall

INTRODUCTION

The mitral valve can be affected by many different disease processes but in developing countries rheumatic fever still predominates. In the USA and Western Europe, rheumatic heart disease is no longer frequent in the young and it has become mainly a disease of the middle-aged and elderly. By contrast, it is still an important cause of disability and death in all age-groups in Eastern Europe, Asia, Africa and Central and South America, often affecting children and young adults.

Acquired mitral valvular stenosis is generally regarded to be exclusively rheumatic in origin although the possibility that some cases result from a preceding viral carditis or other cardiac insult has been argued persuasively.[1-3] This is not so with mitral regurgitation: some cases are rheumatic in origin and may be associated with mitral stenosis, but many other processes can upset the complex integrity of the mitral valve and lead to regurgitation. This is not surprising as mitral competence depends upon the normal function of the mitral valve, subvalvar apparatus, left ventricle and mitral valve annulus.

The mitral valve can be rendered stenotic by non-valvular causes, such as vegetations, thrombus or tumour prolapsing into the mitral valve orifice, and by congenital abnormalities of the mitral valve, such as a stenosing supravalvar ring or a parachute mitral valve[4,5] which are rare and nearly always present in childhood but occasionally they are diagnosed for the first time in adult life.

PATHOLOGY

Acute rheumatic valvulitis causes scarring with thickening, shortening and deformity of the mitral valve cusps and retraction of their free margins. Similar inflammatory changes with subsequent fibrosis cause thickening, fusion and shortening of the chordae tendineae (Fig. 28.1). Inflammation along the margins of the valve leaflets leads to fusion of the commissures. In the late stages of the disease calcification frequently occurs in the damaged structures (Fig. 28.2 and 28.3). Whether predominant mitral stenosis or regurgitation or a combination of the two ensues following an attack of acute rheumatic fever depends on the relative degree of cusp fusion and retraction. When commissural fusion is the predominant feature with preservation of the cusps, stenosis results, the mitral valve frequently becoming a funnel-shaped structure. Sometimes, adhesion and shortening of the cusps occur to such an extent that the valve becomes a diaphragmatic structure with a slit in it, often described as the buttonhole or fish-mouth type of mitral stenosis (Fig. 28.4).

When commissures, cusps and chordae are all seriously damaged (Fig. 28.1) and the valve leaflets retract, mitral regurgitation is predominant and often occurs mainly at the posterior (posteromedial) commissure. The posterior cusp becomes drawn down by fibrosis into the left ventricle and may even become adherent to the left ventricular endocardium. The mitral valve ring is also affected and scarring may lead to dilatation of the orifice with interference of the normal muscular systolic contraction of its circumference. The orifice of the valve then becomes so large that the cusps are incapable of closing it. This dilatation of the mitral valve ring may be increased as left ventricular enlargement occurs and stretches the mitral valve ring further.

Other valves may be affected indirectly as a consequence of mitral valve disease. Prolonged and severe pulmonary hypertension may stretch the pulmonary valve ring with subsequent pulmonary regurgitation, and when the right ventricle begins to fail and thereby dilates so the tricuspid valve ring dilates causing functional tricuspid regurgitation.

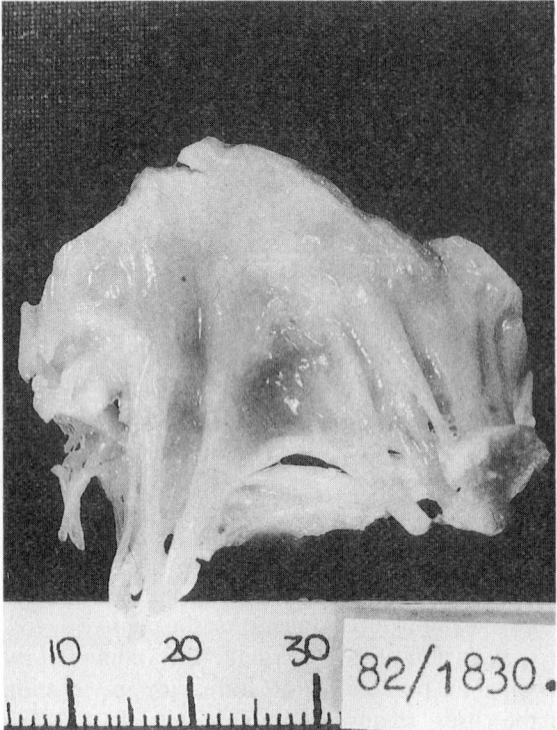

Fig. 28.1. Excised rheumatic mitral valve seen from its ventricular aspect. The chordae on the right are adherent and markedly shortened. The head of the papillary muscle has been excised and is still attached to them. Similar changes are seen in the other chordae (left of picture), but these are less marked. The patient from whom this valve was excised had severe mitral regurgitation and some stenosis.

Both stenosis and regurgitation may lead to considerable dilatation and hypertrophy of the left atrium. Sometimes the left atrium enlarges to enormous proportions; this usually occurs in severe mitral regurgitation but occasionally it can occur in pure mitral stenosis.[6] Thrombus frequently forms behind a stenotic or regurgitant mitral valve within the left atrium and may become adherent to the left atrial wall and calcify (Fig. 28.5).

The left ventricle is both dilated and hypertrophied in cases of predominant mitral regurgitation whereas in cases in which stenosis is the main lesion the left ventricle is either of normal size or smaller than normal. Abnormalities of left ventricular function in mitral valve disease are dealt with in a separate section below. In severe pulmonary hypertension, the right ventricle enlarges and hypertrophies and, once heart failure has developed, usually with significant functional tricuspid regurgitation, the right atrium also dilates.

PATHOPHYSIOLOGY

The normal mitral valve area is between 4 and 6 cm^2. When mitral stenosis is severe, this area is reduced to < 1 cm^2 and sometimes it is as small as 0.5 cm^2. The degree of stenosis determines the haemodynamic disturbances and the clinical manifestations of mitral stenosis; however, there is a wide range of individual response such that the severity of clinical symptoms is not consistently related to the degree of stenosis.

When mitral stenosis is mild to moderate (valve area approximately 1.5 cm^2), there is often little or no increase in left atrial pressure at rest. However, a considerable increase in pressure gradient across the mitral valve is required to obtain adequate forward flow on exercise when the left atrial pressure frequently rises to significant levels (25 mmHg). Once the stenosis is moderate (1–1.5 cm^2), a persisting elevation in left atrial pressure is required to maintain the normal resting cardiac output and further increases occur with exercise. For example, only a moderate degree of exertion may increase the left atrial pressure to 30 or 35 mmHg. When there is severe mitral stenosis (< 1 cm^2), elevation of left atrial pressure to this level is often seen at rest. Such pressures cannot be tolerated by normal lungs, but the slow progression in the rise of pressure over months or years causes changes in the pulmonary capillaries and alveolar walls that limit the risk of exudation of fluid into the alveoli.

While the patient remains in sinus rhythm and mitral stenosis is mild to moderate, cardiac output

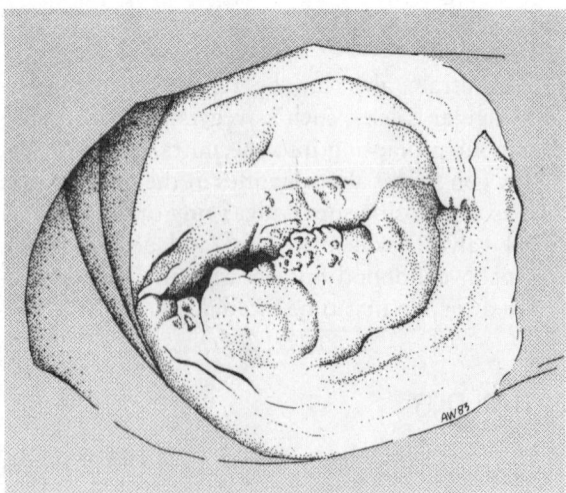

Fig. 28.2. The typical appearances of a stenotic calcified mitral valve. The orifice is slit-like but it is irregular due to the calcific deposits.

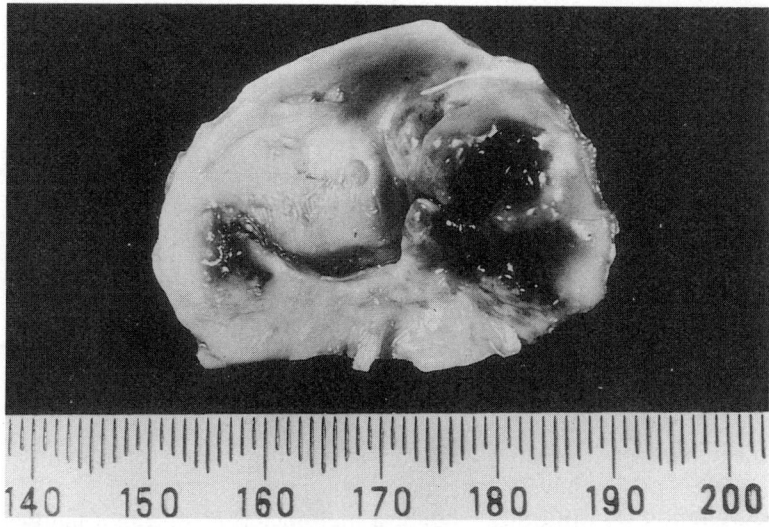

Fig. 28.3. Pathological specimen showing similar changes to those in Fig. 28.2. There are gross calcific deposits seen on the right-hand side of the valve. The dark area associated with this is adherent blood clot.

is normal at rest, although it does not rise normally with exercise. Once a patient develops atrial fibrillation or the degree of stenosis becomes more severe, cardiac output at rest falls below normal. Furthermore, the capacity of the heart to increase its cardiac output during exercise is significantly reduced and there may be no increase whatsoever. Reduction of cardiac output leads to an increased arteriovenous oxygen difference because the body's demand for oxygen can be met only by greater oxygen extraction in the tissues rather than increased oxygen uptake and increased peripheral blood flow.

To some extent, changes in left atrial function compensate for the effects of mitral stenosis. The left atrium hypertrophies, and if sinus rhythm persists left atrial contraction becomes more important than usual in maintaining cardiac output. Unfortu-

nately, the left atrial musculature is often affected by fibrosis from the previous rheumatic fever; consequently, its capacity for compensation is less than that of a normal left atrium. The loss of atrial contraction with the onset of atrial fibrillation has been reported to result in a 20% reduction in cardiac output at a similar heart rate.[7,8]

The left atrial pressure pulse in mitral stenosis often has a characteristic shape. The hypertrophy of the left atrium leads to a high dominant 'a' wave while sinus rhythm persists. The descent from the 'v' wave (Fig. 28.6) ('y' descent) is slow due to obstruction of left atrial emptying, and more sustained than usual because left ventricular filling continues during late diastole. Once atrial fibrillation occurs, the 'a' wave disappears (Fig. 28.7). Even when there is no significant mitral regurgita-

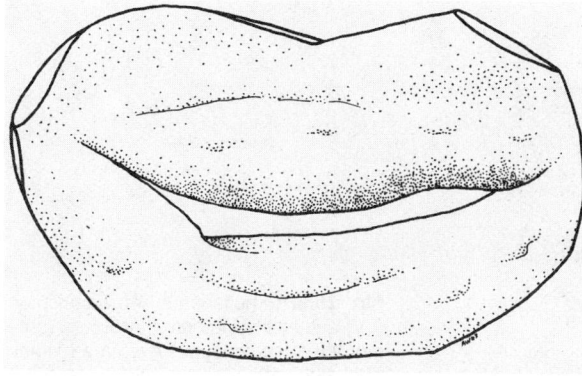

Fig. 28.4. The slit-like buttonhole appearance of the mitral valve often seen in mitral stenosis.

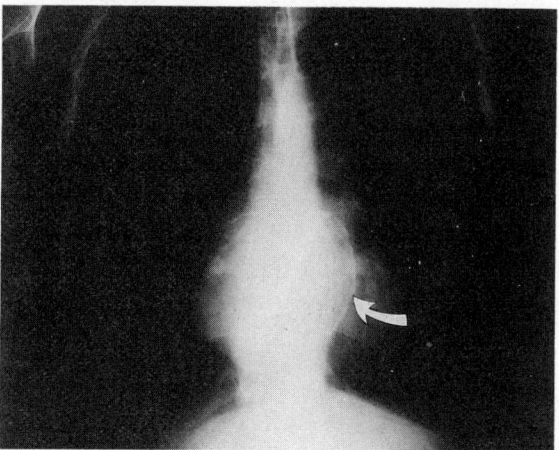

Fig. 28.5. Penetrated chest X-ray showing extensive calcification outlining the border of the left atrium in a patient with longstanding rheumatic mitral valve disease.

tion, the 'v' wave may be well seen (Figs 28.6 and 28.7) and occasionally attain the shape or contour usually associated with severe pure mitral regurgitation. However, in rheumatic mitral regurgitation (unlike severe mitral regurgitation of other aetiology), a giant 'v' wave is unusual in the left atrial pressure trace because there is often some associated mitral stenosis which has an obstructive effect on the backward transmission of the 'v' wave from the left ventricle to the left atrium, and because the capacitance effect of a very large left atrium damps the waveform. When mitral regurgitation predominates over mitral stenosis, the 'y' descent from the 'v' peak may be fast and there is a rise in the atrial pressure during diastasis similar to that seen in the normal subject.

The pathophysiology of pure mitral regurgitation is discussed in detail below (see p. 757). In general, the pathophysiology of rheumatic mitral regurgitation is similar to that of pure mitral regurgitation except frequently there is some associated mitral stenosis which tends to limit the degree of mitral regurgitation. Furthermore, when managing patients with rheumatic heart disease, it should be borne in mind that left ventricular function may have been impaired by the preceding rheumatic fever.

VENTRICULAR FUNCTION

The discussion below encompasses rheumatic and non-rheumatic mitral valve disease.

MITRAL STENOSIS

Abnormalities of both systolic and diastolic left ventricular function have been described in mitral stenosis. The diastolic abnormalities are much more prominent because the primary problem in mitral stenosis is obstruction to left ventricular diastolic inflow.

Systolic function

Systolic abnormalities of left ventricular function may be global or localized. In most studies, it has been found that a variable proportion (38%,[9] 31%,[10] 12%[11]) of patients with mitral stenosis have a left ventricular ejection fraction of < 50%. In other studies, a high incidence of abnormalities of regional wall motion which occur in both the postero-basal and the antero-lateral aspects of the ventricle, has been shown. Although the postero-basal abnormalities are regarded as being the most common (occurring in 20 of 25 patients in one study),[12] the results of a recent study have suggested a similar incidence of antero-lateral abnormalities.[13] The *postero-basal* abnormalities are thought to be due to tethering of that part of the ventricular wall by subvalvar fibrosis and possibly due to atrophy of immobilized muscle in this area, although alterations in left ventricular filling or other unknown mechanisms may also contribute. The *antero-lateral* changes have been ascribed to right ventricular overload affecting left ventricular performance.[14] Global reduction in left ventricular

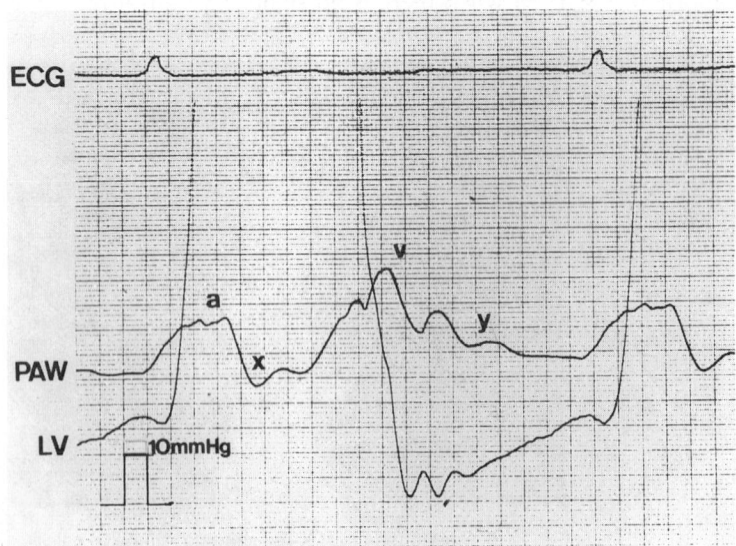

Paper speed 100 mm/sec

Fig. 28.6. Simultaneous left ventricular (LV) and indirect left atrial pressure (pulmonary artery wedge–PAW) in a patient with sinus rhythm and mitral stenosis. The 'y' descent is slow although interrupted by an oscillation in the pressure trace. Both 'a' and 'v' waves are prominent.

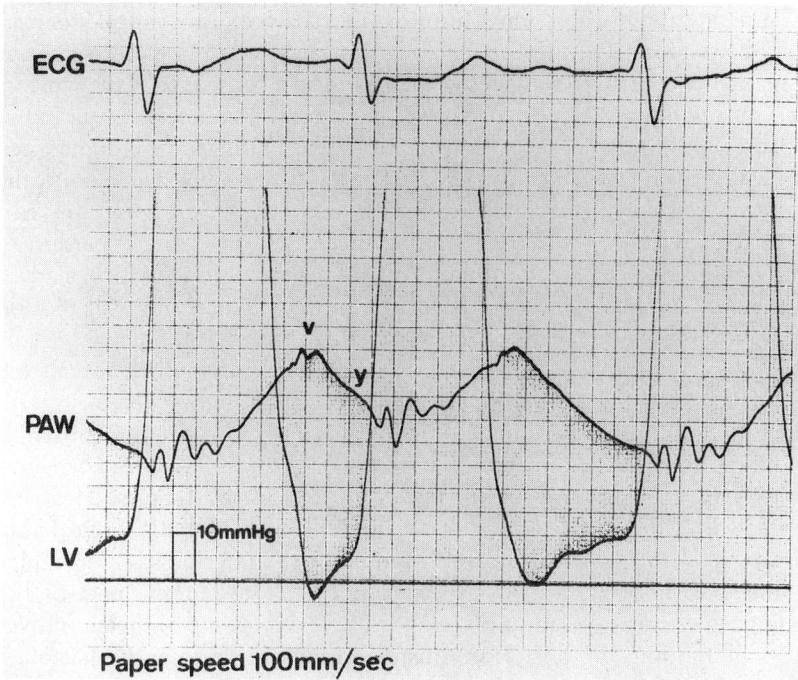

Fig. 28.7. Simultaneous recording of the left ventricular (LV) and pulmonary artery wedge pressure (PAW) in a patient with severe mitral stenosis and atrial fibrillation. The PAW trace shows a prominent 'v' wave and a slow 'y' descent. The end-diastolic gradient varies according to the cycle length. Following an RR interval of approximately 500 ms, the gradient is 30 mmHg (first beat). When the RR interval is 650 ms (right-hand beat), the gradient has fallen to 20 mmHg.

function has been attributed to the deleterious effects of the rheumatic process on the left ventricular myocardium and myocardial atrophy[15] resulting from reduced left ventricular work. There is disagreement over whether there is a correlation between the presence of global and regional abnormalities.[10,13] Abnormalities of other ejection phase indices, such as the velocity of circumferential fibre shortening, stroke work index and volume index, have also been described.[10,16–18]

In addition to the explanations put forward above, it is likely that alterations in left ventricular loading play an important part in these abnormalities. Indeed, it has been found that many of the abnormalities of systolic variables disappear when patients are corrected for abnormalities of loading.[10,19] This is not surprising since ejection phase indices are highly dependent on preload and afterload,[20] both of which are abnormal in mitral stenosis. The limitation of preload due to the stenotic mitral valve is obvious. Increased afterload (high end-systolic wall stress) may occur as a result of both reduced end-systolic wall thickness (via the Laplace relationship, see p. 473 and the increased peripheral resistance that occurs in patients who have severe mitral stenosis[10] as a result of peripheral arteriolar constriction induced by low cardiac output. Finally, alterations of left ventricular end-diastolic pressure are often difficult to interpret as

an index of left ventricular function because they may be altered by the changes in right ventricular pressure and volume which are common in severe mitral stenosis.[14,21]

Abnormalities of systolic function are rarely a clinical problem once mitral stenosis is relieved by surgery. Occasionally, however, poor systolic left ventricular function may contribute to reduced cardiac output in the early post-operative phase.

Diastolic function

Diastolic abnormalities of left ventricular function in mitral stenosis are universal. Obstruction to left ventricular inflow by the stenotic valve has several important effects. The peak filling rate of the left ventricle is considerably reduced (falling from the normal value of 600–800 ml/s to 200–500 ml/s)[22,23] and the normal filling pattern of the left ventricle is also disturbed. The distinct early rapid filling phase of the left ventricle, which is normally followed by slower mid and late diastolic filling, is lost and, instead, if mitral stenosis is severe, diastolic filling proceeds at an almost uniform rate throughout diastole. This occurs because the stenotic valve prevents early rapid inflow and the high pressure gradient that persists across the mitral valve causes filling to continue into late diastole when it would normally have almost ceased. The mid and late diastolic filling tails off at a rate that depends inversely on the severity of obstruction. Late in diastole, if sinus rhythm is maintained, a small increase in the velocity of transmitral flow usually occurs as a result of atrial systole (Fig. 28.8).

If the motion of the left ventricular walls during diastole reflected inflow alone, a slow generalized outward wall motion would be expected. What actually happens is the rate of outward wall motion in each individual area of the ventricle is normal or only slightly reduced but the normal co-ordination of left ventricular relaxation, which causes outward wall motion throughout the ventricle to occur almost synchronously to accommodate rapid filling, is lost.[22] Instead, rapid outward wall motion is staggered, occurring first in the anterior wall, then the cardiac apex and finally the inferior wall. This staggering of outward wall motion slows the overall increase in left ventricular volume. In some patients, the rapid outward wall motion in one part of the ventricle is accompanied by inward wall motion elsewhere producing a change in left ventricular shape rather than volume. The mechanisms underlying the abnormalities of left ventricular wall motion and shape in diastole are complex, and only partly understood. The interplay between the physical restriction of inflow into the left ventricle caused by the stenotic valve and the forces responsible for left ventricular filling is probably important. Rapid thinning of the left ventricular wall in early diastole, once thought to be due to the inflow of blood into the ventricle, has been shown in other conditions, for example, ischaemic heart disease,[24,25] to be largely independent of inflow and probably the result of a combination of active relaxation and the restoring forces built up in the ventricle during the previous systole. If inflow through the mitral valve is unrestricted, these restoring forces result in wall motion that can be translated into an increase in left ventricular

volume. If inflow is restricted, as in mitral stenosis, the capacity to translate these forces into volume change is reduced and as a consequence they distort the ventricle. The pattern of temporal staggering of outward wall motion is an exaggeration of that seen in normal ventricles and probably depends on the architecture of the ventricle.[26] This concept is reinforced by the occurrence of an identical pattern of incoordination in other conditions, which lead to incoordinate left ventricular diastolic wall motion e.g. ischaemic heart disease.[24,25]

The M-mode echocardiogram, which reveals the base of the left ventricle, is able to demonstrate a striking reduction in the rate of left ventricular dimension change in early diastole which correlates well with the severity of mitral stenosis. This correlation, although clinically useful,[27,28] is probably fortuitous. Thinning of the inferior left ventricular wall occurs at a normal rate but the part of the septum visualized by the M-mode beam moves posteriorly instead of anteriorly in early diastole[27] such that the peak rate at which the two structures separate from each other is markedly reduced.

Right ventricular function

The study of right ventricular function is extremely difficult because of the complicated shape of the right ventricle. Consequently, although right ventricular function must be abnormal in many patients with mitral stenosis and pulmonary hypertension, there have been very few studies performed. Recently, estimates of right ventricular ejection fraction in mitral stenosis, both at rest and on exercise, have been reported.[29,30] These suggest that in moderate mitral stenosis right ventricular performance is normal, but that, in more severe stenosis, exercise causes an abnormal fall in right ventricular ejection fraction which correlates with the degree to which resting pulmonary vascular

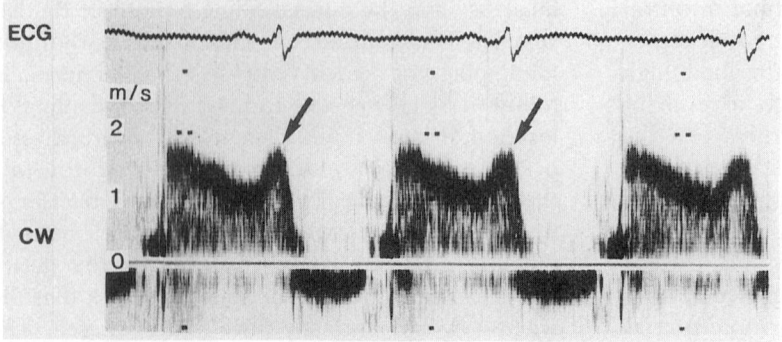

Fig. 28.8. Continuous wave Doppler recording from a patient with moderately severe mitral stenosis who is in sinus rhythm. As this recording was obtained from the cardiac apex, the diastolic mitral flow is towards the transducer. In early diastole, the velocity of flow across the valve is increased and slowly declines as diastole progresses. There is a further acceleration in flow (arrows) at end-diastole due to atrial contraction.

resistance is increased. Following successful surgical relief of mitral stenosis, the normal exercise-induced increase in right ventricular ejection fraction, seen in milder case,. is restored, suggesting that the pre-operative abnormalities of function result from increased right ventricular afterload rather than an abnormality of right ventricular contractility. As mentioned above, alterations in both left ventricular end-diastolic pressure and changes in regional wall motion, particularly in the antero-lateral aspect of the ventricle, may be secondary to changes in right ventricular pressure and volume.[14,21]

MITRAL REGURGITATION

As the effects of acute and chronic mitral regurgitation and left ventricular function are different, they are discussed separately.

Acute mitral regurgitation

If sudden disruption of the mitral valve apparatus occurs, the left ventricle is unprepared for this catastrophe and initially has a normal muscle mass. Regurgitation of blood into the left atrium causes a sharp rise in left atrial pressure and as a result left ventricular preload rises. This increase in preload stretches the left ventricle so that end-diastolic volume rises slightly and the myocardial sarcomeres function at or near their maximum diastolic length.[31] This increase in muscle stretch increases systolic shortening via the Frank–Starling mechanism. At the same time, there is some decrease in left ventricular afterload because some of the stroke volume is ejected into the left atrium, which has a relatively lower impedance than the aorta.[32] This reduction in afterload is much greater than the increase in preload and consequently the end-systolic volume decreases considerably more than the end-diastolic volume increases. The combination of a slightly increased end-diastolic volume and a considerably reduced end-systolic volume increases both ejection fraction and stroke volume. Forward cardiac output is also maintained, by increased heart rate. However, when regurgitation is severe, stroke volume does not increase sufficiently to compensate for the volume of blood regurgitated into the left atrium and cardiac output falls. The results of experimental studies of myocardial contractile function in acute mitral regurgitation suggest that it is normal.[31] However, when mitral regurgitation is very severe, the metabolic changes

of heart failure and pulmonary oedema ultimately lead to a reduction in contractile function. The pathophysiology is often more complicated than this, particularly when the underlying cause of mitral regurgitation is ischaemic. In such patients, the extent to which myocardial perfusion is impaired will have a powerful effect on the response of the ventricle to increased demands.

Chronic mitral regurgitation

When mitral regurgitation develops slowly or when a patient survives acute mitral regurgitation without requiring surgery, various adaptations of left ventricular and left atrial structure and function occur to compensate for the regurgitation.

The volume-overloaded left ventricle enlarges and the most prominent change is an increase in end-diastolic volume, which is not a marked feature in *acute* mitral regurgitation. The end-systolic volume increases slightly or remains normal such that the overall ejection fraction stays in the normal range or is slightly increased.[33] The normal or slightly increased ejection fraction occurring from an increased end-diastolic volume is sufficient to produce a significant increase in stroke volume, which compensates for the leak into the left atrium while still providing an adequate forward cardiac output.

As well as becoming enlarged, the left ventricle also hypertrophies.[34] This hypertrophy has three main effects.

1 A moderate increase in wall thickness occurs, which tends to normalize wall stress (via the Laplace relationship), that would otherwise rise as left ventricular dimension increased. This is of considerable importance because it allows oxygen consumption, which depends principally on wall stress and heart rate, to remain within the normal range.

2 As the muscle hypertrophies, additional sarcomeres are added in series; this, in combination with some rearrangement and slippage of myofibres, maintains sarcomere length at or near normal.[31] This is important because the left ventricle then retains normal or near-normal preload reserve, i.e. an increase in preload can increase sarcomere length further and thereby increase myocardial performance, when needed, by the Frank–Starling mechanism.

3 Increased muscle mass increases the force of contraction.

Systolic function

Assessment of systolic function in mitral regurgitation is extremely difficult. Ejection phase indices, for example, ejection fraction, fractional shortening and the velocity of circumferential fibre shortening, are particularly unreliable because they are sensitive to afterload which is greatly reduced as a result of the low impedance run-off into the left atrium.[35] As a result, they often remain in or above the normal range well after myocardial dysfunction has begun to develop.[33,36,37] Once these parameters of left ventricular function are reduced, contractility is nearly always seriously impaired. It has been suggested that the end-systolic volume index (the end-systolic volume normalized for body surface area) is better than the ejection fraction as a predictor of irreversible left ventricular damage.[38] Unlike ejection fraction, it is not sensitive to preload. However, it remains very sensitive to afterload, the main abnormality of loading in mitral regurgitation, and the results of another study[33] have found it to be equally unreliable as a measure of left ventricular function.

Right ventricular function

Little is known about right ventricular function in mitral regurgitation. As with mitral stenosis, the right ventricular ejection fraction has been shown to correlate with pulmonary artery pressure and it is a good predictor of exercise tolerance and symptoms.[39] A low right ventricular ejection fraction seems to be a strong predictor of a poor prognosis, but the effect of surgery on prognosis once this deterioration has occurred is not known.

PULMONARY HYPERTENSION

Pulmonary hypertension is a characteristic feature of rheumatic mitral valve disease and is usually most marked when mitral stenosis is the predominant lesion. There are at least three components involved in the genesis of pulmonary hypertension in this condition.

1 Passive backward transmission of pressure via the left atrium and pulmonary circulation.
2 Pulmonary arteriolar constriction which seems to be activated by pulmonary venous hypertension (reactive pulmonary hypertension).
3 Obliterative changes in the pulmonary arteries and arterioles as a complication of longstanding

hypertension. Atheromatous changes may occur if pulmonary hypertension has been particularly severe and longstanding. There may also be a further increase in pulmonary vascular obstruction due to thrombosis in situ and pulmonary thrombo-embolic disease occurring as a complication of low cardiac output.

Pulmonary hypertension leads to right ventricular hypertrophy which initially maintains cardiac output. Eventually, the right ventricle begins to dilate, together with the tricuspid valve ring, leading to tricuspid regurgitation.

PULMONARY FUNCTION

Changes in pulmonary function occurring in mitral valve disease are discussed in detail in Chapter 56. The effects of chronically raised left atrial pressure on the lungs produce marked pathological changes in their parenchyma and vasculature. These changes increase lung stiffness, reduce lung volumes, obstruct air flow and alter gas transfer, and must inevitably contribute to symptoms. The additive effect of cigarette smoking is also important and has only recently received attention.

EXERCISE IN MITRAL STENOSIS

If mitral stenosis is significant, exercise causes a sharp rise in left atrial pressure, pulmonary artery pressure and right ventricular systolic pressure, and in some patients right atrial pressure rises as well.[29,40] These pressure changes are due to augmented venous return but result in little or no increase in forward cardiac output because, although they increase the pressure gradient across the stenosed mitral valve, the diastolic time available for left ventricular filling is also curtailed considerably by the increased heart rate, particularly when the patient is fibrillating, and because increased flow is related to the square root of the pressure increase and consequently a large rise in pressure gradient produces a disproportionately small rise in flow. Pulmonary vascular resistance does not change but the increased afterload on the right ventricle may cause its ejection fraction to fall.[29,30] Oxygen extraction in the periphery increases because there is little increase in the cardiac output and therefore the arteriovenous oxygen difference increases. The clinical consequence of these changes is dyspnoea because the raised left atrial pressure causes pulmonary congestion or even oedema, and fatigue and tiredness on exercise are common features since the cardiac output does not rise.

Recently, isometric exercise (handgrip) during cardiac catheterization has been suggested as a method for distingishing between patients with mitral stenosis who have normal and those who have compromised left ventricular function.[41] Patients in whom the ratio of end-systolic pressure to stroke volume increases and ejection fraction remains unchanged during this manoeuvre are assumed to have normal left ventricular function, and they show a marked improvement in exercise tolerance following surgery. In contrast, those patients in whom the ratio of end-systolic pressure to stroke volume does not increase and the left ventricular ejection fraction falls may not derive benefit from mitral valve surgery because of poor pre-operative left ventricular function.

EXERCISE IN MITRAL REGURGITATION

Patients with mitral regurgitation do not enjoy the same protection from the effects of exercise as patients with severe aortic regurgitation.[42] In aortic regurgitation, the increase in heart rate associated with exercise reduces the total duration of diastole per unit time and, consequently, the amount of regurgitation. In contrast, systole remains at a fairly constant length and therefore, with increased heart rate, it occupies an increased amount of unit time. As a result, mitral regurgitation is not reduced by an increase in heart rate. Altered left ventricular loading occurs during exercise and its effects on left ventricular function and the degree of regurgitation are complex. Increased venous return raises left atrial pressure and therefore left ventricular preload; consequently, there is a modest increase in end-diastolic volume while end-systolic volume falls because the inotropic state of the left ventricle is enhanced during exercise and because peripheral resistance and hence afterload usually falls. Although increased end-diastolic volume will stretch the mitral valve ring and increase its effective regurgitant orifice, this is offset by the fall in peripheral resistance which tends to divert blood into the aorta and away from the left atrium. Therefore, the end result in moderate mitral regurgitation is that stroke volume increases but regurgitant fraction changes little.[42] Once mitral regurgitation becomes more advanced and left ventricular function is compromised, the left ventricle is likely to dilate further with exercise, thereby causing greater stretching of the mitral valve ring and a more marked regurgitation. Furthermore, under these circumstances, peripheral resistance will tend to fall less than is usual because it is countered by the high sympathetic tone engendered by reduced cardiac output. Once mitral regurgitation becomes severe, the increase in cardiac output that occurs during exercise is less, there is a greater rise in left atrial pressure, with consequent pulmonary congestion and dyspnoea, and mitral regurgitation may actually increase because of alterations in left ventricular volume and loading.

The use of exercise and other forms of cardiovascular stress to detect early left ventricular dysfunction and the possible response to valve replacement has been explored far less in mitral than in aortic regurgitation. Huikiri et al. used isometric exercise (handgrip) in patients with mitral regurgitation.[43] This raised mean aortic pressure and hence afterload and, as expected, led to an increase in end-systolic volume and wall stress with a reduction in ejection fraction. The extent to which ejection fraction fell when this stimulus was used pre-operatively correlated well with the fall in ejection fraction that occurred in individual patients following mitral valve replacement. This result is logical since the magnitude of the increase in systolic wall stress during pre-operative isometric exercise and at rest following valve replacement were similar. In view of the difficulties in deciding at what point in the natural history of mitral regurgitation changes in left ventricular function are beginning to become irreversible, further application of this type of investigation in the future may help to indicate the appropriate timing of mitral valve surgery and predict its outcome.

CLINICAL FEATURES

SYMPTOMS

Stage of complete compensation

The signs of mitral stenosis usually do not emerge for at least 2 years after an episode of rheumatic fever; this time-interval is necessary for sufficient fibrosis and distortion of the valve to occur. By contrast, rheumatic mitral regurgitation is often present immediately after the episode of rheumatic fever; however, it may appear later and often increases in severity years after the event.

Even when physical signs develop, many patients with rheumatic valve disease remain completely asymptomatic for a long time. Once symptoms appear, they often do so insidiously with dyspnoea getting worse slowly over many years. However, particularly in pure mitral stenosis, additional stresses on the circulation, such as those imposed by intercurrent infection, the onset of atrial fibrillation and pregnancy, may all precipitate the sudden onset of severe dyspnoea with pulmonary congestion and oedema. Some patients remain remarkably free of symptoms until right-sided heart failure develops, but such cases are rare.

Stage of left atrial and pulmonary venocapillary hypertension

Dyspnoea

Shortness of breath is the most frequent symptom in rheumatic mitral valve disease and is often the presenting complaint. It is usually induced by exertion, but when mitral valve disease is very advanced it may occur at rest. The dyspnoea results from pulmonary congestion, interstitial oedema and chronic changes in the lung secondary to venocapillary hypertension. These changes make the lungs stiffer than usual and thereby they interfere with the mechanics of breathing and impair gas exchange.

Orthopnoea sometimes accompanied by paroxysmal nocturnal dyspnoea are usually late features which imply the presence of chronic interstitial oedema. Occasionally they are the presenting features of the disease. The relationship between the degree of pulmonary congestion and the extent of dyspnoea varies considerably from patient to patient. Patients in whom dyspnoea is provoked only on exertion of moderate or severe degree, usually have a resting pulmonary capillary pressure of < 20 mmHg, although this may rise to much higher levels on exercise. Occasionally, patients with severe resting pulmonary hypertension have relatively few symptoms.

Acute pulmonary oedema may occur in rheumatic mitral valve disease but it is relatively uncommon in the absence of a provoking factor, such as the recent onset of atrial fibrillation, the cardiovascular stress of pregnancy or an intercurrent chest infection. Other precipitating factors may include excessive administration of intravenous fluids, premenstrual fluid retention, pulmonary embolism or anaemia.

Fatigue

Fatigue is common in all forms of mitral valve disease and in some patients it is a more marked feature than dyspnoea on exertion. It is a difficult symptom for the patient to quantify and for the doctor to assess.

Palpitation

Palpitation is a common and sometimes early symptom of mitral valve disease. Initially, it is usually the result of atrial ectopic beats; later, the commonest cause is atrial fibrillation either in paroxysms or as a sustained arrhythmia. Many patients with atrial fibrillation, however, are unaware of its presence, particularly when the rate is well controlled by medical therapy. The awareness of atrial fibrillation is increased on exercise.

Haemoptysis

Haemoptysis has been recorded in 10% of patients with mitral stenosis; it is much less common in patients who have mitral regurgitation. It can occur at any stage of the illness and may occasionally be the presenting complaint. Usually the degree of haemoptysis is slight; occasionally it may be very severe. There are many possible causes of haemoptysis in mitral valve disease. In some patients, red cells are extravasated into the alveoli and then coughed up causing the sputum to be frankly bloody or pink and frothy. In severe and longstanding mitral stenosis, the bronchial veins may become varicose and can occasionally rupture to produce profuse haemoptysis. Pulmonary embolism is not infrequent in advanced mitral stenosis and may lead to haemoptysis. Finally, haemoptysis may be due to some other concomitant condition, such as bronchiectasis, tuberculosis or a pulmonary neoplasm.

Cough

Cough is a frequent symptom and is often associated with dyspnoea. It may occur at rest or be exacerbated by exercise. It is usually worse at night, when pulmonary congestion also tends to increase. Cough also occurs as the result of intercurrent bronchitis which is particularly common in mitral valve disease, especially when the patient is a smoker. On occasions, the cough occurs in the absence of either pulmonary congestion or intercurrent infection and may be due to the pressure of an enlarged left atrium on the bronchial tree.

Angina pectoris

Vague pain in the precordium is quite common in rheumatic mitral valve disease and frequently it cannot be explained. However, definite angina pectoris is also encountered even in the absence of coronary arterial disease. The incidence with which angina is reported in rheumatic mitral valve disease has increased over the years. In 1955, Stuckey reported an incidence of 8.5%,[44] whereas in 1984 Ramsdale found angina in 28% of patients with mixed mitral valve disease.[45] There are several possible explanations for these differences. With the recent introduction of coronary artery surgery, angina has been more diligently sought prior to surgery in patients with valve disease in case coronary artery bypass grafting needs to be carried out at the same time as valve surgery. Furthermore, patients presenting with mitral valve disease in Western cardiological practice have become older and the incidence of coronary disease is age-related. Finally, modern series tend to include some patients in whom the mitral valve disease is non-rheumatic and may have an ischaemic aetiology.

Angina may be the direct result of coincident coronary disease (62% of the patients with angina and mitral valve disease in Ramsdale's studies[45]); in others, it may be due to coronary embolism[46] and patients with severe pulmonary hypertension may develop angina in the absence of coronary artery disease. Finally, if angina is a prominent symptom, it is important to suspect and exclude the possibility of severe co-existent aortic stenosis. As many as 20% of patients with a combination of coronary and mitral valve disease do not have angina.[45]

Hoarseness (Ortner's syndrome)

Hoarseness may occur but it is an unusual symptom of mitral valve disease. It is usually intermittent initially, but may progress to complete aphonia. It is due to left vocal chord paralysis secondary to a left recurrent laryngeal nerve lesion. Although Ortner, in the original description of this syndrome, attributed the recurrent laryngeal nerve lesion to pressure on the nerve by the enlarged left atrium, the results of more recent studies suggest that the true mechanism of the nerve lesion is likely to be compression of the nerve between the dilated left main pulmonary artery and the aorta or aortic ligament.[47,48] A similar syndrome can occur in other conditions in which pulmonary artery pressure is grossly elevated and the left main pulmonary artery dilated, for example, primary pulmonary hypertension, atrial septal defect and obstructive airways disease.

Dysphagia

Although dysphagia may occasionally result from pressure of the dilated left atrium on the oesophagus, it is uncommon. When dysphagia occurs in a patient with rheumatic mitral valve disease, it is more commonly caused by oesophagitis, cardiospasm and neoplasm of the oesophagus.

PHYSICAL SIGNS

General appearance

The most striking feature is the malar flush. This is a cyanotic flush over the cheek bones and is seen most often in patients with longstanding mitral valve disease, particularly when the predominant lesion is mitral stenosis. Although most commonly seen in rheumatic mitral valve disease, it is not a specific feature and can be seen in any type of heart disease that reduces cardiac output and causes pulmonary congestion. When the mitral valve disease is particularly advanced, or if it is associated with pulmonary disease, the patient may show central cyanosis due to inadequate gas exchange in the lungs, and peripheral cyanosis due to poor peripheral flow.

Inspection and palpation

In children, the precordium may be deformed so that it bulges over the enlarged heart; this is not seen in adults. When the main lesion is mitral stenosis, there is usually little that is abnormal on inspection, although occasionally, when pulmonary hypertension is severe, right ventricular pulsation is visible to the right of the sternum, or occasionally in the epigastrum. On palpation, right ventricular hypertrophy and dilatation is easily appreciated as a parasternal heave. The apex beat is often characteristic in mitral stenosis. It has a sharp tapping nature; the tapping corresponds to the first heart sound. Occasionally, the opening snap can also be appreciated by palpation as a precordial shock between the apex beat and the left sternal edge. Severe pulmonary hypertension may lead to a palpable impulse from the pulmonary artery at the upper left sternal border and the pulmonary component of the second heart sound may also be felt at this site. When mitral regurgitation is the predominant lesion, the features of right ventricular hypertrophy are less marked but left ventricular hypertrophy and enlargement occur causing the apex beat to be displaced downwards and to the left which may be visible; it is usually easily appreciated by palpation as a diffuse heaving sensation in the left lower chest.

It may be possible to palpate the mitral murmurs as thrills, and in patients with mitral regurgitation a third heart sound may also be palpable. All apical events are most easily felt with the patient tilted to the left so that the heart is in closer contact with the chest wall.

Pulse and blood pressure

When rheumatic mitral valve disease is mild, the pulse is generally normal. Once stenosis becomes severe, the arterial pulse is of small volume and atrial fibrillation is usually present. If severe mitral regurgitation is the predominant lesion, the pulse volume is also small but its quality is much more collapsing and sharp because the ejection of blood into the aorta is curtailed by the simultaneous rapid leak into the left atrium. The blood pressure is usually normal unless the disease is severe in which case it is often slightly diminished.

Auscultation–mitral stenosis

Auscultation in mitral stenosis (Fig. 28.9) is often aided by turning the patient onto their left side. This tends to bring out mid-diastolic murmurs and pre-systolic murmurs which may be difficult to hear. Furthermore, mild exercise just prior to examination may accentuate the murmurs in a patient in whom the diagnosis is suspected but there is doubt about the auscultatory findings.

First heart sound

Characteristically, the first heart sound, heard at the cardiac apex, is loud and has a sharp or snapping quality. It is often accompanied by a palpable shock (the tapping apex beat). This loud first heart sound in mitral stenosis probably occurs as follows: as left ventricular inflow is obstructed, flow through the mitral valve continues until the end of diastole; as a result, the mitral valve cusps remain open until the time of left ventricular contraction and then close abruptly from a widely open position causing a loud first heart sound. In a normal subject, the valve cusps have already begun to drift together at the end of diastole because by this time the rate of filling is slow. If the valve cusps are rigid, either due to

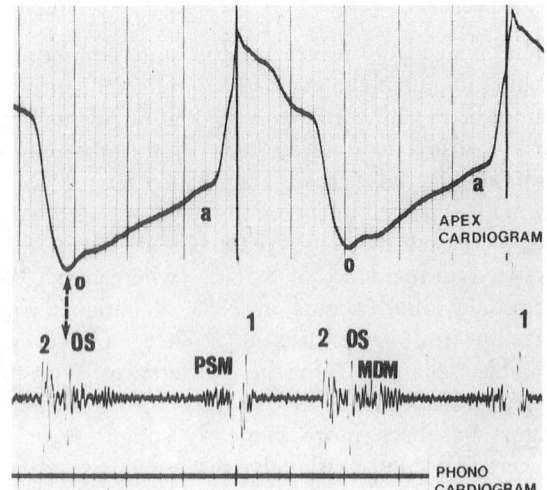

Fig. 28.9. Phonocardiogram and apex cardiogram of a patient with mitral stenosis who is in sinus rhythm. The opening snap (OS) coincides with the 'O' point of the apex cardiogram and is followed by the mid-diastolic murmur (MDM). There is a pre-systolic murmur (PSM) which merges into the first heart sound which is accentuated. The 'a' wave of the apex cardiogram is hardly noticeable. This is because the stenotic mitral valve prevents the rise in atrial pressure, caused by atrial systole, being conducted to the left ventricle and cardiac apex. The mid-diastolic murmur occupies only half of diastole and the opening snap is relatively late (approximately 0.1 s after S_2—the vertical heavy lines are at 0.2-s intervals). Both features suggest that mitral stenosis is mild.

fibrosis or calcification, the first heart sound is soft or absent.

Second heart sound

The second heart sound is normal in mitral stenosis until the pulmonary artery pressure begins to rise. Once this occurs, the pulmonary component of the second heart sound becomes loud and may be somewhat delayed. Occasionally, it may be difficult to differentiate the pulmonary component of the second heart sound from an early opening snap.

Opening snap

The opening snap is a short, sharp, high-pitched click which usually occurs between 0.08 and 0.11 s after the beginning of the second heart sound. Occasionally, it is palpable as well as audible. It is caused by the sudden tensing of the mitral valve cusps as they are opened rapidly by the large pressure gradient between left atrium and left ventricle. The interval between the second heart sound and the opening snap gives some guide to the severity of mitral stenosis. As the atrioventricular pressure difference increases, so the valve opens earlier and therefore the opening snap occurs earlier.[49,50] In atrial fibrillation, the interval between the second heart sound and the opening snap varies with the preceding cycle length. The opening snap is usually best heard between the lower left sternal border and the cardiac apex. However, it may be audible over quite a large area of the chest including the upper left sternal border and pulmonary area. When this is the case, it may be difficult to distinguish it from the pulmonary component of the second heart sound. Occasionally, an opening snap that radiates to the apex may be confused with the third heart sound, although usually this is at a lower pitch and occurs later than the opening snap. Once the mitral valve becomes rigid due to calcification and fibrosis, the opening snap, like the loud first heart sound, disappears.

Mid-diastolic murmur

The mid-diastolic murmur is the most characteristic auscultatory feature of mitral stenosis. When present, it begins immediately after the opening snap. In general, the length of the mid-diastolic murmur is a guide to the severity of mitral stenosis: murmurs extending only a short distance after the opening snap occur in mild cases of mitral stenosis; filling occurring for the length of diastole from the opening snap to the next first heart sound is present in severe cases. Patients with mild mitral stenosis may have no mid-diastolic murmur but simply an opening snap and pre-systolic murmur (see below). Occasionally, patients are seen in whom mitral stenosis is very severe, and transmitral flow has fallen considerably because of the severity of stenosis. In these patients, there may be no obvious abnormal auscultatory signs and as a consequence they are often very difficult to diagnose.

Pre-systolic murmur

The presence of a pre-systolic murmur suggests the diagnosis of mitral stenosis. Although it may be of low pitch and rumbling, like the mid-diastolic murmur, it is often of higher frequency and blowing. The crescendo accentuation of this pre-systolic murmur merges into the snapping first heart sound. The inexperienced auscultator can easily misinterpret the pre-systolic murmur as systolic. This murmur is usually well localized at the cardiac apex and can be overlooked unless carefully sought. The presence or absence of a pre-systolic murmur bears little relationship to the severity of mitral stenosis and often

the loudest pre-systolic murmurs are heard in patients with mild disease. Although its presence depends to a large extent on the pre-systolic flow across the mitral valve induced by atrial systole, this murmur can rarely be heard in patients who are in atrial fibrillation.

Auscultation—mitral regurgitation

When mitral regurgitation is the predominant lesion, the most important auscultatory finding is a loud systolic murmur. The first heart sound is of normal or decreased intensity and the opening snap is absent. The systolic murmur usually commences immediately after the first heart sound, persists until the aortic component of the second heart sound or just beyond (Fig. 28.10) and is often of an even intensity throughout systole. Occasionally, it may rise to a crescendo, but this is never as marked as it is non-rheumatic mitral regurgitation. More rarely, the murmur is decrescendo. Usually the murmur is high pitched and blowing rather than harsh and rasping, as it may be in non-rheumatic mitral regurgitation. The murmur is usually loudest at or near the cardiac apex, radiates to the axilla and, particularly in the presence of a giant left atrium, may extend to be heard at the right of the sternum. When mitral regurgitation is severe, a large quantity of blood has to flow into the left ventricle from the left atrium during diastole (the normal forward flow

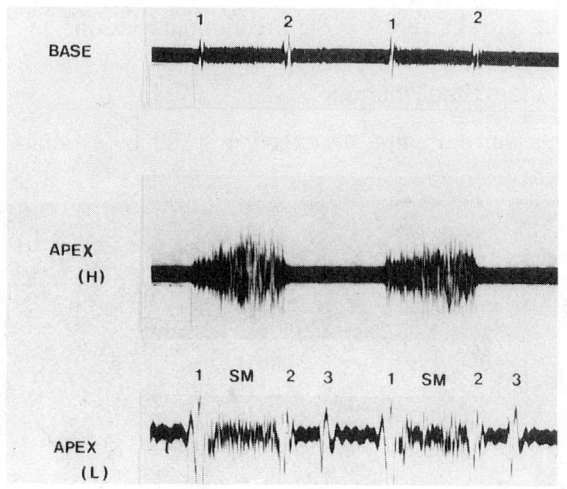

Fig. 28.10. Phonocardiogram from a patient with severe mitral regurgitation (recordings made from the base of the heart and at the cardiac apex at two frequencies: H, high; L, low. There is a pan-systolic murmur (SM) and a loud third heart sound (3). A mid-diastolic murmur was not recorded in this patient.

plus the blood that regurgitated in the previous cardiac cycle). This large flow across the mitral valve often produces a mid-diastolic murmur of moderate length, even if there is no associated mitral stenosis. The rapid inflow also causes a sudden tensing of the left ventricle and leads to a third heart sound (Fig. 28.10). The presence of these two physical signs is a useful guide to the severity of mitral regurgitation, although occasionally both may be absent when mitral regurgitation is severe.

Auscultation—mixed stenosis and regurgitation

Any combination of the features described for the isolated lesions may occur. The relative predominance of the various signs may give a clue to the main lesion, although the clinical impression in mixed mitral valve disease is sometimes very misleading. It is unusual to hear an apical third heart sound if there is any significant mitral stenosis because it prevents the rapid inflow into the left ventricle necessary to produce this physical sign. When most physical signs suggest that the main problem is mitral stenosis but a systolic murmur is present at the apex, careful consideration must be given to either an aortic or tricuspid origin for this murmur as both may be more prominent at the cardiac apex than in their more customary sites. In general, signs other than auscultation are more helpful in deciding the relative contribution of stenosis and regurgitation. A diffuse heaving cardiac apical impulse tends to favour mitral regurgitation, whereas marked signs of pulmonary hypertension and a parasternal heave often suggest that mitral stenosis is the predominant lesion.

Graham Steell murmur

This murmur, first described in 1889 by Graham

Steell as "the murmur of high pressure in the pulmonic artery", is a soft blowing high-pitched diastolic murmur heard in the pulmonary area in patients with severe pulmonary hypertension. It must be distinguished from the murmur of aortic regurgitation; clinically, this can be extremely difficult as the characteristic peripheral signs of aortic regurgitation may be masked by co-existent mitral stenosis. However, this distinction can now be made easily since the advent of the Doppler technique which is extremely sensitive and reliable in detecting both pulmonary and aortic regurgitation (Fig. 28.11).

COMPLICATIONS

The most important complications of rheumatic mitral valve disease are cardiac failure (see natural history below), atrial fibrillation, systemic embolization and infective endocarditis.

ATRIAL FIBRILLATION

Atrial fibrillation is common in patients with significant rheumatic mitral valve disease, and its frequency increases as the condition becomes more severe. The onset of atrial fibrillation is often preceded by frequent atrial premature contractions. These do not cause any serious problems, but the patient may experience occasional palpitations. The onset of atrial fibrillation is usually accompanied by a sudden haemodynamic and symptomatic deterioration. The cardiac output in atrial fibrillation is about 20–25% lower than that in sinus rhythm at the same rate.[8] The occurrence of atrial fibrillation is closely related to left atrial size. Less than 3% of patients with an echocardiographic atrial dimension

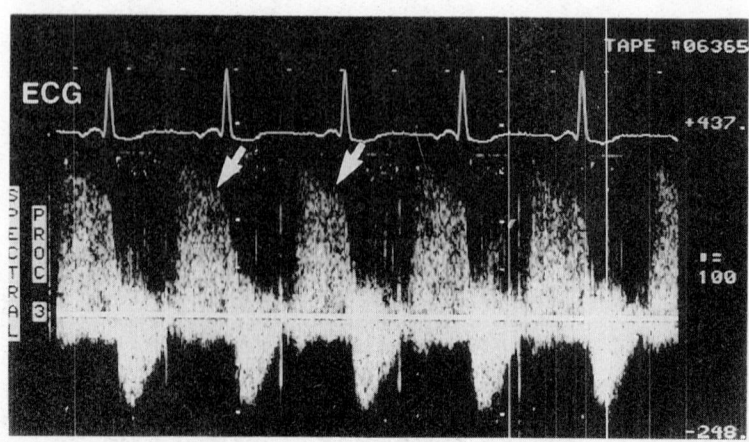

Fig. 28.11. Continuous wave Doppler recording from the left parasternal border in a patient with pulmonary regurgitation secondary to pulmonary hypertension resulting from mitral stenosis. The regurgitant jet due to pulmonary regurgitation (arrows) is towards the transducer.

of < 4 cm are in atrial fibrillation compared with more than 80% of patients over the age of 40 years who have a left atrial dimension of > 4.5 cm.[51] The incidence of atrial fibrillation increases with age and is usually present by the age of 35 or 40 years but this may simply reflect more longstanding disease leading to greater left atrial dimensions. Rheumatic involvement of the left atrial wall may also contribute to the development of atrial fibrillation.[52] Although atrial fibrillation is sometimes paroxysmal in its early stages, it almost invariably becomes established within weeks or months of the first episode.

Atrial flutter and supraventricular tachycardia sometimes occur as a result of rheumatic mitral valve disease, but they are considerably less common than atrial fibrillation. The management of atrial fibrillation is discussed in Chapter 23.

SYSTEMIC EMBOLIZATION

Systemic embolization is an extremely serious complication of rheumatic mitral valve disease and may lead to death. Before anticoagulant therapy and valve surgery became available, it caused 25% of deaths in this condition.[53,54] Systemic emboli usually originate from the left atrium, particularly from its appendage. At surgery, thrombi are frequently found in these sites and are more frequent in patients with mitral stenosis (43%) than in those with mitral regurgitation (8.5%).[55] These differences in surgical findings are reflected in the clinical situation: systemic embolization is more common in patients with predominant mitral stenosis than in those with predominant mitral regurgitation; nevertheless, it remains a significant hazard for patients with mitral regurgitation.

Systemic embolization is most common in patients with advanced disease, atrial fibrillation and a large left atrial appendage. It may occur, however, in patients with only mild-to-moderate mitral valve disease who are still in sinus rhythm, and occasionally it is the presenting manifestation before exercise tolerance is limited. Approximately 20% of patients with rheumatic mitral valve disease experience systemic embolization at some time during the course of their illness and in 25% of patients the emboli are recurrent. The most extensive study of systemic embolization in patients with rheumatic mitral valve disease was carried out by Szekely who followed 750 patients with rheumatic mitral valve disease over 5833 patient-years.[56] He concluded that the incidence of systemic embolization was

approximately 1.5% per patient-year, 80% of patients affected by embolization are in atrial fibrillation and atrial fibrillation increases the risk of embolization by sevenfold. He also showed that there was a strong temporal relationship between the onset of atrial fibrillation and the occurrence of emboli: 33% of emboli occurred in the first month after the onset of atrial fibrillation and 66% in the first year.

Approximately 50% of detected systemic emboli appear in the cerebral circulation[57] and, although the neurological deficit may be temporary, some patients do not recover fully. Systemic emboli may cause myocardial infarction by obstructing a coronary artery, threaten the viability of a limb or the gut, particularly in the elderly in whom collateral flow to these areas may be poor, and can lead to hypertension via renal infarction. Another manifestation is abdominal pain due to splenic infarction. Autopsy studies have shown that clinically silent emboli, mainly to the spleen or kidney, are not uncommon.

The thrombi found in the left atrium at surgery are usually small ovoid friable masses, but occasionally large organized thrombi can occur when there is severe mitral stenosis or as a complication of prosthetic mitral valves. These large thrombi may be pedunculated (Fig. 28.12) or free-floating (Figs 28.13 and 23.14) and can obstruct the mitral valve orifice further—the so-called 'ball valve' thrombus (Fig. 28.15). Since these thrombi are frequently mobile, symptoms may change in severity according to the patient's position. Usually, when a clot is of sufficient size to produce such symptoms death follows soon unless the condition is relieved by surgery.[58] Indeed, the results of a recent study suggest that if such a thrombus is found it should be regarded as a surgical emergency (Fraser A., personal communication). The most important condition to be differentiated is a left atrial myxoma. This behaves in a similar manner giving rise to systemic emboli and often obstructs the mitral valve (Fig. 28.16). The echocardiographic appearances of the intra-atrial mass may be similar, although in a patient with a ball valve thrombus due to mitral stenosis the severely stenotic mitral valve is usually easily detected by echocardiography. Patients with left atrial myxoma often have other clinical features, such as fever and a high erythrocyte sedimentation rate, that suggest the true diagnosis. Differentiation of these two conditions is of little clinical significance because both necessitate surgical removal as a matter of urgency. Occasionally, a large vegetation due to bacterial endocarditis may

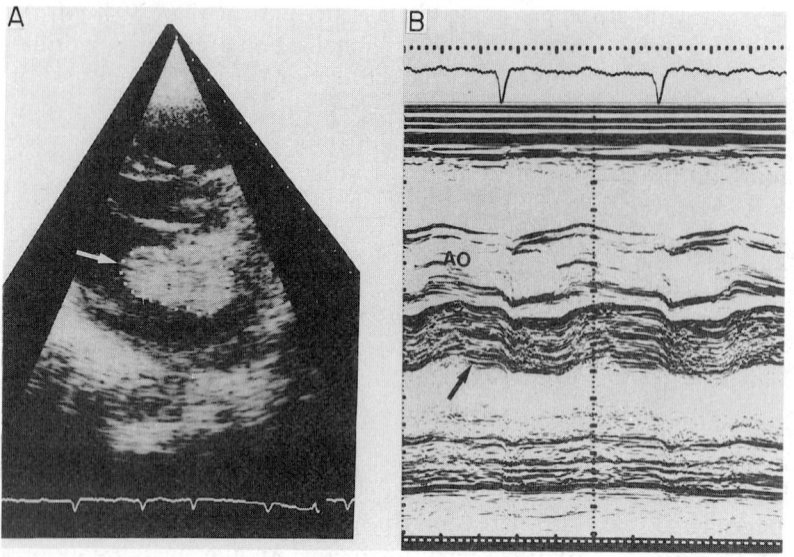

Fig. 28.12. (A) Cross-sectional echocardiogram (long-axis parasternal view) and (B) M-mode echocardiogram of the aorta and left atrium in a patient with a pedunculate left atrial thrombus. The thrombus (arrow) is clearly seen on the cross-sectional echocardiogram as a mass attached to the left atrial wall just below the aortic root. The M-mode detects this thrombus as a mass of echoes (arrow) just below the aortic root (AO). (Courtesy of Dr A. Fraser.)

cause similar clinical and echocardiographic features.

Clot adherent to the left atrial wall can calcify and become apparent on the chest X-ray; this makes surgical procedures on the mitral valve more difficult than usual.

INFECTIVE ENDOCARDITIS

Infective endocarditis is an important complication of rheumatic mitral valve disease. It occurs more often in patients with pure or predominant mitral regurgitation than in those with pure mitral stenosis. All patients with rheumatic mitral valve disease should be regarded as being at risk and receive antibiotic prophylaxis before dentistry or any other procedure likely to cause bacteraemia. It is important that the possibility of endocarditis is always considered when patients with mitral valve disease suffer systemic embolization or become non-specifically unwell in the absence of the classic features of endocarditis.

MITRAL RESTENOSIS

Following mitral valvotomy, 20% of patients require re-operation within 5 years and by 10 years this figure has risen to 60%.[59] Not all these operations are required because of true restenosis; some are necessary because the initial operation was inadequate,[6] because significant mitral regurgita-

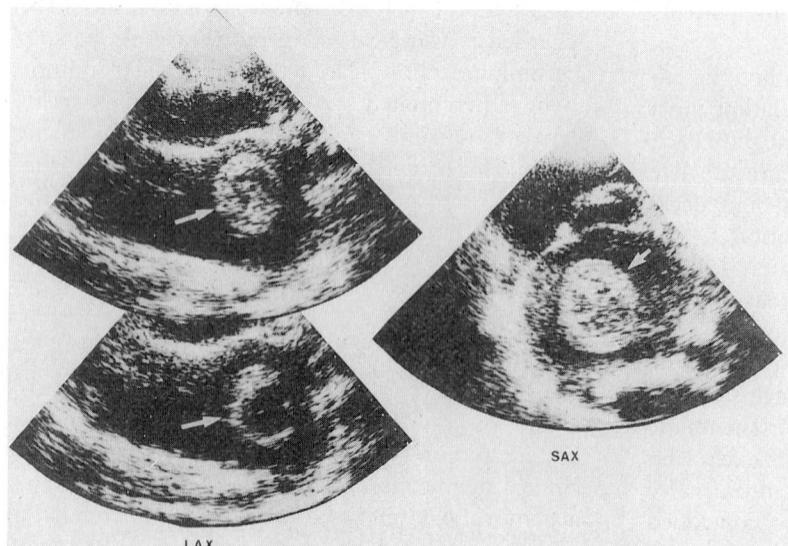

Fig. 28.13. Cross-sectional echocardiograms in both the parasternal long-axis (LAX) and short-axis (SAX) views from a patient with a left atrial thrombus. The mobile thrombus (arrow) which did not appear to be attached to the left atrial wall, is clearly seen. The thrombus varies in echo density from place to place, and slight alteration of the angulation of the echo beam in the long-axis parasternal view emphasizes this variation. (By courtesy of Dr A. Fraser.)

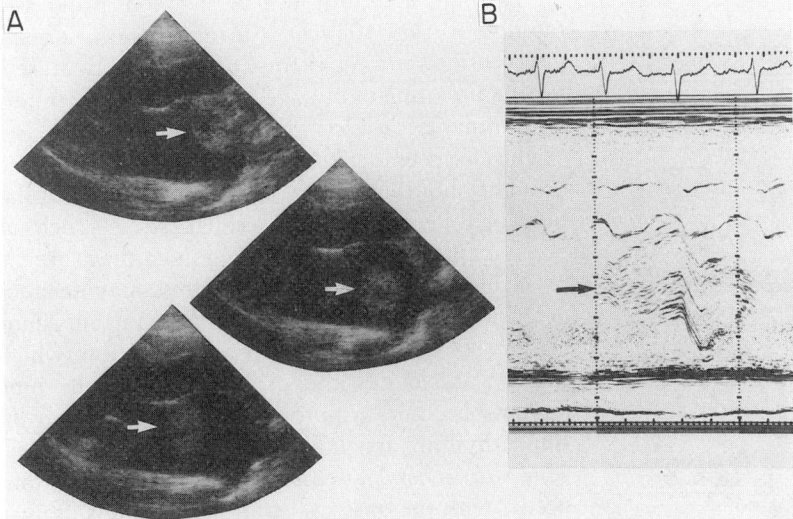

Fig. 28.14. Cross-sectional echocardio-gram in the long-axis parasternal view (A) and an M-mode echocardiogram through the left atrium (B) in a patient with a very mobile left atrial thrombus. The considerable movement of the thrombus, which appears to bounce around the left atrium (arrows), is seen in the cross-sectional echocardiogram and the opacity recorded by the M-mode in the left atrium (arrow) is due to the throm-bus passing through the echo beam. This movement was not related to the cardiac cycle. (By courtesy of Dr A. Fraser.)

tion occurs at or after valvotomy, and because significant aortic valve disease develops at a later date. If the initial operation is adequate and there is no associated aortic valve disease, many patients obtain prolonged relief from mitral valvotomy, often exceeding 10–15 years.[59]

NATURAL HISTORY AND PROGNOSIS

It is difficult to ascertain the natural history of rheumatic mitral valve disease. Although there are large follow-up studies available dating from the era before effective mitral valve surgery,[61,62] the relevance of these data has been reduced by subsequent socio-economic changes, the introduction of more effective medical treatment for congestive heart failure and endocarditis, the prevention of recurrent

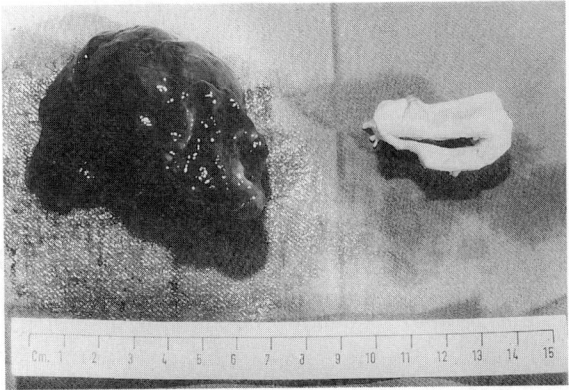

Fig. 28.15. Pathological specimen of a large left atrial thrombus removed at operation (left) and the stenotic mitral valve from the same patient (right).

attacks of rheumatic fever with penicillin and the more widespread use of anticoagulants. These changes mainly affect cardiological practice in the developed world; at present, there are striking differences in the natural history of rheumatic mitral valve disease between developed and underdeveloped countries. In underdeveloped countries, rheumatic mitral valve disease is a serious problem in the young, often running a rapid and fatal course. By contrast, in developed countries, clinically apparent attacks of rheumatic fever are infrequent and rheumatic mitral valve disease tends to present in the fourth or fifth decades of life; it runs a much slower course, and the prognosis is improved by surgical intervention. The more aggressive nature of rheumatic mitral valve disease in underdeveloped countries may be explained by a greater frequency of recurrent attacks of acute rheumatism, and increased individual susceptibility.

Although recurrent attacks of rheumatic fever are important in increasing the amount of cardiac damage and accelerating the progression of disease, mitral valve lesions commonly progress in severity in the absence of recognizable attacks of recurrent carditis. This progression occurs at a variable rate. It has been suggested that the initial rheumatic lesion produces turbulence within the heart which leads to a non-specific and progressive response of fibrosis and deformity of the valves.[63]

MITRAL STENOSIS

A large follow-up series of patients with symptomatic mitral stenosis, conducted in the pre-surgery era, showed that after an average follow-up of 18 years,

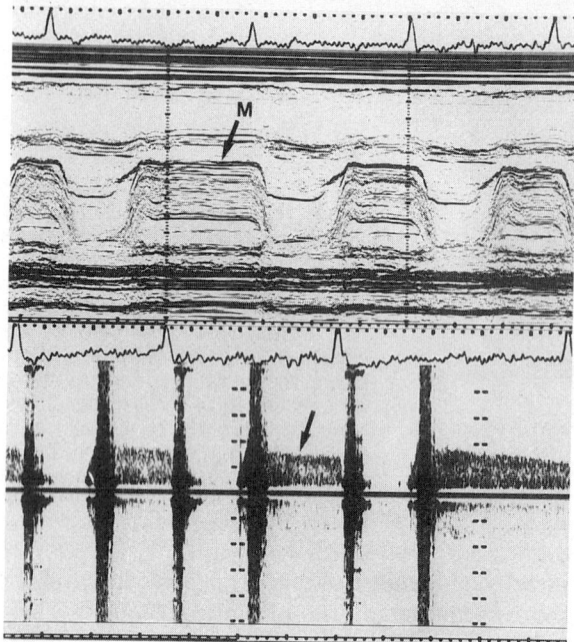

Fig. 28.16. M-Mode echocardiogram (upper panel) and continuous wave Doppler recording of blood flow through the mitral valve (lower panel). The Doppler recording was obtained from the cardiac apex. The M-mode echocardiogram shows the characteristic appearances of a left atrial myxoma (M) and the continuous wave Doppler recording shows an increased velocity of transmitral flow (arrow) throughout diastole which has a similar appearance to the flow pattern of severe mitral stenosis. The heavy deflections on the Doppler trace before and after transmitral flow are due to movement of the myxoma being detected by the Doppler technique.

83% of the patients were dead.[64] In this study, survival of patients was significantly influenced by the degree of functional impairment present when they were enrolled. After only 5 years, 85% of the patients who were initially in NYHA class IV were dead compared with only 18% of patients originally in NYHA class III. In another more recent study of medically treated patients with mitral stenosis of varying severity, 5-year mortality was found to be 20% and 10-year mortality was 40%.[65] These results and those of other studies have suggested that, as well as the severity of symptoms, the onset of atrial fibrillation, congestive heart failure, increased heart size and embolization all indicate a poor prognosis. This high mortality can be significantly reduced by surgical treatment.[66]

The course of rheumatic mitral stenosis shows considerable individual variation. In developed countries, a typical sequence of events would be as follows: the patient remains asymptomatic for 10–20 years following an acute attack of rheumatic fever, then deterioration begins and progresses rapidly over 5–10 years if there is no surgical intervention. Some patients, however, may present for the first time in old age[67] or remain only mildly symptomatic for a long time.

The first evidence of deterioration is often brought about either by the onset of atrial fibrillation or by some cardiovascular stress, such as pregnancy, chest infection or a non-cardiac surgical procedure. This cardiovascular stress may produce deterioration while the patient remains in sinus rhythm or may induce atrial fibrillation which rapidly accelerates the problem. Although some patients become symptomatic while remaining in sinus rhythm, atrial fibrillation eventually supervenes in most patients. The deterioration that occurs with the onset of atrial fibrillation is dramatic, but it can be partly reversed by controlling heart rate and clearing pulmonary congestion with diuretics. Once this point in the illness has been reached, however, the course is usually one of decline, although a patient may be sufficiently well controlled on medical therapy in atrial fibrillation to avoid mitral valve surgery for several years. Deferring surgery for too long may lead to suboptimal surgical results.

In patients with mitral stenosis treated medically, death is usually cardiovascular.[64] Congestive failure and low cardiac output are the commonest modes of death followed in frequency by thrombo-embolic events and infective endocarditis. In patients with surgically treated mitral stenosis, death may occur from these causes but patients often survive mitral stenosis to die from other common causes, such as atherosclerotic heart disease and neoplasia.

MITRAL REGURGITATION

There are similar differences in the natural history of mitral regurgitation in underdeveloped and developed regions of the world. Severe pure rheumatic mitral regurgitation is rarely seen in Western cardiological practice but it is quite common in young patients in underdeveloped countries.

The results of studies performed prior to the advent of effective surgery suggest that the annual mortality from regurgitant rheumatic mitral valve lesions is approximately one-third of that in patients with stenotic lesions.[68,69] These figures may be misleading because the classification of patients was made on clinical grounds. Some patients with severe regurgitant lesions who may have a poor prognosis have a mid-diastolic murmur and it is likely that in the past, many such patients were wrongly excluded from groups of patients with mitral regurgitation. Despite this, rheumatic mitral regurgitation appears to follow a more benign course than mitral stenosis, unless it is complicated by further attacks of acute rheumatism, endocarditis or chordal rupture.[70] Patients with mitral regurgitation who are asymptomatic or mildly symptomatic may lead normal lives for many years. The more benign course of mitral regurgitation probably results from the fact that, as the lesion becomes chronic, the left atrium slowly dilates and acts as a capacitance chamber which accommodates the blood regurgitating through the mitral valve without a significant rise in pressure and therefore ameliorates pulmonary congestion and pulmonary hypertension and their consequences. In comparison, in acute severe mitral regurgitation, the left atrium is usually small and affords no such protection.

As in mitral stenosis, the onset of atrial fibrillation produces a deterioration in patients with mitral regurgitation. However, this is not usually as marked, because left ventricular filling is not so dependent on the length of diastole when there is no significant mitral stenosis, and the large left atrium prevents a rapid rise in left atrial pressure when fibrillation begins and hence protects the lungs.

Although the natural history of regurgitation is more benign than that of stenosis, patients with significant regurgitation deteriorate steadily and eventually die of the disease if treated medically. Munoz et al.[66] found a 5-year survival rate of only 45% in patients with medically treated severe regurgitation; the prognosis of patients with severe mitral regurgitation is substantially improved by surgery.

In mitral regurgitation, the onset of atrial fibrillation, cardiac failure and embolization are all adverse prognostic factors. The heart size on the chest X-ray increases earlier and has less prognostic significance than it does in mitral stenosis. Infective endocarditis is a much more common complication and is a serious risk even in patients who have only a mild regurgitant lesion. Although embolization is a serious complication, it occurs much less frequently than it does in stenotic lesions.

MIXED LESIONS

The outlook in mixed lesions is extremely variable and depends on the relative extent of regurgitation and stenosis. In patients with balanced stenosis and regurgitation, the risk of endocarditis probably approaches that of pure regurgitation whereas the risk of embolization approaches that of pure stenosis.

REFERENCES

1. Ward, C. A reappraisal of the clinical features in acute and chronic heart disease: Etiological implications. *Am. Heart J.* 1979; 98: 298–306.
2. Ward, C. and Ward, A.M. Virus antigen demonstrated in valvular heart disease. *Lancet* 1974; i: 755–6.
3. Burch, G.E. and Colcolough, H.L. Pathogenesis of "rheumatic heart disease": Critique and theory. *Am. Heart J.* 1970; 80: 556.
4. Shore, J.D., Sellers, R.D., Anderson, R.C. *et al*. The developmental complex of "parachute mitral valve", supravalvular ring of left atrium, subaortic stenosis and coarctation of the aorta. *Am. J. Cardiol.* 1963; 11: 714.
5. Khandheria, B.K., Tajik, A.J. *et al*. Supravalvular stenosing ring of left atrium in a 31 year old patient: A case illustrating value of two-dimensional and Doppler echocardiography. *Echocardiography* 1985; 2: 337–40.
6. De Sanctis, R.W., Dean, D.C. and Bland, E.F. Extreme left atrial enlargement. Some characteristic features. *Circulation* 1964; 29: 14.
7. Mitchell, J.H. and Shapiro, W. Atrial function and the hemodynamic consequences of atrial fibrillation in man. *Am. J. Cardiol.* 1969; 23: 556.
8. Stott, D.K., Marpole, D.G.F., Bristow, J.D. *et al*. The role of atrial transport in aortic and mitral stenosis. *Circulation* 1970; 41: 1031.
9. Kennedy, J.W., Yarnell, S.R., Murray, J.A. and Figley, M.M. Quantitative angiocardiography. IV. Relationships of left atrial and ventricular pressure and volume in mitral valve disease. *Circulation* 1970; 21: 817.
10. Gash, A.K., Carabello, B.A., Cepin, D. and Spann, J.F. Left ventricular ejection performance and systolic muscle function in patients with mitral stenosis. *Circulation* 1983; 67: 148–54.
11. Holzer, J.A., Karliner, J.S., O'Rourke, R.A. and Peterson, K.L. Quantitative angiographic analysis of left ventricle in patients with isolated rheumatic mitral stenosis. *Br. Heart J.* 1973; 35: 497.
12. Heller, S.J. and Carleton, R.A. Abnormal left ventricular contraction in patients with mitral stenosis. *Circulation* 1970; 42: 1099.
13. Colle, P., Rahal, S. *et al*. Global left ventricular function and regional wall motion in pure mitral stenosis. *Clin. Cardiol.* 1984; 7: 573–80.
14. Curry, G.C., Eliott, L.P. and Ramsey, H.W. Quantitative left ventricular angiographic findings in mitral stenosis. *Am. J. Cardiol.* 1972; 29: 621–7.
15. Dodge, H.T., Kennedy, J.W. and Peterson, J.L. Quantitative angiographic methods in the evaluation of valvular heart disease. *Prog. Cardiovasc. Dis.* 1973; 16: 1.
16. Horwitz, L.D., Mullins, C.B., Payne, P.M. and Curry, G.C. Left ventricular function in mitral stenosis. *Chest* 1973; 64: 609.
17. Bolen, J.L., Lopes, M.G., Harrison, D.C. and Alderman, E.L. Analysis of left ventricular function in response to afterload changes in patients with mitral stenosis. *Circulation* 1975; 52: 894.
18. Kasalicky, J. Hurych, J. *et al*. Left heart haemodynamics at rest and during exercise in patients with mitral stenosis. *Br. Heart J.* 1968; 30: 188.
19. Ahmed, S.S., Regan, T.J., Fiore, J.J. and Levinson, G.E. The

status of the left ventricular myocardium in mitral stenosis. *Am. Heart J.* 1977; **94**: 28.

20. Quinones, M.A., Gaasch, W.H. and Alexander, J.K. Influence of acute changes in pre-load, after-load, contractile state and heart rate on ejection phase and isovolumic indices of myocardial contractility in man. *Circulation* 1976; **53**: 293.

21. Bove, A.A. and Santamore, W.P. Ventricular interdependence. *Prog. Cardiovasc. Dis.* 1981; **23**: 365.

22. Hui, W.K.K., Lee, P.K., Chow, J.S.F. and Gibson, D.G. Analysis of regional left ventricular wall motion during diastole in mitral stenosis. *Br. Heart J.* 1983; **50**: 321–329.

23. Hammermeister, K.E. and Warbasse, J.R. The rate of change of left ventricular volume in man. II. Diastolic events in health and disease. *Circulation* 1974; **49**: 739–47.

24. Gibson, D.G., Traill, T.A. and Brown, D.J. Changes in left ventricular free wall thickness in patients with ischaemic heart disease. *Br. Heart J.* 1977; **39**: 1312–8.

25. Greenbaum, R.A. and Gibson, D.G. Regional non-uniformity of left ventricular movement in man. *Br. Heart J.* 1981; **45**: 29–34.

26. Gibson, D.G., Greenbaum, R.A., Marier, D.L. and Brown, D.J. Clinical significance of early diastolic changes in left ventricular wall thickness. *Eur. Heart J.* 1980; **1** (Suppl. A): 157–63.

27. Hall, R., Austin, A. and Hunter, S. M-mode echogram as a means of distinguishing mild and severe mitral stenosis. *Br. Heart J.* 1981; **46**: 486–91.

28. Furukawa, K., Matsuura, P. *et al.* Use of digitised left ventricular echocardiograms in assessment on mitral stenosis. *Br. Heart J.* 1979; **42**: 176–81.

29. Cohen, M., Horowitz, S.F., Machac, J. *et al.* Response to exercise in isolated mitral stenosis. *Am. J. Cardiol.* 1985; **55**: 1054–8.

30. Wroblewski, E., James, F., Spann, J.F. and Bove, A.A. Right ventricular performance in mitral stenosis. *Am. J. Cardiol.* 1981; **47**: 51–5.

31. Ross, J. Jr, Sonneblick, E.H., Taylor, R.R. and Covell, J.W. Diastolic geometry and sarcomere lengths in the chronically dilated canine left ventricle. *Circ. Res.* 1971; **28**: 49–61.

32. Urschell, C.W., Covell, J.W., Sonneblick, E.H. *et al.* Myocardial mechanics in aortic and mitral valvular regurgitation. The concept of instantaneous impedance as a determinant of the performance of the intact heart. *J. Clin. Invest.* 1968 **47**: 867–883.

33. Carabello, B.A., Nolan, S.P. and McGuire, L.B. Assessment of pre-operative left ventricular function in patients with mitral regurgitation: Value of the end-systolic wall stress-end-systolic volume ratio. *Circulation* 1981; **64**: 1212–7.

34. Grossman, W., Jones, D. and McLaurin, P. Wall stress and patterns of hypertrophy in the human left ventricle. *J. Clin. Invest.* 1975; **56**: 56–64.

35. Braunwald, E. Mitral regurgitation—physiological, clinical and surgical considerations. *N. Engl. J. Med.* 1969; **281**: 425.

36. Eckberg, D.L., Gault, J.H., Bouchard, R.L. *et al.* Mechanics of left ventricular contraction in chronic severe mitral regurgitation. *Circulation* 1973; **47**: 1252–1259.

37. Osbakken, M.D., Bove, A.A., and Spann, J.F. Left ventricular regional wall motion and velocity of shortening in chronic aortic and mitral regurgitation. *Am. J. Cardiol.* 1981; **47**: 1005–9.

38. Borow, K.M., Green, L.H., Mann, T. *et al.* End-systolic volume as a predictor of post-operative left ventricular function in volume overload from valvular regurgitation. *Am. J. Med.* 1980; **68**: 655–63.

39. Hochreiter, C., Niles, N., Devereux, R.B. *et al.* Mitral regurgitation: relationship of non-invasive descripters of right ventricular performance to clinical and hemodynamic findings and to prognosis in medically and surgically treated patients. *Circulation* 1986; **5**: 900–12.

40. Gorlin, R., Sawyer, C.G., Haynes, F.W. *et al.* Effects of exercise on circulatory dynamics in mitral stenosis III. *Am. Heart J.* 1951; **41**: 192–203.

41. Huikiri, H.V. and Takkunen, J.T. Value of isometric exercise testing during cardiac catheterization in mitral stenosis. *Am. J. Cardiol.* 1983; **52**: 540–3.

42. Levinson, G.E., Frank, M.J. and Schwartz, C.J. The effect of rest and physical effort on the left ventricular burden of mitral and aortic regurgitation. *Am. Heart J.* 1970; **80**: 791–801.

43. Huikuri, H.V., Ikaheimo, M.J., Linnalusto, M.M.K. and Takkunen, J.T. Left ventricular response isometric exercise and its value in predicting the change in ventricular function after mitral valve replacement for mitral regurgitation. *Am. J. Cardiol.* 1983; **51**: 1110–5.

44. Stuckey, D. Cardiac pain in association with mitral stenosis. *Br. Heart J.* 1955; **17**: 397–408.

45. Ramsdale, D.R., Bennett, D.H., Bray, C.L. *et al.* Angina, coronary risk factors and coronary artery disease in patients with valvular heart disease. A prospective study. *Eur. Heart J.* 1984 **5**: 716–726.

46. Oakley, C., Yusuf, R. and Hollman, A. Coronary embolism and angina in mitral stenosis. *Br. Heart J.* 1961; **23**: 357.

47. Stocker, H.H. and Enterline, M.D. Cardiovocal syndrome: Laryngeal paralysis in intrinsic heart disease. *Am. Heart J.* 1958; **56**: 51–59.

48. Dorward, A.J. and Kerr, J.W. Left vocal cord paralysis and chronic obstructive airways disease. *Br. J. Dis. Chest* 1982; **76**: 306–8.

49. Yigitbasi, O., Nalbantgil, I., Birand, A. and Terek, A. O-I/IIA-OS formula for predicting left atrial pressure in mitral stenosis. *Br. Heart J.* 1970; **32**: 547–550.

50. Ebringer, R., Pitt, A. and Anderson, S.T. Haemodynamic factors influencing opening snap interval in mitral stenosis. *Br. Heart J.* 1970; **32**: 350–354.

51. Henry, W.L., Morganroth, J., Pearlman, A.S. *et al.* Relation between echocardiographically determined left atrial size and atrial fibrillation. *Circulation* 1976; **53**: 273–9.

52. Bailey, G.W.H., Braniff, B.A., Hancock, E.W. and Cohn, K.E. Relation of left atrial pathology to atrial fibrillation in mitral valvular disease. *Ann. Intern. Med.* 1968; **69**: 13–20.

53. Neilson, C.H., Galea, E.G. and Hossack, K.F. Thromboembolic complications of mitral valve disease. *Aust. N.Z. J. Med.* 1978; **8**: 372–6.

54. Daley, R., Mattingly, T.W., Holt, C.L. *et al.* Systemic arterial embolism in rheumatic heart disease. *Am. Heart J.* 1951; **42**: 566–81.

55. Janton, O.H., Heidorn, G. *et al.* The clinical determination of mitral insufficiency when associated with mitral stenosis. *Circulation* 1954; **10**: 207–12.

56. Szekely, P. Systemic embolisation and anticoagulant prophylaxis in rheumatic heart disease. *Br. Med. J.* 1964; **1**: 1209–12.

57. Jordon, R.A., Scheifley, C.H. and Edwards, J.E. Mural thrombus and arterial embolization in mitral stenosis. A clinicopathologic study of fifty-one cases. *Circulation* 1951; **3**: 363–7.

58. Lie, J.T. and Entman, M.L. "Hole in one" sudden death: Mitral stenosis and left atrial thrombus. *Am. Heart J.* 1976; **91**: 798–804.

59. Heger, J.J., Wann, L.S., Weyman, A.E. *et al.* Long term changes in mitral valve area after successful mitral commissurotomy. *Circulation* 1979; **59**: 443–8.

60. Higgs, L.M., Glancy, D.L., O'Brien, K.P. *et al.* Mitral Stenosis: An uncommon cause of recurrent symptoms following mitral commissurotomy. *Am. J. Cardiol.* 1970; **26**: 34–7.

61. Bland, E.F. and Jones, T.D. Rheumatic fever and rheumatic heart disease. A twenty year report on 1,000 patients

followed since childhood. *Circulation* 1951; **4**: 836–43.

62. Joint report United Kingdom and United States. The natural history of rheumatic fever and rheumatic heart disease. Ten year report of a cooperative clinical trial of ACTH, cortisone and aspirin. *Circulation* 1965; **32**: 457–76.

63. Selzer, A. and Cohn, K.E. Natural history of mitral stenosis: A review. *Circulation* 1972; **45**: 878–90.

64. Oleson, K.H. The natural history of 271 patients with mitral stenosis under medical treatment. *Br. Heart J.* 1962; **24**: 349–57.

65. Rapaport, E. Natural history of aortic and mitral valve disease. *Am. J. Cardiol.* 1975; **35**: 221–7.

66. Munoz, S., Gallardo, J., Diaz-Gorrin, J.R. and Medina, O. Influence of surgery on the natural history of rheumatic mitral and aortic valve disease. *Am. J. Cardiol.* 1975; **35**: 234–42.

67. Klovstad, O. Mitral stenosis in patients over the age of seventy. *Acta Med. Scand.* 1956; **156** (Suppl. 319): 99–103.

68. Wilson, M.G. The life history of systolic murmurs in rheumatic heart disease. *Prog. Cardiovasc. Dis.* 1962; **5**: 145–51.

69. Wilson, M.G. and Lim, W.N. The natural history of rheumatic heart disease in the third, fourth and fifth decades of life. *Circulation* 1957; **16**: 700–12.

70. Allen, H., Harris, A. and Leatham, A. Significance and prognosis of an isolated late systolic murmur. *Br. Heart J.* 1974; **36**: 525–32.

Chapter 29

Non-rheumatic Mitral Valve Disease

Roger Hall

INTRODUCTION

The mitral valve apparatus is complex and therefore it is not surprising it can fail in many different situations leading to mitral regurgitation. Nowadays most mitral regurgitation is non-rheumatic, e.g. Selzer and Katayama found that 87% of the patients with mitral regurgitation whom they studied were non-rheumatic.[1] Although it is convenient to classify the different types of mitral regurgitation according to the part of the mitral valve affected (Table 29.1), this is an oversimplification because many conditions involve more than one part of the valve, for example, mitral valve prolapse affects the annulus, leaflets and chordae whereas ischaemic heart disease may produce mitral regurgitation as a consequence of poor left ventricular function, increased left ventricular size leading to annular dilatation, and papillary muscle dysfunction or rupture. The relative frequency of the different causes of mitral regurgitation depends on the population investigated. In the developed world, where the population includes a large number of elderly people with a high incidence of coronary artery disease, the two commonest causes of mitral regurgitation are chordal rupture and ischaemic heart disease. Mitral regurgitation may occur acutely or be chronic and slowly increase in severity over a variable period of time. The causes of these two clinically different situations are summarized in Tables 29.1 and 29.2.

AETIOLOGY AND PATHOLOGY

FUNCTIONAL MITRAL REGURGITATION

If the left ventricle dilates for any reason, the mitral valve annulus also increases in size and this eventually leads to mitral regurgitation. In addition to annular dilatation, disturbance of the alignment and function of the papillary muscles and chordae may also contribute to this 'functional' mitral regurgitation. Most often, functional mitral regurgitation is an expression of very severe left ventricular dysfunction and the patient does not benefit from its surgical correction. The degree of functional mitral regurgitation decreases with effective medical treatment, particularly with vasodilators and after correction of the primary cause if this is possible, e.g. severe aortic regurgitation or stenosis.

ISCHAEMIC HEART DISEASE

Ischaemic heart disease may cause mitral regurgitation in a number of ways.[1,2] In this setting, mitral regurgitation is often very mild and of no clinical

Table 29.1. Non-rheumatic mitral regurgitation.

Part of the mitral valve affected	Chronic	Acute
Annulus	Dilatation secondary to increased left ventricular size or mitral valve prolapse	Subacute
	Destruction:	
	Connective tissue disorder	
	Abscess	+
	Calcification	
Leaflet	Congenitally abnormal, e.g. cleft	
	Damage or deformity:	
	Infection	+
	Connective tissue disease	
	Idiopathic	
	Trauma/tumour	+
Chordae and papillary muscle	Congenital anomalies	
	Papillary muscle rupture or dysfunction (ischaemic)	+
	Disruption by endocarditis or trauma	+
	Chordal rupture	+

Table 29.2. Acute mitral regurgitation.

Papillary muscle malfunction
Partial or complete rupture complicating acute myocardial infarction
Severe ischaemic dysfunction

Chordal rupture
Spontaneous or traumatic
Mitral valve prolapse (floppy valve)
Infective endocarditis

Mitral valve cusp malfunction
Myxomatous change (mitral valve prolapse and floppy valve) often with chordal rupture
Perforation by infective endocarditis

Mitral prosthetic leak
Partial detachment (± infective endocarditis)
Cusp perforation or rupture (degeneration or infective endocarditis in a tissue valve)
Major mechanical failure (e.g. strut fracture)
Jammed mechanical valve (thrombus, vegetation or spontaneous—usually produce combined stenosis and regurgitation)

significance, but it is probably extremely common, having been described in 30% of patients undergoing coronary artery surgery.[3]

Papillary muscle rupture

The rarest but most dramatic form of mitral regurgitation in ischaemic heart disease is due to acute papillary muscle rupture occurring during the course of acute myocardial infarction.[4] Fortunately, this occurs in less than 1% of patients. When it does occur, it affects the postero-medial papillary muscle more frequently (2.5 times) than it does the antero-lateral papillary muscle.[5] Rupture usually occurs early in the course of infarction (within the first few hours or days) and leads to sudden and very severe left heart failure and low cardiac output associated with a loud systolic murmur. Patients with complete rupture of the papillary muscle rarely survive long enough to get to surgery and those who are operated on successfully usually have partial papillary muscle rupture with several of the heads of the papillary muscle detached but others remaining intact. The important differential diagnosis is from a ventricular septal defect, the other important cause of acute left ventricular failure and a loud systolic murmur occurring during the course of acute myocardial infarction.

Papillary muscle dysfunction

Mild degrees of mitral regurgitation due to papillary muscle dysfunction are said to be common in the early stages of acute myocardial infarction. This diagnosis is usually based on the finding of an apical systolic murmur during the first few days after infarction. In one study of 200 patients, 117 had this clinical finding.[6] Although many of these patients may have papillary muscle dysfunction, it may be difficult to differentiate a systolic murmur due to mitral regurgitation from a pericardial rub; other patients will have had minor degrees of mitral regurgitation before the infarction, possibly due to the ubiquitous mitral valve prolapse; in some, the murmur will be due to mild tricuspid regurgitation. Despite these reservations, mild degrees of mitral regurgitation are common in this situation and the results of pathological studies show that there is some ischaemic necrosis involving the papillary muscles in as many as 30% of patients who have experienced myocardial infarction.

The concept of papillary muscle dysfunction is easily appreciated by the clinician but much more difficult to reproduce experimentally. In experimental models, damage to the papillary muscle alone does not usually lead to significant mitral regurgitation, and considerable dysfunction of the myocardium underlying the papillary muscle is needed before regurgitation occurs.[7,8] This experimental finding is borne out by the clinical findings. Echocardiography of patients with new systolic murmurs developing during infarction[9] shows that left ventricular function is nearly always severely deranged, with abnormal function of the left ventricular wall below one or both of the papillary muscles.

Mitral regurgitation of this type is often transient resolving within a few days or weeks after infarction. Occasionally, however, it is sufficiently severe during the acute phase of infarction or the early recovery phase to require further investigation with a view to immediate valve replacement or repair. Pre-operative assessment of such patients is difficult as left ventricular function may be at least moderately impaired, some of this impairment may be reversible by grafting of the diseased arteries supplying non-infarcted muscle and the fresh infarct itself may increase surgical problems and mortality. A further small group of patients exhibit progressively increasing mitral regurgitation in the first few weeks or months following infarction. If untreated, these patients have a high mortality. It is difficult to predict which patients will go on to develop this situation but every patient with a significant murmur and symptoms or signs that suggest pulmonary congestion during the acute phase of infarction needs to be followed closely after myocardial infarction.

Dilated left ventricle

When ischaemic heart disease severely disturbs left ventricular function and causes left ventricular dilatation mitral regurgitation is common.

MITRAL VALVE PROLAPSE

This cause is discussed in detail below.

CHORDAL RUPTURE

Chordal rupture is an extremely important cause of mitral regurgitation. It is erroneous to regard it as an ischaemic manifestation. *There is no link between ischaemic heart disease and chordal rupture.* It is generally a condition of late middle- and old age and is one of the commonest causes of haemodynamically significant mitral regurgitation. It may be secondary to several conditions (Tables 29.1 and 29.2) but most clinical cases are either of unknown aetiology or occur in association with idiopathic mitral valve prolapse and 'floppy' mitral valves.[10] It occurs five times more commonly in men than in women.[10] In idiopathic cases, the pathological basis of rupture is not clear and, although ultrastructural abnormalities have been described,[11] some authorities regard the chordal changes as being secondary to fibrotic changes in the papillary muscle leading to increased tension on the chordae.[12] In patients with mitral valve prolapse and floppy valves, the myxomatous changes seen in the valve leaflets extend into the chordae and presumably weaken them. Chordal rupture has a wide spectrum of clinical presentations. If several important chordae rupture at the same time, the effect is of sudden acute mitral regurgitation. This can occur in the idiopathic form and in association with a floppy valve or be due to another cause such as bacterial endocarditis. More often, chordae snap a few at a time and, as the total number of ruptured chordae increases, mitral regurgitation becomes progressively worse. There may be a stepwise increase in clinical severity, paralleling the temporal pattern of chordal rupture.

THE FLOPPY MITRAL VALVE

The stretched voluminous cusps of the floppy mitral valve often leak severely when the chordae are still

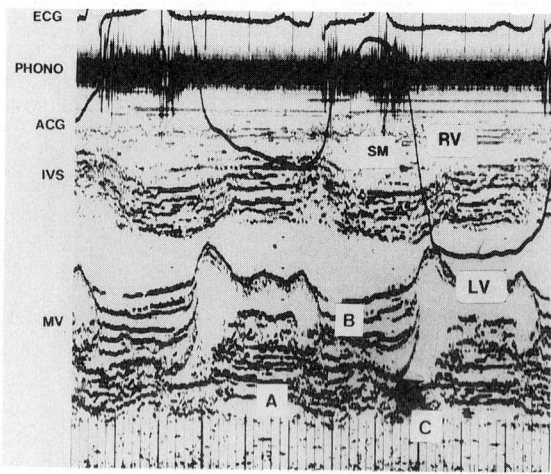

Fig. 29.1. M-Mode echocardiogram and phonocardiogram (PHONO) from a patient with a floppy mitral valve and chordal rupture causing severe mitral regurgitation. The echocardiogram shows an extremely abnormal mitral valve (MV). There are multiple echoes from the mitral valve during diastole (A) and systole (B) due to the chaotic movement of the unsupported voluminous mitral valve cusps and chordae. At end-systole (C), further backward prolapse of the mitral valve is seen. The phonocardiogram shows a pan-systolic murmur (SM) which is considerably accentuated towards the end of systole. This accentuation coincides with the further late systolic prolapse (c) of the mitral valve. There is also an apexcardiogram (ACG) on this recording. LV, left ventricle; RV, right ventricle; IVS, interventricular septum.

intact, but this kind of regurgitation is usually made worse by the commonly associated chordal rupture (Fig. 29.1).

INFECTIVE ENDOCARDITIS

Infective endocarditis should always be suspected when there is a sudden worsening of mitral regurgitation or when it develops as a new feature. Infective endocarditis usually produces regurgitation by perforation of the valve cusps, but chordal rupture due to erosion of the chordae tendinae by the infective process is also important as are papillary muscle damage and involvement of the mitral valve annulus.[13,14]

CALCIFICATION OF THE MITRAL VALVE ANNULUS

The mitral valve annulus often calcifies in the elderly (Fig. 29.2) and calcification is more frequent in women than men.[15–17] Usually, it is a degenerative change but its frequency is increased in certain situations, for example, chronic renal failure with secondary hyperthyroidism, co-existent aortic ste-

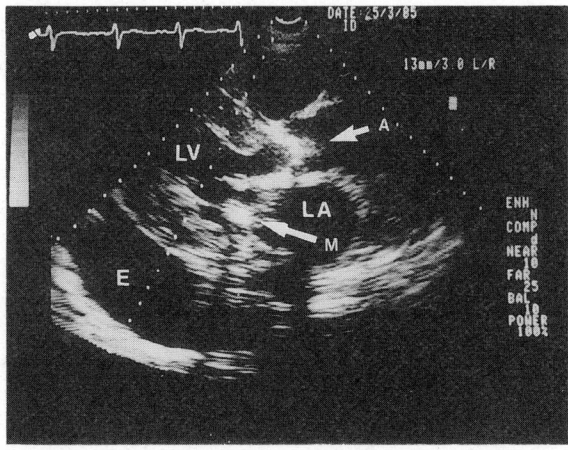

Fig. 29.2. Cross-sectional echocardiogram (parasternal long-axis view) from a patient with calcification of the mitral valve annulus (M). This patient also had calcific aortic stenosis with a thickened aortic valve (A) and a pleural effusion (E). LV, left ventricle; LA, left atrium.

nosis, hypertension, diabetes mellitus, mitral valve prolapse, hypertrophic cardiomyopathy, Marfan's syndrome and Hurler's syndrome.[17–19] Usually, it has little or no functional significance but occasionally leads to mild or severe mitral regurgitation[16] presumably because calcification in the annulus prevents its normal pre-systolic and systolic contraction which helps maintain the competence of the mitral valve. Even more rarely, it can lead to significant mitral stenosis,[20] and very occasionally, the calcification extends into the conducting system and disturbs its function.

HYPERTROPHIC CARDIOMYOPATHY

Many patients with hypertrophic cardiomyopathy have mitral regurgitation.

RARE CAUSES

There is a wide variety of congenital and acquired conditions that can lead to mitral regurgitation some of which are listed in Table 29.1. Some can be extremely bizarre, such as the case described by Wenkebach of a young man who shot himself in the chest, survived the wound but died of progressive heart failure 10 years later. Post-mortem showed a bullet hole in the anterior cusp of the mitral valve.[1] Many of the causes of mitral regurgitation and their pathological and clinical features have been comprehensively reviewed by Selzer[1] and Roberts.[21]

PATHOPHYSIOLOGY

The pathophysiological effects that result from mitral regurgitation are variable and depend on the acuteness of onset, the severity and duration of regurgitation and the adaptive changes that occur in left ventricular and left atrial function. The amount of regurgitation depends on the relative impedance offered to flow from the left ventricle in systole by the left atrium and aorta and on the size of the 'regurgitant orifice'. Both vary with the loading conditions of the left ventricle; therefore, the degree of mitral regurgitation in an individual patient *can vary considerably* over time. For example, if afterload rises due to an increase in peripheral vascular resistance, flow into the left atrium is encouraged and, in addition, left ventricular dimensions may increase causing the mitral valve annulus to increase in size leading to a larger regurgitant orifice. Consequently, raised left ventricular afterload will increase mitral regurgitation, whereas therapeutic measures that reduce peripheral resistance and thus left ventricular afterload will decrease it. Changes in left ventricular preload also alter the degree of mitral regurgitation but less dramatically and rather more unpredictably than changes in afterload, for example, left atrial pressure (preload) will tend to increase left ventricular filling and therefore end-diastolic dimension thereby increasing the effective regurgitant orifice; however, this may be negated because increased left atrial pressure may itself reduce the degree of regurgitation by decreasing the pressure gradient between left ventricle and left atrium during systole. This effect is particularly marked in acute severe mitral regurgitation; the large 'v' wave that occurs in the left atrial pressure trace towards the end of systole (Fig. 29.3) significantly decreases the pressure gradient between left ventricle and left atrium and therefore reduces the amount of regurgitation in late systole. This is illustrated by the sudden late systolic fall in the velocity of severe mitral regurgitation seen on Doppler traces (Fig. 29.4).

Other factors may cause mitral regurgitation to change dramatically over a short period of time. A sudden change in left ventricular function induced by acute ischaemia can markedly increase the severity of mitral regurgitation,[1] and alterations in left ventricular haemodynamics during exercise may also suddenly increase the severity of regurgitation particularly in patients in whom myocardial ischaemia develops.

The time at which mitral regurgitation occurs

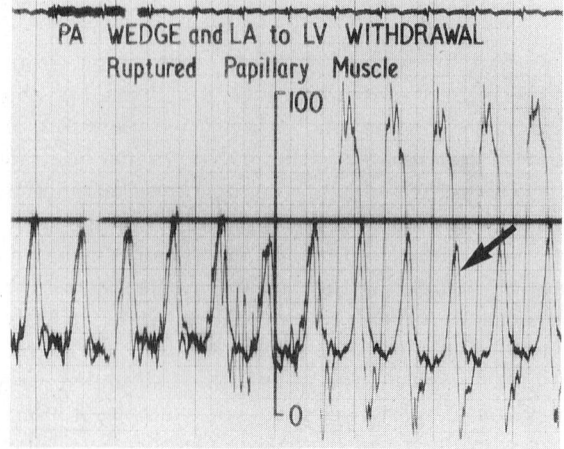

Fig. 29.3. Pressure recordings from a patient with acute mitral regurgitation due to a ruptured papillary muscle. At the left-hand side of the recording, there are simultaneous tracings from the pulmonary artery wedge and left atrium, which are almost identical. On the right-hand side of the recording, the catheter in the left atrium has been withdrawn to the left ventricle and the left ventricular and pulmonary artery wedge pressures are recorded simultaneously. The 'v' wave in the pulmonary artery wedge pressure (arrow) and left atrium is tall and sharp. This 'v' wave is approximately 60 mmHg.

during systole is variable. When the subvalvar apparatus is disrupted, the degree of regurgitation often increases as systole progresses, but in some patients as much as 30% of the total amount of mitral regurgitation can occur during the pre-ejection phase of systole, i.e. before the aortic valve opens, because in this early phase of systole, ejection into the left atrium is favoured because the aortic valve is still closed.

If cardiac output is to be maintained in mitral regurgitation, and the heart rate is normal, left ventricular stroke volume must be increased. One of the reasons why mitral regurgitation is often well tolerated is that the left ventricle is able to do this additional work at low cost in terms of energy consumption. Because wall stress is not increased, myocardial oxygen consumption, which depends mainly on wall stress and heart rate, is not increased.[22,23]

ACUTE MITRAL REGURGITATION

Acute mitral regurgitation of any severity causes a sudden rise in left atrial pressure since the unprepared left atrium is of normal size and compliance. The systolic ejection of blood into the left atrium produces a large sharp 'v' wave which may be as high as 60–80 mmHg (Fig. 29.3), but is more

usually in the region of 30 to 40 mmHg. If the pulmonary vascular resistance is low, this 'v' wave may be transmitted back as far as the pulmonary artery and, even more rarely, left atrial blood is forced back through the pulmonary circulation and detected as a step-up in oxygen saturation at this site. The latter situation may lead to the erroneous diagnosis of a left-to-right shunt at pulmonary artery level. Furthermore, a 'v' wave transmitted back from the left atrium to the pulmonary artery (Fig. 29.5) may cause early closure of the pulmonary valve which is probably of little or no consequence.[24] The diversion of blood into the left atrium in early systole shortens left ventricular ejection time, and may cause early closure of the aortic valve.[25]

Left ventricular stroke volume is augmented by the altered loading conditions. Increased preload increases stroke volume by encouraging left atrial filling whereas decreased afterload contributes by reducing end-systolic volume. Sinus tachycardia occurs via reflexes responding to decreased blood pressure, cardiac output, raised left atrial pressure and hypoxia. The immediate clinical effect of the sudden rise in left atrial pressure with the onset of acute mitral regurgitation is the development of pulmonary oedema and congestive heart failure may ensue.

If the left ventricle is normal before the onset of acute mitral regurgitation, it is frequently able to maintain the resting cardiac output at least in the

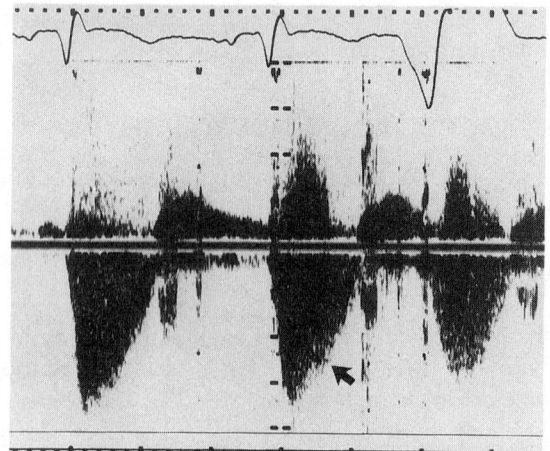

Fig. 29.4. Continuous wave Doppler tracing of mitral valve flow obtained from the cardiac apex. A strong systolic jet due to mitral regurgitation is seen. This tracing shows a fall in velocity in late systole (arrow) because the pressure gradient between left ventricle and left atrium is reduced at this point in the cardiac cycle by a large 'v' wave in the left atrium. These appearances are characteristic of severe mitral regurgitation.

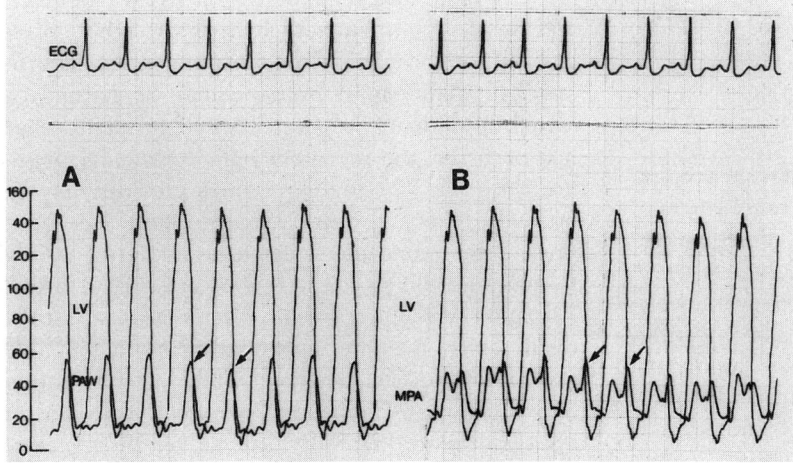

Fig. 29.5. (A) Simultaneous recording of pulmonary artery wedge (PAW) and left ventricular pressure. There is a sharp 'v' wave (arrows) due to acute mitral regurgitation secondary to papillary muscle rupture. In (B), the pulmonary artery pressure (MPA) and left ventricular (LV) pressure are recorded simultaneously. The 'v' wave recorded in (A) can be seen in the pulmonary artery trace (arrows).

early stages, unless mitral regurgitation is particularly severe (for example, rupture of a papillary muscle), by a combination of an increase in stroke volume and in sinus tachycardia. However, if the ventricle is already damaged by infarction and mitral regurgitation is severe, the ventricle is unable to handle the volume load and becomes acutely dilated with reduced wall motion and a subsequent fall in cardiac output. However, if hypoxia due to pulmonary oedema is severe, even initially normal left ventricular function will eventually deteriorate.

CHRONIC MITRAL REGURGITATION

Even quite severe mitral regurgitation is well tolerated if it develops slowly. This is because adaptive mechanisms allow cardiac output to be maintained with only moderate increases in intracardiac pressures. This compensation is achieved by adaptations in left ventricular and left atrial function.

The left ventricle is able to maintain the extra work involved without much increase in energy consumption (see above) and, although the increased stroke volume required to maintain cardiac output is achieved initially by increased systolic emptying of the left ventricle, as time passes the chronic volume overload increases left ventricular end-diastolic volume and causes left ventricular hypertrophy, and left ventricular end-systolic volume returns to normal or increases slightly. This rise in left ventricular volume is accompanied by an increased compliance and consequently left ventricular end-diastolic pressure remains normal de-

spite the increased left ventricular end-diastolic volume. This adaptation allows large volumes of blood to be handled without a large increase in left atrial pressure and therefore without pulmonary congestion. Initially, left ventricular systolic function is normal but, if mitral regurgitation is severe and longstanding, eventually it begins to deteriorate. This deterioration is particularly difficult to detect because ejection phase indices often remain normal long after left ventricular contactility has begun to fall. Left ventricular function in mitral regurgitation is discussed in more detail in Chapter 21. Once left ventricular systolic function is sufficiently poor to cause a fall in ejection fraction, the situation is very serious; such patients rarely gain any benefit from correction of their mitral regurgitation and, as further left ventricular dilatation progressively occurs, the mitral regurgitation becomes more severe.

Changes in left atrial function are also important. Many patients with chronic mitral regurgitation develop marked left atrial dilatation although this rarely reaches the magnitude that may be seen in chronic *rheumatic* mitral regurgitation. This considerable left atrial enlargement allows severe regurgitation to occur into the left atrium with only a moderate rise in left atrial pressure and consequently the lungs are protected and the 'v' wave is not usually as prominent as it is in severe *acute* mitral regurgitation. However, there are patients with chronic mitral regurgitation in whom the left atrium remains small and hypertrophies considerably. In this situation, left atrial pressure tends to be higher and the 'v' wave more prominent.

CLINICAL FEATURES

ACUTE MITRAL REGURGITATION

Symptoms

The symptoms of acute mitral regurgitation are the result of a sudden rise in left atrial pressure causing pulmonary congestion. The patient becomes aware of dyspnoea either at rest or on slight exertion, orthopnoea is common and in the more severe cases paroxysmal nocturnal dyspnoea also occurs. Cough, particularly at night, is also an important symptom of this pulmonary congestion, and frothy sputum, sometimes coloured pink by extravasated red blood cells, may also occur. The onset of this breathlessness may be so acute that the clinician suspects that the onset of symptoms marks the time at which the affected part of the mitral valve apparatus gave way. This sudden onset of symptoms is particularly characteristic of mitral regurgitation due to papillary muscle rupture complicating myocardial infarction. More often, symptoms develop progressively over the course of a few days or even weeks. Some patients with acute mitral regurgitation do not present until the full picture of congestive heart failure has developed. Chest pain is not usually a prominent feature, unless coronary artery disease is either the underlying cause or co-existent.

Signs

When the onset of acute mitral regurgitation is particularly sudden, for example, when papillary muscle rupture appears in the context of acute myocardial infarction, the clinical picture is dominated by sudden cardiovascular collapse, poor peripheral perfusion and pulmonary oedema. The patient appears centrally and peripherally cyanosed, is breathless at rest and often coughs up copious pinky frothy sputum. Other patients with acute mitral regurgitation do not present quite so abruptly, but develop dyspnoea either at rest or on mild exertion over a few hours or days. If there is delay between the onset of acute regurgitation and clinical presentation, the features of congestive heart failure may also be present. In both situations, crepitations are usually present either at the lung bases or throughout the lung fields.

The blood pressure is usually normal or slightly reduced unless the onset is extremely acute in which case marked hypotension is common. The arterial pulse is rapid and regular, with a sharp character, and the degree of sinus tachycardia roughly correlates with the degree of the haemodynamic disturbance. Jugular venous pressure may be normal or raised. In patients in whom acute regurgitation has just occurred and in whom right ventricular pressure is normal, the jugular venous pressure may be normal. If acute mitral regurgitation has been present for some days, congestive failure usually follows and therefore the venous pressure is raised. Palpation of the precordium often reveals a systolic thrill which may be accompanied by a palpable gallop rhythm at the apex which itself is often hyperdynamic. The extent to which the cardiac apex is displaced laterally depends on the degree of chronic regurgitation preceding the onset of acute mitral regurgitation. Generally, if there was little or none, apical displacement is only slight. Once congestive heart failure has occurred and the right ventricle has had time in which to adapt, a parasternal heave may be present, but is not common; even when this has not occurred, palpable expansion of the left atrium, due to the 'v' waves transmitted back into it from the ventricle, may sometimes be detected at the left sternal border.

On auscultation, a loud and often harsh apical systolic murmur is the characteristic finding. This murmur tends to become louder as systole progresses but often fades away towards the second heart sound because of the early equalization of left atrial and left ventricular pressures when the mitral leak is very large. These characteristics sometimes lead to a crescendo–decrescendo type of murmur which can be confused with aortic stenosis. A loud gallop is frequent; there is often a fourth heart sound,[27,28] and the rapid inflow back to the left ventricle of the regurgitated blood from the previous systole produces a third heart sound which may be accompanied by a short mid-diastolic flow murmur. Murmurs due to non-rheumatic mitral regurgitation, whether acute or chronic, may radiate widely in the chest, and, as this radiation may be to the base of the heart and to the neck, this is a further cause of confusion with aortic stenosis. The best means of differentiating the murmur of mitral regurgitation from that of aortic stenosis is by the character of the carotid pulse which is slow rising in aortic stenosis and sharp in mitral regurgitation.[29,30] The direction of radiation of the murmur may suggest which part of the mitral valve apparatus has given way. When there is damage to the posterior mitral valve leaflets, the murmur tends to radiate to the base of the heart and may be heard in the neck;[29] this is believed to be the result of the regurgitant jet striking the atrial septum which is continuous with the posterior aortic wall.[30] Damage to the anterior mitral valve leaflet tends to produce murmurs that radiate into the back and may even be heard on top of the head.[31]

CHRONIC MITRAL REGURGITATION

Symptoms

Chronic mitral regurgitation may be asymptomatic for a long time. Often the first symptom noted by the patient is dyspnoea on exertion accompanied by fatigue which becomes progressively more severe. This progression may take place over weeks, months or even years. The dyspnoea is the result of pulmonary congestion and is often accompanied by other congestive symptoms, for example, cough, orthopnoea and paroxysmal nocturnal dyspnoea. Eventually, if congestive heart failure develops, ankle swelling, abdominal swelling and discomfort may all become prominent features. Chest pain is an unusual symptom unless there is co-existing coronary artery disease. If a sudden exacerbation of symptoms occurs during the course of chronic mitral regurgitation, the possibility of infective endocarditis should be considered.

Signs

The physical signs of chronic non-rheumatic mitral regurgitation are usually similar regardless of aetiology. The blood pressure is normal and pulse is either normal or sharp in character; the patient is usually in sinus rhythm but may develop atrial fibrillation. On palpation of the precordium, the main abnormality is the heaving apical impulse due to left ventricular enlargement. This is usually displaced to the left and downwards. A pre-systolic apical impulse (and a fourth heart sound) are uncommon in chronic mitral regurgitation but a diastolic impulse may be felt at the apex, due to ventricular filling, coinciding with the third heart sound. Similarly, systolic and diastolic thrills corresponding to the characteristic murmurs may be felt at the cardiac apex. In patients in whom pulmonary hypertension has developed, a parasternal impulse due to right ventricular hypertrophy and dilatation may be present and sometimes a palpable impulse felt at this site is caused by systolic expansion of an extremely large left atrium.

The clinical hallmark of mitral regurgitation is a systolic murmur. When the mitral regurgitation is mild, the murmur is frequently limited to the later part of systole. If preceded by a click, such a murmur is likely to be due to mitral valve prolapse, but similar late systolic murmurs, usually without a click, can occur in all forms of mild non-rheumatic mitral regurgitation and are particularly frequent when mitral regurgitation is due to mild papillary muscle dysfunction. Occasionally, patients with mild mitral regurgitation have a systolic murmur that continues throughout systole, but this is usually of moderate intensity and not associated with evidence of cardiac enlargement (see above) or other auscultatory signs which suggest that mitral regurgitation is severe (see below). When mitral regurgitation is severe, the murmur is usually, but not always, pan-systolic. Although in some patients the murmur remains of equal intensity throughout systole, in many there is a marked crescendo towards the second heart sound and it may continue for a short time after the second heart sound. It is unlike the murmur of chronic rheumatic mitral regurgitation which tends to be of equal intensity throughout systole. Mitral systolic murmurs of whatever cause are usually best heard at the cardiac apex and radiate to the axilla. Occasionally, as with acute regurgitation, unusual radiation may occur and lead to confusion with aortic stenosis (see above). The rapid inflow of blood into the left ventricle in diastole, resulting from the return of blood regurgitated in the previous systole to the left ventricle, often leads to a third heart sound accompanied by a mid-diastolic flow murmur. A third heart sound and a mid-diastolic murmur are useful clinical indicators that mitral regurgitation is severe, but significant mitral regurgitation can occur in their absence.

Rarely, the systolic murmur of mitral regurgitation is either absent or insignificant when the regurgitant lesion is severe.[32] Obviously, it is extremely difficult to make the correct diagnosis in such cases, but the possibility of a silent mitral regurgitant lesion should always be suspected in a patient with severe symptoms, a chest X-ray suggesting raised left atrial pressure and an echocardiogram showing hyperdynamic left ventricular wall motion. The Doppler technique will always reveal the presence of mitral regurgitation but cardiac catheterization *may* be necessary to quantify its severity.

When mitral regurgitation is mild, the first and second heart sounds are normal. When it is severe, the first heart sound may be soft and the second heart sound widely split. This wide splitting has been ascribed to the aortic valve closure occurring early because the duration of left ventricular ejection is curtailed as a result of the ease with which the left ventricular stroke volume is ejected into the left atrium in early and mid-systole. Some authors have disputed this.[1]

COMPLICATIONS

The most important complications of non-rheumatic mitral valve disease are the same as those of rheumatic mitral valve disease although the frequency with which each complication occurs in the two conditions, and even in different types of non-rheumatic mitral valve disease, may vary. Accurate figures for the incidence of these complications cannot be given because the age structure of the patients and the aetiology and severity of the regurgitation differ widely in the various reported series.

PULMONARY OEDEMA AND HEART FAILURE

Pulmonary oedema and heart failure result either from acute mitral regurgitation occurring in a previously normal heart or when the compensatory mechanisms for chronic mitral regurgitation can no longer prevent a significant rise in left atrial pressure which leads to pulmonary congestion. Although response to medical therapy may be good, particularly if the condition is chronic, occurrence of these complications must be regarded as an indication that mitral valve replacement should not be delayed for long. Despite this, some patients are encountered in whom initial treatment of such an episode is followed by a long period of satisfactory progress on medical therapy.

The occurrence of pulmonary oedema and heart failure are not so ominous if there is a transient precipitating factor. For example, dramatic improvement may occur once the rate of atrial fibrillation has been controlled or if the precipitating factor is reversible or transient, e.g. anaemia, pregnancy, thyrotoxicosis, major non-cardiac surgery or an intercurrent infection.

ATRIAL FIBRILLATION

The majority of patients with non-rheumatic mitral regurgitation are in sinus rhythm,[1] but atrial fibrillation is common (it occurs in possibly 30% of patients), particularly when mitral regurgitation is longstanding and the heart size is increased. The relationship between chronicity and heart size in atrial fibrillation is not surprising in view of the finding that in all types of heart disease the occurrence of fibrillation is more strongly related to left atrial size than to aetiology.[33] Although atrial fibrillation may produce a sudden symptomatic deterioration, it is generally better tolerated by patients with mitral regurgitation, of whatever cause, than those with mitral stenosis. Controlling the ventricular rate often produces a considerable clinical improvement, and it is rarely worthwhile to convert atrial fibrillation to sinus rhythm while leaving significant mitral regurgitation uncorrected because fibrillation soon recurs. Exceptions to this recommendation are discussed under medical management of mitral valve disease (see p. 768).

SYSTEMIC EMBOLIZATION

Although systemic embolization is less common in non-rheumatic than in rheumatic mitral valve disease, it occurs sufficiently frequently to be an important problem. Its occurrence should always suggest the possibility of infective endocarditis. As in rheumatic heart disease, the occurrence of systemic embolization occurs almost exclusively in patients who are fibrillating (90% of episodes), and it is much more likely to occur soon after the onset of atrial fibrillation; the risk of embolization in the first week after the onset of atrial fibrillation in patients with 'mitral valve disease' of an unspecified type[33] was found to be 38% as compared with an additional 34% risk over the next 10 years.

INFECTIVE ENDOCARDITIS

Infective endocarditis is an extremely important complication of non-rheumatic mitral regurgitation. It should always be suspected in a patient who shows an unexpected clinical deterioration, who is non-specifically unwell or who sustains a systemic embolus. Mitral regurgitation need not be severe to predispose to infective endocarditis and therefore patients with any degree of mitral regurgitation should be regarded as being at risk and receive suitable antibiotic prophylaxis.

NATURAL HISTORY AND PROGNOSIS

As non-rheumatic mitral regurgitation has so many

different aetiologies,[1] it is highly unlikely that the natural history of a similar degree of mitral regurgitation will also be similar regardless of cause. The large number of causes also means that the natural history information available for any one aetiology is often extremely limited.

In general, mild mitral regurgitation has an excellent prognosis and frequently causes no clinical problems;[34,35] however, there are exceptions. Once mild mitral regurgitation occurs in a patient with infective endocarditis, the regurgitation may rapidly worsen because further valve destruction occurs during the course of the illness. Similarly, in patients with Marfan's syndrome, the connective tissue abnormality means that once the regurgitant lesion begins to be clinically obvious the already weakened mitral valve structures become more distorted and more regurgitant. Furthermore, patients with mild mitral regurgitation due to the mitral valve prolapse syndrome may go on to develop a floppy mitral valve, which may leak significantly, and chordal rupture can lead to a rapid increase in the severity of mitral regurgitation. The natural history of mitral valve prolapse and floppy mitral valve are discussed on page 790.

The difficulties in establishing the true natural history of non-rheumatic mitral regurgitation are complicated because, prior to the advent of successful surgery, many series of patients with mitral regurgitation, deemed to be rheumatic, contained an unknown number of patients who actually had non-rheumatic mitral regurgitation. In addition, many of the conditions nowadays regarded as significant causes of mitral regurgitation were unrecognized. For these reasons, information on the natural history of medically treated patients with non-rheumatic mitral regurgitation from the pre-surgical era is scanty and, now that mitral valve surgery is widely available and usually employed in such patients, it is unlikely to be forthcoming.

The information available on medically treated patients shows that prognosis depends on the severity of the mitral regurgitation. Rapaport[36] reported a 5-year survival of 80% and a 10-year survival of 60% in medically treated patients with mitral regurgitation due to a variety of causes. Munoz et al.[37] studied more disabled patients and found a 5-year survival rate of only 45%. Left ventricular enlargement and reduced cardiac output seem to predict a poor prognosis.[38] In the context of rheumatic heart disease, mitral regurgitant lesions are known to have a much better prognosis than mitral stenosis, and it is probable that many other

patients with mitral regurgitation share this better prognosis, reflecting the ability of the left ventricle to do volume work at only a small cost in terms of oxygen consumption (see above). Indeed, most clinicians are familiar with occasional patients with very severe mitral regurgitation who do well for prolonged periods on medical therapy.[1]

Although it is difficult to define the natural history of mitral regurgitation in specific lesions, certain situations deserve mention. If mitral regurgitation is secondary to poor left ventricular function, and particularly if the underlying cause is ischaemic heart disease, the prognosis is usually poor with progressive heart failure and death usually occurring within 1 year. Similarly, rupture of a major portion of the papillary muscle generally has a poor prognosis unless successful surgery is undertaken at a very early stage. Occasionally, however, patients with rupture of part of the papillary muscle may present months after infarction.[1] It is probable that patients with complete papillary muscle rupture secondary to myocardial infarction only survive for minutes or hours unless urgent surgical intervention is undertaken. In contrast, the prognosis of dysfunction rather than ruptured papillary muscles occurring during infarction is very variable.[39,40] Trivial regurgitation occurring during the course of myocardial infarction has little effect on prognosis. If moderate or severe regurgitation occurs within days or weeks of infarction, follow-up studies from the era before effective surgical treatment suggest that if the patient survives the acute phase of infarction the normal course is steadily downhill with congestive heart failure being a common sequel in the following weeks or months. Consequently, such a patient needs to be considered for mitral valve surgery urgently, although the outcome of mitral valve surgery in ischaemic mitral regurgitation is generally less good than that in patients who are free of ischaemic heart disease. This is because of the complex interplay of three important variables: the extent of regurgitation, the extent of left ventricular dysfunction and the extent of coronary artery disease. Another situation which may have a characteristic natural history is mitral regurgitation due to chordal rupture. It can follow several different courses. It may present for the first time with sudden acute mitral regurgitation due to rupture of one or more major supporting chordae. These patients may stabilize on medical treatment initially but frequently need surgery at an early stage. Other patients with chordal rupture deteriorate slowly as regurgitation becomes more severe due to the sequential rupture of minor chordae, each supporting only a small part of the mitral valve. This deterioration can sometimes be step-wise, each downward step probably coinciding with the rupture of a few more chordae. These patients may develop quite severe chronic mitral regurgita-tion which they will be able to tolerate for a prolonged period while receiving medical treat-ment.

The natural history and prognosis of mitral regurgitation can be summarized as follows. Mild mitral regurgitation usually has an excellent prog-nosis and even quite severe mitral regurgitation can be tolerated by some patients for a prolonged period. However, if severe regurgitation is allowed to persist for too long before surgical correction is undertaken, irreversible changes in left ventricular function may occur. Without surgical intervention, the course of severe mitral regurgitation is steady deterioration, which may be stepwise in patients who experience sequential rupture of the chordae tendineae; it is most rapid in patients in whom the underlying cause of mitral regurgitation is myocar-dial ischaemia.

MITRAL VALVE PROLAPSE

The commonest cause of malfunction of the mitral valve is prolapse of part or all of one or both of its cusps towards the left atrium during systole. The extent of this prolapse is extremely variable, as are the physical signs and haemodynamic effects that it produces. Frequently, it is of little or no clinical or haemodynamic significance and simply represents an interesting and sometimes confusing ausculta-tory or echocardiographic finding. Occasionally, however, it assumes clinical importance because it causes haemodynamically significant mitral reg-urgitation, acts as the site for infective endocarditis or is associated with significant arrhythmias.

Although usually idiopathic, mitral valve pro-lapse occurs as a feature of several syndromes in which a widespread abnormality of collagen is well documented, e.g. the Marfan and Ehlers–Danlos syndromes (Fig. 29.6).[41,42] Furthermore, abnorma-lities of left ventricular and papillary muscle func-tion, for example, in ischaemic heart disease, may allow prolapse of part of the mitral valve towards the left atrium during systole with or without mitral regurgitation.

IDIOPATHIC MITRAL VALVE PROLAPSE

Definition

Considerable confusion surrounds the definition of mitral valve prolapse mainly because the criteria used for diagnosis are very variable. In some studies, the diagnosis has been based purely on auscultatory findings, in others, on echocardiog-raphic grounds alone, and in some series it has been made on the basis of both echocardiographic and physical findings. Furthermore, some series com-prise patients presenting with cardiological symp-toms whereas others are derived from population surveys of healthy subjects. To add to this confu-sion, the echocardiographic findings, often thought to be diagnostic, may be unreliable and have poor reproducibility.[43] For example, bowing of the

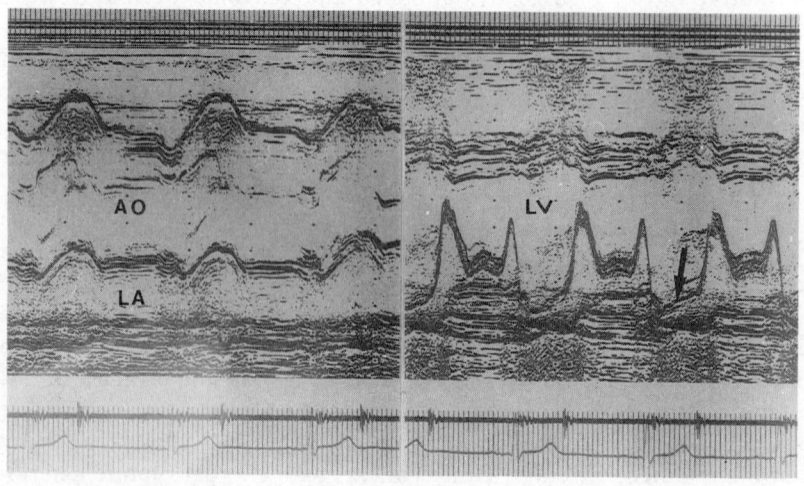

Fig. 29.6. M-Mode echocardiograms of the aorta and left atrium (left) and mitral valve and left ventricle (right) from a patient with Marfan's syndrome. The aorta is grossly dilated (approximately 5 cm). There is pan-systolic prolapse of the mitral valve (arrow). LV, left ventricle; LA, left atrium; Ao, aorta.

mitral valve cusps towards the left atrial side of the valve annulus during systole is thought by some authors to be diagnostic of this condition. In studies of young subjects without cardiac signs or symptoms between the ages of 10 and 18 years, the incidence of this echocardiographic finding may be as high as 30%.[44] Under these circumstances, it is unreasonable to regard such a finding as abnormal.

This diagnostic difficulty has been recognized and recommendations have been made with regard to patients with only trivial echocardiographic abnormalities and without physical signs as being normal.[45] Clinical sense can be made of the situation if the following guidelines are always considered.

1 Minor auscultatory (for example, an isolated click) or minor echocardiographic findings (slight bowing of the mitral valve leaflets beyond the mitral valve annulus on the cross-sectional echocardiogram) should be regarded as normal.

2 Associated features, such as minor echocardiographic abnormalities or minor arrhythmias, should be regarded sceptically unless appropriate control subjects have been included in the study.

3 The subjective nature of many of the echocardiographic criteria, often regarded as diagnostic, and their dependence on image quality as well as their poor reproducibility must always be borne in mind.

4 Data derived from patients with idiopathic mitral valve prolapse must not be extrapolated to the secondary forms of mitral valve prolapse which may arise from any condition that disturbs the integrity of the complicated mitral valve apparatus.

A variety of names have been given to this syndrome which are often descriptive and sometimes quaint (Table 29.3). The term 'floppy mitral valve' is usually reserved for the most extreme form of mitral valve prolapse in which the chordae are grossly elongated, the valve voluminous and there is usually severe mitral regurgitation.

Table 29.3. Synonyms for mitral valve prolapse.

Click syndrome
Click–murmur syndrome
Barlow's syndrome
Systolic click–late systolic murmur syndrome
Overshooting mitral leaflets
Floppy valve syndrome
Billowing posterior leaflet syndrome
Ballooning of the mitral valve leaflets
Auscultatory–electrocardiographic syndrome

Prevalence

Mitral valve prolapse is common and probably the single most frequent cause of abnormal auscultatory signs in the heart. Its exact prevalence is very difficult to determine because of the major differences between studies.[46–49] These differences include variation in diagnostic criteria, in methods of selection, and differences in the age, race and sex of the patients. Despite these problems, a reasonable conclusion from the published surveys is that its incidence is approximately 6% in adult women, who comprise two-thirds of subjects, and approximately 2% in adult men.[50,51] The sex and age of the patients studied seem to have an important effect. Results of the Framingham study[51] show that in women the incidence falls steadily with increasing age: in the third decade, the incidence was 16.9%, in the fifth decade it was 12.2%, in the seventh decade it was 4.4.% and when the patients studied were over 80 years of age the incidence was only 1.4%. In contrast, the incidence of mitral valve prolapse in men remained at approximately 3% regardless of age. As a result, in older patients, the incidence was similar in the two sexes. The reason for the falling incidence in women is unknown but it seems likely that the high incidence reported in young females may reflect the detection of a normal variant of mitral valve motion.

Inheritance

Mitral valve prolapse shows a definite familial incidence, being reported in between 25 and 50% of first-degree relatives over the age of 20 years.[53,54] Although an autosomal dominant mode of inheritance with incomplete penetrance and increased expressivity in females has been suggested, as yet there is no convincing evidence to support this hypothesis.

Pathology

As already suggested, many patients who are diagnosed as having mitral valve prolapse, particularly when young, may be normal; there are no pathological studies to confirm or refute this suggestion. Most pathological material has been obtained from patients with the more severe degrees of mitral valve prolapse, which has often led to a floppy mitral valve requiring mitral valve replacement. The common factor in valves obtained from patients with all degrees of the syndrome is myxomatous degeneration of the mitral valve cusp tissue.[55–57] This degeneration is a loss or disruption of the normal valve architecture with considerable increase of the ground substance but without significant inflammatory change. A normal valve leaflet has at its centre the *fibrosa*, a dense continuous sheet of collagen, which inserts into the valve ring and fibrous skeleton of the heart and gives the valve cusp its strength. On the atrial side, there is the *spongiosa* which is made of myxomatous (acid mucopolysaccharide) tissue. In mitral valve prolapse, this layer is greatly increased in thickness and may invade and interrupt the fibrosa thereby weakening the valve. Although in early reports it was suggested that these changes were more common in the posterior mitral valve leaflet, the results of recent studies have indicated that involvement of both anterior and posterior cusps is the commonest situation. As the condition becomes more advanced, the mitral valve leaflets stretch and become slightly thickened and voluminous.

Similar myxomatous degeneration also affects the mitral valve annulus and the chordae tendineae. This results in considerable stretching of the mitral valve annulus[58] and a loss of its normal systolic contraction, and an elongation of the chordae tendineae, which are also thin and fragile such that chordal rupture is a common complication. Occasionally, the chordae are thickened and may adhere to the left ventricular myocardium.

In addition to myxomatous degeneration of the mitral valve, similar changes have been described in the tricuspid valve in 25–50% of patients in whom the mitral valve is affected[55,59,60] and these changes are also well documented in the aortic valve.[61,62] The changes in the tricuspid and aortic valves are much less frequently of sufficient degree to lead to haemodynamic disturbances.

Pathological changes in the heart muscle are not prominent features in mitral valve prolapse, although areas of superficial fibrous thickening may occur on the endocardium of the ventricle, probably as a result of friction from contact with abnormal chordae and valve cusps.

Although there is no doubt that myxomatous degeneration is the histological hallmark of mitral valve prolapse, there is dispute over whether the prolapse itself is the cause or the result of this abnormality,[50] which cannot be resolved on present evidence. If myxomatous degeneration is the primary process, its cause has not yet been established. If it is a secondary effect, not universally accepted primary abnormality has been established although

several suggestions have been put forward, which include regional contraction abnormalities in the left ventricle that disturb papillary muscle function and may be the result of some unspecified type of localized cardiomyopathy. Coronary artery anomalies have been suggested as a cause, for example, congenital absence of the atrioventricular groove branch of the circumflex artery leading to regional myocardial ischaemia. These proposed mechanisms depend upon the presence of regional wall motion abnormalities; however, widely differing contraction abnormalities have been described and a high frequency of normal left ventricular contraction patterns has been reported, findings that do not provide support for these proposals.

Although it is highly unlikely that coronary disease is the universal underlying factor in idiopathic mitral valve prolapse, angiographically detectable prolapse of the mitral valve can occur when papillary muscle function is disturbed by ischaemia. This type of prolapsing mitral valve, however, tends to produce a different clinical picture. There is rarely a mid-systolic click, although late systolic murmurs are not uncommon, and the echocardiogram does not show characteristic changes of mitral valve prolapse. The occasional reports of associations between coronary artery disease and mid-systolic clicks are no more frequent than would be expected by the chance coincidence of two such common conditions. The apparent paradox between angiographically documented prolapse and the absence of physical signs has led Jeresaty[50] to postulate that, although valve motion into the left atrium during systole is common in patients with abnormal left ventricular function due to coronary artery disease, these patients lack the elongated chordae and redundant valve tissue required to produce the characteristic auscultatory and echocardiographic findings of idiopathic mitral valve prolapse.

Clinical features

The vast majority of patients with idiopathic mitral valve prolapse are asymptomatic. When symptoms do occur, it is frequently difficult to ascertain whether they are due to mitral valve prolapse or to a chance finding. This is because many series which give the incidence of symptoms are derived from patient populations referred to cardiological centres because of symptoms thought to be of a cardiovascular nature. These studies rarely include appropriate contol subjects such as patients without findings of mitral valve prolapse but with similar symptoms. Consequently, symptoms in patients with mitral valve prolapse are of two types. First, symptoms that are non-specific and occur commonly in patients wih and without mitral valve prolapse. Such symptoms tend to be ascribed to mitral valve prolapse if auscultatory or echocardiographic evidence of this condition is found; confirmation that they are no more than a chance association is often lacking. Second, symptoms that are more specifiic, and a reasonable link between mitral valve prolapse and the symptoms can be established.

Non-specific symptoms

Chest pain   In most series, chest pain is the most common symptom,[50,63] however it is also the most frequent reason for referral of patients without obvious cardiological disease to cardiological clinics. Unfortunately, no study to date has been designed to include a suitable control group to help assess the significance of such pain or its true relationship to mitral valve prolapse. Although pain reported by patients with mitral valve prolapse is often disabling, it rarely has the classical features of pain due to myocardial ischaemia. It tends to be unrelated to exercise, sharp in character, situated in the left breast and is often unrelieved by nitrates. Although some authors ascribe these pains to papillary muscle ischaemia caused by abnormal traction of the chordae, or even coronary spasm, the dissimilarity to all other forms of ischaemic pain make this explanation unlikely. In a small number of patients with mitral valve prolapse and normal coronary arteries, the pain may have all the classic features of angina pectoris. It is difficult to be sure of its significance in the context of mitral valve prolapse. As echocardiographic and auscultatory findings of mitral valve prolapse are so common and tend to occur most often in women, this may simply be a chance association of the syndrome of angina with normal coronary arteries (a condition most commonly seen in women) and mitral valve prolapse. Regardless of whether there is a causal relationship between chest pain and mitral valve prolapse, some patients are disabled by this symptom and it usually proves resistant to treatment.

Dyspnoea, fatigue and dizziness in the absence of significant mitral regurgitation or arrhythmias The symptoms of dyspnoea, fatigue and dizziness, like the chest pain associated with mitral valve prolapse, are non-specific and their true relationship

to mitral valve prolapse is impossible to determine. Dyspnoea and fatigue have been reported in up to 60% of patients presenting with idiopathic mitral valve prolapse and half of these patients had no evidence of mitral regurgitation. In some patients, dyspnoea and fatigue has been attributed to hyperventilation,[64] and anxiety combined with psychoneurotic disturbance has been reported in a large proportion of such patients (15–38%).[64,65] Dizziness, which cannot be explained, and palpitations occurring when the 24-h electrocardiogram shows sinus tachycardia have also been reported.

Specific symptoms

Palpitations, dizziness and syncope associated with arrhythmias Palpitation is usually associated with arrhythmias and is a common presenting symptom, occurring in more than 40% of patients in hospital-based referral series. These palpitations are frequently trivial but occasionally arrhythmias may be serious and troublesome (see below).

Exertional dyspnoea associated with significant mitral regurgitation In a small number of patients with mitral valve prolapse, mitral regurgitation progresses and becomes haemodynamically significant producing all the usual symptoms that would be expected under these circumstances. There are three main ways in which mitral regurgitation becomes significant. First, progressive stretching of the valve cusps, chordae and mitral annulus may led to the true floppy valve. Second, chordal rupture often associated with the floppy valve worsens mitral regurgitation. Third, valve disruption may occur as a result of infective endocarditis. When mitral regurgitation occurs as the result of the first mechanism, symptoms tend to be slowly progressive whereas chordal rupture or valve disruption due to infective endocarditis may often produce a rapid progression of symptoms.

EXAMINATION

General

Although many patients with idiopathic mitral valve prolapse appear to be normal on general examination, a variety of minor differences in bodily habitus and the musculoskeletal system have been described[63,66,67] and are summarized in Table 29.4. The suggestion that many, or perhaps all, of

Table 29.4. Abnormalities of body habitus and the musculo-skeletal system in mitral valve prolapse.

Straight back syndrome
Pectus excavatum and thoracic asymmetry
High arch palate
Disproportionately long arms
Articular hypermobility
Hypomastia

these abnormalities represent a forme fruste of a more major collagen abnormality such as Marfan's syndrome is now thought to be unlikely,[63] but they may represent as yet uncharacterized minor syndromes resulting from collagen abnormalities of which mitral valve prolapse is a component.

Cardiovascular system

Unless there is haemodynamically significant mitral regurgitation, the only cardiovascular abnormalities are auscultatory and consist of a mid- or late systolic click or clicks, with or without a systolic murmur.

Clicks

The clicks that occur in the mitral valve prolapse syndrome are non-ejection, i.e. they occur later in systole (Fig. 29.7) than aortic and pulmonary ejection clicks. These clicks were long thought to be extracardiac in origin. In 1963, however, they were shown by Barlow[68] to be associated with mitral valve prolapse; later studies using intracardiac phonocardiography confirm that they originate from the mitral valve.[69] Mid–late systolic clicks vary considerably among patients, and in the same patient with time. They may appear and disappear as the patient changes posture. They are usually brief, staccato and high frequency but occasionally they may have the quality of normal heart sounds and can be distinguished from these heart sounds only by their timing. Their presence can lead to confusion particularly for the inexperienced auscultator. The most common mistake is to identify the mid-systolic click as the second heart sound and the normal second heart sound as the third heart sound. Alternatively, the three sounds may be misinterpreted as a first sound, a second heart sound and an opening snap or a first heart sound followed by a widely split second heart sound. Less often, particularly when they occur early in systole, they are mistaken for aortic or pulmonary ejection sounds. Occasionally, multiple clicks may make a crunching

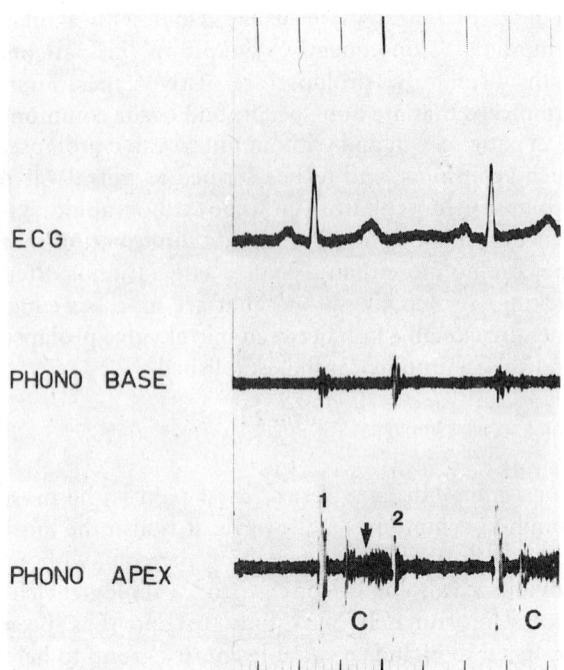

Fig. 29.7. Simultaneous electrocardiogram (ECG) and phonocardiogram (PHONO) from a patient with mitral valve prolapse. The phonocardiogram recorded from the apex shows a mid-systolic click (C). This is followed by a systolic murmur (arrow) which stretches from the click to the second heart sound (2). The first heart sound is also shown (1).

sound which is very difficult to distinguish from the systolic component of the pericardial rub; however, the diastolic component, usually present when the cause of the sound is pericardial, is missing. From time to time, a similar sound is made either by pulmonary oedema in the lingula being pressed against the chest wall with each heart beat or by air (usually as the result of trauma) in the mediastinum.

Murmurs

Late systolic   Many patients have only a click or clicks. Once mitral regurgitation occurs, a late systolic murmur is heard (Figs 29.7 and 29.8) which usually follows the click but may start before it. When mitral regurgitation becomes more severe, the click moves to be heard earlier in systole and the murmur becomes longer and louder. Murmurs, like clicks, are variable even in the same patient and may be revealed or altered by various manoeuvres (see below). The late systolic murmur may peak at or before the second heart sound. Although it is usually of high frequency in character, the murmur may occasionally have a loud honking or whooping sound in late systole. As for other auscultatory

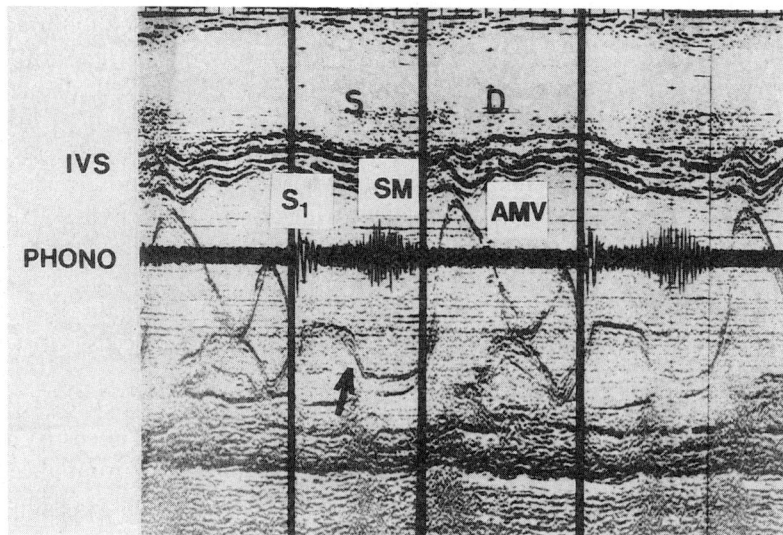

Fig. 29.8. Simultaneous M-mode echocardiogram and phonocardiogram (PHONO) (recorded at the apex) from a patient with mitral valve prolapse. The echocardiogram shows late systolic prolapse of the mitral valve (arrow) and this coincides with the late-systolic murmur (SM) shown on the phonocardiogram. There is no electrocardiogram on this tracing, and systole and diastole are shown by the heavy vertical line. S, systole; D, diastole; S_1, first heart sound; AMV, anterior mitral valve leaflet; IVS, interventricular septum.

features of mitral valve prolapse, this is highly variable and has been attributed to resonance in the mitral valve caused by a thin regurgitant jet striking it at a particular angle.[70] This dramatic noise may sometimes occur only with an arrhythmia and can be loud enough for the patient to hear it. A late systolic murmur without a click is a non-specific finding which is common in other types of mild mitral regurgitation.

Pan-systolic murmur Pan-systolic murmurs are associated with more severe mitral valve prolapse and mitral regurgitation. Once the murmur becomes pan-systolic, it tends to drown the clicks and the only non-invasive evidence that the patient has mitral valve prolapse is echocardiographic. Pan-systolic murmurs tend to peak either in mid–late systole or at the second heart sound. They rarely have a constant intensity throughout systole (Fig. 29.1).

Silent mitral valve prolapse A small proportion of patients (10–15%) have no abnormal auscultatory findings despite definite echocardiographic evidence of prolapse.[50]

Mechanism of clicks and murmurs

The click coincides with the point at which maximum mitral valve prolapse occurs.[71,72] When there are multiple clicks, this is probably due to the asynchronous tensing of different scallops of the mitral valve leaflet. The click itself has been attributed to sudden tensing of the chordae,[73] valve

leaflets[72] or vibrations of the whole heart caused by deceleration of the blood in the left ventricle as the mitral valve apparatus arrests its progress towards the left atrium.[74] Murmurs occur once the redundant valve leaflets become incompetent and allow mitral regurgitation.

Effect of manoeuvres on clicks and murmurs

The timing and extent of mitral valve prolapse depend on left ventricular dimensions and contractility and therefore manoeuvres that alter either of these will tend to alter the timing or intensity of clicks and murmurs. It has been suggested that in any individual mitral valve prolapse occurs at a particular left ventricular volume.[71,75] As a consequence, manoeuvres that increase left ventricular dimensions at end-diastole or reduce contractility will cause the necessary volume to be reached later and consequently the click and murmur will occur later. Conversely, reduced left ventricular end-diastolic volume or increased contractility will cause the prolapsed volume to be reached earlier leading to an earlier click and longer murmur. This explanation may be an oversimplification but it fits with what happens with common manoeuvres (Table 29.5). Many of these manoeuvres, particularly the simple one of standing the patient, are of little clinical relevance but they may help to clarify physical signs which are difficult to detect in the resting supine patient.

Significant mitral regurgitation

The features of significant mitral regurgitation

associated with mitral valve prolapse and the floppy mitral valve are identical to those occurring in other forms of non-rheumatic mitral regurgitation.

Investigations

Most patients with mitral valve prolapse have normal electrocardiograms. Infero-lateral ST/T-wave abnormalities, often with some sagging of the ST segment combined with normal, biphasic or frankly inverted T waves, have been reported in as many as 30% of patients in hospital-based series,[72] and in approximately 15% of patients identified in screening studies.[46,49] As with many of the symptoms attributed to mitral valve prolapse, the significance and true relationship to mitral valve prolapse of these abnormalities are difficult to establish. Many of these changes may be the reasons why a patient was referred for cardiological assessment; moreover, this type of electrocardiographic abnormality is frequently found in young and nervous but otherwise normal individuals. Despite these reservations, there appears to be a definite correlation between abnormalities on the resting electrocardiogram and significant ventricular arrhythmias (see below). The electrocardiographic abnormalities can often be normalized by beta-blockade,[73] a feature not unique to the electrocardiographic changes seen in mitral valve prolapse. This has been attributed to reduced prolapse due to increased left ventricular end-diastolic volume,[50] or to a correction of 'autonomic imbalance'—a vague concept.[47] Prolongation of the QT interval has been reported but its incidence is probably very low.[50,72] There is little or no correlation between ST/T-wave abnormalities in patients with mitral valve prolapse and symptoms or the severity of mitral regurgitation.

Once significant mitral regurgitation occurs, the expected electrocardiographic changes of left atrial and ventricular hypertrophy may become apparent.

Chest X-ray

The cardiac contour and lung fields are normal unless haemodynamically significant mitral regurgitation is present.

Exercise stress testing and radionuclide scintigraphy

Exercise stress testing produces a high incidence of positive tests (> 1 mm ST-segment depression) in patients with mitral valve prolapse and normal coronary arteries. The incidence of such 'false positive' tests has been reported to be as high as 53%[76] and may be higher when there are abnormalities on the resting electrocardiogram. Under these circumstances, exercise testing is unlikely to be a successful method of ascertaining whether chest pain is due to co-existent coronary disease. Exercise thallium scintigraphy seems to be a more reliable technique of identifying coronary disease in the presence of mitral valve prolapse,[77] although some workers have reported a high incidence of defects both at rest and on exercise in the absence of coronary artery disease. This area needs further investigation.

During exercise testing, abnormalities on the resting electrocardiogram may either intensify or disappear, and can reappear in a more pronounced form during the recovery phase. On occasions, exercise may reveal significant arrhythmias.[77]

Echocardiography and Doppler

Echocardiography is the technique of choice for diagnosing mitral valve prolapse (Figs 29.8–29.10). It should be remembered, however, that approximately 15% of patients in whom mitral valve prolapse is definitely identified by echocardiography will have no auscultatory signs and, conversely, between 10 and 25% of patients with characteristic mid-systolic clicks and late systolic murmurs have no echocardiographic abnormality.[79,80] The main echocardiographic features on which the diagnosis depends have been described in detail in Chapter 13. It is of paramount importance that echocardiograms are of high quality and the echocardiographic findings are considered in the context of the clinical situation. Doppler will detect mitral regurgitation and identify its timing and duration (Fig. 29.11). It may also indicate the degree of severity.

Angiography and haemodynamics

In the absence of significant mitral regurgitation, intracardiac haemodynamics are normal. Global left ventricular function is generally normal. Various local abnormalities of left ventricular function have been reported, many of which are of doubtful significance. A fairly constant finding, however, is a systolic inward protrusion of the inferior wall of the left ventricle just below the mitral valve.[50] This seems to be related to prolapse because it has been shown to disappear following mitral valve replacement.[80]

Left ventricular angiography can identify mitral valve prolapse (Fig. 29.12). All parts of the normal mitral valve show some convexity towards the left

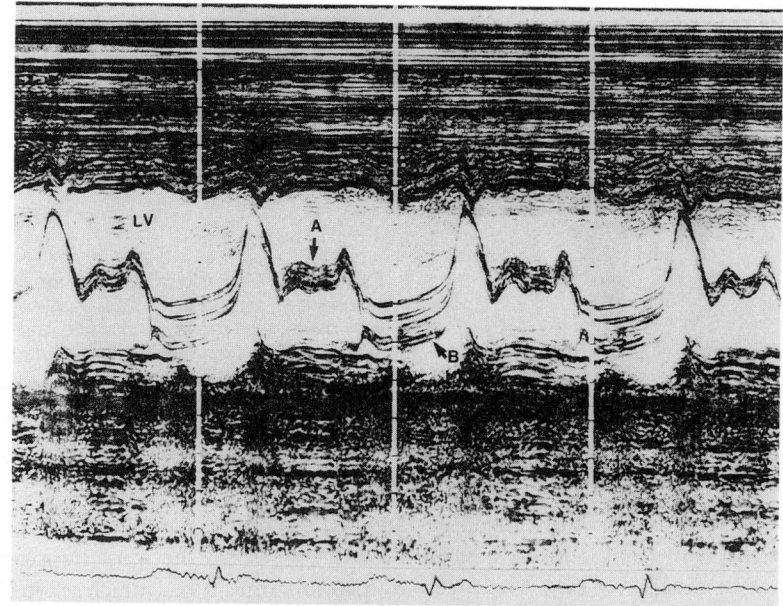

Fig. 29.9. M-Mode echocardiogram of the mitral valve from a patient with mitral valve prolapse, which shows several characteristic features. The excursion of the anterior cusp of the mitral valve is wide and when the valve is fully open it comes into contact with the interventricular septum. There is apparent thickening of the anterior cusp of the mitral valve (A) due to the redundant valve tissue, and there is also pan-systolic 'hammocking' of the mitral valve (B).

atrium in systole and consequently the diagnosis of mitral valve prolapse, particularly when it is slight, tends to be subject to considerable interobserver variability. The normal anterior mitral valve leaflet is anatomically and angiographically a single flap, whereas the normal posterior leaflet has three scallops: the postero-medial scallop, the middle scallop and the antero-lateral scallop. Angiography demonstrates prolapse or bulging of one or more of these four components towards the left atrium in systole with or without mitral regurgitation. The scallops of the posterior mitral valve leaflet are best seen in the right anterior oblique projection, although the aortic root may partly obscure the antero-lateral and middle scallops. The anterior leaflet is best seen in the left anterior oblique or left lateral view and visualization in the left anterior oblique view can often be improved by adding 30° of caudal tilt. In this projection, a large redundant anterior mitral valve cusp may appear as a filling defect in the left ventricular outflow tract in diastole and bulge backwards into the left atrium in systole. The anterior leaflet can also sometimes be identified in the right anterior oblique projection and may be confused with the antero-lateral scallop of the posterior cusp. In the left anterior oblique projection, the scallops of the posterior cusp are often superimposed.

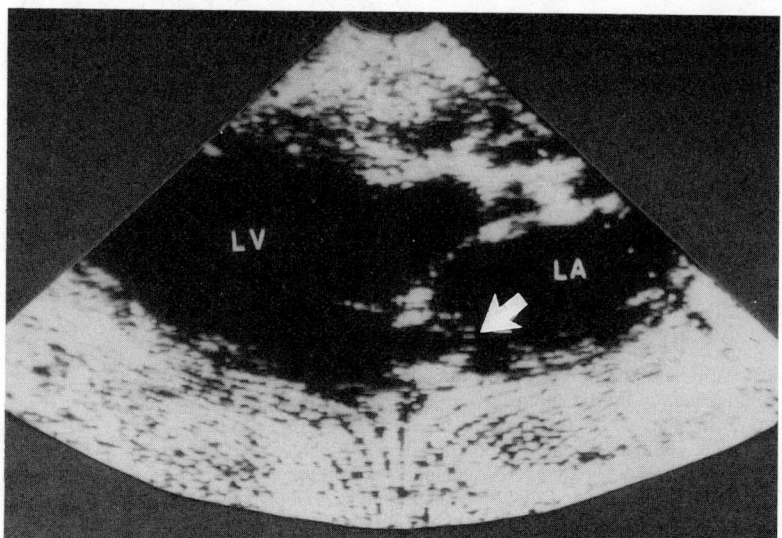

Fig. 29.10. Cross-sectional echocardiogram (long-axis parasternal view) from a patient with severe mitral valve prolapse. This recording was taken in systole, and the posterior cusp of the mitral valve can be seen bulging back into the left atrium well beyond the mitral valve annulus (arrow). Abbreviations: LV, left ventricle; LV, left atrium.

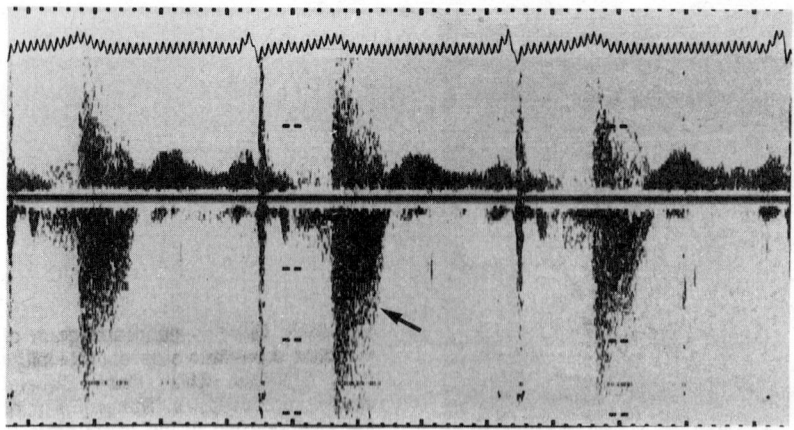

Fig. 29.11. Continuous wave Doppler recording of mitral valve flow in a patient with mitral valve prolapse causing late-systolic mitral regurgitation. The jet due to mitral regurgitation (arrow) can be seen to occur in late systole and follow the QRS of the electrocardiogram by a considerable interval.

Left ventricular dysfunction associated with coronary artery disease may disturb mitral valve movement and lead to appearances similar to those seen in mild-to-moderate idiopathic mitral valve prolapse; however, it cannot be confused with severe mitral valve prolapse in which the enormous redundant prolapsing mitral valve cusps are easily recognized.

Natural history and complications

The prognosis of patients with idiopathic mitral valve prolapse is good, but a few patients develop serious complications,[82] of which the most important are severe mitral regurgitation, infective endocarditis, serious arrhythmias and sudden death, and stroke. If a patient has only an isolated click, the prognosis is exceptionally good[80,84] because significant mitral regurgitation or infective endocarditis rarely develop[85,86] and severe arrhythmias are extremely uncommon. All complications are much more likely to occur if there is echocardiographic evidence of redundant mitral valve leaflets.[84]

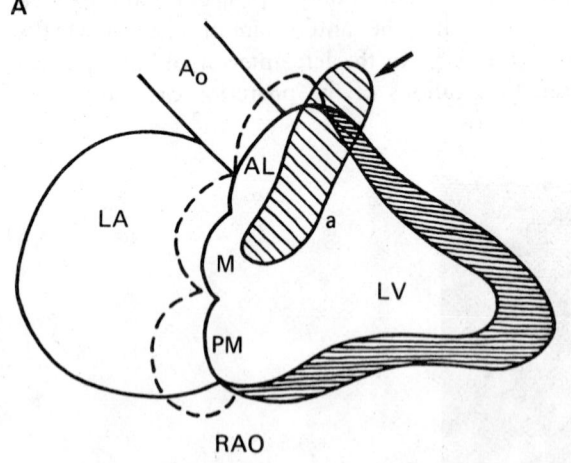
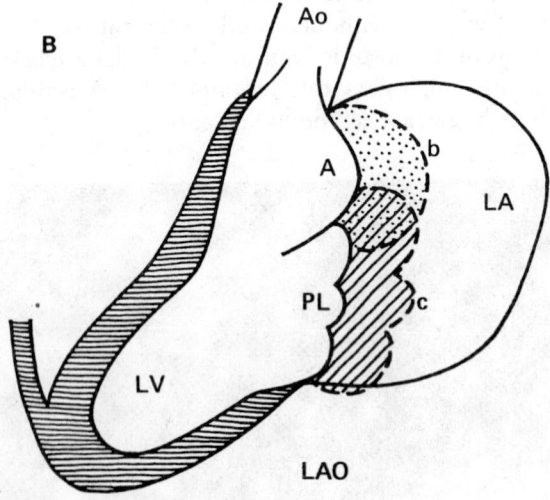

Fig. 29.12. Schematic drawings of the angiographic appearances of mitral valve prolapse. (A) Right anterior oblique view (RAO). In this view, the three scallops of the posterior cusp may be seen. PM, postero-medial; M, middle; AL, antero-lateral. The dotted lines show the direction in which prolapse occurs. The anterior leaflet is mainly behind the left ventricular shadow and is shown by the cross-hatched area (a). Occasionally, prolapse may be seen above the left ventricular shadow (arrow). LV, left ventricle; LA, left atrium; Ao, aorta. (B) Left anterior oblique view (LAO). The stippled area (b) is the position in which prolapse of the anterior cusp (A) is seen and the cross-hatched area (c) the position in which prolapse of the posterior cusp (PL) is observed.

Mitral regurgitation

Only a small number of patients develop severe mitral regurgitation and it is often impossible to predict which patients this will affect.[87] Progression to significant mitral regurgitation, needing mitral valve replacement, has been shown to be more likely within a 6-year follow-up period if the left ventricular dimensions are increased when the patient is first seen.[84] There is a lack of reliable information about the natural history of mitral regurgitation in mitral valve prolapse. It is generally assumed that the floppy mitral valve is the end result of mitral valve prolapse that has been present since an early age. Long-term follow-up data to substantiate this assumption are lacking, although patients in whom there is a steady progression from click and late systolic murmur with no evidence of haemodynamic disturbance to a pan-systolic murmur and severe mitral regurgitation associated with a floppy mitral valve have occasionally been documented. Available follow-up data suggest that steadily progressive mitral regurgitation due to a floppy mitral valve is less common than sudden worsening of mitral regurgitation due to either chordal rupture or valve damage resulting from infective endocarditis. However, this observation may not be valid because most follow-up studies are of short duration and, therefore, it is more likely that sudden and dramatic events will be detected rather than steadily progressive disease. Chordal rupture may occur before the valve becomes grossly distorted and voluminous, although patients undergoing surgery who have a true floppy mitral valve frequently show chordal rupture.[88] Chordal rupture may often be progressive, occurring in a stepwise fashion rather than being sudden and overwhelming. It is probable that the rupture of a few chordae increases the tension on the remaining chordae making them more prone to rupture. It is of interest that patients with mitral valve prolapse and mild-to-moderate mitral regurgitation who have little or no haemodynamic embarrassment frequently have echocardiographic evidence of chordal rupture.[89]

With the decline in incidence of rheumatic mitral regurgitation, floppy valves are becoming one of the commonest causes of pure mitral regurgitation requiring mitral valve surgery, and such valves often show chordal rupture (40–80% of valves at surgery).[26,62,90]

Infective endocarditis

Infective endocarditis is not a significant risk if a patient has only a click or no abnormal auscultatory signs,[85] although infective endocarditis has been reported in this situation.[86] Once mitral valve prolapse is more severe, it is an important underlying cause of infective endocarditis, and antibiotic prophylaxis should be advised.[91] It is impossible to define the risk of endocarditis in a patient with mitral valve prolapse, but it is probably very low considering the widespread prevalence of undiagnosed mitral valve prolapse in the population and the relative rarity of infective endocarditis. Mitral valve prolapse has been reported as the underlying cause in as many as 11% of patients in whom infective endocarditis is proven.[92]

Stroke and transient ischaemic attacks

An unusually high incidence of mitral valve prolapse has been reported in young patients (< 45 years of age) with stroke;[93,94] this risk appears to be higher if there is prolapse of both the mitral and aortic valves.[95] Emboli originating at areas of endothelial damage on the atrial surface of the valve near its attachment to the atrial wall and caused by the valve's abnormal structure and mobility have been postulated as the cause. However, some workers have been unable to document an increased incidence of mitral valve prolapse in young patients with stroke.[96] The lack of an association in more elderly patients does not mean that mitral valve prolapse is not the cause of some cerebral events in these patients, it may simply reflect the overwhelmingly greater incidence of stroke due to atherosclerotic and hypertensive disease.

Arrhythmias and sudden death

Minor arrhythmias, such as atrial and ventricular ectopic beats and short runs of supraventricular tachycardia, have all been reported as occurring more frequently in patients with mitral valve prolapse than in normal subjects. The results of recent studies with adequate control subjects have suggested, however, that such arrhythmias may be no more common in patients with mitral valve prolapse than in suitable symptom-matched control subjects presenting in a cardiological clinic.[97,98]

More serious arrhythmias, such as ventricular tachycardia and even ventricular fibrillation leading to sudden death, have been reported in association with mitral valve prolapse.[99,100] The risk of such arrhythmias is extremely low in patients with only a click or no abnormal auscultatory findings. As with many other features of this condition, the significance of mitral valve prolapse in the genesis of these arrhythmias is difficult to assess because of the heterogeneity of reported cases, the differences in case selection and the absence of adequate control data.[101] Some authors have reported that an abnormal resting electrocardiogram, a common finding in patients with mitral valve prolapse, is significantly associated with an increased incidence of significant ventricular arrhythmias,[102] although other authors have not been able to confirm this.[103] Furthermore, recent work by Kligfield *et al.*[95] who studied two groups of patients, one with mitral valve prolapse and the other without mitral valve prolapse but with a similar degree of mitral regurgitation, showed that the incidence of complex arrhythmias, including ventricular tachycardia, was increased in the two groups to a similar extent. The conclusion was that mitral valve regurgitation, a factor often ignored in studies of arrhythmias in mitral valve prolapse, may be important in causing these arrhythmias rather than the mitral valve prolapse *per se*.

Despite the absence of a definite link between mitral valve prolapse and significant arrhythmias, certain patients may be at high risk. In view of reports of serious arrhythmias and sudden death, further investigation is justified in an attempt to identify these patients. A reasonable approach is to carry out ambulatory electrocardiographic monitoring and exercise testing in patients who have a history of sustained tachycardia, definite dizziness or syncope, or an abnormal resting electrocardiogram. However, it should be remembered that the latter finding is extremely common. If these investigations reveal significant arrhythmias, they should be treated conventionally and investigated further if necessary. An increased incidence of concealed bypass tracks and also the Wolff–Parkinson syndrome has been reported in association with mitral valve prolapse.[104]

Diagnosis

Often the physical signs of mitral valve prolapse are so characteristic that there is no doubt about the diagnosis. Occasionally, however, clicks due to mitral valve prolapse may be misinterpreted (see above) or systolic clicks due to other causes may be mistakenly ascribed to mitral valve prolapse. Ejection sounds from the aortic or pulmonary valve are unlikely to be confused by the experienced auscultator because they occur earlier in systole and do not move in position in the cardiac cycle with the

manoeuvres summarized in Table 29.5 Occasionally, other conditions can lead to mid-systolic clicks but they are rarely confused with mitral valve prolapse. These are summarized in Table 29.6. In general, a combination of clinical auscultation, manoeuvres to alter the position of the click, the type of associated murmur and the echocardiographic findings makes the differentiation straightforward.

Management and treatment

Patients who are asymptomatic, have a mid-systolic click, or a click followed by a short murmur, and normal left ventricular dimensions on echocardiography do not require any special treatment other than advice about antibiotic prophylaxis against infective endocarditis. Although the risk of endocarditis is minimal in patients with a click and no murmur, it is impossible to be sure at which stage, if at all, such patients will develop mild mitral regurgitation and, as this may occur when the patient is no longer under medical follow-up, it is reasonable to give all patients this advice. Physicians vary in their views about follow-up of such patients. In general, the long-term course of patients with a click and short murmur is so benign that long-term supervision is hardly worthwhile and such patients will usually present themselves again once symptoms recur.

If the patient has any features which suggest they may be at 'high risk' of serious arrhythmias, it is reasonable to investigate them further (see above) to ascertain whether arrhythmias are present. Arrhythmias are treated conventionally, but it is worth remembering that beta-adrenergic blockers may be more effective in treating ventricular arrhythmias associated with mitral valve prolapse than those in other groups of patients.[105,106] Digitalis should be

---

Table 29.5. Effect of manoeuvres on the click and murmur in mitral valve prolapse.

Manoeuvre	Click	Murmur
Standing and inspiration	Earlier	Louder and longer
Squatting	Later	Softer and shorter
Valsalva:		
Strain phase	Earlier	Variable
Release phase	Later	Variable
Amyl nitrate	Earlier	Initially softer then louder and longer
Beta-blockade	Later	Softer and shorter

Table 29.6. Causes of systolic clicks other than mitral valve prolapse. (*NB* All causes are rare except for aortic and pulmonary ejection sounds.)

Aortic and pulmonary ejection sounds
Left-sided pneumothorax (often in diastole as well)
Small ventricular septal defect with aneurysm of the septum
Following mitral valvotomy
Calcified left atrial myxoma
Hypertrophic cardiomyopathy

used with care when treating superventricular arrhythmias in mitral valve prolapse because of its potentially dangerous effects in patients with pre-excitation, a condition that has been described to be unusually common in patients with mitral valve prolapse.[104] It has been suggested in some reports that mitral valve replacement will cure severe arrhythmias and, although this recommendation has not been substantiated as yet,[107] it is an attractive idea in view of the recent evidence that arrhythmias are correlated with the severity of mitral regurgitation rather than mitral valve prolapse *per se*.[96]

Treatment of chest pain

Chest pain associated with mitral valve prolapse is often extremely resistant to treatment. Conventional anti-anginal treatment is frequently ineffective, although beta-blockade may be helpful, possibly because of its ability to increase left ventricular size and reduce contractility thereby decreasing the degree of prolapse, in addition to suppressing arrhythmias and having an anxiolytic effect. As mitral valve prolapse is so common and the pain associated with it is often difficult to treat, it is worth considering the other treatable non-cardiac causes for the pain (for example, musculoskeletal or gastro-intestinal) before attributing it to mitral valve prolapse.

Stroke and transient ischaemic attacks

The correct treatment in this situation is not known. Most physicians avoid full anticoagulation, with its accompanying risk, because its value is unproven; antiplatelet agents are used in the hope that they will be effective. However, in patients with established atrial fibrillation, particularly when there is significant mitral regurgitation, full anticoagulation is indicated.

Mitral regurgitation

Treatment of significant mitral regurgitation does not differ in any respect from that of any other form of non-rheumatic mitral regurgitation.

MITRAL VALVE PROLAPSE SECONDARY TO OTHER CONDITIONS (Table 29.7)

Connective tissue disorder

Mitral valve prolapse is common in several connective tissue disorders (Table 29.7). In Marfan's syndrome (Fig. 29.6), the prevalence of echocardiographic prolapse has been reported to be as high as 91%,[41] with 46% of these patients exhibiting the murmurs of mitral regurgitation and/or systolic clicks. These patients also frequently develop aortic mitral regurgitation which may be severe. Mitral valve prolapse should be carefully sought in patients with any evidence of connective tissue disorder; these patients should be followed because mitral regurgitation often develops, sometimes over only a few years, to reach considerable severity. Conversely, patients with apparently isolated 'idiopathic mitral valve prolapse' should be examined carefully for signs of connective tissue disorder.

Thyroid disease

The association between mitral valve prolapse and thyroid disease is probably confined to patients with auto-immune hyperthyroidism rather than other forms of thyrotoxicosis.[108,109] The association has not been satisfactorily explained, although a common auto-immune mechanism and similar histocompatibility antigens in the two conditions have been suggested.[63]

Table 29.7. Some conditions reported in association with mitral valve prolapse.[18,63]

Definite link	Probable chance association
Connective tissue disorders:	Rheumatic mitral valve
Marfan's syndrome	
Ehlers–Danlos syndrome	Ventricular septal defect
Osteogenesis imperfecta	Ebstein's and Uhl's anomalies
Pseudoxanthoma elasticum	Transposition of great vessels
Von Willebrand's syndrome	Primary pulmonary hypertension
Atrial septal defect (secundum)	Emphysema
Prolapse of a *normal* mitral valve:	Muscular dystrophy
(a) coronary disease	Noonan's and Turner's syndromes
(b) hypertrophic cardiomyopathy	
Auto-immune thyroid disease	Acromegaly

Other cardiac abnormalities

The high prevalence of mitral valve prolapse in the population means that chance associations with other conditions must be common and may explain the sporadic reports of mitral valve prolapse associated with a variety of congenital defects.[62] However, mitral valve prolapse seems to be unexpectedly common in patients with secundum atrial septal defect. Estimates of its incidence vary from 17 to over 30%.[110,111] Systolic clicks, although not infrequent, seem to occur less commonly than in other forms of prolapse and pan-systolic murmurs are more frequent than late systolic murmurs. The association between atrial septal defect and mitral valve prolapse has never been satisfactorily explained, although the small left ventricular dimensions and distorted left ventricular shape that occur with atrial septal defects may be important. Closure of atrial septal defects may correct this abnormality and there is some evidence that mitral valve prolapse disappears concurrently.[112,113] Patients with uncomplicated atrial septal defects do not require antibiotic prophylaxis for infective endocarditis but this should be considered in patients with associated mitral valve prolapse. The combination of a prolapsing mitral valve and the secundum atrial septal defect has to be distinguished from a primum atrial septal defect with its commonly associated mitral valve abnormalities. This distinction can often be achieved clinically; if this is not possible, echocardiography usually resolves any doubts.

In ischaemic heart disease and hypertrophic cardiomyopathy, angiographic evidence of definite prolapse of the mitral valve towards the left atrium during systole is common. However, in both conditions, clicks of the type occurring in 'idiopathic mitral valve prolapse' are rare, probably because this auscultatory sign is produced by redundant valve tissue and chordae neither of which are present in these two conditions.[50] Although typical mid-systolic clicks are unusual in hypertrophic cardiomyopathy, clicks occurring earlier in systole and associated with systolic anterior motion of the mitral valve are well documented.[114] In both ischaemic heart disease and hypertrophic cardiomyopathy, mitral valve prolapse is almost certainly secondary to abnormalities of left ventricular size and function.

TRICUSPID VALVE PROLAPSE

Cross-sectional echocardiographic studies have shown that tricuspid valve prolapse occurs in between 20 and 40% of patients who exhibit prolapse of the mitral valve.[115–117] In general, echocardiographically detectable tricuspid valve prolapse seems to be associated with the more clinically severe form of mitral valve prolapse. This may be because tricuspid involvement is a marker of a more extensive myxomatous process. Tricuspid valve prolapse may produce right-sided clicks and murmurs; significant tricuspid regurgitation is produced only rarely.

AORTIC VALVE PROLAPSE

Aortic valve prolapse can be detected as a diastolic bowing of the aortic valve towards the left ventricular cavity in diastole on cross-sectional echocardiography in 20% of patients with mitral valve prolapse.[115] In about one-third of these patients, there is also some echocardiographically detectable aortic root dilatation. This abnormality is rarely of clinical significance, although a small number of patients develop mild aortic regurgitation, and it may form the site of infective endocarditis.

REFERENCES

1. Selzer, A. and Katayama, F. Mitral regurgitation: Clinical patterns, pathophysiology and natural history. *Medicine* 1972; 51: 337–66.
2. Fox, A.C., Glassman, E. and Isom, O.W. Surgically remediable complications of myocardial infarction. *Prog. Cardiovasc. Dis.* 1979; 21: 461–84.
3. Gahl, K., Sutton, R., Pearson, M. *et al*. Mitral regurgitation in coronary heart disease. *Br. Heart J.* 1977; 39: 13.
4. Cederqvist, L. and Soderstrom, J. Papillary muscle rupture in myocardial infarction. A study based upon an autopsy material. *Acta Med. Scand.* 1964; 176: 287–92.
5. Sanders, R.J., Neuburger, K.T. and Ravin, A. Rupture of papillary muscle: occurrence of rupture of posterior muscle in posterior myocardial infarction. *Dis. Chest* 1957; 31: 316–23.
6. Heikkila, J. Mitral incompetence as a complication of acute myocardial infarction. *Acta Med. Scand.* 1967; 475 (Suppl.): 1–149.
7. Tsakiris, A.G., Rastelli, G.C., Des Amorim, D. *et al*. Effect of experimental papillary muscle damage on mitral valve closure in intact anaesthetized dogs. *Proc. Mayo Clin.* 1970; 5: 275.
8. Miltal, A.K., Langston, M., Cohn, E.E. *et al*. Combined papillary muscle and left ventricular wall dysfunction as a cause of mitral regurgitation. *Circulation* 1971; 44: 174–80.
9. Godley, R.W., Wann, L.S., Rogers, E.W. *et al*. Incomplete mitral leaflet closure in patients with papillary muscle dysfunction. *Circulation* 1981; 63: 565–71.
10. Grenadier, E., Keidar, S., Sahn, D.J. *et al*. Ruptured mitral chordae tendinae may be a frequent and insignificant complication in the mitral valve prolapse syndrome. *Eur. Heart J.* 1985; 6: 1006–15.

11. Scott-Jupp, W., Barnett, N.L., Gallagher, P.J. et al. Ultrastructural changes in spontaneous rupture of mitral chordae tendinae. J. Pathol. 1981; 133: 185–201.
12. Gallagher, P.J., Caves, P.K. and Stinson, E.B. Pathological changes in spontaneous rupture of chordae tendinae. Ann. Cir. Gynaecol. 1977; 66: 135,
13. Buchbinder, N.A. and Roberts, W.C. Left sided valvular infective endocarditis. Am. J. Med. 1972; 53: 20.
14. Roberts, W.C. and Buchbinder, N.A. Healed left sided infective endocarditis. A clinico-pathological study of 59 patients. Am. J. Cardiol. 1976; 40: 876.
15. Pomerance, A. Pathological and clinical study of calcification of the mitral valve ring. J. Clin. Pathol. 1970; 23: 354.
16. Korn, D., DeSantis, R.W. and Sell, S. Massive calcification of the mitral annulus. N. Engl. J. Med. 1962; 267: 900.
17. DePace, N.L. et al. Rapidly progressive, massive mitral annular calcification. Occurrence in a patient with chronic renal failure. Arch. Intern. Med. 1981; 141: 166.
18. Jeresaty, R.M. Mitral valve prolapse. New York: Raven Press, 1979, p.139.
19. Wanderman, K.L. and Margulis, G. Co-existence of hypertrophic obstructive cardiomyopathy and mitral annular calcification: proposed etiologic relationship. Isr. J. Med. Sci. 1979; 15: 422.
20. Osterberger, L.E., Goldstein, S., Khaja, S. and Lakier, J.B. Functional mitral stenosis in patients with massive mitral annular calcification. Circulation 1981; 64: 472–6.
21. Roberts, W.C., Dangel, J.C. and Bulkley, B. Non-rheumatic valvular cardiac disease: A clinico-pathologic survey of 27 different conditions causing valvular dysfunction. In: Likoff, W.C., (ed) Cardiovascular Clinics, 5: Vol. 2, Valvular Heart Disease. Philadelphia, 1973, p.334.
22. Eckberg, D.L., Gault, J.H., Bouchard, R.L. et al. Mechanics of left ventricular contraction in chronic severe mitral regurgitation. Circulation 1973; 47: 1252.
23. Urschel, C.W., Covell, J.W. et al. Effects of acute valvular regurgitation of the oxygen consumption on the canine heart. Circ. Res. 1968; 23: 33.
24. Grosse, R., Strain, J. and Cohen, M.V. Pulmonary arterial V waves in mitral regurgitation: Clinical and experimental observations. Circulation 1984; 69: 214–22.
25. Brigden, W. and Leatham, A. Mitral incompetence. Br. Heart J. 1953; 15: 55.
26. DePace, N.L., Nestico, P.F. and Morganroth, J. Acute severe mitral regurgitation. Pathophysiology, clinical recognition, and management. Am. J. Med. 1985; 78: 293.
27. Ronan, J.A., Steelman, R.B. et al. The clinical diagnosis of acute severe mitral insufficiency. Am. J. Cardiol. 1971; 27: 284.
28. Cohen, L.S., Mason, E.T. and Braunwald, E. Significance of an atrial gallop sound in mitral regurgitation. A clue to the diagnosis of ruptured chordae tendinae. Circulation 1967; 35: 112.
29. Thomas, J.B. Mitral insufficiency due to rupture of chordae tendinae simula-aortic stenosis. Am. Heart J. 1966; 71: 12.
30. Alitman, L. et al. Mitral regurgitation mimicking aortic stenosis. Am. J. Cardiol. 1978; 42: 1044.
31. Merendino, K.A. and Hessel, E.A. The 'murmur on top of the head' in acquired mitral insufficiency. JAMA 1967; 199: 142.
32. Aravanis, C. Silent mitral insufficiency. Am. Heart J. 1965; 70: 620.
33. Henry, W.L., Morganroth, J., Pearlman, A.S. et al. Relation between echocardiographically determined left atrial size and atrial fibrillation. Circulation 1976; 53: 273–9.
34. Allen, H., Harris, A. and Leatham, A. Significance and prognosis of an isolated late systolic murmur: A 9–22 years follow-up. Br. Heart J. 1974; 36: 525.
35. Leatham, A. and Brigden, W. Mild mitral regurgitation and the mitral prolapse fiasco. Am. Heart J. 1980; 99: 659.
36. Rappaport, E. Natural history of aortic and mitral valve disease. Am. J. Cardiol. 1975; 35: 234–42.
37. Munoz, S., Gallardo, J., Diaz-Gorrin, J.R. and Medina, O. Influence of surgery on the natural history of rheumatic and aortic valve disease. Am. J. Cardiol. 1975; 35: 235.
38. Hammermeister, K.E., Fisher, L., Kennedy, J.W. et al. Prediction of late survival in patients with mitral valve disease from clinical, haemodynamic and quantitative angiographic variables. Circulation 1978; 57: 341.
39. DeBusk, R.F. and Harrison, D.C. The clinical spectrum of papillary muscle disease. N. Engl. J. Med. 1969; 281: 1458–67.
40. Waller, B.F. Non-rheumatic causes of pure mitral regurgitation. Practical Cardiol. 1985; 11: 69–84.
41. Brown, O.R., DeMots, H., Kloster, F.E. et al. Aortic root dilatation and mitral valve prolapse in Marfan's syndrome. Circulation 1975; 52: 651–7.
42. Call, T., Leier, C. and Wooley, C. Cardiac defects in the Ehlers–Danlos syndrome (Abstract). Circulation 1977; 55:56 (Suppl. II); 69.
43. Wan, L.S., Gross, C.M., Wakefield, R.J. and Kalbfleisch, J.H. Diagnostic precision of echocardiography in mitral valve prolapse. Am. Heart J. 1985; 109: 803–8.
44. Warth, D.C., King, M.E. et al. Prevalence of mitral valve prolapse in normal children. J. Am. Coll. Cardiol. 1985; 5: 1173–7.
45. Perloff, J.K. Evolving concepts of mitral valve prolapse. N. Engl. J. Med. 1982; 307: 369–70.
46. Procacci, P.M., Savran, S.V., Schrieter, S.L. et al. Prevalence of clinical mitral valve prolapse in 1169 young women. N. Engl. J. Med. 1976; 294: 1086–8.
47. Brown, O.R., Kloster, F.E. and DeMots, H. Incidence of mitral valve prolapse in the asymptomatic normal (Abstract). Circulation 1975; 52 (Suppl. II): 77.
48. Thompson, W.P. and Levine, S.A. Systolic gallop rhythm: A clinical study. N. Engl. J. Med. 1935; 213: 1021–5.
49. Markiewicz, W., Stoner, J., London, E. et al. Mitral valve prolapse in one hundred presumably healthy young females. Circulation 1976; 53: 464–73.
50. Jeresaty, R.M. Mitral valve prolapse. New York: Raven Press, 1979.
51. Savage, D.D., Garrison, R.J., Devereux, R.B. et al. Mitral valve prolapse in the general population: Epidemiologic features. The Framingham Study. Am. Heart J. 1983; 106: 571–6.
52. Devereux, R.B., Perloff, J.K., Reichek, N. and Josephson, M.E. Mitral valve prolapse. Circulation 1976; 54: 3–14.
53. Weiss, A.N., Mimbs, J.W., Ludbrook, P.A. and Sobel, B.E. Echocardiographic detection of mitral valve prolapse. Exclusion of false positive diagnosis and determination of inheritance Circulation 1975; 52: 1091–6.
54. Chan, W.W., Chan, F.L., Wong, P.H. and Chow, J.S. Familial occurrence of mitral valve prolapse: Is this related to the straight back syndrome? Br. Heart J. 1983; 50: 97–110.
55. Pomerance, A. Ballooning deformity (mucoid degeneration) of atrioventricular valves. Br. Heart J. 1969; 31: 343–51.
56. King, B.D., Clark, M.A., Baba, N. et al. "Myxomatous" mitral valves: Collagen dissolution as the primary defect. Circulation 1982; 66: 288–96.
57. Roberts, W.C. Morphologic features of the normal and abnormal mitral valve. Am. J. Cardiol. 1983; 51: 1005–8.
58. Ormiston, J.A., Shah, P.M., Tei, C. and Wong, M. Size and motion of the mitral valve annulus in man. II Abnormalities in mitral valve prolapse. Circulation 1982; 65: 713–9.
59. Read, R.C., Thal, A.P. and Wendy, V.E. Symptomatic valvular myxomatous transformation (the floppy valve

syndrome): A possible Forme Fruste of the Marfan Syndrome. *Circulation* 1965; **32**: 897–910.

60. Maranhao, V., Gooch, A.S., Yang, S.S. *et al.* Prolapse of the tricuspid leaflets in the systolic murmur–click syndrome. *Cathet.,Cardiovasc. Diag.* 1975; **1**: 81–90.

61. Kern, W.H. and Tucher, B.L. Myxoid changes in cardiac valves: Pathologic, clinical and ultrastructural studies. *Am. Heart J.* 1972; **84**: 294–301.

62. McKay, R. and Yacoub, N.H. Clinical and pathological findings in patients with "floppy" valves treated surgically. *Circulation* 1973; **47**:48 (Suppl. III): 63–73.

63. Malcolm, A.D. Mitral valve prolapse associated with other disorders. Casual coincidence, common link or fundamental genetic disturbance? *Br. Heart J.* 1985; **53**: 353–62.

64. Hancock, E.W. and Cohn, K. The syndrome associated with mid-systolic click and late systolic murmur. *Am. J. Med.* 1966; **41**: 183–96.

65. Jeresaty, R.M. Mitral valve prolapse–click syndrome. *Prog. Cardiovasc. Dis.* 1973; **15**: 623–52.

66. Beighton, P. Mitral valve prolapse and a Marfanoid habitus. *Br. Med. J.* 1983; **284**: 920.

67. Rosenberg, C.A., Derman, G.H., Grabb, W.C. and Buda, A.J. Hypomastia and mitral valve prolapse: Evidence of a linked embryologic and mesenchymal dysplasia. *N. Engl. J. Med.* 1983; **309**: 1230–2.

68. Barlow, J.B., Pocock, W.A., Marchand, P. and Denny, M. The significance of late systolic murmurs. *Am. Heart J.* 66: 443–52.

69. Ronan, J.A., Perloff, J.K. and Harvey, W.P. Systolic clicks and the late systolic murmur. Intra cardiac phonocardiographic evidence of their mitral valve origin. *Am. Heart J.* 1965; **70**: 319–25.

70. Cobbs, B.W. Clinical recognition and medical management of rheumatic heart disease and other acquired valvular heart disease. In: Husrt, J.W., Logue, R.B., Schlant, R.C. and Wenger, N.K., eds. *The Heart*, 3rd edn. New York: McGraw-Hill, pp.883–9.

71. Lima, S.D., Lima, J.A.C., Pyeritz, R.E. and Weiss, J.L. Relation of mitral valve prolapse to left ventricular size in Marfans syndrome. *Am. J. Cardiol.* 1985; **55**: 739–43.

72. Barlow, J.B. and Pocock, W.A. The problem of non-ejection systolic clicks and associated mitral systolic murmurs: Emphasis on the billowing mitral leaflet syndrome. *Am. Heart J.* 1975; **90**: 636–55.

73. Abinader, E.G. Adrenergic beta blockade and ECG changes in the systolic click murmur syndrome. *Am. Heart J.* 1976; **91**: 297–302.

74. Winkle, R.A., Lopes, M.G., Fitzgerald, J.W. *et al.* Arrhythmias in patients with mitral valve prolapse. *Circulation* 1975; **52**: 73–81.

75. Winkle, R.A., Goodman, D.J. and Popp, R.L. Simultaneous echocardiographic–phonographic recordings at rest and during amyl nitrite administration in patients with mitral valve prolapse. *Circulation* 1975; **51**: 522.

76. Massie, B., Botvinick, E.H., Shames, D. *et al.* Myocardial perfusion scintigraphy in patients with mitral valve prolapse. *Circulation* 1978; **57**: 19–26.

77. Tabbe, V., Schicha, H., Neumann, P. *et al.* Mitral valve prolapse in the ventriculogram: scintigraphic, electrocardiographic and haemodynamic abnormalities. *Clin. Cardiol.* 1985; **8**: 341–7.

78. Sloman, G., Wong, M. and Walker, J. Arrhythmias of exercise in patients with abnormalities of the posterior leaflet of the mitral valve. *Am. Heart J.* 1972; **82**: 312–7.

79. DeMaria, A.N., Neumann, A., Lee, G. *et al.* Echocardiographic identification of the mitral valve prolapse syndrome. *Am. J. Med.* 1977; **62**: 819–29.

80. Malcolm, A.D., Bonghaner, D.R., Kostuk, W.J. *et al.* Clinical features and investigative findings in presence of mitral leaflet prolapse. Study of 85 consecutive patients. *Br. Heart J.* 1976; **38**: 244–56.

81. Cobbs, B.W. and King, S.B. Ventricular buckling: A factor in the abnormal ventriculogram and peculiar haemodynamics associated with mitral valve prolapse. *Am. Heart J.* 1977; **93**: 741–58.

82. Appelblatt, N.H., Willis, P.W., Lenhart, J.A. *et al.* Ten to 40 year follow-up of 69 patients with systolic click with or without apical late systolic murmur (Abstract). *Am. J. Cardiol.* 1975; **35**: 119.

83. Mills, P., Rose, J., Hollingsworth, B.A. *et al.* Long-term prognosis of mitral valve prolapse. *N. Engl. J. Med.* 1977; **297**: 13–8.

84. Nishimura, R.A., McGoon, M.D., Shub, C. *et al.* Echocardiographically documented mitral valve prolapse. Long-term follow-up of 237 patients. *N. Engl. J. Med.* 1985; **313**: 1305–9.

85. Barlow, J.B. and Pocock, W.A. Mitral valve prolapse, the specific billowing mitral leaflet syndrome, or an insignificant non-ejection systolic click. *Am. Heart J.* 1979; **97**: 277–85.

86. Lachman, A.S., Bramwell-Jones, D.M., Lakier, J.B. *et al.* Infective endocarditis in the billowing mitral leaflet syndrome. *Br. Heart J.* 1975; **37**: 326–30.

87. Atlas, P., Yahini, J.H., Palant, A. *et al.* Chordal rupture: A common complication of myxomatous degeneration of the mitral valve. *Isr. J. Med. Sci.* 1976; **12**: 1320–4.

88. Tresch, D.D., Doyle, T.P., Bonchek, L.I. *et al.* Mitral valve prolapse requiring surgery. Clinical and pathological study. *Am. J. Med.* 1985; **78**: 245.

89. Grenadier, E., Keider, S., Sahn, D.J. *et al.* Ruptured mitral chordae tendinae may be a frequent and insignificant complication in the mitral valve prolapse syndrome. *Eur. Heart J.* 1985; **6**: 1006–15.

90. Salomon, N.W., Stinson, E.B., Griepp, R.B. *et al.* Surgical treatment of degenerative mitral regurgitation. *Am. J. Cardiol.* 1976; **38**: 463–8.

91. Clemens, J.D., Horwitz, R.K., Jaffe, C.C. *et al.* A controlled evaluation of the risk of bacterial endocarditis in persons with mitral valve prolapse. *N. Engl. J. Med.* 1982; **307**: 776–81.

92. Corrigall, D., Bolen, J., Hancock, E. and Popp, R.L. Mitral valve prolapse and infective endocarditis. *Am. J. Med.* 1977; **63**: 215–22.

93. Kostuk, W.J., Boughner, D.R., Barnett, H.J.M. and Silver, M.D. Strokes: A complication of mitral leaflet prolapse? *Lancet* 1977; **2**: 313–6.

94. Barnett, H.J.M., Boughner, D.R., Taylor, D.W. *et al.* Further evidence relating mitral valve prolapse to cerebral ischaemic events. *N. Engl. J. Med.* 1980; **302**: 139–44.

95. Barletta, G.A., Gagliardi, R., Benvenufi, L. and Fantina, F. Cerebral ischaemic attacks as a complication of aortic and mitral valve prolapse. *Stroke* 1985; **16**: 219–23.

96. Egeblad, H. and Sorenson, P.S. Prevalence of mitral valve prolapse in younger patients with cerebral ischaemic attacks. *Acta Med. Scand.* 1984; **216**: 385–92.

97. Kligfield, P., Hochreiter, C. *et al.* Complex arrhythmias in mitral regurgitation with and without mitral valve prolapse: Contrast to arrhythmias in mitral valve prolapse without mitral regurgitation. *Am. J. Cardiol.* 1985; **55**: 1545–9.

98. Kramer, H.M., Kligfield, P., Devereux, P. *et al.* Arrhythmias in mitral valve prolapse: Effect of selection bias. *Ann. Intern. Med.* 1984; **144**: 2360–4.

99. Ritchie, J.L., Hammermeister, K.E. and Kennedy, J.W. Refractory ventricular tachycardia and fibrillation in a patient with the prolapsing mitral leaflet syndrome: successful control with overdrive pacing. *Am. J. Cardiol.* 1976; **37**: 314–6.

00. Jeresaty, R.M. Sudden death in the mitral valve prolapse–

click syndrome. *Am. J. Cardiol.* 1976; **37**: 317–8.

101. Chesler, E., King, R.A. and Edwards, J.E. The myxomatous valve and sudden death. *Circulation* 1983; **3**: 632–9.

102. Campbell, R.W.F., Godman, M.G., Fiddler, G.I. *et al.* Ventricular arrhythmias in syndrome of balloon deformity of mitral valve. Definition of possibly high risk group. *Br. Heart J.* 1976; **38**: 1053–7.

103. DeMaria, A.N., Amsterdam, E.A., Vismara, L.A. *et al.* The mitral valve prolapse syndrome. *Ann. Intern. Med.* 1976; **84**: 656–60.

104. Josephson, M.E., Horowitz, L.N. and Kastor, J.A. Paroxysmal supraventricular tachycardia in patients with mitral valve prolapse. *Circulation* 1978; **57**: 111–5.

105. Winkle, R.A., Lopes, M.G., Fitzgerald, J.W. *et al.* Propranolol for patients with mitral valve prolapse. *Am. Heart J.* 1977; **93**: 422–7.

106. Gooch, A.S., Vicencio, F., Maranhao, V. and Goldberg, H. Arrhythmias and left ventricular asynergy in the prolapsing mitral leaflet syndrome. *Am. J. Cardiol.* 1972; **29**: 611–20.

107. Campbell, R.W.F. Arrhythymias in mitral valve prolapse. *Practical Cardiol.* 1972; **8**: 124–35.

108. Channick, B.J., Adlin, E.V., Marks, A.D. *et al.* Hyperthyroidism and mitral valve prolapse. *N. Engl. J. Med.* 1981; **305**: 497–500.

109. Brauman, A., Algom, M., Gilboa, Y. *et al.* Mitral valve prolapse in hyperthyroidism of two different origins. *Br. Heart J.* 1985; **53**: 497–500.

110. Leachman, R.D., Cokkinos, E.V. and Cooley, D.A. Association of ostium secondum atrial septal defect with mitral valve prolapse. *Am. J. Cardiol.* 1976; **38**: 167–9.

111. Owens, J.P., Williams, R.G. and Fellows, K.E. Prolapsing mitral leaflet associated with secundum atrial septal defect (Abstract). *Circulation* 1974; **50** (Suppl. III): 240.

112. Angel, J., Soler-Soler, J., Gareia Dol Castillo, H. *et al.* The role of reduced left ventricular end-diastolic volume in the apparently high prevalence of mitral valve prolapse in atrial septal defect. *Eur. J. Cardiol.* 1980; **11**: 341–55.

113. Ballester, M., Presbitero, P., Foale, R. *et al.* Prolapse of the mitral valve in secumdum atrial septal defect: A functional mechanism. *Eur. Heart J.* 1983; **4**: 472–6.

114. Sze, K.C. and Shah, P.M. Pseudo-ejection sound in hypertrophic subaortic stenosis. *Circulation* 1976; **54**: 504–9.

115. Morganroth, J., Jones, R.H., Chen, C.C. and Naito, M. Two-dimensional echocardiography in mitral, aortic and tricuspid valve prolapse. *Am. J. Cardiol.* 1980; **46**: 1164–77.

116. Werner, J.A., Schiller, N.B. and Prasquier, R. Occurrence and significance of echocardiographically demonstrated tricuspid valve prolapse. *Am. Heart J.* 1978; **96**: 180–6.

117. Brown, A.K. and Anderson, V. Two-dimensional echocardiography and the tricuspid valve. Leaflet definition and prolapse. *Br. Heart J.* 1983; **49**: 495–500.

Chapter 30

Acute Rheumatic Fever

S.J. Hutchison

EPIDEMIOLOGY

Although the incidence of acute rheumatic fever and its sequel, chronic rheumatic heart disease, has declined in Western Europe and North America the disease remains common in Eastern Europe and is increasing in Asia. Worldwide, it remains the single most important cause of valvular heart disease.

The falling incidence of rheumatic fever (which pre-dated the antibiotic era) has been best documented in Denmark, where the disease has been notifiable for over 100 years (Fig. 30.1).[1] The annual incidence, which was 200 per 100 000 in 1862 had fallen to 11 per 100 000 by 1962. Similar changes occurred in other Western nations: there were 81 deaths notified as resulting from acute rheumatic fever in England and Wales in 1944, 64 in 1954, 7 in 1964 and 4 in 1975.

The many reasons for this decline are interrelated. It is likely that an improvement in social conditions, in particular, the reduction of overcrowding, has been the major factor, as inadequate housing is probably the major reason for the magnified risk of streptococcal infection in certain

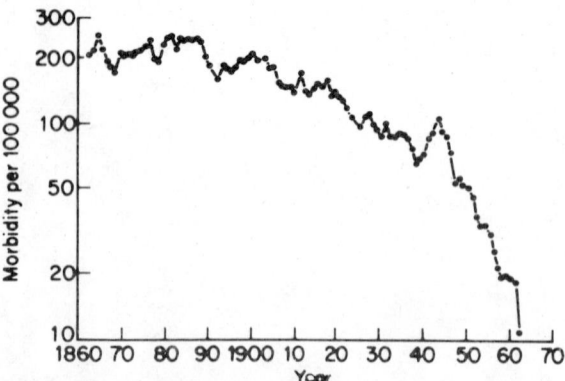

Fig. 30.1. The incidence of rheumatic fever in Denmark between 1862 and 1962. (Reproduced with permission from the *American Heart Journal.* Di Sciascis and Taranta, *Am. Heart J.* 1980; **99**: 635.[1])

disadvantaged populations. Additional factors contributing to the abrupt decrease in acute rheumatic fever since 1940 may include use of antibiotics,[2] reduced virulence of the streptococcus and improved delivery of health care.[3] However, streptococcal pharyngitis has remained common among populations in which rheumatic fever has become rare.[4]

The modest contribution of medical advances to the decline in acute rheumatic fever is underlined by a recent resurgence in the USA.[5] In the area around Salt Lake City, the number of cases increased 8-fold between 1984 and 1985.[6] This increase, which has mainly affected middle-class white subjects, has not been explained convincingly, but seems to be associated with a particular strain of streptococcus.

In the 1930s, rheumatic fever was considered to be rare in tropical countries. Today, the prevalence is increasing. This is likely to be a genuine increase rather than the result of improved diagnosis: in a review of 4800 post-mortem examinations reported from Calcutta in 1930 only one case of rheumatic endocarditis was found.[7] The rapid urbanization and extreme overcrowding that have occurred in many of the larger cities probably explain the increase in rheumatic fever, which remains relatively uncommon in rural areas.[8]

Parallel changes have occurred in the pattern of chronic rheumatic heart disease. In Western countries, it is rarely seen in young people; most patients are over 50 years old having had an acute attack (often subclinical) some 40 years before; by contrast, in Asia, Africa, Eastern Europe and South America, rheumatic valve disease is common in the young. In Peru and Pakistan, 5% of school-age children have evidence of rheumatic valve disease and in Thailand as many as 20% may be affected.[9]

AETIOLOGY AND PATHOGENESIS

Rheumatic fever is a sequel to group A streptococcal pharyngitis. Although one-third of sufferers give no history of sore throat and have negative throat and blood cultures, there is invariably a streptococcal antibody response.[10] Epidemiological studies, particularly in military institutions, have shown a clear relationship between streptococcal infection and subsequent rheumatic fever.[11] Perhaps the most convincing evidence of the link is the effectiveness of penicillin in preventing initial and recurrent attacks of rheumatic fever.[12,13] However, not all strains of group A streptococci are rheumatogenic; those which cause rheumatic fever do not induce glomerulonephritis,[14] and vice versa.

There is strong evidence that rheumatic fever results from a hyperimmune reaction. In general, patients with rheumatic fever are hyperimmune to all streptococcal products. The strength of antibody response is a major determinant of the attack rate of rheumatic fever following streptococcal infection: strong antibody responses are associated with a 5% attack rate whereas the attack rate is < 1% in those who mount a weak antistreptococcal antibody response.[15]

Carbohydrate in the cell wall of group A streptococci (N-acetylglucosamine) shares antigenic characteristics with heart valve glycoprotein, antibodies to this and other shared antigens may be found in patients with rheumatic fever.[16] There is also activation of cellular immunity; lymphocytes sensitized to cardiac antigens are found in the myocardium.

Although it is clear that rheumatic fever has an immune basis, it is not certain whether the pathogenesis reaction is that of auto-immunity or of bacterial allergy.

PATHOLOGY

Acute rheumatic fever is characterized by diffuse inflammatory reactions in the skin, joints and heart. Small blood vessels are commonly involved but thrombotic lesions do not occur. When there is cardiac involvement, the picture is invariably a pancarditis.

The histological hallmarks of rheumatic fever are the Aschoff nodules, which are found in the interstitium of the myocardium, particularly in the interventricular septum and posterior left atrium and ventricle. They are seldom found in valves. The characteristic granulomatous nodules, which are about 1 mm across, are present about 1 month after the onset of illness. They consist of multinucleate giant cells, lymphocytes and plasma cells around an amorphous core. Aschoff nodules are usually situated around small blood vessels. In addition to these specific features, a diffuse inflammatory myocarditis is often present.

In the acute stage, valvular lesions are relatively slight, the cusps are thickened with small warty vegetations ('verrucae') consisting of fibrin along the lines of closure. The mitral valve is most often affected. On microscopic examination, there is a non-specific inflammatory infiltrate. Within a few days, the valves become vascularized. Progressive scarring may then occur.

The pericardium is thickened and is covered in a fibrinous exudate; it may contain a serosanguinous effusion. Histological findings are of a non-specific inflammatory infiltrate. In survivors, pericarditis usually resolves completely and, although adhesions may develop, pericardial constriction does not occur.

CLINICAL FEATURES

Rheumatic fever most commonly occurs between the ages of 5 to 15 years with the peak at around 8 years. There is an equal sex incidence, although females are more susceptible to chorea. Typically, the illness starts 2–3 weeks after an episode of pharyngitis. Arthritis is usually the most prominent feature, although the clinical picture is variable. The diagnosis may be difficult, not least to a generation of doctors who have never seen the condition.[17]

GENERAL SYMPTOMS

The initial symptoms are often vague with non-specific features of anorexia, weight loss and listlessness being common. Fever is almost invariable but is often mild tending to peak when the arthritis flares up. Pyrexia usually subsides within 2–3 weeks, although there may be a transient 'rebound' after 4–6 weeks in treated patients. The temperature mirrors disease activity in the untreated, but it is suppressed by salicylates and steroids and thus cannot be used as an index of disease activity in the treated patient. Sweating is common and there is usually a sinus tachycardia. Nausea, vomiting and abdominal pain may occur, particularly in children. Epistaxis was a common occurrence in the past, but is rarely reported today.

Arthritis occurs in 75% of patients, becoming more common with increasing age. It is often symmetrical, particularly affecting the larger joints.

The knees, ankles, wrists and shoulders are the most frequently involved, although any joint can be affected. Typically, several joints are involved in quick succession, resulting in the classical picture of 'flitting polyarthritis'. The severity of arthritis is variable, but there is usually pain and swelling of the joint which feels warm and is tender (q.v. arthralgia). An individual joint is seldom inflamed for more than a week and there is rarely any residual deformity.

Subcutaneous nodules, which are present in around 10% of cases, were once regarded as being pathognomonic of rheumatic fever, however they may also occur in rheumatoid arthritis and systemic lupus erythematosus. They are painless firm round subcutaneous lesions 0.5–2 cm in diameter, which usually occur over bony prominences and tendons and are not attached to the overlying skin. Other sites include the back of the hand and foot, the patella, the elbow and vertebrae. Nodules tend to appear in crops and may persist for up to 1 month.

Erythema marginatum is characteristic of rheumatic fever, although it has been reported in staphylococcal sepsis and in drug reactions. It occurs in 8% of cases. The rash consists of pink circumscribed circles with pale centres which spread serpiginously and may appear and disappear within hours. Lesions are painless and do not itch. Erythema marginatum affects the trunk and proximal extremities, but never the face. It may relapse intermittently for several months after other features of rheumatic fever have resolved.

Sydenham's chorea (St Vitus' dance) is a neurological manifestation of the rheumatic process. Although it may occur in the absence of other features, it is often associated with subcutaneous nodules, and is frequently associated with carditis; chorea never occurs with arthritis. After puberty, the condition is seen only in females. The onset is insidious, the child appears clumsy initially, the characteristic purposeless non-repetitive involuntary movements gradually becoming more apparent. Grimacing, slurred speech and emotional lability may be observed. Choreiform movements disappear during sleep. Chorea may last from 1 week to up to 2 years, but on average it persists for 3 months.

CARDITIS

Carditis is the most important manifestation of rheumatic fever. It complicates about 55% of initial attacks, and, in contrast to the arthritis, is common-er in younger patients. Although serious long-term cardiac problems may result from scarring of the valves, in the acute phase carditis is usually asymptomatic.

The main clinical criteria for the diagnosis of carditis are organic murmurs, cardiomegaly, pericardial friction and congestive heart failure. Tachycardia and a systolic murmur do not necessarily imply cardiac involvement.[18]

Endocarditis, with valvular involvement, is suggested by the appearance of murmurs; 75% of all patients who develop carditis have murmurs within the first week of illness.[19] An apical pan-systolic murmur suggests mitral regurgitation either due to valvular inflammation or to functional regurgitation associated with left ventricular dilatation caused by myocarditis. Organic systolic murmurs tend to be longer and louder than non-organic ones and have a high-pitched blowing quality. An apical mid-diastolic murmur (the Carey Coombs murmur) is often present in the early stages. It is usually soft, transient and low pitched. Although its presence tends to confirm the significance of an apical systolic murmur, in isolation it does not necessarily indicate involvement of the mitral valve. Aortic diastolic murmurs often do not regress following the acute attack.

Pericarditis occurs in about 10% of cases. It is said to be particularly common in severe carditis and is usually found in patients who die. Pericardial pain and friction are usually accompanied by an increase in fever and there may be associated pleurisy. Symptoms last from 1 to 4 days. Effusions are usually small and seldom cause tamponade. Myocardial involvement is suggested by cardiac dilatation. This is best detected by chest X-ray or echocardiogram. Progressive cardiac enlargement suggests severe myocarditis and indicates a poorer prognosis.

Heart failure is the least common but most serious manifestation of carditis, occurring in 5–10% of cases. Severe cardiac failure is more frequent in recurrent than initial attacks. When heart failure occurs in a young patient with previously well-compensated rheumatic valve disease, a recurrence of carditis should be suspected.

Although first degree heart block is very common (even in the absence of clinical carditis), second and third degree atrioventricular block are very rare. Serious arrhythmias are very unusual.

LABORATORY INVESTIGATIONS

Although there is no definitive test for rheumatic fever, laboratory investigations are helpful in establishing that there was preceding streptococcal infection and in documenting an inflammatory response.

EVIDENCE OF STREPTOCOCCAL INFECTION

By the time rheumatic fever has developed, only about 25% of throat swabs yield streptococci. Specific antibodies are more important diagnostically as they reach a peak after the onset of rheumatic fever and confirm definite preceding infection rather than transient carriage of streptococci. Provided the onset of rheumatic fever can be clearly defined, raised antistreptolysin O titres are invariable. The highest antistreptolysin O titres occur 2–3 weeks after the onset of rheumatic fever, usually coinciding with the most active phase of the polyarthritis. Titres decline over the next few months. Other raised antibody titres include anti-DNAse B, anti-hyaluronidase and anti-streptosyme (ASTZ). The latter is a very sensitive measure of the streptococcal immune response and a low titre is helpful in excluding a diagnosis of rheumatic fever since it makes recent streptococcal infection very unlikely.

ACUTE PHASE REACTANTS

Although non-specific, the white count, erythrocyte sedimentation rate and C-reactive protein are virtually always raised. To some extent, they can be used to monitor disease activity, although the erythrocyte sedimentation rate may fall and the C-reactive protein rise further simply as the result of cardiac failure rather than altered disease activity.

ANAEMIA

A mild-to-moderate normochronic normocytic anaemia is common. Its severity reflects that of the rheumatic fever. Anaemia is corrected (partially or completely) by anti-inflammatory treatment, especially the use of steroids.

ELECTROCARDIOGRAPHIC CHANGES

Prolongation of the PR interval, occasionally up to 0.4 s, is common and, in isolation, should not be taken as evidence of carditis. Minor ST-segment changes are frequently found and ST-segment elevation may occur with pericarditis.

THE DIAGNOSIS OF RHEUMATIC FEVER

There is no definitive test for rheumatic fever and the diagnosis depends upon a combination of clinical features and laboratory findings. The diagnostic criteria proposed by Duckett Jones in 1944 have been widely accepted and were updated in 1965 and 1984 (Table 30.1).[20–22] In addition to evidence of antecedent streptococcal infection, two major or one major and two minor manifestations are considered to indicate a high probability of acute rheumatic fever.

Isolated chorea or carditis may occur some months after streptococcal infection, when antibody titres have returned to normal. In these circumstances, the diagnosis may be accepted without the criteria being fulfilled.[22]

There are many causes of polyarthritis, so it is essential that the antistreptolysin O and, if possible, the anti-DNAse B titres should be measured. Similarly, it is important to ascertain the extent of cardiac involvement; confusion is most likely to occur when fever occurs in a patient with pre-existing murmur which may be functional or congenital in origin.

COURSE AND PROGNOSIS

The usual duration of a rheumatic attack is about 3

Table 30.1. Duckett Jones criteria for the diagnosis of rheumatic fever. For **diagnosis**, the presence of:
- 2 major criteria **or**
- 1 major and 2 minor criteria

plus evidence of streptococcal infection is required.

Major
Carditis
Polyarthritis
Chorea
Erythema marginatum
Subcutaneous nodules

Minor
Clinical:
  Previous rheumatic fever
  Arthralgia
  Fever
Laboratory:
  Acute phase reactants
  Prolonged PR interval

Evidence of streptococcal infection
Antistreptolysin O and other antibodies
Positive throat culture
Recent scarlet fever

months. When there is severe carditis, activity may continue for 6 months, cases in whom it persists for longer are classified as having 'chronic rheumatic fever'. This occurs in less than 5% of cases.

RECURRENCE

Whereas only around 3% of those with epidemic streptococcal pharyngitis develop rheumatic fever, such an infection is associated with a recurrence rate of around 65% in a patient who has previously had rheumatic fever. The risk of recurrence declines with the time between attacks. Recurrence is always due to re-infection and may be prevented by the prophylactic administration of antibiotics with anti-streptococcal activity.

CARDITIS

Recurrent attacks are more likely to cause cardiac failure and death than are initial attacks. However, carditis is seldom a feature of recurrence unless it was present in the first episode. The prognosis is excellent for those who escape carditis; in the United Kingdom–United States Cooperative study,[23,24] 94% of those without organic murmurs in the acute phase were free of heart disease at 10-year follow-up. In the same study, 30% of those showing evidence of heart failure acutely were completely healed at 5 years and 40% at 10 years.

In another study, the severity of carditis was related to subsequent valve disease. No evidence of heart disease was found at follow-up in 151 patients without carditis on admission for rheumatic fever, but residual heart disease was found in 73% of those with mild carditis and 100% of those with severe carditis.[25]

In Western countries, long-term prognosis has improved because the disease itself seems to have moderated and also because antibiotic prophylaxis has prevented subsequent attacks. In the cooperative study previously cited,[24] only 3.8% of children died during a 10-year follow-up.

TREATMENT

There is no specific treatment for rheumatic fever. Therapy is aimed at the relief of symptoms and the limitation of cardiac damage. During the acute phase, bed rest is necessary; this should be continued until fever has subsided. Rest is particularly important for patients with carditis. If possible, specific treatment should be delayed until a diagnosis has been established.

When the diagnosis is made, penicillin is given to eradicate any residual streptococcal infection, although evidence of such infection is usually lacking.

Salicylates and corticosteroids are valuable agents of symptomatic treatment, but there is little evidence that either shortens the course of rheumatic fever or prevents progression to chronic valvular damage. Generally, salicylates alone are used for arthritis, steroids being added if aspirin is inadequate or if there is severe carditis. The dose of acetylsalicylic acid is 50 mg/kg in children and 6–9 g every 4 h in adults over 70 kg. Large doses may cause salicylate poisoning or fluid overload in children. Prednisone can be added in a dose of 40–60 mg/day, the dosage should be gradually reduced as soon as there is evidence of control of rheumatic activity.

PREVENTION

PREVENTION OF THE INITIAL ATTACK[26]

The best prevention is improved social conditions. Acute rheumatic fever can be prevented if the initial streptococcal infection is treated promptly. Hence, mass penicillin prophylaxis can halt epidemics of streptococcal sore throat and subsequent rheumatic fever. The most effective treatment is a single intramuscular dose of benzathine penicillin G (1.2 megaunits (600 000 units) for those < 30 kg). Alternatives include oral penicillin V 500 000 units b.d. for 10 days and erythromycin for those allergic to penicillin.

PREVENTION OF RECURRENT ATTACKS[26]

Patients who have suffered from rheumatic fever require preventative therapy. Once-monthly intramuscular benzathine penicillin 1.2 megaunits is the most effective prophylaxis.[27] Oral penicillin or sulphadiazine are alternatives.

Prophylaxis should be started when the diagnosis of acute rheumatic fever is made and continued for at least 5 years or until the patient reaches the early 20s, whichever is longest.

REFERENCES

1. Di Sciascis, D. and Taranta, A. Rheumatic fever in children. *Am. Heart J.* 1980; **99**: 635–58.

2. Hassell, B.F., Chute, C.G., Walker, A.M. and Kurland, G.S. Penicillin and the marked decrease in morbidity and mortality from rheumatic fever in the United States. *N. Engl. J. Med.* 1988; **318**: 280–6.

3. Gordis, L. Effectiveness of comprehensive care program in preventing rheumatic fever. *N. Engl. J. Med.* 1973; **289**: 331–5.

4. Bisno, A.L. The rise and fall of rheumatic fever. *JAMA* 1985; **254**: 538–41.

5. Hosier, D.M., Craenen, J.M., Teske, D.W. and Wheller, J.J. Resurgence of acute rheumatic fever. *Am. J. Dis. Child.* 1987; **141**: 730–3.

6. Versy, L.G., Wiedmeier, S.E., Orsmond, G.S. *et al.* Resurgence of acute rheumatic fever in the intermountain area of the United States. *N. Engl. J. Med.* 1987; **316**: 421–7.

7. Rogers, L. Cited in Clarked, V.G. The geographic distribution of rheumatic fever. *J. Trop. Med. Hygiene* 1930; **33**: 252–60.

8. Argarwal, B.L. Rheumatic heart disease unabated in tropical countries. *Lancet* 1981; **2**: 910–1.

9. World Health Organisation. Community control of rheumatic fever in developing countries. 1: A major health problem. *WHO Chronicle* 1980; **34**: 336.

10. Stollerman, G.H. The epidemiology of primary and secondary rheumatic fever. In: Uhr, J.W., ed. *Streptococcus rheumatic fever and glomerulonephritis*. Baltimore: Williams and Wilkins, 1964, p. 311.

11. Rammelkamp, C.H. Jr. The epidemiology of streptococcal infections. *Harvey Lect.* 1955–56; **51**: 113.

12. Taranta, A. Rheumatic fever in children and adolescents: A long term epidemiological study of subsequent prophylaxis; streptococcal infection and sequelae: IV: relation of rheumatic fever recurrence rate per streptococcal infection to the titers of streptococcal antibodies. *Ann. Intern. Med.* 1960; **60**(Suppl. 5): 47–57.

13. Taranta, A., Kleinberg, E., Feinstein, A.R., Wood, H.F., Tursky, E. and Simpson, R. Rheumatic fever in children and adolescents: A long term epidemiological study of subsequent prophylaxis; streptococcal infection and sequelae: V: Relation of the rheumatic fever recurrence rate per streptococcal infection to pre-existing clinical features of the patients. *Ann. Intern. Med.* 1960; **60**(Suppl. 5): 58–67.

14. Martin, D.R. Streptococci and rheumatic fever: a review. *N.Z. Med. J.* 1984; **97**: 629–30.

15. Stetson, C.A. Relation of antibody response to rheumatic fever. In: McCarty, M., ed. *Streptococcal infections*. New York: Colombia University Press, 1954, pp. 208–218.

16. Zabriskie, J.B. Rheumatic fever; the interplay between host genetics and microbe. *Circulation* 1985; **71**: 1077–86.

17. Bland, E.F. Rheumatic fever: the way it was. *Circulation* 1987; **76**: 1190–5.

18. Lessot, M. and Brigden, W. Systolic murmurs in healthy children and children with rheumatic fever. *Lancet* 1975; **2**: 673–7.

19. Massell, B.V., Flyer, D.C. and Roy, S.B. The clinical picture of rheumatic fever. Diagnosis, prognosis, course and therapeutic implications. *Am. J. Cardiol.* 1958; **1**: 436–49.

20. Jones, T.D. The diagnosis of rheumatic fever. *JAMA* 1944; **126**: 481–4.

21. Jones criteria (revised) for guidance in the diagnosis of rheumatic fever. *Circulation* 1965; **32**: 664–8.

22. Ad Hoc Committee to revise the Jones Criteria (Modified) of the council in rheumatic fever and congenital heart disease of the American Heart Association. Jones Criteria (revised) for guidance in the diagnosis of rheumatic fever. *Circulation* 1984; **69**: 203A.

23. United Kingdom and United States joint report on rheumatic fever. The treatment of acute rheumatic fever in children. A cooperative clinical trial of ACTH, cortisone and Aspirin. *Circulation* 1955; **11**: 343–77.

24. United Kingdom—United States joint report on rheumatic heart disease. The evolution of rheumatic heart disease 5 year report of a cooperative clinical trial of ACTH, cortisone and Aspirin. *Circulation* 1960; **22**: 503–15.

25. Feinstein, A.R., Zagala, J.G. and Spagnuolo, M. The pattern of symptoms, pre-treatment interval and prognosis of acute rheumatic fever. *Ann. Intern. Med.* 1962; **57**: 563–71.

26. Committee of Rheumatic Fever and Infective Endocarditis of the Council on Cardiovascular Disease in the Young. Prevention of rheumatic fever. *Circulation* 1984; **70**: 1118A.

27. Frankish, J.D. Rheumatic fever prophylaxis. *N.Z. Med. J.* 1984; **97**: 674.

Chapter 31

Diagnosis, Investigation and Medical Management of Rheumatic and Non-rheumatic Mitral Valve Disease

Roger Hall

DIAGNOSIS

Mitral stenosis

The clinical diagnosis of mitral stenosis normally depends on the detection of characteristic physical signs. Non-invasive investigations including the chest X-ray, the electrocardiogram and ultrasound usually readily confirm the physical findings. Occasionally, however, there may be difficulties. Sometimes, the pre-systolic murmur, a prominent feature particularly in patients with mild mitral stenosis, may be mistaken for a systolic murmur, especially by the inexperienced auscultator, and lead to an erroneous diagnosis of mitral regurgitation or aortic stenosis.

Although the physical signs of mitral stenosis are often characteristic, several other conditions may lead to physical signs that may mimic some or all of those of mitral stenosis (Table 31.1). The most important of such conditions are aortic regurgitation with an Austin Flint murmur, atrial myxoma, tricuspid stenosis, atrial septal defect and, occasionally, pulmonary disease. The main features of these conditions are summarized in Table 31.2. These problems of differentiation have become considerably easier to resolve since the widespread introduction of high-quality non-invasive imaging of the heart, using cross-sectional echocardiography (Figs 31.1 and 31.2), and the assessment of the velocity of flow across the cardiac valves using Doppler ultrasound.

In addition to the conditions in which the physical signs of mitral stenosis may be mimicked, there are several diagnostic problems that may be difficult to resolve by clinical examination.

1 *An associated pan-systolic murmur.* Such a murmur heard at the cardiac apex and often

suspected on clinical grounds to be due to mitral regurgitation may be due to tricuspid regurgitation[1] as functional tricuspid regurgitation is a common sequel to pulmonary hypertension developing as a consequence of mitral stenosis. Occasionally, the differentiation between mitral and tricuspid regurgitation can be made on clinical grounds. The murmur is more likely to be due to mitral regurgitation if other clinical evidence supports this diagnosis, for example, a diffuse heaving cardiac apical impulse displaced to the left, a murmur that radiates to the axilla, and evidence of cardiac enlargement on the chest X-ray. If the murmur is loudest at the left sternal border, increased by inspiration and associated with a parasternal heave and 'v' waves in the jugular venous pressure, it is much more likely to be due to tricuspid regurgitation. This differentiation, however, is complicated because tricuspid murmurs can often be well heard at the apex,[1] whereas mitral murmurs may radiate to the left sternal border, and the two situations may often co-exist. Therefore, although it may be possible to differentiate tricuspid and mitral regurgitation on clinical grounds, the most accurate method of differentiation is use of the Doppler technique to identify the regurgitant jet or jets.

2 *Associated aortic valve disease.* It may be extremely difficult to assess the severity of aortic valve disease when it co-exists with severe mitral stenosis because the upstream mitral stenotic lesion limits flow across the aortic valve and makes the physical signs of aortic valve disease, which depend on flow across the aortic valve, less prominent. Although a normal echocardiographic and Doppler study of the aortic valve rules out associated aortic valve disease, the

Table 31.1. Conditions in which physical signs may mimic mitral stenosis.

Physical sign	Condition	Comment
Loud first sound	Hyperkinetic circulation	Mitral valve wide open at the end of diastole and slammed shut
Opening snap (OS)	Tricuspid stenosis	True OS
	Pure mitral regurgitation	Rare – true OS
	Constrictive pericarditis	Loud, early S_3
	Atrial myxoma	'Tumour plop'
Mid-diastolic rumble ± pre-systolic accentuation	Tricuspid stenosis	
	Aortic regurgitation (Austin Flint murmur)	Common
	Acute rheumatic fever	Disappears after acute episode
	Atrial myxoma	
	Hypertrophic cardiomyopathy	Uncommon
	Cor triatriatum	Uncommon
	Increased flow across atrioventricular valve:	
	1 regurgitation	Atrial septal defect
	2 L–R shunt	most likely to cause confusion

assessment is much more difficult when some degree of aortic valve disease is present. Despite the array of modern non-invasive techniques, it may still be difficult to define the severity of the aortic valve lesion because restricted flow across the aortic valve reduces the gradient, irrespective of the method of measurement, and therefore the severity of stenosis cannot be assessed accurately without the use of cardiac catheterization to measure the valve area. Although there are techniques for measuring aortic valve area using Doppler, as yet none has been validated in the complicated setting of mixed valve lesions. Similarly, non-invasive estimates of the severity of aortic regurgitation are often inaccurate because the degree of volume overload of the left ventricle due to a particular amount of aortic regurgitation is decreased by the reduction in forward flow caused by the mitral valve. Assessment of aortic regurgitation in this situation is further compli-cated because Doppler assessment of aortic regurgitation is only semi-quantitative.

3 *A high-pitched early diastolic murmur.* In a patient with mitral stenosis, a high-pitched early diastolic murmur at the cardiac base may be either the Graham Steell murmur of pulmonary regurgitation secondary to pulmonary hyperten-sion or that due to aortic regurgitation. Certain clinical features may help to differentiate be-

tween the two. If there is obvious evidence of pulmonary hypertension and no associated peripheral signs of aortic regurgitation, it is likely that the murmur is pulmonary in origin. An increase in the intensity of the murmur with inspiration also strongly favours a pulmonary origin. Similarly, associated physical signs of aortic regurgitation favour an aortic origin for the murmur, but it should be borne in mind that the two murmurs may co-exist. The differentia-tion of early diastolic murmurs due to pulmon-ary and aortic regurgitation is of considerable clinical significance. If the murmur is due to pulmonary regurgitation, this will nearly always resolve after successful mitral valve surgery. By contrast, an early diastolic murmur due to aortic regurgitation although it may be quite soft could signify severe aortic regurgitation masked by the downstream lesion. If such aortic regurgitation is ignored at surgery, a patient who had under-gone a successful mitral valve replacement is left with significant aortic regurgitation which may impair recovery. Although the echocardiogram may help in the differentiation, it has been superseded by the Doppler technique which can detect both pulmonary and aortic regurgitation with a high degree of accuracy.

4 *Silent mitral stenosis.* Occasionally, patients with mitral stenosis have no detectable murmurs.[2] The murmurs of mitral stenosis

Table 31.2. Differential diagnosis of mitral stenosis.

Condition	Features mimicking mitral stenosis	Differentiation

Austin Flint murmur	Apical MDM
	Pre-systolic accentuation may be present
		No OS
		
		Echo and Doppler:
		  normal left ventricle
		  MV and septal vibration
		  no MV gradient

Left atrial myxoma	Apical MDM OS may be mimicked by tumour 'plop' which is usually of lower frequency than OS Apical SM due to valve destruction may be present	Systemic illness, raised ESR Symptoms (particularly dyspnoea and syncope) brought on by changing posture suggest diagnosis Echo establishes the diagnosis
Tricuspid stenosis	OS and MDM may be apical but usually loudest at LSB	Marked elevation of JVP with slow 'y' descent Lack of pulmonary congestion and right ventricular enlargement Accentuation of MDM by inspiration Echo and Doppler establish diagnosis

Atrial septal defect	PV enlargement with parasternal heave
	Pulmonary congestion and plethora on chest X-ray
	Wide splitting of S_2 may mimic OS
	MDM from flow over tricuspid valve (decreases as shunt falls with normal PA pressure)
		Enormous hilar shadows on chest X-ray
		Partial RBBB
		
		Echo:
		  Very large right ventricle
		  Normal mitral valve
		  May show ASD and Doppler detects flow across ASD

MDM, mid-diastolic murmur; OS, Opening snap; SM, systolic murmur; LSB, left sternal border; PA, pulmonary artery; MV, mitral valve; ESR, erythrocyte sedimentation rate; JVP, jugular venous pressure; RBBB, right bundle branch block; ASD, atrial septal defect.

become soft or inaudible because the flow across the valve is low, and the large right ventricle may push the left ventricle and mitral valve posteriorly in the chest away from the chest wall. Although such patients are rare, it is extremely important to recognize their condition because they are frequently diagnosed as having intractable and untreatable cor pulmonale; if the true diagnosis can be established, mitral valve surgery is often beneficial. Mitral stenosis should always be suspected in any patient with unexplained pulmonary hypertension, particularly if they are in atrial fibrillation and the chest X-ray shows upper lobe blood diversion. Echocardiography and the Doppler technique nearly always resolve this question. Occasionally, mitral valve disease with inconspi-

cuous signs may be confused with other forms of pulmonary disease. The large hilar shadows resulting from pulmonary congestion in patients with mitral valve disease may be mistaken for hilar adenopathy, and, even more rarely, a dilated aneurysmal pulmonary vein can form a smooth mass easily mistaken for a pulmonary neoplasm (Fig. 31.3). If the hilar shadows are particularly prominent in a patient with suspected mitral valve disease the alternative diagnosis of atrial septal defect should always be considered (see Table 31.1).

MITRAL REGURGITATION

The diagnosis of mitral regurgitation is usually straightforward and depends on the presence of an

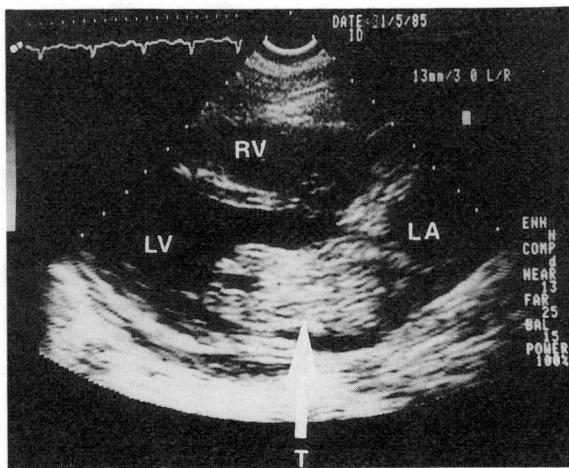

Fig. 31.1. Cross-sectional echocardiogram (parasternal long-axis view) from a patient with a left atrial myxoma (T) who was thought prior to echocardiography to have mitral valve disease. LA, left atrium; LV, left ventricle; RV, right ventricle.

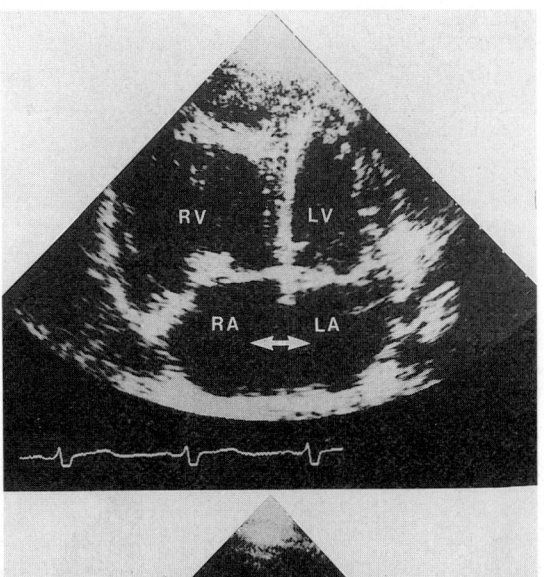

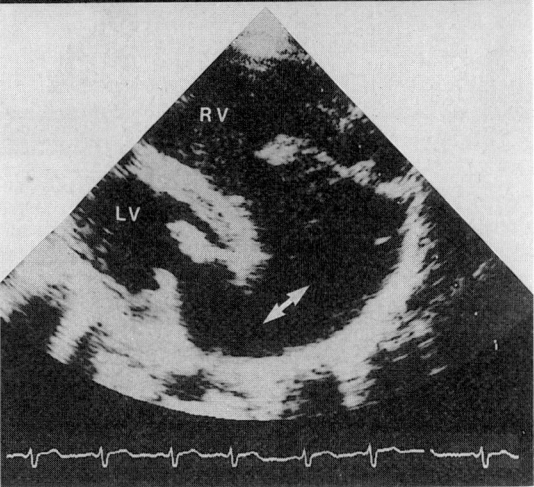

Fig. 31.2. Cross-sectional echocardiograms from a patient with a large atrial septal defect. The defect is seen in the apical four-chamber view (above) and is confirmed in the sub-xiphoid long-axis view (below) when the defect is at right angles to the echo-beam. The defect is marked by the arrows. Note the enormous dilatation of the right ventricle (RV). LA, left atrium; RA, right atrium; LV, left ventricle.

apical pan-systolic murmur, combined with a third heart sound and mid-diastolic murmur and left ventricular enlargement when the lesion is moderate or severe. If mitral regurgitation is rheumatic in origin, the echocardiogram invariably shows thickened mitral valve disease; when mitral regurgitation is non-rheumatic, the echocardiogram may often define the underlying cause, although significant mitral regurgitation can occur through an echocardiographically normal mitral valve. Clinically silent mitral regurgitation may occur, but it is uncommon.[3]

Usually, the main distinction that has to be made is between the different causes of mitral regurgitation, however, mitral regurgitation must also be differentiated from other important causes of a systolic murmur heard best at the cardiac apex, including tricuspid regurgitation (see above), aortic stenosis, hypertrophic cardiomyopathy and ventricular septal defect. All of these conditions can be distinguished by echocardiography and the Doppler technique.

Aortic stenotic murmurs are often well heard at the cardiac apex. As their crescendo/decrescendo nature is different to the constant character of the pan-systolic murmur caused by rheumatic mitral regurgitation, it is unlikely that confusion between the two conditions will occur. However, non-rheumatic mitral regurgitation often produces harsh murmurs which do not extend as far as the second heart sound and they are easily confused with those of aortic stenosis. The carotid pulse is the most

useful physical sign for distinguishing between these two conditions. In aortic stenosis, it is slow rising and often small in volume, unless the patient is elderly and has sclerotic vessels; in mitral regurgitation, it is either normal or sharp in character. Although radiation of the murmur may be helpful, it can also lead to confusion because mitral regurgitant murmurs may radiate to the cardiac base or even the neck, particularly when due to chordal rupture, and aortic murmurs very frequently radiate to the cardiac apex and are often loudest at this site, particularly in the elderly with co-existent lung disease in whom the cardiac apex is the only site at which the heart is in continuity with the chest wall.

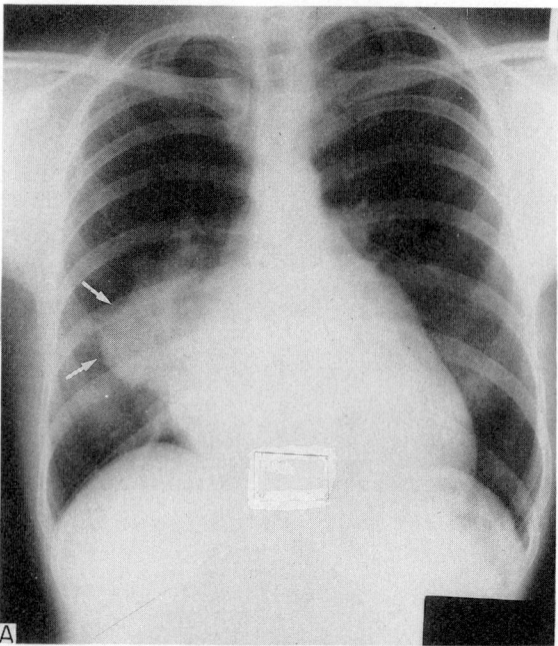
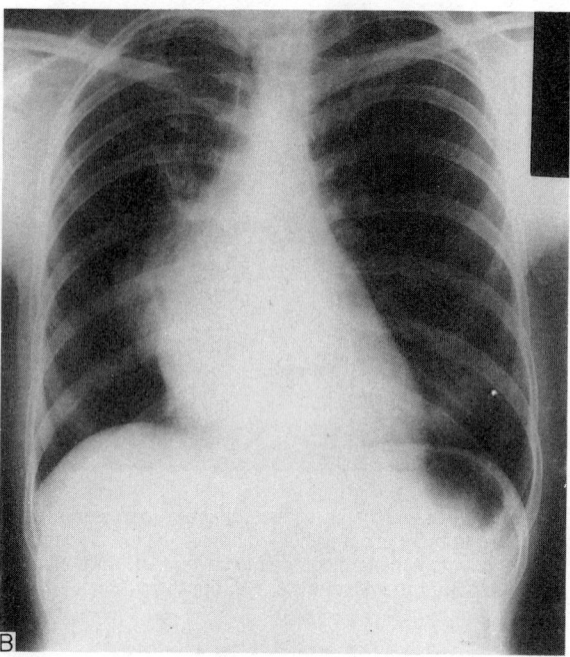

Fig. 31.3. (A) Chest X-ray showing a mass in the right lung field that was due to aneurysmal dilatation of a pulmonary vein in a patient with severe mitral stenosis. (B) Further film taken a year later following successful mitral valve replacement. The mass has decreased in size considerably.

If differentiation is difficult, on clinical grounds, the use of echocardiography or Doppler makes the distinction clear.

Although the systolic murmur of hypertrophic cardiomyopathy is commonly confused with that of aortic stenosis, it can occasionally be mistaken for mitral regurgitation (which is often present in this condition). If there is doubt over whether a systolic murmur is due to either aortic or mitral valve disease, the diagnosis of hypertrophic cardiomyopathy should be considered. It may be impossible on clinical grounds to differentiate the murmur of hypertrophic cardiomyopathy from that of mitral regurgitation, but the diagnosis is suggested by gross left ventricular hypertrophy on the electrocardiogram; echocardiography combined with the Doppler technique usually makes the distinction without difficulty. An important but rare situation is that of a left atrial myxoma which, instead of producing the usual physical signs that lead to confusion with mitral stenosis, destroys the mitral valve and causes mitral regurgitation. The true diagnosis in these patients is usually revealed only by echocardiography; fortunately, this technique is reliable.

A small ventricular septal defect may cause a loud harsh systolic murmur which theoretically can cause confusion with mitral regurgitation. In practice, confusion hardly ever occurs because the murmur is often well localized at the left sternal border and, although harsh and loud, it is not accompanied by any of the other physical signs or by the haemodynamic disturbance to be expected in a patient with mitral regurgitation generating such a loud murmur. Differentiation is easily made using ultrasound; the echocardiogram reveals a normal left ventricle and mitral valve and the pulsed and colour Doppler techniques allow the site of the ventricular septal defect to be defined in most patients. When small, the defect itself is rarely seen on the echocardiogram.

Clinical differentiation of mitral regurgitation of differing aetiology

It is often difficult, or impossible, to discover the underlying cause of mitral regurgitation by clinical means alone. A diagnosis of rheumatic mitral regurgitation may be suggested by a history of rheumatic fever and this suspicion is strengthened if there is evidence of disease of more than one valve. The diagnosis is also favoured if the murmur is high pitched and blowing and of fairly constant intensity throughout systole. By contrast, murmurs which are rough and of an intensity that varies during systole and possibly occupy only part of systole favour a diagnosis of non-rheumatic mitral regurgitation. A mid/late-systolic click or clicks suggest the possibility of mitral valve prolapse or a floppy valve. Associated clinical features may also give a clue to the underlying cause, for example, evidence of a recent myocardial infarction, coronary disease, Marfan's syndrome or infective endocarditis. Although such clinical features suggest the possible underlying cause, they are often unreliable and the distinction of one type of mitral regurgitation from another is best achieved by echocardiographic imaging of the mitral valve and left ventricle and Doppler studies (Figs 31.4 and 31.5).

The differentiation of cases with functional mitral regurgitation due to poor left ventricular function from those in which mitral regurgitation is the primary abnormality is important. Generally, this is not difficult because there are other features to suggest the cause of left ventricular dysfunction, for example, extensive ischaemic heart disease; both clinical and non-invasive features reveal poor left ventricular function. Sometimes it may be difficult to distinguish the end-stage of mitral regurgitation which has led to significant deterioration in left ventricular function from functional regurgitation but this is of little practical importance. When left ventricular function has reached this stage, correction of the mitral valve regurgitation is not likely to be beneficial because, although the mitral valve may be rendered competent, left ventricular function remains poor and may deteriorate further once the afterload on the left ventricle is increased by the presence of a competent mitral valve. Patients are sometimes encountered in whom an intermediate

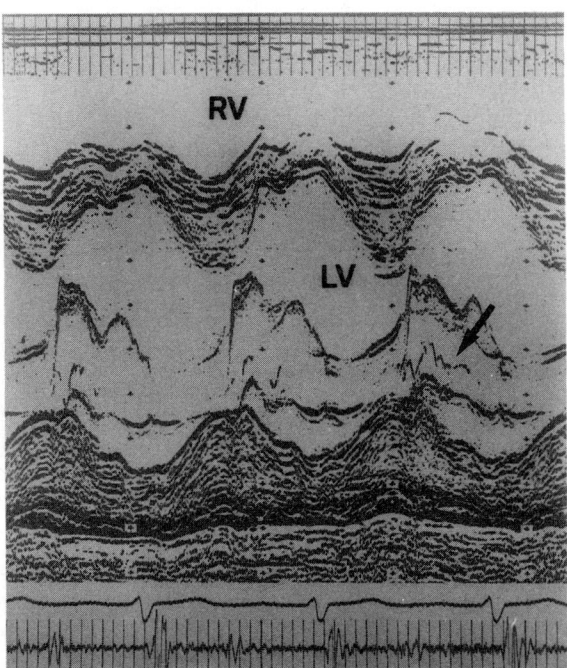

Fig. 31.5. M-Mode echocardiogram showing the left ventricle (LV) and mitral valve in a patient with mitral regurgitation due to chordal rupture. The LV shows very vigorous wall motion and there are fine echoes close to mitral valve (arrow) which are produced by the ruptured chordae and the unsupported edges of the mitral valve, RV, right ventricle.

situation is seen: left ventricular function is somewhat diminished and there is a moderate degree of mitral regurgitation. If such patients are symptomatic, it is difficult to decide on the appropriate management. If mitral valve surgery is needed but postponed, left ventricular function may deteriorate further, whereas if poor left ventricular function is the main problem a competent mitral valve may confer no benefit and could make the condition worse. These patients require a full assessment using both non-invasive and invasive techniques; however, doubt may remain about the best therapeutic approach even when all investigations are complete.

Distinction of acute mitral regurgitation from ventricular septal defect in acute myocardial infarction

When a patient develops a loud harsh systolic murmur, usually with cardiovascular deterioration, during the course of an acute myocardial infarction, acute mitral regurgitation must be differentiated from ventricular septal defect. This can be extremely difficult on clinical grounds, but it can usually be established by bedside investigation. The most

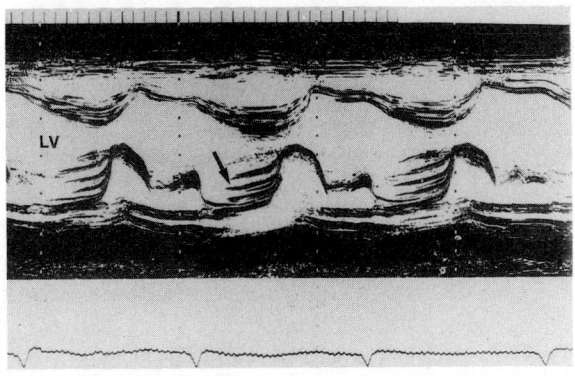

Fig. 31.4. M-Mode echocardiogram of the left ventricle (LV) and mitral valve from a patient with mitral regurgitation due to a floppy mitral valve. The prolapsing, thickened valve is shown clearly (arrow).

important investigations are cross-sectional echo-cardiography, which may show either the ventricular septal defect or a flail cusp with attached chordae and papillary muscle, and Doppler ultrasound.[4-7] Echocardiography in this setting can be technically difficult; it must be remembered that a ventricular septal defect can be in an unusual situation in the septum and be seen only when the ventricular septum is imaged as fully as possible, particularly towards its posterior aspect (Fig. 31.6). Septal defects shown by echocardiography are often ragged irregular holes which may cross the septum obliquely and be associated with small aneurysms within the septum. Septal movement near the defect is often bizarre. The use of contrast echocardiography[8] may help to define a ventricular septal defect in those patients in whom it is not visualized directly, but it has been superseded by the Doppler technique. This shows turbulent flow localized to the right ventricle in patients with

ventricular septal defect (Fig. 31.7) and to the left atrium in patients with mitral regurgitation. In addition to ultrasound investigations, bedside catheterization with a Swan–Ganz catheter can be used since it is rapidly available in most coronary care units. Comparison of the oxygen saturations in the superior vena cava and pulmonary artery will detect a ventricular septal defect.[9] Although the step-up is usually large and the diagnosis easy, there are two potential problems. First, backward transmission of the 'v' wave caused by severe acute mitral regurgitation to the pulmonary artery[10] (see Chapter 29) is associated with the reflux of oxygenated blood into the pulmonary artery.[11] This can

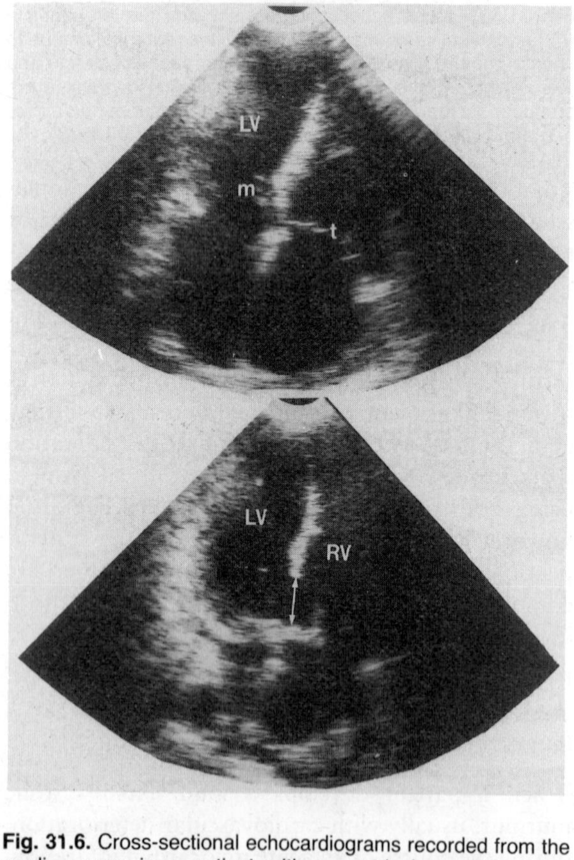

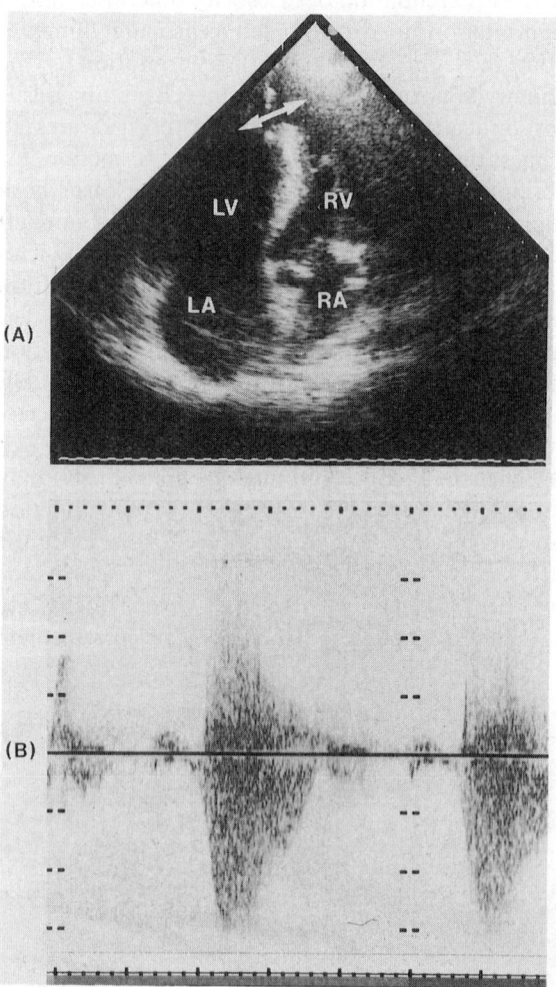

Fig. 31.7. (A) Cross-sectional echocardiogram (apical four-chamber view) and (B) continuous wave Doppler from a patient with a ventricular septal deftect in the distal part of the septum following myocardial infarction (arrow). The Doppler recorded the rapid flow through the defect when directed from the parasternal window. LV, left ventricule; RV, right ventricle; LA, left atrium; RA, right atrium.

Fig. 31.6. Cross-sectional echocardiograms recorded from the cardiac apex in a patient with a ventricular septal defect following acute myocardial infarction. The standard four-chamber view does not show the defect (above), but when the echo beam is directed more posteriorly the defect is seen (arrow). LV, left ventricle; RV, right ventricle; m, mitral valve; t, tricuspid valve.

usually be overcome by sampling in the right ventricle in which there will be a step-up due to the ventricular septal defect but not one due to mitral regurgitation with reflux into the pulmonary artery. Second, when left atrial pressure is particularly high in the setting of acute mitral regurgitation, left-to-right shunting may occasionally occur at atrial level through a patent foramen ovale. Further complications can be introduced: associated tricuspid regurgitation may carry oxygenated blood, which entered the right ventricle through the ventricular septal defect, back into the right atrium to result in a step-up in oxygen saturation at this level. In practice, these problems are of minor importance. The additional finding of a giant 'v' wave in the pulmonary artery trace is strongly in favour of mitral regurgitation. Although the diagnosis may be undecided before catheterization and angiography, this is rare and ultrasound and bedside right heart catheterization nearly always provide the diagnosis within minutes.

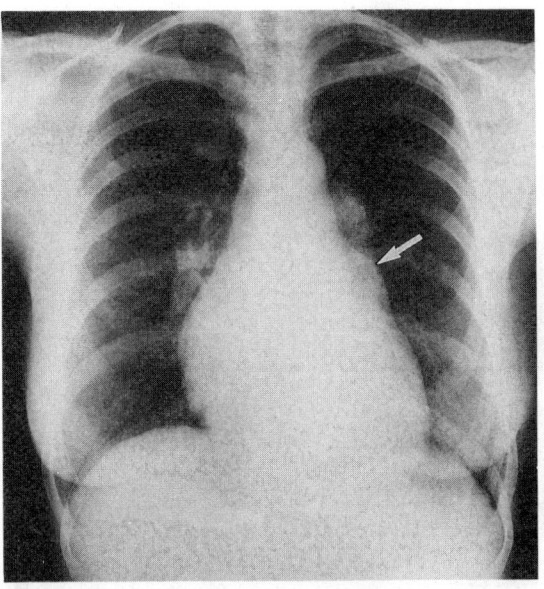

Fig. 31.8. Chest X-ray from a patient with mitral stenosis showing a prominent left atrial appendage (arrow).

INVESTIGATION

CHEST X-RAY

Mitral stenosis

The X-ray appearances vary with the stage and severity of the stenotic lesion. When mitral stenosis is mild, the chest X-ray may be completely normal. Once the lesion becomes more severe, the first abnormality to appear is left atrial enlargement which is almost invariable when haemodynamically significant mitral stenosis is present.[12] On the postero-anterior chest film, the first sign of left atrial enlargement is enlargement of the left atrial appendage which may appear as a prominent hump on the left cardiac border (Fig. 31.8). Once the pulmonary artery pressure begins to rise, the pulmonary artery shadow is also enlarged. The two shadows (pulmonary artery and left atrial appendage) in combination tend to straighten or give a convexity to the normally concave mid left heart border and produce the so-called 'mitralized' cardiac contour (Fig. 31.9). Enlargement of the left atrium itself may also be appreciated on a penetrated postero-anterior film of the chest or on the lateral view (Fig. 31.10). As mitral stenosis becomes more severe, right ventricular enlargement occurs and, once functional tricuspid regurgitation is present, the right atrium may also increase in size.

Left ventricular enlargement is not a feature of mitral stenosis. In addition to the changes in cardiac contour, calcification of the mitral valve may be detected by a penetrated postero-anterior chest film or on the lateral X-ray, but it is more obvious on fluoroscopy.[13] Calcification of the mitral valve tends to increase with age; in a study of juvenile mitral stenosis in India,[14] calcification was found at surgery in only 1 of 23 patients under the age of 20 years. If calcification is sufficiently severe to be detected by X-ray, there is often associated mitral regurgitation.[15] Calcification may also be seen in the left atrial wall probably in thin layers of organized thrombus. This calcification is often 'shell like' and can be seen outlining the left atrial wall.[16]

Characteristic changes also occur in the lung fields. As mitral stenosis becomes more severe, pulmonary venous hypertension and pulmonary arterial hypertension occur and are reflected in the chest X-ray. The first change seen is 'upper lobe blood diversion'. Early tomographic X-ray studies[17] and more recent studies[18,19] using perfusion or ventilation lung scanning demonstrate that blood flow and ventilation are increased in the upper lobes and reduced in the lower lobes when compared with normal.

There is a rough correlation between the level of mean pulmonary artery pressure and both the size of the main pulmonary arteries and the extent of attenuation or 'cut-off' of the peripheral pulmonary

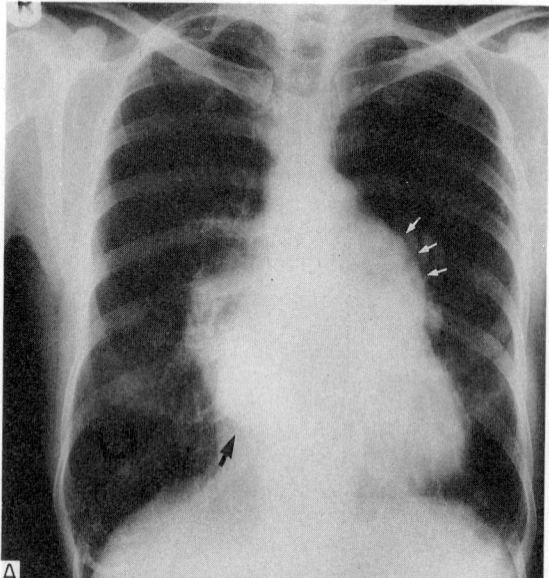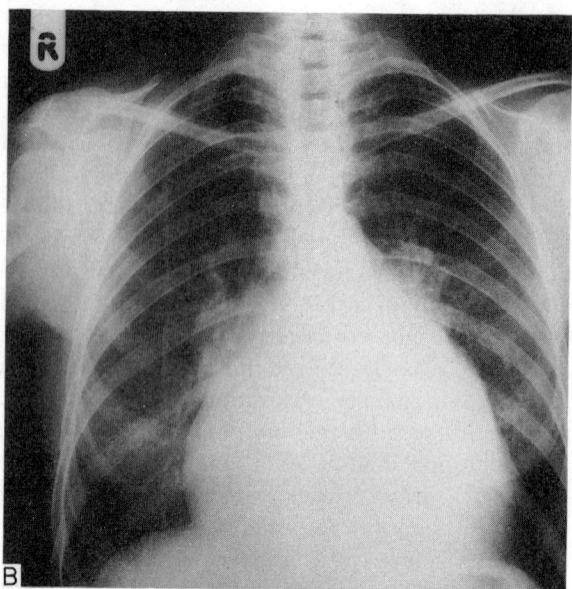

Fig. 31.9. Chest X-rays from two patients with mitral valve disease. (A) A prominent bulge can be seen on the left heart border made up of the combined shadows of the enlarged main pulmonary artery and the left atrial appendage. There is also a double shadow within the heart shadow (black arrow) due to the enlarged left atrium. This patient had pure mitral stenosis and as a result the overall heart size is only moderately increased (cf. B). (B) The typical straightening of the left heart border often seen in mitral valve disease. This patient had significant mitral regurgitation as well as stenosis and the overall heart size is increased due to the combination of left atrial and ventricular enlargement.

arteries.[20] When pulmonary hypertension is severe and longstanding, the main pulmonary artery and its major branches occupying the hilar can be extremely prominent.[21] Pulmonary venous congestion, particularly in the upper lobes, is the only evidence of pulmonary venous hypertension until the level of pressure reaches that at which pulmonary oedema occurs. In mitral stenosis, the chronic changes in the lung capillaries mean that the pressure needed to produce pulmonary oedema is higher than normal. As a consequence, pulmonary oedema is uncommon, although it may occur when there is a sudden deterioration in haemodynamics, for example, with the onset of atrial fibrillation. Under these circumstances, frank pulmonary oedema may develop but often there is diffuse oedema in the lungs which produces a different radiographic picture with general haziness and blurring of vascular definition. Raised left atrial pressure is also associated with Kerley B lines; occasionally, Kerley A lines may become apparent. The presence of Kerley B lines is strongly related to left atrial pressure;[22] they are seen in less than 30% of patients with mitral stenosis if the left atrial pressure is < 20 mmHg but in 70% of patients in whom it exceeds this level.

Other changes may occur in the lung fields. Pulmonary haemosiderosis was a characteristic finding in mitral stenosis. Nowadays, with surgical relief of mitral stenosis performed at a relatively early stage, this X-ray finding is becoming uncommon. Similarly, small ossific nodules in the lung, which are also associated with longstanding pulmonary congestion, are now far less common than formerly.[23]

Mitral regurgitation

Chronic mitral regurgitation of whatever aetiology produces similar chest X-ray findings. Left atrial enlargement is an early feature, as in mitral stenosis, but it rarely occurs in isolation and is usually associated with generalized cardiac enlargement with a leftward displacement and rounding of the cardiac apex due to left ventricular hypertrophy.[24] Left ventricular enlargement may also be visible on the lateral chest film. Longstanding severe mitral regurgitation may sometimes lead to left atrial enlargement considerably in excess of that usually seen with mitral stenosis (unless the mitral stenosis is associated with an atrial septal defect—Lutembacher's syndrome). The occurrence of

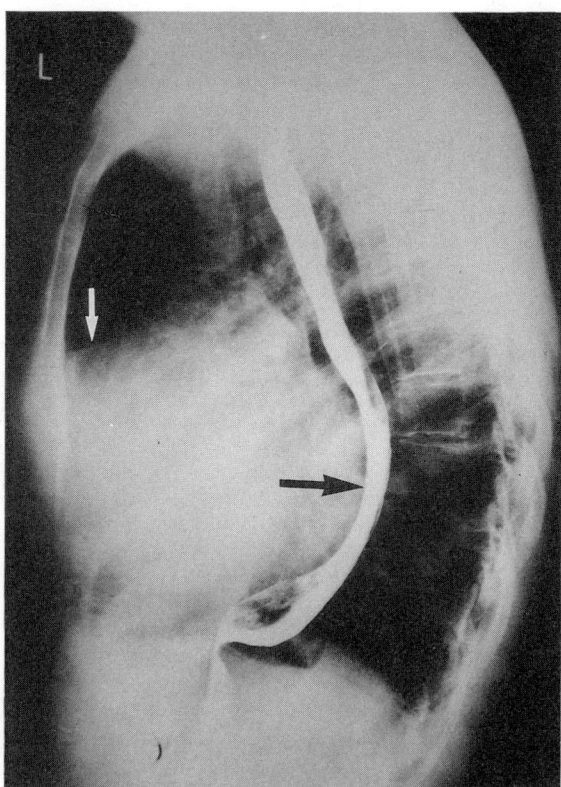

Fig. 31.10. Lateral chest X-ray showing left atrial enlargement (black arrow). There is also right ventricular enlargement which fills in the retrosternal space (white arrow). There is barium in the oesophagus.

marked left atrial enlargement strongly suggests that regurgitation is the predominant lesion in patients with mixed mitral valve disease.

Although pulmonary venous hypertension and increased pulmonary vascular resistance occur in mitral regurgitation, they are not as prominent as in mitral stenosis and, therefore, the changes in the lung fields although similar, are generally less marked.

The X-ray appearances of acute non-rheumatic mitral regurgitation are very different from those of chronic rheumatic mitral regurgitation of whatever aetiology. The heart size may be only slightly increased, as there is often insufficient time between the onset and clinical presentation for marked cardiac enlargement to occur. The most striking features are the marked lung field changes due to pulmonary venous hypertension and pulmonary oedema.

It is not possible to distinguish between the different causes of mitral regurgitation from the chest X-ray. However, if mitral regurgitation appears to be clinically severe and the chest X-ray findings not particularly marked, a non-rheumatic cause is more likely. Increase in cardiac size on the chest X-ray usually indicates progression in severity of the lesion regardless of its aetiology.

Mixed stenosis and regurgitation

In rheumatic mitral valve disease, any combination of stenosis and regurgitation can occur. In general, predominant stenosis is suggested by a small ventricular mass, left atrial enlargement and marked lung field changes, whereas predominant regurgitation is indicated by a greater degree of cardiomegaly and less marked changes in the lung fields. Evenly balanced but severe degrees of stenosis and regurgitation in combination may produce enormous hearts with striking changes in the lung field on the chest X-ray.

ELECTROCARDIOGRAM

The electrocardiogram is a useful but non-specific indicator of the severity of mitral valve lesions. In *mitral stenosis*, the sequence in which electrocardiographic changes occur mirrors the sequence of pathophysiological change. In the early stages of mitral stenosis, the only changes detected on the electrocardiogram are usually those of left atrial hypertrophy (Fig. 31.11); once surgery is required, electrocardiographic evidence of left atrial hypertrophy is present in as many as 90% of patients remaining in sinus rhythm.[25] As stenosis becomes more severe and leads to pulmonary hypertension, electrocardiographic evidence of right ventricular hypertrophy may appear (Fig. 31.11). However, patients may have severe mitral stenosis with little or no evidence of right ventricular hypertrophy on the electrocardiogram because it is an extremely insensitive detector of right ventricular hypertrophy.[26] A rightward shift in the QRS axis usually precedes overt evidence of right ventricular hypertrophy.

The characteristic electrocardiographic changes associated with left atrial hypertrophy, right ventricular hypertrophy and right atrial hypertrophy (see below) are described in detail in Chapter 9. It is worth noting that the broadened and often notched P wave in lead II that occurs as a result of left atrial hypertrophy and is referred to as 'P mitrale' is a non-specific finding which may occur in association with left atrial hypertrophy of any cause. If there is electrocardiographic evidence of right atrial hyper-

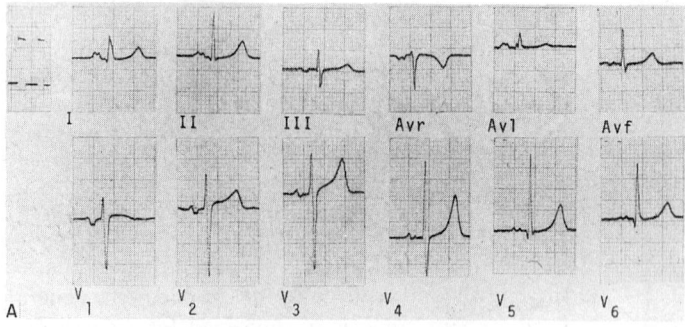

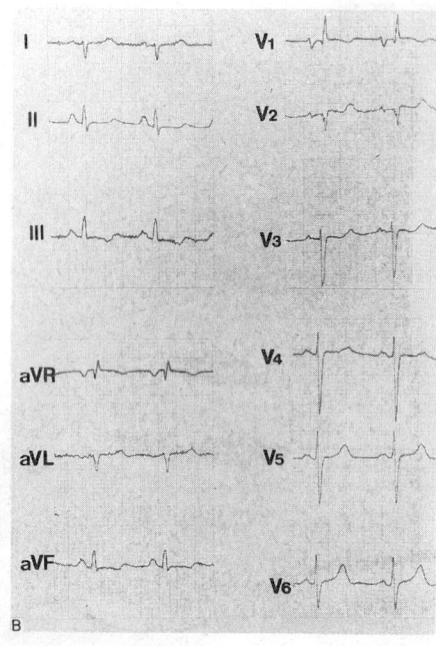

Fig. 31.11. Electrocardiograms from two patients with mitral stenosis. (A) The only abnormality is the broad notched P wave seen best in leads I and II (P mitrale) and the large negative component to the P wave in lead V₁. Both these changes are characteristic of left atrial hypertrophy. (B) This patient had far more advanced mitral stenosis and pulmonary hypertension. There is evidence of left atrial hypertrophy (large negative component to the P wave in lead V₁) but the most striking change is right-axis deviation and right ventricular hypertrophy (dominant R wave in V₁ and deep S wave in V₅ and V₆).

trophy, it may be the result of longstanding mitral stenosis leading to tricuspid regurgitation (as mentioned above); however this situation is unusual and its presence should lead to co-existent tricuspid stenosis or lung disease being suspected.

Atrial fibrillation is common in mitral stenosis, and frequent atrial ectopic beats should be regarded as a warning that the onset of atrial fibrillation is imminent. The onset of atrial fibrillation is strongly related to atrial size.[27,28]

Left atrial hypertrophy and atrial fibrillation are also common in *mitral regurgitation*. However, electrocardiographic evidence of right-axis deviation and right ventricular hypertrophy is much less common: pulmonary vascular resistance is generally not elevated to the same extent as in mitral stenosis and moderate right ventricular hypertrophy rarely produces any characteristic electrocardiographic changes, because of the insensitivity of the electrocardiogram to right ventricular hypertrophy[26] and because the left ventricular hypertrophy, which occurs in mitral regurgitation, tends to balance the electrical changes produced by any right ventricular hypertrophy.

Although electrocardiographic evidence of left ventricular hypertrophy may occur when mitral regurgitation is severe, hypertrophy is rarely as marked as it is in patients with aortic valve disease and frequently it is absent. The results of one study of the relative frequency of ventricular hypertrophy in mitral regurgitation[29] suggested that left ven-

tricular hypertrophy alone is seen in between 40 and 50% of patients, biventricular hypertrophy can be detected in 5–10% of patients, right ventricular hypertrophy alone occurs in 15% of patients, but 30% show no evidence of ventricular hypertrophy.

In acute mitral regurgitation, the electrocardiogram is frequently normal showing only sinus tachycardia, although evidence of 'left atrial hypertrophy' can be seen in the early stages and probably reflects elevated left atrial pressure rather than true hypertrophy of the atrial wall. Occasionally, in acute rheumatic and non-rheumatic mitral regurgitation, the electrocardiogram provides a clue to the aetiology of regurgitation when it is ischaemic by revealing either recent or old myocardial infarction or definite ischaemic changes.

Any combination of the electrocardiographic changes described above for pure stenotic and regurgitant lesions can be seen in patients with mixed mitral valve lesions. Left atrial hypertrophy and atrial fibrillation are particularly frequent because they are features of both stenosis and regurgitation. A rightward axis or evidence of right ventricular hypertrophy tends to favour a predominantly stenotic lesion but does not rule out predominant regurgitation; however, left ventricular hypertrophy strongly favours a predominantly regurgitant lesion and is extremely uncommon in pure mitral stenosis in the absence of systemic hypertension or aortic valve disease.

Aortic and mitral valve lesions frequently occur

in combination and their effects on the electrocardiogram are complicated. Left ventricular hypertrophy resulting from aortic valve lesions may balance the right-axis deviation and right ventricular hypertrophy due to mitral valve disease. As a result, the electrocardiogram may underestimate the extent of both right and left ventricular hypertrophy. In addition, mitral stenosis masks electrocardiographic changes due to aortic valve disease because the amount of left ventricular hypertrophy resulting from a particular degree of aortic stenosis or regurgitation is limited by the reduced amount of forward blood flow permitted by the stenotic mitral valve. This effect is often slight in aortic stenosis because the left ventricle still performs an appreciable degree of pressure work even when the forward flow is reduced. In contrast, the effect in aortic regurgitation is more striking because the volume load from the left ventricle is considerably reduced by the co-existent mitral stenosis. Therefore, less left ventricular hypertrophy occurs with the same degree of aortic valve disease if there is co-existent severe mitral stenosis.

ULTRASOUND

The use of ultrasound in mitral valve disease has been discussed in detail in Chapters 13 and 14. The use of these techniques in mitral valve disease has become so refined that cardiac catheterization rarely has to be undertaken to establish a diagnosis.

In mitral stenosis, the echocardiographic appearances of the mitral valve are characteristic and well known and frequently allow an accurate assessment of the severity of mitral stenosis (Fig. 31.12).[30] With the additional application of the Doppler technique (Fig. 31.13),[31] the pliability and thickness of the mitral valve and the degree to which the subvalvar apparatus is involved can also be assessed (Fig. 31.14). This information may allow the surgeon to plan either mitral valvotomy or a repair procedure in preference to replacement of the mitral valve.[32]

Echocardiography will always identify a rheumatic valve causing regurgitation and can often reveal other causes, for example, mitral valve prolapse, floppy mitral valve, chordal rupture or infective endocarditis. Other patients with obvious mitral regurgitation detected both clinically and by Doppler will have echocardiographically normal mitral valves.

An important application of ultrasound in mitral valve disease is the assessment of left ventricular function. Generally, left ventricular function is

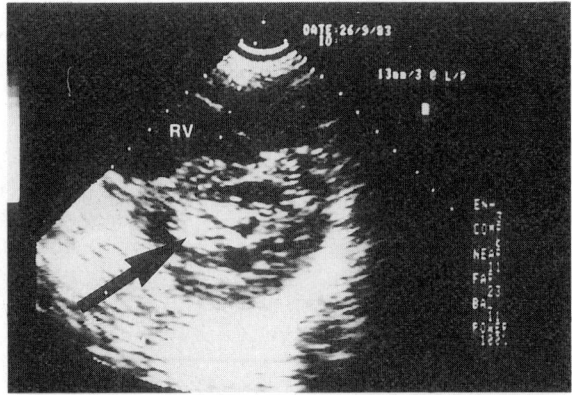

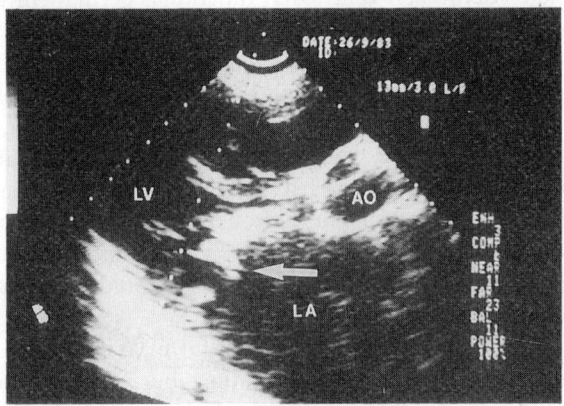

Fig. 31.12. Cross-sectional echocardiograms from a patient with severe mitral stenosis. The parasternal short-axis view (above) shows the slit-like mitral valve orifice in cross-section (arrow) and the parasternal long-axis view (below) demonstrates that the anterior leaflet of the valve (arrow) is grossly thickened and that there is considerable left atrial enlargement. LA, left atrium; LV, left ventricle; AO, aorta; RV, right ventricle.

altered only slightly by mitral stenosis, although occasionally patients with significant mitral stenosis have left ventricular dysfunction due to another cause. Under these circumstances, echocardiography is a sensitive way of detecting the associated abnormality. In mitral regurgitation, assessment of left ventricular function has a wider and more important role. It may help in the assessment of severity; if mitral regurgitation is haemodynamically significant, there is usually some increase in left ventricular dimensions and wall motion is vigorous (Fig. 31.15). It is also important in the follow-up of patients with mitral regurgitation and may help decide the correct time for surgery. As for patients with aortic regurgitation, patients with severe mitral regurgitation may be asymptomatic for a long time. It is important that deteriorating left ventricular function is detected non-invasively at an early stage so that surgical intervention can be under-

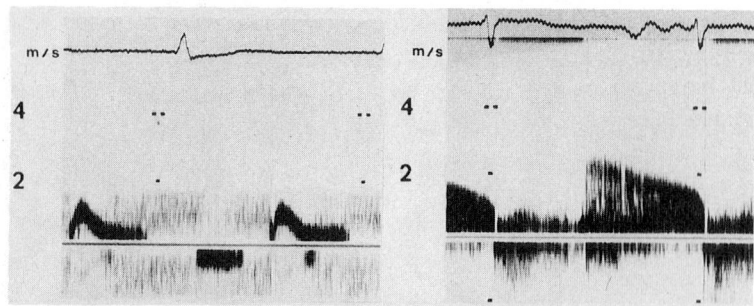

Fig. 31.13. Continuous wave Doppler recordings of mitral valve flow obtained from the apex in a normal subject (left) and a patient with mitral stenosis (right). In the normal subject, the flow velocity is normal and falls as soon as rapid left ventricular filling has finished in early diastole. By contrast, in the patient with mitral stenosis the flow velocity is much higher (> 2 m/s) and although declining slightly remains high throughout diastole.

taken before left ventricular function is permanently damaged. This application of ultrasound in mitral regurgitation is imprecise. The extent of wall motion gives only a rough guide to the severity of mitral regurgitation, and there is no general agreement about the echocardiographic parameters that denote a decrease in left ventricular function that is likely to be permanent, although, if left ventricular end-diastolic diameter is > 8 cm or end-systolic diameter is > 5.5 cm, surgery should not be delayed.[33]

The Doppler technique is useful in assessing the severity of mitral regurgitation but it is often semiquantitative (Fig. 31.16). Accuracy is likely to improve as ultrasound techniques which assess regurgitation by a combination of imaging, and Doppler to measure aortic and mitral valve flow, are investigated further and validated.[34,35] These methods depend on the antegrade diastolic flow across the mitral valve (MF) being the product of the regurgitant flow from the previous systole and the forward cardiac output which is equivalent to the aortic systolic flow (AF). Therefore, the regurgitant flow is equal to MF—AF as long as there is no aortic regurgitation. Mapping and assessment of the regurgitant jet using Doppler colour flow mapping may also prove useful for assessing severity.

Despite the current rapid improvement of Doppler techniques, clinical evaluation combined with echocardiography and the chest X-ray remains of paramount importance in determining the severity and clinical significance of mitral lesions.

Although there are problems in quantifying the severity of mitral regurgitation, both imaging and Doppler techniques are invaluable in distinguishing mitral regurgitation from other causes of systolic murmurs which may be confused with it. Finally, a modern application of Doppler, the measurement of pulmonary artery pressure, is useful in the overall assessment of patients with mitral valve disease.

PULMONARY FUNCTION TESTING

Mitral valve disease may disturb respiratory function and at times it may be difficult to distinguish the effects of mitral valve disease from those of primary lung disease (for detailed discussion, see Chapter 56).

CARDIAC CATHETERIZATION AND ANGIOGRAPHY

The place of cardiac catheterization and angiography in mitral valve disease has changed considerably in the last 10 years. The introduction of high-quality echocardiographic imaging combined with the Doppler technique has enabled an accurate assessment of the severity of mitral valve lesions without resorting to invasive techniques in all but a few patients.[36] There is no evidence that the assessment obtained by invasive techniques is more accurate than that obtained from high-quality ultrasound except in occasional cases of mitral regurgitation of questionable severity. In patients in whom high-quality images cannot be obtained, cardiac catheterization should be undertaken to establish the nature of the valve lesion and its severity. More often, however, cardiac catheterization is used to assess the state of the coronary arteries in patients in whom the valve diagnosis is already certain from non-invasive investigations. Coronary artery disease in valvular heart disease is discussed in detail in Chapter 33. Generally, left ventricular function can be assessed from non-invasive tests, but occasionally cardiac catheterization is required.

When catheterization is used to establish the diagnosis and severity of a mitral valve lesion, mitral stenotic lesions are assessed by the pressure gradient and flow across the mitral valve and regurgitant lesions from angiography although pressure traces may be helpful.

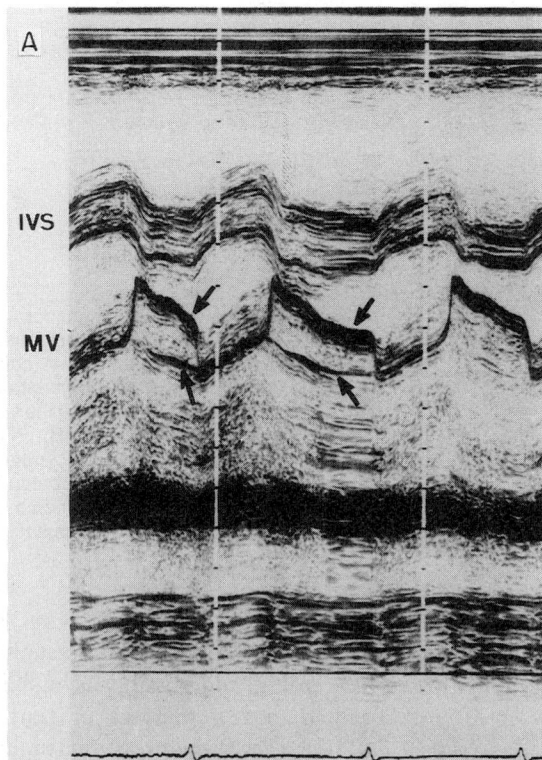

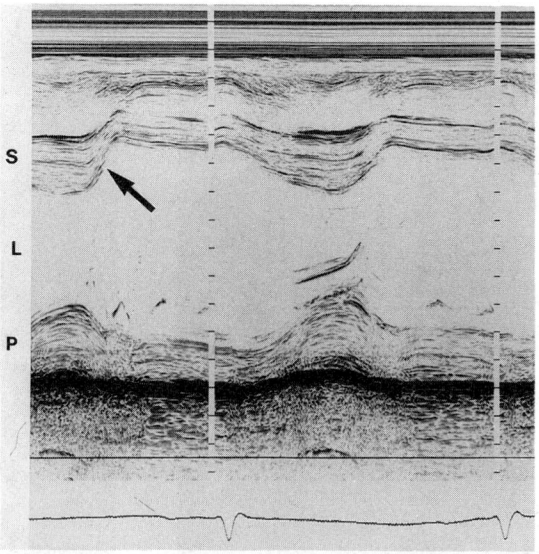

Fig. 31.15. M-Mode echocardiogram showing the left ventricle of a patient with severe mitral regurgitation. The left ventricle is enlarged and shows vigorous wall motion due to the volume overload. There is a rapid anterior motion of the septum in early diastole that is often seen in this situation and is due to rapid left ventricular filling (arrow). S, interventricular septum; L, left ventricle; P, posterior wall of the left ventricle.

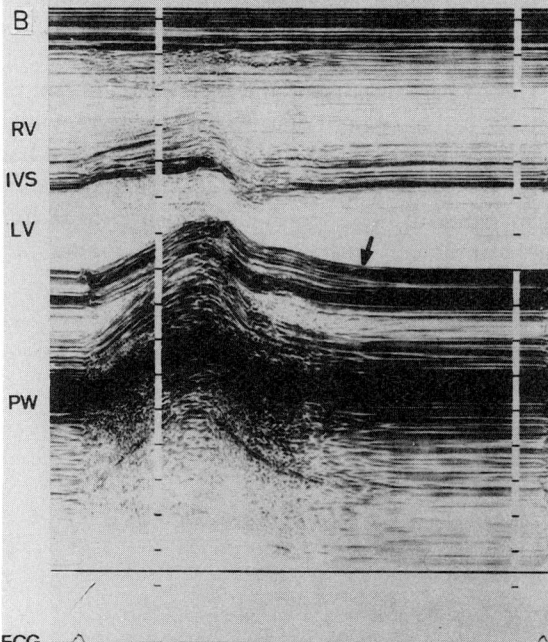

Fig. 31.14. M-Mode echocardiograms from a patient with mitral stenosis. (A) This view shows the mitral valve; the cusps are thin but show the typical pattern of motion seen in mitral stenosis. The posterior cusp is tethered to the anterior cusp and does not move posteriorly in diastole. (B) When the echo beam is directed down towards the left ventricle, it can be seen that although the valve cusps are thin and mobile there is gross thickening of the subvalvar structures (arrow). RV, right ventricle; IVS, interventricular septum; LV, left ventricle; MV, mitral valve; PW, posterior wall of the LV.

In mitral stenosis, the pressure gradient across the mitral valve is assessed by simultaneous recording of left atrial pressure, obtained directly by transseptal catheterization or indirectly as the pulmonary capillary wedge pressure, and the left ventricular pressure usually obtained by retrograde catheterization of the left ventricle. If cardiac output is normal and the pressure gradient between the left atrium and left ventricle in diastole is considerable (for example, a mean pressure gradient > 15 mmHg or end-diastolic gradient > 5–10 mmHg at a normal heart rate suggest significant stenosis), pressure recordings alone can be used to assess the severity of mitral stenosis satisfactorily (Figs 31.17 and 31.18). If there is a significant increase or decrease in cardiac output, the pressure gradient alone may be misleading because it depends on the severity of stenosis and on the flow across the valve in diastole. In the absence of significant mitral regurgitation, the diastolic flow across the mitral valve equals the cardiac output. For example, if the cardiac output is very low, even severe mitral stenosis may produce only a small gradient. The reverse occurs when the cardiac output is high, for example, in anaemia or thyrotoxicosis. Under these circumstances it is safer to calculate mitral valve area using the Gorlin formula or one of the other formulae that have been

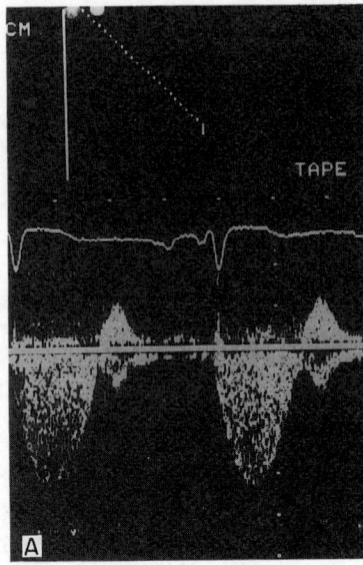

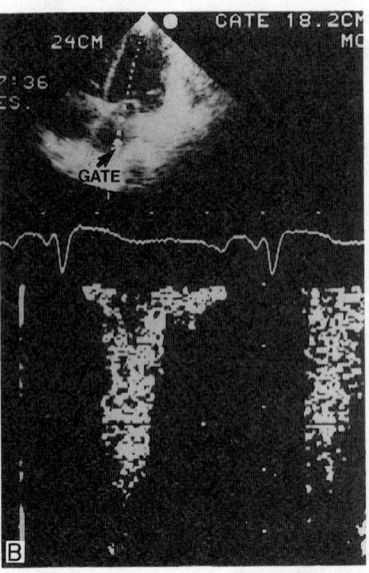

Fig. 31.16. Doppler recordings from a patient with severe mitral regurgitation (recorded from the apex). The continuous wave (A) detects the regurgitant jet which can be tracked back into the left atrium using the pulsed mode (B). The Doppler sample volume (gate —upper part of B) is at the back of the left atrium and the regurgitant jet is still detected at this point indicating that the regurgitation is severe.

proposed more recently.[37] The calculation of valve area can be misleading if it is not performed with considerable care. It requires accurate measurement of the pressure and cardiac output and it may be of limited value because of the many assumptions involved.[37]

In some patients with mitral stenosis, the resting haemodynamics are unimpressive but a low level of exercise, which increases the cardiac output slightly, leads to a large rise in left atrial pressure and the pressure gradient across the mitral valve, as the pressure gradient is roughly proportional to the square of the flow. If there is doubt over the haemodynamic significance of mitral stenosis or whether it is causing symptoms, exercise on a catheter table is worthwhile;[38] the pressure usually rises quickly to > 25 mmHg, and possibly as high as 40 or 50 mmHg, with a few minutes of gentle exercise. At the end of exercise, the pressure usually falls rapidly to its resting level. If the left atrial pressure does not rise significantly on exercise, the mitral stenosis is unlikely to be clinically significant.

The other important measurement in mitral stenosis is that of pulmonary artery pressure, which used to be regarded as one of the variables that had to be known before a decision about surgery could be made; with the anaesthetic and surgical techniques available 20 years ago, a very high pulmonary

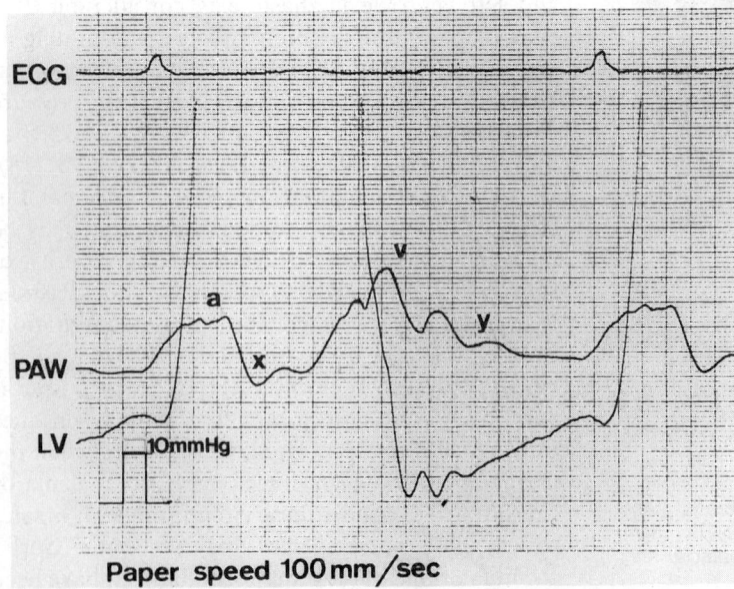

Fig. 31.17. Pressure traces obtained at catheterization from a patient with mitral stenosis who is in sinus rhythm. There is a pressure gradient between the left ventricle (LV) and pulmonary artery wedge (PAW) throughout diastole. Both the 'a' and 'v' waves are well seen. The 'y' descent from the 'v' wave is slow although it is interrupted by an artefactual oscillation in the pressure trace.

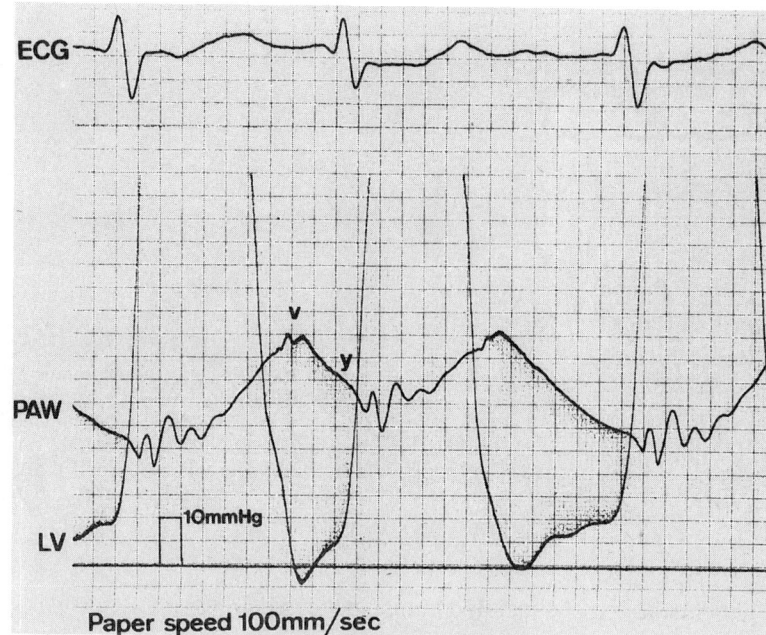

ECG

PAW

LV

10mmHg

Paper speed 100mm/sec

Fig. 31.18. Simultaneously recorded left ventricular (LV) and pulmonary artery wedge (PAW) pressures in a patient with mitral stenosis who is in atrial fibrillation. Note that the pressure gradient at the end of diastole varies according to the RR interval; with the shorter cycle (left), it is about 30 mmHg whereas with the longer cycle (right) it is about 17 mmHg.

artery pressure carried a considerably increased operative risk. Although nowadays this does not appear to be the case, patients who have considerable pulmonary hypertension pre-operatively tend to experience a more stormy course after operation. The assessment of pulmonary artery pressure is also important in deciding whether tricuspid regurgitation is organic or functional (see 'Associated tricuspid valve disease' below).

In mitral regurgitation, there is usually a moderate degree of pulmonary hypertension but the pulmonary artery pressure does not reach the levels often seen in severe mitral stenosis. The left atrial (or pulmonary capillary wedge pressure) usually shows a dominant 'v' wave caused by the regurgitant jet (Fig. 31.19). In chronic rheumatic mitral

regurgitation, the 'v' wave, although often prominent,[39] is usually not as large or as sharp as that in the acute forms of non-rheumatic mitral regurgitation. One reason for this is that the 'v' wave is damped by the large volume of blood already present in the enormously enlarged left atrium. When combined mitral stenosis and regurgitation is present, there is a diastolic gradient across the mitral valve and both the 'a' and 'v' waves in the left atrial trace may be prominent (Fig. 31.20).

In mitral stenosis and in mitral regurgitation, left ventricular end-diastolic pressure is usually normal until a late stage in the disease. In some patients with mitral stenosis, especially if extensive subvalvar fibrosis is present, the left ventricular end-

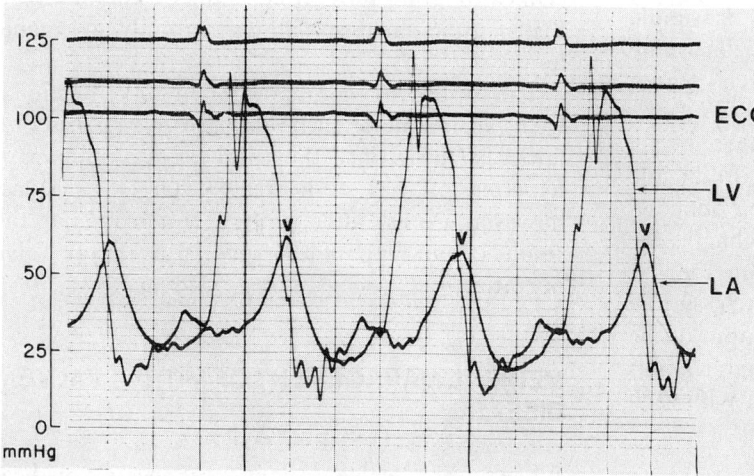

125

100

75

50

25

0
mmHg

ECG

LV

LA

Fig. 31.19. Simultaneous left ventricular (LV) and left atrial (LA) pressures recorded in a patient with severe mitral regurgitation. The LA trace shows a prominent 'v' wave of about 60 mmHg. The left ventricular end-diastolic pressure is elevated to > 30 mmHg.

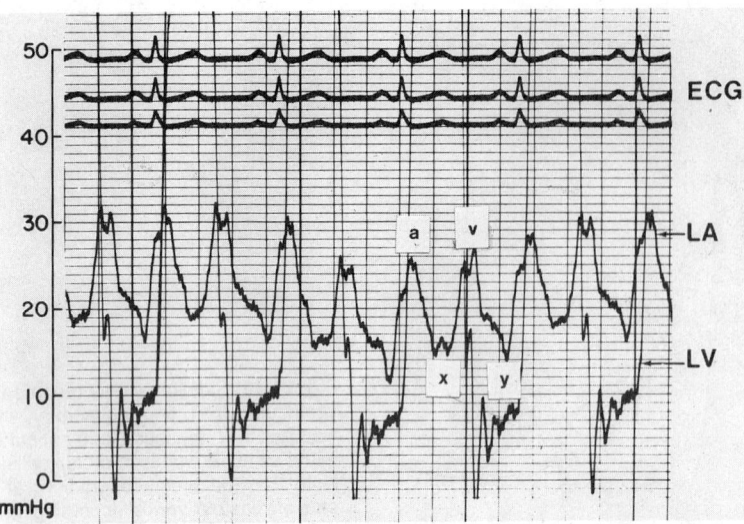

Fig. 31.20. Simultaneous left ventricular (LV) and left atrial (LA) pressures recorded from a patient with combined mitral stenosis and regurgitation. There is a pressure gradient between the LV and LA throughout diastole and both the 'a' and 'v' waves in the LA trace are prominent.

diastolic pressure may be raised; in such patients, it may be particularly difficult to assess the severity of mitral stenosis.[40] Once significant deterioration of left ventricular function occurs in mitral regurgitation, the end-diastolic pressure rises. This is a late sign and should be regarded as an indication that mitral valve replacement or repair should not be delayed.

Left ventricular angiography provides some helpful information in mitral stenosis. The mitral valve is often seen in silhouette and its thickness and mobility can sometimes be distinguished. The left ventriculogram is extremely important in the catheter assessment of mitral regurgitation: it may show an abnormality of the mitral valve, for example, thickening due to the rheumatic process or prolapse of the valve cusps; and it demonstrates the reflux of dye from the left ventricle to the left atrium (Fig. 31.21). The degree of mitral regurgitation can be assessed in two ways. Most commonly, a simple visual scale (usually out of 4) is used to determine whether the mitral regurgitation is trivial, mild, moderate or severe. This method is known to be extremely inaccurate and not particularly reproducible.[41] A more accurate and a reproducible assessment of mitral regurgitation can be obtained by calculating the regurgitant fraction, which is the amount of blood that regurgitates from the left ventricle into the left atrium with each systole expressed as a percentage of the total output of the left ventricle, i.e. the amount that regurgitates plus the amount that is ejected into the aorta with each systole.

Associated tricuspid valve disease

One of the most difficult distinctions to make in the clinical study of valvular heart disease is that between organic and functional tricuspid regurgitation. Statistically, the overwhelming majority of regurgitant tricuspid lesions are functional, i.e. due to stretching of the tricuspid valve ring secondary to right ventricular dilatation resulting from pulmonary hypertension. If, at catheterization, the right ventricular pressure is normal or only slightly elevated (peak systolic pressure < 40 mmHg), the regurgitation is likely to be organic. If the right ventricular pressure is high, the lesion may be either organic or functional. This distinction frequently cannot be made at catheterization (or there is a significant diastolic gradient at catheterization recorded by Doppler) and the only solution is inspection of the tricuspid valve at surgery.[36] If the echocardiogram shows thickening or immobility of the tricuspid valve, it is almost certainly an organic lesion.

This distinction is important in that functional tricuspid lesions often resolve, for example, severe mitral stenosis once the cause of the pulmonary hypertension has been treated. Organic lesions, however, persist after surgery and may mar the result of an apparently successful mitral valve operation.

MEDICAL MANAGEMENT OF MITRAL VALVE DISEASE

When mitral valve lesions are severe, medical

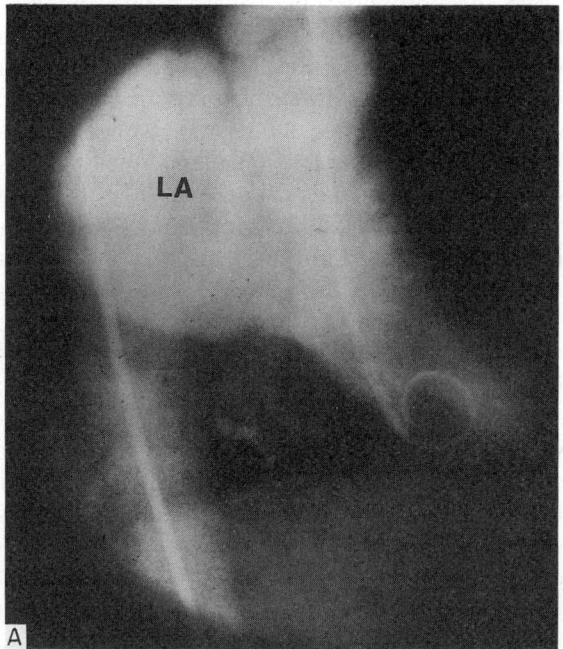 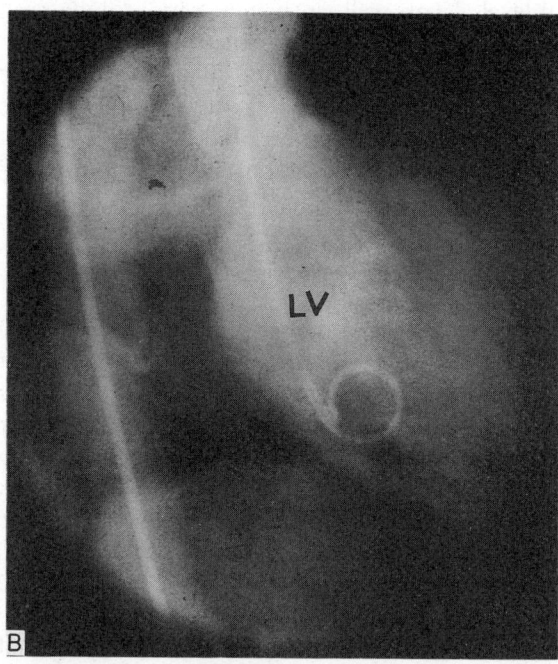

Fig. 31.21. Left ventriculogram from a patient with severe mitral regurgitation. (A) The first systolic frame after the injection of contrast. There is already complete opacification of the left atrium indicating that the regurgitation is very severe. The left ventricle is contracting vigorously; this can be seen by the large change in left ventricular size between the systolic (A) and diastolic (B) frames. LV, left ventricle; LA, left atrium.

management has a limited but important role; ultimately, the only solution is often surgical. Indeed, postponement of surgical intervention for too long may impair the result. However, not every patient has mitral valve disease sufficiently severe to require surgery; many patients, particularly those with mild mitral stenosis or a moderate degree of mitral regurgitation, may remain well on medical therapy for many years. The long-term problems of valve replacement must be borne in mind and carefully considered when there is a temptation to recommend surgery in the mildly symptomatic patient in whom there is no evidence of the development of serious complications, such as significant pulmonary hypertension or deteriorating left ventricular function.

CONTROL OF HEART RATE IN ATRIAL FIBRILLATION

The onset of atrial fibrillation is a significant event in the course of mitral valve disease; in many patients, it is the first sign of clinical deterioration. The high intrinsic heart rate of untreated atrial fibrillation has a particularly damaging effect in mitral stenosis (although it also produces deteriora-tion in mitral regurgitation) because it reduces the length of diastole per unit time and therefore the time available for left ventricular filling. This is obviously deleterious since left ventricular filling is already impaired even at a normal heart rate. Furthermore, the contribution of atrial contraction in augmenting left ventricular filling is also lost. As all mitral valve prostheses are at least mildly stenotic,[42] patients who have undergone mitral valve replacement are also vulnerable to rapid heart rates.

The resting heart rate can usually be controlled using digitalis but sometimes adequate doses cannot be administered without incurring toxic side-effects. In these patients, the addition of a beta-blocker (e.g. propranolol or atenolol) or a calcium antagonist (e.g. verapamil or diltiazem[43,44]) may help to control the heart rate. The slight negative inotropic effect of these agents is usually outweighed by their beneficial effect on heart rate, particularly on exercise. However, it is wise to be cautious because both verapamil and diltiazem may raise the level of digoxin in the blood.[45] Although amiodarone also slows atrial fibrillation and does not have a signi-ficant negative inotropic effect, it may profoundly disturb anticoagulation[46] and increase serum digoxin levels,[47] as well as having serious long-term side-effects,[48] therefore, it is best avoided if possible. In some patients, although digitalis controls the resting heart rate, it exerts little influence on the heart rate during exercise. Under these circumstances, additional medication with a calcium antagonist or beta-blocker may be very beneficial.

CONVERSION OF ATRIAL FIBRILLATION TO SINUS RHYTHM

Restoration of sinus rhythm by direct current cardioversion or pharmacologically with agents such as quinidine or disopyramide may confer significant clinical benefit on patients who develop atrial fibrillation as a result of mitral valve disease. Nowadays, cardioversion is preferred because it has a higher initial success rate. Before cardioversion is undertaken, several factors must be considered, the most important of which are the chances of success in the short and the long term and the potential benefits and risks. Information to guide the clinician in this situation is scanty but it has been well reviewed by Mancini and Goldberger.[49] The chances of lasting success are less if atrial fibrillation is longstanding (i.e. it has been present for > 1 year) and if the patient has haemodynamically severe mitral valve disease. The results are likely to be particularly unsatisfactory if the left atrial dimension measured echocardiographically is > 5 cm; in these circumstances, only 10% of patients are likely to have remained in sinus rhythm 6 months after conversion and up to 30% will experience systemic embolism at or soon after conversion.[50] The long-term success rate (at 1 year) also seems to be lower in patients with predominant mitral regurgitation (20–25%) than in those with stenosis (50–55%) possibly because the left atrium is larger.

In practice, there are three situations in which conversion of atrial fibrillation to sinus rhythm is likely to be useful in mitral valve disease: firstly, when atrial fibrillation develops in the presence of only mild or moderate valve disease and the left atrial dimension is not > 5 cm on M-mode echocardiography; second, following successful surgical correction of the mitral valve lesion, particularly if fibrillation has been present for only a short time before surgery; and, third, it is sometimes worth attempting in patients who have severe mitral valve disease and particularly poor haemodynamics in whom mitral valve surgery is not possible.

As conversion to sinus rhythm is often an elective procedure, it is important that the risks are mini-

mized, the most important being systemic embolization at or soon after conversion, or in association with the recurrence of fibrillation, and the initiation of a dangerous arrhythmia by the procedure itself. Most of the available information suggests it is prudent to administer anticoagulants to all patients for at least 2 weeks before cardioversion and for a week or so after cardioversion because the restoration of atrial function may dislodge thrombus present in the left atrium either at the time of conversion or as atrial function recovers after the procedure. Moreover, the risk of reversion to atrial fibrillation, with the attendant risk of embolization, is highest soon after the procedure. In patients in whom atrial fibrillation is likely to recur, for example, those in whom the underlying mitral valve disease has not been corrected, many clinicians would continue antiocoagulation indefinitely following conversion. In patients in whom a surgical procedure other than valve replacement has been performed to alleviate mitral valve disease, i.e. valvotomy or mitral valve repair, and left atrial size is not greatly increased, anticoagulants can be discontinued once sinus rhythm has been re-established for several weeks. The need for long-term anticoagulation in patients with prosthetic valves is discussed elsewhere (Chapter 35). The risk of serious arrhythmias being induced by cardioversion is highest if there is digitalis toxicity. As these arrhythmias can be fatal[51] (ventricular fibrillation or ventricular tachycardia), digitalis should be discontinued prior to the procedure. In patients who are taking digoxin and have no evidence of toxicity, the drug should be discontinued 48 h before the procedure; if there is any evidence of toxicity or if the patient is taking a long-acting cardiac glycoside such as digitoxin, a longer period is required. It is essential that the serum potassium level is known to be normal before direct current cardioversion is carried out.

Following conversion to sinus rhythm, long-term quinidine or disopyramide may enhance the maintenance of sinus rhythm, however, chronic treatment with quinidine can potentiate digoxin toxicity and be hazardous.[52] Perhaps the most effective drug for maintaining sinus rhythm is amiodarone, but as it potentiates the effects of anticoagulants and digoxin and occasionally extreme toxicity with long-term use [46–48] it should be avoided unless there is a strong clinical indication. Amiodarone is beneficial in patients with severe mitral valve lesion in whom surgery cannot be undertaken but who are expected to benefit from conversion to sinus rhythm; it can be initiated prior to direct current cardioversion and continued after the procedure. If given in this way, it considerably enhances the chances of short- and long-term success in such patients.

ANTICOAGULANTS IN MITRAL VALVE DISEASE

Systemic embolization is a common complication of mitral valve disease; it is the first manifestation in up to 12.5% of cases of rheumatic mitral valve disease.[53] As systemic embolization is potentially disastrous, anticoagulation should be considered in all patients. Although many features of systemic embolization have already been described those that are central to the understanding of the use of anticoagulants are reiterated here. Systemic embolization can occur in patients in sinus rhythm, but it is strongly associated with the presence of atrial fibrillation.[54] The risk of embolization is highest soon after the onset of atrial fibrillation; although embolization is more common in patients with mitral stenosis, its incidence in patients with mitral regurgitation and atrial fibrillation is sufficiently high to be a significant problem. Furthermore patients with mechanical prosthetic valves are at a high risk of embolization and valve thrombosis if they are not receiving adequate anticoagulation. The risk of embolization is increased if left atrial size (as assessed by M-mode echocardiography) is > 4.5 cm.[50]

Although there have been no randomized trials of anticoagulation in mitral valve disease, there is convincing evidence that it substantially reduces embolic events, embolic deaths and recurrent emboli by at least 60%.[54–56] This considerable benefit has to be weighed against the risk of bleeding conferred by chronic anticoagulation. The overall incidence of haemorrhagic complications in anticoagulated patients with valve disease is between 1 and 2% per annum and the risk of death from haemorrhage has been estimated at 0.17% per annum.[57,58] (The initial figures were obtained from large groups of patients with prosthetic valves and extrapolated to patients with diseased native valves.) The use of antiplatelet agents in mitral valve disease and in patients with prosthetic valves is contentious:[59] there is some evidence[60–62] that the addition of an antiplatelet agent, such as aspirin, dipyridamole or sulphinpyrazone, to an anticoagulant regimen may further reduce the incidence of emboli; there is no convincing evidence that antiplatelet agents alone are effective.[63]

Mitral valve disease in atrial fibrillation

Anticoagulants should be given to patients with mitral valve disease in atrial fibrillation, unless specifically contra-indicated, particularly if there has been a recent embolus (there is a 30–65% chance of another within the next few months[54]), the onset of atrial fibrillation is recent or the rhythm disturbance is paroxysmal. However, the risk of anticoagulation may sometimes outweigh the risk of embolism, particularly in patients of extremely advanced age, of gross obesity, who have severely impaired liver function (especially alcoholics who tend to comply poorly and have fluctuating liver function) or who have suffered recent serious bleeding (gastro-intestinal or cerebrovascular).

Mitral valve disease in sinus rhythm

The risk of embolism in patients with mitral valve disease in sinus rhythm is much lower (probably 25% of the risk of atrial fibrillation)[64] consequently a more selective policy can be employed; anticoagulation is generally given to patients who have had a previous embolism or in whom the left atrium is enlarged. An enlarged left atrium may warn of impending atrial fibrillation with a high risk of embolization at or near the time of onset. A reasonable policy is to anticoagulate routinely when the left atrial dimension is > 4.5 cm,[50] although in patients who have bioprosthetic valves some authors have recommended anticoagulation in those with a left atrial dimension of > 5.5 cm.[65] Generally, the threshold for anticoagulation is lower in patients with predominantly stenotic as opposed to predominantly regurgitant lesions.

Prosthetic valves

Anticoagulation in patients with prosthetic valves is discussed in detail in Chapter 35.

Anticoagulants and direct current conversion in mitral valve disease

Anticoagulation is generally necessary prior to direct current cardioversion (see above).

Anticoagulants during pregnancy in patients with mitral valve disease or mitral valve prostheses

This is a particularly troublesome aspect of the management of mitral valve disease and is discussed in Chapter 58.

Management of patients who develop embolization while receiving anticoagulation

The management of patients who suffer embolization while receiving anticoagulants can be a difficult clinical problem. The quality of previous anticoagulant control should be checked. If it was inadequate, more careful attention to the level of anticoagulation may solve the problem. If it was adequate, then an antiplatelet agent (preferably dipyridamole or sulphinpyrazone) can be added to the regimen as there is some evidence that this combination is more effective at reducing embolic risk than anticoagulation alone.[60-62]

Other measures may reduce the risk. If the patient has hemodynamically significant mitral valve disease, valvotomy or mitral valve repair should be considered as a way of reducing the embolic risk,[64] although the need for anticoagulation will often continue after the operation. If the valve is unsuitable for a conservative operative procedure, the appropriate management is not straightforward because of the embolic risk associated with a prosthetic valve. However, as long as the valve is causing a significant haemodynamic problem, it is likely that the chance of recurrent embolism will be reduced by replacing the valve. If valve replacement is undertaken in a patient who has suffered several embolic episodes despite adequate anticoagulation, many surgeons would prefer to use a tissue rather than a mechanical prosthesis. If the valve is only mildly diseased, it is unlikely that valve replacement will reduce the occurrence of emboli. Finally, some patients with mechanical mitral valves have recurrent emboli despite anticoagulation; re-replacement with a tissue valve will often solve the problem.

OTHER MEDICAL THERAPY IN MITRAL VALVE DISEASE

Diuretic therapy

Patients with mitral valve disease in whom either pulmonary or peripheral oedema without effusions into the pleural and peritoneal cavities have developed can receive considerable benefit from diuretic therapy. Quite often moderate degrees of fluid retention can be eliminated with considerable clinical benefit to the patient; however, once mitral valve disease has reached this stage, surgical intervention must be considered. In some patients with severe disease, it may be impossible to eliminate all accumulated fluid without producing gross electrolyte abnormalities and a reduced cardiac output; in such patients, the need for mitral valve surgery is even more urgent. Occasionally, there are patients in whom adequate diuretic therapy will reduce right ventricular size sufficiently for a functionally regurgitant tricuspid valve to become competent again. This is often accompanied by a considerable increase in cardiac output and clinical improvement.

Peripheral vasodilators

When mitral stenosis is the predominant lesion, peripheral vasodilators are of no clinical use and they may lead to hypotension which could be fatal in the severely ill patient because the vasoconstriction, which has maintained blood pressure, is abolished, the cardiac output cannot increase because of the stenotic mitral valve orifice and, as a result, the blood pressure falls disastrously.

In contrast, patients with mitral regurgitation of whatever aetiology often undergo considerable haemodynamic and symptomatic improvement on vasodilator therapy for two reasons. First, reduced peripheral vascular resistance decreases left ventricular afterload and therefore some of the left ventricular output destined for the left atrium is re-directed into the peripheral circulation. Second, reduced peripheral resistance reduces left ventricular size and with it 'the effective regurgitant orifice' of the mitral valve.[66] Considerable experience has been acquired with the administration of arterial vasodilators,[67] of which hydralazine, a pure arteriolar dilator, is the most convenient to use. Recently, angiotensin converting enzyme inhibitors, such as captopril and enalapril, have been used effectively in patients with mitral regurgitation.[68] Medication with these agents should be started cautiously in hospital because it can result in severe initial hypotension, especially in severely ill patients, and can also disturb renal function particularly when the patient is already receiving large doses of diuretic agents. Although vasodilators may greatly improve the clinical condition of a patient with mitral regurgitation, their prescription usually indicates that mitral valve replacement should be performed unless contra-indicated for another reason.

Balloon valvuloplasty

Recently, balloon dilatation of the mitral valve has been introduced as a means of treating mitral stenosis.[69-71] Much of the work exploring the potential of this technique has involved co-operation between workers at centres in developed countries who have supplied the necessary technical guidance and workers at centres in underdeveloped countries where mitral stenosis remains common but which have fewer facilities for expert surgical treatment.[70,71] Balloon valvuloplasty has the obvious advantage of being cheaper than surgery, and it can be used in situations where surgery is either not available or not appropriate. Despite these advantages, more experience with this technique is needed before its place in the overall management of mitral stenosis can be defined.

The following technique has been used in most of the studies performed.[70] First, the left atrium is entered by a standard trans-septal puncture with a long sheath lying over the trans-septal catheter. The sheath is left in the left atrium and the trans-septal catheter is withdrawn. An end-hole flow-directed catheter is introduced via the sheath into the left atrium, which is then passed through the stenotic mitral valve to the left ventricle and onwards via the aortic valve to the ascending and finally the descending aorta. Next, a long (400 cm) exchange guidewire is introduced through this catheter, which is then withdrawn together with the trans-septal sheath leaving the wire in place running from its point of insertion in the femoral vein to the descending aorta via the inferior vena cava, right atrium, left atrium, mitral valve, left ventricle, aortic valve and ascending aorta. As the hole made by the trans-septal puncture is usually too small to allow the passage of the large balloon catheters needed to dilate the mitral valve, it has to be enlarged by passing an 8-mm balloon over the wire until it lies across the interatrial septum and inflating it with contrast material. This small balloon is then withdrawn and replaced with a larger balloon catheter, e.g. with a 20 or 25 mm inflated diameter, which is passed over the guidewire until it lies across the mitral valve orifice where it is inflated by hand about 3–4 atmospheres of pressure) several times to dilate the valve. This technique can be modified slightly to allow two balloons to be positioned across the valve which can then be inflated at the same time thereby achieving greater dilatation of the valve.[71]

Initial results with this technique have shown that satisfactory dilatation of the valve is achieved in about 80% of patients who experience a marked improvement in both haemodynamics and symptoms. Surgery is needed in the remaining patients because distortion of the subvalvar appartatus of the mitral valve (chordae tendineae, papillary muscles and adjacent left ventricular wall) is an important part of the stenotic process and cannot be expected to be improved by inflating a balloon in the valve orifice. Increasing experience has shown that an important factor determining success is the use of sufficiently large dilating balloons alone or in combination. In skilled hands, there seems to be remarkably little risk. In the largest series (35 patients) reported to date,[71] there was only one death and this occurred in an elderly patient with very severe mitral stenosis following mitral valve replacement undertaken immediately after balloon valvuloplasty had failed. Successful dilatation causes a mild degree of mitral regurgitation in 40% of patients, but significant regurgitation is rare.[71] The hole produced in the interatrial septum may leave a trivial left-to-right shunt.[71] Another potential complication is the release of a systemic embolus from the left atrium during the procedure. This can be minimized by excluding patients with echocardiographic evidence of left atrial thrombus, by using systemic heparinization during the procedure and by giving anticoagulants to patients with atrial fibrillation for several weeks before the procedure. Complete heart block, which may be either permanent or transient, is another rare complication.

Despite these encouraging initial results, most of the patients treated so far have been highly selected often by using most of the criteria for closed mitral valvotomy, i.e. sinus rhythm, pliable valves and lack of previous embolism. However, good results have been obtained in patients with calcified valves who are in atrial fibrillation,[71] who may have a far higher incidence of complications than has yet been reported for the more highly selected patients who comprise the majority of those treated so far. Before the place of the technique in the management of patients with mitral valve disease can be defined, the results must be compared with those of the established and excellent surgical techniques already available. This caution is particularly pertinent in more elderly patients who may have calcified valves and are in atrial fibrillation because the risks are potentially the greatest and the experience is least in such patients. A reasonable approach is to use the technique as an alternative to closed mitral valvotomy in patients who satisfy all the criteria for the latter procedure and in patients in whom these criteria are not satisfied only if there is a strong contra-indication to surgery, e.g. advanced respiratory disease or other debilitating non-cardiac disease. This cautious attitude may change when more experience is available, particularly in the more complicated type of patient and when there is evidence that the procedure produces acceptable long-term results.

REFERENCES

1. Aravanis, C. and Michaelides, G. Tricuspid insufficiency masquerading as mitral insufficiency in patients with severe mitral stenosis. *Am. J. Cardiol.* 1967; **20**: 417–22.
2. Levine, S.A. and Love, D.E. Mitral stenosis without murmurs. *Cardiologia* 1952; **21**: 598–611.
3. Aravanis, C. Silent Mitral Insufficiency. *Am. Heart J.* 1965; **70**: 620.
4. Erbel, R., Schweizer, P., Bardos, P. and Meyer, J. Two-dimensional echocardiographic diagnosis of papillary muscle rupture. *Chest* 1981; **79**: 595–7.
5. Mintz, G.A., Victor, M.F., Kottler, M.N. *et al.* Two-dimensional echocardiographic identification of surgically correctable complications of acute myocardial infarction. *Circulation* 1981; **64**: 91–6.
6. Drobac, M., Gilbert, D., Howard, R. *et al.* Ventricular septal defect after myocardial infarction. Diagnosis by two-dimensional echocardiography. *Circulation* 1983; **67**: 335–41.
7. Miyatake, K., Okamato, M., Kinnoshita, N. *et al.* Doppler echocardiographic feature of ventricular septal rupture in myocardial infarction. *J. Am. Coll. Cardiol.* 1985; **5**: 182–7.
8. Jennings, K., Evemy, K. and Hunter, S. Cross-sectional echocardiography and exercise testing following myocardial infarction. In: Hunter, S. and Hall, R. (eds) *Echocardiography II.* Edinburgh: Churchill Livingstone, 1984.
9. Meister, S.G. and Helfant, R.H. Rapid bedside differentiation of ruptured intraventricular septum from acute mitral insufficiency. *N. Engl. J. Med.* 1972; **287**: 1029.
10. Gross, R., Strain, J. and Cohen, M.V. Pulmonary arterial V waves in mitral regurgitation: clinical and experimental observations. *Circulation* 1984; **69**: 214–22.
11. Tatooles, C.J., Gault, J.H., Mason, B.T. and Ross Jr, J. Reflux of oxygenated blood into the pulmonary artery in severe mitral regurgitation. *Am. Heart J.* 1968; **75**: 102.
12. Chen, J.T.T., Behar, V.S., Morris, J.J. *et al.* Correlation of roentgen findings with hemodynamic data in pure mitral stenosis. *Am. J. Roentgenol. Radium Ther. Nucl. Med.* 1968; **102**: 280–92.
13. Woodruff, J.H. Calcified heart valves. A comparison of methods for their demonstration. *Radiology* 1962; **79**: 384–8.
14. Roy, S.B., Bhatia, M.L., Lazaro, E.J. and Ramalingaswami, V. Juvenile mitral stenosis in India. *Lancet* 1963; **ii**: 1193–6.
15. Janton, O.H., Heidorn, G. *et al.* The clinical determination of mitral insufficiency when associated with mitral stenosis. *Circulation* 1954; **16**: 207–12.
16. Vickers, C.W., Kincaid, O.W., Ellis, F.H. and Bruwer, A.J. Left atrial calcification. *Radiology* 1959; **72**: 569–75.
17. Lavender, J.P., Doppman, J., Shawdon, H. and Steiner, R.E. Pulmonary veins in left ventricular failure and mitral stenosis. *Br. J. Radiol.* 1962; **35**: 293–302.
18. Anderson, L.H., Johansen, J.K. and Hyldebrandt, N. Regional pulmonary blood flow in mitral disease studied by Xenon radiospirometry. *Br. Heart J.* 1976; **38**: 573–9.
19. Dawson, A., Rocamara, J.M. and Morgan, J.R. Regional lung function in chronic pulmonary congestion with and without mitral stenosis. *Am. Rev. Resp. Dis.* 1976; **113**: 51–9.
20. Aber, C.P., Campbell, J.A. and Meecham, J. Arterial patterns in mitral stenosis. *Br. Heart J.* 1963; **25**: 109–18.
21. Lavender, J.P. and Doppman, J. The hilum in pulmonary venous hypertension. *Br. J. Radiol.* 1962; **35**: 303–13.
22. Melhem, R.E., Dunbar, J.D. and Booth, R.W. 'B' lines of Kerley and left atrial size in mitral valve disease: their correlation with mean left atrial pressure as measured by left atrial puncture. *Radiology* 1961; **76**: 65–9.
23. Galloway, R.W., Epstein, E.J. and Coulshed, N. Pulmonary ossific nodules in mitral valve disease. *Br. Heart J.* 1961; **23**: 297–307.
24. Priest, E.A., Finlayson, J.K. and Short, D.S. The X-ray manifestations in the heart and lungs of mitral regurgitation. *Prog. Cardiovasc. Dis.* 1962; **5**: 219–29.
25. Rios, J.S. and Goo, W. Electrocardiographic correlate of rheumatic valvular disease. In: Likoff, W., ed. *Cardiovascular Clinics, Vol. 5 Valvular Heart Disease.* 1973, p.248.
26. Flowers, N.C. and Horan, L.G. Subtle signs of right ventricular enlargement and their relative importance. In: Sclant, R.C. and Furst, J.W., eds. *Advances in electrocardiography.* New York: Grune and Stratton, 1972, p. 297.
27. Probst, P., Goldschlager, N. and Selzer, A. Left atrial size and atrial fibrillation in mitral stenosis: Factors influencing their relationship. *Circulation* 1973; **48**: 1282.
28. Henry, W.L., Morganroth, J., Pearlman, A.S. *et al.* Relation between echocardiographically determined left atrial size and atrial fibrillation. *Circulation* 1976; **53**: 273–9.
29. Bentoviglio, L.G., Uricchio, J.F., Waldow, A. *et al.* An electrocardiographic analysis of mitral regurgitation. *Circulation* 1956; **18**: 572.
30. Martin, R.P., Rakowski, H., Kleiman, J.H. *et al.* Reliability and reproducibility of two-dimensional echocardiographic measurement of the stenotic mitral valve orifice area. *Am. J. Cardiol.* 1979; **43**: 560–8.
31. Hatle, L., Brubakk, A., Tromsdal, A. and Angelsen, B. Non-invasive assessment of pressure drop in mitral stenosis by Doppler ultrasound. *Circulation* 1978; **40**: 131–40.
32. Dernevik, L., Brorsson, L., Walletin, I. and William-Olsson, G. Improved results of closed commissurotomy for mitral stenosis using ultracardiography as selection ground. *Acta Med. Scand.* 1981; **210**: 283–6.
33. Peterson, K.L. Timing of surgical intervention in chronic mitral regurgitation. *Herz* 1986; **11**: 63–73.
34. Zhang, Y., Ihlen, H., Myhre, E. *et al.* Quantification of mitral regurgitation by Doppler echocardiography. *Eur. Heart J.* 1987; **8** (Suppl. C): 59–62.
35. Pearlman, A.S. and Oho, C.M. The use of Doppler techniques for quantificative evaluation of valvular regurgitation. *Eur. Heart J.* 1987; **8** (Suppl. C): 35–43.
36. Hall, R.J.C., Kadushi, O.A. and Evemy, K. Need for cardiac catheterisation in assessment of patients for valve surgery. *Br. Heart J.* 1983; **49** 268–75.
37. Odemuyiwa, O. and Hall, R.J.C. Assessing the severity of valve stenosis. *Br. Heart J.* 1986; **55**: 117–9.
38. Gorlin, R., Sawyer, C.G., Haynes, F.W. *et al.* Effects of exercise on circulatory dynamics in mitral stenosis III. *Am. Heart J.* 1951; **41**: 192–203.
39. Pizzarello, R.A., Turnier, J. *et al.* Left atrial size, pressure and V wave height in patients with isolated pure mitral regurgitation. *Cathet. Cardiovasc. Diag.* 1984; **10**: 445–54.
40. Traill, T.A., Sutton, M.G. St J. and Gibson, D.G. Mitral stenosis with high left ventricular diastolic pressure. *Br. Heart J.* 1979; **41**: 405–11.
41. Croft, C.H., Lipscomb, K., Mathis, K. *et al.* Limitations of qualitative grading in aortic or mitral regurgitation. *Am. J. Cardiol.* 1984; **53**: 1593–8.
42. Ubago, J.L., Figueroa, A., Colman, T. *et al.* Hemodynamic factors that affect calculated orifice areas in the mitral Hancock xenograft valve. *Circulation* 1980; **61**: 388–94.
43. Klein, H.O., Panzer, H., DiSengi, E. *et al.* The beneficial effects of verapamil in chronic atrial fibrillation. *Arch.*

Intern. Med. 1979; **139**: 747–9.

44. Theissen, K., Haufe, M. *et al.* The effect of the calcium antagonist diltiazem on atrioventricular conduction in chronic atrial fibrillation. *Am. J. Cardiol.* 1985; **55**: 98–102.

45. Klein, H.O., Lang, R., Weiss, E. *et al.* The influence of verapamil on serum digoxin concentration. *Circulation* 1982; **65**: 998–1003.

46. Raeder, E.A., Podrid, P.J. and Lown, B. Side effects and complications of amiodarone therapy. *Am. Heart J.* 1985; **109**: 975–83.

47. Moysey, J.O., Jaggaro, N.S.U., Grundy, E.N. *et al.* Amiodarone increases plasma digoxin concentrations, *Br. Med. J.* 1981; **282**: 272.

48. Darmenta, J.I., van Zandwick, N. *et al.* Amiodarone pneumonitis—three further cases with a review of published reports. *Thorax* 1984; **39**: 57–64.

49. Mancini, G.B.J. and Goldberger, A.L. Cardioversion of atrial fibrillation: consideration on embolization, anticoagulation, prophylactic pacemaker and long term success. *Am. Heart J.* 1982; **104**: 617–21.

50. Henry, W.L., Morganroth, J., Pearlman, A.S. *et al.* Relation between echocardiographically determined left atrial size and atrial fibrillation. *Circulation* 1976; **53**: 273–9.

51. Kleiger, R. and Lown, B. Cardioversion and digitalis. II Clinical studies. *Circulation* 1966; **33**: 878–87.

52. Doering, W. Quinidine–digoxin interaction. Pharmokinetics, underlying mechanism and clinical implications. *N. Engl. J. Med.* 1979; **301**: 400–4.

53. Wood, P.H. *Diseases of the heart and circulation*. London: Eyre and Spottiswood, 1968.

54. Szekely, P. Systemic embolism and anticoagulant prophylaxis in rheumatic heart disease. *Br. Med. J.* 1964; **1**: 209–12.

55. Adams, G.F., Merret, J.D., Hutchinson, W.M. and Pollock, A.M. Cerebral embolism and mitral stenosis: survival with and without anticoagulants. *J. Neurol. Neurosurg. Psychiatr.* 1974; **37**: 378–83.

56. Fleming, H.A. and Bailey, S.M. Mitral valve disease, systemic embolism and anticoagulants. *Postgrad. Med. J.* 1971; **47**: 599–604.

57. Rahimtoola, S.H. Valvular heart disease: a perspective. *J. Am. Coll. Cardiol.* 1983; **1**: 199–215.

58. Edmunds Jr, L.H. Thrombotic complications of current valvular prostheses. *Ann. Thorac. Surg.* 1982; **34**: 96–106.

59. Goodnight, S.H. Antiplatelet therapy for mitral stenosis? *Circulation* 1980; **62**: 466–8.

60. Steele, P. and Rainwater, J. Favorable effect of sulfinpyrazone on thromboembolism in patients with rheumatic heart disease. *Circulation* 1980; **62**: 462–5.

61. Arrants, J.E. and Hairston, P. Use of persantin in preventing thromboembolism following valve replacement. *Am. J. Surg.* 1972; **38**: 432–5.

62. Dale, J., Myhre, E., Storstein, O. *et al.* Prevention of arterial thrombo-embolism with acetylsalicylic acid: a controlled clinical study in patients with aortic ball valves. *Am. Heart J.* 1977; **94**: 101–11.

63. Mok, C.K., Boey, J., Wang, R. *et al.* Warfarin versus dipyridamole–aspirin and pentoxifylline–aspirin for the prevention of prosthetic heart valve thromboembolism: A prospective randomized clinical trial. *Circulation* 1985; **72**: 1059–63.

64. Coulshed, N., Epstein, E.J., McKendrick, C.S. *et al.* Systemic embolism in mitral valve disease. *Br. Heart J.* 1970; **32**: 26–34.

65. Pumphry, C.W., Fuster, V. and Cheseboro, J.H. Systemic thrombo-embolism in valvular heart disease and prosthetic heart valves. *Mod. Concepts Cardiovasc. Dis.* 1982; **51**: 131–136.

66. Yoran, C., Yellin, E.L., Becker, K.R.N. *et al.* Mechanisms of reduction of mitral regurgitation with vasodilator therapy. *Am. J. Cardiol.* 1979; **43**: 773–7.

67. Greenberg, B.H., DeMots, H., Murphy, E. and Rahimtoola, S.H. Arterial dilators in mitral regurgitation: effects on rest and exercise haemodynamics and long term clinical follow-up. *Circulation* 1982; **65**: 181–7.

68. Heck, I., Schmidt, J., Mattern, H. *et al.* Reduktion der regurgitation bei aorten—und mitral insuffizienz durch captopril im akut—und langzeitversuch. *Schweiz. Med. Wschr.* 1985; **115**: 1615–8.

69. Inoue, K., Owani, T., Nakamura, T. *et al.* Clinical application of transvenous mitral commissurotomy by a new balloon catheter. *J. Thorac. Cardiovasc. Surg.* 1984; **87**: 394–402.

70. Lock, J.E., Khalilullah, M., Shrivastava, S., Bahl, V. and Keane, J.F. Percutaneous catheter commissurotomy in rheumatic mitral stenosis. *N. Engl. J. Med.* 1985; **313**: 1515–8.

71. Palacios, I., Block, P.C., Brandi, S. *et al.* Percutaneous balloon valvotomy for patients with severe mitral stenosis. *Circulation* 1987; **75**: 778–84.

Chapter 32

Other Valve Disorders: (a) Tricuspid, Pulmonary and Mixed Lesions, (b) Prosthetic Valves

Roger Hall

ACQUIRED LESIONS OF THE TRICUSPID AND PULMONARY VALVES

TRICUSPID VALVE DISEASE

Organic disease affects the tricuspid valve much less commonly than it does the mitral and aortic valves, but 'functional' tricuspid regurgitation secondary to right ventricular dilatation resulting from pulmonary hypertension of any cause is common. Congenital abnormalities of the tricuspid valve are important and are discussed elsewhere (Chapter 25).

Tricuspid stenosis

Tricuspid stenosis is nearly always rheumatic in origin, but rheumatic tricuspid valve disease is relatively uncommon when compared with rheumatic aortic and mitral valve disease. It is clinically significant in 3–5% of all cases of rheumatic heart disease,[1] although some evidence of organic tricuspid valve disease is found at autopsy in 10–25% of cases.[2] Rheumatic tricuspid valve disease is much more common in women than in men.

Occasionally, a functional stenosis of the tricuspid valve occurs because the valve is obstructed by a primary tumour (e.g. a right atrial myxoma), vegetations or, much more rarely, a sarcoma or a secondary deposit from a tumour, such as a hypernephroma or a thyroid carcinoma. The tricuspid lesion caused by the carcinoid syndrome is often a mixture of stenosis and regurgitation resulting from the valve becoming thickened and fixed in a mid position (Fig. 32.1),[3] and the tricuspid valve can be stenosed when it is involved with a more generalized process such as endomyocardial fibrosis or fibro-elastosis.

Pathology

Rheumatic tricuspid stenosis results from fusion of the commissures between the valve cusps to produce a diaphragm-like structure, which tends to fibrose or calcify to a much lesser degree than a rheumatic mitral or aortic lesion of similar severity. In severe cases, the aperture of the valve is often less than 1 cm.[2]

Pathophysiology

When the tricuspid valve is significantly stenosed, the right atrium hypertrophies and is able to produce a large 'a' wave in the right atrium and the systemic venous pulse which is augmented by inspiration.

A pressure gradient develops across the valve but frequently this is small, and tricuspid stenosis can be regarded as being present when the mean diastolic pressure gradient across the tricuspid valve is as little as 2 mmHg. The right atrial pressure depends upon the severity of stenosis and the right ventricular diastolic pressure. Once the tricuspid valve orifice area falls below 1.3 cm,[2] the mean right atrial pressure is nearly always > 10 mmHg, even in the presence of normal right ventricular pressures; such a pressure is likely to be associated with peripheral oedema and hepatic enlargement.

The restriction of flow through the heart by the stenotic tricuspid valve prevents the cardiac output rising normally with exercise; when the lesion becomes advanced, cardiac output at rest may also be reduced. Tricuspid stenosis frequently occurs in association with significant mitral valve disease and modifies the haemodynamic effects of the mitral lesion by restricting forward flow into the right ventricle and lungs. Consequently, it is unusual for a patient to have severe pulmonary hypertension when significant tricuspid stenosis is present, and pulmonary congestion, haemoptysis and other pulmonary manifestations of mitral stenosis are often less marked than when a mitral lesion of similar severity occurs in isolation.

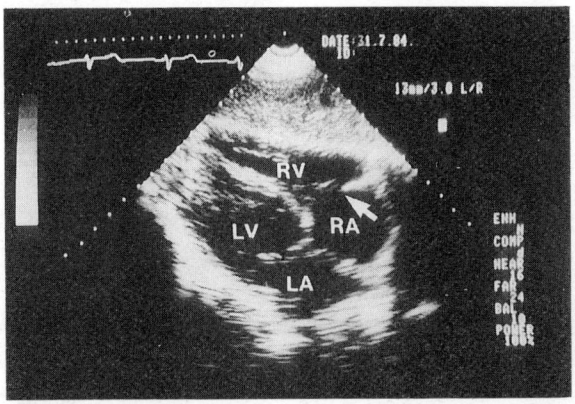

Fig. 32.1. Cross-sectional echocardiogram from a patient with carcinoid heart disease (sub-xiphoid four-chamber view). The tricuspid valve is considerably thickened and stuck in a mid-position throughout the cardiac cycle (arrow). RV, right ventricle; RA, right atrium; LV, left ventricle; LA, left atrium.

Clinical features

The main symptoms of tricuspid stenosis are related to the limitation of forward flow by the tricuspid valve which results in increased tiredness and reduced effort tolerance and venous congestion which causes symptoms related to right-sided heart failure, for example, ankle swelling, hepatic discomfort and abdominal swelling. Venous congestion may also lead to a feeling of uncomfortable fullness and fluttering in the neck and face, particularly on exercise or when bending. The presence of tricuspid stenosis in patients with significant mitral valve disease tends to ameliorate some of the effects of mitral valve disease and, in particular, symptoms such as breathlessness, orthopnoea and paroxysmal dyspnoea that are related to pulmonary congestion.

Owing to the common association of significant mitral valve disease with tricuspid stenosis, the physical signs of significant tricuspid stenosis are often overlooked because they are overshadowed by those of mitral stenosis. The patient is usually in sinus rhythm, but the pulse is often of small volume and the pulse pressure low. Examination of the jugular venous pulse reveals a prominent 'flicking' 'a' wave which may reach the angle of the jaw when the lesion is severe, and there is a slow and often scarcely appreciable 'y' descent.[3,4] When atrial fibrillation develops, the 'a' wave is lost but the slow 'y' descent may still be discernible. Precordial palpation in tricuspid stenosis is often unremarkable, but occasionally pulsation due to the huge right atrium can be felt over the right precordium and a mid-diastolic thrill accompanying the mur-

mur of tricuspid stenosis may also be present at this site. Palpation over the liver may reveal a pre-systolic impulse, coinciding with the 'a' wave, in severe cases. Frequently, the palpatory features of associated mitral stenosis are present.[5]

On auscultation, a mid-diastolic murmur is heard in the tricuspid area or at the lower left sternal edge. This murmur may have a rumbling quality, like that of mitral stenosis, but it is often of a higher frequency and may be scratchy; it is increased by inspiration and frequently shows pre-systolic accentuation when the patient is in sinus rhythm.[1,2,4,6] The first heart sound is often split due to delay of the tricuspid component; the second heart sound may be relatively soft. An opening snap may be present, which it is usually difficult to distinguish from that of mitral stenosis although it occurs slightly later[4,7] and may be more prominent to the right of the lower part of the sternum.

Investigations

Electrocardiogram The only characteristic electrocardiographic finding in tricuspid stenosis is evidence of right atrial hypertrophy. This is revealed by tall sharply peaked P waves (3 mm or more in height) best seen in leads II, III, aVF and V_1 (Fig. 32.2).[4,6,7] The QRS complex is more often of small amplitude but otherwise normal unless influenced by associated mitral valve disease.

Chest X-ray The characteristic feature of tricuspid stenosis is marked enlargement of the right atrium, although changes associated with mitral valve disease are common (Fig. 32.3).

Echocardiography and Doppler The main echocardiographic changes in tricuspid valve disease are described in Chapter 13. Often, the tricuspid valve is difficult to image using M-mode echocardiography (Fig. 32.4), but it can usually be seen using the cross-sectional technique.[8] Usually, the best views are obtained from the apical or subcostal approach, although frequently only two of the cusps (anterior and septal) can be seen. The detection of thickening and limitation of cusp movement is not specific to rheumatic tricuspid valve disease, but the detection of a tricuspid valve with a restricted and a doming movement towards the right ventricle in diastole makes the diagnosis likely (Fig. 32.5). Other causes of thickening of the tricuspid valve often have different appearances, for example, the carcinoid syndrome produces thickened and immobile tricus-

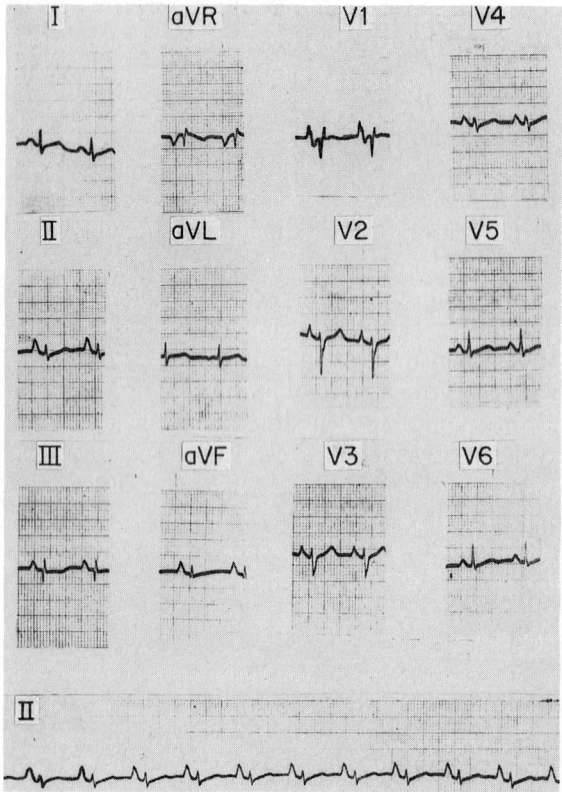

Fig. 32.2. Electrocardiogram from a patient with tricuspid stenosis. This trace demonstrates severe right atrial hypertrophy demonstrated by the sharp upright P waves particularly noticeable in leads II and V_1. In lead II, the P wave is more than 4 mm in height. There are no other significant abnormalities in the electrocardiogram. The electrocardiogram was recorded at a normal standardization, i.e. 10 mm = 1 mV.

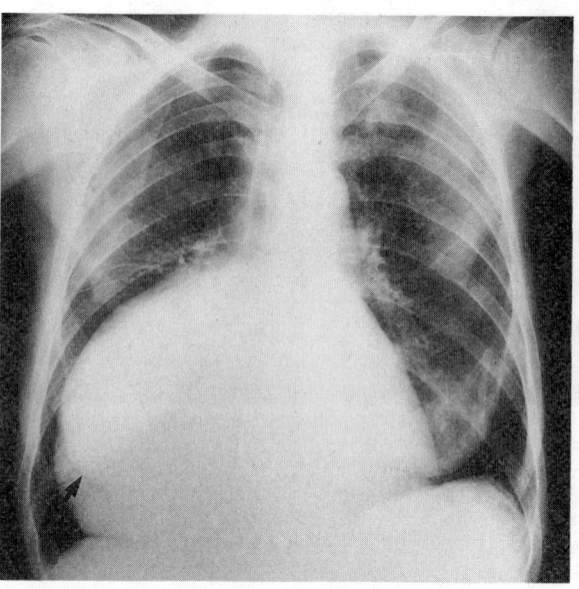

Fig. 32.3. Chest X-ray showing gross right atrial enlargement in a patient with tricuspid valve disease. The apparent double shadow (arrow) in the left lower part of the chest X-ray is due to a breast shadow superimposed on the cardiac shadow and not left atrial enlargement.

pid valve leaflets which appear to be stuck in a mid-position rather than showing diastolic doming (Fig. 32.1).[3] The severity of tricuspid stenosis is best defined using the Doppler technique (Fig. 32.4). Although experience with the Doppler technique in this condition is limited because of its low incidence, the available information suggests there is a good correlation between pressure gradients obtained using the Doppler technique and those obtained with cardiac catheterization.[9,10]

Cardiac catheterization

Simultaneous measurement of pressure in the right atrium and pressure in the right ventricle reveals the diastolic pressure difference across the tricuspid valve, which is often small. When it exceeds 2 mmHg, some degree of tricuspid stenosis is usually present. These small pressure differences require accurate measurement which can be difficult.

Perhaps the best technique is to insert two catheters into the right atrium and ascertain whether they record identical pressures at this site. One is then advanced into the right ventricle and the pressure gradient between the two is measured. Severe stenosis, i.e. a valve area is $< 1\text{cm}^2$, usually leads to a mean gradient > 5 mmHg. The gradient across the valve is increased by inspiration and also on exercise,[1,5] both of which increase flow across the valve. As is the case with all mixed stenotic and regurgitant lesions, associated tricuspid regurgitation increases the diastolic gradient because, in addition to the forward cardiac output, the blood regurgitated during the previous systole has to return to the right ventricle during the next diastole. Calculation of tricuspid valve area is usually done using the Gorlin formula and constants initially derived for the mitral valve. The reliability of applying such assumptions to the tricuspid valve is unproven (and never likely to be proved).

Injection of contrast into the right atrium will reveal enormous enlargement of the chamber, thickening of the tricuspid valve and a thin jet of contrast entering the right ventricle via the stenotic orifice during diastole.

Management

Diuretic therapy will help to eliminate the retained

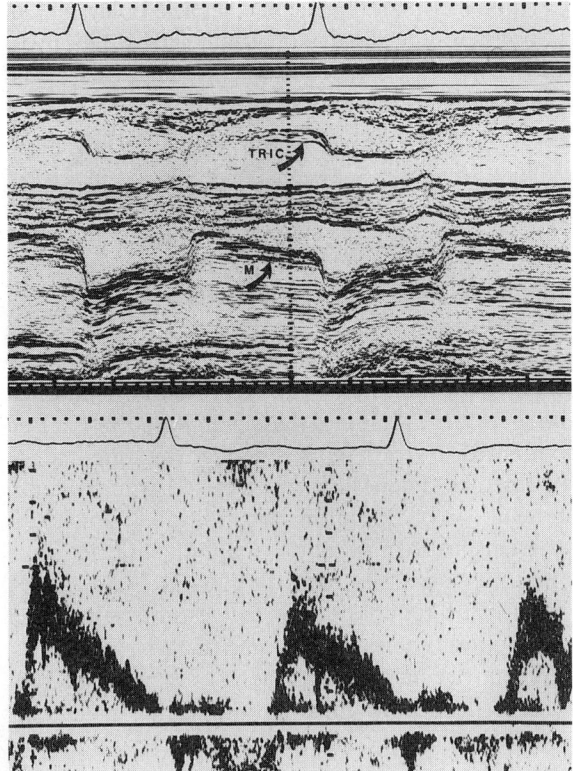

Fig. 32.4. Upper panel: M-mode echocardiogram from a patient with mitral and tricuspid stenosis. The movement of the mitral (M) and tricuspid (TRIC) valve cusps (arrows) are similar. Lower panel: Continuous wave Doppler recording from the same patient recorded across the tricuspid valve. There is a significant gradient in early and mid-diastole but by end-diastole the gradient has fallen to zero. These Doppler findings are consistent with moderate tricuspid stenosis. The peak velocity of the tricuspid valve is only 1 m/s but the rate of decline of velocity is much slower than normal.

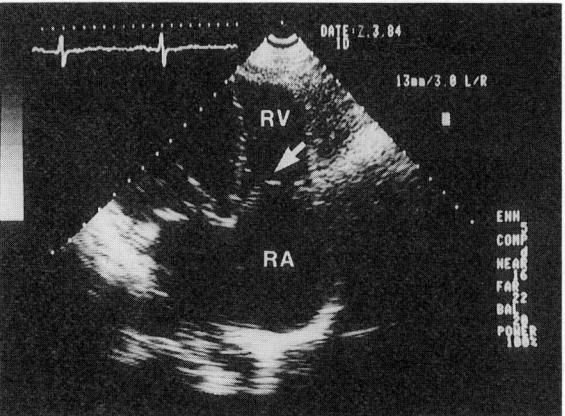

Fig. 32.5. Cross-sectional echocardiogram from a patient with rheumatic tricuspid stenosis (apical four-chamber view). The tricuspid valve can be seen doming (arrow). This recording was taken towards the end of diastole. RA, right atrium; RV, right ventricle.

fluid, and arrhythmias are managed in the same way as those in mitral valve disease. If the tricuspid valve lesion is severe, surgery is needed and usually tricuspid valve replacement has to be performed.[11] Open commissurotomy is occasionally successful but is often an unsatisfactory procedure. In general, a pressure gradient across the tricuspid valve of 5 mmHg or a tricuspid valve orifice estimated as $< 2\text{cm}^2$ is sufficient to indicate the need for surgery. Tricuspid lesions alone only rarely necessitate surgery, and most operations on the tricuspid valves are performed at the same time as surgery for other valve lesions, particularly those affecting the mitral valve.

Tricuspid regurgitation

Isolated organic disease of the tricuspid valve causing regurgitation is extremely rare, but it may be seen in carcinoid heart disease,[3] in infective endocarditis and following trauma.[12] Generally, isolated tricuspid regurgitation can occur to myxomatous changes in the structure of the tricuspid valve associated with Marfan's syndrome or in patients with tricuspid valve prolapse,[13] but it is rarely very severe in such cases.

The majority of cases of tricuspid regurgitation are 'functional'. They occur secondary to right ventricular dilatation which in turn increases the size of the tricuspid valve annulus. Any cardiac or pulmonary condition that imposes a load on the right ventricle by producing an increased pulmonary vascular resistance can cause tricuspid regurgitation, and, in addition, but more rarely, other causes of right ventricular dilatation have the same effect, for example, right ventricular infarction,[14,15] cardiomyopathy and congenital abnormalities (e.g. Uhl's anomaly).

Pathology and pathophysiology

Organic lesions of the tricuspid valve cause regurgitation because damaged tricuspid valve leaflets are unable to coapt properly. The right ventricular volume overload produced by tricuspid regurgitation causes further dilatation of the tricuspid valve ring as a secondary event. When tricuspid regurgitation is functional, regurgitation occurs because the normal tricuspid valve leaflets are unable to coapt properly due to the dilatation of the valve ring supporting them. Furthermore, reduced ventricular contractility decreases the amount of systolic reduction in tricuspid annulus area that normally occurs. The severity of tricuspid regurgitation depends on the degree to which the diameter of the tricuspid annulus is increased in systole, the contractility of the right ventricle and the relative impedance imposed on the right ventricle by the pulmonary circuit and the regurgitant tricuspid valve. Changes in pulmonary vascular resistance can produce marked changes in the amount of tricuspid regurgitation. For example, if pulmonary vascular resistance increases on exercise or during an episode of pulmonary infection or infarction, the amount of tricuspid regurgitation increases considerably. By contrast, tricuspid regurgitation occurring during an episode of fluid retention may resolve once the fluid retention has been treated successfully by medical means.[16] Furthermore, successful correction of mitral valve lesions by surgery often leads to a complete resolution of functional tricuspid regurgitation. When tricuspid regurgitation is severe, the regurgitant flow across the tricuspid valve may greatly exceed forward flow. Consequently the cardiac output can be reduced despite an increase in the output of the right ventricle by as much as 50% above normal.[17] Tricuspid regurgitation leads to dilatation of the right atrium, distension of the great veins and liver engorgement, resulting in disturbed liver function and cardiac cirrhosis. Considerable venous back-pressure is generated which promotes the formation of peripheral oedema, pleural effusions and ascites.

Clinical features

When tricuspid regurgitation occurs in isolation, symptoms are related to inadequate forward flow and to the effects of a greatly increased venous pressure. The main symptoms are tiredness on exertion, peripheral oedema, hepatic enlargement, leading to abdominal pains which may be aggravated by exercise, and also anorexia, nausea and vomiting due to gastro-intestinal engorgement. Uncomfortable abdominal swelling due to ascites occurs and some patients experience unpleasant facial congestion, particularly when bending over, which is due to the very high venous pressure. A few patients develop dyspnoea, not as a result of pulmonary congestion but secondary to large pleural effusions or ascites.

Far more often, pulmonary regurgitation is functional and, although the symptoms mentioned above are troublesome, the clinical picture is often dominated by pulmonary congestion due to the left-sided cardiac lesion which is the primary cause of the underlying pulmonary condition. Occasionally, tricuspid regurgitation may ameliorate these symptoms because forward flow into the lungs, which leads to pulmonary congestion, is reduced once pulmonary regurgitation occurs.

When tricuspid regurgitation is advanced, there is a loss of lean body mass although the weight may change little as fluid accumulation makes up for this loss. Patients may be cachetic, jaundice occurs as a result of liver congestion and cyanosis is also common. At least 80% of cases are in atrial fibrillation with a pulse which is of normal character but small in volume.

The most striking, and diagnostic, feature in the cardiac examination is the presence of systolic pulsation in the jugular veins. The normal 'x' descent disappears and is replaced by a prominent systolic ('cv') wave which has a very sharp 'y' descent (Fig. 32.6). This is also transmitted to the liver which is enlarged and pulsates in systole. Precordial palpation usually reveals a parasternal heave due to an enlarged right ventricle, and systolic

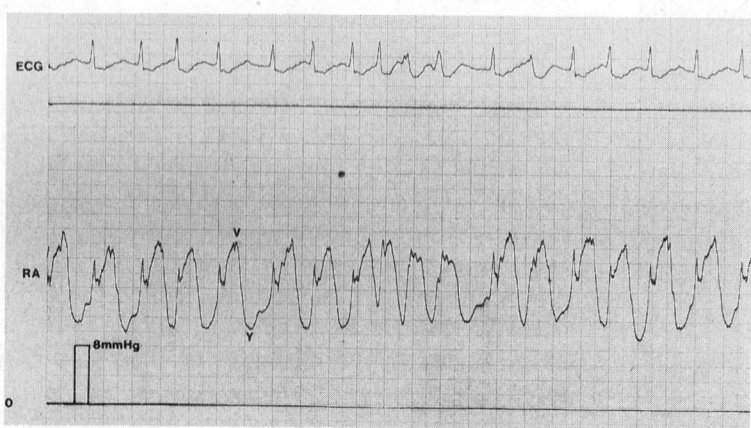

Fig. 32.6. Pressure trace from the right atrium of a patient with tricuspid regurgitation. Note the prominent 'v' wave and the sharp 'y' descent. The peak of the 'v' wave is approximately 20 mmHg.

pulsation may also be detectable at the right sternal edge due to systolic expansion of the right atrium.[17] a systolic thrill may be present in the tricuspid area but this is unusual.

The characteristic murmur of tricuspid regurgitation is pan-systolic and usually best heard to the left of the sternum in the fourth intercostal space. The murmur often increases in intensity with inspiration and occasionally is heard only on inspiration. Once atrial fibrillation develops, there may be a considerable variation in the intensity of the murmur from cycle to cycle. In some patients with severe tricuspid regurgitation, *no murmur* is audible and the diagnosis is made solely on the abnormalities seen in the venous pulse. A mid-diastolic murmur and a third heart sound originating from the right ventricle are often heard at the left sternal border when regurgitation is severe. In patients with slight tricuspid regurgitation, the systolic murmur may be heard only in early systole.

Ascites is frequently present and may be gross, peripheral oedema is usual in patients with moderate or severe regurgitation and pleural effusions are common.

Investigations

Electrocardiogram Tricuspid regurgitation does not produce any characteristic alterations in the electrocardiogram. The main changes usually relate to the primary process leading to functional tricuspid regurgitation.

Chest X-ray The chest X-ray findings in tricuspid regurgitation reflect the volume load on the right heart, with evidence of considerable right ventricular and right atrial enlargement (Fig. 32.3).

Echocardiography and Doppler The characteristic echocardiographic features of tricuspid regurgitation are discussed in detail in Chapter 13. When tricuspid regurgitation of whatever cause occurs, the echocardiogram reveals right ventricular dilatation and septal motion is usually reversed (Fig. 32.7).[18,19] These changes are non-specific and can be seen in any of the other causes of right ventricular volume overload, for example, atrial septal defect (Fig. 32.8).

In functional tricuspid regurgitation, the valve cusps, if visualized, usually appear as normal. When tricuspid regurgitation is organic, the echocardiogram may reveal the cause, for example, vegetations in infective endocarditis (Fig. 32.9), a congenital abnormality of the tricuspid valve, such as Ebstein's anomaly, or thickening of the valve due to rheumatic involvement or the carcinoid syndrome. Among patients with rheumatic heart disease in whom echocardiographic thickening of the tricuspid valve is detected, approximately 75% will have tricuspid regurgitation alone and only 20% will have significant tricuspid stenosis.[8] Occasionally, tricuspid valve prolapse is detectable, but it should be remembered that the diagnostic criteria for this condition are even less well defined than those for mitral valve prolapse (Chapter 29) and this diagnosis should be made only with extreme caution.

As the features of tricuspid regurgitation detected by conventional echocardiography are non-specific, other techniques have been employed to improve diagnosis. Contrast echocardiography has been used widely,[20,21] but it can be difficult to interpret and occasionally significant degrees of regurgitation may be missed. The most important advance in the assessment of tricuspid regurgitation was the introduction of the Doppler technique (Fig. 32.10).[21] This method is highly sensitive in detecting tricuspid regurgitation; it has shown that mild degrees of tricuspid regurgitation are extremely common even in normal subjects. The assessment of the severity of tricuspid regurgitation may be very difficult. At present, the best guides to severity are the intensity of the regurgitant signal and the distance which turbulence can be traced back into the proximal chamber (the right atrium) using the pulsed mode. If tricuspid regurgitation is present, the Doppler technique can be used to assess right ventricular systolic pressure (Fig. 32.10) which may assist in the distinction between organic or functional tricuspid regurgitation. Regurgitation occurring in the presence of a normal right ventricular systolic pressure is nearly always organic, but if the right ventricular systolic pressure is elevated regurgitation may be either functional or organic.

Cardiac catheterization If tricuspid regurgitation is haemodynamically important, the right atrial pressure is always increased substantially with a prominent systolic pressure wave (Fig. 32.6). The right ventricular end-diastolic pressure is raised in most cases of tricuspid regurgitation whether organic or functional in origin. The right atrial pressure is often seen to rise with inspiration and, on exercise, it fails to fall, as it does in normal subjects, but stays at the same level or increases.[22] When tricuspid regurgitation is extremely severe, the pressure tracing in the right atrium may resemble

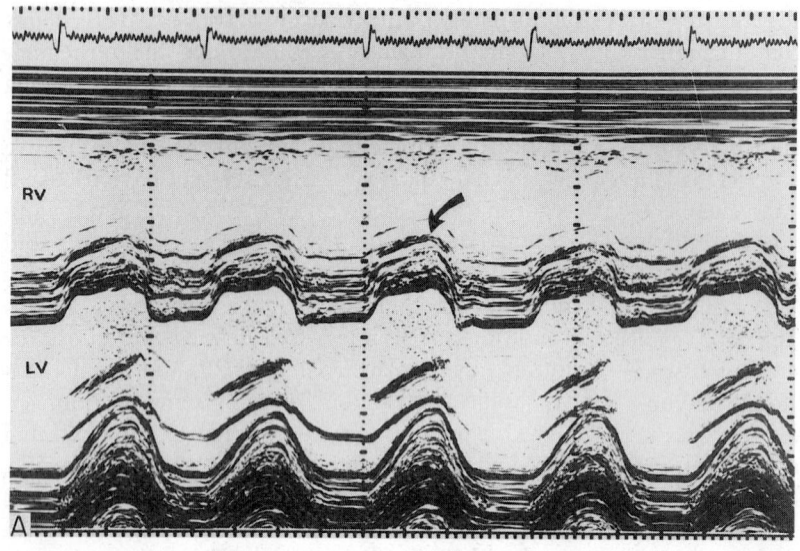

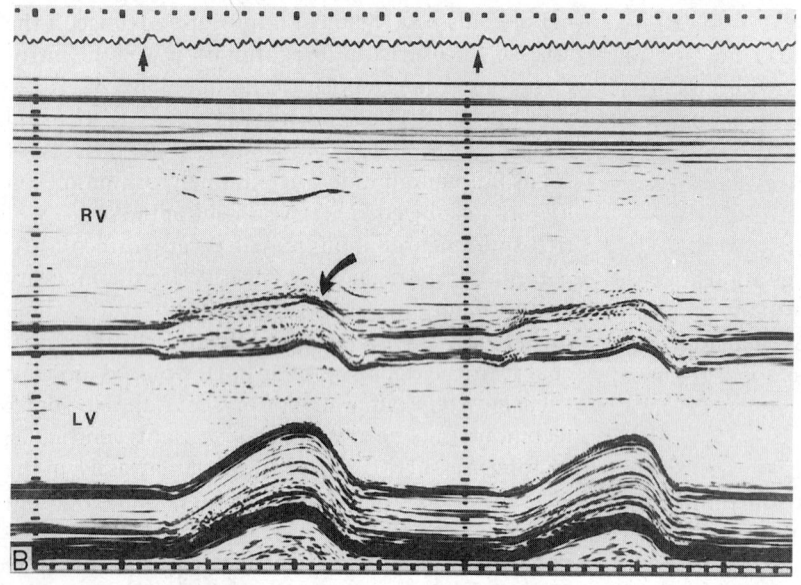

Fig. 32.7. M-Mode echocardiograms from patients with tricuspid regurgitation. Note that the septum moves paradoxically in both cases. At the point shown by the curved arrows, the septum should be moving posteriorly, i.e. inwards towards the left ventricle at the same time as the posterior wall moves inward. There is also right ventricular enlargement which is more marked in (B) than in (A). The small arrows in (B) denote the onset of the QRS which is not shown particularly clearly on the electrocardiogram. RV, right ventricle; LV, left ventricle.

that in the right ventricle.[23,24] Although right ventricular angiography reveals whether significant tricuspid regurgitation is present, this technique is rarely required because the diagnosis can usually be based on clinical findings, the Doppler assessment and the prominent 'v' wave in the right atrium. As the angiographic catheter has to traverse the tricuspid valve to enter the right ventricle, spurious tricuspid regurgitation may occur although it is often slight.

Management

Isolated organic tricuspid regurgitation, even when quite severe, is often well tolerated, for example in drug addicts with tricuspid valve endocarditis. These patients may have reasonable exercise tolerance even after the tricuspid valve has been excised, rather than replaced, to eradicate infection. Generally, however, mild-to-moderate organic tricuspid regurgitation leads to some fluid accumulation in the form of ascites and peripheral oedema, which can usually be eliminated with diuretic therapy. If the patient is in atrial fibrillation, digitalis is also required. If such measures fail to control the patient's symptoms, tricuspid valve replacement may be required.

Functional tricuspid regurgitation frequently resolves if the primary cause is treated successfully. If

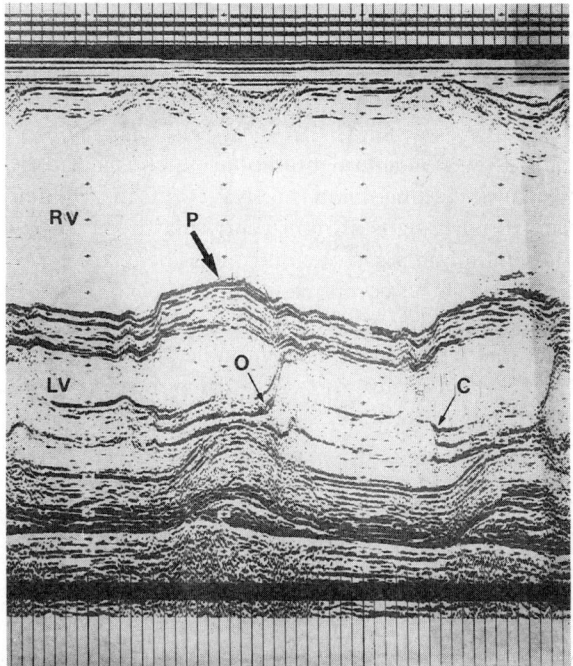

Fig. 32.8. M-Mode echocardiogram from a patient with an atrial septal defect. The right ventricle (RV) is grossly enlarged whereas the left ventricle (LV) is of normal size. There is paradoxical septal motion (P). This is similar to the paradoxical septal motion seen in tricuspid regurgitation and shown in Fig. 32.7, although the right ventricular dilatation is more marked. There is no electrocardiogram on this trace and for this reason the beginning (O) and end (C) of diastole are shown to allow timing of events.

mitral valve surgery is being undertaken in a patient who also has functional tricuspid regurgitation, a tricuspid annuloplasty may reduce or abolish the tricuspid regurgitation and facilitate post-operative recovery. If tricuspid annuloplasty is not done but mitral valve surgery is successful, the right ventricular size decreases steadily following operation and the tricuspid valve often becomes competent again within a few weeks.

In patients in whom functional tricuspid regurgitation is due to left ventricular dysfunction other than mitral valve disease, the regurgitation may disappear if left ventricular failure can be ameliorated satisfactorily with diuretics, digitalis and vasodilators; surgery to the tricuspid valve is never undertaken because it is unlikely to be successful while the primary cause persists and furthermore it might exacerbate symptoms by increasing right ventricular ejection into the lungs. Sometimes, the regression and disappearance of functional tricuspid regurgitation is an important turning point in the recovery of patients with cardiac failure because once the tricuspid valve becomes competent, cardiac output increases and consequently the remaining oedema is more easily dispersed once renal perfusion has improved.

ACQUIRED PULMONARY VALVE DISEASE

Acquired pulmonary valve disease is uncommon and only rarely of clinical significance. By contrast, pulmonary stenosis is one of the commonest congenital heart lesions, and although it is nearly always detected in childhood occasional cases present in adult life.

Acquired pulmonary stenosis and right ventricular outflow obstruction

Obstruction to right ventricular outflow at the

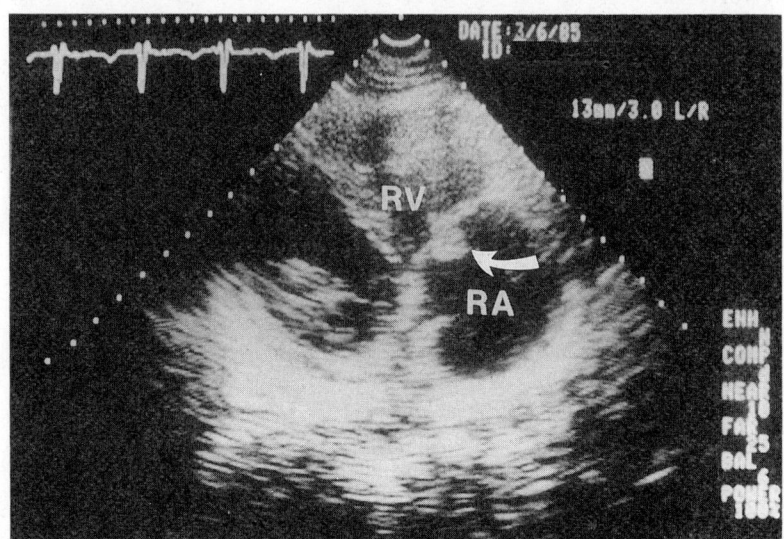

Fig. 32.9. Cross-sectional echocardiogram from a patient with infective endocarditis involving the tricuspid valve. This is an oblique apical view showing the right ventricle (RV) and right atrium (RA) clearly. There is a large vegetation on the tricuspid valve (arrowed). The tricuspid valve is closed because this recording was obtained during systole.

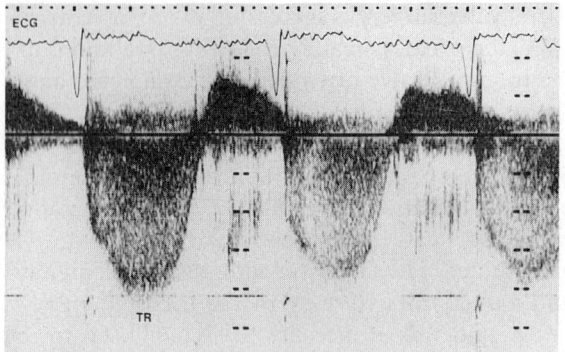

Fig. 32.10. Continuous wave Doppler recording in a patient with severe functional tricuspid regurgitation (TR) (secondary to mitral stenosis). The regurgitant jet has a velocity of approximately 4 m/s giving a systolic gradient of 64 mmHg ($4V^2$) between the right ventricle and right atrium during systole. The right atrial pressure at this time was 10 mmHg. Therefore, the right ventricular systolic pressure and thus the pulmonary artery pressure was approximately 74 mmHg.

pulmonary valve level is extremely rare and rheumatic pulmonary valve disease is very uncommon. The most frequent cause is carcinoid heart disease. In this condition, fibrotic tissue involves the outflow tract to the right ventricle and the pulmonary valve ring, with fusion and retraction of the valve cusps leading to right ventricular outflow obstruction. In addition, the tricuspid valve is often involved and may be both stenotic and regurgitant. These pulmonary and tricuspid valve lesions often result in marked right heart failure, but right heart failure can also occur in the absence of severe valve lesions because of fibrosis of the endocardium and myocardium of the right ventricle and right atrium.[3]

Other rare causes of right ventricular outflow obstruction at or around the pulmonary valve can occur[25–33] and are summarized in Table 32.1. Occasionally, in such conditions, acquired pulmon-

---

Table 32.1.   Causes of acquired right ventricular outflow obstruction.

Intrinsic
Thickened, immobilized valve (e.g. carcinoid, calcification in renal failure)
Pulmonary/right ventricular emboli
Vegetations
Intracardiac tumours, e.g. right ventricular myxoma

Extrinsic compression
Mediastinal tumours and glands (e.g. carcinoma of bronchus and lymphoma)
Pericardial tumours (e.g. mesothelioma)
Aortic aneurysm

---

ary stenosis is the dominant clinical feature but more often it is overshadowed by other more prominent clinical features of the particular condition. The physical signs depend on the severity of the pulmonary stenosis; if it is severe, most of the features of congenital pulmonary stenosis will be present including giant 'a' waves in the jugular venous pulse, signs of right ventricular hypertrophy and a pulmonary systolic murmur. The character of the pulmonary component of the second heart sound, its timing and the presence of a pulmonary ejection sound are all very variable and depend on the level and nature of the obstruction to the right ventricular outflow.

Diagnosis and investigation

The possibility of acquired pulmonary stenosis and right ventricular outflow obstruction is usually suggested by the unexpected finding of clinical and electrocardiographic features of right ventricular hypertrophy and a systolic murmur in the pulmonary area. The chest X-ray usually has no distinctive features but it may reveal the primary process, for example, a mediastinal tumour or aortic aneurysm.

Ultrasound may be very helpful. Many cases of acquired right ventricular outflow obstruction in adults are secondary to other conditions and cross-sectional echocardiography may reveal the primary condition, e.g. a large vegetation on the pulmonary valve, a mass in the right ventricular outflow tract or evidence of extrinsic pressure narrowing the right ventricular outflow or pulmonary arteries. Whatever the cause of right ventricular outflow obstruction, the cross-sectional echocardiogram will show right ventricular hypertrophy. This may be extreme if the cause of right ventricular outflow obstruction is hypertrophic cardiomyopathy.[11] When the underlying condition involves the pulmonary valve, the abnormality is usually detected, for example, in the carcinoid syndrome, the pulmonary valve cusps are frequently thickened and immobile and appear to be fixed in a half-open position. Doppler ultrasound is also very helpful;[34,35] regardless of the cause of outflow obstruction, it will reveal an increased velocity of flow across the obstruction from which the severity can be calculated using the modified Bernoulli equation (Fig. 32.11). Furthermore, associated tricuspid or pulmonary regurgitation allows an indirect assessment of right ventricular pressure and pulmonary artery pressure (Fig. 32.10).

Cardiac catheterization may be needed to confirm

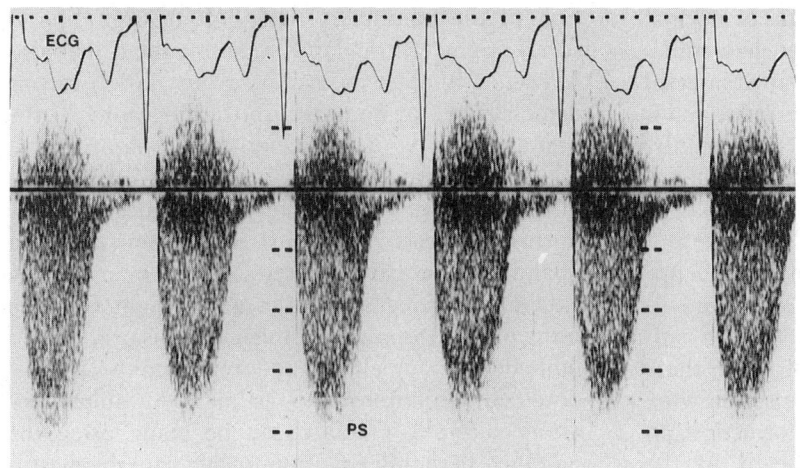

Fig. 32.11. Continuous wave Doppler recording obtained from the left parasternal region in a patient with pulmonary stenosis. The peak velocity (PS) is approximately 4 m/s which is equivalent to a gradient of 64 mmHg acorss the patient (pressure gradient $= 4V^2$).

the pressure gradient across the right ventricular outflow tract, although when an intracardiac tumour is suspected considerable care should be taken in case catheter manipulation displaces tumour tissue in such a way as to worsen obstruction of the right ventricular outflow tract or some of the tumour embolizes into the pulmonary arteries. If inadequate ultrasound images are available, angiography may be needed to define the precise anatomical site of obstruction.

Management

The treatment of acquired pulmonary stenosis depends on the underlying disorder. Thus, appropriate therapy for infective endocarditis, pulmonary embolism and a compressing tumour may cause the degree of stenosis to lessen but occasionally surgical relief of the obstruction may be helpful, for example, in carcinoid heart disease or with certain types of tumour.

Acquired pulmonary regurgitation

Recently, the use of the Doppler technique has revealed that mild pulmonary regurgitation is relatively common in normal subjects. This mild pulmonary regurgitation does not lead to any abnormal physical signs and it is of no clinical importance. Pulmonary regurgitation secondary to dilatation of the pulmonary valve ring is common in patients with pulmonary hypertension *due to any cause*, but it may also occur when dilatation of the pulmonary valve ring occurs in the absence of pulmonary hypertension, for example, idiopathic dilatation of the pulmonary trunk[36-39] which has

been regarded as a forme fruste of Marfan's syndrome.[40] Pulmonary regurgitation can also occur as a result of absent, fenestrated or supernumary pulmonary valve leaflets,[40] anomalies usually associated with other congenital lesions of which Fallot's tetralogy is the most important. Other causes of pulmonary regurgitation in the absence of pulmonary hypertension are infective endocarditis,[42] particularly in drug addicts, and, extremely rarely, rheumatic involvement of the pulmonary valve.[43] Quite frequently, a minor degree of pulmonary regurgitation is present after surgery on the pulmonary valve, particularly following corrections of complex congenital heart lesions such as Fallot's tetralogy. In most cases, pulmonary regurgitation does not impose an important burden on the circulation, but if it is severe it may contribute to the development of right ventricular failure and lead to functional tricuspid regurgitation.

Generally, the clinical picture is dominated by co-existing disorders, of which pulmonary hypertension is the most common. The commonest physical finding is a pulmonary diastolic murmur, the features of which differ depending on whether the regurgitation is associated with pulmonary hypertension, but which, regardless of cause, is accentuated by inspiration.[44] The Graham Steell murmur, which is characteristic of pulmonary hypertension, is usually of high frequency, begins with the second heart sound and progressively diminishes thereafter,[45] and although usually loudest in the pulmonary area it can easily be confused with the murmur of aortic regurgitation. Use of the Doppler technique distinguishes between the two conditions. The diastolic murmur of pulmonary regurgitation occurring with a normal pulmonary artery pressure has different characteristics. There is often a short but definite interval between the second heart sound and its onset and it is predominantly mid diastolic. Occasionally, however, it closely follows the pulmonary component of the second heart sound and has a crescendo–decrescendo configuration. It is often of a medium frequency, unlike the high-frequency murmur of pulmonary regurgitation secondary to pulmonary hypertension. If systolic flow is sufficiently high across the pulmonary valve or if there is a minor degree of stenosis, for example, following surgery for right ventricular outflow obstruction, an ejection systolic murmur is also heard in the pulmonary area. This type of murmur is unusual when regurgitation is minor and particularly when it results from pulmonary hypertension.

When pulmonary regurgitation is severe, other physical signs may develop. The jugular venous pressure will usually reveal a striking 'a' wave produced by forceful right atrial contraction occurring against the impedance of the hypertrophied right ventricle. If sufficient right ventricular dilatation occurs to cause tricuspid regurgitation, the characteristic physical signs of the latter will also occur.

In patients with idiopathic dilatation of the pulmonary artery, an ejection click in early systole is characteristic and precedes the pulmonary systolic murmur. A similar ejection sound is frequently heard in patients with pulmonary hypertension of any aetiology.

Diagnosis and investigation

Pulmonary regurgitation is usually suspected from the presence of an early diastolic murmur heard in the pulmonary area and confirmed using the Doppler technique. If the underlying cause is pulmonary hypertension, the electrocardiogram often reveals right ventricular hypertrophy. In the absence of pulmonary hypertension, the electrocardiographic appearances may be those of 'partial right bundle branch block'. The commonest feature on the chest X-ray is dilatation of the main pulmonary artery; when the lesion is severe, there may be evidence of right ventricular enlargement. Other radiological features reflect concomitant lesions.

Echocardiography (see also Chapter 13) will reveal increased pulmonary artery dimensions[27] when pulmonary regurgitation is secondary to either pulmonary hypertension or idiopathic dilata-

tion of the pulmonary artery; if regurgitation is severe, right ventricular volume overload will also be seen. Although pulmonary regurgitation can be demonstrated by contrast echocardiography,[47] it is best detected with the Doppler technique,[34,48,49] which is extremely sensitive and capable of detecting minor degrees of pulmonary regurgitation in normal subjects. Attempts have been made to quantify pulmonary regurgitation by mapping the extent of the regurgitant jet in the right ventricle using pulsed Doppler, but the method is probably of limited accuracy. If a good regurgitant signal is obtained, a non-invasive estimate of pulmonary artery diastolic pressure can be made using the modified Bernoulli equation to calculate the diastolic pressure difference between pulmonary artery and right ventricle (Fig. 32.12).[34] Cardiac catheterization is rarely necessary in cases of pulmonary regurgitation; however, if it is undertaken, pulmonary regurgitation secondary to pulmonary hypertension is usually found to be associated with systolic pulmonary artery pressures > 70 mmHg. If pulmonary regurgitation is severe, the pulmonary artery diastolic pressure will be low and may even approach the right ventricular end-diastolic pressure (which is raised).

Management

Pulmonary regurgitation seldom requires treatment in its own right. The relief of pulmonary hypertension, for example, by mitral valve surgery, usually corrects or reduces the degree of pulmonary regurgitation. Occasionally, pulmonary valve replacement may be justified in patients in whom pulmonary regurgitation is sufficiently severe to produce right-sided heart failure.[50]

COMBINED VALVULAR LESIONS

Lesions of more than one cardiac valve often occur in rheumatic heart disease but they may also be seen in other conditions, such as infective endocarditis, certain varieties of congenital heart disease and some connective tissue disorders. The description that follows relates mainly to chronic rheumatic heart disease but the underlying principles can be applied to valve diseases of any type occurring in combination. References 51–55 refer generally to mixed valve lesions and contain useful information about these conditions.

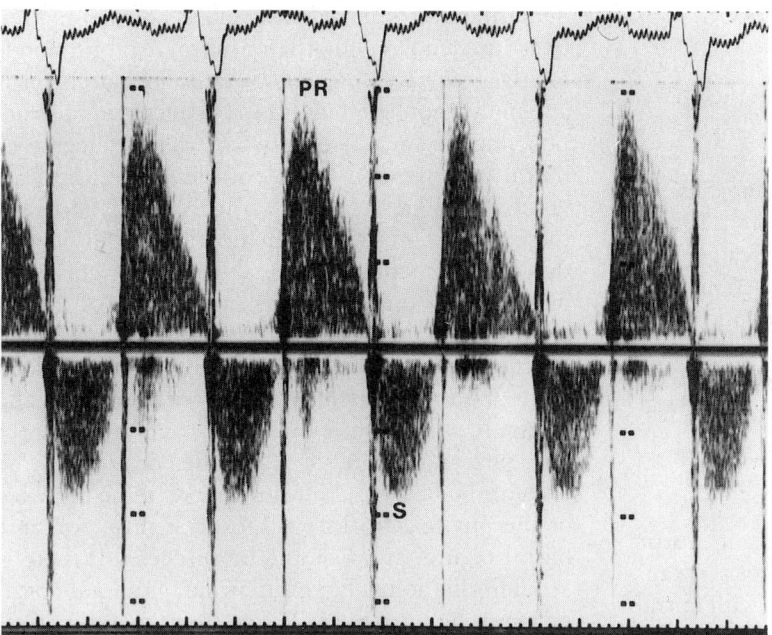

Fig. 32.12. Continuous wave Doppler recordings obtained from the left parasternal region in a patient with pulmonary regurgitation (PR). The systolic velocity across the pulmonary valve (S) is slightly increased (approximately 2 m/s). This is owing to the increased flow back across the pulmonary valve in systole due to the regurgitation. The peak velocity of pulmonary regurgitation is high (approximately 3 m/s). In this patient at the beginning of diastole, there is a pressure difference between the pulmonary artery and right ventricle of approximately 36 mmHg suggesting mild-to-moderate pulmonary hypertension. This was confirmed at cardiac catheterization.

MITRAL STENOSIS AND AORTIC REGURGITATION

Mild-to-moderate aortic regurgitation complicates a high proportion of cases of rheumatic mitral valve disease. Indeed, a soft aortic diastolic murmur can be heard in about 75% of all cases of rheumatic mitral valve disease; however, only in about 10% is the aortic regurgitation of sufficient severity to be a major factor in the overall clinical situation.[51]

Mild aortic regurgitation leading to a soft early diastolic murmur at the left sternal edge is most often confused with the murmur of pulmonary regurgitation but the latter is unlikely to occur in the absence of severe pulmonary hypertension. Use of the Doppler technique, which reliably identifies and distinguishes both lesions, has made this differentiation very much easier.

Often, when severe aortic regurgitation is present in a patient with significant mitral stenosis, the peripheral physical signs of aortic regurgitation are sufficiently characteristic to allow it to be diagnosed with certainty on clinical and non-invasive grounds, despite the coincident mitral lesion. In patients with very severe mitral stenosis or in whom aortic regurgitation is only moderate, it may be more difficult to assess the severity of aortic regurgitation because the restricted forward flow caused by mitral stenosis tends to mask the more florid signs of aortic regurgitation which depend on a large volume load on the left ventricle and a high flow across the aortic valve. If there is any doubt about the severity of aortic regurgitation in a patient who also has mitral stenosis, cardiac catheterization should be undertaken. Aortography may reveal the true situation, but it may also underestimate the severity of the lesion because the restricted forward flow also reduces the amount of blood (and thus contrast) regurgitating into the left ventricle in the same way that it diminishes the physical signs. Often the surgeon, given prior warning, will have to assess the aortic valve lesion on the operating table. In cases of doubt, it is usually better to undertake double valve replacement than to leave possibly severe aortic regurgitation uncorrected.

A common problem in the clinical assessment of combined mitral stenosis and aortic regurgitation is the evaluation of mid-diastolic and pre-systolic murmurs at the cardiac apex which may result from either lesion. The Austin Flint murmur due to aortic regurgitation may be identical to that of mitral stenosis although it is not usually associated with an opening snap or accentuation of the first heart sound. Furthermore, patients with aortic regurgitation alone are rarely in atrial fibrillation. The use of echocardiographic imaging and Doppler ultrasound are of great value: mitral stenosis can be readily excluded by the presence of an echocardiographically normal mitral valve across which there is no significant diastolic pressure gradient on Doppler recordings.

MITRAL STENOSIS AND AORTIC STENOSIS

Pure aortic stenosis rarely occurs as an important lesion when many valves are involved by rheumatic heart disease, but if this situation does occur its features are often atypical and the diagnosis may be overlooked.[52–55] Usually, the characteristics of associated mitral stenosis are preserved and there is little difficulty in diagnosing this clinically. The stenosed mitral valve, however, decreases the forward output into the aorta across the stenotic aortic valve, consequently the characteristic systolic murmur of aortic stenosis may be *soft or absent* despite significant narrowing, and the characteristic features of the aortic stenotic pulse may be difficult to appreciate or absent because of the very small forward flow.

The danger of overlooking significant aortic stenosis in the presence of mitral stenosis means that the proper evaluation of all patients with mitral valve disease must include careful assessment of the aortic valve. This can be achieved with a combination of echocardiographic imaging of the valve itself and measurement of the aortic valve gradient using the Doppler technique. If doubts remain after non-invasive assessment, cardiac catheterization should be undertaken. It is important to remember that the low left ventricular stroke volume caused by mitral stenosis will reduce the pressure gradient across the aortic valve because this depends on the severity of the stenosis and on the flow across the valve. For this reason, *it is essential* that both cardiac output and pressure gradient are measured so that the aortic valve area can be calculated. Similarly, gradients assessed by Doppler will underestimate the severity of stenosis when forward flow is reduced and under these circumstances use of a Doppler technique to assess *valve area* is desirable.

Very occasionally, the reverse can occur and mitral stenosis may be overlooked in a patient in whom aortic stenosis is clinically obvious. This possibility should be suspected if atrial fibrillation is present, if there is obvious pulmonary hypertension or if there has been systemic embolization. The routine use of echocardiography and Doppler in patients with valve disease should prevent this mistake being made.

AORTIC STENOSIS AND MITRAL REGURGITATION

Functional mitral regurgitation often complicates the late stages of aortic stenosis once left ventricular dilatation has occurred. However, the combination of aortic stenosis and organic mitral regurgitation is relatively uncommon; but when it does occur, it is an unpleasant combination: the outflow obstruction due to aortic stenosis worsens the degree of mitral regurgitation while both lesions reduce forward flow. The main reason why the diagnosis of these two lesions in combination is often difficult is that it is sometimes impossible to distinguish the murmur of aortic stenosis from that of mitral regurgitation. Aortic stenotic murmurs are often heard best near the cardiac apex whereas mitral regurgitant murmurs, particularly of non-rheumatic origin, may be of the ejection type and radiate from the apex to the left sternal border or even to the base of the heart and into the neck. In the presence of the physical features of aortic stenosis, organic mitral regurgitation should be suspected if there is atrial fibrillation, a large left atrium or a loud apical pan-systolic murmur radiating into the axilla. Calcification of the mitral valve and left ventricular dilatation also suggest the possibility of a significant mitral valve lesion. Conversely, in the presence of the typical features of mitral regurgitation, concomitant aortic stenosis should be suspected if the systolic murmur radiates into the neck, if the pulse is slow rising or if there is calcification of the aortic valve seen on the lateral chest X-ray or by fluoroscopy.

Fortunately, many of the difficulties in diagnosis are solved readily by ultrasound. Echocardiographic imaging reveals the degree of left ventricular dilatation and of hypertrophy and will show thickening and immobility of the aortic valve. A regurgitant mitral valve may appear echocardiographically normal although the abnormality causing regurgitation may be detected. The Doppler technique will identify the presence of mitral regurgitation, indicate its severity and also allow the gradient across the aortic valve to be assessed with accuracy. Occasionally, particularly in patients who yield less than perfect echo and Doppler tracings, cardiac catheterization may be needed to resolve these problems.

AORTIC REGURGITATION AND MITRAL REGURGITATION

Although the combination of pure aortic regurgitation and pure mitral regurgitation is relatively uncommon in rheumatic heart disease, combined mixed lesions in which aortic regurgitation predominates over aortic stenosis and mitral regurgitation predominates over mitral stenosis are relatively frequent. The combination of pure aortic and mitral regurgitation is common in Marfan's syndrome. Clinically, the diagnosis of these two lesions in combination is not usually difficult, but it may be hard to assess the relative severity of the aortic and mitral lesions. Ultrasound may be helpful, but cardiac catheterization is frequently required, although its interpretation may be complicated or unsatisfactory because mitral regurgitation of at least moderate degree can occur secondary to the left ventricular dilatation produced by aortic regurgitation. Occasionally, the surgeon has to decide at operation whether the mitral regurgitation is organic or functional.

TRIPLE VALVE DISEASE

Organic aortic and mitral valve disease occurring in combinations are frequently complicated by functional tricuspid regurgitation. Organic lesions of all three valves are less common; when they do occur, it is most common for there to be mixed stenotic and regurgitant lesions at all three sites. As this is relatively rare, it is frequently not recognized clinically because the tricuspid valve lesion is assumed to be functional. Careful inspection of the neck veins revealing some evidence of stenosis at the tricuspid valve (a slow 'y' descent) may provide the necessary clue.

In nearly all cases of triple valve disease, the mitral valve lesion is the easiest to diagnose; it may obscure the aortic valve lesion and frequently overshadows the tricuspid valve lesion. The scratchy diastolic murmur of tricuspid stenosis may be masked by a mitral diastolic murmur radiating to the left sternal border or by an aortic regurgitant murmur heard at the same site. A significant degree of tricuspid stenosis should be suspected in a patient who *remains in sinus rhythm* despite right-sided failure, mitral valve disease and a large heart. The use of ultrasound with careful examination of all three cardiac valves yields a large amount of useful information but cardiac catheterization is often required to define the lesions precisely before considering surgery.

MITRAL AND TRICUSPID VALVE DISEASE

A combination of mitral valve disease with functional tricuspid valve disease is extremely common. Combined mitral and tricuspid stenosis can be difficult. Clinically one or the other predominates (usually the tricuspid) but the echo and Doppler nearly always resolve the problem immediately.

MEDICAL ASPECTS OF PROSTHETIC HEART VALVES

NORMAL FUNCTION

The physical signs of normally functioning prosthetic valves depend on the type of valve and its position.

Mitral prostheses

Mechanical mitral prostheses produce a sharp click when they open and when they close. The interval between the aortic component of the second heart sound and the opening sound of the mechanical valve gives an indication of left atrial pressure in a similar way to the timing of the opening snap of mitral stenosis, i.e. the later the opening sound, the lower the opening (left atrial) pressure. The closing sound of the mechanical prosthesis replaces the normal mitral component of the first heart sound. The loudness and sonic characteristics of the clicks vary with the type of prosthesis and the thickness of the patient's chest wall. As well as the opening and closing sounds, there is frequently a soft apical early systolic murmur which may represent slight mitral regurgitation but it is a normal finding.

Tissue valves in the mitral position may generate a definite opening sound, but this is not always the case, their closing sound is often indistinguishable from the normal mitral component of the first heart sound. A perfectly functioning mitral tissue prosthesis often produces no murmur, but a soft systolic murmur possibly due to a trivial degree of regurgitation through the valve or a minor degree of obstruction in the left ventricular outflow by the valve stent[56] is common even with normal valve function. A short soft rumbling diastolic murmur at the apex due to turbulent flow through the prosthetic valve is heard fairly frequently even when the prosthesis is functioning normally.

Tricuspid prostheses

Tricuspid prostheses produce similar physical findings to those of mitral prostheses except that the tricuspid events occur slightly earlier, are best heard at the left lower sternal edge and are accentuated by inspiration.

Aortic prostheses

Aortic mechanical prostheses produce a sharp opening sound which occurs in the usual position in the cardiac cycle for an aortic ejection sound, i.e. soon after the first heart sound. The closing sound replaces the aortic component of the second heart sound and is usually loud. Normally, a tissue prosthesis does not produce an opening sound and its closing sound makes up the aortic component of the second heart sound. A short mid-systolic murmur, which is usually soft, is a normal finding in the aortic area with all types of aortic valve prostheses.

ABNORMAL VALVE FUNCTION

If a patient with a prosthetic heart valve shows cardiovascular deterioration, dysfunction of the prosthetic valve *should always be suspected* as a potential cause. Other important possibilities are ventricular dysfunction, the development or progression of ischaemic heart disease or the deterioration of another valve.

Like the valves they replace, prosthetic valves may leak, become stenosed/obstructed or infected.[57] Systemic embolization is a serious problem which is discussed in detail in Chapter 35. Whenever an embolism occurs, the possibility of endocarditis (emboli occur in 30% of cases of prosthetic endocarditis) or thrombus obstructing the prosthetic valve should be considered (Fig. 32.13).

Leaking prosthetic valves

When regurgitation occurs with a mechanical valve,

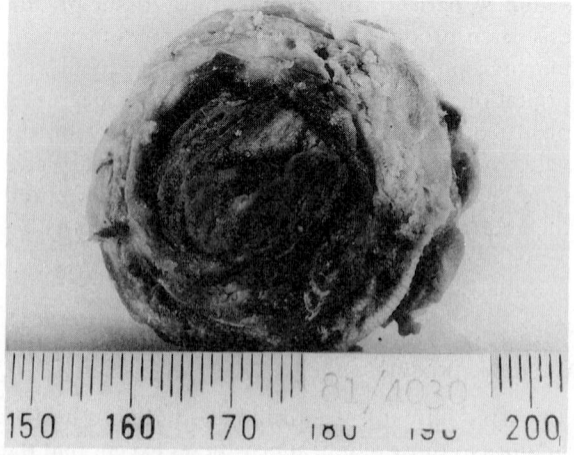

Fig. 32.13. Thrombosed mitral valve seen from its ventricular aspect. Both the disc and valve ring are completely encased and immobilized by thrombus. By courtesy of Mr C. Hilton.

it is nearly always around (paraprosthetic) rather than through the valve, although occasionally the latter can occur with very old and worn valves. Paraprosthetic leaks also occur around tissue valves but these valves are also prone to leak through the valve orifice because of damage to the cusps from infection as well as from degeneration and rupture secondary to wear and tear and accelerated by calcification.

Minor paraprosthetic leaks are not uncommon with both types of valve and generally they do not cause problems; occasionally, a small high-pressure jet leads to mechanical haemolysis which may become clinically serious.

Severe *paraprosthetic* regurgitation usually develops within the first six months after surgery and it is most likely to occur when the conditions under which the valve replacement was undertaken were not favourable, i.e. replacement of a heavily calcified or infected valve. Despite their high incidence during the early phase after cardiac surgery, paraprosthetic leaks can occur at any stage, and as they are often associated with infective endocarditis this diagnosis should always be suspected.

Occasionally, prosthetic valve leakage is due to the sudden mechanical failure of the valve, such as the escape of the occluding ball or the rupture of a strut and escape of the disc held within it.[59,60]

The diagnosis of leaks either through or around *prosthetic aortic valves* is usually easy. The clinical features are those of aortic regurgitation. It should be remembered that, as in native aortic regurgitation, sudden malfunction of a prosthetic valve may lead to a low-output state and overwhelming pulmonary oedema with little or no murmur.

The diagnosis of *mitral paraprosthetic leaks* can be extremely difficult. Although the characteristic physical signs of mitral regurgitation may be present, it is not unusual for torrential paraprosthetic mitral regurgitation to produce either a *very soft murmur or no murmur at all*.[61] Consequently, the true diagnosis is often missed.

Obstructed prosthetic valves

Stuck disc

Sudden life-threatening obstruction of a prosthetic valve is a rare complication, mainly confined to disc valves, in which the disc sticks, usually in mid position, resulting in a combination of severe obstruction and regurgitation. Thrombus surrounding the prosthesis often collects predominantly in the smaller of the two orifices and immobilizes the valve. Recent improvements in valve design have reduced this risk.

If the valve sticks suddenly, it leads to dramatic clinical deterioration with a low-output state and pulmonary oedema. Usually the most striking physical sign is the absence of normal valve clicks, and there may be associated bizarre systolic, diastolic or continuous murmurs. Occasionally valve clicks persist but this is uncommon. Major peripheral embolism often occurs and may be part of the presenting episode. The diagnosis is usually made with ease using echocardiography, Doppler and fluoroscopy (see below).

Other forms of valve obstruction

All prosthetic valves are mildly obstructive and the degree to which they obstruct the circulation depends on their size and type. Once in position, mechanical valves produce a constant obstruction throughout their life, whereas tissue valves tend to become stiffer as they age,[62] which process is hastened by calcification, particularly in children and young adults (see Chapter 35).[63] If calcification is present a moderate degree of obstruction usually associated with some regurgitation occurs. Stiffened or degenerating tissue valve cusps may tear and produce severe regurgitation, often with a particularly loud, high-pitched or whooping murmur. Once there is evidence of a torn valve cusp, the progression of regurgitation is often rapid and early re-replacement of the valve should be considered.

Although obstruction of a prosthetic valve most often results from thrombus accumulating in the valve orifice, vegetations due to infective endocarditis can produce the same effect but this is rare.[64]

Diagnosis of prosthetic valve dysfunction

Diagnosis of prosthetic valve dysfunction depends on a high index of suspicion. Dysfunction should be suspected in any patient with a prosthetic valve who shows cardiovascular deterioration. The physical signs may suggest the diagnosis but further investigations are often required.

X-ray screening

Several abnormalities can be revealed by X-ray screening. Excessive hingeing of the whole prosthesis (either mechanical or tissue) suggests a major dehiscence.[53] If a mechanical valve is obstructed or jammed, this will usually be detected by fluoros-copy; most modern disc valves have a radiopaque ring incorporated into the disc, and the ball and cage of other mechanical prostheses are usually radiopaque. It should not be forgotten, however, that in patients with a very low cardiac output for some other reason, disc or ball movement may be severely reduced simply by the low flow across the valve. Fluoroscopy may reveal calcification in malfunctioning tissue valves.

Ultrasound

The introduction of ultrasound has proved extremely useful in assessing prosthetic valve malfunction. Even when working perfectly, mitral prostheses are all obstructive[65–67] and cause slow left ventricular filling usually combined with abnormal movement of the interventricular septum.[67,68] These alterations vary with the type of valve and are most marked with Starr–Edwards prostheses. Abnormalities of left ventricular filling can be identified by measuring the rate of change of left ventricular dimension in early diastole from digitized M-mode echocardiograms.[67,68] This technique requires high-quality echoes and considerable operator experience. It is of only limited value in diagnosing valve obstruction because it is difficult to distinguish pathological valve obstruction from the considerable obstruction caused by a normally functioning valve. However, the technique is of considerable value in patients with a leaking mitral prosthesis (see Chapter 35), in whom the rate of change of left ventricular dimension in early diastole is normal or increased. A further characteristic of a leaking mitral prosthesis is that the usually reversed septal motion returns to normal (Fig. 32.14). Indeed *normal* septal motion in a patient with a mitral valve replacement should always be viewed with suspicion. Finally, when the leak is large, left ventricular wall motion may be extremely vigorous.

Echocardiography can often identify the individual leaflets of tissue valves and show their movement or lack of it, for example, immobilized, calcified cusps or torn flailing leaflets (Fig. 32.15). In contrast, although echocardiography can reveal the motion of the moving parts of mechanical valves, it is often impossible to define the structure of the valve precisely because the strong reflections from the prosthetic material distort the images (Fig. 32.16). Most of the information about the function of a mechanical prosthesis is obtained indirectly from the left ventricular wall motion or derived from the Doppler technique.

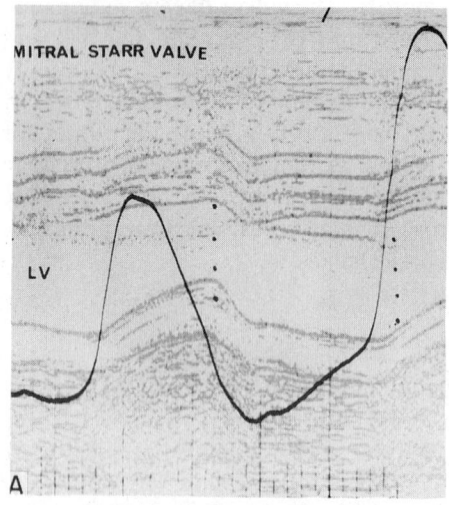

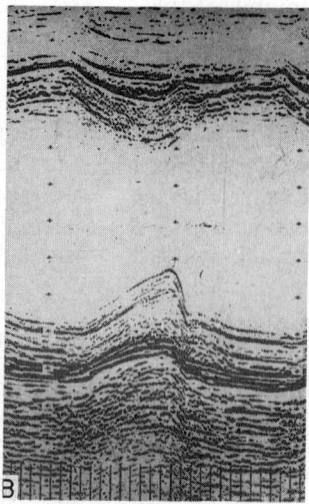

Fig. 32.14. M-Mode echocardiograms obtained from (A) a patient with a normally functioning mitral Starr–Edwards prosthesis and (B) a patient with the same type of prosthesis and a large paraprosthetic leak. In (A), septal motion is reversed whereas in (B) septal motion is normal. LV, left ventricle.

The Doppler technique has proved extremely valuable as a means of diagnosing all forms of prosthetic malfunction.[69–72] As regurgitation occurring through or around a mitral prosthesis may be extremely difficult to detect clinically, the introduction of a non-invasive technique to help make this diagnosis is particularly welcome. The extent of mitral regurgitation is assessed in the same way as in other clinical circumstances. Sometimes, a mechanical prosthesis can intervene between the Doppler probe and the paraprosthetic jet thereby preventing the jet from being detected (Fig. 32.17);[73] to avoid this, multiple views and a careful search using pulsed Doppler is necessary. Recent work with colour Doppler[74] shows that this technique often identifies leaking prostheses, and an indication of the severity of the leak can be gained from the extent of turbulence in the left atrium. Doppler can also be used to detect obstruction at a mitral prosthesis. Although most mitral prostheses have a gradient in early diastole (Fig. 32.17), this has usually disappeared by the end of diastole when the valve is functioning normally. When the valve is obstructed, the gradient persists throughout diastole, the pressure half-time is prolonged and the

Fig. 32.15. Cross-sectional echocardiogram of a mitral valve bioprosthesis (short-axis parasternal view). One cusp of the valve was calcified and immobile (the triangular white shadow marked by the curved arrow). The other two valve cusps were uncalcified and mobile. The posterior aspect of the valve is shown by the smaller arrow.

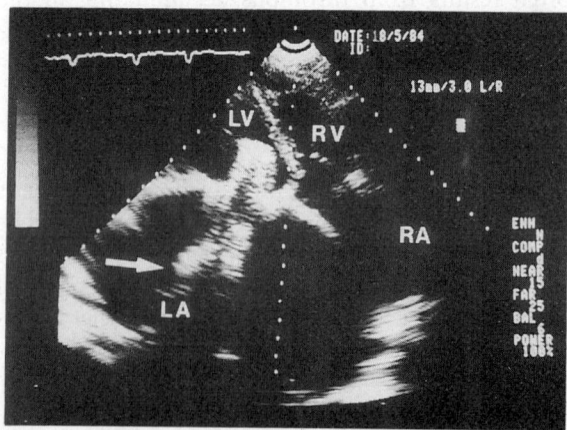

Fig. 32.16. Cross-sectional echocardiogram from a patient with a mitral Starr–Edwards prosthesis (apical four-chamber view). The arrow shows echoes that suggest there may be a mass in the left atrium (LA) but this is artefactual and due to reverberations from the prosthetic valve. LV, left ventricle; RV, right ventricle; RA, right atrium.

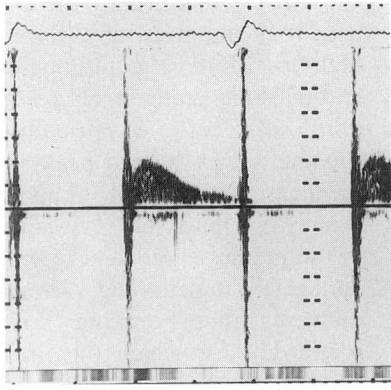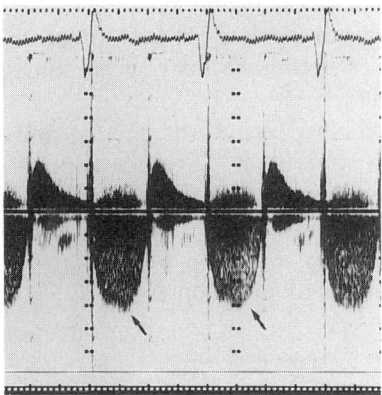

Fig. 32.17 Two continuous wave Doppler recordings obtained from a patient with a disc-type mechanical prosthesis in the mitral position. Both recordings were obtained from the cardiac apex. The recordings are at different paper speeds. In (A), the appearances suggest normal prosthetic valve function with a small increase in flow velocity at the beginning of diastole and no significant increase of velocity at the end of diastole. There is no systolic signal recorded. The recording in (B) was obtained from the same patient at the same time as that in (A) by shifting the position of the transducer. In (B), there is a strong mitral regurgitant jet detected (arrows) due to severe paraprosthetic mitral regurgitation. This jet was not recorded in (A) because the mechanical structure of the prosthetic mitral valve came between the echo probe and the regurgitant jet.

Doppler pattern resembles that of significant mitral stenosis (Fig. 32.18).

Obstructed aortic valve prostheses are less common than obstructed mitral prostheses. Echocardiographic assessment is not very helpful in this situation apart from being able to demonstrate the immobilization of a disc or ball. Generally, Doppler is of far more use in assessing the degree of outflow obstruction (Fig. 32.19). The clinical situation when aortic prostheses leak differs from that when mitral prostheses are incompetent. This type of leak is very rarely clinically silent and as a rule the physical signs usually associated with regurgitation through a native valve are present. In addition the echocardiogram will show left ventricular volume overload and vigorous wall motion. Occasionally, sudden dehiscence of a prosthesis produces physical signs similar to those of acute aortic regurgitation. Under these circumstances, early mitral valve closure may be seen. The Doppler technique will identify aortic

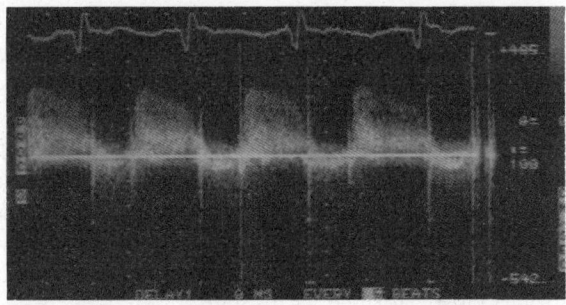

Fig. 32.18. Continuous wave Doppler recording obtained from a patient with an obstructed (by thrombus) mitral disc valve. This recording was obtained from the apex. There is a jet of increased velocity present which persists throughout diastole and has an appearance similar to that seen in severe mitral stenosis. This pattern should be compared with the normal pattern of diastolic flow through this type of valve as shown in Fig. 32.17A. In this particular patient, there is also a suggestion of some mitral regurgitation, and the mitral valve clicks are still recorded by the Doppler preceding and following the diastolic jet.

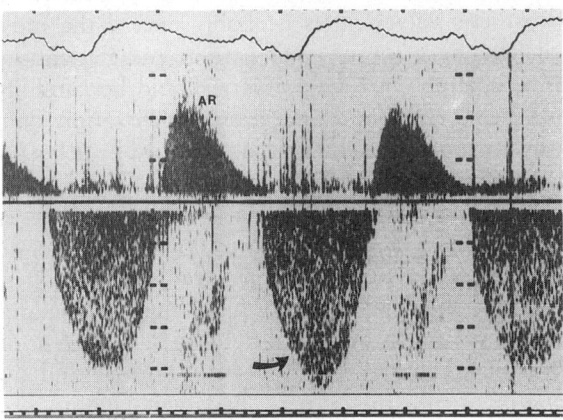

Fig. 32.19. Continuous wave Doppler recording obtained from the apex in a patient with an obstructed Starr–Edwards aortic prosthesis. There is a high-velocity jet (> 4 m/s) across the aortic prosthesis (arrow). This suggests a gradient of about 70 mmHg across this valve which was obstructed by thrombus. There is also evidence of some aortic regurgitation (AR).

regurgitation without difficulty and mapping of the regurgitant jet using either pulsed-mode Doppler or the colour Doppler technique may give some indication of severity.

In the past, combined echocardiography and phonocardiography were used[75,76] to assess prosthetic valve function; however, as these techniques are difficult to employ and of limited reliability they have been superseded by a combination of cross-sectional echocardiography and Doppler.

Cardiac catheterization

Occasionally, catheterization is required if non-invasive assessment is inconclusive. In general tissue valves can be treated as native valves, for example, aortic valve prostheses can be crossed retrogradely, but the catheterization of patients with mechanical valves is much more difficult. Although mechanical valves can be crossed retrogradely, often with some difficulty, the presence of the catheter in the valve immediately produces severe regurgitation which profoundly affects the haemodynamic situation in general. There is also a small danger that the catheter may become wedged in a disc prosthesis. Normally, when assessing aortic prosthetic function, it is better to enter the left ventricle by the trans-septal route, via the left atrium, or to carry out a direct left ventricular puncture, which is extremely easy and safe in experienced hands and particularly useful in patients with aortic and mitral mechanical prostheses; under which circumstances, the left ventricle is essentially closed to useful anterograde or retrograde entry. There are many other problems in catheterizing a patient with prosthetic valves—it is probably one of the most challenging areas of adult cardiac catheterization. Investigations in such patients should be carefully planned beforehand and the catheterization data used *in combination* with that obtained by echocardiography and Doppler assessment.

If catheterization is being carried out, it is important that pressure and flow data are as accurate as possible. Pressure gradients are often present across the normally functioning aortic and mitral prostheses and the difference in the extent of the pressure gradient between a normal and an abnormal prosthesis may be small. Pulmonary wedge measurement, which tends to overestimate left atrial pressure and therefore the degree of valve obstruction, may be too inaccurate to be clinically acceptable.[77] The mean pressure gradient across a normally functioning mitral valve prosthesis (this can also be detected by the Doppler technique) is usually in the range of 2–8 mmHg, but may be as high as 10 mmHg, although there is rarely an end-diastolic gradient at a normal (60–70 beats/min) heart rate. A normally functioning aortic prosthesis may have a peak systolic pressure gradient across it in systole of up to 40–50 mmHg, but usually it is much less.[72] Because there is an overlap in the pressure gradients found over normally and abnormally functioning valves, more sophisticated methods incorporating flow have been put forward,[66] for which the preliminary results are encouraging.

Treatment

Minor prosthetic valve dysfunction is often well tolerated. Small paraprosthetic leaks are not uncommon and the Doppler technique may detect them in between 10 and 18% of patients who have a prosthesis whether tissue or mechanical.[70] The detection of a new prosthetic or paraprosthetic leak should always raise the possibility of infective endocarditis. Under some circumstances, minor leakage can quickly progress to more major problems, particularly in patients with endocarditis or when there is a tear in a leaflet of a tissue valve that may extend rapidly. This type of regurgitation, particularly of mitral valves, produces bizarre high-pitched murmurs. If such a murmur is detected, early surgery should be considered.

Moderate degrees of prosthetic malfunction can often be treated conservatively. However, some patients become rapidly unwell and need urgent surgery, such as those in whom the disc valve is stuck or jammed. These patients often need to be taken directly from the emergency department, where they present, to the operating theatre. Catheterization is unnecessary in most cases. Major dehiscence of a prosthetic valve is of similar urgency. As many patients with prosthetic endocarditis also need surgery within a matter of hours or days, they should be managed in a centre where cardiac surgery is performed. Although there have been reports of successful thombolytic therapy of jammed disc valves, surgery is generally the preferred course of action.

Prosthetic valve endocarditis

Prosthetic valve endocarditis is discussed in detail on page 865.

Haemolysis

Haemolysis, often severe enough to cause a moderate degree of anaemia, can occur with any type of prosthetic valve. Its incidence has fallen considerably with the improvements in prosthetic valve design; in the past, it occurred with normally functioning valves whereas now it is usually associated with prosthetic malfunction. Significant haemolysis is most frequently associated with a paraprosthetic leak; even if the leak is haemodynamically slight, severe haemolysis can still occur as the red cells are broken up in turbulent flow through the leak.

The haematological features of haemolysis caused by a prosthetic valve are well known. The most prominent are those of a normocytic normochromic anaemia, with fragmented red cells seen in the peripheral blood film; there is usually a persistent reticulocyte response. The presence of intravascular haemolysis is easily confirmed by the measurement of the lactate dehydrogenase level, which is always extremely high. Mild jaundice is common. Other features of this type of intravascular haemolysis can be found in any standard textbook of haematology.

Treatment depends on the degree of haemolysis and anaemia. Compensation for mild-to-moderate haemolysis is normally achieved by increased bone-marrow activity. Such patients often run out of folic acid and need supplements to bring the haemoglobin level back to normal. If the haemolysis is severe enough to need transfusion, re-replacement of the valve is often the only sensible course of action, although in some patients who are either too elderly or unwell to undergo re-replacement repeated transfusion may be necessary. Generally, iron therapy is not required; given chronically, it may lead to iron overload, particularly if it is combined with repeated transfusions. It is sensible to check serum iron and iron capacity occasionally and use the results as a guide to iron therapy.

REFERENCES

1. Kitchen, A. and Turner, R. Diagnosis and treatment of tricuspid stenosis. *Br. Heart J.* 1964; **26**: 354.
2. Bousvaros, G.A. and Stubinger, D. Some auscultatory and phonocardiographic features of tricuspid stenosis. *Circulation* 1964; **29**: 26.
3. Callahan, J.A., Wroblewski, E.M., Reeder, G.S. *et al.* Echocardiographic features of carcinoid heart disease. *Am. J. Cardiol.* 1982; **50**: 762–8.
4. Perloff, J.K. and Harvey, W.P. Clinical recognition of tricuspid stenosis. *Circulation* 1960; **52**: 346.
5. Reichek, N., Shelbourne, J.C. and Perloff, J.K. Clinical aspects of rheumatic valvular disease. *Prog. Cardiovasc. Dis.* 1973; **15**: 491.
6. Killip, T. and Lucas, D.S. Tricuspid stenosis: clinical features in 12 cases. *Am. J. Med.* 1958; **24**: 836.
7. Gibson, R. and Wood, P. The diagnosis of tricuspid stenosis. *Br. Heart J.* 1955; **17**: 552.
8. Daniels, S.J., Mintz, G.S. and Kotler, M.N. Rheumatic tricuspid valve disease. Two dimensional echocardiographic, hemodynamic and electrocardiographic correlations. *Am. J. Cardiol.* 1983; **51**: 492.
9. Hatle, L. In: Hatle, L. and Anglesen, B. *Doppler Ultrasound in Cardiology. Physical principles and clinical applications*, 2nd edn. Philadelphia: Lea and Febiger, 1985.
10. Veyrat, C., Kalmanson, D., Farjon, M. *et al.* Noninvasive diagnosis and assessment of tricuspid regurgitation and stenosis using one and two-dimensional echo pulsed Doppler. *Br. Heart J.* 1982; **47**: 596.
11. Thorburn, C.W., Morgan, J.J., Shanahan, M.X. and Chang, V.P. Long-term results of tricuspid valve replacement and the problem of prosthetic valve thrombosis. *Am. J. Cardiol.* 1983; **51**: 1128.
12. Morgan, J.R. and Forker, A.D. Isolated tricuspid insufficiency. *Circulation* 1971; **43**: 559.
13. Chen, C.C., Morganroth, J., Mardelli, J.R. and Naito, M. Tricuspid regurgitation in tricuspid valve prolapse demonstrated with contrast cross sectional echocardiography. *Am. J. Cardiol.* 1980; **46**: 983.
14. Zone, D.D. and Botti, R.E. Right ventricular infarction with tricuspid insufficiency and chronic right heart failure. *Am. J. Cardiol.* 1976; **37**: 445.
15. McAllister Jr., R.G., Friesinger, G.C. and Sinclair-Smith, B.C. Tricuspid regurgitation following inferior myocardial infarction. *Arch. Intern. Med.* 1976; **136**: 95.
16. Korner, P. and Shillingford, J. Tricuspid incompetence and right ventricular output in congestive heart failure. *Br. Heart J.* 1957; **19**: 1.
17. Reichek, N., Shelburne, J.C. and Perloff, J.K. Clinical aspects of rheumatic valve disease. *Prog. Cardiovasc. Dis.* 1973; **15**: 491.
18. Weyman, A.E., Wann, S., Feigenbaum, H. and Dillon, J.C. Mechanism of abnormal septal motion in patients with right ventricular volume overload. *Circulation* 1976; **54**: 179.
19. Feneley, M. and Gavaghan, T. Paradoxical and pseudoparadoxical interventricular septal motion in patients with right ventricular volume overload. *Circulation* 1986; **74**: 230–8.
20. Meltzer, R.S., van Hoogenhuyze, D., Serruys, P.W. *et al.* Diagnosis of tricuspid regurgitation by contrast echocardiography. *Circulation* 1981; **63**: 1093–9.
21. Skjaerpe, T. and Hatle, L. Diagnosis of tricuspid regurgitation. Sensitivity and Doppler ultrasound compared with contrast echocardiography. *Eur. Heart J.* 1985; **6**: 429–36.
22. Lingamneni, R., Cha, S.D., Maranhao, V. *et al.* Tricuspid regurgitation: clinical and angiographic assessment. *Cathet. Cardiovasc. Diag.* 1979; **5**: 7.
23. McCord, M.C. and Blount Jr., S.G. The hemodynamic pattern in tricuspid valve disease. *Am. Heart J.* 1952; **44**: 671.
24. Hansing, C.E. and Rowe, G.G. Tricuspid insufficiency: a study of hemodynamics and pathogenesis. *Circulation* 1972; **45**: 793.
25. Gottsegen, G., Wessely, J., Arvay, A. and Tamesvari, A. Right ventricular myxoma simulating pulmonary stenosis. *Circulation* 1963; **27**: 95.
26. Babcock, K.B., Judge, R.D. and Bookstein, J.J. Acquired pulmonic stenosis. *Circulation* 1962; **26**: 931.
27. Leise, G.J., Brainard, S.C. and Goto, U. Giant blood cyst to the pulmonary valve. *N. Engl. J. Med.* 1963; **269**: 465.
28. Waldhausen, G.A., Lombardo, C.R. and Morrow, A.G. Pulmonic stenosis due to compression of the pulmonary

artery by an intra-pericardial tumor. *J. Thorac. Surg.* 1959; 37: 679.

29. Shaver, V.C., Bailey Jr., W.R. and Marrangoni, A.G. Acquired pulmonary stenosis due to external cardiac compression. *Am. J. Cardiol.* 1965; 16: 1965.

30. Schrire, V., Beck, W. and Barnard, C.N. Aneurysm of the ascending aorta obstructing right ventricular outflow and producing severe "pulmonary stenosis". *Am. Heart J.* 1963; 65: 396.

31. Seymour, J., Emanuel, R. and Pattinson, N. Acquired pulmonic stenosis. *Br. Heart J.* 1968; 30: 776.

32. Alday, L.W. and Moreyra, E. Calcific pulmonary stenosis. *Br. Heart J.* 1973; 35: 887.

33. Taylor, R.R., Bernstein, L. and Jose, A.D. Obstructive phenomena in ventricular hypertrophy. *Br. Heart J.* 1964; 26: 193.

34. Hatle, L. and Angelsen, B. (eds) *Doppler Ultrasound in Cardiology; Physical principles and clinical applications*, 2nd edn. Philadelphia: Lea and Febiger, 1985.

35. Lima, C.O., Sahn, D.J. *et al.* Non-invasive prediction of transvalvular pressure gradient in patients with pulmonary stenosis by quantitative 2-dimensional echo Doppler studies. *Circulation* 1983; 67: 866–71.

36. Criscitiello, M.G. and Harvey, W.P. Clinical recognition of congenital pulmonary valve insufficiency. *Am. J. Cardiol.* 1967; 20: 765.

37. Schloff, L.D. and Wang, Y. Congenital isolated pulmonic regurgitation. *Chest* 1969; 55: 254.

38. Rosketh, R. Isolated pulmonic valvular regurgitation: report on 9 new cases. *Acta Med. Scand.* 1969; 185: 489.

39. Brayshaw, J.R. and Perloff, J.K. Congenital pulmonary insufficiency complicating idiopathic dilatation of the pulmonary artery. *Am. J. Cardiol.* 1962; 10: 282.

40. Edwards, J.E. Congenital pulmonary vascular disorders. In: Moser, K.M. ed. *Pulmonary Vascular Diseases*. New York: Marcel Dekker, 1979.

41. Roberts, W.C., Dangel, J.C. and Bulkey, B.H. Non-rheumatic valvular cardiac disease; a clinico-pathological survey of 27 different conditions causing valvular dysfunction. In: Likoff, W. (ed.) *Cardiovascular Clinics*, Vol. 5, No. 2. *Valvular Heart Disease*. Philadelphia: F.A. Davis. 1973, p.334.

42. Levin, H.S., Runca, V., Wooley, C.F. and Ryan, J.M. Pulmonic regurgitation following staphylococcal endocarditis. *Circulation* 1964; 30: 411.

43. Vela, J.E., Conteras, R. and Sosa, F.R. Rheumatic pulmonary valve disease. *Am. J. Cardiol.* 1969; 23: 12.

44. Bousvaros, G.A. and Deuchar, D.C. The murmur of pulmonary regurgitation which is not associated with pulmonary hypertension. *Lancet* 1961; ii: 962.

45. Steell, G. The murmur of high pressure in the pulmonary artery. *Medical Chronicle, Manchester* 1888; 9: 182.

46. Weyman, A.E., Dillon, J.C., Feigenbaum, H. and Chang, S. Pulmonary valve echo motion in pulmonary regurgitation. *Br. Heart J.* 1975; 37: 1184–90.

47. Gulace, G., Savoia, M.T., Ravizza, P. *et al.* Contrast echocardiographic features of pulmonary hypertension and regurgitation. *Br. Heart J.* 1981; 46: 369–73.

48. Waggoner, A.D., Quinones, M.A., Young, J.B. *et al.* Pulsed Doppler echocardiographic detection of right-side valve regurgitation. *Am. J. Cardiol.* 1981; 47: 279–86.

49. Patel, A.K., Rowe, C.G., Dhanani, S.P. *et al.* Pulsed Doppler echocardiography in diagnosis of pulmonary regurgitation: its value and limitations. *Am. J. Cardiol.* 1982; 49: 1801–5.

50. Emery, R.W., Landes, R.G., Moller, J.H. and Nicolhoff, D.M. Pulmonary valve replacement with a porcine aortic heterograft. *Ann. Thorac. Surg.* 1979; 27: 148.

51. Segal, B., Harvey, W.P. and Hufnagel, C.A. Clinical study of 100 cases of severe aortic insufficiency. *Am. J. Med.* 1956; 21: 200.

52. Honey, M. Clinical and haemodynamic observations on combined mitral and aortic stenosis. *Br. Heart J.* 1961; 23: 545.

53. Reid, J.M., Stevenson, J.G., Barclay, R.S. and Welsh, T.M. Combined aortic and mitral stenosis. *Br. Heart J.* 1962; 24: 509.

54. Schattenburg, T.T., Titus, J.L. and Parkin, T.W. Clinical findings in acquired aortic stenosis. Effect of disease of other valves. *Am. Heart J.* 1967; 73: 322.

55. Terzaki, A.K., Cokkinos, D.V., Leachman, R.D. *et al.* Combined atrial and aortic valve disease. *Am. J. Cardiol.* 1970; 25: 588.

56. Eldar, M., Motro, M., Rath, S. *et al.* Systolic closure of aortic valve in patients with prosthetic mitral valves. *Br. Heart J.* 1982; 48: 48.

57. Oakley, C.M. Long-term complications of valve replacement. *Br. Med. J.* 1982; 284: 995–7.

58. Richardson, J.V., Karp, R.B., Kirklin, J.W. and Dismukes, W.E. Treatment of infective endocarditis: a 10 year comparative analysis. *Circulation* 1978; 58: 589–97.

59. Davies, P.K., Myers, J.L., Pennock, J.L. and Thiele, B.L. Strut fracture and disc embolization in Björk–Shiley mitral valve prostheses: Diagnosis and management. *Ann. Thorac. Surg.* 1985; 40: 65–8.

60. Odell, J.A., Durandt, J., Shama, D.M. and Vythilingum, S. Spontaneous embolization of a St Jude prosthetic mitral valve leaflet. *Ann. Thorac. Surg.* 1985; 39: 569–72.

61. Miller, H.C., Gibson, D.G. and Stephens, J.D. Role of echocardiography and phonocardiography in diagnosis of mitral paraprosthetic regurgitation with Starr–Edwards prostheses. *Br. Heart J.* 1973; 35: 1217–25.

62. Oyer, P.E., Miller, D.C., Stinson, E.B. *et al.* Clinical durability of the Hancock porcine bioprosthetic valve. *J. Thorac. Cardiovasc. Surg.* 1980; 80: 824–33.

63. Curcia, C.A., Commerford, P.J., Rose, A.G. *et al.* Calcification of gluteraldehyde preserved porcine xenografts in young patients. *J. Thorac. Surg.* 1980; 81: 621–31.

64. Bortolotti, U., Thiene, G., Milano, A. *et al.* Pathological study of infective endocarditis on Hancock porcine bioprostheses. *J. Thorac. Cardiovasc. Surg.* 1981; 81: 934–42.

65. Lurie, A.J., Miller, R.R., Maxwell, K.S. *et al.* Hemodynamic assessment of the glutaraldehyde/preserved porcine heterograft in the aortic and mitral position. *Circulation* 1977; 56 (Suppl. II): 104–10.

66. Czer, L.S.C., Gray, R.J., Bateman, T.M. *et al.* Hemodynamic differentiation of pathologic and physiologic stenosis in mitral porcine bioprostheses. *J. Am. Coll. Cardiol.* 1986; 7: 284–94.

67. Sutton, M.G. St. J., Traill, T.A., Ghaffaur, A.S. *et al.* Echocardiographic assessment of left ventricular filling after mitral valve surgery. *Br. Heart J.* 1977; 39: 1283–91.

68. Dawkins, K.D., Cotter, L. and Gibson, D.G. Assessment of mitral Björk–Shiley prosthetic dysfunction using digitised M-mode echocardiography. *Br. Heart J.* 1984; 51: 168–74.

69. Veyrat, C., Witchitz, S., Lessana, A. *et al.* Valvular prosthetic dysfunction: localisation and evaluation of the dysfunction using the Doppler technique. *Br. Heart J.* 1985; 54: 273–84.

70. Williams, G.A. and Labovitz, A.J. Doppler hemodynamic evaluation of prosthetic (Starr–Edwards and Björk–Shiley) and bioprosthetic (Hancock and Carpentier–Edwards). *Am. J. Cardiol.* 1985; 56: 325–32.

71. Holen, J., Simonsen, S. and Froysaker, T. An ultrasound Doppler technique for the non-invasive determination of the pressure gradient in the Björk–Shiley mitral valve. *Circulation* 1979; 59: 436–44.

72. Holen, J., Simonsen, S. and Froysaker, T. Determination of pressure gradient in the Hancock mitral valve from non-invasive ultrasound Doppler data. *Scan. J. Clin. Lab. Invest.* 1981; 41: 177–83.

73. Sprecher, D.L., Adamick, R., Adams, D. and Kisslo, J. In vitro color flow, pulsed and continuous wave Doppler ultrasound masking of flow by prosthetic valves. *J. Am. Coll. Cardiol.* 1987; 9: 1306–10.
74. Stewart, W.J., Agler, D.A., Koch, J.M. and Currie, B.J. Color flow mapping diagnosis and localization of paravalvular aortic regurgitation. *Circulation* 1987; 76 (Suppl. IV): 448.
75. Mintz., G.S., Carlson, E.B. and Kottler, M.N. Comparison of non-invasive techniques in the evaluation of the non-tissue cardiac valve prostheses. *Am. J. Cardiol.* 1982; 49: 39.
76. Brodie, B.R., Grossman, W., McLaurin, L. *et al.* Diagnosis of prosthetic mitral valve malfunction with combined echocardiography. *Circulation* 1976; 53: 93.
77. Schoenfeld, M.H., Palacios, I.F., Hutter, A.M. *et al.* Underestimation of prosthetic valve areas: role of transseptal catheterization in avoiding unnecessary repeat mitral valve surgery. *J. Am. Coll. Cardiol.* 1985; 5: 1387–92.

Chapter 33

Coronary Artery Disease in Patients with Valve Disease

Roger Hall

Coronary artery disease occurs in patients with valvular heart disease at about the same frequency as it does in the general population from which these patients were drawn.[1-3] In Western populations, this incidence is approximately 30%.[3,4] It was suggested in some early reports[5] that aortic valve disease had a protective effect on the coronary arteries, but the results of more recent studies indicate that this is not the case and the incidence is similar in aortic and mitral valve disease.[3] As the incidence of coronary artery disease varies widely among different populations and increases rapidly with age, the incidence of coronary artery disease in patients with valve disease will vary considerably from population to population. In underdeveloped countries where coronary artery disease is rare and patients with valve disease are young, coronary disease co-existing with valve disease is not a serious problem.

Angina pectoris is a poor predictor of the presence of coronary artery disease in patients with valvular heart disease; conversely, the absence of angina does not predict its absence. Some authors have suggested that coronary artery disease is very rare in patients with aortic stenosis who do not have angina,[6] but others have found significant stenoses in the coronary arteries in as many as 25% of such patients who are free of angina.[7] As angina is a common symptom of aortic valve disease in the absence of coronary artery disease, it is not surprising that the results of all studies have shown angina to be more common in aortic valve disease than in mitral valve disease (50% of patients with aortic valve disease and 30% of patients with mitral valve disease);[3] angina is less often due to coronary artery disease in aortic (33%) than mitral valve disease (85%).[2] In recent large studies, it has been shown that the likelihood of the presence of coronary artery disease can be assessed in patients with valvular heart disease with a high degree of accuracy using risk factor analysis.[3] The risk factors analysed were smoking, hypertension, family history, obesity, diabetes mellitus and hyperlipidaemia. It was shown that if *angina is absent*, the overall risk of coronary artery disease is 19% but in patients with *neither angina nor a coronary risk factor* this incidence is reduced to 3%. Age is also an important variable as the incidence of coronary artery disease rises steadily with age, for example, in one study from the North East of England, coronary disease was detected in only 5% of patients below the age of 50 years but in 36% over the age of 60.[8]

SIGNIFICANCE OF CORONARY HEART DISEASE IN VALVULAR HEART DISEASE

Information about the significance of coronary artery disease in patients with valvular heart disease is far from complete. If the significance of coronary artery disease is to be assessed, it is important to know its effect on the early mortality of valve operations, whether the combined procedures of coronary artery grafting and valve replacement carry a higher or lower risk of mortality than valve replacement alone and whether coronary artery grafting at the time of valve replacement improves long-term prognosis. It is particularly desirable to obtain such information in patients who have asymptomatic coronary artery disease. In patients who are symptomatic, it is logical to undertake coronary angiography and to graft the lesions detected in this way at the same time as performing valve replacement. In patients who are asymptomatic, the quest for coronary artery lesions may be the only reason for invasive investigation prior to valve surgery now that the non-invasive assessment of valve lesions is so accurate.

As the available information suggests that the situation is different in aortic and mitral valve disease, they are discussed separately.

AORTIC VALVE DISEASE

With modern surgical techniques, the mortality of aortic valve replacement does not seem to be affected by concomitant coronary artery grafting.[9,10] Kirklin and Kouchoukos[10] have reviewed this matter in considerable detail and summarised the argument for and against coronary artery grafting in patients with asymptomatic coronary artery disease. They concluded that at present there is no evidence either to support or to contra-indicate the routine use of combined coronary artery surgery and aortic valve replacement. Although late mortality in patients undergoing aortic valve replacement is strongly influenced by coronary artery disease,[11] there is no evidence that coronary artery grafting reduces this late mortality and in one report[12] it was found that coronary artery grafting did not confer prognostic benefit on such patients.

MITRAL VALVE DISEASE

In mitral valve disease the situation is much more complicated because in many patients the mitral valve lesion is the consequence of coronary artery disease. The results of many studies have shown the combined procedure of coronary artery grafting and mitral valve replacement carries a much higher mortality than mitral valve replacement alone. The Coronary Artery Surgery Study (CASS) demonstrated a 23.7% operative mortality for the combined procedure carried out in 15 centres between 1975 and 1978.[13] Recently, better results have been reported with mortality rates as low as 7.3%,[14] but other contemporary series have suffered mortality rates as high as 19%.[15] The wide variation in mortality reported probably results mainly from considerable differences among the patients in terms of age, severity of coronary artery disease, left ventricular function, and so on. Surgery carried out as an emergency in patients with ischaemic mitral regurgitation carries a mortality in the range of 20–30% whereas for elective procedures mortality may be as low as 4–7%.[4,16]

When mitral regurgitation is due to myocardial ischaemia, revascularization performed at the same time as correcting the mitral valve lesion is logical. The appropriate management in patients with coronary artery disease and non-ischaemic mitral regurgitation is more difficult. If the coronary artery disease is symptomatic it is reasonable to recommend coronary artery surgery; if it is asymptomatic, coronary artery surgery should only be performed if it would significantly reduce operative mortality or improve long-term prognosis. At present, it is impossible to answer these questions as no prospective randomized trial has been performed and it is unlikely that such a trial will ever be carried out. However, a recent extremely detailed study[4] was designed in an attempt to clarify some of these issues. Analysis of patients matched retrospectively for the severity of their valve and coronary lesions who underwent either mitral valve replacement alone or mitral valve replacement with myocardial revascularization suggested that coronary artery grafting improved the short- and the long-term results. The difficulty inherent in the analysis of results in patients undergoing different procedures who are retrospectively matched means that these results should be interpreted with caution.

CONCLUSIONS

Many uncertainties remain in this area. The significance of asymptomatic coronary artery disease and its effect on surgical results remain largely unknown. Owing to the implications of screening every patient for coronary artery disease in terms of the use of catherization facilities, a reasonable approach is that employed by Ramsdale et al.[3] Using risk factor analysis, these workers were able to identify with coronary angiography a group of patients in whom the chance of coronary artery disease is extremely low. It would seem unreasonable to pursue coronary disease in such patients.

REFERENCES

1. Ramsdale, D.R., Bennett, D.H., Bray, C.L. et al. Coronary arteriography prior to valve replacement. Eur. Heart J. 1981; 2: 83–6.
2. Morrison, G.W., Thomas, R.D., Grimmer, S.F.M. et al. Incidence of coronary artery disease in patients with valvular heart disease. Br. Heart J. 1980; 44: 630–7.
3. Ramsdale, D.R, Bennett, D.H., Bray, C.L. et al. Angina, coronary risk factors and coronary artery disease in patients with valvular disease. A prospective study. Eur. Heart J. 1984; 5: 716–26.
4. Czer L.S.C., Gray, R.J., DeRobertis, M.A. et al. Mitral valve replacement: impact on coronary artery disease and determinants of prognosis after revascularization. Circulation 1984; 70 (Suppl. I): 198–207.
5. Nakib, A., Lillehei, C.W. and Edwards, J.E. The degree of coronary atherosclerosis in aortic valve disease. Arch. Pathol. 1965; 80: 517–20.
6. Exadactylos, K.N., Sugrue, D.D. and Oakley, C.M. Prevalence of coronary artery disease in patients with isolated aortic valve stenosis. Br. Heart J. 1984; 51: 121–4.
7. Green, S.J., Pizzarello, R.A., Padmanabahn, V.T. et al.

Relation of angina pectoris to coronary artery disease in aortic valve stenosis. *Am. J. Cardiol.* 1985; **55**: 1063–5.

8. Hall, R.J.C., Kadushi, O.A. and Evemy, K. Need for cardiac catheterisation in assessment of patients for valve surgery. *Br. Heart J.* 1983; **49**: 268–75.

9. Bonnow, R.O., Kent, K.M., Rossing, D.R. *et al.* Aortic valve replacement without myocardial revascularization in patients with combined aortic valvular and coronary artery disease. *Circulation* 1981; **63**: 243–51.

10. Kirklin, J.W. and Kouchoukos, N.T. Aortic valve replacement without myocardial revascularization. *Circulation* 1981; **63**: 252–3.

11. Richardson, J.V., Kouchoukos, N.T., Wright, J.O. and Kaarp, R.B. Combined aortic valve replacement and myocardial revascularization: results in 220 patients. *Circulation* 1979; **59**: 75.

12. Jang, G.C. and Hancock, E.W. Aortic stenosis and coronary artery disease: long term survival after valve replacement (Abstract). *Am. J. Cardiol.* 1979; **43**: 368.

13. Kennedy, J.W., Kaiser, G.C., Fisher, L.D. *et al.* Clinical and angiographic predictors of operative mortality from the Collaborative Study in Coronary Artery Surgery (CASS). *Circulation* 1981; **63**: 793.

14. Little, B.W., Cosgrove, D.M., Gill, C.C. *et al.* Mitral valve replacement combined with myocardial revascularization: early and late results for 300 patients. 1971–1983. *Circulation* 1985; **71**: 1179–90.

15. Kabbini, S.S., Bashour, T.T., Hanna, E.S. and Ellertsen D. Risk of combined coronary artery bypass and mitral valve replacement. *Tex. Heart Inst. J.* 1984; **11**: 348–51.

16. Yardar, K.S., Ross, J.K., Monro, J.L. and Shore, D.F. Study of the risk factors related to early mortality following combined mitral valve replacement and coronary artery bypass grafting. *Thorac. Cardiovasc. Surg.* 1985; **33** 16–9.

Chapter 34

Infective Endocarditis

Roger Freeman and Roger Hall

INTRODUCTION

Infective endocarditis is one of the most serious complications of valvular heart disease and if left untreated it almost invariably leads to death. A strict definition of infective endocarditis could be confined to infection of heart valves, septal defects and mural endocardium. In practice, it includes infection on arteriovenous shunts, arterio-arterial shunts and coarctations, as the clinical picture is often indistinguishable. This wider definition will be adopted throughout this chapter.

INCIDENCE AND EPIDEMIOLOGY

The incidence of infective endocarditis is difficult to determine as it is not a notifiable disease. Estimates vary from 0.3 to 3 per thousand hospital admissions.[1] These figures are almost certainly an underestimate because many cases die undiagnosed outside hospital. A study of a community of 1.2 million people in South East Scotland over 4 years revealed an incidence of 16 cases per million per annum.[2] This is also likely to be an underestimate since undiagnosed and un-notified cases must have occurred during this period.

Many of the factors leading to imprecision in the estimates of incidence are obvious. They include inadequate case definition, inclusion and exclusion of culture-negative cases, failure to obtain autopsy confirmation of diagnoses based on clinical suspicion alone, and the unknown number of cases which may have been inadvertently cured by antibiotic therapy given for other reasons.

In recent study by the British Cardiac Society and the Royal College of Physicians, an attempt was made to define the current incidence and mortality of the disease in Great Britain and to identify possible measures by which they might be reduced.[3] In a single year, 582 episodes of infective endocarditis were identified, occurring in 577 patients. There was a male preponderance of 2:1, also a common finding in other studies. One hundred and thirty-seven cases occurred in patients who had pre-existing rheumatic heart disease. A further 108 patients had congenital heart disease, and other cardiac abnormalities, chiefly mitral valve prolapse and calcific disease of the aortic valve, were found in another 145. Ninety-seven patients had had previous valve replacement. One hundred and eighty-three patients were not thought to have had any previous cardiac abnormality. Infection occurred most commonly on the aortic valve. In 27 patients the aortic and the mitral valves were involved.

It has been suggested in several studies that the pattern of endocarditis may be changing. Pelletier and Petersdorf reviewed the American experience of infective endocarditis since the 1950s.[4] They noticed a decline in the incidence of rheumatic valvular heart lesions as the main predisposing cause and the emergence of a significant number of cases of endocarditis occurring in association with lesions such as mitral valve prolapse, calcification on the mitral valve annulus, aortic valve disease in the elderly and hypertrophic cardiomyopathy (Fig. 34.1). Several series reported from single centres have indicated an increase in the incidence of acute infective endocarditis due to *Staphylococcus aureus*, often associated with cardiac surgery, intravenous drug abuse or the widespread use of intravascular access technology (Fig. 34.2).[5]

The mean age of patients with infective endocarditis has risen over the last few decades, possibly as the result of the longer life-expectancy of patients with predisposing heart disease, the decline of rheumatic fever and the rising incidence of degenerative aortic valve disease in an aging population.

MICROBIOLOGY

The traditional classification of infective endocardi-

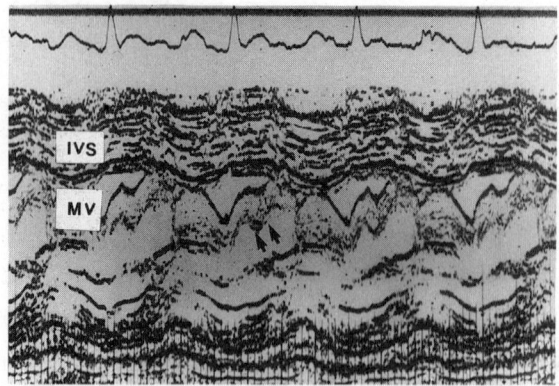

Fig. 34.1. M-Mode echocardiogram from a patient with hypertrophic obstructive cardiomyopathy and infective endocarditis on the mitral valve. The fuzzy echoes due to a vegetation attached to the mitral valve (MV) are shown (arrows). IVS, interventricular septum.

tis into acute (short history, rapid progression and association with *Staph. aureus*, *Streptococcus pneumoniae*, *Neisseria gonorrhoeae* or *Streptococcus pyogenes*) and subacute (a prolonged course of weeks to months, predisposing heart lesion and associations with viridans or faecal streptococci) was based on the untreated disease. Therapy has altered this natural history and these terms are less valid, although the broad concepts remain appropriate. Nowadays, the practice is to refer to infective endocarditis by the name of the aetiological organism, e.g. staphylococcal endocarditis and streptococcal endocarditis.

In Table 34.1, the commoner organisms implicated in infective endocarditis are listed. Although virtually every organism can cause endocarditis, it is clear that staphylococci and streptococci are the predominant causative agents. As it is unusual for streptococci to cause uncomplicated bacteraemia, it has been postulated that they possess a facility to adhere to cardiac endothelium which commoner organisms, such as Gram-negative bacilli, do not.[6] This concept of 'bacterial stickiness' has been supported by its association with certain properties of the commonest streptococci isolated from infective endocarditis, notably the ability to produce dextran from sucrose.

Before discussing the individual organisms of infective endocarditis, it is necessary to outline the nature of the bacteraemia. In infective endocarditis, the bacteraemia is constant and the number of organisms per ml is low (1–30 bacteria/ml).[7] The density is not related to periods of fever. Therefore, if the first culture is positive, it is likely that all

subsequent samples will be positive. Conversely, if the first few samples are negative, undue persistence in sampling is unlikely to be rewarded. There are only two exceptions to this: first, intermittently positive cultures may occur in right-sided disease and, second, recent antibiotic therapy may be an indication to extend the numbers of cultures, although it has been shown that the likelihood of recovering an organism is only slightly reduced by antibiotic therapy given within the preceding two weeks.[7] The overall strategy should be to obtain three separate cultures over a period of a few hours.

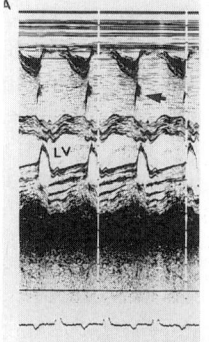
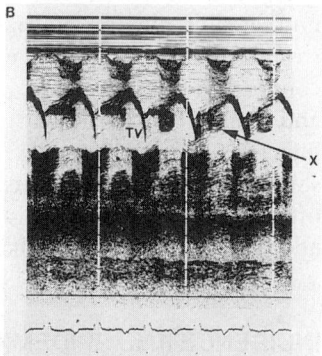

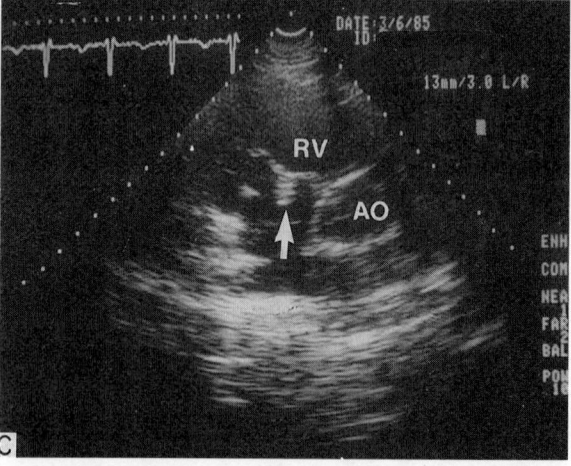

Fig. 34.2. M-Mode (A and B) and cross-sectional echocardiogram (C: short-axis parasternal view) from a patient with infective endocarditis on the tricuspid valve. In (A), the vegetation on the tricuspid valve can be seen within the right ventricular cavity (arrow). In (B), when the transducer is tilted to image the tricuspid valve, the vegetation attached to the tricuspid valve (X) can be seen more clearly. TV, tricuspid valve; LV, left ventricle. In (C), the vegetation can be seen attached to the atrial aspect of the tricuspid valve. Endocarditis occurred in this patient as a consequence of an indwelling catheter in the right atrium used for chemotherapy. The infecting agent was *Staph. epidermidis*. RV, right ventricle; AO, aorta.

Table 34.1. The distribution of the commoner isolates in blood culture-positive infective endocarditis.[a]

Organism group	Distribution (%)
Streptococci:	60–80
'Viridans' group	30–40
Enterococci	10
Other streptococci	20–30
Staphylococci:	10–30
Staphylococcus aureus	9–27
Coagulase-negative staphylococci	1– 3
Other bacteria and organisms:	3–10
Gram-negative bacilli, haemophili, anaerobes, fungi, rickettsia	

[a] Adapted from Kaye, D. *Infective Endocarditis*. Baltimore: University Park Press, 1976, p. 47.

This will allow the recognition of skin contamination (one positive amongst several samples) and will yield the causative organism from all cultures in the vast majority of cases. Stubbornly negative cultures in a clinically suggestive setting should prompt a logical approach rather than futile repeat sampling (see later).

SPECIFIC ORGANISMS

Streptococci

Streptococci account for 60–80% of culture-positive cases of infective endocarditis streptococcus. 'S viridans' is usually quoted as the leading streptococcal agent. In fact, no such organism has ever existed, the term implying an alpha-haemolytic streptococcus other than *Strept. pneumoniae*. This 'rag-bag' group can be properly speciated into many entities, such as *Strept. mutans*, *Strept. salivarius*, *Strept. sanguis* and *Strept. milleri*. They originate mainly in the upper respiratory or upper alimentary tracts. Although most are sensitive to penicillin, resistant strains can occur, therefore identity alone should not be used as a guide to treatment (see later).

Faecal streptococci (often called enterococci) are the next largest group to account for culture-positive cases of infective endocarditis. The broadest definition of these organisms is that of belonging to Lancefield's group D. Various species have now been recognized and include *Strept. faecalis* (more than one variety), *Strept. faecium*, *Strept. durans* and *Strept. bovis*. *Streptococcus bovis* merits a special note because it is often just as sensitive to penicillin as 'S. viridans' and, therefore, combination therapy with an aminoglycoside may not be required. It is another example wherein the identity of the organism may not be the most reliable guide to treatment. Also, *Strept. bovis* endocarditis has a strong association with mucus-producing diseases of the colon, especially adenocarcinoma, ulcerative colitis and polyposis.[8] Such conditions must be sought, especially as the endocarditis sometimes occurs months and years before the colonic symptoms. Faecal streptococci originate from the alimentary, urinary and genital tracts.

Faecal streptococci occasionally cause acute infective endocarditis but more typically they produce a subacute picture, as does the viridans group. Abscess formation is rare in streptococcal infective endocarditis but if it does occur it is almost always due to the faecal group. Streptococci other than of the viridans or faecal group account for the remainder of cases of streptococcal infective endocarditis. *Streptococcus pyogenes*, now a rare cause, may cause acute fulminant disease attacking a previously normal heart.

Staphylococci

Staphylococcus aureus is the only common cause of acute endocarditis in the modern era. It frequently attacks normal hearts during *Staph. aureus* septicaemia. Abscess formation, both intracardiac and metastatic, is common. Associations with prosthetic valves and the right-sided infective endocarditis of drug abuse have led to an increase in the incidence of *Staph. aureus* infective endocarditis. Although it is often related to an operation, prosthetic implant or other breach of the integument, there is some evidence that *Staph. aureus* can 'spontaneously' invade during acute virus infections.

Coagulase-negative staphylococci are commonly associated with infections on prostheses and other intravascular devices. They usually cause a subacute picture and require a predisposed heart to initiate infective endocarditis.

Pneumococci and gonococci

These organisms each formerly accounted for 10% of cases of infective endocarditis. Pneumococcal infective endocarditis is usually acute and fulminant, but it is now rare. It is possible that many cases are now inadvertently cured by therapy for pneumonia. Gonococcal infective endocarditis is also now rare but it deserves mention because of its association with right-sided valve disease.

Other bacteria

Many other bacteria have been shown to cause infective endocarditis, but it is noteworthy that such organisms as Gram-negative bacilli rarely do so in comparison to their frequency as causative agents of septicaemia. One theory is that the large numbers required to initiate infective endocarditis kill the patient before endocarditis can begin.[9] Other more fastidious Gram-negative bacilli, such as haemophili and *Brucella*, occasionally cause infective endocarditis and may require special culture techniques.

Fungi

Candida, *Aspergillus* and *Histoplasma* spp. are the main fungal causes of infective endocarditis. It is important to note that all *Candida* spp. and not just *C. albicans* can do so. For yeasts and yeast-like fungi, ordinary blood culture methods are usually successful but aspergillus infective endocarditis always gives sterile blood cultures. In fungal endocarditis, large emboli frequently occur and culture of these after surgical removal is often a good way of isolating the fungus, especially in aspergillus infective endocarditis. Strong associations with broad-spectrum antibiotics, corticosteroids, prosthetic valves, intravascular access devices, cytotoxic agents and drug abuse suggest the possibility of fungal infective endocarditis.

Other micro-organisms

Rickettsia and *Chlamydia* spp. have been associated with a particularly chronic form of infective endocarditis in which the initial acute infection may precede the infective endocarditis by months or years. Neither type of organism is cultivable by conventional methods but serological tests will confirm the diagnosis. In Q fever, infective endocarditis antibodies to phase I and phase II antigens are found in distinction to the acute self-limiting disease in which only phase II antibody is produced. It is worth noting that serological testing will always confirm or exclude brucella infection.

Claims that cell wall-deficient bacteria are implicated in infective endocarditis continue to be made. There is no evidence that such bacteria can initiate infective endocarditis and their involvement in recurrences is debatable.

Finally, mixed infection in infective endocarditis is remarkably rare (1–2% of all cases).

ENDOCARDITIS WITH STERILE BLOOD CULTURES

The reported incidence of sterile blood cultures in a clinical setting strongly suggestive of infective endocarditis ranges from 7 to 28%.[10] This variability partly implies that the definitions of infective endocarditis and a sterile culture differ from series to series. Three possibilities should be considered: prior antibiotic therapy, in which case extended culturing, possibly with attempted neutralization of the given agent, may be worthwhile; those causes of infective endocarditis in which conventional cultures will always be negative should be excluded, for example, fungal infective endocarditis, Q fever, chlamydial infective endocarditis and infective endocarditis due to very fastidious organisms requiring special techniques; and the sterile thrombotic endocarditis which can complicate various cachectic states, especially terminal malignant disease, should be considered. This condition, often called marantic endocarditis, may exhibit nearly all the features of true infective endocarditis. Its association with the underlying diseases will usually suggest the diagnosis.

If the above conditions are excluded, the incidence of truly sterile cultures in infective endocarditis will be low but not non-existent. It seems clear, from occasional positive cultures when valve replacement has occurred early in the course of the disease, from studies in experimental models and from the results of quantitative studies of the bacteraemias of infective endocarditis, that faecal streptococcal infective endocarditis is a form of the disease in which cultures are most likely to be negative. Accordingly, most clinicians plan 'blind' treatment on the basis that culture-negative infective endocarditis is probably due to a faecal streptococcus.

PORTALS OF ENTRY

Bacteria must gain access to the circulation for infective endocarditis to occur. Normally, bacteraemias are cleared from the blood by the fixed reticulo-endothelial systems of the liver and spleen within a very short time. Arteriovenous connections that allow blood to bypass the splanchnic bed may prolong bacteraemia, whereas pre-existing specific antibody will shorten it.

UNPROVOKED BACTERAEMIA

Unprovoked bacteraemia has been demonstrated in normal individuals and is almost certainly much more common than is realised. It is said to occur in 11%[11] of patients with acute peri-apical abscesses[12] and 9% of patients with chronically infected tonsillar fossae.[13] Spontaneous bacteraemia may also occur in patients with pneumococcal pneumonia and staphylococcal sepsis.

PROVOKED BACTERAEMIA

Simple manipulation of infected foci such as boils, polyps and teeth will produce transient bacteraemias. Similarly, traumatic procedures involving mucosae with a resident bacterial flora will result in a short-lived bacteraemia, particularly in procedures involving the oropharynx. Tooth-brushing, chewing hard materials or dental irrigation have all been shown to provoke bacteraemia in 20–40% of instances.[14,15] The organisms liberated may contain any or all of the resident flora, including anaerobes and actinomyces. The frequency of bacteraemia increases in proportion to the degree of dental trauma and is much higher in those with infection, for instance, periodontitis. Oropharyngeal organisms may also be released after other procedures involving the upper respiratory tract, for instance, bronchoscopy, intubation and tonsillectomy.

Operations, manipulations and instrumentation of the gastro-intestinal and genito-urinary tracts all release bacteria. In this instance, the streptococci liberated will be of the faecal variety, but anaerobes, particularly bacteroides, and Gram-negative bacilli may also be given access to the bloodstream. Vaginal delivery and the insertion of intra-uterine contraceptive devices[16] have both been shown to cause transient bacteraemias.

Finally, intravenous drug abuse is frequently complicated by the direct inoculation of infected material into the blood. The unsterile nature of this procedure and the sources of material employed sometimes mean that very unusual organisms, especially fungi, are favoured. However, even the carefully controlled use of indwelling intravascular devices in medical therapy presents a portal of entry for micro-organisms, and the prolonged use of simple devices such as plastic intravenous catheters

has been the cause of bacteraemias leading to infective endocarditis.

PREDISPOSING LESIONS

Although it has been suggested that embolization of micro-organisms to the interstitium of the valve can initiate endocarditis, most authorities have accepted that implantation of organisms onto the endothelial surface is the mechanism whereby infective endocarditis begins. Experimental work strongly suggests that thrombus formation precedes this implantation so that the sterile thrombotic lesion is 'seeded' at the time of bacteraemia.[17]

Sterile thrombi can form on prosthetic valves and other implants and commonly complicate the low-grade inflammatory lesions found in rheumatic fever, and following myocardial infarction and, occasionally, the rare degenerative lesions of Marfan's syndrome and auto-immunity. The common sites of thrombus formation in marantic endocarditis parallel the sites of infective endocarditis as does the distribution of verrucae in acute rheumatic fever. Thus, in both infective endocarditis and acute rheumatic fever the atrial surface of the mitral valve and the ventricular surface of the aortic valve are the main sites; the mitral and aortic valves are most commonly involved while the tricuspid and pulmonary valves are very rarely affected.

Infective endocarditis occurs at a site where blood passes through a narrow orifice at great speed, travelling from an area of high pressure to one of low pressure. The resulting fall in lateral pressure may decrease intimal perfusion, favouring the development of infective endocarditis. The lesions of infective endocarditis are usually found immediately distal to a coarctation, in the pulmonary artery when the ductus is infected, or on the right side of a ventricular septal defect. Infective endocarditis rarely occurs when there is only a small pressure gradient, as in atrial septal defect. Occasionally in infective endocarditis satellite lesions occur where the infected stream impinges onto an area of mural endocardium or may seed from the aortic to the mitral valve because an aortic regurgitant jet strikes the anterior mitral valve cusp.

A hyperdynamic circulatory state can initiate thrombotic and, therefore, subsequent infective endocarditis. Large arteriovenous fistulae, such as those used in haemodialysis, may produce thrombotic lesions on the aortic valve in patients without prior heart disease. Subsequent infection on the fistula is then complicted by infective endocarditis on the aortic valve.

There is no simple explanation for the ability of virulent pathogens such as *Staph. aureus* to initiate infective endocarditis in normal hearts. The severe stress associated with septicaemia may induce thrombotic lesions which then become infected. Stress is known to initiate both thrombotic and infective endocarditis in animal models.[9] Infective endocarditis is found in two-thirds of autopsies performed on patients dying of acute staphylococcal septicaemia.[18]

UNDERLYING HEART DISEASE

Rheumatic heart disease is still the commonest underlying heart lesion in infective endocarditis, accounting for 40–60% of all cases. Before the therapeutic era, this figure was higher and might be expected to decline further in the future. Rheumatic disease of the heart is commoner in women than in men with the exception of isolated aortic disease. The distribution of infective endocarditis complicating rheumatic disease follows this pattern. Rheumatic disease is rarely the underlying lesion in right-sided infective endocarditis.

Congenital heart disease underlies infective endocarditis in up to 20% of cases. Certain forms of congenital disease are much more likely to be complicated by infective endocarditis than others. Patent ductus arteriosus, ventricular septal defect, coarctation of the aorta and the tetralogy of Fallot are the principal lesions involved. The common factor is the high-to-low pressure gradient and consequent haemodynamic turbulence.

Up to 40% of patients have no previously known heart disease. Such patients comprise two subgroups: those in whom the underlying heart disease has not been apparent until revealed by infective endocarditis, e.g. mild rheumatic heart disease, mild forms of mitral valve prolapse and, the most important example, a congenital bicuspid aortic valve, which often remains clinically silent until infective endocarditis supervenes, and those who had normal hearts prior to infective endocarditis. In these patients, the infective endocarditis is acute and the pathogen virulent, typically *Staph. aureus* (50% of infective endocarditis due to *Staph. aureus* occurs on normal hearts[10]).

The last group of patients with pre-existing lesions of the heart often complicated by infective endocarditis is those with intracardiac prosthetic material. With the increase in cardiac surgery in recent years, between 15 and 30% of all cases of endocarditis seen in Western cardiological practice are of this type.

PATHOGENESIS OF INFECTIVE ENDOCARDITIS

The pathogenesis of the various manifestations of infective endocarditis depends primarily on whether the disease is destined to follow an acute or subacute course. In acute endocarditis, the picture is one of a fulminant septicaemic illness and in the modern era it closely coincides with that of acute *Staph. aureus* septicaemia. Destruction within the heart, metastatic abscess formation and the manifestations of disseminated coagulopathy are all changes caused by the organisms directly. Early immunological changes take place, and nephritis is present.

In subacute infective endocarditis, the prolonged course of the illness produces an opportunity for further pathological processes to evolve. The lesions and processes relate to: developments at the initial site (the vegetation); 'mechanical' consequences of the vegetation, both local and systemic; and the immunological consequences of a longstanding infective process.

The vegetation grows in shape and size as a result of further deposition of platelets and fibrin (Fig. 34.3). Paradoxically, although located within the main bloodstream, the vegetations are relatively avascular. Suppuration does not occur, and the organisms in this privileged site develop almost like colonies on a culture plate. Sometimes, the vegetation becomes large enough to occlude the valve orifice. Damage to the annulus, fistulae, damage to the conduction pathways and rupture of the chordae tendineae may all follow local extension of the infection.

Vegetations containing necrotic material are very friable (Fig. 34.3) and pieces often break off and enter the systemic circulation as infected emboli. It should be remembered that in right-sided disease infected emboli will enter the pulmonary bed. In subacute endocarditis, the relatively avirulent organism loses its protection from the normal host defences once the embolus lodges in the tissues and is rapidly destroyed. Hence, the septic embolus often results in a sterile infarct. In acute endocarditis, however, metastatic abscess formation is common.

The local and embolic consequences of infective endocarditis can explain the changing murmurs, the

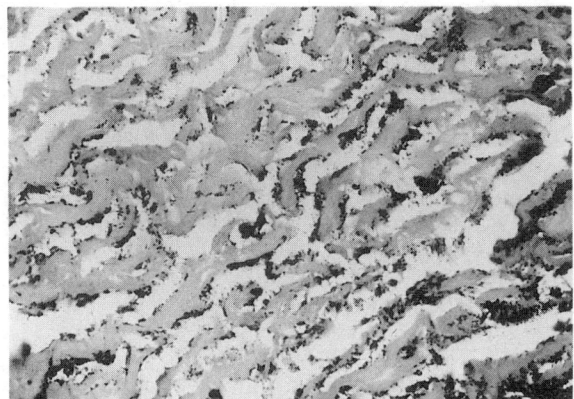

Fig. 34.3. The microscopic appearances of a vegetation. Clumps of bacteria (black dots) can be seen enmeshed in strands of fibrin.

arrhythmias, heart failure, neurological syndromes and distant abscess formation seen.

Much recent interest has centred on the third type of process that occurs in infective endocarditis—the immunological consequences. The body, unable to mount a suppurative or granulomatous reaction to the privileged site of the infection, responds by producing large amounts of humoral antibody. The vegetation acts as an antigen which is surrounded by antibody. Immune complexes result and are found in the glomeruli of patients with nephritis in subacute infective endocarditis. Similar deposits are now thought to be the basis of Roth's spots, Osler's nodes and other vasculitic and petechial lesions of the skin.

The manufacture of large amounts of antibody produces a dysglobulinaemia which leads to the raised erythrocyte sedimentation rate and the falsely

positive tests for rheumatoid factor. It also plays a significant role in the development of the normyocytic normochromic anaemia characteristic of subacute infective endocarditis. The lack of a stimulus to mount a large inflammatory reaction is the reason why a neutrophil leucocytosis is not a prominent feature. Prolonged stimulation of the reticuloendothelial system may be the cause of the monocytosis (histiocytosis) often seen in the peripheral blood.[9]

PATHOLOGY

INTRACARDIAC PATHOLOGY

The hallmark of infective endocarditis is the vegetation (Figs. 34.3 and 34.4). Vegetations may be single or multiple and vary widely in their size and macroscopic appearance. They are usually found on the atrial surfaces of atrioventricular valves but on the ventricular aspects of semilunar valves. Histologically, a vegetation is an amorphous mass of fibrin, platelets, white and red blood cells and aggregations of bacteria (Fig. 34.2). Suppuration is rare within the vegetation, but at the base of the valve and in the annulus abscess formation extending into adjacent tissues may damage surrounding structures (e.g. conduction tissue), impair function (e.g. myocardial abscess) or lead to fistula formation. Aneurysms may be formed on the valve or annulus and may erode into the sinus of Valsalva. Rupture of the chordae tendineae and papillary muscles can occur; fistulous tracts to the pericardium and to other cardiac chambers sometimes result.

Nowadays, in surgical specimens, the beginnings of healing are often seen. Fibrosis and organization within the valvular lesions occur and even calcification and re-endothelialization can be detected.

Myocarditis is common, although not much is known of its pathogenesis. Direct embolization, toxin production and immune complex deposition have all been suggested as mechanisms. Clearly demarcated myocardial abscesses are seen in up to 20% of patients with infective endocarditis coming to autopsy. Rarely, myocardial infarction distal to a blocked coronary artery occurs (Fig. 34.5).

EXTRACARDIAC PATHOLOGY

Emboli

Autopsy evidence of embolism in infective endocar-

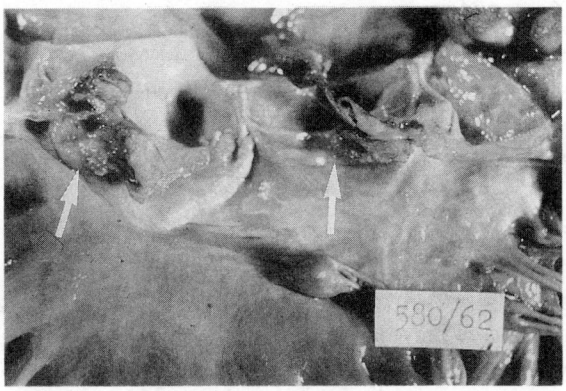

Fig. 34.4. Pathological specimen showing infective endocarditis of the aortic valve. A large vegetation is attached to one of the cusps (left-hand arrow) and an eroded and torn cusp is also demonstrated (right-hand arrow).

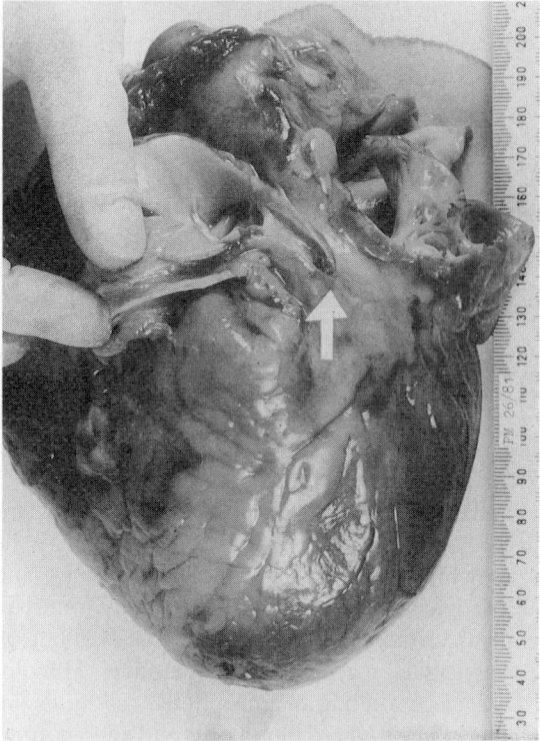

Fig. 34.5. Pathological specimens of a patient who died of infective endocarditis. A large piece of vegetation which has embolized into a coronary artery is shown (arrow).

ditis occurs in 50% of cases. Any organ or tissue can be involved. In many cases, the lesion is clearly due to physical emboli and the histology is typical of the resultant infarction, sometimes complicated by suppuration. However, it is now thought that many lesions are due to the deposition of immune complexes; they show a characteristic vasculitic reaction with endothelial and intimal cell proliferation and certain of them have become regarded as typical of infective endocarditis (see below).

Lesions of the skin

The commonest skin lesion is a petechial rash. It is not certain whether this rash is due to embolization or is vasculitic. Most evidence favours the latter. So-called splinter haemorrhages seen beneath the nails are probably petechial, whereas other manifestations, such as Osler's nodes and Janeway lesions, are probably immunologically mediated, although bacteria have been isolated from them.

Lesions of the spleen

The spleen is almost always enlarged in infective

endocarditis, the degree being directly related to the duration of the illness. Microscopically, there is generalized hyperplasia of the lymphoid tissue and reticulo-endothelial elements. Embolic infarction, occasionally complicated by abscess formation, is relatively common, and rupture, usually secondary to suppuration, can occur with resultant peritonitis.

Lesions of the lung

Changes in the lung are virtually restricted to patients with right-sided infective endocarditis. Pneumonia, pulmonary embolism and lung abscesses secondary to infected emboli occur.

Lesions of the peripheral vascular system

The important lesion of infective endocarditis specific to the vascular system is the mycotic aneurysm. This lesion was formerly attributed to embolic occlusion of the vasa vasorum. More recently, the damage has been thought to be due to the deposition of immune complexes. Lesions are typically located at bifurcations or wherever vessels undergo sharp changes of direction. Cerebral vessels are the most commonly involved, accounting for roughly half of those recognized; abdominal sites make up the majority of the remainder and the vessels in limbs account for about 10% of the total. The overall incidence of mycotic aneurysms is difficult to ascertain but they are noted in 10–15% of autopsies performed on patients with infective endocarditis.

Lesions of the eye

Petechiae commonly occur in the anterior portions of the eye and in the retina. Roth's spots are probably due to infarction of the neural layer of the retina.

Lesions of the central nervous system

In addition to vasculitic lesions and the mycotic aneurysms previously described, the brain may suffer infarction due to emboli. Mycotic aneurysms may rupture, leading to subarachnoid haemorrhage and other vascular catastrophes. Single or multiple brain abscesses may occur due to septic embolism. Rarely, purulent meningitis may occur.

Lesions of the kidney

Renal complications include metastatic abscesses, embolic infarction and three varieties of glomerulonephritis. The pathology of the first two lesions (abscess and infarction) is discussed above. All three nephritides are now considered to be immunologically mediated.

Focal glomerulonephritis ('flea-bitten kidney') used to be thought to be the result of embolization. However, the fibrinoid necrosis, polymorph infiltration and adjacent endothelial and mesangial proliferation suggest that it is immunologically mediated.

Diffuse glomerulonephritis occurs less frequently than focal glomerulonephritis, although they may co-exist in the same patient. If renal failure occurs, it is usually associated with diffuse glomerulonephritis affecting every glomerulus and characterized by cellular hyperplasia throughout the glomerular tufts.

Membranoproliferative glomerulonephritis is characterized by florid mesangial proliferation. It is associated with staphylococcal infection and not with other infecting agents.

In all forms of glomerulonephritis complicating endocarditis, suitable techniques will show the deposition of immune complexes, immunoglobulins and complement typical of immune complexes.

CLINICAL FEATURES

GENERAL

Subacute infective endocarditis usually presents insidiously with symptoms that are frequently mistaken for those of influenza. The most frequent complaints are of malaise, low-grade fever and weight loss often accompanied by sweating, headache, joint and muscle pains and backache.[2,19,20] The onset of the acute form of the illness is much more dramatic. The patient becomes suddenly ill with high fever, chills, sweating and dyspnoea, which may be accompanied by the symptoms and signs of heart failure of acute onset if valve destruction is severe. Death may occur within a few days.

Before effective treatment was available, the subacute form of illness followed a stuttering course for many months. The patient became progressively weaker and thinner, with fever that was sometimes continuous, and often accompanied by rashes and eventually by features of cardiac failure. Death was inevitable. Nowadays, most cases are diagnosed before death but occasionally infective endocarditis is detected for the first time at autopsy.[2]

Although subacute endocarditis usually presents with a history of general ill-health, occasionally its initial manifestations are those of one of its complications, an embolic manifestation being the most frequent (see below).[2,21,22]

The physical signs at presentation depend to a large extent on the duration of illness. Many of the features which used to be regarded as classical are observed only in patients with longstanding disease; nowadays, they are seen in a smaller proportion of patients.

On general examination, the patient usually appears pale and unwell often with evidence of weight loss. The pallor is due to a combination of anaemia and general ill-health. In the past, it was frequently accompanied by pigmentation, which is now rarely seen. Some patients have none of these features when they present because the history is short and they are diagnosed quickly because of a high index of suspicion possibly aroused by knowledge of a preceding cardiac condition.

Clubbing of the fingers and toes, like pigmentation, is a feature of longstanding illness and is infrequently seen these days. Although patients often complain of non-specific joint pain, there are rarely any abnormal physical signs in the joints.

Petechiae are an important physical finding, occurring in from one-third to two-thirds of cases.[19] They are often found on skin of the legs and chest, mucous membranes and ocular fundi and are most commonly detected in the conjunctiva, particularly of the lower lid. They may occur in crops that come and go or singly. They are usually small and may have a pale centre. In the ocular fundi, they are 1 mm or so across, and if they have a white centre they are known as Roth's spots. Roth's spots are rare. Although localized blotchy erythematous rashes can occur at any site on the body, which last for a few days and then disappear, they are less common than petechial haemorrhages.

An important but quite uncommon skin manifestation of subacute bacterial endocarditis is the Osler's node. This is a small swollen area about the size of a pea which is exquisitely tender. It occurs most often in the pads of the fingers or toes and on the thenar or hypothenar eminences; it last for a few days and then disappears often to recur elsewhere on the body. Its presence strongly suggests a diagnosis of infective endocarditis. It is seen most often in patients with longstanding illness. Before effective therapy became available, Osler's nodes were de-

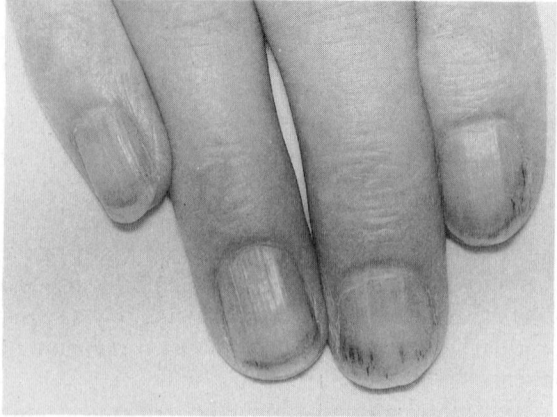

Fig. 34.6. Splinter haemorrhages in a patient with infective endocarditis.

tected in 50% of cases but in recent studies their incidence has been reported to be as low as 5%.[2] An even rarer manifestation is the Janeway lesion, an erythematous or haemorrhagic lesion which may be raised and nodular occurring on the palms of the hands or the soles of the feet. This lesion is painless.

Finally splinter haemorrhages beneath the finger and toe nails are frequent (Fig. 34.6). They have been erroneously regarded as a specific feature of endocarditis. They occur frequently in normal subjects, they are particularly common in patients who do manual work, and they have been reported in up to 10% of patients without endocarditis who have been admitted to hospital.[23]

CARDIAC FEATURES

The cardiological features of infective endocarditis are very variable and superimposed on those of any underlying cardiac condition. They result from the general ill-health engendered by the condition, the destruction of cardiac valves and the involvement of the myocardium and occasionally the pericardium.

General ill-health

General ill-health, anaemia and fever usually produce a moderate resting tachycardia, which, combined with the increased cardiac output from the fever and anaemia, augments flow across cardiac valves and thus may change the character of murmurs even if the valve lesion itself has not been exacerbated. However, it is wise to regard a change in the character of murmur as being due to valve destruction until proved otherwise.

Destruction of valves

In the early stages of the illness, infected valves may function normally. As a consequence, a murmur may not be present despite the classical presentation of infective endocarditis being one of general ill-health plus a cardiac murmur. In a series reported by Smith *et al.*, 81% of cases presented with a cardiac murmur and a further 15% developed one during their stay in hospital.[2] Other workers have reported similar findings.[19] As valve destruction in infective endocarditis is usually progressive, the appearance of a murmur or a changing murmur is an important sign. By far the most common situation during the course of the illness is for a regurgitant murmur, usually suggesting aortic or mitral regurgitation, to appear or to become more prominent. In 36% of the patients described by Smith *et al.*, a murmur appeared or changed during the course of the illness.[2]

Heart failure may appear or worsen during the course of infective endocarditis because a heart which is already compromised by a chronic valve lesion is further stressed by anaemia and fever and regurgitant lesions become more severe due to valve destruction. A deterioration in haemodynamics with the onset of cardiac failure should always be suspected as being due to valve destruction and is often an indication for early surgical intervention.

Valve destruction (Fig. 34.4) can occur extremely rapidly, particularly in patients with acute infective endocarditis. As this condition often occurs on previously normal valves, the patient tolerates new and severe regurgitant lesions poorly as compensatory hypertrophy and chamber dilatation to accommodate valve regurgitation has no time in which to develop. Acute pulmonary oedema may develop. When infective endocarditis, whether subacute or acute, suddenly destroys the integrity of one of the aortic valve cusps causing acute aortic regurgitation the true situation may be difficult to establish from the physical signs.[24,25] These patients usually present with severe heart failure, pulmonary oedema and a loud gallop rhythm; the murmur due to the aortic regurgitation may be soft or undetectable because the overwhelming regurgitation occurs into a small and unprepared left ventricle (unless there has been prior chronic aortic regurgitation). The torrential reflux in early diastole rapidly raises the pressure within the unprepared left ventricle to that of the aorta, consequently backflow of blood into the left ventricle occurs only briefly and therefore does not lead to a particularly prominent murmur. The heart rate is usually extremely fast such that a short, soft, early diastolic murmur cannot be distinguished from the loud third heart sound which is normally also present. A high index of clinical suspicion, combined with echocardiography (see later), usually leads to the correct diagnosis. Severe regurgitation without characteristic murmurs may also occur in patients with prosthetic heart valves (see below). Acute regurgitation through the mitral valve is not as difficult to diagnose. A loud systolic murmur is usually present in addition to severe acute pulmonary oedema. Finally, infective endocarditis of the tricuspid valve often produces significant tricuspid regurgitation sometimes without obvious heart murmurs.

Involvement of myocardium and pericardium

Although cardiac failure is most commonly due to destruction of valves and the consequent regurgitation, it may be caused or exacerbated by myocardial damage. Vegetations from valve cusps, usually the aortic, can embolize into the coronary arteries (Fig. 34.5). Small emboli may produce diffuse myocardial damage. Large emboli lead to myocardial infarction which may have all the classical features of myocardial infarction due to coronary disease. Myocardial function may also be compromised by intramyocardial abscesses resulting from spread of infection directly from the infected valve. Patients with such abscesses often appear particularly unwell and continue to be febrile despite appropriate antibiotic therapy. If an intramyocardial abscess extends to the intraventricular septum, the conducting system is frequently affected. Initially, this leads to a lengthening of the PR interval on the electrocardiogram, and may go on to bundle branch block (usually left) and sometimes complete heart block. Disturbances of conduction occur in between 10 and 20% of cases of infective endocarditis and suggest extensive spread of infection.

Pericardial involvement is much rarer. Occasionally, a suppurative pericarditis accompanied by all the classical physical signs and symptoms of pericarditis may occur if an abscess in the myocardium extends into the pericardial cavity. This is particularly sinister suggesting severe myocardial damage and often leading to death. Occasionally, a more benign form of pericarditis with pericardial effusion occurs (Fig. 34.7); it resolves spontaneously if the infective endocarditis is treated successfully. The cause is unknown but it is probably a manifestation of the altered immune state of the patient.

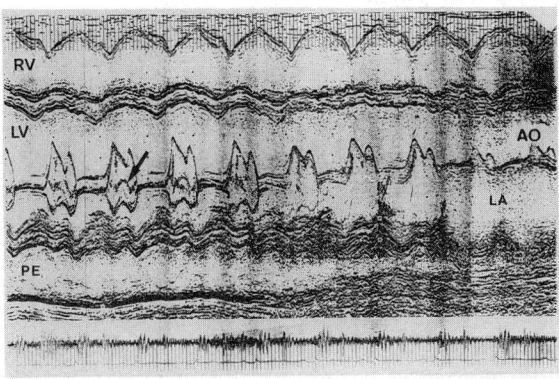

Fig. 34.7. M-Mode echocardiogram from a patient with infective endocarditis involving the mitral valve. The echoes due to the vegetation on the mitral valve are seen within the mitral valve echo (arrow). There is also a sizeable pericardial effusion seen both anteriorly and posteriorly (PE), which occurred as a complication of the pericarditis. Aspiration of this pericardial effusion produced sterile serosanguinuous fluid. RV, right ventricle; LV, left ventricle; AO, aorta; LA, left atrium.

Equally rarely, pleural effusions may occur as a similar type of manifestation.

EMBOLIZATION

Systemic emboli may be the initial manifestation of endocarditis or they may occur during the course of the illness.[19,21] When a patient who has a known cardiac condition which predisposes to bacterial endocarditis experiences a systemic embolus, the possibility of infective endocarditis should always be considered. Emboli can occur to any site in the body and may be clinically silent. The most important sites are the brain, causing acute neurological disturbances, the kidney, producing sudden loin pain, the spleen, producing left subcostal pain often made worse by respiration, or the eye, resulting in unilateral blindness. Occasionally, large emboli, which are particularly associated with fungal endocarditis, may occlude the vessel to a limb. Embolic manifestations are an important presenting feature. Schnurr et al. reported cerebral emboli as the presenting feature in 15% of cases and other systemic emboli in 7%.[21]

Although embolism is usually systemic, patients who have endocarditis on right-sided heart lesions or involving a ventricular septal defect often experience pulmonary emboli and these may be a presenting feature. Acute endocarditis at these sites is usually due to the staphylococcus and the infected emboli may lead to multiple lung abscesses.

OTHER FEATURES

Central nervous system

Cerebral symptoms are the presenting manifestation in about 20% of cases.[26] They may take the form of a definite meningitis, encephalitis or cerebral abscess but more often they are non-specific. The most frequent cerebral manifestations are acute confusion and stupor, which is particularly common in the elderly and represents a difficult diagnostic problem. Elderly patients frequently have little or no fever as a result of their endocarditis, and both confusion and cardiac murmurs are common in these patients in the absence of infective endocarditis.

Renal and splenic involvement

Both the kidneys and spleen are frequently involved in this illness but rarely produce any obvious clinical signs or symptoms.

The most common form of renal involvement is glomerulonephritis due to the deposition of immune complexes (see above). This leads to microscopic haematura which have been reported in between 20 and 93% of patients.[21] Impairment of renal function is usually mild, but if the disease is longstanding patients can develop severe renal failure. Embolization to the kidneys is less frequent and does not usually affect enough of the renal blood supply to impair renal function but it does lead to loin pain and haematuria.

When infective endocarditis is longstanding, the spleen is frequently enlarged, but nowadays *clinically obvious* splenic enlargement is an unusual feature. Emboli to the spleen may produce sudden left subcostal pain and a localized rub (discussed above).

Mycotic aneurysm

Mycotic aneurysms often produce no clinical symptoms or signs. They may occasionally rupture, the clinical consequences of which depend on the site. Rupture of an intracranial aneurysm usually has disastrous and rapidly fatal results.

CLINICAL FEATURES OF INDIVIDUAL TYPES OF ENDOCARDITIS

Although the clinical features of endocarditis are usually similar regardless of the infecting organism,

endocarditis occurring as a result of certain organisms in particular situations have some individual features that are worth noting (Table 34.2). Prosthetic endocarditis is of particular importance because it can be difficult to diagnose and has a poor prognosis. It is discussed separately below.

ENDOCARDITIS IN INTRAVENOUS DRUG ABUSERS

Infective endocarditis is a common and often fatal complication of intravenous drug abuse.[25] The

Table 34.2. Endocarditis due to particular agents.

Agent	General features	Clinical features
Fungal[62–66]	1. *C. albicans and Aspergillus* Often after valve surgery (30% later than 6/12) Other predisposing factors: – intracardiac cannulae – pacing wires – steroid therapy – ? antibiotics Concomitant bacterial infective endocarditis (19%) 2. *Candida* (non-albicans) Often intravenous drug abuse	May attack normal valves Myocardial involvement (abscesses, etc.) Large systemic emboli a feature Therapy difficult and mortality high; Surgery often required particularly with prosthetic valves
Q Fever[46]	Contact with farm animals (not always) Males 2 × females Diagnosis by serology	Aortic valve commonly involved Liver involvement by organism common Thrombocytopenia and purpura common May need prolonged (or indefinite) therapy
Brucella[55]	Contact with cattle or goats; usually farmers or veterinary surgeons	Predilection for aortic valve Tricuspid endocarditis not uncommon Aneurysm of sinus of Valsalva with intramyocardial spread common
Staphylococcus aureus	Commonest agent in intravenous drug abusers Important in prosthetic endocarditis; therefore routine prophylaxis needed at surgery	Nearly always produces an 'acute endocarditis' May attack normal valves May be rapidly fatal

diluent for the injected drug is often heavily contaminated by bacteria or fungi. Infection acquired in this way frequently affects the right-sided heart valves; involvement of the tricuspid valve is a particularly common feature. Often such cases go undiagnosed if there is no murmur because other features of infective endocarditis may be difficult to detect in the generally debilitated drug abuser. Pulmonary embolism from the infected right-sided valve is common and its occurrence in a known intravenous drug abuser should raise the possibility of endocarditis.[27] The range of infecting organisms is different from that occurring in other types of endocarditis. Stimmel and Dack[28] found that *Staph. aureus* was responsible for 47% of cases, *Pseudomonas* species caused 19% of infections, and candida infections account for 5% of cases. Mixed infections may occur. In certain areas, particular organisms may be prominent, for example, the incidence (8%) of *Serratia marcescens* in San Francisco.[29]

A similar type of right-sided endocarditis occurs in patients with indwelling right atrial cannulae particularly when patients are immunologically compromised, for example when such lines are used in patients with leukaemia.

PROSTHETIC VALVE ENDOCARDITIS

Prosthetic valve endocarditis is an important condition because nowadays between 15 and 30% of all cases of endocarditis occur on prosthetic valves.[22] The risk of endocarditis is highest soon after surgery (Fig. 34.8) with a peak occurring at about three weeks.[30] In the most detailed study to date, the risk during the first year after surgery was 3.1%.[31] This high early risk probably results from a combination of infection introduced at the time of surgery and bacteraemia associated with monitoring and infusion lines used in the peri-operative period, and this risk is substantially higher in patients receiving mechanical prostheses.[30,31] The overall incidence of endocarditis during the next four years is much lower (2.6%) than that during the first year.[31]

Endocarditis occurring in the first 2 months after surgery is considered to differ from that occurring later, although the bacteriology of cases occurring up to one year after operation tends to support a more prolonged influence of surgery.[31] A common infecting agent during the first year is the methicillin-resistant *Staphyloccus epidermidis*. This organism may colonize the patient following surgery as a result of prophylactic antibiotics used

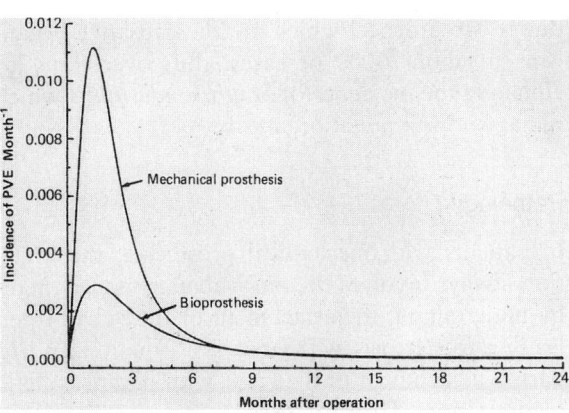

Fig. 34.8. Hazard function for prosthetic valve endocarditis in patients with mechanical and bioprostheses. Note the early peak and the increased incidence in patients with mechanical prostheses. (Reproduced by permission of the American Heart Association from Ivert T.S.A. *et al., Circulation* 1984, **69**: 223–32.)

to cover the period of surgery and remain as the predominant skin commensal for some time thereafter. While it persists, it is likely to be the causative agent in any episodes of infective endocarditis that occur. Other important causative organisms early after surgery are faecal streptococci and diphtheroids.

Infective endocarditis occurring late after operation (sometimes many years) behaves in a similar manner to that on native valves, and the organisms implicated are generally the flora of infective endocarditis on native valves although coagulase-negative staphylococci still occur more often than in other situations.

Although the results of early studies suggested that aortic prostheses carried a higher risk than mitral prostheses, in the largest study to date no such difference was found.[31] Further findings from the same study showed that elderly patients and those with multiple valve prostheses have a particularly high risk and that valve replacement for active endocarditis of a native valve carries an increased risk of early prosthetic valve endocarditis.

Bacteriology

The most frequent organism in both early and late endocarditis is *Staph. epidermidis* (30% of cases). In early endocarditis, other organisms, which are not frequently seen later, are important, including *Staph. aureus* (15%), aerobic Gram-negative organisms (20%) and fungi (14%) (*Candida* and *Aspergillus* spp.). In contrast, late endocarditis is often due to streptococci which are the causative organisms in about 40% of cases, thus overtaking or equalling the incidence of *Staph. epidermidis* which remains a prominent organism.

Pathology

In patients with mechanical prostheses, the infection always involves the paravalvular tissues thereby undermining the attachment of the valve, often leading to necrosis with abscess formation and to partial detachment of the valve with paraprosthetic regurgitation. These abscesses may extend further into the myocardium to cause myocardial damage and fistulae as in other forms of infective endocarditis although such events are more common in prosthetic endocarditis. In addition, vegetations may obstruct the valve itself, a complication occurring more frequently with mitral than aortic prostheses. The relative incidence of these complications is shown in Table 34.3.[32–35]

Infective endocarditis involving tissue valves follows a similar pattern, but paravalvular involvement with its potential for extension into the myocardium and valve detachment occurs at about half the frequency of that with mechanical prostheses (30–40% of cases).[36] In approximately 50% of cases, infection is limited to the valve leaflets which are often eroded or perforated or, less commonly, partially obstructed by vegetations.[37]

Clinical features and diagnosis

The diagnosis of prosthetic valve endocarditis requires a high index of suspicion. The diagnosis should be suspected in any patient with a prosthetic valve who has unexplained fever, embolization, a new murmur or generalized ill-health. New murmurs may not occur, particularly in the early stage before valve detachment occurs. Even then, severe regurgitation, particularly through or around the mitral valve, may not produce *any significant heart murmur*.

As for endocarditis affecting native heart valves, blood cultures are the mainstay of diagnosis. Fungal precipitins should be measured in view of the relatively high incidence of fungal infection in this group of patients, and Q fever should always be borne in mind. The high incidence of *Staph. epidermidis* is a particularly important feature. In prosthetic valve endocarditis, this organism should not be dismissed as a contaminant. Echocardiography is not particularly useful in patients with mechanical valves because vegetations are often not visible, but vegetations on tissue prostheses can frequently be identified.

Mortality is extremely high, ranging between 30 and 50%;[22,30] it is probably twice as high for early cases than for late cases,[22] because the infecting organisms are often virulent and difficult to treat. Fungal endocarditis is virtually confined to early cases.

Treatment

The first phase of treatment in any patient who is not haemodynamically compromised is appropriate antibiotic therapy. The recent trend towards early surgery in infective endocarditis has been particularly marked in the context of prosthetic endocarditis. In some centres, this approach has radically reduced mortality (from 60 to 23% in one series[38]). Many different indications for surgery have been suggested but the most important are listed in Table 34.4). Although 10 days of antibiotic therapy prior to surgery is often thought to be desirable, surgery should not be delayed if there is *any evidence* that the patient's condition is worsening, as postoperative endocarditis is remarkably uncommon even when the period of pre-operative antibiotic therapy has been brief.[22,32] Surgical mortality in this context has been reported to be no higher than that in patients with a similar degree of haemodynamic disturbance but who do not have endocarditis.[39] This observation needs to be confirmed.

Conclusion

Prosthetic endocarditis is common and a high index of suspicion is needed for its diagnosis. Because mortality is so high and as it may be lowered by timely surgery, all patients with this condition should be managed in a centre where cardiac surgery is available.

Table 34.3. Complications of prosthetic valve[a] endocarditis.[32–35]

Valve ring abscess	66%
Myocardial abscess	40%
Valve obstruction by vegetations	16%
Purulent pericarditis	6%

[a] Data refer to mechanical valves.

Table 34.4. Indications for surgery in infective endocarditis.

Indication	Native valve	Prosthetic valve[a]
Haemodynamic deterioration	+ +	+ +
Myocardial invasion or abscess	+ +	+ +
Signs of infection not resolving on medical therapy or relapse after adequate therapy	+ +	+ +
Fungi	+	+ +
Large vegetations on echo	(+)	(+)
New regurgitant murmur without haemodynamic deterioration	0	+ (early infection with agents which are not highly sensitive to antibiotics (+))
Systemic emboli	+	+

[a] Threshold for operation generally much lower with prosthetic endocarditis.
Key: (+), uncertain, an indication in some centres; +, sometimes required; + +, nearly always required.

NON-BACTERIAL THROMBOTIC ENDOCARDITIS

The term non-bacterial thrombotic endocarditis was introduced in 1936 by Gross and Friedberg to describe verrucous endocardial lesions occurring in a wide variety of chronic infections and wasting diseases, especially neoplasia and chronic leukaemia.[40] This condition is sometimes known as marantic thrombotic endocarditis. It is probably inappropriate to use the term endocarditis for this condition since it leads to little or no inflammatory reaction in the heart. A more appropriate term is non-bacterial endocardial thrombosis. These thrombi produce vegetation-like lesions which are sometimes minute but may be large and pedunculate. They can involve the mitral, aortic and tricuspid valves. Initially they consist of platelets and fibrin, but eventually they may become fibrotic.

The chief importance of this condition lies in its propensity to become colonized by bacteria and lead to infective endocarditis,[41] but even when not infected the vegetations may embolize to the brain, viscera, extremities and lungs and may also cause

petechiae on skin and mucous membranes.[42] Coronary emboli leading to myocardial infarction have been reported in up to 9% of patients.[43] Although some of the features of this condition simulate infective endocarditis, fever is usually absent and blood cultures are negative. The erythocyte sedimentation rate is often normal although it may be raised due to the underlying condition. A cardiac murmur is present in approximately 30% of cases. Non-bacterial endocardial thrombosis has been reported as a complication of most chronic illnesses and also in association with endocardial pacing electrodes and indwelling central venous lines and Swan–Ganz catheters.[44]

INVESTIGATIONS

Urine microscopy remains a useful but often neglected investigation. Microscopic haematuria is common, occurring in up to 90% of cases. There may also be casts in the urine as a result of the immune-complex glomerulonephritis.

There is usually a mild-to-moderate degree of anaemia which is usually of the normocytic normochromic type. The white blood cell count is often moderately raised (usually 12 000–14 000) with an increase in the number of neutrophils, but it may be normal. The erythrocyte sedimentation rate is invariably raised,[1,19] hyperglobulinaemia is common and the occurrence of a false-positive rheumatoid factor is not infrequent.[19,45]

The most important investigation is that of blood culture (discussed in detail elsewhere). Occasionally, important bacteriological information is obtained by culture and microscopic examination of material taken at valve surgery, or from a systemic embolus that has had to be removed. The latter is particularly important in fungal endocarditis which commonly leads to large peripheral emboli and is often difficult to diagnose by blood culture.

In certain specific situations, other blood tests are helpful. Q fever,[46] psittacosis[47] and brucella infections are usually diagnosed by characteristic serology and the diagnosis of fungal endocarditis is often dependent on identifying specific precipitins in the blood.

ELECTROCARDIOGRAM

An electrocardiogram should be performed every few days in patients with bacterial endocarditis. The occurrence of conduction abnormalities, most often first degree heart block but sometimes left bundle branch block or complete heart block, strongly suggest the possibility of intramyocardial spread of the infection with abscess formation near the conducting tissue. This is particularly sinister and requires urgent surgery.

ECHOCARDIOGRAM

The echocardiogram has proved invaluable in the diagnosis and the management of infective endocarditis. A detailed description of the changes occurring in endocarditis is given in Chapter 13. The most important features are reviewed below.

Echocardiography helps in the diagnosis of endocarditis, mainly by the detection of vegetations. It may be the only way in which intramyocardial spread of infection can be detected, and it contributes to the assessment of valve damage and haemodynamic disturbance produced by endocarditis. It often reveals the cardiac lesion that predisposed to infective endocarditis.

The minimum size of vegetation that can be detected by echocardiography is about 2 mm in diameter; most vegetations > 5 mm in diameter will be visualized. Vegetations may be attached to the surface of the valve or to the neighbouring endocardium. Echocardiography detects the former much more easily than the latter. Vegetations have a characteristic appearance, particularly on M-mode echocardiography in which they appear shaggy due to their rapid oscillation (Figs 34.1 and 34.9). Although their appearance is more characteristic on the M-mode than on the cross-sectional echocardiogram, the latter technique is much more sensitive in detecting vegetations (Fig. 34.10): M-mode echocardiography detects vegetations in approximately 50–60% of patients whereas cross-sectional echocardiography detects them in 70–80% of patients.[48,49]

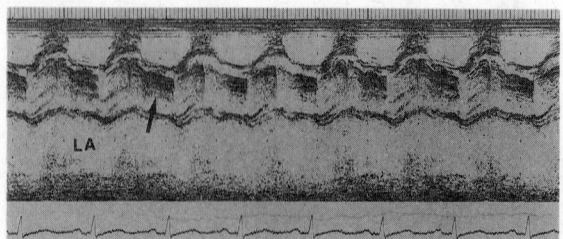

Fig. 34.9. M-Mode echocardiogram showing the aorta and left atrium (LA) of a patient with infective endocarditis involving the aortic valve. The vegetations on the aortic valve (arrow) produce prominent fuzzy echoes which have the M-mode characteristics of a vegetation.

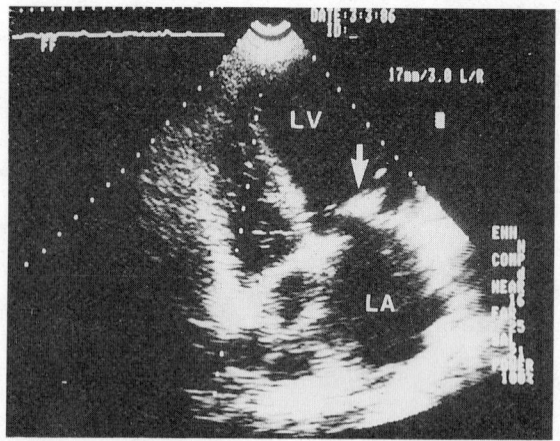

Fig. 34.10. Cross-sectional echocardiogram from a patient with infective endocarditis (apical four-chamber view). There is a large vegetation attached to the anterior cusp of the mitral valve (arrow). LV, left ventricle; LA, left atrium.

Echocardiography often fails to identify vegetations associated with right-sided endocarditis or on prosthetic valves.[50] Strong reflections from the prosthetic valve tend to overshadow the more delicate reflections from the vegetations. Detection tends to be better when the patients have larger vegetations, which occur in more advanced cases. During the first 2 weeks of the infection, vegetations tend to be small and are very rarely detected. Most studies of echocardiography in endocarditis have been reported from surgical referral centres. As these centres manage more advanced cases, the rate at which vegetations are detected is probably considerably higher than that in a district general hospital where early cases are diagnosed and treated before the vegetations enlarge and become visible.

Although the echocardiographic appearances of vegetations are often characteristic, occasionally mobile clots, tumours and redundant or exceptionally mobile valve tissue may be misdiagnosed as vegetations (Fig. 34.11). Finally, as vegetations frequently persist for a long time after endocarditis has been satisfactorily treated, the detection of a vegetation does not necessarily indicate that the patient has active endocarditis (Fig. 34.12).

Many of the problems with echocardiography can be resolved by using multiple views and a combination of cross-sectional and M-mode techniques.

Echocardiography is the best and often the only method available of detecting the extension of infection from its primary site into the surrounding tissues of the heart to form abscesses (Fig. 34.13).

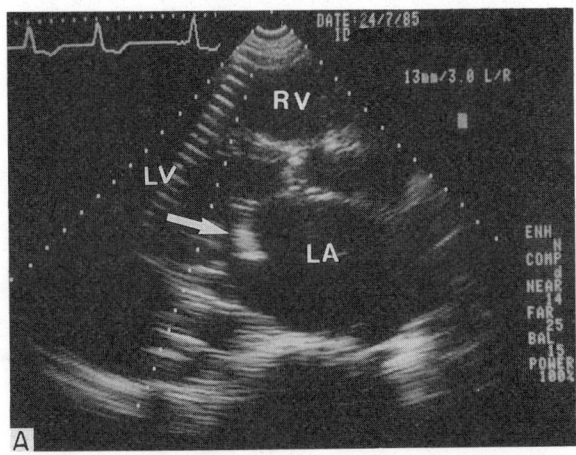
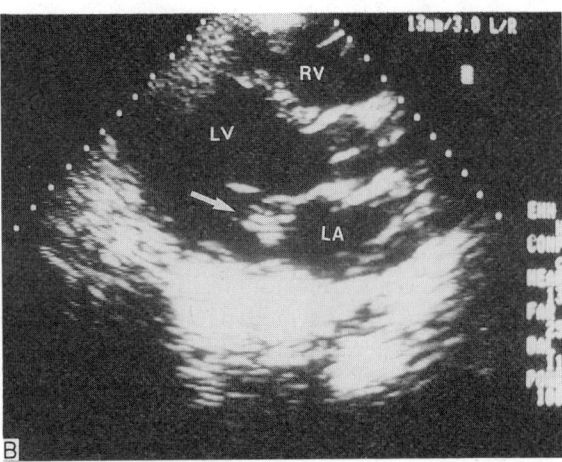

Fig. 34.11. Cross-sectional echocardiogram from a patient with infective endocarditis (A) and a patient with mitral valve prolapse and chordal rupture (B). The appearances on the cross-sectional echocardiogram (arrows) of the vegetation and of the redundant valve tissue and ruptured chordae are similar. LV, left ventricle; RV, right ventricle; LA, left atrium.

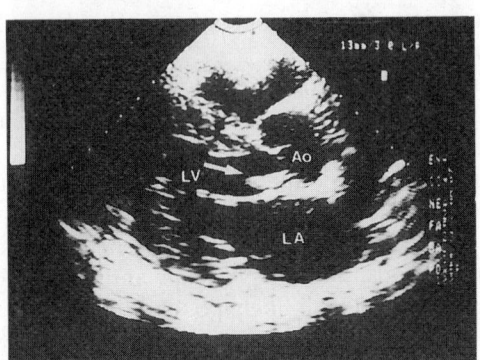

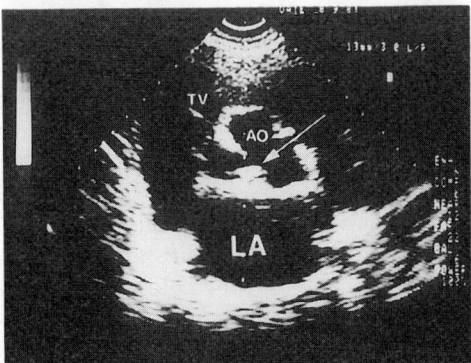

Fig. 34.12. Cross-sectional echocardiogram from a patient who had recovered from an attack of infective endocarditis some years before. A vegetation (arrow) is seen attached to the aortic valve in both the parasternal long-axis (upper panel) and parasternal short-axis (lower panel) views. AO, aorta; LV, left ventricle; LA, left atrium; TV, tricuspid valve.

Although abscesses may sometimes be detected by M-mode echocardiography, cross-sectional echocardiography is superior in this context[51]. It also allows close follow-up of the haemodynamic effects of endocarditis. Increasing ventricular size and changes in ventricular function can be detected and this information is valuable when making decisions about the timing of surgery.

Echocardiography is particularly helpful in the diagnosis of severe acute aortic regurgitation which

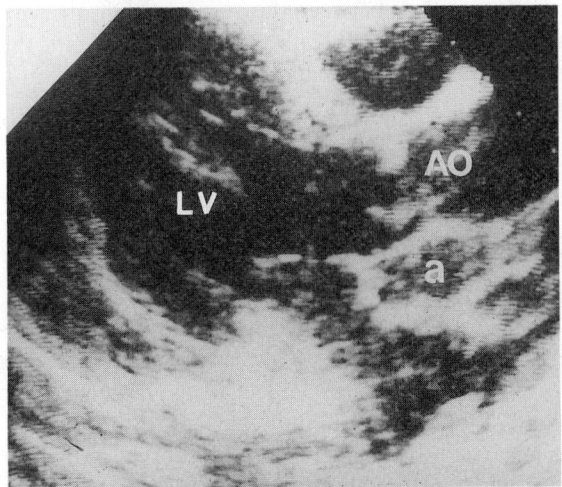

Fig. 34.13. Cross-sectional echocardiogram (parasternal long-axis view) showing a large abscess (a) posterior to the aortic root (AO). LV, left ventricle.

leads to premature closure of the mitral valve.[24,25] This phenomenon can only be detected with certainty using the M-mode technique which is far superior to cross-sectional echocardiography when determining the timing of cardiac events. The mechanisms underlying premature mitral valve closure are discussed in detail in Chapter 27.

Patients with endocarditis in whom vegetations are detected echocardiographically have a much higher incidence of haemodynamic deterioration, unresolved infection and embolization than those in whom vegetations are not detected, probably because vegetations are more easily detected when they are large and large vegetations occur in advanced disease. Despite this, up to 70% of patients in whom vegetations are detected by echocardiography do well on medical therapy.[52]

Recently, the detection of vegetations has improved considerably with the introduction of trans-oesophageal echocardiography.[53] In this technique, the echo transducer can be placed closer to the heart valves than when it is used on the exterior chest wall. Consequently, imaging is done in the near field of the echo transducer and resolution is much higher. Although this technique needs further evaluation and is available only in certain specialist centres, it appears to be extremely promising as a way of significantly increasing the echo detection of vegetations (possibly in as many as 90% of cases) and may be particularly valuable in prosthetic endocarditis.

Recently, we have found computed tomographic scanning to be a useful technique for the detection of intracardiac abscesses, missed by echo (e.g. in the para-aortic area between the aorta and left atrium), and extracardiac abscesses (e.g. splenic). In the future, magnetic resonance imaging will be helpful in detecting abscesses.

CARDIAC CATHETERIZATION

There are very few applications for cardiac catheterization in infective endocarditis. The passage of a catheter through a valve covered by friable vegetations is likely to be disastrous in view of the high risk of embolism. In the past, aortography was necessary to define aneurysms and abscesses associated with aortic valve endocarditis, but nowadays cross-sectional echocardiography gives superior results to those of angiography and the associated risk is less.

DIAGNOSIS

The diagnosis of infective endocarditis depends on a high index of suspicion, particularly in the elderly, who may have no fever and in whom heart murmurs of no haemodynamic significance are common, and in high-risk patients, such as those with prosthetic valves or intravenous drug abusers in whom endocarditis commonly occurs without significant cardiac murmurs. A high-risk group who are becoming particularly prominent are immunocompromised patients, for example, those on chemotherapy for leukaemia in whom chronic indwelling vascular devices are frequently used to facilitate venous access.

The mainstay of diagnosis is the blood culture and, in certain situations, measurement of specific precipitins or antibodies, e.g. Q fever and fungal endocarditis. The echocardiogram is an extremely helpful investigation,[54] however, the absence of vegetation does not exclude the diagnosis, particularly in the early stages of the condition, and vegetations may still be present from a previous episode of endocarditis, in patients who do not have active infection.[52]

Diagnosis is particularly difficult in the so-called culture-negative cases. These patients have a clinical picture which is so suggestive of endocarditis that it cannot be ignored, and often they have vegetations detected on echocardiography.[54] Such patients may require treatment, despite the absence of positive blood culture, initially with an antibiotic regime designed to cover all likely possibilities; in a patient who is deteriorating clinically, surgery may be necessary to eradicate the undefined infection.

DIFFERENTIAL DIAGNOSIS

As endocarditis does not have any clinical features that are absolutely characteristic, its differential diagnosis is wide.

The most important conditions likely to masquerade as infective endocarditis are chronic infective diseases, such as tuberculosis or brucellosis which itself may cause infective endocarditis,[55] and chronic inflammatory conditions of a non-infective nature, such as collagen vascular disease and occult neoplasia. Lymphomas are particularly likely to produce a clinical picture that can be confused with endocarditis.

Cardiac tumours, of which left atrial myxoma is the most common, can produce an illness very similar to that of infective endocarditis, with evidence of chronic inflammatory disease, weight loss, fever and murmurs. Fortunately, echocardiography usually resolves uncertainty about the diagnosis.

Patients who have undergone cardiac surgery and develop a post-cardiotomy syndrome may have a persistent fever which can be difficult to differentiate from endocarditis. The occurrence of precordial discomfort, which is uncommon in endocarditis, and small bilateral pleural effusions possibly with evidence of pleurisy are features that may aid in differentiation. Ultimately, repeated negative blood cultures and an absence of vegetations on echocardiography are the most helpful ways of differentiating the post-cardiotomy syndrome from infective endocarditis.

NATURAL HISTORY AND PROGNOSIS

Until effective antibiotic therapy became available, the mortality from infective endocarditis was nearly 100%. Nowadays, eradication of infection can be achieved in over 90% of patients, but considerably fewer survive the illness because death is often not due to uncontrolled infection but to complications, such as heart failure, embolic episodes and renal failure. These complications may persist and worsen after active infection has been controlled. Widely differing figures for mortality have been reported from series of patients with infective endocarditis occurring on native heart valves and diagnosed during life. The joint report of the British Cardiac Society and the Royal College of Physicians Research Unit found a mortality of only 14.4% but the authors suggested that there was serious underreporting.[3] A much higher overall mortality is reported in most series. Schnurr et al. reported a 35% mortality in 70 patients with infective endocarditis;[21] cardiac failure was the commonest cause of death (19 of 25 deaths), followed in frequency by embolic phenomena, problems at surgery or renal failure. Certain features have been identified as likely to lead to an adverse outcome, including increasing age, infection with Staph. aureus and cardiac failure. In contrast to the high overall mortality that occurs in series comprising patients with different types of endocarditis, the classic form of subacute bacterial endocarditis caused by 'Streptococcus viridans' carries a much lower mortality of between 10 and 15% provided that the diagnosis is made and treatment is instituted before serious complications occur.

Series in which patients are diagnosed during life will inevitably lead to an underestimate of the overall mortality from this disease. Smith et al. tried to find all the cases of endocarditis occurring in South East Scotland over a 4-year period. They discovered a small number of patients in whom the diagnosis was first made at necropsy;[2] including these patients, they found that of 78 patients identified 37 died as a result of the illness (46%). Infective endocarditis remains a serious condition with a high mortality. The commonest cause of death is cardiac failure, on which early surgery is likely to have a significant effect. Special types of endocarditis, particularly those occurring on prosthetic valves (between 15 and 30% of all cases), continue to have a very high mortality. Bayliss et al. reported a 45% death rate in early cases and a 24% death rate in cases diagnosed more than 1 year after operation.[3] It seems likely that early surgery will reduce this mortality and the results contained in some reports confirm this possibility.[38]

Relapses of infection usually occur within the first 4 weeks after antibiotic treatment is discontinued, but they may develop as late as 3 months later. If a clinical and bacteriological cure appears to be present 6 months after treatment, this nearly always denotes permanent recovery from the given attack. Although the long-term outlook is favourable once the patient recovers from endocarditis without developing heart failure, renal failure, embolic complications or free aortic regurgitation, sometimes unexpected late deterioration occurs. Garvey and Neu[56] reported that 25% of patients leaving hospital, apparently cured, died during the next 7 years.

TREATMENT OF INFECTIVE ENDOCARDITIS

Treatment of infective endocarditis depends greatly on the recovery of the causative organism and careful examination of its sensitivity to antibiotics. Cure demands the eradication of every single living organism from the site of the infective endocarditis by the use of bactericidal drugs without assistance from the body defences. 'Ordinary' sensitivity tests do not reliably determine whether the antibiotic effects they detect are the result of killing the organism or merely the inhibition of growth. In infective endocarditis it is usually necessary to determine the minimum inhibitory concentration (MIC) and minimum bactericidal concentration (MBC) of the drug against the isolate for each case. Experimental work has shown that if levels 4–8 times the MIC/MBC are achieved in the serum sufficient drug will penetrate to the centre of the vegetations to produce cure. It has also been shown experimentally that the duration of treatment should be at least 10–14 days because a small subpopulation of organisms may survive in the presence of the antibiotic for this period before finally succumbing.[57]

STREPTOCOCCAL ENDOCARDITIS

It is unwise to rely on the identity of the streptococcus to guide therapy. Penicillin-resistant 'viridans' streptococci occur and penicillin-sensitive enterococci exist (*Strept. bovis*). In general, the dividing line between streptococci susceptible to killing by penicillins acting alone and those requiring the synergic effect of a penicillin-aminoglycoside combination is the MIC to penicillin of 0.1 mg/l. Although it has been argued that combination therapy should be given to all cases, exposure to the toxic side-effects of aminoglycosides should be limited to those patients in whom it is necessary. Therefore, if the MIC to penicillin is < 0.1 mg/l, the infective endocarditis should be treated with penicillin alone.[58] Treatment with penicillin entails prolonged parenteral therapy (28 days), and phlebitis is a problem. Sodium load can be significant at high dosage and neurotoxicity (myoclonus, grand mal fits and coma) can occur. For these reasons, intravenous ampicillin, 2 g every 6 hours for 2 weeks, followed by oral amoxycillin, 500 mg every 6 hours for 2 weeks, can be used instead, thereby obviating both these problems. The activity of ampicillin and amoxycillin against enterococci is probably greater than that of penicillin.

If an aminoglycoside is required, the usual choice is gentamicin. As only low serum levels are necessary (2–3 mg/l) to achieve synergy, it is permissible to underdose the patient, for example, to give 80 mg intravenously every 12 hours despite normal renal function, and so avoid toxicity. Although gentamicin seems to produce satisfactory synergy in almost all instances, streptomycin will not and netilmicin apparently fails to synergize on *Strept. faecium* strains.[58] In faecal streptococcal infective endocarditis gentamicin should be given for 28 days along with intravenous ampicillin (2 weeks) and oral amoxycillin (2 weeks).

In the first few days of therapy, the combination is often given until the MIC result is known, at which time the gentamicin can be withdrawn if appropriate. Considerable debate now centres on the course to be adopted when penicillin tolerance is detected (MIC < 0.1 mg/l, MBC much higher). Such strains, nearly always those of *Strept. sanguis*, are killed very slowly by penicillin; combination therapy may be necessary to achieve cure.

STAPHYLOCOCCUS AUREUS ENDOCARDITIS

Most cases of *Staph. aureus* endocarditis are due to methicillin-sensitive strains, in which case the mainstay of treatment is one of the isoxazolyl penicillins (flucloxacillin, cloxacillin, nafcillin) given in large intravenous doses (2 g) every 6 hours for 2 weeks, followed by a further 2 weeks of oral therapy at a dose of 1 g every 6 hours. Opinions differ over the value in combining this with a second drug such as fusidic acid or clindamycin. Flucloxacillin monotherapy is probably as effective as combination treatment.[59] The use of aminoglycosides in *Staph. aureus* infective endocarditis should be avoided because of the high risk of renal damage. If infective endocarditis due to a methicillin-resistant strain occurs, the drug of choice is vancomycin, 1 g IV every 12 hours; in cases of penicillin-allergy and in strains where beta-lactam tolerance is detected, an alternative regime of oral rifampicin 600 mg every 12 hours together with oral erythromycin 500 mg every 6 hours can be used.

COAGULASE-NEGATIVE STAPHYLOCOCCAL ENDOCARDITIS

As sensitivity tests on coagulase-negative staphylococci are among the most unpredictable used in infective endocarditis, recommendations are difficult to make. The combination of oral rifampicin, 600 mg every 12 hours, and oral erythromycin, 500 mg every 6 hours, is the initial regime of choice, although it is essential that detailed sensitivity testing is carried out; the regime may require modification depending on the test results.

OTHER ORGANISMS

It is impossible to list all the possible regimes occasionally necessary for the more unusual causes of infective endocarditis, many of which are anecdotal. However, logical changes have occurred in the treatment of rickettsial infective endocarditis, once thought to be incurable because only bacteriostatic drugs could be used. Recently, co-trimoxazole and also rifampicin-containing regimes have been used to treat this condition and there is now a prospect of medical cure.

PENICILLIN ALLERGY

It is always difficult to deny patients with the common forms of infective endocarditis the benefits of the penicillin group of drugs. Although alternatives can be used, the penicillins remain the mainstay of treatment. The majority of patients classified as allergic to penicillin are not found to be so when a history is obtained. However, those patients who have histories of urticarial eruptions or angioneurotic oedema are at obvious risk. A simple method of 'de-sensitization' (i.e. induction of tolerance) can be used successfully in most cases and then penicillin can be prescribed.[59]

ADJUNCTIVE TESTS

Tests of the ability of the patient's serum to kill the isolated organism are often performed during treatment (back-titrations, killing levels, cidal levels, Schlichter's test) and satisfactory titres are taken to indicate adequate therapy of the infective endocarditis. Such tests have the advantage of assessing the efficacy of a synergic combination. Whether such tests reliably indicate cure is debatable, but they are often a good guide to finding the cause of a continuing fever or other problem occurring during treatment. If inadequate therapy is excluded, common causes include abscess formation, drug fevers, venous thrombosis extending from the site of venous cannulae used for antibiotic administration and unrelated concurrent infections.

SURGERY IN INFECTIVE ENDOCARDITIS

Certain criteria are accepted as indications for surgery (Table 34.4), including dehiscence of the valve, uncontrollable left ventricular failure, evidence of annular abscess formation (usually manifest as conduction abnormalities) and recurrent major embolism. The presence of prosthetic material, the nature of the infecting organism, especially *Staph. aureus*, and more recently the presence of a large vegetation on echocardiography have been proposed as indications for surgery. The validity of these proposals has yet to be confirmed, but one reason for this variability in surgical indications could be that patients with different stages of the disease present at different centres. In at least one centre at which patients with *Staph. aureus* infective endocarditis on prosthetic valves presented within 4 days of the onset, medical cure was found to be possible in the majority of cases.[59] The commoner

experience of presentation later in the disease may explain the higher incidence of suppuration and therefore of surgery in most other centres.

Surgery has an important role in the management of infective endocarditis. It can be life-saving, particularly in patients with aortic valve endocarditis in whom the rupture of a cusp may lead to sudden severe irreversible heart failure. Surgery also has an important role in the treatment of patients with increasing haemodynamic deterioration due to valvular regurgitation and in those who have an intramyocardial spread of infection. As delay in such patients may lead to disastrous results, surgery should be undertaken earlier rather than later. In the past, attempts were made to give adequate courses of antibiotics before operation, but the additional haemodynamic deterioration that occurred during this time was often disastrous; moreover, the risk of infection following surgery, even after a brief period of antibiotic therapy, is low. Other indications for surgery in infective endocarditis are reviewed in Table 34.4. Surgery has a particularly important place in the treatment of prosthetic valve endocarditis, which is discussed elsewhere and summarized in Table 34.4.

PREVENTION OF INFECTIVE ENDOCARDITIS

There is considerable debate about the prevention and prophylaxis of infective endocarditis. The best approach to prevention would be the correction of all the cardiovascular defects on which infective endocarditis can arise, not only is this impossible, it has other major disadvantages. Prevention of the initiating bacteraemia is the most practical approach. However, the elimination of predisposing lesions can be pursued in a limited manner, the commonest example being the ligation of a patent ductus arteriosus.

Prophylaxis based on prevention of bacteraemia can be effective only in those patients in whom an episode of bacteraemia can be predicted. The earlier account of unprovoked bacteraemias and of bacteraemias due to such normal events as chewing indicates that many bacteraemias must occur which cannot be predicted and, therefore, prevented. Similarly, as chemoprophylaxis cannot be applied to those not known to be at risk of infective endocarditis, it is clear that even the best prophylaxis schemes can cover only a fraction of the potential problem. Studies in animal models have suggested that the prophylactic regimes commonly used for many years may not produce the desired effect.[60] Finally, there is no proof that antibiotic prophylaxis, correctly administered at times of predictable bacteraemia in subjects at risk, works. Prevention of bacteraemia may be demonstrable but demonstrating the prevention of infective endocarditis is almost impossible.

Two other factors are relevant. First, patients with predisposing heart lesions must be educated in the need for good dental care and prophylaxis and of the times at which it should be offered. Although it is reasonable to hope that the level of awareness in doctors, dentists and surgeons will be sufficient to ensure that appropriate patients are always identified at appropriate times, mistakes will occur. A card issued to every patient at risk, identifying that risk and stating the regimens to be given, is the safest system. The patient should be instructed to show the card to every physician, surgeon or dentist under whose care he or she may be and to ensure that enquiry is made of the cardiological unit whenever doubt exists. Second, it has been shown that the incidence of bacteraemia following trauma of contaminated mucosae and areas of localized infection can be decreased by using techniques that minimize damage to soft tissue, for instance, in dentistry, endodontic procedures are preferred to extractive measures in patients at risk.

There is no evidence to support the procedure of total dental clearance in order to reduce the incidence of infective endocarditis. It is much resented by patients and should not be undertaken.

ANTIBIOTIC PROPHYLAXIS FOR INFECTIVE ENDOCARDITIS

Three principles govern antibiotic prophylaxis. First, the antibiotic(s) chosen must be appropriate to the likely offending organism to be killed. It is important to note that not all released organisms are likely to initiate infective endocarditis. On native valves, prophylaxis is directed against streptococci and Staph. aureus. Second, the antibiotic regimen should be such that sufficient drug enters the blood and remains there for the required time to combat the bacteraemia. Third, the drug must be introduced in as short a time as possible before the onset of the bacteraemia to avoid the creation of a bacterial flora resistant to the drug. Failure to observe this last principle vitiates the whole technique.

Many different schemes have been proposed for antibiotic prophylaxis, that outlined in Table 34.5 has the merit of employing a well-tolerated oral drug whenever possible.

Prophylaxis for patients with predisposing lesions during pregnancy consists of appropriate use of the dental regimes when needed plus the use of the genito-urinary regime at the onset of the second stage of labour.

Prophylaxis is not routinely given for cardiac

Table 34.5. Scheme for antibiotic prophylaxis of infective endocarditis.

Situation	Regimen recommended
Dental procedures (extraction, scaling or surgery). Native valve. No antibiotics in last 4 weeks.	*Local anaesthesia*: 3 g amoxycillin,[a,b,c] orally, 1 h before procedure. *General anaesthesia*: 3 g amoxycillin,[a,b,c] orally, 4 h before procedure, then 3 g orally 6 h later. If oral route denied, 1 g amoxycillin[c] i.m. immediately prior, then 500 mg i.m. 6 h later
Dental procedures in patients sent to hospital: **1** General anaesthesia and antibiotics in last month **2** General anaesthesia and prosthetic valve **3** Previous infective endocarditis	1 g amoxycillin[c] i.m. plus 80 mg gentamicin i.m. immediately before anaesthesia or procedure. Then 500 mg amoxycillin[c] orally 6 h later
Surgery or instrumentation of upper respiratory tract. Native valve	1 g amoxycillin i.m. immediately before anaesthesia or procedure. Then 500 mg amoxycillin[c] i.m. 6 h later
Surgery or instrumentation of upper respiratory tract. Prosthetic valve	1 g amoxycillin[c] i.m. plus 80 mg gentamicin i.m. immediately before anaesthesia or procedure. Then 500 mg amoxycillin[c] i.m. 6 h later
Genito-urinary surgery or instrumentation	1 g amoxycillin[c] i.m. plus 80 mg gentamicin i.m. immediately before anaesthesia. Then 500 mg amoxycillin[c] i.m. or orally 6 h later

[a] A specially formulated 3-g sachet of amoxycillin is available for these procedures, where indicated.
[b] In children under 10 years of age, half the adult dose of amoxycillin should be given and gentamicin, where indicated, at 2 mg/kg.
[c] In patients allergic to penicillins or in those receiving continuous penicillin prophylaxis for rheumatic fever, erythromycin may be substituted for the oral amoxycillin at a dose of 500 mg in adults and 20 mg/kg in small children. In regimes specifying parenteral amoxycillin, allergic subjects should receive i.v. vancomycin 500 mg (20 mg/kg in children) in place of the i.m. amoxycillin.

catheterization. In open-heart surgery, narrow-spectrum prophylaxis to cover staphylococci and diphtheroids is afforded by intravenous flucloxacillin (or nafcillin) (2 g) at induction of anaesthesia, followed by 500 mg every 6 hours until all major lines are removed.[61]

REFERENCES

1. Blount, J.G. Bacterial endocarditis. *Am. J. Med.* 1965; **38**: 909–22.
2. Smith, R.H., Radford, D.J., Clark R.A. and Julian D.G. Infectious endocarditis: A survey of cases in the South East region of Scotland between 1969 and 1972. *Thorax* 1976; **31**: 373.
3. Bayliss, R., Clark, C., Oakley, C.M. *et al.* Incidence, mortality and prevention of infective endocarditis. *J. R. Coll. Physicians Lond.* 1986; **20**: 15.
4. Pelletier, L.L. and Petersdorf, R.G. Prevention of infective endocarditis. In: Julian, D.G. and Humphries, J.O'N., eds. *Preventive Cardiology*. London: Butterworths, 1983, p. 88.
5. Uwaydah, M.M. and Weinberg, A.N. Bacterial endocarditis—a changing pattern. *N. Engl. J. Med.* 1965; **273**: 1231–5.
6. Bisno, A.L. Antimicrobial prophylaxis of infective endocarditis. In: Bisno, A.L., ed. *Treatment of Infective Endocarditis*. New York: Grune and Stratton, 1981, Ch. 17.
7. Werner, A.S., Cobbs, C.G. and Kaye, D. Studies on the bacteraemia of bacterial endocarditis. *JAMA* 1967; **202**: 199–203.
8. Wilson, W.R. and Garaca, J.E. Antimicrobial therapy for penicillin-sensitive streptococcal endocarditis. In: Bisno, A.L., ed. *Treatment of Infective Endocarditis*. New York: Grune and Stratton, 1981, Ch. 4.
9. Levison, M.E. Pathogenesis of infective endocarditis. In: Kaye, D., ed. *Endocarditis*. Baltimore: University Park Press, 1976, pp. 29–41.
10. Lerner, P.I. and Weinstein, L. Infective endocarditis in the antibiotic era. *N. Engl. J. Med.* 1966; **274**: 323–31.
11. Okell, C.C. and Elliot, S.D. Bacteraemia and oral sepsis with special reference to the etiology of subacute endocarditis. *Lancet* 1935; **2**: 869–74.
12. Elliot, S.D. Bacteraemia and oral sepsis. *Proc. R. Soc. Med.* 1939; **32**: 747–54.
13. Elliot, S.D. Bacteraemia following tonsillectomy. *Lancet* 1939; **2**: 589–92.
14. Cobe, H.M. Transitory bacteraemia. *Oral Surg.* 1954; **7**: 609–15.
15. Berger, S.A., Weitzman, S. and Edberg, S.C. Bacteraemia after using an oral irrigation device. *Ann. Intern. Med.* 1974; **80**: 510–1.
16. Cobbs, C.G. IUD and endocarditis. *Ann. Intern. Med.* 1973; **78**: 451.
17. Durack, D.T. and Beeson, P.B. Experimental bacterial endocarditis. I. Colonization of a sterile vegetation. *Br. J. Exp. Pathol.* 1972; **53**: 44–9.
18. Rogers, D.E. *Staphylococcal infections*, Disease-a-month series. Chicago: Year Book, April 1958, pp. 23–4.
19. Lerner, P.I. and Weinstein, L. Infective endocarditis in the antibiotic era. *N. Engl. J. Med.* 1966; **274**: 199, 259, 323, 388.
20. Holler, J.W. and Pecora, A.S. Back-ache in bacterial endocarditis. *N. Y. State J. Med.* 1962; **70**: 1903.
21. Schnurr, L.P., Ball, A.P., Geddes, A.M. *et al.* Bacterial endocarditis in England in the 1970's. A review of 70 patients. *Q. J. Med.* 1977; **46**: 499.
22. Karchmer, A.W. Treatment of prosthetic valve endocarditis. In: Sand, M.A., Kaye, D. and Root, R.T., eds. *Endocarditis*. New York, Edinburgh, London and Melbourne: Churchill Livingstoke, 1984.
23. Kilpatrick, Z.M., Greenberg, P.A. and Ganford, J.P. Splinter hemorrhages—their clinical significance. *Arch. Intern. Med.* 1965; **115**: 730.
24. Wise, J.R. Jr, Bentall, H.H., Cleland, W.P. *et al.* Urgent aortic valve replacement for acute aortic regurgitation due to infective endocarditis. *Lancet* 1971; **2**: 115.
25. Mann, T., McLaurin, L., Grossman, W. and Craige, E. Assessing the haemodynamic severity of acute aortic regurgitation due to infective endocarditis. *N. Engl. J. Med.* 1975; **108**: 293.
26. Greenlee, J.E. and Mandell, G.L. Neurological manifestations of infective endocarditis. A review. *Stroke* 1973; **4**: 958.
27. Banks, R., Fletcher, R. and Ali, N. Infective endocarditis in heroin addicts. *Am. J. Med.* 1973; **55**: 444.
28. Stimmel, B. and Dack, S. Infective endocarditis in narcotic addicts. In: Rahimtoola, S.H., ed. *Infective Endocarditis*. New York: Grune and Stratton, 1978, p. 195.
29. Rapaport, E. The changing role of surgery in the management of infective endocarditis (Editorial). *Circulation* 1978; **58**: 598.
30. Ivert, T.S.A., Dismukes, W.E., Cobbs, C.G. *et al.* Prosthetic Valve Endocarditis. *Circulation* 1984; **69**: 223–32.
31. Calderwood, S.B., Swinski, L.A., Waternaux, C.M. *et al.* Risk factors for the development of prosthetic valve endocarditis. *Circulation* 1985; **72**: 31–7.
32. Richardson, J.V., Karp, R.B., Kirklin, J.W. and Dismukes, W.E. Treatment of infective endocarditis: a 10-year comparative analysis. *Circulation* 1978; **58**: 589–97.
33. Dismukes, W.E., Karchmer, A.W. and Buckley, M.J. Prosthetic valve endocarditis: analysis of 38 cases. *Circulation* 1973; **48**: 365–77.
34. Anderson, D.J., Bulkly, G.H. and Hutchins, G.M. A clinicopathologic study of prosthetic valve endocarditis in 22 patients: morphologic basis for diagnosis and therapy. *Am. Heart J.* 1977; **94**: 325–32.
35. Arnett, E.N. and Roberts, W.C. Prosthetic valve endocarditis. Clinicopathologic analysis of 22 necropsy patients with active infective endocardiotic involving natural left-sided cardiac valves. *Am. J. Cardiol.* 1976; **38**: 281–92.
36. Baumgartner, W.A., Miller, D.C., Reitz, D.A. *et al.* Surgical treatment of prosthetic valve endocarditis, *Ann. Thorac. Surg.* 1983; **35**: 87.
37. Bortolotti, U., Thiene, G., Milano, A. *et al.* Pathological study of infective endocarditis on Hancock porcine bioprostheses. *J. Thorac. Cardiovasc. Surg.* 1981; **81**: 934–42.
38. Saffle, J.R., Gardner, P., Schoenbaum, S.C. and Wild, W. Prosthetic valve endocarditis: the case for prompt valve replacement. *J. Thorac. Cardiovasc. Surg.* 1977; **73**: 416–20.
39. Wison, W.R., Danielson, G.K., Giuliani, E.R. *et al.* Cardiac valve replacement in congestive heart failure due to infective endocarditis. *Proc. Mayo Clin.* 1979; **54**: 223–6.
40. Gross, L. and Friedberg, C. Non-bacterial thrombotic endocarditis. *Arch. Intern. Med.* 1936; **58**: 620.
41. Durack, D.T. and Beeson, P.B. Pathogenesis of infective endocarditis. In: Rahimtoola, S.H., ed. *Infective Endocarditis*. New York: Grune and Stratton, 1978.
42. Deppisch, L.M. and Fayemi, A.O. Non-bacterial thrombotic endocarditis. *Am. Heart J.* 1976; **92**: 723.
43. Fayemi, A.O. and Deppisch, L.M. Coronary embolism and myocardial infarction associated with non-bacterial thrombotic endocarditis. *Am. J. Clin. Pathol.* 1977; **68**: 393.
44. Greene, J.F. and Cummings, K.C. Aseptic thrombotic endocardial vegetations. A complication of indwelling pulmonary artery catheters. *JAMA* 1973; **225**: 1525.

45. Messner, R.P., Laxdal, T., Quie, P.G. and Williams Jr, R.C. Rheumatoid factors in subacute bacterial endocarditis—Bacterium, duration of disease, or genetic predisposition? *Ann. Intern. Med.* 1968; **746**: 68.
46. Turck, W.P.G., Howitt, G., Turnberg, L.A. *et al.* Chronic Q fever. *Q. J. Med.* 1976; **45**: 193.
47. Levison, D.A., Guthrie, W., Ward, C. *et al.* Infective endocarditis as part of psittacosis. *Lancet* 1971; **2**: 844.
48. Kisslo, J., Guadalajara, J.F., Stewart, J.A. *et al.* Echocardiography in the diagnosis and management of infective endocarditis. *Herz* 1983; **8**: 271.
49. Smith, M.D., Kwan, O.L. and DeMaria, A.N. The role of echocardiography in the diagnosis and management of infective endocarditis. *Practical Cardiol.* 1984; **10**: 78.
50. Martin, R.P., Meltzer, R.S., Chia, B.L. *et al.* Clinical utility of two dimensional echocardiography in infective endocarditis. *Am. J. Cardiol.* 1980; **46**: 379.
51. Scanlan, J.G., Seward, J.B. and Tajik, A.J. Valve ring abscesses in infective endocarditis: visualization with wide angle two-dimensional echocardiography. *Am. J. Cardiol.* 1982; **49**: 1794.
52. Stewart, J.A., Slimperi, D., Harris, P. *et al.* Echocardiographic documentation of vegetative lesions in infective endocarditis: clinical implications. *Circulation* 1980; **61**: 374.
53. Erbel, R., Rohmann, S., Drexter, M. *et al.* Diagnostic value of transoesophageal echocardiography in infective endocarditis (Abstract). *Circulation* 1986; **74** (Suppl. II): 55.
54. Rubenson, D.S., Tucker, C.R., Stinson, E.B. *et al.* The use of echocardiography in diagnosing culture-negative endocarditis. *Circulation* 1981; **64**: 641.
55. Peery, T.M. and Belter, L.F. Brucellosis and heart disease. II. Fatal brucellosis: A review of the literature and a report of new cases. *Am. J. Pathol.* 1969; **36**: 673.
56. Garvey, G.J. and Neu, H.C. Infective endocarditis: an evolving disease. A review of endocarditis at the Columbus Presbyterian Medical Center. 1968–1973. *Medicine* 1978; **57**: 105.
57. Karchmer, A.W. Issues in the treatment of endocarditis caused by viridans streptococci. In: Bisno, A.L., ed. *Treatment of Infective Endocarditis.* New York: Grune and Stratton, 1981, pp. 31–59.
58. Moellering, R.C., Korzeniowski, O.M., Sande, M.A. and Wennersten, C.B. Species-specific resistance to antimicrobial synergism in *Streptococcus faecium* and *Streptococcus faecalis. J. Infect. Dis.* 1979; **140**: 203–8.
59. Freeman, R., Jones, M.R. and Gould, F.K. Treatment of *Staphylococcus aureus* endocarditis: An analysis based on 25 proven cases. *Eur. Heart J.* 1986; **7**: 679–84.
60. Durack, D.T. Experience with prevention of experimental endocarditis. In: Kaplan, E.L. and Taranta, A.V., eds. *Infective Endocarditis*, American Heart Association Monograph No. 52. Dallas: American Heart Association, 1977, p. 28.
61. Freeman, R. and Gould, F.K. Antibiotic prophylaxis for cardiac surgery. *Perfusion* 1986; **1**: 75–9.
62. McLeod, R. and Remington, J.S. Fungal endocarditis. In: Rahimtoola, S.H., ed. *Infective Endocarditis.* New York: Grune and Stratton, 1978, p. 211.
63. Rubinstein, E., Noriega, E.R., Simberkoff, M., Fahal Jr, J.J. Tissue penetrations of amphotericin B in candida endocarditis. *Chest* 1974; **66**: 376.
64. Craddock, P.R., Yawata, Y., Silvis, S. and Jacob, H. Phagocyte dysfunction induced by intravenous hyperlimentation. *Clin. Res.* 1973; **21**: 597.
65. Robboy, S.J., Salisbury, K., Ragsdale, B. *et al.* Mechanism of Aspergillus-induced microangiopathic hemolytic anemia. *Arch. Intern. Med.* 1971; **128**: 790.
66. Utley, J.R., Mills, J. and Roe, B. The role of valve replacement in the treatment of fungal endocarditis. *J. Thorac. Cardiovasc. Surg.* 1975; **69**: 255.

Chapter 35

Surgery for Valvular Heart Disease

David J. Wheatley

Diseases affecting heart valves may result in valve stenosis causing obstruction to forward blood flow or valve incompetence causing regurgitation of blood, or a combination of both. Techniques that correct valve malfunction, whether by repair or replacement, have an important role in the management of valvular heart disease. These techniques are now routine, but refinements and improvements continue to be made.

Although the operation of closed mitral commissurotomy had become well established by the late 1950s, it was not until the advent of safe techniques of cardiopulmonary bypass that a direct approach was possible to allow repair or replacement of diseased heart valves. Prosthetic heart valves have been available for over 25 years[1] and, broadly speaking, can be categorized as mechanical or tissue prostheses.[2-4]

Probably over one million heart valves have now been replaced;[1] currently, in the USA, more than 30 000 valve operations[5] and in the UK about 5000 operations[6] are performed annually. Although surgical treatment is not yet devoid of problems, it has transformed the outlook for most patients with valvular heart disease.

PATHOPHYSIOLOGICAL ASPECTS OF VALVULAR HEART DISEASE

Surgical management of patients with valvular heart disease depends very much on the nature of the pathology; indications for surgery, its timing, and its risks are directly related to the pathophysiological effects of the abnormal valve on the heart, lungs and other viscera.

AORTIC VALVE

Congenital abnormalities of the aortic valve may be encountered surgically at any age and it may be impossible to distinguish between a congenital and an acquired cause for the commonly encountered, heavily calcified, stenotic aortic valve in the elderly.

A bicuspid aortic valve may be stenotic at birth due to commissural fusion but, more commonly, it becomes stenotic in later life due to calcification which stiffens the leaflets. Stenosis of the aortic valve in children may be due to a variety of pathologies. The most severe is hypoplastic left heart syndrome (in which the underdeveloped aortic valve is merely part of a more widespread abnormality), incompatible with prolonged extrauterine life. Underdevelopment of the aortic root, often with commissural fusion, requires a surgical procedure to enlarge the aortic root in addition to relief of the valve stenosis itself. The simpler forms of stenosis are due to commissural fusion of either bicuspid or three-leaflet valves, where the tissues are usually thin and pliable and amenable to commissural division.

The aortic valve may be incompetent due to prolapse of a leaflet inadequately supported as a result of sub-aortic ventricular septal defect. The aortic valve in truncus arteriosus is frequently incompetent but, because of the early age at presentation, is often not amenable to surgical treatment.

Abnormalities of collagen, such as occur in Marfan's syndrome, may affect the aortic valve annulus, usually together with the aortic root. This causes progressive dilatation of the aortic root and valve annulus and results in aortic incompetence.

The most common acquired condition affecting the aortic valve is rheumatic fever. The surgeon rarely sees the acute, oedematous, inflamed valve, although commissural fusion or aortic valve annular dilatation may require surgical intervention in florid manifestations of the disease. Longstanding rheumatic change in the aortic valve may result in the fusion of commissures causing stenosis, fibrosis, stiffening and shrinkage of the leaflets leading to a combination of stenosis and incompetence and, less often, predominant retraction of the free edges of the leaflets leading to incompetence alone (Fig. 35.1). Increasing calcification in the valve leaflets and annulus, often extending down onto the anterior leaflet of the mitral valve, is common by the time the valve is seen at surgery.

Aortic incompetence as a result of syphilis is rarely seen now. Dissection of the ascending aorta (type A) may lead to aortic incompetence as a result of the undermining of commissural support and prolapse of the valve leaflets. Other uncommon causes of aortic valve abnormality include aortic sclerosis, systemic lupus erythematosus and ankylosing spondylitis.[7]

Infective endocarditis may affect any abnormal heart valve, including the normally functioning bicuspid valve, and occasionally even an apparently anatomically normal valve. It produces vegetations on the valve and it may lead to systemic embolism and extension of infection into the valve annulus and surrounding tissues.

The main pathophysiological consequence of aortic valve disease relevant to surgical management is its adverse effect on the balance of myocardial oxygen supply and demand.[8] Hypertrophied left ventricular myocardium has to depend for its perfusion on a shorter diastolic period with stenotic lesions or a lowered diastolic perfusion pressure with regurgitant lesions. This has important implications for anaesthetic and peri-operative management.

MITRAL VALVE

Congenital mitral stenosis is very rare. Incompetence is a common feature of ostium primum and atrioventricular canal defects.

Rheumatic fever is the commonest cause of acquired mitral valve disease. The valve may become incompetent in the acute phase due to annular dilatation with inflammatory thickening of the leaflets but this rarely presents to the surgeon.

Chronic rheumatic fever may cause fusion of the commissures and very little abnormality in the leaflets or chordae tendineae; such pliable valves are ideal for commissurotomy. More extensive involvement results in fusion and thickening of the chordae which retract with time and pull the leaflets down into the ventricle causing the characteristic funnel-shaped valve. Thickening due to fibrosis causes loss of pliability of the leaflets which contributes to stenosis and regurgitation. Calcification is common and increases with time, affecting the commissures, the valve leaflets and the valve annulus (Fig. 35.2).

Floppy mitral valves show myxomatous degeneration of the collagen in the valve, which may be due to a genetically determined abnormality of collagen synthesis. Most frequently it occurs in isolation but may be seen in conditions such as Marfan's syndrome, in which more widespread abnormalities of collagen occur in the cardiovascular system and elsewhere. The mitral leaflets are voluminous and prolapse into the atrium. Dilatation of the mitral annulus or rupture of chordae may occur and result in mitral incompetence (Fig. 35.3).

Ischaemic mitral incompetence is a complex and varied condition occurring as a consequence of coronary disease. It may result from damage to a papillary muscle due to infarction, either with rupture of a muscle tip, or with loss of contractility of papillary muscle and the surrounding myocardium as a result of the infarct. Alternatively, ischaemic dysfunction of the papillary muscle and its surrounding myocardium, or generalized dilatation and distortion of the extensively infarcted or scarred left ventricle, may result in mitral incompetence.[9]

The abnormal mitral valve may be affected by

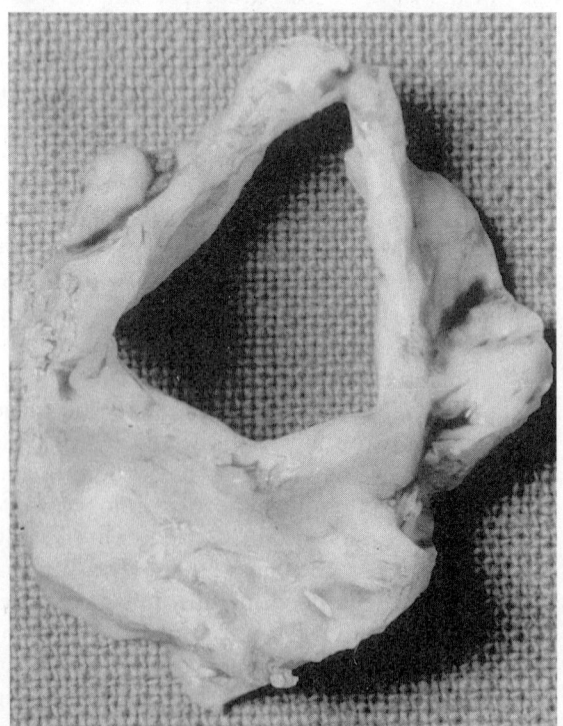

Fig. 35.1. A surgically resected aortic valve showing features of chronic rheumatic disease.

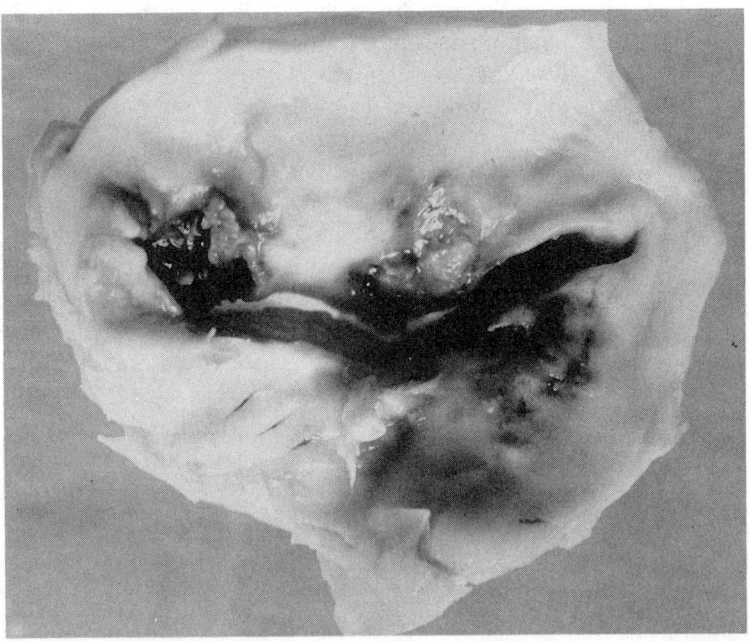

Fig. 35.2. A surgically resected mitral valve showing features of chronic rheumatic disease. There is ulceration over calcific areas.

infective endocarditis, acute or subacute, bacterial or fungal. Vegetations may break off the leaflets and embolize; leaflet destruction leads to rapid progression of mitral regurgitation.

From a surgical viewpoint, the major pathophysiological effects of mitral valve disease of relevance are those on the lungs, the right side of the heart and the liver.[8] Passive pulmonary congestion may result in pulmonary oedema, an important consideration in the indications for surgery, and also limits the patient's ability to cope with changes in posture and fluid balance, of relevance to anaesthetic and operative management. Active pulmonary arteriolar vasoconstriction may exacerbate pulmonary hypertension with mitral disease and increase the risks of surgery. The main effect on the right side of the heart of relevance in surgery is that on the tricuspid valve, which may become functionally regurgitant due to dilatation of its annulus and the increased right ventricular systolic pressure. This frequently requires surgical correction by annuloplasty at the time of mitral valve surgery. The effects of passive congestion of the liver include derangements of clotting mechanisms.

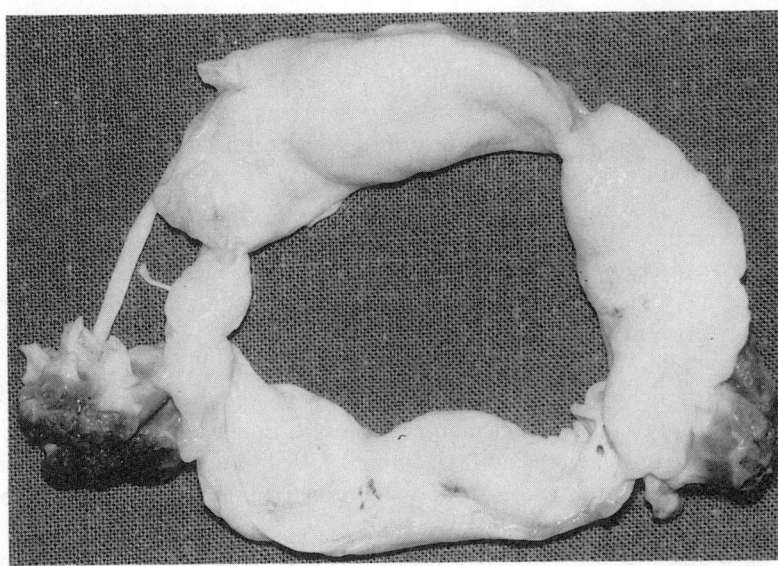

Fig. 35.3. A surgically resected floppy mitral valve.

TRICUSPID VALVE

Tricuspid valve abnormalities may be part of complex congenital conditions, such as Ebstein's anomaly, atrioventricular canal defects and tricuspid atresia. Although the tricuspid valve may be involved in the rheumatic process, organic disease is relatively uncommon. Tricuspid valve involvement is more frequently a functional incompetence consequent on organic rheumatic mitral valve disease with pulmonary hypertension, high right ventricular systolic pressure and dilatation of the tricuspid annulus being the cause of tricuspid regurgitation.

PULMONARY VALVE

The pulmonary valve is rarely affected by acquired lesions. Simple commissural fusion is seen in congenital stenosis. More complex forms of hypoplasia or dysplasia occur and pulmonary valve abnormalities are part of a more extensive abnormality in pulmonary atresia and tetralogy of Fallot.

INVESTIGATIONS AND INDICATIONS FOR SURGERY

Rational evaluation of the need for surgery, its nature, timing and conduct, as well as subsequent management, require knowledge of the severity of haemodynamic disturbance caused by the abnormal heart valve, the pathological effects on the myocardium, lungs and other viscera, the nature of the causative pathology and its natural history,[10] as well as an awareness of the problems and results of surgery.

Much of this information can be obtained from a good history and physical examination and confirmed by relatively simple, non-invasive means including electrocardiography, radiology and echocardiography. The need for cardiac catheterization arises when the history or physical findings are equivocal, where multiple valve involvement is suspected, or where significant coronary artery disease may be present.

The need for coronary angiography may arise in patients with valvular heart disease in whom appropriate non-invasive means of assessment, such as exercise testing, are not possible. In practice, this means undertaking coronary angiography in patients with aortic valve disease who present with angina pectoris. It is wise to undertake coronary angiography even when the severity of aortic stenosis may be deemed adequate to explain the angina, particularly in populations where coronary disease is prevalent, as co-existing coronary disease may be present.

The need for coronary angiography arises less frequently in patients with mitral valve disease; it is required in the presence of angina pectoris. If mitral incompetence is judged to have an ischaemic basis, coronary angiography is an integral part of the investigation. In populations with a high prevalence of coronary artery disease, particularly in which there are coronary risk factors, this study should be undertaken in those over an arbitrary age of 45–50 years when valvular surgery is contemplated.

The indications for valvular heart surgery are relatively well established.[8] In general, surgery is indicated for relief of symptoms and in the expectation of favourably modifying the natural history. The risk of the particular intervention required must be taken into account. The risk of surgery is generally lower in less severely disabled patients than in those toward the end of their natural history.

AORTIC VALVE DISEASE

Aortic stenosis, once it becomes symptomatic, has a poor natural history and, therefore, surgery is indicated in all patients with symptoms attributable to a stenotic aortic valve. When symptoms are absent, clinical signs of severe stenosis together with electrocardiographic evidence of left ventricular hypertrophy or strain, a systolic pressure gradient of 50 mmHg or greater at rest, or a valve area (where calculated) of 1cm^2 or less are generally indications for surgery, although clinical assessment may modify the decision as, for example, in the elderly individual who is free of symptoms.

Aortic regurgitation may be present for many years with little deterioration. Surgery is indicated in the presence of New York Heart Association (NYHA) class III or IV symptoms. Those who are symptom-free or mildly symptomatic with evidence of increasing or severe left ventricular enlargement on radiological or echocardiographic criteria, or left ventricular hypertrophy on echocardiography, should be further investigated to determine left ventricular dimensions and ejection fraction. A left ventricular end-systolic dimension > 55 mm, an ejection fraction < 45% and a left ventricular end-systolic volume > 70 ml/m^2 indicate the need for surgery.[11]

As with mitral valve disease, haemodynamic

deterioration in the course of infective endocarditis, or prosthetic valve dysfunction, is an indication for surgical intervention.

MITRAL VALVE DISEASE

Mitral stenosis in symptomatic patients generally requires surgery, particularly in younger patients in whom operation is likely to have a low risk and the valve is often amenable to repair. The risk of systemic embolism is always present in mitral valve disease, particularly when atrial fibrillation is present; this risk increases with advancing age. It is difficult to evaluate the influence of mitral valvotomy on the subsequent risk of thrombo-embolism and claims have varied; it would appear to provide only partial protection from further thrombo-embolism.[12] An effective repair is likely to give greater protection than replacement with a prosthetic valve. Thus, if thrombo-embolism is the predominant presenting problem, a decision for surgery is influenced by the likelihood of a valve-conserving operation being possible.

It is possible to manage patients with mitral stenosis for many years by medical means, but this often results in unnecessary physical limitation. The recommendation for surgery takes account of many factors, such as age and symptomatic status, radiological, echocardiographic and haemodynamic data and the likelihood of valve conservation being feasible. When symptoms are of NYHA class III or class IV, there is little difficulty in recommending surgery. A history of episodes of pulmonary oedema suggests the need for surgery. Radiological evidence of pulmonary congestion and findings on cardiac catheterization suggesting a mitral valve area of $<$ 1.5 cm^2, a mean pressure drop across the mitral valve of $>$ 5 mmHg at rest, a left atrial pressure (assessed directly or indirectly) $>$ 18–20 mmHg and a systolic pulmonary artery pressure $>$ 50 mmHg indicate a recommendation for surgery. The best non-invasive criterion in the assessment of the severity of mitral stenosis is the use of Doppler echocardiography, where a mitral pressure half-time of $>$ 200 ms would suggest the need for mitral valve surgery.

For mitral regurgitation, the indications for surgery are based on symptomatic criteria and on evaluation of the pathological changes in the left ventricle. Those patients with NYHA class III or class IV symptoms require surgery. In those who are symptom-free or mildly symptomatic, evidence of increasing left ventricular enlargement on radiolo-

gical or echocardiographic criteria, the appearance of left ventricular hypertrophy on electrocardiography, a left ventricular end-systolic dimension of $>$ 50 mm and an end-systolic volume of $>$ 60 ml/m^2 or a reduction in ejection fraction below normal suggest the need for surgery.[11]

Haemodynamic deterioration in patients with endocarditis is a further indication for surgery, as is significant prosthetic valve malfunction.

TRICUSPID VALVE DISEASE

Isolated acquired tricuspid valve disease is extremely uncommon and is usually due to infective endocarditis in intravenous drug abusers in whom excision of the valve may be indicated as part of the eradication of infection. In rheumatic valvular disease, tricuspid involvement is virtually always accompanied by organic disease of the left-sided valves; it is usually a functional abnormality secondary to pulmonary hypertension but is occasionally organic in nature. The indications for surgery are those that apply to the left-sided valves, and evidence of tricuspid stenosis or regurgitation requires inspection of the tricuspid valve with appropriate correction.

PULMONARY VALVE DISEASE

Surgical relief of pulmonary stenosis is indicated when the systolic pressure drop across the valve is $>$ 40 mmHg. This can usually be estimated with Doppler echocardiography. Many centres are now obtaining good results with balloon valvuloplasty and the need for surgery for simple lesions may decline.[13] The more complex forms of pulmonary stenosis require correction as part of the surgical management of conditions in which right ventricular outflow tract obstruction is a component.

OPERATIVE PROCEDURE

Anaesthetic technique has the aim of attaining analgesia and muscle relaxation, and at the same time maintaining a favourable balance between myocardial oxygen supply and requirement. This is particularly important in aortic valve disease, where the pathophysiological effects militate against this balance. The maintenance of normal blood pressure, ventricular filling pressure and pulse rate is required. In practice, this involves control of pre-induction anxiety, care in maintaining fluid balance and oxygenation, and avoidance of myocardial depressant drugs.

AORTIC VALVE SURGERY

Closed procedures on the aortic valve

Closed procedures for aortic valve disease have never been as successful as similar procedures on the mitral valve, and are now virtually obsolete. However, it is of interest that the concept has been revived in the form of transarterial balloon dilatation of the stenosed aortic valve. Although the procedure is not without risk and may not be particularly effective,[14] it does offer an option for treating poor risk patients considered unlikely to survive aortic valve replacement surgery.

Open procedures on the aortic valve

Aortic valve surgery requires exposure of the heart by vertical sternotomy, and cardiopulmonary bypass is used. The valve is exposed by incising into the aortic root after cross-clamping the ascending aorta.

Valve conservation

Procedures that allow the aortic valve to be repaired are feasible less often than they are for the mitral valve. The commonest procedure is that of aortic valvotomy in which fused commissures are divided to relieve severe stenosis.[15] The operation is most applicable to children, in whom the tissues are unlikely to be calcified and valve replacement is rarely a practical option. Care is required to avoid creating regurgitation by excessive commissural mobilization.

Where aortic regurgitation is caused by prolapse of an aortic leaflet due to proximity to an underlying ventricular septal defect, competence can be restored at the time of closure of the ventricular septal defect by shortening the free edge of the elongated leaflet. This is achieved either by excising a triangular segment in the mid portion of the leaflet,[16] or by plicating the free edge along the edge,[17] or at each end.[18] More extensive procedures to conserve diseased aortic valves consist of decalcification to restore mobility,[19] repair of perforations due to endocarditis and plication of the dilated annulus.[16]

Valve replacement

Where the valve is heavily calcified or extensively fibrosed (Fig. 35.1), replacement is the only practical option. The valve leaflets are excised, during which great care is necessary to avoid calcific debris escaping into the left ventricular cavity or the left coronary artery. The prosthesis is anchored with multiple interrupted sutures placed securely through the annulus (Fig. 35.4). The inaccessibility of the aortic valve usually makes continuous suture techniques difficult. Following closure of the aortotomy, care is required to achieve filling of the heart with blood and to remove intracardiac air.

The small aortic root. An important practical problem arising with aortic valve replacement is the patient with a small aortic root where the size of prosthesis that can be inserted might be anticipated to cause residual obstruction. In practice, valves 19 and 21 mm in diameter are often unsatisfactory, although this depends on the type of prosthesis and the size of the patient.[20] There are several techniques appropriate for managing the small aortic root.

1   *Posterior division of the annulus* is the simplest and most widely used technique. The aortotomy incision is extended across the aortic annulus, either at the mid point of the non-coronary sinus into the origin of the mitral valve[21] or at the left/non-coronary commissure into the anterior mitral leaflet,[22] and a gusset of pericardium or

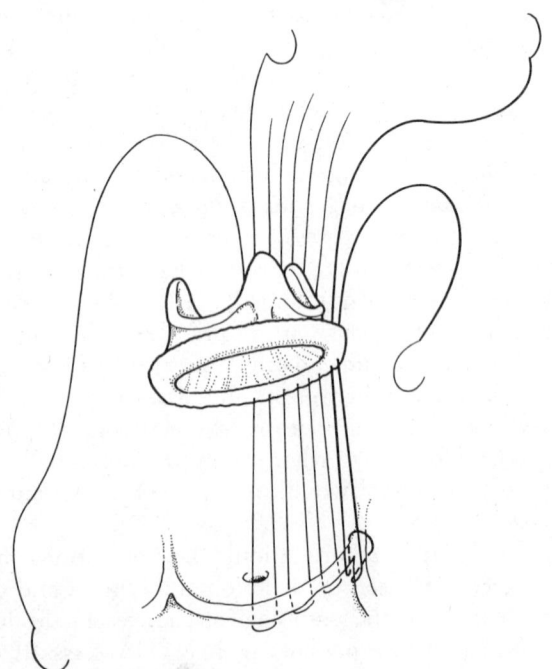

Fig. 35.4. Aortic valve replacement. Interrupted sutures are placed through the valve annulus and the sewing ring of a suitably sized prosthesis.

Dacron is sewn into the lower part of the incision to widen the annulus.

2 *Anterior division of the annulus*, in which the interventricular septum is exposed by a right ventriculotomy and incised from the aorta across the right coronary sinus and annulus. A double patch of Dacron is used to repair the openings in the septum and right ventricle. This technique is relatively uncommon and is probably safer in children than in adults.[23]

3 *Excision of the aortic root*, together with any obstructive subvalvular fibrous tissue, and replacement with an aortic root allograft and its valve have been advocated by Ross.[24]

4 *Insertion of a valved conduit* from the left ventricular apex to either the descending or the ascending aorta, provided that a competent native valve can be left *in situ*.[25]

Sub-aortic stenosis. Apart from congenital sub-aortic obstructions that require excision, the interventricular septum below the stenotic aortic valve may sometimes be sufficiently hypertrophied to represent a degree of left ventricular outflow tract obstruction. Although its recognition preoperatively and at operation is difficult and may be subjective, it can be relieved by incising for several millimetres into the septum (myotomy) away from the area of conducting tissue.

MITRAL VALVE SURGERY

Closed mitral commissurotomy

Closed mitral commissurotomy still has an important role in countries where cardiopulmonary bypass facilities are scarce and where rheumatic mitral valve disease is commonly seen in relatively young patients.[26] It is important to select patients who have physical signs of pliable valves and in whom calcification and regurgitation are either absent or minimal. Ideally, the patient should be in sinus rhythm because the advent of atrial fibrillation increases the risk of atrial appendage thrombosis.

The operation does not need cardiopulmonary bypass and has a low operative risk. The heart is exposed by left lateral thoracotomy and the mitral valve is palpated by a finger inserted via an incision made in the left atrial appendage, with appropriate snare or purse-string suture to minimize blood loss. Although it is often possible to induce some separation of fused commissures by finger pressure, it is more effective to achieve this with a dilator,

inserted via a small stab incision at the left ventricular apex and guided into the mitral orifice before being opened. There is little interference with the heart's action, and results are usually good.[27]

Although balloon valvuloplasty of the stenotic mitral valve has been reported, it has not been validated as an alternative to surgical commissurotomy as yet.

Open procedures on the mitral valve

Vertical sternotomy with cardiopulmonary bypass and exposure of the mitral valve through a left atrial incision allows the surgeon to evaluate the valve pathology carefully and repair or replace the diseased valve.

Valve conservation

The likelihood of being able to repair and conserve the natural valve depends very much on the patient population; this largely accounts for differences in reported practice. Division of fused commissures under direct vision is relatively simple and can be accomplished with greater certainty than at closed commissurotomy.

Specialized techniques[16,28] are required in more extensive reparative surgery, including the restoration of competence to regurgitant valves by achieving a more normal annular shape and size (prosthetic ring annuloplasty). Several types of semi-rigid rings are available for this purpose, the best-known example being the Carpentier ring. The surgeon anchors an appropriately sized ring to the dilated annulus with interrupted sutures in such a way as to restore normal size and shape to the annulus (Fig. 35.5). This procedure is often combined with division of fused commissures, shortening of elongated chordae, resection of flail or redundant segments of valve leaflets, sometimes with transplantation of segments of one leaflet with its chordae to the other.[16] Provided that the procedure is undertaken in patients with appropriate pathology by experienced surgeons, valve repair is preferable to valve replacement, because it carries lower operative mortality and has better long-term results without the need for anticoagulants.[29,30]

Valve replacement

If the pathology of the valve makes a conservative procedure impractical (Fig. 35.2), the valve is excised close to the annulus and the chordae are divided at their origin from the papillary muscles.

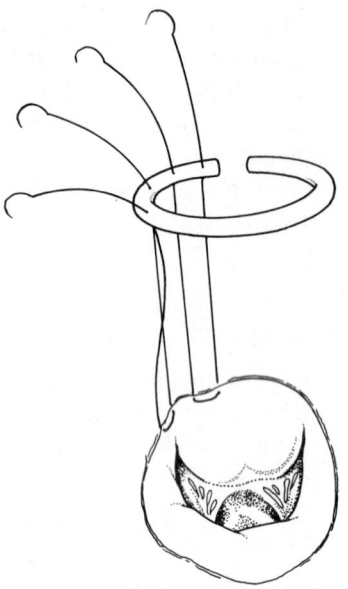

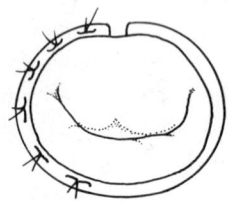

Fig. 35.5. Mitral annuloplasty. A prosthetic ring is placed with interrupted sutures through the dilated annulus to restore normal annular dimensions.

Where the posterior leaflet is retracted, particularly if it is adherent to the ventricular wall, it may be left in place. An appropriately sized prosthesis is inserted with anchoring sutures being placed through the valve annulus (Fig. 35.6). Individual practice varies and the pathology also influences technique chosen. Readily accessible valves with a tough fibrous annulus can often be more speedily replaced with a continuous suture technique. Where access is poor and the annulus calcified or friable, the use of multiple interrupted sutures gives a more secure result.[31]

With any open valve procedure, it is essential to remove any tissue or thrombus from the left atrium to avoid systemic embolism, and care is required to ensure filling of the heart with blood and removal of air prior to allowing the heart to eject before discontinuing cardiopulmonary bypass.

Repair versus replacement of the mitral valve

All prostheses have disadvantages and known complications. It is well recognized that natural valves can give satisfactory haemodynamic function even in the presence of significant anatomical abnormality. There is therefore obvious potential benefit in repairing rather than replacing the mitral valve.

When the abnormality is confined to fusion of commissures without heavy calcification, division of these fused commissures is relatively simple and safe and frequently restores normal function. Such valves can be anticipated with reasonable certainty in patients with a loud first sound, an opening snap,

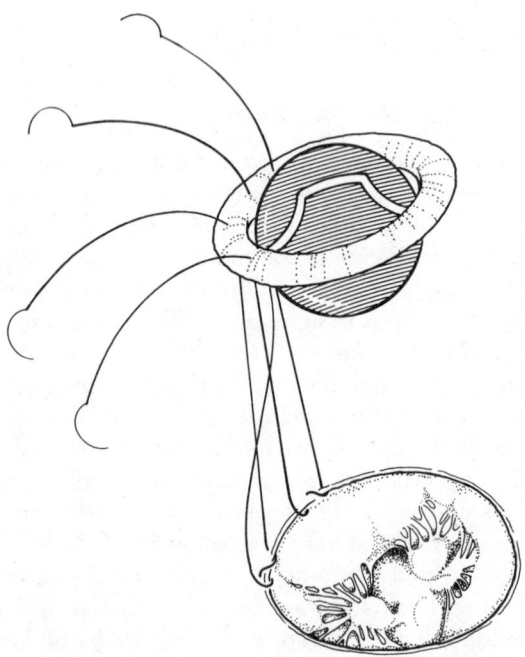

Fig. 35.6. Mitral valve replacement. Interrupted sutures are placed through the annulus and the sewing ring of the prosthesis.

no systolic murmur and absence of calcification on radiological screening or ultrasound evaluation. Patients with this type of pathology are usually encountered in regions where rheumatic fever is endemic and are often young. In these circumstances, closed commissurotomy is the preferred option. Where cardiopulmonary bypass facilities are readily available, these patients are probably better managed by open commissurotomy because of the more complete separation that can be achieved.

The possibility of repairing the mitral valve in patients in whom regurgitation is the major problem depends on the pathology: if annular dilatation is the main cause, insertion of an annuloplasty ring is likely to give good results; if there is prolapse of a leaflet, chordal shortening may be successful; if there is an excess of redundant leaflet tissue (floppy valve), the chances of achieving a repair are lessened. Chordal rupture affecting up to one-third of the anterior leaflet can often be treated by excision and transfer of a segment of the posterior leaflet with its chordae to fill the defect. Excision of a segment of the posterior leaflet can usually be treated by direct suturing and shortening of the annulus by anchoring to an annuloplasty ring.[16] All these procedures require that the valve be assessed following its repair to judge competence and, if this is not satisfactory, the valve should be excised and replaced.

Where there is heavy calcification or where fibrous thickening of the leaflets has resulted in excessive stiffness, repair techniques are generally not applicable. Inevitably, there is a degree of subjectivity in making decisions regarding repair.

Valve replacement and valve repair should not be seen as competing options — repair is preferable but not always feasible or appropriate. Thus, it is difficult to draw conclusions when comparing the results of the two approaches, but there is good evidence of the superiority of valve repair over valve replacement with a variety of prostheses in terms of prosthesis-related mortality and morbidity up to 7 years post-operatively.[30,32–37]

COMBINED AORTIC AND MITRAL VALVE SURGERY

Surgery for both the aortic and mitral valves is required frequently, particularly in patients with chronic rheumatic valvular heart disease. The principles of surgery for individual aortic and mitral valve replacement still apply. It is usual practice to excise the aortic valve first (the aortic root needs to be opened at an early stage to give access to the coronary ostia to ensure accurate delivery of cardioplegic solution and it is convenient to remove the aortic valve at this stage, particularly if it is heavily calcified, to minimize any risk of retained calcific debris). The mitral valve is then repaired or replaced as appropriate and aortic valve replacement follows. If there is an aortic valve prosthesis already in place, the rigidity it causes tends to limit access to the mitral annulus in the sub-aortic region, hence the preference for replacing the mitral before the aortic valve in double-valve replacement.

TRICUSPID VALVE SURGERY

Fulminant or intractable endocarditis with recurrent septic pulmonary emboli in intravenous drug abusers has been treated by excision of the tricuspid valve and removal of infected vegetations.[38] Cardiopulmonary bypass is required, and the tricuspid valve is approached through a right atrial incision. The operation is often hazardous in these ill patients but the absence of a tricuspid valve is often relatively well tolerated. Once infection has been treated, a second operation may be required to insert a tricuspid valve prosthesis. Unfortunately, the likelihood of recurrent endocarditis is extremely high if intravenous drug abuse continues. Optimal treatment in this group of patients remains undecided; at least one group of workers has reported good results with immediate tricuspid valve replacement with a prosthesis.[39]

More commonly, the surgeon encounters tricuspid regurgitation in patients who require mitral or mitral and aortic valve replacement. The degree of tricuspid regurgitation can be judged at operation by the presence of a dilated and hypertrophied right atrium and palpation of a regurgitant jet by a finger inserted into the right atrium. This also helps to distinguish a dilated annulus from organic disease prior to commencing cardiopulmonary bypass. Once the mitral and aortic valves have been dealt with appropriately, the tricuspid valve is exposed by an incision in the right atrium, and the pathology is accurately assessed.

If annular dilatation is the basis of regurgitation, this is repaired by the operation of tricuspid annuloplasty. Several techniques are available. In the De Vega technique,[40] a continuous suture is placed through the base of the posterior and anterior tricuspid leaflets (avoiding the base of the septal leaflet which does not stretch and which is close to conducting tissue) and pulled tight enough to produce an annulus of a more normal size, thus restoring competence to the valve (Fig. 35.7). Techniques for placing an annuloplasty ring, such as the Carpentier ring,[41] are similar to those used for the mitral valve.

If fusion of commissures has resulted in stenosis, division is often satisfactory. Where the valve is fibrosed, stiff and retracted, replacement may be the only option. The anterior and posterior leaflets are resected close to the annulus. It is important to leave a good rim of septal leaflet as this allows sutures to be placed in this region without the risk of interfering with conducting tissue. Either multiple interrupted sutures or a combination of interrupted and continuous sutures are used to anchor an appropriately sized prosthesis. Care is required to avoid impingement of the prosthesis posts on the interventricular septum if a bioprosthesis is used, or disc impingement if a tilting disc valve is used. Tricuspid valve replacement is not ideal and should be undertaken only for significant organic disease where conservative techniques are inappropriate. On the other hand, the annuloplasty techniques for functional regurgitation are quick to perform and largely trouble-free.

PULMONARY VALVE SURGERY

When surgical pulmonary valvotomy is undertaken, a vertical sternotomy incision is used, cardiopulmonary bypass is required and the pulmonary valve is approached via an incision in the main pulmonary artery. Fused commissures are divided out to the annulus. The consequences of surgically induced regurgitation are minor. It is important to ensure that this procedure has relieved the obstruction by checking the pressure drop across the valve after discontinuing cardiopulmonary bypass. Residual

obstruction may be present as a result of subvalvar muscular hypertrophy and this may require localized resection.

CONCOMITANT PROCEDURES

Coronary artery surgery may be required in addition to valve replacement, in which case the order of procedures depends on the extent of the coronary revascularization required. Retraction of the heart with a prosthesis in place is undesirable, particularly in the presence of a mitral bioprosthetic valve where perforation of the ventricular wall can occur. It is wisest to construct the distal coronary anastomoses prior to replacing the valve(s) in most instances. This also gives the opportunity of administering cardioplegic solution into the grafts for additional myocardial protection.

Aortic valve replacement may need to be combined with resection of the ascending aorta where aneurysm or dissection is present. Dacron tubes with prosthetic valves already sewn to one end are available which assist rapid replacement of the valve and aortic root.

HEART VALVE PROSTHESES

Since the 1950s, many different types of heart valve prostheses have been developed and used. All have had shortcomings and many are now obsolete.[42] Throughout the development of such prostheses, there has been broad separation into mechanical devices, manufactured from a variety of materials (e.g. metallic alloys, silicone rubber or carbon) and not resembling natural valves, and biological valves made from human or animal tissue, mimicking the natural aortic valve.[2] In general, all prostheses function less well haemodynamically than normal

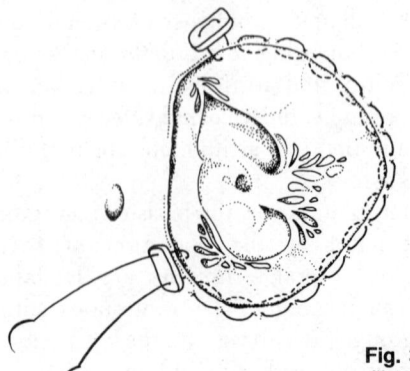

Fig. 35.7. Tricuspid annuloplasty. The De Vega technique for reducing the size of a dilated annulus with a double suture placed through the base of the anterior and posterior leaflets.

valves. An indication of how stenotic prosthetic valves are is obtained by comparing the normal adult aortic valve area of about 3 cm² and the normal adult mitral valve area of 4–6 cm² with the effective orifice area of the presently available valve prostheses. Only the bileaflet valves would appear to approach normal values. Caged ball, tilting disc and biological valves have values half or less than half of those of natural valves.[43] Mechanical prostheses have a high risk of thrombo-embolism which necessitates indefinite anticoagulation; biological valves have a lower thrombo-embolic risk and may be used without anticoagulation, although their durability is limited.

HYDRODYNAMIC PERFORMANCE OF HEART VALVE PROSTHESES

Laboratory performance of prosthetic heart valves *in vitro* has been studied in a number of centres. Although there are well-recognized difficulties in simulating the clinical environment for which the valves are intended,[44] useful data are available from a number of well-established pulsatile test rigs now in use.

In general, earlier studies concentrated on pressure drop at varied forward flow, but it is apparent that regurgitant flow during valve closure is also a significant factor in valve performance. The two aspects have been expressed in a combined fashion as total transvalvar energy loss.[45] In Fig. 35.8, the energy loss for 23-mm aortic mechanical prostheses (three tilting disc and two bileaflet prostheses) is shown at various simulated cardiac outputs during forward flow phase, during the closing phase, and when the valve is closed. Energy loss with the valve closed represents a relatively large proportion of total energy loss, particularly at the lower cardiac outputs. Energy loss due to forward flow increases with cardiac output, corresponding to an increased pressure drop at higher flow.

In Fig. 35.9, a different pattern of energy loss for the larger 29-mm mitral mechanical prostheses (three tilting disc, two bileaflet and one caged ball) is shown. Energy loss during forward flow is a small proportion of total energy loss for all valves, with the exception of the caged ball valve which at higher flows develops a relatively large pressure drop. There is a much greater energy loss during valve closure with these larger valves, representing regurgitation of fluid during the period that the leaflets are coming into apposition. This corresponds to the observation in clinical practice when left ventricu-

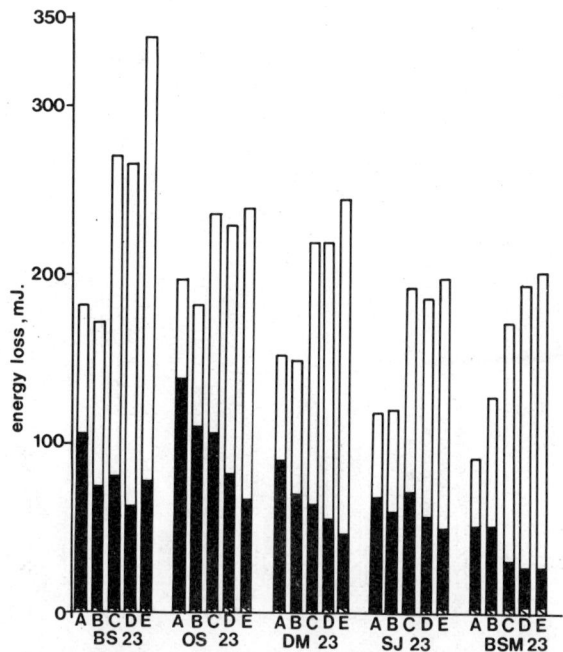

Fig. 35.8. Energy loss for 23-mm aortic mechanical prostheses. In (A)–(E), increasing flow rates are shown. BS, Björk–Shiley convexo-concave valve; OS, Omniscience valve; DM, Duromedics bileaflet valve; SJ, St Jude Medical bileaflet valve; BSM, Björk–Shiley monostrut valve. □, forward flow; ■, closed; □, closing.

lography often demonstrates reflux of radiopaque medium back into the atrium during prosthetic valve closure. Energy loss due to leakage through the closed valve is less significant in the mitral position because of the shorter duration of systole. It is also apparent that in the surgical choice of valve size, attempts to place the largest possible prosthesis in the mitral position may not be advantageous, taking into account closing energy loss.

Earlier designs of aortic bioprosthetic valves created relatively high pressure drops.[46] The mitral tilting disc valves and bileaflet mechanical valves currently available appear to have comparable and satisfactory performance.[47] Of the newest bioprosthetic valves, the porcine valves show the largest pressure drop during forward flow, although the total energy loss of this valve is similar to that of pericardial valves.[45]

Experimental studies of flow patterns through valve prostheses show that there is considerable disturbance of flow with development of shear forces as assessed by Doppler anemometry,[48,49] and this may have practical value in future valve design.

In Fig. 35.10, the mean pressure difference is plotted against forward flow for the commonly used porcine, pericardial and mechanical prostheses.[50]

When evaluated only in terms of pressure drop

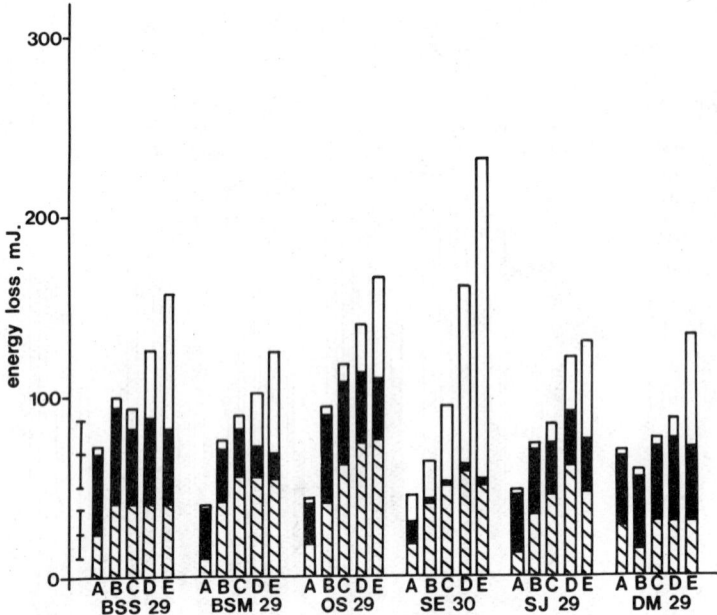

Fig. 35.9. Energy loss for 29-mm mitral mechanical prostheses. In (A)–(E) increasing flow rates are shown. BSS, Björk–Shiley convexo-concave valve; BSM, Björk–Shiley monostrut valve; OS, Omniscience valve; SE, Starr–Edwards caged ball valve; SJ, St Jude bileaflet valve; DM, Duromedics bileaflet valve. □, forward flow; ■, closed; □, closing.

during forward flow, mechanical valves appear to have the best performance. However, consideration of total transvalvar energy loss has shown that overall energy losses are similar for many of the porcine, pericardial and mechanical prostheses, and this is reflected in satisfactory haemodynamic performance.

BIOLOGICAL VALVES

The aortic valve transplanted from a cadaver (allograft) was the first clinically used biological valve and it still has a place. Difficulty in procurement led to many ingenious alternatives, such as the use of autogenous fascia lata mounted on a frame to mimic an aortic valve. Interest waned when poor results became evident. The application of glutaraldehyde tanning to biological tissue led to the development of the glutaraldehyde-prepared porcine aortic valve prosthesis and the glutaraldehyde-preserved pericardial prosthesis; these two types of biological valve are the most widely used in clinical practice today.

The allograft aortic valve

Pioneered independently by Ross[51] and Barratt-Boyes[52] in 1962, transplantation of the allograft aortic valve has given good long-term results when used to replace the aortic valve.[53] A variety of methods of sterilization have been used, exposure to a mixture of antibiotics being the current method.

Cryopreservation is now used to allow prolonged storage before use.[54] Insertion is technically difficult, experience being required to suture the valve into place without distortion. Mounting of such valves on a frame for insertion into the mitral

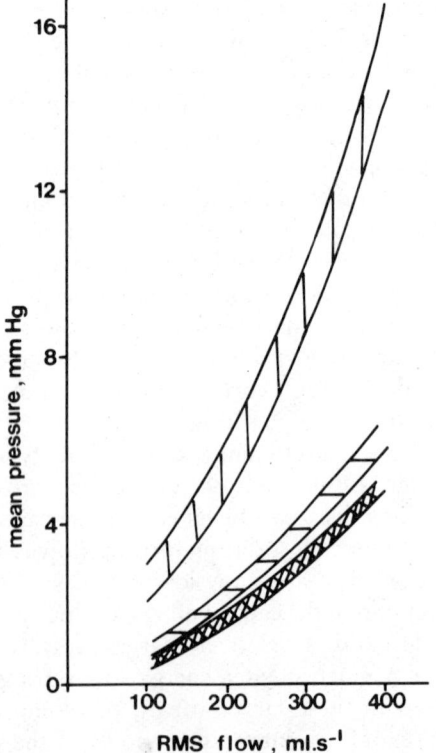

Fig. 35.10. Mean pressure difference across porcine ▥, pericardial ▤, and mechanical tilting disc or bileaflet valves ▨.

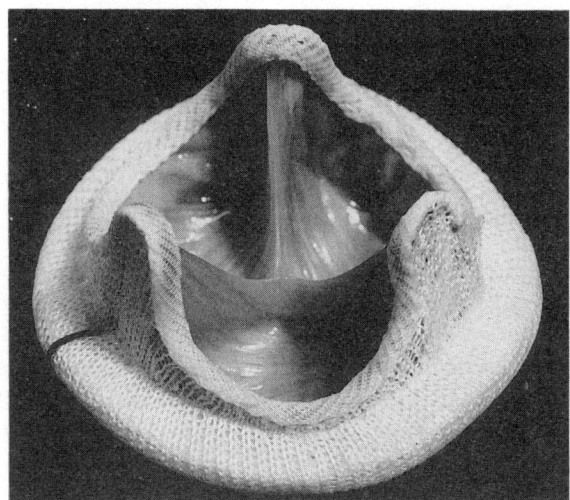

Fig. 35.11. Carpentier–Edwards porcine bioprosthetic valve.

position has been less successful. Aortic valve replacement with an allograft valve gives certainty of freedom from thrombo-embolism and normal haemodynamic function if accurately inserted, but the likelihood of degenerative change increases after 8–10 years.[53]

Glutaraldehyde-treated porcine valves

Currently, several glutaraldehyde-treated porcine valves are available, the best known being the Carpentier–Edwards (Fig. 35.11) and the Hancock bioprostheses.[55] The porcine aortic valve is mounted on a suitable frame with sewing ring to allow insertion into the aortic, mitral or tricuspid position. Haemodynamic performance is satisfactory in the larger sizes, but the smaller sizes are mildly stenotic. Thrombo-embolic risk is small and the valves can be used without anticoagulants, although in practice with mitral valve replacement the presence of atrial fibrillation often needs anticoagulation.

Glutaraldehyde-treated pericardial valves

Several glutaraldehyde-treated pericardial valves have been available until recently, the best known being the Ionescu–Shiley pericardial bioprosthesis (Fig. 35.12).[56] However, this valve is no longer available. Three leaflets fashioned from glutaraldehyde-treated bovine pericardium are mounted on a three-pronged frame in order to simulate a natural aortic valve. The valve can be used in appropriate sizes and orientation to replace aortic, mitral or

tricuspid valves. Haemodynamic performance is excellent, allowing prostheses of small size to be used with satisfactory results.[57] Thrombo-embolic risk is small, and anticoagulants are not required in the absence of other indications.

MECHANICAL VALVES

Since the late 1950s, a large variety of mechanical valves have been used for heart valve replacement. Many design concepts have been tried, often with a poor haemodynamic performance, an unacceptable risk of thrombo-embolism, a tendency to cause haemolysis, or the risk of mechanical dysfunction. The haemodynamic performance of the valves currently available is generally excellent. Long-term anticoagulation is required for all mechanical valves and, provided satisfactory control is maintained, thrombo-embolic rates are low. Durability is superior to that of biological valves, although occasional mechanical disruption has occurred with some designs.[58]

Caged ball valves

A caged ball valve consists of a circular valve seat with a cage to restrain a spherical occluder. The best known example is the Starr–Edwards valve (Fig. 35.13).[59] There have been many modifications to the original valve design but the most successful version has an uncovered stellite cage restraining a silastic rubber occluder. Haemodynamic performance is not ideal, the central occluder causing a degree of stenosis, and the bulk of the cage may impinge on the ventricular walls when used for

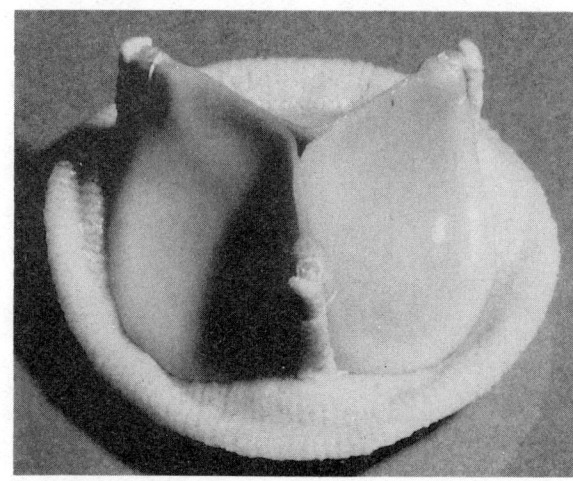

Fig. 35.12. Ionescu–Shiley pericardial bioprosthetic valve.

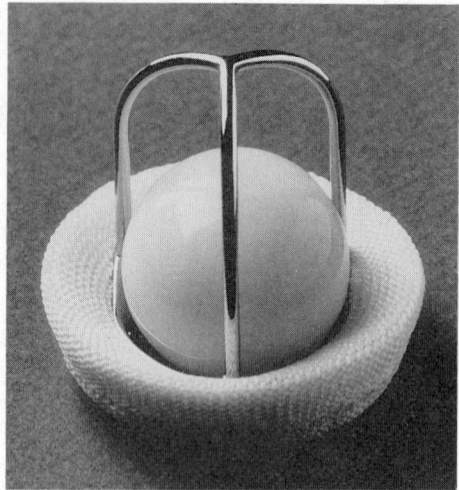

Fig. 35.13. Starr–Edwards caged ball valve.

mitral valve replacement in patients with small ventricles.

Tilting disc valves

Tilting disc valves are composed of a circular valve seat having a tilting disc occluder with some form of restraining struts. The best known is the Björk–Shiley valve in which there have been modifications to the composition of the disc (initially delrin, later carbon), modifications to the shape of the disc (initially flat, later convexo-concave), and modifications of the restraining struts (Fig. 35.14).[60]

Bileaflet valves

Bileaflet valves consist of a circular valve seat with

two semicircular occluding leaflets. This gives the advantage of a low profile height and the risk of disc entrapment is reduced. A popular valve of this type is the St Jude Medical valve, made of pyrolytic carbon (Fig. 35.15).[61,62]

THE CHOICE OF VALVE PROSTHESIS

The choice of valve prosthesis is often dictated by the individual surgeon's background and training and differences of opinion about policy for rational choice remain. These differences of opinion arise because there are particular problems with all types of valve prostheses, none is ideal, and it is difficult to make comparisons of the complications and the advantages among different types of valve.[63] There is no scientific method for deciding whether the indefinite requirement for anticoagulants (with their disadvantages) with mechanical valve use is preferable to the greater likelihood of repeat surgery (with its risks) when bioprosthetic valves are used. However, there are certain categories of patients in whom reasonable agreement as to the choice of prosthesis exists.

Bioprosthetic valves unsuitable

Accelerated calcification in glutaraldehyde-treated bioprosthetic valves has been shown to occur in patients under the age of 20 years.[64] There is evidence that an increased risk of accelerated calcification persists in patients up to the age of 35 years, although to a lesser extent.[55]

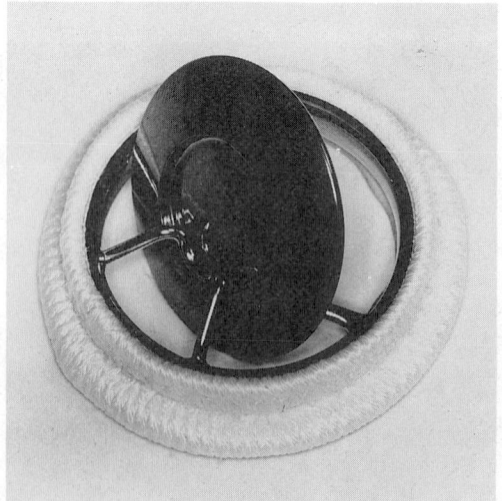

Fig. 35.14. Björk–Shiley tilting disc valve.

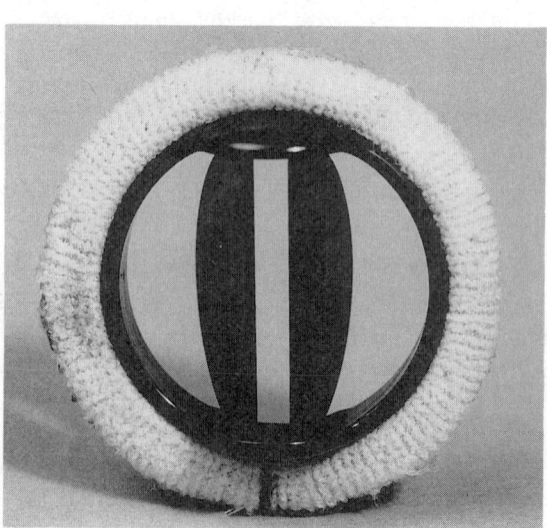

Fig. 35.15. St Jude Medical bileaflet valve.

Mechanical valves unsuitable

Mechanical valves are clearly unsuitable for patients with well-defined contra-indications to anticoagulant treatment, such as active chronic peptic ulceration, or those unlikely to be amenable to adequate anticoagulant control.

In women in whom future pregnancy is likely, it is probably wisest to use a tissue valve in view of the teratogenic risk of warfarin and the hazards of pregnancy in anticoagulated patients. Unfortunately, such patients will be young and therefore have the risk of accelerated bioprosthetic calcification.[65,66]

Audible prosthetic sounds are a small disadvantage of some mechanical valves in some patients.

Choice of prosthesis debatable

Patients not in the categories discussed above are likely to do equally well, at least in the medium term, with either mechanical or biological valves. Although there are numerous reports of outcome in large series of patients from many centres for different valves, it is difficult to make valid comparisons between prostheses because of such variables as patient population and age, selection and management policy.

Workers at several centres have reported experience with biological and mechanical valves used in broadly similar, although not randomly allocated, patient groups.[67-70] In these studies, glutaraldehyde-prepared porcine valves have been compared with mechanical valves. In general, follow-up is still in the intermediate range and little information is available beyond 10 years. Up to this stage, however, there is no clear evidence in favour of either mechanical or biological valves in terms of patient survival. In all studies, anticoagulants have been used with mechanical valves which understandably gives a small anticoagulant-related risk, whereas anticoagulants are often not used with biological valves. Some groups report a significantly higher rate of thrombo-embolism in the mechanical group,[67,68] but others have found no significant difference.[69,70] Re-operation for valve failure is significantly higher for biological valves where follow-up extends beyond 5 years and it must be anticipated that increasing follow-up will demonstrate a greater divergence between re-operation rates in the two groups.

Experience in Glasgow extending to over 8 years[71] of 774 patients with Björk–Shiley mechanic-al valves and 620 patients with Carpentier–Edwards porcine valves has shown similar late mortality (3.1% and 3.0% per patient-year for mechanical and biological valves, respectively), similar thrombo-embolic rate (1.4% and 1.6% per patient-year, respectively), similar valve failure rate (0.78% and 0.68% per patient-year, respectively) and similar symptomatic improvement.

It is not difficult to find evidence of satisfactory performance of any type of valve from the many reported series.[72-77] The choice of valve for the individual patient will be carefully considered by the surgeon/physician and many factors govern valve selection. It is therefore difficult to decide where the reported satisfactory performance of an individual valve is due to its inherent properties, or whether good results are a consequence of judicious valve–patient matching. Perhaps the optimal way of objectively assessing one valve against another is use in a randomized prospective trial in which selection bias is abolished.[78] Recent evidence from one such British study[79] tends to support the contention that there is little to choose in the medium term between mechanical and biological valves; in 540 patients randomly allocated to receive a mechanical valve (Björk–Shiley) or a porcine bioprosthetic valve, similar rates of 7-year actuarial survival, thrombo-embolism and re-operation were found.

Although it is perhaps an oversimplification to consider the decision regarding biological or mechanical valve use only in terms of the drawbacks of indefinite anticoagulation compared with the likelihood of re-operation, this is an important aspect best resolved by discussion with the individual patient. It would seem logical to use mechanical valves where there is likely to be a continued indication for anticoagulant use. Thus, the patient with longstanding atrial fibrillation who requires mitral valve replacement may very reasonably be offered a mechanical valve in preference. For patients requiring aortic valve replacement or those requiring mitral valve replacement and still in sinus rhythm, the choice of a biological valve is entirely reasonable provided that the likelihood of re-operation is accepted. It is not attractive to have to commence permanent anticoagulation in elderly patients and the policy of using biological valves after an arbitrary age of perhaps 65 years has merit.

ANTICOAGULATION WITH PROSTHETIC HEART VALVES

It is well recognized that thrombo-embolic complications are a risk in heart valve replacement surgery. These complications can be grouped as follows.

1   Small early systemic emboli which may arise from the sewing ring and which may be expected to lessen as incorporation of the sewing ring occurs; these are seen with both mechanical and biological valves.
2   Systemic emboli which appear to arise from the presence of the prosthesis itself, explained partly by the shear stresses developed in relation to the valve, partly by areas of relative stasis in blood flow around components of the valve, and partly by the presence of a foreign surface. These thrombi are a continuing risk and are more likely to arise with mechanical than with biological valves.
3   Thrombotic obstruction which interferes with valve function is caused by the same factors as systemic emboli and has a propensity to occur more frequently with mechanical valves.

Biological valves

The allograft valve is devoid of thrombo-embolic complications when used as a free graft to replace the aortic valve.[53]

Pericardial and porcine bioprosthetic valves are recognized to be less thrombogenic than mechanical valves.[80] However, small early emboli may occur and for this reason administration of anticoagulants for the first 6–12 weeks post-operatively is advisable. Thrombo-emboli may arise from the atrium when atrial fibrillation is present and, in these circumstances, indefinite anticoagulation is probably indicated.

Mechanical valves

Anticoagulation reduces the risk of thrombo-embolic complications to acceptably low levels,[81] generally below 2% per patient-year for aortic prostheses and 4% per patient-year for mitral prostheses. Experience of using mechanical valves without anticoagulation is limited but the thrombo-embolic rate would appear to be 3–6 times higher than that with anticoagulants.[81] Attempts to manage patients with mechanical valves with antiplatelet drugs alone (aspirin and dipyridamole) have

generally resulted in a higher thrombo-embolic complication rate than when anticoagulants are used.[80,82–84]

Where anticoagulation is impractical, the St Jude valve at least has been shown to function in the aortic position with a relatively low risk of thrombotic obstruction.[85]

In general, all patients with mechanical valves should receive anticoagulants. It is reasonable to consider a policy of using antiplatelet drug therapy alone in patients over 70 years, or in children, and only valves in the aortic position should be treated in this way, although inevitably this entails an increased risk.[86]

In summary, anticoagulants should be used:

1   with biological valves for the first 6–12 weeks and thereafter only if other indications for continued anticoagulation exist. In practice, the commonest such indication is the presence of atrial fibrillation;
2   with all mechanical valves, with the possible exception of aortic valves in children, the elderly or in those in whom anticoagulation is impractical, provided that antiplatelet therapy is substituted.

Anticoagulation therapy

Anticoagulation is usually achieved by oral anticoagulants, such as warfarin (coumadin), which act slowly by inhibiting synthesis of vitamin K-dependent clotting factors. Intravenous therapy with heparin is used in special circumstances where oral anticoagulation is contra-indicated (e.g. in pregnancy). It produces rapid and effective anticoagulation but requires in-patient treatment.

Following valve replacement, oral anticoagulation therapy is started as soon as the patient can swallow and the mediastinal drains have been removed – normally the first post-operative day. The total anticoagulant effect following a single dose of warfarin is not reached for several days and may require several weeks to stabilize. The greatest variable affecting blood anticoagulation with warfarin is the response of the individual patient to the drug.

Anticoagulant complications

Fatal bleeding complications due to long-term anticoagulation have been reported to occur at the rate of 0.1%–0.2% per patient-year.[81] Non-fatal complications are 2–3 times more common. Fatal complications most frequently involve the central nervous system. Non-fatal bleeding usually involves the genito-urinary and gastro-intestinal tracts. Complications occur more frequently when patients become over-anticoagulated (e.g. when other drugs interfere with warfarin control). Thrombo-embolic events may occur despite seemingly adequate anticoagulation with warfarin and in these circumstances an antiplatelet drug (dipyridamole) should be added to the regimen.[80]

Laboratory control of anticoagulation

All patients taking warfarin require monitoring of anticoagulation, initially every second day until a safe and effective maintenance dose is established, and then every 2 or 3 months. The most common method for establishing the degree of anticoagulation with warfarin is by the prothrombin time test (PTT). Results may be expressed as the prothrombin ratio, prothrombin activity or prothrombin index. Standardization of this test has resulted in expression of the results as the International Normalised Ratio (INR), formerly the British Corrected Ratio (BCR). The therapeutic range for warfarin lies between 3 and 4 times the control value for patients with mechanical valves. Some laboratories check anticoagulation with the Thrombotest (therapeutic range 5–10%), or with the Capillary Clotting Time (therapeutic range 50–77 s).

Heparin control is maintained by the Activated Partial Thromboplastin Time (APPT), therapeutic range 1.5–2.5 × control.

COMPLICATIONS OF PROSTHETIC VALVES

All currently available prosthetic valves have associated complications, their frequency and nature varying with different types of valves.

Complications with biological valves

Tissue failure

Allograft valves were the first biological valves to be used clinically. Their major drawback was soon seen to be tissue failure which began to reach unacceptable levels by 5–7 years after implantation. Preparation methods were blamed and antibiotic sterilization has apparently improved the longevity of these valves. Late degeneration, however, remains the major problem. The leaflets of the valve tend to become thin, atropic and often perforate.

Calcification occurs predominantly in the supporting rim of allograft aorta. Degeneration is usually gradual, giving adequate warning for re-operation. For the allograft valve in the aortic position, Yacoub's group report freedom from valve failure at 5 years as 90% and at 10 years 72%.[53]

Glutaraldehyde-prepared porcine bioprostheses develop leaflet calcification, probably related to areas of abnormal mechanical stress; the leaflets may become progressively stiffer and more stenotic or, more commonly, they tear close to sites of calcification producing regurgitation (Fig. 35.16). These changes generally begin to manifest themselves in a significant number of valves between 5 and 10 years,[55,87] although earlier failures of this nature have been reported, particularly when the valves are used in children in whom accelerated calcification is very common.[64]

Two reports[55,87] of long-term follow-up of patients undergoing valve replacement with porcine bioprostheses have shown similar rates of freedom from degeneration or primary tissue failure at 10 years. In contrast to previously reported experience,[88] no statistically significant differences in failure rates between mitral and aortic valves were found, a finding confirmed by others.[68] These reports disclose actuarial freedom from degeneration at 10 years of 71%[55] and 69%[87] for aortic bioprostheses and 71%[55] and 70%[87] for mitral bioprostheses.

In both series, age was a major determinant of failure. Magilligan[55] reports 55% freedom from degeneration at 10 years in patients under 35 years of age, whereas for those over 35 years there was 80% freedom from degeneration. In Gallo's

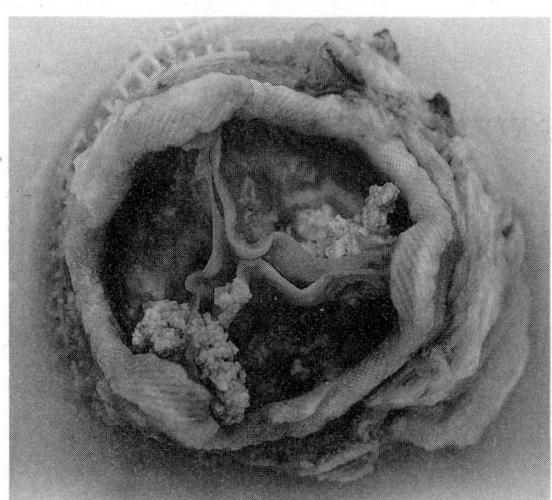

Fig. 35.16. Explanted calcified porcine bioprosthetic valve.

series,[87] incidence of valve failure was related to age such that in the 21–30 year age-group, 26% of mitral and 42% of aortic valves failed in 10 years, whereas in the 61–70 year age-group the corresponding figures were 11% and 0%. Cohn[89,90] has reported 10-year actuarial freedom from failure of 86% for aortic and 82% for mitral porcine bioprostheses, where the mean age of the patients studied was 60 years and 58 years, respectively, in the aortic and mitral valve replacement groups.

Further striking evidence for the high incidence of degeneration of porcine bioprosthetic valves in children comes from Antunes and Santos[91] who reported survival free from degeneration of only 20% at 6 years for patients 20 years of age or younger. In contrast, Pupello et al.[92] have reported a 97% freedom from valve failure at 9 years in a group of patients over 70 years of age undergoing valve replacement with porcine bioprostheses.

A significant proportion of glutaraldehyde-prepared pericardial bioprostheses also develop calcification after 5–10 years.[93] In addition, there is an incidence of premature tissue failure in the absence of calcification, which may be related to design.[94] As with other bioprostheses, there is also a risk of accelerated calcification in children.[95] Ionescu[96] has reported actuarial freedom from primary tissue failure at 10 years of 88% for mitral pericardial bioprostheses and 85% for aortic pericardial bioprostheses. In a report from the Texas Heart Institute[97] of 2701 patients undergoing valve replacement with Ionescu–Shiley pericardial bioprostheses and followed for a maximum of 5 years, freedom from primary tissue failure was reported to be 94% for mitral and 89% for aortic pericardial prostheses at 5 years. Patients under the age of 20 years had an actuarial probability of freedom from degeneration at 5 years of only 38%, whereas those over 60 years had a 93.5% actuarial probability of freedom from degeneration.

In a large series of valve replacement in children (the majority aged between 11 and 15 years) using porcine and pericardial bioprostheses, Odell et al.[95] found that the bovine pericardial prostheses calcified even earlier than the porcine valves: in those undergoing mitral valve replacement, actuarial analysis revealed only 32.5% survival free from calcification at 4 years in those receiving porcine prostheses and 2.3% in those receiving bovine pericardial prostheses.

The recognition of tissue failure in biological valves may be easy in patients who show symptomatic deterioration and who develop new murmurs. It is usually a gradual occurrence but patients may present with sudden incapacity and the onset of a murmur which may even be apparent to the patient. Early tissue deterioration that has not produced symptomatic change may be recognized when new murmurs appear (e.g. a diastolic murmur with an aortic prosthesis or a systolic murmur with a mitral prosthesis). Earlier detection of tissue degeneration may be possible by ultrasound investigation when an increasing pressure gradient may be detectable or evidence of calcification is seen.

Deterioration in the aortic allograft may continue over several years with apparently slow progression; with the glutaraldehyde-prepared bioprosthetic valves, there may be sudden deterioration due to valve leaflet tearing, and early surgical intervention to replace such prostheses is advisable once tissue failure becomes evident.

Thrombo-embolism

The free allograft valve used in the aortic position is devoid of thrombo-embolic complications.[53]

Although glutaraldehyde-prepared porcine and pericardial prostheses are not devoid of the risk of thrombo-embolism, the thrombogenicity of these valves is sufficiently low to allow them to be used without anticoagulants (in the absence of other sources for thrombo-embolism) with results that are comparable to those obtained using mechanical prostheses with anticoagulation.[81]

Overall freedom from thrombo-embolism with porcine bioprosthetic valves has been reported at 84% and over 90% at 10 years.[55,68] In a comparative study of aortic valve replacement with mechanical and porcine valves, Perier et al.[67] showed a 95% actuarial freedom from thrombo-embolism at 8 years for the porcine valve (without anticoagulants), compared with 81% and 84%, respectively, for the Starr–Edwards and Björk–Shiley mechanical valves. One report has suggested that the pericardial bioprosthesis may be superior to the porcine bioprosthesis in having a reduced risk of thrombo-embolism in the mitral position.[98]

Based on a study of the literature, Edmunds[81] has calculated the incidence of thrombo-emboli to be < 2% per patient-year for aortic biological valves without anticoagulation. For mitral bioprostheses, both with and without anticoagulation, the thrombo-embolic rate is approximately 4% per patient-year. The first few weeks after implantation is the time of greatest risk.

Management of thrombo-embolism may require

specific treatment depending on the site of the embolus (e.g. embolectomy for embolus to the limbs or supportive treatment for major cerebral embolus). If anticoagulants have not been used, it is wise to commence anticoagulation; if the patient was adequately anticoagulated at the time of the embolus, antiplatelet drugs may be added to the treatment regimen.

Thrombotic complications on the valve itself are not commonly recognized, but immobilization of a leaflet by thrombus may occur and simulates tissue failure in its effects.

Endocarditis

There is a small risk of infection occurring on any prosthetic valve, as with abnormal natural valves. With biological valves, endocarditis presents with systemic effects as well as early, and often severe, haemodynamic upset as leaflet tissue is destroyed by infection.

Prosthetic valve endocarditis is a serious complication with high mortality. Arbitrarily, it is defined as early (within 60 days of operation) or late to distinguish infection that may have been related to operation. The routine use of prophylactic antibiotics in the peri-operative period is intended, at least in part, to reduce this hazard. There does not appear to be a difference between mechanical or bioprosthetic valves, nor between aortic and mitral valves, in the risk of developing this complication.[99–101]

In a large series of patients receiving a variety of mechanical and biological valves in all positions, the risk of developing prosthetic valve endocarditis was reported as 3.1% at 1 year and 5.7% at 5 years.[99] Experience at Glasgow has shown a similar rate of endocarditis in bioprosthetic and mechanical valves of 0.8% and 0.6% per patient-year, respectively.[71]

Recognition depends on having a high index of suspicion whenever there is an unexplained pyrexial illness in patients with prosthetic valves. Diagnosis is made by the findings of new or changing cardiac murmurs, peripheral emboli or splinter haemorrhages, or haematuria. The diagnosis is suggested by echocardiographic demonstration of leaflet vegetations and confirmed by blood culture.

Management includes early intravenous antibiotic therapy once blood cultures have been taken and modification as necessary, depending on culture and sensitivity testing.

Surgical intervention for prosthetic valve en-docarditis may be required after successful treatment of the infection with antibiotics if a haemodynamic abnormality remains.

For active infection, it has been increasingly recognized that earlier surgical intervention can improve results. Indeed, there is considerable risk in continued antibiotic management in the absence of good evidence of a response. With mechanical valves in particular, it is possible for large peri-annular abscesses to develop without deterioration in valve function; surgery to remove infected tissue and prosthesis may result in cure.

A review[101] of major series indicates an overall mortality of 61.4% where management was with antibiotics alone, compared with an overall mortality of 38.5% for those having valve replacement. There is a risk of recurrent infection on the replacement valve. The risk of infection on a prosthetic valve inserted in patients with active native or prosthetic valve endocarditis has been reported to be between 0 and 20%.[101,102] Sweeney et al.[102] showed a greater incidence of recurrent endocarditis with bioprostheses than mechanical prostheses when replacing native or prosthetic valves with active infection.

In general, the indications for surgical intervention in prosthetic valve endocarditis are haemodynamic deterioration manifested by heart failure due to valve dysfunction, evidence of uncontrolled infection after 5–7 days of appropriate antibiotic management, major systemic embolism, the onset of conduction abnormalities or changes in the radiological silhouette of the heart, suggestive of extending peri-annular abscess. Fungal infection or infection with *Staphylococcus aureus* carries a very high mortality with medical therapy alone and early surgery is recommended.[101]

The appearances of infected prosthetic valves are frequently alarming at the time of surgery; large friable vegetations, extensive detachment of the prosthesis and paravalve abscess are commonly encountered, all of which lend weight to the policy of early surgical intervention.

Paravalve leak

Paravalve leak may occur with any prosthesis and is not strictly a complication of the prosthesis itself.

Haemolysis

Haemolysis may occur in the presence of paravalve leak (or with haemodynamic malfunction in a failing bioprosthesis), but is not a complication of normally functioning bioprosthetic valves.

Complications with mechanical valves

Mechanical failure

Failure of the components of mechanical valves is exceedingly rare.[58,103] Its occurrence is usually fatal. Patients presenting with rapid deterioration, often with loss of valve clicks, have been identified. Radiological screening confirms the diagnosis and emergency surgery is occasionally life-saving.[104]

Thrombo-embolism

Thrombo-embolism and the need for permanent anticoagulation are the major drawbacks to the use of mechanical valves. At present, none of the mechanical valves can be recommended for use without anticoagulants, although the St Jude valve has been used in the aortic position with antiplatelet drugs alone with reasonably satisfactory results.[85,86]

Thrombosis may occur on or around the valve and extend to interfere with movement of its components.[105–110] Thus, thrombosis of a prosthetic valve may present with rapidly developing stenosis and regurgitation depending on the manner in which the occluder becomes restricted (Fig. 35.17). Often, thrombosis of a valve develops when anticoagulation is poorly controlled, but this is not invariably the case. There is usually a change in prosthetic sounds and often a loss of the normal clicks. Radiological screening is of great help in diagnosis if the occluder has a radiopaque marker.

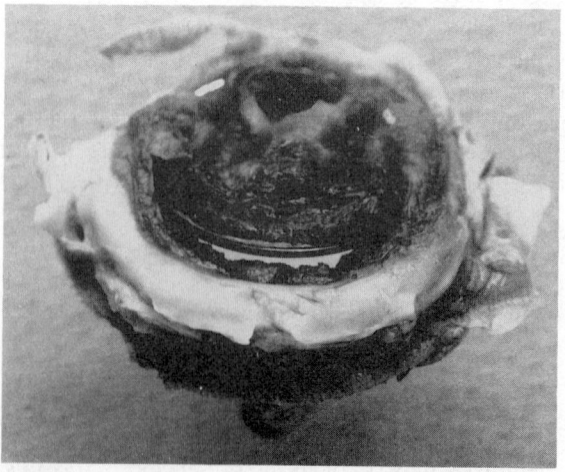

Fig. 35.17. Explanted thrombosed mechanical tilting disc valve.

Urgent surgery to replace the thrombosed prosthesis is the preferred treatment. However, streptokinase may have a role as an initial treatment in critically ill patients, particularly for the tricuspid valve.[105] Surgery with thrombectomy of the prosthesis alone has been reported.[110]

Recognition of thrombo-embolism is not always easy. Reported series often give incomplete information and there is lack of standardization in terminology.[78,111] Unless patients are asked the appropriate questions at follow-up, the true incidence of thrombo-embolic complications is unlikely to be known.[111] Cerebral embolism can be defined as all new focal neurological symptoms, including blackouts, strokes, abnormalities of vision, numbness and weakness. Episodes of embolism to limbs may be clinically apparent, but undoubtedly small emboli may escape detection or recognition.

Edmunds[81] has compiled detailed tables of the reported thrombo-embolic rates with a large number of prosthetic valves. The incidence of thrombo-emboli would appear to be less than 2% per patient-year for the best aortic mechanical valves and about 4% per patient-year for the best mitral mechanical valves.

Endocarditis

Endocarditis is a complication common to mechanical and bioprosthetic valves and has already been discussed. Although the risk of prosthetic valve endocarditis is similar for both types of valves,[99] the presentation may differ. Haemodynamic deterioration, when it occurs with mechanical valves, is usually due to severe paravalve leak, the consequence of infective destruction of the annulus; peri-annular abscesses may develop causing severe structural disruption of the heart in spite of the valve apparently continuing to work well. In contrast, in tissue valves leaflet destruction may cause haemodynamic failure at an earlier stage.

Paravalve leak

Paravalve leak occurs with both mechanical and biological valves,[71] and appears to be largely a technical problem unrelated to the particular type of prosthesis. Kirklin's group[112] showed an actuarial freedom from periprosthetic leak, in the absence of infection, of 98.5% at 5 years. In Cohn's series,[89,90] there was no difference in the occurrence of paravalve leak between mechanical and biological prostheses, although Hammond et al.[68] found a significantly increased incidence of re-operation for paravalve leak with mechanical valves.

Haemolysis

Current designs of mechanical prostheses rarely cause clinically significant haemolysis in the absence of paravalve leak. Detection of sub-clinical levels of haemolysis by measurement of serum lactic dehydrogenase activity and the haptoglobin level is possible with all types of current mechanical valves.[113]

OUTCOME OF SURGERY FOR VALVULAR HEART DISEASE

For the patient, physician and surgeon considering surgery for valvular heart disease, it is natural that there will be concern about the risk of death or complication associated with operation. It is important, therefore, to have an idea of the likely hazards as well as the factors which influence these risks.

Although it is conventional to refer to operative risk, hospital (or 30-day) risk and late-risk, it has been pointed out[112] that this is an artificial division and Kirklin's group have encouraged the concept of regarding the risk of death as a hazard function present from the time of operation (and highest in the early period, corresponding to hospital mortality) and which continues, albeit at a decreasing level, indefinitely.

The hazard of any particular operation is frequently assessed on the basis of reports in surgical literature, which may reflect the better results, as there is often an understandable lack of incentive to report the less good. It is also often assumed that present-day practice gives improved results when compared with those of earlier practice.

In considering the history of cardiac surgery, it is true that operative mortality for valvular heart disease has improved considerably since early 'pioneering' experience. Operative mortality for aortic valve replacement has been quoted at 10–30% between 1969 and 1975, but at < 5% for more recent practice.[114] However, this assertion is based on isolated reports from leading centres, which may not be representative, and does not compare the same centres' practice in the two different time-frames.

In examining this question, Kirklin's group[115] compared the results in their own institution for mitral valve replacement in 478 patients operated

on between 1975 and 1979 with a later group of 341 patients operated on between 1979 and 1983. Patients in the later group had a slightly, but inconclusively, lower survival rate at 2 weeks and at 4.5 years than those in the earlier group. Based on detailed analysis of patient characteristics and operative management, they suggest that continuing delay in advising mitral valve replacement, as well as continued imperfection in methods of myocardial protection, were the likely reasons for lack of improvement in results.

A report of experience in 72 Veterans Administration medical centres in the USA[116] has shown a fall in operative mortality from 9.5% in 1975 to 3.0% in 1984 for isolated aortic valve replacement, although there is no discernible trend for isolated mitral valve replacement (13.7% early in this 10-year review period, and 12.4% in 1984). Similarly, at the Cleveland Clinic, a comparison of hospital mortality for combined aortic valve replacement/coronary grafting showed an improvement from 5.9% for the period 1967–1981 to 3.4% for their subsequent practice, whereas that for combined mitral valve replacement/coronary grafting remained virtually unchanged at 7%.[117]

Consideration of operative mortality (defined as death at or within 30 days of operation) for valve surgery in the UK shows that, although mortality for double and aortic valve replacement declined over the years 1977–1982, that for mitral valve replacement remained virtually unchanged.[6] It is perhaps naïve to assume that current practice necessarily reflects a continuing trend towards improvement in mortality and reduced risk.

Undue emphasis on operative mortality may be misplaced if it inhibits acceptance for surgery of older, more ill patients, or those with multiple pathology for whom medical therapy may have little further to offer; the acceptance of such patients in greater numbers may explain part of the continuing operative mortality.

A detailed analysis[112] of death and other time-related events after valve replacement in the period 1975–1979 has given insight into outcome and risk factors. Of 1533 patients (842 aortic valve, 478 mitral valve and 213 combined aortic and mitral valve replacements), 4.4% died in hospital after operation. Older age was an incremental (although not strong) risk factor for early death; aortic incompetence, mitral stenosis and/or mitral incompetence were also risk factors. Pre-operative functional status as documented by NYHA class was a risk factor for early death, as were longer cross-clamp time and combined valve procedures. Reduction in early risk, therefore, might be expected by improving myocardial protection and surgical techniques.

MORTALITY RISK ASSOCIATED WITH SURGERY

Closed mitral commissurotomy

In the Western world, closed mitral commissurotomy is uncommon today. It forms less than 5% of the total valvular heart surgery undertaken in the UK at present. The risk of early mortality associated with closed procedures on the mitral valve is low, being in the range of 1–2% in current British practice.[118]

In countries where resources for cardiac surgery are limited and the prevalence of rheumatic fever in young patients is high, this operation still has a considerable role. In 654 patients having closed mitral valvotomy from 1965 to 1977 in Cape Town,[119] operative mortality was 2.97%. A report from Vellore, India, of 3724 patients having closed mitral valvotomy between 1956 and 1980 shows an operative mortality of 3.8%.[26]

Conservative procedures on the mitral valve

For mitral stenosis, open commissurotomy (or valvotomy) has become more popular than closed operation in many centres. The procedure is undoubtedly safer than isolated mitral valve replacement. Open mitral valvotomy can be performed with an operative mortality of 2% or less.[120]

Open valvotomy can be achieved reasonably safely even in the presence of severe subvalvar changes, as reported by Nakano's group,[121] who performed open valvotomy on 53 patients with such changes with 2 operative deaths. Further evidence for the safety of this operation, even with quite severely diseased valves, is provided by a group in Spain reporting on 81 patients who had densely scarred or partially calcified valves and underwent open mitral commissurotomy without operative death.[122]

For mitral regurgitation, mitral valve repair is preferable to replacement, but it is not always feasible. Despite the greater technical difficulties that the procedure may present, in centres undertaking this form of surgery in reasonable numbers, the mortality is low, particularly in those in whom associated procedures on other valves or myocar-

dial revascularization are not required. In 1090 patients operated on between 1969 and 1982 for isolated mitral valve repair, Carpentier's group[16] reports a mortality of 3.6%. A mortality of 4.3% (1.8% in the 56 patients having isolated mitral valve repair) in 117 patients undergoing mitral valve reconstruction from 1980 to 1985 is reported by workers at the Cleveland Clinic.[32] In their experience[123] of mitral valve repair for mitral insufficiency using the Puig–Massana–Shiley annuloplasty ring, workers at the Texas Heart Institute report an operative mortality of 6.3% in 126 patients operated on between 1982 and 1984; of these, 44 had mitral valve repair alone, and operative mortality was 2.3%.

Mitral valve replacement

Recent reports of operative mortality for isolated mitral valve replacement suggest this to be in the range of 2–10%.[71,89,103,115,124–126] British practice for the 5 years from 1980 to 1984 shows a mortality in the region of 7% for isolated mitral valve replacement.[118]

Figures taken from large series or from national statistics give a guide to average mortality. However, these figures include patients who are recognizably at high risk, such as those with advanced disease, multiple pathology, or who are older. There will also be a large group of people who do not have such risk factors, in whom results will be better than indicated by the average figures.

The nature of mitral dysfunction may influence the risk, mitral regurgitation carrying a higher mortality[124] than mitral stenosis in some series (13% compared with 8% in one series),[125] although not in others (7.2% compared with 7.0%).[126] An ischaemic basis for mitral regurgitation is widely recognized to confer an increased risk.[115,125,126]

Patients nearing the end of the natural history of their condition and displaying features of advanced disease, such as NYHA class IV dyspnoea, tricuspid regurgitation, hepatic dysfunction or cardiac cachexia, are at increased risk.[124] Severe pulmonary hypertension is usually an accompaniment of severe disease, but of itself it does not appear to confer increased operative risk.[124] In a report of 1329 patients undergoing isolated mitral valve replacement either with Starr–Edwards mechanical or with porcine xenograft valves,[125] it was shown that overall mortality was 10 ± 1%, and that advanced disability (high NYHA classification), pre-operative myocardial infarction, hepatic dysfunction, greater age, renal dysfunction, mitral regurgitation and angina pectoris were correlated with higher operative mortality. The implication for practice is that if surgical management is judged to be likely in an individual patient care should be taken to intervene before the patient's condition deteriorates to the stage of advanced disease, thereby improving not only the immediate operative mortality, but also late survival.[89,112]

Increasing age is associated with an increased risk, the effect being noticeable after about 60 years of age,[79,124,125] although good results have been reported for patients over 70 years.[127] Murphy et al.[128] found male sex to be associated with increased operative mortality for aortic and mitral valve replacement in their analysis of possible risk factors, although a similar analysis in another study of isolated mitral valve replacement surgery did not find an influence of gender on operative mortality.[125]

When surgery is undertaken as an emergency or urgently, the risk is increased. This usually reflects the severity of pathology present and the patient's general resultant condition. Thus, surgery for infective endocarditis on the mitral valve carries a higher risk if it has to be undertaken as an emergency.

Aortic valve replacement

The hospital mortality for isolated aortic valve replacement in recent years has been variously reported as 5.8%,[129] < 5%,[114] 2%,[130] and 1%.[90] British practice over the 5 years from 1980 to 1984 shows mortality for aortic valve replacement to be about 5%.[118]

A review from the Stanford group of 1479 patients undergoing isolated aortic valve replacement between 1967 and 1981[131] revealed an overall operative mortality of 7 ± 1%. Where the valve lesion was aortic regurgitation, mortality was 10 ± 2%, in aortic stenosis it was 6 ± 1%, and in combined aortic stenosis and regurgitation 5 ± 2%. After multivariate analysis, functional class emerged as the strongest statistical determinant of operative mortality, along with renal dysfunction, atrial fibrillation and the nature of valve dysfunction (aortic regurgitation being stronger than aortic stenosis). Older age was a weaker, but significant, determinant of operative mortality.

The results of a similar, but more recent, study from Toronto[114] suggested that the nature of the aortic valve disease did not influence hospital mortality and, with the advent of non-invasive methods of investigation and earlier referral of patients with aortic regurgitation, including those who may be asymptomatic, mortality had fallen. In common with other workers,[90,132] the Toronto group thought that better methods of myocardial protection had improved results.

Further evidence for improvement in the outcome of surgery for chronic aortic regurgitation by earlier operation is provided by a comparison between practice in 1970–1974 and 1975–1979.[130] Not only was there a decrease in early mortality (2.0% compared with 3.5%) but there was also an improvement in 5-year survival (90.6% compared with 80.1%).

Patients presenting for isolated aortic valve replacement often do so at an advanced age. The influence of age on the risk of hospital mortality is therefore an important consideration. In the Toronto study,[114] age was identified as the most important independent risk factor for operative mortality: it was shown that patients who died were older than survivors and none of the 52 patients under 50 years of age died. Patients between 50 and 65 years had a lower mortality (0.8%) than patients older than 65 years (5%) and patients between 82 and 85 years had a predicted mortality between 15 and 22%. The likelihood of more advanced disease and other pathologies in older patients may partly explain this finding, which has been confirmed in other studies. Arom et al.[132] reported an operative mortality of 9.8% for aortic valve replacement in 41 patients over 70 years of age, but only 1% in 99 patients under 70 years.

In general, therefore, an operative mortality for isolated aortic valve replacement in those under 70 years and not at the end of their natural history should be in the range of 1–5% for current practice. Advanced age is likely to be the most important factor increasing risk in present practice. This risk should not be prohibitive, and for those in their 70s should not exceed 10%. The major factor likely to result in excessive risk is poor pre-operative state at all ages. The need for additional procedures, most commonly coronary surgery, should not add undue extra risk.

Multiple valve procedures

The risks associated with single-valve procedures also apply to multiple-valve procedures,[112] but the more prolonged operation required adds to the hazard, particularly where problems are encountered in myocardial protection. If the tricuspid valve is involved in association with mitral disease, it usually reflects advanced disease and hence poorer operative outcome. An increased mortality for double-valve as compared with single-valve replacement has been reported from many centres,[103,133] although it is not universal.[62]

British practice over the 5 years from 1980 to 1984 shows an average mortality for aortic and mitral valve procedures (usually, but not always, valve replacement) to be around 9.5%, compared with 5% for aortic valve replacement and 7% for mitral valve replacement. For mitral and tricuspid procedures (usually tricuspid repair), mortality was about 17%, reflecting the more advanced pathology of those requiring such procedures.[118]

In a prospective study of 90 patients undergoing multiple valve procedures, tricuspid regurgitation and aortic stenosis were shown to be independent predictors of both post-operative low-output syndrome and hospital mortality.[134] Other factors that adversely influence hospital mortality are pre-operative functional class,[135,136] urgency of operation[135] and age.[136] The most important factor in improved operative mortality over the years appears to be the better clinical status of patients referred for surgery.[136]

Valve replacement combined with coronary grafting

Coronary disease and aortic valve disease may co-exist and are not causally related. Where significant obstruction at the origin of major vessels is demonstrated, coronary bypass grafting should be added to valve replacement. The major risk factors are similar to those for coronary surgery: impaired ventricular function, increasing age and female sex.

It is apparent that aortic valve replacement can be combined with coronary surgery with only a modest increase in hospital mortality resulting. Thus, Cohn's group,[90] in reporting experience for 1983, disclosed a mortality for aortic valve replacement alone of 1%, and 4.4% for aortic valve replacement combined with coronary grafting. For the period 1978–1981, workers at the Cleveland Clinic reported an operative mortality of 3.4% for combined aortic valve replacement and coronary artery surgery.[137]

Mitral valve disease may co-exist with coronary disease without causal relationship. It may also be a consequence of ischaemia or disruption of the papillary muscle mechanism; in these circumstances, surgery carries a high risk, although it is usually the only option to give the patient any

prospect of survival. When not causally related, coronary disease and mitral valve disease can be treated surgically; hospital mortality has been reported in the range of 14–24%.[117] Workers at the Cleveland Clinic report a 7.3% hospital mortality, identifying poor ventricular function and left main coronary disease as major risk factors.[117]

Patients having combined mitral and coronary surgery have a higher hospital mortality than those with either coronary or mitral pathology alone undergoing appropriate surgery. However, in patients in whom mitral pathology and significant coronary disease co-exist, the combined procedure has a lower hospital mortality than isolated mitral surgery in such patients.

Repeat operations

Whenever the heart is exposed for a second or even third time, the adhesions between the heart and the pericardium or posterior aspect of the sternum pose hazards as they increase the risk of injury to the heart and great vessels during sternotomy and exposure of the heart. Although careful dissection under vision makes safe re-entry reasonably likely, there is always an additional risk to re-operation. In a review of a large series of 1000 re-operations at the Cleveland Clinic,[138] 277 were for replacement of an existing prosthesis (the remainder following coronary surgery or conservative mitral surgery). Catastrophic haemorrhage at re-sternotomy was seen in a small proportion. The major factor contributing to higher operative risk appeared to be advanced age, although impaired left ventricular function and significant coronary disease adversely influenced risk. First re-operation for aortic valve surgery was associated with a hospital mortality of 11%, and second re-operation a mortality of 13%. In mitral valve surgery, mortality was 10% for the first re-operation and 12% for second re-operation. Few patients required more than two re-operations; those who did had a considerably increased mortality, a finding which was confirmed by Kirklin's group.[139] In a review of 200 aortic valve replacements, overall operative mortality was 5%, mortality was 3.9% in those having first time re-replacement, rising to 15% in the group undergoing second or third re-replacement.

LATE OUTCOME OF SURGERY

There is widespread acceptance that surgery considerably improves the outlook for life-expectancy. Most of the available information about the natural history of valvular heart disease has been derived from the era before surgical treatment was available. It is now impossible to compare the outlook in surgically treated patients with a matched control series. Indeed, it has been pointed out[10] that there are difficulties in comparing different series of untreated patients: for instance, 66% dying within 10 years of diagnosis of mitral stenosis in one series contrasts with only 7% dying within a similar time in another series. The difference would appear to lie in the different stages of the disease at which first diagnosis is made.

The poor natural history of mitral stenosis is well documented and is unlikely to be seen in contemporary Western practice. There may be many years of survival free of symptoms. When patients present in NYHA functional class III, survival rates of 62% and 38% at 5 and 10 years, respectively, have been estimated, which contrasts with 5-year survival of 15% in class IV patients. Once symptoms arise, progression to death occurs over relatively few years. Survival statistics for mitral insufficiency appear to be similar.

Aortic regurgitation is known to have a long course in many cases. The major problem is the myocardial damage that occurs, which impairs longevity following surgical correction. Half of patients diagnosed as having haemodynamically significant aortic insufficiency are still alive at 10 years after diagnosis. The onset of congestive heart failure heralds rapid deterioration. By contrast, the natural history of symptomatic aortic stenosis is much worse, with life-expectancy being on average < 5 years.

Late survival after valve replacement

A review of reports of outcome in the surgical literature is often hampered by lack of detail regarding pre-operative symptomatic status; however, most reports of surgery for valve replacement are of patients with relatively severe symptoms. Bloomfield et al.[79] report their experience in patients undergoing mitral valve replacement, of whom 59% pre-operatively were in NYHA class III or class IV (32% being in class V at some time), and found a 7-year actuarial survival of 56.7%; in patients undergoing aortic valve replacement, of whom 47% were in class III or class IV pre-operatively (28% in class V at some time), there was a 7-year actuarial survival of nearly 70%.

A better outlook was reported by Sethia et al.[103] who found a 10-year actuarial survival of about

70% and 90% for mitral and aortic valve replacement, respectively. Pre-operatively, 72% of all their patients were in class III or class IV. Other groups[55,69,73] have reported 5-year survival rates of 80% and over, and 10-year survival rates of 60–86% for mitral, aortic and double-valve replacement.

Starr's group[59] have drawn attention to the influence of time-frame on long-term outcome. They reviewed long-term survival with the Starr-Edwards ball valve in the mitral position, and showed that a major improvement occurred after 1973 in thrombo-embolic complication rates. It is possible that similar improvements are occurring in long-term survival for valve surgery generally. Gersh et al.[136] reporting on the long-term follow-up of 91 patients undergoing triple valve replacement, noted a 5-year survival of 81% in those undergoing surgery after 1975, compared with a 5-year survival of 52% in those having the same procedure before 1975. Their overall results show that long-term outcome is influenced by pre-operative functional class: survival at 5 years in class II or class III patients was 80% and 59% at 10 years, whereas for those in pre-operative class IV, the figures are 59% and 45%, respectively. However, Kirklin's group[115] were unable to show a difference in actuarial survival at 4.5 years for a group of patients having mitral valve replacement between 1975 and 1979 compared with a later group having surgery between 1979 and 1983. The results in this group also demonstrate poorer pre-operative functional class to be associated with poorer 5-year survival.

When coronary surgery is combined with aortic valve surgery, pre-operative left ventricular function is the major influence on late survival. The group at the Cleveland Clinic have reported a 10-year survival of 55% The majority of late deaths were cardiac in nature; in this series, survival to 4.5 years was best in those receiving biological aortic valve prostheses.[137]

When coronary surgery is combined with mitral valve surgery, late survival is less good, workers at the Cleveland Clinic reporting a 10-year survival of 31%. Left ventricular dysfunction was a major adverse factor and those receiving bioprostheses without warfarin had better survival and fewer cardiovascular events.[117]

Symptomatic status after valve replacement

Although medical management of atrial fibrillation can improve symptomatic status in patients with valvular heart disease, there is generally continuing deterioration once symptoms have become apparent. All surgical series of valve replacement report improvement, which is often striking. In Cohn's study of the results of mitral valve replacement,[89] 46% of patients were in functional class III and 53% in class IV before surgery; after surgery, 69% were in class I, 26% in class II and 5% in class III. Such improvement in symptomatic status appears to be well maintained. Thus, Sethia[103] reports 91% of patients to be in class I or class II at a mean follow-up period of 5.2 years (range 4–14 years). The Edinburgh randomized study reported by Bloomfield[79] showed a highly significant improvement in functional class for all patients following surgery, and this remained so throughout the follow-up period.

Outcome after conservative surgery

Conservative procedures may be expected to avoid the complications associated with the implantation of prostheses. Such procedures are not always applicable but, when they are, the results appear to be excellent. For closed mitral valvotomy, a procedure still widely applicable in many countries, excellent long-term results have been reported. In their review of 3724 patients, John et al.[26] report actuarial survival as 95, 93.1, 89.5 and 84.2% at 6, 12, 18 and 24 years, with good sustained symptomatic improvement. Only 130 patients had been submitted to re-operation for restenosis. Commerford[118] disclosed a higher rate of restenosis in his series. At 6 years, 72% of patients were surviving without re-operation. At 12 years, overall cumulative survival was 78% and 47% were surviving without re-operation.

Good long-term results for mitral valve reconstruction by open operation have been reported with an actuarial survival rate of 82% at 9 years (including hospital mortality) with 70% of patients in NYHA class I.[140] When compared with broadly similar patients undergoing mitral valve replacement with porcine or mechanical valves, Perier et al.[30] showed a better outcome in the group undergoing repair, with lower early and late mortality and lower risk of complications. Excellent results are also reported for mitral valve reconstructive surgery by Cosgrove et al.;[32] 2-year actuarial survival was 90.6%, and 96.2% of survivors were in NYHA functional class I or class II.

Causes of late mortality

The cause of late death following surgery for valvular heart disease may be related to the prosthesis (embolus, death at re-operation), cardiac, related to valvular heart disease (dysrhythmia, myocardial failure), cardiac not related to valvular heart disease, or it may be due to non-cardiac causes. Starr's group[59] indicated that only 16% of late deaths could be shown to be prosthesis-related (there was a 14% incidence of sudden death and a further 35% were cardiac deaths). In the Edinburgh study,[79] 30 of the 113 late deaths were considered to be prosthesis-related and included re-operation, endocarditis, thrombo-embolism and anticoagulant complications. Nashef et al.[71] report an incidence of 27% for prosthesis-related mortality, although it is possible that the prosthesis could have been implicated in some of the 23% of patients dying from unknown causes. In Cohn's 12-year comparison of porcine and mechanical mitral valves,[89] 97 of the 155 late deaths were found to be cardiac in nature, including congestive cardiac failure, myocardial ischaemia, re-operation for valve dysfunction and sudden death (presumed arrhythmia). Thrombo-embolism and haemorrhage accounted for 15 cases.

Prosthesis-related death accounts for only a proportion of late mortality, which partly explains the finding of little difference in long-term outcome for different valve prostheses. Furthermore, the finding of a large proportion of sudden late deaths, cardiac in nature but not prosthesis-related, does suggest that earlier intervention in the natural history of valvular heart disease would result in better late surgical outcome.

Surgery has an important role in the management of valvular heart disease and has transformed the outcome for the majority of patients. Intervention at the appropriate time in the natural history, i.e. before secondary pathological sequelae have caused permanent deterioration in myocardium, lungs or other organs, has been shown to result in lower operative risk, enhanced late survival and better symptomatic improvement. When valves can be conserved rather than replaced, the outcome is better than when a prosthesis is required. For most patients, there is little to choose between available prostheses in terms of overall survival and symptomatic improvement, although the nature of prosthesis-related complications differs. Such complications contribute only partly to late deterioration and death. The surgical treatment of valvular disease in children, in whom prostheses are unsatisfactory, is still a problem. The generally excellent outcome, particularly in adults, of surgery for valvular heart disease may be expected to improve further with the benefit of past clinical experience and with refinements in prosthetic valves.

REFERENCES

1. Roberts, W.C. The silver anniversary of cardiac valve replacement (editorial). *Am. J. Cardiol.* 1985; **56**: 503.
2. Wheatley, D.J. Valve prostheses. In: Jamieson, S.W. and Shumway, N.E, eds. *Cardiac Surgery* (Rob & Smith's *Operative Surgery* series, general eds Dudley, H. and Carter, D). 4th edn. London: Butterworths, 1986, p.415.
3. Wheatley, D.J. Mechanical prosthetic heart valves. *Current Opinion in Cardiology* 1986; **1**: 738.
4. Duran, C.G. Tissue valves. *Current Opinion in Cardiology* 1986; **1**: 730.
5. Rutkow, I.M. Thoracic and cardiovascular operations in the United States, 1979 to 1984. *J. Thorac. Cardiovasc. Surg.* 1986; **92**: 181.
6. English, T.A.H., Bailey, A.R., Dark, J.F. and Williams, W.G. The UK Cardiac Surgical Register, 1977–1982. *Br. Med. J.* 1984; **289**: 1205.
7. Roberts, W.C. Valvular, subvalvular and supravalvular aortic stenosis. Morphologic features. *Cardiovasc. Clin.* 1973; **5**: 97.
8. Braunwald, E. Valvular heart disease. In: Braunwald E., ed. *Heart disease. A textbook of cardiovascular medicine*, 2nd edn. Philadelphia: W.B. Saunders & Co, 1984, p.1063.
9. Davies, M.J. The pathology of the mitral valve. In: Ionescu, M.I. and Cohn, L.H., eds. *Mitral valve disease. Diagnosis and Treatment*. London: Butterworths, 1985, p.27.
10. Rapaport, E. Natural history of aortic and mitral valve disease. *Am. J. Cardiol.* 1975; **35**: 221.
11. Barratt-Boyes, B.G. The timing of operation in valvular insufficiency. *J. Cardiac Surg.* 1987; **2**: 435.
12. Smith, W.M., Neutze, J.M. Barratt-Boyes, B.G. and Lowe, B. Open mitral valvotomy. Effect of pre-operative factors on result. *J. Thorac. Cardiovasc. Surg.* 1981; **82**: 738.
13. Kan, J.S., White, R.I., Mitchell, S.E. and Gardener, T.J. Percutaneous balloon valvuloplasty: a new method for treating congenital pulmonary valve stenosis. *N. Engl. J. Med.* 1982; **307**: 540.
14. McKay, R.G., Safian, R.D., Lock, J.E. *et al*. Assessment of left ventricular and aortic valve function after aortic valvuloplasty in adult patients with critical aortic stenosis. *Circulation* 1987; **75**: 192.
15. Dobell, A.R.C., Bloss, R.S., Gibbons, J.E. and Collins, G.F. Congenital valvular aortic stenosis. Surgical management and long-term results. *J. Thorac. Cardiovasc. Surg.* 1981; **81**: 916.
16. Carpentier, A. Cardiac valve surgery—the "French correction". *J. Thorac. Cardiovasc. Surg.* 1983; **86**: 323.
17. Spencer, F., Doyle, E., Danilowich, D., Bahnson, H. and Weldon, C. Long-term evaluation of aortic valvuloplasty for aortic insufficiency and ventricular septal defect. *J. Thorac. Cardiovasc. Surg.* 1973; **65**: 15.
18. Trusler, G., Moes, C. and Kidd, B. Repair of ventricular septal defect with aortic insufficiency. *J. Thorac. Cardiovasc. Surg.* 1973; **66**: 394.
19. King, R.M., Pluth, J.R., Giuliani, E.R. and Piehler, J.M. Mechanical decalcification of the aortic valve. *Ann. Thorac. Surg.* 1986; **42**: 269.
20. Rahimtoola, S.H. The problem of valve prosthesis-patient mismatch. *Circulation* 1978 **58**: 20.
21. Blank, R.H., Pupello, D.F., Bessone, L.N., Harrison, E.E. and Sbar, S. Method of managing the small aortic annulus during valve replacement. *Ann. Thorac. Surg.* 1976; **22**: 356.
22. Manouguian, S. and Seybold-Epting, W. Patch enlargement of the aortic valve ring by extending the aortic incision into the anterior mitral leaflet. *J. Thorac. Cardiovasc. Surg.* 1979; **78**: 402.
23. Misbach, G.A., Turley, K., Ullyot, D.J. and Ebert, P.A. Left ventricular outflow enlargement by the Konno procedure. *J. Thorac. Cardiovasc. Surg.* 1982; **84**: 696.
24. Somerville, J. and Ross, D. Homograft replacement of aortic root with reimplantation of coronary arteries. Results after one to five years. *Br. Heart J.* 1982; **47**: 473.
25. Cooley, D.A., Norman, J.C., Reul Jr, G.J., Kidd, J.N. and Nihill, M.R. Surgical treatment of left ventricular outflow tract obstruction with apicoaortic valved conduit. *Surgery* 1976; **80**: 674.
26. John, S., Bashi, V.V., Jairaj, P.S. *et al*. Closed mitral valvotomy: Early results and long-term follow-up of 3724 consecutive patients. *Circulation* 1983; **68**: 891.
27. Gautam, P.C., Coulshed, N., Epstein, E.J., Llewellyn, M.J., Vargas, E. and Tallis, R.C. Preoperative clinical predictors of long term survival in mitral stenosis: analysis of 200 cases followed for up to 27 years after closed mitral valvotomy. *Thorax* 1986; **41**: 401.
28. Nunley, D.L. and Starr, A. The evolution of reparative techniques for the mitral valve. *Ann. Thorac. Surg.* 1984; **37**: 393.
29. Spencer, F.C., Colvin, S.B., Culliford A.T. and Isom O.W. Experiences with the Carpentier techniques of mitral valve reconstruction in 103 patients (1980–1985). *J. Thorac Cardiovasc. Surg.* 1985, **90**: 341.
30. Perier, P., Deloche, A., Chauvaud, S. *et al*. Comparative evaluation of mitral valve repair and replacement with Starr, Björk, and porcine valve prostheses. *Circulation* 1984; **70** (Suppl. I): I–187.
31. Dhasmana, J.P., Blackstone, E.H., Kirlin, J.W. and Kouchoukos, N.T. Factors associated with periprosthetic leakage following primary mitral valve replacement: with special consideration of the suture technique. *Ann. Thorac. Surg.* 1983; **35**: 170.
32. Cosgrove, D.M., Chavez, A.M., Lytle, B.W. *et al*. Results of mitral valve reconstruction. *Circulation* 1986; **74** (Suppl. I): I–82.
33. Oury, J.H., Peterson, K.L., Folkerth, T.L. and Daily, P.O. Mitral valve replacement versus reconstruction: an analysis of indications and results of mitral valve procedures in a consecutive series of 80 patients. *J. Thorac. Cardiovasc. Surg.* 1977; **73**: 825.
34. Duran, C.G., Pomar, J.L., Revuelta, J.M. *et al*. Conservative operation for mitral insufficiency—critical analysis supported by post-operative hemodynamic studies in 72 patients. *J. Thorac Cardiovasc Surg.* 1980; **79**: 326.
35. Yacoub, M., Halim, M., Radley-Smith, R., McKay, R, Nijueld, A. and Towers, M. Surgical treatment of mitral regurgitation caused by floppy valves: repair versus replacement. *Circulation* 1981; **64** (Suppl. II): II–210.
36. Oliveira, D.B.G., Kawkins, K.D., Kay, P.H. and Paneth, M. Chordal rupture: comparison between repair and replacement. *Br. Heart J.* 1983; **50**: 318.
37. Adebo, O.A. and Ross, J.K. Surgical treatment of ruptured mitral valve chordae: a comparison between valve replacement and valve repair. *Thorac. Cardiovasc. Surg.* 1984; **32**: 139.
38. Arbulu, A. and Asfaw, I. Tricuspid valvulectomy without prosthetic replacement. Ten years of clinical experience. *J. Thorac. Cardiovasc. Surg.* 1981; **82**: 684.
39. Stern, H.J., Sisto, D.A., Strom, J.A. *et al*. Immediate tricuspid valve replacement for endocarditis. *J. Thorac.*

Cardiovasc. Surg. 1986; **91**: 163.

40. De Vega, N.G. La anuloplasty selectiva, regulable y permanente. *Rev. Esp. Cardiol.* 1972; **25**: 555.

41. Carpentier, A., Deloche, A., Dauptain, J. *et al.* A new reconstructive operation for correction of mitral and tricuspid insufficiency. *J. Thorac. Cardiovasc. Surg.* 1971; **61**: 1.

42. Silver, M.D., Datta, B.N. and Bowes, V.F. A key to identify heart valve prostheses. *Arch. Pathol.* 1975; **99**: 132.

43. Morgan, R.J., Davis, J.T. and Fraker, T.D. Current status of valve prostheses. *Surg. Clin. North Am.* 1985; **65**: 699.

44. Tindale, W.B., Black, M.M. and Martin, T.R.P. In vitro evaluation of prosthetic heart valves: anomalies and limitations. *Clin. Phys. Physiol. Meas.* 1982; **3**: 115.

45. Walker, D.K., Scotten, L.N. and Brownlee, R.T. New generation tissue valves. Their in vitro function in the mitral position. *J. Thorac. Cardiovasc. Surg.* 1984; **88**: 573.

46. Yoganathan, A.P., Woo, Y.-R., Sung, H.-W., Williams, F.P., French, R.H. and Jones, M. In vitro hemodynamic characteristics of tissue bioprostheses in the aortic position. *J. Thorac. Cardiovasc. Surg.* 1986; **92**: 198.

47. Scotton, L.N., Racca, R.G., Nugent, A.H., Walker, D.K. and Brownlee, R.T. New tilting disc cardiac valve prostheses. In vitro comparison of their hydrodynamic performance in the mitral position. *J. Thorac. Cardiovasc. Surg.* 1981; **82**: 136.

48. Chandran, K.B., Khalighi, B. and Chen, C.J. Experimental study of physiological pulsatile flow past valve prostheses in a model of the human aorta. I. Caged ball valves. *J. Biomech.* 1985; **18**: 763.

49. Chandran, K.B., Khalighi, B. and Chen, C.J. Experimental study of physiological pulsatile flow past valve prostheses in a model of the human aorta. II. Tilting disc valves and the effect of orientation. *J. Biomech.* 1985; **18**: 773.

50. Fisher, J., Reece, I.J. and Wheatley, D.J. In vitro evaluation of six mechanical and six bioprosthetic valves. *Thorac. Cardiovasc. Surg.* 1986; **34**: 157.

51. Ross, D.N. Homograft replacement of the aortic valve. *Lancet* 1972; **2**: 487.

52. Barratt-Boyes, B.G. Homograft aortic valve replacement in aortic incompetence and stenosis. *Thorax* 1964; **19**: 131.

53. Penta, A., Qureshi, S., Radley-Smith, R. and Yacoub, M.H. Patient status 10 or more years after 'fresh' homograft replacement of the aortic valve. *Circulation* 1984; **70** (Suppl. I): I–182.

54. Angell, W.W., Angell, J.D., Oury, J.H., Lamberti, J.J. and Grehl, T.M. Long-term follow-up of viable frozen aortic homografts: A viable homograft valve bank. *J. Thorac. Cardiovasc. Surg.* 1987; **93**: 815.

55. Magilligan, D.J., Lewis, J.W., Tilley, B. and Peterson, E. The porcine bioprosthetic valve. 12 years later. *J. Thorac. Cardiovasc. Surg.* 1985; **89**: 499.

56. Brais, M.P., Bedard, J.P., Goldstein, W. *et al.* Ionescu–Shiley pericardial xenografts: follow-up of up to 6 years. *Ann. Thorac. Surg.* 1985; **39**: 105.

57. Becker, R.M., Strom, J., Frishman, W. *et al.* Hemodynamic performance of the Ionescu-Shiley valve prosthesis. *J. Thorac. Cardiovasc. Surg.* 1980; **80**: 613.

58. Mok, C., Lee, J.W.-T., Kong, S.-M. and Hui, K.K.-K. Experience with outlet strut fracture of the Björk–Shiley convexo-concave mitral valve prosthesis. *Am. Heart J.* 1985; **110**: 814.

59. Cobanoglu, A., Grunkemeier, G., Aru, G.M., McKinley, C.L. and Starr, A. Mitral replacement: clinical experience with a ball valve prosthesis. Twenty five years later. *Ann. Surg.* 1985; **202**: 376.

60. Bjork, V.O. and Lindblom, D. The monostrut Bjork–Shiley heart valve. *J. Am. Coll. Cardiol.* 1985; **6**: 1142.

61. Czer, L.S.C., Matloff, J., Chaux, A., DeRobertis, M.,

Yoganathan, A. and Gray, R.J. A 6 year experience with the St Jude Medical Valve: Hemodynamic performance, surgical results, biocompatibility and follow-up. *J. Am. Coll. Cardiol.* 1985; **6**: 904.

62. Arom, K.V., Nicoloff, D.M., Kersten, T.E., Northrup, W.F. and Lindsay, W.G. Six years of experience with the St Jude Medical valvular prosthesis. *Circulation* 1985; **72** (Suppl. II): II–153.

63. Anonymous. Which heart valve prosthesis (Editorial)? *Lancet* 1985; **2**: 756.

64. Elliott, M.J. and de Leval, M. Valve replacement in children. *World J. Surg.* 1985; **9**: 568.

65. Larrea, J.L., Nunez, L., Reque, J.A., Aguado, M.G., Matarros, R. and Minguez, J.A. Pregnancy and mechanical valve prostheses: A high risk situation for the mother and fetus. *Ann. Thorac. Surg.* 1983; **36**: 459.

66. Salazar, E., Zajarias, A., Gutierrez, N. and Iturbe, I. The problem of cardiac valve prostheses, anticoagulants, and pregnancy. *Circulation* 1984; **70** (Suppl. I): I–169.

67. Perier, P., Bessou, J.P., Swanson, J.S. *et al.* Comparative evaluation of aortic valve replacement with Starr, Bjork, and porcine valve prostheses. *Circulation* 1985; **72** (Suppl. II): II–140.

68. Hammond, G.L., Geha, A.S., Kopf, G.S. and Hashim, S.W. Biological versus mechanical valves. Analysis of 1,116 valves inserted in 1,012 adult patients with a 4,818 patient-year and a 5,327 valve-year follow-up. *J. Thorac. Cardiovasc. Surg.* 1987; **93**: 182.

69. Martinell, J., Fraile, J., Artiz, V., Moreno, J. and Rabago, G. Long-term comparative analysis of the Bjork–Shiley and Hanock valves implanted in 1975. *J. Thorac. Cardiovasc. Surg.* 1985; **90**: 741.

70. Douglas, P.S., Hirshfeld Jr, J.W., Edie, R.N., Harken, A.H., Stephenson, L.W. and Edmunds Jr, L.H. Clinical comparison of St Jude and porcine aortic valve prostheses. *Circulation* 1985; **72** (Suppl. II): II–135.

71. Nashef, S.A.M., Sethia, B., Turner, M.A., Davidson, K.G., Lewis, S. and Bain, W.H. Bjork–Shiley and Carpentier–Edwards valves: A comparative analysis. *J. Thorac. Cardiovasc Surg.* 1987; **93**: 394.

72. Damle, A., Coles, J., Teijeira, J., Pelletier, C. and Callaghan, J. A six-year study of the Omniscience valve in four Canadian centres. *Ann. Thorac. Surg.* 1987; **43**: 513.

73. Fessatidis, I., Hackett, D., Oakley, C.M., Sapsford, R.N. and Bentall, H.H. Ten-year clinical evaluation of isolated mitral valve and double-valve replacement with the Starr–Edwards prostheses. *Ann. Thorac. Surg.* 1987; **43**: 368.

74. Harlan, B.J., Smeloff, E.A., Miller Jr, G.E. *et al.* Performance of the Smeloff aortic valve beyond ten years. *J. Thorac. Cardiovasc Surg.* 1986; **91**: 86.

75. Hall, K.V., Nitter-Hauge, S and Abdelnoor, M. Seven and one-half years' experience with the Medtronic-Hall valve. *J. Am. Coll. Cardiol.* 1985; **6**: 1417.

76. Colombo, T., Donatelli, F., Quaini, E., Vitali, E. and Pellegrini, A. Results of heart valve replacement with the Sorin prosthesis. *Texas Heart Inst. J.* 1987; **14**: 77.

77. Revuelta, J.M. and Duran, C.M. Performance of the Ionescu-Shiley pericardial valve in the aortic position: 100 months clinical experience. *Thorac. Cardiovasc. Surg.* 1986; **34**: 247.

78. Gersh, B.J., Fisher, L.D., Schaff, H.V. *et al.* Issues concerning the clinical evaluation of new prosthetic valves. *J. Thorac. Cardiovasc. Surg.* 1986; **91**: 460.

79. Bloomfield, P., Kitchin, A.H., Wheatley, D.J., Walbaum, P.R., Lutz, W. and Miller, H.C. A prospective evaluation of the Bjork–Shiley, Hancock, and Carpentier–Edwards heart valve prostheses. *Circulation* 1986; **73**: 1213.

80. Stein, P.D., Collins Jr, J.J. and Kantrowitz, A. Antithrombotic therapy in mechanical and biological prosthetic heart valves and saphenous vein bypass grafts. *Chest*

1986; **89**: 46S.

81. Edmunds Jr, L.H. Thromboembolic complications for current cardiac valvular prostheses. *Ann. Thorac. Surg.* 1982; **34**: 96.

82. Baudet, E.M., Oca, C.C., Roques, X.F. *et al.* A 5½ year experience with the St Jude Medical cardiac valve prosthesis. Early and late results of 737 valve replacements in 671 patients. *J. Thorac. Cardiovasc. Surg.* 1985; **90**: 137.

83. Brott, W.H., Zajtchuk, R., Bowen, T.E., Davia, J. and Green, D.C. Dipyridamole-aspirin as thromboembolic prophylaxis in patients with aortic valve prostheses. Prospective study with the Model 2320 Starr–Edwards prosthesis. *J. Thorac. Cardiovasc. Surg.* 1981; **81**: 632.

84. Moggio, R.A., Hammond, G.L., Stansel Jr, H.C. and Glenn, W.W.L. Incidence of emboli with cloth-covered Starr–Edwards valve without anticoagulation and with varying forms of anticoagulation. Analysis of 183 patients followed for 3½ years. *J. Thorac. Cardiovasc. Surg.* 1978; **75**: 296.

85. Ribeiro, P.A., Zaibag, M.A., Idris, M. *et al.* Antiplatelet drugs and the incidence of thromboembolic complications of the St Jude Medical aortic prosthesis in patients with rheumatic heart disease. *J. Thorac. Cardiovasc. Surg.* 1986; **91**: 92.

86. Bradley, L.M., Midgley, F.M., Watson, D.C., Getson, P.R. and Scott, III L.P. Anticoagulation therapy in children with mechanical prosthetic cardiac valves. *Am. J. Cardiol.* 1985; **56**: 533.

87. Gallo, I., Nistal, F. and Artinano, E. Six- to ten-year follow-up of patients with the Hancock cardiac bioprosthesis. Incidence of primary tissue failure. *J. Thorac. Cardiovasc. Surg.* 1986; **92**: 14.

88. Bolooki, H., Mallon, S., Kaiser, G.A., Thurer, R.J. and Kieval, J. Failure of Hancock xenograft valve: Importance of valve position (4- to 9-year follow-up). *Ann. Thorac. Surg.* 1983; **36**: 246.

89. Cohn, L.H., Allred, E.N., Cohn, L.A. *et al.* Early and late risk of mitral valve replacement. A 12 year concomitant comparison of the porcine bioprosthetic and prosthetic disc mitral valves. *J. Thorac. Cardiovasc. Surg.* 1985; **90**: 872.

90. Cohn, L.H., Allred, E.N., DiSesa, V.J., Sawtelle, K., Shemin, R.J. and Collins Jr, J.J. Early and late risk of aortic valve replacement. A 12 year concomitant comparison of the porcine bioprosthetic and tilting disc prosthetic aortic valves. *J. Thorac. Cardiovasc. Surg.* 1984; **88**: 695.

91. Antunes, M.J. and Santos, L.P. Performance of glutaraldehyde-preserved porcine bioprosthesis as a mitral valve substitute in a young population group. *Ann. Thorac. Surg.* 1984; **37**: 387.

92. Pupello, D.F. Bessone, L.N., Blank, R.H., Lopez-Cuenca, E., Hiro, S.P. and Ebra, G. The porcine bioprosthesis: Patient age as a factor in predicting failure. In: Bodnar E. and Yacoub M., eds. *Biologic and bioprosthetic valves.* New York: Yorke Medical Books, 1986, p.130.

93. Walley, V.M. and Keon, W.J. Patterns of failure in Ionescu–Shiley bovine pericardial bioprosthetic valves. *J. Thorac. Cardiovasc. Surg.* 1987; **93**: 925.

94. Wheatley, D.J., Fisher, J., Reece, I.J., Spyt, T. and Breeze, P. Primary tissue failure in pericardial heart valves. *J. Thorac. Cardiovasc. Surg.* 1987; **94**: 367.

95. Odell, J.A., Gillmer, D., Whitton, I.D., Vythilingum, S.P. and Vanker, E.A. Calcification of tissue valves in children: Occurrence in porcine and bovine pericardial bioprosthetic valves. In: Bodnar E. and Yacoub M., eds. *Biologic and bioprosthetic valves.* New York: Yorke Medical Books, 1986, p.259.

96. Ionescu, I.M. Long-term durability of the pericardial valve. *Z. Kardiol.* 1986; **75** (Suppl. 2): 207.

97. Cooley, D.A., Ott, D.A., Reul Jr, J., Duncan, J.M. Frazier,

O.H. and Livesay, J.J. Ionescu–Shiley bovine pericardial bioprostheses: clinical results in 2,701 patients. In: Bodnar, E. and Yacoub, M., eds. *Biologic and bioprosthetic valves.* New York: Yorke Medical Books, 1986, p.177.

98. Gonzalez-Lavin, L., Tandon, A.P., Chi, S. *et al.* The risk of thromboembolism and hemorrhage following mitral valve replacement. A comparative analysis between the porcine xenograft valve and Ionescu–Shiley bovine pericardial valve. *J. Thorac. Cardiovasc. Surg.* 1984; **87**: 340.

99. Calderwood, S.B., Swinski, L.A., Waternaux, C.M., Karchmer, A.W. and Buckley, M.J. Risk factors for the development of prosthetic valve endocarditis. *Circulation* 1985; **72**: 31.

100. Baumgartner, W.A., Miller D.C. Reitz, B.A. *et al.* Surgical treatment of prosthetic valve endocarditis. *Ann. Thorac. Surg.* 1983; **35**: 87.

101. Cowgill, L.D., Addonizio, V.P., Hopeman, A.R. and Harken, A.H. A practical approach to prosthetic valve endocarditis. *Ann. Thorac. Surg.* 1987, **43**: 450.

102. Sweeney, M.S., Reul, G.J., Cooley, D.A. *et al.* Comparison of prosthetic and mechanical valve replacement for active endocarditis. *J. Thorac. Cardiovasc. Surg.* 1985; **90**: 676.

103. Sethia, B., Turner, M.A., Lewis, S. *et al.* Fourteen years' experience with the Bjork–Shiley tilting disc prosthesis. *J. Thorac. Cardiovasc. Surg.* 1986; **91**: 350.

104. Khalil, Y., Sethia, B., Quin, R.O. and Bain, W.H. Disc and strut embolisation after minor strut fracture in a Bjork–Shiley mitral valve prosthesis. *Thorax* 1985; **40**: 158.

105. Boskovic, D., Elezovic, I., Boskovia, D., Simin, N., Rolovic, Z. and Josipovic, V. Late thrombosis of the Bjork–Shiley tilting disc valve in the tricuspid position. Thrombolytic treatment with streptokinase. *J. Thorac. Cardiovasc. Surg.* 1986; **91**: 1.

106. Ryder, S.J., Bradley, H., Brannan, J.J., Turner, M.A. and Bain, W.H. Thrombotic obstruction of the Bjork–Shiley valve: the Glasgow experience. *Thorax* 1984; **39**: 487.

107. Prabhu, S., Friday, K.J., Reynolds, D., Elkins, R. and Lazzara, R. Thrombosis of aortic St Jude valve. *Ann. Thorac. Surg.* 1986; **41**: 332.

108. Wright, J.O., Hiratzka, L.F., Brandt, B. and Doty, D.B. Thrombosis of the Bjork–Shiley prosthesis. Illustrative cases and review of the literature. *J. Thorac. Cardiovasc. Surg.* 1982; **84**: 138.

109. Arom, K.V., Nicoloff, D.M., Kersten, T.E., Lindsay, W.G. and Northrup, W.F. St Jude Medical prosthesis: valve-related deaths and complications. *Ann. Thorac. Surg.* 1987; **43**: 591.

110. Venugopal, P., Kaul, U., Iyer, K.S. *et al.* Fate of thrombectomized Bjork–Shiley valves. A long-term cinefluoroscopic, echocardiographic, and hemodynamic evaluation. *J. Thorac. Cardiovasc. Surg.* 1986; **91**: 168.

111. McGoon, D.C. The risk of thromboembolism following valvular operations: how does one know? (Editorial). *J. Thorac. Cardiovasc. Surg.* 1984; **88**: 782.

112. Blackstone, E.H. and Kirklin, J.W. Death and other time-related events after valve replacement. *Circulation* 1985; **72**: 753.

113. Khayat, M.C., Piard, J., Zerr, C. and Khayat, A. Hemolysis following cardiac valve replacement. In: Horstkotte, D. and Loogen, F., eds. *Update in Heart Valve Replacement.* New York: Springer–Verlag, 1986, p.97.

114. Christakis, G.T., Weisel, R.D., Fremes, S.E. *et al.* Can the results of contemporary aortic valve replacement be improved? *J. Thorac. Cardiovasc. Surg.* 1986; **92**: 37.

115. Ferrazzi, P., McGiffin, D.C., Kirklin, J.W. *et al.* Have the results of mitral valve replacement improved? *J. Thorac. Cardiovasc. Surg.* 1986; **92**: 186.

116. Takaro, T., Ankeney, J.L. Laning, R.C. and Peduzzi, P.N. Quality control for cardiac surgery in the Veterans Administration. *Ann. Thorac. Surg.* 1986; **42**: 37.

117. Lytle, B.W., Cosgrove, D.M. and Gill, C.G. Mitral valve replacement combined with myocardial revascularisation: early and late results for 300 patients, 1970 to 1983. *Circulation* 1985; 71: 1179.

118. *Returns of the UK Cardiac Surgical Register, 1980–1984.* London: The Society of Thoracic and Cardiovascular Surgeons.

119. Commerford, P.J., Hastie, T. and Beck, W. Closed mitral valvotomy: actuarial analysis of results in 654 patients over 12 years and analysis of pre-operative predictors of long-term survival. *Ann. Thorac. Surg.* 1982; 33: 473.

120. Lower, R.R. and Ducey, K.F. Open mitral valvotomy. In: Ionescu, M.I. and Cohn, L.H., eds. *Mitral valve disease. Diagnosis and Treatment.* London: Butterworths, 1985, p.153.

121. Nakano, S., Kawashima, Y., Hirose, H. *et al.* Long-term results of open mitral commissurotomy for mitral stenosis with severe subvalvular changes: A 10 year evaluation. *Ann. Thorac. Surg.* 1984; 37: 159.

122. Eguaras, M.G., Montero, A., Moriones, I. *et al.* Conservative operation for mitral stenosis with densely fibrosed or partially calcified valves. An eight year evaluation. *J. Thorac. Cardiovasc. Surg.* 1987; 93: 898.

123. Murphy, J.P., Sweeney, M.S. and Cooley, D.A. The Puig–Massana–Shiley annuloplasty ring for mitral valve repair: Experience in 126 patients. *Ann. Thorac. Surg.* 1987; 43: 52.

124. Christakis, G.T., Kormos, R.L. Weisel, R.D. *et al.* Morbidity and mortality in mitral valve surgery. *Circulation* 1985; 72 (Suppl. II): II–120.

125. Scott, W.C., Miller, D.C., Haverich, A. *et al.* Operative risk of mitral valve replacement: discriminant analysis of 1329 procedures. *Circulation* 1985; 72 (Suppl. II): II–108.

126. Sethi, G.K., Miller, D.C., Soutchek, J. *et al.* Clinical, haemodynamic, and angiographic predictors of operative mortality in patients undergoing single valve replacement. *J. Thorac. Cardiovasc. Surg.* 1987; 93: 884.

127. Hochberg, M.S., Derkac, W.M., Conkle, D.M., McIntosh, C.L., Epstein, S.E. and Morrow, A.G. Mitral valve replacement in elderly patients: Encouraging postoperative clinical and hemodynamic results. *J. Thorac. Cardiovasc. Surg.* 1977; 77: 422.

128. Murphy, D.A., Levine, F.H., Buckley, M.J. *et al.* Mechanical valves: A comparative analysis of the Starr–Edwards and Bjork–Shiley prostheses. *J. Thorac. Cardiovasc. Surg.* 1983; 86: 746.

129. Hartz, R.S., Fisher, E.B., Finkelmeier, B. *et al.* An eight-year experience with porcine bioprosthetic cardiac valves. *J. Thorac. Cardiovasc. Surg.* 1986; 91: 910.

130. Turina, J., Turina, M., Rothlin, M. and Krayenbuehl, H.P. Improved late survival in patients with chronic aortic regurgitation by earlier operation. *Circulation* 1984; 70 (Suppl. I): I–147.

131. Scott, W.C., Miller, D.C., Haverich, A. *et al.* Determinants of operative mortality for patients undergoing aortic valve replacement. Discriminant analysis of 1,479 operations. *J. Thorac. Cardiovasc. Surg.* 1985; 89: 400.

132. Arom, K.V., Nicoloff, D.M., Lindsay, W.G., Northrup, W.F. and Kersten, T.E. Should valve replacement and related procedures be performed in elderly patients? *Ann Thorac. Surg.* 1984; 38: 466.

133. Daenen, W., Nevelsteen, A., van Cauwelaert, P., de Maesschalk, E., Willems, J. and Stalpaert, G. Nine years' experience with the Bjork–Shiley prosthetic valve. Early and late results of 932 valve replacements. *Ann. Thorac. Surg.* 1983; 35: 651.

134. Teoh, K.H., Christakis, G.T., Weisel, R.D. *et al.* The determinants of mortality and morbidity after multiple-valve operations. *Ann. Thorac. Surg.* 1987; 43: 353.

135. Kara, M., Langlet, F., Blin, D. *et al.* Triple valve procedures: An analysis of early and late results. *Thorac. Cardiovasc. Surg.* 1986; 34: 17.

136. Gersh, B.J., Schaff, H.V., Vatterott, P.J. *et al.* Results of triple valve replacement in 91 patients: perioperative mortality and long-term follow-up. *Circulation* 1985; 72: 130.

137. Lytle, B.W., Cosgrove, D.M., Loop, F.D. *et al.* Replacement of aortic valve combined with myocardial revascularisation: determinants of early and late risk for 500 patients. *Circulation* 1983; 68: 1149

138. Lytle, B.W., Cosgrove, D.M., Taylor, P.C. *et al.* Reoperations for valve surgery: Perioperative mortality and determinants of risk for 1,000 patients, 1958–1984. *Ann. Thorac. Surg.* 1986; 42: 632.

139. Wideman, F.E., Blackstone, E.H., Kirklin, J.W., Karp, R.B., Kouchoukos, N.T. and Pacifico, A.D. Hospital mortality of re-replacement of the aortic valve. Incremental risk factors. *J. Thorac. Cardiovasc. Surg.* 1981; 82: 692.

140. Carpentier, A., Chauvaud, S., Fabiani, J.N. *et al.* Reconstructive surgery of mitral valve incompetence. Ten-year appraisal. *J. Thorac. Cardiovasc. Surg.* 1980; 79: 338.

Chapter 36

Myocarditis

W.A. Littler

Myocarditis is the presence of inflammatory foci in the myocardium. An internationally accepted histological definition is that

> "myocarditis is characterised by an inflammatory infiltrate and by injury to adjacent myocardial cells that is not typical of infarction".[1]

The clinical consequences of myocarditis are governed by the degree and extent of myocardial damage. That myocarditis may occur without being detected has been demonstrated in several ways. Evidence of myocarditis has been found in autopsy studies of a large number of patients in whom it could not have been suspected clinically.[2] Histological evidence of myocarditis has also been found in a surprisingly high proportion (5%) of apparently healthy young adults dying in air crash and road traffic accidents.[3] Electrocardiographic evidence of myocarditis has been seen in almost 50% of patients with mild influenza and has also been reported in patients without cardiac symptoms or signs during *Mycoplasma* and echovirus infections.[4] Viruses have been detected unexpectedly in myocardial biopsies either by culture or by electron microscopy.

The overt clinical picture of myocarditis includes fever, pericardial chest pain and 'flu-like' symptoms, such as headache, sore throat, malaise, generalized aches, vomiting and diarrhoea. Physical examination may reveal lymphadenopathy, arrhythmias, cardiomegaly, a pericardial friction rub, pulmonary oedema or congestive heart failure. Sudden death is not uncommon in such patients.[5]

As the symptoms and signs are non-specific, a diagnosis of myocarditis involves a high index of suspicion and clinical awareness. Laboratory tests may demonstrate a raised erythrocyte sedimentation rate, leucocytosis and raised levels of cardiac enzymes.

The electrocardiogram is often abnormal but not specific; atrioventricular block, including complete heart block, bundle branch block, atrial fibrillation, both atrial and ventricular premature contractions and ventricular tachycardia are all seen. Abnormal Q waves, ST-segment elevation and T-wave inversion may simulate the changes of myocardial infarction. The chest radiograph shows cardiomegaly involving all chambers in the majority of cases. Echocardiography may reveal chamber dilatation and ventricular dysfunction including segmental wall motion abnormalities whilst a pericardial effusion is common. Radionuclide studies confirm poor cardiac function and may sometimes reveal segmental wall motion abnormalities. Gallium-67 has been shown to be an 'inflammation avid' isotope which may be taken up by the myocardium in cases of myocarditis.

Haemodynamic studies and angiography demonstrate a non-specific picture of heart failure. Autopsy may reveal a flabby heart with all four chambers dilated and sometimes hypertrophied. The myocardium may show patchy discolouration and haemorrhagic areas. Histological changes will depend upon the duration of the condition and sometimes on the specific cause of the myocarditis. Acute phase changes may include a monocytic infiltration with necrosis and myocytic degeneration whilst chronic fibrosis and hypertrophy may be discerned.

VIRAL MYOCARDITIS

Almost all viral infections have been shown to involve the heart but enterovirus, particularly Coxsackie B viruses, are considered to account for most causes of acute cardiac disease.[6] The majority of patients with acute viral myocarditis recover completely, a few die suddenly and some progress to a more chronic form of myocardial disease. Subclinical myocarditis may be of more importance than a brisk overt infection in the development of long-term sequelae. Viruses are seldom demonstrated in the myocardium, either by electron microscopy or immunofluorescence. Serological tests may demonstrate increased levels of virus titres. Molecular genetic techniques have shown that the DNA of some viruses is present in heart muscle cells.

The clinical diagnosis of myocarditis is suggested by preceding viral illness, electrocardiographic changes, changes in heart size on the chest radiograph and in conjunction with a rise in viral titres.[7] Histological confirmation of myocarditis may be provided by endomyocardial biopsy. Olsen has suggested that three phases may be seen, depending on the stage of the illness when the biopsy is obtained.[8]

1   Acute (active) phase. The chief histological features include widening of the interstitium with inflammatory cells and intimate contact with adjacent myocardium fibres which show extensive fraying (Fig. 36.1).
2   Healing (resolving) phase. The inflammatory cells are no longer in intimate contact with adjacent myocardial fibres which now have smooth contours.
3   Healed (resolved) phase. There is an increase in interstitial fibrous tissue with few inflammatory cells (Fig. 36.2).

There are undoubtedly problems in making a diagnosis of myocarditis by endomyocardial biopsy. These have been clearly presented by Billingham.[9] She considers that such a diagnosis should be made conservatively by the pathologist, particularly because of the influence of clinical bias. Mistakes occur because pathologists fail to recognize the number of lymphocytes that occur in the interstitium of normal myocardium. Although non-inflammatory interstitial cells may be misinterpreted as lymphocytes, qualitative evidence of interstitial leucocyte infiltration should be sought, a lymphocyte count of > 5 per high power field has been suggested as of diagnostic significance.

VIRAL MYOCARDITIS AND DILATED CARDIOMYOPATHY

It is debatable whether hearts from patients with persisting disease following viral myocarditis can be distinguished pathologically from those from patients with congestive cardiomyopathy. Some claim to be able to make this distinction but this may depend on the stage at which the heart is examined. At least in chronic Chagasic heart disease microscopic features may be indistinguishable from those of congestive cardiomyopathy.

The hypothesis that myocarditis may lead to congestive cardiomyopathy has been tested in other ways. Patients with congestive cardiomyopathy have been studied for evidence of past infection, and long-term sequelae of viral myocarditis in animals have been sought.[10] Similar work has suggested that viral and chlamydial infections may cause acquired valvular heart disease. High antibody titres to Coxsackie B virus have been found in a greater proportion of patients with congestive cardiomyopathy than in controlled populations. Antibodies to echo- and herpesviruses were also more common but not significantly so. Antibodies to *Chlamydia psittaci* have been found in patients with primary myocardial disease but a miscellany of disorders were studied and most of the patients had heart disease prior to developing antibodies. Positive *Treponema*

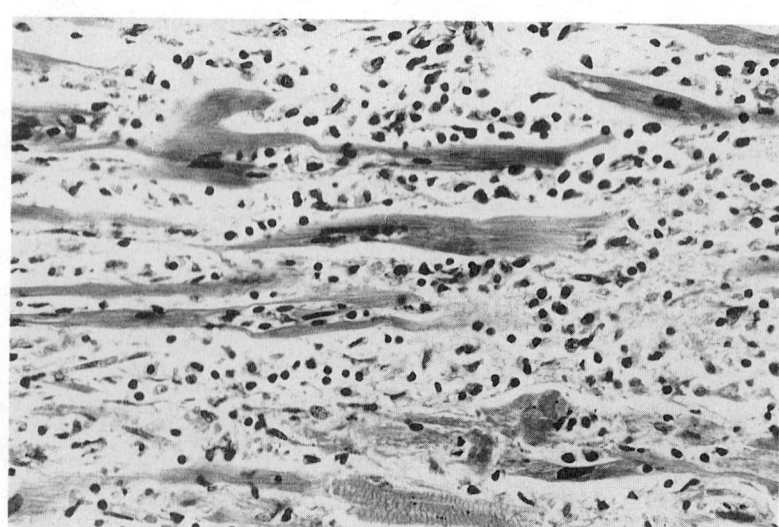

Fig. 36.1. Histology of viral myocarditis: mononuclear cellular infiltrate with myocardial damage. (H&E stain.)

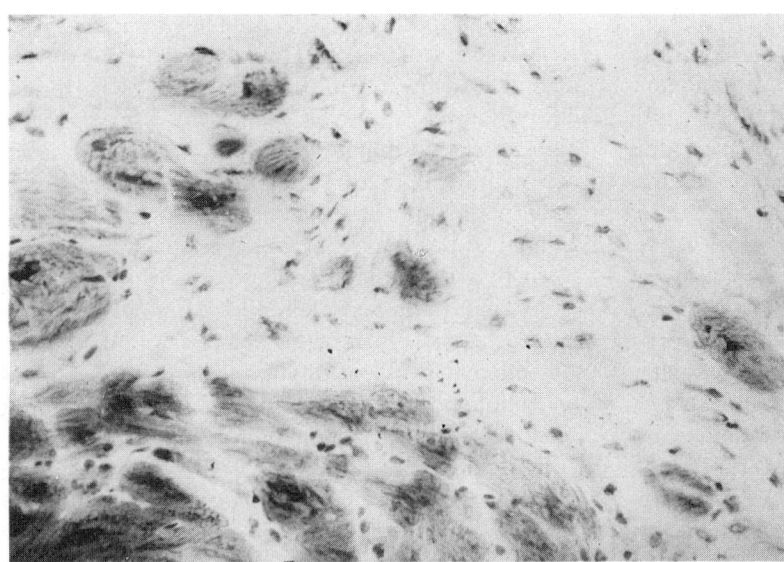

Fig. 36.2. Histological section showing fibrous scarring following virus myocarditis. (H&E stain.)

serology has been found in Jamaican patients with cardiomegaly of unknown origin.[11] Similar patients in Cameroon have exhibited antibodies to *Trypanosoma* antigens.[12] However, the control groups in both studies were not strictly comparable.

Cambridge *et al.* reported that 50 patients with congestive cardiomyopathy exhibited neutralizing antibody to Coxsackie B virus to a titre of 1024 or more.[13] Only one of 50 control subjects who had other cardiac disorders exhibited a similar titre. A fourfold rise in titre was rarely seen, but titres of 512 or more are considered to be strongly suggestive of recent infection and tend to remain raised for many months. High titres were most often found in patients who have been ill for < 1 year. In those with symptoms of < 6 months' duration, a high titre was more commonly found if there was an initial febrile illness. The relationship of high titre to a short history may explain the lack of evidence of Coxsackie virus. Endomyocardial biopsies were taken from 18 patients in the series of Cambridge and co-workers including 3 of the 5 with symptoms of < 6 months' duration and an initial febrile illness. No histological evidence of myocarditis and no viral particles were seen. Viral cultures taken from 12 of the 18 biopsies were negative. Viral antigens were also not detected in myocardial biopsies of 20 patients with dilated cardiomyopathy studied by Kawai. The results of these studies suggest, therefore, that congestive cardiomyopathy follows viral myocarditis but is not due to the continued presence of virus within the myocardium.

Cellular immunity in congestive cardiomyopathy

Antibodies and cell-mediated immunity are important protective mechanisms against infection.[14] When these mechanisms themselves are responsible for tissue damage and destruction, this is known as hypersensitivity. Cell-mediated (or delayed) hypersensitivity usually involves T-lymphocytes and non-specific inflammatory cells.

Abnormalities of cellular immunity are known to occur in heart diseases. In rheumatic fever, marked cellular hypersensitivity has been demonstrated to streptococcal cell membranes, specifically to group A streptococci, which persists for as long as 5 years after the acute attack; patients with streptococcal sore throats do not demonstrate this reactivity.[15] In Chagas' disease (which presents a similar clinical picture to that of congestive cardiomyopathy in its chronic stage) cytotoxic T-lymphocytes are directed to both the parasite, *Trypanosoma cruzi*, and the heart muscle cells.[16] Cellular hypersensitivity has also been demonstrated in ischaemic heart disease. It is not known whether these abnormalities are the result or cause of myocardial damage in these conditions.

It has been suggested that in congestive cardiomyopathy the normal cell-mediated immune process may be deficient and allow virus damage to occur that would not have occurred otherwise (as in subacute sclerosing panencephalitis). In studies by Das and his colleagues, 28 and 42% of patients with congestive cardiomyopathy had abnormal cell-mediated responses compared with < 11% of normal control subjects; however, the mean values for each patient group studied showed that patients with other heart diseases had impaired cell-mediated responses and the mean values were not significantly different from those in the patients with congestive cardiomyopathy.[17] Similarly, in tests conducted by the same authors who were seeking prior cellular sensitization to human heart antigen, up to 25% of patients with congestive cardiomyopathy had results suggesting such previous sensitization but up to 52% of patients with ischaemic heart disease showed a similar result.[18] These findings suggest that the abnormalities of cellular immunity found in congestive cardiomyopathy are not specific but may be secondary to cardiac damage rather than primarily involved in pathogenesis.

To date, the work on cellular immunity has failed to demonstrate a uniform abnormality in congestive cardiomyopathy which might be implicated in aetiology. Subgroups of patients have shown abnormalities, but results are conflicting and may reflect secondary immunological abnormalities occurring as a result, rather than a cause, of congestive cardiomyopathy. These results may be further confounded by lack of 'blindness', repeated observations and several observers in the experimental procedures employed.

ENDOMYOCARDIAL BIOPSY

Percutaneous transvascular catheter biopsy techniques are now firmly established as a diagnostic investigation in patients with suspected heart muscle disease.[19,20]

The cardiac bioptome was originally developed and pioneered in Japan in the early 1960s by Sakakibara and Konno;[21] Richardson later adapted endoscopic forceps for intracardiac use, producing the King's bioptome.[22] The development of cardiac transplantation led to the modification of the Japanese bioptome to a shorter and more flexible instrument (the Caves–Schultz instrument) for use in the jugular vein/right ventricle to detect the early morphological changes associated with rejection.[23]

Cardiac biopsy is a simple technique. The bioptome is introduced percutaneously via a femoral vein or internal jugular vein for right ventricular biopsy or via a femoral artery for the left ventricle. Cardiac biopsy specimens are usually obtained from the right ventricular septum or the inferior surface of the left ventricle. There are few satisfactory

studies comparing the potential advantages of right versus left ventricular biopsy and no clear advantage is evident. Obviously, it is better to perform a biopsy on the ventricle in which the disease process appears predominantly, but ultimately the choice lies with the operator. Cardiac biopsy is a relatively safe procedure in experienced hands. Reported complications have included cardiac perforation with or without tamponade, pericarditis, arrhythmias and pulmonary emboli. Although multiple biopsy samples may be obtained, sampling error is an inherent problem of the technique and normal morphological appearances of the biopsy cannot exclude disease elsewhere in the myocardium therefore caution should be exercised in interpretation. Biopsy specimens may be subjected to a variety of analyses, including histology, histochemistry, immunology and viral culture.[24]

The indications for biopsy and the diagnostic yields that can be expected are controversial despite its increasing popularity. The two firmly established indications for its performance are to assess rejection of the transplanted heart and to assess anthracycline (usually Adriamycin) induced cardiomyopathy. Cardiac biopsy has been used in an attempt to define the nature of cardiomyopathy; diagnostic usefulness has ranged from 10 to 75%. As dilated cardiomyopathy does not have sufficient characteristic histological features to warrant a precise pathological diagnosis, it remains in effect a diagnosis of exclusion. To determine the prognosis of patients with dilated cardiomyopathy, a points system was devised whereby the degenerative changes found in the biopsy specimens were evaluated. Although there was a trend for groups of patients with more severe degenerative changes to have a poorer prognosis, the prognosis for any individual patient was impossible to assess.[25]

Difficulties in diagnosing myocarditis clinically are well recognized but the use of cardiac biopsy has enabled a diagnosis of myocarditis to be based on histological examination.[26] The timing of the biopsy following a viral illness has been shown to influence the ability to detect myocardial information. Billingham has demonstrated the difficulties in diagnosing acute myocarditis, particularly for the unwary and inexperienced pathologist, difficulties that, in her opinion, have lead to the over-diagnosis of the disease. The Dallas Myocarditis Panel set forth useful criteria and guidelines in an attempt to classify the morphological diagnosis of myocarditis. Their definition of myocarditis follows:

"Myocarditis is characterized by an inflammatory infiltrate and by injury to adjacent myocytes that is not characteristic of acute infarction. Primary forms of myocarditis are idiopathic, whereas secondary forms have an identifiable cause."

The diagnostic categories of myocarditis are given in Table 36.1.

Morphological examination of biopsies from some patients clinically suspected of having dilated cardiomyopathy has revealed the presence of myocarditis. The significance of these findings has caused considerable argument. The morphological diagnosis of myocarditis is difficult to make; the presence of inflammatory cells within the myocardium is not sufficient of itself to sustain the diagnosis. The question of when to designate a patient's biopsy 'healed myocarditis' or dilated cardiomyopathy can be difficult and there is overlap between these two conditions. Billingham has demonstrated that hearts removed at transplantation from patients with end-stage cardiomyopathy have a significant cellular infiltrate, varying between 3 and 30 foci. On biopsy, an inflammatory infiltrate in the absence of hypertrophy or interstitial fibrosis does not cause a problem in diagnosing myocarditis but co-existent hypertrophy does.

TREATMENT OF VIRAL MYOCARDITIS

General measures

It is probably wise to admit patients suspected of having myocarditis to hospital. Experimental studies suggest restricting the activities of patients, preferably with complete bed rest. Specific complications such as arrhythmias, heart block or heart failure should be treated with the appropriate conventional therapy. Anticoagulants should be considered in view of the increased risk of intracardiac thrombus and potential emboli. The use of a specific antiviral treatment has not yet been evaluated.

Immunosuppressive therapy

Although controversial, the evidence that auto-immune mechanisms may be implicated in the production of myocardial necrosis after viral infections has suggested a role for immunosuppressive drugs in the treatment of myocarditis. In several small series of cases of myocarditis, the patients have responded to steroids and azathioprine, showing not only clinical and haemodynamic improvement but histological evidence of healing as detected on serial cardiac biopsy specimens.[27,28] Although these results are encouraging, such studies have been open, uncontrolled and have examined only small numbers of patients to be accepted without further validation. Furthermore, they have been conducted against the background of the natural history of viral myocarditis which is that the majority of patients get better anyway. It should also be borne in mind that the results of animal studies indicate immunosuppressive therapy might be detrimental in the acute stage.[29]

Owing to the potential adverse effects of immunosuppressive therapy, Billingham recommends that a cardiac biopsy should be performed to confirm the diagnosis of myocarditis.[26] However, as only about one-third of clinically suspected cases

---

Table 36.1. Inflammatory myocarditis.

Bacterial
Diphtheria
Brucellosis
Clostridia
Infective endocarditis
Meningococcus
Salmonella
Streptococci
Tuberculosis
Typhoid

Fungal
Actinomycosis
Aspergillosis
Blastomycosis
Candidiasis
Coccidioidomycosis
Cryptococcosis
Histoplasmosis

Spirochaetal
Leptospirosis
Relapsing fever
Syphilis

Protozoal
Trypanosomiasis (Chagas' disease)
African trypanosomiases
Toxoplasmosis
Malaria

Metazoal
Cysticercosis
Echinococcosis (hyatid disease)
Schistosomiasis
Trichinosis

Rickettsial
Typhus: Scrub
        Rocky Mountain spotted fever
Q fever

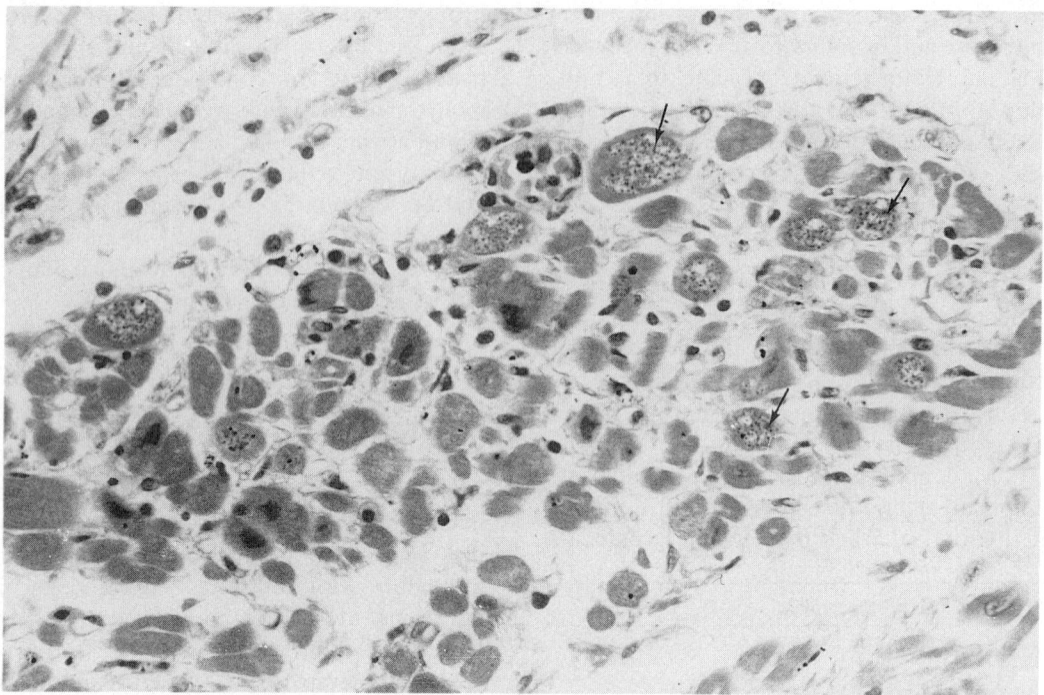

Fig. 36.3. Chagas' disease. Myocardial fibres are cut in transverse sections and many of them contain parasites (seen as black dots which are arrowed). (Courtesy Dr C.E. Edwards.)

show the appropriate morphological changes the decision is not necessarily made any easier. Until controlled studies are conducted in which a clear benefit to patients treated with immunosuppressive therapy can be demonstrated, it would be wise to exercise caution in the use of these drugs. Cardiac transplantation offers the most realistic hope of saving patients who have uncontrollable myocarditis.

INFLAMMATORY MYOCARDITIS

In inflammatory myocarditis, almost all micro-organisms appear to be capable of producing myocardial damage, either by direct invasion of the myocardium, through the production of toxins, or by vascular occlusion.[30] Infectious myocarditis (Table 36.1) is, with a few exceptions, a relatively uncommon problem in the UK, although there is much geographical variation on a global scale. Symptoms are often few and death rarely occurs in the acute illness; evidence of myocarditis usually appears in the convalescent phase of the disease.

INFECTIVE MYOCARDITIS

Bacterial myocarditis may result from either the

presence of organisms in the myocardium or from toxin production. In general cardiac symptoms are not a major part of the illness, but when cardiac involvement occurs it can produce serious morbidity and mortality. Most of the infections will cause changes on the electrocardiogram ranging from ST–T wave changes, conduction abnormalities to atrial and ventricular arrhythmias, which may account for sudden death in these patients. Pericarditis with or without an effusion may often accompany myocardial involvement. Diphtheria is rarely seen in the UK these days.[31] Cardiac involvement occurs in up to 25% of cases as a result of exotoxin production. The toxin results in fatty degeneration of myocytes with myolysis and interstitial inflammation. Cardiac involvement is the commonest cause of death which can result from acute circulatory collapse in the early stages or heart failure and conduction problems later.

Chagas' disease (Fig. 36.3) is the commonest cause of chronic heart disease in Central and South America.[32] *Trypanosoma cruzi* is transmitted to man in the faeces of an insect vector (triatomes) during blood feeding. The disease is traditionally divided into an acute and a chronic phase which are separated by a period of time averaging 20 years. The acute illness includes symptoms and signs of generalized infection whereas signs of myocarditis include cardiomegaly, heart failure and electro-cardiographic abnormalities. Pericardial effusions and intracardiac thrombus may be demonstrated by echocardiography during this phase.

The most common clinical signs of human chronic Chagas' disease are cardiomegaly, cardiac failure, conduction disturbances and characteristic findings in the electrocardiogram of right bundle branch block, left anterior hemi-block, premature ventricular contractions and T-wave inversion. The clinical picture resembles closely that of dilated cardiomyopathy. Syncope and sudden death are not infrequent.

Involvement of the hollow viscera such as the oesophagus and colon may accompany cardiac involvement. In this disease, degeneration of intramural ganglia and lesions of the cardiac nerves are the outstanding pathological features. Experimental evidence provides support for the notion that mammalian cells might share common antigens with T. cruzi and so an anti-parasite response could give rise to an auto-immune reaction involving uninfected host cells. It has been suggested that T. cruzi antigens can bind to mammalian cell surfaces thereby rendering them potential targets for the host's immune response to the parasite.

Toxoplasmosis is caused by an intracellular protozoan Toxoplasma gondii. In the UK, the dog is the most likely source of this infection, which most commonly produces eye and brain damage. Cardiac involvement is uncommon and may be found in the immune-compromised patient.[33] Myocarditis and pericarditis may both occur, giving rise to arrhythmias and atrioventricular conduction abnormalities, and occasionally heart failure. Most commonly, the only manifestation of the condition is an abnormality in the electrocardiogram, particularly of the ST segment and T waves.

Fungal infections of the myocardium usually occur in those patients who have serious predisposing disease, such as malignancy or a compromised immune system.[34] Often, the infection is spread directly from the thorax or mediastinum and first involves the pericardium further spreading to the myocardium producing caseous necrosis. Arrhythmias and T-wave changes are often the only sign of involvement.

Hydatid disease is caused by Echinococcus granulosus and the heart is involved in between 0.5 and 2% and of echinococcal disease. Humans act as an intermediate host and myocardial problems occur as a result of cyst formation, usually in the left ventricle. Cardiac involvement is usually solitary without other viscera being involved; in the absence of complications, no symptoms occur. Symptoms are often the result of the local effect of large cardiac cysts and include ventricular premature contractions, arrhythmias and conduction abnormalities. Rupture of the cysts may produce chest pain, pericarditis or sudden death due to anaphylactic shock.

Treatment of patients with infective myocarditis will include general measures applied to any infection, such as palliation of fever, myalgia and arthralgia. Specific antibiotic therapy must be given for the particular infection; complications such as heart failure, arrhythmias and heart block are treated in the appropriate manner.

TOXIC MYOCARDITIS

In toxic myocarditis, drugs, chemicals, physical agents, animal and insect toxins may all produce changes in the myocardium which are best described as myocarditis (Table 36.2).

Drug-induced toxic myocardial changes are becoming an increasing problem; such changes may produce either a toxic or a hypersensitivity reaction. Billingham has written an excellent review of this problem and demonstrated how drug-induced myocarditis and hypersensitivity can be distinguished morphologically.[35]

The clinical manifestations of toxic myocarditis have many features in common. Electrocardiographic abnormalities are by far the commonest manifestation of the condition and include T-wave inversion, ST-segment shifts, QT-interval prolongation, arrhythmias and conduction disturbances. Sudden death may sometimes occur, presumably on the basis of an arrhythmia.

Many of these agents are myocardial depressants and may produce hypotension, heart failure or circulatory collapse which in the case of hypersensitivity reactions may be sudden.

IDIOPATHIC MYOCARDITIS

Many cases of a similar nature have been reported as idiopathic myocarditis, giant cell myocarditis or Fiedler's myocarditis.[36] The condition(s) is of unknown aetiology; the myocardium contains inflammatory cells consisting of lymphocytes, plasma cells and macrophages but the characteristic cells are multinucleated giant cells. The condition usually

Table 36.2. Toxic myocardial diseases.

Drugs associated with toxic myocarditis

Arsenicals
Amphetamines
Antihypertensive agents
Anthracyclines
Barbiturates
Catecholamines
Cyclophosphamide
Emetine
Fluorouracil
Histamine-like drugs
Lithium
Paraquat
Phenothiazines
Quinidine
Theophylline

Drugs associated with hypersensitivity myocarditis

Horse serum
Isoniazid
Methyldopa
Penicillin
Phenindione
Phenylbutazone
Streptomycin
Sulphonamides
Tetanus toxoid
Tetracyclines
Thiazide diuretics

Other causative agents

Carbon monoxide
Fluorinated hydrocarbons (aerosol propellants)
Scorpion stings
Wasp and spider stings
Snake bites
Radiation (therapeutic)
Heat stroke
Hypothermia

has a rapid onset with fever, chest pain, dyspnoea and hypotension, often deteriorating to heart failure and death. The ventricles are usually found to be dilated with intracardiac thrombus and widespread necrotic areas.

REFERENCES

1. Olsen, E.G.J. Dilated cardiomyopathy, myocarditis and the bioptome. *Br. Med. J.* 1986; 293: 90–1.
2. Gore, I. and Saphir, O. Myocarditis: A classification of 1402 cases. *Am. Heart J.* 1947; 34: 827–30.
3. Stevens, P.J. and Ground, K.E.U. Occurence and significance of myocarditis in trauma. *Clin. Aviation Aerospace Med.* 1970; 41: 776–80.
4. Lewes, D., Rainfall, D.J. and Lane, W.E. Symptomless myocarditis and myalgia in viral and *Micoplasma pneumoniae* infections. *Br. Heart J.* 1974; 36: 924–32.
5. Kawai, C., Matsumori, A., Kitaura, Y. and Takatsu, T. Viruses in the heart: viral myocarditis and cardiomyopathy. In: Yu, P.M. and Goodwin, J.F. eds. *Progress in Cardiology.* Philadelphia: Lea and Febiger, 1978, pp. 141–62.
6. Woodruff, J.F. Viral myocarditis: A review. *Am. J. Pathol.* 1980; 101: 427–79.
7. Abelmann, W.H. Clinical aspects of viral cardiomyopathy in myocardial diseases. In: Fowler, N.O. ed. *Myocardial Disease.* New York and London: Grune and Stratton, 1973.
8. Olsen, E.G.J. Histological aspects of viral myocarditis and its diagnostic criteria. In: Sakiguchi, M., Olsen, E. and Goodwin, J.F. eds. *Myocarditis and Related Disorders.* Tokyo, Berlin, Heidelberg and New York: Springer Verlag, 1985, pp. 130–2.
9. Billingham, M.E. The diagnostic criteria of myocarditis by myocardial biopsy. In: Sakiguchi, M., Olsen, E. and Goodwin, J.F. eds. *Myocarditis and Related Disorders.* Tokyo, Berlin, Heidelberg and New York: Springer Verlag, 1985, pp. 133–7.
10. Kawai, C. Idiopathic cardiomyopathy. A study on the infectious immune theories and cause of the disease. *Jap. Circ. J.* 1971; 35: 765–70.
11. Stewart, K.L. and Bras, G. Prognosis of idiopathic cardiomegaly in Jamaica with reference to coronary arteries and other factors. *Br. Heart J.* 1971; 33: 187–93.
12. Blackett, K. and Ngu, J.L. Immunologic studies in congestive cardiomyopathy in Cameroon. *Br. Heart J.* 1976; 38: 605–11.
13. Cambridge, C., MacArthur, C.G.C., Waters, A.P. *et al.* Antibodies to Coxsackie B virus in congestive cardiomyopathy. *Br. Heart J.* 1979; 41: 692–6.
14. Brown, D.L. Interpretation of test of immune function. In: Lachman, P.J. and Peters, D.K. eds. *Clinical Aspects of Immunology.* Oxford: Blackwell Scientific Publications, 1982, pp. 414–42.
15. Read, S.E., Fischetti, V.A., Utermohlen, V., Falk, R.E. and Zabriskie, J.B. Cellular reactivity studies to streptococcal infections and rheumatic fever. *J. Clin. Invest.* 1974; 54: 439.
16. Teixeira, A.R.L., Teixeira, G., Macedo, V. and Prata, A. *Trypanosoma cruzi*-sensitised T-lymphocytes mediated Cr release from human heart cells in Chagas' disease. *Am. J. Trop. Med. Hyg.* 1978; 27: 1097.
17. Das, S.K., Petty, R.E., Meengs, W.A. and Tubergen, D.G. Studies of cell-mediated immunity in cardiomyopathy. In: Sekiguchi, M. and Olsen, E.G.S. eds. *Cardiomyopathy.* Tokyo and Baltimore: University of Tokyo Press, 1980, pp. 375–7.
18. Das, S.K., Stein, L.D., Reynolds, R.T., Thebert, P. and Cassidy, J.T. Immunological studies in cardiomyopathy and pathophysiological implications. In: Goodwin, J.F., Hjalmarson, A. and Olsen, E.G.J. eds. *Congestive Cardiomyopathy.* Molnar, Sweden: A.B. Hassle, 1981, pp. 87–93.
19. Olsen, E.G.J. Diagnostic value of endomyocardial bioptome. *Lancet* 1974; 1: 658–60.
20. McKay, E.H., Littler, W.A. and Sleight, P. Critical assessment of diagnostic value of endomyocardial biopsy. *Br Heart J.* 1978; 40: 69–78.
21. Sakakibara, S. and Konno, S. Endomyocardial biopsy. *Jap. Heart J.* 1962; 3: 537–43.
22. Richardson, P.J. King's endomyocardial bioptome. *Lancet* 1974; 1: 660–1.
23. Caves, P.K., Schultz, W.P. and Dong, D. Jr *et al.* New instrument for a transvenous cardiac biopsy. *Am. J. Cardiol.* 1974; 33: 264.
24. Ewer, M.S. and Ali, M.K. Cardiac biopsy: A review of the procedure, complications and its indications. *Prac. Cardiol.* 1981; 7: 143–54.
25. Breithardt, G., Juhn, H. and Knieriem, H.J. Prognostic

significance of endomyocardial biopsy in patients with con-
gestive cardiomyopathy. In: Kaltenbech, M., Loogen, F. and
Olsen, E.G.J. eds. *Cadiomyopathy and Myocardial Biopsy.*
Berlin: Springer Verlag, 1978, pp. 258–70.

26. Mason, J.W., Billingham, M.E. and Ricci, D.R. Treatment
of acute inflammatory myocarditis assisted by endomyocardial biopsy. *Am. J. Cardiol.* 1980; **45**: 1037–44.

27. O'Connell, J.B., Robinson, J.A., Henkin, R.E. and Guller,
R.M. Immunosuppressive therapy in patients with conges-
tive cardiomyopathy and myocardial uptake of Gallium 67.
Circulation 1982; **64**: 780–6.

28. Daly, K., Richardson, P.J., Olsen, E.G.J. *et al.* Acute
Myocarditis. Role of histological and virological examination in the diagnosis and assessment of immunosuppressive
treatment. *Br. Heart J.* 1984; **51**: 30–6.

29. Kilbourne, E.D., Wilson, C.B. and Perrier, D. The induction
of gros myocardial lesions by Coxsackie (Pleurodynia) virus
and cortisone. *J. Clin. Invest.* 1956; **35**: 362–70.

30. Gore, R. Myocarditis in infectious diseases. *Am. Pract.*
1947; **1**: 292.

31. Riley, H.D. Jr and Weaver, T.S. Cardiovasicular and nervous system complications in diphtheria. *Am. Pract.* 1952;
3: 536.

32. Amorim, D.S. Chagas' disease. *Prog. Cardiol.* 1978; **8**: 235.

33. Theologides, A. and Kennedy, B.J. Toxoplasmic myocarditis
and pericarditis (Editorial). *Am. J. Med.* 1969; **47**: 169.

34. Walsh, T.J., Hutchins, G.M., Bulkley, B.H. and Mendel-
sohn, G. Fungal infections of the heart: Analysis of 51
autopsy cases. *Am. J. Cardiol.* 1980; **45**: 357.

35. Billingham, M.E. Pharmacotoxic myocardial disease in endomyocardial study. In: Sakiguchi, M., Olsen, E. and Goodwin, J.F. *Myocarditis and Related Disorders.* Tokyo, Berlin,
Heidelberg, New York: Springer Verlag, 1985, pp. 278–82.

36. Ferrans, V.J., Rodrigues, E.R. and McAllister, H.A. Jr.
Granulomatous inflammation of the heart. In: Sakiguchi,
M., Olsen, E. and Goodwin, J.F. eds. *Myocarditis and
Related Disorders.* Tokyo, Berlin, Heidelberg, New York:
Springer Verlag, 1985, pp. 262–70.

Chapter 37

Dilated Cardiomyopathy

W.A. Littler

DEFINITION

Dilated cardiomyopathy is a syndrome of congestive heart failure not associated with coronary artery disease. The cardiomyopathies are diseases of heart muscle and the dilated form probably represents the end-stage of a wide range of disorders (Table 37.1). Before making such a diagnosis, the physician should take care to exclude pre-existing hypertension, valvular heart disease, vascular shunts and coronary artery disease.

The terminology dilated (congestive) cardiomyopathy implies the fundamental pathophysiological abnormalities, viz. marked dilatation of both ventricles with severe impairment of systolic function and a high end-diastolic pressure. Such a condition may be associated with multisystem disorders and is usually classified as specific heart muscle disease or secondary cardiomyopathy. More commonly, no specific cause is found but conditioning factors such as hypertension, alcohol, current or recent pregnancy may be evident or elicited from the history. Primary or idiopathic cardiomyopathy is the definition usually applied to this group.

Table 37.1. Aetiology of dilated cardiomyopathy.

Idiopathic
Alcohol
Viral infections
Pregnancy: puerperium

Infectious
Toxins
Drugs (toxicity, hypersensitivity)
Deficiency states
Metabolic problems
Endocrine disorders
Collagen diseases

Familial
Muscular dystrophies

INCIDENCE

The true incidence of dilated cardiomyopathy is unknown. Torp has found an incidence of 7.5 cases per 100 000 inhabitants per year from a study conducted in Malmö in southern Sweden. Malmö has a stable population of one-quarter of a million inhabitants, is served by only one hospital and has a post-mortem rate of about 90%.

A retrospective study was carried out to assess the incidence of cardiomyopathy in western Denmark (population 2.8 million) during a 2-year period (1980–1981). An overall incidence of dilated cardiomyopathy was calculated as 7.3 per 100 000 population per year. A family history of dilated cardiomyopathy was noted in 28% of patients. More recently, Williams and Olsen found a prevalence of 8.3 cases per 100 000 of population in two regions in England covering a total sample of nearly one million inhabitants. The study was undertaken by means of questionnaires sent to general practitioners. The incidence of dilated cardiomyopathy may be higher in Third World countries, comprising perhaps one-third of all cases of congestive heart failure.

CLINICAL FEATURES

Brandenburg has suggested that dilated cardiomyopathy may be observed in three stages: asymptomatic, moderately severe disease and severe disease. In clinical practice, few patients are seen in the asymptomatic stage, except by chance or on routine medical screening when cardiomegaly may be observed on a chest X-ray (Fig. 37.1) or an electrocardiogram reveals some abnormality.

Most patients present when symptomatic, usually with some degree of heart failure. The earliest symptoms include effort dyspnoea, nocturnal cough or tiredness. As ventricular function deteriorates,

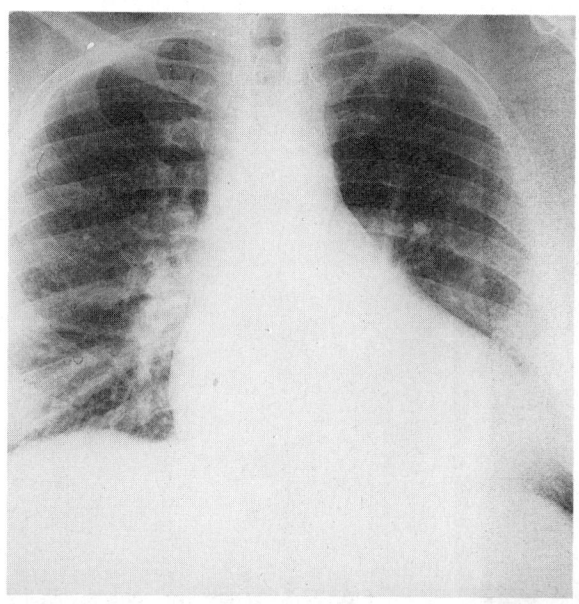

Fig. 37.1. Chest radiograph in a patient with congestive cardiomyopathy showing generalized cardiomegaly and pulmonary congestive changes.

orthopnoea and paroxysmal nocturnal dyspnoea develop, progressing to symptoms of right heart failure such as tiredness, peripheral oedema, abdominal distension and jaundice.

Approximately 20% of patients relate the onset of their symptoms to a 'flu-like' illness or a chest infection which has led to the belief that infection is a predominant cause of cardiomyopathy. Alternatively, the symptoms of heart failure have been misinterpreted as being those of a chest infection; on the other hand, an infection could simply be the precipitating factor for an already compromised heart which then fails.

Atypical or true anginal pain has been reported in about 10% of patients; some workers believe it is more common than this. It may sometimes be confused with hepatic pain which results from liver congestion.

Symptoms may occur as a result of the complications of cardiomyopathy. Systemic emboli are not infrequent with an incidence of approximately 6% per year. Pulmonary embolism also occurs either from a deep venous thrombosis or from the right ventricle, the latter source has been particularly recognised since the advent of two-dimensional echocardiography. Although arrhythmias are quite common, they are not particularly symptomatic; atrial fibrillation is found in up to 20% of patients and ventricular arrhythmias in up to 80% when

ambulatory electrocardiographic monitoring has been used.

There are no specific physical signs of dilated cardiomyopathy; the signs are those of low-output cardiac failure and include poor peripheral circulation, raised jugular venous pressure, dependent oedema, sinus tachycardia with a small-volume pulse and narrow pulse pressure, cardiac enlargement involving both ventricles, gallop rhythm with third and/or fourth heart sounds and murmurs of mitral and/or tricuspid incompetence. The lungs may reveal bilateral crepitations or pleural effusions; abdominal examination may indicate hepatomegaly and ascites.

INVESTIGATIONS

ELECTROCARDIOGRAM

There are no specific findings on the electrocardiogram and the changes may sometimes simulate those found in coronary artery disease. Findings include left ventricular hypertrophy, left bundle branch block, generalized ST–T changes, poor R-wave progression in the precordial leads, pathological Q waves (pseudo-infarction), frequent ventricular extrasystoles and atrial fibrillation. As already mentioned, ambulatory electrocardiographic monitoring may show a high incidence of atrial and ventricular arrhythmias which may account for the incidences of sudden death.

His-bundle electrocardiography has demonstrated atrioventricular prolongation, although atrioventricular block is not a particularly common feature of this condition.

CHEST X-RAY

Cardiomegaly is a consistent feature and involves all four chambers giving a globular appearance to the cardiac silhouette which may be indistinguishable from that seen in pericardial effusion. The lung fields may show pulmonary venous congestion, pleural effusions or less frequently alveolar oedema.

ECHOCARDIOGRAPHY

The typical appearance in a case of dilated cardiomyopathy is that of dilated ventricles with generalized reduced wall motion (Fig. 37.2), increased end-systolic and end-diastolic diameters and reduced ejection fraction (Fig. 37.3). The left atrium

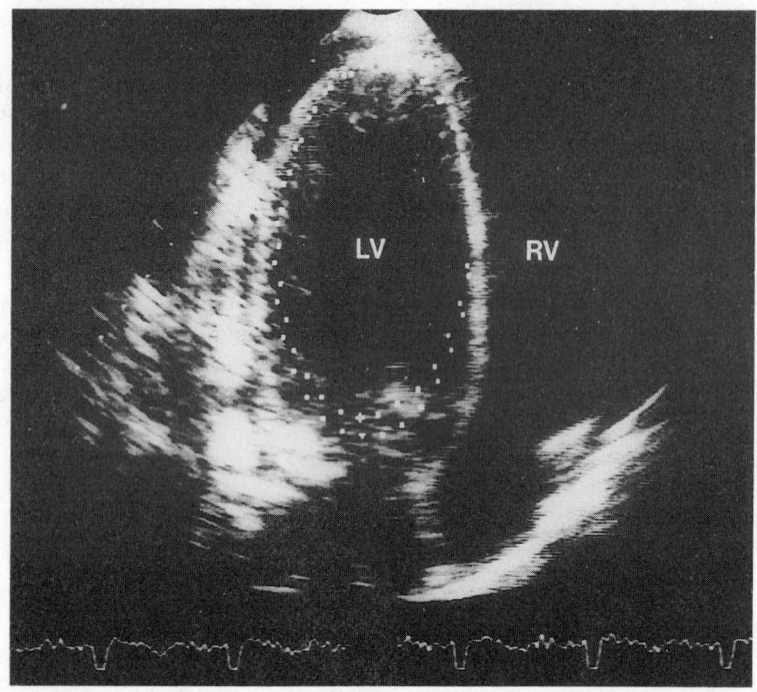

Fig. 37.2. Congestive cardiomyopathy. Two-dimensional echocardiogram of the left ventricle (LV). RV, right ventricle; ■ + ■ systolic frame; ■ ▼ ■ diastolic frame. Ejection fraction = 11%.

may be enlarged. Ventricular wall thickness is usually normal, although the calculation of ventricular mass may be increased as there is considerable dilatation. Mural thrombus may be found in either the left or the right ventricle (Fig. 37.4).

SYSTOLIC TIME-INTERVALS

Systolic time-intervals usually demonstrate decreased left ventricular ejection time and a prolonged pre-ejection period.

RADIONUCLIDE IMAGING

Radionuclide imaging may show biventricular dilatation and a global decrease in contractility, especially of the left ventricle. Thallium-201 scintigraphic studies have demonstrated that reversible images are non-specific, occurring in both ischaemic and idiopathic dilated cardiomyopathy. However, reversed distribution defects (worsening of images from exercise to redistribution) are more in keeping with ischaemic aetiology, as is a fixed defect of > 40% of the outer left ventricular perimeter.

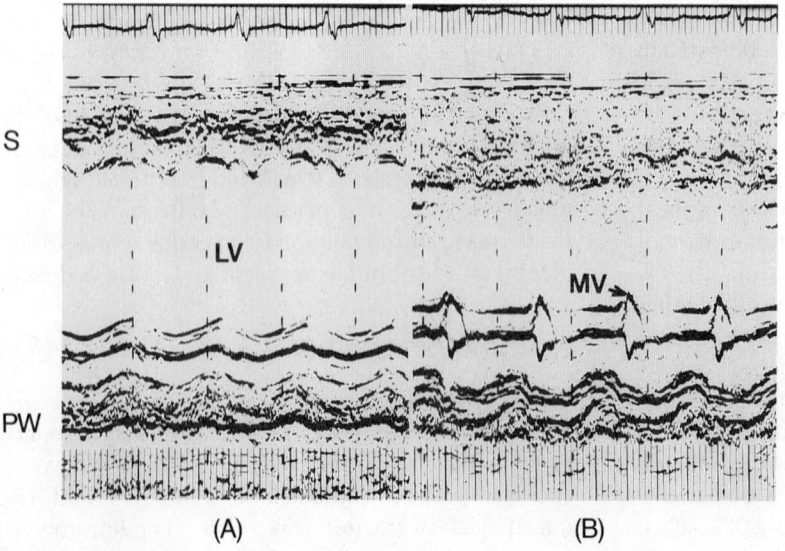

(A)   (B)

Fig. 37.3. Congestive cardiomyopathy. M-Mode echocardiogram of the left ventricle at the level of the chordae just below the mitral valve (A) and at the level of the mitral valve (B). The left ventricle is markedly dilated with poor systolic contraction. The mitral valve opening is reduced and shows early diastolic closure consistent with the high left ventricular diastolic pressure. S, septum; PW, posterior left ventricular wall; LV, left ventricular cavity; MV, mitral valve.

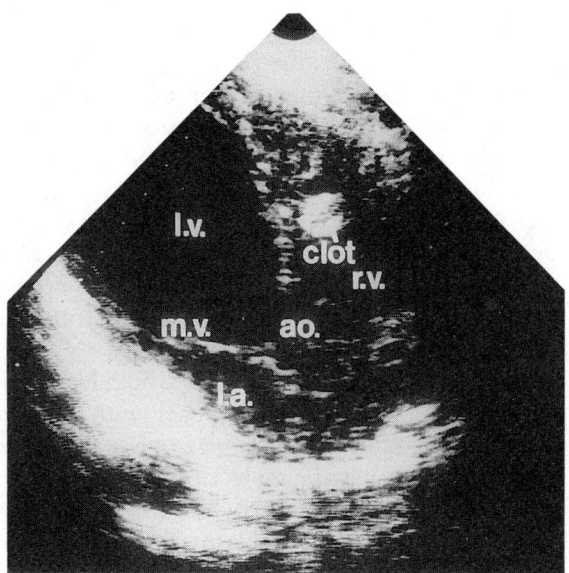

Fig. 37.4. Dilated cardiomyopathy. Two-dimensional echocardiogram (apical four-chamber view) showing an apical clot in the right ventricle (r.v.). l.v., left ventricle; m.v., mitral valve; l.a. left atrium; ao., aorta.

CARDIAC CATHETERIZATION

The principal findings on cardiac catheterization are those of raised filling pressures, a reduced cardiac output and ejection fraction. Angiography reveals a dilated left ventricle, usually without evidence of localized wall motion abnormalities (although this is not invariable), and on occasion mitral regurgitation. The coronary arteries are usually normal. If atheroma is present, it is incompatible with the global dysfunction of the ventricle.

ENDOMYOCARDIAL BIOPSY (see Chapter 36)

Although a biopsy may be useful in excluding a particular cause of heart muscle disease, there are no specific histological findings in dilated cardiomyopathy (Fig. 37.5).[8]

PROGNOSIS

The prognosis of dilated cardiomyopathy is variable; the general outlook is poor.[9] Death is most commonly from worsening heart failure, but a significant number of patients die suddenly. Studies are mainly based on retrospective group analysis from which it is difficult to make any comments on an individual patient. Less than half the patients survive for more than 5 years from the time of diagnosis; often, a majority of the deaths occur within the first 2 years. The prognosis appears to be most closely linked with ventricular function. Those patients with dilated hearts on chest X-ray and echocardiography who are subsequently shown to have a high left ventricular end-diastolic pressure and low cardiac index do badly. In the experience of some workers, biventricular failure is more predictive of early death than left-sided failure alone. Group data indicate that older patients (> 55 years) have the worst prognosis, although in clinical practice some of the most rapid deaths occur in younger patients. Associated arrhythmias, such as atrial fibrillation or ventricular tachycardia, have not been found independently to worsen prognosis in some studies, although the incidence of sudden death in cardiomyopathy varies widely, being as high as 46% in one series. Meinertz *et al.* studied

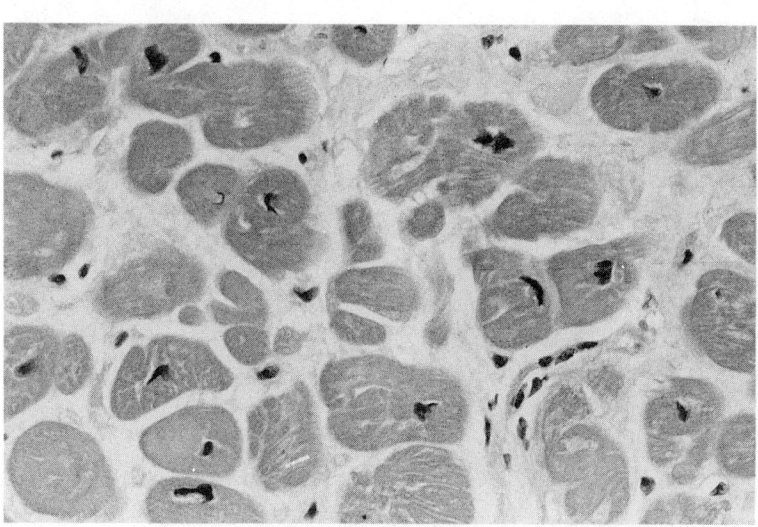

Fig. 37.5. Dilated cardiomyopathy. Myocardial fibres cut in transverse section are enlarged with 'smudging' of the nuclei. There is an increase in interstitial fibrous tissue. (Courtesy Dr C.E. Edwards.)

the incidence and prognostic significance of ventricular arrhythmias using ambulatory electrocardiographic monitoring in 74 patients with idiopathic dilated cardiomyopathy who were followed for a mean of 11 months.[10] Frequent ventricular premature beats (> 1000 per 24 h) were present in 35%, complex ventricular beats (Lown grade 3 or 4) in 87% and non-sustained ventricular tachycardia in 49%. Nineteen of these patients died, 7 of heart failure and 12 suddenly. Those who died suddenly had significantly more episodes of ventricular tachycardia, ventricular pairs or total ventricular premature beats when compared with those who died from heart failure and those who survived. It was argued that patients with idiopathic dilated cardiomyopathy whose left ventricular ejection fraction was < 40% and who had frequent episodes of ventricular tachycardia or ventricular pairs detected by 24-hour ambulatory monitoring had a high risk of dying. The presence of left ventricular hypertrophy in conjunction with dilatation improves prognosis, the implied mechanism being a reduction in ventricular stress.

In several studies, endomyocardial biopsies have been used in an attempt to obtain a more definite index of prognosis. The results are variable, sometimes contradictory and provide no conclusive evidence that this investigation has any advantage over simpler non-invasive assessments of ventricular size and function.

PATHOLOGY

At autopsy, the appearance of the dilated cardiomyopathic heart is globular, soft, flabby and pale and there is usually dilatation of all four chambers (Fig.37.6); the heart is heavier than normal, but dilatation tends to mask the hypertrophy that is present. The endocardium is often thickened and mural thrombus is found attached in more than 60% of cases. Light microscopy and electron microscopy reveal abnormalities nonspecific to dilated cardiomyopathy but which if present support the diagnosis. Some workers believe that more severe changes correspond with the severity of disease.

On light microscopy, there may be both hypertrophy and attenuation of myofibres with nuclear changes associated with hypertrophy. In some areas, myofibres may be replaced by fibrous tissue; interstitial fibrosis is increased. Electron microscopy reveals degenerative changes in myocardial cells, myofibrillar disarray, interstitial fibrosis and varying degrees of hypertrophy. No histochemical, enzymological or ultrastructural abnormality is diagnostic of dilated cardiomyopathy.[9]

PERIPARTUM CARDIOMYOPATHY

Most observers identify this cardiomyopathy presenting as congestive cardiac failure or cardiac symptoms late in pregnancy or during the puerperium in the absence of any of the commonly recognized causes of heart disease. It is not known whether pregnancy plays a specific role in this cardiomyopathy or whether pregnancy is a nonspecific precipitating event in the history of a woman with pre-existing heart disease.[11,12]

It is difficult to assess the true prevalence of this condition; it has been reported most frequently

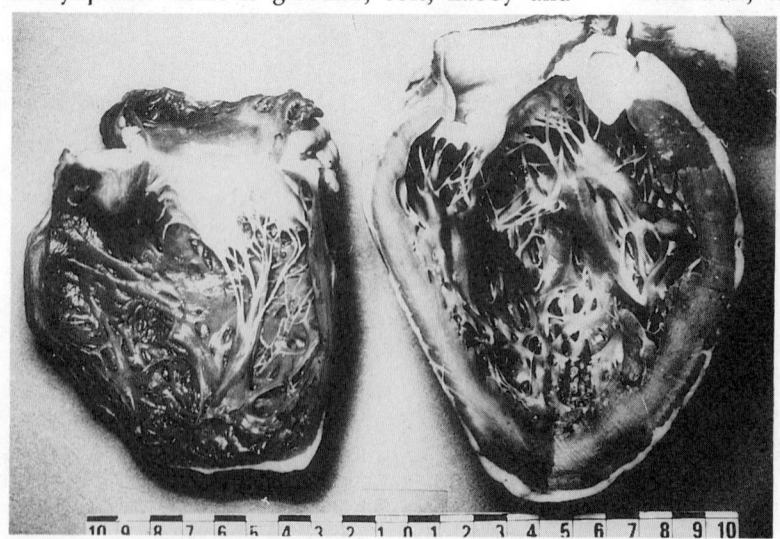

Fig. 37.6. The right and left ventricles are markedly dilated in congestive cardiomyopathy.

among black subjects, but it affects all races, and particularly those in the lower socio-economic groups. The reported incidences range from 1:1300 to 1:4000 pregnancies.

Aetiological and conditioning factors may include malnutrition, myocarditis (Coxsackie B) and immunological abnormalities. It appears to be commoner in older multiparous women, particularly those who have a twin pregnancy or one complicated by toxaemia. In Africa, more than 50% of cases are associated with hypertension, perhaps in combination with alcohol intake and malnutrition.[13,14] The highest incidence in the world is among the Hausa of Northern Nigeria, but this has been related to the local custom of postpartum body heating together with an excessive consumption of salt (up to 450 mmol/day) with the aim of increasing the production of breast milk. The reason why dilated cardiomyopathy should emerge in late pregnancy is not known. One suggestion is that there is an increased afterload imposed on the heart during late pregnancy due to the rise in the peripheral resistance, and labour increases the stress on the heart coupled with the sudden increase in the venous return following delivery. All these factors may be precipitant in a previously precariously balanced situation.

There is considerable uniformity in the clinicopathological features of peripartum cardiomyopathy which are identical to those of dilated cardiomyopathy. Congestive cardiac failure is common, and embolic episodes are frequent. Examination reveals a large heart with triple rhythm and a sinus tachycardia.

The prognosis appears to be related to heart size; in those in whom heart size returns to normal within 6 months of delivery the prognosis is good, although the condition may recur in future pregnancies. Mortality ranges from 20 to 60% in those who continue to have cardiomegaly 6 months after delivery.

The management of heart failure is the same as that described for dilated cardiomyopathy. The role of therapeutic abortion or the indications for early induction of labour or Caesarean section should be determined in each individual case in close collaboration with obstetric colleagues.

ALCOHOLIC CARDIOMYOPATHY

Heart failure associated with excessive alcohol consumption was first recognized over 100 years ago.[15] Probably 1–2% of chronic alcoholics develop heart failure. The extent of cardiac involvement varies greatly among individuals with a similar intake of alcohol, and it is not yet clear whether ethanol has a direct toxic effect on the myocytes. Some authors believe that alcoholic cardiomyopathy is a form of dilated cardiomyopathy, in which alcohol is one of several causal or conditioning factors, rather than a separate entity. Alcoholic cardiomyopathy usually occurs in the absence of other features of alcoholism and alcoholic liver disease and the patients are usually well nourished.[16–18]

Alcohol causes transient changes in the normal heart and circulation.[19] Studies in animals and man have demonstrated the development and reversibility of haemodynamic and biochemical abnormalities following short-term ingestion of alcohol. The main effect of alcohol is loss of cardiac contractility. Alcohol inhibits mitochondrial respiration and the activity of enzymes in the tricarboxylic acid cycle, and it interferes with calcium uptake and binding by mitochondria and sarcoplasmic reticulum. However, as reduced calcium uptake and binding have been noted in most types of severe cardiac failure, they are not specific effects of alcohol.[20]

Alcoholism may affect the heart in one of several other ways. A high incidence of arrhythmias, particularly atrial fibrillation, has been noted in alcoholics, especially during 'binge drinking', in the absence of overt manifestations of cardiomyopathy. Cardiac beriberi is associated with thiamine (vitamin B_1) deficiency and produces heart failure. It used to be seen far more commonly than nowadays in derelict alcoholics who were usually heavy beer drinkers, many of whom had had a previous gastrectomy. 'Beer cobalt cardiomyopathy', a relatively fulminant condition, originally reported in Quebec, was due to cobalt poisoning from excessive consumption of beer to which cobalt chloride had been added as a froth stabilizer.[21] Cobalt given to rabbits has been reported to cause extensive myocardial damage.

Alcoholic (dilated) cardiomyopathy may present incidentally as cardiomegaly on a chest X-ray or with symptoms of heart failure. The recognition of excessive alcohol intake is clearly of overriding importance in making a diagnosis. 'Excessive' has been defined as a daily intake > 110 ml.

The symptoms, physical findings and investigations are generally indistinguishable from those in patients with dilated cardiomyopathy of indeterminate cause.[22] Effort dyspnoea is the commonest symptom and cardiomegaly the commonest sign. The echocardiogram may show left ventricular hypertrophy with abnormal T waves. So-called 'dimpled' T waves are no longer thought to be specific for alcoholic cardiomyopathy. Echocardiography and ventricular contrast or isotope studies reveal enlarged poorly contracting ventricular cavities.

Non-specific morphological criteria have been defined for distinguishing the alcoholic from the idiopathic form of cardiomyopathy. Differences have been claimed as a result of enzymatic and immunological studies of endomyocardial biopsies. In one study, the content of lactate dehydrogenase was higher in patients with alcoholic cardiomyopathy when compared with those who had idiopathic cardiomyopathy; the activity of enzymes, such as creatinine phosphokinase and alpha-hydroxybutyric dihydrogenase, was also found to be raised in the alcoholic heart muscle. Patients with alcoholic cardiomyopathy have been found to have a negative myocardial antimyolemmal antibody test but increased binding of IgA to heart muscle. Other workers have not been able to confirm this and it is unlikely that any such findings are specific.

Many studies have demonstrated reversibility of heart failure with abstention from alcohol; however, further deterioration occurs if consumption continues.[23] Abstinence was followed by an 80% likelihood of long-term survival in one study. The primary aim of therapy is alcohol withdrawal and abstinence combined with supportive therapy for heart failure and arrhythmias. As relapses are common, rehabilitation programmes should be encouraged.

RIGHT VENTRICULAR DILATED CARDIOMYOPATHY

Oakley and her colleagues have described a predominantly right-sided cardiomyopathy; severe dilatation of the right ventricle was the hallmark of the condition, left ventricular function being relatively well preserved.[24] Such a condition was considered to be one end of the spectrum of clinical and pathological features of idiopathic dilated cardiomyopathy. Patients tend to be young and male; clinically, palpitations and syncope are the commonest symptoms. Sudden death is common. Physical signs include third or fourth heart sounds, a right ventricular impulse and right-sided heart failure.

The electrocardiogram usually reveals some form of right ventricular abnormality, including right bundle branch block, right ventricular hypertrophy, right-axis deviation and T-wave inversion of the right precordial leads.

Arrhythmias are common, accounting for the symptoms of palpitation and syncope.[25] Ventricular tachycardia which typically has a left bundle branch block pattern on the surface electrocardiogram is common. Electrophysiological studies and endomyocardial mapping have demonstrated the right ventricular origin of this tachycardia and also that the ventricular tachycardia may degenerate into ventricular fibrillation.

Cross-sectional echocardiography, radionuclide angiography and ciné-angiography all demonstrate the extreme dilatation and poor function of the right ventricle whereas left ventricular function is seen to be relatively normal. Necropsy and endomyocardial biopsy studies have demonstrated areas of endocardial fibrosis in the right ventricle; histological examination has shown numerous foci of fibrous replacement in both ventricles.

Distinguishing right ventricular dilated cardiomyopathy from conditions causing abnormalities of the right heart, such as congenital lesions, or those causing selective right ventricular dysfunction, such as right ventricular dysplasia, is important. The possibility of right ventricular dilated cardiomyopathy should be considered in any young patient presenting with syncope or ventricular tachycardia. Treatment is aimed at control of arrhythmias as assessed by ambulatory electrocardiograms or electrophysiological studies. Effective drug therapy can be gauged only from a small number of cases in the literature; amiodarone is commonly used.[25] In refractory cases, endocardial excision has been performed with apparent success.

TREATMENT

HEART FAILURE

The conventional management of heart failure in dilated cardiomyopathy is discussed in Chapter 5.

Particular measures will be dictated by the stage of disease at which the patient is seen and by the specific complications; for example, a patient found on routine examination to have cardiomegaly may require no treatment but if an ambulatory electrocardiogram reveals significant ventricular arrhythmias anti-arrhythmic drugs may be required.

At some stage, the management of heart failure will be necessary. For patients presenting with congestive heart failure, the role of general measures such as rest in bed, fluid and salt restriction and oxygen therapy should not be ignored or underplayed. Congestive cardiac failure is a complex pathophysiological process with both central and peripheral haemodynamic abnormalities combined with altered neurohumeral mechanisms.

Diuretics are the mainstay of treatment, increasing the excretion of water and excessive sodium found in cardiac failure. Loop diuretics, such as frusemide, are the treatment of choice, and these should be combined with potassium supplements or a potassium-sparing diuretic to avoid hypokalaemia. Careful monitoring of renal function is necessary when large doses of diuretics are employed.

The role of cardiac glycosides, such as digoxin, remains controversial in the patient with heart failure who is in sinus rhythm; its role in the patient with atrial fibrillation is well established.[26] Digoxin is a weakly positive inotropic drug with a narrow toxic/therapeutic ratio but it is probably of benefit in patients with heart failure who have large dilated hearts.[27] The role of the newer inotropic drugs in the treatment of dilated cardiomyopathy has yet to be established.

The rationale of vasodilator therapy in heart failure is that vasoconstriction in arteries and veins increases both preload and afterload which impairs cardiac performance.[28] Venodilators, such as nitrates, arterial dilators, such as hydralazine, and mixed dilators, such as prazosin, have all been shown to be effective in relieving symptoms in some patients with dilated cardiomyopathy; there is no clear evidence that any of these agents increase the life-expectancy of such patients. The combination of hydralazine and isosorbide dinitrate was shown to reduce significantly mortality in patients with chronic congestive cardiac failure when compared with placebo.[28] This study has been criticized because 50% of the treatment group were not receiving maximum therapy throughout the study and those patients randomized did not have severe low-output cardiac failure because 1-year mortality on placebo was 19%.[29]

Converting enzyme inhibitors which inhibit the conversion of angiotensin I to angiotensin II are becoming increasingly popular in the management of congestive cardiac failure. Drugs such as captopril and enalapril produce significant haemodynamic improvement at rest and during exercise; a recent report suggests that enalapril may reduce mortality in such patients.[30]

BETA-BLOCKING DRUGS IN DILATED CARDIOMYOPATHY

Patients with end-stage heart failure have been shown to have 'down-regulation' of the beta-adrenoceptors together with a lack of responsiveness. The elevated levels of circulating catecholamines found in these patients is thought to be the cause. Objective evidence of improvement with prolonged survival has been obtained in open studies performed by Swedberg and his colleagues using beta-blocking drugs in some patients with dilated cardiomyopathy, whereas the patients' conditions deteriorated when the beta-blockers were withdrawn.[31,32] Other workers, using double-blind crossover study protocols, have not confirmed these findings.[33] The routine use of beta-blockers is not advised until this controversy has been resolved.

PREVENTION AND TREATMENT OF ARRHYTHMIAS

Ventricular arrhythmias are commonly recorded by the ambulatory electrocardiogram in patients with dilated cardiomyopathy and are of prognostic significance. In a recent prospective study, Neri and his colleagues studied 65 patients with dilated cardiomyopathy, of whom 41 received amiodarone (200–400 mg daily).[34] A significant reduction of ventricular arrhythmias was seen in 70% of these patients over a 3-year period. In the whole series, 4 sudden deaths occurred, none of which were in the amiodarone-treated patients. Amiodarone has the advantage over other anti-arrhythmic agents, such as disopyramide, in that it does not have a negative inotropic effect. Ambulatory electrocardiographic monitoring, rather than sophisticated intracardiac electrophysiological studies, is probably the most convenient way of assessing the presence of ventricular arrhythmias and their response to treatment with anti-arrhythmic drugs.

PREVENTION AND TREATMENT OF EMBOLISM

Patients with dilated cardiomyopathy have an increased risk from both systemic and pulmonary emboli. Patients particularly at risk include those in atrial fibrillation, those in whom intracardiac clot can be demonstrated by echocardiography and those confined to bed with severe congestive cardiac failure. Oral anticoagulants should be used in selected patients with careful attention paid to the control of anticoagulation.

CARDIAC TRANSPLANTATION

For patients who have chronic heart failure as a result of dilated cardiomyopathy, cardiac transplantation offers the best chance of long-term survival with a substantial improvement in the quality of life. Survival at 1 year is currently 80%, and 60% at 3 years (see Chapter 6).

REFERENCES

1. Goodwin, J.F. The frontiers of cardiomyopathy. *Br. Heart J.* 1982; **48**: 1–18.
2. Torp, A. Incidence of congestive cardiomyopathy. *Postgrad. Med. J.* 1978; **54**: 435–7.
3. Bagger, J.P., Baandrup, U., Rasmussen, K. *et al.* Cardiomyopathy in western Denmark. *Br. Heart J.* 1984; **52**: 327–31.
4. Williams, G. and Olsen, G.J. Prevalance of an overt dilated cardiomyopathy in two regions of England. *Br. Heart J.* 1985; **54**: 153–5.
5. Johnson, R.A. and Palacios, I. Dilated cardiomyopathies of the adult. *N. Engl. J. Med.* 1982; **307**: 1051–119.
6. Fuster, V., Gersh, B.J., Giuliani, E.R. *et al.* The natural history of idiopathic dilated cardiomyopathy. *Am. J. Cardiol.* 1981; **47**: 525–31.
7. Marriott, H.J.L. Electrocardiographic abnormalities, conductions disorders and arrhythmias in primary myocardial disease. *Prog. Cardiovasc. Dis.* 1964; **7**: 99–114.
8. Olsen, E.G.J. The pathology of cardiomyopathies: A critical analysis. *Am. Heart J.* 1979; **98**: 385–92.
9. Engler, R., Ray, R., Higgins, C.B. *et al.* Clinical assessment and follow up of functional capacity of patients with chronic congestive cardiomyopathy. *Am. J. Cardiol.* 1982; **49**: 1832–7.
10. Meinertz, T., Hofmann, T., Kasper, W. *et al.* Significance of ventricular arrhythmias in idiopathic dilated cardiomyopathy. *Am. J. Cardiol.* 1984; **53**: 902–7.
11. Stuart, K.L. Cardiomyopathy of pregnancy in the puerperium. *Q. J. Med.* 1968; **37**: 463–78.
12. Brown, A.K., Douks, N., Riding, W.D. and Wynn-Jones, E. Cardiomyopathy in pregnancy. *Br. Heart J.* 1967; **29**: 387–39.
13. Falase, A.O. Peripartum heart disease. In: Sakiguchi, M., Olsen, E.G.J. and Goodwin, J.F. eds. *Myocarditis and Related Disorders.* Tokyo, Berlin, Heidelberg, New York: Springer-Verlag, 1985, pp. 232–5.
14. Davidson, M.N. and Parry, E.H. *Peripartum cardiac failure in cardiovascular disease in the tropics.* London: British Medical Association, 1974, pp. 199–208.
15. Walsag, W.A. *A practical treatise on the diseases of the heart and great vessels including the principles of their physical diagnosis.* London: Smith Elder, 1873.
16. Alderman, E.L. and Coltart, D.J. Alcohol and the heart. *Br. Med. Bull.* 1982; **38**: 77–80.
17. Anonymous. Alcoholic heart muscle disease. *Br. Med. J.* 1979; **2**: 1457.
18. Komajda, M., Richard, J.L., Bouhour, J.B. *et al.* Dilated cardiomyopathy and the level of alcohol consumption: A planned multicentre case control study. *Eur. Heart J.* 1986; **7**: 512–9.
19. Knochel, J.P. Cardiovascular effects of alcohol. *Ann. Intern. Med.* 1983; **98A**: 849–54.
20. Bing, R.J. Cardiac metabolism and its contributions to alcoholic heart disease and myocardial failure. *Circulation* 1978; **58**: 965–70.
21. Alexander, C.S. Cobalt in the heart. *Ann. Intern. Med.* 1969; **70**: 411–3.
22. Demakis, J.G., Proskey, A., Rahimtoola, S.H., Sutton, G.C., Gunnar, R.M. and Tobin, J.R. The natural course of alcoholic cardiomyopathy. *Ann. Intern. Med.* 1974; **18**: 293–7.
23. Kino, M., Nakayama, Y., Har, M. *et al.* Factors discriminating survivors and non-survivors in alcoholic heart disease. In: Sakiguchi, M., Olsen, E.G.J., Goodwin, J.F. eds. *International Symposium on Cardiomyopathy in Myocarditis.* Tokyo, Berlin, Heidelberg and New York: Springer-Verlag, 1985, pp. 301–5.
24. Fitchett, D.H., Sugrue, D.D., MacArthur, C.G. and Oakley, C.M. Right ventricular dilated cardiomyopathy. *Br. Heart J.* 1984; **51**: 25–9.
25. Rowland, E., McKenna, W.J., Sugrue, D.D., Barclay, R., Foale, R.A. and Krikler, D.A. Ventricular tachycardia of left bundle branch block configuration in patients with isolated right ventricular dilatation. Clinical and electrophysiological features. *Br. Heart J.* 1984; **51**: 15–24.
26. John, G.D. and McDevitt, D.J. Is maintenance digoxin necessary in patients with sinus rhythm? *Lancet* 1979; **i**: 567–70.
27. Lee, D.C. Heart failure in out-patients: A randomised trial of digoxin versus placebo. *N. Engl. J. Med.* 1982; **306**: 699–701.
28. Franciosa, J. Effectiveness of long-term vasodilator administration in the treatment of chronic left ventricular failure. *Prog. Cardiovasc. Dis.* 1982; **24**: 219–330.
29. Kohn, J.N., Archibald, D.G., Ziesca, G.S. *et al.* Effect of vasodilator therapy on mortality in chronic congestive heart failure. *N. Engl. J. Med.* 1986; **314**: 1547–52.
30. The Consensus Study Trial Group. Effects of enalapril on mortality in severe congestive heart failure: Results of the cooperative North Scandinavian Enalapril Survival Study. *N. Engl. J. Med.* 1987; **316**: 1429–35.
31. Swedberg, K., Hjalmarson, A., Waggstein, E. and Wallentin, I. Beneficial effects of long-term beta blockade in congestive cardiomyopathy. *Br. Heart J.* 1980; **44**: 117–33.
32. Swedberg, K., Hjalmarson, A., Waggstein, F. and Wallentin, I. Adverse effects of beta blockade withdrawal in patients with congestive cardiomyopathy. *Br. Heart J.* 1980; **44**: 134–42.
33. Skram, H. and Fitzpatrick, D. Beta-blockade for dilated cardiomyopathy; the evidence against therapeutic benefit. *Eur. Heart J.* 1983; **4**(Suppl. A): 179.
34. Neri, R., Mestroni, L., Salvi, A., Pandullo, C. and Camerini, K. Ventricular arrhythmias in dilated cardiomyopathy; efficacy of amiodarone. *Am. Heart J.* 1987; **113**: 707–15.

Chapter 38

Restrictive Cardiomyopathy

W.A. Littler

Restrictive cardiomyopathy may be due to several pathological conditions involving the endocardium and/or myocardium which reduce ventricular diastolic compliance and restrict inflow of blood. Stroke volume is accommodated by the stiffened ventricle only through an abnormal rise in diastolic pressure which accounts for the congestive symptoms and characteristic haemodynamic signs. Specific causes include endomyocardial fibrosis, Loeffler's endomyocardial disease, amyloidosis, sarcoidosis and haemochromatosis. In many cases, the condition is associated with non-specific ventricular hypertrophy and/or fibrosis.[1] Symptoms are non-specific, the commonest reported being of left and/or right ventricular failure including fatigue, atypical chest pain and symptoms arising from arrhythmias.

Physical findings are variable and depend upon the relative involvement of the ventricles and the atrioventricular valves. The best recognized clinical picture is that produced by right ventricular involvement with a high jugular venous pressure exhibiting both Friedreich's and Kussmaul's signs. A third (or diastolic) heart sound is audible, and there may be hepatomegaly and ascites.[2] The clinical picture is indistinguishable from that produced by constrictive pericarditis.

Involvement of the left side does not produce the picture of 'constriction'; signs may be few and include a third heart sound and the murmur of mitral regurgitation. The electrocardiographic and radiographic findings are non-specific.

Echocardiography is most useful in aiding diagnosis. It may exclude pericardial pathology such as thickening, calcification or an effusion, all of which produce a similar clinical picture. An abnormal filling pattern, associated with small cavities, and septal and ventricular hypertrophy, is highly suggestive of restrictive cardiomyopathy. The myocardium may produce bright echoes; this granular 'sparkle' is seen in certain infiltrations such as amyloidosis, haemochromatosis or excessive fibrosis.

The haemodynamic pattern of restrictive cardiomyopathy is that of elevated filling pressures in the ventricles whilst systolic function is preserved and closely simulates that of constriction (Fig. 38.1).[3] The characteristic pressure tracing reveals the 'square-root' sign due to the rapid rise and abrupt plateau in the early diastolic phase of ventricular pressure. Ventricular angiography may produce particular appearances with some of the specific infiltrations.

EOSINOPHILIC ENDOMYOCARDIAL DISEASE

ENDOMYOCARDIAL FIBROSIS AND LOEFFLER'S ENDOMYOCARDITIS PARIETALIS FIBROPLASTICA

Although originally considered as separate entities, endomyocardial fibrosis and Loeffler's endoymocarditis parietalis fibroplastica are now thought to be part of a single spectrum whereby eosinophilia and cardiac damage are closely associated.[4] Endomyocardial fibrosis occurs sporadically throughout the world but is endemic in the rainforest belt of Africa, in India and in parts of South America. In sporadic cases, blood eosinophilia is common, whereas it is a variable finding in endemic areas.[5] It should be noted that the geographical areas in which the endemic cases occur have a high incidence of infectious diseases which result in an eosinophilia. Spry, Olsen and their colleagues have greatly clarified the pathology of endomyocardial fibrosis and Loeffler's endomyocarditis and brought attention to the cardiotoxic role of the eosinophil in these conditions.[6] The macroscopic appearance of the heart in endomyocardial fibrosis is that of hypertrophied ventricles with cavities which can be either dilated or reduced in size and immense thick-

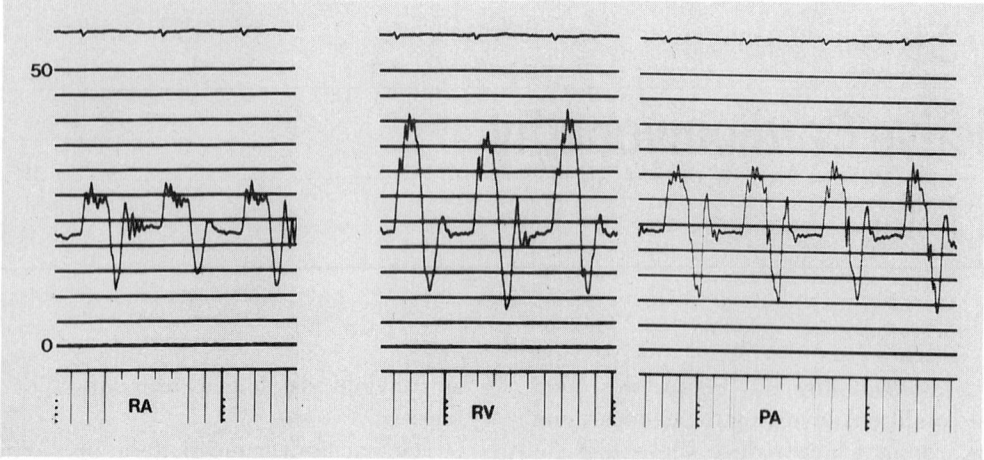

Fig. 38.1. Amyloid heart disease. Cardiac catheterization pressure data showing equal diastolic pressures throughout the right heart with an early rapid rise in diastolic pressure in the right ventricle (RV) consistent with a restrictive cardiomyopathy. RA, right atrium; PA, pulmonary artery.

ening of the endocardium. Strands of this endocardial thickening are seen to extend into the inner third of the underlying myocardium. According to Olsen, both ventricles are involved in about 51% of cases, the left ventricle alone in 38% and the right ventricle alone in 11%. The atrium may also be involved, but not as an isolated feature. On closer inspection, the cavity obliteration is seen to involve the posterior papillary muscles, the chordae tendineae and the valve cusp of the mitral apparatus. Superimposed thrombus is frequently found in advanced cases; this may be calcified.

Histologically, Olsen found layers of collagen beneath the thrombus whereas the deepest layer consisted of granulated tissue made up of loose connective tissue, blood vessels and inflammatory cells.

Subsequent work based on cases of endomyocardial fibrosis associated with eosinophilia led Olsen to describe three stages in the pathological process. The first stage showed signs of myocarditis and arteritis and was reached within 6 weeks. Thrombotic features were prominent in the second phase which was reached in less than 1 year; the third and final phase consisted of a predominantly fibrotic reaction which was present at about 2 years. Loeffler's endomyocarditis is seen as an aggressive more rapidly progressive form of the disorder and the differences between this and endomyocardial fibrosis without eosinophilia may relate to the hypereosinophilic syndrome.

The cardiotoxicity of the eosinophils has been characterized by Spry and his colleagues.[7] Three observations are of critical importance: first there is the consistent clinical finding that a high blood eosinophilia is associated with endomyocardial disease; second, the development of heart disease in these cases is associated with the presence of degranulated eosinophils in the blood and tissue together with an increase in serum levels of eosinophilic granule basic protein; third, it has been shown that low concentrations of these proteins will injure isolated myocytes *in vitro*. There appears to be a specific toxic effect of eosinophilic cationic protein on the plasma membrane and on the enzymes pyruvate dehydrogenase and 2-oxoglutarate dehydrogenase, which are inhibited.[8]

It would appear that in temperate zones hypereosinophilia, from whatever cause, leads to damage of the endomyocardium rather rapidly. In endemic areas, endomyocardial fibrosis is produced by the same process but in a slower fashion, possibly because the eosinophilia is not as intense or simply because the cases have not been studied early enough for the acute phase to be detected.

The clinical picture depends on the extent to which the individual ventricle or both ventricles is/are affected.[9] Fatigue and dyspnoea are the commonest symptoms; the physical signs may be those of constriction if the right side is involved, but may present as mitral regurgitation if the left ventricle alone is affected. There are no specific findings on the electrocardiogram, but left ventricular hypertrophy and atrial enlargement are frequently found. The chest X-ray is also non-specific. The lack of pericardial calcification may help to distinguish from constrictive pericarditis although a strip of linear calcification of thrombus within the ventricle is sometimes seen and may be misinterpreted as being pericardial.[10]

Echocardiography is useful in making the diagnosis, showing hyperdynamic ventricles with diminished cavity size and large atria. The obliteration of the apices of the ventricles by echogenic masses is well demonstrated on a four-chamber view and close inspection may reveal posterior fibrotic thickening of the mitral and/or the tricuspid valve.[11]

Angiography confirms the echocardiographic appearances. Goodwin has likened the ventricular appearance to a 'boxing glove' because the obliterated apices give rise to a cut-off picture.

Direct histological evidence of the pathology can be obtained by endomyocardial biopsy although extreme caution should be taken on the left side for fear of dislodging thrombus and causing a systemic embolus.

TREATMENT

The standard therapeutic approach to the management of various aspects of the condition, such as heart failure or arrhythmias, should be undertaken. However, two specific points require mention. First, treatment of the hypereosinophilic syndrome may require steroids and cytotoxic drugs to reduce the severity of tissue injury, and leukopharesis and plasma exchange may be necessary to reduce the eosinophil count.[12] It is advisable to give anticoagulants at this stage because of the thrombo-embolic problems. Second, cardiac surgery for endomyocardial fibrosis involves removal of the fibrotic and thrombotic endocardial tissues with replacement or repair of the involved mitral and/or tricuspid valves. In follow-up studies of patients treated in this way, there has been no evidence of local recurrence but the long-term outlook is not yet known.[13]

AMYLOID HEART DISEASE

Amyloidosis is not a single disease entity but a variety of different disease processes resulting in the deposition in various tissues of twisted beta-pleated sheet fibrils formed from different proteins by several pathogenic mechanisms.[14] The amyloid fibril has the structure of a beta-sheet not normally found in mammalian tissue. Two major proteins have been obtained from amyloid fibril preparations: immunoglobulin amyloid fibril protein (AL), consist-

ing of lambda or kappa light polypeptide chains of immunoglobulin proteins, and amyloid fibril protein (AA). The cell (or cells) of origin of this class of protein is not known, but it is probably derived from larger proteins by proteolytic digestion.

Amyloid fibrils are deposited extracellularly and first appear in the walls of small blood vessels. This siting suggests that constituents of plasma which escape from small blood vessels are converted to amyloid fibrils by digestive enzymes of phagocytic cells. These inert fibrils cause the enlargement of organs, giving them a rubbery consistency, which eventually causes pressure atrophy and death. The main clinicopathological classification of amyloid deposition divides the acquired systemic amyloidoses into 4 groups.

1 Primary (idiopathic), which has no preceding or concurrent disease, is made up of AL fibrils and is laid down preferentially in mesenchymal tissues, especially the heart and cardiovascular system.
2 Amyloid associated with multiple myeloma made up of AL fibrils.
3 Secondary amyloid associated with co-existing chronic inflammatory or infectious diseases consisting of AA fibrils is laid down preferentially in a parenchymal organ such as the spleen.
4 Tumour-forming amyloid consisting of localized amyloid masses and probably related to the primary type.

In addition, several systemic and localized heredo-familial syndromes of amyloid deposition involving various organs have been described in various geographical areas. The heart may be involved in all types of amyloidosis but commonly in the primary form and when it is associated with multiple myeloma. Brandt *et al.* found 90% of patients with these types of amyloidosis have cardiac involvement, whereas only 54% of patients with secondary amyloidosis had cardiac involvement.[15] Senile cardiac amyloidosis has been reported to have an overall incidence of 2%. In this condition, amyloid first involves the atrial myocardium, then the ventricles and finally the aortopulmonary tree.

Restrictive cardiomyopathy may be caused by amyloid deposition in the heart: amyloid is deposited sub-endocardially and irregularly between the myocardial fibres rendering the myocardium thick and firm with ventricular cavities of normal or small size. Amyloid is frequently deposited in the conducting tissue. The symptoms and signs tend to be dictated by the pattern of amyloid deposition in the heart. Cardiac failure is the commonest presentation; it may simulate constrictive pericarditis or present with arrhythmias or conduction defects.[16] Amyloidosis gives rise to low voltages on the electrocardiogram with poor R-wave progression in the precordial leads (Fig. 38.2), sometimes simulating myocardial infarction. Conduction abnormalities or arrhythmias may be present. The chest X-ray may reveal only slight cardiomegaly. Child *et al.* have listed the echocardiographic features which include symmetrically uniform thickening of the ventricular walls with hypokinesia and systolic thickening of the interventricular septum and left ventricular posterior wall (Fig. 38.3).[17] The ventricular cavities are small or normal; the indices of left ventricular performance are decreased. Finally, the abnormal texture of the myocardium may give a granular sparkle to the echocardiogram.

The haemodynamic and angiographic findings are not specific and have already been discussed. Endomyocardial biopsy may enable a tissue diagnosis to be made.

The prognosis is extremely poor, with death occurring between 1 and 2 years after diagnosis; no effective treatment is available other than cardiac transplantation. If digitalis is prescribed, it should be used cautiously because amyloid fibrils bind the drug, thereby increasing the likelihood of heart block. Diuretics may cause volume depletion and cardiovascular collapse.

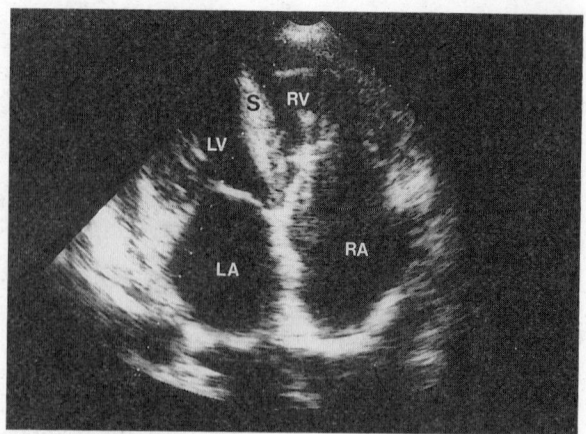

Fig. 38.3. Amyloid heart disease. Two-dimensional echocardiogram (apical four-chamber view) showing a glistening, hypertrophied interventricular septum(s), left ventricular posterior wall hypertrophy, increased width and density of the interatrial septum and a small left ventricular cavity. LV, left ventricle; LA, left atrium; RV, right ventricle; RA, right atrium. (Courtesy Dr M.K. Davies).

SARCOID HEART DISEASE

Sarcoidosis has been defined as the presence in all of several affected organs or tissues of epithelial tubercles without caseation. The cause of this granulomatous disorder is not known.[18] Although clinical cardiac involvement is low in those suffering from systemic sarcoidosis (estimated at 1.5%), there is a much higher incidence of cardiac sarcoid in those

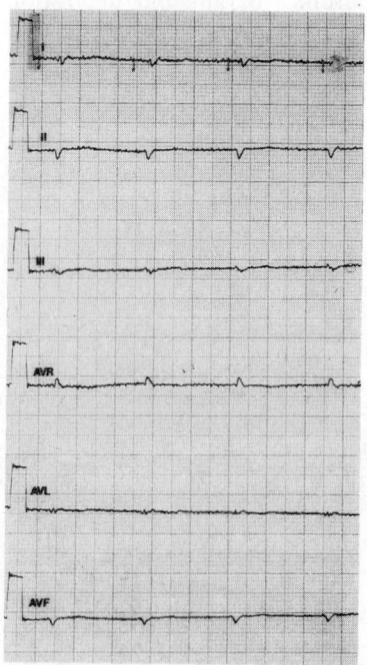

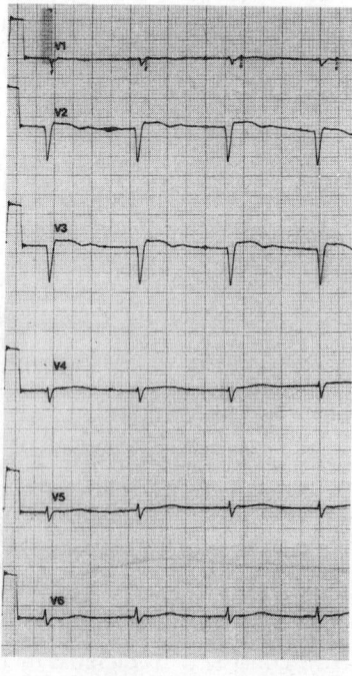

Fig. 38.2. Amyloid heart disease. 12-Lead electrocardiogram recorded at normal standardisation and showing low voltages.

dying of sarcoidosis. Over the past 15 years, Fleming has done much work on the clinical manifestations of this condition.[19,20]

The heart usually looks flabby with areas of infiltration scattered throughout the myocardium, particularly the left ventricular free wall, the papillary muscles, which are often completely replaced by granulomatous tissue, and the interventricular septum, which may be thinned or even aneurysmal from resulting fibrosis. The conducting system is often extensively replaced. The epicardium and the pericardium may be involved. Japanese workers have described acute and chronic forms of cardiac sarcoidosis.[21] Two types of acute histology are seen: an 'exudative' type with lymphocytic infiltration and oedema and a 'granulomatous' type, in which granulomata with epithelial cells predominate. These two types are associated with systemic disease and multisystem involvement and follow a subacute course.

The two types of chronic histology are fibrosis with or fibrosis without the presence of giant cells; these types follow a more insidious course. Diffuse interstitial fibrosis may give rise to generalized hypokinesia of the ventricles or localized focal contraction abnormalities.

The cardiac involvement may produce several clinical features.[22] The cardiomyopathy may have restrictive or congestive features due to the increased stiffness of the myocardium and the diminished systolic function. Arrhythmias, heart block and mitral regurgitation have been well documented. There is a high incidence of sudden death in cases of cardiac sarcoid (estimated at 60%) and this is often the first symptom. Table 38.1 is taken from Fleming's collection of 197 cases in the UK. The electrocardiogram is not specific and may include arrhythmias, conduction disturbances or

heart block; a pattern simulating myocardial infarction may be seen. The chest X-ray may give a clue to the diagnosis if there is bilateral lymphadenopathy or pulmonary involvement. Certain echocardiographic features, focal left ventricular wall motion abnormalities, particularly in the basal portion of the ventricular septum and free wall, may implicate cardiac sarcoid. Diffuse left ventricular hypokinesia with focal abnormalities in the antero-apical regions has also been described although this is not specific. In thallium radionuclide studies, segmental filling defects representing areas of infiltration of the myocardium have been documented.

The prognosis of cardiac sarcoidosis is very variable and has been poorly documented in published reports. Fleming believes the only way to make the diagnosis is to 'think of it' constantly in otherwise unexplained cases of cardiac disorder. A histological confirmation should be sought but endomyocardial biopsies are subject to considerable sampling errors; in autopsy-proven cases, 30% of biopsies are negative in the right ventricle and 53% are negative in the left ventricle.

The treatment will involve conventional therapy for such complications as heart failure and arrhythmias; a pacemaker may be necessary to treat heart block. Fleming believes that steroids should not be withheld,

"if in doubt use steroids – you cannot afford not to".

Steroids promote healing; occasionally, healing may be complicated by the development of an aneurysm in the left ventricle, the septum or the great vessels.

IRON STORAGE DISEASE IN THE HEART

Both haemochromatosis and haemosiderosis may be associated with the deposition of iron in the heart. Usually, when the myocardium is involved, other tissues, such as liver, spleen, pancreas and bone marrow, are already saturated with iron. Cardiac muscle has a greater affinity for iron than skeletal or smooth muscle. Iron is initially deposited in the perinuclear region of the myocardial fibre, but subsequently the whole fibre becomes involved. Cardiac dysfunction depends on the quantity of iron deposited in individual myocardial fibres and the number of fibres affected. Degeneration and loss of myocardial fibres leads to fibrosis with the resultant cardiac dilatation.

Cardiac failure is the predominant clinical pic-

Table 38.1. **Cardiac features of sarcoidosis at time of presentation in 197 cases (after Fleming).**

Features	No. of cases
Ventricular ectopic beats, ventricular tachycardia	77
First degree heart block and bundle branch block (especially right bundle branch block)	71
Complete heart block	42
Supraventricular arrhythmias	47
Sudden death	34
Myocardial disease	31
Simulating myocardial infarction	13
Pericarditis	4
Road-traffic/accident (valve involvement infrequent)	3

ture, although a restrictive cardiomyopathy may be seen early in the course of haemochromatosis. In a series of 1018 histologically proven cases of haemochromatosis, 31% had fatal cardiac failure. Atypical chest pain and transient arrhythmias, particularly atrial, occur but heart block is less common than arrhythmias.[23] There are no specific features, either clinically or on investigation, with reference to the heart alone, although the total clinical picture should suggest the diagnosis. Treatment will include the conventional measures for specific cardiac problems, such as heart failure and arrhythmias; repeated venesection and the use of chelating agents may be of general benefit.

CARCINOID HEART DISEASE

The carcinoid syndrome is an endocrine manifesta-

tion of neoplastic enterochromaffin cells.[24] The humoral consequences of enterochromaffin carcinoid tumours include cutaneous flushing, diarrhoea, valvar lesions of the right side of the heart, bronchoconstriction and facial telangectasia. The carcinoid syndrome is a rare cause of acquired cardiac disease, but cardiac involvement is a common cause of death.

Carcinoid tumours are primary tumours of the gastro-intestinal tract found predominantly in the appendix, which rarely arise from extraportal sites, such as the ovaries and lungs.[25] Serotonin overproduction, as manifested by excessive urinary excretion of its metabolite, 5-hydroxyindoleacetic acid (5HIAA), is the diagnostic hallmark of the carcinoid syndrome. Ileal tumours metastasize to the liver which results in 5-hydroxytryptamine and vasodilator peptides being released into the hepatic

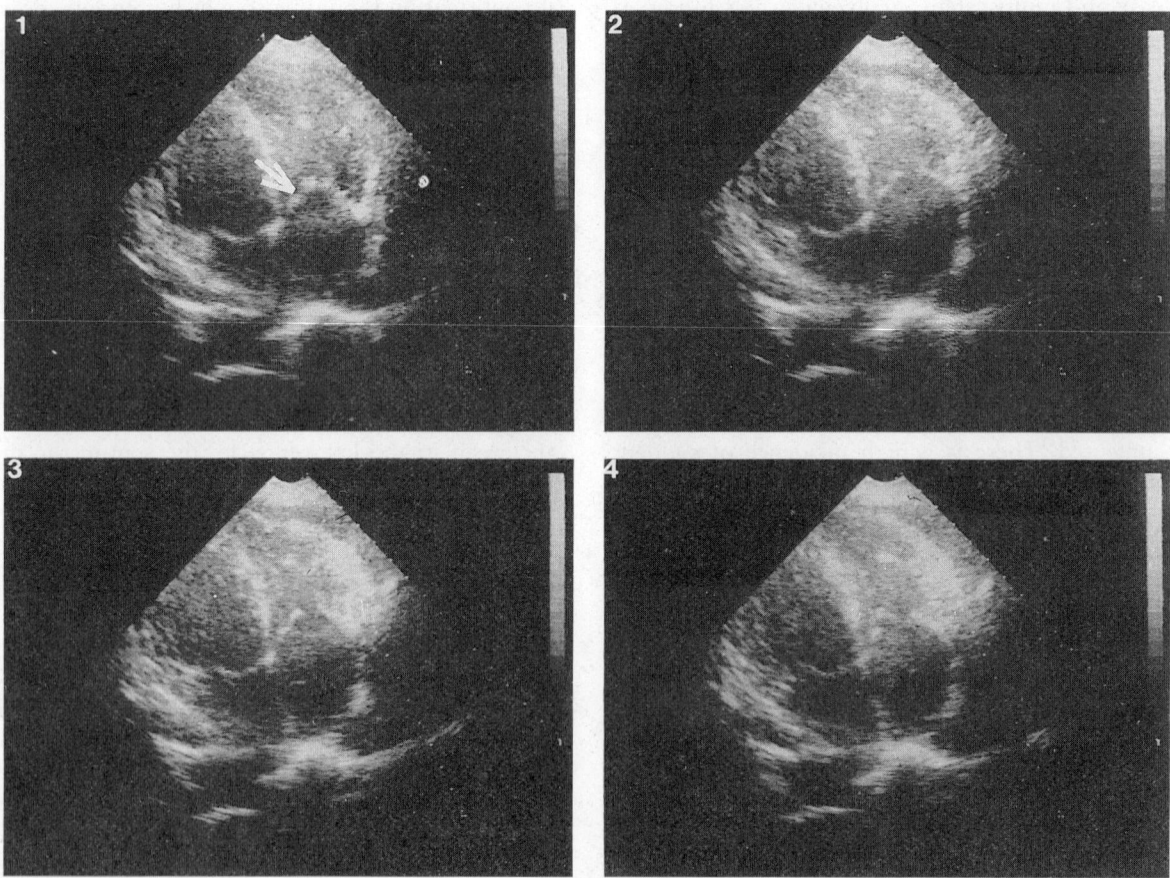

Fig. 38.4. Carcinoid heart disease. Cross-sectional echocardiogram in four-chamber view showing consecutive systolic frames (right ventricle on right of each frame). At the beginning of systole (1), the right ventricle and right atrium are enlarged compared with the left ventricle and left atrium. The tricuspid valve is irregularly thickened and has a high reflectance compared with the mitral valve but the leaflets are coapted. As systole proceeds and the right ventricular cavity dimensions decrease (2,3), the tricuspid valve leaflets lose their coaption and the tricuspid valve opens to reach a maximum at end-systole (4). The septal leaflet is relatively immobile (1, arrow). The mitral valve is normal and remains closed throughout the systole.

veins, thereby escaping degradation by the hepatic enzymes. The rare carcinoid tumours that arise from the ovaries and lungs release their endocrine mediators directly into the systemic circulation and can cause the carcinoid syndrome before metastasizing.

Cardiac involvement occurs in at least 50% of cases; right-sided involvement predominates with hepatic metastases, but lung carcinoids can produce left-sided cardiac lesions.[26] Plaques of pearly grey fibrous tissue are found on the endocardium, the endocardial surfaces of valves, the venae cavae and the coronary sinus. These plaques are probably the consequence of endocardial injury by vaso-active substances. Histologically, they consist of smooth muscle cells embedded in a stroma rich in acid mucopolysaccharides and collagen. The commonest cardiac lesions are a combination of tricuspid incompetence and tricuspid stenosis with pulmonary stenosis with or without pulmonary incompetence. The physical signs reflect the particular pattern of cardiac involvement; cardiac failure is a common mode of death. The diagnosis of carcinoid syndrome is made from the history and confirmed by an elevated 24-h excretion of 5HIAA in the urine. Liver ultrasonography may demonstrate tumour deposits; liver biopsy may produce a positive tissue diagnosis.

There are no specific electrocardiographic or chest radiographic appearances in carcinoid heart disease. Cross-sectional echocardiography may be very useful in making the diagnosis of cardiac involvement.[27] The tricuspid leaflets may be thickened in a nodular fashion and have a high reflectance. The septal leaflet is usually immobile and foreshortened, and the valve may be fixed in a semi-open position throughout the cardiac cycle. Another mechanism causing tricuspid regurgitation is the deposition of carcinoid tissue on the chordae tendineae and papillary muscles, producing thickening and a shortening and then traction on the valve leaflets as the right ventricular configuration changes during systole (Fig. 38.4).[28] The right atrium may be dilated. The pulmonary valve may be similarly uniformly thickened and immobile. The prognosis is variable, but cardiac involvement is inevitably fatal. Apart from symptomatic cardiac treatment, valve replacement has an important role in alleviating symptoms.[29] The distressing generalized symptoms of carcinoid heart disease may be palliated by resection of much of the metastatic tumour mass from the liver; resection may also delay the development of cardiac valvular lesions.

Specific pharmacological treatment is available for the unique form of carcinoid syndrome seen in a small subset of patients with tumours of gastric origin in whom flushing attacks can be prevented by a combination of H_1; and H_2-histamine antagonists. Trials of somatostatin analogues in the treatment of this condition are now being undertaken. Although some evidence suggests that serotonin may contribute to the valvular lesion, the mediator responsible for the pathogenesis of the lesions of the cardiac endocardium is not known.

REFERENCES

1. Benotti, J.R., Grossman, W. and Cohn, E.F. Clinical profile of restrictive cardiomyopathy. *Circulation* 1980; **61**: 1206–12.
2. Oakley, C.M. Clinical recognition of cardiomyopathies. *Circ. Res.* 1974; **35**(Suppl. II): 152.
3. Davis, J. In: Goodwin, J.F. ed. *Restrictive Cardiomyopathy in Heart Muscle Disease*. Lancaster: MTP Press Ltd, 1985, pp. 87–94.
4. Brockington, I.F. and Olsen, E.G.J. Loeffler's endocarditis and Davis' endocardial fibrosis. *Am. Heart J.* 1973; **85**: 308–22.
5. Davis, J., Spry, C.J.F., Vijayaraghava, G. and de Souza, J.A. A comparison of the clinical and cardiological features of endomyocardial disease in temperate and tropical regions. *Postgrad. Med. J.* 1983; **59**: 178–83.
6. Olsen, E.G.J. and Spry, C.J.F. The pathogenesis of Loeffler's endomyocardial disease and its relationship to endomyocardial fibrosis. *Prog. Cardiol.* 1979; **8**: 281–303.
7. Spry, C.J.F. and Tai, P.C. Studies on blood eosinophils II; patients with Loeffler's cardiomyopathy. *Clin. Exp. Immunol.* 1976; **24**: 423–34.
8. Spry, C.J.F., Tai, P.C., Davies, J., Olsen, E.G.J. and Goodwin, J.F. The role of eosinophils in myocarditis. In: Boulte, H.D. ed. *Viral Heart Disease*. Berlin, Heidelberg, New York and Tokyo: Springer Verlag, 1984, pp. 83–6.
9. Spry, C.J.F., Davis, J., Tai, P.C., Olsen, E.G.J., Oakley, C.M. and Goodwin, J.F. Clinical features of 15 patients with a hypereosinophilic syndrome. *Q. Gen. Med.* 1983; **52**: 1–22.
10. Davis, J., Spry, C.J.F., Sapsford, D.R. *et al.* Cardiovascular features of 11 patients with eosinophilic endomyocardial disease. *Q. J. Med.* 1983; **52**: 23–39.
11. Davis, J., Gibson, D.G., Foale, R. *et al.* Echocardiographic features of eosinophilic endomyocardial disease. *Br. Heart J.* 1982; **48**: 434–40.
12. Davis, J. and Spry, C.J.F. Plasma exchange in leucophoresis in the hypereosinophilic syndrome. *Ann. Intern. Med.* 1982; **6**: 791.
13. Davis, J., Sapsford, R., Brooksby, I. *et al.* Successful surgical treatment of two patients with eosinophilic endomyocardial disease. *Br. Heart J.* 1981; **46**: 73–81.
14. Glenner, G.C. Amyloid deposits in amyloidosis. *N. Engl. J. Med.* 1980; **302**: 1283–333; 1292–343.
15. Brandt, K., Cathcart, E.S. and Cohen, A.S. A clinical analysis of the course and diagnosis of 42 patients with amyloidosis. *Am. J. Med.* 1968; **44**: 955.
16. Oakley, C.M. Amyloid heart disease. In: Goodwin, J.F. ed. *Heart Muscle Disease*. Lancaster: MTP Press Ltd, 1985, pp. 141–53.
17. Child, J.S., Levisman, J.A., Abbas, A.S. and MacAlpine, R.N. Echocardiographic manifestations of infiltrated car-

diomyopathy: A report of 7 cases due to amyloid. *Chest* 1976; **70**: 726–31.

18. Scadding, J.G. *Sarcoidosis*. London: Eyre and Spottiswoode, 1967, p. 291.
19. Fleming, H.A. and Bailey, S.M. Sarcoid heart disease. *J. R. Coll. Phys. Lond.* 1981; **15**: 245–53.
20. Fleming, H.A. Sarcoid heart disease. *Br. Heart J*. 1974; **36**: 54–68.
21. Sakiguchi, M., Umao, U., Imai, M., Furuei, T. and Mikami, R. Clinical and histological profile of sarcoidosis of the heart and acute idiopathic myocarditis. Concepts through a study employing endomyocardial biopsy: I sarcoidosis. *Jap. Circ. J*. 1980; **44**: 249–63.
22. Roberts, W.C., McAllister, J. and Ferrans, A.J. Sarcoidosis of the heart. A clinico-pathological study of 35 necrotic patients (group 1) and review of 78 previously described necropsy patients (group 2). *Am. J. Med.* 1977; **63**: 86–108.
23. Buja, L.M. and Roberts, W.C. Iron in the heart. Etiology and clinical significance. *Am. J. Med.* 1971; **51**: 209–21.
24. Grahame-Smith, D.G. The carcinoid syndrome. *Am. J. Cardiol.* 1968; **21**: 376–87.
25. Oates, J.A. The carcinoid syndrome. *N. Engl. J. Med.* 1986; **315**: 702–3.
26. Roberts, W.C. and Msjaerdisma, A. The cardiac disease associated with the carcinoid syndrome (carcinoid heart disease). *Am. J. Med.* 1964; **36**: 5–34.
27. Howard, R.J., Dropac, M., Ryder, W.D. *et al*. Carcinoid heart disease; diagnosis by two dimensional echocardiography. *Circulation* 1982; **66**: 1059–65.
28. Davies, M.K., Lowry, P.J. and Littler, W.A. Cross sectional echocardiography featuring carcinoid heart disease. A mechanism for tricuspid regurgitation syndrome. *Br. Heart J*. 1984; **51**: 355–7.
29. Hendel, N., Lecke, P. and Richards, J. Carcinoid heart disease: eight years survival following tricuspid valve replacement at pulmonary valvotomy. *Ann. Thorac. Surg.* 1980; **30**: 391–5.

Chapter 39

Hypertrophic Cardiomyopathy

William J. McKenna

Reports of individual patients who undoubtedly had hypertrophic cardiomyopathy appear over 100 years ago in the literature.[1,2] The first systematic characterization of such patients, however, was not reported until 1958 when the pathologist Donald Teare described asymmetric hypertrophy in the hearts of 9 adolescents and young adults who had died suddenly.[3] Detailed clinical characterization and the recognition of the familial nature of the condition followed shortly.[4] In the literature, more than 60 names have been given to the condition.[5] This multiplicity of terms reflects different views of the pathophysiology of hypertrophic cardiomyopathy, which are a function of the techniques used for assessment. In the 1960s, a left ventricular outflow tract gradient that was increased following administration of catecholamine and reduced after administration of phenylephrine was considered to be the essential feature of the condition (Fig. 39.1); thus, idiopathic hypertrophic subaortic stenosis,

obstructive cardiomyopathy and muscular subaortic stenosis were early names applied to the condition. Subsequently, it was recognized that the majority of patients do not have left ventricular gradients.[6] In the 1970s, M-mode echocardiography became widely available. This permitted visualization of the upper anterior septum and left ventricular posterior wall,[7–9] the thickest and thinnest myocardial segments, and, thus, the asymmetric nature of the condition was re-affirmed; some investigators proposed that asymmetric septal hypertrophy (ASH) was the pathognomonic feature of the condition.[10] With the subsequent development of two-dimensional echocardiography and nuclear magnetic resonance imaging, the broader spectrum of the condition is now appreciated.[11–14] The majority of patients have asymmetric septal hypertrophy; however, hypertrophy may be symmetric or confined to the left ventricular free wall, posterior wall and rarely to the right ventricle.

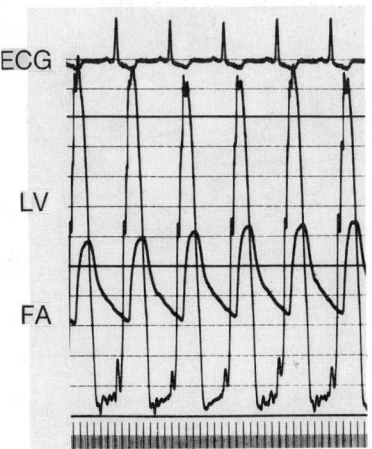
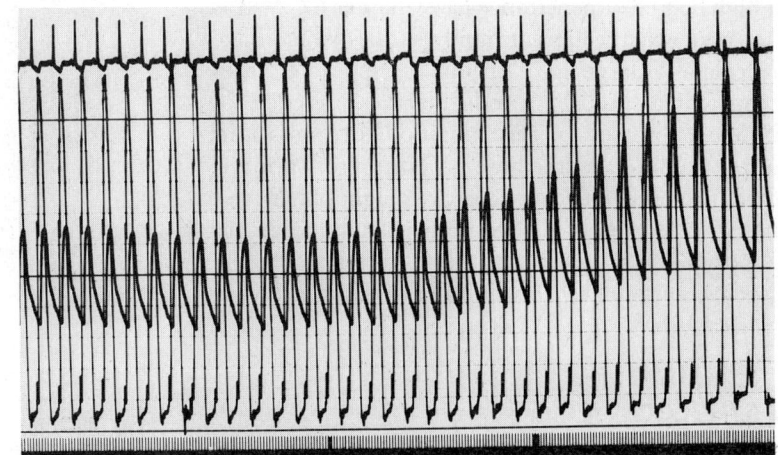

Fig. 39.1. Left ventricular (LV) and femoral artery (FA) pressure traces. The peak aortic pressure is 230 mmHg and there is a peak-to-peak left ventricular to aortic gradient of 120 mmHg. Left, during the infusion of phenylephrine, the aortic pressure is increased in association with a reduction in the left ventricular gradient and an increase in left ventricular end-diastolic pressure. On the right administration of phenylephrine helps differentiate the functional gradient of hypertrophic cardiomyopathy from the fixed obstruction of valvular aortic stenosis.

DEFINITION

Currently, hypertrophic cardiomyopathy is defined as an idiopathic heart muscle condition characterized by a hypertrophied and non-dilated left and/or right ventricle in the absence of a cardiac or systemic cause.[5,15,16] This definition of unexplained myocardial hypertrophy is useful in the clinical and prognostic assessment of patients and is now widely accepted. It must be recognized, however, that such a diagnosis of exclusion often presents problems. Does the young adult with a blood pressure of 160/95 mmHg and 2-cm left ventricular hypertrophy have one or two diseases? Is 2.5-cm hypertrophy a physiological response in a highly trained athlete? Such diagnostic difficulties, which are not uncommon, illustrate the limitations of the current definition of hypertrophic cardiomyopathy and underscore the need to determine the molecular basis of the condition and to find pathognomonic, genetic, immunological or metabolic markers.

EPIDEMIOLOGY

Hypertrophic cardiomyopathy has been described in Western, African and Asian populations.[5,17–20] In a study by workers at the Mayo Clinic of residents in Olmstead County, Minnesota, the incidence of unexplained left ventricular hypertrophy was 3 per 100 000 per year and the prevalence was 20 per 100 000 general population.[21] Hypertrophic cardiomyopathy appears to be a genetic disease with autosomal dominant transmission and a high degree of penetrance (see Chapter 67).[22] It is not clear whether recent family studies which have revealed a large proportion of sporadic cases (approximately 50%) indicate the presence of different diseases, of new mutations or limitations of the studies;[23,24] the high proportion of sporadic cases probably reflects insensitive diagnostic criteria based on secondary changes rather than the primary abnormality as well as other limitations of the studies, particularly the inability to assess multiple generations.

PATHOLOGY

MACROSCOPIC

The description of a disease may reflect the pinhole through which a condition is viewed; even the pathologist may have been influenced by the clinician's ante-mortem diagnosis.[25] Although asymmetric septal hypertrophy was emphasized in Teare's original pathological report (Fig. 39.2)[3] and by subsequent M-mode echocardiographic studies,[7–10] hypertrophic cardiomyopathy can occur in many other forms.[11–13] It is now clear that hypertrophic cardiomyopathy may involve the left, right or both ventricles.[26,27] Hypertrophy is usually symmetric in the right ventricle,[27] but in the left ventricle it may be symmetric or asymmetric, involving the septum, free wall, posterior wall or occasionally being isolated to the distal ventricle.[11–13,28] Another macroscopic finding is a patch of endocardial thickening just below the aortic valve resulting from contact with the anterior mitral leaflet in patients with reduced left ventricular dimensions, particularly that of the outflow tract.[28] Occasionally, the disease is found in hearts that do not appear to have any macroscopic abnormality, are not hypertrophied and do not have increased muscle mass.[29] Such patients highlight a limitation of the current definition based on the demonstration of unexplained left ventricular hypertrophy, indicating that hypertrophy may be a secondary rather than a primary abnormality.

HISTOLOGY

The histological findings in hypertrophic car-

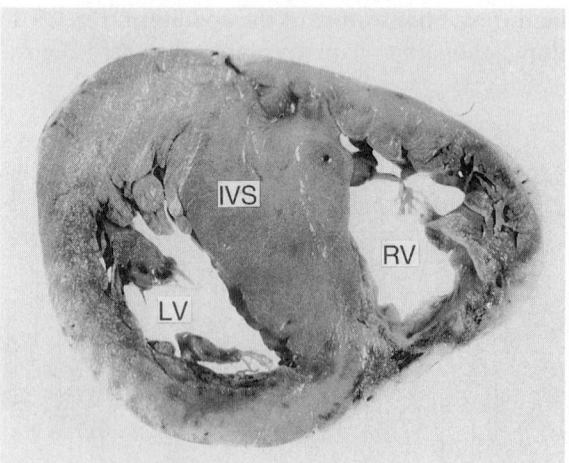

Fig. 39.2. Macroscopic section of the heart of patient 5 from Teare's original report.[3] She died suddenly, aged 21 years, while running to catch a bus. There is marked anterior and posterior septal hypertrophy with relative sparing of the left ventricular free and posterior walls. There is also moderate right ventricular hypertrophy, best demonstrated in the right ventricular outflow tract area. LV, left ventricle; RV, right ventricle; IVS, interventricular septum. (By courtesy of Professor M.J. Davies.)

diomyopathy are distinctive (Pl. 39.1) and provide an almost specific morphology.[30] Within areas of affected myocardium, there is considerable interstitial fibrosis with gross disorganization of the muscle bundles resulting in a characteristic whorled pattern.[31] The cell-to-cell orientation of muscle cells is lost (disarray) and there is disorganization of the myofibrillar architecture within a given cell.[32] Myocardial cells are wide, short and often bizarre in shape. Foci of disorganized cells are often interspersed among areas of hypertrophied muscle cells that are otherwise normal in appearance. Although these changes are diagnostic, they are not completely specific because there is some malarrangement, but no other histological abnormality, found at the junction of the septum with the anterior and posterior walls of the left ventricle in normal subjects,[33] and congenitally abnormal hearts may also show fibre disarray.[34] Although the absolute specificity of these histological changes has been a matter of controversy, experienced pathologists agree that given the whole heart at autopsy the diagnosis is not usually difficult to make.[28,30]

PATHOPHYSIOLOGY

Myocardial disarray and hypertrophy, hyperdynamic systolic function and impaired diastolic function account for many of the clinical features of hypertrophic cardiomyopathy. The extent and distribution of myocardial disarray are determined at post-mortem; at present, they cannot be readily assessed during life. It is probable that the disorganized architecture with abnormal myofibre and myofibrillar alignment provides a substrate for electrical instability and contributes to diastolic abnormalities.[29] However, the precise relation of myocardial disarray with spontaneous arrhythmia and the threshold for ventricular fibrillation have not been established. The severity of myocardial hypertrophy can be readily assessed with two-dimensional echocardiography. It is uncertain whether the development of myocardial disarray and of myocardial hypertrophy are unrelated responses to a molecular or a developmental abnormality or are contingent upon each other.[35] The recognition of patients who have severe left ventricular hypertrophy and minimal disarray and those who have severe disarray and minimal hypertrophy is consistent with the former hypothesis.[29]

Most patients have evidence of hyperdynamic systolic function with rapid, early and near complete ventricular emptying.[4,36] As left ventricular hypertrophy is usually prominent, such changes may be secondary to myocardial hypertrophy; some patients, however, have hyperdynamic systolic function with minimal hypertrophy suggesting the presence of other abnormalities, such as altered handling of calcium by the myocardium.[37-40] Approximately 30% of patients with hyperdynamic systolic function have recordable gradients at rest between the body and outflow tract of the left ventricle; an additional 20–25% develop such a gradient following manoeuvres that increase myocardial contractility or result in a decrease in ventricular volume with reduced afterload or venous return.[41] The mechanism and significance of such gradients have been subjects of controversy.[42,43] Many workers have claimed that the development of a left ventricular gradient in close temporal association with the development of systolic anterior motion of the mitral valve and a fall in peak aortic velocity represents impediment or obstruction to left ventricular emptying.[42] Another interpretation of these findings is that they are generated by a dynamic left ventricle that has almost completely emptied.[43] Interpretation of the significance of a left ventricular gradient in an individual patient requires knowledge of the relative volume ejected by the onset of the gradient.[44,45] In the majority of patients with resting left ventricular gradients, at least 70% of stroke volume has already been ejected by the onset of the gradient.[45-47] Although it is fascinating, the argument about left ventricular gradients has dominated many investigators' approach to hypertrophic cardiomyopathy to the detriment of more important issues, for example, the mechanism and prevention of sudden death and the molecular genetics and pathophysiology of the condition.

Diastolic abnormalities are common, although less obvious.[36,48-50] The period during which the heart is isovolumic (end-systole and early diastole) is prolonged, filling is slow and the proportion of filling volume that results from atrial systolic contraction may be increased. Occasionally, there is early rapid filling with restrictive physiology which resembles the situation in patients with constrictive pericarditis or endocardial fibrosis. It is seldom possible to identify the predominant pathophysiological mechanism of altered diastolic function because most patients have myocardial hypertrophy, evidence suggestive of ischaemia and architectural abnormalities including myocardial disarray and fibrosis.

CLINICAL FEATURES

HISTORY

The evidence suggests that hypertrophic cardiomyopathy is a Mendelian disorder with autosomal dominant inheritance. There is therefore no major sex preponderance, although the condition is more often diagnosed in younger men and older females. Symptomatic presentation may be at any age with breathlessness on exertion, chest pain, syncope or sudden death. Occasionally, hypertrophic cardiomyopathy is found at autopsy in a stillborn or presents during infancy with cardiac failure which is usually fatal.[51] In children and adolescents, the diagnosis is most often made during screening of siblings and offspring of affected family members.[52,53] Paroxysmal symptoms or mild impairment of exercise tolerance are often present but in the absence of a murmur may not elicit a diagnostic cardiac evaluation. Approximately 50% of consecutive adult patient populations present with symptoms,[41] whereas in the remainder the diagnosis is made during family screening or following the detection of an abnormality on physical, electrocardiographic or echocardiographic examination.

Approximately 50% of patients experience dyspnoea,[4,41] thought to be a consequence of elevated left ventricular diastolic, left atrial and pulmonary venous pressures resulting from impaired ventricular relaxation and filling. However, in a recent study, there was no relationship between an objective measurement of maximal exercise capacity and pulmonary capillary wedge pressures, indicating that, as for patients with cardiac failure, other mechanisms such as control of muscle energetics and blood flow and central perception of breathlessness may be important.[54] Approximately 50% of patients complain of chest pain which is exertional, atypical or both in similar proportions of patients.[41,55] Atypical pain may have no obvious precipitant; more commonly, it follows exercise or anxiety-related tachycardia when it persists for up to several hours after the stress has been removed without enzymatic evidence of myocardial damage.[55] Speculation over the mechanism of chest pain in hypertrophic cardiomyopathy continues; the increased metabolic demand of the greatly increased muscle mass in association with decreased diastolic perfusion of sub-endocardial layers, resulting from a relative increase in coronary impedance from poorly relaxing muscle and from narrowed small intramural coronary arteries, may contribute to it.[56] Approximately 15–25% of patients have experienced syncopal episodes and in only a minority are there findings suggestive of an arrhythmia or evidence of overt conduction disease.[41,57] In most patients, the mechanism cannot be determined. The surgical experience of workers at Düsseldorf is of interest. After successful myotomy/myectomy, their results have shown a greatly reduced incidence of syncope and sudden death; these findings are consistent with a haemodynamically related mechanism.[57,58] However, the view that syncope is related to an inability to increase cardiac output during exercise appears to be too simplistic: syncopal episodes can occur at rest or during normal daily activities and can develop in patients whose cardiac output response during exercise is normal.[59] Rarely, patients present with symptoms attributable to left or right heart failure with paroxysmal nocturnal dyspnoea, cough, ascites or peripheral oedema. Thus, there is a wide spectrum of clinical presentation in hypertrophic cardiomyopathy, from severe cardiac failure in infancy to an incidental finding that may occur at any age.

PHYSICAL EXAMINATION

In the majority of patients with hypertrophic cardiomyopathy, the physical examination is unremarkable and the detection of abnormalities is dependent on the elucidation of subtle physical signs. The majority of patients have a rapid upstroke arterial pulse, best felt in the carotid area, which reflects dynamic left ventricular emptying. In children and adolescents, this pulse may be difficult to distinguish from normality, whereas in the elderly, the normal pulse transmitted by non-compliant atheromatous vessels may appear to have a rapid upstroke. The majority of patients also have a forceful left ventricular cardiac impulse, best appreciated on full held expiration in the left lateral position. In about one-third of patients the jugular venous pulse may demonstrate a prominent 'a' wave reflecting diminished right ventricular compliance secondary to right ventricular hypertrophy. The first and second heart sounds are usually normal, and, unless patients are in atrial fibrillation, there is either a loud fourth heart sound, reflecting increased atrial systolic flow into a non-compliant ventricle, or a palpable atrial beat reflecting forceful atrial systolic contraction which may or may not be associated with significant forward flow of blood. The most obvious physical sign in hypertrophic cardiomyopathy is an ejection systolic murmur present only in those patients (one-third) who have a resting left ventricular outflow tract gradient. This murmur starts well after the first heart sound and ends well before the second. It is best heard at the left sternal border radiating towards the aortic and mitral areas but not into the neck or the axilla. The intensity of outflow tract murmurs varies with changes in ventricular volume; it can be increased by physiological and pharmacological manoeuvres that decrease afterload or venous return (amyl nitrate, standing, Valsalva) and decreased by man- oeuvres that increase afterload and venous return (squatting, phenylephrine). Occasionally, ejection systolic murmurs are associated at their onset with an ejection sound. The majority of patients with a left ventricular gradient also have mild mitral regurgitation which may be difficult to distinguish by auscultation. Doppler examination reveals that mitral regurgitation usually begins just before (30– 40 ms) the onset of the gradient and continues for the duration of systole. Radiation of the systolic murmur to the axilla is often the best auscultatory clue to the presence of co-existent mitral regurgita- tion. Occasionally, mitral regurgitation may be moderate to severe either alone or in association with a left ventricular outflow tract gradient. A mid-diastolic rumble may occasionally result from increased transmitral flow in patients with severe mitral regurgitation; more commonly, it occurs in isolation, presumably reflecting inflow tract turbu- lence. Early diastolic murmurs of aortic incompe- tence may develop following surgical myotomy/ myectomy or infective endocarditis involving the aortic valve. Although such murmurs are rare in the absence of such complications, they appear to occur more commonly than would be expected by chance and may reflect traction of the non-coronary cusp of the aortic valve by the septum. An ejection systolic murmur in the pulmonary area, reflecting right ventricular outflow tract obstruction, is also rare; when present, it is usually associated with severe biventricular hypertrophy and is more commonly seen in the young.[52,53]

DIAGNOSIS

The diagnosis of hypertrophic cardiomyopathy is based upon the demonstration of unexplained myocardial hypertrophy, which is best done using two-dimensional echocardiography; ideally, measurements of wall thickness should exceed two standard deviations for age-, sex- and size-matched populations. This latter consideration may be im- portant as myocardial mass increases with both age and size. In practice, in an adult of normal size, the presence of a left ventricular myocardial segment of 1.5 cm or greater in thickness is usually considered to be diagnostic.[11–13] Isolated right ventricular hypertrophic cardiomyopathy is extremely rare. When the classical clinical features, including a left ventricular outflow tract murmur, are present or when more subtle clinical features are associated with a positive family history of the condition, echocardiography may serve only to confirm the diagnosis. More often, however, the history, physic- al examination and electrocardiogram are equivocal and not diagnostic, and reliance is placed on the two-dimensional echocardiographic findings.

In children and adolescents, myocardial hypertro- phy often develops during growth spurts.[60] Thus, a negative diagnosis made before adolescent growth has been completed must be tempered by the proviso for a subsequent re-assessment. In adults, however, the development of left ventricular hyper- trophy *de novo* has not been reported. In the elderly, physical signs may be misleading because inelastic arteries may give rise to a large-volume rapidly rising pulse, and the systolic murmurs of aortic sclerosis or stenosis, mitral regurgitation and mitral valve prolapse from chordal rupture or papillary muscle dysfunction are common and may resemble the systolic murmur of hypertrophic car- diomyopathy. Also, the left ventricular outflow tract murmur typical of hypertrophic car- diomyopathy often decreases or disappears with age and gradual deterioration in left ventricular systolic function. Thus, in the elderly, the electrocardiogram and in particular the echocardiogram become very important diagnostically.[61] Practical problems in diagnosis often arise in highly trained athletes and in patients with mild hypertension in whom the hypertrophic response appears greater than ex- pected from the apparent stimulus. Highly trained athletes normally have an increase in muscle mass with an upward shift of about 3 mm in the bell-shaped curve for the distribution of left ven- tricular wall thickness.[62] The determinants of the hypertrophic response in a patient with hyperten- sion, including the duration and severity of previous hypertension, are seldom known. In both groups of subjects, the diagnosis of hypertrophic car- diomyopathy is more dependent on the total clinical picture. For example, an athlete who has concentric 1.7 cm left ventricular hypertrophy and a family history of hypertrophic cardiomyopathy or the physical signs of a left ventricular outflow tract gradient with a small left ventricular cavity probably does have hypertrophic cardiomyopathy, whereas an athlete who has a negative family history, normal left ventricular cavity dimensions and no evidence of a gradient is unlikely to have hypertrophic cardiomyopathy. In a middle-aged or elderly hypertensive with mild symmetrical left ventricular hypertrophy, it may not be clinically important whether one or two diseases are present. The diagnostic decision in the young athlete, however, could have a significant effect on his/her future lifestyle.

INVESTIGATIONS

Cardiological evaluation of patients with hypertrophic cardiomyopathy is performed to confirm or make the diagnosis, to characterize the functional and morphological features in order to guide symptomatic therapy, and to assess the risk of complications, particularly that of sudden death.

ELECTROCARDIOGRAPHY

The 12-lead electrocardiogram is normal in 5% of symptomatic patients and in 25% of asymptomatic patients, particularly those who are young.[4,63] At the time of diagnosis, 10% of patients are in atrial fibrillation, 20% have left axis deviation and 5% have right bundle branch block pattern.[41,63] The majority of patients have an intraventricular conduction delay, but complete left bundle branch block pattern is rare. It may develop following surgery and is occasionally seen in the elderly. ST-segment depression and T-wave changes are the most common abnormalities and are usually associated with voltage changes of left ventricular hypertrophy and/or deep S waves in the anterior chest leads V_1–V_3.[63] Occasionally, giant negative T waves are seen.[19] Repolarization changes alone or isolated voltage criteria for left ventricular hypertrophy are unusual. Approximately 20% of patients have abnormal Q waves either inferiorly (2,3 and aVF) or less commonly in leads 1–aVL and V_4–V_6 or in anteroseptal leads V_1–V_3. The distribution of the PR interval is similar to that in the normal population but occasionally a short PR interval may be associated with a slurred upstroke to the QRS complex, similar to that seen in the Wolff–Parkinson–White syndrome. At electrophysiologic-al study, such changes are not usually associated with evidence of pre-excitation although patients with hypertrophic cardiomyopathy and accessory pathways have been described.[64] P-wave abnormalities of left and/or right atrial overload are common reflecting the difficulties faced by the atria in emptying their contents into poorly relaxing, stiff ventricles. As there are so many electrocardiographic abnormalities, there is no electrocardiogram typical of hypertrophic cardiomyopathy; a useful rule is to consider the diagnosis whenever the electrocardiogram is bizarre, particularly in younger patients.

In adults, arrhythmias are common during 48-hour ambulatory electrocardiographic monitoring.[65,66] Non-sustained ventricular tachycardia (Fig. 39.3) is detected in 25–30% of patients. Although this arrhythmia is invariably asymptomatic, its presence represents an approximately sevenfold increased risk of sudden death over those patients with hypertrophic cardiomyopathy who do not have non-sustained ventricular tachycardia.[66–68] Established atrial fibrillation is detected in 10–15% of consecutive patient populations; a further 30–35% will have episodes of paroxysmal atrial fibrillation or supraventricular tachycardia.[65,66] Sustained supraventricular arrhythmias (> 30 s) are poorly tolerated unless the ventricular response is controlled; they carry an increased risk of embolism. In contrast, most children and adolescents are in sinus rhythm and arrhythmias during ambulatory electrocardiographic monitoring are uncommon (Table 39.1).[69] The increased incidence of supraventricular arrhythmias with age is not surprising as the development of these arrhythmias is related to increased echocardiographic left atrial dimensions and increased left ventricular end-diastolic pressure, both of which increase with age.[65,66] The aetiology of non-sustained ventricular arrhythmias is not known but it may relate to myocyte necrosis and myocardial fibrosis which appear to be related to age. The occurrence of documented sustained ventricular tachycardia is extremely rare (3 cases).[70] The optimal duration and the method of electrocardiographic monitoring to detect asymptomatic but prognostically important ventricular arrhythmia depend upon the frequency with which episodes occur. Ventricular arrhythmias have been shown to have a marked biological variability; at initial evaluation of a patient, 5 days of electrocardiographic monitoring is necessary to ensure at least a 75% chance of not missing non-sustained ventricu-

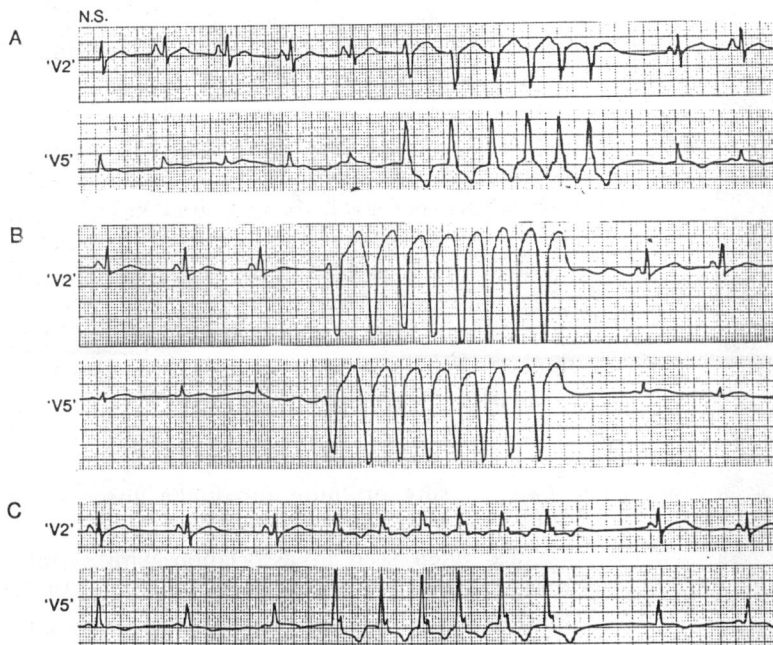

Fig. 39.3. Simultaneous two-channel ambulatory electrocardiographic recordings from a patient with hypertrophic cardiomyopathy. Some of the characteristic features of ventricular tachycardia in hypertrophic cardiomyopathy are shown. The episodes are multiform, initiated by a late coupled ventricular extrasystole and are neither sustained nor excessively fast. (Reproduced with permission from McKenna *et al.*, *Am. J. Cardiol.* 1984; **54**: 802–10.[114]

lar tachycardia.[71] The recommendation of 48 h represents a pragmatic compromise which is unlikely to give rise to an important sampling error.[68,71]

CHEST X-RAY

The chest X-ray may be normal or show evidence of left and/or right atrial or left ventricular enlargement; if left atrial pressure has been chronically elevated, there may be redistribution of blood flow to upper lung zones with interstitial changes including Kerley B lines. Mitral valve annular calcification is not uncommon. Aortic valve calcification is not seen; when present, it suggests a diagnosis of aortic stenosis rather than one of hypertrophic cardiomyopathy.

TWO-DIMENSIONAL ECHOCARDIOGRAPHY/DOPPLER

In hypertrophic cardiomyopathy, two-dimensional echocardiography has replaced the M-mode technique in the assessment of the severity and distribution of myocardial hypertrophy because of its capacity to visualize the entire heart rather than just the upper anterior septum and posterior wall. It is now recognized that left ventricular hypertrophy may be symmetric or asymmetric and localized to the septum, the free wall but most commonly to both the septum and free wall with relative sparing of the posterior wall (Fig. 39.4). In Japan, 'apical' hypertrophic cardiomyopathy appears to be common;[19,20] in the West, hypertrophy confined to the apex is rare, although approximately 10% of patients have left ventricular hypertrophy which is maximal in the distal ventricle from the level of the papillary muscle down to the apex (Fig. 39.5).[13] Approximately one-third of patients also have hypertrophy of the right ventricular free wall (Fig. 39.6); the severity of right ventricular hypertrophy is strongly related to the severity of left ventricular hypertrophy.[27] Typically, left ventricular end-

Table 39.1. The incidence of arrhythmia in relation to age in 177 patients with hypertrophic cardiomyopathy.

	Age (year)				
	≤ 15 (n = 20)	16–20 (n = 50)	31–45 (n = 32)	46–60 (n = 52)	> 60 (n = 23)
Atrial fibrillation	0	0	2 (6%)	4 (8%)	2 (9%)
Supraventricular tachycardia	1 (5%)	8 (16%)	12 (40%)	17 (35%)	8 (38%)
Ventricular tachycardia	0	8 (16%)	10 (31%)	14 (27%)	6 (26%)

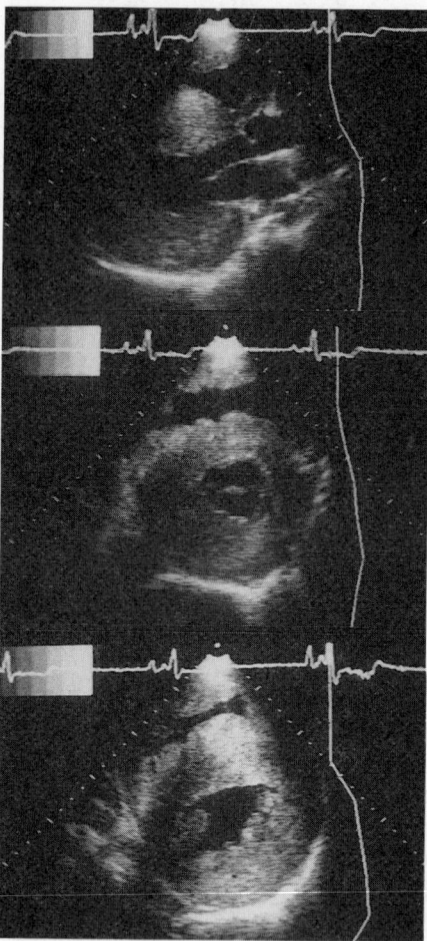

Fig. 39.4. Two-dimensional echocardiographic views from an adolescent with hypertrophic cardiomyopathy. In the upper panel, a diastolic long-axis view shows severe upper septal and left ventricular posterior wall hypertrophy of approximately 4 cm. Left atrial dimension is not increased. In the middle and lower panels, short-axis views are recorded at mitral valve (middle) and papillary muscle level (lower) showing severe symmetric left ventricular hypertrophy.

systolic and end-diastolic dimensions are reduced, and the left atrial dimension is increased. The left ventricular outflow tract appears narrowed, particularly when there is gross upper septal hypertrophy, and right ventricular dimensions are normal while indices of systolic function, such as ejection fraction and velocity of fibre shortening are increased. Colour Doppler provides a sensitive method of detecting left ventricular outflow tract turbulence and when combined with continuous wave Doppler the peak velocity of left ventricular blood flow can be measured and left ventricular outflow tract gradients calculated by the modified Bernoulli equation:[72,73]

$$\text{Pressure gradient (mmHg)} = 4V_{max}^2$$

Doppler-calculated gradients correlate well with those measured invasively. When the calculated outflow tract gradient is > 30 mmHg, systolic anterior motion of the mitral valve is usually present.[74,75] This is best demonstrated on M-mode recordings which have the advantage of being able to time cardiac events when recorded at fast paper speed. Measurement of the time from the onset of systolic anterior motion of the mitral valve (SAM) to the onset of SAM–septal contact (x) and the duration of SAM–septal contact (y) provides another reliable non-invasive method for estimation of the pressure gradient:[76,77]

$$\text{Gradient} = (y/x)\,25 + 25 \text{ mmHg}$$

Early closure or fluttering of the aortic valve leaflets and Doppler evidence of mitral regurgitation are often seen in association with systolic anterior motion of the mitral valve (Fig. 39.7). Contrary to earlier reports in the literature, systolic anterior motion of the mitral valve is found in other conditions associated with left ventricular hypertrophy and hyperdynamic systolic performance.[78]

EXERCISE TESTING

Maximal exercise testing is simple, non-invasive and provides useful functional and possibly prognostic information. When used in association with respiratory gas analysis, it provides an objective assessment of exercise capacity which can be monitored serially. Maximal oxygen ventilatory capacity (Vo_2max) is moderately reduced even in patients who claim their exercise tolerance is not limited.[54] Careful measurement of the blood pressure every minute or, if possible, continuously during exercise reveals that approximately one-third of patients have an abnormal blood-pressure response with drops of 25–150 mmHg from peak recordings.[59] In the majority, such changes are asymptomatic but preliminary observations suggest that they are likely to be of prognostic significance. The mechanism of the hypotensive response during exercise in hypertrophic cardiomyopathy is not known but it may be related to altered baroreflex control of blood flow.[59] ST-Segment changes of > 2 mm from baseline are documented in 25% of patients and associated with symptoms of angina. The relation of such changes to ischaemia and thallium defects requires further evaluation and their prognostic significance has yet to be determined.[79]

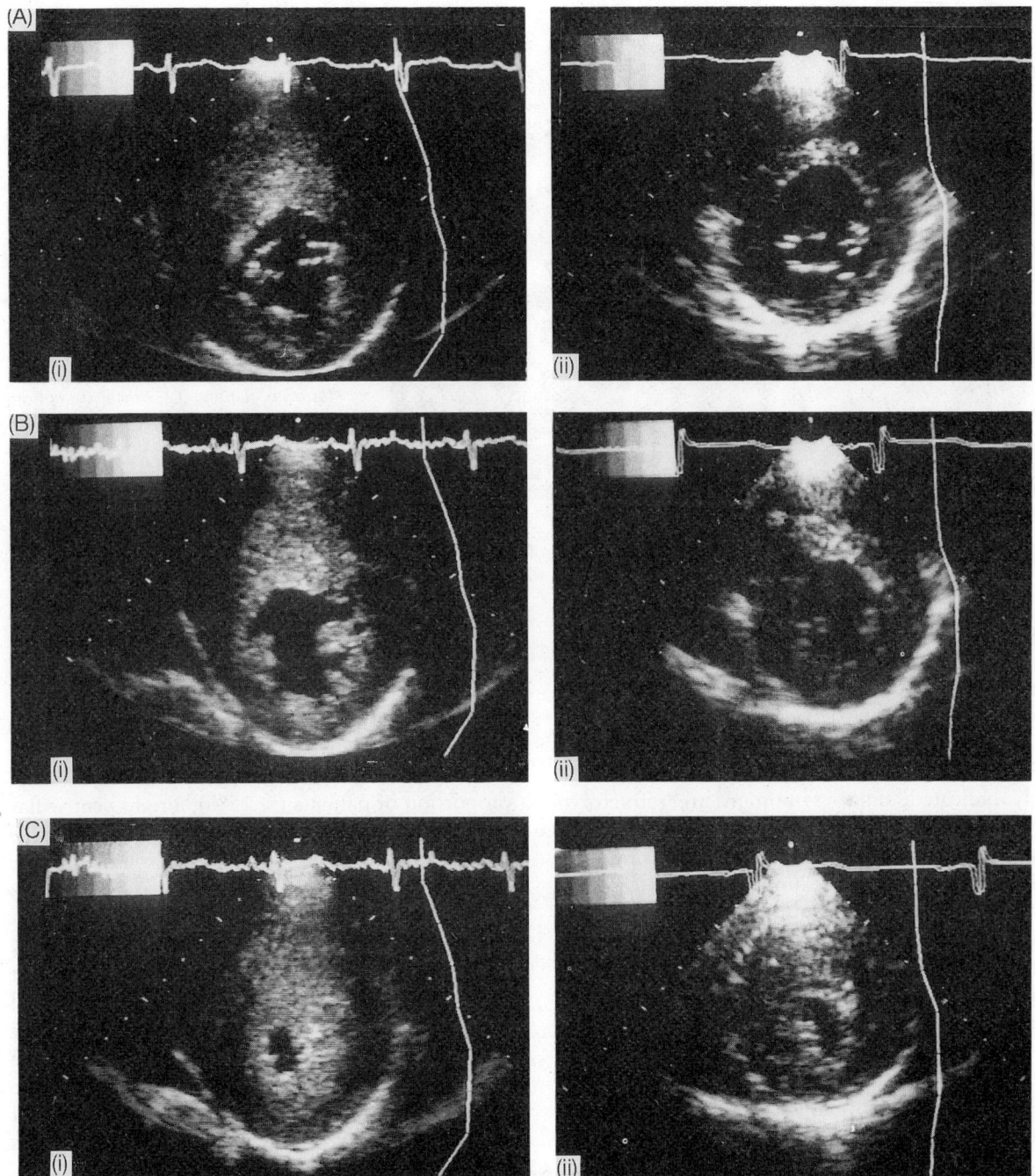

Fig. 39.5. On the left (i) are short axis views recorded at mitral valve tip level (A), papillary muscle level (B) and in the distal ventricle (C) revealing severe asymmetric septal hypertrophy. At mitral valve and papillary muscle level the hypertrophy is most marked in the upper anterior and posterior septum and there is relative sparing of the left ventricular free and posterior walls. On the right (ii) are short-axis two-dimensional echocardiographic recordings at comparable levels (A–C) from mitral valve to the apex of the left ventricle in a patient whose hypertrophy is largely confined to the distal ventricle. There is no left ventricular hypertrophy at the level of the mitral valve tip. (By courtesy of Dr P. Nihoyannopoulos.)

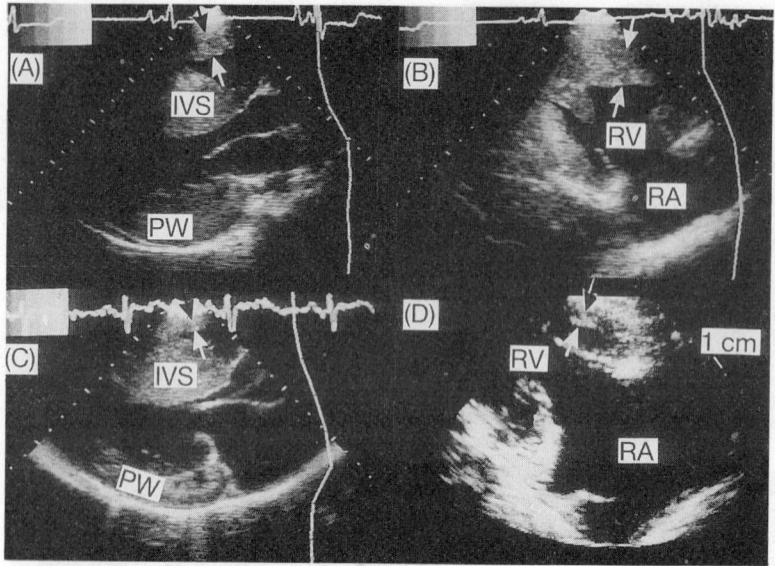

Fig. 39.6. Long-axis (A) and tricuspid inflow tract (B) views from a patient with severe right ventricular hypertrophy (arrows). (C) and (D), similar views from a patient with moderate (1 cm) right ventricular hypertrophy. IVS, interventricular septum; PW, posterior wall; RA, right atrium; RV, right ventricle. (By courtesy of Dr P. Nihoyannopoulos.)

CARDIAC CATHETERIZATION

The combination of two-dimensional echocardiography and Doppler has replaced cardiac catherization with haemodynamic measurements and angiography as the method of assessing left ventricular structure and function in patients with hypertrophic cardiomyopathy. It is not necessary to perform cardiac catheterization for diagnosis; it is rarely indicated, unless symptoms are refractory and the direct measurement of cardiac pressures may be informative, particularly in assessing the severity of mitral regurgitation. However, cardiac catheterization for the purpose of performing coronary arteriography is often necessary in patients older than 40 years of age who have significant angina or ST-segment changes during exercise. Typically, left ventricular end-diastolic pressure, the mean left atrial pressure and mean pulmonary capillary wedge pressure are elevated as consequences of abnormal left ventricular diastolic filling and reduced compliance.[4] Cardiac output may be reduced, normal or occasionally increased.[4] In approximately one-third of patients, there is a pressure gradient at rest between the body and outflow tract of the left ventricle. Such gradients are usually relatively stable but may be labile, and intraventricular pressures of up to 300 mmHg have been recorded.[80] When such a gradient is present, the arterial pressure trace may occasionally demonstrate a spike and dome configuration.[80] In a small proportion of patients (< 15%), a right ventricular infundibular gradient of > 10 mmHg may be recorded.[4] Typically, right ventricular end-diastolic and mean right atrial pressures are mildly to moderately elevated.

Left ventricular angiography reveals an abnormally shaped ventricle which typically ejects at least 75% of its contents in association with mild mitral regurgitation (Fig. 39.8). Papillary muscles may occasionally be very prominent and obliterate the left ventricular cavity in late systole. Usually, the coronary arteries are large in calibre. The left anterior descending and septal perforator arteries

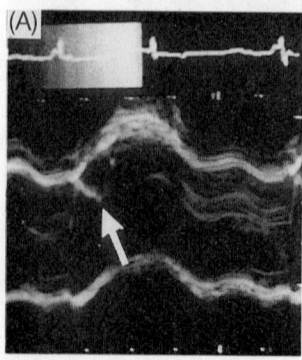

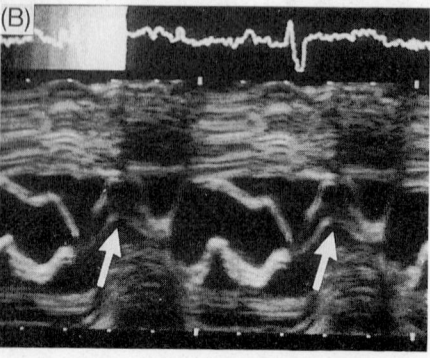

Fig. 39.7. M-Mode echocardiographic recordings of the aortic valve (left) and mitral valve (right). There is early systolic closure of the aortic valve and systolic anterior motion of the mitral valve (arrows) with systolic contact of the anterior mitral valve leaflet with the septum. These are features associated with left ventricular outflow tract gradients. (By courtesy of Dr P. Nihoyannopoulos.)

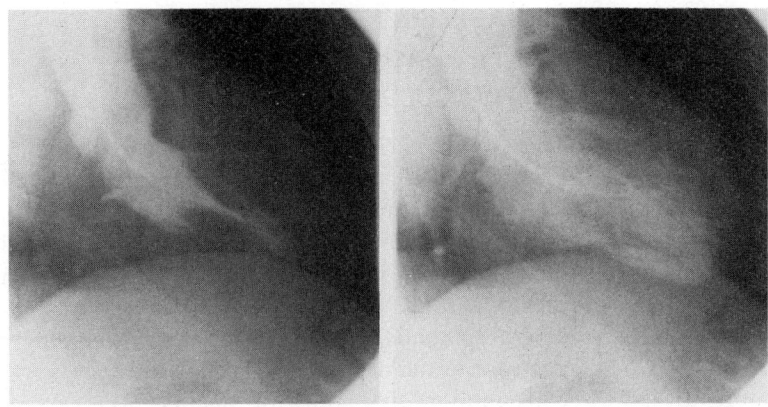

Fig. 39.8. End-systolic (left) and end-diastolic (right) frames from a left ventricular angiogram in the right anterior oblique projection in a patient with hypertrophic cardiomyopathy. There are prominent papillary muscles with a very small residual end-systolic volume.

may demonstrate phasic narrowing during systole in the absence of fixed obstructive lesions; such changes do not relate to symptoms.[81]

NATURAL HISTORY

The natural history of hypertrophic cardiomyopathy is one of slow progression of symptoms, gradual deterioration in left ventricular function and a significant incidence of sudden death which occurs at all ages.[82] Data from tertiary referral centres indicate that the annual mortality from sudden death in adults is about 2.5%, whereas in children and adolescents it is at least 6%[41,83,84] and even greater in those who have recurrent syncope or a family history of malignant hypertrophic cardiomyopathy.[52,53,85,86] Although the mortality figures from non-referral hospitals are lower, the risk of sudden death is still present.[87] In 'low risk' children and adolescents in whom the diagnosis of hypertrophic cardiomyopathy was made during routine family screening or who came to medical attention because of paroxysmal symptoms or an asymptomatic murmur, the annual mortality was approximately 4% in two consecutive patient populations between 1960 and 1985;[69,85] autopsy studies reveal that unsuspected hypertrophic cardiomyopathy is the commonest cause of sudden death in competitive athletes.[88,89]

Symptomatic deterioration is usually slow and associated with a gradual reduction in left ventricular systolic performance; it does not usually cause significant limitation of lifestyle or pose a major therapeutic problem. Occasionally, however, symptomatic deterioration may be associated with progressive myocardial wall thinning presumably reflecting myocyte necrosis and fibrosis which causes severe reduction in left ventricular systolic performance and/or diastolic fillings.[90] In such patients, end-diastolic volume increases but even in the end-stages it rarely exceeds normal limits; thus, such patients resemble those who have dilated cardiomyopathy only in the degree of impairment of systolic performance. Occasionally, patients who experience such a deterioration may present with a clinical picture resembling that of restrictive cardiomyopathy with grossly enlarged atria, signs of right heart failure and relative preservation of left ventricular systolic performance.

Data from serial electrocardiograms revealed increased QRS voltage in 20% of adults suggesting that left ventricular hypertrophy was progressive in a subset of patients.[91] Serial echocardiographic assessment of adults, however, has not confirmed these electrocardiographic findings.[92] The development of atrial fibrillation has long been considered to be associated with dramatic symptomatic deterioration and to indicate a poor prognosis.[80,93] A recent retrospective study revealed that 5-year survival in those with atrial fibrillation was similar to that of age- and sex-matched patients who remained in sinus rhythm and, if the ventricular response was controlled and emboli prevented, symptomatic status remained stable.[94] Indeed, most patients who develop atrial fibrillation have previously had a palpable atrial beat in the absence of a fourth heart sound reflecting forceful atrial contraction but minimal atrial systolic contribution to filling volume.

PROGNOSIS

The major problems in the management of hypertrophic cardiomyopathy are the identification of high-risk patients and the prevention of sudden death. In adults, the presence of non-sustained ventricular tachycardia during electrocardiographic monitoring is associated with, although probably does not cause, sudden death and it is the best single marker of high risk with a sensitivity of 69% and a specificity of 80%.[66–68] However, the positive predictive accuracy of ventricular tachycardia as a marker is low (22%) reflecting the fact that most patients with ventricular tachycardia do not die suddenly and thus further risk stratification of this subgroup would be helpful because a policy of aggressive therapy may include patients at relatively lower risk.[68] In adults, no other clinical feature is associated with or predictive of sudden death including symptoms, left ventricular wall thickness, filling pressures or the presence of a left ventricular gradient.[41,89] Children and adolescents who have experienced recurrent syncope and those who have two or more siblings with hypertrophic cardiomyopathy who have died suddenly are clearly at increased risk.[85,86] The majority of young patients who die suddenly, however, have not experienced syncope nor do they have a malignant family history.[69,85] The young pose problems in terms of both identification and therapy. Most are asymptomatic, many are athletic; even those at apparently low risk have an annual mortality from sudden death of 4%. The recommendation for those with marked hypertrophy, significant gradients, arrhythmias or adverse family history to abstain from competitive sports is precautionary but often imposes a significant limitation on the lifestyle of a child, adolescent or young adult.[95]

The ability to identify patients who are at increased risk is dependent upon understanding the likely mechanisms of sudden death. There is evidence to suggest that haemodynamic deterioration with reduced stroke volume following a physiological tachycardia,[96] an arrhythmia[69,97] or reduction in venous return or hypotension developing in the presence of a normal stroke volume but altered baroreflex control of peripheral blood flow are all possible initiating mechanisms.[59] The outcome, survival versus sudden death, must be influenced by the underlying electrical stability of the myocardium which it is reasonable to speculate is related to the extent of myocardial disarray. In adults, non-sustained ventricular tachycardia is a marker of electrical instability; in the younger patients, no such marker has been identified.

MANAGEMENT

SYMPTOMATIC TREATMENT: PHARMACOLOGICAL

The goal of therapy is to improve symptoms and prevent complications, in particular sudden death. Beta-adrenoceptor blockers, particularly propranolol, and calcium antagonists, especially verapamil, are the mainstay of symptomatic pharmacological therapy. Both propranolol and verapamil have several potentially beneficial actions including a decrease in the determinants of myocardial oxygen consumption and thus of angina pectoris and blunting of the heart-rate response during exercise to provide increased time for filling at equivalent workloads in those with poor relaxation and slow filling. Both agents exert a negative inotropic effect reducing hyperdynamic systolic function and left ventricular gradients;[98,99] it is also claimed they improve diastolic filling, verapamil by improving relaxation[36,39,50,100] and propranolol by increasing compliance.[101] Such changes appear to occur in some patients receiving propranolol;[101] the effect of verapamil is more consistent and associated with increased exercise duration in about two-thirds of patients.[36,39] Both propranolol and verapamil are usually well tolerated and the beneficial effects outweigh the unwanted effects. None of the side-effects of propranolol are serious; however, the suppressant effect of verapamil on impulse formation and atrioventricular nodal conduction may cause problems in patients with unsuspected pre-existing conduction disease, and its vasodilatory and negative inotropic effects have resulted in acute pulmonary oedema and death.[102] It is not clear which patients are at particular risk of developing such detrimental haemodynamic effects from verapamil; the recommendation to avoid giving verapamil to patients who are obviously at high risk with increased filling pressures, paroxysmal nocturnal dyspnoea or orthopnoea would eliminate those patients in most need of therapy.[102] In practice, both drugs are effective but it is safer to use propranolol. If it is ineffective, verapamil can then be tried; in high-risk patients, verapamil should be started in hospital. The results of preliminary studies with diltiazem are consistent with those in the extensive clinical experience with verapamil.[103] Nifedipine has also been shown to improve diastolic function by increasing compliance without significantly altering systolic performance;[104] however, the clinical experience has been disappointing and complicated by the effects of peripheral vasodilatation.[105] The potential role of beta-blockers with intrinsic sympathomimetic activity in patients with impaired diastolic function has not been assessed.

SYMPTOMATIC TREATMENT: SURGICAL

Surgery offers another major therapeutic option with a reported experience in over 1000 patients.[82,106] The majority of patients operated upon have had a left ventricular outflow tract gradient and been refractory to medical therapy. The commonest operation has been to remove a segment of the upper anterior septum (myotomy/myectomy) via a transaortic approach. Transventricular approaches have also been used but are associated with a higher incidence of late complications, particularly of cardiac failure. Despite this large experience, even in the most experienced hands, the operation carries a peri-operative mortality of 5–10%.[83] Successful surgery confers symptomatic and haemodynamic (reduced left ventricular gradient and filling pressures) improvement and is a useful therapeutic alternative for patients who are refractory to medical therapy. It is not known which patients will die and why others benefit; the optimal patient population for myotomy/myectomy has not been identified. Mitral valve replacement has also been advocated; excellent results have been achieved in young and elderly patients who have had severe mitral regurgitation.[107]

DYSPNOEA

Therapy depends on the predominant mechanism of dyspnoea. It is not clear whether characterization of patients in relation to the predominant diastolic abnormality (relaxation versus compliance) will aid the selection of drugs likely to be beneficial. In patients with slow filling that continues throughout diastole, beta-blockers and verapamil are appropriate. Conversely, those with rapid early filling may benefit from a relative tachycardia and do better without negative chronotropic agents. Diastolic function can be characterized by cardiac output pacing studies or non-invasively by assessment of the proportion of filling volume under the radionuclide time–activity curve[108] or from digitized M-mode echocardiographic tracings.[48–50] When dyspnoea is associated with significant obstruction, i.e. at least 50% of stroke volume in the left ventricle at the onset of the gradient,[46] verapamil in high doses (240–480 mg daily) and, failing this, myotomy/

myectomy may be beneficial. Occasionally, dyspnoea is associated with severe mitral regurgitation and responds well to mitral valve replacement. In the assessment of patients with clinical and Doppler evidence of mitral regurgitation, an elevated pulmonary capillary wedge pressure with a prominent 'v' wave may result from a diseased and non-compliant left atrium in the absence of significant mitral regurgitation, and left ventricular angiography in sinus rhythm without ventricular ectopic beats may be particularly important to assess the severity of mitral regurgitation. Endocarditis is a rare complication; it occurs in patients with left ventricular outflow tract turbulence and/or mitral regurgitation.[109] It may involve the mitral or aortic valve and is usually associated with increased dyspnoea. Antibiotic prophylaxis is important in appropriate patients.

CHEST PAIN

When chest pain is severe, associated with significant ST-segment changes during exercise or refractory to therapy, the performance of coronary arteriography is warranted. The results of coronary artery bypass grafting in hypertrophic cardiomyopathy are excellent even when additional procedures are performed (myotomy/mitral valve replacement).[110] Exertional chest pain usually responds to therapy with propranolol or verapamil but when it is refractory very high doses of these agents (propranolol 480 mg daily, verapamil 720 mg daily) have been beneficial.[111,112] Atypical chest pain may persist long after the initial stimulus has been removed, presumably because a new dynamic situation has developed.[73] Short-acting nitrates, diuretics and high-dose verapamil may be useful in selected patients perhaps by reducing filling pressures and improving coronary flow to subendocardial layers.[55] When severe chest pain is associated with significant obstruction, high-dose verapamil, disopyramide[113] or myectomy may be beneficial. Experience with disopyramide is limited but, in a small group of patients with reduced exercise capacity and left ventricular outflow tract obstruction, left ventricular gradients and filling pressures were reduced and symptoms of angina and dyspnoea were improved.[113]

ARRHYTHMIA

Arrhythmias are a common complication of hypertrophic cardiomyopathy, and supraventricular arrhythmias are particularly associated with embolic complications. Once atrial fibrillation is established, treatment with anticoagulants and digoxin with or without verapamil or beta-blockers is appropriate. The aim of therapy is to control the ventricular response and prevent emboli. Most patients who develop atrial fibrillation during electrocardiographic monitoring are unaware of changes from sinus rhythm to atrial fibrillation as long as the ventricular response is well controlled and this is consistent with the loss of a forceful atrial contraction (palpable atrial beat) which does not contribute significantly to filling volume (no fourth heart sound). In a minority, the loss of atrial systolic contribution to filling volume is important; in these patients, electrical cardioversion can be facilitated by 6 weeks' therapy with amiodarone (300 mg daily) if pharmacological cardioversion does not occur first.[114] The role of conventional class I agents in aiding cardioversion and the maintenance of sinus rhythm is uncertain. Sustained (> 30 s) episodes of paroxysmal atrial fibrillation or supraventricular tachycardia are relatively uncommon but represent a risk of haemodynamic collapse and emboli. Amiodarone in low doses (1000–1400 mg weekly) is effective in suppressing such episodes and also provides control of the ventricular response should breakthrough occur;[114] it is not known whether amiodarone attenuates the subsequent development of established atrial fibrillation. Non-sustained episodes of supraventricular arrhythmia are common but usually asymptomatic and have a variable relation to the subsequent development of established atrial fibrillation.[95] Anti-arrhythmic therapy is not usually warranted; the precise risk of emboli and of the development of sustained episodes or established atrial fibrillation remains uncertain. Episodes of non-sustained ventricular tachycardia are common but are rarely symptomatic and therapy is warranted only if prognosis can be shown to be improved (see below).

PREVENTION OF SUDDEN DEATH

Management of adults is facilitated by the identification of a relatively sensitive and specific marker of increased risk, non-sustained ventricular tachycardia during electrocardiographic monitoring,[68] and the use of amiodarone (maintenance dose 200–300 mg daily with plasma concentrations of 0.5–1.5 mg/l) is associated with improved survival when compared with well-matched historical control subjects (Fig. 39.9).[115] With plasma concentra-

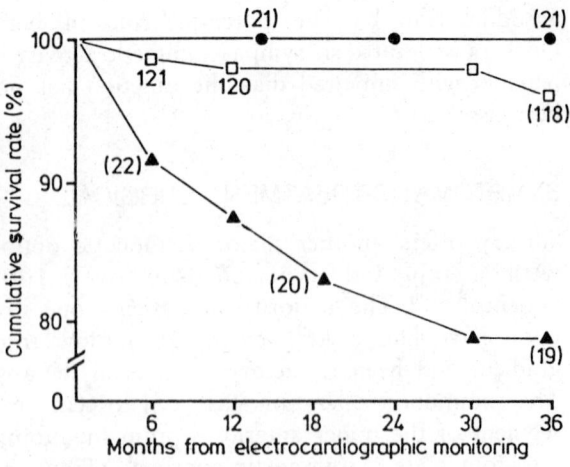

Fig. 39.9. Cumulative survival in 24 patients with ventricular tachycardia treated with conventional anti-arrhythmic agents (triangle), 21 with ventricular tachycardia treated with amiodarone (circle) and 123 without ventricular tachycardia (open square). (Reproduced with permission from McKenna *et al.*, *Br. Heart J.* 1985; **53**: 412–6.[115]

tions of amiodarone of < 1.5 mg/l, serious side-effects are rare, although photosensitivity and sleep disturbance are common and may be troublesome.[114,116] The management of young patients with hypertrophic cardiomyopathy is less clear. In 15 high-risk children and adolescents with recurrent syncope, out-of-hospital ventricular fibrillation or a malignant family history, empirical use of very low-dose amiodarone (plasma concentrations of 0.5 mg/l) was associated with no deaths at 3 years compared with an annual mortality of about 4% in apparently low-risk young patients who did not have arrhythmias, syncopal episodes or an adverse family history.[69] These data require confirmation with larger numbers and longer follow-up. Currently, young patients who do not have obvious risk factors may either receive no treatment or be given propranolol or verapamil for symptoms. Neither of these agents prevents sudden death. Until practical management guidelines are established, young patients with hypertrophic cardiomyopathy should undergo risk factor characterization, in relation to likely mechanisms of sudden death, at a specialist centre.

REFERENCES

1. Liouville, H. Retrecissement cardiaque sous aortique. *Gaz. Med. Paris*. 1869; 24: 161.
2. Hallopeau, L. Retrecissement ventriculo-aortique. *Gaz. Med. Paris* 1869; 24: 683.

3. Teare, D. Asymmetrical hypertrophy of the heart in young adults. *Br. Heart J.* 1958; **20**: 1–8.

4. Braunwald, E., Lambrew, C., Rockoff, S. *et al.* Idiopathic hypertrophic subaortic stenosis. I. Description of the disease based upon an analysis of 64 patients. *Circulation* 1964; **29** (Suppl. 4): III–119.

5. Maron, B.J. and Epstein, S.E. Hypertrophic cardiomyopathy: a discussion of the nomenclature. *Am. J. Cardiol.* 1979; **43**: 1242–4.

6. Criley, J.M., Lewis, K.B., White, R.I. *et al.* Pressure gradients without obstruction. A new concept of "hypertrophic subaortic stenosis". *Circulation* 1965; **32**: 881–7.

7. Abbasi, A.S., MacAlpin, R.N., Eber, L.M. and Pearce, M.L. Echocardiographic diagnosis of idiopathic hypertrophic cardiomyopathy without outflow obstruction. *Circulation* 1972; **46**: 897–904.

8. Shah, P.M., Gramiak, R., Adelman, A.G. and Wigle, E.D. Role of echocardiography in diagnostic and hemodynamic assessment of hypertrophic subaortic stenosis. *Circulation* 1971; **44**: 891–8.

9. Tajik, A.J. and Giuliani, E.R. Echocardiographic observations in idiopathic hypertrophic subaortic stenosis. *Mayo Clin. Proc.* 1974; **49**: 89–97.

10. Henry, W.L., Clark, C.E. and Epstein, S.E. Asymmetric septal hypertrophy: echocardiographic identification of the pathognomonic anatomic abnormalities of IHSS. *Circulation* 1973; **47**: 225–33.

11. Maron, B.J., Gottdiener, J.S. and Epstein, S.E. Patterns and significance of distribution of left ventricular hypertrophy in hypertrophic cardiomyopathy: a wide angle, two dimensional echocardiographic study of 125 patients. *Am. J. Cardiol.* 1981; **48**: 418–28.

12. Maron, B.J., Gottdiener, J.S., Bonow, R.O. and Epstein, S.E. Hypertrophic cardiomyopathy with unusual location of left ventricular hypertrophy undetectable by M-mode echocardiography: identification by wide-angle two-dimensional echocardiography. *Circulation* 1981; **63**: 409–18.

13. Shapiro, L.M. and McKenna, W.J. Distribution of left ventricular hypertrophy in hypertrophic cardiomyopathy: a two-dimensional echocardiographic study. *J. Am. Coll. Cardiol.* 1983; **2**: 437–44.

14. Been, M., Kean, D., Smith, M.A., Douglas, R.H.B., Best, J.J.K. and Muir, A.L. Nuclear magnetic resonance in hypertrophic cardiomyopathy. *Br. Heart J.* 1985: **54**: 48–52.

15. Report of the WHO/ISFC task force on the definition and classification of cardiomyopathies. *Br. Heart J.* 1980; **44**: 672–3.

16. Goodwin, J.F. The frontiers of cardiomyopathy. *Br. Heart J.* 1982; **48**: 1–18.

17. Steingo, L., Dansky, R., Pocock, W.A. and Barlow, J.B. Apical hypertrophic nonobstructive cardiomyopathy. *Am. Heart J.* 1982; **104**: 635–7.

18. Seftel, H.C. Cardiomyopathies in the Johannesburg Bantu. *S. Afr. Med. J.* 1973; **47**: 321–4.

19. Yamaguchi, H., Ishimura, T., Nishiyama, S. *et al.* Hypertrophic nonobstructive cardiomyopathy with giant negative T waves (apical hypertrophy); ventriculographic and echocardiographic features in 30 patients. *Am. J. Cardiol.* 1979; **44**: 401–12.

20. Kawai, C. Studies on cardiomyopathy in Japan. In: Sekiguchi, M. and Olsen, E.G.J. eds. *Clinical, pathological and theoretical aspects.* Tokyo: University of Tokyo Press, 1980, pp. 3–10.

21. Codd, M.B., Sugrue, D.D., Gersh, B.J. and Melton, L.J. Epidemiologic features of idiopathic dilated cardiomyopathy and hypertrophic cardiomyopathy: a population based study in Olmstead County, Mn, 1975–1984. *Circulation* 1989; (in press).

22. Clark, C.E., Henry, W.L. and Epstein, S.E. Familial prevalence and genetic transmission of idiopathic hypertrophic subaortic stenosis. *N. Engl. J. Med.* 1973; **289**: 709–14.

23. Maron, B.J., Nichols, P.F., Pickle, L.W., Wesley, Y.F. and Mulvihill, J.J. Patterns of inheritance in hypertrophic cardiomyopathy: Assessment by M mode and two dimensional echocardiography. *Am. J. Cardiol.* 1984; **53**: 1087–94.

24. Greaves, S.C., Roche, A.H.G., Neutze, J.M., Whitlock, R.M.L. and Veale, A.M.O. Inheritance of hypertrophic cardiomyopathy: a cross sectional and M mode echocardiographic study of 50 families. *Br. Heart J.* 1987; **58**: 259–66.

25. Darsee, J.R. The hypertrophic heart syndromes: a glance at the chromosome. *Am. Heart J.* 1981; **101**: 124–6.

26. Pomerance, A. and Davies, M.J. Pathological features of hypertrophic obstructive cardiomyopathy (HOCM) in the elderly. *Br. Heart J.* 1975; **37**: 305–12.

27. McKenna, W.J., Kleinebenne, A., Nihoyannopoulos, P. and Foale, R.A. Echocardiographic measurement of right ventricular wall thickness in hypertrophic cardiomyopathy: relation to clinical and prognostic features. *J. Am. Coll. Cardiol.* 1988; **11**: 147–53.

28. Davies, M.J. Colour Atlas of Cardiovascular Pathology. In: Curran, R.C. ed. *Oxford Colour Atlases of Pathology.* London: Harvey Miller Ltd, 1986, pp. 100–25.

29. McKenna, W.J., Nihoyannopoulos, P. and Davies, M.J. Hypertrophic cardiomyopathy without hypertrophy: a description of two families with premature cardiac death and myocardial disarray in the absence of increased muscle mass (Abstract). *Circulation* 1988; **78** (Suppl. 2): 375.

30. Davies, M.J. The current status of myocardial disarray in hypertrophic cardiomyopathy. *Br. Heart J.* 1984; **51**: 361–63.

31. Maron, B.J., Anan, T.J. and Roberts, W.C. Quantitative analysis of the distribution of cardiac muscle cell disorganization in the left ventricular wall of patients with hypertrophic cardiomyopathy. *Circulation* 1981; **63**: 882–94.

32. Ferrans, V.J., Morrow, A.G. and Roberts, W.C. Myocardial ultrastructure in idiopathic hypertrophic subaortic stenosis: a study of operatively excised left ventricular outflow tract muscle in 14 patients. *Circulation* 1972; **45**: 769–92.

33. Becker, A.E. and Caruso, G. Myocardial disarray. A critical review. *Br. Heart J.* 1982; **47**: 527–38.

34. Bulkley, B.H., Weisfeldt, M.L. and Hutchins, G.M. Asymmetric septal hypertrophy and myocardial fibre disarray: features of normal and developing malformed hearts. *Circulation* 1978; **57**: 520–6.

35. Perloff, J.K. Pathogenesis of hypertrophic cardiomyopathy: Hypotheses and speculations. *Am. Heart J.* 1981; **101**: 219–26.

36. Bonow, R.O., Rosing, D.R., Bacharach, S.L., Green, M.V., Kent, K.M., Lipson, L.C., Maron, B.J., Leon, M.B. and Epstein, S.E. Effects of verapamil on left ventricular systolic function and diastolic filling in patients with hypertrophic cardiomyopathy. *Circulation* 1981; **64**: 787–96.

37. Kaltenbach, M., Hopf, R. and Kelle, M. Calcium-antagonistische Therapie bei hypertroph-obstruktiver Kardiomyopathie. *Dtsch Med. Wochenschr.* 1976; **101**: 1284–7.

38. Goodwin, J.F. and Krikler, D.M. Arrhythmia as a cause of sudden death in hypertrophic cardiomyopathy. *Lancet* 1976; **2**: 937–40.

39. Lorell, B.H. Use of calcium channel blockers in hypertrophic cardiomyopathy. *Am. J. Med.* 1985; **78**(Suppl. 2B): 43–54.

40. Pearce, P.C., Hawkey, C., Symons, C. and Olsen, E.G.J. Role of calcium in the induction of cardiac hypertrophy and myofibrillar disarray. Experimental studies of a possible cause of hypertrophic cardiomyopathy. *Br. Heart J.* 1985; **54**: 420–7.

41. McKenna, W.J., Deanfield, J., Faruqui, A., England, D., Oakley, C. and Goodwin, J. Prognosis in hypertrophic cardiomyopathy: Role of age and clinical, electrocardiographic and hemodynamic features. *Am. J. Cardiol.* 1981; **47**: 532–8.

42. Wigle, E.D., Henderson, M., Rakowski, H. and Wilansky, S. Muscular (hypertrophic) subaortic stenosis (hypertrophic obstructive cardiomyopathy): the evidence for true obstruction to left ventricular outflow. *Postgrad. Med. J.* 1986; **62**: 531–6.

43. Criley, J.M. and Siegel, R.J. Obstruction is unimportant in the pathophysiology of hypertrophic cardiomyopathy. *Postgrad. Med. J.* 1986; **62**: 515–29.

44. Siegel, R.J. and Criley, J.M. Comparison of ventricular emptying with and without a pressure gradient in patients with hypertrophic cardiomyopathy. *Br. Heart J.* 1985; **53**: 283–91.

45. Sugrue, D.D., McKenna, W.J., Dickie, S., Myers, M.J., Lavender, J.P., Oakley, C.M. and Goodwin, J.F. Relation between left ventricular gradient and relative stroke volume ejected in early and late systole in hypertrophic cardiomyopathy. *Br. Heart J.* 1984; **52**: 602–9.

46. Yonezawa, Y., Dickie, S., Nihoyannopoulos, P., Lavender, J.P., Oakley, C.M. and McKenna, W.J. Significance of left ventricular gradient in hypertrophic cardiomyopathy (Abstract). *Br. Heart J.* 1987; **57**: 581.

47. Murgo, J.P., Alter, B.R., Dorethy, J.F., Altobelli, S.A. and McGranahan, G.M. Jr. Dynamics of left ventricular ejection in obstructive and nonobstructive hypertrophic cardiomyopathy. *J. Clin. Invest.* 1980; **66**: 1369–82.

48. Sutton, StJ. M.G., Tajik, A.J., Gibson, D.G., Brown, D.J., Seward, J.B. and Giuliani, E.R. Echocardiographic assessment of left ventricular filling and septal and posterior wall dynamics of idiopathic hypertrophic subaortic stenosis. *Circulation* 1978; **57**: 512–20.

49. Sanderson, J.E., Traill, T.A., Sutton, StJ. M.G., Brown, D.J., Gibson, D.G., Goodwin, J.F. Left ventricular relaxation and filling in hypertrophic cardiomyopathy. An echocardiographic study. *Br. Heart J.* 1978; **40**: 596–601.

50. Hanrath, P., Mathey, D.G., Siegert, R. and Bleifeld, W. Left ventricular relaxation and filling pattern in left ventricular hypertrophy. An echocardiographic study. *Am. J. Cardiol.* 1980; **45**: 15–23.

51. Maron, B.J., Tajik, A.J., Ruttenberg, H.D. *et al.* Hypertrophic cardiomyopathy in infants: Clinical features and natural history. *Circulation* 1982; **65**: 7–17.

52. Fiddler, G.I., Tajik, A.J., Weidman, W.H., McGoon, D.C., Ritter, D.G. and Giuliani, E.R. Idiopathic hypertrophic subaortic stenosis in the young. *Am. J. Cardiol.* 1978; **42**: 793–9.

53. Maron, B.J., Henry, W.L., Clark, C.E., Redwood, D.R., Roberts, W.C. and Epstein, S.E. Asymmetric septal hypertrophy in childhood. *Circulation* 1976; **53**: 9–19.

54. Frenneaux, M.P., Porter, A., Caforio, A.L.P., Odawara, H., Counihan, P.J. and McKenna, W.J. Determinants of exercise capacity in hypertrophic cardiomyopathy. *J. Am. Coll. Cardiol.* 1989; (in press).

55. Cannon, R.O., III, Rosing, D.R., Maron, B.J. *et al.* Myocardial ischemia in patients with hypertrophic cardiomyopathy: contribution of inadequate vasodilator reserve and elevated left ventricular filling pressures. *Circulation* 1985; **71**: 234–43.

56. Maron, B.J., Wolfson, J.K., Epstein, S.E. and Roberts, W.C. Intramural ("small vessel") coronary artery disease in hypertrophic cardiomyopathy. *J. Am. Coll. Cardiol.*

1986; **8**: 545–57.

57. Loogen, F., Kuhn, H., Gietzen, F., Lösse, H.D., Schulte, H.D. and Bircks, W. Clinical course and prognosis of patients with typical and atypical hypertrophic obstructive and with hypertrophic non-obstructive cardiomyopathy. *Eur. Heart J.* 1983; **4**(Suppl. F): 145–53.

58. Borggrefe, M., Lösse, B., Loogen, F., Schulte, H. and Bircks, W. The influence of myotomy/myectomy on arrhythmias in hypertrophic cardiomyopathy (Abstract). *Circulation* 1986; **74**(Suppl. II): II–227.

59. Frenneaux, M.P., Counihan, P.J., Webb, D. and McKenna, W.J. Evidence for an abnormal vasodilator response in hypertrophic cardiomyopathy (Abstract). *J. Am. Coll. Cardiol.* 1989; (in press).

60. Maron, B.J., Spirito, P., Wesley, Y. and Arce, J. Development and progression of left ventricular hypertrophy in children with hypertrophic cardiomyopathy. *N. Engl. J. Med.* 1986; **315**: 610–4.

61. McKenna, W.J. and Kleinebenne, A. Hypertrophic cardiomyopathy in the elderly. In: Coodley, E.L., ed. *Geriatric Heart Disease.* Littleton: PSG Publishing Company, Inc., 1985, pp. 260–8.

62. Shapiro, L.M., Kleinebenne, A. and McKenna, W.J. The distribution of left ventricular hypertrophy in hypertrophic cardiomyopathy: comparison to athletes and hypertensives. *Eur. Heart J.* 1985; **6**: 967–74.

63. Savage, D.D., Seides, S.F., Clark, C.E. *et al.* Electrocardiographic findings in patients with obstructive and non obstructive hypertrophic cardiomyopathy. *Circulation* 1978; **58**: 402–8.

64. Krikler, D.M., Davies, M.J., Rowland, E., Goodwin, J.F., Evans, R.C. and Shaw, D.B. Sudden death in hypertrophic cardiomyopathy: Associated accessory atrioventricular pathways. *Br. Heart J.* 1980; **43**: 245–51.

65. Savage, D.D., Seides, S.F., Maron, B.J., Myers, D.J. and Epstein, S.E. Prevalance of arrhythmias during 24 hour electrocardiographic monitoring and exercise testing in patients with obstructive and non obstructive hypertrophic cardiomyopathy. *Circulation* 1979; **59**: 866–75.

66. McKenna, W.J., England, D., Doi, Y.L., Deanfield, J.E., Oakley, C.M. and Goodwin, J.F. Arrhythmia in hypertrophic cardiomyopathy. 1. Influence on prognosis. *Br. Heart J.* 1981; **46**: 168–72.

67. Maron, B.J., Savage, D.D., Wolfson, J.K. and Epstein, S.E. Prognostic significance of 24-hour electrocardiographic monitoring in patients with hypertrophic cardiomyopathy: a prospective study. *Am. J. Cardiol.* 1981; **48**: 252–7.

68. McKenna, W.J. Sudden death in hypertropic cardiomyopathy: Identification of the "high risk" patient. In: Brugada, P. and Wellens, H.J.J. eds. *Cardiac Arrhythmias: Where to go from here?* Mount Kisco, New York: Futura Publishing Co., 1987, pp. 353–65.

69. McKenna, W.J., Franklin, R.C.G., Nihoyannopoulos, P., Robinson, K.R. and Deanfield, J.E. Arrhythmia and prognosis in infants, children and adolescents with hypertrophic cardiomyopathy. *J. Am. Coll. Cardiol.* 1988; **11**: 147–53.

70. Alfonso, F., Frenneaux, M.P., Cripps, T.R., Rowland, E., McKenna, W.J. Clinical sustained monomorphic ventricular tachycardia in hypertrophic cardiomyopathy: Association with left ventricular apical aneurysm. *Br. Heart J.* 1989; **61**: 171–81.

71. Mulrow, J.P., Healy, M.J.R. and McKenna, W.J. Variability of ventricular arrhythmias in hypertrophic cardiomyopathy and implications for treatment. *Am. J. Cardiol.* 1986; **58**: 615–8.

72. Maron, B.J., Gottdiener, J.S., Arce, J., Rosing, D.R., Wesley, Y.E. and Epstein, S.E. Dynamic subaortic obstruction in hypertrophic cardiomyopathy: analysis by pulsed Doppler echocardiography. *J. Am. Coll. Cardiol.* 1985; **6**:

1–15.

73. Yock, P.G., Hatle, L. and Popp, R.L. Patterns and timing of Doppler-detected intracavity and aortic flow in hypertrophic cardiomyopathy. *J. Am. Coll. Cardiol.* 1986; **8**: 1047–58.

74. Doi, Y., McKenna, W.J., Gehrke, J., Oakley, C.M. and Goodwin, J.F. M-mode echocardiography in hypertrophic cardiomyopathy: diagnostic criteria and prediction of obstruction. *Am. J. Cardiol.* 1980; **45**: 6–14.

75. Gilbert, B.W., Pollick, C., Adelman, A.G. *et al.* Hypertrophic cardiomyopathy: subclassification by M mode echocardiography. *Am. J. Cardiol.* 1980; **45**: 861–72.

76. Pollick, C., Morgan, C.D., Gilbert, B.W., Rakowski, H. and Wigle, E.D. Muscular subaortic stenosis: the temporal relationship between systolic anterior motion the anterior mitral leaflet and the pressure gradient. *Circulation* 1982; **66**: 1087–94.

77. Pollick, C., Rakowski, H. and Wigle, E.D. Muscular subaortic stenosis: the quantitative relationship between systolic anterior motion and the pressure gradient. *Circulation* 1984; **69**: 43–9.

78. Maron, B.J. and Epstein, S.E. Hypertrophic cardiomyopathy. Recent observations regarding the specificity of three hallmarks of the disease: asymmetric septal hypertrophy, septal disorganization and systolic anterior motion of the mitral valve. *Am. J. Cardiol.* 1980; **45**: 6–14.

79. O'Gara, P.T., Bonow, R.O., Maron, B.J., Damske, B.A., Van Lingen, A., Bacharach, S.L. and Epstein, S.E. Myocardial perfusion abnormalities in patients with hypertrophic cardiomyopathy: with Thallium-201 emission computed tomography. *Circulation* 1987; **76**: 1214–23.

80. Wigle, E.D., Sasson, Z., Henderson, M.A., Ruddy, T.D., Fulop, J., Rakowski, H. and Williams, W.G. Hypertrophic cardiomyopathy. The importance of the site and the extent of hypertrophy. A review. *Prog. Cardiovasc. Dis.* 1985; **28**: 1–83.

81. Brugada, P., Bar, F.W.H.M., de Zwaan, C., Roy, D., Green, M. and Wellens, H.J.J. "Sawfish" systolic narrowing of the left anterior descending coronary artery: An angiographic sign of hypertrophic cardiomyopathy. *Circulation* 1983; **67**: 191–7.

82. McKenna, W.J. and Goodwin, J.F. The natural history of hypertrophic cardiomyopathy. *Curr. Prob. Cardiol.* 1981; **VI**: 5–26.

83. Maron, B.J., Merrill, W.H., Freier, P.A. *et al.* Long-term clinical course and symptomatic status of patients after operation for hypertrophic subaortic stenosis. *Circulation* 1978; **57**: 1205–13.

84. Loogen, F., Kuhn, H. and Krelhaus, W. Natural history of hypertrophic obstructive cardiomyopathy and effect of therapy. In: Kaltenbach, M., Loogen, F. and Olsen, E.G.J., eds. *Cardiomyopathy and myocardial biopsy.* Berlin: Springer-Verlag, 1978, pp. 286–99.

85. McKenna, W.J. and Deanfield, J.E. Hypertrophic cardiomyopathy: an important cause of sudden death. *Arch. Dis. Child.* 1984; **59**: 971–5.

86. Maron, B.J., Lipson, L.C., Roberts, W.C., Savage, D.D. and Epstein, S.E. "Malignant" hypertrophic cardiomyopathy: identification of a subgroup of families with unusually frequent premature death. *Am. J. Cardiol.* 1978; **41**: 1133–40.

87. Wahedra, D., Gunnar, R.M. and Scanlon, P.J. Prognosis in hypertrophic cardiomyopathy with asymmetrical septal hypertrophy. *Postgrad. Med. J.* 1985; **61**: 1107–9.

88. Maron, B.J., Roberts, W.C., McAllister, H.A., Rosing, D.R. and Epstein, S.E. Sudden death in young athletes. *Circulation* 1980; **62**: 218–29.

89. Maron, B.J., Roberts, W.C. and Epstein, S.E. Sudden death in hypertrophic cardiomyopathy: A profile of 78 patients. *Circulation* 1982; **65**: 1388–94.

90. Spirito, P., Maron, B.J., Bonow, R.O. and Epstein, S.E. Occurrence and significance of progressive left ventricular wall thinning and relative cavity dilatation in patients with hypertrophic cardiomyopathy. *Am. J. Cardiol.* 1987; **59**: 123–9.

91. McKenna, W.J., Borggrefe, M., England, D., Deanfield, J., Oakley, C.M. and Goodwin, J.F. The natural history of left ventricular hypertrophy in hypertrophic cardiomyopathy: an electrocardiographic study. *Circulation* 1982; **66**: 1233–40.

92. Spirito, P. and Maron, B.J. Absence of progression of left ventricular hypertrophy in hypertrophic cardiomyopathy. *J. Am. Coll. Cardiol.* 1987; **9**: 1013–7.

93. Glancy, D.L., O'Brien, K.P., Gold, H.K. and Epstein, S.E. Atrial fibrillation in patients with idiopathic hypertrophic subaortic stenosis. *Br. Heart J.* 1970; **32**: 652–9.

94. Robinson, K., Frenneaux, M.P., Stockins, B., Karatasakis, G., Poloniecki, J.D. and McKenna, W.J. Atrial fibrillation in hypertrophic cardiomyopathy. A longitudinal study.

95. Maron, B.J., Gaffney, F.A., Jeresaty, R.M., McKenna, W.J. and Miller, W.W. Bethesda Conference No 16: "Cardiovascular Abnormalities in the Athlete: Recommendations regarding eligibility for competition". Task Force II: Hypertrophic cardiomyopathy and other myopericardial diseases; mitral valve prolapse. *J. Am. Coll. Cardiol.* 1985; **6**: 1215–7.

96. McKenna, W.J., Harris, L. and Deanfield, J. Syncope in hypertrophic cardiomyopathy. *Br. Heart J.* 1982; **47**: 177–9.

97. Stafford, W.J., Trohman, R.G., Bilsker, M., Zaman, L., Castellanos, A. and Myerburg, R.J. Cardiac arrest in an adolescent with atrial fibrillation and hypertrophic cardiomyopathy. *J. Am. Coll. Cardiol.* 1986; **7**: 701–4.

98. Goodwin, J.F., Shah, P.M., Oakley, C.M., Cohen, J., Yipintosi, T. and Pocock, W. The clinical pharmacology of hypertrophic obstructive cardiomyopathy. In: Wolstenholme, G.E.W. and O'Connor, M., eds. *Cardiomyopathies.* Ciba Foundation Symposium. London: J & A Churchill, 1964, pp. 189–213.

99. Rosing, D.R., Kent, K.M., Maron, B.J. *et al.* Verapamil therapy: A new approach to the pharmacologic treatment of hypertrophic cardiomyopathy. I. Hemodynamic effects. *Circulation* 1979; **60**: 1201–7.

100. Betocchi, S., Bonow, R.O., Bacharach, S.L., Rosing, D.R., Maron, B.J. and Green, M.V. Isovolumic relaxation period in hypertrophic cardiomyopathy: assessment by radionuclide angiography. *J. Am. Coll. Cardiol.* 1986; **7**: 74–81.

101. Alvares, R.F. and Goodwin, J.F. Non-invasive assessment of diastolic function in hypertrophic cardiomyopathy on and off beta adrenergic blocking drugs. *Br. Heart J.* 1982; **48**: 204–12.

102. Epstein, S.E. and Rosing, D.R. Verapamil: Its potential for causing serious complications in patients with hypertrophic cardiomyopathy. *Circulation* 1981; **64**: 437–41.

103. Suwa, M., Hirota, Y. and Kawamura, K. Improvement in left ventricular diastolic function during intravenous and oral diltiazem therapy in patients with hypertrophic cardiomyopathy: an echocardiographic study. *Am. J. Cardiol.* 1984; **54**: 1047–53.

104. Paulus, W.J., Lorell, B.H., Craig, W.E., Wynne, J., Murgo, J.P. and Grossman, W. Comparison of the effects of nitroprusside and nifedipine on diastolic properties in patients with hypertrophic cardiomyopathy: altered left ventricular loading or improved muscle inactivation? *J. Am. Coll. Cardiol.* 1983; **2**: 879–86.

105. Betocchi, S., Cannon, R.O. III, Watson, R.M., Bonow, R.O., Ostrow, H.G., Epstein, S.E. and Rosing, D.R. Effects of sublingual nifedipine on hemodynamics and systolic and diastolic function in patients with hypertrophic car-

diomyopathy. *Circulation* 1985; **72**: 1001–7.

106. Kirklin, J.W. and Barratt-Boyes, B.G. *Cardiac Surgery*. New York: John Wiley and Sons, 1986, pp. 1013–30.

107. Cooley, D.A., Leachman, R.D. and Wukasch, D.C. Diffuse muscular subaortic stenosis: Surgical treatment. *Am. J. Cardiol.* 1973; **31**: 1–6.

108. Bonow, R.O., Frederick, T.M., Bacharach, S.L., Green, M.V., Goose, P.W., Maron, B.J. and Rosing, D.R. Atrial systole and left ventricular filling in hypertrophic cardiomyopathy: effect of verapamil. *Am. J. Cardiol.* 1983; **51**: 1386–91.

109. Chagnac, A., Rudniki, C., Loebel, H. and Zahavi, I. Infectious endocarditis in idiopathic hypertrophic subaortic stenosis: Report of three cases and review of the literature. *Chest* 1982; **81**: 346–9.

110. Gill, C.C., Duda, A.M., Kitazume, H., Kramer, J.R. and Loop, F.D. Idiopathic hypertrophic subaortic stenosis and coronary atherosclerosis. Results of coronary artery bypass alone and myectomy combined with coronary artery bypass. *J. Thorac. Cardiovasc. Surg.* 1982; **84**: 856–60.

111. Frank, M.J., Abdulla, A.M., Canedo, M.I. and Saylors, R.E. Long-term medical management of hypertrophic obstructive cardiomyopathy. *Am. J. Cardiol.* 1978; **42**: 993–1001.

112. Kaltenbach, M. and Hopf, R. Use of calcium channel blockers in the treatment of hypertrophic cardiomyopathy. *Practical Cardiol.* 1984; **10**: 197–215.

113. Pollick, C. Muscular subaortic stenosis. Hemodynamic and clinical improvement after disopyramide. *N. Engl. J. Med.* 1982; **307**: 997–9.

114. McKenna, W.J., Harris, L., Rowland, E., Kleinebenne, A., Krikler, D.M., Oakley, C.M. and Goodwin, J.F. Amiodarone for long-term management of hypertrophic cardiomyopathy. *Am. J. Cardiol.* 1984; **54**: 802–10.

115. McKenna, W.J., Oakley, C.M., Krikler, D.M. and Goodwin, J.F. Improved survival with amiodarone in patients with hypertrophic cardiomyopathy and ventricular tachycardia. *Br. Heart J.* 1985; **53**: 412–6.

116. Harris, L., McKenna, W.J., Rowland, E. and Krikler, D.M. Side effects of long-term amiodarone therapy. *Circulation* 1983; **67**: 45–51.

Chapter 40

Genetics of Cardiomyopathy and the Genetics and Clinical Features of Rare Inherited Diseases of the Myocardium

John Burn and C.P. Bennett

The provision of a precise definition for the term 'cardiomyopathy' has proved difficult. Very often in clinical practice 'cardiomyopathy' is used for any heart disease that cannot be given a better term. Perhaps the best definition is that of the WHO/ISFC:[1] a cardiomyopathy is "heart muscle disease of unknown cause". However, this definition implies that the cause is understood in a condition, such as heart muscle disease occurring in hyperparathyroidism, which is not included by this definition as a cardiomyopathy. This definition, however, is preferable to other definitions founded on a belief that the mechanism of heart muscle disease can be ascribed to 'structural defects', 'inadequate energy supply' and 'abnormal membrane system with ineffective activation–contraction coupling' and that cardiomyopathies can be effectively classified into these groups.[2]

In broad terms, heart muscle disease leads to thickening, dilatation or stiffening. In the first part of this chapter, the inheritance of these three abnormalities will be discussed in this order (their order of importance to the geneticist; the clinical manifestations of these three types of abnormality are discussed elsewhere). In view of the indistinct boundary between cardiomyopathy and other 'specific' heart muscle diseases section II reviews other genetic and acquired forms of heart muscle disease as a source for further reading.

GENETICS OF CARDIOMYOPATHY

HYPERTROPHIC CARDIOMOPATHY

In this section, the inheritance of hypertrophic cardiomyopathy will be described; the clinical features of the condition are discussed in Chapter 39. In 1958, Teare[3] described a large pedigree in which the distinctive disorder hypertrophic cardiomyopathy appeared to be segregating as an autosomal dominant trait. Although it was not the first pathological description of this condition, this report was responsible for attention being focused on hypertrophic cardiomyopathy which is often fatal and is relatively common. Bennett et al.[4] reported a clinical prevalence of 3.2 per 100 000 population, but many other cases are subclinical. In a pathological survey in Iceland, the prevalence was found to be 33 cases per 100 000.[5] After the initial suggestion of dominant inheritance, further extensive family studies revealed a more complex situation. Emanuel et al.[6] found other family members to be affected in less than half of the hypertrophic cardiomyopathy families they studied; on the basis of families with normal parents and multiple affected sibs, these workers suggested that hypertrophic cardiomyopathy could be a recessive trait.

The advent of echocardiography in the early 1970s revealed the error of this interpretation. Asymptomatic relatives with asymmetric septal hypertrophy and systolic anterior movement of the mitral valve were identified. It was subsequently found that asymmetric septal hypertrophy could occur in a variety of other clinical situations and in trained athletes but within hypertrophic cardiomyopathy pedigrees a person with asymmetric septal hypertrophy was as likely to have children with hypertrophic cardiomyopathy as a person who had the full clinical disease.[7] In other words, asymmetric septal hypertrophy and hypertrophic cardiomyopathy were different manifestations of

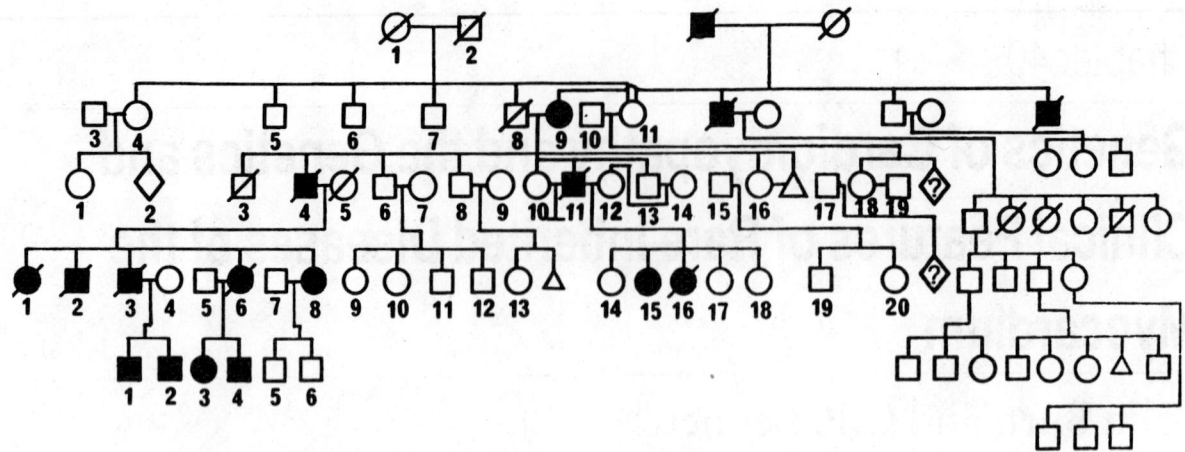

Fig. 40.1. The original pedigree of Teare *et al.* extended with data kindly provided by Professor J. Renwick and Dr W. McKenna. Dominant transmission is apparent although with variable expression.

the same genetic disorder. This is 'variable expression', a frequent finding in families with single gene defects (see Chapter 47).

A dominant gene defect which does not reduce a person's ability to procreate (genetic fitness) is transmitted to half of their offspring. If the mutation rate in the gene is low, one or other parent of the affected person would be expected to be carrying the gene and to have passed it on to half the patient's brothers and sisters. In this 'ideal' situation half of the first degree relatives would be found to be affected. With the exception of the study by Clarke *et al.*,[8] most authors have reported evidence of hypertrophic cardiomyopathy, usually clinically mild, in about 1 in 5 first degree relatives.

The most comprehensive family study performed to date is that of Maron *et al.*[9] Of 298 first degree relatives of a series of 70 patients, 53 (18%) met the criteria of diagnosis, principal among which was a septal thickness > 15 mm in adults or in excess of the 95% confidence limit for children. In 19 first degree relatives, there was doubt about the diagnosis; 226 were adjudged to be unaffected. In the latter group, 27 (9% of all first degree relatives) had abnormal electrocardiographs and were under 40 years of age. As electrocardiographic abnormalities of a similar type are seen in overt cases, it is possible that these relatives were minimally affected. It is noteworthy that among 30 pedigrees with 2 or more affected relatives and parents who could be examined, all were consistent with autosomal dominant inheritance. A large recent study from New Zealand has produced comparable results.[10] These data, together with those from the large pedigrees with affected individuals in several generations,

such as reported in the original study of Teare (Fig. 40.1) and that of Haugland *et al.*,[11] argue strongly for a single dominant gene.

Two factors that may account for part of the shortfall in affected relatives are the influences of sex and age.[9] Overall 27% of male relatives were affected as compared with 16% of females. This male excess is likely to represent an indirect effect of male status on expression of the disease. Even more striking was the evidence of the effect of age: 18 of 45 parents (40%) were affected, compared with 26 of 112 (23%) sibs and 20 of 139 (14%) offspring. It is likely that in many individuals the disease does not become apparent until well into adult life.

Recent advances in molecular biology make feasible the localization of any major single gene defect (see Chapter 47). One approach in this situation involves linkage analysis. Genes close together on the same chromosome tend to be inherited together. If one is the disease gene and the other is a polymorphic (variable) marker, such as a blood group or HLA, it is possible to identify a particular copy of the marker gene, or allele, consistently travelling with the disease in each family. If the marker gene employed is on a different chromosome, no such linkage will be evident because the disease gene in the parent will be as likely to be transmitted with either copy of the marker gene.

If genes are on the same chromosome but are physically separated, there is a chance that they will be separated by cross-overs. At meiosis (egg/sperm formation), matching pairs of chromosomes are arranged side by side to allow separation from each other in order to form gametes. Typically , at least one chiasma forms; these result from breakage in the matching chromosome pair and exchange of the end pieces. A marker and disease gene on either side of such a break point would be separated in the offspring. Thus, the marker will 'cross over' to the other member of the chromosome pair. The further apart are the disease gene and marker gene, the greater the likelihood that they will be separated. If, for example, the disease gene and marker were transmitted together in 90% of cases in a family, and in 10% a cross-over occurred, it could be concluded that the two were on the same chromosome but were separated by 10 map units. The demonstration of linkage would make it likely that hypertrophic cardiomyopathy is the result of a homogeneous single gene disorder and would open the way to investigation of the disease by the reverse route of first localizing the gene then analysing its structure. This general approach to aetiology is a cause of great excitement in genetic research. Gene probes which detect variations in DNA sequence now provide an almost limitless range of markers while sequencing techniques are being developed that will allow large sections of DNA to be analysed base by base. It is being suggested that knowledge of the complete gene sequence of the human genome is less than 20 years away.

There are many problems to be overcome before the 'gene' for hypertrophic cardiomyopathy can be discovered. There may be several different genes involved in the basic defect of the heart muscle, mutation at any of which could cause the disease. The report by Branzi et al.[12] of a recessive pedigree was not particularly convincing because a non-penetrant disease gene in one parent, or even non-paternity, could account for hypertrophic cardiomyopathy in a sib pair.[13]

Even if inheritance is always dominant, it need not be the same gene in all families. In this situation, a linkage analysis that combines data from many families would not be successful; however, given the large number of early deaths in hypertrophic cardiomyopathy families, such pooling of data is essential.

Two approaches other than linkage analysis may lead to the gene. The first involves identification of any child with a chromosome deletion and hypertrophic cardiomyopathy as part of the clinical picture. One such report has appeared; a child with a deletion of chromosone 11[14] was described as having hypertrophic cardiomyopathy. Although this may prove to be an inaccurate or coincidental observation, it is worthy of note that a similar

observation led to the localization of the gene for familial adenomatous polyposis on chromosome 5.

The other, and potentially most profitable, approach is the employment of candidate genes. Over 1000 genes have now been characterized, and the number is growing rapidly. As genes involved in heart function become known, these can be analysed in families with hypertrophic cardiomyopathy to see if affected individuals always inherit the same copy. A single cross-over can effectively exclude a particular gene as being the cause in that family. As yet application in hypertrophic cardiomyopathy has been limited, but an illustration of its use in dominant supravalvular aortic stenosis is shown in Fig. 40.2. As our knowledge of the basic pathology is so limited, the choice of candidate genes is difficult. Myocardial disarray, although not exclusive to hypertrophic cardiomyopathy,[16] is typically extensive and present in almost all cases examined, which makes it likely that the primary pathology involves the genes responsible for the orderly pattern of myocardial muscle. Pearce et al.[17] have obtained evidence to suggest that experimental production of high intracellular calcium in the rat can produce myocardial disarray and hypertrophy; this finding suggests that genes involved in fetal calcium homeostasis are worthy of study. Similarly, the association of hypertrophic cardiomyopathy with Noonan's syndrome (see Chapter 47), lentiginosis,[18] neurofibromatosis and phaeo-

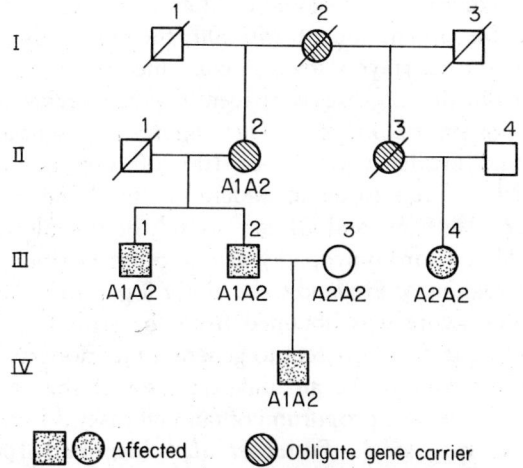

Fig. 40.2. The candidate gene approach of testing likely genes in affected families.[15] There was evidence to suggest that a defect in the calcitonin gene might be responsible for supravalvular aortic stenosis. A polymorphism with the calcitonin probe produced two alleles A1 and A2. In the family illustrated, one of the affected individuals must have inherited the disease with A1 and another with A2. In this family, the gene defect is very unlikely to involve the calcitonin gene.

chromocytoma[19] may reflect a disturbance of the embryonic neural crest mediated through either the effects of cell migration into the heart or the effects of abnormal catecholamine production.

DILATED CARDIOMYOPATHY

The WHO/ISFC Task Force[1] has defined dilated cardiomyopathy as being recognized by dilatation of the left or right ventricle or both ventricles. The clinical features of dilated cardiomyopathy are discussed in Chapter 37. Dilatation often becomes severe and is invariably accompanied by hypertrophy. Systolic ventricular function is impaired and congestive heart failure may supervene. Presentation with disturbances of ventricular or atrial rhythm is common, and death may occur at any stage (see Chapter 37 for further clinical details).

Although a clinical distinction between hypertrophic cardiomyopathy and dilated cardiomyopathy is occasionally not clear, the observation that hypertrophic cardiomyopathy is hereditary in a substantial proportion of probands whereas familial dilated cardiomyopathy is very rarely reported suggests a difference in the underlying cause. The aetiology of dilated cardiomyopathy varies throughout the world and an underlying cause can sometimes be identified (see below). There remains a group of idiopathic dilated cardiomyopathies, the genetics of which is dealt with in this section.

The incidence of idiopathic dilated cardiomyopathy was assessed in Malmö, Sweden;[20] in a stable population of 250 000, the diagnosis of dilated cardiomyopathy was confirmed in 59 cases and a further 35 cases were identified by a review of the post-mortem reports. These figures represent an annual incidence of 5 per 100 000 population, which is likely to be an underestimate of the true figure. Williams and Olsen[21] found the prevalence of dilated cardiomyopathy at one point in time in two regions of England to be about 8 per 100 000; as this figure was obtained from the replies to a postal questionnaire sent to general practitioners; it is also likely to be an underestimate of the true prevalence. The proportion of familial cases is likely to be very small. Fuster et al.[22] identified 104 patients who were seen at the Mayo clinic between 1960 and 1973 as having dilated cardiomyopathy, of whom 2 had a family history of the condition; a similar review at the Mayo clinic from 1976 to 1982 yielded 169 patients under the age of 50 years, of whom 11 had a family history (2 of whom were brothers). The results in these reports give an

estimate of familial dilated cardiomyopathy at between 2 and 6%.

Dilated cardiomyopathy has been reported as being inherited in autosomal recessive, dominant and X-linked forms. A review of 65 families with idiopathic cardiomyopathy in Japan[23] indicated that the consanguinity rate among parents of affected individuals was high. This suggests an autosomal recessive gene in a large proportion of Japanese dilated cardiomyopathy families.

Ibsen et al.[24] reported a family in which 3 of the 6 sibs were affected; they investigated the maternal side of the family because of a family history of heart disease. No other family members were shown to have dilated cardiomyopathy; although 3 relatives had died of heart disease several years earlier, the records were inadequate to assess the cause of death. The pattern of disease in this family would be consistent with autosomal recessive inheritance.

Dominantly inherited dilated cardiomyopathy has been reported in a large pedigree[25] which showed male-to-male transmission. Evidence of a more generalized skeletal myopathy, only detectable on biopsy, was also found.

Berko and Swift[26] reported a large pedigree in which dilated cardiomyopathy was inherited as an X-linked disorder, affecting the males at an earlier age and who had a worse prognosis than the females. It is possible that this was an autosomal dominant condition with, by chance, no male-to-male transmission and a sex difference in expression, although considering the size of the family this is an unlikely interpretation. These authors cite the original report by Evans in 1949[27] as containing an example of X-linked inheritance, but this should be disregarded because the family referred to by Evans showed unequivocal evidence of hypertrophic cardiomyopathy.

Michels et al.[28] reported 10 families from their consecutive series of patients at the Mayo Clinic. They noted that because of the nature of the data collection the inheritance patterns could not be determined with certainty. Five of the families showed affected members in consecutive generations; the others could have been dominantly inherited and in one family there appeared to be non-penetrance in the second generation. Voss[29] reported a family with dilated cardiomyopathy which manifested itself in the latter part of the pregnancy and in the puerperium in most of the women. The family tree is interesting in that of the 8 offspring only 2 were boys both of whom died at an early age of unknown causes and that 2 of the 6 females were unaffected. This could be an autosomal dominant pattern of inheritance with the observed family arising by chance or it could be an X-linked condition fatal to males and expressed in the females only at times of physiological stress.

O'Connell[30] reported on two families who had familial dilated cardiomyopathy and evidence of myocarditis. Both families exhibited a dominant type of inheritance with male-to-male transmission. One individual responded dramatically to immuno-suppressive treatment, suggesting an immunological factor in gene expression.

RESTRICTIVE CARDIOMYOPATHY

Restrictive cardiomyopathy is dealt with in Chapter 38. There is no clear evidence of a genetic cause of the primary form.

DISEASES WITH HEART MUSCLE INVOLVEMENT: CLINICAL FEATURES AND INHERITANCE

INBORN ERRORS OF METABOLISM WITH CARDIAC INVOLVEMENT

A wide variety of genetic metabolic defects may be associated with cardiac dysfunction. In general, those that are best understood are rare, affect children rather than adults and affect predominantly other organ systems, particularly the skeletal muscle. These disorders are worthy of attention because they provide insights into the metabolic functions of the heart and are thus likely to help our understanding of the pathogenesis of cardiomyopathy in adult life.

The metabolic disorders with cardiac involvement are listed in Table 40.1; selected examples are discussed below.

Carbohydrate metabolism—glycogenoses

Cardiac dysfunction plays a minor part in most of the 8 disorders in this group; hypoglycaemia and skeletal muscle anomalies characterize most of the forms. The exception is Pompe's disease.

Pompe's disease: Type II glycogenosis

This autosomal recessive disorder results from deficiency of the lysosomal enzyme acid maltase (amylo–1,4–glucosidase). Interruption of the secondary pathway of glycogen breakdown in the lysosomes results in rapid accumulation within these organelles of structurally normal glycogen. The pathological features of this lysosomal storage in the heart and conduction tissue have been the subject of detailed study.[31,32] In the classic form, profound hypotonia and macroglossia accompany massive enlargement of the heart (Fig. 40.3). All chambers are involved as is the conduction tissue with shortening of the PR interval. Outflow obstruction is a common late feature and death is usual in the first 2 years of life.[33] Vacuolated lymphocytes in the peripheral blood provide a useful clue to the diagnosis which is confirmed by skeletal muscle biopsy; this reveals a vacuolated myopathy due to glycogen deposits. Enzyme assay on lymphocytes is definitive and also forms the basis of pre-natal diagnosis on amniotic fibroblasts or chorionic villi. Rarer childhood and adult forms are recognized in which a mild skeletal myopathy is the presenting feature. The heart is not involved in the adult form. No therapy is available for type II glycogenosis.

Defects in intermediary metabolism

Carnitine and fatty acids

Cardiac muscle is heavily dependent on beta-oxidation of fatty acids as an energy source. Recent advances in the understanding of this biochemical pathway have begun to clarify a spectrum of clinical disorders with cardiac involvement. The co-factor carnitine has attracted particular attention. Carnitine is essential for the transfer of long chain fatty acyl groups into the mitochondrial matrix. Carnitine deficiency with a lipid storage myopathy was described originally by Engel and Angelini in 1973.[36] Clinically, three forms have been reported: myopathic, as in the original report, systemic[37] and cardiomyopathic.[38] In all three types, the carnitine tissue concentration has been shown to be reduced, but the cause is uncertain.

As a variety of metabolic errors may lead to depletion of carnitine, it is likely that many cases of carnitine deficiency are secondary. Five mechanisms for primary deficiency have been proposed:[39]

1 defective synthesis;
2 abnormal renal handling;
3 defective transport into cells;
4 increased carnitine degradation;
5 abnormal intestinal absorption.

Table 40.1.   **Metabolic diseases associated with heart muscle disease.**

Glycogen storage disease (GLD)

Pompe's disease GLD IIA
(acid maltase deficiency)
(alpha-1,4-glucosidase deficiency)[31–33]

Autosomal recessive
Lysosomal storage of glycogen, hypotonia,
extreme cardiomegaly, short PR interval, death
by end of second year

Cori's disease GLD III
(Debrancher deficiency)
(amylo-1,6-glucosidase deficiency)[34]

Autosomal recessive
Hepatomegaly, hypoglycaemia muscle
weakness. Glycogen in the myocardium may
lead to progressive cardiac failure

Andersen's disease GLD IV
(Brancher deficiency)
(alpha-1,4-glucan:alpha-1,4-glucan-6-
glucosyl-transferase deficiency)[35]

Autosomal recessive
Hepatosplenomegaly, hypotonia
developmental delay. Early death due to liver or
cardiac failure. Cardiac dilatation without
glycogen deposition in myocardium

Defects in intermediary metabolism
Carnitine deficiency

Primary carnitine deficiency (defects possible
in synthesis, renal handling, transmembrane
transport, rate of degradation and intestinal
transport)[36–42]

May present with slowly progressive muscle
weakness; systemic form with encephalopathy
and non-ketotic hypoglycaemia;
cardiomyopathic with hypertrophy dilatation
and depressed contractility dysrhythmias, giant
T waves 50% familial, heterogeneous with
possible autosomal recessive forms and
possible mitochondrial transmission

Non-genetic secondary carnitine deficiency[43]

Malnutrition, total parenteral nutrition, renal
dialysis. Renal Fanconi syndrome, cirrhosis
pregnancy, thyroid, adrenal, pituitary
insufficiency, valproic acid therapy

Fatty acid metabolic defects
Long chain acyl CoA dehydrogenase
deficiency[45]

Autosomal recessive
General muscle weakness, failure to thrive,
non-ketotic hypoglycaemia, hypertrophic
cardiomyopathy and reduced contractility. May
resolve, possibly due to L-carnitine therapy

Multiple acyl CoA dehydrogenase deficiencies
(Glutaricaciduria type II)[46]

X-linked
Metabolic acidosis, hypoglycaemia hypotonia,
hepatomegaly, foul odour, fatty change in
myocardium at autopsy

Carnitine octanoyltransferase deficiency[49]

Autosomal recessive
Encephalopathy, hypotonia, cardiomyopathy

Organic acidaemias
Beta-ketothiolase deficiency[50]

Probably autosomal recessive
Attacks of vomiting, lethargy, ketosis, acidosis.
May develop rapidly progressive congestive
cardiomyopathy

Pyruvate metabolic defects
Pyruvate dehydrogenase (PDH) deficiency
(intramitochondrial conversion of pyruvate to
acetyl CoA)[51]

Autosomal recessive
Features vary with level of residual enzyme
activity. Milder forms present with
spinocerebellar degeneration plus non-
obstructive cardiomyopathy in about one-third
of cases

Pyruvate carboxylase deficiency
(intramitochondrial)[52,53]

Similar to PDH
Similar metabolic profile of lactic acidosis with
normal pyruvate/lactate ratio. May respond to
high-fat low-carbohydrate diet with co-factors
thiamine, lipoate and biotin

Table 40.1. continued.   Metabolic diseases associated with heart muscle disease.

Defective mitochondrial electron transport

Complex I NADH–CoQ reductase deficiency[54]	Autosomal recessive Variable features include attacks of muscle weakness, mental confusion, ophthalmoplegia, lactic acidosis. Ragged red fibres, lipid storage and para-crystalline mitochondrial inclusions on biopsy. One adult male had hypertrophic cardiomyopathy. Secondary carnitine deficiency may contribute
Complex II–III succinate cytochrome C oxidoreductase deficiency[55]	Carnitine deficiency, lactic acidosis. Potential for cardiac involvement but not yet reported
Complex III Cytochrome 6 deficiency[56]	All sporadic to date. Could be mitochondrial or nuclear genome defect Rapidly fatal histiocytoid cardiomyopathy with ventricular hypertrophy and severe dysrhythmias
Complex IV cytochrome C oxidase deficiency[57]	Possible mitochondrial inheritance Variable features. Lactic acidosis, muscle weakness and renal defects in some. In others, failure to thrive, hypotonia and hypertrophic cardiomyopathy

Metabolic storage diseases

Mucopolysaccharidoses (MPS)

MPS 1H (Hurler's syndrome) Alpha-L-iduronidase deficiency[58]	Autosomal recessive Dwarfism, coarse facies, corneal clouding. Progressive retardation dysostosis multiplex hepatosplenomegaly. Death by 10 years in most cases. Myocardial failure due to valve dysfunction, hypertension, coronary artery disease, infiltration by storage cells, foci of fibrosis
MPS II (Hunter's syndrome) Iduronate sulphatase deficiency[59]	X-linked recessive Severe type A similar to Hurler syndrome but without corneal clouding. Milder type B later onset of similar features including ventricular hypertrophy, thickened valves, coronary arterial narrowing
MPS VI Maroteaux–Lamy syndrome N-Acetyl-galactosamine 4 sulphatase (arylsulphatase B) deficiency[60]	Autosomal recessive Three forms, most severe closely resembles Hurler syndrome but with normal intelligence

Mucolipidoses (ML)

MLII (I-cell disease) N-Acetyl glucosamine-I-phosphotransferase deficiency[61]	Autosomal recessive Early severe mental retardation, hernias, coarse face, hyperplastic gums, dysostosis multiplex. Cardiomegaly, valve thickening, infiltration of myocardium with vacuolated fibroblasts

Glycoproteinoses

Fucosidosis Alpha-L-fucosidase deficiency[62]	Autosomal recessive Severe type I psychomotor regression by second year, coarse face, hepatomegaly spasticity. Cardiomegaly, extrasystoles, bundle branch block, myocardial cells distorted by lamellar storage material

Table 40.1. continued.   Metabolic diseases associated with heart muscle disease.

Mannosidosis Alpha-mannosidase deficiency[63]	Autosomal recessive Severe type I early death preceded by mental and motor retardation, coarse face, flat nasal bridge, prognathism, gingival hyperplasia, spoke-like posterior cataract, hepatosplenomegaly mild skeletal changes with lax joints. Lysosomal deposition of oligosaccharides throughout heart
Lipidoses GM1 Gangliosidosis Generalized gangliosidosis[64]	Autosomal recessive Severe form: rapidly progressive motor and mental retardation, cherry red macular spots. Mild form: juvenile onset, ataxia, seizures, spastic quadriplegia; adult onset, cerebellar dysarthria in second decade, followed by spasticity and ataxia. Gangliosides and keratan sulphate accumulate in multiple organs, including heart but cardiac symptoms are unusual
Tay–Sachs disease Hexosaminidase A deficiency[65]	Autosomal recessive Severe form onset 3–6 months, exaggerated startle response, neurologial regression, cherry red macular spots. Death third year by which time deafness, blindness, spasticity and seizures are apparent. Juvenile form presents with ataxia, leads to death by 15 years. Adult form, onset as late as 3rd decade characterized by spinocerebellar degeneration weakness and fatiguability. Gangliosides accumulate in the heart but cardiac symptoms are rare.
Sandhoff's disease Hexosaminidase A and B deficiency[66]	Autosomal recessive Clinical features closely resemble features of Tay–Sachs disease but cardiac involvement greater; GM2 gangliosides and globosides in all cardiac tissues. Mitral valve leaflets and chordae tendineae thickened. Hypertrophy of myocardial tissue. Narrowing of coronary arteries by internal fibroblast proliferation
Fabry's disease Alpha-galactosidase A deficiency[67,68]	X-linked Protean features such as acroparaesthesiae, cutaneous angiokeratomata, corneal dystrophy, cataract, progressive renal failure, strokes. Milder features in female carriers. Cardiac features include aortic stenosis, mitral insufficiency, dysrhythmia, angina pectoris, hypertension. Left ventricular hypertrophy may be secondary or primary due to storage cells containing glycosphingolipids
Gaucher's disease Glucosylceramide lipidosis Glucocebrosidase deficiency[69]	Autosomal recessive Type I: late onset, hepatosplenomegaly, hypersplenism, aseptic necrosis of bone, pulmonary hypertension. Type II: acute neuronopathic–early CNS degeneration leading to death in first year. Type III: mixed features with death due to neurological degeneration in second or third decade. Cardiac signs and symptoms are unusual but all show myocardial infiltration with Gaucher cells (characteristic macrophages which stain strongly for acid phosphatase)

Table 40.1. continued.   Metabolic diseases associated with heart muscle disease.

Neimann–Pick disease Sphingomyelin lipidosis Sphingomyelinase deficiency[70]	Autosomal recessive Four types distinguished on clinical grounds based on relative involvement of nervous system and viscera. Hepatosplenomegaly, pulmonary infiltrates. Severe CNS involvement and early death in type A; type B lacks CNS changes; type C mixed picture; type D (Novo Scotia) resembles type C but shows normal enzyme activity. Widespread foam cells contain coalesced lipid-laden lysosomes. Pseudohypertrophy of the myocardium has been described
Farber's lipogranulomatosis Ceramidase deficiency[71]	Autosomal recessive Variable age of onset, a few reach adulthood. Failure to thrive, painful joints deformed by peri-articular nodules, hoarse cry. Severe pulmonary involvement. Cardiac murmurs due to valve involvement. Extensive myocardial infiltration by lipid-laden cells but rarely produces overt cardiac disease
Miscellaneous metabolic diseases Primary amyloidosis[72]	Autosomal dominant Wide variety of presentations include peripheral neuropathy, renal disease, ophthalmic signs and cardiac disease. Congestive heart failure common. ECG may resemble myocardial infarction. Appearances of restrictive pericarditis and hypertrophic cardiomyopathy common. Atrial dilatation is very common. Heavy sub-endocardial infiltration causes restrictive features
Haemochromatosis[73]	Autosomal recessive: gene linked to HLA on chromosome 6 Typical features diabetes, liver disease, skin pigmentation. Cardiac features prominent in 15% at presentation. Iron deposition within myofibres leads to dilatation of ventricles with concentric thickening and reduced compliance. Arrhythmias are common. Features are mimicked by haemosiderosis due to repeated transfusion. Treatment is with venesection and desferrioxamine
Refsum's disease (Phytanic acid storage disease) (Heredopathia atactica polyneuritiformis) Phytanic acid alpha-hydroxylase deficiency[74]	Autosomal recessive Retinitis pigmentosa, peripheral neuropathy, cerebellar ataxia. In severe cases, ophthalmoplegia, ptosis and facial weakness occur. Cardiovascular involvement typical, conduction defects may cause sudden death. Atrophic cells and fibrosis seen in myocardium. Cardiomyopathy due to phytanic acid storage is a rare complication. Dietary restriction of phytanic acid beneficial

Table 40.1. continued.   **Metabolic diseases associated with heart muscle disease.**

Acute intermittent porphyria[75]	Autosomal dominant Defective haem synthesis with variety of symptoms in porphyric crises triggered by a variety of drugs, e.g. barbiturates. Neuropsychiatric symptoms and peripheral neuropathy predominate. Photosensitivity, a major feature of variegate porphyria, is not prominent. In crises, hypertension and tachycardia occur. Histologically, pigment deposition in myocardial fibres leads to loss of nuclei and striations

The patient in the original report by Engel and Angelini[36] was subsequently shown to have impaired uptake of carnitine by muscle;[40] in healthy muscle, the carnitine concentration is 60 times the level in plasma.

Between 96 and 99% of the carnitine crossing the glomeruli is re-absorbed by the kidney tubules. In the case of carnitine deficiency associated with familial cardiomyopathy described by Waber *et al.*,[41] carnitine excretion was greater than that seen in control subjects, despite low plasma levels. Caution is needed, however, in the interpretation of these results. One of the patients with systemic carnitine deficiency and excess renal clearance described by Engel *et al.*[42] was subsequently shown to have carnitine deficiency secondary to medium chain acyl CoA dehydrogenase deficiency.[39] The metabolic defects associated with secondary carnitine deficiency are reviewed in the following sections.

Deficiencies of acyl CoA dehydrogenases

The first step in beta-oxidation of acyl CoA esters involves three enzymes acting on short, medium and long chain forms. A major consequence of a deficiency of one of these enzymes is non-ketotic hypoglycaemia. With the exception of the report cited above,[39] cardiac involvement is not a feature of the deficiency of the short or medium chain forms.[44] Major cardiac involvement occurs in the rare long chain acyl CoA dehydrogenase deficiency; in addition to non-ketotic hypoglycaemia occurring with fasting and general muscle weakness, hypertrophic cardiomyopathy may occur before the age of 6 months, with a propensity to cardiac arrest.[45] Resolution of heart disease can occur but it is not clear whether it is the result of dietary intervention (low-fat high-carbohydrate diet with L-carnitine supplements) or spontaneous.

Carnitine therapy In cases of primary carnitine deficiency, and in some cases of secondary deficiency, such as those associated with acyl CoA dehydrogenase deficiencies, oral therapy with L-carnitine is indicated. Therapy may be life-saving in cases of cardiac involvement. It is administered 3–4 times daily in a dose of 50–100 mg/kg/day for 3–6 months as a therapeutic trial.[38,41,47]

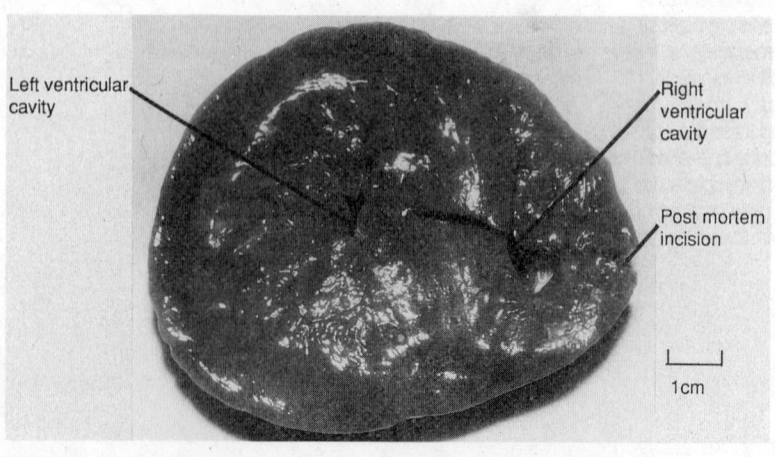

Left ventricular cavity

Right ventricular cavity

Post mortem incision

1cm

Fig. 40.3. A cross-section of the heart of an infant who died from Pompe's disease. Note the gross thickening of the ventricular wall leading to almost complete obliteration of the ventricular cavity.

In view of the availability of therapy, investigation of cardiomyopathy should include measurement of fasting plasma carnitine (normal range: 25–65 μM in females; 30–70 μM in males). Most individuals with carnitine deficiency have impaired renal tubal re-absorption (< 90% that of creatinine) assessed on mass spectrometry of a 24-h sample. Elevated levels of urinary dicarboxylic acids suggest the use of alternative pathways of lipid metabolism. Skeletal muscle biopsy is valuable for the measurement of tissue carnitine levels and to seek evidence of mitochondrial disorder, including ragged red fibres.

The number of transferase enzymes involved in transport and reversible binding of carnitine is not known. Carnitine acetyl transferase deficiency has been reported in one adult who had a restrictive cardiomyopathy.[48] Sansaricq et al.[49] reported siblings with encephalopathy, hypotonia and cardiomyopathy thought to be due to deficiency of carnitine octanoyl transferase deficiency. L-Carnitine therapy is not effective in these disorders.

Organic acidaemias

Many of the metabolic defects result in a metabolic acidosis in which organic acids are excreted in the urine. One of these, beta-ketothiolase deficiency, the details of which are given in Table 40.1, may produce a rapidly progressive dilated cardiomyopathy.[50] Treatment comprises restriction of protein and isoleucine intake.

Pyruvate metabolism

Pyruvate dehydrogenase and pyruvate carboxylase catalyse the conversion of pyruvate to acetate and oxaloacetate, respectively, both of which are essential components of the Krebs cycle. Their deficiency leads to chronic lactic acidosis as excess pyruvate is converted to lactate. Both enzymes are located in the mitochondria. Severe deficiency of both enzymes results in intractable metabolic acidosis and early death and is associated with the pathological changes of subacute necrotizing encephalomyelopathy (Leigh's disease) in young infants. Milder forms present with spinocerebellar degeneration and in this group cardiac involvement is prominent.[51–53] Over half the infants and almost one-third of older cases displayed hypertrophic cardiomyopathy. Asymmetric septal thickening is common but dynamic subaortic obstruction is not seen, thereby distinguishing the changes clinically

from those of idiopathic hypertrophic cardiomyopathy.

Lactic acidosis is characteristic with elevated serum and urinary pyruvate and alanine. Estimation of the levels of lactate and pyruvate should form part of the investigation of patients who have idiopathic non-obstructive cardiomyopathy, particularly when developmental delay or neurological degeneration are present. To exclude any underlying metabolic cause, urinary amino and organic acids should be assayed before proceeding to enzyme assay in fibroblasts.

No specific therapy is available, but oral supplements of the co-factors thiamine, lipoate and biotin may occasionally have dramatic beneficial effects.

Defects of mitochondrial electron transport

The mitochondrial electron transport chain comprises a series of four polypeptide-containing complexes embedded in the inner wall of the mitochondria. Their transfer of electrons to oxygen permits the controlled release of energy; their deficiency has a profound impact on muscle function. Severe defects are rapidly fatal, but milder forms present with muscle weakness, exercise intolerance and, in some cases, cardiomyopathy. For example, Busch et al.[54] described a 46-year-old man with echocardiographic features of hypertrophic cardiomyopathy, characterized by septal thickening, and evidence of ventricular strain on the electrocardiogram, in whom a complex I (NADH-CoQ reductase) deficiency was demonstrated. Secondary carnitine deficiency may occur with respiratory chain defects. Further details of this important category of metabolic defect are given in Table 40.1.

Metabolic storage diseases

A variety of inborn errors of metabolism result in the accumulation of waste products. Those involving the heart are listed in Table 40.1, according to the nature of the chemical defect (mucopolysaccharidoses, mucolipidoses, glycoproteinoses and lipidoses). One unusual disorder that may present to the cardiologist managing adult patients is Fabry's disease.

Fabry's disease (angiokeratoma corporis diffusum)[67,68]

Fabry's disease results from the intracellular accumulation of the neutral glycolipid ceramide trihexoside. This is due to a deficiency of the enzyme alpha-galactosidase A, also known as ceramide trihexosidase. As the gene for this enzyme is on the X chromosome, the disorder is seen typically in males, although some carrier females display cutaneous and ocular features.

Cardiac involvement is a constant feature, with histological evidence of involvement of all the structures of the heart. Light microscopy reveals intracytoplasmic bodies measuring up to 3 μm in diameter which, in osmium-fixed sections, stain intensely with toluidine blue. Birefringence is seen on polarized microscopy. The cytoplasmic deposits appear as vacuoles in paraffin-fixed sections and as lamellar myelin-like membranes on electron microscopy. Left ventricular hypertrophy results from primary deposition in the myocardium; it can also be secondary to aortic stenosis and severe hypertension. Involvement of the conduction tissue may result in impaired pacemaker function, atrial fibrillation and conduction disturbances. The electrocardiogram reveals ST- and T-wave changes and a short PR interval. Mitral valve regurgitation may result from valve involvement or be secondary to ventricular disease.

The extracardiac features are protean. The classic cutaneous feature is diffuse angiokeratomata: small dark red spots seen most often at the umbilicus, on the genitalia and over the lower extremities. Neurological features include crises of burning pain, acroparaesthesiae and psychiatric disturbances. In the eye, corneal dystrophy and posterior cortical cataracts occur. Renal deposits result in progressive renal failure, a common cause of death, and contribute to the severe hypertension. Vascular involvement is severe. Involvement of the coronary and cerebral vessels is a common cause of death in early-to-mid adult life.

Once suspected on clinical grounds, the diagnosis may be confirmed by enzyme assay on leucocytes or fibroblasts. Pre-natal diagnosis in carrier females is available on cultured amniocytes. Aggressive antihypertensive therapy is indicated. Coronary artery bypass surgery and renal transplantation may prolong life. Transplantation does not supply sufficient enzyme to reverse the metabolic defect, however; attempts at enzyme replacement have not been successful.

NEUROMUSCULAR DISEASES WITH HEART INVOLVEMENT

Several neuromuscular diseases, particularly those that involve primary myopathic processes, are associated with disease of the heart muscle. Many

of those that involve single gene defects will soon be understood as metabolic disorders, as is now the case with Duchenne muscular dystrophy, but it is reasonable to examine them separately from the perspective of those enzyme defects that have been elucidated to date. A summary of the diseases discussed in this section is given in Table 40.2; the more important diseases are also discussed below.

Duchenne muscular dystrophy

Duchenne muscular dystrophy is the commonest muscular dystrophy. It is characterized by onset of symptoms usually before the fourth year, rarely as late as the seventh, with symmetric and, at first, selective involvement of the muscles of the pelvic and pectoral girdles. Hypertrophy of the calf and certain other mucles is apparent at some stage of the disease in almost every case. The weakness shows relentless progression, leading to inability to walk within 10 years of onset and later to contractures and thoracic deformity. There is frequent, but not invariable, intellectual involvement, with affected individuals having a mean IQ of between 70 and 85. Death by the second or third decade is usually due to respiratory failure, with or without infection; less commonly, it is due to cardiac failure. Incidence at birth is between 18 and 30 per 100 000 liveborn males; prevalence varies from 1.9 to 4.8 per 100 000 population.[76]

The finding of a grossly elevated serum creatine kinase in a young boy with proximal muscle weakness makes the diagnosis highly likely. In the early stages, the creatine kinase level may be 100–300 times that of normal. Muscle biopsy provides definitive evidence. Initial features are of excess endomysial connective tissue and large hyaline muscle fibres. Later, variation in fibre size, fat replacement, active muscle necrosis, phagocytosis and regeneration are conspicuous.

Cardiac involvement is probably invariable, but may not be apparent in the early stages.[77] Persistent sinus tachycardia is common and sudden cardiac arrest may occur,[78] but chronic cardiac failure is rare. Pathological examination of the myocardium reveals variation in the size of the cardiac fibres; frequently, atrophic fibres and, occasionally, hypertrophic fibres are present. Myocardial replacement by interstitial fibrosis, particularly of the posterior wall of the left ventricle, is characteristic, together with fatty infiltration and fibrosis of the sinus and atrioventricular nodes. Degeneration of Purkinje fibres and arteriopathy of small intramural coron-

Table 40.2. **Neuromuscular diseases associated with cardiac disease.**

Duchenne muscular dystrophy[76–91]	X-linked recessive defect in dystrophin gene at Xp21 Proximal selective myopathy with pseudohypertrophy onset under 5 years, death by 25 years due to relentless muscle wasting. Markedly elevated serum creatine kinase levels. Invariable cardiac involvement with interstitial fibrosis, fatty infiltration and fibrosis of conduction tissue, degeneration of Purkinje fibres and intramural arteriopathy
Becker muscular dystrophy[91–96]	Milder deficiency of dystrophin, same gene as Duchenne Prominent calf hypertrophy and proximal myopathy. Variable onset, usually adolescence and early adulthood. Extensive fibrosis and infiltration of myocardium. Overt failure in under 10%
Emery–Dreifuss muscular dystrophy[97,98]	X-linked recessive, rare Joint contractures, diffuse slowly progressive weakness. Invariable atrial standstill by third decade. Prominent atrophy of cardiac muscle fibres and extensive myocardial fibrosis
Myotonic dystrophy Steinert's disease[99–101]	Variable autosomal dominant gene on chromosome 19 Grip myotonia, peripheral weakness, ptosis, expressionless face, frontal balding and testicular atrophy, cataracts, mental apathy and frequent retardation. Frequent conduction defects. Diffuse myocardial changes may resemble patchy myocarditis and lead to congestive failure late in disease
Facioscapulohumeral muscular dystrophy[102]	Usually autosomal dominant Variable slowly progressive with initial weakness in facial and shoulder girdle muscles. Symptomatic cardiac disease is rare but at necropsy slight myocardial fibrosis and fibre loss are seen
Nemaline myopathy[103]	Dominant and recessive forms Thin weak muscles, elongated face, high palate, variable skeletal deformities. 3–5 mm rods under sarcolemma in skeletal and cardiac muscle. Cardiomyopathy with biventricular insufficiency in adult cases
Centronuclear (myotubular) myopathy[104]	Possibly recessive but inheritance unclear Often severe generalized weakness with ptosis, ocular palsy and dysphagia. Congestive failure, aortic stenosis, ventricular hypertrophy and arrhythmias are described
Friedreich's ataxia[105–109]	Autosomal recessive, gene on chromosome 9 Onset usually in second decade of progressive spinocerebellar degeneration. Concentric hypertrophy of the heart with ECG changes in over half of cases. End-stage development of dilatation associated with congestive failure

Table 40.2. continued. Neuromuscular diseases associated with cardiac disease.

Structural mitochondrial diseases
(see also metabolic mitochondrial disorders, Table 40.1)

Kearns–Sayre syndrome (Ophthalmoplegia plus)[110]	?Mitochondrial inheritance ?nuclear genome Progressive ophthalmoplegia, pigmentary degeneration of retina, atrioventricular block. Other possible features include short stature, slow neurological degeneration. Despite involvement of mitochondria and conduction defects, myocardial dysfunction is not a major problem
X-linked cardiomyopathy with abnormal mitochondria[111]	Probable X-linked inheritance Rapidly progressive congestive heart failure in infancy. Marked hypertrophy and dilatation of cardiac chamber with endocardial fibro-elastosis. Mitochondria from heart and several other tissues show circularly arranged cristae dense bodies and glycogen deposits
Congenital cataract and mitochondrial myopathy[112]	Probable autosomal recessive Early cataracts, hypertrophic cardiomyopathy, metabolic acidosis and lactic acidaemia on exercise. Myopathic EMG, lipid droplets, excessive glycogen and excess mitochondria with abnormal cristae on skeletal muscle biopsy
Juvenile spinal muscular atrophy Kugelberg Welander disease[113]	Recessive and dominant forms Onset 2–15 years of anterior horn cell disease leading to denervation, atrophy most obvious in pelvic girdle muscles. Atrial arrhythmias and cardiomegaly with occasional heart failure described

ary arteries further complicate the picture.[79] The fibrosis of the left ventricular free wall and conducting tissue results in characteristic electrocardiographic changes:[80] tall R waves in the right precordial leads and deep Q waves in the limb leads and left precordial leads. It has been suggested that this pattern is of diagnostic value in distinguishing Duchenne muscular dystrophy from the rarer autosomal recessive form of juvenile muscular dystrophy.[81]

Echocardiography in affected boys has revealed a reduction in the rate of diastolic relaxation, but otherwise myocardial function appears to be relatively well preserved.[82–84] In boys with thoracic distortion, a very high incidence of mitral valve prolapse is seen,[85,86] which may be due, in part, to myopathic involvement of papillary muscle.[87]

Recently, dramatic progress has been made in the understanding of Duchenne muscular dystrophy at the molecular level.[88–90] The gene is on the X chromosome at band p21; it codes for a large structural protein which has been given the name dystrophin. The precise function of this protein remains unclear, but it is thought to be located in the cell membrane. It has been shown to present in a large range of tissues; its concentration in cardiac muscle is similar to that in skeletal muscle. By weight, dystrophin makes up only one two-hundred-thousandth of the muscle yet its absence has a major impact on function. In boys with Duchenne muscular dystrophy, the protein is either absent or present in only very small quantities. In at least 70% of cases, a deletion is demonstrable in the gene structure. The high frequency of deletions is related to the unique nature of the dystrophin gene, which has been shown to be made up of a large number of short coding sequences separated by long stretches of non-coding, or intervening, sequences. The result is that the gene has a total length of over 2 million base pairs, making it the largest human gene. (By comparison, the β-globin gene is only 1600 base pairs in length, *see* Chapter 67).

Becker muscular dystrophy

Clinical weakness in Becker muscular dystrophy

begins in the legs, typically in the second decade with associated calf hypertrophy. Cardiac disease has been estimated to occur in about a half of affected males.[91] Extensive fibrosis and fatty replacement of the myocardium are prominent histologically;[87] they lead to chamber dilatation and muscle flabbiness. Overt cardiac failure affects fewer than 10% of individuals, and is usually a late feature, although in occasional families severe heart involvement occurs early.[92]

The distribution of muscle weakness in Becker muscular dystrophy mirrors that seen in Duchenne muscular dystrophy. Linkage studies have shown that the two disorders map to the same chromosomal location.[93] As expected, subsequent analysis using the gene probes specific for the 'Duchenne' gene showed that Becker muscular dystrophy results from defects in the same gene.[94] In some cases of Becker muscular dystrophy, large segments of the gene are deleted, but the nature of the deletion is such that some dystrophin is produced.[95]

It may be argued that the two clinical terms are a false dichotomy and that Xp21 dystrophy should be the term used to describe this spectrum of disability, which is in part due to the degree of impairment of dystrophin production. The basis for clinical differences is not yet fully understood; within families, affected males with the same deletion may show wide variation in clinical features with onset occurring from teenage years to late middle-age.[96]

Emery–Dreifuss muscular dystrophy[97,98]

Emery–Dreifuss muscular dystrophy, first described in 1966, is a rare disorder caused by a defect in a gene on the long arm of the X chromosome. It deserves mention because cardiac problems are a predominant feature. Pathological changes in the heart affect both the conduction tissue and the myocardium. Atrophy of cardiac muscle fibres and extensive fibrosis are the principal microscopic features.

The typical presentation is of a mild diffuse muscular weakness, which is slowly progressive from childhood. Contractures develop early, particularly at the elbows and neck. Conduction defects are invariable, leading to atrial standstill by middle life. Palpitations, bradycardia, syncope or stroke may be the presenting features in the third decade. Atrial fibrillation, nodal rhythm with absent P waves, right bundle branch block and ventricular hypertrophy are some of the electrocardiographic features described.

Myotonic dystrophy

Myotonic dystrophy occurs in about 1 in 20 000 people. It displays a wide variety of clinical presentations and may involve significant cardiac disease in adulthood.

The term myotonia refers to the inability of contracted muscles to relax promptly, a sign noted particularly on shaking hands. In the overt case, peripheral weakness with wasting of the sternomastoid muscles, ptosis, dysarthria and mental apathy become evident in the second to fourth decades. An expressionless face, cataracts, diabetes mellitus and in the male frontal balding and testicular atrophy may complicate the clinical picture. Mental retardation may be a feature, particularly in children who have the severe congenital form which presents with profound hypotonia from birth. The disorder is autosomal dominant and results from a defect in a gene on chromosome 19, close to the centromere and the Apo C2 gene, which may be used in pre-natal diagnosis as a linked marker.[99] As an autosomal dominant disorder, the disease presents, in some form, in half of the offspring of a gene carrier. The severe congenital form is seen only in children who inherit the gene from an affected mother. The reason for this difference is obscure; some form of materno–fetal interaction may be involved. Pre-natal diagnosis has greater relevance for carrier females because about 1 in 5 of carrier offspring will have the severe form of the disease.

Investigation of close relatives relies on clinical examination, electromyography, and slit lamp examination to identify lens opacities. In recent studies, the value of electrocardiography has been demonstrated. In a consecutive hospital series of 65 patients,[100] significant abnormalities were revealed in 6 of 17 (35%) mild cases, 12 of 24 (50%) moderate cases and 23 of 24 (96%) severely affected cases. Atrioventricular block and left anterior hemiblock were the most common features in the mildly and moderately affected patients. Atrial fibrillation and atrial flutter, pathological Q waves and abnormalities of repolarization were observed in patients with severe disease. A review of the literature had suggested that only 1 in 6 patients had cardiac symptoms. The results of this study have confirmed that cardiac disease is common and that it relates in severity to the neurological disease. Sudden unexpected death is more common in patients with myotonic dystrophy than in the general population, which is presumably related to the conduction defects. Electrocardiography is, therefore, of diagnostic and prognostic value in all suspected cases.

Congestive cardiac failure may occur late in the disease and is associated with patchy myocarditis. Of greater practical significance are the pulmonary abnormalities. Chronic aspiration due to defective swallowing and oesophageal motility combine with varying degrees of diaphragmatic involvement to produce respiratory insufficiency. These predispose to recurrent chest infections. A third, poorly understood, factor, is a tendency to alveolar hypoventilation which can cause hypercapnia, hypoxaemia and a reduced response to inspired carbon dioxide in those with advanced disease. The combination of disordered function of conduction tissue, myocardium and lungs accounts for the considerable increase in anaesthetic risk in these patients.

Friedreich's ataxia

This autosomal recessive disorder is rare, affecting about 1 in 50 000 of the population. Cerebellar ataxia is the predominant feature; it begins before puberty and is relentlessly progressive.

In the original report of 1863, 3 of the 6 cases had cardiac hypertrophy. The results of subsequent studies have confirmed that this feature is present in about half of the affected individuals. Asymmetric hypertrophy is described, the thickening usually being concentric. Pathological examination reveals severe myocardial damage with diffuse fibrosis, small cell infiltration and atherosclerotic obstructive lesions of small and medium-sized branches of the coronary arteries. These changes are different from the fibre disarray seen in the familial form of hypertrophic cardiomyopathy. This distinction is important in view of the recent localization of the gene for Friedreich's ataxia to chromosome 9. This discovery is unlikely to contribute to the search for the gene for hypertrophic cardiomyopathy.

It is estimated that congestive cardiac failure is the cause of death in at least half of the cases. Berg et al.[107] described a sib pair, both of whom developed symptomatic cardiac involvement prior to the onset of ataxia. In classic cases, dysarthria, muscle weakness, diminished vibration and position sense and areflexia beginning in the legs are cardinal features. Secondary features include extensor plantar responses, pes cavus, scoliosis, nystagmus and diabetes mellitus.

The overall clinical picture in Friedreich's ataxia, its mode of inheritance and various reports of abnormal metabolites suggest an enzyme defect, perhaps involving intermediary metabolism, which should be identified quickly once the gene is characterized.

Mitochondrial diseases

The major disorders involving mitochondria are dealt with in Table 40.1. As yet, metabolic abnormality has not been elucidated in some disorders where structural anomalies of the mitochondria are apparent. Three rare disorders in this category are given in Table 40.2: Kearns–Sayre syndrome[110], X-linked cardiomyopathy with abnormal mitochondria[111] and congenital cataract and mitochondrial myopathy.[112]

Tuberous sclerosis[114–117]

This highly variable autosomal dominant condition derives its name from the 'potato-like' tumours that develop in the brain. The gene has been localized to the long arm of chromosome 9.

Mental retardation and seizures occur in the classic case. Calcification of the cerebral lesions results in periventricular and subependymal opacities on the computer tomographic scan. The typical skin lesion is the 'ash leaf' patch, a small area of depigmentation best seen under ultraviolet Wood's light. The other cutaneous features are facial adenoma sebaceum, periungual fibromata and areas of thickened red skin known as shagreen patches. Ocular examination reveals retinal phacomata, and benign mass lesions occur in several organs. Angiomyolipomata of the kidney are reported in over half of the gene carriers.[114]

Cardiac rhabdomyomata were present in the original case and have been reported frequently in subsequent pathological series. These derive from cardiac muscle and are regarded as fetal hamartomata. Histologically, the cells are filled with glycogen and have nuclei that are either peripheral or connected to the cell wall by strands of cytoplasm (spider cells). The 'tumours' are not encapsulated but merge into surrounding myocardium. Encapsulated cardiac lipomata are also reported.

Cardiac tumours are seen in about half of the cases and may cause severe obstructive symptoms in infants leading to early demise.[115,116] Their recognition on fetal echocardiography provides one means of pre-natal diagnosis. Linked DNA markers should soon be available as an alternative method of pre-natal diagnosis.

SYSTEMIC DISEASES

Direct and indirect involvement of the heart is seen in a wide variety of systemic acromegaly and thyroid disease, collagen vascular diseases and infiltrative diseases, such as sarcoidosis and myeloma. These diseases are discussed elsewhere, together with the wide range of drugs, toxins and infections that may adversely influence the myocardium. Brief summaries are provided in Tables 40.3 and 40.4.

MISCELLANEOUS SYNDROMES

A variety of rare syndromes may include cardiomyopathy as a feature. To provide a reference source, several of these syndromes are summarized in Table 40.5.

SUMMARY

Disease of heart muscle is of major clinical import-

Table 40.3. **Systemic diseases with direct or indirect cardiac involvement.**

Endocrine disease

Acromegaly[118]	Growth hormone excess, usually due to pituitary adenoma leads to generalized soft tissue and membranous bone overgrowth with muscle weakness. Cardiovascular disorder may be secondary to hypertension, diabetes mellitus, hyperthyroidism and coronary artery disease. Primary cardiomyopathy occurs in under 5% with ventricular hypertrophy myocarditis and subsequent interstitial fibrosis
Hyperparathyroidism[119]	Parathyroid hormone (PTH) excess usually due to adenomata leads to hypercalcaemia and bone disease. Left ventricular hypertrophy in some form is almost invariable and may mimic hypertrophic cardiomyopathy. The positive inotropic effect of PTH is blocked by verapamil suggesting effect may be mediated via calcium flux. Hypercalcaemia from other causes does not cause hypertrophy
Hyperthyroidism[120,121]	Excess production of thyroid hormone results in elevated metabolic rate and widespread systemic effects. Atrial arrhythmias and congestive cardiac failure may occur in the absence of overt systemic signs. Cardiac hypertrophy mimicking hypertrophic cardiomyopathy may occur. Fetal rat exposure to thyroid hormone produced fibre disarray and hypertrophy. Increased incidence of a history of hyperthyroidism among patients with hypertrophic cardiomyopathy has led to suggestion that the endocrine disturbance may expose a predisposition to hypertrophic cardiomyopathy
Hypothyroidism[122]	Underproduction of thyroid hormone may be due to primary defect or auto-immune disease. Pericardial effusions and abnormal left ventricular function are seen in adults. In longstanding cases, asymmetric septal hypertrophy, responsive to therapy, is described. Histologically, fibre disarray is slight. Vacuolization of muscle fibres distinguishes change from classic hypertrophic cardiomyopathy

Table 40.3. continued.   Systemic diseases with direct or indirect cardiac involvement.

Auto-immune diseases

Systemic lupus erythematosus[123]	An acute and/or chronic complex auto-immune disease of skin, joints, serous membranes, central nervous system, kidneys and other organs. Pericarditis in 20–30% clinically and 75% on echo. Myocarditis common but usually silent. Less obvious with advent of steroid therapy. In chronic phase, degenerating myocardial and inflammatory cells, patchy fibrosis and scarring
Dermatomyositis/polymyositis[124]	Symmetric weakness, limb girdle and neck flexor muscles progressing over weeks or months; necrosis, regeneration, perifascicular atrophy, perivascular inflammatory exudate in skeletal muscle +/– lilac discoloration of eyelids and joint erythema. ECG changes in 19%; congestive failure in < 10%. In some series, cardiac disease reported more commonly. Changes may mimic skeletal muscle
Rheumatoid arthritis[125]	Acute or chronic symmetric polyarthritis with synovial hypertrophy and effusions with subcutaneous nodules, weight loss and lassitude; vasculitis and pulmonary disease common. Pericarditis in over half of cases, non-specific valvulitis, non-specific inflammatory changes and granulomata in myocardium

Table 40.4.   Infections, drugs and toxins that adversely affect the myocardium.

Infectious diseases associated myocardial involvement[127]	Drugs associated with myocardial damage[128]
Bacteria	*Hypersensitivity myocarditis*
Diphtheria	Acetazolamide
Streptococcus	Amitriptyline
Meningococcus	Amphotericin B
Leptospirosis	Carbamazepine
	Chloramphenicol
Viruses	Indomethacin
Coxsackie A and B	Isoniazid
Echovirus	Methyldopa
Poliovirus	*Para*-aminosalicylic acid
Dengue	Penicillin
Yellow fever	Phenindione
Influenza	Phenylbutazone
Herpes simplex	Phenytoin
Chicken pox	Smallpox vaccine
Epstein–Barr	Spironolactone
Cytomegalovirus	Streptomycin
Mumps	Sulphonamides
Rabies	Tetracyclines
	Thiazide diuretics
Rickettsiae	Tetanus toxoid
Chlamydia (psittacosis)	
Coxiella (Q fever)	*Toxic myocarditis*
Scrub typhus	Antimony
Rocky mountain spotted fever	Anthracycline antibiotics
	Arsenicals
Protozoa	Barbiturates
Chagas' disease	
Toxoplasmosis	

Table 40.4. continued.   Infections, drugs and toxins that adversely affect the myocardium.

Caffeine
Catecholamines
Cyclophosphamide
Emetine
5-Fluorouracil
Lithium carbonate
Hydralazine
Paraquat
Phenothiazines
Plasmocid
Quinidine
Rapeseed oil

Endocardial Fibrosis
Serotonin
Methysergide
Mercury
Busulfan

Toxins[129]
Antimony
Arsenic
Arsine gas
Cobalt

Ethyl alcohol
Iron
Lead
Mercury
Scorpion venom

Infiltrative diseases and malignancy
Sarcoidosis
Hand–Schüller–Christian disease
Wegener's granulomatosis
Leukaemia
Myeloma
Phaeochromocytoma

Deficiency states
Beriberi (thiamine deficiency)
Kashan disease (selenium deficiency)
Kwashiorkor
Potassium deficiency
Magnesium deficiency

Physical insult[129]
Mediastinal irradiation

Table 40.5.   Miscellaneous syndromes that have cardiomyopathy as a feature.

Berardinelli syndrome (generalized lipodystrophy) Seip syndrome[130]	Autosomal recessive Lipo-atrophy, phallic hypertrophy, hepatomegaly, hyperlipaemia, corneal opacities, large superficial veins. Cardiomegaly
Fenichel syndrome[131]	Autosomal dominant Slowly progressive humeropelvic weakness, joint contractures in childhood. Cardiomyopathy in early adult life
Jeune thoracic dysplasia[132]	Autosomal recessive Severe rib shortening, short limbs, polydactyly, glomerulonephritis. Cardiomyopathy
LEOPARD syndrome (acronym)[18]	Autosomal dominant Multiple lentigines, ocular hypertelorism, abnormal genitalia, retardation, deafness. Electrocardiographic anomalies, pulmonary stenosis (?overlap with Noonan)
Malouf syndrome[133]	Autosomal recessive Hypergonadotrophic hypogonadism due to ovarian dysgenesis, ptosis, prominent nasal bones, congestive cardiomyopathy
Najjar syndrome[134]	Recessive—3 brothers, ?autosomal, ?X-linked Hypospadias, small penis, mental retardation. Congestive cardiomyopathy
Noonan's syndrome[135]	Autosomal dominant Short, retarded, down-slanting palpebral fissures, low set ears, short/webbed neck, cryptorchidism, pectus excavatum/carinatum. Pulmonary valve stenosis atrial septal defect, hypertrophic cardiomyopathy

---

Table 40.5. continued.   Miscellaneous syndromes that have cardiomyopathy as a feature.

Sacks' syndrome[136]	Probably variable Primary testicular failure, collagenomas of the scalp. Congestive cardiomyopathy, mainly right heart with tricuspid incompetence
Rigid spine syndrome[137]	Onset in childhood or early adulthood of restricted flexion and overextension of spine. Loss of adipose tissue and reduced muscle bulk but retained power. Single report of associated hypertrophic cardiomyopathy

---

ance yet it is all too often categorized as cardiomyopathy of unknown cause without adequate investigation. In this chapter, the focus has been on genetic aspects of cardiomyopathy and on the wide variety of associated diseases that should be considered during investigation. A detailed family history and a search for disease in other organs are essential to investigation. The close relationship between skeletal muscle and cardiac muscle is reflected in the numerous diseases that may afflict both tissues. It is worthy of note that the skeletal musculature is readily accessible to detailed assessment including biopsy. Increasing specialization in medicine may separate 'heart doctors' from 'muscle doctors' and 'metabolic doctors', yet there is much to be gained from close co-operation among these specialists in the evaluation of the patient with cardiomyopathy.

REFERENCES

1. WHO/ISFC. Report of the WHO/ISFC Task Force on the definition and classification of the cardiomyopathies. *Br. Heart J.* 1980; **44**: 672–3.
2. Taylor, W.J. Genetic aspects of the cardiomyopathies. In: Steinberg, A.G., Bearn, A.G., Motulsky, A.G. and Childs, B., eds. *Progress in Medical Genetics. V. Genetics of Cardiovascular Disease.* London: W.B. Saunders, 1983, pp.163–90.
3. Teare, D. Asymmetric hypertrophy of the heart in young adults. *Br. Heart J.* 1958; **20**: 1–8.
4. Bennett, C.P., Burn, J. and Moore, G. Prevalence of hypertrophic cardiomyopathy in the Northern region of England. *J. Med. Genet.* 1987; **94**: 243.
5. Bjarnason, I. and Hallgrimsson, J. Hypertrophic cardiomyopathy. An autopsy study of the years 1966–78. *Icelandic Med. J.* 1980; **66**: 205–9.
6. Emanuel, R., Withers, R. and O'Brien, K. Dominant and recessive modes of inheritance in idiopathic cardiomyopathy. *Lancet* 1971; ii: 1065–7.
7. Emanuel, R., Marcomichelakis, J., Withers, R. and O'Brien, K. Asymmetric septal hypertrophy and hypertrophic cardiomyopathy. *Br. Heart J.* 1983; **49**: 309–16.
8. Clarke, C.E., Henry, W.L. and Epstein, S.E. Familial prevalence and genetic transmission of idiopathic hypertrophic subaortic stenosis. *N. Engl. J. Med.* 1973; **289**: 709–14.
9. Maron, B.J., Nichols, P.F. III, Pickle, L.W., Wesley, Y.E. and Mulvihill, J.J. Patterns of Inheritance in hypertrophic cardiomyopathy: assessment by M-Mode and two dimensional echocardiography. *Am. J. Cardiol.* 1984; **53**: 1087–94.
10. Greaves, S.C., Roche, A.H.G., Neutze, J.M., Whitlock, R.M.L. and Veale, A.M.O. Inheritance of hypertrophic cardiomyopathy: a cross sectional and M-mode echocardiographic study of 50 families. *Br. Heart J.* 1987; **58**: 259–66.
11. Haugland, H., Ohm, O.-J., Boman, H. and Thorsby, E. Hypertrophic cardiomyopathy in three generations of a large Norwegian family: a clinical, echocardiographic and genetic study. *Br. Heart J.* 1986; **55**: 168–75.
12. Branzi, A., Romeo, G., Specchia, S. *et al.* Genetic heterogeneity of hypertrophic cardiomyopathy. *Int. J. Cardiol.* 1985; **7**: 129–33.
13. Burn, J. The genetics of hypertrophic cardiomyopathy. *Int. J. Cardiol.* 1985; **7**: 135–8.
14. Gilgenkrantz, S., Vigneron, C., Gegoire, M.J., Penot, C. and Raspiller, A. Association of del (11) (p14.1–p12) Aniridia, catalase deficiency and cardiomyopathy. Chromosome 11 deletion case. *Am. J. Med. Genet.* 1982; **13**: 39–49.
15. Bennett, C.P., Burn, J., Moore, G.E., Chambers, J., Williamson, R. and Wilkinson, J. Exclusion of calcitonin as a candidate gene for the basis defect in a family with autosomal dominant supravalvular aortic stenosis. *J. Med. Genet.* 1988; **25**: 311–2.
16. Pearce, P.C., Hawkey, C., Symons, C. and Olsen, E.G.J. Role of Calcium in the induction of cardiac hypertrophy and myofibrillar disarray. Experimental studies of a possible cause of hypertrophic cardiomyopathy. *Br. Heart J.* 1985; **54**: 420–7.
17. Becker, A.E. and Caruso, G. Myocardial disarray. A critical review. *Br. Heart J.* 1982; **42**: 527–38.
18. St John Sutton, M.G., Tajik, A.J., Guiliani, E.R., Gordon, H. and Daniel, W.P. Hypertrophic obstructive cardiomyopathy and lentiginosis. A little known neural ectodermal syndrome. *Am. J. Cardiol.* 1981; **47**: 214–7.
19. Fitzpatrick, A.P. and Emanuel, R.W. Familial neurofibromatosis and hypertrophic cardiomyopathy. *Br. Heart J.* 1988; **60**: 247–51.
20. Torp, A. Incidence of congestive cardiomyopathy. *Postgrad. Med. J.* 1978; **54**: 435–7.
21. Williams, D.G. and Olsen, E.G.J. Prevalence of overt dilated cardiomyopathy in two regions of England. *Br. Heart J.* 1985; **54**: 153–5.
22. Fuster, V., Gersh, B.J., Giuliani, E.R., Tajik, A.J., Brandenburg, R.O. and Frye, R.L. The natural history of idiopathic dilated cardiomyopathy. *Am. J. Cardiol.* 1981; **47**: 525–31.
23. Yamaguchi, M., Toshima, H. and Yanase, T. Genetic

heterogeneity of idiopathic cardiomyopathies. *Jap. Circulation J.* 1978; **42**: 1131–2.

24. Ibsen, H.H.W., Baandrup, V. and Simonsen, E.E. Familial right ventricular dilated cardiomyopathy. *Br. Heart J.* 1985; **54**: 156–9.

25. Gardner, R.J.M. and Hanson, J.W. *Am. J. Med. Genet.* 1987; **27**: 61–71.

26. Berko, B.A. and Swift, M. X linked dilated cardiomyopathy. *N. Engl. J. Med.* 1987; **316**: 1186–91.

27. Evans, W. Familial cardiomegaly. *Br. Heart J.* 1949; **11**: 68–82.

28. Michels, V.V., Driscoll, D.J. and Miller, F.A. Familial aggregation of idiopathic dilated cardiomyopathy. *Am. J. Cardiol.* 1985; **55**: 1232–3.

29. Voss, E.G., Reddy, C.V.R., Detrano, R., Virmani, R., Zabriskie, J.B. and Fotino, M. Familial dilated cardiomyopathy. *Am. J. Cardiol.* 1984; **54**: 455–7.

30. O'Connell, J.B., Fowles, R.E., Robinson, J.A., Subramanian, R., Henkin, R.E., Gunnar, R.M. Clinical pathologic findings of myocarditis in two families with dilated cardiomyopathy. *Am. Heart J.* 1984; **107**: 127–35.

31. Ehlers, K.H., Hagstrom, J.W.C., Lukas, D.S., Redo, S.F. and Engle, M.A. Glycogen storage disease of the myocardium with obstruction to left ventricular outflow. *Circulation* 1962; **25**: 96–109.

32. Bharati, S., Serratto, M., DuBrow, I., Paul, M.H., Swiryn, S., Miller, R.A., Rosen, K. and Lev, M. The conduction system in Pompe's disease. *Pediatric Cardiology* 1982; **2**: 25–32.

33. Ruttenberg, H.D., Steidl, R.M., Carey, L.S. and Edwards, J.E. Glycogen storage disease of the heart. Hemodynamic and angiographic features in two cases. *Am. Heart J.* 1964; **67**: 469–80.

34. Olson, L.J., Reeder, G.S., Noller, K.L., Edwards, W.D., Howell, R.R. and Michels, V.V. Cardiac involvement in glycogen storage disease III: Morphologic and biochemical characterisation with endo-myocardial biopsy. *Am. J. Cardiol.* 1984; **53**: 980–1.

35. Reed, G.B., Dixon, J.F.P., Newstein, H.B., Donnell, G.N. and Landing, B.H. Type IV glycogenosis. *Lab. Invest.* 1968; **19**: 546–57.

36. Engel, A.G. and Angelini, C. *Science* 1973; **179**: 899–902.

37. Karpati, G., Carpenter, S., Engle, A.G., Watters, G., Allen, J., Rothman, S., Klassen, G. and Mamer, O.A. *Neurology* 1975; **25**: 16–24.

38. Tripp, M.E., Katcher, M.L., Peters, H.A., Gilbert, E.F., Arya, S., Hodach, R.J. and Shug, A.L. Systemic carnitine deficiency presenting as familial endocardial fibroelastosis. *N. Engl. J. Med.* 1981; **305**: 385–90.

39. Turnbull, D.M. and Sherratt, H.S.A. Mitochondrial myopathies: Defects in B oxidation. *Biochem. Soc. Trans.* 1985; **13**: 645–8.

40. Rebouche, C.J. and Engle, A.G. *J. Clin. Invest.* 1984; **73**: 857–67.

41. Waber, L.J., Valle, D., Neill, C., DiMauro, S. and Shug, A.L. Carnitine deficiency presenting as familial cardiomyopathy: A treatable defect in carnitine transport. *J. Pediatr.* 1982; **101**: 700–5.

42. Engle, A.G., Rebouche, C.J., Wilson, D.M., Glasgow, A.M., Romshe, C.A. and Cruse, R.P. Primary systemic carnitine deficiency II. Renal handling of carnitine. *Neurology* 1981; **31**: 819–25.

43. Pierpont, M.E. and Tripp, M.E. Abnormalities of intermediary metabolism. In: Pierpont, M.E. and Moller, J.H., eds. *Genetics of Cardiovascular disease.* Boston: Martinus Nijhoff, 1986, pp.193–214.

44. Turnbull, D.M., Bartlett, K., Stevens, D.L., Alberti, K.G.M.M., Gibson, G.J., Johnson, M.A., McCulloch, A.J. and Sherratt, H.S.A. Short chain acyl-CoA dehydrogenase deficiency associated with a lipid-storage myopathy and secondary carnitine deficiency. *N. Engl. J. Med.* 1984; **311**: 1232.

45. Hale, D.E., Batshaw, M.L., Coates, P.M., Frerman, F.E., Goodman, S.I., Singh, I. and Stanley, C.A. Long chain acyl coenzyme A dehydrogenase deficiency: An inherited cause of non-ketotic hypoglycaemia. *Pediatr. Res.* 1985; **19**: 666–71.

46. Rhead, W.J. and Amendt, B.A. Electron-transferring flavoprotein deficiency in the multiple acyl-CoA dehydrogenation disorders glutaric aciduria type II and ethylmalonic-adipic aciduria. *J. Inherit. Metab. Dis.* 1984; **7**: 99–100.

47. Tripp, M.E. and Shug, A.L. Long term management problems in carnitine deficient cardiomyopathy. *Pediatr. Res.* 1985; **19**: 135A.

48. Tripp, M.E., Lennon, D.L., Stratman, F.W., Hodach, R.J. and Shug, A.L. Restrictive cardiomyopathy with preclinical myopathy: Metabolic and morphologic findings. *Clin. Res.* 1982; **30**: 227A.

49. Sansaricq, C., Kaufmann, R., DiMauro, S., Schacht, R.G., Greco, A. Goldstein, F., Naylor, E.W., Bazaz, G. and Snyderman, S.E. Mixed form of carnitine deficiency with dicarboxylic aciduria unresponsive to carnitine. *Pediatr. Res.* 1983; **17**: 295A.

50. Henry, C.G., Strauss, A.W., Keating, J.P. and Hillman, R.E. Congestive cardiomyopathy associated with B ketothiolase deficiency. *J. Pediatr.* 1981; **99**: 754–7.

51. Robinson, B.H. Inborn errors of pyruvate metabolism. *Biochem. Soc. Trans.* 1983; **11**: 623–6.

52. Rutledge, J.T., Haas, J.E., Monnat, R. and Milstein, J.M. Hypertrophic cardiomyopathy is a component of subacute necrotizing encephalomyelopathy. *J. Pediatr.* 1982; **101**: 706–10.

53. Boyer, S.H., Chisholm, A.W. and McKusick, V.A. Cardiac aspects of Friedreich's ataxia. *Circulation* 1962; **25**: 493–9.

54. Busch, H.F.M., Scholte, H.R., Arts, W.F. and Luyt-Houwen, I.E.M. A mitochondrial myopathy with a respiratory chain defect and carnitine deficiency. In: Busch, H.F.M., Jennekens, F.G.I. and Scholte, H.R., eds. *Mitochondria and muscle diseases.* Beetsterwaag, Netherlands: Mefar, 1981, pp.207–11.

55. Behbehani, A.W., Goebel, H., Osse, G., Gabriel, M., Langenbeck, V., Berden, J., Berger, R. and Schutgens, R.B. Mitochondrial myopathy with lactic acidosis and deficient activity of muscle succinate cytochrome-c-oxidoreductase. *Eur. J. Pediatr.* 1984; **143**: 67–71.

56. Papadimitriou, A., Neustein, H.B., DiMauro, S., Stanton, R. and Bresolin, N. Histiocytoid cardiomyopathy of infancy: Deficiency of reducible cytochrome b in heart mitochondria. *Pediatr. Res.* 1984; **18**: 1023–8.

57. Sengers, R.C., Trijbels, J.M., Bakkeren, J.A.J.M., Ruitenbeek, W., Fischer, J.C., Janssen, A.J.M., Stadhouders, A.M. and Orhaak, H.J. Deficiency of cytochromes b and aa3 in muscles from a floppy infant with cytochrome oxidase deficiency. *Eur. J. Pediatr.* 1984; **141**: 178–80.

58. Renteria, V.G., Ferrans, V.J. and Roberts, W.C. The heart in the Hurler syndrome: Gross histologic and ultrastructural observations in five necropsy cases. *Am. J. Cardiol.* 1976; **38**: 487–501.

59. Emanuel, R.W. Gargoylism with cardiovascular involvement in two brothers. *Br. Heart J.* 1954; **16**: 417–22.

60. Maroteaux, P. and Lamy, M. Hurler's disease, Morquio's disease and related mucopolysaccharidoses. *J. Pediatr.* 1965; **67**: 312–23.

61. Neufeld, E.F. and McKusick, V.A. Disorders of lysosomal enzyme synthesis and localisation: I-cell disease and pseudo Hurler polydystrophy. In: Stanbury, J.B., Wyngaarden, J.B., Fredrickson, D.S., Goldstein, J.L. and Brown, M.S. eds. *The metabolic basis of inherited disease*

5th edn. New York: McGraw Hill, 1983, pp.778–87.

62. Durand, P., Borrone, C. and Della Cella, G. Fucosidosis. *J. Pediatr.* 1969; **75**: 665–74.

63. Desnick, R.J., Sharp, H.L., Grabowski, G.A., Brunning, R.D., Quie, P.G., Sung, J.H., Gorlin, R.J. and Ikoune, J.U. Mannosidosis: clinical morphologic immunologic and biochemical studies. *Pediatr. Res.* 1976; **10**: 985–95.

64. O'Brien, J.S. The gangliosidoses. In: Stanbury, J.B., Wyngaarden, J.B., Fredrickson, D.S., Goldstein, J.L. and Brown, M.S., eds. *The metabolic basis of inherited disease*, 5th edn. New York: McGraw Hill, 1983, pp.945–69.

65. Rodriguez-Torres, R., Schneck, L. and Kleinberg, W. Electrocardiographic and biochemical abnormalities in Tay–Sachs disease. *Bull. N.Y. Acad. Med.* 1971; **47**: 717–30.

66. Blieden, L.C., Desnick, R.J., Carter, J.B., Krivit, W., Moller, J.H. and Sharp, H.L. Cardiac involvement in Sandhoff's disease. Inborn error of glyco-sphingolipid metabolism. *Am. J. Cardiol.* 1974; **34**: 83–8.

67. Colucci, W.S., Lorell, B.H., Schoen, F.J., Warhol, M.J. and Grossman, W. Hypertrophic obstructive cardiomyopathy due to Fabry's disease. *N. Engl. J. Med.* 1982; **307**: 926–8.

68. Becker, A.E., Schoorl, R., Balk, A.G. and Van der Heide, R.M. Cardiac manifestations of Fabry disease. *Am. J. Cardiol.* 1975; **36**: 829–35.

69. Sack, G.H. Clinical diversity in Gaucher's disease. *Johns Hopkins Med. J.* 1980; **146**: 166–72.

70. Westwood, M. Endocardial fibroelastosis and Niemann–Pick disease. *Br. Heart J.* 1977; **39**: 1394–6.

71. Abdul-Haj, S.K., Martz, D.G., Douglas, W.E. and Greppert, J.L. Farber's disease. *J. Pediatr.* 1962; **61**: 221–32.

72. Roberts, W.C. and Waller, B.F. Cardiac amyloidosis causing cardiac dysfunction: analysis of 54 necropsy patients. *Am. J. Cardiol.* 1983; **52**: 137–46.

73. Easley, R.M. Jr, Schreiner, B.F. Jr and Yu, P.N. Reversible cardiomyopathy associated with hemochromatosis. *N. Engl. J. Med.* 1972; **287**: 866–867.

74. Refsum, S. Heredopathia atactica polyneuritiformis (Refsum disease). In: Dyck, P.J., Thomas, P.K., Lambert, E.H. and Bunge, R.P., eds. *Peripheral neuropathy*, 2nd edn. Philadelphia: W.B. Saunders, 1984, pp.1680–3.

75. Stein, J.A. and Tschudy, D.P. Acute intermittent porphyria. A clinical and biochemical study of 46 patients. *Medicine (Baltimore)* 1970; **49**: 1–16.

76. Walton, J.N. and Gardner Medwin, D. The muscular dystrophies. In: Walton, J.N., ed. *Disorders of voluntary muscle*, 5th edn. Edinburgh: Churchill Livingstone, 1988, pp.519–68.

77. Slucka, C. The electrocardiogram in Duchenne progressive muscular dystrophy. *Circulation* 1968; **38**: 933.

78. Berenbaum, A.A. and Horowitz, W. Heart involvement in progressive muscular dystrophy. Report of a case with sudden death. *Am. Heart J.* 1956; **51**: 622.

79. Perloff, J.K., de Leon, A.C. Jr and O'Doherty, D. The cardiomyopathy of progressive muscular dystrophy. *Circulation* 1966; **33**: 625–48.

80. Perloff, J.K., Roberts, W.C., de Leon, A.C. and O'Doherty, D. The distinctive electrocardiogram of Duchenne's progressive muscular dystrophy. *Am. J. Med.* 1967; **42**: 179.

81. Emery, A.E.H. Abnormalities of the electrocardiogram in hereditary myopathies. *J. Med. Genet.* 1972; **9**: 8–12.

82. Kovick, R.B., Fogelman, A.M., Abbasi, A.S., Peter, J.P. and Pearce, M.L. Echocardiographic evaluation of posterior left ventricular wall motion in muscular dystrophy. *Circulation* 1975; **52**: 447.

83. Ahmad, M., Sanderson, J.E. and Dubowitz, V. Echocardiographic assessment of left ventricular function in Duchenne's muscular dystrophy. *Br. Heart J.* 1978; **40**: 734.

84. Goldberg, S.J., Stern, L.Z., Feldman, L., Allen, H.D., Sahn, D.J. and Valdes-Cruz, L.M. Serial two-dimensional echocardiography in Duchenne muscular dystrophy. *Neurology* 1982; **32**: 1101–5.

85. Danilowicz, D., Rutkowski, M., Myung, D. and Shively, D. Echocardiography in Duchenne muscular dystrophy. *Muscle Nerve* 1980; **3**: 298–303.

86. Hunsacker, R.H., Fulkerson, P.K., Barry, F.J., Lewis, R.O., Leier, C.V. and Unverferth, D.V. Cardiac function in Duchenne's muscular dystrophy. *Am. J. Med.* 1982; **73**: 235–8.

87. Sanyal, S.K. and Johnson, W.W. Cardiac conduction abnormalities in children with Duchenne's muscular dystrophy. *Circulation* 1982; **66**: 853–63.

88. Monaco, A.P., Neve, R.L., Colletti-Feener, C., Bertelson, C.J., Kurnit, D.M. and Kunkel, I.M. Isolation of candidate cDNA's for portions of the Duchenne muscular dystrophy gene. *Nature* 1986; **323**: 646–50.

89. Koenig, M., Hoffman, E.P., Bertelson, C.J., Monaco, A.P., Feener, C. and Kunkel, L.M. Complete cloning of the Duchenne muscular dystrophy (DMD) cDNA and preliminary genomic organisation of the DMD gene in normal and affected individuals. *Cell* 1987; **50**: 509–17.

90. Chelly, J., Kaplan, J.-C., Maire, P., Gautron, S. and Kahn, A. Transciption of the dystrophic gene in human muscle and non-muscle tissues. *Nature* 1988; **333**: 858–60.

91. Bradley, W.G., Jones, M.Z., Mussini, J.-M. and Fawcett, P.R.W. Becker-type muscular dystrophy. *Muscle Nerve* 1978; **1**: 111–32.

92. Mabry, C.C., Roeckel, I.E., Munich, R.L. and Robertson, D. X linked pseudohypertrophic muscular dystrophy with late onset and slow progression. *N. Engl. J. Med.* 1965; **273**: 1062–70.

93. Kingston, H.M., Thomas, N.S.T., Pearson, P.L., Sarfarazi, M. and Harper, P.S. Genetic linkage between Becker muscular dystrophy and a polymorphic DNA sequence on the short arm of the X chromosome. *J. Med. Genet.* 1983; **20**: 255–8.

94. Kunkel, L.M. and 75 co-authors. Analysis of deletions in DNA from patients with Becker and Duchenne muscular dystrophy. *Nature* 1986; **322**: 73–7.

95. Monaco, A.P., Bertelson, C.J., Liecht-Gallati, S., Moser, H. and Kunkel, L.M. A molecular mechanism for the clinical difference between Duchenne and Becker muscular dystrophy. *N. Engl. J. Med.* 1988; in press.

96. Forrest, S.M., Cross, G.S., Speer, A., Gardner-Medwin, D., Burn, J. and Davies, K.E. Preferential deletion of exons in Duchenne and Becker muscular dystrophies. *Nature* 1987; **329**: 638–40.

97. Hopkins, L.C., Jackson, J.A. and Elsas, L.J. Emery–Dreifuss humeroperoneal muscular dystrophy. An X-linked myopathy with unusual contractures and bradycardia. *Ann. Neurol.* 1981; **10**: 230–7.

98. Thomas, P.K., Calne, D.B. and Elliot, C.F. X-linked scapuloperoneal syndrome. *J. Neurol. Neurosurg. Psychiatr.* 1972; **35**: 209–15.

99. Harper, P.S. Myotonic disorders. In: Walton, J.N., ed. *Disorders of voluntary muscle*. Edinburgh: Churchill Livingstone, 1988, pp.569–87.

100. Olofsson, B.-O., Forsberg, H., Andersson, S., Bjerle, P., Henriksson, A. and Wedin, I. Electrocardiographic findings in myotonic dystrophy. *Br. Heart J.* 1988; **59**: 47–52.

101. Rausing, A. Focal myocarditis in familial dystrophica myotonica. *Br. Heart J.* 1972; **34**: 1292–4.

102. Ziter, F.A. and Tyler, F.H. Neuromuscular disorders. In: Pierpont, M.E.M. and Moller, J.H., eds. *Genetics of cardiovascular disease*. Boston: Martinus Nijhoff, 1987, pp.241–63.

103. Meier, C., Voellmy, W., Gertsch, M., Zimmerman, A. and Geissbuhler, J. Nemaline myopathy appearing in adults as

cardiomyopathy: a clinicopathologic study. *Arch. Neurol.* 1984; **41**: 443–5.

104. Verhiest, W., Brucher, J.M., Godderis, P., Lanweryns, J. and De Geest, H. Familial centronuclear myopathy associated with 'cardiomyopathy'. *Br. Heart J.* 1976; **38**: 504–9.

105. Gottdiener, J.S., Hawley, R.J., Maron, B.J., Bertorini, T.F. and Engle, W.K. Characteristics of the cardiac hypertrophy in Friedreich's ataxia. *Am. Heart J.* 1982; **103**: 525–31.

106. Smith, E.R., Sangalang, V.E., Heffernan, L.P. *et al.* Hypertrophic cardiomyopathy: the heart disease in Friedreich's ataxia. *Am. Heart J.* 1977; **94**: 428–34.

107. Berg, R.A., Kaplan, A.M., Jarrett, P.B. and Moltham, M.E. Friedreich's ataxia with acute cardiomyopathy. *Am. J. Dis. Child.* 1980; **134**: 309–3.

108. Williamson, R. Gene for Friedreich's ataxia is located on chromosome 9. Presented at the European Society of Human Genetics Meeting in Cardiff, 1988.

109. Sanchez-Casis, G., Cote, M. and Barbeau, A. Pathology of the heart in Friedreich's ataxia: review of the literature and report of one case. *Canad. J. Neurol Sci.* 1976; **3**: 349–54.

110. Butler, I.J. and Gadoth, N. Kearn–Sayre's syndrome: A review of a multisystem disorder of children and young adults. *Arch. Intern. Med.* 1976; **136**: 1290–3.

111. Neustein, H.B., Lurie, P.R., Dahms, B. and Takahashi, M. An X-linked recessive cardiomyopathy with abnormal mitochondria. *Pediatrics* 1979; **64**: 24–9.

112. Sengers, R.C.A., Stadhouders, A.M., Lakwijk-Vondrovicova, E., van Kubat, K. and Ruitenbeek, W. Hypertrophic cardiomyopathy associated with a mitochondrial myopathy of voluntary muscles and congenital cataract. *Br. Heart J.* 1985; **54**: 543–7.

113. Tanaka, H., Nobuhiro, U., Yoshifumi, T., Kudo, A., Ohkatsu, Y., Kanehisa, T. Cardiac involvement in the Kugelberg-Welander syndrome. *Am. J. Cardiol.* 1976; **38**: 528–32.

114. Chouko, A.M., Weiss, S.M., Stein, J.H. and Ferris, T.F. Renal involvement in tuberous sclerosis. *Am. J. Med.* 1974; **56**: 124–32.

115. Bass, J.L., Breningstall, G.N. and Swaiman, K.F. Echocardiographic incidence of cadiac rhabdomyoma in patients with tuberous sclerosis. *Am. J. Cardiol.* 1985; **55**: 1379–82.

116. McAllister, H.A. and Fenoglio, J.J. Rhabdomyoma, tumours of the cardiovascular system. In: *Atlas of tumour pathology*, 2nd Series, Fascicle 15. Bethesda, MD: Armed Services Institute of Pathology, 1978, pp.25–31.

117. Yates, J. Localisation of the gene for tuberous sclerosis to the long arm of chromosome 9. Presented European Society of Human Genetics, 1988.

118. Hayward, R.P., Emanuel, R.W. and Nabarro, J.D.N. Acromegalic heart disease: influence of treatment of the acromegaly on the heart. *Q. J. Med.* 1987; **237**: 41–58.

119. Symons, C., Fortune, F., Greenbaum, R.A. and Dandona, P. Cardiac hypertrophy, hypertrophic cardiomyopathy and hyperparathyroidism—an association. *Br. Heart J.* 1985; **54**: 539–42.

120. Symons, C. Thyroid heart disease. *Br. Heart J.* 1979; **41**: 257–62.

121. Bell, R., Barber, P.V., Bray, C.L. and Beton, D.C. Incidence of thyroid disease in cases of hypertrophic cardiomyopathy. *Br. Heart J.* 1978; **40**: 1306–9.

122. Altman, D.I., Murray, J., Milner, S., Dansky, R. and Levin, S.E. Asymmetric septal hypertrophy and hypothyroidism in children. *Br. Heart J.* 1985; **54**: 533–8.

123. Ansari, A., Larson, P.H. and Bates, H.D. Cardiovascular manifestations of systemic lupus erythematosus: current perspective. *Prog. Cardiovasc. Dis.* 1985; **27**: 421–34.

124. Gottdiener, J.S., Sherbel, H.S., Hawley, R.J. and Engel, W.K. Cardiac manifestations in polymyositis. *Am. J. Cardiol.* 1978; **41**: 1141–9.

125. Jayson, M.I.V. and Grennan, D.M. Clinical features of rheumatoid arthritis. In: Weatherall, D.J., Ledingham, J.G.G. and Warrell, D.A., eds. *Oxford textbook of Medicine*, 2nd ed. Oxford: Oxford University Press, 1987, pp.16.3–16.8.

126. Schultheiss, H.-P., Schutze, K., Kuhl, V., Ulrich, G. and Klingenberg, M. The ADP/ATP carrier as a mitochondrial auto-antigen. Facts and Perspectives. *Ann. N.Y. Acad. Scl.* 1986; **488**: 44–64.

127. Oakley, C.M. Specific heart muscle disorders. In: Weatherall, D.J., Ledingham, J.G.G. and Warrell, D.A., eds. *Oxford Textbook of Medicine*, 2nd edn. Oxford: Oxford University Press, 1987, pp.13.196–13.209.

128. Ettedgui, J.A. Cardiological aspects of systemic disease. In: Anderson, R.A., Macartney, F.J., Shinebourne, E.A., Tynan, M. (eds.) *Paediatric Cardiology* Edinburgh: Churchill Livingstone, 1987, pp.1245–7.

129. Goodwin, J.L., Roberts, W.C. and Wenger, N.K. Cardiomyopathy. In: Hurst, J.W., ed. *The Heart.* 1982, pp.1299–262.

130. Berardinelli, W. An undiagnosed endocrinometabolic syndrome: report of two cases. *J. Clin. Endocrinol. Metab.* 1954; **14**: 193–204.

131. Fenichel, G.M., Chul Sul, Y., Kilroy, A.W. and Blouin, R. An autosomal-dominant dystrophy with humeropelvic distribution and cardiomyopathy. *Neurology* 1982; **32**: 1299–401.

132. Tahernia, A.C. and Stamps, P. 'Jeune syndrome' (asphyxiating thoracic dystrophy). Report of a case, a review of the literature, and an editor's commentary. *Clin. Pediatr.* 1977; **16**: 903–8.

133. Malouf, J., Alan, S., Kanj, H., Mufarrij, A., Kaloustian, V., M der. Hypergonadotrophic hypogonadism with congestive cardiomyopathy. An autosomal recessive disorder. *Am. J. Med. Genet.* 1985; **20**: 483–9.

134. Najjar, S.S., Der Kaloustian, V.M. and Nassif, S.I. Genital anomaly, mental retardation and cardiomyopathy: A new syndrome? *J. Pediatr.* 1973; **83**: 286–8.

135. Duncan, W.J., Fowler, R.S., Farkas, L.G. *et al.* A comprehensive scoring system for evaluating Noonan's syndrome. *Am. J. Med. Genet.* 1981; **10**: 37–50.

136. Sacks, H.N., Crawley, I.S., Ward, J.A. and Fine, R.M. Familial cardiomyopathy: hypogonadism and collagenoma. *Ann. Intern. Med.* 1980; **93**: 813–7.

137. Colver, A.F., Steer, C.R., Godman, M.J. and Uttley, W.S. Rigid spine syndrome and fatal cardiomyopathy. *Arch. Dis. Child.* 1981; **56**: 148–51.

Chapter 41

Pericardial Diseases

Celia Oakley

Introduction

Pericardial disease has been known since at least the time of Galen. The physical signs of acute pericarditis, "adherent pericardium", pericardial tamponade and constrictive pericarditis were worked out in the nineteenth century. Pericardiectomy for chronic constrictive pericarditis was the first, 'cardiac' operation, becoming performed quite commonly in the 1940s for constriction of tuberculous origin.

As tuberculosis is now rare in the indigenous population of the UK and the use of antibiotics has also reduced the incidence of acute purulent pericarditis, patients with pericardial diseases comprise only a small number of those seen by the cardiologist. Cardiac surgical units carry out 1 pericardiectomy for every 200–300 coronary artery bypass operations performed. Pericardial disease, however, forms a major part of the fascinating cardiology of other specialities, particularly rheumatology and oncology.

As bacterial pericarditis became rare, acute 'benign' pericarditis of presumed viral origin was recognized; occasionally, this progresses rapidly to constriction of which it is now the commonest 'cause'. The syndrome of *relapsing pericarditis* was first recognized after the Second World War in soldiers with retained shrapnel. Subsequently, with the advent of closed mitral valvotomy, the *post-cardiotomy syndrome* became recognized, and then the *post-myocardial infarction syndrome of Dressler*. It is now clear that any pericarditis may be followed by a relapsing course of presumed immunological origin.

From its inception, echocardiography was a reliable means of recognizing pericardial effusion; it has also clarified the pathophysiology of tamponade.

Anatomy

The serous pericardium is a delicate invaginated sac, the 'joint space' in which the heart moves. The parietal pericardium has an outer layer, the fibrous pericardium, which is tough and unyielding. The visceral pericardium is reflected over the heart forming its outer layer. The pericardial space contains up to 50 ml of clear fluid similar to lymph. The pericardium is bordered anteriorly by the sternum, posteriorly by the oesophagus and descending aorta, laterally by the lungs and inferiorly by the diaphragm to which the fibrous pericardium is attached. Superiorly, the pericardium is reflected off the ascending aorta just below the aortic arch and half way down the superior vena cava below the entry of the azygos vein. The main pulmonary artery and the proximal left and right branches are enclosed within it, as are the proximal portions of the pulmonary veins. A layer of adipose tissue of varying amount separates the myocardium from the visceral pericardium and this is a useful marker when examining the pericardium by computed tomography. The arterial supply to the pericardium arises from the internal mammary arteries and the descending thoracic aorta and it receives the phrenic, sympathetic and vagus nerves.

Function

The pericardium does not seem to be very important in health because in congenital total absence of the pericardium no circulatory disturbance occurs[1]. The pericardium can be seen to exercise a restraining function[2] limiting cardiac dilatation in acute cardiac failure[3], such as mitral regurgitation following sudden chordal rupture, right ventricular infarction and acute massive pulmonary embolism[4]. In experiments in dogs, the pericardium appears to limit cardiac dilatation whenever ventricular diastolic pressures are elevated acutely. It also determines a certain ventricular interdependence[5], thus right ventricular distension limits left ventricular compliance[6]. The fibrous pericardium plays an important role in protecting the heart from the spread of infection from adjacent structures.

Congenital defects of the pericardium

Total absence of the pericardium is rare[1] and often associated with other congenital cardiac or pulmonary defects. Partial defects are nearly always on the left side and they vary from small to complete. Patients with complete absence of the left pericardium may be asymptomatic but some give a history of recurrent chest infection, chest discomfort or dyspnoea. The heart is usually displaced to the left with prominence of the main pulmonary artery segment on the chest radiograph. Partial defects are usually found accidently when herniation of the left atrial appendage through the defect may simulate a tumour radiologically. Echocardiography[7] or a computed tomography scan allows identification of the cause of the mass.

Sudden death has been reported in patients with partial defects secondary to herniation with strangulation of the heart, but, in patients with the complete defect, cardiac catheterization has usually demonstrated normal function.

Pericardial cysts

Pericardial cysts (spring-water cysts) are rare. They do not cause symptoms and are usually discovered accidentally as smooth round masses usually occupying the left or right costophrenic angle[8]. Computed tomography scans show them well. They may or may not communicate with the pericardium. Diagnostic aspiration reveals clear limpid fluid; no treatment is necessary.

PERICARDIAL SYNDROMES (TABLE 41.1)

ACUTE PERICARDITIS

Precordial pain, pericardial friction and concordant ST-segment elevation on the electrocardiogram are the cardinal features of acute pericarditis[6]. The possible causes are numerous (Table 41.2).

Symptoms

Precordial pain is usually associated with fever. The

Table 41.1. Pericardial syndromes.

Acute pericarditis
Relapsing pericarditis
Subacute constrictive – effusive pericarditis
Tamponade
Chronic pericardial effusion
Constrictive pericarditis

pain may be mild or severe. It may be similar to the pain of myocardial infarction except that it is exacerbated by inspiration. In other cases, it is felt only on deep inspiration. The pain is substernal, radiating to the neck and shoulders. It can be predominately epigastric simulating an acute abdomen. It is characteristically increased by coughing, swallowing or movement, eased by sitting up and leaning forward or even by adopting the Mohammedan prayer position. The pain is conveyed by the left phrenic nerve and also the left stellate ganglion. Dyspnoea may result from rapid shallow breathing

Table 41.2. Important causes of acute pericarditis.

1 Idiopathic (previously called acute benign)
2 Infections
   Viral: Coxsackie group B
                     Echovirus type 8
                     Mumps
                     Ebstein–Barr
                     Varicella
                     Rubella
   Bacterial: Pneumococcus
                     Meningococcus
                     Haemophilus
                     Gonococcus
                     Tuberculous
   Fungo-bacterial: Actinomyces
                     Nocardia
   Fungal: Candida
                     Histopolasma
   Parasitic: *Entamoeba histolytica*
                     Echinococcus
                     Toxoplasma
3 Immunological
   Post infarction (Dressler's syndrome)
   Post-cardiotomy syndrome
   Relapsing pericarditis
   Associated with the connective tissue disorders:
      Rheumatic fever
      Systemic lupus erythematosus
      Rheumatoid arthritis
      Scleroderma
      Mixed connective tissue disease
      Polyarteritis and the Churg–Strauss variant
      Wegener's granulomatosis
4 Neoplastic
5 Post-irradiation
6 Traumatic
7 Uraemic

caused by the pleuritic component. Other constitutional symptoms such as sweating, anorexia and fatigue are usual.

Physical signs

The pericardial friction rub results from grating of the roughened epicardial and parietal pericardial surfaces with movement of the heart. The rub is characteristically superficial, scratchy and intensified by pressure on the sternum. It is out of phase with the heart sounds, usually both systolic and diastolic, but occasionally only systolic, and usually loudest on inspiration. It may be transient or intermittent. If a large effusion develops, the rub may disappear but it may persist. There may be tachycardia but no pulsus paradoxus or rise in venous pressure unless some degree of tamponade occurs. It is rarely necessary to tap the effusion therapeutically.

Investigations

1   The chest radiograph may be normal but the heart shadow may be slightly enlarged if >250 ml of fluid are present. Sometimes there are pulmonary shadows or pleural effusions.
2   The electrocardiogram usually shows characteristic changes even though the pericardium itself is electrically silent. The ST-segment elevation which is nearly always present is a current of injury (Fig. 41.1) from the superficial layers of the myocardium. As acute pericarditis is usually diffuse, the changes are characteristically generalized and concordant but this is not invariable. The QRS complex is normal unless accumulation of pericardial fluid results in reduced voltage. With healing, the ST segment becomes iso-electric often with T-wave inversion which is usually transient but sometimes permanent even in the absence of sequelae such as constriction. Disturbances of rhythm may also result from the associated myocarditis with excessive sinus tachycardia or bradycardia, paroxysmal atrial fibrillation, flutter or supraventricular tachycardia.

The ST-segment changes have to be distinguished from the normal variant pattern, most often seen in young black males, in which ST-segment elevation results from early repolarization, from the short QT interval seen in hypercalcaemia and, most importantly, from the changes in early myocardial infarction of which ST-segment elevation is the earliest sign. However, in early infarction the changes are regional and rapidly followed by loss of R-wave height with the appearance of pathological Q and Pardee waves in which the ST segment becomes convex upwards with commencing T-wave inversion.
3   Cross-sectional echocardiography permits detection, quantification and serial evaluation of the pericardial effusion, as well as of left and right ventricular function. The pericardium itself is invisible. Characteristically, there is an echo-free space anterior and posterior to the heart whose size varies with the heart beat and also cyclicly if the effusion is large due to the heart swinging within the fluid sack. When the effusion is very fibrinous, the space may not be echo free but it remains recognizable. The space should be visible both anteriorly and posteriorly, otherwise error may come from excessive epicardial fat or an enlarged thymus anteriorly or from a pleural effusion or giant left atrium posteriorly.

Relation of acute pericarditis to subsequent dilated cardiomyopathy

It is remarkable that acute pericarditis of presumptively and sometimes proven viral origin, although typically associated with superficial myocarditis, the cause of the electrocardiographic changes, is not usually accompanied by evidence of a generalized myocarditis. Depression of left and/or right ventricular function is uncommon; it is not part of the typical picture of idiopathic pericarditis. This observation is at variance with the notion that many cases of dilated cardiomyopathy result from previous viral myocarditis, although by analogy with meningitis and encephalitis the pericardium or myocardium might become infected or diseased without necessary involvement of both structures. As the pericardium is electrically silent, the electrocardiogram should remain normal if acute pericarditis did not involve the myocardium. The fact that the myocardium is involved is shown by the electrocardiogram and by release of CPK MB iso-enzyme[9]. It is therefore surprising how infrequently evidence of old pericarditis is found in cases of dilated cardiomyopathy. (See specific forms of pericarditis.)

RELAPSING PERICARDITIS

Relapsing pericarditis may follow pericarditis of

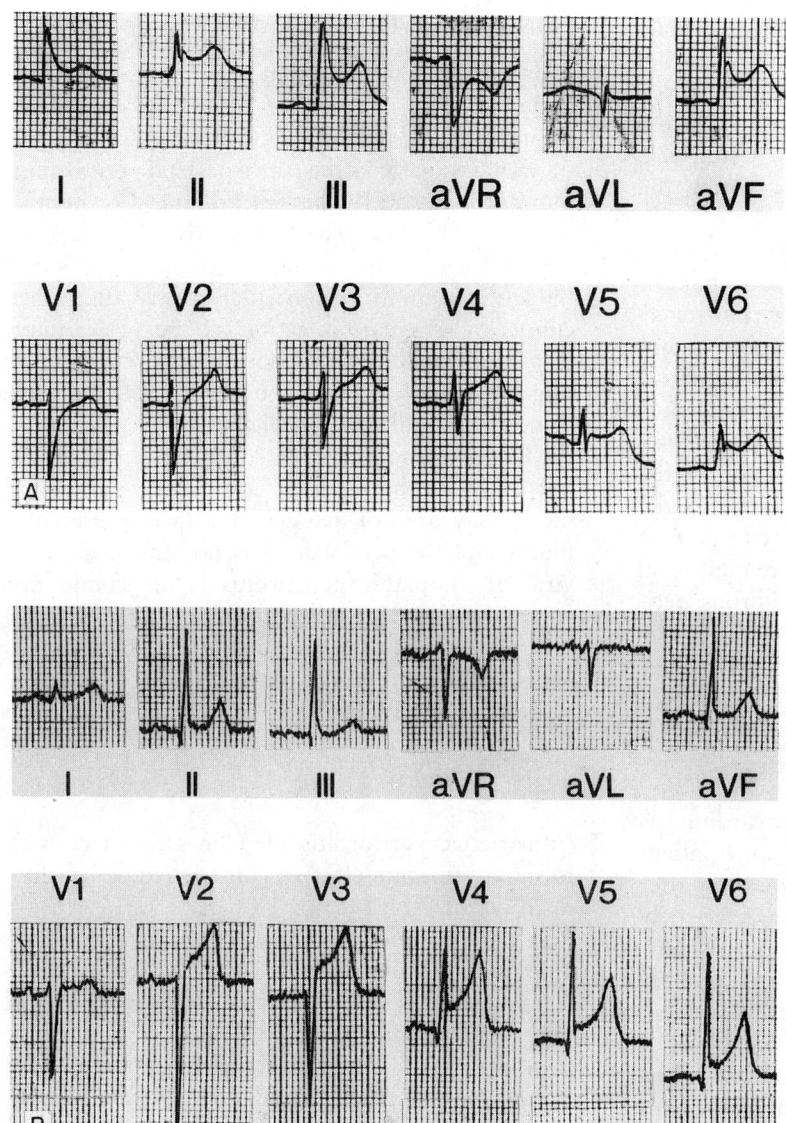

Fig. 41.1. The electrocardiogram in acute pericarditis. (A) Concordant concave upward ST-segment elevation is seen in all the surface leads with reciprocal ST-segment depression in aVR. In contrast, in (B), from a case of early acute anterior myocardial infarction, ST-segment elevation can be seen in leads V_2-V_6 but not in the standard and unipolar leads and there has already been loss of R-wave voltage from leads V_2 and V_3.

any cause or it may develop without an initiating acute illness. It may follow idiopathic pericarditis, myocardial infarction, infective endocarditis[10] or any form of cardiac surgery, complicate uraemic pericarditis or follow irradiation or trauma.

When the syndrome follows acute pericarditis or cardiac surgery, it is usually easily recognized, but in the absence of an acute precipitating cause relapsing pericarditis may be mistaken for unstable angina pectoris or even ulcer dyspepsia. When it follows myocardial infarction, it may simulate extension or recurrence of infarction. The pain may be severe or experienced only on effort, precipitated by chest wall movement and deep breathing, or simulating effort angina. A rub may be present; if

so, it may be very transient. The electrocardiogram may show recurrence of acute changes, the chest X-ray may show linear deflation or small effusions.

Although benign, the recurrent chest pain may be disabling, depressing and seemingly intractable[11]. Mild cases can be quenched by adequate aspirin in doses of 600 mg, three-hourly whilst the pain lasts or by colchicine 1 mg followed by 500 µg two- or three-hourly until the pain goes or vomiting occurs. Indomethacin can be useful, taken regularly to prevent recurrence, but it is not usually as effective in treating acute attacks. Severe attacks need treatment with steroids, but it is most important to give the patient only enough for a short course, as maintenance dosage does not prevent relapse and nearly always leads to increasing dosage with its attendant problems. A commencing dose of between 40 and 60 mg of prednisolone daily for 2 days should be followed by rapidly decreasing dosage to 0 over the next 10 days. Using this approach, there is virtually no risk from the steroids, which are usually effective in the relief of pain and resolution of the flare-up. For intractable relapsing pericarditis, some workers advocate pericardiectomy, but it may fail to prevent recurrence. Although the cause of relapsing pericarditis is not known, it may result from misrecognition of native autolysing myocardial protein as foreign and thus be immunologically based. If this is the case, removal of the parietal pericardium and even of the epicardium would not cure the condition. In the long term, resolution usually occurs;[11] constriction does not occur probably because recurrent effusion prevents adherence and stretches the fibrous pericardium.

EFFUSIVE CONSTRICTIVE PERICARDITIS

When thickening of the visceral pericardium is associated with pericardial effusion[12,13], the patient will have persistent cardiac compression even after pericardiocentesis. The condition characteristicly occurs during the evolution of tuberculous pericarditis but may follow idiopathic pericarditis, mediastinal irradiation or occur in neoplastic involvement of the pericardium. The patient will complain of shortness of breath, fatigue, and sometimes oedema and precordial discomfort. Examination reveals pulsus paradoxus and a raised venous pressure with prominent x and y descents. The heart sounds are normal or diminished. There may be a friction rub or a third heart sound.

Chest radiographs usually show an enlarged cardiac silhouette. The electrocardiogram shows reduced voltage and changes similar to those found in constrictive pericarditis. Echocardiography reveals the effusion plus signs of constriction such as rapid outward posterior wall movement to a plateau and features of a low cardiac output. Treatment is specific for the underlying disorder, such as antituberculous chemotherapy and pericardiectomy. Removal of the visceral pericardium is required. In neoplastic disease, the treatment may be local installation of chemotherapeutic agents or monoclonal antibodies followed by pericardiectomy.

CONSTRICTIVE PERICARDITIS

Constriction develops when scarring of the parietal and/or visceral pericardium results in compression of the heart and restriction of cardiac filling. Usually the condition affects the entire parietal pericardium, but not necessarily the epicardium. Constriction may rarely be localized, particularly when there is a calcified constricting band which may develop in the left or right atrioventricular groove after tuberculous or pyogenic infection of the pericardium. Rarely, isolated constriction of the superior or inferior vena cava may occur or of the right ventricular outflow tract. Tuberculosis used to be the most common cause of constrictive pericarditis, but many of the cases of constrictive pericarditis seen today are not associated with any preceding illness and the pericardium is not calcified. Acute viral or idiopathic pericarditis is the commonest preceding event[14]. Rheumatoid arthritis, mediastinal irradiation, chronic uraemia and cardiac surgery account for some of the other cases.

Some important causes of constrictive pericarditis are shown in Table 41.3.

Symptoms

Constrictive pericarditis may be seen in classical form, as subacute effusive constrictive pericarditis, or in occult form[15].

In mild or moderate constriction, the complaints are usually non-specific with loss of previous stamina, fatigue and exertional dyspnoea. In more severe cases, patients complain of swelling of the abdomen, and sometimes swelling of the feet. Cough and shortness of breath may predominate and, although orthopnoea may be mentioned, paroxysmal nocturnal dyspnoea is rare[16,17].

Physical signs

Patients with severe constriction appear to be ill, having lost flesh. They are peripherally vasoconstricted because of a low cardiac output, and have a prominent abdomen caused by hepatomegaly and ascites. The blood pressure is usually low, with a

---

Table 41.3. **Causes of constrictive pericarditis.**

Post viral or idiopathic
Tuberculous
Post pyogenic
Rheumatoid (or rarely other connective tissue disorders)
Post irradiation
Post cardiac surgery
Neoplastic

narrow pulse pressure and pulsus paradoxus in about half the patients, but this is rarely as florid as in tamponade.

The venous pressure is raised with a marked M shape due to exaggerated x and y descents. The x descent may predominate because there is no tricuspid regurgitation. In patients with atrial fibrillation, the y descent is most prominent, but the lack of a visible expansile v wave also indicates the absence of significant tricuspid regurgitation. The venous pressure rises on inspiration (Kussmaul's sign). This sign is not specific for constrictive pericarditis and occurs also in most other types of congestive failure. The prominent y descent was described by Friedreich and the sometimes dominant x descent by Ronald Gibson. The liver is enlarged and often said to be non-pulsatile (it is pulsatile, however, because the hepatic veins are in free communication with the right atrium). Its pulsation is not as great as that in tricuspid regurgitation. There may be ascites associated with the high venous pressure, exacerbated sometimes by hypo-albuminaemia particularly in children who may have a protein-losing enteropathy[18]. The cardiac impulse is usually impalpable but there may be a short diastolic impulse terminating in a palpable third heart sound. Typically, there is an early high-frequency third sound[19], best heard at the left sternal edge with timing similar to the opening snap of mitral stenosis i.e. between 60 and 100 ms after aortic closure. In very severe constriction, no third heart sound can be heard because it is even earlier blending with pulmonary closure. The second heart sound is usually widely split[16] because aortic closure happens early due to the greatly shortened left ventricular ejection time. Inspiratory splitting is exaggerated because right ventricular filling is increased and left ventricular filling is diminished more than normal on inspiration due to flattening of the ventricular septum towards the left ventricle.

In the American literature, the third heart sound is often described as a pericardial knock[21], but the sound arises within the heart and is related to the early abrupt cessation of rapid diastolic filling of the ventricles. Murmurs are uncommon, but localized pericardial constriction, narrowing the left or right atrioventricular groove, may be associated with mid-diastolic murmurs simulating mitral or tricuspid stenosis. Rarely, patients with constrictive pericarditis may have a mitral regurgitant murmur due to splinting of the annulus. Such mitral regurgitation may disappear after successful pericardiectomy. In general, however, absence of murmurs is one of the features which helps in the differentiation of constrictive pericarditis from restrictive cardiomyopathy and endomyocardial fibrosis (Table 41.4).

Investigations

Chest radiography usually shows a heart of normal

Table 41.4. Differential diagnosis of constrictive pericarditis from endomyocardial fibrosis and amyloid heart disease.*

	Constriction	Endomyocardial fibrosis	Amyloid	Primary restrictive cardiomyopathy
Pulsus paradoxus	+	0	0	0
Kussmaul's sign	+	+	+	+
Third heart sound	+	+	0	+
Murmurs	0	+	0	±
Pulmonary artery pressure	<50 mmHg	>50 mmHg	>50 mmHg	>50 mmHg
Wedge pressure (LVEDP)	<20	>20	>20	>20
LVEDP − RVEDP	< 5	> 5	> 5	> 5
End-diastolic pressure equalization in all four chambers	+	0	0	0
Two-dimensional echo	Abnormal septal movement. Premature opening of pulmonary valve	Apical obliteration, increased endocardial echoes	Thickened left and right ventricles. Thickened atrial septum and valves	Like constriction but often very large right ± left atrium
Echo Doppler	Usually no abnormal reflux	Mitral and tricuspid regurgitation	Usually no abnormal reflux	Tricuspid reflux
Computed tomography scan	Thick pericardium, sigmoid ventricular septum	± Effusion	± Effusion	Looks normal except for atrial size

*NB None of these distinctions is absolute.

size, but the silhouete may be enlarged if the pericardial thickening is gross or associated with effusion. In addition, a high diaphragm from ascites may increase the apparent size of the heart and the cardiothoracic ratio. Prominence of the superior vena cava and azygos vein reflect the high venous filling pressure. Pericardial calcification is most marked in the dependent portions of the heart around the apex and posteriorly; it is best seen on lateral views (Fig. 41.2). It usually indicates a tuberculous cause for the constriction but calcification also occurs after pneumococcal or other purulent pericarditis and in post-traumatic cases. Less than 30% of recent cases have shown pericardial calcification, most of whom were middle-aged or old. Calcification of the pericardium does not invariably indicate constriction and may be seen with similar distribution and of presumptive origin in some patients with no evidence of constriction. The lungs are usually clear, but may show evidence of pulmonary venous congestion in very severe cases. There may be pleural effusions.

The electrocardiogram is nearly always abnormal and, although there are no specific abnormalities, certain changes are characteristic. 'Step-ladder' P waves (like a reversed dome and dart in petit mal epilepsy) may be seen in about half of the patients who are in sinus rhythm. The mean frontal QRS axis is usually towards the right and the horizontal axis is deflected somewhat posteriorly with S waves as far as V6 in the chest leads. The voltage is low and there are usually non-specific inverted T waves (Fig.41.3).

Echocardiography which reveals the effusion in subacute effusive constrictive pericarditis does not show pericardial thickening in most cases of constriction. The ventricles are small and active, with normal or reduced wall thickness. The left ventricular posterior wall shows rapid abruptly curtailed outward movement in diastole followed by a plateau coincident with the third heart sound. Inspiratory premature opening of the pulmonary valve may be seen;[22] septal movement is abnormal with diastolic flattening seen on the short-axis view of the left ventricle, and marked exaggeration of this movement on inspiration with displacement towards the left ventricle can be seen on M-mode[23].

Measurement of systolic time-intervals reveals a normal pre-ejection period to ejection time ratio (PEP/LVET) but this does not distinguish constrictive pericarditis from restrictive cardiomyopathy and there may still be difficulty at this point in deciding whether the restrictive syndrome results from pericardial, endocardial or endomyocardial disease (Table 41.4).

Although computed tomography has little place yet in the diagnosis of heart disease, it is very useful in the non-invasive recognition of pericardial disease (and aortic dissection). The computed tomography scan is superior to echocardiography in the visualization of thickening of the pericardium[24]. This is usually clearly visible[25] with a high-density line of thickening around the heart which contrasts with the inner low-density epicardial fat layer (Fig.41.4). If pericardial fluid is present, this will also be visualized. The inferior vena cava is seen to be dilated; the ventricular septum loses its normal bowing towards the right ventricle and has an abnormal sinusoidal shape which is also characteristic of constriction. Electrocardiographic gating, contrast enhancement and modern fast scanners have greatly improved the quality of the images.

Differential diagnosis

Cardiac catheterization is unnecessary in typical cases of constrictive pericarditis; computed tomography scanning can make the differentiation from restrictive cardiomyopathy in difficult cases. Typically, it reveals similarity of the diastolic pressures in all four chambers to within a millimetre or two except in cases of left or right atrioventricular groove constriction.

The right ventricular diastolic pressure is always very high in constriction; if it is not, the diagnosis is likely to be wrong (unless the patient has undergone excessive diuresis).

The shape of the diastolic pressure in the left and right ventricles produces the well-known 'square root' sign with a low early diastolic pressure and rapid rise to a high plateau but this is not specific. The beginning of the plateau coincides with cessation of outward posterior wall movement on the echo and with the third heart sound.

The response to a Valsalva manoeuvre is a square wave as in heart failure. In restrictive cardiomyopathy, endomyocardial fibrosis and amyloid heart disease, the left-sided diastolic pressures are usually considerably higher than those on the right (Table 41.4). Moreover, pulmonary hypertension is common in myocardial disease secondary to the much higher left atrial pressure, whereas in constrictive pericarditis it is rare for the left atrial pressure to rise high enough to generate pulmonary hypertension. Despite this, differentiation still causes difficulty.[26]

The echocardiographic features of infiltrative

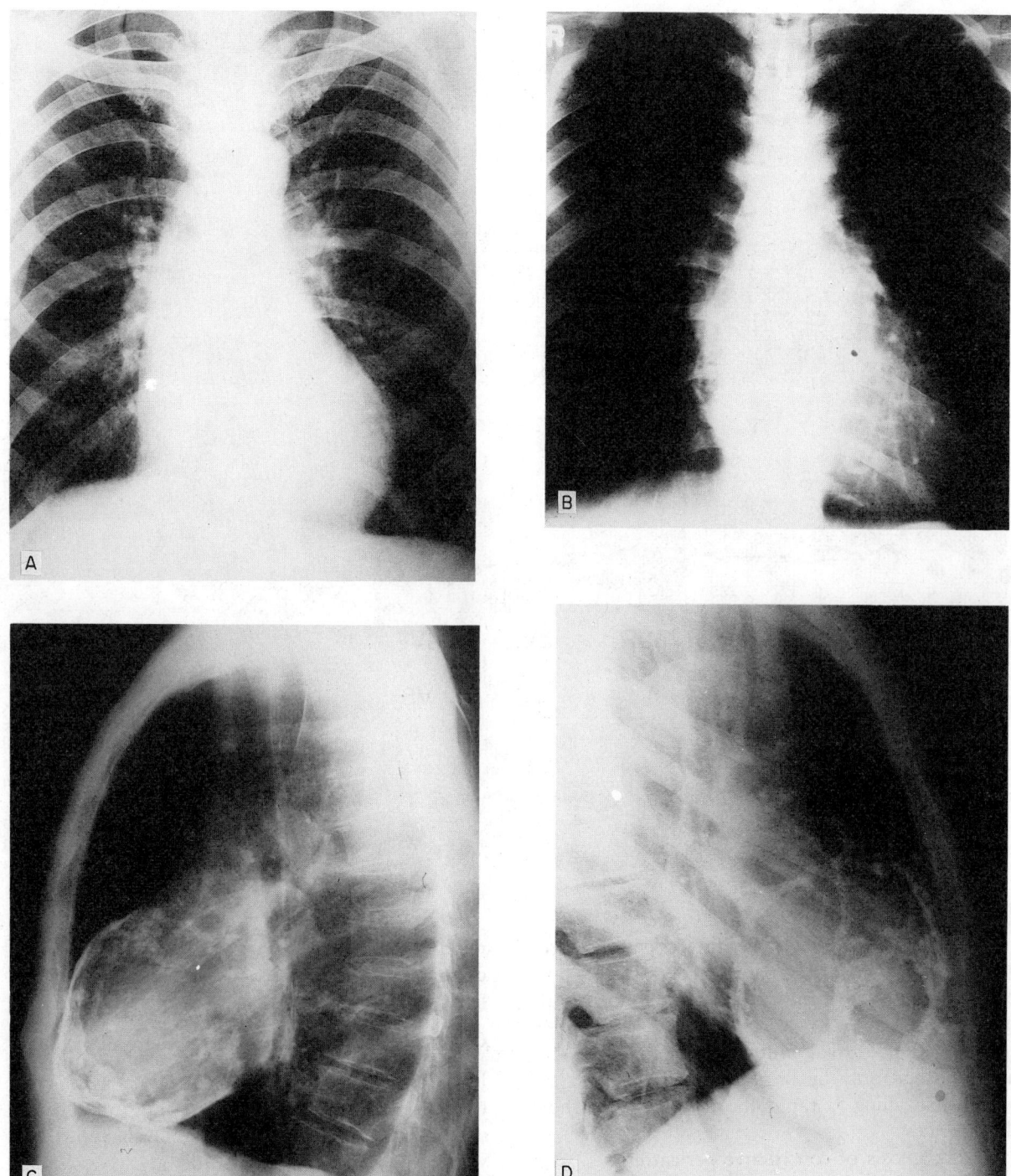

Fig.41.2. Chest radiograph in tuberculous calcific constrictive pericarditis. Normal (A) and over-penetrated (B) postero-anterior views. Calcification of the pericardium is only just visible even in the over-penetrated view but it is grossly obvious on both the left (C) and right lateral (D) views *NB* (A), (B) and (D) are from the same patient; (C) is from a different patient.

myocardial disease, particularly amyloid heart disease, are characteristic and very reliable. Finally, endomyocardial biopsy may be useful in demonstrating myocardial disease by revealing amyloid or

haemochromatosis as the cause of the restrictive cardiomyopathy.

Elevation or reduction of the venous filling pressure causes little change in the output; treat-

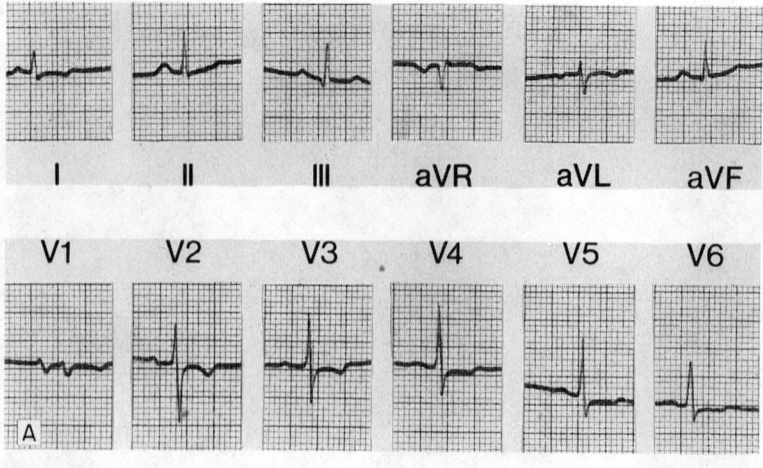

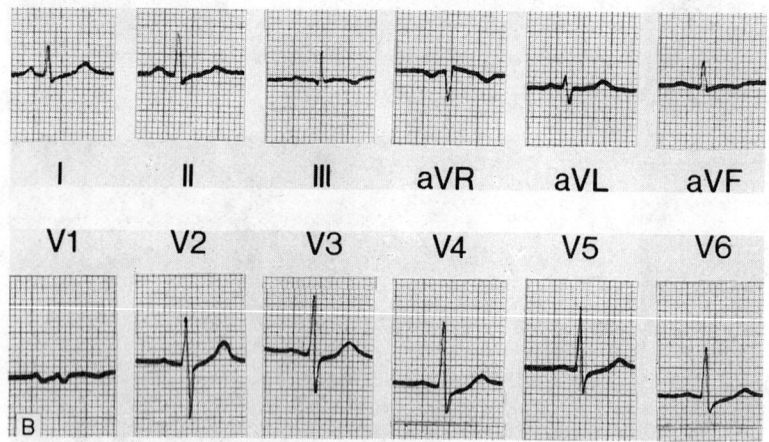

Fig.41.3. The electrocardiogram in constrictive pericarditis. (A) Atrial enlargement with step ladder P-waves in leads II and aVR. The QRS voltage is low and there are generalized repolarization changes. (B) After pericardiectomy, electrocardiogram has returned almost to normal except for T-wave inversion in leads III and aVF.

ment with diuretics may lower the venous pressure sufficient to make the patient comfortable but excessive dosage can cause marked postural hypotension.

Increase of cardiac output on effort can be accomplished only by increasing the rate and as ventricular filling is rapid the tachycardia is not detrimental.

The diagnosis of constrictive pericarditis is easy in the face of a high M shaped venous pressure with rapid x and y descents, a small heart, a third heart sound and no evidence of left ventricular disorder on the electrocardiogram. Clinically difficult cases can usually be diagnosed by a combination of echocardiography, computed tomography scan, haemodynamic measurements and biopsy.

Exploratory thoracotomy should no longer be necessary in any patient as the final method of making the distinction between restrictive cardiomyopathy and constrictive pericarditis.

Occult constrictive pericarditis

In classic constrictive pericarditis, it is obvious that the patient's heart is not functioning properly. In occult constriction, the patient may have no convincing signs of a cardiac disorder and yet complain of easy fatiguability and other non-specific symptoms. Exercise testing may reveal an excessive heart-rate response and the value for MVo_2 will be less than expected for the patient's age and build. Moreover, examination of the patient immediately after exercise will reveal an undue rise in venous pressure and the appearance of a crisp early third heart sound. These features may alert the cardiologist to the probable diagnosis despite normal clinical

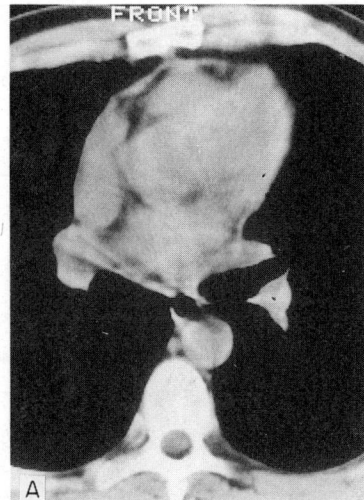
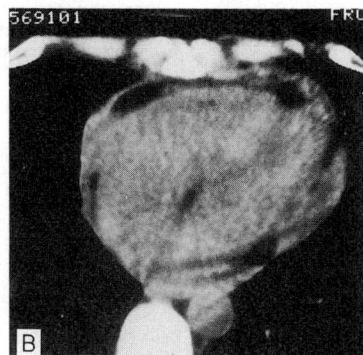
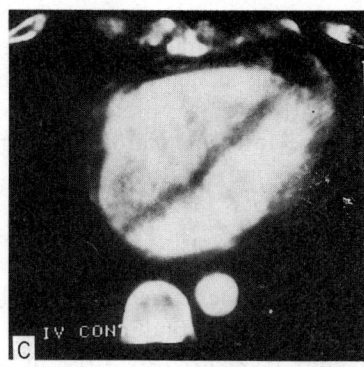

Fig.41.4. Computed tomograms of the thorax. (A) Constrictive pericarditis, showing the dense and thickened pericardium outlined by the epicardial fat layer. (B) Effusive constrictive pericarditis in which the pericardium is thickened but there is also a pericardial effusion (from a case of tuberculous pericarditis). (C) is from the same patient as (B) and shows straightening of the ventricular septum which has lost its normal bowing towards the right ventricle.

findings at rest, normal chest X-ray and normal or non-specific electrocardiogram. A computed tomography scan should be the next diagnostic test performed and may make the diagnosis incontrovertible.

Recent interest in this syndrome and its recognition has led to the suggestion that the constriction may be revealed by a fluid challenge during catheterization[15]. Occult constriction will be apparent from a brisk rise in the diastolic pressures which will equalize in the four cardiac chambers even if they were normal before the infusion. It has been suggested that the performance of pericardiectomy then carries a very low risk with a high possibility of curing the patient's symptoms.

Pericardiectomy

Pericardiectomy has been available for nearly half a century. When this procedure was first performed, mortality was high because of the advanced state of the patients with chronic ascites, jaundice and cachexia. In advanced cases, the operative mortality may still be as high as 40%. Death is usually due to a low cardiac output[27] or liver failure. Most surgeons use a median sternotomy but some still favour an anterolateral thoracotomy. Cardiopulmonary bypass is not essential, but it may be chosen for patients likely to require removal of the visceral pericardium because of the risk of perforating the cavity.

Pericardiectomy involves removal of the pericardium from the anterior and inferior surfaces of the right ventricle and the anterolateral, apical and diaphragmatic surfaces of the left ventricle including the left atrioventricular groove. It is not necessary to remove the pericardium from the atria, venae cavae or pulmonary veins except very rarely when pressure gradients have demonstrated focal constriction at these sites.

In tuberculous constriction, the visceral pericardium is invariably involved with fingers of fibrosis extending down into an atrophied myocardium. The lack of a plane of dissection makes the operation difficult and tedious. In most cases of idiopathic non-calcific constriction, the heart bulges out after an incision is made in the parietal pericardium and the visceral pericardium does not need to be touched, but it always has to be dissected off in cases of tuberculous origin.

Constriction does not seem to recur; if it seems as if it has, this semblance is usually due to poor myocardial function with persistence of the restrictive picture caused by restriction of filling at myocardial level, often coupled with poor systolic function.

Surgery on patients who are in New York Heart Association classes I or II carries an operative mortality of about 1%, abolishes all of the symptoms and confers a normal life-expectancy[27].

Either formal pericardiectomy or limited pericardial resection using a subxiphoid approach[28] is needed for most patients with chronic or recurrent effusive pericardial disease including patients with underlying malignancy[29,30]. When feasible, total pericardiectomy is preferred, except in patients who have relapsing pericarditis or asymptomatic chronic lax effusions.

CARDIAC TAMPONADE

When cardiac tamponade develops in a hospital patient with a condition known to carry risk, it is readily recognized by a rise in heart rate, a fall in arterial pressure with pulsus paradoxus, a rise in venous pressure and a quiet heart with faint heart sounds and usually no added sounds or murmurs although a friction rub may be heard. When tamponade occurs in a previously fit individual, although the signs are the same, it is frequently fatal because it may be missed especially if chest pain is absent.

Tamponade may occur in pericarditis of any origin (Table 41.5). It is relatively uncommon in idiopathic or viral pericarditis, post-myocardial infarction pericarditis and in pericarditis associated with connective tissue disorders and uraemia. It is usual in acute bacterial, tuberculous and malignant pericarditis. Acute haemopericardium may cause tamponade as in cardiac rupture following myocardial infarction or when an aortic dissection ruptures into the pericardium. It is a relatively common early complication of cardiac surgery. Pericardial tumours such as mesothelioma and lymphoma may present with tamponade, as may metastatic carcinoma.

Chronic tamponade may occur in tuberculosis, uraemia and after irradiation.

Symptoms

Patients with acute tamponade complain of shortness of breath but they may not have chest pain. In chronic tamponade, the predominant symptoms are weakness, dyspnoea, weight loss and sweating.

Physical signs

Tachycardia is always present and pulsus paradoxus. This may be so gross that the rhythm is thought to be irregular because the pulse becomes impalpable on inspiration. The heart rate is fast and blood pressure and pulse pressure low. The venous pressure is high, with prominent x but absent y descents and may increase markedly on inspiration. The liver will be enlarged in chronic tamponade.

Table 41.5.   Important causes of cardiac tamponade.

1	Infective:	
	Acute purulent	
	Tuberculous	
2	Haemorrhagic:	
	Dissection of the aorta	
	Post-infarction rupture:	anticoagulant induced
		cardiac rupture
	Traumatic:	stab wounds
		iatrogenic – cardiac catheter
		central venous line
		post cardiac surgery
	Uraemic	
3	Neoplastic:	
	Primary mesothelioma	
	Lymphoma	
	Secondary carcinoma	
4	Serous:	
	Viral or idiopathic	
	Systemic lupus erythematosus or drug-induced lupus syndrome (rare)	
	Rheumatoid and other connective tissue disorders (rare)	

The heart sounds are quiet but there may be a friction rub.

Pulsus paradoxus is an exaggeration of the normal respiratory variation in arterial pressure in which there is an increase of venous return to the right ventricle on inspiration and diminished inflow to the left ventricle so that the left ventricular stroke volume declines[31]. In tamponade there is also inspiratory increase of blood flow into the right ventricle but this is accommodated at the expense of left ventricular volume because the total diastolic volume of the heart cannot increase. The ventricular septum can be seen on echo to move sharply posteriorly and to bulge into the left ventricular cavity greatly reducing its size (Fig.41.5). The result is a gross reduction in left ventricular stroke volume. Pulsus paradoxus may also occur in asthma and in shock, but it is never as marked as it is in tamponade.

The heart sounds are usually faint and occasionally they are cyclically variable. Pericardial friction is heard in up to 50% of cases and may be caused by friction between the parietal pericardium and the pleura as the parietal and visceral pericardium are widely separated. The rub may be augmented on inspiration (pleuropericardial).

Investigations

The chest radiograph usually shows an enlarged heart but a normal heart shadow does not exclude tamponade. The lungs are clear without congestive

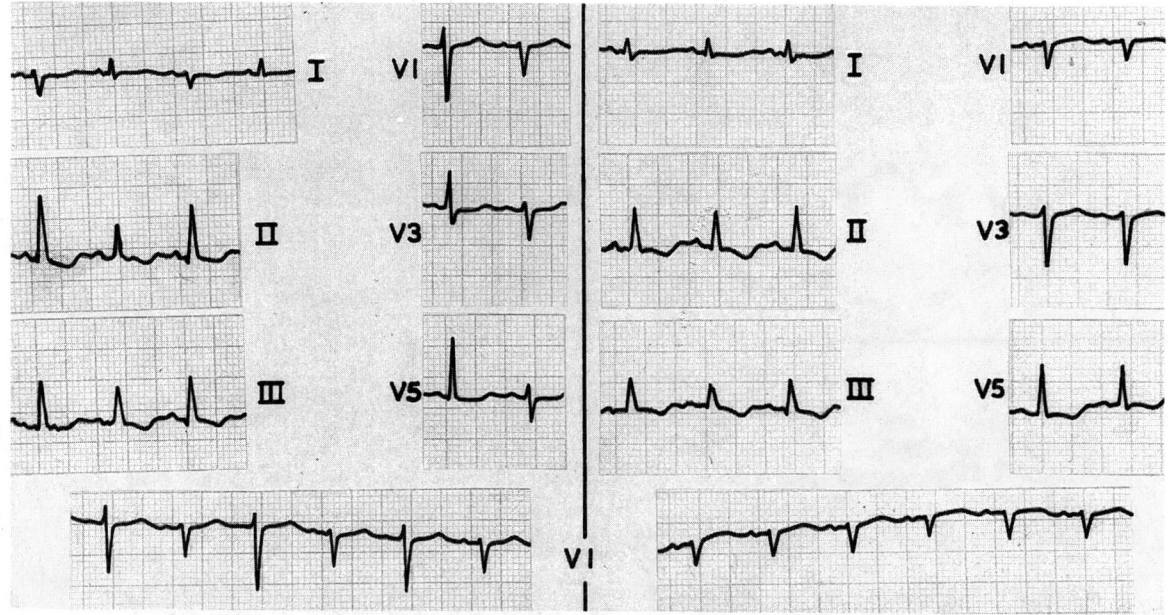

Fig.41.5. The electrocardiogram in cardiac tamponade. On the left, marked electrical alternans is present with a change in electrical axis affecting both the frontal and horizontal planes. On the right, after pericardiocentesis, although the voltage remains low, the electrical alternans has disappeared.

changes. The outline of the heart is smooth with obliteration of the angles. Very occasionally, on a lateral chest film, the epicardial line of fat may be seen well within the edge of the cardiac outline.

The electrocardiogram shows tachycardia and low voltage and may show electrical 'alternans' (Fig.41.5), but as this is caused by the heart swinging about alternation may not be precise.

In typical cases of acute cardiac tamponade, the diagnosis is obvious. Urgent pericardiocentesis is needed. Echocardiography is a rapid and reliable means of confirming the diagnosis of tamponade (Fig.41.6) and can also be used to guide the aspiration particularly if the fluid is loculated as in neoplastic effusions or post-myocardial infarction. In the latter, if a point of actual cardiac rupture has been sealed by pericardial adherence, introduction of the needle at that point would result in immediate entry into the ventricular cavity.

Pathophysiology of cardiac tamponade

The intrapericardial pressure is normally several mmHg lower than the diastolic pressure in either ventricle. When a pericardial effusion accumulates rapidly, the intrapericardial pressure rises abruptly cancelling out the usual diastolic transmural distending pressure which normally aids ventricular

filling. This causes diastolic collapse of the walls of the right and left atria and right ventricle, visible on echocardiography[32], and greatly limits cardiac filling (Fig.41.7). During systolic ejection, the volume of the heart decreases causing an abrupt fall in intrapericardial pressure, thereby allowing the right atrium to fill replenishing the total cardiac volume until the pericardial pressure rises again.[33] This accounts for the steep x descent in the venous pulse. After opening of the tricuspid valve, only a small volume enters the right ventricle before the transmural distending pressure is again abolished, therefore the diastolic y descent of the venous pulse is very small and the typical venous pulse in tamponade is high with exaggerated x but attenuated y descents. Measurement of superior vena caval flow velocity by Doppler ultrasound can be used at the bedside in the diagnosis of tamponade[35].

Inspiration is usually accompanied by an increase in right ventricular diastolic volume with a decrease in left ventricular volume, and increased flow into the right atrium from the systemic veins. On inspiration, intrapericardial pressure falls, and inflow to the right ventricle increases, but is accommodated by a marked reduction in left ventricular volume caused by the flattening and displacement of the septum. Left ventricular stroke volume falls abruptly but rises again in expiration

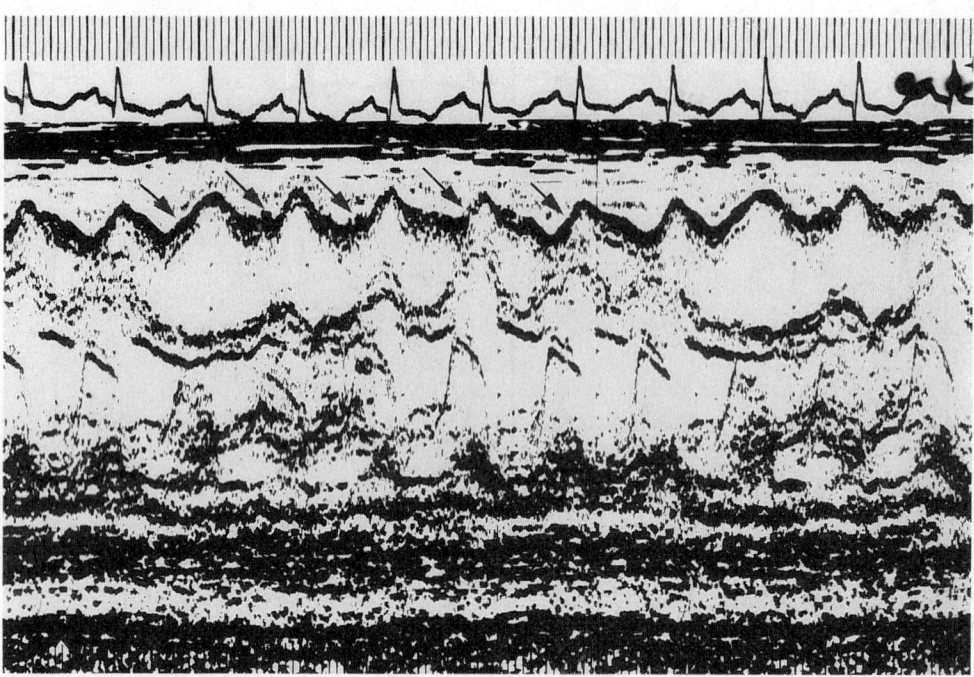

Fig.41.6. M-Mode echocardiogram from a case of cardiac tamponade showing a fibrinous pericardial effusion anteriorly and diastolic collapse of the right ventricle (arrowed). On inspiration, the ventricular septum moves posteriorly causing marked reduction in the size of the left ventricular cavity. The pericardial effusion is well seen anteriorly. ACW, anterior chest wall; PE, pericardial effusion; AW of RV, anterior wall of right ventricle; RV, right ventricular cavity; VS, ventricular septum; AMVL, anterior mitral valve leaflet; PW of LV, posterior wall of left ventricle.

when the septum moves back and venous return from the lungs is augmented (Fig.41.6). In the experimental animal, diastolic collapse visible on echo precedes the appearance of pulsus paradoxus[36] and therefore it is a useful sign of impending tamponade and the need for pericardiocentesis (Fig.41.7).[37]

Left ventricular stroke output may be further reduced during inspiration through the Starling mechanism, when diminished left ventricular myocardial fibre stretch is followed by a weaker contraction. The peripheral vascular resistance is high with increased adrenergic and angiotensin release[38] and inhibition of atrial natriuretic peptide secretion[39].

Pericardiocentesis

Whenever possible, pericardiocentesis should be performed in the cardiac catheterization laboratory. Ideally, simultaneous measurement of intracardiac pressures during pericardiocentesis permits the continuous assessment of a patient's haemodynamic state. Without cardiac catheterization, pericardiocentesis with fluoroscopy and electrocardiographic control (using the aspiration needle as a

chest lead electrode) plus ultrasonic visualization provides maximum patient safety. The use of cardiac ultrasound allows the amount and location of the fluid to be seen and the aspirating catheter to be guided. This is particularly useful when the fluid is loculated. Electrocardiographic guidance alone will at least allow the immediate recognition of a current of injury on contact with the myocardium and also the recognition of which structure the needle has touched. In tamponade, right and left ventricular diastolic pressures and right and left atrial pressures are similar and equal to the intrapericardial pressure. With aspiration of fluid, the intrapericardial pressure falls, the y descent reappears in the right atrial pressure tracing and the right and left ventricular diastolic pressures separate. As more fluid is withdrawn, the raised right atrial and right ventricular diastolic pressures fall to normal and the arterial pressure rises. The exaggerated swings of the ventricular septum cease and the inspiratory fall in arterial systolic pressure and in pulse pressure (pulsus paradoxus) disappears as left ventricular stroke volume becomes better maintained during inspiration.

The safest route for pericardiocentesis is the sub-xiphoid approach and the patient is positioned

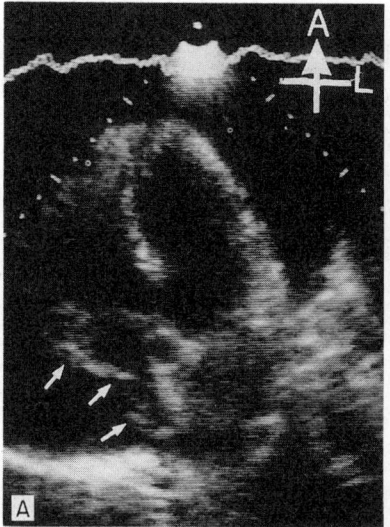
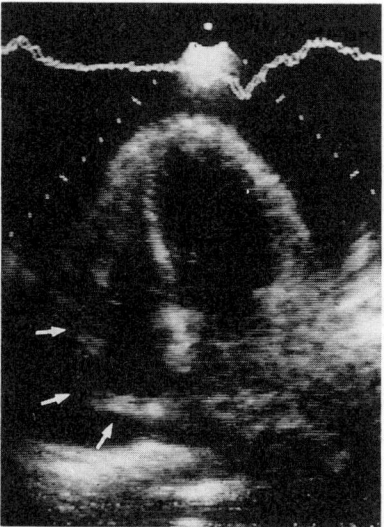

Fig.41.7. Cross-sectional echocardiography in cardiac tamponade. (A) Apical four-chamber view with diastolic collapse of the right atrial wall (arrowed). (B) Diastolic collapse of the right ventricular outflow tract in parasternal long-axis views. The top arrow in each frame shows the free wall of the right ventricle and the bottom arrow indicates the large pericardial effusion.

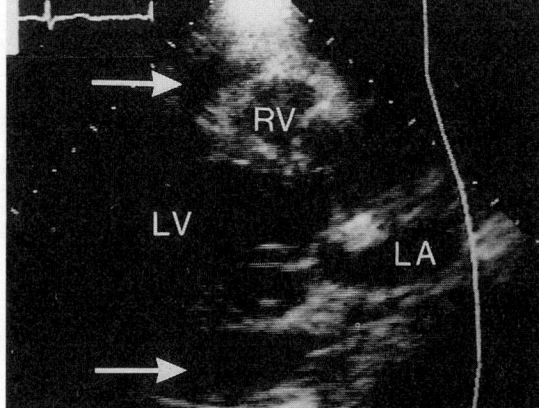
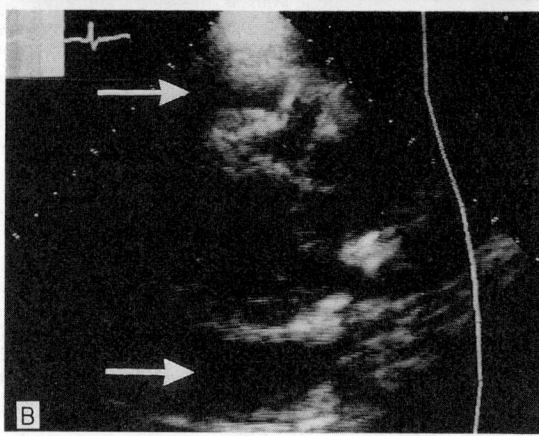

anaesthetic is injected as the needle is advanced upwards posteriorly and medially towards the inferior surface of the right atrium. The V lead of the electrocardiogram is attached to the hub of the needle for recording. The needle is advanced until it is felt to pierce the pericardium and fluid is aspirated. If ST-segment elevation appears on the electrocardiogram or ventricular ectopic beats are seen, the needle is withdrawn, whilst attempting to aspirate. If no fluid is obtained, the needle is withdrawn completely, flushed and the procedure repeated inserting the needle with some slight change in direction.

When fluid is flowing, the syringe is removed from the needle and a short guidewire introduced through the needle, the needle withdrawn and a short soft catheter equipped with multiple side-holes passed by the Seldinger technique over the wire into the pericardial space. This enables the pericardial fluid to be drained completely without risk of needle trauma to the myocardium. The catheter can also be used to explore the pericardial space in cases of suspected tumour and to inject air or contrast. It is traditional to inject air which allows good visualization of the thickness of the pericardium and the presence of any solid masses when radiographs are exposed with the patient in different postures (Fig.41.8). The catheter can be left *in situ* and continuous drainage provided[40]. Chemotherapeutic agents or cytotoxic drugs can be instilled as indicated.

All the pericardial fluid that has been removed should be sent to the laboratory for bacteriology and cytology.

sitting up so that the fluid pools inferiorly. This approach is extrapleural and avoids the coronary arteries. After local anaesthesia, which should be liberal, a small cut is made in the skin below and to the left of the xiphoid process. After spreading the subcutaneous tissues, a long thin-walled 16-gauge short-bevelled needle is inserted and further local

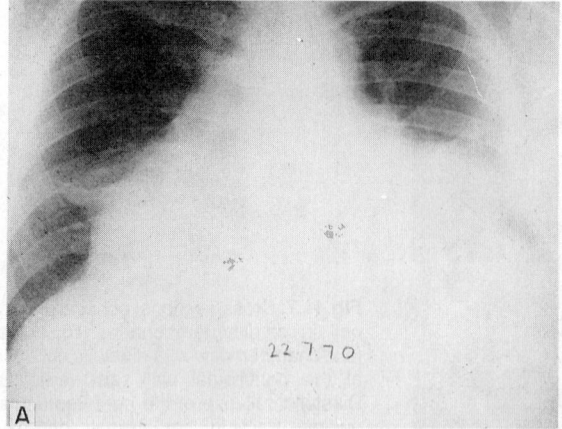

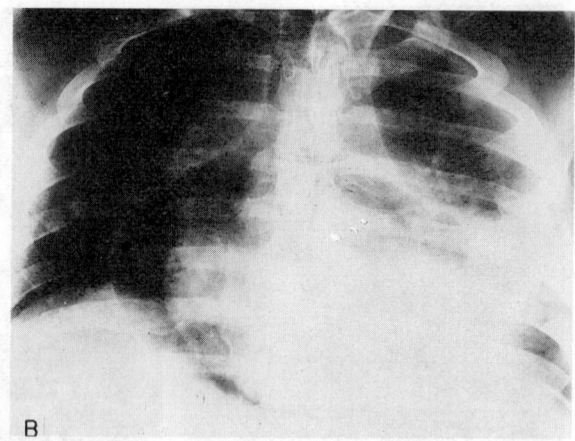

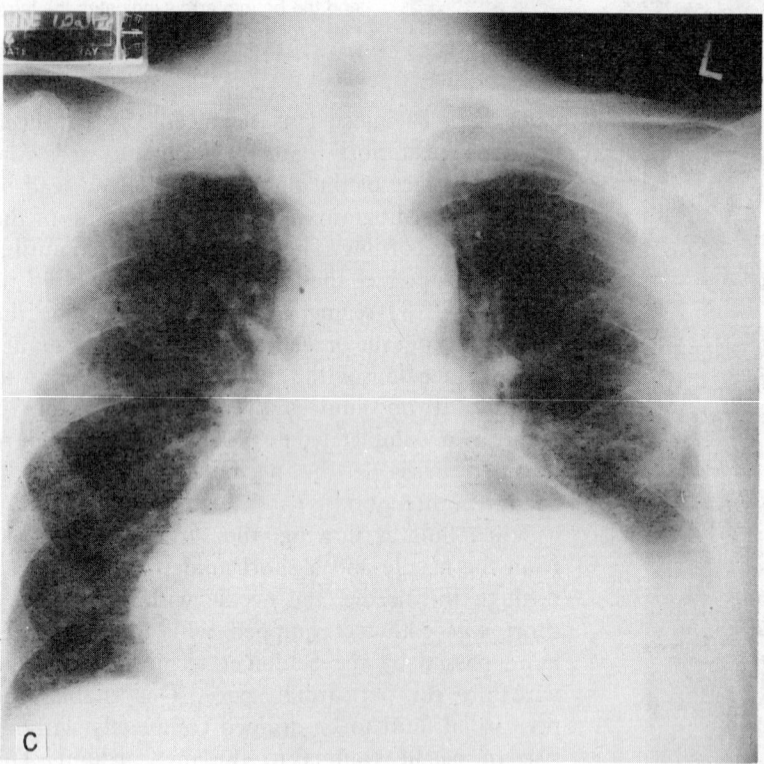

Fig.41.8. (A) Chest radiograph from a patient with a massive haemopericardium. (B) The appearance after air replacement with the patient on his left side. The pericardium is thin. (This patient had had an inferior infarct and fluid could not be obtained from the subxiphoid approach but was obtained by aspiration from a right parasternal site.) (C) Upright postero-anterior chest radiograph from a patient with a chronic lax effusion after aspiration of clear serous fluid and air replacement. The pericardium is slightly thickened.

CHRONIC PERICARDIAL EFFUSION WITHOUT COMPRESSION

A large lax pericardial effusion may cause few symptoms and be an unexpected finding on the chest X-ray, or it may give rise to aching in the chest, dysphagia, hoarseness or hiccup. It may follow acute pericarditis of any cause but commonly there is no history (Table 41.6). The effusion will have accumulated slowly allowing the pericardium time to expand without a rise of intrapericardial pressure. Myxoedema and amyloid heart disease should be considered in older patients.

The physical signs may be sparse with normal arterial pressure without pulsus paradoxus and normal venous pressure with x and y descents. The cardiac impulse is impalpable and the heart sounds may be faint or variable. Classically, there may be crackles or a patch of dullness below the left scapula (Ewart's sign).

Radiography of the chest shows an unexpectedly massive cardiac silhouette of smooth outline with-

Table 41.6. Chronic pericardial effusion.

Idiopathic
Post pericarditic
Post infarction
Post irradiation
Myxoedema
Amyloid
Chylous effusion

out indentations and the lung fields are clear and free from congestive changes (Fig.41.8). Very rarely, a sub-epicardial layer of fat may be seen well inside the cardiac outline. This is best looked for in a lateral view.

The electrocardiogram is likely to show generalized low voltage, but may be otherwise normal or show flat or inverted T waves secondary to the presumed previous acute pericarditis.

Echocardiography provides immediate recognition of pericardial effusion. It allows verification of the presence or absence of tamponade in chronic lax effusions.

SPECIFIC FORMS OF PERICARDITIS

ACUTE VIRUS AND IDIOPATHIC PERICARDITIS

Apart from Coxsackie virus group B and echovirus type 8, several other viruses less commonly cause acute pericarditis including mumps and influenza virus, Epstein–Barr virus, hepatitis B and rubella[41]. Chickenpox may be complicated by severe pneumonia and acute pericarditis, whereas infectious mononucleosis and rickettsia infection[43] may cause either myocarditis or acute pericarditis. The effusion may be small and fibrinous. Much less commonly, it may be large and progress to tamponade. Progression to constriction can occur rapidly following the acute illness. Idiopathic pericarditis is indistinguishable clinically from acute viral pericarditis and is almost certainly caused by unrecognized viruses.

Many of the viruses that can cause acute pericarditis have also been associated with acute myocarditis, but it is remarkably uncommon for patients with acute viral pericarditis to show evidence of associated myocarditis or for acute pericarditis to progress to dilated cardiomyopathy. Nevertheless, the possibility of underlying myocarditis should be borne in mind as there has been at least one fatality caused by acute dilatation of the heart after pericardiocentesis in acute pericarditis with unrecognized myocarditis.

Both the visceral and the parietal pericardium are involved. Beneath the visceral pericardial membrane, the epicardium is almost invariably involved and this results in the typical electrocardiographic changes. The effusion is serous exudate, usually fibrinous and rarely haemorrhagic, containing neutrophils in the early stages and later a predominance of lymphocytes. Resolution may be associated with the formation of thick adhesions between the pericardial layers resulting in constrictive pericarditis. Calcification is rare. The symptoms of pericarditis may follow an influenza-like illness and are associated with the recurrence of fever.

Virus is only rarely isolated from pharynx, stool, blood or pericardial fluid and the diagnosis of virus pericarditis is usually made by excluding other causes and by a rise in serial covalent neutralizing antibody. In one large study of 231 cases, aetiology was established in only 15% despite every effort including cultures of the pericardial fluid isolates of the virus from pharyngeal swab or stool, and convalescent serology.[44] Infectious mononucleosis is recognized by associated sore throat and lymphadenopathy plus positive heterophil antibody and monospot tests.

Differential diagnosis

In the differential diagnosis, it is important to exclude purulent pericardial effusion, tuberculous pericarditis, connective tissue disorder, particularly systemic lupus erythematosus or rheumatoid arthritis, neoplasm and acute anterior myocardial infarction.

Other laboratory findings include a leucocytosis, raised erythrocyte sedimentation rate and C-reactive protein. There may also be a slight elevation of cardiac enzyme levels. If the enzyme titres rise to high levels, a diffuse myocarditis[45] or myocardial infarction should be suspected. The electrocardiographic changes in early acute anterior myocardial infarction may be mistaken for acute pericarditis, or acute pericarditis may develop after a 'missed' inferior infarct. Intravenous thrombolytic therapy may be instituted on a mistaken diagnosis of infarction with potentially disastrous results[46,47].

The outcome is usually complete recovery in 1–2 weeks or at longest 1 month. The possible complications are:

1 early tamponade;
2 associated myocarditis;
3 constriction;
4 relapsing pericarditis;

5 dilated cardiomyopathy.

Constriction or a relapsing course are the commonest complications. Patients with relapsing pericarditis eventually recover completely (the pericarditis does not become constrictive.

Treatment

Treatment is symptomatic. The patient is helped by rest in bed and should be admitted to hospital. The patient will be most comfortable sitting up and leaning forward with elbows on a bed table, avoiding any unnecessary movement. Aspirin or other non-steroidal anti-inflammatory drugs usually provide rapid relief. Steroids are probably unwise during the acute phase, but may be necessary if this is followed by relapses.

TUBERCULOUS PERICARDITIS

When acute tuberculous pericarditis is seen in the UK, the patient is usually an Asian immigrant and may be middle-aged. The pericardium is usually affected by direct spread from paratracheal lymph nodes or in the young by early haematogenous spread from primary infection.

Acid-fast bacilli are numerous within the pericardial fluid during the acute phase. The effusion is usually serous, but may be blood-stained, and has a high protein content. The cell content is initially polymorphonuclear but later lymphocytic.

Tamponade may occur and it is common for an effusive constrictive process to develop followed by replacement of the effusion with fibrous scar tissue and eventually calcification (Fig.41.2). Constriction is the most frequent outcome of the illness.

The diagnosis may be made during the acute phase, but it is not uncommon for patients with constrictive pericarditis of undoubted tuberculous origin to give no history of an acute episode, or indeed, of known tuberculous infection at any time.

The illness may be severe or subacute with constitutional symptoms, low-grade fever, malaise, anorexia, weight loss and sweating. Associated pulmonary tuberculous infiltration is not usually present. The patient may have no pericardial pain but there may be diffuse precordial discomfort.

The physical signs may include a rub, evidence of cardiac compression or frank tamponade.

Tuberculous pericarditis should be suspected particularly in a patient with pyrexia of unknown origin and unexplained cardiomegaly or electrocardiographic abnormality, paticularly if the patient is Asian or immunosuppressed.

Diagnosis

A tuberculin skin test is usually positive but occasionally it is negative during the acute illness only subsequently becoming strongly positive. The diagnosis is made by isolation of the mycobacterium from the pericardial fluid or from a pericardial biopsy. To improve the chances of a bacteriological diagnosis, all the pericardial fluid that can be aspirated should be sent to the laboratory so that it can be spun down, stained and examined by microscopy and then cultured. Neither a negative pericardial effusion or biopsy nor a subsequent negative culture excludes a tuberculous origin. When there is doubt, antituberculous drugs should be prescribed to patients who are more ill than is usual in viral pericarditis, in whom a tuberculin skin test is strongly positive and in whom bacteriological proof is still awaited. Very few patients with idiopathic or viral pericarditis are likely to be mistakenly treated as tuberculous.

Treatment

The use of prednisolone in addition to antituberculous drugs has been controversial because it has not been possible to prove whether the addition of steroids improves the chances of healing without constriction. However, steroids are generally prescribed. Development of constriction is recognized by the combination of a rise in venous pressure, a reduction of heart size on the chest X-ray, a rise in heart rate and the appearance of pulsus paradoxus.

Initial therapy will be with a three drug regime, such as oral ethambutol with isoniazide plus intramuscular streptomycin and prednisolone. Pericardiectomy will be needed for patients with tamponade, large effusions recurrent after drainage, effusive constrictive pericarditis or constrictive pericarditis. The results of pericardiectomy are much better when it is performed early.

BACTERIAL PERICARDITIS

Purulent pericarditis carries a high mortality. Primary purulent pericarditis has become rare but it is still seen as an acute illness particularly in previously healthy children[48] and young adults following bacteraemia. Haemophilus is an important organism,[49] but purulent pericarditis may be caused by staphylococci or streptococci[50], pneumococci, meningococci or gonococci. A wide range of bacteria, including campylobacter and legionella, may rarely infect the pericardium following bacteraemia[51]. It may complicate immunosuppression including that seen in AIDS[52] or a sterile effusion in rheumatoid arthritis may become secondarily infected. It may also occur following cardiac surgery or in infective endocarditis when it may develop by extension from an aortic root or myocardial abscess or following a septic coronary embolus. A localized pericardial abscess may form[53].

In the past, purulent pericarditis complicated pneumonia as a result of contiguous spread, but this is now uncommon. Rarely, it may complicate sub-diaphragmatic infections as when amoebic liver abscess or echinococcal disease spreads to the pericardium.

The illness is usually fulminant with high fever, rigors, sweating and dyspnoea. The heart rate is rapid but there may be no pain or pericardial rub to bring attention to the pericardium. Tamponade may appear suddenly and be associated with a further abrupt deterioration in an already very sick patient. Primary meningococcal pericarditis may develop early without other evidence of meningococcal septicaemia or meningitis, causing collapse within hours of the development of signs of illness[54,55].

Laboratory findings include a polymorphonuclear leucocytosis with marked leftward shift and toxic changes. The chest radiograph usually shows an enlarged cardiac shadow and may show pneumonia or empyema. The electrocardiogram usually shows typical acute changes.

The development of tamponade may provide the first evidence of pericarditis in so-called 'primary' pericarditis following bacteraemia. The mortality is high simply because the condition may be missed completely. Purulent pericarditis is to be suspected in acutely toxic patients, who may have been previously debilitated, when there is a high fever, dyspnoea, hypotension, a grossly elevated white cell count and cardiomegaly on a chest X-ray. An urgent echocardiogram and pericardiocentesis are required.

The pericardial fluid contains neutrophils, or may be frankly purulent. It may be possible to drain it completely via a pericardial catheter, but if the fluid is thickly purulent it will need surgical drainage. The pericardial fluid will show numerous organisms on Gram-staining and it should be cultured both aerobically and anaerobically. If the Gram-stain is negative, the fluid should be stained for acid-fast bacteria and fungi, and appropriately cultured.

Antibiotic therapy must be accompanied by efficient drainage of the pericardial space, otherwise death from tamponade may still occur. It is not necessary to instil antibiotics directly into the pericardium as high concentrations are achieved from oral or parenteral dosage.

A post-pericarditis syndrome may occur during convalescence with recurrent fever and usually with precordial pain but without recurrence of the severe toxic illness. There may be pleurisy and arthritis as well as recurrent serous pericardial effusion.

Constriction is common after infection by pyogenic organisms and may occur quickly. Surgical pericardiectomy is required without delay.

THE PERICARDIUM IN CONNECTIVE TISSUE DISEASE

The pericardium is involved in many of the connective tissue diseases, but in the majority the involvement is subclinical. There may be a serous effusion or pericardial thickening with adhesions leading to obliteration of the pericardial space, and constrictive pericarditis may occur.

Rheumatoid arthritis

Charcot first observed that pericarditis tends to occur during exacerbation of the arthritis. A healed fibrous pericarditis seen in 30–45% of cases at autopsy is commonest in patients with severe disability and sero-positive disease of long duration.

Immunofluorescence studies have demonstrated the presence of IgG, IgM, rheumatoid factor, IgA, C3 and low complement levels in the pericardial fluid which is a fibrinous exudate with a low level of glucose and a high level of lactic dehydrogenase[56]. Rheumatoid effusions occasionally contain a high concentration of cholesterol.

The frequency of clinical pericarditis is between 2 and 10% of hospital patients with rheumatoid arthritis but much lower in outpatients who have the disease. These patients may have only a friction rub or excess fluid on echo. When echocardiography is carried out routinely in rheumatoid patients, the incidence of otherwise undetectable pericardial effusion rises to as high as 15–50%.

Pain is rare in rheumatoid pericarditis, and the electrocardiogram usually shows either no abnormality or transient T-wave inversion. Large effusions develop only rarely, but tamponade may occur.

Although constrictive pericarditis is not a common complication of rheumatoid pericarditis[58], rheumatoid disease is so common that, given the near disappearance of tuberculous constriction, rheumatoid constriction comes second only to idiopathic presumed post-viral constriction in frequency of occurence (Fig.41.9).

Patients with hot joints and active pericarditis respond well to short courses of prednisolone.

Surgical pericardiectomy may be needed for the rare cases with large effusions or tamponade caused by marked pericardial thickening (chronic effusive constrictive pericarditis)[59].

Constrictive pericarditis may occur at any time during the course of rheumatoid disease and may even precede the onset of arthritis. Rheumatoid factor should be sought in patients with constrictive pericarditis of unknown origin.

Surgical treatment is usually dramatically successful, but if it fails to relieve the signs then underlying constrictive myocardial disease should be suspected. Surgically excised material should be cultured to exclude a tuberculous origin. Very rarely, constriction may be focal in the right or left atrioventricular groove mimicking tricuspid or mitral stenosis.

Juvenile chronic arthritis

Pericardial involvement is common in juvenile chronic arthritis. Acute pericarditis is occasionally the presenting manifestation, particularly in Still's disease, with fever, lymphadenopathy, splenomegaly, pleurisy and sometimes the development of amyloidosis. Prednisolone is used in patients with acute pericarditis, but tamponade[59] or suspicion of a purulent pericarditis provide an absolute indication for pericardiocentesis.

Systemic lupus erythematosus

Pericarditis is common in systemic lupus erythematosus, both clinically and at autopsy when about 50% of patients show evidence of pericardial involvement[60].

The inflammation is blamed on immune complex deposition made visible by immunofluorescent techniques which reveal deposits of IgG, IgM and C3.[61] The fluid may contain antinuclear antibodies, lupus erythematosus cells and high levels of anti-DNA as well as IgM rheumatoid factor.

Pericarditis is most often recognized clinically during acute flares of the disease; it may be painful or painless. Pericardial rubs are common with non-specific T-wave changes on electrocardiogram. Radiological cardiac enlargement may be due to effusion or to depressed myocardial function, and echocardiography may also reveal Libman–Sacks vegetations on the mitral valve, especially in patients with anticardiolipin antibodies. Relapsing

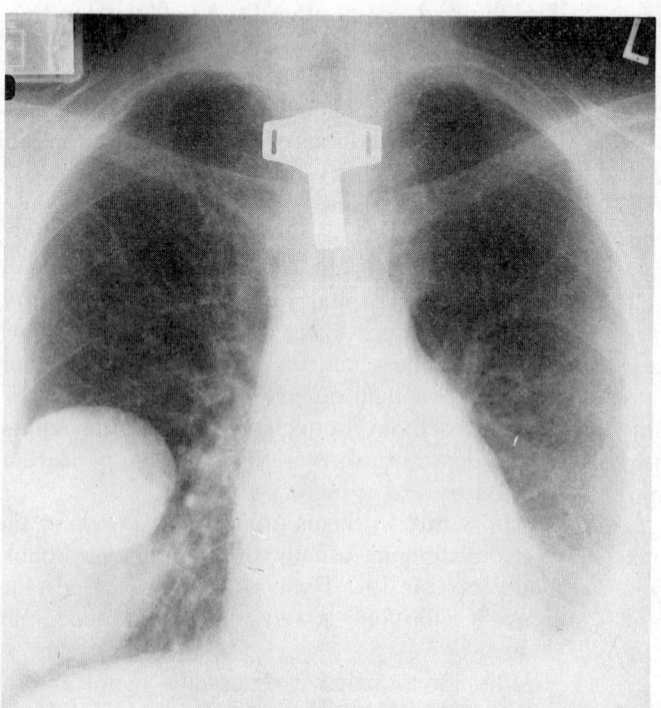

Fig.41.9. Postero-anterior radiograph from a case of severe rheumatoid constriction. It shows a rather small heart with obliteration of the normal contours. There is a left pleural effusion and a loculated right pleural effusion but no pulmonary venous congestion. The patient had a permanent tracheostomy because of arthritis affecting the cricoarytenoid joints.

pericarditis may occur. The incidence of tamponade is low. Constriction is rare. In patients with systemic lupus erythematosus who are receiving immunosuppressive treatment, the development of an infection can mimic a flare of the disease and purulent pericarditis has been reported. Therefore, it is important to obtain fluid for culture, particularly as blood cultures may be sterile even when there are bacteria in the pericardial fluid. *Staphylococcus aureus* infection is most common. It requires appropriate antibiotics and urgent surgical pericardial drainage.

Drug-induced lupus syndromes

Pericarditis is also observed in the drug-induced lupus syndromes (Table 41.7). Most of these are precipitated by hydralazine[62] and procainamide,[63] but other drugs may be implicated including methyldopa[64] minoxidil[65] and methysergide.[66] Methysergide causes a constrictive picture due to a fibrosing mediastinitis. Tamponade may occur in drug-induced lupus syndromes[62].

Scleroderma

Pericarditis is most often subclinical and an autopsy finding but small pericardial effusions are not uncommon[67]. The pericarditis differs from that in rheumatoid disease and systemic lupus erythematosus in showing lack of inflammatory changes and immune complexes. Clinical pericardial disease in scleroderma is usually a late complication of the disease; tamponade[68] and constriction are rare. Electrocardiographic changes are not usually diagnostic, particularly because of the common involvement of the myocardium in the disease.

Table 41.7. **Drug-induced pericarditis.**

---

1 Iatrogenic lupus syndrome
   Commonly: Procainamide
                Hydralazine
   Rarely: Reserpine
                Methyldopa
                Isoniazide
                Diphenylhydantoin
                Minoxidil

2 Adriomycin   (acute early reaction)
   Methysergide (mediastinal fibrosis)
   Penicillin   (acute sensitivity)

3 Constrictive syndrome
   Methysergide (mediastinal fibrosis)

4 Penicillin (acute sensitivity)

Pericarditis does not carry the ominous prognosis of myocardial involvement with heart failure in scleroderma.

The overlap syndromes (mixed connective tissue disease)

Patients with these conditions show clinical characteristics of more than one connective tissue disease with features of systemic lupus erythematosus, scleroderma, dermatomyositis or rheumatoid arthritis. Acute pericarditis or pleurisy is common as a presenting feature of mixed connective tissue disease.

Systemic vasculitides

Pericarditis is uncommon in polyarteritis nodosum, unless the pericarditis associated with uraemia is included, but acute pericarditis may be caused by the vasculitis, in which case there may be a pericardial rub and small effusion. Pericarditis is also rare in Wegener's granulomatosis, the Churg–Strauss variant of polyarteritis nodosa and temporal arteritis[69]. In Takayasu's arteritis, tamponade can occur due to rupture of a coronary artery aneurysm. In Behçet's syndrome, pericarditis has been observed rarely; it is also infrequent in relapsing polychondritis.

Sero-negative spondylo-arthropathies

Pericarditis is not very common in ankylosing spondylitis. It occurs more frequently in Reiter's syndrome,[70] but tamponade and constriction do not seem to occur. Constrictive pericarditis has been reported in psoriatic arthritis.

Whipple's disease

In Whipple's disease, pericarditis and pleurisy may precede other manifestations, or it may be accompanied by a sero-negative migratory arthritis in the absence of gastro-intestinal symptoms[71]. Pericardial involvement in Whipple's disease is found in a high proportion of cases at autopsy.

Recurrent pericarditis may occur in coeliac disease[72] and inflammatory bowel disease[73].

Rheumatic fever

Clinical pericarditis is uncommon in acute rheumatic fever, but when present it often signifies a profound pancarditis. The pericarditis is usually diffuse and fibrous, leading to obliteration of the pericardial space, but not to constriction.

POST-INFARCTION PERICARDITIS

A pericardial friction rub becomes audible in about 10% of patients following acute myocardial infarction, but a localized fibrinous pericarditis overlies almost all transmural infarcts such that the autopsy incidence of previous pericarditis is very much higher[74,75].

Early post-infarction pericarditis

A pericardial rub may complicate infarction at any site and appears within about 12 hours to 2 or 3 days of the onset. It may be associated with the reappearance of chest pain which may mimic extension of infarction, but there is no new enzyme release and no extension of the electrocardiographic change of infarction. The diagnosis of post-infarction pericarditis is suggested by the appearance of a rub and new ST-segment elevation; however, if serial routine two-dimensional echocardiography was carried out on all patients in a coronary care unit, a pericardial effusion would be found at some stage in many patients in whom there is no clinical sign of pericarditis because rubs are evanescent. Only a few of these patients[74] develop Dressler's syndrome. Sometimes atrial arrhythmias may complicate the picture. If the pericardial rub is systolic with no diastolic component, it may suggest the development of mitral regurgitation due to papillary muscle dysfunction, but in contrast there is no accompanying clinical deterioration, no new congestive changes on the chest radiograph and the 'murmur' is evanescent.

The increasing use of thrombolysis and the usual prescription of anticoagulants after successful reperfusion to reduce the risk of re-occlusion highlight the importance of accurate diagnosis of early infarction. The avoidance of thrombolytic agents when the infarct is probably already complete is obvious. Thrombolytic agents have already been given inadvertently to patients with acute pericarditis and it is likely that their use will result in an increase of Dressler's syndrome (qv).

Haemopericardium and cardiac rupture

Pericarditis developing 5–10 days after infarction may be caused by haemorrhage from the infarct site and this can be sufficiently profuse to cause tamponade. Compression of the heart may be localized depending on the site of the haematoma and may simulate tricuspid stenosis[76] or another mechanical fault.

Acute myocardial rupture may occur from 4 days after the onset and cause collapse from tamponade. It is recognized by circulatory arrest with electromechanical dissociation or asystole rather than ventricular fibrillation. Sometimes the extent of rupture of the free wall is small and collapse does not occur because it seals onto the parietal pericardium, with or without tamponade, or a false aneurysm develops. A true aneurysm may rupture in the course of its formation with haemopericardium but pericardial sealing of the hole. When pericardial haemorrhage is massive, death usually follows rapidly despite evacuation of the pericardium but if the patient survives the moment, formal surgical exploration and suturing of the rupture site may be successful[77]. Subacute rupture with only slow haemorrhage into the pericardium may even go undetected if the patient has not had regular electrocardiographic, radiographic and echocardiographic monitoring or the reason for a slow recovery may only be recognized later.

Acute tamponade secondary to cardiac rupture must be differentiated from other causes of cardiogenic shock, such as new myocardial infarction, ventricular septal rupture or mitral regurgitation.

Hypotension with a rise of venous pressure and pulsus paradoxus may follow massive right ventricular infarction. The haemodynamic findings may be hard to separate because pericardial restriction after acute right ventricular failure may lead to equally high diastolic pressures throughout the four cardiac chambers. Echocardiography is able to differentiate.

Chest pain due to post-infarction pericarditis is best treated with aspirin rather than non-steroidal anti-inflammatory drugs or steroids, but all these drugs need to be covered with an H_2-antagonist such as ranitidine because the risk of gastric haemorrhage from acute erosion is high in the post-infarct patient.

The post-myocardial infarction syndrome (Dressler's syndrome)

The post-myocardial infarction syndrome may develop weeks or months after an acute myocardial infarct. Dressler estimated that it occurred in up to 4% of patients[78]. The syndrome does not differ from relapsing pericarditis following cardiac surgery or following acute pericarditis of any cause. It is more common in post-infarct patients who have had a major transmural infarct and pericardial friction than in patients who have had a small or non-Q wave infarct. It is almost certainly of immunological origin, and leakage of blood from the infarct surface may be important. A diminishing incidence of Dressler's syndrome as well as of haemopericardium may be explained by the use of anticoagulants in smaller numbers of coronary care unit patients than formerly. It will be interesting to see if the incidence starts to rise again with the increasing use of thrombolysis and the slight pericardial seepage which may follow percutaneous transluminal coronary angioplasty.

Dressler's syndrome, the post-cardiotomy syndrome and relapsing pericarditis after pericarditis of any cause have a common aetiology. The following features are common to all three conditions.

1 Blood will have entered the pericardial space.
2 There is an interval between the initiating event and the development of the syndrome.
3 Antiheart antibodies can be found.
4 Rapid response to treatment with anti-inflammatory agents.
5 Frequent relapses are common, although each relapse is of diminishing intensity.
6 The pericarditis is usually diffuse with a small to moderate sized effusion and tamponade is rare; pleural effusions commonly occur.
7 Constriction does not occur.

The syndrome may recur and it is usually self-limiting. The interval elapsing between the initiating event and the development of the syndrome means that the patient will already have been discharged from hospital and will have to be re-admitted for diagnostic purposes and observation in case of the development of tamponade. If oral anticoagulants had been given, they should be discontinued. Aspirin in adequate dosage usually reduces the pain; prednisolone may be needed[79], only a short course of which should be given starting with 40–60 mg daily and reducing the dose to stop within 10 days. Colchicine, may be tried for acute flares (1 mg followed by 500 µg every 2–3 h until relief or nausea and vomiting, or a maximum of 10 mg).

POST-CARDIOTOMY PERICARDITIS

About 25% of post-operative cardiac surgical patients may be shown by ultrasound to have a pericardial collection which usually gradually re-solves without incident. It is responsible for the very common finding of an increase in heart size radiographically even up to the time of hospital discharge post-operatively.

Acute haemorrhagic tamponade may occur in the early post-operative period, being recognized by a rise in heart rate with declining blood pressure and pulse pressure and urine output. The patient needs to be returned urgently to theatre, the sternotomy re-opened and the blood removed. A bacterial mediastinitis or pericarditis may occur with fever, tamponade or spread to infect a prosthetic valve. Cardiac tamponade may occur later post-operatively[80] or subacute tamponade may be associated with slow recovery and a rising venous pressure. After diagnostic ultrasound, the fluid can sometimes be evacuated by pericardiocentesis but in most patients there is already a subacute constrictive effusive syndrome requiring return to the operating room. This syndrome is usually caused by a combination of free fluid and organizing thrombus which may be localized.

Rarely, constrictive pericarditis occurs after cardiac surgery; although this is now being reported with increasing frequency, it was first recognized only as recently as 1984[81] and only after coronary artery bypass surgery when it may be a cause of graft occlusion[82]. This is partly because of the increasing number of patients undergoing coronary surgery but also because it may be missed in patients with valvar or other problems in whom a raised venous pressure may be attributed to other causes.

Surgery of post-operative constrictive pericarditis is rendered difficult by the need to avoid the coronary artery bypass grafts.

The incidence was recently estimated at 0.2% of adults who had undergone cardiac surgery. Constriction may occur despite the pericardium not being sutured and, like constriction following acute infective pericarditis, it develops early. It occurs in patients whose post-operative pericardial collection becomes organized; usually, the constriction is already evident at the time of discharge although if the condition is not known and not recognized the patient may not be referred back to the surgical centre until weeks or months after discharge from hospital. In such late cases, constriction may be severe with loss of weight, hepatomegaly and ascites.

Post-operative pericardial constriction is not invariably associated with peri-operative infarction, although this may be the triggering mechanism in some patients. All patients who have undergone cardiac surgery have some blood left in the pericardial space and it may be that the combination of this with a low-grade mediastinal infection may be conducive to the development of constriction, but not all patients show evidence of this.

Uraemic pericarditis

Uraemic pericarditis used to be found in about 50% of renal failure patients who died but the incidence has diminished since treatment with haemodialysis and chronic ambulatory peritoneal dialysis has been available[83].

Many of the features of uraemic pericarditis are unexplained. It may develop in patients despite regular haemodialysis whose serum creatinine and electrolyte levels are close to normal; there is no clear correlation between the presence of pericarditis and the level of blood urea. Pericarditis is less common in patients undergoing chronic ambulatory peritoneal dialysis than in those undergoing haemodialysis. Regular heparinization of the haemodialysis patient may be conducive to haemorrhage into the pericardium which can then give rise to chronic effusion, relapsing pericarditis, tamponade or even constriction. In uraemic pericarditis, the pericardial surfaces are very vascular and bleed easily. Organization may be associated with fibrous adhesions and ultimately with an 'onion peel' constriction. Calcification is uncommon.

Uraemic pericarditis may lead to haemodynamic complications during routine dialysis, patients becoming hypotensive when blood volume diminishes during ultrafiltration.

Patients may have precordial pain, fever and dyspnoea. Echocardiography is useful in documenting the presence and size of effusion, whether tamponade is present or incipient and whether uraemic myocardial failure makes a contribution to the patient's illness.[83]

Uraemic patients are subject to other causes of pericarditis, particularly myocardial infarction, secondary infection of a pericardial effusion, neoplasia and hypothyroidism. As uraemic pericarditis is no longer just a terminal event in end-stage renal failure, it has become more important clinically. About one-third of dialysis patients who have had uraemic pericarditis recover without subsequent problems, about one-fifth develop arrhythmias and hypotension and less than one-tenth develop tamponade or constriction.

No treatment is required for small asymptomatic pericardial effusions in uraemic patients. Large pericardial effusions may need to be tapped or may resolve after an increase in the frequency of dialysis, particularly if this is combined with non-steroidal anti-inflammatory drug therapy. Episodic steroid treatment may be needed when painful pericardial effusion is recurrent[84] and some workers recommend an early pericardiectomy in uraemic patients in order to avoid complications[85]. As the condition resolves without surgery in many patients, pericardiectomy should probably be reserved for patients requiring recurrent pericardiocentesis for tamponade or those who have developed constriction.

Pericardial effusion in myxoedema

Pericardial effusion is said to occur in up to one-third of hypothyroid patients and may be associated also with pleural effusion and ascites due to a combination of salt and water retention and slow lymphatic drainage. The pericardial fluid is straw-coloured with elevated protein and cholesterol concentrations. As it accumulates very slowly, the effusion may become very large containing several litres. Usually, therefore, the effusion is lax and does not cause symptoms; it is detected because of a large heart on radiography and can be confirmed on ultrasound. Tamponade has occasionally been reported[86]. The electrocardiogram is already low voltage and there are no particular features that would allow identification of effusion in hypothyroid patients.

The effusion regresses as thyroid replacement therapy is implemented, but this may take many months. Other causes of chronic lax pericardial effusion are listed in Table 41.6.

Pericardial effusion in amyloid disease

The amyloid heart is typically small with amyloid infiltration between the myofibrils leading to an increase in wall thickness but a diminution in cavity size. Amyloid infiltration of the walls of the small vessels in the epicardium may be associated with pericardial effusion which may be large and usually serous but occasionally blood-stained. In such patients, the cardiac shadow may be enlarged on chest radiograms, the effusion recognized ultrasonically and the condition thought to be one of subacute tamponade or chronic effusive constrictive pericarditis[87]. The possibility of underlying heart disease needs to be considered in patients presenting with large pericardial effusions and in amyloid disease the characteristic thickening of all walls of the heart including the valves and atrial septum seen on echocardiography should prevent error. Aspiration of fluid will not alter the haemodynamics in such cases; the only treatment at present available for patients with advanced amyloid heart disease is transplantation in those who are otherwise reasonably well and not too old.

NEOPLASTIC PERICARDITIS

Primary pericardial neoplasms are rare but include primary mesothelioma, fibrosarcoma and angiosarcoma. Teratomas may be benign or malignant. Primary pericardial neoplasms may present with effusion, constriction, arrhythmia or rarely with symptoms caused by compression of one of the cardiac chambers, the superior vena cava or the aorta, simulating aortic stenosis.

Hodgkin's and non-Hodgkin's lymphoma, Burkitt's lymphoma and lymphoblastic lymphoma may occasionally present with pericardial effusion and tamponade[88].

Metastatic carcinoma is the commonest cause of malignant pericarditis, the most frequent being, in order of occurrence, cancer of the lung, breast, stomach and colon. Sarcomas and melanomas may also involve the pericardium. Clinical presentation is usually with tamponade.

Haemorrhagic pericardial effusion due to malignant infiltration of the pericardium may cause rapid development of cardiac tamponade, or subacute compression of the heart may be the first symptom of malignancy[89,90,91]. Complete tumour encasement of the heart may occur in mesothelioma causing the clinical features of constrictive pericarditis.

Malignant pericarditis is frequently an incidental finding at autopsy in patients with cancer and has often been asymptomatic during the patient's life.

Patients who have had previous irradiation may develop non-malignant pericarditis with effusion and tamponade or with constriction. Surgical treatment may be required; pericardiectomy may also help to palliate the symptoms of patients with active pericardial malignancy[30].

Immunosuppression for advanced malignant disease may be complicated by opportunistic infections which may involve the pericardium.

POST-IRRADIATION PERICARDITIS

Megavoltage therapy for the treatment of Hodg-kin's lymphoma, non-Hodgkin's lymphoma and carcinoma of the breast or lung can damage the heart and pericardium. Evidence of damage may appear within weeks or even up to years later (Table 41.8). In modern radiotherapy techniques, the heart is shielded thereby reducing the risk of radiation injury to it.

Pathology

The early acute inflammatory pericarditis is associated with an exudative effusion which may be blood-stained and contains lymphocytes and fibrin. The inflammation may resolve or it may organize, obliterating the pericardial space and sometimes going on to constriction[92]. Sometimes a chronic effusive constrictive pericarditis or a chronic lax effusion develops[93]. Radiation may also damage the coronary arteries and the myocardium causing acute myocardial depression and eventual myocardial fibrosis. Radiation coronary arteritis may be followed by changes similar to those of atheroma; there may be damage to valves, particularly the tricuspid valve. Patients with the most severe form of pericardial injury, namely fibrosis and constriction, are the most likely to have myocardial fibrosis, but radiation-induced coronary artery occlusion may be seen in the absence of detectable pericardial damage. All of the various pericardial syndromes can follow irradiation of the mediastinum (Table 41.7). Acute pericarditis can develop within 3 or 4 weeks of the onset of radiotherapy and be associated with fever, pericardial rub, electrocardiographic changes and evidence of a pericardial effusion on ultrasound examination. Resolution may occur spontaneously but a relapsing syndrome may follow. Healing with organization may lead to a chronic effusive constrictive pericarditis which may need later pericardiectomy.

Sometimes patients who give no history of acute pericarditis following a course of radiotherapy first

---

Table 41.8. Post-irradiation pericarditis.

Syndromes:
Acute pericarditis
Relapsing pericarditis
Chronic lax pericardial effusion
Effusive constrictive pericarditis
Constrictive pericarditis

Also:
Interstitial myocardial fibrosis
Coronary artery fibrosis

present months or years afterwards with a chronic asymptomatic lax pericardial effusion.

Unlike other causes of constrictive pericarditis, patients with post-radiation constriction may not present for many years, even 20 years after radiotherapy[94].

Differential diagnosis

The main difficulty is differentiation from pericarditis caused by the malignancy treated. However, patients with recurrent malignancy most often present with cardiac tamponade. Constriction may develop if the heart becomes encased in solid tumour.

Traumatic damage to the pericardium

The reader is referred to a comprehensive review of cardiovascular trauma by Cheitlin[95,96].

Blunt trauma may cause myocardial contusion, laceration or actual rupture. Laceration of the pericardium without rupture of the heart can be followed by herniation of the heart and death after an interval. Closed chest cardiac massage may cause myocardial contusion or even infarction with the development of effusion or tamponade. The damage is usually infero-posterior.

Clinical manifestations range from pericardial pain, friction and electrocardiographic changes to haemopericardium and tamponade. Blunt trauma may cause associated structural injury such as ventricular septal rupture, coronary occlusion and true or false aneurysm formation. Relapsing pericarditis may follow traumatic haemopericardium and, rarely, constriction.

The agents of penetrating injury are usually knives or bullets. Stab wounds may seal without consequence, and they can be routinely treated in the emergency room simply by inserting a pericardial drain. However, in developed countries, patients are routinely taken to the operating room. Bullets cause far more destruction; tamponade, cardiac herniation, pericardial infection and constriction may follow.

Chylopericardium

A chylous pericardial effusion may develop after occlusion of the thoracic duct by tuberculosis, malignancy or surgical ligation or rupture; rarely, it is idiopathic[97].

The accumulation of chyle is slow and most patients are asymptomatic with a chronic lax effusion found accidentally. The connection between a damaged thoracic duct and the pericardium can be established by recovery of ingested Sudan red from aspirated pericardial fluid[98].

Mulibrey nanism

Mulibrey nanism, described in 1973, is a rare disorder with autosomal recessive inheritance, the main features of which are dwarfism and severe constrictive pericarditis[99]. The acronym stands for *mu*scle, *br*ain and *ey*es because the patients have hypotonic muscles, a squeaky voice and yellow dots with pigmentary dispersion in the ocular fundi. *Nanos* is from the Greek meaning a dwarf. Pericardiectomy is often necessary in these patients.

REFERENCES

1. Bor, I. and Kafke, V. Aplasia of Pericardium. *J. Cardiovasc. Surg.* 1961; 2: 389.
2. Smiseth, O.A., Frais, M.A., Kingma, I. *et al.* Assessment of pericardial constraint: the relationship between right ventricular filling pressure and pericardial pressure measured after pericardiocentesis. *J. Am. Coll. Cardiol.* 1986; 7: 307.
3. Lee, M.C., LeWinter, M.M., Freeman, G., Shabetai, R. and Fung, Y.C. Biaxial mechanical properties of the pericardium in normal and volume overloaded dogs. *Am. J. Physiol.* 1985; 249: H222.
4. Spodick, D.H. The normal and diseased pericardium: current concepts of pericardial physiology, diagnosis and treatment. *J. Am. Coll. Cardiol.* 1986; 1: 240.
5. Bove, A.A. and Santamore, W.P. Ventricular Interdependence. *Prog. Cardiovasc. Dis.* 1981; 23: 365.
6. Lorell, B.H., Palacios, I., Daggett, W.M. *et al.* Right Ventricular Distension and Left Ventricular Compliance. *Am. J. Physiol.* 1981; 240: 1187.
7. Nicolosi, G.L., Borgoioni, L., Alberti, E. *et al.* M-mode and two-dimensional echocardiography in congenital absence of the pericardium *Chest* 1982; 81: 610.
8. Klatte, E.C. and Yune, H.Y. Diagnosis and treatment of pericardial cysts. *Radiology* 1972; 104: 541.
9. Tiefe, N., Brunn, A.J. and Roberts, R. Elevation of plasma MB creatinine kinase and the development of new Q-waves in association with pericarditis. *Chest* 1980; 77: 438.
10. Ribeiro, P., Shapiro, L., Nihoyannopoulos, P. *et al.* Pericarditis in Infective Endocarditis. *Eur. Heart J.* 1985; 6: 975.
11. Fowler, N.O. and Harbin, A.D. Recurrent acute pericarditis: follow-up study of 31 patients. *J. Am. Coll. Cardiol.* 1986; 7: 300.
12. Hancock, E.W. subacute effusive constrictive pericarditis *Circulation* 1971; 43: 183.
13. Rasaretnam, R. and Chanmugam, D. Subacute Effusive Constrictive Pericarditis. *Br. Heart J.* 1980; 44: 44.
14. Cameron, J., Oesterle, S.N., Baldwin, J.C. and Hancock, E.W. The etiologic spectrum of constricted pericarditis. *Am. Heart J.* 1987; 113: 354.
15. Bush, C.A., Stang, T.M., Wooley, O.G. and Kilman, J. Occult constrictive pericardial disease. Diagnosis by rapid volume expansion and correction by pericardiectomy. *Circulation* 1977; 56: 924.

16. Wood, P. Chronic Constrictive Pericarditis. *Am. J. Cardiol.* 1961; **7**: 48.

17. Hancock, E.W. Constrictive Pericarditis. Clinical clues to Diagnosis. *JAMA* 1975; **232**: 176.

18. Wilkinson, P., Pinto, B. and Senior, J.R. Reversible protein losing enteropathy with intestinal lympangiectasis secondary to chronic constrictive pericarditis. *N. Engl. J. Med.* 1965; **273**: 1178.

19. Mounsey, P. The early diastolic sound of constrictive pericarditis. *Br. Heart J.* 1955; **17**: 143.

20. Beck, W., Shrire, V. and Vogelpoel, L. Splitting of the second heart sound in constrictive pericarditis with observations on the mechanism of pulsus paradoxus. *Am. Heart J.* 1962; **64**: 765.

21. Tyberg, T., Goodyer, A.V.N. and Langou, R.A. Genesis of pericardial knock in constrictive pericarditis. *Am. Heart J.* 1962; **64**: 765.

22. Vandenbossche, J.L., Jacobs, P., Decroly, P., Primo, G. and Englert, M. Significance of inspiratory premature opening of pulmonic valve in constrictive pericarditis. *Am. Heart J.* 1985; **110**: 896.

23. Engel, P., Fowler, N.O., Tei, C et al. M-mode echocardiography in constrictive pericarditis. *J. Am. Coll. Cardiol.* 1985; **6**: 471.

24. Sutton, F.J., Whitely, N.O. and Applefeld, M.M. The role of echocardiography and computed tomography in the evidence of constrictive pericarditis. *Am. Heart J.* 1985; **109**: 350.

25. Levy-Ravetch, M., Auh, Y.O., Rubenstein, W.A., Whalen, P. and Kazarman, E. CT of the pericardial recesses. *Am. J. Roentgenol.* 1985; **144**: 707.

26. Seifert, F.C., Miller, D.C., Oesterle, S.N., Oyer, P.E., Stinson, E.B. and Shumway, N.E. The surgical treatment of constrictive pericarditis: analysis of outcome and diagnostic error. *Circulation* 1985; **72** (Suppl.): 264.

27. McCaughan, B.C., Schaff, H.V., Piehler, J.M. et al. Early and late results of pericardiectomy for constrictive pericarditis. *J. Thorac. Cardiovasc. Surg.* 1985; **89**: 340.

28. Prager, R.L., Wilson, C.H. and Bender, H.W. Jr. The subxiphoid approach to pericardial disease. *Ann. Thorac. Surg.* 1982; **34**: 6.

29. Miller, J.I., Mansour, K.A. and Hatcher, C.R. Jr. Pericardiectomy: Current indications, concepts and results in a university center. *Ann. Thorac. Surg.* 1982; **34**: 40.

30. Piehler, J.M., Pluth, J.R., Schaff, H.V., Danielson, G.K., Orszulak, T.A. and Puga, F.J. Surgical management of effusive pericardial disease: influence of extent of pericardial resection on clinical course. *J. Thorac. Cardiovasc. Surg.* 1985; **90**: 506.

31. McGregor, M. Current Concepts in Pulsus Paradoxus. *N. Engl. J. Med.* 1979; **301**: 480.

32. Fast, J., Wielenga, R.P., Jansen, E. and Schuurmans Stekhoven, J.H. Abnormal wall movements of the right ventricle and both atria in patients with pericardial effusion as indicators of cardiac tamponade. *Eur. Heart J.* 1986; **7**: 431.

33. Tyberg, I.V., Taichman, G.C., Smith, E.R., Douglas, N.W.S., Smiseth, O.A. and Keon, W.J. The relationship between pericardial pressure and right atrial pressure: an intraoperative study. *Circulation* 1986; **73**: 428.

34. Fowler, N.O. and Gabel, M. The hemodynamic effects of cardiac tamponade: mainly the result of atrial, not ventricular, compression. *Circulation* 1985; **71**: 154.

35. Appleton, C.P., Hatle, L.K. and Popp, R.L. Superior vena cava flow velocity patterns can diagnose cardiac tamponade in patients with pericardial effusions. *J. Am. Coll. Cardiol.* 1987; **9**: 118A.

36. Singh, S., Wann, S., Klopfenstein, H.S., Hartz, A. and Brooks, H.L. Usefulness of right ventricular diastolic collapse in diagnosing cardiac tamponade and comparison to

37. Klopfenstein, H.S., Schuchard, G.H., Wann, L.S. et al. The relative merits of pulsus paradoxus and right ventricular diastolic collapse in the early detection of cardiac tamponade: an experimental echocardiographic study. *Circulation* 1985; **71**: 829.

38. Cogswell, T.L., Bernath, G.A., Raff, H., Hoffman, R.G. and Klopfenstein, H.S. Total peripheral resistance during cardiac tamponade: adrenergic and angiotensin roles. *Am. J. Physiol.* 1986; **251**: 916.

39. Osborn, J.L. and Lawton, M.T. Neurogenic antinatriuresis during development of acute cardiac tamponade. *Am. J. Physiol.* 1986; **250**: H195.

40. Kopecky, S.L., Callahan, J.A., Tajik, A.J. and Seward, J.B. Percutaneous pericardial catheter drainage: report of 42 consecutive cases. *Am. J. Cardiol.* 1986; **58**: 633.

41. Fink, C., Schaad, U.B. and Stocker, P.F. Pericarditis complicating rubella. *Schweiz Med. Wochenschr.* 1987; **117**: 28.

43. Maisch, B. Rickettsial perimyocarditis: a follow-up study. *Heart Vessels* 1986; **2**: 55.

44. Permanyer-Miralda, G., Sagrista-Sauleda, J. and Soler-Soler, J. Primary acute pericardial disease: a prospective series of 231 consecutive patients. *Am. J. Cardiol.* 1985; **56**: 623.

45. Karjalainen, J. and Heikkila, J. Acute pericarditis: myocardial enzyme release as evidence for myocarditis. *Am. Heart J.* 1986; **111**: 546.

46. Ferguson, D.W., Dewey, R.D. and Plante, D.A. Clinical pitfall in the non-invasive thrombolytic approach to presumed acute myocardial infarction. *Can. J. Cardiol.* 1986; **2**: 146.

47. Tilley, W.S. and Harston, W.E. Inadvertent administration of streptokinase to patients with pericarditis. *Am. J. Med.* 1986; **81**: 541.

48. Hoier-Madsen, K., Saunamaki, K.I., Wulff, J., Kjoller, S. and Jensen, C. Purulent pericarditis in children. *Scand. J. Thorac. Cardiovasc. Surg.* 1985; **19**: 185.

49. Greenberg, D., Siefkin, A.D., Veliji, M.A. and Hoeprich, P.D. Pericarditis caused by beta-lactamase-producing *Haemophilus influenzae*: report of two cases in adults and review of the literature. *Texas Heart Inst. J.* 1986; **13**: 297.

50. Vigneswaran, W.T., Hardie, R., Ferguson, J.C. and Faichney, A. Cardiac tamponade due to Lancefield group A β haemolytic streptococcal pericarditis. *Thorax* 1985; **40**: 549.

51. Nelson, D.P., Renismer, E.R. and Raffin, T.A. *Legionella pneumophila* pericarditis without pneumonia. *Arch. Intern. Med.* 1985; **145**: 926.

52. Stechel, R.P., Cooper, D.J., Greenspan, J., Pizzarello, R.A. and Tenenbaum, M.J. Staphylococcal pericarditis in a homosexual patient with AIDS-related complex. *N.Y. State J. Med.* 1986; **86**: 592.

53. Johnson, M.A., Hirji, M.K., Hennig, R.C. and Williams, B. Pericardial abscess: diagnosis using two-dimensional echocardiography and CT. *Radiology* 1986; **159**: 419.

54. Braester, A., Nusem, D. and Horn, Y. Primary meningococcal pericarditis in a pregnant woman. *Int. J. Cardiol.* 1986; **11**: 355.

55. Hardy, D.J., Bartholomew, W.R. and Amsterdam, D. Pathophysiology of primary meningococcal pericarditis associated with *Neisseria meningitidis* group C: a case report and review of the literature. *Diagn. Microbiol. Infect. Dis.* 1986; **4**: 259.

56. Quismorio, J.P. Jr. Immune complexes in pericardial fluid in systemic lupus erythematosus. *Arch. Intern. Med.* 1980; **140**: 112.

57. Kirk, J. and Cosh, J. The Pericarditis of Rheumatiod Arthritis. *Q. J. Med.* 1969; **38**: 397.

58. Thadani, U., Iveson, J.M. and Wright, V. Cardiac Tamponade, constrictive pericarditis and pericardial resection in rheumatoid arthritis. *Medicine* 1975; **54**: 261.

pulsus paradoxus. *Am. J. Cardiol.* 1986; **57**: 652.

59. Majeed, H.A. and Kvasnicka, J. Juvenile Rheumatoid Arthritis with Cardiac Tamponade. *Ann. Rheum. Dis.* 1978; 37: 273.

60. Collins, R.L., Turner, R.A., Nomeir, A.M. *et al.* Cardiopulmonary manifestations of systemic lupus erythematosus. *J. Rheumatol.* 1978; 5: 299.

61. Jacobson, E.L. and Reza, M.J. Constrictive pericarditis in systemic lupus erythematosus. Demonstration of immunoglobulins in the pericardium. *Arth. Rheum.* 1978; 21: 972.

62. Carey, R.M., Coleman, H. and Feder, A. Pericardial tamponade: a major manifestation of hydralazine induced lupus syndrome. *Am. J. Med.* 1973; 54: 84.

63. Goldberg, M.J., Husain, M., Wajszczuk, W.J. *et al.* Procaine amide induced lupus erythematosus pericarditis encountered during coronary artery bypass surgery. *Am. J. Med.* 1980; 69: 159.

64. Harrington, T.M. and Davis, D.E. Systemic lupus-like syndrome induced by methyldopa therapy. *Chest* 1981; 79: 696.

65. Bennett, W.M. Pericardial effusions associated with minoxidil. *Lancet* 1977; 2: 1356.

66. Meeran, M.K., Ahmed, A.H., Parsons, F.M. *et al.* Constrictive pericarditis due to methysergide therapy. *S. Afr. Med. J.* 1976; 50: 1595.

67. McWherter, J.E. and Leroy, E.C. Pericardial Disease in Scleroderma (Systemic Sclerosis). *Am. J. Med.* 1974; 57: 566.

68. Uhl, G.S. and Kippes, G.M. Pericardial tamponade in systemic sclerosis (scleroderma). *Br. Heart J.* 1979; 42: 345.

69. Dupond, J.L. and Leconte Des Floris, R. Temporal arthritis manifested as an acute febrile pericarditis. *JAMA* 1982; 247: 2371.

70. Csonka, G.W. and Oates, J.K. Pericarditis and electrocardiographic changes in Reiter's syndrome. *Br. Med. J.* 1957; 1: 866.

71. Vlietstra, R.E., Lie, J.T., Kuhl, W.E. *et al.* Whipple's Disease involving the pericardium. Pathologic confirmation during life. *Aust. N.Z. J. Med.* 1978; 8: 649.

72. Dawes, P.T. and Atherton, S.T. Coeliac disease presenting as recurrent pericarditis. *Lancet* 1981; 1: 1021.

73. Thompson, D.C., Lennard-Jones, J.E., Swarbrick, E.T. and Bown, R. Pericarditis and Inflammatory Bowel Disease. *Q. J. Med.* 1979; 48: 93.

74. Pierard, L.A., Albert, A., Henrard, L. *et al.* Incidence and significance of pericardial effusion in acute myocardial infarction as determined by two-dimensional echocardiography. *J. Am. Coll. Cardiol.* 1986; 8: 517.

75. Galve, E., Garcia-Del-Castillo, H., Evangelista, A., Batlle, J., SclerPermanyer-Miralda, G. and Soler-Soler, J. Pericardial effusion in the course of myocardial infarction—incidence, natural history and clinical relevance. *Circulation* 1986; 73: 294.

76. Silver, M.A., Hilgard, J.G., Murabit, I. and Bloom, K.J. Right atrial tamponade simulating tricuspid stenosis following acute myocardial infarction. *Am. Heart J.* 1986; 111: 984.

77. Pugliese, P., Tommassini, G., Macri, R., Moschetti, R. and Eufrate, S. Successful repair of post-infarction heart rupture. Case report and review of the literature. *J. Cardiovasc. Surg.* 1986; 27: 332.

78. Dressler, W. The Post Myocardial Infarction Syndrome. A report of forty-four cases. *Arch. Intern. Med.* 1959; 103: 28.

79. Stubbs, D.F. Post-acute myocardial infarction symptomatic pericarditis (PAMISP): report on a large series and the effect of methylprednisolone therapy. *J. Int. Med. Res.* 1986; 14 (Suppl. 1): 25.

80. Solem, J.O., Kugelberg, J., Stahl, E. and Olin, C. Late Cardiac Tamponade following open heart surgery. *Scand. J. Thorac. Cardiovasc. Surg.* 1986; 20: 129.

81. Ribeiro, P., Sapsford, R., Evans, T. *et al.* Constrictive pericarditis as a complication of coronary artery bypass surgery. *Br. Heart J.* 1984; 51: 205.

82. Kabbani, S.S., Bashour, T., Ellertson, D.G., Geiger, J., Hanna, E.S. and Cheng, T.O. Constrictive pericarditis following myocardial revascularization: a possible cause of graft occlusion. *Am. Heart J.* 1985; 110: 493.

83. D'Cruz, I.A., Bhatt, G.R., Cohen, H.C. and Glick, G. Echocardiographic detection of cardiac involvement in patients with chronic renal failure. *Arch. Intern. Med.* 1978; 138: 720.

84. Fuller, T.J., Knochel, J.P., Brennan, J.P. *et al.* Reversal of intractable uraemic pericarditis by triamcinolone hexacetomide. *Arch. Intern. Med.* 1976; 136: 979.

85. Koopot, R., Zerefos, N.S. and Lavender, A.R. Cardiac tamponade in uremic pericarditis: surgical approach and management. *Am. J. Cardiol.* 1973; 32: 846.

86. Singh, A. and Krishan, I. Cardiac tamponade due to massive pericardial effusion in myxoedema. *Br. J. Med. Prac.* 1970; 24: 347.

87. Chew, C., Ziady, G., Raphael, M.J. *et al.* The functional defect in amyloid heart disease. *Am. J. Cardiol.* 1975; 36: 438.

88. Haskell, R.J. and French, W.I. Cardiac tamponade as the initial presentation of malignancy. *Chest* 1985; 88: 70.

89. El-Allaf, D., Burette, R., Pierard, L. and Limet, R. Cardiac tamponade as the first manifestation of cardiothoracic malignancy: a study of 10 cases. *Eur. Heart J.* 1986; 7: 247.

90. Malden, L.T. and Tattersall, M.H.N. Malignant effusions. *Q. J. Med.* 1986; 58: 221.

91. Bian, S., Brufman, G., Klein, E. and Hochman, A. The management of pericardial effusion in cancer patients. *Chest* 1977; 71: 182.

92. Scott, O.L. and Thomas, R.D. Late onset constrictive pericarditis after thoracic radiotherapy. *Br. Med. J.* 1978; 1: 341.

93. Masland, D.S., Rotz, C.T. Jr and Harris, J.H. Post-radiation pericarditis with chronic pericardial effusion. *Ann. Intern. Med.* 1968; 68: 97.

94. Applefeld, M.M., Slawson, R.G., Hall-Craigs, M. *et al.* Delayed pericardial disease after radiotherapy. *Am. J. Cardiol.* 1981; 47: 210.

95. Cheitlin, M.D. Cardiovascular Trauma Part I. *Circulation* 1982; 65: 1529.

96. Cheitlin, M.D. Cardiovascular Trauma Part II. *Circulation* 1982; 66: 244.

97. Dunn, R.P. Primary chylopericardium. A review of the literature and an illustrated case. *Am. Heart J.* 1975; 89: 369.

98. Morishita, Y., Taira, A., Furoi, A., Arima, S. and Tanaka, H. Constrictive pericarditis secondary to primary chylopericardium. *Am. Heart J.* 1985; 109: 373.

99. Thoren, C. So-called mulibrey nanism with pericardial constriction. *Lancet* 1973; 2: 731.

Chapter 42

Ischaemic Heart Disease: Risk Factors and Prevention

A.G. Shaper

INTRODUCTION

In the search for the causes of ischaemic heart disease (IHD), attention has been focused on differences (variations) between the characteristics of those who suffer episodes of IHD and those who do not. Comparisons are made between individuals in a community, between population groups within a country, and between countries. Whatever the level of approach, the question has always been much the same: who suffers a heart attack? Those personal and environmental characteristics (factors) most strongly associated with increased risk of IHD have been termed 'risk factors', without necessarily imputing a direct causal relationship between the factor and IHD.

In the earliest studies, subjects who had experienced a myocardial infarction or angina pectoris were compared with control subjects who had not experienced such an event. These retrospective *case–control* studies are liable to considerable bias (error) produced by the very fact of survival, by changes occurring after the IHD event and by the difficulty in choosing appropriate controls. Nevertheless, they provide useful clues to factors that differ between cases and control subjects and which later may be shown to be of importance to the causation of IHD. However, they do not provide reliable quantitative measures of the risk of IHD associated with the factor, nor do they allow the effects of other factors present at the same time to be taken into account. Case–control studies are not unimportant in the search for causes and they remain popular because they can be carried out relatively quickly and without considerable expense. Only rarely do they provide strong evidence of causality and considerable caution should be shown in accepting the claims that may be attached to such studies.

A more sophisticated approach to characteristics that differ between those who develop IHD and those who do not is the *prospective (longitudinal, cohort) study*. This is based on large selected groups of the population in whom the factors of concern are measured and who are then followed for long periods of time. Major IHD events such as myocardial infarction (fatal or non-fatal) or sudden cardiac death will occur in some subjects and several types of analysis can be carried out. Comparisons of risk factor levels can be made between those who manifest major IHD events and those who do not. In addition, the number of cases of major IHD occurring at varying levels of each risk factor can be determined and the possibility of a dose–response relationship explored. If the cohort under study includes subjects with evidence of IHD at entrance into the study, ascertained from the history, standardized chest pain questionnaires or electrocardiography, the *'attack rates'* for each risk factor and for each level of exposure to the risk factor can be calculated. If these subjects are excluded and only those free of pre-existing IHD are analysed, *'incidence rates'* related to the levels of the various risk factors are obtained. This approach of examining each risk factor without regard to the presence of other risk factors, i.e. *univariate*, provides a quantitative assessment of the risk of IHD associated with each level of exposure to the risk factor.

Many of the risk factors are related, for example, obesity and blood pressure, serum cholesterol and serum triglycerides, and all are acting simultaneously on the same individual. Their interactions are complex and often poorly understood. Sophisticated methods of *multivariate* analysis have been developed (multiple logistic regression) which allow for the assessment of the independent effect of each risk factor when all are acting at the same time. Although this approach is statistically sound, it cannot take into account all the complex biological relationships that exist, and thus some factors lose their apparent importance when analysed together with other highly correlated factors. For example, obesity plays an important role in the development of high blood pressure in most populations and it is a risk factor for IHD in univariate analysis. As obesity is correlated with both blood pressure and blood cholesterol levels, in multivariate analysis the competing effects of blood pressure and blood cholesterol render obesity a non-significant risk factor. Clearly, the findings of univariate analysis cannot be completely ignored, particularly when risk factors, such as obesity, play a role in the development of other factors and are involved in the clinical management of increased risk.

A further step in the search for causality is to determine whether the risk factors emerging from these prospective studies and multivariate analyses can adequately account for ('explain') the occurrence rate of IHD. From several studies, it has emerged that the three major independent risk factors—serum total cholesterol, cigarette smoking and raised blood pressure—do not account in statistical terms for more than half of the variation seen between different groups of subjects in their incidence rates of IHD. The assumption has been made that there must be a factor or factors that have at least as much effect on the incidence of IHD as the three established major risk factors combined. Measurement of any one risk factor at one point in time has limited predictive power when one considers the considerable duration of time over which the factors act, their variability during that prolonged period and their complex interactions. Indeed, the proportion of the variance 'explained' by these three key risk factors, measured at one point in time, should be regarded as remarkable under the circumstances! The assumption that there must be a major 'Factor X' as yet undiscovered is tenable but not necessary. The major risk factors, together with several other factors of lesser independent importance, such as physical activity, genetic factors, diabetes mellitus, obesity, emotional and psychological factors, may adequately explain the pathogenesis of IHD. There are large areas of ignorance and uncertainty regarding the mechanisms by which the risk factors operate; it is not reasonable to present IHD as a mystery.

VARIATIONS IN THE FREQUENCY OF ISCHAEMIC HEART DISEASE

The incidence of IHD shows variations on an international scale. In the period following the Second World War (1939–1945), several studies were set in motion, specifically designed to explore the reasons for what appeared to be remarkably wide variations in the occurrence of IHD. In more recent years, interest has been focused on changes in the rates of IHD mortality in different countries and on attempts to explain why the mortality rates have declined considerably in some countries and increased considerably in others. Attempts have been made to use the knowledge about risk factors acquired from observational studies to intervene in order to prevent the occurrence of IHD, some of which have been relatively small and focused on highly specific groups, others have involved very large groups of subjects or whole populations. In considering the role of risk factors, it seems important to look at some of the outcomes of these geographic enquiries and interventions.

THE SEVEN COUNTRIES STUDY

The Seven Countries Study is perhaps the best known of the major international epidemiological investigations. Keys and his collaborators planned a series of prospective studies in countries known to have widely differing mortality rates from IHD and also known to differ in their dietary habits. Their underlying concern was nutritional but the study was a carefully controlled attempt to assess a wide range of risk factors for IHD in geographically and culturally unrelated groups.[1]

There were 16 groups of men aged 40–59 years drawn from seven countries: the USA (1 group), Japan (2), Yugoslavia (5), Finland (2), Italy (3), the Netherlands (1), and Greece (2). More than 12 000 men were examined during the years 1957–62 using standardized methods, exchanging professional personnel among the teams and analysing the data centrally. It was a remarkable feat of co-ordinated collaboration on an international scale. After the initial examination, all the men were followed with particular reference to the development of IHD. Reports on the 5-, 10- and 15-year follow-up periods have been published.

The results of this study remain central to our concepts of the aetiology of IHD. Serum total cholesterol appeared to be a critical factor in determining the community (cohort) level of risk for IHD, and the community level of serum cholesterol was strongly correlated with the percentage of total calories (energy) derived from saturated fats in the diet. Cigarette smoking, hypertension, obesity and physical activity did not appear to explain the differences in IHD incidence rates between these communities. These risk factors appeared to exert an important effect on risk of IHD only in those communities in which the mean serum cholesterol concentration·was raised. For example, Japan, with the lowest incidence of IHD, had a high prevalence of hypertension (systolic blood pressure > 160 mmHg), a high proportion of men smoking cigarettes and a relatively low mean concentration of serum cholesterol. Although Finland had a very high level of physical activity among its cohort, it had the highest incidence rate of IHD; presumably the benefits of physical activity could not outweigh the effects of a high level of serum cholesterol and high rates of cigarette smoking and hypertension in the community. Body mass index (obesity) did not appear to have an independent effect on IHD once other factors had been taken info account.

From studies such as this, certain basic concepts have emerged.

1 There appears to be a specific susceptibility to atherosclerosis and IHD related to the mean level of serum cholesterol in a community.

2 There appears to be an optimum community level of serum cholesterol concentration below which IHD is uncommon, about 5.0 mmol/l (190 mg/dl).

3 Above this optimum level, susceptibility to IHD increases progressively as the concentration of serum˜cholesterol rises.

4 The incidence of IHD in a susceptible community depends to a considerable extent on the prevalence of additional factors, such as cigarette smoking and raised blood pressure.

CHANGES IN MORTALITY RATES FROM ISCHAEMIC HEART DISEASE

The most striking change in IHD mortality rates has been seen in the USA where there has been a steady decline since the late 1960s. Between 1968 and 1976, the mortality rate in the USA had fallen by about 20% and a similar rate of decline has continued up to the present. The IHD mortality rates per 100 000 population (1981) are shown in Fig. 42.1.

There has been considerable argument as to the reasons for the declining mortality rates of IHD in the USA. A crucial question concerns the degree to which the mortality rates have resulted from changes in lifestyle, i.e. diet, smoking, physical activity, or from a reduction in the case-fatality of IHD, to which medical and surgical intervention has contributed. Workers in most of the American

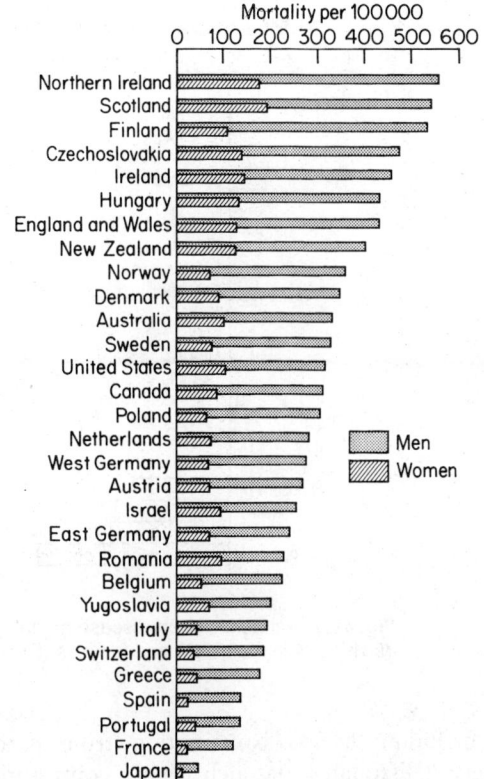

Fig. 42.1. Ischaemic heart disease mortality rates per 100 000 population (1985) for men and women aged 40–69 years.

studies have concluded that improvements in medical and surgical treatment, however beneficial to specific individuals, could not account for the large and consistent reductions in mortality. An analysis of long-term trends of incidence of acute myocardial infarction and case-fatality rates among employees of the Du Pont Company from 1957 to 1983 has clarified this issue.[2] The annual age-adjusted incidence rate fell from 3.2/1000 in 1957–1959 to 2.3 per 1000 in 1981–1983, a 28% decline. The case-fatality rate showed a small decline beginning in 1969, with a marked drop in case-fatality (at 30 days) after 1975. The major decline in case-fatality rates took place well after the decline in incidence had become apparent. The results of this study suggest that the major source of the decline in mortality rate has been the reduction in incidence of the disease, although improved medical/surgical care has probably made some contribution. In another American study, it was estimated that medical management has accounted for about 40% of the decline in the USA, including a 4% contribution from cardiac surgery.[3] In New Zealand, it has been similarly estimated that medical management accounted for about 40% of the decline in mortal-

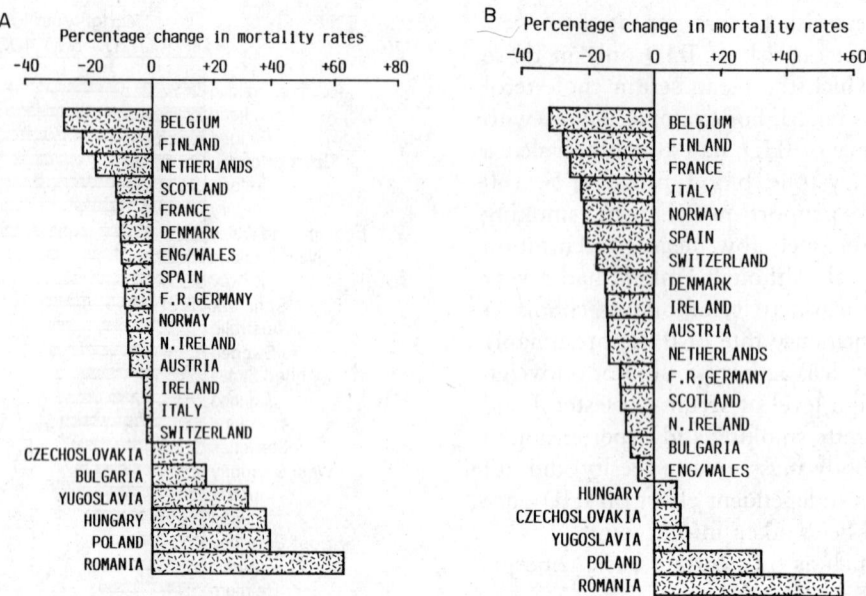

Fig. 42.2. Ischaemic heart disease mortality in Europe. Changes (%) in mortality from 1971–1974 to 1981–1984 in males (A) and females (B) aged 40–69 years.

ity, including a 5% contribution from cardiac surgery.[4] Estimates of such small contributions from cardiac surgery have been challenged; in another New Zealand study, it was estimated that coronary surgery could account for 26–42% of the reduction in IHD deaths.[5] Whatever the outcome of the debate, it is evident that medical/surgical management makes some difference.

A more comprehensive exploration of changing trends in IHD mortality has been carried out with particular reference to changes in risk factor status.[6] Eleven countries are included in the survey and in seven the IHD mortality declined during the 1970s: USA, Australia, New Zealand, Finland, Norway, Belgium and Israel. In the remaining four—Sweden, Poland, Italy and Spain—there had been an increase in male mortality rates from IHD during this period. National efforts towards the prevention of IHD by risk factor modification, i.e. better diet, lower serum cholesterol, less cigarette smoking, more physical activity, better control of hypertension, had been taking place in six of the seven countries showing a decline. In the four countries with rising IHD mortality rates, no discernible change had taken place in dietary habits and, in three of the four, average serum cholesterol concentrations had increased. Overall, there was a strong impression that improvements in IHD risk factor status had run parallel to the declining rates of IHD. The Israelis considered that their decline in mortal-

ity was substantially due to improved medical management of IHD because no changes in diet or smoking had been observed. It is interesting that Sweden is among the group with increasing IHD mortality rates despite its highly advanced medical and surgical treatment of IHD.

Changes in Europe

The changes that have taken place in IHD mortality rates in Europe and Scandinavia over the decade 1971–1974 to 1981–1984 are revealing and give rise to interesting speculation (Fig. 42.2). The largest increases in IHD mortality have taken place in the Eastern European countries and the greatest declines have taken place in countries which have been actively concerned with population strategies directed towards changes in risk factors. Such speculation should give way to comparative certainty when the results of the WHO MONICA (Monitoring the Trends and Determinants in Cardiovascular Diseases) research project are published. This project was designed to measure changes in IHD morbidity and mortality as well as changes in risk factors, lifestyle and medical care in 30 participating countries using standardized methods.

Awareness of the high incidence of cardiovascular disease in Finland as a whole, and in North Karelia in particular, led to a comprehensive, community-based prevention programme to control cardiovascular disease.[7] In the North Karelia project, the aim was to reduce morbidity and mortality from cardiovascular disease by reducing established risk factors (cigarette smoking, serum cholesterol, blood pressure) in the entire community. The early reports indicated that mortality from IHD started to decline faster in North Karelia than in the rest of Finland. The decrease was particularly steep from 2 years after the start of the North Karelia Project. The most recent review shows that the decrease in IHD mortality and cardiovascular mortality was significantly greater in North Karelian men than in the rest of the country. This decrease in mortality was in accord with the greater change in risk factors in North Karelia than in the rest of Finland. This difference in risk factor levels is attributed to the comprehensive intervention carried out in North Karelia since 1972, although the intervention there has influenced developments in the whole country. Finland, Australia and the USA have all shown similar steep declines in cardiovascular mortality and in all these countries the major influence has been attributed to changes in the risk factors.

RISK FACTORS FOR ISCHAEMIC HEART DISEASE

The description of risk factors in relation to IHD that follows is based on information from countries in which the disease is common. In particular, information will wherever possible relate to Great Britain, with supporting data for other countries with a similar incidence of IHD.

AGE

In all countries with a high incidence of IHD, there is a strong and continuous relationship with age. In men and women in Great Britain, mortality rates rise steeply with increasing age, about 15-fold in men from 35–44 to 55–64 years and about 30-fold in women over the same two decades. Although claims have been made for ageing being a risk factor in its own right, the epidemiological evidence strongly suggests that atherosclerosis and IHD are not necessary consequences of growing old. It is far more likely that age represents the accumulated effects of exposure to raised blood lipid levels, raised blood pressure, cigarette smoking and a variety of other factors over a lifetime.

SEX

The difference in the incidence of IHD between men and women is probably one of the most striking characteristics of the disease (Fig. 42.3). Young men (35–44 years) have an IHD mortality rate about 6 times that of women of the same age. A major change takes place between 45 and 55 years of age and further reductions in the difference occur in the next decade. However, only in the ninth decade do women have almost (but not quite) the same mortality rate as men. Although a difference in cigarette smoking is probably the most obvious environmental factor of importance, it seems likely that women are protected to some degree by their hormonal function and that this diminishes progressively during and after the menopause. There is a hypothesis that the protection is not hormonal but is mediated by regular menstrual loss of iron resulting in chronic iron depletion in women relative to age-matched men.[8] The iron depletion is held responsible for a wide range of biological effects ultimately providing protection against IHD. It does not seem likely that this hypothesis will be substantiated and data relating to IHD rates in women who have lost their ovaries at an early age strongly support the hormonal hypothesis.[9]

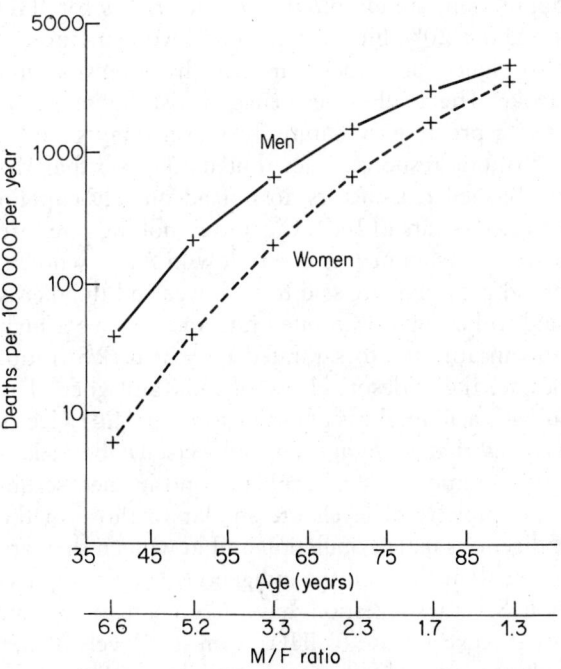

Fig. 42.3. Ischaemic heart disease (ICD 410–414) mortality rates per 100 000 for men and women by age in England and Wales 1984, male to female mortality ratios.

RACE

The wide geographical variations in the patterns of IHD have led to strong statements about racial and genetic factors in the development of the disease. Although there are still some anomalies to be resolved, the evidence suggests that no racial or ethnic group is immune to atherosclerosis and IHD and that race or ethnic group is probably irrelevant to the development of the disease. Some genetic hyperlipidaemas may occur with greater frequency in certain racial groups but as the gross hyperlipidaemas make a very small contribution to the overall risk of IHD in any community the issue is not of great importance. Migration studies and trends with time in rapidly urbanized societies have made it clear that environmental factors (diet, cigarette smoking, patterns of physical activity) are all closely associated with changes in the incidence of IHD. The studies of Japanese subjects in Japan, Hawaii and the USA are good examples of such environmental effects.

Interesting material has been emerging in recent years on the susceptibility to IHD of Asian immigrants to Great Britain from the Indian subcontinent.[10] There are about 1 million Asians (immigrants from the Indian subcontinent) in Great Britain. There is evidence to suggest that they have higher rates of IHD than the rest of the British population; standardized mortality ratios for IHD are about 20% higher in men and women, and are also higher for diabetes mellitus, hypertension and stroke. The available evidence on risk factor status is of a preliminary nature, being on small samples with poor response rates, but it suggests that the established risk factors do not adequately explain this excess rate of IHD. Cigarette smoking rates are lower in Asian men and very low in Asian women, blood pressures are said to be lower and the diet is said to be low in saturated fats and to have a high polyunsaturated to saturated fatty acid (P/S) ratio, despite the widespread use of milk and ghee. The linoleic acid intake is reported as more than twice as high as that in indigenous subjects. Diabetes is a very common clinical problem, and in men serum total cholesterol levels are similar to those in the indigenous male population and in women they are lower than those in the indigenous female population. Several suggestions have been made to account for the excess rate of IHD, from low levels of n-3 polyunsaturated fats to widespread hypothyroidism in Indian women. There is also interest in psychosocial factors relating to the stress of acculturation

and adaptation. Whatever the outcome, studies of incidence and risk are of considerable importance in this large ethnic minority.

BLOOD LIPIDS

In terms of risk of IHD, the serum total cholesterol concentration remains the strongest blood lipid predictor of IHD for communities and for individuals within communities with high frequencies of IHD. Although it is a crude measure, it is an overall indicator of group and individual response to the many dietary and other factors that can influence blood concentrations of cholesterol. Cholesterol and triglycerides, the blood lipids of major interest in atherosclerosis and IHD, are carried in the blood as lipoprotein complexes. There are many ways of classifying the lipoproteins; commonly, it is done on the basis of ultracentrifugation. Depending on their density, there are very low density lipoproteins (VLDL), low density lipoproteins (LDL) and high density lipoproteins (HDL). About two-thirds of the serum total total cholesterol is carried in the LDL fraction and about 20–25% in the HDL fraction. The major atherogenic effect of serum cholesterol is mediated by the LDL cholesterol. High density lipoprotein cholesterol generally has an inverse relationship to the incidence of IHD and is widely regarded as 'protective' cholesterol. The VDL carries triglycerides predominantly; current evidence suggests that its blood concentration is not an independent indicator of the risk of IHD.

The protein components of the lipoprotein complexes (apoproteins) are currently arousing considerable interest and seem to be more refined markers of lipid metabolism and transport.[11] Families of apoprotein are designated by letters, A, B, C, D and E, with each letter having several subclasses. Low density lipoprotein contains mainly apo-B and HDL contains mostly apo-A. Comment will be made later on the value of these apoproteins in the measurement of risk of IHD.

Serum total cholesterol

The evidence that the serum total cholesterol concentration is a strong, independent and consistent predictor of risk of IHD is considerable, if not overwhelming. The many sources of evidence—experimental, pathological, epidemiological and genetic—agree that raised serum cholesterol, predominantly due to high levels of LDL cholesterol, is

a causal factor in atherosclerosis and IHD. There is also good evidence that serum cholesterol may be the most important single factor in determining the risk of IHD, possibly a necessary factor; it can be stated that no community with a low mean level of serum cholesterol has an appreciable incidence rate of IHD.

Recent data on 361 662 men aged 35–57 years taking part in the Multiple Risk Factor Intervention trial (MRFIT) in the USA lend power to the statement that there is a continuous curvilinear relationship between serum cholesterol concentration and IHD mortality.[12] The men in the lowest fifth (below the 20th percentile) of the cholesterol distribution) are regarded as the baseline risk group. Above this level, the risk of IHD increases as the cholesterol level increases. The relative risk for individuals above the 80th percentile (the top 20% of the cholesterol distribution) is 3.4 when compared with men in the lowest fifth (Fig. 42.4).

When the IHD mortality is plotted in a different way and compared with total mortality, the curves are similar (Fig. 42.5), as IHD comprises a considerable proportion of total mortality and may share certain environmental risk factors, particularly diet and cigarette smoking, with the other major mortality group, the cancers. The total mortality curve shows an increase in mortality below the 10th

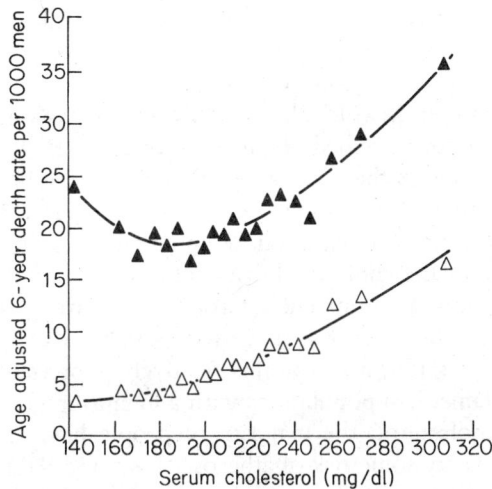

Fig. 42.5. Ischaemic heart disease death rate (△) and total mortality rates (▲) (both age-adjusted) per 1000 men over 6 years, for men screened for MRFIT according to serum cholesterol (each point represents approximately one-twentieth of the 361 662 men).[12]

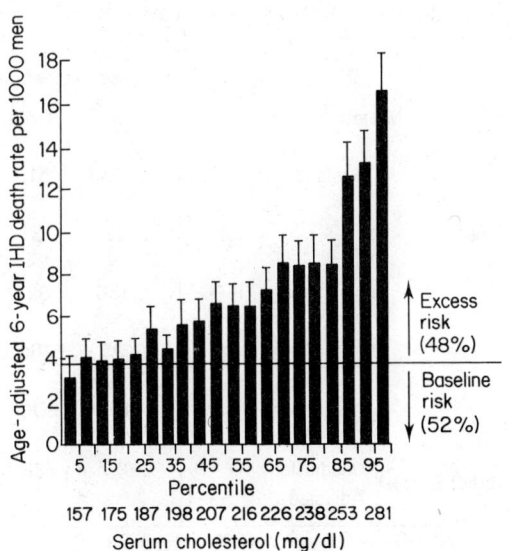

Fig. 42.4. Ischaemic heart disease death rate (age-adjusted) per 1000 men over 6 years for men screened for MRFIT according to serum cholesterol percentile.[12] (Horizontal line represents expected death rate of 3.7 per 1000 men. Area above the line represents excess risk associated with serum cholesterol. T-bars represent upper limit of the 95% confidence interval.)

percentile of the cholesterol distribution, mainly due to an excess of cancer deaths. This finding, drawn from several other studies, has alarmed those who fear that lowering serum cholesterol concentrations could lead to an increase in cancer mortality. The finding is almost certainly due to the cholesterol-lowering effect of cancer. Analysis of the MRFIT data has shown that the association between low serum cholesterol and cancer does not persist beyond 5 years.[13] A Swedish study of 92 000 subjects less than 75 years old, based on health screening and cancer registry data, revealed a *positive* association between serum cholesterol level and the risk of rectal and colon cancer in men.[14] The same trends were seen in women but were not significant. No statistically significant inverse correlations were observed.

British data confirm the critical role of serum cholesterol in risk of IHD. In the Whitehall (London) Study of 17 718 male civil servants aged 40–64 years, the risk gradient was continuous over the whole range of cholesterol concentrations, the lowest mortality being in men with concentrations below the lowest decile.[15] In the British Regional Heart Study of middle-aged men (40–59 years) drawn from 24 towns in England, Wales and Scotland, serum cholesterol was found to have a continuous, curvilinear association with risk of major IHD events, with a relative risk of 3.1 for the top fifth of cholesterol distribution compared with the lowest fifth,[16] a finding very similar to that of

MRFIT. It is evident from all these studies that serum total cholesterol *by itself* is not a very good predictor of coronary heart disease risk in individuals. In MRFIT, the top 20% of the cholesterol distribution yielded about 35% of all IHD deaths occurring in the 6 years of follow-up. In the British Regional Heart Study, 31% of major IHD events occurring in 5 years follow-up came from the top 20% of the cholesterol distribution.

If raised serum cholesterol concentration is as important a factor as suggested (possibly a *sine qua non* of IHD), how can this relatively poor yield be explained? In populations with a high average level of cholesterol, the majority of people have levels that carry some risk of atherosclerosis and IHD. As this risk is so widespread, it may not be obvious. It is then the additional factors, such as cigarette smoking and hypertension, that contribute to the overall incidence of IHD; they may appear to be as important or even more important in determining risk than the underlying lipid abnormality.

High-density lipoprotein cholesterol

Ten years ago, when the first publications appeared showing an *inverse* association between HDL cholesterol and risk of IHD, there was considerable excitement. The results of further studies supported the concept that HDL cholesterol had a 'protective' effect, i.e. low levels were associated with highest risk of IHD, and that this effect was independent of other risk factors. These observations led to the revival of an interest in the role of HDL cholesterol in lipid transport. The concept that HDL or a small subclass within the HDL class plays an important role in mobilizing cholesterol from the tissues, i.e. reverse transport, seems firmly established. In the British Regional Heart Study, the men in the lowest fifth of the HDL cholesterol distribution had a twofold risk of a major IHD event when compared with all other men.[16] Above this lowest fifth, there was little trend of association between HDL cholesterol and risk of IHD. Once other factors such as cigarette smoking, non-HDL cholesterol, body mass index, pre-existing IHD had been taken into account, the increased risk associated with the lowest fifth of HDL cholesterol distribution was much reduced and not statistically significant.

An examination of 7 prospective studies showed that, in 6 of them, the differences in HDL cholesterol between those subjects who suffered a major IHD event and those who did not was relatively small, although the IHD cases *consistently* had lower concentrations of HDL cholesterol than the men who remained free of IHD events (Fig. 42.6).[17] Only in the Tromso study, which was the smallest, was the difference fairly large.

In several studies, full adjustment had not been made for the presence of additional and related risk factors, and the selection of cases in some studies was unusual. For example, in the Framingham study, subjects were selected who had survived the first 20 years of follow-up and who still remained free of any evidence of IHD.

The findings of the British Regional Heart Study have given rise to some uncertainty regarding the independent role of HDL cholesterol in predicting the risk of IHD events.[18] Although the cumulative evidence does indicate a weak inverse relationship with IHD, it would now seem that HDL cholesterol should not be given such a high profile when assessing the risk of an individual. However, its vital role in cholesterol metabolism should not be ignored. (See postscript 1).

Triglyceride

In many univariate analyses, the concentration of serum triglyceride has been shown to be associated with the risk of IHD. The Stockholm Prospective Survey has apparently shown that this relationship is independent of serum cholesterol concentrations. In this study, analysis was carried out using

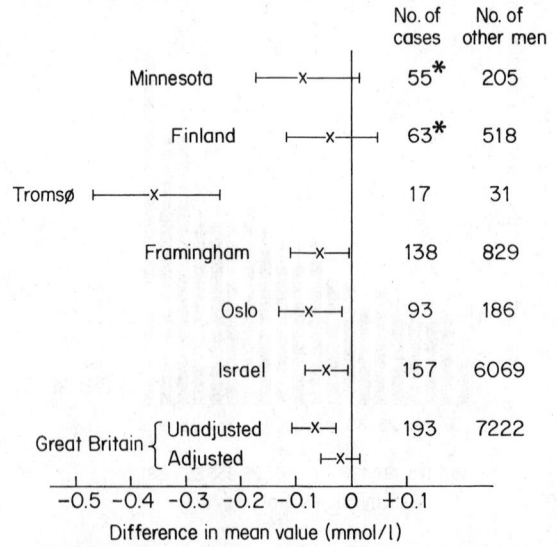

Fig. 42.6. Difference in mean HDL cholesterol concentrations between men developing ischaemic heart disease (cases) and other men in seven prospective studies.[17] Crosses are observed differences in mean HDL cholesterol values, bars are 95% confidence limits. (*Fatal cases only.*) 1 mmol = 38.6 mg/dl.)

arbitrary divisions of concentration for triglycerides and for cholesterol; until the analysis is repeated using continuous variables, these findings must remain open to debate.[19] Serum triglyceride levels are significantly correlated (positively) with body mass index and with serum total cholesterol, and (negatively) with HDL cholesterol. When these relationships are taken into account (in multivariate analyses), triglyceride concentration appears to have no independent relationship with major IHD events.[20] This does not mean that the triglyceride concentration is of no importance in the complex lipid abnormalities associated with atherosclerosis and IHD. There is evidence that certain subclasses of triglyceride-rich lipoproteins, the remnant particles, play a role in the development of atherosclerosis. However, the measurement of triglycerides appears to be of little value as an independent indicator of risk of IHD, although raised levels may be of interest in relation to a wide range of other conditions.

Two recent papers, however, have rekindled interest in serum triglyceride levels as predictors of IHD. The results of the Paris Prospective Study involving 7000 middle-aged civil servants suggest that the level of serum triglyceride is a significant predictor of risk in subjects with *low* serum total cholesterol concentration, i.e. < 5.7 mmol/l (220 mg/dl);[21] the findings of the Framingham study indicate that triglyceride elevations are a highly significant independent risk factor IHD in women and in both sexes those with elevated levels of triglyceride should be considered at risk for IHD if their ratio of total cholesterol to HDL cholesterol ratio is > 3.5, i.e. normal or *high* total cholesterol and low HDL cholesterol.[22] In practice, only 10% of those with elevated levels of triglycerides have such a high total cholesterol/HDL cholesterol ratio. These two studies present opposing views; however, both outcomes could be the result of subgroup analysis without prior hypothesis. (See postscript 1).

DIETARY FACTORS

The literature on the dietary aspects of IHD is immense and complex and can only be summarized with extreme prejudice. However, in this section current views on the nutritional background to atherosclerosis and IHD will be reviewed and the recent recommendations of the European Atherosclerosis Society[23] and the British Cardiac Society[24] will be presented as examples of consensus views on what should be done about dietary factors. These recommendations reflect the current degree of conviction regarding the impact of the dietary factors on IHD.

Fats

There is consistent support for the hypothesis that populations on diets low in saturated fat and dietary cholesterol and with a relatively high P/S ratio exhibit a low incidence of IHD. The evidence is also consistent that populations with high dietary intakes of saturated fat and dietary cholesterol and with low P/S ratios have substantial rates of IHD. In the Seven Countries Study, there is a strong correlation between the 10-year death rate from IHD in the 16 cohorts and the percentage dietary calories supplied by saturated fatty acids. The relationship between the P/S ratio and IHD incidence rates for the seven countries is even stronger (Figs 42.7 and 42.8).

Although comparisons *between* populations have consistently supported the dietary hypothesis, it has been difficult to relate the diets of individuals *within* populations to their individual levels of serum cholesterol or to their risk of major IHD events. In some studies, e.g. the Western Electric Study in Chicago[25] and Civil Servants Study in Britain,[26] it has been possible to relate individual diets to the risk of IHD with results that support the hypothesis regarding saturated fat intake and the dietary P/S ratio. There have been many reviews of the reasons for this difficulty within populations, but paramount amongst the arguments must be the relatively small range of blood cholesterol concentration in communities at high risk and the considerable biological variation in response to any stimulus. Genetic and other factors must play important roles in determining the ultimate blood concentration of cholesterol in individuals exposed to similar food intakes. It would be surprising if the relationship between diet and total cholesterol or between diet and the risk of IHD (with diet and serum cholesterol measured at one point in time) were strong. Diet affects metabolism over a subject's lifetime, whereas serum total cholesterol reflects the current response to diet, and risk of IHD is multifactorially determined. Despite this, the blood levels of cholesterol in relatively small groups of individuals can readily be manipulated in highly predictable ways by making changes in the fat content of the diet. In brief, saturated fats tend to raise and polyunsaturated fats tend to lower the total cholesterol

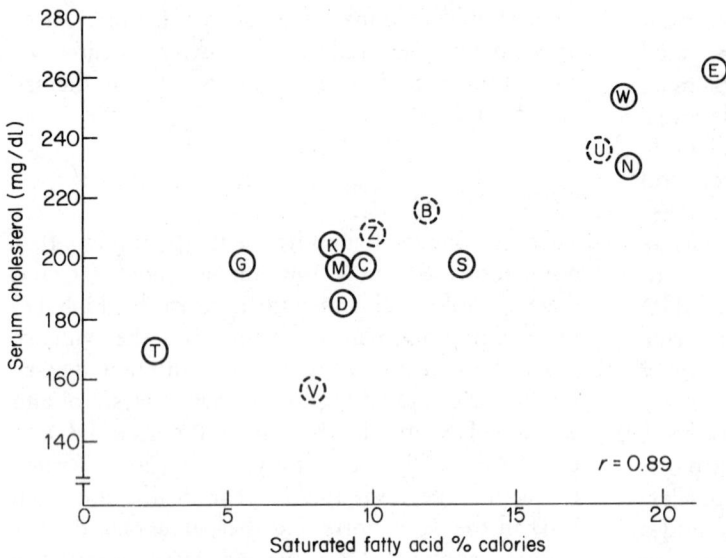

Fig. 42.7. Seven Countries Study. The relationship between dietary saturated fatty acid and serum cholesterol in 14 communities from 7 countries—5-year follow-up (Reproduced from *Circulation* 1970; **41** (Suppl. I): I–1.)

concentration, the latter having half the power of the saturated fats.

In an interesting international collaborative study, the mechanisms of variation of serum cholesterol within populations and between populations were examined; 109 men aged 35–49 years were studied in five centres: Helsinki (Finland), Baix-Camp (Spain), Cape Town (South Africa), Naples (Italy) and Sheffield (England).[27] The emphasis was on LDL cholesterol, the major component of serum total cholesterol and the prime suspect in the aetiology of atherosclerosis and IHD. Within these five nutritionally disparate populations, the

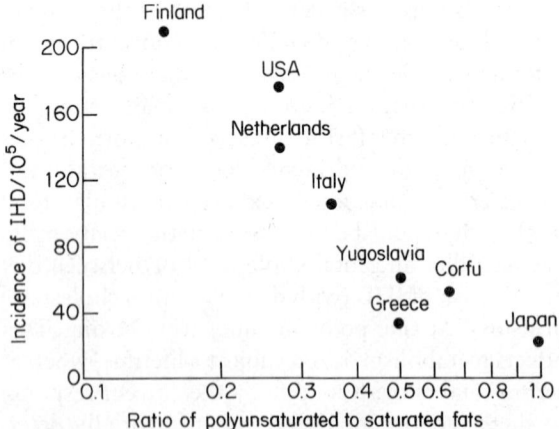

Fig. 42.8. Seven Countries Study. Ratio of polyunsaturated to saturated fats (P/S ratio) and incidence of ischaemic heart disease (per 100 000 per year) in men aged 40–59 years. (Greece = Corfu + Crete, but as data for polyunsaturated fatty acids for Crete were not reliable, data for Corfu are also presented.) (From Shaper, A.G. and Marr, J.W. *Br. Med. J.* 1977; **i:** 867–71.)

highest concentrations of total cholesterol and LDL cholesterol resulted largely from greater *production* of LDL, with slower *catabolism* (breakdown) contributing to their maintenance. Common ('polygenic') hypercholesterolaemia may be attributed to these metabolic differences. Low serum cholesterol and LDL cholesterol result from slower production of LDL and more rapid catabolism. The investigators found significant associations between LDl metabolism and the dietary intake of fatty acids. *Variations in the intake of saturated fats appeared to be the most powerful single dietary determinant of serum cholesterol.* Low density lipoprotein production was directly related to the intake of saturated fatty acids, so that the high mean serum cholesterol seen in populations in which the habitual diet is rich in saturated fatty acids may be explained in part by greater rates of LDL production. The catabolism of LDL was directly related to the intake of mono-unsaturated fatty acids. Thus, the use of olive oil, which has a high content of mono-unsaturated oleic acid, in Mediterranean countries may partly account for the low mean serum cholesterol values in these countries.

A study in 57 healthy Dutch volunteers adds strength to these sophisticated experimental findings.[28] The effects of two strictly controlled diets, one rich in complex carbohydrates, the other rich in olive oil, on serum lipids were studied. Both diets caused a similar fall in serum total cholesterol when compared with a diet high in saturated fatty acids. The olive oil diet, unlike the complex carbohydrate diet, caused a specific fall in non-HDL cholesterol leaving HDL cholesterol and triglyceride levels unchanged. On the complex carbohydrate diet, HDL cholesterol levels fell and triglyceride levels increased over the 36 days of the study.

Fibre

There is some evidence that diets high in fibre, i.e. those fractions of complex carbohydrate that are not digested, are associated with lower total cholesterol concentrations and less incidence of IHD.[29] Whether fibre has any independent or specific role in the aetiology of IHD is not known, because subjects on high-fibre diets are likely to be on diets high in carbohydrates and low in fats. However, as those subjects who wish to reduce their fat intake must increase their carbohydrate intake if they wish to maintain their energy levels, an increased intake of complex carbohydrates is likely to be an intrinsic part of any low-fat diet.

Salt

Although there is a high level of scientific suspicion regarding the role of salt intake in the genesis of raised blood pressure, it is largely based on international studies comparing populations that differ in many ways other than their salt intake.[30] It has proved more difficult to relate current salt intakes in individuals to their current blood pressures, although very large population studies have shown statistically significant correlations, albeit of very small magnitude. Salt intake in most populations is greatly in excess of physiological requirements; major reductions in salt intake would be without harm but whether this would remove the worldwide problem of hypertension is doubtful. However, it must be stated that the results of epidemiological, animal experimental and clinical studies support the hypothesis that salt could be a critical factor in the development of hypertension. As the insult may be delivered at a very early age, subsequent blood pressure increments may be a consequence of the initial rise in blood pressure. There is no suggestion that salt intake *directly* effects atherosclerosis or IHD, but, if it does induce raised blood pressure, it indirectly becomes a potential co-factor in the pathogenesis of IHD.

Sugar

Despite Yudkin's work on sugar and IHD ("pure,

white and deadly"),[31] there is no substantial evidence linking sugar intake to the incidence of IHD.

Alcohol

The most widely accepted view of alcohol is that regular moderate drinking is protective against IHD[32] and that wine in particular may be a factor in producing low rates of IHD in countries such as France.[33] The evidence is complex and does not completely support these simplistic views. Moderate or heavy drinking, i.e. > 6 drinks a day, may raise the blood pressure and it is well established that regular daily drinkers of > 6 drinks a day have a higher proportion of hypertension than any other group (a 'drink' is half a pint of beer or a single tot of spirits or a glass of wine).[34] Despite this, the evidence of a relationship between alcohol intake and IHD is not certain: in some studies an increased incidence of IHD in heavy drinkers was found whereas in others low rates of IHD were found in heavy drinkers. In the British Regional Heart Study, no significant relationship between alcohol intake and the attack rate of IHD was found.[35] However, an univariate analysis, the lowest rates of IHD were seen in men taking 1–2 drinks a day on a regular basis. This group had the lowest proportion of manual workers, the lowest cigarette smoking rate, the lowest blood pressures and the lowest body mass index. They also had the lowest serum triglyceride levels and were amongst the physically most active in leisure time. It seems unlikely that alcohol could be directly responsible for all these effects, and it seems likely that the low rate of IHD reported in light regular drinkers is the outcome of the combined effects of all these advantageous characteristics experienced over a lifetime. (See postscript 2).

Alcohol does increase the HDL cholesterol concentration but only by about 15% in heavy drinkers (> 6 drinks daily). This seems a small benefit, in comparison with the effects of this quantity of alcohol on blood pressure[36] and hepatic enzymes.[37]

Coffee

Interest in coffee as a potential risk factor for IHD has been current for about 15 years; there have been conflicting results from several large prospective studies. In the Tromso[38] and Jerusalem[39] studies, it was suggested that heavy coffee drinking may be responsible for an increase in serum cholesterol concentration of about 0.5 mmol/l; it seems likely that black, strong, boiled ground coffee is particularly responsible for the effects.

The early case–control studies which drew attention to the link between coffee and IHD have received substantial support from two recent prospective studies. The first is based on a prospective study of 1130 male American medical students followed for 19–35 years.[40] After the effects of age, current smoking, hypertension status and baseline level of serum cholesterol had been taken into account, the estimated relative risk for men drinking 5 or more cups of coffee a day was 2.49 (95% confidence intervals 1.08–5.77) compared with men who drank no coffee. The findings support an independent dose–response association of coffee consumption with clinical IHD, consistent with a 2–3-fold elevation in risk among heavy coffee drinkers.

In the second prospective study, initial coffee consumption was examined in relation to 19-year mortality rates in 1910 white American males aged 40–56 years at baseline examination.[41] After adjustment for age, serum cholesterol, diastolic blood pressure and smoking status, mortality was highest in men drinking 6 or more cups of coffee a day, due primarily to an increase in coronary heart disease. The adjusted relative risk compared with those drinking less coffee was 1.71 (95% confidence intervals 1.27–2.30). The association between coffee and coronary heart disease was present in smokers and non-smokers and was not explained by differences in serum cholesterol. The results of these two studies support the hypothesis relating heavy coffee drinking and coronary heart disease; despite the lack of a clear mechanism and the inconsistency in the many studies, these findings cannot be lightly dismissed.

Fish, fatty acids and ischaemic heart disease

Atherosclerosis and IHD are apparently uncommon amongst Eskimos on their traditional diet of seal, caribou and fish; the 'fishy' aspect of their diet has aroused particular attention. The major polyunsaturated fatty acids in the plant foods of the Western world are linoleic acid and its derivative arachidonic acid, polyunsaturates of the n-6 series. In marine animals, the polyunsaturated fats are different, notably eicosapentaenoic acid (20 : 5n-3) and docosahexaenoic acid (22 : 6n-3); their effect on lipoprotein metabolism and on the eicosanoids (prostaglandins, thromboxanes, prostacyclines and leukotrienes) is thought likely to afford protection from IHD.[42] A small Dutch study has suggested that eating relatively small fish meals once or twice a week might help to prevent IHD. In a larger Swedish study a dose–response relationship was found, with the lowest risk in those who had the higher fish intake. However, reports from the USA and Hawaii have produced conflicting results and a Norwegian study did not support the hypothesis. It is clear that the association between fish intake and IHD requires more evidence before it can be properly assessed; in particular to decide whether it is simply a matter of fish eaters taking less meat and dairy products. An experimental study, in which the development of coronary atherosclerosis in hyperlipidaemic swine was prevented by supplementing their diet with cod liver oil suggests a direct effect of marine oils rather than merely a substitution phenemenon.[43] However, it is probably reasonable to replace some of our foods high in saturated fats with fish products.

Linoleic acid in adipose tissue and ischaemic heart disease

The results of population studies suggest that a low proportion of the essential fatty acid linoleic acid (C18 : 2 n-6) in adipose tissue may be associated with an increased risk of IHD. The fatty acid composition of adipose tissue provides a stable indication of long-term dietary habits. A cross-sectional study of healthy middle-aged men from four countries with differing mortality rates from IHD was designed to explore this hypothesis.[44] The proportion of linoleic acid was lowest in men from North Karelia, Finland, where mortality from IHD is highest, and highest in men from Italy, where mortality is lowest. Men from Scotland and South West Finland show intermediate proportions of linoleic acid in adipose tissue and intermediate IHD mortalities. Saturated fatty acid in adipose tissue behaved in the converse manner. In a more recent case–control study, the fatty acid composition of adipose tissue and platelet membranes in subjects with angina pectoris and myocardial infarction was examined.[45] In those with angina pectoris, newly diagnosed by standardized WHO questionnaire, there was a progressive increase in estimated risks as adipose tissue linoleic acid or platelet membrane eicosapentaenoic acid declined. The finding did not hold for those with acute myocardial infarction, and there appeared to be important relationships between linoleic acid and cigarette smoking. Apparently, cigarette smokers had a much lower intake of linoleic acid than non-smokers.

The relevance of these studies is to emphasize the importance of dietary factors in the development of IHD, and to focus attention on the essential linoleic acid of plant origin and the fatty acid derived from fish oil, eicosapentaenoic. Whether these have specific protective effects or whether they reflect the outcome of high saturated fat intakes has yet to be established.

BLOOD PRESSURE

In most communities throughout the world, blood pressure rises with increasing age, although the rate of rise and the level to which the blood pressure rises vary considerably. There are communities in which blood pressure does *not* increase with age; these are almost always unacculturated peoples living rural or nomadic lives away from urbanization and development. These groups tend to be lean, physically active and generally live on a subsistence level of nutrition. It has been suggested that these people, who show no increase in blood pressure with age, are biologically normal and the rising blood pressure seen with age in most communities is biologically abnormal despite its statistical normality, i.e. usualness. In support of this view is the well-established finding that as blood pressure rises there is a steady increase in the rate of several vascular disorders, including hypertensive heart disease, cerebrovascular disease (stroke), IHD and renal disease. In countries where atherosclerosis and IHD are not common, raised blood pressure is one of the most important risk factors for IHD. In countries where atherosclerosis and IHD are common, the levels of blood pressure and the prevalence of hypertension (however defined) may be the same as in countries with high levels of IHD, but nevertheless this does not result in a high rate of atherosclerosis and IHD. Raised blood pressure must be a potent aggravating or precipitating factor in communities with a sufficient degree of atherosclerosis to make them susceptible to the effects of hypertension. More directly, hypertension accelerates existing atherosclerosis and initiates IHD in

highly susceptible communities. The background susceptibility on which hypertension exerts its effects is likely to be a high circulating level of serum total cholesterol.

What levels of blood pressure should be regarded as 'risk factor' levels in communities prone to IHD? In the Framingham study, hypertensive subjects (> 160/95 mmHg) were at twofold risk of IHD when compared with normotensive subjects (< 140/90 mmHg).[46] In the British Regional Heart Study, a twofold increase in risk of a major IHD event was evident at systolic blood pressures > 148 mmHg, with little or no gradient of risk below this level.[16] The highest risk for diastolic pressure was in those with a level > 93 mmHg (phase V); even levels between 72 and 92 mmHg were associated with an increased risk compared with those in the lowest fifth of the blood pressure distribution (< 72 mmHg). It seems clear that in the British population about 40% of middle-aged men have casual systolic blood pressures which carry at least a twofold risk of a major IHD event occurring within the next 5 years (Fig. 42.9).

The debate on the primacy of systolic or diastolic blood pressure measurement in assessing the risk of cardiovascular disease continues. Most authorities recommend the use of the diastolic blood pressure as the index for making a diagnosis of 'hypertension' and for making decisions on management. In virtually all trials of treatment of raised blood pressure, diastolic blood pressure has been used as the criterion for entry into the trial. There is increasing evidence that, at least in middle-aged men, the top quintile of systolic blood pressure may yield a greater percentage of IHD events than the top quintile of diastolic blood pressure and, of the two, systolic blood pressure has the greater independent role.[44]

CIGARETTE SMOKING

It is only in recent years that the public have been made sufficiently aware that cigarette smoking is a risk factor for IHD. The earlier focus on lung cancer

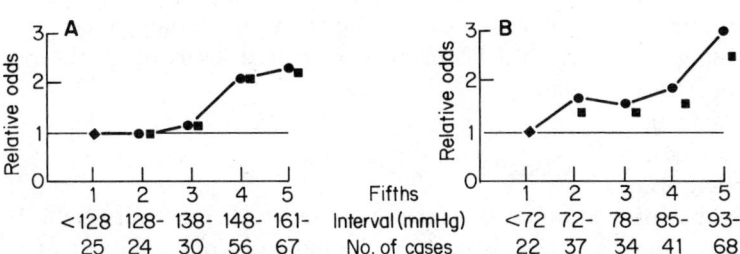

Fig. 42.9. British Regional Heart Study. Relative odds (risk) of a major IHD event over 4 years' follow-up, according to systolic (A) and diastolic (B) blood pressure (by fifths of ranked distribution).[16] ■, adjusted for other risk factors, age, pre-existing IHD; ●, adjusted for age.

and chronic bronchitis obscured the important relationship with coronary artery disease, although the link with peripheral vascular disease was well recognized.

Although cigarette smoking is a potent risk factor for IHD, it is an aggravating or potentiating factor rather than one of primary aetiology. The example of Japan, a country with a very high rate of cigarette smoking and an extremely low rate of IHD, is compelling. However, cigarette smoking acts as a risk factor for IHD only when the internal environment is susceptible. This susceptibility is likely to be associated with high circulating levels of serum total cholesterol and other lipid fractions. This is not to gainsay the importance of cigarette smoking in communities at high risk, but to emphasize the fundamental importance of the hypercholesterolaemia and its related nutritional background.

There is good evidence that men who have only ever smoked a pipe or cigars, a very small group in any community, tend to have the same rates of IHD as men who have never smoked cigarettes.[48] Pipe and cigar smokers who are ex-cigarette smokers tend to have very much higher rates of IHD, more closely linked to their duration of previous cigarette smoking. It has been widely accepted that giving up cigarette smoking leads to a rapid decline in the risk of IHD and much is made of this in anti-smoking literature. Recent data from the British Regional Heart Study shows that ex-cigarette smokers continue to have an increased risk of IHD and that the benefit of giving up cigarette smoking is more gradually acquired and is less complete than is widely accepted.[49] The number of years a man has been smoking cigaretes may be the best measure of this risk of IHD, irrespective of the number of years since giving up smoking. This finding emphasizes the need to persuade individuals not to start smoking, to give up as soon as possible if they are smoking and to cut down on their consumption of cigarettes if they are unable to stop.

DIABETES MELLITUS

In every community with a high incidence of IHD, diabetes mellitus has been shown to be an important risk factor for IHD, its presence increasing the risk at least twofold.[50] In those countries in Africa and Asia where IHD is not common, diabetes mellitus is not associated with an increased risk of IHD. This suggests that diabetes mellitus is not a primary cause of IHD but that it is capable of aggravating the susceptible situation. It has been

suggested that part of the increased risk is due to the high-fat low-carbohydrate diets once commonly used in the management of diabetes mellitus in Western societies. Obesity, a common association of maturity onset diabetes, may also be suspected of playing a role in the excess risk of IHD seen in diabetics, but obesity is common in diabetics in developing countries who do not develop IHD. Whatever the mode of action, which may be linked with the properties of insulin itself, diabetes mellitus increases the risk of IHD and is an important indicator of increased risk of IHD in Great Britain.

FAMILY HISTORY

A history of cardiovascular disease in a close relative, especially IHD before the age of 50 years is an important risk factor for IHD.[51] There is a well-recognized aggregation of risk factors such as hypertension, diabetes mellitus and obesity in families; even high levels of serum cholesterol may cluster in families. The heterogenous form of familial hypercholesterolaemia occurs in about 1 in 500 of the population and only a very small proportion of IHD events are due to this particular genetic abnormality. Most familial clusterings of risk factors and IHD are probably the result of interaction between genetic factors and environmental influences, and it is difficult to determine whether a 'positive family history' has an independent genetic effect. It is unlikely that there is a single specific genetic factor underlying the population problem of IHD. It is far more likely that the genetic component of IHD comprises separate genetic effects on a wide variety of physiological responses.

In the British Regional Heart Study, those men who recalled that a parent had died of 'heart trouble' (other than rheumatic heart disease), high blood pressure or stroke, had an increased risk of developing a major IHD event in the 5 years following screening. The risk was greater if the parent's death occurred under 70 years of age; the effect of both parents having died of 'heart trouble' was multiplicative. Even when the established risk factors were taken into account, the positive parental history carried increased risk, although men with such a history had increased levels of all the risk factors.

OBESITY

In most Western societies, being overweight or obese is perhaps the most obvious indicator of an increased risk of IHD (except the presence of a smoking cigarette!). Being overweight carries about a twofold increase in risk of IHD compared with being in the 'desirable' weight category.[52] However, overweight/obesity is closely associated with increased levels of blood pressure, serum total cholesterol and triglycerides and with decreased levels of HDL cholesterol and physical activity. Once these factors, particularly blood pressure and total cholesterol, have been taken into account in predicting heart attacks, obesity no longer has an independent effect. This does not negate the importance of obesity; it has accompanied the rise in blood pressure and blood lipids over the lifetime of the individuals concerned; however, in middle-age, blood pressure and blood lipids supersede obesity as risk factors for IHD. Obesity remains a visible indicator of increased risk, even if it is not used in statistical calculations of risk profiles. (It should be noted that insurance companies take account of overweight/obesity in their clients—further evidence in support of the importance of obesity with respect to the risk of IHD.)

PHYSICAL ACTIVITY

The weight of evidence from studies of work and leisure activity indicate that sustained regular physical activity affects the development of ischaemic heart disease.[53] It is not clear whether physical activity has to be of sufficient vigour to improve cardiovascular efficiency or whether lower levels are also protective to some degree. Raised levels of the established risk factors can overwhelm the beneficial effects of physical activity, for example, in the Seven Countries Study cohort in North Karelia, Finland, those subjects who had the highest incidence of major IHD events were lumbermen and farmers who had very high levels of physical activity at work. The important role attributed to leisure-time physical activity may reflect the fact that those who pursue vigorous sporting activities for pleasure are likely to have more positive (healthy) attitudes to weight control, diet and cigarette smoking.

Studies on Harvard, USA, graduates show that habitual exercise after leaving college predicts low risk of IHD, independent of smoking, obesity, hypertension or parental death from heart disease.[54] The results of this study also suggest that it is physical activity continued in adult life, rather than student athletic activity, that exerts the strongest influence on IHD risk.

PERSONALITY AND STRESS

It is accepted that severe emotional or physical stress can precipitate a major IHD event in individuals with an advanced degree of coronary atherosclerosis, irrespective of whether they have manifest evidence of established IHD. John Hunter (1728–1794) typifies the effect of emotional stress and he knew well that anger precipitated his episodes of angina pectoris. His final heart attack was precipitated by a violent dispute at the Board of Governers at his teaching hospital. The effects of physical stress are well illustrated by the reports of sudden death occurring during or after squash games, almost always in individuals who have severe coronary artery disease and often with recognized increase in risk factors. Shovelling snow in winter, trying to open jammed window frames or pushing a car are equally illustrative of the lethal effects of physical stress on those with compromised coronary arteries.

However, the fundamental issue is whether emotional stress associated with interpersonal relationships, such as acculturation problems in immigrant groups, loss of support in a community through bereavement, divorce or loss of religious belief, can lead to arterial damage through effects on the body *in the absence* of the standard risk factors.[55]

In the 1950s, Rosenman and Friedman described a personality pattern, Type A, which they concluded was an independent risk factor for IHD. The behaviour pattern of type A individuals is characterized by aggressiveness, ambition and competitiveness, chronic impatience, a strong sense of time urgency and an abrupt manner of speech and movement. In the early studies, using the original interview technique, type A behaviour was found to be an independent risk for IHD. In the Framingham study, the type A personality was found to be an independent risk factor but only for men in non-manual (white-collar) occupations. Later studies, using standard questionnaires instead of the personalized and provocative interview, have not been consistent in their outcome; about half of them have failed to confirm an independent association between type A behaviour and the risk of IHD. In communities like West-coast USA, where Rosenman and Friedman carried out their original work, it would seem a combination of a high prevalence of atherosclerotic coronary artery disease and IHD, combined with a high prevalence of type A personalities, has resulted in an association that has the appearance of independent causality, but it is probably only secondary and precipitant. In the British Regional Heart Study, a simplified method of assessing type A personality (the Bortner questionnaire) was used which showed no relationship between high scores on the Bortner scale (type A) and the attack rate of IHD.[56] There were significant associations with the presence of pre-existing IHD and there was a strong social class trend, with men in the non-manual occupations (social classes I, II and III non-manual) having higher scores for type A than men in manual occupations (social classes III manual, IV and V).

Although an individual's personality may influence the risk of IHD through effects on dietary patterns, smoking, obesity and physical activity and the pattern of response to stress, emotional and physical, may be lethal in a coronary-prone individual, there is little evidence that psychosocial factors in their own right will result in coronary artery damage and IHD.

SOCIAL CLASS AND ISCHAEMIC HEART DISEASE IN GREAT BRITAIN

In Great Britain, IHD mortality rates are higher in manual than in non-manual workers.[57] The British Regional Heart Study includes a representative sample of men from all social classes, derived from all the major geographical regions of Great Britain. At screening, the prevalence rates of IHD were 84% higher for angina pectoris on questionnaire, 40% higher for recall of a doctor-diagnosis of IHD and 24% higher for myocardial infarction or definite myocardial ischaemia on electrocardiogram.[58] Over a 6-year period, the attack rate was 44% higher in the manual workers, which is in rough agreement with the 32% excess mortality for IHD in manual workers reported in the 1981 national statistics. The manual workers had markedly higher rates of cigarette smoking, higher levels of blood pressure, more obesity and less regular physical activity in leisure time. When these differences were taken into account, the excess attack rate was diminished to 24% and was of only marginal statistical significance ($P=0.08$). It seems very likely that these differences in risk factor experience over a lifetime account for a substantial part of the social class difference in morbidity and mortality from IHD in Great Britain. The risk of IHD is high in *all* social classes in Great Britain and there seems little justification for IHD prevention campaigns directed specifically at any one group.

THROMBOSIS AND THROMBOLYSIS

The pathology of IHD has provided good evidence that thrombosis within the coronary arteries plays a crucial role in the initiation of a substantial proportion of major IHD events—myocardial infarction and sudden cardiac death.[59] It also seems likely that fibrin deposition and thrombus formation and incorporation play an important role in the development of the atherosclerotic plaque in the coronary vessels. Fibrinolytic activity, a physiological process by which fibrin is removed from vessel surfaces, is also an important factor in determining whether thrombi, once formed, persist and increase in size or are dissolved. There are important relationships between blood lipids, cigarette smoking, obesity and physical activity patterns on the one hand and thrombogenic and thrombolytic processes on the other. These relationships are complex but suggest that thrombogenesis and thrombolysis may be important *secondary* mechanisms by which the risk factors exert their effect. In international studies comparing communities with marked differences in their incidence of IHD, there are striking differences in fibrinolytic activity and some differences in coagulation factor concentrations.[60,61]

In terms of the assessment of risk, there have been few studies in which coagulation or lysis factors have been measured and their independence explored. In Swedish studies, plasma fibrinogen emerged as a strong univariate risk factor, but it was strongly related to cigarette smoking. After multivariate analysis, the association between fibrinogen and heart attack became non-significant.[62] In an American study of young (under 54 years) survivors of acute myocardial infarction, the results suggested that there was reduced fibrinolytic activity in the patients when compared with the control subjects.[63] However, case–control studies are complicated by problems of hidden confounding variables and such results must be confirmed by data from prospective studies.

Although coagulation/thrombus formation and fibrinolytic activity may be found to be potent risk factors (indicators) for IHD, it is important to determine whether their effects are primary or a response to changes in the established areas of risk, such as cigarette smoking, dietary factors, blood pressure, obesity, physical activity. Data from the Northwick Park Heart Study demonstrate that lifetime duration of cigarette smoking is a determinant of initial plasma fibrinogen levels. It takes over 5 years of non-smoking before levels return to those found in lifelong non-smokers. A switch from cigarettes to cigars was associated with a larger increase in fibrinogen than continuing to smoke cigarettes. A substantial part of the relationship between smoking and IHD appears to be mediated through the fibrinogen concentration.[64]

SEX HORMONES

The ability to menstruate appears to provide an important measure of protection against IHD. Women in their 40s and 50s who are menopausal have 2–3 times the risk of IHD compared with women of the same age who continue to menstruate. In post-menopausal women, the use of exogenous oestrogens (hormone replacement therapy) does not appear to increase the risk of IHD; the results of some studies have suggested that their use might reduce the risk of IHD. The Framingham study showed a 50% increase in the incidence of vascular disease in women taking oestrogen, but only if they were cigarette smokers.[65] In a very large American postal questionnaire study, the risk of IHD in oestrogen users was half that of non-users, even when cigarette smoking and other factors were taken into account.[66]

Oral contraceptives may be associated with an increased risk of cardiovascular events, including stroke and myocardial infarction. The effect is particularly seen in older women (> 35 years) who smoke cigarettes, and also in those with hypertension or a strong family history of vascular disease. Although relative risk in these women may be increased 2–3-fold, the absolute risk is very small. Nevertheless, the use of oral contraceptives in the presence of cigarette smoking and other risk factors, constitutes sufficient risk to warrant advising the use of alternative contraception especially in older women.

EXISTING ISCHAEMIC HEART DISEASE AND THE RISK OF FURTHER MAJOR ISCHAEMIC HEART DISEASE EVENTS

All studies of heart attacks in the community indicate that about half of the individuals with confirmed major IHD events have evidence of preceding IHD, i.e. they may have been told in the past that they have had a heart attack or angina, or evidence may have been uncovered on routine health checks including electrocardiography. One of the strongest risk factors for a major IHD event, either myocardial infarction (fatal or non-fatal) or sudden cardiac death, is pre-existing evidence of IHD.

In the British Regional Heart Study, men who had current angina on standardized WHO chest pain questionnaire had 4 times the risk of a major IHD event in the 5 years following screening when compared with men who had no such symptom.[16] The presence of electrocardiographic evidence of previous definite myocardial infarction increased the risk of IHD 6-fold when compared with those who had a normal electrocardiograph. Similarly, those men who recalled that a doctor had told them that they had IHD (heart attack, angina) had a 6-fold increase of risk. These estimates of risk may be compared with a 2-fold risk in men known to be diabetic or a 50% increase in risk in men with a parent who had died of heart trouble. All these estimates are univariate. When both angina on questionnaire and definite myocardial infarction on electrocardiogram are present and the man recalls a doctor having told him of his condition, the risk is likely to be nearer 20-fold. This estimate of risk does not take into account the presence of other risk factors which may be concurrently present in such individuals.

There are two reasons for dwelling on the increased risk of major IHD events in men with pre-existing evidence of IHD. First, such subjects do not comprise a small subgroup of the population who may be regarded as already receiving special attention; a considerable proportion of the men with current angina on standardized questionnaire are not known to have IHD and about 50% of the men with definite myocardial infarction on electrocardiogram have never had a severe chest pain and are not known to have IHD. Second, symptoms and signs of IHD derived from WHO questionnaire and electrocardiograms were present in 25% of middle-aged men in the British Regional Heart Study, indicating the considerable prevalence of the problem in Great Britain and the impossibility of excluding this large group from consideration of those at high risk.[67,68]

RISK OF ISCHAEMIC HEART DISEASE

PREDICTING A HEART ATTACK

The prediction of major IHD events can be attempted in several ways. The simplest is to measure each separate risk factor and to choose an arbitrary cut-off point in the distribution of that risk factor likely to yield a considerable proportion of all the cases of major IHD occurring in a defined period of time. The Report of the British Cardiac Society Working Party on Coronary Disease Prevention (1987) recommends that

"We should aim at identifying those in the top 20% of the distribution of serum cholesterol concentrations and the top 10% of the distribution of blood pressure for that population for which it is planned to give advice".[24]

The European Atherosclerosis Society (1987) is less specific and their "goal is to recognise most people with levels of risk factors requiring treatment";[23] the list of characteristics includes a family history of premature cardiovascular disease or hyperlipidaemia, the presence of xanthomas or premature corneal arcus, obesity, diabetes, hypertension, smoking and gout. The European Atherosclerosis Society criteria for selective screening may be too all embracing to be practical in Western society. The approach of the British Cardiac Society also has severe limitations; it may encourage widespread measurement of blood cholesterol at considerable cost, probably without great benefit.

The percentage of cases of major IHD occurring in the top fifth of the distribution of several major risk factors, taken from the British Regional Heart Study, is shown in Table 42.1.[69] It is evident that the top fifth of the serum cholesterol concentration will yield only 31% of the cases occurring over a 5-year period of observation and the top 20% of the blood pressure distribution (systolic or diastolic) will yield about 35% of cases. However, it can be seen that age alone, even within this 40–59-year-old group of men, will yield more cases than serum cholesterol. The number of years a man has spent smoking cigarettes provides the best yield (38%). In the light of these findings, an approach to screening for IHD should not be based solely on the level of serum cholesterol or blood pressure.

It has been known for many years that the

prediction of cases of major IHD can be improved by assessing the combined effect of several risk factors acting simultaneously. Workers in the Framingham study produced a small booklet from which individual risk could be determined, using several risk factors including the electrocardiographic findings of left ventricular strain.[70] At the simplest level, it was demonstrated that combinations of risk factors could lead to an 8-fold increase in risk in men whose level of serum cholesterol was above average, who smoked cigarettes and who had hypertension (> 140/90 mmHg) when compared with men whose level of serum cholesterol was below average, who did not smoke and who did not have hypertension.

In the British Regional Heart Study, a similar attempt has been made to combine the effects of the risk factors, including the presence of pre-existing IHD, to achieve the best yield of cases of major IHD occurring in 5 years of follow-up.[69,71] The *full* model used in this multivariate analysis included age, systolic blood pressure, serum total cholesterol, years of cigarette smoking, electrocardiographic findings of myocardial infarction or ischaemia, current angina on WHO questionnaire, recall of a doctor-diagnosis of IHD or diabetes and history of parental death from 'heart trouble'.

Using multiple logistic regression, a sophisticated statistical technique for assessing the independent contribution of each factor to the subsequent risk of IHD, coefficients were derived that gave a weighting to each of the risk factors. Using these coefficients, a score was calculated for each individual based on the level of each of the risk factors and the presence or absence of the other criteria. The number of cases of IHD falling into each fifth of the distribution of the full risk score, the risk rate 1000/year and the percentage yield of cases of major IHD falling into the top fifth are shown in Table 42.2. Compared with 31% yield for the top fifth of serum cholesterol, the full score gives almost twice the yield of cases—59%.

Using the full score in general practice would entail considerable effort because the recording and

Table 42.1. British Regional Heart Study. Relative risk* and percentage of cases in top fifth of the ranked distribution for the principal risk factors.[65] (*Rate in top fifth relative to rate in lowest fifth).

Factor	Relative risk	Cases in top fifth
Age	4.7	34%
Total cholesterol	3.1	31%
Systolic BP	3.0	36%
Diastolic BP	3.1	34%
Body mass index	1.8	28%
'Smoking years'	5.1	38%

Table 42.2. British Regional Heart Study. Full risk score for identifying men at high risk of a major IHD event (270 cases out of 7506 men).[65]

	Distribution					% Cases in top fifth
	1 (Low)	2	3	4	5 (High)	
No. of cases	5	14	34	57	160	59
Risk rate/1000/year	0.7	1.9	4.5	7.6	21.3	

interpretation of an electrocardiogram, and the determining of a serum cholesterol concentration are time-consuming and costly. A modified score has been developed which leaves out the electrocardiogram and the blood cholesterol, and the outcome for this modified score is also presented in Table 42.3

Compared with the full score, the yield of cases in the top fifth fell from 59% to 54%. For all practical purposes, this would seem to be an acceptable loss of discrimination when weighed against the simplicity of the approach. Many screening situations have serum cholesterol estimation readings available and do not wish to exclude it from the scoring system. The intermediate system (with cholesterol) yields 58% of cases of IHD over a 5-year period which is virtually the same as using the full score, i.e. including electrocardiogram.

PREDICTION FOR INDIVIDUALS AND GROUPS

A screening system such as this enables an individual to be placed in a group with a high risk of major IHD; it does not enable a precise prediction to be made that a specific individual will or will not have a major IHD event within a given period of time. Given the variability of the arterial disease and the multiplicity of possible alterations in blood characteristics (particularly thrombogenic and thrombolytic factors), this is not surprising. The scoring system only allows a clinician to estimate an increased probability of an event occurring.

ISCHAEMIC HEART DISEASE WITHOUT RISK FACTORS?

There is a widely held view by cardiologists that they see many patients admitted with heart attacks who do not have identifiable risk factors. In the British Regional Heart Study, there was at least a twofold independent increase in risk associated with any *one* of the following criteria:
1   serum total cholesterol > 6.0 mmol/l;

Table 42.3. British Regional Heart Study. Scoring system (Basic/GP) for identifying men at high risk of a major IHD event based on 5-years follow-up. (Shaper, A.G. *et al. Health Trends* 1987; **19**: 37–39).

Smoking years	× 7.5
Systolic BP	× 4.5
Diagnosis of IHD	+ 265
Diagnosis of diabetes	+ 150
Current angina	+ 150
Parental death from 'heart trouble'	+ 80
	Total

2   systolic blood pressure > 148 mmHg or diastolic blood pressure > 93 mmHg;
3   current cigarette smoking.
Only 5 of the 202 cases in that analysis did not meet any of these three criteria, but in over two-thirds of the cases at least two criteria were present.[16] Of the 5 men who did not meet the above criteria, 3 had evidence of pre-existing IHD. Although episodes of major IHD do occur in individuals who do not meet the criteria for increased risk, they are rare. The belief that major IHD occurs not infrequently in the absence of identifiable risk factors is perpetuated by a failure to recognize that even moderate increases in blood lipids and blood pressure can carry an excess risk of IHD, especially in the presence of a large number of 'smoking years'.

RISK FACTORS AND PRE-EXISTING ISCHAEMIC HEART DISEASE

There has been considerable controversy over whether the established risk factors (cigarette smoking, blood pressure and serum total cholesterol) continue to exert an influence on those men in whom IHD has already developed. It has already been demonstrated that the presence of IHD, in terms of angina, previous myocardial infarction or ischaemia on the electrocardiogram, or recall of a diagnosis of IHD by a doctor constitutes an important risk for subsequent major IHD events. It can be deduced that the independent predictive role of the conventional risk factors *must* be proportionately reduced in those with pre-existing IHD. However, there is convincing evidence that the established risk factors continue to contribute to an increase in risk of subsequent major IHD events, albeit their proportionate contribution to risk is diminished. In the British Regional Heart Study, men with and without pre-existing IHD who become 'cases' (i.e. developed new major IHD events) had similar levels of risk factors.[16] Furthermore, men with pre-existing IHD who remained free of new major IHD episodes over the 5 years of follow-up had *lower* levels of systolic and diastolic blood pressure, lower body mass index, serum total cholesterol, serum triglycerides, a lower percentage of current cigarette smokers and higher concentrations of HDL cholesterol. Multivariate analysis confirmed that when all these effects were considered simultaneously, blood pressure and serum cholesterol continued to make important independent contributions to risk. The implication of these observations is that the management and control of risk factors in men who already have evidence of IHD is as important as it is in men without such evidence. There is evidence from a large Belgian study that the results of risk factor intervention in men with electrocardiographic evidence of IHD was strikingly more effective than in men with a normal electrocardiogram at baseline.[72] (See postscript 3).

REVERSIBILITY OF RISK OF ISCHAEMIC HEART DISEASE

There is evidence that the level of IHD in a community can vary considerably over time, although there are those who attribute all or most of this variation to changes in diagnostic and coding practices, familiarity with the clinical and patholo-gical features of the disease and diagnostic errors in certified causes of death.[73] The mortality from 'arteriosclerotic' heart disease declined sharply in Finland, Norway and Sweden during the Second World War. The decline was associated with a marked reduction in the intake of meat, butter, eggs and other foodstuffs high in saturated fats and cholesterol and was most marked in the urban population, who had little opportunity for obtain-ing food beyond the official rations. In England and Wales during this period, the mortality rates for heart disease, which had been rising steadily, levelled off and did not rise again until after the war. In the USA, unaffected by food restrictions, the mortality rate from heart disease during this period showed a progressive increase.[74] Although this is not 'hard evidence', it is in keeping with the dietary hypothesis of IHD and also suggests that drastic food restrictions are followed fairly closely by changes in mortality rates. Speculation regarding the effects of diet on the thrombogenic and throm-bolytic processes is inevitable, and the data provide interesting circumstantial evidence.

In individuals, there is evidence of considerable variability in the atherosclerotic process over time. Angiographic studies in the USA have shown that in some patients lesions may appear and progress rapidly over a few years, but in many there is slow steady progression of the lesions. Progression of arteriographically demonstrated coronary artery disease correlates strongly with the established risk factors, particularly hypercholesterolaemia.[75] Furthermore, progression of angiographically proved coronary artery disease can be inhibited by drugs that lower the level of serum cholesterol over a prolonged period.

If an extension of lesions is the usual and expected pattern, an arrest of such progression must be regarded as useful in the control of the problem: There have been many trials of diet and/or drugs that lower serum cholesterol, in attempts to reduce femoral or coronary atherosclerosis. Some claims have been made for regression of the disease in these studies, but the criteria for judging regression were variable and success of such studies has been questioned.

Animal studies have provided the strongest evi-dence for the reversibility of atherosclerosis, and although these can never duplicate the process in humans they provide the best available model on which to test the hypothesis. In all the studies reported in pigs and in rhesus monkeys, in which atherosclerosis had been produced, regression has been shown to be possible. Following the dietary production of atherosclerotic lesions, a further period of 1–4 years on a low-fat low-cholesterol diet reduced serum cholesterol to baseline levels. The lesions became smaller, there was a diminution in arterial narrowing and the regressing plaques showed endothelial healing. The implications are that the amount of atherosclerosis and its potential to extend and become complicated can be consider-ably diminished by active encouragement of regression.[76]

THE PREVENTION OF ISCHAEMIC HEART DISEASE

Recently, two important policy statements on the prevention of IHD have been issued, one from the British Cardiac Society (1987)[24] and the other from European Atherosclerosis Society (1987).[23] These differ little in their recommendations from the reports by the Royal College of Physicians of London and the British Cardiac Society (1976),[77] the World Health Organisation (1982)[78] and the Committee on Medical Aspects of Food Policy (1984).[79] What is most important about both the new reports is that they represent an attempt to emphasize that a

> "more positive attitude by cardiologists to the prevention of CHD is urgently needed. Car-diologists and other physicians have a crucial and leadership role in establishing a really effective policy to prevent and reduce CHD."

The active concern and involvement of physicians and cardiologists is important in the prevention of IHD, not only in the management of those with evidence of IHD and those at high risk but also in their support for community and national action towards the reduction in the risks associated with IHD.

Until recently two major strategies have competed for predominance in IHD prevention. The *population* strategy is based on the fact that in most populations at high risk the major risk factors are widespread and most heart attacks occur in those individuals with moderate increases in risk factor levels. In the British Regional Heart Study, for example, 60% of middle-aged men had serum cholesterol levels associated with at least a twofold risk of a major IHD event in the next 5 years, 40% had systolic blood pressure levels carrying this level of risk and 41% were current smokers, with another 35% who were ex-smokers, still carrying a twofold risk of IHD.[16] When combined with a high prevalence of overweight/obesity[52] and very low levels of physical activity, it is clear that only a major national effort to alter the risk factor status of the population over a long period of time can be effective.

In the *individual or high-risk strategy*, the aim is to identify those people in the population who are at particularly high risk of IHD. The argument put forward for this policy is that for those individuals with very high levels of individual risk factors, e.g. severe hypertension, major genetic hyperlipidaemias or marked obesity, the moderate changes in health habits inherent in the population strategy are not adequate and that they require individual therapy in a clinical setting. Although this argument is valid, it does not encompass the main reasons for promoting a high-risk strategy as a *complementary* activity to the population strategy.

1   Risk of IHD does not depend on being in the top fifth (or tenth) of the distribution of any single risk factor. It is based on the combined effects of multiple risk factors acting simultaneously. In the system of scoring for high risk proposed by the British Regional Heart Study, men in the top fifth of the risk score distribution had a risk rate for major IHD events of 20 per 1000 per year. This was 5 times greater than the remaining four-fifths (80%) of the men and 20 times greater than the men in the lowest fifth. However, while 72% of men with current angina (on standardized questionnaire) fell into the top fifth of the risk score distribution, i.e. 'high risk', only 30% of current smokers, 24% of men in the top fifth of the serum cholesterol distribution and 50% of men with systolic blood pressure > 160 mmHg were included in the high-risk (top fifth) category. Although there is

good reason to stop these men smoking, and to reduce the raised serum cholesterol levels and the raised blood pressures, in comparative terms, they are not at high risk of IHD. They may have a higher risk of IHD than men in a Mediterranean country, but in terms of strategy for prevention they do not fall into the category demanding special care and attention from physicians and cardiologists.

2   The high-risk strategy brings to the attention of the doctor (general practitioner, physician, cardiologist) those who are at highest risk of a major IHD event in the near future (within 5 years). Even when the basic (GP) score is used, the high risk group includes almost all men in whom a diagnosis of IHD has already been made, a large proportion of those with electrocardiographic evidence of definite myocardial infarction or ischaemia and those in whom angina is currently present, as well as the men in whom the combination of several risk factors, with or without evidence of pre-existing IHD, renders them at high risk of a heart attack. These individuals are in need of appropriate medical care.

3   The doctor has an appropriate and skilled role to play in the management of these individuals. Such involvement should arouse greater concern for the whole concept of risk factors for IHD and should enhance enthusiasm for supporting other strategies for the prevention of IHD. These include the role of nurses in general practice, the role of nurses in cardiac clinics and the overall community-based strategies for health education.

4   Unless this high-risk strategy is supported by a population strategy, a constant movement of people into the high-risk category will continue to occur. Although the high-risk strategy can prevent or delay episodes of heart attacks, it is capable of making only moderate reductions in overall mortality from IHD. It would be shortsighted to encourage a high-risk strategy unless action was being taken to reduce the inflow of new high-risk subjects by appropriate population-based strategies.

MANAGEMENT OF RISK FACTORS

The report of the British Cardiac Society Working Group on Coronary Heart Disease Prevention (1987) and that of the European Atherosclerosis Society (1987) should be consulted for detailed recommendations.[23–24] The British document is simpler in its approach; that of the European Atherosclerosis Society reflects the fact that it is drawn up by 36 experts from 19 countries and is based on their concordant views. The reader is advised to concentrate only on those recommendations it seems possible to implement. Only two areas will be commented upon, one relating to serum cholesterol and the other to blood pressure.

1   The British Cardiac Society recommend that

"those with blood cholesterol concentrations above 6.5 mmol/l (250 mg/dl) should be given dietary advice. This may need to be combined with drug therapy when the levels are greater than 7.8 mmol/l (300 mg/dl). The aim should be to lower blood cholesterol towards 5.2 mmol/l (200 mg/dl)."

The European Atherosclerosis Society provides a complex table with blood cholesterol and triglyceride levels in combination, providing five categories for management.

Inherent in these recommendations is a requirement for the universal measurement of serum cholesterol (and serum triglyceride) either systematically or opportunistically, on a repeated basis when necessary. As the mean level of serum cholesterol in middle-aged British men is about 6.2 mmol/l, roughly half the male middle-aged population would require dietary advice. As risk of IHD is continuous from levels above 5.0–5.2 mmol/l, this clearly presents a problem for a population-based health education strategy. Furthermore, the majority (76%) of men with serum cholesterol levels > 7.2 mmol/l (i.e. the top 20% of the cholesterol distribution in the British Regional Heart Study) do *not* fall into the high-risk category on the multivariate risk score. To attempt to provide individualized dietary advice from physicians and cardiologists or dietitians would be impossible. However, it would seem reasonable to measure the serum cholesterol in all men falling into the top fifth of the multivariate risk score distribution, to ensure compliance with dietary advice and to monitor progress. The detection of gross hyperlipidaemia in those without obvious clinical syndromes can probably be most economically approached by special attention to those with strong family histories of premature (< 50 years) IHD.

2   The British Cardiac Society recommends that

"those with diastolic pressures above 100 mmHg require treatment and attention to other risk factors."

The report draws attention to the fact that

"lowering of elevated blood pressure by drug therapy has not been shown convincingly to reduce the incidence of myocardial infarction, though the beneficial effects of treatment on the incidence of stroke and cardiac failure are undoubted."

Attitudes to the management of high blood pressure, particularly mild hypertension (90–105 mmHg) have been strongly influenced by the MRC Mild Hypertension Trial which failed to show any effect of drug treatment on the incidence of IHD events.[80] However, it may be important to emphasize that the subjects taking part in this trial were at low risk of IHD, all high-risk subjects (almost 50% of those eligible on grounds of blood pressure levels) had been exluded. Thus, the power of such a study to affect significantly IHD incidence was considerably diminished.

It would seem appropriate to assess an individual's overall risk of IHD in a multivariate way, using the type of scoring system provided by the British Regional Heart Study. Those with mild hypertension who are at high risk of IHD within the subsequent 5 years constitute a different group from those with identical blood pressure levels who are at much lower risk of IHD. This consideration should be taken into account in both the design of clinical trials and their analysis and in individual clinical management. Non-pharmacological measures liable to reduce raised blood pressure should always be considered first and strongly encouraged in those with mild hypertension, i.e. weight reduction, alcohol restriction, salt restriction and perhaps stress-reduction regimes. Even in those subjects with mild hypertension and low risk of IHD, such methods should be recommended to prevent the rise of blood pressure to levels likely to demand pharmacological intervention. In the MRC trial, about 20–25% of those on placebo showed such a rise in blood pressure, possibly the most important observation in the trial but not included as an 'endpoint' of importance.

There seems little to add to what is widely known about stopping cigarette smoking, maintaining a 'desirable' weight, taking regular physical activity in leisure time and adhering to the dietary recommendation widely agreed by almost all authorities. Although these dietary recommendations vary, they all agree on the main themes of reducing saturated fat intake, partial substitution by polyunsaturated fats and the achieving of a dietary P/S ratio nearer to 0.5–0.6 than the current levels of 0.2–0.3

PRIMARY PREVENTION OF HEART ATTACK: THE USE OF ASPIRIN

Attempts at primary prevention of IHD through lipid-lowering drugs are reviewed in Chapter 43. The stated aim of the WHO Clofibrate Study was to determine whether reduction of elevated blood lipids in healthy men would reduce the incidence of IHD; there was no intention to advocate the widespread use of drugs in primary prevention.[81] The Lipid Research Clinics Coronary Primary Prevention Trial of cholestyramine[82] and the Helsinki Heart Study of gemfibrozil[83] had similar aims and the results have shown that reduction of blood cholesterol lowers the incidence of coronary heart disease. The recently reported trials of aspirin in primary prevention were concerned not with lipids but with platelet function and prostacyclin synthesis in the vessel wall, both processes inhibited by aspirin. In a series of studies in the 1970s, aspirin had been shown to reduce significantly cardiovascular morbidity and mortality in patients who had previously experienced a myocardial infarction.[84] For men with cardiovascular disease, the use of aspirin significantly reduced the incidence of transient ischaemic attacks, stroke and death.[85] Two recent reports provide further support for the use of 300 mg aspirin a day in patients requiring *secondary* prevention of cardiovascular disease, provided there are no contra-indications.[86,87] Although this seems to provide conclusive evidence of the efficacy of aspirin in secondary prevention of cardiovascular disease, a determined reduction of risk factors including blood cholesterol may be as effective and carry less risk of side-effects. However, in relation to patient compliance, taking aspirin is easier than adhering to a changed diet.

The issue that remains to be satisfactorily resolved concerns the use of aspirin in the *primary* prevention of IHD. A British randomized open (not blind) trial in 5139 male doctors using 500 mg aspirin a day has reported its findings after 6 years' observation.[88] A non-significant reduction of 10% in total mortality was obtained, but there was no significant difference between the rates of fatal or definite non-fatal myocardial infarction in the aspirin and control groups. The authors note that the confidence intervals of the study do not exclude a beneficial effect of aspirin of about 10–20% and suggest that aspirin may yet be found to be beneficial in apparently healthy people. The reluctance to accept their own findings may be conditioned by their knowledge of the very different results obtained by an American Study reported at about the same time.

The double-blind American Study involved 22 071 male doctors aged 40–84 years and was terminated early because of the large (47%) reduction in the incidence of non-fatal and fatal myocardial infarction in those on 325 mg aspirin on alternate days ($P<0.00001$).[89] There was a small (non-significant) increase in the number of strokes in the aspirin groups with a significant increase in the risk of haemorrhagic stroke in those in the aspirin group, albeit based on a relatively small number of events. The authors consider that the decision to prescribe aspirin for primary prevention of cardiovascular disease must remain an individual judgement in which the benefit of preventing myocardial infarction must be weighed against the well-recognized hazards of gastro-intestinal discomfort and bleeding, and stroke. Considerable caution should be shown before the widespread use of aspirin in primary prevention is advocated.

A major issue in both the UK and American studies is the selective nature of the population samples taking part in the study and the limited grounds on which generalizations of the findings have been applied to the general population. In the UK study, only one-quarter of the doctors approached were eventually recruited to the study and half of them were over 60 years of age at the start of the study. In the American study, only 23% of the 261 248 doctors initially approached were willing to participate and, after exclusions, only 8% of those initially approached took part in the study. The overall cardiovascular death rate in the study was only 12% of that expected in US white men, which further emphasizes the highly selective nature of the sample. Although the biological effects of aspirin might be the same in other populations, the compliance rates and the complications might be very different. It is not reasonable to extrapolate from the findings of the American study to the general male population of America or that of any other country.

REFERENCES

1. Keys, A. *Seven Countries. A multivariate analysis of death and coronary heart disease.* Cambridge, Mass.: Havard University Press, 1980.
2. Pell, S. and Fayerweather, W.E. Trends in the incidence of myocardial infarction and in associated mortality in a large employed population 1957–1983. *N. Engl. J. Med.* 1985; 312: 1005–11.
3. Goldman, L. and Cook, E.F. The decline in ischaemic heart disease mortality rates. An analysis of the comparative

effects of medical intervention and changes in lifestyle. *Ann. Intern. Med.* 1984; **101**: 835–6.

4. Beaglehole, R. Medical management and the decline in mortality from coronary heart disease. *Br. Med. J.* 1986; **292**: 33–5.

5. Neutze, J.M. and White, H.D. What contribution has cardiac surgery made to the decline in mortality from coronary heart disease? *Br. Med. J.* 1987; **294**: 405–9.

6. Pyorala, K., Epstein, F.H. and Kornitzer, M. (eds). Changing trends in coronary heart disease mortality: possible explanations. *Cardiology* 1985; **72**: 5–104.

7. Tuomilehto, J., Gebbers, J., Salonen, J.T., Nissinen, A., Kuulaswa, K. and Puska, P. Decline in cardiovascular mortality in North Karelia and other parts of Finland. *Br. Med. J.* 1986; **293**: 1068–71.

8. Sullivan, J.L. Iron and the sex difference in heart disease risk. *Lancet* 1981; **i**: 1293–4.

9. Colditz, G.A., Willett, W.C., Stampfer, M.J., Rosner, B., Speizer, F.E. and Hennekens, C.H. Menopause and the risk of coronary heart disease in women. *N. Engl. J. Med.* 1987; **316**: 1105–10.

10. Coronary Prevention Group. *Coronary heart disease and Asians in Britain.* CPG and Confederation of Indian Organisations (UK), 1986.

11. Ball, H. and Mann, J.I. Apoproteins: predictors of coronary heart disease? *Br. Med. J.* 1986; **293**: 769–70.

12. Martin, M.J., Hulley, S.B., Browner, W.S., Kuller, L.H. and Wentworth, D. Serum cholesterol, blood pressure, and mortality: implications from a cohort of 361,662 men. *Lancet* 1986; **ii**: 933–6.

13. Sherwin, R.W., Wentworth, D.N., Cutler, J.A., Hulley, S.B., Kuller, L.H. and Stamler, J. Serum cholesterol levels and cancer mortality in 361,662 men screened for the Multiple Risk Factor Intervention Trial. *JAMA* 1987; **257**: 943–8.

14. Tornberg, S.A., Holm, L.E., Carstensen, J.M. and Eklind, G.A. Risks of cancer of the colon and rectum in relation to serum cholesterol and beta-lipoprotein. *N. Engl. J. Med.* 1986; **315**: 1629–38.

15. Rose, G. and Shipley, M. Plasma cholesterol concentrations and deaths from coronary heart disease: 10 year results of the Whitehall Study? *Br. Med. J.* 1986; **293**: 306–7.

16. Shaper, A.G., Pocock, S.J., Walker, M., Phillips, A., Whitehead, T.P. and Macfarlane, P.W. Risk factors for ischaemic heart disease: the prospective phase of the British Regional Heart Study. *J. Epidemiol. Community Health* 1985; **39**: 197–209.

17. Pocock, S.J., Shaper, A.G., Phillips, A.N., Walker, M. and Whitehead, T.P. High density lipoprotein cholesterol is not a major risk factor for ischaemic heart disease in British men. *Br. Med. J.* 1986; **292**: 515–9.

18. Anonymous. HDL and ischaemic heart disease in Britain [Editorial]. *Lancet* 1986; **i**: 481–2.

19. Carlson, L.A., Bottinger, L.E. and Ahfeldt, P.E. Risk factors for myocardial infarction in the Stockholm prospective study: a 14-year follow-up focussing on the role of plasma triglycerides and cholesterol. *Acta Med. Scand.* 1979; **206**: 351–60.

20. Hulley, S.B., Rosenman, R.H., Bawol, R.D. and Brand, R.J. Epidemiology as a guide to clinical decisions: the association between triglyceride and coronary disease. *N. Engl. J. Med.* 1980; **302**: 1383–9.

21. Cambien, F., Jacqueson, A., Richard, J.L., Warnet, J.M., Ducimetiere, P. and Claude, J.R. Is the level of serum triglyceride a significant predictor of coronary death in 'normocholesterolemic' subjects? *Am. J. Epidemiol.* 1986; **124**: 624–32.

22. Castelli, W.P. The triglyceride issue: A view from Framingham. *Am. Heart J.* 1986; **112**: 432–7.

23. European Atherosclerosis Society. Strategies for the prevention of coronary heart disease. *Eur. Heart J.* 1987; **8**: 77–88.

24. Report of British Cardiac Society Working Group on Coronary Disease Prevention. London: British Cardiac Society, 1987.

25. Shekelle, R.B., Shryock, A.M., Paul, O. *et al.* Diet, serum cholesterol and death from coronary heart disease. The Western Electric Study. *N. Engl. J. Med.* 1981; **304**: 65–70.

26. Morris, J.N. and Marr, J.W. Diet and heart: a postscript. *Br. Med. J.* 1977; **2**: 1307–14.

27. International Collaborative Study Group. Metabolic epidemiology of within population and between populations. *Lancet* 1986; **ii**: 991–6.

28. Mensink, R.P. and Katan, M.B. Effect of monounsaturated fatty acids versus complex carbohydrates on high-density lipoproteins in healthy men and women. *Lancet* 1987; **i**: 122–5.

29. Anonymous. The Bran Wagon [Editorial]. *Lancet* 1987; **i**: 782–3.

30. MacGregor, G.A. Salt and blood pressure. In: Yu, P.N. and Goodwin, J.F. eds. *Progress in Cardiology.* Philadelphia: Lea and Febiger, 1986, pp.1–12.

31. Yudkin, J. *Pure, White and Deadly.* London: Davis-Poynter, 1972.

32. Marmot, M.G. Alcohol and coronary heart disease. *Int. J. Epidemiol.* 1984; **13**: 160–7.

33. St Leger, A.S., Cochrane, A.L. and Moore, F. Factors associated with cardiac mortality in developed countries with particular reference to the consumption of wine. *Lancet* 1979; **i**: 1017–20.

34. Klatsky, A.L., Friedman, G.D., Siegelaub, A.B. and Gerard, M.J. Alcohol consumption and blood pressure. Kaiser-Permanente Multiphasic Health Examination data. *N. Engl. J. Med.* 1977; **296**: 1194–200.

35. Shaper, A.G., Phillips, A.N., Pocock, S.J. and Walker, M. Alcohol and ischaemic heart disease in middle-aged British men. *Br. Med. J.* 1987; **294**: 733–7.

36. Bulpitt, C.J., Shipley, M.J. and Semmence, A. The contribution of a moderate amount of alcohol to the presence of hypertension. *J. Hypertens.* 1987; **5**: 85–91.

37. Shaper, A.G., Pocock, S.J., Ashby, D., Walker, M. and Whitehead, T.P. Biochemical and haematological response to alcohol intake. *Ann. Clin. Biochem.* 1985; **22**: 50–61.

38. Arnesen E., Forde, O.H. and Thelle, D.S. Coffee and serum cholesterol. *Br. Med. J.* 1984; **288**: 1960.

39. Kark, J.D., Friedlander, Y., Kaufman, N.A. and Stein, Y. Coffee, tea and plasma cholesterol: the Jerusalem Lipid Research Clinical Prevalence Study. *Br. Med. J.* 1985; **291**: 699–704.

40. La Croix, A.Z., Mead, L.A., Liang, K.Y., Thomas, C.B. and Pearson, T.A. Coffee consumption and the incidence of coronary heart disease. *N. Engl. J. Med.* 1986; **315**: 977–82.

41. LeGrady, D., Dyer, A.R., Shekelle, R.B. *et al.* Coffee consumption and mortality in the Chicago Western Electric Company Study. *Am. J. Epidemiol.* 1987; **126**: 803–12.

42. Sanders, T.A.B. Fish and coronary artery disease. *Br. Heart J.* 1987; **57**: 214–9.

43. Weiner, B.H., Ockere, L.S., Levine, P.H. *et al.* Inhibition of atherosclerosis by cod-liver oil in a hyperlipidaemic swine model. *N. Engl. J. Med.* 1986; **315**: 841–6.

44. Riemersma, R.A., Wood, D.A., Butler, S. *et al.* Linoleic acid content in adipose tissue and coronary heart disease. *Br. Med. J.* 1986; **292**: 1423–7.

45. Wood, D.A., Riemersma, R.A., Butler, S. *et al.* Linoleic and eicosapentaenoic acids in adipose tissue and platelets and risk of coronary heart disease. *Lancet* 1987; **i**: 177–83.

46. Dawber, T.R. *The Framingham Study. The epidemiology of atherosclerotic disease.* Cambridge, Mass.: Harvard University Press, 1980.

47. Lichtenstein, M.J., Shipley, M.J. and Rose, G. Systolic and diastolic blood pressures as predictors of coronary heart disease mortality in the Whitehall Study. *Br. Med. J.* 1985;

291: 243–5.

48. Kaufman, D.W., Palmer, J.R., Rosenberg, L. and Shapiro, S. Cigar and pipe smoking and myocardial infarction in young men. *Br. Med. J.* 1987; **94**: 1315–6.

49. Cook, D.G., Shaper, A.G., Pocock, S.J. and Kussick, S.J. Giving up smoking and the risk of heart attack. A report from the British Regional Heart Study. *Lancet* 1986; ii: 1376–80.

50. Pan, W.-H., Cedres, L.D., Lu, K. *et al*. Relationship of clinical diabetes and asymptomatic hyperglycemia to risk of coronary heart disease mortality in men and women. *Am. J. Epidemiol.* 1986; **123**: 504–16.

51. Perkins, K.A. Family history of coronary heart disease: is it an independent risk factor? *Am. J. Epidemiol.* 1986; **124**: 182–94.

52. Report from the Royal College of Physicians. Obesity. *J. R. Coll. Phys.* 1983; **17**: 1–58.

53. Leon, S. Physical activity levels and coronary heart disease. Analysis of epidemiologic and supporting studies. In: Goldberg, L. and Elliot, D.L., eds. *The Medical Clinics of North America*. Symposium on Medical Aspects of Exercise. Philadelphia: W.B. Saunders, 1985, pp.3–20.

54. Paffenberger, R.S., Hyde, R.T., Wing, A.L. and Steinmetz, C.H. A natural history of athleticism and cardiovascular health. *JAMA* 1984; **252**: 491–5.

55. Review Panel on coronary-prone behaviour and coronary heart disease. Coronary-prone behaviour and coronary heart disease: a critical review. *Circulation* 1981; **63** 1199–215.

56. Johnson, D.W., Cook, D.G. and Shaper, A.G. Type A behaviour and ischaemic heart disease in middle-aged British men. *Br. Med. J.* 1987; **295**: 86–89.

57. OPCS. *Occupational mortality. Decennial supplement, 1979–80. 1980–83. Great Britain*. London: HMSO, 1986.

58. Pocock, S.J., Shaper, A.G., Cook, D.G., Phillips, A.N. and Walker, M. Social class differences in ischaemic heart disease in British men. *Lancet* 1987; i: 197–201.

59. Davies, M.J. and Thomas, A.C. Plaque fissuring: the cause of acute myocardial infarction, sudden ischaemic death and crescendo angina. *Br. Heart J.* 1985; **53**: 363–73.

60. Shaper, A.G., Jones, K.W., Kyobe, J. and Jones, M. Fibrinolysis in relation to body fatness, serum lipids and coronary heart disease in African and Asian men in Uganda. *J. Atherosclerosis Res.* 1966; **6**: 313–27.

61. Meade, T.W., Stirling, Y., Thompson, S.G. *et al*. An international and inter-regional comparison of haemostatic variables in the study of ischaemic heart disease. *Int. J. Epidemiol.* 1986; **15**: 331–6.

62. Wilhelmsen, L., Svardsudd, K., Korsan-Bengtsen, K., Larsson, B., Welin, B. and Tebblin, G. Fibrinogen as a risk factor for stroke and myocardial infarction. *N. Engl. J. Med.* 1984; **311**: 501–5.

63. Hamsten, A., Wiman, B., De Faire, U. and Blomback, M. Increased plasma levels of a rapid inhibitor of tissue plasminogen activator in young survivors of myocardial infarction. *N. Engl. J. Med.* 1985; **313**: 1557–63.

64. Meade, T.W., Imeson, J. and Stirling, Y. Effects of changes in smoking and other characteristics on clotting factors and the risk of ischaemic heart disease. *Lancet* 1987; ii: 986–8.

65. Wilson, P.W.F., Garnson, R.J. and Castelli, W.P. Postmenopausal estrogen use, cigarette smoking and cardiovascular mortality in women over 50 years. The Framingham Study. *N. Engl. J. Med.* 1985; **313**: 1038–43.

66. Stampfer, M.J., Willet, W.C., Colditz, G.A., Rosner, B., Sperzer, F.E. and Hennekens, C.H. A prospective study of postmenopausal estrogen therapy and coronary heart disease. *N. Engl. J. Med.* 1985; **313**: 1044–9.

67. Shaper, A.G., Cook, D.G., Walker, M. and Macfarlane, P.W. Prevalence of ischaemic heart disease in middle-aged British men. *Br. Heart J.* 1984; **51**: 595–605.

68. Shaper, A.G., Cook, D.G., Walker, M. and Macfarlane, P.W. Recall of diagnosis by men with ischaemic heart disease. *Br. Heart J.* 1984; **51**: 606–11.

69. Shaper, A.G., Pocock, S.J., Phillips, A.N. and Walker, M. Identifying men at high risk of heart attack: strategy for use in general practice. *Br. Med. J.* 1986; **293**: 474–79.

70. *Coronary Risk Handbook. Estimating risk of coronary heart disease in daily practice*. New York: American Heart Association, 1973.

71. Shaper, A.G., Pocock, S.J., Phillips, A.N. and Walker, M. A scoring system to identify men at high risk of a heart attack. *Health Trends* 1987; **19**: 37–9.

72. Kornitzer, M., De Backer, G., Dramaux, M. *et al*. Belgian heart disease prevention project: incidence and mortality results. *Lancet* 1983; i: 1066–70.

73. Stehbens, W.E. An appraisal of the epidemic rise of coronary heart disease and its decline. *Lancet* 1987; i: 606–10.

74. Shaper, A.G. National trends in mortality from ischaemic heart disease: implications for prevention. *Lancet* 1986; i: 795.

75. Campean, L., Enjalbert, M., Lesperance, J. *et al*. The relation of risk factors to the development of atherosclerosis in saphenous vein grafts and the progression of the disease in the native circulation. *N. Engl. J. Med.* 1984; **311**: 1329–32.

76. Shepherd, J. and Packard, C.J. Regression of coronary atherosclerosis: is it possible? *Br. Heart J.* 1988; **59**: 149–50.

77. Report of the Joint Working Party of the Royal College of Physicians of London and the British Cardiac Society. Prevention of Coronary Heart Disease 1976. *J. R. Coll. Phys.* 1976; **10**: 213–76.

78. WHO Expert Committee. *Prevention of Coronary Heart Disease*, Technical Report Series No. 678. Geneva: WHO, 1982.

79. DHSS Committee on Medical Aspects of Food Policy: Panel on diet in relation to cardiovascular disease. London: HMSO, 1984.

80. Medical Research Council Working Party. MRC Trial of treatment of mild hypertension: principal results. *Br. Med. J.* 1985; **291**: 97–104.

81. Committee of Principal Investigators. WHO Cooperative trial on primary prevention of ischaemic heart disease with clofibrate to lower serum cholesterol: final mortality follow-up. *Lancet* 1984; ii: 600–4.

82. Lipid Research Clinics Program. The Lipid Research Clinics Coronary Primary Prevention Trial results. The relationship of reduction in incidence of coronary heart disease to cholesterol lowering. *JAMA* 1984; **251**: 365–74.

83. Frick, M.H., Elo, O., Haapa, K. *et al*. Helsinki Heart Study? primary prevention trial with gemfibrozil in middle-aged men with dyslipidemia. *N. Engl. J. Med.* 1987; **317**: 1237–45.

84. Anonymous. Aspirin after myocardial infarction [Leading article]. *Lancet* 1980; i: 1172–3.

85. Canadian Cooperative Study Group. A randomized trial of aspirin and sulfinpyrazone in threatened stroke. *N. Engl. J. Med.* 1978; **199**: 53–9.

86. UK–TIA Study Group. United Kingdom transcient ischaemic attack (UK–TIA) aspirin trial: interim results. *Br. Med. J.* 1988; **296**: 316–20.

87. Antiplatelet Trialists' Collaboration. Secondary prevention of vascular disease by prolonged antiplatelet treatment. *Br. Med. J.* 1988; **296**: 320–31.

88. Peto, R., Gray, R., Collins, R. *et al*. Randomised trial of prophylactic daily aspirin in British male doctors. *Br. Med. J.* 1988; **296**: 313–6.

89. Steering Committee of the Physicians' Health Study Research Group. Preliminary report: findings from the aspirin component of the ongoing physician's health study. *N. Engl. J. Med.* 1988; **318**: 262–4.

90. Pocock, S.J., Shaper, A.G. and Phillips, A.N. Concentrations of high density lipoprotein cholesterol, triglycerides and total cholesterol in ischaemic heart disease. *Br. Med. J.* 1989; **298**: 998–1002.
91. Shaper, A.G., Wannamethee, G. and Walker, M. Alcohol and mortality in British men: explaining the U-shaped curve. *Lancet* 1988; **ii**: 1267–73.
92. Phillips, A.N., Shaper, A.G., Pocock, S.J., Walker, M. and Macfarlane, P.W. The role of risk factors in heart attacks occurring in men with pre-existing ischaemic heart disease. *Br. Heart J.* 1988; **60**: 404–10.

POSTSCRIPT

Three recent papers from the British Regional Heart Study bring the chapter up to date.

1. A reappraisal of the role of blood lipids in predicting major IHD events after 7.5 years follow-up and 443 major IHD events. Serum total cholesterol remains the most important single lipid risk factor for heart attack. HDL-cholesterol is significantly (inversely) associated with IHD risk but is less important than total cholesterol. Triglyceride concentratins do not have predictive power once other risk factors have been taken into account.[90]

2. After 7.5 years follow-up, the 504 deaths from all causes showed a U-shaped relationship with alcohol intake. Cardiovascular deaths showed an inverse relationship with alcohol intake. These relationships were only present in men with cardiovascular or cardiovascular-related doctor-diagnosed illnesses at screening. The data suggest that men with such illnesses move from drinking into non-drinking or occasional drinking categories and that the concept of a 'protective' effect of drinking on mortality is ill-founded.[91]

3. The importance of three risk factors—serum total cholesterol, systolic blood pressure and cigarette smoking—on the risk of new major IHD events in men who already have evidence of IHD was assessed after 7.5 years follow-up. The key finding is that the important association between serum total cholesterol and the risk of heart attack persists in men with pre-existing IHD, including those with definite myocardial infarction. The reduction of serum total cholesterol in these men may be at least as important as it is in men without evidence of IHD.[92]

Chapter 43

Hyperlipidaemias

Gilbert R. Thompson

Hyperlipidaemia plays a crucial causal role in the aetiology of atherosclerosis and coronary heart disease, yet few cardiologists have any formal training in lipidology. In this chapter, a guide to the definition and classification of hyperlipidaemia will be provided and the clinical features and management of those genetic disorders of lipoprotein metabolism that predispose to atherosclerosis will be described.

PLASMA LIPIDS AND LIPOPROTEINS

The major lipids in plasma are cholesterol, triglyceride and phospholipid. Only cholesterol and triglyceride are routinely measured in clinical laboratories, serum values being about 3% higher than those of plasma. All three lipids are present together in lipoprotein particles, in which they are rendered water-miscible by interacting with apolipoproteins (apoproteins). The relative proportions of the major lipids and apoproteins, and the nature of the latter, vary among the different lipoproteins. These are now usually classified according to their density rather than their electrophoretic mobility. Apoproteins, which are designated alphabetically with a numerical suffix, have a key role in regulating lipoprotein metabolism.[1]

Chylomicrons are large particles which contain mainly triglyceride of dietary origin, together with small amounts of cholesterol and certain apoproteins, including $apoB_{48}$ and apoE. They are normally undetectable after a 12-hour fast but their presence increases the triglyceride content of non-fasting samples. The other triglyceride-rich lipoprotein in plasma is very low density lipoprotein (VLDL or preβ-lipoprotein) which transports triglyceride of endogenous origin. These particles are the main determinant of the triglyceride concentration of fasting samples and they also contain appreciable amounts of cholesterol and various apoproteins, including $apoB_{100}$ and apoE. Chylomicrons and VLDL both undergo hydrolysis by the enzyme lipoprotein lipase, to give rise to chylomicron and VLDL remnants (Fig.43.1). These are cleared by the liver but a proportion of VLDL remnants (sometimes called intermediate density lipoprotein or IDL) remains in plasma and undergoes conversion to low density lipoprotein (LDL or β-lipoprotein). Low density lipoprotein carries most of the cholesterol and immunoassayable $apoB_{100}$ present in plasma. Increased levels can result from overproduction via VLDL or from decreased clearance, a process largely mediated by hepatic LDL receptors.[2] High density lipoproteins (HDL or α-lipoprotein) are subdivided into HDL_2 and the smaller HDL_3, women having higher levels of the former than do men. These particles are derived from the liver and the small intestine, as illustrated in Fig. 43.1. They consist mainly of phospholipid and apoproteins, notably apoA-I, together with some cholesterol of tissue origin, which is destined for excretion via the liver.

QUANTIFICATION OF LIPIDS AND LIPOPROTEINS

Because LDL is the main cholesterol-rich lipoprotein in plasma, hypercholesterolaemia commonly indicates an increased number of LDL particles, although it can also result from an increase in HDL. Fasting hypertriglyceridaemia usually indicates an increase in VLDL but, if gross, it is sometimes due to hyperchylomicronaemia. As an increase in LDL has different implications from an increase in HDL, it is important to quantify their respective contributions to total cholesterol. This is usually done by precipitating VLDL and LDL from serum by addition of polyanion–divalent cation mixtures and then measuring the amount of HDL cholesterol in the supernatant. If the values of total and HDL

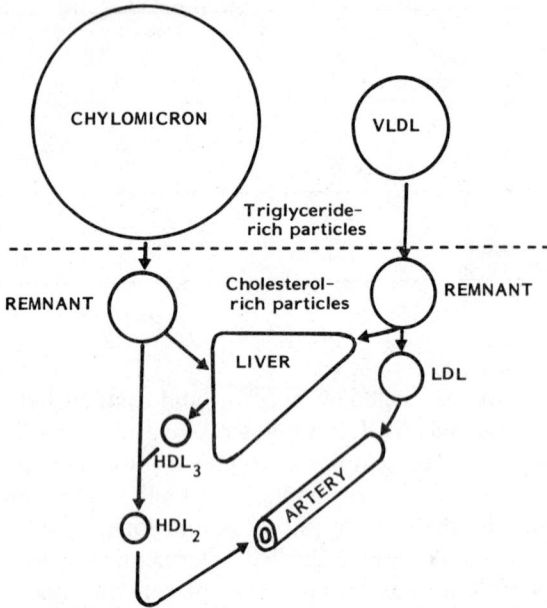

Fig. 43.1. Diagrammatic representation of the conversion of the triglyceride-rich lipoproteins, chylomicrons and VLDL, into remnant particles and thence into the cholesterol-rich lipoproteins, HDL and LDL. The balance between the number of HDL and LDL particles in plasma exerts an important influence on the atherosclerotic process.

cholesterol and of triglyceride are known, it is relatively simple to calculate LDL cholesterol, adapting the formula devised by Friedwald et al.[3]

$$\text{LDL cholesterol}$$
$$= \text{total cholesterol} - \text{the sum of HDL cholesterol}$$
$$- \frac{\text{triglyceride}}{2.2} \quad \text{(mmol/l)}$$

This formula is inaccurate if used on samples that have a triglyceride concentration > 4.5 mmol/l.

Additional information can be obtained by analysing the major apoproteins. Quantification of apoA-I may reveal a deficiency of HDL particles despite a normal HDL cholesterol, and conversely measurement of apoB provides a better index of the number of LDL particles in plasma than does LDL cholesterol.[1] The occurrence of an increase in LDL-apoB despite a normal LDL cholesterol has been termed hyperapoβlipoproteinaemia.[4] Qualitative analysis of apoE phenotypes is also useful, especially in confirming the diagnosis of type III hyperlipoproteinaemia (see below).

DEFINITION OF HYPERLIPIDAEMIA

Hyperlipidaemia may be defined either in statistical terms or according to arbitrary criteria based on the relative risk of coronary heart disease in any given population. The results of most epidemiological studies show positive correlations between coronary heart disease and total or LDL cholesterol and between coronary heart disease and triglyceride, but a negative correlation between coronary heart disease and HDL cholesterol. Although cholesterol and triglyceride levels rise with age the accompanying increase in the risk of coronary heart disease relative to normolipidaemic contemporaries is less marked. Also, at any given level of cholesterol, the risk for men is greater than that for women. These considerations need to be borne in mind when defining hyperlipidaemia. Statistical cut-off levels in a large sample of British men are shown in Fig. 43.2.

The relative risk of coronary heart disease rose steeply in MRFIT when the serum cholesterol exceeded 6.5 mmol/l.[5] This value has been recommended by the British Cardiac Society as the level above which dietary intervention should be instituted and 7.8 mmol/l as the level above which drug therapy might be required.[6] The British Hyperlipidaemia Association Guidelines[7] advocate accept-

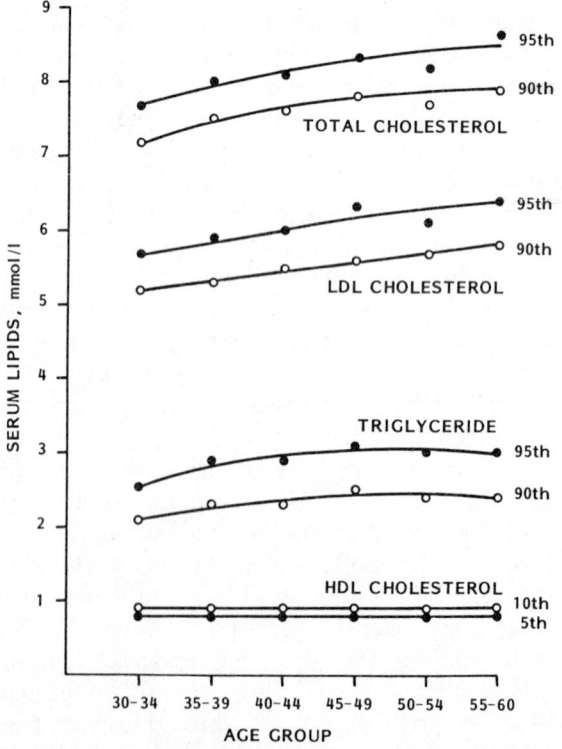

Fig. 43.2. Age-related percentiles of serum lipids and lipoproteins in 6507 men screened at the BUPA Medical Centre, London in 1984. (Courtesy of Dr Carolyn Ritchie, BUPA Medical Research).

ance of 5.2 mmol/l as the optimal level of serum cholesterol for the population at large and also recommend that levels betwen 6.5 and 7.8 mmol/l should normally be treated with diet not drugs, unless the individual concerned has established coronary disease or has undergone coronary artery bypass grafting. However, levels of serum cholesterol above 7.8 mmol/l which fail to respond to dietary intervention and which do not represent hyperalphalipoproteinaemia (HDL cholesterol >2 mmol/l) may necessitate lipid-lowering drug therapy as a primary preventive measure, especially in subjects with a family history of coronary heart disease. The guidelines emphasize that at any given level of serum cholesterol the relative risk of coronary heart disease is less in women than in men and the extent to which risk is reduced by intervention diminishes with increasing age. The need to treat is accentuated if the LDL cholesterol exceeds 5 mmol/l or if the HDL ratio (calculated as HDL cholesterol/total-HDL cholesterol) is below 0.2. Hyperalphalipoproteinaemia is associated with longevity and does not require treatment.

Whether hypertriglyceridaemia plays a causal role in coronary heart disease is debatable and indications for its treatment are less well defined than those for hypercholesterolaemia. However, fasting levels persistently above the 95th percentile (2.5 – 3 mmol/l) are abnormal and probably require treatment, especially if accompanied by a positive family history of coronary heart disease, a decrease in HDL cholesterol or apoA-I or an increase in LDL-apoB. It should be recognized that mild to moderate hypertriglyceridaemia is often iatrogenic, especially in patients on diuretics or beta-adrenergic blockers.

CLASSIFICATION OF HYPERLIPIDAEMIA

Fredrickson et al.[8] described five lipoprotein phenotypes, based on measurement of total cholesterol, triglyceride and LDL cholesterol, aided by lipoprotein electrophoresis. This scheme was later amended by the World Health Organisation to include a sixth phenotype.[9] Despite certain limitations, the WHO classification remains a useful means of indicating which class of lipoproteins is present in excess. Used intelligently it can not only help define the genetic basis of hyperlipidaemia but also provides a guide to therapy. One drawback is that it takes no account of HDL cholesterol, although reduced levels of the latter (hypoαlipoproteinaemia) are associated with increased susceptibility to coronary heart disease.[1]

As shown in Table 43.1, the type I phenotype indicates hypertriglyceridaemia due to hyperchylomicronaemia; in type IIa, hypercholesterolaemia is due solely to an increase in LDL cholesterol whereas in type IIb this is accompanied by mild to moderate hypertriglyceridaemia, due to an increase in VLDL; in type III, serum cholesterol and triglyceride are

---

Table 43.1. **Classification of hyperlipidaemia according to lipoprotein phenotype.**

Type	Plasma (serum) lipids	Lipoprotein abnormality	Primary causes	Secondary causes
I	Hypertriglyceridaemia	Excess chylomicrons	Lipoprotein lipase deficiency, Apo CII deficiency	
IIa	Hypercholesterolaemia	Excess LDL	Familial hypercholesterolaemia,	Hypothyroidism,
IIb	Hypercholesterolaemia + hypertriglyceridaemia	Excess LDL and VLDL	Familial combined hyperlipidaemia	Nephrotic syndrome, Diabetes mellitus, Anorexia nervosa
III	Hypercholesterolaemia + hypertriglyceridaemia	Excess chylomicron and VLDL remnants	Familial type III hyperlipoproteinaemia	Hypothyroidism, Diabetes mellitus, Obesity
IV	Hypertriglyceridaemia ± hypercholesterolaemia	Excess VLDL LDL normal HDL often low	Familial combined hyperlipidaemia, Familial hypertriglyceridaemia	Diabetes mellitus, Chronic renal disease, Alcohol, Diuretics,
V	Hypertriglyceridaemia ± hypercholesterolaemia	Excess chylomicrons and VLDL	Familial hypertriglyceridaemia, Apo CII deficiency	Beta-blockers, Oral contraceptives

both raised, often in equimolar concentrations, due to accumulation of chylomicron and VLDL remnants; in type IV, fasting hypertriglyceridaemia, due to an increase in VLDL, is often accompanied by mild to moderate hypercholesterolaemia but the LDL cholesterol is normal, which distinguishes it from type IIb; in type V, marked hypertriglyceridaemia is due to hyperchylomicronaemia, as in type I, accompanied by an increase in VLDL, as in type IV.

Whatever the phenotype, hyperlipoproteinaemia usually reflects interaction between primary genetic factors and secondary environmental influences, such as diet, drugs or disease. Often the inherited component is polygenically determined and poorly defined but at least three monogenic disorders have now been described. Familial hypercholesterolaemia, usually expressed as a type IIa or sometimes a IIb phenotype, is due to an inherited deficiency or defect of LDL receptors.[10] Familial type III hyperlipoproteinaemia results from inheritance of an abnormal isoform of apoE, although environmental or additional genetic influences must also be present for overt hyperlipidaemia to occur.[11] Familial combined hyperlipidaemia presents with both hypercholesterolaemia and hypertriglyceridaemia (type IIb or IV) and is characterized by the presence of multiple phenotypes (IIa, IIb or IV) in first-degree relatives.[12] Each of these disorders predisposes to atherosclerosis and their clinical features will now be described.

FAMILIAL HYPERCHOLESTEROLAEMIA

This disorder affects approximately 0.2% of the population and is due to inheritance of one mutant gene encoding the LDL receptor (heterozygous familial hypercholesterolaemia), or rarely to inheritance of two mutant alleles (homozygous familial hypercholesterolaemia). The LDL receptor normally has a major role in the catabolism of LDL and thereby regulates its level in plasma. Deficient expression or defective function of LDL receptors in familial hypercholesterolaemia results in accumulation of LDL, causing hypercholesterolaemia from birth. Serum total cholesterol ranges between 8 and 15 mmol/l in adult heterozygotes and between 15 and 25 mmol/l in homozygotes. Triglyceride levels are usually normal in affected children, most of whom exhibit a type IIa phenotype, but a type IIb phenotype is quite common in adults. High density lipoprotein cholesterol is normal or reduced.

A definitive diagnosis of familial hypercholester-

olaemia depends upon identifying the mutant gene or demonstrating a deficiency of LDL receptors in fresh or cultured cells.[13] However, the presence of tendon xanthomata in an individual with a type IIa or IIb phenotype or of a raised LDL cholesterol in someone with a hypercholesterolaemic first-degree relative with tendon xanthomata is presumptive proof of heterozygous familial hypercholesterolaemia. Homozygotes result from unions between two heterozygotes, which are often consanguineous. Criteria for diagnosing familial hypercholesterolaemia in infancy and childhood are described elsewhere.[14]

Homozygous familial hypercholesterolaemia

This rare condition is characterized by extreme hypercholesterolaemia and the early onset of cutaneous planar or tuberose xanthomata, tendon xanthomata and corneal arcus. Atheromatous involvement of the aortic root is evident by puberty, manifested by an aortic systolic murmur without a click, a gradient across the aortic valve and narrowing of the aortic root.[15] Coronary ostial stenosis is commonly seen on angiography or two-dimensional echocardiography.[16] Sudden death from acute coronary insufficiency during the late teens or early twenties used to be the rule but the introduction of plasma exchange has markedly improved survival.[17,18] At post-mortem, the aortic valve, sinuses of Valsalva and ascending arch of the aorta are grossly infiltrated with atheroma. Less severe changes are found in the abdominal aorta, pulmonary artery, carotid arteries and circle of Willis. Histologically, the lesions are typical of advanced atherosclerosis.[19]

The age of onset and severity of cardiovascular involvement depends upon the nature of the gene defect,[20] being earlier and worse when the abnormality is an inability to produce mature receptors (receptor-negative) than when mature but abnormal receptors are formed (receptor-defective). This rather than the sex of the individual or their HDL cholesterol determines the clinical outcome in homozygotes.

The management of homozygous familial hypercholesterolaemia presents a major therapeutic challenge. Dietary and drug regimens have little impact on the hypercholesterolaemia and the same applies to partial ileal bypass. Portacaval shunt occasionally has a dramatic effect but the most reliable means of reducing cholesterol levels is to undertake plasma exchange at two-weekly intervals.[17] This has been shown to be safe for periods of as long as 10 years and to improve prognosis.[18] Liver transplantation remedies the hepatic deficiency of LDL receptors and results in near normal cholesterol levels[21] but necessitates long-term immunosuppression. Although plasma exchange slows down the rate of progression of aortocoronary atherosclerosis,[22] it may be necessary to undertake coronary artery bypass grafting for coronary ostial stenosis and to replace the aortic valve if this becomes significantly fibrosed, which usually involves widening the aortic root first.[23]

Heterozygous familial hypercholesterolaemia

Heterozygous familial hypercholesterolaemia may be detected early when screening the children or siblings in an affected family but often remains undiagnosed until the onset of cardiovascular symptoms in adult life. There is a marked increase in the risk of premature coronary heart disease in males and females, such that the frequency of familial hypercholesterolaemia in patients presenting with myocardial infarction is roughly tenfold greater than that in the population at large.[24] In addition to hypercholesterolaemia, heterozygotes often show visible signs of cholesterol deposition, such as corneal arcus, xanthelasma and tendon xanthomata (Pl. 43. 1a and b). Characteristic sites for the latter are the extensor tendons on the back of the hands and elbows, the Achilles tendon and the patellar tendon insertion into the pre-tibial tuberosity. Some patients exhibit a systolic ejection murmur, indicative of atherosclerotic involvement of the aortic root.

If left untreated 50% of males and 12% of females with heterozygous familial hypercholesterolaemia develop coronary heart disease by the age of 50 years, rising to 85% and 57%, respectively by the age of 60 years.[25] It has been estimated that the onset of coronary heart disease occurs about 20 years earlier than in the remainder of the population.[26] One factor influencing the presence of vascular disease is the HDL cholesterol, high levels being protective;[27] another factor is smoking, the age of onset of coronary heart disease in women with familial hypercholesterolaemia who smoke being similar to that in men.[28]

On angiography, over 70% of male heterozygotes have triple-vessel disease, including 32% with disease of the left main stem.[29] Lesions occur in both the proximal and distal portions of affected vessels compared with normocholesterolaemic smokers, in whom distal lesions affecting a single vessel are quite common. Completely occluded vessels and coronary ectasia were also found to be much commoner in familial hypercholesterolaemic patients. Because of the severity and potentially hazardous nature of coronary disease in this disorder, exercise tests should be performed routinely on all affected adults and coronary angiography should be undertaken urgently if there is any suspicion of myocardial ischaemia.

The treatment of heterozygous familial hypercholesterolaemia usually involves drug therapy although the effects of a low cholesterol, high polyunsaturated:saturated fat ratio diet should always be tried initially and maintained thereafter. If this does not reduce the total cholesterol to < 7 mmol/l and increase the HDL ratio to > 0.2, an anion-exchange resin such as cholestyramine should be given in a dose of 8 g twice or thrice daily. In patients with a type IIb phenotype, this may need supplementing with a triglyceride-lowering agent such as nicotinic acid or one of the fibric acid derivatives. Partial ileal bypass can be useful in patients who are intolerant of resins.[30] The effectiveness of both these approaches is markedly enhanced by concomitant administration of an HMG CoA reductase inhibitor, such as lovastatin (mevinolin),[31] which helps to overcome the compensatory increase in cholesterol syntheses that they cause. Plasma exchange has been used in an attempt to induce regression of coronary disease in heterozygotes,[22] and the recent advent of LDL apheresis, which selectively removes LDL but not HDL,[32] holds greater promise, especially when used in conjuction with a cholesterol synthesis inhibitor. Despite these measures, it will sometimes be necessary to resort to coronary artery bypass grafting, especially in those with left main stem disease. Post-operative control of hypercholesterolaemia is vital if graft atherosclerosis is to be avoided.[23] Familial hypercholesterolaemic patients should never smoke, and if female, should avoid oral contraceptives with a high content of oestrogen.

FAMILIAL TYPE III HYPERLIPOPROTEINAEMIA

This disorder is characterized by the accumulation in plasma of chylomicron and VLDL remnants, which fail to get cleared by the liver because they contain apoE$_2$ instead of the normal isoform, apoE$_3$. Most type III patients are homozygous for apoE$_2$ but some are heterozygous, exhibiting an apoE$_2$/E$_3$ or apoE$_2$/E$_4$ phenotype. Inheritance of the apoprotein abnormality alone, which occurs in 1% of the population, is not sufficient to cause the full clinical picture of the disorder, which occurs in only 1:10 000 individuals, and other factors must also be present, such as obesity, hypothyroidism, diabetes mellitus or the gene for familial combined hyperlipidaemia.[11] Drugs such as beta-blockers and diuretics may have a similar role.

Type III hyperlipoproteinaemia seldom presents in males before puberty; in females, it is rare before the menopause. Clinical features include corneal arcus, xanthelasma, eruptive or tubero-eruptive xanthomata on the knees and elbows and, characteristically, the presence of palmar striae (Pl. 43. 1c). Tendon xanthomata may also occur. Serum cholesterol and triglyceride are both elevated, usually to about 10 mmol/l, and lipoprotein electrophoresis shows the 'broad β' band characteristic of remnant particles. The diagnosis should be confirmed by apoE phenotyping whenever possible. Other abnormalities which often co-exist are hyperuricaemia and glucose intolerance. Vascular disease occurs in over 50% of patients, involving not only the coronary tree but also peripheral and cerebral vessels.[11] The lesions are indistinguishable from those seen in other types of hyperlipidaemia.[33]

Management of type III hyperlipoproteinaemia involves first looking for and remedying any obvious precipitating factor, such as hypothyroidism or diabetes mellitus. Obesity is common and should be treated with a calorie-restricted modified fat diet designed to achieve ideal body weight. In addition, most patients will require therapy with a fibric acid derivative such as bezafibrate or gemfibrozil. Clofibrate is just as effective but has the drawback of increasing the risk of gallstones. Providing body weight can be controlled, administration of one of these drugs will usually result in virtual normalization of serum lipids and rapid regression of cutaneous xanthomata. Anion-exchange resins aggravate the hyperlipidaemia and are contraindicated. Patients who are double heterozygotes for type III hyperlipoproteinaemia and familial hypercholesterolaemia may need a combination of bezafibrate and lovastatin.[31]

FAMILIAL COMBINED HYPERLIPIDAEMIA

Goldstein et al.[12] were the first to describe this disorder which they considered was the commonest cause of hyperlipidaemia in survivors of a myocardial infarct below the age of 60 years. The results of family studies suggested that the disorder was monogenically inherited although its phenotypic expression varied considerably among individuals within a family. Overall, roughly 50% of the relatives of affected subjects were hyperlipidaemic, of whom one-third had hypercholesterolaemia (type IIa), one-third had hypertriglyceridaemia (types IV or V) and one-third had both abnormalities (type IIb). Affected children presented with type IV or IIb phenotypes but not with a type IIa phenotype, differing in this respect from subjects with familial hypercholesterolaemia. The disorder differs also from familial hypertriglyceridaemia in that individuals with the latter condition exhibit type IV or V phenotypes, but never type IIa or IIb phenotypes.

Familial combined hyperlipidaemia has several features in common with hyperapoβlipoproteinaemia, including raised LDL–apoB levels in plasma due to increased synthesis of VLDL–apoB. These findings suggest that the underlying abnormality in both disorders may reside in a genetic defect causing overproduction of $apoB_{100}$. Analysis of restriction fragment length polymorphism at the promoter end of the apoB may provide the answer to this question.

Until a genetic marker becomes available, familial combined hyperlipidaemia will continue to be diagnosed mainly by exclusion. There are no distinctive physical signs, in contrast with familial hypercholesterolaemia or familial hypertriglyceridaemia. Eruptive xanthomata can occur in the latter condition (Pl. 43. 1d) but it carries a much lower risk of coronary heart disease than familial combined hyperlipidaemia.[34] In general, adults with a type IIb phenotype who do not have familial hypercholesterolaemia or any secondary cause can be regarded as having familial combined hyperlipidaemia. The response of such individuals to diet should always be tried first but if inadequate then a fibric acid derivative such as gemfibrozil is often effective.

EFFECT OF TREATING HYPERLIPIDAEMIA ON CORONARY HEART DISEASE

The beneficial effects of lowering serum cholesterol have been demonstrated in several trials of primary prevention of coronary heart disease and of secondary intervention, as reviewed elsewhere.[35] These showed that reducing serum cholesterol on average by just over 1 mmol/l by diet or drugs resulted in significant decreases in the incidence of coronary heart disease and the rate of progression of coron-

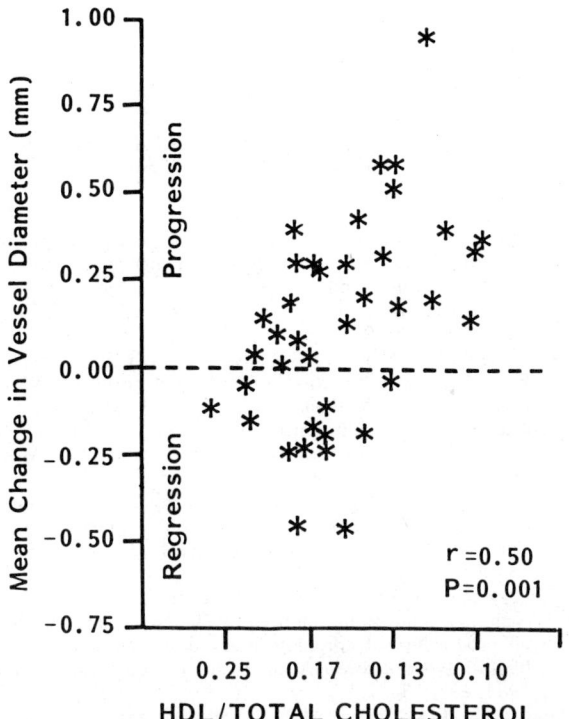

Fig. 43.3. Correlation between change in coronary lesions and the HDL to total cholesterol ratio in patients in the Leiden Intervention Trial. (Reprinted, after modification, by permission of the author and the editor of the *New England Journal of Medicine: N. Engl. J. Med.* 1985; **312**: 805.)

ary lesions. A close relationship was observed between progression or regression of lesions and the ratio of HDL to total cholesterol achieved by diet,[36] as shown in Fig. 43.3. Similarly, the HDL ratio or the ratio of HDL to LDL cholesterol were the best predictors of angiographic change in trials in which cholestyramine[37] or clofibrate and nicotinic acid were used,[38] each of these ratios being negatively correlated with progression of coronary disease. Further reports of the benefits of therapeutic measures that increase HDL cholesterol and decrease LDL cholesterol have recently been published;[39,40] it is hoped that the advent of newer and more potent drugs such as lovastatin and simvastatin will render lipid-lowering therapy an easier and more rewarding endeavour than hitherto.

REFERENCES

1. Thompson, G. Apoproteins: determinants of lipoprotein metabolism and indices of coronary risk. *Br. Heart J.* 1984; **51**: 585–8.
2. Brown, M.S. and Goldstein, J.L. How LDL receptors influence cholesterol and atherosclerosis. *Sci. Am.* 1984; **251**: 52–60.
3. Friedewald, W.T., Levy, R.I. and Fredrickson, D.S. Estimation of the concentration of low-density lipoprotein cholesterol in plasma, without use of the preparative ultracentrifuge. *Clin. Chem.* 1972; **18**: 499–502.
4. Sniderman, A., Shapiro, S., Marpole, D., Skinner, B., Teng, B. and Kwiterovich, P.O. Association of coronary atherosclerosis with hyperapobetalipoproteinemia [increased protein but normal cholesterol levels in human low density (β) lipoproteins]. *Proc. Natl. Acad. Sci. U.S.A.* 1980; **77**: 604–8.
5. Martin, M.J., Hulley, S.B., Browner, W.S., Kuller, L.H. and Wentworth, D. Serum cholesterol, blood pressure and mortality: implications from a cohort of 361 662 men. *Lancet* 1986; **2**: 933–6.
6. The British Cardiac Society Working Group on Coronary Prevention: conclusions and recommendations. *Br. Heart J.* 1987; **57**: 188–9.
7. Shepherd, J., Betteridge, D.J., Durrington, P. *et al*. Strategies for reducing coronary heart disease and desirable limits for blood lipids for blood lipid concentrations: guidelines of the British Hyperlipidaemia Association. *Br. Med. J.* 1987; **295**: 1245–6.
8. Fredrickson, D.S., Levy, R.I. and Lees, R.S. Fat transport in lipoproteins—an integrated approach to mechanisms and disorders *N. Engl. J. Med.* 1967; **276**: 148–56.
9. Beaumont, J.L., Carlson, L.A., Cooper, G.R., Fejfar, A., Fredrickson, D.S. and Strasser, T. Classification of hyperlipidaemias and hyperlipoproteinaemias. *Bull. WHO* 1970; **43**: 891–908.
10. Goldstein, J.L. and Brown, M.S. Familial hypercholesterolemia. In: Stanbury, J.B., Wyngaarden, J.B., Fredrickson, D.S., Goldstein, J.L. and Brown, M.S., eds. *The Metabolic Basis of Inherited Disease*, 5th edn. New York: McGraw Hill, 1983; pp. 672–712.
11. Brown, M.S., Goldstein, J.L. and Fredrickson, D.S. Familial type 3 hyperlipoproteinemia (dysbetalipoproteinemia). In: Stanbury, J.B., Wyngaarden, J.B., Fredrickson, D.S., Goldstein, J.L. and Brown, M.S., eds. *The Metabolic Basis of Inherited Disease*, 5th edn. New York: McGraw Hill, 1983; pp. 655–71.
12. Goldstein, J.L., Schrott, H.G., Hazzard, W.R., Bierman, E.L. and Motulsky, A.G. Hyperlipidemia in coronary heart disease. II. Genetic analysis of lipid levels in 176 families and delineation of a new inherited disorder, combined hyperlipidemia. *J. Clin. Invest.* 1973; **52**: 1544–68.
13. Cuthbert, J.A., East, C.A., Bilheimer, D.W. and Lipsky, P.E. Detection of familial hypercholesterolemia by assaying functional low density lipoprotein receptors on lymphocytes. *N. Engl. J. Med.* 1986; **314**: 879–83.
14. Thompson, G.R. The hyperlipidaemias. In: Lloyd, J.K. and Scriver, C.R., eds. *Genetic and Metabolic Disease in Pediatrics*. London: Butterworths, 1985; pp. 211–33.
15. Allen, J.M., Thompson, G.R., Myant, N.B., Steiner, R. and Oakley, C.M. Cardiovascular complications of homozygous familial hypercholesterolaemia. *Br. Heart J.* 1980; **44**: 361–8.
16. Ribiero, P., Shapiro, L.M., Gonzalez, A., Thompson, G.R. and Oakley, C.M. Cross sectional echocardiographic assessment of the aortic root and coronary ostial stenosis in familial hypercholesterolaemia. *Br. Heart J.* 1983; **50**: 432–7.
17. Thompson, G.R., Lowenthal, R. and Myant, N.B. Plasma exchange in the management of homozygous familial hypercholesterolaemia. *Lancet* 1975; **1**: 1208–11.
18. Thompson, G.R., Miller, J.P. and Breslow, J.L. Improved survival of patients with homozygous familial hypercholesterolaemia treated by plasma exchange. *Br. Med. J.* 1985; **291**: 1671–3.
19. Buja, L.M., Kovanen, P.T. and Bilheimer, D.W. Cellular pathology of homozygous familial hypercholesterolemia.

Am. J. Pathol. 1979; **97**: 327–45.

20. Tolleshaug, H., Hobgood, K.K., Brown, M.S. and Goldstein, J.L. The LDL receptor locus in familial hypercholesterolemia: multiple mutations disrupt transport and processing of a membrane receptor. *Cell* 1983; **32**: 941–51.

21. Bilheimer, D.W., Goldstein, J.L., Grundy, S.M., Starzl, T.E. and Brown, M.S. Liver transplantation to provide low-density-lipoprotein receptors and lower plasma cholesterol in a child with homozygous familial hypercholesterolemia. *N. Engl. J. Med.* 1984; **311**: 1658–64.

22. Thompson, G.R., Myant, N.B., Kilpatrick, D., Oakley, C.M., Raphael, M.J. and Steiner, R.E. Assessment of long-term plasma exchange for familial hypercholesterolaemia. *Br. Heart J.* 1980; **43**: 680–8.

23. Thompson, G.R. and Sapsford, R. Coronary artery bypass grafting and hyperlipidaemia. *Br. Heart J.* 1985; **53**: 237–9.

24. Goldstein, J.L. and Brown, M.S. Hyperlipidemia in coronary heart disease: a biochemical genetic approach. *J. Lab. Clin. Med.* 1975; **85**: 15–25.

25. Slack, J. Risk of ischaemic heart disease in familial hyperlipoproteinaemic states. *Lancet* 1969; **2**: 1380–2.

26. Stone, N.J., Levy, R.I., Fredrickson, D.S. and Verter, J. Coronary artery disease in 116 kindred with familial Type II hyperlipoproteinemia. *Circulation* 1974; **49**: 476–88.

27. Streja, D., Steiner, G. and Kwiterovich, P.O. Plasma high-density lipoproteins and ischaemic heart disease: studies in a large kindred with familial hypercholesterolemia. *Ann. Intern. Med.* 1978; **89**: 871–80.

28. Beaumont, V., Jacotot, B. and Beaumoint, J.-L. Ischaemic disease in men and women with familial hypercholesterolaemia and xanthomatosis. A comparative study of genetic and environmental factors in 274 heterozygous cases. *Atherosclerosis* 1976; **24**: 441–50.

29. Sugrue, D.D., Thompson, G.R., Oakley, C.M., Trayner, I.M. and Steiner, R.E. Contrasting patterns of coronary atherosclerosis in normocholesterolaemic smokers and patients with familial hypercholesterolaemia. *Br. Med. J.* 1981; **283**: 1358–60.

30. Spengel, F.A., Jadhav, A., Duffield, R.G.M., Wood, C.B. and Thompson, G.R. Superiority of partial ileal bypass over cholestyramine in reducing cholesterol in familial hypercholesterolaemia. *Lancet* 1981; **2**: 768–70.

31. Thompson, G.R., Ford, J., Jenkinson, M. and Trayner, I. Efficacy of mevinolin as adjuvant therapy for refractory familial hypercholesterolaemia. *Q. J. Med.* 1986; **60**: 801–9.

32. Yokoyama, S., Hayashi, R., Satani, M. and Yamamoto, A. Selective removal of low density lipoprotein by plasmapheresis in familial hypercholesterolemia. *Arteriosclerosis* 1985; **5**: 613–22.

33. Cabin, H.C., Schwartz, D.E., Virmani, R., Brewer, H.B. and Roberts, W.C. Type III hyperlipoproteinemia: quantification, distribution and nature of atherosclerotic coronary arterial narrowing in five necropsy patients. *Am. Heart J.* 1981; **102**: 830–5.

34. Brunzell, J.D., Schrott, H.G., Motulsky, A.G. and Bierman, E.L. Myocardial infarction in the familial forms of hypertriglyceridemia. *Metabolism* 1976; **25**: 313–20.

35. Thompson, G.R. Evidence that lowering serum lipids favourably influences coronary heart disease. *Q. J. Med.* 1987; **62**: 87–95.

36. Arntzenius, A.C., Kromhout, D., Barth, J.D. *et al.* Diet, lipoproteins and the progression of coronary atherosclerosis. The Leiden Intervention Trial. *N. Engl. J. Med.* 1985; **312**: 805–11.

37. Levy, R.I., Brensike, J.F., Epstein, S.E. *et al.* The influence of changes in lipid values induced by cholestyramine and diet on progression of coronary artery disease: results of the NHLBI type II coronary intervention study. *Circulation* 1984; **69**: 325–37.

38. Nikkila, E.A., Viikinkoski, P., Valle, M. and Frick, M.H. Prevention of progression of coronary atherosclerosis by treatment of hyperlipidaemia: a seven year prospective angiographic study. *B. Med. J.* 1984; **289**: 220–3.

39. Blankenhorn, D.H., Nessim, S.A., Johnson, R.L. *et al.* Beneficial effects of combined colestipol-niacin therapy on coronary atherosclerosis and coronary venous bypass grafts. *JAMA* 1987; **257**: 3233–40.

40. Frick, M.H., Elo, O., Haapa, K. *et al.* Helsinki Heart Study: primary prevention trial with gemfibrozil in middle-aged men with dyslipidaemia. *N. Engl. J. Med.* 1987; **317**: 1237–45.

Chapter 44

The Pathology of Ischaemic Heart Disease

M.J. Davies

The majority of ischaemic heart disease results, directly or indirectly, from the presence of atheroma in the coronary arteries, but rarer conditions such as emboli, arteritis and congenital anomalies can also lead to ischaemic myocardial damage. Atheroma itself is described in Chapter 45; in this chapter, only the sequelae of the basic disease process as it affects the heart will be discussed.

PHYSIOLOGICAL CONSIDERATIONS

The characteristics of myocardial metabolism and blood flow influence the clinical expression of ischaemic damage to the heart. The myocardium generates energy, within the mitochondria, by the aerobic metabolism of glucose and fatty acids to regenerate the high-energy phosphates creatinine and adenosine triphosphate (ATP), which are used, in turn, to generate myocyte contraction by the interaction of calcium ions and adenosine triphosphatase on the myofibrils. A small, but significant, aliquot of energy is used to maintain membrane integrity both within the cell and in relation to the extracellular environment. Sodium, calcium and potassium ions within the cell all have high concentration gradients in relation to the interstitial tissues and the maintenance of these gradients requires energy expenditure.

Cardiac muscle is required to contract and relax constantly but, intermittently, it is also required to increase both the rate and force of contraction, for example, during physical exercise. The abstraction of oxygen from the blood by the myocardium is high at rest. Increased energy demand by the myocardium therefore cannot be met by increasing the oxygen extraction, yet myocardial muscle cells have a limited capacity for anaerobic energy production. An increased energy demand can be met only by a rapid rise in blood flow making the myocardium particularly vulnerable to any factor that limits such an increase.

Intramyocardial blood flow occurs during diastole, flow in systole being prevented by the compressive effect of ventricular contraction. The epicardial arteries are not subject to this compression and fill in systole. As the ventricular myocardium relaxes in diastole, blood is sucked into the intramyocardial vessels from the epicardial coronary arteries and aortic root. When ventricular contraction begins, blood is squeezed from the myocardium into the coronary sinus and, for a brief period, flow is reversed in the epicardial arteries.

Myocardial blood flow is directly proportional to diastolic pressure and inversely proportional to vascular resistance.[1,2] Myocardial oxygen consumption is the predominant determinant of myocardial blood flow (metabolic regulation) and little variation follows changes in perfusion pressure alone (autoregulation). Flow is controlled by variations in tone in the small resistance vessels within the myocardium thus the increase of intramyocardial blood flow on exercise is brought about largely by a decrease of vascular resistance within the myocardium.[3]

The epicardial coronary arteries are regional, i.e. each major branch supplies one segment of the myocardium. Under artificial conditions in the dead human heart, low viscosity media injected down one coronary artery orifice will emerge, eventually, from the other orifice. In man, as well as experimental animals such as the pig, sudden ligation of a major coronary artery branch often leads to death of a segment of myocardial muscle; it is in this sense that coronary arteries are regarded as regional end-arteries. In smaller animals, such as rodents, intramyocardial anastomotic flow is so great that ligation of one coronary artery does not lead to regional myocardial necrosis.

ANATOMY OF THE CORONARY ARTERIES

There is a basic pattern to the coronary artery

anatomy in man, but also considerable individual variation in detail. Most individuals possess two coronary arteries opening from the right and left aortic sinuses, respectively. The level at which the arteries arise, in relation to the junction between the aortic sinuses and the aorta (supra-aortic ridge), varies. Most ostia are a few millimetres above this ridge but an origin a centimetre or more into the aorta or from the sinus itself is not unusual. The main left coronary artery varies considerably in length, being at one extreme over a centimetre in length to, at the other extreme, being absent; in this latter case, the left anterior descending and left circumflex arteries open from the left aortic sinus by separate orifices.

The branches of the left anterior descending artery supply the anterior two-thirds of the interventricular septum and the anterior wall of the left ventricle, comprising at least 50% of the overall mass of the left ventricular myocardium. The first septal perforating branch running into the interventricular septum is constant in position but the other branches of the left anterior descending artery vary in pattern; there may be a division into two relatively large arteries immediately after the first septal branch or a single artery may pass to the apex of the ventricle.

The left circumflex artery passes laterally in the left atrioventricular groove, and branches supply the lateral wall of the left ventricle, including the antero-lateral papillary muscle.

The right coronary artery runs in the atrioventricular groove around the right ventricle to reach the posterior wall of the left ventricle supplying the postero-medial papillary muscle in most cases. The right ventricular myocardium is supplied by branches of the right coronary artery, the first of which, the conus branch, in approximately 30% of hearts has a small separate orifice in the right aortic sinus.

The right and left circumflex arteries are inversely related as regards size, and in the proportion of the posterior wall of the left ventricle that each supplies. The term dominance is used to express this relation. In right dominant individuals (70% approximately), the posterior descending artery is derived from the right coronary artery; in left dominant individuals, it is derived from the left circumflex artery. The posterior descending coronary artery supplies the posterior third of the ventricular septum by perforating branches which meet the corresponding branches of the left anterior descending coronary artery. At the apex of the left ventricle, the anterior and posterior descending artery meet. In many

hearts, the anterior descending artery is longer than the posterior descending artery and turns the apex to supply a portion of the posterior wall of the left ventricle. Dominance, as defined so far, is absolute and can be determined at a glance from angiographs or by dissection of the coronary arteries. However, the blood supply to the posterior wall of the left ventricle is also important and here dominance can be used in a relative rather than an absolute sense. The right coronary artery, after giving origin to the posterior descending branch may extend across onto the posterior wall of the left ventricle. If it does, branches supply the left ventricular myocardium until the point at which the termination of the left circumflex artery is met in the atrioventricular groove. In extreme cases, the left circumflex artery is absent and the right coronary continues to supply the whole lateral wall of the left ventricle. At the other extreme, the left circumflex artery crosses the posterior crux of the heart to reach and supply the right ventricle, the right coronary artery being represented only by the conus branch opening directly from the aorta.

The posterior medial papillary artery is supplied by whichever artery, right or, more rarely, left circumflex, has reached the posterior aspect of the left ventricle. The most representative situation is for the left anterior descending artery to supply over 50% of the left ventricular mass, comprising the anterior two-thirds of the septum and the anterior wall, for the right coronary artery to supply the posterior third of the interventricular septum and about half the posterior wall including the papillary muscle, comprising 20–30% of the left ventricular mass, and for the left circumflex artery to supply the lateral wall including the anterolateral papillary muscle making up 10–20% of the left ventricular mass.

INTRAMYOCARDIAL BLOOD FLOW

In the normal human myocardium, a branching system of arteries runs from the epicardium to the endocardium. The main trunks of this intramyocardial system measure 1–2 mm in diameter and are regarded as a continuation of the epicardial conduction vessels but they do have high medial muscle to lumen diameter ratios. Smaller branches of this system measuring 0.1–0.5 mm in diameter are believed to contribute 25% of resistance to flow, the remainder being due to smaller pre-capillary arterioles. A second separate intramyocardial arterial system supplies the trabeculated sub-endocardial myocardium.[4] Straight, non-tapering and non-branching, arteries up to a millimetre in diameter pass direct from the epicardium to the endocardium.

CONTROL OF VASOMOTOR TONE

The epicardial arteries are capable of undergoing a wide variation in lumen diameter resulting from alterations in medial smooth muscle tone. Medial smooth muscle cells are arranged in a regular circumferential manner; in contrast, intimal smooth muscle cells are haphazardly arranged, being concerned with the synthesis of connective tissue components of the intima rather than contraction. Sympathetic and parasympathetic nerve fibrils ramify in the adventitia of the epicardial and intramyocardial arteries but do not enter the media itself.[5] There is evidence for rhythmic basal tone, dependent on calcium, which is modified by mediators diffusing into the media to react with specific receptors on smooth muscle cells. In addition to the adrenergic constrictor and dilator receptors, other normal mediators include neuropeptide Y released from sympathetic nerves and the vasodilator neuropeptides, vaso-intestinal peptide and calcitonin gene-related peptide. Direct infusion of these neuropeptides into human coronary arteries can be used to confirm their actions.[6]

Endothelial cells in arteries down to 20 μm in diameter also release a labile non-prostanoid product, endothelial derived relaxant factor, possibly nitric oxide, which has potent vasodilator effects based on stimulating guanylate cylase in the smooth muscle cell.[7,8] Small amounts of endothelial derived relaxant factor are released constantly; reduced oxygen tension, viscous drag of blood flow, increased pulsatile pressure and a wide range of substances including acetylcholine, substance P and 5-hydroxytryptamine all increase the amount released. The vasodilatory effect of such substances as acetylcholine and serotonin is based on release of endothelial derived relaxant factor and, in the absence of a normal endothelial surface, these substances have a directly constrictor affect on smooth muscle cells. It is not known if differences exist in the innervation or receptor status of the epicardial and intramyocardial arteries of different regions. The very close relation between intramyocardial blood flow and demand, which can vary from beat to beat, is thought to be dependent on local autoregulation of capillaries mediated by factors such as oxygen tension and adenine nucleotides released by myocytes.

THE PATHOLOGY OF ANGINA

STABLE ANGINA

Numerous angiographic studies *in vivo*[9] have shown that patients whose pain is predictable and provoked by a constant level of cardiac work have segments of high-grade stenosis in one or more epicardial coronary arteries. In this context, significant means a reduction of more than 50% in the diameter of the vessel lumen when compared with an adjacent reference segment of 'normal' artery and corresponds to a reduction by 75% in the cross-sectional area of the lumen. The evidence for regarding this degree of stenosis as significant is derived from the practical clinical experience of symptomatic as compared with asymptomatic patients and the theory of flow in tubes. At a standard perfusion pressure, flow begins to fall sharply when the lumen is narrowed by 75% in cross-sectional area from which degree onward there is a significant drop of pressure across the stenosis.[10,11] Work *in vitro* also suggests that the length of the stenotic segment and the number of stenotic segments existing in series, in the same artery, also influence flow by progressively increasing turbulence.[12]

An atheromatous plaque causing this degree of obstruction will have converted a low-resistance conduction vessel into one with significant resistance to flow. To some extent, this can be offset by a compensatory fall in resistance within the distal intramyocardial vessels. However, there will be a point at which this vasodilatory capacity within the myocardium is exhausted and the stenosis due to atheroma in the epicardial arteries becomes flow limiting, usually on exercise.

Autopsy studies of patients who had stable angina in life have confirmed the presence of multiple segments of stenosis, usually in more than one major coronary artery.[13–15] When compared with clinical angiographic studies, pathological studies show a far higher proportion of main left coronary artery stenosis and of involvement of all three coronary arteries. This reflects the inevitable bias of studying dead subjects; clinical series will contain more patients with single-vessel disease. A finding common to both clinical and pathological studies is that patients with stable exertional angina have well-preserved myocardial function although many of these individuals will have had episodes of previous infarction.

The morphology of the stenotic arterial segments in patients with stable angina is important as an aid to understanding both the disease and the results of angioplasty.

At autopsy, the appearances of coronary stenoses are best appreciated by examining arteries which have been distended at physiological pressure during fixation. In such arteries, the lumen is seen to be approximately circular in shape suggesting that the slit and star-shaped lumens, often illustrated in the literature, are to a great extent artefacts of collapsed arteries.[16]

Stenoses can be classified by their possession of certain basic characteristics; atheromatous plaques may be concentric (Fig. 44.1) or eccentric (Fig. 44.2) with regard to the residual lumen and may be fibrous or contain, in addition, a variable amount of lipid.[17] Plaques that are situated eccentrically with respect to the residual lumen allow the retention of an arc of normal medial muscle on the opposite wall of the vessel (Fig. 44.2). The greater the arc of normal vessel wall that surrounds the residual lumen the greater will be the capacity for variations in muscle tone to produce significant alterations in resistance across the stenosis. It has been calculated that with plaques causing > 75% cross-sectional area stenosis, if the arc of normal vessel wall occupies > 16% of the circumference of the residual lumen of the artery, normal variation in

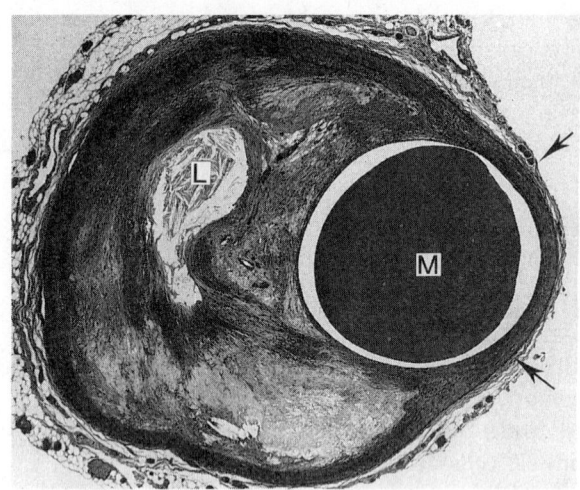

Fig. 44.2. Eccentric stenosis. The lumen containing angiographic media (M) is displaced from the mid-line of the vessel. The intimal thickening, containing a small amount of lipid (L), is eccentric leaving an arc of normal vessel wall (arrows) opposite the plaque.

smooth muscle tone could significantly reduce blood flow.[18–20] An unknown factor in such calculations is the rigidity of the atheromatous plaque which may vary depending on the amount of collagen relative to that of lipid. The shape of the lumen in arteries distended after death at postmortem, and therefore in the total absence of muscle tone, is round; however, in life the presence of rigid eccentric plaques may alter this shape. The degree to which the shape of the lumen deviates from circular would vary with medial tone and it would be D-shaped or oval rather than crescentic in shape.[16]

Beneath atheromatous plaques, the media undergoes striking atrophy[21] and the internal elastic lamina is often disrupted (Fig. 44.3). In concentric stenoses, the majority of the medial muscle is lost therefore and this factor, associated with the thickened and rigid intima, precludes any variation in lumen cross-sectional area. Clinical angiographic studies confirm that a high proportion of eccentric stenoses can be varied in degree by drugs, such as ergonovine and nifedipine, but concentric stenoses remain unaltered.[22]

Patients with coronary atheroma therefore can have stenotic segments that are fixed in the degree of stenosis and those that have the potential for undergoing some degree of alteration. The proportion of the two types of stenosis, fixed or variable, has been reported in several pathological series with divergent results. In some series, variable stenosis

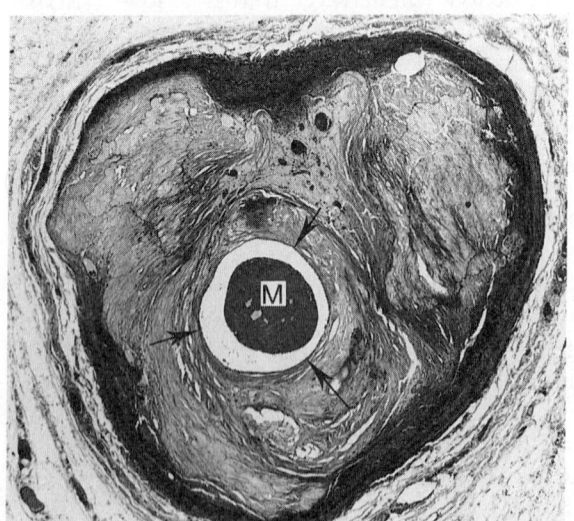

Fig. 44.1. Concentric stenosis. The lumen (arrows) is placed centrally and contains angiographic media (M) which shrinks away from the vessel wall in processing the tissue for histology. The stenosis is due to fibrous thickening of the intima.

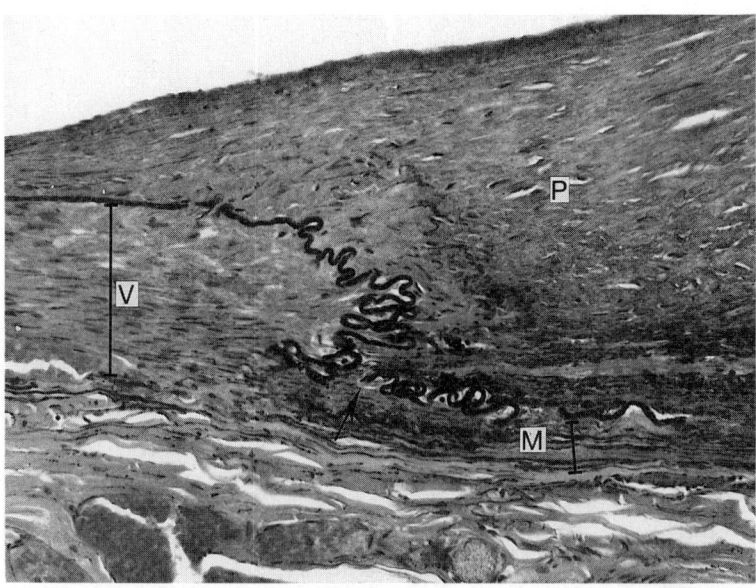

Fig. 44.3. Medial attenuation in atheroma. The media (M) behind an atheromatous plaque (P) which has ruptured the internal elastic lamina (arrow) is markedly thinned as compared to adjacent areas of more normal vessel wall (V).

has been found to be predominant;[19,23] in others, it is rare.[15] There is however immense individual variation from patient to patient, and group data are biased by the selection of different types of patient and clinical presentations. However, it is certain that some patients with stable angina will have no segments of variable high-grade stenosis whereas others will have many. In a pathological study confined to patients with stable angina and excluding those with diabetes, it was found that 56% of patients had at least one segment of eccentric high-grade stenosis with the potential for variation. In a small subset of patients, all the high-grade lesions were eccentric in type.[17] Eccentric stenosis is more common with moderate rather than very high grades of obstruction, thus the majority of patients with exertional angina will have segments of variable stenosis in series with higher grade fixed lesions.

Plaques may also be purely fibrous (Fig. 44.1) or contain a pool of extracellular lipid encapsulated within the intima (Figs. 44.4 and 44.5). The lipid pool varies considerably in volume and contains a complex mixture of cholesterol and its esters which may be semi-fluid at body temperature making the use of the word 'pool' apposite.[24] The lipid within the intima is separated from the arterial lumen by a cap of fibrous tissue.

In addition to stenoses formed by different permutations of the basic characteristics of eccentric or concentric and fibrous or lipid, the majority of patients with stable exertional angina also have one or more arterial segments in which the lumen is occluded by connective tissue within which there is more than one new vascular channel (Fig. 44.6). This appearance is regarded as indicative of recanalization, by organization, of an originally occlusive thrombus.[25] Segments in which the lumen is totally occluded by fibrous tissue but within which recanalization has not occurred are also thought to indicate old occlusive thrombi. The presence of such recanalized arterial segments is not confined to patients with old myocardial infarction; in one pathological study of patients with stable angina, 85% of patients with healed infarcts were found to have such stenoses, and 65% of such patients without healed infarcts had similar arterial lesions.[17]

It is possible in a large group of patients with stable angina to give the overall prevalence of each type of stenotic lesion: 40% of high-grade stenoses are associated with a large lipid pool, conversely 60% are purely fibrous. Such data, however, mask the considerable variation in the types of stenosis found in different individuals. Most patients will have both lipid and fibrous plaques in varying proportions but a minority lie at the extremes and have all fibrous or all lipid lesions.

Other morphological features of stenotic segments, regarded as of possible functional significance include vascularization of the intima, calcification and inflammatory cell infiltration in the adventitia. Thickening of the intima, whether focal, as in the formation of atheromatous plaques, or more diffuse, leads inevitably to the appearance of new capillary vessels within the vessel wall itself. In

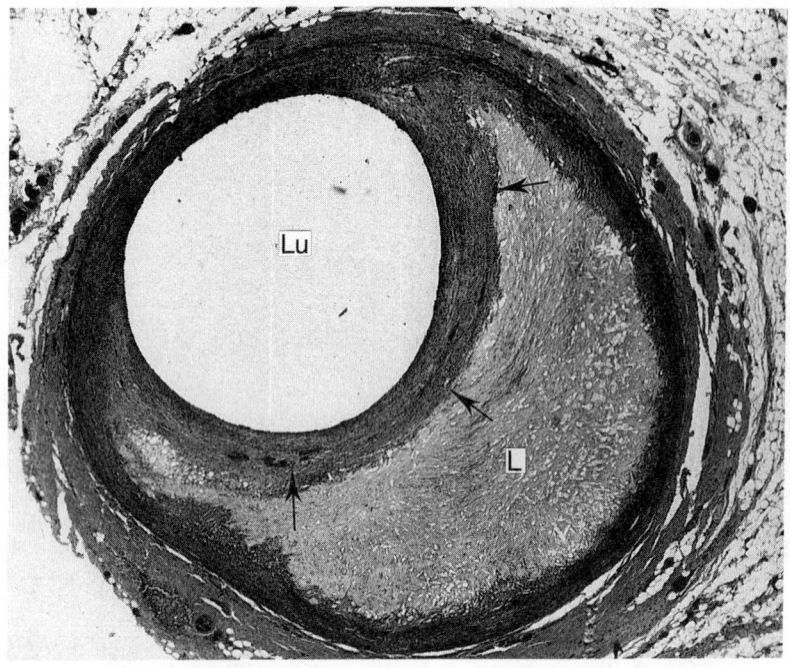

Fig. 44.4. Eccentric stenosis due to a lipid-rich plaque. There is eccentric thickening of the intima displacing the lumen from the mid-line. The intima contains a crescentic paler staining area of lipid (L) spearated from the lumen (LU) by a cap of fibrous tissue (arrows).

normal human coronary arteries, the intima and media are avascular structures but beneath atheromatous plaques new capillaries extend into the media from the adventitia, breach the internal elastic lamina and reach the intima. This enhanced network of small vessels in the adventitia beneath the plaques causing stenosis can be easily identified in angiograms, during life and at autopsy.[26]

Calcification of atheroma occurs either as a shell within the collagen of the intima (Fig. 44.7) at the base of plaque or as irregular nodules within the lipid pool itself. Neither form of calcification is directly related to the degree of stenosis and, to some extent, each is related to age. The calcification has little functional significance other than hindering dissection of the coronary arteries by surgeons or pathologists. Coronary artery calcification, visi-

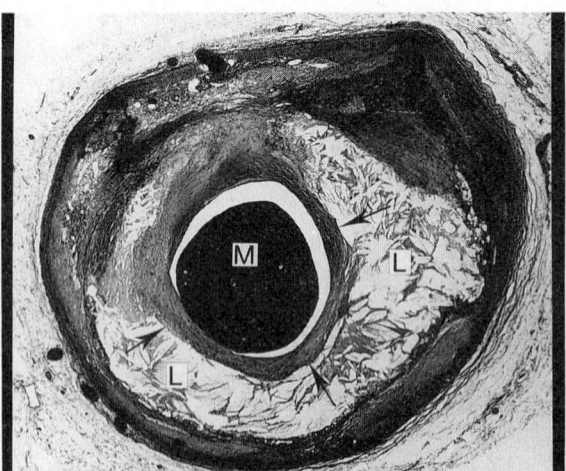

Fig. 44.5. Concentric stenosis due to lipid-rich atheroma. The lumen containing angiographic media (M) is placed centrally. The intima contains a large lipid pool (L) which surrounds most of the circumference of the vessel wall. The lipid mass is separated from the lumen by an intact fibrous cap (arrows).

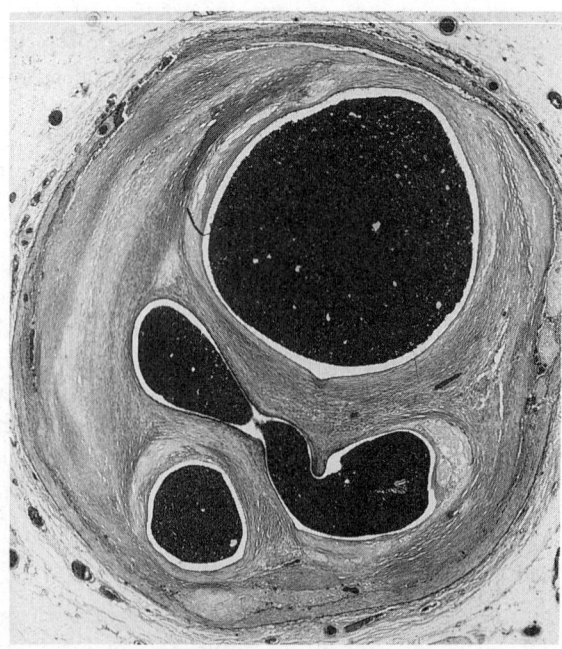

Fig. 44.6. Recanalization. The original lumen contains four new vascular channels each containing angiographic media.

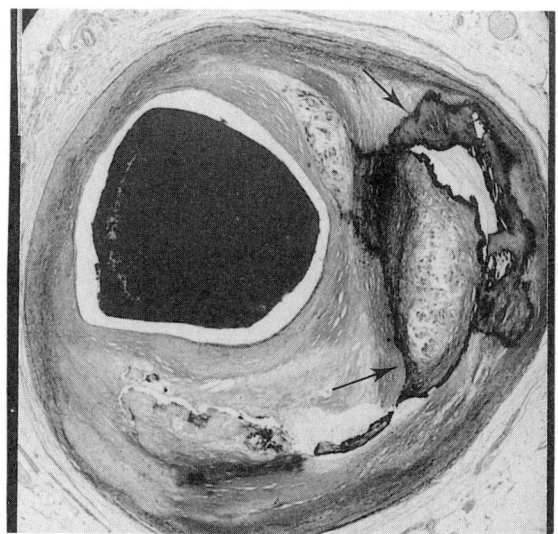

Fig. 44.7. Calcification in atheroma. There is an eccentric predominantly fibrous plaque within which calcification (arrows) has occurred.

ble in life on radiography, has little relevance except in younger patients in whom extensive calcification indicates diffuse atheroma and therefore a strong likelihood of significant stenosis being present.

In some patients, there is a heavy infiltrate of chronic inflammatory cells in the adventitia adjacent to atheromatous plaques. Such infiltrates vary in severity among individuals and have been taken to indicate some form of immune-mediated damage to the vessel wall as a component of atheroma itself.[27] A more tenable explanation in most instances is a secondary response to lipid released from the plaque, and a large population of B lymphocytes reactive to lipoprotein has been found to be present.[28] Some forms of immune damage to the vessel wall do lead to an accelerated intimal proliferation with secondary lipid accumulation and very diffuse 'atheroma'. In such cases, the whole vessel wall is involved and the media destroyed by an inflammatory infiltrate, a picture seen in some patients with scleroderma and ankylosing spondylitis, but this type of immune damage is not present in the majority of patients who have coronary atheroma.

Endothelial status in human atheroma

An intact normal endothelial surface influences blood flow by the prevention of platelet activation and by the production of a smooth muscle relaxant factor (endothelial derived relaxant factor). Animal models of atheroma induced by high-lipid diets[29,30] illustrate that endothelial cell abnormalities are present over raised lesions. These abnormalities consist of retraction and loss of endothelial cells to expose the collagen of the underlying intima and are associated with both monocyte migration and platelet adhesion. Knowledge of the status of the endothelial covering of the surface of human atheromatous lesions is scanty. The assessment of endothelial integrity demands instant perfusion fixation; post-mortem or endarterectomy specimens are thereby precluded. However, there is accumulating evidence, both morphological and functional, of the presence of abnormalities of the endothelium over plaques in man, identical to those found in experimental atheroma (Fig. 44.8) that lead to the adhesion of platelets.

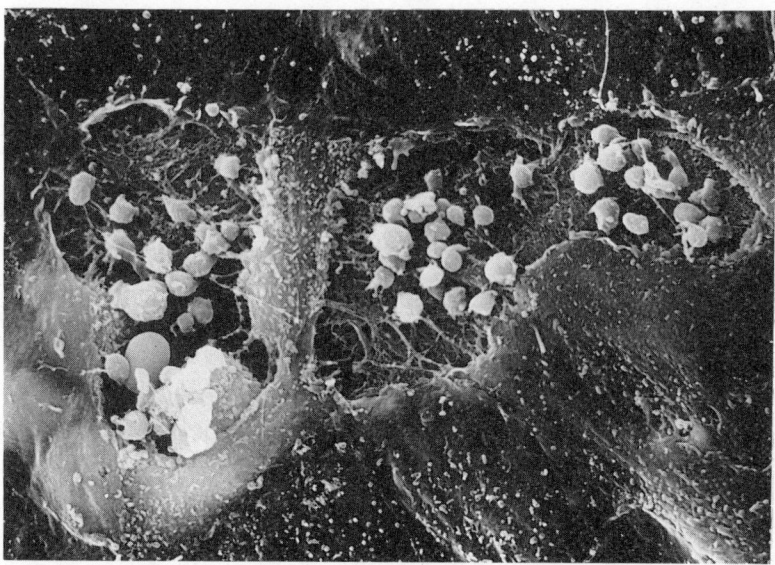

Fig. 44.8. Endothelial damage in atheroma. Scanning electron microscopic appearances of the endothelium over a human coronary artery atheromatous lesion. There is focal loss of endothelium leading to platelet adhesion to underlying intimal components.

Acetylcholine infused into atheromatous human coronary arteries induces constriction rather than the normal dilatation dependent on the release of endothelial derived relaxant factor suggesting a functional abnormality of the endothelial surface.[31]

UNSTABLE ANGINA

Thrombosis in relation to coronary atheroma

There is now overwhelming evidence to implicate thrombosis forming over an atheromatous plaque as one precipitator of acute ischaemic events including unstable angina, acute infarction and sudden death. Thrombosis may form as a result of either superficial loss of the endothelial surface over an atheromatous lesion or deep intimal injury in the process known as fissuring, cracking or rupture of an atheromatous plaque. The latter process is a complication of plaques in which lipid is contained within a space or cleft in the fibrous tissue of the intima. As this lipid, consisting of a complex mixture of cholesterol esters and fatty acids, is thought to be semi-fluid at body temperature, the term 'pool' is used. The lipid is separated from the lumen of the artery by the fibrous tissue of the innermost layer of the intima over which is an endothelial layer. Breaks through the fibrous cap of the plaque allow blood from the lumen of the artery to enter deep into the intima, a process described as 'dissecting' haemorrhage.[32] Many red blood cells accumulate within the lipid pool but the reaction of the platelets with both lipid and exposed collagen leads,

additionally, to a large mass of predominantly platelet thrombus *within* the intima itself (Fig. 44.9). The result is a sudden increase in the volume, and change in configuration, of the plaque and therefore of the degree of arterial obstruction. The change has been identified as leading to abrupt changes in plaque morphology on angiography; typical appearances designated as type II occur.[33,34] Type II stenoses have a ragged outline often with undercut or concave edges which contrast with the smooth oval narrowings (type I) caused by static plaques (Fig. 44.10).

At this stage, the plaque may re-stabilize and re-seal by organization of the break with fibrous tissue but inevitably it will have grown rapidly in size. Such plaques contain a large mass of thrombus deep within the intima. Alternatively, the fissured plaque may not re-seal and thrombus begins to project from the fissure into the lumen, initially not causing total occlusion. Such mural non-occlusive thrombi (Fig. 44.11) are a potential source of small emboli (Fig. 44.12), consisting largely of aggregated platelets, into the distal myocardium. Mural thrombi may grow ultimately to occlude the lumen (Fig. 44.13).

It is a misconception that plaque fissuring is always a catastrophic event. Plaque fissures are a common complication of atheromatous plaques containing lipid and act as a stimulus for plaque growth and the formation of thrombus in the lumen. The strength of the stimulus and the magnitude of the thrombotic response are determined by many additional factors.

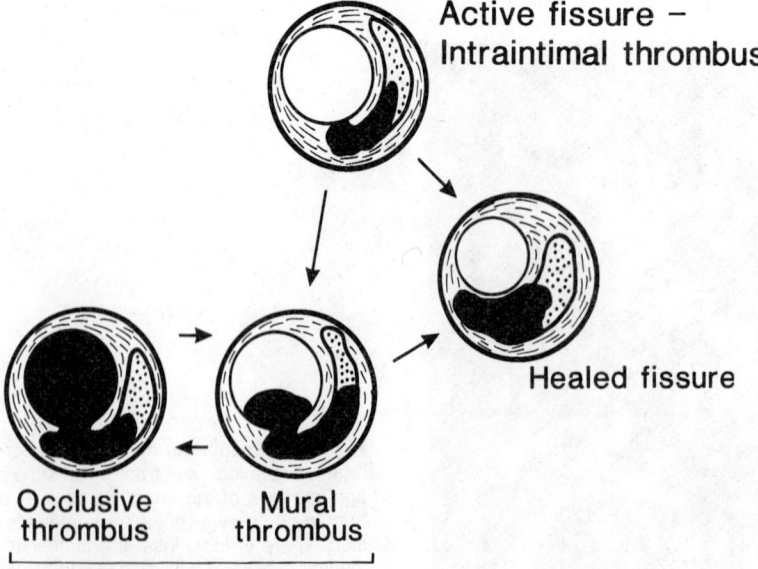

Active fissure –
Intraintimal thrombus

Healed fissure

Occlusive thrombus   Mural thrombus

Intraluminal thrombus

Fig. 44.9. Sequelae of plaque fissuring. Diagrammatic representation of the relation between plaque fissuring, intraintimal and intraluminal thrombus formation.

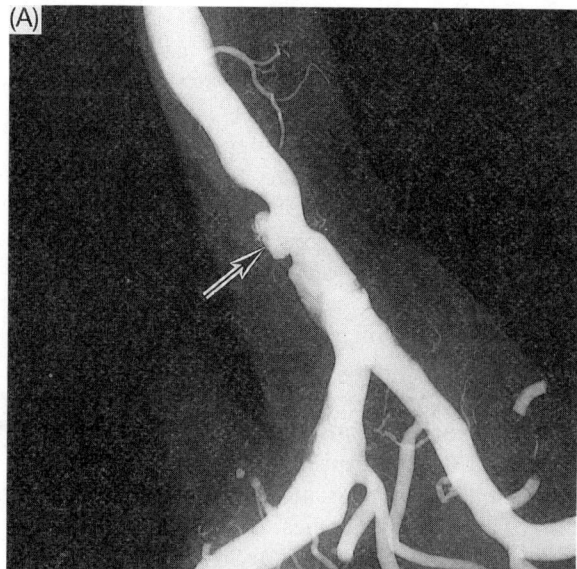

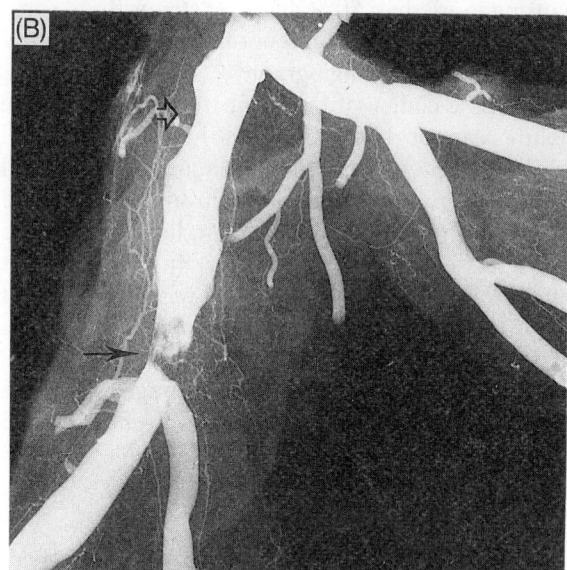

Fig. 44.10. (A) Angiogram of type II stenosis. The stenosis has a ragged outline and overhanging edges (arrows). The appearances are typical in both clinical and post-mortem angiograms of a plaque fissure with loss of the whole cap (ulceration). (B) Angiogram of type II stenosis. Post-mortem angiogram of a type II stenosis (arrow) with a large intraluminal filling defect. Histological confirmation as plaque fissure with large mural thrombus. More proximally in the artery there is a typical smooth type I stenosis (double arrow).

Plaque fissuring is a complication of plaques that have undergone 'atheronecrosis' i.e. there is the formation of a space or cleft within the intima containing lipid. The space is created by death of macrophages releasing lipid and there may be an additional element of destruction of the connective

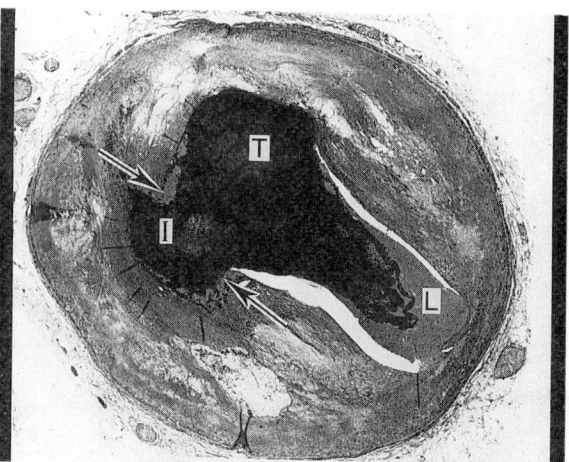

Fig. 44.11. Non-occlusive mural thrombus. A mass of dark-staining thrombus has a portion contained within the intima (I) which protrudes through a break in the intima (arrows) and has a second layer component (T) which protrudes into the lumen (L) containing angiographic medium.

tissue of the intima by release of enzymes such as elastase.[35] The size and depth of the mass of lipid within the intima vary widely and will directly influence the size of the intramural thrombus; large intra-intimal thrombi can form only within large lipid pools. Some fissures are confined to lifting a shallow surface layer of intima, others extend deep into the intima.

Examination of control hearts taken from subjects who had a non-cardiac cause of death shows that minor episodes of plaque fissuring are present, albeit not common. The incidence is directly related

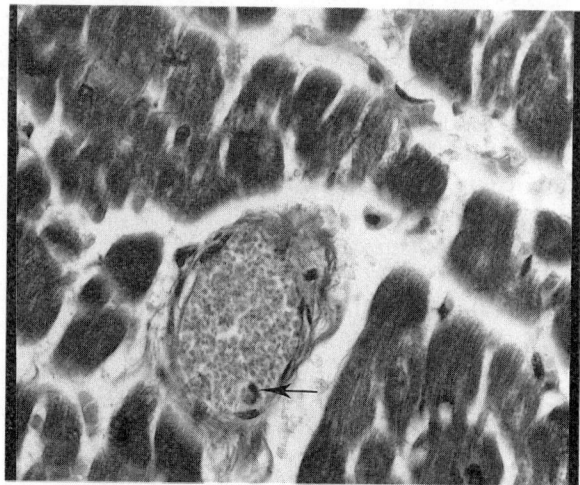

Fig. 44.12. Intramyocardial platelet emboli. A small artery within the myocardium is completely occluded by a mass of platelets recognizable as punctate bodies smaller than a single white cell (arrow) which is also present.

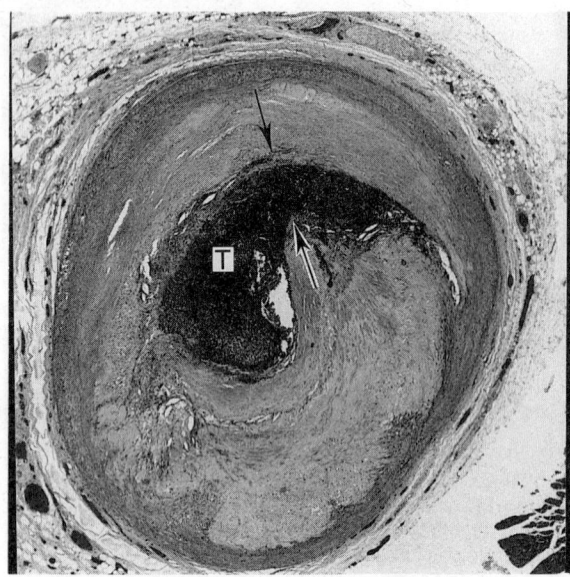

Fig. 44.13. Occlusive thrombus. The dark-staining thrombus (T) is comma shaped. The tail is within the intima and protrudes through a break in the cap (arrows) where the head occludes the lumen. Pre-existing high-grade stenosis due to intimal fibrosis was present.

to the number of plaques in the coronary arteries and thus is far higher in patients with known atheroma-related risk factors, such as hypertension or diabetes mellitus. In these control hearts, fissures are small (Fig. 44.14), often superficial, associated with the formation of intra-intimal but not intraluminal thrombi and many appear to have spontaneously re-sealed from the lumen. The implication of this finding is that minor episodes of plaque fissuring are a significant cause of plaque growth thereby contributing to the development of stable angina. Patients in whom stable angina is of sudden onset have probably suffered a fissure in which the amount of thrombus incorporated within the plaque led to sufficient increase in stenosis to limit flow. Angiographic studies have shown that plaque growth in patients developing stable angina is often episodic.[36]

In patients who develop acute symptoms as a result of plaque fissuring, either the degree of plaque expansion due to incorporated thrombus has been large or superadded thrombosis has developed within the lumen. Breaks into a large lipid pool deep within the intima are more likely to lead to significant plaque growth than small breaks into clefts in the intima close to the endothelial surface.

Some of the factors that militate for the development of intraluminal thrombi are known and others

are speculative.[37] The magnitude of the plaque event varies; at one extreme, the fissures are measured in micrometres, at the other in millimetres and lipid is extruded into the lumen itself. Such major events probably lead to thrombosis; Falk[38] in a study of occlusive coronary thrombi found a high incidence of lipid extrusion into the lumen. Minor fissures may invoke thrombosis in the lumen if the thrombotic potential of the patient is enhanced or the fibrinolytic activity reduced. Reduction in flow over the lesion will also enhance a trend toward intraluminal thrombosis, and it is associated with high degrees of pre-existing stenosis, a large intra-intimal thrombotic mass radically altering plaque configuration, local spasm or reduced distal run-off as a result of microvascular damage in the myocardium. Although a significant degree of pre-existing stenosis is common with occlusive thrombosis,[39] many will develop over plaques that were not causing more than 50% diameter stenosis and some over plaques which would not have been previously visible on clinical angiography.[40]

The time-course of the events following a plaque fissure cannot be ascertained by morphological methods. The sequence of a plaque fissure, mural thrombus and finally occlusive thrombus, as judged by symptoms and angiography, in life can progress or regress over days. It seems certain that the onset of infarction does not coincide with the time of fissuring as the thrombotic sequence will take at least hours to develop.

Very little is known about the pathogenesis of the fracture of the fibrous cap. It has been suggested

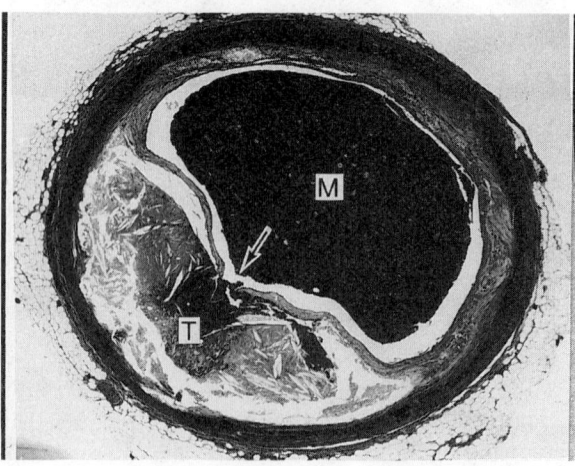

Fig. 44.14. Plaque fissure. A small mass of thrombus (T) within a lipid-rich plaque underlies a small fissure in the plaque cap (arrow). No intraluminal thrombus is present. The arterial lumen contains angiographic medium (M).

that surges in haemodynamic pressure are responsible and case-reports record the sudden onset of symptoms on exercise.[41,42] Such rapid onset of pain would imply massive plaque events and the relevance to less catastrophic degrees of fissuring is unclear. Local spasm could be another factor initiating fissuring by flexing the plaque itself or exerting stress on the junction of the cap with adjacent normal intima. Some of the caps that have undergone fissuring are thinned and infiltrated by macrophages suggesting a dissolution of structural proteins, whereas in others an apparently solid collagenous cap has simply broken suggesting a mechanical process.

The pre-eminence of plaque fissuring as a cause of coronary thrombosis must not obscure the existence of other local causes usually associated with endothelial loss and very superficial intimal damage. Thrombi may form over intact plaques particularly at points of high-grade stenosis[43] and have been related to endothelial damage as a result of turbulent flow. Although usually small and mural in type, a proportion of these thrombi do grow to cause complete occlusion. Similar mural thrombi form in areas of intima which are diffusely infiltrated by lipid-containing macrophages. The intimal surface appears to become eroded with loss of the endothelial lining and mural thrombus forms intimately mixed with very fine strands of collagen and lipid-filled macrophages. This type of thrombus may also become occlusive, particularly in small arteries such as the posterior descending or left marginal branches. The type of atheroma present in both familial hyperlipidaemia and diabetes is particularly prone to this form of thrombosis.

Pathological basis of transient reductions in blood flow in ischaemic heart disease

Several clinical conditions are associated with episodes of transient myocardial ischaemia at rest for which a major precipitating factor appears to be a reduction in myocardial blood flow, in which the ischaemia is not of sufficient duration to result in damage to the myocardium. Such transient episodes may not be associated with pain (silent ischaemia). The clinical conditions range from the crescendo type of unstable angina through variant angina of the Prinzmetal type to episodes of silent ischaemia at rest detected by Holter monitoring in patients whose clinical picture is otherwise that of stable exertional angina. The prognosis of these conditions is very diverse and it seems unlikely that a single pathophysiological mechanism can be responsible. Two basic mechanisms are thought to exist, vasospasm and thrombosis, but in any individual patient it may be difficult to ascertain which is predominant.

Thrombosis and unstable angina

Patients with the crescendo form of unstable angina in whom the pain is unpredictable, comes on at rest and increases in severity or frequency are known to have a substantial risk of developing acute infarction or dying suddenly, but in the majority the symptoms ultimately settle and patients may be left with exertional angina or recover completely. Angiographic studies in such patients initially showed that the extent and severity of atheroma was no different to that in patients with stable angina.[44,45] Unstable angina, however, is characterized by the possession of an eccentric stenotic lesion with irregular or concave outlines,[33,46,47,48] over which an intraluminal filling defect thought to represent thrombus is common.[49] Post-mortem studies[34,50] and angioscopy[51] have shown that these appearances indicate a fissured plaque with overlying thrombus. The attacks of pain may be mediated by intermittent complete occlusion with spontaneous lysis restoring antegrade flow within a few minutes, by superimposed local vascular spasm or by distal platelet emboli, mechanisms which are not exclusive. Experimental production of intimal damage by angioplasty in the pig, simulating plaque fissuring in man, showed that the deeper the injury the greater the deposition of platelets at the site. The severity of vasoconstriction at the site correlated closely with the extent of platelet deposition. Mild deposition of platelets was reduced by pretreatment with aspirin but more severe degrees were uninfluenced.[52] Partial obstruction of the canine coronary artery producing mural non-occlusive thrombus[53] is associated with focal ischaemic myocardial damage and platelet thrombi confined to the territory downstream of the arterial lesions.

In man, there is pathological evidence of intramyocardial platelet emboli in up to 40% of fatal cases of crescendo unstable angina.[54,55] Such emboli are specific for segments of myocardium downstream of arteries containing fissured plaques, confirming the embolic nature of platelet masses in the myocardium. Peak excretion of metabolites of thromboxane[56] coincide with episodes of pain, suggesting that thrombosis and platelet activation have a role in precipitating ischaemic attacks. Circulating levels of fibrinopeptide A are significantly higher in patients with unstable angina than in those with stable angina which suggests that thrombin generation is occurring.[57]

Angina due to vasospasm

Spasm of focal segments of the coronary artery tree is responsible for the attacks of rest pain and ST-segment elevation typical of the Prinzmetal type of variant angina.[58] Many of the patients have co-existent atheroma, either with an irregular outline to the lumen or additional fixed stenosis on angiography; to date, none of the pathological studies have reported totally normal vessels free from atheroma in Prinzmetal's angina.[59] The focal nature of the spasm in most cases suggests there must be a local reason for enhanced medial tone; there is some tenuous evidence of a more generalized smooth muscle abnormality in an association with oesophageal spasm, migraine and Raynaud's phenomenon.[60-63] Undoubted cases of rest pain due to spasm, at the site of a high-grade stenosis due to an eccentric plaque, are described. In one case, the arterial lesion responsible was excised at the time of inserting vein grafts thereby establishing its nature beyond doubt.[18] Such work indicates that, for unknown reasons, a particular atheromatous lesion has acquired a hypersensitivity to vasoconstrictor stimuli. One possibility is that the endothelium at this site is deficient in the production of endothelial derived relaxant factor. Experimental atherosclerosis, in which endothelial damage is known to occur, increases the arterial sensitivity to vasoconstrictor stimulation[64,65] and in human coronary atherosclerosis the normal vasodilator action of intracoronary acetylcholine is paradoxically converted to vasoconstriction.[31] Alternative explanations for focal vascular hypersensitivity include infiltration of the adventitia by chronic inflammatory cells either interfering with the neural release of mediators[66] or by the release, from mast cells in the adventitia, of histamine and leucotrienes which act directly on medial smooth muscle.[67] These hypotheses concerning the role of adventitial chronic inflammatory cells are based on autopsies of single cases; it is not clear why all stenoses that have such an adventitial infiltrate do not show the same phenomenon.

ACUTE MYOCARDIAL INFARCTION

The term myocardial infarction, when used correctly, means necrosis of myocytes due to a reduction or cessation in the blood supply. Providing that the subject, whether an experimental animal or a human being, survives a period of 8–12 h after the inception of infarction the resulting pattern of necrosis can be recognized morphologically as a loss of enzyme activity in the non-viable myocardium. It must be emphasized that morphological methods of recognizing irreversible necrosis depend on a sufficient survival period for structural changes to develop; in experimental studies, in which conditions of fixation can be made optimal, a minimum of 4–6 h is required. Any infarct can be categorized as regional (Fig. 44.15), i.e. encompassed within the territory of myocardium supplied by one major coronary artery, or diffuse (Fig. 44.16). Any infarct can also be categorized as sub-endocardial or transmural (Figs 44.17–44.18). In addition to areas of infarction that are visible macroscopically, in slices of myocardium stained for enzyme activity, there are microscopic foci of necrosis which can also be categorized as regional or diffuse in distribution. There is clinical and experimental evidence that there are separate pathogenetic mechanisms for these different forms of necrosis, the majority of which can be categorized as regional transmural (RTM), regional sub-endocardial (RSE), diffuse sub-endocardial (DSE) or microscopic.

The clinical correlations of these patterns is more difficult; the pathologist can detect amounts of

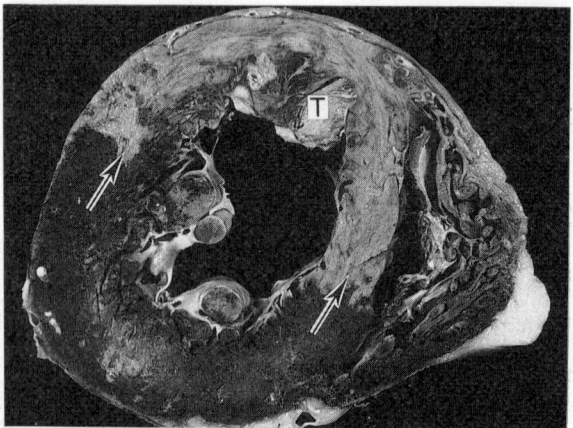

Fig. 44.15. Regional transmural infarction. Anterior transmural infarction of 50% of the total left ventricular myocardium due to occlusion high in the left anterior descending artery. The infarct (arrows) is clearly demarcated and occupies the whole anterior wall of the left ventricle and the anterior two-thirds of the interventricular septum. Mural ventricular thombus (T) is present over the infarct. The myocardium has been stained to demonstrate succinic dehydrogenase activity; normal myocardium stains darkly, infarcted muscle remains pale due to enzyme loss.

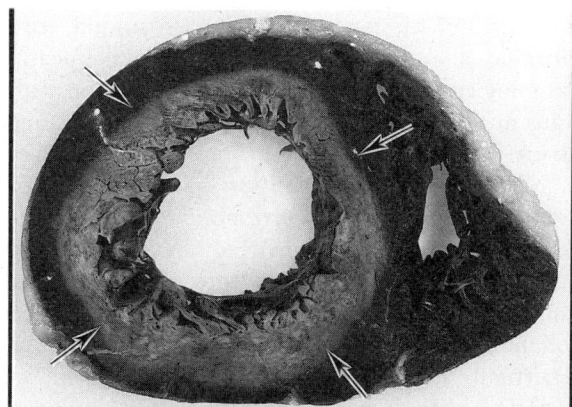

Fig. 44.16. Diffuse sub-endocardial infarction. There is a circumferential loss of enzyme activity in the inner half (arrows) of the whole left ventricular myocardium.

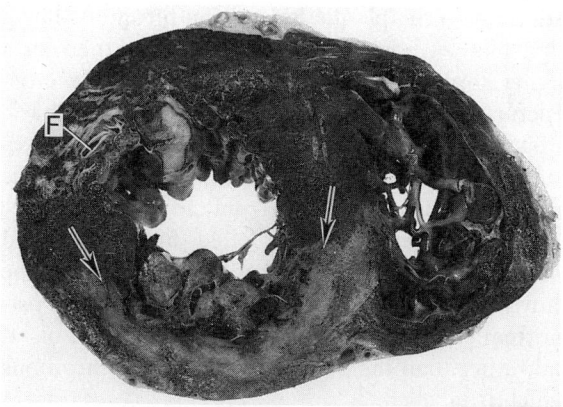

Fig. 44.18. Regional transmural infarction. There is a localized area of enzyme loss (arrows) in the postero-inferior region of the left ventricle, as in Figure 44.17, in the region supplied by the right coronary artery. The infarct is transmural but in contrast to figure 44.15 occupies <30% of the total left ventricular mass. An old fibrous scar (F) is also present.

myocardial necrosis not apparent on electrocardiography in life. Electrocardiographic changes are accurate in determining the regional distribution of necrosis but, although emphasis is often placed on the distinction between Q and non-Q wave infarction, implying that it distinguishes transmural from non-transmural infarction, pathological studies[68,69] show this assumption to be invalid. Microscopic foci of necrosis probably occur in patients with ST-segment changes, but how long such elevation or depression must persist to indicate at least some myocytes have undergone necrosis is not known. ST-segment elevation is thought to indicate sub-epicardial ischaemia, ST-segment depression sub-endocardial ischaemia; the formal proof of this is tenuous.

PATHOGENESIS OF INFARCTION IN MAN

Clinical angiographic studies of Q wave regional infarction in man show that within the first hour the subtending artery is totally occluded in over 90% of cases, but subsequently re-opens spontaneously in up to 30% of cases by 12 h.[70–72] Fibrinolytic therapy will restore antegrade flow in many more cases and, during this re-opening phase, filling defects within the lumen thought to represent thrombus are often present. In the re-opened vessel, a stenosis with a type II configuration is present suggesting an underlying fissured plaque.[46] The efficacy of thrombolytic therapy in restoring flow suggests thrombosis is the major element in the occlusion, although co-existent spasm may be present.[73] Pathological studies confined to regional transmural infarcts[74–76] have revealed that the supplying artery is totally occluded in over 90% of cases, suggesting that persistent occlusion is related to greater risk of a fatal outcome possibly because of larger infarct size. Reconstruction of the micro-anatomy of these occlusive thrombi[38,77,78] confirms there is an underlying fissured plaque in the majority of cases. At the proximal end of the occlusion *within* the intima, there is a mass of predominantly platelet thrombus which is contiguous through a fissure in the cap with the main mass of thrombus within the lumen.

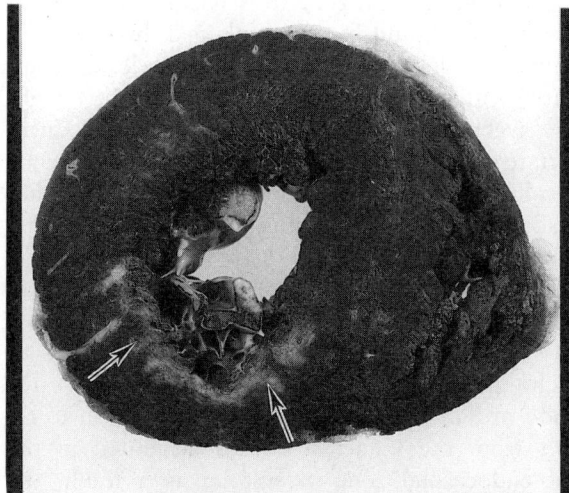

Fig. 44.17. Regional sub-endocardial infarction. There is a localized area of enzyme loss (arrows) in the postero-inferior region of the left ventricle in the region supplied by the right coronary artery. The infarct is not transmural and involves only a small proportion of the total left ventricular mass. There is additional necrosis of the anterior papillary muscle.

Adjacent to the plaque fissure, the thrombus has a high platelet content but more distally there is a higher fibrin and red blood cell content. The microstructure of the thrombus is consistent with a phasic progression and the distal propagation is of a 'stasis' type, suggesting growth after the vessel was occluded. Clinical evidence from radiolabelling supports this view. Radiolabelled fibrinogen and platelets given after the onset of infarction can be shown to localize in the occluded artery.[79,80] Postmortem studies, however, show that it is the distal tail rather than the proximal head of the thrombus which is labelled.[81]

The magnitude of the fissure varies; at one extreme the amount of intra-intimal thrombosis and size of the fissure is small, needing reconstruction from serial histological sections for its detection, while at the other extreme the plaque cap is lost over a centimetre and fragments of intima and extruded lipid are mixed with thrombus occluding the lumen. The arterial events taking place within the first hour of the inception of infarction are complex and it may be an oversimplification to regard occlusion of the lumen by thrombus itself as the sole mechanism by which antegrade flow is prevented. Local vascular spasm at the site can be demonstrated angiographically and occlusion is often intermittent.[82] A fall in myocardial perfusion could follow both micro-emboli and ischaemic damage to capillaries within the myocardium. It seems certain that the cycle is initiated by events related to endothelial and intimal damage over a plaque invoking thrombosis.

A minority of occlusive thrombi associated with regional infarcts in man are not underlain by a fissured plaque. In smaller vessels, such as the left marginal and posterior descending arteries, thrombosis develops at points of high-grade stenosis over intact plaques without deep intimal injury. In some of these, infiltration of the endothelium and intima by lipid macrophages is present, a phenomenon known to be associated with thrombus in experimental atheroma. This form of thrombosis may represent loss of the endothelial layer and superficial damage to the intima exposing collagen to platelets. Only in small arteries or at points of high-grade stenosis is the stimulus for thrombosis sufficient to produce occlusion. The difference in the potential ability to form large thrombi of superficial and deep intimal injury has been shown also in experimental models.[52]

Autopsy studies show that regional subendocardial (non-transmural) infarction in man is not uncommon, particularly in association with unstable angina or in sudden ischaemic death. Pathological studies confirm that, in common with transmural infarction, there is a recent plaque fissure in the supplying artery. In contrast to transmural infarction, there is a far lower incidence of total occlusion[83] and a corresponding higher incidence of the distal segment of the artery being patent and filling either by antegrade flow over mural thrombus or more rarely by well-developed collateral flow.[68,84] Distal propagation of thrombus is virtually never found in non-transmural infarction. This pathological distinction is very similar to that found between Q- and non-Q-wave infarction on clinical angiography; rich collateral development is common in the latter situation.[85] This is also in accord with the view that in non-transmural infarction there remains viable myocardium at risk if further acute thrombotic episodes develop in the same artery. However, many non-Q-wave infarcts are found to be transmural at autopsy and vice versa. There are also differences in the histological structure of transmural and non-transmural infarction; the latter is far more frequently made up of coalescence of focal areas of necrosis of different ages.

Diffuse (non-regional) sub-endocardial necrosis may occur in man in the absence of any structural coronary artery obstruction and reflects an overall fall in myocardial perfusion accentuated in its affect on the sub-endocardial zone. The vulnerability of the sub-endocardial zone to ischaemic damage can be confirmed, and in part explained, by studies in animal models. Sub-endocardial muscle, as compared with sub-pericardial muscle, has a 20% higher oxygen utilization per gram of tissue, produces lactate and undergoes necrosis first under ischaemic conditions and, in conscious animals, has a higher resting blood flow.[2] Significant decreases in aortic diastolic pressure, reduction in diastolic duration and increase in left ventricular diastolic pressure all produce a decrease in the proportion of total flow entering the sub-endocardial muscle and signs of ischaemia. The physiological basis of subendocardial underperfusion has been shown to result from the higher pressures generated in the sub-endocardial zone in systole; as a result, the intramyocardial vessels of this zone are empty and offer greater impedance to reflow in diastole.[2] Subendocardial necrosis in man may also occur in carbon monoxide poisoning and prolonged hypoglycaemia. In association with coronary atheroma in man, diffuse sub-endocardial necrosis is common in end-stage triple-vessel disease particularly when small vessels are involved as in diabetes mellitus and hypercholesterolaemia. Diffuse sub-endocardial necrosis may also be superimposed on regional infarction complicated by cardiogenic shock. The central zones of the papillary muscles are the most vulnerable component of the sub-endocardial tissues and undergo necrosis first. At autopsy, many patients with a large regional infarct can be observed to have recent necrosis of the centre of the contralateral papillary muscle.

Multifocal microscopic foci of necrosis are of diverse origin. In the sub-endocardial zone, they appear to represent an early stage of more confluent necrosis and are almost ubiquitous at the margins of larger areas of infarction. In the sub-pericardial zone, microscopic foci of necrosis are related to the occurrence of intramyocardial platelet emboli.[54,55] Any patient dying after prolonged hypoxia or hypotension will have microscopic foci of necrosis as a preliminary stage of diffuse non-regional ischaemic damage. In severe left ventricular hypertrophy, microscopic foci of necrosis are common without obvious impairment of coronary blood flow or hypoxia. High catecholamine levels, both iatrogenic or natural, as in raised intracranial pressure, are also causes of small foci of myocardial necrosis. The 'myocarditis' reported to occur in patients with phaeochromocytomas reflects similar small foci of necrosis due to high levels of catecholamine.

SUDDEN ISCHAEMIC CARDIAC DEATH

When sudden natural death occurs within 6 h of the onset of symptoms in an individual not previously known to have ischaemic heart disease, coronary atheroma is found to be the direct cause of death in about 70% of cases in men. The incidence approaches 85% in individuals known previously to have ischaemic disease. However, in those who die suddenly *from* ischaemic disease, about 50% have not been known to suffer from ischaemic heart disease. Ambulatory monitoring and resuscitation of sudden death victims in ischaemic disease show that the onset of ventricular fibrillation is the common precipitating event for death. The study of resuscitated victims has also revealed that only a proportion of them, between 25 and 50%, will develop a clinically demonstrable infarct.[86] Sudden death, therefore, is not synonymous with death from early myocardial infarction, although there is a persistent belief that it is. Data which have been claimed as showing a peak of deaths in the first few minutes of infarction are suspect because, within this time-interval, there can be no certainty that acute infarction is present. Clinical studies show no difference in the extent or distribution of atheroma in patients who die suddenly from ischaemic heart disease as compared with those who die of acute infarction after 6 h.[87] An angiographic study of resuscitated patients within a mean of 2.3 h of the onset of symptoms showed 56 of 78 (72%) to have a thrombotic occlusion.[87]

Detailed pathological studies of sudden ischaemic death suggest that victims fall into one of two basic groups. In the first, there is an acute arterial lesion, usually a fissured plaque, over which either mural or occlusive thrombus has formed.[88] Recent myocardial necrosis may be demonstrable histologically. In this group, the onset of ventricular fibrillation reflects an acute ischaemic myocardium and the pathological process present in the subjects with acute coronary thrombi is essentially identical to that found in patients with unstable angina and acute infarction. In these patients, prodromal symptoms, albeit not recognized as indicating heart disease by the patient before the final attack, are not uncommon. In the second group, advanced coronary stenosis is present in association with old myocardial scarring; often, significant left ventricular hypertrophy is also present and frequently acute coronary thrombi are absent.[89–91] Re-entrant arrhythmias in a scarred poorly functioning left ventricle are likely precipitating events for ventricular fibrillation in this latter group.

Divergent opinions exist on the relative frequency of the two basic groups. Three recent pathological series[88,92,93] highlight the pre-eminence of the thrombotic group in sudden ischaemic death overall, a view substantiated by an angiographic study in survivors of sudden ischaemic death.[87] Other series in which the majority of patients are known to have ischaemic disease or old infarction and who die without any prodromal warning will contain a higher proportion of patients with widespread arterial stenosis and no acute coronary thrombi.[89–91] Patient selection predetermines the type of vascular pathology found in sudden ischaemic death.

THE MYOCARDIUM IN ISCHAEMIC HEART DISEASE

METABOLIC AND STRUCTURAL CONSEQUENCES OF EXPERIMENTAL CORONARY ARTERY OCCLUSION

Animal models provide insight into the structural and metabolic events that occur in human disease.[94–96] A limitation of these models is that they represent an abrupt cessation of coronary flow rather than the intermittent obstruction which precedes the final occlusion in human infarction.[82]

The experimental model used most frequently is ligation of the left circumflex coronary artery in the anaesthetized dog. Within 1 or 2 min of ligation, a portion of the lateral wall of the left ventricle ceases to contract. A majority of the dogs survive but a minority develop increasing numbers of ventricular ectopic beats which culminate in the sudden onset of ventricular fibrillation. In those that survive a minimum of 8–12 h, autopsy reveals an area of infarcted muscle in the lateral wall of the left ventricle. The size of the infarct varies depending on the degree of collateral formation which existed previously and on the basic coronary artery anatomy.[97]

Functional changes

Myocardial ischaemia can be defined as a level of ATP consumption above that which can be produced at a particular coronary blood flow.[3] The characteristics of myocardial metabolism mean that such ischaemia is translated into structural damage within a relatively short time. Within 20 s following complete coronary occlusion, systolic contraction declines and ceases by 1–2 min. The electrocardiogram changes by 30 s. If flow is re-established within 20–40 min, necrosis can be totally prevented; if flow is not re-established, some myocyte necrosis is inevitable.

Biochemical changes

Seconds after coronary arterial occlusion tissue oxygen levels fall in the affected segment of myocardium and mitochondrial aerobic glycolysis ceases.[3] Anaerobic glycolysis becomes the only source of new high-energy phosphates using glycogen as a substrate. Creatinine phosphate levels fall to virtually zero within 2–3 min and are the first back-up system to regenerate ATP from adenosine diphosphate (ADP) by donation of a high energy phosphate group. Adenosine triphosphate levels within the cell begin to fall significantly only after 2–3 min and cannot therefore be the immediate cause of cessation of contraction which begins to decline within 20 beats of the induction of ischaemia.[3] Intracellular acidosis appears within this time-span and may directly affect contractile protein reaction with calcium. Intracellular acidosis, in part, reflects lactate production from glycogen stores; the depletion of stainable glycogen granules is the first morphological evidence of ischaemia. Phosphate also accumulates within the myocyte very rapidly following the breakdown of creatinine phosphate.

Within seconds of ischaemia, there is also evidence of a membrane functional abnormality with loss of intracellular potassium ions probably responsible for the rapid development of alterations in the configuration of the action potential. The intracellular sodium levels do not change initially. Brief periods of ischaemia can be reversed without leading to tissue necrosis. The best indication of irreversible cell damage is disruption of the cell membrane; such changes can be detected by electron microscopy after 40 min of ischaemia.[96] The biochemical events leading to the transition from reversible to irreversible ischaemia are as yet not known. It is tempting to postulate that membrane integrity is energy dependent and that irreversible damage is the result of the loss of control of intracellular ionic and osmolar homeostasis. However, the degree of necrosis does not directly correlate with levels of ATP and, although restoration of ATP production is a necessary prerequisite for survival, it is not the key factor. The increasing acidosis and calcium accumulation within the myocyte activates phospholipases in the cell membrane, but such changes are probably very late and associated with the development of structural changes. The rise in intracellular calcium is due to an increased influx; an excess of intracellular calcium is known to inhibit mitochondrial ATP production and to destabilize membranes.

Structural changes following experimental infarction

Ultrastructural changes can be observed within the reversible phase of ischaemia, including mitochondrial swelling and glycogen depletion. Within 40 min of total occlusion the changes are more severe, including disruption of cristae within swollen mitochondria, sarcoplasmic swelling, clumping of chromatin within the nuclei and total loss of glycogen. Irreversible change is regarded as certain once granular electron-dense deposits of calcium appear within mitochondria and there are breaks in the cell membrane.

Although ultrastructural changes occur within 40 min of occlusion, changes visible on light microscopy cannot be recognized before at least 4–8 h has elapsed. The first recognizable histological feature is an accumulation of polymorphs within the interstitial tissues which may start as early as 4 h and last for up to 3 days. Beyond this time, macrophages are the dominant cells. Individual muscle cells become hypereosinophilic (coagulative necrosis) with nuclear pyknosis followed by loss of cross-striations and by 4–5 days they have disintegrated to be phagocytosed by macrophages. Perfusion within the central zone of an infarct is absent due to persistent occlusion of the major artery and destruction of the capillary bed by the necrotic process. Thus, within this central zone, the changes described above are retarded or absent. Repair of these infarcts is dependent on a rim of granulation tissue at the junction with viable tissue which contains intact perfused capillaries. Fibroblasts extend inward into the infarct from about 7–10 days; the whole process takes up to 8 weeks to produce a solid mass of fibrous tissue.

Evolution of acute infarction and reperfusion injury

Experimental models provide an opportunity to study the evolution of infarction by removing the arterial clip at varying times and re-establishing flow; sacrifice 4 days later allows the extent of necrosis to be identified on light microscopy. Such work reveals that infarction is not an instantaneous process in which all the myocardial cells at risk undergo death at the same moment. Infarcts reperfused after intervals longer than 6 h are no different morphologically to those that have not been reperfused. The infarct is transmural, extending from endocardium to pericardium. Comparison of nonperfused and reperfused infarcts at time-intervals up to a maximum of 6 h after occlusion shows that re-establishing blood flow reduces the infarct size by a factor related to time. This reduction in size is in the depth to which infarction extends through the wall from the sub-endocardial zone and not in the centrifugal extent of the infarct.[94,95] Limitation of infarction by reperfusion within the period from 40 min to 4–6 h is therefore due to sparing of the sub-pericardial zone; this has given rise to the concept that infarction spreads as a wavefront through the ventricular wall from endocardium to pericardium over 6 h. Although there has been much clinical interest in the concept of reduction in infarct size in man by reperfusion, the failure of reperfusion of experimentally induced infarction to limit spread in a lateral direction strongly suggests that a similar phenomenon will exist in man. The therapeutic hope must be to reduce the number of infarcts that progress to become transmural.

A comparison of infarcted areas that have been reperfused with those in which flow was not re-established reveals significant functional and structural differences.[96] Within minutes of reperfusion, the myocardial muscle cells undergo explosive swelling due to water entering the cell. Calcium ions also pour into the cell invoking supercontraction of sarcomeres forming 'contraction bands' within the cell, recognizable on light microscopy (Fig. 44.19). This tonic contracture often disrupts the cell leading to extrusion of mitochondria into the interstitial spaces. Contraction band necrosis is recognizable histologically within 20 min of the onset of infarction in contrast to the traditional form of 'coagulative' necrosis (Fig. 44.20) which requires survival for at least 4–6 h before it is recognizable.

The mechanisms of cell death in reperfused myocardium are of major interest because in the experimental animal control of some of these is associated with an increase in the proportion of myocardium at risk that can be salvaged.[98]

Reactive free radicals toxic to cell membranes and organelles are known to develop in ischaemic myocardium;[99] further production occurs on reperfusion. Potential sources include the myocytes, polymorphs and endothelial cells. Myocyte damage releases complement activation factors[100] leading to adhesion of polymorphs to capillary endothelium and their passage into the interstitial tissues. This accumulation of polymorphs in the tissue is the first morphological feature of necrosis recognizable on light microscopy in both human and experimental infarction. Polymorphs within the tissues release cytoxic factors including free radicals such as oxygen and enzymes such as elastase. Reperfusion is also associated with evidence of microvascular damage which may result in a progressive decrease in blood flow (no-reflow phenomenon) in areas of ischaemic damage following reperfusion.[101] At a structural level, this is associated with the obliteration of the capillary lumen by endothelial swelling and the formation of plugs of polymorphs and red

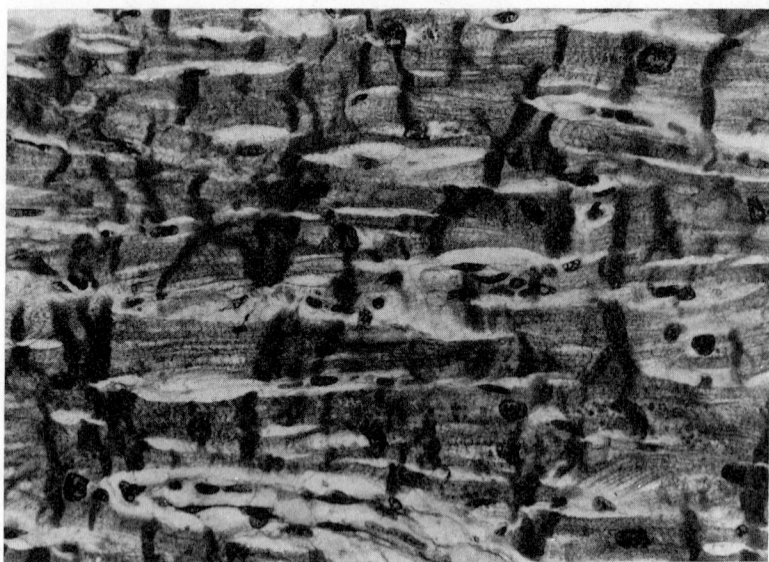

Fig. 44.19. Contraction band necrosis. Within the myocytes, focal hypercontraction has produced darkly staining bands of conglomerated myofibrils.

blood cells. Interstitial haemorrhage and oedema are present reflecting capillary damage. In man and in animals, a characteristic macroscopic appearance of haemorrhagic infarction is produced. The mechanism of endothelial damage may involve interactions with neutrophils and also production of free radicals within the endothelium itself; in animal experiments, a range of scavengers or inhibitors of free radical production[102] will reduce the degree of vascular damage, as judged by endothelial swelling and the number of polymorph plugs, as well as reducing infarct size. The concordance of these two effects makes it difficult to determine if the protective effect is primarily on the myocyte or on the vasculature. Agents suggested to be protective in experimental infarction include perfluorochemicals,

adenosine, superoxide dismutase, catalase and xanthine oxidase inhibitors such as allopurinol.

Reperfusion has been regarded as a 'double-edged sword',[103] it reduces infarct size while causing further myocyte death mediated, at least in part, by microvascular damage. However, in man, there is no evidence that reperfusion ever causes lateral extension of infarction outside the area at risk or that the repair processses involving organization and fibrosis differ in the haemorrhagic infarcts typical of reperfusion.[104] Animal models are of interest because it is possible that procedures developed experimentally, such as intracoronary infusion of free radical scavengers, could be used, immediately after restoration of flow by thrombolysis, to improve the salvage of myocardium in man.

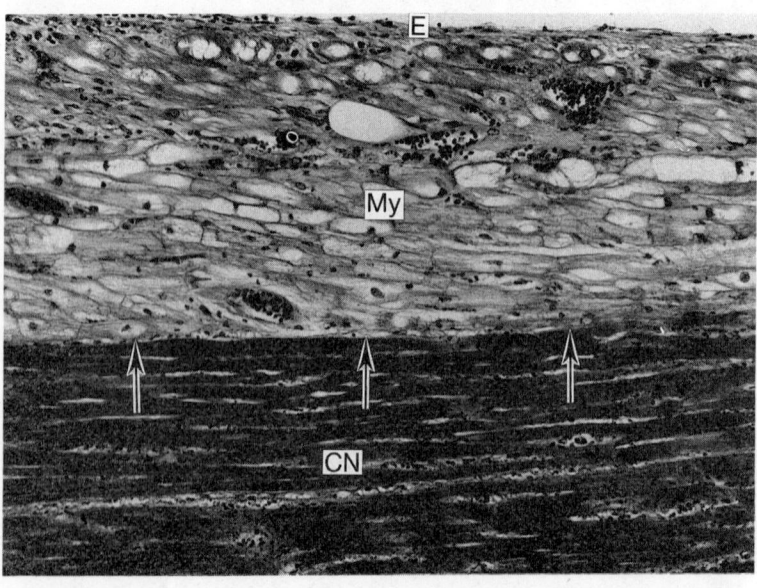

Fig. 44.20. Coagulative necrosis and myocytolysis. Within an area of infarction, the deepest myocytes show coagulative necrosis (CN) and have lost all nuclear structure but the myofibrillary structure remains. No contraction bands are present. The most superficial myocytes (arrows) in the zone immediately beneath the endocardium (E) are still viable with nuclei present but the cytoplasm is empty of myofibrils giving the cell a vacuolated ghost appearance known as myocytolysis (My).

Morphological changes in human myocardial infarction

The microscopic appearances of human myocardial infarcts are complex. Some regional infarcts are a single contiguous area of necrosis, although there is always some irregular mixture with focal areas of viable myocardium on the lateral margins. A surviving sub-endocardial band of muscle up to 10 cells in thickness is also almost universal. The central zone of such infarcts comprises totally necrotic myocytes with no vascular perfusion. In contrast, other infarcts appear to represent the confluence of multifocal areas of necrosis of different ages. Such appearances suggest that in some cases arterial obstruction is complete and sudden whereas in others it is staccato in origin with repeated episodes of occlusion and reperfusion. Although there are complicated classifications of the microscopic changes designed to date exactly the onset of infarction,[105] they provide only a rough approximation because the process of necrosis does not involve every myocardial cell at risk at the same moment and the reparative process does not proceed at an identical rate throughout the infarcted area.

Coagulation necrosis (Fig. 44.20) is the typical appearance of myocardial muscle cells, as seen in well-established regional transmural infarction following complete cessation of blood flow to the area. The muscle cells become hypereosinophilic but otherwise appear little affected until 24 h, following which the cross-striations vanish and the myofibrils begin to coalesce as granular debris. The earliest histologically recognizable change at 12–24 h is the accumulation of polymorphs within the interstitial tissue.

In contraction band necrosis (Fig. 44.19), dense eosinophilic transverse bands are present within the muscle cell. These represent telescoped sarcomeres and the cell is often greatly shortened in length. Such cells are often contiguous at the intercalated disc with an apparently normal cell. This form of necrosis is more common in situations in which flow is known to have been restored; in man, as in the experimental model, this probably represents a reperfusion phenomenon.

In any area of necrosis, a distinction has to be made between those instances in which the whole tissue is dead, including the stroma and vascular component and those in which only the muscle cells have died. In the former, often known as colliquative necrosis and usually found in the centre of regional transmural infarcts, the reparative process

takes place only at the margins where the infarct abuts on to tissue with viable stroma and vessels. Amorphous hyaline muscle fibres, which have undergone little change other than total loss of striations, and nuclei may persist for many weeks or months incarcerated in the centre of such infarcts. From 3–5 days, macrophages, fibroblasts and capillaries begin to extend into the infarct from the periphery. Collagen deposition begins by 7–10 days and may take many weeks to transform the infarct into a fibrous scar. The ingrowth of capillaries into the area of infarction is mediated by release, within the infarct, of a myocardial angiogenesis factor closely related in structure to angiogenesis factors elaborated by tumour cells.

In areas of infarction in which the stroma has not undergone necrosis, the reparative process is far more rapid. In part, this may be due to the smaller size of the foci of necrosis but it is also due to the presence of viable stromal cells within the area. In such areas, the myofibrillary structure of the muscle is lost leading to the formation of hyaline masses after which macrophages appear within the sheath of the original muscle cells. The stroma collapses and coalesces to allow some proliferation of collagen to leave ultimately a small focal scar (Fig. 44.21) often containing some residual lipofuscin. Microscopic focal areas of acute necrosis in which the stroma has survived are common in ischaemic heart disease, particularly at the margins of large areas of necrosis. They are also characteristic of micro-embolic myocardial damage. Such foci are also found in severe cardiac hypertrophy irrespective of the presence or absence of significant coronary atheroma; a range of factors, including excess catecholamine levels, thyrotoxicosis and potassium deficiency can lead to similar foci.

Myocytolysis (Fig. 44.20) is a further expression of ischaemic damage to myocardial muscle cells. The cells become large and vacuolated often to the point at which virtually no myofibrils remain. At the same time, the nuclei persist and mitochondrial enzyme activity remains. The appearance is often seen immediately beneath the endocardium or around blood vessels within areas which otherwise show conventional coagulative necrosis. The change is thought to indicate muscle cells which have lost the ability to maintain normal ionic gradients with the interstitial fluid and are only just viable. There is some evidence, based on biopsies taken at the time of aortocoronary bypass grafting, that myocytes showing moderate degrees of myocytolysis can revert to normal over a prolonged

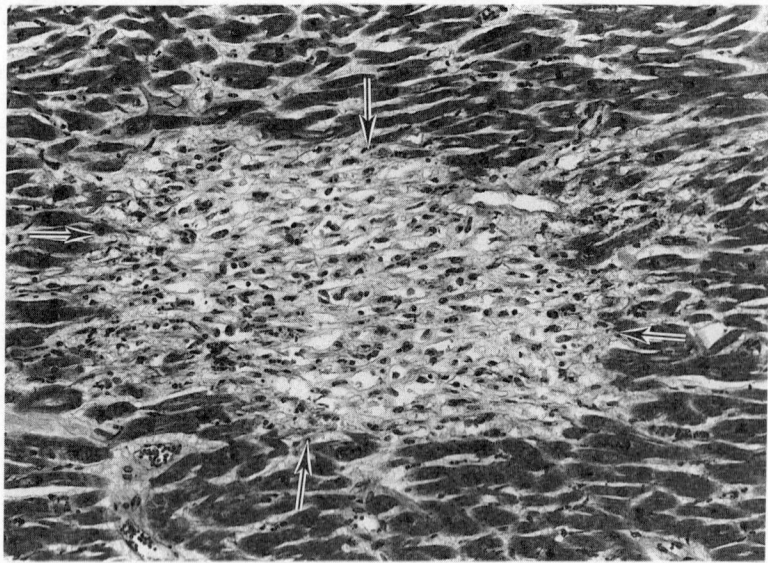

Fig. 44.21. Focal microscopic ischaemic scarring. A small focus of necrosis (arrows) which can be contained within a low-power microscopic field is present. The myocytes have undergone lysis leaving a lattice of surviving stromal cells within which macrophages have accumulated. The stroma ultimately condenses to form a small fibrous scar.

period; this finding forms a potential morphological basis for a chronic stunned or hibernating myocardium in which function returns after revascularization.[106]

FACTORS INFLUENCING INFARCT SIZE

Thrombotic occlusion of a coronary artery leads to a segment of myocardium supplied by that artery being 'at risk'. The actual mass of muscle that has undergone infarction by 6–12 h, however, may be significantly less than the mass at risk originally. In man, blood flow may be restored in an antegrade manner by spontaneous or iatrogenic lysis of the occluding thrombus; this mechanism may be a major factor in the production of non-transmural rather than transmural infarction. Infarct size is also influenced by the degree of collateral flow. There are considerable interspecies differences in the degree to which collateral flow exists in normal hearts. The importance of collaterals can be judged by the relation of time with the proportion of the area of myocardium at risk that has undergone necrosis when a major coronary artery is ligated. In the guinea-pig, collateral flow is so rich that no infarction develops. In the pig, the area at risk is virtually all irreversibly damaged by 1 h; in the dog, 6 h is needed for an equivalent degree of necrosis to occur. Man lies somewhere between these two extremes.[107] Collaterals develop following the creation of a pressure gradient between two vascular beds. In the pig, such collaterals develop in the sub-endocardial zone of the myocardium; in the dog, they are epicardial. In man, collateral develop-

ment is more likely to occur in patients who have stenosis that pre-dates the development of thrombosis; at its maximal level, it may completely prevent infarction following complete occlusion of a major coronary artery. In man, collateral development takes place on the epicardial surface, where enlarged rather tortuous vessels develop linking separate regional territories, and by a sub-endocardial plexus of thin-walled vessels joining the straight and branching intramyocardial system. In extreme cases, a complete circumferential ring of thin-walled vessels develops in the sub-endocardial zone of the left ventricle. However, despite the presence of well-developed collateral vessels, minimal resistance is considerably higher than that in a normal vascular bed. Canine collateral vessels develop a new medial muscle coat with vasoconstrictor responses; however, nothing is known about the responses of human collaterals. In man, when antegrade flow is re-established, by organization of thrombi, through segments of artery occluded for some time or by vessels in the adventitia, collateral flow probably develops far too slowly to influence infarct size. Such means of re-establishing flow, however, may influence whether post-infarct angina develops. Collateral flow can be reliably demonstrated at post-mortem only by angiography, consequently it is not widely studied by pathologists.

FACTORS INFLUENCING PROGNOSIS AFTER REGIONAL TRANSMURAL INFARCTION

The concept of intensive care in the first 48 h of acute myocardial infarction is dependent on the recognition of ventricular fibrillation followed by resuscitation and defibrillation; in effect, sudden deaths are avoided. By 48 h, the risk is virtually over providing no further ischaemic myocardial necrosis occurs. Infarct size, i.e. the proportion of the total left ventricular muscle mass which is infarcted, is directly related to the mortality and morbidity of acute infarction. The incidence of serious ventricular arrhythmias is also related to infarct size, but even small infarcts can cause sudden death.[108] Cardiogenic shock is a major cause of mortality at present and tends to occur in patients whose infarcts involve > 40% of the total left ventricular muscle mass.[109-112] It is these patients who enter a vicious cycle of hypoperfusion and progressive sub-endocardial infarction. The remaining causes of mortality and morbidity are due to certain specific complications.

ARRHYTHMIAS IN ACUTE MYOCARDIAL INFARCTION

Acute sinus node dysfunction is commonly seen in the acute stages of infarction and reflects a multifactorial problem which resolves in the majority of cases. The range of putative mechanisms are well reviewed by James.[113] They include occlusion either proximal to or within the nodal artery. Although such instances have been described,[113,114] they are rare. Infarction of the node and surrounding atrial muscle is also described. The node is immediately adjacent to the pericardium and will be involved *pari passu* in any pericarditic process. The reversibility of sinus node dysfunction in most cases of acute infarction suggest that factors such as local hypoxia, acidosis and hyperkalaemia are pre-eminent rather than actual structural damage. Atrial fibrillation has similar associations but is significantly more common if atrial infarction is present.

CONDUCTION DEFECTS IN ACUTE INFARCTION

The pathogenesis, pathology and prognosis of atrioventricular block complicating postero-inferior infarction differ from those of anterior infarction.

In posterior infarction, the clinical features suggest that the phenomenon is one of reversible nodal dysfunction. Pathological studies show that there is an occlusion, due to thrombosis, in the artery giving rise to the nodal supply.[115] The thrombus, however, very rarely extends into the nodal artery itself and, in most instances, the node does not have histolo-

gical evidence of gross ischaemic damage; indeed, the majority of patients who survive revert to sinus rhythm. The mechanism of the nodal inhibition have been postulated to be due to temporary hypoxia or to excess potassium ions released from adjacent necrotic myocardium. This necrotic myocardium could lie within the adjacent atrial muscle[116] or the upper interventricular septum, whose venous drainage passes back across the central fibrous body and through the nodal area. The rare cases of permanent nodal damage following posterior infarction are associated with occlusion of the nodal artery itself probably by emboli from more proximal thrombi. The size of a posterior–inferior infarct does not seem to be involved in the pathogenesis of atrioventricular block.

In contrast, anterior infarction causes atrioventricular block by involving both bundle branches, either in potentially reversible hypoxic damage including myocytolysis or frank necrosis. As the infarcts must be far larger to affect both branches, they carry a worse prognosis. The high incidence of necrosis of the bundle branches is associated with a significant risk of residual conduction defects in those who do survive.

PATHOLOGICAL COMPLICATIONS OF ACUTE INFARCTION

Infarct distension or expansion

Stretching and thinning of the infarcted tissue within the first few days is associated with a high mortality and may progress to cardiac rupture (Fig. 44.22).[117] Such distension is a feature of anterior transmural infarcts[118] that involve > 10% of the total left ventricular mass; distension carries a high risk of developing mural thrombus. The enlargement of the infarct is due to combinations of simple stretching and tearing or sliding of muscle bundles relative to each other. The importance of such distension is that a permanent globular dilatation of the ventricle may result with detrimental effects, on both left ventricular contraction and mitral valve function. Expansion is negatively related to pre-existing left ventricular hypertrophy.[118]

External cardiac rupture

Pericardial tamponade resulting from external cardiac rupture is responsible for 10–20% of the fatality of myocardial infarction; it has been estimated to be the most common cause of death after

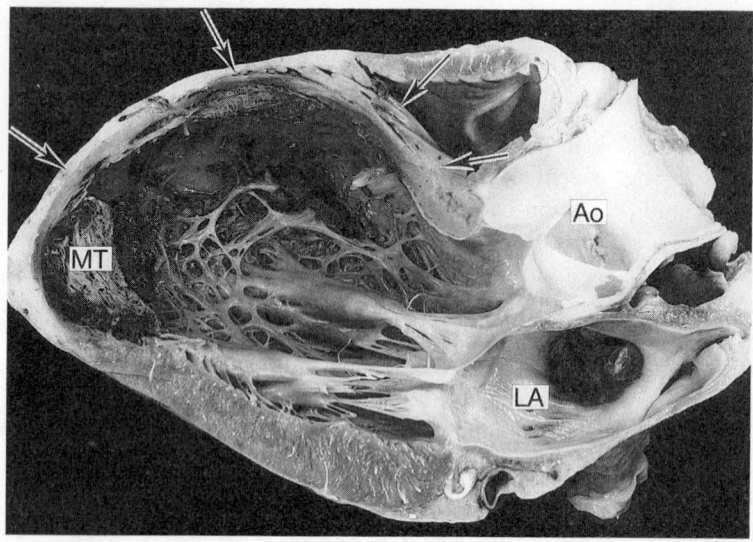

Fig. 44.22. Acute infarct expansion. Long-axis transection of a heart in which an anterior infarct has undergone expansion leading to marked thinning of the ventricular wall and an outward bulge (arrows). Mural thrombus (MT) is present at the apex. Ao, aorta; LA, left atrium.

ventricular arrhythmias and cardiogenic shock. Rupture is a complication of transmural infarction but there is no direct relation between infarct size and cardiac rupture,[112] which is relatively more common in older women.[119]

The mechanism of myocardial rupture[120] is not clear but there are at least two variants. In some cases, there is a slit-like tear between viable and non-viable muscle in an infarct that has not undergone distension. Such rupture can occur within the first 2 days. In other infarcts that have undergone expansion, the endocardium is torn with extravasation of blood between muscle bundles and layers; this form of rupture, preceded by infarct distension, occurs typically from the 5th to the 10th day. One report links accumulation of eosinophils within the infarct with an increased risk of rupture.[121]

Modern resuscitation procedures with vigorous external cardiac massage has created a problem for pathologists. In some such cases, the infarct is found to be split but only 200–300 ml of blood are present in the pericardial sac and there is the possibility the rupture is an agonal iatrogenic phenomenon.

Ventricular septal defects

Transmural infarcts of the interventricular septum may rupture leading to the sudden acquisition of a left-to-right shunt at ventricular level. Septal rupture is a complication of both antero-septal and postero-septal infarction.[122] In the former case, the arterial occlusion is characteristically in the left anterior descending coronary artery, above the first septal branch, in a patient who has not had previous symptoms of angina and in whom collateral flow is

minimal. The resulting infarct is large. This, in association with the haemodynamic burden of a shunt, causes a high mortality. The shunt takes place initially through a ragged hole ranging from 1 to 3 cm^2 in size. It is rare for patients to survive; it is usually those with smaller defects, who will develop a smoothed-edged hole as the infarct heals. In antero-septal infarction, the defect is in the anterior or apical portion of the ventricular septum on the left side and opens into the right ventricular outflow or apex of the right ventricle. In postero-septal infarction, ventricular septal defects occur behind the posterior medial papillary muscle on the left side and open into the right ventricle close to the septal cusp of the tricuspid valve. These defects have a strong association with aneurysms of the posterior wall of the left ventricle and with right ventricular infarction. Subsequent external rupture of the same posterior infarct that induced a septal shunt a day or two before is well recognized. It is difficult to assess the true relative frequency of anterior and posterior septal defects because in autopsy studies approximately equal numbers have been reported whereas in clinical series the preponderance of anterior septal defects has been stressed. This difference may reflect the greater ease with which the anterior septal defect can be clinically diagnosed and surgically repaired.

Papillary muscle infarction

Necrosis of the papillary muscles is very common during acute infarction, being present to some degree in from 15 to 30% of anterior and up to 50% of posterior infarcts.[123] The greater frequency of posterior medial papillary muscle infarction reflects the blood supply from the right coronary artery whereas the antero-lateral group of papillary muscles is predominantly supplied by the left circumflex artery, a less common site of thrombosis than the right coronary artery. Papillary muscle infarction complicates both regional sub-endocardial and transmural infarction and is responsible for transient mitral regurgitation in the acute phase. In a tiny minority, < 1% of all fatal infarcts, a portion or all of a papillary muscle avulses. In the most severe form, the whole papillary muscle ruptures and the stump attached to the chorda passes in a flail-like motion across the mitral valve orifice associated with torrential mitral regurgitation. Rupture of a subhead of a papillary muscle, to which only one or two chordae are attached, is less catastrophic and leads to prolapse of a portion of cusp only. Partial tears may heal to leave an elongated papillary muscle with a central fibrous isthmus. Rupture of the posterior papillary muscle is 4–7 times more frequent than the rupture of the antero-lateral papillary muscle, but in neither case is the infarct necessarily large or transmural.[124–126] There is a distinctive syndrome of rupture of the antero-lateral papillary muscle causing death from rapid onset of torrential mitral regurgitation due to a very small localized infarct resulting from thrombosis of the marginal branch of the left circumflex coronary artery.

Right ventricular infarction

In isolation, right ventricular infarction is very rare, but it may occur in patients with ischaemic heart disease who have pre-existing severe right ventricular hypertrophy. Between 20 and 50% of patients with postero-inferior infarcts of the left ventricle have some concomitant right ventricular necrosis.[127] The incidence of right ventricular infarction in association with anterior infarction is far lower and many series contain no such cases. The right ventricular myocardium is supplied by the right coronary artery and the more proximal and the more complete the occlusion due to thrombosis the more likely it is for infarction to occur in the right ventricle. The effect of concomitant right ventricular infarction on clinical management has been of considerable interest;[127] it leads to severe heart failure and an enlarged liver without evidence of left-sided failure in the form of pulmonary oedema.

Ventricular aneurysms

The term aneurysm is used inconsistently in clinical *cardiology*, but a working morphological definition is that of a convex protrusion of the ventricular wall composed of collagenous replacement of the myocardium throughout its full thickness.[128] Such ischaemic aneurysms can result only from transmural infarction. There is a wide spectrum from, on the one hand, aneurysms with very diffuse bulges with a wide base to on the other hand very localized saccular bulges with a narrow neck (Figs 44.23–44.25). The clinical presentation of aneurysms is of persistent ventricular arrhythmias, cardiac failure and systemic emboli from mural thrombosis within

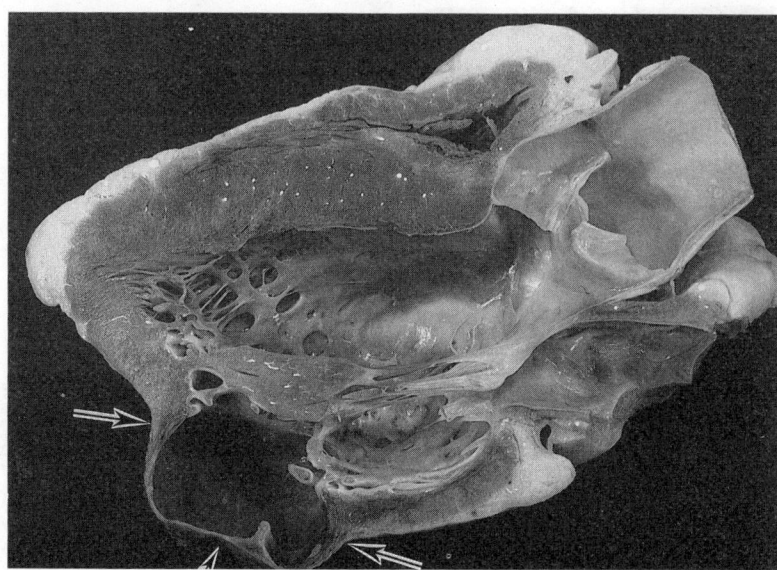

Fig. 44.23. Localized ventricular aneurysm. Long-axis transection of the left ventricle with a discrete aneurysm (arrows) of the inferior wall. The aneurysm sac has a relatively narrow neck.

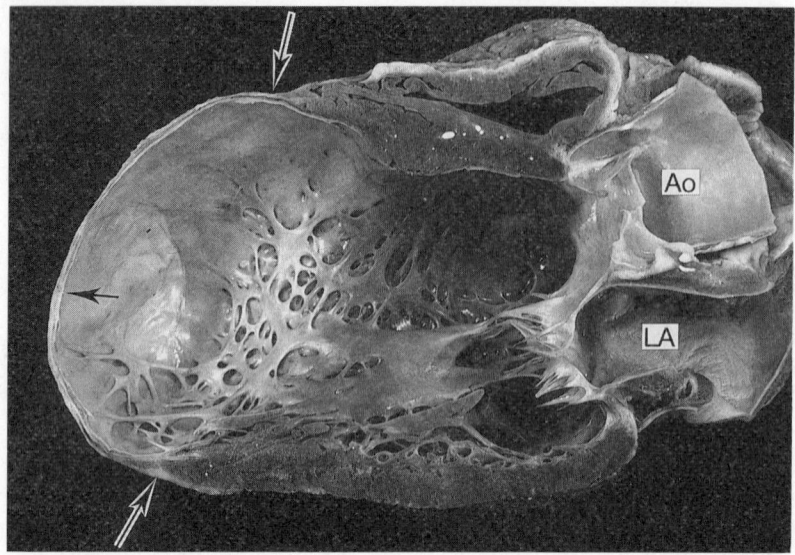

Fig. 44.24. Diffuse apical ventricular aneurysm. Long-axis transection of the left ventricle showing an aneurysm of the anterior apical portion (arrows). The aneurysm has a wide neck and does not contain mural thombus. Ao, aorta; LA, left atrium.

the cavity of the aneurysm, all of which may be correctable by resection of the aneurysm. Late cardiac rupture is rare. The presence of mural thrombus is not constant; aneurysms apparently identical in shape and size may be full of thrombus obliterating the sac, contain some mural thrombus or have no thrombus (Figs 44.23–44.25). The wall of ventricular aneurysms is composed predominantly of collagen but calcification may occur,[129] particularly where the sac is lined by a thin coat of old thrombus. The pathogenesis of aneurysm formation has been regarded either as acute expansion of the necrotic myocardium with subsequent replacement fibrosis stabilizing the new shape or the later expansion of an infarct which had already undergone fibrous replacement. A clinical study using serial two-dimensional echocardiography found aneurysms developed in 35 of 158 patients (22%) with infarction but the reported incidence varies widely. Early aneurysms developed within the period in intensive care in 15 patients and all were anterior and apical. Aneurysms developed within 3 months in a further 14 patients including some on the posterior inferior wall.[130]

A different pathogenesis has been proposed for those aneurysms that have a narrow neck leading to a large fibrous sac which is predominantly outside the ventricle. This may result from a ventricular tear which has led to a sub-pericardial haematoma, stopping just short of rupture into the pericardium

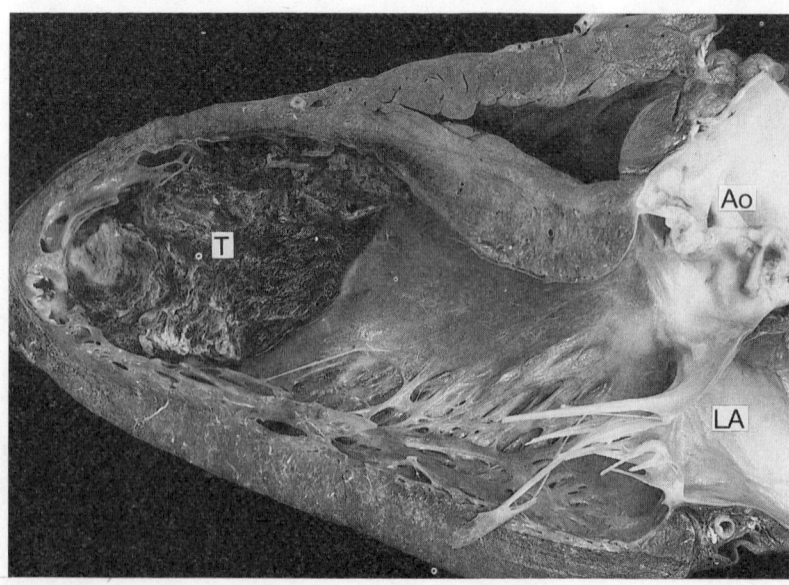

Fig. 44.25. Apical ventricular aneurysm with thrombus. Long-axis transection of the left ventricle showing an anterior apical aneurysm which is completely filled and obliterated by thrombus (T). Ao, aorta; LA, left atrium.

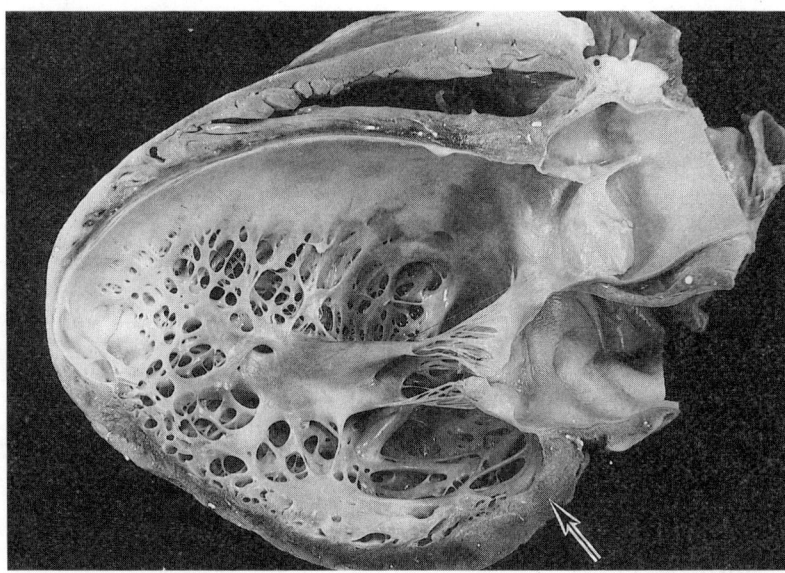

Fig. 44.26. Ischaemic cardiomyopathy. Long-axis transection of left ventricle in ischaemic 'cardiomyopathy'. The ventricle is thin walled and dilated with the endocardium thickened and opaque. The whole left ventricle has become a diffuse aneurysm with only a small portion of the basal posterior wall containing normal myocardium (arrow).

in the acute stage. Organization of the haematoma results in an aneurysmal sac to which the name pseudoventricular aneurysm has been applied[131] because the wall did not derive originally from ventricular myocardium. The distinction between true and pseudoaneurysms is more of theoretical than practical importance and localized saccular aneurysms (Fig. 44.23) are intermediate in appearance between the two forms. Aneurysms with a narrow neck are also found in patients without coronary artery disease and must be presumed to be congenital in origin in this case. Penetrating trauma such as knife wounds also leads to similar aneurysms.

ISCHAEMIC CARDIOMYOPATHY

Cardiomyopathy is usually taken to be indicative of a disease of the myocardium itself, hence the term ischaemic cardiomyopathy is a misnomer. The term is usually applied to chronic heart failure without anginal pain and a dilated left ventricle with generalized hypokinesia simulating an idiopathic dilated cardiomyopathy. The pathology is usually of a dilated left ventricle (Fig. 44.26) with no increase in wall thickness, in which there is no evidence of a previous large regional infarct. There is widespread myocardial fibrosis with scarring throughout the sub-endocardial zone and papillary muscles. The characteristic coronary arterial pathology is of widespread even stenosis in all the epicardial arteries and extreme development of intramyocardial collateral flow. A small minority of patients have

this arterial pattern but very little macroscopic or microscopic scarring, suggesting a chronic 'stunned' myocardium. The reason for absence of pain and large scars in this form of coronary atheroma is not known.

MYOCARDIAL INFARCTION WITH NORMAL CORONARY ARTERIES

The prevalence of patients who develop myocardial infarction and in whom subsequent angiography shows normal coronary arteries is between 1 and 3%.[132] Clinical parameters include young age, a high proportion of women and the absence of classic risk factors of atheroma with the exception of smoking habit. As the number of pathological studies of this entity is very small, it is possible to list only potential mechanisms of action. In some cases, the development of thrombosis is out of proportion with the degree of underlying atheroma so that lysis restores a vessel outline which, at worst, is slightly irregular. The absence of classic risk factors for atheroma would suggest that enhancement of thrombosis is the major factor. Other possible precipitating mechanisms are emboli from minor abnormalities of the aortic or mitral valve and unrecognized coronary artery dissection stopping at the point of subadventitial haematoma without an intimal tear. The majority of cases, however, probably represent spasm and can be regarded as forms of variant angina.[133]

It is difficult to determine the mechanisms of action in patients who have anginal pain but either a normal angiogram or insignificant stenosis (irregular outline, no stenosis > 25% in diameter). In a large study, there was a 20% incidence of normal angiograms and 7% of insignificant stenosis[134] in patients being studied for angina even when patients with Prinzmetal's angina were excluded. The patients with irregular arteries had a signifiantly higher incidence of infarction and sudden death by 10 years when compared with those who had totally normal arteries, but both groups continued to be symptomatic. The origin of the symptoms is ischaemic, as judged by myocardial lactate production, but the cause of the ischaemia is not known. Some patients have been shown to have inappropriate arteriolar constriction within the myocardium reducing the vasodilator reserve; however, in one study no morphological abnormalities were reported within the intramyocardial vessels on biopsy,[135] whereas, in another study, endothelial swelling within capillaries of the myocardium was recorded.[136]

VARIANTS OF ATHEROMATOUS CORONARY ARTERY DISEASE

CORONARY ARTERY LESIONS IN HYPERLIPIDAEMIA

The pattern of aortic and coronary atheroma differs in the five types of genetically determined hyperlipoproteinaemia.[137,138] Type I hyperlipoproteinaemia is not associated with enhanced atheroma. In homozygous type II hyperlipoproteinaemia, there is severe diffuse involvement of the ascending aorta often with heavy calcification superimposed on atheroma. Supra-aortic stenosis, valvar calcification and ostial stenosis may all result. The coronary arteries show widespread stenosis often with diffuse intimal thickening containing numerous foam cells and there is a high incidence of main left disease. Heterozygous type II hyperlipoproteinaemia is closer to 'conventional' coronary atheroma but with a tendency to diffuse intimal disease often with extension into small arteries. In types III and IV hyperlipoproteinaemia, there is an increased risk of ischaemic heart disease but little evidence of atheroma that has features different to those that are usually seen. In secondary hyperlipoproteinaemia, such as found in diabetes mellitus or myxoedema, there is unusually even intimal involvement with abundant lipid containing foam cells. Distal extension to small vessels such as the posterior descending or marginal arteries and even to intramyocardial arteries may occur.

CORONARY OSTIAL STENOSIS

Angiographic studies *in vivo* emphasize the rarity of ostial stenosis and that the majority of cases are found in association with widespread coronary stenosis. Thompson[139] found 27 examples in 2105 angiograms (1.2%) and Miller[140] found 35 in 4000 angiograms (0.8%). In only 10 of these 62 cases was the ostial stenosis isolated; all were relatively young women who had a low incidence of atheroma-related risk factors. These findings led to speculation that isolated ostial stenosis might be due to aortic root dysplasia, intimal hyperplasia or a sphincter-like ring of smooth muscle in the ostium and not due to atheroma. The results of the few pathological studies suggest an unusual distribution of atheroma rather than a different pathogenesis for ostial stenosis.[141] In some pathological series, a very high incidence of ostial stenosis was recorded[142] but in studies in which functional significance was assessed, by use of casts of the aortic root, values very similar to those obtained by clinical angiography were found.

THE PATHOLOGY OF ANGIOPLASTY

Pathological studies suggest two mechanisms exist for successful dilatation by angioplasty of stenoses due to atheroma.[143] In eccentric stenoses, in which there is a segment of normal arterial wall opposite the plaque, the segment of normal wall may be stretched with necrosis and attenuation of the media leaving the plaque itself unaltered. In many cases, however, a second mechanism occurs in which splitting and tearing of the fibrous intima of the plaque enlarges the lumen.[144] The degree of intimal damage and exposure of collagen is considerable underlining the necessity to limit secondary thrombosis by restoring high flow and by use of anticoagulants. Over succeeding days, the intima is smoothed over by a proliferation of cellular fibrous tissue remodelling the torn plaque.[145] Excessive smooth muscle proliferation within this tissue leads to recurrent stenosis in up to 30% of cases. Angioplasty of lipid-rich plaques is associated with extrusion of lipid through the attenuated media to invoke a florid giant cell response within the adventitia. Extrusion of small amounts of lipid into the circulation may also be common and these embolize into the myocardium forming small giant cell granulomas. Major complications of angioplasty involve rupture at the site, either of the normal arterial wall opposite the plaque due to necrosis of the medial muscle or by extrusion of lipid through a very attenuated media. Dissection develops when the intimal tears enter the plane between the intima and media following which an extending intramural haematoma may develop compressing the arterial lumen from the outside. Intimal tears that do not enter the plane between the intima and media do not have the same tendency to extend.

PATHOLOGY OF CORONARY ARTERY BYPASS GRAFTS

All coronary vein grafts in which flow is established develop a new thickened intimal layer by the process of fibromuscular proliferation.[146] The process appears to be inevitable and may be a result of endothelial damage and resultant platelet adhesion releasing mitogenic factors for smooth muscle cells. In keeping with this view the process can be minimized in animals by antiplatelet drugs. As similar intimal changes develop in arteriovenous shunts created for dialysis, it may be a response of venous intima to high flow and pressure. Intimal fibromuscular proliferation begins within 3 days of insertion of the graft and in most patients reaches a steady state by 1 month. A few patients show an exuberant intimal proliferation which may lead to occlusion particularly at anastomotic sites. Use of antiplatelet drugs will improve graft patency within the first year. The degree to which the original media of the vein survives varies widely both within different segments of the same vein and among patients. Where marked medial loss with replacement fibrosis has occurred, chronic dilatation of the graft often develops. Medial loss probably represents damage to the graft at insertion and examination of patent grafts in patients who have died within the first week often show frank necrosis of the graft media.

The early fibromuscular proliferation has no direct link to graft atheroma which is time-related becoming manifest from 3 years onward from insertion.[146] Foam cells begin to accumulate within the most superficial layer of the neo-intima, usually as a diffuse process rather than in discrete plaques; when discrete plaques do form, they relate to ligature sites of side branches. With time, there is a superficial breakdown of the neo-intima and the graft becomes lined by a mixture of foam cells, endothelial cells and strands of fine collagen over which friable thrombus foams. The final stage is

graft occlusion by a mixture of cholesterol and thrombus.[147] There is some clinical evidence that graft atheroma is accelerated by hyperlipidaemia and reduced in patients with normal levels of high density lipoprotein.[148]

NON-ATHEROMATOUS CORONARY ARTERY DISEASE

CONGENITAL ANOMALIES

Origins of both arteries from one aortic sinus or a single coronary orifice have no functional significance except for an artery that passes between the aorta and pulmonary trunk.[149] In this situation, progressive intimal proliferation may occlude the artery possibly due to intermittent external pressure. The artery may be the right coronary originating from the left aortic sinus or the left anterior descending and circumflex artery arising from the right sinus. Arteries crossing from right to left or vice versa behind the aorta have a far lower incidence of intimal proliferation and the only danger of crossing anterior to the pulmonary trunk is inadvertent damage at cardiac surgery. The presence of one orifice in the pulmonary trunk has far more serious sequelae.[150] In patients who survive infancy, a significant left-to-right shunt develops and the artery opening into the pulmonary trunk becomes aneurysmally dilated. Sub-endocardial fibrosis and calcification develop in infancy making early heart failure a common presentation. Late sudden death as the presenting symptom in adult life is also common. Aneurysmal dilatation of a coronary artery also develops with congenital fistulae into atria, ventricles or coronary sinus.

DISSECTION OF CORONARY ARTERIES

Dissecting aneurysms of the ascending aorta may extend into the coronary arteries themselves, a complication that develops more frequently in relation to the right coronary artery. Dissection occurs within the coronary artery as a complication of procedures, such as endarterectomy, insertion of vein grafts, cardiac catheterization and angioplasty, as well as developing spontaneously. The plane in which dissection develops in the coronary arteries is between the media and adventitia rather than intramedially as in dissection of the aorta. A review of less than 100 reported cases of spontaneous dissection in the literature, most of which are case-reports, indicates characteristic features of the process.[151-153] There is a preponderance of women; 40% of cases occur in the puerperium. Presentation is with acute infarction, sudden death or unstable angina, with the left anterior descending artery being affected more commonly than the right, by a ratio of 4:1. Post-mortem studies, however, show that multiple dissections are common suggesting the basis lies in a generalized abnormality of the coronary arteries. Pathological studies also suggest the process begins as a subadventitial haematoma due to bleeding from vessels crossing into the most superficial layer of the media. Such haematomas may compress the arterial lumen leading to ischaemic myocardial damage or may invoke local arterial spasm. Resolution and organization of the haematoma at this stage can lead to a return to normal angiographic appearances. In other cases, the haematoma breaks through into the lumen, by the development of an intimal tear, leading to more major arterial disruption. Medial cystic change analogous to the changes seen in the aortic media with dissection are described inconsistently; an infiltrate of the adventitia with chronic inflammatory cells including eosinophils is frequently described. The basic structure of the media of the coronary arteries is very different from that of the aorta in which elastic tissue rather than smooth muscle predominates and no clear association of coronary artery dissection with diseases that produce cystic medial necrosis in the aorta such as Marfan's syndrome is established. In one case, as yet unconfirmed, fibroblasts in the skin of a patient with spontaneous dissection of a coronary artery in the puerperium had impaired collagen synthesis.[153] No association with coronary atheroma is described. It is not known whether the tendency to coronary dissection is intermittent or persistent. Patients who develop dissection in the puerperium suggest the tendency is intermittent, whereas in patients who develop dissection after apparently routine angiography the tendency may be persistent. A further possibility is that subadventitial haematomas develop after prolonged spasm.

ARTERIAL BRIDGING

At certain points, the epicardial arteries are covered by a layer of superficial epicardial myocardium. The phenomenon occurs in varying degrees in up to 50% of normal hearts. Reports suggest that external compression of the artery during systole can be detected angiographically, can be responsible for temporary occlusion or for myocardial infarction[154] and can play a part in inducing angina in hypertrophied ventricles including hypertrophic cardiomyopathy. However, it must be emphasized that bridging is common in normal hearts.[155] Data exist to show that bridged arterial segments are protected from atheromatous disease.[155]

CORONARY ANEURYSMS

The term coronary aneurysm, aneurysmal dilatation and coronary ectasia are all used to describe different parts of a spectrum running from localized lateral bulges in an otherwise angiographically normal artery through localized areas of dilatation in an artery with areas of stenosis to diffuse dilatation of the whole artery. There is considerable overlap and inconsistency in the use of these terms by different authors but agreement exists that about 1.5% of coronary arteriograms in adults show appearances falling within this spectrum.[156,157] In all cases, the basic pathological process is one of medial destruction but the exact pathogenesis is not known particularly when it is determined solely from angiographic appearances. The commonest form is dilated ectatic segments of artery alternating with stenotic segments suggesting atheroma is responsible.[157] Diffuse initial atheroma does lead to marked medial atrophy but the reason why stenosis should occur in some areas and dilatation in others is not known. Although diffuse ectasia without stenosis is associated with diffuse loss of medial muscle often with some intimal calcification and minor lipid deposition, it is debatable whether this is sufficient evidence to regard the whole process as a variant of atheroma. Diffuse dilatation of one artery in young individuals may represent high flow either due to fistulae into a chamber or the coronary sinus or due to an anomalous origin from the pulmonary artery.

Localized saccular coronary aneurysms represent destruction or loss of the media in part of the circumference of the artery. A minority are due to congenital defects in the media but most represent the end-stage of an arteritic inflammatory process. Classic polyarteritis nodosa affects the coronary arteries as part of a systemic involvement of muscular arteries but in Kawasaki disease the coronary arteries are almost exclusively involved. Kawasaki disease,[158] first described as endemic in Japan, presents as an acute febrile illness in children, associated with a skin rash, oral ulceration and cervical lymphadenopathy. Cardiac involvement may develop after a short latent period and is characterized by coronary aneurysms leading to thrombosis and myocardial infarction as the principal cause of death. Epidemics of the disease are characteristic worldwide and in Japan, and a viral aetiology is likely.[159,160] The coronary arterial involvement may be very widespread leading to early death or less severe leaving residual aneurysm which may be detected by angiography or thrombose to induce infarction in later adult life.[161,162]

REFERENCES

1. Klocke, F.J. Coronary blood flow in man. *Prog. Cardiovasc. Dis.* 1976; **19**: 117.
2. Hoffman, J.I.E. Coronary physiology and pathophysiology. In: Fox, K.M., ed. *Ischaemic Heart Disease*. Lancaster: MTP Press, 1987, p. 69.
3. Poole-Wilson, P.A. Haemodynamic and metabolic consequences of angina and myocardial infarction. In: Fox, K.M., ed. *Ischaemic Heart Disease*. Lancaster: MTP Press, 1987, p. 123.
4. Farrer-Brown, F. Normal and diseased vascular patterns of myocardium of human heart. *Br. Heart J.* 1968; **30**: 527.
5. Burnstock, G. and Griffith, S.G. Neurohumoral control of the vasculature. In: Woolf, N., ed. *Biology and Pathology of the vessel wall—A modern Appraisal*. Eastbourne: Praeger Publ., 1983, p 15.
6. McEwan, J., Larkin, S., Davies, G.J. *et al.* Calcitonin gene related peptide is a potent dilator of human epicardial coronary arteries. *Circulation* 1986; **74**: 1243.
7. Busse, R., Trogisch, G. and Bassenge, E. The role of endothelium in the control of vascular tone. *Basic Res. Cardiol.* 1985; **80**: 475.
8. Anonymous EDRF [Editorial]. *Lancet* 1987; **II**: 137.
9. Weiner, D.A., Ryan, T.J., McGabe, C.H. *et al.* Exercise stress testing. Correlations among history of angina. ST segment response and prevalence of coronary artery disease in the CAS study. *N. Engl. J. Med.* 1979; **301**: 230.
10. Higgins, D., Santamore, W.P., Walinsky, P. and Nemir, P. Haemodynamics of human arterial stenosis. *Int. J. Cardiol.* 1985; **87**: 177.
11. Klocke, F.J. Measurement of coronary blood flow and degree of stenosis: current clinical implications and continuing uncertainties. *J. Am. Coll. Cardiol.* 1983; **1**: 31.
12. Sabbah, H.N. and Stein, P.D. Hemodynamics of multiple versus single 50% coronary arterial stenoses. *Am. J. Cardiol.* 1982; **50**: 278.
13. Roberts, W.C. and Virmani, R. The coronary arteries and left ventricle in clinically isolated angina pectoris—a necropsy analysis. *Am. J. Med.* 1979; **67**: 792.
14. Roberts, W.C. The coronary arteries and left ventricle in clinically isolated angina pectoris. *Circulation* 1976; **54**: 388.
15. Quyyumi, A.A., Al-Rufaie, H.K., Olsen, E.G.J. and Fox, K.M. Coronary anatomy in patients with various manifestations of three vessel coronary artery disease. *Br. Heart J.* 1985; **54**: 362.
16. Thomas, A.C., Davies, M.J., Dilly, S., Dilly, N. and Franc, F. Potential errors in the estimation of coronary arterial stenosis from clinical arteriography with reference to the shape of the coronary arterial lumen. *Br. Heart J.* 1986; **55**: 129.
17. Hangartner, J.R.W., Charleston, A.J., Davies, M.J. and Thomas, A.C. Morphological characteristics of clinically significant coronary artery stenosis in stable angina. *Br. Heart J.* 1986; **56**: 501.
18. Brown, B.G. Coronary vasospasm: observations linking the clinical spectrum of ischemic heart disease to the dynamic pathology of coronary atherosclerosis. *Arch. Intern. Med.* 1981; **141**: 716.
19. Freudenberg, H. and Lichtlen, P.R. Das nomale Wandsegment bei Koronartsemon, eine post mortale studie. *Z. Kardiol.* 1981; **70**: 863.
20. Brown, B., Robson, E.L. and Dodge, H.T. Dynamic mechanisms in human coronary stenosis. *Circulation* 1984; **70**: 917.
21. Isner, J.M., Donaldson, R.F., Fortin, A.H., Tischler, A. and Clarke, R.H. Attenuation of media of coronary arteries in advanced atherosclerosis. *Am. J. Cardiol.* 1986; **58**: 397.
22. Lichtlen, P.R., Rafflenbeul, W. and Freudenberg, H. Patho-anatomy and function of coronary obstructions leading to unstable angina pectoris—anatomical and angiographic studies. In: Hugenholtz, P.G. and Goldman, B.S., eds. *Unstable Angina*. Stuttgart: Schattauer, 1985, p. 81.
23. Saner, H.E., Gobel, F.L., Salomonowitz, E., Erlien, D.A. and Edwards, J.E. The disease free wall in coronary atherosclerosis: Its relation to degree of obstruction. *J. Am Coll. Cardiol.* 1985; **6**: 1096.
24. Lundberg, B. Chemical composition and physical state of lipid deposits in atherosclerosis. *Atherosclerosis* 1985; **56**: 93.
25. Roberts, W.C. and Virmani, R. Formation of new coronary arteries within a previously obstructed epicardial coronary artery (intra-arterial arteries). *Am. J. Cardiol.* 1984; **54**: 1361.
26. Barger, A.C., Beeuwkes, R., Lainey, L.L. and Silverman, K.J. Hypothesis vasa vasorum and neovascularization of human coronary arteries. A possible role in the pathophysiology of atherosclerosis. *N. Engl. J. Med.* 1983; **310**: 363.
27. Davies, D.F., Rees, B.W.G. and Davies, P.T.G. Cows milk antibodies and coronary heart disease. *Lancet* 1980; **1**: 1190.
28. Parums, D.V. and Mitchinson, M.J. Autoallergy in atherosclerosis. *J. Pathol.* 1985; **146**: 245.
29. Faggiotto, A., Ross, R. and Harker, L. Studies of hypercholesterolaemia in the non-human primate. 1. Changes that lead to fatty streak formation. *Arteriosclerosis* 1984; **4**: 323.
30. Ross, R. The pathogenesis of atherosclerosis—an update. *N. Engl. J. Med.* 1986; **314**: 488.
31. Ludmer, P.L., Selwyn, A.P., Shook, T.L. *et al.* Paradoxical vasoconstriction induced by acetylcholine in atherosclerotic coronary arteries. *N. Engl. J. Med.* 1986; **315**: 1046.
32. Fulton, W.F.M. *The coronary arteries: arteriography, microanatomy and pathogenesis of obliterative coronary disease*. Springfield: Charles C. Thomas, 1965, p. 230.
33. Ambrose, J.A., Winter, S.L., Sterna Eng, A., Teicholg, L.E., Gorlin, R. and Fuster, V. Angiographic morphology and the pathogenesis of unstable angina pectoris. *J. Am. Coll. Cardiol.* 1981; **5**: 609.
34. Levin, D.C. and Fallon, J.T. Significance of the angiographic morphology of localized coronary stenoses. Histopathological correlates. *Circulation* 1982; **66**: 136.
35. Mitchinson, M.J. and Ball, R.Y. Macrophages and atherogenesis. *Lancet* 1987; **II**: 146.
36. Singh, R. Progression of coronary atherosclerosis. Clues to pathogenesis from serial coronary angiography. *Br. Heart J.* 1984; **52**: 451.
37. Maseri, A. Pathogenetic mechanism of post infarction angina. *Eur. Heart J.* 1986; **7**(Suppl. C): 3.
38. Falk, E. Plaque rupture with severe pre-existing stenosis

precipitating coronary thrombosis. Characteristics of coronary atherosclerotic plaques underlying fatal occlusive thrombi. *Br. Heart J.* 1983; 50: 127.

39. Falk, E. Thrombosis in unstable angina: pathologic aspects. In: Mehta, L.J. and Conti, R., eds. *Thrombosis and platelets in myocardial ischaemia—Cardiovascular Clinics.* Philadelphia: F.A. Davis & Co., 1987, p. 137.

40. Ambrose, J.A., Winters, S.L., Arora, R.R. *et al.* Angiographic evolution of coronary artery morphology in unstable angina. *J. Am. Coll. Cardiol.* 1986; 7: 472.

41. Ciampricotti, R. and Elgamal, M. Exercise induced plaque rupture producing myocardial infarction. *Int. J. Cardiol.* 1986; 12: 102.

42. Black, A., Black, M.M. and Gensini, G. Exertion and acute coronary artery injury. *Angiology* 1975; 26: 759.

43. Chandler, A.B. Mechanisms and frequency of thrombosis in the coronary circulation. *Thromb. Res.* 1974; 4: 3.

44. Alison, H.W., Russell, R.O., Mantle, J.A., Kouchoukos, N.T., Moraski, R.E. and Rackley, C.E. Coronary anatomy and arteriography in patients with unstable angina. *Am. J. Cardiol.* 1978; 41: 204.

45. Fuster, V., Frye, R.L., Connolly, D.C., Danielson, M.A., Elveback, L.R. and Kurland, L.T. Angiographic patterns early in the onset of coronary syndromes. *Br. Heart J.* 1975; 37: 1250.

46. Ambrose, J.A., Winters, S.L., Arora, B.R. *et al.* Coronary angiography morphology in acute myocardial infarction: Link between the pathogenesis of unstable angina and myocardial infarction. *J. Am. Coll. Cardiol.* 1985; 6: 1233.

47. Ambrose, J.A., Winters, S.L., Arora, R.R. *et al.* Angiographic evolution of coronary artery morphology in unstable angina. *J. Am. Coll. Cardiol.* 1986; 7: 472.

48. Kranjec, I., Delaye, J., Didier, B., Delahaye, F. and Grand, A. Angiographic morphology and intraluminal coronary artery thrombus in patients with angina pectoris: clinical correlations. *Eur. Heart J.* 1987; 8: 106.

49. Moise, A., Theroux, P., Taeymans, Y. *et al.* Unstable angina and progression of coronary atherosclerosis. *N. Engl. J.* 1983; 309: 685.

50. Davies, M.J. and Thomas, A.C. Plaque fissuring—the cause of acute myocardial infarction, sudden ischaemic death and crescendo angina. *Br. Heart J.* 1985; 53: 363.

51. Sherman, C.T., Litvack, F., Grundfest, W. *et al.* Coronary angioscopy in patients with unstable angina pectoris. *N. Engl. J. Med.* 1986; 315: 913.

52. Lam, J.Y.T., Chesebro, J.H., Steele, P.M., Badimon, L. and Fuster, V. Is vasospasm related to platelet deposition? Relationship in a porcine preparation of arterial injury *in vivo. Circulation* 1987; 75: 243

53. Moore, E., Belbeck, L.W., Evans, G. and Pineau, S. Effects of complete or partial occlusion of a coronary artery. *Lab. Invest.* 1981; 44: 151.

54. Davies, M.J., Thomas, A.C., Knapman, P.A. and Hangartner, R. Intramyocardial platelet aggregation in unstable angina and sudden ischemic death. *Circulation* 1986; 73: 418.

55. Falk, E. Unstable angina with fatal outcome: dynamic coronary thrombosis leading to infarction and/or sudden death. *Circulation* 1985; 71: 699.

56. Fitzgerald, D.J., Roy, L., Catella, F. and Fitzgerald, G.A. Platelet activation in unstable coronary disease. *N. Engl. J. Med.* 1986; 315: 983.

57. Serneri, G.G., Gensini, G.F., Carnovali, M. *et al.* Association between time of increased fibropeptide A levels in plasma and episodes of spontaneous angina: a controlled prospective trial. *Am. Heart J.* 1987; 113: 672.

58. Maseri, A., Severi, S., Nes, M.D. *et al.* Variant Angina; one aspect of a continuous spectrum of vasospastic myocardial ischaemia: pathogenetic mechanisms, estimated incidence,

clinical and coronary arteriographic findings in 138 patients. *Am. J. Cardiol.* 1978; 42: 1019.

59. Roberts, W.C., Curry, R.C., Isner, J.M. *et al.* Sudden death in Prinzmetal's angina with coronary spasm documented by arteriography: analysis of three necropsy cases. *Am. J. Cardiol.* 1982; 50: 203.

60. Hillis, D. and Braunwald, E. Coronary artery spasm. *N. Engl. J. Med.* 1978; 299: 695.

61. Rasmussen, K., Ravnbaek, J., Funch-Jensen, P. and Bagger, J.P. Oesophageal spasm in patients with coronary artery spasm. *Lancet* 1986; 1: 174.

62. Robertson, D. and Oates, J.A. Variant angina and Raynaud's phenomenon. *Lancet* 1978; 1: 452.

63. Miller, D., Waters, D.D., Warnica, W. *et al.* Is variant angina the coronary manifestation of a generalized vasospastic disorder? *N. Engl. J. Med.* 1981; 304: 763.

64. Kawachi, Y., Tomoiki, H., Marvoka, Y. *et al.* Selective hypercontraction caused by ergonovine in canine coronary artery under conditions of induced atherosclerosis. *Circulation* 1984; 69: 441.

65. Heistad, D.D., Armstrong, M.L., Marcul, M.L., Piegors, D.J. and Mark, A.L. Augmented responses to vasoconstrictor stimuli in hypercholesterolemic and atherosclerotic monkeys. *Circ. Res.* 1984; 54: 711.

66. Kohchi, K., Takebayashi, S., Hiroki, T. and Nobuyoshi, M. Significance of adventitial inflammation of the coronary artery in patients with unstable angina; results at autopsy. *Circulation* 1985; 71: 709.

67. Forman, M.B., Oates, J.A., Robertson, D. *et al.* Increased adventitial mast cells in a patient with coronary spasm. *N. Engl. J. Med.* 1985; 313: 1138.

68. Levine, H.D. Subendocardial infarction in retrospect: pathologic, cardiographic and ancillary features. *Circulation* 1985; 72: 790.

69. Spodick, D.H. Q wave infarction versus ST infarction. Non-specificity of electrocardiographic criteria for differentiating transmural and non-transmural infarction. *Am. J. Cardiol.* 1983; 51: 913.

70. DeWood, M.A., Spores, J., Notske, R. *et al.* Prevalence of total coronary occlusion during the early hours of transmural myocardial infarction. *N. Engl. J. Med.* 1980; 303: 897.

71. Stadius, M.L., Maynard, C., Fritz, J.K. *et al.* Coronary anatomy and left ventricular function in the first twelve hours of acute myocardial infarction: the Western Washington randomized intracoronary streptokinase trial. *Circulation* 1985; 72: 292.

72. Bertrand, M.E., Lefebvre, J.M., Laisne, C.L. *et al.* Coronary angiography in acute transmural myocardial infarction. *Am. Heart J.* 1979; 97: 61.

73. Maseri, A., Chierchia, S. and Davies, G. Pathophysiology of coronary occlusion in acute infarction. *Circulation* 1986; 73: 233.

74. Davies, M.J., Woolf, N. and Robertson, W.B. Pathology of acute myocardial infarction with particular reference to occlusive coronary thrombi. *Br. Heart J.* 1976; 38: 659.

75. Ridolfi, R.L. and Hutchins, G.M. The relationship between coronary artery lesions and myocardial infarcts: ulceration of atherosclerotic plaques precipitating coronary thrombosis. *Am. Heart J.* 1977; 93: 468.

76. Chapman, I. The cause–effect relationship between recent coronary artery occlusion and acute myocardial infarction. *Am. Heart J.* 1984; 87: 267.

77. Davies, M.J. and Thomas, A. The pathological basis and microanatomy of occlusive thrombus formation in human coronary arteries. *Phil. Trans. R. Soc. Lond.* (Biological) 1981; 294: 255.

78. Horie, T., Sekiguchi, M. and Hirosawa, K. Coronary thrombosis in pathogenesis of acute myocardial infarction. Histopathological study of coronary arteries in 108 nec-

ropsied cases. *Br. Heart J.* 1978; **40**: 153.

79. Erhardt, L.R., Unge, G., and Bowman, G. Formation of coronary arterial thrombi in relation to onset of necrosis in acute myocardial infarction in man. *Am. Heart J.* 1976; **1**: 592.

80. Henriksson, P., Edhag, O., Jansson, B. *et al.* A role for platelets in the process of infarct extension. *N. Engl. J. Med.* 1985; **313**: 1660.

81. Fulton, W.E.M. and Sumner, D.J. I^{125}-labelled fibrinogen, autoradiography and stereo-arteriography in identification of coronary thrombotic occlusion in fatal myocardial infarction. *Br. Heart J.* 1976; **38**: 880.

82. Hackett, D., Davies, G., Chierchia, S. and Maseri, A. High frequency of intermittant occlusion in acute myocardial infarction. *Circulation* 1986; **74** (Suppl. 2): 278.

83. DeWood, M.A., Spores, J., Notske, R.N. *et al.* Nontransmural (subendocardial) myocardial infarction in man: The prevalence of total coronary occlusion. *Am. J. Cardiol.* 1981; **47**: 459.

84. Erhardt, L.R. Clinical and pathological observations in different types of acute myocardial infarction. A study of 84 patients decreased after treatment in coronary care unit. *Acta. Med. Scand.* 1974; Suppl. 560: 1078.

85. Schulza, R.A., Pitt, B., Griffith, L.S.C. *et al.* Coronary arteriography and left ventriculography in survivors of transmural and non-transmural myocardial infarction. *Am. J. Med.* 1978; **64**: 108.

86. Cobb, L.A., Werner, J.A. and Trobaugh, G.B. Sudden cardiac death: 1. A decade's experience with out-of-hospital resuscitation. *Mod. Concepts Cardiovasc. Dis.* 1980; **49**: 31.

87. DeWood, M.A., Spores, J., Notske, R.N. *et al.* Coronary artery occlusion determined early after sudden cardiac death due to myocardial infarction. *J. Am. Coll. Cardiol.* 1985; **5**: 401.

88. Davies, M.J. and Thomas, A. Thrombosis and acute coronary artery lesions in sudden cardiac ischemic death. *N. Engl. J. Med.* 1981; **310**: 1137.

89. Warnes, C.A. and Roberts, W.C. Sudden coronary death: comparison of patients with those without coronary thrombus at necropsy. *Am. J. Cardiol.* 1981; **54**: 1206.

90. Warnes, C. and Roberts, W.C. Comparison at necropsy by age group of amount and distribution of narrowing by atherosclerotic plaque in 2995 five mm long segment of 240 major coronary arteries in 60 men aged 31–70 years with sudden coronary death. *Am. Heart J.* 1984; **108**: 431.

91. Roberts, W.C. and Jones, A.A. Quantitation of coronary arterial narrowing at necropsy in sudden coronary death. Analysis of 31 patients and comparison with 25 control subjects. *Am. J. Cardiol.* 1979; **44**: 39.

92. Van Dantzig, J.M. and Becker, A.F. Sudden cardiac death and acute pathology of coronary arteries. *Eur. Heart J.* 1986; **7**: 987.

93. El-Fawal, M.A., Berg, G.A., Wheatley, D.J. and Harland, A. Sudden coronary death in Glasgow: nature and frequency of acute coronary lesions. *Br. Heart J.* 1987; **57**: 329.

94. Reimer, K.A., Lowe, J.E., Rasmussen, M.M. and Jennings, R.B. The wave front phenomenon of ischemic cell death. I. Myocardial infarct size vs duration of coronary occlusion in dogs. *Circulation* 1977; **56**: 786.

95. Reimer, K.A. and Jennings, R.B. The wave front phenomenon of myocardial ischemic cell death. II Transmural progression of necrosis within the framework of ischemic bed size (myocardium at risk) and collateral flow. *Lab. Invest.* 1979; **40**: 633.

96. Jennings, R.B. and Reimer, K.A. Lethal myocardial ischemic injury. *Am. J. Pathol.* 1981; **102**: 241.

97. Reimer, K.A., Jennings, R.B., Cobb, F.R. *et al.* Animal models for protecting ischemic myocardium—results of

98. Jolly, S.R., Kane, W.J., Bailie, M.B. *et al.* Canine myocardial reperfusion injury: its reduction by the combined administration of superoxide dismutase and catalase. *Circ. Res.* 1984; **54**: 277.

99. McCord, J.M. Oxygen-derived free radicals in post ischemic tissue injury. *N. Engl. J. Med.* 1985; **312**: 159.

100. Rosen, R.D., Swain, J.L., Michael, L.H. *et al.* Selective accumulation of the first component of complement and leucocytes in ischemic canine heart muscle. A possible initiator of an extra myocardial mechanism of ischemic injury. *Circ. Res.* 1985; **57**: 119.

101. Kloner, R.A., Ganote, C.E. and Jennings, R.B. The "no-reflow" phenomenon after temporary coronary occlusion in the dog. *J. Clin. Invest.* 1974; **54**: 1496.

102. Werns, S.W., Shea, M.J., Mitson, S.E. *et al.* Reduction of infarct size by allopurinol in the ischemic reperfused canine heart. *Circulation* 1986; **73**: 518.

103. Braunwald, E. and Kloner, R.A. Myocardial reperfusion: A double edged sword. *J. Clin. Invest.* 1985; **76**: 1713.

104. Roberts, C.S., Schoen, E.J. and Kloner, R.A. Effect of coronary reperfusion on myocardial infarct healing and hemorrhage. *Am. J. Cardiol.* 1983; **52**: 610.

105. Lodge-Patch, I. The aging of cardiac infarcts and its influence on cardiac rupture. *Br. Heart J.* 1951; **13**: 37.

106. Flameng, W., Wouters, L., Sergeant, P. *et al.* Multivarate analysis of angiographic, histologic and electrocardiographic data in patients with coronary heart disease. *Circulation* 1984; **70**: 7.

107. Schaper, W. Natural defence mechanisms during ischaemia. *Eur. Heart J.* 1983; **4**(Suppl. D): 73.

108. Grande, P. and Pedersen, A. Myocardial infarct size: Correlation with cardiac arrhythmias and sudden death. *Eur. Heart J.* 1984; **5**: 622.

109. Page, D.L., Caulfield, J.B., Kastor, J.A., DeSanctis, R.W. and Sanders, C.A. Myocardial changes associated with cardiogenic shock. *N. Engl. J. Med.* 1971; **285**: 133.

110. Alonzo, D.R., Scheidr, S., Post, M. and Kjillip, T. Pathophysiology of cardiogenic shock, quantifications of myocardial necrosis, clinical pathologic and electrocardiographic correlations. *Circulation* 1973; **48**: 588.

111. Gutovitz, A.L., Sobel, B.E. and Roberts, R. Progressive nature of myocardial injury in selected patients with cardiogenic shock. *Am. J. Med.* 1978; **41**: 469.

112. Saffitz, J.E., Fredrickson, R. and Roberts, W.C. Relation of size of transmural acute myocardial infarction to mode of death. *Am. J. Cardiol.* 1986; **57**: 1249.

113. James, T.N. The coronary circulation and conduction system in acute myocardial infarction. *Prog. Cardiovasc. Dis.* 1968; **10**: 410.

114. Cancilla, P.A. and Nicklaus, T.M. Atrial fibrillation with occlusion of the sinus node artery. *Arch. Intern. Med.* 1966; **117**: 422.

115. Becker, A.E. Atrioventricular Conduction disturbances in acute myocardial infarction. In: Davies, M.J., Anderson, R.H. and Becker, A.E., eds. *The Conduction System of the Heart*. London: Butterworths, 1983, p. 161.

116. Bilbao, F.J., Zabalza, I.E., Vilanova, J.R. and Froufe, J. AV block posterior acute myocardial infarction: a clinico-pathological correlation. *Circulation* 1987; **75**: 733.

117. Schuster, E.H. and Bulkley, B.H. Expansion of transmural myocardial infarction: a pathophysiologic factor in cardiac rupture. *Circulation* 1979; **60**: 1532.

118. Pirolo, S., Hutchins, G.M. and Moore, W. Infarct expansion: Pathologic analysis of 204 patients with a single myocardial infarct. *J. Am. Coll. Cardiol.* 1986; **7**: 349.

119. Dellborg, M., Held, P., Swedberg, K. and Anders, V. Rupture of the myocardium: occurrence and risk factors. *Br. Heart J.* 1985; **54**: 11.

120. Becker, A.E. and Vanmantgem, J.P. Cardiac tamponade—

the NHLBI co-operative study. *Circ. Res.* 1985; **56**: 651.

a study of 50 hearts. *Eur. J. Cardiol.* 1975; **3**: 349.

121. Atkinson, J.B., Robinowitz, M., McCallister, H.A. and Virmani, R. Association of eosinophils with cardiac rupture. *Human Pathol.* 1985; **16**: 562.

122. Vlodaver, Z. and Edwards, J.E. Rupture of ventricular septum or papillary muscle complicating myocardial infarction. *Circulation* 1977; **55**: 815.

123. Sanders, C.A., Armstrong, P.W., Willerson, J.T. and Dinsmore, R.E. Aetiology and differential diagnosis of acute mitral regurgitation. *Prog. Cardiovasc. Dis.* 1971; **14**: 129.

124. Nashimura, R.A., Schaff, H.V., Shub, C., Gersh, B.J., Edwards, W.D. and Takik, A.J. Papillary muscle rupture complicating acute myocardial infarction—analysis of 17 patients. *Am. J. Cardiol.* 1983; **51**: 373.

125. Wei, J.Y., Hutchins, G.M. and Bulkley, B.H. Papillary muscle rupture in fatal acute myocardial infarction: A potentially treatable form of cardiogenic shock. *Ann. Intern. Med.* 1979; **90**: 149.

126. Barbour, D.J. and Roberts, W.C. Rupture of a left ventricular papillary muscle during acute myocardial infarction. Analysis of 22 necropsy patients. *J. Am. Coll. Cardiol.* 1986; **8**: 558.

127. Kulbertus, H.E., Rigo, P. and Legrand, V. Right ventricular infarction: pathophysiology diagnosis, clinical course and treatment. *Mod. Concepts Cardiovasc. Dis.* 1985; **54**: 1.

128. Tibbutt, D.A. True left ventricular aneurysm. *Br. Med. J.* 1984; **289**: 450.

129. Roberts, W.C. and Kaufman, R.J. Calcification of healed myocardial infarcts. *Am. J. Cardiol.* 1987; **60**: 28.

130. Visser, C.A., Kan, G., Meltzer, R.S., Koolen, J.J. and Dunning, A.J. Incidence timing and prognostic value of left ventricular aneurysm formation after infarction. *Am. J. Cardiol.* 1986; **57**: 729.

131. Van Tassel, R.A. and Edwards, J.E. Rupture of the heart complicating myocardial infarction. Analysis of 40 cases including nine examples of left ventricular false aneurysm. *Chest* 1972; **61**: 104.

132. Fox, K.M. Myocardial infarction and the normal coronary arteriogram. *Br. Heart J.* 1983; **287**: 446.

133. Legrand, V., Deliege, M., Henrard, L., Boland, J. and Kulbertus, H. Patients with myocardial infarction and normal coronary arteriogram. *Chest* 1982; **82**: 678.

134. Papanicolaou, M.N., Califf, R.M., Hlatky, M.A. *et al.* Prognostic implications of angiographically normal and insignificantly narrowed coronary arteries. *Am. J. Cardiol.* 1986; **58**: 1181.

135. Opherex, D., Zebe, H., Weihe, E. *et al.* Reduced coronary dilatory capacity and ultrastructural changes in the myocardium in patients with angina pectoris but normal coronary arteriograms. *Circulation* 1981; **63**: 817.

136. Mosseri, M., Yarom, R., Gotsman, M.S. and Hasin, Y. Histologic evidence for small vessel coronary artery disease in patients with angina pectoris and patent large coronary arteries. *Circulation* 1986; **74**: 964.

137. Ferrancs, V.J. and Boyce, S.W. Metabolic and familial diseases. In: Silver M.D., ed. *Cardiovascular Pathology.* New York: Churchill Livingstone, 1983; p. 966.

138. Roberts, W.C., Ferrans, V.J., Levy, R.I. and Fredrickson, D.S. Cardiovascular pathology in hyperlipoproteinemias. anatomic observations in 42 necropsy patients. *Am. J. Cardiol.* 1973; **31**: 557.

139. Thompson, R. Isolated coronary ostial stenosis in women. *J. Am. Coll. Cardiol.* 1986; **7**: 997.

140. Miller, A.H., Honey, M. and El Sayed, H. Isolated coronary stenosis. *Cathet. Cardiovasc. Diag.* 1986; **12**: 30.

141. Stewart, J.T., Ward, D.E., Davies, M.J. and Pepper, J.R. Isolated coronary ostial stenosis: observations on the pathology. *Eur. Heart J.* 1987; **8**: 917.

142. Rissanen, V. Occurrence of coronary ostial stenosis in necropsy series of myocardial infarction, sudden death and violent death. *Br. Heart J.* 1975; **37**: 182.

143. Block P.C. Mechanisms of transluminal angioplasty. *Am. J. Cardiol.* 1984; **53**: 69.

144. Colavita, P.G., Ideker, R.E., Reimer, K.A., Hackle, D.B. and Stack, R.S. The spectrum of pathology associated with percutaneous coronary angioplasty during acute myocardial infarction. *J. Am. Coll. Cardiol.* 1986; **8**: 855.

145. Veda, M., Becker, A.E. and Fujimoto, T. Pathological changes induced by percutaneous transluminal coronary angioplasty. *Br. Heart J.* 1987; **58**: 635.

146. Bourassa, M.G., Campeau, L., Lesperance, J. and Solymoss, B.C. Atherosclerosis after coronary artery bypass surgery: results of recent studies and recommendations regarding prevention. *Cardiology* 1986; **73**: 259.

147. Bulkley, B.H. and Hutchins, G.M. Accelerated "atherosclerosis": a morphological study of 91 saphenous vein coronary artery bypass grafts. *Am. J. Cardiol.* 1976; **37**: 124.

148. Neitzel, G.F., Barboriak, J.J., Pintar, K. and Qureshi, I. Atherosclerosis in aorto-coronary bypass grafts. Morphologic study and risk factor analysis 6–12 years after surgery. *Arteriosclerosis* 1986; **6**: 594.

149. Roberts, W.C. Major anomalies of coronary arterial origin seen in adulthood. *Am. Heart J.* 1986; **111**: 941.

150. Levin, D.C., Fellows, K.E. and Abrams, H.L. Haemodynamically significant primary anomalies of the coronary arteries. *Circulation* 1978; **58**: 25.

151. Mathieu, D., Larde, D. and Vasile, N. Primary dissecting aneurysm of the coronary arteries: case report and literature review. *Cardiovasc. Intervent. Radiol.* 1984; **7**: 71.

152. Baker, P.B., Keyhani-Rofagha, S., Graham, R.L. and Sharma, H.M. Dissecting hematoma (aneurysm) of coronary arteries. *Am. J. Med.* 1986; **80**: 317.

153. Bonnet, J., Aumailley, M., Thomas, D., Grosgogeat, Y., Broustet, J.P. and Bricaud, H. Spontaneous coronary artery dissection: case report and evidence for a defect in collagen metabolism. *Eur. Heart J.* 1986; **7**: 904.

154. Felman, A.M. and Baughman, K.L. Myocardial infarction association with a myocardial bridge. *Am. Heart J.* 1986; **111**: 784.

155. Ishll, T., Hosoda, Y., Osaka, T. *et al.* The significance of myocardial bridging on atherosclerosis in the left anterior descending coronary artery. *J. Pathol.* 1986; **148**: 279.

156. Daoud, A.S., Pankin, D., Tulgan, H. and Florentin, R.A. Aneurysms of the coronary artery: Report of 10 cases and review of the literature. *Am. J. Cardiol.* 1963; **11**: 228.

157. Swanton, R.H., Lea-Thomas, M., Coltart, D.J. Jenkins, B.S., Webb-Peploe, M. and Williams, B.T. Coronary artery ectasia—a variant of occlusive coronary arteriosclerosis. *Br. Heart J.* 1978; **40**: 393.

158. Seiguchi, M., Takao, A., Endo, M., Asai, T. and Kawasaki, I. On the mucocutaneous lymph node syndrome or Kawasaki disease. In: Yu, P.N. and Goodwin, J.F., eds. *Progress in Cardiology.* Philadelphia, 1985, p. 97.

159. Yanagawa, H., Nakamura, Y., Kawasaki, T. and Shigematsu, I. Nationwide epidemic of Kawasaki disease in Japan during the winter of 1985–1986. *Lancet* 1986; **ii**: 1138.

160. Shulman, S.T. and Rowley, A.H. Does Kawasaki disease have a retroviral aetiology? *Lancet* 1986; **ii**: 545.

161. Kato, H., Ichinose, E., Yoshioka, F. *et al.* Fate of coronary aneurysms in Kawasaki disease: serial coronary arteriography and long term follow up study. *Am. J. Cardiol.* 1982; **49**: 1758.

162. Brecker, S.J.D., Gray, H.H. and Oldershaw, P.J. Coronary artery aneurysms and myocardial infarction; adult sequlae of Kawasaki disease? *Br. Heart J.* 1987; **59**: 509.

Chapter 45

The Pathogenesis of Atherosclerosis

Elspeth B. Smith

Human arterial lesions exhibit enormous diversity both between individuals and within a single artery. A major problem in understanding their pathogenesis is that it is only possible to speculate about their sequence of development, and the validity of experimental animal models is uncertain.

MORPHOLOGICAL CHARACTERISTICS OF LESIONS

The following descriptions are based on the author's own extensive observations of human *aortic* lesions, which are large enough to allow correlation of morphological and biochemical characteristics. Although there may be some variation in expression in different arteries, it seems unlikely that there are fundamental differences in the underlying pathological processes.

Diffuse intimal thickening

In the aortas of young children, there is virtually no intima; the endothelium is separated from the internal elastic lamina only by occasional collagen fibres and traces of proteoglycan, giving a total thickness of about 10 μm. By the second decade, a sub-endothelial layer of smooth muscle cells (SMC) and collagen develops, and by the end of the third decade the intima is characteristically 50–100 μm in thickness. This thickening seems to continue throughout life, so that in the sixth and seventh decades areas of apparently normal intima are 200–250 μm in thickness. Areas of diffuse intimal thickening are found in the coronary arteries even in the first decade.[1] Diffuse intimal thickening is regarded as a physiological and not a pathological process,[2] but it is within the SMC layer between the endothelium and internal elastic lamina that significant atherosclerotic lesions develop. This layer is missing from all the usual experimental animal models.

Fatty lesions

Classical *fatty streaks* are found in the aortas of some neonates and increase rapidly to reach a maximum extent at about the age of 20 years.[3] Microscopically, they consist of groups of cells filled with large lipid droplets; these groups range in size from two or three cells immediately under the endothelium with little intimal thickening to moderately thickened patches in which the fat-filled cells are in several layers of confluent strands or bunches. *Raised fatty plaques* consist of small focal proliferations containing layers of close-packed fat-filled cells and a central core of extracellular lipid, part of which is probably derived from cells that have disintegrated, thereby releasing their lipid droplets.

In Watanabe heritable hyperlipidaemic rabbits and fat-fed rabbits, the fat-filled cells immediately under the endothelium appear to be macrophages whereas those lying deeper in larger lesions are a mixture of macrophages and SMC.[4] Both types of cell were present in small (< 2 mm) 'fibro-fatty' lesions in human aortas;[5] this is probably also the case for fatty streaks, but so far no definitive quantitative immunological study has been published. Lesions consisting mainly of fat-filled cells do not generally form large stenosing plaques but they may be prone to ulceration, leading to thrombus formation. In cholesterol-fed primates, it was found that endothelial cell continuity was interrupted over fat-filled macrophages so that they became exposed; platelets adhered to the *macrophages*, forming mural thrombi.[6]

Proliferative lesions

Fatty streaks are easily seen as discrete whitish/yellow dots and spots; as they were detected in infants and young children it was long assumed that they were the precursors of all adult lesions. However, it is now widely believed that the key event in the development of stenosing lesions is the

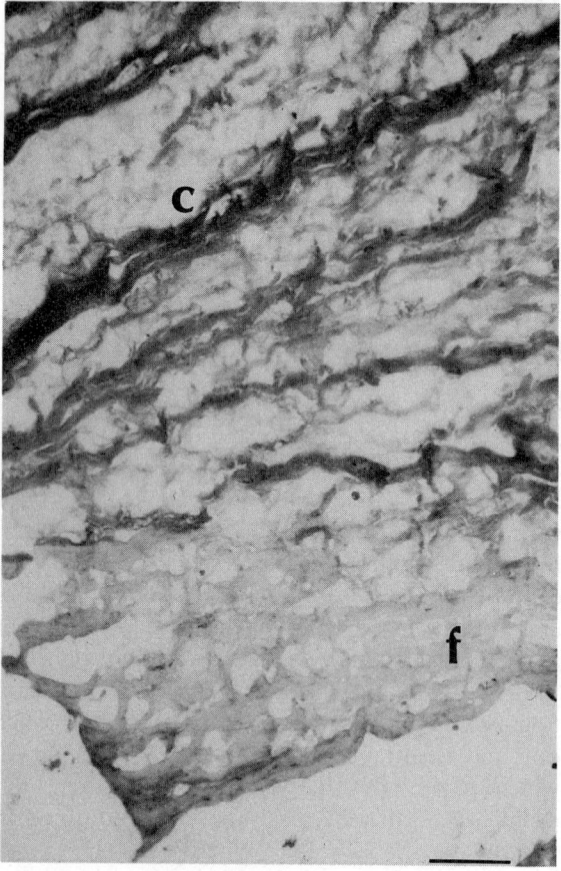

Fig. 45.1. The centre of a large gelatinous lesion (maximum thickness 1500 μm) that was stripped off the media 100 μm above the internal elastic lamina. The dark bands (c) are collagen bundles that show the wide spacing typical of these lesions, and were associated with traces of fine perifibrous lipid; there was no lipid core. The pale area in the centre of the lesion (f) is fibrin. Bar = 100 μm.

focal proliferation of SMC. The early proliferations appear to take the form of *gelatinous lesions*.[7] These are soft translucent elevations of gelatinous texture, frequently neutral in colour and difficult to see with the naked eye. They were described in detail by Virchow[8] but were subsequently largely ignored or missed, perhaps because of the overwhelming emphasis on cholesterol and lipids in atherosclerosis. However, in the 1960s, their morphology and histochemistry were studied by Haust, More and co-workers[9,10] and studies on their biochemistry were started in my laboratory;[7] I have no doubt that they are the main precursors of fibrous plaques. Macroscopically, their appearance is rather uniform but they show great histological diversity; it is not clear if this reflects different modes of initiation or different stages of development. Typically, lesions of 1000–1500 μm in

thickness contain SMCs and thick collagen fibres in linear strands that are widely separated; the interstitial fluid space is increased two- to threefold.[7] Lipid staining (frozen sections) is absent or shows faint diffuse sudanophilia. Stainable fibrin shows great variation: none, bands throughout the lesions, small deposits in the deepest layers (Fig. 45.1), deposits on or just under the surface, and diffuse fibrin-like staining. In some lesions, there are poorly structured areas that seem to be pools of insudated plasma[9,10] and in some perifibrous lipid is associated with the collagen bundles, most frequently in the deeper layers. In some of the smaller lesions, the structure is ill defined; the extracellular matrix fails to give definitive staining for collagen, fibrin or glycosaminoglycan, and the cells are widely separated; it is possible these are very early lesions.

Macroscopically, the larger lesions may have greyish more opaque centres while remaining soft, and translucent round the edges. I have called these *transitional lesions* and assume that they are an intermediate stage between gelatinous lesions and white fibrous plaques. Their water content is lower[11] and, histologically, they are more compact than large gelatinous lesions; in about half the transitional lesions, the central core contains stainable lipid in the form of fine extracellular perifibrous droplets.

Tough white *fibrous plaques* are immediately recognizable macroscopically, but histologically they show marked variation in their content and location of fibrin and lipid. The supposedly typical pattern of a dense collagen cap overlying a central pool of amorphous 'atheroma' lipid occurs in only about half the lesions in the aorta and the coronary arteries[12,13] and in a minority of occlusive lesions in the femoral artery.[14] In the deep layers of the remaining lesions, there may be no lipid staining, traces of perifibrous lipid, abundant perifibrous lipid, either widely distributed or in foci, and small foci of amorphous lipid. The white caps are more uniform and mainly consist of dense collagen with sparse elongated SMCs.

Some proliferative lesions contain no detectable fat-filled cells, some contain occasional scattered single fat-filled cells or small foci of fat-filled cells, most commonly located at the shoulders and the junction of the cap and central lipid core. However, some contain large numbers of fat-filled cells throughout, and are described as *mixed fibro-fatty plaques*. It is not clear if they are primarily fatty streak-type lesions which have undergone an unusual degree of proliferation or SMC proliferations

which have accumulated an unusual number of fat-filled cells. There seems little doubt that fatty streaks and focal SMC proliferations can develop independently, and the mixed lesions may be of two different origins, representing a convergence of the extreme ends of the two spectra. There appear to be two types of foam cell, one type resembling SMC and the other macrophages.[5] The postulated relationship between different types and stages of atherosclerotic lesions is shown diagrammatically in Fig. 45.2.

PATHOGENESIS

A crucial gap in our knowledge is how focal lesions are initiated. Until the initiating processes are understood, attempts at intervention can only be crude, and possibly misdirected.

INITIATING FACTORS FOR FOCAL SMOOTH MUSCLE CELL PROLIFERATION

Endothelial injury

The endothelium presents a non-thrombogenic surface to the circulating blood and, on the basis of studies in the peripheral microcirculation, was also assumed to present a virtually impermeable barrier to large plasma proteins, particularly low density lipoprotein (LDL) which has a molecular mass of approximately 2.5×10^6 Daltons. Consequently, the theory that focal endothelial damage might lead to platelet and fibrin deposition and/or increased permeability to LDL has attracted pathologists for decades, and was forcefully advocated in 1976.[15] The theory rested on two main suppositions: loss of endothelium (i) allowed platelets to adhere to the exposed sub-endothelium where they released a growth factor (platelet-derived growth factor, PDGF) which stimulated SMC to migrate and proliferate, and (ii) allowed LDL to flood into the artery wall where it might lead to deposition of lipid and also stimulate SMC proliferation.

Endothelial denudation and platelet-derived growth factor

There have been numerous experimental studies on the effects of removing endothelium, and the systems used have ranged from widespread denudation by drawing a balloon catheter through the aorta[16] to localized abrasion which may be severe and damage the internal elastic lamina[17] or finely controlled so that endothelial cells can be removed without damage to underlying structures.[18] Extensive and severe mechanical damage seem unlikely to occur spontaneously. Endothelial removal without other damage caused immediate platelet adhesion to the exposed sub-endothelium, but there was no proliferation of SMCs and no intimal thickening even when large areas were removed, requiring up to 8 days for endothelial regeneration. Smooth

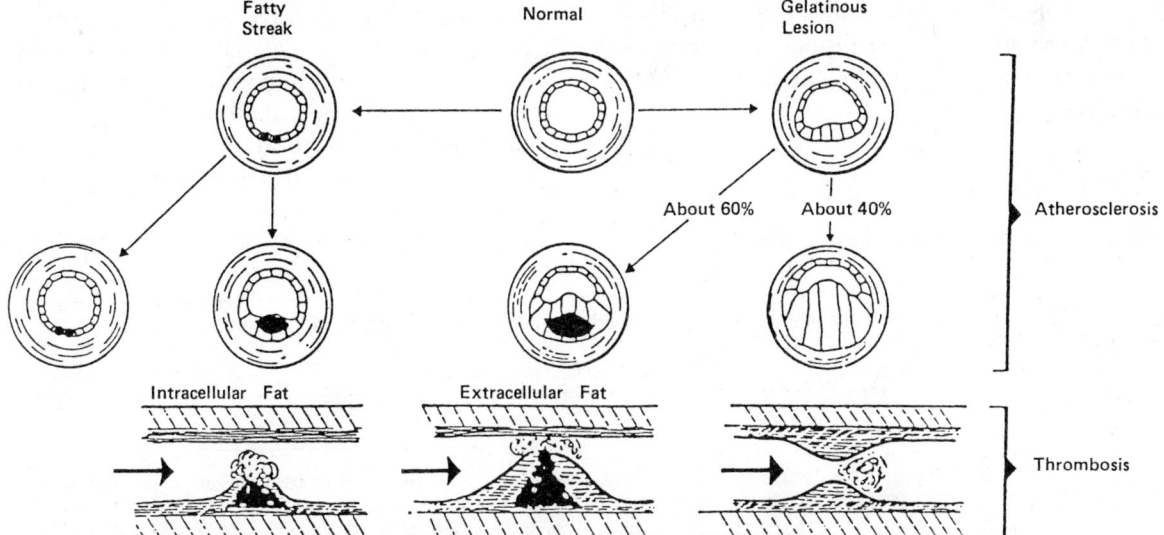

Fig. 45.2. Diagram depicting two separate families of atherosclerotic lesions. On the left, fatty streaks consisting of small groups of cells (probably macrophages) filled with lipid droplets are found at all ages and may develop into small raised lesions containing masses of lipid, mainly intracellular. On the right, focal proliferations of smooth muscle cells, containing no fat-filled cells, are probable precursors of large stenosing fibrous plaques, of which about half accumulate a central core of *extracellular* lipid.

muscle cell proliferation seemed to depend on disruption of the internal elastic lamina (reviewed by Reidy[19]). Furthermore, there is little evidence that endothelial denudation occurs spontaneously. Mechanical removal of endothelium was followed by rapid re-endothelialization.[19] Injury by injection of endotoxin caused increased endothelial cell turnover but no evidence of denudation or increased platelet adherence. As dying cells started to retract it appeared that their neighbours migrated into the space so that the integrity of the monolayer was maintained.[19] In cholesterol-fed animals, fatty lesions developed *before* there was any evidence of endothelial damage; denudation occurred only over advanced lesions, exposing macrophages to which platelets adhered.[6]

In 1974, it was found that whole blood serum stimulated the growth of arterial SMC and fibroblasts in cell culture whereas serum prepared from platelet-poor plasma did not, and the effect was mediated by a growth factor released by the platelets (PDGF).[20,21] This finding was evidence in support of the theory that endothelial damage and platelet adhesion were causative links in atherogenesis, but as research continues the true relationship becomes increasingly unclear. As discussed above, adherence of platelets to sub-endothelium does not lead to SMC proliferation and, *in vitro*, stimulation of proliferation by PDGF seems to occur mainly in cells grown in plastic dishes, with little response from cells grown on a biological matrix.[22,23] Furthermore, it is now clear that PDGF and other growth factors are produced by endothelial cells, macrophages and the SMC themselves.[24,25]

Barrier and transport functions of endothelium

In theory, increased flux of LDL and other plasma macromolecules into the intima could both stimulate SMC proliferation and lead to lipid accumulation. Arterial endothelium is of the continuous type with tight junctions; in this respect, it resembles the capillaries in skin and skeletal, smooth and cardiac muscles.[26] From studies on peripheral lymph, it appears that outward passage of plasma macromolecules across the endothelium is inversely proportional to molecular mass. In human foot lymph, the concentration of albumin was 40% and of LDL only 7% of plasma concentration,[27] suggesting that intact endothelium presents a major barrier to LDL. However, in the diffusely thickened intima of normal human aorta, the concentration of LDL was found to be *higher* than the concentration in the patients' plasma, and there was a *direct* relation between concentration relative to plasma concentration and molecular mass.[28–30] Virtually all plasma proteins seem to be present in intima and, with a few exceptions, their concentration relative to the concentration in plasma shows a linear relation with molecular mass, suggesting that concentration is largely determined by molecular sieving.[30,31]

The LDL in intima may be reversibly or irreversibly complexed with components of the connective tissue matrix, or free in the interstitial fluid. The latter provides the immediate nutrient environment of the SMC and is therefore most likely to influence SMC proliferation and lipid metabolism. Smith and Staples[32] developed a method for collection and assay of arterial interstitial fluid, and in Table 45.1 the concentrations of LDL and other plasma proteins are compared with the concentrations in human foot lymph.[27] In normal intima, the concentration of LDL free in the interstitial fluid is more than twice the concentration in the patients' own plasma; clearly, endothelial denudation or damage is unlikely to allow additional LDL to enter the intima against a twofold concentration gradient. By

Table 45.1. The concentration of plasma proteins in interstitial fluid from human aorta compared with human foot lymph.

		Percentage of plasma concentration			
		Aorta			
	$M_r \times 10^{-4}$	Normal intima ($n = 44$)	Normal media ($n = 11$)	Gelatinous lesions ($n = 28$)	Foot lymph ($n = 5–8$)[27]
LDL	240	216 ± 12^a	0–trace	296 ± 19	7 ± 1
α_2-Macroglobulin	73	115 ± 8	11 ± 2	172 ± 17	9 ± 2
HDL	18 }	48 ± 9	—	73 ± 14	$12–14 \pm 3$
	35 }				
Albumin	6.7	54 ± 3	18 ± 6	59 ± 3	40 ± 12

^{a} Standard error of the mean.

contrast, LDL is virtually excluded from normal media; an intact internal elastic lamina appears to be a major but not complete barrier to outward passage of plasma macromolecules.[33] This explains the apparently different behaviour of capillary and aortic endothelia; macromolecules crossing capillary endothelium can pass with little hindrance back into the lymphatics whereas those crossing aortic endothelium meet an almost impermeable barrier. There is now strong evidence that macromolecules cross the endothelium by transcytosis in vesicles;[26,31,34] this process is bidirectional.[35] The endothelial basement membrane seems to provide a significant molecular sieve; macromolecules entering the sub-endothelial space from the lumen will be carried across it in the transarterial water flow by convective transport which is mainly independent of molecular size, but efflux back into the lumen will involve *diffusion* across the basement membrane, which is highly dependent on size, thus a twofold concentration gradient develops before influx and efflux of the large LDL molecule come into equilibrium.[31,36] The twofold concentration gradient remains constant irrespective of plasma LDL concentration,[32] i.e. high plasma cholesterol levels do not increase 'permeability' but have a major influence on the absolute concentration of LDL in intima.

The SMCs in *normal* adult intima are thus constantly exposed to a high concentration of LDL, but they neither proliferate nor accumulate lipid. The average concentration of LDL in interstitial fluid from gelatinous lesions is 30–40% higher than in adjacent normal intima (Table 45.1) but in 10% of lesions it is actually lower and in a further 20% it is not significantly increased,[37] suggesting that increased 'permeability'/increased LDL concentration cannot be the initiating factors for the focal SMC proliferation.

Addition of LDL to cell and tissue cultures has produced contradictory results. The LDL from hyperlipaemic monkeys and the lowest density fraction of monkey LDL stimulated growth, whereas 'normal' monkey LDL did not.[38,39] Pig cell proliferation was reported to be stimulated 70–80% by an unspecified LDL preparation at about 1% of serum concentration,[40] but in two studies with human SMCs growth was inhibited by LDL at 5 or 10% of serum concentration, but not by 5% whole serum, and the effect was modified by addition of high density lipoprotein (HDL).[41,42] It is, however, increasingly clear that with artificial conditions of culture and non-physiological ratios of serum proteins the response of all cell types may be markedly different from the response of cells *in vivo*.[22,23,43,44]

Modulation of smooth muscle cells

Smooth muscle cells in media have numerous myofilaments and appear to be in a contractile state in which, in culture, they do not migrate or proliferate. Enzyme-dispersed cells seeded at low density undergo spontaneous phenotypic modulation with loss of contractile fibrils and increase in synthetic organelles; in this 'synthetic state', they will proliferate if in a suitable growth medium. If seeded at sufficient density to produce a confluent monolayer within five cell-doublings, they will revert to the original contractile phenotype, but after more than five doublings they remain irreversibly in the synthetic phenotype and are immediately responsive to mitogens such as platelet-derived growth factor. Contractile phenotype cells are not stimulated to proliferate or to modulate to synthetic phenotype by platelet- or plasma-derived factors.[45,46] Phenotypic variation is also found in the arterial wall. In carotid endarterectomy samples, the SMCs at the edges of plaques contained more synthetic organelles than the cells in the underlying media or those in areas of 'normal' diffuse intimal thickening which were not close to plaques.[47,48] It is not clear if the cells in the lesion have exceeded their five doublings and are in an irreversible synthetic state or if a focal stimulus has caused them to modulate. In either case, if they behave like cells in culture they will be more responsive to mitogens than the contractile phenotype cells in normal intima.

Cell transformation

In 1973, Benditt and Benditt[49] demonstrated that the SMCs in human fibrous plaques appear to be monoclonal, suggesting that there has been cell transformation and the plaque is comparable to a benign tumour. Factors that might induce cell transformation have been reviewed by Benditt and Gown,[50] but although the original findings have been consistently confirmed in fibrous plaques there has been continued controversy over whether they are truly monoclonal, i.e. derived from a single cell, or they have become monotypic because one cell type has outgrown the others. Cells from fibrous plaques in culture have not shown growth patterns characteristic of transformed cells,[51,52] and the cells in fibrous plaques show great heterogeneity.[5,53] However, very recently, Penn et al. found strong evidence that human coronary artery plaque DNA contains transforming genes;[54] this finding must stimulate further work using modern methods of cell biology.

Fibrin deposition

The idea that deposition of fibrin in the arterial wall initiates "the atheromatous process" (sic) was put forward by Rokitansky in 1852.[55]

"The deposit is an endogenous product derived from the blood, and for the most part from the fibrin of the arterial blood."

It was rejected on the grounds that the fibrin must be on the surface of the endothelium whereas the lesion was sub-endothelial. In 1913, Anichkov published the results of feeding cholesterol (and milk, meat and egg yolk) to rabbits;[56] since then, the main emphasis has been on the role of cholesterol. However, in 1946, Duguid demonstrated that fibrin may play a major role in the growth of plaques;[57,58] this finding stimulated the performance of numerous experimental studies which showed that fibrin emboli are rapidly covered with endothelium and invaded by SMC which deposit collagen (reviewed in Smith[59]).

Small encrustations, which may be detected only on microscopy, occur quite frequently above apparently normal intima and may consist of mixtures of fibrin, platelets and leucocytes or of almost pure fibrin mesh.[9,10,60] These observations have been confirmed in this laboratory, where we also found, on histological examination, that macroscopic small gelatinous lesions frequently contain partially or wholly incorporated fibrin (Fig. 45.1). Fibrin enhances migration and proliferation of cells in culture, and binds thrombin which is itself a major growth factor;[59,61] fibrin also appears to be a major factor in wound healing, stimulating growth of granulation tissue; it may also be a factor in tumour growth.[59] The fibrin mesh provides a scaffold along which cells migrate. However, there is concomitant fibrinolysis, and fibrin degradation products generated by plasmin degradation of purified fibrin stimulate angiogenesis, DNA synthesis and collagen synthesis in the chick chorioallantoic membrane;[62] they are also chemotactic for leucocytes.[59] Deposition of fibrin on endothelial cells in culture disrupts the monolayer and increases pinocytotic activity and DNA synthesis.[63–65] Fry[36]

points out that a porous layer such as a thrombus will allow a build-up of potentially atherogenic molecules at the lumen–wall interface by sequestering them from the mixing effects of blood flow.

Thus, a small mural encrustation could provide a multifactorial but highly localized atherogenic stimulus. This idea is of particular interest in the light of recent prospective epidemiological studies in which raised levels of fibrinogen and clotting factor VII activity were found to be significant predictors of death from coronary heart disease.[66–69] It will be difficult to determine the role of endothelial 'damage' in localization of the encrustations because fibrin deposition itself 'damages' endothelial cells.[63–65] However, there is increasing evidence that different factors are associated with platelet adherence to and fibrin deposition on the wall; their deposition differs spatially.[70] Moreover, platelet deposition is low at low shear rates and increases with increasing shear rate, whereas the reverse relation is found for fibrin deposition which is maximum at low wall shear rates.[71] Intimal thickening is also greatest in areas of low wall shear and least in areas of high wall shear.[72,73]

INITIATING FACTORS FOR INTRACELLULAR LIPID ACCUMULATION

A major component of the lipid that accumulates in the fat-filled cells of fatty streaks is cholesterol esterified with oleic acid (18:1, n9); most of the cholesterol moiety is derived from plasma LDL, but its lipids have been subjected to extensive reprocessing within the cells. This intracellular lipid differs markedly from the extracellular lipid that accumulates as fine perifibrous lipid droplets in adult normal intima, and which closely resembles plasma LDL (Table 45.2).[28]

In the Watanabe heritable hyperlipidaemic rabbit, most of the fat-filled cells are macrophages;[4] this finding has been reported many times for cholesterol-fed animals. Unfortunately, the proportions of fat-filled macrophages and fat-filled SMCs in human fatty streaks are still not known. On a morphological basis, (light and electron microscopy) Stary[74] reported that in the youngest children fatty streaks consisted of small accumulations of macrophage foam cells, but in other age-groups (up to the age of 29 years) the fat could be contained mainly in lipid-laden SMCs, mainly in macrophages, or more or less equally in both cell types. In an older population, Orekhov et al.[53] reported that most intracellular fat was associated with

Table 45.2. Composition of the lipids in LDL and intima.

	Plasma LDL	Normal intima with perifibrous lipid (age 40–59 years)	Fatty streaks: confluent fat-filled cells
No. of samples (*n*)	22	33	10
Total lipid (mg/100 mg tissue)[a]	—	10.8 ± 2.1[b]	40.0 ± 8.7
Percentage of total lipid:			
Cholesterol ester	58.2 ± 2.2	42.1 ± 5.7	68.7 ± 5.8
Free cholesterol	11.5 ± 1.0	13.0 ± 2.3	10.1 ± 2.9
Phospholipid	20.0 ± 1.5	29.3 ± 3.6	14.8 ± 2.2
Triglyceride	10.2 ± 2.6	15.4 ± 6.1	6.4 ± 2.7
Cholesterol ester fatty acid			
Percentage 18:2 in 18:1 + 18:2 fraction	66.0	58.0	18.6 ± 3.5
Percentage of total:			
16:0	13.7 ± 3.2	14.5 ± 1.5	10.7 ± 3.1
16:1	4.2 ± 0.6	5.5 ± 2.5	7.7 ± 1.5
18:0	2.5 ± 1.0	1.5 ± 1.8	2.0 ± 1.6
18:1	24.1 ± 3.1	28.0 ± 4.4	52.4 ± 4.3
18:2	46.8 ± 6.6	38.6 ± 7.0	12.1 ± 3.0
20:3	Trace	1.0 ± 0.5	5.0 ± 1.7
20:4	5.2 ± 1.2	5.3 ± 1.0	3.6 ± 1.4

[a] Defatted dry tissue.
[b] ± Standard deviation.

stellate cells, which they classified as modified (synthetic state) SMCs. By contrast, using immunocytochemical markers, Gown *et al.*[5] reported that most of the cells in fibro-fatty lesions were macrophages. Identification of the cell types involved is not just of academic interest; the lipid metabolism of SMCs and macrophages is markedly different, therefore failure to identify the cell type complicates attempts to understand why groups of cells, which may be quite isolated, fill themselves with fat.

Lipid metabolism of cells in culture

Smooth muscle cells and fibroblasts

In culture, SMCs and fibroblasts express high affinity receptors that bind LDL; the receptors with bound LDL are then internalized in endocytotic vesicles which fuse with lysosomes. The lysosomal acid hydrolases degrade the apoprotein (apoprotein B) and cleave the cholesterol ester (mainly cholesterol linoleate—18:2, n6), releasing free cholesterol into the cell cytoplasm where it suppresses the cells' own cholesterol synthesis and is incorporated into cell membranes. 'Surplus' free cholesterol activates the microsomal enzyme acyl-CoA:cholesterol acyltransferase, which leads to re-esterification of the cholesterol, mainly with oleic acid (18:1, n9), and

simultaneously, to suppression of re-synthesis of the high affinity binding sites on the cell surface, thus reducing further LDL uptake.[75] The LDL receptor recognizes apoprotein B, which is the only apoprotein in LDL, but it is also present in VLDL (very low density lipoprotein). The LDL receptor also recognizes apoprotein E which occurs in VLDL, chylomicrons and chylomicron remnants, and β–VLDL and HDL_c which are produced by cholesterol feeding.[76] The efficiency of the control mechanism is such that SMCs in culture do not accumulate excess cholesterol even when incubated with high concentrations of LDL or VLDL for long periods; only incubation with LDL modified to increase its *positive* charge (cationized LDL) leads to unregulated uptake by non-specific pinocytosis and accumulation of cholesterol oleate, causing the cells to resemble foam cells.[75]

Macrophages

In marked contrast to SMCs, macrophages express few receptors for normal plasma LDL or VLDL, and incubation *in vitro* with these lipoproteins does not lead to binding and internalization or stimulation of cholesterol oleate synthesis or accumulation.[77] If, however, LDL is acetylated by treatment with acetic anhydride, which increases its *negative* charge, it is rapidly bound by a specific acetyl-LDL receptor on the macrophage, internalized, the cholesterol esters hydrolysed and the cholesterol re-esterified with oleic acid. Thus, macrophages handle acetyl-LDL in the same way as SMCs handle native LDL but with the striking difference that there is no feedback control of receptor numbers, thus they continue to accumulate cholesterol oleate until they come to resemble foam cells. Acetylation, which is unlikely to occur *in vivo*, blocks positive charges in the lysine groups, thus increasing the net negative charge on the LDL molecule, and this seems to be a requirement for recognition by the macrophage receptor; it also *blocks* recognition by the LDL receptor on SMC so that uptake of acetyl-LDL by SMCs is inhibited. Malondialdehyde is produced by platelets and also reacts with the lysine groups, converting LDL to a form that is taken up by the acetyl-LDL receptor but it seems unlikely that the reaction could occur *in vivo*. Oxidation of LDL also leads to uptake by macrophages[78] but there is no direct evidence that this occurs *in vivo*; the only naturally occurring plasma lipoproteins that bind to macrophage receptors are β-VLDL, chylomicrons and an abnormal VLDL found in some hypertriglyceridaemic patients; it is of particular interest that the binding of all these lipoproteins is increased by incubation with thrombin.[79] Thrombin is sequestered in fibrin,[59,61] and fibrin degradation products are chemotactic for macrophages,[59] suggesting that fibrin deposition might also play a role in initiating fatty streaks.

However, it is difficult to reconcile these findings *in vitro* with events in the arterial wall. Fatty streaks develop in healthy children and young adults who do not have any known lipoprotein abnormalities. The fat-filled cells appear to be taking up and degrading LDL, because in their immediate vicinity the concentration of LDL is greatly reduced when compared with that of adjacent normal intima.[28,37] In some early lesions, we have found that the interstitial fluid is totally depleted of LDL, suggesting that it is degraded at a faster rate than it enters the intima (Table 45.3). The net negative charge on LDL in the interstitial fluid from fatty streaks shows no consistent difference from LDL in adjacent normal intima.[80]

PROGRESSION OF LESIONS

Development of gelatinous lesions

The soft translucent gelatinous lesions, which seem

Table 45.3. The concentrations of LDL and albumin in fatty streaks expressed as percentage of the concentrations in adjacent normal intima.

	LDL	Albumin
Whole intimal tissue (n = 14)	28 ± 5	69 ± 13
Interstitial fluid:		
Lipid mainly intracellular (n = 4)	Trace	91 ± 19
Intra- and extracellular lipid (n = 4)	35 ± 5	137 ± 36

to be the earliest manifestations of focal SMC proliferation, range in size from barely detectable spots, about 2 mm in diameter and 100–200 μm thicker than the adjacent normal intima, to massive elevations, about 5 cm in length and up to 2000 μm in thickness. They vary greatly in cellularity and collagen content, but all are characterized by a very high water content, and thus conform to Haust's description of 'insudation lesions'.[9,10] On average, their water content was found to be about twice that of normal intima, but in some individual samples it was up to five times greater.[81,82] Histologically, there appears to be increased 'interstitial space' between the strands of collagen and SMCs, but Smith and Ashall[81] found almost equal increases in the volume of the interstitial fluid containing the plasma macromolecules (distribution volume) and the volume of water from which plasma macromolecules were excluded (exclusion volume); this latter compartment presumably represents water associated with collagen fibres and proteoglycans, and intracellular water. It is possible that intracellular water may increase disproportionately because proliferating SMCs not only increase in number but also in size, many of them becoming polyploid.[83] The *concentration* of LDL and other plasma proteins in the interstitial fluid is not necessarily higher than that in normal intima (see p. 1071), but the *total amount* present in the expanded interstitial fluid space is greatly increased (Table 45.4)[37,81,82] In many lesions, there is no increase in non-LDL-bound cholesterol and little stainable lipid, either intra- or extracellular.[7,82] In addition to LDL, the interstitial fluid contains high concentrations of fibrinogen and fibrin degradation products but the amount of fibrin is variable: in some lesions, it is a major component whereas in others it is quite low.[84–86] It is not clear if the fibrin is deposited from the interstitial fluid *in situ*, as occurs in inflammatory exudates, or if it represents incorporated mural encrustation; Woolf identified platelet antigens deep in fibrous plaques, which

Table 45.4. Relation between the content and distribution of water and the concentration and total content of LDL in intima.

| | Total tissue water (mg/100 mg dry tissue) | | Concentration of LDL | |
	Distribution volume	Exclusion volume	Interstitial fluid (% plasma concentration)	Tissue (μl PS[a]/100 mg dry tissue)
Normal intima	397	369	226	860
Proliferative lesions:				
Gelatinous	644	614	330	2024
Transitional	255	463	432	1085
White fibrous (caps only)	129	364	118	128

[a] μl of the patients' serum from which the LDL was derived.

presumably derived from mural encrustation, but he also observed fine diffusely distributed fibrin within gelatinous lesions.[87]

For these large lesions to develop, cell proliferation must not only be initiated, but also sustained. We have examined intimal extracts for mitogenic activity using the chick chorio-allantoic membrane in an attempt to avoid some of the artefacts that arise with cultured cells. Extracts of gelatinous lesions consistently stimulated DNA synthesis,[88] and preliminary fractionation experiments suggested that the stimulatory activity was associated with the fibrinogen/fibrin degradation products fraction.

Transitional lesions

In the human, it is possible only to speculate that one type of lesion progresses into another, but some gelatinous lesions have slightly firmer greyish centres and may show some stainable lipid; I postulate that abruptly raised soft grey lesions represent a transitional stage between gelatinous lesions and fibrous plaques. In about half these lesions, there is virtually no stainable lipid; in the remainder, there is an accumulation of fine extracellular lipid droplets associated with collagen bundles, mainly in the deeper layers. Biochemically, a major difference between gelatinous and transitional lesions is their water content (Table 45.4). The distribution volume, which is approximately equivalent to interstitial fluid space, decreases in transitional lesions to about one-third of the volume in gelatinous lesions, but the concentration of LDL in the interstitial fluid increases (Table 45.4). Taking all gelatinous and transitional lesions together, there is a significant negative regression of LDL concentration in interstitial fluid on distribution volume (b = −0.53, $P < 0.01$). There was an elevenfold differ-

ence between the gelatinous lesion with the largest distribution volume and the lower layers of the transitional lesion with the smallest distribution volume; in the latter, the concentration of LDL in the interstitial fluid was eleven times that in the patient's plasma.[81] If the assumption that transitional lesions progress to fibrous plaques is correct, about half the lesions in this lower layer would become filled with stainable extracellular lipid droplets. In the low lipid white fibrous caps of plaques, the interstitial fluid space is very small and the concentration of LDL low, suggesting that the LDL is unable to penetrate the densely packed collagen (Table 45.4).

Thus, in the development of large space-occupying lesions, there seems to be an initial phase of simultaneous proliferation and retention of large amounts of fluid and other plasma constituents, followed by a movement of water out of the interstitial fluid compartment, leaving highly concentrated macromolecules which, in addition to LDL, include fibrinogen and other components of the haemostatic system. However, there is no information about either the factors producing the oedema, which differs from inflammatory oedema in that no microvessels are involved, or the factors leading to the withdrawal of water. There is no direct evidence that LDL level influences the proliferative phase, but it probably has a secondary effect on the way in which the lesion develops because the higher the level of plasma LDL the greater will be the amount of LDL cholesterol trapped in the lesion.

Lipid deposition in plaques

It is widely assumed that the pool of 'atheroma' lipid under about half the white fibrous plaques is derived from disintegration of fat-filled SMCs or macrophages, but epidemiological, topographic, morphological and chemical studies all suggest that this is not correct.[28,80,85,87–89] As mentioned previously (p. 1073), the lipid in fat-filled cells of fatty streaks is characterized by a high proportion of *cholesterol oleate*, which arises from hydrolysis of the cholesterol esters of LDL followed by re-esterification with oleic acid. In marked contrast, the lipid that accumulates as fine extracellular droplets, which are perifibrous in ageing normal intima and some gelatinous and transitional lesions and massed together in developed fibrous plaques, is characterized by a high proportion of *cholesterol linoleate*, and closely resembles the lipid of LDL with the exception that there is a marked increase in the proportion of free (unesterified) cholesterol in larger lesions.[28] Chemical analysis of layers isolated from mixed plaques by microdissection suggests that the characteristic cholesterol oleate-rich lipid in fat-filled cells does not undergo change when the cells disintegrate, and extracellular accumulation of LDL-type lipid occurs even in lesions rich in fat-filled cells.[92] The proportion of free cholesterol increased with increasing lesion size both in the presence and absence of fat-filled cells; it is not clear if this represents hydrolysis of cholesterol ester or direct deposition of free cholesterol. Free cholesterol deposition has been reported to occur before accumulation of cholesterol ester in the cholesterol-fed rabbit.[93,94]

Interactions of low density lipoprotein and the connective tissue matrix

Direct deposition of extracellular lipid from LDL seems to occur in proliferative lesions, but the mechanism involved is not known. The amount of LDL present in the lesion, which is related to plasma LDL concentration, is not the only factor involved because apparently similar transitional or fibrous plaques may occur in adjacent positions in the same aorta, one containing abundant lipid and another containing virtually none.

The main connective tissue component of intima is collagen, which comprises about 25% of normal intimal dry weight. Its concentration increases by about 20% in gelatinous lesions but more than doubles in white fibrous plaques.[95] Together, type I and type III collagens comprise 80–90% of the total, and although there has been considerable disagreement it now seems probable that they occur in close proximity.[96] On light microscopy, I have observed great variation in the thickness of collagen

bundles and in the intensity of their reaction with the Van Gieson stain and with Sudan stains for lipid; thick strongly staining bundles are most likely to be sudanophilic. Lipid droplets have been demonstrated within collagen bundles by electron microscopy.[97]

Elastin is the main component of aortic media, where it is arranged in thick concentric laminae[87] which seem to present a major barrier to the outward passage of large macromolecules, particularly those of LDL.[32,33] In diffuse intimal thickening in the ageing human aorta, there is frequently a zone of variable thickness at the intimal–medial junction containing fragmentary elastic laminae, and these are particularly associated with accumulation of perifibrous lipid.[95,97] The elastin molecule has hydrophobic zones which are presumably associated with the lipid binding, but its role in sequestrating lipid in plaques is not clear. On histological staining of human arteries, elastin appears to be a minor component of the inner intima, where plaques develop; in advanced plaques, the elastin-rich inner media may be involved, but this seems to be secondary to lipid accumulation in the low-elastin inner intima. In the lipid-rich core of plaques, lipid at the cap–core junction was found to be mainly associated with collagen and at the core–media junction it was associated with both collagen and elastin.[91]

The 'ground substance' of the connective tissue matrix consists of a three-dimensional network of proteoglycans. The proteoglycans consist of a core protein to which many chains of acidic glycosaminoglycan are covalently linked, and although the glycosaminoglycans comprise only about 2% of normal intimal dry weight they probably exert a significant influence on the compartmentalization of water and molecular sieving within the intima. On a dry weight basis, total GAGs decrease by about 10% in gelatinous lesions, but the water content of the lesion doubles, therefore the concentration of the gel is greatly reduced.[81,95,98] Like heparin, the proteoglycans *in vitro* have anticoagulant activity and inhibit thrombin-induced platelet aggregation.[98] The isolated GAGs also form dissociable ionic complexes with LDL *in vitro* at high concentrations of calcium ions,[99,100] and it is postulated that this is a factor determining the high concentration of LDL in intima. However, we have been unable to find any evidence of specific reversible binding on comparison of the ratios of LDL to other macromolecules in interstitial fluid and whole tissue,[37] and LDL was not released when glycosaminoglycans were degraded by incubating intimal tissue with chondroitinase ABC.[101]

Interactions of low density lipoprotein and fibrin

Endogenous LDL decreases on incubation of finely minced intima at pH < 5.5;[102] at higher values of pH, there is much less destruction, and in a few samples an increase in LDL was observed, suggesting that a tightly bound fraction was being released.[102] The obvious implication seemed to be that LDL was bound to glycosaminoglycan, but incubation of the tissue with chondroitinase ABC did not release significant amounts of LDL, whereas incubation with proteolytic enzymes released large amounts from some lesions, and the most effective protease was the fibrinolytic enzyme, plasmin.[101] On rocket immuno-electrophoresis in agarose, the released LDL showed little difference from the freely mobile LDL in fresh tissue, but on iso-electric focusing in polyacrylamide gel (PAG) it appeared to be a larger molecule, suggesting that it is an aggregated form of LDL.[101,103] The apo-B moiety can also be extracted from tissue with detergents.[104]

With enzyme release and detergent release, the highest ratios of bound to free LDL occurred in lesions that had accumulated substantial amounts of cholesterol. The highest concentrations of plasmin-releasable LDL were found in lipid-rich areas of large translucent gelatinous lesions (Table 45.5); in these areas, fibrin accounted for more than one-quarter of the total dry weight. It seems probable that these lesions were in a state of rapid progression; frequently, the lipid-rich area, which was not always in the central core region, appeared

macroscopically bright translucent yellow and histologically the lipid was in the form of very abundant perifibrous lipid. Although the highest concentrations of plasmin-releasable LDL occurred in lesions with a high fibrin content, within that group of lesions there was no quantitative correlation between the concentrations of bound LDL and fibrin.[105] Within a tissue sample, LDL release paralleled release of fibrin degradation products, but their ratios differed by a factor of ten between different samples,[101] and bound LDL was low in thrombi but it increased with increasing endothelialization and collagen invasion.[105]

From these studies, it is clear that, although fibrin seems to be associated with lipid accumulation, the relationship is not simple. Histologically, it often appears that lipid staining is associated with collagen invading the fibrin mesh, suggesting that LDL might be bound at the collagen–fibrin interface or linked through fibronectin, which is abundant in thrombi and can be crosslinked by factor XIII with fibrin, collagen and proteoglycan.[106] Plasmin is a non-specific serine protease and degrades fibronectin, thus the LDL could be released from fibronectin and not from fibrin. By contrast, purified collagenase releases fibronectin from connective tissues, but has little effect on fibrin. Smith and Ashall[106] found that incubation of normal intima and lesions with purified collagenase released large amounts of fibronectin but very variable amounts of LDL, which showed no correlation with fibronectin release. Thus, the mechanism by which large amounts of LDL-derived lipid are deposited in some proliferative plaques is not yet known.

Table 45.5. **Free and plasmin-releasable LDL in lesions.**

	Concentration (mg/100 mg lipid-extracted dry tissue)			
		LDL		
	Fibrin	Free	Released by plasmin	Residual cholesterol
Normal intima (n = 12)	2.0	5.2	0.8	3.2
Low lipid gelatinous lesions (n = 15)	5.1	15.7	1.5	5.3
Large gelatinous plaques:				
Low lipid caps and sides (n = 10)	10.3	12.3	2.9	9.4
Lipid-rich areas (n = 22)	28.3	8.5	16.5	106.1
White fibrous plaques:				
Caps (n = 11)	3.8	2.5	0.8	7.8
Lipid-rich core (n = 23)	6.9	2.1	3.9	78.3

Haemostatic factors in intima

Morphologically, the fibrin in lesions shows great variation. It may occur in layered bands, suggesting successive incorporation of mural thrombi, in niduses of fibrin mesh, and as diffuse staining or widely distributed flecks; the extent to which fibrin is deposited by clotting of fibrinogen within the intima is not clear. In normal intima, the relative retention of prothrombin is greater than predicted from its molecular mass and plasma concentration; in the lipid-rich centres of plaques, which are also rich in fibrin, retention of prothrombin relative to antithrombin III increased fivefold when compared with normal intima.[59,85] Fibrinogen appears to clot in intima minced without EDTA, and this is most marked in plaque centres.[89]

Most of the antigen present in intima appears to be prothrombin, but in preliminary studies using SDS–PAG electrophoresis and immunoblotting a weak band migrating as thrombin was found in intimal extracts prepared in the presence of EDTA and protease inhibitors (E.B. Smith, unpublished observations). Thus, some thrombin is present and, in addition to clotting fibrinogen, could act as a growth factor for SMCs and as a chemo-attractant for monocyte macrophages within the intima.[61]

In contrast to the ubiquitous abundance of prothrombin, factor VIII antigen was detected in only about half the samples investigated, including the deep layers of lesions which did not contain any endothelium;[85] most surprisingly, plasminogen antigen was recovered from only about 30% of intimal samples.[107] Plasminogen concentration seemed to be associated with the aorta and not with particular types of lesion; it was absent in all the patients who died following myocardial infarction and half the patients dying from other causes, but there was no difference in plasma plasminogen levels between those with and those without aortic plasminogen. Absence of plasminogen was also associated with increased involvement with atherosclerosis, suggesting that failure to lyse fibrin resulted in increased lesion formation. Thus, arterial intima seems to have a high potential for fibrin deposition coupled with a low potential for fibrin removal.

The ultimate fate of lesions

The extent to which intact space-occupying lesions interfere with coronary blood flow is not entirely clear. Studies in primates suggest that intimal thickening is accompanied by increase in vessel size (measured as length of the internal elastic lamina) such that the actual lumen is not greatly changed (see p. 1080). Obvious problems arise when there is calcification, which changes the rheology of the vessel, and ulceration or rupture, which increases the probability of thrombus formation.

The calcium content of arteries increases with age, even in the absence of atherosclerosis, and seems to be closely associated with elastin,[87,108] but the focal calcification of lesions shows great variation among individuals, and as yet no clear understanding of the factors involved has been gained.[109,110] Calcification of lesions is frequently associated with a high lipid content, and in aorta it occurs most commonly in the lower abdominal segment, but there is no constant relationship with severity of atherosclerosis. It is not uncommon to find ulceration at the edge of a plate of hard calcium.

Plaque rupture and ulceration are discussed in Chapter 44 in relation to predisposing factors and their role in coronary artery occlusion.

INTERRELATION OF HAEMOSTATIC FACTORS AND LIPOPROTEINS IN MYOCARDIAL INFARCTION AND ATHEROGENESIS

The epidemiology of conventional risk factors for myocardial infarction and the pathology of coronary artery occlusion are discussed in Chapters 42 and 44; the purpose of this section is to re-emphasize the complexity of the interrelation of clotting, lipids, atherogenesis and coronary occlusion.

The end-point in most clinical intervention trials and epidemiological studies is acute myocardial infarction, and the major cause of infarction is thrombotic occlusion of the coronary arteries (Chapter 44). Thus, the end-point is a thrombotic episode, but measurements of haemostatic function were not made in virtually any of the large intervention trials, and were included in only four of the many prospective epidemiological studies.[66–69] In these studies, fibrinogen levels were significantly greater in men who developed coronary heart disease than in healthy survivors, and in most of the groups studied the impact of fibrinogen level was greater than the impact of total cholesterol level. In the Northwick Park study,[69] the level of activated factor VII was also significantly raised in cases of fatal coronary heart disease but not in non-fatal cases; decrease in fibrinolytic activity was of borderline significance. Increasing levels of fibrinogen increase platelet aggregation, but this did not show an independent association with coronary heart disease.[69,111]

Haemostatic function is linked with the conventional risk factors for coronary heart disease. Fibrinogen levels show significant positive correlations with cholesterol level and hyperlipidaemia, age, smoking, obesity and social class.[112–115] The proportion of factor VII in the activated state is increased in hyperlipidaemia and acute fat feeding, and decreases on treatment of the hyperlipidaemia.[115–117] Fibrin and cholesterol deposition in the lesion seem to be linked, so that hypercoagulability and hypercholesterolaemia may be a potent combination for accelerating atherogenesis, whereas the hypercoagulability factor is most likely to increase the risk of thrombotic occlusion.

ANIMAL MODELS

One reason for our poor progress in understanding atherogenesis is the lack of a suitable animal model or, perhaps, the use of an inappropriate model. 'Experimental atherosclerosis' has become synonymous with cholesterol and/or high fat feeding, but the predominantly macrophage foam cell lesions produced bear little resemblance to the lesions found in the average adult human. In recent detailed reviews and critiques of cholesterol feeding in experimental atherogenesis and resultant vascular complications,[118,119] Stehbens concludes that

"human atherosclerosis and the lesions produced by the dietary overload of cholesterol and fats are not one and the same disease. Many investigators are seemingly unaware of the extent of these differences, but to overlook them and to accept the experimental lesions as atherosclerotic . . . is misleading and misrepresenting the facts."

The development of lesions in response to levels of cholesterol that are ridiculously high with the cholesterol carried in abnormal lipoproteins is unlikely to mirror the development of lesions in the average human being, and the regression of these lesions when lipid levels are returned to normal is even more unlikely to provide a model for regression in human subjects in whom it is not clear whether hyperlipidaemia is the primary initiating factor.

Experimental studies to answer specific questions

The foregoing does not mean that animal experiments have no place in atherogenesis research. On the contrary they can be of great importance in answering specific questions, provided the structural difference from human arteries, i.e. almost total absence of a sub-endothelial intimal layer, is fully appreciated when interpreting results. Some selected examples are listed below.

Endothelial function

As discussed previously (p. 1069), selective endothelial damage has demonstrated that endothelial denudation is unlikely to be an initiating factor in atherogenesis.[18,19] Total removal of endothelium followed by partial re-growth has provided a model for its barrier function. In de-endothelialized regions, which were covered with a layer of proliferated SMCs, there was rapid entry of LDL, but equally rapid re-equilibration with plasma; in re-endothelialized regions, which were also thickened, LDL entry was slower, but it was then retained within the intima.[120]

Transendothelial transport of low density lipoprotein

Despite the difficulties presented by the virtual absence of an intimal layer, elegant studies in rabbits have demonstrated that vesicular transcytosis of LDL across the endothelium does not require the LDL receptor,[26,34,121] is bidirectional, and that only part of the LDL that enters is degraded.[35] These experimental results elucidate the finding in human arteries that influx greatly exceeds accumulation.[122]

The fate of thrombi

Emboli consisting of platelet-rich thrombi and pure fibrin are invaded by SMCs and collagen and become indistinguishable from fibrous plaques.[59] The same sequence was observed in large endogenous thrombi, and the lesions accumulated cholesterol even in normocholesterolaemic rabbits.[123]

Studies in primates

Particular insights derived from the many primate studies include differences in the types of lesion induced by different dietary fats,[124] and the magnitude of the difference in response of individual animals to the same diet. In a series of 236 cynomolgus macaques, Malinow found serum cholesterol levels ranging from 150 to 1100 mg/100 ml.[125] Rhesus monkeys on the same diet showed sixteenfold differences in amount of coronary atherosclerosis, but artery size measured as the area within the internal elastic lamina increased with intimal thickness, such that the area of the lumen was not decreased.[125] Age has been shown to influence the type of lesion produced; in response to the same diet, mainly fatty streaks developed in young animals, whereas proliferative lesions developed in the older animals, possibly reflecting some degree of diffuse intimal thickening, so that the older arteries were more like those in humans.[126]

Atherosclerosis-susceptible and atherosclerosis-resistant pigeons

White Carneau pigeons develop atherosclerosis spontaneously on a normal diet, and are highly susceptible to cholesterol feeding whereas the Show Racer breed is resistant to atherosclerosis. If differences in the two breeds could be pinpointed, it might increase our understanding of atherogenesis, but so far no differences in accepted risk factors, such as blood pressure, total plasma cholesterol level or distribution and composition of plasma lipoproteins, have been found.[127] Both breeds of pigeon lack specific high affinity LDL receptors, thus they resemble patients with familial hypercholesterolaemia or Watanabe heritable hyperlipidaemic rabbits, but on normal diets their serum cholesterol levels are low—about 100 mg/100 ml.[128] On cholesterol feeding, both breeds develop comparable hypercholesterolaemia and very high levels of β-VLDL, but the severity and extent of atherosclerosis in the Show Racer breed is only one-quarter of that in the White Carneau; there was no correlation of severity with β-VLDL or HDL levels either within or between breeds. The β-VLDL from both breeds was taken up to the same extent by macrophages.[129] The difference must lie either in the genetic constitution of the artery wall itself or in risk factors, possibly haemostatic factors, that have not yet been measured.

MONITORING PROGRESSION AND REGRESSION OF ATHEROSCLEROSIS IN HUMAN ARTERIES

With increasing refinement of angiographic techni-

ques and of non-invasive techniques such as ultrasound, it is becoming increasingly possible to follow the natural history of human atherosclerotic lesions directly. These techniques do not have the ability to reveal the nature of the lesions, but they provide information on the time-course of their growth in relation to other factors. Of the completed studies, the majority were on patients who had undergone previous coronary artery bypass grafting and the purpose of performing repeated angiograms was primarily to locate graft occlusions and new arterial stenoses and occlusions rather than to study the natural history of lesions.[130] Nevertheless, this material has produced useful insights; in bypassed arteries, progression of atherosclerosis is greatly accelerated,[131,132] presumably because of the reduction in flow leading to an increased tendency to thrombosis.[133] Fibrin deposition and intimal thickening are increased in areas of low wall shear.[71–73] Risk factors for progression of lesions are not the same as the risk factors for occlusion, and in most studies lipoprotein levels have not shown a significant correlation with either progression or occlusion.[130,134] There are now numerous intervention trials in progress, mainly directed at the investigation of the effect of lipid-lowering regimes on lesions. So far, the results have been mixed; there has been little evidence of regression, but the rate of progression may have been slightly decreased in some studies.[135]

REFERENCES

1. Smith, E.B. From the fatty streak to the calcified lesion. In: Born, G.V.R., Catapano, A.L. and Paoletti, R., eds. *Factors in Formation and Regression of the Atherosclerotic Plaque.* NATO Advanced Study Institutes, Series A, Vol. 51. New York: Plenum Press, 1982, p. 45.
2. Geer, J.C. and Haust, M.D. *Smooth Muscle Cells in Atherosclerosis.* Basel: S. Karger, 1972.
3. Holman, R.L. Atherosclerosis—a pediatric nutrition problem? *Am. J. Clin. Nutr.* 1967; 20: 5.
4. Tsukada, T., Rosenfeld, M., Ross, R. and Gown, A.M. Immunocytochemical analysis of cellular components in atherosclerotic lesions. Use of monoclonal antibodies with the Watanabe and fat-fed rabbit. *Arteriosclerosis* 1986; 6: 601.
5. Gown, A.M., Tsukada, T. and Ross, R. Human atherosclerosis. II. Immunocytochemical analysis of the cellular composition of human atherosclerotic lesions. *Am. J. Pathol.* 1986; 125: 191.
6. Faggiotto, A., Ross, R. and Harker, L. Studies of hypercholesterolaemia in the non-human primate. 1. Changes that lead to fatty streak formation. *Arteriosclerosis* 1984: 4: 323.
7. Smith, E.B. Identification of the gelatinous lesion. In: Schettler, G., Gotto, A.M., Middlehoff, G., Habernicht, A.J.R. and Jurutka, K.R., eds. *Atherosclerosis VI.* Berlin: Springer-Verlag, 1983, p. 170.
8. Virchow, R. *Gesammelte Abhandlungen zur Wissenchasf-*

tlichen Medicin. Frankfurt AM: Meidinger, 1856, p. 496.

9. Haust, M.D. The natural history of human atherosclerotic lesions. In: Moore, S., ed. *Vascular Injury and Atherosclerosis*. New York: Marcel Dekker, 1981. p. 1.

10. Haust, M.D. The morphogenesis and fate of potential and early atherosclerotic lesions in man. *Human Pathol.* 1971; 2: 1.

11. Smith, E.B. and Ashall, C. Low density lipoprotein concentration in interstitial fluid from human atherosclerotic lesions. *Biochim. Biophys. Acta* 1983; 754: 249.

12. Panaganamala, R.V., Greer, J.C., Sharma, H.M. and Cornwell, D.G. The gross and histologic appearance and the lipid composition of normal intima and lesions from human coronary arteries and aorta. *Atherosclerosis* 1974; 20: 93.

13. Hangartner, J.R.W., Charleston, A.J., Davies, M.J. and Thomas, A.C. Morphological characteristics of clinically significant coronary artery stenosis in stable angina. *Br. Heart J.* 1986; 56: 501.

14. Ross, R., Wight, T.N., Strandness, E. and Thiele, B. Human atherosclerosis 1. Cell constitution and characteristics of advanced lesions of the superficial femoral artery. *Am. J. Pathol.* 1984: 114: 79.

15. Ross, R. and Glomset, J.A. The pathogenesis of atherosclerosis. *N. Engl. J. Med.* 1976; 295: 369 and 420.

16. Baumgartner, H.R. and Studer, A. Folgen des Gefaesskatheterismus am normo- und hypercholesterolinaemischen Kaninchen. *Pathologia et Microbiologia* 1966; 29: 393.

17. Bjorkerud, S. Atherosclerosis initiated by mechanical trauma in normolipidaemic rabbits. *J. Atheroscler. Res.* 1969; 9: 209.

18. Reidy, M.A. and Schwartz, S.M. Endothelial regeneration: III. Time course of intimal changes after small defined injury to rat aortic endothelium. *Lab. Invest.* 1981; 44: 301.

19. Reidy, M.A. A reassessment of endothelial injury and arterial lesion formation. *Lab. Invest.* 1985; 53: 513.

20. Ross, R., Glomset, J., Kariya, B. and Harker, L. A platelet-dependent serum factor that stimulates the proliferation of arterial smooth muscle cells in vitro. *Proc. Nat. Acad. Sci., U.S.A.* 1974; 71: 1207.

21. Kohler, N. and Lipton, A. Platelets as a source of fibroblast growth-promoting activity. *Exp. Cell. Res.* 1974; 87: 297.

22. Gospodarowicz, D. and Tauber, J.-P. Growth factors and the extracellular matrix. *Endocrinol. Rev.* 1980; 1: 201.

23. Gospodarowicz, D. Growth factors and their action in vivo and in vitro. *J. Pathol.* 1983; 141: 201.

24. Ross, R. Growth factors, platelets, macrophages and atherosclerosis. In: Fidge, N.H. and Nestel, P.J., eds. *Atherosclerosis VII*. Amsterdam: Elsevier Science Publishers, 1986, p. 355.

25. Nilsson, J. Growth factors and the pathogenesis of atherosclerosis. *Atherosclerosis* 1986; 62: 185.

26. Simionescu, M. and Simionescu, N. Ultrastructure of the microvascular wall: functional correlations. In: Renkin, E.M. and Michel, C.C., eds. *Handbook of Physiology*. Section 2, the Cardiovascular System, Volume IV, Microcirculation, part 1. Bethesda: American Physiological Society, 1984, p. 41.

27. Reichl, D., Rudra, D.N., Myant, N.B. and Pflug, J.J. Further evidence for the role of high density lipoprotein in the removal of tissue cholesterol *in vivo*. *Atherosclerosis* 1982; 44: 73.

28. Smith, E.B. The relationship between plasma and tissue lipids in human atherosclerosis. *Advances Lipid Res.* 1974; 12: 1.

29. Hoff, H.F., Gaubatz, J.W. and Gotto, A.M. Apo-B concentration in the normal human aorta. *Biochem. Biophys. Res. Commun.* 1976; 85: 1424.

30. Smith, E.B. Endothelium and lipoprotein permeability. In: Woolf, N., ed. *Biology and Pathology of the Vessel Wall*. Eastbourne: Praeger, 1983, p. 279.

31. Smith, E.B. Some of the accumulating evidence from human artery studies of what gets transported and what accumulates relative to atherogenesis. In: Glagov, S., ed. *Evolution of the Human Atherosclerotic Plaque*. Berlin: Springer–verlag, 1989.

32. Smith, E.B. and Staples, E.M. Plasma protein concentrations in interstitial fluid from human aortas. *Proc. R. Soc. Lond. B* 1982; 217: 59.

33. Smith, E.B. and Staples, E.M. Distribution of plasma proteins across the human aortic wall: barrier functions of endothelium and internal elastic laminae. *Atherosclerosis* 1980; 37: 579.

34. Vasile, E., Simionescu, M. and Simionescu, N. Visualization of the binding, endocytosis and transcytosis of low-density lipoprotein in the arterial endothelium in situ. *J. Cell Biol.* 1983; 96: 1677.

35. Carew, T.E., Pittman, R.C., Marchand, E.R. and Steinberg, D. Measurement in vivo of irreversible degradation of low density lipoprotein in the rabbit aorta. *Arteriosclerosis* 1984; 4: 214.

36. Fry, D.L. Problems and progress in understanding "endothelial permeability" and mass transport in human arteries. In: Glagov, S., ed, *Evolution of the Human Atherosclerotic Plaque*. Berlin: Springer–verlag, 1989.

37. Smith, E.B. and Ashall, C. Low density lipoprotein concentration in interstitial fluid from human atherosclerotic lesions: relation to theories of endothelial damage and lipoprotein binding. *Biochim. Biophys. Acta* 1983; 754: 249.

38. Dzoga, K. and Wissler, R.W. Stimulation of proliferation in stationery primary cultures of monkey aortic smooth muscle cells. Part 2: Effect of varying concentrations of hyperlipemic serum and low density lipoproteins of varying dietary fat origins. *Atherosclerosis* 1976; 24: 515.

39. Fless, G.M., Kirchhausen, T., Fischer-Dzoga, K., Wissler, R. and Scanu, A.M. Relationship between the properties of the apo-B containing LDL of normolipidaemic Rhesus monkeys and their mitogenic action on arterial smooth muscle cells grown in vitro. In: Gotto, A.M., Smith, L.C. and Allen, B., eds. *Atherosclerosis V*. New York: Springer-Verlag, 1980, p. 607.

40. Mey, J., Lehman, R. and Hauss, W.H. Effects of low density lipoproteins, staphylolysin, glucocorticoid, D-penicillamine, and the combined application of glucocorticoid and staphylolysin on the proliferative activity of cultured aortic smooth muscle cells of the minipig. *Exp. Molec. Pathol.* 1978; 28: 119.

41. Hessler, J.R., Robertson, A.L. and Chisolm, G.M. LDL-induced cytotoxicity and its inhibition by HDL in human vascular smooth muscle and endothelial cells in culture. *Atherosclerosis* 1979: 32: 213.

42. Wosu, L., Parisella, R. and Kalant, N. Effect of low density lipoprotein on glycosaminoglycan secretion by cultured human smooth muscle cells and fibroblasts. *Atherosclerosis* 1983; 48: 205.

43. Henriksen, T., Evensen, S.A. and Carlander, B. Injury to human endothelial cells in culture induced by low density lipoproteins. *Scand. J. Clin. Lab. Invest.* 1979; 39: 361.

44. Tauber, J.-P., Cheng, J. and Gospodarowicz, D. Effect of high and low density lipoproteins on proliferation of cultured bovine vascular endothelial cells. *J. Clin. Invest.* 1980; 66: 696.

45. Chamley-Campbell, J., Campbell, G.R. and Ross, R. The smooth muscle cell in culture. *Physiol. Rev.* 1979; 59: 1.

46. Chamley-Campbell, J., Nestel, P. and Campbell, G.R. Smooth muscle reactivity in atherogenesis: LDL metabolism and response to serum mitogens differ according to

phenotype. In: Born, G.V.R., Catapano, A.L. and Paoletti, R., eds. *Factors in Formation and Regression of the Atherosclerotic Plaque*. NATO Advanced Study Institutes Series A, Vol. 51. New York: Plenum Press, 1982, p. 115.

47. Mosse, P.R.L., Campbell, G.R., Wang, Z.L. and Campbell, J.H. Smooth muscle phenotypic expression in human carotid arteries. I. Comparison of cells with diffuse intimal thickenings adjacent to atheromatous plaques with those of the media. *Lab. Invest.* 1985; 53: 556.

48. Mosse, P.R.L., Campbell, G.R. and Campbell, J.H. Smooth muscle phenotypic expression in human carotid arteries, II. Atherosclerosis-free diffuse intimal thickenings compared with the media. *Arteriosclerosis* 1986; 6: 664.

49. Benditt, E.P. and Benditt, J.M. Evidence for a monoclonal origin of human atherosclerotic plaques. *Proc. Nat. Acad. Sci. U.S.A.* 1973; 70: 1753.

50. Benditt, E.P. and Gown, A.M. Atheroma: the artery wall and the environment. *Int. Rev. Exp. Pathol.* 1980; 21: 55.

51. Eskin, S.G., Sybers, H.D., Lester, J.W., Navarro, L.T., Gotto, A.M. and DeBakey, M.E. Human smooth muscle cells cultured from atherosclerotic plaques and uninvolved vessel wall. *In Vitro* 1981; 17: 713.

52. Ross, R., Wight, T.N., Strandness, E. and Thiele, B. Human atherosclerosis 1. Cell constitution and characteristics of advanced lesions of the superficial femoral artery. *Am. J. Pathol.* 1984; 114: 79.

53. Orekhov, A.N., Andreeva, E.R., Krushinsky, A.V. *et al.* Intimal cells and atherosclerosis. *Am. J. Pathol.* 1986; 125: 402.

54. Penn, A., Garte, S.J., Warren, L., Nesta, D. and Mindich, B. Transforming gene in human atherosclerotic plaque DNA. *Proc. Nat. Acad. Sci. U.S.A.* 1986; 83: 7951.

55. Rokitansky, C. *A Manual of Pathological Anatomy*, Vol. IV. London: Sydenham Society, 1852.

56. Klimov, A.N. and Nagornev, V.A. N.N. Anichkov and his contribution to the doctrine of atherosclerosis. In: Fidge, N.H. and Nestel, P.J., eds. *Atherosclerosis VII*. Amsterdam: Excerpta Medica, 1986, p. 371.

57. Duguid, J.B. Thrombosis as a factor in the pathogenesis of coronary atherosclerosis. *J. Pathol. Bacteriol.* 1946; 58: 207.

58. Duguid, J.B. Thrombosis as a factor in the pathogenesis of aortic atherosclerosis. *J. Pathol. Bacteriol.* 1948; 60: 57.

59. Smith, E.B. Fibrinogen, fibrin and fibrin degradation products in relation to atherosclerosis. *Clin. Haematol.* 1986; 15: 355.

60. Jorgensen, L., Packham, M.A., Rowsell, H.C. and Mustard, J.F. Deposition of formed elements of blood on the intima and signs of intimal injury in the aorta of rabbit, pig and man. *Lab. Invest.* 1972; 27: 341.

61. Bar-Shavit, R. and Wilner, G.D. Mediation of cellular events by thrombin. *Int. Rev. Exp. Pathol.* 1986; 29: 213.

62. Thompson, W.D., Evans, A.T. and Campbell, R. The control of fibrogenesis: stimulation and suppression of collagen synthesis in the chick chorioallantoic membrane with fibrin degradation products, wound extracts and proteases. *J. Pathol.* 1986; 148: 207.

63. Kadish, J.L., Butterfield, C.E. and Folkman, J. Effect of fibrin on cultured vascular endothelium. *Tissue Cell* 1979; 11: 99.

64. Schleef, R.R. and Birdwell, C.R. Biochemical changes in endothelial cell monolayers induced by fibrin deposition *in vitro*. *Arteriosclerosis* 1984; 3: 14.

65. Weimar, B. and Delvos, U. The mechanism of fibrin-induced disorganisation of cultured human endothelial cell monolayers. *Arteriosclerosis* 1986; 6: 139.

66. Wilhelmsen, L., Svardsudd, K., Korsan-Bengsten, K., Larsson, B., Welin, L. and Tibblin, G. Fibrinogen as a risk factor for stroke and myocardial infarction. *N. Engl. J. Med.* 1984; 311: 501.

67. Stone, M.C. and Thorp, J.M. Plasma fibrinogen—a major coronary risk factor. *J.R. Coll. Gen. Pract.* 1985; 35: 565.

68. Kannel, W.B., Castelli, W.P. and Meeks, S.L. Fibrinogen and cardiovascular disease (Abstract). In: *34th Annual Scientific Session*. American College of Cardiology, 1985.

69. Meade, T.W., Brozovic, M., Chakrabarti, R.R. *et al.* Haemostatic function and ischaemic heart disease: principal results of the Northwick Park heart study. *Lancet* 1986; ii: 533.

70. Muller-Mohnssen, H. and Schauerte, W. Hydrodynamic conditions of fibrin thrombus formation. In: Muller-Berghaus, G., Scheefers-Borchel, U., Selmayr, E. and Henschen, A. *Fibrinogen and its Derivatives*. Amsterdam: Elsevier Science Publishers, 1986, p. 169.

71. Weiss, H.J., Turitto, V.T. and Baumgartner, H.R. Role of shear rate and platelets in promoting fibrin formation on rabbit subendothelium. *J. Clin. Invest.* 1986; 78: 1072.

72. Ku, D., Giddens, D.P., Zarins, C.K. and Glagov, S. Pulsatile flow and atherosclerosis in the human carotid bifurcation. *Arteriosclerosis* 1985; 5: 293.

73. Friedman, M.H., Deters, O.J., Bargeron, C.B., Hutchins, G.M. and Mark, F.F. Shear-dependent thickening of the human arterial intima. *Atherosclerosis* 1986; 60: 161.

74. Stary, H.C. Macrophages in coronary artery and aortic intima in atherosclerotic lesions of children and young adults up to age 29. In: Schettler, G., Gotto, A.M., Middelhoff, G., Habenicht, A.J.R. and Jurutka, K.R., eds. *Atherosclerosis VI*. Berlin: Springer-Verlag, 1983, p. 462.

75. Goldstein, J.L. and Brown, M.S. The low density lipoprotein pathway and its relation to atherosclerosis. *Annu. Rev. Biochem.* 1977; 46: 897.

76. Mahley, R.W., Rall, S.C., Innerarity, T.L. and Weisgraber, K.H. Apoliprotein E and cholesterol metabolism. In: Schettler, G., Gotto, A.M., Middlehof, G., Habenicht, A.J.R. and Jurutka, K.R. *Atherosclerosis VI*. Berlin: Springer-Verlag, 1983, p. 489.

77. Brown, M.S. and Goldstein, J.L. Lipoprotein metabolism in the macrophage. *Annu. Rev. Biochem.* 1983; 52: 223.

78. Steinberg, D. Arterial lipoprotein metabolism in relation to the pathogenesis of atherosclerosis. In: Fidge, N.H. and Nestel, P.J. eds. *Atherosclerosis VII*. Amsterdam: Excerpta Medica, 1986, p. 345.

79. Gianturco, S.H. and Bradley, W.A. The β-VLDL pathway of macrophages. In: Fidge, N.H. and Nestel, P.J., eds. *Atherosclerosis VII*. Amsterdam: Excerpta Medica, 1986, p. 495.

80. Smith, E.B. and Ashall, C. Variability of the electrophoretic mobility of low density lipoprotein—Comparison of interstitial fluid from human aortic intima, and serum. *Atherosclerosis* 1983; 49: 89.

81. Smith, E.B. and Ashall, C. Compartmentalisation of water in human atherosclerotic lesions. *Arteriosclerosis* 1984; 4: 21.

82. Smith, E.B. Intimal lipids and associated changes in intimal composition. In: Glagov, S., ed. *Evolution of the Human Atherosclerotic Plaque*. Berlin: Springer-verlag, 1989.

83. Owens, G.K. and Schwartz, S.M. Alteration in vascular smooth muscle mass in the spontaneously hypertensive rat: role of cellular hypertrophy, hyperploidy and hyperplasia. *Circ. Res.* 1982; 51: 280.

84. Smith, E.B., Alexander, K.M. and Massie, I.B. Insoluble "fibrin" in human aortic intima. Quantitative studies on the relationship between insoluble "fibrin", soluble fibrinogen and LD-lipoprotein. *Atherosclerosis* 1976; 23: 19.

85. Smith, E.B. and Staples, E. Haemostatic factors in human aortic intima. *Lancet* 1981; i: 1171.

86. Smith, E.B. and Walker, J.E. Soluble fibrin/fibrinogen related antigen in human intima in relation to atherogenesis. In: Lane, D., Henschen, A. and Jasani, K., eds. *Fibrinogen, fibrin formation and fibrinolysis*. Berlin, New

York: Walter de Gruyter & Co., 1986, p. 363.

87. Woolf, N. *Pathology of Atherosclerosis.* London: Butterworth Scientific, 1982.

88. Thompson, W.D., McGuigan, C.J., Snyder, C., Keen, G.A. and Smith, E.B. Mitogenic activity in human atherosclerotic lesions. *Atherosclerosis* 1987; **66**: 85.

89. Smith, E.B. from the fatty streak to the calcified lesion. In: Born, G., Catapano, A.L. and Paoletti, R., eds. *Factors in Formation and Regression of the Atherosclerotic Plaque.* NATO Advanced Study Institutes Series A, Vol. 51. New York: Plenum Press, 1982, p. 45.

90. Cornhill, J.F. Topographic distribution of human atherosclerotic lesions. In: Glagov, S., ed. *Evolution of the Human Atherosclerotic Plaque.* Berlin: Springer-verlag, 1989.

91. Bocan, T.M.A., Schifani, T.A. and Guyton, J.R. Ultrastructure of the human aortic fibro-lipid lesion. Formation of the atherosclerotic lipid-rich core. *Am. J. Pathol.* 1986; **123**: 413.

92. Smith, E.B. and Slater, R.S. The microdissection of large atherosclerotic plaques to give morphologically and topographically defined fractions for analysis. Pt 1. The lipids in the isolated fractions. *Atherosclerosis* 1972; **15**: 37.

93. Kruth, H.S. Subendothelial accumulation of unesterified cholesterol. An early event in atherosclerotic lesion developoment. *Atherosclerosis* 1985; **57**: 337.

94. Simionescu, N., Vasile, E., Lupu, F., Popescu, G., and Simionescu, M. Accumulation of extracellular cholesterol-rich liposomes in the arterial intima and cardiac valves of the hyperlipidemic rabbit. *Am. J. Pathol.* 1986; **123**: 109.

95. Smith, E.B. Acid glycosaminoglycan, collagen and elastin content of normal artery, fatty streaks and plaques. In: Wagner, W.D. and Clarkson, T.B., eds. *Arterial mesenchyme and Arteriosclerosis.* Advances in Experimental and Medical Biology, Vol. 43. 1974, p. 125.

96. Mayne, R. Collagenous proteins of blood vessels. *Arteriosclerosis* 1986; **6**: 585.

97. Guyton, J.R., Bocan, T.M.A. and Schifani, T.A. Quantitative ultrastructural analysis of perifibrous lipid and its association with elastin in nonatherosclerotic human aorta. *Arteriosclerosis* 1985; **5**: 644.

98. Berenson, G., Radhakrishnamurthy, B., Srinivasan, S.R. and Vijayagopal, P. Arterial wall proteoglycans-biologic properties related to pathogenesis of atherosclerosis. In: Fidge, N.H. and Nestel, P., eds. *Atherosclerosis VII.* Amsterdam: Excerpta Medica, 1986, p. 417.

99. Bihari-Varga, M. and Vegh, M. Quantitative studies on the complex formed between aortic and mucopolysaccharides and serum lipoproteins. *Biochim. Biophys. Acta* 1967; **144**: 202.

100. Inverius, P.-H. The interaction between human plasma lipoproteins and connective tissue glycosaminoglycans. *J. Biol. Chem.* 1972; **247**: 2607.

101. Smith, E.B., Massie, I.B. and Alexander, K.M. The release of an immobilized lipoprotein fraction from atherosclerotic lesions by incubation with plasmin. *Atherosclerosis* 1976; **25**: 71.

102. Smith, E.B. and Massie, I.B. Destruction of endogenous low density lipoproteins in incubated intima. *Atherosclerosis* 1977; **26**: 427.

103. Smith, E.B., Dietz, H.S. and Craig, I.B. Characterisation of free and tightly bound lipoprotein in intima by thin layer isoelectric focussing. *Atherosclerosis* 1979; **33**: 329.

104. Hoff, H.F., Heideman, C.L., Gaubatz, J.W., Scott, D.W., Titus, J.L. and Gotto, A.M. Correlation of apoprotein B retention with the structure of atherosclerotic plaques from human aortas. *Lab. Invest.* 1978; **38**: 560.

105. Smith, E.B., Staples, E.M. Dietz, H.S. and Smith, R.H. Role of endothelium in sequestration of lipoprotein and fibrinogen in aortic lesions, thrombi and graft pseudo-intimas. *Lancet* 1979; **ii**: 812.

106. Smith, E.B. and Ashall, C. Fibronectin distribution in human aortic intima and atherosclerotic lesions: concentration of soluble and collagenase-releasable fractions. *Biochim. Biophys. Acta* 1986; **880**: 10.

107. Smith, E.B. and Ashall, C. Fibrinolysis and plasminogen concentration in aortic intima in relation to death following myocardial infarction. *Atherosclerosis* 1985; **55**: 171.

108. Partridge, S.M. and Keeley, F.W. Age-related and atherosclerotic changes in aortic elastin. In: Wagner, W.D. and Clarkson, T.B., eds. *Arterial Mesenchyme and Arteriosclerosis.* Advances in Experimental and Medical Biology, Vol. 43. 1974, p. 173.

109. Daoud, A.S. Significance of calcification in human lesions. In: Glagov, S., ed. *Evolution of the Human Atherosclerotic Plaque.* Berlin: Springer-verlag, 1989.

110. Anderson, H.C. Mechanics of calcification in atherosclerosis. In: Glagov, S., ed. *Evolution of the Human Atherosclerotic Plaque.* Berlin: Springer-verlag, 1989.

111. Meade, T.W., Vickers, M.V., Thompson, S.G., Stirling, Y., Haines, A.P. and Miller, G.J. Epidemiological characteristics of platelet aggregability. *Br. Med. J.* 1985; **290**: 428.

112. Korsan-Bengsten, K., Wilhelmsen, L. and Tibblin, G. Blood coagulation and fibrinolysis in a random sample of 788 men 54 years old: II. Relations of the variables to "risk factors" for myocardial infarction. *Thromb. Diath. Haemor.* 1972; **28**: 99.

113. Meade, T.W., Chakrabarti, R., Haines, A.P., North, W.R.S. and Stirling, Y. Characteristics affecting fibrinolytic activity and plasma fibrinogen concentrations. *Br. Med. J.* 1979; **i**: 153.

114. Markowe, H.L.J., Marmot, M.G., Shipley, M.J. *et al.* Fibrinogen: a possible link between social class and coronary heart disease. *Br. Med. J.* 1985; **291**: 1312.

115. Elkeles, R.S., Chakrabarti, R., Vickers, M., Stirling, Y. and Meade, T.W. Effect of treatment of hyperlipidaemia on haemostatic variables. *Br. Med. J.* 1980; **281**: 973.

116. Simpson, H.C.R., Meade, T.W., Stirling, Y., Mann, J.I., Chakrabarti, R. and Woolf, L. Hypertriglyceridaemia and hypercoagulability. *Lancet* 1983; **i**: 786.

117. Miller, G.J., Martin, J.C., Webster, J. *et al.* Association between dietary fat intake and plasma Factor VII coagulant activity—a predictor of cardiovascular mortality. *Atherosclerosis* 1986; **60**: 269.

118. Stehbens, W.E. An appraisal of cholesterol feeding in experimental atherogenesis. *Prog. Cardiovasc. Dis.* 1986; **29**: 107.

119. Stehbens, W.E. Vascular complications in experimental atherosclerosis. *Prog. Cardiovasc. Dis.* 1986; **29**: 221.

120. Falcone, D.J., Hajjar, D.P. and Minick, C.R. Lipoprotein and albumin accumulation in re-endothelialized and de-endothelialized aorta. *Am. J. Pathol.* 1984; **114**: 112.

121. Wiklund, O., Carew, T.E. and Steinberg, D. Role of the low density lipoprotein receptor in penetration of low density lipoprotein into rabbit aortic wall. *Arteriosclerosis* 1985; **5**: 135.

122. Stender, S. and Hjelms, E. In vivo influx of free and esterified plasma cholesterol into human aortic tissue without atherosclerotic lesions. *J. Clin. Invest.* 1984; **74**: 1871.

123. Weigensberg, B.I., Lough, J. and More, R.H. Biochemistry of atherosclerosis produced by cholesterol feeding, thrombosis and injury. *Exp. Molec. Pathol.* 1982; **37**: 175.

124. Wissler, R.W. and Vesselinovitch, D. Diet and experimental atherosclerosis. In: Chavez, A., Bourges, H. and Basta, S., eds. *Nutrition: Volume 1. Review of Basic Knowledge.* Basel: S. Karger, 1975, p. 333.

125. Malinow, M.R. and Blaton, V.H. *Regression of Atherosclerotic Lesions.* NATO Advanced Study Institutes Series A, Vol. 79. New York: Plenum Press, 1984, p. 79.

126. Weingand, K.W., Clarkson, T.B., Adams, M.R. and Bostrom, A.D. Effect of age and/or puberty on coronary artery atherosclerosis in cynomolgus monkeys. *Atherosclerosis* 1986; **62**: 137.

127. St Clair, R.W. Metabolic changes in the arterial wall associated with atherosclerosis in the pigeon. *Fed. Proc.* 1983; **42**: 2480.

128. St Clair, R.W., Leight, M.A. and Barakat, H.A. Metabolism of low density lipoproteins by pigeon fibroblasts and aortic smooth muscle cells. *Arteriosclerosis* 1986; **6**: 170.

129. St Clair, R.W., Randolph, R.K., Jokinen, M.P., Clarkson, T.B. and Barakat, H.A. Relationship of plasma lipoproteins and the monocyte macrophage system to atherosclerosis severity in cholesterol-fed pigeons. *Arteriosclerosis* 1986; **6**: 614.

130. Anonymous. The progression of atherosclerosis. *Lancet* 1985; **i**: 791.

131. Cosgrove, D.M., Loop, F.D., Saunders, C.L., Lytle, B.W. and Kramer, J.R. Should coronary arteries with less than fifty percent stenosis be bypassed? *J. Thorac. Cardiovasc. Surg.* 1981; **82**: 520.

132. Loop, F.D. Progression of coronary atherosclerosis. *N. Engl. J. Med.* 1984; **311**: 851.

133. Spray, T.L. and Roberts, W.C. Status of the grafts and the native coronary arteries proximal and distal to coronary anastomotic sites of aorto-coronary bypass grafts. *Circulation* 1977; **55**: 741.

134. Insull, W. Ultrasound carotid lesions and risk factors in men. In: Glagov, S., ed. *Evolution of the Human Atherosclerotic Plaque*. Berlin: Springer-verlag, 1989.

135. Nikkila, E.A. Lipoproteins and progression of coronary artery disease. In: Fidge, N.H. and Nestel, P.J., eds. *Atherosclerosis VII*. Amsterdam: Excerpta Medica, 1986, p. 85.

Chapter 46

Coronary Blood Flow and Myocardial Ischaemia

Stuart M. Cobbe

INTRODUCTION

The heart is an aerobic organ. Unlike skeletal muscle, which may accumulate an oxygen debt on exercise to be repaid later at rest, cardiac muscle is in continuous use and must keep its energy supply in balance with its metabolic demands at all times. Anaerobic glycolysis, even under conditions of maximum stimulation in experimental models, cannot provide more than 18% of the rate of aerobic adenosine triphosphate (ATP) production of a working normoxic heart.[1] As cardiac metabolism is almost exclusively aerobic under normal circumstances, myocardial oxygen consumption (MVo_2) provides a simple readily measured index of the metabolic activity of the heart.

Measurement of MVo_2 is undertaken by application of the Fick principle:

$$MVo_2 = \text{Total coronary blood flow} \times \text{Arteriovenous oxygen difference} \quad \text{(equation 46.1)}$$

The majority of the coronary blood flow empties via the coronary sinus, although a small percentage drains directly into the right atrium via the Thebesian veins. The oxygen extraction across the coronary vascular bed is high even under resting conditions, and little additional oxygen supply to the myocardium can be obtained by increasing extraction. For this reason, changes in MVo_2 dictate rapid and substantial changes in coronary blood flow, as will be discussed below. Failure of coronary blood flow to supply sufficient oxygen and metabolic substrate to satisfy the requirements of the myocardium, and to remove the end-products of metabolism, results in myocardial ischaemia. The term hypoxia is used when impairment of myocardial oxygen supply occurs as a result of reduced arterial oxygen saturation, a condition normally associated with an *increase* in coronary blood flow.

DETERMINANTS OF MYOCARDIAL OXYGEN CONSUMPTION

The oxygen consumption of the heart is determined by the sum of the metabolic processes undertaken by the myocardial cell. These may be summarized as follows.

1 Basal metabolism.
2 Generation of action potential.
3 Activation, maintenance and reversal of active state (calcium cycling).
4 Tension development.
5 Contractile work (shortening).

The factors responsible for variation in MVo_2, and their relative importance, have been extensively studied and reviewed.[2] The total MVo_2 of the heart at a physiological workload is 8–15 ml/min/100 g, of which basal metabolism comprises about 2 ml/min/100 g, as determined in quiescent hearts.[3] The oxygen consumption required for myocardial depolarization is small, being about 0.04 ml/min /100 g at a heart rate of 100 beats/min, or approximately 0.5% of the total MVo_2.[4]

It is clear, therefore, that the principal determinants of the metabolic rate of the cardiac myocyte must be related to the processes of tension development and shortening or, in the case of the whole heart, to pressure generation and ejection. Extensive investigation has been undertaken to identify the indices of mechanical activity that most closely correlate with oxygen consumption. Based on simple mechanics, it might be expected that left ventricular minute work (the product of heart rate, stroke volume, and developed pressure) would accurately characterize MVo_2. However, careful studies by Sarnoff and his group, using isolated dog hearts in which heart rate, cardiac output and arterial pressure could be independently varied, demonstrated that left ventricular minute work correlated poorly with MVo_2, while the area under the left ventricular pressure curve per minute (tension–time index) was related to MVo_2 under differing conditions of heart rate, cardiac output and afterload.[2,5,6] Subsequently, left ventricular wall stress, or tension, has been identified as a superior index to pressure[7,8] (Table 46.1). Wall tension, derived from the relationship of the intraventricular pressure and volume (Laplace equation) is expressed by the equation:

$$\text{Stress} = \frac{\text{Intraventricular pressure} \times \text{Intracavity radius}}{\text{Ventricular wall thickness}} \quad (\text{equation } 46.2)$$

In studies in intact hearts, tension (or pressure) generation has been identified as a major determinant of MVo_2. Such observations have been confirmed in isolated papillary muscles, when oxygen consumption at a given preload is increased with increasing afterload, and is maximal when afterload is equal to preload (i.e. under isometric conditions). However, when shortening is allowed to occur at the same level of tension development as the isometric contraction (afterloaded isotonic contraction), a further increase in oxygen consumption occurs. Thus, in addition to the oxygen consumed during tension generation, there is an additional oxygen requirement associated with shortening (Fenn effect).[9]

A further independent determinant of MVo_2 is the inotropic state of the myocardium which may be assessed by the peak velocity of contraction or ejection. Inotropic state can be altered by catecholamines, calcium, other drugs with positive or negative inotropic effects, or by changes in heart rate. Under these circumstances, major changes in MVo_2 are seen independent of tension–time index (Fig. 46.1).[10,11] For a given level of MVo_2, an inverse

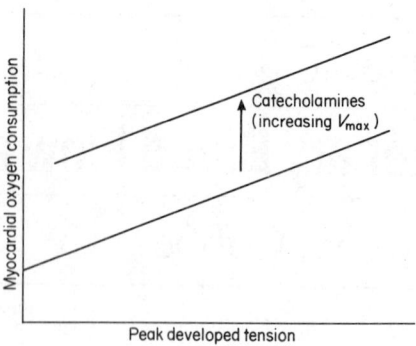

Fig. 46.1. Diagram showing the linear relationship between peak developed tension and myocardial oxygen consumption (MVo_2). The intercept on the y axis represents basal MVo_2. At any given level of developed tension, MVo_2 may be increased by increasing the velocity of contraction (V_{max}) by inotropic stimulation. (After Graham *et al. J. Clin. Invest.* 1968; **47**: 375–85.

relationship exists between peak developed tension and shortening velocity (V_{max}).[12] The effect of catecholamine stimulation on MVo_2 is almost entirely determined by its effect on V_{max}, although there may be a small oxygen-wasting effect on intermediary metabolism.[13]

The third major determinant of MVo_2 after tension development and inotropic state is heart rate. In one sense, this is self-evident, because MVo_2 is the product of stroke oxygen consumption and heart rate. However, increasing heart rate also exerts a positive inotropic influence (Bowditch effect) which will alter MVo_2 independently.[14]

Other, less important, determinants of MVo_2 include the energy required for generation, maintenance and reversal of the active state.[15,16] These processes involve the release and re-uptake of stored calcium ions from the sarcoplasmic reticulum. Release occurs in response to the increase in cytoplasmic calcium activity mediated by the inward calcium current at the onset of the action potential, whereas active re-uptake of calcium into the sarcoplasmic reticulum brings about relaxation. Variations in myocardial substrate, from predominant glucose consumption to free fatty acid consumption, cause an increase in MVo_2, probably related to a degree of uncoupling of oxidative phosphorylation.[17]

The discussion thus far has centred on the determinants of MVo_2 considered in isolation. In the intact animal or in man, however, different determinants of MVo_2 may have opposing effects. A simple example is the effect of inotropic stimulation in the normal and dilated heart. The effect of catecholamines in the normal heart will be to

---

Table 46.1. **Determinants of myocardial oxygen consumption.**

Major

1 Left ventricular wall tension
2 Inotropic state
3 Heart rate

Minor

4 Basal metabolism
5 Generation of action potential
6 Calcium uptake and release
7 Substrate

increase V_{max} and heart rate, with little if any effect on left ventricular end-diastolic volume. There will be therefore a substantial increase in MVo_2. In contrast, although inotropic stimulation of the failing heart will tend to increase MVo_2 by the same mechanisms, a reduction in chamber size will reduce wall stress and thus reduce MVo_2. The algebraic sum of these opposite influences will be impossible to predict, but may result in a small increase, no change or a small decrease in MVo_2. These observations should be borne in mind in clinical practice or clinical research; an attempt to estimate changes in MVo_2 from the easily measured product of heart rate and systolic blood pressure (rate–pressure product, an approximation of tension–time index) may be misleading if changes in ventricular volume or inotropic state are not considered.

A further observation of clinical relevance which can be deduced from the relationship between wall stress and MVo_2 (equation 46.2) is that an increase in the pressure work of the heart results in a greater demand on MVo_2 than an increase in volume work. Thus, whereas wall stress (and hence MVo_2) is directly proportional to peak intraventricular pressure, it is only proportional to the cube root of intraventricular volume (since $V = 4/3\ \pi r^3$ or $r \propto \sqrt[3]{V}$, where V is the ventricular volume and r its radius). The abnormal wall stress associated with an increased intraventricular pressure may be corrected by a compensatory increase in wall thickness (equation 46.2). This relationship explains why lesions associated with an increase in the pressure work of the left ventricle (e.g. systemic hypertension, aortic stenosis) elicit a greater degree of hypertrophy and increase in wall thickness than volume-overload lesions, such as aortic and mitral regurgitation.

CORONARY BLOOD FLOW

The function of the coronary circulation is to supply oxygenated arterial blood and metabolic substrates

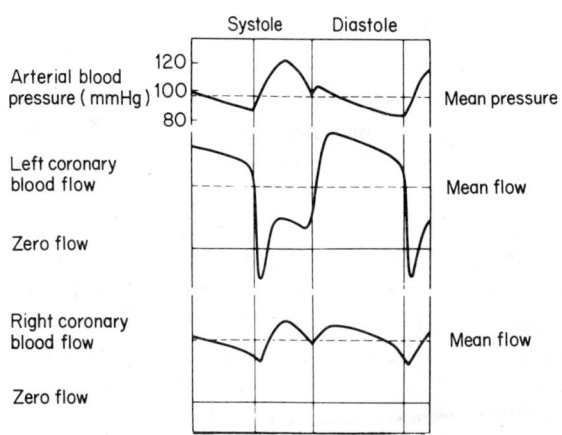

Fig. 46.2. Relationship between coronary blood flow and arterial pressure. The majority of left coronary flow occurs during diastole. (Reproduced with permission from Hutton, I. Physiology of myocardial perfusion. In: Wheatley, D.J. ed. *Surgery of Coronary Disease*. London: Chapman & Hall, 1986, pp. 41–9.)

to the myocardium and to remove end-products of metabolism. Myocardium contractile function is closely dependent on coronary flow, and reductions of as little as 10–20% will impair systolic function.[18,19] The intimate relationship between coronary blood flow and MVo_2 is implicit in the Fick equation (equation 46.1) because the only variable that can dissociate the two is the arteriovenous oxygen difference, which remains within narrow limits in the heart. The determinants of coronary blood flow are listed in Table 46.2. Although the majority of coronary arterial flow occurs during diastole, it has been demonstrated that about 20–30% occurs in systole[20] (Fig. 46.2). The diastolic coronary driving pressure is derived by subtracting the right atrial pressure from the aortic diastolic pressure. In view of the autoregulatory properties of the coronary vasculature (see below), it is only at very low levels of aortic diastolic pressure that total coronary driving pressure becomes limiting. Of course, regional reduction in driving pressure may occur in the presence of a coronary artery stenosis.

The term extravascular pressure describes the myocardial compressive forces that may cause collapse of arterioles and capillaries and thus interfere with flow. This phenomenon is maximal during systole, although coronary driving pressure is also greater during systole than diastole. In aortic stenosis, left ventricular cavity and intramyocardial pressures exceed coronary driving (aortic systolic) pressure, and may cause a reversal in epicardial coronary flow. During diastole, extravascular press-

---

Table 46.2. Determinants of coronary blood flow.

1 Driving pressure
   (aortic diastolic pressure – right atrial pressure)
2 Extravascular pressure
3 Diastolic time per minute
4 Coronary vascular resistance

ure is related to the left ventricular diastolic pressure. When the latter is elevated, in left ventricular failure, the driving force for diastolic coronary flow will be determined by the difference between aortic and left ventricular, rather than right atrial, pressure.

As the majority of coronary flow occurs during diastole, the total diastolic time per minute is a determinant of coronary flow. During tachycardia, the duration of diastole is abbreviated relative to systole, hence the diastolic time per minute falls. The indices of driving force, tissue compression and diastolic time have been combined to produce a 'diastolic pressure–time index' (DPTI), which has been used as an index of myocardial oxygen supply, and related to tension–time index as an index of oxygen demand. As discussed below, coronary flow is autoregulated over a wide range, and thus flow becomes directly proportional to pressure (or DPTI) only below the autoregulatory range.[21]

CONTROL OF CORONARY VASCULAR RESISTANCE

The majority of the variation in coronary blood flow under physiological conditions is achieved by alterations in coronary vascular resistance. Thus, while resting left ventricular coronary blood flow is around 70–90 ml/min/100 g, this value can be increased by excitement, exercise or vasodilators to levels of 350–400 ml/min/100 g. These changes are brought about by a 4–5-fold reduction in coronary vascular resistance. The ratio between resting and maximal coronary blood flow, or between resting and minimal coronary vascular resistance, expresses

Table 46.3. Factors affecting coronary vascular resistance.

1 Increased MV_{O_2} — metabolic vasodilatation
2 Reduced arterial oxygen content — hypoxic vasodilatation
3 Reduced coronary arterial flow
4 Pressure autoregulation
5 Neurohormonal effects
6 Pharmacological agents

the vasodilator capacity, or coronary reserve, of the heart.[22]

The mechanisms responsible for changes in coronary vascular resistance under physiological and pathological conditions continue to be of enormous interest to both cardiovascular physiologists and cardiologists. The three principal aspects of the control of coronary vascular resistance are metabolic regulation, pressure autoregulation and the effect of neurohormonal influences (Table 46.3).

METABOLIC REGULATION (Fig. 46.3)

The intimate relationship between myocardial oxygen consumption and coronary blood flow has already been mentioned, and has been extensively reviewed.[23–25] The relationship between MV_{O_2} and coronary blood flow can be demonstrated in isolated denervated hearts, and is thus intrinsic to the heart. Metabolic control of coronary blood flow may be regarded as a system of dynamic vasodilatation which operates against a tonic vasoconstriction. Thus, resting coronary resistance is 4–5 times that which can be achieved by maximal dilatation. Increases in coronary blood flow will arise not only

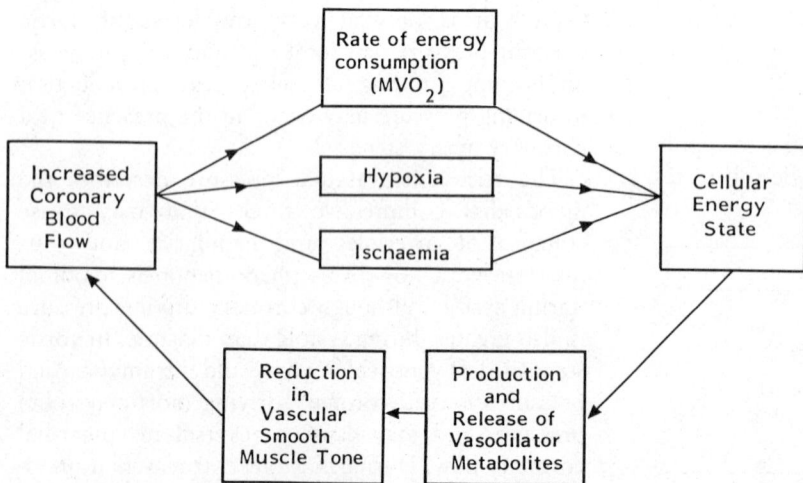

Fig. 46.3. Mechanism of metabolic flow regulation in response to increased MV_{O_2}, arterial hypoxaemia or ischaemia.

as a result of an increase of the determinants of MVo_2 mentioned earlier in the chapter, but also in the presence of a reduced arterial oxygen content (hypoxia). Vasodilatation occurs after transient coronary occlusion and results in a reactive hyperaemia during which the 'flow debt' is repaid. Finally, metabolic vasodilatation may occur distal to the flow-limiting stenosis in an attempt to maintain coronary flow.

Much research has centred on the metabolic 'signal' generated in the myocardium that links metabolic rate with coronary flow, and on the substance(s) responsible for transmission of this signal to the vascular smooth muscle. The most likely metabolic signal would appear to be the energy state of the cell as expressed by the cytosolic ATP potential:[25]

$$\frac{[ATP]}{[ADP]\ [P_i]}$$

Where Pi is the concentration of inorganic phosphate.

One theory assumes that control of coronary vascular resistance occurs by local oxygen consumption transiently exceeding supply, or by cyclical closure of coronary resistance vessels resulting in areas of local hypoperfusion. Both mechanisms result in a reduction in ATP potential, which generates the signal for vasodilatation and reperfusion of the segment (microhypoxia model).[26] An alternative hypothesis is based on the observation that the cytosolic ATP potential of the normally perfused heart may fall simply as a result of an increase in cardiac workload, without oxygen supply being limited (normoxia model).[25] Irrespective of the mechanism, a reduction in cytosolic ATP potential may be the signal for the release of vasodilator metabolites (adenosine, carbon dioxide, potassium ions) from the cell, which will adjust local oxygen supply to demand.

PRESSURE AUTOREGULATION

A corollary of the fact that coronary blood flow is under metabolic control is that flow is insensitive to changes in driving pressure (pressure autoregulation).[27] This property is common to other organs under predominantly metabolic flow control, e.g. brain, skeletal muscle. Pressure autoregulation is difficult to demonstrate in the intact heart, because changes in aortic pressure will alter not only coronary driving pressure but also MVo_2, and

thus produce an indirect metabolic change in coronary blood flow. Experimental studies in which coronary arteries have been selectively cannulated, and perfusion pressure altered independent of aortic pressure, have demonstrated autoregulation over a range of 60–140 mmHg. Autoregulation to an abrupt change in coronary pressure results in a return to the previous flow rate within 10 s, although some oscillation, typical of a negative feedback system, may persist. Above and below the limits of autoregulation, a more linear change of flow with pressure is seen.

One complication in the study of autoregulation is that changes in coronary perfusion pressure result in small directionally similar increases in MVo_2 (Gregg phenomenon).[28] The most likely explanation for the Gregg phenomenon (garden-hose effect) is that increased vascular turgor within the myocardium causes increase in sarcomere length which results in enhanced contractile function and oxygen consumption. The magnitude of the Gregg effect appears to be greatest when autoregulation is absent.

MECHANISMS OF AUTOREGULATION

Despite intensive investigation, no single metabolite or mechanism has been shown unequivocally to link increased myocardial oxygen consumption with coronary vasodilatation. The problems of idenfication of the vasodilator signal are partly methodological, but may also be explained on the basis of the interaction of several mechanisms, each quantitatively insufficient alone to account for the observed changes.

Adenosine

The coronary vasodilator properties of adenosine have long been recognized,[29] and increased adenosine production has been identified during hypoxic vasodilatation and ischaemia.[30–32] Inverse correlation was demonstrated between coronary resistance and tissue and coronary venous adenosine concentrations in vitro,[32] and increased adenosine concentrations have been measured in the coronary venous effluent of patients during pacing-induced myocardial ischaemia.[33] Olsson and Bunger[25] have reviewed the mechanisms of adenosine synthesis and identified linkage between the rate of cytosolic adenosine production and cytosolic AMP concentration, which is itself related to cytosolic ATP potential. This model allows for the generation of adenosine in response to increased workload as well as during hypoxia or ischaemia. Adenosine leaves the cell via a carrier mechanism and by passive diffusion, and exerts its vasodilator activity on vascular smooth muscle. Although adenylate cyclase stimulatory (A_2) receptors have not been identified in coronary resistance vessels, considerable indirect evidence supports their role in adenosine-mediated vasodilatation.[25]

Definitive proof of the adenosine hypothesis requires correlation between adenosine concentrations at the vascular receptor and coronary vascular resistance. This is currently impossible to obtain as indirect estimates of adenosine concentration at the receptor by measurement of total tissue adenosine, or adenosine concentrations in coronary venous effluent, epicardial superfusate or cardiac lymph, are beset with methodological problems, not least of which is the active metabolism of adenosine by endothelial cells. Furthermore, infusion of the enzyme adenosine deaminase, which rapidly destroys adenosine, does not abolish pressure autoregulation,[34] although it does reduce reactive hyperaemia.[35] It is arguable that the enzyme did not destroy all available adenosine, or that destruction of adenosine simply results in a compensatory increase in other mechanisms.

Adenosine triphosphate

Adenosine triphosphate is a potent vasodilator like adenosine; it is also released from myocytes during hypoxia.[36] Quantification of its physiological role is likely to be even more difficult than that for adenosine, in view of the rapid degradation of ATP.

Oxygen

In view of the central role of oxygen in myocardial metabolism, a direct relation between partial pressure of oxygen (Po_2) and control of coronary blood flow is plausible. Except under conditions of arterial desaturation, Po_2 at the arteriolar wall will be normal. However, tissue Po_2 is substantially lower than arterial Po_2 (normally 20 mmHg) and is influenced by metabolic factors or ischaemia. Values of tissue Po_2 approximate closely to those of venous Po_2, which has been closely correlated with pressure and metabolic autoregulation by several authors.[37,38] Although isolated rabbit coronary artery strips are insensitive to hypoxia down to levels of Po_2 of 5–10 mmHg, addition of adenosine 10^{-7} mol/l results in a linear relation between tension and Po_2 between 10 and 100 mmHg.[39] More recently, hypoxia has been shown to stimulate release of endothelium-derived relaxing factor.[40] Thus, a potential mechanism exists whereby Po_2 could directly influence smooth muscle tone and coronary vascular resistance.

Carbon dioxide and hydrogen ions

Carbon dioxide is a powerful vasodilator,[41] which is produced in equimolar quantities to oxygen consumption during aerobic metabolism. The gas is freely diffusible between the intracellular and extracellular spaces, and is a clear candidate for a role as metabolic regulator. However, so far, no quantitative studies have been undertaken to verify such a role. Carbon dioxide is rapidly hydrated within cells to carbonic acid, and its effects may be mediated via intracellular acidosis. It is noteworthy that the vasodilator effects of adenosine are enhanced at low pH.[42]

Potassium

Potassium efflux from the myocardial cell occurs with each action potential, and a transient directionally similar change in potassium efflux occurs with changes in heart rate or contractile force.[43] Potassium efflux from the cell occurs during ischaemia and hypoxia,[44] and cellular potassium balance has been linked mathematically to ATP potential.[25] An increase of perfusate potassium concentration in isolated hearts causes a dose-dependent coronary vasodilatation.[45] Thus, potassium could act as a mediator of coronary vasodilatation. However, whereas an increase in heart rate results in a persistent increase in coronary flow, the increase in potassium efflux is only transient.

Thus, although potassium efflux might act in the initiation of metabolic coronary vasodilatation, it is not responsible for its maintenance.

Prostaglandins

Prostaglandins are known to be synthesized by coronary endothelium, and are powerful coronary vasodilators. Although autoregulation in isolated buffer-perfused rabbit hearts is dependent on plasma to provide substrate for prostaglandin synthesis,[46] this is not the case in other species or blood-perfused hearts.[27] Inhibitors of prostaglandin synthesis (e.g. indomethacin) do not interfere with autoregulation and may improve it.[38] Thus, there is little evidence to implicate prostaglandins in physiological flow control.

Myogenic hypothesis

The myogenic hypothesis was put forward by Bayliss[47] and modified by Folkow.[48] It was proposed that vascular resistance is proportional to transmural microvascular pressure as a result of the direct effect of intravascular pressure on arteriolar smooth muscle. According to this hypothesis, an increase in intravascular pressure would elicit vasoconstriction, and a decrease vasodilation. This mechanism could account for pressure autoregulation, but it is difficult to envisage the link between the degree of stretch of vascular smooth muscle and the metabolic state of the myocardium. Nevertheless, the myogenic hypothesis may account for the tonic vasoconstriction of the coronary bed against which metabolic vasodilators may act.

Endothelium-derived relaxing factor

Endothelium-derived relaxing factor is released by endothelium and mediates the vasodilator properties of numerous agents, such as acetylcholine, ADP, ATP, bradykinin and substance P.[49] It is a substance of enormous physiological and pharmacological interest; its ubiquity raised the possibility of its involvement in metabolic control of coronary blood flow. Two observations potentially of relevance to coronary flow regulation have been made. First, release of endothelium-derived relaxing factor is stimulated by hypoxia,[40] which could provide a link between tissue Po_2 and vasomotor control. Second, an increase in flow, and particularly pulsatile flow, elicits both endothelium-derived relaxing factor and prostaglandin release.[50] This observation is of interest, because flow-induced release of enothelium-derived relaxing factor and prostaglandin could enable a transient stimulus such as potassium efflux to produce a vasodilatation of longer duration. Inhibition of tonic endothelium-derived relaxing factor release as a result of vasoconstriction could result in further constriction, thus providing a putative mechanism for the myogenic hypothesis.

It must be emphasized that the above suggestions are at present speculative, but it is likely that further evidence of the possible role of endothelium-derived relaxing factor in coronary flow regulation will soon be available.

NEUROHORMONAL INFLUENCES

Ultrastructural and histochemical studies of the coronary vasculature have demonstrated areas of dense innervation, particularly of intimal cushions and in the pre-capillary region. The existence of adrenergic and cholinergic fibres has long been recognized, but evidence of other transmitters, such as purines, 5-hydroxytryptamine and various peptides, is accumulating.[51] The physiological role of coronary innervation is unclear. Stimulation of cardiac sympathetic nerves results in an alpha-receptor-mediated vasoconstriction, which can be demonstrated only when the inotropic and chronotropic effects of sympathetic stimulation, and their resultant increase in MVo_2, are blocked. Selective chemical sympathectomy results in an increase in local myocardial flow, suggesting that the coronary circulation is under tonic alpha-adrenergic constrictor influence.[53] The quantitative importance of the autonomic nervous system, however, appears to be small in relation to metabolic regulation of coronary vascular resistance.

Vagal stimulation or infusion of acetylcholine results in endothelium-mediated coronary vasodilatation.[49,54] An interesting observation has been that, if endothelium is absent, acetylcholine causes a paradoxical vasoconstriction.[49] Deficiency or malfunction of the endothelium is a feature of coronary atherosclerosis; it provides an explanation for the observation that infusions of acetylcholine result in vasodilatation in normal epicardial coronary arteries but vasoconstriction at atheromatous stenoses.[55]

The role of peptides in the control of coronary tone is at present putative. Both neuropeptide Y and calcitonin-gene related peptide are found in perivascular nerves. Infusion of neuropeptide Y causes coronary vasoconstriction,[56] whereas calcitonin gene-related peptide induces dilatation.[57] Angiotensin II has also been shown to cause coronary vasoconstriction, which may be of pathological significance in conditions associated with stimulation of the renin–angiotensin system, such as acute myocardial infarction and cardiac failure.[58]

REGIONAL AND TRANSMURAL VARIATIONS IN CORONARY FLOW

Considerable clinical and experimental evidence has demonstrated that the properties of the coronary circulation are not uniform either regionally or transmurally. There are major differences between the right and left ventricles with regard to oxygen consumption, transmural pressure and coronary vascular resistance. Within the left ventricle, sub-endocardial muscle has a 20% greater oxygen consumption, but a lower tissue and venous Po_2 than sub-epicardial muscle.[27,59] The levels of various metabolic intermediates suggest that there is relatively less oxygen delivery to the sub-endocardium than to the sub-epicardium. Although regional flow measurements with radioactive microspheres show no transmural flow differences under control conditions, a reduction in coronary flow results in a preferential fall in sub-endocardial as compared with sub-epicardial flow.[60] This fall is associated with a loss of autoregulation of sub-endocardial flow, which becomes directly dependent on coronary driving pressure. Under these circumstances, an increase in ventricular diastolic pressure as a result of ischaemic left ventricular dysfunction may exacerbate the reduction in sub-endocardial flow. These mechanisms underline the common pathological observations that, following a coronary occlusion, myocardial necrosis is most extensive in the sub-endocardium.

EFFECTS OF ISCHAEMIA AND REPERFUSION ON MYOCARDIAL CONTRACTILE FUNCTION

SYSTOLIC FUNCTION

The importance of coronary blood flow to the mechanical function of the heart has been known since 1698, when Chirac noted that coronary artery ligation in the dog caused a rapid failure of the heart beat.[61] Experimental studies have demonstrated an impairment in mechanical function after reductions of only 10–20% in coronary blood flow.[18,19] The time-course of the decline in systolic function during ischaemia will depend on the degree of flow reduction, the determinants of myocardial oxygen demand (see above) and, in isolated preparations, on the temperature. The mechanical function of isolated hearts often demonstrates an almost instantaneous change attributable to an alteration in preload,[64] which will be discussed later. Developed tension then declines steadily, and is usually <10% of control within 10–14 min.[63,65] The impairment of systolic function comprises a reduction in the rate of tension development (V_{max}) and a shortening in the duration of the contraction, usually measured as a reduction in time to peak tension (TPT) (Fig. 46.4). The shortening of TPT in ischaemia occurs within 30 s, and is not attributable to the shortening in action potential duration, which follows a slower time-course.[63]

Changes of systolic function in regional myocardial ischaemia are analogous to those in isolated hearts, but the interaction between ischaemic and non-ischaemic areas is important. Coronary occlusion results in a rapid loss of segmental contraction[62] with a shortening in TPT.[66] Contraction is more severely depressed in the sub-endocardial than the sub-epicardial layers of the ischaemic area.[67] If ischaemia is sufficiently severe to result in complete loss of contraction, the ischaemic area then undergoes passive expansion (dyskinesis) during systole.[62,66,68] The overall im-

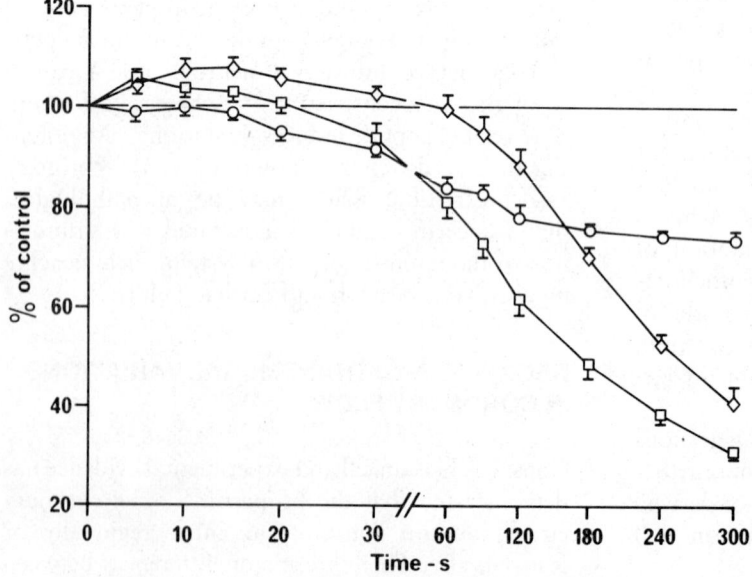

Fig. 46.4. Time-course of changes in developed tension (□), rate of tension development (◇) and time to peak tension (○) at the onset of ischaemia in isolated heart muscle. (Reproduced with permission from Cobbe, S.M. and Poole-Wilson, P.A. *J. Mol. Cell. Cardiol.* 1980; **12**: 745–60.[65])

pact of a coronary occlusion on left ventricular function depends on the extent of the ischaemic area. If it is small, there will be little change in the mechanical properties of the non-ischaemic myocardium or in global cardiac function,[66,69] whereas extensive area of ischaemia may elicit compensatory hyperkinesis in the normal area, which may or may not be sufficient to maintain cardiac output and blood pressure. The presence of previous myocardial infarction or other abnormalities of function will impair the ability of the non-ischaemic ventricle to maintain overall left ventricular function.

DIASTOLIC FUNCTION

Changes in diastolic function of- ischaemic heart muscle lag behind those in systolic function. Thus, resting tension in isolated heart muscle remains at or below control levels until contraction has virtually ceased, but then increases gradually.[63] The increase in resting tension is greater in low-flow than in zero-flow ischaemia.[65] Studies of diastolic function in regional ischaemia indicate an initial increase in end-diastolic segment length in the ischaemic area as a result of passive stretching.[69] The degree of passive distension of the ischaemic segment steadily falls from 1 to 6 h after occlusion, irrespective of any recovery in contraction.[70] The process of infarct stiffening or contraction persists in the canine model for up to 4 weeks, and results in a reduction in the diastolic compliance of the ventricle.[71] This mechanism reduces the amount of energy wasted by the normal myocardium in distending the infarct,[72] although it also results in an increase in left ventricular end-diastolic pressure for a given end-diastolic volume. The opposite process, namely thinning and passive expansion of the infarct, is recognized in experimental and clinical studies. Infarct expansion results in progressive impairment of global left ventricular function and the development of cardiac failure.[73,74]

REPERFUSION

The ability of ischaemic myocardium to recover contractile function if its blood supply is restored has long been recognized and is fundamental to modern cardiac surgery and to attempts at reperfusion in acute myocardial infarction. The extent to which function will recover depends on the duration and severity of the ischaemic insult.[65,75] Reperfusion after occlusions of up to 30 min in

canine experiments is normally followed by substanial if not complete recovery.[76] During recovery, there is an action potential-independent lengthening in TPT and in the duration of the active state which may result in the reperfused segment still contracting during the isovolumic relaxation period.[68] If ischaemia is sufficiently severe or prolonged to have resulted in an increase in resting tension (contracture), the extent of recovery of systolic function is reduced, and reperfusion results in a further increase in resting tension associated with calcium influx into myocardial cells.[77] Increased myocardial resting tension, along with endothelial cell damage and swelling, result in an increase in coronary vascular resistance which may prevent effective reperfusion of severely damaged areas—the 'no reflow phenomenon'.[78,79]

The maximum period of ischaemia from which full recovery can occur appears to be 40–60 min in the dog model.[75] Reperfusion after longer periods of ischaemia results in very little early recovery in contractile function, although it is now recognized that slow recovery over a period of weeks can occur.[76,80] Even after brief occlusions, full recovery can be very gradual, while repeated short occlusions, each in itself insufficient to cause permanent damage, may result in myocardial necrosis.[81] The term 'stunned myocardium' has been used to describe the phenomenon of prolonged dysfunction in viable myocardium after reperfusion.[82]

Although animal experiments would suggest that the maximum period of ischaemia from which full recovery can occur is about 1 h, this figure should be extrapolated to man with great caution. The duration of coronary occlusion beyond which reperfusion will be ineffective depends on the extent of coronary collateral flow, the determinants of myocardial oxygen consumption and the possibility that clinical coronary occlusion may be a stuttering process, unlike the abrupt ligation of a coronary artery in an experimental model.[83] Thus, whereas optimum results from thrombolytic therapy in man have been obtained within 1 h of the onset of chest pain, there is a reduction in mortality when therapy is given at 6–9 h[84] and possibly up to 24 h after the onset of symptoms.[85]

BIOCHEMICAL CHANGES IN ISCHAEMIC MYOCARDIUM

By definition, ischaemia is a condition in which coronary blood flow is insufficient to meet the metabolic needs of the tissue. The onset of ischaemia at rest is normally associated with an absolute reduction in coronary blood flow. This results simultaneously in a reduced delivery of oxygen and metabolic substrate to the myocardium, and impaired washout of the end-products of metabolism. Ischaemia is to be contrasted with hypoxia, in which a reduction in oxygen supply to the myocardium is produced by reduction in arterial Po_2. This is often combined, in experimental studies, with substrate-free perfusion or the use of metabolic inhibitors. Under hypoxic conditions, coronary vasodilatation occurs and will result in an *increased* coronary blood flow with enhanced washout of metabolites. Thus, the biochemical consequences of myocardial ischaemia and arterial hypoxaemia are different.[1]

Interruption of coronary blood flow in dogs results in a rapid fall in tissue Po_2 to < 5 mmHg.[86] At this level, production of ATP by oxidative phosphorylation is severely depressed but not abolished. Residual collateral flow in experimental regional ischaemia[87] or flow rates as low as 4% of control in global ischaemia supply sufficient oxygen for some continued oxidative metabolism. At 4% of control flow, the rate of oxidative ATP production was 13% of normal in one study.[1] The contribution of enhanced glycolysis to energy production in ischaemia is small. Apart from a possible brief increase in the first minute,[87] glycolytic flux in severe ischaemia is equal to or less than that in normal tissue, unlike the enhanced anaerobic glycolysis that occurs during hypoxic perfusion.[1] Oxidation of free fatty acids is proportionately more inhibited than that of glucose during ischaemia, and results in the accumulation of long chain fatty acyl-CoA, which is incorporated into triglyceride at the expense of ATP.[87]

The alterations in energy metabolism described above result in a dramatic fall in the rate of ATP production. Continued ATP consumption results in a breakdown of ATP and increased levels of ADP and inorganic phosphate. Tissue levels of ATP fall relatively slowly, however, because ATP is regenerated from a 'buffer' store of creatine phosphate (CP) by the reaction:

$$\text{CP} + \text{ADP} \underset{\text{phosphokinase}}{\overset{\text{Creatine}}{\rightleftharpoons}} \text{ATP} + \text{Creatine}$$

However, the cytosolic ATP potential

$$\frac{[\text{ATP}]}{[\text{ADP}][\text{P}_i]}$$

falls, and it may be that this value, or some derivative such as the thermodynamic ATP affinity,[89] is a better index of cellular energy state than [ATP] alone.

Ischaemia results not only in impairment of oxygen and substrate supply and utilization, the consequences of which are described above, but also in impaired washout of metabolites and their accumulation within the cell. An increased concentration of inorganic phosphate and fatty acyl-CoA has already been mentioned.[89,90] The other major metabolites that accumulate in the cell are lactate and hydrogen ions. Lactate production occurs as an end-result of glycolysis, because pyruvate cannot enter the Krebs cycle when oxidative phosphorylation is inhibited. The rate of lactate production declines with reduction in coronary flow, but the actual tissue concentration increases as a result of impaired washout.[91] Hydrogen ions are generated via numerous mechanisms in ischaemia.[93,93] Residual oxidative phosphorylation results in carbon dioxide generation, with the resultant production of hydrogen and bicarbonate ions under the influence of carbonic anhydrase. Anaerobic glycolysis to lactate, breakdown and re-synthesis of triglycerides and ATP hydrolysis all generate hydrogen ions, whereas ATP re-synthesis from creatine phosphate consumes them.[89]. A fall in tissue pH, an indirect measurement of intracellular pH, occurs within 5 s of the onset of ischaemia,[65] while the reduction of intracellular and extracellular pH is of the order of 0.85–1.70 pH units after 1 h (Fig. 46.5).[94,95]

MECHANISM OF CONTRACTILE FAILURE IN ISCHAEMIA

MECHANICAL AND ELECTRICAL CHANGES

Several hypotheses have been advanced to account for the rapid mechanical failure observed in ischaemic myocardium. Although major biochemical changes undoubtedly occur, it may be that the earliest decline in contraction arises as a result of a reduction in vascular and hence tissue turgor distal to a coronary occlusion, causing a diminished preload.[64] This mechanism, described as the garden-hose effect, is particularly evident in isolated whole-heart models.[96,97] Its significance *in vivo* remains to be established. Major changes in action potential configuration occur during ischaemia, involving reduction in membrane potential, action potential amplitude and upstroke velocity, shorten-

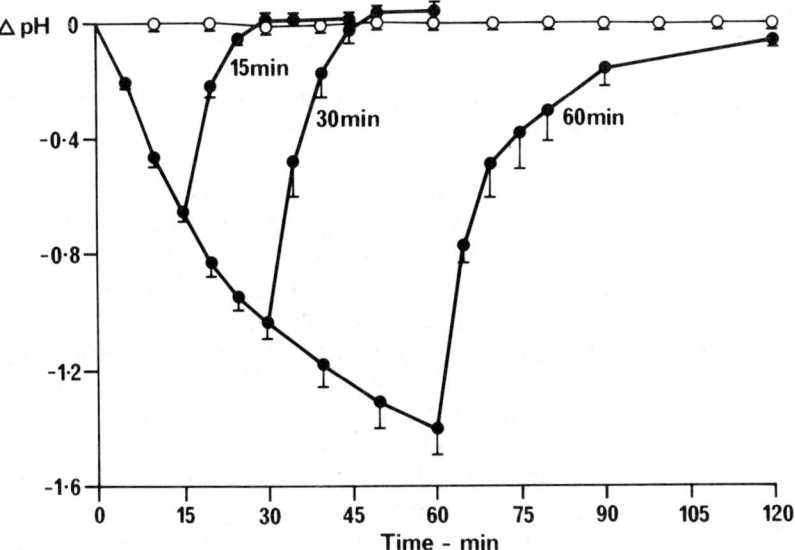

Fig. 46.5. Changes of tissue pH during ischaemia and reperfusion in isolated heart muscle. There was a fall of 1.0 pH unit after 30 min. ●, total ischaemia; ○, control. (Reproduced with permission from Cobbe, S.M. and Poole-Wilson, P.A., *J. Mol. Cell. Cardiol.* 1980; **12**: 745–60.[65])

ing of action potential duration and slowing of conduction, with the ultimate development of inexcitability.[98] The time-course of these electrical changes, however, is much slower than that of mechanical failure. Thus, contractile failure cannot be attributed to electrical inexcitability. Furthermore, even the shortening in TPT during ischaemia precedes the shortening of action potential duration.[63]

BIOCHEMICAL CHANGES

Many biochemical causes have been proposed for the contractile failure of ischaemic myocardium. For a given biochemical mechanism to be considered relevant, it must be shown to exert a negative inotropic effect on heart muscle, to be initiated sufficiently early in the time course of ischaemia, to precede or parallel the fall in contractility and to be of sufficient magnitude to account for the degree of contractile failure. No single mechanism has yet been found to satisfy all these criteria; it is likely that ischaemic contractile failure has a multifactorial basis.

Changes in adenosine triphosphate concentration

Although a reduction in ATP concentration would appear to be an obvious mechanism of contractile failure, the studies of cellular ATP levels have consistently shown falls of only 20% or so from the normal levels of 5–8 mmol/l at a time of severe depression of contractility.[89,90] These levels remain well above the concentrations required for half-maximal activation of the principal ATP-consuming enzymes of the sarcolemma, sarcoplasmic reticulum or myofibrils. Substantially lower levels of total tissue ATP (1.5–2.0 mmol/l) have been found in normally functioning muscle from non-ischaemic areas.[99] Adenosine triphosphate levels are maintained by the buffering effect of creatine phosphate whose concentration falls rapidly to <20% of normal.[99] There is a rapid increase in the concentrations of ADP and inorganic phosphate, and it has been suggested that the impairment of cellular energy supply may be better correlated with the ratio:

$$\frac{[ATP]}{[ADP] [P_i]}$$

than with [ATP] alone.[89] A further suggestion has been that critically low ATP concentrations at certain key sites within the cell may occur as a result of impaired transfer of high-energy phosphates from the mitochondria to the cytosol, and that the extent of ATP depletion in these compartments is underestimated in the measurement of mean tissue ATP concentration.[99,100] Adenosine triphosphate depletion at the myofibrils would result in the early development of rigor, which is not a feature of ischaemic mechanical failure.[101] Similarly, impairment of uptake of calcium into the sarcoplasmic reticulum as a result of ATP depletion would result in an increased diastolic calcium concentration and hence an early rise in resting tension. In contrast, a reduced inward calcium current has been shown to be triggered by a fall in cytoplasmic ATP concentration, and is reversed by injection of ATP into the cell.[102] Reduction of calcium influx would result in a depression of tension development without immediate effects on resting tension. However, the magnitude of reduction of ATP concentration needed to depress calcium influx is greater than that occurring in ischaemia.

Thus, despite its plausibility, no definite evidence exists to confirm the role of high-energy phosphate depletion as a primary cause of contractile failure.

Oxygen

There is no evidence that a reduction in cellular P_{O_2} exerts a *direct* negative inotropic effect. Cardiac muscle cells from which the cell membrane has been removed will contract in the absence of oxygen, provided that calcium and ATP are present.[103]

Inorganic phosphate

The accumulation of inorganic phosphate as a result of ATP hydrolysis during ischaemia has been mentioned, and concentrations of up to 20–40 mmol/l have been estimated.[89,90] Such levels could result in the binding of intracellular calcium, which will reduce calcium availability at the myofibrils, and also generate hydrogen ions.[97] Phosphate ions exert a pronounced effect on myofibrillar sensitivity to calcium ions.[104] The localization and time-course of phosphate accumulation are not precisely known from experimental studies, and thus the role of phosphate is at present uncertain.

Fatty acids, lactate

The concentration of these metabolites rises during ischaemia, and fatty acids and lactate are capable of binding calcium and thus reducing calcium availability at the myofibril. The rates of accumulation of fatty acyl-CoA and lactate are not sufficiently well defined to assess the quantitative significance of this mechanism.

Potassium

Extracellular potassium concentration rises to a level of 10–12 mmol/l within 5–10 min of the onset of ischaemia.[44] However, perfusion of isolated muscle with potassium concentrations of this level leads to only minor reductions in contraction in comparison to the changes occurring in ischaemia.[105]

Acidosis

Intracellular acidosis has long been known to exert a negative inotropic action without increasing resting tension.[106] In view of the demonstration of substantial acidosis during ischaemia, competitive inhibition of the action of calcium ions by hydrogen ions at one or more sites of excitation–contraction coupling has been proposed as a major mechanism of pump failure.[97,107] Intracellular acidosis reduces calcium ion influx via the inward calcium current, an effect which is reversed by increasing the level of extracellular calcium ions,[108] which also restores contractility to normal.[109] Acidosis increases the rate and amount of calcium ion binding to sarcoplasmic reticulum.[110] Finally, hydrogen ions competitively depress the sensitivity of myofibrils to calcium ions, resulting in a reduction of tension generation and ATPase activity.[111,112] Overall, a reduction of intracellular pH by 0.4 units has been estimated to reduce developed tension by 50%.[113]

It has been established that tissue pH, an indirect measure of intracellular pH, falls within 5 s of the onset of ischaemia,[65] whereas a fall of 0.5 units in intracellular pH occurs after 5 min.[95] Comparison of the rate of fall of pH and tension in ischaemia suggests that a substantial proportion of the early fall in contractility may be attributed to acidosis.[65] The fact that the pH-tension relationship may be perturbed by experimental interventions such as catecholamines or calcium depletion[114] emphasizes the likelihood of multiple mechanisms responsible for contractile failure.

BIOCHEMICAL CHANGES DURING PROLONGED ISCHAEMIA

The biochemical changes discussed above are responsible for the early decline of contraction in ischaemia, at a time when reperfusion will result in full recovery of mechanical function. During this period, no ultrastructural damage to the cell membrane, sarcoplasmic reticulum or myofibrils is apparent[115] and isolated preparations of sarcoplasmic reticulum and myofibrils demonstrate normal function *in vitro* when exposed to normal intracellular ionic and ATP concentrations.[116,117] Prolonged ischaemia results in the development of defects in the cell membranes, swelling of mitochondria and the aggregation of nuclear chromatin.[115] The causes of irreversible damage are poorly understood, but activation of lysosomal enzymes at low intracellular pH[118] and disruption of lipid bilayer membranes by the detergent effects of fatty acid–calcium 'soaps' are possible mechanisms.

NON-ATHEROSCLEROTIC CAUSES OF MYOCARDIAL ISCHAEMIA

The majority of clinical manifestations of myocardial ischaemia are associated with atherosclerotic narrowing of epicardial coronary arteries. There exists, however, a significant minority of patients with symptoms of effort angina or of atypical chest pain despite normal coronary angiographic appearances. Coronary spasm is an important cause of such symptoms, and is discussed in Chapter 47. Angina with normal coronary arteries may also occur as a result of abnormal myocardial oxygen demand secondary to increased wall stress, or from impaired perfusion as a result of excessive hypertrophy jeopardizing sub-endocardial flow or of increased extravascular coronary resistance due to tissue compression during systole (e.g. aortic stenosis) or diastole (e.g. left ventricular failure) (Table 46.4). Diffuse small-vessel disease may occur in diabetic micro-angiopathy and in vasculitic conditions such as systemic lupus erythematosus. After exclusion of these conditions, there remains a substantial number of patients with the clinical syndrome of 'angina with normal coronary arteries'.

The problem of patients with angina and normal coronary arteries was identified soon after the widespread introduction of coronary arteriography.[119] The study of this problem has been bedevilled by the heterogeneity of the patient group. Published series have included patients with classical effort angina responsive to nitrates as well as those with atypical or rest pain,[120,121] many of whom may have a non-cardiac cause for their pain. Some authors have studied only those patients with significant ST-segment depression on exercise testing,[122–124] whereas other series have included only a small proportion of patients with a positive exercise electrocardiogram.[125–127] The presence of hypertensive heart disease is another confounding factor because coronary vasodilator reserve is impaired in this condition.[128] In one series, 61% of the patients were hypertensive;[129] other studies have excluded such patients.[123] The term 'syndrome X', first coined in 1973,[130,131] describes those patients who have anginal chest pain, normal coronary arteriography and ST-segment depression on exercise testing or atrial pacing, in whom alternative causes of chest pain have been excluded.

Overall, patients with angina and normal coronary arteries have a good prognosis for survival, comparable to that of the general population.[120,132] A substantial proportion of patients become asymptomatic after angiography, and the incidence of myocardial infarction on follow-up is low. However, significant numbers of patients remain disabled by chest pain. A high incidence of psychiatric morbidity has been identified in this group,[133] but it is not known if this is the cause or result of their continuing symptoms.

PATHOPHYSIOLOGY

The underlying cause(s) of syndrome X remain to be established. Endocardial biopsy showed no evidence of microvascular disease in one study,[134] although another series of atypical patients with arrhythmias and conduction disturbance demonstrated hyperplastic fibromuscular thickening of small arteries.[135] The functional defect has been suggested to be in medium-sized intramural arteries of 100–500 μm in diameter.[136] Unfortunately, these cannot be visualized by coronary arteriography or biopsy, and post-mortem data are not available. Although other mechanisms for syndrome X have been proposed, such as an abnormality of the oxyhaemoglobin dissociation curve[137] or myocardial hypoxia,[138] there is no evidence in support of these hypotheses.

The underlying basis of the chest pain in syndrome X appears to be ischaemia secondary to an abnormal vasodilator reserve. Regional perfusion defects with impaired ^{133}Xe clearance were iden-

Table 46.4. Possible causes of angina with normal coronary arteriogram.

Coronary artery spasm

Mitral valve prolapse

Left ventricular hypertrophy:
  Hypertension
  Aortic stenosis
  Aortic regurgitation
  Hypertrophic cardiomyopathy

Right ventricular hypertrophy:
  Tetralogy of Fallot
  Pulmonary hypertension

Elevated left ventricular diastolic pressure

Small-vessel disease:
  Arteritis
  Diabetic micro-angiopathy

Syndrome X

tified at rest in 50% of patients in one series;[122] a more characteristic feature has been the presence of normal or only mildly abnormal resting coronary blood flow and coronary vascular resistance, but an impairment of maximal vasodilator reserve in response to dipyridamole or angiographic contrast.[129,134] In one study, mean coronary blood flow rose by a factor of only 2.0 in patients with angina and normal coronary arteries as compared with 3.8 in normal subjects and 1.9 in patients with occlusive coronary artery disease.[134] Even a proportion of patients who have chest pain but a normal exercise test have an impaired vasodilator response to atrial pacing.[126] The incidence of regional perfusion defects identified by exercise ^{201}Tl imaging in patients with angina and normal coronaries ranges from 16 to 22%, of which about two-thirds of the defects are reversible.[123,129,139]

Evidence that the ST-segment depression and flow restriction of syndrome X is associated with biochemical and functional indices of myocardial ischaemia has been sought. Several studies have demonstrated reduced lactate extraction or frank lactate production during pacing-induced chest pain,[125,127,130,134] although no reduction in coronary sinus oxygen saturation was found despite ST-segment depression in one pacing study.[140] An abnormal response of overall left ventricular ejection fraction on exercise has been reported in 28–55% of patients in various studies,[121,123,127,129] associated with patterns of regional and global wall motion abnormalities. Left ventricular segments demonstrating abnormal ^{201}Tl uptake or regional wall motion abnormalities on exercise have been correlated with impaired vasodilator reserve in the subtending artery.[129] Reduced left ventricular filling rates have suggested diastolic as well as systolic abnormalities.[127] However, resting left ventricular end-diastolic pressure is not increased in syndrome X,[134] and monitoring of pulmonary artery end-diastolic pressure as an indirect index of left ventricular filling pressure has failed to demonstrate any increase in association with exercise-induced or spontaneous episodes of ST-segment depression.[124] These observations suggest that the overall severity of ischaemia and left ventricular dysfunction associated with a given degree of ST-segment depression is less in syndrome X than those in occlusive coronary artery disease.

Ambulatory electrocardiographic monitoring in patients with syndrome X demonstrated that only 25% of episodes of chest pain were associated with ST-segment depression.[141] Of the episodes of ST-segment depression, 52% were asymptomatic. Many episodes were not preceded by increases in heart rate, and may thus represent primary reductions in flow rather than increases in myocardial oxygen demand. Episodes of ST-segment depression occur predominantly during the daytime.[124,141]

TREATMENT

Few studies of the effect of therapy in these patients exist. In a retrospective study, Kemp et al.[120] reported that 51% of patients obtained prompt relief and a further 28% slow relief from nitrates. Propranolol produced some diminution in the frequency and severity of chest pain in 60% of patients, particularly those with effort-related chest pain. Calcium-channel blockers (nifedipine or verapamil) were shown in a double-blind study[142] to reduce the frequency of episodes of chest pain by 37%, and glyceryl trinitrate consumption by 42%.

REFERENCES

1. Neely, J.R., Liedtke, A.J., Whitmer, J.T. and Rovetto M.J. Relationship between coronary flow and adenosine triphosphate production from glycolysis and oxidative metabolism. In: Roy, P.E. and Harris, P., eds. *Recent Advances in Studies on Cardiac Structure and Metabolism. The Cardiac Cytoplasm*, Vol. 8. Baltimore: University Park Press, 1975, p. 301.
2. Braunwald, E. Control of myocardial oxygen consumption *Am. J. Cardiol.* 1971; 27: 416–32.
3. McKeever, W.P., Gregg, D.E. and Canney, P.C. Oxygen uptake of the nonworking left ventricle. *Circ. Res.* 1958; 6: 612–23.
4. Klocke, F.J., Braunwald, E. and Ross, Jr J. Oxygen cost of electrical activation of the heart. *Circ. Res.* 1965; 18: 357–65.
5. Sarnoff, S.J., Braunwald, E., Welch, G., Case, R.B., Stainsby, W.N. and Macroz, R. Hemodynamic determinants of oxygen consumption of the heart with special reference to the tension–time index. *Am. J. Physiol.* 1958; 192: 148–56.
6. Braunwald, E., Sarnoff, S.J. and Case, R.B. Hemodynamic determinants of coronary flow: effect of changes in aortic pressure and cardiac output on the relationship between myocardial oxygen consumption and coronary flow. *Am. J. Physiol.* 1958; 192: 157–63.
7. Monroe, R.G. and French, G.M. Left ventricular pressure–volume relationships and myocardial oxygen consumption in the isolated heart. *Circ. Res.* 1961; 9: 362–74.
8. Rodbard, S., Williams, C.B., Rodbard, D. and Berglund, E. Myocardial tension and oxygen uptake. *Circ. Res.* 1964; 14: 139–49.
9. Coleman, H.N., Sonnenblick, E.H. and Braunwald, E. Myocardial oxygen consumption associated with external work. The Fenn effect. *Am. J. Physiol.* 1969; 217: 291–6.
10. Krasnow, N., Rolett, E.L. and Yurchak, P. Isoproterenol and cardiovascular performance. *Am. J. Med.* 1964; 37: 514–25.
11. Sonnenblick, E.H., Ross, Jr J., Covell, J.W. *et al.* Velocity of contraction as a determinant of myocardial oxygen

consumption. *Am. J. Physiol.* 1965; **209**: 919–27.

12. Graham, T.P., Covell, J.W., Sonnenblick, E.H., Ross, Jr J. and Braunwald, E. The control of myocardial oxygen consumption: Relative influence of contractile state and tension development. *J. Clin. Invest.* 1968; **47**: 375–85.

13. Klocke, F.J., Kaiser, G.A., Ross, Jr J. *et al*. Mechanism of increase of myocardial oxygen uptake produced by catecholamines. *Am. J. Physiol.* 1965; **209**: 913–8.

14. Boerth, R.C., Covell, J.W., Pool, P.E. *et al*. Increased myocardial oxygen consumption and contractile state associated with increased heart rate in dogs. *Circ. Res.* 1969; **24**: 725–34.

15. Monroe, R.G. Myocardial oxygen consumption during ventricular contraction and relaxation. *Circ. Res.* 1964; **14**: 294–300.

16. Pool, P.E. and Sonnenblick, E.H. The mechanochemistry of cardiac muscle: l. The isometric contraction. *J. Gen. Physiol.* 1967; **50**: 951–65.

17. Henderson, A.H., Craig, R.J., Gorlin, R. and Sonnenblick, E.H. Free fatty acids and myocardial function in perfused rat hearts. *Cardiovasc. Res.* 1970; **4**: 466–72.

18. Vatner, S.F. Correlation between acute reductions in myocardial blood flow and function in conscious dogs. *Circ. Res.* 1980; **47**: 201–7.

19. Gallagher, K.P., Kumada, T., Koziol, J.A., McKown, M.D., Kemper, W.S. and Ross, Jr J. Significance of regional wall thickening abnormalities relative to transmural myocardial perfusion in anesthetized dogs. *Circulation* 1980; **62**: 1266–73.

20. Gregg, D.E. Physiology of the coronary circulation. *Circulation* 1963; **27**: 1128–37.

21. Buckberg, G.D., Fixler, D.E., Archie, J.P. and Hoffman, J.I.E. Experimental subendocardial ischemia in dogs with normal coronary arteries. *Circ. Res.* 1972; **30**: 67–81.

22. Tauchert, M. and Hilger H.H. Application of the coronary reserve concept to the study of myocardial perfusion. In: Schaper, W., ed. *The Pathophysiology of Myocardial Perfusion*. Amsterdam: Elsevier/North Holland, 1979, pp. 141–67.

23. Schaper, W. Regulation of coronary blood flow. In: Schaper, W., ed. *The Pathophysiology of Myocardial Perfusion*. Amsterdam: Elsevier/North Holland, 1979, pp. 171–98.

24. Feigl, E.O. Coronary phsyiology. *Physiol. Rev.* 1983; **63**: 1–205.

25. Olsson, R.A. and Bunger, R. Metabolic control of coronary blood flow. *Prog. Cardiovasc. Dis.* 1987; **29**: 369–87.

26. Bardenheuer, H. and Schrader, J. Supply-to-demand ratio for oxygen determines formation of adenosine by the heart. *Am. J. Physiol.* 1986; **250**: H173–80.

27. Dole, W.P. Autoregulation of the coronary circulation. *Prog. Cardiovasc. Dis.* 1987; **29**: 293–323.

28. Gregg, D.E. The effect of coronary perfusion pressure or coronary flow on oxygen usage of the myocardium. *Circ. Res.* 1963; **13**: 497–500.

29. Drury, A.N. and Szent-Gyorgyl, A. The physiological activity of adenine compounds with especial reference to their action upon the mammalian heart. *J. Physiol. (Lond.)* 1929; **68**: 213–37.

30. Berne, R.M. Cardiac nucleotides in hypoxia—Possible role in regulation of coronary blood flow. *Am. J. Physiol.* 1963; **204**: 317–22.

31. Olsson, R.A. Changes in content of purine nucleosides in canine myocardium during coronary occlusion. *Circ. Res.* 1970; **26**: 301–6.

32. Schrader, J., Haddy, F.J. and Gerlach, E. Release of adenosine, inosine and hypoxanthine from the isolated guinea pig heart during hypoxia, flow-autoregulation and reactive hyperemia. *Pflugers Arch.* 1977; **369**: 1–6.

33. Fox, A.C., Reed, G.E. and Grassman, E. Release of adenosine from human hearts during angina induced by rapid atrial pacing. *J. Clin. Invest.* 1974; **53**: 1447–57.

34. Dole, W.P., Yamada, N., Bishop, V.S. *et al*. Role of adenosine in coronary blood flow regulation after reductions in perfusion pressure. *Circ. Res.* 1985; **56**: 517–24.

35. Saito, D., Steinhart, C.R., Nixon, D.G. *et al*. Intracoronary adenosine deaminase reduces canine myocardial reactive hyperemia. *Circ. Res.* 1981; **49**: 1262–7.

36. Paddle, B.M. and Burnstock, G. Release of ATP from perfused heart during coronary vasodilatation. *Blood Vessels* 1974; **11**: 110–9.

37. Drake-Holland, A.J., Laird, J.D., Noble, M.I.M. *et al*. Oxygen and coronary vascular resistance during autoregulation and metabolic vasodilatation in the dog. *J. Physiol. (Lond.)* 1984; **348**: 285–99.

38. Dole, W.P. and Nuno, D.W. Myocardial oxygen tension determines the degree and pressure range of coronary autoregulation. *Circ. Res.* 1986; **59**: 202–15.

39. Gellai, M., Norton, J.M. and Detar, R. Evidence for direct control of coronary vascular tone by oxygen. *Circ. Res.* 1973; **32**: 279–89.

40. Busse, R., Trogisch, G. and Bassenge, E. The role of endothelium in the control of vascular tone. *Basic Res. Cardiol.* 1985; **80**: 475–90.

41. Clancy, R.L. and Gonzalez, N.C. Effect of respiratory and metabolic acidosis on coronary vascular resistance. *Proc. Soc. Exp. Biol. Med.* 1975; **148**: 307–11.

42. Raberger, G., Schutz, W. and Kraupp, O. Coronary reactive hyperemia and coronary dilator action of adenosine during normal respiration and hypercapnic acidosis in the dog. *Clin. Exp. Pharmacol. Physiol.* 1975; **2**: 373–82.

43. Kline, R.P. and Morad, M. Potassium efflux in heart muscle during activity: Extracellular accumulation and its implications. *J. Physiol.* 1978; **280**: 537–58.

44. Hill, J.L. and Gettes, L.S. Effect of acute coronary artery occlusion on local myocardial extracellular K^+ activity in swine. *Circulation* 1980; **61**: 768–78.

45. Bunger, R., Haddy, F.J., Querengasser, A. *et al*. Studies of potassium induced coronary dilation in the isolated guinea pig heart. *Pflugers Arch.* 1976; **363**: 27–31.

46. Moretti, R.L., Abraham, S. and Ecker, R.R. The stimulation of cardiac prostaglandin production by blood plasma and its relationship to the regulation of coronary flow in isolated isovolumic rabbit hearts. *Circ. Res.* 1976; **39**: 231–8.

47. Bayliss, W.M. On the local reactions of the arterial wall to changes in internal pressure. *J. Physiol. (Lond.)* 1902; **28**: 220–31.

48. Folkow, B. Intravascular pressure is a factor regulating the tone of the small vessels. *Acta Physiol. Scand.* 1964; **17**: 289–310.

49. Furchgott, R.F. The role of endothelium in the responses of vascular smooth muscle to drugs. *Ann. Rev. Pharmacol. Toxicol.* 1984; **24**: 175–97.

50. Rubanyi, G.M., Romero, J.C. and Vanhoutte, P.M. Flow-induced release of endothelium-derived relaxing factor. *Am. J. Physiol.* 1986; **250**: H1145–59.

51. Burnstock, G. Cholinergic and purinergic regulation of blood vessels. In: Bohr, D.F., Somlyo, A.D., Spaeks, H.W. and Geiger, S.R., eds. *Handbook of Physiology, Section 2: The Cardiovascular System, Vol. II: Vascular Smooth Muscle*. Baltimore: Waverley Press and American Physiological Society, 1980, pp. 567–612.

52. Feigl, E.O. Carotid sinus reflex control of coronary blood flow. *Circ. Res.* 1968; **23**: 223–37.

53. Holtz, J., Mayer, E. and Bassenge, E. Demonstration of alpha-adrenergic coronary control in different layers of canine myocardium by regional myocardial sympathectomy. *Pflugers Arch.* 1977; **372**: 187–94.

54. Feigl, E.O. Parasympathetic control of coronary blood

flow in dogs. *Circ. Res.* 1969; **25**: 509–19.

55. Ludmer, P.L., Selwyn, A.P., Shook, T.L. *et al.* Paradoxical vasoconstriction induced by acetylcholine in atherosclerotic coronary arteries. *N. Engl. J. Med.* 1986; **315**: 1046–51.

56. Clarke, J., Davies, G.J., Kerwin, R. *et al.* Coronary artery infusion of Neuropeptide Y in patients with angina pectoris. *Lancet* 1987; **1**: 1057–9.

57. McEwan, J., Larkin, S., Davies, G.J. *et al.* Calcitonin gene-related peptide: A potent dilator of human epicardial coronary arteries. *Circulation* 1986; **74**: 1243–7.

58. Ertl, G. Coronary vasoconstriction in experimental myocardial ischaemia. *J. Cardiovasc. Pharmacol.* 1987; **9** (Suppl. 2): S9–17

59. Weiss, H.R., Neubauer, J.A., Lipp, J.A. *et al.* Quantitative determination of regional oxygen consumption in the dog heart. *Circ. Res.* 1978; **42**: 394–401.

60. Guyton, R.A., McClenathan, J.H., Newman, G.E. *et al.* Significance of subendocardial ST-segment elevation caused by coronary stenosis in the dog. *Am. J. Cardiol.* 1977; **40**: 373–80.

61. Chirac, P. *De motu cordis, adversaria analytica* 1698: 121 Cited by Porter, W.T. *J. Physiol.* 1894; **15**: 121–38.

62. Tennant, R. and Wiggers, C.J. The effect of coronary occlusion on myocardial contraction. *Am. J. Physiol.* 1935; **112**: 351–61.

63. Shine, K.I., Douglas, A.M. and Ricchiuti, N. Ischemia in isolated interventricular septa: mechanical events. *Am. J. Physiol.* 1976; **231**: 1225–32.

64. Apstein, S., Ahn, J., Brent, B.N., Briggs, L. and Shapiro. H.M. Ischemic "pump" failure: evidence for a mechanical non-metabolic initial cause. *Circulation* 1979; **60** (Suppl. II): II-114.

65. Cobbe, S.M. and Poole-Wilson, P.A. The time of onset and severity of acidosis in myocardial ischaemia. *J. Mol. Cell. Cardiol.* 1980; **12**: 745–60.

66. Tomoda, H., Parmley, W.W., Fujimura, S. and Matloff, F.M. Effects of ischemia and reoxygenation on the regional myocardial performance of the dog. *Am. J. Physiol.* 1971; **221**: 1718–21.

67. Kirk, E.S., Turbow, M., Urschel, C.W. and Sonnenblick, E.H. Non-uniform contractility across the heart wall caused by redistribution of coronary flow (Abstract). *J. Clin. Invest.* 1970; **49**: 51A.

68. Forrester, J.S., Wyatt, H.L., Da Luz, P.L., Tyberg, J.V., Diamond, G.A. and Swan, H.J.C. Functional significance of regional ischemic contraction abnormalities. *Circulation* 1976; **54**: 64–70.

69. Heyndrickx, G.R., Millard, R.W., McRitchie, R.J., Maroko, P.R. and Vatner, S.F. Regional myocardial functional and electrophysiological alterations after brief coronary artery occlusion in conscious dogs. *J. Clin. Invest.* 1975; **56**: 978–85.

70. Lavallee, M., Cox, D., Patrick, T.A. and Vatner, S.F. Salvage of myocardial function by coronary artery reperfusion 1, 2 and 3 hours after occlusion in conscious dogs. *Circ. Res.* 1983; **53**: 235–47.

71. Vokonas, P.S., Pirzada, F.A., Hood, Jr W.B. Experimental myocardial infarction. XII. Dynamic changes in segmental mechanical behavior of infarcted and non-infarcted myocardium. *Am. J. Cardiol.* 1976; **37**: 853–9.

72. Swan, H.J.C., Forrester, J.S., Diamond, G., Chatterjee, K. and Parmley, W.W. Hemodynamic spectrum of myocardium infarction and cardiogenic shock: A conceptual model. *Circulation* 1972; **45**: 1097–110.

73. Pfeffer, J.M., Pfeffer, M.A. and Braunwald, E. Influence of chronic captopril therapy on the infarcted left ventricle of the rat. *Circ. Res.* 1985; **57**: 84–95.

74. Hochman, J.S. and Bulkley, B.H. Myocardial infarct extension and expansion. In: Califf, R.M. and Wagner,

G.S., eds. *Acute Coronary Care: Principles and Practice.* Boston: Martinus Nijhoff, 1985, pp. 449–58.

75. Jennings, R.B. Relationship of acute ischemia to functional defects and irreversibility. *Circulation* 1976; **53** (Suppl. 1): 26–9.

76. Puri, P.S. Contractile and biochemical effects of coronary reperfusion after extended periods of coronary occlusion. *Am. J. Cardiol.* 1975; **36**: 244–51.

77. Henry, P.D., Shuchleib, R., Davis, J., Weiss, E.S. and Sobel, B.E. Myocardial contracture and accumulation of mitochrondrial calcium in ischemic rabbit heart. *Am. J. Physiol.* 1977; **233**: H677–84.

78. Willerson, J.T., Watson, J.T., Hutton, I., Templeton, G.H. and Fixler, D.E. Reduced myocardial reflow and increased coronary vascular resistance following prolonged myocardial ischemia in the dog. *Circ. Res.* 1975; **36**: 771–81.

79. Kloner, R.A., Ganote, C.E. and Jennings, R.B. The "no reflow" phenomenon after temporary coronary occlusion in the dog. *J. Clin. Invest.* 1974; **54**: 1496–508.

80. Bush, L.R., Buja, L.M., Samowitz, W. *et al.* Recovery of left ventricular segmental function after long-term reperfusion following temporary occlusion in conscious dogs. *Circ. Res.* 1983; **53**: 248–63.

81. Geft, I.L., Fishbein, M.C., Ninomiya, K. *et al.* Intermittent brief periods of ischemia have a cumulative effect and may cause myocardial necrosis. *Circulation* 1982; **66**: 1150–3.

82. Braunwald, E. and Kloner, R.A. The stunned myocardium: Prolonged, post-ischemic ventricular dysfunction. *Circulation* 1982; **66**: 1146–9.

83. Hackett, D., Davies, G.J., Chierchia, S. and Maseri, A. High frequency of intermittent coronary occlusion in acute myocardial infarction. *Circulation* 1986; **74** (Suppl. II): 278.

84. Gruppo Italiano per lo Studio Della Streptochinasi Nell' Infarto Miocardico (GISSI). Effectiveness of intravenous thrombolytic treatment in acute myocardial infarction. *Lancet* 1986; **1**: 297–301.

85. Yusuf, S., Collins, R., Peto, R. *et al.* Intravenous and intracoronary fibrinolytic therapy in acute myocardial infarction: Overview of results on mortality, reinfarction and side-effects from 33 randomised controlled trials. *Eur. Heart J.* 1985; **6**: 556–85.

86. Sayen, J.J., Sheldon, W.F., Peirce, G. and Kuo, P.T. Polarographic oxygen, the epicardial electrocardiogram and muscle contraction in experimental acute regional ischaemia of the left ventricle. *Circ. Res.* 1958; **6**: 779–98.

87. Opie, L.H. Effects of regional ischemia on metabolism of glucose and fatty acids: relative rates of aerobic and anaerobic energy production during myocardial infarction and comparison with effects of anoxia. *Circ. Res.* 1976; **38** (Suppl. 1): 52–68.

88. Scheuer, J. and Brachfeld, N. Myocardial uptake and fractional distribution of palmitate–1–C^{14} by the ischemic dog heart. *Metabolism* 1966; **15**: 945–54.

89. Allen, D.G. and Orchard, C.H. Myocardial contractile function during ischemia and hypoxia. *Circ. Res.* 1987; **60**: 153–68.

90. Kubler, W. and Katz, A.M. Mechanism of Early "Pump" Failure of the Ischemic Heart. Possible role of adenosine triphosphate depletion and inorganic phsophate accumulation. *Am. J. Cardiol.* 1977; **40**: 467–71.

91. Neely, J.R., Rovetto, M.J., Whitmer, J.T. and Morgan, H.E. Effects of ischemia on ventricular function and metabolism in the isolated working rat heart. *Am. J. Physiol.* 1973; **225**: 651–8.

92. Gevers, W. Generation of protons by metabolic processes in heart cells. *J. Mol. Cell. Cardiol.* 1977; **9**: 867–74.

93. Wilkie, D.R. Generation of protons by metabolic processes other than glycolysis in muscle cells: A Critical review. *J. Mol. Cell. Cardiol.* 1979; **11**: 325–30.

94. Jacobus, W.E., Taylor, G.J., Hollis, D.P. and Nunnally, R.L. Phosphorus nuclear magnetic resonance of perfused working rat hearts. *Nature* 1977; **265**: 756–8.

95. Garlick, P.B., Radda, G.K. and Seeley, P.J. Studies of acidosis in the ischemic heart by phosphorus nuclear magnetic resonance. *Biochem. J.* 1979; **184**: 547–54.

96. Arnold, G., Kosche, F., Meissner, E., Neitzert, A. and Locher, W. The importance of the perfusion pressure in the coronary arteries for the contractility and oxygen consumption of the heart. *Pflügers Arch.* 1968; **299**: 339–56.

97. Poole-Wilson, P.A., Fleetwood, G. and Cobbe, S.M. Early contractile failure in myocardial ischaemia — role of acidosis. In: Refsum, H., Jynge, P., Mjos, O.D., eds. *Myocardial ischaemia and protection*. Edinburgh: Churchill Livingstone, 1983, pp. 9–17.

98. Janse, M.J. and Kleber, A.G. Electrophysiological changes and ventricular arrhythmias in the early phase of regional myocardial ischemia. *Circ. Res.* 1981; **49**: 1069–81.

99. Gudbjarnason, S., Mathes, P. and Ravens, K.G. Functional compartmentation of ATP and creatine phosphate in Heart Muscle. *J. Mol. Cell. Cardiol.* 1970; **1**: 325–39.

100. Vial, C., Font, B., Goldschmidt, D., Pearlman, A.S. and Delaye, J. Regional myocardial energetics during brief periods of coronary occlusion and reperfusion: comparison with S-T segment changes. *Cardiovasc. Res.* 1978; **12**: 470–6.

101. Katz, A.M. and Tada, M. The "stone heart": a challenge to the biochemist. *Am. J. Cardiol.* 1972; **29**: 578–80.

102. Taniguchi, J., Noma, A. and Irisawa, M. Modification of the cardiac action potential by intracellular injection of adenosine triphosphate and related substances in guinea pig single ventricular cells. *Circ. Res.* 1983; **53**: 131–9.

103. Fabiato, A. and Fabiato, F. Calcium release from the sarcoplasmic reticulum. *Circ. Res.* 1977; **40**: 119–29.

104. Kentish, J.C. The effects of inorganic phosphate and creatine phosphate on force production in skinned muscles from rat ventricle. *J. Physiol.* 1986; **370**: 585–604.

105. Weiss, J. and Shine, K.I. Extracellular potassium accumulation during myocardial ischemia: implications for arrhythmogenesis. *J. Mol. Cell. Cardiol.* 1981; **13**: 699–704.

106. Klug, F. Ueber den Einfluss gasartiger Korper auf die Function des Froschherzens. *Archiv fur Anatomie und Physiologie, Physiologische Abtheilung* 1879; 435–78.

107. Katz, A.M. and Hecht, H.N. The early "pump" failure of the ischemic heart. *Am. J. Med.* 1969; **47**: 497–502.

108. Kohlhardt, M., Haap, K. and Figulla, H.R. Influence of low extracellular pH upon the Ca inward current and isometric contractile force in mammalian ventricular myocardium. *Pflügers Arch.* 1976; **366**: 31–8.

109. Williamson, J.R., Safer, B., Rich, T., Schaffer, S. and Kobayashi, K. Effects of acidosis on myocardial contractility and metabolism. *Acta Med. Scand.* 1975; Suppl. **587**: 95–111.

110. St Louis, P.J. and Sulakhe, P.V. Adenosine triphosphate-dependent calcium binding and accumulation of guinea-pig cardiac sarcolemma. *Can. J. Biochem.* 1978; **54**: 946–56.

111. Fabiato, A. and Fabiato, F. Effects of pH on the myofilaments and the sarcoplasmic reticulum of skinned cells from cardiac and skeletal muscles. *J. Physiol.* 1978; **276**: 233–55.

112. Kentish, J. and Nayler, W.G. Effect of pH on the Ca^{2+} dependent ATPase of rabbit cardiac and white skeletal myofibrils. *J. Physiol.* 1977; **265**: 18–19P.

113. Poole-Wilson, P.A. Measurement of myocardial intracellular pH in pathological states. *J. Mol. Cell. Cardiol.* 1978; **10**: 511–26.

114. Couper, G.S., Weiss, J., Hiltbrand, B. and Shine, K.I. Extracellular pH and tension during ischemia in the isolated rabbit ventricle. *Am. J. Physiol.* 1984; **247**: H916–27.

115. Jennings, R.B. and Ganote, C.E. Structural changes in myocardium during acute ischaemia. *Circ. Res.* 1974; **35** (Suppl. III): 156–72.

116. Lee, K.S., Ladinsky, H. and Stuckey, J.M. Decreased Ca^{2+} uptake by sarcoplasmic reticulum after coronary occlusion for 60 and 90 minutes. *Circ. Res.* 1967; **21**: 439–44.

117. Katz, A.M. The contractile proteins of the heart. *Physiol. Rev.* 1970; **50**: 63–158.

118. Dehaan, R.L. and Field, J. Mechanism of cardiac damage in anoxia. *Am. J. Physiol.* 1959; **197**: 449–53.

119. Likoff, W., Segal, B.L. and Kasparian, H. Paradox of normal selective coronary arteriograms in patients considered to have unmistakable coronary heart disease. *N. Engl. J. Med.* 1967; **276**: 1063–6.

120. Kemp, H.G., Vokonas, P.S., Cohn, P.F. and Gorlin, R. The anginal syndrome associated with normal coronary angiograms. Report of a six year experience. *Am. J. Med.* 1973; **54**: 735–42.

121. Favoro, L., Caplin, J.L., Fettiche, J.J. and Dymond, D.S. Sex differences in exercise induced left ventricular dysfunction in patients with syndrome X. *Br. Heart J.* 1987; **57**: 232–6.

122. Korhola, O., Valle, M., Frick, M.H., Wiljasalo, M. and Riihimaki, E. Regional myocardial perfusion abnormalities on Xenon-133 imaging in patients with angina pectoris and normal coronary arteries. *Am. J. Cardiol.* 1977; **39**: 355–9.

123. Berger, H.J., Sands, M.J., Davies, R.A. *et al.* Exercise left ventricular performance in patients with chest pain, ischemic-appearing exercise electrocardiograms and angiographically normal coronary arteries. *Ann. Intern. Med.* 1981; **94**: 186–91.

124. Levy, R.D., Shapiro, L.M., Wright, C., Mockus, L. and Fox, K.M. Syndrome X: the haemodynamic significance of ST segment depression. *Br. Heart J.* 1986; **56**: 353–7.

125. Boudoulas, H., Cobb, T.C., Leighton, R.F. and Wilt, S.M. Myocardial lactate production in patients with angina-like chest pain and angiographically normal coronary arteries and left ventricle. *Am. J. Cardiol.* 1974; **34**: 501–5.

126. Cannon, R.O., Watson, R.M., Rosing, D.R. and Epstein, S.E. Angina caused by reduced vasodilator reserve of the small coronary arteries. *J. Am. Coll. Cardiol.* 1983; **1**: 1359–73.

127. Cannon, R.O., Bonow, R.O., Bacharach, S.L. *et al.* Left ventricular dysfunction in patients with angina pectoris, normal epicardial coronary arteries, and abnormal vasodilator reserve. *Circulation* 1985; **71**: 218–26.

128. Strauer, B.E. Ventricular function and coronary hemodynamics in hypertensive heart disease. *Am. J. Cardiol.* 1979; **44**: 999–1006.

129. Legrand, V., Hodgson, J.M., Bates, E.R. *et al.* Abnormal coronary flow reserve and abnormal radionuclide exercise test results in patients with normal coronary angiograms. *J. Am. Coll. Cardiol.* 1985; **6**: 1245–53.

130. Arbogast, R. and Bourassa, M. Myocardial function during atrial pacing in patients with angina pectoris and normal coronary arteriograms. *Am. J. Cardiol.* 1973; **32**: 257–63.

131. Kemp, H.G. Left ventricular function in patients with the anginal syndrome and normal coronary arteriograms. *Am. J. Cardiol.* 1973; **32**: 375–6.

132. Bemiller, C.R., Pepine, C.J. and Rogers, A.K. Long-term observations in patients with angina and normal coronary arteriograms. *Circulation* 1973; **47**: 36–43.

133. Bass, C., Wade, C., Hand, D. and Jackson, G. Patients with angina with normal and near normal coronary arteries: clinical and psychosocial state 12 months after angiography. *Br. Med. J.* 1983; **287**: 1505–8.

134. Opherk, D., Zebe, J., Weihe, E. *et al.* Reduced coronary dilatory capacity and ultrastructural changes of the myocardium in patients with angina pectoris but normal coronary arteriograms. *Circulation* 1981; 63: 817–25.

135. Mosseri, M., Yarom, R., Gotsman, M.S. and Hasin, Y. Histologic evidence for small-vessel coronary artery disease in patients with angina pectoris and patent large coronary arteries. *Circulation* 1986; 74: 964–72.

136. Epstein, S.E. and Cannon R.O. Site of increased resistance to coronary flow in patients with angina pectoris and normal epicardial coronary arteries. *J. Am. Coll. Cardiol.* 1986; 8: 459–61.

137. Eliot, R.S. and Bratt, G. The paradox of myocardial ischemia and necrosis in young women with normal coronary arteriograms. Relation to abnormal hemoglobin-oxygen dissociation. *Am. J. Cardiol.* 1969; 23: 633–8.

138. Neill, W.A., Kassebaum, D.G. and Judkins, M.P. Myocardial hypoxia as the basis for angina pectoris in a patient with normal coronary arteriograms. *N. Engl. J. Med.* 1968; 179: 789–92.

139. Meller, J., Goldsmith, S.J., Rudin, A. *et al.* Spectrum of exercise thallium-201 myocardial perfusion imaging in patients with chest pain and normal coronary angiograms. *Am. J. Cardiol.* 1979; 43: 717–23.

140. Crake, T., Crean, P., Shapiro, L.M., Canepa-Anson, R. and Poole-Wilson, P.A. Continuous recording of coronary sinus oxygen saturation during atrial pacing in patients with and without coronary artery disease or with syndrome X (Abstract). *Br. Heart J.* 1987; 57: 67.

141. Kaski, J.C., Crea, F., Ninoyannopoulos, P., Hackett, D. and Maseri, A. Transient myocardial ischemia during daily life in patients with syndrome X. *Am. J. Cardiol.* 1986; 58: 1242–7.

142. Cannon, R.O., Watson, R.M., Rosing, D.R. and Epstein, S.E. Efficacy of calcium channel blocker therapy for angina pectoris resulting from small-vessel coronary artery disease and abnormal vasodilator reserve. *Am. J. Cardiol.* 1985; 56: 242–6.

Chapter 47

The Pathophysiology and Investigation of Chronic Stable Angina

G.J. Davies

INTRODUCTION

Angina pectoris is one possible manifestation of ischaemic heart disease. Stable angina pectoris refers to stability in the frequency and duration of attacks of angina and implies that a certain period of observation has elapsed during which it can be assessed. It reflects the stability of the underlying pathophysiological process. However, as myocardial ischaemia can present in other ways or be silent, the actual degree of instability of myocardial ischaemia and of the process giving rise to it may be greater than that suggested by the pattern of angina pectoris.

PATHOPHYSIOLOGY

Myocardial ischaemia will occur whenever the demand of the myocardium for oxygen is greater than that which can be delivered by the coronary blood flow. There is thus a balance between myocardial oxygen demand and coronary blood flow. A transient attack of myocardial ischaemia therefore may be caused by either a transient reduction of coronary blood flow below the resting level or a transient increase in myocardial oxygen demand without an appropriate increase in coronary blood flow (Fig. 47.2).

Transient decreases in coronary blood flow can be caused by coronary vasoconstriction[1], coronary thrombosis,[2] platelet aggregation[3] and presumably other, as yet unknown, mechanisms. These mechanisms are usually associated with spontaneous attacks of angina pectoris and attacks that are unpredictable in occurrence and their relationship to precipitating factors.[4] Coronary constriction is the cause of the reductions that precipitate the

spontaneous attacks of myocardial ischaemia seen in Prinzmetal's variant angina.[5] Platelet aggregation and thrombosis usually give rise to unstable angina or evolving myocardial infarction.[6,7] All these mechanisms may also operate in chronic stable angina but to a lesser degree than in variant angina, unstable angina and myocardial infarction. Their effects in chronic stable angina will be discussed below.

The predominant mechanism operating in chronic stable angina is an increase in myocardial oxygen demand in the presence of a fixed coronary luminal narrowing which imposes a fixed upper limit on the extent to which the coronary flow can increase in response to demand (Fig. 47.1), i.e. a

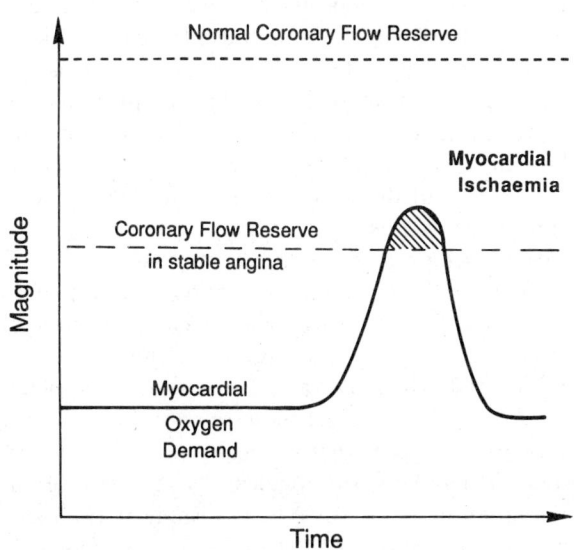

Fig. 47.1. Diagram to illustrate the mechanism of myocardial ischaemia in effort angina, assuming the coronary flow reserve to be constant. When the myocardial oxygen demand exceeds (e.g. on exercise) the level of oxygen supply that can be provided within the limits of the coronary flow reserve, myocardial ischaemia follows.

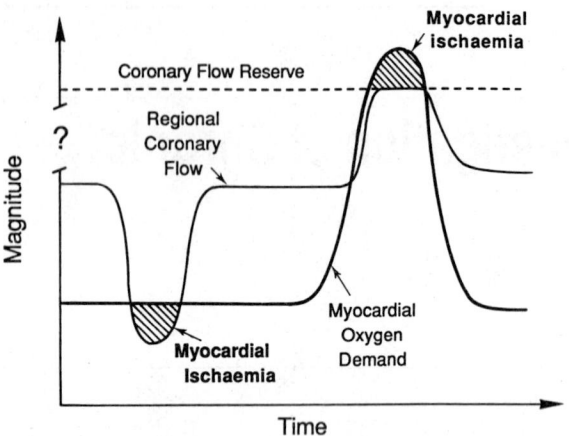

Fig. 47.2. Diagram to illustrate the mechanisms of myocardial ischaemia which may occur in patients with a dynamic component to their coronary blood supply, assuming a constant coronary flow reserve. In addition to the mechanism illustrated in Fig. 47.1, myocardial ischaemia can be precipitated by a fall in regional coronary flow, due to coronary constriction, thrombosis or other mechanism.

limit on the coronary flow reserve.[8] The stability is determined by the nature of the coronary luminal stenosis which is almost invariably atheromatous. The transient nature of the attacks of myocardial ischaemia and of angina pectoris is determined by the increases in myocardial oxygen demand.

ATHEROMATOUS STENOSIS

Fixed stenosis in a coronary artery is usually due to the presence of an atheromatous plaque. In patients with angina pectoris, atheromatous stenosis (or occlusion) is usually found in the proximal or middle segment of at least one large coronary branch. The plaque may involve the whole circumference of the wall at that point, giving rise to concentric stenosis, or it may spare an arc of variable length to form an eccentric stenosis.[9]

In general, the angina is more disabling with lower exercise capacity when stenosis occurs in larger coronary branches, when the stenosis is very severe and when several large coronary branches are involved. However, these relationships are not very precise, such that extensive severe coronary stenosis may be found incidentally at post-mortem examination in persons who displayed no manifestations of coronary disease in life.[10] Conversely, isolated single-vessel coronary stenosis of modest severity may become clinically manifest when vasoconstriction or thrombosis supervenes.[11] Although these mechanisms usually give rise to the syndrome of unstable angina, vasoconstriction may combine

with atheromatous stenosis to give the clinical picture of stable angina but with a variable effort tolerance and a tendency to occasional apparently spontaneous attacks (Fig. 47.3).

CORONARY FLOW RESERVE

Coronary flow reserve is a term used to indicate the amount by which coronary arterial flow can be increased in response to maximal coronary arterial and arteriolar dilatation, i.e. when coronary vascular resistance is at its minimum. In normal adult subjects, maximum coronary flow is 3–4 times greater than the resting value, i.e. the coronary flow reserve is very great. Atheromatous stenosis imposes a limitation on the coronary flow reserve which increases in magnitude as the severity of the stenosis increases. A limitation sufficiently great as to be associated with effort angina is not usually present until the stenosis reaches > 70% of the luminal diameter.[12] Reduction in resting coronary

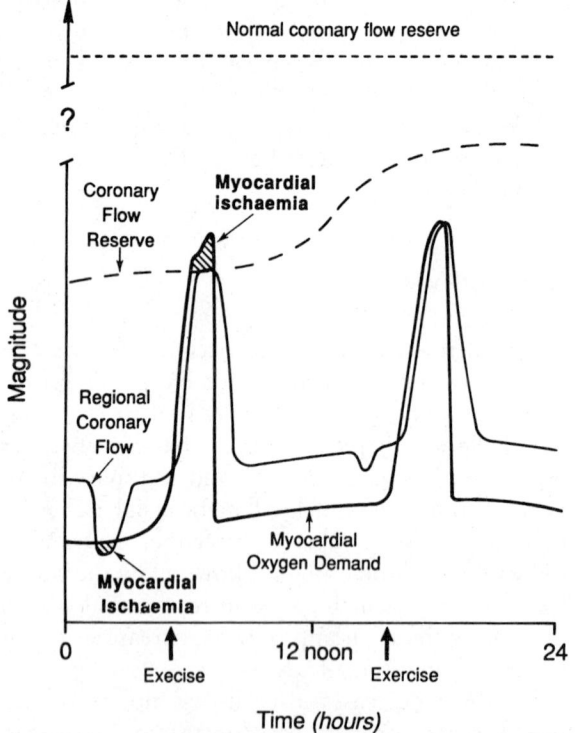

Fig. 47.3. Diagram to illustrate the circumstances found in the majority of patients with chronic angina. Coronary flow reserve probably varies over any 24-h period so that similar increases in myocardial oxygen demand may or may not lead to myocardial ischaemia. The resting level of myocardial oxygen demand and coronary flow probably also vary during this period. Furthermore, transient reductions of coronary flow may occur and may occasionally be so profound that ischaemia occurs even when resting myocardial oxygen demand is at its lowest.

flow, i.e. zero coronary flow reserve, requires the presence of a stenosis of > 90% of coronary luminal diameter.

In the presence of a sufficient fixed limitation of coronary flow reserve, the level of myocardial oxygen demand that can be met will also be fixed and therefore such patients will have a fixed limit on their exercise capacity, a certain level of activity always inducing myocardial ischaemia often accompanied by angina pectoris.

MYOCARDIAL OXYGEN DEMAND

The demand of the myocardium for oxygen is determined by the level of the heart rate, the level of the systemic vascular resistance, the volume of the ventricular cavities, the myocardial mass and the myocardial contractility.

CORONARY SPASM

Dynamic changes in coronary vasomotor tone may be a contributory factor to episodes of myocardial ischaemia in chronic stable angina.[13] However, in occasional patients, abnormally intense vasoconstriction (spasm) occurs transiently causing focal occlusion or near-occlusion of a major coronary vessel leading to transient but massive regional myocardial ischaemia.[14] These patients characteristically present with episodes of spontaneous angina, occurring at rest, and with greater frequency during the night or the early hours of the morning. During an attack of pain, the electrocardiogram shows regional ST-segment elevation (Fig. 47.4), and formal exercise testing often reveals good effort tolerance. This syndrome has been termed 'variant angina' and was first described by Prinzmetal in 1959.[5] The cause of this focal coronary spasm is not known but its mechanism appears to differ from the 'physiological' vasoconstriction seen in other forms of ischaemic heart disease.

In its pure form, variant angina appears to be uncommon, accounting for < 1% of angina cases. However, the difficulty in detecting such spontaneous phenomena would indicate that its true incidence might be higher. In a suspected case, 24-h ambulatory electrocardiographic monitoring will facilitate the detection of spontaneous attacks of ischaemia by ST-segment analysis. The detection of spontaneous ST-segment elevation and the demonstration of good effort tolerance in a patient with a classic history are sufficient to establish the diagnosis. When spontaneous attacks of myocardial ischaemia cannot be demonstrated by a standard 12-lead electrocardiogram or by ambulatory electrocardiographic monitoring and the attacks of chest pain are infrequent, it may be necessary to perform provocative tests. The most potent stimulus to spasm in these patients is ergometrine which is administered at the time of routine coronary arteriography.[15] Spasm is seen as a focal occlusion of a coronary branch and is rapidly relieved by the intracoronary or intavenous administration of glyceryl trinitrate or isosorbide dinitrate (Fig. 47.5). Such investigations should be applied only to the most difficult diagnostic problems and be per-

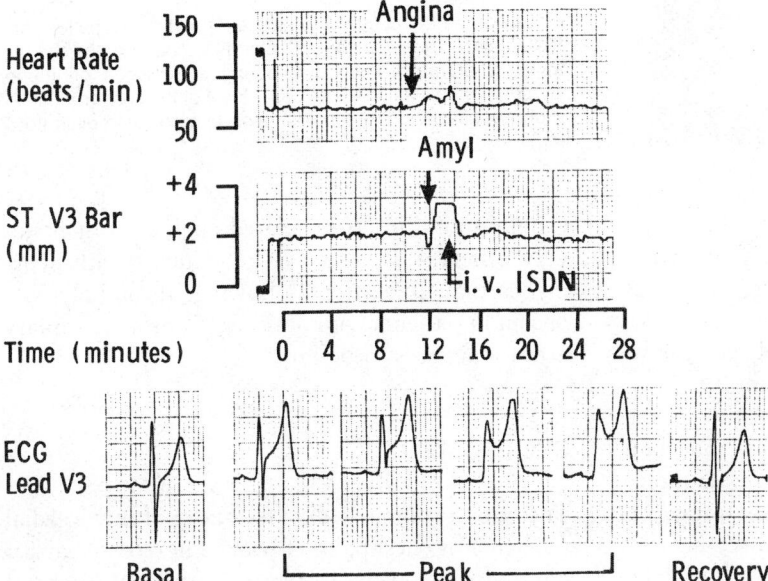

Fig. 47.4. Lead V_3 of the electrocardiogram showing spontaneous ST-segment elevation accompanied by angina pectoris, in a patient with Prinzmetal's variant angina. The continuous plot of the heart rate shows no change in rate from its resting value prior to the onset of angina. There is a small increase consequent to the administration of amyl nitrate.

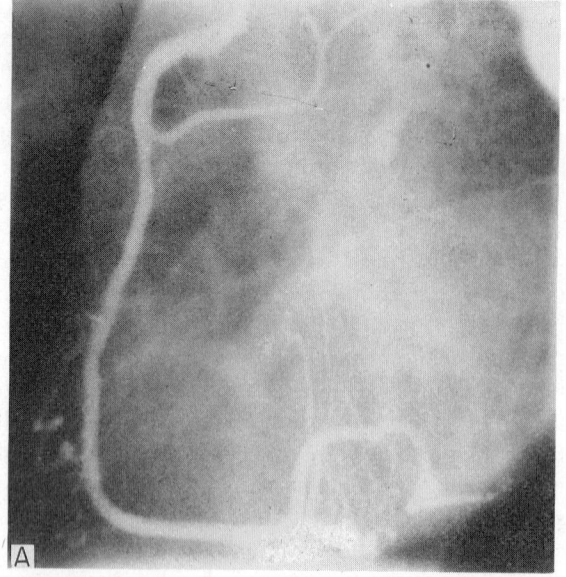

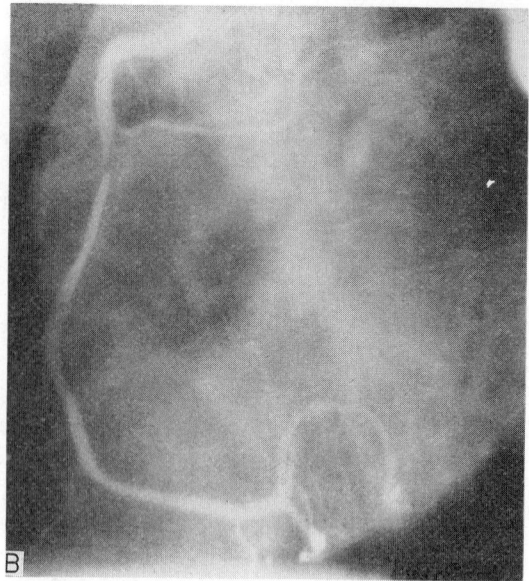

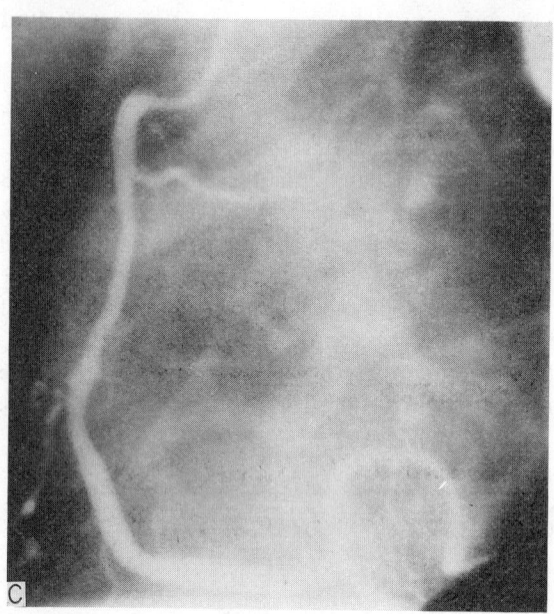

Fig. 47.5. (A) Basal right coronary arteriogram in a patient with Prinzmetal's variant angina. (B) Coronary spasm at the site of a trivial atheromatous stenosis during an episode of inferior ST-segment elevation at rest. (C) Relief of the spasm within 20 s of the intracoronary administration of isosorbide dinitrate (2 mg).

formed at specialized centres where there are doctors with expertise in this field. The administration of ergometrine is contra-indicated in those patients shown by Holter monitoring to have frequent attacks and in those who have a low threshold to ischaemia on exercise testing.

In most patients with variant angina, the spasm occurs at the site of an atheromatous plaque but usually the degree of stenosis due to the plaque is not very severe and is commonly in the range of 30–60% of the diameter of the normal segment.[16] This severity of stenosis is considerably less than

usually found in effort-related angina but it is not very different to that seen in patients with acute myocardial infarction following thrombolysis.[17] Spasm in patients with absolutely normal coronary arteries appears to be rare.

SYMPTOMS

The most common manifestation of myocardial ischaemia is chest pain. However, in recent years, it has become well recognized that myocardial ischaemia may be painless[18] and, furthermore, that this entity is quite common. Painless does not mean symptomless, and other symptoms may be associated with myocardial ischaemia, such as dyspnoea, diaphoresis, palpitation and syncope.

CHEST PAIN

Typically, the character of the pain is variously described as 'tight', 'heavy', 'constricting', 'a compression' or 'a tight band around the chest'. The perception of pain differs from one individual to another as does the patient's ability to describe clearly the character of the pain. When asked what the pain is like, the patient will frequently reply: 'Terrible!' It is then worth asking, 'What does the pain *feel* like, what kind of pain or sensation is it, exactly?', whereupon a more precise description will be obtained from most patients.

The site of chest pain is typically central, retrosternal, often radiating into the neck and to the arms. The left arm is more frequently involved than the right, the pain being localized to the upper arm, forearm or hand or may be present in the entire upper limb. Occasionally, the pain may be predominantly epigastric, interscapular or felt only in the mandible, gums, throat or neck. Thus, angina pectoris may sometimes be confused with pain originating from the stomach, gallbladder, teeth or ear.

Factors that may precipitate an attack of myocardial ischaemia in patients with chronic stable angina are mainly those that are associated with elevated levels of myocardial oxygen demand. The most common factor is effort, thus attacks of angina pectoris are frequently effort related, the pain following the onset of effort and resolving within a few minutes of rest. This close relationship with effort makes angina easy to recognize even when the character and radiation of the pain is atypical. As pain is an inconsistent and relatively late manifestation of myocardial ischaemia,[19] it is unusual to elicit a history of pain commencing after just a few steps, the lowest effort tolerance being comparable to 25–50 m walking on level ground before angina appears. Under certain circumstances, such as anxiety,[20] exposure to cold[21] and after meals,[22] pain may become manifest earlier. In the absence of these additional factors, which may increase myocardial oxygen demand, some patients exhibit a remarkably consistent effort tolerance such that their angina always begins at a certain fixed distance and this may remain constant from day to

day over a period of months or even years. In these cases, it is likely that severe atheromatous stenosis is the major determinant of their angina, coronary vasomotion playing only a minor role such that the attacks occur whenever myocardial oxygen demand rises above a certain level.

In other patients, however, effort tolerance is variable even when other factors determining myocardial oxygen consumption are not operating.[23] Thus, a patient may experience angina at 100 m on level ground on one day and yet the next day may be able to walk an almost unlimited distance and walk briskly uphill with no symptoms. Furthermore, these patients may occasionally suffer spontaneous attacks when they are resting and in a relaxed state of mind or may be awoken from sleep by angina. A circadian variation in effort tolerance has been demonstrated in several studies of effort angina.[24] This variability in effort tolerance is due to transient changes in coronary flow reserve and the spontaneous attacks of angina to a transient fall in coronary arterial flow below the resting level.[25] The cause of these changes in coronary flow is likely to be coronary vasoconstriction although whether this is at the site of the atheromatous stenosis, elsewhere in the epicardial arterial segment, in the intramyocardial arteries or in the arterioles is not yet established. It is possible for dynamic changes in calibre to occur even at the site of an atheromatous stenosis,[26,27] particularly when the stenosis is eccentric in which case there is an arc of arterial wall containing smooth muscle.

Cold exposure is a potent stimulus to the occurrence of angina[21] operating both by increasing myocardial oxygen demand due to increased systemic vascular resistance and left ventricular dilatation and by reflex coronary arterial constriction which decreases coronary flow reserve. Chronic stable angina pectoris is thus often more severe in the winter months with an increased frequency and severity of attacks, particularly in patients who have severely impaired left ventricular function because cold-induced ventricular dilatation is more marked in these patients. Not infrequently, patients report angina precipitated by mere exposure to cold without significant effort, such as that induced by a blast of cold air on opening an outside door. The stimuli of effort and cold are additive in the induction of angina such that angina may be rapidly precipitated by such circumstances as pushing a car in freezing weather in an attempt to start it or shovelling snow off a drive.

Anxiety may also induce attacks of angina[20]

mainly by catecholamine-induced increases in myocardial oxygen demand but also by alpha-adrenoreceptor-mediated coronary vasoconstriction. Anxiety levels vary considerably from individual to individual, as does the coronary arterial response to anxiety; therefore, its contribution to symptomatology in patients with ischaemic heart disease is variable. Nevertheless, it may provoke attacks of angina at rest in patients with chronic stable angina and its effect may summate with other stimuli, such as effort, cold and meals, to induce attacks on minimal exertion. A typical situation would be that of running through snow to catch a train in order to attend an important business meeting.

Meals may also reduce the threshold for angina,[28] although the mechanism has not been elucidated. Redistribution of the cardiac output in favour of the gastro-intestinal tract and to the detriment of myocardial vascular territories has been postulated as one such mechanism. However, it is not clear whether this is mediated through neural or through humoral mechanisms as nervous connections exist between the upper gastro-intestinal tract and the heart, and, furthermore, certain peptides produced in the gastro-intestinal tract are known to affect vascular smooth muscle.[29] The typical history is one of reduced effort tolerance, limited by angina, noticeable at 0.5–1 h after a meal. This appears to be the case even when an attempt is made to exercise immediately after a meal. Typically, these patients have extensive coronary artery disease with proximal occlusion or severe stenosis of several major coronary artery branches and hence a low coronary flow reserve. Furthermore, they often have severe impairment of left ventricular function and therefore may give a history of angina with low effort tolerance with further impairment after meals. Occasionally, patients report angina at rest after meals with an effort tolerance that is moderate or good and not necessarily associated with extensive coronary disease. In these patients, changes in coronary vasomotor tone may be operating as an important mechanism in the induction of myocardial ischaemia. When this pain is epigastric and lower retrosternal in site, it may easily be confused with upper gastro-intestinal pain.

Rarely, postural changes may precipitate an attack of angina. The most frequent example of this is angina decubitus, in which angina occurs on reclining, to be relieved by sitting up or standing. These patients are characterized by low coronary flow reserve and therefore they have very low effort tolerance and invariably have extensive coronary artery disease.

The duration of angina attacks in patients with chronic stable angina depends to a large extent on the duration of the stimulus. Low-grade chest discomfort can be well tolerated by some individuals, particularly when the significance of the discomfort has not been appreciated. However, severe and extensive myocardial ischaemia will be poorly tolerated and lead to avoidance of the stimulus. The latter, however, may be difficult to achieve, particularly when anxiety is the predominant operating mechanism. When the stimulus is removed, for example, when the patient with effort-induced angina rests, pain usually subsides rapidly, disappearing completely in only a few minutes. When myocardial ischaemia is profound and extensive, the pain may subside slowly taking up to 10 or 15 min to resolve completely. Although it is generally not the case, myocardial infarction is sometimes precipitated by exertion,[30] cold or anxiety and, in the event of angina persisting for > 15 min, it is reasonable to suppose that acute myocardial infarction is likely and therefore to institute appropriate emergency therapy.

Removal of the stimulus is not the only mechanism by which myocardial ischaemia can be relieved. Certain substances, such as adenosine, are released by ischaemic tissue and can induce coronary arterial and arteriolar dilatation. Such negative feedback mechanisms may protect the individual against myocardial infarction. Certain clinical phenomena which suggest the activity of a negative feedback loop can be observed in clinical practice. An example is the 'walk-through' phenomenon in which angina occurs during exertion only to resolve during continued exertion of at least equal severity. Thereafter, the patient may be able to walk a considerable distance without recurrence of angina or may again experience angina after a short interval. A related phenomenon is that of 'second wind'; the patient experiences angina on effort which is relieved by a short period of rest and subsequently can walk a very long distance, even at a brisk pace, without experiencing angina. A typical situation would be that of a workman who regularly experiences angina on setting out to walk to work early in the morning; after a short rest, the angina completely resolves and does not recur as he completes his journey. Furthermore, due to the circadian variation in the angina threshold, he may be able to carry out his work during the remainder of the day without experiencing further angina.

DYSPNOEA

The perception of pain varies greatly among individuals as does their interpretation of the same sensation and their ability to describe that sensation. Thus, a feeling of tightness in the chest described by one patient as pain will be described by another as shortness of breath, particularly if it occurs on exertion and thus impairs the effort capacity of that patient.

It should also be remembered that pain is a late and inconsistent manifestation of acute myocardial ischaemia and that regional impairment of left ventricular function is an early manifestation. If the acute ischaemic region of the left ventricle is large or there are other, chronic, regional abnormalities of contraction due to previous myocardial infarction or global abnormalities of ventricular function such as hypertrophy, a rapid rise in left ventricular diastolic pressure will ensue and, simultaneously, a rise in left atrial and pulmonary venous pressures. Under these circumstances, the patient will develop dyspnoea as the first manifestation of myocardial ischaemia and this will quickly resolve as the myocardial ischaemia resolves on resting or when some other stimulus is removed. In other words, acute left ventricular failure accompanies acute myocardial ischaemia and will be transient if the myocardial ischaemia is transient. The rate of development of left ventricular failure depends on the extent to which left ventricular function is impaired by the combination of acute myocardial ischaemia and chronic myocardial pathology. If the rate is rapid or if the development of pain is impaired, dyspnoea may occur as the first manifestation of ischaemia. Myocardial ischaemia should always be considered in the differential diagnosis of patients presenting with dyspnoea, particularly when there is no obvious pulmonary cause.

In certain groups of patients, acute myocardial ischaemia is more likely to be painless and therefore to present as dyspnoea. The most common groups are the elderly and those subjects who have diabetes mellitus.[31] Furthermore, in these groups, even the severe persistent myocardial ischaemia associated with myocardial infarction is frequently painless.[32]

DIAPHORESIS

The marked impairment of left ventricular function that commonly occurs during acute severe myocardial ischaemia is associated with a fall in stroke volume which may be only partly compensated by reflex tachycardia and therefore a fall in cardiac output ensues. Further reflex sympathetic stimulation occurs which may be associated with profuse sweating and intense cutaneous vasoconstriction giving rise to cold clammy skin. This is the clinical picture of cardiogenic shock but it is transient, a reversible consequence of acute myocardial ischaemia. In some patients, this may be the presenting symptom.

SYNCOPE

Although it occurs more commonly in the presence of more severe ischaemia, as in unstable angina and acute myocardial infarction, syncope is an occasional feature of an attack of myocardial ischaemia in patients who have chronic stable angina. It may have several possible mechanisms, including transient reduction in cardiac output due to severe left ventricular failure in patients with extensive ischaemia and previously impaired left ventricular function, transient asystole due to sinus node arrest or complete atrioventricular block, or tachyarrhythmia, particularly ventricular fibrillation. Perhaps the most common cause, however, is the self-administration of rapid acting nitrates taken to relieve an attack of angina. Nitrates cause marked venodilatation with consequent peripheral venous pooling of blood.[33] This venous pooling, exaggerated by standing, causes a marked fall in venous return to the heart at a time when the left ventricle may not have fully recovered from ischaemia. There is consequently a dramatic fall in cardiac output and in systemic arterial pressure leading to syncope.

FATIGUE

The impaired increase of cardiac output or even reduction in cardiac output occurring during effort-induced myocardial ischaemia, by causing skeletal muscle ischaemia, can lead to transient muscular fatigue which may occasionally be a prominent symptom of myocardial ischaemia. The lack of a close correlation between the pulmonary venous pressure and dyspnoea may suggest that the latter symptom may also be partly related to muscular fatigue.

INTERMITTENT CLAUDICATION

Coronary artery disease and peripheral vascular disease frequently co-exist; patients frequently experience both angina and intermittent claudication. However, the onset of these symptoms is commonly synchronous and this is probably due to ischaemia of the leg muscles precipitated by the transient fall in cardiac output occurring during a transient attack of myocardial ischaemia in the presence of peripheral arterial stenosis. The myocardial ischaemia may be painless resulting in claudication as the limiting symptom.

ASYMPTOMATIC TRANSIENT MYOCARDIAL ISCHAEMIA ('SILENT' ISCHAEMIA)

In recent years, it has become increasingly clear that asymptomatic transient myocardial ischaemia is a common phenomenon.[34] The existence of asymptomatic myocardial infarction was previously well established.[35] Studies of Prinzmetal's variant angina, based on continuous electrocardiographic and haemodynamic monitoring, have shown the existence of asymptomatic episodes and provided the haemodynamic evidence that these were attacks of myocardial ischaemia and not just electrical events.[36] In patients whose angina is predominantly spontaneous, numerous asymptomatic episodes may occur; on average 70% of their attacks are symptomless.[36] This is also the case in patients with predominantly exertional angina who comprise the majority of the population with chronic stable angina.[37] The extent to which symptomless ischaemia occurs in the general population is unknown but the occurrence of positive exercise electrocardiographic results in occasional subjects undergoing routine health checks has established the existence of this entity. Although false-positive results may occur, a significant proportion of these patients have associated atheromatous coronary artery disease, and the ischaemic nature of the electrocardiographic changes can be verified by assessment of left ventricular function and regional myocardial perfusion during exercise.

The reasons why some episodes of myocardial ischaemia are symptomatic and others are symptomless are not clear. A certain duration and extent of myocardial ischaemia are required to produce symptoms. In this respect, episodes of ischaemia < 3 min in duration are invariably symptomless.[19,25] Furthermore, ischaemic episodes that are not very severe or involve only a small mass of myocardium, as evidenced by elevations of left ventricular end-diastolic pressure of < 7 mmHg, are almost invariably symptomless. However, in the case of episodes which are of greater duration and severity, some are symptomatic and others are symptomless.[19] The reason for this is not clear but it does not appear to be related to the severity and duration of ischaemia or the rate or degree of ventricular dilatation.[19] Diabetic subjects and the elderly have an impaired appreciation of pain. Furthermore, it is widely accepted that individuals differ greatly in their ability to perceive pain. Several studies have provided evidence that patients with painless ischaemia have a higher threshold for the perception of pain than those with painful ischaemia[38] and that these two groups of patients show differences in personality (see Chapter 70).[39]

PHYSICAL SIGNS

In patients with chronic stable angina, physical signs are relatively infrequent and therefore the diagnosis is usually made on the basis of meticulous history-taking. However, the importance of physical signs is not lessened by their infrequency and therefore clinicians should be vigilant in their detection.

GENERAL EXAMINATION

Evidence of anaemia[40] and thyrotoxicosis[41] should be sought as conditions that might unmask occult coronary artery disease causing angina. Evidence of systemic conditions that may be associated with coronary lesions should be sought, such as systemic lupus erythematosus,[42] polyarteritis nodosa,[43] other types of vasculitis and Kawasaki's disease.[44] Manifestations of hyperlipidaemia may be present, namely xanthelasma and xanthomas of the Achilles tendon, the triceps insertion into the olecranon process and the extensor tendons of the fingers.

Inspection of the chest may reveal a median sternotomy scar from previous coronary artery bypass surgery and inspection of the lower limbs evidence of saphenous venectomy.

CARDIOVASCULAR EXAMINATION

Other cardiac conditions that may cause angina, apart from atheromatous coronary disease, may be present and therefore complete cardiovascular examination is essential (see Chapter 8). These conditions include severe aortic stenosis,[45] pulmonary stenosis,[46] pulmonary hypertension,[47] Eisenmenger's syndrome,[48] anomalous coronary artery[49] and coronary arteriovenous fistula.[50] It is also necessary to consider other conditions associated with pain that has certain features of angina pectoris but may not be quite typical. These are the cardiomyopathies, particularly hypertrophic cardiomyopathy,[51] and mitral valve prolapse,[52] which is otherwise known as floppy mitral valve or Barlow's syndrome. Typically, patients with hypertrophic cardiomyopathy have a brisk upstroke of the arterial pulse, an accentuated left ventricular impulse with a palpable atrial impulse and, on auscultation, a prominent fourth heart sound and a long systolic murmur which is harsh in quality and best heard at the left sternal edge and apex. Mitral valve prolapse is associated with one or more mid-systolic clicks with or without a crescendo late-systolic murmur.

Certain physical signs, which may be found in patients with ischaemic heart disease associated with atheromatous coronary artery disease, are discussed below.

The arterial pulse

The arterial pulse is most commonly normal.

However, in patients treated by beta-adrenergic blockade, the resting pulse rate may be low, frequently < 60 beats/min, and may show only a modest increase on exercise. When there is severe impairment of left ventricular function, either transiently, in the case of an attack of angina, or consistently, in the case of extensive myocardial scarring, the pulse volume is usually small, reflecting the small stroke volume, and the pulse is narrow. Occasionally, pulsus alternans will be detected. Left ventricular failure will usually be associated with sinus tachycardia of a variable degree, which is less marked in those patients receiving beta-adrenergic blocking agents.

Although most patients with chronic stable angina are in consistent sinus rhythm and consequently have a virtually regular pulse, a few are in chronic atrial fibrillation or are subject to paroxysms of atrial fibrillation and therefore may have a pulse that is irregularly irregular, of variable volume and rate and with a rate deficit from heart to radial pulse. Although supraventricular and ventricular extrasystoles are common in chronic ischaemic heart disease, they are not normally noticed by the patient as palpitation. They may occur as single

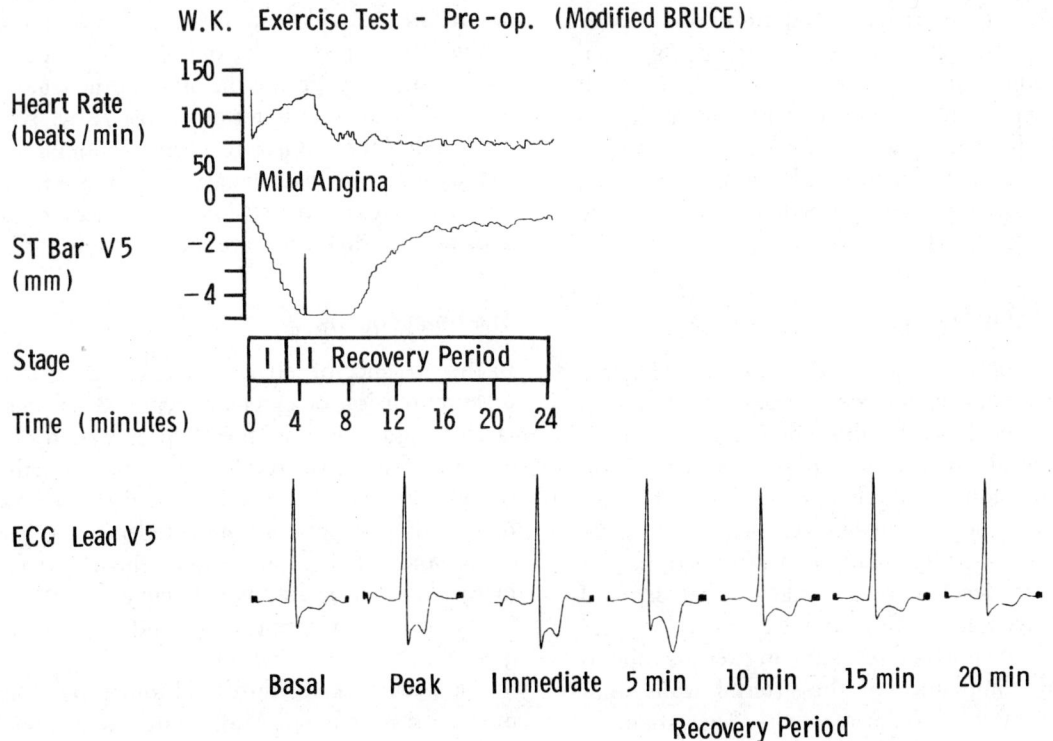

Fig. 47.6. Exercise electrocardiogram. The sequential changes in lead V_5 are shown from basal, through peak exercise and immediately post exercise to the 20th min of the recovery period. More than 4 mm (0.4 mV) of ST-segment depression occurs at peak exercise as shown in the continuous plot of ST-segment level.

extrasystoles with any frequency, which may be regular or exhibit any degree of irregularity. They may also occur in couplets, triplets or runs of four or more, in which case they are given the term tachycardia. This very varied combination of extrasystoles gives rise to a pulse pattern that may differ widely not only among patients, but also in an individual patient over time. The extrasystoles may be detected at the wrist as a transient weakness or absence of the pulse, as pulsus bigeminus or they may be indistinguishable from atrial fibrillation. Supraventricular and ventricular extrasystoles cannot be distinguished by examination of the arterial pulse. Tachycardias may be induced by effort, particularly when myocardial ischaemia occurs, and a rapid, regular or irregular, pulse persisting after effort may be indicative of this. Rapid ventricular tachycardia or ventricular fibrillation will be associated with pulselessness and loss of consciousness.

The jugular venous pulse

In the absence of arrhythmia and when myocardial function is normal, the jugular venous pulse is normal. However, when myocardial function is grossly abnormal, particularly in the presence of previous right ventricular infarction, the venous pressure may be elevated. The waveform is often unremarkable but prominence of the 'v' wave will be apparent in the presence of tricuspid regurgitation due to tricuspid valve ring dilatation or papillary muscle dysfunction. Changes in waveform will occur in the presence of arrhythmias but these are discussed elsewhere.

The blood pressure

Hypertension is a major risk factor for ischaemic heart disease and therefore it is frequently found in patients with chronic stable angina.[53] The blood pressure level should be carefully recorded on several occasions in these patients. Patients with hypertension, because of left ventricular hypertrophy and increased left ventricular afterload, have a greater basal level of myocardial oxygen demand for any given heart rate and experience greater increases in their blood pressure on exercise, due to a lack of compliance of the arterial walls and, perhaps, greater arteriolar reactivity. They are more likely to develop myocardial ischaemia and suffer attacks of angina pectoris than other patients who have a similar degree of coronary narrowing, either fixed or dynamic, but no hypertension.

In patients in severe cardiac failure, either chronic or precipitated by acute severe myocardial ischaemia, hypotension may occur with marked reduction in pulse pressure, and occasionally pulsus alternans may be detected during the measurement of blood pressure. Hypotension may also occur in response to the administration of rapid-acting nitrates, and postural hypotension may be a feature of those patients with severe impairment of left ventricular function who are receiving vasodilator therapy.

The cardiac impulse

In the majority of patients with chronic stable angina, the cardiac impulse is normal. However, those with hypertension may have a forceful apex beat, perhaps with a palpable atrial beat, due to left ventricular hypertrophy. Patients with extensive left ventricular damage due to an old myocardial infarction may have a displaced diffuse apex beat with or without an atrial impulse. Recent or old anterior myocardial infarction may cause parasternal pulsation which represents the transmitted impulse imparted by the dyskinetic anterior left ventricular wall. In the presence of a left ventricular aneurysm, a double impulse may be found, not only temporally but spatially, one impulse occurring at the left sternal edge and the other at the true cardiac apex. Mitral regurgitation caused by papillary muscle dysfunction is rarely severe enough to make the cardiac impulse dynamic. Severe mitral regurgitation and extensive left ventricular damage causing ring dilatation are incompatible.

The heart sounds

In the presence of left ventricular hypertrophy due to hypertension or extensive regional left ventricular function abnormalities such as would occur in extensive old myocardial infarction, a fourth heart sound is frequently detectable. A third heart sound might also be present and reflects the lack of compliance of the scarred left ventricle. The sinus tachycardia associated with incipient left ventricular failure, in the presence of added heart sounds, gives rise to gallop rhythm.

The occurrence of third and fourth heart sounds may be transient when associated with attacks of myocardial ischaemia. Furthermore, severe depression of left ventricular function, whether acute or chronic, may be associated with a reduced intensity of the first and second heart sounds.

Particularly in acute myocardial ischaemia in the territory of the right coronary artery, a third heart sound of right ventricular origin or a fourth heart sound of right atrial origin may be detected.

Cardiac murmurs

Dilatation of the mitral valve ring in patients with severely impaired left ventricular function causes mitral regurgitation and the typical soft blowing pan-systolic murmur, which is of maximum intensity at the apex and radiates to the axilla. Posterior papillary muscle dysfunction, which commonly occurs in patients with postero-inferior myocardial infarction, is usually associated with a crescendo late-systolic murmur, which may be slightly rough in character and is audible at the apex but often radiates to the left sternal edge and to the base of the heart where its intensity may be maximal. In some cases, the systolic murmur may be long, commencing soon after the first heart sound and continuing up to the second heart sound. Even when virtually pan-systolic, it maintains a rough quality and can be mistaken for the murmur of a ventricular septal defect.

The mitral murmurs may be transient,[54] precipitated by acute myocardial ischaemia, and disappear within seconds, minutes or hours of its resolution.

DIFFERENTIAL DIAGNOSIS

The character, radiation and temporal characteristics of the pain and its close relationship to effort may be sufficient to warrant a firm diagnosis of angina pectoris. Physical examination will clarify whether the angina is due to atheromatous coronary artery disease and the extent to which other systemic diseases, such as vasculitis, or other cardiovascular diseases, such as aortic stenosis, may be contributory causes.

When the history is not typical, for example, when the pain is described as burning or sharp, when it is very transient or lasts for many hours or when it is predominantly epigastric, interscapular, inframammary, brachial, pharyngeal or mandibular in site, other conditions should be considered, such as other heart diseases, including hypertrophic cardiomyopathy and mitral valve prolapse, pericarditis, pericardial effusion and aortic aneurysm, and a variety of miscellaneous conditions, including gastric ulcer, hiatus hernia, cholelithiasis, chronic pancreatitis, dental caries, cervical or thoracic nerve root compression, brachial neuralgia, intercostal myalgia, costochondritis, pleurisy and pain related to recent cardiothoracic surgery.

It is important to remember that the more serious causes of chest pain should be considered first. For example, myocardial ischaemia should be excluded as a cause of chest pain before hiatus hernia is considered as a serious possibility. Unfortunately, angina pectoris is frequently considered to be indigestion not only by patients but also by physicians.

Myocardial ischaemia can be frequently confused with peptic ulcer pain because it may give rise to epigastric pain, particularly when the ischaemia is in the diaphragmatic wall of the heart as in patients with right coronary artery or circumflex coronary artery lesions. Furthermore, the ischaemia may be temporally related to meals, as described above.

It should also be remembered that the patient may be experiencing more than one kind of pain, one or none of which may be due to myocardial ischaemia. The ischaemic pain may appear to the patient to be of less importance than the other pain and described as a mere chest discomfort. Occasionally, the patient will forget to mention the ischaemic pain, which had been noted by the general practitioner and was the reason for hospital referral, and be intent on describing the intricate details of the other pain. Specific inquiry should be made regarding other types of chest pain.

On the basis of the history and the physical examination, an estimation of the probability of the patient having ischaemic heart disease can be made; for example, in a patient with effort-related constricting retrosternal pain, it will be high; in a patient with episodes of sharp 'stabbing' left inframammary pain lasting < 5 s it will be low. It is then possible to decide on the best strategy of investigation and of treatment bearing in mind the disadvantages related to each.

INVESTIGATIONS

The aim of investigation is threefold:
1 to establish the diagnosis of ischaemic heart disease and its relationship to the patient's symptoms;
2 to find out the mechanisms determining the attacks of myocardial ischaemia and angina pectoris;
3 to assess the severity of the problem. These aspects will be relevant to treatment and an assessment of prognosis.

THE CHEST X-RAY

Although the majority of patients will have a normal heart size, those with previous myocardial infarction or associated conditions, such as hypertension, may show left ventricular enlargement, which can be detected on the lateral X-ray and, on the postero-anterior film, together with left atrial enlargement, as an increase in heart size. The presence of left ventricular aneurysm may give rise to a localized prominence of the lower left heart border on the postero-anterior film. In patients with severe left ventricular dysfunction, left atrial enlargement may be more pronounced with evidence of left ventricular failure provided by distension of the upper lobe pulmonary veins, fluid in the horizontal fissure, pleural effusion, Kerley B lines, the 'bat's wing' appearance of interstitial pulmonary oedema or florid alveolar oedema.

The presence of sternal wires will indicate previous relevant cardiac surgery. Radiopaque markers in the region of the ascending aorta, best seen on the lateral X-ray, indicate the presence of coronary vein grafts. Metallic clips in the line of the internal mammary artery indicate the use of this vessel as a graft to a coronary artery, most likely the left anterior descending artery. The presence of prosthetic heart valves should be sought.

THE RESTING 12-LEAD ELECTROCARDIOGRAM

The presence of pathological Q waves on the resting electrocardiogram, indicative of previous myocardial infarction, will suggest the presence of ischaemic heart disease with a high degree of probability increasing the possibility that the pain is angina pectoris. The occurrence of a regional reduction of R-wave voltage, of symmetrical T-wave inversion and of planar or downsloping ST-segment depression are also indicative of, but less specific for, ischaemic heart disease. It should be remembered that other conditions, such as the cardiomyopathies and infiltrative disorders affecting the myocardium, will often give rise to pathological Q waves and other QRS complex, ST-segment and T-wave abnormalities. Other electrocardiographic abnormalities which may be found in patients with angina pectoris are non-specific for ischaemic heart disease and include left bundle branch block, right bundle branch block, anterior or posterior hemiblock, bifascicular block, various degrees of atrioventricular block, atrial fibrillation,

atrial flutter, atrial and ventricular extrasystoles and ventricular tachycardia.

A firm diagnosis can be made when a transient ST-segment change is found on the 12-lead electrocardiogram recorded during and following an episode of chest pain or other symptom thought to be due to myocardial ischaemia. As patients with chronic stable angina may experience episodes at rest, either spontaneous or provoked by anxiety, cold or meals, the diagnostic opportunity that an episode of pain presents should be grasped and an electrocardiogram recorded. These opportunities may occur in the outpatient clinic, but are particularly likely to occur during hospital admission for investigation.

THE EXERCISE TEST

As angina pectoris is commonly effort related, a formal exercise test is routinely used as a provocative manoeuvre to induce myocardial ischaemia. The protocol is terminated when the symptom of which the patient was complaining has occurred, when myocardial ischaemia has been detected or at the patient's request. The electrocardiogram is usually used for the detection of myocardial ischaemia but other techniques which assess ventricular function or regional myocardial perfusion can be used.

Exercise protocols

Either a bicycle ergometer or a motor-driven treadmill can be used for graded exercise, although the latter is in more widespread use. Several treadmill protocols are available, but the most commonly used are the Bruce,[55] modified Bruce and Naughton protocols. In the Bruce and the modified Bruce protocols, 3-min stages are used and in the Naughton protocol 2-min stages are employed; in all three protocols, the combination of increasing inclines and speeds is utilized to achieve increasing workloads which can be expressed as multiples of basal metabolic rate (mets). Arterial blood pressure, measured with a manual or automatic sphygmomanometer, is recorded at the end of each stage of the test. A vigorous exercise protocol, such as the Bruce, is appropriate for apparently healthy individuals, apart from those who are elderly; a less vigorous protocol, such as the modified Bruce, is appropriate for those with known cardiac disease or who have a high probability of ischaemic heart disease. Elderly patients should be subjected to a slowly increasing workload, as employed in the Naughton protocol.

Lead systems

The electrocardiogram is used to detect acute myocardial ischaemia which is defined as planar or downsloping ST-segment depression (Fig. 47.6) or elevation of > 0.1 mV, measured 80 ms after the J point. Normalization of previously inverted T waves is frequently a manifestation of myocardial ischaemia but it is less specific. Upsloping ST-segment depression is non-specific and usually occurs in normal subjects at high heart rates.

To obtain high-quality recordings, silver–silver chloride electrodes should be used which provide good skin contact by means of a liquid conductor. The sites of electrode application should be cleaned with ethyl alcohol and the superficial keratinized layer of the epidermis removed by gentle abrasion with an emery board or vigorous rubbing with gauze.

If only single-channel recording is available, the most widely used lead system is a modified bipolar lead V_5 (CM_5) with the positive electrode placed in the fifth intercostal space at the left anterior axillary line and the negative electrode placed at the manubrium. This lead system is reported to detect 89% of the electrocardiographic abnormalities detected by 12-lead recordings.[56] When a two-channel recorder is available, an additional inferior lead (II, III or aVF) increases the diagnostic power. A three-channel recorder will allow the recording of an inferior lead, modified V_3 and V_5 throughout exercise. Most modern systems use a treadmill and computer processing of the electrocardiographic signals. Three leads can be monitored continuously and a complete 12-lead electrocardiogram recorded at 1-min intervals. Signal averaging allows the display of a continuously updated electrocardiographic complex, together with display of the heart rate and maximum ST-segment shift. At the end of the test, a computerized plot of heart rate, blood pressure and ST-segment level against time is produced, with computer-averaged electrocardiographic complexes showing the ST-segment change and QRS morphology at 1-min intervals from the basal state, throughout exercise and recovery (Fig. 147.6, p. 1111). Complete non-averaged 12-lead electrocardiograms can also be obtained at any stage.

Endpoints

The test is terminated when an ST-segment shift > 0.2 mV occurs, in the event of chest pain, dyspnoea, muscular fatigue or other symptom or on achieving a heart rate 85–90% of the maximum predicted for that patient's age and sex. Other indications for termination of the test include a fall in systolic blood pressure during exercise or the development of a serious dysrhythmia.

A positive exercise test confirms the occurrence of myocardial ischaemia, particularly when it is associated with typical angina pectoris. If the patient's usual pain is similar to that experienced during the exercise test or if the patient describes typical angina pectoris, it can be assumed that the pain of which the patient complains is due to myocardial ischaemia and that the patient has ischaemic heart disease. However, in some patients, ischaemic heart disease is confirmed by a positive exercise test but their pain is not caused by myocardial ischaemia.

It should be remembered that ST-segment change is a manifestation of myocardial ischaemia and not a direct consequence of coronary artery disease. Although myocardial ischaemia is usually associated with coronary artery disease, this relationship is not invariable. Therefore, when a positive exercise test is found in a patient with no structural coronary abnormality, it cannot be assumed to be a false-positive test; it may represent myocardial ischaemia even though the mechanism seems obscure. However, if the exercise electrocardiogram is used solely to detect 'significant' atheromatous coronary stenosis, the sensitivity of the test is 55–70% and the specificity 85–95%.[57]

As intramyocardial pressure is greater in the sub-endocardial layer and perfusion pressure is lower, ischaemia usually develops first in this layer, giving rise to ST-segment depression on the electrocardiogram which is therefore the most common electrocardiographic manifestation of myocardial ischaemia during exercise testing. However, ST-segment elevation is occasionally seen,[58,59] indicating extensive ischaemia across that segment of the ventricular wall, which usually happens when active reduction of coronary flow reserve occurs during exercise or when regional coronary flow falls below the resting level, perhaps with transient complete coronary occlusion. The most likely mechanism for this is coronary vasoconstriction and is most prevalent in patients with variant angina.

The site of the ST-segment changes on the electrocardiogram often indicates the site of myocardial ischaemia in the heart, particularly when the maximum ST-segment change is in leads V_1–V_4, indicating antero-septal ischaemia, or in leads II, III and aVF, indicating inferior wall ischaemia. It should be borne in mind that anterior ST-segment depression may occasionally be due to transmural posterior wall ischaemia and that inferior ST-segment depression may occasionally be due to transmural high lateral wall ischaemia, although the latter will be apparent from the presence of ST-segment elevation in leads I and aVL. ST-segment depression localized to leads I, aVL, V_5 and V_6 may indicate lateral wall ischaemia but it is often the extension of ischaemic changes in other vascular territories.

The number of electrocardiogram leads showing ST-segment change is a poor indicator of the size of the ischaemic region because the various aspects of the heart are not evenly examined by the recording leads. However, the occurrence of marked ST-segment depression in all the chest leads and in lead I and aVL strongly suggests the presence of significant stenosis of the mainstem of the left coronary artery or left coronary disease of equivalent importance.

Bayes' theorem

If exercise testing is used as a means to detect atheromatous coronary artery disease, false-negative tests are frequently found in groups of patients with a high incidence of coronary disease, for example, those with typical angina or previous myocardial infarction. Conversely, false-positive tests are frequent in groups of patients with a low incidence of coronary disease, for example, those with atypical chest pain and asymptomatic individuals.

Bayes' theorem[60,61] states that the probability of the presence or absence of coronary disease depends partly on the prevalence of the disease and partly on the likelihood ratio of the exercise test. The likelihood ratio is the probability that the test results are true, the greater the ratio the more it is likely that the test will be accurate. The ratio is derived as follows:

$$\text{Sensitivity (of test)} = \frac{\text{True positives}}{\text{True positives} + \text{False negatives}}$$

$$\text{Specificity (of test)} = \frac{\text{True negatives}}{\text{True negatives} + \text{False positives}}$$

$$\text{Likelihood ratio for an abnormal test} = \frac{\text{Sensitivity}}{1 - \text{Specificity}}$$

$$\text{Likelihood ratio for a normal test} = \frac{\text{Specificity}}{1 - \text{Sensitivity}}$$

As an example, a middle-aged man with a history suggestive of angina and a normal resting electrocardiogram would have a pre-test risk of 67% of having coronary artery disease. With a multiple-lead system, the likelihood ratio for a positive test is 3.58 and for a negative test, 5.43. Applying Bayes' theorem would increase the probability of coronary disease to 88% for a positive test and reduce it to 32% for a negative test.

Coronary flow reserve

The exercise electrocardiogram provides not only diagnostic information but also an assessment of the patients' coronary flow reserve, particularly when frequent recordings of the systemic arterial pressure are made throughout the test using a sphygmomanometer. The blood pressure should be recorded at rest, in both the lying and standing positions, just before the end of each exercise stage, at the time of 0.1-mV ST-segment depression or elevation, at the cessation of exercise and at 3-min intervals during the recovery phase. If possible, additional recordings should be made at 1-min intervals throughout the exercise period. The single most important recording is that taken at the point of significant ST-segment change because this represents a fixed point for comparing the exercise performance of different patients and for serial testing in individual patients.

As heart rate and arterial blood pressure are the main determinants of myocardial oxygen consumption, the product (known as the double product) of the values of these two parameters at the point of 0.1-mV ST-segment change indicates the amount of heart work that just fails to elicit an adequate increase in regional coronary arterial flow and, therefore, the coronary flow reserve of that patient. Although heart rate and blood pressure are not the only determinants of myocardial oxygen consumption, the double product at the onset of ischaemia is a useful index of coronary flow reserve under most circumstances. A low coronary flow reserve as indicated, for example, by significant ST-segment depression at a heart rate of 95 beats/min and systolic blood pressure at 130 mmHg is usually associated with severe stenosis in the proximal segments of the coronary arterial tree, often involving more than one major coronary branch. Patients with severe left coronary main stem stenosis frequently exhibit low effort tolerance, demonstrable by exercise testing. In patients with extensive coronary disease, particularly those with main stem stenosis, the extensive myocardial ischaemia induced by exercise may depress left ventricular function to such an extent that the blood pressure falls during the exercise test. In the event of a fall in blood pressure during exercise, the test should be terminated immediately. A high double product at the onset of significant ST-segment change, for example, a heart rate of 150 beats/min and systolic blood pressure of 190 mmHg, indicates a good coronary flow reserve. This good effort tolerance is frequently found in patients who have single-vessel disease, but this relationship is not invariable because patients with extensive atheromatous coronary disease may have high or normal effort tolerance, particularly when a collateral circulation has developed. The mismatch often found between the extent of atheromatous coronary disease and effort tolerance is probably due to dynamic changes in coronary arterial calibre.

Variation in coronary flow reserve, reflected as a variation in effort tolerance, is common in patients with chronic stable angina.[62] Not only is there circadian variation but also variation from day to day and over longer time-intervals. Furthermore, the variable effect of drugs over short and long periods will affect the effort tolerance. In certain patients, therefore, it may be necessary to perform more than one test prior to treatment to obtain sufficient information on which to base management.

Relevance of exercise testing to treatment

Drugs for the treatment of effort-related angina pectoris may improve effort tolerance in two ways, thereby increasing the patient's capacity for physical work and recreational exercise.

1 They may delay the point at which the heart rate and blood pressure rise to the level at which coronary flow reserve is exhausted, by reducing either the resting level of these parameters or their rate of rise, or both.

2 They may increase the coronary flow reserve, mainly by coronary vasodilatation, allowing a greater level of heart rate and blood pressure to be achieved without the development of myocardial ischaemia.

Whatever their mechanism of action, drugs are more likely to render a patient asymptomatic if the coronary flow reserve, indicated by the double product at the onset of ischaemia, is high prior to treatment. Surgery or angioplasty is not often required at this stage. However, patients with low effort tolerance prior to treatment are much more likely to require early angioplasty or surgery for persistent symptoms, depending on their response to drugs. Furthermore, this group is likely to contain those patients with left main stem stenosis or severe proximal triple-vessel stenosis for whom surgery is required to improve prognosis.

If a very variable coronary flow reserve has been found prior to treatment or a dramatic increase in coronary flow reserve is induced by the administration of a coronary vasodilator drug,[63] calcium antagonists and nitrates assume greater importance in the drug treatment of that patient because coronary vasoconstriction is likely to be contributing to the genesis of the ischaemic attacks. However, if the patient's coronary flow reserve varies little on sequential testing, with a poor response of the coronary flow reserve (indicated by little change in the double product at the point of significant ST-segment change) to coronary vasodilators, the emphasis of treatment will be on beta-blockade to prevent a significant rise in myocardial oxygen demand.

Occasionally, exercise testing will induce typical angina pectoris but no significant ST-segment change. In other patients, resting electrocardiographic abnormalities, such as conduction defects and extensive QS complexes, will render the electrocardiogram virtually useless as a means of detecting ischaemia. The interpretation of exercise-induced electrocardiographic changes will be difficult in the presence of other resting abnormalities, such as left ventricular hypertrophy, or the effect of digitalis therapy. In these patients, a different indicator of myocardial ischaemia is required. Changes in left ventricular function induced by myocardial ischaemia can be detected by echocardiography[64] or radionuclide imaging; perhaps the most common technique currently in use is electrocardiogram gated technetium-labelled blood pool imaging.[65] Regional myocardial perfusion can be directly assessed by gamma-camera or positron-camera imaging of the myocardial distribution of short-lived radionuclides. Of these latter techniques, the most widely available and most commonly used is thallium-201 myocardial perfusion imaging.[66]

TECHNETIUM-99M BLOOD POOL IMAGING

The principle of this technique is to label the red cells; approximately 370 MBq of technetium-99m is administered intravenously between 20 and 30 min after the intravenous administration of sodium stannous pyrophosphate. After a further 15 min, when labelling is complete, with the patient supine in the semi-reclining position on a table equipped for bicycle exercise, the gamma camera is positioned in the left anterior oblique projection over the thorax and a resting scan is obtained. An acquisition period of about 4 min will usually be sufficient to obtain a series of 16 images of the cardiac chambers spanning one cardiac cycle. This can be displayed in ciné mode for the assessment of regional wall motion and from which can be obtained a time–activity curve representing left ventricular volume changes throughout the cardiac cycle allowing the calculation of ejection fraction. After the resting acquisition, bicycle exercise is commenced, during each stage of which a further scan is obtained. Exercise-induced myocardial ischaemia can be detected, by its effect on myocardial contraction, as the development of a regional wall motion abnormality or as a reduction in left ventricular ejection fraction. It should be remembered, however, that the scans represent the average left ventricular function during the acquisition period and consequently very transient changes may not be detected. The sensitivity of the technique, combined with electrocardiographic recording, in the detection of coronary artery disease is greater than that of exercise electrocardiography alone.

THALLIUM-201 MYOCARDIAL PERFUSION IMAGING

Thallium-201 is a potassium analogue which, following intravenous injection, is rapidly cleared from the blood and enters viable cells throughout the body.[67] It is particularly taken up by myocardial cells and the early myocardial activity is related both to the mass of viable myocardium and to the magnitude of the coronary blood flow. Regional defects of myocardial thallium-201 activity may be due to either old myocardial infarction or acute myocardial ischaemia.[68] After the initial cellular uptake of the tracer, redistribution occurs which becomes significant beyond 30 min after the tracer's administration. This will lead to tracer uptake in a previously ischaemic segment of myocardium.

In order to detect acute myocardial ischaemia, the isotope is injected intravenously during suspected myocardial ischaemia, e.g. during exercise-induced chest pain or electrocardiographic change. In the case of exercise or other provocative test, it is continued for 1 or 2 min to allow clearance of the majority of the tracer from the blood and accumulation of the tracer in the perfused myocardium. The exercise is then stopped and the patient positioned under a gamma camera. Imaging is begun about 10 min after the injection of thallium and repeated in several projections, each image requiring approximately 2 min. The imaging series is then repeated approximately 4 h later when redistribution of tracer is complete. A regional defect of trace uptake detectable only on the initial images indicates acute myocardial ischaemia. A regional defect present on the initial and redistribution images indicates either myocardial infarction, recent or old, or another cause of myocardial necrosis or scarring.

There are several limitations of thallium myocardial perfusion imaging. Uptake of tracer in the liver may obscure the detection of inferior wall ischaemia. As the uptake of thallium into the myocardium is not linearly proportional to flow (a 40% increase in uptake requires a 100% increase in flow), myocardial ischaemia of lesser severity may not be detected. Furthermore, myocardial ischaemia associated with ST-segment depression, as is usually seen in patients who have chronic stable angina, is sub-endocardial and therefore confined to a layer of variable thickness, which may be below the limit of the spatial resolution of a gamma camera and, additionally, may be obscured by overlying layers of normally perfused myocardium. Therefore, negative myocardial perfusion scans can be obtained in some patients with positive exercise electrocardiograms. Nevertheless, unequivocally positive thallium myocardial perfusion scans can be obtained in many instances and provide a valuable secondary technique if the exercise electrocardiogram is unhelpful. The sensitivity of the technique for the detection of coronary artery disease, combined with electrocardiographic recording is greater than that of exercise electrocardiography alone.[69]

CARDIAC CATHETERIZATION

In patients with chronic stable angina, cardiac catheterization involves the insertion of a cardiac catheter into the femoral artery, using the Seldinger technique, or into the brachial artery, by arteriotomy, and its advancement to the heart to record pressures and to obtain a left ventriculogram and right and left coronary arteriograms.

Pressures

From the left ventricular and aortic pressure recordings, essential information can be obtained: the aortic pressure, the left ventricular end-diastolic pressure and the presence and magnitude of any systolic pressure gradient across the aortic valve (indicative of aortic stenosis). The left ventricular end-diastolic pressure is normally < 13 mmHg but it will be elevated in the presence of abnormal left ventricular function. Furthermore, increased amplitude of the 'a' wave may be seen, reflecting increased force of left atrial contraction due to lack of left ventricular compliance.

Left ventriculogram

A left ventriculogram is obtained, in the adult of average size, by the pressurized injection of approximately 30 ml of radiopaque contrast material through the cardiac catheter into the left ventricle, and a recording is made on ciné film. Ideally, recordings should be made in both the right anterior oblique and left anterior oblique projections to allow assessment of all aspects of the left ventricle. For routine clinical purposes, analysis is by inspection; it may reveal an abnormal contraction and relaxation pattern, regional akinesia or dyskinesia, suggestive of a previous myocardial infarction, a dyskinetic region with a narrow base, consistent with an aneurysm, or dilatation with global abnormality of contraction, compatible with widespread myocardial scarring or other diffuse myocardial abnormality. Mitral regurgitation may be found as a jet of contrast material entering the left atrium, due to mitral ring dilatation or ischaemic papillary muscle dysfunction.

More precise evaluation can be obtained by computer-assisted analysis, which requires the recording of a reference grid of known dimensions at the time of cardiac catheterization. Parameters that can be derived from such analysis include the ejection fraction, volume changes throughout the cardiac cycle and the percentage shortening of the left ventricular diameter at various levels within the ventricle and of the long axis of the ventricle. The simplest parameter describing the overall left ventricular function and that most commonly used is the ejection fraction.

Coronary arteriography

Detailed morphological information can be obtained by coronary arteriography. This involves the ciné recording of 3–10 ml of contrast injected by hand through specially designed catheters in the right and left coronary arteries. At least two (orthogonal) projections are required to assess the right coronary artery and at least four are required to assess the left.

Typically, in a patient with effort angina and a positive exercise test, at least one severe atheromatous stenosis will be found, usually in the proximal portion of a major branch. Particularly in those patients who have low effort tolerance, as demonstrated by exercise testing, many significant stenoses may be found, often involving two or three major branches and sometimes involving the main stem of the left coronary artery (Fig. 47.7).

Occasionally, the severity of stenosis will be much less than expected, and in these cases it is likely that transient decreases in coronary calibre or transient increases in coronary vascular resistance

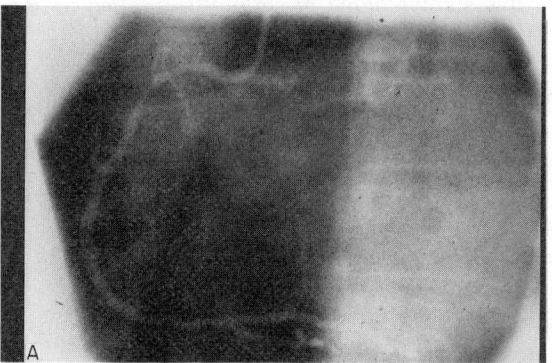

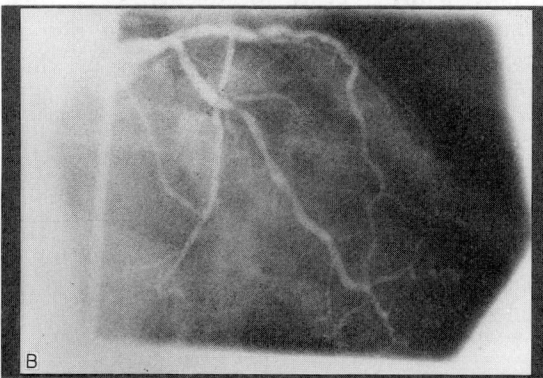

Fig. 47.7. (A) Right and (B) left coronary arteriograms of a patient with chronic stable angina and consistently low effort tolerance. There is diffuse irregularity of the right coronary artery with a proximal severe stenosis. The left coronary artery shows irregularity in the proximal portion of its major branches with a severe stenosis proximally in the left anterior descending artery and also in the proximal part of the circumflex artery.

are contributing to the impaired effort tolerance. For these patients, performance during the exercise test may be dramatically improved by vasodilator drugs.[70]

Indications for coronary arteriography

The information derived from coronary arteriography is complementary to that derived from the history, physical examination and non-invasive investigations; it is important for the assessment of prognosis and the planning of treatment. The overall annual mortality of patients with chronic stable angina is approximately 4%[71,72] and the mortality of diagnostic cardiac catheterization is about 0.1%. However, it should be remembered that the latter is an overall figure and relates mainly to a high-risk subgroup which includes those patients in heart failure, those with unstable angina and those with consistently very low effort tolerance. Despite the safety of coronary arteriography and the value of the information it provides, it is not mandatory for all patients with suspected or known chronic stable angina. It should be applied only to certain subgroups:

1 those with angina that does not respond satisfactorily to drug therapy;
2 those with a positive exercise test at low workload;
3 those who are unable to tolerate the necessary drugs, for whom surgery or angioplasty would provide an alternative form of treatment;
4 those in whom arteriography is required for diagnostic reasons, because of atypical symptoms or equivocal results of non-invasive tests;
5 those patients being investigated by cardiac catheterization for other types of cardiac disease, particularly if they are in the age-group in which coronary disease is common or if they have angina or chest pain which may be of ischaemic origin.

Age is obviously important, and in patients beyond the age of 70 years coronary arteriography should not be undertaken routinely; consideration should be given to the general physical condition of the patient, to the severity of symptoms and to the initial response to drug therapy.

RELEVANCE OF INVESTIGATION TO TREATMENT

There are three major forms of treatment available: drugs, coronary angioplasty and bypass grafting. If a diagnosis of angina pectoris can be made on clinical grounds, drug treatment can be commenced pending the results of investigation.

Following investigation, drug therapy will be required in virtually all patients. Unless there is a contra-indication, it is reasonable to use beta-adrenergic blockade with a long-acting preparation. This will reduce the myocardial oxygen demand for a given level of exercise and therefore increase the duration of exercise that is angina-free. This can be expected to relieve effort-induced angina in the majority of patients who have good coronary flow reserve, i.e. a high double product at the onset of ischaemia on pre-treatment exercise testing. However, if there is residual angina, particularly with occasional spontaneous attacks, a calcium antagonist or nitrate should be added to the regimen; if necessary, both types of drug can be added. In the event of persistent angina, coronary angioplasty or surgery must be considered, depending on the coronary anatomy. Patients with a low coronary flow reserve, as evidenced by formal exercise testing, are less likely to experience sufficient relief of their angina even with maximal drug therapy and are more likely to have extensive atheromatous coronary artery disease—the majority of surgical candidates are in this group. An indication of their likely response to drug therapy can be obtained, if resources allow, by comparing the results of two exercise tests, one performed with the patient off all therapy and the other performed after the acute administration of a calcium antagonist or nitrate. A marked increase in the coronary flow reserve in response to these vasodilators suggests a good response to their chronic administration. A poor response indicates that the severity of the angina can be completely ascribed to severe atheromatous coronary artery disease and, if it cannot be controlled by beta-blockade, it is very likely that coronary angioplasty or surgery will be required.

Although the therapeutic approach should be largely determined by symptoms and functional testing, there are certain morphological patterns that indicate a poor prognosis and therefore arteriographic findings may sometimes dictate the need for surgery, for example, stenosis of the main stem of the left coronary artery and severe proximal stenosis of the three major coronary artery branches. Coronary arteriography is also required to determine the most suitable form of mechanical intervention, either coronary angioplasty or coronary artery bypass surgery.

When planning the therapeutic strategy, clinicians must take into account not only the factors described above but also the risk involved in performing coronary artery bypass surgery. One of the important determinants of this risk is myocardial function; therefore, particular attention should be paid to the left ventriculogram and further information obtained by two-dimensional echocardiography. In general, peri-operative mortality is significantly greater in those patients whose left ventricular ejection fraction is < 30%. However, this risk should be considered with respect to the known natural history of that condition. Thus, severe impairment of left ventricular function is rarely an absolute contra-indication to coronary artery bypass surgery. The situation is different in the presence of heart failure. If the left ventricular or congestive cardiac failure is due to chronic myocardial damage without contribution from acute myocardial ischaemia or valvular abnormality, the peri-operative mortality rate is exceedingly high and represents a contra-indication to coronary artery bypass surgery. In these circumstances, intensive drug therapy is required for both heart failure and myocardial ischaemia. In the younger patient who has heart failure resistant to drugs, consideration should be given to cardiac transplantation (see Chapter 6).

NATURAL HISTORY OF CHRONIC STABLE ANGINA

The term 'chronic stable angina' implies a reasonably favourable outcome when compared with the other subgroups of ischaemic heart disease. In the case of effort-related angina of more than 3 months' duration the overall outlook in terms of mortality and the occurrence of myocardial infarction appears to be reasonably good. The annual mortality rate has been estimated at 4%[71,73] and the annual incidence of acute myocardial infarction at 2.2%. Recent clinical research into acute myocardial infarction indicates that acute thrombotic coronary occlusion does not necessarily occur at the site of severe atheromatous coronary stenosis and that the residual stenosis after successful thrombolysis varies greatly in severity from patient to patient.[74] These findings indicate that many patients suffering acute myocardial infarction do not have a flow-limiting atheromatous stenosis and they are in keeping with the clinical observation that the majority of patients with acute myocardial infarction do not have a history of chronic stable effort angina.

Although the prognosis in chronic stable angina is quite good overall, subgroups of patients can be identified who have a poorer prognosis. One subgroup can be identified on the basis of exercise testing; it comprises those patients who develop myocardial ischaemia at a very low level of the heart rate–blood pressure product and do so consistently on repeat exercise testing.[75] Another subgroup can be identified by coronary arteriography; it consists of those patients with severe atheromatous stenosis of all the major coronary artery branches (triple-vessel disease) and those with left main stem stenosis.[76] A third subgroup consists of those patients who have substantial impairment of left ventricular function, as evidenced by an ejection fraction of < 30% calculated from the left ventriculogram. The three subgroups of low effort tolerance, widespread coronary stenosis and impaired left ventricular function overlap to a large extent.

POST-INFARCTION ANGINA

In the early weeks following acute myocardial infarction, between 16 and 30% of patients will begin to experience effort angina[77] which, in the majority, will be found to be stable with the passage of time. Painful or painless ST-segment changes will be found in approximately 70% of patients on formal exercise testing, which are most likely to be due to acute myocardial ischaemia when the involved electrocardiogram leads are outside the territory of infarction. The significance of exercise-induced painless ST-segment changes within the territory of infarction is less certain; they may be related to geometric changes in the region of the myocardial scar. However, infarction is not usually uniform throughout the thickness of the left ventricular wall, patches of viable myocardium remain, and coronary patency, either spontaneous or due to thrombolysis, is common after myocardial infarction.[78] Therefore, acute effort-induced myocardial ischaemia within the infarct region is not an unreasonable possibility as an explanation of these acute electrocardiographic changes.

The mechanism of effort-induced myocardial ischaemia in these patients appears to be similar to that found in other patients with chronic stable angina, predominantly an increase in myocardial oxygen demand in the presence of a coronary flow reserve limited by a fixed coronary stenosis. The nature of this fixed coronary stenosis is, however, not clear. Although atheroma accounts for part of it, many such patients did not suffer with effort angina prior to the myocardial infarction and the stenosis at coronary angioplasty often presents little resistance to the passage of the balloon catheter, suggesting that recent thrombus might contribute to the severity of stenosis. Furthermore, the severity of residual coronary stenosis after thrombolysis in these patients is variable and frequently < 50% of the luminal diameter.

The principles of the treatment of post-infarction effort angina are similar to those of chronic stable angina without infarction described above. A large proportion of patients who have suffered a recent infarct but have no history of previous infarction have single-vessel disease and, in the event of patency of that vessel, are candidates for coronary angioplasty should their angina not be easy to control with drugs. In patients with persistent complete coronary occlusion with or without multi-vessel disease in whom the angina is difficult to control with drugs, coronary artery bypass grafting may be required. This should be postponed for at least 6 weeks after the onset of myocardial infarction, if circumstances permit, because peri-operative mortality is significantly greater in the early post-infarction period.[79]

RECURRENT ANGINA AFTER SURGERY

Coronary artery bypass surgery relieves angina completely in about 85% of patients and leads to improvement in approximately 10%.[80] Among the former group, angina can occasionally occur when the patient engages in exceptional physical exercise and many of these patients will have a positive exercise test for myocardial ischaemia, unaccompanied by pain, at a high workload.

Recurrent angina may be related to early graft stenosis or occlusion, typically within 6 months of surgery, or late stenosis or occlusion, most frequently between 7 and 10 years after surgery.[81-83] Early occlusion is mainly due to low flow secondary to distal coronary disease or supply to an infarcted region or is caused by intra-operative technical factors. Late stenosis or occlusion is caused by the development of atherosclerosis in the graft or in the vessel it supplies. In addition, there is a more consistent occurrence of post-operative angina related to either the failure to bypass a significant coronary stenosis or the development of stenosis in branches unaffected at the time of surgery.

Graft or native vessel stenosis and occlusions may be silent and unassociated with myocardial ischaemia or infarction, due to the presence of collateral blood supply. When this is inadequate, the patient may present with chronic stable angina, unstable angina or acute myocardial infarction. Those with chronic stable angina need not necessarily be investigated by coronary arteriography unless it is clear that, because of failure to respond adequately to drug therapy, coronary angioplasty or repeat surgery may be required. In general, repeated coronary artery bypass surgery is less desirable than first-time surgery because of its higher operative mortality and reduced effectiveness in the relief of angina.[84]

Initial investigation is very similar to that of other patients who have chronic stable angina and includes the recording of resting and exercise 12-lead electrocardiograms. Although the grafted heart has many potential routes of blood supply, in patients presenting with angina, the native vessels and most of the grafts may be occluded and it is therefore conceivable that the continued survival of the patient depends virtually on one diseased graft. Particular caution should be taken with the invasive investigation of previously grafted patients presenting with unstable angina or with crescendo effort angina and those previously grafted patients with chronic stable angina who, on formal exercise testing, are found to have a very low threshold for myocardial ischaemia. These patients should be on maximal drug therapy with appropriate doses of nitrates, calcium antagonists and beta-adrenergic blocking agents prior to cardiac catheterization and should be given adequate sedative pre-medication to cover the procedure.

CONCLUSION

A clear understanding of the pathogenetic mechanisms involved in chronic stable angina together with careful history-taking, physical examination and a logical sequence of investigation will lead to rational decisions on treatment and thereby to the optimal management of these patients.

REFERENCES

1. Maseri, A., Severi, S., De Nes, M., L'Abbate, A., Chierchia, S., Marzilli, M., Ballestra, A.M., Parodi, O., Biagini, A. and Distante, A. Variant angina: one aspect of a continuous spectrum of vasospastic myocardial ischemia. Pathogenetic

mechanisms, estimated incidence, clinical and coronarographic findings in 138 patients. *Am. J. Cardiol.* 1978; **42**: 1019.

2. Sherman, C.T., Litvack, F., Grundfest, W. *et al.* Coronary angioscopy in patients with unstable angina pectoris. *N. Engl. J. Med.* 1986; **315**: 913.

3. Folts, J.D., Crowell, E.B. and Rowe, G.C. Platelet aggregation in partially obstructed vessels and its elimination with aspirin. *Circulation* 1976; **54**: 365–70.

4. Maseri, A., L'Abbate, A., Pesola, A., Ballestra, A.M., Marzilli, M., Maltinti, G., Severi, S., De Nes, D.M., Parodi, O. and Biagni, A. Coronary vasospasm in angina pectoris. *Lancet* 1977; **i**: 713–7.

5. Prinzmetal, M., Kennamer, R. and Merliss, R. Angina pectoris. I. A variant form of angina pectoris. *Am. J. Med.* 1959; **27**: 375–88.

6. Mandelkorn, J.B., Wolf, N.M., Singh, S. *et al.* Intracoronary thrombus in non-transmural myocardial infarction and in unstable angina pectoris. *Am. J. Cardiol.* 1983; **52**: 1.

7. Rentrop, K., Blanke, H., Karsh, K., Wiegand, V., Kostering, H., Oster, H. and Leitz, K. Acute myocardial infarction: intracoronary application of nitroglycerine and streptokinase. *Clin. Cardiol.* 1979; **2**: 354–63.

8. Robinson, B.F. Relation of heart rate and systolic blood pressure to the onset of pain in angina pectoris. *Circulation* 1967; **35**: 1073.

9. MacAlpin, R. Contribution of dynamic vascular wall thickening to luminal narrowing during coronary arterial constriction. *Circulation* 1980; **61**: 296.

10. Maseri, A. Pathogenetic mechanisms of angina pectoris: expanding views. *Br. Heart J.* 1980; **43**: 648–60.

11. Maseri, A., Chierchia, S. and L'Abbate, A. Pathogenetic mechanisms underlying the clinical events associated with atherosclerotic heart disease. *Circulation* 1980; **62** (Suppl. V): 3–13.

12. McMahon, M., Brown, B., Cukingnan, R., Rolett, E., Bolsen, E., Frimer, M. and Dodge, H. Quantitative coronary arteriography: measurement of the "critical" stenosis in patients with unstable angina and single vessel disease without collaterals. *Circulation* 1979; **60**: 106–13.

13. Crea, F., Margonato, A., Kaski, J.C., Rodriguez-Plaza, L., Meran, D.O., Davies, G., Chierchia, S. and Maseri, A. Variability of results during repeat exercise stress testing in patients with stable angina pectoris: role of dynamic coronary flow reserve. *Am. Heart J.* 1986; **112**: 249–54.

14. Uthurralt, N., Davies, G.J., Parodi, O., Bencivelli, W. and Maseri, A. Comparative study of myocardial ischaemia during angina at rest and on exertion using thallium-201 scintigraphy. *Am. J. Cardiol.* 1981; **48**: 410–7.

15. Screoder, J., Bolen, J., Quint, R., Clark, D., Hayden, W., Higgins, C. and Wexler, L. Provocation of coronary spasm with ergovine maleate: a new test with results in 57 patients undergoing coronary arteriography. *Am. J. Cardiol.* 1977; **46**: 487–91.

16. Scholl, J.M., Benacerra, F.A., Ducimetiere, P., Chabas, D., Brau, J., Chapelle, J. and Thery, J.C. Compensation of risk factors in vasospastic angina without significant fixed coronary narrowing to significant fixed coronary narrowing and no vasospastic angina. *Am. J. Cardiol.* 1986; **57**: 199.

17. Serruys, P., Arnold, A., Brower, R., deBono, D., Bokslag, M., Lubsen, J., Reiber, J., Rutsch, W., Uebis, R., Vahanian, A. and Verstraete, M. Effect of continued rt-PA administration on the residual stenosis after initially successful recanalization in acute myocardial infarction—a quantitative angiocardiography study of a randomised trial. *Eur. Heart J.* 1987; **8**: 1172–81.

18. Guazzi, M., Fiorentim, C., Polese, A. and Magrini, F. Continuous electrocardiographic in Prinzmetal's variant angina pectoris. A report of four cases. *Br. Heart J.* 1970; **32**: 611–6.

19. Davies, G.J., Bencivelli, W., Fragasso, G., Chierchia, S., Crea, F., Crowe, J., Pratt, T., Morgan, M., Crean, P. and Maseri, A. Sequence and magnitude of ventricular volume changes in painful and painless myocardial ischaemia. *Circulation* 1988; **78**: 310–319.

20. Schiffer, F., Hartley, L.H., Schulman, C.L. and Abelmann, W.H. Evidence for emotionally induced coronary arterial spasm in patients with angina pectoris. *Br. Heart J.* 1980; **44**: 62.

21. Feldman, R.L., Whittle, J.C., Marx, J.D., Pepine, C. and Conti, R. Regional coronary hemodynamic responses to cold stimulation in patients without variant angina. *Am. J. Cardiol.* 1982; **49**: 655–73.

22. Goldstein, R.W., Redwood, D.R., Rosing, D.R., Beiser, G.D. and Epstein, S.E. Alterations in the circulatory response to exercise following a meal and their relationship in postprandial angina pectoris. *Circulation* . 1971; **44**: 90.

23. Starling, M.R., Moody, M., Crawford, M.I., Levi, B. and O'Rourke, R. Repeat treadmill exercise testing: variability of results in patients with angina pectoris. *Am. Heart J.* 1984; **107**: 298.

24. Chierchia, S., Smith, G., Morgan, M., Gallino, A., Deanfield, J., Croom, M. and Maseri, A. Role of heart rate in pathophysiology of chronic stable angina. *Lancet* 1984; **ii**: 1353.

25. Chierchia, S., Brunelli, C., Simonetti, J., Lazzari, M. and Maseri, A. Sequence of events in angina at rest: primary reduction in coronary flow. *Circulation* 1980; **61**: 759–68.

26. Brown, B.G., Lee, A.B., Bolson, E.L. and Dodge, H.T. Reflex constriction of significant coronary stenosis as a mechanism contributing to ischemic left ventricular dysfunction during isometric exercise. *Circulation* 1984; **70**: 18.

27. Brown, B.G., Bolson, E.L. and Dodge, H.T. Dynamic mechanisms in human coronary stenosis. *Circulation* 1984; **70**: 917.

28. Figueras, J., Singh, B.N., Ganz, W. and Swan, H.J.C. Haemodynamic and electrocardiographic accompaniments of resting post-prandial angina. *Br. Heart J.* 1979; **42**: 402–9.

29. Polak, J.M., Pearse, A.G.E., Garaud, J.-C. and Bloom, S.R. Cellular localisation of a vasoactive intestinal peptide in the mammalian and avian gastro-intestinal tract. *Gut* 1974; **15**: 720–4.

30. Harper, R.W., Kennedy, G., DeSanctis, R.W. and Hutter, A.M. Jr. The incidence and pattern of angina prior to acute myocardial infarction. A study of 577 cases. *Am. Heart J.* 1979; **97**: 178–83.

31. Chiariello, M., Indolfi, C., Catecchia, M.R., Sifola, C., Romano, M. and Condorelli, M. Asymptomatic transient S-T changes during ambulatory ECG monitoring in diabetic patients. *Am. Heart J.* 1985; **110**: 529–32.

32. Kannel, W.B. and Abbott, R.D. Incidence and prognosis of unrecognized myocardial infarction. An update on the Framingham study. *N. Engl. J. Med.* 1984; **311**: 1144–7.

33. Frishman, W.H. Pharmacology of the nitrates in angina pectoris. *Am. J. Cardiol.* 1985; **56**: 81–90.

34. Schang, S.J. and Pepine, C.J. Transient asymptomatic S-T depression during daily activity. *Am. J. Cardiol.* 1977; **39**: 396–402.

35. Guazzi, M., Magrini, F., Fiorentini, C. and Polese, A. Clinical electrocardiographic and haemodynamic effects of long term use of propranolol in Prinzmetal's variant angina pectoris. *Br. Heart J.* 1971; **33**: 889–94.

36. Chierchia, S., Lazzari, M., Simonetti, I. and Maseri, A. Haemodynamic monitoring in angina at rest. *Herz* 1980; **5**: 189–98.

37. Deanfield, J.E., Maseri, A. and Selwyn, A.P. Myocardial ischaemia during daily life in patients with stable angina: its relation to symptoms and heart-rate changes. *Lancet* 1983; **11**: 753–8.

38. Glazier, J.J., Chierchia, S., Brown, M.J. and Maseri, A. Importance of generalized defective perception of painful stimuli as a cause of silent myocardial ischemia in chronic stable angina pectoris. *Am. J. Cardiol.* 1986; **58**: 667–72.

39. Fields, H.L. and Basbaum, A.I. Endogenous pain control mechanisms. In: Wall, P.D. and Melzack, R., eds. *Textbook of Pain*. Edinburgh: Churchill Livingstone, 1984.

40. Grattinger, J.S., Parsons, R.L. and Campbell, J.A. A correlation of clinical and hemodynamic studies in patients with mild and severe anemia with and without congestive failure. *Ann. Intern. Med.* 1963; **58**: 617.

41. Resnekov, L. and Falicov, R.E. Thyrotoxicosis and lactate producing angina pectoris with normal coronary arteries. *Br. Heart J.* 1977; **39**: 1051–57.

42. Meller, J., Conde, C.A., Deppisch, L.M., Donoso, E. and Dack, S. Myocardial infarction due to coronary atherosclerosis in three young adults with systemic lupus erythematosus. *Am. J. Cardiol.* 1975; **35**: 309.

43. Holsinger, D.R., Osmundson, P.J. and Edwards, J.E. The heart in Periarteritis Nodosa. *Circulation* 1962; **25**: 610.

44. Daniels, S.R., Specker, B., Capannari, T.E., Schwartz, D.C., Burke, M. and Kaplan, S. Correlates of coronary artery aneurysm formation in patients with Kawasaki's disease. *Am. J. Dis. Child.* 1987; **141**: 205–7.

45. Moraski, R.E., Russell, R.O., Mantle, J.A. and Rockley, C.E. Aortic Stenosis, Angina Pectoris, Coronary Artery Disease. *Cathet. Cardiovasc. Diag.* 1976; **2**: 157.

46. Wood, P. Pulmonary stenosis with normal aortic root. In: *Diseases of the Heart and Circulation*, 3rd edn. London: Eyre and Spottiswoode, 1968, p.503.

47. Sleeper, J.C., Orgain, E.S. and McIntosh, H.D. Primary pulmonary hypertension. Review of clinical features and pathologic physiology with a report of pulmonary hemodynamics derived from repeat catheterization. *Circulation* 1962; **26**: 1358–9.

48. Wood, P. Eisenmenger's syndrome or pulmonary hypertension with a revised shunt. In: *Diseases of the Heart and Circulation*, 3rd edn. London: Eyre and Spottiswoode, 1968, p. 475.

49. Cheitlin, M.D., McAllister, H.A. and deCastro, C.M. Myocardial infarction without atherosclerosis. *JAMA* 1975; **231**: 951.

50. Rubio, P.A., Al-Bassam, M.S. and Shaw, L.B. Fistula between the left anterior descending coronary artery and the pulmonary artery causing angina in two middle-aged patients. *South. Med. J.* 1987; **80**: 518–9.

51. Ouzts, H.G., Turner, J.L., Douglas, J.S. Jr and Hurst, J.W. Prolonged chest pain suggesting myocardial infarction in patients with hypertrophic cardiomyopathy. In: Hurst, J.W., ed. *Update 111: The Heart*. New York: McGraw-Hill, 1980, p.139.

52. Nakhjavan, F.K., Natarajan, G., Seshachary, P. and Goldberg, H. The relationship between prolapsing mitral valve leaflet syndrome and angina and normal coronary arteriograms. *Chest* 1976; **70**: 706–10.

53. Samuelson, O., Wilhelmsen, L., Pennert, K. and Berglund, G. Angina Pectoris, Intermittent Claudication and Congestive Heart Failure in Middle-aged Male Hypertensives. *Acta Med. Scand.* 1987; **221**: 23–32.

54. Gahl, K., Sutton, R., Pearson, M. Caspari, P., Lairet, A. and McDonald, L. Mitral regurgitation in coronary heart disease. *Br. Heart J.* 1977; **39**: 13.

55. Bruce, R.A., Blackman, J.R., Jones, J.W. and Strait, G. Exercise testing in adult normal subjects and cardiac patients. *Paediatrics* 1963; **32**: 742–756.

56. Blackburn, H. *et al.* The standardization of the exercise ECG. A symptomatic comparison of chest lead configurations employed for monitoring during exercise. In: Simonson, E., ed. *Physical Activity and the Heart*. Springfield, Illinois: Charles C. Thomas, 1967.

57. Helfant, R.H. *et al.* Exercise related ventricular premature complexes in coronary heart disease. *Ann. Intern. Med.* 1974; **80**: 589.

58. Chahine, R.A., Raezner, A.E. and Ischimori, T. The clinical significance of exercise-induced ST segment elevation. *Circulation* 1976; **54**: 209.

59. Ellestad, M.H. ECG patterns and their significance. In: *Stress Testing. Principles and Practice*, 3rd edn. Philadelphia: F.A. Davis, 1986, p. 223.

60. Diamond, G.A. *et al.* Application of conditioned probability analysis to the clinical diagnosis of coronary artery disease. *J. Clin. Invest.* 1980; **65**: 1210–20.

61. Rifkin, R.D. and Hood, N.B. Bayesian analysis and electrocardiographic exercise stress testing. *N. Engl. J. Med.* 1977; **297**: 681–6.

62. Maseri, A. Mixed angina pectoris. *Am. J. Cardiol.* 1985; **56**: 30E.

63. Brown, B.G., Bolson, E., Petersen, R.B., Pierce, C.D. and Dodge, H.T. The mechanisms of nitroglycerin action; stenosis vasodilation as a major component of the drug response. *Circulation* 1981; **64**: 1089–92.

64. Robertson, W.S., Feigenbaum, H., Armstrong, W.F., Dillon, J.C., O'Donnell, J. and McHenry, P.W. Exercise echocardiography, a clinically practical addition in the evaluation of coronary artery disease. *J. Am. Coll. Cardiol.* 1983; **2**: 1085.

65. Borer, J., Bacharach, S.L., Green, M.V., Kent, K.M., Epstein, S.E. and Johnston, G.S. Real-time radionuclide cineangiography in non-invasive evaluation of global and regional left ventricular function at rest and during exercise in patients with coronary artery disease. *N. Engl. J. Med.* 1977; **296**: 839.

66. Bailey, I.K., Griffith, L.S.C., Rouleau, J., Strauss, H.W. and Pitt, W. Thallium-201 myocardial imaging at rest and during exercise. Comparative sensitivity to electrocardiography in coronary artery disease. *Circulation* 1977; **55**: 79.

67. Weich, H.F., Strauss, H.W. and Pitt, B. The extraction of thallium-201 by the myocardium. *Circulation* 1977; **56**: 188.

68. Leibowitz, E., Greene, M.W., Bradley-Moore, P., Atkins, H., Ansari, A., Richards, P. and Belgrave, E. 201-Thallium for medical use. *J. Nucl. Med.* 1973; **14**: 421.

69. Rigo, P., Bailey, I.K., Griffith, L.S.C., Pitt, B., Barrow, R.D., Wagner, H.N. Jr and Becker, L.C. Value and limitations of segmental analysis of stress thallium myocardial imaging for localization of coronary artery disease. *Circulation* 1980; **61**: 973.

70. Stone, P.H., Antman, E.M., Muller, J.E. and Braunwald, E. Calcium channel-blocking agents in the treatment of cardiovascular disorders. Part 11. Haemodynamic effects and clinical applications. *Ann. Intern. Med.* 1980; **93**: 886.

71. Kannel, W.B. and Feinlieb, M. Natural history of angina pectoris in the Framingham study. Progress and survival. *Am. J. Cardiol.* 1972; **29**: 154.

72. Reeves, T.J., Oberman, A., Jones, W.B. and Sheffield, L.T. Natural history of angina pectoris. *Am. J. Cardiol.* 1974; **33**: 423–30.

73. Proudfit, W.J., Brushke, A.V.G., MacMillan, J.P., Williams, G.W. and Sones, F.M. Jr. Fifteen year survival study of patients with obstructive coronary artery disease. *Circulation* 1983; **68**: 986.

74. Brown, B., Gallery, C., Badger, R., Kennedy, J., Mathey, D., Bolson, E. and Dodge, H. Incomplete lysis of thrombus in the moderate underlying atherosclerotic lesion during intracoronary infusion of streptokinase for acute myocardial infarction: quantitative angiographic observations. *Circulation* 1986; **73**: 653–61.

75. Cole, J.R. and Ellestad, M.H. Significance of chest pain during treadmill exercise: correlation with coronary events. *Am. J. Cardiol.* 1978; **41**: 227.

76. Stone, P.H., LaFolette, E.L. and Cohn, K. Patterns of

exercise treadmill test performance in patients with left main coronary artery disease: detection dependent on left coronary dominance or coexistent right dominant coronary artery disease. *Am. Heart J.* 1982; **104**: 13.

77. Bosch, X., Theroux, P., Waters, D.D., Pelletier, G.B. and Roy, D. Early post-infarction ischemia: clinical, angiographic and prognostic significance. *Circulation* 1987; **75**: 988.

78. DeWood, M.A., Spores, J., Notske, R., Mouser, L.T., Burroughs, R., Golden, M.S. and Lang, H.T. Prevalence of total coronary occlusion during the early hours of transmural myocardial infarction. *N. Engl. J. Med.* 1980; **303**: 897.

79. Kennedy, J.W., Kaiser, G.C., Fisher, L.D., Fritz, J.K., Nyers, W., Mudd, J.G. and Ryan, T.J. Clinical and angiographic predictors of operative mortality from the collaborative study in coronary artery surgery (CASS). *Circulation* 1981; **63**: 793.

80. Rutherford, J.D., Whitlock, R.M.L., McDonald, B.W., Barratt-Boyes, B.G. and Kerr, A.R. Multivariate analysis of the long-term results of coronary artery by-pass grafting performed during 1976 and 1977. *Am. J. Cardiol.* 1986; **57**: 1264.

81. CASS Principal Investigators and their Associates: Coronary Artery Surgery Study (CASS): A randomized study of coronary artery by-pass surgery. Quality of life in patients randomly assigned to treatment groups. *Circulation* 1983; **68**: 951.

82. Haltgren, H.M., Peduzzi, P., Detre, K., Takaro, T. and the study participants: The five-year effect of by-pass surgery on relief of angina and exercise performance. *Circulation* 1985; **72** (Suppl. V): 79.

83. Campeau, L., Enjalbert, M., Lesperance, J., Vaislic, C., Grondin, C.M., Bourassa, M.G. Atherosclerosis and late closure of aortocoronary saphenous vein grafts: sequential angiographic studies at 2 weeks, 1 years, 5 to 7 years and 10–12 years after surgery. *Circulation* 1983; **68** (Suppl. II): 1.

84. Foster, E.D., Fisher, L.D., Kaiser, G.C. and Myers, W.O. Comparison of operative mortality and morbidity for mitrial and repeat coronary artery by-pass grafting: The Coronary Artery Study (CASS) registry experience. *Ann. Thorac. Surg.* 1984; **38**: 563–70.

Chapter 48

The Treatment of Chronic Stable Angina

K.M. Fox

The use of nitrates for the relief of angina pectoris was first described in 1857 by Lauder Brunton;[1] in 1879, William Murrel demonstrated that glyceryl trinitrin had similar effects.[2] For almost 100 years after Lauder Brunton's description, sublingual nitrates were the mainstay of treatment. However, in the early 1960s, the introduction of beta-adrenoceptor blocking drugs and, later, calcium antagonists has almost revolutionized the treatment of patients with chronic stable angina pectoris. Also, in the last 25 years, the management of these patients has changed dramatically with the introduction of coronary artery bypass graft surgery and coronary angioplasty.

As considerable advances have been made in our understanding of the pathophysiology of stable angina (see Chapter 47), it is now possible to direct treatment at the underlying cause by selecting the appropriate therapy or combination of therapies; the symptoms of the majority of patients with chronic stable angina can be successfully treated and many individuals are able to resume a normal active life. However, our understanding of the effects of these therapies on prognosis is less clear.

The pathophysiology of angina pectoris has been described in Chapter 47. When selecting treatment for patients with angina pectoris, it is important to bear in mind the principal mechanisms leading to the development of myocardial ischaemia: increases in myocardial oxygen demand in the presence of fixed atherosclerotic narrowing, alterations in coronary tone in the presence of atherosclerotic disease, in which both increased myocardial oxygen demand and a reduction in coronary blood flow will have an important role and, finally, coronary spasm in patients with normal coronary arteries, in which a reduction in coronary blood flow predominates. It is also important to be aware that more than one mechanism may occur in any one patient. Although the general aim of the investigation of patients with angina pectoris (see Chapter 47) is to establish a diagnosis, investigation should also be specifically directed in an attempt to identify the appropriate pathophysiological mechanisms in each individual and assess the severity of any derangements so that a full anatomical and physiological profile is assembled. On the basis of this information, the appropriate treatment can be selected.

MEDICAL TREATMENT

Before starting treatment for angina, a general assessment of risk factors and adverse features of lifestyle, including cigarette smoking, hyperlipidaemia, hypertension, obesity and lack of physical activity, should be made. Appropriate advice on the importance of these risk factors and treatment, where necessary, are essential in the medical management of angina pectoris. It is also important that the physician is aware of the adverse interactions between some of these risk factors and commonly used treatments, for example, smoking decreases the efficacy of certain anti-anginal drugs, particularly beta-blockers and calcium antagonists,[3] and hyperlipidaemia may cause premature coronary artery bypass graft occlusion.

The aim of medical treatment is to reduce myocardial oxygen requirements or to increase myocardial perfusion. Often, it may be possible to achieve both aims. However, in patients in whom the overriding mechanism is fixed obstructive coronary disease and increases in myocardial oxygen demand predominate, drugs that reduce myocardial oxygen requirements are to be preferred; in contrast, if patients have coronary spasm in the presence of normal coronary arteries, drugs that relieve spasm and increase coronary blood flow will be the most appropriate.

NITRATES

Nitrates (nitroglycerine, isosorbide dinitrate) were initially introduced in a sublingual form, which is still the first line of therapy in all patients with angina pectoris. Sublingual nitrates work rapidly, i.e. within minutes, and the effect lasts for about 30–45 min. Profound relief of symptoms is the result of a series of events: initially, there is smooth muscle relaxation with reduction in afterload, followed by profound venodilatation causing the pooling of blood peripherally which reduces the filling pressure of the left ventricle;[4–6] this reduced filling pressure has two important consequences—a reduction in myocardial wall stress and in myocardial oxygen consumption, and a fall in left ventricular end-diastolic pressure, which facilitates greater capillary blood flow to the ischaemic area. Nitrates may also improve oxygenation and nutrient flow to areas of myocardial ischaemia; sub-endocardial oxygenation is enhanced, collateral flow increases and there may be a redistribution of coronary flow towards ischaemic zones of the myocardium.[7,8] Finally, nitrates cause dilatation of the large coronary arteries,[9,10] a particularly important effect in variant angina in which coronary spasm is the predominant mechanism and also where alterations in coronary tone influence the threshold of the onset of angina.[11–13] This effect is probably not important in patients with fixed obstructive coronary disease.

Sublingual nitrates or those in aerosol form[14,15] should be offered to all patients with angina pectoris irrespective of the underlying pathophysiology because these drugs will have beneficial effects on all of the known pathophysiological mechanisms. In addition, patients should be instructed to use sublingual nitrates prophylactically, i.e. if they are about to undertake any activity that is likely to induce chest pain. Recent evidence has suggested that glyceryl trinitrin and isosorbide dinitrate may be degraded to inactive compounds when carried in plastic bottles and exposed to sunlight. For patients who use sublingual nitrates only infrequently, the use of a nitroglycerine or isosorbide dinitrate spray may be preferable because this formulation is stable for up to 2 years.

In recent years, many nitrate delivery systems have been developed for chronic prophylactic use (Table 48.1),[16] including the transmucosal or buccal preparations of nitroglycerine,[17,18] the oral preparations of isosorbide dinitrate, sustained released isosorbide dinitrate and sustained release isosorbide mononitrate.[19] Various transcutaneous preparations have also been developed, such as nitroglycerine and isosorbide dinitrate ointment, nitroglycerine cream and nitroglycerine discs or patches. For patients with unstable angina, intravenous nitroglycerine and isosorbide dinitrate are also available. Although sublingual nitroglycerine has an onset of action within 5 min, with a peak action within 10 min and a duration of action of about 30–35 min, the buccal preparations may have a duration of action lasting up to 5 h. Oral isosorbide dinitrate and oral nitroglycerine have an onset of action of about 15–45 min, with a peak action of 45 min to 2 h and a duration of action of up to about 6 h. The nitroglycerine discs or transdermal nitrates have an onset of action of about 30–60 min, with a peak action of 60 min to 3 h and a duration of action covering 24 h.

Isosorbide dinitrate was introduced as a long-acting therapy; if given in large enough doses, therapeutic blood levels are obtained. Isosorbide dinitrate is extensively metabolized in its first pass through the liver; its bioavailability is about 25%. The drug is metabolized to two pharmacologically active components, 5-mononitrate and 2-

Table 48.1. **Nitrate delivery systems.**[a]

Delivery system	Onset of action (min)	Peak action (min)	Duration
Sublingual nitroglycerine	2–5	4–8	10–30 min
Lingual nitroglycerine spray	2–5	4–8	10–30 min
Sublingual isosorbide dinitrate	5–20	15–60	45–120 min
Buccal nitroglycerine	2–5	4–10	30–300 min
Oral isosorbide dinitrate	15–45	45–120	2–6 h
Oral nitroglycerine	20–45	45–120	2–6 h
Oral isosorbide mononitrate	15–45	45–120	6–10 h
Nitroglycerine discs	30–60	60–180	Up to 24 h

[a] From: Abrams, J. The use of nitroglycerine and long-acting nitrates in angina pectoris. In: Weiner, D.A. and Frishman, W.H., eds. *Therapy of Angina Pectoris*. New York/Basel: Marcel Dekker.

mononitrate. The results of the use of oral long-acting nitrates are conflicting, and it has become clear that patients can develop at least partial tolerance to this therapy.[20,21] The mechanism of nitrate tolerance is not understood. However, it is thought that nitrates act by stimulating the production of cyclic guanosine monophosphate in smooth muscle which leads to dilatation. This may cause decreased entry of calcium into the muscle cell or increased uptake of calcium by the sarcoplasmic reticulum. Continued administration of nitrate may lead to a deficiency of reduced sulphydryl groups which are necessary for the production of guanosine monophosphate. The ease of induction of nitrate tolerance appears to be related to the dose, the duration of action and the number of daily nitrate doses administered. Nitrate formulations that provide sustained and constant plasma nitrate levels for many hours seem to be more likely to induce tolerance.[22,23] The results of recent studies have shown that tolerance develops very rapidly, probably within 24 h, although the degree of tolerance does vary among patients. However, after the drug is discontinued, tolerance appears to be abolished quickly, probably within about 18 h of drug withdrawal. Thus, in single-dose studies of long-acting nitrates, exercise tolerance and the time to the onset of angina were prolonged;[24] in studies involving the prolonged use of long-acting nitrates for 1 week or longer, the beneficial effects are not as marked. It is possible that by manipulating the release of isosorbide dinitrate pharmacologically and by appropriate dosage, such that a nitrate-free period occurs during the night, the problem of tolerance may be obviated.

In view of the problems of the uncertain bioavailability of isosorbide dinitrate, oral preparations of the 5-mononitrate have been developed. Isosorbide-5-mononitrate, which has a plasma half-life of 4.2 h, does not undergo significant first pass metabolism and has a predictable systemic bioavailability. The use of the skin or the buccal mucosa as a site of absorption also avoids the effects of first pass hepatic metabolism. Although transdermal and buccal nitrates provide prolonged effective action, these preparations are also subject to the possible development of tolerance in the same way as oral isosorbide dinitrate. However, the use of a nitrate-free interval between dosing is an effective means of overcoming the development of tolerance.

Individual patient sensitivity to organic nitrates is extremely variable and unpredictable. Some pa-

tients are very responsive to nitrates and will develop headaches, hypotension and dizziness when given them in low doses, whereas others are either relatively or completely resistant to the effects of nitrate and require very large doses. Nitrate dosage should be titrated for each individual patient, starting with a small dose which should be increased until the desired clinical effect has been achieved or until side-effects occur. Although long-acting nitrates may be effective in patients who have angina due to increases in myocardial oxygen demand, nitrates are specifically indicated in those who have coronary vasospasm, particularly in the presence of normal coronary arteries, and in those who have severe left ventricular dysfunction[25] or mitral regurgitation.[26] Long-acting nitrates have been shown to be beneficial in patients with heart failure, and the exercise-induced increases in left ventricular end-diastolic pressure and pulmonary artery pressure are attenuated following nitrate administration in patients with angina. These effects of nitrates in patients with mitral regurgitation may be helpful because nitrates can improve forward cardiac performance at the expense of the mitral regurgitant fraction.

The most common side-effects of nitrate administration include headache, dizziness, overt fainting and nausea. The headache may simply be a feeling of throbbing or fullness in the head, but some patients complain of such severe headaches that the further use of nitrates is impossible. Most of these symptoms usually attenuate or disappear during chronic therapy and often it is worthwhile counselling the patient to persevere with nitrate therapy for about 7 days to see if these side-effects become tolerable. Alternatively, a small reduction in the nitrate dosage may be adequate to lessen these effects.

Methaemaglobinaemia is a possible adverse consequence of chronic high-dose nitrate administration.[27] The importance of this finding is not known. Topical nitrates can cause a rash or dermatitis; if so, this form of therapy should be discontinued.

BETA-ADRENOCEPTOR BLOCKING AGENTS

In patients in whom an increase in myocardial oxygen demand in the presence of atherosclerotic narrowing of the coronary arteries is the prominent mechanism for producing angina pectoris, beta-blockers have been proved to be effective.[28,29] Beta-blockers act by blocking the beta-1 receptor; some beta-blockers also block the beta-2 receptor and all beta-blockers have some effect on the beta-2 receptor.[30] Blockade of the beta-1 receptor slows the heart rate and reduces myocardial contractility; both these effects will reduce myocardial oxygen demand. Beta-blockers may also reduce myocardial oxygen demand by altering the metabolic substrate used by the heart.[31] Although the clinical importance of this effect is not known, theoretically the shift in substrate for myocardial metabolism from free fatty acids to carbohydrates would decrease myocardial oxygen consumption while causing lactate production to revert to extraction.[32]

Although beta-blockers are used as first-line agents in most patients with chronic effort-related angina, a few patients who have ischaemic heart disease and overt heart failure, beta-blockers can increase myocardial oxygen requirements of the heart by increasing left ventricular fibre length and left ventricular end-diastolic pressure. Increases in left ventricular end-diastolic pressure could limit an already compromised sub-endocardial blood flow and these factors could offset the beneficial reductions in heart rate and blood pressure. Thus, beta-blockers should be avoided in patients with either overt or incipient left ventricular failure; if their use is necessary, extreme caution should be exercised.

Coronary blood flow

Theoretically, beta-blockers decrease coronary blood flow.[33] The reduction of cardiac output by beta-blockers may lead to an increase in vascular resistance; in circumstances of increased myocardial oxygen demand, this is unlikely to be detrimental, but more an autoregulatory response of the coronary circulation to the reduction of oxygen demand produced by the beta-blocker. In coronary spasm, however, beta-blockade may aggravate the spasm and symptoms directly, which may be via a beta-1 or beta-2 effect, and indirectly because by blocking both beta-1 and beta-2 receptors alpha activity will be unopposed and lead to vasoconstriction. In patients who have coronary spasm and normal coronary arteries, therapy with nitrates and calcium antagonists is more appropriate.

Beta-blockers have several miscellaneous effects, the importance of which has yet to be investigated. Propranolol has been shown to inhibit platelet aggregation;[34] the mechanism by which inhibition is achieved is not known; the clinical importance of this effect is also not known. It has been claimed that propranolol shifts the oxygen dissociation curve to the right,[35] although the therapeutic benefit of such an effect has yet to be determined.

The first beta-blocker to be used in routine clinical practice was propranolol. Black's original studies suggested that a reduction in sympathetic stimulation would reduce myocardial oxygen demand and its importance in the development of myocardial ischaemia. Since that time, many beta-blockers have become available, each with different ancillary properties. Selection of the appropriate beta-blocker in an individual patient will depend on the ancillary properties required.

Adrenaline and noradrenaline are important regulators of cardiovascular function. In 1948, Ahlquist characterized the receptors relative to the action of adrenaline and noradrenaline and defined them as alpha- and beta-adrenoreceptors.[37] The original concept that adrenoreceptors were static entities has been shown to be incorrect and it is now clear that an apparent increase in the number of beta-adrenoceptors, which can cause a supersensitivity to beta-receptor agonists, may be induced by chronic exposure to beta-receptor antagonists.[38] This up-regulation of the beta-receptor may explain the phenomenon of beta-blocker withdrawal which occurs in some patients following the sudden cessation of beta-blockade. With chronic beta-blocker therapy, the number of available beta-receptors is increased; when beta-blockers are suddenly stopped, an increased pool of sensitive receptors are open to stimulation by endogenous

Table 48.2. Pharmacodynamic properties of some commonly used beta-blocking drugs.[a]

Beta-blocker	β_1 selectivity	Partial agonist activity	Membrane stabilizing activity
Acebutolol	+/−	+/−	+/−
Atenolol	+	−	−
Celiprolol[b]	+/−	−	−
Labetalol[c]	−	−	−
Metoprolol	+	−	−
Nadolol	−	−	−
Oxprenolol	−	+	−
Pindolol	−	+	+/−
Sotalol[d]	−	−	−
Timolol	−	−	−

[a] From: Frishman, W.H. Beta adrenergic blockade for the treatment of angina pectoris. In: Weiner, D.A. and Frishman, W.H., eds. *Therapy of Angina Pectoris.* New York/Basel: Marcel Dekker.
[b] Celiprolol has peripheral alpha-blocking activity.
[c] Labetalol also has alpha-blocking activity.
[d] Sotalol has type III anti-arrhythmic activity.

catecholamines.[39] This may precipitate angina pectoris or even acute myocardial infarction.

Cardioselectivity (Table 48.2)

Cardioselective beta-blockers preferentially block the beta-1-receptor, although any cardioselective beta-blocker will also affect the beta-2-receptor to some degree. Non-selective beta-blockers block both beta-1- and beta-2-receptors. In patients with angina, only blockade of the beta-1-receptor is required; in most cases, blockade of the beta-2-receptor is of little importance. In patients who have reversible airways disease, blockade of the beta-2-receptor could be deleterious causing increased airways obstruction due to smooth muscle constriction, and patients with asthma should not be treated with a non-selective beta-blocker;[40] it is probably advisable not to use a beta-blocker in any patient who has significant airways obstruction.

Stimulation of the beta-2-receptors by the hepatocytes results in gluconeogenesis, and therefore hypoglycaemia, which might be important in patients with insulin-dependent diabetes, may be prolonged by the use of non-selective beta-blocking drugs.[41] Diabetic patients therefore may be more conveniently treated with a cardioselective beta-blocker.

Patients with Raynaud's phenomenon and peripheral vascular disease may benefit from the use of a cardioselective beta-blocker as opposed to one that blocks the beta-2-receptor because blockade of the beta-2-receptor will cause increased peripheral vascular resistance.[30] In such patients, however, it may be more sensible to consider the use of a calcium antagonist.

Partial Agonist Activity (Table 48.2)

In addition to blocking the beta-receptors, some beta-blockers are sympathetic agonists.[30,42] Thus, when sympathetic tone is low, their agonist properties are more important in comparison to their beta-receptor blocking activity; when sympathetic tone is high, such as during exercise or excitement, the agonist properties are of only minor importance when compared with the beta-receptor blocking activity. The agonist effect varies among beta-blockers; some, such as atenolol, have no partial agonist activity whereas others have the stimulating effect attainable with isoprenaline (oxprenolol about 10% and pindolol 35%). It has been suggested that partial agonist activity may be useful in those patients with angina who also have poor left ventricular function, reversible airways disease or peripheral vascular disease.[42] However, in such patients, it would probably be better to use a calcium antagonist.

The important effect of beta-blockers which have partial agonist activity is that, in contrast to those which do not have this property, the resting heart rate will not be significantly reduced and it is only on exercise when the heart rate increase will be attenuated that the effect of beta-blockade will become apparent.[42,43] Consequently, the maximum exercise-induced heart rate that can be achieved on a beta-blocker with or without partial agonist activity will not differ. However, at night, when the levels of endogenous catecholamines are low, a beta-blocker with partial agonist activity will cause a slight tachycardia which could be detrimental in those patients who have nocturnal angina.[44]

Lipid Solubility (Table 48.3)

Beta-blockers may be either lipophilic (propranolol/metoprolol) or hydrophilic (atenolol).[40] The lipophilic beta-blockers are well absorbed orally, and undergo hepatic metabolism. However, because of their hepatic metabolism, the potential exists for drug interactions. In general, these have been of little importance except in those patients who smoke cigarettes. Cigarette smoking induces the generation of drug-metabolizing enzymes in the liver so that the effective plasma level of a drug such as propranolol will be reduced.[3]

As lipophilic beta-blockers cross the blood–brain barrier more easily, the tendency to suffer neurological side-effects, such as nightmares and tiredness, will be greater in patients treated with such beta-blockers.

Hydrophilic beta-blockers are poorly absorbed from the gut and consequently they have a longer duration of action; they are more appropriate for single daily dosage. As they are excreted unchanged by the kidney, hydrophilic beta-blockers may be the agents of choice in patients with hepatic dysfunction.

In contrast, in patients with renal failure, the lipophilic beta-blockers are more appropriate. Although hydrophilic beta-blockers do not cross the blood–brain barrier, side-effects such as tiredness do occur although probably not as frequently as with the lipophilic beta-blockers.

Table 48.3. **Pharmacokinetic properties of some commonly used beta-blocking drugs.**[a]

Beta-blocker	Extent of absorption (% of dose)	Interpatient variations in plasma levels	Lipid solubility	Predominant route of elimination
Acebutolol	70	7-fold	Moderate	Renal
Atenolol	50	4-fold	Weak	Renal
Celiprolol	30	3-fold	Weak	Renal
Labetalol	> 90	10-fold	Weak	Hepatic
Metoprolol	> 90	7-fold	Moderate	Renal
Nadolol	30	7-fold	Moderate	Renal
Oxprenolol	90	5-fold	Moderate	Hepatic
Pindolol	> 90	4-fold	Moderate	Renal
Propranolol	> 90	20-fold	High	Hepatic
Sotalol	70	4-fold	Weak	Renal
Timolol	> 90	7-fold	Weak	Renal

[a] From: Frishman, W.H. Beta adrenergic blockade for the treatment of angina pectoris. In: Weiner, D.A. and Frishman, W.H., eds. *Therapy of Angina Pectoris.* New York/Basel: Marcel Dekker.

Membrane stabilizing activity (Table 48.2)

Membrane-stabilizing activity is a property of several beta-blockers (metoprolol, oxprenolol, propranolol), but in the doses used in clinical practice it is of no practical importance.[45]

Alpha-adrenergic blocking activity

Labetalol is a non-selective beta-blocker (beta-1 plus beta-2 effects) which also blocks the alpha-adrenoreceptors (its alpha-blocking effects are about one-quarter of its beta-blocker effects) leading to a reduction in peripheral resistance. Labetalol has been widely used for the treatment of hypertension; the results of recent studies suggest that it is also beneficial in the treatment of angina although whether the alpha-blocking effects confer any benefit additional to that obtained from the beta-blocking effects has not been demonstrated.[46,47]

Pharmacokinetics

The pharmacokinetics of the various beta-blocking drugs differ markedly depending on the degree of their lipid solubility, which leads to differences in the completeness of gastro-intestinal absorption, the extent of first pass hepatic metabolism, penetration into the brain, the concentration in the heart, the rate of hepatic biotransformation and the rate of renal clearance of the drug and its metabolites.[48] In addition, the protein binding, the extent of distribution and the pharmacological activity of the metabolites of the various beta-blockers may differ.

Thus, the extent of absorption (e.g. atenolol 50%, propranolol > 90%, metoprolol > 90%) and the degree of bioavailability (e.g. atenolol 50%, propranolol 30%, metoprolol 50%) of each drug will differ greatly. Large interpatient variations in plasma levels may occur (atenolol fourfold, propranolol twentyfold, metoprolol sevenfold—see Table 48.3). Protein binding also varies (atenolol 5%, metoprolol 12%, propranolol 93%). Absorption is usually via the small intestine although hydrophilic agents will be completely absorbed on passage through the gut and eliminated unchanged by the kidney. The bioavailability of hydrophilic agents is fairly constant and they have a flat dose–response curve.

The duration of action of the various beta-receptor antagonists differs greatly. Those that are rapidly absorbed from the gut and undergo hepatic metabolism, such as propranolol, oxprenolol and labetalol, have elimination half-lives of about 3–4 h, whereas beta-blockers excreted by the kidney, such as atenolol, have an elimination half-life of 6–9 h. Beta-blockers with elimination half-lives of 3–4 h must be given 2 or 3 times a day, whereas atenolol can be given once daily. Long-acting preparations of the shorter acting beta-blocking drugs are now available, in which the beta-blocker forms part of a soluble matrix inside a tiny spheroid made up of an insoluble membrane; gastro-intestinal fluid enters the spheroids and the drug is released along a concentration gradient into the gut lumen and from thence into the bloodstream. The absorption of the drug is not dependent on gastric acidity or enzyme action.

Side-effects

Most patients who have chronic effort-related angina will tolerate beta-blocking drugs. However, up to 10% of patients have tolerable side-effects, including fatigue, depression, gastro-intestinal disturbances and loss of libido. Beta-blocking drugs should be avoided in those patients who have severely compromised left ventricular function, heart block, asthma or peripheral vascular disease.

CALCIUM ANTAGONISTS

Flekenstein conferred the term 'calcium antagonist' on those compounds that inhibited the slow influx of calcium, which is necessary for the contraction of myocardial and vascular smooth muscle cells.[49,50] He recognized that the coronary and peripheral vasodilative effects of these drugs, together with their negative inotropic effects, were likely to be of benefit in the treatment of angina pectoris. Subsequent experience has confirmed his initial suggestions; calcium antagonists are now important drugs particularly in the treatment of patients with coronary spasm and those in whom alterations in coronary tone may influence the threshold to the onset of angina.[51,52] Furthermore, the smooth muscle relaxation and reduction of afterload induced by calcium antagonists, together with their negative inotropic effects, will reduce myocardial oxygen consumption, an action that renders them suitable for use in patients with chronic stable effort-related angina pectoris.

Three calcium antagonists are in routine clinical use; several more are in preparation and about to be introduced into clinical practice. Unlike the beta-blockers, structurally the calcium antagonists are a heterogeneous group of compounds with important differences in pharmacological action (Tables 48.4 and 48.5).

Verapamil

Verapamil, which was the first calcium antagonist to be clinically available, is a papaverine derivative. It is rapidly absorbed from the gut, and peak blood levels are reached within about 2 hours of oral dosing.[53,54] It is extensively metabolized in the liver, the systemic availability of the oral dose being about 20%. However, liver metabolism varies from day to day and hepatic clearance of the drug is reduced during consecutive oral dosings up to at least 7 doses. The major N-demethylated metabolite of verapamil, nor-verapamil, is less potent haemodynamically than it is electrophysiologically when compared with the parent compound. Sustained release formulations have now been developed and are available for clinical use.

Verapamil has profound effects on cardiac pacemaker tissue, slowing conduction through the atrioventricular node. The sino-atrial node may also be affected with a small slowing in the resting heart rate, although usually the resting heart rate is not affected. Verapamil causes significant depression of ventricular muscle and it probably has the greatest negative inotropic effects of the three calcium antagonists clinically available. It causes coronary and peripheral smooth muscle relaxation which lead to an increase in coronary blood flow and a reduction in afterload.[55]

Nifedipine

Nifedipine belongs to the dihydropyridine class of calcium blocking drugs. More than 90% is absorbed after oral ingestion and it is almost completely bound to plasma proteins and rapidly inactivated via hepatic oxidative biotransposition.[56,57] Its principal metabolite has little or no pharmacological activity. Capsules containing nifedipine in solution are rapidly absorbed and peak

Table 48.4. **Pharmacodynamics of some commonly used calcium antagonists.**[a]

Calcium antagonist	Coronary vasodilatation	Peripheral vasodilatation	Heart rate	Atrioventricular conduction
Nifedipine	↑	↑↑	0/↑	0
Verapamil	↑	↑	0/↓	↓
Diltiazem	↑	↑	0/↓	0/↓

[a] From: Weiner, D.A. and Klein, M.D. Calcium antagonists for the treatment of angina pectoris. In: Weiner, D.A. and Frishman, W.H., eds. *Therapy of Angina Pectoris.* New York/Basel: Marcel Dekker.

Table 48.5. Pharmacokinetics of some commonly used calcium antagonists.[a]

Calcium antagonist	Absorption (%)	Oral elimination half-life (h)	Oral onset of action (min)	Metabolism
Nifedipine	> 90	2.5–5	20	Hepatic
Verapamil	> 90	3–7	30	Hepatic (> 70% first pass)
Diltiazem	> 90	4–6	20	Hepatic (> 50% first pass)

[a] From: Weiner, D.A. and Klein, M.D. Calcium antagonists for the treatment of angina pectoris. In: Weiner, D.A. and Klein, M.D., eds. *Therapy of Angina Pectoris.* New York/Basel: Marcel Dekker.

blood levels are reached within approximately 1.5 h; plasma elimination occurs at approximately 2.5 h.

Nifedipine is the most potent of the calcium antagonists, causing smooth muscle relaxation which results in a reduction of afterload and an increase in coronary blood flow.[55] This drug has little or no effect on sino-atrial or atrioventricular nodal conduction; smooth muscle relaxation tends to cause a reflex increase in the mean heart rate. In common with other calcium antagonists, nifedipine has negative inotropic effects, which are less marked than those of verapamil.[56]

Diltiazem

Diltiazem is a benzothiazepine with calcium channel blocking activity.[59] Like verapamil and nifedipine, it is rapidly absorbed after oral ingestion, hepatically metabolized and saturates the hepatic metabolic pathways resulting in non-linear kinetic effects and an apparent increase in bioavailability.

The effects of diltiazem are similar to those of verapamil in that it affects both sino-atrial and atrioventricular nodal conduction.[60] Also, diltiazem causes coronary and peripheral smooth muscle relaxation which leads to an increase in coronary blood flow and a reduction in afterload. The net effect on heart rate will be either non-existent or a slight slowing. Diltiazem has a negative inotropic effect which is more marked than that of nifedipine.

New calcium antagonists

Many new calcium antagonists are being evaluated and they will shortly be introduced into clinical practice. Gallopamil has a similar pharmacological structure to verapamil; nicardipine, naludipine, nisoldipine, amlodipine and nimodipine are all dihydropyridines similar to nifedipine. It is claimed that these newer calcium antagonists will have more favourable pharmacokinetic profiles, and it is suggested that some will be more organ specific. Further studies will be necessary before these claims can be substantiated.

Side-effects

Although the calcium antagonists are a heterogeneous group, they have similar side-effects; the severity and frequency of these effects vary with the drug given and among patients. Vasodilatory side-effects are not infrequent and include flushing, palpitation, dizziness or headache; peripheral oedema is reported with nifedipine. Gastro-intestinal symptoms such as constipation and nausea occur most frequently with verapamil. Many of these side-effects, particularly those due to vasodilatation, may become less apparent within about 1 week of dosing and patients should be encouraged to continue treatment for at least this period of time.

Occasional patients with angina pectoris treated with calcium antagonists have experienced a deterioration in their symptoms.[61,62] Although the exact cause of this is not known, coronary steal, hypotension or, as in the case of nifedipine, tachycardia may adversely affect myocardial oxygen demand and coronary blood flow. With all these agents, it is important to start treatment with a low dose and to titrate the dose for each patient according to symptomatic relief and drug tolerance.

In patients with atrioventricular block, verapamil and diltiazem should be avoided. Patients with incipient or overt left ventricular failure should not be treated with verapamil; although nifedipine causes negative inotropic effects, the marked smooth muscle relaxation it induces will tend to render this drug useful in such patients.

COMBINATION THERAPY

Calcium antagonists with beta-blockers

In many studies, additional beneficial anti-anginal effects have been reported when a beta-blocker is used in combination with a calcium antagonist.[63–65] These effects are due to an additional reduction in the rate–pressure product both at rest and on exercise. In addition, synergy between the two classes of drug may abolish the potentially detrimental effects of each. Thus, any increases in heart rate that may occur with nifedipine treatment will be prevented by the use of a beta-blocking drug; any increase in peripheral resistance and a possible fall in coronary blood flow that may occur on beta-blockade will be prevented by the effects of the calcium antagonist.

Beneficial effects have been reported when a beta-blocker has been used in combination with any of the three calcium antagonists, but potential adverse side-effects would be most likely to occur with a combination of beta-blocker and verapamil or diltiazem.[66,67] In patients with underlying sick sinus syndrome or atrioventricular conduction disease, the combination of a beta-blocker and verapamil should be avoided.[68] Patients who have left ventricular dysfunction may develop overt cardiac failure if given the combination of a beta-blocker and a calcium antagonist. However, the frequency of adverse reactions with these combinations can be minimized by careful screening of the patients for cardiac failure, poor left ventricular function, hypotension and conduction system disease. Care should also be taken when using other drugs that may have independent negative inotropic effects, particularly anti-arrhythmic agents.

Nitrates and calcium antagonists

The calcium antagonists and nitrates have many similar clinical properties and both sets of agents will reduce myocardial oxygen demand by reducing afterload and increasing coronary blood flow.[69] In contrast to calcium antagonists, nitrates also possess venodilating effects, which may be particularly useful in a patient who has left ventricular dysfunction.

The combination of a calcium antagonist and a nitrate may cause adverse effects if the patient is hypotensive; if a nitrate is combined with nifedipine, a reflex tachycardia may be induced.

Nitrates and beta-blockade

The combination of a nitrate and beta-blocker has been shown to be effective in the management of patients with chronic stable angina and those who have mixed angina with alterations in coronary tone.[70] This combination may be particularly useful in those with mildly compromised left ventricular function in whom the beta-blocker alone would have adverse effects and also in those in whom an alteration in coronary tone may be important. Side-effects may occur due to hypotension.

Triple therapy

Increasing numbers of patients are now being treated using the combination of a beta-blocker, calcium antagonist and nitrate. This combination may be theoretically attractive and some workers hope that a synergistic benefit may be obtained in terms of reduction in myocardial oxygen demand and increases in coronary blood flow, but current evidence does not support this strategy; in a recent study, no additional benefit was obtained either in terms of exercise tolerance or angina frequency by adding a third drug to the regimen.

PERCUTANEOUS TRANSLUMINAL CORONARY ANGIOPLASTY

The use of transluminal angioplasty to dilate the peripheral arterial narrowings of the femoral and iliac arteries was first described by Dotter and Judkins in 1964.[71] In 1977, Grüntzig demonstrated that this technique could be used to dilate localized atherosclerotic narrowings of the coronary arteries.[72,73]

Technological advances in guidewires and balloons, together with much improved operator expertise, have dramatically expanded the application of this technique; in 1987, approximately 200 000 angioplasties were performed in the USA.

TECHNIQUE

The specific details are described in Chapter 16. In brief, the coronary artery is selectively catheterized and a specially designed guidewire is passed through the coronary artery narrowing. The balloon is passed over the guidewire and across the lesion and then inflated (Fig. 48.1). The balloon is inflated several times; the inflation pressure and the

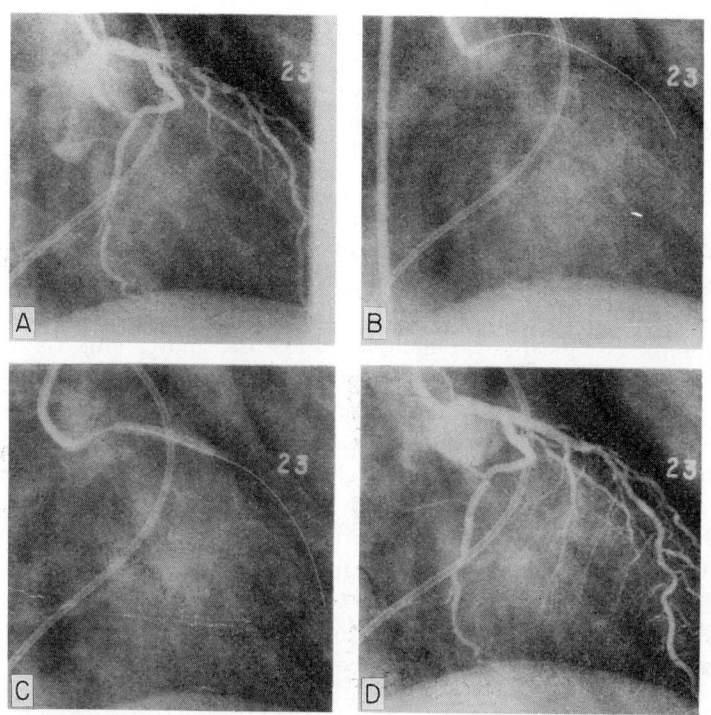

Fig. 48.1. (A) Left coronary arteriogram showing a severe stenosis of the left anterior descending coronary artery. (B) The guidewire has been passed across the stenosis in the left anterior descending coronary artery. (C) The balloon has been inflated in the area of the stenosis of the left anterior descending coronary artery. (D) Left coronary arteriogram following balloon inflation showing a successfully dilated left anterior descending coronary artery. (By courtesy of Dr M. Raphael.)

duration of inflation will depend on the nature of the lesion being dilated.

Concomitant drug therapy is used in most units to improve the success rate and reduce the complications of this procedure. At most units, patients will be started on a calcium antagonist, if they are not already on this therapy 24–48 h before the procedure; this treatment will be continued for 1–6 months after the procedure. Heparin is usually given during the procedure, and, either prior to angioplasty or immediately afterwards, some form of antiplatelet agent such as aspirin or aspirin and dipyridamole, will be used at most centres. Intracoronary nitrates are given in some centres before the guidewire manipulation is performed and particularly if there is any evidence of coronary spasm occurring at any time during the procedure.

MECHANISM OF ACTION

Grüntzig's initial description 'like a footprint in the snow' reflected his belief that the atheroma was being squashed by the inflation of the balloon. Initial attempts involving histopathological examination of autopsy material suggested that vascular damage occurred with dissection and rupture,[74] but autopsy studies have marked limitations; animal work has shown that there is no neo-intimal fracture of the concentric cellular lesions, whereas in eccentric cellular lesions stretching and thinning

of the non-involved vessel appears to occur. Further experimental studies support the hypothesis that angioplasty may work to a large extent by stretching of the vessel and not by plaque compression or embolization.[75] Also, minor areas of dissection are often present at the time of successful angioplasty and are seen to heal over in the subsequent months.

INDICATIONS

The indications for coronary angioplasty have increased dramatically; originally, only isolated proximal lesions of the major coronary arteries were attempted. With increasing operator experience and technological developments, multiple lesions in one or several coronary arteries are now being tackled successfully.[76] Although symmetric non-calcified lesions used to be the initial indication, today asymmetric calcified lesions and even branch stenoses submitted to double-balloon techniques can be successfully dilated. Although dilatation of the left anterior descending artery is the most straightforward, dilatations of the circumflex and right coronary arteries are now routinely undertaken.

RESULTS

Successful angioplasty is associated with a marked relief of symptoms together with a significant reduction or sometimes abolition of objective evidence of exercise-induced ischaemia. In the NHLBI registry of angioplasty performed between 1979 and 1982 on 3248 patients (3567 angioplasties) an improvement in luminal diameter of 20% was achieved in 70% of patients.[77-79] These results, however, included those of many operators who were still within their learning curve; more recently, success rates of 90% have been reported by experienced operators in patients who have single-vessel disease. Although the success rate of dilatation of lesions of the left anterior descending coronary artery remains the highest, with improved guide catheters, guidewires and balloons, similar results are beginning to be obtained for dilatations of the left circumflex and right coronary arteries.

In recent years, angioplasty of total vessel occlusion has been undertaken (Fig. 48.2).[80] Although the results were not as good as those in patients with stenosis, primary success was demonstrated in 40 of 76 consecutive patients (53%); no deaths related to the procedure and no perforations occurred. Dilatation of an occluded vessel is more likely to be successful if the clinical history is short, there is no previous history of infarction and the occlusion occurs in a short non-visualized segment.

Coronary angioplasty may also be used to dilate stenoses in coronary artery bypass grafts.[81] Although it is usually easy to perform dilatation of graft stenoses the long-term results are not as good as those obtained in the dilatation of native coronary arteries because restenosis occurs more frequently. Recently, the dilatation of internal mammary artery grafts has been successful with resolution of the patients' symptoms and no complications.[82] Dilatation of native coronary disease in patients who have undergone coronary artery bypass surgery is increasingly being undertaken in patients who develop angina in the early or late post-operative stages.

Left main coronary artery stenosis is usually considered to be a contra-indication to balloon angioplasty because of the serious risks involved with either early or late vessel occlusions. Stertzer et al. have performed 20 left main dilatations over 20 years and there have been no deaths or complications related to the procedure during this time.[83] However, such procedures should be considered only if the myocardium is protected by the presence of a patent bypass graft or a good collateral blood supply or if the operator is very experienced and bypass surgery is contra-indicated.

The results of multiple-vessel dilatations are continually improving with increasing operator experience and better guidewire and catheter technology. In the NHLBI registry, the initial results in 234 patients in whom angioplasty of multiple lesions was attempted (52%) displayed a similar learning curve to those of angioplasty for single-vessel disease. In more recent series, a success rate of almost 90% has been reported in patients with multivessel disease when the operator is experienced.[76] Most authors indicate that an increasing proportion of patients undergoing angioplasty have multivessel disease, and careful use of non-invasive and invasive investigational techniques should provide the operator with guidance about the most critical lesions requiring dilatation.

The results of single- and multivessel angioplasty in experienced hands would appear to be similar to those of coronary artery bypass grafting, although as yet there are no data comparing these techniques. Currently, clinical trials are being organized in which the results of coronary angioplasty and coronary artery bypass grafting will be compared. The rate of serious complications in the NHLBI registry was 9%, surgery was performed in 6.6%, death related to the procedure occurred in 0.9%, mortality in those suffering myocardial infarction was 8.4% and in those requiring surgery it was 4.4%. Of the 1418 patients followed for 1 year, 2.7% had died, and restenosis occurred in 34% within 6 months.

To a large extent, these figures reflect the learning curve of many operators, but it is clear that even in the most experienced hands it is essential to have coronary artery bypass grafting available on site when coronary angioplasty is performed.

Restenosis is a frequent complication, even in experienced hands; it accounts for around 20–30% of cases of the recurrence of symptoms within 6 months. The use of antiplatelet agents and anticoagulants to reduce the frequency of restenosis is being investigated; mechanical means (stents) are also being subjected to clinical investigation.[84] The use of laser angioplasty to aid dilatation and to prevent restenosis is still at an experimental stage.[85]

CORONARY ARTERY BYPASS GRAFTING

The specific details and results of coronary vein graft surgery and internal mammary implantation are dealt with in Chapter 52. Approximately 70% of patients whose symptoms are resistant to medical therapy will be rendered free of pain following coronary artery bypass surgery.[86] There is also evidence that in certain subgroups of patients with angina pectoris, coronary artery bypass grafting may prolong life.

The first study in which the relative prognoses of medical and surgical therapy were assessed in a randomized manner was the Veterans Administration Study in which 1015 male patients were recruited over a 5-year period at 13 centres.[87,88] The study was performed at a time when surgical mortality was high, particularly at some centres where the surgeons were less experienced, and the data are usually analysed on the basis of 686

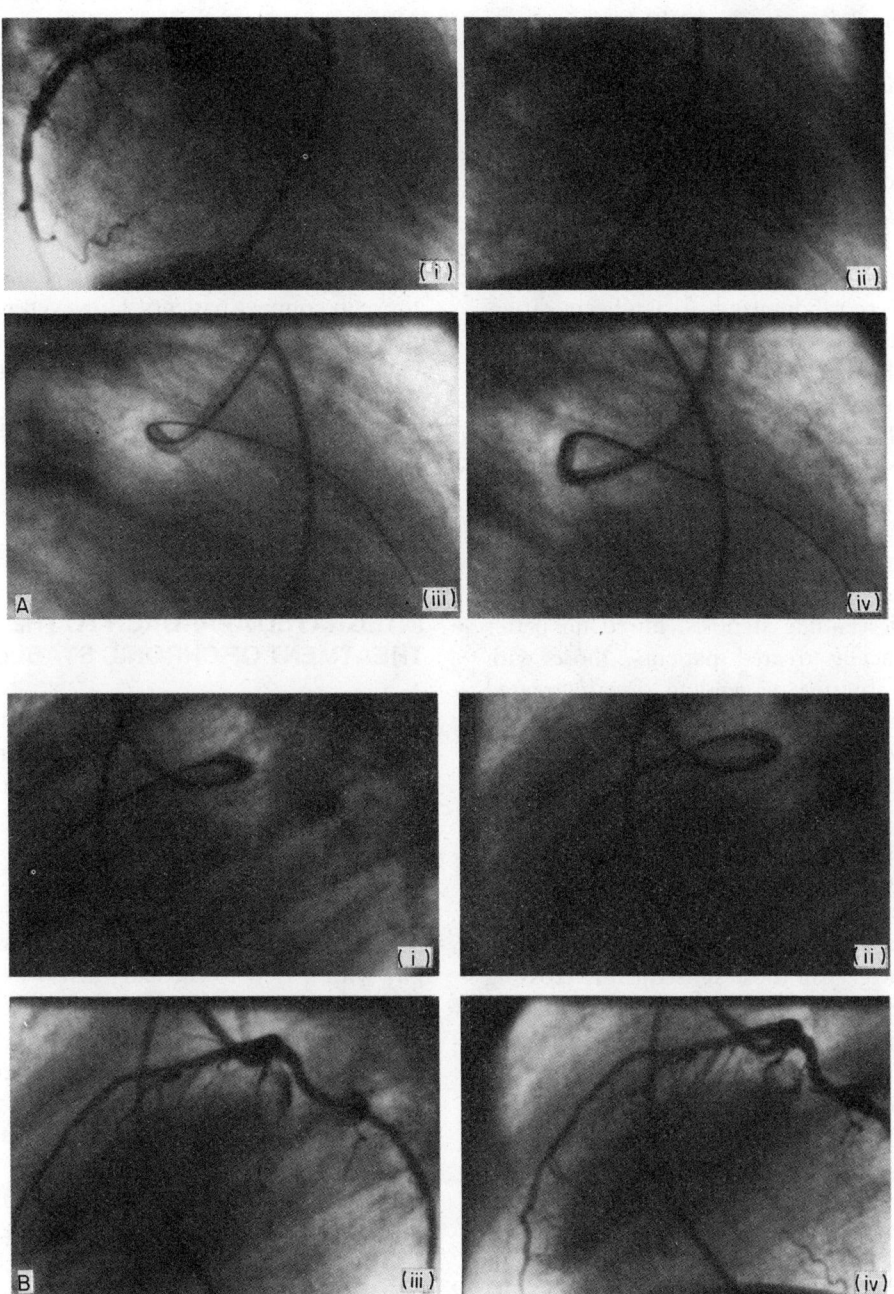

Fig. 48.2. (A) Left coronary arteriogram in the left anterior oblique projection showing an occluded left anterior descending coronary artery (i). The guide catheter has been placed in the left coronary ostium (ii) and the guidewire is subsequently passed across the area of occlusion (iii). Following this, the balloon catheter is passed over the guidewire across the area of occlusion (iv). (B) The balloon catheter has been passed across the area of occlusion of the left anterior descending coronary artery (i) and inflated (ii). Subsequent coronary arteriograms demonstrate a widely patent left anterior descending coronary artery (iii and iv). (By courtesy of Dr M. Raphael.)

patients who were randomized between 1972 and 1974. The study population comprised patients who were relatively symptomatic. A highly significant difference in mortality was found in patients who had left main disease: at 4 years, mortality was 33% for those who had been treated medically compared with 7% for those who had been treated surgically.

The study population of the European Coronary Artery Surgery Study comprised men under the age of 65 years in whom surgery was not deemed essential on account of their symptoms, but who had angina and angiographic evidence of coronary artery disease in 2 or 3 major coronary arteries;[89] resting ejection fractions were > 50%. A total of 768 patients were randomized. A significant difference, in favour of surgery, was found in those patients with three-vessel disease: in patients undergoing surgery, survival at 5 years was 94% and at 8 years it was 91.8%; in medically treated patients it was 82.4 and 76.7%, respectively. The results of this study also emphasized the importance of disease in the proximal left anterior descending coronary artery: although surgically treated patients with two-vessel disease, but without proximal left anterior descending stenosis, faired no better than the medically treated patients, those with proximal left anterior descending disease treated surgically did. Several other non-angiographic variables that were predictive of a better result following surgery were identified, including the presence of ST-segment depression greater than or equal to 1.5 mm. At 5 years, 46% of patients treated surgically were free of symptoms compared with 20% of those treated medically; most of the apparent change in the medical group could be attributed to surgery in those subsequently crossing over from medical therapy.

The Coronary Artery Surgery Study comprised 2095 patients who had either mild angina or who were asymptomatic following an acute myocardial infarction.[90] Patients with left main stem stenosis were excluded. Impairment of left ventricular function was not a contra-indication to surgery providing heart failure was not present and the left ventricular ejection fraction was at least 35%. Of the 2095 patients whom it was considered possible to randomize, only 780 were eventually randomized to either medical or surgical treatment. In contrast to the European study, analysis at 5 years showed that there was no difference in survival between medically and surgically treated patients (92 and 95%, respectively). Overall, there was no significant difference between medically treated patients and surgically treated patients with three-vessel disease. However, of the 160 patients who had an ejection fraction of between 35 and 50%, the 7-year mortality was 30% in the medically treated group and 16% in the surgically treated group; about half of this subset had three-vessel disease in whom the differences were even more marked (surgical mortality at 7 years was 12% and medical mortality at 7 years was 35%). At 5 years, 55% of surgical patients were free of anginal symptoms, and had a small increase in exercise time.

Although there has been no randomized trial of surgery in elderly patients, analysis of the CASS registry suggests that the results would be similar to those in younger patients. However, it is difficult to draw too many conclusions about surgery in the elderly from these studies because patient selection must have varied among different centres and different physicians. Despite this reservation, the results do suggest that, provided the elderly patient is fit for surgery, an operation can be performed at an acceptable risk.

INTEGRATED APPROACH TO THE TREATMENT OF CHRONIC STABLE ANGINA

Nowadays, medical therapy, percutaneous transluminal coronary angioplasty and coronary artery bypass grafting must be considered together in an integrated approach to treatment. The use of non-invasive investigations, particularly exercise testing and gated blood pool scanning at rest and on exercise, should be used to define those patients at risk who should be considered for early angiography with a view to coronary artery bypass grafting or coronary angioplasty. Patients whose lifestyle is severely limited or who are unable to tolerate drug therapy should be considered for coronary angioplasty or coronary artery bypass grafting. Those patients who have mild symptoms but a significant stenosis of the left main stem are candidates for coronary artery bypass surgery. Patients who have three-vessel disease, particularly those whose exercise test is positive at a low level of exercise, and impaired left ventricular function or proximal left anterior descending coronary artery stenosis should be considered as candidates for coronary artery bypass surgery even if their symptoms are mild.

It is now clear that symptoms will recur in about 50% of patients 7–10 years after coronary artery bypass grafting. Therefore, it is reasonable to consider the use of coronary angioplasty initially, particularly in the younger patient, even if only to delay the first and subsequent operations. Coronary angioplasty should also be considered in the elderly in whom the operative risks may be higher. In those patients whose symptoms recur following coronary artery bypass grafting, angina can often be more easily controlled with medical therapy, or coronary angioplasty may be considered.

REFERENCES

1. Brunton, T.L. On the use of nitrate of amyl in angina pectoris. *Lancet* 1857; **2**: 97.
2. Murrell, W. Nitroglyerine as a remedy for angina pectoris. *Lancet* 1879; **1**: 80.
3. Deanfield, J., Wright, C., Krikler, S., Ribeiro, B. and Fox, K. Cigarette smoking and the treatment of angina pectoris with propranolol, atenolol and nifedipine. *N. Engl. J. Med.* 1984; **310**: 951.
4. McGregor, M. Pathogenesis of angina pectoris and role of nitrates in relief of myocardial ischemia. *Am. J. Med.* 1983; **74** (6B): 21.
5. Greenberg, H., Dwyer, E.M., Jameson, A.G. and Pinkernell, B.H. Effects of nitroglycerin on the major determinants of myocardial oxygen consumption. *Am. J. Cardiol.* 1975; **36**: 426.
6. Tauchert, M., Jansen, W., Osterspey, A., Fuchs, M., Homback, V. and Hilger, H.H. Dose dependence of tolerance during treatment with mononitrates. *Z. Kardiol.* 1983; **72** (Suppl. 3): 218.
7. Horwitz, L.D., Gorlin, R., Taylor, W.J. and Kemp, H.G. Effects of nitroglycerin on regional myocardial blood flow in coronary artery disease. *J. Clin. Invest.* 1971; **50**: 1578.
8. Cohen, M.V., Downey, J.M., Sonnenblick, E.H. and Kirk, E.S. The effects of nitroglycerin on coronary collaterals and myocardial contractility. *J. Clin. Invest.* 1973; **52**: 2836.
9. Brown, G., Bolson, E., Petersen, R.B., Pierce, C.D. and Dodge, H.T. The mechanisms of nitroglycerin action. Stenosis vasodilatation as a major component of drug response. *Circulation* 1981; **64**: 1089.
10. Conti, C.R., Feldman, R.L., Pepine, C.J., Hill, J.A. and Conti, J.B. Effect of glyceryl trinitrate on coronary and systemic hemodynamics in man. *Am. J. Med.* 1984; **74** (6B): 28.
11. Maseri, A. The changing face of angina pectoris: Practical implications. *Lancet* 1983; **1**: 746.
12. Hill, J.A., Feldman, R.L., Pepine, C.J. and Conti, C.R. Randomized double-blind comparison of nifedipine and isosorbide dinitrate in patients with coronary arterial spasm. *Am. J. Cardiol.* 1982; **49**: 431.
13. Ginsburg, R., Lamb, I., Schroeder, J.S., Hu, M. and Harrison, D.C. Randomized double-blind comparison of nifedipine and isosorbide dinitrate therapy in variant angina pectoris due to coronary arterial spasm. *Am. Heart J.* 1982; **103**: 44.
14. Parker, J.O., van Koughnett, K.A. and Farrell, B. Nitroglycerin lingual spray: clinical efficacy and dose–response relation. *Am. J. Cardiol.* 1986; **57**: 1.
15. Frishman, W.H. and Teicher, M. Nitroglycerin lingual spray. *Cardiovasc. Rev. Rep.* 1989; **7**: (in press).
16. Abrams, J. Nitrate delivery systems in perspective: A decade of progress. *Am. J. Med.* 1984; **76** (6A): 38.
17. Abrams, J. New nitrate delivery systems. Buccal Nitroglycerin. *Am. Heart J.* 1983; **105**: 848.
18. Greengart, A., Lichstein, E., Hollander, G., Bolton, S. and Sanders, M. Efficacy of sustained-release buccal nitroglycerine in patients with angina pectoris. *Chest* 1983; **83**: 473.
19. Abrams, J. Usefulness of long-acting nitrates in cardiovascular disease. *Am. J. Med.* 1978; **64**: 183.
20. Abrams, J. Nitrate tolerance and dependence. *Am. Heart J.* 1980; **99**: 113.
21. Thandani, U., Fung, H., Darke, A.C. and Parker, J.O. Oral isosorbide dinitrate in angina pectoris: Comparison of duration of action and dose response relation during acute and sustained therapy. *Am. J. Cardiol.* 1982; **49**: 411.
22. Parker, J.O. and Ho-Leung Fung. Transdermal nitroglycerin in angina pectoris. *Am. J. Cardiol.* 1984; **54**: 471.
23. Sullivan, M., Sawides, M., Abouantowm, S., Madsen, E.F. and Froelicher, V. Failure of transdermal nitroglycerin to improve exercise capacity in patients with angina pectoris. *J. Am. Coll. Cardiol.* 1985; **5**: 1220.
24. Glancy, D.L., Richter, M.A., Ellis, E.V. and Johnson, W. Effect of swallowed isosorbide dinitrate on blood pressure, heart rate and exercise capacity in patients with coronary artery disease. *Am. J. Med.* 1977; **62**: 39.
25. Packer, M. New perspectives on therapeutic application of nitrates as vasodilator agents for severe chronic heart failure. *Am. J. Med.* 1983; **73**: 61.
26. Sniderman, A.D., Marpole, D.G.F., Palmer, W.H. and Fallen, E.L. Response of the left ventricle to nitroglycerin in patients with and without mitral regurgitation. *Br. Heart J.* 1974; **36**: 357.
27. Arsura, E., Lichstein, E., Guadagnino, V., Nucchi, V., Sanders, M., Hollander, G. and Greengart, A. Methemoglobin levels produced by organic nitrates in patients with coronary artery diseaase. *J. Clin. Pharmacol.* 1984; **24**: 160.
28. Kirk, E.S. and Sonnenblick, E.H. Newer concepts in the pathophysiology of ischemic heart disease. *Am. Heart J.* 1982; **103**: 756.
29. Frishman, W.H. Multifactorial actions of beta-adrenergic blocking drugs in ischemic heart disease: Current concepts. *Circulation* 1983; **67** (Suppl. I): 11.
30. Frishman, W.H. Beta-adrenoceptor antagonists new drugs and new indications. *N. Engl. J. Med.* 1981; **305**: 500.
31. Opie, L.H. Myocardial infarct size. Part 2. Comparison of anti-infarct effects of beta-blockade, glucose insulin, potassium, nitrates and hyaluronidase. *Am. Heart J.* 1980; **100**: 531.
32. Mueller, H.S., Ayres, S.M., Religa, A. and Evans, R.G. Propranolol in the treatment of acute myocardial infarction: Effect on myocardial oxygenation and hemodynamics. *Circulation* 1974; **49**: 1078.
33. Downey, J.M. An evaluation of the coronary constriction following propranolol. *Eur. J. Pharmacol.* 1977; **46**: 119.
34. Weksler, B., Gillick, M. and Pink, J. Effect of propranolol on platelet function. *Blood* 1977; **49**: 185.
35. Oski, F., Miller, L., Delivoria-Papadopoulous, M., Manchester, J.H. and Shelbourne, J.C. Oxygen affinity in red cells. Changes induced in vivo by propranolol. *Science* 1972; **175**: 1372.
36. Black, J.W. Ahlquist and the development of beta adrenoceptor antagonists. *Postgrad. Med. J.* 1976; **52** (Suppl. 4): 11.
37. Ahlquist, R.P. A study of adrenotropic receptors. *Am. J. Physiol.* 1948; **53**: 586.
38. Lefkowitz, R. Direct binding studies of adrenergic receptors: Biochemical, physiologic, and clinical implications. *Ann. Intern. med.* 1979; **91**: 450.
39. Shand, D.G. and Wood, A.J.J. Propranolol withdrawal syndrome—Why? *Circulation* 1978; **58**: 202.
40. Cruickshank, J.M. The clinical importance of cardioselectivity and lipophilicity in beta blockers. *Am. Heart J.* 1980; **100**: 2160.

41. Kendall, M.J. Are selective beta adrenoceptor blocking drugs an advantage? *J. R. Coll. Phys.* 1981; **15**: 33.

42. Frishman, W. Pindolol: A new beta-adrenoceptor antagonist with partial agonist activity. *N. Engl. J. Med.* 1983; **308**: 940.

43. Harry, J.D. The demonstration of atenolol as a beta adrenoceptor blocking drug in man. *Postgrad. Med. J.* 1977; **54** (Suppl. 3): 65.

44. Quyyumi, A.A., Wright, C., Mockus, L. and Fox, K. Effect of partial agonist activity in beta blockers in severe angina pectoris: a double blind comparison of pindolol and atenolol. *Br. Med. J.* 1984; **289**: 951.

45. Opie, L.H. Drugs and the heart. 1. Beta-blocking agents. *Lancet* 1980; **1**: 693.

46. Frishman, W. and Halprin, S. Clinical pharmacology of the new beta-adrenergic blocking drugs. Part 7. New horizons in beta-adrenoceptor blocking therapy: Labetalol. *Am. Heart J.* 1979; **98**: 660.

47. Michelsen, E.L. and Frishman, W.H. Labetalol: An alpha and beta-adrenoceptor blocking drug. *Ann. Intern. Med.* 1981; **99**: 553.

48. Conolly, M.E., Kersting, F. and Dollery, C.T. The clinical pharmacology of beta adrenoceptor blocking drugs. *Prog. Cardiovasc. Dis.* 1976; **19**: 203.

49. Fleckenstein, A. Specific inhibitors and promoters of calcium action in the excitation contraction coupling of heart muscle and their role in the prevention of production of myocardial lesions. In: Harris, P. and Opie, L., eds. *Calcium and the Heart*. London and New York: Academic Press, 1970/71, pp. 135–88.

50. Fleckenstein, A. Specific pharmacology of calcium in myocardium cardiac pacemakers and vascular smooth muscle. *Am. Rev. Pharmacol. Toxicol.* 1977; **17**: 149.

51. Engel, H.J. and Lichtlen, P.R. Beneficial enhancement of coronary blood flow by nifedipine. Comparison with nitroglycerin and beta blocking agents. *Am. J. Med.* 1981; **71**: 658.

52. Maseri, A. and Chierchia, S. A new rationale for the clinical approach to the patient and angina pectoris. *Am. J. Med.* 1981; **71**: 639.

53. Weiner, D.A. and Klein, M.D. The efficacy of verapamil for the treatment of various angina syndromes. *Cardiovasc. Rev. Rep.* 1983; **4**: 1163.

54. Hamann, S.R., Blouin, R.A. and McAllister, R.G. Jr. Clinical pharmacokinetics of verapamil. *Clin Pharm.* 1984; **9**: 26.

55. Braunwald, E. Mechanism of action of calcium-channel blocking agents. *N. Engl. J. Med.* 1982; **307**: 1618.

56. Kleinbloesem, C.H., van Brummelen, P., van de Linde, J.A., Voogd, P.J. and Breimer, D.D. Nifedipine: Kinetics and dynamics in healthy subjects. *Clin. Pharmacol. Ther.* 1984; **35**: 742.

57. Traube, M., Hongo, M., McAllister, R.G. Jr and McCallum, R.W. Correlation of plasma levels of nifedipine and cardiovascular effects after sublingual dosing in normal subjects. *J. Clin. Pharmacol.* 1985; **25**: 125.

58. Findlay, I.N., Dargie, H.J., Gillen, G. and Elliott, A.T. The treatment of angina pectoris with calcium channel blockers; efficacy and effect on cardiac function. *J. Am. Coll. Cardiol.* 1984; **3**: 482.

59. Sprith, M.S.A., Erghese, C.P., Shand, D.G. and Prtichett, E.L.C. Pharmacokinetic and pharmacodynamic effects of diltiazem. *Am. J. Cardiol.* 1983; **51**: 1369.

60. Chaffman, M. and Brogden, R.N. Diltiazem—A review of its pharmacological properties and therapeutic efficacy. *Drugs* 1985; **29**: 387.

61. Jariwalla, A.G. and Anderson, E.G. Production of ischaemic cardiac pain by nifedipine. *Br. Med. J.* 1978; **1**: 1181.

62. Deanfield, J., Wright, C. and Fox, K.M. Treatment of angina pectoris with nifedipine: the importance of dose titration.

63. Leon, M.B., Rosing, D.R., Bonow, R.O. and Epstein, S.E. Clinical efficacy of verapamil alone and combined with propranolol in treated patients with chronic stable angina pectoris. *Am. J. Cardiol.* 1981; **48**: 131.

64. Dargie, H.J., Lynch, P.G., Krikler, D., Harris, L. and Krikler, S. Nifedipine and propranolol; a beneficial drug interaction. *Am. J. Med.* 1981; **71**: 676.

65. Kenny, J., Kiff, P., Holmes, J. and Jewitt, D.E. Beneficial effects of diltiazem and propranolol, alone and in combination, in patients with stable angina pectoris. *Br. Heart J.* 1985; **53**: 43.

66. Kieval, J., Kirsten, E.B., Kessler, K.M., Mallin, S.M. and Myerburg, R.J. The effects of intravenous verapamil on hemodynamic status of patients with coronary artery disease receiving propranolol. *Circulation* 1982; **65**: 653.

67. Strauss, W.E., Egan, T., McIntyre, K.M. and Parisi, A.F. Combination therapy with diltiazem and propranolol: Precipitation of congestive heart failure. *Clin. Cardiol.* 1985; **8**: 363.

68. Winniford, M.D., Markham, R.V., Jr, Firth, B.G., Nicod, P. and Hillis, L.D. Hemodynamic and electrophysiologic effects of verapamil and nifedipine in patients on propranolol. *Am. J. Cardiol.* 1982; **50**: 704.

69. Hill, J.A., Feldman, R.L., Pepine, C.J. and Conti, C.R. Randomized double-blind comparison of nifedipine and isosorbide dinitrate in patients with coronary arterial spasm. *Am. J. Cardiol.* 1982; **49**: 431.

70. Parmley, W.W. The combination of beta-adrenergic blocking agents and nitrates in the treatment of stable angina pectoris. *Cardiol. Rev. Rep.* 1982; **3**: 1425.

71. Dotter, C.G. and Judkins, M.P. Transluminal treatment of atherosclerotic obstruction: Description of a new technique and a preliminary report of its application. *Circulation* 1964; **30**: 654.

72. Gruentzig, A.R. Transluminal dilation of coronary artery stenosis. *Lancet* 1978; **1**: 263.

73. Gruentzig, A.R., Senning, A. and Siegenthaler, W.E. Nonoperative dilation of coronary artery stenosis; Percutaneous transluminal coronary angioplasty. *N. Engl. J. Med.* 1979; **301**: 61.

74. Block, P.C., Myler, R.K., Stertzer, S. and Fallon, J.T. Morphology after transluminal angioplasty in human beings. *N. Engl. J. Med.* 1981; **305**: 382.

75. Sanborn, T.A., Faxon, D.P., Haudenschild, C., Gottinsman, S.B., Ryan, T.J. The mechanism of transluminal angioplasty: evidence for formation of aneurysms in experimental atherosclerosis. *Circulation* 1983; **68**: 1136.

76. Vliestra, R.E., Holmes, D.R. Jr, Reeder, G.S. *et al.* Balloon angioplasty in multivessel coronary artery disease. *Proc. Mayo Clin.* 1983; **58**: 563.

77. Detre, K.M., Mylery, R.K., Kelsey, S.F., Van Raden, A.A., To, T. and Mitchell, H. Baseline characteristics of patients in the National Heart, Lung and Blood Institute Percutaneous Transluminal Coronary Angioplasty Registry, *Am. J. Cardiol.* 1984; **53**: 7C.

78. Cowley, M.J., Danos, G., Kelsey, S.F., Van Radan, M. and Detre, K.M. Acute coronary events associated with percutaneous transluminal coronary angioplasty. *Am. J. Cardiol.* 1984; **53**: 12C.

79. Danos, G., Cowley, M.J., Janke, L., Kelsey, S.F., Mullen, S.M. and Van Radan, M. In hospital mortality rate in the National Heart, Lung and Blood Institute Percutaneous Transluminal Coronary Angioplasty Registry. *Am. J. Cardiol.* 1984; **53**: 17C.

80. Kereiakes, D.J., Selmon, M.R., McAuley, B.J., McAuley, D.B., Sheehan, D.J. and Simpson, J.B. Angioplasty in total coronary artery occlusion: experience in 76 consecutive patients. *J. Am. Coll. Cardiol.* 1985; **6**: 526.

81. Corbelli, J., Franco, I., Hollman, J., Simpfendorfer, C. and

Br. Med. J. 1983; **286**: 1467.

Galan, K. Percutaneous transluminal coronary angioplasty after previous coronary artery bypass surgery. *Am. J. Cardiol.* 1985; **56**: 398.

82. Kereiakes, D.J., George, B., Stertzer, S.H. and Myler, R.K. Percutaneous transluminal angioplasty of left internal mammary artery grafts. *Am. J. Cardiol.* 1985; **55**: 1251.

83. Stertzer, S.H., Myler, R.K., Insel, H., Wallsh, E. and Rossi, P. Percutaneous transluminal coronary angioplasty in left main stem coronary stenosis: a 5-year appraisal. *Int. J. Cardiol.* 1985; **9**: 149.

84. Sigwart, U., Puel, J., Mirkovitch, V., Joffere, F. and Kappenherger, L. Intravascular stents to prevent occlusion and restenosis after transluminal angioplasty. *N. Engl. J. Med.* 1987; **316**: 701.

85. Choy, D.S.J., Stertzer, S., Rotterdam, H.Z., Sharrock, N. and Kaminow, I.P. Transluminal laser catheter angioplasty. *Am. J. Cardiol.* 1982; **50**: 1206

86. Rahimtoola, S.H. Coronary bypass surgery for chronic angina—1981: a perspective. *Circulation* 1982; **65**: 225.

87. Detre, K., Hultgren, H. and Takaro, T. Veterans Administration cooperative study of surgery for coronary arterial occlusive disease III methods and baseline characteristics, including experience with medical treatment. *Am. J. Cardiol.* 1977; **40**: 212.

88. The Veterans Administration Coronary Artery Bypass Surgery Cooperative Study Group. Eleven-year survival in the Veterans Administration randomized trial of coronary bypass surgery for stable angina. *N. Engl. J. Med.* 1984; **311**: 1333.

89. Long-term results of prospective randomised study of coronary artery bypass surgery in stable angina pectoris. *Lancet* 1982; **2**: 1173.

90. CASS Principal Investigators and their Associates. Coronary Artery Surgery Study (CASS): a randomized trial of coronary artery bypass surgery. Survival data. *Circulation* 1983; **68**: 939.

Chapter 49

The Pathophysiology, Investigation and Treatment of Unstable Angina

Nicholas Brooks

INTRODUCTION

Cardiac pain occurring without provocation, an abrupt worsening of previously stable angina or the first episode of anginal pain is experienced by up to 60% of patients during the hours or days preceding an acute myocardial infarction; similar premonitory symptoms herald many instances of sudden coronary death. Such clinical presentations consequently came to be recognized as reflecting an unstable phase of coronary heart disease with an unpredictable, and potentially poor, prognosis.

Numerous terms have been used to subdivide the condition according to its initial clinical manifestations, but it seemed logical, and has become customary, to include them all within the single diagnosis of unstable angina. In one respect, this unification is unhelpful because it links clinical syndromes (and, probably, pathophysiological processes) generally associated with a favourable short-term prognosis with those accompanied by a relatively high risk of progression to myocardial infarction or death. It is principally for these high-risk patients that a more urgent policy of investigation and treatment is indicated than is appropriate for patients with 'stable' angina.

DEFINITION AND PRESENTATION

Unstable angina is a clinical diagnosis defined broadly as new angina or angina that is worsening in its frequency, severity or duration.

There are three characteristic presentations: the recent onset of effort angina (recent onset angina), an abrupt worsening of previously stable angina ('progressive' angina) and angina at rest, occurring without provocation (rest angina).

These presentations are not always distinct: recent onset angina may be rapidly progressive or present with pain at rest, and progressive angina in a patient with previously 'stable' angina may evolve into rest angina, with pain occurring on miminal provocation and persisting for progressively longer periods. Recent onset angina has been defined arbitrarily as angina that has developed within the preceding 4 weeks,[1] although in the absence of a progressive increase in severity or its occurrence at rest, there is little justification for regarding it as an unstable manifestation of coronary heart disease. Rest angina may be relieved by sublingual nitrate therapy or it may be prolonged and unresponsive to nitrates. It may occur as a single episode simulating a myocardial infarction, or there may be repeated attacks. In practice, prolonged (i.e. lasting >15 min) recurrent cardiac pain at rest is the condition that poses particular clinical problems beyond those of the management of chronic angina, and is the main subject of this chapter.

A negative component of the definition is that there should be no evidence of myocardial infarction; however, a rise in cardiac enzymes to twice the upper limit of normal is generally considered not to preclude the diagnosis. Moreover, it is important to emphasize that unstable angina may occur in the early recovery phase of a myocardial infarction.

VARIANT ANGINA

A specific category of rest angina, variant angina, was described originally by Prinzmetal.[2] The condition is characterized by recurrent attacks of angina at rest accompanied by ST-segment elevation and, often, an increase in R-wave amplitude on the electrocardiogram, which are relieved within 5 min by nitroglycerin. Typically, the patient has a relatively well-preserved exercise capacity. The attacks tend to be clustered in the early morning, and periods of disease activity may be followed by months or years of freedom from symptoms.

Clinically, variant angina may be indistinguishable from 'ordinary' rest angina, and it is debatable whether there is any justification for making the distinction in a patient with major atherosclerotic coronary disease. In patients who are found subsequently to have normal coronary arteries or minor disease, in whom spasm may be demonstrated or provokable, the clinical distinction from unstable angina is useful because there are implications for treatment. However, as the condition presents with angina at rest and is accompanied by a substantial risk of progression to myocardial infarction, and it is not possible to distinguish clinically those with severe underlying coronary disease from patients with mild disease or normal coronary arteries,[3] it is logical to consider variant angina as part of the spectrum of unstable angina.

PATHOLOGY AND PATHOPHYSIOLOGY

The paroxysms of myocardial ischaemia associated with unstable angina are thought to result from a spectrum of pathophysiological mechanisms, the relative importance of each varying among patients and, probably, within an individual patient at different times. However, the condition appears to be initiated, almost invariably, by a specific process—the sudden disruption of an atherosclerotic plaque.

PATHOLOGICAL CHANGES IN THE CORONARY ARTERIES

Pathological studies of patients who have died suddenly after the development of symptoms of unstable angina have disclosed coronary arterial changes identical to those found in patients who have died from an acute myocardial infarction. The characteristic finding is a fissured atheromatous plaque, within which can be found evidence of haemorrhage and thrombosis. Typically, the intramural head of the thrombus consists of layers of aggregated platelets of different age, suggesting a progressive, stepwise development; this head is continuous with a tail, consisting predominantly of fibrin with enmeshed red blood cells, which projects into the arterial lumen. Intramyocardial platelet aggregates and atheromatous particles may be found in arterioles downstream from the plaque,

and are often accompanied by areas of micro-infarction; such peripheral embolization might account for arrhythmias and sudden death in patients with symptoms of unstable angina.[4–6]

The cause of the plaque disruption is unknown, but it seems likely to be a physical rather than a biological phenomenon; the constant bending and twisting of the coronary arteries during the cardiac cycle may account partly for the frequency of plaque disruption in these vessels compared with those of similar size in other parts of the body exposed to comparable haemodynamic stresses. Haemorrhage into the plaque might be the initiating event, although intramural blood is thought in most instances to have arisen from the arterial lumen after disruption of the intima has occurred.

Contact of blood with the contents of the plaque, which are often rich in lipid, would result in platelet adhesion and aggregation and account for the formation of the mural thrombus. The platelet activation, biochemical evidence of which can be detected in patients with unstable angina,[7,8] might activate the intrinsic coagulation pathway and cause superimposition of the fibrin–red cell thrombus.

PATHOPHYSIOLOGY OF THE MYOCARDIAL ISCHAEMIA

Myocardial ischaemia in patients with angina at rest usually results from a transient reduction in regional myocardial blood flow rather than, as had previously been thought, from an increase in myocardial oxygen consumption in the presence of a critical 'fixed', obstruction to blood flow. In haemodynamic studies, it has been shown that ischaemic left ventricular dysfunction and ST-segment displacement on the electrocardiogram precede the development of chest pain and any increase, which commonly occurs secondarily, in heart rate or blood pressure or both.[9,10]

Intermittent ('dynamic') coronary obstruction superimposed on a fixed stenosis accounts for several observations that had been difficult to reconcile with the view that angina occurring at rest is caused solely by a static reduction in coronary flow reserve of such severity that a small increase in myocardial oxygen consumption (as might result from a slight increase in heart rate) could precipitate myocardial ischaemia. The principal inconsistencies with this concept are the overall comparability in the extent of coronary artery obstruction in patients with stable and unstable angina,[11–13] that in up to a quarter of patients who have had coronary angiograms before and after the development of unstable angina the appearances are unchanged[14] (and at least 10% of patients have normal angiograms[15]), the well-preserved exercise capacity of many patients who have recovered from an episode of unstable angina, the relative tolerance to pacing-induced tachycardia,[16] and, finally, the occurrence of cardiac pain associated with heart rates and blood pressures below those observed at other times but in the absence of myocardial ischaemia.

However, symptoms consistent with the definition of unstable angina can result from severe 'fixed' coronary arterial obstruction. This may develop over many years from a gradual progression of coronary atherosclerosis, and is suggested by a history of progressively (rather than abruptly) increasing effort angina, eventually culminating in pain at 'rest' although in fact precipitated by the slightest physical or emotional stimulus. Alternatively, a sudden increase in obstruction may result from plaque rupture, with or without superimposed thrombosis.

The two mechanisms are not mutually exclusive, and in many patients it is likely that intermittent flow reduction and low coronary reserve operate together to cause rest angina. Moreover, even in patients in whom dynamic coronary obstruction is thought to be the primary abnormality, the importance of changes in myocardial oxygen consumption should not be discounted. Any increase in cardiac work accompanying a period of reduced flow will increase the imbalance between myocardial oxygen supply and demand and intensify the resulting myocardial ischaemia.

Dynamic coronary obstruction may be caused by recurrent episodes of thrombosis followed by fragmentation and distal embolization, or vasospasm. Both mechanisms may operate in some patients.

Thrombosis

The fundamental role of thrombosis in the genesis of unstable angina is supported primarily by its almost invariable presence, in pathological specimens and in life, when it can be observed angioscopically in patients with angina at rest but not in those with stable angina.[17] Second, myocardial infarction, which is a principal complication of unstable angina, is known to be precipitated by thrombosis in most cases, and, finally, antithrombotic therapy is the only treatment that has been shown to reduce both the mortality and the incidence of myocardial infarction associated with unstable angina.[18-20]

An attractive hypothesis, for which there is some supporting evidence, is that haemorrhage into the plaque consequent upon its acute rupture results in a rapid increase in encroachment on the coronary artery lumen and the abrupt appearance or worsening of effort angina; and that should intraluminal thrombosis occur, it is associated with the development of angina at rest or, if the thrombus occludes the artery for any length of time, with myocardial infarction.

Spasm

Atherosclerotic plaques tend to develop eccentrically around the arterial circumference, leaving an arc of normal wall which may be able to lengthen or shorten in response to changes in tone of the medial smooth muscle.[21,22] Energy loss (reflected by pressure drop) in a stenosis is related to the fourth power of its radius, such that, once an atherosclerotic obstruction has become severe, a further slight reduction in diameter from shortening of the muscle of the disease-free arc could cause a dramatic reduction in distal perfusion.[23] Such shortening might be part of a process affecting the whole artery, or it might be localized to the region of the plaque; it has been shown angiographically that the residual lumen associated with up to 70% of coronary stenoses can be increased or decreased by pharmacological interventions known to relax or constrict the vascular smooth muscle of the coronary arteries.[24,25] An important aspect of the concept is that, with a severe atherosclerotic (or atherosclerotic plus thrombotic) stenosis, muscle shortening within the physiological range could result in a critical reduction in the residual lumen, and a supraphysiological contraction—spasm—could superimpose severe obstruction on an initially mild stenosis.

Direct evidence for the pathogenetic role of spasm is derived from angiographic observations of total or sub-total coronary artery occlusion, which can reverse spontaneously or in response to a vasodilator, during attacks of rest angina.[26] In many patients, vascular occlusion and myocardial ischaemia can be provoked by the administration of ergometrine, which is a powerful constrictor of the coronary artery smooth muscle.

The term 'vasotonic' angina encompasses the wide spectrum of spasm that may be encountered in stable and unstable angina.[27] At one extreme is the patient who has little or no angiographic evidence of atheromatous coronary disease in whom myocardial ischaemia is caused entirely by severe spasm of the affected vessel; at the other, is the patient with a sub-total occlusion from atheromatous plaque (with or without superimposed thrombus) in whom a slight shortening of the disease-free arc is sufficient to cause a critical reduction in myocardial blood flow.

The cause of coronary arterial smooth muscle contraction in unstable (and stable) angina is not known, but recent experimental evidence suggests that the essential trigger might be the damage to the vascular endothelium at the site of the disrupted atheromatous plaque. Arterial vasoconstriction is normally opposed by release of an endothelium-derived relaxing factor, and loss of the endothelium results in a vasoconstrictor response to certain stimuli that would normally cause vaso-dilatation.[28–31] Platelet activation is accompanied by the release of vaso-active materials, including thromboxane A_2, serotonin, and platelet-derived growth factor,[32] and the endothelial disruption, therefore, might account for thrombosis and vaso-spasm in unstable angina.

In variant angina, spasm may be mediated by stimulation of alpha-adrenergic receptors.[33]

Resolution of unstable angina

Two mechanisms could account for recovery from unstable angina. Spontaneous fibrinolysis of the thrombus may be followed by healing of the plaque with restoration of endothelial integrity and an adequate coronary lumen. In support of this suggestion is the angiographic observation of 're-modelling', with improvement in the residual lumen of some coronary lesions weeks or months after successful thrombolytic treatment during evolving myocardial infarction. Alternatively, repeated myocardial ischaemia might result in the development of a collateral circulation adequate to maintain myocardial viability despite the persistence of a high-grade coronary obstruction; angiography in patients who have recovered from an episode of unstable angina often shows an occluded artery with collateral filling of its distal branches, and normal contraction of the compromised region of myocardium.

PROGNOSIS

The complications of unstable angina are myocardial infarction and sudden death.

Reports of overall mortality in the first year after an episode of unstable angina have ranged from 4 to 18%, with infarction occurring in from 7 to 17% within the first month,[34,15] although the results from the majority of studies of medically treated patients,[35–37] and the control group mortality in two trials of aspirin therapy,[19,20] suggest a 1-year mortality of 8–15% and an incidence of myocardial infarction of 8–13% at 1 month and of 10–14% within 1 year.

Apart from chance, the differences in published mortality and incidence of infarction can be ascribed to variations in the criteria used for the diagnosis of unstable angina, to the inclusion or exclusion of patients who are found to have had an infarction soon after presentation, to their origin (those referred directly from their general practitioners probably having a more favourable prognosis than those transferred to a secondary referral centre after initial treatment has been ineffective) and, possibly, to different methods of treatment.

Myocardial infarction is most likely to occur within the first few hours of presentation with unstable angina,[38] and in many patients it will develop too soon to be amenable to any form of therapeutic intervention short of immediate revascularization. (Such patients tend to be regarded retrospectively as having had a myocardial infarction from the outset rather than unstable angina.) After a lapse of 3–4 months, the risk of death or infarction is little different to that of patients who have stable coronary disease of comparable severity. A significant proportion of patients, up to one-third, can be expected to become free of symptoms by the end of this period, most of them becoming so within the first few days.

Although there is a considerable element of unpredictability over the prognosis for a patient with unstable angina, certain clinical characteristics are helpful in assessing the individual risk and useful when deciding on the most appropriate management. Continuing episodes of myocardial ischaemia (painful or painless) reflected by electrocardiographic changes after admission to hospital are an adverse sign and are associated with an overall rate of death plus non-fatal infarction of 14–20% within the first 3 months.[15,35,39–42] A history of previous myocardial infarction and clinical evidence of left ventricular dysfunction also indicate a relatively poor prognosis; if an infarction develops in such patients, it is less likely to be survived than in patients who do not have pre-existing myocardial damage. Patients in whom severe angina develops within about 4 weeks of a myocardial infarction are particularly likely to experience complications; in one study, 56% died within 6 months.[43] Finally, patients who had chronic angina before the development of unstable angina are likely to continue with undiminished symptoms after recovery from the unstable episode, and the long-term prognosis is worse than for those with a short history, presumably because patients with a long history are likely to have more extensive coronary disease.

Patients with effort angina of recent onset generally have a favourable immediate prognosis, little different from that of patients with chronic effort angina; in the absence of additional adverse features, the diagnosis of unstable angina is inappropriate.

PROGNOSIS OF VARIANT ANGINA

The overall prognosis of variant angina is not greatly different from that associated with other forms of unstable angina, with death occurring in about 5% and infarction in about 20% within the first year;[44,45] these complications, however, are concentrated to an even greater extent within the first 3 months, with survival beyond this time being associated with a favourable medium-term outlook. As in the more usual form of unstable angina, complications are most likely to affect patients who have frequent episodes of ischaemia, severe coronary disease or impaired left ventricular function. Patients with normal or minimally diseased coronary arteries have an excellent prognosis once the acute symptoms have subsided.[46] There is some evidence that treatment with calcium antagonist drugs improves the outcome.[45]

DIAGNOSIS

The diagnosis of unstable angina is made from the recognition of ischaemic cardiac pain (a process requiring differentiation from other causes of chest pain), and the exclusion of myocardial infarction.

HISTORY

As in the diagnosis of effort angina, the site,

character and distribution of the pain are helpful, but its occurrence at rest and the inconsistent influence of or resistance to nitrate therapy may eliminate two of the more helpful diagnostic features of ischaemic cardiac pain. Patients with previous stable angina can often judge whether their pain is similar in character to that which was formerly induced by effort, although anxiety can readily result in the mistaken attribution of chest pain from other causes to their known heart disease.

Many patients with 'stable' coronary disease experience marked variations in exercise tolerance with the time of day, temperature and in relation to eating; these features should not be regarded as manifestations of unstable angina. Similarly, attacks of angina occurring with emotional stress or wakening the patient from sleep, although usually associated with extensive coronary disease, may recur over long periods and do not of themselves justify a diagnosis of unstable angina. The hallmark of the transition from stable to unstable angina is a sudden change in its severity and in the circumstances in which it occurs.

PHYSICAL EXAMINATION

Physical examination in a patient with unstable angina is frequently normal. There may be signs of left ventricular dysfunction or overt heart failure from previous infarction; occasionally a fourth or, exceptionally, a third heart sound may be audible during but not between episodes of chest pain. It is important to measure the blood pressure, to search for evidence of peripheral or cerebrovascular disease and to examine for signs of non-coronary heart disease or extracardiac disease which might mimic unstable angina.

INVESTIGATION

The electrocardiogram

The electrocardiogram is of crucial importance, both diagnostically, because certain abnormalities reflect a high probability of the existence of underlying myocardial ischaemia (and, therefore, of coronary heart disease), and prognostically, because the outlook is worse for patients with an abnormal than with a normal recording. Whenever possible, the electrocardiogram should be recorded during an episode of pain.

The characteristic electrocardiographic findings are transient ST-segment depression, with or without associated T-wave changes or, less frequently, ST-segment elevation. Depression and elevation of the ST-segment may occur at different times in the same patient. These changes may be recorded in the absence of chest pain; continuous electrocardiographic monitoring has shown that such episodes, indicative of myocardial ischaemia ('silent ischaemia'), may occur very much more frequently than those associated with pain. In one study, 80% of ischaemic episodes, some of which were prolonged, were painless.[47]

Changes in the T-wave are less specific for myocardial ischaemia than ST-segment depression or elevation, but they are commonly observed in patients with unstable angina. Deep symmetrical inversion (which may be persistent), or a combination of augmentation and peaking (usually transient), are characteristic, but the changes can be subtle, and 'minor' T-wave abnormalities can be of great diagnostic value. Sometimes, ischaemic T-wave changes are accompanied by marked prolongation of the QT interval. A potentially misleading appearance can occur if the 'baseline' electrocardiogram shows T-wave flattening or inversion, which becomes 'normalized' during episodes of ischaemia. It is important to emphasize that persistent T-wave inversion, in the absence of a rise in cardiac enzymes, does not indicate that 'subendocardial' myocardial infarction has occurred.

Arrhythmias occur in 15–30% of ischaemic episodes, most commonly ventricular premature beats and most seriously ventricular fibrillation. In patients with variant angina, profound bradycardia (usually due to atrioventricular block) or ventricular tachycardia may cause syncope. Occasionally, episodes of ischaemia are accompanied by the development of transient bundle branch block.

The presence of pathological Q waves indicative of previous myocardial infarction provides strong evidence of coronary heart disease and, therefore, circumstantial evidence in support of a diagnosis of unstable angina in a patient with a suggestive history.

Exercise testing

A persistently normal electrocardiogram, during and between episodes of chest pain, is strong evidence against, but does not preclude, a diagnosis of unstable angina.

In certain circumstances, notably when a patient is seen after a single episode of chest pain which does not recur and the electrocardiogram is normal, exercise-induced ST-segment depression (or a reversible defect on the thallium scan) may support a retrospective diagnosis of unstable angina, by suggesting the presence of underlying coronary disease. Conversely, a completely normal exercise test in these circumstances militates against the presence of important coronary artery disease. Exercise testing is not helpful in making a diagnosis when the resting electrocardiogram is abnormal; it is contraindicated in patients with continuing evidence of recurrent myocardial ischaemia.

Once the acute illness has resolved, the exercise test may be valuable in the selection of patients for coronary arteriography and, for those in whom angiography has been carried out, it provides complementary information helpful in determining the need for myocardial revascularization. A test accompanied by angina, ST-segment depression or both appears to be predictive of future symptoms, myocardial infarction and the need for myocardial revascularization.[48]

Cardiac enzymes

Cardiac enzymes should be measured on admission to hospital, and then daily until the acute symptoms have resolved. The results are not helpful in planning initial therapy, and can give only a retrospective diagnosis of myocardial infarction.

A small rise in enzyme concentration, reflecting minor myocardial necrosis, commonly occurs; and it can be difficult to decide whether a patient who has been free of pain for several hours but in whom a modest enzyme release has occurred should be regarded as having had a small but complete infarction, or remains at risk of sustaining further myocardial damage. If rest pain recurs, the patient has unstable angina regardless of the enzyme level and requires appropriate treatment; in occasional patients, myocardial infarction occurs episodically over hours or days; theoretically, such an evolution might be amenable to therapeutic intervention and could be regarded, if it could be recognized in advance, as a form of unstable angina.

Coronary arteriography

The diagnosis of unstable angina is based on clinical and electrocardiographic criteria, but coronary arteriography provides invaluable information in many patients. The indications for angiography are discussed in the section on management.

About 90% of patients who have angina at rest

accompanied by repolarization abnormalities on the electrocardiogram will be found to have coronary artery disease. Overall, the extent of the disease, in terms of the number of affected vessels and the severity of obstruction, is similar in patients with stable and unstable angina.[11-13]

Even in patients with multivessel disease, it is generally possible, by combining analysis of the angiographic appearances with electrocardiographic localization of the affected region of myocardium, to identify the lesion responsible for the acute ischaemia.[13]

Filling defects in relation to the stenosis, sometimes associated with persistent staining of contrast medium, or occlusions with a convex border indicate intraluminal thrombus.[49,50] The frequency with which thrombus is visualized appears to be related to the recency of the symptoms of unstable angina; in one study, it was identified in association with over 50% of angina-producing stenoses when angiography was carried out within 24 h of the last episode of chest pain, whereas it was detected in less than one-third of those investigated between 24 h and 14 days.[51]

In addition to the visualization of thrombus, it can be possible to identify the complicated atheromatous plaque itself. High-resolution images of the 'culprit lesion' in patients with unstable angina or recent infarction may show scalloping, irregularity or definite clefts indicative of surface ulceration. These features are observed rarely in patients with stable angina.[13,51,52]

In patients who have previously undergone angiography, the responsible lesion may be at the site of an old stenosis or it may have arisen in an arterial segment that was apparently normal at the time of the first angiogram. The angiogram following the development of unstable angina, however, appears unchanged in up to 25% of patients.[14]

The left ventriculogram

The left ventricular angiogram may show normal contraction or any degree of impairment, as in patients with stable angina. If it is recorded during, or even within several hours of, an episode of ischaemia, contraction may be depressed, with recovery of normal function after resolution of the ischaemia, either spontaneously or as a result of surgical revascularization or angioplasty. It is important to consider the possibility that apparently severe left ventricular dysfunction may be reversible in patients who seem to carry an unacceptable risk

for surgical treatment, particularly if there are no Q waves on the electrocardiogram and there is no history of previous infarction.

DIFFERENTIAL DIAGNOSIS

Differentiation from myocardial infarction

When a patient is first seen during or soon after a single episode of prolonged chest pain, it may be impossible to differentiate unstable angina from acute myocardial infarction. The duration of continuous pain is surprisingly unhelpful because that resulting from unstable angina may last for >1 h and, when one episode of ischaemia is followed closely by another, the patient may consider that the pain has lasted for several hours. Conversely, the pain from an acute myocardial infarction may fluctuate, or resolve rapidly in <1 h.

Fortunately, it is unimportant if the diagnosis of rest angina has to be revised to myocardial infarction subsequently, because the initial treatment of unstable angina is appropriate for that of acute infarction; this error is generally preferable to the mistaken diagnosis of infarction which might result in the treatment for unstable angina being withheld. If a high index of suspicion of unstable angina is maintained when the electrocardiographic signs of a possible infarction are equivocal, up to a quarter of patients initially diagnosed as having unstable angina will be found to have had a myocardial infarction at the time of their presentation, or within the first few hours of hospital admission.

Chest pain from non-coronary heart disease

Cardiac conditions other than those associated with coronary artery disease may cause chest pain that can be confused with that of unstable angina.

Cardiomyopathy, particularly of the hypertrophic type, may present with anginal pain on effort or at rest; in this condition, the repolarization abnormality (sometimes with additional Q waves) which is almost invariably present on the electrocardiogram reinforces the error. Evidence of unexplained left ventricular hypertrophy should lead to suspicion of the diagnosis which, once considered, is easily confirmed by echocardiography.

The pain from acute pericarditis is more likely to be mistaken for that of myocardial infarction than for that of unstable angina. The pleuritic character is nearly always helpful, and the condition may be accompanied by fever and signs of a systemic disease of which the pericarditis is a manifestation. The presence of a pericardial rub is of great diagnostic value. The ST-segment elevation associated with pericarditis typically involves multiple leads, whereas that from myocardial ischaemia is usually localized to anterior, inferior or inferolateral leads. Subsequent evolution of the changes (rapid resolution in unstable angina or gradual T-wave inversion with pericarditis) should clarify the diagnosis.

Other cardiac conditions associated with angina rarely cause rest pain; its occurrence, for example, in a patient with aortic stenosis strongly indicates the co-existence of coronary artery disease.

Extracardiac disease

Oesophageal pain arising from reflux disease, abnormal motility or both may be indistinguishable from ischaemic cardiac pain, and acid reflux may be provoked by effort, precisely mimicking previous effort angina.[53,54] Particular difficulty occurs when one of these conditions co-exists with coronary heart disease; 'ischaemic' changes on the electrocardiogram may cause further confusion.

A common diagnostic error is to mistake biliary colic for unstable angina; the development of jaundice or the discovery of gallstones after the performance of a normal coronary arteriogram in a patient presumed to have had rest angina often serves to remind the cardiologist of an earlier, and similarly embarrassing, occasion. A helpful feature is that biliary colic almost invariably radiates to the back between the scapulae; this feature occurs less commonly in angina.

In certain circumstances, almost any disease of the spine, nerve roots, mediastinal structures (including the aorta), chest wall or upper abdominal viscera may mimic unstable angina, as indeed the pain from such disorders may be confused with that from acute myocardial infarction.

MANAGEMENT

The objectives of the management of unstable angina are to abolish the episodes of myocardial ischaemia (both symptomatic and asymptomatic) and prevent death and the development of myocardial infarction.

GENERAL MEASURES

Patients with unstable angina are most safely managed in hospital, ideally in a coronary care unit. Initial assessment should include a search for conditions that might aggravate myocardial ischaemia: in particular, anaemia, heart failure or hypertension. Rest, in order to minimize myocardial oxygen consumption, should be advised until the acute symptoms have subsided; smoking must be forbidden.

DRUG THERAPY

Two main categories of drug therapy are helpful in the treatment of unstable angina.

1   Agents with a primarily anti-ischaemic effect: nitrates, beta-adrenoceptor blockers and calcium antagonists.
2   Anti-thrombotic agents: heparin and the orally active vitamin-K antagonists, aspirin and fibrinolytic agents.

Nitrates, beta-blockers, and calcium antagonists are effective in reducing the frequency and severity of the episodes of myocardial ischaemia.

Concern that beta-blockers might worsen the ischaemia in some patients, by transforming sympathetic stimulation of the coronary circulation from a mixed vasodilator-vasoconstrictor (beta + alpha) to a purely vasoconstrictor (alpha) response, was reinforced by a study of patients with predominantly vasotonic angina,[55] but this effect can be countered by the addition of a calcium antagonist to the beta-blocker regimen.[56] Beta-blocker therapy is probably more effective first-line treatment for unstable angina than that with a calcium antagonist, but the combination of both is better than the administration of either alone.[38,41,42]

The results of several studies have suggested that conventional anticoagulant therapy improves the prognosis for patients with unstable angina; although none of these trials satisfies the current criteria for a reliable unbiased trial (and some are seriously deficient), taken collectively they indicate a beneficial effect from these agents.[18,57–60]

There is compelling evidence for the value of aspirin therapy. In two large randomized controlled trials, a reduction of over 50% in the rates of death and non-fatal myocardial infarction with aspirin treatment, from 3 months to 2 years after an episode of unstable angina, was found.[19,20] Daily doses of 325 mg and 1300 mg appear to be comparably effective, but the lower dose is less liable to cause gastro-intestinal side-effects which necessitate the withdrawal of the drug. It is not known whether an even smaller dose would be equally or more effective.

At present, the place of thrombolytic therapy in the management of unstable angina is poorly defined, although evidence of its value in acute myocardial infarction and recognition of the importance of thrombosis in the pathogenesis of unstable angina suggest that it might prove to be of value. In one small trial, intravenous streptokinase administered over 24 h, followed with warfarin anticoagulation, was associated with the occurrence of fewer cardiovascular complications during 3–6 months' follow-up than that in a similar number of patients who were randomized to receive only warfarin.[61] Intracoronary streptokinase administration can decrease the severity of coronary obstruction and improve the clinical state in some patients with unstable angina;[62] it can lyse occlusive thrombi in patients who have rest pain after a recent myocardial infarction.[63]

Ideally, the treatment of unstable angina would be tailored individually according to the underlying pathophysiology in each case; but as it is not always possible, even after coronary arteriography has been carried out, to determine with any confidence the relative importance of fixed coronary obstruction, spasm and thrombosis, all possibilities must be covered. The combination of all three classes of anti-anginal agent, plus aspirin or heparin, can be expected to minimize cardiac work and myocardial oxygen consumption, to improve myocardial blood flow in patients with vasotonic angina and to diminish the tendency for thrombosis.

Therefore, unless contra-indicated, all patients who have unstable angina should receive a beta-blocker, regular nitrate therapy, a calcium antagonist and aspirin. In patients with variant angina in whom angiography has confirmed the presence of mild atherosclerotic coronary obstruction, the beta-blocker can be omitted.

If the patient has chest pain at the time of presentation, this and subsequent episodes should be treated with a nitrate, administered either sublingually or intravenously. If this therapy is not rapidly effective, the dose should be repeated and morphine (or an alternative analogue) given intravenously in small doses, titrated against the pain. If there is a tachycardia, intravenous administration of a beta-blocker should be considered.

Prophylactic therapy should be commenced as soon as these initial measures have been implemented.

Long-term nitrate therapy can be administered sublingually, orally, in a variety of preparations, or transdermally. The different preparations and methods of administration affect principally the frequency with which the agent has to be administered; none has a clear advantage over the others in terms of prophylactic anti-anginal action. Glyceryl trinitrate or isosorbide dinitrate should be given by continuous intravenous infusion if the ischaemic episodes are not rapidly brought under control; the dose can be increased until the angina is controlled or the blood pressure falls unacceptably thereby causing symptomatic hypotension. Once the patient has been free of recurrent pain for 12–24 h, the infusion can be gradually withdrawn and replaced by oral or transdermal treatment.

The dose of beta-blocker should be increased until the heart rate has fallen to <60 beats/min; as agents with partial agonist activity do not usually slow the resting heart rate, they are unsuitable for use in patients with unstable angina. Water-soluble agents have an advantage in that the optimal dose varies relatively little among patients, but they have the disadvantage of a longer half-life such that, if an adverse effect does develop, it will persist for longer than that resulting from a lipid-soluble drug which has a short half-life.

No single calcium antagonist is clearly superior to the others in the treatment of unstable angina, although individual circumstances may determine a specific choice. Verapamil and diltiazem exert an additive effect with beta-adrenoceptor blockade in depressing sino-atrial and atrioventricular conduction, and the combination can cause severe bradycardia even in patients with previously normal conduction. These drugs given separately or in combination with a beta-blocker should be avoided in patients with evidence of sino-atrial or atrioventricular block. The combination of verapamil with a beta-blocker is probably the most likely to depress left ventricular function and is contra-indicated in patients who have heart failure. Nifedipine is highly satisfactory in combination with a beta-blocker; it does not affect conduction and is unlikely to depress left ventricular contraction, but it should not be used without a beta-blocker because of its tendency to provoke a reflex tachycardia[42] and the suspicion that it may increase the risk of infarction.[38]

The combination of two vasodilators with a beta-blocker is liable to cause hypotension, and therefore, the initial doses should be small. Subsequent doses can be increased, and brought forward in time if necessary.

It is logical to start aspirin treatment immediately, but, as there is a danger of increased blood loss

in the event of surgical treatment being required, it can be argued that its administration should be delayed until the acute symptoms have settled. However, many surgeons are prepared to accept this slight risk, and, if 'medical' bleeding is excessive in a patient receiving aspirin, it can be controlled by transfusion of fresh blood or platelets. The risk of gastric haemorrhage can be minimized by prescription of an 'enteric-coated' or buffered aspirin preparation, and use of no more than a single tablet of 325 mg daily.

If aspirin is contra-indicated and the patient continues to have angina at rest, intravenous heparin anticoagulation should be considered.

FURTHER MANAGEMENT

With this regimen of rest and multiple drug therapy, ischaemic episodes will decline sharply in the majority of patients, and 50–80% can be expected to become asymptomatic within the first 48 h; the mortality during this period is low, and many patients will have no further rest pain after admission to hospital. For these patients, the risk of infarction is relatively small (although it may occur unpredictably after several days of freedom from symptoms) and further treatment should be based on the same principles as those that guide the management of any other patient with coronary heart disease. The mobilization of patients is the same as that for those who have had an uncomplicated myocardial infarction.

Patients who continue to experience recurrent episodes of myocardial ischaemia for >24–48 h, after hospital admission and the institution of medical therapy should be considered for revascularization. Although a more conservative approach, with a longer trial of medical therapy, is appropriate for elderly or otherwise frail patients, they should not be denied a coronary arteriogram if intractable angina persists, because treatment by angioplasty may be feasible.

Indications for coronary arteriography

Knowledge of the location, severity, and extent of coronary disease and insight into the pathophysiology of the myocardial ischaemia are valuable for determining immediate and long-term management; the performance of coronary angiography can be justified in essentially all patients with, or who have recently recovered from, unstable angina. This approach is not always practical, however; in

these circumstances, an attempt should be made to select for angiography those most likely to be candidates for surgical treatment or angioplasty, or those for whom the findings are otherwise likely to have a crucial influence on management.

Angiography is indicated for patients who continue to have unprovoked episodes of myocardial ischaemia which are not promptly relieved by sublingual nitrates for >24–48 h after the commencement of medical treatment; in these circumstances, it should be performed with the intention of an early recourse to myocardial revascularization if the findings are appropriate. If facilities permit, it is helpful to have the patient's permission to proceed directly from angiography to angioplasty.

Elective angiography, after the acute symptoms have subsided, should be considered in the following patients.

1 Those with long standing effort angina, particularly if their earlier symptoms were sufficiently severe to have justified myocardial revascularization.
2 Those with a previous myocardial infarction, or with clinical evidence of left ventricular dysfunction, unless the dominant problem is heart failure.
3 Those in whom an exercise test, carried out after the acute symptoms have settled, discloses electrocardiographic (or scintigraphic) evidence of severe myocardial ischaemia at a low workload. (In the future, it is possible that ambulatory ST-segment analysis will provide a better indication than exercise testing of the propensity to develop myocardial ischaemia during everyday life and, therefore, it will serve as a valuable investigation in judging the need for angiography.)
4 Those thought to have had variant angina.
5 Those in whom there is uncertainty about the diagnosis.

MYOCARDIAL REVASCULARIZATION—SURGERY OR ANGIOPLASTY

Aortocoronary bypass surgery or, if the coronary arteriographic findings are suitable, angioplasty is indicated for patients who continue to have recurrent episodes of myocardial ischaemia despite optimal medical therapy.

Precisely when medical therapy should be regarded as having failed is arbitrary, and the decision must be influenced by the clinical setting. For example, early revascularization would be advisable for a high-risk patient who has had previous angina or myocardial infarction, with severe and widespread repolarization changes on the electrocardiogram during pain, and in whom angiography has shown coronary lesions compromising an extensive area of myocardium, whereas a further period of medical treatment would be appropriate for a low-risk patient who has a short history and a single lesion in a distal coronary branch, particularly if angioplasty is not feasible. In patients with diffuse coronary disease, for whom satisfactory revascularization cannot be anticipated with any confidence, it may be advisable to persist with medical therapy over a prolonged period, because the unstable angina will eventually subside, although there is a risk that it will do so only after the occurrence of a myocardial infarction.

Coronary angioplasty

Coronary angioplasty is immediately and dramatically effective in relieving the myocardial ischaemia in selected patients who have unstable angina which has proved refractory to medical treatment.[64-66] The risk of the procedure is low; a mortality rate of <1% and an incidence of infarction of <10% have been reported consistently by workers at centres where considerable experience has been accumulated. Angioplasty seems to be preferable to surgery for patients in whom the coronary anatomy is suitable, although no formal comparisons of the two techniques have been made.

The principal limitations of angioplasty are the unsuitability of some patients and the high rate of recurrent stenosis. Early experience suggested that lesions associated with unstable angina were more liable to restenose after angioplasty than those in patients with stable angina;[67-69] although this has not been confirmed by the more recent reports, among lesions with superimposed spasm (as in variant angina), restenosis occurs in at least 50%.[70,71] The risk of acute coronary occlusion during angioplasty is greater in patients with unstable angina than in those with stable angina; this is likely to be related to the pre-existing arterial injury and the presence of thrombus.

Angioplasty is ideally suited to the patient with a single accessible angina-producing lesion and no significant disease in the remaining coronary circulation. In patients with multiple vessel disease, dilatation of the responsible stenosis alone is effective in abolishing the unstable state,[65,66] but residual effort angina may be troublesome,[66] and

unless the other lesions can be dilated (either at the initial or, more safely, at a subsequent procedure) surgical treatment might be preferable. Moreover, there is evidence that failure to achieve complete revascularization has an adverse influence on the long-term prognosis of surgically treated patients with coronary disease;[72,73] this provides an additional argument in favour of operative treatment for patients with multivessel disease in whom it is not possible to dilate by angioplasty all the significant lesions.

Coronary artery bypass surgery

Aortocoronary bypass surgery is a highly effective treatment for patients with unstable angina who are unsuitable for angioplasty; patients who have undergone surgery are less likely to have residual effort angina than those managed conservatively. However, the operative risk is higher than that for patients with stable angina,[74-76] and a policy of early surgery for all patients with suitable coronary anatomy has not been shown to confer any advantage over medical therapy in terms of survival or the incidence of myocardial infarction. This applies even to patients with proximal lesions in the left anterior descending coronary artery who have been perceived to be at high risk,[74,77] although there is some evidence that the risk associated with impaired left ventricular function is reduced by surgical treatment,[76] as in patients with stable angina. These conclusions are based on the findings of trials in which the surgery was carried out mainly in the mid and late 1970s, and although surgical techniques may have improved since that time such that a lower operative mortality and incidence of perioperative infarction might now be anticipated, medical treatment has also improved with the introduction of calcium antagonists and recognition of the value of aspirin therapy; in view of the low risk during the first few days of conservative management, there is no reason to review the general policy of an initial period of intensive medical treatment, followed by coronary bypass grafting for patients who fail to respond and are unsuitable for angioplasty.

Coronary bypass operations carried out on patients with unstable angina who have recently had a myocardial infarction are particularly hazardous. At most centres, the overall operative mortality approaches 10%,[78,79] but the risk is probably related more to the severity of impairment of left ventricular function than to the recency of the infarction,[79] and remarkably good results from surgical treatment have been reported in these circumstances.[80–82]

UNSTABLE ANGINA IN PATIENTS WITH HEART FAILURE

Patients with unstable angina accompanied by heart failure, particularly those who have had a recent myocardial infarction, have a poor prognosis. The general principles of management are the same as those for patients who do not have heart failure, but certain modifications may be required.

Treatment with a beta-blocker is possible and desirable in patients with mild or moderate heart failure, although it may be necessary to intensify the diuretic therapy; an ideal measure in these circumstances is to combine the beta-blocker with a nitrate infusion. The addition of a calcium antagonist should be made cautiously (unless there is a strong suspicion of variant angina in which case it should be given instead of the beta-blocker) because of the risk of causing further myocardial depression. When left ventricular function is so severely compromised as to preclude treatment with a beta-blocker, intensive nitrate therapy, combined with nifedipine or one of the newer and possibly less depressant dihydropyridine calcium antagonists, should be employed.

Surgical treatment or, ideally, angioplasty is indicated for refractory unstable angina; although the risk is higher in these circumstances than in patients with preserved ventricular function, the benefits from successful revascularization may be correspondingly greater. Peri-operative use of the intra-aortic balloon pump may increase the safety of aortocoronary bypass or angioplasty.

Angina at rest accompanied by heart failure and hypotension poses a difficult therapeutic problem. Swan–Ganz catheterization of the pulmonary artery can be helpful because it allows optimization of the left ventricular filling pressure (and cardiac output) by the manipulation of diuretic and vasodilator therapy and, if necessary, by volume expansion. If there is a realistic prospect of myocardial revascularization, insertion of an intra-aortic balloon pump should be considered, because mechanical circulatory assistance usually results in rapid control of the heart failure and the unstable angina and allows surgical treatment or angioplasty to be carried out more safely.

TREATMENT OF VARIANT ANGINA

Variant angina associated with mild coronary disease should be treated medically, with nitrates and a calcium antagonist in full dosage. When severe 'fixed' obstructions are present in the coronary circulation and the angina is refractory to medical therapy, surgical treatment is effective[83] and preferable to angioplasty because the latter, although effective in the short term, is particularly liable to be complicated by restenosis[70,71]

FOLLOW-UP

Medical treatment should not necessarily be continued indefinitely in patients who remain asymptomatic and are able to return to normal activity after a first episode of unstable angina, although if exercise testing provokes electrocardiographic evidence of myocardial ischaemia it may be advisable to continue the beta-blocker. As yet, there is no evidence that long-acting nitrates or calcium antagonists confer any benefit on asymptomatic patients, other than those with variant angina. On the basis of the results of the Canadian study, aspirin should be continued[20] for at least 2 years, perhaps indefinitely.

Patients with variant angina, in whom angiography has shown normal coronary arteries or mild disease and total suppression of the ischaemic episodes has been achieved, can have their treatment withdrawn after about 1 year, although careful follow-up is advisable as there is a definite risk of recurrence.[84]

Medically treated patients with residual effort angina should be treated, and assessed for revascularization, using the same criteria as those used for any other patient with chronic coronary disease.

REFERENCES

1. Conti, C.R., Brawley, R.K., Griffiths, L.S.C. *et al.* Unstable angina pectoris: morbidity and mortality in 57 consecutive patients evaluated angiographically. *Am. J. Cardiol.* 1973; **32**: 745–50.
2. Prinzmetal, M., Kennamer, R., Merliss, R., Wada, T. and Bor, N. Angina pectoris. I. A variant form of angina pectoris: preliminary report. *Am. J. Med.* 1959; **27**: 375–88.
3. Bott-Silverman, C. Heupler, F.A. Jr and Yiannikas, J. Variant angina: comparison of patients with and without fixed severe coronary disease. *Am. J. Cardiol.* 1984; **54**: 1173–5.
4. Davies, M.J. and Thomas, A.C. Plaque fissuring—the cause of acute myocardial infarction, sudden ischaemic death, and crescendo angina. *Br. Heart J.* 1985; **53**: 363–73.

5. Falk, E. Unstable angina with fatal outcome: dynamic coronary thrombosis leading to infarction and/or sudden death. Autopsy evidence of recurrent mural thrombosis with peripheral embolization culminating in total vascular occlusion. *Circulation* 1985; **71**: 699–708.

6. Davies, M.J., Thomas, A.C., Knapman, P.A. and Hangartner, J.R. Intramyocardial platelet aggregates in patients with unstable angina suffering sudden ischaemic cardiac death. *Circulation* 1986; **73**: 418–27.

7. Hirsh, P.D., Hillis, L.D., Campbell, W.B., Firth, B.G. and Willerson, J.T. Release of prostaglandins and thromboxane into the coronary circulation in patients with ischaemic heart disease. *N. Engl. J. Med.* 1981; **304**: 685–91.

8. Fitzgerald, D.J., Roy, L., Catella, F. and Fitzgerald, G.A. Platelet activation in unstable coronary disease. *N. Engl. J. Med.* 1986; **315**: 983–9.

9. Guazzi, M., Polese, A., Fiorentini, C., Magrini, F., Olivari, M.T. and Bartorelli, C. Left and right heart haemodynamics during spontaneous angina pectoris. Comparison between angina with ST segment depression and angina with ST segment elevation. *Br. Heart J.* 1975; **37**: 401–13.

10. Chierchia, S., Brunelli, C., Simonetti, I., Lazzari, M. and Maseri, A. Sequence of events in angina at rest: primary reduction in coronary flow. *Circulation* 1980; **61**: 759–68.

11. Fuster, V., Frye, R.L., Connolly, D.C., Danielson, M.A., Elveback, L.R. and Kurland, L.T. Arteriographic patterns early in the onset of the coronary syndromes. *Br. Heart J.* 1975; **37**: 1250–5.

12. Balcon, R., Brooks, N., Warnes, C. and Cattell, M. Clinical spectrum of unstable angina. In: Rafflenbeul, W., Lichtlen, P.R. and Balcon, R., eds. *Unstable Angina Pectoris, International Symposium, Hanover 1980.* New York: Thieme–Stratton, 1981; pp.42–44.

13. Ambrose, J.A., Winters, S.L., Stern, A. *et al.* Angiographic morphology and the pathogenesis of unstable angina pectoris. *J. Am. Coll. Cardiol.* 1985; **5**: 609–16.

14. Moise, A., Theroux, P., Taeymans, Y. *et al.* Unstable angina and progression of coronary atherosclerosis. *N. Engl. J. Med.* 1983; **309**: 685–9.

15. Gazes, P.C., Mobley, E.M. Jr, Faris, H.M. Jr, Duncan R.C. and Humphries, G.B. Preinfarctional (unstable) angina—a prospective study—ten year follow-up. *Circulation* 1973; **48**: 331–7.

16. Berndt, T.B., Fitzgerald, J., Harrison, D.C. and Schroeder, J.S. Hemodynamic changes at the onset of spontaneous versus pacing-induced angina. *Am. J. Cardiol.* 1977; **39**: 784–8.

17. Sherman, C.T., Litvak, F., Grundfest, W. *et al.* Coronary angioscopy in patients with unstable angina pectoris. *N. Engl. J. Med.* 1986; **315**: 913–9.

18. Telford, A.M. and Wilson, C. Trial of heparin versus atenolol in prevention of myocardial infarction in intermediate coronary syndrome. *Lancet* 1981; i: 1225–8.

19. Lewis, H.D. Jr, Davis, J.W., Archibald, D.G. *et al.* Protective effects of aspirin against acute myocardial infarction and death in men with unstable angina. *N. Engl. J. Med.* 1983; **309**: 396–403.

20. Cairns, J.A., Gent, M., Singer, J. *et al.* Aspirin, sulfinpyrazone or both in unstable angina. Results of a Canadian multicenter trial. *N. Engl. J. Med.* 1985; **313**: 1369–75.

21. Freudenberg, H. and Lichtlen, P.R. The normal wall segment in coronary stenosis—a postmortem study. *Z. Kardiol.* 1981; **70**: 863–9.

22. Saner, H.E., Gobel, F.L., Salomonowitz, E., Erlien, D.A. and Edwards, J.E. The disease free wall in coronary atherosclerosis: its relation to degree of obstruction. *J. Am. Coll. Cardiol.* 1985; **6**: 1096–9.

23. Brown, B.G., Bolson, E.L. and Dodge, H.T. Dynamic mechanisms in human coronary stenosis. *Circulation* 1984; **70**: 917–22.

24. Lichtlen, P.R., Raffenbeul, W. and Freudenberg, H. Pathoanatomy and function of coronary obstructions leading to unstable angina pectoris: anatomical and angiographic studies. In: Hugenholz, P.G. and Goldman, B.S. eds. *Unstable angina.* Stuttgart: Schattauer, 1985; pp.81–93.

25. Brown, B.G., Response of normal and diseased epicardial coronary arteries to vasoactive drugs: quantitative arteriographic studies. *Am. J. Cardiol.* 1985; (Suppl. E): 23E–29E.

26. Maseri, A., L'Abbate, A., Pesola. A. *et al.* Coronary vasospasm in angina pectoris. *Lancet* 1977; **1**: 713–7.

27. Maseri, A., Severi, S., DeNes, M. *et al.* 'Variant' angina: one aspect of a continuous spectrum of vasospastic myocardial ischemia. *Am. J. Cardiol.* 1978; **42**: 1019–35.

28. Furchgott, R.F. Role of endothelium in responses of vascular smooth muscle. *Circ. Res.* 1983; **53**: 557–73.

29. Griffith, T.M., Edwards, D.H., Collins, P., Lewis, M.J. and Henderson, A.H. Endothelium-derived relaxant factor. *J. R. Coll. Phys. Lond.* 1985; **19**: 74–9.

30. Kawachi, Y., Tomoike, H., Marnoka, Y. *et al.* Selective hypercontraction caused by ergonovine in the canine coronary artery under conditions of induced atherosclerosis. *Circulation* 1984; **69**: 441–50.

31. Ludmer, P.L., Selwyn, A.P., Shook, T.L. *et al.* Paradoxical vasoconstriction induced by acetylcholine in atherosclerotic coronary arteries. *N. Engl. J. Med.* 1986; **315**: 1046–51.

32. Berk, B.C., Alexander, R.W., Brock, T.A., Gimbrone, M.A. Jr and Webb, R.C. Vasoconstriction: a new activity for platelet-derived growth factor. *Science* 1986; **232**: 87–90.

33. Yasue, H., Touyma, M., Kato, H., Tanaka, S. and Akiyama, F. Prinzmetal's variant form of angina as a manifestation of alpha-adrenergic receptor-mediated coronary artery spasm: documentation by coronary arteriography. *Am. Heart J.* 1976; **91**: 148–55.

34. Duncan, B., Fulton, M., Morrison, S.L. *et al.* Prognosis of new and worsening angina. *Brit. Med. J.* 1976; **1**: 981–5.

35. Krauss, K.R., Hutter, A.M. and DeSanctis, R.W. Acute coronary insufficiency. Course and follow-up. *Circulation* 1972; **XLV and XLVI** (Suppl. I): 66–71.

36. Heng, M.-K., Norris, R.M., Singh, B.N. and Partridge, J.B. Prognosis in unstable angina. *Br. Heart J.* 1976; **38**: 921–5.

37. Mulcahy, R., Al Awadhi, A.H., de Buitleor, M., Tobin, G., Johnson, H. and Contoy, C. Natural history and prognosis of unstable angina. *Am. Heart J.* 1985; **109**: 753–8.

38. The Holland Interuniversity Nifedipine/Metoprolol Trial (HINT) research group. Early treatment of unstable angina in the coronary unit: a randomised double-blind, placebo-controlled comparison of recurrent ischaemia in patients treated with nifedipine or metoprolol or both. *Br. Heart J.* 1986; **56**: 400–13.

39. Johnson, S.M., Mauritson, D.R., Winniford, M.D., Willerson, J.T., Firth, B.G., Carg, J.R. and Hillis, L.D. Continuous electrocardiographic monitoring in patients with unstable angina pectoris: identification of high risk sub-group with severe coronary disease, variant angina, and/or impaired early prognosis. *Am. Heart J.* 1982; **103**: 4–12.

40. Gottlieb, S.O., Weisfeldt, M.L., Ouyang, P., Mellits, E.D., and Gerstenblith, G. Silent ischaemia as a marker for early unfavourable outcomes in patients with unstable angina. *N. Engl. J. Med.* 1986; **314**: 1214–9.

41. Gerstenblith, G., Ouyang, P., Aschuff, S.C. *et al.* Nifedipine in unstable angina. A double-blind, randomized trial. *N. Engl. J. Med.* 1982; **306**: 885–9.

42. Muller, J.E., Turi, Z.G. Pearle, D.L. *et al.* Nifedipine and conventional therapy for unstable angina pectoris: a randomized, double-blind comparison. *Circulation* 1984; **69**: 728–39.

43. Schuster, E.H. and Bulkley, B.H. Early post-infarction angina. Ischaemia at a distance and ischaemia in the infarct zone. *N. Engl. J. Med.* 1981; **305**: 1101–5.

44. Severi, S., Davies, G., Maseri, A., Marzullo, P. and

L'Abbate, A. Long-term prognosis of "variant" angina with medical treatment. *Am. J. Cardiol.* 1980; **46**: 226–32.

45. Waters, D.D., Miller, D.D., Szlachicic, J. *et al.* Factors influencing the long-term prognosis of treated patients with variant angina. *Circulation* 1983; **68**: 258–65.

46. Freedman, S.B., Richmond, D.R., Alwyn, M. and Kelly, D.T. Late follow-up (41 to 102 months) of medically treated patients with coronary artery spasm and minor atherosclerotic coronary obstructions. *Am. J. Cardiol.* 1986; **57**: 1261–3.

47. Nademanee, K., Intarachot, V., Singh, P.N., Josephson, M.A. and Singh, B.N. Characteristics and clinical significance of silent myocardial ischaemia in unstable angina. *Am. J. Cardiol.* 1986; **58**: 26B–33B

48. Butman, S.M., Olson, H.G., Gardin, J.M., Piters, K.M., Hullett, M. and Butman, L.K. Submaximal exercise testing after stabilization of unstable angina pectoris. *J. Am. Coll. Cardiol.* 1984; **4**: 667–73.

49. Holmes, D.R., Hartzler, G.O., Smith, H.C. and Fuster, V. Coronary artery thrombosis in patients with unstable angina. *Br. Heart J.* 1981; **45**: 411–6.

50. Zack, P.M., Ischinger, T., Aker, V.T., Dincer, B. and Kennedy, H.L. The occurrence of angiographically detected intracoronary thrombus in patients with unstable angina pectoris. *Am. Heart J.* 1984; **108**: 1408–11.

51. Capone, G., Wolf, N.M. and Meister, S.G. Frequency of intracoronary filling defects by angiography in angina pectoris at rest. *Am. J. Cardiol.* 1985; **56**: 403–6.

52. Wilson, R.F., Holida, M.D. and White, C.W. Quantitative angiographic morphology of coronary stenoses leading to myocardial infarction or unstable angina. *Circulation* 1986; **73**: 286–93.

53. Alban Davies, H., Jones, D.B. and Rhodes, J. "Oesophageal angina" as the cause of chest pain. *JAMA* 1982; **248**: 2274–8.

54. Schofield, P.M., Bennett, D.H., Jones, P.E. *et al.* Exertional gastro-oesophageal reflux. A mechanism for symptoms in patients with angina pectoris and normal coronary angiograms. *Br. Med. J.* 1987; **294**: 1459–61

55. Robertson, R.M., Wood, A.J., Vaughn, W.K. and Robertson, D. Exacerbation of vasotonic angina pectoris by propranolol. *Circulation* 1982; **65**: 281–5.

56. Tilmant, P.Y., Lablanche, J.M., Thieuleux, F.A., Dupuis, B.A. and Bertrand, M.E. Detrimental effect of propranolol in patients with coronary artery spasm countered by combination with diltiazem. *Am. J. Cardiol.* 1983; **52**: 230–3.

57. Nichol, E.S., Phillips, W.C. and Casten, G.G. Virtue of prompt anticoagulant therapy in impending myocardial infarction: Experiences with 318 patients during a 10-year period. *Arch. Intern. Med.* 1959; **50**: 1158–73.

58. Wood, P. Acute and subacute coronary insufficiency. *Br. Med. J.* 1961; **i**: 1779–82.

59. Beamish, R.E. and Storrie, V.M. Impending myocardial infarction: recognition and management. *Circulation* 1960; **21**: 1107–15.

60. Vakil, R.J. Preinfarction syndrome – management and follow-up. *Am. J. Cardiol.* 1964; **14**: 55–63.

61. Lawrence, J.R., Shepherd, J.T., Bone, I., Rogen, A.S. and Fulton, W.F.M. Fibrinolytic therapy in unstable angina pectoris. A controlled clinical trial. *Thromb. Res.* 1980; **17**: 767–77.

62. Vetrovec, G.W., Leinbach, R.C., Gold, H.K. and Cowley, M.J. Intracoronary thrombolysis in syndromes of unstable ischaemia: angiographic and clinical results. *Am. Heart J.* 1982; **104**: 946–52.

63. Shapiro, E.P., Brinker, J.A., Gottlieb, S.O., Guzman, P.A. and Bulkley, B.H. Intracoronary thrombolysis 3 to 13 days after acute myocardial infarction for post-infarction angina pectoris. *Am. J. Cardiol.* 1985; **55**: 1453–8.

64. deFeyter, P.J., Serruys, P.W., van den Brand, M. *et al.* Emergency coronary angioplasty in refractory unstable angina. *N. Engl. J. Med.* 1985; **313**: 342–6.

65. Wohlgelernter, D., Cleman, M., Highman, A. and Zaret, B.L. Percutaneous transluminal coronary angioplasty of the "culprit lesion" for management of unstable angina pectoris in patients with multivessel coronary artery disease. *Am. J. Cardiol.* 1986; **58**: 460–4.

66. deFeyter, P.J., Serruys, P.W., Arnold, A. *et al.* Coronary angioplasty of the unstable angina related vessel in patients with multiple vessel disease. *Eur. Heart J.* 1986; **7**: 460–7.

67. Kent, K.M., Bentiviglio, L.G., Block, P.C. *et al.* Long term efficacy of PTCA: report from the NHL&BI PTCA registry. *Am. J. Cardiol.* 1984; **53**: 27C–31C.

68. William, V.L. PTCA – a 1985 perspective. *Circulation* 1985; **71**: 189–92.

69. Leingruber, P.P., Roubin, G.S., Hollman, J. *et al.* Restenosis after coronary angioplasty in patients with single vessel disease. *Circulation* 1986; **73**: 710–7.

70. David, P.R., Waters, D.D., Scholl, J.-M. *et al.* Percutaneous transluminal coronary angioplasty in patients with variant angina. *Circulation* 1982; **66**: 695–701.

71. Leisch, F., Schutzenberger, W., Kerschner, K. and Herbinger, W. Influence of a variant angina on the results of percutaneous transluminal coronary angioplasty. *Br. Heart J.* 1986; **56**: 341–5.

72. Lawrie, G.M., Morris, G.C., Silvers, A. *et al.* Influence of residual disease after coronary bypass on the 5-year survival rate of 1274 men with coronary artery disease. *Circulation* 1982; **66**: 717–23.

73. Cosgrove, D.M., Loop, F.D., Lytle, B.W. *et al.* Determinants of 10-year survival after primary myocardial revascularization. *Ann. Surg.* 1985; **202**: 480–90.

74. Russell, R.O., Resnekov, L., Wolk, M. *et al.* Unstable angina pectoris: National Co-operative Study Group to compare surgical and medical therapy. II. In-hospital experience and initial follow-up results in patients with one, two and three vessel disease. *Am. J. Cardiol.* 1978; **42**: 839–48.

75. McCormick, J.R., Schick, E.C. Jr, McCabe, C.H., Kronmal, R.A. and Ryan, T.J. Determinants of operative mortality and long term survival in patients with unstable angina. The CASS experience. *J. Thorac. Cardiovasc. Surg.* 1985; **89**: 683–8.

76. Luchi, R.J., Scott, S.M., Deupree, R.H. *et al.* Comparison of medical and surgical treatment for unstable angina pectoris. Results of a Veterans Administration Cooperative Study. *N. Engl. J. Med.* 1987; **316**: 977–84.

77. Russell, R.O. Jr, Resnekov, L., Wolk, M. *et al.* Unstable angina pectoris: National Co-operative Study Group to compare medical and surgical therapy. IV. Results in patients with left anterior descending coronary artery disease. *Am. J. Cardiol.* 1981; **48**: 517–24.

78. Baumgartner, W.A., Borkon, A.M., Zibulewsky, J. *et al.* Operative intervention for post-infarction angina: results and long-term follow-up. *Ann. Thorac. Surg.* 1984; **38**: 265–7.

79. Breyer, R.H., Engelman, R.M., Rousou, J.A. and Lemeshow, S. Postinfarction angina: an expanding subset of patients undergoing coronary artery bypass. *J. Thorac. Cardiovasc. Surg.* 1985; **90**: 532–40.

80. Jones, E.L., Waites, T.F., Craver, J.M. *et al.* Coronary bypass for relief of persistent pain following acute myocardial infarction. *Ann. Thorac. Surg.* 1981; **32**: 33–43.

81. Williams, D.B., Ivey, T.D., Bailey, W.W., Ivey, S.J., Rideout, J.T. and Stewart, D. Postinfarction angina: results of early revascularization. *J. Am. Coll. Cardiol.* 1983; **2**: 859–64.

82. Singh, A.K., Rivera, R., Cooper, G.N. and Karlson, K.E. Early myocardial revascularization for postinfarction angina: results and long-term follow-up. *J. Am. Coll. Cardiol.* 1985; **6**: 1121–5.

83. Schick, E.C. Jr, Davis, Z., Lavery, R.M. *et al.* Surgical therapy for Prinzmetal's variant angina. *Ann. Thorac. Surg.* 1982; 33: 359–64.
84. Previtali, M., Panciroli, C., Ardissino, D., Chimienti, M., Angoli, L. and Salerno, J.A. Spontaneous remission of variant angina documented by Holter monitoring and ergonovine testing in patients treated with calcium antagonists. *Am. J. Cardiol.* 1987; 59: 235–40.

Chapter 50

Myocardial Infarction

Michael C. Petch

INTRODUCTION

Myocardial infarction is necrosis of heart muscle due to interruption of its blood supply. The usual cause is occlusion of a major coronary artery by thrombus superimposed on an atheromatous plaque.

This hypothesis was proposed many decades ago and has withstood various challenges. For example the discovery that ^{131}I-labelled fibrinogen (given to establish the diagnosis of leg vein thrombosis in patients suffering from myocardial infarction) became incorporated into the coronary thrombus in those patients who died, was thought to indicate that the thrombus had been formed after the event. Subsequently it was realized that thrombus is dynamic and is constantly being lysed and reformed. More recent studies in humans undergoing coronary arteriography during the early stages of myocardial infarction have confirmed both the truth of the original hypothesis and the dynamic nature of the coronary thrombus.[1] Although the term coronary thrombosis went out of fashion as a result of the above findings, it remains an accurate, albeit less good description, of the pathological events. The term myocardial infarction is also to be preferred because the thrombus may undergo spontaneous lysis, while the infarct continues to evolve.

There are other, less common causes of myocardial infarction. The first, coronary embolism, is usually identified in patients already suffering from heart disease, commonly those with valve disease and atrial fibrillation. It may be underdiagnosed. Secondly, myocardial infarction may result from disease of the coronary ostia. Syphilitic aortitis is now very rare, but other forms of aortitis may obstruct the coronary blood supply, as may dissection of the aortic root; it is surprising how often the coronary arteries are spared in this condition.

Thirdly, cardiac trauma may cause infarction either by direct contusion of the myocardium or by tearing of the coronary arteries. Fourthly, there are congenital anomalies of the coronary arteries which render the myocardium ischaemic and thus liable to infarction; most anomalies seem to present with progressive myocardial failure rather than the clinical picture of infarction, although the latter can occur through a steal phenomenon or through some other mechanism, such as embolism from thrombus in a coronary artery aneurysm. Fifthly, the coronary arteries may be thickened or inflamed as in Takayasu's disease. Sixthly, myocardial infarction may be iatrogenic today. Damage to the coronary artery by instrumentation during angioplasty or coronary bypass surgery is a familiar and not uncommon event.

Finally, myocardial infarction is well described in patients who are subsequently shown to have patent coronary arteries with no lesion identifiable on angiography. In these patients the mechanism remains speculative. A few may have severe pressure overload, as in aortic stenosis, causing infarction particularly in the subendocardium through hypoperfusion. Others may have had thrombi which have undergone lysis. Some may have had coronary spasm, although spasm of arteries in other vascular beds is a very rare cause of permanent tissue damage unless the spasm is recurrent or provoked by some noxious stimulant. This may explain the occurrence of myocardial infarction in some heavy smokers.[2] The most plausible explanation, however, is that thrombus formation and subsequent lysis occur on an area of endothelial ulceration which does not encroach on the lumen sufficiently to be apparent at angiography. Both coronary embolism and myocardial infarction in patients with normal coronary arteries are so rare compared with the usual mechanism that throughout this chapter it is, unless otherwise stated, assumed that myocardial infarction is due to atheromatous disease of the coronary artery.

Myocardial infarction is often fatal. Indeed before Herrick's classic description of the disease,[3] coronary thrombosis leading to myocardial infarction was thought to be always fatal. Death occurs suddenly and is usually due to ventricular fibrillation.[4] Subsequent investigation of those patients who have been resuscitated from ventricular fibrillation before they reach hospital has shown that only two-thirds go on to develop the typical features of myocardial infarction.[5] The other third do not, although approximately 75% have coronary artery disease. This finding gives the layman's term 'heart attack' a new and useful meaning in that it describes both the victims of sudden cardiac death and those with myocardial infarction who survive to reach hospital. Any discussion of the incidence of myocardial infarction must take account of both entities.

INCIDENCE

The precise incidence of myocardial infarction is difficult to establish because the victim may die suddenly, or may live and reach hospital with the characteristic features of the disease, or he may not seek medical help at all and only be recognized by subsequent enquiry. The Framingham survey suggested that approximately one-third of episodes of myocardial infarction were silent.[6] In the British Regional Heart Study only one-half of the men with definite myocardial infarction on their electrocardiogram gave a history of cardiac pain.[7] Thus the estimated incidence of myocardial infarction will depend to some extent upon the nature of the study.

Tunstall-Pedoe and his colleagues in their classic work in Tower Hamlets in East London found that the incidence of heart attacks (sudden death and myocardial infarction) in the community was 1 per 100 per year in men aged 45–64 years.[8] In those who had previous evidence of cardiovascular disease the figure was 12 times greater: 1 per 100 per month. These figures are especially valuable because they are easy to commit to memory. The work confirmed a previous finding in Edinburgh[9] that most deaths tend to occur early; of those who are dead at 28 days, 60% died within the first hour, compared with 45% in the earlier study. This obviously makes it difficult to provide a figure for the overall mortality rate for myocardial infarction

because some of those who died suddenly would not have developed infarction. However, the mortality rate at 28 days for heart attacks can be estimated and is around one-third, 38% in the Tower Hamlets study, 29.5% in the Edinburgh study, 36% in a study from the Grampian Region of Scotland,[10] and a surprising 50% in a study from Teeside in North East England.[11]

The *incidence* of myocardial infarction has been the subject of a number of studies in this country. In Edinburgh 1858 suspected acute heart attacks were documented in subjects under the age of 70 years in 1 year in a population of approximately 500 000 persons[9] giving an incidence for men under age 70 years of 8.4 per 1000. In Oxford, 357 episodes occurred in 1 year, giving a lower incidence for men under age 70 of 4.5 per 1000 in a population of some 375 000.[12] These estimates are equivalent to annual attack rates of 15.5 per thousand for men aged 40–69 in Edinburgh and 16.7 per thousand for men aged 40–69 in Oxford. These compare with the attack rate in the Tower Hamlets study of 10 per 1000 per year for men aged 45–64 and 4.89 per 1000 per year for the total population found in Teeside.[11] The morbidity statistics from general practice agree well with the above in that the episode rate was 12.4 for men aged 45–64 years per 1000 per year (4.3 for the total population).[13] Myocardial infarction is therefore common, more so in the North of Great Britain than the South, the incidence being around 10 per 1000 middle aged men per year or 4 per 1000 population.

The *prevalence* of myocardial infarction in the community has been estimated from a survey of civil servants[14] and the British Regional Heart Survey.[15] Both examined middle-aged men. The prevalence rates were 6.5% and 9.1% based on questionnaires; 3.1% had definite electrocardiographic evidence of myocardial infarction in the Regional Heart Study.

These figures show a reasonable measure of agreement, bearing in mind the diverse methods of study and the geographical variation in the incidence of myocardial infarction. Throughout the world, the incidence parallels the incidence of cardiovascular disease (see also Shaper, Chapter 42). In the United Kingdom deaths from stroke and cardiovascular disease are twice as common in the West of Scotland as the South East of England.[16] The British Regional Heart Study is examining this observation and has drawn attention to the wide range of blood pressure levels and smoking habits.[17] Race is another factor: men of Indian extraction have a higher risk than the Caucasian men; men of Caribbean origin have a lower risk.[8]

In the United Kingdom approximately 160 000 deaths a year are due to coronary artery disease. Scotland and Northern Ireland now share with Finland the unwelcome distinction of having the highest incidence in the world (see Shaper, Chapter, 42 Fig. 42.1). The factors associated with this world variation have been the subject of intense study over many decades. In general the incidence of coronary heart disease is highest in industrialized countries. Those with a low standard of living are spared— Japan is an interesting exception. In some countries, for example the United States, the incidence has fallen markedly, and this is accompanied by a decline in cigarette smoking and the consumption of animal fat products. There has been little change in the United Kingdom, whose incidence of myocardial infarction, high prevalence of risk factors, and complacency give cause for concern.

PATHOPHYSIOLOGY

The pathology of myocardial infarction is described earlier (see Chapter 44). The initiating event is a critical reduction in the lumen of one or more coronary arteries. In general this is caused by thrombus formation on the surface of a plaque of atheroma, which might itself exhibit evidence of instability, such as fissuring. The underlying atheroma is usually sufficient to produce a severe stenosis of the lumen, as has been shown both by postmortem studies and by angiography following successful thrombolytic treatment. The reduction of the arterial lumen may permit infarction to occur without the addition of thrombus, especially if other coronary arteries are diseased.

Ligation of a coronary artery in a dog leads to a well described sequence of events. There is rapid decline in myocardial oxygen tension, accompanied by loss of contractile performance; the affected area appears cyanotic and bulging. Shortly afterwards the ST segment of the electrocardiogram begins to rise and arrhythmias develop leading to ventricular fibrillation. Biochemical changes include the early loss of high energy phosphates, intracellular acidosis, and the accumulation of calcium ions. These changes lead to irreversible myocardial damage within 3–4 minutes; repeated brief periods of ischaemia may have a cumulative effect.[18,19] Changes in the cardiac ultrastructure which may be observed after 20 minutes, and so gross pathologic-

al changes, which develop after 6 hours (see above), occur relatively late.

In man the coronary obstruction is often very different. Routine coronary arteriography following myocardial infarction has shown that 1% of patients have disease of the left mainstem, 9% have three-vessel disease, 26% two-vessel disease and 58% single-vessel disease.[20] Myocardial infarction in man, unlike in the experimental animal, is an untidy, stuttering, affair. The site and severity of the atheroma in the arteries supplying the zone of infarction, the possibility of spontaneous lysis,[21] the dynamic nature of the occluding thrombus, the presence of separate lesions both in the supplying artery and in other coronary arteries, the existence of a collateral supply, the myocardial oxygen need and other less obvious factors, such as anaemia and oxygen tension of the arterial blood, will all affect the site and extent of infarction. There can often be difficulty in deciding in clinical practice whether infarction has occurred.

The extent of myocardial infarction is most important. Larger infarcts not only give rise to more profound physiological changes but are also attended by a worse prognosis. Small infarcts have little effect on cardiac function. There is a good relationship between the amount of left ventricular damage and the resulting physiology; less than 10% loss and there is merely some reduction in left ventricular ejection fraction, 15% loss is associated with elevation of filling pressure, 25% loss results in clinical cardiac failure, and 40–50% results in cardiogenic shock.[22,23] The site of the infarct also has some effect on the physiological changes. Atrial infarction is a recognizable pathological entity which has little physiological effect. Right ventricular infarction occurs in inferior infarction and may give rise to a disproportionate elevation of the venous pressure compared with the left heart filling pressure; this is one of the causes of a low cardiac output and low pulmonary capillary wedge pressure. However the bulk of the damage is usually inflicted on the left ventricular myocardium. The infarcted zone becomes akinetic and stiff as the myocardium becomes oedematous, necrotic, and infiltrated by inflammatory cells. All but the smallest infarct will thus cause a rise in left ventricular filling pressure, reduction in ejection fraction and stroke volume, and some reduction in cardiac output, depending upon the extent of the compensatory tachycardia.

The subendocardial zone of the left ventricle is more vulnerable to ischaemia than the epicardial zone. This is because subendocardial perfusion is more easily compromised by an elevated left ventricular diastolic pressure. At post mortem it is possible to identify hearts in which the infarct is confined to the subendocardial zone and contrast these with hearts in which the infarct is transmural. There is a relationship between these two types of infarct and the electrocardiographic appearances; the subendocardial infarct tends only to have ST segment and T wave changes, whereas the transmural infarct is associated with Q waves. There is also a tendency for subendocardial infarcts to occur in the presence of multi-vessel coronary disease, sometimes without a complete occlusion[24] whereas transmural infarcts are caused by complete occlusion of a major coronary artery with little or no evidence of collateral channels. This pathological distinction between subendocardial and transmural infarction has some value, but it is open to criticism[25] and is overshadowed by the importance of infarct size.

Coronary collateral vessels have a role in limiting infarct size. Myocardial collaterals are present from birth but enlarge in response to chronic ischaemia. The rate at which they develop and their functional importance in curtailing the effects of coronary obstruction are uncertain. But their value is suggested by the following: there is an inherent likelihood that collaterals will have a protective effect, clinical observation suggests that younger men who have not had the opportunity to develop such collaterals are more prone to suffer massive infarcts, and myocardial infarcts are smaller following coronary bypass surgery. These considerations, coupled with the nature of the arterial pathology, determine not only the size of the infarct but also the extent of any residual myocardial ischaemia. An area of ischaemia—that is, myocardium at risk from infarction which survives albeit with a reduced blood supply—has been shown in experimental animals to exist around the infarct. These areas are important because their survival will ultimately affect the size of the infarct and thus the fate of the patient.

Myocardial infarction has an effect throughout the body. Elevation of the pulmonary venous pressure leads to interstitial oedema and hypoxaemia. Reduction in cardiac output will result in decreased perfusion of other organs, e.g. kidney, causing a reduction in urine output. Catecholamine secretion is enhanced. Carbohydrate tolerance is impaired and may bring to light occult diabetes mellitus. Platelet activity is increased.

CLINICAL FEATURES

Many attempts have been made to identify immediate precipitating factors in myocardial infarction. Patients themselves often look back on events leading up to the attack and can point to circumstances which they consider relevant. When this is done in a more formal manner no pattern emerges, or at least none that can withstand scientific scrutiny, but myocardial infarction does seem to occur more commonly after acute psychological stress, such as bereavement. Moreover physical activity is more likely to be associated with the onset of symptoms of myocardial infarction than would be expected by chance. Most episodes start between the hours of 6.00 a.m. and noon;[26,27] the reason for this circadian rhythm remains obscure, although surges in heart rate, blood pressure, and increases in coronary tone may play a role.

Prodromal symptoms are another contentious issue. Some studies show that some two-thirds of patients admit to symptoms such as chest discomfort, dyspnoea or undue fatigue in the weeks before myocardial infarction.[28] Any such study is necessarily retrospective and the predictive value of these symptoms is likely to be small, but if a patient is known to suffer from coronary heart disease, a crescendo of his familiar symptoms should be taken very seriously.

Chest pain is the classic symptom of myocardial infarction. Typically the pain is precordial, with radiation to the neck, lower (not upper) jaw, left and, less frequently, right arm and sometimes through to the back. The pain is described as crushing, gripping, like a weight on the chest, or like a tight band. The pain is seldom sharp or localized. Usually the pain is severe and is associated with a sensation of difficulty in breathing. Sweating, malaise, nausea and vomiting are common and vomiting is an especially useful diagnostic aid.[29] Syncope may occur through a variety of mechanisms, most commonly vagal stimulation, but also by vasodilatation as a result of consuming several tablets of glyceryl trinitrate. Apprehension and fear of impending doom are common.

Many patients do not present this typical picture, as Herrick[3] recognized:

> A study of cases of this type shows that nearly all are in men past the middle period of life. Previous attacks of angina have generally been experienced, though as shown by my first case, the fateful thrombosis may bring on the first seizure. The seizure is described by patients who have had

previous experience with angina, as of unusual severity, and the pain persists much longer. In some instances there has been no definite radiation of the pain as to the neck or left arm, though this may have been a feature of other anginal attacks, and the pain, as in these two cases, may be referred to the lower sternal region or definitely to the upper abdomen. Cases with little or no pain have been described . . . nausea and vomiting, with belching of gas, are common.

This description can hardly be bettered.

Elderly patients are more likely to present with atypical symptoms[30] such as the sudden development of lassitude and lack of interest or the onset of cardiac failure. In patients who are unwell for other reasons, for example following abdominal surgery, virtually any unexpected constitutional disturbance should raise the possibility of myocardial infarction, particularly if the patient is at risk by virtue of having a history of cardiovascular disease. Among the atypical features of myocardial infarction is pain that mimics the pain of previous visceral disease, so patients with a history of peptic ulceration may first experience cardiac pain in the epigastric region. The diagnosis may also be difficult to establish in patients who have undergone coronary bypass surgery because the cardiac pain may be different and confused with chest wall pain. Patients with myocardial infarction will occasionally present with one of the complications of the disease such as stroke through cerebral embolism from a mural thrombus in the left ventricle. The diagnosis is often made on the electrocardiogram, for example in men who undergo health screening because of their employment.

The prevalencce of atypical symptoms goes some way towards explaining why so many episodes of myocardial infarction are wrongly thought to be silent. Patients and their medical advisers are blinkered by the traditional, textbook description of the event (see above), and the diagnosis goes unrecognized.

On examination, patients appear frightened, unwell, pale, and sweaty. Restlessness in an attempt to find a comfortable position is usual, unlike those with an attack of angina, who will sit very still. Frequently patients will clutch or massage their precordium and describe their pain with a clenched fist. Patients in pain who indicate the site of their pain with a finger tip may well not have myocardial infarction.

The heart rate is often slow, initially, as a result of vagal stimulation, but subsequently a tachycardia is usual due to sympathetic over-activity resulting from a combination of myocardial damage and central mechanisms. The blood pressure is usually normal, but will be raised when fever and anxiety dominate the picture. In patients who have previously had hypertension, the pressure will commonly fall to normal and remain within the normal range for some months. The character of the arterial pulse is usually normal, but a small volume pulse and low blood pressure are found in patients with more severe myocardial damage. The venous pressure is usually normal; elevation reflects a raised right atrial and right ventricular diastolic pressure. This is generally a manifestation of congestive failure and does occur in patients with left heart failure; occasionally it may be due to right ventricular infarction. The cardiac impulse feels abnormal whenever there is significant haemodynamic deterioration in ventricular performance. The abnormality may be subtle and is often not detected initially (for example, the development of an atrial filling wave), or the abnormality may be obvious, as occurs some days after an extensive area of infarction when an abnormal impulse, moving out of phase with the apex beat, can be palpated bulging paradoxically during systole. Such an abnormality is best felt above the normal apex beat well to the left of the sternum. The auscultatory features echo these signs with an atrial (fourth) sound being common and a ventricular (third) sound being evident in patients with moderate ventricular impairment. Both sounds take time to develop and are best heard at the cardiac apex or over the paradoxical segment if such exists. An abnormal cardiac impulse and gallop rhythm are the best clinical guides to the extent of cardiac damage; the development of cardiac failure rarely occurs without their being present. The first and second heart sounds are normal. An ejection murmur is often heard. This finding is commonplace in normal subjects in the age-group who are at risk from myocardial infarction. The cause is some stiffening of the aortic valve leaflets with resulting turbulence of blood in the aortic root during systole. The murmur is best heard at the left sternal edge but may be maximal at the apex in those subjects with deep chests whose lung tissue is interposed between the aorta and the stethoscope. This is a potential source of confusion in patients who develop complications of myocardial infarction, such as mitral regurgitation or ventricular septal defect; these should give rise to pansystolic murmurs but the diagnosis can be extremely difficult in a sick patient with a tachycardia.

Another auscultatory feature is the pericardial friction rub, which is often evanescent. Normally the rub is very high pitched, has both systolic and diastolic components, and is best heard at the lower left sternal edge with the patient sitting up and leaning forwards. If only a systolic component is present, confusion can again occur.

Fever develops within 24 to 48 hours and generally settles within one week. Abnormal signs in other systems are mostly the result of complications of myocardial infarction. Tachypnoea is due to fear or left ventricular failure. The respiratory rate remains fast if the cause is failure and then fine inspiratory crackles are heard at the lung bases. Both the rate and the extent of the crackles reflect the severity of the failure. Cheyne–Stokes respiration is seen in patients who are gravely ill and in some who have received more than adequate doses of opiates. Hepatosplenomegaly and peripheral oedema are features of right heart failure and are unusual. Neurological examination is normal unless there is coexisting cerebrovascular disease, but both this and an examination of the peripheral pulses should be undertaken so that any change, due to systemic embolism, can be detected. Retinopathy and albuminurea may indicate pre-existing hypertension.

INVESTIGATIONS

A 12-lead electrocardiogram is the first and most important investigation in patients suspected of having myocardial infarction. The initial electrocardiogram may be normal, as it was in 11% of cases described by McGuiness et al.,[31] but this initial electrocardiogram is vital because any subsequent change, such as T wave flattening, carries greater significance if the abnormality is seen to evolve and perhaps regress. A normal electrocardiogram must not be taken to rule out the diagnosis, and the patient should not be reassured if the clinical suspicion of myocardial infarction is high. Rather, a normal electrocardiogram should be regarded as an indication for energetic treatment to minimize cardiac damage.

The electrocardiographic changes of myocardial infarction in man were first described by Pardee in 1920, and his name is still given to the characteristic symmetrical T wave inversion of infarction.[32] The typical changes of acute infarction include ST segment elevation and the development of Q waves in addition to the T wave inversion (Fig. 9.32, p. 177). The diagnosis can be established from the initial electrocardiogram in about half of the patients but with serial tracings the diagnostic accuracy rises to 83%.[31]

The earliest change in man during acute myocardial infarction is elevation of the ST segment. This may be considerable and can be associated with peaking of the T wave to such an extent that the normal QRS–T configuration is transformed into a bizarre, almost rectangular shape in which the normal depolarization sequence is hardly recognizable. However, these so-called hyperacute changes are not usually seen, and a more common pattern is less marked convex elevation of the ST segment (Fig. 9.26, p. 172). This is due to the current of injury, which has both diastolic and systolic components. During diastole the infarcted area is depolarized and thus electrically negative relative to the surrounding myocardium. Current therefore flows towards the electrodes over the infarcted area, resulting in depression of the diastolic TQ segment, but since this is automatically corrected by the electrocardiographic amplifiers the shift appears as ST segment elevation. This traditional explanation has been supplemented by the concept of a systolic current flowing towards the resting electrode and due to some continuing electrical activity in the infarcted area which can allow early repolarization or incomplete depolarization. The ST segment elevation is seen in the electrodes overlying the infarcted area; reciprocal ST segment depression may be seen in the other leads (Fig. 9.33, p. 178). If the infarct is localized to the subendocardial region, the ST segment elevation is seen only in lead aVR—the other leads show ST segment depression.

The development of pathological Q waves is the third electrocardiographic criterion of infarction (Figs 9.29 and 9.30, p. 174). These are effectively electrical windows in the myocardium, which allow the recording electrode to 'see' the wave of depolarization in the ventricular muscle opposite to the infarct, for example, the posterior wall in cases of anterior infarction. Q waves were accepted as the hallmark of transmural infarction, but the pathological correlation is imperfect and today the terms Q or non-Q myocardial infarction are to be preferred. Pathological Q waves are generally at least 40 milliseconds in duration and 25% or more of the height of the ensuing R wave.

A more subtle electrocardiographic change of infarction is loss of R waves. This can be recognized if previous electrocardiograms are available but can sometimes assist in the diagnosis of infarction even in the absence of previous tracings. For example, if the normal R wave progression in amplitude from V1–V6 is interrupted, infarction can be inferred, especially if there is accompanying ST segment and T wave change.

The rate at which the changes of acute infarction evolve vary from individual to individual, so it is difficult to determine the timing of infarction. Usually the ST segment will rise in hours and return to normal in days. As this occurs, so the T wave inversion becomes apparent, although it is often perceptible at an earlier stage as a negative deflection following the elevated ST segment. Persisting ST segment elevation usually indicates more extensive infarction, with possible aneurysm formation. Q waves appear slightly later and persist longer although even they may disappear.

The location of these changes approximates to the location of the infarct as follows: septal—V1 and V2; anterior—V3 and V4 (Fig. 9.35, p. 180); lateral I, aVL, V5 and V6; inferior—II, III and aVF (Fig. 9.34, p. 179). Posterior infarction is recognizable by a tall R wave in V1 in association with inferior or lateral infarction (Fig. 9.39, p. 184); right ventricular infarction should be suspected in inferior and septal infarction and can be recognized by characteristic changes in the right chest leads, V4R, and so on.

Often the electrocardiographic changes of infarction are atypical and do not permit localization. The diagnosis then rests on the history and other findings. Atypical electrocardiographic changes include non-specific ST segment and T wave change; these are commonly seen in patients who have had previous myocardial infarction or bypass surgery when the pre-existing myocardial damage and coronary collateral circulation will modify both the extent and localization of the electrocardiographic change. A problem also exists in patients with conduction defects. In right bundle branch block initial depolarization is unaltered and the pattern of infarction is still identifiable, but in left bundle branch block the pattern of infarction is masked and the diagnosis is unreliable. Either form of bundle branch block, especially the left and its subdivisions, may be due to infarction and a change in electrocardiogram when associated with the typical clinical picture may be taken as evidence of the diagnosis. The delta wave of the Wolff–Parkinson–White syndrome likewise masks the Q wave of infarction, but ST segment and T wave

changes may allow the diagnosis to be established.

U wave inversion is well recognized in myocardial infarction.[33]

LABORATORY INVESTIGATIONS

Myocardial infarction causes intracellular enzymes to escape into the blood stream, where increased concentrations can be detected and so aid the diagnosis. Most laboratories measure creatine kinase (CK) and its cardiospecific isoenzyme (MB), aspartate transaminase (AST, formerly serum glutamic oxalo-acetic transaminase hence SGOT) and lactic dehydrogenase (LDH). LDH has five isoenzymes, of which LDH_1 is mostly cardiac and has hydroxybutyric dehydrogenase (HBD) activity, so this property is measured in some laboratories. The speed of release of these enzymes varies. Some increase in CK activity can be detected within 4 hours of the onset of symptoms, whereas AST peaks at 2 days and LDH may remain elevated for 1 week or more.[34] It is important to recognize that none of these enzymes, with the exception of CK–MB, is specific to the heart. Thus muscle damage will elevate CK levels and make the estimation of little value in some situations, for example following cardiac surgery. Even an intramuscular injection of an opiate can raise the enzyme activity to at least twice its normal level.[35] Similarly liver damage, perhaps caused by alcohol, may elevate the AST, and haemolysis of the blood sample will elevate the serum LDH activity. Nevertheless the intelligent use of these changes in enzyme levels in the peripheral blood can be of great assistance in confirming the diagnosis of infarction. It is unnecessary to measure all three enzymes routinely, but three samples taken on consecutive days is a usual recommendation; the most useful enzyme will depend on the time at which the patient is seen during his illness.

Myoglobin can be detected in the serum following myocardial infarction. It appears quickly, within 4 hours in 89% of patients.[36] It is also a smaller molecule than the cardiac enzymes and is excreted relatively quickly so that the early peak disappears within 24 hours. The appearance of myoglobin in staccato bursts may be further evidence that infarction in man is an intermittent event.[37] The estimation of myoglobin may be a useful research tool, but its use in diagnosis is superfluous. Other biochemical changes include hyperglycaemia in response to stress, hypokalaemia, which may be pronounced in patients taking diuretics and which may be a factor in the genesis of arrhythmias, and alterations in the serum lipids.[38] Although tradition dictates that the estimation of serum lipids should be deferred for 4 weeks, the value of knowing a patient's serum cholesterol when the time comes for giving dietary advice on discharge is such that there is much to be said for measuring this in a blood sample taken within 24 hours when any change in serum cholesterol is modest.[39]

Haematological changes include an early leukocytosis, the white count usually returning to normal within 1 week, and a modest rise in erythrocyte sedimentation rate, which may remain elevated for several weeks. Reduced fibrinolytic capacity has been described.[40]

IMAGING TECHNIQUES

An early chest X-ray is valuable because pulmonary congestion can be detected. This is an important sign in determining prognosis, but the delay between the rise in left ventricular filling pressure and the appearance of congestive changes must be remembered. Likewise the fall in filling pressures in response to treatment may not be accompanied by clearing of the lung fields for several hours, or even days if there is frank pulmonary oedema. Changes in the heart size in what are generally portable films are unhelpful; cardiomegaly at this stage reflects previous cardiac damage through hypertension or infarction. X-ray screening of the heart has been superseded by more modern imaging techniques, but if screening is undertaken, an area of paradoxical left ventricular wall motion can be appreciated in patients with moderate to large infarcts. Computerized tomography is also little practised at this stage unless some other intrathoracic pathology is strongly suspected. However, if it is undertaken, the infarcted area can be visualized as a thin, bulging segment of the left ventricular wall.[41]

Cross-sectional echocardiography is proving to be a valuable imaging technique especially when combined with Doppler estimation of blood flow. The necessary apparatus has the advantage of being cheap, mobile and easier to use than other imaging techniques. However, echocardiography suffers from the disadvantage that satisfactory images cannot be obtained in all patients, only 91% in skilled hands.[42] The greatest value at present is the ability of Doppler echocardiography to detect the complications of myocardial infarction, particularly

ventricular septal rupture and mitral regurgitation. Following ventricular septal rupture, identification of blood flow across the septum and measurement of right ventricular cavity size allow the degree of shunting to be estimated, while visualization of left ventricular wall movement provides a reasonable guide to left ventricular function.[43] Mitral regurgitation can likewise be detected and shown to be remarkably common following infarction;[44] so much so that minor degrees of regurgitant flow are probably of little clinical significance. Cross-sectional echocardiography has yet to realize its full potential in the cardiac care unit. The ability to undertake repeated studies in complete safety without moving the patient should allow the effects of infarction on left ventricular performance to be monitored in detail. The spontaneous recovery of normal wall motion[45] and early aneurysm formation[46] have already been described. The problem to date has been the lack of any objective measurements; the extent of abnormal wall motion and any subsequent change are subjective judgements, although attempts are being made to overcome this.[47]

A further finding on cross-sectional echocardiography is the frequent presence of left ventricular mural thrombus. Thrombi are seldom seen following inferior infarction but have been demonstrated in 46% of patients with anterior infarcts and associated apical akinesis or dyskinesis.[48] Of 119 patients with left ventricular thrombus studied by Visser and his colleagues systemic embolism occurred in 26; mobile and protruberant thrombi were more likely to embolize.[49]

Scintigraphy (see Chapter 19) is useful in myocardial infarction in three ways. First, technetium-99m pyrophosphate accumulates in acutely infarcted tissue. Secondly, thallium-201 is taken up by normal myocardium so that defects can usually be taken to represent areas of infarction. Thirdly, blood pool imaging with technetium-99m, either using the first pass or equilibrium method, provides an excellent measure of left ventricular performance.

Infarct-avid or 'hot spot' scintigraphy can identify quite small localized infarcts. Uptake of technetium-99m pyrophosphate is detectable at 4 hours, reaches a peak at 48 hours and disappears after about 7 days. This process is slower in large infarcts and may be protracted if extension of the original infarct occurs. Problems in interpretation arise when the abnormal image is not focal but diffuse; such a pattern can occur in a variety of myocardial disorders, including unstable angina; it has been described in subjects with no apparent heart disease. The technique has not been used routinely in the diagnosis of myocardial infarction because serial enzyme and electrocardiographic recordings are quite sufficient. There are, however, special circumstances where the technique may establish a diagnosis, for example following cardiac surgery,[50] and where right ventricular infarction is suspected.[51]

Thallium-201 is likewise little used in the routine diagnosis of acute infarction although perfusion defects can be found in 82% of patients.[52] Defects disappear with time, but a normal study within 24 hours of the onset of symptoms makes the diagnosis of myocardial infarction very unlikely. Defects are also seen in patients with unstable angina and may persist after the pain has settled. Probably the greatest value of the technique lies in excluding infarction and in identifying areas of residual myocardial ischaemia following infarction—areas which render the patient liable to infarct extension or post-infarct angina. Similar information may however be acquired more simply by exercise electrocardiography (see below).

Blood pool imaging is the best method of quantifying ventricular function following cardiac infarction. Because left ventricular function is one of the most important determinants of prognosis, this technique is of considerable value. Both left ventricular ejection fraction and wall motion abnormalities can be measured; if the technique is combined with exercise, additional areas of ischaemia can be identified. Blood pool imaging is therefore the most useful and most widely used of all the nuclear techniques, because it accurately identifies the degree of left ventricular dysfunction, differentiates global impairment from aneurysm formation, and localizes areas of ischaemia. The study is generally best undertaken shortly before the patient leaves hospital.

Other nuclear techniques are available. Pulmonary scintigraphy (ventilation/perfusion scanning) is the investigation of choice in suspected pulmonary embolism, but most other techniques have an application in research but not yet in clinical practice. Among the most exciting is the study of myocardial blood flow and metabolism using positron emission tomography.

Magnetic resonance imaging of the heart is yet another and expensive method of detecting and localizing myocardial infarction.[53] Its value lies not so much in its imaging capability but than in its ability to measure blood flow, characterize tissue, and, by spectroscopy, to study biochemical changes in the myocardium.[54] These may well prove to be powerful research tools in the study of myocardial ischaemia and possibly in the estimation of infarct size.[55]

Conventional contrast angiography of the heart may be undertaken during acute myocardial infarction with little increased risk.[1] Once this fact had been demonstrated the procedure became widely used by investigators seeking to minimize myocardial loss during infarction. This led to some profitable research and helped to establish the feasibility of intracoronary thrombolysis, although the procedure is accompanied by some increase in morbidity, mainly due to ventricular fibrillation, and cannot be recommended as routine. Rather coronary arteriography and left ventricular angiography should be reserved for those victims of myocardial infarction who stand to gain most from interventions such as angioplasty or surgery. The chief indication is recurrent cardiac pain, either rest pain or easily provoked angina during mobilization. This indication may be refined by early exercise testing. The other major indication is to confirm the presence of one or more of the complications of myocardial infarction, such as ventricular septal rupture.

HAEMODYNAMIC MONITORING

All patients with myocardial infarction should have their blood pressure monitored. This can be easily accomplished by sphygmomanometry. Whether venous catheterization aids the understanding of uncomplicated myocardial infarction is doubtful. If it is to be undertaken, there is little point in only measuring central venous pressure because the result may be misleading in this disease, which affects primarily the left ventricle but which can also cause profound and unsuspected disturbances of right ventricular function.

Swan and Ganz and their colleagues invented a balloon-tipped catheter which can float through the right heart into the pulmonary wedge position.[56] The modern catheter incorporates a thermistor so that cardiac output may be measured by the thermodilution technique. This has improved our understanding of the haemodynamic consequences of myocardial infarction and allowed the recognition of haemodynamic subsets, which correlate well with the clinical picture and with prognosis[57]

(Table 50.1). This investigation is of considerable value in severe or complicated cases of myocardial infarction since it enables appropriate treatment to be given. An example of this might be the administration of fluid to a patient in subset 3 who was receiving treatment with diuretics.

How much haemodynamic monitoring is undertaken must depend upon the resources of the cardiac care unit and the likely benefits. No firm guidance can be given.

DIFFERENTIAL DIAGNOSIS

CARDIAC PAIN WITHOUT INFARCTION

Cardiac pain without infarction is much the most common differential diagnosis. To some extent differentiation is unimportant because all patients with cardiac pain should be managed alike at first. The problem is usually encountered in a patient who is known to have ischaemic heart disease and who presents with 30 minutes or more rest pain. The problem is compounded because most diagnostic tests cannot distinguish between prolonged myocardial ischaemia with recovery and small areas of myocardial necrosis. In either case the electrocardiographic ST segment and T wave changes may revert to normal quite quickly. Also there is evidence from experimental animals including primates that creatine kinase activity and its MB isoenzyme may be markedly increased following 15 minutes of coronary occlusion without there being any subsequent evidence of myocardial necrosis.[58] Furthermore nuclear techniques give a positive result for either prolonged ischaemia or infarction. Thus the distinction between unstable angina and a small cardiac infarct becomes impossible. Both conditions probably reflect instability of an atheromatous plaque in a coronary artery (see Chapter 44) and both conditions should therefore be taken very seriously. To try to decide whether a given patient has had angina or a possible myocardial infarct is unsound on pathophysiological grounds and irrelevant to management. The only purpose is for epidemiological data gathering.[59]

CHEST PAIN ? CAUSE

Chest pain of questionable cause is the third most common final diagnosis in patients admitted to a cardiac care unit under the care of an honest physician, 13% in one series.[60] These authors made the point that the diagnosis is not one to be ashamed of. The physician should take all reasonable steps to exclude myocardial ischaemia and some of the diagnoses listed below, but having done so he should have confidence in his clinical judgement. The diagnosis carried an excellent prognosis in the series quoted above and no mortality after one year of follow-up.

Naturally the chest pain must have some cause in these patients. Chest wall pain is a good diagnosis. Many of the musculoskeletal elements of the chest wall are liable to hurt, especially after exercise involving the thorax and arms. Even unaccustomed running may leave the precordial area sore because the rate and depth of respiration have induced some muscular stiffness. Tietze's syndrome or costochondritis is common in middle-aged persons and is usually recognized during an attack because the affected joint is tender on palpation. Pain from the cervical spine may be felt mainly in the precordium and may be reproduced by neck movement. Chest wall pain may cause the patient to alter his normal rhythmic breathing pattern. Hyperventilation—perhaps dysventilation would be a better description—is not a diagnosis but a response to some other process, often chest wall pain, but also angina, pulmonary congestion, etc.

Occasionally when the physician has pondered on these thoughts the rash of herpes zoster appears.

PERICARDITIS

Pericarditis can be very difficult to differentiate. In practice clinicians rely on probability, as always. A young person with no risk factors for coronary heart disease who develops cardiac-like pain following a coryzal illness is likely to have pericarditis whereas an older man with a full house of risk factors who develops cardiac-like pain is likely to have myocardial ischaemia. In typical cases pericar-

Table 50.1. Mortality rates in clinical and haemodynamic sub-sets (after Forrester).

Subset	Pulmonary congestion[a]	Peripheral hypoperfusion[b]	Percentage mortality	
			Clinical	Haemodynamic
I	−	−	1	3
II	+	−	11	9
III	−	+	18	23
IV	+	+	60	51

[a] Pulmonary-capillary pressure > 18 mmHg
[b] Cardiac index < 2.2 litres/min/m²

dial pain is like cardiac pain in most respects but is eased by sitting up and leaning forward. This characteristic posture immediately suggests the diagnosis. Movement, respiration and swallowing make the pain worse. On auscultation a soft rub is heard at the lower left sternal edge.

Pericarditis commonly complicates myocardial infarction (see below). A diagnostic problem therefore arises in patients who suffer a recurrence of chest pain following the initial event. There is no certain way of distinguishing the two because the physical findings and acute ST segment elevation on the electrocardiogram are common to both. Subsequent investigation, including serial electrocardiograms, cardiac enzymes, and in this instance, infarct-avid scintigraphy, should enable the distinction to be made, although the results of these investigations may come too late to affect management, which therefore has to be based on clinical judgement. An identical diagnostic problem exists in patients following coronary by-pass surgery.

AORTIC DISSECTION

The pain and circulatory collapse of aortic dissection may mimic myocardial infarction. The pain however should have a tearing or stabbing quality and may often originate in the back. Bizarre evanescent symptoms reflecting a transient loss of blood supply to certain organs may assist in the diagnosis. For example if the dissection involves the aortic arch, a hemiparesis or cold white arm may result. If the signs persist or if a carotid, brachial, or femoral pulse is absent, the diagnosis is more certain. However, caution is necessary because the pulses may be very difficult to palpate in a sick hypotensive patient, and may be thought to vary when the truth of the matter, as revealed by subsequent post mortem, is that the patient had an extensive infarct and widespread arterial atheroma.

Dissection back into the aortic root may cause aortic regurgitation, pericarditis, tamponade, and cardiac infarction, the mechanisms being respectively separation of the aortic valve leaflets from their supporting wall, leakage of blood into the pericardium, and damage to the coronary ostia. The development of aortic regurgitation is a strong pointer to the diagnosis, as is a high venous pressure in cases of tamponade. Only CT scanning and aortography can establish the diagnosis with certainty.

Aortic dissection carries a very high early mortality which can be improved by emergency surgical repair. If the clinical suspicion is strong, immediate transfer to a cardiac surgical unit is indicated. Preliminary investigation should be confined to a chest X-ray, which should show widening of the mediastinum, and an electrocardiogram, which should be near normal. In suspected acute dissection, emergency aortography is essential; other, less invasive investigations introduce a delay which may prove fatal. In subacute or chronic dissection, cross-sectional echocardiography, digital subtraction angiography or CT scanning may establish the diagnosis.

PULMONARY EMBOLISM

Acute pulmonary embolism does not usually provoke severe precordial pain. The usual presentation is with pleuritic pain in small pulmonary emboli, and circulatory collapse in cases of massive embolism. The clinical setting is helpful. The patient is typically in hospital recovering from a surgical operation or medical illness such as myocardial infarction. Confusion arises because the symptoms and signs may be transient, the electrocardiographic changes may mimic those of myocardial ischaemia, and the enzymes, aspartate transaminase and lactic dehydrogenase may appear in the blood. Because the condition is potentially lethal, pulmonary scintigraphy is indicated whenever the diagnosis is suspected.

Recurrent pulmonary thrombo-embolism is a special and rather uncommon diagnostic problem in which the features of pulmonary hypertension and right heart failure predominate.

OTHER PULMONARY PATHOLOGY

Many other disorders of the lungs, pleura and mediastinum can cause confusion, particularly in patients known to have coronary heart disease. These disorders include spontaneous pneumothorax, pneumonia, and carcinoma of the bronchus with infiltration into the mediastinum and pericardium. Most can usually be differentiated on clinical grounds with a few appropriate investigations such as a chest X-ray.

GASTROINTESTINAL DISORDERS

Oesophageal pain can be severe enough to mimic the pain of myocardial infarction. Rupture or perforation so that the oesophageal contents leak into the mediastinum is uncommon but may provoke collapse. Usually there are diagnostic pointers such as protracted vomiting or dysphagia. There may be a paucity of other gastrointestinal symptoms, no signs, and no definite abnormalities on investigation. It may be a common cause of undiagnosed chest pain. Peptic ulceration, cholecystitis, oesophageal reflux and virtually any pathology of the upper gastrointestinal tract may initially suggest myocardial infarction. Most pathologies can easily be differentiated, but functional disorders may cause considerable uncertainty.

Many case reports testify to the numerous disorders that simulate myocardial infarction. Most are caused by other cardiac or cardiovascular pathologies. No reader should think that a case is unique because it has been omitted in this account.

COMPLICATIONS

The complications of myocardial infarction can be classified as arrhythmias, 'mechanical', miscellaneous, and infarct extension.

ARRHYTHMIAS

The overall incidence of arrhythmias in myocardial infarction is very high (see Table 50.2).[61–63]

Sinus tachycardia is the most common rhythm in patients arriving at hospital. It is due to sympathetic stimulation and is a result of pain, fear, and impaired left ventricular function. Persisting sinus tachycardia suggests left ventricular failure and a poor prognosis. With the advent of mobile coronary care units it was realized that sinus bradycardia is a very frequent early arrhythmia.[64,65] It is more common and more persistent in patients with inferior infarcts. This might argue in favour of a direct mechanism, namely, ischaemia of the sinus node, but the rhythm can be corrected by atropine and thus seems likely to be mediated by the vagus nerve. Its significance is twofold: the bradycardia will reduce myocardial work, and it may permit the development of more sinister ventricular arrhythmias.[66]

Atrial extrasystoles are common and benign. Supraventricular tachycardia and atrial flutter are unusual. Atrial fibrillation is the most important of the supraventricular arrhythmias.[61,63] Although atrial ischaemia is a logical and demonstrable cause of atrial arrhythmias,[67] raised atrial pressures and older age are the most important associated features.[68] This implies that atrial fibrillation reflects more extensive cardiac damage, so the higher mortality rate associated with this arrhythmia is not unexpected. An established atrial arrhythmia will result in loss of atrial transport and cause a further deterioration in cardiac output in those patients with impaired left ventricular function. Atrial fibrillation may be benign when associated with pericarditis and no haemodynamic deterioration.

Nodal rhythm is generally a benign escape rhythm secondary to sinus bradycardia. Accelerated nodal rhythm and tachycardia are described but have no particular significance.

Ventricular extrasystoles are extremely common in acute myocardial infarction. In the early days of coronary care units the idea that certain manifestations of ventricular ectopic activity presaged ventricular fibrillation gained wide acceptance. Considerable effort was expended in trying to identify and treat these warning extrasystoles which were described as having the following characteristics: more than 5 per minute, variable shape, early coupling interval (R on T phenomenon) and salvoes. Subsequent research has shown that ventricular fibrillation is just as likely to occur in those patients who exhibit these features as in those who do not.[61] Ventricular fibrillation is generally initiated by a ventricular extrasystole, but although this has been said to occur early (R on T) in the first 12 hours following myocardial infarction,[69] others have found no relationship to the coupling interval.[70] Ventricular extrasystoles therefore have little predictive value when they occur in the first

Table 50.2. Arrhythmias detected by ECG monitoring in a coronary care unit in 1000 consecutive patients with infarction 1967–71 (after Norris).

Arrhythmia	Incidence (%)	Mortality (%)
All ventricular ectopics	57	19
i Salvoes (runs)	17	35
ii Bigemini	7	36
iii R on T	6	41
iv Vent. Es. not i, ii or iii	36	15
Ventricular tachycardia	10	55
Ventricular fibrillation	8	61
Accelerated idioventricular rhythm	9	19
Atrial fibrillation	11	28
Atrial flutter	3	24
Paroxysmal supraventricular tachycardia	3	37
Sinus tachycardia	41	26
Sinus bradycardia	25	9
All cases		18

few hours following myocardial infarction, but when they occur later they are associated with a worse prognosis.[71] Whether they are an independent risk factor for cardiac death or whether they merely reflect more extensive ventricular damage remains uncertain.

Ventricular tachycardia may be a benign early finding or a sinister development if it occurs more than 24 hours after infarction.[61] The early type is rarely sustained and seldom degenerates into ventricular fibrillation. The late type is usually associated with more extensive ventricular damage and a poor prognosis.[72] Accelerated idioventricular rhythm is also seen in the early hours following infarction and is benign; often the rate is similar to the sinus rate, so that the ventricular focus becomes apparent during periods of sinus bradycardia; it may be related to reperfusion of myocardium.

Ventricular fibrillation occurring early in myocardial infarction without haemodynamic disturbance is termed primary, whereas ventricular fibrillation occurring in association with left ventricular failure or cardiogenic shock is termed secondary. The distinction is useful because the former group does well following defibrillation whereas the latter does not.[73] It is now recognized that virtually all patients who are resuscitated out of hospital are victims of ventricular fibrillation and about three-quarters have coronary heart disease.[5] But only one-quarter or so go on to develop myocardial infarction. Thus ventricular fibrillation is the usual mode of death in coronary heart disease and the term primary ventricular fibrillation has been extended to cover both those who go on to develop infarction and those who do not. The incidence of ventricular fibrillation in association with infarction is highest at the onset of the attack and declines rapidly thereafter—a fact that has stimulated the growth of mobile coronary care units and coronary ambulances. Primary ventricular fibrillation is equally common in anterior and inferior infarction,[63] and the overall incidence in the coronary care unit is about 10%.

Asystole is the ultimate event and is generally seen after resuscitation attempts. It is the usual cause of death in patients with heart block.

Heart block is a result of damage to the conduction tissue and can occur at any level. The conduction system receives a dual blood supply.[74] The sino-atrial and atrioventricular nodes are supplied by branches of the right coronary artery in 80% of cases; the His–Purkinje network in the ventricular septum is supplied mainly by the perforating branches of the left anterior descending coronary artery. Occlusion of the former can cause conduction disturbances with little overall myocardial damage but occlusion of the latter must cause more extensive septal infarction for the conduction disturbance to occur. This helps to explain why first degree and second degree Wenckebach block have the following features: they are usually seen in association with inferior infarcts, the QRS complex is narrow, the block seldom lasts more than 3 days and rarely progresses to complete atrioventricular block, haemodynamic deterioration is rare. Second degree block Mobitz type II usually complicates anterior infarction with damage to the conduction system below the atrioventricular node; the QRS complex is usually broad, sudden progression to complete AV block is not uncommon, and the prognosis is poor. The differences reflect the site and extent of the infarct. If complete heart block develops, there are similar differences but also in inferior infarction the ventricular rate is generally adequate at 40–70 per minute and recovery in a week is usual, whereas in anterior infarction the rate is slower and the patients commonly die, even with pacing.[61]

Both right and left bundle branch block are occasional findings in myocardial infarction and both carry a high mortality, 65% and 47% respectively;[61] this is a manifestation of the extensive ventricular damage rather than the conduction defect itself. Left posterior and anterior hemiblock are also unusual; the former is often associated with right bundle branch block and carries a poor prognosis,[75] whilst the latter is usually an isolated abnormality which is not accompanied by a worse prognosis.[76]

These conduction abnormalities develop 12 to 72 hours after infarction and are therefore not due to the initial ischaemic insult. Most patients recover. Thus the precise pathological basis is uncertain, but hydropic degeneration and other reversible lesions have been described in the conduction system.[74,77]

In general any disturbance of cardiac rhythm will not only have an adverse effect on cardiac performance but will diminish myocardial efficiency and hence increase myocardial oxygen consumption, thus exacerbating ischaemia.

MECHANICAL

The consequence of any myocardial infarct is left ventricular failure. This may be no more than a transient and undetectable impairment in left ventricular performance, or there may be frank left ventricular failure leading to pulmonary oedema or, at worst, cardiogenic shock. To these varying degrees of pump failure must be added the anatomical faults: left ventricular aneurysm formation; ventricular rupture, either of the free wall leading to tamponade or of the septum leading to a left to right shunt; and papillary muscle damage leading to mitral regurgitation.

Minor degrees of left ventricular failure are common in myocardial infarction. The patient becomes short of breath. More severe degrees cause distressing dyspnoea with orthopnoea, cough and haemoptysis. On examination the patient has tachypnoea, fine inspiratory basal crackles, and the features of left ventricular damage including a dyskinetic cardiac impulse, gallop rhythm, tachycardia, and low blood pressure. A chest X-ray confirms the diagnosis by showing pulmonary congestion and, in severe cases, septal lines. The haemodynamic changes are described above.

Cardiogenic shock is an extreme form of left ventricular failure which, when rigidly defined, carries a mortality rate approaching 100%. As described above, there is extensive ventricular damage and generally three-vessel coronary artery disease with involvement of the left anterior descending.[78] The patient is restless and pale, with a cold, clammy skin. The pulse is thready, and the systolic blood pressure is by definition less than 80 mmHg systolic. The clinical features of a severely damaged left ventricle, with pulmonary oedema and oliguria are invariable. This complication affects some 10–15% of patients with myocardial infarction[79] and is now the commonest mode of death in patients who reach hospital. It often complicates the other anatomical faults described above.

A ventricular aneurysm is difficult to define in life. The pathological definition is a thin-walled bulge or outpouching of the left ventricular chamber.[80] This may be visualized by angiography as a diastolic deformity of the left ventricular outline which becomes more marked during systole i.e. there is paradoxical or dyskinetic wall movement. However, to some extent all full-thickness infarcts exhibit this abnormal pattern of contraction; how big the bulge has to be before it becomes an aneurysm is a subjective judgement. Radionuclide angiography, which can be more readily quantified, may provide a more accurate definition.[81] Nevertheless there are some bulges which by any definition constitute a ventricular aneurysm and develop in 10–15% of patients.[79] There is a

suggestion from gated blood pool scintigraphy that the deformity of the left ventricular wall may occur within the first two days of infarction but the traditional concept is of a slower 'blow-out'.[82] Aneurysms are more common in the antero-apical segments perhaps because the left ventricular wall is thinner in these sites or perhaps as a result of forces generated within the left ventricle during systole. These true aneurysms of the left ventricle can be distinguished at surgery from false aneurysms in which left ventricular rupture has occurred and the wall of the aneurysm is formed by a mixture of parietal pericardium, inflammatory and thrombotic material.

Cardiac rupture, that is, rupture of the left ventricular free wall, is found in about 3% of patients dying from myocardial infarction in hospital[83] and 8% overall.[84] The victim succumbs rapidly from tamponade. One-quarter of the deaths occur within 24 hours and three-quarters by the end of the first week. Rupture may complicate silent infarction and present as sudden death. This complication tends to occur more frequently in the elderly, in women, and in those who have had high blood pressure. The reason why some hearts rupture is not understood, but the site of rupture is generally in the ischaemic zone between the healthy myocardium and the necrotic zone so shearing forces may be a factor. The infarct is invariably transmural but its size is unimportant; the location is usually the lateral or anterior wall of the left ventricle in the territory of the left anterior descending coronary artery.[85]

Ventricular septal rupture is less common; it is seen in about 1% of patients coming to post mortem.[86] This complication may be seen after anterior or inferior infarction and any portion of the muscular septum may be involved. Typically the patient appears to be recovering some days after his myocardial infarct when he deteriorates into a low output state. A new pansystolic murmur is heard. The differential diagnosis at this stage is papillary muscle rupture leading to mitral regurgitation. Many clinical features have been described to differentiate these two conditions: the murmur should be loudest and may be associated with thrill at the lowest left sternal edge in ventricular septal rupture whilst it radiates to the axilla in mitral regurgitation, the venous pressure is more likely to be elevated in ventricular septal rupture, rupture is more likely to complicate anterior infarction whereas mitral regurgitation is more common in inferior infarction, the chest X-ray should assist by revealing plethora or congestion. In practice the patient's posture is generally most helpful: if he is lying back on the pillows, ventricular septal rupture is likely, if he is sitting up short of breath, mitral regurgitation is the usual diagnosis. The prognosis is poor although individuals may survive for many years.[87] The most important factor in determining prognosis is, as always, the extent of the infarct and the state of the left ventricle. The volume of left to right shunting is important in the short term. Both these features and the site of septal rupture may be visualized by Doppler echocardiography, which is the investigation of choice in this condition. Cross-sectional echocardiography alone is less sensitive.[43] When it is combined with Swan–Ganz catheterization, patients can be classified into prognostic groups:[57] those with a poor prognosis demonstrate the following features: cardiac index less than 1.75 l/min/m^2, poor right ventricular function on echocardiography, right atrial pressure exceeding 12 mmHg. Gradual deterioration leading to death within a few weeks or less is the usual outcome.

Papillary muscle rupture is another rare complication of myocardial infarction which presents in a manner similar to ventricular septal rupture.[88] If the patient survives, it may be distinguished by the features described above and in such cases the rupture is usually partial. Papillary muscle rupture usually complicates inferior myocardial infarction. Doppler echocardiography is invaluable in establishing the diagnosis.[44] Complete rupture with overwhelming mitral regurgitation is probably always fatal.[89]

These various mechanical complications of myocardial infarction often coexist in the same patient. This is not surprising because all tend to occur in the victims of transmural infarcts. In practice the formation of a left ventricular aneurysm with rupture leading to cardiogenic shock is a familiar and generally hopeless complication.

MISCELLANEOUS

Thrombo-embolism is the most important of the miscellaneous conditions. The changes associated with cardiac infarction include a reduced cardiac output, venous stasis, and altered platelet behaviour as shown by increased stickiness *in vitro* and the liberation of substances such as beta-thromboglobulin *in vivo*.[90] Two conditions of Virchow's triad are thus met, and the third condition is satisfied by the infarcted heart muscle. Both

peripheral venous thrombosis and cardiac thrombi are common.

Venous thrombosis may be detected in the calf muscle in about one-third of patients with myocardial infarction using the technique of ^{131}I fibrinogen scintigraphy.[91,92] Thrombi are detected most commonly in older patients and those with heart failure. They seldom propogate beyond the calf veins[93] and most lyse spontaneously. These thrombi may be confirmed at post mortem but can rarely be detected clinically. If evidence of pulmonary embolism is looked for at post mortem, it can be found in 28% of patients who have not received anticoagulants.[94] Earlier accounts suggested an incidence of over 20%,[95] and massive pulmonary embolism in 10% of deaths following myocardial infarction.[96] Most recent reports suggest a much lower incidence, with only 1% of deaths being due to this cause.[97] This dramatic difference is probably due to the modern policy of early mobilization, which contrasts markedly with the former practice of advising several weeks' bed rest. The occurrence of right atrial and ventricular thrombus leading to pulmonary embolism, while possible in theory, is decidedly rare.

Left ventricular mural thrombus is commonly detected by cross-sectional echocardiography (see above) and this finding corroborates the post mortem evidence: 44% of 924 in one series[96] had mural thrombi overlying the infarct. Systemic emboli may be found in 10% of patients dying after acute myocardial infarction, with about half lodging in the cerebral circulation.[98] Clinical stroke has been described in 1.7%[99] and 3.4%[100] of patients; those with larger infarcts are at greatest risk. Emboli to other organs are described in individuals but their incidence is very low indeed, for example limb artery occlusion occurs in less than 1%.[100]

Pericarditis is an invariable pathological finding in all cases of transmural infarction. The diagnosis may be suspected in life by the development of pericardial pain, and confirmed by the finding of a pericardial rub. In one prospective study a pericardial rub was heard in 15% of patients.[101] The rub is usually an incidental finding heard within the first 48 hours, not accompanied by symptoms. It carries no particular significance but tends to occur more commonly in larger, transmural infarcts and may be associated with atrial fibrillation and more prolonged fever.

The post-myocardial infarction syndrome described by Dressler[102] is a special form of pericarditis, pleurisy, and prolonged fever occuring some weeks later. It has been described in 3% of patients,[103] but this would seem to be an overestimate; no cases were found in 282 patients with proven myocardial infarction in Dressler's own hospital in 1980.[104] A high erythrocyte sedimentation rate is characteristic and a high titre of heart reactive antibodies may be found.[105] The cause is unknown but these features suggest an autoimmune mechanism. Reactivation of a previous viral infarction has been suggested, but the idea that the syndrome may be related in some way to the presence of blood in the pericardium has strongest support; this circumstance is common to all conditions in which Dressler's syndrome occurs.[106] It would also fit with the notion that the syndrome has become less common as the use of oral anticoagulants has declined.[104]

Vague aches and pains in the chest are common following myocardial infarction. There is no evidence that they are due to a mild form of Dressler's syndrome.[107] They are probably just due to a heightened awareness of normal musculoskeletal discomfort but persistent pains in the left mammary region may be attributable to anatomical deformation; an explanation which patients find helpful but for which there is no shred of evidence. The Guillain–Barré syndrome has been described.[108]

Most patients who suffer myocardial infarction exhibit psychological changes, initially variable levels of anxiety and subsequently depression. Frank psychiatric illness is unusual and is generally a manifestation of a previous morbid state which has been exacerbated by the experience of a severe illness and the coronary care unit. Loss of confidence and depression usually respond to counselling by nursing and medical staff without resort to drug therapy.

INFARCT EXTENSION

Some patients will suffer recurrence of cardiac pain and infarction during their hospital stay. The incidence of this complication is difficult to identify because the diagnosis depends upon the criteria used. Persisting chest pain may be a legacy of the original insult and thus an unreliable guide to reinfarction. Likewise the electrocardiographic criterion of ST segment shift is common and has been estimated to occur in 86% of patients in one series;[109] this is probably an overestimate. Secondary peaks of creatine kinase have been described in as many as 62% of patients following myocardial infarction,[110] again suggesting that infarct exten-

sion is very common. However both these techniques are open to criticism: ST segment changes may merely indicate ischaemia and not infarction, and creatine kinase may be liberated from other sources.[111] Using plasma CK MB isoenzyme and myoglobin to identify secondary peaks, Marmor and his colleagues estimated the incidence of infarct extension to be 17%,[112] a credible figure which is close to the pathological estimate of 20%.[113]

Infarct extension is more likely to occur following subendocardial infarction and is more common in fat women. The mortality rate for patients who experience this complication is doubled.[112] Most patients dying from cardiogenic shock have evidence of infarct extension.[114] The average time between the initial infarct and recurrence or extension is 10 days.[112] Recurrent cardiac pain is the cardinal feature.

PROGNOSIS AND INFARCT SIZE

The older the patient and the larger the infarct, the poorer is the short term prognosis.[61] This statement applies to the patient with myocardial infarction who escapes early sudden death due to ventricular fibrillation. The overall hospital mortality has gradually fallen over the years, mainly due to the more effective treatment of arrhythmias, but it remains high. In Norris's series[61] the mortality figures were 26% in 1966–67 and 14% in 1977–79. Most deaths happen after the first day and are due to the mechanical complications described above. Once the patient has left hospital, an additional factor in determining the long term prognosis is the extent and severity of coronary artery disease.

The importance of the age of the patient and the size of the infarct in determining prognosis is theoretically likely and demonstrable in practice. Early investigators lacked a direct measure of infarct size and used indirect manifestations such as the presence of left ventricular failure or hypotension. They were able to derive prognostic indices using simple clinical criteria, and were able to categorize patients according to their risk of dying. The first such index was described by Peel[115] who gave high scores to the following criteria: age over 65 years, previous history of infarction, shock, severe failure, rhythms other than sinus, and Q waves or bundle branch block on the electrocardiogram. Killip[116] and Norris[117] devised similar indices with greater predictive power. Other predictors, such as respiratory rate or ventricular gallop rhythm, electrocardiographic criteria, and haemodynamic variables (see above) can be used, but all reflect the same underlying problem—the amount of myocardium lost through infarction. The better early survival of patients with subendocardial infarction compared with those with transmural infarction is well recognized[118] and is probably due to less myocardial loss. Similarly, the poor early prognosis of patients who experience extension of the original infarct[112,119] is a reflection of further myocardial loss. It is cumulative myocardial loss that matters rather than the loss associated with the acute event, hence the importance of previous myocardial infarction in the history.

Because infarct size is so important in determining prognosis, much effort has been devoted to the search for a test that will measure this. Ideally the test should be accurate, reproducible, repeatable and capable of predicting ultimate infarct size. Unfortunately, none of the tests currently available is adequate. One of the simplest is electrocardiographic mapping of the ST segment elevation using multiple precordial leads.[120] The results, however, are too variable to be of any use for this purpose.[121,122] The evolution of Q waves or loss of R wave is more accurate, at least in patients with uncomplicated anterior infarcts.[123] Better still is the use of plasma creatine kinase activity.

In myocardial infarction in experimental animals, the depletion of myocardial creatine kinase activity correlates well with the histological change and the total amount of enzyme activity in the serum.[124] The dynamics of enzyme release can be subjected to mathematical analysis and the limitations of this estimate of infarct size are fully appreciated,[61] but this is currently the best method available. Both total enzyme release into the plasma as calculated from the area under the time–activity curve[125] and the peak of activity obtained from 4-hourly blood samples[126,127] correlate well with prognosis.

Cardiac scintigraphy may also be used to estimate infarct size. Larger infarcts as judged by technetium-99m pyrophosphate[128] or thallium–201 scintigrams[129] carry a worse prognosis, but these methods are not sufficiently quantifiable to hold much promise at present. Although it does not measure infarct size directly, blood pool imaging does allow the degree of left ventricular impairment to be accurately estimated and measures such as the ejection fraction correlate well with other prognostic indices.[130] Whether a scintigraphic technique or one of the new imaging methods will provide a better estimate of infarct size remains to be seen. At present the peak creatine kinase level in the plasma is the most useful guide for everyday purposes.

Following discharge from hospital, survivors of myocardial infarction have a higher risk of dying than the general population. In the Framingham survey the mortality rate was 5% per annum over the ensuing 10 years.[131] A similar risk has been described by others; for example the 5-year survival rate for males was 70% in the 420 patients in the Edinburgh series.[132] The coronary prognostic index of Norris retains its predictive value for at least 6 years, indicating the importance of myocardial damage as one determinant.[133] Left ventricular ejection fraction is also a good predictor whether measured by conventional or radionuclide angiography:[134–136] Fioretti found that the mortality rate for 214 survivors was 13% in hospital with an additional 9% by one year. Those with the lowest (< 20%) ejection fraction had a mortality rate of 33%, for those with ejection fractions ranging from 20–39%, it was 14%, and for those with an ejection fraction over 40% it was 3%.[137] Impaired left ventricular function is the probable explanation for the paradoxical finding that patients with hypertension have a relatively good prognosis following myocardial infarction since they would have better left ventricular function as compared to those with a low blood pressure.

The other major determinant of survival following hospital discharge is the number of diseased coronary vessels.[134] This is to be expected: it has long been known that prognosis in coronary heart diseaase is dependent upon the extent of arterial disease[138] as well as the ventricular damage. Any coronary stenoses additional to the disease of the vessel supplying the infarct allows the possibility of further myocardial ischaemia. Similarly an incomplete coronary obstruction giving rise to subendocardial infarctions will allow an area of residual ischaemia. Infarction of this may account for the fact that the mortality at one year is comparable to that of patients with transmural infarction.[118] Residual myocardial ischaemia may be identified by exercise testing. Theroux studied 210 patients following uncomplicated myocardial infarction and found one-year mortality rates of 27% in those with ST segment changes on their electrocardiogram and 2.1% in those without.[139] Other parameters such as poor workload achieved or an inadequate blood pressure response also have predictive value.[137,140] Other techniques such as thallium-201 scintigraphy tell the same story; that residual ischaemia is an important determinant of late prognosis.[141] Although other workers have not been able to reproduce Theroux's remarkable results, patients at higher risk of subsequent cardiac events can be identified by exercise testing.[142,143]

Either ventricular damage or myocardial ischaemia can render the patient susceptible to arrhythmias. Ventricular arrhythmias detected by ambulatory electrocardiography are associated with a worse prognosis,[135] and although these have been claimed to have an independent predictive value, it seems likely that they merely reflect the extent of myocardial pathology.[61] It is also difficult to believe that electrophysiological testing will gain ground as a superior method of assessing risk following myocardial infarction, although it has been suggested.[144]

The relative merits of these sophisticated tests over simple clinical variables such as a history of previous infarction is being debated.[145] No definite guidelines are available, but gated blood pool imaging is the best method of quantifying left ventricular performance and exercise electrocardiography is the simplest method of demonstrating reversible myocardial ischaemia after infarction.

MANAGEMENT

The high early mortality from ventricular fibrillation during acute myocardial infarction provided the stimulus for attempts at resuscitation in the community. The pioneers of this approach to management were Pantridge and his colleagues in Belfast.[146] Whilst the prime purpose of their mobile coronary care unit was to provide facilities for defibrillation, they were also able to learn much about the events taking place in the critical first hour or so following infarction. They showed not only that patients' lives could be saved but also that early relief of pain and correction of bradycardia could be achieved. Their ability to respond quickly, with the ambulance reaching the patient within 15 minutes of receiving a call in 85% of cases, was perhaps a major factor in their success.

However, the use of hospital-based doctors and nurses was relatively inefficient. Cobb and his colleagues in Seattle developed this approach by training and equipping 'paramedics' in the local fire service. This allowed an even quicker response time, averaging 3 minutes. A further development in Seattle was an extensive campaign of public education in the techniques of cardiopulmonary resuscita-

tion; by 1979 nearly half of the victims of cardiac arrest for whom resuscitation attempts had been initiated by bystanders survived to leave hospital.[5]

In England the existence of a well-organized ambulance service led Chamberlain to train a group of men and equip two vehicles with equipment for defibrillation. In 2253 calls they took a median time of 5 minutes to reach a patient, attempts at resuscitation were made in 207, of whom 160 had ventricular fibrillation; 27 survived to leave hospital.[147] Other workers, for example Norris in Auckland, New Zealand,[61] had had similar success. The principle of coronary care outside hospital is widely accepted and has been adapted to suit local needs, for example by using general practitioners in the Grampian Region of Scotland.[148] However, it is unlikely to enjoy universal success. In London, one effort was thwarted by traffic. In Nottingham[149] no benefit was found, although their response time was relatively slow. Despite these failures patients can be resuscitated from ventricular fibrillation outside hospital, and attempts to achieve this must be encouraged.

The provision of a special area within a hospital where patients could be monitored and resuscitated from ventricular fibrillation was proposed by Julian.[150] This remains the chief justification for coronary care units, but there are additional advantages for the management of patients with suspected myocardial infarction: other complications, notably arrhythmias, can be detected early and treated; facilities for temporary cardiac pacing and bedside haemodynamic monitoring can be provided; and measures designed to reduce infarct size can be explored. In practice this means that so many patients with unstable angina or difficult arrhythmias are admitted to coronary care units that in some hospitals the term cardiac care unit is preferred. Whatever the unit is called it must engender an atmosphere of calm assurance and should therefore be separate, even if only by one wall, from a general intensive care unit where patients are recovering from road traffic accidents and the effects of major surgery. The existence of a cardiac care unit within a hospital also encourages a higher standard of education about cardiac disorders among doctors and nurses with the result that resuscitation attempts in other parts of the hospital are more likely to be successful.

The need for all patients suffering from myocardial infarction to be admitted to hospital has quite properly been challenged. In a trial in South West England,[151] 1895 men under the age of 70 years with probable or definite infarction were studied but 1445 were excluded from randomization, most of them being admitted to hospital; women were also excluded 'because home care for most would be difficult for social reasons'. Less than half the randomized patients were seen within 3 hours of the onset of symptoms. Twelve per cent of those treated at home had died by 28 days compared with 14% of those treated in hospital. A survey from Teeside in the North East of England drew similar conclusions[11] about the lack of effects that hospital treatment had on the natural history of acute myocardial infarction and a second randomized study from Nottingham in the East Midlands of England[152] also found no difference in mortality for patients treated at home (13%) or in hospital (11%). In this latter study, only 500 calls were received in 4 years and only 150 patients were randomized; it has been suggested that only a minority of patients with myocardial infarction were seen and that only patients at low risk from ventricular fibrillation were treated.[61] The home versus hospital debate has been effectively stilled by an admirable paper from Rawles and Kenmure,[153] who pointed out that the wrong question was being asked. Immediate coronary care is humane and saves lives. It must be encouraged, and as a corollary hospital cardiac units must be equipped to receive the survivors. Patients seen later do not stand to gain by hospital admission.

Most of the delay in admitting patients to a cardiac care unit has been due to failure of the patient to recognize the cause of his symptoms and of his doctor to respond quickly. The latter delay is now less, but even so many patients are only identified as suffering from myocardial infarction several hours or days after the event. When this happens, and especially when the infarct is uncomplicated and the patient elderly, there are very good grounds for managing him at home. The domiciliary service provided by physicians in the United Kingdom can provide support for the general practitioner in this decision and in his management of the patient.

LIMITATION OF INFARCT SIZE

The importance of the size of the infarct in determining prognosis was discussed earlier in this chapter. The idea that the ultimate size of an infarct may be reduced by treatment is a relatively new concept which derives from animal experiments. To be effective any such treatment must be given soon after the onset of ischaemia—the earlier the better. It has become apparent that the treatment does not have to be given within a few mintues in order to salvage myocardium. This is due to a number of factors, including first the existence of a border-zone of ischaemic or 'jeopardized' myocardium between the healthy and infarcted zone; secondly the surprising length of time that it takes the myocardium to become irreversibly necrotic as opposed to being merely stunned; thirdly the often patchy nature of infarction in man, depending as it does on the suddenness of coronary occlusion and the adequacy of a collateral supply; and fourthly the other determinants of myocardial oxygen demand such as left ventricular diastolic pressure.

The earliest attempts to salvage myocardium during acute infarction involved the use of hyaluronidase,[154] which was thought to enhance the diffusion of nutrients into the ischaemic zone. Some success has been reported using hyaluronidase preparations,[155,156] but its use has not gained wide acceptance. Likewise corticosteroids were suggested in the hope that these agents might stabilize lysosomal and other sub-cellular membranes, thus limiting tissue damage.[157] Again some success was reported but there was concern about the deleterious effects, including a possible increase in the incidence of cardiac rupture.[158] The administration of a regime comprising glucose/insulin/potassium enjoyed a vogue on the theoretical ground that it would facilitate glycolysis; again no convincing benefit could be demonstrated.[159] The use of intra-aortic balloon counter pulsation was another logical idea[160] which proved difficult to implement in practice.

In theory, any agent which reduces myocardial work during acute infarction might limit the final size of an infarct. The two approaches which have shown promise are beta-adrenergic blockade and nitrate-induced vasodilatation. However, it is important to recollect the difficulties encountered in measuring infarct size (see above). Clinical endpoints such as death are not adequate for this purpose since any beneficial effect might have a different mechanism such as protection against ventricular fibrillation. The best methods available at present are a reduction in creatine kinase (and its MB isoenzyme) release; reduction in scintigraphic indices of infarction such as fixed thallium-201 defects; or preservation of left ventricular function as judged by techniques such as radionuclide estimates of ejection fraction and wall movement.

Norris and his colleagues were the first to show the beneficial effect of intravenous propranolol in reducing creatine kinase levels in patients with myocardial infarcts, but this was only when the drug was administered within 4 hours of the onset of symptoms.[161] The results of this randomized trial have been extended and an improvement in left ventricular function has been shown.[162] Similar results have been reported using timolol,[163] atenolol,[164] and metoprolol.[165] However, some studies have shown no benefit; for example Roberts and his colleagues,[166] using propranolol, were unable to show any difference in plasma creatine kinase MB activity in the control and treated groups. Most of the unsuccessful trials are open to criticism, and in the Roberts trial less than 2% of patients were treated within 4 hours of the onset of symptoms.

The use of intravenous nitrates can have beneficial haemodynamic effects in patients suffering acute myocardial infarction but the evidence for a reduction in infarct size is less convincing. Following intravenous nitroglycerin, one study[167] has shown lower creatine kinase and CK MB levels and another has shown smaller thallium-201 defects.[168] Two multicentre randomized trials using sodium nitroprusside also showed lower peak creatine kinase values in the treated groups.[169,170]

The place of emergency coronary by-pass grafting in limiting infarct size has been explored. The procedure can certainly be performed without undue risk,[171] but the wisdom of this approach has been criticized[172] and its application would always remain limited to those centres capable of undertaking cardiac surgery. It is never likely to be available quickly enough for the vast majority of patients.

THROMBOLYSIS

The indirect approaches to limiting infarct size have been superseded by a direct attack on the blocked coronary artery which formerly supplied the infarcted area. DeWood and his colleagues paved the way for this approach when they demonstrated the relative safety of acute coronary arteriography and the thrombotic nature of the final obstruction.[1] Rentrop and his colleagues then showed that intracoronary streptokinase could lyse the thrombus and reopen the artery.[173,174] The logistic difficulties in getting the patient to the cardiac catheter laboratory and selectively infusing streptokinase into the affected vessel were formidable, but several groups of workers showed that this approach was at least feasible and that subsequent left ventricular performance[175,176] and myocardial perfusion[177] was better in those patients with reopened arteries than in those whose arteries remained occluded. Three randomized controlled trials of intracoronary streptokinase were then undertaken in America.[178–180] The largest,[180] including 250 patients from Western Washington, revealed fewer deaths at 30 days in the treated group but no difference in left ventricular ejection fraction. Neither of the other two smaller studies showed a reduction in early mortality, but one[179] did show an improvement in subsequent left ventricular performance. One of the differences in these three trials is the time from the onset of symptoms to treatment: this was longer in the negative studies (the average delay of just 4 hours in the study which did show benefit[179]). The Netherlands Interuniversity study also showed improved survival[181] and left ventricular performance[181] in those patients randomized to receive intracoronary streptokinase. These were interpreted as emphasizing the importance of early reperfusion, something that would always be difficult to achieve as long as treatment depended upon a cardiac catheter laboratory. Interest therefore turned to the use of intravenous streptokinase, which had earlier been shown to be successful in reducing hospital mortality in acute myocardial infarction.[183]

Blocked coronary arteries can be reopened by intracoronary streptokinase in about 70% of patients; about 10% recanalize spontaneously.[180] Intravenous streptokinase also reopens blocked arteries,[184] but the success rate is somewhat lower 35%[185] to 49%.[186] Nevertheless intravenous streptokinase can be given earlier—by any doctor—and it avoids the risks of catheterization. Three large studies have examined this approach. The Italian study (GISSI), involving 11 700 patients, showed a reduction in mortality at 21 days, the advantage being chiefly in those patients who received treatment within 3 hours; infarct size was not measured.[187,188] In the smaller ISAM study, involving 1700 patients, infarct size was reduced as judged by the area under the CK–MB curve and by an improvement in left ventricular ejection fraction 3–4 weeks later.[189] Mortality was lower although the difference did not achieve statistical significance. A New Zealand study of 219 patients has also confirmed the improvement in left ventricular function.[190] The third, and largest study, the second International Study of Infarct Survival (ISIS-2), has convincingly established the value of early intravenous streptokinase.[190] Of 17 187 cases of suspected myocardial infarction the 5-week vascular mortality was reduced from 12.0% to 9.2% in those receiving 1.5 MU streptokinase. Most benefit was seen in those treated within 4 hours of the onset of symptoms, but surprisingly some benefit was seen up to 24 hours. ISIS-2 also examined the role of aspirin: 162.5 mg given in enteric-coated tablets for 5 weeks was accompanied by a similar reduction in mortality from 11.8 to 9.4%. The effect appeared to be additive so that those who received both treatments had a mortality rate of only 8% compared with 13.2% among those allocated to neither. Follow-up of patients given intravenous streptokinase is limited so far but in the GISSI study the improvement in survival was maintained at 1 year.[188]

There were certain differences in the design of these studies: for example the GISSI study was open, and ISIS-2 did not require ECG change but GISSI did. However, the overall conclusion is inescapable: early intravenous streptokinase saves lives in acute myocardial infarction and is to be strongly recommended. Such treatment is not without risk, notably bleeding. Therefore patients with, for example, recent peptic ulceration or stroke were, and should always be, excluded. Arterial puncture should be avoided and venepuncture minimized. If the diagnosis is wrong, streptokinase may be inadvertently given to patients with aortic dissection or pericarditis; however, in the clinical trials streptokinase appeared to be remarkably safe. The percentage incidence of complications in ISIS-2 was: hypotension and bradycardia 10.0, allergic reaction 4.4, minor bleed 3.6, major bleed requiring transfusion 0.5. Major catastrophes such as intracerebral haemorrhage were even rarer: 0.1%.

Streptokinase is antigenic, and its thrombolytic action is generalized and relatively brief. The next step in this approach has been therefore to search for a clot-specific thrombolytic agent. Tissue type plasminogen activator (rt–PA) is one such agent that has been developed by recombinant DNA technology. Reopening of coronary arteries has been demonstrated in 60–75% of patients[185,192–4] without depletion of circulating fibrinogen levels. Randomized trials[185,195] of intravenous streptokinase versus rt-PA have confirmed that the latter is more effective in re-opening occluded coronary arteries: 35% versus 60% in the TIMI trial[185] and 70% versus 55% in the European study.[195] In the TIMI trial bleeding was equally frequent in the two groups although less severe with rt–PA; the need to avoid invasive procedures was emphasized.[196] The large (5011 patients) Anglo–Scandinavian study (ASSET)[197] has examined the effect of 100 mg rt–PA plus heparin in suspected myocardial infarction and has shown a significant reduction in one-month mortality from 9.8 to 7.2%. Bleeding complications were not uncommon: 6.3% overall, of which 1.4% were major. The European Co-operative Study Group[198] examined 100 mg rt–PA plus heparin and aspirin in 721 patients and showed a significant reduction in mortality in the treated group: 2.8% compared with a control of 5.7% at 14 days. Infarct size was smaller and left ventricular function was better amongst the survivors. Unfortunately rt–PA remains very expensive. An alternative agent is anisoylated plasminogen streptokinase activator complex, (previously called APSAC and now anistreplase) which becomes concentrated at the site of recent thrombus, thus reducing the systemic effects; early reports have shown promising results with reperfusion rate of 60–65%.[199,200] A randomized double-blind placebo-controlled trial of this agent, given within 6 hours of the onset of myocardial infarction, has shown a reduction in 30-day mortality from 12.2 to 6.4% with a similar trend at one year and few adverse reactions.[201]

Whatever thrombolytic agent is used there is always an increased incidence of ventricular arrhythmias. These 'reperfusion' arrhythmias were well described in animal experiments. They are common and generally benign, taking the form of ventricular extrasystoles or accelerated idioventricular rhythm. Ventricular fibrillation was reported in 6% in one series,[180] but there was no difference between control and treated patients; ventricular arrhythmias are very common at this stage of infarction.

Successful coronary thrombolysis might be expected to limit infarction but leave an area of ischaemia; the obstructing thrombus is lysed but the underlying atheromatous stenosis remains. In some studies this idea is supported because of a higher incidence of reinfarction,[181] angina, and reversible thallium-201 perfusion defects,[202] in patients successfully treated by streptokinase. Moreover the residual stenosis is usually severe.[203] Such findings prompted the thought that thrombolytic therapy should be combined with angioplasty of the affected vessels in order to prevent recurrent ischaemia. This notion was encouraged by an early study which showed that emergency coronary angioplasty undertaken instead of intracoronary streptokinase resulted in a less severe residual stenosis; subsequent scintigraphy showed less peri-infarction ischaemia.[204] However, studies on both sides of the Atlantic which have examined the practice of immediate angioplasty following intravenous thrombolysis using rt–PA have now shown that angioplasty confers no advantage;[205,206] any theoretical gain is offset by bleeding problems and re-occlusion with recurrent ischaemia.

Thrombolytic therapy has thus ushered in a new era of coronary care. Any hospital admitting patients with acute myocardial infarction must have an efficient receiving service so that thrombolytic treatment can be given as quickly as possible following the onset of symptoms. The only real contra-indications are factors predisposing to bleeding or, in the case of streptokinase, previous treatment. Advanced age does not matter: 10% of the patients in the GISSI study were over 75 years. Men and women benefit equally. The presence of shock is not a contra-indication. Most authorities prefer to see some confirmatory electrocardiographic evidence of myocardial ischaemia but this is not mandatory. Ideally treatment should be started as early as possible, and most benefit is seen in those patients receiving treatment within 4–6 hours. Measurable benefits include reduction in infarct size, improvement in left ventricular function, and lower mortality in the treated patients.

The choice of thrombolytic agent cannot be finally agreed until the results of further trials are available. Such trials to compare streptokinase, rt–PA, and anistreplase (GISSI-2 and ISIS-3) are under way or planned. However, streptokinase is still the agent of choice because neither of the others is clearly superior and both are more expensive. In patients who have previously received streptokinase, rt–PA should be given. The question of adjuvant therapy is also unclear, with the exception of aspirin, which can be firmly recommended on the strength of the findings in ISIS-2. Heparin seems to confer no additional benefit and may increase the risk of bleeding. Beta blockade and nitrates are probably best reserved for patients who show evidence of recurrent ischaemia, either painful or silent. Emergency coronary angiography is not necessary and should be reserved for patients who do not settle with medical therapy. Delayed, elective angioplasty or bypass surgery seems to be safer than emergency procedures.

The next phase will be to administer thrombolytic treatment before hospital admission, either at home or in the ambulance. One such study is

already taking place using anistreplase (EMIP) and others will undoubtedly follow. The vehicle for administering thrombolytic treatment will depend upon local resources but may include coronary ambulances or general practitioners. At present the best advice for patients with suspected myocardial infarction is to take an aspirin and get to hospital as quickly as possible.

MANAGEMENT OF THE UNCOMPLICATED CASE

Patients seen soon after the onset of symptoms should be admitted to a coronary care unit. Those seen later can be cared for at home if the circumstances are suitable. It is not possible to give firm guidance about what constitutes early or late but a few hours is certainly early. The coronary care unit should provide facilities for continuous electrocardiographic monitoring, defibrillation and resuscitation, temporary pacing, haemodynamic monitoring, and so on. The unit should be staffed by nurses and managed in consultation with a physician experienced in cardiovascular medicine.

Relief of pain and anxiety is the first priority in patients suffering from myocardial infarction. Diamorphine or morphine is best for this purpose and may be combined with a drug such as prochlorperazine if nausea and vomiting are troublesome. Diazepam is a useful sedative, and nitrazepam is valuable for night sedation. Relief of myocardial ischaemia using thrombolytic agents, nitrates and beta-blockade is important in improving prognosis and may assist in relieving pain. Drug therapy can never replace the explanation and reassurance that nurses and doctors are able to provide at this stage. The advice may be supplemented by explanatory booklets. The risk of primary ventricular fibrillation is so small after 48 hours that patients can be discharged to the general ward. The role of a progressive care area is still uncertain. If it is available next to the coronary care unit, it provides a level of care intermediate between the coronary care unit and the general ward. This can certainly be justified in complicated cases and may be helpful for uncomplicated cases if further observation, for example by electrocardiographic telemetry, is desirable. Much will depend upon the size of the population served and other local factors.

The posture of the patient should be determined by his comfort rather than by any medical criterion. Becoming upright early prevents loss of vascular reflexes.[207] The evils of prolonged bed rest have been well described[208] and mobilization at 48 hours is recommended. Previous advice to rest for several weeks following infarction was based on a knowledge of the pathological changes taking place in the infarcted myocardium. Physicians knew that necrotic muscle predominated for 2 weeks and was only gradually replaced by scar tissue after this time; they feared that early mobilization might increase cardiac work and induce further damage. Although this view can still attract support,[209] studies have shown no increase in complications or mortality when a policy of early mobilization and discharge is followed.[210–212] However, these studies are small and one trial showed slightly better survival in the second and third years following infarction when mobilization began later.[213] The lack of proof of benefit of prolonged rest, together with the documented hazards of such a policy, including a high incidence of venous thrombo-embolism, and the practical consideration of keeping an apparently fit patient in bed for more than a few days is sufficient justification for a policy of early mobilization. Early discharge at 7–14 days is a logical consequence of this policy.

Oxygen might in theory improve myocardial oxygenation but there is no evidence that it helps unless there is hypoxaemia.[214] The routine use of anticoagulant therapy can also be advanced on theoretical grounds in that it will prevent venous thrombo-embolism, diminish the risk of left ventricular mural thrombus and systemic embolism, and partly arrest the propagation of the coronary arterial thrombus.

There is persuasive evidence that anticoagulant drugs reduce the mortality rate in patients with myocardial infarction during their hospital stay.[215] The incidence of cerebral embolism is reduced,[216] but in all trials the risk of bleeding is increased. Because physicians perceive themselves as more culpable when iatrogenic complications ensue, anticoagulant drugs are often not given. A compromise is to give low dose heparin (5–10 000 units every 8–12 hours) and to continue this until the patient is fully ambulant. This regime can certainly reduce the incidence of calf vein thrombosis[217] and can therefore be recommended. Studies of its effect on systemic embolism are lacking. A reasonable policy is to reserve full anticoagulation for those at high risk from thrombo-embolism such as those with heart failure, obesity, left ventricular aneurysm. There is no evidence that 'anti-platelet' drugs influence the outcome of patients with myocardial infarction despite the proven long term value of aspirin in patients with unstable angina.[218] In the absence of contra-indication, aspirin 75–150 mg per day might reasonably be given to patients with non-Q-wave infarction once the low dose heparin has been stopped, the rationale being that these patients may yet develop an occlusive coronary thrombus.

The merits of long term beta-blockade are discussed in the next chapter. If beta-adrenergic antagonists are to be given, they should be given early, when the deleterious effects of sympathetic stimulation are most likely to occur. Early beta blockade can help limit infarct size (see above), and can reduce the incidence of ventricular arrhythmias,[219] including ventricular fibrillation;[220] it can prevent the progression of threatened to completed infarction.[221,222] Although many patients will not be suitable for this form of treatment and many physicians will remain nervous about it, there is a good case to be made for giving intravenous beta-blocking drugs to patients seen early after the onset of symptoms and to continue such treatment until hospital discharge. A priori the case would seem to be strongest in those with marked sympathetic overactivity manifested through signs such as systolic hypertension, although there is no proof of this. The possibility exists that beta blockade is the modern equivalent of prolonged bed rest.

Other cardiovascular drugs, for example nifedipine,[223] have been suggested and tried in acute myocardial infarction but none is of proven value.

MANAGEMENT OF COMPLICATIONS

MANAGEMENT OF ARRHYTHMIC COMPLICATIONS

Cardiac arrhythmias that cause the patient's condition to deteriorate must be treated energetically. There can be no argument about the need of cardioversion in a collapsed patient with ventricular tachycardia or fibrillation, but for many arrhythmias the need for treatment is debatable. Fashion has oscillated between prophylactic regimes designed to suppress all potentially harmful arrhythmias and a policy of masterly inactivity based on the fact that all anti-arrhythmic drugs can cause arrhythmias and/or depress ventricular function. Any dogmatic assertion about the treatment of cardiac arrhythmias would be imprudent.

Sinus tachycardia may be a manifestation of pump failure in which case anti-arrhythmic treatment is inappropriate. If sinus tachycardia is due to sympathetic overactivity, beta blockade is advisable. Most supraventricular arrhythmias require no treatment. Atrial fibrillation with a fast ventricular response is often associated with extensive infarction and poor left ventricular function, and then digoxin is appropriate. If there is severe haemodynamic deterioration, cardioversion will be necessary. There may be an increased risk of ventricular fibrillation if cardioversion is undertaken when the patient has already received digoxin. If this is considered likely, verapamil can be used to slow the ventricular rate.

Ventricular extrasystoles do not require treatment, unless they are sufficiently frequent to cause haemodynamic deterioration. Efforts to identify and treat all ventricular arrhythmias in the hope of preventing ventricular fibrillation are now no longer deemed necessary. Occasionally ventricular tachycardia can be well tolerated. If treatment of ventricular extrasystoles or well tolerated ventricular tachycardia is required, lignocaine is the drug of choice. Usually ventricular tachycardia—and always ventricular fibrillation—require DC cardioversion. A shock of 100–200 Joules is highly effective in primary ventricular fibrillation.

The prevention of ventricular arrhythmias has been described in a well-designed and often quoted trial by Lie et al.[224] An initial bolus of 100 mg lignocaine followed by an infusion of 3 mg/minute prevented ventricular fibrillation. As always there was a price to be paid: in this example, a 15% incidence of side-effects mainly affecting the central nervous system. In view of this and the success of cardioversion in primary ventricular fibrillation, the use of prophylactic lignocaine hardly seems warranted. Lignocaine, however, should be administered following cardioversion. For recurrent ventricular fibrillation bretylium may be useful and this drug enjoys official support in the United States.[225] The duration of treatment is not decided because the genesis of arrhythmias in acute myocardial infarction almost certainly differs from that in chronic ischaemia. Thus when the acute event has passed there may be no need for long-term anti-arrhythmic drugs. The safest policy is stop the lignocaine infusion after a few days and monitor the patient carefully with ambulatory electrocardiography before discharge from hospital. Electrophysiological testing may be helpful. If the patient remains well and no sinister arrhythmia is encountered, no specific anti-arrhythmic treatment is required.

Refractory ventricular arrhythmias, particularly those that occur after the first day or two, are more difficult to manage. They often reflect severe ventricular damage. Lignocaine may be ineffective. Often the best therapeutic approach is to improve ventricular function, but if this fails, procainamide or disopyramide may be tried. The large number of different drugs that have been used to treat refractory ventricular arrhythmias is a tribute to their toxicity or lack of efficacy and the poor prognosis of the underlying condition. Disopyramide, mexiletine, phenytoin and tocainide all have their advocates. At present amiodarone appears more promising; in view of the pharmacokinetics of this drug a massive loading dose may be necessary. Overdrive pacing (that is, pacing the heart at rates that will suppress the ventricular arrhythmia) is generally a desperate measure but can be tried in conjunction with anti-arrhythmic drugs when all else fails. If possible, dual chamber pacing should be undertaken to maintain atrioventricular synchrony. Surgery for refractory ventricular arrhythmias in acute infarction cannot be recommended without a very full trial of medical therapy and therefore should not be undertaken at this stage.

Sinus bradycardia and transient sinus arrest with a slow nodal escape rhythm generally respond to atropine. Care must be taken to avoid overdosage or an alarming tachycardia may supervene. Second-degree heart block in association with inferior infarction is also benign. When complete heart block arises, no treatment may be necessary if the ventricular rate is adequate and the patient has no symptoms. The rate may be increased by atropine. Symptomatic patients should be paced. In anterior infarction complete heart block must be treated by pacing. Even with this form of treatment mortality remains around 90%. The development of bundle branch block may suddenly progress to ventricular asystole and loss of consciousness. This sequence of events is very difficult to predict and so any patient with anterior infarction with conduction defects beyond axis deviation should have a temporary pacemaker inserted.

MANAGEMENT OF MECHANICAL COMPLICATIONS

Minor degrees of left ventricular failure and pulmonary congestion are common in myocardial infarction. Often no treatment is required. However, if the patient is short of breath or pulmonary congestion is apparent on the chest X-ray, diuretics such as frusemide should be given, at first intravenously and later orally. Chronic potassium loss is best minimized by the concomitant administration of a potassium-sparing diuretic such as amiloride rather than by giving potassium supplements.

More severe degrees of pump failure should be treated by the addition of vasodilator drugs. Although many such drugs are available, nitrates are to be preferred because of their short duration of action. The ability of sodium nitroprusside to lower left ventricular filling pressure and to reduce pulmonary congestion is well documented.[57] It must be protected from light and there has been anxiety about the accumulation of cyanide in the body, so glyceryl trinitrate and isosorbide dinitrate have largely replaced sodium nitroprusside. Both drugs can be highly effective in the patient with pulmonary congestion and systemic vasoconstriction. The hazards of vasodilator therapy include hypotension and collapse, so treatment must be administered with caution. Initial intravenous therapy can be followed by the use of oral isosorbide dinitrate and oral or cutaneous glyceryl trinitrate.

The management of sick patients is facilitated by haemodynamic monitoring. Although some parameters, such as heart rate, blood pressure and urine flow, can be measured easily, others, such as pulmonary capillary wedge pressure and cardiac output, can only be obtained by Swan–Ganz catheterization. Younger patients with the mechanical complications of infarction should be treated vigorously, whereas older patients with global impairment of left ventricular function need not necessarily be treated thus. A knowledge of the pulmonary capillary wedge pressure and cardiac output is vital to the proper management of sick patients to identify those whose filling pressures are low, to monitor the effects of vasodilator therapy, and so on.

Very sick patients—those tending towards or actually suffering from cardiogenic shock—require rapid assessment and energetic treatment. In addition to the measures outlined above an early attempt to assess the outcome of treatment is essential. This can be achieved by careful clinical assessment. If the patient is suffering from cardiogenic shock following several myocardial infarcts with no surgically correctable lesion, the prognosis is hopeless, but if the patient has ventricular septal rupture with good residual left ventricular function, there is hope of successful repair and resuscitative measures should be pursued. Doppler echocardiography is extremely helpful in this assessment.

The use of inotropic drugs in sick and very sick patients is controversial. Beta-adrenergic agonists increase myocardial oxygen consumption and lactate production[226] and increase infarct size in experimental animals,[227] and in theory their use must be deprecated. In practice, however, beta stimulation of the heart may be the only way of maintaining the circulation and then these agents will have to be used. Noradrenaline, adrenaline, isoprenaline, dobutamine, and dopamine have all been tried. None is clearly superior. Dobutamine[228] and dopamine are fairly cardioselective and will have a positive inotropic effect; in addition dopamine will produce vasodilatation of the splanchnic and renal beds and will thus increase urine output. Digoxin is very little used for its inotropic effect in acute infarction.[229]

The poor results of drug treatment in patients with low output states following myocardial infarction have prompted the development of mechanical devices to assist the circulation. The best and most widely used of these devices is intra-aortic balloon counter pulsation. The advantages include improved coronary perfusion, decreased afterload and hence reduced myocardial oxygen consumption.[230] Not surprisingly this form of treatment by itself does not improve outcome[231] and it should be reserved for patients with the mechanical defects of ventricular septal rupture or mitral regurgitation that are amenable to surgical correction.[232] Even then any delay in undertaking definitive treatment is regrettable and it is often best to take the patient straight to the operating theatre if feasible. The use of counter pulsation is thus limited to patients whose condition needs to be stabilized before transfer to a cardiac surgical centre.

Surgery has an established role in the correction of ventricular septal rupture and mitral regurgitation following myocardial infarction. Both conditions carry a very high mortality if left untreated. Early surgery can be life saving. Those who are more likely to benefit from surgical treatment can be identified by haemodynamic and echocardiographic criteria (see above). The timing of surgery has been the subject of debate. It has been argued that deferring the operation allows some resolution of myocardial necrosis so that repair is easier, but a more usual experience is that patients often run a complicated course, with the development of renal failure, pneumonia, etc., so that immediate surgery is preferable. The results in selected patients can be very gratifying (see Wheatley, Chapter 52). Anecdotal reports testify to the occasional success of surgery in myocardial rupture.[233]

Revascularization for left ventricular pump failure in myocardial infarction is an ambitious surgical approach. Of 50 patients treated in this way, 15 died within 30 days of surgery and a further 11 died later.[234] These results are an improvement on the natural mortality, which exceeds 90%, but the tremendous cost and limited availability of this form of emergency surgery will restrict its application to a handful of patients. This also applies to the artificial heart and transplantation,[235] at least in 1989.

MANAGEMENT OF OTHER COMPLICATIONS

Thrombo-embolism must be treated by anticoagulants (the routine use of anticoagulants is discussed above). Pericarditis should be treated with anti-inflammatory analgesic drugs and is not a contra-indication to anticoagulation. The occasional patient with Dressler's syndrome may require treatment with corticosteroids but most respond to anti-inflammatory analgesics.

RISK STRATIFICATION

Once a patient is identified as having suffered from myocardial infarction his prognosis is determined by his age, the amount of myocardium lost, and the extent of the coronary artery disease. Age is very important: the first-year mortality for patients under 45 years is 6.2%; for those over 70 years it is 24.4%[236]. Age is irreversible, but myocardial loss and the extent of coronary disease can be assessed both by the clinical features and by various investigative techniques. The subsequent prognosis can thus be gauged; this tactic has become known as risk stratification.[135,237] The risk is not static: assessment of risk starts when the patient is first seen, goes on while he is being managed in the coronary care unit, and is finalized at the time of discharge from hospital. The last stage is discussed in Chapter 51, but the concept is so important that it should be considered here with particular reference to patients at risk from re-infarction.

For patients following myocardial infarction, the risk of subsequent events is a spectrum. At one extreme there is the elderly person with previous infarction whose myocardium is largely replaced by fibrous and necrotic tissue: left ventricular function is very poor, malignant ventricular arrhythmias are commonplace, and the prognosis is very poor

indeed. Further investigation would be unkind and superfluous. At the other extreme is the young person with a small infarct, very little myocardial loss, normal ventricular function, no arrhythmias, and an excellent prognosis. Such a patient also requires little further investigation. Between these two ends of the spectrum lies the majority of patients. They have varying degrees of myocardial loss and residual ischaemia that can be characterized by further investigation as outlined below.

Although it has been customary to undertake risk stratification following discharge from hospital, this policy is mistaken. Some 10–15% of patients will die in the first year following infarction. Half of these deaths will occur within the first 3 months[238,239] and one-third within the first 6 weeks.[240] The moment of discharge is arbitrary and certainly does not separate safe and unsafe periods of convalescence. The risk of further cardiac events following infarction gradually declines from the onset of symptoms. Thus, as stated above, risk stratification must be a continuous process with clinical assessment taking place daily and the timing of investigations should be judged according to the patient's state and local circumstances. Definitive guidelines cannot be given, but certain rules are dictated by common sense: exercise testing should not be undertaken in patients with heart failure, and patients at high risk from ventricular fibrillation should not be removed from the coronary care unit.

The prognosis following uncomplicated myocardial infarction is good, but some patients, particularly those with non-Q wave infarction, are liable to further ischaemic events. These may occur at any time following the initial infarct and may happen suddenly. Victims of subendocardial infarction have a good initial prognosis but are just as likely as those with transmural infarcts to suffer further cardiac events.[118] Patients with this type of infarction should undergo further testing in an attempt to identify those at risk in the ensuing weeks and months. For this purpose, exercise testing is valuable and this policy may be reasonably extended to all those patients with uncomplicated infarction, unless there is some contra-indication such as locomotor disability.

Exercise testing is generally undertaken on a treadmill using a relatively mild protocol such as the Naughton or modified Bruce. Observations should include the patient's condition (presence of dyspnoea, angina, and so on), heart rate, blood pressure, and electrocardiogram with special attention to the ST segment and development of arrhythmias. There

is debate about whether the test should be symptom-limited or sub-maximal and whether it should be performed before or after hospital discharge. The first point is rather subjective and depends on the enthusiasm of the attending staff. The best compromise is probably to take the patient to the onset of symptoms but not beyond. The second point is being resolved in favour of a predischarge test, partly because it is more convenient for the patient and partly because a test performed after discharge will miss those who have already suffered their further cardiac event during that time. A further advantage of exercise testing before discharge is that the patient and his physician can derive comfort from a negative test at a good workload and plan a more rapid convalescence.

Most studies of exercise testing following cardiac infarction have examined electrocardiographic ST segment depression. If this parameter is used alone, false negatives and positives occur. The value of the exercise test may be enhanced by taking into account other observations such as the development of angina, duration of test, speed of recovery and the adequacy of the blood pressure and heart rate response. Thallium-201 scintigraphy may also be used for this purpose but probably adds little prognostic information.[242]

An early low-level exercise test can be recommended for those patients following small uncomplicated infarcts with no evidence of left ventricular failure. The test may be particularly helpful in patients with subendocardial infarction. A negative test implies a good prognosis with no need for further investigation or treatment. An early return to full activities can be permitted. The development of angina or electrocardiographic ST segment depression implies continuing myocardial ischaemia. The patient should be treated by beta blockade and equipped with nitrates. Early follow-up, in practice within 4 weeks is advisable. Further investigation with a view to angioplasty or bypass surgery may be desirable.

Recurrent cardiac pain during the hospital stay is a sinister symptom. The patient who seems to make a good recovery from the initial event and progresses from the coronary care unit only to return a few days later with more chest pain is probably extending his infarct and worsening his prognosis. Every effort must be made to prevent this; if it does occur, it must be treated energetically. The difficulties in recognizing this complication are considerable because patients commonly experience chest pains of pericardial or musculoskeletal origin at this stage,

but the patient should be returned to the coronary care unit, and beta blockade, nitrates, and heparin should be administered. If the pain recurs, early angiography is recommended.

Angina developing during mobilization should also be regarded as an indication for angiography, especially when it occurs despite full medical therapy. Exercise testing is superfluous. Both recurrent rest pain and angina suggest continuing myocardial ischaemia and thus, in all probability, viable myocardium supplied by compromised coronary circulation. Ischaemic myocardium can exist either around the infarct zone or remote from the infarct. With the former a single coronary artery may be diseased, and perhaps not totally occluded; with the latter multivessel coronary disease is the rule. Attempts have been made to identify ischaemia 'at a distance' from the early electrocardiograms. Often the localized electrocardiographic changes of acute infarction are accompanied by reciprocal changes in the other leads. This can be recognized, for example, as ST segment depression in the precordial leads on patients with inferior infarction. Although this finding reflects more severe left ventricular damage[243] and a higher frequency of complications,[244] it does not necessarily predict concomitant disease in the coronary artery supplying the reciprocal territory.[245] The value of this finding is therefore that it defines a group of patients who require more careful observation and perhaps a longer hospital stay, rather than a need for angiography.

Patients with moderate or large infarcts, especially those with previous infarction, have sustained more myocardial loss and are therefore more prone to develop left ventricular failure. They, too, may have residual areas of myocardial ischaemia which must be conserved but the chief problem is to identify those at risk from left ventricular failure. It can be very difficult to decide, on clinical grounds alone, how much myocardium has been lost. Radionuclide ventriculography is by far the best tool for this purpose. Cross-sectional echocardiography may supplant this, but at present the difficulty of obtaining good quality records in all patients, coupled with the lack of quantification, makes radionuclide ventriculography superior.

Ideally radionuclide ventriculography should be performed near the coronary care unit. Accurate estimates of left ventricular function are then available early in the hospital course and the patient's management can be altered accordingly. Although the prognostic indices discussed above define populations of patients, there are always exceptions. It is not uncommon for an apparently sick patient who seems to have electrocardiographic evidence of extensive infarction to have surprisingly good left ventricular function on investigation. The potential for a full recovery implies a greater need for further investigation and more vigorous treatment. A policy of early radionuclide ventriculography also allows improvement in left ventricular function to be documented. A further advantage is that the risk of subsequent left ventricular failure, and so the need for diuretic therapy etc. can be assessed. Patients with good left ventricular function with an ejection fraction of over 0.4 should have some form of exercise testing to define areas of ischaemia. Those with an ejection fraction of under 0.35 should not usually undergo exercise testing initially but should be treated with diuretics and vasodilators to reduce left ventricular workload. Ambulatory electrocardiography should be considered.

Arrhythmias are very common following myocardial infarction. Complex ventricular arrhythmias such as runs of ventricular tachycardia are associated with a higher risk of subsequent death; 15% at 12 months in one study compared with 5% in patients with no, or just simple, ventricular extrasystoles.[246] The difficulty is that these arrhythmias correlate with poor left ventricular function and are not a strong independent predictor of prognosis.[246–248] Hence information derived from ambulatory electrocardiography may add little to risk stratification. Moreover attempts to suppress ventricular arrhythmias may be fraught with problems because the negative inotropic and pro-arrhythmic effect of anti-arrhythmic drugs may actually make the patient worse. The best policy may be to improve ventricular function by vasodilator therapy, although there is as yet no firm evidence for this. What evidence there is suggests that beta blockade may be helpful because propranolol seems to reduce mortality even in patients who had heart failure following myocardial infarction;[249] the same study has found that propranolol does not preferentially reduce the risk of sudden death in patients with complex ventricular arrhythmias.[250]

Programmed ventricular stimulation has also been suggested as a method of identifying patients at high risk following myocardial infarction.[144] This technique is certainly beyond the scope of most hospitals and seems unlikely to be widely used. It has yet to be shown that induceable ventricular arrhythmias or the existence of 'late potentials' derived from the surface electrocardiogram are anything more than another manifestation of a severely damaged left ventricle.

The techniques of exercise testing, radionuclide ventriculography, cross-sectional echocardiography, and ambulatory electrocardiography are subordinate to clinical judgement. Risk stratification must always start with a history, physical examination, and the evaluation of simple investigations such as a resting electrocardiogram. etc. This should be undertaken by a physician with special training and experience in cardiovascular disease. 'Non-invasive' investigations should be readily available, with the proviso that if radionuclide ventriculography is not available, cross-sectional echocardiographic assessment of left ventricular function may provide a reasonable alternative. Coronary arteriography is not recommended as a routine.

The indications for coronary arteriography are discussed in Chapter 15. After myocardial infarction the chief indication is recurrent cardiac pain, either pain at rest or induced by exercise. To this should be added those with a strongly positive exercise test and some, but not all, of those patients with the 'mechanical' complications of infarction. As described above, some patients with mitral regurgitation or ventricular septal rupture can be referred for surgery on the strength of the echocardiographic findings, but most patients with refractory left ventricular failure or aneurysm formation will require coronary arteriography and left ventricular angiography. Patients with these mechanical complications form a minority. Most will require coronary arteriography because they have evidence of continuing myocardial ischaemia and stand to gain from coronary angioplasty or bypass surgery. The timing of investigation must depend on local circumstances but any delay may be deleterious.

Finally the value of risk stratification should be re-examined in the light of the foregoing discussion. Patients with poor left ventricular function have a poor prognosis. These patients can be identified but their left ventricular damage cannot be corrected. Nevertheless a negative approach to this dilemma is unwarranted. Many pharmacological agents are available to improve left ventricular function; new agents are undergoing trial. Careful follow-up and guidance about lifestyle are necessary. Patients and their relatives usually appreciate a frank discussion of the prognosis. Retirement from work on medical grounds can be financially advantageous. A restricted lifestyle should be advised. The clinical impression that limiting physical activities improves survival may have physiological justification in that cardiac work is reduced. There is always room for an optimistic approach, because individuals with poor left ventricular function may defy the gloomy statistical prognosis. The physician giving such advice must have his facts correct. The evidence for poor left ventricular function must not be based solely on clinical impression and a recollection of the patient's state on admission to hospital.

At the other end of the spectrum lies the patient with good left ventricular function and one or more critical coronary stenoses. Too often he identifies himself by dropping dead or being re-admitted to hospital with massive re-infarction. Not all such patients can be recognized, but some can: they have recurrent cardiac pain in hospital and/or a strongly positive exercise test. Although no study is available to show that the prognosis of these patients is improved by more aggressive treatment, medical therapy including beta blockade, nifedipine, and nitrates can be recommended. Physicians should have a low threshold for recommending angiography in this group of patients.

REFERENCES

1. DeWood, M.A., Spores, J., Notske, R. Prevalence of total coronary occlusion during the early hours of transmural myocardial infarction. N. Engl. J. Med. 1980; 303: 897–902.
2. McKana, W.J., Chew, C.Y.E., Oakley, C.M. Myocardial infarction with normal coronary angiogram possible mechanism of smoking risk in coronary artery disease. Br. Heart J. 1980; 43: 493–8.
3. Herrick, J.B. Clinical features of sudden obstruction of the coronary arteries. J. Am. Med. Assoc. 1912; 49: 2015–20.
4. Adgey, A.A.J., Nelson, P.G., Scott, M.E. et al. Management of ventricular fibrillation outside hospital. Lancet 1969; 1: 1169–71.
5. Cobb, L.A., Werner, J.A., Trobaugh, G.B. Sudden cardiac death. 1 A decade's experience with out-of-hospital resuscitation. Mod. Concepts Cardiovasc. Dis. 1980; 49: 31–6.
6. Kannel, W.B. and Abbott, R.D. Incidence and prognosis of unrecognised myocardial infarction: an update on the Framingham study. N. Engl. J. Med. 1984; 311: 1144–7.
7. Shaper, A.G., Cook, D.G., Walker, M., McFarlane, P.W. Recall of diagnosis by men with ischaemic heart disease. Br. Heart J. 1984; 51: 606–11.
8. Tunstall-Pedoe, H., Clayton, D., Morris, J.N., Brigden, W., McDonald, L. Coronary heart attacks in East London. Lancet 1975; 2: 833–8.
9. Armstrong, A., Duncan, B., Oliver, M.F. Natural history of acute coronary heart attacks. A community study. Br. Heart J. 1972; 34: 67–80.
10. Pai, G.R., Haites, N.E., Rawes, J.M. One thousand heart attacks in Grampian: the place of cardiopulmonary resuscitation in general practice. Br. Med. J. 1987; 294: 352–4.
11. Colling, A., Dellipiani, A.W., Donaldson, R.J., McCormack, P. Teeside coronary survey: an epidemiological study of acute attacks of myocardial infarction. Br. Med. J. 1976; 2: 1169–72.
12. Kinlen, L.J. Incidence and presentation of myocardial infarction in an English community. Br. Heart J. 1973; 35: 616–22.
13. Royal College of General Practitioners. Morbidity Statistics from General Practice 1971–72. Second National Study. London: HMSO, 1979.
14. Reid, D.D., Hamilton, P.J.S., Keen, H., Brett, G.Z., Jarrett, R.J., Rose, G. Cardiorespiratory disease and diabetes among middle-aged male civil servants. Lancet 1974; 1: 469–73.
15. Shaper, A.G., Cook, D.G., Walker, M., MacFarlane, P.W. Prevalence of ischaemic heart disease in middle aged British men. Br. Heart J. 1984; 51: 595–605.
16. Pocock, S.J., Shaper, A.G., Cook, D.G. et al. British Regional Heart Study: geographical variations in cardiovascular mortality; and the role of water quality. Br. Med. J. 1980; 280: 1243–9.
17. Shaper, A.G. and Pocock, S.J. Editorial: Risk factors for ischaemic heart disease in British men. Br. Heart J. 1987; 57: 11–16.
18. Braunwald, E. and Kloner, R.A. The stunned myocardium: prolonged, postischaemic ventricular dysfunction. Circulation 1982; 66: 1146–9.
19. Geft, I.L., Fishbein, M.C., Ninomiya, K. et al. Intermittent brief periods of ischaemia have a cumulative effect and may cause myocardial necrosis. Circulation 1982; 66: 1150–3.
20. Roubin, G.S., Harris, P.J., Bernstein, L., Kelly, D.T. Coronary anatomy and prognosis after myocardial infarction in patients 60 years of age and younger. Circulation 1983; 67: 743–9.
21. Huey, B.L., Gheorghiade, M., Crampton, R.S. Acute non-Q wave myocardial infarction associated with early ST segment elevation: evidence for spontaneous coronary reperfusion and implications for thrombolytic trials. J. Am. Coll. Cardiol. 1987; 9: 18–25.
22. Page, D.L., Caulfield, J.B., Kaston, J.A., DeSanctus, R.W., Sanders, C.A. Myocardial changes associated with cardiogenic shock. N. Engl. J. Med. 1971; 285: 133–7.
23. Scheidt, S., Ascheim, R., Killip, T. Shock after acute myocardial infarction. A clinical and hemodynamic profile. Am. J. Cardiol. 1970; 26: 556–64.
24. DeWood, M.A., Stifter, W.F., Simpson, C.S. et al. Coronary arteriographic findings soon after non-Q-wave myocardial infarction. N. Engl. J. Med. 1986; 315: 417–23.
25. Phibbs, B. 'Transmural' versus 'subendocardial' myocardial infarction: an electrocardiographic myth. J. Am. Coll. Cardiol. 1983; 1: 561–4.
26. Myers, A. and Dewar, H.A. Circumstances attending 100 sudden deaths from coronary artery disease with coronary necropsies. Br. Heart J. 1975; 37: 1133–43.
27. Muller, J.E., Stone, P.H., Turi, Z.G. et al. Circadian variation on the frequency of onset of acute myocardial infarction. N. Engl. J. Med. 1985; 313: 1315–22.
28. Stowers, M. and Short, D. Warning symptoms before major myocardial infarction. Br. Heart J. 1970; 32: 833–8.
29. Ingram, D.A., Fulton, R.A., Portal, R.W., Aber, C.P. Vomiting as a diagnostic aid in acute ischaemic cardiac pain. Br. Med. J. 1980; 281: 636–8.
30. Aronow, W.S., Starling, L., Etienne, F. et al. Unrecognized Q-wave myocardial infarction in patients older than 64 years in a long term health care facility. Am. J. Cardiol. 1985; 56: 483.
31. McGuiness, J.B., Begg, T.B., Semple, T. First electrocardio-

gram in recent myocardial infarction. *Br. Med. J.* 1976; **2**: 449–51.

32. Pardee, H.E.B. An electrocardiographic sign of coronary artery obstruction. *Arch. Intern. Med.* 1920; **26**: 244–57.
33. Lepeschlein, E. The U wave of the electrocardiogram. *Mod. Concepts Cardiovasc. Dis.* 1969; **38**: 39–45.
34. Hearse, D.J. Myocardial enzyme leakage. *J. Mol. Med.* 1977; **2**: 185–200.
35. Scott, B.B., Simmons, A.V., Newton, K.E., Payne, R.B. Interpretation of serum creatine kinase in suspected myocardial infarction. *Br. Med. J.* 1974; **2**: 691–3.
36. McComb, J.M., McMaster, E.A., MacKenzie, G., Adgey, A.A.J. Myoglobin and creatine kinase in acute myocardial infarction. *Br. Heart J.* 1984; **51**: 189–94.
37. Kagen, L., Scheidt, S., Butt, A. Serum myoglobin in myocardial infarction: The 'staccato phenomenon'. Is myocardial infarction in man an intermittent event? *Am. J. Med.* 1977; **62**: 86–92.
38. Fyfe, T., Baxter, R.H., Cochran, K.M., Booth, E.M. Plasma-lipid changes after myocardial infarction. *Lancet* 1971; **2**: 997–1001.
39. Jackson, R., Scragg, R., Marshall, R., White, H., O'Brien, K., Small, C. Changes in serum lipid concentrations during first 24 hours after myocardial infarction. *Br. Med. J.* 1987; **294**: 1588–9.
40. Hamsten, A., Wiman, B., de Faire, U., Blomback, M. Increased plasma levels of a rapid inhibition of tissue plasminogen activation in young survivors of myocardial infarction. *N. Engl. J. Med.* 1985; **313**: 1557–63.
41. Masuda, Y., Yoshida, H., Morooka, N., Watanabe, S., Inagaki, Y. The usefulness of X-ray computed tomography for the diagnosis of myocardial infarction. *Circulation* 1984; **70**: 217–25.
42. Visser, C.A., Kan, G., Lie, K.I., Becker, A.E., Durrer, D. Apex two dimensional echocardiography. Alternative approach to quantification of acute myocardial infarction. *Br. Heart J.* 1982; **49**: 461–7.
43. Recusani, F., Raisasro, A., Sgalambro, A. *et al.* Ventricular septal rupture after myocardial infarction: diagnosis by two-dimensional and pulsed Doppler echocardiography. *Am. J. Cardiol.* 1984; **54**: 277–81.
44. Loperfido, F., Biasucci, L.M., Pennestri, F. *et al.* Pulsed Doppler echocardiographic analysis of mitral regurgitation after myocardial infarction. *Am. J. Cardiol.* 1986; **58**: 692–7.
45. Kumar, A., Minagoe, S., Chandraratna, P.A.N. Two dimensional echocardiographic demonstration of restoration of normal wall motion after acute myocardial infarction. *Am. J. Cardiol.* 1986; **57**: 1232–5.
46. Visser, C.A., Kan, G., Meltzer, R.S., Kooler, J.J., Dunning, A.J. Incidence timing and prognostic value of left ventricular aneurysm formation after myocardial infarction: a prospective, serial echocardiographic study of 158 patients. *Am. J. Cardiol.* 1986; **57**: 729–32.
47. Kan, G., Visser, C.A., Lie, K.I., Durrer, D. Measurement of left ventricular ejection fraction after acute myocardial infarction. A serial cross sectional echocradiographic study. *Br. Heart J.* 1984; **51**: 631–6.
48. Asinger, R.W., Mikell, F.L., Elsperger, J., Hodges, M. Incidence of left ventricular thrombosis after acute transmural myocardial infarction. Serial evaluation by two dimensional echocardiography. *N. Engl. J. Med.* 1981; **305**: 297–302.
49. Visser, C.A., Kan, G., Meltzer, R.S., Dunning, A.J., Roclandt, J. Embolic potential of left ventricular thrombus after myocardial infarction: a two dimensional echocardiographic study of 119 patients. *J. Am. Coll. Cardiol.* 1985; **5**: 1276–80.
50. Platt, M.R., Paskey, R.W., Willerson, J.T., Bonte, F.J., Shapiro, W., Sugg, W.L. Technetium stannous pyrophos-phate myocardial scintigrams in the recognition of myocardial infarction in patients undergoing myocardial revascularisation. *Ann. Thorac. Surg.* 1976; **21**: 311–7.

51. Sharpe, D.N., Botvinick, E.M., Shames, D.M. *et al.* The non-invasive diagnosis of right ventricular infarction. *Circulation* 1978; **59**: 483–90.
52. Wackers, F.J.T., Sokole, E.B., Samson, G., van der Schoot *et al.* Value and limitations of thallium-201 scintigraphy in the acute phase of myocardial infarction. *N. Engl. J. Med.* 1976; **295**: 1–5.
53. Filipchuk, N.G., Peshock, R.M., Malloy, C.R. *et al.* Detection and localisation of recent myocardial infarction by magnetic resonance imaging. *Am. J. Cardiol.* 1986; **58**: 214–9.
54. Pohost, G.M., Canby, R.C. Nuclear magnetic resonance imaging: current applications and future prospects. *Circulation* 1987; **75**: 88–95.
55. Been, M., Smith, M.A., Ridgeway, J.P. *et al.* Characterisation of acute myocardial infarction by gated magnetic resonance imaging. *Lancet* 1983; **2**: 348–50.
56. Swan, H.J.C., Ganz, W., Forrester, J.S. *et al.* Catheterisation of the heart in man with the use of a flow-directed balloon-tipped catheter. *N. Engl. J. Med.* 1970; **283**: 447–51.
57. Forrester, J.S., Diamond, G., Chatterjee, K., Swan, H.J.C. Medical therapy of acute myocardial infarction by application of hemodynamic subsets. *N. Engl. J. Med.* 1976; **295**: 1356–62 and 1404–13.
58. Heyndrickz, G.R., Amano, J., Kenna, T. *et al.* Creatine kinase release not associated with myocardial necrosis after short periods of coronary artery occlusion in conscious baboons. *J. Am. Coll. Cardiol.* 1985; **6**: 1299–303.
59. Rowley, J.M. and Hampton, J.R. Diagnostic criteria for myocardial infarction. *Br. J. Hosp. Med.* 1981; **26**: 253–8.
60. Wilcox, R.G., Roland, J.M., Hampton, J.R. Prognosis of patients with 'chest pain ?cause'. *Br. Med. J.* 1981; **282**: 431–3.
61. Norris, R.M. *Myocardial infarction*. Edinburgh: Churchill Livingstone, 1982.
62. Julian, D.G., Valentine, P.A., Miller, G.G. Disturbances of rate rhythm and conduction in acute myocardial infarction. *Am. J. Med.* 1964; **37**: 915–27.
63. Meltzer, L.E. and Kitchell, J.B. The incidence of arrhythmias associated with acute myocardial infarction. *Prog. Cardiovasc. Dis.* 1966; **9**: 50–63.
64. Adgey, A.A.J., Alley, J.D., Geddes, J.S., James, R.G.G., Webb, S.W., Zaidi, S.A. Acute phase of myocardial infarction. *Lancet* 1971; **2**: 501–4.
65. Grauer, L.E., Gershen, B.J., Orlando, M.M., Epstein, S.E., Bradycardia and its complications in the pre-hospital phase of acute myocardial infarction. *Am. J. Cardiol.* 1973; **32**: 607–11.
66. Zipes, D.P. The clinical significance of bradycardic rhythms in acute myocardial infarction. *Am. J. Cardiol.* 1969; **24**: 814–25.
67. Hod, H., Lew, A.S., Keltai, M. *et al.* Early atrial fibrillation during evolving myocardial infarction: a consequence of impaired left atrial perfusion. *Circulation* 1987; **75**: 146–50.
68. Sugiura, T., Iwasaka, T., Ogawa, A. *et al.* Atrial fibrillation in acute myocardial infarction. *Am. J. Cardiol.* 1985; **56**: 27–9.
69. Adgey, A.A.J., Devlin, J.E., Webb, S.W., Mulholland, H.C. Initiation of ventricular fibrillation outside hospital in patients with acute ischaemic heart disease. *Br. Heart J.* 1982; **47**: 55–61.
70. El-Sherif, N., Myerburg, R.J., Scherlag, B.J. *et al.* Electrocardiographic antecedents of primary ventricular fibrillation. Value of the R-on-T phenomenon in myocardial infarction. *Br. Heart J.* 1976; **38**: 415–22.

71. Moss, A.J., De Camilla, J.J., Davis, H.P., Bayer, L. Clinical significance of ventricular ectopic beats in the early post-hospital phase of myocardial infarction. *Am. J. Cardiol.* 1977; **39**: 635–40.

72. Bigger, J.T. jr, Weld, F.M., Rolnitzky, L.M. Prevalence, characteristics and significance of ventricular tachycardia (three or more complexes) detected with ambulatory electrocardiography recording in the late hospital phase of acute myocardial infarction. *Am. J. Cardiol.* 1981; **48**: 815–23.

73. Lie, K.I., Lien, K.L., Durrer, D. Management in hospital of ventricular fibrillation complicating acute myocardial infarction. *Br. Heart J.* 1978; **40** (suppl.): 78–82.

74. Sutton, R. and Davies, M. The conduction system in acute myocardial infarction complicated by heart block. *Circulation* 1968; **38**: 987–92.

75. Rizzon, P., Rossi, L., Baissus, C., Demoulin, J.C., Di Biase, M. Left posterior hemiblock in acute myocardial infarction. *Br. Heart J.* 1975; **37**: 711–20.

76. Buyukozturk, K., Korkut, F., Meric, M., Deligonul, U., Ozkan, E., Oxcan, R. Prognostic significance of isolated left anterior hemiblock and left axis deviation in the course of acute myocardial infarction. *Br. Heart J.* 1977; **39**: 1192–5.

77. Becker, A.E., Lie, K.I., Anderson, R.H. Bundle branch block in the setting of acute anteroseptal myocardial infarction. Clinicopathological correlation. *Br. Heart J.* 1978; **40**: 773–82.

78. Wackers, F.J., Lie, K.I., Becker, A.E., Durro, D., Wellens, H.J.J. Coronary artery disease in patients dying from cardiogenic shock or congestive heart failure in the setting of acute myocardial infarction. *Br. Heart J.* 1976; **38**: 906–10.

79. Rackley, C.E., Russell, R.O. jr, Mantle, J.A., Moraski, R.E. Cardiogenic shock: Recognition and management. *Cardiovasc. Clinc.* 1975; **7**: 251.

80. Abrams, D.L., Edelist, A., Luria, M.H., Meller, A.J. Ventricular aneurysm: A reappraisal based on a study of 65 autopsied cases. *Circulation* 1963; **27**: 164–9.

81. Ormerod, O.J.M., Barber, R.W., Stone, D.L., Taylor, N.C., Wraight, E.P., Petch, M.C. Improved selection of patients for aneurysmectomy by combined phase and amplitude analysis of gated cardiac scintigraphy. *Eur. Heart J.* 1985; **6**: 921–9.

82. Meizlish, J.L., Berger, H.J., Plankey, M., Errico, D., Levy, W., Zaret, B.L. Functional left ventricular aneurysm formation after acute anterior transmural myocardial infarction. Incidence, natural history and prognostic implications. *N. Engl. J. Med.* 1984; **311**: 1001–6.

83. Vroom, R.J.A.F. Myocardial rupture after acute myocardial infarction [letter]. *Br. Heart J.* 1984; **51**: 98.

84. Bates, R.J., Beutler, S., Resnekov, L., Anagnostopoulos, C.E. Cardiac rupture—challenge in diagnosis and management. *Am. J. Cardiol.* 1977; **40**: 429–37.

85. Braunwald, E. *Heart disease*. Philadelphia: W.B. Saunders, 1984.

86. Vlodavv, Z. and Edwards, J.E. Rupture of ventricular septum or papillary muscle complicating myocardial infarction. *Circulation* 1977; **55**: 815–22.

87. Fleming, H.A. Ventricular septal defect and mitral regurgitation secondary to myocardial infarction. A case treated medically with long survival. *Br. Heart J.* 1973; **35**: 344–6.

88. Nishinmura, R.A., Schaff, M.V., Shub, C., Gersh, B.J., Edwards, W.D., Tajik, A.J. Papillary muscle rupture complicating acute myocardial infarction: analysis of 17 patients. *Am. J. Cardiol.* 1983; **51**: 373–7.

89. Wei, J.Y., Hutchins, G.M., Buckley, B.H. Papillary muscle rupture in fatal acute myocardial infarction. *Ann. Intern. Med.* 1979; **90**: 149–53.

90. Smitherman, T.C., Milam, M., Woo, J., Willerson, J.T., Frenkel, E.P. Elevated beta thromboglobulin in peripheral venous blood of patients with acute myocardial ischaemia: direct evidence for enhanced platelet reactivity in vivo. *Am. J. Cardiol.* 1981; **48**: 395–402.

91. Murray, T.S., Lorimer, A.R., Cox, F.C., Laurie, T.D.V. Leg-vein thrombosis following myocardial infarction. *Lancet* 1970; **2**: 792–3.

92. Maurer, B.J., Wray, R., Shillingford, J.P. Frequency of venous thrombosis after myocardial infarction. *Lancet* 1971; **2**: 1385–7.

93. Kakkar, V.V. Venous thrombosis after myocardial infarction [letter]. *Lancet* 1972; **1**: 258–9.

94. Hilder, T., Ivesen, K., Raaschou, F., Schwartz, M. Anticoagulants in acute myocardial infarction. *Lancet* 1961; **2**: 237–30.

95. Eppinger, E.C., Kennedy, J.A. The cause of death in coronary thrombosis, with special reference to pulmonary embolism. *Am. J. Med. Sci.* 1938; **195**: 104–6.

96. Hellerstein, H.K., Martin, J.W. Incidence of thromboembolic lesions accompanying myocardial infarction. *Am. Heart J.* 1947; **33**: 443–52.

97. Norris, R.M., Samuel, N.L. Predictors of late hospital death in acute myocardial infarction. *Prog. Cardiovasc. Dis.* 1980; **23**: 129–40.

98. Davies, M.J., Woolf, N., Robertson, W.B. Pathology of acute myocardial infarction with particular reference to occlusive coronary thrombi. *Br. Heart J.* 1976; 659–64.

99. Thompson, P.L., Robinson, J.S. Stroke after myocardial infarction: relation to infarct size. *Br. Med. J.* 1978; **2**: 457–9.

100. Wright, I.S., Marple, C.D., Beck, D.F. Anticoagulant therapy of coronary thrombosis with myocardial infarction. *J. Am. Med. Assoc.* 1948; **138**: 1074–9.

101. Lein, K.L., Lie, K.I., Durrer, D., Wellens, H.J.J. Pericarditis in acute myocardial infarction. *Lancet* 1975; **2**: 1004–6.

102. Dressler, W. The post-myocardial infarction syndrome: a report of forty four cases. *Arch. Intern. Med.* 1959; **103**: 28–42.

103. Welin, L., Vedin, A., Wilhelmsson, C. Characteristics, prevalence and prognosis of postmyocardial infarction syndrome. *Br. Heart J.* 1983; **50**: 140–5.

104. Lichstein, E., Arsura, E., Hollander, G., Greengart, A., Sanders, M. Current incidence of postmyocardial infarction (Dressler's) syndrome. *Am. J. Cardiol.* 1982; **50**: 1269–71.

105. Van der Geld, H. Anti-heart antibodies in the postpericardiectomy and the postmyocardial infarction syndromes. *Lancet* 1964; **2**: 617–21.

106. Lessof, M. Immunological reactions in heart disease. *Br. Heart J.* 1978; **40**: 211–4.

107. Williams, R.K.T., Nagle, R.E., Thompson, R.A. Postcoronary pain and the postmyocardial infarction syndrome. *Br. Heart J.* 1984; **51**: 327–9.

108. McDonagh, A.J.G., Dawson, J. Guillain–Barré syndrome after myocardial infarction. *Br. Med. J.* 1987; **294**: 613–4.

109. Reid, P.R., Taylor, D.R., Kelly, D.T. *et al.* Myocardial infarct extension detected by precordial ST segment mapping. *N. Engl. J. Med.* 1974; **290**: 123–8.

110. Mathey, D., Bleifeld, W., Buss, H., Hanrath, P. Creatine kinase release in acute myocardial infarction: correlation with clinical, electrocardiographic, and pathological findings. *Br. Heart J.* 1975; **37**: 1161–8.

111. Kottinen, A., Somer, H. Specificity of serum creatine kinase isoenzymes in diagnosis of acute myocardial infarction. *Br. Med. J.* 1973; **1**: 386–9.

112. Marmor, A., Sobel, B., Roberts, R. Factors presaging early recurrent myocardial infarction ('extension'). *Am. J. Cardiol.* 1981; **48**: 603–10.

113. Hutchins, G.M., Bulkley, B.H. Infarct expansion versus

extension: two different complications of acute myocardial infarction. *Am. J. Cardiol.* 1978; **41**: 1127–32.

114. Alonso, D.R., Scheidt, S., Post, M., Killip, T. Pathophysiology of cardiogénic shock quantification of myocardial necrosis, clinical, pathological and electrocardiographic correlation. *Circulation* 1973; **48**: 588–96.

115. Peel, A.A.F., Semple, T., Wang, I., Lancaster, W.M., Dall, J.L.G. A coronary prognostic index for grading the severity of infarction. *Br. Heart J.* 1962; **24**: 745–60.

116. Killip, T. and Kimball, J.T. Treatment of myocardial infarction in a coronary care unit. A two year experience with 250 patients. *Am. J. Cardiol.* 1967; **20**: 457–64.

117. Norris, R.M., Brandt, P.W.T., Caughey, D.E., Lee, A.J., Scott, P.J. A new coronary prognostic index. *Lancet* 1969; **1**: 274–8.

118. Hutter, A.M., DeSactis, R.W., Flynn, T., Yeatman, L.A. Nontransmural myocardial infarction: A comparison of hospital and late clinical course of patients with that of matched patients with transmural anterior and transmural inferior myocardial infarction. *Am. J. Cardiol.* 1981; **48**: 595–602.

119. Marmor, A., Geltman, E.M., Schechtman, K., Sobel, B.E., Roberts, R. Recurrent myocardial infarction: clinical predictors and prognostic implications. *Circulation* 1982; **66**: 415–21.

120. Maroko, P.R., Libby, P., Covell, J.W., Sobel, B.E., Ross, J. Braunwald, E. Praecordial S–T segment elevation mapping: an atraumatic method for assessing alterations in the extent of myocardial ischaemic injury. *Am. J. Cardiol.* 1972; **29**: 223–30.

121. Norris, R.M., Barratt-Boyes, C., Herg, M.K., Singh, B.N. Failure of S–T segment elevation to predict severity of acute myocardial infarction. *Br. Heart J.* 1976; **38**: 85–92.

122. Selwyn, A.P., Ogunro, E.A., Shillingford, J.P. Natural history and evaluation of S–T segment change and MB CK release in acute myocardial infarction. *Br. Heart J.* 1977; **39**: 988–94.

123. Selwyn, A.P., Ogunro, E., Shillingford, J.P., Loss of electrically active myocardium during anterior infarction in man. *Br. Heart J.* 1977; **39**: 1186–91.

124. Shell, W.E., Kjekshus, J.K., Sobel, B.E. Quantitative assessment of the extent of myocardial infarction in the conscious dog by means of analysis of serial changes in serum creatine phosphokinase activity. *J. Clin. Invest.* 1971; **50**: 2614–25.

125. Sobel, B.E., Bresnahan, G.R., Shell, W.E., Yoder, R.D. Estimation of infarct size in man and its relation to prognosis. *Circulation* 1972; **46**: 640–8.

126. Fiolet, J.W.T., Ter Welle, H.F., van Capelle, F.J.L., Lie, K.I. Infarct size estimation from serial CK MB determinations: peak activity and predictability. *Br. Heart J.* 1983; **49**: 373–80.

127. Hindman, N., Grande, P., Harrell, F.E. *et al.* Relation between electrocardiographic and enzymatic methods of estimating acute myocardial infarct size. *Am. J. Cardiol.* 1986; **58**: 31–5.

128. Holman, B.L., Chisholm, R.J., Braunwald, E. The prognostic implications of acute myocardial infarct scintigraphy with 99m Tc-pyrophosphate. *Circulation* 1978; **57**: 320–6.

129. Silverman, K.J., Becker, L.C., Balkley, B.H. *et al.* Value of early thallium-201 scintigraphy for predicting mortality in patients with acute myocardial infarction. *Circulation* 1980; **61**: 996–1003.

130. Sanford, C.F., Corbett, J., Nicol, P. Value of radionuclide ventriculography in the immediate characterisation of patients with acute myocardial infarction. *Am. J. Cardiol.* 1982; **49**: 637–44.

131. Kannel, W.B., Sorlie, P., McNamara, P.M. Prognosis after initial myocardial infarction: The Framingham study. *Am.*

J. Cardiol. 1979; **44**: 53–9.

132. Kitchin, A.H., Pocock, S.J. Prognosis of patients with acute myocardial infarction admitted to a coronary care unit. 11 survived after hospital discharge. *Br. Heart J.* 1977; **39**: 1167–71.

133. Norris, R.M., Caughey, D.E., Mercer, C.J., Scott, P.J. Prognosis after myocardial infarction. Six year follow up. *Br. Heart J.* 1974; **36**: 786–90.

134. Sanz, G., Castaner, A., Betriu, A. *et al.* Determinants of prognosis in survivors of myocardial infarction. A prospective clinical angiographic study. *N. Engl. J. Med.* 1982; **306**: 1065–1070.

135. The Multicenter Postinfarction Research Group. Risk stratification and survival after myocardial infarction. *N. Engl. J. Med.* 1983; **309**: 331–6.

136. Dewhurst, N.G., Muir, A.L. Comparative prognostic value of radionuclide ventriculography at rest and during exercise in 100 patients after first myocardial infarction. *Br. Heart J.* 1983; **49**: 111–21.

137. Fioretti, P., Browis, R.W., Simmons, M.L. *et al.* Prediction of mortality in hospital survivors of myocardial infarction. Comparison of predischarge exercise testing and radionuclide ventriculography at rest. *Br. Heart J.* 1984; **52**: 292–8.

138. Proudfoot, W.L., Bruschke, A.V., Somes, F.M. jr. Natural history of obstructive coronary artery disease: ten year study of 601 non-surgical cases. *Prog. Cardiovasc. Dis.* 1978; **21**: 53–78.

139. Theroux, P., Waters, D.D., Halphen, C., Debaisjeux, J.C., Mizgala, H.F. Prognostic value of exercise testing soon after myocardial infarction. *N. Engl. J. Med.* 1979; **301**: 341–5.

140. Waters, D.D., Bosch, X., Bouchard, A., *et al.* Comparison of clinical variables and variables derived from a limited predischarge exercise test as predictors of early and late mortality after myocardial infarction. *J. Am. Coll. Cardiol.* 1985; **5**: 1–8.

141. Leppo, J.A., O'Brien, J., Rothendler, J.A., Getchell, J.D., Lee, V.W. Dipyridamole – thallium-201 scintigraphy in the prediction of future cardiac events after myocardial infarction. *N. Engl. J. Med.* 1984; **310**: 1014–18.

142. Handler, C.E. Exercise testing early after myocardial infarction: discussion paper. *J. Roy. Soc. Med.* 1983; **76**: 569–73.

143. Williams, W.L., Nair, R.C., Higginson, L.A.J., Baird, M.G., Allan, K., Beanlands, D.S. Comparison of clinical and treadmill variables for the prediction of outcome after myocardial infarction. *J. Am. Coll. Cardiol.* 1984; **4**: 477–86.

144. Cobbe, S.M. Electrophysiological testing after acute myocardial infarction. *Br. Med. J.* 1986; **292**: 1290–1.

145. Fioretti, P., Browis, R.W., Simmons, M.L. *et al.* Relative value of clinical variables, bicycle ergometry, rest radionuclide ventriculography and 24 hour ambulatory electrocardiographic monitoring at discharge to predict 1 year survival after myocardial infarction. *J. Am. Coll. Cardiol.* 1986; **8**: 40–9.

146. Partridge, F. Flying squad services; in acute myocardial infarction. Julian D.G., Oliver, M.F. (eds). Edinburgh: Livingstone, 1968.

147. Briggs, R.S., Brown, P.M., Crabb, M.E. *et al.* The Brighton resuscitation ambulances: a continuing experiment in prehospital care by ambulance staff. *Br. Med. J.* 1976; **2**: 1161–5.

148. Pai, G.R., Haites, N.E., Rawles, J.M. One thousand heart attacks in Grampian: the place of cardiopulmonary resuscitation in general practice. *Br. Med. J.* 1987; **294**: 352–4.

149. Hampton, J.R. Importance of patient selection in evaluating a cardiac ambulance service. *Br. Med. J.* 1976; **1**: 201–3.

150. Julian, D.G. Treatment of cardiac arrest in acute myocardial ischaemia and infarction. *Lancet* 1961; **2**: 840–4.

151. Mather, H.G., Pearson, N.G., Read, K.L.Q. *et al.* Acute myocardial infarction: home and hospital treatment. *Br. Med. J.* 1971; **2**: 334–8.

152. Hill, J.D., Hampton, J.R., Mitchell, J.R.A. A randomised trial of home versus hospital management for patients with suspected myocardial infarction. *Lancet* 1978; **1**: 837–41.

153. Rawles, J.M., Kenmure, A.C.F. The coronary care controversy. *Br. Med. J.* 1980; **281**: 783–6.

154. De Oliveira, J.M., Carballo, R., Zimmerman, H.A. Intravenous injection of hyaluronidase in acute myocardial infarction; preliminary report of clinical and experimental observations. *Am. Heart J.* 1959; **57**: 712–22.

155. Saltissi, S., Robinson, P.S., Coltart, D.J., Webb-Peploe, M.M., Croft, D.N. Effects of early administration of a highly purified hayluronidase preparation (GL enzyme) on myocardial infarct size. *Lancet* 1982; **1**: 867–70.

156. MILIS study group. Hyaluronidase therapy for acute myocardial infarction: results of a randomised, blinded, multicenter trial. *Am. J. Cardiol.* 1986; **57**: 1236–43.

157. Brachfeld, N. Maintenance of cell viability. *Circulation* 1969; **40** (suppl 4): 202–15.

158. Morrison, J., Reduto, L., Pizzarello, R., Geller, K., Maley, T., Gulotta, S. Modification of myocardial injury in man by corticosteroid administration. *Circulation* 1976; **53** (suppl 1): 200–3.

159. Heng, M.K., Norris, R.M., Singh, B.N., Barratt-Boyes, C. Effects of glucose and glucose–insulin–potassium on haemodynamics and enzyme release after acute myocardial infarction. *Br. Heart J.* 1977; **39**: 748–57.

160. Amsterdam, E.A., Banas, J., Criley, J.M. *et al.* Clinical assessment of external pressure circulatory arrest in acute myocardial infarction. Report of a co-operative clinical trial. *Am. J. Cardiol.* 1980; **45**: 3490–56.

161. Peter, T., Norris, R.M., Clarke, E.D. Reduction of enzyme levels by propranolol after acute myocardial infarction. *Circulation* 1978; **57**: 1091–5.

162. Norris, R.M., Sammel, N.L., Clarke, E.D., Brandt, P.W.T. Treatment of acute myocardial infarction with propranolol. Further studies on enzyme appearance and subsequent left ventricular function in treated and control patients with developing infarcts. *Br. Heart J.* 1980; **43**: 617–22.

163. The International Collaborative Study Group. Reduction of infarct size with early use of timolol in acute myocardial infarction. *N. Engl. J. Med.* 1984; **310**: 9–15.

164. Yusuf, S., Ramsdale, D., Peto, R. *et al.* Early intravenous atenolol treatment in suspected acute myocardial infarction, preliminary report of a randomised trial. *Lancet* 1980; **2**: 273–6.

165. Kjalmusson, A., Herlitz, J., Holmberg, S. *et al.* The Goteborg metoprolol trial. Effects on mortality and morbidity in acute myocardial infarction. *Circulation* 1983; **67** (suppl 1): 26–32.

166. Roberts, R., Croft, C., Gold, H. Effects of propranolol on myocardial infarct size in a randomized blinded multicenter trial. *N. Engl. J. Med.* 1984; **311**: 218–25.

167. Bassman, W.D., Passek, D., Seidel, W., Kaltenbach, M. Reduction of CK and CK–MB indices of infarct size by intravenous nitroglycerin. *Circulation* 1981; **63**: 615–22.

168. Becker, L.C., Balkley, B.J., Pitt, B. Enhanced reduction of thallium-201 defects in acute myocardial infarction by nitroglycerin treatment. Initial results of a prospective randomised trial. *Clin. Res.* 1978; **26**: 219A.

169. Durrer, J.D., Lie, K.I., van Capelle, F.J.L., Durrer, D. Effect of sodium nitroprusside on mortality in acute myocardial infarction. *N. Engl. J. Med.* 1982; **306**: 1121–8.

170. Cohn, J.N., Franciosa, J.A., Francis, G.S. *et al.* Effect of short-term infusion of sodium nitroprusside on mortality rate in acute myocardial infarction complicated by left ventricular failure. *N. Engl. J. Med.* 1982; **306**: 1129–35.

171. Phillips, S.J., Kongtahworn, C., Zeff, R.H. *et al.* Emergency coronary artery revascularisation: a possible therapy for acute myocardial infarction. *Circulation* 1979; **60**: 241–6.

172. McIntosh, H.D., Buccino, R.A. Editorial. Emergency coronary artery revascularisation of patients with acute myocardial infarction. You can ... but should you? *Circulation* 1979; **60**: 247–50.

173. Rentrop, R.K., De Vivie, E.R., Karsch, K., Kreuzer, H. Acute coronary occlusion with impending infarction as an angiographic complication relieved by a guidewire recanalization. *Clin. Cardiol.* 1978; **1**: 101–7.

174. Rentrop, P., Blanke, H., Karsch, K.R., Kaiser, H., Kostering, H., Leitz, K. Selective intracoronary thrombolysis in acute myocardial infarction and unstable angina pectoris. *Circulation* 1981; **63**: 307–17.

175. Reduto, L.A., Smalling, R.W., Freund, G.C., Gould, K.L. Intracoronary infusion of streptokinase in patients with acute myocardial infarction: effects of reperfusion on left ventricular performance. *Am. J. Cardiol.* 1981; **63**: 403–11.

176. Mathey, D.G., Kuck, K.H., Tilsner, V., Krebber, H.J., Bleifeld, W. Non-surgical coronary artery recanalisation in acute transmural myocardial infarction. *Circulation* 1981; **63**: 489–97.

177. Markis, J.E., Malagold, M., Parkes, J.A. *et al.* Myocardial salvage after intracoronary thrombolysis with streptokinase in acute myocardial infarction. Assessment by intracoronary thallium-201. *N. Engl. J. Med.* 1981; **305**: 777–82.

178. Khaja, F., Walton, J.A., Brymer, J.F. *et al.* Intracoronary fibrinolytic therapy in acute myocardial infarction. *N. Engl. J. Med.* 1983; **308**: 1305–11.

179. Anderson, J.L., Marshall, H.W., Bray, B.E. *et al.* A randomized trial of intracoronary streptokinase in the treatment of acute myocardial infarction. *N. Engl. J. Med.* 1983; **308**: 1312–8.

180. Kennedy, J.W., Ritchie, J.L., Davis, K.B., Fritz, J.K. Western Washington randomized trial of intracoronary streptokinase in acute myocardial infarction. *N. Engl. J. Med.* 1983; **309**: 1477–82.

181. Simoons, M.L., van der Brand, M., de Zwann, C. *et al.* Improved survival after early thrombolysis in acute myocardial infarction. *Lancet* 1985; **2**: 578–81.

182. Res, J.C.J., Simoons, M.L., van der Wall, E.E. *et al.* Long term improvement in global left ventricular function after early thrombolytic treatment in acute myocardial infarction: report of a randomised multicentre trial of intracoronary streptokinase in acute myocardial infarction. *Br. Heart J.* 1986; **56**: 414–21.

183. European Working Party. Streptokinase in recent myocardial infarction: controlled multicentre trial. *Br. Med. J.* 1971; **3**: 325–31.

184. Schroder, R., Biamino, G., von Leitner, E.R. *et al.* Intravenous short-term infusion of streptokinase in acute myocardial infarction. *Circulation* 1983; **67**: 536–48.

185. The TIMI Study Group. The thrombolysis in myocardial infarction (TIMI) trial: Phase I findings. *N. Engl. J. Med.* 1985; **312**: 932–6.

186. Spann, J.F., Sherry, S., Carabello, B.A. *et al.* Coronary thrombolysis by intravenous streptokinase in acute myocardial infarction: Acute and follow-up studies. *Am. J. Cardiol.* 1984; **53**: 655–661.

187. GISSI. Effectiveness of intravenous thrombolytic treatment in acute myocardial infarction. *Lancet* 1986; **1**: 397–402.

188. GISSI. Long-term effects of intravenous thrombolysis in acute myocardial infarction: Final report of the GISSI study. *Lancet* 1987; **2**: 871–4.

189. The ISAM Study Group. A prospective trial of intravenous streptokinase in acute myocardial infarction (ISAM).

Mortality, morbidity, and infarct size at 21 days. *N. Engl. J. Med.* 1986; **314**: 1465–70.

190. White, H.D., Norris, R.M., Brown, M.A. *et al.* Effect of intravenous streptokinase on left ventricular function and early survival after acute myocardial infarction. *N. Engl. J. Med.* 1987; **317**: 850–5.

191. ISIS-2 Collaborative Group. Randomised trial of intravenous streptokinase, oral aspirin, both, or neither among 17,187 cases of suspected myocardial infarction: ISIS-2. *Lancet* 1988; **2**: 349–60.

192. Van de Werf, F., Bergmann, S.R., Fox, K.A.A. *et al.* Coronary thrombolysis with intravenously administered human tissue-type plasminogen activator produced by recombinant DNA technology. *Circulation* 1984; **69**: 605–10.

193. Verstraete, M., Bleifeld, W., Brower, R.W. *et al.* Double-blind randomised trial of intravenous tissue-type plasminogen activator versus placebo in acute myocardial infarction. *Lancet* 1985; **2**: 965–9.

194. Collen, D., Topol, E.J., Tievenbrunn, A.J. *et al.* Coronary thrombolysis with recombinant human tissue-type plasminogen activator: a prospective randomised, placebo-controlled trial. *Circulation* 1984; **70**: 1612–17.

195. Verstraete, M., Bernard, R., Bury, M. Randomised trial of intravenous recombinant tissue-type plasminogen activator versus intravenous streptokinase in acute myocardial infarction. *Lancet* 1985; **1**: 842–47.

196. Rao, A.K., Pratt, C., Berke, A. *et al.* Thrombolysis in myocardial infarction trial: Phase I: Hemorrhagic manifestations and changes in plasma fibrinogen and fibrinolytic system in patients treated with recombinant tissue plasminogen activator and streptokinase. *J. Am. Coll. Cardiol.* 1988; **11**: 1–11.

197. Wilcox, R.G., Olsson, C.G., Skene, A.M., von der Lippe, G., Jensen, G., Hampton, J.R. Trial of tissue plasminogen activator for mortality reduction in acute myocardial infarction. *Lancet* 1988; **2**: 527–30.

198. Van de Werf, F. and Arnold, A.E.R. Intravenous tissue plasminogen activator and size of infarct, left ventricular function and survival in acute myocardial infarction. *Br. Med. J.* 1988; **297**: 1374–8.

199. Ikram, S., Lewis, S., Bucknall, C. *et al.* Treatment of acute myocardial infarction with anisoylated plasminogen streptokinase activator complex. *Br. Med. J.* 1986; **293**: 786–9.

200. Anderson, J.L. Development and evaluation of anisolyated plasminogen streptokinase activator complex (APSAC) as a second generation thrombolytic agent. *J. Am. Coll. Cardiol.* 1987; **10B**: 22–7.

201. AIMS Trial Study Group. Effect of intravenous APSAC on mortality after acute myocardial infarction: preliminary report of a placebo-controlled clinical trial. *Lancet* 1988; **2**: 545–9.

202. Melin, J.A., de Coster, P.M., Renkin, J., Detry, J.M.R., Beckers, C., Col, J. Effect of intracoronary thrombolytic therapy on exercise-induced ischaemia after myocardial infarction. *Am. J. Cardiol.* 1985; **56**: 705–11.

203. Satter, L.F., Pallas, R.S., Bond, O.B. *et al.* Assessment of residual coronary arterial stenosis after thrombolytic therapy during acute myocardial infarction. *Am. J. Cardiol.* 1987; **59**: 1231–3.

204. O'Neill, W., Timmis, G., Bourdillon, P. *et al.* A prognostic randomised clinical trial of intracoronary streptokinase versus coronary angioplasty therapy of acute myocardial infarction. *N. Engl. J. Med.* 1986; **314**: 812–28.

205. Topol, E.J., Califf, R.M., George, B.S. *et al.* A randomised trial of immediate versus delayed elective angioplasty after intravenous tissue plasminogen activator in acute myocardial infarction. *N. Engl. J. Med.* 1987; **317**: 582–9.

206. Simoons, M.L., Arnold, A.E.R., Betriu, A. Thrombolysis with tissue plasminogen activator in acute myocardial

infarction: no additional benefit from immediate percutaneous coronary angioplasty. *Lancet* 1988; **1**: 197–202.

207. Convertimo, V., Hung, J., Goldwater, D., DeBusk, R.F. Cardiovascular responses to exercise in middle-aged men after 10 days of bedrest. *Circulation* 1982; **65**: 134–30.

208. Asher, R. The dangers of going to bed. *Br. Med. J.* 1947; **2**: 967–8.

209. Evans, D.W. Early ambulation after myocardial infarction. *J. Roy. Coll. Phys. (London)* 1983; **17**: 217–9.

210. Tucker, H.H., Carson, P.H.M., Bass, N.M., Sharratt, G.P., Stock, J.P.P. Results of early mobilization and discharge after myocardial infarction. *Br. Med. J.* 1973; **1**: 10–13.

211. Lamers, H.J., Drost, W.S.J., Kroon, B.J.M., van Es, L.A., Meilink-Hoedemaker, L.J. Early mobilisation after myocardial infarction: a controlled study. *Br. Med. J.* 1973; **2**: 257–9.

212. Hayes, M.J., Morris, G.K., Hampton, J.R. Comparison of mobilisation after two and nine days in uncomplicated myocardial infarction. *Br. Med. J.* 1974; **2**: 10–13.

213. West, R.R., Henderson, A.H. Randomised multicentre trial of early mobilisation after uncomplicated myocardial infarction. *Br. Heart J.* 1979; **42**: 381–5.

214. Editorial. Oxygen in myocardial infarction. *Br. Med. J.* 1976; **1**: 731–2.

215. Chalmers, T.C., Matta, R.J., Smith, H., Kunzler, A.M. Evidence favoring the use of anticoagulants in the hospital phase of acute myocardial infarction. *N. Engl. J. Med.* 1977; **297**: 1091–6.

216. Medical Research Council Working Party. Assessment of short-term anticoagulant administration after myocardial infarction. *Br. Med. J.* 1969; **1**: 335–42.

217. Wray, R., Maurer, B., Shillingford, J. Prophylactic anticoagulant therapy in prevention of calf-view thrombosis after myocardial infarction. *N. Engl. J. Med.* 1973; **288**: 815–7.

218. Petch, M.C. Editorial. Aspirin for unstable angina. *Br. Med. J.* 1986; **293**: 1–2.

219. Rossi, P.R.F., Yusuf, S., Ramsdale, D., Furze, L., Sleight, P. Reduction of ventricular arrhythmias by early intravenous atenolol in suspected acute myocardial infarction. *Br. Med. J.* 1983; **286**: 506–10.

220. Norris, R.M., Brown, M.A., Clarke, E.D. *et al.* Prevention of ventricular fibrillation during acute myocardial infarction by intravenous propranolol. *Lancet* 1984; **2**: 883–6.

221. Norris, R.M., Clarke, E.D., Sammel, N.L., Smith, W.M. Protective effect of propranolol in threatened myocardial infarction. *Lancet* 1984; **2**: 907–9.

222. Yusuf, S., Peto, R., Bennett, D. *et al.* Early intravenous atenolol treatment in suspected acute myocardial infarction. *Lancet* 1980; **2**: 273–6.

223. Wilcox, R.G., Hampton, J.R., Banks, D.C. *et al.* Trial of early nifedipine in acute myocardial infarction: the Trent Study. *Br. Med. J.* 1986; **293**: 1204–8.

224. Lie, K.I., Wellens, H.J., Van Capelle, F.J., Durrer, D. Lidocaine in the prevention of primary ventricular fibrillation. *N. Engl. J. Med.* 1974; **291**: 1324–6.

225. Jaffe, A.S. Cardiovascular Pharmacology. 1. Proceedings of the 1985 National Conference on standards and guidelines for cardiopulmonary resuscitation and emergency cardiac care. *Circulation* 1986; **74** (suppl 4): 4 70–4.

226. Mueller, H., Ayres, S.M., Gianelli, S. jr, Conklin, E.F., Mazzara, J.T., Grace, W.J. Effect of isoprotenalol, 1-norepineptsine, and intra-aortic counterpulsation on haemodynamics and myocardial metabolism in shock following acute myocardial infarction. *Circulation* 1972; **45**: 335–51.

227. Maroko, P.R., Kjekshus, J.K., Sobel, B.E. *et al.* Factors influencing infarct size following experimental coronary artery occlusions. *Circulation* 1971; **43**: 67–82.

228. Gillespie, T.A., Ambos, H.D., Sobel, B.E., Roberts, R.

Effects of dobutamine in patients with acute myocardial infarction. *Am. J. Cardiol.* 1977; **39**: 588–94.

229. Marcus, F.I. Editorial. Use of digitalis in acute myocardial infarction. *Circulation* 1980; **62**: 17–0.

230. Mueller, H., Ayres, S.M., Conklin, E.F. *et al.* The effects of intra-aortic counterpulsation on cardiac performance and metabolism in shock associated with acute myocardial infarction. *J. Clin. Invest.* 1971; **50**: 1885–1900.

231. O'Rourke, M.F., Norris, R.M., Campbell, T.J., Chang, V.P., Sammel, N.L. Randomised controlled trial of intra-aortic balloon counterpulsation in early myocardial infarction with acute heart failure. *Am. J. Cardiol.* 1981; **47**: 815–20.

232. Gold, H.K., Leinbach, R.C., Sanders, C.A., Buckley, M.J., Mundith, E.D., Austen, W.G. Intra-aortic balloon pumping for ventricular septal defect or mitral regurgitation complicating acute myocardial infarction. *Circulation* 1973; **47**: 1191–6.

233. Eisenmann, B., Barciss, P., Pacifico, A.D. *et al.* Anatomic, clinical and therapeutic features of acute cardiac rupture. *J. Thorac. Cardiovasc. Surg.* 1978; **76**: 78–82.

234. Laker, H., Rosenkrantz, E., Buckberg, G.D. Surgical treatment of cardiogenic shock after myocardial infarction. *Circulation* 1986; **74** (suppl): III 11–6.

235. Griffith, B.P., Hardesty, R.L., Kormos, R.L., *et al.* Temporary use of the Jarvik-7 total artificial heart before transplantation. *N. Engl. J. Med.* 1987; **316**: 130–4.

236. Holt, B.D., Gilpin, E.A., Henning, H. *et al.* Myocardial infarction in young patients: an analysis by age subsets. *Circulation* 1986; **74**: 712–21.

237. Bigger, J.T. jr, Heller, C.A., Wenger, T.L., Weld, F.M. Risk stratification after acute myocardial infarction. *Am. J. Cardiol.* 1978; **42**: 202–10.

238. Co-operative Study. Death rate among 759 patients in first year after myocardial infarction. *J. Am. Med. Assoc.* 1966; **197**: 906–8.

239. Medical Division, Royal Infirmary, Glasgow. Early mobilisation after uncomplicated myocardial infarction: prospective study of 538 patients. *Lancet* 1973; **2**: 346–9.

240. De Feyter, P.J., van Eenige, M.J., Dighton, D.H., Visser, F.C. Prognostic value of exercise testing, coronary angiography and left ventriculography 6–8 weeks after myocardial infarction. *Circulation* 1982; **66**: 527–36.

241. Gibson, R.S., Beller, G.A., Gheorghiade, M. The prevalence and clinical significance of residual myocardial ischaemia 2 weeks after uncomplicated non-Q wave infarction: a prospective natural history study. *Circulation* 1986; **73**: 1186–98.

242. Epstein, S., Palmeri, S.T., Patterson, R.E. Evaluation of patients after acute myocardial infarction. Indications for cardiac catheterisation and surgical intervention. *N. Engl. J. Med.* 1982; **307**: 1487–92.

243. Gibson, R.S., Crampton, R.S., Watson, D.D. *et al.* Precordial ST-segment depression during acute inferior myocardial infarction: clinical scintigraphic and angiographic correlations. *Circulation* 1982; **66**: 732–41.

244. Gelman, J.S., Saltups, A. Precordial ST segment depression in patients with inferior myocardial infarction: clinical implications. *Br. Heart J.* 1982; **48**: 560–5.

245. Odemuyiura, O., Pearl, I. Albers, C., Hall, R. Reciprocal ST depression in acute myocardial infarction. *Br. Heart J.* 1985; **54**: 479–83.

246. Moss, A.J., Davis, H.T., DeCamilla, J., Bayer, L.W. Ventricular ectopic beats and their relation to sudden and non-sudden cardiac death after myocardial infarction. *Circulation* 1979; **60**: 998–1003.

247. Schulze, R.A. jr, Strauss, H.W., Pitt, B. Sudden death in the year following myocardial infarction: relation to ventricular premature contractions in the late hospital phase and left ventricular ejection fraction. *Am. J. Med.* 1977; **62**: 192–9.

248. Mukharji, J., Rude, R.E., Poole, K.L. *et al.* Risk factors for sudden death after myocardial infarction: two year follow up. *Am. J. Cardiol.* 1984; **54**: 31–36.

249. Chadda, K., Goldstein, S., Byington, R., Curb, J.D. Effect of propranolol after acute myocardial infarction in patients with congestive heart failure. *Circulation* 1985; **73**: 503–10.

250. Friedman, L.M., Byington, R.P., Capone, R.J. *et al.* Effect of propranolol in patients with myocardial infarction and ventricular arrhythmia. *J. Am. Coll. Cardiol.* 1986; **7**: 1–8.

Chapter 51

Prognosis, Risk Stratification and Rehabilitation after Acute Myocardial Infarction

D.G. Julian

PROGNOSIS AND RISK STRATIFICATION

The chief determinants of prognosis after recovery from the acute phase of myocardial infarction appear to be age, the severity of myocardial damage sustained during the recent and previous infarctions, the severity of residual coronary artery disease and instability of ventricular rhythm. Our knowledge of prognosis, however, is largely based on information acquired many years ago, and it seems probable that long-term survival after myocardial infarction is now substantially better than it was in the 1960s and early 1970s. In the Minnesota Heart Survey[1], it was reported that 4-year survival for men was 35% better in 1980 than it was in 1970, and for women it was 27% better.

OVERALL MORTALITY

The mortality in the first year after recovery from acute infarction is about 10–15%[2–4], the most dangerous period being during the first month, when many patients experience re-infarction, ventricular fibrillation or death from cardiac failure. The mortality rate thereafter is lower, averaging about 5–10% per annum[2–4].

AGE

Age is a powerful predictor of survival, in the acute phase of infarction and subsequently. Norris and his colleagues[4] reported a mortality rate at 3 years of 14% for those patients under 50 years of age, 26% for those aged 50–59 years, 38% for those aged 60–69 years and 43% for those aged 70–79 years. Comparable mortality rates at 6 years were 26, 40, 51 and 67%.

GENDER

Overall, women have a worse long-term prognosis than men, but this can be partly or completely explained by the older age on average of women who sustain infarcts.[4]

PREVIOUS HISTORY OF ISCHAEMIC HEART DISEASE

Prognosis is substantially worse in those patients who have had chronic angina prior to infarction or who have had a previous infarction. Thus, in the series of Norris et al,[2] the mortality of patients with previous infarction was 50% at 3 years and 64% at 6 years. Comparable figures for those without previous evidence of ischaemic heart disease were 23 and 38%, and in those with preceding angina they were 31 and 49%, respectively.

COMPLICATIONS DURING THE ACUTE EVENT

Patients whose in-hospital course is complicated by cardiac failure, severe angina or ventricular tachycardia have a substantially worse subsequent prognosis than those whose course is uncomplicated. About 15–30% of all infarct patients have a complicated in-hospital course.[5] In the series of Saunamaki and Andersen,[6] patients with complicated infarction had a mortality of 20% at 1 year, and 49% at 4.5 years, whereas patients with an uncomplicated course had a mortality of 7% at 1 year and 23% at 4.5 years.

Pulmonary oedema during the acute event is particularly sinister. In Norris's series,[6] 64% of patients so affected were dead within 3 years, and 80% were dead within 6 years.

ROUTINE ELECTROCARDIOGRAM

Abnormalities on the 12-lead electrocardiogram, such as QRS score, ST-segment depression and prolongation of the QT interval, are associated with a relatively poor prognosis but their presence seems to add little to information gained from the clinical variables mentioned above.[9]

Particular interest has been focused on the so-called 'sub-endocardial' or non-Q-wave infarction. Although the in-hospital mortality of such cases is low, the longer term prognosis seems to be at least as bad as that of Q-wave (or 'transmural') infarction. Madigan et al.[8] observed an incidence of unstable angina of 46% and an incidence of Q-wave infarction of 21% after a mean follow-up of 10.6 months. Norris et al.[4] reported that the 6-year mortality was the same in survivors of 'transmural' and of 'sub-endocardial' infarctions.

LEFT VENTRICULAR DYSFUNCTION

Cardiac enlargement, as shown radiologically, is an indicator of poor prognosis; mortality is about twice as great in patients who have this feature as it is in those who do not. Probably the best single indicator of survival is the left ventricular ejection fraction, which can be measured by left ventriculography at cardiac catheterization or by radionuclide angiography. As shown particularly clearly by the Multicenter Postinfarction Research Group,[9] 1-year mortality rises steeply as ejection fraction falls below 40%; an ejection fraction < 30% is associated with a fivefold risk of death. However, Fioretti et al.[10] have suggested that resting radionuclide ventriculography adds little to the information that can be obtained from clinical features and exercise electrocardiography, and it should be limited to patients not eligible for exercise testing.

ANGINA PECTORIS IN THE EARLY POST-INFARCTION PERIOD

The prognostic significance of post-infarction angina probably depends on the time at which it occurs relative to the infarction and on whether the ischaemia from which it derives is from the area of the infarction or from a more remote area, the latter being more sinister. New or progressive angina developing while the patient is still resting after the infarction carries a much worse outlook than exercise-induced pain occurring at a later stage when the patient has become more active. In the Multicenter Postinfarction Research Group report,[8] there was a 30-month mortality of 11% in those who developed angina for the first time after infarction compared with 15% in those who had not experienced angina either before or after the infarction. By contrast, those that had suffered from chronic angina prior to the infarction had a mortality of 17% if they did not have pre-discharge angina, whereas mortality was 23% if pre-discharge angina was experienced.

The significance of angina following thrombolysis has yet to be defined.

SILENT ISCHAEMIA

Transient ST-segment changes unaccompanied by angina are common in the convalescent period, but their importance as independent risk factors has yet to be established.

EXERCISE STRESS TESTS

Exercise stress can be used to detect myocardial ischaemia and left ventricular dysfunction, as revealed by the electrocardiogram, thallium scintigraphy and radionuclide angiography.

Exercise tests after infarction may be performed before discharge (usually 7–21 days after the onset of symptoms) or at a subsequent follow-up. The advantages of pre-discharge tests are that they provide evidence of risk at a critical time in the patient's convalescence, they are easier to organize and they act as a guide to the rate at which rehabilitation can proceed. Usually, they are limited in duration (e.g. 8 min) and in workload. However, some patients are not fit enough to perform a submaximal exercise test at this time; more information may be forthcoming from a maximal symptom-limited exercise test at 4–6 weeks. Patients who are not fit for pre-discharge exercise testing have a poor prognosis.[11,12]

There have been conflicting reports over the prognostic significance of ST-segment depression during the exercise test. The most striking findings have been those of Theroux et al.[13] who reported a 1-year mortality rate of 27% in 64 patients with exercise-induced ST-segment depression of 1 mm or more, compared with a rate of 2% in those without this finding. Other workers have failed to find any prognostic significance in ST-segment changes,[6,14,15] although such changes are certainly predictive of angina and the likelihood of coronary surgery or angioplasty being undertaken in the succeeding months.[16]

There have also been conflicting reports over the significance of ventricular arrhythmias on exercise testing, but Saunamaki and Andersen[6] provide good evidence of the adverse prognosis of patients who have such arrhythmias, particularly if they are combined with a poor haemodynamic response. The length of time for which a patient is able to exercise on testing and the haemodynamic response to this exercise appear to be better predictors of mortality than the occurrence of ST-segment depression. Krone et al.[16] undertook pre-discharge exercise tests in 667 patients; those in whom the systolic blood pressure did not increase above 110 mmHg had a 1-year mortality of 18% compared with 3% in those in whom it did. The 1-year mortality was 8% in those who could not complete a 9-min exercise test, but 3% in those who could.

Radionuclide exercise ventriculography can be used to identify high-risk patients who have residual ischaemia and multivessel coronary disease, because in such patients there is a tendency for the ejection fraction to fall and for wall motion abnormalities to develop in areas remote from the infarction.[17] Exercise thallium-201 scintigraphy has also been found to be of value in identifying high-risk patients after myocardial infarction. Gibson et al.[18] reported that about 50% of patients who had suffered an apparently uncomplicated myocardial infarction and who demonstrated multiple defects, delayed redistribution of thallium or abnormal lung uptake experienced cardiac death, recurrent infarction or severe angina at a mean follow-up of 15 months, compared with 6% of those who did not have these abnormalities. Dipyridamole scintigraphy may also be used to identify high-risk patients, and it is particularly valuable in those who are unable to exercise.[19]

VENTRICULAR ARRHYTHMIAS

Ventricular arrhythmias are common in the convalescent phase after myocardial infarction. Dynamic electrocardiography has demonstrated that 10–16 days after myocardial infarction about 10% of patients have ventricular tachycardia and 20–25% have 10 or more ventricular ectopic beats per hour.[20] There is a strong relationship between complex ventricular arrhythmias and subsequent death, the strongest association being with ventricular tachycardia. Complex arrhythmias are also related to the severity of left ventricular dysfunc-

tion, and it is not entirely clear to what extent the bad prognostic significance of arrhythmias is related to this association. However, in the Multicenter Postinfarction Research Group study,[9] it was found that frequent ventricular ectopic beats, repetitive ectopic beats and left ventricular ejection fraction were each independently associated with mortality. These findings have led Bigger et al.[21] to suggest that dynamic electrocardiography provides uniquely valuable data and, at present, it is not possible to select patients for monitoring on the basis of impaired left ventricular function. Other workers have questioned the necessity of obtaining such information, particularly in those who have good left ventricular function, bearing in mind the doubtful value of anti-arrhythmic therapy in this population.

INVASIVE ELECTROPHYSIOLOGY

The results of several studies have provided evidence that programmed stimulation yields valuable prognostic information (see also Chapter 11). Denniss and associates[22] reported that programmed ventricular stimulation could identify a subset of patients at high risk in whom mortality was 26% in 1 year, compared with a mortality of 6% in other patients. These workers consider that the provocation of ventricular tachycardia is a strong indicator of subsequent sudden death, but other workers have not found this to be so. It would seem that there are other less complicated methods of establishing prognosis, but programmed stimulation may be of great value in studying patients who spontaneously experience life-threatening arrhythmias and in assessing their responsiveness to treatment.

SIGNAL AVERAGING

Signal averaging (see Chapter 23) has been used to record 'late potentials' in post-infarct patients. Some workers have found them to be a sensitive marker of subsequent recurrent ventricular tachycardia and sudden death, but as they are a frequent finding in these patients they have a low specificity.

CORONARY ARTERIOGRAPHY

Coronary arteriography provides valuable information about prognosis after myocardial infarction but ejection fraction is a much more powerful determinant of prognosis than the number of vessels involved. In the study of Sanz et al.,[23] the prognosis was good in patients with three-vessel disease if the ejection fraction was normal, whereas the prognosis was poor if the ejection fraction was low, even in those with one-vessel disease.

MULTIPLE RISK FACTOR ANALYSIS

The prognosis can best be assessed in an individual by taking a number of factors into account. Much effort has gone into defining the relative importance of the various risk indicators and formulating prognostic indices based on them.[24] These are invaluable for research, but are cumbersome to use in practice. What emerges from virtually all the studies is the importance of age, previous myocardial infarction, pump failure during the acute attack, left ventricular dysfunction, recurrent ventricular tachycardia and the presence of easily provoked myocardial ischaemia.

RISK STRATIFICATION AS A BASIS FOR MANAGEMENT

It is logical to base the investigation and treatment of the patient in the convalescent period after myocardial infarction on the expected natural history, with regard to both morbidity and mortality. The patient who has had a complicated course during the acute illness should be assessed very carefully. Exercise testing may not be feasible, but left ventricular function should be studied, with particular attention being paid to the possibility of identifying a remediable abnormality, such as a ventricular aneurysm. If cardiac failure can be brought under control, consideration should be given to the use of beta-adrenergic blockers, even though these drugs may precipitate a recurrence of heart failure in a few patients.

If possible, patients who have made an apparently satisfactory recovery should be submitted to a pre-discharge exercise test, provided there are no contra-indications. Those who are unable to complete a low-level exercise test, who quickly develop ST-segment depression, or who have a severely impaired blood pressure response to exercise should be evaluated with respect to the need for further investigations, including coronary angiography. In some of these cases, coronary artery surgery or angioplasty will be indicated; in others, beta-blockers will be the most appropriate therapy.

REHABILITATION

The purpose of rehabilitation after myocardial infarction is to restore the patient to as full a life as possible. During rehabilitation, physical, psychological and social factors that may determine a patient's prognosis, and which are often interrelated,[25] must be taken into account.

EXERCISE

All patients require advice and help with regard to the return to physical activity. As discussed in Chapter 50, the timing and speed of mobilization depends upon the complications that have occurred in the acute phase. Many patients can start walking gently in 2–3 days, and can be ascending a few stairs by the end of 1 week. However, those who have been in cardiac failure or who have had serious arrhythmias may need prolonged rest. Many patients fall into an intermediate category; their rate of progress must be closely observed so that, if they develop symptoms, appropriate measures can be taken.

A group exercise programme can be initiated in hospital by a physiotherapist. If possible, a low-level exercise test should be carried out prior to hospital discharge. This has been shown to be safe if the patient is free of rest pain and cardiac failure, and provided that the electrocardiogram and blood pressure are carefully monitored throughout the test.[26,27] Patients who can complete such a test without the occurrence of pain or electrocardiographic changes and, during the test, can raise their systolic blood pressure by 15 mmHg or more may rapidly increase their physical activity. Those who cannot fulfil these criteria require careful re-evaluation, consideration for therapeutic interventions and closer attention during the process of rehabilitation.

The pre-discharge exercise test usually serves to reassure the patient and his or her relatives, because it gives them an indication of the patient's physical capabilities, as well as providing the doctor with information that is valuable in planning future management policy. Prior to returning home, each patient should be given individual advice about the amount and type of exercise that can be undertaken and the rate at which this can be increased.

EXERCISE TRAINING

Although the benefits of exercise training in terms

of prognosis are disputed, an exercise training programme does accelerate the return to general fitness and, in many cases, the return to work. This benefit is probably unrelated to any direct effect on the heart, but rather due to a training effect on the periphery,[28] with increased oxygen extraction by skeletal muscle, a decrease in peripheral vascular resistance and a better distribution of the cardiac output on exercise. Exercise training leads to a feeling of well-being, and may increase the threshold at which effort induces angina. Although many patients succeed in regaining a satisfactory level of activity on their own initiative, most of them probably benefit from a formal rehabilitation programme under the supervision of trained paramedical personnel, such as occupational therapists, in association with doctors, nurses and physiotherapists. Ideally, this should start about 2 weeks after discharge, with attendance for sessions two to three times a week for 2 or 3 months. The effect of the exercise on symptoms and the cardiac rate and rhythm should be monitored; there is a small but definite risk of inducing ventricular fibrillation during or after an exercise session; resuscitatory facilities (including a defibrillator) must be immediately available.

The exercise test results should act as a guide to the amount of exercise that can be undertaken; exercise, at least during the earlier stages after infarction, should be dynamic rather than isometric.

PSYCHOSOCIAL REHABILITATION

Failure in rehabilitation after myocardial infarction is probably more often due to psychological problems than to physical disability. Mayou et al.[29,30] found that 30% of survivors of infarction had moderate to serious psychological disturbance 2 months after the event, with little improvement at 1 year.

Anxiety is a natural response to a serious illness and it is common in the initial period after a myocardial infarction. It may be aggravated by the intensive care environment, unless the medical and nursing staff provide strong and continuing reassurance. Further anxiety can occur at the time of transfer to the general ward and at hospital discharge, but it can generally be avoided by appropriate explanation and counselling. It is essential that the spouse and other close associates understand the psychological as well as physical problems that the patient encounters. Most patients lose their excessive anxiety as they return to a normal life; those that do not have often had psychological disturbances prior to the infarct. Some patients benefit from the use of tranquillizing agents, but these should be discontinued as soon as possible.

Depression may begin by about the third day in hospital, but it is more likely to become a serious problem after the patient returns home. It often presents as weakness and fatigue; these symptoms may be wrongly interpreted as manifestations of cardiac failure. Irritability and withdrawal are other common features about which those who live with the patient should be warned. Depression is a major factor in delaying return to full activity; its early recognition is important because it becomes more difficult to treat at a later stage. Explanation and reassurance may help to mitigate depression, particularly if the patient can be brought to appreciate its usually limited duration.

Denial, defined as "the conscious or unconscious repudiation of all or a portion of the total available meaning of an illness in order to allay anxiety and to minimise emotional stress", is common in the acute and in the later phases of myocardial infarction.[31] It may make it easier for patients to cope with the initial illness, but subsequently they may feel more vulnerable to anxiety and depression when the physical or social problems of convalescence have to be faced.

Help with domestic, financial and occupational problems is often required. Although much is to be gained in the convalescent period by group education and discussion, most patients need individual advice with regard to their specific problems. It does not necessarily matter which member of the team is responsible for assessment and counselling, but for each case a particular individual should be made responsible, who can ensure that other relevant personnel, such as occupational therapists, social workers or psychologists, are involved as necessary.

SEXUAL ACTIVITY

The physical component of sexual intercourse involves an expenditure of energy about equivalent to walking upstairs, but emotional factors greatly enhance this. Patients are usually fit to return to sexual activity about 6–8 weeks after infarction, but they should be counselled to avoid intercourse if angina or breathlessness are readily induced.

RETURN TO WORK

To many, return to work is the gold standard of rehabilitation, and it is certainly an important end-point for those who were previously employed. Most patients who have not suffered severe myocardial damage can go back to work in about 8 weeks if they have a light job, and in 10–12 weeks if their work is heavier. However, those whose work has involved strenuous physical activity usually cannot return to their previous position; re-employment is also difficult for certain occupations such as public service drivers, heavy goods vehicle drivers and airline pilots. In such cases, the social worker should be involved at an early stage, so that alternative forms of employment can be discussed.

In many cases, failure to return to work is due to the patient's anxiety or depression or to lack of suitable advice from the doctor. Frequently, poor communication between the hospital and general practitioner is to blame; each may wait for the other to make the decision about when the patient is fit to resume work.

Important as return to gainful employment may be, it is not necessarily the best index of successful rehabilitation.[32] Some patients, although fully recovered, may opt for early retirement. Others may be keen to go back quickly but then fail to work effectively; it is common for such individuals to leave their jobs subsequently.

DRIVING

Car driving is an important aspect of the normal life for many individuals and it can be resumed when the risks of doing so seem to be small. Most post-infarction patients can take up driving again 4–8 weeks after the event, but the length of this period must be determined by the risk of sudden death or of the provocation of symptoms in the individual concerned. It is unwise to allow the early return to driving of those with persistent serious arrhythmias, cardiac failure or angina that is easily provoked. In general, drivers of heavy goods vehicles or public service vehicles cannot return to their occupations, but professional drivers of smaller vehicles may be able to do so.

SECONDARY PREVENTION AFTER INFARCTION

Owing to the substantial risk of re-infarction and of death within the months following a myocardial infarction, much attention has been paid to the possibility of preventing these events, either by modification of the patient's lifestyle or by pharmacological means.

SMOKING

It has not been possible to conduct a randomized study of stopping smoking after infarction, but there is impressive evidence to suggest that to do so greatly improves a patient's prognosis. Mulcahy et al.[33] reported that, at 5-year follow up, 28.8% of those who continued to smoke after an acute coronary episode had died whereas only 14.6% of those who gave up died. In a long-term follow-up study in Gothenburg,[34] there was a cumulative mortality rate of 14% at 5 years and of 16% at 7.5 years in those who stopped smoking, compared with 29% and 49%, respectively, in those who continued to smoke, notwithstanding the fact that those who stopped had evidence of having sustained more severe infarcts.

HYPERTENSION

There has been no formal trial of antihypertensive treatment following myocardial infarction. Hypertension is not an important risk factor early after infarction, but it becomes so after 3 years.[4] It therefore seems logical to treat hypertension in survivors of myocardial infarction particularly to prevent the development of cardiac failure.

HYPERLIPIDAEMIA

Hyperlipidaemia is a relatively weak prognostic factor after myocardial infarction; there is little evidence of benefit from the use of lipid-lowering agents after infarction.[35] In the Coronary Drug Project,[36] nicotinic acid in a dosage of 3 g/day was associated with a reduced incidence of non-fatal myocardial infarction, but there was no difference in mortality and there was a higher incidence of arrhythmias and gastro-intestinal side-effects when compared with control subjects receiving placebo. In all the trials performed to date, however, there has been only a minor overall effect of treatment on lipids, and most of the trials have been small. As it is probable that hyperlipidaemia has a long-term adverse effect on the progression of coronary artery disease, it would seem wise to institute a lipid-lowering diet in all hyperlipidaemic survivors, not only for their own benefit but also to encourage their families, who may be at increased risk of ischaemic heart disease, to eat a healthier diet. Those whose lipid levels remain high despite dietetic measures may require hypolipidaemic drug therapy.

EXERCISE TRAINING

Exercise training is an important component of rehabilitation after myocardial infarction. Although it improves exercise tolerance, it is not clear if it reduces the risk of re-infarction and death. It has proved difficult to undertake controlled trials of exercise training because many patients do not comply with their exercise regimen; when considered in isolation, none of the trials has shown a convincing benefit. However, May et al.[35] have pointed out that if the results of several large trials are pooled, there is a survival advantage of 25–35% in subjects who exercise.

MODIFICATION OF BEHAVIOUR PATTERN

Following their observations relating type A behaviour to the development of coronary heart disease, Friedman et al.[37] have reported a lower mortality in patients counselled to modify their behaviour when compared with that of other groups of control subjects who did not receive such advice. Other workers have not been able to confirm these findings.

MULTIPLE RISK FACTOR INTERVENTION

It seems likely that a comprehensive approach to risk factor control would have more effect than the modification of only one factor. Evidence for this assertion is provided by the study of Kallio et al.[38] performed in Finland. Patients were randomised to be looked after by either their personal physicians or a special clinic, at which they received health education and took part in a formal physical education programme. The latter group had a lower mortality; in particular, the incidence of sudden deaths was reduced. A similar study conducted in Sweden, however, did not show a reduction in mortality with risk factor intervention.[39]

BETA-ADRENOCEPTOR BLOCKING DRUGS

There is now convincing evidence from a large number of trials that beta-blocking drugs started in the convalescent period after myocardial infarction reduce mortality. Although most of the individual trials were too small to demonstrate an effect, pooling of the results of all the trials does indicate a reduction in mortality of about 20–25%.[35,40] The most significant results have been obtained with timolol,[41] propranolol[42] and metoprolol.[43] In the Norwegian trial of timolol,[41] treatment was started with 5 mg b.d. 7–28 days after the onset of myocardial infarction, and increased to 10 mg b.d. if possible. The patients were followed for 12–33 months. During this period, 152 (17.5%) of the 939 patients receiving placebo died compared with 97 (10.6%) of the 945 receiving timolol ($P=0.003$). In the Beta-block Heart Attack trial[42] of propranolol (180–240 mg daily), 3837 patients were randomly allocated to receive active agent or to receive placebo for a mean of 24 months. Mortality in the control group was 9.5% compared with 7% in the treatment group ($P=0.006$). In the Gothenburg study of metoprolol,[43] treatment was started in the acute phase of myocardial infarction (median time after onset of symptoms 11 h) and continued for 3 months. The mortality was 8.6% for patients receiving placebo and 5.3% for those receiving metoprolol. The failure to achieve significance in trials of other agents (e.g. sotalol, oxprenolol and pindolol) may have been due to trial design or chance.

Some subsets of patients seem to benefit more than others; those who have experienced electrical or mechanical complications during the acute event are most likely to benefit (although they are at greater risk of adverse effects), whereas the prognosis of those who have had an uncomplicated course is not greatly affected.[44]

Opinions differ over the indications for the prophylactic (as opposed to the therapeutic) use of beta-blockers after myocardial infarction. Some cardiologists prescribe them for all patients for whom they are not contra-indicated; others reserve them for the relatively high-risk patient who has either had a complicated infarction or who shows signs of readily induced myocardial ischaemia.

It is not known for how long beta-blocker therapy should be maintained; the evidence suggests that it should be continued for at least 3 years.

CALCIUM ANTAGONISTS

The use of calcium antagonists following infarction has been studied less than that of beta-blockers; as yet, it is not possible to draw conclusions about their effectiveness in the prevention of re-infarction or death. Furthermore, as they differ markedly among themselves, findings relating to one agent may not apply to the others. The results of a trial with verapamil,[45] started in the acute phase following infarction and continued for 6 months thereafter, did not show any benefit with treatment. It has been claimed that diltiazem was successful in preventing re-infarction in patients who had non-Q wave infarcts,[46] but the design and analysis of this trial have been questioned. More recently, in the Multicenter Diltiazem Post-infarction Trial (MDPIT),[47] involving more than 3000 patients, there was no overall benefit to patients who took this drug; indeed, there was a significantly higher mortality in those receiving diltiazem who had suffered pulmonary congestion during the acute event. By contrast, those who had not had this complication appeared to benefit.

ANTICOAGULANTS

Anticoagulants have been extensively tested in post-infarction patients, but most of the studies were carried out before much experience had been gained of clinical trials in this context. Consequently, sample size was often too small or true randomization was not achieved. Furthermore, the quality of anticoagulant control was not good by current standards. In the five major trials reviewed by May et al.,[35] a total of 2327 patients were recruited; there was no significant reduction in mortality in any of the trials. The Sixty Plus Reinfarction trial[48] differed from the other trials in that it tested the discontinuation of anticoagulants in patients over the age of 60 years who had been on this therapy for at least 6 months. The incidence of re-infarction was significantly lower in those who continued anticoagulants than in those who stopped.

PLATELET-ACTIVE DRUGS

There have been several trials of aspirin and other platelet-active agents, including dipyridamole and sulphinpyrazone, after infarction. None of these trials has shown a significant reduction in mortality, but most have shown lower re-infarction rates. In the Persantine–Aspirin Reinfarction Study Part II (PARIS II),[49] there was a significant reduction in coronary events (mainly non-fatal infarction) in the group receiving the two drugs, but only a non-significant reduction in mortality. The accumulated evidence from these studies and those of unstable angina suggests that aspirin and, perhaps, the other platelet-active agents reduce the risk of myocardial infarction, but their effect on mortality is slight. The most appropriate dose of aspirin has yet to be established, but 300 mg a day or given on alternate days seems adequate and causes few adverse effects.

ANTI-ARRHYTHMIC DRUGS

Trials with phenytoin, mexiletine, tocainide and aprindine have not shown a reduction in mortality with treatment in post-infarction patients.[35] In several of these trials, the mortality in the treated group was higher, albeit insignificantly.

CLINICAL MANAGEMENT OF THE POST-INFARCTION PATIENT

ANGINA PECTORIS

Angina pectoris affects about one-third of patients in the post-infarction period; it occurs about twice as frequently in those who have had chronic angina as it does in those who were previously free of this symptom. It is particularly likely to occur in those who have had successful thrombolysis. Angina may be due to several different causes, including severe residual stenosis in the infarct-related artery, stenoses in other arteries and disorders of coronary vasomotor tone, which seem to be common in the weeks following myocardial infarction.[50]

If angina occurs only on exercise, its management depends upon its severity and response to treatment. In most cases, it is appropriate to prescribe beta-blockers and short-acting nitrates, reserving long-acting nitrates and calcium antagonists for those who require additional therapy. An exercise test either before discharge or at 1 month is valuable in assessing whether further investigation is necessary in these patients. If the test causes angina or gross ST-segment changes at a low workload, or if the haemodynamic response is poor, invasive investigation should be considered, because it is likely that the patient will be a candidate for coronary artery bypass surgery or angioplasty in the forthcoming months.

The occurrence of unstable angina during convalescence is serious, whether it is manifested as chest pain at rest or as deteriorating exertion-induced angina. If it does not respond rapidly to medical treatment, immediate coronary angiography should be undertaken with a view to possible angioplasty or surgery.

DYSPNOEA AND CARDIAC FAILURE

Many patients are slightly breathless when they first start walking after a few days' bed rest; this is often due to physical deconditioning and improves with increasing activity. Some, however, are markedly dyspnoeic once the acute event is over, and a few have the features of right-sided heart failure, with raised venous pressure, hepatomegaly and peripheral oedema. In most such cases, there has been extensive myocardial damage; the patient is often elderly, having suffered one or more previous infarctions. Before the assumption is made that there is irremediable myocardial failure, it is essential to ensure that a surgically correctable abnormality has been excluded. The most important of these is a ventricular aneurysm, but mitral regurgitation and ventricular septal rupture may also be responsible for cardiac failure at this time.

Ventricular aneurysm

A ventricular aneurysm may be defined as an area of the left ventricular wall that moves in a paradoxical (or dyskinetic) manner, being displaced outwards during systole. The wall may be entirely fibrous or it may contain a small amount of residual muscle tissue. Its presence exerts harmful effects because of the loss of contractile tissue and because the remaining myocardium wastes energy in producing the futile outward movement. Also, ventricular aneurysms are often associated with malignant ventricular tachycardia or ventricular fibrillation, although such arrhythmias tend to start in adjacent myocardium rather than in the aneurysmal tissue itself. Aneurysms nearly always contain clot, which may cause systemic embolization.

In many cases, an aneurysm is suspected on physical examination, if the paradoxical movement can be palpated or visualized on the chest wall. The abnormal motion may be seen at the apex, but it can often be detected medial to this, because aneurysms in the septal region cause a systolic movement in the left parasternal region. A posterior aneurysm may displace the right ventricle forward in the parasternal area in systole. Aneurysms seldom occur in the absence of Q- wave infarction, and a common finding is that ST-segment elevation persists after the acute phase of the infarction is over. This feature, however, is neither very sensitive nor very specific.

In a minority of affected patients, a characteristic bulge may be seen protruding beyond the cardiac border on the chest X-ray (see Fig. 12.39). Although M-mode echocardiography is not a suitable technique for the diagnosis of ventricular aneurysms, the cross-sectional method allows the visualization of aneurysms in most cases. It also provides information on mural thrombi and the state of the remaining myocardium, an important appraisal when surgery is being considered.

Probably, the best non-invasive method of diagnosis is gated blood pool imaging. With this technique, an aneurysm can usually be delineated and its size estimated; other aspects of myocardial function can also be evaluated.

Even though non-invasive techniques permit the diagnosis in most cases, cardiac catheterization is necessary to demonstrate the coronary arteries; it is customary to perform left ventriculography at the same investigation. If serious arrhythmias are a complication, an electrophysiological examination may also be undertaken.

If an aneurysm is responsible for major symptoms, surgery should be undertaken if it is feasible. If the aneurysm is a chance finding in a relatively asymptomatic patient, surgery is usually not indicated, but the patient should be kept under observation, and consideration given to instituting anticoagulant therapy.

Mitral regurgitation

Mitral regurgitation may complicate myocardial infarction, either because of necrosis of papillary muscles or because of dilatation of the annulus, as a consequence of dilatation of the ventricle. If a papillary muscle ruptures completely, mitral regurgitation is catastrophic and usually fatal. Lesser degrees of papillary muscle disruption are not uncommon in patients with chronic ischaemic heart disease, but they tend to be associated with quite severe myocardial damage. Echocardiography is valuable in defining the cause of the mitral regurgitation if mitral valve prolapse can be demonstrated. Mitral valve repair or replacement may be required but the mortality of such operations is high.

Global left ventricular dysfunction

Cardiac failure after myocardial infarction is usually due to extensive myocardial damage. In such cases, the heart is dilated, and the diffuse and feeble apex beat is displaced laterally and downwards. A third sound is common, and there may be the systolic murmur of mitral regurgitation. The electrocardiogram may show evidence of one or more previous myocardial infarctions, but sometimes exhibits only non-specific ST-segment and T-wave changes. The chest X-ray usually shows some cardiomegaly, and echocardiography and nuclear imaging confirm that the heart is diffusely enlarged and contracting poorly. The ejection fraction is commonly < 40%, and may be only 10–15%.

Surgery (other than transplantation) does not have a place in the treatment of such patients, unless life-threatening arrhythmias, or severe co-existent angina, are present. Essentially, medical treatment is similar to that for other causes of myocardial failure, diuretics being first-line drug therapy supplemented, if necessary, by digitalis and vasodilator drugs. The results of the Consensus trial[51] suggest that angiotensin converting enzyme inhibitors may be of particular value in advanced cases, improving both symptoms and prognosis.

ARRHYTHMIAS

Arrhythmias are common in the convalescent period although in most cases they are asymptomatic. Their detection and management are discussed in Chapter 23.

POST-MYOCARDIAL INFARCTION SYNDROME

The post-myocardial infarction syndrome, first described by Dressler,[52] is characterized by fever, pericarditis and pleurisy; it occurs from one week to some months after the myocardial infarction. Although it has been reported as affecting about 3% of cases, it now seems to be much rarer. Often, a patient who appears to have been making a satisfactory recovery can develop malaise, a fever and a typical pericardial or pleural pain, accompanied by corresponding rubs. The condition is self-limited, usually subsiding within 1 or 2 weeks. Its mechanism is not known; it has been attributed to an auto-immune phenomenon, activation of a viral infection or a reaction to previous haemorrhagic effusion. It may be confused with a recurrent myocardial infarction or pulmonary infarction. The electrocardiogram (which may reveal the ST-segment elevation of pericarditis), the enzyme tests and chest X-ray are helpful in diagnosis, and echocardiography may show a pericardial effusion. Most cases respond promptly to treatment with aspirin or non-steroidal anti-inflammatory agents, but in more resistant cases steroids are effective.

THE SHOULDER–HAND SYNDROME

The features of the shoulder–hand syndrome are pain and stiffness in one or both shoulders, accompanied to a varying degree by pain, swelling and vasomotor changes in the hands.[53] The syndrome starts 2–12 weeks after myocardial infarction and may last for some months. It seems to be much less common now than formerly; it is likely that disuse, associated with immobility, is an important factor in its genesis. It usually responds satisfactorily to physiotherapy and treatment with steroids.

REFERENCES

1. Gomez-Marin, O., Folsom, A.R., Kottke, T.E. *et al.* Improvement in long-term survival among patients hospitalized with acute myocardial infarction, 1970 to 1980: the Minnesota Heart Survey. *N. Engl. J. Med.* 1987; **316**: 1353.
2. Kitchin, A.H. and Pocock, S.J. Prognosis of patients with acute myocardial infarction admitted to a coronary care unit. II: Survival after hospital discharge. *Br. Heart J.* 1977; **39**: 1167.
3. Pohjola, S., Siltanen, O. and Romo, M. Five year study of 728 patients after myocardial infarction. *Br. Heart J.* 1980; **43**: 176.
4. Norris, R.M., Caughey, D.E., Deeming, L.W., Mercer, C.J. and Scott, P.J. Prognosis after myocardial infarction. Six-year follow-up. *Br. Heart J.* 1974; **36**: 786.
5. Beller, G.A. and Gibson, R.S. Risk stratification after myocardial infarction. *Mod. Concepts Cardiovasc. Dis.* 1986; **55**: 5.
6. Saunamaki, K.I. and Andersen, J.D. Clinical significance of the ST-segment response and other early exercise variables in uncomplicated vs complicated myocardial infarction. *Eur. Heart J.* 1987; **8**: 603.
7. Fioretti, P., Tijssen, J.G.P., Azar, A.J. *et al.* Prognostic value of predischarge 12 lead electrocardiogram after myocardial infarction compared with other routine clinical variables. *Br. Heart J.* 1987; **57**: 306.
8. Madigan, N.P., Rutherford, D.B. and Frye, R.H. The clinical course, early prognosis and coronary anatomy of subendocardial infarction. *Am. J. Med.* 1976; **63**: 634.
9. Multicenter Postinfarction Research Group. Risk stratification and survival after myocardial infarction. *N. Engl. J. Med.* 1983; **309**: 331.
10. Fioretti, P., Brower, R.W., Simoons, M.L. *et al.* Relative value of clinical variables, bicycle ergometry, rest radionuclide ventriculography and 24 hour ambulatory monitoring at discharge to predict 1 year survival after myocardial infarction. *J. Am. Coll. Cardiol.* 1986; **8**: 40.
11. Fioretti, P., Brower, R.W., Simoons, M.L. *et al.* Prediction of mortality during the first year after acute myocardial infarction from clinical variables and stress test at hospital discharge. *Am. J. Cardiol.* 1985; **55**: 1313.
12. DeBusk, R.F., Kraemer, H.C., Nash, E., Berger, W.E. and Lew, H. Stepwise risk stratification soon after myocardial infarction. *Am. J. Cardiol.* 1983; **52**: 1161.
13. Theroux, P., Waters, D.D., Halphen, C., Debaisieux, J.C. and Mizgala, H.F. Prognostic value of exercise testing soon after myocardial infarction. *N. Engl. J. Med.* 1979; **301**: 3.
14. Weld, F.M., Chu, K., Bigger, J.T. Jr and Rolnitzky, L. Risk stratification with low-level exercise testing 2 weeks after myocardial infarction. *Circulation* 1981; **64**: 306.
15. Jennings, K., Reid, D.S., Hawkins, T. and Julian, D.G. Role

of exercise testing after myocardial infarction in identifying candidates for coronary artery surgery *Br. Med. J.* 1984; **288**: 185.

16. Krone, R.J., Gillespie, J.A., Weld, F.M., Miller, J.P. and Moss, A.J. The Multicenter Postinfarction Research Group. Low-level exercise testing after myocardial infarction: usefulness in enhancing clinical risk stratification. *Circulation* 1985; **71**: 80.

17. Morris, D.D., Rozanski, A., Berman D.S. *et al.* Noninvasive prediction of the angiographic extent of coronary artery disease after myocardial infarction. Comparison of clinical, bicycle exercise, electrocardiography and ventriculographic parameters. *Circulation* 1984; **70**: 192.

18. Gibson, R.S., Taylor, G.J., Watson, D.D. *et al.* Predicting the extent and location of coronary disease during the early post-infarction period by quantitative thallium-201 scintigraphy. *Am. J. Cardiol.* 1981; **47**: 1010.

19. Leppo, J.A., O'Brien, J., Rothendler, J.A., Getchell, J.D. and Lee, V.W. Dipyridamole-thallium-201 scintigraphy in the prediction of future cardiac events after acute myocardial infarction. *N. Engl. J. Med.* 1984; **310**: 1014.

20. Bigger, J.T. Jr, Fleiss, J.L., Kleiger, R., Miller, J.P. and Rolnitzky, L.M. The relationship between ventricular arrhythmias, left ventricular dysfunction and mortality in the 2 years after myocardial infarction, *Circulation* 1984; **69**: 250.

21. Bigger, J.T. Jr, Coromilas, J., Rolnitzky L.M. and Weld, F.W. Ventricular arrhythmias after myocardial infarction: significance of findings in 24 hour ECG recordings. In: Kulbertus, H.E., ed. *Medical Management of Cardiac Arrhythmias.* Edinburgh: Churchill Livingstone, 1986.

22. Denniss, A.R., Baaijens, H., Cody, D.V. *et al.* Value of programmed stimulation and exercise testing in predicting one-year mortality after myocardial infarction. *Am. J. Cardiol.* 1985; **56**: 213.

23. Sanz, G., Castener, A., Betriu, A. *et al.* Determinants of prognosis in survivors of myocardial infarction. *N. Engl. J. Med.* 1982; **306**: 1065.

24. Norris, R.M., Caughey, D.E., Deeming, L.W., Mercer, J.C. and Scott, P.J. Coronary prognostic index for predicting survival after recovery from acute myocardial infarction. *Lancet* 1970; **2**: 485.

25. Wenger, N.K. Rehabilitation of the coronary patient: status 1986. *Prog. Cardiovasc. Dis.* 1986; **29**: 181.

26. Hamm, L.F., Stull, G.A. and Crow, R.S. Exercise testing early after myocardial infarction: Historic perspective and current uses. *Prog. Cardiovasc. Dis.* 1986; **28**: 463.

27. Naughton, J.P. and Hellerstein, H.K. (eds). *Exercise testing and exercise training after myocardial infarction.* New York: Academic Press, 1973.

28. Detry, J.M.R., Rousseau, N., Vandenbroucke, G., Kusumi, F., Brasseur, L.A. and Bruce, R.A. Increased arteriovenous oxygen difference after physical training in coronary heart disease. *Circulation* 1971; **49**: 1971.

29. Mayou, R.A., Williamson, B. and Foster, A. Outcome two months after myocardial infarction. *J. Psychosom. Res.* 1978; **22**: 439.

30. Mayou R.A, Foster A, Williamson B. Psychosocial adjustment of patients one year after myocardial infarction. *J. Psychosom. Res.* 1978; **22**: 447.

31. Froese, A, Vasquez, E., Cassem, N.H. and Hackett, T.P. Validation of anxiety, depression and denial scales in a coronary care unit. *J. Psychosom. Res.* 1974; **18**: 137.

32. Cay, E.L., Vetter, N.J., Philip, A.E. and Dugard, P. Return to work after a heart attack. *J. Psychosom. Res.* 1973; **17**: 231.

33. Mulcahy, R., Hickey, N., Graham, I.M. and McKenzie, G. Factors affecting the 5 year survival rate of men following acute coronary disease. *Am. Heart J.* 1977; **93**: 556.

34. Aberg, A., Bergstrand, R., Johansson, S. *et al.* Cessation of smoking after myocardial infarction. *Br. Heart J.* 1983; **49**: 416.

35. May, G.S., Eberlein, K.A., Furberg, C.D., Passamani, E.R. and DeMets, D.L. Secondary prevention after myocardial infarction: A review of long-term trials. *Prog. Cardiovasc. Dis.* 1982; **24**: 331.

36. The Coronary Drug Project Research Group. Clofibrate and niacin in coronary heart disease. *JAMA* 1975; **231**: 360

37. Friedman, M., Thoresen, C.E., Gill, J.J. *et al.* Feasibility of altering type A behaviour pattern after myocardial infarction. *Circulation* 1982; **66**: 83.

38. Kallio, V., Hamalainen, H., Hakkila, J. and Luurila, O.J. Reduction in sudden deaths by a multifactorial intervention programme after acute myocardial infarction. *Lancet* 1979; **2**: 1091.

39. Vedin, A., Wilhelmsson, C., Tibblin, G. and Wilhelmsen, L. The post-infarction clinic in Goteborg, Sweden. *Acta Med. Scand.* 1976; **200**: 453.

40. Yusuf, S., Peto, R., Lewis, J., Collins, R. and Sleight, P. Beta Blockade during and after myocardial infarction: an overview of the randomized trials. *Prog. Cardiovasc. Dis.* 1985; **27**: 335.

41. The Norwegian Multicenter Study Group. Timolol-induced reduction in mortality and reinfarction in patients surviving myocardial infarction. *N. Engl. J. Med.* 1981; **304**: 801.

42. Beta-blocker Heart Attack Study Group (BHAT). A randomized trial of propranolol in patients with acute myocardial infarction. 1. Mortality results. *JAMA* 1982; **247**: 1707.

43. Hjalmarson, A., Elmfeldt, D., Herlitz, J. *et al.* Effect on mortality of metoprolol in acute myocardial infarction: a double-blind randomized trial. *Lancet* 1981; **2**: 823.

44. Furberg, C.D., Hawkins, C.M. and Lichstein, E. Effect of propranolol in postinfarction patients with mechanical and electrical complications. *Circulation* 1983; **69**: 761.

45. Danish Study Group on Verapamil in Myocardial Infarction. Verapamil in acute myocardial infarction. *Eur. Heart J.* 1984; **5**: 516.

46. Gibson, R.S., Boden, W.E., Theroux, P. *et al.* Diltiazem and reinfarction in patients with non-Q wave infarction. *N. Engl. J. Med.* 1986; **315**: 423.

47. Multicenter Diltiazem Post-infarction Trial Research Group. The effect of diltiazem on mortality and reinfarction after myocardial infarction. *N. Engl. J. Med.* 1988; **319**: 385.

48. Sixty-Plus Reinfarction Study Group. A double-blind trial to assess long-term oral anticoagulant therapy in elderly patients after myocardial infarction. *Lancet* 1980; **ii**: 989.

49. Klimt, C.R., Knatterud, G.L., Stamler, J. and Meier, P. Persantine-Aspirin Reinfarction Study. Part II. Secondary coronary prevention with persantine and aspirin. *J. Am. Coll. Cardiol.* 1986; **7**: 251.

50. Bertrand, M.E., La Blanche, J.M., Timant, P.Y., Thieuleux, F.A., Delforge, M.R. and Chahine, R.A. The provocation of coronary artery spasm in patients with recent transmural infarction. *Eur. Heart J.* 1982; **4**: 532.

51. Consensus Trial Study Group. Effects of enalapril on mortality in severe congestive heart failure. *N. Engl. J. Med.* 1987; **316**: 1429.

52. Dressler, W. A post-myocardial infarction syndrome. *JAMA* 1956; **160**: 1379.

53. Edeiken, J. Shoulder–hand syndrome following myocardial infarction with special reference to prognosis. *Circulation* 1957; **16**: 14.

Chapter 52

Surgery in Ischaemic Heart Disease

David J. Wheatley

There have been many attempts to intervene surgically in patients with manifestations of ischaemic heart disease, beginning early this century. The more logically conceived attempts were aimed at improving non-coronary collateral flow to the myocardium. Pericardial abrasion, wrapping of omentum around the heart and implantation of the distal end of a pedicle containing the internal mammary artery into the myocardium (Vineberg procedure) were the most notable of these procedures.[1] The imprecision of the available diagnostic techniques, the dubious physiological basis of many of the operations and their unpredictable clinical results combined to bring these procedures into disrepute.

With the development of selective coronary arteriography in the early 1960s, it became possible to demonstrate coronary arterial anatomy and pathology in patients with manifestations of ischaemic heart disease.[2] It was then feasible to devise operations to remove or bypass coronary obstructions. In the late 1960s, Favaloro, Johnson and Cooley were among the first to report large series of patients having aortocoronary bypass operations in which autologous saphenous vein was used.[3–5] In 1968, Green and his group[6] reported results for bypassing coronary obstructions with the internal mammary artery. Surgical resection of aneurysms of the left ventricle,[7] closure of perforations of the infarcted interventricular septum[8] and replacement of the mitral valve with ischaemic papillary muscle rupture[9] had been firmly established by this time. Although there continue to be refinements and developments, most current surgical management of ischaemic heart disease consists of applying these techniques alone or in combination.

Such has been the popularity of surgery for ischaemic heart disease in recent years that in the USA alone in 1983, 191 000 coronary operations were performed, and it was estimated 250 000 operations would be performed in 1986.[10] Although practice in most other countries is not at this level, there is general recognition that coronary surgery could have a greater role. For the UK, the requirement for coronary surgery has been estimated at a minimum of 300 operations annually for each million of population.[11]

CURRENT INTERVENTIONS FOR ISCHAEMIC HEART DISEASE

Restoration of normal myocardial perfusion

Intervention is intended to augment the supply of blood to coronary arteries distal to coronary obstruction in patients who have impaired myocardial perfusion; the aim is to restore normal homogeneous myocardial perfusion at rest and on exercise.

Surgery does this by *coronary artery bypass grafting* (aortocoronary bypass grafting, saphenous vein bypass grafting, internal mammary bypass grafting). The principle of such surgery is the construction of an effective strategically placed collateral circulation to the coronary arterial tree distal to obstruction. This is achieved by the insertion of autologous saphenous vein conduits between the ascending aorta and the coronary tree or by anastomosis of the internal mammary arteries to the coronary vessels.

Direct removal of obstructive atheromatous disease from within the coronary artery, *endarterectomy*, is generally a less satisfactory approach, although it often has a place in coronary surgery where scope for bypassing an obstruction is limited by the small size of distally placed branches or where a particularly long segment of artery is totally occluded. It is almost always combined with bypass grafting to the restored coronary lumen.

The more recent application of *percutaneous transluminal coronary angioplasty* for directly modifying obstructive atheromatous lesions and restoring normal myocardial perfusion by less invasive means than surgical operation is an attractive development that must be considered in the overall approach to intervention in ischaemic heart disease.

Improvement in left ventricular geometry

In patients in whom ischaemic heart disease has manifested itself as myocardial infarction followed later by myocardial fibrosis and aneurysm formation, surgery has a role in restoring improved cardiac function in those with severe effort dyspnoea by the creation of a more normal left ventricular geometry—*left ventricular aneurysmectomy* or *aneurysmorrhaphy*.

Repair for acute ischaemic myocardial disruption

Acute myocardial infarction may be complicated by rupture of the interventricular septum, resulting in left-to-right shunting of blood, or of the papillary muscle, resulting in mitral regurgitation. The prognosis is extremely poor and surgery has a role in salvaging many such patients by closing the site of myocardial perforation or by replacing the flail mitral valve.

Removal of ischaemic dysrhythmic foci

Much less commonly, surgery with intra-operative mapping and ablation has a role in the management of refractory dysrhythmias associated with ischaemic myocardial fibrosis.

THE ROLE OF SURGERY

Surgical intervention in ischaemic heart disease represents only one of several possible options, which may include reassurance of the patient, observation, various pharmacological regimes, modifications in lifestyle and coronary angioplasty. Each may have a role in the individual.

There have been important developments in both medical and surgical management of ischaemic heart disease in the past two or three decades, and advances continue to be made. It is not surprising, therefore, that popular perceptions of indications for surgery in ischaemic heart disease are constantly evolving.[12]

In considering surgery in ischaemic heart disease, it is necessary to take account of *symptomatic status* and *natural history*. In general, surgery is indicated in patients in whom it is judged likely to produce a better, more complete or more lasting improvement in symptomatic status than the available medical therapy, or in those in whom medical therapy has had limited success or has produced undesirable side-effects. Surgery is also indicated when it is anticipated that it will result in a better prognosis than medical therapy.

INDICATIONS FOR SURGERY

Surgery for chronic stable angina

Surgery may be indicated for symptoms in patients in whom angina is severe, is causing undue anxiety or is interfering with lifestyle to an extent unacceptable to the patient, despite adequate medical therapy, and in whom coronary arteriography has demonstrated significant obstruction (loss of 50% or more of diameter) of one or more major coronary arteries. The location and extent of angiographically demonstrable coronary disease, objective evidence of exercise-induced myocardial ischaemia, the effect of maximal medical therapy, the possible role of coronary angioplasty and the risk of surgery in the particular patient (having regard to likely nature of surgery, the age and medical background of the patient) are all factors that will influence the final decision.

Although coronary angiography is an essential investigation in making the final decision regarding coronary surgery (or percutaneous transluminal coronary angioplasty) and in planning its conduct, the facilities for such investigation may not always be readily available; the cost, the need for hospitalization and the small associated hazard are further factors to be considered before making a decision to proceed to angiography. The results of exercise electrocardiography may be helpful in this context. A strongly positive test reached at low workload, failure to increase pulse rate and blood pressure or a fall in blood pressure on exercise indicates the likelihood of severe coronary disease or left ventricular dysfunction, and makes the need for angiography clear. Conversely, the achievement of high work levels with a normal exercise electrocardiogram suggest a good prognosis and mild disease and, in such patients, medical measures may be indicated in the absence of angiography.

Surgery for prognostic considerations

The presence of obstructive coronary artery lesions

may be demonstrated in patients not complaining of severe angina. This may arise as a result of investigation of patients with valvular heart disease, as a result of investigation of a patient with mild or atypical angina, or previous myocardial infarction, or where there is a strong family history of premature coronary artery disease. The response to exercise testing is particularly helpful in deciding the need for coronary angiography and possible surgical intervention. Ischaemic electrocardiographic changes, failure to increase heart rate or blood pressure on exercise and hypotension occurring at low work levels are indicators of strategically important or widespread coronary disease, or of poor left ventricular function, with poor prognosis. Such findings are an indication for coronary arteriography. Where there is significant obstruction of the left main coronary artery or proximal obstruction of all three major coronary arteries (right, circumflex and anterior descending), surgery is generally indicated, irrespective of the symptomatic state. The quality of left ventricular function has little influence on this recommendation. If left ventricular function is good, the operative hazard is low. However, it is in the patients with poor left ventricular function and three-vessel disease that the greatest potential long-term survival benefit is obtained from surgical treatment in spite of the increased operative hazard.

Significant proximal stenosis (proximal to the first septal perforator) of the anterior descending artery, together with significant proximal obstruction of another major coronary vessel (two-vessel disease including anterior descending), should probably be regarded in the same manner as three-vessel disease.

Where there is angiographically less extensive proximal disease (one-vessel or two-vessel excluding proximal anterior descending disease), there is no evidence for improved survival benefit from surgical treatment as compared with medical treatment, and the indication for surgery in this group of patients is dependent on angina not responding satisfactorily to adequate medical therapy, or intolerance of medical therapy.

The risk of surgery is increased when ventricular function is severely compromised (ejection fraction < 30% with generalized hypokinesia, left ventricular end-diastolic pressure > 20 mmHg at rest). The increased risk may be worth accepting in view of the potential long-term benefit. Consideration should be given to the relative predominance of angina or dyspnoea in the history, the demonstration of late filling of perfusion defects on thallium scanning and the nature of the coronary vessels.

Surgery for unstable angina

In general, where pain is of recent onset, is changing in pattern, or occurring at rest or with minimal provocation, investigation should be undertaken with a view to possible coronary surgery because coronary lesions that carry a high risk of myocardial infarction may be present. It is preferable to control symptoms by intensive medical means prior to surgery, although, if such measures fail, surgery should be undertaken promptly, provided there are appropriate angiographic criteria as described above.

Surgery in myocardial infarction

Limitation of evolving infarction

Early in the onset of acute myocardial infarction (usually within the first 4–6 h), while pain is still present, a policy of urgent coronary angiography followed by prompt coronary artery bypass surgery for revascularization of the infarct-related vessel, as well as any other jeopardized vessels, has been practised in a number of centres.[13,14] Phillips[15] and Berg[16] have been among the pioneers of early surgical intervention for acute evolving infarction. Besides having low hospital mortality rates, they report good long-term benefit with evidence of salvage of left ventricular myocardium. Phillips' group[14] reported a 3.5% hospital mortality rate in patients undergoing surgery for acute evolving infarction; all deaths occurred in the 95 patients who were in cardiogenic shock and none occurred in the 185 haemodynamically stable patients. Kirklin et al.[17] have reported excellent results in 35 patients 1–2 years after coronary artery bypass grafting undertaken within 48 h of the onset of acute myocardial infarction: there was 1 hospital death; 1-year overall actuarial survival was 94%, and 82% of survivors had no post-operative angina. Such surgical treatment for 'evolving infarction' is dependent on the ready availability of resources for angiography and surgery at all times.

The practice of early intervention to restore patency to the infarct-related vessel in the early stage of myocardial infarction with thrombolytic therapy offers a more feasible option for clinicians at most centres.[18] Once thrombolysis in an occluded infarct-related artery has been achieved, a residual high-grade stenosis is often seen.[13] This may be amenable to balloon dilatation but, if not, aortocoronary bypass grafting may be carried out within the following few days to reduce the risk of re-occlusion.

The nature and timing of intervention in acute myocardial infarction remain uncertain and further experience is required. Early thrombolysis, supplemented as necessary by percutaneous transluminal coronary angioplasty, would seem the most appropriate early intervention. Those who remain unstable may require emergency coronary surgery; those who are stable should be assessed for provokable ischaemia at about 10 days. Where this can be demonstrated, the decision is made for revascularization, either by balloon angioplasty or by coronary surgery as appropriate.[13]

Intervention for early post-infarction angina

Where there is an occurrence of angina in the early post-infarction period while the patient is still hospitalized, prompt investigation is indicated with a view to surgical intervention for prognostic considerations. Such patients have been shown to be at considerable risk of early death and recurrent infarction or unstable angina.[19] Surgery may be undertaken with reasonable safety (with operative mortality reported between 0 and 9%) even within a few days of infarction if considered necessary on the basis of the severity of angina, the lack of response to medical therapy and the extent of angiographically demonstrable disease.[20–22]

DiSesa et al.[23] have shown that myocardial revascularization early (within 2 weeks) after acute transmural infarction can have a low risk. The 20% mortality for such early surgery was confined to those patients with cardiogenic shock. For all patients operated on within 6 weeks of infarction, there was an actuarial probability of survival at 1 year of 96% and at 5 years of 83%.

Based on a review of 174 patients undergoing revascularization for evidence of ischaemia within 7 weeks of acute myocardial infarction, Hochberg et al.[24] concluded that revascularization is safe at any stage in those with an ejection fraction > 50%, but where ejection fraction is < 50% surgery should be delayed for at least four weeks.

Surgery for prognostic implications in early post-infarction period

Routine investigation of patients surviving myocardial infarction with a view to identifying a high-risk subgroup[25] is practised during the convalescent phase by workers at a number of centres. Where exercise-induced electrocardiographic evidence of myocardial ischaemia or poor exercise tolerance during the convalescent period following myocardial infarction has resulted in coronary angiography being undertaken, surgical intervention is indicated when left main, three-vessel, or two-vessel disease, including proximal anterior descending artery disease, is present. Surgery is not indicated if the sole or predominant abnormality is in the infarct-related vessel with akinesis or hypokinesis in the infarcted territory. Such patients may subsequently develop ventricular aneurysm and be potential candidates for surgery at a later stage.

Acute myocardial disruption complicating infarction

Surgery has an important role in the management of the complications of myocardial infarction.[26] In the acute phase, perforation of the interventricular septum may occur in a region of necrotic myocardium. This adds the haemodynamic burden of left-to-right shunting to an already compromised heart and pulmonary circulation; it is usually rapidly fatal. Surgery for the closure of the interventricular septal defect may salvage many of these patients. Similarly, replacement of a flail mitral valve resulting from papillary muscle infarction and rupture may be life-saving.

Myocardial scarring

Acute myocardial infarction may be followed after several months by the development of a weak and expanding scar in the left ventricle which results in a left ventricular aneurysm. If such aneurysm is large and causing symptoms or signs of left ventricular failure, resection is indicated, combined if necessary with bypass grafting of stenosed coronary arteries.[27]

Mitral insufficiency may occur in chronic ischaemic heart disease. When myocardial ischaemia affects the papillary muscles and the adjacent free wall myocardium, there may be sufficient loss of mitral tension during systole to cause mitral insufficiency. This is curable by revascularization surgery. When the papillary muscle and adjacent myocardium is scarred, the mitral leaflets may be pulled into the ventricle, and the resultant mitral insufficiency may be sufficiently severe to result in breathlessness and pulmonary congestion. Similarly, diffuse myocardial scarring may result in a dilated ventricle and dilatation of the mitral annulus may cause insufficiency. Care is required to distinguish between mitral insufficiency and poor left ventricular function as the cause of such patients' breathlessness. Mitral valve replacement is the only way of treating mitral insufficiency where myocardial scarring is the basis. Surgical risks are increased over those for non-ischaemic valvular disease, and revascularization of major jeopardized coronary arteries should be combined with valve replacement.

Occasionally, myocardial scar is the source of dysrhythmia. When refractory to drug management, surgery with ablation of dysrhythmic foci as located by mapping may be indicated.[28]

Contra-indications

It is uncommon for the quality of the distal coronary vessels to be so poor that coronary surgery is unequivocally contra-indicated, but where most of the jeopardized major coronary vessels are diffusely diseased over much of their epicardial course, or are very narrow (less than 1.5 mm in diameter), the likelihood of being able to achieve satisfactory bypass grafting is much reduced, and coronary surgery may be contra-indicated.

Similarly, the degree of left ventricular dysfunction is not usually so severe as to unequivocally contra-indicate surgery, but where breathlessness is the predominant feature (unless there is a left ventricular aneurysm amenable to resection) poor left ventricular function with ejection fraction < 20% is generally a contra-indication.

General contra-indications to surgery may include senility, advanced pulmonary, renal or hepatic disease and malignancy judged likely to have a rapidly fatal outcome.

The role of percutaneous transluminal coronary angioplasty

The role of percutaneous transluminal coronary angioplasty is not yet fully defined. Where the facilities and expertise for this form of treatment exist, it is reasonable to recommend coronary angioplasty in those patients with suitable lesions, particularly where there are only one or two discrete lesions in the coronary tree, and where these are not close to major branches or bifurcations, in the hope of avoiding or postponing surgery. Urgent surgical intervention is occasionally required for acute complications of balloon angioplasty, where there has been occlusion of a vessel due to thrombo-

sis or dissection, and consists of aortocoronary bypass grafting to the jeopardized vessels.[29,30] Elective surgery may be required when balloon angioplasty fails to dilate coronary stenoses adequately.

TECHNIQUES OF SURGERY

Pre-operative preparation

Patients should be admitted a day before surgery to allow them to become familiar with their surroundings and to have post-operative management explained. Anxiety is an understandable and potentially dangerous emotion in these patients. The opportunity to have the hospital course explained and to see others who are awaiting or have recently been through the operation often does much to allay fears.

Many patients will be on beta-blocking therapy, and this should be maintained until the day of surgery.[31] Nitrate therapy is continued up to the time of surgery and the use of nitroglycerine ointment at the time of pre-medication is of value.[32] Intravenous nitrate therapy is maintained until the commencement of cardiopulmonary bypass in those patients with unstable angina. The aim is to have patients free of pain overnight and prior to anaesthesia.[33]

Routine clinical examination is undertaken to identify any condition that may require prior management. A pre-operative chest X-ray is made and a 12-lead electrocardiogram is recorded. Measurement is made of serum electrolytes, urea, indices of hepatic function, haemoglobin, white cell count and erythrocyte sedimentation rate. Skin of the chest, abdominal wall, groins and legs is shaved and washed. Night sedation and pre-medication (usually with a benzodiazepine) is prescribed.

Anaesthesia

During anaesthesia and surgery, the balance between myocardial oxygen supply and demand may readily be altered unfavourably by tachycardia, hypertension, hypotension, inadequate oxygenation or the use of myocardial depressant drugs. Ischaemic myocardial injury may therefore occur during the phase of anaesthetic induction or during the preparatory stages of operation, unless care is taken to maintain a stable and satisfactory physiological state.

Induction of anaesthesia and intubation of the

trachea for institution of intermittent positive pressure ventilation is undertaken in a quiet environment with monitoring of pulse rate, blood pressure and electrocardiogram to ensure that tachycardia, hypotension or hypertension, and possible consequent myocardial ischaemia are avoided. Choice of anaesthetic agents will vary with different practices. Intubation is usually undertaken with the aid of muscle relaxants once hypnosis has been achieved and the patient has been breathing oxygen for a few minutes. Intravenous drugs are usually used as the main anaesthetic agents, because inhalational agents depress the myocardium and require special arrangements for administration during cardiopulmonary bypass. A combination of an opiate and a benzodiazepine is usually satisfactory.[33]

Monitoring

Haemodynamic status is monitored throughout the peri-operative period by having a continuous oscilloscope display of the electrocardiogram. Blood pressure is recorded with an automatic blood-pressure cuff monitor until an intra-arterial blood pressure recording is available from a percutaneously inserted radial artery cannula. At some centres, pulmonary artery or pulmonary arterial wedge pressure is recorded; although ideal, this is usually not essential for routine practice but it is a wise precaution in those patients with unstable angina or poor left ventricular function. The simpler, although less appropriate, recording of central venous pressure at least gives some guide to general circulatory filling. Measurement of urine output from a bladder catheter is a further guide to the state of tissue perfusion. At some centres, a cerebral function monitor is used to indicate the state of cerebral activity as an indicator of cerebral perfusion during cardiopulmonary bypass.

Adequacy of ventilation and tissue perfusion is monitored by regular measurement of arterial blood gas and acid–base balance. Serum potassium and packed cell volume are measured at intervals and correction is applied as necessary during cardiopulmonary bypass and in the early post-operative period. Body temperature (usually nasopharyngeal) and blood temperature are monitored. Measurement of myocardial temperature from an intramyocardial temperature probe inserted into the septum is undertaken in some centres to ensure that adequate myocardial cooling has been achieved and maintained during cardioplegic myocardial protection, although this procedure is not without pitfalls and inconvenience.

OPERATIVE TECHNIQUE

Surgical exposure and preparation

Vertical sternotomy provides the standard approach to the heart. When it is intended to use the internal mammary artery as a conduit, the dissection of one or both of these vessels within a pedicle of surrounding tissue is undertaken as soon as the sternum has been divided longitudinally in the midline. Some 15–30 min may be required for the division of branches and safe isolation of each internal mammary artery pedicle without injury to the artery. The artery is left intact, conducting blood at this stage.[34,35]

When saphenous vein is required for use as a conduit, the dissection of the vein and division of its branches is undertaken at the same time as sternotomy and preparation for cardiopulmonary bypass. Usually the long saphenous system is harvested, either below the knee or from the thigh, aiming for a vein of uniform calibre and a diameter of 3–5 mm. The presence of varicosities or previous removal of vein increase the difficulties of surgery and may require the use of the lesser saphenous vein or the generally less satisfactory arm veins. Artificial conduits remain disappointing in this application and are rarely used.

Institution of cardiopulmonary bypass with cannulation of the ascending aorta and right atrium or venae cavae should be achieved without handling the heart unduly and avoiding any interference with the ventricles. The avoidance of periods of hypotension or hypertension, even if transitory, does much to reduce the risk of peri-operative infarction.

Repeat coronary surgery requires care in separation of the heart from the overlying sternum, with gradual division of the sternum from the xiphisternum towards the suprasternal notch. Adhesions between the heart and overlying pericardium or sternum require to be divided with care.[36] Because of the risk of liberation of atheromatous debris and its embolization into the coronary tree, it may be advisable to ligate any severely diseased, but still patent, vein grafts at an early stage before handling the grafts or the heart in patients having repeat coronary surgery.[37]

Cardiopulmonary bypass and myocardial protection

The general principles of cardiopulmonary bypass and myocardial protection applicable to all cardiac surgery are followed. There are many safe techniques of cardiopulmonary bypass and of managing the myocardium for provision of the necessary conditions for coronary surgery.[38,39] Avoidance of imbalance between coronary supply and myocardial work in the preparation of the patient for cardiopulmonary bypass is particularly important, and in practice this means not handling the heart while it is working and avoiding blood loss, together with adequate analgesia and ventilation. During the period that coronary anastomoses are being constructed, or myocardial scar is being resected, the heart is made ischaemic by applying a cross-clamp to the ascending aorta. This stops myocardial perfusion from the cardiopulmonary bypass circuit. Protection of the ischaemic myocardium is obtained by a combination of cooling of the myocardium, to reduce basal metabolic activity, and prompt electromechanical arrest of the heart, to conserve high-energy phosphate stores. This is achieved by infusion into the aortic root (and hence the coronary tree) of a cold (4–10°C) potassium-containing crystalloid cardioplegic solution, or chilled blood with added potassium. Non-coronary collateral blood supply is often well developed in patients with coronary artery disease, and this may create difficulties due to the presence of blood in the operative field when the coronary artery is opened and, more importantly, may wash out cardioplegic solution and speed re-warming of the cold myocardium when cold cardioplegic techniques are used for myocardial protection. It is usual practice to use hypothermic cardiopulmonary bypass, lowering the patient's blood temperature to between 20 and 28°C, depending on the anticipated length of the procedure. This allows the cardiopulmonary bypass flow rate to be reduced from 2.4 l/m²/min to levels half or two-thirds of this rate and it is of particular help as an adjunct to cold cardioplegic techniques.[40,41]

Coronary artery bypass grafting

The decision about which coronary arteries should be bypassed is largely made on the basis of the coronary arteriographic appearances. The surgeon has very limited scope for evaluating the status of the coronary vessels as far as their lumen is concerned—the proximal left system is inaccessible, and the appearance and feel of coronary arteries is sometimes misleading because considerable amounts of visible and palpable atheroma may be present without undue encroachment on the lumen. In general, coronary arteries jeopardized by ste-noses of > 50% loss of lumen diameter are bypassed, provided that the distal vessels are judged to be > 1 mm in diameter. The surgeon selects segments of coronary arteries that are relatively straight, free from disease and distal to known stenoses for the construction of an anastomosis with the graft conduit. Commonly, grafts are inserted into the anterior descending artery, the distal right or posterior descending artery, and a lateral branch of the circumflex (the main circumflex usually being difficult to expose is best managed by bypassing to a large branch). Large diagonal branches of the anterior descending artery, multiple lateral branches of the circumflex or intermediate branches may all be grafted if they are proximally jeopardized and of adequate size.

The sequence of constructing the graft-to-coronary anastomoses is a matter of surgical preference and it is influenced by the technique of myocardial management. The distal anastomoses may be performed first, followed by anastomosis of the grafts to the ascending aorta, or the proximal anastomoses may be constructed first as soon as suitable distal targets are confirmed. In view of the more delicate nature of the internal mammary arteries and their vulnerability to injury with manipulation of the heart, it is usual practice to complete any vein conduit grafting first. The internal mammary artery pedicle is distally transected and the adequacy of its size and blood flow is judged prior to anastomosis. This is a subjective assessment because flow in the vessel is often not high on cardiopulmonary bypass when systemic pressure may be low, and the cold environment may encourage spasm of the internal mammary artery.

All anastomoses should be made with the aid of magnification and the use of a fine-suture technique. Usually 6/0 or 7/0 polypropylene suture material is used for the coronary anastomoses and 6/0 or 5/0 material for the aortic anastomoses. A continuous suture technique is rapid and haemostatic (Fig. 52.1). For anastomoses to very small vessels, and often for anastomosis of the internal mammary artery to the coronary artery, an interrupted suture technique may be preferred as greater precision may be achieved with less risk of injury to the smaller vessels (Fig. 52.2). Anastomosis of the proximal ends of vein grafts to the ascending aorta is made with the use of a side-biting clamp. This allows a fold of aorta to be excluded from the circulation, and suitably placed holes can be made to create openings for anastomosis with the vein grafts (Fig. 52.3).

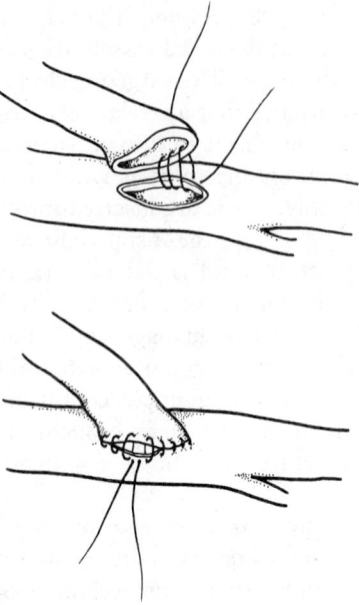

Fig. 52.1. Anastomosis of vein conduit to coronary artery. The end of the vein is bevelled to match the longitudinal coronary arteriotomy. Magnification and fine-suture technique are essential to achieve accuracy, with a haemostatic junction and absence of narrowing. The native coronary artery is left undisturbed on the epicardium and the presence of a bypass graft should not impinge on its lumen.

Care is required in judging the length and course of the grafts to avoid kinking or undue tension. It may be possible to anastomose a single saphenous vein conduit or an internal mammary artery to more than one distal coronary artery—sequential grafting or 'jump' grafting. This has the advantages of better utilization of existing conduit and a reduction in the number of anastomoses to the ascending aorta, and it may improve the late patency of anastomoses to smaller vessels which would otherwise be poor prospects for individual bypass grafting.[42-44]

When the anastomoses have been completed, the patient is weaned from cardiopulmonary bypass once full systemic re-warming has been achieved and the heart is beating well in a regular rhythm. The chest is closed once haemostasis has been confirmed, leaving chest drains in the pericardial and anterior mediastinal spaces. The leg wounds at vein donor sites are sutured.

Endarterectomy

When coronary arteries are totally occluded over a long segment or where there is extensive atheroma making the vessel wall very thick and liable to disintegration during sewing, the atheromatous material may be removed by the technique of endarterectomy to leave a patent lumen. This is generally less satisfactory than bypass grafting to an undisturbed vessel with a reasonably normal lumen and should therefore be undertaken only when there are no suitably sized distal branches. Endarterectomy is achieved by incising into the artery and using a blunt dissecting probe to develop a cleavage plane between the atheromatous core and the atrophied outer layer of media. With skill and luck, a long segment can be disobliterated by gentle traction on the core, although the risk of it breaking off and leaving a flap that may lift and occlude the

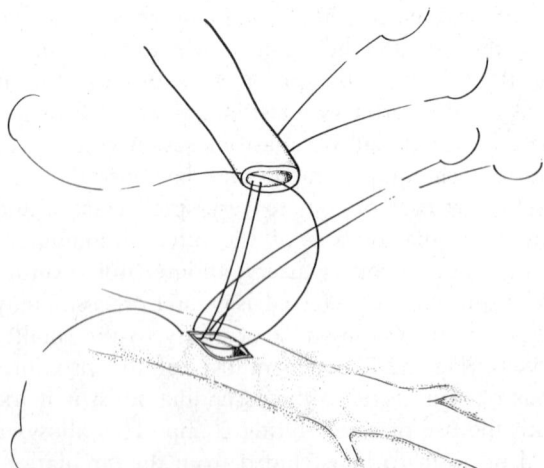

Fig. 52.2. The interrupted suture technique is particularly applicable to small vessel anastomoses, especially when using the internal mammary artery as a conduit.

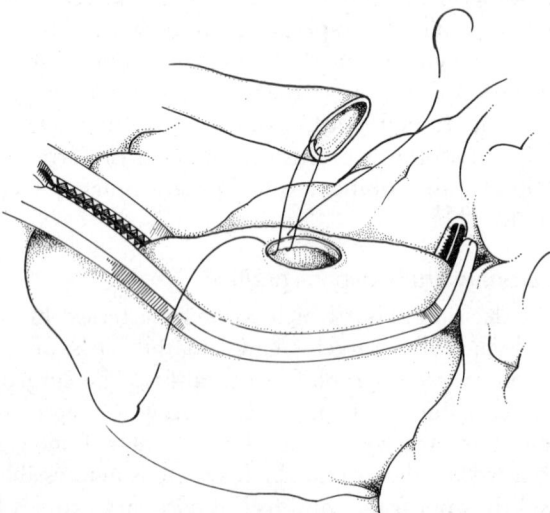

Fig. 52.3. Anastomosis of a vein conduit to the ascending aorta. A side-biting clamp allows exclusion of a fold of aorta. A hole is made in the aorta and the continuous-suture technique is used for anastomosis.

lumen is the main anxiety with this procedure. In the event of this happening, the vessel requires to be opened further distally for the core to be retrieved and removed. A bypass graft is constructed to the site of endarterectomy, even if proximal dissection is successful in totally disobliterating the artery, because re-occlusion of endarterectomized vessels is a hazard if the arterial opening is merely closed.[45–49]

Management of left ventricular aneurysm and scar

For those patients in whom resection of a left ventricular aneurysm is indicated, the techniques for cardiopulmonary bypass and myocardial protection are the same as for coronary revascularization. Particular care is needed to avoid manipulation of the ventricles until the ascending aorta has been cross-clamped, in view of the risk of dissemination of mural thrombus which so often lines such aneurysms. During coronary revascularization surgery, if ventricular scar is encountered, even where its resection is not indicated, there is a risk of mural thrombus being present, and a limited opening into the ventricle through the scar is a wise precaution to allow any such thrombus to be removed.

True aneurysm of the left ventricle is virtually always the consequence of transmural infarction, which is followed by fibrosis of the necrotic myocardium and gradual stretching and expansion of the fibrotic region.[50] Half of these aneurysms contain thrombus, often in layers, usually firmly adherent to the fibrotic endocardial surface of the aneurysm, and spontaneous systemic embolization is uncommon.[51] Adhesions are frequently present between the epicardial surface of the aneurysm and the overlying pericardium. The wall of the aneurysm consists of dense fibrous tissue which is thin, being only 3 or 4 mm thick, although true left ventricular aneurysms rarely rupture. At the margins of the aneurysm, the fibrotic tissue merges fairly abruptly into normal myocardium, the transition being readily identified at surgery. The majority of true left ventricular aneurysms seen in surgical practice are located in the antero-apical region of the left ventricle in the territory of the anterior descending artery. The aneurysm typically spares the papillary muscles and involves the anterior half or two-thirds of the interventricular septum. They are commonly due to isolated disease of the anterior descending artery, although they may be seen with multivessel disease. When these aneurysms become

large enough, they impair left ventricular function, wall tension increases and there is an increase in oxygen demand in the myocardium. The aneurysm is akinetic and there is a compensatory increase in movement of the rest of the ventricular wall. Congestive cardiac failure, angina and, less frequently, recurrent ventricular dysrhythmias are the main consequences. Symptomatic left ventricular aneurysms have a poor prognosis, with a 5-year mortality of 80–90% being reported.[52,53]

At surgery, true left ventricular aneurysms are recognized by the presence of adhesions over an akinetic scarred antero-apical region of the left ventricle. When the heart is empty and non-working on cardiopulmonary bypass, the aneurysmal area will often collapse inward. On cutting into the region, once the aorta has been cross-clamped to reduce the risk of embolizing thrombus, the dense nature of the fibrous tissue is readily appreciated; lining thrombus and relatively clear demarcation of scar from myocardium, and the typical location of the aneurysm in the territory of the anterior descending artery, make surgical confirmation of the diagnosis clear.

The aneurysm is opened and thrombus removed. Much of the thin scar is resected, leaving a rim of scar tissue at the neck of the aneurysm near the junction with normal myocardium, to allow secure suturing. Conventionally, the resultant defect in the left ventricle has been closed by suturing the two sides together in a linear fashion, using strips of Teflon felt to reduce the risk of suture tearing.[54] A newer concept has been described[55] in which a more normal ventricular geometry is restored by suturing a strong non-absorbable patch of Dacron, of dimensions judged to correspond to the original infarct that gave rise to the aneurysmal scar, into the neck of the aneurysm. Strong sutures are passed through the repairing patch and the full thickness of the ventricular wall at the boundary of scar and normal myocardium and tied over reinforcing Teflon felt buttresses. These procedures for resection of left ventricular aneurysm and restoration of an improved left ventricular geometry may be combined with coronary artery bypass grafting if remaining myocardium is supplied by coronary arteries jeopardized by stenoses of 50% or greater loss of lumen diameter.

False aneurysm is encountered infrequently in surgical practice. It is a consequence of rupture in an infarcted area of the free wall of the left ventricle. If such rupture is limited in size and allows gradual leakage of blood, there may be time for the development of pericardial adhesions which will contain the thrombus and prevent fatal cardiac tamponade. The wall of such false aneurysms consists only of thrombus and pericardium, and fatal extension or rupture is common.[56] Their location in areas other than the territory of the anterior descending artery may lead to a suspicion of the false nature of the aneurysm; the finding of a narrow neck, and absence of a dense fibrotic wall merging with normal myocardium, makes surgical recognition possible. The principles of repair are similar to those for true aneurysm.

Difficulty may arise when there is angiographic demonstration of an area of abnormally moving ventricular wall, which bulges on systole and appears to move inward in diastole. Such areas vary in size and locality, and may appear as paradoxically moving or dyskinetic areas, and have been termed *functional aneurysms*.[54] They may represent anatomically normal but ischaemic (and therefore non-contractile) myocardium at the time of investigation, or they may represent areas of diffuse fibrous tissue interspersed with myocardium. The anatomically normal, but ischaemic, areas are rarely identifiable at surgery because normal contraction occurs in the absence of physiological stress. Their treatment is usually accomplished by coronary artery bypass grafting. Areas of diffuse fibrous tissue intermingled with myocardium are usually not associated with overlying adhesions and are often contractile to some extent (unlike a true aneurysm which is non-contractile); the abnormal area can be seen to contain a mixture of fibrous and muscle tissue and to merge gradually with more normal myocardium. Resection of such areas is not indicated, although in view of the possibility of thrombus being adherent to the endocardial surface it is wise to open such areas by a short incision to remove any such thrombus. The thicker and less fibrous nature of a functional aneurysm, as compared with that of a true aneurysm, is then appreciated.

Management of ischaemic ventricular septal rupture

Rupture of the infarcted ventricular septum is relatively rare, occurring in less than 2% of patients with acute infarction. Rupture usually occurs within the first week of infarction.[57] Its occurrence is accompanied by a rapid deterioration in the haemodynamic status of the patient with the appearance of a precordial systolic murmur. With-

out surgery prognosis is poor.[58]

Surgical management is the only prospect for salvaging such patients. Investigation to confirm the diagnosis and to differentiate from acute papillary muscle rupture with mitral regurgitation, as well as to evaluate the state of the coronary arteries, is a matter of urgency. Right-heart catheterization may confirm the diagnosis by showing a step-up in oxygen saturation at ventricular level. Echocardiography will usually differentiate ventricular septal rupture from mitral insufficiency. Coronary arteriography, with left ventriculography, gives the most complete information, allowing assessment of the need for concomitant coronary artery bypass grafting and location of the interventricular septal defect. The presence of cardiogenic shock and pulmonary oedema increases the hazard and impairs the quality of such investigations. Intra-aortic balloon counterpulsation and endotracheal intubation with intermittent positive pressure ventilation are of value in these circumstances.

A small proportion of patients with rupture of the ventricular septum may survive in a reasonable haemodynamic state for several weeks, and they represent a very favourable group for surgical correction. However, the majority rapidly develop cardiogenic shock with hypotension, cold, pale skin, oliguria and rising blood urea, loss of mental alertness and increasing evidence of pulmonary oedema. Inotropic drugs, diuretics, intra-aortic balloon counterpulsation and intermittent positive pressure ventilation should be used only to allow investigation and preparation for surgery. A fatal outcome is likely without operation. Ventricular function is usually good, with the area of infarction being relatively limited and a large left-to-right shunt being responsible for most of the haemodynamic deterioration.

The heart is approached by vertical sternotomy, and hypothermic cardiopulmonary bypass with cardioplegic myocardial protection is used. The ventricular perforation is approached by incising through the adjacent infarcted left ventricular free wall, which is recognizable by its appearance and tendency to retract inward into the cavity of the decompressed left ventricle. The incision is thus parallel to the anterior descending artery for anterior septal rupture, and parallel to the posterior descending artery for inferior or posterior septal rupture.

The rupture of the septum is readily identifiable from the left side of the septum (and is frequently obscured by trabeculae on the right side). Necrotic muscle is excised. The defect in the ventricular septum is repaired by placing a patch of Teflon felt on the left side of the septum. This is anchored to the viable muscle of the septum with strong interrupted mattress sutures, each passing through the septum and through a pledget of Teflon on the right ventricular side to reduce the risk of the sutures cutting through the myocardium. For anterior infarcts, the free-wall incision is closed after trimming away necrotic muscle, using thick sutures passed through viable muscle, with Teflon buttresses to prevent sutures from cutting out. For inferior infarcts, closure of the free ventricular wall incision usually requires insertion of a patch of Dacron, because pulling the edges together creates undue tension on the sutures.

If coronary angiography has demonstrated significant stenoses in major coronary vessels, bypass grafting is undertaken. The infarct-related artery is usually incorporated in the repair of the septal defect and is not amenable to bypass grafting. Air is removed from the heart prior to weaning from cardiopulmonary bypass.

Management of ischaemic mitral valve dysfunction

A degree of mitral valve incompetence is often present in the acute phase of myocardial infarction. It is usually mild and resolves spontaneously, there being no physical disruption of the mitral papillary apparatus. Mitral annular dilatation, retraction of papillary muscles by a dilating left ventricle, or ischaemic paralysis of a papillary muscle can be the basis of the regurgitation.[59] In 1 or 2% of patients with myocardial infarction, severe mitral incompetence occurs as a result of rupture of a necrotic papillary muscle (usually the posteromedial papillary muscle) being involved in inferior infarction. As with rupture of the ventricular septum, papillary muscle rupture usually occurs within the first week following myocardial infarction, and it produces rapid deterioration in haemodynamic status. Prognosis is poor without surgical treatment.[26]

The appearance of a systolic murmur in a patient who was relatively well following acute myocardial infarction, associated with severe pulmonary oedema and cardiogenic shock, signals the onset of the condition. Confirmation of the diagnosis and differentiation from ventricular septal rupture must be established urgently. Tracheal intubation with intermittent positive pressure ventilation and intra-aortic balloon counterpulsation may be necessary. Echocardiography will usually make the diagnosis

clear and allows some assessment of ventricular function. Coronary arteriography is necessary to assess the state of the coronary arteries and to plan concomitant bypass grafting. Urgent surgery is required. Hypothermic cardiopulmonary bypass with cardioplegic myocardial protection is used. The left atrium is opened anterior to the right pulmonary veins and the mitral valve is exposed. The degree of rupture varies from complete avulsion of an entire papillary muscle to less extensive disruption involving a few chordae inserting into a papillary muscle tip. Repair of such lesions is not practical and replacement with a prosthetic valve is required. The normal leaflet and annular tissues do not hold sutures well, and pledgeted interrupted sutures are often required to reduce the risk of paravalve leaks. Bypass grafting of significantly stenosed coronary arteries is undertaken at the same time. Distal graft–coronary anastomoses are constructed after excision of the mitral valve. Proximal graft–aorta anastomoses are constructed following insertion of the prosthetic valve and removal of air from the heart during the re-warming phase of cardiopulmonary bypass.

POST-OPERATIVE MANAGEMENT FOLLOWING SURGERY FOR ISCHAEMIC HEART DISEASE

The principles of post-operative management are common to all cardiac surgical procedures.[60,61] Patients are returned to the intensive care or recovery area with drains in place in the pericardial and anterior mediastinal spaces to prevent accumulation of blood, which oozes from the exposed tissues and sometimes from suture lines on the heart or great vessels. Monitoring is continued to ensure that haemodynamic state can be continuously assessed. Mechanical ventilation is usually continued for several hours until the effects of anaesthesia have completely worn off and to ensure good expansion of the lungs and adequate ventilation. Appropriate analgesia is given.

Changes in haemodynamic state may require correction of blood loss, fluid imbalance or electrolyte alteration. Hypertension is common following coronary artery bypass grafting and this is controlled by intravenous infusion of sodium nitroprusside or nitrates. The aim is to avoid imbalance between myocardial work and myocardial oxygen supply; hence, hypotension, hypertension and tachycardia are treated promptly. Hypertension is common in the first 12–24 h after coronary surgery; management with nitroprusside or nitrate infusion is usually satisfactory. When hypertension persists beyond this time, it should be treated with a beta-blocking drug. In those patients known to be hypertensive prior to surgery, previous treatment is resumed.

Complications are treated as they occur. The commonest such problems are bleeding (which may require re-opening of the chest) and low cardiac output state (which may require inotropic support or intra-aortic balloon counterpulsation).

Pre-operative drug therapy for angina is not resumed, provided that the technical aspects of surgery are satisfactory.

At many centres, the post-operative use of aspirin, and sometimes also dipyridamole, is advised for the first 6–12 months to improve graft patency. It is particularly in the early months that such intervention may be of value. There is general agreement that aspirin (in low dosage of 80 or 100 mg/day) is of value, although the evidence for the effectiveness of dipyridamole is not clear.[62–65]

As atherosclerosis may progress in the native circulation and in the vein grafts, it is particularly important to modify any recognized risk factors, such as hyperlipidaemia, that may have been discovered in the pre-operative assessment.[66]

Post-operative wound discomfort, particularly discomfort or numbness related to the vein donor site, and general tiredness, weakness and breathlessness consequent on cardiopulmonary bypass usually take several weeks to clear. Occasionally sternal discomfort persists. In the absence of wound infection and failure of sternal union, such discomfort is often relieved by removal of the sternal wires. The sternum may fail to unite, particularly in the overweight patient, and especially when chest infection causes coughing and increased respiratory effort. The sternal wires may break or, more commonly, they cut through one-half of the divided sternum. Respiratory movements and lifting the arms or moving in bed become painful. Once the possibility of wound infection has been excluded, the sternum should be re-wired, placing new wires well round the sternum rather than through the bone. Long-term swelling of the ankles, in the absence of right heart failure, may be due to the removal of large sections of the saphenous system in the presence of venous disease or varicosities affecting the remaining veins. Prolonged use of support stockings may be helpful. Ideally, a programme of supervised graded physical training to regain physical fitness and restore confidence is desirable.

There is an incidence of major cerebral deficit following coronary surgery of about 1%,[67] manifesting itself as delay in regaining consciousness, stroke or fits. Among the more likely explanations are impaired perfusion during cardiopulmonary bypass in the presence of unsuspected cerebral arterial disease, cerebrovascular embolism of thrombus lining an akinetic area of left ventricular endocardium or cerebrovascular embolism of atheromatous material from the ascending aorta. However, in recent years, there has been concern about the more common finding of minor degrees of neuropsychiatric abnormality, presenting as difficulty in concentration, memory loss, depression or loss of intellectual skills.[68,69] Such findings are relatively common and may be transient. They are usually ascribed to the effects of cardiopulmonary bypass and are not specific to coronary surgery.

EARLY OUTCOME OF SURGERY IN ISCHAEMIC HEART DISEASE

The majority of surgical procedures for ischaemic heart disease have become routine and largely trouble-free. Death associated with coronary surgery is usually the consequence of failure of the myocardium to support a viable systemic circulation after operation (as a result of diffuse myocardial injury or segmental peri-operative myocardial infarction) or the consequence of cerebrovascular accident or cerebral injury. In current practice, haemorrhage, post-operative tamponade or dysrhythmia, respiratory insufficiency or infection, and other major sepsis are relatively infrequent causes of death. However, each of these may represent a risk to the surgical patient, whether complete recovery occurs or whether there is lasting morbidity or impaired prognosis as a consequence.

Risk factors for death, low output state and peri-operative infarction are relatively clearly defined for coronary surgery. Risk factors for other complications are well recognized, although often not as accurately defined, and include conditions such as diabetes mellitus, chronic bronchitis, chronic renal failure, cerebrovascular disease and peripheral vascular disease.

Mortality associated with coronary artery bypass surgery

Death associated with surgery is conventionally described as operative death, hospital death (usually defined as within 30 days of surgery) and late death.

Kirklin's group[70] has suggested that death is more logically regarded as a risk, or hazard function, that is constantly present, at a higher level in the immediate peri-operative period, and which persists for a considerable time after operation albeit at a decreasing level.

As is commonly the case with surgical practice, the results of surgery are often better in individual reported series (where operative mortality varies from 0 to 1 or 2%) than in large collected reviews or randomized trials. Thus, workers at the Cleveland Clinic reported[71] an operative mortality of 1.4% for 3540 patients receiving vein grafts for aortocoronary bypass during the period 1980–1982, and of 0.2% for 3565 patients receiving at least one internal mammary artery graft during the same period. An overall operative mortality of 2.2% was reported[72] in a series of 833 patients having internal mammary artery grafting alone or in combination with vein grafting between 1968 and 1981; however, when those having associated procedures performed, or those in NYHA class IV were excluded, the operative mortality for the remaining 750 patients was 0.4%. Five hundred patients having coronary artery bypass surgery with intermittent cross-clamping between 1983 and 1985 had a hospital mortality of 1%.[73]

A detailed report[74] on the results of coronary surgery in 7139 patients having surgery between August 1975 and December 1978 in 15 centres in the USA as part of a collaborative study—Coronary Artery Surgery Study (CASS)—has given good insight into the risk factors for coronary surgery.

The operative risk for each individual patient was estimated from the pooled operative experience for each of the participating centres. Comparison was then made between observed operative mortality (defined as death occurring after commencement of operation and before discharge from hospital) and the expected operative mortality. For the 6176 patients having isolated coronary artery bypass grafting, the overall hospital mortality was 2.3%. Although the actual operative mortality varied from 0.3 to 6.4%, calculation of the observed to expected mortality ratio suggested that the variation in actual mortality concealed an even greater variation in the risk between the best and poorest reported results. Thus, the techniques used and experience of workers at the centre have an influence on mortality risk, separate from the influence of risk to be anticipated by variation in patient characteristics.

Risk factors

In CASS, the most important patient characteristics predictive of an increased operative mortality for isolated coronary artery bypass surgery were age, female sex, severe left main coronary disease (defined as 90% or more stenosis) and poor left ventricular function.

Thus, for those under 60 years, overall operative mortality was 1.4%; for those over 60 years, it was 4.2%. Overall operative mortality for men was 1.8% and for women it was 4.5%.

The severity of coronary disease as defined by its distribution and degree of stenosis did have an influence on mortality from surgery, but the effect was most pronounced for left main coronary stenosis of > 50%, particularly where the left system was dominant. The operative mortality differed relatively little for one-vessel, two-vessel or three-vessel disease (1.4, 2.1 and 2.8%, respectively).

Indicators of poor left ventricular function, such as poor wall motion score, raised end-diastolic pressure or râles, were predictive of increased operative mortality. In this study, wall motion score was estimated and was shown to influence operative mortality from 1.7% with a score of normal to 9.1% with the poorest score for wall motion.

In CASS, operative mortality for patients with varying severity of angina differed little: for class I, II or III stable angina it was 1.7%; for those with class IV, it was 4.3%; for those with unstable angina, it was 3.5%.

Surgery on an emergency or urgent basis had a higher operative mortality than elective surgery (1.4% for elective surgery in 4190 men, and 3.8% for emergency or urgent surgery in 1007 men).

For UK practice for the 7-year period 1977 to 1982, the reported operative mortality for isolated coronary artery bypass surgery declined from 6.4% in 1977 to 3.2% in 1982,[75] suggesting that British practice by 1982 was achieving similar results to practice at the CASS centres a few years earlier in the USA.

There is little evidence to suggest that the risks are very different for contemporary surgery. There is even a possibility that results are generally less good now, because at many centres patients who are older and at greater risk have been accepted for surgery, and it may be argued that percutaneous transluminal angioplasty has removed from surgical practice some of the relatively better surgical risk patients.

Experience at the Cleveland Clinic from 1980 to

1982[71] showed that pre-operative congestive cardiac failure, female gender, emergency surgery, increasing age, abnormal electrocardiogram, incomplete revascularization and the use of veins only (rather than veins and internal mammary artery grafts) were incremental risk factors. It was possible to identify a low-risk group of 3538 patients (by excluding those requiring emergency surgery, females, those over 65 years of age, those with pre-operative congestive cardiac failure and those with incomplete revascularization) in whom operative mortality was 0.6% if vein grafts only were used and 0.1% if internal mammary grafts were included in their revascularization.

In an analysis[76] of 1980 patients having coronary artery bypass surgery between 1982 and 1984, female sex, pre-operative left ventricular ejection fraction and urgency of operation were identified as independent risk factors for operative mortality. Overall operative mortality was 3.5%. Patients undergoing urgent revascularization had an operative mortality of 8.5%. The highest predicted mortality (49%) was in women with an ejection fraction < 20% undergoing urgent surgery.

Based on surgical experience between 1976 and 1982 in 466 patients with ejection fractions < 40%, an operative survival rate of 89% was reported[77] in patients with ejection fractions from 20 to 39%, compared with an operative survival rate of only 63% for those whose ejection fractions were < 20%.

Peri-operative myocardial infarction

Peri-operative myocardial infarction is the most important complication of coronary artery bypass surgery: it is the usual cause of operative and early hospital death and low cardiac output state; it is associated with poorer long-term symptomatic outcome and survival. Schaff et al.[78] examined the influence of peri-operative myocardial infarction on late survival in 9777 patients having surgery between 1974 and 1979; 5.7% of the patients were diagnosed as having definite or probable myocardial infarction (the incidence did decrease during the period studied). Actuarial survival at 1, 3 and 5 years was significantly greater in patients without infarction (96, 94 and 90% versus 78, 74 and 69%).

The incidence of peri-operative myocardial infarction is difficult to assess because definition depends on the sensitivity of the methods used for diagnosis. In a study of 50 patients,[79] peri-operative infarction was diagnosed in 14% using a combination of serial electrocardiography, pre- and post-operative technetium scanning, gated radionuclide ventriculography and measurement of myocardial enzyme release. Fennel et al.[80] confirmed that a greater incidence of peri-operative infarction is found when multiple diagnostic techniques are used. They also showed that unstable angina was the only significant predictor for peri-operative infarction and peri-operative infarction was associated with significantly greater mortality.

Early reported experience suggested a peri-operative infarction rate of between 10 and 30%.[78] With advances in anaesthetic and peri-operative management and myocardial protective techniques, the rate is probably in the region of 5% in surgery for stable angina in current practice.[78]

Teoh et al.[76] showed that urgent revascularization in patients refractory to medical therapy for unstable angina carried a higher risk, reporting an overall incidence of peri-operative myocardial infarction of 8.6% in 1980 patients undergoing coronary surgery between 1982 and 1984.

As a general guide for contemporary practice, a hospital mortality of 1–2% or less should be attainable in males under 65 years of age, in whom left ventricular function is normal or near-normal and severe left main stenosis is not present. For females, the mortality may be twice this figure. With age above 65 years, and with poor left ventricular function, particularly in the presence of severe left main stenosis, mortality may be about 10% or more, depending on the severity of left ventricular dysfunction. When surgery is undertaken as an urgent or emergency procedure, the risk is increased.

Repeat operations

Repeat coronary surgery is being undertaken with increasing frequency. It has been estimated that about 7% of patients will require re-operation for graft failure or progression of native coronary disease within 10 years of primary operation.[81] Of the first 1000 patients undergoing revascularization between 1971 and 1978 at the Cleveland Clinic, 9.7% had re-operation at a mean of 6.9 years.[82]

Hospital mortality and morbidity are increased when compared with those for primary operations (5.3% versus 3.1% hospital mortality in the CASS experience).[83] An overall operative mortality of 3.4% for 1500 coronary re-operations undertaken between 1967 and 1984 has been reported from the

Cleveland Clinic. Left main stenosis, class III or IV symptoms, advanced age and incomplete revascularization were identified as predictors of increased hospital mortality.[84]

Left ventricular aneurysm resection

Surgery carries a higher mortality when angiographic evidence of left ventricular aneurysm is present. In the CASS experience,[85] 467 patients with angiographically documented left ventricular aneurysm had surgery (coronary artery bypass grafting with or without aneurysm resection) with an overall operative mortality of 7.9%. When bypass grafting alone was performed, mortality was 7%; when left ventricular aneurysm was resected in addition to bypass grafting, mortality was 9%, although the difference was not significant. This compares with the reported 2.4% overall operative mortality for patients undergoing coronary artery surgery in the entire CASS registry.

The functional status of residual left ventricular muscle not involved in the aneurysm has predictive value in determining hospital mortality for surgery.[86,87]

A 15% hospital death rate was reported by Barratt-Boyes et al. for a series of 113 patients over a 13-year experience.[88] Poor NYHA class, severe congestive heart failure and extensive coronary disease increased the risk of hospital death.

A review of 244 patients operated on for left ventricular aneurysm between 1971 and 1980[27] showed a hospital mortality of 10.6%. When left ventricular aneurysmectomy was combined with operations on the heart valves, or with closure of ventricular septal defect, the hospital mortality was 20%. Workers at the Cleveland Clinic have reported a hospital mortality for the period 1972–1976 of 3.3% for left ventricular aneurysmectomy alone, and 3.8% when combined with coronary artery grafting.[89] Jatene[55] has reported a hospital mortality in 214 patients having conventional left ventricular aneurysmectomy of 11.6%; this decreased to 4.3% in a more recent group of 508 patients having reconstruction to restore a more normal left ventricular geometry, and isolated left ventricular aneurysmectomy carried a 2.3% hospital mortality compared with 5.0% when concomitant revascularization was required.

Closure of post-infarction ventricular septal defect

Hospital mortality has been shown to depend on the urgency with which surgery is required, reflecting the clinical state of the patient. In the Stanford experience, there was a hospital mortality of 35% if surgery was required within 3 weeks of infarction and of 7% if surgery could be deferred beyond 3 weeks.[90] Daggett et al[91] reported an operative mortality of 25% in patients undergoing surgery since 1975.

Replacement of mitral valve for papillary muscle rupture

The clinical condition of patients with papillary muscle rupture is usually very poor and hence surgery carries considerable risk. It is a rare complication; reports of surgical experience are sparse, and often comprise only a small number of patients. However, 81% hospital survival (13 of 16 patients) has been reported for mitral valve replacement in such patients by Killen et al. (with 75% actuarial 5-year survival)[92] who suggest early diagnosis followed by prompt surgical intervention to be the most appropriate and beneficial therapy.

SYMPTOMATIC RESULTS OF CORONARY ARTERY BYPASS SURGERY

Angina is the usual symptom for which coronary artery bypass surgery is undertaken, and symptomatic benefit is therefore most frequently measured in terms of angina-free status. This is inevitably a subjective assessment and is influenced by drug therapy, patient expectations and modifications in lifestyle that an event such as surgery may initiate.

Other measures of symptomatic improvement are even more difficult to assess. Return to work, reduction in anxiety, improved mood and increased family, sexual and job satisfaction have all been used as indicators of symptomatic benefit from coronary surgery, but the results are sometimes conflicting, difficult to evaluate and influenced by too many factors to be able to draw unequivocal conclusions easily.[93-98]

It is widely recognized that surgery offers the most effective treatment for severe angina and that symptomatic results of surgery are generally very good, with 60–80% of patients being symptom-free after surgery, at least for the first few years, and most of the remainder being improved.[99-102] Furthermore, reported results from individual series, as is commonly the case with surgical results, are generally better than those of randomized studies.

The European prospective randomized study of coronary surgery in stable angina (based on practice of 1973–1976 in 768 men)[103] showed that the surgically allocated group had 56% of patients with 'mild' angina and 44% with 'moderately severe' angina. At 1 year, 83% of the surgical group were improved and 58% were angina-free; in the medically allocated group, 45% were improved and 14% were angina-free at 1 year. Twenty-two per cent of the surgical and 76% of the medical group were receiving beta-blocking drug treatment at 1 year.

Influence of age

Although hospital mortality has been shown to be a little higher in those over 65 years, extremely satisfactory symptomatic results can be obtained. A non-randomized study from the CASS registry[104] of 1491 patients 65 years of age or over indicated that improvement of angina by surgery was comparable to results achieved in younger patients.

Influence of gender

Reported hospital mortality for coronary artery bypass surgery is higher in women than in men.[105–108] Symptomatic benefit from surgery would also appear to be poorer in women. A report[106] of 1089 patients having primary elective coronary surgery between 1978 and 1985 indicated that 5-year event-free survival (absence of cardiac death, absence of myocardial infarction and absence of recurrent angina) was 67% for men and 43% for women.

While reporting similar 5- and 10-year survival rates (90.6% and 78.6%, respectively, for women; 93% and 78.2%, respectively, for men), workers at the Cleveland Clinic noted lower overall graft patency rates in women after a mean interval of 2 years (76.4% compared with 82.1% in men), and poorer symptomatic benefit (60.5% compared with 71.5% of men free of angina at 5 years).[105]

Influence of poor ventricular function

Symptomatic improvement in angina is also seen in those with poor left ventricular function undergoing surgery, although it would appear that the poor long-term survival when ejection fraction is < 20% limits lasting improvement to those with ejection fractions between 20 and 40%.[77]

Repeat coronary surgery

The symptomatic status of patients following re-operation is generally not as favourable as that for patients following primary surgery. In the Cleveland Clinic experience, only about half of the survivors of re-operation were symptom-free beyond 5 years, although very few of those with recurrent angina had more than mild symptoms up to 10 years after re-operation.[84]

Adequacy of revascularization

If coronary artery bypass surgery is undertaken in a technically satisfactory manner, with appropriately placed grafts achieving restoration of normal myocardial perfusion at rest and on exercise, there is every reason to expect that angina will be abolished. Recurrence of angina is then dependent on graft occlusion and progression of disease in the coronary arteries, both of which are known to occur.

Post-operative symptomatic status is well recognized to correlate with the adequacy of revascularization and graft patency. Thus, Cukingnan et al.[108] showed in a study of 83 patients at 1 year after surgery that there was an overall patency rate of 86% and that 71% of patients were asymptomatic. Complete revascularization resulted in a higher rate of symptomatic improvement than incomplete revascularization, and better patency rate was associated with greater symptom relief. Lavee et al.[109] showed that of 366 patients who had coronary surgery in 1980–1982, 120 had incomplete segmental revascularization with a mean of 3.4 grafts per patient and at just over 1 year after surgery 54% were totally free from symptoms. Two hundred and forty-six had complete segmental revascularization with a mean of 4.0 grafts per patient and 68% were totally free from symptoms at a similar post-operative interval.

Graft patency

When used as an aortocoronary bypass conduit, vein patency has been shown to decrease with time.[110,111] It has been estimated that there is a 7–15% early closure rate (within 6 months) due to thrombosis, thereafter a 2% per year attrition rate until the seventh year, followed by a 5% per year attrition rate from the seventh to the twelfth year. Only 38–45% of vein grafts are reported to be open with a normal appearance at 10 years. Progression of disease in the native coronary arteries has also been noted and contributes to increasing recurrence of angina in the post-operative period.[110] In a study of 1179 vein grafts,[111] occlusion was shown in 10% at 1 month, in 17% at 1 year and in 26% at 5 years. A normal angiographic appearance at 1 year had no prognostic value for findings at 5 years. Grondin's group[110] has reported vein patency rates of 76.4% at 1 year and of 52.8% at 10 years.

All longer term reports reflect the progression of graft and native vessel disease in recurrence of angina. The Texas Heart Institute series[112] of 22 284 patients undergoing surgery from 1970 to 1981 showed actuarial freedom from angina at 3 years after coronary surgery to be 67.4%, but only 35.4% at 10 years.

Endarterectomy

It is recognized that grafting to an endarterectomized coronary artery is less satisfactory than grafting to an undisturbed distal vessel. Workers at most centres report peri-operative infarction to be more common when endarterectomy has been performed—twice as high as for routine bypass grafting in the experience of one centre.[45] Shumway's group[46] has documented distal right coronary endarterectomy to be associated with a greater probability of peri-operative myocardial infarction than grafting to unendarterectomized vessels (16 versus 8% incidence). Overall survival rates and long-term functional results in their experience did not differ.

Patency rates of grafts to endarterectomized segments are probably not as good, although Keon[45] reports 85% patency at a mean follow-up of just over 1 year. Kamath et al.[49] have reported early patency of grafts to endarterectomized arteries to be 87.3% compared with 91.1% for conventional vein grafts in the same patients and they showed a very low peri-operative infarction rate. Yacoub's group has reported early patency rates of grafts to endarterectomized vessels to be 85%, with 77% patency after 1 year.[47] They have reported endarterectomy of the left coronary system to have similar patency rates to the endarterectomized right coronary system and to be associated with a peri-operative myocardial infarction rate of 12%.[48]

Internal mammary artery grafting

A report from the Cleveland Clinic[113] highlighted a growing body of opinion[114–117] regarding the superiority of the internal mammary artery as a conduit for coronary surgery, which has been reported to have a patency rate at 7–10 years of 85–95% when used as a conduit for coronary revascularization. In the Cleveland Clinic report, 2306 patients who had an internal mammary artery used as one of the conduits for revascularization were compared with 3625 patients who had only saphenous vein used as the conduit. There was a better outlook for the patients in whom internal mammary artery was used, reflected in a better 10-year actuarial survival (93.4 compared with 88%); in those having only vein conduits, there was a greater risk of death (1.61 times greater), a greater risk of late myocardial infarction (1.41 times greater), a greater risk of hospitalization (1.25 times greater), a greater risk of cardiac re-operation (2.0 times greater—an indicator of symptomatic status) and a greater risk of all late cardiac events (1.27 times greater). The striking difference in late development of atherosclerosis in internal mammary artery conduits and saphenous vein conduits is now well recognized and the Cleveland Clinic report provides evidence that this difference does translate into differences in late clinical course, for both symptomatic status and survival.

Exercise tolerance

Patients treated by coronary artery bypass grafting can usually be shown to be able to increase their exercise capacity to a level greater than that before surgery.[103,118,119] The rate–pressure product, duration of exercise, maximum heart rate response and incidence of ischaemic electrocardiographic changes have all been shown to improve after successful surgery.[120,121] Good correlation has been shown between adequacy of revascularization and exercise achievement and electrocardiographic response.[122–124]

Left ventricular function

Revascularization surgery can be expected to improve ischaemic myocardial dysfunction, but to have no effect on myocardial dysfunction due to scar. There is also the possibility of peri-operative myocardial infarction impairing left ventricular function. Thus, little change in resting levels for left ventricular end-diastolic pressure or ejection fraction is reported.[125] However, significant improvements have been reported in left ventricular function during exercise, particularly when myocardial scarring is minimal and revascularization and graft patency are satisfactory.[126,127] Lim et al.[128] demonstrated a fall in left ventricular ejection fraction from 60 to 53% on exercise before surgery, and an increase from 60 to 63% after surgery. In addition, a higher workload and rate–pressure product were achieved. Rankin's[129] group in a study of 149 patients having pre- and post-operative left ventriculography showed that reversible ischaemic myocardial dysfunction appeared to be common in those having coronary artery bypass grafting. They report improved regional wall motion after successful revascularization in 40% of their patients who had unstable angina and 34% in those with stable angina. They also showed that left ventricular aneurysm resection significantly enhanced left ventricular performance.

Myocardial perfusion studies

Since the theoretical aim of revascularization surgery is to restore homogeneous myocardial perfusion at rest and on exercise, it is to be expected that successful surgery would result in normal perfusion being demonstrable to viable myocardium. The presence of normal or improved scintigraphic myocardial imaging appearance is usually associated with patent grafts.[130–132]

LATE SURVIVAL FOLLOWING CORONARY ARTERY BYPASS SURGERY

Evidence of the influence of coronary surgery on long-term survival is based on past practice, and both medical and surgical practice continue to evolve. The achievement of greater diagnostic precision, better peri-operative management and more complete and lasting revascularization, particularly by more frequent use of the internal mammary artery as a conduit, may reasonably be expected to result in better late surgical outcome in the future. Indeed, improved early and late survival has been documented for more recent practice when compared with earlier practice,[112,133] although at least one major recent study has failed to demonstrate any important differences with increasing experience for the period from 1970 to 1980.[134]

Randomized prospective clinical trials comparing medical and surgical management of coronary disease have given some insight into the potential impact of surgery on the disease. However, these trials apply to limited groups of patients, are based on early and possibly less effective practice and their interpretation has often caused controversy.

The extent and distribution of coronary disease, and the functional state of the left ventricle, are major determinants of survival, both in unoperated and in operated patients. The interpretation of survival data from natural history studies is complex, and requires consideration of lead-time bias, referral bias and incidence–prevalence bias.[135,136] In addition, the presence of severe angina, which presumably reflects the physiological impact of anatomically demonstrable disease, the presence of electrocardiographic evidence of exercise-induced ischaemia and poor exercise tolerance are adverse prognostic factors.[137–141]

In the *European Prospective Randomized Study* of patients with mild-to-moderate angina and good left ventricular function, the outcome in 394 patients allocated to surgical management was compared with that in 373 patients allocated to medical management.[96]

It was shown that three-vessel disease (defined as > 75% obstruction) was associated with an 8-year survival of 73% in the medical group and of 91% in the surgical group. Surgery conferred a survival benefit in those with three-vessel disease and in those with two-vessel disease where one of the vessels was the proximal anterior descending artery. Eight-year survival in surgically managed patients with three-vessel disease was at least as good as that of patients with less extensive disease regardless of its management.[96]

The *Veterans Administrative Cooperative Study* of a group of male patients treated between 1972 and 1974 included 91 patients with left main coronary stenosis of 50% or greater; 2-year survival in this group was 71% for medically allocated and 92% for surgically allocated patients.[142] There is general agreement now that survival in patients with left main coronary disease is poor with medical management, and survival with surgical treatment is comparable to survival for three-vessel disease with surgical management.

The *Coronary Artery Surgery Registry* contains data on 24 959 patients.

In 12 778 patients treated medically, 5-year survival for one-, two- and three-vessel disease was 89, 82 and 63%, respectively.[143]

Five-year survival for 8971 surgically treated patients in the CASS registry for one-, two- and three-vessel disease was 93, 92 and 88%, respectively.[144] As with unoperated coronary disease, survival in these surgically treated patients was influenced by the functional state of the left ventricle. Those with normal or near-normal left ventricular function had a 5-year survival of 92%, those with moderate impairment 80%, and those with poor ventricular function 65%.

A more recent study[145] of 13 476 patients from the Coronary Artery Surgery Study registry showed 5-year survival free of sudden death to be 94% for medically treated patients and 98% for surgically treated patients. Reduction in risk of sudden death by surgical treatment was most pronounced in high-risk patients.

The much smaller group of 780 patients randomized to either medical or surgical management in the *Coronary Artery Surgery Study* showed no significant difference in 5-year survival, regardless of the extent of disease.[146,147] The estimated annual mortality rate in patients allocated to medical therapy was 1.6% and in those allocated to surgical therapy was 1.1%. This indicates that the randomization was made in a group of patients who had an inherently good prognosis and it may not represent the majority of patients.

Indeed, evidence of the importance of severity of angina at commencement of treatment in determining subsequent survival, is provided by a study of 4209 patients from the CASS registry[148] in which 5-year survival is compared for different symptomatic categories. In those with Class I and Class II angina and normal left ventricular function, 5-year survival was 93% or greater, regardless of the extent of coronary involvement or the method of treatment. Five-year survival of surgically treated patients with class III or IV angina and normal left ventricular function was similar (92% or greater) regardless of the number of vessels involved. Five-year survival in medically treated patients with class III or IV angina and normal left ventricular function was poorer (74% with three-vessel disease). When left ventricular function was abnormal, those with three-vessel disease and class III or IV angina had a 5-year survival of 82% in the surgical group and of 52% in the medical group.

Reports from a number of other centres show broadly similar results for late outcome for coronary surgery.[112,123,133,134,149,150] It would appear that the prognosis for survival following coronary artery surgery in present practice is generally very good. Symptomatic status and functional state of the left ventricle are important indicators of prognosis in those who have had coronary surgery. The number of diseased vessels bypassed has little influence on long-term outcome. For patients with three-vessel disease and good left ventricular function, 5-year survival might be expected to be in the vicinity of 90% and 10-year survival 50–75%.

Prognosis would also appear to be satisfactory in those over 65 years of age.[104] Rahimtoola et al.[151] have shown 5- and 10-year survival rates for those aged 65 years and older to be 81 and 65%, respectively, in a study of 1304 patients aged between 65 and 84 years. They concluded from their experience that immediate and long-term results of coronary artery bypass surgery in these patients are similar to those seen in younger patient groups. Both immediate and long-term results are not quite as favourable for women as for men.[105,106]

Influence of graft conduit fate on survival

Saphenous veins are subject to progressive intimal proliferation and occlusion when used as conduits for coronary surgery.[110,111] The contrasting observation of excellent late patency of the internal mammary artery when used as a conduit for coronary surgery—a patency at 7–10 years of 85–95%—prompted a review of experience at the Cleveland Clinic.[113] Comparison was made between 2306 patients receiving an internal mammary graft to the anterior descending artery alone or in combination with other saphenous vein grafts, and 3625 patients who had only saphenous vein grafts. Ten-year actuarial survival (excluding hospital deaths) was 86.6% in those receiving an internal mammary graft and 75.9% in those receiving only saphenous vein grafts; in patients with single-vessel disease, 10-year survival was 93.4 and 88%, respectively; for patients with two-vessel disease 10-year survival was 90 and 79.5%, respectively; for those with three-vessel disease it was 82.6 and 71%, respectively. The use of the internal mammary artery graft was associated also with a higher actuarial freedom from late myocardial infarction, hospitalization for cardiac causes and cardiac re-operation.

These findings are supported by those of Green's group[152] in their 15-year follow-up of 748 consecutive patients having coronary bypass procedures; 532 patients had bypass grafting with either one or two internal mammary artery grafts (with or without additional saphenous vein grafts) and they were compared with 216 patients having saphenous vein grafts alone. Those having internal mammary grafts were shown to have better cumulative survival (72% at 14 years compared with 57% in those having vein grafts only), lower early recurrence of angina, fewer myocardial infarctions, fewer reoperations and better event-free survival. The 38 patients having double internal mammary grafts had the best late results.

Late results following ventricular aneurysmectomy

Best results are obtained when there is only disease of the anterior descending artery and the myocardium (apart from the aneurysm) is normal. Such patients can be expected to be relieved of angina or symptoms of left ventricular failure in the great majority of instances. A 7-year survival of 69% has been reported for those with one-vessel disease having aneurysmectomy only, of 65% for those with multiple-vessel disease having aneurysmectomy and complete revascularization and of 51% for those with multiple-vessel disease having aneurysmectomy but being incompletely revascularized. Incomplete revascularization and preoperative congestive heart failure were identified as adversely influencing long-term survival.[89]

In Olearchyk's series,[27] an actuarial 10-year survival of 69% is reported for the 218 patients having left ventricular aneurysmectomy combined with coronary bypass grafting. In the 26 patients having aneurysmectomy alone (either because the left anterior descending artery alone was involved or because other vessels were not considered graftable), actuarial survival at 10 years was 56.8%.

Of 1161 patients with angiographically documented left ventricular aneurysm from the CASS registry, 6-year survival in those treated medically was similar to 6-year survival in those treated surgically (67 and 69%, respectively). However, the definition of aneurysm used in this report included any protrusion from the expected angiographic outline of the ventricular chamber displaying either akinesis or dyskinesis. This would encompass 'functional aneurysms' and areas of partial thickness scar. Thus, as a group, the patients reported in this study are not directly comparable to groups reported in most surgical series. The report did show that surgical therapy conferred improved survival on those patients with three-vessel disease who were in subgroups at moderate and high risk.[85]

In the series reported by Barratt-Boyes,[88] significant right coronary stenosis and severely impaired contractility of the postero-basal segment were predictors of late death. An 8-year actuarial survival of 45% is reported for this series.

Excellent late survival is reported for the operation proposed by Jatene,[55] which aims to conserve normal left ventricular geometry: late mortality in 508 patients operated on between 1977 and 1983 is reported as 3.5%.

Late results for repair following ischaemic myocardial disruption

Patients surviving surgery for post-infarction ventricular septal defect have relatively good long-term survival. Eighteen of the 28 patients treated since 1975 in the Massachussetts General Hospital are reported to be long-term survivors, 7 of whom are in NYHA class I, 8 are in class II and 3 are in class III.[58] Gaudiani et al. have reported a 5-year actuarial survival of 88% for hospital survivors in their series.[90]

Long-term outlook for survivors of mitral valve replacement for ischaemic papillary muscle rupture has also been reported to be good. Results are dependent on the status of left ventricular function. A 5-year actuarial survival of 75% has been reported following surgery for ischaemic papillary muscle rupture.[92]

CONCLUSION

Although modern techniques of surgery for ischaemic heart disease have only been developed over the past two decades, surgery now has a well-established role. The indications for surgery, its associated hazards and the results to be expected are well defined. Interventions such as percutaneous transluminal coronary angioplasty and more widespread use of internal mammary artery conduits for revascularization are likely to have a beneficial impact in the future, expanding further the role of intervention and improving the outcome for patients with coronary disease. Although the optimal management for acute myocardial infarction is not yet established, techniques for active intervention are promising.

Surgery should be regarded as only one of the options available in the management of patients with manifestations of coronary disease. Rational and effective application of surgery requires consideration of all the available therapeutic options by cardiologist and surgeon, with continuing reassessment of the outcome, and evaluation of new methods of treatment as they become available.

REFERENCES

1. Vansant, J.H. and Muller, W.H. Jr. Surgical procedures to revascularize the heart. A review of the literature. *Am. J. Surg.* 1960; **100**: 572.

2. Sones, F.M. Jr and Shirey, E.K. Cine coronary arteriography. *Mod. Conc. Cardiovasc. Dis.* 1962; **31**: 735.

3. Effler, D.B., Favaloro, R.G. and Groves, L.K. Coronary artery surgery utilizing saphenous vein graft techniques. Clinical experience with 224 operations. *J. Thorac. Cardiovasc. Surg.* 1970; **59**: 147.

4. Johnson, W.D., Flemma, R.J., Lepley, D. Jr and Ellison, E.H. Extended treatment of severe coronary artery disease: a total surgical approach. *Ann. Surg.* 1969; **170**: 460.

5. Cooley, D.A., Dawson, J.T., Hallman, G.L. *et al.* Aortocoronary saphenous vein bypass: Results in 1492 patients, with particular reference to patients with complicating features. *Ann. Thorac. Surg.* 1973; **16**: 380.

6. Green, G.E., Stertzer, S.H. and Reppert, E.H. Coronary arterial bypass grafts. *Ann. Thorac. Surg.* 1968; **5**: 443.

7. Cooley, D.A. and DeBakey, M.E. Surgical considerations of intrathoracic aneurysms of aorta and great vessels. *Ann. Surg.* 1952; **135**: 660.

8. Cooley, D.A., Belmonte, B.A., Zeis, L.B. and Schur, S. Surgical repair of ruptured interventricular septum following acute myocardial infarction. *Surgery* 1957; **42**: 930.

9. Austen, W.G., Sanders, C.A., Averill, J.H. and Friedlich, A.L. Ruptured papillary muscle. *Circulation* 1965; **32**: 597.

10. Rutkow, I.M. Thoracic and cardiovascular operations in the United States, 1979 to 1984. *J. Thorac. Cardiovasc. Surg.* 1986; **92**: 181.

11. Anonymous. Consensus development conference: coronary artery bypass grafting (Editorial). *Br. Med. J.* 1984; **289**: 1527.

12. Manley, J.C. Indications for surgery. In: Wheatley, D.J. ed. *Surgery of coronary artery disease.* London: Chapman and Hall, 1986, p. 209.

13. Braunwald, E. The aggressive treatment of acute myocardial infarction. *Circulation* 1985; **71**: 1087.

14. Phillips, S.J. Intervention in acute ischaemia: surgery in evolving acute infarction. In: Wheatley, D.J. ed. *Surgery of coronary artery disease.* London: Chapman and Hall, 1986, p. 489.

15. Phillips, S.J., Kongtahworn, C., Zeff, R.H. *et al.* Emergency coronary artery revascularisation: A possible therapy for acute myocardial infarction. *Circulation* 1979; **60**: 241.

16. Berg, R. Jr, Selinger, S.L., Leonard, J.J., Grunwald, G.P. and O'Grady, W.P. Immediate coronary artery bypass for acute evolving myocardial infarction. *J. Thorac. Cardiovasc. Surg.* 1981; **81**: 493.

17. Kirklin, J.K., Blackstone, E.H., Zorn, G.L. *et al.* Intermediate-term results of coronary artery bypass grafting for acute myocardial infarction. *Circulation* 1985; **72**(Suppl. II): II–175.

18. Rentrop, K.P. Thrombolytic therapy in patients with acute myocardial infarction. *Circulation* 1985; **71**: 627.

19. Schuster, E.H. and Bulkley, B.H. Early postinfarction angina: Ischemia at a distance and ischemia in the infarct zone. *N. Engl. J. Med.* 1981; **305**: 1101.

20. Fudge, T.L., Harrington, O.B., Crosby, V.G. *et al.* Coronary artery bypass after recent myocardial infarction. *Arch. Surg.* 1982; **117**: 1418.

21. Williams, D.B., Ivey, T.D., Bailey, W.W. *et al.* Postinfarction angina: Results of early revascularization. *J. Am. Coll. Cardiol.* 1983; **2**: 859.

22. Jones, E.L., Waits, T.F., Craver, J.M. *et al.* Coronary bypass for relief of persistent pain following acute myocardial infarction. *Ann. Thorac. Surg.* 1981; **32**: 33.

23. DiSesa, V.J., O'Neil, A.C., Bitran, D., Cohn, L.H., Shemin, R.J. and Collins, J.J. Jr. Aggressive surgical management of post-infarction angina: Results of myocardial revascularization early after transmural infarction. *Texas Heart Inst. J.* 1985; **12**: 333.

24. Hochberg, M.S., Parsonnet, V., Gielchinsky, I., Hussain, S.M., Fisch, D.A. and Norman, J.C. Timing of coronary revascularization after acute myocardial infarction. Early and late results in patients revascularized within seven weeks. *J. Thorac. Cardiovasc. Surg.* 1984; **88**: 914.

25. Rogers, W.J., Smith, L.R., Oberman, A. *et al.* Surgical vs nonsurgical management of patients after myocardial infarction. *Circulation* 1980; **62**(Suppl. I): I–67.

26. Hanson, E.C. and Daggett, W.M. Surgery for the complications of myocardial infarction. In: Wheatley, D.J., ed. *Surgery of coronary artery disease.* London: Chapman and Hall, 1986, p. 503.

27. Olearchyk, A.S., Lemole, G.M. and Spagna, P.M. Left ventricular aneurysm. Ten years' experience in surgical treatment of 244 cases. Improved clinical status, hemodynamics, and long-term longevity. *J. Thorac. Cardiovasc. Surg.* 1984; **88**: 544.

28. Cox, J.L. The status of surgery for cardiac arrhythmias (Editorial). *Circulation* 1985; **71**: 413.

29. Reul, G.J., Cooley, D.A., Hallman, G.L. *et al.* Coronary artery bypass for unsuccessful percutaneous transluminal coronary angioplasty. *J. Thorac. Cardiovasc. Surg.* 1984; **88**: 685.

30. Page, U.S., Okies, J.E., Colburn, L.Q., Bigelow, J.C., Salomon, N.W. and Krause, A.H. Percutaneous transluminal coronary angioplasty. A growing surgical problem. *J. Thorac. Cardiovasc. Surg.* 1986; **92**: 847.

31. Jones, E.L., Kaplan, J.A., Dorney, E.R. *et al.* Propranolol therapy in patients undergoing myocardial revascularization. *Am. J. Cardiol.* 1976; **38**: 696.

32. Hardarson, T., Henning, H. and O'Rourke, R.A. Prolonged salutary effects of isosorbide dinitrate and nitroglycerin ointment on regional left ventricular function. *Am. J. Cardiol.* 1977; **40**: 90.

33. Campbell, D. and Macdonald, D.J.F. Preoperative management and anaesthesia for coronary artery surgery. In: Wheatley, D.J. ed. *Surgery of coronary artery disease.* London: Chapman and Hall, 1986, p. 247.

34. Green, G.E. Technique of internal mammary–coronary artery anastomosis. *J. Thorac. Cardiovasc. Surg.* 1979; **78**: 455.

35. Loop, F.D. Technique for performance of internal mammary artery–coronary artery anastomosis. *J. Thorac. Cardiovasc. Surg.* 1979; **78**: 460.

36. Culliford, A.T. and Spencer, F.C. Guidelines for safely opening a previous sternotomy incision. *J. Thorac. Cardiovasc. Surg.* 1979; **78**: 633.

37. Keon, W.J., Heggtveit, H.A. and Leduc, J.B. Perioperative myocardial infarction caused by atherothromboembolism. *J. Thorac. Cardiovasc. Surg.* 1982; **84**: 849.

38. Sethia, B., Wheatley, D.J. and Taylor, K.M. Short review: The current status of cardiopulmonary bypass. *Life Support Systems* 1983; **1**: 271.

39. Weisel, R.D., Hoy, F.B.Y., Baird, R.J. *et al.* Comparison of alternative cardioplegic techniques. *J. Thorac. Cardiovasc. Surg.* 1983; **86**: 97.

40. Hearse, D.J., Braimbridge, M.V. and Jynge, P. *Protection of the ischemic myocardium: Cardioplegia.* New York: Raven Press, 1981.

41. Goor, D.A., Mohr, R. and Lavee, J. Enhanced protection of myocardial function by systemic deep hypothermia during cardioplegic arrest in multiple coronary bypass grafting. *J. Thorac. Cardiovasc. Surg.* 1982; **84**: 237.

42. Brower, R.W., Van Bijk, K.F., Spek, J. and Bos, E. Sequential versus conventional coronary artery bypass

graft surgery in matched patient groups. *Thorac. Cardiovasc. Surg.* 1981; **29**: 158.

43. Tector, A.J., Schmahl, T.M., Canino, V.R., Kallies, J.R. and Sanfilippo, D. The role of the sequential internal mammary artery graft in coronary surgery. *Circulation* 1984; **70**(Suppl. I) I–222.

44. Kamath, M.L., Matysik, L.S., Schmidt, D.H. and Smith, L.L. Sequential internal mammary artery grafts. Expanded utilization of an ideal conduit. *J. Thorac. Cardiovasc. Surg.* 1985; **89**: 163.

45. Keon, W.J. Manual coronary endarterectomy and revascularization: Improving techniques and results. *Ann. Thorac. Surg.* 1981; **32**: 427.

46. Miller, D.C., Stinson, E.B., Oyer, P.E. et al. Long-term clinical assessment of the efficacy of adjunctive coronary endarterectomy. *J. Thorac. Cardiovasc. Surg.* 1981; **81**: 21.

47. Halim, M.A., Qureshi, S.A., Towers, M.K. and Yacoub, M.H. Early and late results of combined endarterectomy and coronary bypass grafting for diffuse coronary disease. *Am. J. Cardiol.* 1982; **49**: 1623.

48. Qureshi, S.A., Halim, M.A., Smith, P. and Yacoub, M.H. Endarterectomy of the left coronary system. Analysis of a 10 year experience. *J. Thorac. Cardiovasc. Surg.* 1985; **89**: 852.

49. Kamath, M.L., Schmidt, D.H., Pedraza, P.M. et al. Patency and flow response in endarterectomized coronary arteries. *Ann. Thorac. Surg.* 1981; **31**: 28.

50. Johnston, J.B., Lamb, A.C. and Wright, J.S. Ventricular aneurysm after infarction. Pathological and surgical features. *J. Thorac. Cardiovasc. Surg.* 1969; **58**: 14.

51. Cabin, H.S. and Roberts, W.C. Left ventricular aneurysm, intra-aneurysmal thrombus and systemic embolus in coronary heart disease. *Chest* 1980; **77**: 586.

52. Schlichter, J., Hellerstein, H.K. and Katz, L.N. Aneurysm of heart: correlative study of 102 proved cases. *Medicine* 1984; **33**: 43.

53. Bruschke, A.V., Proudfit, W.L. and Sones, F.M. Jr. Progress study of 590 consecutive non-surgical cases of coronary disease followed five–nine years. II. Ventriculographic and other correlations. *Circulation* 1973; **47**: 1154.

54. Cosgrove, D.M. and Loop, F.D. Ventricular aneurysm. In: Wheatley, D.J. ed. *Surgery of coronary artery disease.* London: Chapman and Hall, 1986, p. 449.

55. Jatene, A.D. Left ventricular aneurysmectomy. Resection or reconstruction. *J. Thorac. Cardiovasc. Surg.* 1985; **89**: 331.

56. Rittenhouse, E.A., Sauvage, L.R., Mansfield, P.B. et al. False aneurysm of the left ventricle. Report of four cases and review of surgical management. *Ann. Surg.* 1979; **189**: 409.

57. Radford, M.J., Johnson, R.A. and Daggett, W.M. Ventricular septal rupture: A review of clinical and physiologic features and an analysis of survival. *Circulation* 1981; **64**: 545.

58. Heitmiller, R., Jacobs, M.L. and Daggett, W.M. Surgical management of postinfarction ventricular septal rupture. *Ann. Thorac. Surg.* 1986; **41**: 683.

59. Gahl, K., Sutton, R., Pearson, M., Caspari, P., Lairet, A. and McDonald, L. Mitral regurgitation in coronary heart disease. *Br. Heart J.* 1977; **39**: 13.

60. Hinds, C.J. Current management of patients after cardiopulmonary bypass. *Anaesthesia* 1982; **37**: 170.

61. Kirklin, J.K. and Kirklin, J.W. Management of the cardiovascular subsystem after cardiac surgery. *Ann. Thorac. Surg.* 1981; **32**: 311.

62. Chesebro, J.H., Clements, I.P., Fuster, V. et al. A platelet-inhibitor drug trial in coronary artery bypass operations. Benefit of perioperative dipyridamole and aspirin therapy on early postoperative vein graft patency. *N. Engl. J. Med.* 1982; **307**: 74.

63. Mayer, J.E. Jr, Lindsay, W.G., Castaneda, W. and Nicoloff, D.M. Influence of aspirin and dipyridamole on patency of coronary artery bypass grafts. *Ann. Thorac. Surg.* 1981; **31**: 204.

64. Pirk, J., Vojacek, J., Kovac, J., Fabian, J. and Firt, P. Improved patency of the aortocoronary bypass by anti-thrombotic drugs. *Ann. Thorac. Surg.* 1986; **42**: 312.

65. Brown, B.G., Cukingnan, R.A., DeRouen, T. et al. Improved graft patency in patients treated with platelet-inhibiting therapy after coronary bypass surgery. *Circulation* 1985; **72**: 138.

66. Campeau, L., Enjalbert, M., Lesperance, J. et al. The relation of risk factors to the development of atherosclerosis in saphenous-vein bypass grafts and the progression of disease in the native circulation. A study 10 years after aortocoronary bypass surgery. *N. Engl. J. Med.* 1984; **311**: 1329.

67. Bojar, R.M., Najafi, H., DeLaria, G.A., Serry, C. and Goldin, M.D. Neurological complications of coronary revascularization. *Ann. Thorac. Surg.* 1983; **36**: 427.

68. Treasure, T. Cerebral complications of cardiac surgery (Comment). *Current Medical Literature—Cardiovascular Medicine* 1985; **4**: 33.

69. Shaw, P.J., Bates, D., Cartlidge, N.E.F. et al. Long-term intellectual dysfunction following coronary artery bypass graft surgery: A six month follow-up study. *Q. J. Med.* 1987; **62**: 259.

70. Blackstone, E.H. and Kirklin, J.W. Death and other time-related events after valve replacement. *Circulation* 1985; **72**: 753.

71. Cosgrove, D.M., Loop, F.D., Lytle, B.W. et al. Does mammary artery grafting increase surgical risk? *Circulation* 1985; **72**(Suppl. II): II–170.

72. Olearchyk, A.S. and Magovern, G.J. Internal mammary artery grafting. Clinical results, patency rates, and long-term survival in 833 patients. *J. Thorac. Cardiovasc. Surg.* 1986; **92**: 1082.

73. Bonchek, L.I. and Burlingame, M.W. Coronary artery bypass without cardioplegia. *J. Thorac. Cardiovasc. Surg.* 1987; **93**: 261.

74. Kennedy, J.W., Kaiser, G.C., Fisher, L.D. et al. Multivariate discriminant analysis of the clinical and angiographic predictors of operative mortality from the Collaborative Study in Coronary Artery Surgery (CASS). *J. Thorac. Cardiovasc. Surg.* 1980; **80**: 876.

75. English, T.A.H., Bailey, A.R., Dark, J.F. and Williams, W.G. The UK Cardiac Surgical Register, 1977–1982. *Br. Med. J.* 1984; **289**: 1205.

76. Teoh, K.H., Christakis, G.T., Weisel, R.D. et al. Increased risk of urgent revascularization. *J. Thorac. Cardiovasc. Surg.* 1987; **93**: 291.

77. Hochberg, M.S., Parsonnet, V., Gielchinsky, I. and Hussain, S.M. Coronary artery bypass grafting in patients with ejection fractions below forty percent. Early and late results in 466 patients. *J. Thorac. Cardiovasc. Surg.* 1983; **86**: 519.

78. Schaff, H.V., Gersh, B.J., Fisher, L.D. et al. Detrimental effect of perioperative myocardial infarction on late survival after coronary artery bypass. Report from the Coronary Artery Surgery Study – CASS. *J. Thorac. Cardiovasc. Surg.* 1984; **88**: 972.

79. McGregor, C.G.A., Muir, A.L., Smith, A.F. et al. Myocardial infarction related to coronary artery bypass graft surgery. *Br. Heart J.* 1984; **51**: 399.

80. Fennell, W.H., Chua, K.G., Cohen, L. et al. Detection, prediction, and significance of perioperative myocardial infarction following aorta-coronary bypass. *J. Thorac. Cardiovasc. Surg.* 1979; **78**: 244.

81. Loop, F.D., Lytle, B.W., Gill, C.C., Golding, L.A.R.,

Cosgrove, D.M. and Taylor, P.C. Trends in selection and results of coronary reoperations. *Ann. Thorac. Surg.* 1983; **36**: 380.

82. Cosgrove, D.M., Loop, F.D., Lytle, B.W. *et al.* Predictors of reoperation after myocardial revascularization. *J. Thorac. Cardiovasc. Surg.* 1986; **92**: 811.

83. Foster, E.D., Fisher, L.D., Kaiser, G.C. and Myers, W.O. Comparison of operative mortality and morbidity for initial and repeat coronary artery bypass grafting: The Coronary Artery Surgery Study (CASS) Registry experience. *Ann. Thorac. Surg.* 1984; **38**: 563.

84. Lytle, B.W., Loop, F.D., Cosgrove, D.M. *et al.* Fifteen hundred coronary reoperations. Results and determinants of early and late survival. *J. Thorac. Cardiovasc. Surg.* 1987; **93**: 847.

85. Faxon, D.P., Myers, W.O., McCabe, C.H. *et al.* The influence of surgery on the natural history of angiographically documented left ventricular aneurysm: the Coronary Artery Surgery Study. *Circulation* 1986; **74**: 110.

86. Lee, D.C., Johnson, R.A., Boucher, C.A. *et al.* Angiographic predictors of survival following left ventricular aneurysmectomy. *Circulation* 1977; **56**(Suppl. II): II–12.

87. Burton, N.A., Stinson, E.B., Oyer, P.E. and Shumway, N.E. Left ventricular aneurysm. Preoperative risk factors and longterm results. *J. Thorac. Cardiovasc. Surg.* 1979; **77**: 65.

88. Barratt-Boyes, B.G., White, H.D., Agnew, T.M., Pemberton, J.R. and Wild, C.J. The results of surgical treatment of left ventricular aneurysms. An assessment of the risk factors affecting early and late mortality. *J. Thorac. Cardiovasc. Surg.* 1984; **87**: 87.

89. Cosgrove, D.M., Loop, F.D., Irarrazaval, M.J. *et al.* Determinants of longterm survival after ventricular aneurysmectomy. *Ann. Thorac. Surg.* 1978; **26**: 357.

90. Gaudiani, V.A., Miller, D.C., Stinson, E.B. *et al.* Postinfarction ventricular septal defect: argument for early operation. *Surgery* 1981; **89**: 48.

91. Daggett, W.M., Buckley, M.J., Akins, C.W. *et al.* Improved results of surgical management of post-infarction ventricular septal rupture. *Ann. Surg.* 1982; **196**: 269.

92. Killen, D.A., Reed, W.A., Wathanachersen, S., Beauchamp, G. and Rutherford, B. Surgical treatment of papillary muscle rupture. *Ann. Thorac. Surg.* 1983; **35**: 243.

93. Anderson, A.J., Barboriak, J.J., Hoffman, R.G. and Mullen, D.C. Retention or resumption of employment after aortocoronary bypass operations. *JAMA* 1980; **243**: 543.

94. Kornfeld, D.S., Heller, S.S., Frank, K.A. *et al.* Psychological and behavioural responses after coronary artery bypass surgery. *Circulation* 1982; **66**(Suppl. III): III–24.

95. Bass, C. Psychosocial outcome after coronary artery bypass surgery. *Br. J. Psychiatr.* 1984; **145**: 526.

96. Varnauskas, E. and the European Coronary Surgery Study Group. Survival, myocardial infarction, and employment status in a prospective randomized study of coronary bypass surgery. *Circulation* 1985; **72**(Suppl. V): V–90.

97. Oberman, A., Wayne, J.B., Kouchoukos, N.T., Charles, E.D., Russell, R.O. and Rogers, W.J. Employment status after coronary artery bypass surgery. *Circulation* 1982; **65**(Suppl. II): II–115.

98. Smith, H.C., Hammes, L.N., Gupta, S., Vlietstra, R.E. and Elveback, L. Employment status after coronary artery bypass surgery. *Circulation* 1982; **65**(Suppl. II): II–120.

99. Spencer, F.C. Surgical management of coronary artery disease. In: Sabiston, D.C. and Spencer, F.C. eds. *Gibbon's Surgery of the Chest, Vol. II*, 4th edn. Philadelphia: W.B. Saunders, 1983, p. 1441.

100. Manley, J.C. Results of coronary surgery. In: Wheatley, D.J. ed. *Surgery of coronary artery disease*. London: Chapman and Hall, 1986, p. 625.

101. Hurst, J.W., King, S.B., Walter, P.F., Freisinger, G.C. and Edwards, J.E. Atherosclerotic coronary heart disease: angina pectoris, myocardial infarction and other manifestations of myocardial ischemia. In: Hurst, J.W. ed. *The heart. Arteries and veins*, 5th edn. New York: McGraw-Hill, 1982, p. 1009.

102. Cohn, P.F. and Braunwald, E. Chronic ischaemic heart disease. In: Braunwald, E., ed. *Heart disease. A textbook of cardiovascular medicine*, 2nd edn. Philadelphia: W.B. Saunders, 1984, p. 1334.

103. European Coronary Surgery Study Group. Long-term results of prospective randomised study of coronary artery bypass surgery in stable angina pectoris. *Lancet* 1982; ii: 1173.

104. Gersh, B.J., Kronmal, R.A., Schaff, H.V. *et al.* Comparison of coronary artery bypass surgery and medical therapy in patients 65 years of age or older. A nonrandomized study from the Coronary Artery Surgery Study (CASS) Registry. *N. Engl. J. Med.* 1985; **313**: 217.

105. Loop, F.D., Golding, L.R., Macmillan, J.P., Cosgrove, D.M., Lytle, B.W. and Sheldon, W.C. Coronary artery surgery in women compared with men: analyses of risks and long-term results. *J. Am. Coll. Cardiol.* 1983; **2**: 383.

106. Richardson, J.V. and Cyrus, R.J. Reduced efficacy of coronary artery bypass grafting in women. *Ann. Thorac. Surg.* 1986; **42**(Suppl.): S16.

107. Gardner, T.J., Horneffer, P.J., Gott, V.L. *et al.* Coronary artery bypass grafting in women. A ten-year perspective. *Ann. Surg.* 1985; **201**: 780.

108. Cukingnan, R.A., Carey, J.A., Wittig, J.H. and Brown, B.G. Influence of complete coronary revascularization on relief of angina. *J. Thorac. Cardiovasc. Surg.* 1980; **79**: 188.

109. Lavee, J., Rath, S., Tran-Quang-Hoa, *et al.* Does complete revascularization by the conventional method truly provide the best possible results? *J. Thorac. Cardiovasc. Surg.* 1986; **92**: 279.

110. Grondin, C.M., Campeau, L., Lesperance, J., Enjalbert, M. and Bourassa, M.G. Comparison of late changes in internal mammary artery and saphenous vein grafts in two consecutive series of patients 10 years after operation. *Circulation* 1984; **70**(Suppl. I): I–208.

111. Fitzgibbon, G.M., Leach, A.J., Keon, W.J., Burton, J.R. and Kafka, H.P. Coronary bypass graft fate. Angiographic study of 1,179 vein grafts early, one year, and five years after operation. *J. Thorac. Cardiovasc. Surg.* 1986; **91**: 773.

112. Hall, R.J., Elayda, MacA. A., Gray, A. *et al.* Coronary artery bypass: long-term follow-up of 22,284 consecutive patients. *Circulation* 1983; **68**(Suppl. II): II–20.

113. Loop, F.D., Lytle, B.W., Cosgrove, D.M. *et al.* Influence of the internal-mammary-artery graft on 10-year survival and other cardiac events. *N. Engl. J. Med.* 1986; **314**: 1.

114. Okies, J.E., Page, U.S., Bigelow, J.C., Krause, A.H. and Salomon, N.W. The left internal mammary artery: the graft of choice. *Circulation* 1984; **70**(Suppl. I): I–213.

115. Tector, A.J. Fifteen years' experience with the internal mammary artery graft. *Ann. Thorac. Surg.* 1986; **42**(Suppl.): S22.

116. Tector, A.J., Schmahl, T.M. and Canino, V.R. Expanding the use of the internal mammary artery to improve patency in coronary artery bypass grafting. *J. Thorac. Cardiovasc. Surg.* 1986; **91**: 9.

117. Loop, F.D., Lytle, B.W., Cosgrove, D.M., Golding, L.A.R., Taylor, P.C. and Stewart, R.W. Free (aorta-coronary) internal mammary artery graft. Late results. *J. Thorac. Cardiovasc. Surg.* 1986; **92**: 827.

118. Hultgren, H.N., Peduzzi, P., Detre, K., Takaro, T. and the Study Participants. The 5 year effect of bypass surgery on relief of angina and exercise performance. *Circulation*

1985; 72(Suppl. V): V–79.

119. Peduzzi, P., Hultgren, H., Thomsen, J. and Detre, K. Ten year effect of medical and surgical therapy on quality of life. Veterans Administration Cooperative Study of Coronary Artery Surgery. *Am. J. Cardiol.* 1987; 57: 1017.

120. Lawrie, G.M., Morris, G.C. Jr, Howell, J.F. *et al.* Results of coronary bypass more than 5 years after operation in 434 patients. Clinical, treadmill exercise and angiographic correlations. *Am. J. Cardiol.* 1977; 40: 665.

121. Rahimtoola, S.H. Postoperative exercise response in the evaluation of the physiologic status after coronary bypass surgery. *Circulation* 1982; 65(Suppl. II): II–106.

122. Serruys, P.W., Rousseau, M.F., Cosyns, J., Ponlot, R., Brasseur, L.A. and Detry, J.-M.R. Haemodynamics during maximal exercise after coronary bypass surgery. *Br. Heart J.* 1978; 40: 1205.

123. Schaff, H.V., Gersh, B.J., Pluth, J.R. *et al.* Survival and functional status after coronary artery bypass grafting: Results 10–12 years after surgery in 500 patients. *Circulation* 1983; 69(Suppl. II): II–200.

124. Frick, M.H., Harjola, P.-T. and Valle, M. Persistent improvement after coronary bypass surgery: ergometric and angiographic correlations at 5 years. *Circulation* 1983; 67: 491.

125. Cheseboro, J.H., Ritman, E.L., Frye, R.L., Smith, H.C., Vlietstra, R.E. and Pluth, J.R. Left ventricular performance before and after aortocoronary artery bypass surgery. *Circulation* 1982; 65(Suppl. II): II–98.

126. Carroll, J.D., Hess, O.M., Hirzel, H.O., Turina, M. and Krayenbuehl, H.P. Left ventricular systolic and diastolic function in coronary artery disease: effects of revascularization on exercise-induced ischemia. *Circulation* 1985; 72: 119.

127. Brundage, B.H., Massie, B.M. and Botvinick, E.H. Improved regional ventricular function after successful surgical revascularization. *J. Am. Coll. Cardiol.* 1984; 3: 902.

128. Lim, Y.L., Kalff, V., Kelly, M.J. *et al.* Radionuclide angiographic assessment of global and segmental left ventricular function at rest and during exercise after coronary bypass graft surgery. *Circulation* 1982; 66: 972.

129. Rankin, J.S., Newman, G.E., Muhlbaier, L.H., Behar, V.S., Fedor, J.M. and Sabiston, D.C. Jr. The effects of coronary revascularization on left ventricular function in ischemic heart disease. *J. Thorac. Cardiovasc. Surg.* 1985; 90: 818.

130. Ritchie, J.L., Narahara, K.A., Trobaugh, G.B., Williams, D.L. and Hamilton, G.W. Thallium-201 myocardial imaging before and after coronary revascularization. Assessment of regional myocardial blood flow and graft patency. *Circulation* 1977; 56: 830.

131. Schmidt, D.H., Blau, F.M., Hendrix, L.J., Kamath, M.L. and Ray, G. Myocardial perfusion after aortocoronary bypass surgery: meaurements at rest and after administration of isoproterenol. *Circulation* 1985; 71: 767.

132. Wainwright, R.J., Roper, B., Maisey, D.A. and Sowton, E. Exercise thallium-201 myocardial scintigraphy in the followup of aortocoronary bypass graft surgery. *Br. Heart J.* 1980; 43: 56.

133. Cobanoglu, A., Freimanis, I., Grunkemeier, G. *et al.* Enhanced late survival following coronary artery bypass graft operation for unstable versus chronic angina. *Ann. Thorac. Surg.* 1984; 37: 52.

134. Adler, D.S., Goldman, L., O'Neil, A. *et al.* Longterm survival of more than 2,000 patients after coronary artery bypass grafting. *Am. J. Cardiol.* 1986; 58: 195.

135. Goldman, L., Mudge, G.H. Jr and Cook, E.F. The chang-
ing "natural history" of symptomatic coronary artery disease: basis versus bias. *Am. J. Cardiol.* 1983; 51: 449.

136. Julian, D.G. The practical implications of the coronary artery surgery trials. *Br. Heart J.* 1985; 54: 343.

137. Cohn, P.F., Harris, P., Barry, W.H., Rosati, R.A., Rosenbaum, P. and Waternaux, C. Prognostic importance of anginal symptoms in angiographically defined coronary artery disease. *Am. J. Cardiol.* 1981; 47: 233.

138. Bruce, R.A., DeRouen, T., Peterson, D.R. *et al.* Noninvasive predictors of sudden cardiac death in men with coronary heart disease: predictive value of maximal stress testing. *Am. J. Cardiol.* 1977; 39: 833.

139. McNeer, J.F., Margolis, J.R., Lee, K.L. *et al.* The role of the exercise test in the evaluation of patients for ischemic heart disease. *Circulation* 1978; 57: 64.

140. Bonow, R.O., Kent, K.M., Rosing, D.R. *et al.* Exercise-induced ischemia in mildly symptomatic patients with coronary artery disease and preserved left ventricular function. *N. Engl. J. Med.* 1984; 311: 1339.

141. Gohlke, H., Samek, L., Betz, P. and Roskamm, H. Exercise testing provides additional prognostic information in angiographically defined subgroups of patients with coronary artery disease. *Circulation* 1983; 68: 979.

142. Takaro, T., Hultgren, H.N., Detre, K.M. and Peduzzi, P. The Veterans Administration Cooperative Study of stable angina: current status. *Circulation* 1982; 65(Suppl. II): II–60.

143. Loop, F.D. CASS continued. *Circulation* 1985; 72(Suppl. II); II–1.

144. Myers, W.O., Marshfield, W.I., Davis, K., Foster, E.D., Maynard, C. and Kaiser, G.C. Surgical survival in the Coronary Artery Surgery Study (CASS) Registry. *Ann. Thorac. Surg.* 1985; 40: 245.

145. Holmes, D.R. Jr, Davis, K.B., Mock, M.B. *et al.* The effect of medical and surgical treatment on subsequent sudden cardiac death in patients with coronary artery disease: A report from the Coronary Artery Surgery Study. *Circulation* 1986; 73: 1254.

146. CASS principal investigators and their associates. Coronary Artery Surgery Study (CASS): a randomized trial of coronary artery bypass surgery. Survival data. *Circulation* 1983; 68: 939.

147. Weinstein, G.S. and Levin, B. The Coronary Artery Surgery Study (CASS). A critical appraisal. *J. Thorac. Cardiovasc. Surg.* 1985; 90: 541.

148. Kaiser, G.C., Davis, K.B., Fisher, L.D. *et al.* Survival following coronary artery bypass grafting in patients with severe angina pectoris. An observational study. *J. Thorac. Cardiovasc. Surg.* 1985; 89: 513.

149. Hammermeister, K.E., DeRouen, T.A. and Dodge, H.T. Comparison of survival of medically and surgically treated coronary disease in patients in Seattle Heart Watch: a nonrandomized study. *Circulation* 1982; 65(Suppl. II): II–53.

150. Lawrie, G.M., Morris, G.C., Calhoon, J.H. *et al.* Clinical results of coronary bypass in 500 patients at least 10 years after operation. *Circulation* 1982; 66(Suppl. I): I–1.

151. Rahimtoola, S.H., Grunkemeier, G.L. and Starr, A. Ten year survival after coronary artery bypass surgery for angina in patients aged 65 years and older. *Circulation* 1986; 74: 509.

152. Cameron, A., Kemp, H.G. Jr and Green, G.E. Bypass surgery with the internal mammary artery graft: 15 year follow-up. *Circulation* 1986; 74 (**Suppl. III**): III–30.

Chapter 53

Hypertension

J.I.S. Robertson and S.G. Ball

INTRODUCTION

Hypertension or, more explicitly, high blood pressure, despite its implications being better understood than even a decade ago, remains to many clinicians enigmatic. Arterial blood pressure, albeit often measured under quite casual circumstances, and usually by indirect rather than direct methods is a powerful indicator of the risks of a range of cardiac and vascular complications, namely the malignant phase of hypertension, hypertensive heart failure, stroke, coronary artery disease and progressive impairment of renal function. Appropriate blood pressure reduction, by pharmacological or other means, may correct, prevent or delay the appearance of many of these hypertension-related disorders. Thus, there is a strong case for identifying persons with even symptomless and mild blood pressure elevation.[1]

Although the matter was disputed for several years, it is now accepted that the distribution of blood pressure values, systolic and diastolic, within any population is continuous, with no division other than arbitrary, between 'hypertension' and normal blood pressure. The distribution curve is roughly bell-shaped, slightly but definitely skewed towards the upper end (Fig. 53.1). The distribution of risk follows the blood pressure curve and is also continuous, there being no point of cut-off where risk ceases. This raises crucial issues in the practicalities and economics of preventive anti-hypertensive therapy. At the highest blood pressure levels, there are small numbers of persons at high risk; as lower, but above average, blood pressures are considered, there is a very much larger population in which, overall, the cardiovascular risks although distinct are much more modest.

This concept of the continuous distribution of blood pressure values within populations, and the corresponding continuous distribution of the danger of complications, is central to the principles of preventive antihypertensive therapy.[2] In most cases, hypertension is not a disease in the traditional sense, but rather an indicator of risk. Although hypertension may come to light because of its adverse vascular effects, notably on the eye, brain, kidney or heart, or, in the case of secondary hypertension, from features of the disease causing the raised pressure, the great majority of cases are largely devoid of clinical symptoms or signs, and hypertension is often discovered at routine blood pressure measurement.

PRIMARY ('ESSENTIAL') AND SECONDARY HYPERTENSION

Raised arterial pressure may sometimes result from an evident anatomical, biochemical or pathological abnormality. Many of these are potentially correctable, in some instances by surgical means. Such forms of hypertension are termed 'secondary'.* Although secondary hypertension tends to be seen often in specialized centres, it is uncommon in the population at large. In unselected groups of hypertensive subjects, whatever definition of hypertension is taken, at most 5%, and probably nearer 1%, of all cases are secondary. Therefore, the main concern clinically is with primary or 'essential' hypertension, and the greater emphasis of this chapter, and epidemiological considerations, will deal with essential hypertension. Traditionally, essential hypertension has been defined as raised

---

* There are identifiable causes of secondary hypertension. However, the usage occasionally perpetrated in medical writing: "hypertension due to a secondary cause" is internally contradictory, and betrays confusion of thought. The phrase should be eschewed.

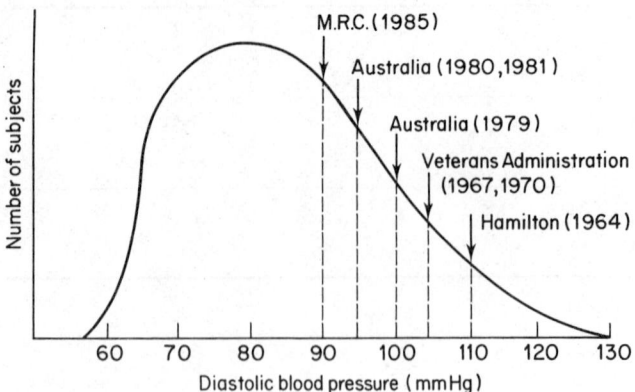

Fig. 53.1. Schematic representation of the distribution of diastolic pressures within an adult Westernized population. Also shown are the thresholds of presenting diastolic pressure above which a protective effect of antihypertensive drug therapy has been seen in various controlled trials. For further details see references 62, 63 and 74. (Reproduced from Robertson, J.I.S., *Eur. Heart J.* 1988; **9** (Suppl. G): 41 by kind permission of the Editor.

arterial pressure without evident cause. This traditional view has been challenged in recent years, since there has been increasing recognition of the constitutional, dietary and environmental factors involved in raising arterial pressure.[3]

EPIDEMIOLOGY OF ESSENTIAL HYPERTENSION

In Western or Westernized populations, the characteristic continuous pattern of blood pressure values, systolic and diastolic, has already been described, with the upper end of the distribution skewed. In such populations, blood pressure also typically rises with age. The age-related increase in systolic pressure continues until late in life, whereas diastolic tends to level off, or even to fall slightly, after 50 years.

This characteristic pattern of blood pressure is not universal. Scattered throughout the world are communities in which the rise of blood pressure with age is absent or slight, and in consequence the prevailing level of blood pressure is on average low.[1–3] These communities have attracted much attention because of the possibility of identifying the factors responsible for the failure of blood pressure to rise with age. Herein could be important clues to the aetiology and prevention of hypertension in the Western world. The diversity of location of these peoples deserves emphasis: they occur in Pacific islands, parts of Africa, Asia and New Guinea, the Andean highlands and the South American jungle. Nevertheless, they usually share common features, any or all of which might be relevant to their low blood pressure.

They tend to be isolated, small in population and with a strong intracommunal interdependence. Food supplies are short, often frankly deficient, and generally low in sodium and high in potassium content. Physical activity tends to be high. Economy is usually simple, often having no involvement with a monetary system. In many, but not all, there is a high ambient temperature.

There seems little doubt of environmental influences in the development of high blood pressure, because migration from such communities to more Westernized societies tends to be accompanied by a rise in arterial pressure. This was seen for example in Tokelauans, whose blood pressure rose on migrating from their Pacific islands to New Zealand. Although genetic factors are needed, these require to interact with the appropriate environmental stimuli before hypertension develops. Unfortunately, the studies on migrants have been less revealing than might have been hoped, because with movement from a primitive to a more developed culture, usually more than one, and often many, of the possibly relevant factors change.

GENETIC INFLUENCES IN ESSENTIAL HYPERTENSION

The importance of genetic factors in the pathogenesis of essential hypertension is indicated by the similarity of blood pressure values between close ('first degree') relatives, such as between siblings, and between parents and children.[2] These similarities are usually described by correlation coefficients of the order of 0.2–0.3. Although such relationships are highly significant, there is dispute over whether they are sufficiently close to indicate more powerful genetic than environmental influences. In one interesting Swedish study,[4] although the results confirmed significant correlations between the blood pressures of siblings, and of mothers and their children, no such relationship was found between the pressures of children and their putative fathers. This divergence was interpreted as perhaps indicating genetic transmission of the prevailing blood pressure via the distaff line; certainly a more prominent maternal than paternal influence. An alternative explanation is that maternity is more definitely established than paternity.

Although the majority of workers now favour the genetic link in essential hypertension as multifactorial in nature, the possibility is not excluded of the existence of only one or two genes having a major influence and yet still giving rise to the continuous distribution of blood pressure values evident in population surveys.[5]

SOCIAL INFLUENCES IN ESSENTIAL HYPERTENSION

Social factors are not easily disentangled from other pathogenic influences. Blood pressures are consistently higher in persons from the lower socioeconomic classes, and stroke and coronary artery disease are accordingly commoner.[6] The poorer classes have, however, concurrently higher average bodyweight, greater consumption of alcohol and tobacco, and more exposure to noise, any or all of which might raise arterial pressure. In Birmingham, blacks of West Indian origin were found to have a greater prevalence of hypertension than were Asians; the extent to which this reflects social or genetic influences is unknown.[7]

An interesting example of social factors was seen in the Tokelauan migrant study. Those migrants who, in New Zealand, remained involved with their Pacific native culture, showed less of a rise of blood pressure than did their fellow-countrymen who became more integrated into New Zealand society.[2]

PHYSICAL ACTIVITY AND BLOOD PRESSURE

Circumstantial evidence from epidemiological studies, that physical exercise *per se* can reduce arterial pressure, has been confirmed in controlled trials. This effect could largely result from diminished sympathetic activity. It appears to be independent of weight change, and opens new preventive and therapeutic strategies.[8]

DIETARY ASPECTS OF PATHOGENESIS, PREVENTION AND TREATMENT

Epidemiological evidence directed attention to diet-

ary factors as being perhaps relevant to the pathogenesis, prevention and treatment of hypertension. These various aspects interrelate and therefore will be considered together.[3,8–11]

BODYWEIGHT AND ITS REDUCTION

There is extensive epidemiological evidence testifying to an association between bodyweight and raised blood pressure.[9] This has been confirmed by intra-arterial blood pressure recording, and is not an artifact of imprecise blood pressure measurement with too small a sphygmomanometer cuff on a fat arm, although contamination of the data could have arisen in some studies from this cause. It is known that children who gain weight most rapidly, especially in their teens, show generally the most rapid age-related rise in blood pressure and are likely to have higher pressures as adults. It has also been proposed that congestive heart failure, ventricular arrhythmias and sudden death might be especially frequent in obese hypertensive subjects. However, there is no good evidence that obese hypertensives are at greater risk than lighter subjects who have similar levels of blood pressure.

The cause of the higher blood pressures associated with obesity is not understood. The degree of blood pressure elevation relates more closely to central body fat than to peripheral fat. There is evidence of increased sympathetic activity in obese hypertensive subjects. Obese hypertensives have been compared with obese normotensives and found to have higher extracellular and interstitial fluid volumes; by contrast, plasma volume, total body water and cardiac output did not differ significantly between the groups. Obese hypertensives have been reported as having an increased pulse wave velocity, and thus probably diminished arterial compliance.

The results of several trials have confirmed an antihypertensive effect of weight reduction, an effect that seems to be independent of dietary sodium restriction.

DIETARY SODIUM

The notion that an excessive intake of sodium chloride in the diet might be important in the pathogenesis of hypertension has been a controversial issue for many years.[9–11] Closely linked are proposals that sodium restriction could be valuable in both the prevention and treatment of hypertension. There is a wealth of conflicting, although often strongly suggestive, epidemiological evidence, which the present authors consider to be inconclusive, concerning the pathogenic importance of dietary sodium intake.

In particular, although measurements of both total exchangeable and total body sodium correlate positively and significantly with arterial pressure in untreated essential hypertension, in mild (and presumably early) hypertension, body sodium content is deficient. Only with more severe disease and with ageing is body sodium increased. These aspects are discussed further on page 1236). The observations imply that sodium restriction would be expected to lower the blood pressure only in the later and more severe cases. Recent data suggest that, if sodium is relevant in the genesis of hypertension, sodium chloride is more potent than are other sodium salts; however, a pressor effect of grossly excessive intake of sodium bicarbonate has been recorded.[11]

Therapeutic sodium chloride restriction has led to conflicting reports in various clinical trials. However, modest and acceptable dietary salt restriction, down to about 70–100 mmol/day, can be effective in some patients. Although the value of such therapy is more obvious as an adjunct to drug treatment, it is often worthy of trial. However, the broad-scale restriction of dietary salt intake in hypertension, either as a preventive or therapeutic measure, cannot be recommended on present evidence.

DIETARY POTASSIUM

The epidemiological observation of low blood pressure in communities with a high average potassium intake has been mentioned. Following from this, there have been several studies in which potassium supplementation has been tried therapeutically in patients with essential hypertension.[9] The results of such intervention studies have been conflicting, and it has been suggested that in part confusion may have resulted from errors in experimental design, and from inadequate statistical power. In one recent trial, it was shown that the addition of potassium chloride 65 mEq/day in patients with essential hypertension lowered blood pressure significantly, by an average of 7/3 mmHg. The magnitude of such effects has been considered by some too small to be of great therapeutic value. Moreover, there is concern about the side-effects, especially abdominal pain and diarrhoea, that such treatment may cause. Additionally, hyperkalaemia

could result from potassium supplementation in subjects with renal impairment.

DIETARY CALCIUM

Despite strong advocacy of calcium deficiency as an important cause of hypertension, and for calcium supplementation in treatment, the apparent importance of the role of dietary calcium has receded rather than advanced in recent years.[9] The theoretical and experimental studies underlying the concepts have been severely criticized, and the results of several careful trials have failed to show an effect of calcium supplementation on blood pressure.

ALCOHOL

There is clear evidence of the association between alcohol consumption and hypertension.[9] Although the relationship is seen more clearly with higher alcohol intake, it is also apparent with the consumption of as little as 30–40 g/day. The pressor effect of alcohol disappears within a few days of abstinence, an observation that indicates a causal relationship as well as providing encouragement therapeutically. Alcohol restriction effectively reduces blood pressure independently of falls in bodyweight. Limitation of alcohol intake could be important therapeutically in other ways: heavy drinkers are less likely to be aware that they have hypertension, less likely to comply with treatment, and less likely to be adequately controlled on therapy.

The aetiology of alcohol-related hypertension remains obscure. The acute ingestion of alcohol does not alter plasma concentrations of renin, adrenaline, noradrenaline or cortisol. However, chronic alcohol ingestion can be associated with cortisol excess and can mimic Cushing's syndrome (p. 1270).

Alcohol consumption has been associated with a small but significant fall in plasma calcium concentration. It has been suggested tentatively that alcohol may raise blood pressure acutely by a vasoconstrictor effect possibly mediated by a shift in intracellular calcium.

CAFFEINE

Coffee drinking has been reported to elevate blood pressure acutely, particularly when combined with cigarette smoking. However, not all studies have confirmed this.

VEGETARIAN DIET

An ovolactovegetarian diet has been shown marginally to lower blood pressure in comparison with an omnivorous diet. The effect cannot be attributed to changes in bodyweight or to sodium or potassium intake. The modest results and the strong possibility that patients would not comply with this therapy suggest that this is unlikely to be a rewarding strategy.

The dietary, behavioural and environmental influences outlined here are not comprehensive. Nevertheless, they emphasize that, even with a genetic predisposition, the development of hypertension is not inevitable.[3] Thus, although the term 'essential' or 'primary' hypertension retains its valuable descriptive role, it should not discourage appropriate preventive or therapeutic efforts.

HORMONAL CHANGES IN ESSENTIAL HYPERTENSION

A variety of hormonal systems can influence arterial pressure both acutely and chronically. These systems are relevant to a consideration of essential hypertension; also, several are more directly involved with a number of syndromes of secondary hypertension (see later, in the respective sections). The possibility that hormonal alterations might be concerned fundamentally with the pathogenesis of essential hypertension has attracted repeated attention, although so far no clear evidence of pathogenic involvement has emerged. Hitherto, most interest has been focused on the strictly endocrine aspects of these hormones, i.e. their actions as chemical messengers within the circulation. Although their local autocrine and paracrine functions have long been recognized, and have been considered to be phylogenetically the oldest, they have been largely neglected until recent years. Increasing interest in autocrine and paracrine aspects has been re-awakened, especially in relation to the possible pathogenesis of essential hypertension.[12]

CATECHOLAMINES

Plasma concentrations of noradrenaline and adrenaline are often taken as indicators respectively of sympathetic nerve activity and of adrenal medullary secretion. The approximate nature of such estima-

tions deserves emphasis. Values are influenced by discharge and secretion rates, uptake, metabolism and excretion, and through these by exercise, body posture, mental stress, sodium balance, smoking and age.[13–15]

Plasma noradrenaline has been shown in some but not all studies to rise with age, and this may have suggested wrongly a causal relationship of noradrenaline with arterial pressure. This remains controversial. Plasma adrenaline does not seem to change with age, and thus reports of a correlation of plasma adrenaline with arterial pressure may indicate a pathogenic connection, although interpretation is doubtful. A further attractive possibility is of repeated elevation of circulating adrenaline, released in a susceptible individual from the adrenal medulla, to be taken up in sympathetic nerve terminals, and later to stimulate neurotransmitter release, and to act also as a co-transmitter with noradrenaline. There have been speculations that such a mechanism may initiate essential hypertension. Both in the rat and man, infused adrenaline can lead to neurotransmitter release and/or to elevation of arterial pressure.[15,16] However, in mildly hypertensive patients, many of whom were presumably in the early stages of the disorder, no evidence of excessive noradrenaline or adrenaline secretion was found in comparison with matched normotensive control subjects.[17]

THE RENIN–ANGIOTENSIN SYSTEM

Renin, an enzyme elaborated in and released from the kidney, reacts with a circulating substrate, angiotensinogen, splitting off an inactive decapeptide, angiotensin I. In turn, angiotensin I is cleaved by angiotensin converting enzyme ('ACE'), two amino acid residues are removed, and the principal active component of the system, the octapeptide angiotensin II, is formed (Fig. 53.2).[18]

Angiotensin II has a range of actions within the circulation. It raises arterial pressure via an acute and a slower mechanism; it stimulates the sympathetic nervous system at various levels, while inhibiting vagal tone; it has a range of direct effects on the kidney; it can promote thirst; and it stimulates the secretion of both antidiuretic hormone and aldosterone. The neural effects are discussed in more detail on page 1233.

All of these actions are directed to sustaining arterial pressure and the circulation, and the renin–angiotensin system can be seen as protecting the organism against salt and fluid loss or deprivation.

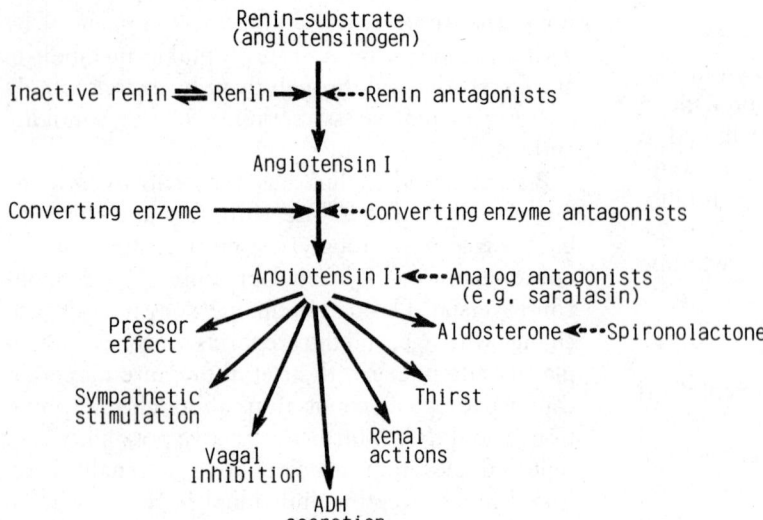

Fig. 53.2. Outline of the renin–angiotensin system, showing some of the principal actions of angiotensin II. Also shown are sites of action of drugs antagonizing the system.

For example, plasma renin is increased by sodium restriction and depressed by sodium loading.

Plasma renin declines progressively with age, and this decline is more marked in essential hypertension. However, the sensitivity of the aldosterone response to angiotensin II is relatively enhanced in essential hypertension, so that the concurrent fall in plasma aldosterone is proportionately less marked.

Plasma renin may sometimes be high in malignant hypertension or with renal artery stenosis.

Increased evidence suggests the presence of a local tissue renin–angiotensin system in the heart and in arterial walls.[19,20] The full significance of this remains to be explored.

ATRIAL NATRIURETIC PEPTIDE

Atrial natriuretic peptide (ANP) is elaborated in and released from cardiac atria; higher amounts are found usually in the right than the left atrium. Smaller quantities are found in the ventricles. It is cleared from the circulation by the liver and kidneys.[21,22] Atrial natriuretic peptide has potent diuretic and natriuretic effects, it relaxes vascular smooth muscle, it inhibits vasoconstriction caused by noradrenaline or angiotensin II, and it reduces the secretion of both renin and aldosterone.

Atrial natriuretic peptide can be seen as counterpoised against the renin–angiotensin system and thus as protecting the organism against fluid overload. In cardiac impairment, peripheral plasma concentrations of atrial natriuretic peptide correlate with right atrial pressure and pulmonary artery wedge pressure, findings consistent with the notion that increase in atrial pressure stimulates atrial natriuretic peptide secretion.[21,22]

Weak, but significant, correlations between plasma atrial natriuretic peptide and systemic arterial pressure have been found in patients with essential hypertension, notably in the presence of left ventricular hypertrophy. This has been interpreted as showing decreased ventricular compliance in hypertension, leading to increased atrial work and a rise in mean atrial pressures. Usually, changes in circulating atrial natriuretic peptide and angiotensin II are inversely related. However, both may be recruited in cardiac failure, atrial natriuretic peptide to promote water and electrolyte excretion and the renin–angiotensin system to assist renal function in the presence of a reduced renal blood flow.[22–25] Atrial natriuretic peptide may additionally act as a neurotransmitter (see p. 1235).

ANTIDIURETIC HORMONE

Posterior pituitary antidiuretic hormone (vasopressin) possesses pressor and antidiuretic properties, and has been repeatedly considered as perhaps being involved in the pathogenesis of essential hypertension.[26] However, physiological variations in plasma vasopressin appear to take place at levels below the threshold concentrations required to affect arterial pressure directly.

Plasma vasopressin values in patients with uncomplicated essential hypertension are in the same range as those in normotensive control subjects. Plasma vasopressin, however, may be elevated in patients with malignant hypertension and in severe cases of hypertension with renal artery stenosis; in these circumstances, stimulation of vasopressin secretion is probably caused by very high plasma concentrations of angiotensin II. Long-term exposure to elevated plasma levels of vasopressin does not lead to hypertension, as shown by the normal age-adjusted blood pressure values seen in a series of patients with bronchial carcinoma and excess vasopressin secretion.

However, very marked elevation of vasopressin, as following haemorrhagic hypotension, may help to sustain arterial pressure in these extreme circumstances.

SEROTONIN (5-HYDROXYTRYPTAMINE)

The possibility that circulating serotonin has a pressor role has long been controversial.[27] Little or no serotonin circulates free in plasma, as the amine is avidly taken up by several mechanisms and especially by platelets. Thus, if it is to be invoked in the pathogenesis of hypertension by a peripheral action, it has to be released from platelets into plasma at the periphery. This could occur in the presence of peripheral vascular disease, with associated platelet aggregation and breakdown, or if the capacity of platelets to take up or retain serotonin were impaired. There is evidence that both of these mechanisms may obtain in clinical hypertension, and are more marked with age. Furthermore, in the presence of endothelial damage, the vasoconstrictor effect of any free serotonin will be enhanced. It has been shown that the arterial contraction induced by serotonin is increased with age. Thus, serotonin could have a peripheral hormonal pressor effect, although this is inherently difficult to establish clinically. The neurotransmitter[13,14] and vascular hypertrophic roles of serotonin are discussed respectively on pages 1233 and 1234, and 1242.

CORTICOSTEROIDS

These are considered on pages 1256, and 1268–1273.

NEUROLOGICAL ASPECTS OF ESSENTIAL HYPERTENSION

In recent years, there has been a rapidly expanding growth in knowledge and, to a lesser extent, understanding of neurological involvement in essential hypertension. An extended treatment of the data is beyond the scope of this chapter, although it may be appropriate to indicate certain especially interesting areas of research.

NEUROTRANSMITTERS AND BLOOD PRESSURE CONTROL[28–32]

The 'classic' neurotransmitters of the autonomic nervous system are acetylcholine and noradrenaline. However, other catecholamines such as adrenaline and dopamine may act as transmitters. Moreover, numerous non-adrenergic and non-cholinergic neurones exist within the central nervous system and at the level of the blood vessel. Transmitter substances include the amines like serotonin (5-hydroxytryptamine), the excitatory amino acid glutamate and the inhibitory amino acid alpha-aminobutyric acid, and the purines. In addition, an extensive array of peptides containing up to 40 amino acid residues has been shown to be associated with various established or putative neurotransmitters (Table 53.1).

Neurones contain more than one transmitter

The classic concept of one neurotransmitter for each type of neurone no longer holds. Neurones can be defined by from 2 to 6 substances. Knowledge of the distribution of these proposed neurotransmitters far outweighs any understanding of their

Table 53.1. 'Classical' neurotransmitters and some associated peptides.

Transmitter	Associated peptides
Acetylcholine	Calcitonin gene-related peptide Vaso-active intestinal polypeptide Substance P Enkephalin
Noradrenaline	Neuropeptide Y Vasopressin Enkephalin
Adrenaline	Neuropeptide Y Substance P Neurotensin
Dopamine	Cholecystokinin Neurotensin
5-Hydroxytryptamine (serotonin)	Substance P Thyrotrophin releasing hormone Cholecystokinin Encephalin
Alpha-aminobutyric acid	Neuropeptide Y Cholecystokinin Vaso-active intestinal polypeptide Encephalin Somatostatin Substance P Galanin
Glycine	Neurotensin

function and particularly of their relevance to blood pressure control. The proportions of putative transmitter substances in single nerve fibres appear to vary among different organs, species and physiological conditions. However, it is not clear to what extent such differences indicate lack of precision and sensitivity of techniques of identification, rather than reflecting truly physiologically relevant distinctions.

Co-existence of multiple messengers

Co-existing neurotransmitter substances could be released differentially and have actions both pre- and post-synaptically. Peptides appear at least in some tissues to be stored exclusively in large dense core vesicles (of diameter around 100 nm or 1000 Å) whereas classic transmitters occur in these and smaller vesicles (50 nm or 500 Å), offering potential for selective release. Effects in different situations might depend on the distribution of appropriate pre- and post-synaptic receptors and their coupling through several second messenger systems to function. Substance P, for example, may exert growth-stimulating effects on smooth muscle cells if co-released with noradrenaline. The immediate vasoconstrictor effect of noradrenaline might then be combined with the more prolonged effect of the peptide.

Co-existence of transmitters in the central nervous system

The C_1-adrenergic neurones which, when stimulated, increase sympathetic activity and raise blood pressure, contain a peptide that resembles neuropeptide Y. Serotonin-containing neurones in the lower medulla of the brain, which have been implicated in cardiovascular control, contain also both substance P and thyroid-releasing hormone-like peptides. Intracerebroventricular injection of substance P in experimental animals increases blood pressure, probably by enhancing sympathetic outflow. In contrast, when this peptide is injected into the nucleus of the tractus solitarius in rats, it decreases sympathetic discharge and causes hypotension and bradycardia. Evidence for co-existence of peptides and classic transmitters in the central nervous system is legion.

Co-existence of transmitters in the peripheral nervous system

Numerous peptides are found within the sympathe-

tic and parasympathetic systems. Neuropeptide Y, calcitonin gene-related peptide, vaso-active intestinal polypeptide and the tachykinins seem to be the most widely distributed in the nerves serving the cardiovascular system.

Neuropeptide Y

Neuropeptide Y (NPY) is a peptide of 36 amino acids which has a direct non-adrenergic but calcium-dependent vasoconstricting action on coronary and cerebral vessels. It may also potentiate the vasoconstricting effect of a number of transmitters and inhibit the pre-junctional release of noradrenaline. Noradrenaline may similarly inhibit the release of the neuropeptide. Field stimulation of the vas deferens releases not only noradrenaline and NPY but also the purine adenosine triphosphate (ATP). Different functions have been attributed to these three transmitters which are co-stored and may be released from single rather than separate neurones. ATP triggers the initial twitch phase, noradrenaline the slow second phase, of muscle contraction and neuropeptide Y has been postulated to potentiate the post-junctional noradrenaline and ATP responses, and to inhibit the pre-junctional release of both.

Purinergic nerves

Burnstock and his colleagues have provided strong evidence to support the concept of purinergic nerves.[31] Two subclasses of purinergic receptor have been identified. The P_1-receptors act via cyclic adenosine monophosphate (cAMP) and their stimulation modulates adrenergic and cholinergic neurotransmission. The P_2-receptors are found post-synaptically on smooth muscle cells and their stimulation causes vasoconstriction. Like serotonin (5-hydroxytryptamine), ATP may cause vasodilatation by releasing endothelial-derived relaxing factor. It also appears to be a co-transmitter with noradrenaline in nerves supplying the tail artery of the rat, and impairment of its inhibitory effect on noradrenaline release (thereby effectively increasing sympathetic stimulation) has been described in the spontaneously hypertensive rat.

Calcitonin gene-related peptide

Calcitonin gene-related peptide is a peptide of 37 amino acids found predominantly in the central nervous system. It has potent vasodilating effects which may in part be mediated through an endothelial-dependent mechanism.

Angiotensin II

The possible role of angiotensin II in circulatory regulation is discussed at length elsewhere in the chapter (p. 1231). Among its many actions, it interacts with the sympathetic and parasympathetic nervous systems. It appears to increase the synthesis of noradrenaline, while facilitating the release and blocking re-uptake of the catecholamine at nerve endings. Angiotensin II has a vagal inhibitory action.

The renin–angiotensin system is represented in its entirety within the central nervous system. Angiotensin II receptors and immunoreactive cells have been identified in areas implicated in cardiovascular control, and increased angiotensin II binding has been reported in some brain areas of the spontaneously hypertensive rat when compared with control animals.[32] The importance of angiotensin II as a neurotransmitter, local hormone or circulating factor in the development of hypertension is not known. A large body of evidence supports the view that, at least in one of these roles, this peptide is important in blood pressure control.

Atrial natriuretic peptide

The gene coding for atrial natriuretic peptide is expressed in the brain as well as in cardiac tissue. The highest concentration of atrial natriuretic peptide-like immunoreactive material appears to surround the hypothalamus but nerve fibres apparently containing atrial natriuretic peptide have been noted in several other regions including the nucleus of the tractus solitarius. Depolarization of hypothalamic tissue *in vitro* releases atrial natriuretic peptide, indicating a possible neurotransmitter role. Thus, again, a circulating peptide may also play a role as neurotransmitter.[29]

Probable role of neuronal peptides

It seems likely that numerous peptides act not only as circulating hormones but also as neurotransmitters or as modulators of neurotransmission. Several seem to be located to specific afferent and efferent nerves involved with cardiovascular regulation. Their physiological role and relevance to the development of increased blood pressure remain to be elucidated.

CENTRAL NERVOUS CONTROL OF BLOOD PRESSURE

The expansion of knowledge of the diversity of neurotransmitters and hence of neurones possessing apparently distinct chemical coding has provided new impetus to long-continued studies which have concentrated on the topographical location of pressor and depressor pathways within the central nervous system and especially within the brainstem.[13–15] The rapid development of this field offers the promise of antihypertensive drug design with the specific purpose of altering the actions of the heart, blood vessels and endocrine, paracrine or autocrine glands.

BAROREFLEX FUNCTION

It is now increasingly accepted that the arterial and cardiac baroreceptors, whose efferent function is variously mediated by changes in autonomic nervous activity and possibly hormonal secretion, are concerned principally with short-term circulatory control, i.e. over seconds and minutes. The baroreceptors, however, have little influence on the long-term level of the prevailing tessitura of blood pressure, i.e. that range in which pressure mostly lies, because their discharge threshold is adjusted to major shifts in resting blood pressure.[8]

ION TRANSPORT ACROSS CELL MEMBRANES IN ESSENTIAL HYPERTENSION

This is an area in which interest and experimentation has receded in recent years. In the early 1980's there was intense effort expended in studies of ion transport across cell membranes and especially the cell membranes of human erythrocytes and leucocytes. These blood cells provided readily accessible material that should have reflected any widespread functional tissue disturbances perhaps responsible for increases in blood pressure in response to the relevant environmental stimuli. Although, as Bianchi especially has pointed out,[33] such studies were soundly based, they have not thus far been useful in the classification of patients or in providing the expected insight at the cellular level into the fundamental pathophysiology of essential hypertension. However, the employment of these approaches in animal models, in which the genetic background can be more easily controlled, continues to be pursued with enthusiasm, and still offers the possibility of major understanding of pathophysiology in hypertension.

CELLULAR SODIUM AND CALCIUM METABOLISM: CIRCULATING DIGITALIS-LIKE SUBSTANCES

It has been proposed that, if there were an inherited or acquired defect in renal sodium excretion, endogenous digitalis-like substances could be released into the circulation. By diminishing renal tubular sodium reabsorption, sodium and water excretion would be promoted by such substances. Concurrently, there would be induced increased intracellular vascular smooth muscle sodium and calcium, with a rise in tone, and enhanced contractile response. Thus, hypertension could result.

Increased digitalis-like activity has been reported by several investigators in the plasma and urine of patients with essential hypertension, and in the plasma of some strains of genetically hypertensive rat. The significance of such findings is not yet known.[34,35]

WHOLE-BODY SODIUM AND POTASSIUM CONTENT IN ESSENTIAL HYPERTENSION

In patients with untreated essential hypertension, average values for both total body and total exchangeable sodium and potassium are normal. However, overall, body sodium content is correlated positively, and body potassium negatively, with arterial pressure. Body sodium is reduced in mild, and expanded in more severe, essential hypertension. These relationships are more apparent in men than in women. Further, the correlation with potassium is more marked in younger patients who have milder hypertension, and that with sodium is more prominent in older and more severely affected patients.[11]

The mechanisms underlying these changes are not fully understood, but it has been proposed that essential hypertension may be initiated by a mechanism that is independent of sodium retention (perhaps involving potassium) and which therefore leads to initial sodium depletion, probably because of pressure natriuresis. Some possibilities have already been discussed. Later in the course of the disease, perhaps as a consequence of hypertension-induced renal changes, there is a tendency to sodium retention. These observations have obvious relevance to arguments concerning the role of dietary sodium restriction in the treatment or prevention of essential hypertension (see p. 1229 and 1230).

INTEGRATED CONTROL OF THE CIRCULATION

The various endocrine, paracrine, autocrine, neurological, structural, cellular, and metabolic accompaniments of essential hypertension have, for ease of description, been described largely in isolation one from another. Although this is unavoidable for didactic purposes, it obscures to some extent the critical interactions between these fundamentally interdependent systems. The integrative approach has been especially emphasized by some recent authors, notably Korner[8] and Bianchi.[36] The latter has described the need to consider all levels of organization within the animal in studying the pathogenesis and evolution of hypertension: genetic, molecular, subcellular, cellular, tissue, organ and whole body. As already recognized, such an approach is more readily rewarding in sub-human animal models of hypertension, where genetic control can be strict. In man, the inherited basis of hypertension, although undeniable, is genetically less pure, and abnormalities at the various organizational levels are less clear, although still discernible. However difficult it may be to achieve, the approach does offer the possibility of designing antihypertensive drugs that are directed at rectifying a specifically relevant causative abnormality.

ARTERIAL CHANGES IN HYPERTENSION

Hypertension is associated with, and causes, progressively severe changes in the arteries, both large and small. These changes will be described first, and a more detailed description will follow of the way in which the arterial lesions affect those organs that sustain the greatest damage due to high blood pressure—the eyes, brain and kidneys.[37,38] In the brain and kidneys, distinct functional, as well as pathological, consequences arise from the arterial lesions of hypertension. The cardiac features of hypertension will be described separately.

Hypertensive changes occur in arteries of all sizes, from the aorta to the arterioles. Such widespread structural alterations comprise hypertensive arteriosclerosis. Arterial lesions derive from two main causes: high blood pressure as such, and flow disturbances. The former appear to be more closely related to diastolic; the latter to systolic hypertension.

LARGE ARTERIES

In large and medium-sized arteries (> 1 mm in diameter), the internal elastic lamina is thickened and new layers are formed, especially towards the intima. Smooth muscle becomes hypertrophied. In the later stages, elastic tissue can break up and be partially reabsorbed; there may be some replacement of hypertrophied smooth muscle by fibrous tissue. The vessels become dilated, thickened and rigid, and are frequently tortuous. Loss of distensibility and compliance in lage arteries is associated with increased responses to constrictor stimuli, disproportionate elevation of systolic pressure, flow disturbance, endothelial lesions and atheroma formation. Atheroma, which is especially prominent in large arteries, is described in Chapter 45. Such lesions occurring in the cerebral, cervical, coronary and renal arteries are of special concern. Hypertension-associated changes in the large arteries often proceed also to the formation of saccular or fusiform aneurysms. Less commonly, but more seriously, dissecting aneurysm may occur in hypertension; it is not unusual in patients with aortic coarctation. A tear in the intima, often transverse, permits blood to dissect through the media. The protean clinical features of dissecting aortic aneurysm, its diagnosis and treatment are discussed in detail on page 1352.

SMALL ARTERIES

The pattern of change in small arteries (of 1 mm diameter or less) is different. Medial hypertrophy occurs, as in the larger arteries, but there is a more pronounced intimal thickening resulting from concentric increase in the connective tissue.

In these smaller arteries, there is progressive hyaline arteriosclerosis which eventually may involve the entire circumference apart from the endothelium. In contrast to the larger arteries, the lumen of the smaller arteries narrows, with important pathophysiological consequences. In the later stages, endothelial lesions also are found. Microaneurysms, which can occur spontaneously, develop more readily with raised arterial pressure. They can be seen in the retina on ophthalmoscopy and are of particular importance in the region of the basal ganglia, pons and cerebellum, where they are termed Charcot–Bouchard aneurysms, and can be the site of haemorrhage.

The structural change in smaller arteries, particularly the medial hypertrophy and the luminal narrowing that occurs in consequence, has been studied especially by Folkow and his colleagues.[39] Resistance to flow varies with the fourth power of the luminal radius, and it has been emphasized that such hypertension-induced alterations will lead to narrowing of the lumen, even at maximal dilatation, and therefore to progressively and markedly increased vascular resistance which will thus reinforce the elevation of arterial pressure. It is also likely that the upward re-setting of the limits of autoregulation of blood flow via various organs that occurs in hypertension, and has been particularly well studied in the brain, results from such structural changes in small arteries, with the consequent narrowing of the lumen. It appears that these structural changes in resistance vessels contribute to persistence of hypertension in secondary hypertensive syndromes even after the causal lesion has been corrected. This vascular hypertrophy in hypertension may result not only from mechanical influences; as will be discussed subsequently, other factors, possibly biochemical or nervous, may be involved.

MALIGNANT PHASE

The most severe vascular lesions resulting from hypertension occur in the malignant phase, and this condition deserves detailed exposition. Malignant ('accelerated') phase hypertension is the most severe of the arterial complications associated with a raised blood pressure. Untreated, it is inevitably fatal, usually within months. It is encountered most often at the highest levels of blood pressure, although it may supervene at rather lower values if the increase in blood pressure occurs rapidly.

The characteristic lesion of the malignant phase is necrosis ('fibrinoid necrosis' or 'plasmatic vasculosis') of small arteries and arterioles, which disrupt as a consequence of the very high blood pressure. Necrotic changes occur in already thickened and often hyaline arteriolar walls.

The vascular endothelium breaks and plasma insudates into the media. Thrombotic occlusion of the lumen may occur, leading to infarction in the organ involved. At other sites, the vascular constriction and structural narrowing, which are the early consequences of hypertension, are overcome and the vessels become overdistended and permeable. Thus, malignant hypertension leads in affected organs to a mixture of ischaemia in some areas and overperfusion in others.

Hypertensive encephalopathy, in which headache, confusion, coma and fits may be added to other features of the malignant phase, is a consequence of the systemic arterial pressure exceeding the upper limit of cerebral autoregulation, with consequent cerebral overperfusion and oedema.

The frequency with which different organs are involved in the malignant phase varies among species. In man, the kidney, brain and retina are especially susceptible, with the pancreas, heart and gut also liable to involvement.

It requires emphasis that the malignant phase may supervene in hypertension of whatever aetiology—it is a consequence of very severe hypertension and the speed with which the pressure has risen. It is not a disease in its own right. Of all the known causes of hypertension, only aortic coarctation has been suggested as being immune to the complication of malignant hypertension, although even in coarctation at least one example of the malignant phase has been described.[40]

This concept of the malignant phase being simply a consequence of very severe hypertension has important therapeutic consequences. Most, if not all, of the pathological accompaniments of the malignant phase can be arrested or corrected with appropriate antihypertensive treatment.

CONSEQUENCES OF HYPERTENSIVE DISEASE IN THE EYE, BRAIN AND KIDNEY

The mechanism(s) by which raised blood pressure, and especially the arterial lesions that are its consequences, affect three organs that show particular susceptibility to such disease, and which manifest important clinical features as a result, will now be considered.

THE EYE

The fundus oculi provides the opportunity for the direct inspection of arteries by means of the ophthalmoscope. Detailed study of the eye allows the clinician to assess the evolution and severity of hypertension-associated arterial disease.

In the early stages, the initial arterial consequences of hypertension are shown as thickening, irregularity and tortuosity of the retinal arteries. Occasionally, emboli may be seen traversing the retinal circulation. Central or sectorial retinal arterial or venous occlusions can accompany high blood pressure and may readily be diagnosed ophthalmoscopically.

The most striking retinal appearances accompany the malignant phase of hypertension. The onset of the malignant phase can be recognized ophthalmoscopically by the appearance of bilateral retinal exudates, which may be circumscribed ('hard') or fluffy ('cotton-wool'), haemorrhages, and, in the later stages, papilloedema and retinal oedema (Pl.53.1A). For many years, several workers made a distinction between those patients in whom retinal haemorrhages and exudates were present, but in whom the optic disc was not swollen (and who were termed by them as having 'accelerated hypertension'), and those in whom papilloedema was also apparent. The term 'malignant hypertension' was reserved for the latter cases. There is now extensive evidence that renal arterial fibrinoid necroses are present even when retinal haemorrhages and exudates short of papilloedema have arisen, and the urgency of therapy is or should be as immediate. Thus, irrespective of the presence of optic disc swelling, 'accelerated' and 'malignant' hypertension are now regarded as identical.[2,41]

The above terminology overlaps the classification of Keith, Wagener and Barker[42] which is also extensively employed, especially in North America. This classification, although much criticized,[43] does have the merit of emphasizing the importance of fundoscopy in assessing the progressive arterial disease of advancing hypertension: group I patients, with the mildest disease, show only minor narrowing or sclerosis of the retinal vessels; group II patients show more severe sclerotic changes; group III patients have retinal haemorrhages, exudates and oedema in addition to the arterial irregularities of group II; and, in group IV, swelling of the optic discs is also evident.

The pathology of the retinal lesions in malignant hypertension has been well studied. Arteriolar leakage is demonstrable on fluorescein angiography. Focal micro-infarction in the inner two-thirds of the retina gives rise to the 'cotton-wool' exudates in the nerve fibre layer, and these exudates comprise the swollen bulbous ends of axons (cytoid bodies) containing both normal and degenerate organelles. 'Hard' exudates are caused by the accumulation of plasma and lipid in the outer plexiform layer of the retina in the 'watershed' zone between the retinal and choroidal circulations. In severe cases, they form a characteristic 'star' around the macula. Haemorrhages from pre-capillary arteries and from capillaries tend to be flame shaped in the nerve fibre layer, and rounded ('blot' haemorrhages) in the outer plexiform layer. Micro-aneurysms appear as small evaginations in the capillary wall, and occur when the endothelial cells or pericytes are destroyed by ischaemia. Papilloedema is the result of massive interference with axoplasmic flow at the disc. Elschnig's spots are small white areas in the fundus resulting from depigmentation in infarcted areas of the pigment epithelium. The various lesions of the malignant phase resolve with effective antihypertensive treatment. The ocular lesions, which are often accompanied by marked visual disturbances, can clear completely in weeks or months (Pl.53.1A,B).

THE BRAIN

Physiological changes: autoregulation of cerebral blood flow

The arterial and arteriolar wall hypertrophy in hypertension is probably a major cause of the upward re-setting of the limits of systemic arterial pressure between which cerebral blood flow is kept constant ('autoregulation of cerebral blood flow') (Fig. 53.3). The upward shift of the upper limit of such autoregulation almost certainly has a protective effect, limiting the likelihood of cerebral over-perfusion and oedema, and thus of hypertensive encephalopathy, in the event of marked elevation of systemic arterial pressure. However, the upward shift also of the lower limit of cerebral autoregulation means that in hypertension, if the blood pressure is suddenly lowered, for example, by overzealous drug administration, cerebral under-perfusion, ischaemia and possibly infarction can occur at higher absolute levels of pressure than

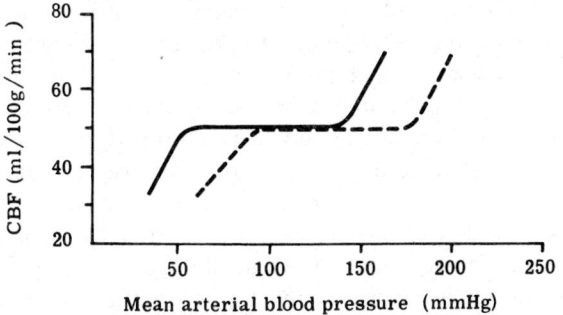

Fig. 53.3. Diagram showing the limits of autoregulation of cerebral blood flow in a normal person (continuous line) and patient with hypertension (dotted line). Cerebral blood flow is held constant over wide limits of systemic arterial pressure. If the systemic blood pressure exceeds the upper limit of autoregulation, the brain will be overperfused and become oedematous. If the pressure falls below the lower limit of autoregulation, cerebral ischaemia and possible infarction will result. Reproduced by permission from Graham, D.I. *et al.* In: *Handbook of Hypertension, Vol. 1: Clinical Aspects of Essential Hypertension*, p.174.

would be the case in normal subjects. This has important implications for antihypertensive therapy, especially in the elderly subject.

Pathological changes

Stroke

Hypertension as such is a major cause of primary intracerebral haemorrhage which accounts for some 20% of strokes. About 80% of such bleeds occur in the cerebral hemispheres, 10% in the brainstem and 8% in the cerebellum. Many of these events occur at the site of micro-aneurysms of the intracranial arteries.

The majority (more than 80%) of strokes result from cerebral infarction, for which hypertension is an important but less direct predisposing factor. Plaques of atheroma may cause cerebral infarcts, either by leading to progressive occlusion of arteries or by acting as a source of emboli, composed variously of atheromatous debris and cholesterol crystals, or mixtures of fibrin, leucocytes and platelets.[38]

The rarer cerebral and cerebellar infarcts that can result from sudden blood pressure reduction and consequent cerebral ischaemia have already been mentioned. They occur at the 'watershed' zones between the areas of distribution of major cerebral arteries.

Transient ischaemic attacks

Transient ischaemic attacks are defined as reversible disturbances of cerebral function lasting < 24 h. They can result from temporary arterial occlusion by embolism, from external compression of an artery, especially if it is already the seat of disease, or from sudden hypotension, for example, due to cardiac arrhythmia. It has been estimated that some 30% of transient ischaemic attacks evolve to a major stroke within 5 years. It is further considered that hypertension is a potent factor predisposing to such an adverse sequel.

Subarachnoid haemorrhage

The role of hypertension in the causation of subarachnoid haemorrhage is uncertain, although associations have been reported between subarachnoid haemorrhage and coarctation of the aorta, polycystic kidneys or fibromuscular hyperplasia of the renal arteries. However, in these conditions, the link may be a disorder of mesodermal development rather than one of raised blood pressure. Nevertheless, prognosis following subarachnoid rupture of a saccular aneurysm is worse in a hypertensive patient, and appropriate antihypertensive therapy is needed.

Dementia

The association between dementia and hypertension is often obscure. However, so-called multi-infarct dementia, in which progressive deterioration of mental function is accompanied by focal neurological signs, is usually associated with hypertension, and patients could benefit from antihypertensive therapy.

THE KIDNEY

Physiological changes

In the kidney, arterial and arteriolar narrowing in hypertension has been invoked as the cause of the upward re-setting of the levels of systemic arterial pressure that can induce natriuresis ('pressure natriuresis'). Guyton and his colleagues[44] have discussed the importance of the consequent tendency for salt and water retention to occur unless the kidney is perfused at higher arterial pressure. Thus, the 'renal barostat' has been regarded by some workers as representing an extension of the concept of arterial and arteriolar wall hypertrophy in hypertension which could be especially relevant to the pathogenesis of the raised arterial pressure.

Pathological changes

Renal lesions occurring in the malignant phase of hypertension are serious. In a majority of patients, the kidney sustains most of the consequences of the malignant phase, with extensive and progressive fibrinoid necrosis of afferent glomerular arterioles, glomerular infarction and consequent renal impairment. Thus, in malignant hypertension, provided the course is not terminated abruptly by a catastrophic cerebral lesion or by cardiac failure, left untreated the patient will eventually succumb to renal failure. The urinary accompaniments of renal lesions of the malignant phase are proteinuria, haematuria and granular casts.

Short of the malignant phase, the clinical effects of hypertension on the kidney are not prominent. However, the decline in renal function with age is faster in the presence of a raised arterial pressure.[45] It is possible that effective antihypertensive therapy

could slow down this progressive renal impairment.

Atheroma of the renal artery is the commonest cause of renal artery stenosis (see p. 1260).

THE HEART IN HYPERTENSION

LEFT VENTRICULAR HYPERTROPHY

An early and consistent feature of hypertension is left ventricular hypertrophy. This appears to be closely akin both in its genesis and rate of development to the medial hypertrophy of small arteries and arterioles already described. There may also be similarities between the heart and small blood vessels in the regression of hypertrophy with treatment of hypertension.[46–48]

The increase in left ventricular mass in hypertension is associated with enlargement of cardiac myocytes but does not involve an increase in their numbers. Greater wall thickness without enlargement of the ventricular cavity is called concentric hypertrophy. Enlargement of the ventricular cavity without increase in the ratio of wall thickness to chamber size despite an increase in left ventricular mass is called eccentric hypertrophy. It has been speculated that, although left ventricular hypertrophy may initially be adaptive and hence beneficial, later, increased collagen deposition will reduce ventricular compliance and impair left ventricular relaxation lusitropy and filling. End-diastolic pressure consequently is elevated, and plasma ANP increased. Left ventricular hypertrophy in hypertension has been found to be accompanied by a reduction in adrenoceptor numbers, and in these circumstances there may be a greater dependence on the Frank–Starling mechanism than on neurohumoral factors to maintain cardiac function. Herein, it is supposed, lies a major reason for progression to cardiac failure in hypertension. Because coronary filling is mainly during diastole, and may be impaired with left ventricular hypertrophy, subendocardial ischaemia is frequent. Cardiac impairment in hypertension may also be a partial consequence of hypertrophy of the media of coronary arterioles or of coronary arteriolar fibrinoid necrosis in the malignant phase. Another possible contributory factor is multifocal ventricular myocardial necrosis, which can be caused by high circulating concentrations of angiotensin II or catecholamines.[49]

In some patients with mild hypertension and little evidence of left ventricular hypertrophy, it appears that the pressure load is supported by increased myocardial contractility rather than by ventricular hypertrophy. Concentric hypertrophy is characteristic of established hypertension without cardiac impairment. Eccentric hypertrophy is associated with less complete systolic emptying. The haemodynamic consequences of these functional changes are discussed below.

It has long been known that left ventricular hypertrophy in hypertension, assessed electrocardiographically, is associated with increased morbidity and mortality. More recent and more accurate methods of measuring left ventricular dimensions, for example, echocardiography, have reinforced these findings. Ventricular ectopic rhythms are more prevalent in the presence of hypertensive left ventricular hypertrophy.

The mechanical effect of blood pressure elevation in the genesis of hypertensive left ventricular hypertrophy, although important, is only one of several factors involved. Numerous studies have failed to show a close correlation between the arterial pressure and the extent of cardiac hypertrophy, although the relationship becomes closer if blood pressure measurements are made over 24 h rather than single readings are utilized. Blood viscosity is also correlated with left ventricular hypertrophy. The possible neural and humoral influences are discussed on page 1242.

HAEMODYNAMIC CHARACTERISTICS OF HYPERTENSION[50,51]

The haemodynamic accompaniments of hypertension are in conformity with the structural and functional changes in resistance vessels and the heart already described. In young subjects with borderline and often very labile hypertension, interindividual variations in haemodynamics may be considerable.

More consistent findings are apparent in young adults with established hypertension (> 140/90 mmHg) that remains uncomplicated. In these subjects, the characteristic pattern is a high cardiac index with an elevated heart rate, and a numerically normal calculated total peripheral resistance.

Later in the course of the disease, the dominant haemodynamic disturbance is an increase in total peripheral resistance; at this stage, cardiac index is lower than that in normotensive control subjects and lower than in the usually younger milder hypertensives. Heart rate may still be slightly elevated. With increasing severity of hypertension and the onset of organ damage, there is a markedly increased total peripheral resistance, a decrease in cardiac index and a reduced stroke volume.

Regional measurements have shown that in established hypertension there is an increased vascular resistance across the kidneys, liver and skeletal muscle. As previously mentioned, the coronary vascular reserve is characteristically reduced, in proportion to the severity of the hypertension. The more serious supervention of atheromatous coronary artery stenosis is discussed below.

PATHOLOGICAL CARDIAC CHANGES

Cardiac failure

The subtle and pervasive effects of hypertension on left ventricular morphology and function, the increased workload imposed directly by the raised arterial pressure, the decline in ventricular adrenoceptor numbers, the diminution in coronary reserve, and possible myocardial necrotic lesions provide substantial reasons for the supervention of cardiac failure in this condition. Three decades ago, before the widespread availability of effective antihypertensive drug treatment, cardiac failure was one of the most common complications of hypertension, and one of the most frequent causes of death in that condition. It is now much rarer. It is especially likely to appear in the malignant phase, where the occasional occurrence of fibrinoid necroses in the coronary arterial tree may also contribute; however, the major cause is almost certainly the extremely high systemic arterial pressure.

Coronary artery atheromatous disease

Coronary artery atheroma is one of the most frequent accompaniments of raised arterial pressure. It has come into increasing prominence in recent years with greater attention being paid to mild elevation of blood pressure. In the lower ranges of hypertension, coronary disease predominates over stroke and cardiac failure in frequency. There is a strong correlation between high blood pressure and atheromatous coronary artery disease. The association was for long assumed to be causal, but failure of antihypertensive therapy appreciably to diminish deaths from coronary events has cast doubt on this assumption. Other possible reasons for this therapeutic failure are discussed on pages 1244 and 1245.

CAUSES OF CARDIAC AND VASCULAR HYPERTROPHY IN HYPERTENSION

The importance of the progressive cardiac structural and functional changes in the evolution of hypertension and its complications should be clear from the foregoing account. The concurrent loss of distensibility and compliance in large arteries leads to disproportionate elevation of systolic pressure, turbulence of flow, endothelial damage and atheroma formation, while progressive hypertrophy of the media of resistance vessels is similarly crucial to the increasing severity of the hypertension and its circulatory pattern as well as to the sequential changes in renal function with the advance of the disease.

Although the mechanical effect of elevation of arterial pressure as such provides a stimulus to cardiac and vascular muscular hypertrophy, and thus to further progression of the hypertension, reasons have been advanced for its inadequacy as a sole explanation.[12,47] Extensive efforts have been devoted to the elucidation of additional stimuli. In this connexion, most workers have regarded such influences as probably affecting the heart and resistance vessels alike.

Blood viscosity is one probable stimulus. There are numerous other vascular growth factors, demonstrable or speculative, around which an extensive literature has accumulated.[8,12,47,52] These include enhanced sympathetic activity, with consequent elevation of adrenaline and/or noradrenaline locally or within the circulation, corticosteroids, serotonin (5-hydroxtryptamine), angiotensin II, either in peripheral blood or generated within the heart or blood vessels, growth hormone, insulin, somatomedin C, platelet-derived growth factor, endothelial-derived growth factor, epidermal-derived growth factor, monocyte-derived growth factor, β-transforming growth factor, heparin, bradykinin, prostaglandins, vasopressin, thyroid hormone and substance P.

Numerous attempts have been made in recent years to identify and to utilize drugs in the treatment of hypertension that would be useful not only in lowering blood pressure but also in arresting and more particularly reversing left ventricular and resistance vessel hypertrophy, and thus in remodelling the left ventricle and enhancing its functional characteristics while improving arterial compliance. Such approaches are as yet rudimentary, but the results of both human and animal studies have indicated that the centrally acting agents methyldopa and reserpine, calcium antagonists of classes I and II, converting enzyme inhibitors and serotonin antagonists could be particularly useful. By contrast, vasodilators such as hydralazine, alpha-adrenergic blockers, such as prazosin or trimazosin, and diuretics have appeared less so.[47] Although this is an active field of research that offers much promise, the supposed differential benefit of various drug classes remains in many respects uncertain.

FACTORS INFLUENCING THE COMPLICATIONS OF HYPERTENSION

Although raised blood pressure *per se* and accompanying flow turbulence have been considered herein as principal causes of the complications of that disease, these are affected by several additional factors. Some have already been mentioned in relation to cardiac hypertrophy. There are several other important influences.[1,2]

AGE

Advancing age predisposes to stroke, cardiac failure, coronary heart disease and progressive renal failure. Concomitant hypertension, probably independently, compounds the risk. However, the malignant phase, alone among the complications of hypertension, is less likely to occur after the age of 60 years than before.

GENDER

For any given blood pressure value, the complication attack rate is higher in men than in women both before and during treatment.[53] This does not indicate that women are immune to the consequences of high blood pressure. Hypertensive women are at risk when compared with their sisters who have lower blood pressure values, but in absolute terms much less so than are men with comparable blood pressure. The male to female differential risk is less marked, but still distinct, after the menopause.

SOCIAL CLASS

Social class (and also some behavioural accompaniments of social differentiation, such as smoking) markedly affect not only the prevalence but also the consequences of high blood pressure. Ménard and his colleagues[6] have testified to, for example, the more ready access of members of the higher social classes to the medical care of hypertension and thus presumably to a more satisfactory response to treatment. By contrast, social class was not found to be related to risk among treated hypertensive patients in the Glasgow Blood Pressure Clinic.[54]

RACE

Racial differences, which often tend to be associated with social class, demonstrate variations in the pattern of hypertension-related complications. In an English study, it was shown that, when correction was made for differences in social class, there were distinctions in the pattern of hypertension-related complications in whites, blacks (mainly of West Indian origin) and Asians (mainly from the Indian subcontinent). The West Indians had proportionately more strokes and fewer heart attacks than did the whites or Asians. Both non-white groups had a higher prevalence of diabetes mellitus.[7]

SMOKING

Of all the factors influencing the frequency and pattern of hypertension-related diseases, cigarette smoking is pre-eminent. Smoking is such a powerful independent risk factor for cardiovascular disease that it may overwhelm a raised blood pressure in importance.[55–58] Smoking greatly compounds the effects of high blood pressure *per se*. For example, the incidence of the malignant phase is more frequent, and its prognosis, even when treated, is distinctly poorer in smokers than in non-smokers. Renal artery stenosis is more prevalent in smokers. Hypertension-related stroke and coronary disease are also much more frequent in smokers, irrespective of treatment.

SERUM CHOLESTEROL

Serum cholesterol is an independent risk factor for cardiovascular disease, and thus the complications of hypertension increase in proportion to the level of serum cholesterol.

OBESITY

Although obesity can lead to or worsen hypertension, while bodyweight reduction can aid blood pressure control, it remains uncertain whether obesity is additionally, and independently, a risk factor for cardiovascular complications.[3,9]

URIC ACID

There is no conclusive evidence that either spontaneous or diuretic-induced elevation of serum uric acid in hypertension worsens vascular risk.[59,60]

DIABETES MELLITUS

Diabetes mellitus is associated with vascular lesions, and thus the co-existence of diabetes with hypertension increases the risk of vascular disease. Diabetes also introduces problems into the management of hypertension, because certain classes of drugs, notably thiazide diuretics and beta-adrenoceptor blocking agents, can impair glucose tolerance, and destabilize diabetic control.

COMPOUNDING OF RISK

The manner in which additional factors can compound the cardiovascular dangers of hypertension is shown in Fig. 53.4.

INCIDENCE OF THE MALIGNANT PHASE

In Sweden and in Australia, there has been an apparent decline in the incidence of the malignant phase of hypertension in the past decade. The reasons for this change are not understood, but one possibility[61] is more effective screening, prevention and therapy. No such decline is evident in Great Britain; although exact figures are difficult to obtain, there is clearly no shortage of patients who have malignant hypertension in cities such as Birmingham and Glasgow.[55,57]

BENEFITS FROM TREATING HYPERTENSION

The various cardiovascular complications associated with raised systemic arterial pressure are described in detail elsewhere (p. 1237–42). Specifically, they comprise the malignant phase (including hypertensive encephalopathy), cardiac failure, stroke, coronary heart disease and progressive impairment of renal function. Antihypertensive therapy is directed to the prevention or correction of these disorders. The effectiveness of treatment has been evaluated with progressive refinement since the introduction of drugs capable of lowering

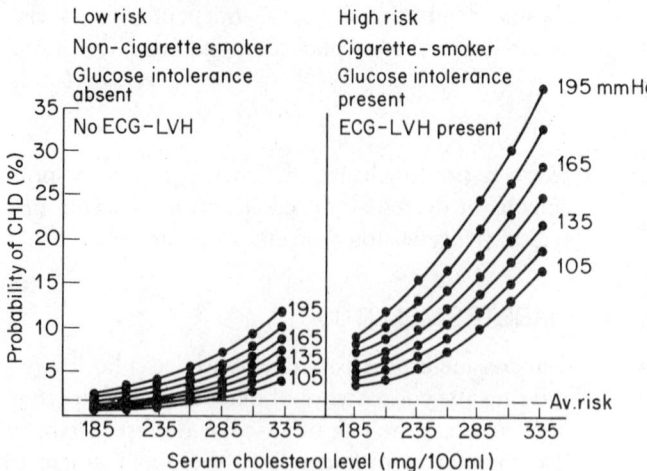

Low risk
Non-cigarette smoker
Glucose intolerance absent
No ECG-LVH

High risk
Cigarette-smoker
Glucose intolerance present
ECG-LVH present

Fig. 53.4. The interaction of several risk factors with systolic arterial pressure in relation to the development of coronary heart disease. The information is taken from the 16-year follow-up in 40-year-old men, and indicates the risk of developing coronary disease in 6 years. (Reproduced from Kannel, W.B. and Stokes, J. Hypertension as a Cardiovascular Risk Factor. In: *Handbook of Hypertension, Vol. 6: Epidemiology of Hypertension*, p.25, by permission of the authors and the publishers, Elsevier, Amsterdam.) 185 mg/100 ml (4.8 mmol/l), 335 mg/100 ml (8.7 mmol/l) serum cholesterol.

arterial pressure in the 1950s. From that time, virtually all of the progress in this respect has been derived from pharmacological treatment. Although there has been steady and increasing interest in non-pharmacological means of blood pressure reduction, such approaches have so far had limited application, and their effect in obviating complications has not been assessed.[3,8–10]

For many years, it was assumed that the complications were the result of high blood pressure as such, and that treatment should therefore be directed at lowering the raised pressure by whatever means available. Recently, there has been increasing interest in possible ancillary benefits of certain drug classes beyond their ability to lower blood pressure. There has also been some caution in assigning potential benefit to newly introduced types of agent, for example, converting enzyme inhibitors or calcium antagonists, because these have not been employed in trials evaluating benefit with blood pressure reduction. Most intervention studies have been focused on diastolic rather than systolic blood pressure in assessing benefit, although it is now clear that systolic blood pressure is at least as important in indicating cardiovascular risk. Furthermore, as the incidence of complications is, for any level of blood pressure at any age, lower in women than in men, evidence of benefit is less clear in women.[53] Moreover, some trials have included only men.

Very soon after the availability of antihypertensive drugs, it became evident that these could correct both the malignant phase (provided that this had not progressed to severe renal failure) and hypertensive heart failure.[62] These benefits were sufficiently clear to preclude the need for formal controlled studies. The demonstration of benefit

from the prophylactic treatment of hypertension required controlled clinical trials (Fig. 53.1), and these have been conducted with progressive refinement since the pioneering study of Hamilton *et al.* in 1964.[63] These various studies have, despite their several faults, lowered the threshold of presenting diastolic pressure (fifth phase), above which a protective effect may be discerned, to 90 mmHg.[62] With such a low threshold at which, at least statistically, benefit can be seen, the advantages at the lower levels of raised pressure are numerically modest, despite the increasingly large numbers of subjects qualifying potentially for therapy.

Hypertensive subjects between the ages of 60 and 79 years have also been shown to have a reduced incidence of complications with treatment, although there is a suggestion that, within this range, the older the subject the less effective is drug therapy. It remains uncertain whether those over 80 years would benefit.[64] Moreover, despite the evident risks accompanying a raised systolic pressure, no advantage has yet been seen from treating elderly subjects with systolic pressures in the range 170–279 mmHg but who have a diastolic pressure below 90 mmHg, so-called 'systolic only' hypertension.

The principal benefits that have emerged from the controlled intervention trials are prevention of stroke and of cardiac failure, and a decline in the progression of renal impairment. Thus far, by contrast, no good evidence of protection against coronary artery disease has been seen, despite the clear association between hypertension and coronary disease. This is a particularly important defect because, in considering progressively milder hypertension, coronary artery disease and its sequelae increasingly predominate over other complications.

Several possible reasons for the failure of antihypertensive drug therapy appreciably to influence ischaemic heart disease have been considered.[65,66] Perhaps most germane is that therapy has focused on high blood pressure as such, to the neglect of related disorders such as left ventricular hypertrophy and reduced large arterial compliance. Thus less impact has been made on atheromatous complications. Among other possibilities are that the relationship with hypertension may not be causal, that because coronary disease is multifactorial in pathogenesis, moderating just one of these factors, hypertension, may have limited influence on the disease, that the vascular pathology differs substantially from that of stroke and hence is less susceptible to treatment, that in the various trials treatment may not have been initiated early enough or have been continued for long enough to show benefit, or that some of the drugs used to treat hypertension may also have some adverse influences in relation to coronary artery disease. In this last connection, the thiazide diuretics, which have been used in nearly all the major studies, have come particularly under suspicion.[67-69] They can provoke a range of complex ventricular ectopic rhythms, which might possibly predispose to sudden death in susceptible individuals, they impair glucose tolerance, and they distort plasma lipids in a manner considered to be potentially adverse. Other workers[70] have interpreted the results of recent trials as freeing diuretics from taint.

Additional evidence from retrospective studies, which has not been fully accepted, has indicated that, in hypertensive patients who already have coronary artery disease, lowering of the diastolic pressure too far (below about 85 mmHg) may increase the risk of coronary events in comparison with more modest blood pressure reduction.[71,72] The arguments advanced in this connexion are that coronary filling is dependent on diastolic pressure and thus, if the latter falls too low in the presence of a coronary artery stenosis, myocardial oxygenation is readily impaired, especially because in the coronary arterial circulation oxygen extraction is already near its maximum.[73]

Despite the successes of antihypertensive drug therapy, several reports have shown that, in treated hypertensive subjects, cardiovascular risk remains worse than that in control populations. In large measure, this is attributable to the failure appreciably to moderate the consequences of coronary artery disease, the possible reasons for which have been considered above. It is likely also that more frequent benefit has been obtained with haemorrha-

gic than with atheromatous stroke. Another potential contributing factor is that reduction of blood pressure, in many clinics, has been inadequate.[72]

The notion that certain drug classes might possess particular adverse properties, notably that thiazides might have demerits in relation to coronary artery disease, although still extant, remains unproven. Similarly, the possession of specific beneficial properties by some agents, although being enthusiastically examined, remains equivocal. For example, the suggestion in two trials[74,75] that beta-adrenoceptor blocking drugs might protect against coronary artery disease in non-smoking men was not borne out in a third study.[76] Similarly, the notion that thiazides might be especially protective in relation to stroke has not been confirmed.[77] The difficulties in achieving a working consensus is emphasized by two related studies in which cardioselective beta-blockers were compared with thiazide diuretics in hypertensive men. In one trial, employing both atenolol and metoprolol,[76] there was no evident superiority of beta-blockade. In the other related study, using only metoprolol, beta-blockade, for similar blood pressure reduction, was associated with significantly fewer cardiovascular complications than was thiazide treatment.[77]

Although the presence of risk factors for cardiovascular complications additional to hypertension is usually taken to increase the urgency of therapy, treatment appears, conversely, to be less effective in correcting or arresting their progress in these circumstances.

ANTIHYPERTENSIVE THERAPY

Until recent years, antihypertensive therapy was based on the assumption that all methods were equally efficacious in correcting or preventing complications, given that the blood pressure was lowered.[78] Thus, treatment might be surgical, pharmacological or non-pharmacological. One of the earliest pieces of evidence that the malignant phase was simply a complication of high blood pressure, albeit a very severe one, and not a disease entity in its own right, was that it might be corrected irrespective of the method of blood pressure reduction employed (Pl. 53.1A, B).

SURGICAL THERAPY

The surgical treatment of essential hypertension (as contrasted with the surgical correction of a specific lesion causing secondary hypertension) is now of historic interest only. Such measures included bilateral dorsolumbar sympathectomy and adrenalectomy. These were formidable surgical procedures, with a high rate of complications and usually unpleasant side-effects. However, they did demonstrate the value of blood pressure reduction in correcting the most severe complications of high blood pressure, such as the malignant phase and hypertensive heart failure, thereby providing a basis for the use of drug therapy.

ANTIHYPERTENSIVE DRUGS

The use of antihypertensive drugs has dominated the treatment of hypertension for the past four decades and will provide the mainstay of therapy in the immediate future at least,[79] although non-pharmacological means are being increasingly enthusiastically explored.[9,10] Details of the wide range of individual drugs and of dosage are given in the Appendix to the book.

Autonomic ganglion-blocking agents

The development of the earliest effective antihypertensive drugs, the autonomic ganglion blocking agents, followed logically from bilateral dorsolumbar sympathectomy. The introduction of these agents represented one of the major therapeutic advances this century.[78] However, the sympathetic blockade meant that ganglion blockers, to be effective, had a marked postural hypotensive effect; their parasympathetic blocking actions induced constipation, dryness of the mouth and occasional paralytic ileus.

Adrenergic neuron-blocking drugs

Their successors, the sympatholytic agents such as bretylium, guanethidine, bethanidine and debrisoquine are highly concentrated in adrenergic neurons, blocking neurotransmitter release. Thus, they combined the disadvantages of unopposed parasympathetic discharge with sympathetic blockade. Their administration was therefore characterized by postural hypotension and diarrhoea.

Both the ganglion blockers and the adrenergic neuron blocking agents have now passed out of clinical use.

Centrally acting drugs

This class now contains principally three drugs, alpha-methyldopa (methyldopa), clonidine and reserpine. These agents have important similarities and differences of action.

Methyldopa

Methyldopa has been most valuable in the treatment of hypertension and, despite its obsolescence, remains widely used. Its mode of action remains imperfectly understood. Methyldopa was thought to lower blood pressure by inhibiting the enzyme dopa-decarboxylase, thereby limiting the generation of catecholamines. Additionally, with methyldopa therapy, noradrenaline in sympathetic nerve terminals is replaced by alpha-methyl-noradrenaline, a much weaker agonist than noradrenaline itself and thus a so-called 'false transmitter'. Third, the methyldopa metabolite, alpha-methyl noradrenaline, has central nervous system effects, prominent among which is probably alpha-2 adrenergic agonism, depressing sympathetic nerve discharge. All three of these actions could contribute to the reduction of arterial pressure.

Methyldopa lowers blood pressure, with a mild but usually distinct additional fall in pressure on standing. Heart rate is modestly slowed.

Side-effects include drowsiness, dryness of the mouth, nasal stuffiness, postural hypotension, rashes and diarrhoea. Rarer but more serious is toxic hepatitis, which occurs in one of two forms, either early or during chronic therapy. Haemolytic anaemia may also be a problem. The initial days and weeks of treatment with methyldopa can be accompanied by salt and water retention, which may limit the antihypertensive effect (so-called 'false tolerance'). This often requires methyldopa to be given in combination with a diuretic to obtain the best therapeutic result.

Methyldopa has been extensively employed in the treatment of pregnancy hypertension, and the demonstration of this aspect of its safety is reassuring. It was also tried and its value shown as a supplementary drug in the European trial of antihypertensive treatment in the elderly, and in the Australian and the British trials of mild hypertension treatment.[62]

Marked rebound hypertension when methyldopa is discontinued is not usually a feature, and this is an important aspect of distinction and advantage in comparison with clonidine.

Clonidine

The mode of action of this drug appears to be a

centrally mediated alpha-2 adrenergic agonism, which depresses sympathetic discharge. Clonidine effectively lowers arterial pressure with, like methyldopa, a distinct reduction of heart rate but probably less of a postural component. The most prominent side-effects are somnolence, dryness of the mouth and constipation. If clonidine therapy is suddenly stopped, there follows excessive sympathetic discharge for 1–2 days, with a surfeit of circulating catecholamines, tachycardia, rebound hypertension and headache. The attack has all the features of a paroxysm of phaeochromocytoma, which it closely resembles pathophysiologically. These attacks can be treated by promptly re-starting clonidine, or, as for phaeochromocytoma, giving alpha-blockers alone, or both alpha- and beta-adrenergic antagonists. More recently, clonidine has been given transdermally rather than orally, an adhesive polymer designed to release clonidine over 1 week being applied to the chest or upper arm. However, skin reactions have been reported in up to 25% of patients given clonidine by patch application. Rebound hypertension has been noted after removal of the clonidine patch.

Reserpine

Reserpine is a rauwolfia alkaloid that depletes noradrenaline stores in sympathetic nerve terminals both within the central nervous system and peripherally. The effect is cumulative and may persist for several weeks after stopping therapy.

Blood pressure lowering is accompanied by some cardiac slowing, but there is minimal postural hypotensive effect.

Side-effects include nasal stuffiness, diarrhoea, drowsiness, lethargy and occasional frank depression.

Although its use is widespread in some countries, notably the USA, Germany and Switzerland, reserpine has never been widely employed in Great Britain, largely because of the depression it may cause, although this is an unusual occurrence at the doses now prescribed.

Diuretics

The antihypertensive effect of the orally acting diuretics has been shown for all of the commonly used thiazides and related drugs, as well as for the more powerful loop diuretics frusemide, ethacrynic acid and xipamide, and the potassium-conserving agents amiloride, spironolactone, canrenoate and triamterene. Generally, the longer acting thiazides, such as bendrofluazide or hydrochlorothiazide, which do not have an abrupt and severe diuretic effect, makes them the most appropriate in the treatment of essential hypertension, unless there are particular features such as renal or cardiac impairment or resistant hypertension which require a loop diuretic. The potassium-conserving agents also have an antihypertensive action, and have been employed as monotherapy in essential hypertension. More usually, however, potassium-conserving drugs are reserved for use in conjunction with a thiazide, when they add to the blood pressure lowering action while helping to sustain plasma potassium. In addition, potassium-conserving diuretics are invaluable as pre-operative therapy in patients with aldosterone-secreting tumours. This use is described in detail on page 1269.

The mode of action of diuretics in lowering arterial pressure in essential hypertension remains uncertain. One obvious possibility is a diuretic and natriuretic effect, with reduction of plasma volume. Although this is plausible, and consistent with the sustained elevations of renin and angiotensin II diuretics produce, it has been difficult to confirm clinically. In one experimental study of chlorothiazide in the spontaneously hypertensive rat,[80] the blood pressure reduction and diminution of exchangeable sodium were dissociated. Exchangeable body potassium content is lowered, together with plasma potassium concentration, with long-term diuretic treatment of essential hypertension. Diuretic-induced loss of sodium and water from the wall of resistance vessels could alter the wall to lumen ratio and facilitate blood pressure reduction. A further possibility is that diuretics lower blood pressure by causing, via a direct effect on arterial smooth muscle, vasodilatation in resistance vessels. This notion is given some credence by the observation that a closely related but non-diuretic drug, diazoxide, is a powerful vasodilator.

The wide range of diuretics available, and their doses, are summarized in the Appendix to this book. Diuretics, and especially the thiazides, have provided the backbone of therapy in all of the major therapeutic trials, and experience of several decades of their use, together with their comparative cheapness, has given a confidence in their employment to many physicians, who regard them as often the first choice in hypertensive treatment. However, the thiazides carry a substantial burden of side-effects, endorsed by findings from the same trials as have confirmed their value. They impair glucose tolerance, they raise serum uric acid and cause gout, they are associated with hypokalaemia and ventricular ectopic activity, the latter more often in older patients, they elevate serum cholesterol, they can depress plasma sodium, they cause muscle cramps, constipation and lethargy, and they provoke male sexual impotence.[67-69] More rare but serious problems are bone marrow depression, hepatitis and necrotizing vasculitis. In some trials, the dose of thiazide was too high; more modest doses would alleviate certain of the problems.

Several of the above side-effects are shared by the loop diuretics, but generally the metabolic disturbances with these agents are less marked than those with the thiazides.

With the use of potassium-conserving agents, hyperkalaemia is a potential danger, especially if there is impairment of renal function. In addition, flatulence has been reported with amiloride, impotence, gynaecomastia, menstrual irregularities and peptic ulceration with spironolactone, and rashes and megaloblastosis with triamterene.

Vasodilators

Dilatation in resistance vessels is a feature of the action of several classes of antihypertensive agent. However, the term is usually reserved for those drugs that cause vasodilatation by a presumed direct action on vascular smooth muscle.

Hydralazine

Hydralazine especially has been a mainstay of antihypertensive therapy for many years, often being given in conjunction with a diuretic and beta-adrenergic blocking agent as 'standard triple therapy'. The full potential of this drug was realized only after the introduction of the beta-blockers, with their action in slowing heart rate. Before that, tachycardia reflexly caused by the vasodilatation limited the application of hydralazine. Postural hypotension is unusual.

Hydralazine can cause fluid retention, and if doses in excess of 200 mg are given daily a syndrome akin to lupus erythematosus can occur, with features of fever, weight loss, joint pains, arthritis and rashes; more rarely, splenomegaly, pleurisy and pericarditis occur. The haemoglobin level may fall, lupus cells may appear in the blood and the erythrocyte sedimentation rate is increased. Renal involvement is unusual. Individuals who acetylate hydralazine only slowly are particularly prone to this syndrome, which has been estimated

to appear in as many as 12% of women and 3% of men during long-term treatment. Sometimes, hirsutism can occur.

Hydralazine, however, remains a most valuable drug and, in one comparative trial of a range of adjuncts to beta-blocker plus thiazide treatment, it was found to be best in terms of efficacy and side-effects.

Minoxidil

A much more powerful vasodilator is minoxidil, reserved for resistant hypertension, in which it is very effective. This drug causes more marked fluid retention and tachycardia than does hydralazine, and therefore should be given in conjunction with a beta-blocker and a loop diuretic. In patients unable to tolerate a beta-blocker for any reason, methyldopa or an angiotensin converting enzyme (ACE) inhibitor or verapamil can sometimes control minoxidil-induced tachycardia.

A major disadvantage of minoxidil treatment is hirsutism. This can lead to refusal to take the drug, despite its efficacy, particularly by female patients.

Diazoxide

Diazoxide, a powerful vasodilator, although very effective, is now little used because it causes, almost always, diabetes mellitus. Other side-effects include tachycardia and hirsutism.

Beta-blockers

The antihypertensive effect of the beta-adrenoceptor blocking agents was discovered by an astute clinical observation.[81] Their mode of action remains obscure. With the thiazide diuretics they are the agents of first choice for many physicians, and they have the additional advantage of combining well with diuretics. The triple combination with a diuretic and a vasodilator, such as hydralazine, is often a standard form of treatment.

A range of beta-adrenoceptor blocking agents has been used in the treatment of hypertension, which vary widely in their individual characteristics (see Appendix to the book). The common feature apparently necessary for blood pressure reduction is beta-1-receptor antagonism.

At least four possible modes of action of beta-blocking agents have been considered in attempting to explain their ability to lower arterial pressure: a central nervous system effect diminishing sympathetic outflow; reduction in cardiac output; diminution of renin secretion; and a pre-synaptic action inhibiting neurotransmitter release. None is entirely convincing as a single explanation.[81,82]

A central nervous effect may contribute but, as a wide range of beta-adrenoceptor blocking agents lower arterial pressure irrespective of their capacity to enter the brain, this seems at best to provide only a partial explanation.

The possibility that beta-blockers could reduce blood pressure by diminishing cardiac output has been studied in detail by several workers. When a drug such as propranolol is administered, there is an initial fall in cardiac output and in arterial pressure, with a rise in calculated peripheral resistance. With continued therapy, although blood pressure stays down, cardiac output increases once more and peripheral resistance falls. Thus, there is evidently no simple relationship between any changes in cardiac output and alterations in arterial pressure.

Renin secretion from the kidney is partially under adrenergic control, being stimulated by beta-adrenergic agonism and inhibited by alpha-adrenergic agonism. Thus, most beta-blockers have an inhibitory effect on renin release, and plasma angiotensin II falls in consequence. Since in many patients with hypertension, as well as in normal subjects, peripheral concentrations of plasma angiotensin II are within a range having a direct immediate effect on arterial pressure, any inhibition of renin secretion induced by beta-blockade must make a contribution to the fall in blood pressure. The results of several studies have demonstrated a correlation between blood pressure reduction achieved by beta-blockers and changes in plasma renin. However, this seems unsatisfactory as a full explanation for the mode of action of this class of drugs. For example, pindolol, a beta-blocker with marked intrinsic sympathomimetic activity, has been shown to lower arterial pressure while plasma renin levels are rising. Further, the inhibitory effect of beta-blockade on renin release is limited, and is readily overcome, for example, by concurrent diuretic administration or by upright tilting, although blood pressure reduction is sustained through such manoeuvres.

A fourth possibility links the antihypertensive action of beta-blockers to the proposed pre-synaptic pressor effect of catecholamines, especially adrenaline. It has been suggested that circulating adrenaline can be taken up and accumulate in sympathetic nerve terminals, subsequently being released and, by stimulating pre-synaptic beta-2-receptors, promoting the discharge of neurotransmitter noradrenaline, thus elevating arterial pressure.[15,16] Stored adrenaline may also be released as a co-transmitter. Beta-blockers could inhibit this effect. However, it is not clear why a beta-2-dependent mechanism should explain the antihypertensive action clearly linked to beta-1 antagonism.

The beta-adrenoceptor blocking drugs have become established, together with the thiazides, as one of the two major classes of drug employed in the therapy of hypertension. They lower blood pressure rapidly, and maintain control indefinitely, with little or no postural component. Heart rate is reduced (an effect that is less marked with those beta-blockers possessing intrinsic sympathomimetic action). Beta-blockers can be hazardous in patients with impending cardiac failure, although this may be less of a problem with those newer beta-blockers having vasodilator properties.

Side-effects are not negligible, and can vary greatly among patients. They include physical and mental fatigue, bad dreams, nausea, rashes, impotence and cold extremities. Beta-blockers are unsafe in patients who have reversible airflow obstruction, especially asthma; as selectivity is relative only, so-called beta-1-selective agents, even when possessed also of partial beta-2 agonism, should not be given to such subjects. As insulin secretion is partly under beta-adrenergic control, beta-blockers could destabilize control of diabetes mellitus, although these drugs have been widely used in such patients without apparently causing major problems. However, tachycardia and other features of hypoglycaemia can be obscured. Bradycardia caused by beta-blockers can also mask internal bleeding.

Despite the problems and the continuing uncertainties concerning their mode of action, the beta-blockers have made, and will continue to make, a major contribution to the treatment of hypertension. A wide range of such drugs have been, and continue to be, developed.

Alpha-blockers

Alpha-adrenergic blockade was initially unimpressive in the treatment of essential hypertension. Non-selective agents such as phentolamine had a modest and poorly sustained antihypertensive effect, and could provoke marked postural hypotension, tachycardia and diarrhoea.

An important advance was the development of prazosin, a selective post-synaptic alpha-1-blocking agent. At first, the mode of action of prazosin was not clearly understood. Further agents have been developed along the prazosin genealogy, including the longer acting drugs terazosin and doxazosin.

The major problem with agents such as prazosin is frequent and unpredictable severe hypotension following the first dose when other than very small quantities are administered. With continued treatment mild postural hypotension can occur, and heart rate may be elevated. These features have limited the popularity of this drug class, especially in older patients, although side-effects are otherwise light, and the lack of disturbance of serum lipids has been regarded as an advantage.

Indoramine is a different alpha-1-blocking antihypertensive agent. Drowsiness, nasal stuffiness and dryness of the mouth are reported.

Alpha-blockers are generally utilized as supportive therapy, rather than as monotherapy, in essential hypertension. Their use in phaeochromocytoma is described on page 1279.

Calcium antagonists

This large and heterogeneous group of drugs has become increasingly employed in the treatment of hypertension in recent years.

Several groups of agent have been recognized[83] and include class I agents, typified by verapamil, class II agents, the dihydropyridines typified by nifedipine, class III agents, typified by diltiazem, and class IV agents, typified by flunarizine. Classes I–III contain those drugs most valuable in treating hypertension. These agents preferentially block the transport of calcium into the cells of vascular smooth muscle, and the myocardium. They act mainly by lowering peripheral vascular resistance.

Class I

Verapamil lowers blood pressure without a postural effect. Verapamil depresses atrioventricular conduction, and heart rate is reduced. It must be used cautiously, if at all, in combination with beta-blockers, because profound bradycardia or cardiac arrest may occur, especially in older patients. The other principal complication is constipation.

Class II

Thus far, the dihydropyridines have been the most extensively used calcium antagonists in the treatment of hypertension, and a wide range has been introduced (see Appendix to the book). Individual drugs differ in the extent of arterial dilatation achieved in various organs. A considerable problem

with these agents is their usually rapid absorption and short duration of action. Thus, if a sufficient dose to give a prolonged effect is administered, excessively high blood levels can occur, with marked side-effects. Attempts have been made to produce sustained-release formulations, which should enhance the convenience of use and limit the occurrence of side-effects.

The effect of nifedipine is enhanced by concurrent cimetidine. The main adverse reactions comprise headache, nausea and tachycardia, which are prominent in the early days and weeks of therapy and tend to subside later, facial flushing, which may persist, and ankle oedema not usually associated with appreciable weight increase.

An attractive feature of some of the class II calcium antagonists is an early modest diuresis and natriuresis. This seems not to be sustained, and no significant diminution in bodyweight or of total body sodium was demonstrable at the third month in one study of nicardipine.[84]

Class III

Despite combining the range of side-effects seen with calcium antagonists of classes I and II, these are usually less severe with diltiazem. However, rashes have proved troublesome.

Drugs acting on the renin system

Of the several classes of drugs that have been designed to act against the renin–angiotensin system (Fig. 53.2), only the orally effective angiotensin converting enzyme inhibitors have so far become established in the therapeutic repertory.

Angiotensin II analogue antagonists

Peptide analogues and thus competitive antagonists of angiotensin II, typified by saralasin, require to be given intravenously. Although these agents have been useful in clarifying the physiology and pathophysiology of the renin–angiotensin system, they have little therapeutic value.

Renin inhibitors

Inhibitors of the enzyme renin offer considerable therapeutic promise, especially because renin is a fastidious substrate-specific enzyme; its inhibition should provide a precise means of lowering angiotensin II. Although parenterally administered renin inhibitors have been tested in man,[85] and shown to be effective, orally active preparations of this kind have yet to be developed.

Angiotensin converting enzyme inhibitors

The orally active inhibitors of angiotensin converting enzyme have provided the major impetus to this area of therapy. A range of these agents is now available.[86] Some, such as captopril and lisinopril, are ingested in the active form; others, like enalapril and ramipril, are administered as a largely inactive pro-drug, which is then de-esterified in the liver to the active form (enalaprilat and ramiprilat, respectively). All four of these agents depend mainly on the kidney for elimination, and the dose needs to be lowered in the presence of renal functional impairment. All have been shown in man to cause dose-dependent falls in circulating plasma angiotensin II; this appears to be a major, but not necessarily the sole, mode of action in lowering blood pressure. Reduction of angiotensin II formation in other tissues, notably in arterial smooth muscle, could also be important. There are converse increases in the circulating concentrations of the enzyme renin and of the precursor peptide angiotensin I.

Angiotensin converting enzyme is furthermore capable of breaking down kinins into smaller peptide fragments. Thus, angiotensin converting enzyme inhibition may lower blood pressure not only by limiting the generation of angiotensin II, but also by promoting the accumulation of kinins in various tissues. Such kinin accumulation could contribute to certain of the side-effects of angiotensin converting enzyme inhibitors.

The use of angiotensin converting enzyme inhibitors in essential hypertension will be considered here; their employment in renovascular hypertension is described on page 1265.

Considerable evidence exists that in many patients with essential hypertension, peripheral plasma concentrations of angiotensin II are within a range that has a direct effect on arterial pressure. Angiotensin converting enzyme inhibitors cause an immediate reduction in blood pressure, in proportion to the fall in plasma angiotensin II they induce. The longer term elimination by angiotensin converting enzyme inhibition of other physiological actions of angiotensin II, such as sympathetic stimulation, promotion of aldosterone secretion, and possibly diminution of angiotensin II generation in cardiac and arterial walls, causes further blood pressure lowering. The initial fall in pressure is usually modest, as most patients with essential hyperten-

sion have low levels of plasma renin and angiotensin II. However, in elderly patients, steep and severe falls in pressure have been reported occasionally with the initial dose of angiotensin converting enzyme inhibitor, despite low pre-treatment plasma renin values. Angiotensin converting enzyme inhibitors do not usually cause postural hypotension or changes in heart rate, although sometimes sinus tachycardia does occur, especially with conjoint diuretic use.

As diuretics cause rises in renin and angiotensin II, which then limit their antihypertensive effect, the combination of a diuretic with an angiotensin converting enzyme inhibitor, the latter lowering circulating angiotensin II, is efficacious. The concurrent administration of angiotensin converting enzyme inhibitors with a thiazide is thus a valuable approach to the treatment of essential hypertension. Similar considerations have led to the use of dietary salt restriction with angiotensin converting enzyme inhibition. Severe and previously intractable hypertension has also been reported often as responding to the combination of angiotensin converting enzyme inhibitor with loop diuretic.

As aldosterone secretion is largely under the regulatory control of angiotensin II, plasma levels of aldosterone will typically with angiotensin converting enzyme inhibition remain low even with concurrent diuretic therapy. Thus, hypokalaemia does not usually develop, and neither potassium supplements nor potassium-conserving diuretics are usually needed with this combination. Indeed, their administration with angiotensin converting enzyme inhibition might provoke dangerous hyperkalaemia, especially in the presence of renal impairment. Renal impairment may also be worsened if aggressive diuretic therapy is combined with angiotensin converting enzyme inhibition.

Angiotensin converting enzyme inhibitors have also been reported as combining effectively with calcium antagonists or with ketanserin in treating only partially responsive cases of hypertension. The combination of angiotensin converting enzyme inhibitor with beta-blocker, by contrast, would be expected to be less potent, possibly because these two drug classes partly share a mode of action in suppressing the renin system. However, in some reports, an added lowering of pressure when combining these two classes of drug has been described.

Side-effects shared by angiotensin converting enzyme inhibitors as a class include cough, which occurs in some 5% of patients, urticarial or morbilliform rash, headache, syncope, Raynaud's phenomenon, and, more rarely, angioneurotic oedema, this last appearing usually early in therapy. Side-effects apparently peculiar to captopril were seen most often when large doses of the drug were employed, and have become less prominent or absent since the dose was limited to 150 mg/day, with further limitation in the presence of renal impairment. It is suspected that these captopril-specific side-effects may be due to the presence of a sulphydryl group in the captopril molecule. They include taste loss or disturbance, proteinuria (with occasional instances of nephrotic syndrome), leucopenia, and Guillain–Barré neuropathy. The sulphydryl group may confer on captopril its property to generate prostacyclin which may prove beneficial.

Caution is needed in introducing angiotensin converting enzyme inhibitors in patients likely to have high plasma levels of renin and angiotensin II, because a steep initial fall in blood pressure may occur in these circumstances. If diuretics (with or without additional drugs) are being given, it is advisable, wherever possible, to withdraw them before initiating angiotensin converting enzyme inhibition. Elderly subjects may be susceptible to first-dose hypotension with angiotensin converting enzyme inhibitors, apparently irrespective of the plasma renin value. Reducing the dose, or selecting a drug with a short action, such as captopril, is unlikely to prevent first-dose hypotension but may limit the duration.

To counterbalance these various side-effects and dangers, angiotensin converting enzyme inhibitors seem often to be well accepted by many patients.

Serotonin antagonists

Only one specific serotonin (5-hydroxytryptamine) antagonist, ketanserin, has thus far been used in the treatment of clinical hypertension.[27] Although it is effective, its place in the therapeutic repertory is not yet established and its mode of action not fully elucidated.

Serotonin is a powerful peripheral vasoconstrictor, which can additionally amplify the constrictor effect of other agents, such as angiotensin II and noradrenaline. Furthermore, serotonin can cause platelet aggregation. These various peripheral actions of serotonin are mediated by the serotonin type-2 (S_2) receptor. Ketanserin is a specific antagonist of the type-2 receptor, and is devoid of agonist effect. It possesses some alpha-blocking

action, which may be relevant clinically.

The mode of action of ketanserin in lowering blood pressure is disputed. A central effect is not excluded. A major influence of a change of baroreceptor function is unlikely. Some alpha-1-blockade can occasionally be demonstrated, especially during prolonged therapy; however, blood pressure lowering has been shown in the absence of demonstrable alpha-blockade. It has been proposed that a combination of powerful S_2 blockade with some weaker alpha-1-blockade may be needed for blood pressure reduction.

Ketanserin given orally has a gradually increasing effect on blood pressure over 2–3 months. Blood pressure reduction is also often greater in older subjects. There is little or no postural effect, and first-dose hypotension seems rare. The drug does not cause changes in serum electrolytes or urea, although minor increases in serum creatinine have been reported in some series.

Ketanserin does have mild class III anti-arrhythmic action and has been shown in both volunteers and patients with hypertension to prolong the QT interval in a dose-related fashion. As, in these circumstances, potassium depletion could predispose to ventricular rhythm disorders, it seems prudent when combining ketanserin and diuretic therapy to include a potassium-conserving agent. For similar reasons, the drug should be used with caution if there is atrioventricular block of grade II or higher, or with anti-arrhythmic agents. Other side-effects include drowsiness, which is usually most prominent in the early days of treatment then receding, dizziness, dryness of the mouth and mild pedal oedema.

'Stepped care' and the concept of drug combinations

In the 1970s, both the World Health Organization and the American Heart Association set out detailed proposals for what came to be termed 'stepped care' in the treatment of hypertension.[2,87] In these schedules, drugs were introduced in set combinations, additions being made to therapy as needed in order to reduce the arterial pressure adequately. These stepped care programmes served well in encouraging and instructing practitioners in the therapy of hypertension, and the ways in which drugs with different modes of action could usefully be combined. However, such formal programmes of treatment are now not as popular.[62,70,87] A more enlightened and enterprising approach is progressively being adopted, with drugs being selected with the specific needs of the individual patient in mind. If a drug given alone is ineffective, the present tendency is to withdraw it and replace it with an alternative, also given as monotherapy. There is increasing reluctance to proceed to multiple drugs in combination unless a distinct need has been demonstrated.

However, it has also to be recognized that the use of two agents together can minimize the side-effects that one drug alone, in larger dose, might impose. Further, an additional agent can eliminate an adverse effect imposed by a previous one; a typical example would be the fluid retention due to methyldopa being corrected by the introduction of a diuretic.

Few physicians now favour the administration of drugs more than once or twice daily, and elaborate titration is to be avoided if possible. Agents that can be given in one or two increments have obvious attractions.

For these reasons, prejudices of only a few years ago against fixed drug combinations, made up in a single preparation, are declining. Many doctors and patients appreciate the rationale and simplicity of such an approach.

It is useful in these circumstances to indicate which drugs when given together are likely to be effective, and which are contra-indicated. A more detailed summary is provided in the Appendix to the book.

Twin combinations likely to be useful include beta-blocker plus diuretic, beta-blocker plus class 2 (dihydropyridine) calcium antagonist, beta-blocker plus prazosin, beta-blocker plus ketanserin, angiotensin converting enzyme inhibitor plus diuretic, angiotensin converting enzyme inhibitor plus calcium antagonist, angiotensin converting enzyme inhibitor plus ketanserin and diuretic plus methyldopa. Combinations less likely to be effective are beta-blocker plus angiotensin converting enzyme inhibitor, and diuretic plus dihydropyridine calcium antagonist. Contra-indicated either because the drugs are too similar in action and/or because the combination might be dangerous are methyldopa, clonidine and reserpine in any conjoint grouping because of their common central effects, angiotensin converting enzyme inhibitors and potassium-conserving diuretics, because of the danger of hyperkalaemia, and verapamil and beta-blocker, because of the danger of cardiac conduction defects.

Should a triple grouping be necessary, one of the best established is that comprising beta-blocker, diuretic and hydralazine (so-called 'standard triple therapy'). In more resistant patients, minoxidil may be substituted for hydralazine, but the diuretic then needs to be a powerful 'loop' agent; an ordinary thiazide will usually be insufficient to counteract the fluid retention caused by minoxidil. The combination of beta-blocker plus diuretic plus prazosin has also been shown to work well.

NON-PHARMACOLOGICAL METHODS OF BLOOD PRESSURE REDUCTION

Several dietary means of lowering high blood pressure have already been discussed on pages 1229–31.[3,8–10] These include the established benefits of weight reduction and of restriction of alcohol intake, the more questionable value of a vegetarian diet, of restriction of caffeine and sodium intake, or of supplementation of potassium and calcium ingestion. The feasibility and efficacy of a multiple dietary approach has been shown in a 4-year trial of weight reduction, sodium restriction and alcohol restriction. Compliance was good, and blood pressure was lowered, although not as effectively as in a control group of patients who remained on antihypertensive drugs.[9]

Certain other non-pharmacological approaches to treatment deserve mention. Physical exercise has been demonstrated to cause a distinct and probably clinically valuable reduction of blood pressure.[8] This effect is independent of any associated weight reduction. A variety of psychological measures, including Yoga, transcendental meditation, relaxation training, and so-called 'biofeedback' techniques, have been shown, at least in the short term, and with dedicated exponents, to lower high blood pressure.[1,2] On present evidence, the use of such methods long term or for wide-scale therapy is more questionable. However, these approaches deserve further attention.

The role of cigarette smoking, and of cessation of smoking, in hypertension and its therapy is important and complex. Smoking greatly compounds the adverse cardiovascular effects of hypertension and minimizes the benefits of therapy.[53–58] For a given blood pressure level, smokers are more likely than non-smokers to suffer a stroke or heart attack, or to enter the malignant phase of hypertension. Prognosis after these events is also worse in smokers than in non-smokers. Smokers are more likely than non-smokers to have renal artery stenosis. These are all powerful reasons for combining strong anti-smoking measures with antihypertensive treatment.

However, although smoking raises blood pressure acutely, particularly if combined with the drinking of coffee, smokers tend otherwise to have lower blood pressures than non-smokers. This may be partly explained by lower bodyweight in smokers.

SECONDARY FORMS OF HYPERTENSION

Secondary hypertension comprises a variety of disparate conditions, which, despite their rarity in comparison with primary or essential hypertension, are often of compelling interest because they may help to clarify the pathophysiology of raised arterial pressure. These conditions are usually therapeutically rewarding because either the raised blood pressure responds to removal or correction of the primary abnormality or, as for example, in Conn's syndrome or phaeochromocytoma, antihypertensive drugs acting specifically against the hormone produced to excess are effective.

In unselected populations of hypertensive patients, probably no more than 1–5% of cases are secondary,[2] although a much higher proportion of a particular disease may be seen in a specialized centre.

Two most interesting aspects of secondary hypertension, first noted by Pickering,[43] are that virtually every form of secondary hypertension can enter the malignant phase, and that the hypertension may persist in a substantial proportion of cases even after the primary cause has been removed or corrected. Persistent hypertension is probably due in part to hypertension-induced changes, including structural thickening in the wall of resistance vessels (see p. 1237), and alterations in the kidney (see p. 1240). Renal functional impairment in any form of secondary hypertension usually presages a less satisfactory fall in blood pressure after correction of the causal abnormality.

The main forms of secondary hypertension are listed in Table 53.2.

DRUG-INDUCED HYPERTENSION

HORMONAL CONTRACEPTIVES AND CONJUGATED OESTROGENS

The most numerous of the drug-induced forms of hypertension and almost certainly the commonest of all the secondary hypertensive syndromes is that caused by hormonal contraceptives.[88] Raised blood

Table 53.2.   **Causes of secondary hypertension.**

1 Drug induced:
   Hormonal contraceptives and conjugated oestrogens
   Liquorice; carbenoxolone
   Pressor amines and monoamine oxidase inhibitors
   ACTH and corticosteroids
2 Coarctation of the aorta (see also Chapter 25)
3 Hypertension of renal origin: renal and renal arterial diseases
4 Adrenocortical disorders
   Primary aldosterone excess: Conn's syndrome and related diseases
   Cushing's syndrome
   Inborn errors of corticosteroid biosynthesis
5 Phaeochromocytoma
6 Acromegaly
7 Thyroid disease
   Thryotoxicosis
   Hypothyroidism
8 Gordon's syndrome
9 Intracranial tumour
10 Pregnancy-induced hypertension (see also Chapter 59)

pressure due to the administration of conjugated oestrogens to post-menopausal women should also be considered in this context.

Compounds used

Two kinds of oestrogen are generally employed in combined oestrogen–progestagen oral contraceptives, ethinyloestradiol or its 3-methyl ether, mestranol. The progestagens used are various derivatives either of 19-nortestosterone (norethynodrel, norethisterone, ethynodiol diacetate, lynestrol or norgestrel) or of 17-hydroxyprogesterone (megestrol acetate, medroxyprogesterone acetate or chlormadinone acetate). The derivatives of nortestosterone may partly be metabolized to oestrogenic substances.

Early preparations contained 100 μg of oestrogen and from 1 to 4 mg of progestagen. Subsequently, and progressively, the dose of oestrogen has been reduced to 50, 35, 30 and 25 μg; in some preparations, the dose of progestagen also has been lowered, for example, to 150 μg of norgestrel.

A triphasic low-dose combination tablet containing ethinyl oestradiol and laevonorgestrel has been formulated, containing of each, respectively, 30 μg and 50 μg for the first 6 days of the menstrual cycle, rising to 40 μg and 75 μg for the next 5 days, and progressing to 30 μg and 125 μg for the next 10 days. Progestagen-only preparations are less reliable contraceptives. Examples in use are ethynodiol diacetate 500 μg, laevonorgestrel 30 μg, norgestrel 75 μg and norethisterone 350 μg.

Blood pressure changes

The balance of current opinion indicates that the magnitude of any blood pressure increase is in proportion to the dose of oestrogen. There is no good evidence that progestagen-only preparations can influence blood pressure.

Virtually all women who take the combined oestrogen–progestagen pill show a rise in arterial pressure. This is usually mild, although it has been estimated that some 5% of pill-takers show blood pressure levels exceeding 140/90 mmHg, which could represent a considerable increase in young women. A few susceptible individuals show a more marked rise in pressure and the malignant phase of hypertension is a well-recorded complication with oral contraceptives containing 50 or 30 μg of oestrogen.[89]

In women on the pill, blood pressure usually rises steadily for the first 6 months, then settles to a plateau which is maintained while therapy continues. In one early prospective study, average rises of 12 mmHg systolic and 8 mmHg diastolic at 5 years were shown. On stopping the pill, pressures usually subside to control values within 3–6 months.

Predisposing factors

It has been suggested that women with a genetic predisposition to essential hypertension are more at risk of a severe rise in blood pressure on the pill, although this is not well substantiated. Women with pre-existing hypertension do not seem to be more susceptible. Black American women have been reported to be less prone to develop hypertension with oral contraceptive use. There is no good evidence of a correlation with pregnancy-induced hypertension, social class or cigarette smoking.

Complications

Progress into the malignant phase carries the attendant serious consequences of this complication whatever the underlying cause. The risks of the commoner more mild elevations of arterial pressure are less certain, but cannot be regarded with complacency, especially when accompanied by the other sequelae of oral contraception, which include distortion of the plasma lipid pattern, impairment of glucose tolerance, and changes in the blood coagulation system. There has been much concern about the possible long-term vascular consequences of oral contraceptive therapy. There is evidence that cardiovascular mortality is increased 5-fold in young women taking oestrogen–progestagen oral contraceptives, and 10-fold in those so treated for 5 or more years. Smoking compounds these risks.

Although data are scanty, it is likely that in some women, elevation of blood pressure, at least to an extent, may persist after stopping the pill. If so, this brings pill-induced hypertension into conformity with the general rule that, in secondary hypertension, the blood pressure of many patients fails to return to the level in age- and sex-matched normal subjects even after the initial cause of the hypertension has been corrected.[43]

Mechanism of blood pressure rise

Oestrogens cause a rise in the level of plasma renin-substrate (angiotensinogen) concentration. As there is no consistent compensatory fall in the plasma concentration of the enzyme renin, plasma levels of angiotensin II, a powerful vasoconstrictor, rise. This has been shown to occur in the absence of changes in total body sodium and must therefore contribute to blood pressure elevation.[90] However, it is not known how important this mechanism is in the majority of instances. Although plasma aldosterone would be expected to rise in association with any increase in plasma angiotensin II, and such changes have been reported, there is no good evidence of sodium or water retention that can consistently explain the blood pressure increase, or of expanded extracellular fluid or plasma volume. The changes in pressure do not usually correlate with changes in bodyweight. Other suggested mechanisms, not as yet fully explored, are increased sympathetic nerve activity, changes in circulating noradrenaline and alterations in the proportions or quantities of prostaglandins.

Management

All women undertaking oestrogen–progestagen oral contraceptive therapy, and all post-menopausal women starting conjugated oestrogens, should have their blood pressure measured before commencing therapy, and at intervals no greater than every 3 months while receiving treatment.

In the event of marked blood pressure elevation, therapy should be changed to a progestagen-only pill, or to an alternative form of contraception. Blood pressure should be monitored carefully to confirm a fall to normal limits; if this has not occurred within 6 months of discontinuation, a search should be made for an additional or alternative form of secondary hypertension. If blood pressure remains high 6 months after stopping the pill and in the absence of evidence of secondary hypertension, the patient should receive drug treatment as for essential hypertension.

A woman who develops malignant hypertension while receiving an oral contraceptive should have this stopped forthwith and should be treated urgently with antihypertensive drugs. After blood pressure has been adequately controlled for 6 months, treatment should be carefully withdrawn and the blood pressure monitored. In the event of sustained blood pressure elevations, long-term antihypertensive treatment will be necessary.

It is not appropriate for a woman to continue to take an oestrogen–progestagen oral contraceptive while remaining hypertensive and thus to require concomitant antihypertensive therapy.

LIQUORICE AND CARBENOXOLONE

Causative compounds

Extracts of liquorice, a substance prepared from the root of the plant *Glycyrrhiza glabra*, contain glycyrrhizinic acid, a compound with mineralocorticoid activity. Carbenoxolone, the semi-synthetic hemisuccinate derivative of glycyrrhizinic acid, is a drug employed to speed the healing of peptic ulcers.

Persons who ingest large quantities of liquorice-containing sweets or beverages, and susceptible individuals taking carbenoxolone or liquorice, may develop mineralocorticoid hypertension.[91] Some patients may be especially sensitive to the biochemical changes and to the blood pressure increases. More generally, it has been found that 300 mg/day of carbenoxolone regularly induces metabolic and blood pressure changes, whereas 20 mg/day does not.

Pathophysiology

The pathophysiology is intriguing. Mineralocorticoid receptors cannot, *in vitro*, distinguish between mineralocorticoids such as aldosterone and glucocorticoids like cortisol. However, *in vivo*, mineralocorticoid receptors in the kidney are selective for aldosterone. This selectivity appears to be due to the presence of the enzyme 11 β–hydroxysteroid dehydrogenase (11 β–OHSD), which converts cortisol to inactive cortisone, and so effectively diverts cortisol from the mineralocorticoid receptors. Liquorice inhibits 11 β–OHSD, and thus permits cortisol to bind to, and activate, mineralocorticoid receptors in the kidney.[131]

Clinical and biochemical features

The pattern and biochemical accompaniments of this condition closely resemble those of an aldosterone-secreting tumour, except that aldosterone secretion and plasma aldosterone concentration are low. The raised blood pressure is characteristically associated with hypernatraemia, hypokalaemia, increased body sodium and diminished body potassium content, and depression of plasma renin, angiotensin II and aldosterone.[92] The hypokalaemia may be accompanied by muscular weakness, paraesthesiae, polyuria, cardiac arrhythmias and, occasionally, red urine because of the presence of myoglobin.

Diagnosis and management

Any patient with hypertension, especially if this is associated with hypokalaemia, should be questioned concerning possible ingestion of liquorice or carbenoxolone. If these substances are being taken, they should be discontinued and the patient reassessed initially after 3–4 weeks. It may take 6–8 weeks before the biochemical abnormalities and the blood pressure have been corrected. Even if blood pressure does not return to normal values, control with antihypertensive drugs should be facilitated.

PRESSOR AMINES AND MONOAMINE OXIDASE INHIBITORS

Occasional examples have been reported of patients developing hypertensive crises following the ingestion of a large dose of a pressor amine such as phenylpropanolamine or dextroamphetamine.[93]

Concurrent administration of monoamine oxidase inhibitors for the treatment of mental ailments can greatly enhance the risk. Monoamine oxidase inhibitors interfere with the breakdown of endogenous catecholamines, such as adrenaline and noradrenaline, as well as of administered amines. The risks are not confined to concurrent abuse of drugs. A number of foods contain large quantities of tyramine, which can accumulate when monoamine oxidase inhibitors are also taken. Thus, patients on these drugs should be warned of the dangers of eating ripe cheese, meat extracts, broad beans, ripe grapes and chocolate.

HYPERTENSION DUE TO ACTH OR CORTICOSTEROID THERAPY

The rare abnormalities of corticosteroid biosynthesis (see p. 1274) demonstrate the ability of increased adrenocorticotrophin (ACTH) to raise arterial pressure. The effect of exogenous ACTH has been extensively studied in experimental animals, notably the sheep.[94] Administration of ACTH to man also raises arterial pressure,[95] an effect dependent on an intact adrenal cortex, because it does not occur in patients with Addison's disease. This potential hazard of long-term therapeutic administration of ACTH should always be borne in mind, and regular checks of arterial pressure be made.

The development of hypertension in Cushing's syndrome (see p. 1270) similarly suggests the ability of corticosteroids, such as cortisol, to induce hypertension in man. This has been demonstrated experimentally,[95] and the similarity of the responses in volunteers to cortisol and ACTH suggests that cortisol is largely responsible for the effects of ACTH. The results of other work, however, have suggested that this is not a common clinical therapeutic problem. In one study of 195 patients who were receiving low doses of prednisone or prednisolone for the treatment of asthma or rheumatoid arthritis, neither an excessive prevalence of hypertension nor features of mineralocorticoid excess were found.[96]

NON-STEROIDAL ANTI-INFLAMMATORY DRUGS

These agents can induce hypertension and interfere with antihypertensive therapy. Indomethacin has been studied in most detail.[97] The mechanism is thought to be a result of diminution of prostaglandin production, possibly resulting in alterations of the renal circulation, of the regulation of extracellular fluid volume or of vascular tone.

COARCTATION OF THE AORTA

Coarctation of the aorta is fully discussed in Chapter 25; only certain aspects will be mentioned here.

PATHOGENESIS OF HYPERTENSION

The cause of the hypertension in coarctation of the aorta is disputed, although several theories have been advanced. Of these, the most plausible is that mechanical factors predominate. Birkenhäger and de Leeuw[98] have summarized these as follows. Initially, there is vascular resistance because of aortic narrowing, thus diverting blood to the upper part of the body, with hypoperfusion of the lower part. A consequent increase in cardiac output then delivers more blood to the distal parts, but provides excessive circulation in terms of metabolic requirements to regions above the coarctation. As a result, the excessively perfused tissues increase their vascular resistance ('autoregulation') until a normal blood flow is restored. Thus, more blood passes via the coarctation and the collaterals to the lower parts of the body. Depending on the requirements of tissues distal to the narrowing, cardiac output may remain elevated or revert to normal. In either event, the increased vascular resistance above the coarctation is responsible for proximal hypertension. As Birkenhäger and de Leeuw point out,[98] although this hypothesis is attractive, there are few convincing data to support or refute it.

An alternative or additional theory proposes that renal ischaemia causes increased release of renin from the kidneys. According to this notion, pathogenesis would be similar to that in bilateral renal artery stenosis (see p. 1266). In the latter model, plasma renin is elevated only transiently, whereas in the established condition there is sustained expansion of body sodium content. In human coarctation, peripheral plasma levels of renin, and renal vein renin values, are normal, as would be expected. There is, however, evidence that renin release in coarctation is hyper-responsive to stimuli such as orthostasis or sodium deprivation. Relevant measurements of body sodium content are wanting. In experimental aortic constriction with resultant hypertension in animal models, the renin system is stimulated transiently, values later declining into the normal range. Transplantation of a kidney from below to above the aortic narrowing can correct the hypertension. For this theory, there is only slender evidence in favour and little against it.

DIAGNOSIS

Although diagnosis should be made in infancy or childhood, some cases can escape detection until adult life. Thus, coarctation of the aorta, despite its rarity, must be considered in every patient of any age presenting with hypertension. Detection is usually straightforward. Concurrent palpation of the radial and femoral pulses, which should always be performed, reveals the femoral as feeble although often easily palpable, with a delayed summit. Chest radiography will show, in nearly every patient over the age of 6 years, notching of the lower borders of the ribs resulting from enlarged collateral arteries, together probably with left ventricular enlargement. Once suspected, collateral arteries, with pronounced pulsation, can be felt and seen especially over the back of the thorax.

The arterial pressure in the upper limbs is elevated, the systolic to a greater degree than the diastolic. If the aortic constriction lies proximal to the origin of the left subclavian artery, blood pressure will be lower, and the pulse more feeble, in the left arm than the right.

Blood pressure measurement in the leg is performed by auscultation of the popliteal artery in the popliteal fossa, employing an appropriately large cuff to compress the thigh. Systolic pressure always, and diastolic usually, is lower in the legs than in the arms. The pulse pressure is diminished below the coarctation.

COMPLICATIONS

Coarctation is the one form of hypertension, primary or secondary, that is rarely complicated by the malignant phase. However, one very suggestive example has been reported, with the ocular lesions and impaired vision correcting after surgical treatment and relief of the hypertension.[40] It is possible that, because the condition is present from birth or earlier, the arteries exposed to the hypertension have adequate time in which to adapt to the raised pressure. Following surgical repair of coarctation, fibrinoid arterial necroses may develop within a few days at sites previously distal to the aortic narrowing, and now subjected to higher pressures. These lesions do not develop post-operatively above the site of the previous coarctation.

PROGNOSIS OF HYPERTENSION

Coarctation of the aorta conforms to the general

Table 53.3.   Classification of renal hypertension.

Unilateral renal disease
1 Renin-secreting tumour
2 Renovascular hypertension: renal artery stenosis or occlusion
3 Other forms of unilateral renal disease:
      Hypertensive small vessel damage
      Renal arteriovenous fistula
      Chronic pyelonephritis
      Interstitial nephritis
      Radiation nephritis
      Hydronephrosis
      Tuberculosis
      Renal carcinoma
      Nephroblastoma
      Single or multiple renal cysts
      Ask–Upmark kidney
      Page kidney

Bilateral renal disease
1 Bilateral renal artery stenosis
2 Primary parenchymal renal disease:
      Polycystic disease
      Glomerulonephritis (acute or chronic)
      Interstitial nephritis
      Pyelonephritis
3 Radiation nephritis
4 Diabetic nephropathy
5 Hypertension-dependent nephrosclerosis
6 Nephropathy from analgesic abuse

---

rule that after correction of the causal abnormality in secondary hypertension, blood pressure remains elevated in a substantial proportion of cases.[43]

HYPERTENSION OF RENAL ORIGIN

Renal hypertension can usefully be considered under two main headings: that due to unilateral renal disease and that in which the raised blood pressure is associated with bilateral renal abnormalities. In unilateral renal disease, it is suggested that the pathogenesis shares a common path, namely stimulation, by whatever mechanism, of hypersecretion of renin by the afflicted kidney. In bilateral renal disease, overall impairment of kidney function provides the principal mechanism of the raised arterial pressure, although in some cases hypersecretion of renin may be an additional factor. Moreover, raised arterial pressure does lead to intrarenal vascular damage, with consequent acceleration of renal functional decline. The classification of renal forms of hypertension is given in Table 53.3.

HYPERTENSION WITH UNILATERAL RENAL DISEASE[99]

RENIN-SECRETING TUMOUR

This rare condition has excited interest disproportionate to its frequency because it offers insight into the pathophysiology of hypertension resulting solely from hypersecretion of renin. As it is proposed that the common pathogenetic route of most, if not all, forms of hypertension resulting from unilateral renal disease is overproduction of renin, secretion of which has been stimulated in one way or another by the lesion, close study of patients with renin-secreting tumour is merited. Moreover, the condition is eminently treatable in its own right.

Pathology

The classic and commonest form of the disease is a benign renal haemangiopericytoma of the renin-producing cells of the juxtaglomerular apparatus (Fig. 53.5). However, more rarely, renin hypersecretion with hypertension has been observed with a variety of other neoplasms, arising both within and outside the kidney, including Wilm's tumour, renal carcinoma, pulmonary carcinoma and pancreatic adenocarcinoma.

Pathophysiology

The principal features of the condition are the result of excessive secretion of renin from the tumour. The syndrome is characterized by hypertension with elevated peripheral plasma levels of renin and of its product the peptide angiotensin II, with consequent secondary aldosterone excess and thus low plasma potassium concentrations.

Renin-secreting tumour, particularly the classic variety haemangiopericytoma, provides critical evidence of the relationship between chronic elevation of renin, and hence of angiotensin II, and hypertension. The analysis of such cases strongly indicates that, with prolonged exposures to high peripheral plasma concentrations of angiotensin II, much higher levels of arterial pressure are achieved than by the short-term elevation of angiotensin II to similar values.[100] Thus, herein is clinical evidence of the slow, as well as of the fast, pressor effect of angiotensin II, now well established in experimental animals. This phenomenon is compatible with the often slow return of blood pressure to normal values when patients or animals with hypertension due to excess of circulating angiotensin II are treated long term with angiotensin II antagonists or converting enzyme inhibitors.

These observations also have important implications for the much commoner clinical hypertensive syndromes resulting from hypersecretion of renin, notably renovascular hypertension.

The classic benign haemangiopericytoma is preponderant in children or young adults, which can be an important diagnostic clue.

Clinical features

In many patients, the history and physical findings are unremarkable, the condition being revealed often following the discovery of hypertension at routine examination. However, some of the rarer malignant renin-secreting neoplasms may manifest evidence of the primary or secondary carcinoma, with the renin excess and hypertension being noted subsequently.

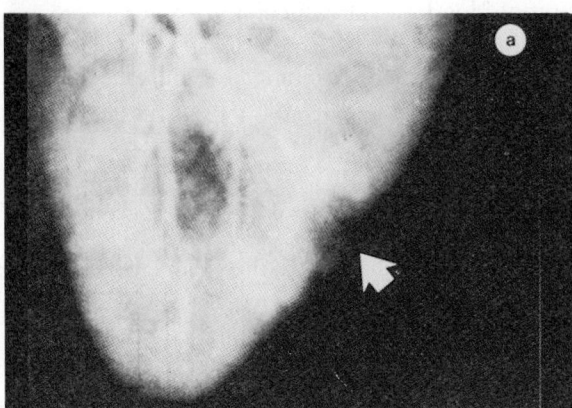
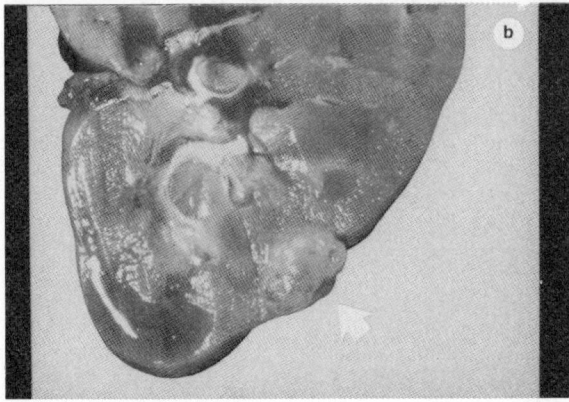

Fig. 53.5. Renin-secreting tumour shown (a) at selective left renal angiography and (b) after nephrectomy. (Reproduced from Mackay, A. *at el.* In: *Handbook of Hypertension, Vol. 2: Clinical Aspects of Secondary Hypertension*, p.33, by permission of the publishers, Elsevier, Amsterdam.)

Diagnosis

In a patient with hypertension and hypokalaemia, and with concurrent elevation of plasma renin and aldosterone, once the more common forms of aldosterone excess, such as that induced by diuretic therapy or resulting from renal artery stenosis or the malignant phase, have been excluded, the possibility of renin-secreting tumour should be considered, especially in a young patient. Untreated, the raised arterial pressure may lead to the various sequelae of that condition, including progression to the malignant phase.

Estimation of renin in renal venous blood is critical, but it should be emphasized that, in contrast to renal artery stenosis, renal blood flow on the affected side is not usually reduced, and thus a high rate of renin secretion, in a patient with renin-secreting tumour, can be reflected in only a modest differential in renin values in the two renal veins. This is an important point because in several instances the difference, albeit genuine, has been close to the limit of discrimination of the relevant assay method.

In two reported cases, one of a renal carcinoma and one of a pancreatic adenocarcinoma, the tumours secreted excess of inactive renin while active renin values were variously normal or high. Thus, in rare cases, the diagnosis may be missed unless both inactive and active renin are assayed in plasma.

The tumour may be localized definitively by selective angiography.

Treatment

Local excision, if possible, or unilateral nephrectomy is usually curative. In the case of the more varied and rarer malignant neoplasms causing this condition, outcome is less certain.

Medical treatment can be useful pre-operatively or as definitive therapy in a patient with an inoperable or metastasizing renin-secreting neoplasm. An orally active angiotensin converting enzyme inhibitor will prevent the excessive formation of angiotensin II from the secreted renin, and should limit or correct the hypertension, aldosterone excess and hypokalaemia.

RENOVASCULAR HYPERTENSION

By definition, this is hypertension resulting from narrowing of one or both renal arteries. Full confirmation of this condition clinically requires restoration of blood pressure to normal following surgical relief of the renal artery constriction or removal of the afflicted kidney. However, in some patients, correction of a stenosis may not return blood pressure to normal, particularly if the hypertension has persisted over a long time. This is the result, at least in some patients, of hypertension-induced lesions in the contralateral kidney, and occasional instances have been reported in which, following correction of a unilateral renal artery stenosis, blood pressure fell only when the contralateral kidney was excised. This latter procedure is unlikely to be undertaken today, with the availability of orally acting converting enzyme inhibitors.

It must be emphasized that the co-existence of hypertension with renal artery stenosis does not establish renovascular hypertension. In addition to the two relationships mentioned above, there is the possible development of renal artery stenosis because of pre-existent hypertension. Further, a patient with essential hypertension could develop significant renal artery stenosis with further elevation of blood pressure; a conjunction of a common condition with a rare one. Lastly, it should be pointed out that the findings of clinical and post-mortem studies have shown anatomical renal artery stenosis in up to 46% of normotensive subjects. Evidently, the co-existence of a renal artery lesion with high blood pressure is not always easily interpreted.

Accurate estimation of the frequency of renal artery stenosis as a cause of hypertension is difficult; patients tend to be selected and referred preferentially to a centre where clinicians have an interest in the condition, and this distorts the apparent prevalence. In retrospective surveys of hypertensive populations, prevalence rates have been variously quoted at 2–30%; a prevalence of 6% was found in a prospective study of an unselected hypertensive population. Speculative estimates have suggested that up to 920 000 people in the USA and 200 000 in the UK could have potentially curable hypertension associated with a renal artery stenosis.

Causes of renal artery stenosis

Clinical renal artery stenosis may result from various lesions.

Atheroma

The commonest clinical cause of renal artery stenosis, accounting overall for about two-thirds of cases, is atheroma or a combination of atheroma with thrombus formation either at the origin of the main renal artery, along the proximal third of the renal artery, or at the first bifurcation of the main renal artery. Dilatation of the artery immediately distal to the stenosis is not unusual. A collateral circulation may often develop via the inferior adrenal, peri-ureteric or other vessels. Atheromatous renal artery disease occurs predominantly in older men who are cigarette smokers. They often show atheromatous disease at other sites.

Fibromuscular hyperplasia

About one-third of cases of renal artery stenosis are due to fibromuscular hyperplasia. This lesion predominantly affects women. On average, patients with fibromuscular hyperplasia present some 10 years earlier in life than do patients with atheromatous lesions. There is less frequent involvement of arteries at other sites, although an association with cigarette smoking has been reported, as with atheromatous renal artery stenosis.

The middle and distal thirds of the main renal artery are principally involved, the right side more often than the left. Other arteries that may be implicated are the iliacs, mesenteric, carotids and coronaries, in that order.

Although the classic arteriographic appearance of this lesion is of a 'string of beads' affecting an appreciable length of artery, fibromuscular hyperplasia can present as a single discrete renal artery stenosis with post-stenotic dilatation.

The pathogenesis of fibromuscular hyperplasia is disputed.

Other causative lesions

A variety of conditions has been reported as occasionally causing renal artery stenosis, including phaeochromocytoma of the renal hilum, haematomas, diaphragmatic crura and sympathetic chains. Accidental trauma can lead to renal artery stenosis or occlusion.

Pathophysiology

The pathophysiology of hypertension resulting from renal artery stenosis is complex, and not all details have been settled more than 50 years after Goldblatt's classic studies.[100]

There are two distinct varieties of the condition. The commoner clinical version has a unilateral renal artery stenosis, the opposite kidney and its artery remaining intact, known experimentally as 'one-clip, two-kidney' hypertension. The second, and rarer, model has either bilateral renal artery stenosis or stenosis of the artery to a sole remaining kidney, known experimentally as 'one-clip, one-kidney' hypertension.

Unilateral stenosis, with contralateral side normal

The pathogenesis of 'one-clip, two-kidney' hypertension has been divided into three phases that merge into one another. The initial phase is rarely seen clinically. In this first phase, lasting for a few days at most, plasma renin, angiotensin II and blood pressure rise together. There is good evidence that at this stage the blood pressure is elevated by the immediate direct pressor effect of angiotensin II. Relief of the stenosis, or removal of the affected kidney, promptly returns the plasma concentrations of renin and angiotensin II and the blood pressure to normal.

Within days or weeks, depending on the species, phase I is succeeded by phase II, in which, although blood pressure remains high, there is, proportionately, less marked elevation of plasma renin and of angiotensin II than in phase I. For years this led to doubts about the relevance of the renin–angiotensin system to pathogenesis in phase II. However, extensive experimental and clinical evidence has shown that the renin–angiotensin system is responsible for sustaining the hypertension in this second phase, despite the less marked elevation of circulating renin and of angiotensin II than those in phase I. An important parallel has been drawn with the disproportionate elevation of blood pressure in relation to circulating angiotensin II seen in the established chronic hypertensive state of renin-secreting tumour. In many patients in the second phase of renovascular hypertension, circulating levels of renin and angiotensin II may be only marginally elevated, or even in the upper part of the normal range. Nevertheless, correction of the stenosis, excision of the afflicted kidney or the administration of antagonists of the renin–angiotensin system can alleviate the hypertension. Evidently, slow, as well as fast, components of the pressor action of angiotensin II are involved in phase II.

Months or years later, phase II of renovascular hypertension is succeeded by phase III. In phase III, surgical relief of the renal arterial lesion or removal of the affected kidney does not correct the hypertension. It is likely that the renin–angiotensin system is no longer involved in phase III, and antagonists of the renin–angiotensin system similarly do not lower the blood pressure. Clinical recognition of phase III is important, in order to avoid unnecessary surgical intervention.

Stenosis with a single kidney

The second and rarer 'one-clip, one-kidney' variety of hypertension shows transient elevations of circulating renin and angiotensin II, for only 1 or 2 days in experimental animals. The established condition shows normal or near-normal plasma renin values. There is, however, expansion of body sodium content, which presumably is a main mechanism responsible for the hypertension.[101] This condition will be considered in more detail on page 1266.

Clinical features[99,102]

Renovascular hypertension is largely devoid of specific symptoms. However, in up to 20% of patients, the malignant phase may have supervened and given rise to visual disturbance, other neurological features, such fits or clouding of consciousness, hypertensive heart failure, headache or nocturia.

A few patients with a severe unilateral renal artery stenoses or thrombosis develop a characteristic and striking constellation of features including polyuria, polydipsia, weight loss and rapidly advancing sodium and potassium depletion. Malignant phase hypertension is usually also present. Plasma renin, angiotensin II, aldosterone and vasopressin values are very high, and plasma sodium and potassium low. This is the 'hyponatraemic hypertensive syndrome' which will advance rapidly to a fatal conclusion unless the stenosis is relieved, the affected kidney is removed, or the gross excess of circulating angiotensin II is corrected by the administration of a converting enzyme inhibitor.

Patients with sudden occlusion of a renal artery or one of its main branches may develop infarction of renal tissue, with consequent loin pain and haematuria. Such a lesion may supervene on a previously occult renal artery stenosis. Alternatively, the infarct may be the consequence of abdominal trauma or a deceleration injury, or there may be evidence of a source of embolus, such as cardiac arrhythmia or endocarditis.

Physical signs similarly may be lacking. An abdominal or loin bruit may arise from turbulent blood flow across a renal artery stenosis, and a bruit audible in both systole and diastole is held to be particularly suggestive. Abdominal bruits have been reported in up to 58% of patients with demonstrable renal artery stenoses but may also occur frequently in subjects with aortic atheroma and no renal arterial lesion. An abdominal bruit must therefore be regarded as an unreliable sign of renal artery stenosis.

Investigation

Investigative procedures in suspected cases of renovascular hypertension have usefully been divided into screening, diagnostic and prognostic tests. Some procedures can provide information related to more than one of these categories.

SCREENING FOR RENOVASCULAR HYPERTENSION

History and physical signs

Although specific symptoms and signs are unusual, there are certain groups of patients in whom a particular suspicion of renal artery stenosis should be entertained, and who therefore merit further investigation. Such patients are considered either to be more likely to harbour the lesion, or to benefit particularly from its diagnosis and treatment.

1 Patients under 45 years of age with moderate to severe hypertension (diastolic pressure in excess of 100 mmHg), especially if they are cigarette smokers.

2 Patients compliant with medical treatment whose blood pressure control unaccountably deteriorates.

3 Hypertensive patients with unexplained overall renal impairment. These could have either bilateral renal artery stenosis or stenosis of the artery to a sole kidney.

4 Patients with renal impairment whose renal function deteriorates further with effective antihypertensive drug therapy, recovering as treatment is withdrawn. This could readily occur in a patient with bilateral renal artery stenosis or with stenosis of the artery of a single kidney. If this occurs with the use of a converting enzyme inhibitor or beta-blockers, the circumstance is even more suggestive.

5 Patients with the malignant phase of hypertension, because up to 20% of patients with renal artery stenosis present in this fashion.

6 Patients with a loin or abdominal bruit, despite the unreliability of this sign.

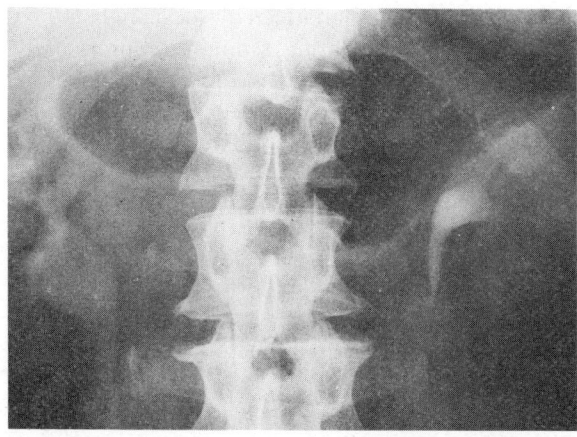

Fig. 53.6. Intravenous urography in a hypertensive man with left renal artery stenosis, showing on the affected side hyperconcentration of dye with evidence of reduced urine flow. These appearances can easily lead to suspicion being directed towards the normal kidney (in this case that on the right).

Screening tests

Intravenous urography   In unselected hypertensive patients, intravenous urography yields few abnormalities, and its value has been questioned.

The characteristic features of this disease on pyelography are usually fourfold. The affected kidney is usually smaller, although the right kidney can normally be as much as 1.5 cm shorter than the left. On the affected side, there is delayed appearance of contrast in the first minutes after injection, with later hyperconcentration. There is usually evidence of reduced urine volume, despite the hyperconcentration, on the affected side (Figs 53.6 and 53.7). On the normal, but not on the affected, side, there may be disappearance or fading of contrast after the administration of a water load. It is important that these last three features are appreciated; suspicion can easily focus on the good kidney, which can then be inappropriately attacked surgically. More rarely, in the presence of a very severe stenosis or occlusion, dye may fail to appear at all stages on the affected side. Renal size may also be reduced on the afflicted side. The value of intravenous pyelography as a screening test may be lost in those patients with bilateral renal artery stenosis.

Ultrasound   Abdominal ultrasound can demonstrate disproportionate kidney size.

Intravenous angiography   The advent of intravenous angiography, combined with digital subtraction methods, has greatly facilitated screening for renal artery stenosis, permitting in many cases not only the detection but also the localization and definition of the lesion. Nevertheless, many surgeons would require the superior definition provided by selective angiography before undertaking surgery.

Isotope renography   In the past, this procedure enjoyed a vogue as a screening test, despite the occurrence of a substantial proportion of both false-negative and false-positive results. It has also been combined with intravenous urography. The role of renography nowadays is more appropriately directed to assessing the severity of a renal artery stenosis.

Plasma renin estimation   An elevated value for plasma renin in peripheral blood has been regarded as indicative of renovascular hypertension. However, many patients with this condition have circulating concentrations of both renin and angiotensin II that are only marginally elevated, or in the upper part of the overall normal range. Therefore, this indicator should be regarded as only a tenuous lead.

More recently, this test has been expanded and refined, by measuring plasma renin following the administration of the fast-acting angiotensin converting enzyme inhibitor captopril. It has been reported that, following captopril, patients with renal artery stenosis show a more marked rise in plasma renin than do those with essential hypertension, with virtually complete separation of the two groups. Other workers, however, have not been

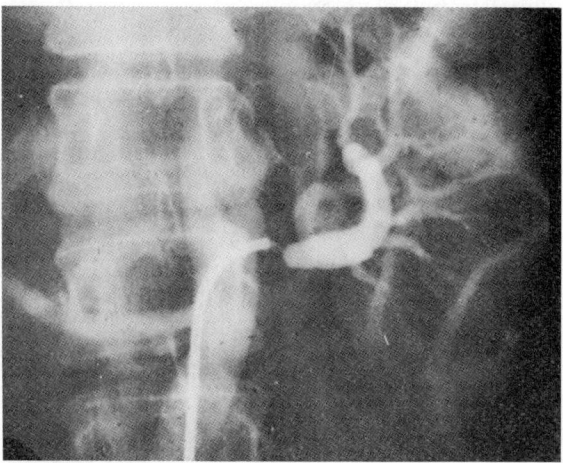

Fig. 53.7. Selective left renal arteriogram in the patient illustrated in Fig. 53.6, showing atheromatous stenosis at origin of the left renal artery. The right renal artery is normal.

able to confirm these findings, and have queried the reliability of the procedure.[102]

Diagnosis of renovascular hypertension

Radiological tests Of the screening procedures enumerated above, intravenous angiography and, not rarely, intravenous urography may permit diagnosis of renal artery stenosis, but not necessarily of renovascular hypertension. However, intra-arterial angiography will usually be required to provide the detail needed to guide the surgeon (Fig. 53.7). Isotope renography has progressed in recent years so that a quantitative assessment of both the extent of reduction of renal plasma flow and the glomerular filtration rate may be made non-invasively.

Bilateral ureteric catheter studies Bilateral ureteric catheterization provides the most detailed functional and diagnostic information in unilateral renal artery stenosis. The procedure is no longer popular because it is time-consuming and expensive, requires expert urological skils, calls for saddle-block anaesthesia, is uncomfortable for the patient and may be complicated by loin or bladder pain, haematuria or urinary infection.

Typical features of unilateral renal artery stenosis are, on the affected side, reduction in urine flow and urinary sodium concentration, enhanced concentrations of creatinine and, if administered, inulin and *para*-aminohippurate (PAH), with reduced clearances of creatinine, inulin and PAH.

Few patients if any, remain in whom the precise details provided by this procedure are needed.

Renal vein renin estimation Comparison of the values of renin (less commonly of angiotensin II) in the two renal veins is a widely employed confirmatory procedure.

Increased values of renin on the affected side are the result of increased renin secretion and diminution of renal plasma flow; renin secretion is usually suppressed on the contralateral normal side, with renin values in renal venous plasma being closely similar to those in the aorta.

In the steady state, increased renin secretion alone cannot in unilateral renal artery stenosis raise the renal vein renin ratio to $> 1.5 : 1$. Values higher than this reflect also reduction of renal blood flow on the affected side, and the procedure has been used to estimate changes in blood flow. The ratio of renin in renal venous plasma on the affected compared with the unaffected side can be raised transiently by stimulating renin secretion acutely; this has been performed as an aid to diagnosis employing various procedures such as orthostasis or the administration of vasodilators or converting enzyme inhibitors.

Prognostic indicators

Many procedures, the majority of very dubious origin, have been employed to attempt the prediction of blood pressure reduction after successful relief of the stenosis.

Clinical features A poor outcome in terms of blood pressure reduction is more likely with older age, longstanding hypertension, cigarette smoking, atheroma, vascular disease at other sites, renal impairment and male sex. Conversely, a better result may be expected with youth, fibromuscular hyperplasia, good renal function and female sex.

Renin estimation High levels of renin in peripheral blood and also a high renal vein renin ratio have been claimed to herald a good prognostic outcome. Suppression of renin release by the unaffected kidney has also been deemed an encouraging feature. However, none of these has been reliably consistent.

Ureteric catheterization studies Ureteric catheterization studies have not proved reliable indicators of surgical success.

Antagonists of the renin–angiotensin system The immediate blood pressure fall following acute administration of antagonists of angiotensin II, such as saralasin, or of converting enzyme inhibitors, such as captopril, has been widely employed. However, our experience and that of other workers has demonstrated the fallibility of this approach, with the acute blood pressure fall in such circumstances variously over- and underestimating the long-term outcome following relief of the stenosis. This is not surprising in view of the pathophysiological considerations discussed already.

However, at least two groups of workers have reported that the long-term blood pressure response (i.e. over several weeks) to orally active converting enzyme inhibitors predicts well, in absolute terms, both for systolic and diastolic pressures, the long-term outcome following operative intervention. This finding is in accord with pathophysiological notions, and, although the findings have not been universally acclaimed, they deserve further critical evaluation.[102]

TREATMENT OF RENOVASCULAR HYPERTENSION[102]

Operative intervention

The two main reasons for operative relief of renal artery stenosis are to lower arterial pressure or to improve renal function. To these may be added a much rarer indication, where the cause of the renal artery narrowing requires excision in its own right, e.g. phaeochromocytoma involving the renal hilum.

As the kidney distal to the stenosis is protected from the effects of systemic hypertension, in most cases this kidney has potentially excellent function. Such considerations make a strong case for operative relief of a renal artery constriction as the treatment of choice. Although both unilateral nephrectomy or reconstruction can relieve high blood pressure, the former consistently diminishes, whereas the latter enhances, overall renal function.

The foregoing comments emphasize that nephrectomy should be avoided if at all possible. However, there are circumstances in which nephrectomy or heminephrectomy is indicated, such as an obviously shrunken kidney or part of the kidney, or in which there exist severe technical problems of aberrant or friable renal arteries, multiple intrarenal branch lesions or renal artery aneurysm. There are also rare cases in which successful reconstruction of a renal artery stenosis fails to relieve hypertension, which is corrected only after the contralateral kidney, the seat of hypertension-induced renal changes, has been removed.

Conservative surgical procedures include endarterectomy with or without patch angioplasty, splenorenal, hepatorenal, iliac–renal or superior mesenteric–renal arterial anastomosis, aortorenal bypass grafting employing Dacron velour, saphenous, ovarian or testicular vein or splenic or hypogastric artery, or autotransplantation to usually the internal iliac artery.

The introduction of extracorporeal methods for reconstructing extensive renal and intrarenal vascular disease has in recent years greatly enhanced the scope and success of these procedures, notably bypass grafting and autotransplantation.

At one time, revascularization techniques carried an anatomical failure rate of 18–45%. However, surgical expertise and especially the use of extracorporeal reconstruction methods have considerably improved these figures, at least in centres where there is extensive experience.

Comparison of the results of surgical 'successes' and 'failures' among centres is difficult because of differing criteria adopted by various authors. Most include a category of 'partial success', in which, although blood pressure has not been lowered to normal, control with drugs has been easier, and/or the burden of side-effects of medical therapy was lighter. We defined a successful outcome, in terms of blood pressure reduction, as the lowering of pressure to within one standard deviation of age- and sex-adjusted values observed in the general population.[99]

Despite the differences of definition, some worthwhile comparisons of outcome among different centres can be made. In a review of 25 series in which 2430 patients were operated upon between 1961 and 1983, 46% of patients were regarded as having a successful operation, 34% were regarded as improved, and 20% of the operations were judged as failures. Diverse surgically managed forms of hypertension yielded overall success rates that are not dissimilar, ranging from 40 to 65%,

The assessment of the success or otherwise of operation to improve renal function is readily achieved. However, no large series in which patients were operated upon specifically for this reason appear to have been reported. It deserves emphasis that normal renal function can be restored even after several weeks of main renal arterial occlusion, especially if an extensive collateral blood supply has developed. Nevertheless, acute renal artery occlusion, if diagnosed, is a surgical emergency.

Transluminal angioplasty

Percutaneous transluminal angioplasty has steadily gained in popularity in recent years as an alternative to surgical intervention for renal artery stenosis. Under local anaesthesia, a pre-shaped Teflon catheter, usually with an internal diameter of some 1.8 mm, is inserted into the femoral artery and passed to the renal artery, where its position is confirmed by the injection of contrast. Through this outer catheter is then passed a second catheter with a double lumen and with an external diameter of 1.3 mm. One lumen is for inflating a terminal balloon, the other opens at the catheter tip. Once suitably situated, the balloon is repeatedly inflated to 5–6 atm for 3–5 s until there is angiographic evidence of relief of the stenosis and the pressure drop across the site of the lesion has been eliminated or substantially alleviated. Anticoagulants are usually administered after the procedure. Improved outcome can in future be expected, with the more enlightened use of antiplatelet agents.

Not all renal arterial lesions are amenable to angioplasty. The most suitable are proximal, accessible, discrete, concentric non-calcified lesions. In general, fibromuscular hyperplastic stenoses do better than do atheromatous lesions.

Complications include pain, segmental or total renal infarction, renal failure, intimal dissection leading to worsening of the stenosis, retroperitoneal bleeding, balloon rupture with embolization of the fragments, and inability to remove the balloon with consequent need for surgery.

Facilities for open surgery must always be available when practising balloon angioplasty.

Medical treatment

Stimulation of the renin–angiotensin system is almost certainly responsible for the initiation and, in both phase I and phase II of renovascular hypertension, the maintenance of the raised blood pressure. Only in phase III, which is unresponsive to surgical measures, is the renin–angiotensin system probably no longer relevant.

Thus, it is to be expected that in both phase I and phase II of renovascular hypertension the administration of agents that neutralize the effects of the renin–angiotensin system would alleviate the hypertension.

The orally active converting enzyme inhibitors are most suitable for long-term treatment, and the fall in blood pressure after several weeks of pre-operative therapy with such agents has been taken by some workers as a good index of the likely blood pressure response following operation. The efficacy of converting enzyme inhibitors can be enhanced by adding a diuretic or a calcium antagonist.

However, as well as being responsible probably for the maintenance of systemic hypertension in this disease, important intrarenal compensatory actions of angiotensin II occur in the kidney beyond the stenosis, helping that kidney, despite the reduction in perfusion, to an extent to sustain glomerular filtration rate, the capacity to excrete urea and the pressure in the main renal artery distal to the stenosis. These compensatory effects will be diminished or lost with angiotensin converting enzyme inhibition; moreover, there are fears that there may be with such medical treatment not only reversible diminution of unilateral renal function, but also on occasion occlusion of the renal artery.

For these reasons, many physicians are reluctant to employ angiotensin converting enzyme inhibitors, other than briefly, in patients with hypertension accompanied by renal artery stenosis. There is particular concern that their use in patients with bilateral renal artery stenosis may regularly provoke renal failure. The conjoint administration of diuretics almost certainly enhances the risks in both unilateral and bilateral renal artery narrowing.

Fears have also been expressed concerning the possible dangers of beta-adrenoceptor blockers in this condition, because these agents also in part work via the renin–angiotensin system, inhibiting renin secretion. However, these drugs less potently interfere with the renin system, and the risks are probably less than those associated with angiotensin converting enzyme inhibitors.

The above considerations do not preclude the use of either angiotensin converting enzyme inhibitors, alone or in combination, or beta-blockers in the long-term treatment of renovascular hypertension in patients unsuitable or unwilling to undergo operation. However, it has to be recognized that such an approach cannot improve, and will almost certainly worsen, the already compromised function of the diseased kidney. Moreover, with bilateral renal artery stenosis, and especially if diuretics are also administered, renal failure can readily be provoked.

OTHER FORMS OF UNILATERAL RENAL DISEASE WITH HYPERTENSION

A wide variety of unilateral renal lesions may occur with hypertension (see Table 53.3) and, at least in some instances, blood pressure may be lowered following removal of the affected kidney. It has been proposed that the common pathogenetic pathway is stimulation of renin secretion by the lesion. If this is so, these patients should show, as in renal artery stenosis or renal renin-secreting tumour, differential renin values in renal venous blood, and also probably a fall in blood pressure with pre-operative administration of angiotensin converting enzyme inhibitors. The number of conditions listed in Table 53.3, give an idea of the protean variety of modes of presentation. Many of these conditions require nephrectomy irrespective of hypertension; consequently, any fall in blood pressure resulting from surgical intervention may often be regarded as a bonus.

The reader is referred to specialist texts for a

detailed account of these lesions. Two require brief elucidation here.

Ask–Upmark kidney

This rarity consists of apparently congenital unilateral renal lobular hypoplasia, with small blind-ending recesses in the renal pelvis. Pyelonephritis may complicate the pathology. The condition is found predominantly in young females and often progresses to the malignant phase.

Page kidney

Page described a form of experimental hypertension induced by cellophane wrapping of the kidney, with consequent perinephritis, capsular fibrosis and subcapsular ischaemia. Clinically, this term has been applied to capsular fibrosis and hypertension resulting from a perirenal haematoma.

HYPERTENSION WITH BILATERAL RENAL DISEASE

As indicated in Table 53.3, hypertension can complicate a range of renal parenchymal disorders, particularly if overall renal functional impairment supervenes. Hypertension is also seen in association with bilateral renal artery stenosis.

BILATERAL RENAL ARTERY STENOSIS

Pathophysiology

The pathophysiology in this condition is essentially similar to that in which there is narrowing of the artery of a single remaining kidney. The experimental model of the latter is known as 'one-clip, one-kidney' hypertension, and has been extensively studied. In this model, peripheral levels of plasma renin are raised only transiently after application of the clip, and then subside to normal or subnormal levels. Body sodium content expands, and this expansion is sustained with persistent hypertension.[101] There is, however, disagreement over whether there is a correlation between the degree of expansion of body sodium and the severity of the hypertension. Nevertheless, it is probable that sodium retention makes at least a contribution to the raised arterial pressure.

Diagnosis

The clinical diagnosis of either bilateral renal artery stenosis or of stenosis of the artery to a single kidney is based, first, on the features suggestive of renal artery stenosis set out above. Second, hypertension resistant to drug therapy should raise this possibility. Third, if the overall renal function is already compromised and/or if renal function deteriorates as systemic blood pressure is lowered with drugs, especially angiotensin converting enzyme inhibitors, the possibility of either bilateral renal artery stenosis or of renal artery stenosis to a single kidney should be seriously considered, and arteriographic studies of the renal arteries conducted as outlined earlier.

Treatment

Treatment consists, wherever possible, of relief of the stenosis or stenoses, either surgically or by transluminal angioplasty, because prevention or relief of renal failure is paramount. Such correction of the stenosis or stenoses often also controls the hypertension. Although reduction of blood pressure is possible in some patients with the use of drugs without operation, renal function in these circumstances must be carefully and regularly monitored. It is axiomatic that no patient should be subjected to regular haemodialysis for renal failure unless the possibility of correctable bilateral renal artery stenoses (or of renal artery stenosis in a single kidney), with potential restoration of renal function, has been excluded. This is important not least because the kidney distal to a renal artery stenosis is largely protected from damage due to hypertension.

BILATERAL PARENCHYMATOUS RENAL DISEASE

Pathology

As indicated in Table 53.3, a diverse range of bilateral renal diseases can be associated with hypertension, and detailed description of these is beyond the scope of this chapter. Diagnoses include bilateral polycystic disease, which is inherited as a Mendelian dominant disorder, acute and chronic glomerulonephritis, interstitial nephritis, pyelonephritis, radiation nephritis, analgesic nephropathy and diabetic nephropathy. Although all of these can cause elevation of arterial pressure, hypertension-dependent nephrosclerosis may add to renal damage and accelerate the rate of deterioration of renal function and the rise of blood pressure. These concepts emphasize the need for prompt recognition and treatment of hypertension. Terminally, when both kidneys are shrunken and scarred, it may be almost impossible to differentiate the initial abnormality from lesions resulting from hypertension.

Pathophysiology

In some instances, the pathophysiological mechanism underlying the hypertension is hypersecretion of renin caused by the renal lesions. In these circumstances, pathogenesis is basically similar to that in many cases of unilateral renal disease (Table 53.3). This could and does occur, for example, in both acute and chronic glomerulonephritis. More often, however, hypertension with bilateral renal disease is accompanied by, and dependent upon, renal impairment. In these latter circumstances, fluid and sodium retention are almost certainly important influences in the causation of raised arterial pressure. Significant correlations have been described between the severity of hypertension and total exchangeable sodium in series of patients with chronic renal failure.[103] The renin–angiotensin system then may provide an additional or alternative factor in some cases.[104]

Other mechanisms that have been proposed, but which are less clearly defined, are increases in plasma noradrenaline and deficiencies of vasodepressor prostaglandins and of kinins.

Treatment

In patients who have hypertension accompanying bilateral renal disease, but who do not require regular dialysis for renal impairment, antihypertensive drug therapy may suffice. Care should be taken so that overzealous blood pressure reduction with drugs does not provoke renal failure. Angiotensin converting enzyme inhibitors in particular may effectively control the blood pressure, especially if there is evidence of hypersecretion of renin; however, these drugs are also prone to cause renal failure, notably if given together with aggressive diuretic therapy.

In patients who are hypertensive and require regular dialysis, blood pressure can usually be controlled by the removal of water and sodium at dialysis, with the addition of antihypertensive drugs if necessary.

Rarely, patients are encountered in whom the intrinsic renal lesion responds to the removal of sodium at dialysis with gross hypersecretion of renin. Thus, there is a resulting marked excess of circulating angiotensin II, with severe and worsening hypertension, raised plasma aldosterone and often intolerable thirst. Formerly, bilateral nephrectomy was required in such patients in order to control the hypertension and other features.[104] Plasma angiotensin II can now be lowered with the use of angiotensin converting enzyme inhibitors. Care must be taken in introducing these agents, however, because, with a very high plasma angiotensin II concentration, its sudden reduction may lead to severe hypotension.

ADRENOCORTICAL DISORDERS

PRIMARY ALDOSTERONE EXCESS; CONN'S SYNDROME AND RELATED DISORDERS[105]

The classic form of mineralocorticoid excess with hypertension is true Conn's syndrome, due to an aldosterone-secreting adenoma of the adrenal cortex. It is an interesting rarity that may be mimicked by several other conditions which have similarities, affinities and also important differences.

Pathology

A classification of the conditions that will be considered in this section is presented in Table 53.4. All are characterized by aldosterone excess and low plasma renin.

Pathophysiology

Aldosterone is a powerful mineralocorticoid secreted by the zona glomerulosa of the adrenal cortex. Its main action is on distal nephrons to promote

---

Table 53.4. Classification of primary aldosterone excess.

1 Conn's syndrome: aldosterone-secreting adrenocortical adenoma; true primary hyperaldosteronism

2 Aldosterone-secreting carcinoma (usually adrenocortical; rarely ovarian)

3 Angiotensin-responsive aldosterone-secreting tumour[106]

4 Glucocorticoid-remedial hyperaldosteronism[11]

5 Idiopathic hyperaldosteronism ('pseudo-primary' hyperaldosteronism or 'non-tumorous hyperaldosteronism'). This is now considered to be part of a continuum with essential hypertension and distinct from primary hyperaldosteronism

sodium reabsorption in exchange for potassium and hydrogen ions. Aldosterone secretion is normally regulated principally by the renin–angiotensin system and, in most physiological and pathophysiological circumstances, plasma renin, angiotensin II and aldosterone levels move in conjunction. By contrast, in the syndromes described herein, aldosterone excess is accompanied by depression of the renin–angiotensin system.

CONN'S SYNDROME: ALDOSTERONE-SECRETING ADRENOCORTICAL ADENOMA

Aldosterone-secreting adrenocortical adenoma is an interesting rarity, probably representing no more than 0.1% of the hypertensive population. It may present at any age, more often in women than in men. Adrenocortical adenoma can be associated with parathyroid adenoma.

Pathology

Most tumours are roughly spherical, of 2 cm or less in diameter (Fig. 53.8). They usually project from the adrenal but can be wholly intraglandular. The cut surface is typically golden yellow. The left gland is affected more often than the right. Bilateral tumours are sometimes found. The hypertension is accompanied by hypokalaemia, contraction of body potassium content, extracellular alkalosis, hypernatraemia and expansion of body sodium. If diuretics have been given, muscle weakness, polyuria, nocturia and polydipsia may be present. Most patients, however, are devoid of symptoms.

Diagnosis

Although low plasma (or serum) potassium concen-

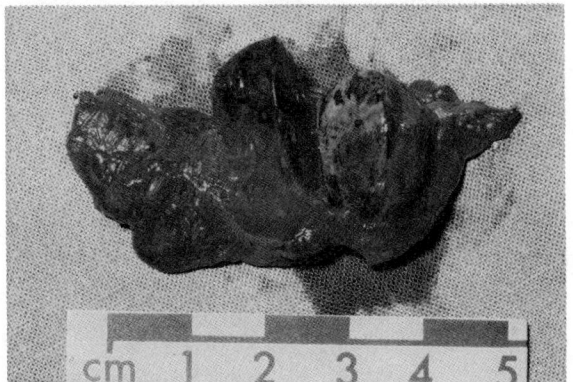

Fig. 53.8. Aldosterone-secreting adrenocortical adenoma of the adrenal cortex after removal.

tration usually provides the initial clue, it must be recognized that on occasions this feature may be masked by a low dietary sodium intake, or by the use of forearm muscular exercise to aid venepuncture.

Despite the low prevailing plasma renin concentrations, and hence angiotensin II concentrations, aldosterone is unresponsive to administered angiotensin II or by stimulating an increase in endogenous angiotensin II by the assumption of the upright posture. These tests have been used as an aid to diagnosis. Once suspected, diagnosis can be further pursued by locating an adrenocortical tumour on computed tomography, adrenal ultrasonography or adrenal scintillation scanning, of which computed tomography is the most sensitive and precise. Confirmation by bilateral adrenal vein sampling may be undertaken. This will reveal high plasma aldosterone values on the suspect side; at the same procedure, adrenal venography can confirm the presence and location of the adenoma. This procedure has been superseded in recent times by computed tomography; however, it may be useful in, for example, the presence of bilateral lesions with only one functional tumour.

Treatment

Pre-operative treatment with a potassium-conserving diuretic (spironolactone up to 300 mg/day or amiloride up to 75 mg/day) will correct the various biochemical abnormalities (apart from aldosterone excess) and lower the raised arterial pressure. The magnitude of blood pressure reduction during 4–6 weeks of treatment with these agents has been taken to predict the subsequent response to surgical removal of the adenoma.

Blood pressure returns to strictly normal age- and sex-matched values in only about 50% of cases, even though operation has corrected the aldosterone excess. Blood pressure reduction tends to be less adequate in patients with renal functional impairment. In the event of persistent elevation of arterial pressure after operation, treatment is as for essential hypertension.

ALDOSTERONE-SECRETION CARCINOMA

Pathology

An aldosterone-secreting carcinoma is most often of adrenocortical origin, but it can also arise in the ovary.

Clinical features

Aspects additional to those of the more usual Conn's syndrome should raise the possibility of carcinoma. Fever, muscle weakness and a large abdominal or pelvic mass may be alerting features. Excessive secretion of corticosteroids in addition to aldosterone is common, and occasionally the predominant mineralocorticoid may be 11-deoxycorticosterone or corticosterone. Prompt surgical excision is indicated.

ANGIOTENSIN-RESPONSIVE ADRENOCORTICAL ADENOMA

This variant has only recently been recognized,[106] and may be distinguished from true Conn's syndrome by showing a rapid rise in plasma aldosterone in response to either infused angiotensin II or orthostasis. The pathways of aldosterone biosynthesis are believed to be distinct from those of classic Conn's syndrome. As blood pressure may be adequately lowered by excision of the adenoma, it is important to distinguish this variant from non-tumorous aldosterone excess, which does not respond well to adrenal surgery.

GLUCOCORTICOID-REMEDIABLE HYPERALDOSTERONISM

In this rare, and often familial, form of aldosterone excess,[11] the administration of glucocorticoids, such as dexamethasone (2 mg/day), produces a sustained reversal of all the abnormalities, usually within 2 weeks or slightly longer. Aldosterone secretion may in this syndrome be unusually sensitive to ACTH, and it has been suggested that the aldosterone may arise from the zona fasciculata rather than the glomerulosa. In this disorder, surgical exploration has usually revealed adrenocortical zona glomerulosa hyperplasia, without tumour.

IDIOPATHIC ALDOSTERONISM (SOMETIMES TERMED 'PSEUDO-PRIMARY' ALDOSTERONE EXCESS OR 'NON-TUMOROUS PRIMARY HYPERALDOSTERONISM')

This condition, once confused with Conn's syndrome, is now believed to be part of the same continuum as essential hypertension. The confusion arose because, in essential hypertension, plasma renin falls progressively with the course of the disease, whereas the aldosterone response to angiotensin II becomes more pronounced. Thus, some patients with essential hypertension, with low renin and rather high aldosterone levels, increasingly resemble, at least superficially, true Conn's syndrome. Hypokalaemia, contraction of body potassium, hypernatraemia and expansion of body sodium are all less marked than in patients with aldosterone-secreting adenoma. These quantitative differences have formed the basis of multifactorial statistical tests to differentiate idiopathic aldosteronism from Conn's syndrome.[107] The greatest danger of diagnostic confusion is likely to be with the newly recognized angiotensin-responsive adrenocortical adenoma.[106] In patients with idiopathic aldosteronism of this kind, specific adrenocortical lesions are wanting, and the response to surgery is usually poor. These cases should be treated medically, including, if appropriate, potassium-conserving diuretics.

CUSHING'S SYNDROME

This condition results from an excess of glucocorticoids, notably cortisol. Hypertension is said to be a feature in about 75–85% of patients.[108]

Pathology

The various causes of Cushing's syndrome are given in Table 53.5. Primary pituitary disease or dysfunction of the hypothalamic–pituitary axis accounts for some 70% of all cases, excess ACTH or corticotrophin-releasing hormones produced by various other tumours for about 12%, and adrenal tumours for about 12%.

Pathophysiology

The pathogenesis of hypertension in Cushing's

Table 53.5.   Classification of Cushing's syndrome.

1 Primary anterior pituitary disease with excess secretion of adrenocorticotrophic hormone (corticotrophin; ACTH). This may be a consequence of dysfunction of the hypothalamic–pituitary axis or associated with micro-adenomata of the anterior pituitary

2 Ectopic neoplasm (often bronchial carcinoma) producing excess ACTH or more rarely corticotrophin-releasing hormones

3 Adrenal benign or malignant neoplasm producing excess glucocorticoids

4 Therapeutic administration of ACTH or glucocorticoids (see page 1256)

5 Alcoholism

syndrome is not fully elucidated. Several possibilities have been proposed.

Pressor action of cortisol

Cortisol is a weak mineralocorticoid, and two characteristic features of mineralocorticoid-induced hypertension, renin suppression and hypokalaemia, are usually lacking in Cushing's syndrome. Nevertheless, the administration of cortisol, or of ACTH with consequent elevation of plasma cortisol, to normal volunteers raises blood pressure, causes antinatriuresis, expands plasma and extracellular fluid volumes, while depressing renin and elevating atrial natriuretic peptide.[95]

Increased production of more potent mineralocorticoids

Potent mineralocorticoids, such as deoxycorticosterone or aldosterone, may be secreted if there is an adrenocortical tumour or the disease results from excess of ACTH. However, ACTH administration to normal volunteers causes only a transient rise in plasma aldosterone, and associated features of mineralocorticoid excess are usually lacking in Cushing's syndrome.

Increased renin-substrate (angiotensinogen)

Plasma renin-substrate levels rise with cortisol administration and thus can be high in Cushing's syndrome. In the absence of corresponding suppression of plasma renin concentration, plasma angiotensin II should increase and could raise arterial pressure. This possibility has so far been inadequately explored.

Increased vascular response to various vasoconstrictors, such as angiotensin II and catecholamines

This possibility awaits critical evaluation.

Clinical features

Cushing's syndrome may be suspected because of the appearance of the patient (Fig. 53.9). There is characteristically a 'moon face', a 'buffalo hump' over the thoracic spine, wasting of muscles and skin, with livid striae in the latter, bruises, and abdominal obesity. Diabetes mellitus is a frequent complication. There may be osteoporosis with spontaneous fractures. Psychiatric disturbances occur in some 40% of patients. Subjects with ACTH excess secreted from a malignant neoplasm are more likely to show hypokalaemic alkalosis.

Diagnosis

In patients suspected of suffering from Cushing's syndrome, it is necessary first to confirm the diagnosis and then to identify the causative abnormality. A detailed history should suffice in subjects being treated with ACTH or exogenous corticosteroids.

A Cushing-like syndrome may be encountered in alcoholics, who can have high plasma cortisol levels. Such subjects should be investigated further after 4 weeks' abstention from alcohol.

Screening tests

Plasma cortisol suppression by dexamethasone
Dexamethasone 1 mg is taken by mouth at bedtime, and a plasma sample drawn for cortisol estimation at between 08 00 and 09 00 hours the next day. A raised plasma cortisol value (variously > 3–10

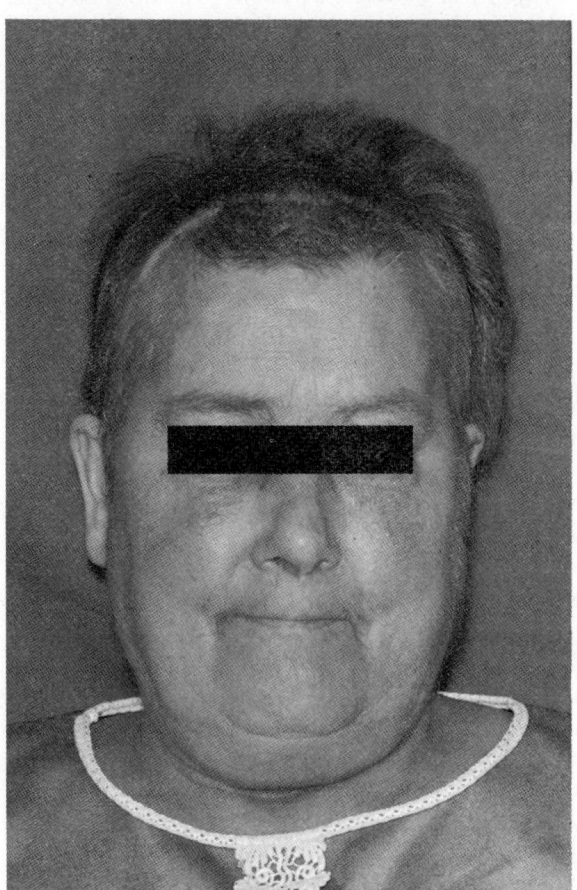

Fig. 53.9. Patient with Cushing's syndrome showing typical facies. The responsible lesion was an anterior pituitary adenoma which had been removed surgically shortly before this photograph. The craniotomy scar is evident.

μg/100 ml or 80–280 nmol/l depending on the laboratory) indicates Cushing's syndrome.

This test may be compromised by the concomitant use of drugs that enhance the rate of inactivation of exogenous dexamethasone and thereby limit the suppression of endogenous ACTH. These agents include diphenylhydantoin, barbiturates, tolbutamide, rifampicin and alcohol.

Patients with endogenous psychiatric depression may also fail to respond to dexamethasone. This can raise difficult diagnostic problems because, conversely, patients with Cushing's syndrome also often have, in consequence, psychiatric disturbances.

Mental stress for any reason may override the suppression by dexamethasone of pituitary ACTH secretion. Many subjects find hospital admission stressful, and for this reason the test may be more valuable when conducted on outpatients.

Urinary free cortisol excretion   The normal upper limit of urinary free cortisol of around 100 μg/24 h varies slightly among laboratories. Measurement of urinary free cortisol in either a 24 h or early morning urine sample is more sensitive and specific than the plasma cortisol suppression test. Measurements made in urine represent an integrated response to plasma concentrations during the collection period and are affected by factors that influence circulating levels.

Low-dose dexamethasone suppression test   Dexamethasone 0.5 mg is given every 6 h for 2 days and either 24-h urinary hydroxycorticoids or free cortisol are assayed. Raised values suggest the diagnosis. Although this test may improve discrimination when compared with the plasma cortisol suppression test or the measurement of urinary free cortisol, overlap is seen between values in Cushing's syndrome and those in normal subjects.

Differential diagnostic tests

Plasma ACTH assay   The availability of a reliable assay for plasma ACTH can greatly facilitate differential diagnosis. Plasma ACTH values are raised if the cause of the disease is hypersecretion of ACTH from a pituitary or ectopic lesion or administration of exogenous ACTH. By contast, plasma ACTH values are low if the causative lesion is an adrenocortical tumour producing an excess of glucocorticoids.

As the demonstration of an undetectable level is often clinically important, meticulous attention to detail is needed. Blood should be sampled in the morning, when ACTH is normally high. Later in the day, ACTH is often undetectable in normal subjects because of limitations of current assay methods.

High-dose dexamethasone suppression test   Dexamethasone 2.0 mg is administered every 6 h for 2 days, and 24-h urinary 17-hydroxycorticosteroids or free cortisol are assayed. Some 40% of patients with ACTH excess of either pituitary or ectopic origin may show suppression of urinary corticoid excretion, although this rarely occurs if the causative lesion lies in the adrenal cortex. This test is less specific than plasma ACTH assay, and it is now obsolescent.

Metyrapone test   Most patients with pituitary Cushing's disease will respond with a rise in ACTH if cortisol synthesis is inhibited. Metyrapone inhibits 11-β-hydroxylase and causes a fall in plasma cortisol. Patients with ectopic tumours or primary adrenal lesions show no response. Metyrapone can be given orally or intravenously and the ACTH response measured directly or by collecting urine over 24 h for assessing excretion rates of precursors of 11-deoxycortisol or 17-oxogenic steroids.

Anatomical localization of the lesion

Computerized tomography   This technique is now well established in the identification and delineation of pituitary and adrenal tumours, and it has substantially replaced arteriography and pneumoencephalography.

Scintigraphy   Adrenocortical scintigraphy with radio-labelled cholesterol compounds, can identify an adrenocortical tumour and quantify the extent of adrenal dysfunction.

Ultrasound   Adrenocortical lesions may be identified non-invasively by ultrasound.

Regional venous sampling   Sampling from veins at various sites, with plasma ACTH assay, has been used to help localize a source of ectopic ACTH secretion.

Treatment

Pituitary Cushing's syndrome

Surgery of pituitary gland Pituitary tumours responsible for Cushing's syndrome may be resected surgically, via either a trans-sphenoidal or trans-frontal (Fig. 53.9) approach. In the absence of a large or invasive tumour necessitating near total hypophysectomy, the objective is to correct hyperfunction without causing local damage or long-term endocrine defect. In occasional patients with pituitary Cushing's syndrome, cure has been achieved by hypophysectomy even when no pituitary tumour has been found.

Irradiation Pituitary tumours may be irradiated externally, or implanted, for example with yttrium-90 or gold-198. This method is decreasing in popularity because of a slow onset of action and a low cure rate. Results from different centres are variable.

Drug therapy The administration of either bromocriptine or cyproheptadine may suppress excessive pituitary ACTH secretion, but the effect of these drugs is usually only temporary. Alternatively, drugs suppressing adrenocortical steroid synthesis, such as mitotane, metyrapone, aminoglutethimide, ketoconazole or trilostane, have been employed, often in conjunction with external irradiation.

Adrenal surgery Although bilateral adrenalectomy can 'cure' Cushing's syndrome of pituitary origin, the subsequent appearance or the progressive enlargement of a pituitary tumour with grossly excessive ACTH output in some 40% of patients (Nelson's syndrome) makes this an unattractive procedure. Lifelong steroid replacement therapy is also needed.

Adrenal Cushing's syndrome

Surgery

When the primary pathology, adenoma or carcinoma, arises in the adrenal gland, surgical excision is required.

Drug treatment

Agents that interfere with corticosteroid biosynthesis (such as mitotane, metyrapone, aminoglutethi-mide, ketoconazole and trilostane mentioned above) can be employed.

Ectopic ACTH secretion

Cushing's syndrome resulting from ectopic ACTH secretion is often the result of a carcinoma arising in some distant tissue. Excision or irradiation of the primary lesion, which usually requires therapy in its own right, is necessary. Such measures are often inadequate, and adrenal surgery, or the administration of drugs inhibiting corticosteroid biosynthesis, may then be needed to alleviate the accompanying features of Cushing's syndrome.

Prognosis

It will be evident from the diversity of abnormalities that can cause Cushing's syndrome that the efficacy of therapy in correcting glucocorticoid excess and its consequences will vary widely. Even when the biochemical abnormalities are fully corrected, Cushing's syndrome conforms to the general rule that, in secondary hypertension, removal or correction of the primary lesion restores blood pressure to age- and sex-adjusted normal values in only a proportion of cases.[43] The approach to treatment of residual hypertension is as that for essential hypertension.

INBORN ERRORS OF CORTICOSTEROID BIOSYNTHESIS[109]

17-α-hydroxylase deficiency

This very rare hypertensive syndrome is of considerable interest, not least because of the light it sheds on the role of adrenocorticotrophic hormone (ACTH) in the pathogenesis of hypertension.[109,110]

The basic defect is lack of the enzyme 17-α-hydroxylase, which results in deficiencies of adrenal steroid synthesis. Both androgens and oestrogens are subnormal; thus, genetic males present as pseudohermaphrodites, and females fail to develop secondary sexual characteristics.

Central to the pathogenesis of the hypertension is a deficiency also of cortisol biosynthesis, leading to excess secretion of ACTH and hence to an overproduction of ACTH-dependent mineralocorticoids, notably deoxycorticosterone, 11-hydroxydeoxy-corticosterone, corticosterone and 11-hydroxy-corticosterone. Sodium is retained and potassium lost. Plasma potassium is reduced, plasma sodium tends to be raised and there is extracellular alkalosis. Plasma renin and angiotensin II fall, and consequently aldosterone levels also are low.

Treatment with dexamethasone lowers the excessive ACTH secretion, the ACTH-dependent mineralocorticoids drop to normal values and blood pressure falls, while renin, angiotensin II and aldosterone rise into the normal range. The sodium and potassium balance is restored, and plasma sodium, potassium and bicarbonate concentrations are corrected.

11-β-Hydroxylase deficiency

This congenital defect of the enzyme 11-β-hydroxylase also leads to deficient biosynthesis of cortisol and hence to overproduction of ACTH. Androgen secretion is unimpaired, thus male patients show precocious sexual development, whereas females are virilized. The site of enzymic defect means that secretion rates of both corticosterone and aldosterone are impaired. Deoxycorticosterone, however, is produced in excess, leading to sodium retention, potassium depletion, hypokalaemia and hypernatraemia, lowering of plasma renin and angiotensin II levels, and hypertension.

In this disease, treatment with dexamethasone corrects the excess of ACTH, lowers the secretion of deoxycorticosterone, restores sodium and potassium balance, returns the suppressed plasma renin and angiotensin II levels into the normal range, and alleviates the hypertension.

PHAEOCHROMOCYTOMA[111]

Phaeochromocytoma is a rare cause of hypertension.

Pathology

The term phaeochromocytoma denotes, strictly, a tumour of neural crest ectodermal origin with an affinity for chromium salts. Chromaffin cells form the adrenal medulla, are distributed adjacent to sympathetic ganglia and nerves, especially in association with nerve plexuses, and are found also in the organ of Zuckerkandl, a fetal structure lying anterior to the abdominal aorta near the origin of the inferior mesenteric artery.

Phaeochromocytomas are tumours of the chromaffin cells, and although the majority lie in the adrenal medulla, they may be widely distributed at other sites where chromaffin cells occur, such as the organ of Zuckerkandl, adjacent to sympathetic ganglia and, less often, in apposition to sympathetic nerve plexuses in the neck, chest, urinary bladder, rectum, testes or ovaries.

More than 97% of all phaeochromocytomas lie within the abdomen. Over 90% arise in the adrenal glands, the right being affected more often than the left; 10% of these adrenal tumours are bilateral.

Malignant phaeochromocytoma

Malignant phaeochromocytomas are rare, and difficult to identify as such histologically. The diagnosis therefore depends on the discovery of metastases. The occurrence of multiple tumours and of local invasion by benign phaeochromocytomas further confounds confirmation of malignancy.

Familial phaeochromocytoma

In some 10% of all cases, phaeochromocytoma is familial, inherited via a dominant gene with a high degree of penetrance. Diagnosis is often made earlier than in sporadic cases, usually before the age of 40 years. Bilateral adrenal tumours are found in 10% of these patients.

More than half of the cases of familial phaeochromocytomas are not associated with evidence of other endocrine gland involvement. In the remainder, there are concomitant tumours that may afflict the parathyroid and thyroid (multiple endocrine neoplasia, 'MEN' type 2). The medullary thyroid carcinoma characteristic of 'MEN' type 2 can be highly malignant, invading locally as well as metastasizing.

Catecholamine-induced cardiomyopathy

Excessive secretion of catecholamines can cause multiple necroses of ventricular myocardial cells and thus lead to cardiac failure or arrhythmias.[49]

Other associations

Five per cent of phaeochromocytomas are associated with neurofibromatosis, although < 1% of patients with neurofibromatosis have phaeochromocytoma. Familial phaeochromocytoma is not especially associated with neurofibromatosis. There is a rare association of phaeochromocytoma with von Hippel–Lindau disease.

Pathophysiology

Secretion of catecholamines

Phaeochromocytomas can secrete excessive noradrenaline and adrenaline, together with the catecholamine precursors dopamine and dopa. Noradrenaline is the hormone predominantly released, and seems to be ubiquitous in non-familial phaeochromocytomas. Adrenaline is secreted by a smaller proportion of cases and rarely, if ever, alone; adrenaline-secreting tumours occur only occasionally outside the adrenal gland.

Secretion of other hormones

Primitive cells of neural crest origin may populate a range of endocrine and other tissues, and can elaborate various hormones and hormone precursors. Thus, neuro-endocrine tumours can secrete adrenocorticotrophic hormone, melanin-stimulating hormone, encephalin, calcitonin, somatostatin, vaso-active intestinal peptide, neuropeptide–Y, or serotonin in conjunction with catecholamines.

Clinical features

The clinical features of phaeochromocytoma result principally from the release of catecholamines, either continuously or paroxysmally, into the circulation. Hypertension is the aspect most likely, but by no means exclusively, to bring the patient to investigation. The elevation of arterial pressure can be intermittent or sustained, or episodes of severe hypertension may be superimposed on a background of continuously elevated blood pressure. The pattern of circulatory disturbance varies with the type of underlying catecholamine excess.

Noradrenaline causes peripheral vasoconstriction, elevation of both systolic and diastolic pressures, and reflex bradycardia; adrenaline raises systolic pressure, lowers the diastolic and increases heart rate. Paradoxically, tachycardia is reported with tumours apparently secreting noradrenaline almost exclusively. Postural hypotension occurs in some patients. Hypotension can also occasionally follow a paroxysm in which noradrenaline has been predominantly released.

Other clinical manifestations are protean, especially given the range of hormones other than catecholamines that may be secreted, and a wide variety of conditions that can simulate phaeochromocytoma (Table 53.6). The diagnosis is held to be particularly likely in a thin hypertensive patient who experiences paroxysmal severe throbbing headache, marked sweating, palpitations, and a sense of impending doom.

Table 53.6. Manifestations of phaeochromocytoma and conditions simulating or associated with the disease.

Manifestations:
Headache
Palpitation
Anxiety
Sweating
Tremor
Weight loss
Nausea
Abdominal/chest pain
Vomiting
Constipation
Polyuria/polydipsia
Heat intolerance
Thyroid swelling
Cold extremities
Raynaud's phenomenon
Hypertension (sustained ±paroxysms or intermittent)
Orthostatic hypotension
Paradoxical response of blood pressure to beta-blockers
Tachycardia
Bradycardia
Arrhythmias
Pallor
Flushing
Ashen cyanosis
Glycosuria
Fever
Retinopathy and other complications of hypertension, e.g. stroke, cardiac failure, renal failure
Conditions simulating:
Anxiety
Hypoglycaemia
Diabetes
Migraine
Thyrotoxicosis
Bacterial endocarditis
Menopause
Eclampsia
Carcinoid syndrome
Porphyria
Important associations:
Multiple endocrine neoplasia
von Hippel–Lindau disease
Cardiomyopathy
Neurofibromatosis

Diagnosis

Diagnosis is furthered by demonstrating an excess of catecholamines and/or metabolites in the urine, or of catecholamines in plasma. The methods available, and the relevant normal ranges, will obviously vary considerably among centres. One of us has earlier reviewed the extensive literature on this topic.[111]

Valuable, but not infallible, guidance is obtained by demonstrating an excess of urinary noradrenaline, adrenaline, and of the metabolites vanilmandelic acid (VMA) and normetanephrine. It is important to recognize that drugs such as methyldopa, L-dopa, labetalol and phenothiazines can interfere with some methods used for assaying urinary normetanephrine. Moreover, various phenolic acids in addition to VMA appear in the urine, often derived from dietary components such as coffee, tea, bananas, chocolate, vanilla and citrus fruits, and also from aspirin. The development of improved assays for plasma and urinary catecholamines in recent years has increasingly displaced measurements of urinary metabolites, and impressive diagnostic information has been obtained via plasma or urine noradrenaline and, less often, adrenaline assay. The concentrations of catecholamines or of metabolites in urine reflect those in the circulation in most circumstances, an exception being a phaeochromocytoma situated in the bladder.

Refinement has come with the clonidine suppression test. In this, the alpha-agonist clonidine (300 μg) is administered, and blood samples are drawn 1, 2 and 3 h later for catecholamine assay. Clonidine suppresses sympathetic activity, and so reduces plasma levels of noradrenaline in normal subjects and in patients with essential hypertension. However, no such lowering of plasma noradrenaline is observed after clonidine administration in patients with phaeochromocytoma. This test has been further refined by giving clonidine before retiring at night and making an overnight urine collection for adrenaline and noradrenaline assay.[112] As sympathetic activity is low during the night, this allows excellent separation of catecholamine secretion from a tumour from that of normal production. There is the additional advantage that methods for measuring the usually high amounts in urine are easier than plasma assays.

Modern biochemical methods have largely eliminated the use of earlier pharmacological tests based on either the hypertensive reaction to a catecholamine-releasing agent, such as histamine, tyramine or glucagon, or the hypotensive response to phentolamine. Such procedures are not consistently reliable and can be dangerous.

Localization of the tumour

Computer-assisted tomography

Once phaeochromocytoma is diagnosed, it is necessary to localize the tumour as a prelude to surgery.

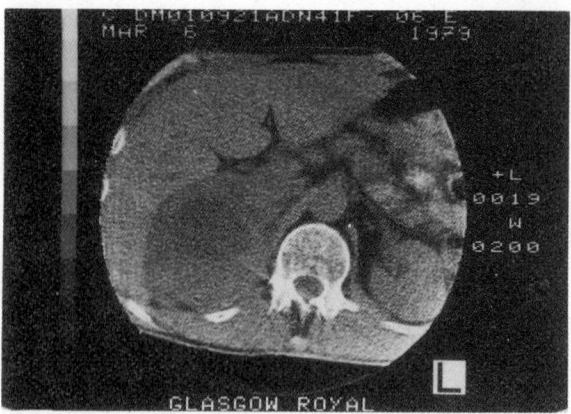

Fig. 53.10. Tumour of Fig. 53.10 shown on computed tomography to be an 8.1 × 9.1 cm mass in the region of the right adrenal gland and indenting the liver. (Reproduced from Ball, S.G. In: *Handbook of Hypertension, Vol. 2: Clinical Aspects of Essential Hypertension*, p.238, by permission of the publishers, Elsevier, Amsterdam.

The advent of computed tomography has greatly facilitated the detection of phaeochromocytomas. This method can reliably identify lesions as small as 1 cm in diameter and probably less (Fig. 53.10). Computed tomography is best suited to the detailed scanning of a selected region under suspicion, but it may not be practicable to apply the technique, with its high resolution, to a wide area. However, as 97% of phaeochromocytomas lie within the abdomen and 90% in the adrenal glands, a scan is likely to find most tumours.

Ultrasound

Ultrasound is a simple and safe method capable of detecting tumours as small as 3 cm in diameter (Fig. 53.11). However, a negative scan is unhelpful;

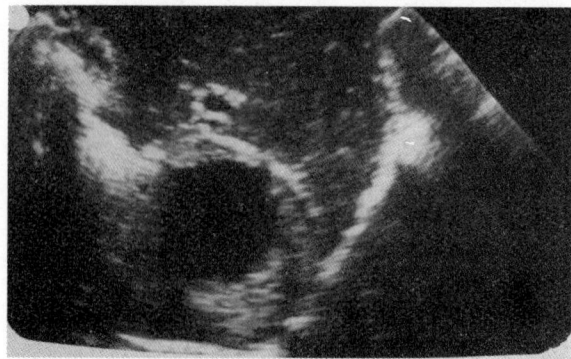

Fig. 53.11. Abdominal ultrasound showing a mass 8 cm in diameter thought to be a phaeochromocytoma with central necrosis lying above the right kidney. (Reproduced from Ball, S.G. In: *Handbook of Hypertension, Vol. 2: Clinical Aspects of Essential Hypertension*, p.238, by permission of the publishers, Elsevier, Amsterdam.)

further, most clinicians would like reassurance that, despite the certain presence of a tumour in one adrenal, there is not a second smaller lesion on the opposite side.

Regional venous sampling

Sampling of blood at various sites in the vena cava, with catecholamine measurement, may be especially useful in identifying the territory in which a phaeochromocytoma lies, if out with the adrenal glands.

Scintigraphy

Scintigraphic images using ^{133}I-metaiodobenzyl-guanidine have been obtained with both intra- and extra-adrenal lesions. However, the role of this method has not yet been clearly defined.

Arteriography

Arteriography is a sensitive method for the localization of phaeochromocytoma, but its value even in difficult cases has been largely supplanted by computed tomography. Moreover, the injection of contrast material can provoke catecholamine release and a hypertensive crisis; therefore, this approach should not be made until the patient is fully controlled medically with both alpha- and beta-antagonists. Even so, marked rises in blood pressure can occur, and nitroprusside for infusion should be available.

Treatment

The great majority of phaeochromocytomas are amenable to resection. Nevertheless, full medical control is a mandatory prelude to surgery, and it is also required in patients who have metastasizing, inoperable, or recurrent tumours.

Medical treatment

Medical therapy is based on the administration of both alpha- and beta-blocking drugs in order to antagonize the effects of excess catecholamines at various sites. Full alpha-adrenergic blockade is advisable before beta-blockers are administered, to limit the risk of hypertensive crises that might otherwise occur.

The non-competitive ('insurmountable') alpha-antagonist phenoxybenzamine is traditionally given, once the diagnosis is seriously entertained, because its use will be unlikely to compromise modern diagnostic procedures. Phenoxybenzamine should be given orally, starting at 10 mg/day, and proceeding to the maximum tolerated dose, which usually lies between 20 and 40 mg/day. The drug is best given in divided doses with food, because various gastro-intestinal disturbances are common side-effects, and, in this way, they may be lessened.

The non-selective alpha-antagonist phentolamine has a shorter duration of action than phenoxybenzamine; it can also cause gastro-intestinal upsets. Phentolamine, either by mouth or intravenously, has been given as supportive therapy to phenoxybenzamine.

The use of competitive alpha-antagonists, such as prazosin or indoramine, is more limited, but seems logical. Large doses may be needed and first-dose hypotension could be a problem.

Once alpha-adrenergic antagonism is fully established, a non-selective beta-blocker, such as propranolol, is given to control tachycardia and to minimize the risk of arrhythmias. Patients with cardiac failure not consequent upon hypertension may respond adversely to beta-blockade, and caution is needed in these circumstances.

The combined alpha- and beta-antagonist labetalol has been successfully used in the pre-operative control of patients with phaeochromocytoma. However, the beta-adrenergic antagonism of this drug predominates over its alpha-antagonist action, which is not the most appropriate balance.

In some patients, the maximum tolerated doses of alpha- and beta-adrenergic antagonists may be inadequate to control hypertension and/or cardiac arrhythmias, especially if massive quantities of catecholamines are released paroxysmally. In such patients, the drug alpha-methylparatyrosine, an inhibitor of the enzyme tyrosine hydroxylase and thus an agent limiting catecholamine biosynthesis at the stage of conversion of tyrosine to dopa, has successfully been employed.

Operation for phaeochromocytoma

Patients coming to surgery should be fully controlled with medical therapy as outlined. However, further gross release of catecholamines with hypertension can occur at operation. Intra-arterial pressure monitoring is mandatory, and the anaesthetist should be prepared to manage such crises by the intravenous administration as necessary of sodium nitroprusside, which, although a non-specific agent, has been successfully used to control hypertension at operation, or of noradrenaline. Blood pressure may fall precipitously at the time the tumour is isolated from the circulation.

Prognosis

Sustained hypertension following removal of a phaeochromocytoma may occur. Provided excision of all tumorous tissues has been achieved and catecholamine output has returned to normal, treatment thereafter is as that for essential hypertension.

PHAEOCHROMOCYTOMA IN PREGNANCY

The presence of phaeochromocytoma complicating pregnancy poses severe problems of diagnosis and management. In the first two trimesters, medical preparation and surgery are generally favoured, whereas in the third trimester medical treatment with combined Caesarian section and tumour removal may be appropriate. Individual circumstances vary widely. The safety of the mother has to be weighed against the viability of the fetus. The combined alpha- and beta-blocker labetalol and a range of other beta-blockers have been extensively used in hypertensive pregnant patients without detectable adverse fetal effects and therefore they are suitable drugs to be used in the treatment of a pregnant woman with phaeochromocytoma. Experience with phenoxybenzamine is more limited. Concerns about adverse drug effects and irradiation accompanying diagnostic procedures recede after the early developmental phase.

ACROMEGALY

Acromegaly is the result of excessive production of growth hormone in an adult.[113]

Pathology

The usual cause of acromegaly is a tumour of the anterior pituitary gland producing an excess of the peptide growth hormone. Ectopic production can also occur with tumours of the bronchus, breast or ovary.

Pathophysiology

Growth hormone has direct effects on target tissues, and indirect effects mediated by the generation of various low molecular weight growth factors, the somatomedins. Acromegaly may also comprise part of the multiple endocrine neoplasia ('MEN') type I syndrome, in which there are tumours afflicting the pituitary, parathyroids and pancreatic islets.

Growth hormone has been implicated in the cardiac and vascular hypertrophy of hypertension. The marked excess of pituitary growth hormone characteristic of acromegaly has been thought to be responsible for the high incidence of cardiovascular complications in this disease (see p. 1242).[8,12,52]

Long-term exposure to excess of circulating growth hormone leads to a series of mainly anabolic reactions and to diabetogenic effects.

Clinical features

Acromegalic subjects have a distinctive facial appearance, with broadening of the nose, protrusion of the lower jaw, prominent lips and thickened, coarse skin (Fig. 53.12). The hands and feet are enlarged, with an excess of soft tissue. Patients often report an increase in their required size of gloves and shoes, and that rings are difficult to put on or remove. These features result from bony enlargement together with an increase in interstitial oede-

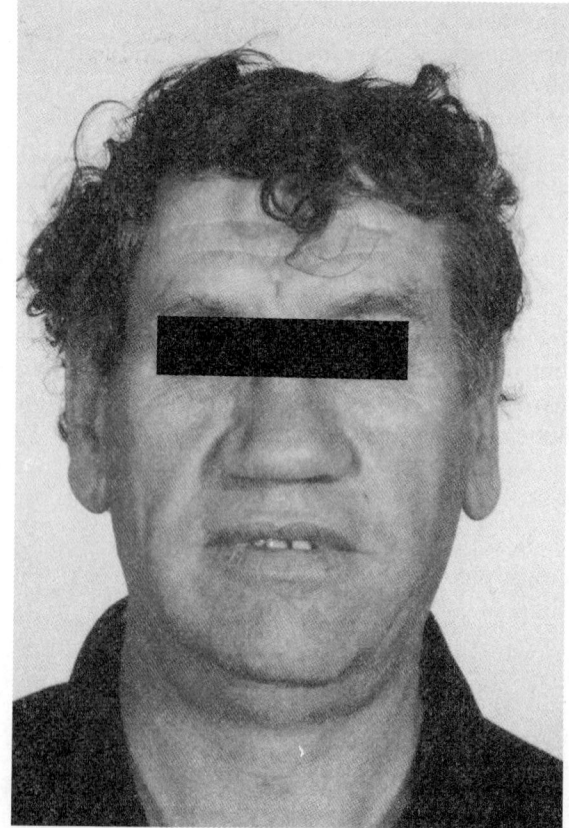

Fig. 53.12. Patient with acromegaly showing typical facies.

ma fluid rich in hyaluronates. Awareness of a change in appearance by the patient or relatives, or recognition of the characteristic features when seeking advice for other problems often lead to diagnosis.

Other symptoms include excessive sweating, headache, lethargy, weakness, paraesthesiae, impotence or menstrual irregularities. Arthritis may develop in an unusual site because of degenerative changes in the hyperplastic articular cartilage.

Radiology may reveal a lower jaw prominence, big paranasal sinuses, tufting of terminal phalanges, and enlargement of the heart and abdominal viscera.

In addition to these consequences of growth hormone excess, there may be features directly consequent on the presence of an expanding pituitary tumour. These include headache, contraction of visual fields and diplopia. Compression of normal pituitary tissue may produce hypopituitarism.

Hypertension

Accurate estimates of the prevalence of hypertension in acromegaly are difficult to make because of varied definitions of 'hypertension' and of methods of blood pressure measurement. However, raised arterial pressure is frequent in association with acromegaly, and possibly affects between 20 and 50% of patients. An important pathogenic influence could be growth hormone-stimulated hypertrophy of arterial smooth muscle and hence elevated peripheral resistance and rapid worsening of hypertension. Moreover, cardiomegaly, cardiac failure and arterial disease are probably disproportionately prominent, even allowing for the increased prevalence of hypertension, in part because of associated acromegalic myocardial hypertrophy, cardiomyopathy or diabetes mellitus. The hypertension associated with acromegaly may be caused or worsened by expansion of body sodium content, which has been reported in several series, and can be significantly correlated with the severity of the hypertension.[114] Plasma volume has also been found to be increased in acromegaly with hypertension. It has been supposed that growth hormone has a direct action on the kidney promoting salt and water retention, but this has not been fully elucidated. In conformity with the reported expansion of body sodium and plasma volume, plasma renin values are low. Aldosterone secretion and plasma concentrations are also usually low or normal. Catecholamines are unaltered.

Diagnosis

The diagnosis of acromegaly can be made by observation of the clinical and radiological features described above. Confirmation is by demonstrating an excess of plasma growth hormone which is not diminished by a glucose load; during a standard glucose tolerance test, growth hormone should normally fall to a plasma concentration below 4 milliunits/l (2 ng/ml). High-resolution computed tomography identifies the tumour and reveals its extent.

Treatment

The pituitary tumour may be removed surgically or irradiated. The drug bromocriptine has also been given to suppress growth hormone secretion, and it can sometimes reduce tumour size. However, values of plasma growth hormone during bromocriptine treatment, although lowered, remain generally higher than after surgery or irradiation. Long-acting analogues of somatostatin can also be used.

Prognosis

The general tenet that following correction of a condition responsible for secondary hypertension, blood pressure returns to age- and sex-matched normal values in only a proportion of cases[43] is well illustrated by acromegaly, in which blood pressure frequently remains high following therapy to the pituitary tumours, and after correction of elevated plasma growth hormone and of expansion of body sodium content.

Treatment of hypertension thereafter is with antihypertensive drugs as in essential hypertension, and should be particularly thorough in view of the high prevalence of hypertension-associated cardiomegaly, cardiac failure and arterial atheroma in this condition.

THYROID DISEASE

THYROTOXICOSIS[115]

Elevation of the systolic pressure (> 150 mmHg) occurs in at least 50% of patients with thyrotoxicosis, returning to age- and sex-matched normal values with treatment. A raised diastolic pressure, by contrast, is unusual. Untreated thyrotoxicosis is characterized by a raised cardiac output, decreased peripheral resistance and an expanded blood volume.

HYPOTHYROIDISM[115]

With thyroid deficiency, several investigators have found both systolic and diastolic pressures to be increased, and that hypothyroidism can exacerbate pre-existent essential hypertension. Adequate therapy lowers the raised pressure. However, an increased prevalence of hypertension in hypothyroidism has not been confirmed by all workers.

Elevated blood pressure in hypothyroidism could be a consequence of the increased noradrenergic activity that has been demonstrated in this condition. Cardiac output and blood volume are typically low, and total peripheral resistance is markedly increased.

GORDON'S SYNDROME

Gordon's syndrome is a rare condition characterized by hypertension, hyperkalaemia and acidosis in the absence of renal failure.[116,117] It has been proposed that the basic defect is a congenital abnormality of renal tubular function leading to sodium retention and hypervolaemia. An alternative proposal is that atrial natriuretic peptide is insufficiently elevated. Plasma concentrations of renin and angiotensin II are depressed, although aldosterone levels may be normal. Associated features can include short stature, hypoplastic upper lateral incisor teeth, cardiac valvular lesions and intellectual impairment.

The condition may be familial, although the genetic base is not elucidated. Recognition of this rarity is clinically important because the hypertension and biochemical abnormalities can readily be corrected by treatment with a thiazide diuretic, by dietary sodium restriction, or by a combination of the two.

INTRACRANIAL TUMOUR

An acute rise in blood pressure together with slowing of the heart rate may result from sudden expansion of an intracranial lesion and is termed the Cushing reflex.

More rarely, hypertension may be caused by a slowly growing intracranial tumour, usually situated in the posterior fossa.[118] Several reported cases of this kind have shown evidence of hypersecretion of catecholamines, and the distinction from phaeochromocytoma is difficult. The presence of

papilloedema with only a few or no retinal haemorrhages or exudates, the converse of that characteristic of the malignant phase, can alert physicians to this important rarity.

THE DETECTION, ASSESSMENT AND CONTROL OF HYPERTENSION

CLINICAL FEATURES IN HYPERTENSION

The majority of subjects with essential hypertension will be free of symptoms and clinical signs. These features appear only with the pathological involvement of various organs, particularly the heart, brain, eye and kidney (see p. 1238–41). Thus, the clinical evaluation of the hypertensive patient is directed particularly to the detection and assessment of such organ modification and damage, with the recognition of evidence of secondary forms of hypertension. The appreciation of hypertension is dependent on supplementary investigations of varying complexity.

SCREENING FOR HYPERTENSION

As raised arterial pressure is not usually accompanied by symptoms or signs, if it is to be detected and preventive therapy initiated, asymptomatic subjects need to be screened.[1,2] If a formal screening programme is undertaken, for example, by inviting inhabitants of a town to attend at a specified date and time, coverage up to about 80% is usually achieved. Alternatively, if a general practitioner takes the opportunity of routinely measuring blood pressure whenever he or she sees a patient, for whatever reason, coverage of around 80% is attained within 3 years. Almost 100% coverage can be achieved if the practitioner invites all patients on list to attend for screening. It is therefore recommended that general practitioners should make every effort to record the blood pressure of all patients on their list and to update the information regularly. Blood pressure measurement in children should not be neglected, and, for example, can be part of routine medical examinations in schools. Those with above-average blood pressure in childhood are more likely to progress to distinct hypertension later in life.

BLOOD PRESSURE MEASUREMENT

Routine measurement[119]

The measurement of blood pressure, although simple, is prone to inaccuracies. Incorrect readings can easily lead to errors of diagnosis and thus to inappropriate or deficient therapy.

For routine clinical use, a mercury sphygmomanometer is preferable to an aneroid model. The mercury and glass should be clean, and the meniscus clearly visible at zero before inflation. An aneroid machine should be calibrated regularly against a mercury instrument. The cuff, consisting of an inflatable bladder within a restrictive cloth sheath, should be sufficiently long to wrap around the arm fully, and to be firmly secured. The inflatable bladder should not be too short or too narrow, otherwise the blood pressure will be overestimated. The bladder length should be at least 80%, and the bladder width at least 40%, of the arm circumference. The centre of the bladder should be marked on the cuff so that it may be placed accurately over the brachial artery. The bladder must be capable of smooth swift inflation and the release valve (very frequently a faulty part) should permit smooth deflation.

Measurements in children under 5 years of age cannot accurately be made using conventional equipment.

It is recommended that before blood pressure is measured, the subject sit or lie quietly for 5 min. The procedure should be explained, emphasizing that it may be necessary to repeat the measurement several times, and especially warning that minor discomfort may be caused. Even so, higher values are likely to be obtained in many subjects initially, with lower readings after several visits and familiarity with the procedure. Conversation should be avoided during the measurement.

In hypertensive patients, and particularly when assessing drug therapy, it is advisable to measure the pressure after at least 5 min of lying (or sitting), and again after 1 min of standing.

The arm should be close to horizontal and supported so that it is at the level of the midsternum.

With the subject in a suitably warm environment, the arm should be freed from restrictive clothing and the point of maximal pulsation of the brachial artery just above the antecubital fossa identified. A cuff of the dimensions already defined should be applied to the upper arm, and firmly secured.

Preferably, the tubing should be at the upper (axillary) side of the cuff so as not to interfere with auscultation. The lower edge of the cuff should be at least 2 cm above the site over the brachial artery identified for auscultation. The mercury column must be vertical and at eye level.

Systolic pressure should be estimated by palpation before using the stethoscope. For this purpose, the brachial or radial artery is palpated and the bladder inflated until the pulse is obliterated. This gives a measure of the systolic pressure, and enables the observer to avoid errors associated, for example, with a 'silent gap' with no Korotkoff sounds on auscultation at less than systolic pressure. The cuff is then deflated.

A stethoscope is applied gently over the site of the brachial artery previously identified, care being taken to avoid contact with the cuff. The bladder is inflated to a pressure about 10 mmHg above the previously determined systolic pressure, and deflated at an even rate of 2–3 mmHg per second. The point at which clear repetitive tapping sounds are heard is the systolic pressure; the point at which these suddenly fade is the fourth phase diastolic value; the point at which the sounds disappear is the fifth phase diastolic. The fifth phase is now used routinely in clinical practice in preference to the fourth phase, which is usually slightly higher than true (intra-arterial) diastolic pressure. However, fourth phase measurements are valuable in some circumstances, for example, pregnancy, or in occasional subjects where the sounds may continue down to a cuff pressure near zero.

At an initial visit, blood pressure should be measured in both arms and if an appreciable difference exists (e.g. > 20 mmHg systolic or 10 mmHg diastolic), the arm with the higher reading should be used on that and subsequent occasions. Aortic coarctation proximal to the origin of the subclavian artery may be responsible for substantially lower pressures in the left arm.

It is emphasized that blood pressure is continuously variable, being influenced, *inter alia*, by the circumstances of measurement, ambient temperature, meals, drinks, smoking, anxiety, the season of the year, and, especially, antihypertensive drugs.

There is a further aspect of blood pressure measurement that may be particularly relevant in elderly subjects. Not rarely, owing to extensive sclerosis in large arteries, they are resistant to compression by a sphygmomanometer cuff. This may give a spurious impression of severe hypertension and has been termed 'pseudohypertension', with a difference between cuff and intra-arterial values as great as 50 mmHg. Osler's manoeuvre consists of assessing whether the pulseless radial or brachial artery, distal to a point of occlusion achieved manually or by cuff compression, remains palpable. If it does, the patient is likely to manifest falsely high sphygmomanometric readings.

'Random-zero' sphygmomanometer

In epidemiological surveys and therapeutic trials, it is important for the observer to avoid preferentially recording certain terminal digits. Milllimeters of mercury expressed with a terminal number of 0 or 5 tend to be especially favoured in 'open' pressure measurements. One method of partially circumventing this problem is to use a 'random-zero' sphygmomanometer.[120] This is a conventional instrument in which, before each measurement, a wheel is spun that re-sets the mercury meniscus to a point above zero unknown to the observer. After measurements have been made, this random addition to the value is ascertained, and then subtracted from the measured reading to obtain the correct value. This instrument is readily portable and simple to use, being basically an orthodox mercury sphygmomanometer.

'Rose box'

The more elaborate device of Rose, Holland and Crowley ('Rose box')[121] is now less favoured, despite its accuracy, because it is heavy and therefore difficult to transport, it requires a special technique of operation and hence some training in its use, and it needs more frequent maintenance.

Automated sphygmomanometers and 24-h recording[122]

In recent years, there has been increasing availability of light portable automated blood pressure monitoring equipment. This has permitted 24-h evaluation of pressure in the circumstances of normal daily life, away from the clinic, and has provided a wealth of epidemiological and therapeutic information.

Continuous intra-arterial recording is now less often employed than formerly, mainly because of worries about its safety. Nevertheless, this approach yielded valuable data and gave insight into many new areas of hypertension research.

Although the modern non-invasive methods of continuous blood pressure recording have progressed rapidly, there remain concerns about their reliability under some circumstances, especially on movement and exercise, with arrhythmias or bradycardia, and because the noise and discomfort accompanying cuff compression can interefere with sleep.

These techniques have consistently shown that end-organ involvement in hypertension correlates more closely with the whole-day blood pressure measurement than with values obtained in the clinic or surgery. This is especially true of those patients prone to experience an alarm reaction in the presence of a doctor. A subject not infrequently shows high blood pressure readings in the clinic, although 24-h records obtained in everyday surroundings are unremarkable. Treatment is not usually indicated in such cases. Twenty-four hour recordings are also invaluable in permitting accurate assessment of the duration and magnitude of efficacy of antihypertensive therapy.

THE INVESTIGATION OF HYPERTENSION

The purpose of investigating a subject with hypertension is fourfold:
1   to detect organ damage consequent upon the hypertension;
2   to diagnose a possible underlying cause for the raised blood pressure;
3   to identify other risk factors;
4   to recognize concomitant diseases that might influence the treatment of hypertension.

The tempo and extent of such investigation will vary greatly. Furthermore, the thoroughness of such procedures will be greater in certain occupational groups, for example, airline pilots.[123] The present account will be concerned with the initial stages of investigation. If evidence of secondary hypertension

Table 53.7. Evidence of additional risk factors to hypertension likely to be obtained from the history, physical examination or initial investigations.

History	Examination	Investigation
Family history of diabetes mellitus	Obesity	Diabetes mellitus
Family history of hypertension or its consequences, e.g. stroke		Hypercholesterolaemia
Smoking		
Alcohol intake		
Oral contraceptives		
Gout		

Table 53.8. **Evidence of hypertensive organ damage as obtained from the history, physical examination or investigation.**

Organ	History	Examination	Investigation
Heart	Chest pain Breathlessness	Cardiomegaly Cardiac failure	Electrocardiogram Echocardiogram Chest X-ray Angiography
Brain	Transient ischaemic attacks Strokes Fits	Focal neurological signs	Electro-encephalogram Computed tomography scan
Blood vessels	Claudication	Absent or decreased peripheral pulses	Arteriography
Eyes	Transient visual disturbance Persistent visual disturbance Retinal vascular occlusion	Arterial changes	Fluorescein angiography
Kidney	Nocturia Polyuria Haematuria Myoglobinuria	Anaemia Skin pigmentation	Anaemia Serum urea, creatinine, electrolytes Urinary blood, protein, casts Intravenous urography Digital subtraction angiography Abdominal ultrasound

is found, the diagnosis should be pursued as detailed in the section dealing with the particular disorder. Some of the main features to be sought in relation to risk factors, organ damage and aetiology are given in Tables 53.7–53.9.

Table 53.9. **Evidence of underlying cause of hypertension as obtained from history or clinical examination.**

History	Clinical examination
Oral contraceptive use	Appearance, e.g. Cushing's
Liquorice ingestion	syndrome or acromegaly
Non-steroidal anti-inflammatory	Evidence of thyroid disorder
drugs	Signs of catecholamine excess
ACTH or corticosteroid use	Multiple neurofibromatoma
Analgesic abuse	Abdominal or loin bruit
Alcohol excess	Enlarged kidneys
'4 Ps' of phaeochromocytoma	Femoral delay
(pain (headache), palpitations,	
perspiration, pallor)	
Polyuria, nocturia or haematuria	
Past renal trauma	
Muscular weakness due to	
hypokalaemia	
Personal or family history of	
polycystic renal disease or	
phaeochromocytoma or of multiple	
endocrine neoplasia	

History

The history-taking should include specific enquiries about a possible family history of hypertension or its consequences, or of familial diabetes mellitus, renal disease or multiple endocrine neoplasia. The patient's smoking and drinking habits should be ascertained, and whether excessive ingestion of liquorice is likely. Medication of any kind should be noted, in particular, the taking of oral contraceptives, ACTH or corticosteroids, non-steroidal anti-inflammatory agents, or analgesics.

Organ damage may be sustained in the heart, reflected by anginal pain or dyspnoea, the brain, indicated by an account of stroke, fits or transient ischaemic attacks, the eyes, manifest by unilateral or bilateral transient or persistent visual disturbance, and the kidneys, as shown by nocturia, polyuria or haematuria. Alternatively, these latter features may indicate a renal lesion responsible for hypertension. An account of possible previous renal trauma should be sought. The physician should enquire for symptoms of intermittent claudication. Symptoms of muscular weakness or polyuria or nocturia may indicate potassium depletion. Features of phaeochromocytoma often emerge in the history, and especially the 'four Ps' pain (usually headache), palpitation, perspiration and pallor.

Clinical examination

Obesity is the main risk indicator likely to be revealed clinically, albeit a controversial one.[9,124]

Possible organ involvement and damage from hypertension should be fully explored on clinical examination. Cardiomegaly may be recognized at the bedside. In more advanced cases, frank cardiac failure may be apparent, with raised central venous pressure, and peripheral or pulmonary oedema. Focal neurological signs may indicate brain lesions. Peripheral vascular disease may be indicated by diminished or absent arterial pulses. Detailed examination of the optic fundi should be undertaken in every hypertensive patient and will indicate the extent of arterial involvement, whether sectorial arterial or venous occlusion has occurred, and if lesions of the malignant phase or of diabetes mellitus are present. The physician should not disdain the use of short acting pupillary-dilating eyedrops, which should always be available.

A diverse range of conditions possibly responsible for secondary hypertension can be revealed or indicated at the bedside. Thyroid disease, Cushing's syndrome or acromegaly may often be immediately apparent. Excessive thinness may suggest thyrotoxicosis or phaeochromocytoma. Multiple cutaneous neurofibromata may accompany simple phaeochromocytoma or multiple endocrine neoplasia. The femoral pulses should be felt in every hypertensive patient irrespective of age. Delay and usually diminution will indicate aortic coarctation. An abdominal or loin bruit can signify renal artery stenosis. Renal enlargement may be due to a tumour or to polycystic disease.

Special tests

The lengths to which special tests should be pursued in patients with raised blood pressure raises many issues, political, social, moral and economic as well as medical. Our personal views are offered here. The principles outlined should be modified for the individual patient and local circumstances. It should be remembered that, in unselected cases, secondary forms of hypertension are rare. Most physicians would feel uncomfortable without some of the simpler basic tests; few would or should be happy to advocate a lifetime of antihypertensive therapy without, for example, measuring serum electrolytes, urea and creatinine, or testing the urine.

A constant problem is a decision on the lengths to which more detailed investigation should be undertaken. Extensive tests may not always be in the interest of the patient. They must be done in the event of malignant hypertension after initially controlling blood pressure or if clear hints of secondary hypertension emerge from the history, clinical examination or routine investigations. Otherwise, no absolute rules can be given. More detailed investigation is indicated in the circumstances listed in Table 53.10, arranged roughly in declining order of importance.

Electrocardiography

The criteria whereby left ventricular hypertrophy may be recognized electrocardiographically are discussed in Chapter 9. The presence of ST/T wave changes, so called 'strain' pattern is of particular concern because of its prognostic implication. Electrocardiography can also reveal or indicate ischaemic heart disease.

Echocardiography

Echocardiography is now widely available and provides more reliable evidence of cardiac hypertrophy than does electrocardiography.

Chest radiography

Chest radiography is a less dependable means of assessing cardiac involvement, but, nevertheless, it should usually be included among the routine tests in hypertension.

Urine examination

Dipstick testing is simple and sensitive. It can be done easily in all patients, it will identify some diabetic subjects and it may alert the physician to a primary renal problem. Dipstick testing is sensitive

---

Table 53.10.   Indications for more thorough investigation of hypertension.

1. Clear evidence of secondary hypertension on history, clinical examination or routine tests
2. Malignant phase hypertension
3. Abnormal urinary analysis
4. Raised serum urea or creatinine
5. Diastolic pressure > 120 mmHg
6. Sudden deterioration of blood pressure control
7. Failure of hypertension to respond to three drugs given in combination
8. Youth (< 45 years)
9. Certain occupational groups (e.g. aircrew)

particularly to albumin, but not to Bence Jones proteose; 150 mg/l will give a 'trace' of protein on testing and is about the upper limit of normal for 24-h excretion.

Stick testing requires lysis of cells to expose the haem pigments to the test area and thus to give a positive reaction to blood.

Microscopy of a fresh urine sample is needed to confirm the presence of red cells. A few may be present in normal urine, which may of course be contaminated at menstruation.

Red cell casts indicate glomerular bleeding and thus continuing glomerulonephritis or vasculitis; they may occur also together with granular casts in malignant hypertension. Red cell casts imply a renal cause for haematuria. However, it must be emphasized that the urine may be normal even with significant renal disease.

Blood sampling

Blood should be taken for estimation of haemoglobin and for white cell counting. Measurement should also be made of serum urea, creatinine, potassium, sodium and uric acid. Forearm muscular exercise must not be employed as an aid to venepuncture, as this will raise serum potassium concentration and may obscure diagnostically important hypokalaemia. Hypokalaemia may also disappear if dietary sodium intake is deficient.

Elevation of serum urea or creatinine will indicate renal impairment. Hypokalaemia may be a consequence of aldosterone excess, or of other forms of mineralocorticoid-induced hypertension, as for example in liquorice ingestion.

Aldosterone excess may be secondary to stimulation of the renin–angiotensin system. Most often, this is the result of prior diuretic therapy but it also may occur with renovascular hypertension or the malignant phase. With secondary hyperaldosteronism, plasma sodium, as well as potassium, tends to be low. Conversely, with primary aldosterone excess, for example, that due to an aldosterone-secreting tumour, and other forms of mineralocorticoid hypertension, such as liquorice ingestion or 17-α-hydroxylase deficiency, the renin–angiotensin system is suppressed, and an elevation of serum sodium accompanies the hypokalaemia.

Elevation of serum potassium may be the result of renal failure, particularly if potassium-sparing agents have been given inappropriately. It is also a feature of the rare Gordon's syndrome.

Abdominal ultrasound   This non-invasive test can often provide useful information on the kidney or adrenal gland.

Intravenous urography

Intravenous urography was once regarded as part of the routine investigation of hypertension. However, several detailed studies have demonstrated that this expensive test, which is not without its discomforts and occasional hazards, is rarely informative in unselected patients.[125] Thus, intravenous urography (or other radiological investigation of the renal tract) is now reserved for those patients in whom there is a particular indication.

MANAGEMENT OF HYPERTENSION

The pursuit and treatment of the various forms of secondary hypertension are detailed in the relevant sections. The great majority of cases, however, will have primary (essential) hypertension, and it is with the management of these patients that we are concerned in this section.

Indications for investigation and treatment: comparative urgency

Hypertensive encephalopathy is an immediate medical emergency.

Malignant ('accelerated') hypertension, with retinal haemorrhages and exudates, irrespective of the presence of papilloedema, requires admission forthwith to hospital for treatment and subsequent investigation.

Severe hypertension, with a fifth phase diastolic pressure > 120 mmHg, especially if accompanied by other features, such as cardiac or renal functional impairment, marked proteinuria, diabetes mellitus or organ damage attributable to the raised blood pressure, requires prompt and thorough investigation, and early initiation of antihypertensive therapy.

Most subjects found on screening to have a raised blood pressure will show more mild hypertension and will be free of symptoms. In many of these, the pressure will subside on subsequent visits, or may not be raised during 24-h recording. Thus, not all subjects identified on screening will require treatment. The British Hypertension Society has proposed guidelines for management in these cases.[126] Those found to have a diastolic pressure > 100 mmHg and whose pressure remains above 100 mmHg with observation over 3–4 months should receive pharmacological treatment; those whose diastolic pressure lies in the range 95–99 mmHg over this period should not usually be treated, but should be carefully followed at intervals of 3–6 months; those whose blood pressure falls to values < 95 mmHg should have their blood pressure measured annually.

These broad therapeutic indications can be refined. Treatment will more readily be started if there is echocardiographic or electrocardiographic evidence of left ventricular hypertrophy, or in the presence of additional cardiovascular risk factors, such as glucose intolerance, hypercholesterolaemia or a family history suggestive of hypertension or its complications. Nevertheless, therapy prevents morbidity less effectively once complications have appeared. The need for drug treatment is less pressing in women than in men.[53]

Predominantly systolic pressure elevation is a feature especially of ageing. Although systolic pressure is a risk indicator, so far none of the trials has shown convincing evidence of benefit from treating isolated systolic hypertension; thus, no firm recommendations on this issue are presently possible. However, pharmacological intervention is indicated if predominant or isolated systolic hypertension is accompanied by symptoms or signs attributable to the raised pressure. Moreover, many physicians will wish to treat patients if the systolic pressure remains above 190 mmHg.

There is currently no evidence of benefit in treating asymptomatic hypertension in persons over 80 years of age.[62,64,26]

In a borderline case, in which neither the physician nor the patient is anxious to start drug treatment, a trial of non-pharmacological therapy alone is worthwhile.

Objective of treatment

The objective of treatment should be a diastolic pressure of 85–90 mmHg in the absence of unacceptable side-effects. Patients should be warned against heavy alcohol intake and, if indicated, dietary weight reduction should be advised. In some patients, restriction of sodium chloride intake to 70–100 mmol/day may help and, if tolerated, is worthy of trial. Moreover, as cigarette smoking compounds the cardiovascular and cerebrovascular risks of hypertension, *all* patients should be warned to stop smoking. Adequate daily physical exercise should also be encouraged.

Choice of drug therapy (see also sections on individual drugs)

Most trials of antihypertensive therapy undertaken in adequate numbers of patients suggest that overall there is little to choose between one form of therapy and another in efficacy. In particular, suggestions that certain classes of drug possess differential efficacy according to the age of the patient are not, at least so far, well substantiated.[127]

There is no good evidence presently available to support the claims that diuretics and calcium antagonists are more effective, and beta-blockers and converting enzyme inhibitors less so, in older patients. The response of an individual's blood pressure to any particular agent cannot readily be predicted.[127] Beta-antagonists, however, may be less effective in reducing systolic blood pressure than alternative agents.[128] This probably relates to their mode of action which induces slowing of the heart and reduction of cardiac output with little effect on arterial compliance or peripheral resistance.

Side-effects or properties other than pressure reduction do separate the different groups of drugs and here it is possible for the clinician to select, or more usually avoid, certain agents in individual patients. Beta-antagonists must not be used in an asthmatic subject but they are an obvious choice in those with angina of effort. Tiredness and breathlessness seem less troublesome with the beta-1-selective than with non-selective beta-blockers and are increasingly preferred. Thiazide diuretics would be avoided normally in those patients with diabetes mellitus.

The older patient

Special problems may be encountered in older patients and these issues will govern the choice of drug and its dose.[127,129] Older patients tend to be lighter, and to have progressive impairment of renal and hepatic function. Thus, drug doses should usually be less with advancing years. Sexual interest and function tend to decline with age, and drugs that exacerbate this trend, for example, thiazides, centrally acting agents or beta-blockers, should be employed cautiously. Postural hypotension may be a feature of ageing, and drugs that worsen this, such as methyldopa or prazosin, should be used with care. First-dose hypotension with prazosin may be especially hazardous in the elderly. Rarely, in old patients, and apparently irrespective of plasma renin level, first-dose hypotension may occur with angiotensin converting enzyme inhibitors. Diuretics, especially loop diuretics, can provoke urinary retention in older men with prostatic enlargement. Verapamil may cause or worsen constipation or cardiac conduction defects; it is regarded by many physicians as a drug unsuitable for the older patient. Agents such as methyldopa, clonidine or reserpine, which can cause depression or worsen mental confusion, should also be used with caution in the elderly. Particularly in older patients, who may have atheromatous changes in the arteries supplying the brain, blood pressure reduction should be gradual, preferably over several weeks, rather than sudden. Ketanserin has been suggested as attractive in this respect. Occult renal artery stenosis will also be more likely to be present in the elderly. The use of angiotensin converting enzyme inhibitors can in these circumstances, by removing the compensatory intrarenal actions of angiotensin II, lead to a loss or decline of function in the affected kidney.

Subjects over the age of 60 years comprise a large and rapidly expanding subgroup of the hypertensive population. Treatment requires careful attention to the needs of each individual. Chronological age is an imperfect indicator of biological age; senility and decrepitude cannot be extrapolated from the birthdate.

Education of the patient and of relatives

It is most important that the patient, as well as all concerned with the patient's care, such as a responsible relative in the case of an elderly subject, understand fully the purpose of antihypertensive treatment, that it is preventive rather than therapeutic, and lifelong. A common misconception is that drug treatment may be stopped once the pressure has been controlled.

Initiation of therapy in patients with mild-to-moderate hypertension

A small dose of a beta-antagonist or diuretic is usually chosen as first-line therapy. Typical regimes would start with atenolol 50 mg or bendrofluazide 2.5 mg once daily. Most of the likely effect will be achieved by the end of 1 month, but blood pressure reduction can be more gradual with some agents such as serotonin antagonists. Thus, continuation of therapy for at least up to 3 months before increasing the dose is advisable unless there are special reasons for haste. The dose of atenolol can be raised to 100 mg or of bendrofluazide to 5 mg. If

pressure still remains inadequately controlled, one drug can be exchanged for the other. However, more than 70% of patients seem to require two agents given together for adequate control of pressure, and often therefore the diuretic and beta-blocker will need to be combined.

There are several alternative two-drug combinations discussed in detail on pages 1252–53, Beta-antagonists or angiotensin converting enzyme inhibitors are effective at blocking the tachycardia sometimes associated, particularly with the initial pressure reduction, with a vasodilating drug like nifedipine. Patients with angina and hypertension might benefit from a beta-antagonist–calcium antagonist combination; those with heart failure not related to the hypertension as such to a diuretic with angiotensin converting enzyme inhibitor. Any antihypertensive drug, but especially those that act primarily as vasodilators, may in occasional patients cause unwanted precipitous falls in blood pressure. Such occurrences can be especially hazardous in older patients. Diuretics should be stopped for a few days before adding an angiotensin converting enzyme inhibitor to the regimen; however, adding a diuretic to an angiotensin converting enzyme inhibitor is not usually associated with a severe initial fall in pressure.

Currently, physicians are moving increasingly to extensive exploration of alternative two-drug regimes rather than proceeding to a third agent in a 'stepped care' approach. If a third drug is required, a vasodilating agent is usually added to the beta-blocker–diuretic combination. Direct-acting vasodilators like hydralazine, alpha-1-antagonists such as prazosin or a class II calcium antagonist such as nifedipine are commonly used.

Resistant hypertension[130]

Resistant hypertension can be defined arbitrarily as the persistence of a diastolic pressure > 110 mmHg despite the prescription of three drugs in combination. Hypertension resistant to therapy may result from poor compliance, inadequate dosing, fluid retention induced by treatment, an antihypertensive effect of concomitant therapy, undetected secondary hypertension or, rarely, from genuine drug refractoriness.

Poor compliance

Poor compliance with therapy is frequently found to underlie inability to control the blood pressure. Failure of the pulse rate to slow in a patient ostensibly taking a beta-blocker should alert the physician. Asking for tablets to be brought to the clinic may help identify some problems. Older patients may be forgetful and thus comply poorly.

Reversion to a simpler, rather than advance to a more complex, therapeutic regime often improves control. The less often patients need to take medication the better; compliance tends to diminish when dosing becomes more frequent than twice daily. Direct confrontation is sometimes useful; asking if the tablets are 'difficult to take for some reason' or enquiring about specific side-effects may help without endangering the doctor–patient relationship. Only occasional patients are frankly perverse (Fig. 53.13). Informing patients of their blood pressure reading and re-confirming the need for therapy sometimes improves control. Overzealous pressure reduction may induce symptoms and less than satisfactory pressure control may have to be accepted. Systolic pressure elevation especially in older patients may be particularly difficult to control without inducing distressing side-effects. A reasonable aim is to achieve the best pressure control possible without side-effects unacceptable to either patient or doctor.

Concomitant treatment

Concurrent administration of non-steroidal anti-inflammatory drugs, such as indomethacin, can attenuate the effect of hypotensive agents, and is often overlooked.[97]

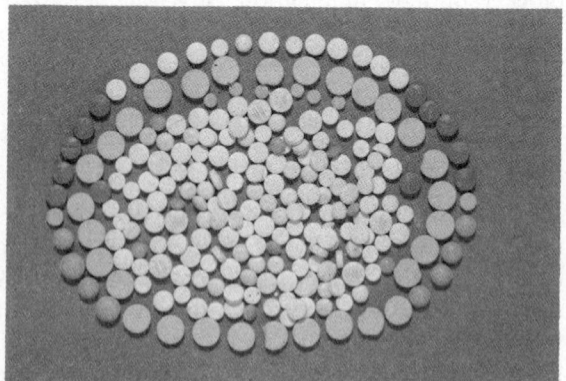

Fig. 53.13. Collection of uneaten antihypertensive drugs recovered from the locker of a 16-year-old girl with apparent drug-resistant hypertension (diastolic pressures 120–150 mmHg). She was observed to be taking tablets into her mouth, then surreptitiously spitting them out. Following further discussions, blood pressure was controlled at around 120/90 mmHg on atenolol 100 mg plus bendrofluazide 10 mg daily. (Reproduced from Mackay, A. *et al.* In: Jewell, J.P., ed. *Advanced Medicine*, Vol. 17, p.39, by permission of the publishers, Pitman Medical, London.)

Adequate dosage

It is not rare for a range of drugs to be prescribed together, but in inadequate doses. This should be checked.

Need for diuretic

Several classes of antihypertensive drug cause sodium and water retention, which attenuates their effect. Adding, or raising the dose of, diuretic can often then be effective.

Undetected secondary hypertension

Patients resistant to therapy should always be investigated adequately to exclude an underlying cause.

Treatment of resistant hypertension

Truly resistant hypertension can require aggressive therapy. A diuretic should always be included.[130] The powerful vasodilator minoxidil is particularly effective but always needs the conjoint use of a loop diuretic to prevent fluid retention and of a drug, typically a beta-blocker to control tachycardia. Moreover, minoxidil is not acceptable to the majority of women because of hypertrichosis. Alternatively, large doses of loop diuretic combined with an angiotensin converting enzyme inhibitor will often achieve control.

Parenteral antihypertensive treatment

Parenteral therapy is rarely needed and can be dangerous, but it is necessary in the rare situation of hypertensive encephalopathy. Intravenous nitroprusside offers the most easily controlled way of reducing pressure, but it requires careful monitoring. Rapid reduction of pressure may also be achieved by intravenous hydralazine, given as small boluses or by constant infusion. Labetalol and atenolol can also be used intravenously to lower blood pressure over some hours.

Follow-up

Once adequate control is achieved with therapy, blood pressure checks every 3 or 6 months are adequate for many patients. Such visits are useful to reinforce instructions, advice and encouragement, to ensure optimal pressure control and to check on renal function and possible alterations of serum potassium. Home blood pressure monitoring is appropriate for some patients, although it is important to avoid the development of an unrealistic and obsessional attitude to control of blood pressure. The ideal outcome is a subject free of symptoms, side-effects and anxiety, who has a diastolic pressure < 90 mmHg.

REFERENCES

1. Robertson, J.I.S. Hypertension: primary and secondary prevention. In: Julian, D.G. and O'Neal Humphries, J.N. (eds). *Preventive Cardiology*. London: Butterworths, 1983, pp. 62–85.
2. Gross, F.H. and Robertson, J.I.S. (eds). *Arterial Hypertension*. London: Pitman Medical, 1979.
3. Beilin, L.J. Epitaph to essential hypertension: a preventable disorder of known aetiology? *J. Hypertens.* 1988; 6: 85.
4. Bengtsson, B., Thulin, T. and Schersten, B. Familial resemblance in casual blood pressure: a maternal effect? *Clin. Sci.* 1979; 57 (Suppl. 5): 279.
5. Cruz-Coke, R. Genetic aspects of essential hypertension. In: Robertson, J.I.S. (ed). *Handbook of Hypertension Vol. I: Clinical Aspects of Essential Hypertension*. Amsterdam: Elsevier, 1983, pp. 21–29.
6. Ménard, J., Degoulet, P., Chatellier, G., Devries, C., Plouin, P., Lang, T., Fouriaud, C. and Jaquine- Salord, M. Influence of educational and sociocultural factors on hypertension care. *J. Hypertens.* 1985; 3 (Suppl. 2): 45.
7. Cruickshank, J.K., Beevers, D.G., Osbourne, V.L., Haynes, R.A., Corlett, J.C.R. and Selby, S. Heart attack, stroke, diabetes and hypertension in West Indians, Asians and Whites in Birmingham, England. *Br. Med. J.* 1980; 281: 1108.
8. Korner, P.I. Integrative neurohumoral control of the circulation. *Australian Soc. Exp. Biol. Proc.* 1988; 1: 151.
9. Ramsay, L.E. Dietary aspects of prevention and treatment of hypertension. *Curr. Opin. Cardiol.* 1987; 2: 758.
10. Swales, J.D. Non-pharmacological antihypertensive therapy. *Eur. Heart J.* 1988; 9 (Suppl. G): 45.
11. Robertson, J.I.S., Fraser, R., Richards, A.M., Murray, G.D., Harrap, S.B., Lever A.F. and Kassirer, J. Salt, volume and hypertension: causation or correlation? *Kidney Int.* 1987; 32: 590.
12. Frohlich, E.D. The mosaic of hypertension: past, present and future. *J. Hypertens.* 1988; 6 (Suppl. 4): 2.
13. Chalmers, J.P. and West, M.J. The nervous system in the pathogenesis of hypertension. In: Robertson, J.I.S. (ed). *Handbook of Hypertension, Vol. I: Clinical Aspects of Essential Hypertension*. Amsterdam: Elsevier, 1983, pp. 64–96.
14. Chalmers, J.P., Kapoor, V., Mills, E., Minson, J., Morilak, D., Morris, M. and Pilowsky, P. Neurotransmitters and the control of blood pressure. *Australian Soc. Exp. Biol. Proc.* 1988; 1: 159.
15. Ball, S.G. Catecholamines in hypertension. *Curr. Opin. Cardiol.* 1986; 1: 622.
16. Blankestijn, P.J., van den Meiracker, A., Man in't Veld, A.J., Boomsma, F., Ritsema van Eck, H.J., Tulen, J., Moleman, P. and Schalekamp, M.A. Support for adrenaline-hypertension hypothesis: 18-hour pressor effect after 6 hours adrenaline infusion. *Lancet* 1988; ii: 1386.
17. Brown, M.J., Causon, R.C., Barnes, V.F., Brennan, P. and Greenberg, G. Urinary catecholamines analyses in essential hypertension: results of 24-hour urine catecholamine from patients in the Medical Research Council Trial for mild hypertension and matched controls. *Q. J. Med.* 1985; 57: 637.
18. Brown, J.J., Leckie, B.J., Lever, A.F., McIntyre, G., Morton, J.J., Semple, P.F. and Robertson, J.I.S. The renin-angiotensin system and the regulation of the circulation. In: Robertson, J.I.S. (ed). *Handbook of Hypertension Vol. I. Clinical Aspects of Essential Hypertension*. Amsterdam: Elsevier, 1983, pp. 278–323.
19. Swales, J.D., Abramovici, A., Beck, F., Bing, R.F., Loudon, M. and Thurston, H. Arterial wall renin. *J. Hypertens.* 1983; I (Suppl. 1): 17.
20. Jin, M., Wilhelm, M.J., Lang, R.E., Unger, T., Lindpaintner, K., Ganten, D. Endogenous tissue renin–angiotensin systems: from molecular biology to therapy. *Am. J. Med.* 1988; 84 (Suppl. 3A): 28.
21. Laragh, J.H. Atrial natriuretic hormone, the renin-aldosterone axis, and blood–pressure–electrolyte homeostasis. *N. Engl. J. Med.* 1985; 313: 1330.
22. Richards, A.M., Cleland, J.G.F., Tonolo, G., McIntyre, G.D., Leckie, B.J., Dargie, H.J., Ball, S.G. and Robertson, J.I.S. Plasma α-natriuretic peptide in cardiac impairment. *Br. J. Med.* 1986; 293: 409.
23. Robertson, J.I.S. and Richards, A.M. Cardiac failure, the kidney, renin and atrial peptide. *Eur. Heart J.* 1988; 9 (Suppl. H): 11.
24. Montorsi, P., Tonolo, G., Polonia, J., Hepburn, D. and Richards, A.M. Correlates of plasma atrial natriuretic factor in hypertension. *Hypertension* 1987; 10: 570.
25. Richards, A.M., Tonolo, G., Tree, M., Robertson, J.I.S., Montorsi, P., Leckie, B. and Polonia, J. Atrial natriuretic peptides and renin release. *Am. J. Med.* 1988; 84 (Suppl. 3A): 112.
26. Padfield, P.L. and Morton, J.J. Antidiuretic hormone and hypertension. In: Robertson, J.I.S. (ed). *Handbook of Hypertension Vol. I: Clinical Aspects of Essential Hypertension*. Amsterdam: Elsevier, 1983, pp. 348–64.
27. Vanhoutte, P., Amery, A., Birkenhäger, W., Breckenridge, A., Bühler, F., Distler, A., Dormandy, J., Doyle, A.E., Frohlich, E., Hansson, L., Hedner, T., Hollenberg, N., Jensen, H., Lund-Johansen, P., Meyer, P., Opie, L., Robertson, J.I.S., Safar, M., Schalekamp, M.A., Symoens, J., Trap-Jensen, J. and Zanchetti, A. Serotonergic mechanisms in hypertension: focus on ketanserin. *Hypertension* 1988; 11: 111.
28. Hökfelt, T., Millhorn, K., Seroogy, K., Tsuro, Y., Ceccatelli, S., Lindh, B., Meister, B., Melander, T., Schalling, M., Bartfai, T. and Terenius, L. Coexistence of peptides with classical neurotransmitters. *Experientia* 1987; 43: 768.
29. Kabge, R.E., Unger, T. and Ganten, D. Atrial natriuretic peptide: a new factor in blood pressure control. *J. Hypertens.* 1987; 5: 255.
30. Warthon, J. and Gulbenkian, S. Peptides in the mammalian cardiovascular system. *Experientia* 1987; 43: 821.
31. Kasakov, L., Ellis, J., Kirkpatrick, K., Milne, P. and Burnstock, G. Direct evidence for concomitant release of noradrenaline, adenosine S^1-triphosphate and neuropeptide Y from sympathetic nerves supplying the guinea-pig vas deferens. *J. Aut. Nerv. Syst.* 1988; 22: 75.
32. Gutkind, J.S., Kurihara, M., Castren, E. and Saavedra, J.M. Increased concentration of angiotensin II binding sites in selected brain areas of spontaneously hypertensive rats. *J. Hypertens.* 1988; 6: 79.
33. Bianchi, G. Ion transport across blood cell membranes in essential hypertension. *Curr. Opin. Cardiol.* 1986; 1: 634.
34. Bianchi, G., Cusi, D. and Vezzoli, G. Role of cellular sodium and calcium metabolism in the pathogenesis of essential hypertension. *Sem. Nephrol.* 1988; 8: 110.
35. Wauquier, I., Pernollet, M.G., Grichois, M.L., Lacour, B., Meyer, P. and Devynck, M.A. Endogenous digitalis-like circulating substances in spontaneously hypertensive rats. *Hypertension* 1988; 12: 108.

36. Bianchi, G. The kidney and hypertension. In: *Future Directions of Cardiovascular Research*. Canberra: National Heart Foundation of Australia, 1988, p. 21.

37. Graham, D.I., Lee, W.R., Cumming, A.M.M., Robertson, J.I.S. and Jones, J.V. Hypertension and the intracranial and ocular circulations: effects of antihypertensive treatment. In: Robertson, J.I.S. (ed). *Handbook of Hypertension, Vol. I: Clinical Aspects of Essential Hypertension*. Amsterdam: Elsevier, 1983, pp. 174–201.

38. Spence, J.D. Antihypertensive drugs and the prevention of atherosclerotic stroke. *Stroke* 1986; **17**: 808.

39. Folkow, B., Hansson, L. and Sivertsson, R. Structural vascular factors in the pathogenesis of hypertension. In: Robertson, J.I.S. (ed). *Handbook of Hypertension, Vol. I: Clinical Aspects of Essential Hypertension*. Amsterdam: Elsevier, 1983, pp. 133–50.

40. Cleland, W.P., Counihan, T.B. and Goodwin, J.F. Coarctation of the aorta. *Br. Med. J.* 1956; **2**: 379.

41. McGregor, E., Isles, C.G., Jay, J.L., Lever, A.F. and Murray, G.D. Retinal changes in malignant hypertension. *Br. Med. J.* 1986; **292**: 233.

42. Keith, N.M., Wagener, H.P. and Barker, N.W. Some different types of essential hypertension: their course and prognosis. *Am. J. Med. Sci.* 1939; **197**: 332.

43. Pickering, G.W. *High Blood Pressure*. 2nd ed. London: Churchill, 1968.

44. Guyton, A.C., Hall, J.E., Lohmeier, T.E., Manning, R.D., Jackson, T.E., Kastner, P.R. and Pan, Y.T. Role of the kidney and volume control in the pathogenesis of hypertension. In: Robertson, J.I.S. (ed). *Handbook of Hypertension, Vol. I: Clinical Aspects of Essential Hypertension*. Amsterdam: Elsevier, 1983, pp. 216–38.

45. Berglund, G., Aurell, M. and Wilhelmsen, L. Renal function in normo- and hypertensive 50-year-old males. *Acta Med. Scand.* 1976; **199**: 25.

46. Messerli, F. and Sclant, R.C. (eds). Left ventricular function in essential hypertension: mechanisms and therapy. *Am. J. Med.* 1983; (Suppl): pp. 1–120.

47. Fouad-Tarazi, M. Structural cardiac and vascular changes in hypertension: response to treatment. *Curr. Opin. Cardiol.* 1987; **2**: 782.

48. Laragh, J.H. Cardiac pathophysiology and its heterogeneity in patients with established hypertensive disease. *Am. J. Med.* 1988; **84** (Suppl 3A): 3.

49. Gavras, H., Kremer, D., Brown, J.J., Gray, B., MacAdam, R.E., Medina, A., Morton, J.J. and Robertson, J.I.S. Angiotensin- and norepinephrine-induced myocardial lesions: experimental and clinical studies in rabbits and man. *Am. Heart J.* 1975; 321.

50. Lund-Johansen, P. The hemodynamics of essential hypertension. In: Robertson, J.I.S. (ed). *Handbook of Hypertension, Vol. I: Clinical Aspects of Essential Hypertension*. Amsterdam: Elsevier, 1983, pp. 151–73.

51. Lund–Johansen, P. The hemodynamics of the aging cardiovascular system. *J. Cardiovasc. Pharmacol.* 1988; **12** (Suppl. 8): 20.

52. Lever, A.F. Slow pressor mechanisms in hypertension: a role for hypertrophy of resistance vessels? *J. Hypertens.* 1986; **4**: 515.

53. Robertson, J.I.S. Hypertension in the female. In: Ginsburg, J. (ed). *Circulation in the Female: From the Cradle to the Grave*. Kirby Lonsdale: Parthenon Press, 1989; 9: pp. 51–62.

54. Isles, C.G., Walker, L.M., Beevers, D.G., Brown, I., Cameron, H.L., Clarke, J., Hawthorne, J., Hole, D., Lever, A.F., Robertson, J.W.K. and Wapshaw, J. Mortality in patients of the Glasgow blood pressure clinic. *J. Hypertens.* 1986; **4**: 141.

55. Isles, C.G., Brown, J.J., Cumming, A.M.M., Lever, A.F., Robertson, J.I.S. and Wapshaw, J. Excess smoking in malignant-phase hypertension. *Br. Med. J.* 1979; **1**: 579.

56. Mackay, A., Brown, J.J., Cumming, A.M.M., Lever, A.F. and Robertson, J.I.S. Smoking and renal artery stenosis. *Br. Med. J.* 1979; **2**: 770.

57. Bloxham, C.A., Beevers, D.G. and Walker, J.M. Malignant hypertension and cigarette smoking. *Br. Med. J.* 1979; **1**: 581.

58. Medical Research Council Working Party. Stroke and coronary heart disease in mild hypertension: risk factors and the value of treatment. *Br. Med. J.* 1988; **296**: 1565.

59. Editorial. Hypertension and uric acid. *Lancet* 1981; i: 365,

60. Editorial. Uric acid in hypertension. *Lancet* 1987; i: 1124.

61. Kincaid-Smith, P. What has happened to malignant hypertension? In: Bulpitt, C. (ed). *Handbook of Hypertension, Vol. 6: Epidemiology of Hypertension*. Amsterdam: Elsevier, 1985, pp. 255–65.

62. Robertson, J.I.S. The large studies in hypertension: what have they shown? *Br. J. Clin. Pharm.* 1987; **24**: 3–14 S.

63. Hamilton, M., Thompson, E.N. and Wisniewski, T.K.M. The role of blood pressure control in preventing complications of hypertension. *Lancet* 1964; i 235.

64. Staessen, J., Fagard, R., Van Hoof, R. and Amery, A. Antihypentive drug treatment in elderly hypertensive subjects: evidence of protection. *J. Cardiovasc. Pharm.* 1988; **12** (Suppl. 8): 33.

65. MacMahon, S.W., Cutler, J.A., Furberg, C.D. and Payne, G.H. The effect of drug treatment for hypertension on morbidity and mortality from cardiovascular disease: a review of randomized controlled trials. *Prog. Cardiol. Dis.* 1986; **29** (Suppl. 3): 99.

66. Robertson, J.I.S. Hypertension and coronary risk: possible adverse effects of antihypertensive drugs. *Am. Heart J.* 1987; **14**: 1051 S.

67. Medical Research Council Working Party. Adverse reactions to bendrofluazide and propranolol following treatment of mild hypertension. *Lancet* 1981; ii: 539.

68. Medical Research Council Working Party. Ventricular extrasystoles during thiazide treatment: substudy of the M.R.C. mild hypertension trial. *Br. Med. J.* 1983; **287**: 1249.

69. Ragnarsson, J., Hardarson, T. and Snorrason, S.P. Ventricular dysrhythmias in middle-aged hypertensive men treated with either a diuretic or a beta-blocker. *Acta Med. Scand.* 1987; **221**: 143.

70. Ramsay, L.E. Mild hypertension: treat patients, not populations. *J. Hypertens.* 1985; **3**: 449.

71. Cruickshank, J.M., Thorp, J.M. and Zacharias, F.J. Benefits and potential harm of lowering high blood pressure. *Lancet* 1987; i: 581.

72. Robertson, J.I.S., and Hansson, L. How well is hypertension treated? *J. Hypertens.* 1986; **4** (Suppl. 6): 638.

73. Strandgaard, S. and Haunso, S. Why does antihypertensive treatment prevent stroke but not myocardial infarction? *Lancet* 1987; ii: 658.

74. Medical Research Council Working Party. M.R.C. Trial of treatment of mild hypertension: principal results. *Br. Med. J.* 1985; **291**: 97.

75. IPPPSH Collaborative Group. Cardiovascular risk and risk factors in a randomized trial of treatment based on the beta-blocker oxprenolol: the International Prospective Primary Prevention Study in Hypertension (IPPPSH). *J. Hypertens.* 1985; **3**: 379.

76. Wilhelmsen, L., Berglund, G., Elmfeldt, D., Fitzsimons, T., Holzgreve, H., Hosie, J., Hornkvist, P., Pennert, K., Tuomilehto, J. and Wede, H. Beta-blockers versus diuretics in hypertensive men: main results of the HAPPHY trial. *J. Hypertens.* 1987; **5**: 561.

77. Wikstrand, J., Warnold, I., Olsson, G., Tuomilehto, J., Elmfeldt, D. and Berglund, G. Primary prevention with metoprolol in patients with hypertension: mortality results

from the MAPHY study. *J. Am. Med. Ass.* 1988; **259**: 1976.

78. Robertson, J.I.S. Traditions of therapy in Britain. In: Ganten, D. (ed). *Antihypertensive Therapeutics.* Heidelberg: Springer-Verlag, 1989 (in press).

79. Hansson, L. Drug treatment of hypertension. In: Robertson, J.I.S. (ed). *Handbook of Hypertension, Vol. I: Clinical Aspects of Essential Hypertension.* Amsterdam: Elsevier, 1983, pp. 397–436.

80. Manhem, P.J.O., Clark, S.A., Brown, W.B., Murray, G.D. and Robertson, J.I.S. Effect of cholorothiazide on serial measurements of exchangeable sodium and blood pressure in spontaneously hypertensive rats. *Clin. Sci.* 1985; **69**: 511.

81. Cruickshank, J.M. and Prichard, B.N.C. *Beta-blockers in Clinical Practice.* Edinburgh: Churchill-Livingstone, 1988, pp. 1–8.

82. Man in't Veld, A.J., Van den Meiracker, A.H. and Schalekamp, M.A. Do beta-blockers really increase vascular resistance? Review of the literature and new observations under basal conditions. *Am. J. Hypertens.* 1988; **1**: 91.

83. Vanhoutte, P.M. The Expert Committee of the World Health Organization on the classification of calcium antagonists. *Am. J. Cardiol.* 1987; **59**: 3A.

84. Murray, T.S., East, B.W. and Robertson, J.I.S. Nicardipine versus propranolol in the treatment of essential hypertension: effect on total body elemental composition. *Br. J. Clin. Pharm.* 1986; **22** (Suppl. 3): 259.

85. Webb, D.J., Manhem, P.J.O., Ball, S.G., Inglis, G., Leckie, B.J., Lever, A.F., Morton, J.J., Robertson, J.I.S., Murray, G.D., Menard, J., Hallett, A., Jones, D.M. and Szelke, M. A study of the renin inhibitor H 142 in man. *J. Hypertens.* 1985; **3**: 653.

86. Robertson, J.I.S., Tillman, D.M., Ball, S.G. and Lever, A.F. Angiotensin converting enzyme inhibition in hypertension. *J. Hypertens.* 1987; **5** (Suppl. 3): 19.

87. Zanchetti, A. Which drug to which patient? *J. Hypertens.* 1985; **3** (Suppl. 2): 57.

88. Weinberger, M.H. and Weir, R.J. Oral contraceptives and hypertension. In: Robertson, J.I.S. (ed). *Handbook of Hypertension, Vol. 2: Clinical Aspects of Secondary Hypertension.* Amsterdam: Elsevier, 1983, pp. 196–207.

89. Hodsman, G.P., Robertson, J.I.S., Semple, P.F. and Mackay, A. Malignant hypertension and oral contraceptives: four cases, with two due to the 30 µg oestrogen pill. *Eur. Heart J.* 1982; **33**: 255.

90. McAreavey, D., Cumming, A.M.M., Boddy, K., Brown, J.J., Fraser, R., Leckie, B.J., Lever, A.F., Morton, J.J., Robertson, J.I.S. and Williams, E.D. The renin-angiotensin system and total body sodium and potassium in hypertensive women taking oestrogen-progestagen oral contraceptives. *Clin. Endocrinol.* 1983; **18**: 111.

91. Nicholls, M.G. and Espiner, E.A. Liquorice, carbenoxolone and hypertension. In: Robertson, J.I.S. (ed). *Handbook of Hypertension, Vol. 2: Clinical Aspects of Secondary Hypertension.* Amsterdam: Elsevier, 1983, pp. 189–95.

92. Beretta-Piccoli, C., Salvade, G., Crivelli, P.L. and Weidmann, P. Body-sodium and blood volume in a patient with licorice-induced hypertension. *J. Hypertens.* 1985; **3**: 19.

93. Simpson, F.O. Non-pharmacological approaches to the treatment of hypertension. In: Robertson, J.I.S. (ed). *Handbook of Hypertension, Vol. 2: Clinical Aspects of Secondary Hypertension.* Amsterdam: Elsevier, 1983, pp. 448–56.

94. Spence, C.D., Coghlan, J.P., Denton, D.A., Mills, E.H., Nelson, M.A., Whitworth, J.A. and Scoggins, B.A. Role of the autonomic nervous system, renin-angiotensin system, and arginine vasopressin during the onset and maintenance of ACTH hypertension in sheep. *Canad. J. Physiol. Pharm.* 1987; **65**: 1739.

95. Connell, J.M.C., Whitworth, J.A., Davies, D.L., Lever, A.F., Richards, A.M. and Fraser, R. Effects of ACTH and cortisol administration on blood pressure, electrolyte metabolism, atrial natriuretic peptide and renal function in normal man. *J. Hypertens.* 1987; **5**: 425.

96. Jackson, S.H.D., Beevers, D.G. and Myers, K. Does long-term low-dose corticosteroid therapy cause hypertension? *Clin. Sci.* 1981; **61** (Suppl. 7): 381.

97. Watkins, J., Abbott, E.C., Hensby, C.N., Webster, J. and Dollery, C.T. Attenuation of hypotensive effect of propranolol and thiazide diuretics by indomethacin. *Br. Med. J.* 1980; **281**: 702.

98. de Leeuw, P.W. and Birkenhäger, W.H. Coarctation of the aorta. In: Robertson, J.I.S. (ed). *Handbook of Hypertension, Vol. 2: Clinical Aspects of Secondary Hypertension.* Amsterdam: Elsevier, 1983, pp. 1–17.

99. Mackay, A., Brown, J.J., Lever, A.F., Morton, J.J. and Robertson, J.I.S. Unilateral renal disease in hypertension. In: Robertson, J.I.S. (Ed). *Handbook of Hypertension, Vol. 2: Clinical Aspects of Secondary Hypertension.* Amsterdam: Elsevier, 1983, pp. 33–79.

100. Robertson, J.I.S., Morton, J.J., Tillman, D.M. and Lever, A.F. The pathophysiology of renovascular hypertension. *J. Hypertens.* 1986; **4** (Suppl. 4): 95.

101. McAreavey, D., Brown, W.B., Murray, G.D. and Robertson, J.I.S. Exchangeable sodium in Goldblatt one-kidney one-clip hypertension in the rat. *Clin. Sci.* 1984; **66**: 545.

102. Glorioso, N., Laragh, J.H. and Rapelli, A. (eds). *Renovascular Hypertension: Pathophysiology, Diagnosis & Treatment.* New York: Raven Press, 1987.

103. Davies, D.L., Schalekamp, M.A., Beevers, D.G., Brown, J.J., Briggs, J.D., Lever, A.F., Medina, A., Morton, J.J., Robertson, J.I.S. and Tree, M. Abnormal relation between exchangeable sodium and renin-angiotensin system in malignant hypertension and in hypertension with chronic renal failure. *Lancet* 1973; i: 683.

104. Brown, J.J., Düsterdieck, G.O., Fraser, R., Lever, A.F., Robertson, J.I.S., Tree, M. and Weir, R.J. Hypertension and chronic renal failure. *Br. Med. Bull.* 1971; **27**: 128.

105. Ferriss, J.B., Brown, J.J., Fraser, R., Lever, A.F. and Robertson, J.I.S. Primary aldosterone excess: Conn's syndrome and similar disorders. In: Robertson, J.I.S. (Ed). *Handbook of Hypertension, Vol. 2: Clinical Aspects of Secondary Hypertension.* Amsterdam: Elsevier, 1983, pp. 132–61.

106. Gordon, R.D., Gomez-Sanchez, C.E., Hamlet, S.M., Tunny, T.J. and Klemm, S.A. Angiotensin-responsive aldosterone-producing adenoma masquerades as idiopathic hyperaldosteronism (IHA: adrenal hyperplasia) or low-renin essential hypertension. *J. Hypertens.* 1987; **5** (Suppl. 5): 103.

107. McAreavey, D., Murray, D.G., Lever, A.F. and Robertson, J.I.S. Similarity of idiopathic hyperaldosteronism and essential hypertension: a statistical comparison *Hypertension* 1983; **5**: 116.

108. Kaplan, N.M. Cushing's syndrome and hypertension. In: Robertson, J.I.S. (ed). *Handbook of Hypertension, Vol. 2: Clinical Aspects of Secondary Hypertension.* Amsterdam: Elsevier, 1983, pp. 208–21.

109. Fraser, R. Inborn errors of corticosteroid biosynthesis: their effects on electrolyte metabolism and blood pressure. In: Robertson, J.I.S. (ed). *Handbook of Hypertension, Vol. 2: Clinical Aspects of Secondary Hypertension.* Amsterdam: Elsevier, 1983, pp. 162–88.

110. Fraser, R., Brown, J.J., Mason, P.A., Morton, J.J., Lever, A.F., Robertson, J.I.S., Lee, H.A. and Miller, H. Severe hypertension with absent secondary sex characteristics due to partial deficiency of steroid 17-α-hydroxylase activity. *J.*

Human Hypertens. 1987; **1**: 53.

111. Ball, S.G., Phaeochromocytoma. In: Robertson, J.I.S. (ed). *Handbook of Hypertension, Vol. 2: Clinical Aspects of Secondary Hypertension.* Amsterdam: Elsevier, 1983, pp. 238–77.

112. MacDougall, I.C., Isles, C.G., Stewart, H., Inglis, G.C., Finlayson, J., Thomson, I., Lees, K.R., McMillan, N.C., Morley, P. and Ball, S.G. Overnight clonidine suppression test in the diagnosis and exclusion of pheochromocytoma. *Am. J. Med.* 1988; **84**: 993.

113. Moore, T.J. and Williams, G.H. Acromegaly and Hypertension. In: Robertson, J.I.S. (ed). *Handbook of Hypertension, Vol. 2: Clinical Aspects of Secondary Hypertension.* Amsterdam: Elsevier, 1983, pp. 222–37.

114. Davies, D.L., Beastall, G.H., Connell, J.M.C., Fraser, R., McCruden, D. and Teasdale, G.M. Body composition, blood pressure, and the renin-angiotensin system in acromegaly before and after treatment. *J. Hypertens.* 1985; **3** (Suppl. 3): 413.

115. Bing, R.F. and Swales, J.D. Thyroid disease and hypertension. In: Robertson, J.I.S. (ed). *Handbook of Hypertension, Vol. 2: Clinical Aspects of Secondary Hypertension.* Amsterdam: Elsevier, 1983, pp. 276–90.

116. Lee, M.R., Ball, S.G., Thomas, T.H. and Morgan, D.B. Hypertension and hyperkalaemia responding to bendrofluazide. *Q. J. Med.* 1979; **48**: 245.

117. Gordon, R.D. and Hodsman, J.P. The syndrome of hypertension and hyperkalaemia without renal failure: long-term correction by thiazide diuretic. *Scott. Med. J.* 1986; **31**: 43.

118. Bell, G.M. and Doig, A. Hypertension and intracranial tumor. In: Robertson, J.I.S. (ed). *Handbook of Hypertension, Vol. 2: Clinical Aspects of Secondary Hypertension.* Amsterdam: Elsevier, 1983, pp. 291–303.

119. Petrie, J.C., O'Brien, E.T., Littler, W.A. and de Swiet, M. British Hypertension Society: Recommendations on blood pressure measurement. *Br. Med. J.* 1986; **293**: 611.

120. Wright, B.M. and Dore, C.F. A random-zero sphygmomanometer. *Lancet* 1970; i: 337.

121. Rose, G.A., Holland, W.W. and Crowley, E.A. A sphygmomanometer for epidemiologists. *Lancet* 1964; i: 296.

122. Weber, M.A. Automatic blood pressure recorders and 24 hour monitoring. *Curr. Opin. Cardiol.* 1987; **2**: 748.

123. Robertson, J.I.S. The management of hypertension in aircrew. *Eur. Heart J.* 1988; **9** (Suppl. G): 41.

124. Anonymous. Sudden cardiac death in obesity and hypertension (Editorial). *Lancet* 1988; i: 628.

125. Atkinson, A.B. and Kellett, R.J. Value of intravenous urography in investigating hypertension. *J. R. Coll. Physic., London* 1974; **8**: 175.

126. Swales, J.D., Ramsay, L.E., Coope, J., Pocock, S., Robertson, J.I.S., Shaper, A. and Sever, P. British Hypertension Society: Recommendations for the treatment of mild hypertension. *Br. Med. J.* 1989; **298**: 694.

127. Robertson, J.I.S., Doyle, A.E. and Vanhoutte, P. (eds). Age-related aspects of antihypertensive therapy: the Corsendonk symposium. *J. Cardiovasc. Pharm.* 1988; **12** (Suppl. 8): pp. 1–182.

128. Ball, S.G. Systolic hypertension: a comparison of the trials with enalapril and beta-antagonists. *Curr. Opin. Cardiol.* 1987; **2** (Suppl. 1): 33.

129. Tuck, M.A. Hypertension in the elderly. *Curr. Opin. Cardiol.* 1987; **2**: 763.

130. Mackay, A., Isles, C., Atkinson, A.B., Brown, J.J., Cumming, A.M.M., Lever, A.F. and Robertson, J.I.S. The treatment of resistant hypertension. In: Jewell, J.P. (ed). *Advanced Medicine, Vol. 17.* London: Pitman Medical, 1981, pp. 39–58.

131. Edwards, C.R.W., Stewart, P.M., Burt, D., Brett, L., McIntyre, M.A., Sutanto, W., Kloet, E.R. and Monder, C. Localization of 11β-hydroxysteroid dehydrogenase: tissue specific protector of the mineralocorticoid receptor. *Lancet* 1988; ii: 986.

Chapter 54

Disorders of the Pulmonary Circulation

R.J.C. Hall and S.G. Haworth

INTRODUCTION

The pulmonary circulation can become disordered in many situations. The common condition of pulmonary thrombo-embolic disease in all its forms and the much rarer entities of primary pulmonary hypertension, involvement of the pulmonary circulation in diseases that also affect the systemic circulation (e.g. collagen vascular diseases) and pulmonary veno-occlusive disease will be discussed in this chapter. Pulmonary hypertension secondary to lung disease or left heart disease which is much more common than any of these abnormalities is dealt with in Chapters 55 and 56.

PULMONARY THROMBO-EMBOLIC DISEASE

DEFINITION

Pulmonary thrombo-embolic disease is any condition in which the pulmonary arteries become obstructed by thrombus. This obstruction is nearly always the result of thrombus that has formed in the venous system or right heart and then embolized into the pulmonary arteries. It is possible that thrombosis *in situ* may sometimes complicate acute pulmonary embolus, chronic thrombo-embolic pulmonary hypertension and primary pulmonary hypertension.

If carefully sought by venography or radio-active fibrinogen scanning, evidence of venous thrombosis is found in at least 70–80% of patients who have sustained a pulmonary embolus;[1,2] in the remainder, it is assumed that all the venous thrombus has already become detached and embolized. As pulmonary embolism is preceded by venous thrombosis, the factors predisposing to the two conditions are, except in special circumstances, the same and still broadly fit Virchow's famous triad of venous stasis, injury to the vein wall and enhanced coagula-

bility of the blood. Often a definite predisposing factor can be identified, although occasionally venous thrombosis and pulmonary embolism occur for no apparent reason. Immobility is an important predisposing factor and seems to be much more powerful when it is combined with trauma, surgery, or some other serious illness that enhances thrombosis. Other factors include neoplasia, cardiac failure, oestrogen-containing oral contraceptives (the new low-oestrogen preparations have reduced this risk substantially) and pregnancy, which combines hormonal changes with venous stasis (pulmonary embolism remains one of the most frequent causes of maternal mortality during both pregnancy and the puerperium[3]). Obesity is also an important risk factor,[4] which may operate alone but often seems particularly potent in combination with another factor such as the contraceptive pill or surgery. Occasionally, thrombo-embolic disease is due to haematological abnormalities which increase clotting such as thrombocythaemia and the rare familial condition of antithrombin III deficiency.[5] Risk factors are summarized in Table 54.1. A risk factor that has emerged in the last few years is thrombosis in association with indwelling catheters in the right heart used for parenteral nutrition, chemotherapy, fluid infusion, pressure monitoring or occasionally pacing. These techniques are often used in debilitated or immobilized patients who already have an increased risk of thrombosis.

Table 54.1. Risk factors for thrombo-embolic disease.

Immobility
Trauma (and surgery)
Neoplasia
Pregnancy and oestrogen-containing contraceptive pill
Reduced cardiac output
Obesity
Clotting abnormalities, e.g. antithrombin III deficiency, thrombocythaemia
Indwelling catheters and pacing electrodes in great veins and right heart

EPIDEMIOLOGY

It is impossible to obtain a true figure for the overall incidence of pulmonary embolism in the population because the clinical diagnosis of both pulmonary embolism and deep vein thrombosis is extremely inaccurate, many events may be asymptomatic, the autopsy rates are low and death certification is inaccurate. Despite these problems, some authors have attempted to estimate the incidence using many tenuous assumptions; for example, Dalen and Alpert[6] suggested that incidence of pulmonary embolism in the USA is 630 000 per year and that this leads to 200 000 deaths. This estimate is likely to be extremely inaccurate because it is based on an assumption that 15% of hospital deaths are due solely to pulmonary emboli whereas in other careful studies the incidence of death in hospital due solely to pulmonary emboli has been found to be < 1%[7] (this figure may also be wrong because of low autopsy rates).

However, it is possible to assess incidence in particular groups at risk. Following surgery, for example, 20–50% of patients develop venous thrombosis; the incidence is highest in those undergoing emergency surgery following trauma, e.g. for hip fractures, and pelvic surgery. Similar figures have been found in other situations of high risk, for example, following myocardial infarction.[8,9] Despite this high incidence of venous thrombosis, only a very small number of these patients suffer a pulmonary embolus and the likelihood of such a complication occuring seems to depend on the site of the deep venous thrombosis. In 80%, the thrombus is confined to the calf veins; in these patients the risk of pulmonary embolism is very low, even if no treatment is given, and long-term post-phlebitic sequelae are rare. In contrast, in the 10% in whom the thrombus extends into the femoral vein or beyond, the incidence of pulmonary embolism and long-term venous sequelae is clinically important.[10]

PATHOLOGY

In the majority of patients with thrombo-embolic disease, the emboli form in the veins of the leg, generally in the sural veins. In cases of massive fatal pulmonary embolism, the emboli often originate from the femoral and iliac veins, frequently beginning in the sinuses of the venous valves.[11] They may also originate in the pelvis, particularly after obstetric and gynaecological procedures, and in the internal jugular vein in the presence of middle-ear sepsis. Thrombosis of the superior vena cava is becoming more common as a result of indwelling central venous catheters, particularly when these are used for hyperalimentation. Recently, the right atrial appendage has been incriminated as a source of emboli in chronic silent thrombo-embolism.[12]

There has been much debate about the relative contributions of mechanical obstruction and pulmonary vasoconstriction to pulmonary artery obstruction. Pathologists usually maintain that mechanical obstruction is sufficient explanation.

In massive pulmonary embolism, the lumen of the pulmonary trunk and/or extrapulmonary arteries is occluded or partially obstructed by thrombi, which may even fill the right ventricular cavity. The presence of organized clot in these and more peripheral arteries indicates that the patient has survived previous thrombo-embolic episodes. To the naked eye, extensive recanalization of organized clot occurring over a long time produces fibrous bands and webs formed of collagen and containing elastic fibres. In thrombo-embolic pulmonary hypertension, the walls of the pulmonary trunk and extrapulmonary arteries are hypertrophied and may contain atherosclerotic plaques.

Within the lung, thrombo-embolic disease is often widespread, but it has a tendency to occur in the posterior basal and apical segments of the lower lobes particularly in the right lung.[13] Pulmonary angiography and post-mortem arteriography show patchy filling defects with obstruction of large arteries, but microscopic examination usually reveals more extensive involvement of the pulmonary arterial bed. Microscopic serial sections[14] show that the obstruction can be localized, such that arteries which are patent in one section of lung tissue are frequently occluded at another point. The presence of recent emboli on top of organizing emboli suggests progressive obstruction by repeated showers of emboli. Organization of the clot begins with infiltration of fibroblasts which deposit collagen and some elastic fibres (Fig. 54.1). The lesion becomes incorporated into the arterial wall, and projects into the lumen as a cushion of intimal fibrosis. The eccentric lesion of thrombo-embolic disease is in marked contrast to the concentric lesion found in primary plexogenic pulmonary arteriopathy (see below). A lumen is nearly always present (Fig. 54.1b). It is usually eccentric, between the thrombus and arterial wall, but it is occasionally central due to central recanalization of the thrombus. With time, the organized thrombus retracts against the arterial wall and the lumen becomes

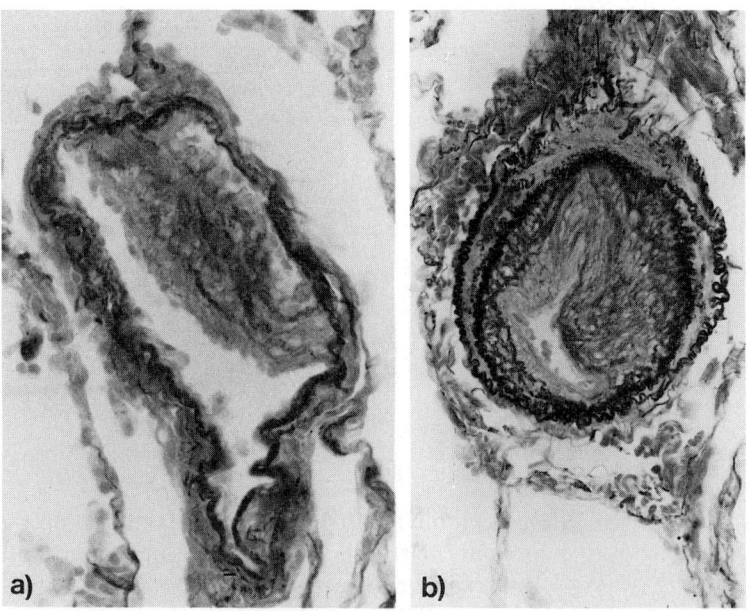

Fig. 54.1. (a) Thrombo-embolic disease: eccentric cushion of intimal fibrosis in alveolar wall artery (× 224). (b) Photomicrograph of a small muscular pulmonary artery containing eccentric intimal fibrosis (× 280).

wider. Part of the rationale for treating patients with thrombo-embolic pulmonary hypertension with anti-thrombotic therapy is to prevent further deposition of thrombi and to allow existing thrombi to retract and recanalize. Recanalization of the lumen in the muscular arteries may produce either fibrous septa or a network of delicate trabeculae (Fig. 54.2). In smaller arteries, either one or more channels or multiple capillary-like spaces appear. Iron pigment is found in early thrombotic lesions.

Pulmonary arterial medial hypertrophy is not usually a feature of thrombo-embolic disease. However, generalized medial hypertrophy can occur when chronic thrombo-embolic disease leads to an increase in pulmonary vascular resistance. Plexiform and dilatation lesions do not occur in

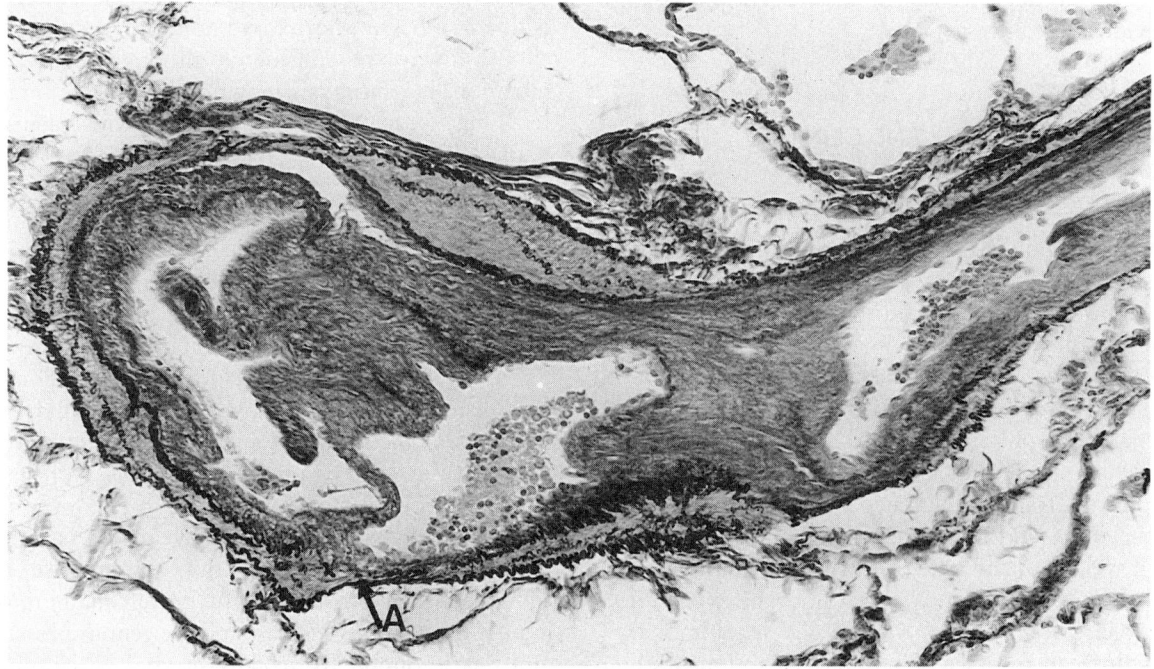

Fig. 54.2. Photomicrograph showing lumen of muscular artery obstructed by strands of fibrous tissue. The media is irregular and atrophied (A) (× 152).

thrombo-embolic disease, although recanalized thrombi can mimic plexiform lesions. Fibrinoid necrosis is rare. Arteritis is an unusual feature and probably results from embolization of infected thrombi.

The pulmonary veins are usually normal. However, many small veins may show an increase in wall thickness and be 'arterialized', particularly in older patients who may have chronic elevation of the left atrial pressure.

Obstruction of the pulmonary arteries is always associated with dilatation of the bronchial circulation and enlargement of the anastomoses between the two circulations. The bronchial circulation offers an alternative source of blood supply and perfuses the distal pulmonary arteries via anastomoses around the necks of the terminal and respiratory bronchioli. In the obstructed arteries, dilated vasa vasorum connect with recanalized channels. Other systemic arteries in the chest wall, diaphragm and mediastinum also contribute to the pulmonary arterial blood supply. The extent of the collateral arterial supply is related to the duration of the thrombo-embolic process. Because of the efficacy of the bronchial artery supply, haemorrhagic infarction with necrosis of lung tissue is relatively uncommon when considered in relation to the high incidence of thrombo-embolic disease. It is most often seen in older patients who are in chronic cardiac failure, but it can also occur in young previously healthy patients.

PATHOPHYSIOLOGY AND CLINICAL FEATURES

The pathophysiology and clinical features of pulmonary embolism are so closely related that they are considered together. The effects of a pulmonary embolus depend mainly on the extent to which the embolus obstructs the pulmonary circulation, the duration over which that obstruction accumulates, and the pre-existing state of the patient, which has been defined only imprecisely. In general, a patient who has pre-existing cardiopulmonary disease or who is old, frail or debilitated will be more sensitive to the effects of an embolus than a patient who has been well until the time of the event. Small emboli are often asymptomatic.[15,16] As both the extent and chronicity of obstruction vary so widely, pulmonary embolus can produce widely differing clinical pictures. It is convenient to consider pulmonary embolus under four main headings (Table 54.2),

Table 54.2. **Classification of pulmonary embolism.**

Pulmonary embolism	History	Degree of pulmonary artery obstruction (%)
Acute minor	Short	< 50
Acute massive	Short	> 50
Subacute massive	Several weeks	> 50
Chronic thrombo-embolic hypertension	Months or years	Usually > 50

but these are arbitrary divisions and some patients do not fit into this classification.

Acute minor pulmonary embolism

If an embolus obstructs a small amount of the pulmonary circulation (< 50%), its effects are dominated by any pulmonary infarction it produces and by the alterations in gas exchange it causes. The patient may occasionally be immediately aware of some slight dyspnoea, possibly on minor exertion, because the affected area of the lung is still ventilated but no longer perfused; normally, the first abnormality the patient notes results from pulmonary infarction. Sharp pleuritic pain develops, often associated with difficulty in breathing induced by inspiratory exacerbation of the pain. In a patient already on anticoagulant therapy for a previous embolus, the possibility that pleuritic pain is due to a haemothorax and not a further embolus should always be considered although this is not common. Haemoptysis may occur from the infarcted lung, with or without accompanying pleuritic pain.

The physical signs are those of pulmonary infarction. The patient is often distressed and breathing shallowly because of the pleuritic pain, but is not usually clinically cyanosed because the disturbance of gas transfer is only slight. The mechanisms causing hypoxaemia in pulmonary embolism are discussed in the section on acute massive pulmonary embolism. Fever is common due to the infarcted lung, and sometimes it is such a prominent feature that differentiation of pulmonary embolism from an infective cause of pleurisy is difficult. The fever and pain often produce a sinus tachycardia. As minor pulmonary embolism does not compromise the right ventricle, cardiac output is well maintained, hypotension does not occur and the venous pressure and heart sounds are usually normal. A common misapprehension is that there is often a loud pulmonary component to the second heart sound;

this is not the case because the right heart pressures are normal. Although atrial fibrillation or other supraventricular tachycardia may occur, these are uncommon. Signs of pulmonary infarction and any associated pleural effusion may be found in the lungs: a mixture of consolidation and effusion, possibly with a pleural rub. They may be unilateral or bilateral and can occur in more than one part of the same lung. In a small percentage of patients (about 20%), there will also be signs of a deep vein thrombosis which sometimes reveal themselves after the pulmonary embolus.

Acute massive pulmonary embolism

This is the most striking form of pulmonary embolism and it is far less common than the minor variety. When > 50% of the pulmonary circulation is suddenly obstructed, the pathophysiology and clinical signs become dominated by the acute and severe derangement of cardiac and pulmonary function. Obstruction of the pulmonary artery causes acute failure of the right heart. Cardiac output falls and the patient suddenly becomes hypotensive. This may occur so rapidly that syncope is either the presenting feature or easily induced by a relatively minor cardiovascular stress, such as sitting up or the vasodilatation consequent on getting into a warm bath. If the degree of obstruction is sufficient, death occurs almost immediately. The right ventricle is a thin-walled structure designed to work against the normally low pulmonary vascular resistance; consequently, it performs poorly against a sudden obstruction. As a result, it dilates, and a moderate rise in the right ventricular systolic and pulmonary artery pressure occurs which rarely exceeds 50 mmHg because the normal right ventricle is unable to generate a higher pressure.[17] The right ventricular end-diastolic pressure and right atrial pressure rise far more as the ventricle fails, and they are often of the order of 15–20 mmHg. Concomitant with these profound circulatory disturbances, the patient becomes severely hypoxaemic;[18] there is a rough correlation between the extent of hypoxaemia and the extent of embolism.[19] Although massive pulmonary embolism without hypoxaemia has been reported,[20] it must be regarded as extremely rare; in our experience of over 300 cases of acute massive pulmonary embolism, we have never encountered such a case.

The mechanisms causing hypoxaemia in pulmonary embolism are not completely understood, mainly because detailed study of respiratory function is difficult in acutely ill patients. the main causes seem to be as follow:[18,21]

1   *Ventilation–perfusion mismatch.* The most obvious abnormality is ventilation of parts of the lung that no longer have a blood supply because of the embolic obstruction. This does not cause hypoxaemia but leads instead to a large physiological dead-space which is still being ventilated; consequently, total ventilation is high as the patient struggles to get enough air to the parts of the lung that are still perfused and is obliged to ventilate lung that is not perfused. Other areas of the lung remain perfused and in fact are relatively overperfused, the ventilation in these areas being insufficient to oxygenate the extra blood flow fully. This leads to hypoxaemia. Overperfusion may also cause some pulmonary oedema in these areas which will further impair oxygenation. Overt pulmonary oedema can occur in the perfused area of lung, but it is a rare clinical manifestation.

2   *Shunting.* Intrapulmonary shunting is an important cause of hypoxaemia in some patients. It occurs through areas of collapse and infarction that are not ventilated but retain some blood flow. This mechanism may become more important a few days after the initial episode as collapse and infarction become more marked. In patients with a patent foramen ovale (5–10% of the population),[22] raised right atrial pressure may open the foramen and cause right-to-left shunting at the atrial level which adds to hypoxaemia.

3   *Low mixed venous oxygen saturation.* The mixed venous oxygen saturation is low due to the reduced cardiac output. This seems to be an important factor generating arterial hypoxaemia because there is insufficient time for this desaturated blood to become fully saturated as it passes through the alveolar capillaries in the overperfused areas of the lung.

4   *Other factors.* A few patients develop bronchospasm[23] as a result of acute massive pulmonary embolism. Constriction of airways in normal areas of the lung near to the embolized segments has also been suggested, but there is no evidence for this mechanism in humans.

The clinical features of acute massive pulmonary embolism can be explained in terms of these pathophysiological changes (Table 54.3). Usually the patient becomes acutely distressed, severely short of breath and syncopal due to the combination of hypoxaemia and low cardiac output, and central anginal-type chest pain may develop due to the combination of hypotension, hypoxaemia and

Table 54.3. **Symptoms and signs of acute massive pulmonary embolism.**

	Symptoms	Signs
Previous minor pulmonary embolism	Pleuritic chest pain, haemoptysis	Pleural rub, signs of pleural fluid and pulmonary consolidation
Severe V/Q disturbance	Dyspnoea, anginal chest pain	Central cyanosis
Obstruction to right ventricular outflow	Postural hypotension, syncope, angina	Hypotension, tachycardia (sinus), peripheral circulatory shutdown and cyanosis; jugular venous pressure increased, S_3 (left sternal border), wide splitting of S_2

increased cardiac work. The physical signs are those of reduced cardiac output: marked sinus tachycardia, hypotension and a cool periphery, sometimes with confusion and oliguria. In addition, the patient is nearly always obviously dyspnoeic, cyanosed both centrally and peripherally and has signs of acute right heart strain, consisting of a raised venous pressure, which is often difficult to appreciate because of the respiratory distress, a gallop rhythm at the right sternal border and a widely split second heart sound due to delayed right ventricular ejection, which is often difficult to detect because of the accompanying tachycardia. The pulmonary component of the second heart sound is not usually loud because the pulmonary artery pressure is only moderately raised. In addition to these features, there may be the additional symptoms and signs of a preceding minor embolus that produced pulmonary infarction. Occasional patients present with severe bronchospasm[23] and may be misdiagnosed as having asthma; very rarely, pulmonary oedema in overperfused areas of lung causes diagnostic confusion.

Subacute massive pulmonary embolism

Subacute massive pulmonary embolism is an uncommon but important condition caused by multiple emboli of moderate or small size that obstruct the pulmonary circulation usually over several weeks. Its main pathophysiological effects are to derange gas exchange and obstruct the right heart. Because this obstruction occurs slowly, there is time

for the right ventricle to adapt and for some hypertrophy to develop; consequently, the right ventricular and pulmonary artery pressures are higher than those in the acute forms of pulmonary embolism.[24] The main symptoms are insidiously increasing dyspnoea, and falling exercise tolerance. There is often an associated cough. Normally, the most prominent physical sign is obvious shortness of breath, either at rest or on only slight exertion, which is out of proportion to all other findings, and there may be central cyanosis. The blood pressure and pulse rates are usually normal because the cardiac output is well maintained. Commonly, the venous pressure is raised and a third heart sound is audible at the right sternal border which may be accentuated by inspiration. The pulmonary component of the second heart sound is sometimes loud.[24] In some cases, all these right heart signs are absent. These clinical features often occur alone, but there may also be symptoms and signs of pulmonary infarction that occurred during the build-up of the obstruction. In advanced cases, right heart failure develops and eventually the cardiac output falls. A further pulmonary embolus may change the clinical picture to one that resembles acute massive pulmonary embolism.

An obvious predisposing factor may be detected (Table 54.1) but is less common than in the acute forms of pulmonary embolism.[24]

Chronic thrombo-embolic pulmonary hypertension

Chronic thrombo-embolic pulmonary hypertension is the least common form of thrombo-embolic disease; it is encountered only very rarely. Large and medium-sized pulmonary vessels become obstructed in a haphazard fashion. It has been assumed that this form of obstruction is the result of recurrent emboli; however, in most cases, the evidence for this mechanism is weak because often there are no identifiable embolic episodes in the history.[25] It is possible that in some cases thrombosis *in situ* may be an important mechanism. The main pathophysiological features are those of impaired gas exchange and obstruction to the output of the right heart, which produce exertional dyspnoea and reduced exercise tolerance with the physical signs of severe pulmonary hypertension (see primary pulmonary hypertension below) combined with cyanosis. As with other causes of severe pulmonary hypertension, there may be classical angina of effort. The pulse rate and blood pressure are normal until a very late stage of the disease. As identifiable episodes of pulmonary infarction are unusual, abnormal physical signs in the lungs are not a feature of this condition. An obvious predisposing factor is often absent, but some patients have longstanding and severe venous thrombosis of the lower limb(s). The illness usually develops slowly over several years and consequently the onset of the symptoms and signs is also insidious. Ultimately, the condition leads to right heart failure and death.[25]

INVESTIGATIONS

Blood gases

The characteristic changes are a reduced Pao_2, caused by V/Q mismatch and shunting of blood through underventilated parts of the lung and a $Paco_2$ that is normal, or is reduced because of hyperventilation.[18] There is a rough correlation between the extent of hypoxaemia and embolism;[19] the Pao_2 is almost never normal on room air in the patient with massive pulmonary embolism (acute, subacute or chronic) but is occasionally normal in cases of minor pulmonary embolism.

Electrocardiogram

Electrocardiographic changes, although common in pulmonary embolism, are usually non-specific.[26] The rhythm is usually sinus. In acute minor pulmonary embolism, there is no real haemodynamic stress and therefore the only finding is sinus tachycardia. In acute massive pulmonary embolism, evidence of right heart strain may be seen, but the classic $S_1Q_3T_3$ pattern (Fig. 54.3) occurs in only a limited number of cases; similar changes are seen in subacute massive pulmonary embolism but they are less common and sometimes the electrocardiogram is normal. In chronic pulmonary embolism, there is nearly always evidence of right ventricular hypertrophy by the time the condition is fully developed.

Chest X-ray

The chest X-ray findings are also non-specific but they may be helpful. A normal film is compatible with all but chronic thrombo-embolic pulmonary hypertension. In all types except chronic thrombo-embolic pulmonary hypertension, the heart shadow is normal and the lung fields may show evidence of pulmonary infarction, either single or multiple: peripheral opacities, sometimes but not always

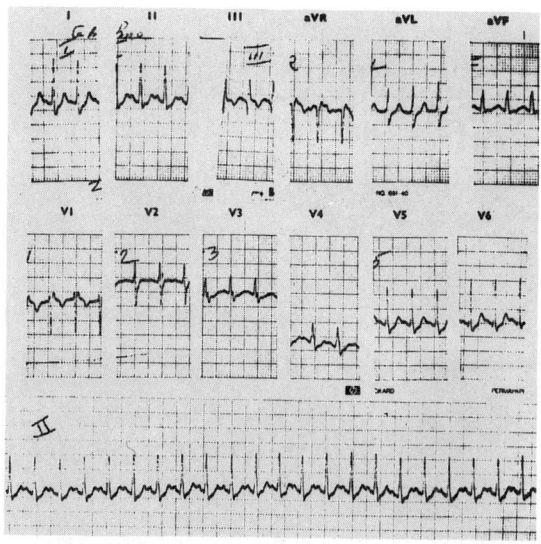

Fig. 54.3. Electrocardiogram of a patient with acute massive pulmonary embolism showing an $S_1Q_3T_3$ pattern and sinus tachycardia.

wedge-shaped, linear shadows, which may radiate out from the hila, pleural effusions and elevation of the diaphragm(s) are the most common signs. In minor pulmonary embolism, the main branches of the pulmonary artery are normal. In acute massive pulmonary embolism, a plump pulmonary artery shadow may be seen particularly in the right hilum but the main pulmonary artery is normal, whereas in subacute massive pulmonary embolism it is occasionally enlarged with the pulmonary artery pressure is elevated. In chronic thrombo-embolic pulmonary hypertension, the main pulmonary artery and the large arteries in the hila are very prominent due to the severe and longstanding pulmonary hypertension (Fig. 54.4) and cardiomegaly is common. It may be possible to detect areas of oligaemia in the parts of the lung affected by emboli[27] (particularly in acute massive pulmonary embolism), but this is difficult, not particularly accurate and almost impossible on the type of portable film that is usually available in the acute situation. Very occasionally, patchy pulmonary oedema is seen on the chest X-ray.

Lung scan

A normal perfusion lung scan excludes the diagnosis because pulmonary embolism of all types produces a defect of perfusion (Fig. 54.5). However, many conditions other than pulmonary embolism, such as tumours, consolidation and chronic obstructive airways disease, can also produce similar

---

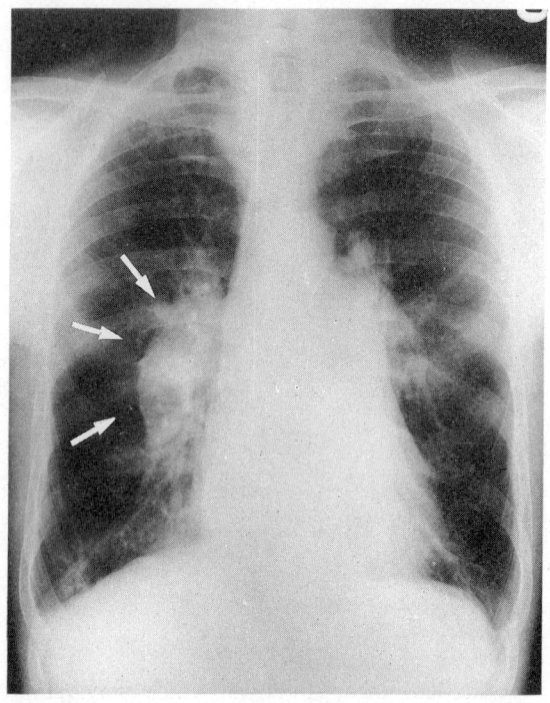

Fig. 54.4. Chest X-ray of a patient with chronic thrombo-embolic pulmonary hypertension showing enlargement of the main pulmonary artery and enormous dilatation of the pulmonary arteries in the hila (arrows).

defects. The addition of a ventilation scan, obtained by the inhalation of a radioactive gas such as krypton or xenon, increases the specificity of this technique. Pulmonary embolism produces a defect of perfusion but not of ventilation (Fig. 54.6); most of the other conditions, such as chronic obstructive airways disease and chest infections, that produce a perfusion defect also impair ventilation such that ventilation and perfusion defects are matched (Fig. 54.7). A defect of perfusion unmatched by one of ventilation is not diagnostic of pulmonary embolism because small defects of this type have been described in normal subjects,[33] but it is highly

suggestive. Pulmonary embolism can also produce perfusion defects that are matched to defects of ventilation when pulmonary infarction has occurred, but in this situation the chest X-ray nearly always shows the infarct. The defects that occur in both acute massive pulmonary embolism and subacute massive pulmonary embolism are always extensive (Fig. 54.8). The diagnostic accuracy of lung scans is greatly enhanced if they are assessed in the light of the clinical picture and chest X-ray findings (Table 54.4).[3,34–38] The ventilation–perfusion lung scan is probably the single most useful investigation in the diagnosis of pulmonary embolism because apart from the pulmonary angiogram, it gives the best information, and it is readily available in most hospitals and carries no risk for the patient.

Lung function tests

In all forms of thrombo-embolic disease, simple spirometry and lung volumes are normal or only mildly disturbed.[28] Such testing is not usually possible or useful in patients with acute pulmonary embolism who are either too distressed or too limited by pleuritic chest pain to perform the tests.[18,21] These tests, however, are very useful for distinguishing patients with chronic thrombo-embolic and subacute massive embolic pulmonary hypertension from those in whom airways obstruction is the true diagnosis.

Similarly, the diffusing capacity for carbon monoxide (transfer factor) can be useful in chronic or subacute situations.[29–31] It is normal or near normal (rarely < 50% of the predicted value) in thrombo-embolic disease, but it is usually grossly reduced when the correct diagnosis is parenchymal lung disease. Findings in primary pulmonary hypertension and Eisenmenger's syndrome resemble those in thrombo-embolic disease.[32]

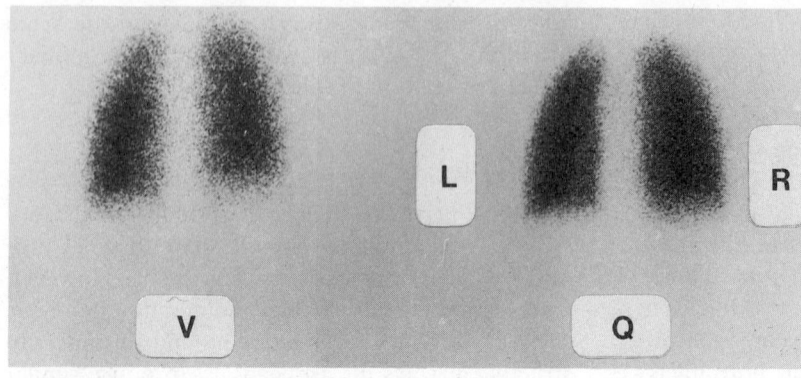

Fig. 54.5. A normal V/Q lung scan (postero-anterior view). Perfusion (Q) on right and ventilation on the left (V).

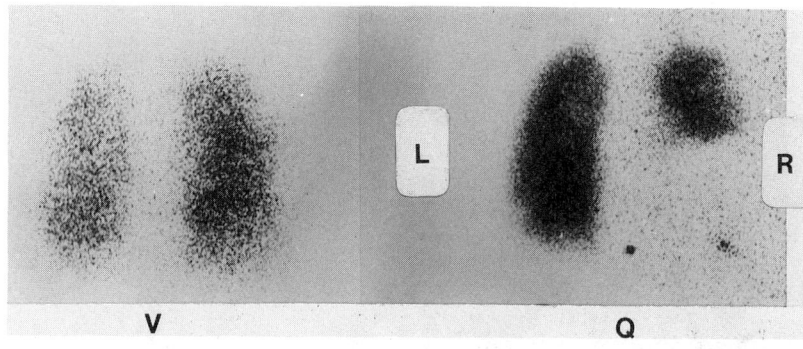

Fig. 54.6. A *V/Q* lung scan showing a single large perfusion defect at the right base with normal ventilation in this area. This defect was due to a single pulmonary embolus.

Right heart catheterization and pulmonary angiography

The changes in the right heart pressures that occur in pulmonary embolism are summarized in Table 54.5. The pulmonary angiogram is the only technique that can diagnose pulmonary embolism with certainty; however, it has disadvantages the most important of which are its limited availability (i.e. only at specialist centres) and a small (< 1%) but definite risk of mortality,[39] which is higher if the pulmonary artery pressure is greatly increased, for example, in chronic thrombo-embolic pulmonary hypertension or primary pulmonary hypertension.[40] To attempt to carry out pulmonary angiography in the X-ray department of a hospital that does not perform cardiac angiography routinely is not recommended because it is essential to apply the skill that arises from the everyday use of invasive cardiology in the acutely ill patient.

Injection of contrast into the main pulmonary artery, combined with 'cut films', is sufficient to delineate the emboli in most cases (Fig. 54.9). When the embolus is small, more specialized methods of investigation may improve diagnostic accuracy,[41] e.g. selective injections into subdivisions of the pulmonary arteries (Fig. 54.10), oblique views and cinéangiography, which has higher definition and can sometimes separate superimposed vessels as they move apart due to the pulsation of the arteries. The angiographic appearances of an embolus are similar in minor, acute massive and subacute massive pulmonary embolism (Fig. 54.11); it appears as a convex filling defect often with a little contrast leaking beyond its edges and the sides of the vessel containing it to give a 'pipe-stem' appearance. The overall perfusion of the affected region is reduced. Miller *et al.*[15] developed a convenient angiographic scoring system to assess the severity of pulmonary embolism using a combination of the number of vessels involved by embolus and the degree to which perfusion is reduced. The appearances are different in chronic thrombo-embolic pulmonary hypertension. Perfusion is patchily decreased but the filling defects are smooth and flat, rather than convex, and completely occlude the vessels which are considerably dilated

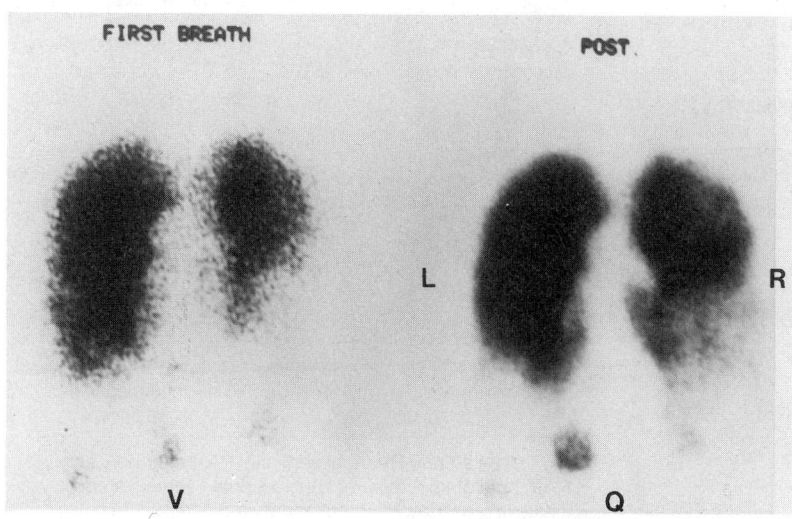

Fig. 54.7. A *V/Q* lung scan showing matching defects of ventilation and perfusion. This was due to severe parenchymal lung disease, mainly at the bases.

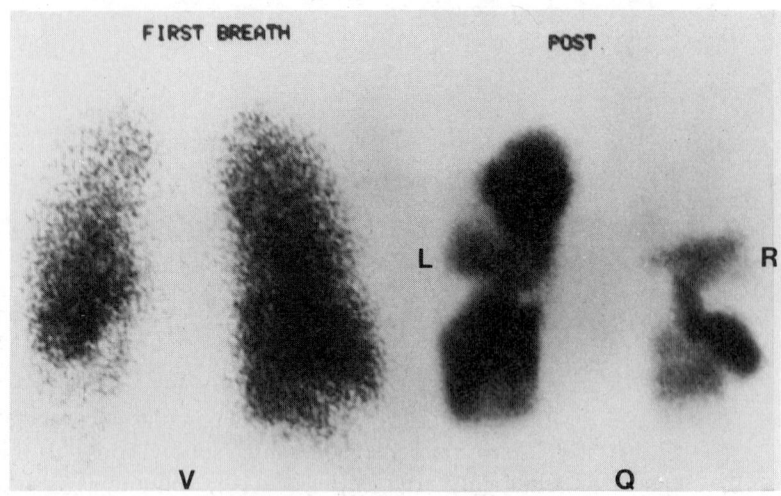

FIRST BREATH

POST

L

R

V

Q

Fig. 54.8. A *V/Q* lung scan showing multiple perfusion defects in both lungs and near normal ventilation. This was due to multiple pulmonary emboli.

proximal to the occlusion.

Early experience using digital subtraction angiography for the diagnosis of pulmonary embolism has been disappointing because definition of the pulmonary vessels is usually poor. More recently, magnetic resonance imaging and computed tomography scanning have both been used to identify pulmonary emboli but their roles in the clinical diagnosis of thrombo-embolic disease are not yet established.

Venography

Venograms will show thrombus in the deep venous system in at least 70% of patients who have sustained a pulmonary embolus, but thrombus will often be present in patients who have not. Consequently, venograms,[1,2] and other methods for detecting thrombus in the deep veins, such as impedance phlebography,[42] have only limited value in making the diagnosis of pulmonary embolism.

Table 54.4. Clinical probability of occurrence of pulmonary embolism.[3,22–26]

	Clinical probability (%)		
V/Q Scan	Low	Medium	High
Low: Matching defects	2	2	2
Medium: Mismatched subsegmental defects (multiple[a])	1	3 (22[a])	40 (70[a])
High: Mismatched segmental or lobar defects (multiple[a])	55	80 (95[a])	95 (100[a])

[a] Multiple defects.

Furthermore, venography is difficult, if not impossible, to carry out in the acutely ill patient.

Echocardiography

Echocardiography may reveal thrombus floating in the right atrium,[43] and in cases of acute massive pulmonary embolism the right ventricle is obviously dilated.[44] The Doppler technique may allow the pulmonary artery pressure to be measured. Ultrasound is of very limited use in the diagnosis of pulmonary embolism but may be helpful in exclud-

Table 54.5. Typical right heart pressures in thrombo-embolic disease.[15–17,52,54]

	Pressures (mmHg)			
	RA	RV	PA	Comment
Minor pulmonary embolism	5	30/0–5	30/15	Normal pressures
Acute massive pulmonary embolism	12	45/0–12	45/20	Severe pulmonary hypertension does not occur. Systolic PAP rarely > 50 mmHg. RAP and RVEDP usually raised
Subacute massive pulmonary embolism	6	70/0–6	70/35	RAP and RVEDP may be raised. RV and PA systolic range 50–90 mmHg
Chronic thrombo-embolic pulmonary hypertension	6	90/0–6	90/50	RAP and RVEDP higher when patient develops congestive cardiac failure

[a] RA, right atrium; RV, right ventricle; PA, pulmonary artery; RAP, right atrial pressure; RVEDP, right ventricular end-diastolic pressure; PAP, pulmonary artery pressure.

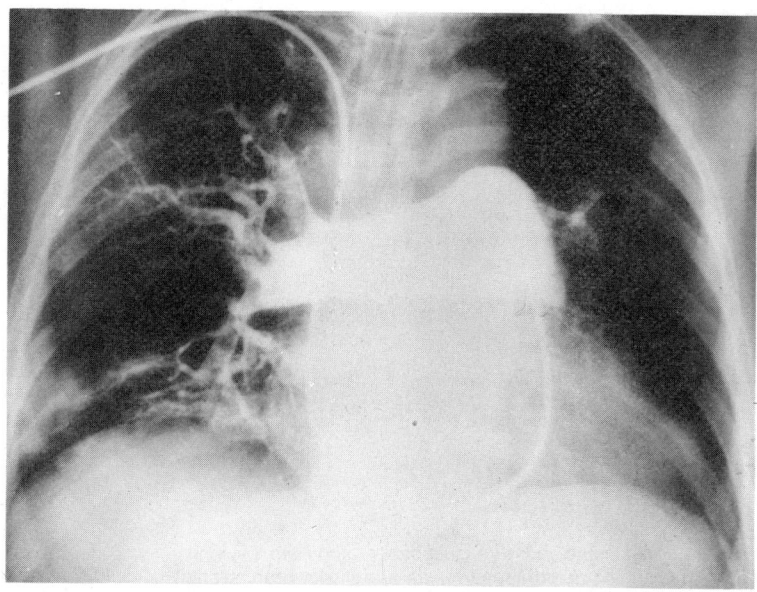

Fig. 54.9. Pulmonary angiogram of a patient with acute massive pulmonary embolism. Injection into the main pulmonary artery showing almost complete obstruction of flow into the left lung and multiple ebmoli in the branches on the right pulmonary artery.

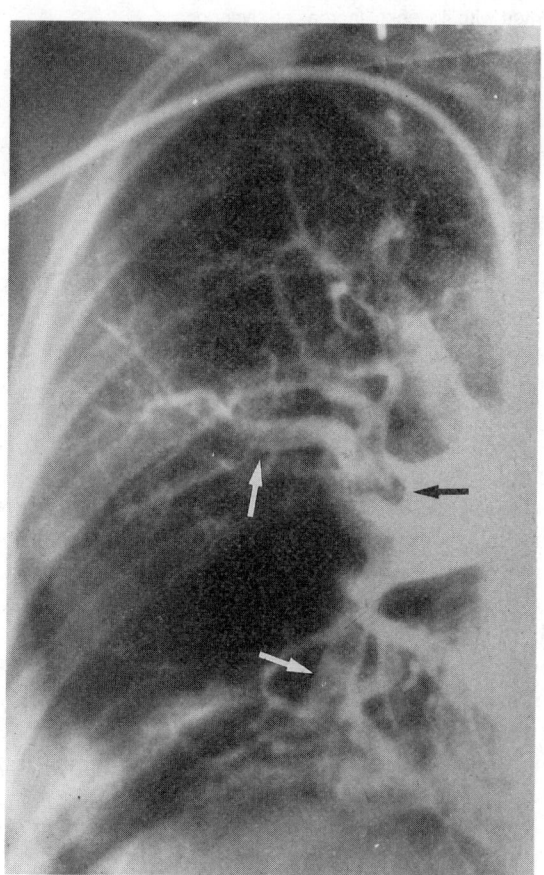

Fig. 54.10. Selective injection into the right pulmonary artery of the same patient as shown in Fig. 54.9 showing improved definition of the multiple emboli present in the main right pulmonary artery (black arrow) and its branches (some of the larger emboli marked by white arrows).

ing or suggesting alternative causes for cardiovascular collapse.

DIAGNOSIS

The clinical diagnosis of pulmonary embolism is often difficult, particularly when there is co-existing pulmonary disease;[45,46] when the diagnosis is based on clinical signs alone, it is notoriously inaccurate.[47,48] The main exception to this is the occasional case of acute massive pulmonary embolism which may be so characteristic that it could be little else. The diagnostic difficulties arise because most of the symptoms and signs are non-specific. It is not surprising that patients with other conditions are diagnosed as having pulmonary embolism and vice versa. The diagnosis requires a high index of clinical suspicion and the judicious use of investigations to confirm or refute these suspicions. Normal blood gases make the diagnosis very unlikely (but not impossible). As electrocardiographic and chest X-ray abnormalities in pulmonary embolism are non-specific, they cannot be used to confirm the diagnosis although they may add to suspicion. The V/Q lung scan is the best technique available for diagnosis in most centres and in many cases either rules out the diagnosis by being normal or suggests a high enough likelihood of pulmonary embolism (Table 54.4) that therapy can be undertaken on the basis of its results. If significant doubt remains after the lung scan, there are two possible approaches: to carry out angiography or to start treatment while

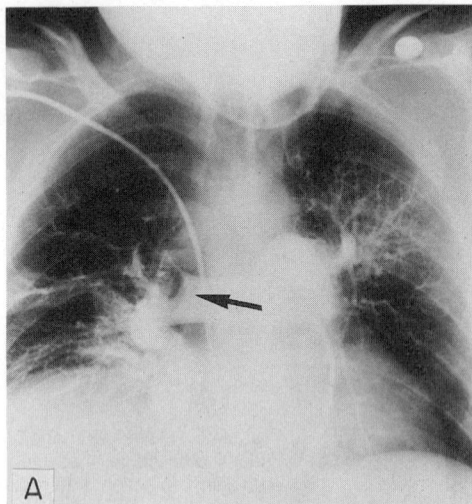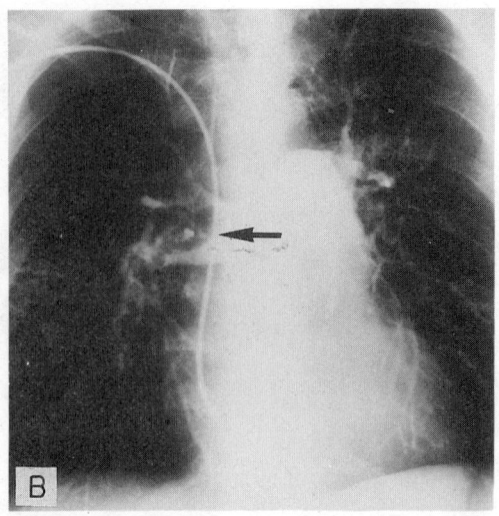

Fig. 54.11. Pulmonary angiograms of patients with acute massive pulmonary embolism (A) and subacute massive pulmonary embolism (B). The angiographic appearances are similar, particularly with respect to the large embolus in the main right pulmonary artery in both cases, despite the very different clinical presentation and haemodynamics. The patient with acute massive pulmonary embolism (A) presented with sudden collapse and a pulmonary artery pressure of 45/20 mmHg; the patient with subacute massive pulmonary embolism (B) presented with 4 weeks' increasing dyspnoea and a pulmonary artery pressure of 85/50 mmHg.

accepting some degree of uncertainty. Outside the USA, the use of angiography to resolve moderate degrees of doubt is not practicable because medical resources are limited and the disease is common. If the degree of doubt is very high or there are other reasons why the diagnosis must be confirmed beyond doubt, for example, when the risks from anticoagulation are higher than normal or when suspected recurrent emboli have led to frequent admissions to hospital often in the absence of any firm evidence of thrombo-embolic disease, the patient should be transferred to a centre where angiography can be performed.

Some authorities have recently advocated strongly the more widespread use of pulmonary angiography,[49] but the value of such an expensive approach is dubious and may have little or no advantage over accepting moderate degrees of doubt and only using angiography in particularly difficult cases.

The diagnosis of chronic thrombo-embolic pulmonary hypertension is usually suggested by a history of progressive dyspnoea and the physical signs of severe pulmonary hypertension, which is also apparent from the electrocardiogram and chest X-ray. The lung scan always shows multiple perfusion defects and normal ventilation, but this does not invariably differentiate it from other causes of severe pulmonary hypertension and angiography

may be necessary (see section on primary pulmonary hypertension).

DIFFERENTIAL DIAGNOSIS

The differential diagnosis is wide.[50] That of acute minor pulmonary embolism consists of all forms of acute respiratory illness that can lead to any combination of pleuritic pain, fever, haemoptysis and dyspnoea; that of acute massive pulmonary embolism includes all conditions that can lead to acute circulatory collapse particularly if they are likely also to cause acute dyspnoea. The conditions that have to be differentiated from subacute massive pulmonary embolism are those that lead to exertional dyspnoea that develops over a few weeks. The most important are cardiac failure and respiratory conditions, such as chronic obstructive airways disease, asthma and fibrosing alveolitis. Rarely, acute pulmonary embolism can produce either pulmonary oedema or bronchospasm which can make diagnosis very difficult.

The differential diagnosis of chronic thrombo-embolic pulmonary hypertension (CTPHT) includes all causes of severe pulmonary hypertension, the most frequent of which are listed in Table 54.6. The most important distinctions are from primary pulmonary hypertension and cor pulmonale.

Distinction from primary pulmonary hyperten-

Table 54.6. Causes of severe pulmonary hypertension.

Cor pulmonale (see Chapter 55)
Chronic thrombo-embolic pulmonary hypertension (CTPHT)
Primary pulmonary hypertension
Pulmonary veno-occlusive disease
Eisenmenger's syndrome
Left heart lesions: mitral valve disease
                    occasionally left ventricular disease
Collagen vascular and allied diseases
Parasites—Schistosoma
Drug induced: Aminorex
              (other appetite suppressants)
              part of 'toxic cooking oil sydrome'
Associated with portal hypertension

sion is discussed below; perhaps the most useful means of achieving this is by lung scanning. The lung scan is nearly always normal or near normal in primary pulmonary hypertension and shows gross widespread perfusion defects with normal ventilation in CTPHT. CTPHT is usually easily distinguished from cor pulmonale by lung function tests (see above). Spirometry and lung volumes are grossly abnormal when airways obstruction is the cause of cor pulmonale; when parenchymal lung disease is the cause, the transfer factor for carbon monoxide is greatly reduced. Spirometry, lung volumes and transfer factor are all normal or only moderately disturbed in CTPHT.

Occasionally, another important distinction has to be made: that from a primary cardiac disorder which has caused severe pulmonary hypertension but in which there are no obvious features pointing to the true diagnosis. The condition most likely to cause such confusion is severe mitral stenosis, which can occasionally occur without either murmurs or obvious pulmonary congestion. More rarely, an atrial septal defect with pulmonary hypertension can produce a similar clinical picture. The echocardiogram will always identify mitral valve disease and will usually identify atrial septal defects.

NATURAL HISTORY AND PROGNOSIS

Minor pulmonary embolism

The early mortality of treated minor pulmonary embolism is extremely low, although in all large series a small number of patients succumb to recurrent large emboli or to haemorrhage due to anticoagulant therapy;[51,52] mortality is usually about 10%. The major risk in the short term is the occurrence of further emboli soon after the initial one. There is very little information about the risk of recurrence in untreated patients, but the original study of Barrit and Jordan[53] showed a recurrence rate in the untreated control group of 35%. This risk is reduced substantially by adequate anticoagulant therapy. Multiple small recurrent emboli occurring for several weeks after the initial episode may cause subacute massive pulmonary embolism, but this is rare.

The long-term prognosis in minor pulmonary embolism is excellent. Once the patient has recovered from the initial event, the normal outcome is complete recovery without any late sequelae. Recurrent emboli months or years after the initial episode are uncommon[25] (the risk is about 0.5% per annum), particularly if the risk factor leading to the initial episode was well defined and transient. The absence of a well-defined risk factor suggests an adverse prognosis because both recurrent pulmonary embolism and occult malignancy are more frequent in such patients.[54] If late recurrence does occur, there is often an identifiable risk factor. These patients often recover completely from the recurrence, but occasionally there is progressive obstruction to the pulmonary circulation that does not resolve after every episode and leads to chronic thrombo-embolic pulmonary hypertension.

Major pulmonary embolism: acute and subacute massive

In the short term, there are several possible outcomes in acute massive pulmonary embolism. Most of the deaths resulting from the initial haemodynamic insult occur either immediately or within a few hours. Those who have such massive obstruction of the pulmonary arteries that cardiac arrest occurs at or soon after onset are unlikely to respond to treatment, but a few can be resuscitated probably because external cardiac massage breaks up clot in the pulmonary arteries, or moves it more peripherally where it obstructs less of the total cross-sectional area of the pulmonary bed. A few patients survive the initial insult but they have profound hypotension which persists and leads to death as long as 24 or 48 h later unless effective treatment is instituted.[55] The patients who survive the initial insult without such severe collapse usually recover over several days without therapy but then run an extremely high risk of a recurrent embolus which often proves fatal.[53] In this group of patients, the main aim of therapy is to prevent further emboli.

In the majority of patients who survive the initial

illness, the long-term prognosis is good.[56,57] As with minor pulmonary embolism, there is a small risk of recurrence particularly if there is a chronic predisposing factor or the patient enters another high-risk situation, for example, further surgery. Chronic thrombo-embolic pulmonary hypertension does not occur as a long-term sequel, irrespective of whether the pulmonary circulation was cleared by surgery or thrombolysis at the time of the initial embolus, except in a very small number of patients. These patients can be recognized at an early stage (2–3 months after the initial event) because their pulmonary artery pressure remains elevated (mean > 30 mmHg), rather than returning to normal, or near normal, as is usual in the vast majority of patients.[58] A few patients with a particularly strong predisposing factor, usually malignant disease, have frequent recurrent emboli despite therapy.

The situation in subacute massive pulmonary embolism is slightly different but, as with the acute forms of the disease, recurrent embolism remains the most important factor influencing the outcome in both the short and the long term. If recurrence occurs early, it may lead to sudden collapse and death or to an exacerbation of dyspnoea and right heart failure. As the individual episodes of embolism are often not distinguishable in this condition it is frequently impossible to be sure that deterioration is the result of a further embolus or simply progressive failure of the right ventricle in the face of an impossible load. There are no data on the natural history of untreated subacute massive pulmonary embolism; even with therapy, it has a high (> 20%) early mortality.[24] Little is known about the long-term prognosis. The results of the only studies that have been performed suggest that if the patient survives the initial episode the outcome is usually good but that chronic thrombo-embolic pulmonary hypertension, although uncommon, may occur.[58] As in other forms of the disease, this risk can be predicated with some accuracy by measuring the pulmonary artery pressure 2–3 months after the onset of the illness. If the mean pulmonary artery pressure is still > 30 mmHg, the risk of chronic thrombo-embolic pulmonary hypertension occurring is high.[58]

Chronic thrombo-embolic pulmonary hypertension

The natural history is one of steady deterioration with worsening right heart failure and cyanosis despite all attempts at therapy, and death usually occurs within a few years of diagnosis.[25] Occa-

sionally, longer survival is seen and there are a few celebrated cases in the literature which are purported to show recovery on long-term anticoagulation.[59,60] but this situation must be regarded as extremely unusual.

TREATMENT

A scheme for the treatment of pulmonary embolism is given in Fig. 54.12, and problems related to therapy have been critically reviewed.[52]

General measures

Patients who are in pain should receive adequate analgesia. If the pain is severe and circulatory embarrassment is only mild, opiates are appropriate, but they should be used with care in the hypotensive patient. If there is hypoxaemia, oxygen in high concentration should be given by face mask. When the cardiac output is reduced, the dilated right ventricle is hypoxic and already near-maximally stimulated by the high level of endogenous catecholamines; it is unlikely to respond to inotropic agents, which may do no more than precipitate arrhythmias. The right atrial pressure should be allowed to remain at a high level (normally 15–20 mmHg) which is necessary if the failing right ventricle is to maintain its output; if the right atrial pressure falls for any reason (e.g. dehydration or bleeding), administration of fluid while monitoring venous pressure may be helpful. Diuretics and vasodilators should be avoided at all times.

Heparin

Heparin is the mainstay of treatment both before the diagnosis has been established and for all patients who do not have severe circulatory embarrassment. The evidence that heparin substantially reduces mortality is good;[53] this is achieved almost entirely by preventing recurrent pulmonary embolism thereby allowing the patient's native thrombolytic mechanisms to destroy the thrombus in the pulmonary arteries. Although heparin has been available for 50 years, there are still some fundamental doubts about the best ways to use it. Dispute continues over whether it should be given by continuous infusion or as intermittent boluses. There is little to choose between the two methods: although haemorrhage may be slightly more common with the bolus technique, this is offset by the

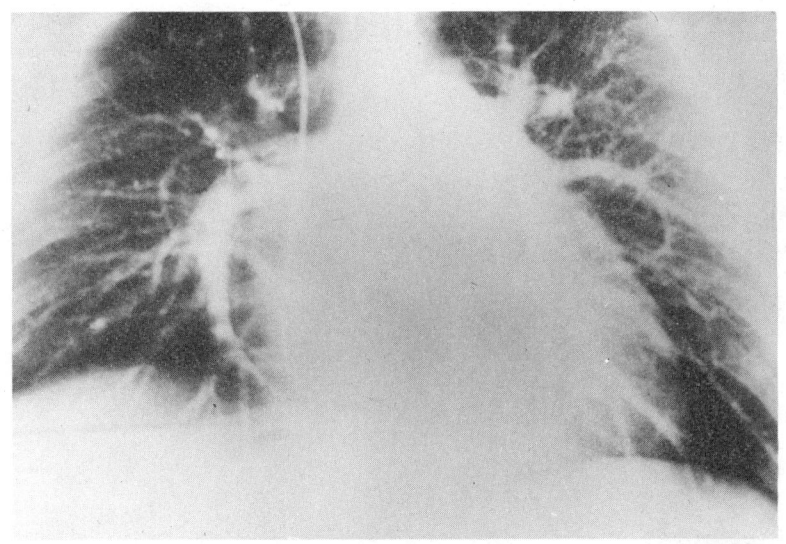

Fig. 54.14. The same patient as shown in Fig. 54.13 following 24 hours' therapy with streptokinase (600 000 units loading dose and 100 000 units per hour following that). Note the considerable improvement of flow to the right lung.

without a loading dose. Immediate heparinization can cause gross over-anticoagulation.

Conventional thrombolytic therapy is effective only when the clot to be lysed is fairly fresh. Once 1 or 2 weeks have passed, the clot contains little or no plasminogen and will not lyse, which explains the disappointing results obtained in patients with subacute massive pulmonary embolism, since the thrombus in these patients is often much older than this. The use of streptokinase, preceded by the infusion of plasminogen to prime the clot for lysis, has been shown to be more effective than streptokinase alone in this situation (Fig. 54.15).[66]

Embolectomy

Pulmonary embolectomy is rarely undertaken for the treatment of acute massive pulmonary embolism although it did enjoy a vogue during the 1970s. The main reason for this is the excellent results obtained in severely ill patients with thrombolytic agents. Emergency embolectomy can be carried out with success only by experienced cardiac surgeons in specialized centres where cardiopulmonary bypass is available. Under these circumstances, the operative mortality is low ($< 10\%$)[63] unless the patient is completely moribund and receiving cardiac massage at the time that the chest is opened; even then, survivors have been reported.[63] Occasional patients are encountered in whom embolectomy is the correct treatment: either those with severe acute massive pulmonary embolism and a strong contra-indication to thrombolytic therapy or those who continue to deteriorate despite thrombolytic agents. The modified Trendelenburg opera-

tion of embolectomy without bypass is rarely successful. Embolectomy employing special catheters, usually inserted via cutdown in the femoral vein, has been used successfully,[67] but such expertise is not widely available and this procedure is rarely indicated.

Embolectomy has also been used in patients with chronic obstruction of the pulmonary arteries and although success has been reported the results are often disappointing.

Oral anticoagulants

Oral anticoagulants have no role in the immediate treatment of pulmonary embolism. Their effectiveness in preventing recurrence is well established and the results of several studies suggest that they should be given for at least 12 weeks following a major thrombo-embolic episode.[68,69] After this time, they can be stopped in most patients. Certain groups of patients require prolonged or even indefinite treatment, including patients with subacute massive pulmonary embolism, particularly when there is no obvious predisposing factor, patients with proven recurrence of either pulmonary embolism or deep vein thrombosis and patients who have chronic thrombo-embolic pulmonary hypertension. The dose should be controlled so that an adequate degree of anticoagulation is maintained; this requires that whatever measure of anticoagulation used (e.g. INR or BCR) is maintained at about 3 times control. The risk of haemorrhage is always present and with long-term therapy the cumulative risk is not inconsiderable. Other side-effects are rare but the wide range of

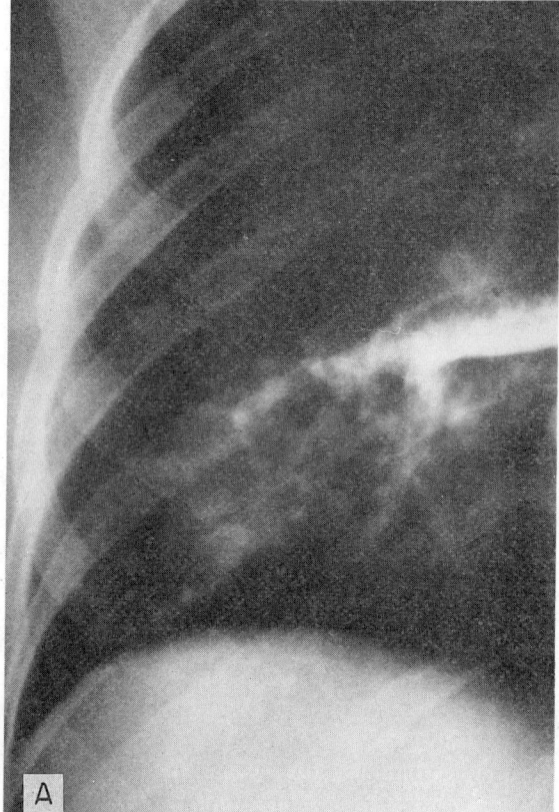 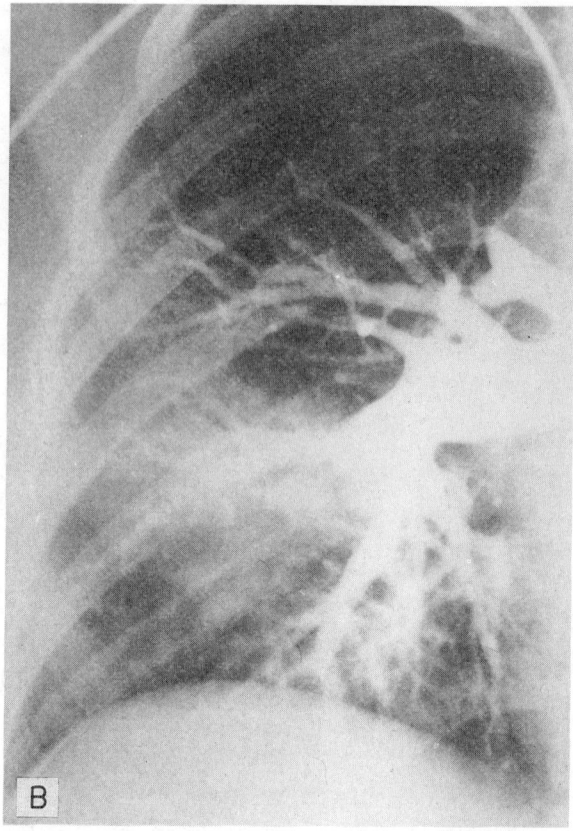

Fig. 54.15. (A) The right pulmonary artery following 48 h of streptokinase therapy in a patient with subacute massive pulmonary embolism. (B) The same vessel immediately after 24 h of combined therapy with streptokinase and plasminogen.

interactions with other drugs should never be forgotten. Perhaps the most common interaction that causes problems is with broad spectrum antibiotics most of which can lead to sudden over-anticoagulation by killing the natural gut flora which are an important natural source of vitamin K.

Low-dose heparin

Low-dose heparin has no place in the management of acute pulmonary embolism because it works by preventing the activation of the coagulation cascade, an event that has already occurred in such patients. It may sometimes be an alternative to the use of oral anticoagulants for preventing recurrent pulmonary embolism after the initial episode[68] has been successfully treated, although there is evidence that it is less effective than the use of coumadin derivatives. Its main use is the prophylaxis of deep vein thrombosis and pulmonary embolism.

Venous interrruption

The use of these procedures has an extremely marked geographical variation: they are widely applied in some centres in the USA whereas they are hardly used in Europe. All these procedures carry a risk of mortality, for example, ligation of the inferior vena cava 15%, plication of the inferior vena cava 7%, and percutaneous insertion of devices in the inferior vena cava 3% and of late complications, of which the severe oedema of the lower limbs associated with ligation of the inferior vena cava is the worst.[70] Devices placed in the inferior vena cava may migrate within and outside the venous system, and pulmonary emboli, either passing through or around the therapeutic obstruction or originating proximally, have been reported with all these measures.[71,72] There is no evidence that they have any advantages for routine prophylaxis following an acute pulmonary embolus because the incidence of recurrence with anticoagulation alone is so low. Their place is in the rare case in which anticoagulation alone fails or when adequate anticoagulation is strongly contra-indicated. Nowadays the method of choice is the pervenous placement of a filter in the inferior vena cava; this technique requires a high degree of skill and it should be attempted by only experienced interventional radiologists or cardiologists.

PROPHYLAXIS OF PULMONARY EMBOLISM

Prophylaxis has received an enormous amount of attention, but the best methods to achieve it remain a matter of dispute. One measure agreed to be simple and effective is early ambulation although it is not well proved scientifically. Once this measure alone has been taken, the incidence of fatal pulmonary embolism is very small. In the low- and average-risk groups, in which measures such as prophylactic low-dose heparin (alone or combined with graded compression stockings) have been shown to reduce the incidence of deep vein thrombosis and possibly that of fatal pulmonary embolism[3,8,73] many thousands of patients have to be treated to prevent one fatality. This type of marginally beneficial but expensive management must be viewed in the overall context of limited health-care resources.

In high-risk patients, among whom those under-going emergency orthopaedic surgery for fractures of the femur probably constitute those with the highest risk because of the combination of trauma quickly followed by surgery, the effectiveness of these measures in preventing pulmonary embolism has not been established despite extensive investigation. This is probably because the clotting cascade has been activated long before the patient reaches medical attention.

A reasonable attitude to adopt at present is to give prophylactic low-dose heparin to patients in the intermediae-risk group, for example, those about to undergo pelvic surgery and planned major orthopaedic surgery, but to withhold it in patients about to undergo other types of planned surgery. In emergency orthopaedic surgery, low-dose heparin is probably pointless although unlikely to do any harm and clinicians hold differing views about its use. In these patients, any suggestion of thrombo-embolism should be treated early and energetically with heparin *in full doses* followed by oral anti-coagulants. The value of other measures, such as anti-embolism stockings alone and devices for maintaining the calf blood flow during surgery is unproven, although firm compressive stockings give symptomatic relief and reduce swelling in patients with severe deep vein thrombosis.

Low-dose heparin is often used in medical patients judged to be at high risk, for example, those with cardiac failure, myocardial infarction or neo-plastic disease who are likely to be immobilized for some time, but there is little or no definitive evidence that it reduces the incidence of fatal pulmonary embolism.

PARADOXICAL EMBOLISM

If an embolus originating in the venous system manages to bypass the lungs, usually via a pre-existing congenital right-to-left shunt, the patient presents with symptoms and signs of systemic embolization. Passage to the left side of the circulation can also occur through communications between the atria[75] which, under normal circumstances, allow either a left-to-right shunt (atrial septal defect) or no shunt at all (patent foramen ovale, present in 5–10% of the population). Para-doxical embolization usually occurs in these circumstances once a prior pulmonary embolus has raised the right atrial pressure thus encouraging right-to-left flow through the interatrial communication.

Although paradoxical embolism is thought to be rare, some workers have suggested that this is only because the possibility is not considered.[22] Treatment is aimed mainly at preventing recurrence. Although it has been suggested that venous interruption is essential,[22,76,77] it is probable that heparin followed by long-term oral anticoagulants is just as effective in most cases. Initial therapy should be cautious. Thrombolytic agents must be avoided if there has been cerebral infarction; under these circumstances, pulmonary embolectomy may be needed if the circulatory effects of the pulmonary embolism are overwhelming. Heparinization is usually safe when cerebral embolism has occurred as long as the usual guidelines for treating any cerebral embolism are followed. If the patient cannot be heparinized, some form of venous inter-ruption should be undertaken (see above).

NON-THROMBOTIC PULMONARY EMBOLISM

A wide variety of substances can occasionally embolize to the lungs and some may produce a characteristic clinical picture.

Fat embolism

Major trauma, usually to the large bones of the leg, the pelvis and soft tissues, may force fat droplets, mainly from the marrow, and some marrow tissue into the blood. Some of this fat may aggregate with red cells, platelets and fibrin to form larger particles and some passes through the lungs so that there is obstruction of both the systemic and pulmonary circulations. The clinical effects are very variable.[78] More than 50% of patients experiencing major trauma have some evidence of fat embolism in the form of a mildly reduced Pao_2. More severe problems occur in 1–5% of trauma patients. Occasionally, the onset is so acute that it occurs within minutes or hours of injury causing unconsciousness, cerebral irritation, profound hypoxemia and acute right heart failure. More often, the onset is delayed for 1–6 days and the main features are fever, tachycardia, coagulation abnormalities combined with evidence of pulmonary and systemic embolization. In the pulmonary circulation, this causes acute right heart failure and reduced cardiac output; pulmonary oedema also occurs as a result of the irritant effects of the fat droplets. The latter in combination with altered pulmonary perfusion causes severe hypoxaemia. The systemic effects are most marked in the cerebral circulation causing cerebral irritation, altered levels of consciousness and convulsions. Petechiae are common, occurring in 25% of case.

Diagnosis depends on a high index of suspicion and exclusion of other important causes of hypoxaemia, right heart failure, reduced cardiac output and disturbed cerebral function. There are no specific tests, but fat in the sputum is consistent with the diagnosis. Therapy is supportive and includes artificial ventilation with positive end-expiratory respiration and a high Fio_2, inotropes, diuretics, etc.

Amniotic fluid embolism

This rare complication should be suspected if sudden cardiorespiratory collapse occurs during labour or soon after.[79] Amniotic fluid as well as fragments of trophoblast and decidual tissue are forced into the circulation by the vigorously contracting uterus and lodge in the lungs causing a syndrome that closely resembles acute massive pulmonary embolism. Treatment is to support the circulation and ventilation as well as possible; there is no effective specific therapy and the mortality is very high (> 80%). Patients who survive the initial event nearly always develop disseminated intravascular coagulation and may develop pulmonary oedema and the adult respiratory distress syndrome.

Air embolism

Air may be introduced into the venous system following trauma to the great veins usually in the neck, as a complication of central venous catheterization[80] and as a complication of a wide variety of surgical procedures, of which neurosurgery performed with the patient in the sitting position perhaps carries the highest risk. Air can enter both the venous and arterial sides of the circulation as the result of penetrating lung trauma,[81] when it may gain access to both bronchial and pulmonary veins. Air may also get into the arterial system as a complication of cardiac surgery, during angiographic procedures in the arterial side of the circulation or in combination with venous air embolism, either by traversing the pulmonary bed[82] or by crossing into the arterial side via a communication such as an atrial septal defect or a patent foramen ovale. Air may also complicate any diagnostic technique that involves the insufflation of gas or air and attempts to speed the rate of intravenous infusion with pressure devices.

When air enters the venous system in any quantity, its most damaging effect is to obstruct the pulmonary circulation, which leads to sudden cardiovascular collapse combined with sudden severe dyspnoea and hypoxaemia due to the sudden reduction of pulmonary perfusion. On examination, the patient is collapsed and dyspnoeic and a loud sucking sound, in time with the cardiac cycle, may be heard without the aid of a stethoscope; on auscultation over the precordium, there is a churnng sound said to resemble the sound of a mill wheel. When air enters the arterial system, some usually finds its way to the cerebral circulation and this results in the main features of sudden confusion, convulsions and loss of consciousness. Often, when air gains access via the venous side of the circulation, the features of pulmonary obstruction are coupled with those of cerebral disturbance because some air gets through to the systemic side of the circulation.

Diagnosis of air embolism depends on an awareness of the possibility, particularly in patients with trauma to the chest and neck who show a degree of collapse out of proportion to their injuries. Although a chest X-ray taken in the left lateral position may show an air–fluid level within the right ventricle and echocardiography can demonstrate the presence of air in the right ventricle, obtaining these investigations is likely to lead to delay which may prove to be fatal. Treatment must be immediate. Placing the patient on the left side with the head down may displace the bubble of air obstructing the right ventricular outflow tract and will also discourage air from entering the cerebral circulation. Attempts should then be made to remove air from the right side of the heart either with a central venous line, Swan–Ganz catheter, direct percutaneous needle puncture of the right ventricle or cardiopulmonary bypass if necessary. Even with prompt treatment, this condition has a mortality that can be as high as 50%, and survivors often have neurological defects.

Septic emboli and infarction

In normal individuals, septic emboli are uncommon. They may sometimes occur as part of pyaemia secondary to serious infection elsewhere, most often in the pelvis or abdomen, for example, an appendix abscess for an abscess associated with diverticular disease or prostatic infection. Infections at these sites are often anaerobic and *Bacteroides* and anaerobic *Streptococci* seem to have a particular ability to invade veins to gain access to the circulation. There is often evidence of septicaemia, and the patient is frequently jaundiced because of hepatic involvement. In the lungs, the septic emboli tends to lodge in the periphery and the pathologist finds firm subpleural nodules. The chest X-ray shows multiple opacities, which can be well defined or rather diffuse, and these may often cavitate.[83] The patient has a mixture of symptoms and signs suggesting both severe infection within the chest and pulmonary arterial obstruction of a variable degree. Sometimes, the infected emboli are large and can reproduce all the features of massive pulmonary embolism, but generally the picture is dominated by the infection and pleurisy. Purulent sputum with or without blood may be expectorated, and when the infection is anaerobic the sputum is 'putrid'.

Very occasionally, septic emboli are secondary to endocarditis either on a ventricular septal defect, when the left-to-right shunt carries the infected material from the defect into the lungs, or on the tricuspid or pulmonary valves. Whether this leads to infection and abscess formation within the lung will depend on the organism involved, for example,

it is unlikely if *Streptococcus viridans* is the infecting organism whereas abscess formation is frequent if the infecting agent is *Staphylococcus aureus*. Lung abscesses are particularly common as a complication of the right-sided endocarditis that occurs in intravenous drug abusers because it is usually due to virulent organisms. This group of patients are also at risk from septic pulmonary embolism originating from septic thrombophlebitis occurring at drug injection sites. Similarly, septic emboli may originate from indwelling venous devices often used to administer cytotoxic therapy to patients with malignant disease who often have the added disadvantage of being immunosuppressed. A small percentage of initially sterile pulmonary infarcts become infected (< 5%). These patients have persistant fever following their infarct and expectorate a mixture of blood and purulent sputum. The lesion may cavitate. Occasionally, *uninfected areas* of infarction may be very persistent and eventually break down leading to the expectoration of large quantities of blood and necrotic material with subsequent cavity formation.

Pulmonary complications of lymphangiography

The oily contrast material used for lymphangiograms sometimes embolizes to the lungs.[84] Reactions to this are usually minor with transient dyspnoea, cough or chest discomfort. A more severe reaction with pulmonary oedema, which may be haemorrhagic, fever and even pulmonary infarction may occur very occasionally.[85] The chest X-ray may show a ground-glass appearance and the transfer factor for carbon monoxide is significantly reduced. Hypoxaemia occurs. The clinical picture usually settles spontaneously over a few days.

Talc embolism

Intravenous drug abusers often inject agents that have been diluted and adulterated with inert particles such as talc. These particles lodge in the small vessels of the lungs and can cause a granulomatous reaction and lead to pulmonary hypertension.

PULMONARY VENO-OCCLUSIVE DISEASE

This is an extremely rare condition. It is of unknown aetiology, although a few cases have been reported in association with other clinical abnormalities including auto-immune disease, viral infection and bone-marrow transplantation, as well as in patients undergoing chemotherapy. It has an equal sex incidence and has been seen most often in children and young adults, although it has been reported in patients as old as 76 years. Many of its most important features have been well reviewed.[86]

PATHOLOGY

The lumen of almost all of the small pre- and intra-acinar veins are narrowed or occluded by loosely organized fibrous tissue. The anastomoses between the pulmonary and bronchial venous systems can also be affected. The obstruction to the small pulmonary veins causes the development of progressive and severe pulmonary hypertension. The pulmonary arteries may show medial hypertrophy, but the arterial lesions are mild when compared with those occurring in primary pulmonary hypertension. Interstitial fibrosis, pneumonia and pulmonary oedema may be extensive.

CLINICAL FEATURES

The main symptom is dyspnoea that steadily progresses in severity and may be associated with orthopnoea, paroxysmal nocturnal dyspnoea and syncope. The physical signs are those of pulmonary hypertension with associated crepitations in the lung fields of 50% of patients.

INVESTIGATIONS

Most cases have a severely reduced Pao_2 and a normal or reduced $Paco_2$. The chest X-ray shows changes of severe longstanding pulmonary hypertension identical to those seen in primary pulmonary hypertension, but in 50% of patients there are also changes that suggest the pulmonary venous pressure is elevated, e.g. pulmonary oedema and Kerley B lines. The electrocardiogram shows increasingly severe right ventricular hypertrophy as the condition advances. Lung scans are nearly always normal. Pulmonary angiography is normal apart from evidence of pulmonary artery dilatation due to the pulmonary hypertension, which often reaches the severity of that in primary pulmonary hypertension. The pulmonary artery wedge pressure is variable; it is usually normal but has been reported to be elevated in some cases. The interpretation of the wedge pressure in this condition is difficult because the disease may be patchy with vessels in some parts of the lung completely occluded while those elsewhere are narrowed or unaffected. The left atrial pressure is normal.

DIAGNOSIS

Diagnosis in life is difficult and can be achieved with certainty only by open lung biopsy. The clinical picture combined with all other tests cannot distinguish this condition from primary pulmonary hypertension unless there is additional evidence of a raised pulmonary venous pressure on the chest X-ray. If there is evidence of pulmonary oedema, with a normal left atrial pressure, it then has to be distinguished from the other rare conditions that may obstruct the pulmonary veins, including mediastinal fibrosis and congenital narrowing of the pulmonary veins.

CLINICAL COURSE

The clinical course is one of progressive deterioration with death usually occurring within 2 years. There is no effective therapy.

PULMONARY HYPERTENSION

There are many causes of pulmonary hypertension (Table 54.6). Pulmonary hypertension, other than that occurring as a result of lung and chest wall disease, proven pulmonary embolic disease, veno-occlusive disease, raised pressure in the left heart and intracardiac shunting, will be discussed in this section. It may be of unknown cause or occur as part of more widespread disease processes or very rarely as the result of ingestion of a toxic agent.

PULMONARY HYPERTENSION OF UNKNOWN AETIOLOGY AND PRIMARY PULMONARY HYPERTENSION

There are three main varieties of pulmonary hypertension of unknown aetiology but their classification is both confused and confusing.[87] Some authorities regard all three types as being primary pulmonary hypertension. This view was put forward in 1975 by a committee of the World Health Organisation,[88] which classified primary pulmonary hypertension into three main pathological types—primary plexogenic pulmonary arteriopathy, recurrent thrombo-embolism and pulmonary veno-occlusive disease (see above). In clinical practice, the term primary pulmonary hypertension is used in the way originally intended by Paul Wood to describe all cases of pulmonary hypertension of unknown aetiology other than those identified in life as due to recurrent thrombo-embolism or pulmonary veno-occlusive disease. About 70% of patients whose condition is defined in this way will have plexogenic arteriopathy (see below), and that of most of the remaining 30% has been attributed, on little evidence, to recurrent micro-emboli.[89] Very occasional patients clinically identified as having primary pulmonary hypertension are shown at post-mortem (or by open lung biopsy) to have pulmonary veno-occlusive disease.

Epidemiology

Primary pulmonary hypertension is a rare condition. It occurs most often in children and young adults and seems to be more frequent in the Indian subcontinent than elsewhere in the world. There is a female preponderance of about 1.7 to 1 which is seen in all age-groups.[103]

Pathology

Pulmonary vascular abnormalities

In primary pulmonary hypertension, all branches of the pulmonary arterial tree in both lungs are involved (Fig. 54.16). Extensive studies by Wagenvoort and Wagenvoort[89] have shown that the lesions in the muscular and more peripheral vessels in primary pulmonary hypertension are like those seen in patients with congenital heart disease and a left-to-right shunt: medial hypertrophy, cellular intimal proliferation and fibrosis, plexiform lesions, dilatation lesions and fibrinoid necrosis.[90] The lesions are usually more severe in primary pulmonary hypertension and the incidence of plexiform lesions, occluded arteries and dilatation lesions is higher.

Pulmonary arterial muscularity

The lungs of all patients with primary pulmonary hypertension show pulmonary arterial medial hypertrophy and the presence of muscle in smaller arteries than normal (extension) (Fig. 54.17). The length of the arterial pathways with the potential to vasoconstrict is thus increased. Examination of lung tissue taken at both thoracotomy and post-mortem shows markedly contracted peripheral pulmonary arteries with a crenulated internal elastic lamina.

Post-mortem studies have shown a close correlation between medial hypertrophy and morphometric estimation of vasoconstriction.[91] It has been suggested that medial hypertrophy is the result of prolonged and intense vasoconstriction in the muscular pulmonary arteries, and vasoconstriction is the primary event in the pathogenesis of plexogenic pulmonary arteriopathy.

At an early stage of the disease, the capillary basement membranes are thickened, widening the blood–gas barrier (Fig. 54.18). Smaller arteries are surrounded by circumferentially arranged collagen fibres, reticulum and pericytes.[92]

Intimal proliferation and fibrosis

Cellular intimal proliferation follows the development of medial hypertrophy. The overlying endothelial cells present an irregular pitted surface to the bloodstream which encourages entrapment of platelets and leucocytes (Fig. 54.19). Widespread concentric intimal proliferation (Fig. 54.20a and b) which later becomes fibrotic is characteristic of primary pulmonary hypertension as opposed to the eccentric intimal proliferation seen in thromboembolic pulmonary hypertension.

Thrombo-embolism can occur in longstanding areas of primary pulmonary hypertension. Of 110 cases of primary pulmonary hypertension, Wagenvoort and Wagenvoort[89] found multiple thrombotic or thrombo-embolic lesions in 6. With the development of obstructive intimal fibrosis, the media begins to atrophy. The media lying beneath areas of intimal fibrosis becomes thin and, in addition, the arteries distal to the obstructed segments become increasingly thin walled. These features may help to explain why in the early reports it was stated that pulmonary arterial wall thickness may be normal in primary pulmonary hypertension, a statement which has since been refuted by many investigators.[89,93] Eventually, long segments of thin-walled arteries form vein-like branches of hypertrophied muscular pulmonary arteries. These vessels become dilated and if large and tortuous they may compose an angiomatoid mass.

Fibrinoid necrosis

This abnormality occurs more commonly in primary pulmonary hypertension than in pulmonary hypertensive congenital heart disease (Fig. 54.20c). Circumstantial and experimental evidence suggests that fibrinoid necrosis may result from intense spastic vasoconstriction.[94] It is associated with

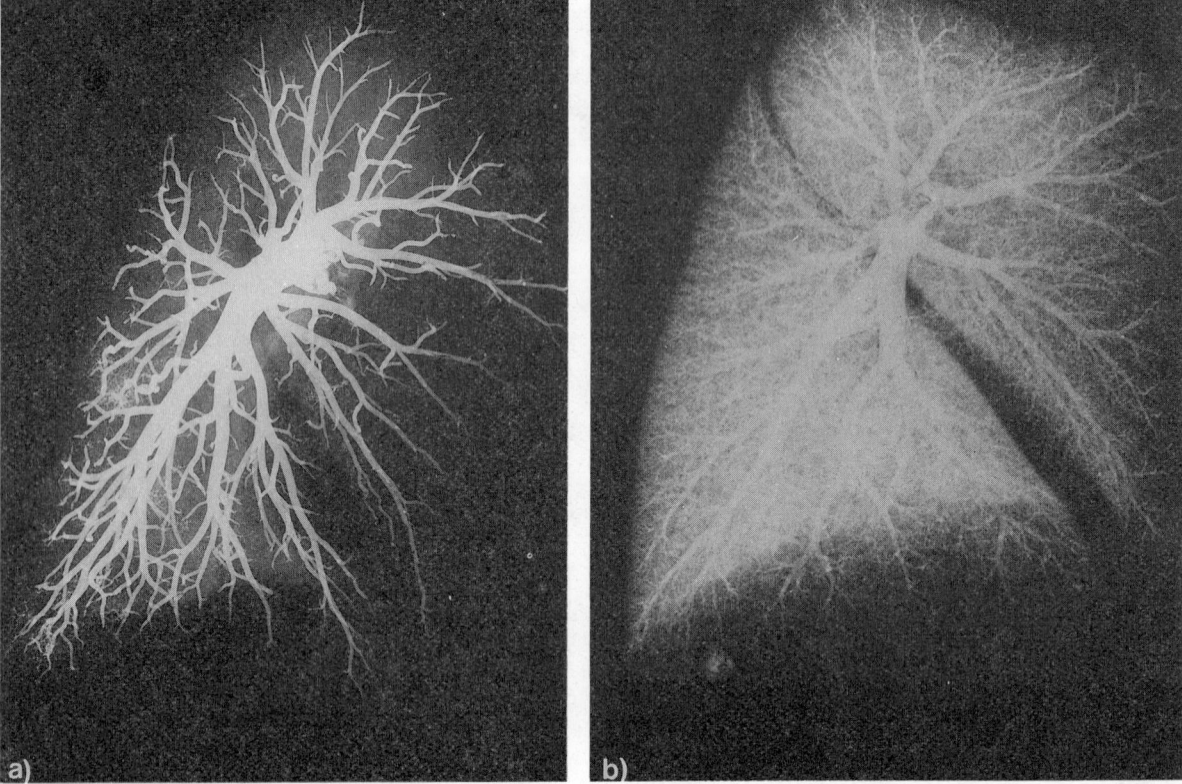

Fig. 54.16. Post-mortem arteriograms of (a) a case of primary pulmonary hypertension and (b) a normal lung, showing a uniform reduction in density of background haze throughout the lung in primary pulmonary hypertension and 'pruning' of the segmental pulmonary arteries and their branches (× 0.47).

severe pulmonary hypertension, where a high level of resting tone is thought to be present. In the laboratory, ingestion of the seeds of the plant *Crotalaria spectabilis* or the pyrrolizidine alkaloids derived from these seeds causes pulmonary hypertension in rats. Fibrin appears to be forced into the arterial wall by sustained constriction and the medial smooth muscle cells show a loss of myofilaments leading to necrosis.[94]

Plexiform lesions

Wagenvoort and Wagenvoort[89] found plexiform lesions in 70% of patients dying with primary pulmonary hypertension. Plexiform lesions occur in arteries of 100–200 μm in diameter. They are usually found in the branches of muscular arteries near their origin from the hypertrophied vessel (Fig. 54.21). When fully developed, a plexus of small channels fills the lumen of the dilated thin-walled muscular artery in which the media shows areas of

fibrinoid necrosis. The plexus consists of strands of proliferating intimal cells which may surround a fibrin clot. Distally, the plexus opens up into a dilated patent thin-walled channel. It is thought that the channels within the plexiform lesions become enlarged with time, as the strands of intimal cells become thinner, less cellular and more fibrous and the fibrin clot disappears. Plexiform lesions are believed to form in arteries affected by necrotizing arteritis.

In primary pulmonary hypertension, the pulmonary veins are usually normal. The pathological lesions seen in primary pulmonary hypertension are indistinguishable from those found in pulmonary hypertensive congenital heart disease and pulmonary hypertension due to appetite suppressants. The diagnosis of primary pulmonary hypertension is therefore one of exclusion.

In primary pulmonary hypertension, the pulmonary trunk and the extrapulmonary and intrapulmonary elastic arteries are usually dilated and

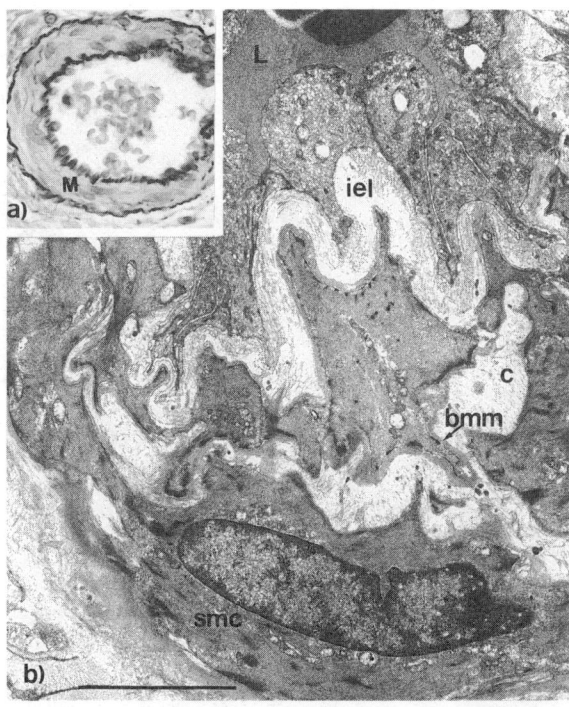

Fig. 54.17. (a) Photomicrograph showing pulmonary arterial medial hypertrophy. M, media (× 162.5). (b) Electron micrograph of a small muscular pulmonary artery showing crenulated internal elastic lamina (iel) and smooth muscle cells (smc) surrounded by a thick layer of basement membrane material (bmm) and widely separated by an increased amount of collagen (c). L, lumen. Bar scale = 5 μm.

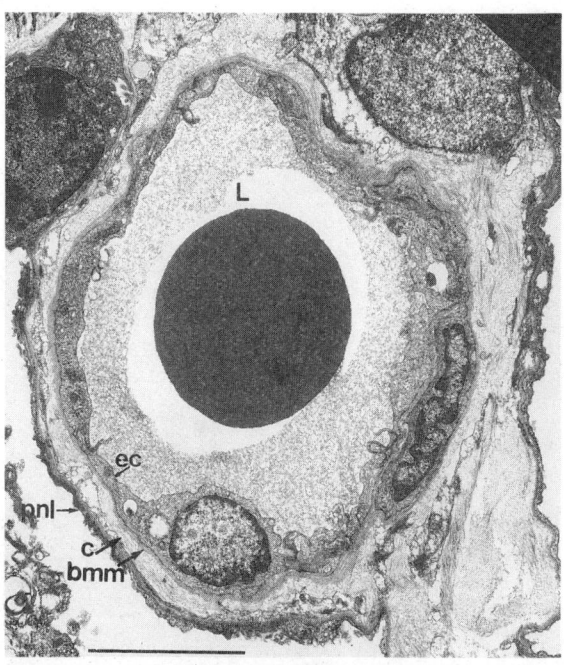

Fig. 54.18. Electronmicrograph of a capillary showing a blood-gas barrier thickened by collagen (c) and basement membrane material (bmm) between endothelial cell (ec) and type I pneumenocyte (pnl). L, lumen containing red blood cell. Bar scale = 5 μm.

abnormally thick walled. Saccular aneurysms can occur. Atherosclerosis is common. Cystic medial necrosis and partial rupture of the pulmonary trunk have been described.[95] The combination of dilated proximal pulmonary arteries and thick-walled obstructed peripheral vessels gives rise to the 'pruned tree' appearance seen on pulmonary angiography or post-mortem arteriography in longstanding cases of primary pulmonary hypertension (Figs 54.16 and 54.22). At autopsy, right ventricular hypertrophy is always present and may be very marked.

Differences in the pathological findings between adults and children

In a recent European study, pulmonary arterial medial hypertrophy was found to be of similar severity in children and adults, plexiform lesions occurred in 53% of children and 68% of adults, and the number of plexiform lesions per cm² of lung tissue was similar in both.[91] However, concentric lamina intimal fibrosis and medial atrophy were more common in adults. Thus, it appears that fibrinoid necrosis and plexiform lesions can precede

widespread fibrotic intimal occlusion as the first sign of irreversible pulmonary vascular disease, particularly in children. There is a high incidence of primary pulmonary hypertension in children living

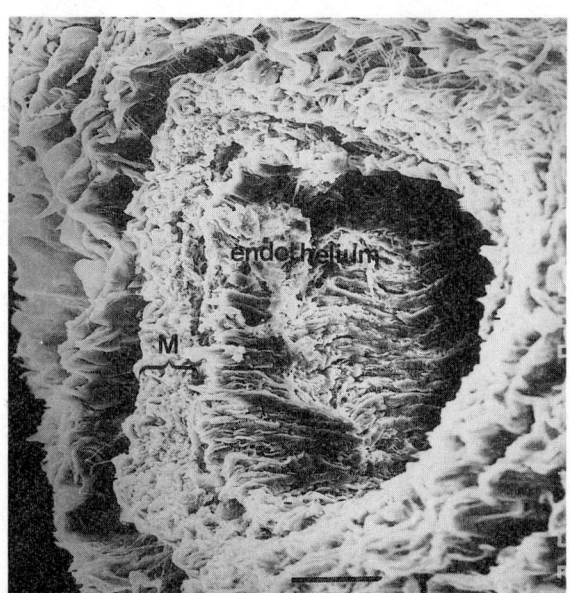

Fig. 54.19. Scanning electronmicrograph on small muscular pulmonary artery shwoing thick media (m) and damaged irregular endothelium. Bar scale = 100 μm.

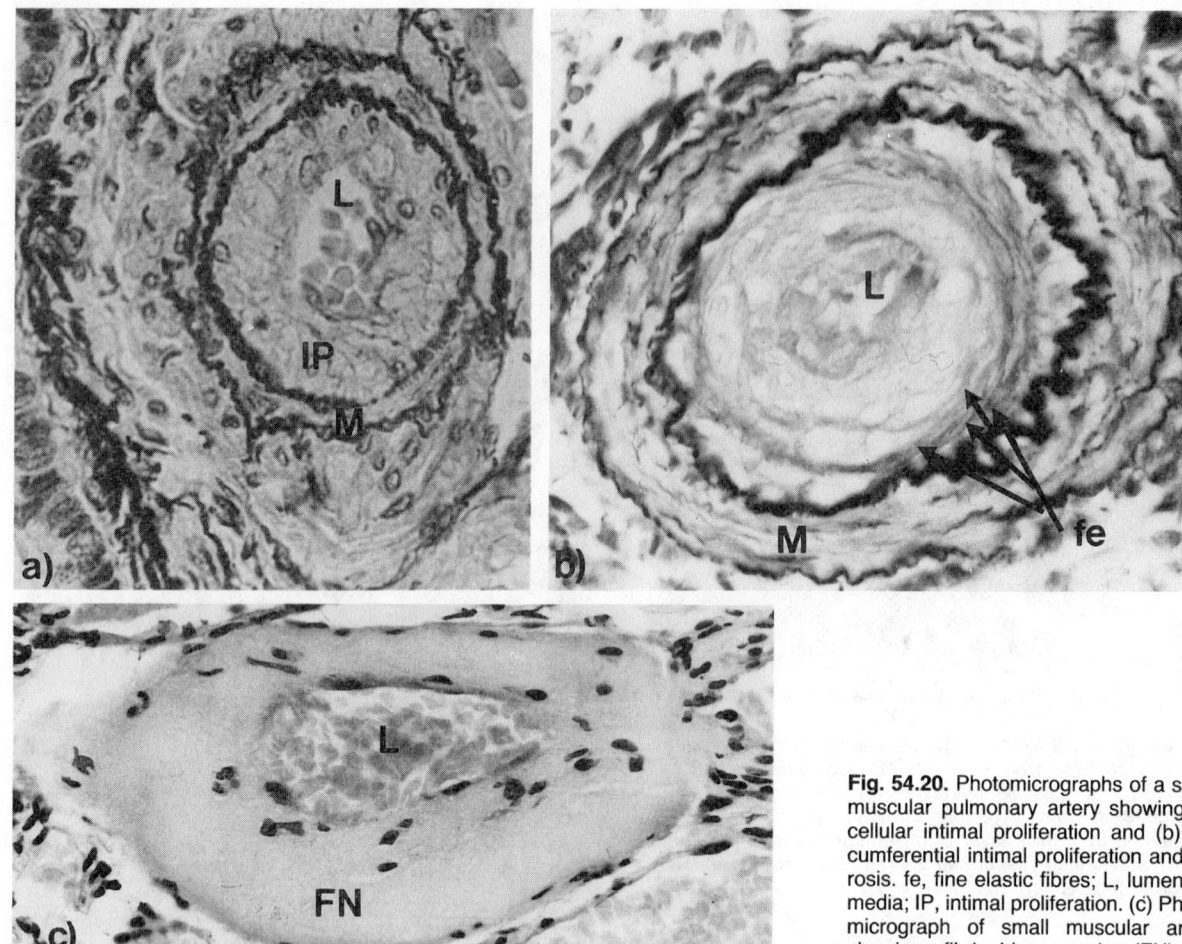

Fig. 54.20. Photomicrographs of a small muscular pulmonary artery showing (a) cellular intimal proliferation and (b) circumferential intimal proliferation and fibrosis. fe, fine elastic fibres; L, lumen; M, media; IP, intimal proliferation. (c) Photomicrograph of small muscular artery showing fibrinoid necrosis (FN) (× 332.5).

in the Indian subcontinent. The majority of children present in their late teenage years and die within 5 years of presentation. The pathological findings are those of an aggressive plexogenic pulmonary arteriopathy, often accompanied by an arteritis.

Correlation between pathological findings and clinical course

Implications for Management Severe pulmonary vascular obliterative disease is present in the majority of patients with primary pulmonary hypertension when they are first seen by a cardiologist. Pulmonary vascular resistance is markedly elevated, patients fail to respond satisfactorily to chronic vasodilator therapy and most die within 3 years of presentation. At autopsy, the pulmonary arteries show fibrotic occlusion, fibrinoid necrosis and plexiform lesions. Occasionally, however, patients die with potentially reversible pulmonary vascular disease,[96] which is particularly true of children. The medial hypertrophy and severe cellular intimal

proliferation which were the only lesions present in an 8-year-old child who died of right heart failure with a history of only 9 months are illustrated in Fig. 54.20a.[97] Thus, some patients with primary pulmonary hypertension die before the pulmonary vascular bed is completely destroyed. Also, patients with this disease occasionally show long-term clinical improvement and, rarely, the disease may regress.[96,98] Regression occurs more frequently in patients who have been taking an anorectic drug than in those in whom there is no identifiable precipitating cause.[99] These observations encourage a more aggressive therapeutic approach in which selected patients are treated with pulmonary vasodilator drugs in the expectation that this will reduce vasoconstriction and prevent the progression of pulmonary vascular disease. An open lung biopsy should help select suitable patients.[87] The biopsy must be taken at sufficient depth to include some of the small muscular pulmonary arteries in which intimal damage first develops.[100]

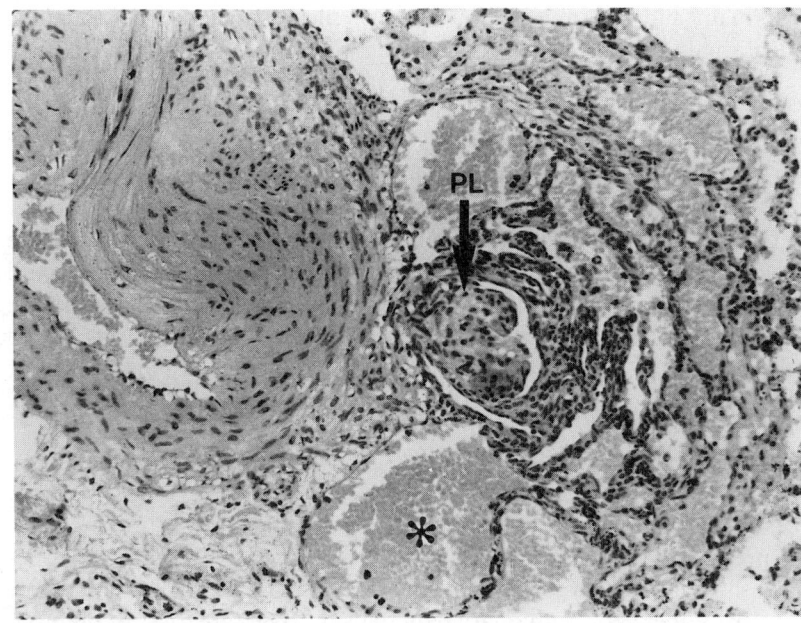

Fig. 54.21. Photomicrograph showing plexiform lesion (PL) in a branch of a muscular pulmonary artery, with dilated thin-walled vessel distal to the lesion (*) (× 70).

Pathophysiology

Obstruction to the pulmonary flow at the level of the small pulmonary arteries reduces cardiac output and leads to severe pulmonary hypertension. The pulmonary artery pressure rises markedly with exercise further impairing the output of the right heart; this may lead to hypotension and exertional syncope. As the disease advances, the right heart fails. Moderate hypoxaemia and hypocapnia are usual although the mechanisms of hypoxaemia are poorly understood.[32] Increased myocardial work and hypoxaemia may cause exertional angina.

Clinical features

The history is one of the insidious onset of exertional dyspnoea which worsens progressively and eventually becomes incapacitating.[96] There is often angina of effort, and exertional syncope may occur. Tiredness, often associated with exertion, is also prominent. The physical signs are those of severe pulmonary hypertension and cyanosis that becomes more prominent on exertion. If a patent foramen ovale is present, cyanosis is particularly marked because elevation of the right atrial pressure leads to right-to-left shunting through the defect. Eventually, right heart failure occurs, often with severe oedema and ascites; it is the commonest mode of death. Some patients do not reach this stage because sudden death occurs first.

Diagnosis

The diagnosis is one of exclusion: primary pulmonary hypertension is regarded as being present if no other cause for severe pulmonary hypertension can be found.

Investigation

Until the disease is advanced, the main changes on

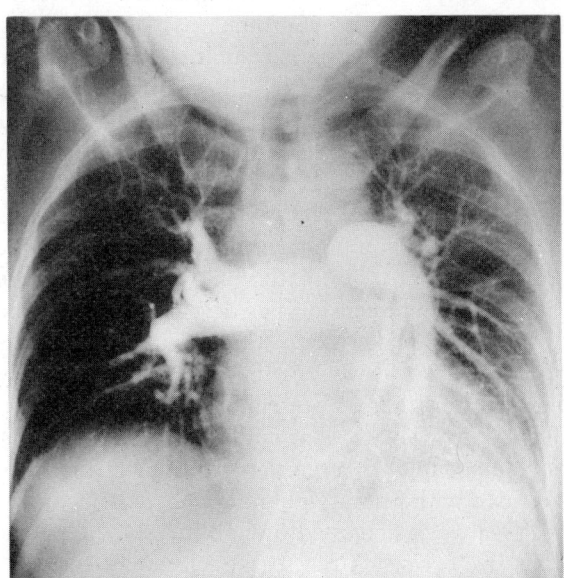

Fig. 54.22. Pulmonary angiogram from a patient with severe primary pulmonary hypertension. There are no filling defects but the vessels taper quickly and are 'pruned' in the peripheral lung field. There is moderate enlargement of the central pulmonary arteries.

the chest X-ray are enlargement of the main and central pulmonary arteries, with a normal or slightly enlarged cardiac shadow. It may be possible to discern 'pruning' of the peripheral pulmonary arteries, although this is an inconstant and difficult sign. Later, as right heart failure develops, the heart size increases. The electrocardiogram is usually grossly abnormal showing marked right ventricular and right atrial hypertrophy. The echocardiogram initially shows slight enlargement of the right ventricle, and increased thickness of its free wall may be seen. Later, the right ventricle enlarges considerably and the left ventricle, which is of normal size, seems to be compressed by it with the interventricular septum showing a flattened appearance. The pulmonary artery pressure can usually be measured non-invasively by the Doppler technique. The lung scan does not show the widespread large defects so characteristic of severe chronic thromboembolic pulmonary hypertension, and is either normal or slightly ragged in appearance.[96]

The arterial Po_2 is usually at least moderately reduced as is the arterial Pco_2. In a series of patients with primary pulmonary hypertension awaiting heart–lung transplantation the average arterial Po_2 was 72 mmHg (range 41–93) and the average arterial Pco_2 was 29 mmHg (range 25–35).[32] Simple spirometry and lung volumes are only slightly disturbed, and there is usually a moderate reduction in the diffusing capacity for carbon monoxide.[29,32] The mechanisms for hypoxaemia in primary pulmonary hypertension are only partly understood but may include reduced oxygen diffusion across thickened capillary basement membranes, minor ventilation/perfusion mismatch and possibly most importantly the oxygen saturation of the venous return may be so low that it cannot be completely oxygenated during its transit through the alveolar capillaries.[101]

The right ventricular systolic and the pulmonary arterial systolic and diastolic pressures are grossly elevated and quite often reach suprasystemic levels. When the disease is advanced and right ventricular failure ensues, the right ventricular end-diastolic and the right atrial pressures rise, and tricuspid regurgitation is common. The pulmonary artery wedge and left-sided intracardiac pressures are normal. Pulmonary angiography (Fig. 54.22) demonstrates dilatation of the large pulmonary arteries. The peripheral vessels appear smooth without filling defects but are narrower than normal towards the chest wall giving the characteristic 'pruned' appearance. Pulmonary arteriography is

not without risk in these patients and should be avoided if possible. The main problem is collapse caused by the vasodilator effects of the contrast material in a patient who has what is essentially a fixed cardiac output. The use of the newer non-ionic contrast media and reducing the volume of contrast to a minimum will decrease the risk but does not completely eliminate it. Occasionally, collapse occurs some hours after an invasive procedure and therefore close observation is required when the patient returns to the ward. It is quite acceptable to omit this investigation if the lung scan is normal or near normal, and there is no echocardiographic evidence of heart disease.

Differential diagnosis

Primary pulmonary hypertension has to be differentiated from other conditions that cause severe pulmonary hypertension. The rare cases of pulmonary hypertension that are possibly associated with the ingestion of a toxic substance can be differentiated only by the history (see below). Features of collagen vascular disease should be sought as should schistosomiasis in patients from areas where the disease is prevalent. Primary lung disease has to be excluded and this is usually achieved easily from clinical assessment and simple respiratory function testing. Sometimes it is difficult to exclude a left-to-right shunt, with severe pulmonary hypertension (Eisenmenger's syndrome), as the underlying cause in a child or young adult. Usually, a large ventricular septal defect, which usually produces no murmur, can be diagnosed from the second heart sound which is single and the echocardiogram which shows the defect. A patent ductus arteriosus, or an aortopulmonary window, causing the same situation is often more difficult to distinguish if the patient has not been seen in the phase before pulmonary hypertension has developed. Often, the only way to make this distinction is by angiography; however, in view of the risks of angiography and the fact that at present little or no effect on therapeutic policy it is usually best avoided. Conditions amenable to surgical correction that may be confused with primary pulmonary hypertension are nearly always suggested by non-invasive investigations (see below). Atrial septal defects presenting in adults do not produce diagnostic problems because the chest X-ray shows much more marked cardiomegaly than occurs in primary pulmonary hypertension and enormous central pulmonary arteries and the defect will usually be seen on the echocardiogram. Very occasionally, left heart lesions can have a clinical picture which is similar to primary pulmonary hypertension. The most important is mitral stenosis which may sometimes produce signs of only severe pulmonary hypertension and no murmurs. The chest X-ray and electrocardiogram usually suggest the left-sided origin of the problems, and ultrasound nearly always confirms the diagnosis. The rare congenital condition of cor triatriatum may behave in a similar fashion. The importance of distinguishing these conditions amenable to surgery from primary pulmonary hypertension is obvious.

Natural history and prognosis

Most patients have symptoms for 2–3 years before the diagnosis is made, and they die, usually from progressive right heart failure, a few years later (median 2.5 years).[96,102,103] Patients who already have evidence of right heart failure at the time of diagnosis, e.g. considerable elevation of the right atrial pressure, usually die within a few months whereas those without these signs may survive for 5 or more years.[102,103] Occasionally, sudden death occurs, particularly on exertion. Very rarely, the patient's clinical state remains stable over many years,[96] and a few cases of regression have been reported.[98]

Treatment

Treatment is unsatisfactory and there is no convincing evidence that medical therapy has any effect on the dismal outlook.[103] General advice to the patient should include avoiding strenuous exercise because the pulmonary artery pressure rises sharply on exercise and syncope or even death may occur. Similarly, pregnancy should be avoided; it is tolerated very poorly and death may occur either during the pregnancy or in labour. Sterilization may be advisable in some patients because of the risk. Some authorities recommend the use of digoxin to stimulate the flagging right heart. Diuretics often reduce dyspnoea, even before the onset of cardiac failure, although the reason for this is not clear. Oral anticoagulation is often used in the hope that it will slow the progression of the condition, either by preventing the recurrent micro-emobli, thought by some authorities to be important in the pathogenesis of some cases, or the large pulmonary emboli occurring secondary to the reduced cardiac output which might make the pulmonary hypertension

worse. Anticoagulation could also reduce thrombosis *in situ* in the diseased pulmonary vessels. Recently, a case of primary pulmonary hypertension, without plexiform lesions but with evidence of thrombosis in small pulmonary arteries on lung biopsy, has been reported which showed partial resolution when treated for 2.5 years with oral anticoagulants.[104] Treatment of primary pulmonary hypertension with vasodilators has been intensively investigated in recent years with generally disappointing results.[105–107] There is no agent that affects specifically the pulmonary vessels and not the systemic vessels. Among the agents that have been used are alpha-blockers, vasodilating antihypertensive agents, such as diazoxide, hydralazine and angiotensin converting enzyme inhibitors, and, more recently, the calcium channel blockers and prostacyclin.[108] Prostacyclin is very expensive and has to be given parenterally. There are reports of occasional resolution of primary pulmonary hypertension occurring at the same time as one of these agents has been administered. Nearly all these unusual cases have a mild form of the condition and it is not clear that there is a true therapeutic effect rather than spontaneous remission. The results of large studies have failed to show that vasodilator therapy produces any improvement in prognosis,[106] although some patients do obtain considerable symptomatic relief and therefore these agents should be tried in all patients. Perhaps the most generally successful agent at present is nifedipine.[103] Although in the past the acute effect of these agents on the pulmonary artery pressure and the pulmonary vascular resistance has been used as a guide to the choice of an agent for chronic use, this type of investigation is probably not necessary because there is no evidence that the results predict which patients will respond to chronic therapy.

Recently, the first really effective form of therapy has appeared in the form of heart–lung transplantation and initial results are encouraging.

COLLAGEN VASCULAR DISEASE

The pulmonary vasculature may become involved in most of the collagen vascular diseases, including polyarteritis nodosa, Wegener's syndrome, allergic vasculitis, Takayasu's disease, scleroderma, dermatomyositis, disseminated lupus erythematosus and rheumatoid arthritis. Often such involvement is minor and the involvement of the pulmonary circulation does not make much impact on the clinical picture. Occasionally, however, the patient

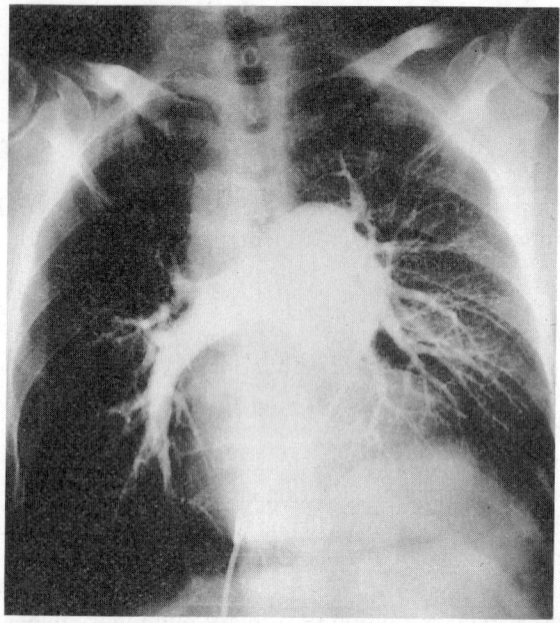

Fig. 54.23. Pulmonary angiogram of a patient with severe pulmonary hypertension complicating systemic sclerosis. There is gross peripheral 'pruning' of the arteries, similar but more pronounced than that seen in Fig. 54.22. There is gross enlargement of the central pulmonary arteries.

develops a syndrome that is clinically indistinguishable from primary pulmonary hypertension.[86] This situation is most often seen in scleroderma (Fig. 54.23) and Takayasu's disease (Fig. 54.24); in both, there is little or no response to therapy with corticosteroids. Suspicion of a link between scleroderma and primary pulmonary hypertension has been suggested on the basis of the very high incidence of Raynaud's phenomenon in patients with primary pulmonary hypertension (10–30%).[109]

Pathology

In polyarteritis nodosa, the lung vessels are involved as part of a generalized vasculitis, and bronchial as well as pulmonary arteries may be diseased. Polymorphonuclear cells and eosinophils infiltrate the arterial wall and the inflammation frequently extends into the surrounding lung tissue.[110] In the acute granulomatous type of disease, nodules develop in which there is a central zone of the fibrinoid material with foreign body giant cells, surrounded by a layer of radially arranged epithelioid cells. The incidence of pulmonary hypertension is low.

In Wegener's syndrome, the changes of polyarteritis nodosa may be widespread within the lungs. In the granulomatous form of the disease, the arteries and veins at the edges of the lesions are infiltrated and finally replaced by granulation tissue. Necrotizing arteritis is also seen in allergic vasculitis. In Takayasu's disease, infiltration of the pulmonary arteries by lymphocytes and histiocytes occasionally leads to pulmonary hypertension which may be severe.[111]

In scleroderma, the lung parenchyma rather than the blood vessels is primarily involved in the disease process, unlike the situation in polyarteritis nodosa. The alveolar walls become thickened by fibrosis and

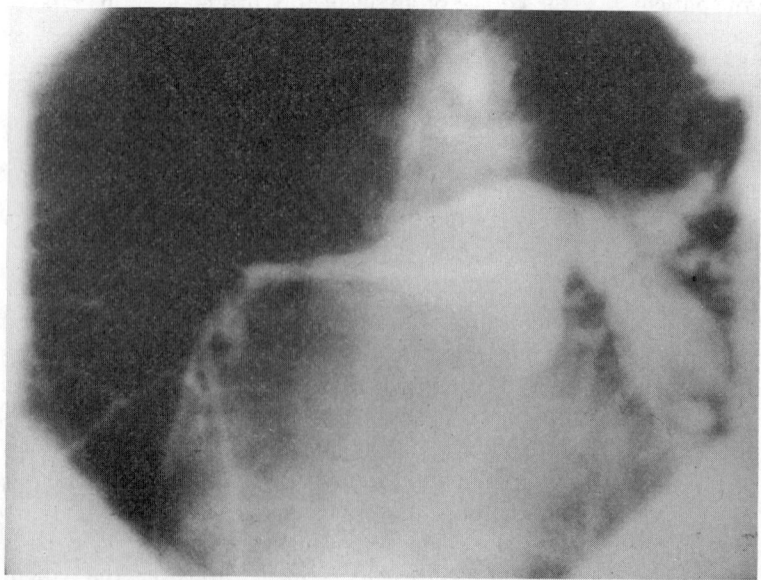

Fig. 54.24. Pulmonary angiogram of a patient with longstanding Takayasu's disease involving the aorta and its branches who developed right heart failure secondary to pulmonary hypertension. There is gross distortion of the arteries with both severe stenosis (right lung) and dilatation (left lung).

may rupture to produce cystic spaces. These changes may eventually lead to a 'honeycomb' lung, in which the outer regions of the lower lobes are particularly severely affected. Vascular changes accompany the parenchymal changes and are particularly severe in the most fibrotic parts of the lung. They may occasionally precede the parenchymal changes and cause pulmonary hypertension. Medial hypertrophy of small muscular pulmonary arteries, organization of thrombi and an increase in vein wall thickness occur, but vasculitis is uncommon. Lung involvement is less common in dermatomyositis than in scleroderma, but the structural abnormalities seen in the lung are similar.

In disseminated lupus erythematosus, pulmonary and or pleural involvement has been described in 50% of patients.[112,113] Fayemi described an acute and chronic form of arteritis.[113] The acute form is associated with fibrinoid necrosis, polymorphonuclear infiltration and a vasculitis. The chronic form is associated with medial hypertrophy and intimal fibrosis. The capillary basement membranes are thickened and the capillaries have the 'wire-loop' appearance of the glomerular capillaries in this condition. Immunohistochemical studies have demonstrated granular deposits of DNA, IgG and C3 complexes on the alveolar capillary basement membrane.[114]

A non-specific pulmonary arteritis is common in rheumatoid arthritis, and the bronchial arteries are also affected. Pulmonary hypertension has been reported. In pulmonary arteries 100–300 μm in diameter, the endothelial cells become separated from the intima by an oedema-filled space, and

intimal proliferation then develops which occludes the lumen. Perivascular fibrosis occurs as part of the fibrotic change occurring in the lung parenchyma surrounding the vessels.[114]

OTHER CAUSES OF PULMONARY HYPERTENSION

Involvement of the lung vasculature in schistosomiasis in any of its three types may lead to pulmonary hypertension, although the clinical picture is usually dominated by the gastro-intestinal, urinary and hepatic features of these conditions. Pulmonary hypertension, when it occurs, is probably multifactorial. Embolism of ova into the lungs obstructs vessels and these ova often lead to granulomatous lesions in the vessel walls or surrounding lung tissue (Fig. 54.25)[115] which may be the result of a delayed type of hypersensitivity.[116] The rare and poorly understood link of severe liver disease and portal hypertension with plexogenic pulmonary hypertension[117] may also play a part since plexiform lesions may occur and on occasion severe pulmonary hypertension is encountered without any ova in the lungs.[118]

Pulmonary hypertension occured as a serious side-effect of the appetite suppressant Aminorex,[99,119] and although an association with other appetite suppressants have been suggested the evidence for this is extremely weak.[120] Although toxins in the diet produce pulmonary hypertension in animals[121] (e.g. *Crotalaria*) there is no evidence for dietary factors producing the condition in humans, although the pulmonary artery pressure is often

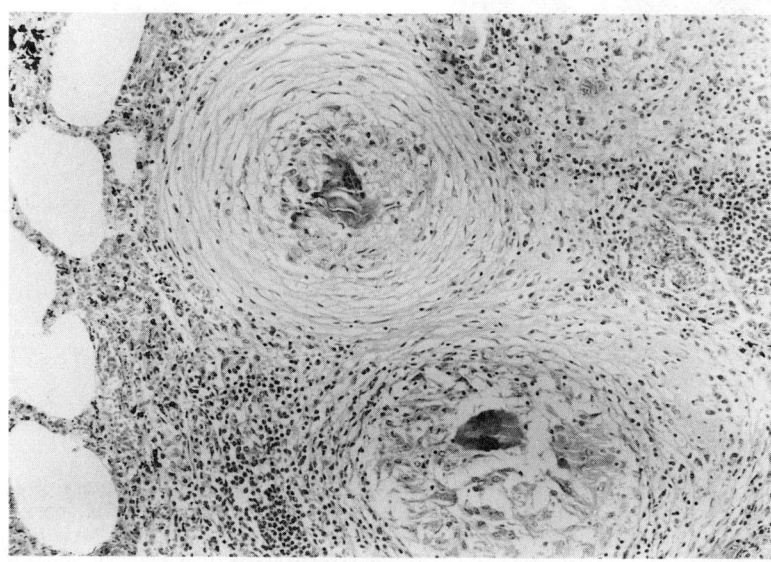

Fig. 54.25. Photomicrograph of *Schistosoma* granulomata in the lung containing remnants of ova and foreign body giant cells ($\times$ 136).

moderately raised in the late stages of the 'toxic cooking oil' syndrome which has recently reached serious proportions in Spain.[122]

PULMONARY ARTERIOVENOUS MALFORMATIONS

Pulmonary arteriovenous malformations result from an abnormality of capillary development in the lungs and are also known as pulmonary arteriovenous fistulae. Their pathological and clinical features have been well reviewed.[123,124] In between 30 and 60% of patients, they occur as part of the syndrome of hereditary haemorrhagic telangectasia, the Osler–Rendu–Weber syndrome; conversely about 15% of patients with this syndrome have pulmonary arteriovenous malformations. They may be single or multiple. Multiple pulmonary arteriovenous malformations are more common in those patients who also have hereditary haemorrhagic telangectasia but they are not confined to this group. They are most often found in the lower lobes, although they may occur in any part of the lung. Generally, they have a single feeding artery, which is a branch of the pulmonary artery, and drain into a pulmonary vein; very rarely, the feeding artery is a systemic bronchial vessel. In the majority, there is a single feeding and draining vessel (Fig. 54.26), but, occasionally, the

architecture of the pulmonary arteriovenous malformation is complex and these vessels are multiple;[125] this feature is of significance when planning therapy (see below). Nearly all of the malformations are a developmental abnormality but a few occur as the result of chest surgery or trauma.

Pathophysiology

The main abnormality is the shunting of blood within the lungs so that it bypasses the alveoli. This produces systemic desaturation, which varies in extent according to the size of the shunt, and leads to bone-marrow stimulation and polycythaemia. Interestingly, the shunt does not lead to an increase in the right heart pressures, and cardiac enlargement is not a feature of this condition.

Clinical features

The classic clinical features are exertional dyspnoea, cyanosis and finger clubbing. Patients with hereditary haemorrhagic telangectasia will often have other symptoms and signs related to vascular abnormalities at other sites. These will include visible telangiectatic lesions most easily seen on the face, particularly around the mouth, and bleeding which can occur from these lesions wherever they

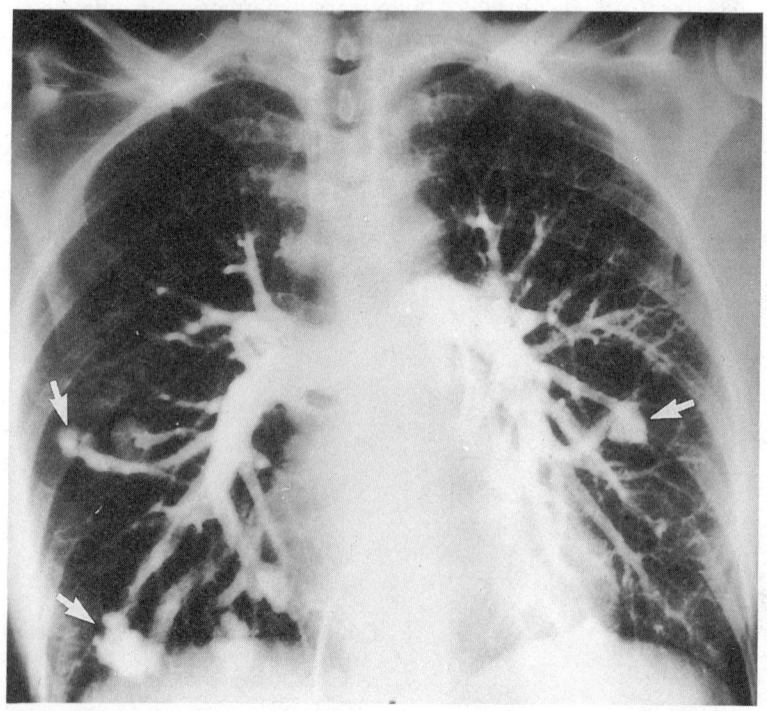

Fig. 54.26. Pulmonary angiogram of a patient with multiple pulmonary arteriovenous malformations. Some of the larger malformations are marked by arrows.

may be, for example, epistaxis, gastro-intestinal bleeding and haematuria. Furthermore, intracerebral bleeding may occur and lesions in other organs, for example, the liver, may increase in size sufficiently to cause significant arteriovenous shunting and a high-output state. Patients with pulmonary arteriovenous malformations of any cause may bleed from them and this may lead to haemoptysis or intrapulmonary bleeding.

Patients with pulmonary arteriovenous malformations often have systemic symptoms such as fatigue and may also have minor, and often transient, cerebral symptoms, which have been attributed to the effects of polycythemia on systemic and cerebral blood flow, respectively. Occasionally, other complications of any right-to-left shunt occur, including paradoxical embolism and an increased risk of cerebral abscess.

In about 30% of patients, a bruit is audible over the site of the fistula; this is normally increased in intensity by inspiration, is often continuous but it may be confined to diastole.

Investigation

Arterial blood gases reveal an oxygen saturation that ranges between 50 and 90%. There is often polycythaemia with haemoglobin values that may be in excess of 20 g/100 ml but patients with hereditary haemorrhagic telangectasia may be anaemic because of haemorrhage, for example, from telangectatic lesions in the gut.

In over 90% of patients, the pulmonary arteriovenous malformation is visible on the chest X-ray as a rounded opacity in the lung field peripheral to the hilar shadows; the feeding and draining vessels may also be visible. A few patients with small pulmonary arteriovenous malformations have normal chest X-rays. Contrast echocardiography is useful because it will define the presence of a right-to-left shunt; if the contrast is injected in the pulmonary artery and detected in the left atrium, the diagnosis of an intrapulmonary shunt is confirmed. It should be borne in mind that this does not necessarily confirm the diagnosis of pulmonary arteriovenous malformation because shunting of this type can occur through areas of infected lung and also via vascular primary or secondary tumours. However, the absence of this finding when high-quality echo images can be obtained makes the diagnosis very unlikely.

Pulmonary angiography is the definitive diagnostic technique in most cases (Fig. 54.26), but in the

Table 54.7. Differential diagnosis of pulmonary arteriovenous malformations.

Condition	Cyanosis	Clubbing	Other
Polycythaemia rubra vera	No[a]	No	—
Cyanotic heart disease	Yes	Yes	Other signs of the cardiac lesions e.g. murmurs and raised heart pressures
Round opacities on the chest X-ray	Rare	Sometimes	Further tests, e.g. CT scan, bronchoscopy needed
Chronic lung disease	Yes	Yes	Lung function severely deranged. Normal with pulmonary arteriovenous malformation

[a] May occur occasionally.

very occasional patient with small malformations confined to the capillary level these will not be seen on angiography. Computer tomographic scanning will also reveal pulmonary arteriovenous malformations, but occasionally it can be misleading.

Right heart pressures are normal.

Diagnosis (Table 54.7)

This condition has to be distinguished from polycythaemia of other varieties, other causes of rounded shadows on the chest X-ray which may, particularly in the case of lung cancer, also produce finger clubbing, and other causes of arterial desaturation, of which cardiac lesions causing right-to-left shunting and chronic lung disease are the most important.

Natural history and prognosis

The prognosis of pulmonary arteriovenous malformations, even without therapy, is generally excellent, but they may cause considerable disability. If serious problems occur, they are always the result of vascular malformations elsewhere, for example, intracranial and gastro-intestinal malformations; rarely, paradoxical embolism into the systemic circulation via a pulmonary arteriovenous malformation or cerebral abscess may have serious and possibly fatal results.

Treatment

If there is significant clinical disability, resection of the malformation may be indicated; this may not be practical if the lesions are multiple. The treatment of choice is usually to obstruct the pulmonary arteriovenous malformation with detachable balloons[125,126] that can be introduced via the systemic venous system using special catheter techniques or metal coils introduced in the same way. These techniques may prove particularly difficult if the pulmonary arteriovenous malformation is complex and has multiple feeding vessels.

REFERENCES

1. Hull, R.D., Hirsch, J., Carter, C.J. *et al.* Pulmonary angiography, ventilation lung scanning, and venography for clinically suspected pulmonary embolism with abnormal perfusion scan. *Ann. Intern. Med.* 1983; 98: 891–9.
2. Corrigan, T.P., Fossard, D.P., Spindler, J. *et al.* Phlebography in the management of pulmonary embolism. *Br. J. Surg.* 1974; 61: 484–8.
3. Benatar, S.R., Immelman, E.J. and Jeffery, P. Pulmonary Embolism. *Br. J. Dis. Chest* 1986; 80: 313–34.
4. Goldhaber, S.Z., Savage, D.D., Garrison, R.J. *et al.* Risk Factors for Pulmonary Embolism. The Framingham Study. *Am. J. Med.* 1983; 74: 1023–8.
5. Winter, J.H., Fenech, A., Ridley, W. *et al.* Familial Antithrombin III Deficiency. *Q. J. Med.* 1982; LI:204 373–95.
6. Dalen, J.E. and Alpert, J.S. Natural History of Pulmonary Embolism. *Prog. Cardiovasc. Dis.* 1975; 17: 259–70.
7. Goldhaber, S.Z. and Hennekens, C.H. Time trends in hospital mortality and diagnosis of pulmonary embolism. *Am. Heart J.* 1982; 104: 305–6.
8. International Multicentre Trial. Prevention of fatal postoperative pulmonary embolism by low dose heparin. *Lancet* 1975; ii: 45–51.
9. Mavor, G.E. and Galloway, J.M.D. The iliofemoral venous segment as a source of pulmonary emboli. *Lancet* 1967; i: 871–4.
10. Moser, K.M. and LeMoine, J.R. Is embolic risk conditioned by location of deep vein thrombosis? *Ann. Intern. Med.* 1981; 94(1): 439–44.
11. Sevitt, S. Pathology and pathogenesis of deep vein thrombosis. In: Poller L. (ed) *Recent Advances in Thrombosis.* Edinburgh and London: Churchill Livingstone, 1973; pp. 17–38.
12. James, T. Thrombi in the antrum atrii dextri of human heart as clinically important source for chronic microembolisation to lungs. *Br. Heart J.* 1983; 49: 122–32.
13. Hamilton, T.R. and Angevine, D.M. Fatal pulmonary embolism in 100 battle casualties. *Military Surgeon* 1946; 99: 450–8.
14. Wagenvoort, C.A. and Wagenvoort, N. *Pathology of pulmonary hypertension.* New York, London: John Wiley and Sons. 1977; pp. 121–5.
15. Williams, J.W., Eikman, E.A. and Greenberg, S. Asymptomatic pulmonary embolism. A common event in high risk patients. *Ann. Surg.* 1982; 195: 323–7.
16. Primm, R.K., Segall, P.H., Alison, H.W. *et al.* Incidence of new pulmonary perfusion defects after routine cardiac catheteristion. *Am. J. Cardiol.* 1979; 43: 529–32.
17. Miller, G.A.H., Sutton, G.C., Kerr, I.H. *et al.* Comparison of streptokinase and heparin in treatment of isolated acute massive pulmonary embolism. *Br. Med. J.* 1971; 2: 681–5.
18. Huet, Y., Lemaire, F., Brun–Buisson, C. *et al.* Hypoxemia in acute pulmonary embolism. *Chest* 1985; 88: 829–36.
19. McIntyre, K.M. and Sasahara, A.A. The hemodynamic response to pulmonary embolism in patients without prior cardiopulmonary disease. *Am. J. Cardiol.* 1971; 28: 288–94.
20. Jardin, F., Bardet, J., Sanchez, A. *et al.* Massive pulmonary embolism without arterial hypoxemia. *Intensive Care Med.* 1977; 3: 77–80.
21. D'Alonzo, G.E., Bower, J.S., DeHart, P. *et al.* The mechanisms of abnormal gas exchange in acute massive pulmonary embolism. *Am. Rev. Resp. Dis.* 1983; 128: 170–2.
22. Meister, S.B., Crossman, W., Dexter, L. *et al.* Paradoxical embolism: Diagnosis during life. *Am. J. Med.* 1972; 53: 292.
23. Windebank, W.J., Boyd, G. and Moran F. Pulmonary thromboembolism presenting as asthma. *Br. Med. J.* 1973; 1: 90.
24. Hall, R.J.C., McHaffie, D., Pusey, C. and Sutton, G.C. Subacute massive pulmonary embolism. *Br. Heart J.* 1981; 45: 681–8.
25. Sutton, G.C., Hall, R.J.C. and Kerr, I.H. Clinical course and late prognosis of treated subacute massive, acute minor and chronic pulmonary thromboembolism. *Br. Heart J.* 1977; 39: 1135–42.
26. Stein, P.D., Dalen, J.E., McIntyre, K.M. *et al.* The electrocardiogram in acute pulmonary embolism. *Prog. Cardiovasc. Dis.* 1975; 17: 247–57.
27. Kerr, I.H., Simon, G. and Sutton, G.C. The value of the plain radiograph in acute massive pulmonary embolism. *Br. J. Radiol.* 1971; 44: 751–7.
28. Colp, C. and Williams, J.R. Pulmonary function following pulmonary embolisation. *Am. Rev. Resp. Dis.* 1962; 85: 799–807.
29. Burgess, H.J. Pulmonary diffusing capacity in disorders of the pulmonary circulation. *Circulation* 1974; 49: 541–50.
30. Jones, N.L. and Goodwin, J.F. Respiratory function in pulmonary embolic disorders. *Br. Med. J.* 1965; 1: 108.
31. Williams, M.H. Jr, Alder, J.J. and Colp, C. Pulmonary function studies as an aid in the differential diagnosis of pulmonary hypertension. *Am. J. Med.* 1969; 47: 378–83.
32. Burke, C.M., Glanville, A.R., Morris, A.J.R. *et al.* Pulmonary function in advanced pulmonary hypertension. *Thorax* 1987; 42: 131–5.
33. Robin, E.D. Overdiagnosis and overtreatment of pulmonary embolism: The emperor may have no clothes. *Ann. Int. Med.* 1977; 87: 775–81.
34. Branch, W.T. Jr and McNeil, B.J. Analysis of the differential diagnosis and assessment of pleuritic chest pain in young adults. *Am. J. Med.* 1983; 75: 671–9.
35. McNeil, B.J. Ventilation perfusion studies and the diagnosis of pulmonary embolism: concise communication. *J. Nucl. Med.* 1980; 21: 319–23.
36. Polak, J.F. and McNeil, B.J. Pulmonary scintigraphy and the diagnosis of pulmonary embolism. A perspective. *Clin. Chest Med.* 1984; 5(3): 457–64.
37. Biello, D.R., Mattar, A.G., McKnight, R.C. and Siegel, B.A. Ventilation perfusion studies in suspected pulmonary embolism. *Am. J. Radiol.* 1979; 133: 1033–7.
38. Cheely, R., McCartney, W.H., Perry, J.R. *et al.* The role of non-invasive testing versus pulmonary angiography in the diagnosis of pulmonary embolism. *Am. J. Med.* 1981; 70: 17–22.
39. Dalen, J.E., Brooks, H.L. and Johnson, L.W. Pulmonary angiography in acute pulmonary embolism: Indications, techniques and results in 367 patients. *Am. Heart J.* 1971; 81: 175–85.

40. Fowler, N.O., Black-Schaffer, B., Scott, R.C. and Gueron, M. Idiopathic and thromboembolic pulmonary hypertension. *Am. J. Med.* 1966; **40**: 331–45.

41. Price, L.R. and Dunn, M. Are modifications necessary in the performance of pulmonary angiograms? *Chest* 1985; **88**: 1–2.

42. Hull, R.D., Hirsh, J., Carter, C.J. *et al.* Diagnostic efficacy of impedance plethysmography for clinically suspected deep vein thrombosis. *Ann. Intern. Med.* 1985; **102**: 21–8.

43. Starkey, I.R. and DeBono, D.P. Echocardiographic identification on right sided cardiac intracavitary thromboembolus in massive pulmonary embolism. *Circulation* 1982; **66**: 1322–5.

44. Bullock, R.E. and Hall, R.J.C. Left ventricular function and mitral valve opening in massive pulmonary embolism: Case report. *Br. Heart J.* 1982; **48**: 413–5.

45. Fanta, C.H., Wright, T.C. and McFadden, E.R. Jr. Differentiation of recurrent pulmonary emboli from chronic obstructive lung disease as a cause of cor pulmonale. *Chest* 1981; **79**: 92–5.

46. Lippman, M. and Fein, A. Pulmonary embolism in the patient with chronic obstructive pulmonary disease. *Chest* 1981; **79**: 39–42.

47. Hildner, F.J. and Ormond, R.S. Accuracy of the clinical diagnosis of pulmonary embolism. *JAMA* 1967; **202**: 115–8.

48. Urokinase Pulmonary Embolism Trial. A National Cooperative Study. *Circulation* 1973; **47 & 48** (Supp. II): 1–108.

49. Menzoian, J.O. and Williams, L.F. Is pulmonary angiography essential for the diagnosis of acute pulmonary embolism? *Am. J. Surg.,* 1979; **137**: 543–8.

50. Hull, R.D., Raskob, G.E. and Hirsh, J. The diagnosis of clinically suspected pulmonary embolism. *Chest* 1986; **89**: Suppl. 417S–25S.

51. Wilson, J.E., Bynum, L.J. and Parkey, R.W. Heparin therapy in venous thromboembolism. *Am. J. Med.* 1981; **70**: 808–16.

52. Hall, R.J.C. Difficulties in the treatment of acute pulmonary embolism. *Thorax* 1985; **40**: 729–33.

53. Barrit, D.W. and Jordan, S.C. Anticoagulant drugs in the treatment of pulmonary embolism: A controlled trial. *Lancet* 1960; **i**: 1309–12.

54. MacIntyre, D., Banham, S.W. and Moran, F. Pulmonary embolism—a long-term follow-up. *Postgrad. Med. J.* 1982; **58**: 222–5.

55. Turnier, E., Hill, J.D., Kerth, W.J. and Gerbode, F. Massive pulmonary embolism. *Am. J. Cardiol.* 1973; **125**: 611–22.

56. Hall, R.J.C., Sutton, G.C. and Kerr, I.H. Long term prognosis of treated acute massive pulmonary embolism. *Br. Heart J.* 1977; **39**: 1128–34.

57. Paraskos, J.D., Adelstein, S.J., Smith, R.E. *et al.* Late prognosis of acute pulmonary embolism. *New Eng. J. Med.* 1973; **289**: 55–8.

58. Riedel, M., Stanek, V., Widimsky and J., Prerovsky, I. Long term follow-up of patients with pulmonary embolism. Late prognosis and evolution of haemodynamic respiratory data. *Chest* 1982; **81**: 151–8.

59. Goodwin, J.F., Harrison, C.V. and Winkel, D.E.L. Obliterative pulmonary hypertension and thromboembolism. *Br. Med. J.* 1966; **1**: 701–11 & 777–83.

60. Wilhelmsen, L., Hagman, M. and Werko, L. Recurrent pulmonary embolism—incidence, predisposing factors and prognosis. *Acta. Med. Scand.* 1972; **192**: 565–75.

61. Decousus, H.A., Croze, M., Levi, F.A. *et al.* Circadian changes in anticoagulant effect of heparin infused at constant rate. *Br. Med. J.* 1985; **290**: 341–4.

62. Bounameaux, H., Vermylen, J. and Collen, D. Thrombolytic treatment with recombinant tissue-type plasminogen activator with massive pulmonary embolism. *Ann. Intern. Med.* 1985; **103**: 64–5.

63. Miller, G.A.H., Hall, R.J.C. and Paneth, M. Pulmonary embolectomy, heparin and streptokinase—their place in the treatment of acute massive pulmonary embolism. *Am. Heart J.* 1977; **93**: 568–74.

64. Tibbut, D.A., Davies, J.A., Anderson, J.A. *et al.* Comparison by controlled clinical trial of streptopkinase and heparin in treatment of life-threatening pulmonary embolism. *Br. Med. J.* 1974; **1**: 343–7.

65. Arnesen, H., Hoiseth, A. and Ly, B.V. Streptokinase or heparin in the treatment of deep venous thrombosis. *Acta. Med. Scand.* 1982; **211**: 65–8.

66. Ellis, D.A., Neville, E. and Hall, R.J.C. Subacute massive pulmonary embolism treated with plasminogen and streptokinase. *Thorax* 1983; **38**: 903–7.

67. Greenfield, L.J., Peyton, M.D., Brown, P.P. and Elkins, R.C. Transvenous management of pulmonary embolic disease. *Ann. Surg.* 1974; **180**: 461–7.

68. Hull, R., Delmore, T., Genton. *et al.* Warfarin sodium versus low-dose heparin in the long-term treatment of venous thrombosis. *New Eng. J. Med.* 1979; **301**: 855–8.

69. Lagerstedt, C.I., Olsson, C.G. *et al.* Need for long-term anticoagulant therapy in symptomatic calf-vein thrombosis. *Lancet* 1985; **211**: 515–8.

70. Bomalski, J.S., Martin, G.J., Hughes, R.L. and Yao, J.S.T. Inferior vena cava interruption in the management of pulmonary embolism. *Chest* 1982; **82**: 767–74.

71. Brewster, D.C. Introduction to symposium on transvenous vena cava interruption. *J. Vasc. Surg.* 1984; **1**: 487–90.

72. Greenfield, L.J. Current indications for and results of Greenfield filter placement. *J. Vasc. Surg.* 1984; **1**: 502–4.

73. Wille-Jorgensen, P., Thorus, J., Fischer, A. *et al.* Heparin with and without graded compression stockings in the prevention of thrombo-embolic complications of major abdominal surgery: A randomised trial. *Br. J. Surg.* 1985; **72**: 579–81.

74. Leonard, R.C.F., Neville, E. and Hall, R.J.C. Paradoxical embolism. A review of cases diagnosed during life. *Eur. Heart J.* 1981; **3**: 362–70.

75. Leonard, R.C.F., Neville, E. and Hall, R.J.C. Paradoxical embolism associated with patent foramen ovale. *Postgrad. Med. J.* 1981; **57**: 717–8.

76. Cheng, T.O. Paradoxical embolism: a diagnostic challenge and its detection during life. *Circulation* 1976; **53**: 565.

77. Laughlin, R.A. and Mandal, S.R. Paradoxical embolisation. *Arch. Surg.* 1977; **112**: 648.

78. Hagley, S.R. The fulminant fat embolism syndrome. *Anaesth. Intens. Care* 1983; **11**: 162–66.

79. Sperry, K. Amniotic fluid embolism. *JAMA* 1986; **255**: 2183–6.

80. Kashuk, J.L. Air embolism after central venous catheterisation. *Surg. Gynaecol. Obstet.* 1984; **159**: 249–52.

81. King, M.W., Aitchison, J.M. and Nel, J.P. Fatal air embolism following penetrating lung trauma. An autopsy study. *J. Trauma* 1984; **24**: 753–5.

82. Butler, D. and Hills, B.A. Transpulmonary passage of venous air emboli. *J. Applied Physiol.* 1985; **59**: 543–7.

83. Jaffe, R.B. and Korschmann, E.B. Septic pulmonary emboli. *Radiology* 1970; **96**: 527–32.

84. Dolan, P.A. Lymphography: complications encountered in 522 examinations. *Radiology* 1966; **86**: 876–80.

85. Silvestri, R.C., Huseby, J.S. *et al.* Respiratory distress syndrome from lymphangiography contrast medium. *Am. Rev. Resp. Dis.* 1980; **122**: 543–9.

86. Case Records of the Massachusetts General Hosp. Case 21—1986. *New Eng. J. Med.* 1986; **314**: 1435–45.

87. Haworth, S.G. Primary pulmonary hypertension. *Br. Heart J.* 1983; **49**: 517–21.

88. Hatano, S. and Strasser, (eds). *Primary pulmonary hyper-*

tension. Geneva: World Health Organisation, 1975.

89. Wagenvoort, C.A. and Wagenvoort, N. Primary pulmonary hypertension: A pathologic study of the lung vessels in 156 clinically diagnosed cases. *Circulation* 1970; **42**: 1163–84.

90. Heath, D. and Edwards, J.E. The pathology of hypertensive pulmonary vascular disease. A description of six grades of structural changes in the pulmonary artery with special reference to congenital cardiac septal defect. *Circulation* 1958; **18**: 533–47.

91. Yamaki, S. and Wagenvoort, C.A. Comparison of primary plexogenic arteriopathy in adults and children: a morphometric study in 40 patients. *Br. Heart J.* 1985; **51**: 428–34.

92. Meyrick, B., Clarke, S.W., Symonds, C. *et al.* Primary pulmonary hypertension: A case report including electron microscopic study. *Br. J. Dis. Chest* 1974; **68**: 11–20.

93. De Navasquez Forbes, J.R. and Holling, H.E. Right ventricular hypertrophy of unknown origin: so called pulmonary hypertension. *Br. Heart J.* 1940; **2**: 177–88.

94. Heath, D. and Smith, P. The electron microscopy of 'fibrinoid necrosis' in pulmonary arteries. *Thorax* 1978; **33**: 579–95.

95. Rawson, A. Incomplete rupture of the pulmonary artery based on cystic medionecrosis. *Am. Heart J.* 1963; **65**: 253.

96. Rozkovec, P., Montanes, P. and Oakley, C.M. Factors that influence the outcome of primary pulmonary hypertension. *Br. Heart J.* 1986; **55**: 449–58.

97. Juaneda, E., Watson, H. and Haworth, S.G. An unusual case of rapidly progressive primary pulmonary hypertension in childhood. *Int. J. Cardiol.* 1985; **78**: 306–9.

98. Bourdillon, P.D.V. and Oakley, C.M. Regression of primary pulmonary hypertension. *Br. Heart J.* 1976; **38**: 264–70.

99. Gurtner, H.P. Pulmonary hypertension 'plexogenic pulmonary arteriopathy' and the appetite depressant drug Aminorex: post or propter? *Bull. Eur. Physiopathol. Respir.* 1979; **15**: 897–923.

100. Haworth, S.G. Pulmonary vascular disease in different types of congenital heart disease. Implications for interpretation of lung biopsy findings in early childhood. *Br. Heart J.* 1984; **52**: 557–71.

101. Dantzker, D.R. and Bower, J.S. Mechanism of gas exchange abnormality in patients with chronic obliterative pulmonary vascular disease. *J. Clin. Invest.* 1979; **64**: 1050–5.

102. Fuster, V., Giuliana, E.R., Bradenbury, R.W. *et al.* The natural history of idiopathic pulmonary hypertension. *Am. J. Cardiol.* 1981; **47**: 422.

103. Rich, S. Primary pulmonary hypertension: Recent advances. *Herz* 1986; **11**: 197–206.

104. Cohen, M., Edwards, W.D. and Fuster, V. Regression in thromboembolic type of primary pulmonary hypertension during 2½ years of antithrombotic therapy. *J. Am. Coll. Cardiol.* 1986; **7**: 177–5.

105. Rich, S., Ganz, R. and Levy, P.S. Comparative actions of hydralazine, nifedipine and amrinone in primary pulmonary hypertension. *Am. J. Cardiol.* 1983; **52**: 1104.

106. Rich, S., Brundage, B.H. and Levy, P.S. The effect of vasodilator therapy on the clinical outcome of patients with primary pulmonary hypertension. *Circulation* 1985; **71**: 1191–6.

107. Rich, S., Martinez, J., Lam, W. *et al.* Captopril as therapy for patients with pulmonary hypertension. The problem of variability in assessing chronic drug therapy. *Br. Heart J.* 1982; **48**: 272.

108. Jones, D.K., Higenbottam, T.W. and Wallwork, J. Treatment of primary pulmonary hypertension with intravenous epoprostenol (prostacyclin). *Br. Heart J.* 1987; **57**: 270–8.

109. Walcott, G., Burchell, H.B., Brown, A.L. Jr. Primary pulmonary hypertension. *Am. J. Med.* 1970; **49**: 70–79.

110. Rose, G.A. and Spencer, H. Polyarteritis nodosa. *Q. J. Med.* 1957; **26**: 43–81.

111. Kawai, C., Ishikawa, K., Kato, M. *et al.* 'Pulmonary pulseless disease': Pulmonary involvement in so called Takayasu's disease. *Chest* 1978; **73**: 651–7.

112. Hejtmancik, M.R., Wright, J.C., Quint, R. and Jennings, F.L. The cardiovascular manifestions of systemic lupus erythematosus. *Am. Heart J.* 1964; **68**: 119.

113. Fayemi, A.O. Pulmonary vascular disease in systemic lupus erythematosus. *Am. J. Clin. Pathol.* 1976; **65**: 284–90.

114. Spencer, H. *Pathology of the lung*, 4th ed. Oxford: Pergamon Press, 1985.

115. Naeye, R.L. Advanced pulmonary vascular changes in schistosomal cor pulmonale. *Am. J. Trop. Med. Hyg.* 1961; **10**: 191.

116. Warren, K.S., Boros, D.L., Le Minh Hang and Mahmoud, A.F. The schistosoma japonicum egg granuloma. *Am. J. Pathol.* 1975; **80**: 279.

117. Kibria, G., Smith, P., Heath, D. and Sagar, S. Observations on the rare association between portal and primary hypertension. *Thorax* 1980; **35**: 945.

118. Rodriguez, H.F., Fernandex-Duran, A., Garcia-Moliner, L. and Rivera, E. Cardiopulmonary schistosomiasis. *Am. Heart J.* 1963; **65**: 253.

119. Kay, J.M., Smith, P. and Heath, D. Aminorex and the pulmonary circulation. *Thorax* 1971; **26**: 262.

120. McMurray, J., Bloomfield, P. and Miller, H.C. Irreversible pulmonary hypertension after treatment with fenfluramine. *Br. Med. J.* 1986; **292**: 239–40.

121. Kay, J.M., Harris, P. and Heath, D. Pulmonary hypertension in rats produced by ingestion of *Crotalaria spectabilis* seeds. *Thorax* 1967; **22**: 176.

122. Lopez-Sendon, J. and Coma-Canella, I. Pulmonary hypertension following ingestion of toxic cooking oil. Symposium on Primary Pulmonary Hypertension. European Society of Cardiology. Vienna, 1982.

123. Moyer, J.H., Glantz, G. and Brest, A.N. Pulmonary arteriovenous fistulas. Physiologic and clinical considerations. *Am. J. Med.* 1962; **32**: 417–34.

124. Dines, D.E., Sewart, J.B. and Bernatza, P.E. Pulmonary arteriovenous fistulas. *Proc. Mayo Clin.* 1983; **58**: 176–81.

125. White, R.I., Mitchell, S.E. *et al.* Angioarchitecture of pulmonary arteriovenous malformations* an important consideration before embolotherapy. *Am. J. Radiol.* 1983; **140**: 681–6.

126. Barth, K.J., White, R.I., Kaufmann, S.L. *et al.* Embolotherapy of pulmonary arteriovenous malformations with detachable balloons. *Radiology* 1982; **142**: 599–606.

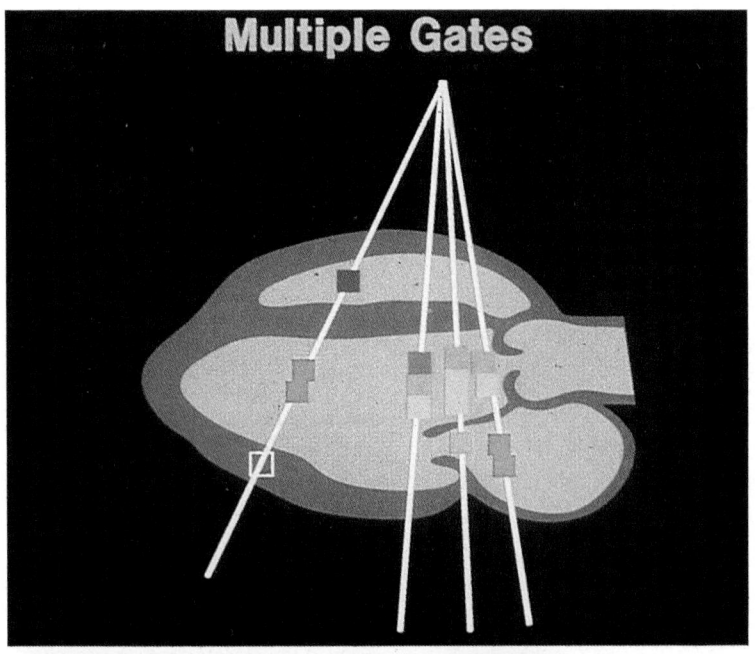

Pl. 14.1. The principle of colour flow mapping, Colour flow mapping is a multigate Doppler technique in which multiple sample volumes are interrogated across a cross-sectional image. These are illustrated by the different coloured areas of interrogation across the image. Because of the multiple sample volumes and the complexity of the subsequent analysis only mean velocity can be derived at each sample side. The direction of flow (red towards the transducer; blue away from the transducer) the mean velocity, and any turbulent flow are then encoded in colour.

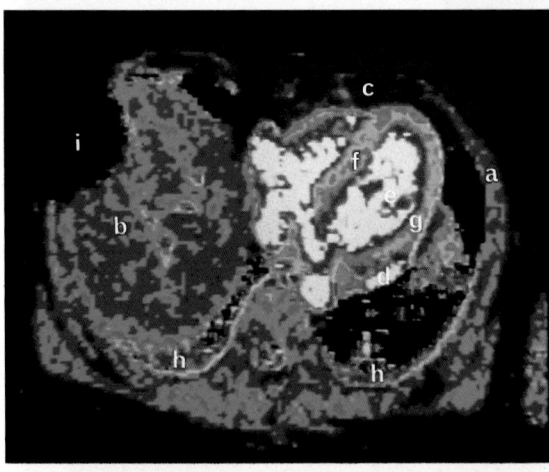

Plates 18.1–18.6 are displayed as colour images. The different colours represent the range of T_1 values so that images consist of T_1 *maps*. Values greater than 600 ms are displayed as white.

Pl. 18.1. Transverse systolic image from a patient with a recent lateral infarct demonstrating: (a) body fat; (b) liver; (c) pericardial fat; (d) pericardial fluid; (e) blood; (f) normal myocardium (septum); (g) abnormal myocardium (lateral wall infarct); (h) small pleural effusions; and (i) artefact from ECG cable.

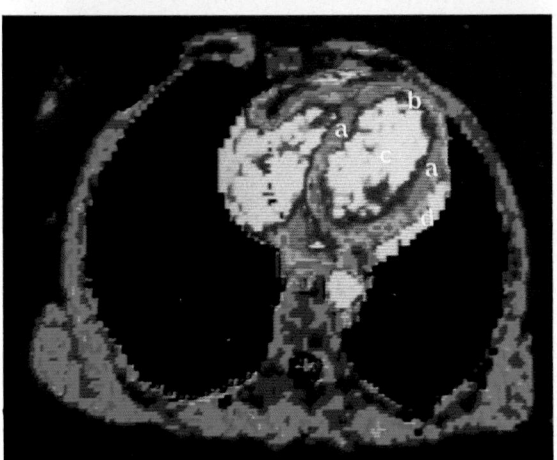

Pl. 18.2. Transverse systolic image in a patient with a recent anterior infarct demonstrating: (a) increased septal, apical and lateral wall T_1; (b) marked apical wall thinning; (c) large end-systolic cavity; and (d) small pericardial collection.

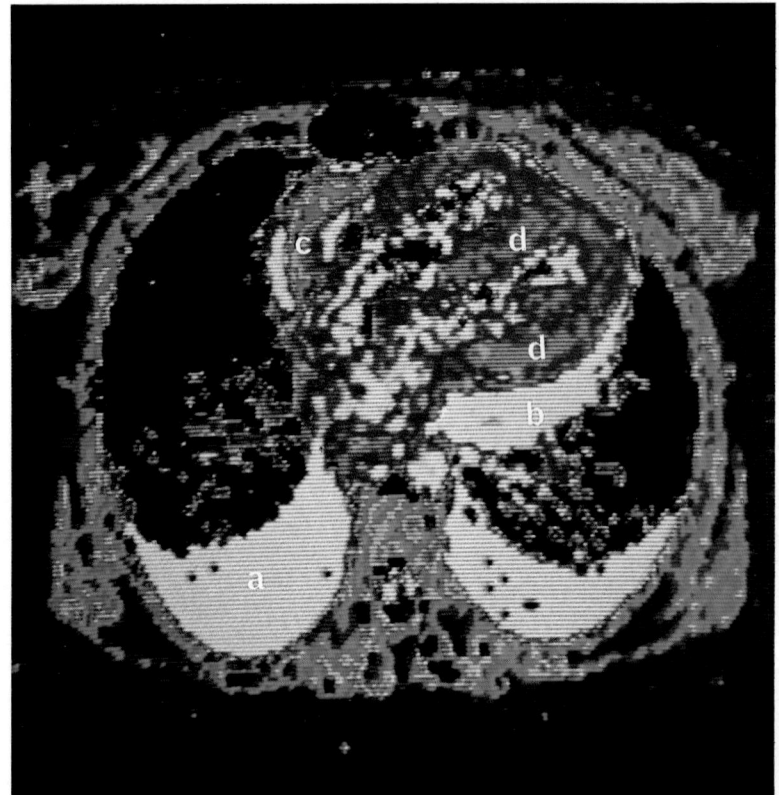

PI. 18.3. (*left*) Transverse image from a patient in heart failure several weeks following cardiac transplantation demonstrating: (a) large pleural effusions; (b) moderate pericardial effusion; (c) marked pericardial thickening; and (d) patchy increase in T_1 throughout the myocardium (patchy necrosis seen histologically).

PI. 18.4. (*below*) Transverse systolic phase image, colour coded for direction and velocity of flow in a normal subject. Flow in the cranial direction is shown in blue (ascending aorta and right ventricular outflow tract). Caudal flow is shown in red (descending aorta). Anatomical and flow images are superimposed in the lower right image.
(Courtesy of Dr J. Ridgway).

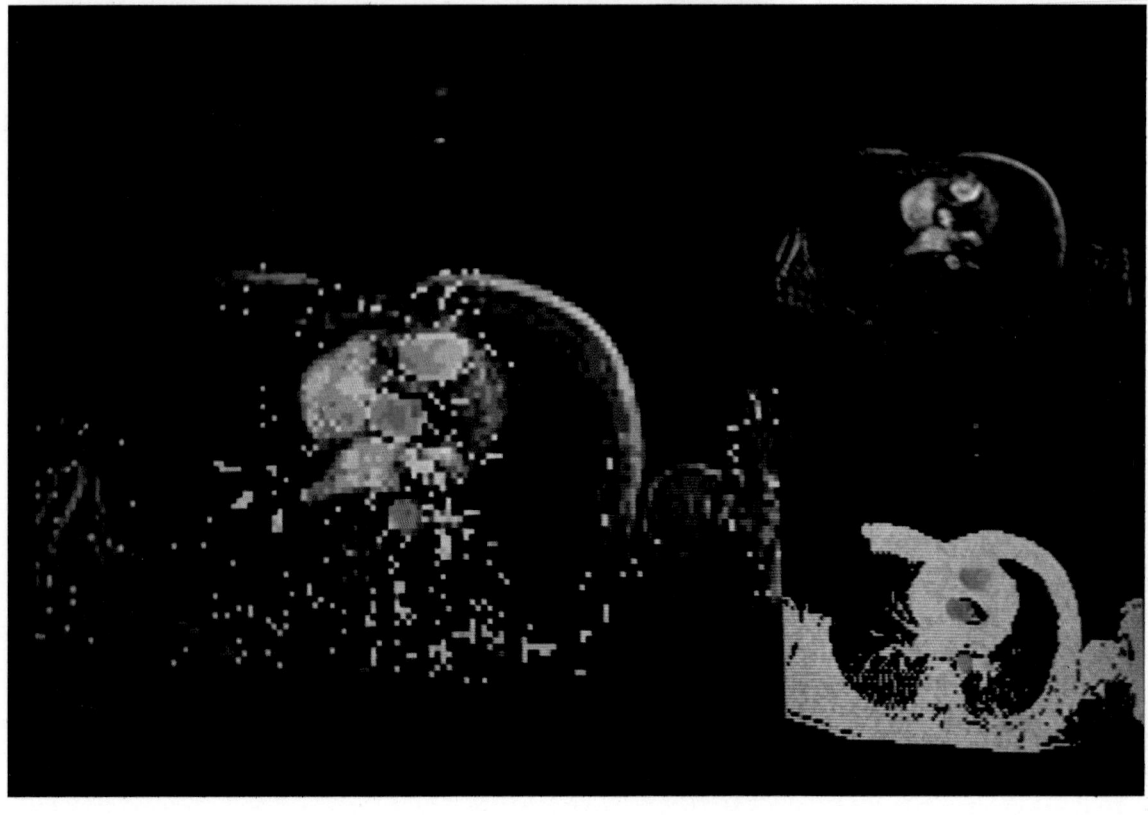

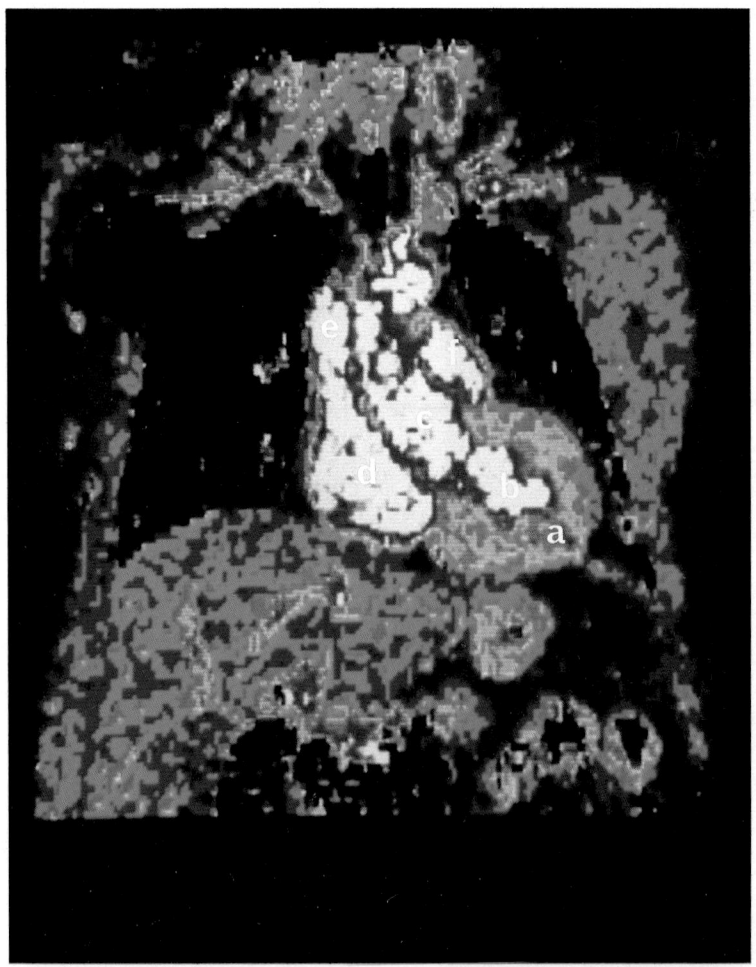

Pl. 18.5. Coronal image in a patient with an inferior infarct demonstrating: (a) raised T_1 in the infero-apical region; (b) left ventricular cavity; (c) aorta; (d) right atrium; (e) superior vena cava; and (f) left atrium.

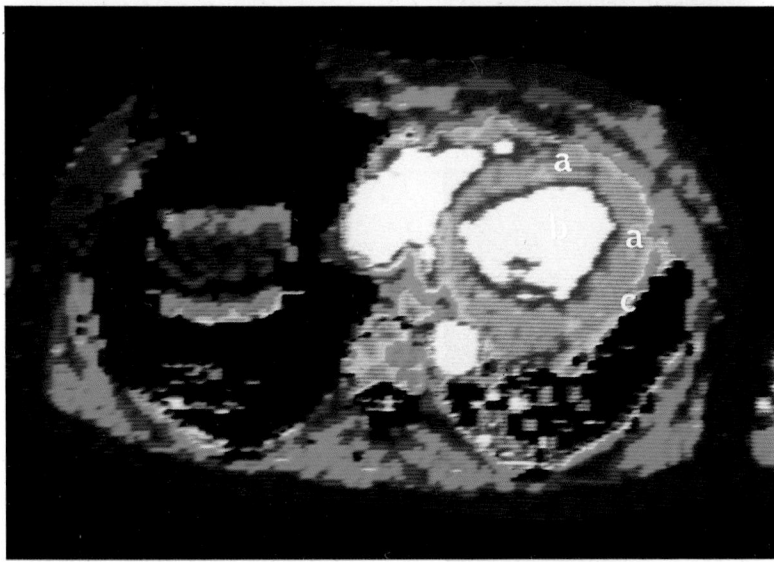

Pl. 18.6. Transverse systolic image in a patient with systemic lupus erythematosus and heart failure demonstrating: (a) uniformly raised T_1 throughout the left ventricular myocardium; (b) dilated left ventricle; and (c) mild left ventricular hypertrophy.

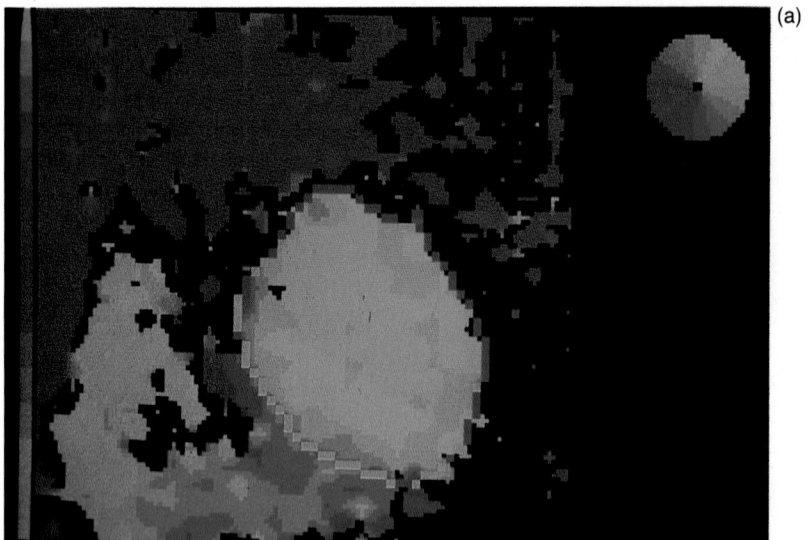

(a)

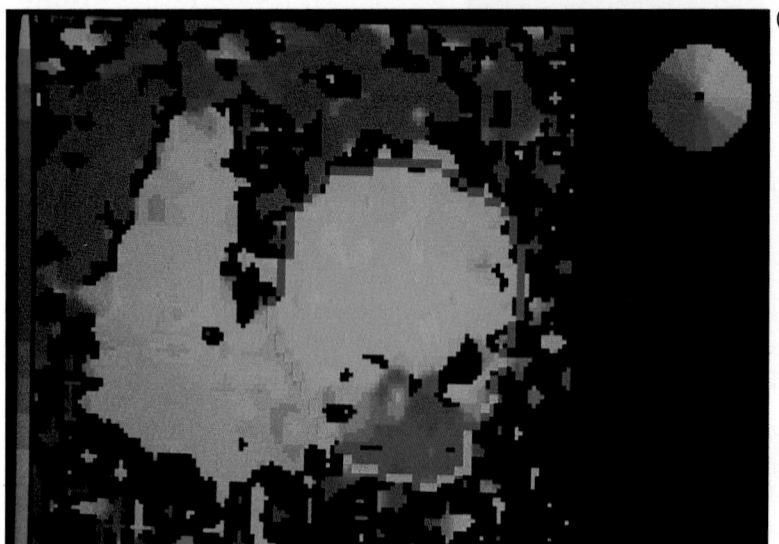

(b)

Pl. 19.1. Phase images from a normal subject (a) and a patient with a dyskinetic apex (b). Each picture cell element (pixel) is assumed to have a sinewave-like change in volume and a phase angle calculated. Synchronous ventricles will have the same colour throughout (a) but the dyskinetic ventricle shows an apical area with a phase angle approximately 180° out of phase with the rest of the ventricle. The colour 'clock' in the top right section gives an indication of phase angle.

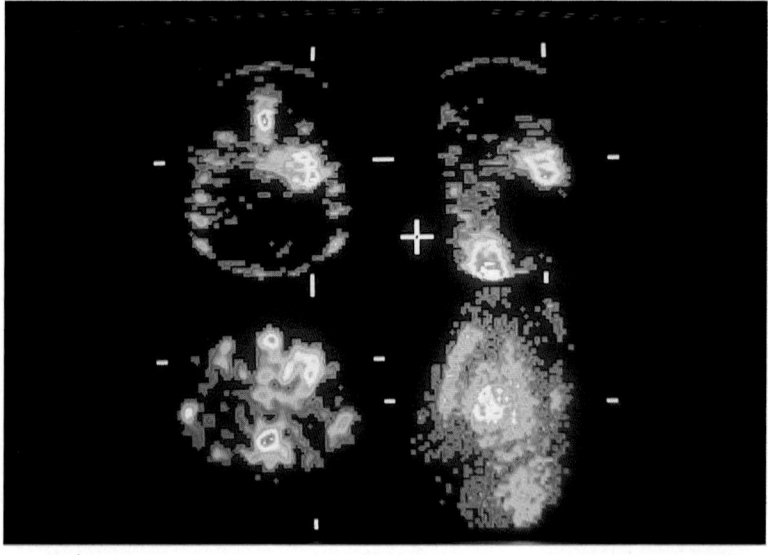

Pl. 19.2. An example of SPECT imaging of pyrophosphate uptake in the myocardium. The bottom right panel is a scout panel. The bottom left panel is the transverse section which shows anteriorly the sternum and posteriorly the spine. The horseshoe-shaped infarct is clearly shown in this transverse section. The pyrophosphate uptake is also clearly demonstrated in the coronal (top left) and sagittal (top right) panels. This patient had sustained a large anteroseptal myocardial infarction.

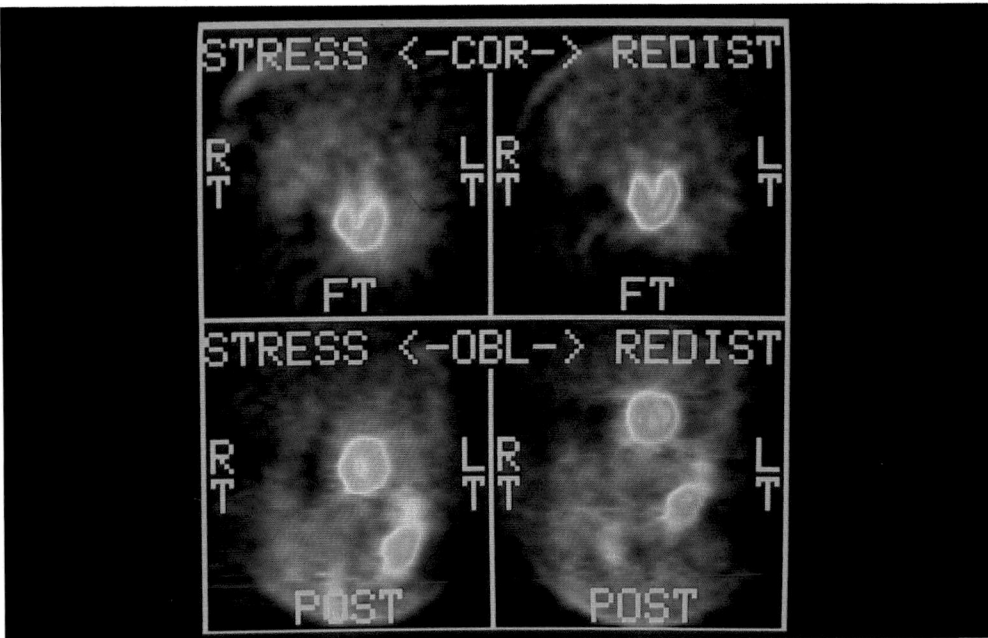

Pl. 19.3. Stress and redistribution thallium SPECT images taken in the coronal and oblique planes along the axis of the heart. There is a significant lack of thallium distribution in the right posterior and apical portions of the ventricle in the stress images with some but not total improvement in the distribution of thallium in the redistribution images.

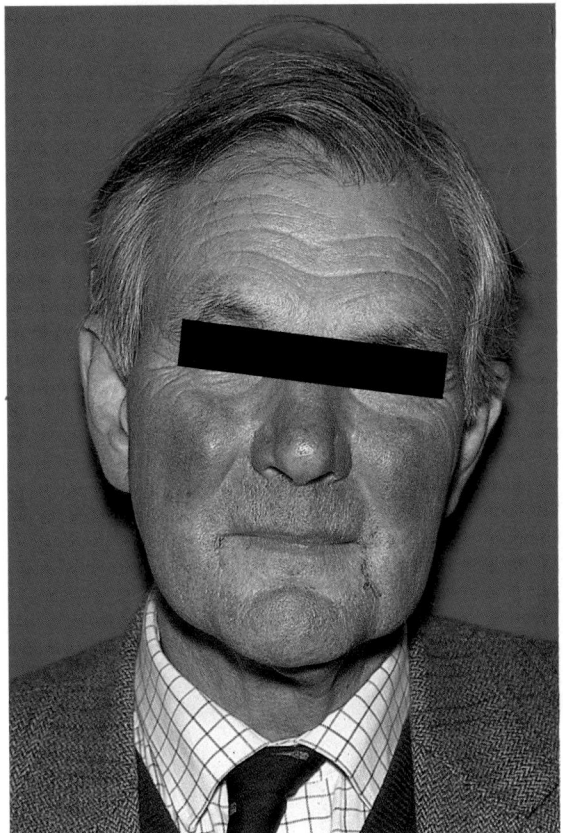

Pl. 23.1. Slate-grey (blue) facial pigmentation in a patient who had taken amiodarone 400 mg daily for several years. After discontinuation of the drug, the discolouration took over 3 years to fade.

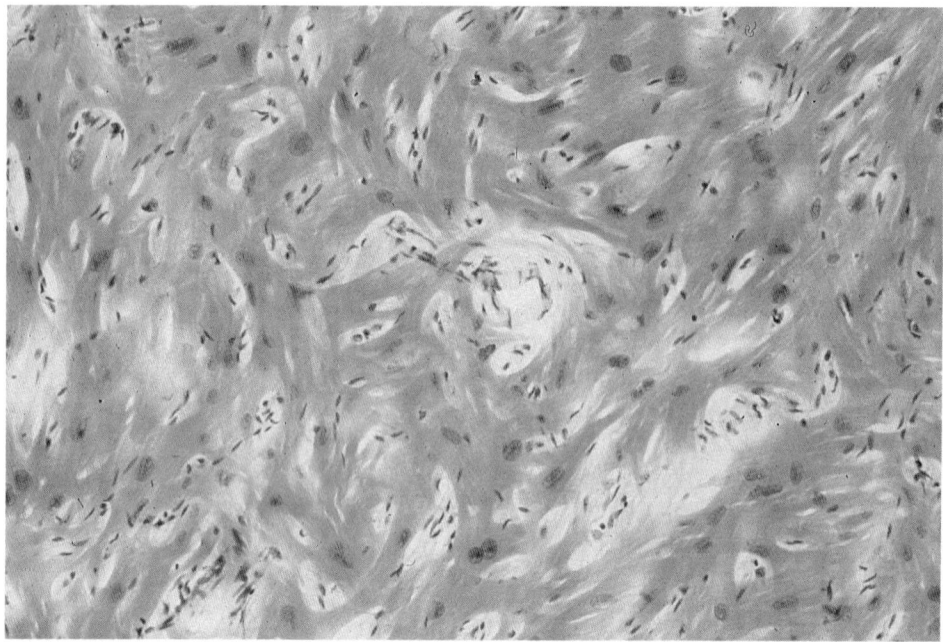

Pl. 39.1. Histological section from the left ventricular myocardium in a patient with hypertrophic cardiomyopathy. The myocardial fibres are irregular in size and appear to radiate out from a central focus and form whorls around foci of loose connective tissue. The nuclei of the myocardial fibres are large and hypochromatic. (Haematoxylin and eosin.) (By courtesy of Professor M.J. Davies.)

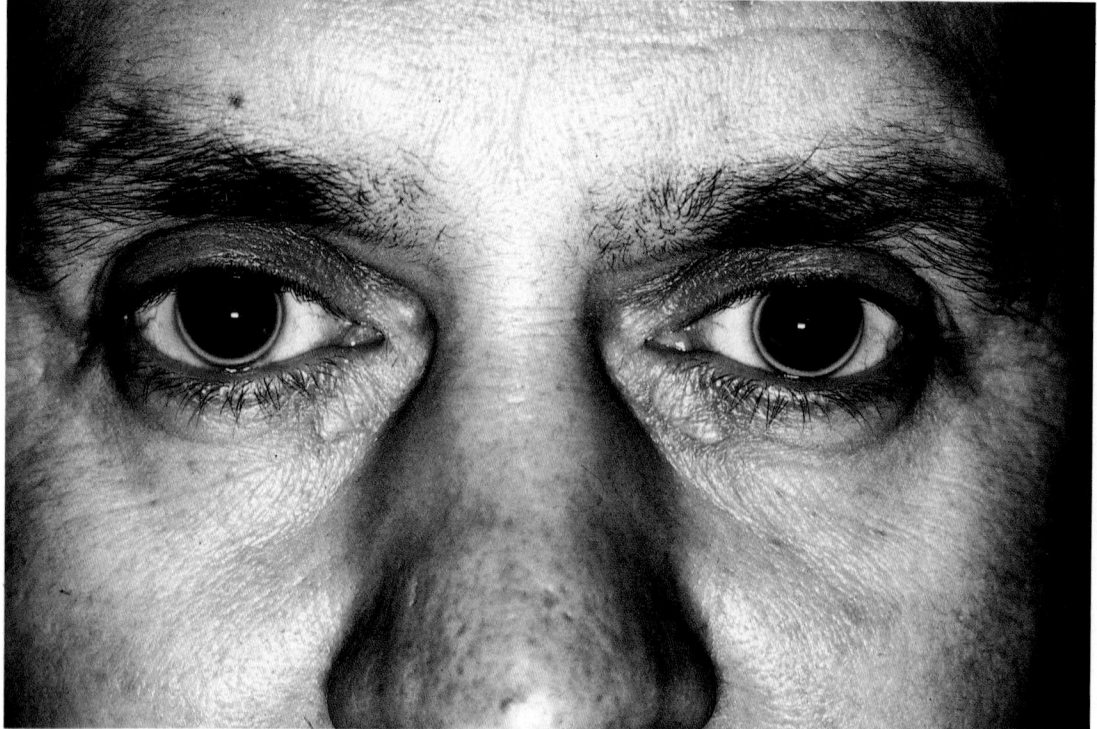

Pl. 43.1. (a) Corneal arcus and xanthelasma in heterozygous familial hypercholesterolaemia

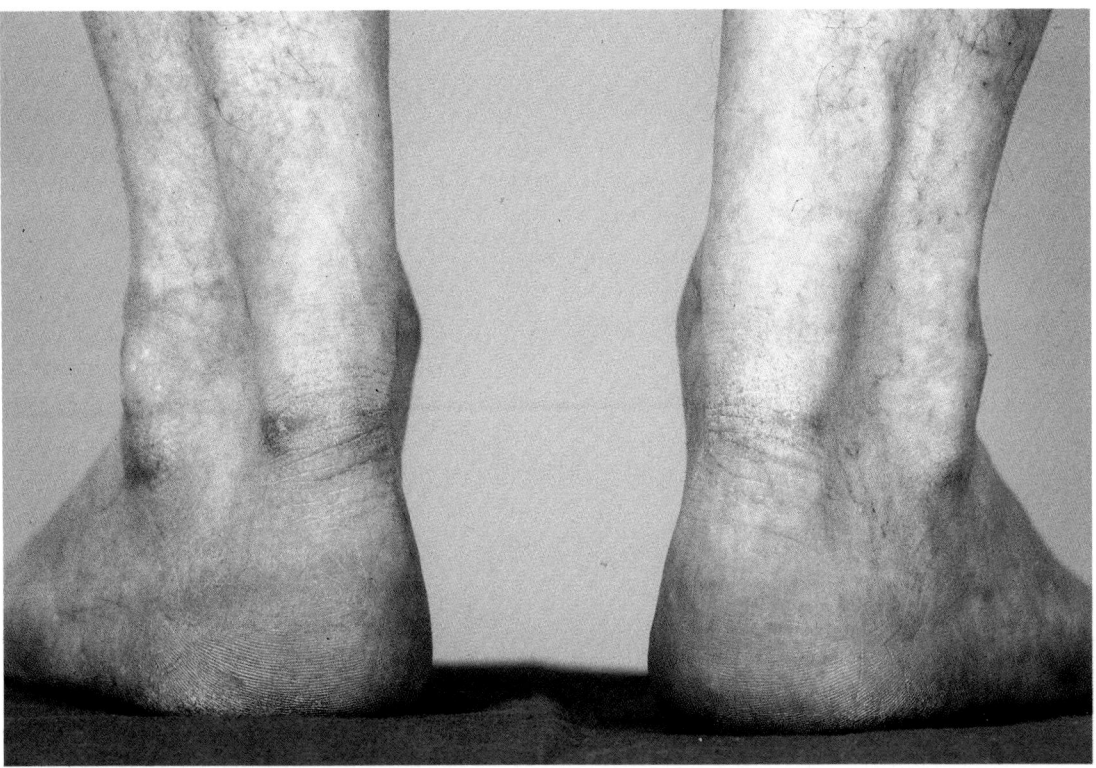

Pl. 43.1. (b) Achilles tendon xanthomata in heterozygous familial hypercholesterolaemia

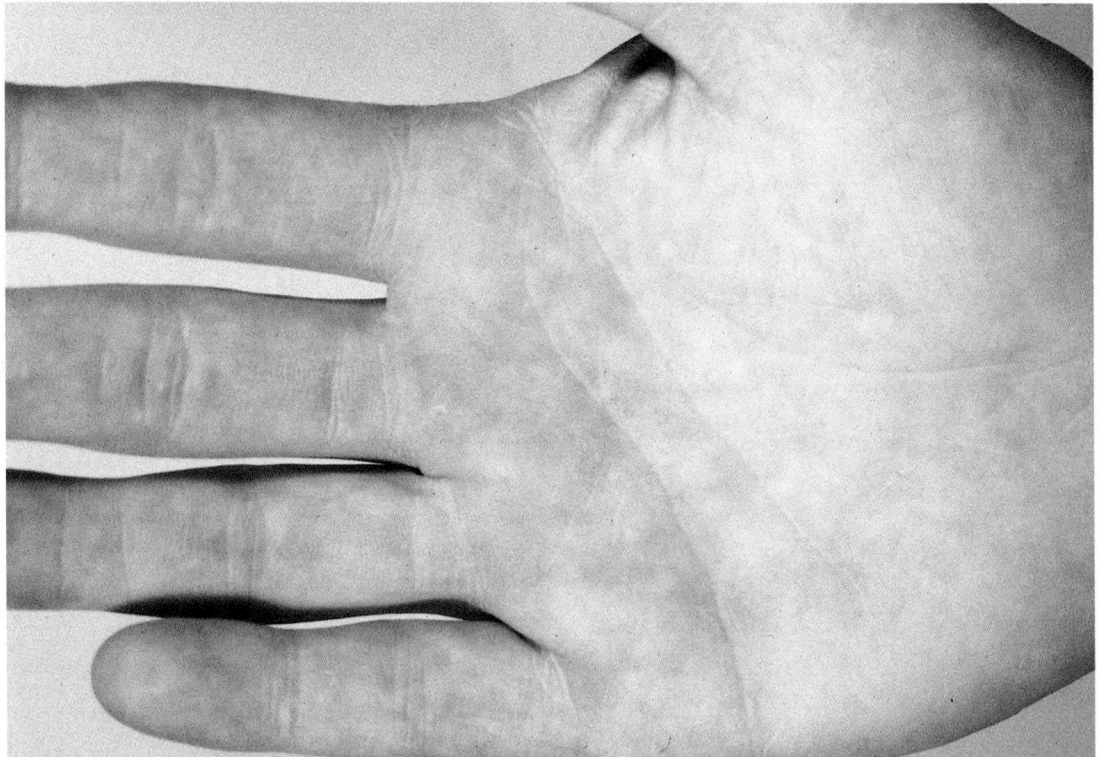

Pl. 43.1. (c) Palmar striae in type III hyperlipoproteinaemia, showing yellowish discolouration of the creases

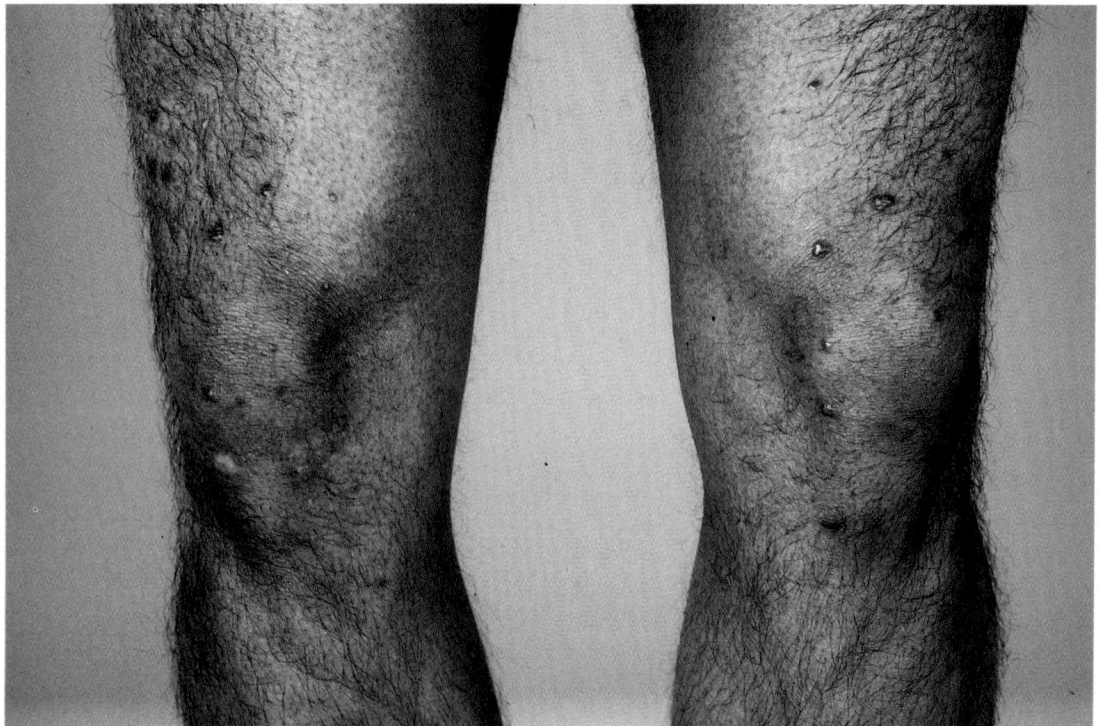

Pl. 43.1. (d) Eruptive xanthomata in an Asian with type V hyperlipoproteinaemia.

(a)

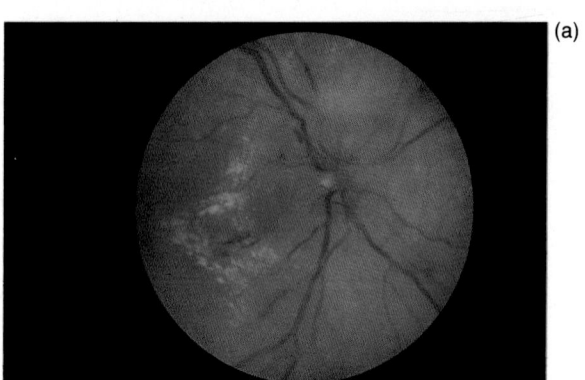

(b)

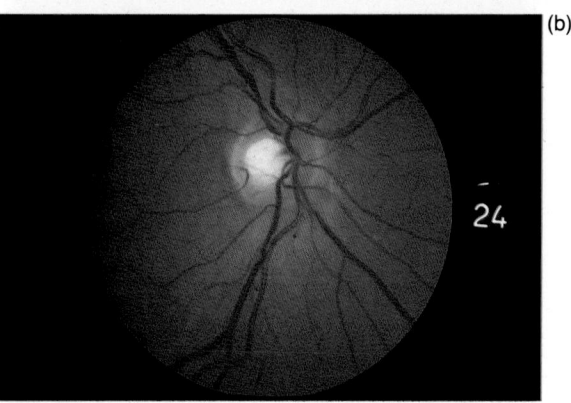

Pl. 53.1. Optic fundus of 35-year-old man presenting with malignant hypertension (blood pressure about 230/130 mmHg). (a) Papilloedema, haemorrhages and exudates can be seen. (b) Two years later, after effective antihypertensive drug treatment (blood pressure about 135/80 mmHg), the papilloedema and retinal lesions have resolved. (Reproduced from Graham, D.I. *et al.* In: *Handbook of Hypertension, Vol. 1: Clinical Aspects of Essential Hypertension*, p.174, by permission of the publishers, Elsevier, Amsterdam.)

Chapter 55

Cor Pulmonale

G.J. Gibson and S.G. Haworth

INTRODUCTION

The reality of an association between cardiac failure and chronic lung disease was a matter of dispute as recently as the 1940s. Detailed pathological[1] and physiological[2,3] studies increased awareness of the association, so that by 1959 a survey of congestive heart failure in the British Midlands showed cor pulmonale as the underlying condition in as many as 35% of patients.[4] Despite greater awareness of the condition, cor pulmonale remains a source of diagnostic confusion in individual patients in whom the presence or severity of the underlying lung disease is frequently unrecognized.

DEFINITION

The definition of cor pulmonale recommended by the World Health Organisation[5] is

> "hypertrophy of the right ventricle resulting from disease affecting the function and/or structure of the lung, except where these pulmonary alterations are the result of diseases that primarily affect the left side of the heart or of congenital heart disease."

In the clinical context, it refers to patients with chronic disease of the lungs, pulmonary vasculature or chest wall, who present with hypoxaemia, usually accompanied by hypercapnia, and transient or persistent ankle oedema and elevation of venous pressure, together with clinical, radiographic or electrocardiographic evidence of right ventricular disease.

The various conditions that can lead to the development of cor pulmonale are listed in Table 55.1. The commonest underlying condition is chronic obstructive pulmonary disease and the major part of this chapter will be devoted to cor pulmonale as seen in patients with chronic obstructive

pulmonary disease. Cor pulmonale due to thrombo-embolic disease or to other primary diseases of the pulmonary vasculature is considered elsewhere (Chapter 54). The remaining causes are briefly discussed later, with emphasis on ways in which the clinical picture differs from cor pulmonale due to chronic obstructive pulmonary disease.

COR PULMONALE IN CHRONIC OBSTRUCTIVE PULMONARY DISEASE

The diagnosis of chronic obstructive pulmonary disease encompasses patients with chronic airways obstruction and varying combinations of chronic obstructive bronchitis and emphysema; the majority of such patients are, or have been, cigarette smokers and they are characterized functionally by evidence of diffuse airway narrowing which shows little spontaneous variability and only small (but not negligible) improvements after exposure to a bronchodilator. Attempts have been made to classify such patients into those with predominantly 'bronchitic' or 'emphysematous' features, with the

Table 55.1. Conditions causing cor pulmonale.

Vascular:	Thrombo-embolic disease
	Primary pulmonary hypertension
Airway diseases:	Chronic obstructive pulmonary disease
	Asthma
	Bronchiectasis
	Cystic fibrosis
Alveolar diseases:	Pulmonary fibrosis
Extrapulmonary:	Pleural symphysis
	Scoliosis
	Thoracoplasty
	Respiratory muscle weakness
	Obesity–hypoventilation syndrome
	Obstructive sleep apnoea syndrome

former usually having more disturbance of arterial blood gases and a tendency to develop clinical evidence of right heart failure at an earlier stage. Typical examples of each type are seen, but many patients have features of both airways disease and alveolar destruction, so that the subdivision is rarely helpful in individual patients.

AETIOLOGY

Cigarette smoking is the most important factor in aetiology; clear evidence of genetic influences applies only to a minority, most notably to patients with α_1, anti-trypsin deficiency. Other as yet unidentified 'host factors' undoubtedly play a part because only 10–20% of heavy cigarette smokers develop disabling airflow limitation.

EPIDEMIOLOGY

The epidemiology of chronic obstructive pulmonary disease and associated cor pulmonale largely mirrors the epidemiology of cigarette smoking. Although historically chronic obstructive pulmonary disease has been associated with large industrial conurbations, the high urban prevalence is largely attributable to variations in social class structure and smoking. The effects of atmospheric pollution *per se* are more difficult to quantify, but most experienced clinicians in large industrial cities are impressed with a decline in the prevalence of cor pulmonale accompanying the improvement in urban atmosphere over the last 25 years. Traditionally, British patients were regarded as 'bronchitic' while their North American counterparts were diagnosed as 'emphysematous'. Detailed comparison[6] has shown that this distinction is essentially semantic.

PATHOLOGY

Cor pulmonale develops in patients with diseases of the lung which either cause chronic alveolar hypoxia or lead to extensive fibrosis and obstruction of the peripheral pulmonary arteries and capillary bed. In hypoxic lung disease, characteristic changes develop in the pulmonary arteries which are similar to those seen in healthy people who live at altitude;[7] pulmonary vascular smooth muscle is increased, but this occurs mainly in the walls of arteries which are close to or within the alveolar walls, in contrast to pulmonary hypertension due to an increase in pulmonary blood flow, or primary pulmonary hypertension, in which the entire arterial pathway is involved. Furthermore, hypoxic lung disease is not associated with the classical intimal changes seen in pulmonary vascular obstructive disease.[8] Pulmonary arterial medial hypertrophy due to hypoxia is presumed to result from prolonged vasoconstriction but the underlying mechanisms are not understood.

In the presence of pulmonary hypertension due to chronic obstructive pulmonary disease, the pulmonary trunk is dilated and hypertrophied as are the intrapulmonary elastic arteries which may also show atheromatous disease. The large muscular pulmonary arteries have a normal or only slightly increased wall thickness. It is the small muscular and pre-capillary arteries that show the distinctive changes (Figs 55.1 and 55.2). The small muscular arteries immediately proximal to and within the respiratory unit show medial hypertrophy.[9] Bundles of longitudinally orientated smooth muscle cells frequently lie within a re-duplicated internal elastic lamina (Fig. 55.2). Pre-capillary vessels, in which it is impossible to discern smooth muscle cells by light microscopy in the normal lung, develop a thick layer of smooth muscle cells in chronic obstructive pulmonary disease (Fig. 55.1). The severity of medial hypertrophy correlates positively with the severity of right ventricular hypertrophy (Fig. 55.3);[10,11] the small arteries with an external diameter of < 250 μm show a greater increase in medial thickness than do larger arteries and muscularity is normal in vessels > 1000 μm in diameter.

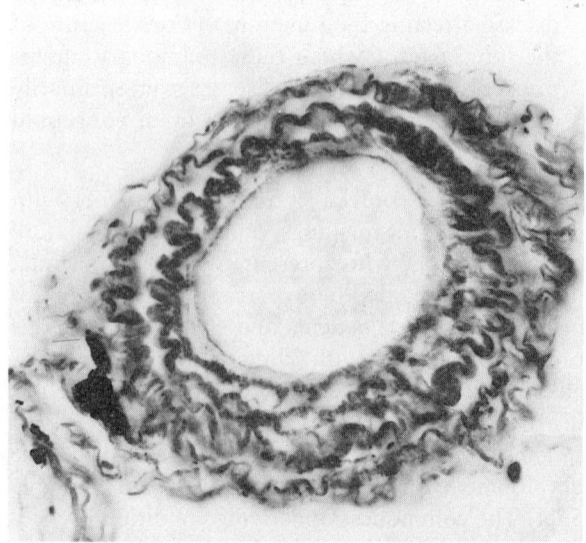

Fig. 55.1. Section through small pulmonary artery (accompanying an alveolar duct) in a patient with chronic obstructive pulmonary disease showing hypertrophy of the media.

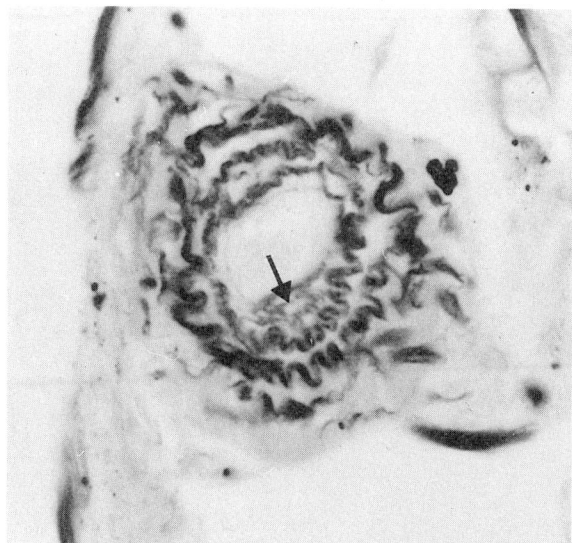

Fig. 55.2. Section through pulmonary arteriole in alveolar wall of a patient with chronic obstructive pulmonary disease showing muscularization of a vessel that is normally thin walled. Arrow indicates a crescent of longitudinal muscle bundles in the intima.

Intimal fibrosis that is eccentric, mild and non-occlusive occurs in chronic bronchitis as a result of the organization of thrombi, generally following a pneumonic episode. The thickness of the peripheral pulmonary vein walls is also increased[10] and muscle extends into more peripheral pulmonary veins than normal, although the changes are less marked than those in the small arteries. Longitudinally orientated smooth muscle cells are sometimes present in the intima. The structural abnormalities found in the veins of patients with chronic alveolar hypoxia resemble those seen in the lungs of normal people living at high altitude.[12] These changes in the pulmonary arteries and veins are widespread in patients with chronic obstructive pulmonary disease but they are accentuated in areas of lung tissue that become chronically infected. It appears that a modest increase in pulmonary arterial pressure and vascular smooth muscle may be tolerated for some time without the mass of the right ventricular muscle being increased.[10] The right ventricle is considered to be hypertrophied when its free wall weighs 80 g or more.[13] When only the right ventricle is hypertrophied, the ratio of the weight of the left ventricle plus that of the septum to the weight of the right ventricle is less than 2:1, but when the left ventricle is also hypertrophied the ratio may be normal.

PATHOPHYSIOLOGY

Autopsy measurements of airways resistance in patients with chronic obstructive pulmonary disease have shown that the main site of the increase is in airways < 2–3 mm in diameter. The distribution of inspired ventilation is demonstrably uneven from an early stage of the disease, leading to local variations in the partial pressures of oxygen and carbon dioxide. Small pulmonary vessels respond to local hypoxia or hypercapnia by vasoconstriction leading to a reduction in local perfusion. This is essentially a compensatory mechanism, tending to minimize the consequences of local hypoventilation on the gaseous composition of blood entering the systemic circulation via the pulmonary veins. Consequently, although radioisotopic scans of ventilation and perfusion in patients with chronic obstructive pul-

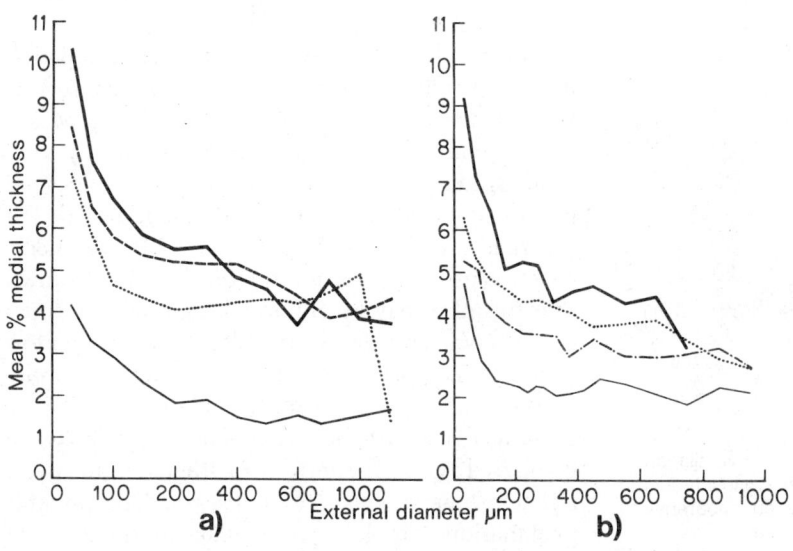

Fig. 55.3. Relationships of pulmonary arterial muscularity (expressed as mean percentage medial thickness related to external diameter) in patients who have (a) cystic fibrosis or (b) chronic obstructive pulmonary disease. Data from patients with and without right ventricular hypertrophy (RVH) are compared with data from normal subjects. (a) —, severe RVH; – –, mild RVH; · · ·, no RVH; —, normal, age 9 years; (b) —, RVH; · · ·, no RVH; – · –, normal, aged; —, normal, young.

monary disease show gross irregularities, they often appear to be reasonably well matched on a relatively crude regional comparison (Fig. 55.4). Within such regions, however, considerable mismatching of ventilation and perfusion occurs, leading to arterial hypoxaemia and sometimes hypercapnia. Although local pulmonary vasoconstriction tends to normalize blood gases, the assumption is that over a prolonged period transient changes in the pulmonary vessels become less reversible. This more permanent arterial and arteriolar constriction, together with loss of the vascular bed due to destructive emphysema, leads to pulmonary hypertension. Initially, this is manifest as a pathological rise in pulmonary artery pressure on exercise[14] and later as persistent elevation at rest. Against a background of mild or moderate elevation of resting pulmonary artery pressure, acute infective episodes leading to 'acute-on-chronic' respiratory failure are associated with further marked rises. Again, these are mediated by worsening hypoxia and hypercapnia and may be ameliorated by enrichment of the inspired air using controlled oxygen therapy.

Cross-sectional studies of groups of patients[15,16] have shown significant inverse correlations of pulmonary artery pressure with the level of arterial oxygenation (Fig. 55.5) and with indices of the severity of airway narrowing, such as FEV_1. Although mean pulmonary artery pressure in the stable state has an important bearing on life-expectancy, its predictive value does not appear to be any greater than that of the FEV_1 or $Paco_2$.[17]

Recent interest in abnormalities of breathing during sleep has led to the performance of nocturnal studies in patients with chronic obstructive pulmonary disease. These show frequent episodes of arterial desaturation which, in general, are related to periods of reduced ventilation (hypopnoea)

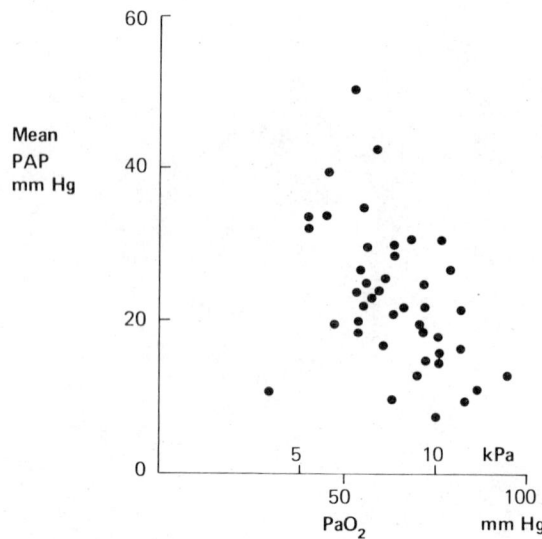

Fig. 55.5. Relationship of mean pulmonary artery pressure (PAP) to arterial Po_2 in 43 patients with chronic obstructive pulmonary disease. (Redrawn, by permission, from *Chest* 1977; **72**: 565–70.[15])

rather than to apnoea; the more severe the waking hypoxaemia the more profound the desaturation during sleep and the more severe the accompanying rises in pulmonary artery pressure.[18]

Elevation of pulmonary artery pressure leads to right ventricular dysfunction. Radionuclide measurements of right ventricular ejection fraction at rest[19,20] show that this is commonly reduced and the degree of abnormality is related to the severity of pulmonary hypertension and of disturbance of arterial blood gases. Therefore, it tends to be most impaired in patients with clinical evidence of cor pulmonale. Typically, the ejection fraction fails to show the normal rise on exercise.

Possible abnormalities of left ventricular function in patients with cor pulmonale are more controversial. Evidence of left ventricular hypertrophy is a fairly common pathological finding, and physiological studies show abnormally high values of pulmonary wedge pressure and sometimes of left ventricular end-diastolic pressure.[21] Measurements of left ventricular ejection fraction[20,22] have shown that this also may be abnormal, especially in those patients whose right ventricular function is most seriously compromised. Abnormalities are more marked and more frequent during exercise, but, in general, left ventricular dysfunction is slight when compared with findings in patients with overt ischaemic or valvular heart disease. One possible explanation for left ventricular dysfunction in

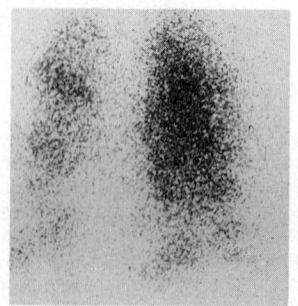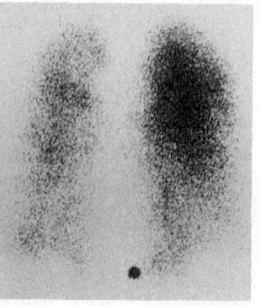

Fig. 55.4. Technetium perfusion (left) and xenon ventilation (right) postero-anterior lung scans in a patient with chronic obstructive pulmonary disease, showing patchy, but apparently well-matched, distribution of the isotopes.

patients with cor pulmonale would be the association of chronic obstructive pulmonary disease and occult ischaemic heart disease via the common aetiological agency of cigarette smoking; radiographic[22] and pathological data[23] suggest that this is the likely mechanism in many instances. Other possible contributory factors include hypoxia and a reduction in left ventricular compliance, consequent on distension of the right ventricle and interventricular septum. Despite these abnormalities, cardiac output at rest and on exercise in patients with cor pulmonale is usually normal.[24] For a given level of exercise, however, the normal cardiac output has to be achieved by an abnormally high cardiac frequency as the stroke volume is reduced.

The cause(s) of fluid retention and oedema in patients with cor pulmonale are not clearly established.[25] The simple explanation of right ventricular 'failure' is not supported by studies of cardiac output nor by the persistence of oedema between exacerbations when pulmonary artery pressures may be only mildly elevated. Interest has focused on the possible role of hypoxaemia and hypercapnia in stimulating the renin–angiotensin system leading to aldosterone excess, but the exact mechanism(s) remain elusive. One important practical point is that in patients with chronic obstructive pulmonary disease, oedema and cor pulmonale the arterial PCO_2 is almost always elevated; this is a sufficiently common association in such patients for the diagnosis of cor pulmonale to be questioned if the $PaCO_2$ is normal.

A further consequence of chronic hypoxaemia is polycythaemia with an approximate inverse relationship between SaO_2 and red cell mass. The associated increase in blood viscosity may increase circulation time sufficiently to outweigh the theoretical benefit of increased oxygen carriage by the blood. It may also contribute to the development of pulmonary hypertension. Isovolaemic reversal of polycythaemia by erythropheresis is associated with falls in systemic and pulmonary resistance and an increase in cardiac output.[26]

Respiratory failure and effects of oxygen

Respiratory failure is a disturbance of gas exchange arbitrarily defined in terms of the level of arterial blood gases: the usual criteria are a $PaO_2 < 8$ kPa (60 mmHg) with or without a $PaCO_2 > 6.5$ kPa (49 mmHg). Hypercapnic respiratory failure (also known as ventilatory failure or type II respiratory failure) is the more relevant to the clinical manifestations of cor pulmonale as these are rarely seen in patients with chronic obstructive pulmonary disease in the absence of carbon dioxide retention. The effect on the pulmonary vessels of increasing the local oxygen tension is to promote vasodilatation. In patients with established cor pulmonale, the acute administration of oxygen during cardiac catheterization usually produces a measurable but small fall in pulmonary artery pressure, and continuous administration over days or weeks results in a larger fall,[27] without complete return to normal levels. However, it is well recognized that uncontrolled oxygen in patients with acute respiratory failure may worsen hypercapnia and lead to a deterioration in conscious level despite improved oxygenation. It is usually assumed that this rise in $PaCO_2$ is a result of hypoventilation and of a reduced drive to breathe, consequent on partial relief of hypoxaemia. An alternative explanation is that relief of pulmonary vasoconstriction by oxygen worsens the local matching of ventilation and perfusion leading to more 'wasted perfusion', thus depriving better ventilated lung of its perfusion, i.e. producing an increase in physiological dead space, so that more ventilation is wasted and the 'effective' alveolar ventilation falls. In recent studies in acute respiratory failure, it has been shown that the simple explanation may be incorrect or incomplete, because the falls in total ventilation when oxygen is given are small, unsustained and not correlated with rises in $PaCO_2$.[28] Whatever the mechanism, the problem in acute respiratory failure is largely circumvented by using masks that operate on the Venturi principle and give only modest increments of inspired oxygen, e.g. 24.5% (which represents an increase in inspired oxygen of only 3.5% above that present in room air). In stable chronic respiratory failure, precise control of the inspired oxygen concentration is much less critical and such patients are increasingly being treated long term with low flow oxygen at 2 l/min by nasal cannulae.

CLINICAL FEATURES

History

When questioned, most patients will admit to chronic cough and sputum for many years; often this is dismissed as a 'smoker's cough' and the patient will have come to regard it as normal. Regular sputum production is initially more troublesome in the winter months with mucoid sputum becoming purulent when infective exacerbations occur. The amount of sputum produced and the frequency of exacerbations bear no relation to the functional deficit. Breathlessness due to chronic obstructive pulmonary disease rarely develops before middle-age, and its presence under the age of 40 years should suggest an alternative diagnosis such as asthma. Typically, it develops insidiously and is gradually progressive over several years, with little variation from day to day. The decline in ventilatory function starts much earlier and indices such as the FEV_1 have usually fallen to 50% or less of the normal value before shortness of breath develops. Most dyspnoeic patients with chronic obstructive pulmonary disease notice wheezing, especially at night or when ventilation is increased by exertion; this is often improved by clearance of secretions. Episodes of shortness of breath and wheezing unrelated to exertion are more suggestive of asthma.

The first indication of cor pulmonale is usually the development of ankle oedema; often, this appears for the first time during an acute infective episode. It may improve after treatment of the infection or with diuretics, only to recur with subsequent infections and later to become more persistent. Occasional patients are seen who develop cor pulmonale insidiously with remarkably few premonitory symptoms. Severe breathlessness is not universal and such patients may have been totally unaware of any disability before the development of fluid retention. Therefore, diagnostic confusion may arise with these patients who present with apparently unexplained cardiac failure; even very severe airways obstruction may be unrecognized unless simple ventilatory tests are applied.

Physical signs

The physical signs of patients with cor pulmonale fall into three groups, those related to airway narrowing, to the blood gas disturbances and to right ventricular dysfunction. The typical patient with chronic airflow obstruction has a hyperinflated chest with an increased antero-posterior diameter. There is often tachypnoea and the accessory muscles (sternomastoids, scalenes) may be visibly contracting; expansion of the ribcage is limited, and a more specific sign is paradoxical inspiratory indrawing of the lower costal margin, resulting from traction on the lower ribs by the flattened diaphragm. If there is very severe airways obstruction, the patient may adopt a characteristic posture,

sitting forward and using the outstretched arms for support. Wheezing may be audible with or without a stethoscope; its detection is a useful guide to the *presence* of airways obstruction, but not to its *severity*. In very severe airway narrowing, wheezing is often absent. Basal crackles are frequently heard and may lead to an erroneous diagnosis of left ventricular failure.

Central cyanosis is the only reliable sign of disturbed blood gases. Classical teaching states that the detection of cyanosis requires a concentration of reduced haemoglobin of 5 g/dl; this is a considerable overestimate as most experienced clinicians can detect central cyanosis in Caucasian patients at a concentration of 3 g/dl or less (3 g/dl corresponds to $Sao_2 < 80\%$ or Pao_2 approximately 6.7 kPa (50 mmHg) if the haemoglobin concentration is normal). The classical signs of hypercapnia, bounding pulse, flapping tremor and papilloedema, may occur but they are inconstant and unreliable.

Cor pulmonale is usually recognized by the combination of bilateral ankle oedema, a right ventricular 'heave' accompanied by a loud pulmonary component of the second cardiac sound and elevation of the venous pressure. Elevation of venous pressure may be a particularly difficult physical sign to elicit in these patients who are often tachypnoeic and vigorously contracting the accessory muscles of respiration. The presence of large 'v' waves in the jugular veins may indicate tricuspid regurgitation due to right ventricular dilatation. This is seen especially during acute exacerbations; the classical pan-systolic murmur and pulsatile liver are less commonly elicited.

INVESTIGATIONS

Radiography

The chest radiograph of a patient with chronic airways obstruction typically shows hyperinflated lungs with diaphragms which are abnormally low and flattened; the lateral radiograph shows an increase in antero-posterior diameter and in the size of the retrosternal airspace. Hyperinflation alone does not imply the presence of emphysema; it is also a frequent finding in patients with asthma, even in those in relative remission. Specific features indicating emphysema include the presence of bullae and marked attenuation of the peripheral pulmonary vessels, but the plain radiograph is relatively insensitive to the presence of emphysema. During infective exacerbations, the radiograph may show areas of consolidation, but most exacerbations are confined to the bronchial tree and are not associated with radiographic shadowing.

Patients with clinical evidence of cor pulmonale usually show cardiomegaly, which typically increases during exacerbations as the right ventricle becomes more dilated. Pulmonary hypertension is manifest as enlargement of the central pulmonary arteries (Fig. 55.6). The presence and severity of pulmonary hypertension can be predicted with reasonable accuracy from the size of these vessels, the most commonly used index being the diameter of the descending branch of the right or left pulmonary artery.[29]

Electrocardiography

The characteristic electrocardiographic features of cor pulmonale include P pulmonale, i.e. a tall P wave > 2.5 mm in height, right-axis deviation on the frontal leads, together with tall R waves in leads V_1 and V_2 and deep S waves in V_5 and V_6 (Fig. 55.7); the T waves in the right precordial leads may be inverted or biphasic. The severity of these abnormalities shows weak correlations with the degree of pulmonary hypertension. Right-axis deviation has been shown to be the most sensitive electrocardiographic indicator of right ventricular hypertrophy in patients with chronic obstructive pulmonary disease.[30] Ventricular or, more commonly, supraventricular ectopic complexes are frequently present.

Respiratory function

The characteristic abnormality of pulmonary mechanics is an obstructive ventilatory defect with reductions in FEV_1, peak expiratory flow and in the

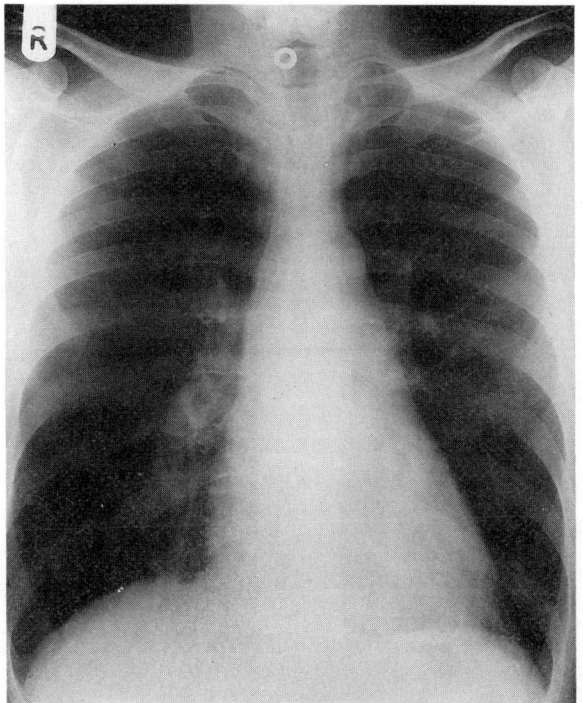

Fig. 55.6. Chest radiograph of patient with chronic obstructive pulmonary disease and cor pulmonale showing overinflated lungs, cardiac enlargement and prominent central pulmonary arteries.

ratio of FEV_1 to vital capacity (FEV_1/VC or FEV_1 %). The vital capacity itself is usually reduced to some extent and residual volume is markedly increased, as also is total lung capacity. The carbon monoxide transfer factor is reduced to a variable degree, the most marked reductions being seen in patients with widespread emphysema. Symptomatic patients usually show a reduction in FEV_1 to less than half of the predicted value.

Arterial blood gases show hypoxaemia and usually hypercapnia. In the patient admitted to hospital

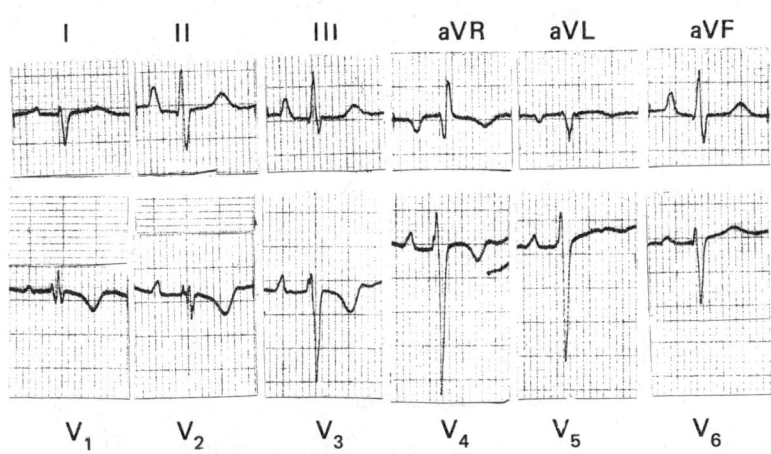

Fig. 55.7. Electrocardiogram of a patient whose radiograph is shown in Fig. 55.6, with cor pulmonale due to chronic obstructive pulmonary disease showing P pulmonale, right-axis deviation, dominant R wave in V_1 and dominant S wave in V_6 and T-wave inversion in leads V_1–V_4.

with 'acute-on-chronic' respiratory failure, values of Pao_2 breathing air are typically between 4.7 and 7.3 kPa (35–55 mmHg) with $Paco_2$ between 6.7 and 9.3 kPa (50–70 mmHg). Values of $Paco_2 > 75$ mmHg (10 kPa) are very unusual unless the patient has received oxygen to breathe. The pH is usually between 7.25 and 7.35 but a proportion of patients have normal or mildly alkalaemic values, which can usually be attributed to the use of diuretics.

Biochemistry

Respiratory acidosis is accompanied by an elevated venous bicarbonate (and reduced chloride) concentration; this, together with hypokalaemia, may be exaggerated by treatment with diuretics or corticosteroids, both of which tend to produce a metabolic alkalosis. Abnormalities of liver function, due to passive congestion, and of renal function, manifested by elevation of blood urea and creatinine, are common in the acute phase. The latter may be exacerbated by treatment with diuretics.

Haematological abnormalities

Elevation of the haemoglobin concentration and haematocrit are common in patients who have been chronically hypoxaemic.

Tests of cardiac function

Echocardiography is often technically difficult in patients with airways obstruction because of lung hyperinflation; features of pulmonary hypertension, right ventricular hypertrophy and dilatation and abnormal septal motion are detectable in some subjects. Radioisotopic imaging of the heart using thallium-201 may show uptake by the hypertrophied right ventricle which is not seen in the normal heart at rest.[19]

Other investigations

Measurement of pulmonary artery pressure is rarely necessary in clinical practice. Nocturnal monitoring of arterial oxygenation shows severe hypoxaemia in many patients, but this adds little information to that obtained from daytime measurements as there is a direct correlation between the two.[18]

DIFFERENTIAL DIAGNOSIS

Differentiation of cor pulmonale due to airways obstruction from primary left ventricular disease can be surprisingly difficult in some patients. Dyspnoea, orthopnoea, wheezing and crackles on auscultation are common to both. Useful distinguishing features on examination are the presence of a third heart sound in left ventricular failure and signs of severe airways obstruction (e.g. costal paradox) and right ventricular hypertrophy in cor pulmonale. On investigation, simple ventilatory tests together with the radiographic and electrocardiographic appearances are usually diagnostic.

Distinction of cor pulmonale due to chronic obstructive pulmonary disease from other causes of right ventricular failure, such as primary pulmonary hypertension, may also be difficult occasionally. Wheezing is not always present in patients with severe chronic obstructive pulmonary disease, but other signs of airways obstruction can be detected and ventilatory tests should be diagnostic. These tests also help to distinguish cor pulmonale due to chronic obstructive pulmonary disease from chronic pulmonary embolic disease; perfusion scans are valuable in the diagnosis of emboli, but confident interpretation often requires a ventilation scan and simple spirometric measurements in addition.

Occasional patients with chronic obstructive pulmonary disease and cor pulmonale are found to have previously unrecognized asthma and the distinction may only be possible after a therapeutic trial of corticosteroids (see below).

COMPLICATIONS

Supraventricular dysrhythmias are relatively common and include atrial fibrillation, atrial flutter and atrial tachycardias with varying degrees of block. These are best treated with either digoxin or a calcium antagonist such as verapamil.

NATURAL HISTORY

The overall 5-year survival of patients with symptomatic chronic obstructive pulmonary disease is about 60%, but once oedema has developed the 5-year survival of untreated patients falls to only 30%. Although pulmonary artery pressure is a predictor of mortality, its predictive value is no better than simple tests such as the FEV_1 and arterial blood gases.[31]

MANAGEMENT

Acute respiratory failure

Most acute exacerbations leading to 'acute-on-chronic' respiratory failure with increased fluid retention are due to bronchial infections and are associated with the production of purulent sputum. The commonest bacterial pathogens are *Streptococcus pneumoniae* and *Haemophilus influenzae*. Antibiotic treatment should be based on this assumption even when bacterial culture of purulent sputum is negative. Appropriate antibiotics include ampicillin, tetracycline and cotrimoxazole for 7–10 days. As long as the patient is able to eat and drink, there is no evidence that treatment with intravenous antibiotics is better than that with oral antibiotics.

Encouraging expectoration is a vital part of treatment. Frequent physiotherapy is desirable during an exacerbation; as well as helping to mobilize secretions, it has the advantage of frequently rousing a drowsy patient.

To achieve bronchodilatation, an inhaled selective β_2 stimulant should be used, e.g. salbutamol or terbutaline, in fairly large doses by nebulization. Monitoring of cardiac rhythm is desirable if the patient has ischaemic heart disease.

Diuretics relieve the discomfort of fluid retention and probably improve pulmonary gas exchange. Large doses are likely to result in a metabolic alkalosis which may exacerbate hypercapnia. A carbonic anhydrase inhibitor, e.g. dichlorphenamide, is occasionally of use in hypercapnia with superadded metabolic alkalosis, especially when the arterial pH is frankly alkaline. It is generally agreed that digitalis is unhelpful unless there is a specific indication, such as uncontrolled atrial fibrillation.

Inspired oxygen should be carefully controlled in the acute situation. This is best achieved by the use of a mask which operates on the Venturi principle (e.g. Ventimask). The higher the initial Pa_{CO_2}, the greater the risk of a progressive rise. Problems rarely occur on 24.5% oxygen; owing to the shape of the oxygen dissociation curve, this small increase in inspired P_{O_2} achieves a useful increase in arterial oxygen saturation and in tissue delivery of oxygen. It is unrealistic and undesirable to aim at a 'normal' level of Pa_{O_2}; values of 55–60 mmHg (7.3–8.0 kPa) are usually acceptable provided the patient does not also have left ventricular disease or hypotension. Oxygen should be given continuously and may be required for several days; it often proves to be a more effective diuretic than large doses of drugs.

In patients who are not improving or who deteriorate, artificial ventilation may have to be considered. This is usually undertaken only in patients whose history suggests a reasonable chance of useful recovery of function and performance. The patient's clinical state and level of consciousness are more appropriate indicators of the need for artificial ventilation than the absolute levels of Pa_{CO_2}. The ventilatory stimulant doxapram is an alternative and often very effective means of management in patients with progressive hypercapnia, and it may allow higher concentrations of oxygen (e.g. 28%) to be given to patients with inadequate oxygenation on 24.5% oxygen.[32] It has to be given by constant intravenous infusion; the dose is titrated against the level of Pa_{CO_2} and the patient's level of consciousness.

Chronic cor pulmonale

Most patients benefit from use of a regular inhaled selective β_2-stimulant because airways obstruction is virtually never totally irreversible. Regular diuretics are indicated in patients with persistent or recurrent oedema. In two large studies, it was established that long-term oxygen used for at least 15 h/day improves the prognosis of patients with chronic obstructive pulmonary disease and chronic hypoxaemia and hypercapnia.[33,34] Initiation of this treatment requires a full assessment of respiratory function and blood gas status when the patient is stable and breathing room air; it is generally agreed that such treatment is not indicated unless the Pa_{O_2} on air is < 8.0 kPa (60 mmHg) and unless the patient has discontinued smoking. The treatment also demands a considerable commitment from the patient to take the oxygen as prescribed. It is usually delivered by nasal cannulae at a flow rate of 2 l/min. This is achieved most conveniently and least expensively using an oxygen concentrator, which, since December 1985, can be prescribed by general practitioners in England and Wales. The value of oxygen for shorter periods or for symptomatic relief is not well established.

Venesection of patients with a markedly elevated haematocrit (> 60%) can produce symptomatic improvement, especially of headaches; in some patients, it also improves exercise capacity. The circulating volume may be maintained by an exchange transfusion in which the blood removed is replaced by dextran[35] or, if appropriate facilities are available, by erythrophoresis.[26]

In general, the long-term use of respiratory stimulant drugs has been disappointing, but the novel agent almitrine (not currently available in the UK) offers a possible new approach. This drug, which is given by mouth, stimulates ventilation via an action of the carotid chemoreceptors, but it appears that its beneficial effects on pulmonary gas exchange are greater than can be explained by an increase in ventilation alone. It may have further direct effects on the pulmonary vasculature, but the mechanism of improvement is not known. It does produce both a sustained increase in PaO_2 and a sustained decrease in $PaCO_2$ at rest and on exercise, but some evidence suggests that this may be at the cost of a modest increase in pulmonary artery pressure.[36] Whether this potential disadvantage outweighs the advantages is not yet clear.

Vasodilators such as hydralazine and nifedipine reduce pulmonary and systemic vascular resistances in patients with cor pulmonale due to chronic obstructive pulmonary disease; although they produce a measurable increase in cardiac output on exercise, there is no good evidence· of an improvement in exercise capacity.[37] Some vasodilators have been shown to result in a deterioration in the matching of ventilation and perfusion in the lungs, with pulmonary vasodilatation leading to diversion of blood to areas of lung with relatively poor ventilation;[38] this potentially deleterious effect is balanced by an improvement in the saturation of mixed venous blood due to the increased cardiac output. At present, these drugs do not have a clearly defined role in the treatment of patients with cor pulmonale due to chronic obstructive pulmonary disease; long-term evaluation is awaited. Early experience with angiotensin converting enzyme (ACE) inhibitors suggests that they may have a useful role in some patients.

OTHER CONDITIONS

ASTHMA

Evidence of cor pulmonale in patients with typical asthma is unusual, although transient electrocardiographic abnormalities are well recognized in acute severe asthma.[39] These abnormalities include P pulmonale, right-axis deviation, right bundle branch block and ST-segment and T-wave changes, suggesting myocardial ischaemia. The appearances are usually transient with the electrocardiogram returning to normal in hours or days. In acute severe asthma, the most notable cardiovascular signs are a tachycardia and pulsus paradoxus. The former is directly related to the severity of hypoxaemia and the latter is thought to be due to limited right ventricular filling because of pericardial stretching in the hyperinflated chest.[40]

Asthma presenting as cor pulmonale is unusual, but a small proportion of patients with severe airways obstruction, fluid retention and signs of right ventricular dysfunction are found to have asthma when appropriately investigated and treated.[41] In particular, the diagnosis should be considered in younger patients, i.e. those under the age of 50 years, presenting with severe airways obstruction.

BRONCHIECTASIS

Extensive bronchiectasis is associated with diffuse airways obstruction and thus may lead to cor pulmonale. Pathologically, bronchiectasis is accompanied by hypertrophy of the bronchial circulation. Large anastomoses develop between bronchial and pulmonary arteries around and beyond the bronchiectatic cavities.[42] The management of cor pulmonale in patients with bronchiectasis is similar to that in patients with chronic obstructive pulmonary disease. A trial of corticosteroids is of particular importance as a proportion of patients with bronchiectasis are asthmatic.

CYSTIC FIBROSIS

Evidence of cor pulmonale is found at autopsy in the majority of patients who die of cystic fibrosis. The pathological features are similar to those in chronic obstructive pulmonary disease with medial hypertrophy of small muscular arteries, the severity of which correlates with the degree of right ventricular hypertrophy (Fig. 55.3).[11] Measurements in life show a reduction in right ventricular ejection fraction, either at rest or on exercise, in most patients with severe airflow obstruction. Abnormalities of left ventricular ejection fraction are found in a smaller proportion, especially on exercise,[43,44] which may be due to abnormal septal motion; in some patients this can be recognized on echocardiography. The management of cor pulmonale in patients with cystic fibrosis is the same as that for cor pulmonale in patients who have other conditions, but the young age of the affected individuals has prompted the performance of heart–lung transplantation in occasional patients. The long-term results of this procedure in such patients are not yet clear.

PULMONARY FIBROSIS

Patients with advanced pneumoconiosis (e.g. progressive massive fibrosis) may develop cor pulmo-

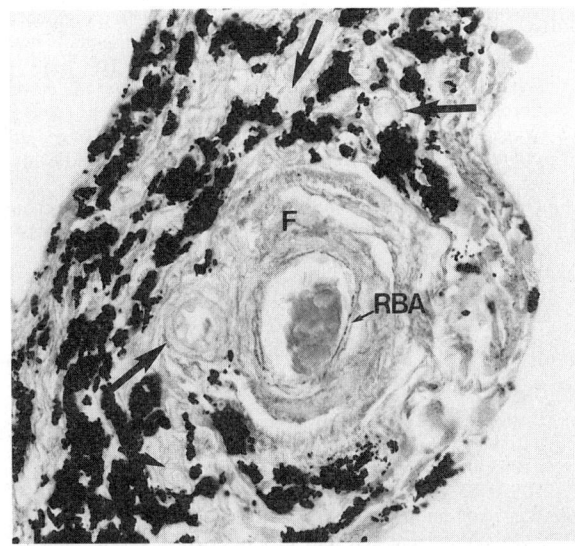

Fig. 55.8. Section of lung from a patient with pneumoconiosis showing silica deposits and fibrosis (F) surrounding a respiratory bronchiolar artery (RBA); other small arteries are indicated by arrows.

nale. The muscular pulmonary arteries within and at the edges of the fibrotic areas show severe medial hypertrophy and intimal fibrosis (Fig. 55.8), they become occluded and finally the pulmonary arterial pressure increases. Anastomoses between pulmonary and bronchial circulations are enlarged.

Radiation and administration of cytotoxic drugs are important causes of lung damage. Excessive radiation causes fibrous thickening of the pleura and connective tissue septa, and peripheral pulmonary arteries and veins develop medial hypertrophy and intimal fibrosis and may become obstructed. Thrombotic changes are common. Cytotoxic drugs can produce an early pneumonitis and vascular damage followed by progressive fibrosis, but sustained pulmonary hypertension is rare.

In patients with cryptogenic fibrosing alveolitis, clinical signs of cor pulmonale are usually late manifestations and associated with severe hypoxaemia and pulmonary hypertension. Granulomatous diseases of the lung, such as tuberculosis and sarcoidosis, produce focal changes and do not usually cause pulmonary hypertension. Particularly in sarcoidosis, however, coalescence and healing of extensive granulomatous areas can lead to widespread fibrosis and impairment of gas exchange. Occasional patients are seen who have advanced sarcoidosis and cor pulmonale associated with grossly distorted lung architecture and the formation of bullae.

Pulmonary artery pressure is the most important determinant of mortality in patients with pulmonary fibrosis.[31] Data on cardiac function in these conditions are limited, but most patients seem to maintain a normal cardiac output at rest and on exercise at the expense of a rapid cardiac frequency and limited stroke volume.[45,46]

CHEST WALL DISEASES

Cor pulmonale develops in some patients with severe scoliosis, some with extensive pleural symphysis (fibrothorax), some following thoracoplasty and some with severe weakness of the respiratory muscles due to various causes.

In scoliosis, the anatomical dimensions of the pulmonary vascular bed are much reduced, but hypoxic vasoconstriction is also important and the level of pulmonary artery pressure is inversely related to Pa_{O_2}. The structural changes are most marked in the compressed lung where the alveoli themselves may be atrophic.[47] Interpretation of the electrocardiogram is complicated by the skeletal deformity: P pulmonale is indicative of pulmonary hypertension but right-axis deviation is unreliable as a guide.[48] Cardiac output is usually normal.[49] Some patients with cor pulmonale and scoliosis develop sleep apnoea or, more commonly, hypopnoea associated with severe nocturnal oxygen desaturation. Although hypercapnia is usually regarded as an ominous feature, the overall prognosis of patients with scoliosis and ventilatory failure is appreciably better than that of patients with chronic obstructive pulmonary disease and an equivalent reduction of FEV_1.[50]

An increasing number of patients is being seen with cor pulmonale as a late consequence of thoracoplasty. Often the symptoms of cor pulmonale develop 15 or 20 years after surgery and most affected patients have some degree of airflow limitation as well as loss of lung volume. Cor pulmonale may also develop in some patients who have a severe restrictive ventilatory defect due to weakness of the respiratory muscles. In such patients, this needs to be distinguished from primary disease of the heart muscle associated with certain myopathies and muscular dystrophies.

In all these examples of cor pulmonale due to 'extrapulmonary' causes of lung volume restriction, treatment is aimed at controlling fluid retention and improving oxygenation. Many patients can also be helped by the regular use of negative pressure ventilation using a cuirass ventilator at night or by the newer technique of intermittent positive pressure ventilation using a nasal mask (nasal IPPV).

SLEEP APNOEA SYNDROMES

The importance of apnoea during sleep was first recognized in grossly obese patients with the 'Pickwickian' syndrome, many of whom present with fluid retention and cardiomegaly. In the most severe cases, hypoxaemia and hypercapnia are present both day and night. Subsequently, many more patients have been recognized who have relatively normal daytime blood gases but frequent episodes of apnoea and arterial desaturation at night; most of these patients with the obstructive sleep apnoea syndrome are not grossly obese. It has been well demonstrated that nocturnal hypoxaemia produces transient and often dramatic rises in pulmonary arterial pressure. Patients with clinical, radiographic and electrocardiographic evidence of cor pulmonale, however, usually have sustained hypoxaemia and/or hypercapnia by day and night; in the majority of such individuals, a degree of diffuse airways obstruction is present and this is an important contributor to the persisting hypoxaemia.[51] Treatment is by weight reduction, control of fluid retention and bronchodilator drugs where appropriate. Many patients with obstructive sleep apnoea are helped by the use of continuous nasal airway pressure (nasal CPAP) at night; in extreme cases, a tracheostomy has been used to bypass the site of upper airway narrowing.

REFERENCES

1. Scott, R.W. and Garvin, C.F. Cor pulmonale: Observations in fifty autopsy cases. *Am. Heart. J.* 1941; **22**: 56–63.
2. Howarth, S., McMichael, J. and Sharpey-Schafer, E.P. Effects of oxygen, venesection and digitalis in chronic heart failure from disease of the lungs. *Clin. Sci.* 1947; **6**: 187–96.
3. Harvey, R.M., Ferrer, M.I., Richards, D.W. and Cournand, A. Influence of chronic pulmonary disease on heart and circulation. *Am. J. Med.* 1951; **10**: 719–38.
4. Stuart-Harris, C.H. A hospital study of congestive heart failure with special reference to cor pulmonale. *Br. Med. J.* 1959; **2**: 201–8.
5. World Health Organisation. *Chronic cor pulmonale.* Report of an expert committee. Geneva: WHO, 1961.
6. Burrows, B., Fletcher, C.M. and Heard, B.E. The emphysematous and bronchial types of chronic airways obstruction. *Lancet* 1966; **1**: 830–5.
7. Heath, D., Smith, P., Rios Dalenz, J., Williams, D. and Harris, P. Small pulmonary arteries in some natives of La Paz, Bolivia. *Thorax* 1981; **36**: 599–604.
8. Heath, D. and Edwards, J.E. The pathology of hypertensive pulmonary vascular disease. A description of six grades of structural changes in the pulmonary artery with special reference to congenital cardiac septal defect. *Circulation* 1958; **18**: 533–47.
9. Dunnill, M.S. An assessment of the anatomical factor in cor pulmonale in emphysema. *J. Clin. Pathol.* 1961; **14**: 246–58.
10. Shelton, D.M., Keal, E. and Reid, L. The pulmonary circulation in chronic bronchitis and emphysema. *Chest* 1977; **71**: 3035.
11. Ryland, D. and Reid, L. The pulmonary circulation in cystic fibrosis. *Thorax* 1975; **30**: 285–92.
12. Wagenvoort, C.A. and Wagenvoort, N. *Pathology of pulmonary hypertension.* London: John Wiley and Sons, 1977, pp. 121–5.
13. Fulton, R.M., Hutchinson, E.C. and Jones, A.M. Ventricular weight in cardiac hypertrophy. *Br. Heart J.* 1952; **14**: 413–20.
14. Burrows, B., Kettel, L.J. and Niden, A.H. Patterns of cardiovascular dysfunction in chronic obstructive lung disease. *N. Engl. J. Med.* 1972; **286**: 912–8.
15. Boushy, S.F. and North, L.B. Hemodynamic changes in chronic obstructive pulmonary disease. *Chest* 1977; **72**: 565–70.
16. Bishop, J.M. and Cross, K.W. Use of other physiological variables to predict pulmonary arterial pressure in patients with chronic respiratory disease. *Eur. Heart J.* 1981; **2**: 509–17.
17. Weitzenblum, E., Hirth, C., Ducolone, A., Mirhom, R., Rasaholinjanahary, J. and Erhart, M. Prognostic value of pulmonary artery pressure in chronic obstructive pulmonary disease. *Thorax* 1981; **36**: 752–8.
18. Fleetham, J.A. and Kryger, M.H. Sleep disorders in chronic airflow obstruction. *Med. Clin. N. Am.* 1981; **65**: 549–61.
19. Matthay, R.A. and Berger, H.J. Cardiovascular performance in chronic obstructive pulmonary diseases. *Med. Clin. N. Am.* 1981; **65**: 489–524.
20. MacNee, W., Xue, Q.F., Hannan, W.J., Flenley, D.C., Adie, C.J. and Muir, A.L. Assessment by radionuclide angiography of right and left ventricular function in chronic bronchitis and emphysema. *Thorax* 1983; **38**: 494–500.
21. Baum, G.L., Schwartz, A., Llamas, R. and Castillo, C. Left ventricular function in chronic obstructive lung disease. *N. Engl. J. Med.* 1971; **285**: 361–5.
22. Steele, P., Ellis, J.H., Van Dyke, D., Sutton, F., Creagh, E. and Davies, H. Left ventricular ejection fraction in severe chronic obstructive airways disease. *Am. J. Med.* 1975; **59**: 21–8.
23. Murphy, M.L., de Soyza, N. and Thenabadu, P.N. Quantitation of fibrosis of the heart in chronic obstructive pulmonary disease with and without cor pulmonale. *Chest* 1983; **84**: 535–8.
24. Light, R.W., Mintz, H.M., Linden, G.S. and Brown, S.E. Hemodynamics of patients with severe chronic obstructive pulmonary disease during progressive upright exercise. *Am. Rev. Resp. Dis.* 1984; **130**: 391–5.
25. Richens, J.M. and Howard, P. Oedema in cor pulmonale. *Clin. Sci.* 1982; **62**: 255–9.
26. Wallis, P.J.W., Skehan, J.D., Newland, A.C., Wedzicha, J.A., Mills, P.G. and Empey, D.W. Effects of erythrapheresis on pulmonary haemodynamics and oxygen transport in patients with secondary polycythaemia and cor pulmonale. *Clin. Sci.* 1986; **70**: 91–8.
27. Bishop, J.M. Cardiovascular complications of chronic bronchitis and emphysema. *Med. Clin. N. Am.* 1973; **57**: 771–80.
28. Aubier, M., Murciano, D., Milic Emili, J. *et al.* Effects of the administration of O_2 on ventilation and blood gases in patients with chronic obstructive pulmonary disease during acute respiratory failure. *Am. Rev. Respir. Dis.* 1980; **122**: 747–54.
29. Matthay, R.A., Schwarz, M.I., Ellis, J.H. *et al.* Pulmonary artery hypertension in chronic obstructive pulmonary disease. *Invest. Radiol.* 1981; **16**: 95–100.
30. Millard, F.J.C. The electrocardiogram in chronic lung disease. *Br. Heart J.* 1967; **29**: 43–50.
31. Bishop, J.M. and Cross, K.W. Physiological variables and

mortality in patients with various categories of chronic respiratory disease. *Bull. Eur. Physiopathol. Respir.* 1984; **20**: 495–500.

32. Riordan, J.F., Sillett, R.W. and McNicol, M.W. A controlled trial of doxapram in acute respiratory failure. *Br. J. Dis. Chest* 1975; **69**: 57–62.

33. Nocturnal Oxygen Therapy Trial Group. Continuous or nocturnal oxygen therapy in hypoxaemic chronic obstructive lung disease. *Ann. Intern. Med.* 1980; **93**: 391–8.

34. Report of the Medical Research Council Working Party. Long-term domiciliary oxygen therapy in chronic hypoxic cor pulmonale complicating chronic bronchitis and emphysema. *Lancet* 1981; i: 681–5.

35. Harrison, B.D.W. and Stokes, T.C. Secondary polycythaemia: its causes, effects and treatment. *Br. J. Dis. Chest* 1982; **76**: 313–40.

36. MacNee, W., Connaughton, J.J., Rhind, G.B. *et al.* A comparison of the effects of almitrine or oxygen breathing on pulmonary arterial pressure and right ventricular ejection fraction in hypoxic chronic bronchitis and emphysema. *Am. Rev. Respir. Dis.* 1986; **134**: 559–65.

37. Dal Nogare, A.R. and Rubin, L.J. The effects of hydralazine on exercise capacity in pulmonary hypertension secondary to chronic obstructive pulmonary disease. *Am. Rev. Respir. Dis.* 1986; **133**: 385–9.

38. Melot, C., Hallimans, R., Naeije, R., Mols, P. and Lejeune, P. Deleterious effect of nifedipine on pulmonary gas exchange in chronic obstructive pulmonary disease. *Am. Rev. Respir. Dis.* 1984; **130**: 612–6.

39. Siegler, D. Reversible electrocardiographic changes in severe acute asthma. *Thorax* 1977; **32**: 328–32.

40. Rebuck, A.S. and Pengelly, L.D. Development of pulsus paradoxus in the presence of airways obstruction. *N. Engl. J. Med.* 1973; **288**: 66–9.

41. Corris, P.A. and Gibson, G.J. Asthma presenting as cor pulmonale. *Br. Med. J.* 1984; **288**: 389–90.

42. Liebow, A.A., Hales, M.R. and Lindskog, G.E. Enlargement of the bronchial arteries and their anastomoses with the pulmonary arteries in bronchiectasis. *Am. J. Pathol.* 1949; **25**: 211.

43. Chipps, B.E., Alderson, P.O., Roland, J.M.A. *et al.* Noninvasive evaluation of ventricular function in cystic fibrosis. *J. Pediatr.* 1979; **95**: 379–84.

44. Benson, L.N., Newth, C.J.L., Desouza, M. *et al.* Radionuclide assessment of right and left ventricular function during bicycle exercise in young patients with cystic fibrosis. *Am. Rev. Respir. Dis.* 1984; **130**: 987.

45. Spiro, S.G., Dowdeswell, I.R.G. and Clark, T.J.H. An analysis of submaximal exercise responses in patients with sarcoidosis and fibrosing alveolitis. *Br. J. Dis. Chest* 1981; **75**: 169–80.

46. Gabriel, S.K. Respiratory and circulatory investigations in obstructive and restrictive lung disease. *Acta Med. Scand.* 1973; Suppl. 546.

47. Davies, G. and Reid, L. Effect of scoliosis on growth of alveoli and pulmonary arteries and on right ventricle. *Arch. Dis. Child.* 1971; **46**: 623–32.

48. Shneerson, J.M., Venco, A. and Prime, F.J. A study of pulmonary artery pressure, electrocardiography and mechanocardiography in thoracic scoliosis. *Thorax* 1977; **32**: 700–5.

49. Bergofsky, E.H. Respiratory failure in disorders of the thoracic cage. *Am. Rev. Respir. Dis.* 1979; **119**: 643–70.

50. Libby, D.M., Briscoe, W.A., Boyce, B. and Smith, J.P. Acute respiratory failure in scoliosis or kyphosis. *Am. J. Med.* 1982; **73**: 532–8.

51. Bradley, T.D., Rutherford, R., Grossman, R.F. *et al.* Role of daytime hypoxaemia in the pathogenesis of right heart failure in the obstructive sleep apnoea syndrome. *Am. Rev. Respir. Dis.* 1985; **131**: 835–9.

Chapter 56

Lung Function in Heart Disease

G.J. Gibson

INTRODUCTION

Cardiac disease and respiratory disease share many clinical features, particularly shortness of breath and wheezing. Furthermore, cardiac disease is frequently associated with measurable abnormalities of respiratory function, and the functional effects may be qualitatively similar to those of primary respiratory disease. However, as there are important quantitative differences between cardiac and respiratory disease, the measurement of respiratory function is often of considerable help in differential diagnosis. Another link between cardiac disease and respiratory function demonstrated in the Framingham and subsequent studies was that a reduced vital capacity appears to be a significant risk factor for myocardial infarction and sudden cardiac death.[1]

RESPIRATORY FUNCTION TESTS

The commonly applied tests of respiratory function are of two main types; those that measure the mechanical performance of the lungs and thorax and those that assess the efficiency of pulmonary gas exchange.[2]

TESTS OF RESPIRATORY MECHANICS

In simple mechanical terms, the lungs consist of distensible elastic structures (the alveoli) subtended by a system of branching tubes (the airways). Inspiration is achieved by contraction of the inspiratory muscles to generate a subatmospheric alveolar pressure which is used to overcome a combination of elastic and resistive forces. The degree of distension and the rate of airflow are determined, respectively, by the elastic properties of the lungs (and also chest wall) and the calibre of the airways. These can be quantified directly by measurements of

pulmonary (and chest wall) compliance and airways resistance; in practice, these variables are measured infrequently. The elastic behaviour of the system can be assessed more easily by measurements of lung volumes (particularly vital capacity) and airway function by calculation of airflow during forced expiration (e.g. FEV_1, peak expiratory flow). In some circumstances, measurement of total lung capacity (TLC, which equals the sum of vital capacity, VC, and residual volume, RV) is also of value. Apart from simplicity of performance and of recording, tests such as the FEV_1 also have the advantage of being relatively independent of effort in that, if a progressively increasing expiratory force is applied, it is met by greater dynamic compression of the intrathoracic airways with consequently little effect on the resulting FEV_1.

Abnormalities of ventilatory function are usually classified as either 'obstructive' or 'restrictive'; in the former, the ratio FEV_1/VC is reduced ($< 75\%$), whereas in the latter the ratio is normal and the FEV_1 and vital capacity are affected in proportion to one another. In the presence of marked airway narrowing, the vital capacity is also reduced, but proportionally less than FEV_1. In most patients with primary airway disease (chronic obstructive pulmonary disease or asthma), the total lung capacity is increased, which implies a considerable increase in residual volume. In patients with 'stiff' lungs, e.g. pulmonary fibrosis or pulmonary oedema, both vital capacity and total lung capacity are reduced.

TESTS OF GAS EXCHANGE

The efficiency of pulmonary gas exchange is assessed by measurement of the carbon monoxide transfer factor (T_LCO, also known as the carbon monoxide diffusing capacity, D_LCO) and of arterial blood gases. The carbon monoxide transfer factor (measured by the single breath method) is a sensitive but non-specific index of the integrity of the alveolar–capillary membrane. It is impaired by several pathological processes, including the effective loss of functioning alveoli, the thickening of the alveolar–capillary membrane or a reduction in the number of functioning pulmonary capillaries. Account can be taken of reductions in the number of functioning alveoli by calculating the carbon monoxide transfer factor per litre of ventilated lung, otherwise known as the transfer coefficient or KCO.

The efficiency of the lungs in taking up oxygen is quantified by measuring the partial pressure of oxygen in arterial blood or non-invasively by use of an ear or pulse oximeter to measure arterial oxygen saturation, the two being related by the haemoglobin–oxygen dissociation curve (Fig. 56.1).

If hypoventilation occurs, the rise in $PaCO_2$ is accompanied by a quantitatively similar fall in PaO_2; conversely, hyperventilation produces a fall in $PaCO_2$ and a rise in PaO_2. Owing to the shape of the haemoglobin–oxygen dissociation curve (Fig. 56.1), however, an increase in PaO_2 above normal is associated with very little increase in arterial oxygen *saturation* or oxygen *content*. The most common pattern of blood gases in disease is the combination of arterial hypoxaemia with a normal or reduced $PaCO_2$. In the majority of conditions, this results from local inequalities of ventilation and perfusion. Most diseases are patchy in their effects. Areas of local airway narrowing or of increased alveolar stiffness impair local ventilation and thus reduce the

ratio of ventilation to perfusion ($\dot{V}/\dot{Q}$); this tends to increase local PCO_2 and reduce local PO_2. At the other end of the spectrum there are alveoli with locally impaired perfusion and hence relatively high $\dot{V}/\dot{Q}$ ratios, which increase local PO_2 and reduce local PCO_2. The net result on arterial blood is an abnormally low PaO_2 and a widening of the normally very small alveolar–arterial oxygen tension difference (AaPo_2 gradient). This occurs because alveoli with high $\dot{V}/\dot{Q}$ ratios cannot improve oxygenation of the blood sufficiently to counter the effects of alveoli with low $\dot{V}/\dot{Q}$ ratios. The alveoli with high $\dot{V}/\dot{Q}$ ratios have a 'dead-space-like' effect and contribute to the physiological dead-space, whereas alveoli with low $\dot{V}/\dot{Q}$ ratios have a 'shunt-like' effect and contribute to the physiological shunt (Fig. 56.2).

The effects of dispersion of $\dot{V}/\dot{Q}$ ratios are minimized when pure oxygen is breathed, because in this condition even a very poorly ventilated alveolus can eventually achieve a high PO_2. In the investigation of arterial hypoxaemia, the patient is given 100% oxygen to breathe in order to calculate the 'anatomical' shunt, i.e. the proportion of the cardiac output that is bypassing gas-containing alveoli. In patients with severe lung disease, adequate equilibration in poorly ventilated alveoli may take 15–20 min. For confident interpretation of the results, it is essential to use a closed system in which 100% oxygen is administered via a mouthpiece and the patient wears a nose-clip. After breathing oxygen in this way, the value for PaO_2 normally exceeds 67 kPa (500 mmHg).

Arterial hypercapnia results when 'effective' alveolar ventilation is less than normal; this does not necessarily imply a reduction in total ventilation, because when the physiological dead-space is very large much of the ventilation is 'wasted'.

Matching of ventilation and perfusion at a regional level can be assessed crudely by routine perfusion and ventilation lung scans. In the normal subject in the upright posture, both ventilation and perfusion per unit volume are greater at the lung bases than at the apices but as the gravitational gradient of perfusion is greater than that of ventilation the $\dot{V}/\dot{Q}$ ratio is higher at the apex than at the base. Lung perfusion usually increases in a linear fashion from the apex to approximately two-thirds of the way down the lung (Fig. 56.3), but at the very base there is a reduction in perfusion, which has been attributed to the effects of increased basal interstitial pressure of the pre-capillary vessels (so-called 'zone 4').[3]

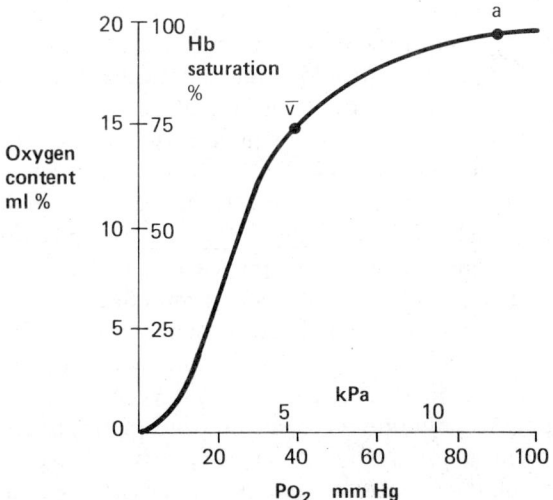

Fig. 56.1. Haemoglobin–oxygen dissociation curve. The ordinate may be plotted in terms of either oxygen content (concentration) or percentage saturation. The values for oxygen content indicated assume a normal haemoglobin concentration. Normal arterial (a) and mixed venous (v̄) values are indicated.

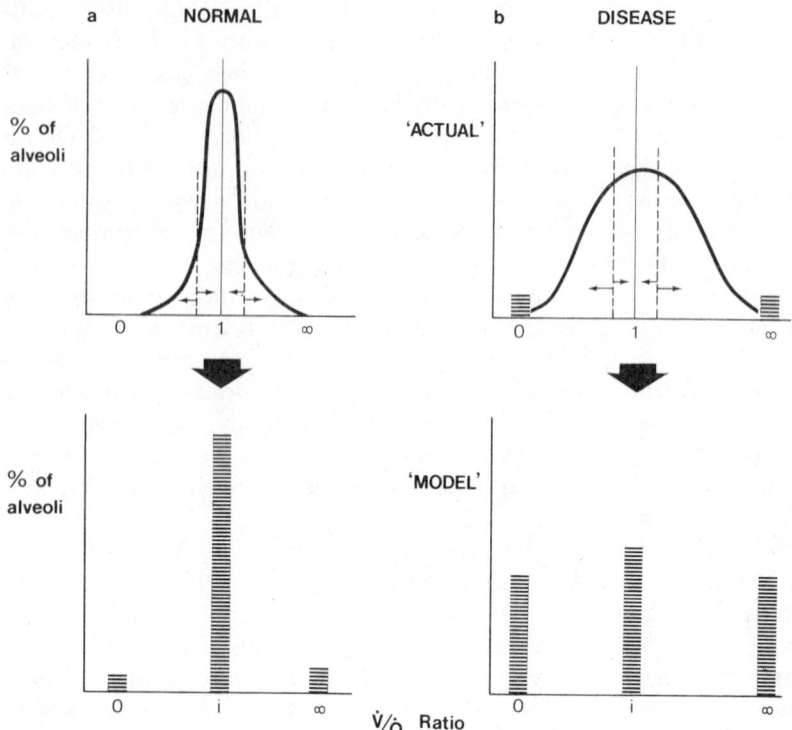

a NORMAL   b DISEASE

% of alveoli

'ACTUAL'

% of alveoli

'MODEL'

$\dot{V}/\dot{Q}$ Ratio

Fig. 56.2. Upper panel: Theoretical distribution of $\dot{V}/\dot{Q}$ ratios in (a) normal and (b) diseased lungs. Lower panel: 'three compartment model' of same lungs in which the distribution of $\dot{V}/\dot{Q}$ ratios is described in terms of a physiological shunt ($\dot{V}/\dot{Q} = 0$), a physiological dead-space ($\dot{V}/\dot{Q} = \infty$) and an 'ideal' alveolar compartment (i). In calculation of the physiological shunt and dead-space, alveoli are effectively partitioned, so that those with lower than average $\dot{V}/\dot{Q}$ ratios contribute to the shunt and those with above average $\dot{V}/\dot{Q}$ ratios contribute to the dead-space. Wider dispersion of $\dot{V}/\dot{Q}$ ratios in disease (right) leads to increases in both of these compartments and a reduction in the 'alveolar' compartment. (Reproduced with permission from Gibson, G.J. *Clinical tests of respiratory function*. London: Macmillan, 1984.[2])

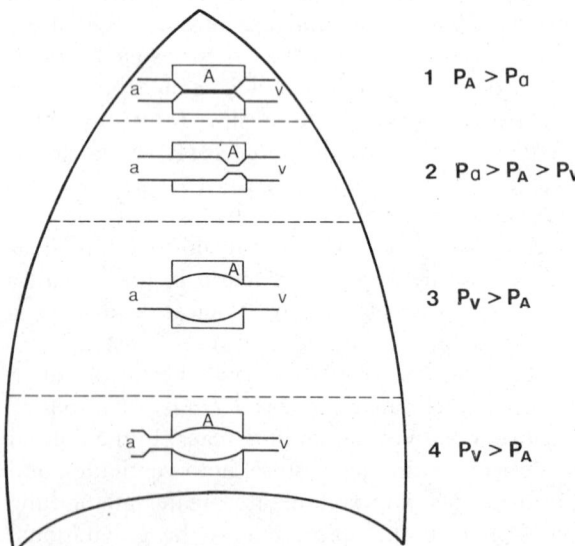

1 $P_A > P_a$

2 $P_a > P_A > P_V$

3 $P_V > P_A$

4 $P_V > P_A$

Fig. 56.3. Effect of gravity on pulmonary perfusion in the upright lung. The lung may be considered as four zones.[3] At rest, there is little perfusion of apical alveoli (zone 1) where pulmonary artery pressure (P_a) is less than the surrounding alveolar pressure (P_A). Both P_a and the outflow pressure (P_V) increase down the lung. Once $P_a > P_A$, flow occurs but if $P_V < P_A$ it is determined, not by the difference ($P_a - P_V$) but by ($P_a - P_A$), as in zone 2. Once $P_V > P_A$ (zone 3), ($P_a - P_V$) becomes the driving pressure. At the lung base (zone 4), flow is reduced probably by the effect of greater local interstitial pressure on pre-capillary vessels.

TESTS OF EXERCISE TOLERANCE

Sometimes, the assessment of ventilatory performance and gas exchange during exercise adds further useful information. The use of exercise testing for assessing electrocardiographic changes is dealt with elsewhere (Chapter 20). Exercise testing allows confirmation of the patient's effort intolerance, observation of the patient when the symptoms are likely to be most troublesome and measurement of various indices that may be helpful in analysing the cause of symptoms. The simplest form of exercise test is to walk the patient along a corridor for 6 or 12 min; use is increasingly being made of these self-paced tests, in which the distance covered by the patient in the time designated is recorded. With more sophisticated methods, ventilation can be measured and, in combination with the measurement of mixed expired gas concentrations, the indices recorded can be related to oxygen consumption. A commonly used method is to exercise the patient at progressively increasing workloads on a treadmill or bicycle ergometer and measure ventilation and cardiac frequency together with oxygen consumption. The intensity of breathlessness can be recorded at each workload using a simple visual analogue score; repeated testing can be used to monitor the effects of therapeutic interventions.

RESPIRATORY FUNCTION IN CARDIAC DISEASE

CARDIAC FAILURE

It is well known that the lungs in patients with cardiac failure are stiff. The vital capacity is reduced by interstitial oedema; if alveolar oedema is also present, the reduction is more severe. Cardiac enlargement also contributes to the loss of lung volume. Even in the absence of radiographic evidence, pulmonary congestion (e.g. after myocardial infarction) produces measurable reductions in vital capacity, and the abnormality may take several weeks to return to normal.[5] 'Cardiac asthma' implies narrowing of the airways due to peribronchial oedema, but in contrast to acute bronchial asthma the FEV_1/VC ratio is only mildly reduced.

Even in uncomplicated myocardial infarction, abnormalities of pulmonary gas exchange occur and can be detected as a widening of the $AaPo_2$ gradient. Patients with pulmonary oedema usually show arterial hypoxaemia with a normal or low value for $Paco_2$. Hypercapnia, however, may also develop, especially in the acute phase of pulmonary oedema in infants or in the elderly. In very sick patients, a metabolic acidosis may develop; when this occurs in combination with a respiratory acidosis, very low values of arterial pH result.[6] The recognition of hypercapnia may have important implications for therapy because if it is present opiate drugs and uncontrolled oxygen, which are standard therapy for patients with left ventricular failure, should be used with caution.

RHEUMATIC HEART DISEASE

Measurements of ventilatory mechanics in patients with mitral valve disease have been made for many years, but in some of the early studies the effects of smoking, particularly in lowering the FEV_1/VC ratio, were not given adequate consideration when the results were interpreted. In non-smoking patients, the FEV_1/VC ratio is normal or only mildly reduced. A reduction in lung compliance is characteristic and this causes a reduction in vital capacity. The residual volume is typically increased, so that the total lung capacity is usually normal,[7] unlike the situation in bronchial asthma or chronic obstructive pulmonary disease, in which the total lung capacity is characteristically increased. An increase in pulmonary capillary blood volume consequent on a high left atrial pressure might be expected to increase the carbon monoxide transfer factor, but,

more commonly, this is reduced, presumably due to a combination of maldistribution of ventilation and pulmonary vascular damage.

The magnitude of the respiratory function abnormalities is related to the degree of narrowing of the mitral valve and the severity of pulmonary hypertension.[7] Raised left atrial pressure produces characteristic abnormalities of the perfusion scan: increased perfusion of the lung apices and reduced perfusion of the bases. These abnormalities have been attributed to increased interstitial oedema at the lung bases; as the shift of perfusion is usually associated with a similar shift in ventilation, the overall regional matching of ventilation and perfusion is retained.[8] Patients with mitral valve disease show excessive ventilation on exercise with a tendency to breathe with a small tidal volume and rapid frequency, presumably due to pulmonary vascular congestion.

After surgical correction of mitral valve disease, improvements in respiratory function have been documented but some abnormalities remain, in particular the reduction in the carbon monoxide transfer factor. Ventilation on exercise improves, and patients are able to achieve a greater workload in a progressive exercise test before the heart rate becomes limiting.[9]

In aortic valve disease, the abnormalities tend to be less marked and may be undetectable unless the pulmonary wedge pressure is increased in which case there is a reduction in lung volumes and in the carbon monoxide transfer factor.[10]

LEFT-TO-RIGHT SHUNTS

The most characteristic abnormality of respiratory function in patients with left-to-right shunts is an increase in the carbon monoxide transfer factor, and in KCO, which tends to be more obvious in patients who have an atrial rather than a ventricular septal defect. It is related to the increase in pulmonary blood flow and an associated expansion of pulmonary capillary blood volume. With the development of pulmonary hypertension, the increase in T_LCO becomes less marked.[11] The effects of a left-to-right shunt on tests of pulmonary mechanics resemble those of mitral stenosis, with a reduction in vital capacity and an increase in residual volume. Despite the abnormally high oxygen saturation of pulmonary arterial blood in patients with left-to-right shunts, a reduction in systemic Pao_2 together with widening of $AaPo_2$ is typical.[12]

RIGHT-TO-LEFT SHUNTS

The most obvious abnormality in patients who have right-to-left shunts is a reduction in arterial oxygen tension, which may be gross. The reduction in oxygen content of arterial blood is partly compensated for by the increase in the haemoglobin concentration but this does not have a significant effect on oxygen partial pressure or percentage saturation. The most important feature of the arterial hypoxaemia of patients with right-to-left shunts is its failure to correct on breathing 100% oxygen; however, some rise in Pao_2 is to be expected because of minimization of the effects of ventilation/perfusion inequalities in the lungs. The problems of the elimination of carbon dioxide are not as well recognized, but the shunted blood contains carbon dioxide at the mixed venous tension, and therefore maintenance of a normal arterial level demands increased ventilation. This can usually be achieved at rest, when most patients have normal or slightly low values of $Paco_2$, but on exercise many patients are unable to maintain the necessary ventilation, which can result in a marked rise in $Paco_2$ accompanied by a fall in Pao_2.[13] Lung perfusion scans in patients with a right-to-left shunt characteristically show uptake of isotope in other organs, particularly the kidneys, liver and spleen, because of direct shunting into the systemic circulation. Presumably because of the associated pulmonary hypertension which is often present, carbon monoxide transfer and KCO are usually reduced and many patients also show evidence of airways obstruction with some reduction in the FEV_1/VC ratio.[14,15]

USE OF TESTS IN DIFFERENTIAL DIAGNOSIS

The commonest problems arise in patients with 'unexplained' exertional dyspnoea. Many such patients presenting to respiratory physicians are found to have cardiological problems; similarly, many others presenting to cardiologists have respiratory problems. In most cases, a careful history, physical examination, chest X-ray and electrocardiogram point to the underlying cause. When the shortness of breath is due to primary airway disease, simple spirometric measurements will usually suffice to make the diagnosis incontrovertible; however, in patients who have asthma, physical examination and simple respiratory function tests performed during remission may be unrewarding. Such pa-

tients should monitor their peak expiratory flow at home twice a day. It may reveal marked variability of airway function and in particular the characteristic asthmatic 'morning dip'. Domiciliary monitoring of peak expiratory flow also allows patients to make measurements if they are woken by an attack of breathlessness and wheezing during the night; if these symptoms are due to 'cardiac asthma', the peak expiratory flow is likely to be only mildly affected. If airway disease has been excluded, interstitial lung disease should also be considered because occasionally this can be present without radiographic evidence; in such patients, measurements of the carbon monoxide transfer factor or ventilatory measurements during exercise may be helpful diagnostically. The performance of a perfusion lung scan should be considered if pulmonary vascular disease is a possible diagnosis because recurrent pulmonary embolism occasionally presents as dyspnoea with no other specific features. If the vital capacity is reduced without apparent cause, measurements of maximum static respiratory pressures are of value in excluding weakness of the respiratory muscles which can occasionally present with dyspnoea. The carbon monoxide transfer factor is a valuable method for assessing global alveolar–capillary function; this and spirometry are the most useful respiratory function tests for the screening of patients who have dyspnoea of uncertain cause.

Some patients whose breathlessness is not otherwise explained are found to have 'psychogenic dyspnoea'. Characteristically, they perform breathing tests erratically, which may be obvious to the technician performing the tests. Typically, they show marked hypocapnia and a respiratory alkalosis; on exercise, they stop at levels of ventilation and heart rate well below those limits predicted by spirometric measurements and age, respectively.

If a progressive exercise test is performed, it is useful to compare the highest measured values of ventilation and heart rate with the predicted maximal values calculated from the FEV_1 and from the age of the subject, respectively. If a patient achieves the predicted maximum heart rate during the test, it is reasonable to conclude that the limit to further exercise is set by the cardiovascular system as it is in normal subjects. In most patients with respiratory disease, exercise is limited by the mechanical performance of the ventilatory system, consequently the patient's maximum exercise ventilation is found to be close to the maximum ventilation predicted from the value of FEV_1. Use is also made of submaximal indices of heart rate and ventilation at standard values of oxygen consumption: cardiac disease is usually accompanied by a relatively greater effect on the heart-rate response and respiratory disease by greater abnormality of the ventilatory response but the distinction is not absolute; in many patients with cardiac disease, ventilation is abnormally high and in many patients with respiratory disease the response of cardiac frequency on exercise is abnormal, perhaps because of unfitness or of abnormalities of right ventricular function.

In patients presenting with right-sided heart failure, tests of ventilatory function allow the recognition of patients with severe chronic obstructive pulmonary disease or asthma resulting in cor pulmonale. In many such patients, severe pathological changes develop insidiously and it is sometimes only the onset of oedema at an advanced stage of the disease that brings the patient to notice. The differential diagnosis of such patients is usually between primary airway disease, mitral valve disease and primary pulmonary hypertension.

In patients with hypoxaemia of uncertain origin, simple respiratory function tests such as spirometry and the carbon monoxide transfer factor are helpful in recognizing or excluding airways obstruction or pulmonary fibrosis. Measurement of the $AaPo_2$ gradient on 100% oxygen is valuable in excluding an anatomical right-to-left shunt but some increase in the gradient on 100% oxygen can be seen in many non-cardiac conditions including severe pulmonary fibrosis, extensive bronchiectasis and hepatic cirrhosis. The 'anatomical' shunt is not necessarily through a single channel but may reflect the presence of many small anastomoses or the effects of numerous small areas of lung that remain perfused but totally unventilated.

REFERENCES

1. Friedman, G.D., Klatsky, A.L. and Siegelamb, A.B. Lung function and risk of myocardial infarction and sudden cardiac death. *N. Engl. J. Med.* 1976; **294**: 1071–5.
2. Gibson, G.J. *Clinical tests of respiratory function.* London, Macmillan, 1984.
3. Hughes, J.M.B., Glazier, J.B., Maloney, J.E. and West, J.B. Effect of lung volume on the distribution of pulmonary flow in man. *Respir. Physiol.* 1968; **4**: 58–72.
4. Jones, N.L. and Campbell, E.J.M. *Clinical exercise testing,* 2nd edn. London: W.B. Saunders, 1982.
5. Hales, C.A. and Kazemi, H. Pulmonary function after uncomplicated myocardial infarction. *Chest* 1977; **72**: 350–8.
6. Avery, W.G., Samet, P. and Sackner, M.A. The acidosis of pulmonary oedema. *Am. J. Med.* 1970; **48**: 320–4.
7. Rhodes, K.M., Evemy, K., Nariman, S. and Gibson, G.J. Relation between severity of mitral valve disease and routine lung function tests in non-smokers. *Thorax* 1982; **37**: 751–5.
8. Dawson, A., Rocamora, J.M. and Morgan, J.R. Regional lung function in chronic pulmonary congestion with and without mitral stenosis. *Am. Rev. Respir. Dis.* 1976; **113**: 51–9.
9. Rhodes, K.M., Evemy, K., Nariman, S. and Gibson, G.J. Effects of mitral valve surgery on static lung function and exercise performance. *Thorax* 1985; **40**: 107–112.
10. Yernault, J.-C. and DeTroyer, A. Mechanics of breathing in patients with aortic valve disease. *Bull. Physiopathol. Respir.* 1980; **16**: 491–500.
11. DeTroyer, A., Yernault, J.-C. and Englert, M. Mechanics of breathing in patients with atrial septal defect. *Am. Rev. Respir. Dis.* 1977; **115**: 413–21.
12. Lees, M.H., Way, R.C. and Ross, B.B. Ventilation and respiratory gas transfer of infants with increased pulmonary blood flow. *Pediatrics* 1977; **40**: 259–71.
13. Davies, H. and Gazetopoulos, N. Dyspnoea in cyanotic congenital heart disease. *Br. Heart J.* 1965; **27**: 28–41.
14. MacArthur, C.G.C., Hunter, D. and Gibson, G.J. Ventilatory function in the Eisenmenger syndrome. *Thorax* 1979; **34**: 348–53.
15. Burke, C.M., Glanville, A.R., Morris, A.J.R., *et al.* Pulmonary function in advanced pulmonary hypertension. *Thorax* 1987; **42**: 131–5.

Chapter 57

Diseases of the Aorta

K.M. Taylor

INTRODUCTION

This chapter is confined to acquired pathology affecting the ascending aorta, transverse arch and descending thoracic aorta. Congenital aortic pathology and aortic valve pathology are dealt with in Chapters 25–27.

The aorta is generally considered to be a relatively simple structure, both anatomically and functionally. However, several pathological conditions are known to affect the thoracic aorta. With the advances in cardiothoracic surgical techniques that have occurred in recent years, the management of acute aortic conditions has changed from a more conservative approach to early and aggressive replacement surgery.

The three main conditions to be considered in this chapter are:
1 aneurysm of the thoracic aorta;
2 dissection of the thoracic aorta;
3 aortitis.

ANEURYSM OF THE THORACIC AORTA

DEFINITION

This condition is characterized by a localized dilatation of the aortic wall. The dilatation may be *fusiform* with true circumferential dilatation or *saccular*, in which a spherical non-circumferential dilatation originates from a narrow neck. The essential requirement for aneurysm development within the thoracic aorta is the presence of pathological weakness within the media of the aortic wall.

AETIOLOGY OF THORACIC AORTIC ANEURYSMS

Conditions leading to medial weakness can be broadly categorized as follows.
1 Atherosclerosis
2 Non-inflammatory medial degeneration
3 Aortitis

Atherosclerosis

Although atherosclerosis of the aorta is widely recognized and an almost inevitable accompaniment of ageing,[1] it is not generally appreciated that atherosclerotic aneurysms are rare in the thoracic aorta, particularly in the ascending aorta. In contrast, below the diaphragm, abdominal aortic aneurysms are almost invariably atheromatous in aetiology. Several authors have stated that atheroma is an intimal disease.[2] Lipoprotein release from within atheromatous plaques may induce secondary macrophage activity with destruction of elastin within the medial layer of the aortic wall.[3] Atherosclerotic aneurysm of the thoracic aorta has been reported in association with hyperlipidaemic syndromes[4] and in patients with longstanding diabetes mellitus.

Non-inflammatory cystic medial degeneration

This description encompasses several different pathological entities including the defined Marfan's syndrome, which accounts for less than 20% of cases of thoracic aneurysm.[2] Thoracic aneurysms occur more frequently in those patients who have idiopathic medial degeneration not associated with the skeletal and ocular manifestations of Marfan's syndrome. In these conditions, the medial degeneration is maximal in the proximal ascending aorta,[5–7] perhaps reflecting the differential collagen cross-link structure between the ascending aorta, the arch and the descending thoracic aorta. Idiopathic medial degeneration has many names including medial arteriopathy, annulo-aortic ectasia and idiopathic aortic dilatation. The term 'forme fruste' Marfan's syndrome has also been used for patients who have localized aortic pathology identical to true Marfan's syndrome, but the use of this term is controversial.

Inflammatory thoracic aortic aneurysms

Aortitis encompasses several conditions in which destruction of the medial layer in the aortic wall is related to chronic inflammation. The following inflammatory agents have been described.
1 Syphilis.
2 Non-syphilitic bacterial aortitis.
3 Non-bacterial aortitis:
   a Takayasu's disease;
   b ankylosing spondylitis;
   c Reiter's syndrome;
   d giant cell arteritis.

In general, aortitis eventually manifests itself in thoracic aortic aneurysm formation. Many of the general features of pathophysiology, diagnosis and treatment of thoracic aneurysms are applicable to the above-mentioned aortitis syndromes, but specific features of these particular syndromes will also be discussed later in this chapter (p. 1359).

PATHOPHYSIOLOGY OF THORACIC AORTIC ANEURYSMS

As previously indicated, the essential abnormality of thoracic aortic aneurysms is weakness of the medial layer of the aortic wall. The severity and extent of the medial weakness may be exacerbated by the presence of systemic arterial hypertension. Once the pathological process of aortic dilatation has begun, the condition tends to be progressive. Increasing dilatation of the thoracic aorta and increasing weakness of the aortic wall continue to progress. Many authors have indicated that the almost inevitable presence of intraluminal clot within the aneurysm, although increasing the risk of distal emboli, may increase the intrinsic strength of the weakened aneurysmal aorta, thereby reducing the incidence of thoracic aneurysm rupture.[5]

Where the proximal ascending aorta is involved, the initiating pathology of medial weakness may be followed through the phase of dilatation with associated aortic valve incompetence. The dilatation and thrombus formation may be associated with systemic arterial embolism, and the underlying weakness of the aortic media may produce rupture or, if associated with hypertension and an intramural tear, with dissection. It should be noted that dissection is not an inevitable consequence of thoracic aneurysm formation. In recent reviews, it has been noted that a substantial proportion of cases of thoracic aortic dissection occur in a structurally normal aorta with no evidence of medial pathology.[2,8,9]

CLINICAL FEATURES OF THORACIC AORTIC ANEURYSMS

The majority of thoracic aneurysms are found by chance, often when a chest X-ray is taken, because the aneurysm sac may develop without any obvious clinical symptoms. The clinical features of thoracic aneurysm are generally related to the following situations.
1 Development of aortic valve regurgitation—clearly this complication is associated with proximal ascending aortic aneurysms.
2 Expansion of the thoracic aneurysm sac–chest pain has been reported in a number of series in association with thoracic aortic aneurysm. The chest pain tends not to be typical of angina and its site may be variable, being felt anteriorly or posteriorly. Lindsay and colleagues have suggested that an acute onset of chest pain may relate to rapid expansion or to potential rupture of the aneurysm sac.[9]
3 Compression or erosion of adjoining structures—the increasing size of the thoracic aortic aneurysm sac may compromise the lumen of the trachea or main bronchi. The presence of the thoracic aortic aneurysm has, in the author's experience, revealed itself by massive haemoptysis with the aneurysm sac eroding into the thoracic oesophagus, or into the trachea or bronchial tree. Finally, if rupture of the aneurysm sac occurs in the proximal ascending aorta within the pericardium, cardiac tamponade may occur.

INVESTIGATION OF THORACIC AORTIC ANEURYSMS

The principles governing the investigation of cases with thoracic aortic aneurysm relate to the following features.
1 Site.
2 Extent.
3 Involvement of aortic valve.
4 Involvement of head and neck vessels.
5 Presence or absence of dissection.

The site and extent of the thoracic aortic aneurysm may be detectable by plain chest X-ray. However, aneurysms of the proximal segment of the ascending aorta may be incorporated within the general cardiac silhouette and thus be difficult to assess (Fig. 57.1). In general, plain chest X-ray must be regarded as insufficient to delineate the features of the thoracic aortic aneurysm as previously

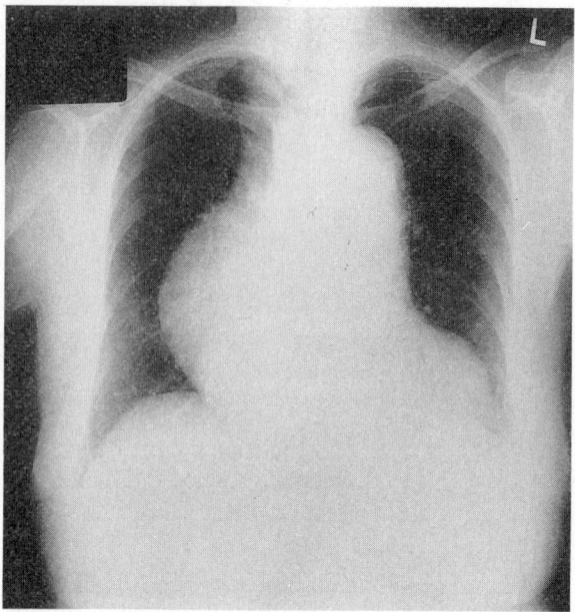

Fig. 57.1. Plain chest X-ray appearances of an ascending aorta aneurysm. The extreme dilatation of the aortic root is seen as an extension of the right heart border. The extent of aneurysmal dilatation on the left side is unclear, due to the underlying cardiac contour.

defined. Increasingly, non-invasive and invasive diagnostic techniques are used. The non-invasive techniques, in addition to plain chest X-ray, include two-dimensional echocardiography and computerized tomography (CT scanning). Both echocardiography and computerized tomography may allow the definition of the site and extent of the thoracic aortic aneurysm.[10–12] In addition to acquiring absolute data, these techniques allow doubtful cases to be assessed sequentially: progressive increase in size and extent of the aneurysm sac may encourage surgical intervention. In addition, cross-sectional echocardiography and computerized tomography may allow identification of the involvement of head and neck vessels. Computerized tomography has been shown to have acceptable definition, particularly with contrast enhancement, to allow the assessment of the presence or absence of dissection and the location of the intimal flap (see Figure 57.2).

Invasive aortic angiography

Most cardiothoracic surgeons will require access to invasive aortography in order to define more accurately the size, extent and associated head and neck vessel involvement of thoracic aortic aneurysms. High-quality definition should be

achieved with angiography, particularly if oblique views opening out the aortic arch are obtained. It should be appreciated, however, that the presence of intraluminal clot on intraluminal angiography may give an underestimate of the size of the aneurysm sac.

INDICATIONS FOR SURGERY IN LOCALIZED SACCULAR AND FUSIFORM THORACIC AORTIC ANEURYSMS

Most authorities would agree that the mere presence of a localized thoracic aortic aneurysm is not in itself sufficient indication to recommend surgical intervention. Indications for surgery include:

1 excessively large aneurysms assessed by ultrasound or aortography;
2 significant symptoms or clinical signs associated with the aneurysm;
3 occurrence of peripheral arterial embolization from clot within the aneurysm sac;
4 co-existent uncontrollable hypertension.

Although the above-mentioned indications are accepted as a consensus view, there has been a trend towards more aggressive surgical intervention whenever thoracic aortic aneurysms of a significant size (i.e. > 5–6 cm in diameter) are identified.

SURGICAL TECHNIQUES FOR LOCALIZED THORACIC AORTIC ANEURYSMS

The essential feature of surgical treatment rests upon excision of the aneurysmal aortic segment and replacement with a synthetic Dacron graft. The surgical techniques required depend very much upon the anatomical site of the aneurysm, being substantially different for ascending aortic aneurysms, arch aneurysms and descending thoracic aortic aneurysms.

Surgical therapy treatment of aneurysms of the ascending thoracic aorta

All procedures are carried out through a median sternotomy, with the patient on cardiopulmonary bypass with cardioplegic myocardial protection.[13–15] The preferred treatment involves excision of the aneurysm and replacement of the ascending aorta with a woven pre-clotted Dacron graft. The graft diameter should be around 25–35 mm. Pre-clotting may be carried out by the simple technique described by Bethea[16] involving exposure of the graft to heparinized blood and subsequent autoclaving

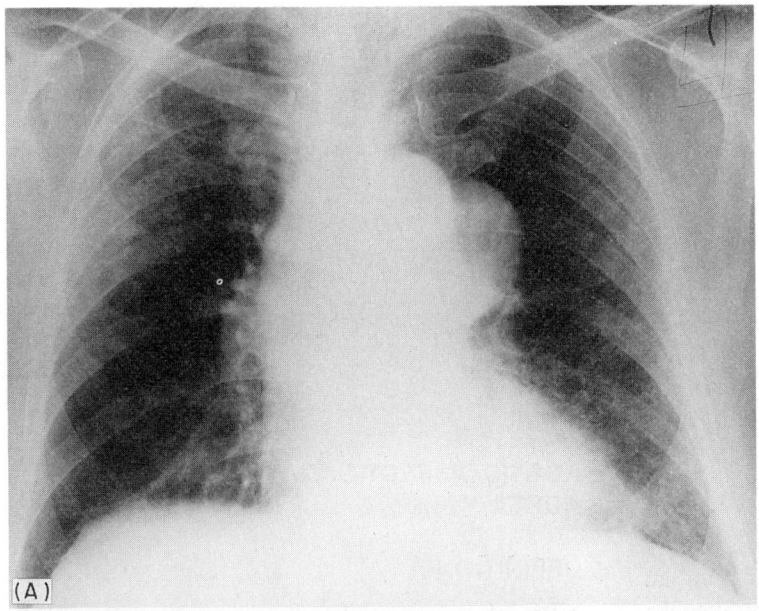

Fig. 57.2. (A) Chest X-ray appearances of saccular aneurysm of the aortic arch. The double shadow at the aortic knuckle is easily seen. (B) Computerized tomographic scan (without contrast enhancement) of the same patient as in (A). The saccular aneurysm of the aortic arch is well visualized. (C) Computerized tomographic scan (with contrast enhancement) of the same patient as in (A) and (B). Contrast enhancement shows that only a small volume of blood passes into the aneurysm sac (the 'finger-like' area of contrast close to the neck of the aneurysm), which suggests that most of the cavity of the aneurysm sac contains organized blood clot.

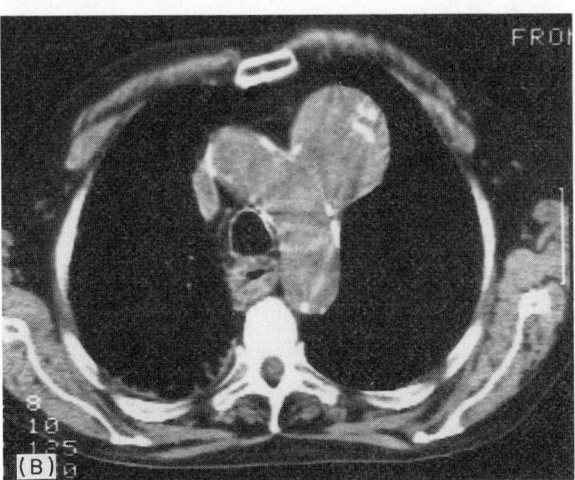

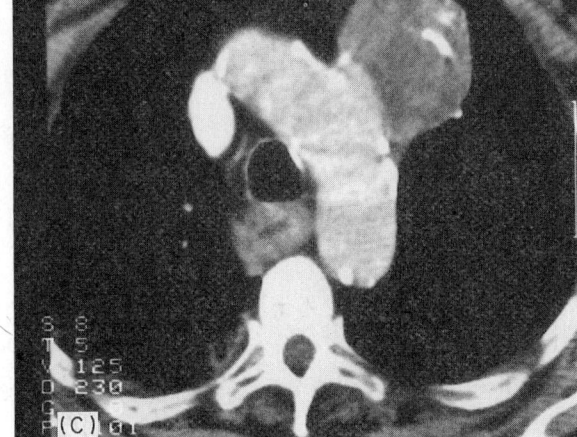

for 3 min. Where the aortic valve annulus is involved in the aneurysmal dilatation, aortic valve replacement, with incorporation or transplantation of the coronary arteries or ostia, is required using either the Bentall technique[17] or that more recently described by Wheat.[18,19]

Small-neck saccular aneurysms of the ascending thoracic aorta may be dealt with by local excision and direct suture or patch replacement of the neck of the aneurysm. Local excision, however, should be reserved for those patients who have good-quality aortic wall tissue immediately adjacent to the neck of the aneurysm sac.

Surgical treatment of the aortic arch aneurysms

Aneurysms involving the aortic arch, with or without the ascending or descending aorta, present a major technical problem. The principal difficulty relates to maintenance of adequate cerebral circulation through the carotid and vertebral arteries. Based on their extensive experience, DeBakey, Crawford and Cooley argue for full resection of the affected aortic arch, Dacron graft replacement of the arch and re-implantation of the head and neck vessels into the graft.[13,15,20,21–23] During the operation, cardiopulmonary bypass is accomplished by veno-caval drainage and arterial return to the femoral artery. Perfusion of the head and neck vessels is achieved by individual cannulation and should be maintained until all distal anastomoses are complete.[14] One alternative technique for resection of arch aneurysms is to employ profound systemic hypothermia (around 15°C core temperature) with a period of total circulatory arrest of approximately 30–45 min.[24] Whatever techniques are used, arch aneurysm surgery is complex and carries a significant mortality even in the most experienced hands.[20]

Surgical treatment of aneurysms of the descending thoracic aorta

Aneurysms arising at, or distal to, the left subclavian artery are best approached through a left lateral thoracotomy, opening the fourth or fifth left intercostal space. Opinions vary regarding the need for cardiopulmonary bypass.[14] Some authorities favour partial bypass with venous drainage from the femoral vein and arterial return to the femoral artery. Others use an heparinized shunt placed between the apex of the left ventricle and the descending thoracic aorta distal to the aneurysm sac (e.g. 9 mm Gott shunt).[25,26] Other experts believe that with sufficient expertise and short clamping times, no form of bypass or shunting is required.[9,27]

The relevant concerns relate, first to the adequacy of blood supply to the spinal cord and the fear of post-operative paraplegia. In addition, the proximal aortic cross-clamp may impose an excessive rise in arterial pressure in the ascending aorta straining a possibly already compromised left ventricle. The complicating effects of collateral vessels encountered, for example, in surgery for coarctation resection do not occur in surgery for descending aortic aneurysms.

The aneurysm is exposed by incising the mediastinal pleura and the proximal and distal ends are controlled with tapes. Clamps are placed across the aorta, proximal and distal to the aneurysm. Femoro-femoral cardiopulmonary bypass is then instituted if cardiopulmonary bypass is to be used. The aneurysm is incised longitudinally and the sac cleared of debris, intraluminal clot, etc. Intercostal arteries opening into the aneurysmal segment are closed by direct suture. The aorta is then divided proximally and distally beyond the limits of the aneurysm and a woven Dacron graft (about 25–35 mm in diameter) is interposed. Additional Dacron collars may be used at the anastomotic sites if the aortic wall is of poor quality. Finally, the trimmed aneurysm sac may be sewn over the graft as an additional haemostatic layer.

ASSESSMENT OF SURGICAL RESULTS IN THORACIC AORTIC ANEURYSMS

Centres at which there is considerable experience in this type of surgery have operative mortality rates for aneurysms of the ascending or descending thoracic aorta of about 15% with a policy of aggressive surgical intervention.[9,13] The operative mortality is substantially higher in patients who have aneurysms involving the transverse arch, particularly if the head and neck vessels are involved. Recurrence of aneurysm, often at anastomotic sites between the Dacron interposition graft and the previously normal aorta, is being increasingly reported and presents a formidable surgical challenge.[20]

AORTIC DISSECTION WITHIN THE THORACIC AORTA

DEFINITION

Aortic dissection within the thoracic aorta is characterized by the creation of a false lumen in the medial layer of the aortic wall, originating at an intimal tear and spreading antegrade or retrograde along the aorta.

It should be noted that the phrase 'dissecting aneurysm' is often used in this condition, although it is not correct. The presence of an aneurysm is not a prerequisite for aortic dissection. In many recent studies, it has been shown that the majority of cases of aortic dissection occur in structurally normal aortas.[8]

AETIOLOGY OF THORACIC AORTIC DISSECTION

The primary abnormality in aortic dissection, the intimal tear, has been shown to be associated with the following aetiological factors.
1   Hypertension.
2   Congenitally abnormal aortic valves.
3   Marfan's syndrome.
4   Coarctation of the aorta.
5   Pregnancy.
Atherosclerosis is often said to be an aetiological factor, but there is little convincing evidence for this. However, intimal tears have been reported in association with descending thoracic aortic dissection.

Of the above-mentioned aetiological factors, the most important is hypertension. Arterial hypertension has been reported in 60–90% of cases of thoracic aortic dissection.[8,28] Although its aetiological significance is well established, the precise mechanism by which systemic hypertension promotes the development of intimal tears is not clear. The initial intimal tear may be produced simply by direct mechanical factors. Davies has recently suggested that the basis of dissection lies in the ease with which the elastic laminae of the aortic media can be cleaved from each other once the intima has been breached.[2] Although it has been suggested that collagen abnormalities within the intima might facilitate the development of intimal tears, there is no convincing evidence for this. Studies of pyridinoline collagen-specific covalent cross-link have revealed no significant differences in the aortas of patients with dissecting aneurysms when compared with normal aortic tissue.[29] Muscle hypertrophy and, possibly associated with this, cross-link enzyme change may occur in the ascending aortas of hypertensive subjects. Clearly, this area requires further investigation. Some authors maintain that the intimal tear is not the primary event, rather that underlying medial weakness and intraluminal haemorrhage create a haematoma within the aortic wall, splitting the medial layer and inducing the dissection process.[28,30] Those who promote this view are in conflict with majority opinion; the results of more recent studies indicate that the majority of dissected aortas have no demonstrable medial layer pathology.[3,8,31,32]

Dissection occurring in association with Marfan's syndrome, however, does represent the situation in which medial pathology is present. The incidence of Marfan's syndrome in series of aortic dissections has varied from 5 to > 15%,[8,33] a relatively small incidence when compared with the major aetiological association between hypertension and aortic dissection. If aortic dissection does occur in association with Marfan's syndrome, the characteristic picture is one of an intimal tear in the posterior wall of the ascending aorta 3–4 cm above the aortic annulus. This dissection occurs in association with the extensive aortic root aneurysm characteristic of Marfan's syndrome.

PATHOPHYSIOLOGY OF THORACIC AORTIC DISSECTION

Dissection of the thoracic aorta is the most common acute aortic pathology. The incidence of this condition in North American practice has been variously reported. Wheat[30] suggested an incidence of 5–10 cases per million population, whereas Miller and colleagues estimate there are 10–20 cases per million per year.[34] It has been calculated that the

condition accounts for almost 5% of cases of sudden death.[35] Whatever the incidence, all experts agree that the condition carries a mortality of 90% within 3 months of onset if the patient does not receive appropriate treatment.[36]

The essential pathological features are as previously indicated.
1 The development of an intimal aortic tear, usually associated with systemic arterial hypertension.
2 Cleavage within the medial layer of the aorta, with the creation of a false lumen, and spread within the medial layer, either antegrade or retrograde, from the site of the intimal tear.

The process of propagation of the false lumen may be extensive and may involve almost the full length of the thoracic and abdominal aorta. The false lumen may rupture into the pericardium with retrograde dissection or, alternatively, into the pleural space. Rupture back into the true lumen of the aorta (the 're-entry' phenomenon) may also occur.[37,38]

The dissection process is not usually circumferential and tends to follow the lateral margin of the ascending aorta and the greater curvature of the aortic arch. Spiralling of the false lumen may occur in the descending aorta. External rupture into the pericardium or the pleural space is the commonest cause of death from aortic dissection. In those patients in whom the dissection process involves the ascending aorta, around 50% have associated aortic valve incompetence. Also, in about 50% of patients, the dissection process occludes arterial branches of the aorta, for example, the carotid arteries, or, in the abdominal aorta, the renal or mesenteric arteries.[39,40]

In some cases, the dissection process does not produce an immediate life-threatening complication, possibly where re-entry into the true lumen occurs. The medial destruction in these patients is often ultimately associated with the formation of saccular aneurysms which may become manifest as late rupture.

CLINICAL FEATURES OF ACUTE DISSECTION OF THE THORACIC AORTA

A history of very severe tearing chest pain in a patient (usually 50–75 years of age) who is significantly hypertensive should raise the suspicion of acute aortic dissection.[41-43] Dissection occurring in younger patients should raise the suspicion of one of the associated aetiologies previously indicated, i.e. Marfan's syndrome,[8,33] pregnancy,[44] aortic coarctation or congenital aortic valve pathology.[45]

The classical symptom of acute aortic dissection is intense chest pain, often described as ripping or tearing in nature, with the pain extending into the interscapular region. In some patients, the pain may be felt solely in the back or even in the epigastric region. This symptomatic presentation requires differential diagnosis, particularly from the conditions of acute myocardial infarction, biliary colic and perforated peptic ulcer.[46,47]

Aortic dissection may occur in the absence of significant pain. This may indicate associated cerebral or spinal cord vessel involvement or may occur when the patient presents with acute syncope.

Physical examination of a patient with suspected aortic dissection should focus on the presence of arterial hypertension, an examination of the peripheral pulses and an assessment of the presence or absence of aortic valve regurgitation.

The persistence of arterial hypertension, sometimes with particularly high levels of arterial blood pressure, helps to exclude major myocardial infarction from the differential diagnosis. Assessment of peripheral pulses may indicate absence or lack of uniformity. Many patients have audible cardiac murmurs, but the detection of the early diastolic murmur of aortic valve regurgitation at the left sternal edge is an important sign.

Assessment of the central nervous system may reveal the presence of a hemiplegia or even a paraplegia. If localized spinal cord damage has occurred, the neurological signs may be less severe.

INVESTIGATION OF THORACIC AORTIC DISSECTION

An important early investigation is the resting electrocardiogram, which should exclude acute myocardial infarction and may confirm the presence of long-standing arterial hypertension by demonstrating left ventricular hypertrophy or even left ventricular strain. Once this important differential diagnosis has been resolved and the clinical suspicion for aortic dissection is high, the formal investigation should focus on three aspects.

1   Confirmation of the presence of aortic dissection.
2   Localization of the site of the intimal tear (the entry point).
3   Assessment of any involvement of the ascending aorta in the dissection process.

A plain postero-anterior chest X-ray may show mediastinal widening, although the absence of this sign does not rule out the diagnosis because mediastinal widening is reported to be present in only 50–60% of cases.[46] Other associated findings may be calcification within the ascending aorta or arch and the possible presence of left pleural infusion.[48,49] If pleural effusion is present, it usually indicates the presence of a sympathetic serosanguineous diffusion; it does not necessarily indicate aortic wall rupture.

Recently, the use of computerized tomographic scanning has, in the author's experience, proved increasingly helpful in the diagnosis and localization of thoracic aortic dissection (see Fig. 57.3).

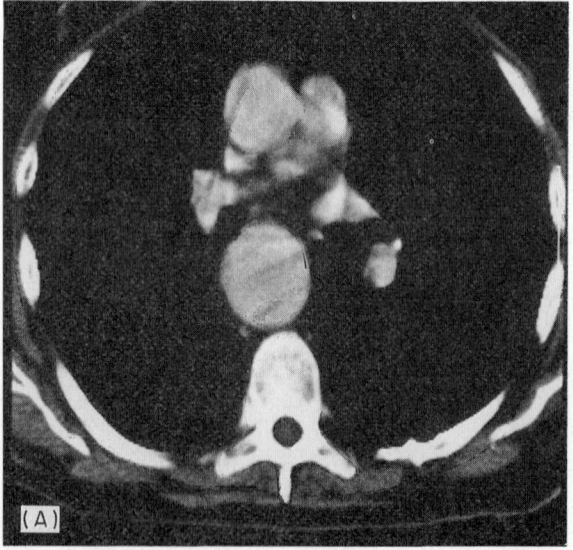

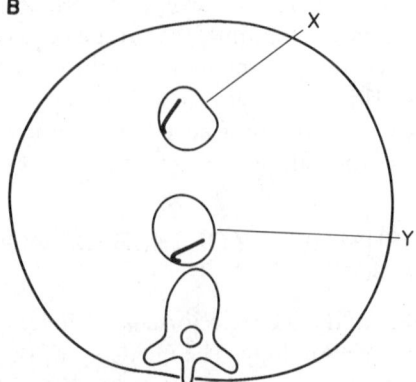

Fig. 57.3. (A) Computerized tomographic scan of aortic dissection. The intimal flap is visible in both the ascending aorta (X) and the descending aorta (Y). (B) Simplified line drawing to show the salient features in (A).

However, the mainstay of investigation remains invasive aortography with views accurately delineating the length of the aorta from the aortic valve to the aortic bifurcation[50-53] (see Fig. 57.4). The principal aortographic features in acute dissection of the aorta include:

1   an appearance of split contrast in the false and true lumens;
2   obvious distortion of the normally smooth intra-aortic contrast;
3   abnormal aortic flow patterns, in particular the demonstration of occluded major aortic vessels, for example, renal or mesenteric arteries. Flow stasis or reversal are also suggestive.

In addition, the following points should be noted:

4   evidence of an intimal flap indicating the site of origin of the acute dissection;
5   the presence of aortic valve regurgitation.

THERAPEUTIC MANAGEMENT OF ACUTE AORTIC DISSECTION

The management of acute aortic dissection involves:

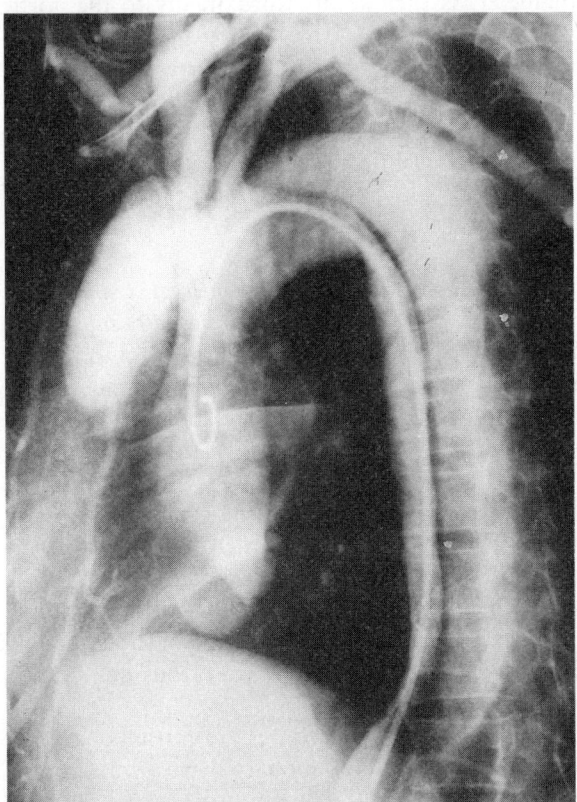

Fig. 57.4. Angiographic features of dissection of the thoracic aorta. The catheter lies in the true lumen of the aorta. The intimal flap and false lumen are clearly seen.

1   drug therapy for all patients to bring about a swift and maintained reduction in arterial hypertension;
2   definition of the site of origin and the extent (both proximal and distal) of the dissection process.

It must be emphasized that the ultimate management choice between continuing medical therapy and referral for surgery relates to the accurate definition of both the originating site and the extent of the dissection process, in particular, the presence or absence of ascending aortic involvement.[43,46,54,55]

First phase hypotensive therapy for all patients with acute aortic dissection

It is vital that once the diagnosis of acute aortic dissection is suspected with a reasonable degree of certainty hypotensive therapy should be instituted. A variety of hypotensive regimes may be employed. One widely favoured regime is to employ sympathetic blockade with a beta-blocker, for example, propranolol, combined with the vasodilatatory effects of sodium nitroprusside infusion.[54,56] The aim in therapy is to reduce the systolic blood pressure to around 100 mmHg. Ideally, the patient should be managed in the intensive care unit; if this is not possible, the patient should be placed in a high dependency unit with careful monitoring of the electrocardiogram, blood pressure and urinary output. Attention should be paid to the continued presence of all peripheral pulses and to the adequacy of peripheral perfusion. Relief of the severe pain associated with acute dissection suggests appropriate initial control of the dissection process. Once control is achieved, definitive aortography may be carried out.

Classification of acute aortic dissection

As previously indicated, management of patients with thoracic aortic dissection depends very much on the site and extent of the dissection process. Confusion exists in the minds of many because of different classification regimes applied to acute aortic dissections. In broad terms, the principal applications in relatively common use are the DeBakey classification (Types 1,2,3) and the AB classification, promoted by the Stanford group. The author's preference is for the AB classification.

DeBakey classification in acute aortic dissection[57,58]

Type 1: Intimal tear in the ascending aorta with dissection continuing around the arch to involve the descending aorta.

Type 2: Intimal tear in the ascending aorta and dissection confined to the ascending aorta.

Type 3: Intimal tear in the descending aorta and dissection confined to the descending and abdominal aorta.

Type AB classification of acute aortic dissection[59,60]

Type A: The dissection process involves the ascending aorta with or without extension into the descending aorta.

Type B: The dissection process involves the descending aorta without involvement of the ascending aorta.

Using the simpler AB classification, type A dissections account for about 66% of cases, type B around 33%.[59,60] The clear differentiation in management is that, as a general rule, type A dissections are most often managed by prompt corrective surgery, whereas the majority of type B dissections are managed initially by vigorous hypotensive medical treatment.

Management of type A acute aortic dissections[57–63]

Type A dissections, i.e. those in which the dissection processes involve the ascending aorta, may have the primary intimal tear in the ascending aorta, the transverse arch or even in the descending aorta. The danger with type A dissections is the possibility of retrograde dissection and fatal tamponade into the pericardial cavity. In the absence of other significant contra-indications, type A dissection patients should proceed to surgery once the diagnosis has been established and their hypertension brought under satisfactory control.

Surgical techniques in type A dissections

The choice of surgical procedure should be determined by the assessment of the following factors.

1 The presence or absence of aortic valve regurgitation. Where the dissection process has produced aortic valve regurgitation, either re-suspension of the native aortic valve or aortic valve replacement should be undertaken. This may be carried out in association with aortic root replacement, where the aortic root is severely affected by the dissection process with or without associated aneurysm formation. Where aortic root replacement is carried out, preservation of the coronary arteries or re-implantation of the coronary arteries into the Dacron graft replacement must be carried out.

2 The quality of the layers of the aortic wall. In some younger patients, the aortic wall layers may have reasonable integrity and the anastomotic sites may safely be secured with over-and-over continuous suture. Where the tissues are friable, some form of buttressing should be carried out. The preferred technique is to use Teflon felt in a 'sandwich' incorporating the aortic wall with or without felt interposition in the false lumen.

In type A dissections, where the dissecting process has resulted in an aortic root aneurysm, an interposition Dacron tube graft is required. Once the true lumen is opened, an assessment of the aortic valve is carried out and aortic valve re-suspension or valve replacement performed as required. The interposition Dacron tube graft (about 30 mm in diameter) is then secured proximally to the aortic valve annulus with incorporation or re-implantation of the coronary arteries. Alternate techniques have been described by Bentall[64–66] and by Wheat.[67] The distal anastomosis is fashioned to the distal end of the ascending aorta after obliterating the false lumen, again using the Teflon strip sandwich technique.

Type A dissection with an intimal tear in the transverse arch or distal to the left subclavian artery. Primary tears in the arch or distal to the left subclavian artery, which dissect retrograde to involve the ascending aorta, are relatively uncommon. The preferred option in such cases is to attempt control of the dissection process with hypotensive therapy as results up to now have been better than those with surgical treatment. If hypotensive therapy does not prevent continued involvement of the ascending aorta, the surgical treatment is simply a segmental replacement of a portion of the ascending aorta with the Dacron tube graft, thus obliterating the passage of the false lumen.

These operative procedures are carried out under conditions of cardiopulmonary bypass with moderate hypothermia to 28°C. Femoro-femoral cannulation may be carried out, although many surgeons prefer venous drainage from the right atrium and arterial return to the femoral artery.

Management of type B acute aortic dissections[57-63,68]

As previously indicated, type B dissections are defined as thoracic aortic dissections that do not involve the ascending aorta. The primary intimal tear is most often just distal to the left subclavian artery, but may originate as far proximal as the transverse aortic arch.

Until recently, traditional management for type B acute dissections was initial medical therapy with hypotensive agents. Surgery was not undertaken primarily unless medical therapy failed to control the dissection process. More recently, this conservative approach has been questioned. The Stanford group have recently reported an aggressive surgical policy towards acute type B dissection, achieving an early mortality of 13 ± 12% whereas the mortality for medical treatment of type B dissections was 39 ± 10%.[55,61]

The traditional medical regime for management of type B aortic dissections should include:

1 continuation of the beta-blocker and the sodium nitroprusside infusion therapy;
2 additional longer-term antihypertensive therapy, for example, methyldopa 250 mg, 4–6 times daily;
3 continual monitoring of electrocardiogram, blood pressure, presence of peripheral pulses and adequacy of renal function;
4 daily chest X-rays and/or ultrasound examinations to assess change in size of the descending thoracic aorta.

In the absence of indications for later surgical intervention, hypotensive drug therapy should be continued on a long-term basis.

Indications for surgical intervention in type B acute dissection

1 *Failure to control the dissecting process.* This would be indicated or suggested by progressive increase in size of the descending thoracic aorta, retrograde process of the dissection to indicate involvement of the ascending thoracic aorta or occurrence of total or significant occlusion of a major aortic arterial branch, for example, renal, mesenteric or iliac arteries.
2 *The appearance of impending aortic rupture.* Suspicion of this complication may be aroused by rapid and significant increase in descending aorta size, the re-appearance of acute chest pain or the appearance of frank blood in the pleural and/or pericardial cavities.

Surgical techniques in type B acute aortic dissection

The site of intimal tear and the extent of the dissection will have been identified by prior aortography. As with descending aortic aneurysms, some surgeons prefer to carry out the operation using femoro-femoral bypass, some with a heparinized left ventriculo-apical to descending aortic shunt and others without bypass or shunt support. Assessment of the quality of the aortic wall layer is as important as in type A dissections and, in addition to the interposition Dacron graft, Teflon felt strips or collars should be used to buttress both anastomotic suture lines.

Results of surgery in acute dissection of the aorta

In a recent review from the Mayo Clinic in North America,[69] workers report their experience of acute ascending aortic dissection (Stanford type A or DeBakey types 1 and 2) from 1962 to 1985. The overall operative mortality was 22%; 39% in patients with acute dissection and 9% in patients with chronic dissection. Within this series, 58% of the patients had aortic valve regurgitation and, of these, the vast majority underwent either re-suspension or replacement of the aortic valve. Late survival rates in this patient population were 63 and 49% at 5 and 10 years, respectively.

There appears to be general agreement among the major reported studies[57-69] that the early mortality among surgically treated patients with acute ascending aortic dissection is about 20–35%. Although this figure is high, it compares very well with a mortality of 85–90% for medically treated patients.

AORTITIS

Aortitis encompasses several divergent pathological conditions, the common feature of all being the involvement of the aortic wall by an inflammatory cell infiltrate. The inflammatory process may be present throughout the layers of the aortic wall, although the involvement of the media tends to be more significant. Ultimately, severe aortitis may manifest itself clinically by aneurysm formation, although some particular aortitis conditions, for example, Takayasu's disease, may have alternative clinical presentations.

AETIOLOGICAL CLASSIFICATION OF AORTITIS

As previously indicated in the section on thoracic aneurysms, conditions producing aortitis may be grouped or classified as follows.

1 Syphilis.
2 Non-syphilitic bacterial aortitis.
3 Non-bacterial aortitis:
    a Takayasu's disease;
    b ankylosing spondylitis;
    c Reiter's syndrome;
    d giant cell arteritis;

In addition to the above, the syndrome of non-specific aortitis is recognized in which thoracic or abdominal aortic aneurysms may develop in the absence of any detectable cause. Although an auto-immune basis has been suggested for the condition, this remains to be proven.

Syphilitic aortitis

The infecting organism in syphilis is the spirochaete, *Treponema pallidum*. The organism is widely distributed through the body being carried in the bloodstream. Aortitis is the principal cardiovascular lesion in established syphilis and the aortic involvement is often localized to the proximal part of the ascending aorta above the aortic valve sinuses. The inflammatory process has been reported more distally in the thoracic and the proximal abdominal aorta. Finally, the syphilitic inflammatory process may involve the aortic valve annulus producing separation of the aortic valve cusps and the commissures and also annular dilatation, aggravating the tendency to aortic valve regurgitation. In addition, the inflammatory process may involve the coronary artery ostea producing ostial stenosis.

The underlying pathological abnormality has been reported as inflammatory involvement within the vasa vasorum in the aortic intima producing areas of necrosis within the aortic wall media. The initial necrotic phase is followed by fibrosis and scar formation, with the fibrosis and distortion also occurring in the intimal layer of the aorta. The resultant abnormalities consequently relate to the effects of medial layer weakening leading to aneurysm formation, to aortic valve disruption and resultant aortic regurgitation and/or to intimal fibrosis, particularly coronary ostial stenosis.

Natural history of syphilitic aortitis

The fully developed syndrome of syphilitic aortitis with aneurysm formation usually presents in the tertiary stage of the disease. Most previous studies indicate a male preponderance with age at presentation of 40–60 years. It should be appreciated that nowadays chronic cardiovascular syphilis is not common in developed countries.

Clinical presentation of syphilitic aortitis

The three commonest presentations are:

1 aortic aneurysm;
2 aortic valve regurgitation;
3 coronary ostial stenosis.

Syphilitic aortic aneurysm. As previously indicated, syphilitic aortic aneurysms occur more often in the proximal ascending thoracic aorta. The aneurysms may be saccular or fusiform. Dissection in association with syphilitic aortitis is extremely rare.

The clinical presentation of the syphilitic aortic aneurysm is usually with symptoms relating to compression of the surrounding viscera,[70] although acute rupture of the aneurysm may be the mode of presentation in a minority. In addition, asymptomatic syphilitic aortic aneurysms may be found on routine chest X-ray. X-ray features suggestive of syphilitic aneurysms include principal involvement of the proximal part of the ascending thoracic aorta without the aortic root dilatation associated with cystic medial necrosis. In addition, calcification is often seen in the wall of syphilitic aneurysms. Once clinical suspicion has been aroused, the anatomy of the aneurysm may be defined by aortography and the underlying aetiology confirmed by serology.

Aortic valve regurgitation. Aortic valve regurgitation is present in about half of the patients presenting with a syphilitic aortic aneurysm.[71] The severity of the aortic valve regurgitation is variable but the degree of left ventricular failure may be relatively greater than the level of aortic regurgitation might suggest.

Coronary ostial stenosis. This particular complication of syphilitic infections is well recognized and may be present in association with aneurysm or aortic regurgitation, although in certain cases it can be present in isolation.[72] The clinical presentation is usually with angina pectoris.

Serological diagnosis in syphilitic aortitis

In suspected cases, a number of antibody-based tests are available, including the Venereal Disease

Reference Laboratory (VDRL) and the Wasser-mann reaction. These are non-specific tests which are most useful in the primary stage of syphilis. False-positive results are an inherent problem of non-specific tests. In addition, the tests may be negative in the late stages of the disease. Where clinical suspicion is strong, it is preferable to carry out one of the specific antibody tests, including the *Treponema pallidum* Immobilization test (TPI), the fluorescent *Treponema* antibody test (FTA) and the Reiter protein complement fixation test.

Once positive serological confirmation of the diagnosis is obtained, antibiotic therapy should be instituted. The drug of choice is penicillin, 2–3 mega units given parenterally, this dose being given every 7 days for 4–6 weeks. Where penicillin allergy or intolerance is present, erythromycin may be used with equal effect.

Surgical treatment for syphilitic aortitis[73,74]

In suitable cases, surgery may be carried out as previously described for ascending thoracic aortic aneurysms. Where aortic regurgitation is present, aortic valve replacement may be undertaken with good results.[73] In conditions of coronary ostial stenosis, some authorities have advised incision of the obstructing tissue from within the aortic root, whereas others have suggested that conventional grafting of the affected coronary arteries is a preferable approach. It should be noted that the patients affected by coronary ostial stenosis may have underlying coronary atherosclerosis.

Non-syphilitic bacterial aortitis

Blood-borne bacteria may produce an acute aortitis in the thoracic aortic wall leading to aneurysm formation. These aneurysms are known as mycotic aneurysms.[75–77] The port of entry may be by spread of bacteria in the vasa vasorum of the aortic wall or from the lumen of the aorta, usually at areas of damaged intima.

The infective organisms will be those of the underlying septicaemia or infective endocarditis. *Salmonella* mycotic aneurysms have also been reported. In the era when thoracic tuberculosis was widespread, tuberculous involvement of the aorta with subsequent aneurysm formation was not infrequently reported.

The treatment for non-syphilitic bacterial aortitis rests upon appropriate antibiotic therapy once cultures and sensitivities of the infective organism

have been obtained. Where aneurysm formation has become established, surgical therapy may be required.[78]

Non-bacterial aortitis

As previously indicated, several non-specific and poorly understood conditions are known to produce a non-bacterial and presumably a non-infective aortitis. Some of the features of these conditions might suggest a rheumatic or auto-immune aetiological association. Within this diverse group, a small number of specific syndromes have been characterized.

Takayasu's aortitis (pulseless disease)

Although Takayasu's aortitis has been described most often in the Oriental population, it does occur in other populations. Most cases present in young females between 20 and 30 years of age.[79] The aetiology of the disease is not known, although Numano has reported the possibility of genetic predisposition.[80]

The essential pathological abnormality is an inflammatory process in all layers of the aortic wall ultimately leading to very severe fibrosis in both intimal and adventitial layers. The medial layer is weakened by the inflammatory process and may develop aneurysm formation in a segmental fashion between the dense and potentially obstructive areas of fibrosis. Involvement of the aortic arch and the brachiocephalic vessels is almost always present. The obstructive nature of the fibrosis in these vessels ultimately leads to loss of radial or carotid pulses. Where the fibrosis is particularly severe, the aorta itself may become significantly narrowed, producing an acquired coarctation syndrome. The pulmonary artery may also be involved and the disease may extend into the abdominal aorta involving the mesenteric and renal arteries.

The disease presents clinically in the inflammatory stage with non-specific features including fever, malaise and weight loss. The erythrocyte sedimentation rate tends to be raised, and non-specific serological abnormalities suggestive of a rheumatoid or auto-immune disorder may be present.

Once the inflammatory phase has passed, the clinical picture slowly but progressively becomes dominated by the consequences of intimal fibrosis and arterial occlusion. Patients may present with angina pectoris due to involvement of the coronary circulation or with symptoms and signs of cerebrovascular or mesenteric vascular insufficiency. Aortic valve regurgitation secondary to fibrotic deformation has been reported.

The ocular features of the disease were first described by Takayasu, a Japanese ophthalmologist. The proliferation of small blood vessels around the optic disc is secondary to retinal ischaemia. Patients may present with a variety of ocular signs and symptoms.

Little success has been reported with any line of therapy in this prolonged and severe condition. Corticosteroids may be used in the acute inflammatory phase. In the chronic phase of arterial obstruction, surgery is rarely of benefit.[81-83]

Aortitis related to ankylosing spondylitis, Reiter's syndrome, etc.

Several conditions including ankylosing spondylitis and Reiter's syndrome (following non-gonorrhoeal urethritis) are known to be associated with an aortitis syndrome similar to that seen with syphilis. The extent of the inflammatory involvement is different from that in syphilis because the pathological process extends into the aortic root and even into the membranous part of the interventricular septum.[84-86]

It has recently been suggested that there may be an aetiological association with one of the histocompatibility leucocyte antigens (HLA-B27)[86]

The clinical features of these conditions are dominated by the development of aortic regurgitation. Echocardiography may reveal that the aortic and mitral valve cusps are involved in the pathological process.[87] Where aortic regurgitation is severe, aortic valve replacement may be indicated.

Giant cell arteritis

The generalized pathological condition of giant cell arteritis (including temporal arteritis and polymyalgia rheumatica) may produce aortic involvement. Giant cell arteritis tends to be a disease of the elderly. It may produce a variety of aortic abnormalities ranging from aneurysm formation through aortic dissection to occlusion of aortic arch vessels.[88] The classical histological feature is the presence of large numbers of giant cells within the aortic wall.

REFERENCES

1. Schilling, F.J., Christakis, G., Hempel, H.H. and Orbach, A. The natural history of abdominal aortic and iliac atherosclerosis as detected by lateral abdominal roentgenograms in 2663 males. *J. Chron. Dis.* 1974; **27**: 37–45.
2. Davies, M.J. Pathology of the aorta. *Curr. Opin. Cardiol.* 1986; **1**: 643–5.
3. Busuttil, R.W., Rinderbriecht, H., Flesher, A. and Carmack, C. Elastase activity: the role of elastase in aortic aneurysm formation. *J. Surg. Res.* 1982; **32**: 214–7.
4. Roberts, W.C., Ferrans, V.J., Levy, R.I. and Fredrickson, D.S. Cardiovascular pathology in hyperlipoproteinemia. Anatomic observations in 42 necropsy patients with normal or abnormal serum lipoprotein patterns. *Am. J. Cardiol.* 1973; **31**: 557–70.
5. Roberts, W.C. The aorta: its acquired diseases and their consequences as viewed from a morphologic perspective. In: Lindsay, J. Jr and Hurst, J.W., eds. *The Aorta.* New York: Grune and Stratton Inc., 1979, p. 51.
6. Hirst, A.E. Jr and Gore, I. Marfan's Syndrome: a review. *Prog. Cardiovasc. Dis.* 1973; **16**: 187–98.
7. Lindsay, J. Jr. Thoracic aneurysms. In: Lindsay, J. Jr and Hurst, J.W., eds. *The Aorta.* New York: Grune and Stratton Inc., 1979, p. 121.
8. Larson, E.W. and Edwards, W.D. Risk factors for aortic dissections: a necropsy study of 161 cases. *Am. J. Cardiol.* 1984; **53**: 849–55.
9. Lindsay, J., DeBakey, M.E. and Beall, A.C. Diseases of the aorta. In: Hurst, J.W., ed. *The Heart.* 5th edn. New York: McGrove Hall, 1982, pp. 1432–57.
10. Dee, P., Granato, J.E. and Gibson, R.S. The CT and ultrasound diagnosis of aortic dissection. *Semin. Ultrasound. CT MR* 1985; **6**: 146–55.
11. Detrano, R., Moodie, D.S., Gill, C.C., Markovich, D. and Simpfendorfer, C. Intravenous digital subtraction aortography in the pre-operative and post-operative evaluation of Marfan's aortic disease. *Chest* 1985; **88**: 249–53.
12. Timmis, A.D., Rosin, M.D. and Rahimtoola, S. Localized aortic dissection with rupture into the right atrium: diagnosis by computed tomography and cardiac catheterization. *Am. J. Cardiol.* 1985; **56**: 204–5.
13. DeBakey, M.E. and Noon, G.P. Aneurysms of the thoracic aorta. *Mod. Conc. Cardiovasc. Dis.* 1975; **44**: 53.
14. Liddicoat, J.E., Bekassy, S.M., Rubio, P.A., Noon, G.P. and DeBakey, M.E. Ascending aortic aneurysms: review of 100 consecutive cases. *Circulation* 1975; **52**(Suppl. 1): 202–9.
15. DeBakey, M.E., McCollum, C.H. and Graham, J.M. Surgical treatment of aneurysms of the descending thoracic aorta. Long-term results in 500 patients. *J. Cardiovasc. Surg.* 1978; **19**: 571.
16. Bethea, M.C. and Reemtsma, K. Graft haemostasis: an alternative to pre-clotting. *Ann. Thorac. Surg.* 1979; **27**: 374.
17. Bentall, H. and DeBono, A. A technique for complete replacement of the ascending aorta. *Thorax* 1968; **23**: 338–9.
18. Koster, J.K. Jr, Cohn, L.H., Mee, R.B.B. and Collins, J.J. Jr. Late results of operation for acute aortic dissection producing aortic insufficiency. *Ann. Thorac. Surg.* 1978; **26**: 461–7.
19. Wheat, M.W. Jr, Harris, P.D., Malm, J.R., Kaiser, G., Bowman, F.O. Jr and Palmer, R.F. Acute dissecting aneurysms of the aorta—treatment and results in 64 patients. *J. Thorac. Cardiovasc. Surg.* 1969; **58**: 344–51.
20. Crawford, E.S., Crawford, J.L., Safi, H.J. and Coselli, J.S. Re-do operations for recurrent aneurysmal disease of the ascending aorta and transverse aortic arch. *Ann. Thorac. Surg.* 1985; **40**: 439–55.
21. Cooley, D.A. and DeBakey, M.E. Surgical considerations of intra-thoracic aneurysms of the aorta and great vessels. *Ann. Surg.* 1952; **135**: 660–80.
22. Cooley, D.A., Ott, D.A. and Reul, G.J. The aortic arch. In: Keen, G., ed. *Operative Surgery and Management.* Bristol:

John Wright & Sons Ltd., 1981, pp. 516–29.

23. Cooley, D.A., Ott, D.A., Frazier, O.H. and Walker, W.E. Surgical treatment of aneurysms of the transverse aortic arch: experience with 25 patients using hypothermic techniques. *Ann. Thorac. Surg.* 1981; **32**: 260–72.

24. Mahfood, S., Qazi, A., Garcia, J., Mispireta, L., Corso, P. and Smyth, N. Management of aortic arch aneurysm using profound hypothermia and circulatory arrest. *Ann. Thorac. Surg.* 1985; **39**: 412–7.

25. Verdant, A. Descending thoracic aneurysmectomy (Letter to the Editor). *Ann. Thorac. Surg.* 1985; **40**: 414.

26. Donahoo, J.S., Brawley, R.K. and Gott, V.L. The heparin-coated vascular shunt for thoracic aortic and great vessel procedures: a ten-year experience. *Ann. Thorac. Surg.* 1977; **23**: 507–13.

27. Crawford, E.S. and Rubio, P.A. Reappraisal of adjuncts to avoid ischaemia in the treatment of aneurysms of the descending thoracic aorta. *J. Thorac. Cardiovasc. Surg.* 1973; **66**: 693–704.

28. Wheat, M.W. Jr. Acute dissecting aneurysms of the aorta: diagnosis and treatment. *Am. Heart J.* 1980; **99**: 373–87.

29. Whittle, M.A., Robins, S.P., Hasleton, P.S. and Anderson, J.C. Biochemical investigation of possible lesions in human aorta that predispose to dissecting aneurysms: pyridinoline crosslinks. *Cardiovasc. Res.* 1987; **21**: 161–8.

30. Wheat, M.W. Jr. Acute dissection of the aorta. In: McGoon, D.C., ed. *Cardiac Surgery.* Philadelphia: F.A. Davis, 1982, pp. 177–96.

31. Eastcott, H.H.G. Aneurysms and the surgeon: an historical review. In: Bergen, J.J. and Yao, J.S.T., eds. *Aneurysms: diagnosis and treatment.* New York: Grune and Stratton, 1983, pp. 3–14.

32. Hasleton, P.S. and Leonard, J.C. Histopathology of the aorta. *Q. J. Med.* 1979; **48**: 63–76.

33. Klima, T., Spjut, H.J., Coehlo, A., Gray, A.G., Wukasch, D.C., Reul, G.J. Jr and Cooley, D.A. The morphology of ascending aortic aneurysms. *Human Pathol.* 1983; **14**: 810–7.

34. Miller, D.C. Acute dissection of the aorta—continuing need for earlier diagnosis and treatment. *Mod. Conc. Cardiovasc. Dis.* 1985; **54**: 51–5.

35. Pepper, J. Investigation and surgery of acquired aortic disease. *Curr. Opin. Cardiol.* 1986; **1**: 652–6.

36. Anagnostopoulos, C.E., Prabhakar, M.J.S. and Kittle, C.F. Aortic dissections and dissecting aneurysms. *Am. J. Cardiol.* 1972; **30**: 263–73.

37. Conston, A.S. Healed dissecting aneurysm. *Arch. Pathol.* 1949; **48**: 309–15.

38. Cassidy, M. and Pinniger, J. Healed dissecting aneurysm. *Br. Heart J.* 1946; **8**: 130–40.

39. Hirst, A.E. Jr, Johns, V.J. Jr and Kime, S.W. Jr. Dissecting aneurysms of the aorta: a review of 505 cases. *Medicine (Baltimore)* 1958; **37**: 217–79.

40. Gore, I. and Hirst, A.E. Jr. Dissecting aneurysm of the aorta. *Prog. Cardiovasc. Dis.* 1973; **16**: 103–11.

41. DeBakey, M.E., Beall, A.C. Jr, Cooley, D.A., Crawford, E.S., Morris, C.G. Jr, Garrett, H.E. and Howell, J.F. Dissecting aneurysms of the aorta. *Surg. Clin. N. Am.* 1966; **46**: 1045–55.

42. DeBakey, M.E., McCollum, C.H., Crawford, E.S., Morris, G.C. Jr, Howell, J., Noon, G.P. and Lawrie, G. Dissection and dissecting aneurysms of the aorta: twenty-year follow-up of 527 patients treated surgically. *Surgery* 1982; **92**: 1118–34.

43. Anagnostopoulos, C.E. *Acute Aortic Dissections.* Baltimore: University Park Press, 1975.

44. Kitchen, D.H. Dissecting aneurysm of the aorta in pregnancy. *J. Obstet. Gynecol. Br. Commwlth.* 1974; **81**: 410–3.

45. Strauss, R.G. and McAdams, A.J. Dissecting aneurysm in childhood. *J. Pediatr.* 1970; **76**: 578–84.

46. Slater, E.E. and DeSanctis, R.W. The clinical recognition of dissecting aortic aneurysm. *Am. J. Med.* 1976; **60**: 625–33.

47. Lindsay, J. Jr and Hurst, J.W. Clinical features and prognosis in dissecting aneurysm of the aorta. A reappraisal. *Circulation* 1967; **35**: 880–8.

48. Beachley, M.C., Ranniger, K. and Roth, F.J. Roentgenographic evaluation of dissecting aneurysms of the aorta. *Am. J. Roentgen. Rad. Ther. Nucl. Med.* 1974; **121**: 617–25.

49. Jang, G.C., Brody, W.R. and Dinsmore, R.E. Radiologic diagnosis in aortic disease. In: Lindsay, J. Jr and Hurst, J.W., eds. *The Aorta.* New York: Grune and Stratton Inc., 1979, p. 296.

50. Seldinger, S.I. Catheter replacement of needle in percutaneous arteriography: a new technique. *Acta. Radiol.* 1953; **39**: 368–76.

51. Dinsmore, R.E., Willerson, J.T. and Buckley, M.J. Dissecting aneurysm of the aorta: aortographic features affecting prognosis. *Radiology* 1972; **105**: 567–72.

52. Wheat, M.W. Jr and Palmer, R.F. Dissecting aneurysm of the aorta. *Curr. Probl. Surg.* 1971; **July**: 1–43.

53. Hayashi, K., Meaney, T.F., Zelch, J.V. and Tarar, R. Aortographic analysis of aortic dissection. *Am. J. Roentgen. Rad. Ther. Nucl. Med.* 1974; **122**: 769–82.

54. Bolooki, H. Management of aortic dissection. *J. Fla Med. Assoc.* 1979; **66**: 1064.

55. Miller, D.C. Acute dissection of the aorta—continuing need for earlier diagnosis and treatment. *Mod. Conc. Cardiovasc. Dis.* 1985; **54**: 51–5.

56. Palmer, R.F. and Lasseter, K.C. Drug Therapy: Sodium nitroprusside. *N. Engl. J. Med.* 1975; **292**: 294–7.

57. DeBakey, M.E., Beall, A.C. Jr, Cooley, D.A., Crawford, E.S., Morris, G.C. Jr, Garrett, H.E. and Howell, J.F. Dissecting aneurysms of the aorta. *Surg. Clin. N. Am.* 1966; **46**: 1045–55.

58. DeBakey, M.E. The development of vascular surgery. *Am. J. Surg.* 1979; **137**: 697–738.

59. Daily, P.O., Trueblood, H.W., Stinson, E.B., Wuerflein, R.D. and Shumway, N.E. Management of acute aortic dissections. *Ann. Thorac. Surg.* 1970; **10**: 237–47.

60. Miller, D.C., Stinson, E.B., Oyer, P.E., Rossiter, S.J., Reitz, B.A., Griepp, R.B. and Shumway, N.E. The operative treatment of aortic dissections: experience with 125 patients over a sixteen year period. *J. Thorac. Cardiovasc. Surg.* 1979; **78**: 365–82.

61. Haverich, A., Miller, D.C., Scott, W.C., Mitchell, R.S., Oyer, P.E., Stinson, E.B. and Shumway, N.E. Acute and chronic aortic dissections—determinants of long-term outcome for operative survivors. *Circulation* 1985; **72**(Suppl. 11): 1122–34.

62. Ergin, M.A., Galla, J.D., Lansman, S. and Griepp, R.B. Acute dissections of the aorta. *Surg. Clin. N. Am.* 1985; **65**: 721–41.

63. DeBakey, M.E., Henly, W.S., Cooley, D.A., Morris, G.C. Jr, Crawford, E.S. and Beall, A.C. Jr. Surgical management of dissecting aneurysms of the aorta. In: Egdahl, R.H. and Mannick, J.A., eds. *Modern Surgery.* New York: Grune and Stratton, 1970, pp. 37–57.

64. Bentall, H. and DeBono, A. A technique for complete replacement of the ascending aorta. *Thorax* 1968; **23**: 338–9.

65. Edwards, W.S. and Kerr, A.R. A safer technique for replacement of the entire ascending aorta and aortic valve. *J. Thorac. Cardiovasc. Surg.* 1970; **59**: 837–9.

66. Kouchoukos, N.T., Karp, R.B. and Lell, W.A. Replacement of the ascending aorta and aortic valve with a composite graft: results in 25 patients. *Ann. Thorac. Surg.* 1977; **24**: 140–8.

67. Wheat, M.W. Jr, Wilson, J.R. and Bartley, T.D. Successful replacement of the entire ascending aorta and aortic valve. *JAMA* 1964; **188**: 717–9.

68. Reul, G.J. Jr, Cooley, D.A., Hallman, G.L., Reddy, S.B., Kyger, E.R. III and Wukasch, D.C. Dissecting aneurysm of the descending aorta: improved surgical results in 91 patients. *Arch. Surg.* 1975; **110**: 632–40.

69. Jex, R.K., Schaff, H.V., Piehler, J.M., Orszulak, T.A., Puga, F.J., King, M., Danielson, G.K. and Pluth, J.R. Repair of ascending aortic dissection. Influence of associated aortic valve insufficiency on early and late results. *J. Thorac. Cardiovasc. Surg.* 1987; **93**: 375–84.

70. Leung, J.S.M., Mok, C.K., Leong, J.C.Y. and Chan, W.C. Syphilitic aortic aneurysm with spinal erosion. Treatment by aneurysm replacement and anterior spinal fusion. *J. Bone Joint Surg.* 1977; **59B**: 89–92.

71. Webster, B., Rich, C. Jr, Dense, P., Moore, J.E., Nicol, C.S. and Padget, P. Studies in cardiovascular syphilis. III. The natural history of syphilitic aortic insufficiency. *Am. Heart J.* 1953; **46**: 117–45.

72. Holt, S. Syphilitic ostial occlusion. *Br. Heart J.* 1977; **39**: 469–70.

73. Grabau, W., Emanuel, R., Ross, D., Parker, J. and Hegde, M. Syphilitic aortic regurgitation. An appraisal of surgical treatment. *Br. J. Vener. Dis.* 1976; **52**: 366–70.

74. Duncan, J.M. and Cooley, D.A. Surgical considerations in aortitis. III. Syphilitic and other forms of aortitis. *Texas Heart Inst. J.* 1983; **10**: 337–41.

75. Bennett, D.E. Primary mycotic aneurysms of the aorta. Report of case and review of the literature. *Arch. Surg.* 1967; **94**: 758–65.

76. Bennett, D.E. and Cherry, J.K. Bacterial infection of aortic aneurysms: a clinico-pathologic study. *Am. J. Surg.* 1967; **113**: 321–6.

77. Jarrett, F., Darling, R.C., Mundth, E.D. and Austin, W.G. Experience with infected aneurysms of the abdominal aorta. *Arch. Surg.* 1975; **110**: 1281–6.

78. Duncan, J.M. and Cooley, D.A. Surgical considerations in aortitis. II. Mycotic aneurysms. *Texas Heart Inst. J.* 1983; **10**: 329–35.

79. Ishikawa, K. Natural history and classification of occlusive thromboaortopathy (Takayasu's Disease). *Circulation* 1978; **57**: 27–35.

80. Numano, F., Tsohisa, I., Maezawa, H. and Juji, T. HL-A antigens in Takayasu's Disease. *Am. Heart J.* 1979; **98**: 153–9.

81. Bloss, R.S., Duncan, J.M., Cooley, D.A., Leatherman, L.L. and Schnee, M.J. Takayasu's arteritis: surgical considerations. *Ann. Thorac. Surg.* 1979; **27**: 574–9.

82. Hwang, T., Alpert, J.N., Cooley, D.A. and Hall, R.J. Takayasu's arteritis: diagnostic considerations and surgical treatment. *Texas Heart Inst. J.* 1983; **10**: 233–47.

83. Moore, J.W., Reardon, M.J., Cooley, D.A. and Vargo, T.A. Severe Takayasu's arteritis of the pulmonary arteries: report of a case with successful surgical treatment. *J. Am. Coll. Cardiol.* 1985; **5**: 369–73.

84. Bulkley, B.H. and Roberts, W.C. Ankylosing Spondylitis and aortic regurgitation. Description of the characteristic cardiovascular lesion from study of eight necropsy patients. *Circulation* 1973; **48**: 1014–27.

85. Good, A.E. Reiter's Disease: a review with special attention to cardiovascular and neurologic sequelae. *Semin. Arth. Rheum.* 1974; **3**: 253–86.

86. Bluestone, R. and Pearson, C.M. Ankylosing Spondylitis and Reiter's Syndrome: their interrelationship and association with HLA B27. *Adv. Intern. Med.* 1977; **22**: 1–19.

87. Labresh, K.A., Lally, E.V., Sharma, S.C. and Ho, G. Jr. Rheumatoid varient diseases. *Am. J. Med.* 1985; **78**: 908–11.

88. Klein, R.G., Hunder, G.G., Stanson, A.W. and Sheps, S.G. Large artery involvement in giant cell (temporal) arteritis. *Ann. Intern. Med.* 1975; **83**: 806–12.

Chapter 58

Pregnancy and Heart Disease

G.D.G. Oakley

INTRODUCTION

Heart disease in the pregnant patient still presents a challenge to those involved with its management. Many familiar problems take on new and unusual aspects when they occur during pregnancy. For instance, over the next 10 years, many girls who have been operated on for complex congenital heart disease will reach reproductive age and little is known about how they will react to pregnancy. Decisions must be made that will affect the welfare of both the mother and the fetus, and the correct management in some situations is still far from clear. In many instances information from the literature is sparse, because at only a few centres are enough patients seen with any given problem to compare different management strategies. Therefore, cardiologists, anaesthetists and obstetricians have to base their management on a sound knowledge of the physiological changes of pregnancy and of the pathology and physiology of the cardiac problems in the mother. Good management can only be achieved by careful reasoning and clinical skills because as yet large multicentre trials have not been performed.

PHYSIOLOGICAL CHANGES DURING PREGNANCY

Physiological changes in the maternal circulation start 10–20 weeks after implantation (or even earlier) and reach a peak at about 30 weeks. These changes are hormonally mediated with oestrogens and prostacyclin playing important roles. Maternal peripheral and pulmonary vascular resistances fall, thus reducing afterload on the heart.[1] Venous return increases with a consequent rise in left ventricular end-diastolic volume, but the filling pressure does not rise because the ventricle becomes more compliant. In late pregnancy the increase in

venous return is sensitive to posture, and a sharp drop in preload due to compression of the inferior vena cava by the gravid uterus may cause hypotension or even syncope. This is easily remedied by turning the subject from the supine to the lateral decubitus position. Blood volume increases by about 40% at 30 weeks and then remains at this level.[2] There is an increase in the volume of plasma and in the number of red cells but the disproportionate increase in plasma leads to a slight haemodilution, i.e. anaemia. These changes are more marked in twin pregnancies. There is an accompanying retention of sodium and water mediated by aldosterone; a little oedema is common.

Cardiac output increases to about 45% above normal levels at 20 weeks. Observations in the later stages of pregnancy have shown either a drop in cardiac output towards term or no change (measurements are very sensitive to posture).[3,4] The increase in cardiac output is due to an increased heart rate and to a larger stroke volume. The blood pressure stays the same or falls slightly because the rise in cardiac output is more than offset by the fall in peripheral vascular resistance. The pulse pressure may increase. These changes and some of the clinical features accompanying them are summarized in Table 58.1.

At the time of labour, further stresses occur. Uterine contractions cause a considerable increase in venous return, and during a contraction cardiac output may rise by a further 20%.[5] Pain causes tachycardia, and analgesia may lead to hypotension. During the puerperium, all these changes regress over about 7 days and with them the physical signs. Nevertheless, this is a surprisingly dangerous period for the cardiac patient for reasons that are not clear. Haemorrhage is the major hazard, particularly if it is compounded by the reduction in peripheral vascular resistance without a concomitant increase in venous return. On the other hand, there are also substantial volume shifts

Table 58.1. Circulatory changes and physical signs during pregnancy.

Circulatory change	Physical signs
Vascular resistance ↓ } Cardiac output ↑	Warm flushed peripheries Bounding pulse
Venous return ↑	Third heart sound
Stroke volume ↑	Dynamic left ventricular impulse Systolic flow murmurs
Heart rate ↑	Tachycardia
Blood volume ↑	Slight elevation of venous pressure 'Tense' soft tissues Peripheral oedema (common)
Arterial blood pressure ↓ or →	None

following delivery and pulmonary oedema may be aggravated by reabsorption of extracellular fluid into a vascular bed the capacitance of which has been reduced by the loss of the fetus and placenta. Release of vena caval obstruction might also increase venous return. The onset of lactation poses a further haemodynamic burden.

CARDIAC DIAGNOSIS IN THE PREGNANT NORMAL PATIENT

SYMPTOMS

The physiological changes of pregnancy often cause a variety of symptoms which may raise the suspicion of organic heart disease. Fatigue is common and chest pain may be caused by oesophageal reflux. As many as 75% of women may complain of dyspnoea, but orthopnoea is rare. Palpitation is very common, due to either an increased awareness of the normal heart beat or ectopic atrial or ventricular activity. Dizziness may be caused by postural hypotension.

SIGNS

The suspicion of symptomatic heart disease may be reinforced by the finding of several characteristic signs. The pulse feels full even though the blood pressure is unchanged. The left ventricle is active but not displaced. Third heart sounds are frequently present whereas fourth heart sounds are not characteristic. A soft early systolic or mid-systolic murmur localized to the left sternal edge is very common. All these changes develop between 12 and 20 weeks and persist for up to 1 week in the puerperium.[6] This clinical picture is usually easy to distinguish

from organic cardiac disease presenting for the first time in pregnancy. The lesions most likely to cause confusion are mild pulmonary stenosis, mild aortic stenosis and atrial septal defect. They seldom give rise to significant problems during pregnancy, but further investigations may be needed to clarify the diagnosis.

INVESTIGATIONS

Chest X-ray

A chest X-ray is not normally performed, especially during the first trimester. The radiation dose to the uterus (5 millirads) however is well below that associated with congenital malformations and the risk of promoting subsequent leukaemia in the offspring is imponderable but miniscule. A chest X-ray should be taken, therefore, if clinically indicated. In normal pregnancy, the heart is slightly enlarged when compared with the heart in the pre-gravid state, but it is still within normal limits. An assessment of pulmonary vascularity is difficult to make unless the subject has taken a deep breath.

Electrocardiogram

There are no characteristic electrocardiographic changes during pregnancy except for a slight shift of the axis to the left which can give rise to a Q3–T3 pattern. This shift does not extend into the abnormal range ($-30°$).

Echocardiography

Echocardiography is the investigation of choice when doubt exists as to the significance of an ejection systolic murmur heard in pregnancy.

MANAGEMENT OF PREGNANCY—GENERAL PRINCIPLES

There has been an increasing tendency towards permitting pregnancy in women who have cardiac disease. Serious cardiac problems that are surgically remediable are best operated on before conception. For a few of the women with severe cardiac disease who conceive accidentally or against medical advice, therapeutic abortion is advisable provided they present early enough; for example, patients with primary pulmonary hypertension, Eisenmenger's syndrome, critical aortic stenosis and possibly

Marfan's syndrome. In the remainder, a rough guide to management and outcome can be gained from functional status. Those in New York Heart Association classes I and II are likely to do well and may require only a short period of bed rest prior to delivery. Exacerbation of symptoms can occur at any stage, however, and close observation in the clinic throughout a patient's pregnancy is desirable. Although the drug treatment of heart failure is along conventional lines, several precautions need to be taken. If digoxin is used, the dose required for a therapeutic effect may be considerably greater during pregnancy; it is essential to monitor digoxin levels carefully. Diuretics should also be used with caution as excessive diuresis will lower cardiac output and reduce uterine blood flow. Diuretics can aggravate the patient's condition if toxaemia is present because this condition is associated with hypovolaemia. Restriction of salt and water and the use of vasodilators is a more logical approach.

MANAGEMENT OF SPECIFIC CARDIAC CONDITIONS

All cardiac conditions pose problems during pregnancy. In Table 58.2, some common cardiac conditions have been grouped into those with higher and those with lower risk.

PULMONARY HYPERTENSION

The lesions carrying the highest risk are undoubtedly primary pulmonary hypertension and Eisenmenger's syndrome. A maternal mortality rate of 30–70% has been reported in Eisenmenger's syn-

Table 58.2. Risk associated with specific cardiac lesions during pregnancy.

High risk
Primary pulmonary hypertension
Eisenmenger's syndrome
Mitral stenosis
Aortic stenosis
Marfan's syndrome

Intermediate risk
Coarctation of the aorta
Cyanotic congenital heart disease without pulmonary hypertension
Hypertrophic cardiomyopathy

Low risk
Mitral regurgitation ⎫
Aortic regurgitation ⎬ (NYHA classes I and II)
Atrial septal defect ⎭
Ventricular septal defect (without pulmonary hypertension)

drome, the early puerperium being a particularly dangerous time.[7,8] Some authors have suggested that sudden collapse of the mother following delivery is due to intravascular thrombosis in pulmonary vessels or pulmonary embolism. Postmortem studies do not confirm this suggestion. A much more plausible therory is that following delivery there is a drop in peripheral vascular resistance and/or a hormonally mediated rise in pulmonary vascular resistance and hence a catastrophic increase in the right-to-left shunting. Such a problem would be greatly exacerbated by haemorrhage or reduction in venous return due to pooling. Resuscitation in this situation is usually unsuccessful; replacement of blood loss combined with inotropic and pressor agent support and oxygen therapy seems the most logical approach. During pregnancy, patients with pulmonary hypertension often develop peripheral venous congestion and oedema. Diuretics should be used with the utmost caution to prevent any undue reduction in right ventricular filling. Patients with pulmonary hypertension should be advised against pregnancy. Sterilization is the best method of contraception. Therapeutic abortion is appropriate in early pregnancy.

MITRAL STENOSIS

Mitral stenosis is poorly tolerated in pregnancy. The increased cardiac output, tachycardia and a predisposition to atrial fibrillation all tend to aggravate the underlying haemodynamic lesion. Mitral stenosis can present for the first time with pulmonary oedema during pregnancy, often in patients who have small hearts and small left atria. At this stage, the characteristic physical signs may be difficult to elicit and a high index of suspicion is needed. The aim of treatment is to control the heart rate with digoxin and beta-adrenergic blocking drugs if appropriate and to treat pulmonary oedema with diuretics. If control is not promptly achieved, it is reasonably safe, for both mother and fetus, to perform closed mitral valvotomy.[9]

AORTIC STENOSIS

It is best to treat significant aortic or pulmonary stenosis before a patient becomes pregnant whenever possible. First principles dictate that very severe aortic stenosis should be particularly difficult to manage in pregnancy and bitter experience bears this out. The transvalvar gradient must increase with the increasing cardiac output and the drop in peripheral vascular resistance.[10] There are marked postural changes in ventricular filling and any consequent drop in blood pressure will reduce coronary perfusion. Prolonged rest seems to be the best method of management, but once heart failure supervenes the outlook is grave and there is no pharmacological agent which can logically be prescribed. It is best to proceed to aortic valve surgery without delay. The role of balloon aortic valvuloplasty in such patients has yet to be determined.

MARFAN'S SYNDROME

Marfan's syndrome with aortic root involvement carries a significant risk of dissection during pregnancy,[11] which could be due, in part, to a specific laxity of elastic tissue that occurs in pregnant women.[12] A widening of the pulse pressure may also be relevant, even though the blood pressure does not usually rise. The number of patients studied so far is not large enough to enable strict management guidelines to be produced, although Pedowitz and Perrell[13] have suggested a set. A good case can be made for advising against pregnancy in those women who have echocardiographic evidence of significant aortic root dilatation, particularly if serial studies have shown that this is progressive. The author currently has two patients who have successfully completed pregnancy following composite aortic graft surgery for Marfan's syndrome.

COARCTATION OF THE AORTA

It has been suggested that coarctation of the aorta is associated with a significantly increased maternal mortality during pregnancy and the puerperium. Rupture of the aorta, cerebral haemorrhage from berry aneurysms, heart failure and endocarditis have all been described.[14] A more critical look at the accumulated evidence, however, would suggest that the risk may have been overstated.[15,16] Obviously, surgical correction prior to pregnancy is desirable, but the risk of rupture is probably not sufficiently high to require termination in those cases of coarctation which present for the first time during pregnancy.

HYPERTROPHIC CARDIOMYOPATHY

There are theoretical reasons why pregnancy might exacerbate the haemodynamic problems of hyper-

trophic cardiomyopathy. In particular, the drop in peripheral vascular resistance and any blood loss at the time of delivery could prove harmful. Also the increased ectopic activity of pregnancy might exacerbate arrhythmias. In fact, pregnancy is well tolerated by women with hypertrophic cardiomyopathy (perhaps this is not too surprising in view of the autosomal dominant mode of inheritance). Although maternal mortality is very low, symptomatic deterioration is common. Diuretics for dyspnoea, beta-adrenergic blocking drugs for angina and anti-arrhythmic medication may be needed for the first time or in increased dosage during pregnancy.[17]

CYANOTIC CONGENITAL HEART DISEASE

Cyanotic congenital heart disease (without pulmonary hypertension) has been included as a fairly low risk lesion for the mother. There is, however, an increased risk of fetal death and premature infants are common. The children are usually of low birthweight despite having larger placentas. Spontaneous abortions are commonest in those mothers who have the greatest degree of cyanosis and highest levels of haematocrit which indicates that failure of oxygen delivery to the growing fetus is the main problem. There are no problems if it is the father who has the cyanotic heart disease. Maternal cyanosis may become worse during pregnancy due to a drop in peripheral vascular resistance and an increased right-to-left shunt.

MITRAL AND AORTIC REGURGITATION

Regurgitation, whether mitral or aortic, in the absence of left ventricular failure, is well tolerated in pregnancy. Cardiac output is maintained by means of tachycardia. Also the reduction in afterload that occurs during pregnancy will reduce the regurgitant fraction. The same observations apply to atrial and ventricular septal defects without pulmonary hypertension.

ISCHAEMIC HEART DISEASE

There are no prospective data on the effect of pregnancy in patients with ischaemic heart disease. Cases of myocardial infarction, of angina and of coronary surgery occurring during pregnancy have been reported. Particular problems may be encountered in patients who have heart failure at the time of delivery. Nitrates are the logical choice of treatment and invasive monitoring may be needed to regulate the dose correctly.[18]

MANAGEMENT OF LABOUR

In general, labour should be managed in accordance with sound obstetric principles notwithstanding the presence of cardiac disease. Spontaneous labour with vaginal delivery is preferable, using forceps only when the second stage is protracted. It is generally desirable to use ergometrine to reduce blood loss during the third stage, but it is contra-indicated in patients who have pulmonary oedema. Antibiotic prophylaxis is of no proven benefit, but it is recommended for patients who have prosthetic heart valves. The British Society for Antimicrobial Chemotherapy suggests a combination of amoxycillin 1 g intramuscularly and gentamicin 120 mg intramuscularly prior to delivery with 0.5 g amoxycillin orally 6 h later. Patients who are allergic to penicillin should receive vancomycin 1 g by slow intravenous infusion over 1 h and intravenous gentamicin 120 mg prior to delivery.

Analgesia is highly desirable at the time of delivery which is best undertaken in the left lateral decubitus position to avoid sudden changes in preload. Epidural anaesthesia should be avoided in those women who might respond badly to sudden hypotension, but it may actually be beneficial in those with heart failure. Invasive haemodynamic monitoring with continuous evaluation of intra-arterial and pulmonary wedge pressures along with fetal monitoring is helpful in the management of patients with critical lesions and heart failure. It enables rapid responses to be made to the marked haemodynamic fluctuations associated with delivery and anaesthesia.[18,19] Caesarian section should be undertaken only for obstetric indications. Circumstances, such as the cardiac state of the mother, the speed of progress of labour, obstetric presentation and the urgency of delivery, will dictate the choice of anaesthesia. Often, better control over haemodynamic variables can be obtained by using a general rather than an epidural anaesthetic.

CARDIAC SURGERY AND PREGNANCY

Closed mitral valvotomy for intractable pulmonary oedema in pregnant patients with mitral stenosis is a life-saving procedure which carries a low fetal and maternal mortality. Early reports of open proce-dures such as valve replacement under cardiopulmonary bypass showed that fetal mortality was as high as 33%, although the maternal mortality was no greater than that in non-pregnant patients.[9] Better results have been published more recently with a fetal mortality of 20% in 68 procedures.[20] Improvements in fetal survival have been attributed to the use of high blood flow and normothermia during bypass. The use of heparin, however, cannot be avoided. The risk to the fetus of maternal cardiopulmonary bypass is considerable, but the condition of a woman with serious valvular lesions may be so intractable as to justify this risk, for example, in cases of aortic stenosis. When Caesarian section is indicated for obstetric reasons, it can be performed at the same time as heart surgery.

ANTICOAGULANTS AND PREGNANCY

There is an increase in maternal coagulability and a decrease in fibrinolytic activity during pregnancy. Thrombo-embolic disease is therefore a real risk in pregnancy and occurs in about 0.2% of pregnant women. It is the second most common cause of maternal death after hypertensive disease. The condition is not frequent enough, however, easily to construct controlled trials so there is no good information about how these patients are best managed. There is no agreement over whether warfarin or heparin is the best anticoagulant to use or which heparin regimen should be followed.[21]

Coumarin anticoagulants are associated with a specific embryopathy, particularly when given from the sixth to the ninth week of pregnancy. Spontaneous abortion is also common at this time and may occur in 30% of mothers taking these drugs. The dangers associated with taking coumarin drugs may extend into the second trimester, but the evidence for this is less strong. In the third trimester, fetal and post-partum haemorrhage may occur. The characteristic embryopathy consists of nasal hypoplasia and stippled epiphyses (chondrodysplasia punctata). Optic atrophy, mental retardation, spasticity or hypotonia occur less frequently. The nasal hypoplasia is manifest by depression of the bridge of the nose. When severe, the nose may appear to be sunk into the face; eventually, reconstructive surgery will be required. When mild, the nose appears to be flattened and upturned. Small nares in the infant may give rise to respiratory problems. Chondrodysplasia punctata is a stippling in uncalcified epiphyseal regions. It is seen on X-rays of the axial skeleton, proximal femurs and the calcanei. Although it may lead to scoliosis, there are often no apparent sequelae.[22,23]

Good control of the international normalised ratio (INR) in the mother does not guarantee against fetal haemorrhage. Warfarin crosses the placenta and has a disproportionate effect on the fetus in whom clotting factors are reduced because the liver is immature. The effect of warfarin can be reversed in the fetus with fresh frozen plasma; vitamin K is effective only in the mother.

It is difficult to assess the risks of heparin administration during pregnancy. The results of retrospective studies would suggest that there is an increased risk of maternal haemorrhage, fetal prematurity, abortion and stillbirth. Heparin in large doses over prolonged periods may cause demineralization of bone. As heparin does not cross the placenta and can be quickly reversed with protamine, there is general agreement that heparin carries less risk than warfarin during pregnancy, especially during the first trimester and around the time of delivery. Heparin is difficult to administer and may not be as effective as warfarin, especially in smaller doses (5000 units twice daily). Various regimens have been suggested, the most widely prescribed being 10 000 units of heparin self-administered subcutaneously twice daily. The dosage is adjusted to maintain the activated partial thromboplastin time at about twice that of the control value.

When making the final decision about anticoagulation during pregnancy, all these points must be taken into account. For a woman with active thrombosis, heparin appears to be the best choice provided she can manage to inject it properly and the therapeutic effect is monitored. Heparin should be given either throughout pregnancy and for 6 weeks of the puerperium or warfarin can be substituted from weeks 13 to 36.

Women with prosthetic valves pose a special problem. It is hoped that the use of biological prostheses will reduce this problem, but women who have tilting disc valves, which in the mitral position are strongly anticoagulant dependent, will need treatment. If heparin is to be used in the first trimester, it would be logical to substitute it before conception otherwise the risk of warfarin embryopathy may not be avoided. These practical problems, combined with the unproved efficacy of heparin in this situation, have led some workers to suggest that warfarin should be continued until shortly before delivery. Patients need to be counsel-

led if this course is chosen. Based on retrospective data, continuous warfarin treatment appears to ensure a completely normal outcome in 2 out of 3 pregnancies. The chances of spontaneous abortion are about 1 in 6, as are the chances of a liveborn infant with embryopathy. As the embryopathy will be trivial in a few of these infants, the chances of a significant defect occurring are about 1 in 8. To some clinicians, this risk is enough to justify the use of warfarin which is easy to administer and of proven efficacy.

SURGICALLY CORRECTED CONGENITAL HEART DISEASE AND PREGNANCY

The effects of some common congenital heart lesions in the mother during pregnancy have been discussed. As the surgical correction of major heart defects has developed greatly over the last two decades, many of these patients are now approaching reproductive age. Experience with some corrected lesions, such as total correction of tetralogy of Fallot, has shown that a good surgical result in the mother is associated with a low risk pregnancy and a healthy child;[24,25] Experience with others is sparse. Theoretically, the drop in pulmonary vascular resistance might be beneficial in women who have Fontan shunts, provided increased ectopic activity does not lead to atrial arrhythmias. The increased cardiac output of pregnancy, however, might exacerbate systemic or pulmonary venous obstruction by the intra-atrial baffle in girls who have transposition of the great vessels and undergone a Mustard correction.

At present, the only general principle is that the surgical result should be optimal prior to pregnancy.[26] Thorough post-operative re-evaluation of these girls, by repeat catheter if necessary, seems to be advisable so that any significant residual defects can be corrected before they embark on raising a family.

Patients with significant congenital heart disease often enquire about the risks of their child being affected. Although there is an increased risk to the child, it is not great. The incidence of congenital heart disease in the general population is about 1%, which rises to about 3–5% if the mother has congenital heart disease. Cono-truncus abnormalities have the strongest familial tendency. In one recent study, the increased risk of the baby being affected was found to be much higher at about 13%.[26] This study included several infants who had ventricular septal defect which closed spontaneously. Concordance between the defect in the mother and child occurred in about 50% of cases. Mothers with aortic stenosis and coarctation had the highest incidence of abnormal infants. Whatever the true incidence of heart defects in the infant, the chances of the child having serious heart disease are low enough to reassure the mother that a future pregnancy is unlikely to be complicated. This advice is not applicable to those patients who have conditions that display a dominant mode of inheritance such as hypertrophic cardiomyopathy, Marfan's syndrome and Friedreich's ataxia.

The echocardiographic detection of serious fetal cardiac malformations at a stage that permits interruption of pregnancy is now feasible. A routine ultrasound scan, available at most centres, will confirm the presence of normally related atria and ventricles with adequate valves. More complex diagnoses require special experience which is available at some referral centres. It is not yet clear who should be referred for this investigation, which will provide reassurance to mothers who have the worst family histories of congenital heart disease.

PERIPARTUM CARDIOMYOPATHY

Peripartum cardiomyopathy is a poorly understood condition; the patient presents with heart failure in the last months of pregnancy or during the 6 months after delivery.[27,28] The clinical features are those of a dilated cardiomyopathy; the diagnosis is made by exclusion of other possible causes of heart failure. Some workers doubt whether this condition is a specific entity and argue that it represents a subclinical cardiomyopathy, or other cardiac disease, aggravated by the haemodynamic stresses of pregnancy.[29] The peak incidence of peripartum cardiomyopathy, however, occurs well into the puerperium, rather than during the last trimester of pregnancy, a finding that does not support this view.

The aetiology of this condition is not known, but the course is rapidly progressive and fatal in up to 50% of cases. Treatment is along conventional lines with diuretics, vasodilators, anticoagulants and anti-arrhythmic drugs in specific cases. Many women recover but there is a tendency for the cardiomyopathy to relapse in subsequent pregnancies. The risk of relapse is probably least in those who have made the most complete recovery from the initial episode. Persistent failure, even if mild, is

a contra-indication to further pregnancy. A specific form of peripartum heart failure is peculiar to women of the Hausa tribe in Nigeria. This appears to be a separate entity and is related to a high salt intake after delivery. It responds well to treatment with diuretics.[30]

ARRHYTHMIAS AND THEIR MANAGEMENT

Pregnancy is associated with an increased ectopic activity, both in the atrium and the ventricle.[31] These ectopic rhythms may prove symptomatic *per se* or they may trigger re-entry tachycardias in susceptible subjects. Isolated ectopic beats seldom need treatment other than reassurance that they are common during pregnancy and do not indicate serious underlying heart disease (given there is no other evidence of this). Re-entry tachycardias, particularly paroxysmal re-entrant atrioventricular tachycardias, are more of a problem. The sudden drop in cardiac output may cause severe dizziness or syncope in the pregnant subject. Cardioversion with intravenous verapamil[32] or direct current countershock[33] is safe and well tolerated. For prophylaxis, beta-adrenoceptor blocking drugs are the treatment of first choice. The earlier reports of placental insufficiency being caused by these drugs have not been confirmed. It is necessary to monitor the babies carefully following delivery because they may develop bradycardia or hypoglycaemia and delayed onset of respiration. These problems are only transient, however, and there is much prospective work attesting to the safety of beta-blockers during pregnancy.[34] There is some evidence to suggest that fetal hypoglycaemia and respiratory distress are less common when a beta-1 selective agent is used.

It is doubtful whether pregnancy *per se* can cause serious ventricular arrhythmias, although in some reports it has been suggested that this is the case. Ventricular tachycardia may occur, however, in patients who have underlying heart disease, e.g. ischaemic heart disease or cardiomyopathy. Lignocaine, quinidine, procainamide and disopyramide are not associated with emybropathy, but the experience with disopyramide is limited. All these drugs cross the placenta, but adverse effects are rare. Large doses of lignocaine may harm the fetus if there is already fetal distress from some other cause. These drugs should be given when indicated for serious maternal arrhythmias. As pregnancy alters the pharmacokinetics of class I agents, it is best, wherever possible, to monitor drug levels when they are given over prolonged periods.[35] Amiodarone has a wide profile of side-effects. It should be reserved for patients who have intractable serious arrhythmias which may worsen during pregnancy. Experience with this drug during pregnancy is limited to a few case-reports. Amiodarone crosses the placenta, as does its desethyl metabolite. It contains a significant amount of iodine which might be expected to cause a fetal goitre. In the reports published so far, the fetus does not appear to be adversely affected by amiodarone even when it is given continuously throughout pregnancy, but caution is necessary when extrapolating from such limited data.[35,36].

All anti-arrhythmic drugs are excreted in breast milk to varying amounts but the dose to the fetus is generally small and adverse effects have not been reported.

CONTRACEPTION IN WOMEN WITH CARDIAC DISEASE

Contraceptive advice is largely a matter of commonsense since there is no published evidence concerning the relative risks of different forms of contraception. The oral contraceptive should not be prescribed to women who have conditions in which thrombosis may occur, e.g. pulmonary hypertension and ischaemic heart disease, conditions with a low cardiac output or cyanotic congenital heart disease associated with a high haematocrit. If an oral contraceptive is used, a low oestrogen or progestogen-only preparation should be favoured. The intra-uterine device carries a theoretical risk of endocarditis in susceptible individuals. Other barrier forms of contraception may be satisfactory; their failure rate would preclude their use in those women in whom pregnancy is absolutely contraindicated, but sterilization should be advised in these cases anyway. Vasectomy avoids all these problems, but as surgical reversal is unreliable the expected lifespan of the man in relation to the prognosis of his wife should be taken into account when considering this option.

SUMMARY

Although historically pregnancy has been forbidden in women with heart disease, the treatment goal in cardiology is to enable patients to lead an active and fulfilling life. For most women, this includes the option of bearing and bringing up children. The modern management of women with heart disease must include provision for pregnancy, and plans to manage an eventual pregnancy may have to be made early during the patient's childhood. The timing of operations for congenital heart disease and the evaluation of results, or the timing of valve surgery and the choice of prosthesis are examples of the variables involved. Contraceptive advice should be given to women who have lesions carrying a higher risk; some conditions may require therapeutic abortion. When pregnancy proceeds despite serious maternal cardiac problems, the best chance of a happy outcome is achieved when cardiologists, anaesthetists and obstetricians work in close cooperation.

REFERENCES

1. Ginsburg, J. and Duncan, S.L.B. Peripheral blood flow in normal pregnancy. Cardiovasc. Res. 1967; 1: 132–7.
2. Pritchard, J.A. Changes in blood volume during pregnancy and delivery. Anesthesiology 1965; 26: 393–9.
3. Bader, R.A., Bader, M.E., Rose, D.J. and Braunwald, E. Hemodynamics at rest and during exercise in normal pregnancy as studied by cardiac catheterization. J. Clin. Invest. 1955; 34: 1534.
4. Ueland, K., Novy, M.J., Peterson, E.N. and Metcalfe, J. Maternal cardiovascular dynamics IV. The influence of gestational age on the maternal cardiovascular response to posture and exercise. Am. J. Obstet. Gynecol. 1969; 104: 856–64.
5. Ueland, K. and Hansen, J.M. Maternal cardiovascular dynamics II. Posture and uterine contractions. Am. J. Obstet. Gynecol. 1969; 103: 1–7.
6. Cutforth, R. and MacDonald, C.B. Heart sounds and murmurs in pregnancy. Am. Heart J. 1966; 71: 741–7.
7. Jones, A.M. and Howitt, G. Eisenmenger syndrome in pregnancy. Br. Med. J. 1965; 1: 1627.
8. Pitts, J.A., Crosby, W.M. and Basta, L.L. Eisenmenger's syndrome in pregnancy. Does heparin prophylaxis improve the material mortality rate? Am. Heart J. 1977; 93: 321–6.
9. Zitnik, R.S., Brandenburg, R.O., Sheldon, R. and Wallace, R.B. Pregnancy and open heart surgery. Circulation 1969; 39 (Suppl.): 257–62.
10. Avias, F. and Pineda, J. Aortic stenosis and pregnancy. J. Reprod. Med. 1978; 20: 229–32.
11. Pyeritz, R.E. Maternal and fetal complications of pregnancy in the Marfan syndrome. Am. J. Med. 1981; 71: 784.
12. Cavanzo, F.J. and Taylor, H.B. Effect of pregnancy on the human aorta and its relationship to dissecting aneurysm. Am. J. Obstet. Gynecol. 1969; 105: 567–8.
13. Pedowitz, P. and Perrell, A. Aneurysms complicating pregnancy, Part 1. Aneurysms of the aorta and its major branches. Am. J. Obstet. Gynecol. 1957; 73: 720–35
14. Mendelson, C.L. Pregnancy and coarctation of the aorta. Am. J. Obstet. Gynecol. 1940; 39: 1014–21.
15. Deal, K. and Wooley, C.F. Coarctation of the aorta and pregnancy. Ann. Intern. Med. 1973; 78: 706–10.
16. Goodwin, J.F. Pregnancy and coarctation of the aorta. Clin. Obstet. Gynaecol. 1961; 4: 645–64.
17. Oakley, G.D.G., McGarry, K., Limb, D.G. and Oakley,

C.M. Management of pregnancy in patients with hypertrophic cardiomyopathy. *Br. Med. J.* 1979; **1**: 1749–50.

18. Hankins, G.D.V., Wendel, G.D., Leveno, K.J. and Stoneham, J. Myocardial infarction during pregnancy: a review. *Obstet. Gynaecol.* 1985; **65**: 139–46.

19. Clark, S.L., Phelan, J.P., Greenspoon, J., Aldah, L.D. and Horenstein, J. Labor and delivery in the presence of mitral stenosis: Central haemodynamic observations. *Am. J. Obstet. Gynecol.* 1985; **152** : 984–8.

20. Becker, R.M. Intracardiac surgery in pregnant women. *Ann. Thorac. Surg.* 1983; **36**: 453–8.

21. Use of anticoagulants in pregnancy. *Drug and therapeutics bulletin.* 1987; **25**: 1–4.

22. Lutz, D.J., Noler, K.L., Spittall, J.A., Danielson, G.K. and Fish, C.R. Pregnancy and its complications following cardiac valve prostheses. *Am. J. Obstet. Gynecol.* 1978; **131**: 460–8.

23. Hall, J.A., Pauli, R.M. and Wilson, K.M. Maternal and foetal sequelae of anticoagulants during pregnancy. *Am. J. Med.* 1980; **68**: 122–40.

24. Singh, H., Bolton P.J. and Oakley, C.M. Pregnancy after surgical correction of tetralogy of Fallot. *Br. Med. J.* 1982; **285**: 168–70.

25. Nissenkorn, A., Friedman, S., Schoufield, A. and Ovadia, J. Fetomaternal outcome in pregnancies after total correction of the tetralogy of Fallot. *Int. Surg.* 1984; **69**: 125–8.

26. Whittemore, R., Hobbins, J.C. and Engle, M.A. Pregnancy and its outcomes in women with and without surgical treatment of congenital heart disease. *Am. J. Cardiol.* 1982; **50**: 641–51.

27. Julian, D.G. and Szekely, P. Peripartum cardiomyopathy. *Prog. Cardiovasc. Dis.* 1985; **27**: 223–40.

28. Homans, D.C. Peripartum cardiomyopathy. *N. Engl. J. Med.* 1985; **312**: 1432–7.

29. Cunningham, F.G., Pritchard, J.A., Hankins, G.D.V., Anderson, P.L., Lucas, M.J. and Armstrong, K.F. Peripartum heart failure: Idiopathic cardiomyopathy or compounding cardiovascular events. *Obstet. Gynaecol.* 1986; **67** : 157–68.

30. Sanderson, J.E., Adesanya, C.O., Anjorin, F.I. *et al.* Post partum cardiac failure—heart failure due to volume overload. *Am. Heart J.* 1979; **97**: 613–7.

31. Mendelson, C.L. Disorders of the heartbeat during pregnancy. *Am. J. Obstet Gynecol.* 1956; **72**: 1268–301.

32. Klein, V. and Repke, J.T. Supraventricular tachycardia in pregnancy: cardioversion with Verapamil. *Obstet. Gynaecol.* 1984; **63**(Suppl. 3): 16.S–18.S.

33. Cullhed, I. Cardioversion during pregnancy. *Acta Med. Scand.* 1983; **214**: 169–72

34. Rubin, P.C. Beta-blockers in pregnancy. *N. Engl. J. Med.* 1981; **305**: 1323–6.

35. Rotmensch, H.H., Elkayaus U., Frishman, W. Antiarrhythmic drug therapy during pregnancy. *Ann. Intern. Med.* 1983; **98**: 487–97.

36. McKenna, W.J., Harris, L., Rowland, E., Whitelaw, A., Storey, G. and Holt, D. Amiodarone therapy during pregnancy. *Am. J. Cardiol.* 1983; **51**: 1231–3.

37. Robson, D.J., Raj, M.V.J., Storey, G.C.A. and Holt, D.W. Use of amiodarone during pregnancy. *Postgrad. Med. J.* 1985; **61**: 75–7.

Chapter 59

Pregnancy Hypertension

E. Malcolm Symonds

HYPERTENSION IN PREGNANCY

Hypertension arising in pregnancy is the commonest complication needing management in obstetric care in the UK. Various attempts have been made to classify the condition, based on the severity of hypertension, the presence of proteinuria and the presence of oedema. However, as each of these signs has a different prognostic significance, they are not of comparable importance. Furthermore, there is a marked difference in perinatal mortality in relation to the level of blood pressure as well as the presence and quantity of the proteinuria. The Committee on Terminology of the American College of Obstetricians and Gynecologists[1] suggested that the following classification should be used.

Gestational oedema: the occurrence of a general successive accumulation of fluid or a weight gain of 2.3 kg (5 lb) or more in 1 week.

Gestational hypertension: the development of hypertension alone, as defined by the term gestational hypertension, carries very little significance in relation to perinatal outcome. Hypertension in pregnancy is defined as a rise in systolic blood pressure of 30 mmHg and a rise in diastolic pressure of 15 mmHg or more. It is also defined in absolute terms as a systolic pressure of at least 140 mmHg or a diastolic pressure of 90 mmHg. The incidence of proteinuria increases with the diastolic pressure; if the diastolic pressure exceeds 115 mmHg, 35% of the women exhibit proteinuria. At the same time, the development of proteinuria denotes the worsening of both maternal and fetal prognosis.

Pre-eclampsia: the development of hypertension with proteinuria and oedema. Proteinuria is defined as the presence of urinary protein in concentrations > 0.3 g/l in a 24-h collection or in concentrations > 1 g/l in a random urine collection on 2 occasions 6 h apart. Although the presence of oedema or features of excessive weight gain is a common manifestation in pre-eclampsia, it does not enhance the diagnostic classification of the condition because it occurs in up to 70% of normal pregnancies. The recent proposals by the International Society for the Study of Hypertension in Pregnancy (ISSHP) recommend exclusion of oedema from the diagnostic classification.

The diagnosis of gestational hypertension and of pre-eclampsia is based on the presence of a normal blood pressure before 20 weeks' gestation.

Eclampsia is defined as the occurrence of fits in the presence of pre-eclampsia.

In addition to these classifications, pregnancy may be complicated by chronic hypertensive disease. Superimposed pre-eclampsia or eclampsia commonly complicates chronic renal or vascular disease and is classified separately. The classification recommended by ISSHP[2] maintains these categories (see Table 59.1) but divides the development of hypertension and proteinuria on a temporal basis by the time of onset of the signs.

RECORDING OF BLOOD PRESSURE

The recommendation by ISSHP for the standard measurement of blood pressure by sphygmomanometry suggests that the patient should lie comfortably on a couch or bed on her right side with a 15–30° tilt and with the arm well supported at the same level as the heart. The tilt is particularly important in late pregnancy because of the effect of the gravid uterus resting on the vena caval trunk. Diastolic blood pressure in pregnancy is taken as the point where the Korotkoff sounds first become muffled. However, if no clear point of muffling is heard, phase V should be recorded instead of phase IV. In carefully controlled prospective studies by Schwartz[3] and MacGillivray,[4] it has been shown significant effect on basal blood pressure levels.

Table 59.1. Classification of hypertensive disorders of pregnancy (ISSHP).

Gestational hypertension and/or proteinuria
Hypertension and/or proteinuria developing during pregnancy, labour or the puerperium in a previously normotensive non-proteinuric woman, subdivided as follows:
1 Gestational hypertension (without proteinuria):
  a developing during pregnancy (antenatal);
  b developing for first time in labour;
  c developing for first time in the puerperium.

2 Gestational proteinuria (without hypertension):
  a developing during pregnancy (antenatal);
  b developing for first time in labour;
  c developing for first time in the puerperium.

3 Gestational proteinuric hypertension (pre-eclampsia):
  a developing during pregnancy (antenatal);
  b developing for first time in labour;
  c developing for first time in the puerperium.

Chronic hypertension and chronic renal disease
Hypertension and/or proteinuria in pregnancy in a woman with chronic hypertension or chronic renal disease diagnosed either before or during or persisting after pregnancy, subdivided as follows.
1 Chronic hypertension (without proteinuria).
2 Chronic renal disease (proteinuria and hypertension).
3 Chronic hypertension with superimposed pre-eclampsia.
   (Proteinuria developing for the first time during pregnancy in a woman with known chronic hypertension).

Unclassified hypertension and/or proteinuria
Hypertension and/or proteinuria either found at first 'booking' examination after the 20th week of pregnancy (140 days) in a woman without known chronic hypertension or chronic renal disease or found during pregnancy, labour or the puerperium where information is insufficient to permit classification. Provisionally regarded as unclassified and subdivided as follows.
1 Unclassified hypertension (without proteinuria).
2 Unclassified proteinuria (without hypertension).
3 Unclassified proteinuric hypertension (pre-eclampsia).

Eclampsia is regarded as one of the complications of the hypertensive disorders of pregnancy and should be included in a separate classification of complications.

that blood pressure falls during the second trimester and is followed by a rise to non-pregnant values in the third trimester. Blood pressure also varies during a 24-h period; during this circadian rhythm in pregnancy, the highest blood pressures occur in the afternoon and early evening. This pattern can be demonstrated in normotensive women and in women with chronic hypertensive disease. In severe pre-eclampsia, there is a reduced fall of blood pressure during sleep and a reversal of the pattern at night. Other factors such as age and race also have a

EPIDEMIOLOGY

There are considerable difficulties in establishing the incidence of gestational hypertension and pre-eclampsia because the classification in reported studies varies greatly and the populations studied often comprise hospital referral populations which do not represent population statistics. High rates of eclampsia and pre-eclampsia occur in primigravidae; this association is particularly apparent in older primigravidae. There are very few total population studies, but the data collected by workers at Aberdeen between 1950 and 1955 suggest that hypertension alone developed in 23% of primigravid women compared with 9.9% in women who were in their third pregnancy; 5.5 and 1.3%, respectively, developed proteinuric hypertension. More recently, Hall and Campbell[5] have reported an apparent increase in the incidence of both gestational hypertension and proteinuric hypertension between 1951 and 1980 from 22.1 and 5.8%, respectively, to 35.9 and 7.5%. The reason for this change is not readily apparent but may be related in part to the quality of obstetric care and to the number of observations made. In general, it seems likely that the overall incidence of gestational hypertension in pregnancy is about 15% in Western European countries; approximately 10% of this population develop proteinuria.

A recent World Health Organisation report[6] on pre-eclampsia in primigravidae in Burma, China, Thailand and Vietnam has revealed marked differences in the incidence of proteinuric hypertension with an incidence of 0.7% in the Vietnamese population and one of 4.7% in China. Davies *et al.*[7] reported the variation in the incidence of pre-eclampsia in different ethnic groups in one city and showed a marked difference under common environmental conditions. Various other conditions, such as multiple pregnancy, diabetes mellitus, severe rhesus iso-immunization and hydramnios, increase the incidence of pre-eclampsia. Chesley's data[8] on eclamptic probands followed for 50 years in a study of the daughters, daughters-in-law, sisters and grand-daughters suggest that severe pre-eclampsia is inherited as a simple autosomal recessive gene but, in view of the changing incidence in many countries and the variations that occur in relation to race and climate, it must be assumed that any genetic factor acts as one that is predisposing rather than as a final determinant.

AETIOLOGY AND PATHOGENESIS

In 1972, Page,[9] in a review of all the various factors known at that time, hypothesized that pre-eclampsia was the result of a chain of reactions which he described as a 'vicious inner circle' of events. It is unlikely any single factor can be considered to be the cause of pre-eclampsia but there may be a series of triggering factors that stimulate or initiate change in a series of reactions in the normal control mechanisms in the regulation of blood flow and blood pressure in the pregnant woman. These factors are generally considered under the three categories of vaso-active substances, haematological changes and the immunological system. The framework of these suggested interactions is shown in Fig. 59.1.

Vaso-active substances

Normal pregnancy is associated with a fall in blood pressure in mid-trimester below the normal non-pregnant values. This fall is associated with a 30–40% increase in cardiac output by 16 weeks' gestation and a progressive increase in plasma volume up to 36 weeks' gestation. Both these factors should increase blood pressure and therefore must be associated with a reduction in total peripheral resistance. With the development of pre-eclampsia, peripheral vascular resistance increases and plasma volume decreases. These changes appear to be mediated through humoral transmission and represent the balance between vasoconstrictor and vasodilator substances.

The renin-angiotensin system

Plasma renin activity and renin concentration increase in normal pregnancy by a factor of two- to threefold in the first trimester and remain elevated,[10] accompanied by a comparable increase in plasma angiotensin II levels. Detailed studies on all these parameters in the immediate period after delivery have shown that the levels fall to non-pregnant values within 2 h but thereafter rise again to full-term pregnant values within the next 2 h and remain elevated over the following week.[11] Plasma renin substrate levels also rise during pregnancy and increase progressively until full term. This appears to be an oestrogen-induced effect. Renin substrate exists in multiple forms and serial studies in normal pregnancy have demonstrated that the percentage of high molecular weight substrate increases throughout pregnancy.[12] The effect of these changes on renin activity is not clearly understood. Plasma levels of angiotensin converting enzyme initially fall in normal pregnancy[10] but rise to the non-pregnant levels in the third trimester. Levels of inactive renin in pregnancy reach their peak at 12–16 weeks of pregnancy and thereafter fall towards term. Inactive renin was first identified in amniotic fluid,[13] and subsequently shown to be present in plasma and to be produced, in conjunction with active renin, by cultures of human chorion. It seems likely that the maternal kidney is the major source of circulating renin in pregnancy and that the fetal kidney is the source of renin in the fetal circulation. Evidence from an anephric fetus showed that the fetal blood contained no active

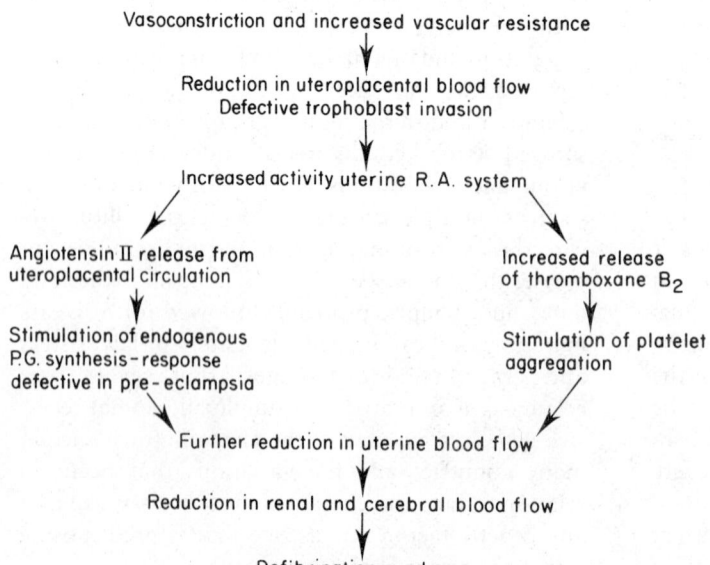

Fig. 59.1. Schematic representation of some major changes in the pathogenesis of pre-eclampsia.

renin[14] and very low concentrations of inactive renin. Cord venous levels of angiotensin are higher than cord arterial levels when the cord samples are obtained following vaginal delivery but the same or similar levels are seen at the time of delivery by elective Caesarean section.

Various sites of renin production have been described in the human female and these include the chorion, myometrium and decidua.[15] Renin has also been demonstrated in seminal fluid and in follicular fluid. Chorion laeve contains very high concentrations of inactive renin and when the tissues are cultured, chorionic cells, which are thought to be cytotrophoblasts, produce both active and inactive renin.[16] Chorion explants incubated in protein-free media have also been shown to generate angiotensin I and the addition of an antirenin to the incubation medium inhibits the generation of angiotensin I.[17] Human myometrium also produces both active and inactive renin in tissue culture and the cells that are renin-positive are generally clustered around the spiral arterioles.[18]

The function of the renin–angiotensin system in the genital tract is still not known and the contribution to the development of pre-eclampsia is obscure. There is general agreement that plasma levels of renin in patients with pre-eclampsia are lower than those in a normotensive population. There are conflicting reports on whether the angiotensin II levels are also low; some authors have reported a positive correlation between circulating angiotensin II levels and diastolic blood pressure. There is also evidence that the concentration of angiotensin II in the uterine venous circulation is increased in women with severe pre-eclampsia. The perfusion of angiotensin II into the peripheral circulation of the pregnant sheep has been shown to increase uterine blood flow initially but in high concentrations there is a subsequent reduction of uterine blood flow.[19] Angiotensin II also promotes the release of vasodilator prostaglandins into the uterine venous circulation and it has been hypothesized that the local release of angiotensin II may stimulate vasodilatation locally but promote a rise in maternal perfusion pressure. These effects are benign if there is an adequate response to the release of local vasodilator prostaglandins. If the response is deficient, an increase in maternal blood pressure will be associated with a reduction in both uterine and renal blood flows.

Angiotensin sensitivity. Pregnancy is associated with a loss of sensitivity to infused angiotensin II. In prospective studies on primigravid women, it has been demonstrated that sensitivity to infused angiotensin II increases to non-pregnant levels before and during the development of pre-eclampsia.[20] An understanding of the mechanism of this change is central to an understanding of the mechanism of the hypertension. It was suggested that progesterone might be the agent of this change and there is some evidence that infused 5, α-hydroxyprogesterone[21] reduces angiotensin II sensitivity in human pregnancy. The response to infused angiotensin II can also be modified by the prior administration of prostaglandin E_1, prostaglandin E_2 and prostacyclin. However, examination of the dose–response curves of angiotensin II infusion in early pregnancy shows a 60% reduction in sensitivity and in the second trimester this reduction is almost 100% (Broughton Pipkin, F. and O'Brien, S., personal communication). It has been demonstrated that this change is based on a shift in the intercept and not a change in the slope of the dose–response curve, which suggests that there is an alteration in angiotensin II vascular receptor activity, but there have been no studies of the maternal vasculature to substantiate this hypothesis.

Eicosanoids

The term 'eicosanoid' refers to all the metabolites of arachidonic acid and therefore includes prostaglandins and thromboxanes. The products exert their actions predominantly at local level and are therefore of particular interest in the regulation of blood flow and blood pressure in pregnancy. Many studies have now been reported on the differences in prostaglandin production and catabolism in pregnancy-induced hypertension. In general, the evidence from fetal and maternal tissues suggests that there is a relative prostacyclin deficiency. The production of prostacyclin by placental, fetal and maternal tissues is reduced during pregnancy-induced hypertension when compared with that in normal pregnancies. It has been suggested that the reduction of prostaglandin I_1 may be associated with a reduction of prostaglandin endoperoxides with increased platelet thromboxane A_2 production and increased levels of its stable hydrolysis product thromboxane B_2.[22] Increased circulating levels of thromboxane are also associated with increased platelet aggregation, a finding that relates to the reduced platelet count and increased tendency to micro-embolization that characterize severe pre-eclampsia. This concept is particularly important because it provides a basis for the prevention of the condition using low-dose aspirin to inhibit thromboxane production. There also appears to be some evidence of essential fatty acid deficiency in pregnancy-induced hypertension which may be related to the development of hypertension.

Catecholamines

Various studies on the role of the sympatho-adrenal system have been reported with widely differing results. These conflicting results may be due, in part, to difficulties of classification but they are also related to differences in the method of measuring the components of the catecholamine system. Measurement of venous plasma levels of noradrenaline and adrenaline indicates reduced, constant or increased levels of catecholamines. There is evidence of enhanced sympathetic reactivity and augmented vascular responses in pregnancy-induced hypertension which may be due to reduced plasma volumes. Some of these responses indicate an inadequate adaptation of the cardiovascular system in pregnancy-induced hypertension.[23]

The kallikrein system

The presence of an active vasodilator system may be especially important in the regulation of blood pressure in pregnancy to counteract the activity of the potent vasoconstrictor effects of the renin–angiotensin system and of some of the eicosanoids. For this reason, the renal kallikrein system is of great importance, but has been considerably underinvestigated, in pregnancy. There are similarities between the renal kallikrein–kinin system and the renin–angiotensin system in that both renin and kallikrein act on a substrate to form a potent vaso-active substance. In the kallikrein system, bradykinin is formed which has a vasodilator effect and also stimulates the production and release of prostaglandin E_2 and prostaglandin I_2. Kallikrein exists in both an active and an inactive form as does renin in the renin–angiotensin system. Low levels of active and inactive urinary kallikrein have been demonstrated in pregnancy characterized by hypertension.[24] These changes cannot be related to other hormonal systems but it is possible that low activity in a vasodilator system may be relevant to the development of hypertension in pregnancy.

Coagulation disorders in pregnancy-induced hypertension

In normal pregnancy, there is an increase in the plasma concentrations of clotting factors with the exception of factors XI and XII. The kallikrein system amplifies factor XII activation and also activates the fibrinolytic and kinin systems. McKay[25] originally described fibrin depositions in the renal glomeruli of women who had fatal eclampsia and suggested that these findings were similar to those seen in the generalized Schwartzmann reaction. An increase in factor VIII-related antigen has been noted in pre-eclampsia, particularly in those cases associated with fetal growth retardation.[26] Factor VIII-related antigen is synthesized by endothelial cells and is released by the aggregation of platelets; these changes in pre-eclampsia may be explained by vascular endothelial damage. The levels of fibrinogen/fibrin degradation products have been extensively studied in pre-eclampsia, and the results vary between studies. Some investigators have found that the levels of urinary fibrinogen degradation products are increased in severe pre-eclampsia, and others have found them to be normal. Platelet counts are lower in pregnancies complicated by pre-eclampsia. In severe pre-eclampsia, thrombocytopenia is associated with elevated levels of liver enzymes and haemolysis and is known as the HELLP syndrome.[27] This syndrome may have a greater tendency to occur in those with severe pre-eclampsia who are being conservatively managed. The configuration of platelets also changes in pre-eclampsia. In normotensive pregnancy, there is a significant negative correlation between platelet count and the percentage of large platelets. In pre-eclampsia, there appears to be no such correlation suggesting an increase in peripheral platelet destruction and fragmentation.

Thromboxane A_2 promotes platelet aggregation and may play a significant role in the various pathological manifestations of pre-eclampsia, particularly as it has been found to be present in excess in fetal and maternal tissues in pre-eclampsia. Prostacyclin has anti-aggregating effects and the relative deficiency of this biochemical in pre-eclampsia would tend to promote platelet aggregation.

Immunological factors

There has been much speculation about the possibility of an immunological basis to the aetiology of pre-eclampsia, particularly in relation to the association with parity. The condition is significantly more common in primigravidae. Also, it appears to occur less frequently in women who have had a miscarriage during their first pregnancy. Pregnancy presents a peculiar immunological challenge to the mother's body because the conceptus carries the immunological characteristics of a foreign body implanted in the uterus. Paternally derived antigens are present on the 8-cell zygote but villous trophoblast fails to express class I or II major histocompatability complex (MHC) antigens at any time.[28] Furthermore, all other trophoblast populations express a form of class I MHC antigens. No trophoblast population has been shown to express class II MHC antigens, a phenomenon that ensures the protection of both the trophoblast and the pregnancy from immune attack.

Paternal specific antibodies are detectable in some women, but their presence varies. Several studies of maternal cell-mediated immunity have been performed; it is currently believed that maternal cell-mediated sensitization to the fetus is not a regular occurrence. The risk of developing pre-eclampsia is not linked with any specific HLA types but there is evidence of excess showing of HLA-A and B antigens among couples where the women develop pre-eclampsia.[29] The complement system is activated in some women with pre-eclampsia; complement deposition can be demonstrated in the uteroplacental bed, the kidneys and the liver. However, it seems likely that the changes in the humoral immune system are non-specific or secondary. There is no definitive evidence of changes in cell-mediated immunity in pre-eclampsia.

PATHOLOGY

The kidney

The major histopathological changes occur in the kidney, the liver and the placenta. The major lesions in the kidney occur in the glomeruli which become swollen and enlarged. Swollen endothelial and mesangial cells encroach on capillary lumina. The enlarged glomerular tufts fill Bowman's space and may protrude into the proximal tubule. The characteristic features are best seen by ultrastructural analysis and exhibit swelling and vacuolization of the capillary endothelial cells. There is a wide variety of vacuoles, some contain lipid and some occur in grape-like clusters. The basement membrane is not thickened and deposits of finely granular electron-dense material may be seen in between the endothelial and mesangial cells. In some cases, the material may consist of fibrin or its precursors or degradation products. The material may also contain proteins such as laminin, type IV collagen,

fibronectin and proteoglycan. There are no significant changes in the tubules.

The liver

Two hepatic lesions have been described in fetal cases of eclampsia. Periportal fibrin deposition and areas of zonal necrosis or infarction are present. Periportal fibrin deposition is probably a consequence of haemorrhage into the base of the liver cell columns. Such haemorrhaging may compress hepatocytes and lead to the necrosis of some cells. These cells are removed by macrophages and the lesions repaired by fibrosis. Fibrin is also deposited within the sinusoids, which may be a consequence of disseminated intravascular coagulation. These hepatic abnormalities are non-specific.

Placenta

The histological abnormalities consistently seen in the villi of the placentae from pre-eclamptic women are an undue prominence and greater number of villous cytotrophoblastic cells with an irregular thickening of the trophoblastic basement membranes. Ultrastructural images confirm the abundance of villous cytotrophoblastic cells with evidence of increased mitotic activity. Some of these cells also show degenerative changes with cytoplasmic rarefaction, organellar swelling and nuclear chromatin condensation. There are small areas of syncytial necrosis and there is often a marked paucity of microvilli on the free surface. Some long syncytial projections extend into intervillous spaces. There is irregular thickening of the trophoblastic basement membrane, and this structure also contains fine microfibrils, collagen fibres, electron-dense fibrillary material and electron-dense inclusions.[30] Most of the changes seen in the villous trophoblast reflect a response to tissue ischaemia. The formation of syncytial protrusions into the intervillous spaces may be a compensatory mechanism to asphyxia in that it increases the surface area of syncytiotrophoblast.

The uteroplacental bed

The changes that occur in the uteroplacental bed during placentation and during the process of placental development in normal pregnancy include extravillous trophoblast migration from the blastocyst to populate the basal decidua; by 10 weeks, some of these cells penetrate the myometrium. The purpose of this invasion appears to be to prepare the decidua and myometrial vessels for subsequent events. During the first trimester, extravillous cytotrophoblast invades the spiral arterioles and migrates down the intima of these vessels. This process results in the loss of normal musculo-elastic material and much of the intima is replaced by fibrinoid material.[31] The vessels become flaccid, sinusoidal channels of low resistance and high flow. A second wave of invasion of a similar type occurs at 16 weeks, reinforcing the changes in the vessel walls. In pre-eclampsia, there is evidence of acute atherosis[32] in the small muscular arteries of the inner myometrium. This is a particular feature of the terminal branches of the radial arteries, which are not involved in the trophoblast-induced physiological changes. There also appears to be defective invasion of trophoblast into the spiral arteries in cases of pre-eclampsia and also in association with intrauterine growth retardation. These changes result in uteroplacental infarcts and the characteristic changes of anoxia that are manifest in the placental villi. The factors that determine the effectiveness of the invasion of extravillous trophoblast are not known; it has been suggested that the phenomenon may be determined by various immunological reactions.

The changes that occur in placentation and the defective vascular development in the uteroplacental bed account for the impairment of fetal growth and sometimes result in asphyxial intrauterine death.

CAUSES OF MATERNAL DEATH

The reports of the Confidential Enquiries into Maternal Deaths in England and Wales,[33] published triennially, have shown that, when taken together, pre-eclampsia and eclampsia are the commonest cause of maternal death in 4 of the 10 reports issued; in the last report (1979–1981), they were ranked number one. The death rate per million births is 19.5. In this last report, of the 20 deaths from eclampsia, 13 resulted from haemorrhage, oedema and infarction of the brain, 4 were due to hepatorenal failure and 3 from other causes. In the 16 deaths associated with pre-eclampsia, 8 were due to hepatic and cardiac complications and 4 were associated with intracranial problems.

DIAGNOSIS AND CLINICAL FEATURES

The symptoms of pre-eclampsia are generally non-specific and late in onset. They include headaches and visual disturbances. The development of persistent epigastric pain is a late and sinister symptom which is often premonitory of the development of eclampsia. The signs of pre-eclampsia include, by definition, the development of hypertension, proteinuria and oedema, which is often associated with excessive weight gain. As the condition worsens, there are signs of hyper-reflexia and subsequently convulsions occur. The differential diagnosis is usually not difficult unless the woman presents with the disease established in the second half of pregnancy having not previously attended for medical care. In other words, the diagnosis is based on the knowledge that the blood pressure and urinalysis were normal in the first 20 weeks of gestation and not on the specificity of the signs and symptoms in the second half of pregnancy. Renal biopsy studies have shown that although 82% of primigravidae with pre-eclampsia exhibit the renal lesions of the disease, it occurs in only 37% of multigravidae in whom the presence of nephrosclerosis and other chronic lesions can be identified.[34]

Pregnancy may also be complicated by essential hypertension, chronic renal disease, phaeochromocytoma, Cushing's syndrome, Conn's syndrome and coarctation of the aorta. Each condition carries its own implications for the pregnancy and for the mother.

In general, the prognoses of mother and child in a pregnancy complicated by renal disease are largely dependent on the degree of impairment of renal function; if creatinine clearance is > 100 ml/min, the outcome is similar to that of a normal pregnancy.

SPECIAL INVESTIGATIONS

There are several specific changes in pre-eclampsia that will enhance the precision of diagnosis: an increased sensitivity to infused angiotensin II, reduced uric acid clearance with raised serum levels, reduced glomerular filtration rate and effective renal plasma flow, increased fibrinogen/fibrin turnover, reduced platelet count and raised liver enzymes. The presence of haemolysis associated with low platelet counts and abnormal liver function tests is referred to as the HELLP syndrome. An assessment of the type of urinary proteins in pre-eclampsia has not been particularly useful in differential diagnosis. In general, glomerular selectivity is poor. Ratios of IgC to transferrin clearance of < 0.15 are not found in pre-eclampsia. Although values > 0.15 are found in pre-eclampsia, they are also found in cases of membranous nephropathy.

POST-PARTUM ASSESSMENT

Persistent hypertension with or without proteinuria at the 6-week visit after delivery should be investigated because it indicates that the hypertension was not due to pre-eclampsia. However, it should be remembered that in most women hypertension does not settle immediately after delivery of the fetus and may take a further 7–10 days before it falls within the normal range. Furthermore, there is evidence that, when compared with a matched control normotensive population, systolic and diastolic pressures are higher in the hypertensive group at 6 weeks' gestation, although the mean values fall within the normal range. If there is a significant degree of hypertension and/or proteinuria at 6 weeks, further investigations should be initiated including urinary cultures, serum electrolytes, urea, creatinine levels and creatinine clearance. An intravenous pyelogram should be performed and, if this is normal, renal biopsy should not be performed. Further investigations of 24-h urinary vanillomandelic acid excretion and magnetic resonance scanning of the adrenals should be performed if there is any suggestion of a phaeochromocytoma.

MANAGEMENT

Mild hypertension

The development of gestational hypertension in the absence of proteinuria tends to occur late in pregnancy and appears to have little effect on fetal growth or perinatal outcome. The objectives of management are:

1 to prevent any damage to the mother or fetus by the effects of reduced uteroplacental and renal blood flow;
2 to prevent, if possible, progression of the condition to the proteinuric phase and to prevent the development of convulsions;
3 to reduce the risks of death and morbidity for both mother and child;
4 to achieve these objectives without worsening the short- and long-term prognosis of the mother.
5 to ensure that any treatment introduced should not have a greater risk for mother and child than the condition itself.

When managing women who have severe pre-eclampsia and eclampsia, the primary objects are different. It is necessary:

1 to control the fits;
2 to control blood pressure;
3 to deliver the child (conservative management is no longer relevant).

One approach to the management of pregnancy-induced hypertension is summarized in Fig. 59.2.

Traditional management dictates that any woman who has been previously normotensive who develops pregnancy-induced hypertension should be admitted to hospital for bed rest and observation. Although it has been claimed that this results in increased uterine and renal blood flow, there is little evidence to support this hypothesis. However, hospital admission does enable the clinician to observe the mother's blood pressure carefully and to test her urine for protein frequently. In this sense, it is a safe and reassuring course to follow, although it is often achieved at the cost of considerable social and psychological disruption. However, several studies have now been reported which have shown that with suitable safeguards, safe outpatient management can be achieved.[35] The introduction of a Day Assessment Unit has been described at the Glasgow Royal Infirmary.[36] Mothers with a past history of pre-eclampsia, pre-existing disease or an abnormality of blood pressure attending an antenatal clinic are referred to the unit for detailed assessment. Blood pressure is checked frequently during the day and urinalysis is performed with Dipstix; urate levels, platelet counts, and fetal growth are monitored and cardiotocography is performed. The patients are admitted to hospital if they show signs of worsening disease. When this policy was adopted, about 75% of the women did not progress to a more severe form of the disease.

Prevention of pre-eclampsia

Until recently, it was believed that eclampsia could be prevented by careful antenatal care and appropriately timed intervention and delivery of the child. However, it seemed unlikely that it would be possible to prevent the development of pre-eclampsia although various attempts have been made, for example, by dietary manipulation of salt intake and essential fatty acid supplementation. In a small placebo-controlled study of the use of low-dose aspirin (60 mg daily) supplementation in women considered to be at high risk of pre-eclampsia because of abnormal angiotensin sensitivity, marked differences in the development of hyperten-

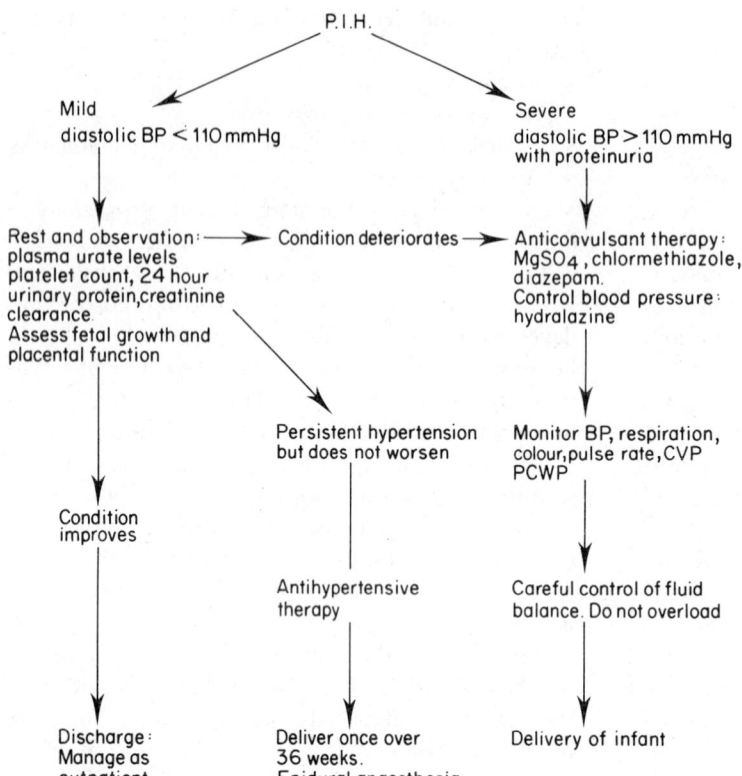

Fig. 59.2. A flow chart for the management of pregnancy-induced hypertension. BP, blood pressure; CVP, central venous pressure; PCWP, pulmonary capillary wedge pressure.

sion were found between the aspirin-treated and the control populations.[37] As the study population was small there is a need for a much larger study to be performed to consolidate these findings. A further study of a high-risk population with aspirin and dipyridamole[38] in a group of 93 multigravidae also showed a significant reduction in the incidence of pre-eclampsia in the treated group.

Diuretics

Plasma volume is reduced in pregnancy-induced hypertension and the administration of diuretics tends to exaggerate this phenomenon. The use of thiazide diuretics to prevent the development of pre-eclampsia has been generally unsuccessful; in a randomized controlled study, the birthweights of infants born to women taking diuretics were found to be significantly less than those of babies born to the control population.[39] Also, diuretics are not valuable in the control of established proteinuric pre-eclampsia.

Antihypertensive therapy

There is continuing debate about the role of antihypertensive therapy in mild pregnancy-induced hypertension; indeed, it is difficult to prove there is

a benefit with therapy in this group of women because the perinatal mortality rate is already low. However, the value of drug therapy in women with mild pregnancy-induced hypertension should be measured by the reduction in the incidence of proteinuric hypertension and a reduction in the length of hospitalization for both the mother and the newborn infant. There is anxiety that lowering the blood pressure may reduce uterine perfusion pressure, but this fear may be unfounded because uteroplacental blood flow depends on the action of the drug on the uterine vasculature. In a large randomized early intervention study of methyldopa in women who developed pregnancy-induced hypertension, there was a significant reduction in the number of mid-trimester abortions and of perinatal deaths.[40] In subsequent randomized studies in which a comparison was made between methyldopa and labetalol[41] and methyldopa and oxprenolol,[42] there was evidence of a reduced incidence of the development of proteinuria in the labetalol- and oxprenolol-treated groups. The results of studies on plasma volume and birthweight have suggested that sympathetic blockade expands plasma volume and results in an increase in the birthweight of the infants.

In a randomized double-blind placebo-controlled

study of atenolol,[43] it was shown that the incidence of subsequent proteinuria is reduced in the treated patients and the length of hospitalization is shortened. It is therefore reasonable to conclude at present that women who develop diastolic pressures in excess of 95 mmHg and who do not respond to rest and conservative management should be treated with methyldopa, labetalol, atenolol or oxprenolol and then monitored carefully. If the hypertension is not controlled by these compounds, hydralazine, administered either orally or systemically, can be added to the regimen; if this fails, delivery is indicated.

Management of severe pre-eclampsia

Severe pre-eclampsia is defined as the development of a diastolic pressure in excess of 110 mmHg and the presence of > 1 g protein/l urine. This is usually accompanied by oliguria with a fall in the output of urine to < 400 ml/h. The major feature of cardiac function in severe pre-eclampsia or eclampsia is an increase in afterload, due to an increase in total systemic vascular resistance. These changes are associated with a reduction in plasma volume. Despite various attempts to correct this situation by volume expansion, volume expansion produces only a slight increase in cardiac output and a transient fall in peripheral resistance. In fact, the intravascular space in eclamptic women is contracted but not underfilled and therefore these women are particularly sensitive to volume expansion. Improperly controlled volume expansion with hyperosmotic fluid, such as a 5% albumin solution, may produce cardiac failure, pulmonary oedema and cerebrovascular accidents. Volume expansion therapy should be attempted only if the pulmonary capillary wedge pressure can be monitored; if this is not possible, central venous pressure should be monitored bearing in mind its accepted limitation. Therapeutic volume expansion should be conducted with great caution. The first stage in management is to prevent or control the development of convulsions. In the USA, this is mainly achieved by the administration of magnesium sulphate. An initial dose of 4 g is given as a 20% solution at a rate of 1 g/min,[44] followed by 10 g in a 50% solution by intramuscular injection into the buttocks; thereafter 5 g by intramuscular injection every 4 h. Injections should be given only if the patella reflex is present and respirations are not depressed. Plasma levels of Mg^{2+} should be kept below 7 mEq/l. In the UK, diazepam is widely used to control convulsions by

giving 10–20 mg in a bolus followed by an infusion of 40 mg in 500 ml of 5% dextrose. Alternatively, after the initial loading dose, therapy can be maintained by intramuscular injections every 4 h. Although diazepam tends to cause hypotonia and hypoglycaemia in the newborn infant,[45] there is no evidence to show that this effect has any long-term consequences. Whichever technique is chosen, it is important that the women can be effectively monitored for colour and respiration; facilities for endotracheal intubation and cardiorespiratory resuscitation should be readily available.

Chlormethiazole is also used to control convulsions; it is administered as a 0.8% solution given rapidly by intravenous infusion until drowsiness is induced. The method has become well established at some centres;[46] it is safe provided it is realized that the therapeutic dose is very close to that which will cause respiratory depression. It is essential that the woman receives nursing care that includes close observations in a good light.

Control of blood pressure

Hydralazine remains the most effective agent available for the control of blood pressure, particularly when the diastolic blood pressure exceeds 110 mmHg. The pattern of administration is a bolus dose of up to 25 mg followed by an infusion of 25–50 mg in 500 ml of Hartmann's solution. The infusion rate should be increased until the diastolic pressure is controlled between 90 and 95 mmHg. During the course of the acute management, fluid therapy should be limited to 60–150 ml/h of Hartmann's solution. Occasionally, additional control of the blood pressure can be achieved with sodium nitroprusside or with a slow calcium channel blocker such as nifedipine.[47]

Once the fits and the blood pressure have been controlled, the fetus should be delivered either by induction and a vaginal delivery or by elective Caesarean section. It has been general policy in the UK to use epidural anaesthesia during labour or for elective Caesarean section provided the platelet count is within safe limits and that there are no other coagulation disorders. Careful attention must be given to the expansion of the vascular bed by pre-loading blood pressure to ensure that unwanted hypotension, which would result in severe reduction of uteroplacental blood flow and hence fetal distress, does not develop.

Post-partum management

Significant hypertension may persist for 7–10 days

1382 PREGNANCY HYPERTENSION

after therapy and convulsions arise *de novo* in about one-third of cases in the first 24 h after delivery. It is therefore essential to maintain a high level of care and observation for the first 48 h after delivery. Antihypertensive therapy should also be maintained and then gradually reduced once the mother's blood pressure appears to have stabilized at a safe level. Rarely, the mother may develop renal failure. The development of oliguria with the production of 300 ml urine/day may be due to hypervolaemia or renal failure but a urine osmolality of 300 mosmol/kg H_2O and urinary sodium > 30 mg/l indicates that the woman has renal failure. It is controversial whether the use of diuretics, such as mannitol and frusemide, can prevent renal failure, but, if there is evidence of hypovolaemia, mannitol can be used to expand plasma volume, and, if there is elevation of central venous pressure, frusemide should be administered to promote a diuresis.

REFERENCES

1. Hughes, E.C. *Obstetric–Gynecologic Terminology*. Philadelphia: Davis, 1972, p. 422.
2. Davey, D.A. and MacGillivray, I. The classification and definition of the hypertensive disorders of pregnancy. *Clin. Exp. Hyp. — Hyp. Preg.* 1987; **B51**: 97.
3. Schwartz, R. The behaviour of the circulation in normal pregnancy. I. Arterial blood pressure. *Arch. Gynakol.* 1964; **199**: 549. Quoted by Hytten, F.E. and Leitch, J. In: *The Physiology of Human Pregnancy*, 2nd edn. Oxford: Blackwell Scientific Publications, 1971.
4. MacGillivray, I., Rose, G.A. and Rowe, D. Blood pressure survey in pregnancy. *Clin. Sci.* 1969; **37**: 395.
5. Hall, M.H. and Campbell, D.M. Geographical epidemiology of hypertension in pregnancy. In: Sharp, F. and Symonds, E.M. eds. *Hypertension in Pregnancy. Proceedings of the Sixteenth Study Group of the Royal College of Obstetricians and Gynaecologists, July 1986*, Vol. 7. London: Royal College of Obstetricians and Gynaecologists, 1987, p. 33.
6. World Health Organisation. *Report of the Study Group on Hypertensive Disorders of Pregnancy*, Technical Report Series No. 758. Geneva: WHO, 1987, p.19.
7. Davies, A.M., Czaczkes, K.W., Sadosky, E., Prywes, R., Weiskopn, P. and Sterk, V.V. Toxaemia of pregnancy in Jerusalem. Epidemiological studies of a total community. *Israel J. Med. Sci.* 1970; **6**: 253.
8. Chesley, L.C. and Cooper, D.W. Genetics of hypertension in pregnancy: possible single gene control of pre-eclampsia and eclampsia in the descendants of eclamptic women. *Br. J. Obstet. Gynaecol.* 1986; **93**: 898.
9. Page, E.W. On the pathogenesis of pre-eclampsia and eclampsia. *J. Obstet. Gynaecol. Br. Cmwlth* 1972; **79**: 883.
10. Oats, J.J.N., Broughton Pipkin, F., Symonds, E.M. and Craven, D.J. A prospective study of plasma angiotensin-converting enzyme in normotensive primigravidae and their infants. *Br. J. Obstet. Gynaecol.* 1981; **88**: 1204.
11. Jadoul, F.A.C., Broughton Pipkin, F. and Lamming, G.D. Changes in the renin-angiotensin-aldosterone system in normotensive primigravidae in the four days after normal spontaneous delivery. *Br. J. Obstet. Gynaecol.* 1982; **89**: 633.
12. Tetlow, H.J. and Broughton Pipkin, F. Changing renin substrates in human pregnancy. *J. Endocrinol.* 1986; **109**: 257.
13. Morris, B.J. and Lumbers, E.R. The activation of renin in human amniotic fluid by proteolytic enzymes. *Biochim. Biophys. Acta* 1972; **289**: 385.
14. Symonds, E.M. and Furler, I. Plasma renin levels in the normal and anephric fetus at birth. *Biol. Neonate* 1973; **23**: 133.
15. Symonds, E.M., Stanley, M.A. and Skinner, S.L. Production of renin by *in vitro* cultures of human chorion and uterine muscle. *Nature* 1968; **217**: 1152.
16. Warren, A.Y., Craven, D.J. and Symonds, E.M. Production of active and inactive renin by cultured explants from the human female genital tract. *Br. J. Obstet. Gynaecol.* 1982; **89**: 628.
17. Craven, D.J., Warren, A.Y. and Symonds, E.M. Generation of angiotensin I by human chorion-decidua *in vitro*. *Am. J. Obstet. Gynecol.* 1983; **145**: 744.
18. Johnson, J., Johnson, I.R., Ronan, J.E. and Craven, D.J. The site of renin in the human uterus. *Histopathology* 1984; **8**: 273.
19. Naden, R.P. and Rosenfeld, C.R. Effect of angiotensin II on uterine and systemic vasculature. *J. Clin. Invest.* 1981; **68**: 468.
20. Gant, N.F., Daley, G.L., Chand, S., Whalley, P.J. and McDonald, P.C. A study of angiotensin II pressor response throughout primigravid pregnancy. *J. Clin. Invest.* 1973; **52**: 2682.
21. Broughton Pipkin, F. Renin angiotensin system in normal and hypertensive pregnancies. In: Rubin, P. ed. *Handbook of Hypertension, Vol. 12, Hypertension in pregnancy*. Amsterdam: Elsevier, 1988, pp. 118–151.
22. Myatt, L. Eicosanoids and blood pressure regulation. In: Sharp, F. and Symonds, E.M. eds. *Hypertension in Pregnancy. Proceedings of the Sixteenth Study Group of the Royal College of Obstetricians and Gynaecologists, July 1986*, Vol 7. London: Royal College of Obstetricians and Gynaecologists, 1987, p. 174.
23. Nisell, H., Lunell, N.O., Hjemdahl, P. and Linde, B. Catecholamines in pregnancy-induced hypertension. In: Sharp, F. and Symonds, E.M. eds. *Hypertension in Pregnancy. Proceedings of the Sixteenth Study Group of the Royal College of Obstetricians and Gynaecologists, July 1986*, Vol. 7. London: Royal College of Obstetricians and Gynaecologists, 1987, p. 187.
24. Karlberg, B.E. and Wichman, K. Hypertension in Pregnancy, Prostaglandins, Kinins and Kallikrein. *Scan. J. Clin. Lab. Invest.* 1984; **44**(Suppl.): 169.
25. McKay, D.G., Merrill, S.J., Weiner, A.E., Hentig, A.E. and Reid, D.E. The pathologic anatomy of eclampsia, bilateral renal corticol necrosis, pituitary necrosis and the acute fetal complications and its possible relationships to the generalised Schwartzman phenomenon. *Am. J. Obstet. Gynecol.* 1953; **66**: 507.
26. Whigham, K.A.E., Howie, P.W., Shah, M.M. and Prentice, C.R.M. Factor VIII related antigen/coagulant activity ratio as a predictor of fetal growth retardation: A comparison with hormone and uric acid measurements. *Br. J. Obstet. Gynaecol.* 1980; **87**: 797.
27. Weinstein, L. Syndrome of hemolysis, elevated liver enzymes, and low platelet count: A severe consequence of hypertension in pregnancy. *Am. J. Obstet. Gynecol.* 1982; **142**: 159.
28. Stirrat, G.M. Immunology of pregnancy. In: Studd, J. ed. *Progress in Obstetrics and Gynaecology*, Vol. 5. Edinburgh: Churchill Livingstone, 1985, p. 1.
29. Redman, C.W.G., Bodmer, J., Bodmer, W.F., Beilin, L.J. and Bonnar, J. HLA antigens in severe pre-eclampsia. *Lancet* 1978; **ii**: 397.

30. MacLennon, A.H., Sharp, F. and Shaw-Dunn, J. The ultrastructure of human trophoblast in spontaneous and induced hypoxia using a system of organ culture: a comparison with ultrastructural changes in pre-eclampsia and placental insufficiency. *J. Obstet. Gynaecol. Br. Cwlth*. 1972; **79**: 113.

31. Pijnenborg, R., Bland, J.M., Robertson, W.B., Dixon, G. and Brosens, I. The pattern of interstitial trophoblastic invasion of the myometrium in early human pregnancy. *Placenta* 1981; **2**: 303.

32. Hertig, A.T. Vascular pathology in the hypertensive albuminuric toxemias of pregnancy. *Clinics* 1945; **4**: 602.

33. Department of Health and Social Security. *Report on Confidential Enquiries into Maternal Deaths in England & Wales, 1979–1981*. London: HMSO, 1986,

34. Fisher, K.A., Luber, A., Spargo, B.H. and Lindheimer, M.D. Hypertension in pregnancy: Clinical-pathological correlations and remote prognosis. *Medicine* 1981; **60**: 267.

35. Matthews, D.D. A randomised control trial of bed rest and sedation of normal activity and non-sedation in the management of non-albuminuric hypertension in pregnancy. *J. Obstet., Gynaecol.* 1977; **84**: 108.

36. Walker, J.J. The case of early recognition and intervention in pregnancy-induced hypertension. In: Sharp, F. and Symonds, E.M. eds. *Hypertension in Pregnancy. Proceedings of the Sixteenth Study Group of the Royal College of Obstetricians and Gynaecologists, July, 1986*, Vol. 7. London: Royal College of Obstetricians and Gynaecologists, 1987, p. 289.

37. Wallenburg, H.C.S., Dekker, G.A., Makovitz, J.W. and Rotmans, P. Low dose aspirin prevents pregnancy induced hypertension and pre-eclampsia in angiotensin sensitive primigravidae. *Lancet* 1986; **i**: 1.

38. Beaufils, M., Uzan, S., Donsimoni, R. and Colau, J.C. Prevention of pre-eclampsia by early anti-platelet therapy. *Lancet* 1985; **i**: 840.

39. MacGillivray, I., Hytten, F.E., Taggart, N. and Buchanan, T.J. The effects of a sodium diuretic on total exchangeable sodium and total body water in pre-eclamptic toxaemia. *J. Obstet. Gynaecol. Br. Cmwlth* 1962; **69**: 548.

40. Redman, C.W.G., Beilin, L.J., Bonnar, J. and Ounsted, M. Fetal outcome in trial of antihypertensive treatment in pregnancy. *Lancet* 1976; **ii**: 753.

41. Lamming, G.D. and Symonds, E.M. Use of labetalol methyldopa in pregnancy induced hypertension. *Br. J. Clin. Pharmacol.* 1979; **8**: 217S.

42. Gallery, E.D.M., Ross, M.R. and Gyory, A.Z. Antihypertensive treatment in pregnancy: analysis of different responses to oxprenolol and methyldopa. *Br. Med. J.* 1985; **291**: 563.

43. Rubin, P.C., Clark, D.M., Sumner, D.J., Steedman, D., Low, R.A. and Reid, J.L. Placebo controlled trial of atenolol in treatment of pregnancy associated hypertension. *Lancet* 1983; **i**: 431.

44. Pritchard, J.A., Cunningham, F.G. and Pritchard, S.A. The Parkland Memorial Hospital protocol for treatment of eclampsia: Evaluation of 245 cases. *Am. J. Obstet. Gynecol.* 1984; **148**: 951.

45. Cree, J.E., Meyar, J. and Hailey, D.M. Diazepam in labour: its metabolism and effect on the clinical condition and thermogenesis of the newborn. *Br. Med. J.* 1973; **4**: 251.

46. Darfour, S.N. and Oduro, K.A. Clinical trial of heminevrin in the treatment of eclampsia. In: Lister, U.M., Dada, T.O. and Frisch, E.T., eds. *Heminevrin Symposium on Convulsive Disorders*. Sweden: A. B. Astra, 1972, p. 99.

47. Walters, B.N.J. and Redman, C.W.G. Treatment of severe pregnancy-associated hypertension with the calcium antagonist nifedipine. *Br. J. Obstet. Gynaecol.* 1984; **91**: 330.

Chapter 60

Systemic Diseases and the Heart

Leonard M. Shapiro

INTRODUCTION

The heart may be involved by a variety of inherited or acquired systemic conditions. There is often marked variability of expression of these diseases: some patients have severe cardiovascular manifestations and few or no systemic manifestations whereas others have severe systemic manifestations and few or no cardiovascular manifestations. The majority of these conditions are disorders of the connective tissue (Marfan's syndrome, osteogenesis imperfecta and homocystinuria) or endocrine systems (thyroid disease, acromegaly and carcinoid disease); rarely, neurological and vascular disorders may also affect the heart.

INHERITED CONNECTIVE TISSUE DISEASE

These disorders may be identified by a known method of inheritance and characteristic abnormality of connective tissue disease. Except for Marfan's syndrome, these disorders are rare and there may be a variety of clinical expressions with the connective tissue of the great arteries, the cardiac valves, the skeleton and skin being involved. In any individual disease or patient, there may be a spectrum of involvement, for example, the characteristic pathological changes may be of minimal cardiological importance, such as mitral valve prolapse or mild aortic root dilatation, or cause severe disease, for example severe aortic and mitral regurgitation, aortic dissection and aneurysm.[1]

MARFAN'S SYNDROME

Marfan's syndrome is named after a Parisian paediatrician who published the first description of the skeletal and ocular manifestations in 1896.[2] The work of Pyeritz and McKusick[3] resulted in a standardized description of the condition and its diagnostic criteria. According to their criteria, two or more clinical manifestations of Marfan's syndrome (see below) must be present to make the diagnosis reasonably certain, at present there is no single reliable test with which to make the diagnosis. In its typical form, Marfan's syndrome occurs in 4–6 per 100 000 of the population, but the *forme fruste* is probably more common.

Inheritance

Marfan's syndrome is usually transmitted as a simple Mendelian autosomal dominant trait with marked variability in clinical expression. In 80–90% of cases, one parent is involved; in the remainder, mutation occurs *de novo*. Mutation is more likely to occur with increasing paternal age.[1]

Pathology

The predominant pathological lesions in patients with Marfan's syndrome are fusiform dilatation or aneurysm of the ascending aorta (35%), aortic dissection (38%) and mitral regurgitation (22%).[3] Dilatation of the pulmonary artery the aortic annulus and the sinuses of Valsalva may also occur. The characteristic histological lesion (not seen in all patients) is cystic medial necrosis with degeneration of elastic elements in the connective tissue. The basic biochemical fault is in the mucopolysaccharide-rich ground substance. The histological appearance is of cystic vacuoles with increased collagen in the tunica media without an inflammatory response. Similar histological features may be observed in the aortic and mitral valves. Macroscopically, the mitral valve may be elongated with fenestration of the leaflets, ballooning and redundant cusps. The chordae tendineae may be thinned and elongated.[1]

Pathophysiology

The cardiovascular manifestations of Marfan's syndrome almost certainly reflect the response of abnormal connective tissue to prolonged haemodynamic stresses. At birth and in infancy, the musculoskeletal features may be prominent, but it is rare to detect the cardiovascular manifestation. With increasing age, dilatation of the proximal aorta leading to aortic regurgitation and dissection of the aorta may occur, both of which may lead to premature death.

Clinical features

Skeletal manifestations

The skeletal manifestations of Marfan's syndrome are probably the most common clinical features and one or more is found in almost all patients. The patients are frequently tall with unusually long arms. The arm span is greater than the subject's height and there is an abnormally low ratio of upper segment (crown to pubic symphisis) to lower segment. The fingers are long with long metacarpals (arachnodactyly). The joints of both upper and lower extremities are excessively mobile and this mobility gives rise to the thumb sign in which the thumb is visible and protrudes beyond the hand when clenched. Sternal deformities include pectus excavatum and pectus carinatum. The spine is frequently abnormal with kyphosis or scoliosis. In the mouth, the characteristic abnormality is a high-arched and narrow palate.

Ocular manifestations

The ocular manifestations include extreme myopia leading to retinal detachment, glaucoma and dislocation and subluxation lenses. The myopia is due to elongation of the globe and flattening of the cornea. Glaucoma and retinal detachment are common following trauma. Weakness of supporting tissues, including the suspensory ligaments of the lens, frequently leads to subluxation. This is best observed on slit-lamp examination.

Cardiovascular manifestations

Depending on the type of presentation, cardiovascular manifestations are present in 30–60% of patients with Marfan's syndrome. The presenting clinical features may be those of aortic dissection with chest pain or of cardiac failure from aortic and/or mitral regurgitation. Anginal-type pain may occur as the result of aortic dissection causing aortic regurgitation or involving the coronary ostia.

There are often loud murmurs, reflecting valvular regurgitation due to stretching, or even rupture, of the valve leaflets. The classic sign of mitral valve prolapse may be present, and infective endocarditis may occur.

DIAGNOSIS

A clinical diagnosis is made when two or more features of Marfan's syndrome are present, although some physicians feel that the presence of an extreme degree of aortic root dilatation is a manifestation of Marfan's syndrome. Echocardiography is of great value in studying patients with Marfan's syndrome. It enables serial evaluation of the size of the aortic root. This is particularly important because some authorities suggest that when the aortic root reaches 6 cm in diameter, aortic root replacement should be undertaken (Fig. 60.1).[6] Echocardiography may also demonstrate mitral valve prolapse and can often show a dissection flap. Supravalvular aortography will demonstrate the typical fusiform dilatation of the ascending aorta and associated aortic regurgitation (Fig. 60.2). Computerized tomography may also help to delineate the aortic lesion (Fig. 60.3).[7] Mitral annular calcification may occur at any early age in patients with Marfan's syndrome.

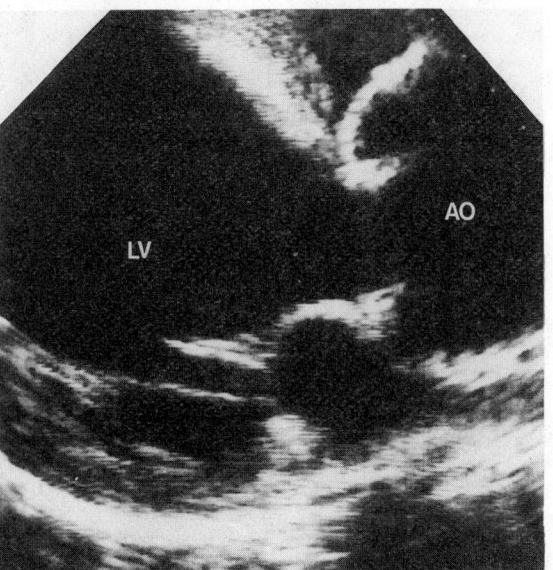

Fig. 60.1. Cross-sectional echocardiogram in a parasternal long-axis view showing a dilated aortic root (AO) in Marfan's syndrome. This patient had moderate-to-severe aortic regurgitation and the left ventricle (LV) is moderately dilated.

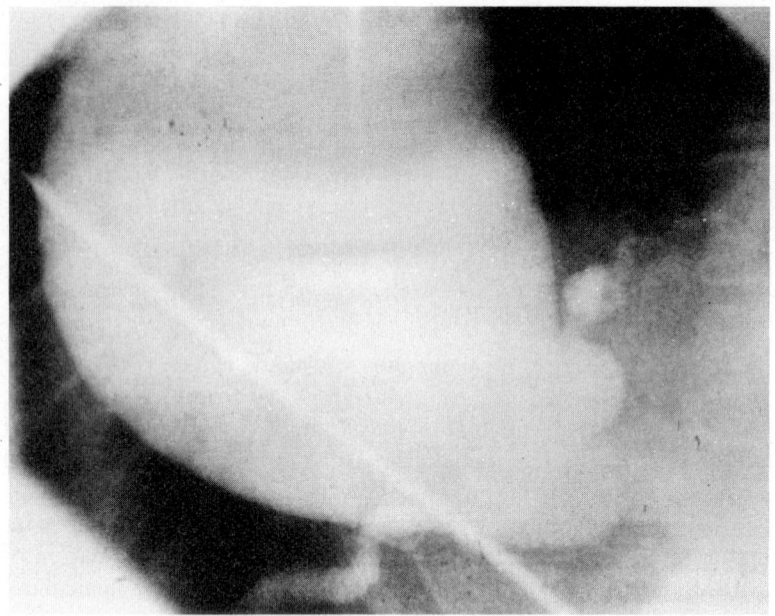

Fig. 60.2. Supraventricular aortogram showing gross dilatation of the ascending aorta in Marfan's syndrome (left anterior oblique projection).

TREATMENT

The treatment of Marfan's syndrome is hampered by the ill-defined nature of the biochemical lesion, and the underlying connective tissue defect influences surgical repair. Patients with cardiac manifestations of Marfan's syndrome have a poor prognosis, 32 years being the average age of death.[8]

Owing to the constant repetitive nature of the haemodynamic stresses on the aorta, it has been suggested that propranolol should be used in patients who manifest the early signs of aortic dilatation.[9] Although this suggestion is attractive, there is currently no conclusive evidence of its efficacy. Although surgical repair of the aortic and mitral valves has been undertaken, it is not without

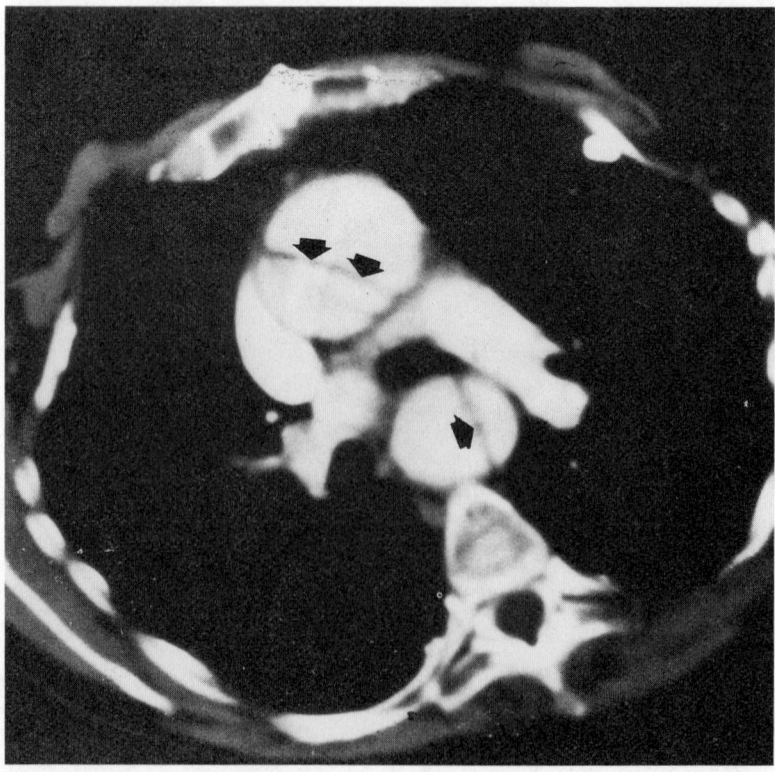

Fig. 60.3. Computerized tomogram through the thorax showing a dissection flap (arrows) in a dilated ascending aorta in a patient with Marfan's syndrome. The intimal tear can also be seen in the descending aorta (arrow). Computerized tomography with contrast enhancement is probably the method of choice for determining the presence of a dissection flap.

difficulty because of the underlying connective tissue defect. Valve replacement and graft reconstruction of the aorta are often followed by valve failure or dislodgement. The usual approach is to undertake replacement of the aneurysmal ascending aorta with a homograft or composite graft containing a prosthetic or xenograft aortic valve. The results of this operation are good.[6] Recurrent dissection and valvular incompetence, together with progressive dilatation of the remaining native aorta, may lead to late complications. It has been advocated that prophylactic surgery in patients with progressive dilatation of the aorta should be undertaken.

EHLERS-DANLOS SYNDROME

The term Ehlers-Danlos syndrome term is applied to a group of diseases that have the clinical features of abnormally extensile and fragile skin, which heals poorly and bruises easily, and hyperextensibility of the joints due to lax ligaments. (Joint mobility is usually grossly abnormal and there may be other musculoskeletal deformities.) Many forms have the additional vascular features of abnormal or prolonged bleeding and rupture of large blood vessels, as well as ocular and spinal manifestations. Each disorder is extremely rare and usually inherited by a well-defined dominant or recessive trait.

The cardiac features are similar to those of Marfan's syndrome, with cystic medial necrosis leading to aortic root dilatation and aortic dissection. Spontaneous rupture and dissection of other large arteries has also been seen.[10] Such patients may die from exsanguination. Vascular rupture may occur with minimal trauma especially secondary to arterial catheterization. Floppy mitral valve and abnormal atrioventricular conduction also occur.[11]

There is no specific treatment for this disease and the aim of treatment is to palliate symptoms.

OSTEOGENESIS IMPERFECTA

This is a group of inherited diseases of the connective tissue which have the common feature of excessive fragility of bone. There are several extra-skeletal manifestations, particularly in the eyes, teeth and heart. There is a variety of forms, but only patients with osteogenesis imperfecta tarda survive to an age at which cardiac disease becomes manifest. In the heart, the pathological features are similar to those in Marfan's syndrome, and cystic medial necrosis may be seen.[12] The disease is inherited as either an autosomal recessive or a dominant gene and has approximately the same incidence as that of haemophilia. In the mild form, which is dominantly inherited, fractures occur on mild trauma. The sclera are characteristically blue and there may be an arcus juvenalis. Dentogenesis imperfecta causes early erosion of deciduous dentition and abnormal staining of the permanent dentition. Osteoporosis is a consistent feature. Aortic regurgitation and mitral valve prolapse and regurgitation are the commonest cardiovascular manifestations. Valve replacement may be performed but there is no specific treatment for the underlying condition and the aim of therapy is to palliate symptoms.[13]

HOMOCYSTINURIA

Homocystinuria is a rare disease with neurological, ocular, skeletal and vascular manifestations which may be similar to those in Marfan's syndrome. The disease is inherited as an autosomal recessive. The biochemical abnormality is a deficiency of cystathionine synthase which causes homocysteine to accumulate leading to excretion of homocysteine in the urine. Homocysteine, which appears to act as a lathyrogen *in vivo*, leads to progressive skeletal deformity. Classic cases have the skeletal manifestations of Marfan's syndrome: often tall with arachnodactyly, a high-arched palate, kyphoscoliosis, pectus excavatum, abnormally lax ligaments and poor muscle development with little subcutaneous fat. There is generalized osteoporosis in contrast to the normal bone structure seen in subjects with Marfan's syndrome. Dislocation of the lens due to weakening of the suspensory ligament occurs predominantly downwards and may lead to glaucoma and cataracts. Myopia, optic atrophy and retinal detachment are often present. Multiple venous and arterial thromboses and emboli may occur; they may be the presenting feature in such patients.[1,14]

The cardiovascular manifestations of homocystinuria are similar to those of Marfan's syndrome; aortic root disease is the commonest manifestation.

As homocysteine gives a positive reaction with cyanide nitroprusside, this can be used to screen subjects for homocystinuria. For a more detailed analysis of urinary amino acids, electrophoretic methods may be used. Dietary restriction of methionine with cystine supplementation and pyridoxamine may be of some help in treatment. The patients who are responsive to pyridoxamine are usually less severely affected by the condition.

HURLER'S SYNDROME

Hurler's syndrome is a severe and typical form of the group of diseases called mucopolysaccharidosis. The enzyme defect is inherited as a recessive trait and gives rise to an accumulation of heparin and dermatan sulphate in the tissues which leads to many clinical abnormalities. The patients have a characteristic appearance with short stature, a thick and short neck and a lumbar gibbus. The abdomen is protruberant with hepatosplenomegaly. The facial features are coarse with a wide bridge to the nose and a large open mouth and tongue. The eyes are prominent and there may be corneal clouding. Deafness is not uncommon. The skull is enlarged. The hands are broad and trident-shaped. The cardiovascular manifestations are striking: thickening of the valves with fibrous nodules along the closure line.[15,16] Valve thickening is due to the presence of classic Hurler cells with granular inclusions and an increase in the extracellular connective tissue matrix. The chordae tendineae are thickened.

The heart is enlarged on cardiac examination and on chest radiography. The electrocardiogram shows left atrial and ventricular hypertrophy. Ventricular hypertrophy with impaired contraction may be demonstrated echocardiographically. Mitral regurgitation, aortic stenosis and regurgitation may all be observed. Currently, there is no specific management for this condition. Cardiac failure and ischaemic heart disease are the most common cardiac features in Hurler's syndrome; the majority of deaths are due to these causes.

ENDOCRINE DISEASE

DIABETES MELLITUS

Diabetes mellitus is a common condition and may affect up to 2% of the Western population. Premature death in diabetes mellitus is largely due to cardiac disease.[1] The majority of these deaths are from accelerated atherosclerosis of the coronary arteries, which is the leading cause of mortality in adult diabetics. Coronary artery disease causes more than three times the number of deaths in diabetics when compared with non-diabetic populations.[18] However, congestive cardiac failure and autonomic neuropathy are also clinically important, but their exact contribution is not known.[19,20] The mortality statistics compiled by the Joslin Clinic, documented in subsequent editions of Joslin's book 1960–85, indicate that considerable changes in the mortality have occurred since the pre-insulin period.[21] Since 1922, mortality from coma, gangrene and infection has fallen sharply whereas mortality due to vascular causes has risen proportionately.[21] By 1956, over half the deaths in the diabetic population of Massachusetts were due to cardiac causes. During this period, the diabetic population had changed to comprise predominantly older, non-insulin-requiring patients who are particularly prone to vascular causes of death. In 1971, Kessler compared the mortality of 21 447 diabetics at the Joslin Clinic with the general Massachusetts population[22] showing that there had been little or no improvement in the survival of diabetic patients (especially those over the age of 30 years) in the past three decades. The standard mortality ratio from coronary artery disease was 1.53 for men and 2.2 for women. When coronary artery disease is eliminated as a cause of death in this population, the mortality reverts to that of the general population.

The effects of hyperglycaemia alone, without frank diabetes, were considered in the Whitehall study in which 18 403 male civil servants aged 40–59 years were followed for 5 years. The degree of glucose intolerance from a 50-g oral glucose tolerance test was related to cardiovascular mortality and morbidity. Any subjects who had 2-h blood glucose greater than 5.9 mmol/l showed a doubling of coronary artery disease mortality independent of age, blood pressure[23] and other risk factors.[24]

In epidemiological studies, several factors that confer an additional risk of coronary artery disease have been identified (see Chapter 42), including age, sex, serum cholesterol, blood pressure and smoking habit. Diabetes and, in particular, hyperglycaemia can be considered as independent risk factors for coronary heart disease. Other abnormalities, such as hyperinsulinaemia, hypercholesterolaemia, hypertriglyceridaemia and abnormal blood coagulation, which are frequently present, may also be important in the development of premature coronary artery disease in diabetic subjects.

For many years, congestive cardiac failure has been reported in diabetics at autopsy; it may occur in up to 50% of such patients.[25] The natural history of congestive cardiac failure was reported for 5209 persons living in Framingham, Massachusetts.[19] After 18 and 20 years' follow-up, diabetic males were found to have a twofold and diabetic females a fivefold increase in congestive cardiac failure when compared with those of non-diabetic men and women, respectively. This excess risk was still evident after excluding other risk factors for atherosclerosis and clinically obvious coronary artery disease.

Autonomic neuropathy may be demonstrated in diabetic patients. It is frequently associated with somatic peripheral neuropathy and presumably has a metabolic origin. Patients who have diabetic autonomic neuropathy with cardiac involvement have a substantially increased risk of sudden cardiac death.[20,26]

Asymptomatic coronary artery disease is common in diabetic subjects and may be found in 10–50% of study populations depending on the method of investigation. In diabetics, pain is a less frequent accompaniment of myocardial infarction than in non-diabetic populations. Retrospective studies[27,28] show that more than 20% of myocardial infarctions are silent and only discovered by routine electrocardiographic testing. Myocardial infarction in diabetics carries a substantially greater mortality than in non-diabetics with an increased risk of between 1.5 and 5. This increased risk is especially prominent in patients who are young, female, hypertensive or obese. Congestive cardiac failure and cardiogenic shock due to ischaemic heart disease are substantially more common in diabetics.[29]

Pathology

The atherosclerotic lesion in diabetes mellitus is histologically no different to that in non-diabetic populations. However, atherosclerosis is more extensive,[30] left main stem lesions are frequent and disease occurs at an earlier age. During the twentieth century, the increase in incidence of coronary atherosclerosis in diabetic subjects has paralleled that in non-diabetic populations and there is a considerable geographical variation in its expression.[31]

Investigation of the coronary artery microvasculature and myocardium is hampered by the lack of a suitable method for studying such structures in life, especially as coronary small vessels cannot be imaged on the X-ray equipment currently available. At autopsy, the hearts of diabetics have more severe hyalinization, increased accumulation of PAS-positive material and greater calcification in intramural coronary arteries than those of non-diabetic hearts and these changes are closely related to the presence of nephropathy, particularly nodular glomerulosclerosis[32,33] In diabetic patients with diabetic nephropathy, the myocardium is fibrotic

and hypertrophied. Small intramural coronary arteries have subintimal and medial thickening due to the accumulation of PAS-positive material. There is an increase in perivascular and interstitial fibrosis and in linear scars.[34] Similar findings have been seen at autopsy of diabetic patients who died from heart failure.[35] Interstitial fibrosis, however, is not pathognomonic of diabetes mellitus and it may be found in a variety of other conditions. Hypertension has an important role in the development of cardiac failure in diabetic patients and it accelerates the development of myocardial fibrosis and scarring.[36] Thickening of the capillary basement membrane is widely accepted as an ultrastructural 'hallmark' of diabetic micro-angiopathy, and it has been demonstrated in diabetics undergoing coronary artery bypass grafting.[37]

The abnormalities that occur in the coronary microcirculation of diabetic patients have been elegantly demonstrated by injecting silicone rubber into the coronary arteries at autopsy.[38] In normal subjects, the coronary arterial system tapers smoothly eventually dividing into numerous capillary loops and arcades. In diabetic subjects, localized saccular aneurysm of the arterioles and capillary limbs are found which are similar to those found in the retina. These occur in any layer of the ventricular myocardium, and are not particularly associated with areas of myocardial fibrosis and degeneration.

Pathogenesis

The mechanisms of the development of atherosclerosis are discussed in Chapter 45. They apply to both diabetic and non-diabetic subjects.

There is substantial clinical and pathological evidence of impaired left ventricular function in diabetic patients, which is most conspicuous in those with longstanding insulin-dependent diabetes who have microvascular complications, especially proliferative retinopathy and nephropathy.[39,40] Owing to the strong association with clinical micro-angiopathy, it is tempting to suggest a causal relationship. The pathological demonstration of micro-angiopathic changes in small coronary arteries, endothelial proliferation with formation of papillary projections and bridges, and eventual occlusion of arterioles suggests that the microvascular changes are important and may lead or be related to the perivascular and diffuse interstitial fibrosis. These pathological features may be comparable with those seen in the diabetic kidney and retina. Capillary basement membrane thickening may also produce ischaemia by separating the myocardium from its blood supply. Metabolic disturbances such as ketone body metabolism, abnormal calcium uptake by the cytoplasmic reticulum and depressed actomycin ATPase may also damage the myocardium.[41]

Clinical features

There are no specific clinical features of heart disease in patients with diabetes mellitus irrespective of whether they have coronary disease, myocardial infarction or congestive cardiac failure, although the presence of co-existing large and small vessel disease elsewhere is frequently evident. The heart is also often involved as a part of a somatic autonomic neuropathy; other important features are postural hypotension, bladder dysfunction, diarrhoea and impotence.

Investigations

Diabetic subjects presenting with heart disease should be investigated according to standard cardiological practice. The results of exercise testing and coronary arteriography have the same implications in a diabetic as in a non-diabetic patient. Non-invasive testing of diabetics has been performed on many occasions to determine the presence of asymptomatic heart disease, which has been found to be common. In several studies, it has been shown that there are so called 'pre-clinical' abnormalities of function of the left ventricle in diabetics.[39,42] These appear to be more prominent in patients who have proliferative retinopathy and nephropathy.

In general, echocardiographic studies have revealed that the left ventricle is of normal size and has normal systolic contraction. Digitized M-mode echocardiography can be used to study left ventricular diastolic properties: measurement may be made of peak rate of left ventricular filling (as cavity dimension increase) and thinning of the posterior wall. The isovolumic relaxation period can be measured from the phonocardiogram and M-mode echocardiogram of the mitral valve. The peak rate of left ventricular filling and wall thinning are generally normal in diabetics who do not have micro-angiopathic complications and patients with coronary artery disease.[40,43,44] In diabetics who have background retinopathy or mild proteinuria, isovolumic relaxation is prolonged; diabetics with

proliferative retinopathy or nephropathy show, in addition, marked reduction in the peak rate of wall thinning and left ventricular filling. In a study of 628 diabetic subjects using resting and exercise electrocardiography and echocardiography, only 25% of patients were found to have no clinical evidence of cardiac disease; heart failure was present in 2%, hypertension in 27% and coronary artery disease in 17%. Only 3% of these patients had marked abnormalities of relaxation and filling in the absence of other evidence of heart disease; most of the subjects were insulin-dependent diabetics with proliferative retinopathy or nephropathy. Therefore, heart disease is common in a diabetic population and usually due to hypertension and coronary artery disease; much less frequently, other functional abnormalities of the left ventricle may be detected.[44]

Coronary artery disease is the major non-renal cause of mortality and morbidity in diabetic patients who have undergone renal transplantation. In patients with diabetic nephropathy, angiographic coronary artery disease may frequently be observed, but an elevated left ventricular end-diastolic pressure or reduced ejection fraction may occur in the absence of coronary stenosis.[45,46]

The diagnosis of diabetic autonomic neuropathy is best made by studying beat-to-beat heart-rate response during the Valsalva manoeuvre, deep breathing and standing and the blood pressure response to sustain handgrip and standing.[26]

Natural history

After suffering a myocardial infarction, diabetic patients have an impaired prognosis. The presence of autonomic neuropathy carries a 2.5-year mortality of 50% compared with that of 15% in diabetics without abnormal tests. Some of these deaths could be attributed to renal failure, but a substantial proportion of subjects died suddenly and unexpectedly the reasons for which are not known.[20,26] It has been known for many years that diabetics with microangiography have impaired long term prognosis. In a 3-year follow-up study in which diabetics who had normal systolic and diastolic left ventricular function were compared with those diabetics who had marked abnormalities of diastolic function, it was found that the latter group had a significantly higher mortality; 3% of those with slow filling and thinning died from heart failure compared with only 2 deaths in the normal function group.[44]

Treatment

Medically, the impact of diabetes mellitus upon the heart may be modified by:

1 the control of risk factors for coronary artery disease: dietary reduction in fat intake, control of hypertension and vigorous avoidance of cigarette smoking;
2 and, possibly, improved diabetic control; the use of antiplatelet agents may influence the deterioration of left ventricular function.

Although diabetic patients with exertional ischaemia often have extensive coronary artery disease,[47] and the early and late mortality rates of coronary artery bypass grafting in such patients are high, this procedure should not be withheld because of the presence of diabetes alone.

THYROID DISEASE

The thyroid gland secretes two biologically active hormones—thyroxine and tri-iodothyronine. The action of these hormones at a cellular level is probably upon the nucleus via the combination of hormone and nuclear protein. The primary effect of this binding is an alteration in protein synthesis. Thyroid hormones probably increase the activity of sodium/potassium ATPase and the increased ATP hydrolysis augments mitchondrial oxygen consumption. Via this mechanism, thyroid hormone has a direct action upon the heart. Experimentally, thyroid hormones have been found to increase heart rate and to augment myocardial contractility.[48] Patients with clinically obvious thyroid disease may present with palpitations and atrial fibrillation, and atrial fibrillation may be the only finding in some elderly patients with thyrotoxicosis.[49,50] Cardiac failure may occur in both hyper- and hypothyroidism.[51]

HYPERTHYROIDISM

Hyperthyroidism is a common condition which occurs much more frequently in women. Oversecretion of thyroid hormone may be due to Grave's disease, in which circulating IgG auto-antibody binds to the thyrotrophin receptor, toxic multinodular goitre or a toxic solitary adenoma.

Clinical features

The clinical features of hyperthyroidism are usually few, but patients may present with fatigue, hyperactivity, insomnia, heat intolerance, palpitations and dyspnoea. There may be an increased appetite with weight loss, diarrhoea, muscle weakness and wasting, tremor and emotional instability. On examination, there may be an increased heart rate, a moist warm skin, systolic hypertension, lid lag and lid retraction, and brisk reflexes. A goitre is often palpable and patients with Grave's disease may have exophthalmus. There may be an active cardiac impulse with loud first and second heart sounds. A third sound is frequently heard. The incidence of mitral valve prolapse is increased in patients with hyperthyroidism.

Investigations

Electrocardiography frequently shows sinus tachycardia with rates up to 130 beats/min. Approximately one-quarter of patients have persistent or paroxysmal atrial fibrillation. Atrial fibrillation is frequently present in elderly patients with hyperthyroidism.[49] It is always worthwhile excluding thyrotoxicosis in patients developing atrial fibrillation for no apparent reason even if there are no clinical features to suggest its presence. If the routine measurements of thyroxine are normal, levels of tri-iodothyronine may reveal the much rarer 'T3-toxicosis'. The TRH test will sometimes reveal thyrotoxicosis which is not apparent from an assay of the blood levels of the thyroid hormones. The chest X-ray shows cardiac enlargement and there may be the accompanying features of cardiac failure. Echocardiography usually shows a hyperdynamic left ventricle with mild left ventricular hypertrophy with no increase in cavity size.[52] Less frequently, there will be dilatation of the left ventricular cavity and left atrial enlargment.

Treatment

Many of the cardiovascular symptoms of thyrotoxicosis are related to increased beta-adrenergic receptor activity. Treatment with beta-adrenergic blocking agents immediately improves the tachycardia, palpitations, tremor, restlessness, muscle weakness and heat intolerance. However, treatment of hyperthyroidism in the long term requires anti-thyroid drugs (e.g. carbimazole), surgery or radioactive iodine. Patients with atrial fibrillation probably do not need cardioversion or anticoagulation initially because the risk of atrial embolization is low and patients often revert to sinus rhythm spontaneously.

Those who do not revert spontaneously should undergo cardioversion once they are euthyriod.

HYPOTHYROIDISM

Destruction of the thyroid gland by inflammatory processes, usually of auto-immune origin, results in a reduced secretion of thyroid hormones. This condition is more common in women and the incidence increases with age until about 60 years of age.

Clinical features

Cold intolerance, dryness of skin, weakness, personality changes and impairment of memory are common. Shortness of breath, heart failure and occasionally palpitations may be prominent. There may be facial puffiness and myxoedema of the lower extremities. Patients may have a yellow hue to their skin due to decreased conversion of carotene into vitamin A. The heart may be pale, flabby and grossly dilated in myxoedema. A pericardial effusion is common. In longstanding severe myxoedema, there is cardiac enlargement, marked bradycardia, weak arterial pulses and hypotension, and distant heart sounds may be heard;[53] however, in the early stages of the disease, such physical signs are seen only rarely.

Investigations

Cardiomegaly on the chest X-ray is a frequent accompaniment, and the enlargement of the heart is usually due to a pericardial effusion. The pericardial effusion can be readily diagnosed by echocardiography.[54] Left ventricular function is usually normal, but may appear to be sluggish on M-mode echocardiography. The electrocardiogram may show a sinus bradycardia with a long QT interval. The P-wave amplitude may be so markedly reduced that it may appear as if there is a nodal bradycardia. It is common to have low QRS voltages due to the pericardial effusion. The ST and T waves may be abnormal. Myxoedema often leads to significant elevation of the serum cholesterol, and the pericardial fluid often contains cholesterol crystals which may give a yellow or 'gold paint' appearance.

Treatment

In patients with myxoedema, treatment with thyroid hormone should be instituted cautiously. In patients who have additional ischaemic heart disease, even greater caution should be exercised over the use of thyroid hormone; it should be introduced more slowly and in lower doses because of the danger of provoking myocardial infarction or congestive heart failure.

As cardiac tamponade is not usually a feature of hypothyroidism, aspiration of the pericardial effusion is only rarely required, even if the effusion is very large; the effusion disappears with thyroid hormone replacement therapy, as do other cardiovascular features of the disease.

ACROMEGALY

Acromegaly is due to an increased secretion of growth hormone from a pituitary adenoma which leads to overgrowth of the skeleton and soft tissues. It is a rare disorder, occurring in only 40 per million of the general population in England and Wales. Excess secretion of growth hormone in the adult leads to bone growth, proliferation of soft tissue and enlargement of the viscera. Most of the affected individuals present with disturbance of the visual field, carpal tunnel syndrome and headaches. Such subjects, particularly the males, have a significantly higher mortality from cardiovascular and cerebrovascular diseases. The heart becomes enlarged. Cardiomegaly was first described in acromegalic patients in 1938[55] and since then it has become apparent that an excess of growth hormone leads to left ventricular hypertrophy. However, the cardiac hypertrophy associated with acromegaly is often of secondary importance to the accelerated atherosclerosis, diabetes mellitus and hypertension that also occur.[56,57]

Clinical features

The clinical manifestations of acromegaly are legion. The classic physical findings are of enlarged hands and feet, macroglossia, displacement of the teeth, coarse facial features and general overgrowth of soft tissues. More specific findings such as carpal tunnel syndrome may also occur. Acromegaly occasionally presents with the cardiovascular manifestations alone, particularly in older patients. Presentation with exertional dyspnoea is not uncommon and may be related to either the heart failure or to severe kyphoscoliosis. Angina pectoris due to the associated coronary atherosclerosis may also be a presenting feature. Systemic hypertension is present in at least 25% of patients with acromegaly, and although only 15–20% of patients with acromegaly have frank diabetes mellitus at least 50% have subclinical glucose intolerance.

Diagnosis

The diagnosis of acromegaly is usually obvious on clinical grounds, but the finding of an elevated fasting serum growth hormone level is pathognomonic especially when it is not suppressed by a glucose load.

The electrocardiogram in acromegaly is non-specific, usually showing the pattern of left ventricular hypertrophy with strain. The echocardiogram reveals left ventricular hypertrophy in up to 90% of patients.[58,59] This could be due to hypertension or associated 'growth hormone cardiomyopathy'. Left ventricular function is usually normal, but, at a later stage, it may deteriorate leading to a reduced ejection fraction. Asymmetrical septal hypertrophy has been reported but it is not common and may simply reflect the septal hypertrophy that occurs in hypertension. There is little or no relationship between the degree of growth hormone excess and the severity of the heart disease.

Natural history

The natural history of acromegaly is variable. Some patients may have a normal lifespan, but others, particularly those with severe heart disease, may die early from myocardial infarction or chronic congestive cardiac failure.

Treatment

The cardiovascular manifestations of acromegaly usually respond to normal therapeutic manoeuvres. Reduction of growth hormone levels to normal by tumour destruction or drug therapy usually has little effect on established cardiac disease.

PHAEOCHROMOCYTOMA

A phaeochromocytoma is a catecholamine-secreting tumour derived from chromaffin cells which were derived from the primitive neural crest cells of the embryo. Chromaffin cells largely arise from the adrenal medulla, but a small percentage arise from extra-adrenal sites, including the abdominal para-aortic sympathetic ganglia, the sympathetic ganglia of the urinary bladder, the thoracic mediastinal ganglia and the bifurcation of the common carotid

artery. Phaeochromocytomas have an extensive blood supply and are usually benign; only 10% are malignant.

The incidence of phaeochromocytoma is not known, but it probably occurs in < 0.1% of patients with hypertension. However, only half of the patients with this condition present with sustained hypertension; in the remainder, the hypertension is paroxysmal.[60]

Most phaeochromocytomas occur sporadically, but in less than 5% of patients there may be a familial association. This may occur as part of the pleuriglandular (multiple endocrine adenoma) syndrome in which there may be an association of phaeochromocytoma, medullary carcinoma of the thyroid, parathyroid adenoma and often neurofibroma of the von Recklinghausen type.

Clinical features

Phaeochromocytoma can be associated with a variety of signs and symptoms; hypertension, either sustained or paroxysmal, is the most important. Typical paroxysms that occur in phaeochromocytoma include hypertension, which may be very severe, headaches, excessive sweating, orthostatic hypotension, flushing or pallor, nausea and abdominal discomfort. A feeling of extreme anxiety is also common during paroxysms. There may be a marked tachycardia or, rarely, reflex bradycardia (secondary to sudden and very severe elevation of blood pressure). Occasionally, a shock-like state may occur during a paroxysm. Acute myocardial infarction, left ventricular failure or cerebral haemorrhage can occur during a paroxysm.

The prolonged and excess cardiac stimulation may result in a 'catecholamine myocarditis' with heart failure.[61] More than half of the patients may have sustained hypertension. There may be a hypermetabolic state with weight loss. Glycosuria is common, but occasionally hypoglycaemia occurs. Paroxysms may be precipitated by certain drugs, in particular, tricyclic antidepressants. Occasionally, bowel movements or palpitation of the abdomen or near the site of a tumour may precipitate paroxysms.

The electrocardiogram is usually abnormal showing sinus tachycardia and left ventricular hypertrophy. T-Wave inversion, which may be widespread, or marked ST-segment depression may be demonstrated.[62] The echocardiogram in phaeochromocytoma usually shows left ventricular hypertrophy with normal function, but occasionally there may be a dilated left ventricle and poor function representing 'catecholamine myocarditis'.

Diagnosis

The diagnosis of phaeochromocytoma is best made by establishing an increased level of urinary, blood or platelet catecholamine. The most widely used screening test is the measurement of vanilmandelic acid (VMA) in 24-h urine samples; a negative result in a hypertensive patient carries a high probability that a phaeochromocytoma is not present. Plasma catecholamine and metanephrine and total catecholamine can also be measured.[63]

Once the diagnosis has been made, the site of the tumour has to be established prior to surgery. Intravenous urography with tomography will identify the tumour in 60–70% of cases. Aortography will demonstrate large vascular tumours, but selective arteriography or adrenal venography and selective caval sampling for catecholamine may be required for accurate delineation. Computerized tomographic scanning may identify tumours as small as 1 cm in diameter and, in particular, it can identify any extramedullary sites. As computerized tomography is able to identify tumours reliably, it has largely replaced invasive tests. Abdominal ultrasound can also be used to identify suprarenal tumours and detect sites of spread within the abdomen. If the phaeochromocytoma is malignant, functional tumour metastases may be localized by scintigraphic imaging with ^{131}I-meta-iodobenzilquardine (I-MIBG) which accumulates in tumour tissues.[64]

Management

Surgical resection of the phaeochromocytoma is usually curative. Certain anaesthetic agents need to be avoided, especially cyclopropane, ether, nitrous oxide and fentanyl as well as morphine and atropine, because all can provoke hyper- or hypotensive crises. Pre-operative alpha-adrenergic blockade for at least 1 week with phenoxybenzamine or prazosin may prevent a pressure crisis. Labetalol, which acts as a combined alpha- and beta-blocker, is also useful pre-operatively in patients in whom complete surgical removal of the tumour is not possible.

CARCINOID HEART DISEASE

In 1954, Thorssen et al. described a syndrome of malignant carcinoid with heart disease.[65] Right-sided valvular dysfunction, facial flushing, abdominal pain, diarrhoea and telangiectasia was observed in a patient with malignant carcinoid deposits in the small intestine which had metastasized to the liver. The vasomotor bronchial constrictor and cardiac manifestations are undoubtedly related to the circulating humoral substances secreted by the tumour. The hormone most likely to be involved is 5-hydroxytryptamine, but other substances including histamine and bradykinin may also be important.

Over half of the tumours arise initially in the appendix, the remainder occur in the large bowel. Although these tumours are present in the large bowel mucosa, they are not obstructive; they do not affect the heart because the humoral substances are metabolized in the liver. When they metastasize to the liver, there is direct stimulation of the heart by 5-hydroxytryptamine. Characteristically, the cardiac lesions are fibrous plaques on the tricuspid and pulmonary valves, which consist of smooth muscle cells embedded in a connective tissue stroma. The endothelium may also become thickened. These plaques may distort the valves and may lead to pulmonary stenosis and tricuspid regurgitation.[66,67] Involvement of a left-sided valve is much less common.

Clinical features

The most common features during an attack are wheezing and flushing. The flushing may be transient and erythematous or violaceous, or prolonged and affect the entire body. Diarrhoea is also common and is episodic and explosive. Peripheral oedema due to cardiac failure and hypoproteinaemia is commonly seen.

The liver is enlarged and irregular due to secondary tumour masses within it. The venous pressure is elevated and a prominent systolic wave can be observed. The murmurs of pulmonary stenosis and tricuspid regurgitation are the most frequently heard, but tricuspid stenosis and left-sided lesions should also be sought.

The electrocardiogram and chest X-ray are nonspecific; the electrocardiogram may show right bundle branch block and the chest X-ray right ventricular hypertrophy and the enlargement of the pulmonary trunk. Echocardiography may be very useful in determining the presence of right-sided valvular lesions. The tricuspid valve has a characteristic appearance with thickened, shortened and rigid leaflets which neither open nor close fully. The features of the pulmonary valve are similar to those of the tricuspid valve.[68] Liver metastases may be detected by ultrasound or computerized tomographic scanning.

In general, the prognosis for patients with carcinoid heart disease is poor; death occurs most commonly from heart failure. Patients with limited liver metastases alone may have prolonged survival, and replacement of the tricuspid or pulmonary valves may be required in severely symptomatic patients.

The symptoms in carcinoid syndrome may be controlled medically. Heart failure is treated conventionally. Intestinal motility can be reduced with codeine phosphate and diphenoxylate. Cyproheptadine is a specific sertonin antagonist and may help to control flushing and diarrhoea. Alpha-adrenergic blocking agents, such as phenoxybenzamine, may also be useful.[69]

REFERENCES

1. McKusick, V.A. *Heritable disorders of connective tissue*, 4th edn. St Louis: C.V. Mosby, 1972.
2. Marfan, A.B. Un cas de deformation congenitale des quatres membres, plus pronouncée aux extremities, caracterisée par l'allongement des os avec un certain degre d'amincussement. *Bull. Sox Clir. Paris* 1896; **13**: 220.
3. Pyreitz, R.E. and McKusick, V.A. Basic defects in the Marfan syndrome. *N. Engl. J. Med.* 1981; **305**: 1101.
6. Grott, V.L., Pyeritz, R.E., McGovern, G.J., Cameron, D.E. and McKusick, V.A. Surgical treatment of aneurysms of the ascending aorta in the Marfan syndrome. *N. Engl. J. Med.* 1986; **314**: 1070.
7. Donaldson, R.M., Olsen, E.G.J., Emanuel, R.W. and Ross, D.N. Management of cardiovascular complications in Marfan's syndrome. *Lancet* 1980; **ii**: 1178.
8. Murdoch, J.L., Walker, B.A., Halpern, B.I. *et al.* Life expectancy and causes of death in Marfan syndrome. *N. Engl. J. Med.* 1972; **286**: 804.
9. Pyertiz, R.E. Propranolol retards aortic root dilatation in Marfan's syndrome (Abstract). *Circulation* 1983; **68**: 365.
10. Madison, W.M., Bradley, E. and Castillo, A. Ehlers–Danlos syndrome with cardiac involvement. *Am. J. Cardiol.* 1963; **11**: 689.
11. Cupo, L.N., Pyeritz, R.E., Olson, J.L. *et al.* Ehlers–Danos syndrome with abnormal collagen fibrils, sinus of Valsalva aneurysms, myocardial infarction, panacinar emphysema and cerebral heterotopias. *Am. J. Med.* 1981; **72**: 1051.
12. Criscitello, M.G., Ronan, J.A., Bestermann, E.M. and Schoenwetter, W. Cardiovascular abnormalities in osteogenesis imperfecta. *Circulation* 1965; **31**: 255.
13. Wood, S.J., Thomas, J. and Braimbridge, M.V. Mitral valve disease and open heart surgery in osteogenesis imperfecta tarda. *Br. Heart J.* 1973; **25**: 103.
14. McCulley, KS. Vascular pathology of homocysteinuria. *Am. J. Pathol.* 1969; **56**: 111.
15. Krovetz, L.J., Lorincz, A.E. and Schiebler, G.L. Car-diovascular manifestations ot the Hurler syndrome. *Circulation* 1965; **31**: 132.
16. Brosius, F.C. III and Roberts, W.C. Coronary artery disease in the Hurler syndrome. *Am. J. Cardiol.* 1981; **47**: 649.
17. West, K.M. *Epidemiology of diabetes and its vascular lesions.* New York: Elsevier North-Holland, 1978.
18. Jarrett, R.J. and Keen, H. Hyperglycaemia and diabetes mellitus. *Lancet* 1976; **ii**: 1009–10.
19. Kannel, W.B. and McGee, D.L. Diabetes and cardiovascular disease. The Framingham Study. *JAMA* 1979; **291**: 2035–7.
20. Ewing, E.P., Campbell, I.W. and Clarke, B.F. The natural history of diabetic autonomic neuropathy. *Q. J. Med.* 1980; **49**: 95–108.
21. Joslin, E.P., Root, H.F., White, P. and Marble, A. *Treatment of diabetes mellitus,* 2nd edn. Philadelphia: Lea and Febiger, 1971.
22. Kessler, I.I. Mortality experience of diabetic patients. *Am. J. Med.* 1971; **51**: 715–8.
23. Fuller, J.H., McCartney, P. and Jarrett, R.J. Hyperglycaemia and Coronary Heart Disease: The Whitehall Study. *J. Chron. Dis.* 1979; **32**: 721–7.
24. Fuller, J.H., Shipley, M.J. and Rose, R. Coronary heart disease risk and impaired glucose tolerance: The Whitehall Study. *Lancet* 1980; **i**: 1373–6.
25. Stearns, S., Schlesinger, M.J. and Rudy, A. Incidence and clinical significance of coronary artery disease in diabetes mellitus. *Arch. Intern. Med.* 1947; **80**: 163–9.
26. Ewing, D.J. Cardiac autonomic neuropathy. In: ed. Jarrett, R.J. *Diabetes and Heart Disease.* Amsterdam: Elsevier, 1984.
27. Margolis, J.R., Kannel, W.B., Feinleib, W. *et al.* Clinical features of unrecognized myocardial infarction—silent and symptomatic. Eighteen year follow up. The Framingham Study. *Am. J. Cardiol.* 1973; **32**: 1–7.
28. Bradley, R.F., and Schonfeld, A. Diminished pain in diabetics with acute myocardial infarction. *Geriatrics* 1962; **17**: 322–6.
29. Dash, H., Johnson, R.A., Dinsmore, R.E. *et al.* Cardiomyopathic syndrome due to coronary artery disease: II Increased prevalence in patients with diabetes mellitus. A matched pair analysis. *Br. Heart J.* 1977; **39**: 740–7.
30. Crall, F.V. and Roberts, W.C. The extramural and intramural coronary arteries in juvenile diabetes mellitus. Analysis of nine necropsy patients 19 to 38 years with onset of diabetes before age 15 years. *Am. J. Med.* 1978; **64**: 221–30.
31. Roberson, W.B. and Strong, J.P. Atherosclerosis in persons with hypertension and diabetes mellitus. *Lab. Invest.* 1968; **18**: 538–43.
32. Ledet, T. Histological and histochemical changes in the coronary arteries of old diabetic patients. *Diabetologia* 1968; **4**: 268–72.
33. Ledet, T. Diabetic cardiomyopathy: Quantative histological studies of the heart from young juvenile diabetics. *Acta Pathol. Microbiol. Scand. (A)* 1976; **84**: 421–8.
34. Rubler, S., Dlugash, J., Vuceoglu, Y.Z. *et al.* New type of cardiomyopathy associated with diabetic glomerulosclerosis. *Am. J. Cardiol.* 1972; **30**: 595–9.
35. Regan, T.J., Lyons, M.M., Ahmed, S.S. *et al.* Evidence for cardiomyopathy in familial diabetes mellitus. *J. Clin. Invest.* 1977; **60**: 885–99.
36. Factor, S.M., Minase, T. and Sonnenblick, E.H. Clinical and morphological features of human hypertensive diabetic cardiomyopathy. *Am. Heart J.* 1980; **79**: 446–58.
37. Fischer, V.W., Barner, H.B. and Leskiw, L. Capillary basal laminar thickness in diabetic human myocardium. *Diabetes* 1979; **28**: 713–9.
38. Factor, S.M., Okum, E.M. and Minase, T. Capillary microaneurysms in the human diabetic heart. *N. Engl. J. Med.* 1980; **302**: 348–8.
39. Seneviratne, B.I.B. Diabetic cardiomyopathy. The pre-

clinical phase. *Br. Med. J.* 1977; **1**: 1444–6.

40. Sanderson, J.E., Brown, D.J., Rivellese, A. *et al.* Diabetic cardiomyopathy: An echocardiographic study of young diabetics. *Br. Med. J.* 1978; **1**: 404–7.

41. Taegtmeyer, H. and Passmore, J.M. Defective energy metabolism of the heart in diabetes. *Lancet* 1984; i: 13–40.

42. Shapiro, L.M., Leatherdale, B.A., Mackinnon, J. *et al.* Left ventricular function in diabetes mellitus: II Relation between clinical features and left ventricular function. *Br. Heart J.* 1981; **45**: 129–32.

43. Shapiro, L.M. Echocardiographic features of impaired left ventricular function in diabetes. *Br. Heart J.* 1982; **47**: 439–41.

44. Shapiro, L.M. A prospective study of heart disease in diabetes mellitus. *Q. J.Med.* 1984; **209**: 55–68.

45. Weinrauch, L., D'Elia, J.A., Healy, R.W. *et al.* Asymptomatic coronary artery disease. *Circulation* 1978; **58**: 1184–90.

46. D'Elia, J.A., Weinrauch, L. and Healy, R.W. Myocardial dysfunction without coronary artery disease in diabetic renal failure. *Am. J. Cardiol.* 1979; **43**: 193–9.

47. Dortimer, A.C., Shenoy, P.N. and Shiroft, R.A. Diffuse artery disease in diabetic patients. Fact or Fiction. *Circulation* 1978; **57**: 133.

48. Morkin, E., Fink, I.L. and Goldman, S. Biochemical and physiological effects of thyroid hormone on cardiac performance. *Prog. Cardiovasc. Dis.* 1983; **23**: 435.

49. Forfar, C. and Toft, A.D. Thyrotoxic atrial fibrillation: an under-diagnosed condition. *Br. Med. J.* 1982; **285**: 909–10.

50. Adlum, E.V., Kessler, R.K., Braitman, L.E. and Denenbery, B.S. Chronic thyroiditis and mitral valve disease. *Ann. Intern. Med.* 1985; **102**: 479–83.

51. Ikram, H. The nature and prognosis of thyrotoxic heart disease. *Q. J. Med.* 1985; **54**: 19–28.

52. Forfar, J.C., Muir, A.L., Sawer, S.A. and Toft, A.D. Abnormal left ventricular function in hypothyroidism. *N. Engl.J.*1982; **307**: 1165.

53. McBrian, D.J. and Hundle, W. Myxoedema and heart failure. *Lancet* 1963; i: 1065.

54. Kerber, R.E. and Sherman, B. Echocardiographic evaluation of pericardial effusion in myxoedema. *Circulation* 1975; **52**: 823.

55. Courville, C. and Mason, V.R. The heart in acromegaly. *Arch. Intern. Med.* 1938; **61**: 704–10.

56. Coggeshall, C. and Root, H.F. Acromegaly and diabetes mellitus. *Endocrinology* 1940; **1**: 26.

57. Souadjian, J.V. and Schirger, A. Hypertension in acromegaly. *Am. J. Med. Sci.* 1967; **254**: 629.

58. Mather, H.M., Boyd, M.J. and Jenkins, J.S. Heart size and function in acromegaly. *Br. Heart J.* 1979; **67**: 697.

59. Savage, D.D., Henry, W.L., Eastman, R.C., Borer, J.S. and Gorden, P. Echocardiographic assessment of cardiac anatomy and function in acromegalic patients. *Am. J. Med.* 1979; **67**: 823.

60. Ram, C.V.S. and Engleman, K. Pheochromocytoma—recognition and management. *Curr. Prob. Cardiol.* 1979; **IV**: 7–34.

61. Van Vliet, P.D., Burchell, H.B. and Titus, J.L. Myocarditis associated with pheochromocytoma. *N. Engl. J. Med.* 1966; **274**: 1102.

62. Cheng, T.O. and Bashour, T.T. Striking electrocardiographic changes with pheochromocytoma. *Chest* 1979; **76**: 600.

63. Zweifler, A.J. and Julius, S. Increased platelet catacholamine content in pheochromocytoma. A diagnostic test in patients with elevated plasma catacholamines. *N. Engl. J. Med.* 1982; **306**: 890.

64. Bravo, E.L. and Gifford, R.W. Pheochromatocytoma: diagnosis, localization and management. *N. Engl J. Med.* 1984; **311**: 1298–303.

65. Thorssen, A., Biorck, G., Bjorkman, G. and Waldenstrom, J. Malignant carcinoid, a clinical and pathological syndrome. *Am. Heart J.* 1954; **47**: 795.

66. Roberts, W.C. and Sjoerdsma, A. The cardiac disease associated with the carcinoid syndrome (carcinoid heart disease). *Am. J. Med.* 1964; **36**: 5–34.

67. Ross, E. and Roberts, W. The Carcinoid Syndrome: Comparison of 21 necropsy subjects with carcinoid heart disease to 15 necropsy subjects without carcinoid heart disease. *Am. J. Med.* 1985; **79**: 339–54.

68. Howard, R., Drobac, M., Rider, W., Keane, T., Finlayson, J., Silver, M., Wigle, E. and Rakowski, H. Carcinoid Heart Disease: Diagnosis by two dimensional echocardiography. *Circulation* 1982; **66**: 1059–65.

69. Roberts, L.J., Marney, S.R. and Oates, J.A. Blockade of the flush associated with metastatic gastric carcinoid by combine H1 and H2 receptor antagonists. *N. Engl. J. Med.* 1979; **300**: 236–8.

Chapter 61

Cardiovascular Manifestations of Collagen Vascular Disease

Ian R. Gray

There is a diverse group of diseases that affect many different systems of the body, particularly joints, skin and connective tissue, which often involve the cardiovascular system as well. They have no common aetiology, but in most of them there is inflammation or degeneration in certain of the smaller arteries. Some cardiac manifestations, like pericarditis and cardiomyopathy, may occur in almost any of these conditions, whereas others, such as the coronary arterial lesions of polyarteritis nodosa or Libman–Sacks endocarditis in lupus erythematosus, are characteristic of a particular disease. Although these diseases and their cardiac features are described separately, they are often less clearly defined than this would imply. The term 'overlap syndrome' and the broad category of 'collagen disease' are sometimes used to designate a clinical picture that has features of more than one of the conditions described in this chapter.

There are two ways in which the advice of the cardiologist is sought in cases of 'collagen disease'. More commonly, the disease has already been recognized and a cardiologist is consulted because symptoms or signs suggesting a cardiac complication have appeared. These cardiac manifestations are seldom florid and the application of appropriate forms of investigation, and their interpretation, is often necessary. Less frequently, a cardiac condition such as pericarditis, heart block or congestive heart failure is the first manifestation of the disease and it is the cardiologist who makes the diagnosis of a collagen disease.

ANKYLOSING SPONDYLITIS

Ankylosing spondylitis is a form of arthritis which mainly involves the spine and sacro-iliac joints. It affects young men and, less often, women. The cause is unknown but its occurrence has a significant association with the presence of the antigen HLA-B27. It runs a prolonged course and often is associated with iritis, and occasionally with characteristic cardiovascular lesions.

The particular form of heart disease that occurs in patients with ankylosing spondylitis affects the aortic valve and the wall of the aorta immediately above the valve.[1] The prevalence of clinically recognized aortic valve disease and aortitis is low, possibly only 1 or 2%.[2] It tends to be found when the disease has been active for many years, so that the incidence is likely to be greater than this when the spondylitis has run its course. There are inflammatory and degenerative changes in all layers of the wall of the aorta immediately above the aortic valve, with dilatation of the valve ring. Also, there is inflammation, fibrous thickening and scarring in the cusps of the aortic valve. These changes, with aortitis, dilatation of the valve ring and scarring of the cusps of the aortic valve, resemble the lesions of syphilitic aortitis and give rise in the same way to aortic regurgitation which may be severe. The inflammatory process occasionally spreads to the base of the anterior cusp of the mitral valve to cause mitral regurgitation.

The other characteristic cardiac manifestation of ankylosing spondylitis is heart block. This is caused by the extension of the inflammation and fibrosis from the aortic root into the muscular septum damaging the bundle of His and its branches. This may give rise to atrioventricular block as well as bundle branch block of all degrees. Among 54 patients with ankylosing spondylitis studied with ambulatory electrocardiography, three had first degree heart block and one had intermittent complete heart block.[3] A search for evidence of ankylosing spondylitis among patients requiring permanent pacing for complete heart block revealed 15 cases of spondylitis among 223 men with pacemakers (7 of the 15 had not previously been diagnosed).[4]

The two principal cardiac complications of ankylosing spondylitis, aortic regurgitation and heart block, often co-exist. Although they tend to occur in patients in whom the spondylitis is easily recognized, this is not always the case. Radiography of the sacro-iliac joints is a simple and reliable means of establishing whether ankylosing spondylitis is the cause of unexplained aortic regurgitation or heart block.

At post-mortem, there is often fibrous obliteration of the pericardial cavity, although clinical manifestations of pericarditis are rare. In a study of 24 patients with ankylosing spondylitis using echocardiography, there were 'abnormal pericardial echoes' in 10, suggesting that symptomless pericardial effusion might be quite common.[5] In another investigation, using M-mode and cross-sectional echocardiography, 30 patients with ankylosing spondylitis were studied, none of whom had clinical evidence of heart or lung disease. There were abnormalities of left ventricular behaviour during early diastole in 16 of them. Myocardium from 28 patients with ankylosing spondylitis, who had died and who did not have ischaemic or valve disease, was studied histologically. There was 'mild, diffuse increase in interstitial connective tissue in the myocardium' which the authors believe could explain their echocardiographic findings.[6] The significance of these findings in clinical or diagnostic terms is not known.

GIANT CELL ARTERITIS

Giant cell arteritis mainly affects the medium-sized arteries and occurs almost exclusively in the elderly. The lesions involve short segments of the arteries and there is cellular infiltration with giant cells, and often thrombosis locally.[7] When the temporal (and often intracranial and retinal) arteries are affected, headache is a prominent symptom and the condition is designated 'temporal arteritis'. When the muscular arteries of the limbs are particularly involved with pain, stiffness and weakness, the condition is called 'polymyalgia rheumatica'. The erythrocyte sedimentation rate is strikingly increased in giant cell arteritis. Symptoms of the condition usually respond quickly and completely to steroid therapy.

The large arteries such as the carotid or femoral vessels are said to be affected in about 10% of cases giving rise to ischaemic manifestations in their distribution.[8] There also may be medial necrosis in the wall of the aorta which can give rise to rupture or dissection of the aorta. Giant cell arteritis often co-exists with arteriosclerotic coronary heart disease, but coronary arteritis is rarely recognized as a cause of coronary occlusion. An autopsy report describes a patient dying of giant cell arteritis in whom characteristic arteritis was found in smaller coronary arteries in addition to atheroma in the main coronary vessels.[9]

POLYARTERITIS NODOSA

The pathological lesion in polyarteritis nodosa consists of necrosis, fibrinoid degeneration and hyalinization in the media of smaller arteries, with perivascular infiltration with mononuclear and polymorphonuclear cells. The lesions are widespread and their distribution is very variable. This explains the diversity of the clinical manifestations of polyarteritis. There usually are general symptoms and signs such as fever, leucocytosis and loss of weight. Proteinuria, hypertension and renal failure occur when the renal arteries are affected; abdominal pain, vomiting and diarrhoea, peripheral neuropathy, dyspnoea and chest pain are frequent symptoms associated with involvement elsewhere.

In a review of 66 patients with polyarteritis nodosa,[10] there was clinical evidence of heart disease in 78%. The commonest cardiovascular features were hypertension in 67% and congestive heart failure in 57%. Chest pain, heart murmurs and pericardial friction were frequent and the electrocardiogram was abnormal in the great majority of cases. At post-mortem, coronary arteritis was found in 62% of cases and myocardial infarction in 62%. The coronary arteritis was found in the main coronary arteries and in the smaller branches. Despite the high incidence of myocardial infarction at autopsy, it was rarely diagnosed clinically. Infarction, however, was believed to play an important role in the cardiac failure which so often occurred. Apart from the ischaemic injury and the frequent left ventricular hypertrophy, acute myocarditis was diagnosed in 2 patients. Pericarditis was a frequent finding at post-mortem; it was sometimes inflammatory in nature and sometimes caused by myocardial infarction or uraemia.

POLYMYOSITIS AND DERMATOMYOSITIS

Polymyositis is a rare disease of unknown cause. It is characterized by inflammatory and degenerative changes, and replacement fibrosis in striated muscle, affecting particularly proximal muscle groups. The condition may also involve the skin when it is designated dermatomyositis. Lesions similar to those in striated muscle can occur in the myocardium. Such inflammation, degeneration and fibrosis constitute a form of cardiomyopathy, manifestations of which may be prominent clinical features of the disease. Extensive replacement fibrosis of the myocardium has been found at autopsy which was responsible for congestive heart failure in life.[11] The fibrosis also may involve the sino-atrial node, and the bundle of His and its branches causing heart block which may require pacing.[12,13] Evidence of pericarditis has been found at autopsy in polymyositis[11] but it is rarely recognized in life.

REITER'S DISEASE

Reiter's disease comprises a triad of arthritis, urethritis and conjunctivitis; sometimes only two of the features are present in a case. The arthritis affects peripheral joints and is self-limited, but may recur over a period of years. Its cause is not known, but it usually affects young men, and often follows bacillary dysentery, non-specific diarrhoea or nongonococcal urethritis. Like ankylosing spondylitis, it has quite a significant association with the presence of the antigen HLA-B27. Cardiac involvement in Reiter's disease is uncommon, and it was not recognized in an analysis of 131 cases in whom there were continuing symptoms over a period of years.[14] Acute pericarditis occasionally occurs together with the arthritis, and a prolonged PR interval is sometimes found on the electrocardiogram.[15] Aortic valve disease occasionally follows Reiter's disease.

A report of three patients with aortic regurgitation who had had Reiter's disease suggests that valve disease is more likely to occur following repeated bouts of arthritis, and there may be a long latent period before evidence of a valve lesion appears. The aortic lesion of Reiter's disease resembles that found in ankylosing spondylitis, with changes in the aortic media, dilatation of the valve ring and scarring in the valve cusps.

RHEUMATOID ARTHRITIS

Although rheumatoid arthritis is predominantly a disorder of the joints, widespread lesions may affect other systems, particularly when the disease is severe and has lasted for a long time. Although cardiovascular involvement seldom plays an important clinical role it is frequently recognized at autopsy.[16] In numerous pathological and clinico-pathological reports, a distinctive pathological picture of rheumatoid heart disease has gradually emerged which differs from that of rheumatic heart disease with which it quite often used to co-exist.[17] The commonest cardiac manifestation of rheumatoid arthritis is pericarditis. There is evidence of healed pericarditis in about 40% of cases of rheumatoid arthritis at post-mortem,[17] and pericardial effusion can be demonstrated by echocardiography in a significant proportion of patients with rheumatoid arthritis during life.[18] Despite this impressive evidence of frequent pericardial involvement, clinically apparent pericarditis is uncommon. There can be acute pericarditis in patients with rheumatoid arthritis presenting with fever, chest pain, pericardial friction and effusion. There may be characteristic electrocardiographic changes, and pericardial effusion can be recognized in a radiograph of the chest or on echocardiography. It is most likely to occur when rheumatoid arthritis is severe and when it affects other systems. Occasionally, however, acute pericarditis can occur when rheumatoid arthritis is not apparently severe, and the diagnosis is made only when evidence of arthritis is sought and its activity confirmed by serological tests. Although acute pericarditis in rheumatoid arthritis nearly always resolves, it occasionally goes on to run a subacute or chronic course. A chronic pericardial effusion with tamponade sometimes develops. The fluid tends to be loculated so that pericardial aspiration is often ineffective, and it may not absorb with steroid therapy. In other cases, there is constrictive pericarditis. Sometimes this occurs as a sequel to acute pericarditis, whereas in other patients the signs of pericardial constriction are found with no history of preceding acute pericarditis.[19]

Steroid therapy is usually effective in treating acute pericarditis or pericardial effusion in rheumatoid arthritis. In patients already taking steroids, a temporary increase in dosage may be equally efficacious. Constrictive pericarditis may require surgical treatment, as may some cases of chronic pericardial effusion.[20] Pericardiectomy can be a formidable undertaking in a frail chronically ill patient who has widespread rheumatoid disease, as the densely fibrous pericardium infiltrates superficial layers of the myocardium.

Granulomatous lesions, typical of rheumatoid disease elsewhere in the body, are occasionally found in the myocardium in patients with rheumatoid arthritis at autopsy.[21,22] These have sometimes given rise to serious cardiac symptoms during life, as in 2 patients[21] in whom extensive granulomata had involved the base of the mitral valve as well as valve cusps and chordae tendineae. Both patients had congestive heart failure with signs of mitral regurgitation. Such severe mitral regurgitation, and rarely aortic valve disease, may require valve replacement. Although clinical and pathological evidence suggests that important valve disease is rare in rheumatoid arthritis, echocardiography has demonstrated that the rate of mitral valve closure during mid-diastole is significantly slowed in the majority of patients with severe rheumatoid disease.[18]

Inflammatory changes in the myocardium are often found at autopsy;[21] focal lesions with plasma cells, lymphocytes and histiocytes are described and occasionally diffuse myocarditis with necrosis of muscle cells which has caused death from heart failure. Arteritis affecting smaller arteries is a feature of severe rheumatoid disease and arteritic lesions of the coronary arteries are sometimes found at autopsy[21] often with similar lesions elsewhere in the body. Such coronary arteritis has occasionally been responsible for cardiac failure and for dangerous disturbances of rhythm and conduction. Amyloid disease sometimes occurs in patients with severe rheumatoid disease and this is yet another possible cause of cardiomyopathy.

SYSTEMIC LUPUS ERYTHEMATOSUS

In this multisystem disease, there is a diffuse and widespread vasculitis caused by the presence of antibodies to components of the nuclei. These give rise to antigen–antibody–complement complexes which can be found in many of the lesions. The syndrome sometimes follows severe infection; it can often be caused by prolonged administration of certain drugs such as hydralazine, procainamide, phenytoin, isoniazide and sulphonamides, but very often no specific cause can be identified. The clinical manifestations of systemic lupus erythematosus are protean and tend to involve skin, joints, brain and kidneys as well as the heart. It occurs much more frequently in women than in men. Prognosis is uncertain: when the kidneys are affected, which is unusual in the drug-induced form, the outlook is much worse than when they are spared; when administration of a drug is recognized as the cause, recovery is likely to follow drug withdrawal.

There is clinical evidence of heart disease in about half of patients with systemic lupus erythematosus: it is often associated with hypertension from renal involvement, but more specific pathological lesions are often encountered.[23] Acute pericarditis is the commonest cardiac lesion to be recognized clinically in systemic lupus erythematosus, and it is sometimes the presenting feature in the absence of other manifestations of the disease. Pericardial effusion may occur and occasionally constrictive pericarditis.

The most characteristic cardiac complication of systemic lupus erythematosus is Libman–Sacks endocarditis,[24] in which there is a verrucose lesion, single or multiple, found on the cusps of the mitral, and sometimes the aortic, valve. There is underlying fibrosis in the valve cusps but seldom enough to cause significant valve stenosis or regurgitation. Indeed, the presence or absence of heart murmurs during life seems to relate poorly with post-mortem evidence of Libman–Sacks endocarditis.[23] Despite the relative frequency of the condition at autopsy (about 10%), it is an uncommon clinical diagnosis. It has been suggested[25] that it is happening less frequently, possibly because of the effect of steroid therapy in lupus erythematosus. The widespread vasculitis of systemic lupus erythematosus may affect the smaller coronary arteries and be accompanied by necrosis and fibrosis in the myocardium. This cardiomyopathy occurs quite frequently. In a haemodynamic study of 5 young women, none of whom had clinical evidence of heart disease,[26] pronounced abnormalities were found which included an increase in left ventricular end-diastolic pressure, a reduction of stroke volume and of myocardial contractility and reduced left ventricular ejection fraction. Coronary blood flow, moderately increased under resting conditions, increased much less than that in normal subjects after vasodilatation induced by dipyridamole.

SYSTEMIC SCLEROSIS (SCLERODERMA)

Systemic sclerosis is a slowly progressive fibrosing condition of the skin and subcutaneous tissues.

Visceral involvement occurs in the course of the disease and may affect the gastro-intestinal tract, particularly the oesophagus, the heart, the lungs and the kidneys. The frequently associated features of calcinosis in the skin of the extremities, Raynaud's phenomenon, oesophageal dyskinesia, sclerodactyly and telangiectasia are summarized in the acronym 'CREST' syndrome. The cause of systemic sclerosis is not known, but the scarring and fibrosis occur as a result of gradual obliteration of smaller blood vessels. Although the cutaneous lesions are distressing and disabling, it is the systemic involvement, particularly of the heart and kidneys, that is likely to prove fatal.

The characteristic cardiac lesion, present in 50% of cases at autopsy,[27] is a cardiomyopathy with ischaemia, areas of infarction, and fibrosis of the myocardium. This is caused by obliterative changes, especially in the intima of the smaller coronary arteries. This may lead to congestive heart failure. The diffuse fibrosis also may involve the conducting tissues to cause heart block.[27] Although systemic sclerosis is usually well established by the time there are signs of cardiac involvement, this is not always the case, and cardiac manifestations sometimes precede skin involvement.[28] Pericarditis, sometimes with effusion, is often found at autopsy but it rarely gives rise to recognizable clinical symptoms.[27]

Hypertension from renal involvement frequently occurs in systemic sclerosis and may be responsible for heart disease. The vascular lesions may occur in pulmonary arterioles giving rise to pulmonary hypertension. In a recent study of 49 patients with systemic sclerosis, definite pulmonary hypertension was reported in 18%[29] (it occurred more frequently in those with CREST syndrome). There are several reports of patients with pulmonary hypertension at systemic level in whom this complication has proved fatal, and in whom attempts have been made to lower the pulmonary vascular resistance with drugs.[30]

TAKAYASU'S ARTERITIS ('PULSELESS DISEASE')

This curious disease of the arteries occurs predominantly in young women, and reports suggest that it is particularly prevalent in the Orient. Its cause is unknown, but an auto-immune aetiology is suspected, and attention has often been drawn to an association with tuberculous infection.[31]

There is a very pronounced proliferation of the intima which may cause severe narrowing or occlusion of an affected artery. Degeneration and fibrosis of the media and adventitia also takes place with obliteration of the vasa vasorum. The disease particularly affects the aortic arch and its branches, but it may involve any part of the aorta from the aortic valve down to its bifurcation. It has been classified into three anatomical varieties:[32] in Type 1, the aortic arch and its branches alone are affected (Fig. 61.1A); in Type 2, the disease involves the thoracic or abdominal aorta (Fig. 61.1B);[33] in Type 3, both the arch and the lower aorta are diseased. Takayasu's arteritis commonly affects the larger

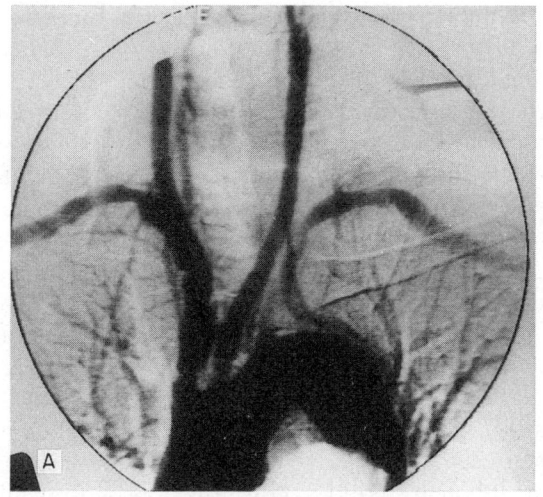
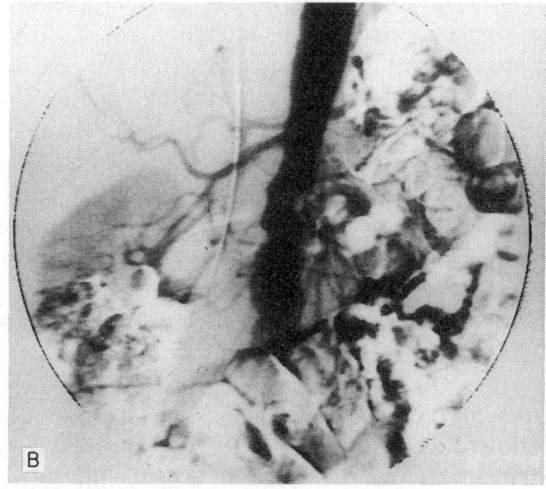

Fig. 61.1. (A) Aortogram showing involvement of the aortic arch and its branches. (B) Aortogram of descending aorta from the same patient as (A). Gross irregularity of the descending aorta is obvious.

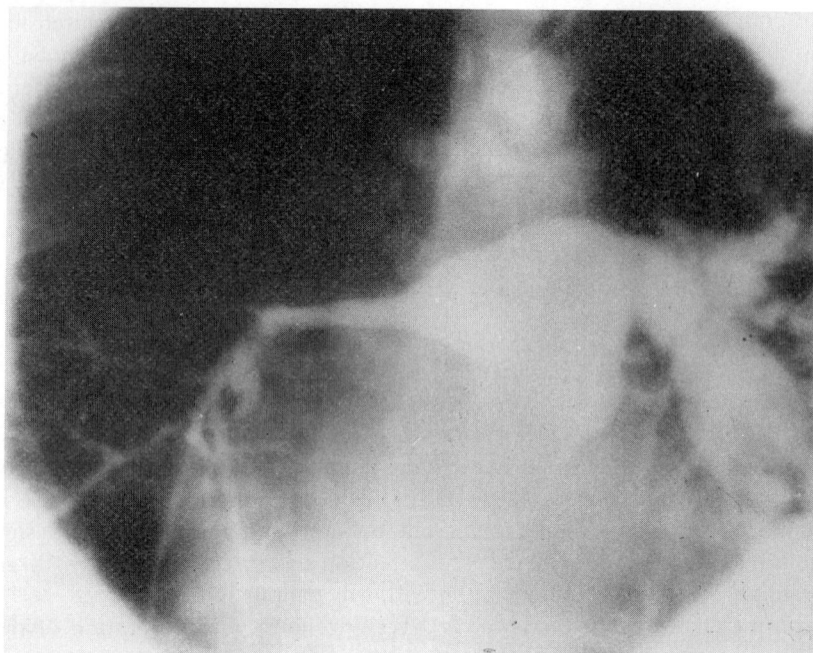

Fig. 61.2. Pulmonary angiogram showing involvement of the pulmonary arteries in Takayasu's Disease. The right pulmonary artery is severely narrowed while the left pulmonary artery is ectatic in its early part.

pulmonary arteries as well (Fig. 61.2); in one series of 22 patients studied by pulmonary angiography 50% of patients were affected.[34]

Takayasu's arteritis, may begin as an acute systemic illness with fever, malaise, increased erythrocyte sedimentation rate, arthralgia and chest pain; congestive heart failure occurs frequently in its early stages.[31] Subsequently, symptoms and signs depend upon the distribution of the arterial lesions. Involvement of the aortic arch and its branches may give rise to visual disturbances, neurological manifestations, syncopal attacks and to claudication in the upper extremities. Examination reveals diminished or absent pulsation of the carotid or brachial pulses and murmurs may be audible in the neck. The characteristic retinopathy, which Takayasu described, is said to be present in about 25% of cases. The aortic valve is sometimes affected, giving rise to systolic and diastolic murmurs, and there can be involvement of the coronary arteries causing angina or myocardial infarction.

When Takayasu's arteritis affects the thoracic or abdominal aorta, the signs may simulate coarctation, with diminished femoral pulses and hypertension.[33] Hypertension is a very common feature of the disease and is usually caused by renal artery involvement. Auscultation along the course of the aorta is likely to demonstrate a murmur at an atypical site, in the lower chest or upper abdomen,

and the usual radiographic features of coarctation will be absent. There are sometimes clinical clues to suggest pulmonary arterial involvement, such as a loud pulmonary second sound, right ventricular hypertrophy on the electrocardiogram or enlargement of the right ventricle or of the main pulmonary artery on the radiograph of the chest.

Other conditions may give rise to what has been described as 'the pulseless syndrome'.[35] Dissecting aneurysm, congenital vascular abnormalities, atheroma, trauma and syphilitic aortitis can occasionally be responsible for such a clinical picture. Clues from the history of the illness and the age of the patient would normally distinguish these from Takayasu's arteritis. The diagnosis of Takayasu's arteritis is established by aortography, and, to establish its extent, the whole length of the aorta should be studied. Right heart catheterization and pulmonary angiography should also be carried out to discover if there is pulmonary artery involvement and pulmonary hypertension.

In some reports, it has been suggested that steroid therapy has a place in the treatment of Takayasu's arteritis. Nakao *et al.* describe remission' in 5 of 29 patients so treated.[31] The chronic course taken by the disease makes such a claim difficult to substantiate, although steroid treatment may be worthwhile if the condition is diagnosed in its early stages when manifestations of systemic illness are still present.

Once the disease is established, it progresses very slowly although the arterial insufficiency may continue to cause disabling symptoms. Congestive heart failure and hypertension will often require appropriate treatment. Disobliteration of occluded vessels has not proved very successful, but surgical procedures, bypassing diseased segments of artery, may be indicated to relieve the effects of arterial obstruction.[36]

REFERENCES

1. Graham, D.C. and Smythe, H.D. The carditis and aortitis of ankylosing spondylitis. *Bull. Rheum. Dis.* 1958; **9**: 171.
2. Ansell, B.M., Bywaters, E.G. and Doniach, I. The aortic lesion of ankylosing spondylitis. *Br. Heart J.* 1958; **20**: 507.
3. Thomsen, N.H., Horslev-Petersen, K., Beyer, J.M. Ambulatory 24 hour continuous electrocardiographic monitoring in 54 patients with ankylosing spondylitis. *Eur. Heart J.* 1986; **7**: 240.
4. Bergfeldt, L., Edhag, O., Vedin, L. and Vallin, H. Ankylosing spondylitis: an important cause of severe disturbances of the cardiac conduction system. *Am. J. Med.* 1982; **73**: 187.
5. Shah, A. and Askari, A.D. Pericardial changes and left ventricular function in ankylosing spondylitis. *Am. Heart J.* 1987; **113**: 1529.
6. Brewerton, D.A., Goddard, D.H., Moore, R.B. *et al.* The myocardium in ankylosing spondylitis. A clinical, electrocardiographic and histopathological study. *Lancet* 1987; i: 995.
7. Hamrin, B., Jonsson, N. and Landberg, T. Arteritis in 'Polymyalgia Rheumatica'. *Lancet* 1964; i: 397.
8. Huston, K.A. and Hunder, G.G. Giant cell (cranial) arteritis: a clinical review *Am. Heart J.* 1980; **100**: 99.
9. Cardell, B.S. and Hanley, T. A fatal case of giant-cell or temporal arteritis. *J. Path. Bact.* 1951; **63**: 587.
10. Holsinger, D.R., Osmundson, P.J. and Edwards, J.E. The heart in periarteritis nodosa. *Circulation* 1962; **25**: 610.
11 Lynch, P.G. Cardiac involvement in chronic polymyositis. *Br. Heart J.* 1971; **33**: 416.
12. Schaumberg, H.H., Nielson, S.L. and Yurchak, P.M. Heart block in polymyositis. *N. Engl. J. Med.* 1971; **284**: 480.
13. Reid, J.M. and Murdoch, R. Polymyositis and complete heart block. *Br. Heart J.* 1979; **41**: 628.
14. Fox, R., Colin, A., Gerber, R.C. and Gibson, D. The chronicity of symptoms and disability in Reiter's symdrome. *Ann. Intern. Med.* 1979; **91**: 190.
15. Csonka, G.W., Litchfield, J.W., Oates, J.K. and Willcox, R.R. Cardiac lesions in Reiter's disease. *Br. Med. J.* 1961; i: 243.
16. Baggenstoss, A.H. and Rosenberg, E.F. Cardiac lesions associated with chronic infectious arthritis. *Arch. Intern. Med.* 1941; **67**: 241.
17. Sokoloff, L. The heart in rheumatoid arthritis. *Am. Heart J.* 1953; **45**: 635.
18. Bacon, P.A. and Gibson, D.G. Cardiac involvement in rheumatoid arthritis. An echocardiographic study. *Ann. Rheum. Dis.* 1974; **33**: 20.
19. Kirk, J. and Cosh, J. The pericarditis of rheumatoid arthritis. *Q. J. Med.* 1969; **38**: 397.
20. Thould, A.K. Constrictive pericarditis in rheumatoid arthritis. *Ann. Rheum. Dis.* 1986; **45**: 89.
21. Lebowitz, W.B. The heart in rheumatoid arthritis (rheumatoid disease). A clinical and pathological study of sixty-two cases. *Ann. Intern. Med.* 1963; **58**: 102.
22. Bonfiglio, T. and Atwater, E.C. Heart disease in patients with seropositive rheumatoid arthritis. A controlled autopsy study and review. *Arch. Intern. Med.* 1969; **124**: 714.
23. Kong, T.Q., Kellum, R.E. and Haserick, J.R. Clinical diagnosis of cardiac involvement in systemic lupus erythematosus. A correlation of clinical and autopsy findings in 30 cases. *Circulation* 1962; **26**: 7.
24. Libman, E. and Sacks, B. A hitherto undescribed form of valvular and mural endocarditis. *Arch. Intern. Med.* 1924; **33**: 701.
25. Doherty, N.D. and Siegel, R.J. Cardiovascular manifestations of systemic lupus erythematosus. *Am. Heart J.* 1985; **110**: 1257.
26. Strauer, B.E., Brune, I., Schenk, A., Knoll, D. and Perings, E. Lupus Cardiomyopathy: cardiac mechanics, haemodynamics and coronary blood flow in uncomplicated systemic lupus erythematosus. *Am. Heart J.* 1976; **92**: 715.
27. Bulkley, B.H., Ridolfi, R.L., Salyer, W.R., Hutchins, G.M. Myocardial lesions of progressive systemic sclerosis. A cause of cardiac dysfunction. *Circulation* 1976; **53**: 483.
28. Goldman, A.P. and Kotler, M.N. Heart disease in scleroderma. *Am. Heart J.* 1985; **110**: 1043.
29. Ungerer, R.G., Tashkin, D.P., Furst, D. *et al.* Prevalence and clinical correlates of pulmonary arterial hypertension in progressive systemic sclerosis. *Am. J. Med.* 1983; **75**: 65.
30. Prouse, P.J., Lahim, A. and Gumpel, J.M. The CREST syndrome—successful reduction of pulmonary hypertension by captopril. *Postgrad. Med. J.* 1984; **60**: 672.
31. Nakao, K., Ikeda, M., Kimata, S. *et al.* Takayasu's Arteritis: Clinical report of 84 cases and Immunological studies of seven cases. *Circulation* 1967; **35**: 1141.
32. Lupi-Herrera, E., Sanchez-Torres, G., Marcushamer, J. *et al.* Takayasu's Arteritis: Clinical study of 107 cases. *Am. Heart J.* 1977; **93**: 94.
33. Sen, P.K., Kinare, S.G., Engineer, S.D., Parulkar, G.B. The Middle Aortic Syndrome. *Br. Heart J.* 1963; **25**: 610.
34. Lupi, H.E., Sanchez, G., Horwitz, S. and Gutierrez, E. Pulmonary Artery Involvement in Takayasu's Arteritis. *Chest* 1975; **67**: 69.
35. Lessof, M.H. and Glynn, L.E. The Pulseless Syndrome. *Lancet* 1959; i: 799.
36. Lande, A., Hard, R., Bole, P. and Guarnaccia, M. Aortic Arch Syndrome (Takayasu's Arteritis): Arteriographic and Surgical Considerations. *J. Cardiovasc. Surg.* 1978; **19**: 507.

Chapter 62

Renal Disease and the Heart

Charles R.V. Tomson and Robert E. Bullock

INTRODUCTION

In this chapter, the effects of heart disease on renal function and the effects of failing renal function and renal replacement therapy on the heart will be discussed.[1] Reference to the renal effects of conditions affecting both organs (including essential hypertension, polyarteritis nodosa, systemic lupus erythematosus, Wegener's granulomatosis, amyloidosis, scleroderma, diabetes mellitus, Fabry's disease, Pompe's disease, primary hyperoxaluria and lecithin cholesterol acyl transferase deficiency) can be found in standard texts. The renal effects of infective endocarditis are discussed in Chapter 34.

RENAL FUNCTION IN HEART DISEASE

ACUTE RENAL FAILURE

Although the frequency of occurrence of acute renal failure due to cardiac disease is difficult to establish, oliguria after myocardial infarction is a well-recognized complication.[2] In a prospective study of hospital-acquired renal insufficiency in a consecutive series of 2216 medical and surgical patients, there were 129 episodes of renal insufficiency, 54 of which were due to decreased renal perfusion; of these, 10 were due to severe congestive heart failure, 4 to cardiogenic shock, and 2 to arrhythmias.[3]

Three patterns of renal injury are described following cardiac surgery: abbreviated acute renal failure, overt acute renal failure and protracted renal failure.[4] The evidence suggests that increasing use of plasma expanders, afterload reduction, vasodilator therapy and dopamine have resulted in the conversion of 'oliguric' to 'non-oliguric' renal failure. Measurements of urinary solute excretion are generally unhelpful in distinguishing between the various phases of post-surgical acute renal failure.

Occasionally, cardiac catheterization can also result in renal failure, either from contrast nephropathy (*vide infra*) or by cholesterol embolism,[5] but this is extremely rare.

RENAL DYSFUNCTION CAUSED BY DRUGS USED IN HEART DISEASE

Diuretics

Hypokalaemia and hypomagnesaemia are well-recognized complications of diuretic use. Diuretic-induced hypovolaemia is a frequent cause of reversible renal impairment, especially when synergistic combinations of thiazide and loop diuretics are used.[6] Thiazide diuretics, particularly when combined with potassium-sparing agents[7] may also impair free water excretion and cause profound and occasionally life-threatening hyponatraemia; this is probably due to a direct effect on tubular function. Heart failure itself can lead to disturbed water excretion, particularly in patients who have pre-existing renal dysfunction.[8] Interstitial nephritis should always be suspected in the presence of an unexplained deterioration in renal function in patients taking diuretics. Fever and eosinophilia are present in one-third of cases.[9] Triamterene frequently causes the appearance of an abnormal urinary sediment and has been implicated in causing nephrolithiasis as well as acute interstitial nephritis, particularly when taken in combination with other diuretics or non-steroidal anti-inflammatory agents.[10]

Hydralazine-induced renal disease

It is now clear that long-term treatment with hydralazine in doses as low as 100 mg/day in women and 200 mg/day in men may cause crescentic glomerulonephritis with haematuria and renal impairment, which may not resolve completely on drug withdrawal.[11]

Angiotensin converting enzyme inhibitors

In conditions in which renal perfusion is impaired, such as renal artery stenosis, some forms of chronic renal failure, and salt depletion as seen in the over-diuresed patient, the maintenance of glomerular filtration is dependent on the intrarenal production of angiotensin II. In these conditions administration of angiotensin converting enzyme inhibitors can cause a marked and not always reversible drop in glomerular filtration rate (Fig. 62.1).[12] A reduction in the levels of angiotensin II can also result in hyperkalaemia.

Angiographic contrast media

Intravenous contrast media are a common cause of renal failure particularly in patients who have pre-existing renal impairment, diabetes mellitus with nephropathy or myeloma.[13] Although renal function recovers in most patients, recovery is not invariable. If a patient at high risk of nephropathy is judged to require angiography, adequate hydration and the avoidance of other nephrotoxic agents are mandatory. The newer lower-osmolarity contrast agents can also cause nephropathy.[14]

HEART DISEASE IN URAEMIA

INTRODUCTION

In the patient without renal disease, many of the clinical signs of heart failure (such as basal crackles, elevated jugular venous pressure and peripheral oedema) used to assess the patient at the bedside are manifestations of renal retention of salt and water secondary to the cardiac disease. In the patient on dialysis, however, salt and water balance is dependent on intake and removal by dialysis, which is relatively unaffected by cardiac function. Therefore,

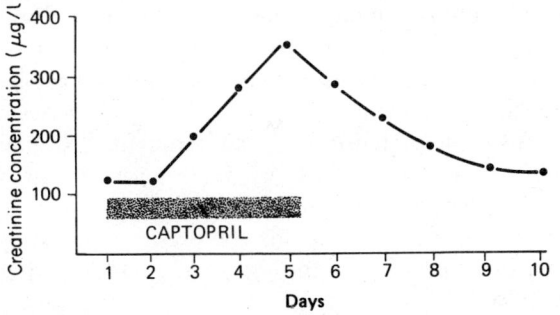

Fig. 62.1. Serial changes in renal function in a patient given captopril.

assessments of cardiac function from clinical signs in these patients must be made with great caution. Judgements about cardiac function are often made with reference to the 'dry weight' of a patient, defined as the weight at which the normo-albuminaemic patient is free of oedema and nor-motensive, and below which persistent cramps and hypotension occur. Most patients are able to say 'where the fluid goes' if they exceed their dry weight, which may give useful clues about cardiac function. However, even these limited assessments are flawed by the assumptions underlying the 'dry weight' prescribed for an individual patient. Blood pressure may take weeks to normalize after correction of fluid overload,[15] and the distinction between 'renin dependent' and 'volume dependent' hypertension can be difficult and made only by cautious experiment.

The effect of electrolyte disturbances on the electrocardiogram are well known. It should also be noted that changes in voltage may occur when altered blood volume leads to alterations in the size of the cardiac chambers. Cardiac enzyme changes should also be interpreted with caution; an abnormal creatine CK-BB band has been described in uraemic patients, lactate dehydrogenase activity is commonly raised, and measurement of aspartate transferase may give falsely low values because uraemic serum may interfere with the assay.

DIALYSIS AND 'ACCELERATED ATHEROSCLEROSIS'

Despite 14 years of debate, the concept that atherosclerosis is accelerated by dialysis remains controversial. In the report from workers at Seattle in which the concept originated,[16] analysis was retrospective and by modern standards the patients were grossly underdialysed. Long-term follow-up, conducted at several centres including Seattle, of patients without evidence of hypertension or cardiovascular disease on starting haemodialysis has shown that survival up to 15 years without development of heart disease is not unusual.[17] These findings suggest that dialysis merely acts as an added 'stress', exposing pre-existing cardiovascular disease. The importance of hypertension as a risk factor is discussed below.

Much depends on how terms are defined. Although 'cardiovascular disease' accounts for 56% of all deaths in European dialysis patients,[18] only one-sixth of these were due to clinically defined 'myocardial infarction and ischaemia', the rest being attributed to hyperkalaemia, unexplained cardiac arrest, cardiac failure attributed to causes other than ischaemia, pulmonary embolism and cerebrovascular disease. It is often difficult to distinguish between these causes of death. However, if the figures are taken at face value, deaths from coronary disease in uraemic patients under 34 years are 150 times more frequent than those in non-uraemic patients of similar age, and cerebrovascular accidents are 250 times more frequent.

Histological studies

Studies of arterial pathology in uraemic patients[19–21] have shown a remarkable lack of lipid accumulation, but prominent calcification of both the media and the intima. The severity of these changes correlates with age and duration of hypertension, but not with serum lipids. Few systematic post-mortem studies have been reported, but the incidence of coronary stenoses does not appear to be particularly high.[22]

Angiographic studies

The evidence available from coronary angiography is limited. In several studies, the incidence of significant coronary artery stenoses and the relationship of such stenoses to symptoms have been examined.[23,24] Angina pectoris is frequent in the absence of stenoses, with an incidence of between 14 and 45%, and may be due to left ventricular hypertrophy, anaemia and increased wall stress leading to myocardial hypoxia. Conversely, the incidence of clinically unsuspected coronary disease is also high. No study has shown a significant association between the presence or severity of disease and the duration of uraemia or time on dialysis, further evidence against the 'accelerated atherosclerosis' hypothesis. Factors associated with the presence of significant stenoses[23] include the presence of angina prior to starting dialysis, male sex (although females are not 'protected' to the same extent as the general population), white race, hypercholesterolaemia and decreased alkaline phosphatase activity (the latter finding remains unexplained). Abnormal left ventricular wall motion is also a strong indicator of coronary disease. Smoking has not been found to be an independent risk factor in any of the angiographic studies. Diabetic patients who have renal failure have a higher incidence of severe atheromatous disease, with an associated poor prognosis, than non-diabetic patients.[25]

Exercise electrocardiography

Exercise electrocardiography has not been formally compared to coronary angiography in uraemic patients and interpretation is complicated by the high incidence of resting electrocardiographic abnormalities and the limitation of exercise tolerance by non-cardiac factors, such as anaemia, myopathy, neuropathy, and poor physical training; however, in a study from Newcastle it was shown that poor exercise tolerance correlated well with the presence of cardiac abnormalities detected by echocardiography and gated radionuclide scanning even in the absence of ST-segment/T-wave changes during exercise.[26]

Epidemiological studies

In epidemiological studies of dialysis patients, it is not possible to distinguish reliably between 'coronary' and 'non-coronary' causes of death, which makes the interpretation of results difficult. The situation is complicated further by the co-existence of numerous potential risk factors and the relatively small numbers involved. In a prospective study of 1453 patients,[27] it was shown that age, male sex, hypertension, low body mass index, and low cholesterol and triglyceride levels were significantly associated with increased cardiovascular mortality; these findings were interpreted as indicating that patients with poor nutrition (and thus low serum lipids) had the poorest survival. The presence of pulmonary oedema at presentation and the presence of ischaemic electrocardiographic changes have been shown to be adverse risk factors for survival in one large series of patients:[28] other factors that had independent prognostic significance included age and duration of diabetes mellitus. Analysis of different dialysis regimes demonstrates increased cardiovascular mortality for techniques that allow increased weight gain between dialyses and are less efficient at the removal of urea.[29] In some series of patients, hypertension[30,31] and smoking[31,32] have also been shown to be risk factors for premature death; hyperparathyroidism has also been shown to be a major risk factor for the presence of dilated cardiomyopathy[33] and left ventricular hypertrophy.[34]

The evidence implicating hyperlipidaemia as a risk factor for death in uraemic patients is extremely limited. As yet, hypertriglyceridaemia, the commonest lipid abnormality in dialysis patients,[35] has not been implicated as a risk factor for death in any of the studies. However, this does not negate the importance of controlling hypercholesterolaemia in patients with ischaemic heart disease.

SPECIFIC CARDIOVASCULAR EFFECTS OF URAEMIA

Left ventricular function in uraemia

Objective evidence of 'abnormal cardiac function' is extremely common in uraemic patients and has been taken by many investigators to imply the existence of 'uraemic cardiomyopathy'. The central feature of this poorly defined entity is the suggestion that myocardial muscular function is impaired by one or more 'uraemic toxins' acting at a cellular level. However, as anaemia,[36] hydration state,[37] hypertension[38] and arteriovenous fistulae (discussed below) may all affect cardiac function, and as these factors co-exist in many patients the clinical definition of 'uraemic cardiomyopathy', if such a condition exists, is very difficult. Changes in cardiac function during dialysis are largely related to changes in loading conditions rather than to improved biochemistry, although it has been shown in one carefully controlled study that increasing the concentration of ionized calcium improves cardiac contractility.[39]

Despite these objections, non-invasive measurements of cardiac function are being increasingly used in the assessment of dialysis patients. Most investigators have agreed that end-diastolic volumes are useful only as an indicator of volume overload. Left ventricular hypertrophy can be reliably diagnosed by echocardiography; it has been shown to relate to hypertension,[26] excessive interdialytic weight gain[37] and hyperparathyroidism.[34] Regression of left ventricular hypertrophy occurs as a result of better fluid balance control with chronic ambulatory peritoneal dialysis and transplantation,[40] but not with long-term haemodialysis. There is less agreement on the most appropriate measurement of systolic function; ejection fraction has been widely used[40] despite its dependence on loading conditions. Indices of diastolic function are frequently abnormal, particularly in patients with left ventricular hypertrophy.[26]

Calcification of conducting tissues

Calcification of cardiac conducting tissues has been

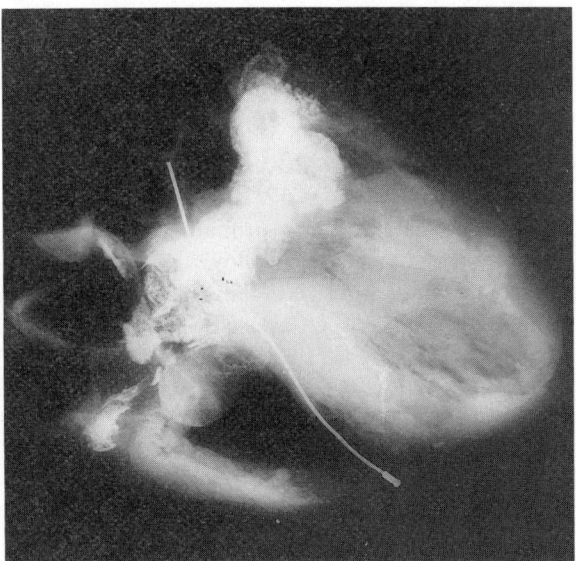

Fig. 62.2. Post-mortem radiograph of the heart of a long-term dialysis patient. Calcific aortic stenosis had been present for several years and permanent pacing had been required 12 months before death because of intermittent complete heart block. (Reproduced by kind permission of Dr H.A. Ellis.)

incriminated as the cause of death in many patients on dialysis,[42,43] who typically present with electrocardiographic conduction disturbances, cardiomegaly, and cardiac failure (Fig. 62.2). Poor control of the calcium/phosphate product, hyperparathyroidism, and intermittent hypercalcaemia and alkalosis as a result of haemodialysis have been implicated as causative factors. Often, such calcification cannot be detected on conventional radiography.

Valvular calcification

Systolic murmurs are common in patients who have renal failure and can frequently be attributed to the functional effects of anaemia and volume overload. However, it is unsafe to assume that such murmurs are innocent, because there is good evidence of an increased incidence of calcific disease especially of the mitral annulus, but also of the aortic valve.[44,45] Such structural alterations may be the substrate for the development of bacterial endocarditis as well as causing myocardial dysfunction. The incidence of calcification increases with time on dialysis; hypertension, poor control of calcium and of phosphate levels, and hyperparathyroidism are predisposing factors,[45] and co-existing vascular calcification is common.

Myocardial oxalosis

It has been suggested that long-term dialysis may be complicated by cardiac deposits of calcium oxalate;[46,47] if severe, such deposits may be associated with heart block or dilated cardiomyopathy. With modern dialysis, this problem is probably confined to patients with primary oxalosis, those with ileal resection (which allows hyperabsorption of oxalate) and those receiving excessive doses of oxalate precursors, such as ascorbate.

Hyperparathyroidism

Hyperparathyroidism is significantly associated with echocardiographic evidence of impaired myocardial function.[33,48,49] Myocardial function may improve after parathyroidectomy[48] or suppression of parathormone secretion by cimetidine,[49] although any improvement is small. As yet, surgical or medical treatment of hyperparathyroidism has not been shown to confer benefit on patients with clinically evident heart disease. The exact mechanism whereby the hormone exerts its supposed myocardial depressant effect is not known, but it may be through interference with the entry of calcium into the myocardial cell. In one epidemiological study, a significant association was found between hyperparathyroidism and left ventricular hypertrophy.[34]

Abnormal pulmonary capillary permeability

Increased pulmonary capillary permeability to albumin appears to be a consequence of fluid overload in uraemia and may permit the development of pulmonary oedema at relatively low pulmonary capillary pressures.[50,51] This does not lead to major clinical problems, and the treatment (removal of fluid by dialysis) remains the same.

Other factors

Cobalt, which was used briefly to treat the anaemia of chronic renal failure, may accumulate in patients who have renal failure and cause a dilated cardiomyopathy.[52] Iron overload is common in multiply transfused patients but there is no evidence that cardiac function is at risk.

ENDOCARDITIS

Infection is second only to cardiovascular disease as a cause of death in patients on renal replacement therapy. Dialysis patients have a high incidence of carriage of *Staphylococcus aureus*, an impaired immune system and arteriovenous fistulae, all of which may predispose to bacterial endocarditis by causing mechanical damage to the heart valves. In addition, they are subject to a high incidence of infection related to external (shunts and temporary subclavian cannulae) or internal vascular access devices. Cardiac murmurs and anaemia frequently occur in renal patients, and infective endocarditis may occur in the absence of fever and of positive blood cultures,[53] making prompt diagnosis difficult. New cardiac murmurs, usually of aortic incompetence, are strongly suggestive of endocarditis, and should not be attributed to volume overload unless endocarditis has been rigorously excluded. *Staphylococcus aureus* is the most common causative agent of endocarditis in uraemic patients; Gram-negative organisms cause 20% of all access site infections, but only rarely do they cause endocarditis.[53] The indications for cardiac surgery are the same as those for patients who do not have renal failure, and if pre- and post-operative dialysis is adequate survival is good.[54]

HEART FAILURE AND ARTERIOVENOUS FISTULAE

Arteriovenous fistulae carry a blood flow of at least 400 ml/min, and if the fistula dilates this may increase to > 1000 ml/min, resulting in high-output cardiac failure,[55] particularly in patients who have pre-existing cardiac disease. An assessment of flow through the fistula may be helpful in deciding whether a particular patient will benefit from a reduction in the size of the fistula; measurement of cardiac output before and after occlusion may also be of value in this context, but changes in heart rate on occlusion of the fistula are not helpful.[55] If peritoneal dialysis is not practicable in patients with pre-existing ischaemic or hypertensive disease, the use of an indwelling venous catheter[56] for haemodialysis access may be preferable.

PERICARDITIS IN RENAL FAILURE

Before regular dialysis was available, the development of pericarditis in a patient with uraemia was a pre-terminal event. This form of pericarditis, classified as 'uraemic pericarditis' in the review by Renfrew *et al.*,[57] is decreasing in incidence with the increasing availability of early dialysis. Diagnosis is usually obvious, with fever, leucocytosis and hypotension occurring in nearly all of the cases; pericardial rubs are frequent (although not universal) and independent of the presence or absence of pericardial fluid.[58] The cause of uraemic pericarditis is not known but it is thought to relate to a generalized serositis caused by 'uraemic toxins', although hypercalcaemia and hyperparathyroidism were implicated in the results from one series.[59] In general, this form of pericarditis responds well to adequate dialysis.

'Dialysis pericarditis'[57] occurs in patients who are well established on dialysis with adequate control of fluid balance and biochemistry. Presentation is similar to that of uraemic pericarditis, with pain, pericardial rub, fever, leucocytosis, mental changes, and hypotension during dialysis. Non-specific electrocardiographic changes are common, as are atrial arrhythmias, but the classical ST-segment changes of pericarditis are present in less than 30% of cases. Tamponade can occur without pulsus paradoxus or Kussmaul's sign, and these signs are likely to be absent in the presence of pre-existing volume overload with elevated left atrial pressure.[60] A prodrome suggesting viral infection is common in this type of pericarditis, and rising titres to influenza and Coxsackie viruses have been detected,[61] but in most cases no cause is discovered. Some cases follow intercurrent illness or surgical operations. Because routine biochemical measurements are not completely satisfactory as a guide to the adequacy of dialysis, differentiation from 'uraemic pericarditis' depends on a trial of intensified dialysis, but in most cases there is little evidence that this alters the course of the disease. Most authorities recommend that haemodialysis be performed with regional heparinization or prostacyclin because of the risk that full heparinization may permit intrapericardial bleeding leading to tamponade, although this complication is probably rare. The theoretical risk of osmotic swelling of the pericardial contents during dialysis has not been confirmed by direct observation and cardiovascular collapse during dialysis is most likely to be due to a decrease in cardiac preload.

For patients who do not respond to increased dialysis there is little agreement on treatment. Anti-inflammatory drugs and systemic steroids are of no proven value. In the hands of its proponents, pericardiocentesis with an indwelling pericardial catheter and regular instillation of large doses (50–100 mg every 6 h) of triamcinolone until the cavity remains dry is highly successful and free of serious complications.[62] The alternatives are placement of a large-bore pericardiostomy tube under local anaesthetic[63] or formal surgical drainage.[64] The final choice will depend largely on local expertise.

CARDIOVASCULAR INSTABILITY DURING HAEMODIALYSIS

Symptomatic hypotension during haemodialysis is common, occurring in up to 25% of all dialyses. It has been ascribed to numerous factors, but the most important seem to be acute volume depletion (particularly seen with dialysis against a dialysate of low sodium concentration and osmolality, permitting increased translocation of water into cells), vasodilatation (which may be due to hyperacetataemia), pre-existing heart disease and autonomic neuropathy.[65] However, recent evidence suggests that left ventricular diastolic dysfunction may contribute to the hypotension, particularly in patients who have left ventricular hypertrophy.[66] Adjustments to dialysate sodium and dialysate temperature may help to prevent the occurrence of hypotension during dialysis, but many patients are eventually converted to either haemofiltration or continuous ambulatory peritoneal dialysis.

CARDIOVASCULAR DISEASE AND SUITABILITY FOR RENAL TRANSPLANTATION

A successful renal transplant may transform the life of the recipient, and costs considerably less than long-term dialysis. However, cadaveric organs are a limited resource and many surgeons are reluctant to 'waste' such resources on patients who have a high risk of post-operative cardiovascular morbidity and mortality, such as diabetics, those with ischaemic heart disease and the elderly. This reluctance must be balanced against the possibility that successful transplantation may improve the manifestations of cardiovascular disease by improving anaemia and improving salt and water balance, and that dialysis is itself a limited resource. Diabetes is a well-recognized risk factor for premature death in uraemic patients, especially in patients > 50 years.[67] Asymptomatic coronary arterial disease is particularly common in diabetic patients and has been shown to have major prognostic significance. However, transplantation improves the prognosis, even that of diabetics who have significant coronary stenoses,[25] and good results have been obtained at several centres without pre-operative angiography.[67,68] In non-diabetic patients, the risk of

Table 62.1. **A guide to drug removal by dialysis.**

Drug	Dose alteration?	Removed by HD*?	Removed by PD*?	Comments
Opiates	?	?	?	Active metabolites of codeine and morphine may accumulate leading to prolonged respiratory depression
Nitrates	No	?	?	
Calcium channel blockers	No	?	?	
Beta-blockers				May decrease renal blood flow — significance uncertain (except nadolol)
Labetolol	No	No	No	
Metoprolol	No	No	No	
Pindolol	No	?	No	
Propanolol	No	No	No	Metabolites interfere with bilirubin estimation
Timolol	No	No	No	
Atenolol	Yes	Yes	?	Increase dose-interval
Acebutolol	Yes	No	?	Some hepatic metabolism occurs
Nadolol	Yes	Yes	?	Increase dose-interval
Sotalol	Yes	Yes	?	Decrease dose. Monitor QT interval
Antihypertensives:				
Indapamide	No	No	?	
Hydralazine	No	No	No	See comments on lupus syndrome
Minoxidil	No	Yes	?	
Prazosin	No	No	No	
Clonidine	Yes	No	?	
Diazoxide	Yes	?	?	Effect unpredictable. Prolonged half-life, decreased protein binding
Methyldopa	Yes	Yes	?	Adjust dose a/c to blood pressure
Nitroprusside	No	Yes	?	Cyanide and thiocyanate toxicity reported: hydroxycobalamin may protect
Angiotensin converting enzyme inhibitors:				
Captopril	Yes	Yes	?	Reduced doses required. Hyperkalaemia can occur
Enalapril	Yes	Yes	Yes	As for captopril
Anti-arrhythmics:				
Amiodarone	No	No	No	
Lignocaine	No	No	?	
Mexilitene	No	No	No	
Phenytoin	No	No	No	Reduced protein binding: serum levels may be misleading. Salivary levels useful
Quinidine	No	Yes	Yes	Some renal excretion: monitor QT interval
Bretylium	Yes	?	?	Avoid
Disopyramide	Yes	Yes	?	See Data Sheet. Monitor serum levels
Flecainide	Yes	?	?	Monitor serum levels
Procainamide	Yes	Yes	?	Active metabolite accumulates
Tocainide	Yes	Yes	?	
Cardiac Glycosides:				
Digitoxin	No	No	No	Only safer than digoxin if serum levels can be monitored
Digoxin	Yes	No	No	Avoid hypokalaemia during dialysis. Decreased volume of distribution: ? decrease loading dose
Diuretics:				
Bumetanide	No	?	?	Higher doses may be needed
Frusemide	No			Higher doses may be needed
Metolazone	No	No	?	Retains efficacy at low glomerular filtration rate
Potassium-sparing agents				High risk of hyperkalaemia — avoid
Thiazides	No	?	?	Ineffective if glomerular filtration rate < 15 ml/min
Theophyllines	No	No	No	

* HD, haemodialysis; PD, peritoneal dialysis.

myocardial infarction is not as great. It is virtually impossible to predict such deaths with accuracy: the presence of angina, of hypertension and of cardiomegaly are of little value.[69] As yet, there is no evidence to support the suggestion that pre-transplant angiography and coronary artery bypass grafting would improve survival in potential transplant recipients.

CARDIOVASCULAR DRUG THERAPY IN URAEMIA

To avoid toxicity, drugs that are normally excreted by the kidneys should be prescribed in decreased dose or with an increased dose-interval to patients who have impaired renal function. Although tubular secretion of some drugs is important, most dose adjustments are made according to creatinine clearance, the measurement of which is notoriously unreliable in outpatients. Creatinine clearance may be more accurately estimated from serum creatinine, age, sex and bodyweight.[70] As the pharmacokinetics of many drugs are not substantially affected by renal failure, such drugs should be given in preference whenever possible. Reference to the Data Sheet for the drug or to one of several authoritative reviews[71,72] is strongly recommended if drugs likely to accumulate are to be used. Data for drug removal by dialysis are incomplete, especially with respect to peritoneal dialysis. A simplified guide to this subject is given in Table 62.1.

REFERENCES

1. O'Rourke, R.A., Brenner, B.M. and Stein, J.H. *The heart and renal disease*. Edinburgh: Churchill Livingstone, 1984.
2. Hutton, I., Pack, A.I., Lindsay, R.M. and Lawrie, T.D.V. Clinical significance of renal haemodynamics in acute myocardial infarction. *Lancet* 1970; ii: 123–5.
3. Hou, S.H., Bushinsky, D.A., Wish, J.B., Cohen, J.J. and Harrington, J.T. Hospital-acquired renal insufficiency: a prospective study. *Am. J. Med.* 1983; 74; 243–8.
4. Myers, B.D. and Moran, S.M. Hemodynamically mediated acute renal failure. *N. Engl. J. Med.* 1986; 314: 97–105.
5. Drost, H., Buis, B., Haan, D. and Hillers, J.A. Cholesterol embolism as a complication of left heart catheterisation. *Br. Heart J.* 1984; 52: 339–42.
6. Ostler, J.R., Epstein, M. and Smoller, S. Combined therapy with thiazide-type and loop diuretic agents for resistant sodium retention. *Ann. Intern. Med.* 1983; 99: 405–6.
7. Tarssanen, L., Huikko, M. and Rossi, M. Amiloride-induced hyponatremia. *Acta Med. Scand.* 1980; 208: 491–4.
8. Mettauer, B., Rouleau, J.-L., Bichet, D., Juneau, C., Kortas, C., Barjon, J.-N. and de Champlain, J. Sodium and water excretion abnormalities in congestive heart failure. *Ann. Intern. Med.* 1986; 105: 161–7.
9. Pusey, C.D., Saltissi, D., Bloodworth, L., Rainford, D.J. and

Christie, J.L. Drug associated interstitial nephritis: clinical and pathological features and the response to high dose steroid therapy. *Q. J. Med.* 1983; 52: 194–211.
10. Spence, J.D., Wong, D.G. and Lindsay, R.M. Effects of triamterene and amiloride on urinary sediment in hypertensive patients taking hydrochlorothiazide. *Lancet* 1985; ii: 73–5.
11. Bjorck, S., Westberg, G. and Svalander, C. Hydralazine-induced glomerulonephritis. *Acta Med. Scand.* 1985; 218: 261–9.
12. Packer, M., Lee, W.H., Yushak, M. and Medina, N. Comparison of captopril and enalapril in patients with severe chronic heart failure. *N. Engl. J. Med.* 1986; 315: 847–53.
13. Talierco, C.P., Vlietstra, R.E., Fisher, L.D. and Burnett, J.C. Risks for renal dysfunction with cardiac angiography. *Ann. Intern. Med.* 1986; 104: 501–4.
14. Smith, H.-J., Levorstad, K., Berg, K.J. and Sveen, K. High dose urography in patients with renal failure. A double blind investigation of iohexol and metrizoate. *Acta Radiol. Diag.* 1985; 26: 213–20.
15. Scharf, S., Wexler, J., Longnecker, R.E. and Blaufox, M.D. Cardiovascular disease in patients on chronic hemodialysis therapy. *Prog. Cardiovasc. Dis.* 1980; 22: 343–56.
16. Lindner, A., Charra, B., Sherrard, D.J. and Scribner, B.H. Accelerated atherosclerosis in prolonged maintenance hemodialysis. *N. Engl. J. Med.* 1974; 290: 697–701.
17. Giordano, C. and Friedman, E.A. (Eds). *Uremia: pathobiology of patients treated for 10 years or more*. Milan: Wichtig, 1981.
18. Brunner, F.P., Brynger, H., Chantler, C., Donckerwolcke, R.A., Hathway, R.A., Jacobs, C., Selwood, N.H. and Wing, A.J. Combined report on regular dialysis and transplantation in Europe, IX, 1978. *Proc. EDTA* 1979; 16: 1–68.
19. Ejerblad, S., Ericsson, J.L.E. and Eriksson, I. Arterial lesions of the radial artery in uraemic patients. *Acta Chir. Scand.* 1979; 145: 415–28.
20. Vincenti, F., Amend, W.J., Abele, J., Feduska, N.J. and Salvatierra, O. The role of hypertension in hemodialysis-associated atherosclerosis. *Am. J. Med.* 1980; 68: 363–9.
21. Ibels, L.S., Alfrey, A.C., Huffer, W.E., Craswell, P.W., Anderson, J.T. and Weil, R. Arterial calcification and pathology in uremic patients undergoing dialysis. *Am. J. Med.* 1979; 66: 790–6.
22. Rostand, S.G., Gretes, J.C., Kirk, K.A., Rutsky, E.A. and Andreoli, T.E. Ischemic heart disease in patients with uremia undergoing maintenance hemodialysis. *Kidney Int.* 1979; 16: 600–11.
23. Rostand, S.G., Kirk, K.A. and Rutsky, E.A. Dialysis-associated ischemic heart disease: insights from coronary angiography. *Kidney Int.* 1984; 25: 653–9.
24. Ikram, H., Lynn, K.L., Bailey, R.R. and Little, P.J. Cardiovascular changes in chronic hemodialysis patients. *Kidney Int.* 1983; 24: 371–6.
25. Khauli, R.B., Steinmuller, D.R., Novick, A.C., Buszta, C., Goormastic, M., Nakamoto, S., Vidt, D.G., Magnusson, M., Paganini, E. and Schreiber, M.J. A critical look at survival of diabetics with end-stage renal disease. *Transplantation* 1986; 41: 598–602.
26. Bullock, R.E., Amer, H.A., Simpson, I., Ward, M.K. and Hall, R.J.C. Cardiac abnormalities and exercise tolerance in patients receiving renal replacement therapy. *Br. Med.J.* 1984; 289: 1479–84.
27. Degoulet, P., Legrain, M., Reach, I., Aime, F., Devries, C., Rojas, P. and Jacobs, C. Mortality risk factors in patients treated by chronic hemodialysis. *Nephron* 1982; 31: 103–10.
28. Hutchinson, T.A., Thomas, D.C., Lemieux, J.C. and Harvey, C. Prognostically controlled comparison of dialysis and renal transplantation. *Kidney Int.* 1984; 26: 44–51.
29. Lowrie, E.G., Laird, N.M., Parker, T.F. and Sargent, J.A.

Effect of the hemodialysis prescription on patient morbidity. *N. Engl. J. Med.* 1981; **305**: 1176–81.

30. Eliahou, H.E., Iaina, A., Reisin, E. and Shapira, J. Probability of survival in hypertensive and nonhypertensive patients on maintenance hemodialysis. *Israel J. Med. Sci.* 1977; **13**: 33–8.

31. Haire, H.M., Sherrard, D.J., Scardapane, D., Curtis, F.K. and Brunzell, J.D. Smoking, hypertension, and mortality in a maintenance dialysis population. *Cardiovasc. Med.* 1978; **3**: 1163–8.

32. Gokal, R., Baillod, R., Bogle, S., Hunt, L., Jakubowski, C., Marsh, F., Ogg, C., Oliver, D., Ward, M. and Wilkinson, R. Multi-centre study of outcome of treatment in patients on continuous ambulatory peritoneal dialysis. *Nephrol. Dial. Transplant.* 1987; **2**: 172–8.

33. Parfrey, P.S., Harnett, J.D., Griffiths, S., Gault, M.H., Barre, P.E. and Guttmann, R.D. Low-output left ventricular failure in end-stage renal disease. *Am. J. Nephrol.* 1987; **7**: 184–91.

34. Harnett, J.D., Parfrey, P.S., Griffiths, S.M., Gault, M.H., Barre, P. and Guttmann, R.D. Left ventricular hypertrophy in end-stage renal disease. *Nephron* 1988; **48**: 107–15.

35. Sakhrani, L. Lipoprotein abnormalities in uremia. In: Nissenson, A.R., Fine, R.N. and Gentile, D.E., Eds. *Clinical Dialysis*. Norwalk, Connecticut: Appleton-Century-Crofts, 1984, pp. 439–50.

36. Neff, M.S., Kim, K.E., Persoff, M., Onesti, G. and Swartz, C. Hemodynamics of uremic anemia. *Circulation* 1971; **43**: 876–83.

37. Golf, S., Lunde, P., Abrahamsen, A.M. and Oyri, A. Effect of hydration state on cardiac function in patients on chronic haemodialysis. *Br. Heart J.* 1983; **49**: 183–6.

38. Ikaheimo, M., Huttunen, K. and Takkunen, J. Cardiac effects of chronic renal failure and haemodialysis treatment. Hypertensive versus normotensive patients. *Br. Heart J.* 1981; **45**: 710–6.

39. Henrich, W.L., Hunt, J.M. and Nixon, J.V. Increased ionised calcium and left ventricular contractility during hemodialysis. *N. Engl. J. Med.* 1984; **310**: 19–23.

40. Deligiannis, A., Paschalidou, E., Sakellariou, G., Vargemezis, V., Geleris, P., Kontopoulos, A. and Papadimitrious, M. Changes in left ventricular anatomy during haemodialysis, continuous ambulatory peritoneal dialysis, and after renal transplantation. *Proc. EDTA–ERA* 1984; **21**: 185–9.

41. Gilmartin, J.J., Duffy, B.S., Finnegan, P. and McCready, N. Non-invasive study of left ventricular function in chronic renal failure before and after haemodialysis. *Clin. Nephrol.* 1983; **20**: 55–60.

42. Terman, D.S., Alfrey, A.C., Hammond, W.S., Donndelinger, T., Ogden, D.A. and Holmes, J.H. Cardiac calcification in uremia. *Am. J. Med.* 1971; **50**: 744–54.

43. Arora, K.K., Lacy, J.P., Schacht, R.A., Martin, D.G. and Gutch, F.G. Calcific cardiomyopathy in advanced renal failure. *Arch. Intern. Med.* 1975; **135**: 603–5.

44. Forman, M.B., Virmani, R., Robertson, R.M. and Stone, W.J. Mitral annular calcification in chronic renal failure. *Chest* 1984; **85**: 367–71.

45. Maher, E.R., Young, G., Smyth-Walsh, B., Pugh, S. and Curtis, J.R. Aortic and mitral valve calcification in patients with end-stage renal disease. *Lancet* 1987; **ii**: 875–7.

46. Fayemi, A.O., Ali, M. and Braun, E.V. Oxalosis in hemodialysis patients. *Arch. Pathol. Lab. Med.* 1979; **103**: 58–62.

47. Salyer, W.R. and Hutchins, G.M. Cardiac lesions in secondary oxalosis. *Arch. Intern. Med.* 1974; **134**: 250–2.

48. Druecke, T., Fauchet, M., Fleury, J., Lesourd, P., Toure, Y., le Pailleur, C., de Vernejoul, P. and Crosnier, J. Effect of parathyroidectomy on left-ventricular function in haemodialysis patients. *Lancet* 1980; **i**: 112–3.

49. Lai, K.N., Fassett, R.G. and Mathew, T.H. Effect of long-term cimetidine treatment on left ventricular function in haemodialysis patients with active hyperparathyroidism. *Br. J. Clin. Pharmacol.* 1982; **13**: 693–7.

50. Gibson, D.G. Haemodynamic factors in the development of acute pulmonary oedema in renal failure. *Lancet* 1966; **iv**: 1217–20.

51. Rackow, E.C., Fein, I.A., Sprung, C. and Grodman, R.S. Uremic pulmonary edema. *Am. J. Med.* 1978; **64**: 1084–8.

52. Curtis, J.R., Goode, G.C., Herrington, J. and Urdaneta, L.E. Possible cobalt toxicity in maintenance hemodialysis patients after treatment with cobaltous chloride: a study of blood and tissue cobalt concentrations in normal subjects and patients with terminal renal failure. *Clin. Nephrol.* 1976; **5**: 61–6.

53. Cross, A.S. and Stiegbigel, R.T. Infective endocarditis and access site infections in patients on hemodialysis. *Medicine* 1976; **55**: 453–66.

54. Connors, J.P. and Shaw, R.C. Considerations in the management of open-heart surgery in uremic patients. *J. Thorac. Cardiovasc. Surg.* 1978; **75**: 400–4.

55. Anderson, C.B., Codd, J.R., Graff, R.A., Groce, M.A., Harter, H.R. and Newton, W.T. Cardiac failure and upper extremity arteriovenous dialysis fistulas. *Arch. Intern. Med.* 1976; **136**: 292–7.

56. Francis, D.M.A., Ward, M.K. and Taylor, R.M.R. Right-atrial catheters for long-term vascular access in haemodialysis patients. *Lancet* 1982; **ii**: 301–2.

57. Renfrew, R., Buselmeier, T.J. and Kjellstrand, C.M. Pericarditis in renal failure. *Ann. Rev. Med.* 1980; **31**: 345–60.

58. Bailey, G.L., Hampers, C., Hager, E.B. and Merrill, J.P. Uremic pericarditis: clinical features and management. *Circulation* 1968; **38**: 582–91.

59. Comty, C.M., Cohen, S.L. and Shapiro, F.L. Pericarditis in chronic uremia and its sequels. *Ann. Intern. Med.* 1971; **75**: 173–83.

60. Reddy, P.S., Curtiss, E.I., O'Toole, J.D. and Shaver, J.A. Cardiac tamponade: hemodynamic observations in man. *Circulation* 1978; **58**: 265–72.

61. Osanloo, E., Shalhoub, R.J., Cioffi, R.F. and Parker, R.H. Viral pericarditis in patients receiving hemodialysis. *Arch. Intern. Med.* 1979; **139**: 301–3.

62. Buselmeier, T.J., Davin, T.D., Simmons, R.L., Najarian, J.S. and Kjellstrand, C.M. Treatment of intractable uremic pericardial effusion; avoidance of pericardiectomy with local steroid instillation. *JAMA* 1978; **240**: 1358–9.

63. Daugirdas, J.T., Leehey, D.J., Popli, S., McCray, G.M., Gandhi, V.C., Pifarre, R. and Ing, T.S. Subxiphoid pericardiostomy for haemodialysis-associated pericardial effusion. *Arch. Intern. Med.* 1986; **146**: 1113–5.

64. Frame, J.R., Lucas, S.K., Pederson, J.A. and Elkins, R.C. Surgical treatment of pericarditis in the dialysis patient. *Am. J. Surg.* 1983; **146**: 800–3.

65. Henrich, W.L. Hemodynamic instability during hemodialysis. *Kidney Int.* 1986; **30**: 605–12.

66. Ritz, E., Ruffmann, K., Rambausek, M., Mall, G. and Schmidli, M. Dialysis hypotension: is it related to diastolic left ventricular malfunction? *Nephrol. Dial. Transplant.* 1987; **2**: 293–7.

67. Legrain, M., Rottembourg, J., Bentchikou, A. Poignet, J.L., Issad, B., Barthelmey, A., Strippoli, P., Gahl, G.M. and de Groc, F. Dialysis treatment of insulin dependent diabetic patients: ten years experience. *Clin. Nephrol.* 1984; **21**: 72–81.

68. Sutherland, D.E.R., Morrow, C.E., Fryd, D.S., Ferguson, R., Simmons, R.L. and Najarian, J.S. Improved patient and primary renal allograft survival in uremic diabetic recipients. *Transplantation* 1982; **34**: 319–25.

69. Gunnarsson, R., Lofmark, R., Nordlander, R., Nyquist, O. and Groth, C.-G. Acute myocardial infarction in renal transplant recipients: incidence and prognosis. *Eur. Heart J.*

1984; 5: 218–21.

70. Cockcroft, D.W. and Gault, M.H. Prediction of creatinine clearance from serum creatinine. *Nephron* 1976; **16**: 31–41.

71. Bennett, W.M., Aronoff, G.R., Golper, T.A., Morrison, G., Singer, I. and Brater, D.C. Drug prescribing in renal failure; dosing guidelines for adults. Philadelphia: American College of Physicians, 1987.

72. Schneller, S.J., Zusman, R.M. and Boucher, C.A. Use of cardiovascular drugs in chronic renal failure. In: O'Rourke, R.A., Brenner, B.M. and Stein, J.H. *The heart and renal disease*. Edinburgh: Churchill Livingstone, 1984, pp. 275–306.

Chapter 63

Left Ventricular Hypertrophy

Leonard M. Shapiro

INTRODUCTION

Detection of left ventricular hypertrophy is essential in the clinical assessment of patients with heart disease. In 1748, Robinson recognized the relationship between increased work and adaptive hypertrophy; left ventricular hypertrophy is commonly seen to be a physiological adaptation to sustained increase in cardiac work.[1] The hypertrophied ventricle is able to perform increased work, but its diastolic and later its systolic properties eventually become impaired and may lead to the syndrome of heart failure.[2,3]

At necropsy, left ventricular hypertrophy may be defined in terms of ventricular weight and muscle thickness. In life, hypertrophy may be defined by electrocardiographic changes (increased QRS voltages with or without repolarization changes), increased wall thickness or muscle mass on echocardiography and, more recently, on magnetic resonance and computer-assisted tomographic scanning. For clinical purposes, a definition of left ventricular hypertrophy is best made echocardiographically and should be compared with ranges of wall thickness and left ventricular mass derived from age- and sex-matched normal control subjects.

Left ventricular hypertrophy is a final common pathway for many physiological and disease processes. It can be usefully distinguished into concentric hypertrophy, in which the left ventricular cavity is not enlarged and wall thickness is increased, and eccentric hypertrophy, in which cavity dilatation is the primary stimulus.[1] During prolonged endurance training, athletes develop mild cavity dilatation and wall thickening. Pressure overload from aortic stenosis and hypertension results in wall thickening without enlargement of the left ventricular cavity. In hypertrophic cardiomyopathy, the left ventricular hypertrophy develops without stimulus and is characteristically but not always asymmetrically distributed. Left ventricular hypertrophy develops in a volume-loaded heart (aortic regurgitation, mitral regurgitation and patent ductus arteriosus) and it is secondary to cavity dilatation and increased stroke volume. Left ventricular hypertrophy also occurs in congestive cardiomyopathy and in the remaining viable muscle following myocardial infarction. These forms of eccentric hypertrophy will not be considered further.

EPIDEMIOLOGY

The results of epidemiological studies have suggested that left ventricular hypertrophy is a common finding. In the Framingham study,[4] the prevalence of left ventricular hypertrophy as assessed by electrocardiography, was compared with that as assessed by echocardiography in a population sample of more than 10 000. Using voltage echocardiographic criteria, left ventricular hypertrophy was found in 1.5% of the population; on M-mode echocardiography, left ventricular hypertrophy was demonstrated in 10%. Prevalence varies with age, from 6% in those younger than 50 years to more than 50% in women over 80 years.[5] The two strongest predictors of left ventricular hypertrophy were age and systolic blood pressure. The prognostic significance of left ventricular hypertrophy was confirmed in this study; it was strongly associated with arrhythmias, and 45% of all cardiovascular deaths were preceded by this electrocardiographic finding.[5]

PATHOLOGY

In compensated pressure-overload hypertrophy, the left ventricular cavity elongates and becomes narrower, and as the mitral ring does not enlarge the increase in wall thickness leads to myocardial encroachment upon the cavity. The cells may be qualitatively normal except for their diameter which can increase from a normal value of 5–7 to 20–30 μm.[2] There may be considerable variations in size between adjacent cells. Cell length increases by addition of sarcomeres, initiated by the proliferation of intercalated discs. There is an increased number of myofibrils which eventually lead to a significant elevation of the ratio of myofibrils to mitochondria. There may be variations in the size of mitochondria with large and very small forms present. Degenerative changes are frequently present in chronic left ventricular hypertrophy, especially when the pressure overload is severe or prolonged, and in hypertrophic cardiomyopathy. There are foci of interstitial fibrosis particularly in proximity to atrophic cells and surrounding blood vessels, and areas of myocardium may be replaced by fibrous tissue.[6,7] Myocardial fibre disarray is a distinctive feature of hypertrophic cardiomyopathy, but the changes of cellular atrophy and fibrous replacement may simulate this appearance in secondary left ventricular hypertrophy.

PATHOPHYSIOLOGY

Mild-to-moderate left ventricular hypertrophy is presumably an adaptive and beneficial mechanism to increase the work capacity of the heart and normalize an increased peak systolic wall stress in pressure overload. However, myocardial cells can hypertrophy beyond an adaptive stage and muscle performance deteriorates. During fetal life, cardiac growth involves myocardial cell hyperplasia (i.e. the number of cells increases). However, soon after birth, no further cell division occurs and cardiac growth, from infancy to adulthood, is associated with cellular enlargement of up to threefold (hypertrophy).[2,3] Therefore, the hypertrophy itself is not associated with a deterioration in function, or at least that which occurs during growth is physiological. This physiological left ventricular hypertrophy is a response to increased preload and is similar to that which occurs in athletes (see later section, p. 1420) or due to a mildly increased workload. It is accompanied by normal or increased contraction, and the peak rate at which ATP is metabolized by myosin is also normal or increased. There is concurrent capillary growth so that a constant density of capillaries in relationship to myocardium is maintained. In pathological hypertrophy, there is left ventricular hypertrophy, a decrease in the rate of ATP hydrolysis and a reduction in capillary density. These changes may be the substrate for later deterioration in ventricular function.

Wall tension is proportional to both the ventricular pressure and the radius of curvature of the ventricular wall. Laplace's law states:

$$\text{Stress} = PR/T$$

where P is pressure, R radius of curvature and T wall tension.

A constant relationship should be observed between systolic pressure generated by the ventricle, ventricular radius and wall thickness. The ratio of wall thickness to ventricular radius is almost linear when compared with systolic left ventricular pressure and it is largely independent of cavity size. Thus, when left ventricular function is normal, peak systolic left ventricular wall stress is normal.[8] Compensatory left ventricular hypertrophy therefore serves to reduce peak systolic wall stress so that systolic force per myocardial fibre is within the normal range. Although ventricular hypertrophy maintains systolic wall stress within normal limits, the remodelling required for this purpose alters the diastolic wall stress and may lead to abnormalities of diastolic function.[9]

CLINICAL FEATURES

The clinical features reflect the underlying aetiology. However, some features are constant and directly related to the left ventricular hypertrophy (see below).

EXERTIONAL DYSPNOEA

Exertional dyspnoea may be due to impairment of the diastolic left ventricular properties, particularly prolongation of isovolumic relation and reduced peak rate of left ventricular filling.

ANGINA

Angina may occur as the result of left ventricular hypertrophy without co-existing coronary artery disease.[10] Studies in hypertrophic cardiomyopathy[11] suggest that patients in whom the peak rate of posterior wall thinning is significantly reduced are at a greater risk of presenting with angina.

PALPITATION

Palpitation may occur in patients with hypertrophied muscle that has a greater ectopy; in addition, atrial enlargement will precipitate atrial tachyarrhythmias.

THE CARDIAC IMPULSE

The cardiac impulse is sustained and a palpable fourth heart sound may be detected. This is particularly accentuated in hypertrophic cardiomyopathy (Fig. 63.1). The first heart sound is quiet due to a high left ventricular end-diastolic pressure. Less commonly, a third heart sound is heard and results from abnormal left ventricular filling. The jugular venous pressure may exhibit an increased 'a' wave, classically thought to reflect septal hypertrophy encroaching upon the right ventricular cavity (the Bernheim effect), but it may be due to the abnormalities of the left ventricle affecting the diastolic behaviour of the right ventricle.

INVESTIGATIONS

ELECTROCARDIOGRAPHY

The electrocardiographic changes in left ventricular hypertrophy include left atrial enlargement, increased QRS voltage, left-axis deviation and repolarization abnormalities. Left atrial enlargement may occur in the absence of other electrocardiographic evidence of left ventricular hypertrophy,

but it is neither specific nor sensitive in its diagnosis. Electrocardiographic QRS voltages bear only a moderate relation to left ventricular mass, and increased voltages are present in many normal young people who have a thin chest wall.[12] However, in the presence of QRS voltages, echocardiographic or necropsy evidence of increased wall thickness is frequently present. Left ventricular hypertrophy is associated with repolarization abnormalities termed 'strain': symmetrical T-wave inversion of the lateral precordial leads.

Such abnormalities have been studied since the early part of this century when Einthoven observed these findings in patients with hypertrophy.[13] This is an important clinical association as this is the most satisfactory electrocardiographic evidence of left ventricular hypertrophy and is frequently used in the decision-making progress in individual patients (Fig. 63.2A). Removal of the cause of hypertrophy often leads to a regression of the T-wave changes particularly in young patients over the ensuing weeks or months (Fig. 63.2B). However, these repolarization changes are non-specific; they also occur in coronary artery disease and following digoxin therapy. Furthermore, they are labile and may occur in otherwise normal subjects in association with ill-defined physiological stimuli such as hyperventilation. In addition, neither the genesis of a normally upright T wave nor that of its inversion in these different conditions has been satisfactorily explained.[14]

Electrocardiographic criteria for a diagnosis of left ventricular hypertrophy with a reasonably high specificity (> 90%) are insensitive (sensitivity <

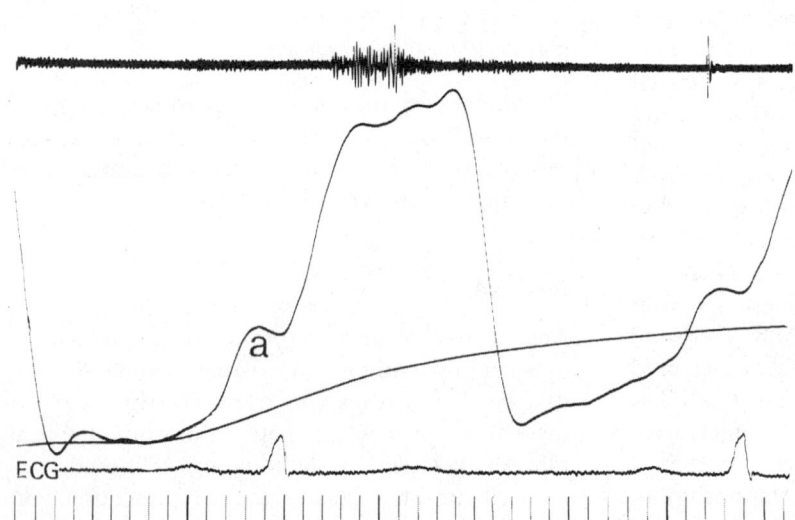

Fig. 63.1. Apexcardiogram in patients with severe left ventricular hypertrophy due to significant aortic stenosis. There is an accentuated 'a' wave which constitutes more than the normal 7% of overall impulse amplitude. In this case it is approximately 30%.

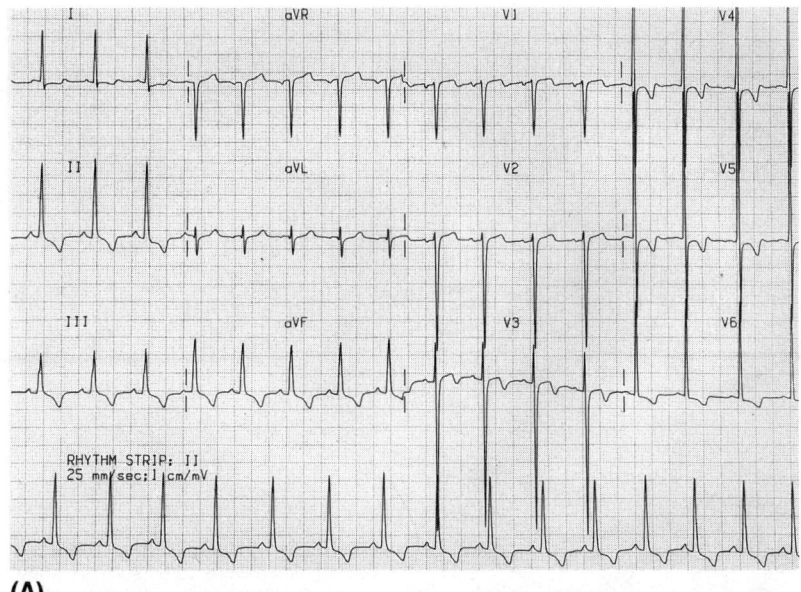

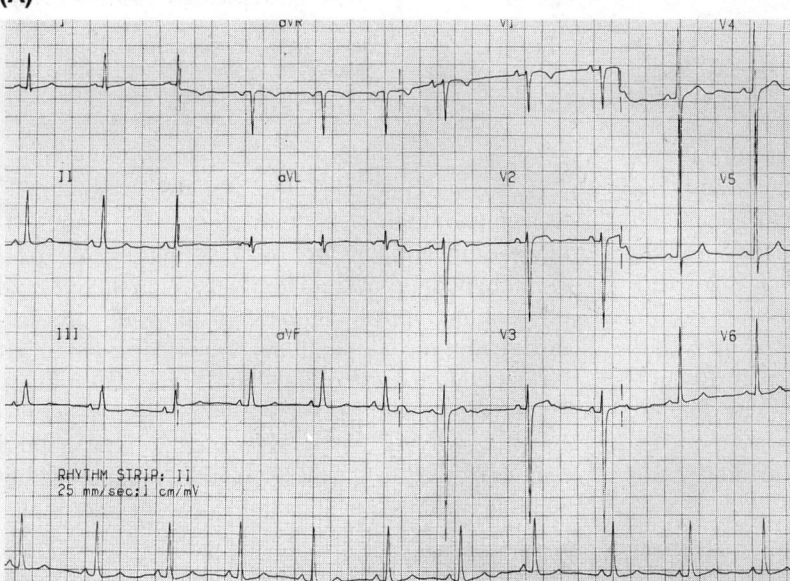

Fig. 63.2. (A) Electrocardiogram of adolescent with severe aortic stenosis. There is left ventricular hypertrophy on voltage criteria. In addition, there is a 'strain' pattern with inferior and lateral ST-segment depression and T-wave inversion. (B) Two months later, following relief of the aortic stenosis, there has been little change in QRS voltage but the repolarization changes have resolved.

50%) in the diagnosis of left ventricular hypertrophy.[15]

CHEST RADIOGRAPHY

Left ventricular hypertrophy without cavity dilatation produces no increase in heart size, but an increase in curvature of the left heart border may suggest the presence of hypertrophy. Upper lobe blood diversion and left atrial enlargement may infer an increased left atrial pressure.

ECHOCARDIOGRAPHY

The M-mode echocardiogram is able to measure

wall thickness around the base of the ventricle (anterior ventricular septum and posterior by the left ventricular wall) (Fig. 63.3). The normal range of wall thicknesses are related to sex and body size, but in adults values range from 0.7 to 1.1 cm. Values in excess of 1.2 cm in the posterior wall and 1.3 cm in the septum may be considered to indicate hypertrophy. From such measurements, left ventricular mass may be calculated by assuming a thickness of myocardium (similar to that measured in the septum and posterior wall), surrounds the left ventricular volume derived from the cube of the left ventricular internal diameter). Although M-mode echocardiography has high spatial and temporal

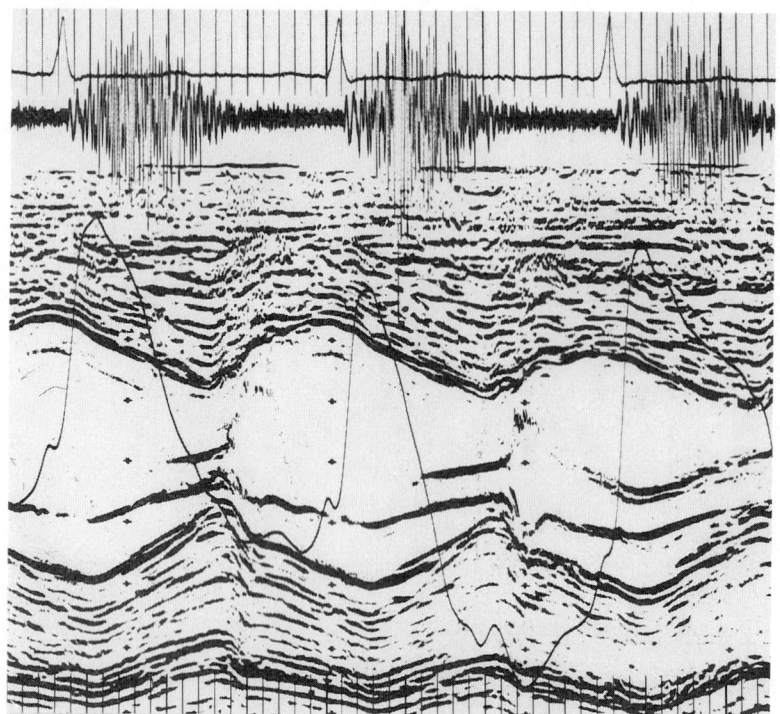

Fig. 63.3. M-Mode echocardiogram in patient with severe aortic stenosis showing marked increase in posterior wall and septal thicknesses resulting in concentric left ventricular hypertrophy. The left ventricular cavity is small, and systolic function normal or supranormal; filling and posterior wall thinning are abnormal.

resolution, cross-sectional echocardiography allows the entire myocardium to be imaged and the presence of localized left ventricular hypertrophy to be detected (Fig. 63.4). This is usually of little importance except in hypertrophic cardiomyopathy where localized hypertrophy may occur in the posterior ventricular septum and cardiac apex and not be detected by the M-mode beam which transects the base of the ventricle.[16,17] The diagnosis of hypertrophic cardiomyopathy is best made by the demonstration of unexplained (primary) left ventricular hypertrophy.[18]

Distribution of hypertrophy

In echocardiographic studies, initially using M-mode echocardiography to diagnose asymmetrical septal hypertrophy and latterly using cross-sectional echocardiography (measurement of wall thickness throughout the left ventricle), the distribution of left ventricular hypertrophy has been determined. Hypertrophy is most often asymmetrical, predominantly involving the interventricular septum and free wall or apex.[16] This asymmetry is most readily demonstrated by an increased ratio of ventricular

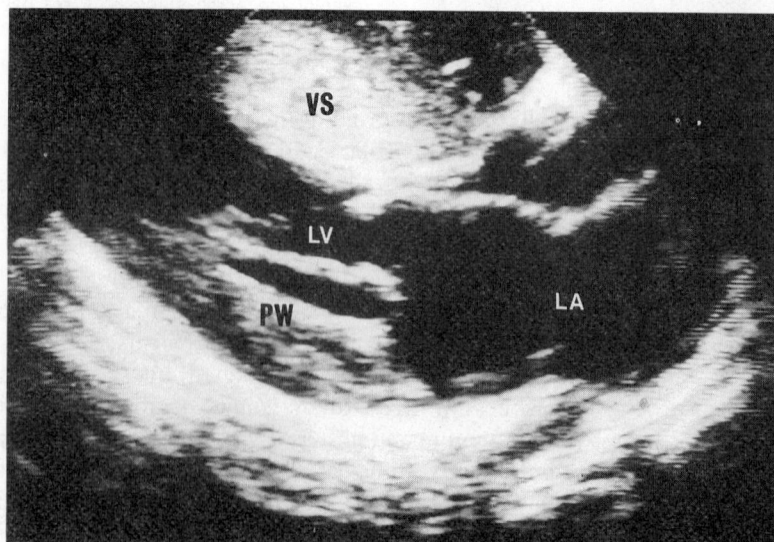

Fig. 63.4. Cross-sectional echocardiography in hypertrophic cardiomyopathy showing the entire interventricular septum (IVS) to be hypertrophied with a small left ventricular cavity (LV) and moderate posterior wall (PW) thickening.

septum to posterior wall. Values > 1.3 or 1.5:1 were initially thought to be specific for the diagnosis of hypertrophic cardiomyopathy,[18] but they may be seen, albeit less commonly, in secondary left ventricular hypertrophy due to a wide variety of causes. Although asymmetrical septal hypertrophy is the most common pattern of hypertrophic cardiomyopathy, in a group of 134 patients with this condition, it was found to be neither sensitive (56%) nor particularly specific (81%); it had a positive predictive value of 83% for hypertrophic cardiomyopathy. However, as the prevalence of the disease is < 1 per 1000 of the normal population, the predictive power of this finding falls to < 3%.[19]

Symmetrical or concentric left ventricular hypertrophy may be found in hypertrophic cardiomyopathy, but this pattern is generally considered to favour the diagnosis of secondary causes of hypertrophy (i.e. aortic stenosis, or hypertension). When left ventricular hypertrophy is caused by aortic stenosis, the severity of hypertrophy correlates with the severity of stenosis and the diagnosis is usually apparent. The finding of moderate or severe hypertrophy in elderly patients, in those with apparently mild hypertension or in highly trained athletes often poses a diagnostic dilemma (see p. 1424). Symmetrical hypertrophy is the predominant pattern in secondary causes, but has a low predictive value in excluding hypertrophic cardiomyopathy. A wall thickness exceeding 2 cm is rarely seen in secondary hypertrophy (11% of patients with aortic stenosis, 8% of hypertensive subjects and no athletes), but occurs in more than one-third of patients with hypertrophic cardiomyopathy.[19] Apical or distal ventricular hypertrophy in hypertrophic cardiomyopathy was first described in Japanese patients,[18] but it also occurs in 10–20% of patients in the West.[17] Hypertrophy may be confined to the apex (associated with symmetrical T-wave inversion on the electrocardiogram), or more commonly it may involve the apex as well as other ventricular regions. This type of hypertrophy does not occur in secondary causes with a pressure overload, or in athletes; it is diagnostic of hypertrophic cardiomyopathy with a sensitivity and specificity approaching 100%. However, apical ventricular hypertrophy is often difficult to diagnose echocardiographically because the apex may be foreshortened by standard ultrasound views and the presence of thrombus may simulate hypertrophy.

LEFT VENTRICULAR FUNCTION

In general, patients with pressure-overload hypertrophy of a concentric nature have values that lie within the normal range for measurements of systolic function, such as ejection fraction or velocity wall motion. This finding is compatible with the homeostatic principle of left ventricular hypertrophy.[20] In some cases, left ventricular ejection may appear to be greater than normal and only in severe longstanding pressure overload does impairment of ejection fraction and cavity dilatation occur. Only exceptionally rarely does cavity dilatation occur in hypertrophic cardiomyopathy and probably never in athletic hypertrophy.

Left ventricular isovolumic relaxation and filling may be measured using digitized M-mode or Doppler echocardiography and contrast or radionuclide angiography. In normal subjects, aortic valve closure (A_2 on the phonocardiogram) precedes minimum left ventricular cavity dimension by 40–60 ms; the onset of mitral valve opening follows immediately afterwards. Isovolumic relaxation (A_2 to mitral valve opening) is largely unrelated to heart rate and may be prolonged in a variety of conditions including left ventricular hypertrophy and coronary artery disease;[21] it is shortened by increasing left atrial pressure[22]. Following mitral valve opening, there is a brief period (120–200 ms) of rapid filling at 450–750 ml/s. This occurs while left ventricular pressure is continuing to fall, there is no atrioventricular pressure difference and coincides with rapid posterior wall thinning. The energy for relaxation and filling is probably generated by elastic forces stored in the myocardium from the previous systole. These diastolic events are complex co-ordinated energy-requiring processes which may be disturbed by ischaemia, fibrosis and changes in myocardial architecture. Diastolic abnormalities are common in left ventricular hypertrophy; they are the most characteristic disturbances of left ventricular function in both primary and secondary forms.[11,21,23]

Delay in mitral valve opening is a manifestation of abnormal and asynchronous relaxation. Left ventricular hypertrophy is characteristically associated with an increased duration of isovolumic relaxation which may be prolonged beyond 100 ms. The delay in mitral valve opening occurs without a change in the relative timing of aortic valve closure and minimum dimension. Therefore, outward motion in some parts of the left ventricle occurs while the mitral valve is still closed. This must be accompanied by inward wall motion elsewhere in the ventricle because the ventricular volume is not changed. This is a period of incoordinate isovolumic relaxation and, in patients with left ventricular hypertrophy, wall motion may be strikingly incoordinate.[21] The peak rate of filling and the peak rate of posterior wall thinning are reduced to below the normal 95% confidence limit in over 50% of patients with left ventricular hypertrophy.[24] The period of early diastolic filling is prolonged and, with the reduction in its rate, it resembles the filling pattern seen in mitral stenosis. The atrial contribution to left ventricular filling may also be accentuated (best demonstrated by Doppler echocardiography or radionuclide angiography). One or more diastolic abnormalities are present in most patients with primary or secondary hypertrophy.

In contrast, athletes who have an equivalent degree of left ventricular hypertrophy to those with aortic stenosis or hypertrophic cardiomyopathy have normal left ventricular diastolic function. Mitral valve opening is normally timed and occurs at minimum dimension, and isovolumic relaxation is of normal duration. The peak rates of filling and posterior wall thinning are normal or accentuated, and the diastolic filling period is often shortened. As these individuals often have a resting bradycardia and only 10–20% of an elongated diastolic period is used for filling, this is presumably a physiological adaptation that allows greater increases in cardiac output during strenuous exercise.[25,26]

ANALYSIS OF MYOCARDIAL TEXTURE

It is possible to derive more information from cross-sectional echocardiography than simply the depth and motion of cardiac structures. The grey-scale intensity gives important clues about the nature of the underlying tissue character.[27] This has been clearly shown in diagnostic ultrasound of the liver, kidney and breast tissues. Simple ultrasound techniques allow for the quantitative assessment of regional echo amplitude and such measurements bear a strong relation to the myocardium collagen content.[28] In normal subjects the values (median pixel count) are low and similar values are found in athletes. In subjects with primary and secondary left ventricular hypertrophy, significantly greater values may be observed. Such changes presumably reflect increased myocardial fibrosis and are strongly associated with a prolongation of isovolumic relaxation, reduced peak rate of filling and an electrocardiographic 'strain' pattern.[26] This method

of investigation may contribute to an understanding of the pathophysiology of left ventricular hypertrophy. The traditional ideas of physiological versus pathological hypertrophy may need to be reconsidered. Physiological hypertrophy in athletes is a simple homeostatic process comprising an increased muscle mass alone whereas pathological hypertrophy is a more complex entity which includes a change in the physical properties of the myocardium.

TREATMENT

Removal of the increased pressure overload usually leads to regression of left ventricular hypertrophy but diastolic function may not recover. Beta-adrenergic blockers may reduce the heart rate thereby allowing a longer time for diastolic filling which is particularly important when diastolic behaviour is abnormal. Beta-adrenergic blockers and calcium antagnoists appear to improve left ventricular filling in patients with hypertrophic cardiomyopathy who show slow filling and to shorten a prolonged isovolumic relaxation time.[29] These actions may have a beneficial effect on symptoms such as breathlessness in patients with left ventricular hypertrophy, but side-effects are common.

In conclusion, left ventricular hypertrophy is a complex process and its physiological form may be differentiated from its pathological form in a variety of ways. Wall thickness should not exceed 2 cm, asymmetrical septal hypertrophy may be seen, but systolic anterior movement of the mitral valve has not been described. The cavity size is normal or increased in athletes and normal or decreased in secondary left ventricular hypertrophy. Systolic function is normal. Athletes, regardless of the degree of left ventricular hypertrophy, have normal diastolic left ventricular function and myocardial texture.

ATHLETE'S HEART

The term 'athlete's heart' is widely used by physicians to describe the cardiovascular effects of long-term training; although this entity is only loosely defined, it should be regarded as a physiological cardiac response. Considerations of athlete's heart should be differentiated from the beneficial effects of moderate occupational or recreational exercise on lowering coronary artery disease risk factors. All forms of exercise increase cardiac output; in particular, endurance sports, such as swimming, running and cycling, demand prolonged periods of high cardiac output at very high cardiac workloads. This leads to a physiological enlargement of the cardiac chambers with an increase in stroke volume and a decrease in heart rate.

Elite or dedicated athletes are a highly selected group of individuals who have outstanding adaptation of skeletal and cardiac muscle. Although Vo_2 max may limit an athlete's ability to achieve competitive status, the limiting factor in whole body exercise may be the capacity of the heart to deliver blood to the active muscles.[30]

PHYSIOLOGY OF CARDIAC ADAPTATION TO EXERCISE

The long-term demand on the heart in athletes may be analogous to pressure or volume overload in disease states. Pressure overload occurs in strength athletes, e.g. weightlifters and shot putters, in whom there are brief increases in cardiac output with greatly increased afterload and systolic blood pressure (values up to 300 mmHg have been recorded) and theoretically this should lead to symmetrical left ventricular hypertrophy.[31,32] Isotonic or endurance sport requires prolonged elevation of cardiac output with little or no increase in afterload; this will result in a volume load upon the heart, which leads to enlargement of the cardiac chambers, especially the left ventricle, and an increased stroke volume.[33] In addition, there is a resting bradycardia and a generalized reduction in heart rate at any level of workload on exercise. The increase in cardiac dimensions may be due to or result from the athlete's bradycardia. The increased myocardial wall stress that would result from increased chamber size is normalized by a moderate increase in wall thickness (Laplace's law, see p. 1415).

The mechanisms of cardiac adaptation are not clear, but they are probably a complicated interaction of biochemical, metabolic and neural factors.

CLINICAL FEATURES

A long period of dedicated athletic training is required for a subject to develop the features of athlete's heart. In subjects who undertake only occasional sporting activity, the cardiac findings described below should be viewed with suspicion because they may reflect a pathological condition, e.g. hypertrophic cardiomyopathy.

The subjects are lean with an increased muscle bulk. The pulse is slow (35–55 beats/min) and there may be an increase in pulse amplitude and systolic blood pressure. The left ventricular cardiac impulse is displaced and may be sustained. Quiet mid-systolic murmurs are not uncommon; third heart sounds and, less commonly, fourth heart sounds may be heard.

INVESTIGATIONS

Electrocardiography

A range of electrocardiographic abnormalities may occur which if discovered at a routine examination may often lead to confusion. More than 50% of athletes have a sinus bradycardia; sometimes rates < 30 beats/min are recorded. Sinus arrhythmia occurs in up to 60% of endurance athletes as compared with about 2% of the normal population (Table 63.1). These changes are attributed to vagotonia and rapidly reverse with the cessation of training.[34] Varying degrees of atrioventricular block may be observed: first degree heart block occurs in up to one-third, Mobitz type I occurs in 10% and Mobitz type II occurs very infrequently (5/12 000); all of these abnormalities reverse on exercise.

The most frequent morphological changes are increased QRS voltages. Electrocardiographic left ventricular hypertrophy (usually measured by $SV_1 + RV_5 > 35$ mV) is seen in up to 85% of athletes (Fig. 63.5). Increased P-wave voltages or notching may also be noticed (Table 63.2).

Abnormalities of repolarization (ST-segment and T-wave changes) are common. ST-segment elevation (V_2–V_4 with J-point elevation) occurs in over 10% of athletes and the frequency of occurrence increases with the intensity of training. ST-segment depression is much less common. The T waves are

Table 63.1. **Electrocardiographic changes in athletes (12-lead and Holter).**[34]

	General population	Athletes
Sinus bradycardia	20%	50–85%
Sinus arrhythmia	2–3%	up to 69%
First degree heart block	> 1%	6–33%
Mobitz type I block	6%	23%
Mobitz type II block	0%	9%

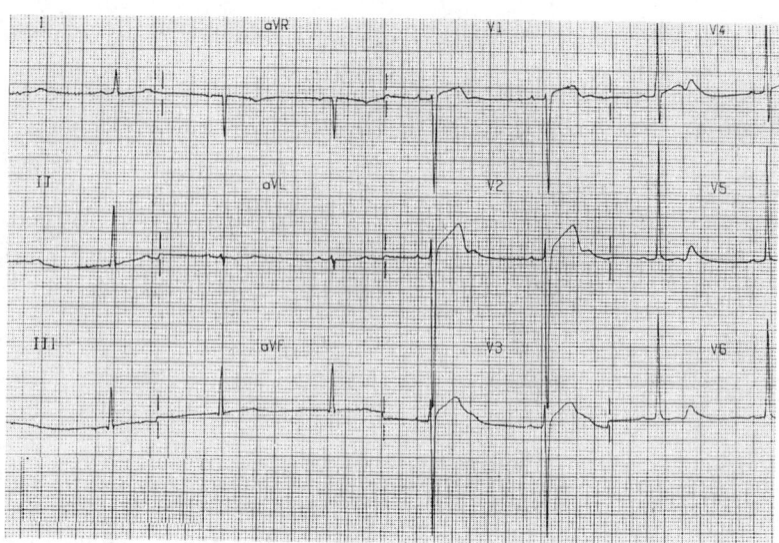

Fig. 63.5. Electrocardiogram in an athlete showing left ventricular hypertrophy, 'J'-point elevation (V_1–V_3) and sinus bradycardia.

often tall and peaked. T-wave inversion (especially biphasic T in V_1–V_5) may be seen fairly frequently (about 10%); if it reverses on exercise, it may be assumed to be physiological. Isolated or symmetrical T-wave inversion is often pathological.[35]

Echocardiography

There are many studies in which comparisons have been made between the echocardiographic left ventricular dimensions and wall thicknesses in athletes and those of normal subjects (see review by Maron[36]). A consistent feature in dynamically trained athletes, when compared with normal age- and sex-matched control subjects, is an increase in left ventricular end-diastolic dimensions (Fig. 63.6). This is a true increase in the cavity size because it is present even after corrections for body surface area have been made.[31,37] Although increase of the end-diastolic dimension is usually within the limits accepted as normal (5.7 cm), occasionally a few athletes (particularly cyclists)[38] have values that lie

outside the normal range.[31] It is probable that the more highly trained a dynamic athlete becomes, especially if training is maintained for many years, the greater the increase in cavity dimension.[38] In dynamic athletes, the posterior wall and septal thicknesses may be within the normal range or mildly elevated but, occasionally, values up to 1.5 cm may be found. Septal hypertrophy of a greater degree than posterior wall hypertrophy (resulting in an increase above the normal septal to posterior wall ratio of 1.3 : 1) may occur in endurance athletes.[35,37] This may also increase as training progresses. As there is an increase in left ventricular cavity size and moderate increases in wall thickness, left ventricular mass is significantly elevated (Fig. 63.7). Values obtained are similar to those found in subjects with moderate-to-severe hypertension and patients with significant aortic stenosis. Increases in left ventricular mass can be detected soon after the onset of training (probably within weeks) and de-conditioning occurs equally rapidly on cessation. The small changes in left ventricular mass seen during conditioning of untrained subjects[39–41] need to be differentiated from the much greater degree of left ventricular hypertrophy seen in elite athletes. This type of more pronounced hypertrophy does not appear to reverse rapidly.

Far fewer studies of power athletes have been performed and the results are conflicting: some workers have demonstrated symmetrical left ventricular hypertrophy without cavity dilatation[32,33,42] whereas the findings of other workers do not appear to support this hypothesis.[31,37,43] It has been suggested that the degree of hypertrophy is inappropriately increased with respect to the level

Table 63.2. Morphological changes of the electrocardiogram in athletes.[34].

	General population	Athletes
ST-Segment elevation	2.4%	10–100%
ST-Segment depression	0%	0–3%
Biphasic T waves	0%	10%
*Electrocardiographic left ventricular hypertrophy	approx. 1	14–85%
Right ventricular hypertrophy	—	18–69%
Right bundle branch block	>1%	13.4%

* $SV_1 + RV_s > 35\,mV$

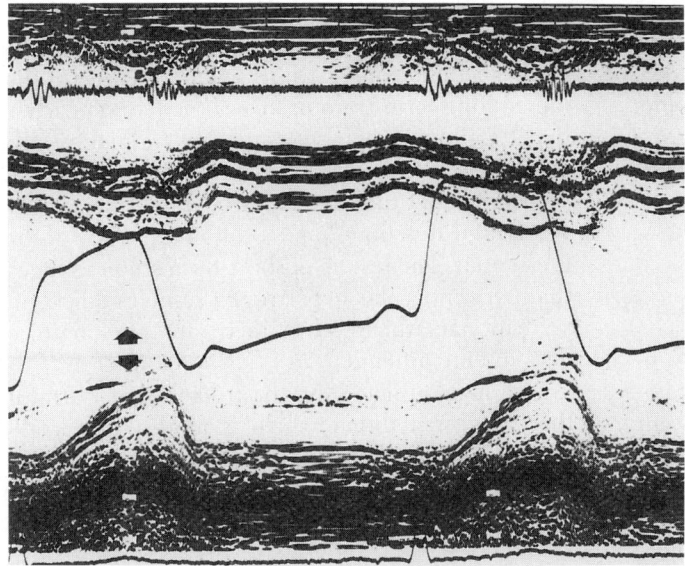

Fig. 63.6. M-Mode echocardiogram in a dynamically trained athlete showing increased cavity size with normal left ventricular function and moderate left ventricular hypertrophy. The arrows indicate 1 cm.

of resting blood pressure and the left ventricular dimension. Another hypothesis is that, when correction is made for the enormous body mass of power athletes, little abnormal hypertrophy can be detected. However, it is rare to find pure power athletes; they tend to belong to a small select group who have a large body mass. Comparisons of matched groups of cyclists and long distance runners confirm that although both runners and cyclists had increased left ventricular diastolic dimensions an increased ratio of wall thickness to left ventricular dimension (representing inappropriate left ventricular hypertrophy) was present only in cyclists. An explanation for these findings is that cyclists have a higher exercising blood pressure than runners[44] which is due to the isometric exercise, performed in the upper portion of the body, of holding the handle bars.

In addition to the factors discussed above, the degree of hypertrophy may vary among individuals undertaking similar training schedules, and there may also be an important hereditary factor.

Left ventricular function

Echocardiographic and radionuclide studies of left ventricular function in athletes have shown that left ventricular ejection fraction or fractional shortening is within or slightly below the normal range, particularly in older athletes. Stroke volume tends to be increased and this is probably explained by the bradycardia and cardiac enlargement. It has been

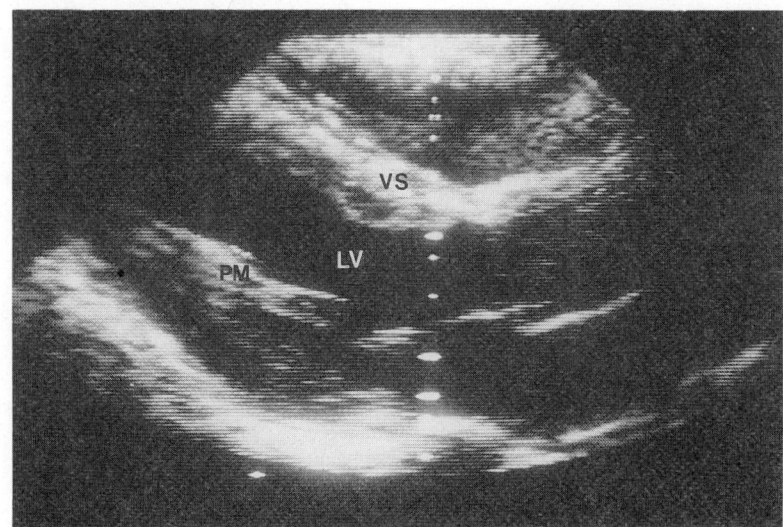

Fig. 63.7. Cross-sectional echocardiogram from a dynamic athlete, parasternal long-axis view, showing left ventricular hypertrophy particularly involving the ventricular septum (VS) and posterior papillary muscle (PM). LV = left ventricle.

suggested that even with physiological hypertrophy left ventricular function may deteriorate during long-term follow-up. Nishimura *et al.*[38] studied professional cyclists and found that the older cyclists had reduced systolic function when compared with the young cyclists. However, the athletic prowess of the older cyclists was not impaired.

DIFFERENTIATION OF ATHLETE'S HEART FROM PATHOLOGICAL HEART DISEASE

Added heart sounds, systolic murmurs, left ventricular hypertrophy, morphological electrocardiographic abnormalities and bradyarrhythmias occur in athletes; they may also be the features of organic heart disease. Sino-atrial disease, hypertrophic cardiomyopathy and valve disease may be simulated, but echocardiography is able to differentiate most of these without difficulty. In addition, diastolic left ventricular function is invariably normal in an athlete's heart (see above).

DANGERS OF TRAINING

Collapse

Collapse is usually due to dehydration and hypovolaemia, especially with hyperpyrexia, in long distance running events; very exceptionally, it may result from myocardial infarction in the presence of normal coronary arteries.

Sudden death

Although each sudden death that occurs during and following exercise is surrounded by considerable publicity, it is extremely rare. Almost all of the cases have an underlying pathological cardiovascular cause, usually hypertrophic cardiomyopathy, coronary artery disease or anomalies of the coronary anatomy.[45]

Chest pain

Chest pain is usually musculoskeletal, but if it is associated with collapse and electrocardiographic changes, especially ST-segment elevation, this may lead to a spurious diagnosis of myocardial infarction.

UNANSWERED QUESTIONS

Epidemiological evidence suggests that moderate exertion has a beneficial effect upon cardiovascular mortality, but there is no such controlled evidence of protection from cardiovascular disease by sustained long-term training. Does the left ventricular hypertrophy following cessation of training resolve and have no sequelae? Studies in older professional cyclists suggest that there may be impairment of left ventricular function[38] and a follow-up study of this is essential. The results of short-term studies suggest that left ventricular hypertrophy resolves quickly in recreational athletes, but there are no long-term data in elite athletes.

Although athlete's bradycardia is not harmful, the sinus arrhythmia which is almost universally present may predispose to systemic emboli;[46] it is possible that it can lead to symptomatic sino-atrial disease in later life which will require pacing.

CONCLUSION

In the last decade, there has been a dramatic increase in the popularity of many forms of sport. This has lead to an increase in the number of individuals presenting to their physicians with the cardiovascular effects of training. An awareness of these cardiovascular changes is vital to ensure that organic heart disease is not spuriously diagnosed. The supposed benefit of exercise training has caused many coronary-prone middle-aged individuals to take up exercise for which they are not adapted; this has led to sudden deaths in a number of cases. Such incidents should not be confused with the cardiovascular effects of training in elite athletes.

REFERENCES

1. Grossman, W. Cardiac hypertrophy: Useful adaptation or pathological process. *Am. J. Med.* 1980; **69**: 576–84.
2. Wikman-Coffelt, J., Parmley, W.W. and Mason, D.T. The cardiac hypertrophy process. *Circ. Res.* 1979; **45**: 697–707.
3. Ford, L.E. Heart size. *Circ. Res.* 1976; **39**: 297–303.
4. Savage, D.D., Abbot, R.D., Paggett, S., Anderson, S.J. and Garrison, R.J. Epidemiologic features of left ventricular hypertrophy in normotensive and hypertensive patients. In: *Cardiac left ventricular hypertrophy.* Boston and The Hague: Martinus Nijoff, 1983, pp. 3–12.
5. Waller, B.F. and Roberts, W.C. Cardiovascular disease in the very elderly. *Am. J. Cardiol.* 1983; **51**: 403–21.
6. Fuster, V., Danielson, M.A., Robb, R.A., Broadbent, J.C., Brown, A.L. Jr and Elveback L.R. Quantitation of left ventricular myocardial fiber hypertrophy and interstitial tissue in human hearts with chronically increased volume and pressure overload.*Circulation* 1977; **55**: 504–8.
7. Moore, G.W., Hutchins, G.M., Bulkley, B.H., Tseng, J.S. and Ki, P.F. Constituents of human ventricular myocardium: tissue hyperplasia accompanying muscular hypertrophy. *Am. Heart J.* 1980; **100**: 610–6.
8. Grossman, W., Jones, D. and McLaurin, L.P. Wall stress and

patterns of hypertrophy in the human left ventricle. *J. Clin. Invest.* 1975; **56**: 56–64.

9. Schwarz, F., Flameng, W., Schaper, J. and Hehrlein, F. Correlation between myocardial structure and diastolic properties of the heart in chronic aortic valve disease. Effects of corrective surgery. *Am. J. Cardiol.* 1978; **42**: 895–903.

10. Marcus, M.L., Doty, D.B., Hiratzka, L.F., Wright, C.B. and Eastham, C.L. Decreased coronary reserve: a mechanism for angina pectoris in patients with aortic stenosis and normal coronary arteries. *N. Engl. J. Med.* 1982; **307**: 1362–6.

11. St John Sutton, M.G., Tajik, A.J., Smith, H.C. and Ritman, E.L. Angina in idiopathic hypertrophic subaortic stenosis: a clinical correlate of regional left ventricular dysfunction: a videometric and echocardiographic study. *Circulation* 1980; **61**: 561–8.

12. Bennett, D.H. and Evans, D.W. Correlation of left ventricular mass determined by echocardiography with vectorcardiographic and electrocardiographic voltage measurements. *Br. Heart. J.* 1974; **36**: 981–7.

13. Einthoven, W., Fahr, G. and deWaart, A. Ueber die Richtung und die manifest Grosse der Potential. *Pflugers Archiv.* 1913; **150**: 275–315.

14. Selzer, A., Naruse, D.Y., York, E. *et al.* Electrocardiographic findings in concentric and eccentric left ventricular hypertrophy. *Am. Heart J.* 1962; **63**: 320–8.

15. Clementy, J. , Bergere, P. and Bricaud, H. Electrocardiogram and vectorcardiogram in the evaluation of left ventricular hypertrophy due to pressure overload. *Eur. Heart J.* 1982; **23**: A37–47.

16. Maron, B.J., Gottdiener, J.S. and Epstein, S.E. Patterns and significance of distribution of left ventricular hypertrophy in hypertrophic cardiomyopathy. *Am. J. Cardiol.* 1981; **48**: 418–28.

17. Shapiro, L.M. and McKenna, W.J. Distribution of left ventricular hypertrophy in hypertrophic cardiomyopathy: A two-dimensional echocardiographic study. *J. Am. Coll. Cardiol.* 1983; **2**: 437–44.

18. Goodwin, J.F. The frontiers of cardiomyopathy. *Br. Heart J.* 1982; **48**: 1–12.

19. Shapiro, L.M., Kleinbenne, A. and McKenna, W.M. The distribution of left ventricular hypertrophy in hypertrophic cardiomyopathy compared to athletes and hypertensives. *Eur. Heart J.* 1985; **6**: 967–74.

20. Spann, J.F., Bove, A.A., Natarajan, G. and Kreulen, T. Ventricular performance, pump function and compensatory mechanisms in patients with aortic stenosis. *Circulation* 1980; **62**: 576–82.

21. Gibson, D.G., Traill, T.A., Hall, R.J.C. and Brown, D.J. Echocardiographic features of secondary left ventricular hypertrophy. *Br. Heart J.* 1979; **41**: 54–9.

22. Mattheos, M., Shapiro, E., Oldershaw, P.J., Sacchetti, R. and Gibson, D.G. Non-invasive assessment of changes in left ventricular relaxation by combined phono-, echo-, and mechanocardiography. *Br. Heart. J.* 1982; **47**: 253–60.

23. Bonow, R.P., Rosing, D.R., Bacharach, S.L., Green, M.V., Kent, K.M., Lipson, L.C., Maron, B.J., Leon, M.B. and Epstein, S.E. Effects of verapamil on left ventricular systolic function and diastolic filling in patients with hypertrophic cardiomyopathy. *Circulation* 1981; **64**: 787–96.

24. Bonow, R.O., Frederick, T.M., Bacharach, S.L., Green, M.V., Goose, P.W., Maron, B.J. and Rosing, D.R. Atrial systole and left ventricular filling in hypertrophic cardiomyopathy. *Am. J. Cardiol.* 1983; **51**: 1386–91.

25. Matsuda, M., Sugishita, Y., Koeseki, S., Ito, I., Akatsuka, T. and Takamatsu, K. Effect of exercise on left ventricular diastolic filling in athletes and non athletes. *J. Appl. Physiol.* 1983; **55**: 323–8.

26. Shapiro, L.M., Moore, R.B., Logan-Sinclair, R.B. and Gibson, D.G. Relation of regional echo amplitude to left ventricular function and the electrocardiogram in left ventricular hypertrophy. *Br. Heart J.* 1984; **52**: 99–105.

27. Logan-Sinclair, R.B., Wong, C.M. and Gibson, D.G. Clinical application of amplitude processing of echocardiographic images. *Br. Heart J.* 1981; **45**: 621–7.

28. Shaw, T.R.D., Logan-Sinclair, R.B., McAnulty, R.J., Surin, C., Heard, B., Laurent, G.J. and Gibson, D.G. Relation between regional echo intensity and myocardial connective tissue in left ventricular disease. *IRCS Med. Sci.* 1982; **10**: 691–2.

29. Hanrath, P., Mathey, D., Kremer, P., Sonntag, F. and Bleifeld, W. Effect of verapamil on left ventricular isovolumic relaxation time and regional left ventricular filling in hypertrophic cardiomyopathy. *Am. J. Cardiol.* 1980; **45**: 1258–64.

30. Saltin, B. Hemodynamic adaptation to exercise. *Am. J. Cardiol.* 1985; **55**: 42.

31. Rost, R. The athletes heart. *Eur. Heart J.* 1982; **3**(Suppl.A): 193–8.

32. Longhurst, J.C., Kelley, A.R., Gonyea, W.J. and Mitchell, J.H. Echocardiographic left ventricular masses in distance runners and weight lifters. *J. Appl. Physiol.* 1980; **48**: 154–60.

33. Morganroth, J., Maron, B.J., Henry, W.L. and Epstein, S.E. Comparative left ventricular dimensions in trained athletes. *Ann. Intern. Med.* 1975; **82**: 521–9.

34. Huston, T.P., Puffer, J.C. and Rodney, W.M. The athletic heart syndrome. *N. Engl. J. Med.* 1985; **313**: 24–9.

35. Oakley, D.G. and Oakley, C.M. Significance of abnormal electrocardiograms in highly trained athletes. *Am. J. Cardiol.* 1982; **50**: 985–9.

36. Maron, B.J. Structural features of the athletic heart as defined by echocardiography. *J. Am. Coll. Cardiol.* 1986; **7**: 190–203.

37. Shapiro, L.M. Physiological left ventricular hypertrophy. *Br. Heart J.* 1984; **52**: 130–5.

38. Nishimura, T., Yamada, Y. and Kawai, C. Echocardiographic evaluation of long-term effects of exercise on left ventricular hypertrophy and function in professional bicyclists. *Circulation* 1980; **61**: 832–40.

39. Shapiro, L.M. and Smith, R.G. Effect of training on left ventricular structure and function: an echocardiographic study. *Br. Heart J.* 1983; **50**: 534–9.

40. Ehsani, A.A., Hagberg, J.M. and Hickson, R.C. Rapid changes in left ventricular dimensions and mass in response to physical conditioning and deconditioning. *Am. J. Cardiol.* 1978; **42**: 52–6.

41. Wieling, W., Borghols, E.A.M., Hollander, A.P., Danner, S.A. and Dunning, A.J. Echocardiographic dimensions and maximum oxygen uptake in oarsmen during training. *Br. Heart J.* 1981; **46**: 190–5.

42. Colan, S.D., Sanders, S.P., MacPherson, D. and Borow, K.M. Left ventricular diastolic function in elite athletes with physiological cardiac hypertrophy. *J. Am. Coll. Cardiol.* 1985; **6**: 545–9.

43. Brown, S., Byrd, J., Jayasinghe, M.D. and Jones, D. Echocardiographic characteristics of competitive and recreational weight lifters. *J. Cardio. Ultrasound.* 1983; **2**: 163–7.

44. Fagard, R., Aubert, A., Staessen, J., Eynde, E.V., Vanhees, L. and Amery, A. Cardiac structure and function in cyclists and runners. Comparative echocardiography study. *Br. Heart J.* 1984; **52**: 124–9.

45. Maron, B.T., Roberts, W.C., McAllister, H.A., Rosing, D.R. and Epstein, S.E. Sudden death in young athletes. *Circulation* 1980; **62**: 218–29.

46. Abdon, N.J., Landin, K. and Johansson, B.W. Athletes bradycardia as an embolising disorder. *Br. Heart J.* 1984; **52**: 660–6.

Chapter 64

Cardiac Tumours

Leonard M. Shapiro

The true incidence of primary cardiac tumours is not known; in autopsy series it ranges from 0.0017 to 0.27%.[1] In comparison with other organs, the heart has a low incidence of primary tumours, possibly due to its motion and static population of myocytes. Despite their rarity, cardiac tumours have been described since the sixteenth century, but only in the 1930s could the diagnosis be made with certainty during life. Much enthusiasm is generated in the diagnosis of primary cardiac tumours because they can masquerade as a variety of much more common cardiac conditions and the possibility of cure by surgical resection.

Metastatic cardiac tumours are much more common and may be found in up to 20% of cases of death from generalized malignancy. The mediastinum is commonly involved by thoracic tumours (especially bronchus and breast), and these spread either via the lymphatics or directly to the heart.[2] In such secondary tumours, the pericardium is often involved initially. Lymphomas, leukaemias and multiple myeloma not infrequently involve the heart with nodular or diffuse infiltration. Few of these present clinically, however.

PATHOLOGY

Both benign and malignant primary cardiac tumours arise from the muscle and connective tissue of the heart. Approximately 75% are benign and the majority of these are myxomas. Other benign cardiac tumours include lipomas, papillary fibroelastomas, rhabdomyomas, fibromas and haemangiomas. The malignant tumours are sarcomas, predominantly rhabdomyosarcoma and angiosarcoma.

MYXOMA

Myxomas are occasionally transmitted as an auto-somal dominant trait although most cases are sporadic.[3] They are usually single, occasionally multiple, of variable size up to 8 cm in diameter and arise in the left atrium much more commonly than in any of the other chambers. Attachment is by a pedicle usually to the interatrial septum in the region of the fossa ovalis (Fig. 64.1). The consistency is gelatinous and polypoid, but they may be firm or even calcified. Histologically, the appearance is one of organized thrombus: uniform, small round cells of polygonal shape are surrounded by a myxomatous stroma.[1,4]

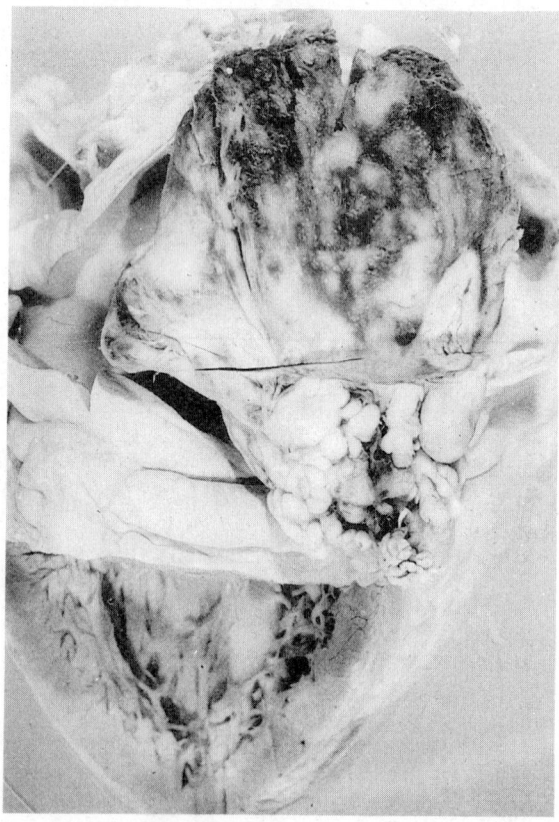

Fig. 64.1. Atrial myxoma showing through the open left atrium. There are islands of mucoid tissue. The tumour is of sufficient mass to obstruct the mitral valve completely.

LIPOMA

Lipomas range in size from 1 to 15 cm and are sessile or intermuscular. The majority are not apparent clinically. Any cardiac chamber or structure may be involved. Histologically, they contain mature fat cells.

RHABDOMYOMA

Rhabdomyomas may be hamartomas. They are the commonest cardiac tumours in children, the majority of whom have tuberose sclerosis.

FIBROMA

Fibromas predominantly occur in the ventricular myocardium of children. They are non-capsulated and resemble fibroids with interlacing bundles of enlongated fibroblasts with connective tissue.

PAPILLOMA

Papillomas are frond-like lesions which may be multiple on the ventricular surfaces of the cardiac valve.

RHABDOMYOSARCOMA

Rhabdomyosarcomas are progressive tumours of striated muscle which usually infiltrate myocardium (especially the right ventricle), but may invade any cardiac chamber (and simulate myxoma) or the pericardium and present with a pericardial effusion.

ANGIOSARCOMA

Angiosarcomas include a variety of tumour types including Kaposi's sarcoma, which is a common finding in patients dying from human immunodeficiency virus and other causes of immunosuppression. There is a male predominance of these tumours, which principally invade the right atrium and interatrial septum. They are necrotic and contain ill-defined vascular spaces and abnormal endothelium.

PATHOPHYSIOLOGY

The effects of the tumour upon its host depend upon its situation and its tendency to obstruct blood flow rather than its histological type. Cardiac tumours obstructing the mitral and tricuspid valves simulate mitral and tricuspid stenosis; polypoid tumours may embolize or give rise to immunological phenomena and invasive tumours mimic myocardial ischaemia or involve the conduction system.

CLINICAL FEATURES

Left atrial myxomas predominantly present with shortness of breath, embolization and syncope; but systemic features may predominate and simulate bacterial endocarditis or systemic lupus erythematosus.[5,6] Right atrial myxomas present with right ventricular failure and pulmonary emboli.[7] Ventricular tumours present with systemic or pulmonary embolization, heart failure or tachy- or bradyarrhythmias.

SYSTEMIC MANIFESTATIONS

The systemic manifestations from a broad array of non-specific findings which include pyrexia, malaise, rash, arthropathy and finger clubbing. These often lead to a clinical diagnosis of bacterial endocarditis or connective tissue disease. The erythrocyte sedimentation rate is frequently raised with a reduced haemoglobin.

EMBOLI

Emboli may arise from thrombus, originating on the surface of the tumour or from the tumour itself. Any type of tumour may embolize, but friable intracavity tumours are particularly liable to do so. Systemic emboli may occlude any major vessel and every effort should be made to recover embolized material and submit this to histological examination.[8] Major pulmonary emboli and secondary cor pulmonale from recurrent emboli may occur and be indistinguishable from venous thrombo-embolism but are extremely rare. Papillomas often present with embolic phenomena without physical signs.

PHYSICAL EXAMINATION

Left atrial myxoma is by far the most frequent tumour seen; mobile pedunculated tumour masses prolapse and partially obstruct the mitral valve. Mitral regurgitation may frequently occur. The signs are of mitral valve disease, which may be intermittent, of sudden onset and related to body position.

The first heart sound is loud and an apical pan-systolic murmur and early diastolic sound (tumour plop) may be heard.[5,6,9] Although this sound does occur later than an opening snap, it may be easily confused with such, especially as a mid-diastolic murmur may follow this sound. In right atrial myxoma, peripheral oedema, hepatomegaly and ascites may be seen. There may be superior vena caval obstruction or gross elevation of the jugular venous pressure with prominent 'a' waves. The 'y' descent may be more rapid than normal.[7] Systolic and diastolic murmurs simulating tricuspid valve disease may be heard and rarely a tumour plop. Occasionally, there are no abnormal physical signs from the heart.[10]

The intracavity component of ventricular tumours may obstruct left ventricular inflow or more commonly left ventricular outflow. This may simulate aortic stenosis, subvalvar aortic stenosis or hypertrophic cardiomyopathy. Intramural spread of tumours may damage the conduction system and lead to complete heart block or produce a variety of atrial and ventricular tachyarrhythmias or impairment of ventricular performance simulating dilated cardiomyopathy or restrictive cardiomyopathy.

Right ventricular tumours also obstruct ventricular inflow and outflow and may present with right heart failure. Both systolic and diastolic murmurs may be heard. The venous pressure is elevated with a prominent 'a' wave and Kussmaul's sign may be evident (Fig. 64.2). Malignant cardiac tumours cannot be readily separated from benign tumours pre-operatively but evidence of local invasion and distant metastasis, bloody pericardial effusion and a rapid increase in heart size suggest malignancy.

DIAGNOSIS AND INVESTIGATION

A high index of clinical suspicion is an important prerequisite for this diagnosis. Cardiac enlargement is frequently demonstrated radiographically and occasional tumour calcification may be observed (Fig. 64.3). Echocardiography has revolutionized the diagnosis of cardiac tumours. Left atrial myxoma was first diagnosed by M-mode echocardiography in 1954, shortly after the introduction of the technique. Cross-sectional echocardiography has improved diagnosis further. The mass is usually well defined and echodense, occasionally with areas of echolucency. The pedicle and its attachments may be visualized (Fig. 64.4). The mobile mass lies within the atrium during systole and prolapses through the valve during diastole (Fig. 64.5). Doppler ultrasound may confirm the presence of valvar obstruction and regurgitation. Computerized tomography or nuclear resonance imaging can also demonstrate the tumour and, in particular, involvement of the pericardium and mediastinum. The echocardiographic differential diagnosis of an intracardiac mass includes vegetations and thrombus as well as tumours. Thrombi usually overlie an area of akinetic myocardium or occur in the fibrillating atria, and are often non-homogeneous immobile masses with a broad base of attachment. Occasionally, however, they are pedunculate and mobile and appear very similar to a myxoma or other tumour. Vegetations are attached to valves or

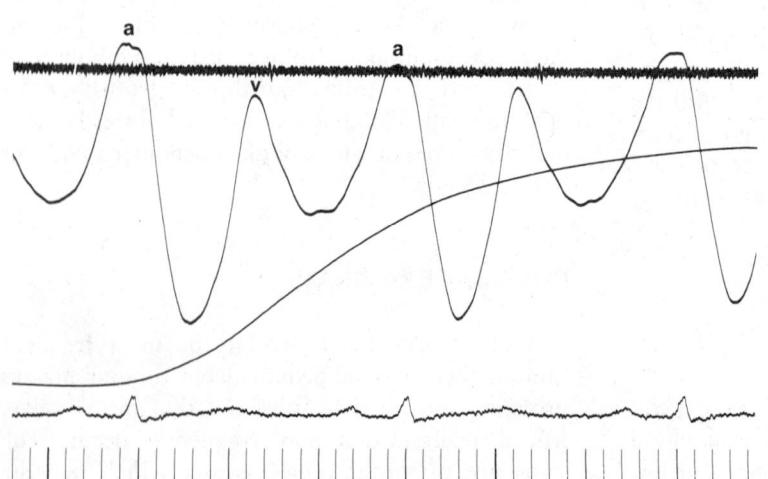

Fig. 64.2. External recording of the jugular venous pulse in a patient with tricuspid valve destruction by intracavity mass. Note the accentuated 'a' wave, which is much more prominent than the 'v' wave.

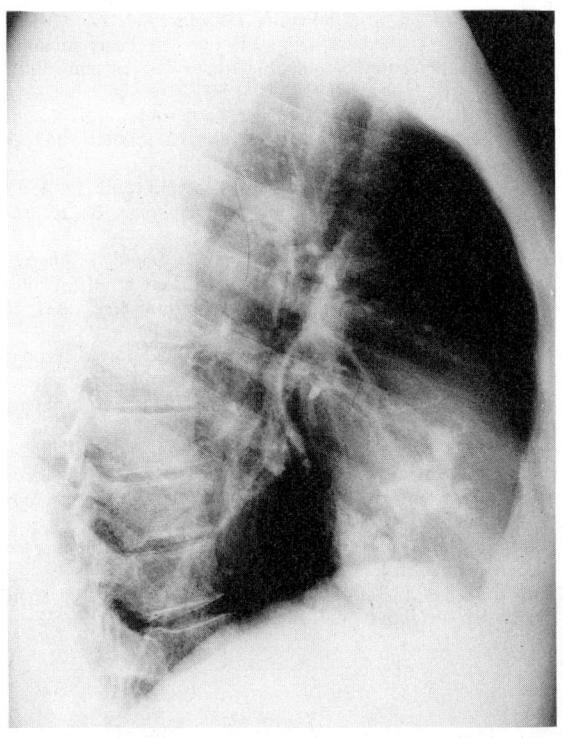

Fig. 64.3. Lateral chest radiograph showing extensive calcification in a benign left ventricular tumour.

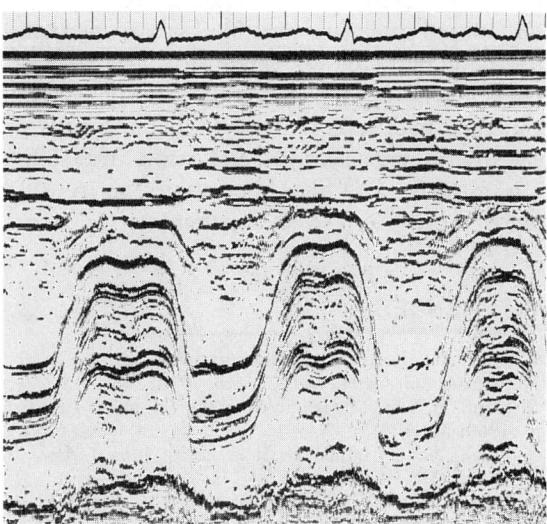

Fig. 64.5. M-Mode echocardiogram showing a left atrial myxoma prolapsing through the mitral valve in diastole.

chordae tendineae. Myxomas usually are mobile with a pedicle and clear site of attachment (Fig. 64.4), and of consistent accoustic properties. Problems may be encountered because intramyocardial tumours appear similar to localized hypertrophy as seen in apical or septal hypertrophic cardiomyopathy. In addition, small tumours, such as mesothelioma, may induce complete heart block by

involving the atrioventricular node but be too small to be detected echocardiographically.

TREATMENT

For most patients who have right or left atrial myxomas, operative excision results in complete cure, although in 1–5% tumour may recur;[12–14] most surgeons advise a wide excision of the base of the tumour to avoid recurrence. Embolization at the time of surgery is a problem and is minimized by gentle handling of the heart and femoro-femoral

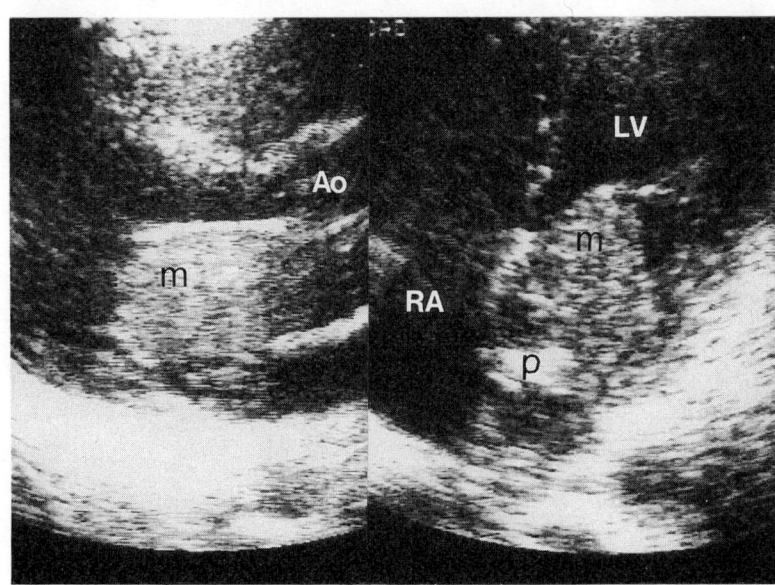

Fig. 64.4. Cross-sectional echocardiogram (parasternal long-axis view, left; apical four-chamber view, right) showing a mobile left atrial myxoma (m) attached by a pedicle (p) to the interatrial septum. Ao, aorta; RA, right atrium; LV, left ventricle.

bypass. Curative surgical excision (of malignant tumours) is often not possible but partial excision may be undertaken for diagnostic purposes and to relieve haemodynamic symptoms. Partial resection combined with radiotherapy or chemotherapy may lead to prolonged survival, and cardiac transplantation may provide the opportunity to resect all malignant tissue in selected patients.

REFERENCES

1. McAllister, H.A. Primary tumours and cysts of the heart and pericardium. *Curr. Prob. Cardiol.* 1979; IV: 1–15.
2. Hanfling, S.M. Metastatic cancer to the heart. *Circulation* 1960; 22: 474–9.
3. Farah, M.G. Familial atrial myxoma. *Ann. Intern. Med.* 1975; 83: 358–61.
4. Hudson, R.E.B. *Cardiovascular Pathology*, Vol. 2. London: Edward Arnold, 1965.
5. Goodwin, J.F. Diagnosis of left atrial myxomas. *Lancet* 1963; i: 464–8.
6. Goodwin, J.F., Stanfield, C.A., Steiner, R.E. *et al.* Clinical features of left atrial myxoma. *Thorax* 1962; 17: 91–110.
7. Massumi, R. Bedside diagnosis of right heart myxomas through detection of palpable tumor shocks and audible plops. *Am. Heart. J.* 1983; 105: 303–7.
8. Silverman, J., Olwin, J.S. and Graettinger, J.S. Cardiac myxomas with systemic embolization. *Circulation* 1962; 26: 99–103.
9. Gershlick, A.H. Leech, G., Mills, P.G. and Leatham, A. The loud first heart sound in left atrial myxoma. *Br. Heart J.* 1984; 52: 403–7.
10. Nihoyannopoulas, P., Veinketesan, P., David, J., Hackett, D., Valantine, H. and Oakley, C.M. Left atrial myxoma: new perspectives in diagnosis of murmur free cases. *Br. Heart J.* 1968; 56: 554–60.
11. Fyke, F.E. III, Seward, J.B., Edwards, W.D. *et al.* Primary cardiac tumors: experience with 30 consecutive patients since the introduction of two-dimensional echocardiography. *J. Am. Coll. Cardiol.* 1985; 5: 1965–73.
12. Hanson, E.C., Gill, C.C., Razavi, M. and Loop, F.D. The surgical treatment of atrial myxomas: clinical experience and late results in 33 patients. *J. Thorac. Cardiovasc. Surg.* 1985; 89: 298–303.
13. Buckley, B.H. and Hutchins, G.M. Atrial myxoma: a fifty year review. *Am. Heart J.* 1979; 97: 639–43.
14. Walton, J.A. Jr, Kahn, D.R. and Willis, P.W. III. Recurrence of a left atrial myxoma. *Am. J. Cardiol.* 1972; 29 872–6.

Chapter 65

Syncope

Richard Sutton

Syncope may be defined as loss of consciousness due to a sudden reduction in cerebral blood flow. It is usually a transient phenomenon, the mechanism of which at cerebral level depends upon the brain cells' need for blood flow carrying those nutrients that provide energy for function.

AETIOLOGY

The causes of syncope are generally considered to be cardiological (Table 65.1) or neurological (Table 65.2). However, a few other conditions must also be considered that cannot readily be classified under either of these categories.

CARDIAC CAUSES

Cardiac causes of syncope may be divided into those that are primarily mechanical and obstructive and those that are primarily disturbances of electrical function. Vascular causes are also largely obstructive in nature.

The majority of the obstructive lesions of the cardiovascular system precipitate syncope during effort when there is an imbalance between the peripheral demand for blood flow in skeletal muscles and the flow that can be delivered by the heart constrained by the obstruction. This is followed by an acute lack of cerebral blood flow and syncope. Obstructive lesions of the cardiovascular system typically include aortic stenosis of all types (supravalvular, valvular and subvalvular), hypertrophic cardiomyopathy, an obstructed prosthetic valve, pulmonary valve and peripheral artery stenosis and tetralogy of Fallot. In tetralogy of Fallot, the problem is enhanced by muscular variability of the calibre of the right ventricular outflow obstruction and by the shunting of blood from the right ventricle to the aorta. Takayasu's disease with its multiple arterial obstructions and pulmonary hypertension may also precipitate syncope by obstruction of blood flow during effort. Pulmonary embolism may

cause syncope, more often at rest than on exercise. In this condition, the mechanism is one of such massive obstruction of the pulmonary arteries as to limit blood flow severely. This may be further compounded by an acute failure of the right ventricle. The presentation of cardiac tamponade is often equally dramatic but the mechanism is dominantly one of external compression of the right heart limiting cardiac output. Cardiac tumours are often pedunculated, the commonest is left atrial myxoma, and may interrupt the circulation intermittently. This picture may be mimicked by a left atrial ball thrombus, a rare complication of rheumatic mitral valve disease with atrial fibrillation. Dissection of the aorta also tends to present at rest in a dramatic and painful manner. The damaged aorta may obstruct aortic flow. Myocardial infarction has been

Table 65.1. The cardiovascular causes of syncope.

1	Cardiac mechanical:	Aortic stenosis
		Hypertrophic cardiomyopathy
		Pulmonary stenosis
		Obstruction of prosthetic valve
		Pulmonary hypertension
		Pulmonary embolism
		Ball thrombus
		Cardiac tumour
		Cardiac tamponade
2	Cardiac electrical:	
	Tachyarryhthmias:	Supraventricular tachycardia
		Ventricular tachycardia
	Bradyarrhythmias:	Sick sinus syndrome
		Atrioventricular block
3	Vascular:	
	Mechanical:	Dissection of the aorta
		Takayasu's disease
		Carotid stenosis
		Vertebrobasilar disease
		Subclavian steal
	Vasospastic:	Migraine
	Intraluminal:	Transient ischaemic attack

Table 65.2. The neurological causes of syncope.

Carotid sinus syndrome
Vasovagal syndrome
Postural or orthostatic hypotension:
    Diabetes mellitus
    Alcohol
    Idiopathic
    Central nervous disorders
    Prolonged bed rest
    Sympathectomy
Glossopharyngeal neuralgia
Cough
Micturition
Defaecation
Deglutition

quoted as a cause of syncope but more recent work suggests that syncope is due to autonomic disturbance, resulting from the pain, or to a complicating arrhythmia. Abnormalities of the cerebrovascular system seldom cause syncope, although they must always be considered. Carotid stenosis usually causes localized central nervous system dysfunction, as does disease of the vertebrobasilar arteries, which is particularly associated with limitation of blood flow to the vestibular apparatus with resulting giddiness (rotational disturbance). The remaining causes involve redistribution of available blood flow away from the cerebral arteries as may occur in subclavian steal, arterial muscular spasm in migraine or temporary occlusion of a cerebral vessel by platelet aggregation, embolism or thrombus.

Venous obstructions are rarely severe enough to limit cardiac output, but the inferior vena caval obstruction that can occur in the supine position in pregnancy may lead to syncope.

Electrical disturbances of cardiac function cause syncope either by a sudden compromise of cardiac efficiency or by its total disruption with either no activity or rapid and completely ineffective activity. Thus, cardiac arrhythmias can be classified as tachyarrhythmias and as bradyarrhythmias, each type being subdivided into those affecting the atria and those affecting the ventricles. It is important to be aware that when cardiac output is compromised by an arrhythmia the presenting features may be modulated by the existence of cerebrovascular disease. Thus, a patient can present cardiac syncope and hemiparesis. The latter manifestation is usually transient but of substantially longer duration than the syncope.

Any atrial tachyarrhythmia including those complicating sick sinus syndrome can lead to syncope. Usually, the faster the conducted atrial rate and the more abnormal the left ventricular function, the more likely it is that syncope will occur. Rates over 200 pulses/min are expected. Ventricular tachycardia is more frequently associated with syncope and fast ventricular rates are more often encountered. Ventricular tachycardia is usually poorly tolerated and may degenerate into ventricular fibrillation. The bradyarrhythmias may be considered to be atrial, all of which are variations of the sick sinus syndrome, and ventricular presenting as defects of atrioventricular conduction. These abnormalities are often transient and may be precipitated by effort where a rising demand in rate leads to fatigue in the affected conduction pathway and resulting asystole. Asystole may also follow the atrial tachyarrhythmias of sick sinus syndrome as the sinus node fails to resume its rhythmic automaticity or the impulse is blocked from reaching the atria and at the same time the autonomic nervous system has affected the atrioventricular node in such a way as to impede its rhythmic escape.

Lastly, syncope in pacemaker patients must be considered. Retrograde atrioventricular conduction may follow ventricular stimulation with resulting atrial contraction during ventricular systole and regurgitation of blood into the pulmonary and systemic veins. This, in turn, leads to ventricular underfilling and occasionally a sufficiently dramatic reduction in cardiac output to cause syncope. Other causes of syncope in pacemaker patients relate to the loss of ventricular capture in pacemaker dependency. This may be caused by inappropriate inhibition of the pacemaker's output, due to electromyographic or electromagnetic interference sensing, by lead fracture, by lead displacement within the ventricle or by a rise in energy requirement for ventricular capture at the electrode–myocardial interface (exit block).

NEUROLOGICAL CAUSES

The neurological causes of syncope are predominantly afflictions of the autonomic nervous system. Central nervous causes of loss of consciousness are numerous and tend to result in prolonged unconsciousness rather than syncope. Some causes especially epilepsy will be discussed under differential diagnosis.

Carotid sinus syndrome is the name given to syncope which is usually typical cardiac syncope and where carotid sinus massage for 6 s results in 3 s or more of asystole and often reproduction of symptoms and where no other cause can be found for syncope. Pure vasodepressor and pure cerebral types of carotid sinus syndrome have been reported but in the author's experience these are extremely rare. However, a vasodepressor component of cardio-inhibitory carotid sinus syndrome is to be expected. Both the lesion and its site in this syndrome are not known. At present, evidence points to the brainstem, in which it is postulated there is excessive 'gain' in the reflex, probably at the level of the vasomotor centre.[1] Recent work has again raised the possibility that minor cardiac pathology at the level of the sinus and atrioventricular nodes might result in local supersensitivity to acetylcholine.[2] Nelson et al.[3] found a high incidence (33%) of inducible monomorphic ventricular tachycardia in patients with apparent carotid sinus syndrome who had additional structural heart disease. These workers postulated that ventricular tachycardia may be the cause of syncope in this subgroup of patients whereas in those who did not have structural heart disease no significant arrhythmias could be induced. Occasionally, the syndrome may seem to be precipitated by a neck tumour. Vasovagal syndrome is the commonest form of syncope. It occurs mainly in young people and is typically associated with warning permitting the sufferer to avoid injury in a fall. Its behaviour is benign and its frequency tends to diminish with age. The condition was first recognized by Sir Thomas Lewis,[4] and was later investigated intensively by Barcroft and others,[5] who showed that the vasodilatation in this syndrome occurs in skeletal muscles in contrast to the splanchnic venodilatation which occurs with carotid sinus massage. Subsequent investigation was aimed at revealing circulatory control mechanisms by study of the vasovagal reaction. Jarisch[6] studying animals, and later Sharpey-Schafer,[7] studying human beings, suggested that the trigger for vasovagal syncope arises from baroreceptors in the left ventricle, although following studies of vasovagal syncope during cardiac catheterization by Glick and Yu,[8] it is suggested that a rise in systemic arterial pressure is the trigger involving arterial baroreceptors. However, the study of Glick and Yu was limited: all reactions took place during instrumentation and in the supine position. Elegant studies by Epstein and co-workers[9] confirmed the vasodilatation in skeletal muscles with accompanying venoconstriction in the skin.

In 1957, Weissler et al.[10] examined some therapeutic approaches, but other workers did not emphasize this aspect of vasovagal syncope until the 1980s when further studies of unexplained syncope revealed that in a significant proportion of patients the cause remained unexplained despite the use of sophisticated diagnostic techniques. Interest is again focused on vasovagal syncope as having a role in the patients who are not diagnosed. Head-up tilt testing to 60° with footplate support, used since the 1920s by physiologists for investigation of the circulation, is now used by clinicians to reveal a variant of vasovagal syncope that occurs in older patients without warning and is therefore frequently associated with injury, called the malignant vasovagal syndrome.[11] These investigations have shown that in a small group of patients, 'unexplained' syncope can be explained by the occurrence of a vasovagal reaction in about two-thirds; more than half of these patients have cardio-inhibition as well as vasodepression. Hormonal changes in vasovagal syndrome have been studied[12] and rises in the levels of adrenaline, vasopressin and angiotensin II occur during phase I of the syncope (as defined by Epstein et al.:[8] gradually falling arterial pressure prior to circulatory collapse) and a rise in the level of pancreatic polypeptide occurs after the onset of phase II. It is possible that certain hormonal changes pre-set left ventricular baroreceptors before they are finally triggered by falling left ventricular volume and possible mechanical stimulation by obliteration of the cavity in systole.

Postural (orthostatic) hypotension occurs in autonomic neuropathies. The most frequently occurring autonomic neuropathies are those of diabetes mellitus and alcohol. There is usually no bradycardia or there may be a failure of the normal slight tachycardia that occurs on adoption of the erect posture. Over and above this lack of tachycardia, there is a failure of the normal autonomic adjustments to the erect posture. A fall in arterial pressure and syncope occur within a few minutes of standing, unlike vasovagal syndrome in which head-up tilting is necessary for more than 20 min and for 1 h to include all cases. Tilt testing, however, may still be valuable in these conditions and in the rare idiopathic dysautomonias such as the Bradbury–Eggleston syndrome,[13] the Shy-Drager syndrome,[14] which appear to be very similar entities, and the familial Riley–Day syndrome.[15] Other neurological conditions may be associated with postural hypotension, including multiple sclerosis, Parkinson's disease, Wernicke's encephalopathy, syringomyelia, demyelinating diseases, brainstem lesions of all pathologies, tabes dorsalis and pernicious anaemia. In addition, both 'detraining' of the autonomic nervous system, which occurs during prolonged bed rest, and abnormal vasomotor control, which may be seen after sympathectomy, may be associated with postural hypotension.

Another group of paroxysmal autonomic disturbances, which is uncommon and poorly investigated, may overlap with vasovagal and carotid sinus syndromes and comprises cough, deglutition, micturition and defaecation syncope and glossopharyngeal neuralgia. In these cases, the act of coughing, swallowing, etc., involves alteration of autonomic control which becomes unbalanced leading to a fall in arterial pressure. Glossopharyngeal neuralgia perhaps is most closely related to carotid sinus syndrome because in both conditions afferent impulses are carried to the brainstem along the glossopharyngeal nerve, and a local tumour has been the trigger for glossopharyngeal syndrome in some cases;[16] moreover, this syndrome has been shown to be associated with sinus arrest and atrioventricular block.[17]

Finally, a number of conditions defy classification into cardiological and neurological categories. These include hyperventilation, hysteria, hypoglycaemia (due to tumour of the islets of Langerhans or drug induced) and conditions induced by drugs that affect autonomic nervous control of the circulation, for example, ganglion-blocking agents, cause arrhythmias, for example, digitalis toxicity giving rise to atrioventricular block or the pro-arrhythmic effect of anti-arrhythmic drugs causing ventricular tachy-arrhythmias, or cause a metabolic disturbance, for example, diuretic induced hypokalaemia. Rarely, phaeochromocytoma, serotonin-secreting tumours or hyperbradykininaemia may lead to syncope.

PRESENTATION

By definition, syncope is of sudden onset and brief duration. However, there are subtle differences which can be detected by careful history-taking from both the patient and an observer of the episode. Cardiovascular obstructive syncope tends to occur on exertion. Cardiac arrhythmic syncope is almost devoid of warning, particularly if the rhythm is bradycardiac: palpitation may be perceived in cases of tachycardia, especially if it is supraventricular. Carotid sinus syndrome has almost no warning, contrary to the impression given by the initial report,[18] and many other subsequent reports, that tight collars and head-rotation are triggers. Vasovagal syndrome in its usual form has a clear pattern,

which has been beautifully described by Lewis[4] and Wayne.[19] Predisposing factors are being out of condition or in ill-health, fatigue, fasting, stuffy rooms, youth, emotion, sight of blood and other medical acts, and pain; the features of an attack are dizziness, nausea, blurring of vision, yawning, pallor, sweating, slow deep respiration, lack of pupillary dilatation, small volume or absent pulse and duration of about 5 min, but up to hours for full recovery. Lewis[4] observed that attacks whilst lying down are very rare, and lack of warning is also rare. However, Lewis's[4] assumption that incontinence and epileptiform convulsions do not occur was not correct.

Within a few minutes of an attack of syncope, the patient typically feels orientated and reasonably well, except for those patients in whom vasodepression is an important component of the syncope, i.e. those with the vasovagal or carotid sinus syndromes. The patient may remain unwell for hours or occasionally completely unconscious for hours leading the author to coin the name hibernation syndrome.[20] Prolonged unconsciousness, bradycardia and hypotension are the features of this syndrome.

History from an observer of syncope is invaluable. In arrhythmic cardiac syncope (Adams–Stokes attack[21]), the patient will be seen to be pallid and, if the attack continues for about 60 s, cyanosed; on recovery, the patient has a bright red flush. If the attack extends into a second minute, incontinence and epileptiform seizures are likely to occur; respiration continues but may be laboured. Estimation of the duration of syncope by observer or patient is likely to be unreliable. The observer can also comment on any visible signs of warning of the attack and the rapidity of re-orientation of the patient afterwards. Patients should be very closely questioned concerning injuries that they may have sustained. Patients who have either vasovagal or carotid sinus syndromes remain pallid for some minutes or hours afterwards and no skin flush is seen. Cardiac syncope is a very frightening symptom and once relieved a sense of well-being and confidence is experienced. In some cases, a total loss of consciousness may not occur but the patient feels that it is imminent; this is called dizziness or pre-syncope. It is a 'floating' phenomenon or a blurring or greying of vision. Rotation is not experienced as part of this symptom. If rotation is experienced, the symptom is giddiness or vertigo which is rarely part of syncope and may occur only if there is localized arterial obstruction in the supply to the vestibular apparatus.

Occasionally, a patient may suffer neurological deficit after syncope which almost always resolves but may take several days to do so. Such features have been described in the sick sinus, carotid sinus and vasovagal syndromes.[11,20] They are assumed to depend largely upon localized cerebrovascular disease, but embolic phenomena coincident with syncope have not been excluded.

Physical examination of syncopal patients may reveal that conditions that are common and easy to diagnose, such as atrioventricular block, an obstructive cardiovascular lesion or gross neurological disturbances, but often there are no abnormal findings.

INCIDENCE

The incidence of syncope is difficult to ascertain because so often it is not reported to a physician and, also, few studies have been performed to assess its contribution to emergency presentations. Up to 30% of apparently healthy adults experience syncope at least once in their lives.[22,23] Over a 4-year period, 121 patients were admitted to the medical services of the University of Pittsburgh for investigation of syncope;[24] 198 (0.8%) of 25 000 emergency room presentations in 1 year in Boston were syncopal.[25] The contributions of the various causes of syncope are even more difficult to assess but most authors agree that vasovagal syncope is the most common: 58% of syncopal patients seen at the Cleveland Cinic over 12 years[19] and 40% in the Boston series.[25] Estimates of the number of these patients who have no diagnosis after detailed investigation vary with the thoroughness of investigation. Excessive investigation was criticized by Kapoor et al.[24] on the basis of a poor cost–benefit ratio. Bloomfield and Miller[26] found as many as 50% of their patients remained undiagnosed.

INVESTIGATION

After full history and physical examination, routine investigations such as the electrocardiogram, chest radiograph and haematology and biochemistry may be ordered. If there are suggestions of a neurological cause at this stage, a neurological consultation is advised which may lead to the performance of an electroencephalogram and computerized tomographic brain scan. However, if a cardiovascular lesion is suggested, appropriate cardiological investigations, such as echocardiography and cardiac catheterization, may be indicated. When neither cardiac nor neurological lesions are obvious and the electrocardiogram is normal or non-diagnostic, 24-h Holter monitoring for one or more periods is the next logical step. This approach may fail to demonstrate the cause of symptoms, the most common reason being the lack of symptoms during the monitoring period. Occasionally, an exercise stress test may precipitate an arrhythmia. Finally, it is necessary to obtain a negative result on carotid sinus massage before the patient can be declared to have unexplained syncope. Two further investigations have been shown to be of value: electrophysiological studies[24,25,27–33] and head-up tilting.[11] The eleven studies quoted comprised 616 patients; electrophysiological study was considered diagnostic in 328 (53%), in whom the induced abnormality was commonly monomorphic ventricular tachycardia and the majority of patients with positive electrophysiological study also had evidence of structural heart disease. There is greater controversy over the use of intravenous drugs to unmask latent conduction defects after electrophysiological study has proved negative; the reliability of this technique has yet to be fully assessed. Of the available anti-arrhythmic drugs, ajmaline has been the most widely used, because it is the least unreliable, and is the subject of a recent report.[37] The author has found flecainide to be the most valuable drug because it combines depression of the sino-atrial node with delay in His–Purkinje conduction in susceptible subjects.[38] However, in none of the studies has a sufficient number of patients been followed for a sufficient length of time for the results to be conclusive.

After all these investigations, some patients may remain undiagnosed.

RECURRENCE OF SYNCOPE

When the cause of syncope is a cardiovascular lesion or a bradycardia that can be readily diagnosed, appropriate treatment usually completely relieves the symptom. All follow-up studies of unexplained syncope indicate that the syncope recurs irrespective of whether it is finally diagnosed and treated appropriately or it remains undiagnosed; however, results in the former group are much more favourable and reported failures occur most often in patients who have not taken medication. In many reports, repeated electrophysiological study to assess drug efficacy has been advised.[27–34] When the data from these reports are pooled, they indicate a recurrence rate of 35% when electrophysiological study was negative over a follow-up of 22.4 months, whereas recurrence after positive electrophysiological study, mainly for ventricular tachycardia, with the majority of patients receiving anti-arrhythmic treatment, was 18% over a follow-up of 24.8 months. Use of the non-invasive technique of signal-averaging of the surface electrocardiogram may predict the likelihood of ventricular tachycardia by identification of late potentials.[38] These figures support the use of electrophysiology study in the investigation and treatment of unexplained syncope but none of these studies used tilt testing. It appears that up to two-thirds of the remaining patients who are undiagnosed by conventional methods and electrophysiology study may be shown to have malignant vasovagal syndrome and possibly half of these may be successfully treated by dual chamber cardiac pacing. When the reason for syncope is obvious on conventional testing, the symptoms can usually be controlled; however, there is a small but clinically significant group of patients who have recurrent syncope after pacing. Full investigation is justified in this group because the syncope is likely to be due either to pacemaker syndrome (atrial contraction during ventricular systole)[39] or to a detectable fault in the pacing system. However, the possibilities of vasovagal syndrome or ventricular tachycardia should not be ignored and tilt testing and electrophysiological study may be necessary.

DIFFERENTIAL DIAGNOSIS

The main challenge to the clinician in the differential diagnosis of syncope is its separation from epilepsy. There is considerable overlap between the two presentations. Again, the value of careful history-taking from patient and observer must be stressed.

Epilepsy offers a very transient warning to the sufferer. Although this is also true of the classic Adams–Stokes attack, it may not be true of tachyarrhythmias, in which there may be palpitation, and of vasovagal syndrome, in which there may be nausea. If the patient relates a rushing noise in the head or a feeling of falling backwards, the attack is most likely to be cardiac. Episodes of pre-syncope may accompany syncope and are unlikely to occur in a patient with epilepsy.

During the attacks, pallor is an invariable feature of cardiac syncope but not of epilepsy. Tongue-biting although not invariable in epilepsy is almost never encountered in syncope. Other features of epilepsy such as pre-ictal amnesia, convulsion and urinary or faecal incontinence may also occur in syncope. In recovery from an attack, orientation is the rule in syncope whereas it is usually impaired in epilepsy for a considerable period. Autonomic disturbances which have a significant vasodepressor component are exceptions to this rule. A medical or paramedical observer may notice a slow or absent pulse. Although the probability of such an observation being made is very low, if it is available, such information cannot be ignored, even in the presence of completely negative investigations, when therapy is determined. It is noteworthy that syncope very rarely occurs during sleeping hours whereas epilepsy may. The only syncope that can occur more often at night than during the day is in a pacemaker patient where the output energy is close to the stimulation threshold. Diurnal variation of threshold is such that the highest levels are experienced during sleeping hours, resulting in a loss of capture when threshold exceeds output. Persistence of a neurological deficit after an attack often leads to a neurological referral but it is important to be aware of cardiogenic neurology.[20] It is also important to be aware of cardiogenic orthopaedics: all too often the patient with a fracture is not questioned about the reason for the fall. Physical examination and investigation may be helpful in the differential diagnosis, but not infrequently the clinician is left after this with a few borderline abnormalities and a decision with regard to treatment mainly to be made on the history. For instance, the electroencephalogram is often slightly abnormal in patients with cardiovascular disease leading to difficulty in interpretation. Drop attacks are frequently confused with syncope. They may be defined as loss of postural tone without loss of consciousness. Their aetiology is obscure. They do not require cardiological investigation or treatment.

MORTALITY

Some cardiovascular causes of syncope, such as aortic stenosis, dissection of the aorta and pulmonary embolism, carry a high mortality. When the picture is clearly one of ventricular tachycardia and appropriate treatment is not given, the mortality is also high. When syncope is more difficult to diagnose and a clear cause is not evident on routine testing, mortality can be as high as 15.5%[40] or 30.6%.[24] Some conditions causing syncope, however, are relatively benign. The mortality of carotid sinus syndrome[1] and even of the malignant variety of the vasovagal syndrome is quite low. Vasovagal syndrome, however, must not be considered as being totally benign and may be the cause of several sudden unexpected deaths; which perhaps equate to Samuel Pepys' record of the weekly bills of mortality published by the Parish Clerks Company in London[22] in the seventeenth century. These lists contain entries such as 'found dead in the street', 'suddenly', 'died of fright' and 'broken heart'.[41]

TREATMENT

The treatment of syncope is largely that of the underlying cause and an appropriate guide to treatment will be found in the sections of this book that deal with each cause. However, certain presentations require specific mention here. The first of these is an appraisal of the need for treatment in patients who have bundle branch block or bifascicular block. In the early 1970s, when the hemiblocks were first recogized[42] and intracardiac electrophysiology with its ability to show delays in His–Purkinje conduction had been introduced, workers were enthusiastic about the possibility of being able to predict from the electrocardiogram and electrophysiology study the need for pacing to prevent syncope.[43] By the mid 1970s after further study, it was realized that greater scepticism should be exercised over the ability of these methods of assessment to predict future developments in conduction system pathology; Dhingra et al.[44] suggested that only patients with syncope and documented serious bradyarrhythmia required pacing. In a later paper, Dhingra and colleagues[45] reported greater predictive accuracy from electrophysiology study by observation of prolongation of the HV interval during rapid atrial pacing in the absence of Wenckebach periodicity at the atrioventricular node. Although they accepted that this finding is rare (15 of 496 patients), two-thirds of the patients in whom it occurred sustained a major morbid event within the 3.5 years of follow-up. Scheinman and co-workers[46] attempted to subdivide the electrophysiology study findings according to severity; in a study of 313 patients, they concluded that HV intervals > 70 ms and especially those > 100 ms were an independent risk factor for progression to high-grade atrioventricular block. Although some of their patients were paced and experienced symptomatic improvement, these patients did not survive for longer than those who were not paced. Emphasis was also placed on appreciation of other causes of syncope in these patients than that of progression to complete block. Ezri et al.[47] stressed the importance of ventricular tachycardia; Morady et al.[48] confirmed this and showed the value of anti-arrhythmic treatment. Thus, if bundle branch block exists in a syncopal patient the conclusion that progression of atrioventricular block is the cause is not justified, but with marked prolongation of HV interval the insertion of a pacemaker is likely to be symptomatically beneficial.

The treatment of youthful vasovagal syndrome is to give an explanation of the problem, its mechanism and its predisposing factors to the patient and also, if possible, to the patient's spouse. It will often be possible for a patient with the help of their spouse to abort an attack by seeking fresh air or lying down. A spouse may recognize the early features of an attack before the patient does. No other treatment is necessary and in the author's experience tilt testing along clinical lines (60° head-up using a footplate) is not helpful.

Treatment of carotid sinus syndrome is most successfully accomplished by use of dual chamber pacing[1] because in this condition the sudden onset of asystole in combination with vasodepression requires atrioventricular stimulation to maximize the falling venous return. Moreover, these patients almost always have normal conduction systems with the ability to conduct a ventricular stimulus retrogradely. This occurrence could not be more adverse. A similar set of problems exists in the cardio-inhibitory malignant vasovagal syndrome, in which dual chamber pacing is also required.[11] The author has been able to document by means of tilt testing malignant vasovagal syndrome in two patients paced ventricularly who had continued syncope. If it proves impossible to achieve a diagnosis in a syncopal patient but evidence points to either atrioventricular block or an autonomic disturbance dual chamber pacing is advised. This advice also applies when pacing is required, albeit rarely, in glossopharyngeal neuralgia, cough syncope, etc.

Treatment of pacemaker syndrome that leads to syncope or pre-syncope demands an up-grade to dual chamber pacing.

REFERENCES

1. Morley, C.A. and Sutton, R. Carotid Sinus Syndrome (Editorial Review). *Int. J. Cardiol.* 1984; **6**: 287.
2. Kaseda, S. and Zipes, D.P. Vagal denervation of canine sinus and atrioventricular nodes creates supersensitive response to Acetylcholine. *J. Am. Coll. Cardiol.* 1988; **11**: 39A
3. Nelson, S.D., Kou, W.H., De Buitleir, M., Di Carlo, L.A. Jr and Morady, F. Value of programmed ventricular stimulation in presumed carotid sinus syndrome. *Am. J. Cardiol.*1987; **60**: 1073.
4. Lewis, T. Vasovagal syncope and the carotid sinus mechanism. *Br. Med. J.* 1932; **1**: 873.
5. Barcroft, H., Edholm, O.G., McMichael, J. and Sharpey-Schafer, E.P. Post haemorrhagic fainting. *Lancet* 1944; **i**: 489.
6. Jarish, A. Vasovagal syncope. *Z. Kreisl. Forsch.* 1941; **23**: 267.
7. Sharpey-Schafer, E.P. Syncope. *Br. Med. J.* 1956; **1**: 506.
8. Epstein, S.E., Stampfer, M. and Beiser, G.D. Role of capacitance and resistance vessels in vasovagal syncope. *Circulation* 1968; **37**: 524.
9. Glick, G. and Yu, P.N. Hemodynamic changes during spontaneous vasovagal reactions. *Am. J. Med.* 1963; **34**: 42.
10. Weissler, A.M., Warren, J.V., Estes, E.H. Jr, McIntosh, H.D. and Leonard, J.J. Vasodepressor syncope. Factors influencing cardiac output. *Circulation* 1957; **15**: 875.
11. Kenny, R.A., Bayliss, J., Ingram, A. and Sutton, R. Head-up tilt: a useful test for investigating unexplained syncope *Lancet* 1986; **ii**: 1352.
12. Sander-Jensen, K., Secher, N.H., Astrup, A., Christensen, N.J., Giese, J., Schwartz, T.W., Warberg, J. and Bie, P. Hypotension induced by passive head-up tilt: endocrine and circulatory mechanisms. *Am. J. Physiol.* 1986; **251**: R742.
13. Bradbury, S. and Egglestone, C. Postural hypotension: a report of three cases. *Am. Heart J.* 1925; **1**: 73.
14. Shy, G.M. and Drager, G.A. A neurological syndrome associated with orthostatic hypotension. *Arch. Neurol.* 1960; **2**: 511.
15. Riley, C.M., Day, R.L., Greeley, D.M. and Longford, W.E. Central autonomic dysfunction with defective lacrimation: report of 5 cases. *Pediatrics* 1949; **3**: 468.
16. Dykman, T.R., Montgomery, F.B., Gerstenberger, P.D., Zieger, H.E., Clutter, W.E. and Cryer, P.E. Glossopharyngeal neuralgia with syncope secondary to tumour: treatment and pathophysiology. *Am. J. Med.* 1981; **71**: 165.
17. Kong, Y., Heyman, A., Entman, M.L. and McIntosh, H.D. Glossopharyngeal neuralgia associated with bradycardia, syncope and seizures. *Circulation* 1964; **30**: 109.
18. Weiss, S. and Baker, J.P. The carotid sinus reflex in health and disease: its role in the causation of fainting and convulsions. *Medicine* 1933; **12**: 297.
19. Wayne, H.H. Syncope: physiological considerations and an analysis of the clinical characteristics in 510 patients. *Am. J. Med.* 1961; **30**: 418.
20. Sutton, R. and Perrins, J. *Cerebral manifestations of episodic cardiac dysrhythmias.* New Jersey: Exerpta Medica, 1978, p. 174,
21. Stokes, W. Observations on some cases of permanently slow pulse. *Dublin Q.J. Med. Sci.* 1846; **2** : 73.
22. Dermskian, G. and Lamb, S.E. Syncope in a population of healthy adults: incidence, mechanisms and significance. *JAMA* 1958; **168**: 1200.
23. Murdoch, B.D. Loss of consciousness in healthy South African men: incidence, causes and relationship to EEG abnormality. *S. Afr. Med. J.* 1980; **57**: 771.
24. Kapoor, W.N., Karpf, M., Maher, Y., Miller, R.A. and Levey, G.S. Syncope of unknown origin: the need for a more cost-effective approach to its diagnostic evaluation. *JAMA* 1982; **247**: 2687.

25. Day, S.C., Cook, E.F., Funkenstein, H. and Goldman, L. Evaluation and outcome of emergency room patients with transient loss of consciousness. *Am. J. Med.* 1982; **73**: 15.
26. Bloomfield, P. and Miller, H. Permanent pacing. *Br. Med. J.* 1987; **295**: 741.
27. DiMarco, J.P., Garan, H., Harthorne, J.W. and Ruskin, J.N. Intracardiac electrophysiological techniques in recurrent syncope of unknown cause. *Ann. Intern. Med.* 1981; **95**: 542.
28. Gulamhusein, S., Naccarelli, G., Ko, P.T., Prystowsky, E.N., Zipes, D.P., Barnett, H.J.M., Heger, J.J. and Klein, G.J. Value and limitations of clinical electrophysiological study in assessment of patients with unexplained syncope. *Am. J. Med.* 1982; **73**: 700.
29. Hess, D.S., Morady, F. and Scheinman, M.M. Electrophysiological testing in the evaluation of patients with syncope of undetermined origin. *Am. J. Cardiol.* 1982; **50**: 1309.
30. Akhtar, M., Shenasa, M., Denker, S., Gilbert, C.T. and Rizwi, N. Role of cardiac electrophysiological studies in patients with unexplained recurrent syncope. *PACE* 1983; **6**: 192.
31. Morady, F., Stein, E., Schwartz, A., Hess, D., Bhandari, A., Sung, R.J. and Scheinman, M.M. Longterm follow-up of patients with recurrent unexplained syncope evaluated by electrophysiological testing. *J. Am. Coll. Cardiol.* 1983; **2**: 1053.
32. Olshansky, B., Mazuz, M. and Martins, J.B. Significance of inducible tachycardia in patients with syncope of unknown origin: a long term follow-up. *J. Am. Coll. Cardiol.* 1985; **5**: 216.
33. Doherty, J.U., Pembrook-Rogers, D., Grogan, E.W., Falcone, R.A., Buxton, A.E., Marchlinski, F.E., Cassidy, D.M., Kienzle, M.G., Almendral, J.M. and Josephson, M.E. Electrophysiologic evaluation and follow-up characteristics of patients with recurrent unexplained syncope and presyncope. *Am. J. Cardiol.* 1985; **55**: 703.
34. Teichman, S.L., Felder, S.D., Matos, J.A., Kim, S.G., Waspe, L.E. and Fisher, J.D. The value of electrophysiologic studies in syncope of undetermined origin: report of 150 cases. *Am. Heart J.* 1985; **110**: 469.
35. Reiffel, J.A., Wang, P., Bower, R., Bigger, J.T. Jr, Livelli, F. Jr, Fernck, K., Gliklich, J. and Zimmerman, J. Electrophysiological testing in patients with recurrent syncope: are results predicted by prior ambulatory monitoring? *Am. Heart J.* 1985; **110**: 1146.
36. Winters, S.L., Stewart, D. and Gomes, J.A. Signal averaging of the surface QRS complex predicts inducibility of ventricular tachycardia in patients with syncope of unknown origin: a prospective study. *J. Am. Coll. Cardiol.* 1987; **10**: 775.
37. Kaul, U., Dey, D., Narula, J., Malhotra, A.K., Talwar, K.K. and Bhatia, M.L. Evaluation of patients with bundle branch block and "unexplained syncope": a study based on comprehensive electrophysiologic testing and ajmaline stress. *PACE* 1988; **11**: 289.
38. Vardas, P., Travill, C., Bayliss, J., Williams, T. and Sutton, R. Intravenous administration of flecainide as a stress test for syncopal patients with normal electrophysiology. *PACE* 1987; **10**: A514.
39. Kenny, R.A. and Sutton, R. Pacemaker syndrome. *Br. Med. J.* 1986; **293**: 902.
40. Silverstein, M.D., Singer, D.E., Mulley, A.G., Thibault, G.E. and Barrett, O. Patients with syncope admitted to medical intensive care units. *JAMA* 1982; **248**: 1185.
41. Pepys, S. Diary 1660–1669. Magdalene College, Cambridge.
42. Rosenbaum, M.B., Elizari, M.V., Lazzari, J.O. *The Hemiblocks.* Oldsmar, Florida: Tampa Tracings, 1970.
43. Scheinman, M., Weiss, A. and Kinkel, F. His bundle recordings in patients with bundle branch block and transient neurologic symptoms. *Circulation* 1973; **43**: 322.

44. Dhingra, R.C., Denes, P., Wu, D., Chuquimia, R., Amat-y-Leon, F., Wyndham, C. and Rosen, K.M. Syncope in patients with chronic bifasicular block: significance, causative mechanisms and clinical implications. *Ann. Intern. Med.* 1974; **81**: 302.

45. Dhingra, R.C., Wyndham, C., Bauernfeind, R., Swiryn, S., Deedwania, P.C., Smith, T., Denes, P. and Rosen, K.M. Significance of block distal to the His Bundle induced by atrial pacing in patients with chronic bifasicular block. *Circulation* 1979; **60**: 1455.

46. Scheinman, M.M., Peters, R.W., Sauve, M.J., Desai, J., Abbott, J.A., Cogan, J., Wohl, B. and Williams, K. Value of the HQ interval in patients with bundle branch block and the role of prophylactic permanent pacing. *Am. J. Cardiol.* 1982; **50**: 1316.

47. Ezri, M., Lerman, B.B., Marchlinski, F.E., Buxton, A.E. and Josephson, M.E. Electrophysiological evaluation of syncope in patients with bifasicular block. *Am. Heart J.* 1983; **106**: 693.

48. Morady, F., Higgins, J., Peters, R.W., Schwartz, A.B., Shen, E.N., Bhandari, A., Scheinman, M.M. and Sauve, M.J. Electrophysiologic testing in bundle branch block and unexplained syncope. *Am. J. Cardiol.* 1984; **54**: 587.

Chapter 66

Trauma to the Heart and Aorta

John H. Dark

INTRODUCTION

Trauma to the heart and any of the great vessels can be readily classified into two categories: penetrating and non-penetrating trauma. They differ greatly in presentation, management and outcome. The former is usually the result of personal violence, and there is broad consensus over treatment, almost regardless of the mechanism of injury. Blunt or non-penetrating trauma has a clinical spectrum that ranges from barely detectable epicardial contusion through discrete coronary and valvar damage to chamber disruption. Related to the extreme end of this spectrum is the well-defined clinical entity of aortic disruption, with reasonable constancy of site, natural history and radiological appearance.

PENETRATING INJURIES OF THE HEART

The repair of a right ventricular stab wound by Rehn[1] in 1897 marked the beginning of cardiac surgery. Although this success ended the prejudice against attempted operation, the salvage rate for such wounds remained at only 50% for the first half of the century. Even in the 1940s, such influential surgeons as Blalock and Ravitch[2] in the USA were in support of performing pericardiocentesis rather than surgery. Experience gained in the Second World War and subsequently of urban violence in the USA[3] has established surgery as the treatment of choice for penetrating trauma. Most recently has come the concept of the warm but otherwise apparently dead patient, who may occasionally be saved by rapid thoracotomy and release of tamponade.[4,5]

INCIDENCE AND AETIOLOGY

Penetrating injuries are usually from knife or gunshot wounds; often they are rapidly fatal. Their incidence and type depends on geography, history and the efficiency of local ambulance services. In Lebanon, in the 1980s, 97% of all chest wounds were due to gunshot or shrapnel.[6] In the USA, the widespread use of handguns results in a preponderance of gunshot wounds over stabbings; but even in urban areas, for patients reaching hospital alive, stab wounds of the heart exceed bullet wounds in a ratio of 3:2.[7] As many as 80% of all patients with penetrating heart injuries die before reaching hospital.[3]

Penetrating cardiac wounds are very rare in mainland Britain. In 1980, only 18 penetrating cardiac injuries were treated by cardiothoracic surgeons in the UK.[8] Even if the number of cases treated by non-cardiac surgeons is taken into account, the total would not rise to more than a few tens annually. In the UK, nearly all penetrating injuries are stab wounds; in 1986, only 8 deaths of any kind were caused by guns in England and Wales.

The experience in Belfast is more similar to that of an American city in that equal numbers of each type of injury are seen at hospital, although the numbers of such cases are very small. Of 158 gunshot wounds of the chest reported by Ferguson and Stephenson, only two involved the heart and pericardium.[9]

PATHOPHYSIOLOGY

The most commonly injured chamber is the right ventricle, the next in order of frequency being the left ventricle, the right atrium and finally the posteriorly placed left atrium.[10] Ventricular wounds may occasionally seal themselves, particularly when the left is penetrated. The coronary arteries can also be injured; the left anterior descending artery is the most commonly involved.[11] The pericardium is invariably damaged, more severely so in cases with gunshot wounds. The extent of pericardial leakage may determine whether tamponade or hypovolaemia dominate the clinical picture. Although any adjacent part of the chest or upper abdomen may be involved, the commonest associated injuries are to the lung.[9]

Intracardiac shunts are found in 2–6% of patients surviving penetrating wounds;[12] the interventricular septum is the commonest site, with the cardiac entry wound usually found on the front of the right ventricle. Less commonly, the communication is between the aorta and right ventricular outflow tract or a coronary artery and a cardiac chamber.[13] Valves may also be damaged, either by direct perforation or division of chordae tendineae and papillary muscles.

Low-velocity weapons, such as airguns may do little more than deposit their pellets in the circulation when they penetrate the heart. Embolus to the lungs or the systemic circulation may result, although the former is more common with perforation of the great veins.[14] The effects of arrow wounds (arrows being lowest velocity weapon likely to penetrate the skin) have recently been reported from Papua New Guinea. In patients who reach medical attention, mediastinitis rather than haemodynamic disturbance dominates the clinical picture.[15]

CLINICAL FEATURES

Any wound of the chest or upper abdomen can potentially involve the heart, but entry wounds between the nipple lines anteriorly are particularly suspicious.[8] Between 10 and 30% of patients will present to hospital *in extremis*, warm with only the slightest signs of life.[5] The management of such patients is discussed below.

A much larger group of patients have definite evidence of serious injury, with signs of tamponade or hypovolaemia. The two frequently coincide, the typical presentation being one of a patient in shock with distended neck veins. Measurement of the central venous pressure is the most useful investigation of tamponade. It may be elevated absolutely, inappropriately elevated in a shocked patient or respond inappropriately to volume expansion. Pulsus paradoxus is also a very useful sign, particularly if a trace of radial artery pressure can be displayed. Faintness of heart sounds is not a reliable sign, and murmurs from associated shunts are rarely heard in the acute phase. If hypovolaemia dominates the picture, there will probably be a detectable haemothorax, which is readily seen on a chest X-ray. Radiology is otherwise unhelpful; in particular, although there may be a slight straightening of the left-heart border, the cardiac outline is generally within normal limits. The electrocardiogram is abnormal in only about 50% of patients. The presence of an effusion may be confirmed on two-dimensional echocardiography, but the measurement of central venous pressure is much more readily available, and contributes quantitative information about the degree of tamponade. Echocardiography with Doppler techniques may identify the site of intracardiac shunts in patients who have them (see Figs 66.1 and 66.2).[16]

The largest group of patients are those who have a penetrating thoracic injury, but no definite evidence of cardiac penetration. They may be in good haemodynamic condition from the start, or respond satisfactorily to basic resuscitation. Many will subsequently demonstrate no cardiac injury. However, some will declare an injury on observation or investigation, and thereby move themselves into the second group of patients described above.

MANAGEMENT AND RESULTS

For the patient reaching hospital warm but without signs of life, immediate opening of the chest to relieve tamponade has a proven place in management. Such patients may make respiratory efforts when intubated and often have good electrocardiographic complexes, despite the absence of a pulse. A left antero-lateral thoracotomy should be made immediately. Preliminary steps other than intubation waste precious time. With the lung retracted, the pericardium is opened in front of the phrenic nerve and the tamponade released. The heart can then be effectively massaged, restoring cerebral perfusion as soon as possible. This can be aided by manually compressing the descending aorta while hypovolaemia is corrected. Stab wounds of the heart can nearly always be controlled by compression using a finger or the palm of the hand until the circulation is stable again.

Survival (to hospital discharge) for these patients ranges from 10[4] to 30%.[17,18] About 60% may be initially resuscitated. Results are best if the patient actually arrests in the ambulance or in the casualty department, 16% and 23%, respectively, in one series.[5] In the same report, there were no survivors in the group who were pulseless at the scene of the incident.[5] Similarly, gunshot victims, even if they reach hospital 'alive', are less likely to survive this sort of intervention. The main reason for success in

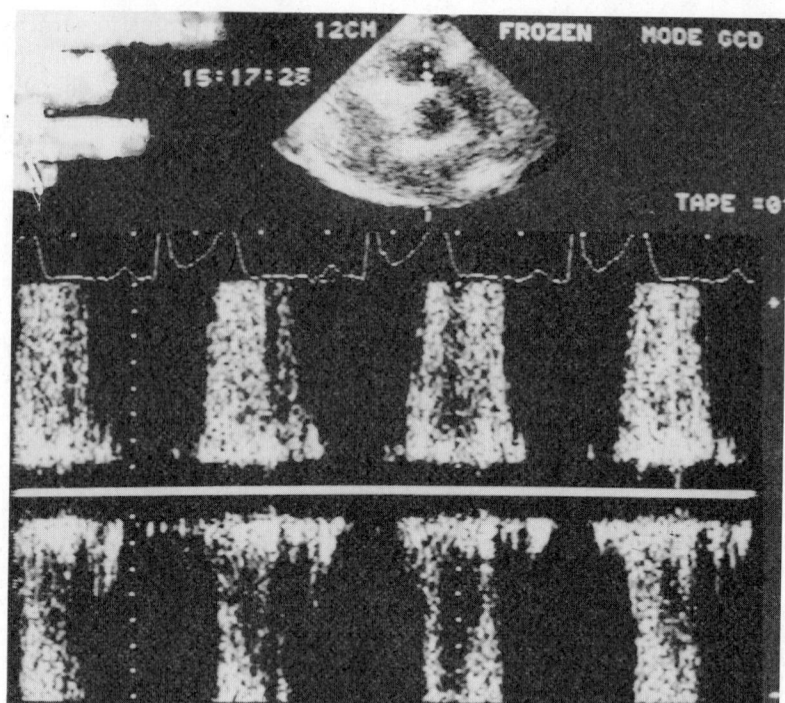

Fig. 66.1. Doppler echocardiographic demonstration of an intracardiac shunt after chest stabbing. The marker in the top display is in the right ventricular outflow tract and at operation there was a fistula from there to the left ventricle.

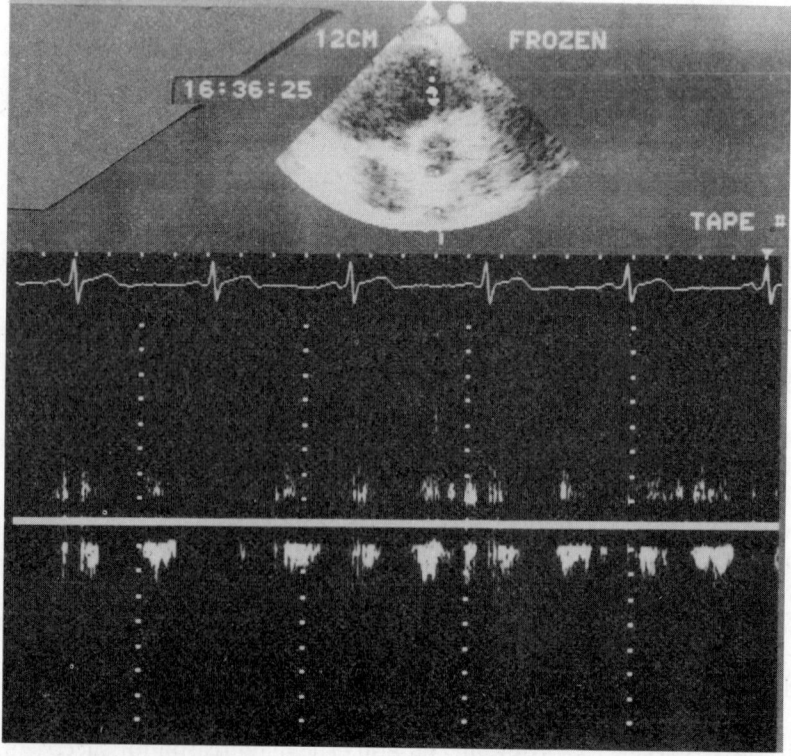

Fig. 66.2. Post-operative Doppler study from the same patient as Fig. 66.1, showing the complete absence of a shunt.

immediate thoracotomy is the relief of tamponade in patients with relatively mild cardiac injury. These circumstances are rarely found after bullet wounds when the pericardium is invariably lacerated and the cardiac injury often severe.

Patients who have definite evidence of serious injury when they reach hospital have a much better outlook[5,17] if they are managed correctly. Some have indications for early thoracotomy: proven tamponade with raised central venous pressure or pulsus paradoxus, or continued blood loss from a chest drain. They should undergo the same urgent left antero-lateral thoracotomy because there is a high risk of catastrophic deterioration. Even in urban areas, they should not be transferred to a cardiothoracic unit because of the inevitable delay, although it may be appropriate for a cardiac surgeon to travel to the patient. Cardiopulmonary bypass facilities are rarely needed, unless there is a through-and-through wound of a cardiac chamber, or major coronary laceration.[7,8] The commonest lesion encountered in the UK will be a single wound on the front of a ventricle. This can usually be controlled by a finger and fairly easily repaired, even on the beating heart, by pledgeted mattress sutures as shown in Fig. 66.3.

For those with stab wounds in this stable group, survival may approach 90 even 100%[5,19] but it falls to around 50% in those with gunshot wounds.[7]

For patients in whom there is a penetrating chest injury, but no definite evidence that the pericardium has been breached, it may be reasonable to transfer them to a cardiothoracic centre if such a centre is nearby. Very few if any such patients should die from their cardiac injury. Although it has been recommended that all wounds between the nipple lines should be explored,[21] it is probably reasonable to observe such patients in an area where rapid thoracotomy can be performed if required.

A very small group of patients will present late, with evidence of intracardiac shunt or valve injury, or have a murmur heard at the time of initial assessment, but never fulfil the criteria for urgent operation. They should be formally assessed from a cardiological standpoint, and the lesion dealt with on its own merits. Thus, a small ventricular septal defect may simply be closely followed without intervention, whereas valvar injury would almost always warrant repair or replacement.

BLUNT INJURIES TO THE HEART

The clinical spectrum of blunt injuries has already

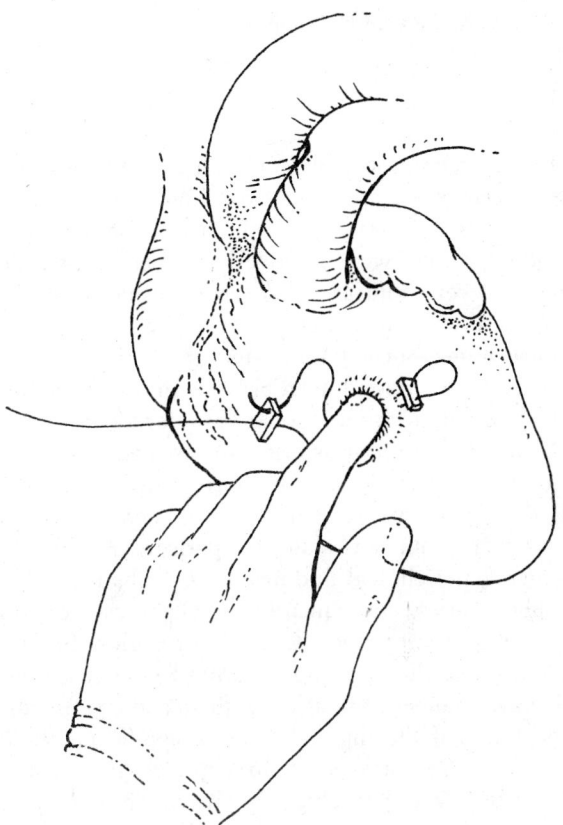

Fig. 66.3. Stab wounds to the front of the heart can often be controlled by a finger until closed with a pledgeted suture.

been mentioned. The exceedingly common myocardial contusion, ranges from a small amount of sub-endocardial bruising to full thickness muscle necrosis which can develop into late rupture or aneurysm formation.[21,22] Most contusions are located anteriorly and result from abrupt backward movement of the sternum. Coronary lesions, which are much rarer, are also located anteriorly, and presumably result from the same mechanism.[23] Sudden compression of the heart between the sternum and the vertebral column is thought to cause the dramatic rises in intraluminal pressure which lead to valve lacerations or even cardiac rupture.

Cardiac injuries of some kind are found in up to 75% of post-mortem examinations of trauma victims.[24] Estimates from the USA suggest an incidence of between 200 000[24] and 900 000 cases per year.[25] If we suppose that only one-tenth of that number occur in the UK (a reasonable estimate, given the relative numbers of road traffic accident victims), the great majority of such injuries must go unrecognized.

MYOCARDIAL CONTUSION

Myocardial contusion is one of the most overlooked diagnoses, the incidence of contusion will depend on how eagerly it is sought. Steering wheel injury is the most common cause, but myocardial contusion has been found after kicks, falls and punches.[24,35] Sub-epicardial brusing is the usual pathological finding, often with an overlying pericarditis. In more severe injuries, there is bruising into the myocardium which may extend down to the endocardium. Such contusions are said to have well-defined edges, but in practice they are difficult to differentiate from myocardial infarctions.

The key symptom is central chest pain, typically unrelieved by nitrates.[26] Inappropriate tachycardia is the most consistent finding, but there may be a gallop rhythm and later a pericardial rub. In general, the clinical findings are overshadowed by other injuries, consequently the electrocardiogram is an important if non-specific investigation. In mild contusions, there are non-specific ST-segment and T-wave changes compatible with an acute pericarditis. Later, if the injury has been significant, there may be the features of an evolving myocardial infarction, with pathological Q waves developing as the ST-segment changes subside. Rhythm changes are common, and typically ventricular with left-sided trauma and atrial if the injury is to the right side of the chest.[24] Over the past few years, measurement of the CK–MB fraction has defined a group of patients who undoubtedly have local cell necrosis. Use of cross-sectional echocardiography will further define a subgroup who have regional impairment of ventricular function (usually the right ventricle). There is a trend towards describing the injury in this group as true myocardial contusion, and referring to the injury in other patients who have only electrocardiographic changes as 'myocardial concussion'.[27] Serious rhythm disturbances and other late sequelae are virtually confined to those patients who have 'contusion' as defined above.[21,27]

Most contusions and concussions are mild and have no sequelae. The chest pain and pericarditis require analgesia, and the patient should be monitored to detect arrhythmias. Complete recovery is the rule. Where there has been myocardial damage, the clinical course resembles myocardial infarction. Depressed cardiac output can be shown, and areas of hypokinesia can be demonstrated on ventriculography,[28] which may be of importance if there are other major injuries and a reason to postpone non-urgent corrective surgery.[29] Any of the complications of myocardial infarction (arrhythmias, pump failure, ventricular aneurysm or even valve dysfunction) can occur, although all are rare. Treatment is along established lines; the long-term prognosis is usually good, because the patient is often young and has an otherwise normal heart.[21,22]

CARDIAC RUPTURE

Cardiac rupture is the commonest lesion found at post-mortem of patients who suffered blunt cardiac injury.[30] Cause of death is either exsanguination (if the pericardium is torn) or tamponade. The four chambers are said to be equally affected,[31] suggesting that the cause is internal hydraulic force. Obviously, severe contusion can progress to rupture. Some of the victims reach hospital alive, where cyanosis of the upper half of the body is a consistent finding.[24] It is probably a *forme fruste* of traumatic asphyxia. Patients with atrial rupture are more likely to reach hospital alive, and tamponade usually, but not always,[32] dominates the clinical picture. The principles of management are as those for penetrating injury, and successful repair of ruptured atria, ventricles, and even both has been recorded.[33] Traumatic ventricular septal defect is found in 5% of post-mortems after lethal cardiac injury.[30] It may also present late,[34] and can be dealt with surgically if required.

CORONARY ARTERY INJURY

These rare lesions were first noted in Parmley's post-mortem series.[30] Laceration is probably the usual injury and results in tamponade. Ligation of the bleeding vessel is unavoidable if the patient comes to thoracotomy in a centre not equipped for immediate aortocoronary bypass surgery.

Thrombosis has also been described, presumably occurring at the site of an intimal tear.[23] In young people, it must be presumed to have been caused by trauma, but in elderly patients it may be impossible to differentiate from classic atherosclerotic myocardial infarction, possibly precipitated by the traumatic episode. Myocardial necrosis tends to be extensive, perhaps because of the lack of a collateral circulation in young adults. Many of the cases described have had ventricular aneurysms or ventricular septal defects,[23] or on one occasion required cardiac transplantation for uncontrollable heart failure.[35] Recanalization of the affected vessel is frequent, perhaps confirming the previous normality of the coronary tree.[36]

CARDIAC VALVE INJURY

Isolated valve injury is relatively uncommon. The aortic valve is the most usual site of injury.[37] The leaflets may be detached or torn. Vertical decelerations are a common cause, and the injury may be a form of the aortic root disruptions seen frequently after aircraft accidents. Diagnosis is suspected from the presence of a regurgitant murmur, and confirmed by aortography, which should be performed to exclude aortic injury. Valve replacement is invariably required if there is significant cardiac embarrassment.

The atrioventricular valves are less frequently damaged; the leaflets may be torn or the papillary muscles infarcted or disrupted. Mitral valve involvement usually results in severe heart failure, with early pulmonary oedema.[38] Although theoretically valve repair is possible, replacement has always been the usual course of action. Damage to the tricuspid valve may be well tolerated and does not always require surgery.[21]

TRAUMATIC RUPTURE OF THE AORTA

Among injuries to the great vessels, post-traumatic disruption of the aorta is prominent because of its frequency and uniformity of appearance. In the classic situation, a severe antero-posterior deceleration causes rupture of the aorta at the isthmus, just distal to the origin of the left subclavian artery. As shown in Fig. 66.4, it is supposed that the relatively mobile heart and great vessels continue to move forward, while the descending aorta is fixed by the intercostal arteries and the surrounding fascia to the vertebral column.[39,40] More than 90% of these injuries occur at the junction of the fixed and mobile portions of the aorta. The tear is usually horizontal, with complete disruption of the intima and media, and survivors have a large haematoma contained by adventitia and the mediastinal pleura.

If the deceleration has been vertical, typically in victims of aircraft accidents but also in those who fall from a great height, the disruption is often found just above the aortic valve. One mechanism of injury can readily be imagined: the blood-filled heart, like a clapper in the bell of the pericardium, continues downwards but the ascending aorta, anchored by the arch vessels cannot follow, and

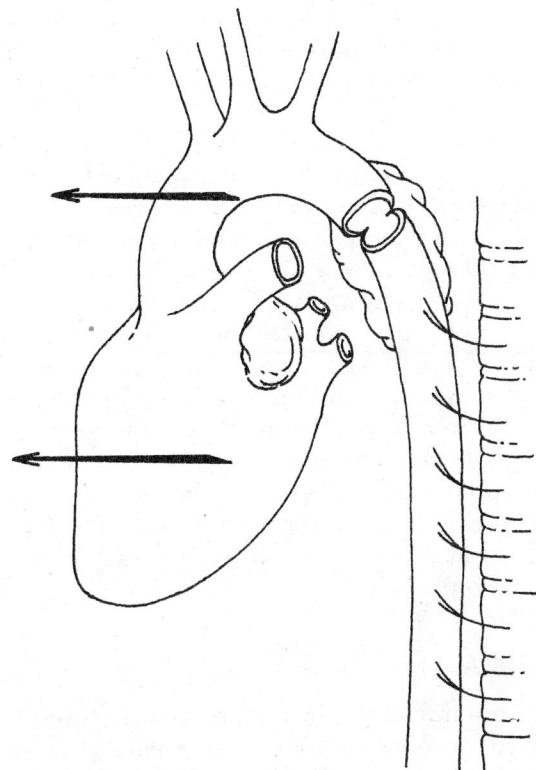

Fig. 66.4. Mechanism of aortic disruption. The descending aorta is fixed to the posterior chest wall, whereas the heart and relatively mobile arch are free to move forward.

rupture occurs at the junction of the two areas.

Other mechanisms suggested include 'bursting' due to an abrupt rise in intraluminal pressure. This explains the invariable intimal tear, but not the preponderance of injury to the aortic isthmus. Direct external injuries have also been recorded, caused by penetration by a spinal vertebra in extreme hyperextension injuries.[39] Finally, in up to 20% of post-mortem series there is more than one tear.[41]

INCIDENCE AND NATURAL HISTORY

Aortic rupture is a relatively common injury, estimated to be the principal cause of death in 10–15% of road traffic accident fatalities.[24,42] Extrapolation of this figure would suggest that in excess of 800 cases a year occur in the UK. Men outnumber women by 2:1 and 90% of the victims are under the age of 45 years. It is twice as common in patients who were ejected from vehicles when compared with those who were not,[41] and although no information is available as yet, seat belt legislation might be expected to reduce the incidence. In one small study from Minnesota, USA, a reduction in speed limits resulted in fewer chest injuries, but there was no change in the number of deaths from cardiac and aortic damage.[43]

The majority of people (80–90%) die at the place where they received the injury, presumably from exsanguination into the pleural space. Of the 15–20% of patients who reach hospital alive, half are dead within 48 h;[44] in Parmley's post-mortem series, 90% were dead within 10 weeks.[40] A small number of patients will develop chronic aneurysms but even they do badly in the long term; 41% die or develop symptoms within 5 years, and that figure rises to 85% after 20 years.[45] Survival curves for operated and non-operated patients separate in favour of the former as soon as they leave hospital. Rupture of the ascending aorta is even more likely to be immediately fatal, and very few such patients reach hospital alive.[40]

CLINICAL FEATURES

The features of aortic rupture may be overshadowed by other injuries to the limbs, head or abdomen. There is always a history of abrupt deceleration, but less than half of the victims have signs of direct trauma to the chest.[24,42] Patients may complain of pain radiating to the back, as in aortic dissection. Paradoxical upper limb hypertension is a common finding, and 30–40% have an 'acute coarctation syndrome', with additional weakness of limb pulses and a posteriorly heard systolic murmur.[46] The expanding haematoma may rarely cause hoarseness, dysphagia or superior vena caval obstruction, and 15% of patients have evidence of a left pleural effusion.

A minority of patients have a complete aortic transection, easily diagnosed by the absence of leg pulses, paraplegia and anuria.

RADIOLOGY

The recognition of rupture of the aorta, or its major branches, depends upon appreciation of the initial abnormality and then referral to aortography. In order to save the 10–15% of patients with aortic rupture who reach hospital alive, the plain chest X-ray must be viewed with a high index of suspicion. As the assessment of portable, supine (or, more often, semi-lordotic) antero-posterior chest films of severely injured patients is very difficult, the literature contains many cases of missed or late

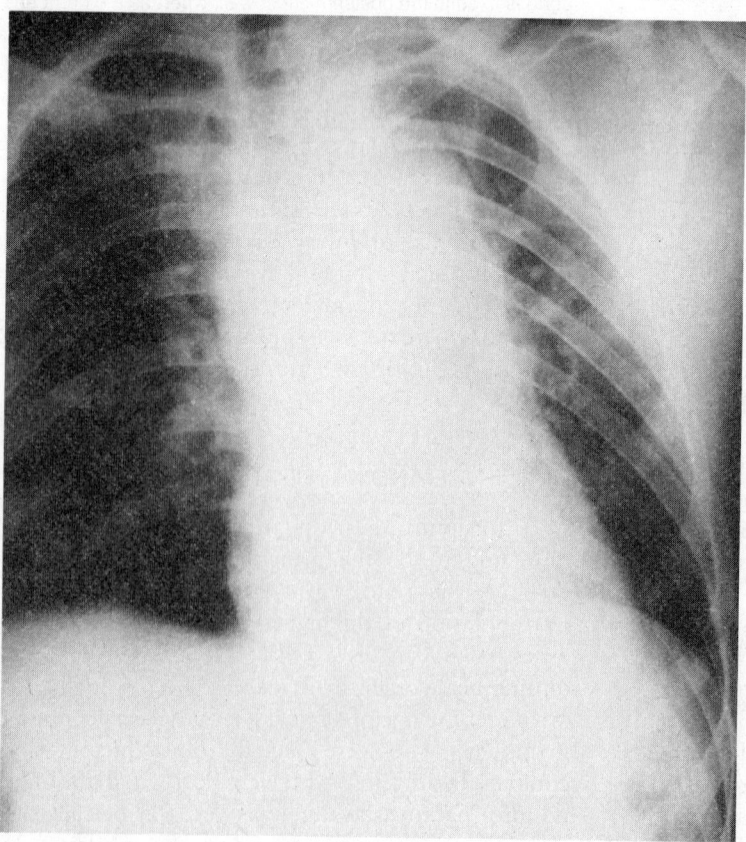

Fig. 66.5. Mediastinal haematoma. Even on this rotated film there is irregularity of the outline of the aortic knuckle and opacification of the subaortic window. Aortography showed aortic disruption.

Table 66.1.   Chest X-ray features of mediastinal haematoma.

1   Wide upper mediastinum (> 8 cm or > 25% of chest diameter)
2   Opacification of subaortic window
3   Downward displacement of left main bronchus
4   String sign: deflection of nasogastric tube to right (Fig. 66.6)
5   Apical cap: haematoma dissecting above apical pleura
6   Left haemothorax, especially in the absence of rib fractures

diagnosis.[39,40] The cardinal feature is mediastinal widening (Fig. 66.5), caused by the haematoma contained in the aortic adventitia. The topic has been reviewed in depth by Woodring and Dillon.[47] Associated 'clues' are listed in Table 66.1 (see also Fig. 66.6). It must be stressed that none of these signs is diagnostic. When present, they serve to raise the suspicion of great vessel injury and as an indication for aortography.

The aortogram is the 'gold standard' investigation of this condition. The typical feature is a pseudo-aneurysm at the isthumus (Fig. 66.7). Extravasation of dye is unusual. There may be intimal tears or even complete occlusion. The precise site will be defined and any further tears identified. A large number of aortograms can be expected to be negative. The proportion will depend on local practice, but in one typical series there was a 12% positive rate.[48] The false-negative rate is very low.[47]

THE PROBLEM OF FIRST RIB FRACTURES

Bony damage to the thoracic inlet, manifest as fractures of the first or second ribs, may directly involve the aortic arch branches, particularly the subclavian arteries. In addition, such fractures of relatively well protected bones are indicators of the severity of blunt trauma. In recognition of these two aspects, at various times it has been recommended that such fractures could be an automatic indication for arch aortography.[49] Other more recent work has refuted this argument,[50] by showing that these fractures were not particularly associated with specific vessel injury. Thus, a reasonable current recommendation would be that in the absence of physical signs or other X-ray abnormality (specifically mediastinal widening) suggesting vessel injury, observation should be adequate.

COMPUTED TOMOGRAPHIC SCANNING

This investigation has not been widely used for the traumatized, as opposed to the dissected, aorta. The diagnostic precision of aortography, particularly for subtle intimal tears, cannot be rivalled by computed tomography. It is most useful in excluding haematoma in patients who have an abnormal mediastinal outline on plain chest X-ray.[51] However, once haematoma is identified, aortography is still required to refute or confirm great vessel damage, and to identify the site of injury accurately.

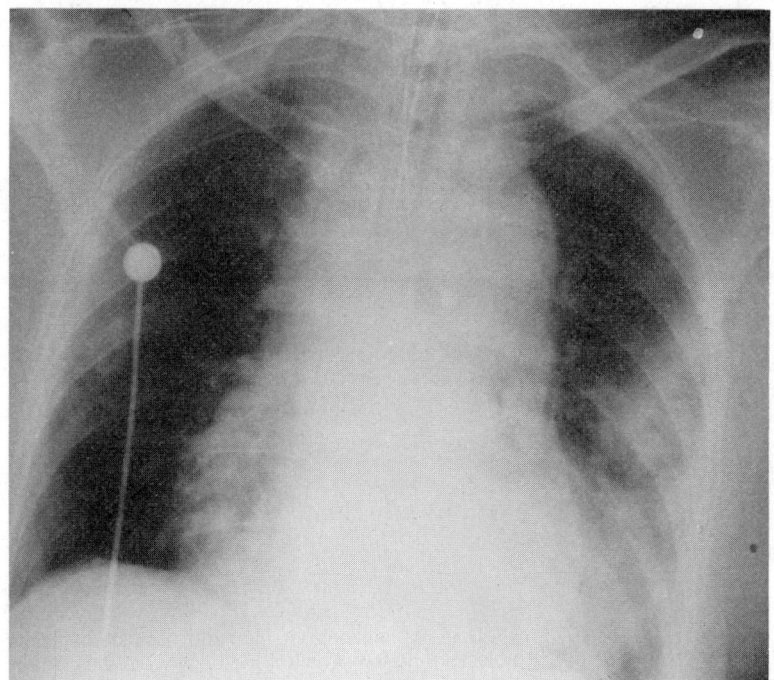

Fig. 66.6. Negative 'string sign'. Although the mediastinum is possibly widened, the radiopaque nasogastric tube in the oesophagus is not displaced. The left main bronchus is also in a normal position. These features indicate that aortic damage is unlikely, but only an aortogram can provide definitive information.

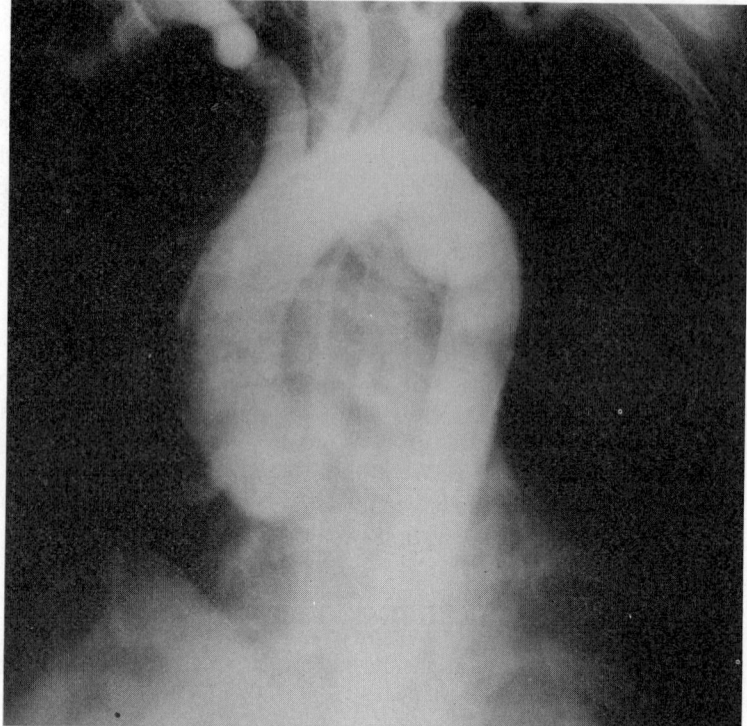

Fig. 66.7. Positive aortogram. The characteristic pseudo-aneurysm is easily seen in this film. There is a little extravasation of dye.

TREATMENT AND OUTCOME

The poor prognosis of aortic disruption has already been stressed; only 10–15% of patients reach hospital alive, and half of them are dead within 48 h if they do not undergo operation. Once the tear is identified, immediate operation is indicated. Virtually all other problems, such as intra-abdominal pathology or limb injuries, should be managed subsequently.[52] Only evacuation of intracranial haematoma should be performed before thoracotomy. Only if the severity of other injuries makes survival unlikely is it reasonable to temporise. In these rare circumstances, management with beta-blockers and antihypertensive agents (as for acute dissection) may have some merit.[53]

A few patients will come to emergency thoracotomy for massive blood loss from the left chest, and have the aortic damage discovered as the source of bleeding.

For the remaining patients, careful consideration should be given to protection of the spinal cord during the mandatory cross-clamp period. One approach is to heparinize the patient formally, and use 'left-heart bypass' from left atrium to femoral artery. It has the advantage that sudden uncontrolled bleeding occurring before the aorta and identi-

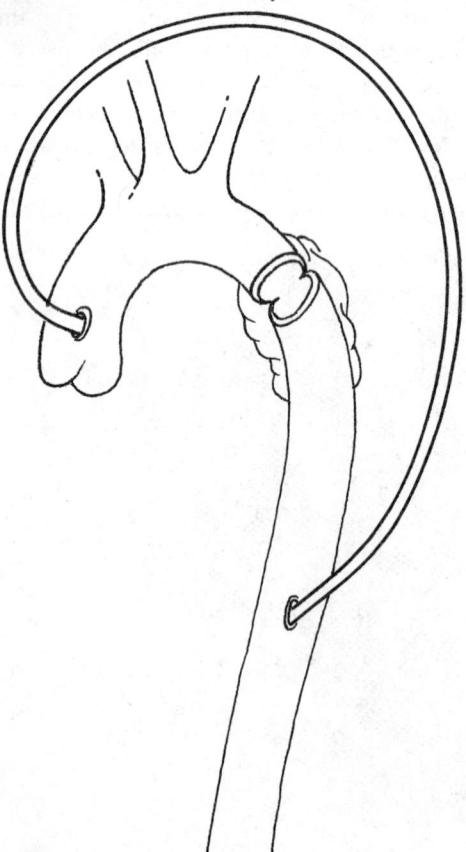

Fig. 66.8. Use of a heparinized shunt to bypass the damaged area, protecting the lower half of the body while the aorta is cross-clamped.

fied beneath the often huge haematoma can be salvaged by auto-transfusion. However, heparinization may exacerbate other injuries. Head injuries, in particular, are very likely to be worsened by uncontrolled intracranial bleeding. An alternative, and now the most frequently used, technique is to employ a heparin-bonded shunt (the so-called 'Gott shunt') to bypass the clamped aorta (Fig. 66.8).[53] Mortality is lower with this method, probably because of a reduction in deaths from other injuries.[52] A third approach is to 'clamp and sew'. It has the advantage of simplicity, and gives good results in the hands of its enthusiasts.[54] Other surgeons have reported a high incidence of spinal cord damage.[55] It is probably a bad choice of technique in the hands of any but the best and fastest surgeons.

Once the aorta is controlled, surgery is straightforward. A short length of a synthetic tube graft is sewn between the two ends of the torn aorta. In some cases, direct anastomosis can be achieved. This may necessitate further dissection of the aorta, but it has the advantage of avoiding foreign material and it requires only a single suture line.[56]

In general, 75–85% of patients can be expected to survive to leave hospital. Most deaths after surgery are the result of associated injuries. The long-term prognosis after satisfactory repair is very good.[45]

REFERENCES

1. Blatchford, J.W. Ludwig Rehn: The first successful cardiorrhaphy. *Ann. Thorac. Surg.* 1985; **39**: 492.
2. Blalock, A. and Ravitch, M.A. A consideration of the non-operative treatment of cardiac tamponade resulting from wounds of the heart. *Surgery* 1943; **14**: 157.
3. Sugg, W.L., Rea, W.J., Ecker, R.R., Rose, E.F. and Shaw, R.R. Penetrating wounds of the heart: an analysis of 459 cases. *J. Thorac. Cardiovasc. Surg.* 1968; **56**: 531.
4. Baker, C.C., Thomas, A.N. and Trunkey, D.D. The role of emergency room thoracotomy in trauma. *J. Trauma* 1980; **20**: 848.
5. Washington, B., Wilson, R.F., Steiger, Z. and Barrett, J.S. Emergency Thoracotomy: A Four Year Review. *Ann. Thorac. Surg.* 1985; **40**: 188.
6. Zakharia, A.T. Thoracic Battle Injuries in the Lebanon War: Review of the Early Operative Approach in 1992 Patients. *Ann. Thorac. Surg.* 1985; **40**: 209.
7. Mandal, A.K., Awariefe, S.O. and Oparah, S.S. Experience in the management of 50 consecutive penetrating wounds of the heart. *Br. J. Surg.* 1979; **66**: 565.
8. Reece, I.J. and Davidson, K.G. Penetrating cardiac injuries in the United Kingdom. *Thorax* 1983; **38**: 81.
9. Ferguson, D.G. and Stevenson, H.M. A review of 158 gunshot wounds to the chest. *Br. J. Surg.* 1978; **65**: 845.
10. Parmley, L.F., Mattingly, T.W. and Manion, W.M. Penetrating Wounds of the Heart and Aorta. *Circulation* 1958; **17**: 953.
11. Rea, W.J., Sugg, W.L., Wilson, L.C., Webb, W.R. and Ecker, R.R. Coronary Artery Lacerations: An analysis of 22 patients. *Ann. Thorac. Surg.* 1979; **7**: 518.
12. Carter, R.L., Albert, A.M. and Glass, B.A. Traumatic ventricular septal defect. *Ann. Thorac. Surg.* 1967; **4**: 256.
13. Thandroyen, F.T. and Mattinson, R.E. Penetrating thoracic trauma producing intracardiac shunts. *J. Thorac. Cardiovasc. Surg.* 1981; **81**: 569.
14. Bernin, C.O., Janqueira, A.R., Hosita, L.T., Birolini, D., Branco, P.D. and de Oliveira, M.R. Bullet emboli from the heart and great veins. *Surg. Gynec. Obstet.* 1983; **156**: 615.
15. Fingleton, L.J. Arrow wounds to the heart and mediastinum. *Br. J. Surg.* 1987; **74**: 126.
16. Goldman, A., Kotler, M.N., Goldberg, S.E., Parameswaran, R. and Parry, W. The uses of two-dimensional doppler echocardiographic techniques preoperatively and postoperatively in a ventricular septal defect caused by penetrating trauma. *Ann. Thorac. Surg.* 1985; **40**: 625.
17. Reece, I.J. and Davidson, K.G. Emergency surgery for penetrating wounds of the heart. *Ann. R. Coll. Surg.* 1983; **65**: 304.
18. Ivatury, R.R., Nallathambi, M.N., Stahl, W.M. and Rohman, M. Penetrating Cardiac Trauma—Quantifying the Severity of Anatomic and Physiologic Injury. *Ann. Surg.* 1987; **205**: 61.
19. Anonymous. Penetrating Cardiac Injuries (Editorial) *Lancet* 1984; **i**: 999.
20. Szentpetery, S. and Lower, R.K. Changing concepts in the treatment of penetrating cardiac injuries. *J. Trauma* 1977; **17**: 457.
21. Frazee, R.C., Mucha, P., Farnell, M.B. and Miller, P.A. Objective evaluation of blunt cardiac trauma. *J. Trauma* 1986; **26**: 510.
22. Liedtke, A.J. and DeMuth, W.E. Non penetrating cardiac injuries: a collective review. *Am. Heart J.* 1973; **86**: 687.
23. Pifarre, R., Grieco, J., Garibaldi, A., Sullivan, H.J., Montoya, A. and Bakhos, M. Acute coronary occlusion secondary to blunt chest trauma. *J. Thorac. Cardiovasc. Surg.* 1982; **83**: 122.
24. Kirsh, M.M. and Sloan, H. *Blunt Chest Trauma.* Boston: Little, Brown and Co., 1977.
25. Jackson, D.H. and Murphy, D.W. Non-penetrating cardiac trauma *Mod. Conc. Cardiovasc. Dis.* 1976; **45**: 123.
26. Saunders, C.R. and Doty, D.B. Myocardial contusion. *Surg. Gynec. Obstet.* 1977; **144**: 595.
27. Tenzer, M.L. The spectrum of myocardial contusion: A review. *J. Trauma* 1985; **25**: 620.
28. Sutherland, G.R., Driedger, A.A., Holiday, R.L., Cheung, H.W. and Sibbald, W.J. Frequency of Myocardial injury after blunt chest trauma as evaluated by radionuclide angiography. *Am. J. Cardiol.* 1984; **52**: 1099.
29. Katz, S., Gimmon, Z. and Appelbaum, A. Cardiac contusion in the patient with multiple injuries. *Injury* 1980–81; **12**: 180.
30. Parmley, F.F., Mannion, W.C. and Mattingly, T.W. Non-penetrating traumatic injury to the heart. *Circulation* 1958; **18**: 375.
31. Bright, E.F. and Beck, C.S. Non-penetrating wounds of the heart: clinical and experimental studies. *Am. Heart J.* 1935; **10**: 293.
32. Sethia, B. Traumatic atrial rupture without haemopericardium. *Injury* 1980–81; **12**: 187.
33. Hendel, P.N. and Grant, A.F. Blunt traumatic rupture of the heart *J. Thorac. Cardiovasc. Surg.* 1981; **81**: 574.
34. Mackintosh, A.F. and Fleming, H.A. Cardiac damage presenting late after road accidents *Thorax* 1981; **36**: 811.
35. Watt, A.H. and Stevens, M.R. Myocardial infarction after blunt chest trauma incurred during rugby football that later required cardiac transplantation. *Br. Heart J.* 1986; **55**: 408.
36. Oren, A., Bar-Shzomo, B. and Stern, S. Acute coronary

occlusion following blunt injury to the chest in the absence of coronary atherosclerosis. *Am. Heart J.* 1976; **92**: 501.

37. Morrit, G.N., Taylor, N.C., Miller, H.M. and Walbaum, P.R. Traumatic aortic regurgitation. *J. R. Coll. Surg. (Edin.)* 1979; **24**: 87.

38. Pellegrini, R.V., Copeland, C.E., DiMarco, R.F. *et al.* Blumt rupture of both atrioventricular valves. *Ann. Thorac. Surg.* 1986; **42**: 471.

39. Sevitt, S. Fatal Road Accidents. *Br. J. Surg.* 1968; **55**: 481.

40. Parmley, L.F., Mattingly, W.T., Manion, W.C. and Jahnke, E.J. Jr. Non-penetrating traumatic injury of the aorta. *Circulation* 1958; **17**: 1086.

41. Greendyke, R.M. Traumatic rupture of the aorta; special references to automobile accidents. *JAMA* 1966; **195**: 527.

42. Kirsh, M.M., Behrendt, D.M., Orringer, M.B. *et al.* The treatment of acute traumatic rupture of the aorta. *Ann. Surg.* 1976; **184**: 308.

43. Alyono, D. and Perry, J.F. Impact of Speed Limit. 1 Chest injuries, review of 966 cases. *J. Thorac. Cardiovasc. Surg.* 1982; **83**: 519.

44. Plume, S. and De Weese, J.A. Traumatic rupture of the Thoracic Aorta. *Arch. Surg.* 1979; **114**: 240.

45. Finkelmeier, B.A., Mentzer, R.M., Kaiser, D.L., Tegtmeyer, C.J. and Nolan, S.P. Chronic traumatic thoracic aneurysm. *J. Thorac. Cardiovasc. Surg.* 1982; **84**: 257.

46. Symbas, P.N., Tyras, D.H., Ware, R.E. *et al.* Traumatic Rupture of the Aorta. *Ann Surg.* 1973; **178**: 6.

47. Woodring, J.H. and Dillon, M.L. Radiographic Manifestations of Mediastinal Haemorrhage from Blunt Chest Trauma. *Ann. Thorac. Surg.* 1984; **37**: 171.

48. Sandor, F. Incidence and significance of traumatic mediastinal haematoma. *Thorax* 1967; **22**: 43.

49. Richardson, J.D., McElvein, R.B. and Trinkle, J.K. First rib fracture: a hallmark of severe trauma. *Ann. Surg.* 1975; **181**: 251.

50. Fisher, R.G., Ward, R.E. and Ben-Menachem, Y. Arteriography and the fractured first rib; too much for too little? *AJR* 1982; **138**: 1059.

51. Toombs, B.D., Sandler, C.M. and Lester, R.G. Computed tomography in chest trauma. *Radiology* 1981; **140**: 730.

52. Pate, J.W. Traumatic Rupture of the Aorta: Emergency Operation. *Ann. Thorac. Surg.* 1985; **39**: 531.

53. Akins, C.W., Buckley, M.J., Daggett, W., McIlduff, J.B. and Austen, W.G. Acute traumatic disruption of the thoracic aorta: A ten year experience. *Ann. Thorac. Surg.* 1981; **31**: 305.

54. Mattox, K.L., Holzman, M., Pickard, L.R., Beall, A.C. and Debakey, M.E. Clamp/Repair: A Safe Technique for Treatment of Blunt Injury to the Descending Thoracic Aorta. *Ann.Thorac. Surg.* 1985; **40**: 456.

55. Katz, N.M., Blackstone, E.H., Kirklin, J.W. and Karp, R.B. Incremental risk factors for spinal cord injury following operation for acute traumatic aortic transection. *J. Thorac. Cardiovasc. Surg.* 1981; **81**: 669.

56. McBride, L.R., Tidik, S., Stothert, J.C. *et al.* Primary repair of traumatic aortic disruption. *Ann. Thorac. Surg.* 1987; **43**: 65.

Chapter 67

Genetics and Heart Disease

John Burn

In 1964, Victor McKusick[1] recalled the observation of the biostatistician Bradford Hill that the practice of medicine could be resolved into three questions: what is wrong (diagnosis), what is going to happen (prognosis) and what can be done about it (treatment)? When dealing with genetic disorders, four further questions emerge: why did it happen (aetiology), will it happen again (recurrence risk in family), will it be as bad (clinical burden) and are there any tests (pre-natal diagnosis)? With the decline in infectious disease and malnutrition in the Western world, the practice of cardiology is now focused on the consequences of malformation, metabolic disorder, auto-immune damage and degenerative disease. Any of these may raise questions of cause, recurrence risk and with increasing frequency, prenatal diagnosis. As it is not possible to provide a comprehensive guide to the genetics of heart disease in a short overview, only selected disorders that illustrate the basic concepts of genetics will be discussed in this chapter because apart from the practical issues of advice to patients and their families, genetics is one of the basic sciences upon which all understanding of disease must rest. The ideas upon which 'gene probes' are based and the rapid advances in molecular genetics will be explored. Through these techniques, the clinical art and basic science of genetics of cardiovascular disease will become united.

SINGLE GENE DEFECTS

The traditional starting point for any discussion of genetics is to review Mendel's classic studies on the pea plant from which were derived the basic laws of single gene inheritance. Shortly after the 'rediscovery' of this work in 1900, Sir Archibold Garrod published his description of alkaptonuria as an autosomal recessive disorder. Garrod quoted the words of William Harvey that

'Nature is nowhere more likely to display her secret workings than in those cases where she. strays from the beaten path'.[2]

This has been particularly true in the elucidation of metabolic disorders in which the recognition that single genes code for single enzymes or, more precisely, single polypeptide chains has made it possible to understand complex biochemical pathways by the investigation of those individuals in whom a gene defect has caused a block at a single step in the pathway. In cardiology, lipid metabolism plays a central role in the pathogenesis of coronary artery disease. Within this complex group of disorders is familial hypercholesterolaemia which will serve as a relevant example for the discussion of single gene inheritance.

FAMILIAL HYPERCHOLESTEROLAEMIA

Familial hypercholesterolaemia (FH) is a rare autosomal recessive disease of childhood which has become a common autosomal dominant disorder of adulthood. This confusing statement is easily understood once it is realized that 'recessive' and 'dominant' are arbitrary terms used by clinicians. The key issue is the importance of a gene to normal bodily function. The majority of the 50 000 or so genes inherited from our parents come in matching pairs, one from the mother and one from the father. The exceptions to this rule, the X-linked genes, will be discussed later. A gene is a coded message made up of a short section of a DNA molecule. The DNA is transcribed to nuclear RNA from which the 'non-coding' intervening sequences are resected to produce messenger RNA. In the cytoplasm, the small transfer RNA molecules, each carrying its amino acid, transfer this burden to the growing polypeptide chain at the ribosome according to the code or base sequence on the messenger RNA. The polypeptide chain then undergoes modification to produce the structural protein, hormone or enzyme. The two copies of the gene normally contribute equal amounts of the final gene product, i.e. the protein. 'Disease' occurs if the quantity of gene product is not equal to the body's need. If an abnormal gene is inherited that is non-functioning, the amount of gene product is halved. If half is enough to allow normal growth and development, as is usually the case, for example, with enzymes, the disease is called recessive because in the carrier, or heterozygote, the presence of a faulty copy of the gene is concealed by the normal allele.* The disease becomes apparent when both partners of a couple carry the faulty gene and each passes it on to a child who, with no functioning copy, manifests the disease.

In subsequent pregnancies, there is a half chance for each parent to pass on the abnormal allele and thus there is a quarter chance of a child receiving a pair of defective genes which will result in disease manifestation.

If 50% production is insufficient for the body's needs, the gene defect causes disease in the *heterozygote* and is then described as dominant. On the rare occasion that two carriers marry and have children, the offspring who are homozygous for the faulty gene would usually have very severe disease.

Individuals homozygous for the FH gene are rare. As a consequence of their extremely high cholesterol levels, they develop symptomatic coronary artery disease in childhood or early adulthood together with generalized atherosclerosis, valvular heart disease due to lipid deposition and extensive xanthomata. Survival beyond 30 years of age is exceptional. The parents of such a child are likely to be clinically normal and the paediatrician would thus be justified in labelling this a rare recessive disorder. As mean adult survival in the population has increased, however, the disadvantage of the FH heterozygotes has become more apparent. Male heterozygotes begin to develop clinical manifestations of ischaemic heart disease from their third decade and, if those affected are not treated, half the men and 1 in 6 of the women will have died by the age of 60 years.[3,4] If, as is usually the case, the skin coloured firm tendon xanthomata on the Achilles tendon and knuckles are not recognized or are not present, the only clinical clue may be a family history of early

coronary deaths. The wider availability of blood lipid analysis has exposed more heterozygote individuals. The typical blood picture is a total plasma cholesterol over 8 mmol/l with an excess of low density lipoprotein (LDL) with or without an excess of very low density lipoprotein (VLDL) (Fredrickson type IIa or IIb). Unfortunately, the blood lipid profile alone is not diagnostic because it overlaps with that of the 'normal' population and ideally a bimodal distribution of cholesterol levels in first degree relatives and/or a three-generation pedigree of early cardiac deaths are needed to verify the diagnosis because the more sophisticated assays of LDL receptors are not widely available.

One in 500 adults in Western populations are heterozygotes for the FH gene defect. If these individuals are considered to have a genetic disease, this constitutes the commonest autosomal dominant disorder in the British population (with the possible exception of mitral valve prolapse if this is also considered to constitute a 'disease'). This figure represents a homozygote frequency of 1 in a 1 000 000 based on the Hardy–Weinberg equilibrium

$$p^2 + 2pq + q^2 = 1$$

where p and q are the gene frequencies for normal and abnormal and the three expressions represent, respectively, the proportions of homozygous normals, of heterozygotes and of homozygotes affected in the population. More simply, each individual has 2 copies of the gene. In the population as a whole, 1 copy of the gene in every 1000 is defective. The chance of having 2 bad copies is 1 in 1000 × 1 in 1000, however, as there are 2 genes per individual there are 2 chances of being a carrier so the carrier rate is 1 in 500.

In 1979, Brown and Goldstein[5] reported that the underlying defect in FH was at the LDL receptor. LDL migrates as the beta band on electrophoresis and comprises cholesterol contained within a protein coat. Chylomicrons are converted in the liver to VLDL. Lypolysis, in the serum, of triglycerides within VLDL converts it to LDL which must be taken up by cells to provide essential cholesterol. This uptake is impaired if there is a deficiency of LDL receptors on the cell surface. The raised serum levels of LDL and cholesterol are a manifestation of this impaired uptake. The genetic fault responsible for FH is in the LDL receptor gene on chromosome 19; to date, at least 12 different mutations have been described in the structure of the gene. Thus, the outward appearance or phenotype of a single

---

* The position of a gene on a chromosome is the gene locus. Matching pairs of chromosomes mean there are two copies of the gene at each locus. Each copy of the gene is called an allele.

genetic disease can result from a host of faulty alleles at the LDL locus: genotypic heterogeneity. The techniques responsible for this advance in understanding are those of recombinant DNA methodology, 'genetic engineering'. All clinicians should make themselves conversant with this area of science whose impact over the next couple of decades on medicine will more than match the development of antibiotics.

The reader interested in exploring this field should consult one of the introductory texts now available such as the excellent work by Weatherall.[6] Those unfamiliar with terms such as restriction fragment length polymorphism should read Appendix 1 of this chapter (p. 1462) which contains a discussion of the underlying principles. Sickle cell disease is used as a model because it is a disorder that has been fully analysed at molecular level, it is of cardiological interest and it is amenable to precise carrier detection and can be diagnosed during the first trimester of pregnancy by the use of either closely linked polymorphic DNA markers or gene probes capable of detecting the actual single base change in the ß-globin gene.[7–9] Sickle cell disease was the first major disorder to yield to this approach; gene defects such as Huntington's chorea[10] can now be tracked in families using these techniques.

The LDL receptor in French Canadians

Hobbs *et al.*[11] have provided an elegant illustration of the power of these techniques in the French Canadian population (Fig. 67.1).

About two-thirds of French Canadians with fami-

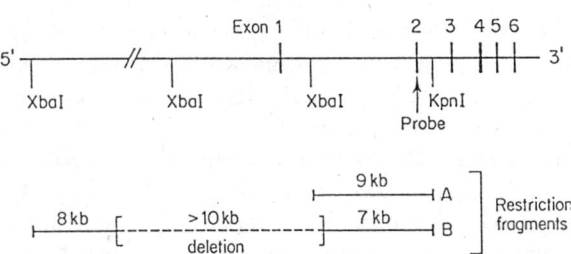

Fig. 67.1. The 6 exons or coding sequences of the LDL receptor are shown, together with the cutting sites for the enzymes XbaI and KpnI. The probe detects the second exon. DNA from normal individuals yields a 9-kb fragment (see A) which is detected by the gene probe. The common mutation in French Canadians involves loss of at least 10 kb, including the first exon of the gene. The result is a non-functioning gene and a 15-kb (7+8) fragment detected by the probe for the second exon (see B). (Reproduced with permission from Hobbs *et al.*, *N. Engl. J. Med.* 1987; **317**: 734–7.[11])

lial hypercholesterolaemia have a null allele, the function of which is destroyed by a 10-kilobase (kb) deletion near the five prime (5′) end of the gene (all genes have a 5′ and a 3′ end). This deletion removes 2 cutting sites for the restriction enzyme Xba1 so that their LDL gene probe, specific to the second coding section of the gene, attached itself to a 15-kb DNA fragment rather than the usual 9-kb fragment. The result is that, within those families with this particular null allele, the presence of the 15-kb band on the DNA blot is clear and specific evidence that they carry the disease gene and such individuals should be treated.

More than 12 genes involved in lipoprotein metabolism have now been localized.[12] It is clear that this complex area will soon yield to the technique of 'reverse genetics' in which the disease process is elucidated by first analysing the underlying gene defect.

COLLAGEN DISORDERS: MARFAN'S SYNDROME

The term Marfan's syndrome has two major weaknesses. The first is historical: Antoine Marfan's original report was of the condition now called congenital contractural arachnodactyly or Beal's syndrome.[13] The second is that the evidence points to an underlying defect in connective tissue, probably the collagen component. Collagen, the most abundant mammalian protein, is the fibrous 'backbone' of mesenchymal tissue, particularly skin, bone tendons, ligaments and blood vessels. The complexity of collagen at the molecular level makes it very unlikely that Marfan's syndrome is a single entity. Even at the clinical level, there is practical danger in adhering too closely to the classic phenotype of arachnodactyly (Fig. 67.2a), slender 'asthenic' build, lens dislocation, pneumothoraces and aortic root dilatation. The patient in Fig. 67.2b had few outward signs of his collagen defect until he developed a dissecting aneurysm.

As more is discovered about collagen pathology, the boundaries between osteogenesis imperfecta, Ehlers–Danlos syndrome, Marfan's syndrome and other collagen disorders become blurred. Maroteaux *et al.*,[14] who have addressed this problem, have begun to group clinical disorders on the basis of predominant areas of involvement—skin, ligament/articular, skeletal and vascular. Marfan's syndrome is considered to be in the last of these groups although it does overlap with the others. For the reader unfamiliar with the biology of collagen, a

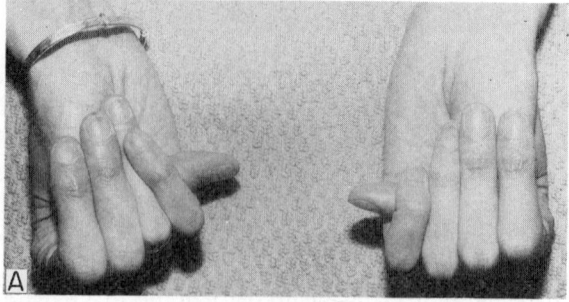

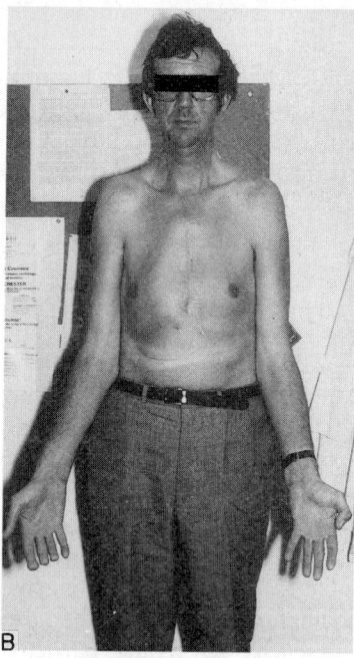

Fig. 67.2. (A) Classic 'Steinberg sign' of Marfan's syndrome—the combination of arachnodactyly and lax joints permits the protrusion of the thumb beyond the ulnar border of the clenched fist. (B) A man with Marfan's syndrome who lacks many of the typical stigmata but who presented for emergency surgery with a dissecting aneurysm.

brief outline has been provided in Appendix 2 (p. 1465).

The large number of defects in collagen formation discovered to date is likely to be only a small percentage of the true total.[15] The most impressive molecular interpretations have been made with other collagen disorders,[16] such as osteogenesis imperfecta, but some progress is being made in Marfan's syndrome. Slow synthesis of type I procollagen in aortic explants,[17] excess excretion of hydroxyproline, suggestive of increased collagen turnover,[18] and defective cross-linking[19] have been reported. The last of these findings raised the possi-

bility of lysyl oxidase deficiency but this has not been confirmed.[20] Similarly, the report[21] of an abnormal insertion in the pro-alpha 2(I) chains suggesting a defect in the COLIA2 gene on chromosome 7 was not confirmed by family linkage studies[22] and may be a coincidental variant.

Ehlers–Danlos (ED) syndrome type IV is better understood. There are at least 10 types of ED; type IV is the very severe form. Sufferers have fragile atrophic skin and a senile appearance called acrogeria, moderate joint laxity, frequent bruising and mitral valve prolapse. The prognosis is poor because of a tendency to intestinal rupture, spontaneous pneumothorax and the rupture of large blood vessels. This description corresponds to the severe autosomal recessive form in which Pope *et al.*[23] demonstrated a total absence of type III collagen. A milder recessive form is known in which some type III collagen is found, and there are 2 clinical forms that behave as dominants, one is a severe arterial type[24] and the other is benign, presenting with acrogeria alone.[25] Defects in the 1(III) gene probably account for most if not all forms of ED IV. As with familial hypercholesterolaemia, the recessive and dominant labels depend on assessment of clinical impact and there is no reason why a defect should not occur in a severe homozygous and a mild heterozygous form in the same pedigree. For example, in a large pedigree of Marfan's syndrome, Chemke *et al.*[26] found a family in which two affected cousins had produced two sibs both of whom had the same severe and ultimately lethal marfanoid features from birth which were almost certainly due to a homozygous collagen defect of the Marfan type.

One interesting aspect of the greater understanding of the molecular structure of collagen is the concept of 'protein suicide'. One of the mutations in the a1(I) gene which produces osteogenesis imperfecta alters the polypeptide chain in such a way that the normal collagen triple helix cannot form. Even though only 1 in 3 of the component alpha chains is abnormal, the majority of triple helical fibres are affected. This provides a molecular model for a dominant gene capable of producing a severe effect despite the presence of a normal allele.[27]

THE X CHROMOSOME AND HUNTER'S SYNDROME

Genes on the X chromosome provide the exception to the rule that genes are inherited in matching pairs. The male receives only one X chromosome and hence only one copy of X-linked genes. The technical term is hemizygosity. Females have two X chromosomes and usually experience no ill-effects from a defective gene on one X due to the 'protective effects' of the other. The impact of X-linked genes in cardiology is limited (excluding the problem of colour blindness which is found in 8% of all males and might impair the employment prospects of some male cardiologists called upon to use the colour flow Doppler technique!). The X-linked muscular dystrophies—Duchenne, Becker and Emery–Dreifuss—all have cardiological implications and are discussed in Chapter 40. For the cardiologist, perhaps the best example of an X-linked disorder is Hunter's syndrome, which is liable in its milder form to present in the adult with valve stenosis and/or incompetence due to the deposition of mucopolysaccharides in cardiac valves. A large Northern pedigree that illustrates the typical pattern of inheritance for an X-linked condition is shown in Fig. 67.3. The other mucopolysaccharidoses (MPS) are autosomal recessive conditions and therefore affect males and females equally. They present in childhood, with the exception of Scheie's syndrome in which the principal features are coarse facies, cloudy corneae, stiff joints, hearing loss, aortic valve defects and occasional hepatomegaly. This clinical condition used to be called type V MPS until it was found by studying the interaction of fibroblasts that the enzyme defect, alpha-iduronidase, was the same as that seen in Hurler's syndrome, in which the symptoms are much more severe. This is a striking example of an allelic variant; different clinical entities resulting from differing defects in the same gene. These two syndromes have been re-named MPS 1(S) and MPS 1(H), respectively.[28]

In females, one X chromosome in each cell is inactivated to achieve a dosage compensation with males, a process called Lyonization. This occurs independently in each cell at the start of differentiation and thereafter the same X chromosome is inactive in that cell line. Occasionally, most of the X chromosomes with the good gene are inactivated and the female carrier manifests the disease. Another cause for females to manifest an X-linked gene is translocation. Mossman et al.[29] reported a girl with Hunter's syndrome who had a translocation between an X chromosome and a number 5 chromosome. Chromosomes often break and, sometimes, the wrong ends are re-affixed during the repair process such that the result of two chromosomes breaking at the same time could be an exchange of the broken pieces. If the X chromosome is involved, cells that inactivate the abnormal X are liable to switch off that part of the other chromosome accidentally attached to the end of the X chromosome, leading to the death of that cell line. Only cell lines in which the normal X is inactivated survive to produce the individual. If the break in the X chromosome damaged a gene, the female, whose cells must all use the translocated X, would manifest the gene defect caused by the break. The case-report described above localized the Hunter's gene precisely to band Xq26. This is one way of mapping the human genome, a process greatly enhanced by the molecular techniques described earlier.

CHROMOSOME DISORDERS

Once the major single gene disorders are understood, the next phase in unravelling the molecular

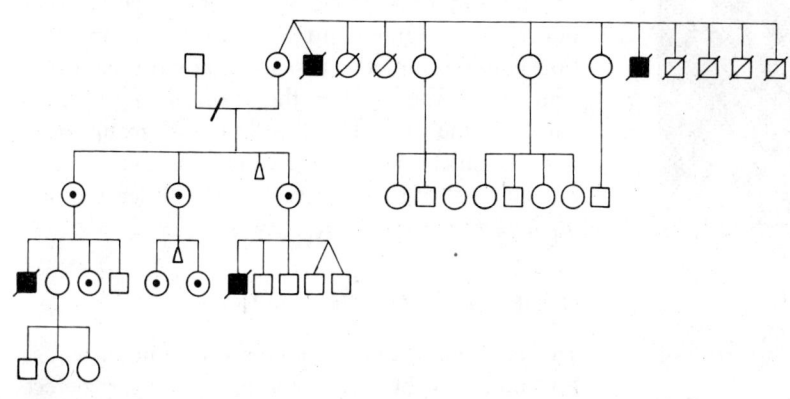

Fig. 67.3. Hunter's syndrome: mucopolysaccharidosis II. A typical X-linked pedigree with affected males linked through unaffected females.

■ Hunters Syndrome
⊙ Carrier female

genetic basis of cardiovascular disease will be the interpretation of the chromosome disorders. Chromosomes come in 23 matching pairs, one of each pair from each parent. Together they contain the body's 'blueprint'. The process of meiosis or reduction division, which produces a gamete with a half (haploid) set, is very prone to error. One in six of all established pregnancies aborts spontaneously. Half of these are chromosomally abnormal. Allowing for losses before a positive pregnancy test is recorded, at least 10%, and quite probably over half, of all human conceptions are chromosomally abnormal; 95% of these miscarry and a substantial proportion of the remainder will not reach adulthood because of the adverse effects of physical and mental malformation produced by the chromosomal abnormality. The physician is rarely called upon to manage a chromosomally abnormal adult.

TURNER'S SYNDROME

An important exception to the above is the female with Turner's syndrome (Fig. 67.4). Although Turner's syndrome was first described by Ullrich[30] in 1930, it gained its eponym from the American physician who described it in 1938.[31] Females with this disorder have only 45 chromosomes in each cell. There is a single X chromosome, the other sex chromosome having been lost. This may have been an X or a Y chromosome. Some affected girls have more complex structural anomalies and some are mosaics in which a proportion of their cells have a full chromosome complement. If the other cell line contains a Y chromosome, it is important to remove the streak gonads in view of the high risk of early malignancy.

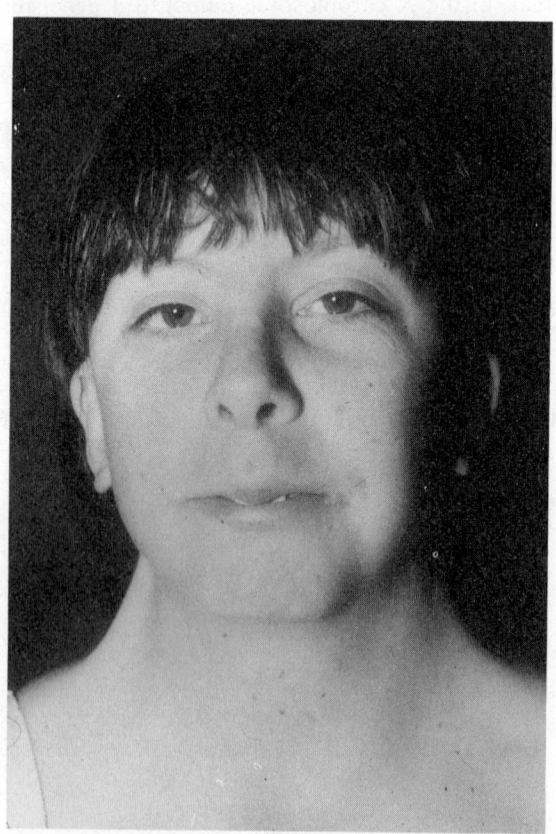

Fig. 67.4. Turner's syndrome: 45X typical webbed neck, partially corrected by surgery (with the common complication of keloid formation at the back of this girl's neck).[38]

Other effects of the 45X karyotype are short stature, 'sexual infantilism', webbing of the neck (pterygium colli) and sometimes other dysmorphic features such as a 'shark mouth' and downslanting palpebral fissures. Any of the above or lymphoedema of the feet occurring in infancy may precipitate medical investigation but a proportion of girls affected come to the attention of the cardiologist because 10% have coarctation of the aorta;[32,33] there are minor valve anomalies on echocardiography in a further 10%. Intelligence is normal, although a proportion have particular problems with spatial understanding. This is in marked contrast to chromosome disorders involving the non-sex chromosomes, or autosomes, in which mental retardation is the rule.

The reason for the relatively mild problems in the 45X female is that all normal females switch off or 'inactivate' one of their X chromosomes at an early stage of development (Lyonization—see above). This prompts the question why the girl with a 45X karyotype should have so many physical problems. One explanation is that normally in the first few cell divisions both X chromosomes are active and may be essential. Furthermore, in the gonads, both X chromosomes are active and are essential for their normal development. In other tissues, X inactivation is not complete. It is now known that several genes near the end of the short arm of the X chromosome (including the Xg blood group locus) remain functional after Lyonization. Presumably one or more of these genes is active in development of the aortic arch.

CONGENITAL MALFORMATIONS

Turner's syndrome represents one 'known cause' for congenital heart defects. In total, heart defects are present in 6–8 per 1000 newborn. Although primarily of interest to the paediatric cardiologist, these patients now survive with increasing frequency into adulthood due to the success of surgical and medical intervention over the last 25 years. A further point to note is recent claims that genetic factors have been underestimated and cardiac malformations may become more common in coming generations. Before addressing this issue, it is necessary to discuss those other categories in which causes are 'known'.

Down's syndrome and other chromosome defects

Based on the birth prevalence of chromosome defects,[34] it can be estimated that up to 10% of heart defects fall into this aetiological category. Trisomy 21 alone accounts for 1 in 20 cardiac malformations.[35] Forty per cent of infants with Down's syndrome have a heart defect, in 40% of whom it is an isolated atrioventricular defect,[36] an abnormality that is rare in other circumstances. This disorder is thought to result from a defect in growth or adhesion of the endocardial cushions which initiate septation of the orifice between the atrium and ventricle of the early heart tube. It is reasonable to assume, therefore, that genes on chromosome 21 are involved in these processes.

All described chromosome defects have been associated with heart defects, from which it may be inferred that a substantial proportion of the 50 000 or so genes in the genome are involved directly or indirectly in heart formation. Chromosome analysis is essential in all cases of heart defect occurring together with other malformations and/or abnormal facies and/or mental retardation. As techniques have advanced in recent years, reports of a normal karyotype that were obtained more than 10 years ago should be treated with caution. Recognition of chromosome abnormality is of particular importance when there is a familial translocation. A large pedigree in which inheritance of an unbalanced translocation has caused multiple cases of malformation is shown in Fig. 67.5.

Environmental insults or teratogens are a cause of a small but important group of heart malformations. The more important examples are listed in Table 67.1.[37] A detailed pregnancy history should provide the diagnosis. Recognition of a characteristic pattern of anomalies, constituting a syndrome, may provide the clue. If an adult with a heart defect fits such an 'environmental' syndrome or if the history reveals an exposure in fetal life, the risks to the patient's offspring should be negligible.

Other syndromes provide the basis for recognition of single gene defects. A mother with the classic facial features of Noonan's syndrome associated with pulmonary stenosis and atrial septal defect is shown in Fig. 67.6A.[38] Both of her daughters inherited the gene and were of short stature (Fig. 67.6B). One had the same heart defects but normal intelligence whereas the other was intellectually handicapped but had a normal heart. As the mother's parents were both normal, it is likely that the copying error that produced the faulty gene occurred at the mother's conception. Even in the absence of such a family history, the syndrome pattern allows recognition of a single gene defect. A list of 25 of the more important cardiac syndromes is given in Table 67.2.[39–63] This list represents only about 15% of the syndromes in the literature which may involve cardiac abnormality. With the continued delineation of syndrome patterns, it is likely that more than 5% of infants with heart defects will fit into a recognized syndrome category.

Among the great majority of cases in which chromosomes are normal and there is no recognized syndrome pattern, the multifactorial model is usually invoked, in which the genetic predisposition is attributed to the additive effect of multiple genes with or without associated environmental triggers. The most common single malformation, persistent ductus arteriosus, is a good illustration of the model. Congenital rubella, birth at high altitude and pre-term delivery are all known to cause this anomaly. In the majority of term infants with a patent arterial duct, however, none of these environmental factors applies and in this group polygenic predisposition provides a good explanation. In the experimental model of certain dog breeds prone to this disorder, Patterson et al.[64] have shown, with breeding experiments, that an abnormality of duct structure controlled by multiple genes is the likely cause. When two dogs with a persistent ductus arteriosus are bred together, 84% of their offspring will cross the disease threshold having either a duct diverticulum with the aortic end of the duct remaining open or a complete persistent opening. In humans, the detailed studies of Zetterqvist[65] have shown that a similar basis applies. The predictions of the polygenic model state that the risk to sibs and offspring should be broadly similar and should approximate to the square root of the population incidence. The risk of recurrence is greater in the relatives of the more severe cases and where there have been two or more affected individuals in the family. Zetterqvist found the square root of the population incidence to be

Table 67.2. **The 'top' 25 syndromes involving cardiac malformations.**

Alagille syndrome
Arteriohepatic dysplasia
At least some cases are autosomal
   dominant
Alagille *et al.*, 1975[39]
	Intrahepatic biliary atresias, embryotoxon of eye (80%),
	   abnormal facies (75%), vertebral anomalies (33%)
		Peripheral pulmonary stenosis

Asymmetric crying face syndrome Sporadic Levin *et al.* 1982	Hypoplasia or absence of depressor angularis oris on one side	Ventricular septal defect

Campomelic dysplasia syndrome
Autosomal recessive
Houston *et al.* 1983[41]
	Polyhydramnios, anterior bowed tibiae, hypotonia, small
	   scapulae, males appear female, cleft palate,
	   micrognathia
		Septal defects, tetralogy of Fallot,
		   aortic stenosis

CHARGE syndrome (acronym)
Unknown—all cases sporadic
Pagon *et al.* 1981[42]
	Colobomata (iris and/or retina), Heart defects, Atresia
	   choanae, Retardation and renal defects, Genitalia
	   small in males, Ears cup-shaped, deafness
		Wide variety including ventricular
		   septal defects, atrioventricular
		   septal defects and tetralogy of
		   Fallot

de Lange syndrome
Sporadic
Ptacek *et al.* 1963[43]
	Synorphrys, thin down-turned upper lip, severe
	   retardation and short stature, malrotation of bowel,
	   micrognathia, severe upper limb reduction defects
		Most often ventricular septal defects

DiGeorge syndrome
Sporadic, more in males? Deletion 22
   in some
Freedom *et al.*, 1972[44]
	Congenital hypoparathyroidism, down-slanting eyes,
	   short philtrum, low-set ears, micrognathia, thymic
	   hypoplasia (defect in fourth branchial arch)
		Outflow defects—interrupted aorta,
		   common arterial trunk, tetralogy of
		   Fallot

Ellis van Creveld syndrome
Chondroectodermal dysplasia
Autosomal recessive
Walls *et al.*, 1959[45]
	Postaxial polydactyly, rhizomelic limb shortening, short
	   ribs, small chest, oral frenulae, natal teeth, nail
	   dysplasia, sparse hair, thin skin
		50% have heart defects, typically
		   common atrium, atrioventricular
		   septal defect

Fetal hydantoin syndrome
Drug disruption
Speidel and Meadow, 1972[46]
	Growth deficiency, microcephaly, mild retardation, broad
	   depressed nasal bridge, hypoplastic nails
		Aortic and pulmonary valve stenosis
		   coarctation, patent arterial duct,
		   septal defects

Fetal alcohol syndrome
Maternal alcohol disruption
Jones *et al.*, 1973[47]
	Short stature, pre-natal onset, short palpebral fissures,
	   hairy forehead, smooth philtrum, thin upper lip,
	   hypoplastic terminal phalanges
		Typically septal defects. One-third of
		   classic cases

Goldenhar syndrome
Sporadic, occasional autosomal
   dominant
Greenwood *et al.*, 1974[48]
	Hemifacial microsomia, epibulbar dermoid, pre-auricular
	   tags, deafness, colobomata of eyelids.
		35% of cases, particularly tetralogy of
		   Fallot

Holt–Oram syndrome
Heart–hand I syndrome
Autosomal dominant, variable
   expression
Smith *et al.*, 1979[49]
	Finger-like hypoplastic to absent thumb, variable
	   hypoplasia first metacarpal, radius or whole limb,
	   narrow shoulders
		Septal defects usual, occasional
		   arrhythmia, hypoplastic distal
		   arteries

Hurler syndrome
   (mucopolysaccharidosis III)
Autosomal recessive—α-iduronidase
   deficiency
Leroy and Crocker, 1966[50]
	Coarse facies, dysostosis multiplex, hepatosplenomegaly,
	   corneal clouding, deafness, mental retardation
		Cardiomyopathy, stenosis and
		   incompetence due to
		   mucopolysaccharide deposition

Jervell and Lange-Nielson syndrome Autosomal recessive Jervell *et al.*, 1966[51]	Deafness–sensorineural, occasional hypochromic anaemia	Conduction defect, long QT interval

Table 67.2. Continued.   The 'top' 25 syndromes involving cardiac malformations.

LEOPARD syndrome (acronym) Autosomal dominant Gorlin et al., 1969[52]	Multiple lentigines, Electrocardiographic anomalies, Ocular hypertelorism, Pulmonary stenosis, Abnormal genitalia, Retardation, Deafness	Electrocardiographic anomalies, pulmonary stenosis (? overlap with Noonan's syndrome)
Maternal diabetes disruption syndrome (Poorly treated) maternal diabetes Rowland et al., 1973[53]	Variety of malformations, sacral agenesis (caudal regression), femoral hypoplasia, cleft palate, vertebral anomalies	Up to 5%—defects include ventricular septal defects and complete transposition
Maternal phenylketonuria disruption syndrome Disruption by high phenylalanine levels in utero Lenke and Levy, 1980[54]	Microcephaly, retardation, short stature, occasional microphthalmos and cleft palate	25% of cases—variety of defects including septal defects and outflow obstruction
Marfan's syndrome Autosomal dominant collagen defect Pyeritz and McKusick, 1979[55]	Arachnodactyly, lens subluxation, tall and slim with scoliosis, herniae, high palate	Aortic dilatation, valve incompetence
Noonan's syndrome Autosomal dominant Duncan et al., 1981[56]	Short, retarded, down-slanting palpebral fissures, low-set ears, short/webbed neck, cryptorchidism, pectus excavatum/carinatum	Pulmonary valve stenosis, atrial septal defect, hypertrophic cardiomyopathy
Pompe's disease Glycogen storage disease type IIA Autosomal recessive acid maltase deficiency Rees et al., 1976[57]	Sever hypotonia, large tonue, hepatomegaly	Progressive cardiac hypertrophy
Rubenstein–Taybi syndrome Sporadic Simpson and Brissenden, 1973[58]	Developmental delay, broad thumbs and great toes, short, small head, down-slanting eyes, beaked nose with downward extension of septum, cryptorchidism	33% ventricular septal defect, persistent arterial duct most common
Smith–Lemli–Opitz syndrome Autosomal recessive Cherstvoy et al., 1975[59]	Mental retardation, microcephaly ptosis, squint, anteverted nostrils, 2/3 syndactyly of toes, broad alveolar ridges, hypospadias, occasional polydactyly	Various cardiac defects reported including atrial and ventricular septal defects and tetralogy of Fallot
Thrombycytopenia–absent radius (TAR) syndrome Autosomal recessive Hall et al., 1969[60]	Bilateral absent radius, ulnar hypoplasia, thumbs present, occasionally (7%) mentally retarded, squint, small jaw	33% have congenital heart defect including tetralogy of Fallot and atrial septal defect
VACTERL association Sporadic ?early general disruption of development Temtamy and Miler, 1974[61]	Acronym: Vertebral anomalies, Anal atresia, Cardiac defects, Tracheo-oEsophageal fistula, Renal anomalies, Limb reduction defects (radial)	Variety of defects: ventricular septal defects most common
Velo-cardio-facial syndrome Shprintzen syndrome Probable autosomal dominant Shprintzen et al., 1981[62]	Cleft palate, nasal voice, square nasal route, mild retardation, short stature, small jaw and head in some, conductive hearing loss	Ventricular septal defect, right aortic arch, tetralogy of Fallot
William's syndrome Sporadic, possible new mutation dominant Burn, 1986[63]	Mild-to-moderate mental retardation, medial eyebrow flare, stellate iris, thick lips, zygomatic flattening, infantile hypercalcaemia	Supravalvar aortic stenosis, peripheral valve stenosis

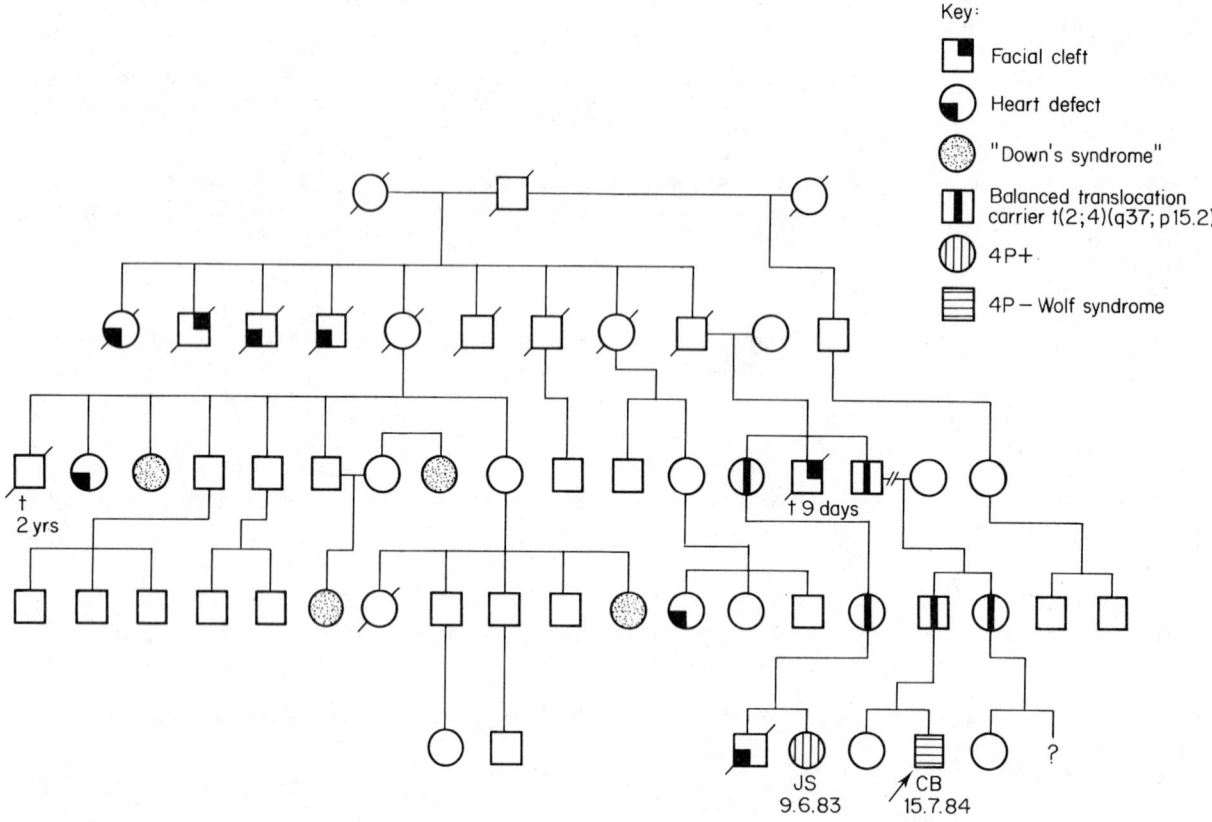

Key:

Facial cleft

Heart defect

"Down's syndrome"

Balanced translocation carrier t(2;4)(q37; p15.2)

4P+

4P − Wolf syndrome

Fig. 67.5. A large pedigree in which inheritance of an unbalanced translocation has caused multiple cases of malformation. As a result of the translocation the end of chromosome 4 has become attached to a chromosome 2. Carriers of the rearrangement are liable to transmit either the long 2 and normal 4 or the normal 2 and short 4. The first would produce trisomy 4p (three copies of the short arm), whereas the latter would be monosomic for 4p. Both forms have occurred in this pedigree. The question mark represents a pregnancy shown to be another trisomy 4p which was terminated. The numerous infants in earlier generations with either facial clefting or heart defects were, almost certainly, affected by unbalanced forms of the same translocation.

2.4%. The recurrence in sibs was 2.3% and in offspring, after excluding 2 syndromic families, it was 2.5%. Families with 2 affected members had a recurrence risk of 10%. At operation, 71 probands were noted to have an unusually wide patent duct; 7 of their 146 offspring were affected (4.8%) whereas the offspring of those probands with a narrow or moderate duct had a recurrence in offspring of only 1.8%. Another rule of polygenic inheritance is the so called Carter effect which states that the risk is greater in the relatives of the more rarely affected sex; in the case of persistent ductus arteriosus where females outnumber males 3 to 1 a greater risk among the relatives of affected males would be expected. Although the figures did not achieve statistical significance, the trend in the data was compatible with this rule also.

For other structural heart defects epidemiological studies have revealed little evidence of environmental insult because the prevalence in different populations is remarkably similar[66] and in longitudinal studies[35,67] it has been shown that the annual incidence remains unchanged over several years. Despite this evidence, some authors have placed great emphasis on environmental insult. The main evidence in support of environmental insult was the observation that in monozygotic (MZ) twins only one of the pair was affected. This argument has been weakened by the demonstration that the MZ twinning process itself is liable to cause one of the pair to have a heart malformation. In two hospital series, Burn and Corney[68] found 50% of the 195 twin pairs with heart defects to be MZ, a figure higher than that expected (35%). A subsequent analysis of heart defects in over 20 000 twins in 5 British twin/malformation studies[69] showed about

Table 67.1.   Some important cardiovascular teratogens.

Teratogen	Frequency of cardiovascular disease (%)	Most common cardiac malformations
Infection		
Rubella	35	Persistent patency of arterial duct; peripheral pulmonary stenosis; septal defects
Drugs		
Alcohol (high intake)	25–30	Septal defects
Hydantoin	2–3	Pulmonary and aortic stenosis coarctation of aorta
Trimethadione	15–30	Complete transposition, Tetralogy of Fallot. Hypoplastic left heart
Thalidomide		Tetralogy of Fallot, septal defects, common arterial trunk
Lithium		Ebstein's anomaly; tricuspid atresia; atrial septal defect
Maternal disease		
Diabetes (poor control)	3–5	Complete transposition; ventricular septal defect; coarctation of aorta
Phenylketonuria	25–50	Tetralogy of Fallot
Systemic lupus erythematosus (Anti Ro-antibody)	20–40	Complete heart block

From Burn *et al.* 1987,[12] after Nora and Nora.[37]

18 per 1000 heart defects among MZ twins, more than twice the prevalence among dizygotic twins and singletons. Thus, the traditional twin method cannot be used to assess the genetic component in singleton heart defects.

There are several possible ways in which the twinning process might be associated with, or cause, heart defects. Haemodynamic disturbance through the placenta is one possibility. Another is the disturbance of laterality. One of the fundamental steps in heart formation is formation of the dextral heart loop—bending of the primitive heart tube towards the right. If this is disturbed in experimental animals, a variety of defects may result, probably due to loss of laminar flow in the two streams of blood with subsequent interference in the septation that normally occurs between the two streams. Several lines of evidence suggest that some form of cell interaction occurs so that the left side acts as a point of reference for all cells lying to the right.[70] Rarely, this process is reversed and the whole structure of the body is reversed (situs inversus). It is possible that in some MZ twins the developmental separation causes the 'right half' to become separated from its point of reference on the left. This 'right-sided' twin may then fail to define clearly the left and right sides with resultant disturbances of the bending process of the heart tube. The mirror image twins in Fig. 67.7, the 'right' half of whom had tetralogy of Fallot, illustrate this hypothesis.

The other main source of evidence in the study of the genetic component of heart defects is the use of family studies. In general, these have shown a recurrence rate in sibs and offspring of about 3–5% which is often quoted as evidence of a polygenic predisposition. It is not proof, however, for two main reasons: heterogeneity and inadequate data. A particular heart defect may be the end result of a variety of single gene and non-genetic disorders. For example, among 100 cases of atrial septal defect, if 10 were new mutation dominant disorders and 20 were due to recessive genes from both parents while the rest were non-genetic, the defect would recur in 5% of offspring and 5% of sibs. In reality, the distinction between 'polygenes' and 'single genes' is probably far from clear.

The published data sets in family studies are often small. In particular, later born sibs, which are less affected by ascertainment bias, and offspring are difficult to collect in large numbers. This is a major problem with more severe defects. In a long-term follow-up study, Whittemore *et al.*[71] found 60 of 372 offspring to have some form of heart defect. Even with critical analysis, this finding could not be reconciled with those of earlier studies.[72] In another recent offspring study from Canada,[73] 40 defects among 385 live offspring (10.4%) were reported. It remains possible that in these studies there is a variety of hidden biases;[74] for example, if parents have a child with a heart defect they may be more inclined to stay close to the major hospital rather than move elsewhere and thus distort the recurrence risk figures. A British collaborative study is now underway in which these possible biases are avoided by tracing all adults from defined surgical units regardless of place of residence. Preliminary data from this study have revealed 7 per 172 (4%) of offspring to be affected.[75]

It is clear that more family studies devoted to specific anatomical defects are needed. A summary of counselling figures arranged according to the

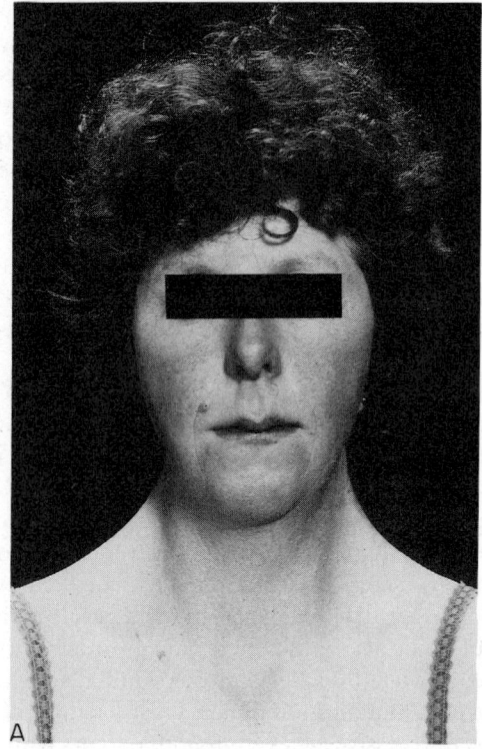
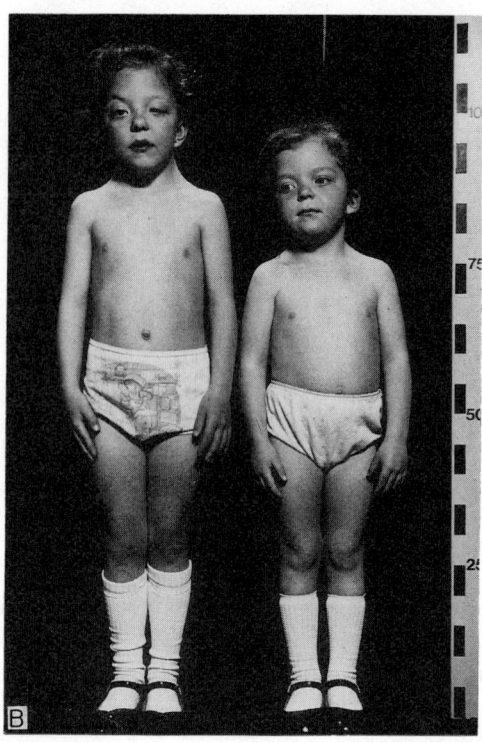

Fig. 67.6. (A) Mother with pulmonary stenosis and atrial septal defect as part of Noonan syndrome. (B) Both daughters are affected by the same gene defect; the older girl had development delay, a webbed neck and short stature but a normal heart, whereas the younger girl is of normal intelligence with short stature and the same heart defects as mother.

sequential segmental classification now employed to describe cardiac anomalies is shown in Table 67.3. The principle is to define situs followed by atrioventricular and ventricular connections followed by associated cardiac anomalies such as septal defects. Table 67.3 is based on traditional family studies. As prospective data from fetal echocardiography allow detailed analysis of subsequent sibs, these figures will need to be revised.[75]

This overview has concentrated on genetic mechanisms. In situations where single gene inheritance is applicable, such as the collagen disorders and certain forms of hyperlipaemia, the knowledge of the precise cause can be applied directly to accurate counselling of patients and their families. When mechanisms are more complex, as with congenital heart defects, counselling must rely on empirical or observational data. As the revolution of the 'new genetics' expands our understanding of the precise causes of such malformations, it is likely that counselling will become more specific and the art and science of genetics will become united across the spectrum of cardiovascular disease.

APPENDIX 1: SICKLE CELL DISEASE AND THE ADVENT OF THE GENE PROBE*

Sickle cell disease is a recessive disorder of haemoglobin structure resulting from a mutation in the beta-globin gene on chromosome 11. A single amino acid substitution (valine for glutamic acid at position 6) causes the haemoglobin molecules to aggregate at low oxygen tension. The red cells take on a 'sickle' shape resulting in cell lysis leading to anaemia, vascular occlusions and consequent multisystem disease. Possession of the gene provides resistance to cerebral malaria; this selective advantage has made the gene exceptionally common in several populations—up to one-third of West African populations are heterozygous and the gene is very common among black Americans in whom it no longer provides any advantage. The disease is thoroughly understood at the molecular level and

---

* Reference numbers used in this Appendix correspond to those in the list relating to the main body of text.

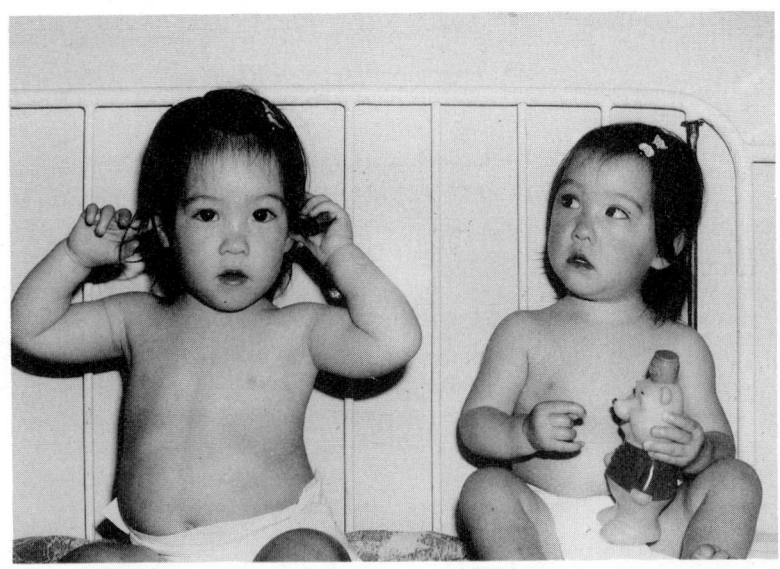

Fig. 67.7. Mono-amniotic twins with mirror imaging for tooth eruption and hair whorl position. The right half of the pair had tetralogy of Fallot. (Reproduced with permission from Burn & Corney[68])

Table 67.3. Recommended counselling figures in families containing a single individual with cardiovascular malformation arranged in order of sequential classification and abstracted from published family studies.[38]

Congenital heart defect	Risk of recurrence (%)	
	Sibs	Offspring
Situs inversus	5	?1
Isomerism	5	?1
Atrioventricular connection		
Double inlet (UVH)	?3	?5
Tricuspid atresia	1	?5
Mitral atresia	2	?5
Ventriculo-atrial connection		
Transposition of the great arteries	2	?5
Truncus arteriosus	1	?5
Pulmonary atresia	1	?5
Aortic atresia	1	?5
(Situs solitus, atrioventricular/ventriculo-atrial concordant)		
Anomalous pulmonary venous return	?3	?5
Secundum atrial septal defect	3	4
Cor triatrium	?3	?5
Atrioventricular septal defect	2	5–10
Ebstein's anomaly	1	?5
(Mitral valve prolapse	50	50)
Ventricular septal defect	3	4
Pulmonary stenosis	2	6
Tetralogy of Fallot	2	4
Aortic stenosis	3	5–10
Coarctation of aorta	2	3
Persistent ductus arteriosus	2.5	3

was the first in which clinical use was made of gene probes.

Each individual receives 23 chromosomes from each parent, 46 in all. Each chromosome contains a molecule of DNA. If the 23 molecules were unravelled and placed end to end, they would measure about 2 m in length. The molecule has a ladder-like structure with the two side-arms of alternating sugar and phosphate molecules linked by 'rungs' of base pairs. The bases are of 4 types: adenine (A), guanine (G), cytosine (C) and thymine (T). The cross-bridges are either A–T or G–C. These base pairs separate easily to allow the molecule to split along its length. Each half of the molecule can act as a template for the production of the other half. This capacity to replicate is the basis of genetic transmission in all life forms. Most of the DNA in the genome has no obvious function. Only about 5% represents coding sequences. In these, the bases are read as triplets: each amino acid is coded for by at least one triplet of bases (codon). With 4 letters, ACGT, there are 64 possible triplets. Two triplets act as full stops and the rest are divided among the 21 amino acids with all but methionine having more than a single codon. Coding sequences are interrupted by one or more intervening sequences (intergenic DNA) in all genes studied to date. These are removed as DNA is transcribed to messenger RNA.

In sickle cell disease, the seventeenth base in the coding sequence is mutated from A to T which alters the sixth amino acid to valine. To detect this error among the 6–7 thousand million base pairs in the whole genome, molecular biologists have several tools, the most important of which are restriction enzymes. These can be thought of as scissors that can read. A particular restriction enzyme will cut a DNA molecule wherever it 'sees' the sequence of bases that comprise its recognition sequence. For example, EcoR1, named after *E. coli* from which it was extracted, will cut DNA, whether it is human or bacterial, at the letter sequence GAACCT. When DNA is extracted from an individual's cells and digested with EcoR1, several million small pieces result which may be spread on an agar plate. The DNA from one person will always be cut into the same array of pieces but these will differ in number and size from another person because of frequent differences in the intergenic DNA where mutations do no obvious harm.

To find the piece or pieces of DNA that comprise the ß-globin gene requires a gene probe, which is a piece of human DNA in single-stranded form (i.e. split lengthways), and made radioactive by incorporation of ^{32}P into its phosphate sugar backbone. The ß-globin gene probe was manufactured by extracting globin RNA from marrow red cell precursors. The enzyme reverse transcriptase, now made famous by the AIDS virus, was then used to convert this RNA into DNA—complementary DNA or cDNA, which is an exact match for the original gene except that the non-coding intervening sequences are missing.

Having produced tiny quantities of ß-globin cDNA, mass production was achieved using plasmid vectors. These are primitive viral-like forms which live as parasites in bacteria. A plasmid is a simple circle of DNA. Laboratory-modified plasmids and *E. coli* are used for safety. The human cDNA is allowed to incorporate into a plasmid by using the same restriction enzyme to open the DNA circle. Using changes in bacterial resistance to identify those bacterial clones whose plasmids contain human DNA, it is possible to culture these clones selectively, and then cut open their plasmids again to release millions of copies of the original human cDNA which can then be used as a diagnostic probe.

When Kan and Dozy[7] used a ß-globin gene probe to highlight by autoradiography the piece of DNA on the agar plate incorporating the ß-globin gene, they found a common polymorphism. Many people had two bands on the gel because on one of the number 11 chromosomes the EcoR1 restriction enzyme fragment, which included the gene, was

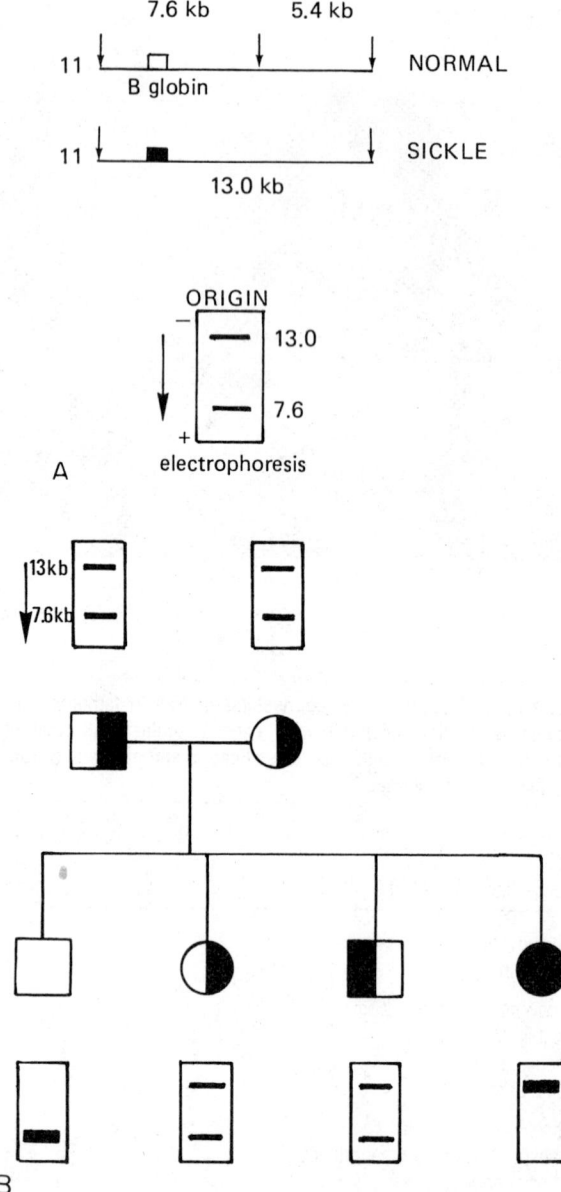

Fig. A67.1. (A) Use of a linked DNA polymorphism to track sickle cell disease. This simplified diagram is based on the original work of Kan and Dozy.[7] The two upper lines represent the piece of DNA in the two number 11 chromosomes which carries the β-globin gene in a patient who is a carrier (i.e. has one normal and one abnormal gene). The arrows indicate the points at which the restriction enzyme EcoR1 cuts this length of DNA. In this carrier of sickle cell disease, the lower chromosome 11 with the mutant gene has a missing cutting site so that the DNA fragment containing the sickle gene is 13 kb in length instead of the more usual 7.6-kb fragment produced from the upper chromosome. When the fragments are separated (below) on the electrophoretic gel and a radioactive β-globin DNA probe is applied, two bands appear. The upper band is the 13-kb fragment which has migrated a shorter distance. Such a 13-kb fragment was rarely present in individuals in whom both β-globin genes were normal (see B). (B) When the DNA pattern is examined in this idealized family, the two carrier parents have the heterozygote pattern with two bands produced by the differing cuttings sites on the two chromosomes. The affected child (bottom right) has received two number 11 chromosomes with the β-globin gene on a 13-kb fragment resulting in a single band on the gene. The normal child on the bottom left has a single band at 7.6 kb, having received the two chromosomes with the extra cutting site. The two carrier children have received one chromosome of each type. Thus, it may be deduced that in this family the abnormal gene is on the chromosome which has the 13-kb fragment and it may be predicted that any future child who has a single 13-kb band will have sickle cell disease. This approach does not detect the fault in the gene itself. The faulty gene is being **tracked** in the family on the basis of the variable cutting sites around the gene. Such variations are called polymorphisms and because the variation depends on the varying fragment size of restriction enzyme digestion the full title of such a variation is a 'restriction fragment length polymorphism' or RFLP.

7600 bases (or 7.6 kb) long whereas the other number 11 chromosome had a missing cutting site so that the ß-globin gene was a fragment 13 kb in length. Although such restriction fragment length polymorphisms (RFLPs) are common, among black Americans of West African descent, almost all homozygotes for the sickle cell gene had only the 13-kb fragment whereas their carrier parents were heterozygous for the RFLP with a slow-moving 13-kb band and a fast-moving 7.6-kb band. The inference was that the original sickle cell mutation in this population had occurred in a number 11 chromosome with the missing cutting site. The RFLP provided a means of tracking the faulty gene. A simplified illustration of the gel pattern and its use in families is shown in Fig. A67.1. For the first time, it was possible to predict the presence of the disease on the basis of the RFLP pattern thus allowing pre-natal diagnosis in the first trimester.

In the case of sickle cell disease, the technique has now been taken further by making use of the fact that the specific base change in sickle cell disease destroys a cutting site for the restriction enzyme Mst II, producing a specific change in the band pattern on the gel.[9] In most diseases, variation of the mutation will make such precision hard to achieve but the idea of tracking a disease gene has wide application. It is even possible when the disease gene product is not known. An important example is Huntingdon's chorea, the gene for which can be tracked in families by closely linked markers on chromosome 4.[10]

APPENDIX 2: THE BIOLOGY OF COLLAGEN

Collagen comprises a triple helix. At least 10 forms

have been described.[15] Nine alpha chains, coded for by distinct genes, make up the 5 major forms of collagen. Of these, types I, III and V are found in blood vessels. Type I collagen has been the subject of most study and comprises triplets of two 1(I) chains and one 2(I) chain—the short hand form being $[1(I)]_2 2(I)$. Every third amino acid is glycine; this is the smallest amino acid and it occupies the limited space where the three chains come together. The 1(I) gene has been mapped to chromosome 17 and is 18 kb in length, more than 10 times bigger than ß-globin. Intervening sequences split the gene into multiple short coding sections called exons. The 2(I) gene is on chromosome 7 and is spread over 38 kb (38 000 bases) with about 50 intervening sequences separating exons each of which is 54 bases long. Most exons in collagen are of this length with the shorter ones all sharing the factor 9, i.e. 'glycine–X–Y', an amino acid structure that is crucial to a viable product and has 9 base pairs coding for the 3 amino acids. The 8-fold reduction in size as the gene is transcribed to messenger RNA is thought to favour recombination and deletion

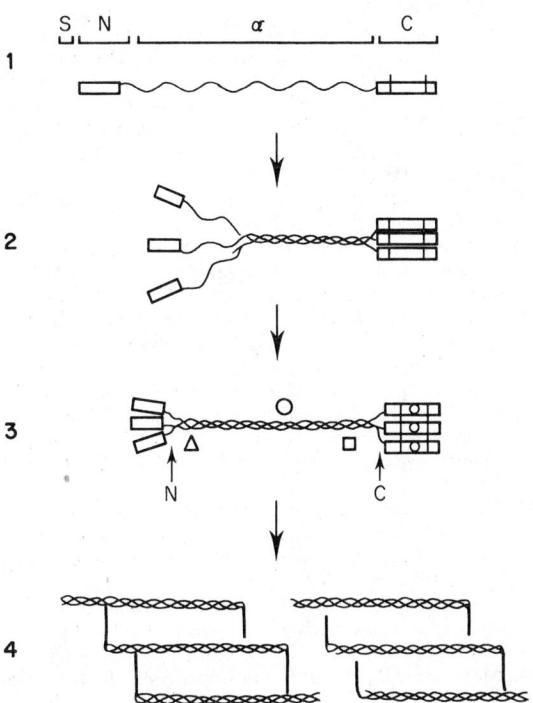

Fig. A67.2. Fibrillogenesis: **1**, pre-procollagen with indication of the various domains (S, signal domain; N, N-pro-peptide; a, alpha chain; C, C-pro-peptide); **2**, triple helix formation; **3**, post-translational modifications ($\triangle$, $\bigcirc$, $\square$) and removal of terminal pro-peptides N and C; **4**, self-assembly into fibrils. (Reproduced with permission from Tsipouras, P. and Ramirez, F. *J. Med. Genet.* 1987; **24**: 2–8.[22]

and provides one explanation for the great variety of collagen mutations now recognized. The procollagens, synthesized in the rough endoplasmic reticulum, have three 'domains': the helix, the COOH terminal and the NH_2 terminal. The latter extensions are needed to align, form and stabilize the triple helix, prevent intracellular fibrogenesis and allow transport. As the chain is synthesized, most of the proline residues in the Y position of the Gly–X–Y triplets are hydroxylated together with a small number of lysine residues which permits later glycosylation. If helix formation is slowed by mutation, hydroxylation and glycosylation may be excessive, a process called overmodification.[16] Fibrillogenesis is shown in Fig. A67.2.

REFERENCES

1. McKusick, V. A genetical view of cardiovascular disease. *Circulation* 1964; 30: 326–57.
2. Garrod, A. The lesson of rare maladies (quotation of Harvey, W., 1657). *Lancet* 1928; i: 1055–9.
3. Slack, J. Risks of ischaemic heart disease in familial hyperlipoproteinaemia. *Lancet* 1969; ii: 1380.
4. Havel, R.J., Goldstein, J.L. and Brown, M.S. Lipoproteins and lipid transport. In: Bondy, P.K. and Rosenberg, L.E., eds. *Metabolic Control and Disease*. Philadelphia: W.B. Saunders, 1980, p. 393.
5. Brown, M.S. and Goldstein, J.L. Receptor mediated control of cholesterol metabolism. *Science* 1976; 191: 150–4.
6. Weatherall, D.J. *The new genetics in clinical practice,* 2nd edn. Oxford: Oxford University Press, 1985.
7. Kan, Y.W. and Dozy, A.M. Antenatal diagnosis of sickle cell anaemia by DNA analysis of amniotic-fluid cells. *Lancet* 1978; ii: 910–1.
8. Burn, J. and Clarke, A.J. Genetic factors in tropical diseases. In: Stanfield, P.J., ed. *Diseases of Children in the Tropics and Subtropics*. London: Edward Arnold (in press).
9. Chang, J.C. and Kan, Y.W. A sensitive new prenatal test for sickle cell anemia. *N. Engl. J. Med.* 1982; 307: 30–2.
10. Gusella, J.F., Wexler, N.S., Conneally, P.M. *et al.* A polymorphic DNA marker genetically linked to Huntington's disease. *Nature* 1983; 306: 234–8.
11. Hobbs, H.H., Brown, M.S., Russell, D.W., Davignon, J. and Goldstein, J.L. Deletion in the gene for the low-density-lipoprotein receptor in a majority of French Canadians with familial hypercholesterolemia. *N. Engl. J. Med.* 1987; 317: 734–7.
12. Burn, J., Durrington, P. and Harris, R. Genetics and cardiovascular disease. In: Rowlands, D.J., ed. *Recent Advances in Cardiology*, Vol. 10. Edinburgh: Churchill Livingstone, 1987, pp. 27–47.
13. Hecht, F. and Beal, R.K. 'New' syndrome of congenital contractural arachnodactyly originally described by Marfan in 1896. *Pediatrics* 1972; 49: 574–9.
14. Maroteaux, P., Frezal, J. and Cohen-Solal, L. The differential symptomatology of errors of collagen metabolism: a tentative classification. *Am. J. Med. Genet.* 1986; 24: 219–30.
15. Human Gene Mapping 8. Eighth International Workshop on Human Gene Mapping, Cytogenetics and Cell Genetics, 1985. Vol. 40, No. 1–4.
16. Prockop, D.J. and Kivirikko, K.I. Heritable diseases of collagen. *N. Engl. J. Med.* 1984; 311: 376–85.
17. Halbritter, R., Aumailley, M., Rackwitz, R., Krieg, T. and Muller, P.K. Case report and study of collagen metabolism in Marfan syndrome. *Klin. Wochenschr.* 1981; 59: 83–90.
18. Kivirikko, K.I. Urinary excretion of hydroxyproline in health and disease. *Int. Rev. Conn. Tiss. Res.* 1970; 5: 93–163.
19. Boucek, R.J., Noble, N.L., Gunja-Smith, Z. and Butler, W.T. The Marfan Syndrome: a deficiency in chemically stable collagen cross-links. *N. Engl. J. Med.* 1981; 305: 988–91.
20. Royce, P.M. and Danks, D.M. Normal lysyl oxidase activity in skin fibroblasts from patients with Marfan's syndrome. *IRCS Med. Sci.* 1982; 10: 41.
21. Byers, P.H., Siegel, R.C., Peterson, K.E. *et al.* Marfan syndrome: abnormal alpha 2 chain in type 1 collagen. *Proc. Natl. Acad. Sci. U.S.A.* 1981; 78: 7745–9.
22. Tsipouras, P. and Ramirez, F. Genetic Disorders of Collagen. *J. Med. Genet.* 1987; 24: 2–8.
23. Pope, F.M., Martin, G.R., Lichtenstein, J.R., Penttinen, R., Gerson, B., Rowe, D.W. and McKusick, V.A. Patients with Ehlers–Danlos Syndrome type IV lack type III collagen. *Proc. Natl. Acad. Sci. U.S.A.* 1975; 72: 1314–6.
24. Beighton, P., Price, A., Lord, J. and Dickson, E. Variants of the Ehlers–Danlos syndrome: clinical, biochemical, haematological and chromosomal features of 100 patients. *Ann. Rheum. Dis.* 1972; 28: 228–45.
25. Pope, F.M., Nichols, A.C., Jones, P.M., Wells, R.S. and Lawrence, D. Eds IV(acrogeria): new autosomal dominant and recessive types. *J. R. Soc. Med.* 1980; 73: 180–6.
26. Chemke, J., Nisani, R., Feigl, A., Garti, R., Cooper, M., Barash, Y. and Duskin, D. Homozygosity for autosomal dominant Marfan Syndrome. *J. Med. Genet.* 1984; 21: 173–7.
27. Spranger, J. The developmental pathology of collagen in humans. In: Gilbert, E.F. and Opitz, F.M., eds. *Genetic aspects of developmental pathology*. Birth Defects Original Articles, Series 23(1), 1987, pp. 1–16.
28. Benson, P.F. and Fensom, A.H. Mucopolysaccharidoses. In: *Genetic Biochemical Disorders*. Oxford Univ. Press, 1985, pp. 8–54.
29. Mossman, J., Blunt, S., Stephens, R., Jones, E.F. and Pembrey, M.E. Hunter's disease in a girl: Association with X:5 chromosomal translocation disrupting the Hunter gene. *Arch. Dis. Child.* 1983; 58: 911–5.
30. Ullrich, O. Uber typische Kombinationsbilder multipler Abartungen. *S. Kinderheilkd.* 1930; 49: 271–6.
31. Turner, H.H. A syndrome of infantilism congenital webbed neck and cubitus valgus. *Endocrinology* 1938; 23: 566–74.
32. Simpson, J.L. *Gonadal dysgenesis in disorders of sexual differentiation etiology and clinical delineation*. New York and London: Academic Press, 1976.
33. Miller, M.J., Geffner, M.E., Lippe, B.M., Itami, R.M., Kaplan, S.A., Disessa, T.G., Isabel-Jones, J.B. and Friedman, M.J. Echocardiography reveals a high incidence of bicuspid aortic valve in Turner syndrome. *J. Pediatr.* 1983; 102: 47–50.
34. Hamerton, J.L., Canning, N., Ray, M. and Smith, S. A cytogenetic survey of 14,069 newborn infants. 1. Incidence of chromosome abnormalities. *Clin. Genet.* 1975; 8: 223–43.
35. Kenna, A.P., Smithells, R.W. and Fielding, D.W. Congenital heart disease in Liverpool 1960–9. *Quart. J. Med.* 1975; 44: 17–44.
36. Park, S.C., Mathews, R.A., Zuberbuhler, J.R., Rowe, R.D, Neches, W.H. and Lenox, C.C. Down's syndrome with congenital heart malformation. *Am. J. Dis. Children* 1977; 131: 29–33.
37. Nora, J.J. and Nora, A.H. Genetic epidemiology of congenital heart diseases. In: Steinberg, A.G., Bearn, A.G., Motulsky, A. *et al.*, eds. *Progress in Medical Genetics*.

V.—*Genetics of Cardiovascular Disease.* London: W.B. Saunders, 1983, pp. 91–137.

38. Burn, J. The aetiology of congenital heart disease. In: Anderson, R.H., Macartney, F.J., Shinebourne, E.A. and Tynan, M., eds. *Paediatric Cardiology.* Edinburgh: Churchill Livingstone, 1987, pp. 15–63.

39. Alagille, D., Odievre, M., Gautier, M. and Dommergues, J.P. Hepatic ductular hypoplasia associated with characteristic facies, vertebral malformations, retarded physical, mental and sexual development and cardiac murmur. *J. Pediatr.* 1975; **86**: 63–71.

40. Levin, B., Burgess, E.A. and Mortimer, P.E. Glycogen storage disease type IV, amylopectinosis. *Arch. Dis. Child.* 1968; **43**: 548–55.

41. Houston, C.S., Opitz, J.M., Spranger, J.W., McPherson, R.I., Reed, M.H., Gilbert, E.F., Herrmann, J. and Schinzel, A. The campomelic syndrome: Review, report of 17 cases, and follow-up on the currently 17-year-old boy first reported by Maroteaux *et al.* in 1971. *Am. J. Med. Genet.* 1983; **15**: 3–28.

42. Pagon, R.A., Graham, J.M., Socana, J. and Yong, S.L. Coloboma, congenital heart disease, and choanal atresia with multiple anomalies: CHARGE association. *Pediatrics* 1981; **99**: 223–7.

43. Ptacek, L.J., Opitz, J.M., Smith, D.W., Gerritsen, T. and Waisman, H.A. The Cornelia de Lange syndrome. *J. Pediatr.* 1963; **63**: 1000–20.

44. Freedom, R.M., Rosen, F.S. and Nadas, A.S. Congenital cardiovascular disease and anomalies of the third and fourth pharyngeal pouch. *Circulation* 1972; **46**: 165–72.

45. Walls, W.L., Altman, D.H. and Winslow, O.P. Chondroectodermal dysplasia (Ellis van Creveld syndrome). Report of a case and review of the literature. *Am. J. Dis. Child* 1959; **98**: 242–8.

46. Speidel, B.D. and Meadow, S.R. Maternal epilepsy and abnormalities of the fetus and newborn. *Lancet* 1972; **ii**: 839–43.

47. Jones, K.L., Smith, D.W., Ulleland, C.N. and Streissguth, A.P. Pattern of malformation in offspring of chronic alcoholic mothers. *Lancet* 1973; **i**: 1267–71.

48. Greenwood, R.D., Rosenthal, A., Sommer, A., Wolff, G. and Craenen, J. Cardiovascular malformations in oculoauriculovertebral dysplasia (Goldenhar syndrome). *J. Pediatr.* 1974; **85**: 816–8.

49. Smith, A.T., Sack, G.H. and Taylor, G.J. Holt–Oram syndrome. *J. Pediatr.* 1979; **95**: 538–43.

50. Leroy, J.G. and Crocker, A.C. Clinical definition of the Hurler–Hunter phenotypes. A review of 50 patients. *Am. J. Dis. Child* 1966; **112**: 518–30.

51. Jervell, A., Thingstad, R. and Endsjo, T.O. The surdocardiac syndrome: three new cases of congenital deafness with syncopal attacks and Q-T prolongation in the electrocardiogram. *Am. Heart J.* 1966; **72**: 582–93.

52. Gorlin, R.J., Anderson, R.C. and Blaw, M. Multiple Lentigenes syndrome. *Am. J. Dis. Child* 1969; **117**: 652–62.

53. Rowland, T.W., Hubell, J.P. and Nadas, A.S. Congenital heart disease in infants of diabetic mothers. *J. Pediatr.* 1973; **83**: 815–20.

54. Lenke, R.R. and Levy, H.L. Maternal phenylketonuria and hyperphenylalaninemia: International survey of treated and untreated pregnancies. *N. Engl. J. Med.* 1980; **303**: 1202–8.

55. Pyeritz, R.E. and McKusick, V.A. The Marfan syndrome: Diagnosis and management. *N. Engl. J. Med.* 1979; **300**: 772–7.

56. Duncan, W.J., Fowler, R.S., Farkas, L.G. *et al.* A comprehensive scoring system for evaluating Noonan's syndrome. *Am. J. Med. Genet.* 1981; **10**: 37–50.

57. Rees, A., Elbl, F., Minhas, K. and Solinger, R. Echocardiographic evidence of outflow tract obstruction in Pompe's disease (glycogen storage disease of the heart). *Am. J. Cardiol.* 1976; **37**: 1103–6.

58. Simpson, N.E. and Brissenden, J.E. The Rubinstein–Taybi syndrome: Familial and dermatoglyphic data. *Am. J. Hum. Genet.* 1973; **25**: 225–9.

59. Cherstvoy, E.D., Lazjuk, G.I., Lurie, I.W., Nedzved, M.K. and Usoev, S.S. The pathological anatomy of the Smith–Lemli–Opitz syndrome. *Clin. Genet.* 1975; **7**: 382–7.

60. Hall, J.G., Levin, J., Kuhn, J.P., Ottenheimer, E.J., van Berkum, K.A.P. and McKusick, V.A. Thrombocytopenia with absent radius (TAR). *Medicine* 1969; **48**: 411–39.

61. Temtamy, S.A. and Miller, J.D. Extending the scope of VATER association. Definition of a VATER syndrome. *J. Pediatr.* 1974; **85**: 345–9.

62. Shprintzen, R.J., Goldberg, R.B., Young, D. and Wolford, L. The velo-cardio-facial syndrome: A clinical and genetic analysis. *Pediatrics* 1981; **67**: 167–72.

63. Burn, J. Williams syndrome. *J. Med. Genet.* 1986; **23**: 389–95.

64. Patterson, D.F. Genetic aspects of cardiovascular development in dogs. In: Van Praagh, R. and Takao, A., eds. *Etiology and morphogenesis of congenital heart disease,* Vol 1. New York: Futura, 1980, pp. 1–20.

65. Zetterqvist, P. *A clinical and genetic study of congenital heart defects.* MD Thesis. Uppsala, Sweden: University of Uppsala Publication, 1972, pp. 1–80.

66. Taussig, H.B. World survey of the common cardiac malformations: developmental error or genetic variant. *Am. J. Cardiol.* 1982; **50**: 544–59.

67. New England Regional Infant Cardiac Programme Report. *Pediatrics* (Supplement) 1980; **65**: 377–461.

68. Burn, J. and Corney, G. Congenital heart defects and twinning. *Acta Genet. Med. Gemellol.* 1984; **33**: 61–9.

69. Burn, J. In: 'Monozygotic twins in contemporary obstetrics and gynaecology' (Ed. G. Chamberlain). London: Butterworths, 1988, pp. 161–176.

70. Corballis, M.C. and Morgan, M.J. On the biological basis of human laterality. Evidence of a maturational left to right gradient. *Behaviour Brain Sci.* 1978; **2**: 261–9.

71. Whittemore, R., Hobbins, J.C. and Engle, M.A. Pregnancy and its outcome in women with and without surgical treatment of congenital heart disease. *Am. J. Cardiol.* 1982; **50**:361–70.

72. Burn, J. Annotation: congenital heart defects—the risks to offspring. *Arch. Dis. Child.* 1983; **58**: 947–8.

73. Rose, V., Gold, R.J.M., Lindsey, G. and Allen, M. A possible increase in the incidence of congenital heart defects among the offspring of affected parents. *Am. Coll. Cardiol.* 1985; **6**: 376–82.

74. Burn, J. "The next lady has a heart defect". (Commentary) *Br. J. Obstet. Gynaecol.* 1987; **94**: 97–9.

75. Burn, J., Coffey, R., Dennis, N., Hunter, S., Somerville, J., Allan, L., Keeton, B., Pembrey, M., Macartney, F.J., Scott, O., Wilkinson, J., Cole, J., Walsh, P., Burn, L.M. and Little, J. Recurrence risks in the offspring of adults born with major heart defects: first results of a British collaborative study. *Br. Heart J.* (submitted for publication).

Chapter 68

Heart Disease in the Elderly

A. John Camm and Anthony Martin

INTRODUCTION

The demographic structure of the population of the Western world is rapidly changing. In 1985, the population of the UK was 55 million, of which 11.4 million were over the age of 60 years and 1.8 million exceeded the age of 80 years.[1] In the USA, there were nearly 29 million people (12% of the population) over 65 years in 1985. This proportion will probably increase to 21% by the year 2030.[2] The sector of the population which will increase most dramatically is that known as the 'oldest old', i.e. those over 85 years, which in the USA is forecast to reach 16 million by 2030.[3] The change in the age distribution of the population is thought to be due to both a declining birth rate and improved survival of the elderly.[4]

In the UK, average life-expectancy has increased dramatically from 40 years in 1841 to 69 years in 1960. Today, the average life-expectancy is 74 years and by the year 2030 it may well be over 77 years. As age advances beyond 65 years, there is an increasingly high prevalence of cardiovascular disease (Table 68.1)[5] and the incidence of malignant disease falls. Heart disease is the commonest cause of death in elderly patients (45% prevalence in those over 65 years).

The elderly section of the population use a disproportionately large part of the medical resources.[6] For example, in the USA, the 12% of the population who are over 65 years consume 30% of the total medical budget (Table 68.2).

CHANGES WITH AGE

Those changes that are dubbed 'normal' in relation to age are a mixture of degenerative and disease processes. Such normal changes may mimic or cause clinical heart disease. Structural and functional changes may be seen.

STRUCTURAL CHANGES

Histological changes

The elderly heart increases in weight.[7] Atrial and ventricular myocardium is progressively replaced with collagen and elastic tissue. Focal amyloid deposits (predominantly in the left atrium), due to a specific fibrillar protein not seen in systemic amyloid, are found in the majority of elderly patients.[8] Brown atrophy, basophilic degeneration and increased sub-epicardial fat are also common features of the old heart. The conduction system becomes fibrotic and the sinus node loses some of its pacemaker cells, and both the sinus and atrioventricular nodes are infiltrated with greater amounts of fatty and collagenous tissue.[9] Coronary arteries become tortuous and develop fibrous and ather-

Table 68.1. Prevalence of heart disease in the elderly (> 65 years).[5]

Condition	Prevalence (%)	
	Male	Female
Coronary heart disease	20	12
Hypertension	10	14
Hypertension with coronary heart disese	7	7
Valvular	4	6
Pulmonary	5	0

Table 68.2. Utilization of cardiology/cardiothoracic facilities in the elderly (> 65 years).[6]

Procedure	Utilization (%)
Coronary angioplasty	25
Cardiac catheterization	33
Coronary artery bypass surgery	36
Cardiac pacemakers	80

omatous plaques. Cystic medial degeneration and inelasticity of the aorta increase with age.

In the normal ageing heart, calcium deposits may be found in the conduction system, valve rings and coronary arteries. Occasionally, heavy aortic cusp calcification may produce clinical aortic stenosis without commissural fusion (senile or degenerative aortic stenosis).[10] Mitral calcification is usually confined to the annulus producing C- or J-shaped radiographic patterns.[11] Systolic murmurs may be associated with this form of calcification. If the calcification extends to the valve cusps, senile mitral stenosis may develop.

Geometrical changes

Epicardial coronary vessels dilate and become tortuous. The left ventricular cavity becomes smaller, its long axis shortens and the aorta dilates. The interventricular septum therefore buckles into a sigmoid-shaped structure deviating to the right at its attachment to the aortic root.[12] At the base of the heart, the septum bulges into the small left ventricular cavity simulating hypertrophic cardiomyopathy. There is progressive thickening of the endocardium, particularly in the higher pressure left heart. The aortic and mitral valve cusps develop fibrous thickening at their margins. The mitral annulus shrinks, and the mitral valve protrudes into the left atrium simulating a floppy mitral valve.[13]

FUNCTIONAL CHANGES

Physiological changes

The variability of heart rate decreases with age, the supine resting heart rate does not slow significantly but the standing rate may slow slightly and the maximal exercise heart rate is certainly reduced in the elderly.[14,15] There is an age-related decrease in stroke volume and cardiac output due to impaired diastolic filling and increased aortic impedance. These changes are most obvious during exercise,[16,17] but some workers have noticed that an increased stroke volume may compensate for a decreased heart rate during exercise.[18] The diastolic impediment to ventricular filling is due to mitral valve sclerosis, myocardial stiffness (increased isovolumic relaxation time) and hypertrophy.[19] Systolic and mean blood pressures are elevated and aortic compliance is reduced in old people.[20] Catecholamine levels are increased in the elderly but the response to beta, and perhaps alpha, stimulation is

reduced.[21] Cardiovascular reflexes, for example, the baroreceptor and Valsalva reflexes, are attenuated as age advances.[22,23]

Pharmacological changes

The management of old people is complicated by their tendency to take numerous pills and potions. Drug interactions are therefore common. In the elderly, there are changes in drug handling (Table 68.3) and changes in the response of the heart and blood vessels to drugs. Drug absorption from the gastro-intestinal tract is reduced, body fat is increased and lean body mass is reduced, plasma volume is reduced and hepatic metabolism and renal clearance are impaired.[24,25]

HYPERTENSION

In young and middle-aged people, the diagnostic criteria, epidemiology and management of hypertension are now well defined, but in subjects over the age of 70 years the situation is much less clear and a matter of some dispute.[26] The potential size of the problem is alarming; the Health and Nutrition Examination Survey in the USA (1977) showed that, if the same criteria for the diagnosis of hypertension were applied to elderly people as are applied to the young, at least 40% of American whites and more than 50% of American blacks would have either systolic hypertension or combined systolic–diastolic hypertension.[27]

Table 68.3. Changed pharmacokinetics of cardiovascular drugs in the elderly.[25]

Drug	Pharmacokinetics
Digoxin	Reduced absorption, volume of distribution and renal clearance Increased plasma half-life
Propranolol	Decreased absorption, hepatic metabolism and receptor sensitivity Increased plasma levels
Beta-agonists	Decreased inotropic and chronotropic effect
Lignocaine	Decreased hepatic metabolism
Quinidine	Decreased renal and hepatic clearance
Procainamide	Decreased hepatic clearance
Disopyramide	Decreased renal clearance
Sotalol	Decreased hepatic clearance
Verapamil	Decreased hepatic clearance

In many of the studies on hypertension in elderly people the concern was to investigate the levels of blood pressure in subjects of different nationalities; the response and level of blood pressure of different ethnic groups may be very dissimilar. Moreover, the majority of large studies of the risk factors and treatment of hypertension were not designed to address the matter in significant numbers of people over the age of 75 years; relatively few people over the age of 70 years have been studied.

THE PATHOPHYSIOLOGY OF HIGH BLOOD PRESSURE IN ELDERLY PEOPLE

Arterial blood pressure is determined by the cardiac output and the peripheral resistance. When measured in the recumbent position, the cardiac output of elderly people falls by as much as 30% when compared with that of young adults.[17] However, most blood pressure readings are taken in the sitting position, in which the cardiac output does not vary much between the young and the old because the expected fall in cardiac output found in the young by moving from the recumbent to the sitting position does not occur to the same extent in the old.[28] During exercise in the elderly, the mean rise in cardiac output is usually lower than that in younger adults.[29] Another determinant of cardiac output is the plasma volume and this does not alter significantly with increasing age.[30] The fall in cardiac output in old age, therefore, must be due to other factors. The left ventricle becomes more rigid as a result of fibrotic changes in elderly people.[29]

Changes in the arterial system with ageing affect three main sites. The walls of major vessels become more rigid due to the loss of the internal elastic lamina. The function of these vessels, which act as a compression chamber, is consequently reduced and the damping effect on the spikes of blood pressure with left ventricular systole is reduced. This leads to a widening of the pulse pressure due to a rise in systolic pressure rather than a fall in the diastolic component.

The peripheral arteries are also affected by an increased atheromatous deposition with ageing. These ageing changes may affect the aortic and carotid baroreceptor reflexes.[31] These atheromatous changes are important because they may contribute to the high incidence of postural hypotension in untreated elderly subjects[32] and exaggerate the response to some antihypertensive medication in these people. The hyaline deposition in the arterioles in elderly people may account for the marked variability in blood-pressure response to various stimuli.[33] Small vessel disease certainly contributes to the progressive renal insufficiency that occurs with increasing age and may have a significant effect on the extracellular and plasma volumes.

THE MEASUREMENT OF BLOOD PRESSURE

The measurement of blood pressure by intra-arterial means has not been used in elderly people in any of the studies performed to date. The information available has been derived, almost exclusively, from studies in which indirect blood pressure measurements were made. The veracity of indirect blood-pressure measurements in elderly people is questionable and may be influenced by several factors, which must be borne in mind when the results of studies are interpreted.

It has long been recognized that the size of the upper arm circumference will affect the blood-pressure reading.[34] Although the arm size can be compensated for by varying the size of the sphygmomanometer cuff, this is often not done in practice. Similarly, the correct positioning of the cuff on the arm is important, but this may not always be easy in fat people.

The effect of blood pressure lability in elderly people may interfere with results. Posture may have considerable effects on the blood pressure of older people, because postural hypotension is known to be common in the old.[32] Sitting and standing blood-pressure readings should always be taken before considering treatment in the elderly.

Atherosclerotic changes occur in the brachial artery and may make the assessment of the diastolic end-point difficult. The rigidity of the sclerosed brachial artery may also introduce errors into the indirect blood-pressure reading because of the need for increased cuff pressure to compress the artery itself. 'Pseudo-hypertension'[35] occurs in older people when there is a large discrepancy between the indirect and direct blood-pressure measurement. This concept has more recently been questioned when it was found that in 40 patients aged between 60 and 80 years there was a close correlation between the indirect and direct measurement of systolic blood pressure and a reasonably close relationship between the two methods of measuring the diastolic pressure, although the indirect measurement was about 9 mmHg higher than the direct reading.[36] However, the great majority of these elderly patients would have been regarded as being normotensive on the basis of their indirect diastolic pressure. Thus, for the present, the problem of assessing the true blood pressure in elderly people with high diastolic pressures by the indirect method remains unresolved.

THE PREVALENCE OF HYPERTENSION AND ITS RELATIONSHIP WITH SURVIVAL

Blood pressure rises with age.[37,38] This continued rise in blood pressure is more marked in the systolic component and after the age of 90 years it tends to fall off. In a group of apparently healthy individuals aged 90 years or over, half of the men and three-quarters of the women had systolic blood pressures > 160 mmHg.[39]

In previous studies of the healthy elderly population, it was considered that the upper limit of normal blood pressure was 160/100 mmHg in men and 170/90 mmHg in women. Some supporting evidence for this came from a study of an elderly population in a London borough, in which it was found that the incidence of electrocardiographic abnormalities was significantly higher when the diastolic blood pressure was > 100 mmHg.[40] The World Health Organisation has recommended that any blood pressure > 160/95 mmHg should be regarded as being hypertensive.

In recent years, more attention has been paid to the problem of systolic hypertension. In the Framingham study in the USA, it has shown that there is a significant relationship between the level of the systolic blood pressure and increased cardiovascular mortality and morbidity, at least in people up to the age of 74 years.[41] The results of this study showed that in men and women the risk of cardiovascular death in subjects between 65 and 74 years of age was twice as high for those with systolic pressures of 160 mmHg or greater than it was for those with pressures of 130 mmHg. Disproportionate systolic hypertension is present in about 45% of patients over the age of 64 years. This is very much higher than would be found in a younger group of patients and it is often resistant to treatment.[42] There is now much information, albeit sometimes contradictory, for the definition and prevalence of hypertension in elderly people. However, the number of studies that have been designed to measure the beneficial effects of treatment of hypertension is small. In two studies from the USA, it has been shown that there was some benefit from reducing elevated levels of diastolic blood pressure in people over the age of 60 years.[43,44] Studies conducted in other parts of the world have produced different results. A trial in Australia in elderly men showed that mortality was increased in the thiazide-treated group.[45] A study of 123 elderly people in British Local Authority Residential Homes suggested that treatment of diastolic blood pressures > 100 mmHg with methyldopa did not reduce the cumulative mortality.[46]

The European Working Party on High Blood Pressure in the Elderly (EWPHE) has recently reported their long-term results of a study started in 1972.[47] In this multicentre study, people over the age of 60 years whose diastolic blood pressure was in the range of 90–119 mmHg were investigated. The treatment regimen was a thiazide diuretic with the addition of methyldopa if necessary; nowadays, this treatment would be regarded as old-fashioned. In the 12 years of recruitment to the study which was conducted at several centres, only 840 patients were admitted. This low level of recruitment over a large age-range does raise doubts about the sample being representative of the hypertensive elderly population in Europe at large. Despite the reservations over the validity of the results of this study, it remains the largest study performed to date.

The results of the EWPHE trial showed that there was no significant effect of treatment on the overall mortality. Similarly, there was no reduction in the mortality from cerebrovascular events. However, there was a significant reduction in the incidence of cardiovascular mortality (27%), cardiovascular events (38%) and non-fatal cerebrovascular events (50%). These results were achieved despite an increase in the level of both biochemical and clinical gout and glucose intolerance in those subjects who were treated.

The original EWPHE trial report left several questions unanswered. Re-analysis of the EWPHE results to take into account age, sex, the presence of cardiovascular complications and the degree of hypertension on entry to the study showed that benefit from therapy occurred at all levels of blood pressure and irrespective of whether cardiovascular events had occurred previously.[48] There was, however, a diminishing benefit of treatment with increasing age and no conclusive benefit was shown in those over 80 years.

ASSESSMENT FOR TREATMENT AND INVESTIGATIONS

A thorough assessment of the general vascular status of the individual should be made, including the palpation of the peripheral pulses and examination of the optic fundi. Osler's manoeuvre can be used to assess the possibility of pseudo-hypertension[49] (in pseudo-hypertension, the radial artery is still palpable when a proximally placed blood-pressure cuff has been inflated above the systolic pressure). Any significant fall in the blood pressure on standing or absence of target organ damage should make the clinician wary of instituting treatment in a person over 70 years.

Apart from a general physical examination, the only investigations that are relevant to elderly people are urinalysis, an electrocardiogram and a chest X-ray, and analysis of the serum urea, electrolytes and creatinine. The finding of a cardiac arrhythmia, especially atrial fibrillation, is important because this may interfere with the accurate assessment of the blood pressure. The finding of left ventricular enlargement will add weight to the need for treatment. The assessment of renal function impairment is important if hypotensive agents, such as angiotensin converting enzyme inhibitors or diuretics, are considered.

The age of the patient and their general well-being are vital in assessing which person should be treated and how vigorously. Statistical evidence points to general guidelines but it is of no value in an individual case. A frail elderly lady of 75 years who has no symptoms but a blood pressure of 220/110 mmHg would not be a candidate for anything but the mildest drug treatment. However, an otherwise fit man of 70 years with angina and the same blood pressure should be treated more vigorously with calcium antagonists or beta-blockade. Quality of the patient's life should be the chief consideration of the physician. There is no evidence that overall mortality is altered by treatment but the diminution of cardiovascular events by modification of the blood pressure will lead to a better quality of life. Conversely, some treatment procedures may cause side-effects that may degrade the quality of life.

MANAGEMENT

Before instituting drug treatment for hypertension, non-pharmacological approaches must be used first.[50] Cessation of smoking, moderation of alcohol consumption, taking regular exercise and weight reduction are essential, where relevant, and should ensure an improved level of physical well-being and at the same time may result in a significant fall in the blood pressure. A low-sodium diet (< 100 mg/day)

should also be advised.[51]

If these simple methods fail to control the pressure, the gentle introduction of drugs in low dosage is appropriate. It is not necessary to be hasty in the reduction of blood pressure in an elderly person; indeed, too rapid a fall in the pressure may lead to serious side-effects and, sometimes, a crucial fall in cerebral perfusion. Despite their known propensity to induce glucose intolerance and elevate serum creatinine, uric acid and cholesterol levels, diuretics remain the first drugs of choice for gentle reduction of the blood pressure.[48] The blood pressure in the majority of patients treated with diuretics will be controlled satisfactorily.[47] Small doses of an intermediate duration diuretic, such as hydrochlorothiazide in a dose of 12.5–25 mg daily, should be used. Larger doses will be no more effective at lowering the blood pressure and will considerably increase the risk of producing hypokalaemia and hypomagnesaemia. The presence of hypomagnesaemia may make it more difficult to correct potassium deficiencies. Hypokalaemia is largely responsible for the production of glucose intolerance associated with diuretic use and hyperosmolar non-ketoacidotic coma is more likely to be related to diuretic use.

Because diuretic therapy is not optimal for elderly subjects, other forms of treatment, including beta-adrenergic blocking agents, calcium channel antagonists and the angiotensin converting enzyme inhibitors, should be considered.[52–54] Adrenergic neurone blocking agents have no place in the treatment of the elderly because of their detrimental effects.

Beta-blocking agents that should be considered for administration to the elderly include atenolol and labetolol (the latter also causes post-synaptic alpha-blockade). Labetolol and pindolol display intrinsic sympathomimetic activity and can be used in subjects who have slow heart rates.[55] The dose of beta-blockers used should be lower than that given to younger adults because these drugs are metabolized more slowly in elderly people. All beta-blockers have the disadvantages of reducing renal blood flow, and inducing left ventricular failure and glucose intolerance. Moreover, they should not be used in patients who have chronic obstructive airways disease.

Calcium channel blockers, such as nifedipine, have a useful hypotensive effect by their direct action on arteriolar smooth muscle. They can be used as monotherapy or in combination with other agents. They have not been associated with either metabolic or electrolyte disturbances. These agents may also be cardioprotective by preventing calcium overload in myocardial and smooth muscle. In common with the beta-blockers, calcium channel antagonists may exert a negative inotropic effect and should be used carefully in elderly people who have left ventricular dysfunction or conduction disorders.

For the last few years, the angiotensin converting enzyme inhibitors have increasingly been used in elderly hypertensives with good effect. These agents reduce preload and afterload. The two most commonly used agents are captopril[56] and enalapril.[57] Both agents may give rise to severe hypotension, especially in patients taking diuretics. They may also cause renal failure and should be used with care in patients who have impaired renal function. The starting dose of enalapril should be 2.5 mg daily and of captopril 12.5 mg twice daily. Patients often respond well to this form of treatment, irrespective of their pre-treatment renin level.

As there is an age-related loss of homeostatic adaptability, elderly people are particularly prone to side-effects from antihypertensive medications. Dizziness and falls are common in the elderly, in part due to reduced carotid and aortic baroreceptor sensitivity, decreased cerebral blood flow autoregulation and limited compensatory cardiovascular responses to reductions in intravascular volume. It is important to monitor carefully drugs that have a tendency to cause postural hypotension, such as nifedipine and the angiotensin converting enzyme inhibitors. It is also important to prevent elderly people taking drugs that are known to aggravate hypertension, such as bronchodilators and decongestants.

CORONARY ARTERY DISEASE

EPIDEMIOLOGY AND RISK FACTORS

Coronary artery disease becomes more common with increasing age.[58] Post-mortem studies indicate that 40–60% of men dying from random causes over the age of 60 years have significant narrowing of at least one coronary artery.[59,60] Epidemiological studies are hampered by the fact that half of the patients who are found at autopsy to have coronary artery disease have a normal electrocardiogram and no history of angina pectoris or myocardial infarction.[61,62] The addition of exercise stress testing and thallium scanning to the diagnostic process increases the diagnostic yield.[63,64] Although such screening of asymptomatic patients might provide more information on the epidemiology of coronary disease, there are no data concerning whether such information would help in reducing subsequent morbidity or mortality. In younger patients, coronary artery disease is predominantly a disease of men, but with increasing age the sex distribution becomes similar. About 10% of men and 5% of women over 70 years of age experience angina; above the age of 80 years, angina occurs in about 10% of each sex.[61] Similarly, myocardial infarction is 4 times more common in men than in women aged 60–69 years, whereas in those over 70 years the sex distribution is approximately 2:1.[65]

Analysis of data from the Coronary Artery Surgery Study (CASS) registry demonstrates that elderly patients have more severe and more extensive coronary artery disease than their younger counterparts.[66] Elderly patients presented significantly less often with atypical chest pains (but this may be because elderly patients with such symptoms were less likely to undergo coronary angiography than their younger counterparts). Ejection fractions were found to be lower in the elderly.

The prognosis for elderly patients with mild coronary artery disease is relatively good, whereas in those with extensive disease it is very poor. The 6-year survival for patients over the age of 65 years who have no significant coronary disease, single-vessel, two-vessel and three-vessel disease was 86, 76, 69 and 40%, respectively. Survival was related to left ventricular ejection fraction.[67]

Conventional risk factors for coronary disease appear to be less applicable in the elderly. Of the conventional risk factors, only elevated levels of triglycerides and the presence of diabetes mellitus in men and systolic hypertension and diabetes mellitus in women aged 70 years were independent predictors of total coronary heart disease manifestations over the ensuing 10 years.[68] It seems unlikely that risk factor intervention in the elderly will significantly reduce the development or progression of coronary disease, and it may be perceived by the patient as significantly reducing their quality of life. Nevertheless, heavy smoking at age 70 years is a significant predictor of total mortality, and advice to stop smoking may still be warranted in the elderly.

MYOCARDIAL INFARCTION IN THE ELDERLY

Although the precise incidence is not known, it is clear that 'silent' myocardial infarction is more common in the elderly and may present with manifestations such as stroke, syncope, abdominal pain, weakness and confusion.[69-71] Routine electrocardiography and cardiac enzymes therefore should be included in the diagnostic work-up of patients presenting with such complaints. Data from the Framingham study suggest that 'silent' myocardial infarction carries the same long-term prognostic significance as symptomatic myocardial infarction.

Co-existing medical diseases and impaired myocardial function are more common in the elderly; therefore it is not surprising that myocardial infarction in the elderly carries a higher mortality than that in younger patients both in the short and long term.[72-75] After myocardial infarction, cardiogenic shock and external cardiac rupture are the commonest causes of death in hospital, and both of these are more common in the elderly.

Clearly, for some elderly patients with myocardial infarction, management at home may be the most appropriate course of action whereas for others modern technology may have a role to play. As the major cause of in-hospital mortality in the elderly is pump failure, efforts aimed at myocardial preservation may have particular relevance. Although intracoronary streptokinase has been shown to be safe in the elderly, reperfusion was less common than in other series of younger patients.[76] The recent large multicentre Italian study (GISSI)[77] and the Anysolated Plasminogen Streptokinase Activator Complex (APSAC) study[78] have demonstrated significant reduction in short- and long-term mortality in younger populations. A large placebo-controlled study using intravenous thrombolytic agents such as tissue plasminogen activator (TPA) or APSAC would be required to determine whether thrombolysis influences prognosis and morbidity in elderly patients with myocardial infarction.

In several studies, it has been suggested that beta-blockers may improve short- and long-term mortality following myocardial infarction, probably as a result of a reduction in cardiac rupture early on and in ischaemia-related arrhythmias later on.[79] However, beta-blockers are not as well tolerated in the elderly and it would be imprudent to extrapolate from the experience gained in younger patients.

THE ROLE OF MEDICAL AND SURGICAL MANAGEMENT

In general, drug therapy is not as well tolerated in the elderly, and this may pose problems in the management of angina. In the absence of a contraindication, beta-blockers should be the first line therapy for angina in the elderly, although the dose should be lower than that given to younger patients (e.g. atenolol 50 mg once daily). In patients with peripheral vascular disease or obstructive airways disease, diltiazem is a useful alternative. Verapamil and nifedipine are generally less effective as monotherapy. Although nitrates are useful when taken sublingually before exercise or to treat an attack of angina, tolerance limits their usefulness for long-term therapy.

When patients are refractory or intolerant to pharmacological therapy, surgery appears to be a useful therapeutic alternative. The peri-operative (30-day) mortality in patients undergoing coronary artery bypass grafting is higher in the elderly: 5.2% in 1086 CASS patients aged over 65 years, compared with 1.9% in patients under 65 years; it was also much higher in those who had rest angina, intercurrent medical illness, smoked cigarettes and had features of congestive heart failure.[66] In addition, neurological complications are much more common in elderly patients undergoing coronary artery bypass grafting.[80] Damage to the watershed area may result in visual agnosia and dyslexia; such abnormalities may be socially devastating and they are not always detected in hospital.

The investigation and management of elderly patients with angina should be based upon the severity of their symptoms. In low-risk older patients in the CASS registry who had mild angina, relatively good left ventricular function and no left main coronary disease, 6-year survival for those treated medically and those treated surgically was almost identical. In such patients with mild symptoms, there would seem to be little benefit in advising coronary artery bypass grafting. Conversely, in elderly patients who had more severe symptoms, left ventricular dysfunction, and extensive coronary disease, 6-year survival was significantly higher and symptoms were fewer in the surgically treated group (despite a relatively high peri-operative mortality).

The treatment of choice for 'suitable' elderly patients with severe angina refractory to medical therapy who have extensive coronary disease and a poor ejection fraction is coronary artery bypass grafting. Unfortunately, in the current financial climate, many surgical centres in the UK are unable to offer such therapy, and some units do not investigate patients over 65 years. Although it is possible to argue about the issue of increasing life-expectancy in the elderly under difficult financial circumstances, such a debate should not extend to the relief of severe angina. Percutaneous transluminal coronary angioplasty may be considered as a cheaper alternative to coronary artery bypass grafting in selected patients, particularly those with severe angina but less extensive disease. Initial angiographic success is achieved in 60–80% of elderly patients undergoing angioplasty. Morbidity and mortality are comparable to those in series of younger patients (mortality < 1%).[81] However, restenosis may be more common in the elderly.[82] Despite the relatively high restenosis rate, long-term symptomatic improvement was obtained in 91% of those in whom angioplasty was initially successful, with 55% remaining asymptomatic in the long term.[83]

Although angioplasty is undoubtedly cheaper than bypass grafting (the procedural cost is less than half of that for coronary artery bypass grafting), when the cost of urgent standby surgery and of re-investigation and intervention in those who relapse is considered, the total yearly cost of angioplasty is almost two-thirds that of bypass grafting.[84] With an increasingly older population, the prevention and management of coronary disease in the elderly will present a major clinical task and financial burden for the future.

HEART FAILURE

The prevalence of heart failure increases with age and therefore it is common in the elderly.[85] Its pathogenesis is the same as that in younger adults but precipitating factors[86] are particularly important (Table 68.4). Systolic, diastolic and high-output failure all occur but diastolic dysfunction is relatively more common in the elderly,[87] presumably due to hypertrophy related to previous hypertension or a mild variant of hypertrophic cardiomyopathy.

CLINICAL FEATURES

In addition to the usual manifestations of heart failure, such as peripheral and pulmonary oedema, atypical presentations are common in the elderly. Thus, Cheyne–Stokes respiration, loss of appetite, nausea, vomiting, loss of weight, confusion, sleepiness, disorientation or unusual weakness may signal the onset of heart failure.[88]

The diagnosis of heart failure should be

Table 68.4. Factors that may precipitate heart failure in the elderly.

Arrhythmias
  Bradycardia
  Tachycardia
  Atrial fibrillation

Systemic disease
  Anaemia
  Infection
  Fever
  Renal failure
  Thyroid disease

Medication
  Beta-blockers
  Calcium antagonists
  Non-steroidal anti-inflammatory drugs

Cardiac disease
  Myocardial infarction
  Valve regurgitation

Toxic causes
  Fluid overload
  Alcohol excess
  High sodium intake

approached with caution because some physical signs are unreliable in the elderly. A fourth heart sound and basilar râles are often heard in normal old people, and ankle oedema in the elderly has many causes other than heart failure. Diagnosis can be facilitated by chest radiography and echocardiography.

MANAGEMENT

Although compliance is usually good in the elderly, co-existing problems, such as disorientation, handicap from stroke and memory impairment, may result in unreliable treatment. Bed rest improves heart failure but it can be dangerous because it encourages venous thrombosis.[85] Passive exercise is recommended until active mobilization is possible. The drug management of heart failure in the elderly is different only in that hypotension and excessive diuresis should be avoided. Digoxin is generally recommended,[89] especially if atrial fibrillation is present,[90] but toxicity may easily occur because of altered pharmacokinetics which are largely due to the reduction in lean body mass and impairment of renal function.[91] The indications for arterial and venous dilators,[92] angiotensin converting enzyme inhibitors[93] and calcium antagonists[94] are similar to those for younger adults with heart failure. Appropriate treatment improves symptoms and enhances survival in elderly patients. However, the overall prognosis is not good; 50% of patients die within 5 years of the diagnosis being made.[85] Age is not an important prognostic factor.[95]

CARDIOMYOPATHY

As age advances, there is progressive stiffening of the myocardium[96] which may give rise to a clinical form of diastolic dysfunction. Classical cardiomyopathies (a generalized myocardial abnormality without apparent cause[97]), such as dilated, hypertrophic and restrictive forms, also occur in the elderly.

DILATED CARDIOMYOPATHY

About 10% of dilated cardiomyopathies occur in subjects over the age of 65 years.[98] It is characterized by systolic failure, and the usual causes include alcoholism, hypertension, irradiation or drug toxicity, for example, with adriamycin. The role of previous myocarditis in the aetiology of dilated cardiomyopathy is not known. Patients present with congestive heart failure, cardiac arrhythmias or sudden death. The diagnosis is best achieved using echocardiography when 4-chamber dilatation is seen.

There is a risk of thrombus formation, which might cause stroke, transient ischaemic attacks or other embolic conditions. Treatment is similar to that of congestive heart failure with the addition of advice about alcohol avoidance and, possibly, anticoagulation, especially when atrial fibrillation is also present.[99]

HYPERTROPHIC CARDIOMYOPATHY

Hypertrophic cardiomyopathy is not rare in the elderly.[100] It is characterized by diastolic ventricular dysfunction in association with hyperdynamic systolic function. It is usually due to an idiopathic or congenital cause. In the elderly, the hypertrophy is often concentric, as opposed to being confined to the septum.[101] Elderly patients with hypertrophic cardiomyopathy may have associated fibrous thickening of the endocardium, and mitral or aortic valve calcification, which complicate the diagnosis. The diagnosis is best made from the echocardiogram, which shows characteristic features including systolic anterior motion of the mitral valve.[102]

The prognosis of hypertrophic cardiomyopathy is better, and the incidence of sudden death is much

reduced, in older patients with this condition.[103,104] Treatment is similar to that given to younger patients.[104,105] Calcium antagonists or beta-blockers constitute primary therapy. Digoxin is used only if fast atrial fibrillation occurs. Anti-arrhythmic agents are usually unnecessary in the elderly, but if ventricular arrhythmias are documented amiodarone is preferred. Treatment with vasodilators and diuretics should be avoided unless congestive heart failure occurs.

Recently, a specific syndrome of 'hypertensive hypertrophic cardiomyopathy' of the elderly has been described.[106] In these cases, the hypertrophic reaction is due to longstanding hypertension.

RESTRICTIVE CARDIOMYOPATHY

This form of myopathy is very rare in the elderly. Although primarily characterized by diastolic dysfunction, systolic heart failure is often associated. Classically, this syndrome results from amyloid infiltration or radiation damage. Senile amyloidosis, in which there is deposition of amyloid, predominantly in the atrial myocardium, is rarely associated with ventricular dysfunction.

VALVULAR AND CONGENITAL HEART DISEASE

The reduction in the incidence of rheumatic heart disease, improvements in cardiological practice and cardiac surgery for the cardiac diseases suffered earlier in life and the generally increased lifespan of the population have changed the spectrum of valve and congenital disease seen in the elderly. Non-invasive techniques, such as echocardiography and Doppler sonography, are now widely available for the diagnosis of these abnormalities. The risks of cardiac surgery have been reduced and there are now new techniques, such as balloon valvuloplasty, for the relief of valvular stenosis.

AORTIC STENOSIS

In the elderly, calcification and fibrosis on the aortic side of a previously normal tricuspid aortic valve is the usual pathology of aortic stenosis and it is thought to result from long-term mechanical stress on the valve cusps.[107] Rheumatic processes, congenital deformity or degeneration of a bicuspid valve are much less common causes. Calcific aortic stenosis occurs in about 1% of the elderly population.[108] There is a risk of sudden death in aortic stenosis in the elderly and when congestive failure occurs the mortality exceeds 50% in 5 years.[108]

Aortic stenosis presents with the classical triad of chest pain, syncope and dyspnoea, but these symptoms are not specific in the elderly because of co-existing cerebral and coronary artery disease.[109] On examination, the usual features may be absent and when present they are not specific. A systolic murmur, fourth heart sound and slow-rising pulse are all common in the elderly because of aortic sclerosis, arterial atheromatous disease and stiff ventricular myocardium. In the elderly, the systolic murmur may be atypical in location and soft rather than harsh. There is usually no ejection click because the valve leaflets are stiff. Physical signs are generally uphelpful.

The chest X-ray may show cardiomegaly and aortic root dilatation, but these features may be masked by kyphoscoliotic changes. The electrocardiogram should show left ventricular hypertrophy but this will also result from hypertension which is common in the elderly and frequently (20%) co-exists with aortic stenosis. Echocardiography[110] will usually demonstrate thickened, calcified and immobile aortic valve cusps and concentric left ventricular hypertrophy. Continuous-wave Doppler recordings may be used to quantify the aortic valve gradient.[111] Cardiac catheterization is indicated for the assessment of coronary anatomy because about 50% of such patients will have significant coronary disease.[112]

The asymptomatic patient with aortic stenosis should be followed with regular echo/Doppler examinations. The registration of a significant aortic gradient or the development of significant symptoms suggests that surgery may be necessary. Medical management may be directed towards the relief of angina, arrhythmias and heart failure but such treatment will not be sufficient in patients who have severe stenosis.

Aortic valve replacement can be undertaken with added risk in elderly patients. Operative mortality is 5–15% in the elderly compared with 1–5% in younger patients.[113] Left ventricular dysfunction, inoperable coronary disease, co-existing diseases and impaired functional, psychological and nutritional status account for the reduced survival of elderly patients. Most surgeons prefer to use tissue valves because they render anticoagulation unnecessary and because elderly patients have a relatively short survival making concerns about bioprosthetic

valve deterioration irrelevant.[114] However, some elderly patients may live for a further 10 years or more and will subsequently require another valve replacement at a very elderly age. Furthermore, only mechanical valves are efficient in the small sizes needed by elderly patients. Balloon dilatation of stenotic aortic valves has been advocated by some workers,[115] but the procedure is only palliative. Only trivial relief of stenosis is achieved and restenosis is common. This form of treatment should be considered if the patient is too sick for surgery or if there are other life-threatening associated conditions.

AORTIC REGURGITATION

The aetiology of aortic valve regurgitation in the elderly is no different from that in the young.[116] Valve regurgitation may occur in a chronic or an acute form. Isolated aortic regurgitation is uncommon in the elderly.

Chronic aortic regurgitation is often well tolerated in the elderly but effort intolerance is usually the first symptom. Physical signs may be misleading because the inelastic vascular system in the elderly may mimic the rapid large-volume pulse of aortic regurgitation. Echo/Doppler studies allow the aortic regurgitation to be quantified, its aetiology to be investigated and the state of the left ventricle to be assessed.[117] The timing of aortic valve replacement is controversial, but such therapy must be considered when there is any sign of left ventricular dysfunction.[118] Post-operative improvement is limited by the extent of left ventricular dysfunction; it is possibly not as good in elderly patients because of the long exposure to the effects of regurgitation.

Acute aortic regurgitation is due to endocarditis or dissection of the aorta. Emergency surgery should be considered for the elderly patient.

MITRAL STENOSIS

Although mitral stenosis usually results from rheumatic fever suffered before the age of 20 years, it may first present in the seventh decade or later with sudden pulmonary oedema, a small heart, atrial fibrillation and characteristic chest X-ray and electrocardiographic features.[119] In elderly patients, there is often no audible diastolic murmur (silent mitral stenosis). Occasionally, the disease may present with a stroke due to embolization. The severity of the disease can be non-invasively assessed using echo/Doppler techniques.[120] Medical management is concentrated on the control of the ventricular rate and anticoagulation. When surgery is necessary, commissurotomy is preferable; if valve replacement must be considered, a bioprosthesis may be preferred to allow management without long-term anticoagulation. Recently, balloon dilatation of the mitral valve has been described.[121] This may provide suitable palliation for elderly patients.

MITRAL ANNULUS CALCIFICATION

Mitral annulus calcification is seen predominantly in elderly patients, occurring in 6% of those over 60 years of age. It is more common in women, in diabetics and in hypertensive subjects. Calcification can be seen as characteristic C- or J-shaped opacities on the lateral chest X-ray. The condition is usually benign but mild mitral regurgitation is common. Occasionally, left ventricular inflow obstruction (functional mitral stenosis) occurs, especially when the left ventricular cavity is small.[122] The calcification may embolize, become a nidus for thrombosis or infection or invade the conduction system. Mitral valve replacement is rarely needed.

MITRAL REGURGITATION

Mitral regurgitation may result when any of the parts of the mitral valve or subvalvar apparatus are defective.[123] The aetiology of mitral regurgitation in the elderly is similar to that in younger patients but ischaemic heart disease, myxomatous degeneration and mitral annulus calcification are relatively more common. The physical features of mitral regurgitation in the elderly are not different to those seen in the young. Accurate diagnosis, including an assessment of aetiology and associated left ventricular function, can be made with the help of echocardiography.[124] Medical management may suffice for many years. Assessment of exercise tolerance is used to help determine the need for surgery but such an investigation may prove difficult to perform in the elderly. When exercise tolerance drops, or left ventricular function fails, surgical replacement should be considered. However, the operative mortality of mitral valve replacement is about 10%.

MITRAL VALVE PROLAPSE

Myxomatous degeneration of the mitral valve cusps gives rise to mitral valve prolapse. In elderly patients with this condition, atrial fibrillation is common but ventricular arrhythmias are rare.[125] Associated chest pain may be related to co-existing coronary disease. Transient ischaemic attacks and mitral prolapse frequently occur together in elderly patients but a causal relationship has not been proved.[126] Left ventricular failure may result if mitral regurgitation is present.[127] Prophylaxis against infective endocarditis is recommended if significant regurgitation is documented.

ATRIAL MYXOMA

Twelve per cent of patients with myxoma are over the age of 70 years.[128] This neoplastic process should be suspected when there are signs of mitral valve disease and peripheral emboli. Management in the elderly patient is no different to that in younger subjects.

PULMONARY AND TRICUSPID VALVE DISEASE

Tricuspid stenosis is rare in the elderly and when present it is usually rheumatic in origin. Tricuspid regurgitation may result from pulmonary hypertension, right heart failure, Ebstein's anomaly or, rarely, carcinoid syndrome.[133] Congenital pulmonary stenosis has not been reported in the elderly.[134] Pulmonary regurgitation frequently results from chronic lung disease or left heart lesions that give rise to pulmonary hypertension.

INFECTIVE ENDOCARDITIS

Elderly patients are frequent victims of infective endocarditis.[129] Its presentation in the elderly may be atypical,[130] with anorexia, nausea and vomiting, pneumonia, confusion, stroke or renal failure. Fever may occur in less than half of the cases and is often a late manifestation. Diagnosis and treatment are similar to those in younger age-groups. In the elderly, the responsible organism is often derived from the gut. Echocardiographic visualization of vegetations is possible in most cases.[131] Antibiotic therapy should be based on the results of blood culture. Standard antibiotic prophylaxis should be offered to elderly patients who have valvular abnormalities.

NON-BACTERIAL THROMBOTIC ENDOCARDITIS

This condition occurs predominantly in elderly

patients who have malignant disease.[132] It mimics infective endocarditis in that strokes, peripheral emboli and murmurs are common although fever and leucocytosis are usually absent. The pathogenesis is not understood but may be related to the hypercoagulable state found with some malignancies. Non-bacterial vegetations which can be visualized on echocardiography are typical. Treatment includes anti-thrombotic therapy, but it is otherwise empirical. The possibility of infective endocarditis must be ruled out.

CONGENITAL HEART DISEASE

Congenital lesions associated with significant haemodynamic impairment are usually diagnosed and treated in early life. However, mild congenital disease may remain undetected or untreated into old age. The most common lesions seen in the elderly are atrial septal defect,[135] bicuspid aortic valve,[136] ventricular septal defect and Ebstein's anomaly. Occasionally, persistent ductus arteriosus, aortic coarctation and tetralogy of Fallot have been discovered. Therapeutic decisions usually concern the necessity and feasibility of correction at an advanced age and the importance of prophylaxis against infective endocarditis. Surgical correction of atrial septal defect and coarctation of the aorta should be considered because operative mortality is very little greater in the elderly and the long-term benefits of surgery may be excellent.[137]

Increasingly, patients who have undergone surgical correction of congenital disease in early life are surviving to old age. Such patients may suffer from arrhythmias, ventricular dysfunction, the effects of incomplete surgical correction or the superimposed problems of coronary artery disease or other degenerative conditions.

CARDIAC ARRHYTHMIAS

As age advances, there is progressive atrophy and fibrosis in the sino-atrial node and specialized conduction system, fibrosis and calcification of the aortic and mitral valve rings, atrial amyloid infiltration, lipofuscin deposition and pathology related to atherosclerotic heart disease and hypertrophy.[138,139] All these changes may contribute to the higher prevalence of arrhythmias in elderly people.

THE RESTING ELECTROCARDIOGRAM

Atrioventricular nodal conduction slows with age, and right bundle branch delay and left fascicular conduction delay are frequent. The upper limit of the PR interval in an elderly subject is 0.22 s, and left-axis deviation of up to −45° is often seen.[140] Slow sinus rates and non-specific T-wave changes are also common.

THE NORMAL RHYTHM ON AMBULATORY MONITORING

It is difficult to identify normal elderly patients because most active elderly people have suffered mild cardiac disease or are taking cardio-active medications. Nonetheless, there have been many attempts to characterize the rhythm of normal old people.[141,142]

Heart rate

There may be a small linear decrease in sinus rate with age.[143] However, sinus arrhythmia, maximum exercise heart rate and heart-rate variability are definitely reduced in old people. Marked bradycardias, such as sinus bradycardia < 40 beats/min and pauses of 2 s or more, are unusual in normal elderly subjects.

Supraventricular rhythms

Atrial premature beats and slow non-sustained atrial tachycardias are common (88%) in the elderly.[142] Atrial fibrillation is probably unusual in the totally normal old person, but it occurs at a prevalence of over 10% in active elderly subjects.[141,144] Often, the ventricular rate during atrial fibrillation is sufficiently slow to avoid the need for rate-control treatment. Atrial flutter and multiform atrial tachycardia are almost always associated with heart disease. Junctional tachycardias are uncommon.

Ventricular rhythms

Ventricular ectopic activity increases with age.[145] About 70% of subjects aged 75 years or more have ventricular ectopic beats.[141] A smaller proportion (< 20%) have frequent ventricular ectopic beats and only a minority have ventricular tachycardia (< 4%). There is little information about the influence of these arrhythmias on prognosis which probably depends on the state of the underlying myocardium Ventricular arrhythmias are more common ir smokers.[142]

SYMPTOMS DUE TO CARDIAC ARRHYTHMIAS

In an elderly population, the spectrum of symptoms related to cardiac arrhythmias is different to that seen in younger patients. Palpitation, an almost invariable symptom related to tachycardia in young adults, is often not noticed by elderly patients. However, the exacerbation of heart failure, dementia, recurrent falls and fractured bones, particularly the neck of the femur, all occur more commonly in the elderly.

SYNCOPE

Syncope occurs at all ages but it is particularly common in the elderly. In one study[146] involving over 700 very old people (mean age 87 years), there was an incidence of 7% per year (23% over 10 years). Of these episodes, at least 21% were due to a cardiovascular cause but the relationship of syncope to arrhythmias was not specified. However, it is difficult to show such a relationship. For example, in a large retrospective study[147] of 1512 patients of all ages who underwent 24-hour electrocardiographic monitoring for the investigation of syncope, this symptom was suffered only 15 times during the period of recording. In 7 cases, an arrhythmic cause was identified. Other common cardiovascular causes of syncope are listed in Table 68.5, some of which are particularly frequent in old age.

Postprandial syncope

Owing to defective blood-pressure control, elderly patients tend to suffer postprandial hypotension and related disturbances of consciousness.[148]

Malignant vasovagal syncope

Another manifestation of poor blood-pressure response is the sudden fall of blood pressure which may occur in elderly people after a sustained upright tilt. Significant bradycardias occur simultaneously with the hypotension.

Carotid sinus syncope

Syncope related to tight collars, neck turning and transient hypertension may be reproduced by caro-

tid sinus massage.[149] This test must be performed, one side at a time, after excluding a carotid bruit, using a non-occlusive, rotatory action. The electrocardiogram, and preferably the blood pressure, should be continuously recorded. A pause in the rhythm (sinus arrest or atrioventricular block) of more than 3 s is usually regarded as positive but unless the test reproduces the patient's symptoms it does not demand treatment.

Sick sinus syndrome

Sick sinus syndrome is the failure of the sinus node to generate or conduct impulses. Clinically, it most commonly presents as persistent sinus bradycardia, intermittent episodes of sinus arrest (or exit block) and bradycardia–tachycardia syndrome (usually the combination of paroxysmal atrial fibrillation and sinus arrest). Atrioventricular conduction disturbances may also be associated with sinus node disease. This condition is best diagnosed by long-term electrocardiographic tape monitoring, but electrophysiological tests may also reveal sinus node abnormalities.

Table 68.5.   Cardiovascular causes of syncope in old age.

Structural cardiovascular disease
  Aortic stenosis
  Hypertrophic cardiomyopathy
  Myocardial infarction
  Atrial myxoma/thrombus
  Pulmonary emboli
  Vertebrobasilar disease

Cardiac arrhythmias
  Sick sinus syndrome
  Atrial fibrillation
  Atrioventricular block
  Ventricular tachycardia
  Torsade de pointes

Drugs
  Diuretics
  Vasodilators
  Antihypertensives
  Antidepressants
  Sedatives
  Anti-arrhythmics

Autonomic/neurogenic
  Defaecation syncope
  Micturition syncope
  Vasovagal syncope
  Carotid sinus syndrome
  Postprandial syndrome
  Cough syncope
  Autonomic neuropathies

Atrioventricular block

In the elderly population, atrioventricular block is most usually due to extensive fibrosis and sclerosis of the intraventricular conduction system. This typically manifests electrocardiographically as Mobitz type II second degree block, fascicular block and complete heart block with wide QRS complexes and a slow ventricular rate. Atrial fibrillation or the sinus mechanism might dominate the supraventricular rhythm. Adams–Stokes attacks occur when the ventricular rhythm slows or stops.

PACEMAKER TREATMENT

A slow symptomatic cardiac rhythm due to chronic cardiac disease should be treated by implantation of a permanent cardiac pacemaker. Cardiac pacing is a cheap, effective and appropriate treatment for patients of all ages, including the very old. Pacemakers improve the longevity of patients with complete heart block, irrespective of their symptomatic status. The lifespan of patients with asymptomatic sinus node disease is not improved by pacing, but symptomatic disease should be treated with a pacemaker rather than drug therapy. Both malignant vasovagal syncope and carotid sinus syndrome may need treatment with an artificial pacemaker.

ANTI-ARRHYTHMIC DRUG TREATMENT

Symptomatic arrhythmias merit treatment. In the elderly population, there is practically no information on which to judge the value of 'prophylactic' therapy for arrhythmias such as ventricular ectopic activity associated with structural heart disease. Anti-arrhythmic drugs are more difficult to handle in the elderly because of their reduced volume of distribution, impaired excretion due to depressed hepatic and renal function, low levels of plasma proteins, and possibly exaggerated cardiac response because of cardiac disease and altered sensitivity. Interactions between anti-arrhythmic drugs and other cardio-active medicaments, such as digoxin, cimetidine, diuretics and beta-blockers, frequently used by elderly patients should be borne in mind.

CONCLUSIONS

The rapidly increasing number of old and very old people is resulting in a dramatic increase in demand for the cardiology facilities necessary for their proper care. In the elderly, degenerative problems must be added to the long list of other diseases that affect younger hearts. The non-invasive methods of diagnosis, such as echocardiography, the expanding range of specific and safe cardio-active drugs and the non-operative techniques for the relief of coronary and valvular stenoses are providing relatively inexpensive and simple methods for the management of cardiac problems in the elderly. It is now clearly recognized that heart disease in the elderly can be as effectively treated as that occurring in young adults. Age does not appear to preclude comprehensive and enthusiastic treatment of cardiovascular complaints.

REFERENCES

1. Craig, J. Changes in the population composition of England and Wales since 1841. Office of Populations Censuses and Surveys. *Population Trends* 1987; **48**: 27–36.
2. Page, L.B. 18th Bethesda Conference: Cardiovascular Disease in the Elderly. Introductory Remarks. *J. Am. Coll. Cardiol.* 1987; **10**: 7A–8A.
3. Binstock, R.H. The oldest old: a fresh perspective on compassionate ageism revisited? *Millbank Mem. Fund Q.* 1985; **63**: 420–51.
4. Rosenwaike, M.A., Yaffe, N. and Sagi, P.C. The recent decline in mortality of the extreme aged: An analysis of statistical data. *Am. J. Public Health* 1980; **70**: 1074–80.
5. Caird, F.L. and Kennedy, R.D. Epidemiology of heart disease in old age. In: Caird, F.I., Dall, F.L.C. and Kennedy, R.D., eds. *Cardiology in Old Age*. New York: Plenum Press, 1976, pp. 1–10.
6. Stason, W.B., Sanders, C.A. and Smith, H.C. Cardiovascular care of the elderly: Economic considerations. *J. Am. Coll. Cardiol.* 1987; **10**: 18A–21A.
7. Baker, P.B., Arn, A.R. and Unverferth, D.V. Hypertrophic and degenerative changes in human hearts with aging. *J. Am. Coll. Cardiol.* 1985; **5**: 536A.
8. Pomerance, A. Pathology of the myocardium and valves. In: Caird, F.I., Dall, J.L.C. and Kennedy, R.D., eds. *Cardiology in Old Age*. New York: Plenum Press, 1976, pp. 57–9.
9. Davies, M.J. Pathology of the conduction system. In: Caird, F.I., Dall, J.L.C. and Kennedy, R.D., eds. *Cardiology in Old Age*. New York: Plenum Press, 1976, pp. 57–9.
10. Surgiura, M., Hiraoka, K., Ohkawa, S. and Shimada, H. A clinico–pathologic study on the heart disease in the aged: The morphologic classification of 1000 consecutive autopsy cases. *Jpn Heart J.* 1963; **16**: 526.
11. Waller, B.F. and Morgan, R. The very elderly heart. In: Waller, B.F., ed. *Contemporary Issues in Cardiovascular Pathology*. Philadelphia: F.A. Davis 1987, p. 361.
12. Goor, D., Lillehei, C.W. and Edwards, J.E. The "sigmoid septum". Variation in the contour of the left ventricular outlet. *Am. J. Roentgenol.* 1969; **107**: 366.
13. Waller, B.F. The old-age heart: Normal aging changes which can produce or mimic cardiac disease. *Clin. Cardiol.* 1988; **11**: 513–7.
14. Kostis, J.B., Moreyra, A.E., Amendo, M.T. *et al.* The effect of age on heart rate in subjects free of heart disease. *Circulation* 1982; **65**: 141–5.

15. Strandell, T. Circulatory studies in healthy old men. With special reference to the limitation of the maximal physical working capacity. *Acta Med. Scand.* 1964; **175** (Suppl. 414): 2–44.

16. Raven, P.B. and Mitchell, J. The effect of aging on the cardiovascular response to dynamic and static exercise. *Aging* 1980; **12**: 269–96.

17. Brandfonbrener, M., Landowne, M. and Shock, N.W. Changes in cardiac output with age. *Circulation* 1955; **12**: 557–66.

18. Rodeheffer, R.J., Gerstenblith, G., Becker, L.C. *et al.* Exercise cardiac output is maintained with increasing age in healthy human subjects: Cardiac dilatation and increased stroke volume compensate for diminished heart rate. *Circulation* 1984; **69**: 202–13.

19. Wei, J.Y. Cardiovascular anatomic and physiologic changes with age. *Topics Geriat. Rehab.* 1986; **2**: 10–6.

20. Yin, F.C.P. The aging vasculature and its effects on the heart. In: *The Aging Heart*. New York: Raven Press, 1980, pp. 137–214.

21. Shimada, K., Kitazumi, T., Sadakane, N. *et al.* Age-related changes of baroreflex function, plasma norepinephrine, and blood pressure. *Hypertension* 1985; **7**: 113–7.

22. Lipsitz, L.A., Maddens, M.E., Pluchino, F.C. *et al.* Effect of advanced age on cardiovascular responses to orthostatic stress. *Gerontologist* 1986; **26**: 58A.

23. Lakatta, E.G. Age-related alterations in the cardiovascular response to adrenergic mediated stress. *Fed. Proc.* 1980; **39**: 3173–7.

24. Greenblatt, D.J., Sellers, E.M. and Shader, R.I. Drug disposition in old age. *N. Engl. J. Med.* 1982; **306**: 1081–8.

25. Opie, L.H. and Mabin, T.A. Medical treatment of cardiovascular disease in the elderly. In: Messerli, F.H., ed. *Cardiovascular Disease in the Elderly*, 2nd edition. Boston: Martinus Nijhoff, 1988, pp. 317–38.

26. Martin, A. Hypertension. In: Martin, A. and Camm, A.J., eds. *Heart Disease in the Elderly*. Chichester: John Wiley and Sons, 1984, pp. 59–78.

27. Health and Nutrition Examination Survey. Blood pressure levels of persons 60–74 years, United States, 1971–1974. *Vital Health Statistics* 1977; **2**: 203.

28. Granath, A., Jonsson, B. and Strandell, T. Studies on the central circulation at rest and during exercise in the supine and sitting body position in old men. *Acta Med. Scand.* 1961; **169**: 125.

29. Strandell, T. Cardiac output in old age. In: Caird, F.I., Dall, J.L.C. and Kennedy, R.D., eds. *Cardiology in Old Age*. New York, Plenum Press, 1976,

30. Maseri, A., Pecorini, V., Toni, P. *et al.* Clinical applications of radiocardiography. *Acta Med. Scand.* 1964; **176**: 769.

31. Gribbin, B., Pickering, T.G., Sleight, P. and Peto, R.C. Effect of age and high blood pressure on baroreflex sensitivity in man. *Circ. Res.* 1971; **29**: 424.

32. Johnson, R.H., Smith, A.C., Spalding, J.M.K. and Wollner, L. Effect of posture on blood pressure of elderly patients. *Lancet* 1965; i: 731.

33. Swales, J.D. Pathophysiology of blood pressure in the elderly. *Age and Ageing* 1979; **8**: 104.

34. O'Brien, E. and O'Malley, K. ABC of blood pressure measurement. *Br. Med. J.* 1979; ii: 920.

35. Spence, J.D., Sibbald, W.J. and Cape, R.D. Pseudohypertension in the elderly. *Clin. Sci. Mol. Med.* 1978; **55** (Suppl. 4): 399s–402s.

36. O'Callaghan, W.G., Fitzgerald, D.J., O'Malley, K. and O'Brien, E. Management of hypertension in the elderly. *N. Engl. J. Med.* 1980; **302**: 1397.

37. Master, A.M., Lasser, R.P. and Jaffe, H.L. Blood pressure in white people over 65 years of age. *Ann. Intern. Med.* 1958; **48**: 284.

38. Anderson, W.F. and Cowan, N.R. Arterial pressure in healthy older people. *Clin. Sci.* 1959; **18**: 103.

39. Danner, S.A., De Beaumont, M.J. and Dunning, A.J. Cardiovascular health in the tenth decade. *Br. Med. J.* 1978; ii: 663.

40. Martin, A. and Millard, P.H. Cardiovascular assessment in the elderly. *Age and Ageing* 1973; **2**: 211.

41. Kannel, W.B. Role of blood pressure in cardiovascular morbidity and mortality. *Prog. Cardiovasc. Dis.* 1974; **17**: 5.

42. Tarazi, R.C. and Gifford, R.W. Clinical significance and management of systolic hypertension. In: Onesti, G. and Brest, A.N., eds. *Hypertension Mechanisms, Diagnosis and Treatment*. Philadelphia: F.A. Davis, 1978.

43. Veterans Administration Cooperative Study Group on Antihypertensive Agents. *Circulation* 1972; **45**: 991.

44. Hypertension Detection and Follow-up Program Cooperative Study Group. Five year findings on the hypertension detection and follow-up program. *JAMA* 1979; **242**: 2562.

45. Morgan, T.O., Adams, W.R., Hodgson, M. and Gibberd, R.W. Failure of therapy to improve prognosis of elderly males with hypertension. *Med. J. Aust.* 1980; **2**: 27.

46. Sprackling, M.E., Mitchell, J.R.A., Short, A.H. and Watt, G. Blood pressure reduction in the elderly: A randomized controlled trial of methyl dopa. *Br. Med. J.* 1981; **283**: 1151–3.

47. Amery, A., Brixko, P., Clement, D. *et al.* Mortality and morbidity results from the European Working Party on High Blood Pressure in the Elderly Trial. *Lancet* 1985; i: 1349–54.

48. Amery, A., Brixko, P., Clement, D. *et al.* Effect of antihypertensive treatment according to age, sex, blood pressure, and previous cardiovascular disease in patients over the age of 60. *Lancet* 1986; ii: 589–91.

49. Messerli, F.H., Ventura, H.O. and Amodeo, C. Osler's maneuver and pseudohypertension. *N. Engl. J. Med.* 1985; **312**: 1348–51.

50. Frohlich, E.D., Gifford, R., Horan, M. *et al.* Non-pharmacologic approaches to the control of high blood pressure. Final report of the Subcommittee on Nonpharmacologic Therapy of the 1984 Joint National Committee on Detection, Evaluation and Treatment of High Blood Pressure. *Hypertension* 1986; **8**: 444–7.

51. The Working Group on Hypertension in the Elderly. Statement on hypertension in the elderly. *JAMA* 1986; **256**: 70–4.

52. Andersen, G.S. Atenolol versus bendrofluazide in middle aged and elderly hypertensives. *Acta Med. Scand.* 1985; **218**: 165–72.

53. Landmark, K. and Dale, J. Antihypertensive, haemodynamic and metabolic effects of nifedipine slow release tablets in elderly patients. *Acta Med. Scand.* 1985; **218**: 389–96.

54. Reid, J.L. Angiotensin converting enzyme inhibitors in the elderly. *Br. Med. J.* 1987; **295**: 943–4.

55. Blowers, A.J. and Melvin, M.A. The use of pindolol in the treatment of essential hypertension: a multi-centre assessment. *Curr. Med. Res. Opin.* 1976; **4**: 368.

56. Jenkins, A.C., Knill, J.R. and Dreslinski, G.R. Captopril in the treatment of the elderly hypertensive patient. *Arch. Intern. Med.* 1985; **145**: 2029–31.

57. Forette, F., Handfield-Jones, R., Henry-Amar, M. *et al.* Traitement de l'hypertension arterielle du sujet age par un inhibiteur de l'enzyme de conversion: l'enalapril. *Présse Med.* 1985; **14**: 2237–41.

58. Kannel, W.B. and Feinleib, M. Natural history of angina pectoris in the Framingham study. *Am. J. Cardiol.* 1972; **29**: 154–63.

59. White, N.K., Edwards, J.E. and Dry, T.J. The relationship

of the degree of coronary atherosclerosis with age in men. *Circulation* 1950; **1**: 645–54.

60. Tejada, C., Strong, J.P., Montenegro, M.R. *et al.* Distribution of coronary and aortic atherosclerosis by geographic location, race and sex. *Lab. Invest.* 1968; **18**: 49–66.

61. Kannel, W.B., Gordon, T. and Offutt, D. Left ventricular hypertrophy by electrocardiogram. Prevalence, incidence, and mortality in the Framingham study. *Ann. Intern. Med.* 1969; **71**: 89–105.

62. Kennedy, R.D., Andrews, G.R. and Caird, F.I. Ischemic heart disease in the elderly. *Br. Heart J.* 1977; **39**: 1121–7.

63. Stone, J.L. and Norris, A.H. Activities and attitudes of participants of the Baltimore Longitudinal Study. *J. Gerontol.* 1966; **21**: 575–80.

64. Gerstenblith, G., Flegg, J.L., Vantosh, A. *et al.* Stress testing redefines the prevalence of coronary artery disease in epidemiologic studies. *Circulation* 1980; **62** (Parts 2, 3): 308.

65. Peel. A.A.T. Age and sex factors in coronary artery disease. *Br. Heart J.* 1955; **17**: 319–20.

66. Gersh, B.J., Kronmal, R.A., Frye, R.L. *et al.* Coronary arteriography and coronary artery bypass surgery: Morbidity and mortality in patients aged 65 years or older. A report from the Coronary Artery Surgery Study. *Circulation* 1983; **67**: 483–91.

67. Mock, M.B., Fisher, L.D., Gersh, B.J. *et al.* Prognosis of coronary heart disease in the elderly patient: The CASS experience. In: Coodley, E.L., ed. *Geriatric Heart Disease.* Littleton: PSG, 1985, pp. 358–63.

68. Agner, E. Natural history of angina pectoris, possible previous myocardial infarction and intermittent claudication during the eighth decade. *Acta Med. Scand.* 1981; **210**: 271–6.

69. Rodstein, M. The characteristics of nonfatal myocardial infarction in the aged. *Arch. Intern. Med.* 1956; **98**: 84–90.

70. Pathy, M.S. Clinical presentation of myocardial infarction in the elderly. *Br. Heart J.* 1967; **29**: 190.

71. Tinker, G.M. Clinical presentation of myocardial infarction in the elderly. *Age and Ageing* 1981; **10**: 237.

72. Kannel, W.B. and Abbott, R.D. Incidence and prognosis of unrecognised myocardial infarction; an update on the Framingham study. *N. Engl. J. Med.* 1984; **311**: 1144–7.

73. Latting, C.V. and Silverman, M.E. Acute myocardial infarction in hospitalized patients over age 70. *Am. Heart J.* 1980; **100**: 311–8.

74. Williams, B.O., Begg, T.X., Semple, T. *et al.* The elderly in a coronary unit. *Br. Med. J.* 1976; **2**: 451–5.

75. Coodley, E.L. and Zebari, D. Characteristics of myocardial infarction in the elderly. In: Coodley, E.L., ed. *Geriatric Heart Disease.* Littleton: PSG, 1985, pp. 334–45.

76. Fuentes, F., Smalling, R.W., Hicks, C.H., Wanta-Matthews, M. and Gould, K.L. Thrombolytic therapy in myocardial infarction of the elderly patient. In: Coodley, E.L., ed. *Geriatric Heart Disease.* Littleton: PSG, 1985, pp. 404–10.

77. Gruppo Italiano per lo Studio della Streptochinasia nell Infarto Miocardico (GISSI). Effectiveness of intravenous thrombolytic treatment in acute myocardial infarction. *Lancet* 1986; **i**: 397–402.

78. AIMS Trial Study Group: Effect of intravenous APSAC on mortality after acute myocardial infarction: Preliminary reports of a placebo-controlled trial. *Lancet* 1985; **i**: 545–9.

79. Sia, S.T.B., Rutherford, J.D., Cook, E.F., Weinstein, M.C. and Goldman, L. Cost-effectiveness of routine beta-blocker therapy following myocardial infarction. *Circulation* 1986; **74** (Suppl. II): 44.

80. Smith, P.L.C., Treasure, T., Newman, F.P. *et al.* Cerebral consequences of cardiopulmonary bypass. *Lancet* 1986; **i**: 823–5.

81. Gersh, B.J., Kronmal, R.A., Schaff, H.V. *et al.* Comparison of coronary artery bypass surgery and medical therapy in patients 65 years of age or older. *N. Engl. J. Med.* 1985; **313**: 217–24.

82. Holmes, D.R. Percutaneous transluminal coronary angioplasty. In: Coodley, E.L., ed. *Geriatric Heart Disease.* Littleton: PSG, 1985, pp. 439–49.

83. Raizner, A.E., Hust, R.G., Lewis, J.M. *et al.* Transluminal coronary angioplasty in the elderly. *Am. J. Cardiol.* 1986; **57**: 29–32.

84. van Halem, C., van den Brand, M., de Feyter, P. *et al.* All inclusive cost comparison PTCA versus CABG versus medical treatment. *Eur. Heart J.* 1987; **8**: 239.

85. Smith, W.M. Epidemiology of congestive heart failure. *Am. J. Cardiol.* 1985; **55**: 3A–8A.

86. Weisfeldt, M.L., ed. *The Aging Heart: Its Function and Response to Stress.* New York: Raven Press, 1980.

87. Soufer, R., Wohlgelernte, D., Vita, N.A. *et al.* Intact systolic left ventricular function in clinical congestive heart failure. *Am. J. Cardiol.* 1985; **55**: 1032–6.

88. Luchi, R.J. and Ware, T. Congestive heart failure. In: Isaacs, B. Ed. *Recent Advances in Geriatric Medicine.* New York: Churchill Livingstone, 1985, pp. 19–36.

89. Ware, J.A., Snow, E., Luchi, J.M. and Luchi, R.J. Effect of digoxin on ejection fraction in elderly patients with congestive heart failure. *J. Am. Geriatr. Soc.* 1984; **32**: 631–5.

90. Lee, D.C.S., Johnson, R.A., Bingham, J.B. *et al.* Heart failure in outpatients: A randomized trial of digoxin versus placebo. *N. Engl. J. Med.* 1982; **306**: 699–705.

91. Greenblatt, D.J., Sellers, E.M. and Shader, R.I. Drug disposition in old age. *N. Engl. J. Med.* 1982; **306**: 1081–8.

92. Chatterjee, K. and Parmley, W.W. Vasodilator therapy for acute myocardial infarction and chronic congestive heart failure. *J. Am. Coll. Cardiol.* 1983; **1**: 133–53.

93. Franciosa, J.A. and Cohn, J.N. Hemodynamic responsiveness to short and long-acting vasodilators in left ventricular failure. *Am. J. Med.* 1978; **65**: 126–33.

94. Agostoni, P.G., DeCesare, N., Doria, E. *et al.* Afterload reduction: a comparison of captopril and nifedipine in dilated cardiomyopathy. *Br. Heart J.* 1986; **55**: 391–9.

95. Franciosa, J.A., Wilerr, M., Ziesche, S. and Cohn, J.N. Survival in men with severe chronic left ventricular failure due to either coronary heart disease or idiopathic dilated cardiomyopathy. *Am. J. Cardiol.* 1983; **51**: 831–6.

96. Gerstenblith, G., Frederiksen, J., Yin, F.C. *et al.* Echocardiographic assessment of a normal adult aging population. *Circulation* 1977; **56**: 273–8.

97. Shad, P.V., Abelmann, W.H. and Gersh, B.J. Cardiomyopathies in the elderly. *J. Am. Coll. Cardiol.* (in press)

98. Fuster, V., Gersh, B.J., Giuliani, E.R. *et al.* The natural history of idiopathic dilated cardiomyopathy. *Am. J. Cardiol.* 1981; **47**: 525–31.

99. Unverferth, D.V., Magorien, R.D. and Leier, C.V. Drug regimens for congestive heart failure. *Geriatrics* 1980; **35**: 26–33.

100. Krasnow, N. and Stein, R.A. Hypertrophic cardiomyopathy in the aged. *Am. Heart J.* 1978; **96**: 326–36.

101. Pomerance, A. and Davies, M.J. Pathological features of hypertrophic obstructive cardiomyopathy (HOCM) in the elderly. *Br. Heart J.* 1975; 37: 305–12.

102. Shenoy, M.M., Khanna, A., Nejat, M. *et al.* Hypertrophic cardiomyopathy in the elderly. *Arch. Intern. Med.* 1986; **146**: 658–61.

103. Shah, P.M., Adelman, A.G., Wigle, E.D. *et al.* The natural (and unnatural) history of hypertrophic obstructive car-

diomyopathy. *Circ. Res.* 1974; **34**: 179–95.

104. McKenna, W., Deanfield, J., Faruqui, A. *et al.* Prognosis in hypertrophic cardiomyopathy: role of age and clinical, electrocardiographic and hemodynamic features. *Am. J. Cardiol.* 1981; **47**: 532–8.

105. Hamby, R.I.´ and Antablian, A. Idiopathic hypertrophic subaortic stenosis in the septuagenerian (Abstract). *Clin. Res.* 1976; **24**: 220A.

106. Topol, E.J., Traill, T.A. and Fortuin, N.J. Hypertensive hypertrophic cardiomyopathy of the elderly. *N. Engl. J. Med.* 1985; **312**: 227–83.

107. Roberts, W.C., Perloff, J.K. and Costantino, T. Severe valvular aortic stenosis in patients over 65 years of age. *Am. J. Cardiol.* 1971; **27**: 497–506.

108. Rapaport, E. Natural history of aortic and mitral valve disease. *Am. J. Cardiol.* 1975; **35**: 221–7.

109. Thompson, M.E. and Shaver, J.A. Aortic stenosis in the elderly. *Geriatrics* 1983; **10**: 50–65.

110. Flohr, K.H., Weir, E.K. and Chesler, E. Diagnosis of aortic stenosis in older age groups using external carotid pulse recording and phonocardiography. *Br. Heart J.* 1982; **45**: 577–82.

111. Currie, P.J., Seward, J.B. and Reeder, G.S. Continuous-wave Doppler echocardiographic assessment of severity of calcific aortic stenosis: A simultaneous Doppler-catheter correlative study in 100 adult patients. *Circulation* 1985; **71**: 1162–9.

112. Brandenburg, R.P. No more routine catheterisation for valvular heart disease? *N. Engl. J. Med.* 1981; **305**: 1277–8.

113. Copeland, J.G., Griepp, R.B., Stinson, E.B. and Shumway, N.E. Isolated aortic valve replacement in patients older than 65 years. *JAMA* 1977; **237**: 1578–81.

114. Kirklin, J.W. The replacement of cardiac valves. *N. Engl. J. Med.* 1981; **304**: 291–2.

115. Cribier, A., Saoudi, N., Berland, J. *et al.* Percutaneous transluminal valvuloplasty of acquired aortic stenosis in elderly patients: an alternative to valve replacement? *Lancet* 1986; **i**: 63–7.

116. Roberts, W.C., Dangel, J.C. and Bulkley, B.J. Nonrheumatic valvular heart disease: A clinicopathologic survey of 27 different conditions causing valvular dysfunction. In: Likoff, W. ed. *Valvular Heart Disease*, Cardiovascular Clinics, Vol. 5. 1973, p. 333.

117. Masuyama, T., Kodama, K., Kitabatake, A. *et al.* Noninvasive evaluation of aortic regurgitation by continuous-wave Doppler echocardiography. *Circulation* 1986; **73**: 460–6.

118. Bonow, R.O., Rosing, D.R., Maron, B.J. *et al.* Reversal of left ventricular dysfunction after aortic valve replacement for chronic aortic regurgitation: Influence of duration of preoperative left ventricular dysfunction. *Circulation* 1984; **70**: 570–9.

119. Selzer, A. and Cohn, K. Natural history of mitral stenosis in review. *Circulation* 1972; **45**: 878–87.

120. Smith, M.D., Handshoe, R., *et al.* Comparative accuracy of two-dimensional echocardiography and Doppler pressure half-time methods in assessing severity of mitral stenosis in patients with and without prior commissurotomy. *Circulation* 1986; **73**: 100–7.

121. Inoue, K., Owaki, T., Nakamura, T., Kitamura, F. and Miyamoto, N. Clinical application of transvenous mitral commissurotomy by new balloon catheter. *J. Thorac. Cardiovasc. Surg.* 1984; **87**: 394–403.

122. Osterberger, L.E., Goldstein, S., Khaja, F. *et al.* Functional mitral stenosis in patients with massive mitral annular calcification. *Circulation* 1981; **64**: 472–87.

123. Kotler, M.N., Mintz, G.S., Parry, W.R. and Segal, B. Bedside diagnosis of organic murmurs in the elderly. *Geriatrics* 1981; **36**: 107–25.

124. Ascah, K.J., Stewart, W.J., Jiang, L. *et al.* A doppler two-dimensional echocardiographic method for quantitation of mitral regurgitation. *Circulation* 1983; **72**: 377–83.

125. Higgins, C.B., Reinke, R.T., Gosink, B.B. and Leopold, G.R. The significance of mitral valve prolapse in middle-aged and elderly men. *Am. Heart J.* 1976; **91**: 292–6.

126. Barnett, H.J.M., Boughner, D.R., Taylor, D.W. *et al.* Further evidence relating mitral valve prolapse to cerebral ischemic events. *N. Engl. J. Med.* 1980; **302**: 139–44.

127. Tresch, D.D., Siegel, R., Keelan, M.H. *et al.* Mitral valve prolapse in the elderly. *J. Am. Geriatr. Soc.* 1979; **27**: 421–4.

128. McAllister, H.A. Primary tumors and cysts of the heart and pericardium. *Curr. Prob. Cardiol.* 1979; **4**: 1–51.

129. Durack, O.T. and Petersdorf, R.G. Changes in the epidemiology of endocarditis. In: Raplam, E.L. and Taronta, A.V., eds. *Infective Endocarditis—An American Heart Association Symposium*. Dallas: American Heart Association, 1977, pp. 3–8.

130. McAnulty, J.H., Rahimtoola, S.H., DeMots, H. and Griswold, H.E. Clinical features of infective endocarditis. In: Rahimtoola, S.H., ed. *Infective Endocarditis*. New York: Grune & Stratton, 1978, pp. 125–48.

131. Reid, C.L. and Rahimtoola, S.H. Infective endocarditis: Role of echocardiography cardiac catheterisation, and surgical intervention. *Mod. Conc. Cardiovasc. Dis.* 1986; **4**: 16–9.

132. Donahoo, J.S., Weiss, J.L., Gardner, T.J. *et al.* Current management of atrial myxoma with emphasis on a new diagnostic technique. *Ann. Surg.* 1979; **189**: 763–8.

133. Hendel, N., Leckie, B. and Richards, J. Carcinoid heart disease: Eight-year survival following tricuspid replacement and pulmonary valvotomy. *Ann. Thorac. Surg.* 1980; **30**: 391–5.

134. Johnson, L.W., Grossman, W., Dalen, J.E. and Dexter, L. Pulmonic stenosis in the adult: Long-term follow-up results. *N. Engl. J. Med.* 1972; **287**: 1159–63.

135. Craig, R.J. and Selzer, A. Natural history and prognosis of atrial septal defect. *Circulation* 1986; **37**: 805–15.

136. Resnekov, L. Congenital heart disease in the adult. *Cardiol. Diag.* 1979; **14**: 21–49.

137. St John Sutton, M., Abdul, T.J. and McGoon, D.C. Atrial septal defect in patients aged 60 years or older: Operative results and long-term postoperative follow-up. *Circulation* 1981; **64**: 402–9.

138. Rossi, L. *Histopathology of cardiac arrhythmias*, 2nd edition. Milan: Casa Editrice Ambrosiana, 1979, pp. 36–8.

139. Fujino, M., Okada, R. and Arakawa, K. The relationship of aging to histological changes in the conduction system of the normal human heart. *Jpn Heart J.* 1983; **24**: 13–20.

140. Mihalick, M.J. and Fisch, C. Electrocardiographic findings in the aged. *Am. Heart J.* 1974; **87**: 117–28.

141. Camm, A.J., Evans, K.E., Ward, D.E. and Martin, A. The rhythm of the heart in acute elderly subjects. *Am. Heart J.* 1980; **99**: 598–603.

142. Fleg, J.L. and Kennedy, H.L. Cardiac arrhythmias in a healthy elderly population. Detection by 24 hour ambulatory electrocardiography. *Chest* 1982; **81**: 302–7.

143. Landowne, M., Brandfonbrener, M. and Shock, N.W. The relation of age to certain measures of performance of the heart and the circulation. *Circulation* 1955; **11**: 567.

144. Patel, K.P. Electrocardiographic abnormalities in the sick elderly. *Age and Ageing* 1977; **6**: 163–7.

145. Glaser, S.P. and Clark, P.I. The rhythm of aging. *Chest* 1982; **81**: 266–7.

146. Lipsitz, L.A., Wei, J.Y. and Rowe, J.W. Syncope in the elderly institutionalised population. *Q. J. Med.* 1985; **55**: 45–54.

147. Gibson, T.C. and Heitzman, M.R. Diagnostic efficacy of 24 hour electrocardiographic monitoring for syncope. *Am. J. Cardiol.* 1984; 53: 1013–7.
148. Lipsitz, L.A., Nyquist, R.P., Wei, J.Y. *et al.* Postprandial reduction in blood pressure in the elderly. *N. Engl. J. Med.* 1983; 309: 81–3.
149. Morley, C.A., Perrins, E.J., Grant, P. *et al.* Carotid sinus syncope treated by pacing. Analysis of persistent symptoms and role of atrioventricular sequential pacing. *Br. Heart J.* 1982; 47: 411–8.

Chapter 69

Environmental and Toxic Heart Disease

A.G. Shaper

INTRODUCTION

The environment includes all those conditions, natural or manmade, that surround us and influence our growth and development, health and disease. The breadth of this definition, which excludes only the truly genetic influences, makes it evident that every disorder included in this textbook will have some environmental factors that relate to its aetiology, pathogenesis and outcome. The broad environmental factors include living conditions, water and food supplies and the climate.

The term toxic or poisonous in relation to heart disease is usually reserved for those environmental factors other than infections that may damage the myocardium or the blood vessels. These include alcohol, as well as a range of chemical substances derived from environmental sources and therapeutic agents administered to patients, for example, poisoning by lead, cobalt, mercury and arsenic, the effects of stings from scorpions, wasps and spiders and the sometimes harmful effects of drugs, such as phenothiazines, emetine, chloroquine, lithium and cyclophosphamide. Even the sulphonamides, penicillin and tetracycline have been incriminated in hypersensitivity responses which damage the myocardium, and the antituberculosis drugs, streptomycin and para-aminosalicylic acid, have been associated on occasions with cardiac dilatation and death.

This chapter will be restricted to a limited number of areas of concern to cardiologists and cardiovascular epidemiologists and which could be of public health concern. As uncertainty predominates in all of these areas (possibly more so than in other areas of cardiovascular medicine), it would be wise for the reader to keep an open mind on many of the conclusions presented in this chapter.

DRINKING WATER AND CARDIOVASCULAR DISEASE

The first report relating cardiovascular mortality to the quality of drinking water came from Japan, where a close association was reported between death rates from apoplexy (cerebrovascular accidents) and the *acidity* of river water used for drinking purposes.[1] The more acid the water, the higher the death rates from apoplexy. The data were examined in detail by Schroeder who found 'a fairly good correlation between deaths from apoplexy and acidity of river water and a better one between death rates from heart disease and water'.[2] The nature of the 'heart disease' is uncertain, but at that time (1950) ischaemic heart disease was extremely uncommon in Japan. Schroeder went on to examine the relationships between cardiovascular mortality and treated water supplies in the USA and found significant negative correlations between water *hardness* and all cardiovascular diseases and less significant correlations with coronary heart disease and strokes.[3] The harder the water, the lower the mortality rate from cardiovascular disease.

In Great Britain, these findings were seen to provide a possible explanation for the marked regional variations in cardiovascular disease mortality which had been recognized for more than a century. Using mortality data for 1948–1954 from the 83 county boroughs of England and Wales, Morris and colleagues found striking negative correlations between water hardness and total cardiovascular mortality and substantial, but less marked, negative correlations with death from cerebrovascular disease and 'myocardial degeneration' for males and females aged 45–64 and 65–74 years.[4] For coronary heart disease, the correlation was significant for men aged 45–64 years but not for older men or for women. There was also a consistently significant negative correlation between water hardness and bronchitis, a finding which aroused suspicion that other factors closely related to both geography and socio-economic circumstances might be confounding the relationship between drinking water and cardiovascular mortality.

A further study was carried out using improved water data and mortality data for 1958–1964 for the 61 county boroughs of England and Wales with a population of 80 000 or more at the 1961 census.[5] The findings were similar to those of the earlier study, except that now the negative correlations between water hardness and coronary heart disease were significant for men and women in both age-groups. This probably reflects the transfer of 'myocardial degeneration' into 'coronary heart disease'.[6] Multivariate analysis showed that the contribution of socio-economic factors to the differences in cardiovascular mortality between the towns was small. Later analyses of the 1948–1954 and the 1958–1964 data showed that rainfall, latitude and water calcium all make significant independent contributions to the explanation of the variations in total cardiovascular mortality between the 61 county boroughs, with broadly similar associations for coronary heart disease and cerebrovascular disease.[7]

Morris and his colleagues then tried to determine whether a change in the hardness of water supply would affect cardiovascular mortality.[8] Their study was based on a comparison of the changes in death rates of towns which had increased their water hardness (n = 5), decreased water hardness (n = 6) or remained unchanged (n = 72) over the 30 years up to 1960. In general, changes in cardiovascular death rates between 1957 and 1961 showed a favourable effect in the towns where the water had become harder and an unfavourable effect in the towns where the water had become softer; non-cardiovascular death rates were not affected. The study seemed to have produced evidence of a direct relationship between cardiovascular death rates and water hardness. The authors considered that 'the technical problems of increasing the hardness of soft water should now be explored'.[8]

Clinical studies were later carried out in 12 towns in England and Wales, 6 with hard water and 6 with soft water, to investigate the clinical and biochemical characteristics of populations with differing water supplies.[9] The soft-water towns all had very soft water (< 40 parts/million total hardness) and had high mortality rates for cardiovascular disease. The hard-water towns all had very hard water (> 250 parts/million total hardness) and low mortality rates for cardiovascular disease. Men in the soft-water towns showed an increase in diastolic blood pressure with increasing age; men in the hard-water towns showed no such increase. The findings suggested that water quality might have some effect on blood pressure but the possibility could not be further explored in this study. Using the same 12 towns, a death certificate study was carried out to assess the contribution made by sudden death to cardiovascular mortality in hard- and soft-water towns.[10] Sudden death, i.e. death within 1 h of the onset of acute symptoms, comprised a greater proportion of male ischaemic heart disease deaths in the soft-water than in the hard-water towns, but this was not statistically significant at the usual arbitrary level.

THE BRITISH REGIONAL HEART STUDY

The British Regional Heart Study (BRHS) was established in 1975 to assess the role of water quality in determining regional variations in cardiovascular mortality and also to determine the extent to which other risk factors could account for the regional variations. In the first phase of the study, cardiovascular mortality data from 253 British towns were related to information on drinking water, climate, air pollution, blood groups and socio-economic factors.[11]

The standardized mortality ratios for all cardiovascular disease (ICD B27–30) for males and females combined, aged 35–74 years are shown in Fig. 69.1. High standardized mortality ratios are seen in Scotland, parts of Lancashire, West Yorkshire and South Wales. This combined standardized mortality ratio has a twofold range from 69 in the London suburbs of Chigwell and Esher to 147 in the Glasgow suburbs of Hamilton and Dumbarton. A map of water hardness shown in Fig. 69.2 indicates that soft waters occur in Scotland, most of Lancashire, West Yorkshire, South Wales, Tyneside and the South West. Except for the South West, all of these areas tend to have higher than average cardiovascular disease mortality. Clearly, there is sufficient relationship between water hardness and cardiovascular mortality to warrant further analysis.

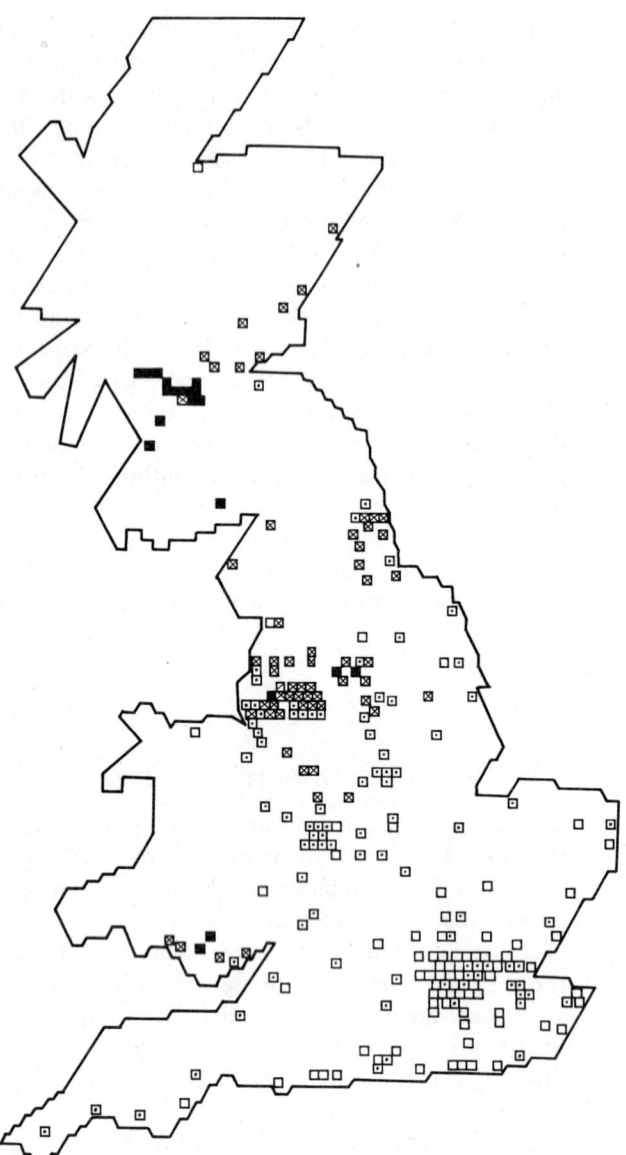

Fig. 69.1. Standardized mortality ratios for cardiovascular disease in men and women aged 35–74 years. □, 60–90; ⊡, 90–110; ⊠, 110–130; ■, 130–150.

EXPLORATION OF THE ASSOCIATION

The association between the standardized mortality ratio and the total hardness for 234 of the towns is shown in Fig. 69.3. Towns with soft water tend to have higher cardiovascular mortality than towns with hard water, with notable exceptions, and there is a wide range of mortality present at any given level of water hardness. Although the data show a significant association between cardiovascular mortality and water hardness ($r = -0.67$), the relationship does not allow for the effect of other factors. In the BRHS, it was noted there were 24 factors, each of which had a marked association ($r > \pm 0.5$) with cardiovascular mortality, including water quality, climate, latitude/longitude, socio-economic factors, blood groups and air pollution. The influence of climate was especially relevant as high rainfall and areas with soft water tended to coincide ($r = 0.70$). Water hardness is only one of the many factors that might influence cardiovascular mortality. It was found that there were 5 variables that collectively had a highly significant relationship with the cardiovascular standardized mortality ratio, namely water hardness (negative), percentage of days with measurable rain (positive), mean early maximum temperature (negative), percentage of manual workers (positive) and percentage car ownership (negative). Each of these variables made a separate and important contribu-

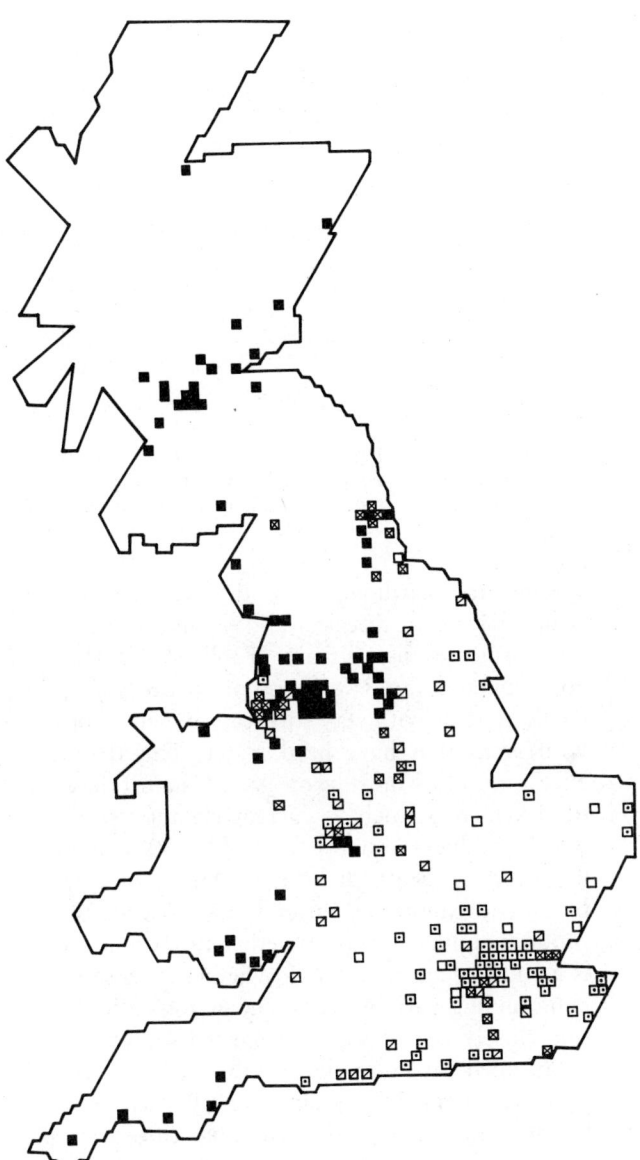

Fig. 69.2. Total water hardness. ■, 0.0–0.8 mmol/l; ⊠, 0.8–1.6 mmol/l; ⌀, 1.6–2.4 mmol/l; ▫, 2.4–3.2 mmol/l; □, 3.2–5.3 mmol/l. *NB*: 1 mmol/l = calcium carbonate equivalent 100 mg/l.

tion to explaining regional variations in cardiovascular mortality. In particular, the effect of water hardness could not be explained by its correlation with rainfall.

The effect of water hardness was not linear, being much greater in the range from very soft to medium-hard water than from medium-hard to very hard water. The mean standardized mortality ratio for cardiovascular disease for towns grouped according to water hardness, both with and without adjustment for the effects of the climate and socio-economic variables, is shown in Fig. 69.4. Adjusting for climatic and socio-economic differences considerably reduced the apparent magnitude of the effect of water hardness. It became clear that

a better understanding would be obtained by considering the effects of hardness on the standardized mortality ratio in two separate intervals, above and below 1.7 mmol/l (170 mg/l calcium carbonate equivalent). A measure of the relative importance of 5 main variables, using standardized regression effects, i.e. the percentage change in standardized mortality ratio for an increase of 1 standard deviation in each variable, is given in Table 69.1.

It can be seen that climate and socio-economic variables have roughly similar effects, although the percentage of manual workers and rainfall seem more important than the other measures. Water hardness below 1.7 mmol/l (very soft to medium-

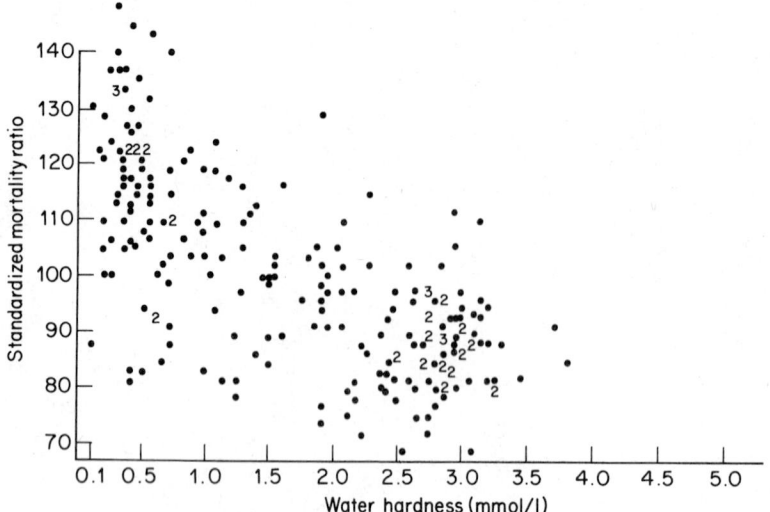

Fig. 69.3. Water hardness plotted against standardized mortality ratio for all men and women aged 35–74 years with cardiovascular disease for each town.

hard water) had the greatest effect; water harder than this had virtually no effect at all on cardiovascular mortality. It can be estimated that the maximal effect of water hardness on cardiovascular mortality lies principally between very soft and medium-hard water and may be of the order of 8% of cardiovascular mortality.[12]

Conclusion

After allowing for climate and socio-economic conditions, there is still a significant negative association between water hardness and cardiovascular mortality in British towns. The effect is specific for cardiovascular disease (stroke and ischaemic heart disease) and is not present for non-cardiovascular disease (Table 69.1). There is approximately an 8% excess of all cardiovascular death in areas with very soft water when compared with areas that have hard water. This degree of excess mortality must be measured against the effect of risk factors, such as current cigarette smoking, which produces about a threefold (300%) increase in coronary heart disease mortality, and raised blood cholesterol and raised blood pressure, which produce similar effects. Whether the 'water factor' is a component of water or whether it represents a confounding variable whose geographical distribution closely resembles water hardness has yet to be determined. It must be emphasized that water hardness, temperature and rainfall *each* play an independent role in determining cardiovascular

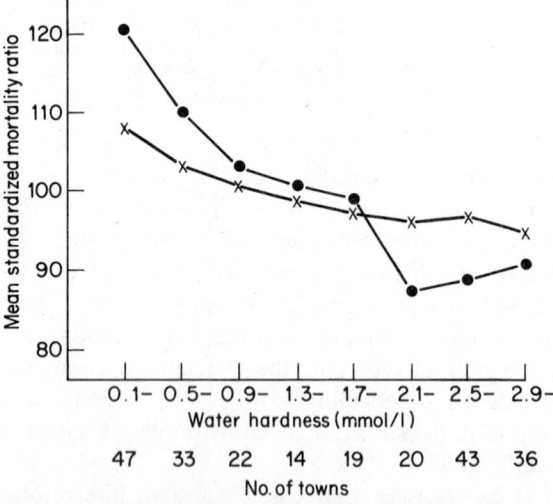

Fig. 69.4. Geometric means of standardized mortality ratio (for all men and women aged 35–74 years with cardiovascular diseases) for towns grouped according to hardness of water. ●, unadjusted; ×, adjusted for climate and socio-economic conditions.

Table 69.1. The effect of 5 key variables on standardized mortality ratios for cardiovascular disease, stroke, ischaemic heart disease and non-cardiovascular disease in men and women aged 35–74 years.

	Standardized regression effects			
Variable	Cardio-vascular disease	Stroke	Ischaemic heart disease	Non-cardio-vascular disease
Water hardness				
up to 1.7 mmol/l	−7.8	−6.8	−8.2	−0.1
over 1.7 mmol/l	−0.8	−3.0	+0.0	+0.0
Rain	+4.1	+4.2	+4.3	+1.8
Maximum temperature	−3.0	−7.5	−2.1	−0.4
Per cent manual workers	+5.1	+6.1	+5.0	+3.5
Car ownership	−2.9	−2.2	−3.2	−6.5

Table 69.2. Correlations of risk factors with ischaemic heart disease mortality, ischaemic heart disease prevalence and water hardness in 24 towns in Great Britain.

	Ischaemic heart disease		Water hardness
	Mortality	Prevalence	
% smoking cigarettes	+0.59	+0.42	−0.22
% manual workers	+0.54	+0.35	0.00
Mean systolic blood pressure	+0.60	+0.47	−0.13
Mean diastolic blood pressure	+0.53	+0.49	−0.17
Mean serum total cholesterol	−0.22	−0.07	−0.33
Mean HDL cholesterol	+0.06	+0.42	−0.44
Mean body mass index	+0.14	+0.18	0.00

mortality in Great Britain. The magnitude of their effects seem small by comparison with the effects of the well-established major personal risk factors, such as smoking, blood cholesterol and blood pressure. Although it is theoretically possible to harden soft water, and this is being done for other reasons in several parts of Scotland e.g. Glasgow, this cannot be justified on the basis of possible effects on cardiovascular disease.[13]

WATER HARDNESS AND PERSONAL RISK FACTORS

It is firmly established that certain factors ('risk factors') are strongly associated with the risk of coronary heart disease in individual men, for example, cigarette smoking, raised blood pressure, raised serum total cholesterol. It seems reasonable therefore to examine the relationship between these risk factors and geographical variations in coronary heart disease mortality and prevalence and between the risk factors and water hardness. Correlations between water hardness and coronary heart disease mortality for men aged 35–64 years in the 24 towns studied in the BRHS for the years 1979–1982 are shown in Table 69.2. Correlations with the prevalence rates of coronary heart disease in the men studied in the 24 towns based on WHO chest pain questionnaire and electrocardiogram findings are also shown.[14]

Clearly, coronary heart disease mortality and prevalence are higher in towns with a higher prevalence of cigarette smokers, higher mean blood pressure and a higher percentage of manual workers. Serum total cholesterol, although a powerful risk factor in individual men, is not associated with geographical variations in coronary heart disease mortality and prevalence, presumably because *all*

towns have a mean level > 6.0 mmol/l, i.e. all are at high risk. The curious association between HDL cholesterol and coronary heart disease might be due to the fact that areas with a high prevalence of coronary heart disease, e.g. Scotland and Northern England, tend to have higher alcohol intakes, which would elevate HDL cholesterol concentrations. The correlation between water hardness and the major risk factors with water hardness are also shown in Table 69.2. Smoking habit, systolic blood pressure and presence of manual workers are only weakly associated with water hardness. If the associations between water hardness and coronary heart disease mortality and prevalence ($r = -0.51$ and -0.46, respectively) are adjusted to take account of these three risk factors, the partial correlations that result ($r = -0.57$ and $r = -0.41$, respectively) are similar to the unadjusted correlations. Therefore, the association of water hardness with coronary heart disease appears to be largely independent of the geographical variation in personal risk factors, at least in the BRHS of middle-aged men.

BLOOD LEAD AND CARDIOVASCULAR DISEASE

Soft waters are corrosive and tend to dissolve metals from distribution pipes. In a survey of Canadian domestic waters, Neri *et al.* have shown that soft tap waters tend to leach copper, zinc and cadmium from piping systems, whereas this does not occur to a significant degree in hard waters.[15] In Great Britain, and particularly in parts of Scotland, it is lead that predominates over other metals in areas with both soft water and lead piping and this makes an important contribution to blood lead concentrations. Lead has long been under suspicion as the possible missing factor in the 'water story', and in the BRHS it was possible to explore this by measuring blood lead in the men from 24 British towns who were screened and then followed for major cardiovascular events.

BLOOD LEAD AND BLOOD PRESSURE

The relationship between blood lead and blood pressure in 7371 men in whom both were measured is shown in Fig. 69.5.[16] The correlation coefficients are small (systolic $r = +0.03$, diastolic $r = +0.01$), although there is a suggestion of a rise in mean systolic blood pressure as blood lead concentration increases. However, other factors affect blood

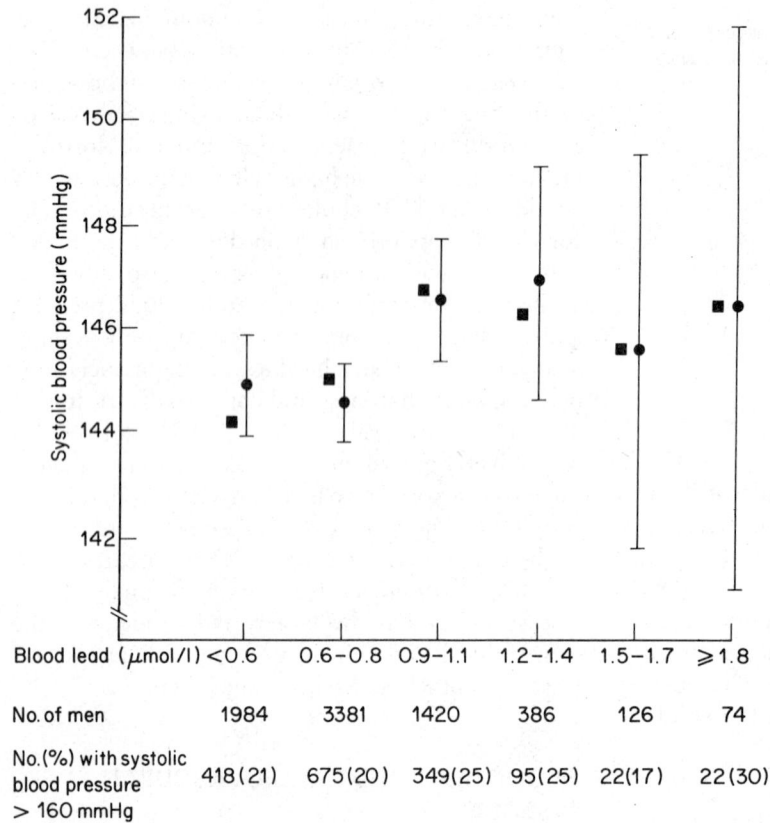

Blood lead (μmol/l)	<0.6	0.6–0.8	0.9–1.1	1.2–1.4	1.5–1.7	≥1.8
No. of men	1984	3381	1420	386	126	74
No.(%) with systolic blood pressure > 160 mmHg	418 (21)	675 (20)	349 (25)	95 (25)	22 (17)	22 (30)

Fig. 69.5. Systolic blood pressure for 7371 middle-aged men categorized according to blood lead concentration. Bars represent 95% confidence limits for unadjusted mean (●); ■, means adjusted for age, town, body mass, alcohol consumption, social class and observer. *NB*: 1 μmol/l lead ≈ 20.7 μg/100 ml.

pressure such as age, body mass index and alcohol intake; alcohol has a substantial association with blood lead concentration as well as with blood pressure. Cigarette smoking, while not affecting blood pressure, is also an important variable associated (positively) with blood lead concentrations. When body mass index, alcohol intake, smoking habit, social class and other factors are taken into account, there is a *weak* positive association between blood lead and both systolic and diastolic blood pressures which cannot be accepted as causal.

OTHER STUDIES OF BLOOD LEAD AND BLOOD PRESSURE

In an American study (United States National Health and Nutrition Examination Surveys—NHANES II), it was concluded that there is an important association between blood lead and blood pressure.[17] This study has been reviewed in detail; its conclusions and extrapolations to public health benefit would appear to be exaggerated.[18] In particular, the estimate of lives saved by removing lead from car exhaust fumes, with consequent effects on blood pressure and thus on ischaemic

heart disease, seem totally unjustified. In two Welsh studies, there was no significant association between blood lead and blood pressure, and no such relationship was found in studies in Canada and Denmark.[19] Although there does appear to be a small increase in blood pressure with increasing blood lead concentrations, the importance of this with respect to cardiovascular disease is not known.

CARDIOVASCULAR EVENTS

The mean blood lead concentrations for 316 men who experienced a new major ischaemic heart disease event following initial screening are shown in Table 69.3, together with those of the 7063 other men.[19] The mean blood lead concentration is significantly higher in the cases with ischaemic heart disease ($P = 0.01$), but this does not take account of important confounding variables, such as cigarette smoking and town of residence. Adjustment for these variables reduces the mean excess in blood lead amongst ischaemic heart disease cases to levels that are no longer significantly different from zero. There do not appear to be any other large-scale prospective epidemiological studies of coronary heart disease and stroke in which blood lead has

Table 69.3. Mean blood lead concentrations in men who experienced a new major ischaemic heart disease event following initial screening compared with those of other men.

	Ischaemic heart disease cases	Other men	Stroke cases	Other men
No. of men	316	7063	66	7313
Mean blood lead (μmol/l)	0.786	0.735	0.808	0.737
Difference in mean ± SE	0.051 ±0.019		0.071 ±0.049	
Difference in means after adjustment for age, smoking years and town ± SE	0.041 ±0.015		0.033 ±0.033	

been included as a potential risk factor. The British data suggest that low-level lead exposure has no important effect on the risk of heart attack or stroke and there is no direct evidence that changing the blood lead level in the population could affect the level of blood pressure or the risk of heart attacks in the population.

WEATHER AND CARDIOVASCULAR DISEASE

COLD WEATHER AND CARDIOVASCULAR MORTALITY

The comprehensive paper by Alderson on 'Season and mortality' provides an important basis of information on this subject. It is a useful contribution to the issue of climatic effects on mortality and deserves to be read in full.[20] In Great Britain, concern regarding increased mortality in the winter months goes back about 150 years, when the Registrar General in 1841 reported on the specific diseases that were particularly influenced by season. He observed that the number of deaths rose when the temperature at night fell below freezing, and rose even more markedly when the mean day and major temperature fell 1 or 2°C below freezing point. There was an immediate rise in mortality with effects continuing for a period of 30–40 days after the extreme cold had passed. The excess mortality was more marked in the elderly, doubling for every 9 years' increase in age beyond the age-group 20–40 years.

The first 'modern' examination of the effect of cold weather on cardiovascular disease was by Rose, who looked at mortality from atherosclerotic heart disease in England and Wales in 1950–1962, in relation to temperature, air pollution and rainfall.[21] During the period studied, the mid-winter peak varied from 20 to 70% above the

mid-summer trough. He concluded that most of the short-term fluctuations in atherosclerotic (ischaemic) heart disease mortality were due to changes in the temperature. Data from England and Wales for 1947–1962 were also examined by Anderson and Le Riche, together with data from Ontario, Canada for 1958–1962.[22] The ratio of the death rate during each month was compared with the mean death ratio for the whole year. In addition, data from Ontario from 1881 and from Australia and Denmark for 1958–1962 were reviewed. Overall, it was concluded that it was seasonal fluctuations in respiratory infections which had an influence on deaths from other causes and that temperature variations would not account for the variations observed. In a later study, Bull demonstrated that the association of deaths from myocardial infarction or stroke with temperature were not due to an association with respiratory or infectious disease.[23]

Stroke mortality was examined in detail using data from London, New York and Tokyo, three cities showing appreciable seasonal variation, which was more marked in London and Tokyo than New York.[24] There was a high correlation between stroke mortality and temperature for Tokyo, an intermediate one for London and a lower correlation for New York. The authors speculated that central heating in New York might protect against the extreme winter temperatures in that city. In a more detailed study, coronary and stroke mortality in American cities in the period 1962–1966 was examined in relation to daily temperature and snowfall.[25] There was an inverse relationship for both coronary heart disease and stroke deaths, with excess deaths being associated with low temperatures 1 or 2 days earlier and with snowfall for 5 or 6 days earlier.

In a study of 114 county and metropolitan

boroughs in England and Wales for 1968–1970 death rates from ischaemic heart disease were examined in relation to rainfall, mean annual temperature and a socio-economic index.[26] The correlation coefficient for temperature as well as those for the other factors were highly significant and the authors suggested that cold and high rainfall precipitated death in subjects with pre-existing ischaemic heart disease. The findings of the BRHS are in substantial agreement with these findings: temperature, rainfall and socio-economic indices as well as water hardness were all found to have significant independent relationships with cardiovascular disease mortality.[11] Further support for the temperature–cardiovascular mortality relationship came from a study of weekly deaths from ischaemic heart disease in Greater London during 1970–1974, with a close association present for all age-groups from 45 to over 75 years.[27] Monthly cardiovascular mortality in England and Wales for 1963–1966 showed significant associations with mean temperatures, particularly in the elderly, and they were more marked with increased duration of temperature change.

MECHANISMS FOR EFFECTS OF COLD ON CARDIOVASCULAR DISEASE

Keatinge and his colleagues have explored the mechanisms that might be responsible for the excess deaths occurring in winter.[28] In experiments on 8 young adults, controlled cold stress was induced for a 6-h period of observation. Systolic and diastolic blood pressures increased by 12 and 18 mmHg, respectively, and pulse rates decreased. There was an increase in platelet, red cell counts and haematocrit during exposure to cold as well as an increase in neutrophil polymorphs. Whole blood viscosity rose by 20% in the cold. Plasma cholesterol in all its fractions increased in concentration. The authors concluded that the increases in platelets, red cells, blood viscosity, arterial pressure and plasma cholesterol could all contribute to the increase in arterial thromboses in cold weather.

HOT WEATHER AND CARDIOVASCULAR MORTALITY

Extremely hot weather may also cause excess mortality from cardiovascular disease, and possibly half of the excess mortality in heatwaves has been ascribed to coronary heart disease and stroke.[29,30] As with excess deaths due to extreme cold, it is the

elderly who are most affected. The problem is far more marked in the USA than in Great Britain, but even in Great Britain there is an increase in mortality associated with heatwaves every few years. The daily deaths that occurred in London during one particular heatwave in 1976, when the outside air temperature reached 34.6°C with a minimal daily temperature of 20.8°C, are shown in Fig. 69.6.[31] Daily deaths from coronary heart disease and stroke almost doubled, peaking about 24 h after the highest minimal temperature and 48 h after the highest maximal temperature. The excess mortality was much larger for the first period of excess temperature than for a second one a few days later. It is suggested that several days of exposure to heat had produced a protective effect of acclimatization.

MECHANISM FOR EFFECT OF HEAT ON CARDIOVASCULAR DISEASE

Keatinge and his colleagues carried out a study of

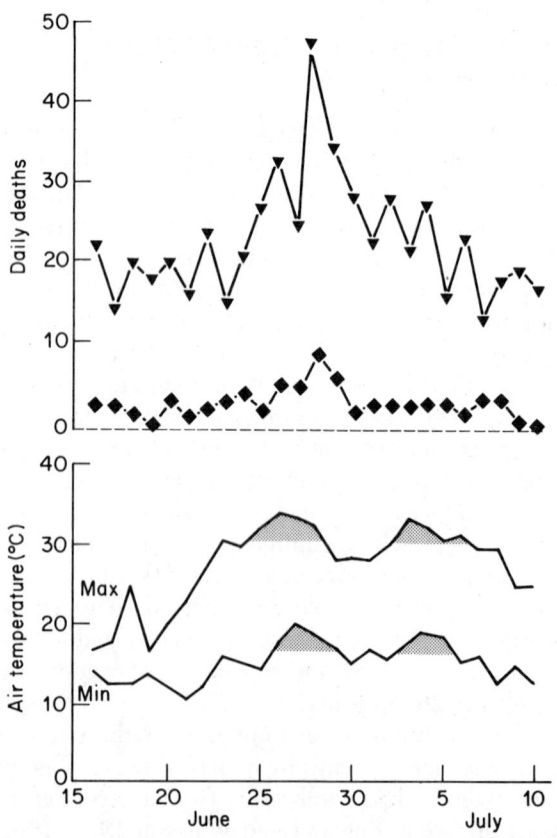

Fig. 69.6. Daily deaths from myocardial ischaemia (▼) and cerebral thrombosis (◆) in Greater London during a brief heatwave. Daily maximal temperatures above 31°C and minimal temperatures above 17°C are blocked in.

the effects of heat on 8 subjects, similar in approach to their work on exposure to cold.[31] The subjects remained in a hot room (temperature between 38.3 and 40.2°C) for 6 h. Heart rate increased by 32 beats/min and arterial blood pressure decreased, particularly on standing. The red blood cell count increased 9% and blood viscosity increased 24%, mostly after the first hour. The platelet count rose 18% and the platelet volume fell, mostly in the first hour. The plasma cholesterol increased 14% without a change in distribution among lipoprotein fractions. The authors consider that these changes could readily account for the increases in deaths from coronary heart disease and stroke. The changes are attributed to the reduction in plasma volume, attributable largely to an almost isotonic net loss of salt and water from the body. However, the increase in platelet count (18%) was double the decrease (9%) in blood volume, indicating release of platelets into the circulation. Keatinge et al. suggest that an increased intake of water with adequate salt intake is desirable and may prevent some of the excess deaths in the elderly during heatwaves.

ALCOHOL AND CARDIOVASCULAR DISEASE

The concern regarding possible toxic effects of alcohol on the heart first arose in the nineteenth century, but only in recent years has it been established that there is a direct effect of alcohol on the heart which may result in a cardiomyopathy (see Chapter 37). There is also evidence regarding the association of heavy alcohol intake or alcoholism on cardiac rhythm, and atrial fibrilation, atrial flutter and heart block have all been described.[32] In this part of the chapter, I will briefly describe the progress made in understanding the relationships between alcohol consumption and blood pressure, stroke and coronary heart disease in recent years. It is not a comprehensive review and should serve only to alert clinicians to the role of alcohol in these disorders and to encourage the recording of the full history of alcohol consumption in subjects with cardiovascular disease.

ALCOHOL, BLOOD PRESSURE AND HYPERTENSION

The first report on an association between alcohol intake and raised blood pressure came from a study of French servicemen in 1915,[33] and this associa-

tion has since been confirmed by the results of the Framingham study[34] and of other large population-based studies in the USA.[35,36] Studies in Great Britain have been based on hospital outpatients[37] and on London-based civil servants,[38,39] groups unlikely to be representative of the general population with respect to their health status or their alcohol consumption. In particular, these latter studies made it extremely difficult to assess the contribution which alcohol intake might make to the prevalence of hypertension in the general community. Nevertheless, the evidence from all these studies is very similar. Alcohol in moderate or large amounts may produce a significant increase in blood pressure and account for a substantial proportion of hypertensive subjects in both the USA and Great Britain.

In the BRHS, alcohol intake was recorded and blood pressure measured in 7735 middle-aged men drawn at random from the registers of one general practice in each of 24 towns in England, Wales and Scotland.[40]

It is evident from Fig. 69.7 that the blood pressure rises with increasing alcohol intake in both weekend and daily drinkers.[41] The findings are independent of the effects of bodyweight (body mass index) or age on blood pressure and occur in manual and non-manual workers. It appears that about 10% of systolic hypertension ($\geqslant$ 160 mmHg) and a similar proportion of diastolic hypertension ($\geqslant$ 90 mmHg) could be attributed to moderate (16–42 drinks/week) and heavy (> 42 drinks/week) drinking patterns.[42]

The need to enquire about alcohol intake in any patient with a raised blood pressure would seem to be imperative. The results of studies in normotensive and hypertensive subjects suggests that the relationship between alcohol and blood pressure depends on intake within the previous 3–4 days[43] and there is evidence that withdrawal of alcohol leads to a lowering of blood pressure.[44,45] Alcohol restriction may have a central role to play in the management of a substantial proportion of hypertensive subjects, and it should certainly be initiated before the use of potent drugs. Abstinence from alcohol for 1 week should be an adequate test of whether it is playing a role in an individual with sustained hypertension.

ALCOHOL AND STROKE

There is remarkably little information available in this area, although a certain amount of attention

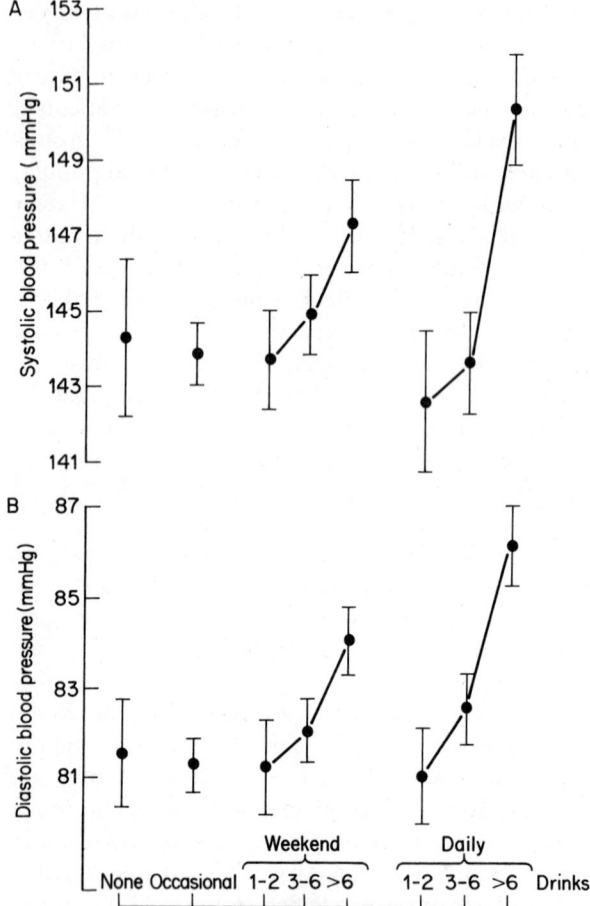

Fig. 69.7. BRHS: systolic (A) and diastolic (B) blood pressure in middle-aged British men by alcohol category.

has focused on stroke associated with 'binge' drinking in young men.[46–48] In some of the larger population-based surveys, the role of regular alcohol intake in the development of cerebrovascular episodes has been examined, and most of the results suggest that there is a positive association.[49–51] Case-control studies have in general suffered from the usual problems of retrospective investigation, although a recent study of this kind has overcome some of the problems.[52] Using non-drinkers as a baseline group, the relative risk of stroke was increased fourfold in men drinking more than 300 g alcohol/week, i.e. about 30 drinks/week. The relationship between alcohol intake and stroke was not linear and it was in only the 'heavy' drinkers that the risk was raised. As this amount is equivalent to 4 drinks/day (2 pints of beer), the validity of the reported intakes could be called into question.

The possible mechanisms by which alcohol may lead to cardiovascular episodes, apart from blood pressure, include vasoconstriction, arrythmias, changes in platelet and red cell aggregation and changes in the haematocrit. Although the findings in this case-control study are strongly suggestive of current alcohol intake being an independent and potentially reversible risk factor in stroke, the results of large prospective studies are needed to support these findings. However, it is good clinical practice to reduce alcohol intake in all subjects with sustained hypertension in order to assess the effect of alcohol on their hypertension. It might be better if hypertensive subjects continued to abstain from drinking alcohol if findings such as these are corroborated.

ALCOHOL AND CORONARY HEART DISEASE

The literature on the relationship between alcohol and coronary heart disease is now considerable, with reports on large-scale prospective studies from the USA, Finland, Sweden, Australia, Japan, Yugoslavia, Puerto Rico and Hawaii. The issue on which most contemporary discussion is centred concerns the possibility that moderate alcohol intake protects against coronary heart disease. Three reviews of this possible beneficial effect of moderate alcohol consumption encompass most of the studies carried out up to 1985.[53–55] Since then, there has been a further report from the Kaiser Permanente Medical Center which supports the view that alcohol protects against coronary heart disease.[56] A further report from the Framingham study based on a 24-year follow-up of the original cohort shows a clear negative association between moderate alcohol consumption and alcohol intake in males, with mortality reduced about 40% in non-smokers and about 50% in heavy smokers at alcohol intakes of 233–355 g/week (30–40 drinks/week).[57] A recently reported study from Alameda County, California, differs from these reports and from the generally accepted belief that alcohol has a protective effect on coronary heart disease.[58] As abstainers differ from drinkers on a number of demographic, physical and psychosocial characteristics, the role of these confounders of the alcohol–mortality association was examined. The authors found that among men only, very heavy drinkers were at significantly greater risk of death from all causes than were lighter drinkers ($P \leq 0.01$). Neither abstainers nor other drinkers were at significantly higher risk of death from coronary heart disease than were the light drinkers.

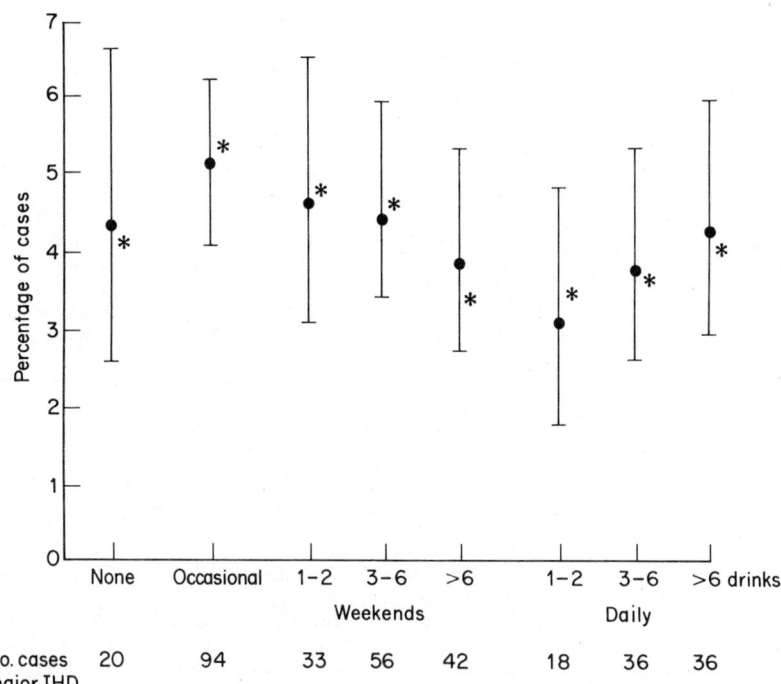

Fig. 69.8. Attack rates (%) of major ischaemic heart disease events in 8 drinking categories. Bars represent 95% confidence limits for unadjusted rates (•); *, rates adjusted for age, smoking years and social class.

No. cases major IHD: None 20, Occasional 94, Weekends 1–2 33, 3–6 56, >6 42, Daily 1–2 18, 3–6 36, >6 drinks 36

"It is important that the ambiguity of findings to date are recognized in order that we may avoid making premature and unwarranted conclusions regarding the potential effects of moderate intake of alcohol." . . . "Therefore it would appear prudent, from a public health perspective, to reserve judgement concerning the protective effects of moderate alcohol consumption."[58]

Results of studies in Great Britain are in agreement with the Alameda County findings, and provide no support for a significant association between alcohol intake and coronary heart disease.[59] After a 6-year follow-up of the 7735 men in the BRHS, 335 men had experienced a myocardial infarction (fatal or non-fatal) or sudden cardiac death. Although no regular association was found between reported alcohol intake and the incidence of such events, the light drinkers had the lowest incidence of such events (Fig. 69.8). This group contained the lowest proportion of current smokers, had the lowest mean blood pressure, had the lowest mean body mass index and contained the lowest proportion of manual workers. There were also other factors that might have been of beneficial importance such as a high proportion of men taking physical exercise in leisure time and the lowest levels of serum triglycerides. All of these characteristics acting in concert were considered more likely to account for the apparent protective effect of alcohol against coronary heart disease than a direct effect of alcohol. It was concluded that compared with the effects of the established risk factors, alcohol seemed to be unimportant in the development of coronary heart disease.[59]

The BRHS, like the Alameda County Study, is very concerned with the nature of abstainers, because the U-shaped curve, upon which the protective effect of alcohol is to a considerable extent based, depends on the higher rates of all-cause and cardiovascular mortality seen in abstainers. In a detailed examination of 'men who do not drink',[60] it was observed that non-drinkers included a large proportion of ex-drinkers who had many characteristics likely to increase their morbidity and mortality. They were older and included an increased proportion of manual workers. They had the same high percentage of current cigarette smokers as moderate/heavy drinkers and a prevalence of obesity and hypertension similar to moderate/heavy drinkers and higher than lifelong abstainers or occasional/light drinkers. The ex-drinkers had the highest prevalence rates of angina and possible myocardial infarction on questionnaire, of myocardial infarction on electrocardiogram and of recall of a doctor-diagnosis of ischaemic heart disease. They also had high rates of recall of high blood pressure, peptic ulcer, diabetes, gallbladder disease and bronchitis. They had the highest rates for regular medical treatment and the highest proportion of men who considered their health to be poor. It is abundantly clear that the general category of non-drinkers should not be used as a baseline against which to measure the effects of alcohol consumption overall.

In a 7.5-year follow-up of the BRHS men, there was a U-shaped relationship between alcohol intake and total mortality and an inverse relationship with cardiovascular mortality. These relationships were only present in men with cardiovascular or cardiovascular-related conditions present at initial examination.[61] The data suggest that the relationships are produced by pre-existing disease and by the movement of men with such disease into non-drinking or occasional drinking categories.[62] The concept of a 'protective' effect of drinking on mortality may be ill-founded.

REFERENCES

1. Kobayashi, J. On geochemical relationship between the chemical nature of river water and death-rate from apoplexy. *Ber. Ohara Inst. Landwirtschaft Biol.* 1957; **11**: 12–21.
2. Schroeder, H.A. Degenerative cardiovascular disease in the Orient. II. Hypertension. *J. Chron. Dis.* 1958; **8**: 312–33.
3. Schroeder, H.A. and Kraemer, L.A. Cardiovascular mortality, municipal water, and corrosion. *Arch. Environ. Health* 1974; **28**: 303–11.
4. Morris, J.N., Crawford, M.D. and Heady, J.A. Hardness of local water-supplies and mortality from cardiovascular disease in the county boroughs of England and Wales. *Lancet* 1961; i: 860–2.
5. Crawford, M.D., Gardner, M.J. and Morris, J.N. Mortality and hardness of local water supplies. *Lancet* 1968; i: 827–31.
6. Clayton, D.G., Taylor, D. and Shaper, A.G. Trends in heart disease in England and Wales 1950–1973. *Health Trends* 1977; **9**: 1–6.
7. Gardner, M.J., Crawford, M.D. and Morris, J.N. Patterns in mortality in middle and early old age in the county boroughs of England and Wales. *Br. J. Prev. Soc. Med.* 1969; **23**: 133–40.
8. Crawford, M.D., Gardner, M.J. and Morris, J.N. Changes in water hardness and local death rates. *Lancet* 1971; ii: 327–9.
9. Stitt, F.W., Clayton, D.G., Crawford, M.D. and Morris, J.N. Clinical and biochemical indicators of cardiovascular disease among men living in hard and soft waters. *Lancet* 1973; i: 122–6.
10. Crawford, M.D., Clayton, D.G., Stanley, F. and Shaper, A.G. An epidemiological study of sudden death in hard and soft water areas. *J. Chron. Dis.* 1977; **20**: 69–80.
11. Pocock, S.J., Shaper, A.G., Cook, D.G. *et al.* British Regional Heart Study: geographic variations in cardiovascular mortality, and the role of water quality. *Br. Med. J.* 1980; **280**: 1243–9.
12. Pocock, S.J., Cook, D.G. and Shaper, A.G. Analysing geographic variations in cardiovascular mortality: methods and results. *J. R. Statist. Soc. A.* 1982; **145**: 313–41.
13. Shaper, A.G., Pocock, S.J., Packham, R.F., Lacey, R.F. and Powell, P. Softness of drinking water and cardiovascular

disease—practical implications of recent research. *Health Trends* 1983; **15**: 22–4.
14. Pocock, S.J., Shaper, A.G. and Powell, P. The British Regional Heart Study: Cardiovascular disease and water quality. In: Calabrese, E.J., Turhill, R.W. and Condie, L. eds. *Inorganics in Drinking Water and Cardiovascular Disease Control*. New Jersey: Princeton Sci. Publ. Co. 1985, pp. 111–27.
15. Neri, L.C., Johansen, H.L. and Talbot, F.D.F. *Chemical contents of cardiovascular drinking-water related to cardiovascular health 1977*. Ottawa: University of Ottawa.
16. Pocock, S.J., Shaper, A.G., Ashby, D., Delves, T. and Whitehead, T.P. Blood lead concentration, blood pressure and renal function. *Br. Med. J.* 1984; **289**: 872–4.
17. Harlan, W.R., Landis, R., Schmouder, R.L., Goldstein, N.G. and Harlan, L.C. Blood lead and blood pressure. *JAMA* 1985; **253**: 530–4.
18. Shaper, A.G. and Pocock, S.J. Blood lead and blood pressure. *Br. Med. J.* 1985; **291**: 1147–9.
19. Pocock, S.J., Shaper, A.G., Ashby, D., Delves, H.T. and Clayton, B.E. The relationship between blood lead, blood pressure, stroke and heart attacks in middle-aged British men. *Environ. Health Perspectives.* 1988; **78**: 23–30.
20. Alderson, M.R. Season and mortality. *Health Trends* 1985; **17**: 87–96.
21. Rose, G. Cold weather and ischaemic heart disease. *Br. J. Prev. Soc. Med.* 1966; **20**: 97–100.
22. Anderson, T.W. and Le Riche, W.H. Cold weather and myocardial infarction. *Lancet* 1970; i: 291–6.
23. Bull, G.M. Meteorological correlants with myocardial and cerebral infarction and respiratory disease. *Br. J. Prev. Soc. Med.* 1973; **27**: 108–13.
24. Sakamoto, M.M. and Katayama, K. Statistical analysis of seasonal variation in mortality. *J. Meteorol. Soc. Jpn* 1971; **49**: 494–509.
25. Rogot, E. and Padgett, S.J. Associations of coronary and stroke mortality with temperature and snowfall in selected areas of the United States 1962–66. *Am. J. Epidemiol.* 1976; **103**: 565–75.
26. West, R.R., Lloyd, S. and Roberts, C.J. Mortality from ischaemic heart disease: associations with weather. *Br. J. Prev. Soc. Med.* 1973; **27**: 36–40.
27. Bainton, D., Moore, F. and Sweetnam, P. Temperature and death from ischaemic heart disease. *Br. J. Prev. Soc. Med.* 1977; **31**: 49–53.
28. Keatinge, W.R., Coleshaw, S.R.K., Cotter, F., Mattock, M.B., Murphy, M. and Chelliah, R. Increases in platelet and red cell counts, blood viscosity and arterial pressure during mild surface cooling: factors in mortality from coronary and cerebral thrombosis in winter. *Br. Med. J.* 1984; **289**: 1405–8.
29. Heyer, H.E., Teng, H.C. and Barris, W. Increased frequency of acute myocardial infarction during summer months in a warm climate. *Am. Heart J.* 1953; **45**: 741–55.
30. Marmot, M. Heat wave mortality in New York City 1949 to 1970. *Arch. Env. Health* 1975; **30**: 130–6.
31. Keatinge, W.R., Coleshaw, S.R.K., Easton, J.C., Cotter, F., Mattock, M.B. and Chelliah, R. Increased platelet and red cell counts, blood viscosity and plasma cholesterol levels during heat stress, and mortality from coronary and cerebral thrombosis. *Am. J. Med.* 1986; **81**: 795–800.
32. Ettinger, P.O., Lyons, M., Oldewartel, M.A. and Regan, T.J. Cardiac conduction abnormalities produced by chronic alcoholism. *Am. Heart J.* 1976; **91**: 66–78.
33. Lian, C. L'alcoolisme, cause d'hypertension arterielle. *Bull. Acad. Med. (Paris)* 1915; **74**: 525–8.
34. Kannel, W.B. and Sorlie, P. Hypertension in Framingham. In: Paul, O., ed. *Epidemiology and Control of Hypertension* Miami: Symposia Specialists, 1975, p. 553.
35. Klatsky, A.L., Friedman, G.D., Siegelaub, A.B. and Gerard,

M.J. Alcohol consumption and blood pressure: Kaiser–Permanente Multiphasic Health Examination Data. *N. Engl. J. Med.* 1977; **296**: 1194–200.

36. Dyer, A.R., Stamler, J., Paul, O. *et al.* Alcohol consumption, cardiovascular risk factors and mortality in two Chicago epidemiologic studies. *Circulation* 1977; **56**: 1067–74.

37. Beevers, D.G. Alcohol and hypertension. *Lancet* 1977; ii: 114–5.

38. Marmot, M.G. and Rose, G. Epidemiology of Hypertension in Cardiology. In: Sleight, P. and Vann Jones, S., eds. *Scientific foundations of Cardiology.* London: W. Heinemann, 1983, pp. 129–36.

39. Bulpitt, C.J., Shipley, M.J. and Semmence, A. The contribution of a moderate intake of alcohol to the presence of hypertension. *J. Hypertens.* 1987; **5**: 85–91.

40. Shaper, A.G., Pocock, S.J., Walker, M., Cohen, W.M., Wale, C.J. and Thomson, A.G. British Regional Heart Study: Cardiovascular risk factors in middle-aged men in 24 towns. *Br. Med. J.* 1982; **283**: 179–86.

41. Shaper, A.G. Coronary Heart Disease: Risks and Reasons p. 32; Current Medical Literature Ltd, London 1988.

42. Shaper, A.G., Wannamethee, G. and Whincup, P. Alcohol, blood pressure and hypertension in British men. *J. Human Hypertension* 1988; **2**: 71–78.

43. Maheswaran, R., Gill, J.S. and Beevers, D.G. The effect of alcohol on blood pressure due to recent alcohol intake. *Clin. Sci.* 1987; **70** (Suppl. 16): 70 .

44. Potter, J.F. and Beevers, D.G. Pressure effect of alcohol in normaltensive and hypertensive subjects. *Lancet* 1984; i: 119–20.

45. Puddey, I.B., Beilin, L.J. and Vandogen, R. Regular alcohol use raises blood pressure in treated hypertensive subjects. *Lancet* 1987; i: 647–53.

46. Hillborn, M. and Kaste, M. Does ethanol intoxication promote brain infarction in young adults? *Lancet* 1978; ii: 1181–3.

47. Lee, K. Alcoholism and cerebrovascular thrombosis in the young. *Acta Neurol. Scand.* 1979; **59**: 270–4.

48. Gill, J.S., Zezulka, A.V. and Beevers, D.G. Stroke affecting young men after alcoholic binges. *Br. Med. J.* 1985; **291**: 1645.

49. Blackwelder, W.C., Yano, K., Rhoads, G.G., Kagan, A., Gordon, T. and Palesch, Y. Alcohol and mortality: the Honolulu Heart Study. *Am. J. Med.* 1980; **68**: 164–9.

50. Kozarevic, D., McGee, D., Vojvodic, N. *et al.* Frequency of alcohol consumption and mortality: the Yugoslavia Cardiovascular Disease Study. *Lancet* 1980; i: 613–6.

51. Donahue, R.P., Abbot, R.D., Reed, D.M. and Yano, K. Alcohol and haemorrhagic stroke and the Honolulu Heart Program. *JAMA* 1986; **255**: 2311–4.

52. Gill, J.S., Zezulka, A.V., Shipley, M.J., Gill, S.K. and Beevers, D.G. Stroke and alcohol consumption. *N. Engl. J. Med.* 1986; **315**: 1041–6.

53. Turner, T.B., Bennett, V.L. and Hernandez, H. The beneficial side of moderate alcohol use. *Johns Hopkins Med. J.* 1981; **148**: 53–63.

54. Marmot, M.G. Alcohol and coronary heart disease. *Int. J. Epidemiol.* 1984; **13**: 160–6.

55. Moore, R.D. and Pearson, T.A. Moderate alcohol consumption and coronary artery disease. A review. *Medicine* 1986; **65**: 242–67.

56. Klatsky, A.L., Armstrong, M.A. and Friedman, G.D. Relations of alcoholic beverage use to subsequent coronary artery disease hospitalization. *Am. J. Cardiol.* 1986; **58**: 710–4.

57. Friedman, L.A. and Kimball, A.W. Coronary heart disease mortality and alcohol consumption in Framingham. *Am. J. Epidemiol.* 1986; **124**: 481–9.

58. Camacho, T.C., Kaplan, G.A. and Cohen, R.D. Alcohol consumption and mortality in Alameda County. *J. Chron. Dis.* 1987; **40**: 229–36.

59. Shaper, A.G., Phillips, A.N., Pocock, S.J. and Walker, M. Alcohol and ischaemic heart disease in middle aged British men. *Br. Med. J.* 1987; **294**: 733–7.

60. Wannamethee, G. and Shaper, A.G. Men who do not drink. *Int. J. Epidemiol.* 1988; **17**: 201–210.

61. Shaper, A.G., Wannamethee, G. and Walker, M. Alcohol and mortality: explaining the U-shaped curve. *Lancet* 1988; ii: 1267–73.

62. Wannamethee, G. and Shaper, A.G. Changes in drinking habits in middle-aged British men. *J. Roy. Coll. G.P's* 1988; **38**: 440–42.

Chapter 70

The Mind and the Heart

Leisa J. Freeman

INTRODUCTION

In 1623, William Harvey stated:

"Every affection of the mind that is attended with either pain or pleasure, hope or fear, is the cause of an agitation, whose influence extends to the heart."

The effect of the mind on the heart has often been ignored in current cardiological practice. It is viewed as vague and subjective, and it cannot be easily quantified. This subject has not been well supported by research; it has been far easier to concentrate on the traditionally accepted risk factors in heart disease: cigarette smoking, hyperlipidaemia and hypertension, which are reasonable and perceptible targets for both primary (i.e. preventive) and secondary therapeutic intervention. There are two reasons why this view is changing:
1   multivariate analysis has demonstrated that the standard risk factors are found in less than half of those who succumb to ischaemic heart disease;
2   the advent of new technology and methodology has meant that a sizeable body of evidence is now accumulating, implicating psychosocial conflict, emotions and behavioural patterns as important risk factors in the pathogenesis of coronary heart disease, sudden death, cardiac arrhythmias and systemic hypertension.

DEFINITION OF PSYCHOLOGICAL STRESS

Stress is a word that produces considerable confusion, since it means stimulus or response to some and interaction, or complex combination of conditions, to others. It is best to appreciate that:

"the environment is a stressor requiring an adaptive response, the measured physiological response as strain, and stress as the psychophysiological degree of response observed during such interactions between subject and environment."

POSTULATED PSYCHOPHYSIOLOGICAL MECHANISMS

Work summarized by Mason[1] and Henry[2] has clearly demonstrated that psychological stress in animals can trigger at least two distinct neuro-endocrine responses. The first is that of the adreno-cortical system, which responds to situations that lead to a high degree of uncertainty; it is linked emotionally with feelings of defeat, despair, loss and isolation. The second is that of the catecholamine fight–flight, sympatho-adrenal medullary system; this system is crucially involved in the response to situations that require attention or vigilance. When the situation involves an aggressive directed attack, noradrenaline (liberated principally at alpha-adrenergic nerve endings and inducing vasoconstriction) is preferentially released; when situations provoking uncertainty and anxiety occur, both adrenaline (principally producing a beta-adrenergic effect increasing heart rate and contractility) and noradrenaline are involved.

In 1969, Carruthers proposed that emotion, acting via the intermediary of enhanced sympathetic activity, resulted in increased mobilization of free fatty acids from adipose tissue; in the absence of metabolic demand, the free fatty acids were converted to triglycerides and were then available to be incorporated into atheroma. In addition, the role of cortisol in response to emotion may be important; it appears to sensitize the heart to the toxicity of noradrenaline, either by increasing its extraneuronal uptake or by interfering with its subsequent degradation by catechol-O-methyl transferase. Emotional stimuli, but not exercise,[3] elicit the potentially detrimental combination of noradrenaline and cortisol, which may account, in part, for the remarkable destructiveness of emotional and sensory stimuli observed in animals, even in those which have normal coronary arteries.

In long-term studies of competing monkeys,

which are not capable of social control, chronic arousal of the sympatho-adrenal medullary and pituitary adrenal cortical systems was produced experimentally. Under such conditions, grossly exaggerated atherosclerosis occurred in these animals, especially when fed high-lipid diets; this compares with the minimal atherosclerosis seen in the relaxed and secure control animals.[4]

ROLE OF THE MIND IN CORONARY ARTERY DISEASE

In the last few years, two particular variables have emerged that appear to enhance the risk of developing coronary heart disease.
1 Psychological stress resulting from interpersonal conflict.
2 Certain personality characteristics which may predispose an individual to becoming more involved in conflict, and will also influence the behavioural response to conflict.

PSYCHOLOGICAL STRESS FROM INTERPERSONAL CONFLICT

Work situation

The way of life associated with an occupation appears to contribute to coronary risks above and beyond the physical labour involved in the job itself. Thus, within the many types of medical practice, the pre-judged 'high-stress' areas of general practice and anaesthesiology have higher coronary prevalence rates (11.9%) when compared with the 'low-stress' areas of pathology and dermatology (3.2%). In addition, it appears that situations involving high demand but low control are particularly important as opposed to situations in which there is high demand (work addict) but a high degree of control.[5]

Family and social situation

In the Whitehall civil servant study, a higher coronary mortality was found in those subjects who also had fewer social supports (i.e. family, friends; were divorced or had marital discord), fewer leisure activities and more adverse experiences at work. These subjects also tended to have a higher fibrinogen level and were in the lower grades of the service.[6] It is difficult to assess the relevance of such findings, since the results of some rehabilitation studies have failed to demonstrate any benefit following counselling and group psychotherapy for such problems.[7]

High life-event change/stress

There is considerable research reported in the literature concerning the association of life-events and heart disease. This suggests that life-changes that deprive individuals of important sources of emotional security, self-esteem or a sense of identity are likely to be followed by a higher than normal risk of cardiovascular disease. Significantly higher life-event scores (illness, divorce, financial change or death of a relative) have been found in the 6 months before a myocardial infarction when compared with the 3 months before that, or the 6 months after myocardial infarction. Similarly, there is an association between bereavement and increased subsequent mortality among spouses or next of kin, such that within 1 year of loss the mortality rate among widowers was 12.2% as compared with 1.2% among matched control subjects.

A recent prospective study further substantiates a causal role for biobehavioural stress in cardiac death. It was shown that high indices of life stress and social isolation, independent of other variables (including education level and the presence of ventricular arrhythmias) are significantly associated with a high risk for cardiac death. In a controlled trial of stress monitoring and subsequent intervention following myocardial infarction (in the survivors at 1 month), a 47% decline in mortality over the first year was found in the psychologically treated group when compared with the control group (no intervention).[9] This remarkable decline, however, has not yet been reproduced.

PERSONALITY CHARACTERISTICS

The coronary-prone behaviour pattern

The type A or coronary-prone behaviour pattern was first formally defined by Rosenman and Friedman, although aspects of the personality had been noted by Osler and Dunbar. Although the Western Collaborative Group studies have demonstrated that the type A behaviour pattern is an independent risk factor in coronary artery disease of the same order of magnitude as blood pressure, serum cholesterol and smoking,[10] there is still considerable debate about this point.

This behaviour pattern may be defined as:

"an action–emotion complex or a chronic incessant struggle to achieve more and more in less and less time, and if required to do so against the opposing efforts of other things or other persons." (Rosenman)

The type A behaviour pattern includes:
1 behavioural dispositions such as ambitiousness, aggressiveness, competitiveness and impatience;
2 specific behaviours, such as muscle tenseness, mental alertness, rapid and emphatic speech stylistics and rapid pace of most activities;
3 emotional responses such as irritation, hostility and anger that is usually covert.

The type A behaviour pattern is a characteristic style of response to an environmental stressor and is enhanced when the stressors threaten the individual with a perceived loss of control over his milieu; it does not appear to be an inherited characteristic.[11] Type A subjects exhibit enhanced secretion of noradrenaline throughout the working day, as well as a greater rise of blood pressure and heart rate in response to many cognitive and physical performance tasks and cold pressor testing (sympathetic nervous function) when compared with type B subjects. Type A subjects also report more stressful life-events and more life events as stressful; active coping is required to deal with this, which is associated with increased noradrenaline excretion and these subjects thus have recurrent chronic activation of the sympatho-adrenal medullary system.[12] Hostility and anger are two specific features that appear to be of great importance.

However, in a recent study, it was also demonstrated that type A patients report more episodes of ischaemia during daily life as painful; type B subjects had a similar incidence of total ischaemic episodes, but over three-quarters of these episodes were painless.[13] This suggests that by virtue of increased reporting of any event, whether somatic or environmental, type A subjects may be considered to be more 'prone' to coronary artery disease and present earlier. Type B behaviour is not merely the absence of type A response, rather, it is a different set of coping behaviours. Thus, the type B individual is more relaxed, unhurried, more easily satisfied and uses an alternative method of coping in daily living which does not often lead to time urgency or competitive hostility. Type B subjects, however, are still subject to heart disease.

The results of the Framingham study in America and the French–Belgian collaborative study in Europe have demonstrated the relationship of the type A behaviour pattern to the prevalence of ischaemic heart disease. There are significant associations between the incidence of both symptomatic and silent myocardial infarction, as well as re-infarction and the type A behaviour pattern. This behaviour pattern is related to the increased reporting of angina pectoris, as well as the earlier recrudescence of angina following coronary artery bypass grafting. The type A behaviour pattern is related to the angiographic severity of disease and to its rate of progression, independent of other risk factors, although this association may only pertain to the type A behaviour pattern as assessed by the structured interview. It does appear possible to modify type A behaviour by counselling and thus reduce the coronary risk.

Personality correlates in angina pectoris

Anxiety, depression, neuroticism and interpersonal problems are frequent precursors of angina pectoris and may have a predictive association with the subsequent development of both angina and coronary death, but not myocardial infarction. In a prospective study, sleep disturbances (waking unrefreshed, long sleep latency) and emotional and physical fatigue appeared to be linked with all presentations of coronary disease.[14]

There appears to be considerable variability in the perception of ischaemic pain; this may be related to personality and possibly to gating mechanisms dependent on beta-endorphin secretion, mediated by higher centres. For example, patients who had totally asymptomatic myocardial ischaemia were found to have a significantly higher threshold to pain perception following electrical skin stimulation, and a greater tolerance of a cold pressor test, when compared with otherwise matched patients who suffered early reproducible angina pectoris. Moreover, the asymptomtic patients had a reduced tendency to complain, with lower scores for nervousness and excitability.[15]

EMOTIONAL STRESS EXACERBATING MYOCARDIAL ISCHAEMIA

The association of mental stress with myocardial ischaemia has been well demonstrated by positron emission tomography, in which perfusion defects occurred in response to mental arithmetic stress tests in 12 of 16 (75%) patients. Chest pain was an associated feature in only four.[16] Radioisotope studies have confirmed these findings and demonstrated that the induction of myocardial ischaemia by mental stress is often of the same magnitude as that induced by exercise.[17] There is now an increasing number of reports linking silent ischaemia, as documented by Holter monitoring, with non-activity pastimes, such as driving and eating, and psychological stress. In a recent study, a period of chronic psychological stress was found to increase significantly the incidence of silent ischaemia in 57% of patients with coronary artery disease when compared with a non-stressful study period. These patients could be identified by higher scores on a psychological distress questionnaire as well as by a higher noradrenaline excretion during stress. Cortisol excretion was higher in all patients during the stressful period of study. Interestingly, the incidence of painful ischaemia was unchanged.[18] A possible mechanism of stress in such situations has been suggested to be one of increased vasomotor tone, mediated via the alpha-adrenergic receptors (noradrenaline transmitters). Certainly, in dogs, behavioural stress produces vasoconstriction by this pathway.[19]

The concept of coronary artery spasm was first presented by Osler in 1910 and described by Prinzmetal in 1959. The pathophysiological mechanisms are not known, although it is clear there are periods of vulnerability and resistance to variable coronary tone. An emotional stress was found to produce ST-segment elevation in 12 men with exertional angina pectoris at heart rates lower than those at which it was provoked on exercise.[20] Spontaneous hyperventilation is a frequent concomitant of emotional stress;[21] it is also a particular laboratory manoeuvre performed to elicit coronary spasm for which it has a sensitivity of 70% and a specificity of 100%. It has been suggested that hyperventilation may represent a trigger mechanism for alteration in coronary tone in daily life, in response to emotional stress.[22]

HYPERVENTILATION SYNDROMES (including Da Costa's syndrome and other functional disorders)

Hyperventilation may be defined as alveolar ventilation in excess of metabolic needs producing fluctuating hypocapnia. In the absence of physiological causes, such as high altitude, and organic causes, such as hyperthyroidism, hyperventilation has been considered to be due to a learnt habit of upper thoracic breathing or to occur in response to an emotional trigger. Typical symptoms affect

many systems, particularly the cardiovascular; chest pain, palpitations and fatigue are among the most common symptoms. Many clinicians find it a difficult syndrome to diagnose, and submit the patient to multiple investigations to screen for organic disease. The inability to take a deep enough breath, frequent sighing, peripheral paraesthesia, especially when associated with the presenting symptom (viz. chest pain), and documentation at some time of hypocapnia ($Pco_2 \leq 30$ mmHg), whether spontaneously or by laboratory provocation, have been suggested as useful hallmarks for diagnosis. Sympathetic hyper-reactivity has been noted; neurotic, dependent and anxious personalities are frequently described with this syndrome, although such an association is not universal and may reflect screening in populations with different principal somatic complaints (e.g. psychiatric or cardiological).

The hyperventilation syndrome was first described in 1871 (Da Costa's syndrome) when chest pain, fatigue and palpitations were the commonest features. It has subsequently been ascribed other terms such as soldier's heart, effort syndrome and neurocirculatory asthenia. There is probably an equal sex distribution, although males are more likely to be screened for organic disease first. A dominant feature of the syndrome is chest pain, which is characteristically described as sharp and stabbing and may be due to intercostal muscle fatigue. It mimics typical angina pectoris; in an uncontrolled study of patients undergoing diagnostic catheterization, such pain was found in 67% of patients who had normal coronary arteriograms. As it may also produce ST-segment depression, it may be implicated in patients who have so-called syndrome X (angina-like chest pain, ST-segment depression with exercise and normal coronary arteriograms ± abnormal myocardial lactate metabolism).

It is also found in as many as 57% of patients with angiographically demonstrated severe coronary artery disease; typical chest pain may frequently be reproduced in these patients, by an overbreathing provocation test. Associated hyperventilation in patients with coronary artery disease is thus a confounding factor in the assessment of the severity of angina pectoris; although ambulatory monitoring has revealed that episodes of both painful and painless ischaemia may be the same in hyperventilators and non-hyperventilators, the former complain of significantly more episodes of chest pain, in the absence of ST-segment shift, than the latter. Thus, on the basis of increased reports of chest pain, although not of documented myocardial ischaemia, hyperventilators are erroneously regarded as having more severe disease. Hyperventilation has also been reported to decrease coronary blood flow in susceptible individuals by a combination of a left shift of the Bohr oxygen dissociation curve, thus rendering oxygen less available to the myocardium, and coronary vasoconstriction, probably mediated by the effect of the alkalosis on the ionized calcium levels.[23,24]

Palpitations in the hyperventilation syndrome are common and most often benign. There have been, however, documented cases in which hyperventilation has produced supraventricular arrhythmias (fibrillation, flutter, supraventricular tachycardia, Wolff–Parkinson–White syndrome) as well as ventricular (ectopy, ventricular tachycardia) arrhythmias.[25] Mitral valve prolapse has been reported in association with both hyperventilation and the hyperkinetic syndrome (a state of high beta-adrenergic drive associated with tachycardia), as well as in stressed, anxious and neurotic individuals. The syndrome is also linked with an increased incidence of both chest pain, palpitations and arrhythmias.[26] The recognition of hyperventilation is important in patients in whom it is the sole cause of functional symptoms and in those with concomitant organic heart disease, because it causes considerable morbidity and confusion and yet is amenable to behavioural training.

THE ROLE OF THE MIND IN HYPERTENSION

Although 'structural autoregulation' in the peripheral vasculature and re-setting of the baroreceptor reflexes may operate to maintain blood pressure, there is increasing evidence to support the role of psychosocial factors in the initiation of hypertension. The suggestion that hurry, worry and anger are important precursors for the development of hypertension was proposed by Brunton as long ago as 1909;[27] over-reaction to "stress or prolonged emotional strain" was listed by Wood in the 1950s as

"the first and foremost of the causes of repetitive or sustained physiological hypertension that could lead to essential hypertension."[28]

The investigation of the role of psychological stress on blood pressure has been confined within epidemiological studies or laboratory reactions to acute stress.[29]

EPIDEMIOLOGICAL

Many attempts have been made to compare the levels of blood pressure between different societies and different cultures. Such attempts are fraught with difficulties due to the varying incidence of hypertension among different populations, and large numbers of confounding factors, all of which contribute to a differing extent. Many workers consider it is only such factors as the diet or the amount of exercise taken, rather than the society in which individuals live, that make important contributions to differences in blood pressure. Nevertheless, it does appear that at least a proportion of the variance may be attributable to cultural ambience; groups with lower blood pressure lead less 'stressful' lives, perhaps the result of maintaining more stable traditional social systems. The results of studies on migration also lend support to the idea that the environment is important, particularly as the behavioural and emotional upheavals involved in migration have been predicted to be of great importance in the development of essential hypertension. Polynesian migrants who moved to New Zealand were found to have significantly higher blood pressures, and this difference persisted after controlling for bodyweight, age and length of stay in New Zealand.[30]

Unlike coronary artery disease, the identification of hypertension is not preceded by a high incidence of stressful life-events, such as divorce and house moves, but by a greater association with prolonged and chronic environmental stress and hypertension. For example, air traffic controllers, who are engaged in a taxing operation that requires constant alertness and carries heavy responsibilities, were shown to have a prevalence of hypertension four times that of second-class airmen, and were more likely to develop hypertension at an earlier age. Two further psychosocial factors, job responsibility and educational achievement, have emerged as significant in the genesis of high arterial pressure; in particular, the discrepancy between these two factors is important, for example, individuals who had achieved a high social and occupational position but had little formal education had a higher blood pressure than individuals in whom the discrepancy was much less.

Vulnerability to hypertension

The results of large studies in which subjects were screened for hypertension have failed to demonstrate a distinctive personality prone to the condition; no consistent association has been found with the type A behaviour pattern. It is frequently noted, however, that hypertensive individuals manifest a desire to please, a wish to be liked but, while outwardly calm, the internal stance is that of supressed anger, tension, suspicion and hostility.[31] The hypertensive patient is thought to struggle with an accumulation of anger and resentment he or she is unable to resolve, and the effect may be mediated via the autonomic system, possibly in association with high renin levels. For men, but not women, conflict over expressing anger has been shown to have at least as strong an effect on blood pressure as other widely acknowledged risk factors for hypertension.

EXPERIMENTAL STUDIES OF PSYCHOLOGICAL STRESS IN HYPERTENSION

Early experimental work by Brod[32] demonstrated how acute emotional stimuli could produce transient elevations of blood pressure in humans, and sustained hypertension often appeared to develop in later life in persons exhibiting such transient hypertension. Normotensive individuals with a family history of hypertension (who are considered to be at high risk) have been found to have exaggerated and prolonged haemodynamic responses to emotional stimuli; more recently such reactive high-risk normal subjects were shown to have sodium and fluid retention following behavioural stress.[33]

Subsequent testing has found that hypertensive subjects, and particularly those who are borderline hypertensives, display a greater haemodynamic reaction to experimental stress than normotensive subjects.[34] Such subjects may also have a heightened emotional lability. The newer techniques of blood pressure monitoring during daily life have demonstrated that the ambulatory readings taken at home and at work correlate more highly with the reactivity of the cognitive stress tasks than with the casual measures of blood pressure obtained in the physician's clinic.[35]

Three mechanisms have been suggested to mediate the effect of behavioural stress in the development of hypertension.

1 A heightened reactivity and overactivity of the autonomic nervous system to stressful tasks or situations, as evidenced by increased 'traffic' in the cardiac sympathetic fibres. As a result, a haemodynamic pattern occurs in which cardiac output is elevated, while peripheral resistance is still in the normal range (abnormally since the raised output 'ought' to be compensated by low vascular resistance).

2 Elevated catecholamine and renin levels in response to psychological stress tests, found in hypertensive patients and frequently in their (as yet) normotensive offspring, but not in normotensive control subjects.

3 An altered renal regulation of sodium with increased retention in response to behavioural stress.

TREATMENT

As psychological stress, autonomic arousal and conditioned learning have been suggested as causes of the elevation of blood pressure particularly in the early stages, various types of behavioural therapy have been applied to hypertensive patients. Nowhere, perhaps, is the effect of the mind on the cardiovascular system so powerfully seen as in the treatment of hypertension, where the placebo effect and the therapeutic expectation of the patient can provoke dramatic short-term responses. The efficacy of treatment is therefore difficult to assess. There have been some controlled investigations of psychological techniques demonstrating long-term reductions in blood pressure, but caution is warranted because many workers have shown that the reduction in blood pressure may not persist beyond 6 months following the cessation of active involvement in relaxation training.

Patel and North have shown the benefit of progressive muscle relaxation, with biofeedback and meditation, in reducing both diastolic and systolic blood pressures;[36] the effect was found to persist at 6 months. Concomitant falls in noradrenaline, renin and dopamine beta-hydroxylase (adrenal medullary enzyme) have also been found.[37] Furthermore, the results of ambulatory monitoring have shown that the reductions in blood pressure are maintained throughout the working day.[38] In a relatively symptomless disorder in which non-compliance and complaints concerning drug side-effects are frequent, non-drug treatment of hypertension is increasingly viewed as important. It may be used as a first step in therapy and also as an adjunct to medication; if non-drug therapy is effective, medication may in consequence be reduced.

THE ROLE OF THE MIND IN ARRHYTHMIAS

Palpitation and tachycardia are among the most

widely recognized effects of emotional stress. Heart rates sometimes exceeding 140 beats/min (often associated with ST-segment depression) and multiple ventricular ectopic beats have been documented in normal subjects whilst driving in heavy London traffic or speaking at medical meetings. In view of the increasing awareness that abnormalities in autonomic neural activity may have a key role in the genesis of certain types of cardiac arrhythmias, it has been postulated that psychological stimuli or extreme stress may induce or lower the 'threshold' for the development of more serious cardiac rhythm disturbances.[39]

SUPRAVENTRICULAR ARRHYTHMIAS

There is some evidence linking supraventricular arrhythmias with psychological stress; atrial fibrillation, supraventricular tachycardia and nodal tachycardia are some of the rhythm disturbances that have been documented in response to laboratory stressors. Some of these have been found to be associated with hyperventilation.[40]

VENTRICULAR ARRHYTHMIAS

In a number of uncontrolled studies and clinical case-reports, an association between ventricular arrhythmias and emotions, resulting from traumatic events or their recall, anxiety, fear, excitement or deliberate induction of stressful states, has been noted. The careful work of Lown and his group has elucidated a definite association between an increase in ventricular premature contractions (mean increase 4 per min) and psychological stress. As it was not possible to produce ectopy in these patients merely by manipulating the peripheral nervous system (e.g. by Valsalva manoeuvre), the important additional component was considered to be enhanced central (cerebrocortical) activity influencing the peripheral sympathetic system.[41] A sustained reduction in ventricular premature contractions, as documented by Holter monitoring, can be produced in some patients by biofeedback and muscular relaxation techniques.[42] Personality inventories, conducted in patients without previous myocardial infarctions and with frequent (> 30 beats/min) ventricular ectopic beats, have demonstrated a significant association between the presence of the arrhythmias and scores of anxiety, depression, social alienation and difficult lifestyles.[43] Depression, in particular, appears to be an independent risk factor for ventricular arrhythmias in patients who

do not have ischaemic heart disease. In patients with ischaemic heart disease, ventricular premature beats have been shown to increase in frequency under stress such as car driving or watching a football game.

A lowered threshold for the development of more serious ventricular arrhythmias, such as ventricular tachycardia and ventricular fibrillation, in response to psychological stress has been clearly shown in animal models.[44] Ambulatory (Holter) studies in man have revealed an association between intense psychological triggers (such as anger, anxiety and bereavement) and the occurrence of ventricular arrhythmia; of 117 patients undergoing prospective investigation of their arrhythmia, 21% suffered ventricular fibrillation or ventricular tachycardia in response to a psychological trigger.[45] It also seems possible that ventricular tachycardia and ventricular fibrillation have different relationships to states of psychological arousal: the precipitation of ventricular tachycardia is associated with surges of anger or fear, whereas ventricular fibrillation occurs after more prolonged emotional states.[46]

LIFE-THREATENING ARRHYTHMIAS ON THE CORONARY CARE UNIT

The patient on the coronary care unit appears to be very vulnerable to psychological stress. For example, episodes of ventricular fibrillation have been noted during ward rounds or with a dramatic arrival in the coronary care unit. Increases in the degree of atrioventricular block have also been found to occur in patients following such simple actions as taking the temperature or pulse. Patients who observe a cardiac arrest in the next bed have also been found to be more acutely prone to ventricular fibrillation as well as to premature beats.

THE ROLE OF THE MIND IN SUDDEN CARDIAC DEATH

Although the process underlying sudden death is most likely (but not ubiquitously) to be due to atherosclerosis, the trigger for the terminal event has not yet been defined; infarction may be found in as few as 17% of cases. A common view implicates psychological stress. Engel describes a series of cases of sudden death which he had gleaned from newspaper reports; he found that in most of them intense displeasure was involved, although in a few intense pleasure had occurred, and all the events had been impossible for the victim to ignore; each victim had responded with overwhelming excitation, or by giving up, or both.

In a few studies, an attempt has been made to determine systematically the prevalence of psychological/psychosocial disturbances associated with sudden death. Despite differences in the methods used and the populations studied, a particular vulnerability to acute psychological factors precipitating sudden cardiac death appeared to be present in at least one-quarter of the patients examined.[47] There are obvious methodological difficulties in the reconstruction of the subjective emotional experiences preceding an unpredictable and usually fatal event. However, in 100 consecutive cases of sudden death, 28 of the victims were found to have experienced moderate or acute emotional stress during the 30 min preceding death; in a further 40 patients, 'substantial' degrees of stress were documented in the 24 h before death. Information came from relatives and others interviewed within 5–10 days of the event.[48]

Although the incidence of sudden death in women is less than that in men ($< 1 : 2$), it has been found that female victims of sudden cardiac death were more often divorced or had a history of bereavement (but not other types of life-change).[49] The factors predicting sudden death in all patients recovering from a myocardial infarction (2 months or more in the past) were found to be depression, extremes of the type A behaviour pattern, and a Sisyphus reaction (exhibited by someone who strives against the odds but with little sense of accomplishment or satisfaction).

The parasympathetic or vagal response to emotional stimuli, producing a decreased heart rate, a fall in arterial pressure and syncope in some individuals, is a familiar syndrome, but there have been a few cases-reports of life-threatening 'vagal reactions' leading to bradycardia and circulatory collapse. Voodoo death may be associated with marked bradyarrhythmias, and Engel has defined the condition in which 'giving up' in the face of emotional arousal and psychological uncertainty predisposes to vasodepressor syncope and sudden death.[50] Persistent bradycardias in middle-aged men have been found to be a risk factor for sudden death.

THE ROLE OF THE MIND IN HEART FAILURE

Myocardial degeneration (both endocardial scar-

ring and cell death) has been reported to occur as a function of frightening sensory stimuli and prolonged psychological stress in laboratory animals with normal coronary arteries. Similar, if not identical, myocardial lesions have been observed in human victims of sudden cardiac death considered to be due to stress, at the Kennedy Space Center.[51] Excessive catecholamine release, in response to the psychological stress, has been suggested as the mediating mechanism, and the term catecholamine/coagulative myocytolysis has been used.

It is considered possible that in some patients the development of dilative cardiomyopathies in the absence of coronary heart disease is linked with psychological/environmental stress and catecholamine cardiotoxicity. As yet, there are no firm prospective data from the Framingham study of a link between psychosocial factors and congestive heart failure. There are, however, many retrospective studies in which it is claimed that emotionally deleterious events precipitate or aggravate congestive failure in up to 49% of patients admitted to hospital.[52] The lack of prospective studies make it very difficult to comment definitively on the possibility of a causal relation between psychological stress and heart failure.

CONCLUSIONS

Although the subject of emotion and the heart remains controversial, with confusing terminology and imperfect methodology, the ability of the human mind to control physiological functions is acknowledged and some justification for its role in the development and exacerbation of cardiovascular disease is perceived. Good clinical evaluation, including the psychosocial history, will enable the thoughtful physician to decide which patients may be more vulnerable. Thereafter, personality traits, areas of psychological stress and individual perception of events can be explored. Methods for dealing with these psychological elements must be incorporated into the management of patients in conjunction with medical and surgical therapy.

REFERENCES

1. Mason, J.W. A review of psychoendocrine research on the pituitary adrenal cortical system and on the sympathetic–adrenal medullary system. *Psychosom. Med.* 1968; 30: 576–607; 631–53.
2. Henry, J.P. and Stephens, P.M. *Stress, health and the social*

environment. A sociobiologic approach to medicine. New York: Springer Verlag, 1977.

3. Steptoe, A. Neural and endocrine factors in cardiovascular control. In: Steptoe, A., ed. *Psychological factors in cardiovascular disorders.* London: Academic Press, 1981; 44–5.

4. Henry, J.P. Mechanisms by which stress can lead to coronary heart disease. *Postgrad. Med. J.* 1986; **62**: 687–93.

5. Karasek R.A., Russell, R.S. and Theorell, T. Physiology of stress and regeneration in job related cardiovascular illness. *J. Human Stress* 1982; **8**: 29–42.

6. Marmot, M.G. Does stress cause heart attacks? *Postgrad. Med. J.* 1986; **62**: 683–6.

7. Mayou, R., MacMahon, D., Sleight, P. and Florencio, M.J. Early rehabilitation after myocardial infarction. *Lancet* 1981; **ii**: 1399–401.

8. Ruberman, W., Weinblatt, E., Goldberg, J.D. and Chaudhary, B.S. Psychosocial influences on mortality after myocardial infarction. *N. Engl. J. Med.* 1984; **311**: 552–9.

9. Frasure-Smith, N. and Prince, R. The ischaemic heart disease life stress monitoring program: Impact on mortality. *Psychosom. Med.* 1985; **47**: 431–45.

10. Rosenman, R.H., Brand, R.J., Jenkins, C.D. Friedman, M. Straus, R. and Wurm, M. Coronary heart disease in the Western Collaborative group study; final follow up of 8½ years. *JAMA.* 1975; **233**: 872–7.

11. Rosenman, R.H. Current status of risk factors and type A behaviour pattern in the pathogenesis of ischaemic heart disease. In: Dembroski, T.M., Schmidt, T.H. and Blumchen, G., eds. *Biobehavioural bases of coronary heart disease.* Basel: Karger, 1983; pp. 5–12.

12. Cooper, T., Detre, T. and Weiss, S. Coronary prone behaviour and coronary disease; a critical review. *Circulation* 1981; **63**: 1199–215.

13. Freeman, L.J. and Nixon, P.G.F. The effect of Type A behaviour pattern on myocardial ischaemia during daily life. *Int. J. Cardiol.* 1987; **17**: 145–54.

14. Jenkins, C.D. Recent evidence supporting psychologic and social risk factors for coronary disease. *N. Engl. J. Med.* 1976; **294**: 987–94; 1033–8.

15. Droste, C. and Roskamm, H. Pain measurements and pain modification by naloxone in patients with asymptomatic myocardial ischemia. *J. Am. Coll. Cardiol.* 1983; **1**: 940–5.

16. Deanfield, J.E., Shea, M., Kensett, M. *et al.* Silent myocardial ischaemia due to mental stress. *Lancet* 1984; **ii**: 1001–4.

17. Rozanski, A., Bairey, N., Krantz, D. *et al.* Mental stress and the induction of silent myocardial ischemia in patients with coronary artery disease. *N. Engl. J. Med.* 1988; **316**: 1088–12.

18. Freeman, L.J., Nixon, P.G.F., Sallabank, P. and Reavely, D. Psychological stress and silent ischemia. *Am. Heart J.* 1987; **114**: 477–82.

19. Billman, G.E. and Randell, D.C. Mechanisms mediating the coronary vascular response to behavioural stress in dogs. *Circulation* 1981; **48**: 214–23.

20. Schiffer, F., Hartley, H., Schulman, C.L. and Abelmann, W.H. Evidence for emotionally induced coronary arterial spasm in patients with angina pectoris. *Br. Heart J.* 1980; **44**: 62–66.

21. Freeman, L.J., Conway, A.V. and Nixon, P.G.F. Physiological responses to psychological challenge in patients considered to have the hyperventilation syndrome—implications for diagnosis and therapy. *J. R. Soc. Med.* 1986; **79**: 76–83.

22. Mortensen, S.A., Nielsen, H. and Grossman, P. Hyperventilation as diagnostic stress test for variant angina and cardiomyopathy: cardiovascular response, likely triggering mechanisms and psychophysiological implications. In: Grossman, P., Janssen, K.H.L. and Vaitl, D., eds. *Cardiorespiratory and cardiosomatic psychophysiology.* London: Plenum Press, 1986, pp. 303–17.

23. Neill, W. and Hattenhauer, M. Impairment of myocardial oxygen supply due to hyperventilation. *Circulation* 1975; **52**: 854–8.

24. Freeman, L.J. and Nixon, P.G.F. Does hyperventilation have any cardiac effect in patients with chest pain. *Br. Heart J.* 1988; **59**: 102.

25. Hisano, K., Matsuguchi, T. and Dotsubo, H. Hyperventilation-induced variant angina with ventricular tachycardia. *Am. Heart J.* 1984; **104**: 423–25

26. Anonymous. Association between arrhythmias and mitral valve prolapse (Editorial). *Arch Int. Med.* 1984; **144**: 2333–4.

27. Brunton, T.L. *Br. Med. J.* 1909; **2**: 64–71.

28. Wood, P. *Diseases of the Heart and Circulation.* London: Eyre and Spottiswoode, 1956.

29. Julius, S. and Cottier, C. Behaviour and hypertension. In: Dembroski, T.M., Schmidt, T.H. and Blumchen, G., eds. *Biobehavioural bases of coronary heart disease.* Basel: Karger, 1983, pp 271–89.

30. Prior, I., Stanhope, J., Evans, J. and Salmon, C. The Tokelau Island Migrant study. *Int. J. Epidemiol.* 1974; **3**: 225–32.

31. Cottingham, E.M., Matthews, K.A., Talbott, E. and Kuller, L.H. Occupational stress, supressed anger and hypertension. *Psychosom. Med.* 1968; **48**: 249–60.

32. Brod, J. Haemodynamic bases of acute pressor reactions and hypertension. *Br. Heart J.* 1963; **25**: 227–31.

33. Light, K.C., Koepke, J.P., Obrist, P.A. and Willis, P.W. Psychological stress induces sodium and fluid retention in men at high risk for hypertension. *Science* 1983; **220**: 429.

34. Cinciripini, P.M. Cognitive stress and cardiovascular reactivity. 1. Relationship to hypertension. *Am. Heart J.* 1986; **112**: 1044–50.

35. Perloff, D., Sokolow, M. and Cowan, R. The prognostic value of ambulatory blood pressures. *JAMA* 1983; **249**: 2792–8.

36. Patel, C. and North, W.R.S. Randomised controlled trial of Yoga and biofeedback in management of hypertension. *Lancet* 1975; **ii**: 93–9.

37. Stone, R. and Deleo, J. Psychotherapeutic control of hypertension. *N. Engl. J. Med.* 1976; **294**: 80–4.

38. Southam, M.A., Agras, W., Taylor, C.B. and Kraemer, H.C. Relaxation training, blood pressure lowering during the working day. *Arch. Gen. Psychiatr.* 1982; **39**: 715.

39. Lown, B., Verrier, R.L. and Corbalan, R., Psychologic stress and theshold for repetitive ventricular response. *Science* 1973; **182**: 834–6.

40. Freeman, L.J., Conway, A.V. and Nixon, P.G.F. Heart rate response, emotional disturbance and hyperventilation. *J. Psychosom. Res.* 1986; **30**: 429–36.

41. Lown, B., deSilva, R.A. and Lenson, R. Roles of psychologic stress and autonomic nervous system changes in provocation of ventricular premature complexes. *Am. J. Cardiol.* 1978; **41**: 979–85.

42. Davidson, D.M., Winchester, M.A., Taylor, C.B., Alderman, E.A. and Ingels, N.B. Effects of relaxation therapy on cardiac performance and sympathetic activity in patients with organic heart disease. *Psychosom. Med.* 1979; **41**: 303–9.

43. Katz, C., Martin, R.D., Landa, B. and Chadda, K.D. Relationship of psychologic factors to frequent symptomatic ventricular arrhythima. *Am. J. Med.* 1985; **78**: 589–94.

44. Lown, B., Verrier, R.L. and Rabinowitz, S.H. Neural and psychologic mechanisms and the problems of sudden cardiac death. *Am. J. Cardiol.* 1977; **39**: 890–902.

45. DeSilva, R.A. and Lown, B. Ventricular premature beats, stress and sudden death. *Psychosomatics* 1978; **19**: 649–53; 656–61.

46. Reich, P. Psychological predisposition to life threatening arrhythmias. *Annu. Rev. Med.* 1985; **36**: 397–405.

47. Rissanen, V., Romo, M. and Siltanen, P. Premonitory

symptoms and stress factors preceding sudden death from ischaemic heart disease. *Acta Med. Scand.* 1978; **204**: 389–96.

48. Myers, A. and Dewar, H.A. Circumstances attending 100 sudden deaths from coronary artery disease with coroner's necropsies. *Br. Heart J.* 1975; **37**: 1133–43.

49. Talbot, E., Kuller, L.H., Perper, J. and Murphy, P.A. Sudden unexpected death in women. Biologic and psychosocial origin. *Am. J. Epidemiol.* 1981; **114**: 671–82.

50. Engel, G.L. Psychologic stress, vasodepressor (vasovagal) syncope and sudden death. *Ann. Intern. Med.* 1978; **89**: 403–12.

51. Eliot, R.S. and Buell, J.C. Role of the central nervous system in sudden cardiac death. In: Dembroski, T.M., Schmidt, T.H. and Blumchen, G., eds. *Biobehavioural bases of coronary heart disease.* Basel: Karger, 1983.

52. Tapp, W.N., Levin, B.E. and Natelson, B.H. Stress induced heart failure. *Psychosom. Med.* 1983; **45**: 171–6.

Chapter 71

Miscellaneous Disorders and Agents Affecting the Heart

David P. Lipkin

PAGET'S DISEASE OF THE BONE

Paget's disease of the bone typically affects the elderly, occurring in 3% of the population.[1,2] The disease is associated with a high-output cardiac state. Increased blood flow occurs through extremities involved in Paget's disease and may be as high as 9 times the normal level.[3,4] It has been assumed that the high flow occurs through the involved bone, but in recent studies in which radioactive technetium-labelled microspheres were injected into the femoral arteries of patients with Paget's disease there was no evidence of arteriovenous shunting.[5] It would appear that the additional blood flow occurs through cutaneous tissue overlying the involved bone possibly secondary to local heat production resulting from the increased metabolic activity of affected bone.[4]

Clinically, a high-output state may be recognized when > 30% of the skeleton is involved. However, echocardiographic abnormalities, including increased left ventricular cavity size and increased left ventricular mass, may be detected when only 15% of the skeleton is involved.[6] Other cardiovascular manifestations of Paget's disease include increased arterial calcification, calcification of the interventricular septum with cardiac conduction abnormalities,[7–9] and calcification of the aortic valve. In a large recent retrospective study, it was shown that Paget's disease is associated with a four-fold increase in the incidence of calcific aortic valve disease, the severity of which is proportional to the extent of the Paget's disease.[10]

Although it is generally unsatisfactory, the treatment of Paget's disease has been documented to be associated with a reduction in cardiac output.

ARTERIOVENOUS FISTULAS

CONGENTIAL ARTERIOVENOUS FISTULAS

Congenital arteriovenous fistulas may be sufficiently large to cause a high-output cardiac state. They frequently involve the vessels of the pelvis and lower extremities. The patient may present with disfigurement, swelling, pain, pulsation, ulceration of the skin, or increased length of the limb. A continuous murmur is heard overlying the fistula. Left heart failure occurs particularly in patients who have larger lesions that involve the pelvis as well as the extremities.[11,12] Fistulous connection may involve any vascular bed, including the internal mammary artery–pulmonary artery connection. Angiography is useful in confirming the diagnosis and in determining the physical extent of the anomaly.

The disease may be diffuse which prevents surgical excision. Embolization of the fistula may replace surgical therapy in many instances.

Hereditary haemorrhagic telangiectasia (Osler–Weber–Rendu disease)

This condition is associated with arteriovenous fistulas, particulary of the lungs and liver. Rarely, arteriovenous fistulas of the liver can be associated with hepatomegaly and abdominal bruits.

Hepatic haemangiomatosis

This is a rare condition which is commonly associated with a high-output state. Hepatic haemangiomas are often associated with cutaneous haemangiomas.

ACQUIRED ARTERIOVENOUS FISTULAS

Acquired arteriovenous fistulas are usually traumatic following gunshot or stab wounds, most frequently to the thigh. Rarely, they may be produced inadvertently during surgery or following cannulation of the femoral artery and femoral vein during cardiac catheterization.

A rare form of acquired arteriovenous fistula results from spontaneous rupture of an aortic aneurysm into the inferior vena cava. Large fistulas may be associated with Wilms' tumour of the kidney and on rare occasions have caused high-output cardiac failure in children.[13] The most frequent form of arteriovenous fistula is produced surgically for haemodialysis patients. In the presence of underlying heart disease and anaemia, these fistulas may cause a sufficiently high-output state to compromise cardiac function and result in heart failure.

GLYCOGEN STORAGE DISEASES

Glycogen storage diseases are the result of a deficiency of one or more of the enzymes involved in the biosynthesis and degradation of glycogen.[14] Cardiac involvement occurs in 3 out of the 8 types of the disease: types II, III and IV. The most common is type II (Pompe's disease) which results from a deficiency of acid maltase, a lysosomal enzyme that hydrolyses glycogen into glucose. Type III disease (Forbe's or Cori's disease) is a result of a deficiency in the debranching enzyme amylo-1,6-glucosidase; type IV (Andersen's disease) is caused by a deficiency in the branching enzyme alpha-1,4-glucan-6-glucosyltransferase.

Pompe's disease is an autosome recessive disorder. Generalized glycogenosis takes place, but occurs especially in the heart, skeletal muscle and liver. The glycogen within cardiac muscle cells is present in excessive amounts. Consequently, the heart enlarges and heart failure may supervene.[15]

PATHOLOGY

The ventricles are massive with thick walls and chambers of normal size. The atria are normal, but the myocardial fibres throughout the heart are enlarged with diffuse and extensive vacuolation, producing a lacework pattern.[16]

CLINICAL FEATURES

Heart failure usually occurs between 2 and 6 months and always before 18 months. Generalized muscle weakness, hypotonia, macroglossia, hyporeflexia, and other neurological deficits are also present.

Sudden death is common in the first year of life, presumably due to an arrhythmia. Death in infancy or early childhood usually occurs due to heart failure or a chest infection. The electrocardiogram shows severe. left ventricular hypertrophy with a short PR interval; pre-excitation and right ventricular hypertrophy may occur. The chest X-ray demonstrates massive generalized cardiac enlargement and pulmonary congestion. The echocardiogram demonstrates grossly thickened ventricular septum and ventricular walls. Systolic anterior motion of the mitral valve has been described, which may result in an outflow tract gradient. Rarely, obstruction to the right ventricular outflow tract may occur.

DIFFERENTIAL DIAGNOSIS

The condition can be differentiated from other causes of severe heart failure, particularly endocardial fibre-elastosis, anomalous left coronary artery and acute myocarditis. Cardiac abnormalities may be confused with those seen in hypertrophic obstructive cardiomyopathy.

DIAGNOSIS

Diagnosis is confirmed by demonstrating the enzymatic deficiency in lymphocytes or in biopsy material from skeletal or cardiac muscle or liver.

TREATMENT

No specific therapy exists. Treatment of heart failure and arrhythmias is required should they develop.

TOXIC, CHEMICAL AND DRUG EFFECTS

SOLVENT ABUSE

Deliberate inhalation of volatile substances, usually halogenated or unsubstituted hydrocarbons, to obtain a 'high' is common among teenage boys and causes important morbidity and mortality; there were 80 deaths from solvent abuse in Britain in

1983.[17] Solvent abuse may cause both acute and chronic cardiotoxicity. Studies of acute toxicity have shown that inhaled volatile hydrocarbons are arrhythmogenic and may induce hypertension.[18] The arrhythmias are more likely to occur during a high catecholamine drive, such as during exercise. Recent anecdotal reports suggest that volatile hydrocarbons such as 1,1,1-trichloroethane (which is found in various glues, typewriter correction fluid, dry-cleaning aids and plastic remover) and toluene (which may be found in glues) can result in a dilated cardiomyopathy. The effects may be potentiated by halothane.[19]

Physicians should consider chronic solvent exposure when treating patients with dilated cardiomyopathy. The anaesthetist should be aware of the potential hazards of using halothane and similar agents in patients who may be solvent abusers.

DOXORUBICIN

Doxorubicin (Adriamycin) is an antineoplastic agent that has broad activity against numerous solid and haematological malignancies. As an anthracycline derivative it possesses significant cardiac toxicity which limits its use.[20] The overall incidence of clinically apparent heart failure in patients treated with doxorubicin is reported to be 7–9%.[21] In one series, however, 21% of asymptomatic patients who had been treated with doxorubicin had an abnormal resting left ventricle ejection fraction.[22] Factors that appear to be associated with a high incidence of cardiomyopathy are a total dose > 550 mg/m^2, prior radiation therapy, pre-existing heart disease, uncontrolled hypertension and treatment with other chemotherapeutic agents.[21,23] The incidence is higher in young children and older adults.[24] Recently, a once-a-week dosing regime (rather than once every 3 weeks) has been shown to reduce the cardiotoxic effects of the drug.[25]

Patients with doxorubicin heart muscle disease usually present with heart failure within days to a few months after the commencement of treatment; rarely, they present a year after therapy has been started.[21] The clinical course varies from acute heart failure and cardiogenic shock to progressive deterioration. A few patients improve and the heart muscle disease regresses with no medical therapy, although the overall mortality rate may be as high as 61%.[21]

Although non-invasive methods have been used to detect early evidence of left ventricular dysfunction, endomyocardial biopsy and histopathological assessment of myocardial damage are thought to be the most reliable methods of measuring myocardial toxicity.[26] However, the validity of the histopathology in determining a safe dose has been challenged.[24] Right-sided heart catheterization with resting and exercise haemodynamics is perhaps the best available method of evaluating dosage safely.[26,27] Electrocardiographic changes have been documented and include non-specific ST–T-wave and QRS changes and, rarely, atrial and ventricular arrhythmias.[21] The appearance of the electrocardiogram has been used as a predictor of cardiac muscle toxicity, but it is unreliable.[23]

DAUNORUBICIN

The overall incidence of heart muscle disease with daunorubicin treatment seems to be slightly less than that with doxorubicin treatment. A total dose < 600 mg/m^2 is associated with an incidence of 1.5%; incidence increases to 12% with a dosage > 1 g/m^2. Children seem to be at a greater risk.[28] Similarly, non-invasive methods of assessing cardiac function may be unreliable for the early detection of cardiac toxicity.[21]

CYCLOPHOSPHAMIDE

High doses of cyclophosphamide have been associated with electrocardiographic changes, congestive heart failure and death from a haemorrhagic myocarditis. A myopericarditis may occur within the first 2 weeks of the initiation of therapy. Impaired systolic function is seen in the majority of patients, which may be reversible, although more than 20% may die.[21]

5-FLUOROURACIL

5-Fluorouracil has rarely been associated with cardiac toxicity, which is manifested by chest pain, arrhythmias and electrocardiographic changes.

PARACETAMOL

Occasionally, an overdose of paracetamol may result in fatty degeneration of the heart and focal myocardial necrosis, although the clinical picture is usually dominated by massive hepatic necrosis.

TRICYCLIC ANTIDEPRESSANTS

The cardiac effects of tricyclic antidepressants in overdose are disturbance in rhythm and abnormalities in atrioventricular conduction. Depression of left ventricular function does not occur.

PHENOTHIAZINES

Phenothiazines in overdose may be associated with atrial and ventricular arrhythmias and sudden death.[29,30] Electrocardiographic changes include the lengthening of the QT interval; T-wave changes may be seen.

LITHIUM

Lithium intoxication may be associated with ventricular arrhythmias, sinus node abnormalities, atrioventricular conduction disturbances and death.[31]

LEAD

Electrocardiographic changes, chest pain, atrioventricular conduction disturbance and overt congestive heart failure may rarely occur in cases of lead poisoning. These changes appear to be reversible.

CARBON MONOXIDE

Cardiac involvement occurs in both acute and chronic carbon monoxide toxicity. Various arrhythmias, including ventricular extra systoles and atrial fibrillation, occur;[32] bradycardia and atrioventricular block may occur. Myocardial ischaemia may be precipitated in patients with coronary artery disease.

PHYSICAL AGENTS

RADIATION

Therapeutic radiation may produce a variety of acute and chronic cardiac complications. It appears that radiation and cancer chemotherapeutic agents may act synergistically in producing myocardial damage.

Although initially the heart was thought to be radioresistant, it is apparent that cardiac effects of radiation therapy are common, and that the pericardium is most commonly involved. Some degree of myocardial fibrosis is frequently seen. Coronary artery disease, conduction system defects and valvular lesions have been described.[33] Heart disease due to radiation therapy usually occurs within 1–2 years of the commencement of therapy, although delayed appearance (after 5 years) of cardiac disease has been more frequently recognized.

The reported incidence of pericardial involvement varies from 2 to 40%.[34–36] In most of the earlier studies, however, an incidence of 6–9% was reported. An asymptomatic pericardial effusion is probably the most common manifestation and frequently occurs in the first year after radiation therapy.[33,34] Cardiac tamponade can occur and may complicate constrictive pericarditis.[33] The treatment includes both non-steroidal anti-inflammatory agents and steroids. Pericardiocentesis and pericardectomy may be indicated.

Some degree of myocardial fibrosis is commonly seen, especially in the right ventricle and the anterior portion of the left ventricle. Significant dysfunction, however, seems to be most common in association with severe pericardial disease. Congestive heart failure may result.

The evidence for the association of radiation and coronary artery disease is circumstantial, but pathological data support an aetiological relationship especially in young patients.[36] The complication may occur some years after radiation therapy and the incidence is unknown. Both small and large vessel disease may occur. Initial damage to capillary endothelium results in rupture and/or thrombosis of those vessels. Unlike a typical atherosclerotic process, there is a greater loss of smooth muscle cells and more frequent adventitial fibrosis.[37] The process is most prominent in the proximal segment of the major coronary arteries.

Valvular regurgitant lesions of no haemodynamic significance have been described in a minority of cases.

HEAT STROKE

Heat stroke results from failure of the thermoregulatory centre following exposure to high temperatures and is manifested by hyperpyrexia and central nervous system dysfunction. Cardiovascular abnormalities are common. Possible aetiological factors include direct thermal injury to the heart, coronary ischaemia due to hypertension secondary to hypovolemia, and metabolic abnormalities resulting from injury to other organs. Pathological changes include dilatation of the right heart chambers. Post-mortem studies have shown haemorrhage into the sub-endocardium and sub-epicardium of the interventricular septum and posterior wall of the left ventricle with necrosis of myocytes and interstitial oedema.

Arrhythmias are unusual, although a sinus tachycardia is usually present. Prolongation of the QT interval, ST-segment and T-wave abnormalities may be seen and may take several months to resolve. Cardiac enzymes may be elevated, reflecting myocardial damage.

HYPOTHERMIA

Hypothermia may occur accidentally and is an important cause of death in cold climates. It is most likely to occur in elderly subjects, alcoholics and patients suffering from hypothyroidism. The effects of hypothermia depend on age and bodyweight.

An early feature of hypothermia is peripheral vasoconstriction with an increase in afterload which results in a rise in blood pressure—an important factor in the genesis of angina pectoris in susceptible individuals. The exposure of normal individuals to hypothermic conditions results in a rise in stroke volume and cardiac output. However, as body temperature drops, cardiac output falls and this is linked to a reduction in systemic blood pressure. Sinus bradycardia and slow atrial fibrillation may develop. Ventricular fibrillation occurs when body temperature falls to 27–30°C.

The electrocardiogram may show a sinus bradycardia with first degree atrioventricular heart block. Muscle tremor is usually aparent. The 'J deflection' point, which occurs at the junction of the QRS complex and the ST segment, is seen in severe hypothermia. It is non-specific and may be seen in other conditions, such as cerebral haemorrhage and trauma.[38,39]

Treatment consists of maintenance of intravascular volume with plasma expanders and intravenous glucose. External warming is contra-indicated because it diverts blood from internal organs to the skin. Patients should be wrapped in a space blanket and if necessary they should be heated internally with warm air, peritoneal dialysis or haemodialysis.

MALNUTRITION

Malnutrition results in a fall in cardiac output which is proportionate to or slightly less than the reduction in total bodyweight. Left ventricular end-diastolic dimensions fall and there is a reduction in cardiac mass.

There is a pronounced sinus bradycardia and decrease in heart size on chest radiography. Systemic blood pressure is reduced and postural hypotension may occur.

The electrocardiogram shows in addition to the bradycardia reduction in the QRS voltages and a tendency to right-axis deviation.

Protein-energy malnutrition covers a spectrum of clinical forms of malnutrition ranging from marasmus to kwashiorkor. Except in famine or war, all forms of malnutrition are commoner in children than in adults. Marasmus is simply semi-starvation. A marasmic child has lost all its subcutaneous fat and much of its muscle.

KWASHIORKOR

The name 'kwashiorkor' derives from Ghana; it was originally introduced by Williams in 1934. In 1968, The Wellcome Trust proposed a classification of protein-energy malnutrition. It is based on two characteristics: the degree of weight deficiency and presence or absence of oedema. Oedema is the only clinical sign essential for the diagnosis of kwashiorkor. It is attributed to protein deficiency alone in the presence of normal intake of calories. Its relationship to protein undernutrition is confirmed by the observation that in most cases the disorder is reversed by the provision of adequate protein in the diet.[40] Kwashiorkor may be precipitated by infection, such as measles, anaemia or electrolyte disturbance.

Clinically, the child may not at first appear to be malnourished. Typically, subcutaneous fat is well preserved, particularly in the buckle pads and the arms and legs. Wasting is most obvious over the trunk. Oedema may be confined to the feet and ankles and is often associated with hypoproteinaemia, although other factors such as variation in tissue pressure, presence of dehydration or the degree of inactivity may also contribute to its presence. Hepatomegaly due to fatty infiltration is a common finding. Other features include dispigmentation and thinning of hair. In African children, the hair may become reddish or straight. The skin is frequently affected with the so-called 'crazy-pavement dermatosis'.[41]

Although manifestations of heart failure are usually absent they may appear rapidly if nutritional deficiency is corrected too enthusiastically or fluid balance is restored too quickly.

Electrocardiographic changes have been reported in most patients with kwashiorkor,[42] but it is not certain that they indicate organic cardiac disease. There may be low-voltage complexes with ST-segment and T- and U-wave abnormalities; T- and

U-wave abnormalities may be reversed by potassium supplementation.[43]

The heart at post-mortem may show hypertrophy and dilatation, and thrombi are frequent.[42] Endocardial fibro-elastosis does not occur.

In severe forms of the disease, the mortality rises to 80%. Death is somtimes sudden due to systemic or pulmonary emboli or conduction abnormalities.[44]

Treatment consists of administration of protein, of which milk is a suitable form. Fluid balance should be corrected slowly, and electrolyte disturbance normalized. Other nutritional deficiences may be present and should be sought and treated.

BERIBERI

Beriberi is due to a deficiency of thiamine. There are four types: acute or wet beriberi, infantile beriberi, chronic or dry beriberi and the Wernicke–Korsakoff syndrome. Thiamine deficiency may be a complication of any disease or treatment that seriously restricts the intake of food. Although beriberi is still encountered in some areas of the Orient, it is recognized in Western countries, particularly in alcoholics who have a poor diet. It may also result from recurrent vomiting as may occur during pregnancy. Dry beriberi is the more common form; it is called 'dry' in contrast to 'wet' because oedema is absent or less obvious—the principal feature being a polyneuropathy. Dry beriberi is the result of a chronic but milder deficiency of thiamine with an intake slightly less than the normal requirement.

'Wet' beriberi usually presents with general malaise and fatigue. Neurological manifestations are uncommon. Many of the cardiovascular manifestations in beriberi probably originate from a fall in peripheral vascular resistance and are similar to those seen in other high cardiac output states. The haemodynamic findings are a high cardiac output and low peripheral vascular resistance.[45] In severe cases, peripheral vascular resistance may fall to 25% of normal and this may be associated with renal vasoconstriction.[46] Peripheral vasodilatation may result from an accumulation of pyruvic acid and lactic acid due to the lack of thiamine which is essential for the production of co-carboxylase, the enzyme required to oxidize pyruvic acid. Myocardial extraction of lactate, pyruvate and oxygen is found to be significantly decreased in thiamine-deficient dogs. In rats, thiamine deficiency results in a decrease in contractility indicated by a diminution in developed isometric tension and in inotropic response to adrenaline.[48]

Physical examination

Physical examination reveals biventricular failure with evidence of peripheral vasodilatation and warm skin, although as heart failure progresses peripheral vasoconstriction occurs. The pulse pressure is wide as is characteristic of a hyperkinetic state.

Electrocardiogram

The electrocardiogram shows non-specific changes with low-voltage QRS complexes and T-wave inversion with prolongation of the QT interval. Sinus tachycardia is usually present.

Chest X-ray

The chest X-ray shows cardiomegaly which may resolve on treatment with thiamine.

Diagnosis

The diagnosis should be considered when heart failure occurs in the presence of dietary deficiency. The diagnosis may be confirmed by measuring red blood cell transketolase. Thiamine pyrophosphate acts as a co-enzyme for transketolase in the pentose phosphate shunt pathway of glucose metabolism. Thiamine deficiency, therefore, leads to a diminished transketolase activity.

Treatment

Beriberi may be a medical emergency. Thiamine is essential and should be given intravenously or intramuscularly in a dose of 25 mg twice a day for 3 days. Dramatic recovery may occur within a few hours with a profuse diuresis which confirms the diagnosis. After 3 days, parenteral treatment, 10 mg 3 times a day, should be given until recovery. Other vitamin and nutritional abnormalities must be corrected and conventional therapy for heart failure is required.

Occasionally, myocardial function does not return to normal. Hypertension and pulmonary oedema may occur, which have been attributed to a sudden increase in peripheral vascular resistance.[48]

OTHER VITAMIN DEFICIENCIES

Deficiencies of other vitamins have not led to specifically definable cardiovascular abnormalities, except for a deficiency in vitamin D accompanied by hypocalcaemia. However, vitamin deficiencies, particularly of the B group, have been diagnosed with increasing frequency in patients with cardiovascular disease. Excessive vitamin D ingestion has resulted in metastatic calcification with gross and microscopic calcific deposits in arterial media, myocardium and cardiac valves.[49] Abnormal vitamin D metabolism may be associated with supravalvular aortic stenosis in children (see Chapter 26).

OBESITY

PHYSIOLOGY

Although the oxygen demands of adipose tissue are relatively low, the increase in body mass leads to a substantial increase in plasma volume and cardiac output, which may approximate to one-half of the total cardiac output at rest.[50]

OBESITY AND HYPERTENSION

Direct intra-arterial pressure measurements indicate that hypertension is not artefactual in obese subjects.[51] However, the use of a small cuff for indirect measurement of blood pressure may result in an overestimation of systolic and diastolic blood pressures. Despite the association of hypertension and obesity, surveys of large numbers of hypertensive patients indicate that the impact of obesity as a risk factor for hypertension is modest.[52] Weight loss is often associated with a significant reduction in blood pressure.[53]

OBESITY AND CORONARY ARTERY DISEASE

Central obesity, as measured by subscapular skinfold thickness, was found to be directly related to the development of coronary heart disease in subjects entered into the Honolulu Heart Program.[54] Interestingly, however, post-mortem studies have shown no effect of obesity on the extent of atherosclerosis.[55] In fact, in extremely obese subjects, virtually no coronary atheroma is found at post-mortem examination.[56]

At present, it appears that the principal link between coronary disease and marked obesity is the extent to which the latter predisposes to hypertension, although further studies are required to clarify the situation.[57]

OBESITY AND CARDIAC MUSCLE DISEASE

In 1933, Smith and Willius described cases of congestive cardiac failure in markedly obese subjects who did not have evidence of hypertension or other cardiovascular disease.[57] Limited observations suggest that the presence of overt congestive heart failure in extremely obese subjects is about 10%.[58] Bodyweight is usually twice the predicted norm, sometimes more, and rapid weight gain may precipitate or exacerbate heart failure. Heart failure is related to increased stroke volume, increased cardiac output and secondary left ventricular hypertrophy, which may be also aggravated by hypertension.[59] Recently, it has been shown that modest weight loss may be associated with a reduction in left ventricular mass and septal and posterial wall thicknesses.[60] Other workers have shown that gross weight loss may be associated with a reduction in left ventricular chamber enlargement and improved systolic function.[61]

The electrocardiogram in obese subjects shows no evidence of ventricular hypertrophy; when left ventricular hypertrophy is present, it usually shows low-voltage complexes with either left- or right-axis deviation.[57]

SLEEP APNOEA AND OBESITY HYPOVENTILATION SYNDROME

A syndrome of hypoventilation, cyanosis and somnolence, with resultant chronic hypoxaemia, hypercapnia, respiratory acidosis and polycythaemia, occurs in about 5% of extremely obese persons.[62] Sleep apnoea results in bouts of hypoxaemia and hypercapnia. Chronic hypoxaemia and hypercapnia stimulate pulmonary vasoconstriction and pulmonary hypertension. Hypoventilation is reversible with weight reduction and the improvement in arterial blood gases is associated with a fall in pulmonary artery pressure.[63]

TREATMENT

Monitored weight reduction is clearly the major target in therapy. Conventional treatment of heart failure may be required.

HAEMATOLOGICAL ABNORMALITIES

ANAEMIA

Abnormal physiology

Cardiac output rises when the haemoglobin level falls below 7 g/dl. Although the pathophysiology of this rise in cardiac output is not understood, it is probably related to a decreased peripheral resistance secondary to a fall in blood viscosity. Patients who are anaemic may develop congestive heart failure but this is rare in the absence of underlying heart disease. Cardiac enlargement and heart failure caused solely by anaemia of chronic blood loss is unlikely unless the heamoglobin level falls below 5 g/dl. Physical examination reveals signs compatible with a high-output state.

Cardiac conditions associated with anaemia

Endocarditis

Anaemia is usual in subacute bacterial endocarditis, especially if the time to diagnosis is delayed. A normochromic normocytic blood film is seen. Features compatible with haemolysis may be seen in acute bacterial endocarditis.

Anaemia associated with prosthetic valves

A chronic low-grade haemolysis may be seen in patients who have prosthetic heart valves, which may be more pronounced if the valve is malfunctioning and regurgitant.

Renal failure

The pathogenesis of anaemia of renal insufficiency is complex. Anaemia may be related to an absolute deficiency of erythropoietin, depression of the marrow due to retention of toxic metabolites, reduced red blood cell survival, occult blood loss and iron deficiency.

Sickle cell disease

Cardiovascular manifestations are due to chronic anaemia, pulmonary arterial thrombosis leading to pulmonary hypertension and myocardial disease caused by thrombosis of small intracardiac blood vessels.[64] Biventricular dilatation and hypertrophy, arteritis with proliferation and thrombosis, and myocardial degeneration, necrosis and fibrosis are seen.

Presentation Congestive heart failure is a late manifestation. Outflow tract and mitral murmurs may be heard. There are no specific electrocardiographic features. Echocardiography in children may show significantly depressed left ventricular performance and hypertrophy.

HAEMOCHROMATOSIS

Physiology and clinical manifestations

Haemochromatosis may be primary or secondary. The primary disorder is more common in males and usually detected in adult life. The disorder is characterized by excessive tissue iron deposition. Iron deposition in the skin is associated with an increase in melanin deposits, resulting in a bronzed pigmentation. Pancreatic involvement results in diabetes mellitus; hepatic involvement results in cirrhosis; involvement of the heart results in myocardial dysfunction. The dominant cardiac abnormalities are heart failure and arrhythmias. Arrhythmias, particularly paroxysmal atrial tachycardia and atrial fibrillation, atrioventricular block and progressive biventricular dilatation may occur. Occasionally, the haemodynamic pattern at cardiac catheterization resembles a restrictive cardiomyopathy.

The electrocardiogram shows diminished QRS voltages, conduction disturbances and non-specific repolarization changes. The chest X-ray shows a large globular heart. Echocardiography in the early stages shows a non-dilated concentrically thickened left ventricle with diminished compliance; late in the illness, the picture is indistinguishable from that of dilated cardiomyopathy.

Diagnosis

Diagnosis is made by finding the excessive iron deposits in marrow aspirates or liver biopsy specimens. The levels of serum iron and serum ferritin are markedly raised. Patients with HLA-A3-B14 appear to have an inherited tendency to increased iron absorption.

Treatment

Treatment involves removal of iron by repeat venesection. The role of chelation remains controversial. A permanent pacemaker may be required to control syncope due to heart block. Death in untreated patients usually occurs within 1–2 years of the onset of cardiac symptoms. Several reports describe patients who have had regression of symptoms, haemodynamic abnormalities and cardiac enlargement with repeated venesection.

Secondary haemochromatosis is seen in patients who have refractory anaemia requiring multiple transfusions. Extensive cardiac siderosis occurs in patients who receive > 100 units of blood. Recently, intensive chelation therapy with desferrioxamine has been shown to reverse left ventricular dysfunction in symptomatic patients with thalassaemia major.[65,66]

POLYCYTHAEMIA

Polycythaemia is characterized by an increase in red cell mass. The most common form of polycythaemia seen in cardiological practice is related to hypoxia, chronic lung disease, or cyanotic congenital heart disease.

Clinical symptoms are related to increased red cell mass and increased blood volume; they include headache, plethora, pruritus, dyspnoea, bleeding, paraesthesia and thrombosis. Angina pectoris and intermittent claudication may occur. Thrombosis has been thought to be related to increased blood viscosity and may occur in coronary and cerebral arteries and less frequently in mesenteric and portal veins.

In cyanotic congenital heart disease, red cell mass increases as resting arterial oxygen saturation falls. Levels of haematocrit as high as 86% may be seen with a red blood cell mass almost 3 times that of normal.[67] Signs and symptoms of hyperviscosity will generally occur when the haematocrit increases above 60%.

Treatment consists of phlebotomy with a plasma expander to alleviate symptoms and prevent thrombotic episodes. Successful surgical correction of the cardiac defect will normalize arterial oxygen saturation and result in a fall in plasma haematocrit levels.

HEPATIC DISEASES

Resting cardiac output may be increased in patients who have liver disease, especially those with nutritional cirrhosis or infectious hepatitis. Rarely, congestive heart failure may develop, but most patients in this group probably die of hepatic failure before heart failure can supervene. Resting cardiac output in patients with infectious hepatitis may be twice that of normal.[68] An echocardiographic study of patients with hepatic cirrhosis demonstrated an increase in cardiac index, left ventricular end-diastolic dimensions and increased left ventricular fractional shortening.[69]

Congestion of the liver in right heart failure causes distension of the liver capsule, which may produce pain and tenderness in the right upper quadrant and occasionally pain on effort which may be confused with angina.

Hepatic disease may be associated with abnormal cardiac funcion as described previously (see section on Anaemia). Alcohol abuse may result in an acute hepatitis or cirrhosis; this may be associated with heart muscle disease and arrhythmias, in particular atrial fibrillation. Haemochromatosis in the UK is perhaps seen most frequently in patients with refractory anaemias, particularly thalassaemia major and has been described previously (see section on haematological disorders).

ACQUIRED IMMUNE DEFICIENCY SYNDROME

Aquired immune deficiency syndrome (AIDS) is associated with serious morbidity and mortality. Data are accumulating to show that the disease affects the heart. Autopsy findings in 41 patients included metastatic Kaposi's sarcoma, non-bacterial thrombotic endocarditis, fibrinous pericarditis and cryptococcal myocarditis. Two patients died of thrombo-embolic disease. These findings suggest that cardiac lesions in AIDS patients relate to both morbidity and mortality.[70]

REFERENCES

1. Brailsford, J.F. Paget's disease of bone. Its frequency, diagnosis and complications. *Br. J. Radiol.* 1938; **11**: 507.
2. Pygott, F. Paget's disease of bone. The radiological incidence. *Lancet* 1957; **i**: 1170.
3. Edholm, O.G. and Howarth, S. Studies on the peripheral circulation in osteitis deformans. *Clin. Sci.* 1953; **12**: 277.
4. Heistad, D.D., Abboud, F.M., Schmid, P.G., Mark, A.L. and Wilson, W.R. Regulation of blood flow in Paget's disease of the bone. *J. Clin. Invest.* 1975; **55**: 69.
5. Rhodes, B.A., Gregson, D.N. and Hamilton, C.R. Jr. Absence of anatomic arteriovenous shunts in Paget's disease of the bone. *N. Engl. J. Med.* 1972; **27**: 686.
6. Arnalich, F., Plaza, I., Sobrino, J.A., Oliver, J., Barbado, J., Pēna, M. and Vazquez, J.J. Cardiac size and function in Paget's disease of bone. *Int. J. Cardiol.* 1984; **5**: 491.
7. Sornberger, C.F. and Smedal, M.I. The mechanism and incidence of cardiovascular changes in Paget's disease (osteitis deformans). A critical review of the literature with case studies. *Circulation* 1952; **6**: 711.
8. Harrison, C.V. and Lennox, B. Heart block in osteitis deformans. *Br. Heart J.* 1948; **10**: 167.

9. King, M., Huang, J.-M. and Glassman, E. Paget's disease with cardiac calcification and complete heart block. *Am. J. Med.* 1969; **46**: 302.

10. Strickberger, S.A., Schulman, S.P. and Hutchins, G.M. Association of Paget's Disease of bone with calcific aortic valve disease. *Am. J. Med.* 1987; **82**: 953.

11. Becker, D.G., Fish, C.R. and Juergren, S.J.L. Arteriovenous fistulas of the female pelvis. *Obstet. Gynecol.* 1968; **31**: 799.

12. Coel, M.N. and Alksne, J.F. Embolisation to diminish high output failure secondary to systemic angiomatosis (Ullman's syndrome). *Vasc. Surg.* 1978; **12**: 336.

13. Sanyal, S.K., Saldivar, V., Coburn, T.P., Wrenn, E.L. Jr. and Kumar, M. Hyperdynamic heart failure due to A-V fistula associated with Wilm's tumour. *Pediatrics* 1976; **57**: 564.

14. Howell, R.R. Glycogen storage diseases. In: Stanbury, J.B., Wyngaarden, J.B. and Frederickson, D.S. eds. *The Metabolic Bases of Inherited Disease*. 3rd ed. New York: McGraw-Hill, 1972, p. 149.

15. Bordiuk, J.N., Logato, M.J., Lovelace, R.E. and Blumenthal, S. Pompe's disease: Electron myographic, electron microscopic and cardiovascular aspects. *Arch. Neurol. (Chicago)* 1970; **23**: 113.

16. Ehlers, K.H., Hagström, J.W.C., Lukas, D.S., Redo, S.F. and Engle, M.A. Glycogen storage disease of the myocardium with obstruction to left ventricular outflow. *Circulation* 1962; **25**: 96.

17. Sourindrhin, I. Solvent misuse. *Br. Med. J.* 1985; **290**: 94.

18. Boon, N.A. Solvent abuse and the heart. *Br. Med. J.* 1987; **294**: 722.

19. McLeod, A.A., Marjot, R., Monaghan, M.J., Hughes-Jones, P. and Jackson, G. Chronic cardiac toxicity after inhalation of 1,1,1-trichloroethane. *Br. Med. J.* 1987; **294**: 727.

20. Unverferth, D.V., Magorien, R.D., Leier, C.V. *et al.* Doxorubicin Cardiotoxicity. *Cancer Treat. Rev.* 1982; **9**: 149.

21. Von Hoff, D.D., Rozencweig, M. and Piccart, M. The cardiotoxicity of anticancer agents. *Semin. Oncol.* 1982; **9**: 23.

22. Dresdale, A., Bonow, R.O., Wesley, T. *et al.* Prospective evaluation of doxorubicin induced cardiomyopathy resulting from post surgical adjuvant treatment of patients with soft tissue sarcomas. *Cancer* 1983; **52**: 51.

23. Minow, R.A., Benjamin, R.S., Lee, E.T. and Gottlieb, J.A. Adriamycin cardiomyopathy—risk factors. *Cancer* 1977; **39**: 1397.

24. Isner, J.M., Ferrans, V.J., Cohen, S.R. *et al.* Clinical and morphologic cardiac finding after anthracycline chemotherapy: Analysis of 104 patients studied at necropsy. *Am. J. Cardiol.* 1983; **51**: 1167.

25. Anders, R.J., Shanes, J.G. and Zeller, F.P. Lower incidence of doxorubicin-induced cardiomyopathy by once-a-week low-dose administration. *Am. Heart J.* 1986; **111**: 755.

26. McKillop, J.H., Bristow, M.R., Goris, M.L., Billingham, M.E. and Bockemeuhl, K. Sensitivity and specificity of radionuclide ejection fractions in duxorubicin cardiotoxicity. *Am. Heart J.* 1983; **106**: 1048.

27. Kantrowitz, N.E. and Bristow, M.R. Cardiotoxicity of antitumor agents. *Prog. Cardiovasc. Dis.* 1984; **27**: 195.

28. Vonhoff, D.D. and Layard, M. Risk factors for development of daunorubicin cardiotoxicity. *Cancer Treat. Rep.* 1981; **61** (Suppl. 4): 19.

29. Fletcher, G.F., Kazamias, T.M. and Wenger, N.K. Cardiotoxic effect of mellaril: Conduction disturbances and supraventricular arrhythmias. *Am. Heart J.* 1969; **78**: 135.

30. Fowler, N.O., McCall, D., Chon, T.C., Holmes, J.C. and Hanenson, I.B. Electrocardiographic changes and cardiac arrhythmias in patients receiving psychotropic drugs. *Am. J. Cardiol.* 1976; **37**: 223.

31. Tilkian, A., Schroeder, J.S., Kao, J. and Hultgren, H. Effect of lithium on cardiovascular performance. Report on extended ambulatory monitoring and exercise testing before and during lithium therapy. *Am. J. Cardiol.* 1976; **38**: 701.

32. Anderson, R.F. Appensenarth, D.C. and De Groot, W.J. Myocardial toxicity from carbon monoxide poisoning. *Ann. Intern. Med.* 1967; **67**: 1172.

33. Hotchkiss, R.S. and Hurst, J.W. Radiation and the heart. In: Hurst, J.W. ed. *Update V: The Heart*. New York: McGraw-Hill. 1981, p. 205.

34. Martin, R.G., Ruckdeschell, J.C., Chang, P., Byhardt, R., Bouchard, R.J. and Wiernik, P.H. Radiation-related pericarditis. *Am. J. Cardiol.* 1975; **35**: 216.

35. Pierce, R.H., Haferman, M.D. and Kagen, A.R. Changes in the transverse cardio-diameter following mediastinal irradiation for Hodgkins disease. *Radiology* 1969; **93**: 619.

36. Stewart, J.R. and Fajardo, L.F. Dose response in human and experimental radiation-induced heart disease. *Radiology* 1971; **99**: 403.

37. Brosius, F.C., Waller, B.F. and Roberts, W.C. Radiation heart disease analysis of 16 young (aged 15 to 33 years) necropsy patients who received over 3,500 rads to the heart. *Am. J. Med.* 1981; **70**: 519.

38. Abbott, J.A. and Cheitlin, M.D. The non-specific camel-hump sign. *JAMA* 1976; **235**: 413.

39. Clements, S.D. and Hurst, J.W. The diagnostic value of the electrocardiographic abnormalities observed in subjects accidentally exposed to cold. *Am. J. Cardiol.* 1972; **29**: 729.

40. Gillanders, A.D. Nutritional heart disease. *Br. Heart J.* 1951; **13**: 11.

41. Higgenson, J., Gillanders, A.D. and Murray, J.F. The heart in chronic malnutrition. *Br. Heart J.* 1952; **14**: 213.

42. Smythe, P.M., Swanepoel, A., Campbell, J.A.H. The heart in kwashiorkor. *Br. Med. J.* 1962; **1**: 67.

43. Swanepoel, A., Smythe, P.M. and Campbell, J.A.H. The heart in kwashiorkor. *Am. Heart J.* 1964; **67**: 1.

44. Sims, B.A. Conducting tissue of the heart in kwashiorkor. *Br. Heart J.* 1972; **34**: 828.

45. Wagner, P.I. Beriberi heart disease. *Am. Heart J.* 1965; **68**: 200.

46. Blackett, R.B. and Palmer, A.J. Haemodynamic studies in high output beriberi. *Br. Heart J.* 1960; **22**: 483.

47. Weiss, S. and Wilkins, R.W. The nature of the cardiovascular system disturbances in nutritional deficiency states (beriberi). *Ann. Intern. Med.* 1937; **11**: 104.

48. Webb, D.I. Beriberi heart disease with acute renal failure. *Arch. Intern. Med.* 1967; **120**: 494.

49. Bauer, J.M. and Freyberg, R.H. Vitamin D intoxication with metastatic calcification. *JAMA* 1946; **130**: 1208.

50. Alexander, J.K., Dennis, E.W., Smith, W.G., Amad, K.H., Duncan, W.C. and Austin, R.C. Blood volume, cardiac output and distribution of systemic blood flow in extreme obesity. *Cardiovasc. Res. Cent. Bull.* 1962; **1**: 39.

51. Nielsen, P.E. and Janniche, H. The accuracy of auscultatory measurement of arm blood pressure in very obese subjects. *Acta Med. Scand.* 1974; **195**: 403.

52. Kannel, W., Brand, N., Skinner, J., Dawber, T. and McNamara, P. Relation of adiposity to blood pressure and development of hypertension. The Framingham Study. *Ann. Intern. Med.* 1967; **67**: 4.

53. Greminger, P., Studer, A., Luscher, T., Mutter, B., Grimm, J., Siegenthaler, W. and Vetter, W. Gewichstreduktion und Blutdruck. *Sch. Med. Wochenschr.* 1982; **112**: 120.

54. Donahue, R.P., Abbott, R.D., Bloom, E., Reed, D.M. and Yano, K. Central obesity and coronary heart disease in men. *Lancet* 1987; i: 819.

55. Montonegro, M.R. and Solberg, L.A. Obesity, body weight, body length and atherosclerosis. *Lab. Invest.* 1968; **18**: 594.

56. Alexander, J.K. and Pettigrove, J.R. Obesity and congestive heart failure. *Geriatrics* 1967; **22**: 101.

57. Alexander, J.K. Obesity of the heart. *Curr. Prob. Cardiol.* 1980; **5**: 1.

58. Alexander, J.K., Amad, K. and Cole, V.W. Observations on

some clinical features of extreme obesity with particular reference to cardiorespiratory effects. *Am. J. Med.* 1962; **32**: 512.

59. Messerli, F.H. Cardmyopathy of obesity—a not so Victorian disease. *N. Engl. J. Med.* 1986; **314**: 378.

60. MacMahon, S.W., Wilcken, D.E.L. and MacDonald, G.L. The effect of weight reduction on left ventricular mass: A randomized controlled trial in young, overweight patients. *N. Engl. J. Med.* 1986; **312**: 334.

61. Alpert, M.A., Terry, B.E. and Kelly, D.L. Effect of weight loss on cardiac chamber size, wall thickness and left ventricular function in morbid obesity. *Am. J. Cardiol.* 1985; **55**: 783.

62. MacGregor, M.I., Block, A.J. and Ball, W.C. Jr. Serious complications and sudden death in the Pickwickian syndrome. *Johns Hopkins Med. J.* 1970; **126**: 297.

63. Kaltman, A.J. and Goldring, R.M. Role of circulatory congestion in the cardiorespiratory failure for obesity. *Am. J. Med.* 1976; **60**: 645.

64. Oliveira, E. and Gomez-Patiño, N. Calcemic cardiomyopathy; Report of a case. *Am. J. Cardiol.* 1964; **13**: 320.

65. Rahko, P.S., Salerni, R. and Uretsky, B.F. Successful reversal by chelation therapy of congestive cardiomyopathy due to iron overload. *J. Am. Coll. Cardiol.* **8**: 436.

66. Marcus, R.E., Davies, S.C., Bantock, H.M. Underwood, S.R., Walton, S. and Huehns, E.R. Desferrioxamine to improve iron overloaded patients with thalassaemia major. *Lancet* 1984; **i**: 392.

67. Rosenthal, A., Button, L.N. and Nathan, D.G. Blood volume changes in cyanotic congenital heart disease. *Am. J. Cardiol.* 1971; **29**: 162.

68. Murray, J.F., Dawson, A.M. and Sherlock, S. Circulatory changes in chronic liver disease. *Am. J. Med.* 1958; **24**: 358.

69. Lewis, B.S., Tur-Kaspa, R. and Lewis, N. Left ventricular function in liver cirrhosis: An echocardiographic study. *Isr. J. Med. Sci.* 1980; **16**: 489.

70. Cammarosano, C. and Lewis, W. Cardiac lesions in acquired immune deficiency syndrome (AIDS). *J. Am. Coll. Cardiol.* 1985; **5**: 703.

Chapter 72

Cardiopulmonary Resuscitation

David Zideman and Tom Evans

Cardiopulmonary resuscitation (CPR) is a treatment sequence that should begin immediately effective cardiac activity has ceased and should be continued until it returns. In its simplest form, it consists of basic life-support, a sequence of actions to be taken when no equipment is available. For advanced life-support, resuscitation with the use of equipment and drugs, there are specific recommendations[1,2] made for ventricular fibrillation, asystole and electromechanical dissociation, the three major arrhythmias associated with cardiac arrest.

BASIC LIFE SUPPORT

The basic life support sequence is:

Airway
Breathing
Circulation

The airway is opened by tilting the head and supporting the jaw. Breathing is checked by looking to see if the chest rises and falls, listening over the victim's mouth and feeling for breathing with the side of the rescuer's face/hand. If no breathing is detected, expired-air resuscitation by the mouth-to-mouth or mouth-to-nose method must be commenced. Two individual breaths of approximately 800 ml are adequate given over 1–1.5 s. Excessive inspiratory force or overventilation will result in

gastric insufflation[3] and may lead to regurgitation of the stomach contents. Following two normal expired-air breaths, the carotid pulse is checked. If no pulse is felt, external chest compressions are performed. Compressions are carried out on the lower third of the sternum (Fig. 72.1) at a rate of 80 per minute alternating every 15 compressions with 2 breaths. This can be reduced to 60 compressions in a ratio of 5 compressions to 1 breath if two rescuers are present.

External closed chest compressions were first described in 1960[4] and became known as standard CPR. In essence, each compression results in the direct compression of the heart between the sternum and the vertebral bodies thus pumping the blood around the circulation. In 1976, Criley found that cardiac arrest patients who were asked to cough repeatedly and vigorously before losing consciousness could maintain a conscious level and a systolic arterial pressure of at least 100 mmHg.[5] More recently, pressure-synchronized cinéangiography in dogs[6] and two-dimensional echocardiography in man[7,8] demonstrated that during external chest compression there was little change in cardiac chamber volume; the aortic and mitral valves open simultaneously during compression whereas the pulmonary valves close during compression and are open during relaxation. In 1980, Chandra and colleagues described 'New CPR'—simultaneous chest compression and ventilation at high airway

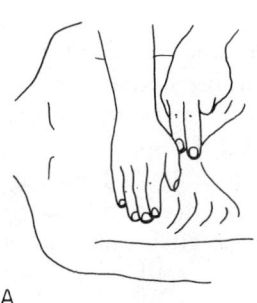
A

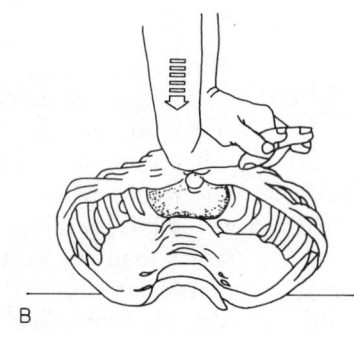
B

Fig. 72.1. External chest compression. (A) Locate the base of the sternum and place one hand two fingers' breadth above this point, over the lower third of the sternum. (B) Place the other hand on top of the first and with elbows straight bring shoulders directly over casualty's chest. Depress and release sternum 4–5 cm at a rate of 80 per minute, alternating every 15 compressions with 2 breaths.

pressures.[9] Despite the raised mean arterial pressure and carotid blood flow attained during this technique, survival rates were poor. It has been suggested that the resultant rise in mean intrathoracic pressure decreases coronary artery blood flow thus extending the size of the infarct.

Other methods of augmenting blood flow have been described: interposed[10] or simultaneous[11] abdominal compression, or the use of military anti-shock trousers.[12] The eventual results in terms of neurological outcome and survival from these and many modifications have been shown to be no better than those of the conventional techniques already described.

BASIC LIFE-SUPPORT WITH ADJUNCTS

A simple saliva filter may reduce the fear of cross-infection of the rescuer. The use of airway adjuncts such as the oropharyngeal airway, the pocket mask together with suction equipment and oxygen therapy may simplify the maintenance of the airway. The addition of defibrillation to these airway procedures can result in the rapid and effective treatment of witnessed or early cardiac arrests. Basic life-support alone is rarely effective without the use of some adjunctive or advanced procedure.

Simple modifications according to the situation of the event are easily added to this basic formula. In a monitored cardiac arrest, it may be more appropriate to begin with external chest compressions. Caldwell et al.[13] showed that mechanical cardioversion, the chest thump, could be effective in the witnessed or monitored cardiac arrest. Miller and colleagues[14] showed that the same technique was not effective in the unwitnessed out-of-hospital event when it was carried out by paramedics.

Basic life-support skills should be taught to trainee nurses, physiotherapists, radiographers, pre-clinical medical students and the general public. Training and practice are necessary to achieve a recognized level of competence in these simple but life-saving manoeuvres.

ADVANCED LIFE-SUPPORT

Advanced life-support is the definitive treatment of cardiac arrest. It will not be effective if basic life-support is not commenced and continued throughout the advanced life-support phase. Cardiopulmonary resuscitation should not be delayed whilst awaiting the arrival of the advanced life-support equipment.

The advanced life-support schedules described (Fig. 72.2) should be regarded as parallel sequences and not necessarily sequential events. They are best performed by a resuscitation team trained in the required techniques.

The airway is secured by intubation of the trachea. Ventilation is established using a self-inflating resuscitation bag adding oxygen to the inspired gases. Intravenous access is established by cannulating a large central vein. In recent studies, it has been shown that there is an appreciable delay in providing effective drug levels when a peripheral vein is used.[15,16] The recommended sites for venous cannulation are the internal or external jugular vein or the subclavian vein. Sub-diaphragmatic veins also provide poor access to the circulation. Lignocaine, adrenaline and atropine can be given down the endotracheal tube when in place.[17] These drugs should be given via a catheter, the tip of which protrudes beyond the end of the tracheal tube. Following instillation into the trachea, 5–10 breaths of hyperventilation will aid distribution of the drug throughout the pulmonary tree and its absorption into the pulmonary circulation.

Direct intracardiac injections cannot be recommended as a method of choice. Sabin et al.[18] showed that most attempts at intracardiac injection missed the heart, entered the right ventricle or lacerated a coronary artery. The administration of drugs by any route should be immediately followed by further chest compressions and the pharmacological effect of the drug confirmed after further time has elapsed.

Drugs used during resuscitation can be divided into two major groups: those that support and improve the circulation and those that control cardiac rhythm (see below).

DRUGS THAT SUPPORT AND IMPROVE THE CIRCULATION

Adrenaline

Adrenaline is a potent alpha- and beta-adrenergic agonist. During cardiac arrest, it improves cerebral and coronary blood flows by preventing arterial collapse and increasing peripheral vasoconstriction. The results of some studies in animals have suggested it is the alpha-adrenergic effect of adrenaline rather than the beta-adrenergic effect that makes ventricular fibrillation more susceptible to direct current countershock.[19]

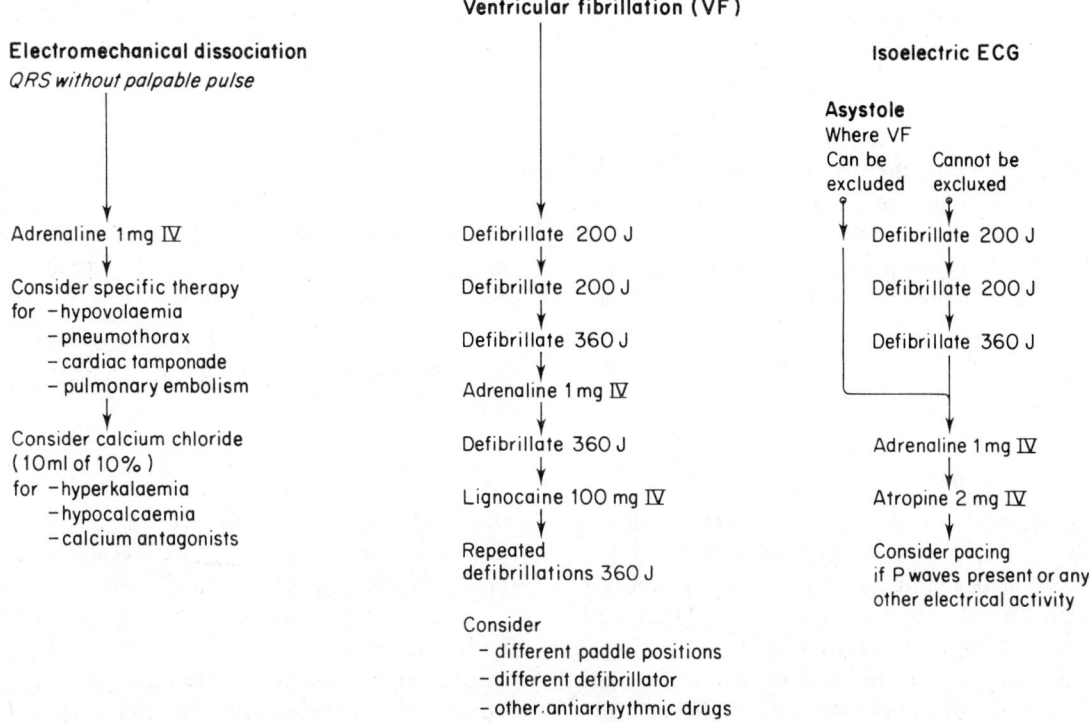

Fig. 72.2. Guidelines for the management of cardiac arrest. Mock-up of 'new' recommendations of Resuscitation Council UK (1989).

Pure alpha-adrenergic agonist drugs, such as phenylephrine or methoxamine, can cause similar peripheral vasoconstriction to adrenaline without producing the myocardial ischaemia of beta-adrenergic receptor stimulation.[20] However, adrenaline has been found to produce a greater increase in cerebral blood flow than the pure alpha-agonists and therefore it is recommended at this time as the catecholamine of choice.

Isoprenaline

Although isoprenaline is a powerful beta-adrenergic agonist, it has been shown to be less valuable than adrenaline during cardiac arrest because it causes peripheral vasodilatation rather than the vasoconstriction required to maintain mean arterial blood pressure and therefore cerebral and coronary blood flows.

The use of isoprenaline is not recommended when the heart has arrested but bolus doses or an isoprenaline infusion may be valuable in severe bradycardias.

Noradrenaline

Noradrenaline is also an adrenergic-receptor agon-

ist with virtually pure alpha-receptor activity. Its effect on blood pressure will depend on the state of the peripheral vascular resistance at the time of administration together with the contractility of the myocardium and the reflex responses monitored by the carotid baroreceptors. Via its alpha effects, it will cause intense vasoconstriction and can shut down essential vascular beds, for example, in the kidney and the gut. This vasoconstriction will cause necrosis of the skin if the drug is extravasated during intravenous administration. Noradrenaline is best administered as an infusion. A suitable initial regimen is to add 4 mg of noradrenaline to 500 ml of 5% dextrose or dextrose saline and the resultant solution titrated to a suitable cardiovascular response. Noradrenaline infusions should be discontinued slowly, not suddenly. Sudden cessation will result in a precipitous fall in blood pressure as the peripheral circulation vasodilates.

Calcium chloride

Calcium, as either the chloride or the gluconate, has been a fundamental drug in resuscitation for many years as a general cardiotonic agent. Much of the evidence has been anecdotal; in recent studies, it has been demonstrated that calcium is of no benefit during resuscitation[21-23] and may be detrimental.[24,25] Calcium, at high ionic levels, may cause coronary artery spasm and may cause tissue damage following anoxia due to the accumulation of the ion intracellularly. Thus, the use of calcium, except in hypercalcaemia or hyperkalaemia, is not recommended.

Studies using calcium channel blockers are currently being evaluated. Although there is evidence to show that they may be of value in minimizing myocardial damage,[26] the evidence is less clear when assessing cerebral protection.[27,28]

Sodium bicarbonate

During cardiopulmonary arrest, ventilatory failure leads to the retention of carbon dioxide and a respiratory acidosis; at the same time, a metabolic acidosis is produced by the generation of lactic acid from hypoxia-induced anaerobic metabolism.

The institution of prompt and efficient ventilation is therefore the key to the correction of this acidosis because it improves oxygenation and reduces the retention of carbon dioxide. Effective circulation of blood and ventilation during cardiopulmonary resuscitation is the treatment required to prevent and manage the acidosis of cardiac arrest.

Sodium bicarbonate reacts with hydrogen ions to form water and carbon dioxide. The major problem is that this reaction generates a lot of carbon dioxide. For each 50 mEq of sodium bicarbonate, 260–280 mmHg of carbon dioxide is produced. Bicarbonate crosses into cells relatively slowly when compared with carbon dioxide and there is therefore a paradoxical deterioration of intracellular acidosis. Metabolic acidosis has been shown experimentally to lower the threshold for the induction of ventricular fibrillation but not to have any effect on the defibrillation threshold;[29] it is doubtful whether metabolic acidosis inhibits the action of catecholamines at the values of pH encountered during cardiac arrest. Sodium bicarbonate has not been shown to facilitate ventricular defibrillation or improve survival after cardiac arrest.

In the past, far too much importance was placed on the use of sodium bicarbonate for the correction of acidosis at the expense of the crucial role of carbon dioxide retention. American and British resuscitation protocols no longer specifically recommend the use of sodium bicarbonate although both suggest that, if standard resuscitation procedures have failed to re-start the heart, its use can be

considered in specific clinical circumstances, such as documented pre-existing metabolic acidosis with or without accompanying hyperkalaemia.

Buffers

The use of buffer solutions such as carbicarb is purely experimental at this time, although the idea of using a buffer that generates less or no carbon dioxide is theoretically attractive.

DRUGS USED TO CONTROL CARDIAC RHYTHM

Lignocaine

This anti-arrhythmic drug reduces automacity of the resting membrane potential[30] and alters the refractory state of the ventricular myocardium.[31]

It is considered a drug of primary importance in the management of ventricular tachycardia and ventricular fibrillation. Although lignocaine decreases the incidence of primary ventricular fibrillation,[32] it elevates the electrical threshold for successful defibrillation.[33] It should therefore be administered prophylactically to stabilize an unstable situation or to prevent the recurrent initiation of ventricular fibrillation. Its use as a direct anti-fibrillatory agent must be questionable.

Bretylium

Bretylium is a post-ganglionic alpha-adrenergic receptor blocker. This action is preceded by a release of catecholamines. Thus, the effect of administering bretylium is a brief period of tachycardia and hypertension followed by a longer period of hypotension. Studies in the use of bretylium have shown it to be favoured as directly anti-fibrillatory.[34] More recent work in survival from cardiac arrest has shown no difference in its effect from that of lignocaine.[35,36] Therefore, it cannot be recommended as a drug of first choice, but it should be considered when lignocaine, together with defibrillation, has failed to convert and maintain an effective cardiac rhythm.

Amiodarone

Another drug now frequently used to treat resistant or recurrent ventricular fibrillation or ventricular tachycardia is amiodarone, a class III agent in the Vaughan Williams' classification. Reports of its value are anecdotal only and as yet there are no formal trials of its efficacy.

Atropine

Atropine is a parasympathetic blocking drug and acts directly to decrease the activity of the vagus nerve and increase the rate of activity of the sinus node. It is considered useful in the management of sinus bradycardia and ventricular asystole.[37,38] Ventricular fibrillation has been observed following the administration of atropine in the process of myocardial ischaemia.[39]

DEFIBRILLATION

Electrical defibrillation is the definitive management of ventricular tachycardia and ventricular fibrillation. A quantity of electrical energy is passed via the chest wall across the heart, depolarizing the myocardial cells and interrupting the random re-polarization of ventricular tachycardia and ventricular fibrillation, thereby allowing a more ordered rhythm to supervene. Rapid early defibrillation is essential in both of these abnormal rhythms.[40] It has been shown that a shock of 175 J is as effective as one of 320 J and that shocks of lower energy are safer.[41] For this reason, the initial energy level presently recommended is 200 J. A second shock at the same energy level was originally believed to deliver more energy because of a decrease in transthoracic resistance following the first shock. However, recent studies have shown that only small insignificant changes actually occur.[42] Nevertheless, on the grounds that two early rapid shocks of 200 J could be effective and yet minimize myocardial damage, the present recommendations have remained. If fibrillation continues, a third shock, and all subsequent defibrillations, should be at 360 J.

Defibrillation should be carried out with paddle electrodes measuring 10 cm in diameter,[43] one applied to the right of the upper sternum just below the clavicle and the other to the mid-axillary line just below the level of the left nipple. An alternative position of anterior/posterior defibrillation should be considered if conventional defibrillation fails.

It must be emphasized that immediately following defibrillation, basic life-support is continued until the electrocardiographic trace returns to the monitor. Prolonged periods of non-activity whilst electrical conversion is attempted are detrimental and will adversely affect the eventual outcome of resuscitation.

Automatic and semi-automatic (automatic advisory) defibrillators

Manual defibrillators require the operator to be able to recognize basic cardiac rhythms and common arrhythmias. They also require a degree of skill to use the controls on the apparatus.

Based on the hypothesis that, especially in ischaemic heart disease, most patients who survive a cardiac arrest are those who have been defibrillated from ventricular fibrillation, defibrillators requiring no knowledge of electrocardiogram interpretation and are simple to use have been designed. These machines allow first responders, such as less highly qualified ambulancemen, first-aiders and nurses at work and doctors who rarely manage a cardiac arrest, to defibrillate a subject.[44–52] The aim is to deliver the first defibrillatory shock as rapidly as possible while recognizing that it is not possible to have highly trained teams, especially out of hospital, with rapid enough response times.

The completely automatic defibrillators merely require adhesive defibrillator pads to be placed on the thorax of the patient and the machine to be activated. The defibrillator will request the operator to stop resuscitation—a verbal command from a voice chip—to allow the electrocardiogram to be analysed without motion artefacts; if the arrhythmia is one requiring defibrillation, i.e. ventricular fibrillation or rapid ventricular tachycardia, the defibrillator will order everyone to 'stand clear', deliver a shock and then recommence its cycle.

Semi-automatic or automatic advisory defibrillators differ from totally automatic defibrillators in that they contain a visual display unit which prompts the rescuer to start the analysis sequence by pressing one button, allows one of two energy levels to be selected and advises the operator to press a defibrillator button if the rhythm requires this. Most devices also have a 'prompting' voice chip; some also display the electrocardiogram and some have an 'override key' facility for a doctor or trained paramedic to convert the system into a 'manual mode'.

Experience in the USA[53] has indicated that after training for 4 h most emergency technicians are able to use these devices safely and effectively, thereby reducing the time to first defibrillation.

Researchers in the USA[52] have conducted pilot studies to investigate the acceptability of automatic defibrillators to spouses and other close relatives of high-risk cardiac patients. It should be clearly understood that patients who are at very high risk of ventricular fibrillation or ventricular tachycardia should be considered for the automatic implantable defibrillator. Many of them would collapse and die unwitnessed or before external defibrillation could be used.

Pacemakers in cardiac arrest

The use of pacemakers, transvenous or trans-cutaneous, in resuscitation has been extensively reviewed.[54] A pacemaker may be of value if the patient has a bradycardia with a cardiac output or if there are P waves on the electrocardiogram indicating complete atrioventricular block with atrial activity. Pacemakers otherwise play no role in the management of combined atrial and ventricular asystole or electromechanical dissociation.[54,55]

In the emergency situation, especially outside hospital, transcutaneous transthoracic pacing may be the method of choice ensuring that the patient is adequately sedated because of the discomfort this may cause.

CARE AFTER RESUSCITATION

The management of cardiac arrest does not end with the restoration of a spontaneous cardiac rhythm with a circulation. Redmond[1] states that the true endpoint is a fully conscious neurologically intact patient who has a spontaneous stable cardiac rhythm and an adequate urine output. Measures to achieve this endpoint may include mechanical ventilation, oxygenation, inotropic and anti-arrhythmic therapy, control of acid–base balance and other techniques to reduce cerebral oedema.

TRAINING AND ORGANIZATION OF RESUSCITATION

In 1987, the Royal College of Physicians of London produced guidelines for the UK.[56] The unit of organization in the National Health Service is the District Health Authority which usually contains a major district general hospital, other smaller hospitals and the community health services. The College recommended that each district health authority should convene a resuscitation committee comprising doctors, nurses, paramedical staff and others with an important role or interest in resuscitation to supervise the training and delivery of resuscitation in that health authority. It also recommended that every district should appoint a resuscitation training officer to execute the policies of the resuscitation committee and to supervise training in basic and advanced life-support.

Resuscitation training officers will usually have a nursing background in either coronary or intensive care or accident and emergency medicine. Some resuscitation training officers have been trained in the ambulance service and, as the advanced life-support training programme spreads in the ambulance service, more appointments from the field seem likely. The College recommended that all staff working in hospitals should be trained in basic life-support. All trained nurses should be able to use airway adjuncts as should certain paramedical staff and all qualified doctors should at the minimum be able to provide basic life-support with airway adjuncts and be able to defibrillate. In teaching hospitals, all pre-clinical medical students should be competent in basic life-support and clinical medical students should be instructed how to use airway adjuncts and defibrillate but should use the latter techniques only under supervision. Advanced life-support techniques beyond those already discussed were considered to be the skills required of the cardiac arrest team leader.

Besides training staff in the skills mentioned above, the resuscitation training officer should regularly organize simulated cardiac arrest scenarios for team practice in different areas of the hospital.

In many parts of the UK, a general practitioner is the first person to respond to a cardiac or respiratory emergency. It has been shown that up to 5% of patients who die following myocardial infarction do so in the presence of their general practitioner. Many could have been successfully resuscitated.[57] Therefore, the training of general practitioners in basic life-support and preferably basic life-support with airway adjuncts and defibrillation skills was encouraged.

In most hospitals, the cardiac arrest team consists of the duty medical and anaesthetic registrars, one or more junior doctors, and nursing staff. Attention must be paid to prompt activation and arrival of the team and the delivery of its equipment to the incident. Special paging devices, emergency telephone numbers and lift override keys in tower blocks play essential parts in this mechanism.[1]

TRAINING AND RETENTION OF SKILLS

It is apparent that simplification of standards and guidelines, course content and the actual time devoted to manikin practice may be important determinants of CPR skills.

Studies of the performance of nurses and pre-registration house officers[57,58] have clearly shown that:

> "experience of attending cardiac arrest calls in hospital is no substitute for formal training sessions with a high practical content."

For advanced cardiac life-support, time spent in simulated cardiac arrest scenarios, an extension of Kaye's 'Mega Code',[59] seems very important.

The availability of realistic training manikins for basic and advanced life-support practice is essential; this topic has been reviewed comprehensively.[1]

RESUSCITATION IN THE COMMUNITY

Up to 60% of deaths resulting from ischaemic heart disease occur in the community.[60,61] These deaths are often sudden within the first hour of an acute myocardial infarction; up to two-thirds occur in the home. It has been known for over 20 years that the vast majority of patients who die develop ventricular fibrillation that is amenable to prompt counter-shock. The results of studies in patients seen by mobile coronary care units, general practitioners and paramedic units all attest to this. There is, however, a narrow time-window within which defibrillation has to be delivered for there to be a good chance of re-starting the heart and producing a neurologically intact survivor. Basic life-support applied by bystanders

> "keeps the brain alive and the heart ready to be defibrillated"[62]

but even with bystander cardiopulmonary resuscitation within 4 min survival from ventricular fibrillation is very poor if defibrillation is not achieved within 8 min. Immediate bystander CPR with early defibrillation has resulted in survival figures of 30–40% in Seattle, USA.[62] When the presenting rhythm outside of hospital is asystole or electromechanical dissociation, survival rates of the order of 1% are to be expected. In communities in which advanced life-support is not practised outside of hospital, patients in whom resuscitation is attempted rarely survive to leave the accident and emergency department, let alone the hospital.[63] In the UK, 'extended training' protocols for the ambulance service are being introduced but the number of crews trained is as yet inadequate, the response times are in general too long and citizen resuscitation training is too patchy for the results to be good. General practitioners in the UK are frequently first

responders. Pai[64] and Colquhoun[65] have clearly demonstrated that trained general practitioners with defibrillators have considerable life-saving potential. With the advent of the automatic and semi-automatic defibrillators, it is likely that less highly trained first responders such as policemen, security guards, occupational health nurses and lay first-aiders may be able to provide defibrillation in addition to basic life-support.

'Telephone cardiopulmonary resuscitation' is a method of immediately instructing a bystander untrained in cardiopulmonary resuscitation. When the bystander dials the emergency number, the ambulance dispatcher/controller will ask the bystander if he or she can perform cardiopulmonary resuscitation. If not, advice and instruction will be offered over the telephone until the ambulance arrives. This method reduces the time during which no resuscitation is given when trained bystanders are not available and has been used with enthusiasm and success particularly in Seattle, USA.[66]

It must never be forgotten that whatever advances in technology or training are made in the hospital environment, most deaths still occur in the community and it is often these patients who respond to CPR and who can be saved.

AUDIT

Resuscitation is a medical/surgical procedure in which electrical, mechanical and pharmacological procedures are employed in an attempt to re-start circulation and respiration. Like any such procedure, good medical practice demands that formal records should be kept. This is also necessary for legal purposes to defend the operators if litigation should ensue.

It is suggested that all hospitals should have a standard recording form for cardiac arrest procedures, which will contain all the necessary demographic, chronological and procedural information. These forms can be used as a basis for research studies to evaluate the outcome of different types of cardiac arrest in different centres or with differing treatment regimens.

ETHICS OF RESUSCITATION

Resuscitation is most appropriate for those patients in whom cardiopulmonary arrest is sudden and unexpected. It is least appropriate for patients who have terminal illnesses in whom death is imminent.[1,67]

The exact ethical issues involved are complex but individual to each case. In the hospital, the consultant or senior registrar looking after the patient may decide after discussion with other doctors, nursing staff and in many instances the patient's relatives and the patient that nature should be allowed to take its course. This decision should be clearly recorded in the patient's notes, signed by the senior doctor and also recorded in the nursing notes. Rarely, the condition of a patient may change so much that the decision needs to be reviewed. Therefore, a time-limit to the validity of the instruction may be a good idea. This instruction is intended as a guideline only; the physician present at the time of a cardiopulmonary arrest may override this instruction if the circumstances of the arrest appear to be different. The instruction is not to institute cardiopulmonary resuscitation. Patients must at all times continue to receive full medical and nursing care, enabling them to die in comfort and with dignity.

REFERENCES

1. Evans, T., ed. *ABC of resuscitation*. London: British Medical Journal, 1986.
2. Standards and guidelines for cardiopulmonary resuscitation and emergency cardiac care. *JAMA* 1986; **255**: 2843–989.
3. Melker, R. Recommendations for ventilation during cardiopulmonary resuscitation. Time for change? *Crit. Care Med.* 1985; **13**: 882–3.
4. Kouwenhoven, W.B., Jude, J.R. and Knickerbocker, G.G. Closed chest cardiac massage. *JAMA* 1960; **173**: 1064–7.
5. Criley, J.M., Blaufuss, A.H. and Kissel, G.L. Cough induced cardiac compression, self induced form of cardiopulmonary resuscitation. *JAMA* 1976; **236**: 1246–50.
6. Nieman, J.T., Rosborough, J.P., Hausknecht, M., Gardner, D. and Criley, J.M. Pressure-synchronized cineangiography during experimental cardiopulmonary resuscitation. *Circulation* 1981; **64**: 985–91.
7. Werner, J.A., Green, H.L., Janko, C.L. and Cobb, L.A. Visualization of cardiac valve motion in man during external chest impression using two dimensional echocardiography. Implications regarding mechanism of blood flow. *Circulation* 1981; **63**: 1417–21.
8. Rich, S., Wix, H.L. and Shapiro, E.P. Clinical assessment of heart chamber size and valve motion during cardiopulmonary resuscitation by two dimensional echocardiography. *Am. Heart J.* 1981; **102**: 368–73.
9. Chandra, N., Rudikoff, M.T. and Weisfeldt, M.L. Simultaneous chest compression and ventilation at high airway pressure during cardiopulmonary resuscitation. *Lancet* 1980; **i**: 175–8.
10. Ralston, S.H., Babbs, C.F. and Niebauer, M.J. Cardiopulmonary resuscitation with interposed abdominal compression in dogs. *Anesth. Analg.* 1982; **61**: 645–51.
11. Rosborough, J.P., Nieman, J.T. and Criley, J.M. Lower abdominal compression with synchronized ventilation: A CPR modality. *Circulation* 1981; **64**: 303.
12. Bircher, N., Safar, P. and Steward, R. A comparison of standard 'MAST'-augmented and open chest CPR in dogs: A preliminary investigation. *Crit. Care Med.* 1980; **8**: 147–52.
13. Caldwell, G., Miller, G., Quinn, E., Vincent, R. and Chamberlain, D.A. Simple mechanical methods of cardioversion: defence of the precordial thump and cough version. *Br. Med. J.* 1985; **13**: 627–30.
14. Miller, J., Tresch, D., Horwitz, L., Thompson, B.M., Aprahamian, C. and Davin, J.C. The Precordial Thump. *Ann. Emergency Med.* 1984; **13**: 791–4.
15. Kuhn, G.J., White, B.C. and Swetman, R.E. Peripheral VS central circulation times during CPR: A pilot study. *Ann. Emergency Med.* 1981; **10**: 417–9.
16. Barson, W.G., Levy, R.C. and Weir, H. Lidocaine levels during CPR: Differences after peripheral venous, central venous and intracardiac injections. *Ann. Emergency Med.* 1981; **10**: 73.
17. Elam, J.O. The intrapulmonary route for CPR drugs. In: Safar, P. and Elam, J.O., eds. *Advances in cardiopulmonary resuscitation*. New York: Springer Verlag, 1977, pp. 132–7.
18. Sabin, H.I., Khanti, K., Coghill, S.B. and McNeill, G.O. Accuracy of intracardiac injections determined by post mortem studies. *Lancet* 1983; **ii**: 1054–5.
19. Redding, J.S. and Pearson, J.W. Evaluation of drugs for cardiac resuscitation. *Anesthesiology* 1963; **24**: 203.
20. Silfvast, T., Saarnivaara, L., Kinnanen, A., Erosno, J., Nick, L., Pesnonen, P. and Luomanmaki, K. Comparison of adrenaline and phenylephrine in out of hospital cardiopulmonary resuscitation. A double blind study. *Acta Anaesthesiol. Scand.* 1985; **29**: 610.
21. Stueven, H., Thompson, B.M., Aprahamian, C. and Darin, J.C. Use of calcium in prehospital cardiac arrest. *Ann. Emergency Med.* 1983; **12**: 136.
22. Stueven, H.A., Thompson, B.M., Aprahamian, C. and Tonsfeldt, D.J. Calcium chloride: Reassessment of use in asystole. *Ann. Emergency Med.* 1984; **13**: 820.
23. Harrison, E.E. and Amey, B.D. Use of calcium in electromechanical dissociation. *Ann. Emergency Med.* 1984; **9**: 358.
24. Dembo, D.H. Calcium in advanced life support. *Crit. Care Med.* 1981; **9**: 358.
25. Carlon, G.C., Howland, W.S., Kahn, R.C. and Schweizer, O. Calcium chloride administration in normocalcemic critically ill patients. *Crit. Care Med.* 1980; **8**: 209.
26. Clarke, R.E., Christlieb, I.Y., Henry, P.D., Fischer, A.E., Nora, J.D., Williamson, J.R. and Sobel, B.E. Nifedipine: A myocardial protective agent. *Am. J. Cardiol.* 1979; **44**: 825.
27. White, B.C., Winegar, C.D., Jackson, R.C., Joyce, K.M., Vigar, D.N., Hoechner, T.J., Krause, G.S. and Wilson, R.F. Cerebral cortical perfusion during and following resuscitation from cardiac arrest in dogs. *A:n. J. Emergency Med.* 1983; **1**: 128.
28. Vaagenes, P., Cantadore, T., Safar, P. and Alexander, H. Effect of lidoflazine on neurological outcome after cardiac arrest in dogs. *Anaesthesiology* 1983; **59**: 100.
29. Minuck, M. and Sharma, G.P. Comparison of THAM and sodium bicarbonate in resuscitation of the heart after ventricular fibrillation in dogs. *Anesth. Analg.* 1977; **56**: 38–45.
30. Rosen, M.R., Hoffman, B.F. and Wit, A.L. Electrophysiology and pharmacology of cardiac arrhythmias V cardiac antiarrhythmic effects of lidocaine. *Am. Heart J.* 1975; **89**: 526.
31. Kupersmith, J. Electrophysiological and antiarrhythmic effects of lidocaine on canine acute myocardial ischaemia. *Am. Heart J.* 1979; **97**: 360.
32. De Silva, R.A., Hennekerns, S.H. and Lown, B. Lignocaine prophylaxis in acute myocardial infarction. An evaluation of randomized trials. *Lancet* 1981; **ii**: 855–8.
33. Tacker, W.A., Niebauer, M.J., Babbs, C.F., Combs, W.J., Hahn, B.M., Barker, M.A., Siepel, J.F., Bowland, J.D. and

Geddes, L.A. The effect of new antiarrhythmic drugs on defibrillation threshold. *Crit. Care Med.* 1980; **8**: 177.

34. Heissenbuttel, R.H. and Bigger, J.T. Bretylium tosylate: a newly available antiarrhythmic drug for ventricular arrhythmias. *Ann. Intern. Med.* 1979; **91**: 229.

35. Haynes, R.E., Chinn, T.L., Copass, M.K. and Cobb, L.A. Comparison of bretylium tosylate and lidocaine in management of out of hospital ventricular fibrillation; a randomized clinical trial. *Am. J. Cardiol.* 1981; **48**: 353.

36. Olson, D.W., Thompson, B.M., Davin, J.C. and Milbrath, M.H. A randomized comparison study of bretylium tosylate and lidocaine in resuscitation of patients out of hospital ventricular fibrillation in a para-medic system. *Ann. Emergency Med.* 1984; **13**: 807.

37. Myerburg, R.J., Estes, D., Zaman, L., Luceri, R.M., Kessler, K.M., Trohman, R.G. and Castellanos, A. Outcome of resuscitation from bradyarrhythmic or asystolic prehospital cardiac arrest. *J. Am. Coll. Cardiol.* 1984; **6**: 1118–22.

38. Stueven, H.A., Tonsfeldt, D.J., Thompson, B.M., Whitcomb, J., Kastenson, E. and Aprahamian, C. Atropine in asystole: Human Studies. *Ann. Emergency Med.* 1984; **13**: 815.

39. Lunde, P. Ventricular fibrillation after intravenous atropine for treatment of sinus bradycardia. *Acta Med. Scand.* 1976; **199**: 369–71.

40. Cobb, L.A. and Hallstrom, A.P. Community-based cardiopulmonary resuscitation: what have we learned. *Ann. N.Y. Acad. Sci.* 1982; **330**: 42.

41. Waever, W.D., Cobb, L.A., Copass, M.K. and Hallstrom, A.P. Ventricular defibrillation—comparative trial using 175-J and 320-J shocks. *N. Engl. J. Med.* 1982; **307**: 1101.

42. Geddes, L.A., Tacker, W.A., Rosborough, J.P., Moore, A.G. and Cabler, P.S. Electrical dose for ventricular defibrillation of large and small animals using precordial electrodes. *J. Clin. Invest.* 1974; **53**: 310.

43. Kerber, R.E., Grayzel, J., Hogt, R., Marcus, M. and Kennedy, J. Transthoracic resistance in human defibrillation. Influence of body weight, chest size, serial shocks, paddle size and paddle contact pressure. *Circulation* 1981; **63**: 676.

44. Eisenberg, M.S., Cummins, R.O., Moore, J. *et al.* Use of automatic external defibrillators in the home. *Crit. Care Med.* 1985; **13**: 946.

45. Eisenberg, M.S., Copass, M.K., Hallstrom, A.P., Blake, B., Bergner, L., Short, F. and Cobb, L. Treatment of out-of-hospital cardiac arrest with rapid defibrillation by emergency medical technicians. *N. Engl. J. Med.* 1980; **302**: 1379–83.

46. Eisenberg, M.S., Hallstrom, A.P., Copass, M.K., Bergner, L., Short, F. and Pierce, J. Treatment of ventricular fibrillation: emergency medical technician defibrillation and paramedic services. *JAMA* 1984; **251**: 1723–6.

47. Cummins, R.O., Eisenberg, M.S., Bergner, L., Hallstrom, A.P., Hearne, T. and Murray, J.A. Automatic external defibrillation: evaluation of its role in the home and in emergency medical services. *Ann. Emergency Med.* 1984; **13**: 798–801.

48. Cummins, R.O. EMT–defibrillation: national guidelines for implementation. *Am. J. Emergency Med.* 1987; **5**: 254–7.

49. Taggarao, N.S., Grainger, R., Heber, M., Vincent, R. and Chamberlain, D. Use of an automated external defibrillator–pacemaker by ambulance staff. *Lancet* 1982; **ii**: 73–5.

50. Gray, A.J., Redmond, A.D. and Martin, M.A. Use of the automatic external defibrillator pacemaker by ambulance personnel: The Stockport experience. *Br. Med. J.* 1987; **294**: 1133–5.

51. Jack, C.M., Hunter, E.K., Pringle, T.H., Wilson, J.T., Anderson, J. and Adgey, A.J. Automatic detection of cardiac arrest rhythms prior to automatic external cardiac defibrillation. *Texas Heart Inst.* 1986; **13**: 419–26.

52. Chadda, K.D. and Kammerer, R. Early experiences with the portable automatic external defibrillator in the home and public places. *Am. J. Cardiol.* 1987; **60**: 732–3.

53. Weaver, W.D., Copass, M.K., Hill, D.L., Fahrenbruch, C., Hallstrom, A.P. and Cobb, L.A. Cardiac arrest treated with a new automatic external defibrillator by out-of-hospital first responders. *Am. J. Cardiol.* 1986; **57**: 1017–21.

54. Zoll, P.M., Zoll, R.H., Falk, R.H. *et al.* External non-invasive temporary cardiac pacing clinical trials. *Circulation* 1985; **71**: 937–44.

55. *Textbook of Advanced Life Support.* American Heart Association, 1987.

56. Resuscitation from cardiopulmonary arrest. Training and Organisation. *J. R. Coll. Phys.* 1987; 1–8.

57. Wynne, G., Marteau, T.M., Johnson, M., Whiteley, C.A. and Evans, T.R. Inability of trained nurses to provide basic life support. *Br. Med. J.* 1987; **297**: 1198–9.

58. Kaye, W., Wynne, G., Marteau, T., Dubin, H.G., Rallis, S.F. and Evans, T.R. Evaluation of an advanced resuscitation training course for pre registration house officers (Abstract). *Br. Heart J.* 1988; **59**: 111.

59. Kaye, W., Linhares, K.C., Breault, R.V. *et al.* The Mega Code for training the advanced life support team. *Heart Lung* 1981; **10**: 860–5.

60. Bainton, C.R. and Peterson, D.R. Deaths from coronary artery disease in persons fifty years of age or younger. A community wide study. *N. Engl. J. Med.* 1963; **268**: 569–75.

61. Armstrong, A., Duncan, B., Oliver, M.F. *et al.* Natural history of acute coronary attacks. A community study. *Br. Heart J.* 1972; **34**: 67–80.

62. Cummins, R.O. and Eisenberg, M.S. Cardiopulmonary resuscitation. American style. *Br. Med. J.* 1985; **291**: 1401–3.

63. Pantridge, J.F. and Adgey, A.A.J. The prehospital phase of acute myocardial infarction. In: Meltzer and Dunning, eds. *Textbook of coronary care.* Amsterdam: Excerpta Medica, 1972.

64. Pai, G.R., Haites, N.E. and Rawles, J.M. One thousand heart attacks in Grampian. The place of cardiopulmonary resuscitation in general practice. *Br. Med. J.* 1987; **294**: 352–4.

65. Colquhoun, M.C. Use of defibrillators by general practitioners. *Br. Med. J.* 1988; **297**: 336.

66. Eisenberg, M.S., Cummins, R.O., Litwin, P., Hallstrom, A. and Hearne, T. Dispatcher cardiopulmonary resuscitation instruction via telephone. *Crit. Care Med.* 1985; **13**: 923–4.

67. Standards and guidelines for cardiopulmonary resuscitation (CPR) and emergency cardiac care (ECC). *JAMA* 1986; **21**: 2905–84.

Chapter 73

The Principles of Pharmacological Therapy for Heart Disease

C.F. George and D.G. Waller

INTRODUCTION

There are three main purposes of cardiovascular drug therapy: curative, the provision of symptomatic relief and prophylaxis. Examples of curative therapy include the use of penicillin and gentamicin for infective endocarditis due to *Streptococcus viridans* and of carbimazole for the control of thyrotoxic heart disease. There are many examples of symptomatic relief in cardiovascular drug therapy including the use of beta-adrenoceptor antagonists, nitrates and/or calcium channel blocking agents for angina pectoris. Symptomatic relief is possible also for the symptoms of heart failure: for example, diuretics for paroxysmal noctural dyspnoea. Finally, examples of preventive therapy include the use of anticoagulants to reduce the risks of thrombo-embolism and of beta-adrenoceptor antagonists to prevent secondary mortality following myocardial infarction.

Because of the high prevalence of cardiac disease in the Western hemisphere, the use of drugs that have an action on the heart and the circulation is widespread.[1] However, the benefits of such treatment are offset by the tendency of such treatments to produce adverse effects.[2,3] The optimum results from the treatment of cardiac disease require careful attention to detail especially dosage adjustment because of individual differences in response. In particular, there is a need to adhere to the principles outlined in this chapter if maximum benefits are to be obtained with the minimum risk of an adverse effect occurring.

MECHANISMS OF DRUG ACTION

A variety of mechanisms of cardiovascular drug action can be defined. Some agents, which include the beta-adrenoceptor antagonists, have a specific action on cell membrane receptors. They block the effects of circulating endogenous substances (ligands) including noradrenaline and adrenaline. They are extremely potent, show biological specificity (having no effect on the contractility of skeletal muscle) and exhibit stereoselectivity. For example, the laevo isomer of propranolol is approximately 120 times more potent than the dextro isomer.[4] Digitalis glycosides are thought also to act by combination with specific membrane-bound receptors,[5] but the endogenous ligand has yet to be identified.

A second mechanism of action is that of enzyme inhibition. A good example is the inhibition of the converting enzyme responsible for the formation of angiotensin II from angiotensin I. The enzyme is located in the cristae terminales within vascular endothelium and is, therefore, concentrated in the lungs. Specific inhibition by either captopril or enalapril (which forms an active metabolite known as enalaprilat) prevents the generation of angiotensin II and reduces the liberation of aldosterone from the adrenal cortex. In addition, there is a reduced breakdown of bradykinin. A second example of cardiovascular drug therapy dependent upon inhibition of a single enzyme pathway can be found in antiplatelet therapy. Thus, acetyl salicyclic acid and sulphinpyrazone both inhibit cyclo-oxygenase within the platelet to prevent the formation of the pro-aggregatory substance, thromboxane A_2.

A third mechanism of action involves interference of transmembrane movement of specific ions, such as sodium. Examples of this category are drugs that have a class I anti-arrhythmic action, e.g. lignocaine. Other agents, e.g. verapamil and diltiazem, affect the slow inward calcium currents responsible for the depolarization of cardiac pacemaking cells in the sino-atrial and atrioventricular nodes.

The three actions described above result from a direct effect of drugs on cardiac and/or vascular tissue. However, therapeutic agents can also have indirect actions to affect the cardiovascular system. These have recently been reviewed by George et al.[6] One example is that of opioid analgesics. By causing constipation, they will result in a Valsalva manoeuvre during defaecation and cause adverse effects in patients with cardiac disease. Finally, it is important to remember that the administration of drugs can also produce psychological actions (the placebo response). Thus, 36% of patients with angina pectoris will show an improvement when given an inert tablet by mouth.[7]

DOSE–EFFECT RELATIONSHIPS

Whatever the precise mechanism of the drug's action, there is usually a relationship between the dose administered and its effect(s). The magnitude of drug action varies according to the logarithm of the dose of drug administered and the free concentration of the drug in plasma water. Excellent examples of this principle can be found in relation to the treatment of angina pectoris and cardiac arrhythmias.

After oral administration of beta-adrenoceptor antagonists, such as propranolol, there is a close relationship between the plasma concentration and the inhibition of submaximal exercise tachycardia.[8–10] Also, following acute administration of five different drugs of this class, a relationship was shown between dose administered and the increase in walking time before the onset of pain.[11] Furthermore, clinical correlations have been observed between the dose of propranolol and the extent of its effects in relieving attacks of angina pectoris.[12] However, there are considerable interindividual differences in response between patients.[12,13] Similarly, in patients with frequent ventricular premature beats, good correlations have been found between the dose of propranolol administered and the proportion of patients responding.[14] Woosley et al. also demonstrated a correlation between the logarithm of the plasma concentration of the drug and the proportion of responders.[14]

For the slow calcium channel antagonist, nifedipine, in stable angina pectoris, despite interindividual differences there is a clear linear relationship, on exercise stress testing, between the logarithm of the mean plasma concentration and average time to the onset of pain and time to the onset of significant ST-segment depression on the electrocardiogram (Fig. 73.1).

The response of atrial fibrillation to digoxin was one of the earliest demonstrations of a concentration–effect relationship. In patients with atrial fibrillation who initially have a fast ventricular response, there is a clear trend for slower ventricular rates after treatment with digoxin to be associated with 'high' plasma drug concentrations and for the highest concentrations to be associated with the presence of clinical signs of toxicity.[15] For other anti-arrhythmic agents, a reliable endpoint may be less easy to define due to the intrinsic variability in arrhythmia frequency. Nevertheless, after intravenous lignocaine, a plasma concentration above 2 µg/ml is probably required to suppress reliably ventricular ectopic beats following acute myocardial infarction[16] whereas concentrations

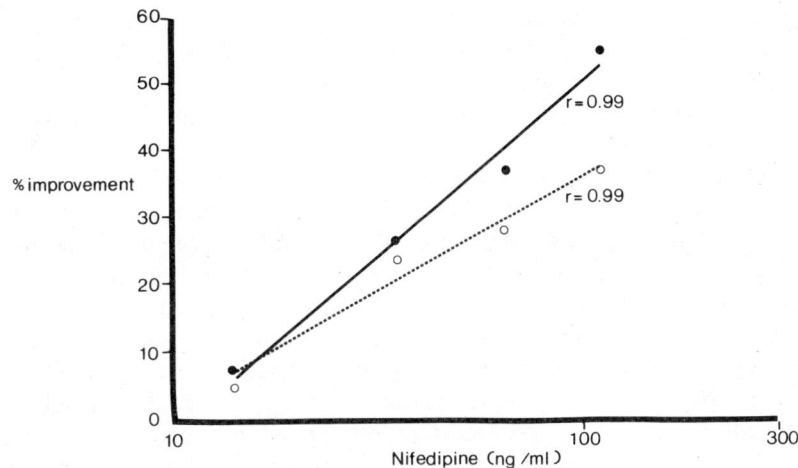

Fig. 73.1. Relationship between plasma nifedipine concentration and percentage improvement in time to onset of significant ST-segment depression in the electrocardiogram (O----O) and anginal pain (●——●) during stress testing. Mean results from 18 patients with stable angina.

above 6 ug/ml usually produce central nervous system side-effects.[17,18] For other drugs, it may be possible to determine a concentration–effect relationship from an alternative endpoint. For example, with verapamil, the most important electrophysiological effect is the slowing of atrioventricular conduction. This is reflected in prolongation of the PR interval on the electrocardiogram, which is closely correlated with plasma drug concentration after both oral and intravenous administration.[19,20]

In view of the importance of plasma drug concentrations in determining the extent of their actions, it is important that the principles underlying pharmacokinetics are understood by those using cardiovascular drugs.

PHARMACOKINETICS

Pharmacokinetics is used to describe the absorption, distribution, metabolism and elimination of drugs. Often mathematical terms are used to describe the rates of such processes. In this chapter, we will describe only those parameters that we consider to be important for practising clinicians.

DRUG ABSORPTION

During long-term therapy, drugs are normally given by the oral route for convenience and because this route offers a wide safety margin. Oral preparations include tablets, capsules and slow-release formulations. Modern pharmaceuticals contain not only a precise amount of the active ingredient but also substances known as excipients which are designed to stabilize the formulation and to ensure that it behaves in a consistent and predictable manner. The *formulation* itself is one of the major factors determining the rate and extent of drug absorption. Some preparations, such as nifedipine capsules, contain the drug substance in liquid form and once the contents have been released absorption is very rapid. This same drug is available in various slow-release forms which ensure a gradual release over a period of time. They reduce the height of the peak plasma concentrations attained, thereby limiting side-effects, such as headache and flushing. But, because the duration of action is limited by the rate of absorption (Fig. 73.2), the drug's effects will persist for a much longer time-interval.

Drugs can be absorbed from most parts of the gastro-intestinal tract. However, palatability and the small surface area make absorption from the

mouth itself impracticable except for a small number of drugs which are highly potent, e.g. nitrates. Apart from acetylsalicylic acid (aspirin) and alcohol, drug absorption from the stomach is poor. This organ has a small surface area and, as most drugs are ionized at the pH of the stomach (<3), in this state they are unable to cross lipoprotein membranes. Thus, for practical purposes, absorption of the drug cannot usually occur until it has left the stomach. Therefore, a second major determinant of the rate of onset of drug action is *gastric emptying*. Gastric emptying is under control of the vagus nerve acting via muscarinic cholinergic receptors. It is accelerated by dopaminergic antagonists, such as metoclopramide,[21] although recent evidence suggests that this effect may be mediated by non-dopaminergic pathways.[22] Further variation in gastric emptying may be related to posture and the effects of gravity.[23] The effects of altering gastric emptying on plasma concentrations and bioavailability of drugs will depend on the rate of drug dissolution in the stomach. Propranolol plasma concentrations are dependent to a small extent on the individual differences in gastric emptying,[24] and after metoclopramide the peak plasma concentration is higher and occurs earlier. Certain drugs used in cardiovascular drug therapy can delay gastric emptying. Examples include atropine, which blocks the muscarinic receptors, and opioid analgesics such as diamorphine used to control pain following a myocardial infarction. Thus, it is hardly surprising that drug absorption is impaired in the first few hours following a myocardial infarction and that orally administered anti-arrhythmic agents may be unsuccessful.

Food may alter the absorption rate of drugs by slowing the rate of gastric emptying.[25,26] This is exemplified by the calcium antagonists, verapamil[27] and nifedipine.[28] The reduced peak plasma concentrations and prolonged (absorption rate-limited) elimination may have implications both for therapeutic action and the incidence of unwanted effects (Fig. 73.3).

After leaving the stomach, the extent of drug absorption from the gastro-intestinal tract depends upon the degree of charge on the drug molecule and its dissolution characteristics in the intestine. Some preparations have a large surface area because of their microcrystalline structure and are well absorbed, e.g. spironolactone (aldactone A). This formulation is some four times better absorbed than its predecessor.[29] Lipid-soluble agents such as propranolol, labetalol and oxprenolol are extremely

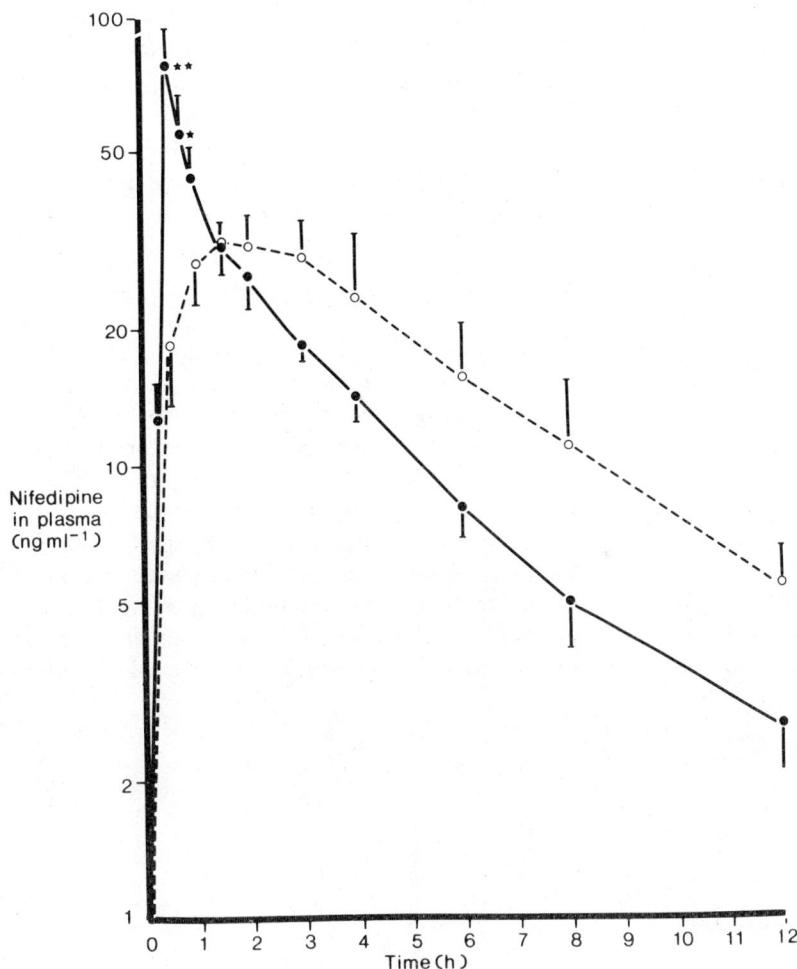

Fig. 73.2. Plasma concentration–time curves after a 10-mg capsule formulation of nifedipine (●——●, $n = 8$) and a 20-mg sustained-release formulation (○---○, $n = 6$) was given to healthy volunteers.

well absorbed (>95%) from the intestine,[30,31] provided that motility of the stomach is normal. However, more ionized compounds including atenolol are absorbed to an extent of <50%.[32] At the other extreme, highly charged molecules such as the aminoglycoside antibiotics such as gentamicin do not undergo significant absorption from the gastro-intestinal tract, and, therefore, must be given by injection, i.e. parenterally.

BIOAVAILABILITY OF ORALLY ADMINISTERED DRUGS

The proportion of a drug that reaches the systemic circulation in an unchanged state is termed its 'bioavailability'. This is normally measured from the concentration–time curve for the drug after two different routes of administration, e.g. oral and intravenous (Fig. 73.4). For some drugs, e.g. the anti-arrhythmic disopyramide, bioavailability is high, averaging 86%.[33] For others, e.g. amiloride,

bioavailability is poor due to incomplete absorption of this highly charged molecule.

Having undergone absorption from the gastro-intestinal tract, drugs then pass in portal venous blood to the liver. Although drugs like propranolol and lignocaine are almost completely absorbed, in the liver they are subject to extensive extraction and metabolism at the first passage which reduces their bioavailability. This process is often referred to as first pass metabolism. More correctly, it should be termed 'pre-systemic drug elimination'.[34] For propranolol, the limited bioavailability can be overcome by increasing the size of the oral dose.[35] By contrast, for lignocaine, pre-systemic metabolism is not readily saturable[36] and it leads to the generation of toxic metabolites. After oral administration of lignocaine, the plasma concentration of its major metabolite, monoethylglycinexylidide, is similar to that of the parent drug.[36] This and the other metabolite, glycinexylidide, may potentiate central nervous system toxicity of lignocaine[37] and produce

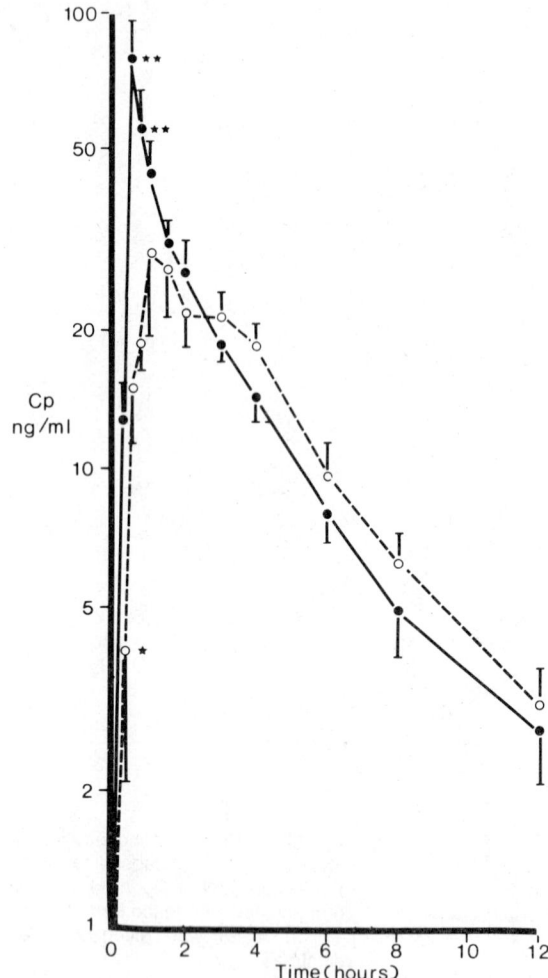

Fig. 73.3. Plasma concentration–time curve after 10-mg capsule formulation of nifedipine was given to 8 healthy volunteers while fasting (●——●) or following a standard breakfast (○– – –○).

propranolol is almost completely absorbed from the gut, this effect is likely to be due to reduced first pass metabolism in the liver, perhaps through increased rates of drug absorption and liver blood flow.[46] In contrast, food has no effect on the bioavailability of sustained release propranolol possibly due to slower delivery to the liver.[47,48]

INTRAVENOUS DOSING

Intravenous dosing has the advantage of rapid onset of action and complete biological availability. An example of the speed of action is shown in Fig. 73.5. Despite its advantages (which include the fact that it is the preferred route for administration of blood and blood products) the intravenous route has many disadvantages, the most important of which is the distribution of drugs in high concentrations to organs that enjoy a rich blood supply, e.g. the brain and heart. Thus, rapid intravenous injection of potassium can cause cessation of cardiac activity

convulsions before therapeutic lignocaine concentrations are achieved.[38] Oral administration of the drug, therefore, is inappropriate and it must be given by parenteral injection, which may be either intravenous or intramuscular.

It is important to consider the potential interaction between food and bioavailability of orally administered drugs. Food may reduce the amount of drug reaching the systemic circulation as is the case with atenolol[39] and captopril.[40] However, the results of a study with captopril[41] suggested there was little difference in the control of blood pressure between administration in the fed and that in the fasted state. In contrast, food enhances the bioavailability of digoxin,[42] dicoumarol,[43] hydrochlorothiazide[44] and propranolol.[45,46] Since

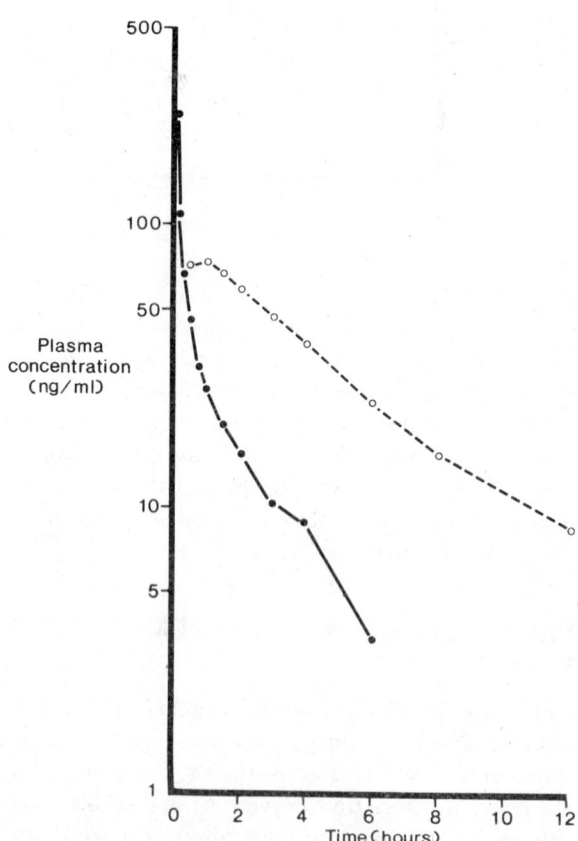

Fig. 73.4. Plasma concentration–time curves after single doses of nifedipine by intravenous (3.5 mg, ●——●) or oral (20 mg, ○----○) routes in a healthy volunteer.

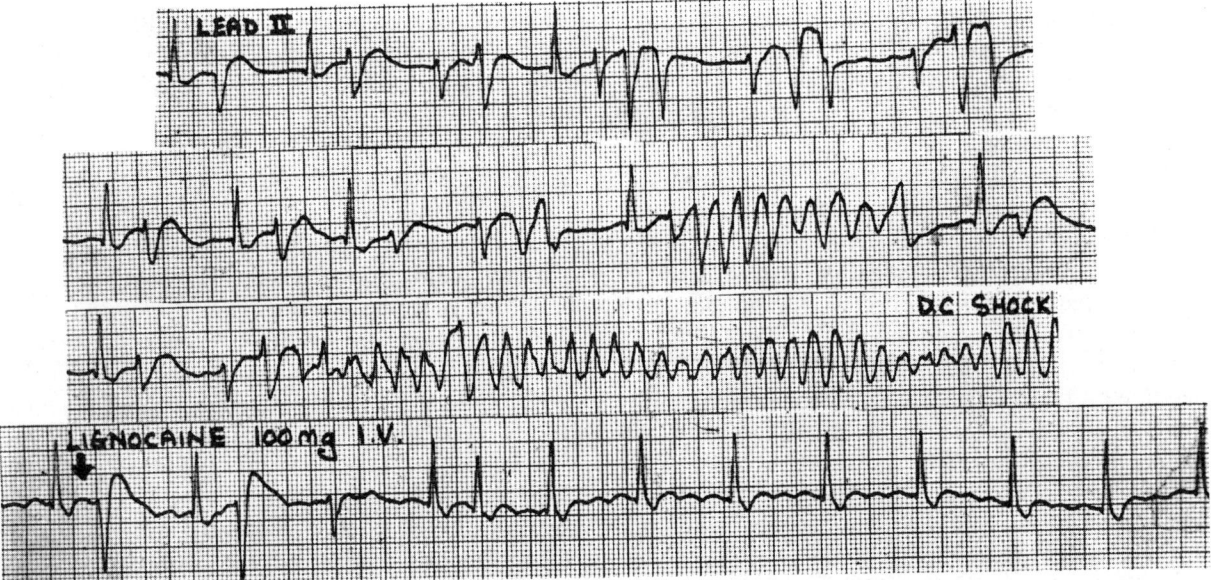

Fig. 73.5. Continuous electrocardiographic recording showing suppression of ventricular ectopic beats by intravenous lignocaine following direct current cardioversion for ventricular fibrillation. (By permission of Dr J.W. Upward.)

and, with the intravenous administration of other drugs, hypotension is quite common.[49] Furthermore, the duration of drug action can be quite short due to redistribution to other tissues. A good example is the return of arrhythmias following an initial intravenous bolus injection of lignocaine.

INTRAMUSCULAR ADMINISTRATION

The intramuscular route offers a slower absorption into the systemic circulation and, therefore, a 'depot effect'. Thus, the duration of action of intramuscular antibiotics of the penicillin and aminoglycoside series is prolonged, as is that of lignocaine (Fig. 73.6).[50,51] The intramuscular route of administration, however, is unsuitable for phenytoin because this drug precipitates out in the muscles; absorption, therefore, is very poor.[52]

TRANSDERMAL ABSORPTION

Interest in the transdermal route for application of drugs has increased in recent years. Cutaneous nitroglycerine for angina was the first example[53] and other drugs have been tested more recently. One advantage of the route is that first pass

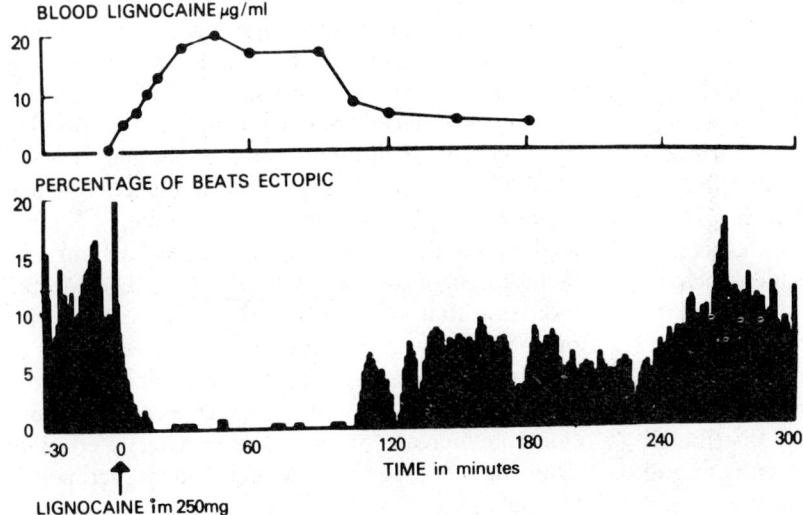

Fig. 73.6. Suppression of premature ectopic beats in a continuous electrocardiographic recording following intramuscular lignocaine. The plasma lignocaine concentrations and percentage of total beats that were ectopic are shown in the upper and lower graphs, respectively. (By permission of Dr D.E. Jewitt.)

metabolism in the liver is avoided, and, if a drug 'reservoir' is used, sustained plasma drug concentrations can be maintained throughout one or more days from a single application. Rate-controlled delivery systems prolong the effects of the drugs that have short half-lives after oral administration, e.g. glyceryl trinitrate. Reducing the frequency of drug administration can also aid compliance, and this is one reason for investigation of transdermal clonidine patches during once weekly application for the control of hypertension.[54,55] Transdermal penetration rates differ widely among drugs, depending on their physicochemical properties[56] and, therefore, not all drugs are suitable for this route of administration. The efficiency of permeability will also depend on the degree of ionization (and thus pH) of the drug, and hydration of the skin. A further complicating factor is the variable permeability of skin at different body sites (and on the same sites in individuals).

DRUG DISTRIBUTION

The extent of drug distribution to the tissues varies according to several factors.

1 The *physicochemical characteristics*. Lipid-soluble agents are able to diffuse freely across cell membranes and into the central nervous system. By contrast, water-soluble agents are less able to traverse membranes and do not concentrate to a significant extent in the tissues.

2 The *molecular weight* of the substance. Heparin is a large highly charged molecule and is confined mainly to the blood volume. By contrast, propranolol which is very lipid soluble has a large distribution volume[31] due to its ability to cross cell membranes and concentrate in the lungs and central nervous system.[57]

3 The extent of *binding to plasma proteins*. Drug that is attached to protein is not available for immediate distribution to the tissues whereas that which is free in plasma water is not only pharmacologically active but also available for distribution and/or metabolism. Acidic molecules such as warfarin tend to bind to basic proteins, especially albumin.[58] By contrast, basic molecules such as propranolol and lignocaine are avidly bound to acidic proteins especially α_1 acid glycoprotein.[59–61]

4 The rate and pattern of drug distribution is influenced by its *method of administration*. Intravenously administered drugs are distributed rapidly to the central circulatory compartment and subsequently redistributed. By contrast, orally administered drugs are more slowly distributed (and in lower concentration) following absorption from the gastro-intestinal tract and passage through the liver.

DRUG METABOLISM

Metabolism is an important method by which the action of many drugs is terminated. Two phases can be recognized: phase I (pre-conjugation) and phase II (conjugation or synthetic). Phase I reactions include oxidation, reduction and hydrolysis, in which chemically reactive groupings are appended or revealed. These groupings may serve for the subsequent attachment of other chemical groupings during phase II metabolism.

Many phase I reactions take place in the so-called mixed function oxidase enzyme systems located in the smooth endoplasmic reticulum (microsomes) of cells. The majority of such cells exist within the liver but other sites at which metabolism can occur include the small intestinal mucosa and lung.[62,63] The hydroxylating enzyme system, cytochrome P_{450}, which carries out most of the phase I oxidative metabolism, is a family of several iso-enzymes with overlapping specificity.[64,65] Their chemical specificity includes stereoselectivity, shown for the metabolism of the enantiomers of warfarin[67,68] and verapamil.[69] Considerable variation in activity of the cytochrome P_{450} system is found between individuals, resulting in differences in the elimination half-life after a single dose and the steady-state plasma concentrations during multiple dosing with many drugs. Thus, several-fold differences in the rate of metabolism have been reported for drugs such as phenytoin,[70] warfarin[71] and propranolol.[72] The activity of these enzymes is in part determined genetically, but environmental factors have important modulatory effects. The amount and activity of the enzyme may be increased by certain drugs known as inducers of microsomal oxidation.[73,74] The activity of different iso-enzymes may not be affected to the same degree by these agents, which include components of tobacco smoke,[75,76] ethyl alcohol and therapeutic agents such as barbiturates, dichloralphenazone and haloperidol.[77] The enzyme induction that occurs after starting treatment with one of these drugs will gradually increase the rate of inactivation of other drugs metabolized by the cytochrome P_{450} system. As a consequence, considerable increases in dose of a previously effective drug may be required to maintain a therapeutic response.[78]

Other drugs inhibit microsomal enzyme metabolism and these include allopurinol, alcohol, dextropropoxyphene and cimetidine.[77,79,80] Again, specificity for particular iso-enzymes may be found.[68]

In addition to the oxidative P_{450} systems, the liver contains flavin enzymes responsible for reduction of azo and nitro groups. The benzodiazepine, nitrazepam, is an example of a drug metabolized by these enzymes. The third type of reaction, hydrolysis, is carried out by various esterases and amidases which metabolize compounds such as procaine and lignocaine. For other compounds, such as sulphinpyrazone,[81] the gut flora are responsible for a considerable degree of pre-systemic metabolism, in addition to degrading hepatic conjugates and contributing to enterohepatic circulation of drugs.[82]

Most phase I reactions lead to a reduction in the activity of the drug molecule but there are exceptions. Among these are formation of 4-hydroxypropranolol[83,84] and of enalaprilat from enalapril.[85] Similarly, hydrolysis of pivampicillin liberates the active molecule, ampicillin,[86] which is used in prophylaxis against infective endocarditis.

Some of the synthetic phase II reactions that can occur are shown in Table 73.1. Some, such as glucuronidation, occur within the microsomal enzyme system within the liver; others involve cell sap enzymes, e.g. N-acetyltransferase which has an important genetic component in its activity. There is polymodal genetic inheritance of this enzyme system so that the majority of individuals are either fast or slow acetylators. Drugs metabolized via this system include procainamide[87] and hydralazine.[87-89] The specific activity of this enzyme system, therefore, will determine the magnitude and duration of the effects of these two drugs. Furthermore,

the incidence of adverse drug reactions, especially the systemic lupus erythematosus syndrome, is affected by the acetylator status.[90-92]

Not all drug metabolism occurs in the liver; drug metabolizing enzymes are found also in the lung and kidney. Enzymes in the gut lumen or mucosal lining may contribute to pre-systemic elimination and are responsible for ester hydrolysis; for example, converting pivampicillin to the active derivative, ampicillin.[86] There is little capacity for other phase I reactions, but conjugation reactions are active, an important example being the sulphation of isoprenaline.[93]

DRUG ELIMINATION

Although drugs can be eliminated to some extent in tears, sweat and breast milk, the most important organ of excretion of water-soluble compounds or metabolites is the kidney.

Renal elimination of drugs

There are three factors affecting the rate and extent of drug excretion in the urine: glomerular filtration, tubular secretion and tubular reabsorption. Glomerular filtration is an important determinant of excretion for water-soluble compounds such as the aminoglycoside antibiotics, certain anti-arrhythmics, such as procainamide and disopyramide, the water-soluble beta-adrenoceptor antagonists, including practolol, atenolol and sotalol, as well as many diuretics, e.g. amiloride. Only the free fraction of drug is available for excretion in this manner. As digoxin is approximately 30% bound to plasma proteins, its removal via the glomeruli

Table 73.1. Synthetic phase II reactions.

	Enzyme	Examples
Glucuronide synthesis	Glucuronyl transferase	Phenytoin Labetalol
Glycine conjugation	Transacylase	Salicylate
Sulphate synthesis	Sulphokinase	Isoprenaline Methyldopa
Methylation	Catechol-O-methyl transferase	Isoprenaline Methyldopa
Acetylation	N-Acetyl transferase	Hydralazine Procainamide
Mercapturic acid synthesis	Glutathione transferase	Paracetamol
Glutamine synthesis	Glutamine transferase	Para-aminosalicylate

approximates to 70% of glomerular filtration rates. Rates of glomerular filtration are increased in thyrotoxicosis and diminished in myxoedema, in many forms of heart disease (cardiac output is reduced) and in old age.[94]

Tubular secretion is responsible for the active elimination of acidic molecules in the urine. This process, which can be blocked by the uricosuric probenecid, is responsible for the very rapid rates of elimination of both penicillins and cephalosporins. Tubular secretion accounts for some of the renal elimination of digitalis glycosides.[95]

Drugs that have reached the distal convoluted tubule may be either charged, e.g. gentamicin and amiloride, or in the non-ionized form, e.g. propranolol, lignocaine and warfarin. Those that are non-ionized are reabsorbed by passive (pH-dependent) diffusion. However, for a small number of cardiovascular-acting drugs, the rate and extent of renal elimination is affected by urinary pH. A good example is quinidine, the excretion of which is facilitated by acidification of the urine.[96]

Biliary elimination of drugs

The biliary excretion of drugs has been the subject of an extensive review by Smith.[82] For drugs to be excreted in the bile, they must have a molecular structure that possesses affinities for both the aqueous and lipid domains of the micelle. Another important determinant of whether a drug is eliminated in bile is its molecular weight. Biliary excretion tends to be relatively unimportant in man because the threshold for elimination by this route lies at a molecular weight of around 500 daltons.[97] Thus, glucuronidation of drugs by the liver has two important consequences. First, glucuronides are strong acids and second the glucuronide grouping increases the molecular weight of the drug by 176 daltons which may facilitate its excretion into the bile. Drugs that undergo excretion by this route include rifampicin and its 25-desacetyl metabolite.[98] Digitoxin is also eliminated in the bile;[99] however, a significant proportion is reabsorbed from the small intestine, a process referred to as enterohepatic recirculation. This has the effect of prolonging its action.

Methods of estimating the rate of drug elimination

The majority of drugs are removed from the body in an exponential fashion, implying that a fixed proportion of the dose is removed in unit time. This type of removal is said to obey first order kinetics. Thus, for these drugs, if the logarithm of their concentration is plotted against time, a straight line relationship will be obtained. The time taken to fall from a concentration of $2x$ to x units can be calculated from this relationship (Fig. 73.7). This gives rise to a measurement known as the half-life. In practice, this is usually estimated from the slope of the regression line and is equal to $-k_{\mathrm{elim}}/2.3$

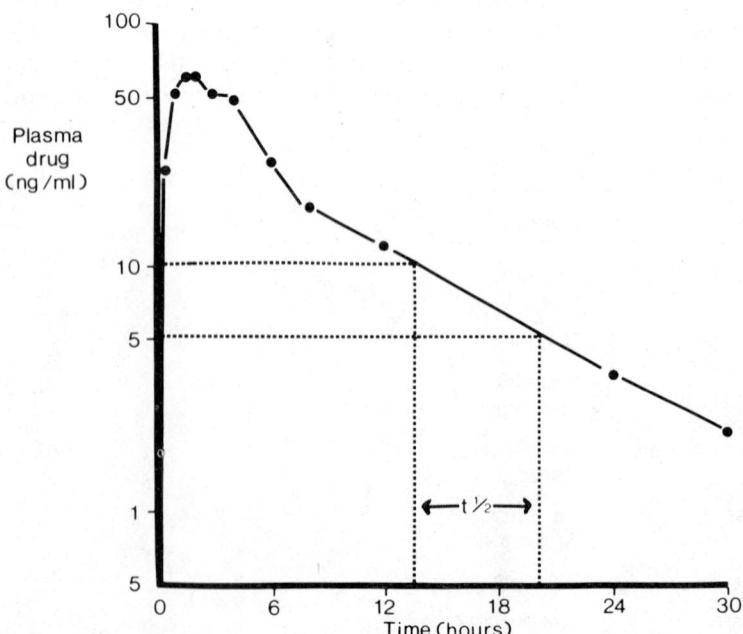

Fig. 73.7. Log plasma concentration plotted against time to show the derivation of plasma elimination half-life after oral administration.

where k_{elim} is the overall first order elimination rate constant and has the dimensions of either minutes or hours and 2.3 represents log e to the base 10; $t_{1/2}$ is then equal to $0.693/k_{elim}$.

This parameter is subject to certain errors in that it assumes that the second phase of the concentration–time curve represents only drug elimination. Not infrequently, particularly after single doses, it is a hybrid representing not only elimination and metabolism but also distribution into the tissues (where access is slow).

With a few drugs, such as phenytoin,[100] the elimination is saturable and linear with time and said to obey zero order kinetics. The relationship between dose and plasma concentration, therefore, is non-linear, but the dose at which saturation occurs shows considerable interindividual variation. The clinical significance of this is that small changes in drug metabolizing capacity can result in marked changes in steady-state serum phenytoin concentrations.

Clearance

Clearance is a more precise estimate of the body's efficiency to remove a drug. This term refers to the total volume of blood or plasma from which a drug is irreversibly removed in unit time.

$$\text{Clearance (C1)} = V_d \times 0.693\, t_{1/2}$$

Alternatively, clearance can be calculated from the ratio of the injected dose to the area under the concentration–time curve from zero to infinite time. Clearance will reflect changes produced by altered protein binding and metabolic capacity which may or may not necessarily be reflected in the $t_{1/2}$.

PLASMA CONCENTRATIONS DURING REGULAR THERAPY

When plasma drug concentrations are closely related to therapeutic effect, the aim of mutliple drug dosing should be to maintain a constant effective plasma concentration between dosing. At 'steady state', the plasma drug concentration will fluctuate around an average value, and the degree of fluctuation will depend on three main factors. The most important determinants are the elimination half-life and the dose interval. The shorter the half-life, the greater the fluctuations in plasma concentrations between dosing. Independently of this, the shorter the dosing interval, the less will be the variability of the plasma concentration around the mean. For

example, giving a single 200 mg dose of a drug with an interval of one half-life between dosing will result in about a 30% variation of plasma concentration at steady state. If two separate doses of 100 mg are given during the same time-interval, that variation will be reduced to about 17%. The third factor is the rate of absorption; slow absorption tends to blunt the fluctuations. Thus, the choice of dosing regimen will depend on drug formulation, the therapeutic to toxic dose ratio and a knowledge of the relationship between plasma concentration and desired effect throughout the dosing interval.

During repetitive dosing a '*steady-state*' plasma concentration will be achieved about 5 half-lives after initiating treatment. For example, if treatment is initiated with digoxin ($t_{1/2}$ 36 h) using a regular maintenance dose, steady-state concentration will be achieved after about 7 days. In contrast, digitoxin with a half-life of 5 days will take approximately 4 weeks to achieve steady state. Therefore, when a rapid onset of action is required and the half-life of the drug is long, it will be necessary to use a loading dose. The appropriate loading dose can be calculated as follows:

$$\text{Loading dose} = 1.44 \times t_{1/2} \times \frac{\text{Maintenance dose}}{\text{Dose-interval}}$$

A single loading dose is often used, but if the drug has a low therapeutic index, such as digoxin, the loading dose may need to be given as a number of smaller doses over a short time-interval.

AGE AND THE RESPONSE TO CARDIOVASCULAR DRUGS

The physiological changes that accompany advancing age may influence the handling of drugs in a variety of ways.[101] Some changes in gastrointestinal function occur in the elderly. The reduced rate of gastric emptying slows the rate but not the extent of digoxin absorption,[102] which will not alter the steady-state concentrations or clinical effect. However, for other drugs, such as aspirin, no effect of age on absorption has been found.[103] Changes in body composition in the elderly, which include reduced plasma albumin, increased fat content and reduced body water, may influence drug distribution. Lipid-soluble drugs, e.g. lignocaine, will tend to have a higher volume of distribution and lower blood levels,[104] whereas the converse is to be expected with a polar drug such as atenolol.[105]

Plasma protein binding, especially to albumin, may be reduced in the elderly. Thus, warfarin binding capacity is reduced with advancing age,[106] but saturation of binding is unlikely at therapeutic blood concentrations. However, the potential for interaction with other drugs that displace warfarin from its binding site is increased.[107]

As liver weight and blood flow fall with age, the plasma concentrations of drugs with high pre-systemic elimination and flow-dependent kinetics will be increased. This explains the higher plasma propranolol concentrations in the elderly after single and multiple dosing.[108-110]

The glomerular filtration rate declines with age,[94] which will reduce the elimination of polar parent drugs, such as digoxin,[111] and of certain active or toxic metabolites, such as the lignocaine metabolite, 4-hydroxyxylidine.[104] It is important to recognize that serum creatinine concentration is a poor guide to glomerular filtration rate in the elderly because creatinine production falls with age. A more accurate measure can be calculated by simple equations, such as that devised by Cockcroft and Gault,[112] which allow prediction of creatinine clearance from age, sex, weight and serum creatinine concentration without the need for urine collection.

Less is understood about receptor sensitivity to drugs in the elderly. Age appears to increase the sensitivity to anticoagulants such as heparin[113,114] and warfarin,[113,114] but complex pharmacokinetic and pharmacodynamic factors are probably involved.[115] Beta-adrenoceptor density decreases linearly with increasing age,[116] which may explain a reduced effect of isoprenaline on heart rate in elderly subjects[117] and the reduced sensitivity of beta-adrenoceptors to inhaled beta-adrenoceptor agonists.[118]

Thus, the effects of age on the response to drugs are variable and frequently unpredictable. For this reason, some general principles should be followed in prescribing for older patients,[101,119] who frequently will also have concurrent disease states that may alter drug handling or effects. The initial doses of most drugs should be smaller than those given to younger patients. If the drug is eliminated slowly, a reduction in individual doses is the most convenient way to achieve this. For drugs that have shorter elimination half-lives, increasing the dosage interval may be more appropriate. The dosage regimen should be as simple as possible to aid compliance (see below) and the requirement for continued treatment needs to be regularly reviewed.

EFFECT OF RENAL IMPAIRMENT ON PHARMACOKINETICS

Reduced renal function is commonly found in patients with hypertension or heart failure. Drugs normally excreted by the kidney will accumulate during repeated dosing in the presence of renal impairment. If a drug is eliminated almost entirely by glomerular filtration, there will be a linear relationship between creatinine clearance and K_{elim}, and a curvilinear relationship between creatinine clearance and half-life. For practical purposes, a substantial prolongation of half-life is found only when renal function is markedly reduced (i.e. a creatinine clearance below about 30 ml/min). In this situation, the drug dose should be reduced or the interval between doses increased.[120,121] The relationship between glomerular filtration rate and drug elimination is less direct if renal tubular or extrarenal drug elimination occurs. Guidance on dosage modification for individual drugs in patients with renal impairment can be found in the British National Formulary.

Other factors also affect drug response in renal impairment. Uraemia may alter drug metabolism, generally having little effect on oxidative reactions but causing impairment of reductive and hydrolytic enzymes.

Plasma protein binding of drugs such as phenytoin also decreases in uraemia,[122] which will increase the apparent distribution volume and decrease total plasma drug concentrations. In contrast, the free fraction, and therefore the active drug, will be increased.

The clinical effects of these changes are difficult to predict but the increased unbound fraction of drug may increase both therapeutic and adverse effects; at the same time, clearance will increase, particularly by liver metabolism. As a result of the altered handling and response to drugs in the presence of considerable impairment of renal function, it is advisable to initiate treatment with smaller drug doses than usual.

CARDIAC DISEASE AND THE RESPONSE TO DRUGS

Despite the obvious importance of the heart in determining regional blood flow, there have been comparatively few well-controlled studies of the effects of cardiac disease on the handling of drugs in the body. However, from the foregoing discussion, it should be apparent that cardiac disease could affect the response to drugs in a number of ways.

1   The bioavailability, half-life or clearance of a drug may change.

2   The response of the end organ (target tissue) may vary.

3   Concurrent drug therapy may influence the response (see below).

In much of the work that has been reported, it has been assumed that patients with cardiac disease represent a homogeneous group. This is clearly erroneous. Response to treatment may vary with the aetiology of the heart disease, its severity and the age of the patient. For example, beta-adrenoceptor antagonists may cause bradycardia, hypotension or cardiac standstill in patients who have suffered a recent myocardial infarction.[123,124] In addition to these obvious factors, response to drugs of the cardiac glycoside series, for example, is influenced also by the oxygen tension of the blood[125] and prevailing concentrations of sodium, potassium, calcium and magnesium;[126,127] but, most important of all, is whether the patient's heart is in sinus rhythm or in atrial fibrillation.

ALTERED PHARMACOKINETICS IN CARDIAC DISEASE

It is well recognized that absorption of drugs from the subcutaneous and intramuscular sites is dependent upon blood flow, but there are comparatively few data to show that splanchnic blood flow has a similar importance for absorption from the gut. Exceptions include studies on various non-dissociable substances examined by Winne and Remischovsky[128] in rat jejunal loops and cardiac glycosides in the guinea-pig.[129] However, there is little published evidence that cardiac decompensation has any effect on drug absorption from the gut.[130] Changes in gastro-intestinal function due to oedema of the bowel wall, reduced splanchnic blood flow and altered gastro-intestinal motility might affect drug absorption. Significant abnormalities have been reported with hydrochlorothiazide,[131] procainamide,[132] metolazone,[133] quinidine[134] and frusemide.[135] For most other drugs, any variations seen in their plasma concentrations relate to differences in their distribution[136,139] or delayed metabolism associated with diminished hepatic blood flow.

Reduced cardiac output in congestive heart failure leads to a proportional reduction in liver blood flow.[138,140] Lignocaine clearance is decreased in this situation[136,139] and steady-state plasma concentrations are inversely proportional to estimated liver blood flow.[138,140] As the extraction of lignocaine by the liver is dependent on flow, the rate of drug delivery is the major determinant of removal. The influence of congestive heart failure on the elimination of flecainide, which is largely excreted unchanged by the kidney, is less marked with only slight reduction of plasma clearance.[141,142]

Following myocardial infarction, changes in acute phase reactant proteins will increase the binding of basic drugs such as lignocaine. Thus, total plasma concentrations may rise, whereas free (and hence active) concentrations do not change significantly.[143] This apparent drug accumulation may make interpretation of plasma drug concentrations more difficult and lead to administration of sub-therapeutic doses of the drug.

ADVERSE EFFECTS OF DRUGS

Adverse or unwanted effects of drugs are common and fall into several categories.

1   The adverse effects may be predictable from the known pharmacological properties of the drug. There are many important examples of this in cardiovascular therapy, such as postural hypotension with vasodilators and bronchospasm induced by beta-adrenoceptor antagonists. This type of unwanted effect can usually be avoided or minimized either by the choice of suitable dosage or by the use of alternative medicines.

2   The unwanted effects may be idiosyncratic and unpredictable. Most such reactions are genetically determined and due to a total or relative deficiency of a certain enzyme, for example, some patients have impaired ability to hydroxylate debrisoquine. In these individuals, hypotension may be profound following a standard oral dose.[144-146] Similar genetic polymorphism occurs in the metabolism of metoprolol. After a single oral dose, the reduction in exercise tachycardia 24 h later is inversely related to the rate of metabolism.[146]

3   The adverse effect may be drug allergy due to an obvious or suspected immunological reaction. These reactions may be immediate (antibody-mediated effects due to IgE) or delayed (involving both antibody- and cell-mediated effects). Immediate hypersensitivity reactions include urticaria, bronchospasm and angioneurotic oedema: if the reaction is severe, anaphylactic shock occurs. An important example of this is seen with penicillin,

occurring minutes after intravenous injection. A less important reaction is more commonly seen with ampicillin, with a skin rash due to delayed cell-mediated immunity, particularly common in patients who have glandular fever. Other examples include haemolytic anaemia with a positive Coombs' test during treatment with methyldopa, and the development of systemic lupus erythematosus with hydralazine or procainamide.

There has been increasing recognition that adverse effects may occur on withdrawal of a therapeutic agent. An early example was the rebound hypertension reported when clonidine was abruptly stopped in hypertensive patients.[147,148] This reaction appears to be due to increased sympathetic activity precipitated by withdrawal of its suppression by the drug. Many other medicines have since been implicated in sudden withdrawal reactions, e.g. the withdrawal of beta-adrenoceptor antagonists in patients who have angina pectoris may lead to unstable angina, the development of ventricular arrhythmias or myocardial infarction.[146,150] The explanations advanced for these effects include the patient becoming accustomed to a greater level of exertion during treatment, and progress of the underlying disease. However, a significant increase or 'up-regulation' of post-synaptic beta-adrenoceptors occurs during long-term treatment with beta-blockade which increases sensitivity to the sympathetic nervous system after withdrawal of the drug.[151] Similar withdrawal reactions have also been reported for calcium antagonists.[152]

It is not always possible to identify patients at risk from adverse reactions. However, certain patients are in high-risk categories. The incidence of adverse reactions is greatest in the very young, due to immature mechanisms for handling drugs and different tissue responsiveness,[153,154] and in the very old. Patients with a history of atopy or previous drug allergy have an increased risk of subsequent allergic drug reactions.[155,156] In patients who have liver or renal disease, adverse reactions are also more common due to altered drug metabolism or drug elimination. Owing to the risk of rebound, care should always be taken when withdrawing long-term treatment from patients with angina or hypertension.

DRUG INTERACTIONS

There are several situations in the treatment of cardiovascular disease when multiple drug therapy may be desirable.

1 A combination of drugs may be necessary to achieve an effect that cannot be attained when using one drug alone. Examples of this are seen in the stepped-care approach for resistant hypertension, and the simultaneous use of more than one antibiotic in the treatment of infective endocarditis.

2 A drug may be given to minimize the side-effect of another, e.g. potassium supplements or a potassium-conserving diuretic in patients receiving loop diuretics.

3 Several diseases may co-exist and require independent treatment, e.g. hypertension, diabetes mellitus and arthritis.

Although multiple drug therapy may be necessary and of benefit to the patient, the risk of unfavourable interactions rises exponentially with the number of drugs given. Fortunately, the majority of these interactions are of little clinical significance. Some interactions in the gastro-intestinal tract have already been considered. A further example is the adsorption of warfarin and digitoxin by cholestyramine.[157]

Interactions may also occur in the circulation, such as those involving competition for protein binding sites, which are important if one drug is highly protein bound with a small free (and thus therapeutically active) fraction and has a narrow therapeutic ratio. Warfarin is up to 98% bound to plasma protein, and an increased anticoagulant effect with haemorrhage may be produced following displacement by drugs such as azapropazone and co-trimoxazole.[158,159] Simple displacement reactions are usually short-lived because the increased free drug is rapidly eliminated by metabolism or excretion. A different type of interaction in the circulation is the prolongation of the elimination half-life and plasma steady-state concentration of lignocaine when propranolol is given. Reduced cardiac output and hence reduced liver blood flow are responsible for this effect.[52]

Important interactions may occur due to changes in liver metabolism. Induction and inhibition of the P_{450} enzyme system by drugs have been considered above. An alteration in the metabolism of warfarin when one of these agents is added to the regime may lead to substantial changes in therapeutic effect. In general, interactions due to enzyme induction require 2–3 weeks to become fully developed, whereas inhibitors of microsomal enzymes usually have an immediate effect.

Adverse pharmacodynamic interactions occur at

Table 73.2. Main uses and parameters of four therapeutic drugs.

Drug	Main cardiac uses (s)	Dose-response	Individual differences	Clearance iv ml/min	$t_{1/2}$ (h)	Vd (l/kg)	Binding (%)	Absorption (%)	Bioavailability (%)
Propranolol	Angina Arrhythmias Hypertension	Yes Yes No	+++ +++ +	≈ 1000	2.3	4.5	96	98+	30[a]
Digoxin	Atrial fibrillation Heart failure	Yes Unclear	+ +/-	175	36	10	30	70	70
Captopril	Hypertension Heart failure	Yes Unclear	+ +/-	900	1.9	0.7	25	70	70
Nifedipine	Angina Hypertension	Yes Yes	++ ++	550	2.0	1.0	93	≃ 100	43

Table 73.2 continued

Drug	Loading dose	Slow release	% renal excretion	% metabolized	Renal disease	Hepatic disease	Age	Other drugs	Smoking
Propranolol	No	Yes	<1	99	Little or no effect	Major effect	Moderate effect or kinetics	Cimetidine increases effect. Indomethacin reduces effect in hypertension	Decreases effect
Digoxin	Yes	No	75	<25	Major effect	No effect	Moderate	Cimetidine no effect. Diuretics enhance effects. Action increased by some anti-arrhythmics and quinine	No known effect
Captopril	No	No	35	65	Moderate effect	Moderate effect to be expected	Probable increase in effect in hypertension	Cimetidine no effect. Diuretics increase effect. Indomethacin decreases effect in hypertension	Not known
Nifedipine	No	Yes	<1	99	No effect	Moderate effect to be expected	Moderate effect on kinetics	Cimetidine increases effects	No effects

[a] Dose dependent.

the site of drug action. One example is the production of asystole due to inhibition of conduction through the atrioventricular node when intravenous beta-adrenoceptor antagonists are given to patients who are receiving verapamil.[150,161] A further example is the observation that many non-steroidal anti-inflammatory drugs can antagonize the natriuretic and hypotensive effects of the benzothiadiazine diuretics.[162]

Interactions should always be considered before prescribing for patients receiving drugs with a narrow therapeutic index, such as warfarin, phenytoin and digoxin. It is not possible, however, to memorize all potential interactions and the possibility of interaction should be considered if any drug has an unexpectedly large effect or if the patient fails to respond to the usual therapeutic dose. Avoidance of interactions by limiting the number of drugs prescribed is probably the most effective preventive action.

COMPLIANCE WITH TREATMENT

Non-compliance with prescribed treatment is common and may explain an apparent failure to respond.[163] The problem is particularly marked in patients who have asymptomatic conditions such as hypertension,[164–166] compliance decreasing with increasing duration of treatment.[164] Compliance is often equally poor in symptomatic conditions such as heart failure and is apparently unrelated to the severity of symptoms.[167] It has been estimated that up to 50% of patients fail to take prescribed medicines regularly,[168,169] and incorrect timing or dosage probably occurs in many others. However, compliance rates for cardiac drugs appear to be higher than those for other groups such as analgesics, antibiotics and sedatives.[170]

The reasons for poor compliance are complex and improvements may require several different approaches. It is important to limit the number of prescribed medicines, because compliance falls when more than three drugs are given.[171] There is less substantial evidence that dose frequency is an important factor in compliance, but reducing administration to once or twice daily is probably beneficial.[172–175] Written reminder letters were found to be of value in elderly hypertensives,[176] but it is important to ensure that any instructions are clearly understandable.[177] Unfortunately, educating the patient about the disease or drug treatment does not appear to influence compliance with long-term treatment.

ADDENDUM

The principles discussed in this chapter are illustrated in relation to four drugs, namely propranolol, digoxin, captopril and nifedipine. Their main uses are tabulated (Table 73.2), together with an indication of whether a dose–response curve exists. Other parameters include the extent of interindividual differences, the pharmacokinetic characteristics of the drugs and how these should determine whether a loading dose is given, and the effects of disease, smoking and concurrent drug therapy.

REFERENCES

1. Ridout, S., Waters, W.E. and George, C.F. Knowledge and attitudes to medicines in the Southampton community. *Br. J. Clin. Pharmac.* 1986; **21**: 701.
2. Williamson, J. Adverse reactions to prescribed drugs in the elderly. In: Crooks, J. and Stevenson, I.H., eds. *Drugs and the Elderly: Perspectives in Geriatric Clinical Pharmacology.* London, Macmillan Press, 1979, p. 239
3. Hurwitz, N. Predisposing factors in adverse drug reactions. *Br. Med. J.* 1969; **1**: 536
4. Howe, R. and Shanks, R.G. Optical isomers of propranolol. *Nature* 1966; **210**: 1336.
5. Schwartz, A., Lindenmayer, G.E. and Allen, J.C. The sodium-potassium adenosine triphosphatase:pharmacological, physiological and biochemical aspects. *Pharmacol. Rev.* 1973; **27**: 3.
6. George, C.F., Swift, C.G. and Challenor, V.F. The effect of commonly used non-cardiac drugs on the heart and circulation. In: Luchi, R.J., ed. *Cardiology in the Elderly.* London: Churchill Livingstone, 1988.
7. Evans, N. and Hoyle, C. The comparative value of drugs used in the continuous treatment of angina pectoris. *Q. J. Med.* 1933; **26**: 311
8. Zacest, R. and Koch-Weser, J. Relation of propranolol plasma level to β-blockade during oral therapy. *Pharmacology* 1972; **7**: 178.
9. Cuthbert, M.F. and Collins, R.F. Plasma levels and ß-adrenoceptor blockade with acebutolol, practolol and propranolol in man. *Br. J. Clin. Pharmac.* 1975; **2**: 49.
10. McDevitt, D.G. and Shand, D.G. Plasma concentrations and the time course of beta-blockade due to propranolol. *Clin. Pharmac. Ther.* 1975; **18**: 708.
11. Thadani, U., Davidson, C., Singleton, W. and Taylor, S.H. Comparison of the immediate effects of five ß-adrenoceptor blocking drugs with different ancillary properties in angina pectoris. *N. Engl. J. Med.* 1979; **300**: 750.
12. Prichard, B.N.C. and Gillam, P.M.S. Assessment of propranolol in angina pectoris. Clinical dose-response curve and effect on electrocardiogram at rest and on exercise. *Br. Heart J.* 1971; **33**: 473.
13. George, C.F., Fenyvesi, T. and Dollery, C.T. In: Davies, D.S. and Prichard, B.N.C., eds. *Biological Effects of Drugs in Relation to their Plasma Concentrations.* London: Macmillan, 1973, p. 123.
14. Woosley, R.L. Kornhauser, D., Smith, R., Reele, S., Higgins, S.B., Nies, A.S., Shand, D.G. and Oates, J.A. Suppression of chronic ventricular arrhythmias with propranolol. *Circulation* 1979; **60**: 819.
15. Chamberlain, D.A., White, R.J., Howard, M.R. and Smith, T.W. Plasma digoxin concentrations in patients

with atrial fibrillation. *Br. Med. J.* 1970; 3: 429.

16. Follath, F., Heierli, B., Ganzinger, U. and Wenk, M. Serumkonzen-trationsmessungen zur Steuerung einer anti-arrhythmischen therapie mit Lidocain. *Sch. Med. Wochenschr.* 1980; 110: 1007.

17. Gianelly, R., von der Groeben, J.O., Spivack, A.P. and Harrison, D.C. Effect of lidocaine on ventricular arrhythmias in patients with coronary heart disease. *N. Engl. J. Med.* 1967; 277: 1215.

18. Harrison, D.C. and Alderman, E.L. Relation of blood levels to clinical effectiveness of lidocaine. In: Scott, D.B. and Julian, D.G. eds. *Lidocaine in the Treatment of Ventricular Arrhythmias.* Edinburgh and London: Livingstone, 1971, p. 178.

19. Eichelbaum, M., Birkel, P., Grube, E., Gutgemann, U. and Somogyi, A. Effects of verapamil on P-R intervals in relation to verapamil plasma levels following single i.v. and oral administration and during chronic treatment. *Klin. Wochenschr.* 1980; 58: 919.

20. Johnston, A., Burgess, C.D. and Hamer, J. Systemic availability of oral verapamil and effect on PR interval in man. *Br. J. Clin. Pharmac.* 1981; 12: 397.

21. Kreel, L., Trott, M. and Howells, T.H. The influence of oral metoclopramide on gastric emptying after a fixed water-load. *Clin. Radiol.* 1972; 23: 213.

22. Bateman, D.N. Studies on the pharmacological control of gastric emptying in man. *Br. J. Clin. Pharmac.* 1985; 20: 339.

23. Tothill, P., McLaughlin, G.P., Holt, S. and Heading, R.L. The effect of posture on errors in gastric emptying measurements. *Phys. Biol. Med.* 1980; 25: 1071.

24. Castleden, C.M., George, C.F. and Short, M.D. Contribution of individual differences in gastric emptying to variability in plasma propranolol concentrations. *Br. J. Clin. Pharmac.* 1978; 5: 121.

25. Minami, H. and McCallum, R.W. The physiology and pathophysiology of gastric emptying in humans. *Gastroenterology* 1984; 86: 1592.

26. Moore, J.G., Christian, P.E., Taylor, A.T. and Alazraki, N. Gastric emptying measurements: delayed and complex patterns without appropriate correction. *J. Nucl. Med.* 1985; 26: 1206.

27. Woodcock, B.G., Kraemer, N. and Rietbrock, N. Effect of a high protein meal on the bioavailability of verapamil. *Br. J. Clin. Pharmac.* 1986; 21: 337.

28. Challenor, V.F., Waller, D.G., Gruchy, B.S., Renwick, A.G. and George, C.F. Food and nifedipine pharmacokinetics. *Br. J. Clin. Pharmac.* 1987; 23: 248.

29. Clark, J.M., Ramsay, L.E., Shelton, J.R., Tidd, M.J., Murray, S. and Palmer, R.F. *J. Pharm. Sci.* 1977; 66: 1429.

30. Paterson, J.W., Conolly, M.E., Dollery, C.T., Hayes, A. and Cooper, R.G. The pharmacodynamics and metabolism of propranolol in man. *Pharmacol. Clin.* 1970; 2: 127.

31. Shand, D.G., Nuckolls, E.M. and Oates, J.A. Plasma propranolol levels in adults with observations in four children. *Clin. Pharmac. Ther.* 1970; 11: 112.

32. Reeves, P.R., McAinsh, J. McIntosh, D.A.D. and Winrow, M.J. Metabolism of atenolol in man. *Xenobiotica* 1978; 8: 313.

33. Whiting, B., Holford, N.H.G. and Sheiner, L.B. Quantitative analysis of the disopyramide concentration-effect relationship. *Br. J. Clin. Pharmac.* 1980; 9: 67.

34. George, C.F., Shand, D.G. and Renwick, A.G. *Presystemic Drug Elimination.* London: Butterworth Medical, 1982.

35. Shand, D.G. and Rangno, R.E. The disposition of propranolol I: Elimination during oral absorption in man. *Pharmacology* 1972; 7: 159.

36. Bending, M.R., Bennett, P.N., Rowland, M. and Steiner, J. Lignocaine pharmacokinetics in man: dose and time

studies. *Br. J. Clin. Pharmac.* 1976; 3: 956P.

37. Drayer, D.E. Pharmacologically active drug metabolites: therapeutic and toxic activities, plasma and urine data in man, accumulation in renal failure. *Clin. Pharmacokinet.* 1976; 1: 426.

38. Boyes, R.N., Scott, D.B., Jebson, P.J., Godman, M.J. and Julian, D.G. Pharmacokinetics of lidocaine in man. *Clin. Pharmac. Ther.* 1971; 12: 105.

39. Melander, A., Stenberg, P., Liedholm, H., Schersten, B. and Wahlin-Boll, E. Food-induced reduction in bioavailability of atenolol. *Eur. J. Clin. Pharmac.* 1979; 16: 327.

40. Williams, G.M. and Sugerman, A.A. The effect of a meal, at various times relative to drug administration, on the bioavailability of captopril. *J. Clin. Pharmacol.* 1982; 22: 18A.

41. Ohman, K.P., Kagedal, B., Larsson, R. and Karlberg, B.E. Pharmacokinetics of captopril and its effects on blood pressure during acute and chronic administration and in relation to food intake. *J. Cardiovasc. Pharmacol.* 1985; 7(Suppl. 1): S20.

42. Johnson, B.F., O'Grady, J., Sabey, G.A. and Bye, C. Effect of a standard breakfast on digoxin absorption in normal subjects. *Clin. Pharmac. Ther.* 1978; 23: 315.

43. Melander, A. and Wahlin, E. Enhancement of dicoumarol bioavailability by concomitant food intake. *Eur. J. Clin. Pharmac.* 1978; 14: 441.

44. Beermann, B. and Groschinsky-Grind, M. Enhancement of the gastrointestinal absorption of hydrochlorothiazide by propantheline. *Eur. J. Clin. Pharmacol.* 1978; 13: 385.

45. Melander, A., Danielson, K., Schersten, B. and Wahlin, E. Enhancement of the bioavailability of propranolol and metoprolol by food. *Clin. Pharmac. Ther.* 1977; 22: 108.

46. McLean, A.J., McNamara, P.J., du Souich, P., Gibaldi, M. and Lalka, D. Food, splanchnic blood flow and bioavailability of drugs subject to first-pass metabolism. *Clin. Pharmac. Ther.* 1978; 24: 5.

47. Byrne, A.J., McNeil, J.J., Harrison, P.M., Louis, W., Tonkin, A.M. and McLean, A.J. Stable oral availability in man of sustained release propranolol when coadministered with hydralazine or food. Evidence implicating substrate delivery rate as a determinant of presystemic drug interactions. *Br. J. Clin. Pharmac.* 1984; 17(Suppl.): 45S.

48. Liedholm, H., Wahlin-Boll, E., Hanson, A. and Melander, A. Influence of food on the bioavailability of 'real' and 'apparent' hydralazine from conventional and slow-release preparations. *Drug Nutrient Interact.* 1983; 1: 293.

49. Greenblatt, D.J. and Koch-Weser, J. Adverse reactions to propranolol in hospitalised medical patients: A report from the Boston Collaborative Drug Surveillance Program. *Am. Heart J.* 1973; 86: 478: 763.

50. Koch-Weser, J. Antiarrhythmic prophylaxis in ambulatory patients with coronary heart disease. *Arch. Intern. Med.* 1972; 129: 763.

51. Valentine, P.A., Frew, J.L., Marshford, M.L. and Sloman, J.G. Lidocaine in the prevention of sudden death in the pre-hospital phase of acute myocardial infarction: A double blind study. *N. Engl. J. Med.* 1974; 291: 1327.

52. Winkle, R.A., Glantz, S.A. and Harrison, D.C. Pharmacologic therapy of ventricular arrhythmias. *Am. J. Cardiol.* 1975; 36: 629.

53. Davis, J.A. and Wiesel, B.H. The treatment of angina pectoris with nitroglycerin ointment. *Am. J. Med.* 1955; 21: 230.

54. Mroczek, W.J., Ulrych, M. and Yoder, S. Weekly transdermal clonidine administration in hypertensive patients. *Clin. Pharmac. Ther.* 1982; 31: 352.

55. Michael, R.C., Jain, A.K., Ryan, J.R. and McMahon, F.G. A study to evaluate the efficacy and side effects of clonidine TTS as initial therapy in mild hypertension. *Clin. Pharmac. Ther.* 1983; 33: 229.

56. Scheuplein, R.J. and Blank, I.H. Permeability of the skin. *Physiol. Rev.* 1971; **51**: 702.

57. Hayes, A. and Cooper, R.G. Studies on the absorption, distribution and excretion of propranolol in rat, dog and monkey. *J. Pharmac. Exp. Ther.* 1971; **176**: 302.

58. O'Reilly, R.A. Interaction of the oral anticoagulant drug warfarin and its metabolites with human plasma albumin. *J. Clin. Invest.* 1969; **48**: 193.

59. Borga, O., Oder-Cederlof, J., Piafsky, K.M. and Sjoquist, F. Plasma protein binding of propranolol in disease states. *Br. J. Clin. Pharmac.* 1977; **4**: 627P.

60. Routledge, P.A., Shand, D.G., Barchowsky, A., Wagner, G. and Stargel, W.W. Relationship between α_1-acid glycoprotein and lidocaine disposition in myocardial infarction. *Clin. Pharmac. Ther.* 1981; **30**: 154.

61. Routledge, P.A. The plasma protein binding of basic drugs. *Br. J. Clin. Pharmac.* 1986; **22**: 499.

62. George, C.F. Drug metabolism by the gastrointestinal mucosa. *Clin. Pharmacokinet.* 1981; **6**: 259.

63. Hook, G.E.R. The metabolic potential of the lungs. In: George, C.F., Shand, D.G., and Renwick, A.G., eds. *Presystemic Drug Elimination*. London: Butterworth Scientific, 1982, p. 117.

64. Guengerich, F.P. Isolation and purification of cytochrome P_{450} and the existence of multiple forms. *Pharmac. Ther.* 1979; **6**: 99.

65. Kato, R. Characteristics and differences in the hepatic mixed function oxidases of different species. *Pharmac. Ther.* 1979; **6**: 41.

66. Lu, A.Y.H. and West, S.B. Multiplicity of mammalian microsomal cytochrome P_{450}. *Pharmac. Rev.* 1979; **31**: 277.

67. Lewis, R.J., Trager, W.F., Chan, K.K., Breckenridge, A., Orme, M., Roland, M. and Schary, W. Warfarin: Stereochemical aspects of its metabolism and the interaction with phenylbutazone. *J. Clin. Invest.* 1974; **53**: 1607.

68. Choonara, I.A., Cholerton, S., Haynes, B.P., Breckenridge, A.M. and Park, B.K. Stereoselective interaction between the R enantiomer of warfarin and cimetidine. *Br. J. Clin. Pharmac.* 1986; **21**: 271.

69. Vogelgesang, B. Echizen, H., Schmidt, E. and Eichelbaum, M. Stereoselective first-pass metabolism of highly cleaved drugs: studies of the bioavailability of (−) and (+) verapamil examined with a stable isotope technique. *Br. J. Clin. Pharmac.* 1984; **18**: 733.

70. Richens, A. and Dunlop, A. Serum phenytoin levels in management of epilepsy. *Lancet* 1975; **ii**: 247.

71. Routledge, P.A., Chapman, P.H., Davies, D.M. and Rawlins, M.D. Pharmacokinetics and pharmacodynamics of warfarin at steady state. *Br. J. Clin. Pharmac.* 1979; **8**: 243.

72. Chidsey, C.A., Morselli, P., Bianchetti, G., Morganti, A., Leonetti, G. and Zanchetti, A. Studies of the absorption and removal of propranolol in hypertensive patients during therapy. *Circulation* 1975; **52**: 313.

73. Ernster, L. and Orrenius, S. Substrate induced synthesis of the hydroxylating enzyme system of liver microsomes. *Fed. Proc.* 1965; **24**: 1190.

74. Remmer, H. and Merker, H.J. Effect of drugs on the formation of smooth endoplasmic reticulum and drug-metabolising enzymes. *Ann. N.Y. Acad. Sci.* 1965; **123**: 79.

75. Jusko, W.J. Role of tobacco smoking in pharmacokinetics. *J. Pharmacokin. Biopharm.* 1978; **6**: 7.

76. Pelkonen, O., Pasanen, M., Kuha, H., Gachalyi, B., Kairaluoma, M., Sotaniemi, E.A., Park, S.S., Friedman, F.K. and Gelboin, H.V. The effect of cigarette smoking on 7-ethoxyresorufin O-deethylase and other monooxygenase activities in human liver: analyses with monoclonal antibodies. *Br. J. Clin. Pharmac.* 1986; **22**: 125.

77. Dollery, C.T., George, C.F. and Orme, M.L.'E. Drug interactions affecting cardiovascular therapy. In: Cluff, L.E. and Petrie, J.C., eds. *Clinical Effects of Interaction Between Drugs*. Amsterdam: Excerpta Medica, 1974, p. 117.

78. Breckenridge, A., Orme, M.L.'E., Davies, L., Thorgeirsson, S.S. and Davies, D.S. Dose-dependent enzyme induction. *Clin. Pharmac. Ther.* 1973; **14**: 514.

79. Bell, J.A., Gower, A.J., Martin, L.E., Milles, E.N.C. and Smith, W.P. Interaction of H_2-receptor antagonists with drug metabolising enzymes. *Biochem. Soc. Trans.* 1981; **9**: 113.

80. Somogyi, A. and Gugler, R. Drug interactions with cimetidine. *Clin. Pharmacokinet.* 1982; **7**: 23.

81. Strong, H.A., Oates, J., Sembi, J., Renwick, A.G. and George, C.F. Role of the gut flora in the reduction of sulfinpyrazone in humans. *J. Pharmacol. Exp. Ther.* 1984; **230**: 726.

82. Smith, R.L. *The Excretory Function of Bile*. London: Chapman and Hall, 1973.

83. Fitzgerald, J.D. and O'Donnel, S.R. Pharmacology of 4-hydroxy-propranolol, a metabolite of propranolol. *Br. J. Pharmacol.* 1971; **43**: 222.

84. Cleaveland, C.R. and Shand, D.G. Effect of route of administration on the relationship between β-adrenergic blockade and plasma propranolol level. *Clin. Pharmac. Ther.* 1972; **13**: 181.

85. Sweet, C.S. and Ulm, E.H. Enalapril. In: Scriabine, A. ed. *New Drugs Annual: Cardiovascular Drugs*, Vol. 2. New York: Raven Press, 1984, p. 1.

86. Lund, B., Kampmann, J.P., Lindahl, F. and Hansen, J.M. Pivampicillin and ampicillin in bile, portal and peripheral blood. *Clin. Pharmac. Ther.* 1976; **19**: 587.

87. Campbell, W., Tilstone, W.J., Lawson, D.H., Hutton, I. and Lawrie, T.D.V. Acetylator phenotype and the clinical pharmacology of slow-release procainamide. *Br. J. Clin. Pharmac.* 1976; **3**: 1023.

88. Talseth, T. Studies on hydralazine 1. Serum concentrations of hydralazine in man after a single dose and at steady state. *Eur. J. Clin. Pharmac.* 1976; **10**: 183.

89. Zacest, R. and Koch-Weser, J. Relation of hydralazine plasma concentrations to dosage and hypotensive action. *Clin. Pharmac. Ther.* 1972; **13**: 420.

90. Evans, D.A.P. Genetic variation in the acetylation of isoniazid and other drugs. *Ann. N.Y. Acad. Sci.* 1968; **151**: 723.

91. Woosley, R.L., Drayer, D.E., Reidenberg, M.M., Nies, A.S., Carr, K. and Oates, J.A. Effect of acetylator phenotype on the rate at which procainamide induces antinuclear antibodies and the lupus syndrome. *N. Engl. J. Med.* 1978; **298**: 1157.

92. Perry, H.M. Jr, Tan, E.M. Carmody, S. and Sakamoto, A. Relationship of acetyl transferase activity to antinuclear antibodies and toxic symptoms in hypertensive patients treated with hydralazine. *J. Lab. Clin. Med.* 1970; **76**: 114.

93. George, C.F., Blackwell, E.W. and Davies, D.S. Metabolism of isoprenaline in the intestine. *J. Pharmac. Pharmacol.* 1974; **26**: 265.

94. Davies, D.F. and Shock, N.W. Age changes in glomerular filtration rate, effective renal plasma flow and tubular excretory capacity in adult males. *J. Clin. Invest.* 1950; **29**: 496.

95. Steiness, E. Renal tubular secretion of digoxin. *Circulation* 1974; **50**: 103.

96. Gerhardt, R.E., Knous, R.F., Thyrum, P.F., Luchi, R.J. and Morris, J.J. Quinidine excretion in aciduria and alkaluria. *Ann. Intern. Med.* 1969; **71**: 927.

97. Hirom, P.C., Milburn, P., Smith, R.L. and Williams, R.T. Species variations in the threshold molecular weight factor

for the biliary excretion of organic amines. *Biochem. J.* 1972; **129**: 1071.

98. Cohn, H.D. Clinical studies with a new rifampicin derivative. *J. Clin. Pharmac.* 1969; **9**: 118.

99. Caldwell, J.H. and Greenberger, N.J. Cholestyramine enhances digitalis excretion and protects against lethal intoxication. *J. Clin. Invest.* 1970; **49**: 16a.

100. Richens, A. Clinical pharmacokinetics of phenytoin. *Clin. Pharmacokinet.* 1979; **4**: 153.

101. Vestal, R.E. Drug use in the elderly: A review of problems and special considerations. *Drugs* 1978; **16**: 358.

102. Cusack, B., Kelly, J., O'Malley, K., Noel, J., Lavan, J. and Horgan, J. Digoxin in the elderly: pharmacokinetic consequences of old age. *Clin. Pharmac. Ther.* 1979; **25**: 772.

103. Castleden, C.M., Volans, C.N. and Raymond, K. The effect of ageing on drug absorption from the gut. *Age and Ageing* 1977; **6**: 138.

104. Nation, R.L., Triggs, E.J. and Selig, M. Lignocaine kinetics in cardiac patients and aged subjects. *Br. J. Clin. Pharmac.* 1977; **4**: 439.

105. Brown, H.C., Carruthers, S.G. and Johnston, G.O. Clinical pharmacological observations on atenolol, a beta-adrenoceptor blocker. *Clin. Pharmac. Ther.* 1976; **20**: 524.

106. Hayes, M.J., Langman, M.J.S. and Short, A.H. Changes in drug metabolism with increasing age 1. Warfarin binding and plasma proteins. *Br. J. Clin. Pharmac.* 1975; **2**: 69.

107. Wallace, S., Whiting, B., and Runcie, J. Factors affecting drug binding in plasma of elderly patients. *Br. J. Clin. Pharmac.* 1976; **3**: 327.

108. Castleden, C.M., Kaye, C.M. and Parsons, R.L. The effect of age on plasma levels of practolol and propranolol in man. *Br. J. Clin. Pharmac.* 1975; **2**: 303.

109. Castleden, C.M., George, C.F. and Short, M.D. Contribution of individual differences in gastric emptying to variability in plasma propranolol concentrations. *Br. J. Clin. Pharmac.* 1978; **5**: 121.

110. Feely, J. and Stevenson, I.H. The effect of age and hyperthyroidism on plasma propranolol steady state concentration. *Br. J. Clin. Pharmac.* 1978; **6**: 446P.

111. Ewy, G.A., Kapadia, G.G., Yao, L., Lullin, M. and Marcus, F.I. Digoxin metabolism in the elderly. *Circulation* 1969; **39**: 449.

112. Cockcroft, D. and Gault, M.H. Prediction of creatinine clearance from serum creatinine. *Nephron* 1976; **16**: 31.

113. Jick, H., Slone, D., Borda, I.T. and Shapiro, S. Efficacy and toxicity of heparin in relation to age and sex. *N. Engl. J. Med.* 1968; **279**: 284.

114. O'Malley, K., Stevenson, I.H., Ward, C.A., Wood, A.J.J. and Crooks, J. Determinants of anticoagulant control in patients receiving warfarin. *Br. J. Clin. Pharmac.* 1977; **4**: 309.

115. Shepherd, A.M.M., Hewick, D.S., Moreland, T.S. and Stevenson, I.H. Age as a determinant of sensitivity to warfarin. *Br. J. Clin. Pharmac.* 1977; **4**: 315.

116. Schocken, D. and Roth, G. Reduced beta adrenergic receptor concentrations in aging man. *Nature* 1977; **267**: 856.

117. Vestal, R.E., Wood, A.J.J. and Shand, D.G. Reduced ß-adrenoreceptor sensitivity in the elderly. *Clin. Res.* 1979; **26**: 181.

118. Ullah, M.I., Newman, G.B. and Saunders, K.B. Influence of age on response to ipratropium and salbutamol in asthma. *Thorax* 1981; **36**: 523.

119. Hall, M.R.P. Drug therapy in the elderly. *Br. Med. J.* 1973; **3**: 382.

120. Bennett, W.M., Aronoff, G.R., Morrison, G., Golper, T.A., Pulliam, J., Wolfson, M. and Singer, I. Drug prescribing in renal failure: dosing guidelines for adults. *Am. J. Kidney Dis.* 1983; **3**: 155.

121. Bennett, W.M. Update on drugs in renal failure. *Adv. Nephrol.* 1986; **15**: 379.

122. Odar-Cederlof, I. and Borga, O. Impaired protein binding of phenytoin in uraemia and displacement effects of salicylic acid. *Clin. Pharmac. Ther.* 1976; **20**: 36.

123. Stock, J.P.P. Beta adrenergic drugs for the clinical management of cardiac arrhythmia. *Am. J. Cardiol.* 1966; **18**: 444.

124. Allen, J.D., Pantridge, J.F. and Shanks, R.G. The effect of practolol on the dysrhythmias complicating acute ischaemic heart disease. *Am. J. Med.* 1975; **58**: 199.

125. Doherty, J.E. and Perkins, W.H. Studies following intramuscular tritiated digoxin in human subjects. *Am. J. Cardiol.* 1965; **15**: 170.

126. Steiness, E. and Olesen, K.H. Cardiac arrhythmias induced by hypokalaemia and potassium loss during maintenance digoxin therapy. *Br. Heart J.* 1976; **38**: 167.

127. Seller, R.H., Greco, J., Banoch, S. and Seth, R. Increasing the inotropic effect and toxic dose of digitalis by the administration of antikaliuretic drugs—Further evidence for a cardiac effect of diuretic agents. *Am. Heart J.* 1973; **90**: 56.

128. Winne, D. and Remischovsky, J. Intestinal blood flow and absorption of non-dissociable substances. *J. Pharm. Pharmac.* 1970; **22**: 640.

129. Haass, A., Lullman, H. and Peters, Th. Absorption rates of some cardiac glycosides and portal blood flow. *Eur. J. Pharmac.* 1972; **19**: 366.

130. Benet, L.Z., Greither, A. and Meister, W. Gastrointestinal absorption of drugs in patients with cardiac failure. In: Benet, L.Z., ed. *The Effect of Disease States on Drug Pharmacokinetics.* American Pharmaceutical Association, Washington, 1976, p. 33.

131. Anderson, K.V., Brettell, H.R. and Aikwa, J.K. C^{14}-labelled hydrochlorothiazide in human beings. *Arch. Intern. Med.* 1961; **107**: 168.

132. Koch-Weser, J. Pharmacokinetics of procainamide in man. *Ann. N.Y. Acad. Sci.* 1971; **179**: 370.

133. Tilstone, W.J., Dargie, H., Dargie, E.N., Morgan, H.G. and Kennedy, A.C. Pharmacokinetics of metolazone in normal subjects and in patients with cardiac or renal failure. *Clin. Pharmac. Ther.* 1974; **16**: 322.

134. Crouthamel, W.G. The effect of congestive heart failure on quinidine pharmacokinetics. *Am. Heart J.* 1975; **90**: 335.

135. Greither, A., Goldman, S., Edelen, J.S., Cohn, K. and Benet, L.Z. Erratic and incomplete absorption of furosemide in congestive heart failure. *Am. J. Cardiol.* 1976; **37**: 139.

136. Thomson, P.D., Rowland, M. and Melmon, K. The influence of heart failure, liver disease and renal failure on the disposition of lidocaine in man. *Am. Heart J.* 1971; **82**: 417.

137. Ilett, K.F., Madsen, B.W. and Woods, J.D. Disopyramide kinetics in patients with acute myocardial infarction. *Clin. Pharmac. Ther.* 1979; **26**: 1.

138. Stenson, R.E. Constantino, R.T. and Harrison, D.C. Interrelationships of hepatic blood flow, cardiac output and blood levels of lidocaine in man. *Circulation* 1971; **43**: 205.

139. Thomson, P.D., Melmon, K.L., Richardson, J.A., Cohn, K., Steinbrunn, W., Cudihee, R. and Rowland, M. Lidocaine pharmacokinetics in advanced heart failure, liver disease and renal failure in humans. *Ann. Intern. Med.* 1973; **78**: 499.

140. Hallkin, R.E., Meffin, P., Melmon, K.L. and Rowland, M. Influence of congestive heart failure on blood levels of lidocaine and its active monodeethylated metabolite. *Clin. Pharmac. Ther.* 1975; **17**: 669.

141. Franciosa, J.A., Wilen, M., Weeks, C.E., Tanenbaum, R., Kvam, C. and Millar, A.M. Pharmacokinetics and

haemodynamic effects of flecainide in patients with chronic low output heart failure. *J. Am. Coll. Cardiol.* 1983; **1**: 699.

142. Conard, G.J. and Ober, R.E. Metabolism of flecainide. *Am. J. Cardiol.* 1984; **53**: 41B.

143. Routledge, P.A., Shand, D.G., Barchowsky, A., Wagner, G. and Stargel, W.W. Relationship between α_1 acid glycoprotein and lidocaine disposition in myocardial infarction. *Clin. Pharmac. Ther.* 1981; **30**: 154.

144. Idle, J.R., Mahgoub, A., Lancaster, R. and Smith, R.L. Hypotensive response to debrisoquine and hydroxylation phenotype. *Life Sci.* 1978; **22**: 979.

145. Silas, J.H., Lennard, M.S., Tucker, G.T., Smith, A.J., Malcolm, S.L. and Marten, T.R. The disposition of debrisoquine in hypertensive patients. *Br. J. Clin. Pharmac.* 1978; **5**: 27.

146. Lennard, M.S., Silas, J.H., Freestone, S., Ramsay, L.E., Tucker, G.T. and Woods, H.F. Oxidation phenotype – A major determinant of metoprolol metabolism and response. *N. Engl. J. Med.* 1982; **307**: 1558.

147. Vanholder, P., Carpenter, J., Schurgers, M. and Clement, D.L. Rebound phenomenon during gradual withdrawal of clonidine. *Br. Med. J.* 1977; **1**: 1138.

148. Hunyor, S.N., Hansson, L., Harrison, T.S. and Hoobler, S.W. Effects of clonidine withdrawal: possible mechanisms and suggestions for management. *Br. Med. J.* 1973; **2**: 209.

149. Mizgala, H.F. and Counsell, J. Acute coronary syndromes following abrupt cessation of oral propranolol therapy. *Circulation* 1974; **49**: 50(Suppl. III): 33.

150. Miller, R.M., Olson, H.G., Amsterdam, E.A. and Mason, D.T. Propranolol withdrawal rebound phenomenon: exacerbation of coronary events after abrupt cessation of antianginal therapy. *N. Engl. J. Med.* 1975; **293**: 416.

151. Rangno, R.E. Beta blocker withdrawal syndrome. In: Kostis, J.B. and De Felice, E.A., eds. *Beta Blockers in the Treatment of Cardiovascular Disease.* Raven Press, New York, 1984, p. 275.

152. Lette, J., Gagnon, R.-M., Lemire, J.G. and Morisette, M. Rebound of vasospastic angina after cessation of long-term treatment with nifedipine. *Can. Med. Assoc. J.* 1984; **130**: 1169.

153. Melmon, K.L. Preventable drug reactions – causes and cures. *N. Engl. J. Med.* 1971; **284**: 1361.

154. Morselli, P.L. Clinical pharmacokinetics in neonates. *Clin. Pharmacokinet.* 1976; **1**: 81.

155. Smith, J.W., Seidl, L.G. and Cluff, L.E. Studies on the epidemiology of adverse drug reactions. *Ann. Intern. Med.* 1966; **65**: 629.

156. Stokes, G.S., Graham, R.M., Gain, J.M. and Davis, P.R. Influence of dosage and dietary sodium on the first-dose effects of prazosin. *Br. Med. J.* 1977; **1**: 1507.

157. Caldwell, J.H. and Greenberger, N. Interruption of the enterohepatic circulation of digitoxin by cholestyramine I. *J. Clin. Invest.* 1971; **50**: 2626.

158. O'Reilly, R.A. Stereoselective interaction of trimethoprim-sulfamethoxazole with the separated enantiomers of racemic warfarin in man. *N. Engl. J. Med.* 1980; **302**: 33.

159. Powell-Jackson, P.R. Interaction between azapropazone and warfarin. *Br. Med. J.* 1977; **1**: 1193.

160. Benaim, M.E. Asystole after verapamil. *Br. Med. J.* 1972; **2**: 169.

161. Boothby, C.G., Garrard, C.S. and Pickering, D. Intravenous verapamil in cardiac arrhythmias. *Br. Med. J.* 1972; **2**: 349.

162. Webster, J. Interactions of NSAID's with diuretics and ß-blockers. Mechanisms and clinical implications. *Drugs* 1985; **30**: 32.

163. Evans, L. and Spelman, M. The problems of non-compliance with drug therapy. *Drugs* 1983; **25**: 63.

164. Hedstrand, H. and Aberg, H. Treatment of hypertension in middle-aged men. *Acta Med. Scand.* 1976; **199**: 281.

165. Langfeld, B.S. Hypertension: deficient care of the medically served. *Ann. Intern. Med.* 1973; **78**: 19.

166. Sackett, D.L., Haynes, R.B., Gibson, E.S., Hackett, B.C., Taylor, D.W., Roberts, R.S. and Johnson, A.L. Randomised clinical trial of strategies for improving medication compliance in primary hypertension. *Lancet* 1975; **i**: 1205.

167. Hulka, B.S., Cassel, J.C., Kupper, L.L. and Burdette, J.A. Communication, compliance and concordance between physicians and patients with prescribed medications. *Am. J. Publ. Health* 1976; **66**: 847.

168. Sackett, D.L. and Haynes, R.B. *Compliance with therapeutic regimes.* Baltimore and London: Johns Hopkins University Press, 1976.

169. Christensen, D.B. Drug-taking compliance. A review and synthesis. *Health Serv. Res.* 1978; **13**: 171.

170. Drury, V.S.M., Wade, O.L. and Woolf, E. Following advice in general practice. *J. R. Coll. Gen. Pract.* 1976; **26**: 712.

171. Haynes, R.B., Sackett, D.L., Taylor, D.W., Roberts, R.S. and Johnson, A.L. Manipulation of the therapeutic regimen to improve compliance conceptions and misconceptions. *Clin. Pharmac. Ther.* 1977; **22**: 125.

172. Ayd, F.J. Jr. Once-a-day neuroleptic and tricyclic antidepressant therapy. *Int. Drug. Ther. Newsletter* 1972; **7**: 33.

173. Brand, F.N., Smith, R.T. and Brand, P.A. Effect of economic barriers to medical care on patients non-compliance. *Publ. Health Rep.* 1977; **92**: 72.

174. Gatley, M.S. To be taken as directed. *J. R. Coll. Gen. Pract.* 1968; **16**: 39.

175. Clinite, J.C. and Kabat, H.F. Improving patient compliance. *J. Am. Pharmac. Assoc.* 1976; **16**: 74.

176. Gabriel, M., Gagnon, J.P. and Bryan, C.K. Improved patient compliance through use of a daily drug reminder chart. *Am. J. Publ. Health* 1977; **67**: 968.

177. Ley, P., Jain, V.K. and Skilbeck, C.E. A method for decreasing patient's medication errors. *Psychol. Med.* 1976; **6**: 599.

Chapter 74

Anaesthesia and Non-cardiac Surgery in Patients with Heart Disease

Robert E. Bullock

INTRODUCTION

Anaesthesia is remarkably safe nowadays with death which is entirely due to anaesthetic mishap occurring only once in 10 000 procedures. Nevertheless, anaesthesia plays a part in 10% of all deaths within 6 days of surgery. Within this population, patients with cardiovascular disease are recognized as a high-risk group. In the recent survey of mortality associated with British anaesthetic practice, Lunn and Mushin reported that cardiovascular disease was the autopsy cause of death in more than half of those who died, and was present preoperatively in two-thirds of the patients whose deaths were totally attributable to anaesthesia.[1]

Attempts have been made to quantify the cardiac risk in non-cardiac surgery. Goldman et al.[2] prospectively studied 1001 patients over the age of 40 years in order to derive a multifactorial index of cardiac morbidity and mortality. They identified 9 independent significant correlates of life-threatening and fatal cardiac complications and assigned to each a point score (Table 74.1). Particularly sinister factors were a myocardial infarction within the preceding 6 months, signs of heart failure and abnormal electrocardiographic rhythms or frequent ventricular ectopic beats. On the basis of the number of points scored, the patient was placed in one of four risk groups, with the recommendation that only life-saving surgery should be performed in the highest risk group. This classification has recently been extended by Detsky et al.[3] using a patient population in which the possibility of cardiac risk had already been identified. A modified index included an improved description of some clinical features, such as angina, and permitted risk calculation for an individual patient. The authors emphasize that cardiac risk calculation can only be

applied within a framework of knowledge of the overall risk for a particular procedure in a specified hospital. Prediction tests cannot guarantee that an operation is free of cardiac risk; over one-third of all severe cardiac complications in this study occurred in patients who had low-risk scores.

The patient undergoing cardiac surgery is anaesthetized and operated on in a specialized environment where expertise, monitoring equipment and post-operative intensive care facilities are all concentrated on the diseased heart, which has been improved by the surgery. The same patient present-

Table 74.1. Multifactorial index score to estimate cardiac risk (after Goldman et al.[2]).

Criteria	Point score
History: Age > 70 years	5
Myocardial infarction in last 6 months	10
Examination: S_3 or raised jugular venous pressure	11
Significant aortic stenosis	3
Electrocardiogram: Rhythm other than sinus	7
> 5 ventricular ectopic beats/min	7
General: Any of the following: Respiratory failure, K^+ < 3.0 mmol, HCO_3 < 20 mmol, renal failure, liver dysfunction, immobilization	3
Surgery: Abdominal, thoracic, aortic	3
Emergency	4
Total possible:	53

Group	Points total	Non-fatal cardiac complications (%)	Cardiac death (%)
I	0–5	0.7	0.2
II	6–12	5	2
III	13–25	11	2
IV	>26	22	56

ing for non-cardiac surgery is at greater risk because the expertise and facilities for cardiac care may not be as good, and surgery subjects the cardiovascular system to stress without any improvement in the underlying cardiac pathology.

ANAESTHETIC DRUGS AND TECHNIQUES

Detailed descriptions of anaesthetic techniques and the cardiovascular pharmacology of anaesthetic agents are available in standard texts.[4,5] For most non-cardiothoracic operations, there is a choice between general anaesthesia with or without endotracheal intubation and artificial respiration, and regional anaesthesia employing a local anaesthetic agent. Both techniques present formidable difficulties and dangers in the sick patient who has co-existing cardiac disease. Regional anaesthesia is currently regaining popularity, but it is still less widely used in the UK than in many other countries. Anaesthetic pre-medication is usually prescribed whatever peroperative technique is to be used, benzodiazepines or opiates commonly being employed to relieve anxiety and to aid the smooth induction of anaesthesia.

GENERAL ANAESTHESIA

General anaesthesia requires the pharmacological induction and maintenance of a triad comprising sleep to prevent awareness and recall, analgesia to abolish the harmful effects of the stress response, and muscular relaxation to stop reflex movements and allow access to the body cavities. For short procedures, all three effects can be achieved by the patient spontaneously breathing a volatile anaesthetic agent, but if this agent has to be used in high concentration in order to obtund the effects of surgical stimuli profound cardiovascular depression will occur (*vide infra*). More usually, a balanced technique consisting of anaesthetic agent, opioid analgesic, and muscle relaxant with artificial ventilation will be employed. A large number of different drugs may be used during an anaesthetic; the pharmacology of the major classes of agent will be briefly reviewed in order to demonstrate how drugs are chosen for the patient with cardiac disease.

Intravenous induction agents

The barbiturates, thiopentone and methohexitone, remain the most popular intravenous agents for rapid smooth induction of the anaesthetic state, but they can cause marked hypotension due to direct myocardial depression if used incautiously. Etomidate causes pain on injection, but it has the least adverse cardiovascular effects of the induction agents currently available and is widely regarded as the drug of choice in the patient with heart disease. Etomidate inhibits adrenocorticoid hormone synthesis,[6] although this does not appear to be clinically important unless administration is prolonged. The new drug propofol is rapidly metabolized and ideal for daycase surgery but is not suitable for most cardiac cases as it causes hypotension.

Anaesthetic gases and vapours

Nitrous oxide is employed in most general anaesthetics. It is a weak analgesic and hypnotic and has often been considered to have no adverse cardiovascular effects. However, its potential for decreasing myocardial contractility and arterial pressure, and raising left ventricular end-diastolic pressure in patients with impaired left ventricular function, is being increasingly recognized.[7] In addition, nitrous oxide causes a marked rise in pulmonary vascular resistance in subjects in whom it is already abnormal.[8]

Three volatile anaesthetic agents are in common use: halothane, enflurane and isoflurane. All have marked cardiovascular side-effects. They decrease mean arterial blood pressure in proportion to their concentration, but the mechanism of each is different. Halothane causes direct myocardial depression and a reduction in cardiac output with no change in systemic vascular resistance, whereas isoflurane is a potent vasodilator with less effect on cardiac output or contractility. The hypotension produced by isoflurane results in a baroreceptor-mediated tachycardia; this is not seen with halothane which inhibits baroreflex control of heart rate and directly depresses the atrial rate, often resulting in bradycardia. Enflurane is usually regarded as intermediate in its actions, depressing contractility and cardiac output and also reducing peripheral resistance. All three agents reduce myocardial oxygen consumption, but because of the bradycardia and marked depression of contractility this reduction in oxygen consumption is most marked with halothane, although it is accompanied by a small rise in left ventricular end-diastolic pressure.

Interactions of the volatile agents

The pharmacological actions of anaesthetic agents are modified by a number of other factors in the anaesthetized patient. The spontaneously breathing patient usually has a mildly elevated level of arterial carbon dioxide which stimulates the heart and preserves cardiac output and blood pressure. Changing to artificial ventilation reduces venous return to the heart by raising intrathoracic pressure, and usually reduces the level of arterial carbon dioxide below normal, resulting in a fall in blood pressure and cardiac output together with peripheral vasoconstriction.

The volatile agents will also interact with the drugs taken by the patient with heart disease. The reduction in contractility caused by beta-blocking drugs will compound that caused by anaesthetic agents and can cause profound myocardial depression. It is thought that part of the reduction in contractility produced by volatile anaesthetics is mediated by alterations in calcium flux, and so we might expect important interactions with calcium channel blocking drugs. The three commonly used anaesthetics, halothane, enflurane and isoflurane, have a similar spectrum of pharmacological actions, respectively, to the three calcium antagonists, verapamil, diltiazem and nifedepine.[9] Halothane like verapamil produces the most myocardial depression and atrioventricular block, whereas isoflurane and nifedepine act predominantly as vasodilators so that additive effects are predicted if the patient receives two drugs with similar cardiovascular properties. Myocardial depression can usually be corrected by infusing calcium, but this does not reverse peripheral vasodilatation or atrioventricular block.

Muscle relaxants

Modern neuromuscular blocking agents, such as suxamethonium, pancuronium, vecuronium and atracurium, have little effect on myocardial contractility or vascular resistance and are generally well tolerated by patients with heart disease. They differ in their effects on heart rate. The short-acting depolarizing agent suxamethonium causes bradycardia which is usually only problematic on repeated administration. The new shorter acting curare-type agents—atracurium and vecuronium—can produce marked bradycardia and occasional asystole. Pancuronium causes a moderate increase in heart rate by a vagolytic action but this is often useful in counteracting the bradycardia produced by other anaesthetic drugs. At the end of surgery, curare-type relaxant drugs are usually reversed with a cholinesterase inhibiting agent, conventionally neostigmine. Because heart cholinesterases are also inhibited, there will be an overactivity of acetylcholine at cardiac receptors and profound bradycardia which must always be counteracted by the simultaneous administration of atropine. Changes in heart rate are always somewhat unpredictable and for some patients with heart disease it may be better to wait for muscle relaxants to wear off spontaneously and support ventilation post-operatively while this is occurring.

Opioid analgesics

The synthetic opioids fentanyl, alfentanil and sufentanil are about 100 times more potent than morphine and they are devoid of the adverse cardiovascular effects of the naturally occurring opiates. In high dosage, they can be used alone to provide anaesthesia with profound analgesia and excellent haemodynamic stability during cardiac surgery, with the abolition of tachycardia and hypertension in response to surgical stimulation.[10] Unfortunately, these high-dose opioid techniques require postoperative ventilatory support and therefore are not suitable for most non-cardiac surgery where the availability of intensive care facilities may be limited. In lower dosage, they form a fundamental part of the balanced anaesthetic technique for patients with heart disease. They are able to reduce the marked haemodynamic responses to laryngoscopy and intubation,[11] and are of sufficiently short duration of action that they can be given during surgery and yet allow the patient to breath unaided at the end of the operation. Respiratory depression persisting after surgery can be reversed with the antagonist naloxone but this is not advisable in patients who have heart disease. Hypertension and pulmonary oedema can be precipitated during sudden reversal of opiates in subjects with normal hearts.[12]

REGIONAL ANAESTHESIA

Local anaesthetic agents can be injected in a variety of sites between the spinal cord and periphery in order to block the conduction of painful stimuli. The avoidance of general anaesthesia has considerable attraction in some patients with heart disease in whom subarachnoid or epidural regional block can be used for surgery to the lower part of the body. Epidural anaesthesia can provide excellent cardiovascular stability for Caesarean section[13] and reduces minute ventilation and oxygen consumption during labour.[14] There are hazards; the cardiovascular toxicity of overdose or inadvertent intravascular injection of local anaesthetics, especially of bupivacaine, will be more serious in the patient who has pre-existing cardiac disease. Epidural and subarachnoid anaesthetics also block sympathetic outflow in the segments anaesthetized. This results in a fall in peripheral vascular resistance in the anaesthetized areas and the ensuing fall in blood pressure can be dramatic and dangerous.

CHOICE OF ANAESTHETIC

Of greatest importance in planning an anaesthetic for a patient with heart disease is the familiarity of the anaesthetist with the chosen technique and a thorough understanding of the pathophysiology of the patient's disease. The anaesthetic agents described are used in conjunction with the administration of familiar cardiovascular drugs, including inotropes, nitrates and beta-blockers, in order to preserve or manipulate blood pressure, heart rate, peripheral vascular resistance and myocardial contractility to achieve optimum conditions to tolerate the stress of surgery. Anaesthetists also make frequent use of vasoconstrictor pressure agents, such as ephedrine and metaraminol, in order to counteract the vasodilating effects of anaesthetic drugs or sympathetic blockade. The anaesthetic for a minor operation in a patient with heart disease will be no simpler or less hazardous than that chosen for a larger procedure.

MONITORING AIDS

A variety of cardiovascular monitoring aids are available in most operating suites. The minimum acceptable standard for any patient having an anaesthetic in the UK is monitoring of the electrocardiogram and blood pressure.[1] In the USA, much more monitoring would be considered mandatory, including a precordial stethoscope and continuous measurement of inspired oxygen concentration. The patient with heart disease undergoing major surgery may have direct pressure recordings from catheters in the radial artery, right atrium or pulmonary artery. The Swan–Ganz catheter can also be used for thermodilution cardiac output measurements and by wedging the balloon the left atrial pressure is estimated. It is now possible to monitor continuous-

ly the adequacy of oxygenation in anaesthetized patients using the pulse-oximeter.[15] This device measures haemoglobin saturation by infrared light absorption on a beat to beat basis and should be particularly useful in the cardiac case in which the avoidance of hypoxia is of paramount importance. Continuous expired carbon dioxide concentration can also be readily measured with the end expiratory level approximating to arterial carbon dioxide tension. Ventilation can be adjusted so that carbon dioxide levels stay within the normal range; hypercapnia predisposes to arrhythmias and causes acidosis whereas too much ventilation results in hypocapnia which depresses cardiac output and causes intense peripheral vasoconstriction.

FLUID AND ELECTROLYTE BALANCE

Large volumes of fluid need to be given during major surgery to maintain extracellular volume, preserve renal function and prevent hypotension. The patient comes to theatre starved and is therefore in negative fluid balance before the operation starts. Evaporative losses from open body cavities are considerable and are at least 4 ml/kg/h during a simple laparotomy. Water vapour is also lost from the respiratory tract to the dry anaesthetic gases when the upper airway is bypassed by endotracheal intubation. Body tissues that are manipulated by the surgeons become oedematous in response to the mild trauma and can absorb large amounts of fluid. Abdominal surgery frequently results in ileus and the accumulation of several litres of fluid in the gut. When all these factors are added together, it is evident that considerable amounts of both crystalloid and colloid may have to be administered in the peri-operative period, even if there has not been overt blood loss.

The major electrolyte of significance to anaesthesia is potassium. In heart disease, hypokalaemia from diuretic therapy is common and predisposes to arrhythmias, especially if the patient is digitalized. Surgery should not be postponed, however, in low-risk patients who are mildly hypokalaemic (K^+ 3.0–3.5 mmol/l) as they do not appear to be at added risk.[16]

PRE-OPERATIVE ASSESSMENT

It is unfortunate that the liaison between physician and anaesthetist all too often fails, through misunderstanding, to achieve the optimum pre-operative assessment of the patient with heart disease presenting for non-cardiac surgery.[17] The anaesthetist who has to administer the anaesthetic should be in the best position to decide the patient's fitness for surgery and the appropriate anaesthetic technique.[18] In order to make these decisions and conduct the anaesthetic safely, the anaesthetist must be provided with detailed information about the extent of cardiac pathology and functional impairment, and assured that the patient is in the best possible condition to face the physiological insult of surgery. All too frequently, the anaesthetist is given an assessment containing comments such as: "Fit for light anaesthetic, monitor the ECG and avoid hypoxia." Such assessments do not give any important information on the severity of disease and its effects on cardiac function, and demonstrates a lack of understanding of modern operating theatre practice. Of equal concern is the possibility that patients may be inappropriately denied surgery which could be carried out with little risk. In turn, anaesthetists cannot escape criticism of their understanding of the manifestations of cardiovascular disease as evidenced by the comment in Lunn and Mushin's report on British anaesthetic mortality:

"... there is little evidence that ischaemic heart disease was always regarded as sufficiently important to justify special precautions."[1]

POST-OPERATIVE CARE

At present, considerable expertise and facilities are employed to care for the patient with heart disease during a non-cardiac operation. As the incidence of peri-operative myocardial infarction is highest on the second or third post-operative day,[19] our objectives may need to be changed. Further improvements in survival are most likely to result from better post-operative care, although this will inevitably be financially expensive. Some patients with bad heart disease are already admitted to the intensive care unit following non-cardiac surgery. These are usually patients who require artificial ventilation with sedation following major surgery. The advantages of this form of treatment are that time is allowed for body temperature, fluid balance and cardiovascular function to be returned towards normal, and for the effects of anaesthetic drugs to wear off before the patient is woken up. Disadvantages are the ever present danger of a hypoxic accident from ventilator failure or disconnection, and the high cost of care on an intensive care unit.

ISCHAEMIC HEART DISEASE

The high prevalence of ischaemic heart disease in the population makes it the most common medical problem seen in anaesthetic practice. Any male presenting for surgery who is over 40 years old should be questioned about symptoms suggesting myocardial ischaemia. Pre-operative stress tests to screen patients for ischaemic heart disease are impracticable in most instances, but the resting electrocardiogram is an inexpensive and useful investigation. Although only a minority of patients with electrocardiographic abnormalities actually develop a peri-operative complication, the presence of ST–T abnormalities, intraventricular conduction defects, signs of past myocardial infarction or left ventricular hypertrophy all appear to identify patients at increased risk.[20,21] On the other hand, a normal electrocardiogram is not reassuring because a substantial number of patients with significant three-vessel coronary disease have a normal resting electrocardiogram.[22]

Chronically administered drug therapy should be continued throughout the peri-operative period.[23] Abrupt cessation of beta-blockers can cause a rebound phenomenon with unstable angina and myocardial infarction,[24] a situation to be avoided in the peri-operative period. There are, however, some difficulties in continuing therapy. Drug levels fall from poor absorption due to nausea, vomiting and ileus. Plasma protein binding of propranolol is increased after surgery, further reducing free drug availability.[25] The most reliable method of maintaining beta-blocker therapy is by a continuous intravenous infusion of propanolol in a dose of 1 mg/kg/day preceded by a loading dose of 0.2 mg/kg.[26] The calcium antagonist nifedipine can be continued by the sublingual route in the presence of poor absorption from the gut. There is no satisfactory intravenous form of nifedipine but verapamil can be given by this route. Nitrates can safely be given by intravenous infusion or by the transcutaneous route.

The results of tests performed to investigate the patient with ischaemia provide important guidelines for peroperative management and should be available to the anaesthetist. The exercise test defines the limits of heart rate and blood pressure that can be sustained safely, and indicates the site on the chest where electrocardiographic signs of ischaemia are most readily detected. An assessment of left ventricular function, whether by angiography, echocardiography or radionuclide scanning, provides important guidance as to whether anaesthetic agents that depress contractility can be employed to maintain anaesthesia or to reduce myocardial work. When formal studies of ventricular function are not available, an assessment has to be made from the patient's history and chest X-ray.

The principles of anaesthetic management for the patient with ischaemic heart disease involve maintaining adequate coronary perfusion whilst reducing myocardial work and ensuring that hypoxia does not occur, thereby minimizing the potential for the development of ischaemia and infarction. The stress of surgery imposes changes similar to those of an exercise stress test, except that during surgery the patient is unable to warn when angina indicates the onset of ischaemia. Careful monitoring of blood pressure, heart rate and the electrocardiogram is therefore mandatory, with monitoring of central venous pressure and Swan–Ganz pulmonary artery catheterization in selected cases.

The balance of myocardial oxygen supply and demand has to be maintained during anaesthesia.[27] Untoward increases in blood pressure and heart rate in response to surgical stimuli increase myocardial work and are prevented initially by deepening anaesthesia and giving additional opioid analgesia, and then by the use of beta-blockers and hypotensive agents. Where left ventricular function is known to be good, the myocardial oxygen requirement can be further reduced by anaesthetic agents, such as halothane and enflurane, that reduce myocardial contractility. Oxygen supply is ensured by maintaining the diastolic coronary perfusion pressure gradient; tachycardia and hypotension must be avoided and left ventricular end-diastolic volume and pressure must be kept low by guarding against vasoconstriction or fluid overload.

Despite careful anaesthetic management, many patients still demonstrate electrocardiographic evidence of ischaemia. Nitroglycerine infusion is effective in reducing the incidence of peroperative ischaemia but only if given in a dose of 1.0 μg/kg/min.[28–30] The percutaneous application of nitrates is popular because of its simplicity, but it is doubtful if absorption will be adequate especially if skin blood flow is reduced by cold, hypocapnia or pain.

The relationship between peri-operative myocardial ischaemia and post-operative myocardial infarction has been explored in patients undergoing coronary artery bypass grafting.[31] A positive correlation was demonstrated, and the quality of anaesthesia in terms of control of blood pressure

and avoidance of tachycardia appeared to be important. The peri-operative infarction rate differed among the 9 anaesthetists in the study who used a variety of anaesthetic techniques. Recently, more sensitive techniques of assessing left ventricular function have been applied during anaesthesia, but none of the studies has shown that detecting and treating wall motion abnormalities affect the outcome of surgery.[32] Thallium scintigraphy can demonstrate a high incidence of new perfusion defects following the haemodynamically stressful procedure of endotracheal intubation.[33] These abnormalities can persist into the post-operative period causing prolonged left ventricular dysfunction,[34] which is not seen in patients who have normal hearts.[35]

PERI-OPERATIVE MYOCARDIAL INFARCTION

The incidence of peri-operative myocardial infarction has been investigated in a number of studies,[19,21,36–38] in which has been demonstrated the considerably increased risk for patients with coronary artery disease, especially if non-cardiac surgery is performed in the first 6 months following a previous myocardial infarction. A retrospective survey[19] of 32 877 patients who were operated on at the Mayo Clinic during the years 1966 to 1968 revealed that among the 422 patients who had suffered a previous myocardial infarction the peri-operative re-infarction rate was 6.6%. This is more than 50 times the peri-operative infarction rate of 0.13% in those who do not have a history of prior myocardial infarction. If surgery occurred within 3 months of a myocardial infarct, the re-infarction rate was 37%, falling to 16% for operation between 3 and 6 months, and to 5% if surgery was delayed for at least 6 months. The myocardial infarct does not usually occur during the operative procedure; the highest number occurred on post-operative day 3 of the study. Mortality from re-infarction was very high at 54%. A subsequent study from the same clinic for the period 1974 to 1975[36] produced similar results. Risk factors were identified as pre-operative hypertension, intra-operative hypotension and thoracic or upper abdominal surgery lasting for more than 3 h.

In a prospective survey in Helsinki,[37] 214 patients identified as having a pre-operative myocardial infarct or electrocardiographic abnormalities suggesting left ventricular hypertrophy or subendocardial injury, underwent major non-cardiac surgery under general or regional anaesthesia.

There was a peri-operative infarction rate of 17.7% resulting in a mortality rate of 32%; 85% of infarctions occurred within the first 3 post-operative days. The prospective design of the study, in which daily electrocardiograms were recorded, illustrated the high incidence of 'silent' infarction; 37% of infarcts occurred without clinical symptoms. Additional risk factors associated with increased infarction rates included pre-operative hypertension and intra-operative hypotension, but the age and sex of the patient, anaesthetic technique, type and length of surgery and presence of pre-operative angina or diabetes mellitus were not significant.

These and similar results clearly indicate that elective surgery should be delayed for 6 months following a myocardial infarction. The re-infarction occurs typically on the first to third post-operative day, it carries a high mortality, and may not be painful. Post-operative symptoms of diffuse unlocalized pain, dyspnoea, hypotension and arrhythmias in a patient at risk are very likely to be due to myocardial infarction.[38] Post-operative myocardial infarction is a rare complication in patients who have no evidence of previous heart disease.

It is possible that aggressive haemodynamic monitoring, with pulmonary artery catheters, and prompt treatment to maintain haemodynamic stability can lessen the re-infarction rate. Rao et al.[39] reported an overall re-infarction rate of 1.9%; re-infarction rates were 5.7% and 2.3% when the previous infarction was 0–3 months old and 3–6 months old, respectively. These findings need to be substantiated before these techniques can be more generally applied because such techniques demand a prolonged expensive post-operative admission to the intensive care unit in order to achieve the improved results.[40]

The magnitude of surgery and the amount of post-operative physiological disturbance are almost certainly important despite the fact that these variables are not always identified as risk factors. Some minor surgery can be performed safely in patients with prior infarction, as illustrated by Becker in his series[41] of 288 ophthalmic operations using retrobulbar local anaesthetic block and 26 performed under general anaesthesia, in which not one of the patients suffered a re-infarction.

OPERATIVE RISK IN PATIENTS WITH PREVIOUS CORONARY ARTERY BYPASS

Patients who have had coronary artery bypass grafting appear to be at reduced risk when they have subsequent non-cardiac surgery. At present, it is not certain whether this improved safety is simply the result of high-risk patients dying during their bypass surgery, or whether it reflects a genuine protective effect of the myocardial revascularization.[42] In several studies, very low complication rates have been reported which indicates that the risk of operation is as good in patients who have had successful coronary artery bypass grafting as it is in those without coronary artery disease,[43] and myocardial revascularization prior to major surgery is recommended.[44,45] However, this problem has not been studied in a randomized clinical trial and until such results are available coronary artery bypass surgery should not be used prophylactically before other surgery, unless the patient requires bypass surgery for the normal indications of relief of symptoms or improved prognosis. Wherever possible, the subsequent elective non-cardiac surgery should be delayed for 6 weeks.[43]

HYPERTENSION

Pre-operative hypertension has been identified as a predictor of post-operative morbidity.[38] Most anaesthetists now believe that moderate or severe hypertension should be controlled before patients come to elective surgery in order to reduce peri-operative risk and ease anaesthetic management. The topic is still controversial; the evidence has recently been critically reviewed with the conclusion that no data definitively establish whether pre-operative treatment of hypertension reduces peri-operative risk.[46]

Patients with untreated hypertension are less tolerant of anaesthesia than those whose hypertension is well controlled.[47] Blood pressure fluctuates much more in the untreated patient in response to stressful stimuli, such as endotracheal intubation and surgical incision, and to the hypotensive effects of intravenous induction agents, with the possibility of resulting myocardial ischaemia. As one of the aims of modern anaesthetic practice is to maintain cardiovascular parameters as near to normal as possible, the increase in the stability of the blood pressure during surgery brought about by the treatment of hypertension is assumed to be beneficial.[48] Benefit also accrues from acute treatment of hypertension with beta-blockers immediately before surgery.[47] Other authors state that elective surgery in the absence of ideal blood pressure control need not subject the patient to added risk provided the diastolic blood pressure does not exceed 110 mmHg and the intra-operative and post-operative blood pressure is closely monitored and treated to maintain stability.[49]

Antihypertensive medication used to be discontinued before elective surgery because of concern about the possible interaction of hypotensive drugs with anaesthetic agents leading to severe hypotension and myocardial depression. Nowadays, our familiarity with the drugs has shown these fears to be unfounded provided the blood pressure and electrocardiogram are closely monitored during anaesthesia. Current opinion is strongly in favour of continuing medication up to, and including, the day of operation.[23]

ARRHYTHMIAS

Cardiac arrhythmias are reported to occur in up to 84% of anaesthetized patients, ventricular arrhythmias being more common (60%) in patients with heart disease.[50] Anaesthesia is classically associated with ventricular tachyarrhythmias generated by the older halogenated volatile anaesthetic agents which sensitize the myocardium to endogenous catecholamines. This was almost certainly the mechanism of collapse and death under light chloroform anaesthesia. Modern drugs cause less sensitization and an understanding that light planes of anaesthesia and carbon dioxide retention are potent stimulators of dangerous ventricular arrhythmias has virtually removed this hazard. The anaesthetist is more likely to be concerned with bradyarrhythmias resulting from depression of atrioventricular conduction (halothane) or direct vagal-type stimulation (opiates, muscle relaxants) and consequently atropine is usually incorporated into the anaesthetic cocktail.

The arrhythmogenic properties of anaesthetic agents on the normal heart are well known but there have been no studies of the effects of anaesthetic and adjuvant drugs on abnormal electrophysiological mechanisms.[51] Prevention and management are empirical and the use of anti-arrhythmic drugs is based on data and experience gained in the coronary care unit and cardiac catheterization laboratory. It is essential that abnormalities likely to cause peri-operative arrhythmias are diagnosed and fully investigated pre-operatively because some, such as the prolonged QT interval syndromes,[52] can cause life-threatening arrhythmias. The anaesthetist must be briefed about the

likely problems and the appropriate therapy.

The interaction of anaesthetic drugs with chronic anti-arrhythmic therapy appears uncommon, although the adrenergic blocking effects of amiodarone are unmasked by anaesthesia and haemodynamically significant bradycardia can occur which may require pacing.[53]

Some particular forms of surgery have a propensity to generate arrhythmias. Dental extractions are well known in this respect, probably in part because of the light planes of anaesthesia used. Although the arrhythmias are usually transient, they could be important in the cardiac patient. Operations on the lungs or oesophagus are likely to result in per-operative or post-operative atrial fibrillation and many anaesthetists and surgeons use prophylactic digitalization in the older patient.[54]

HEART-BLOCK

Conduction defects are often a source of concern to the anaesthetist. The presence of symptoms due to bradycardia and the severity of associated heart disease are guides to the requirements for peri-operative temporary pacing, but symptomatic patients require permanent generators which are usually inserted before elective surgery. Temporary pacing is advised in patients who have acquired complete, and Mobitz type II, heart block because powerful vagal stimuli and temporary disturbance of atrioventricular conduction are common during anaesthesia and surgery, even in normal hearts. Congenital heart block does not usually require pacing for surgery. My personal practice is to assess the heart-rate response to exercise and atropine to establish that some pharmacological control of heart rate will be possible during anaesthesia. Patients with bifascicular block are not now considered at serious risk of progressing to complete heart block under anaesthesia, and temporary pacing is not recommended.[55,56]

PACEMAKERS

The modern permanently implanted pacemaker that is functioning normally pre-operatively will usually continue to do so during non-cardiac surgery.[57] However, problems continue to be reported in the literature[58] and several precautions must be taken to ensure that pacing continues during the use of diathermy.[59] Electromagnetic interference can be collected by the pacing lead and with a VVI generator can cause pacemaker inhibition, reversion to asynchronous mode, or change of pacing rate.[57] Programmable pacemakers can be either transiently or more permanently re-programmed during the application of diathermy. Placing a magnet over the generator will convert demand devices to fixed rate and eliminate inhibition, but the response of programmable devices depends on the type of generator. When electrocautery is used in close proximity to the pacing system, large amounts of energy can be delivered to the tip of the electrode resulting in myocardial burns and a change in threshold, or in ventricular fibrillation.[58]

Peri-operative precautions should include the following.

1   The surgical and anaesthetic team need to be informed of the characteristics of the pacing device, its response to the application of a magnet, and the patient's underlying rhythm.

2   The function of the pacing system should have been checked recently.

3   Diathermy should be used as little as possible and at low energies; however, many surgical procedures, especially neurosurgical and urological, cannot be performed without the extensive use of electrocautery.

4   Bipolar diathermy is to be preferred because with this technique the patient's body does not form part of the electrical circuit.

5   If unipolar diathermy is used, the indifferent electrode should be as far from the pacemaker generator as possible, and should not be located between the active electrode and the pacemaker.

6   A magnet should be available to convert appropriate pacemaker generators to fixed rate.

7   During surgery, the electrocardiogram must be monitored, but as diathermy also often causes interference on the electrocardiogram monitor trace an alternative method of assessing the pulse must also be used.

8   Atropine, isoprenaline and a defibrillator should be available to deal with serious arrhythmias.

9   Pacemaker function and programming should be checked post-operatively.

Major surgery may require the use of invasive monitoring lines, although the presence of the pacemaker itself is not an indication for additional monitoring. Measurement of central venous pressure should not cause problems, but the passage of a pulmonary artery catheter through the right heart could theoretically cause pacemaker dislodgement or catheter entanglement. It has been suggested that dislodgement of the endocardial electrode is unlikely if it has been in place for more than 4 weeks, and that a pacing Swan–Ganz catheter should be used in the presence of a new pacing system.[57]

VALVE DISEASE

Stenotic valvular lesions are, as a general rule, more hazardous than regurgitant lesions during anaesthesia and surgery. A thorough assessment of the severity of the valvular lesion and of ventricular function should be conducted pre-operatively so that appropriate anaesthesia, monitoring and post-operative care can be planned. The anaesthetist must ensure that antibiotic prophylaxis against endocarditis is prescribed before dental, genito-urinary, bowel and biliary surgery (see Chapter 34). Anaesthetic techniques can also result in bacter-aemia; an incidence of 21% was reported after nasotracheal intubation, which warrants antibiotic prophylaxis.[60]

AORTIC VALVE DISEASE

Clinically significant aortic stenosis is identified as a risk factor in the Goldman scoring system.[2] Patients with aortic stenosis must be anaesthetized in a manner that preserves coronary perfusion through the hypertrophied ventricular muscle. Hypotension therefore must be avoided because it reduces diastolic coronary perfusion. Hypertension in response to surgical stress can cause sub-endocardial ischaemia and also needs to be prevented by adequate anaesthesia and analgesia. Sinus rhythm must be maintained because these patients deteriorate rapidly if arrhythmias occur. Cardiac output should be maximized by an appropriately high preload in the presence of a stiff hypertrophied ventricle and by the avoidance of myocardial depressant drugs. The patient with aortic regurgitation is best managed with a higher than normal heart rate, which reduces diastolic time for regurgitant ventricular dilatation, and cautious vasodilatation to increase forward flow. Myocardial depressant anaesthetic drugs should again be avoided because left ventricular function is frequently impaired.

MITRAL VALVE DISEASE

The most important goal in anaesthetizing a patient with mitral stenosis is the maintenance of a normal heart rate. Tachycardia seriously reduces cardiac output by limiting diastolic ventricular filling time. Left atrial pressure should be kept at near maximal levels to aid flow across the stenotic valve. This must be achieved by avoiding hypovolaemia from either blood loss or the vasodilating effects of anaesthetic agents. Great care is needed because pulmonary oedema and right ventricular failure are easily precipitated. Pulmonary vascular resistance is elevated and factors that increase it further, such as hypoxia, acidosis and nitrous oxide, should be avoided. Anaesthetic considerations for patients with mitral regurgitation follow similar arguments as those for aortic regurgitation.

HYPERTROPHIC OBSTRUCTIVE CARDIOMYOPATHY

Patients with hypertrophic obstructive cardio-myopathy appear to tolerate anaesthesia and non-cardiac surgery quite well. Thompson et al. have reported a series of 35 patients who underwent 56 major surgical procedures without a peri-operative death.[61] Intra-operative administration of beta-blockers was necessary to control arrhythmias in 7 of the patients, and in 11 a vasoconstrictor was given to combat hypotension and decrease the gradient across the outlet obstruction. Haemodyna-mic management aims to minimize the systolic pressure gradient between the left ventricle and aorta. Spinal anaesthesia is best avoided because of the rapid and unpredictable onset of hypotension due to sympathetic blockade.[62] General anaesthesia should include a volatile anaesthetic, such as halothane, to reduce contractility and thus keep the left ventricular outflow gradient as low as possible. A high preload is required to maintain adequate filling of the stiff thick-walled ventricle.

ANTICOAGULANTS

Short-term withdrawal of anticoagulants from patients with prosthetic heart valves appears to be relatively safe and is essential for many operations, for example, neurosurgery. Tinker and Tarhan reported 159 patients who had valve prostheses, mainly Starr valves, and underwent 180 non-cardiac operations.[63] Anticoagulants were with-drawn in 87% of cases, such that the prothrombin time was within 20% of normal in 69% of patients. There were no cases of peri-operative thrombo-embolism, and although 10% of cases had a thrombo-embolic event during follow-up the earliest event occurred 14 months after the tempor-

ary cessation of anticoagulation. Katholi et al. also reported the safety of temporary discontinuation of anticoagulation with Starr aortic prostheses, but there were 2 fatal peri-operative thrombo-embolic events in 10 patients who had Shiley disc mitral prostheses; Katholi et al. recommended reversal of anticoagulants immediately before surgery with early post-operative heparinization in these cases.[64] Serious haemorrhage occurred in half of the patients in whom anticoagulants were continued up to the time of surgery. With the above exception, the usual method of withdrawing anticoagulants is to discontinue oral treatment a few days before the proposed surgery, and re-start treatment 2 days after surgery. In the emergency situation, fresh frozen plasma is given to replace clotting factors. Vitamin K reversal is not recommended as a routine measure because it leads to difficulties in re-establishing anticoagulation post-operatively. Sudden cessation of anticoagulant treatment does not lead to a rebound hypercoagulable state.[65] The extent to which normal coagulation needs to be restored depends on the type of surgery to be undertaken. Dental surgery and other minor proce-dures can be safely undertaken in many patients without having to withdraw therapy.[66]

Many patients who have had cardiac surgery take antiplatelet agents. Prolonged bleeding with sul-phinpyrazone and dipyridamole during non-cardiac surgery does not appear to have been reported, but aspirin causes problems which can be corrected by platelet transfusion.[67]

The role of anticoagulant prophylaxis against venous thrombosis and pulmonary embolism is discussed in Chapter 54.

EISENMENGER'S SYNDROME AND INTRACARDIAC SHUNTS

Anaesthesia for patients with haemodynamically significant intracardiac shunting poses difficulties because of the propensity of anaesthetic drugs and procedures to alter the proportion or direction of the shunt. These problems are most obvious in the patient with Eisenmenger's syndrome who not uncommonly survives into adulthood and will occasionally present for incidental surgery. An increasing number of such patients are becoming pregnant and require anaesthesia for delivery. Eisenmenger's syndrome is one of the most difficult and dangerous conditions with which the anaesthe-tist has to deal. It is usually assumed on theoretical grounds that there would be a high mortality due to anaesthesia especially in view of the reported 27% maternal mortality.[68] A review by Lumley et al.[69] published in 1977 gave a different view; 16 patients underwent general anaesthesia 18 times and although there were 3 post-operative deaths they did not appear to be related to anaesthesia and the authors concluded that general anaesthesia was not as serious a risk as had been previously thought.

The management of general anaesthesia in these patients consists primarily of the choice of technique that does not increase right-to-left shunting and exacerbate hypoxia.[70] Many anaesthetic drugs can interfere with the balance between pulmonary and systemic vascular resistance either by causing a fall in peripheral resistance (e.g. halothane, isoflurane) or by increasing pulmonary vascular resistance (e.g. nitrous oxide, ergometrine). Systemic vasoconstrictor drugs (e.g. metaraminol) may have to be used to maintain systemic vascular resistance, but they may also affect the pulmonary circulation.[69,71] The pulmonary vascular resistance in Eisenmenger's syndrome is normally regarded as fixed and not susceptible to reduction by drugs or oxygen, but in an isolated case-report[72] improvement with high concentrations of inspired oxygen has been documented and this should always be used. Artificial ventilation can be deleterious if high intrathoracic pressures are used, which result in reduced pulmonary blood flow.

Spinal or epidural regional anaesthesia can be used for surgery to the lower part of the body, including Caesarean section,[73] but inadvertent hypotension due to autonomic blockade could be difficult to control and result in profound hypoxia. Epidural analgesia is recommended for pain relief in labour.[72]

Careful monitoring is essential during any procedure and should include intra-arterial blood pressure measurement and pulse oximetry. Central venous pressure measurement should also be considered because an increase in right atrial pressure in the presence of a high fixed pulmonary vascular resistance will increase right-to-left shunt whereas a decrease in venous return would lower pulmonary and systemic blood flow, both of which result in decreased systemic oxygen saturation. The hazards of pulmonary artery catheterization are increased in these patients and may outweigh the benefits of the additional information gained from this procedure.[70]

Careful attention must be given to fluid replacement because the patients are intolerant of both blood loss and dehydration. Additional dangers include systemic air embolism from either open veins in the surgical field or bubbles in intravenous infusions. The high haematocrit predisposes to thrombosis and low-dose heparin may be appropriate. Antibiotic prophylaxis against bacterial endocarditis must be prescribed (see Chapter 34).

SURGERY IN PATIENTS WITH A CARDIAC TRANSPLANT

The patient who has a transplanted heart appears to tolerate surgery and anaesthesia well, unless the heart is damaged by rejection.[74-76] The transplanted heart is denervated and so responds atypically to surgical stress and the autonomic effects of anaesthetic agents. It does not respond to atropine but can be stimulated with inotropic and chronotropic catecholamines, which should be at hand during surgery. Hypovolaemia, from either blood loss or vasodilatation caused by anaesthetic agents, is poorly tolerated. The electrocardiogram may be difficult for the non-specialist to interpret due to the presence of activity from the donor and the recipient sino-atrial nodes.

Long-term immunosuppression creates several difficulties for the anaesthetist. The patient has an increased susceptibility to infection and extra care must be taken when inserting intravascular catheters and endotracheal tubes. Additional perioperative steroid cover will be required. As cyclosporin A is nephrotoxic and raises serum potassium levels, it is essential to maintain a good urine output during surgery.

REFERENCES

1. Lunn, J.N. and Mushin, W.W. *Mortality Associated with Anaesthesia.* London: Nuffield Provincial Hospitals Trust, 1980.
2. Goldman, L., Caldera, D.L., Nussbaum, S.R. et al. Multifactorial Index of Cardiac Risk in Noncardiac Surgical Procedures. *N. Engl. J. Med.* 1977; **297**: 845.
3. Detsky, A.S., Abrams, H.B., Forbath, N., Scott, J.G. and Hilliard, J.R. Cardiac Assessment for Patients Undergoing Noncardiac Surgery. *Arch. Intern. Med.* 1986; **146**: 2131.
4. Kaplan, J.A. *Cardiac Anesthesia*, Vol. 2. Cardiovascular Pharmacology. New York: Grune & Stratton, 1983.
5. Miller, R.D. *Anaesthesia Vol. I, II, III*, 2nd edn. New York: Churchill Livingstone, 1986.
6. Moore, R.A., Allen, M.C., Wood, P.J., Rees, L.H. and Sear, J.W. Peri-operative endocrine effects of Etomidate. *Anaesthesia* 1985; **40**: 124.
7. Eisele, J.H., Reitan, J.A., Massumi, R.A., Zelis, R.F. and Miller, R.R. Myocardial Performance and N_2O Analgesia in Coronary Artery Disease. *Anesthesiology* 1976; **44**: 16.

8. Schulte-Sasse, V., Hess, W. and Tarnow, J. Pulmonary vascular responses to nitrous oxide in patients with normal and high pulmonary vascular resistance. *Anesthesiology* 1982; 57: 9.

9. Jones, R.M. Calcium Antagonists. *Anaesthesia.* 1984; 39: 747.

10. Bovill, J.G., Warren, P.J., Schuller, J.L., Van Wezel, H.B. and Hoeneveld, M.H. Comparison of Fentanyl, Sufentanil and Alfentanil Anaesthesia in Patients undergoing Valvular Heart Surgery. *Anesth. Analg.* 1984; 63: 1081.

11. Black, T.E., Kay, B. and Healy, T.E.J. Reducing the haemodynamic responses to laryngoscopy and intubation. A comparison of alfentanil with fentanyl. *Anesthesia* 1984; 39: 883.

12. Prough, D.S., Roy, R., Bumgarner, J. and Shannon, G. Acute Pulmonary Oedema in Healthy Teenagers following Conservative Doses of Intravenous Naloxone. *Anesthesiology* 1984; 60: 485.

13. Veland, K., Ahamatsu, T.J., Eng, M., Bonica, J.J. and Hansen, J.M. Maternal Cardiovascular Dynamics. VI Cesarian section under epidural anaesthesia without epinephrine. *Am. J. Obstet. Gynecol* 1972; 114: 775.

14. Hagerdal, M., Morgan, C.W., Sumner, A.E. and Gutsche, B.B. Minute Ventilation and Oxygen Consumption during Labour with Epidural Analgesia. *Anesthesiology* 1983; 59: 425.

15. Taylor, M.B. and Whitwam, J.G. The current status of pulse oximetry. Clinical value of continuous non-invasive oxygen saturation monitoring. *Anaesthesia* 1986; 41: 943.

16. Vitez, T.S., Soper, L.E., Wong, K.C. and Soper, P. Chronic hypokalemia and intraoperative dysrhythmias. *Anesthesiology* 1985; 63: 130.

17. Wells, P.H. and Kaplan, J.A. Optimal Management of Patients with Ischemic Heart Disease for Noncardiac Surgery by Complementary Anesthesiologist and Cardiologist Interaction. *Am. Heart J.* 1981; 102: 1029.

18. Downing, J.W. and Tinker, J.H. Fitness for Anaesthesia: Who Decides? *Lancet* 1987; i: 387.

19. Tarhan, S., Moffitt, E.A., Taylor, W.F. and Guiliani, E.R. Myocardial infarction after general anaesthesia. *JAMA* 1972; 220: 1451.

20. Cavliner, N.H., Fisher, M.L., Plotnick, G. *et al.* The pre-operative electrocardiogram as an indicator of risk in major non-cardiac surgery. *Can. J. Cardiol.* 1986; 2: 134.

21. Mauney, F.M. Jr, Ebert, P.A. and Sabiston, D.C. Jr. Post-operative Myocardial Infarctions. *Ann. Surg.* 1970; 172: 497.

22. Benchimol, A., Harris, C.L., Desser, K.B., Kwee, B.T. and Promisloff, S.D. Resting Electrocardiogram in Major Coronary Artery Disease. *JAMA* 1973; 224: 1489.

23. Nimmo, W.S., Jones, R.M., Grant, I.S. and Ramsey, L.E. Should a Fasting Patient Receive His Medication? *Survey Anesthesiol.* 1986; 30: 382.

24. Miller, R.R., Olsen, H.G., Amsterdam, E.A. and Mason, D.T. Propanolol-withdrawal rebound phenomenon. Exacerbation of coronary events after abrupt cessation of anti-anginal therapy. *N. Engl. J. Med.* 1975; 293: 416.

25. Feely, J., Forrest, A., Gunn, A., Hamilton, W., Stevenson, I. and Crooks, J. Influence of surgery on plasma propanolol levels and protein binding. *Clin. Pharmacol. Ther.* 1980; 28: 759.

26. Villers, D., Pinaud, L.J., Bourin, M. *et al.* Propanolol postoperative maintenance by continuous infusion. *Anesthesiology* 1984; 60: 594.

27. Laver, M.B. Myocardial Ischaemia. Dilemma between information available and information demand. *Br. Heart J.* 1983; 50: 222.

28. Coriat, P., Daloz, M., Bousseau, D., Fusciardi, J., Echter, E. and Viars, P. Prevention of Intraoperative Myocardial Ischemia during noncardiac surgery with intravenous nitro-

glycerin. *Anesthesiology* 1984; 61: 193.

29. Fusciardi, J., Godet, G., Bernard, J.M., Bertrand, M., Kieffer, E. and Viars, P. Roles of fentanyl and nitroglycerin in prevention of myocardial ischemia associated with laryngoscopy and tracheal intubation in patients undergoing operations of short duration. *Anesth. Analg.* 1986; 65: 617.

30. Thomson, I.R., Mutch, W.A.C. and Culligan, J.D. Failure of Intravenous Nitroglycerine to Prevent Intraoperative Myocardial Ischaemia during Fentanyl–Pancuronium Anesthesia. *Anesthesiology* 1984; 61: 385.

31. Slogoff, S. and Keats, A.S. Does Perioperative Myocardial Ischaemia Lead to Postoperative Myocardial Infarction. *Anesthesiology* 1985; 62: 107.

32. Merin, R.G., Lowenstein, E. and Gelman, S. Is anaesthesia beneficial for the ischemic heart? *Anesthesiology* 1986; 64: 137.

33. Kleinman, B., Henkin, R.E., Glisson, S.N. *et al.* Qualitative Evaluation of Coronary Flow During Anesthetic Induction Using Thallium-201 Perfusion Scans. *Anesthesiology* 1986; 64: 157.

34. Coriat, P., Fauchet, M., Bousseau, D. *et al.* Left Ventricular Dysfunction After Non-cardiac Surgical Procedures in Patients with Ischaemic Heart Disease. *Acta Anaesthesiol. Scand.* 1985; 29: 804.

35. Touze, M.D., Pinaud, M., Rozo, L., Souron, R. and Nicolas, F. Echocardiography and Left Ventricular Function on Recovery from Anaesthesia in Patients with Coronary Artery Disease. *Acta Anaesthesiol. Scand.* 1983; 27: 149.

36. Steen, P.A., Tinker, J.H. and Tarhan, S. Myocardial Reinfarction after Anesthesia and Surgery. *JAMA* 1978; 239: 2566.

37. Van Knorring, J. Postoperative Myocardial Infarction: A Prospective Study in a Risk Group of Surgical Patients. *Surgery* 1981; 90: 55.

38. Eerola, M., Eerola, R., Kaukinen, S. and Kaukinen, L. Risk Factors in Surgical Patients with Verified Pre-operative Myocardial Infarction. *Acta Anaesthesiol. Scand.* 1980; 24: 219.

39. Rao, T.L., Jacobs, K.H. and El Etr, A.A. Re-Infarction Following Anesthesia in Patients with Myocardial Infarction. *Anesthesiology* 1983; 59: 449.

40. Lowenstein, E., Yusuf, S. and Teplick, R.S. Perioperative Myocardial Reinfarction: A Glimmer of Hope—A Note of Caution. *Anesthesiology* 1983; 59: 493.

41. Becker, C.L., Tinker, J.H., Robertson, D.M. and Vlietstra, R.E. Myocardial infarction following local anaesthesia for ophthalmic surgery. *Anesth. Analg.* 1980; 59: 257.

42. Mahar, L.J., Steen, P.A., Tinker, J.H., Vliestra, R.E., Smith, H.G. and Pluth, J.R. Perioperative myocardial infarction in patients with coronary artery disease with and without aorto-coronary artery bypass grafts. *J. Thorac. Cardiovasc. Surg.* 1978; 76: 533.

43. Crawford, E.S., Morris, C.G., Howell, J.F., Flynn, W.F. and Moorhead, D.T. Operative Risk in Patients with Previous Coronary Artery Bypass. *Ann. Thorac. Surg.* 1978; 26: 215.

44. Prorok, J.J. and Trostle, D. Operative Risk of General Surgical Procedures in Patients with Previous Myocardial Revascularization. *Surg. Gynecol. Obstet.* 1984; 159: 214.

45. McCullom, C.H., Garcia-Rinaldi, R., Graham, J.M. and DeBakey, M.E. Myocardial Revascularization Prior to Subsequent Major Surgery in Patients with Coronary Artery Disease. *Surgery* 1977; 81: 302.

46. Roizen, M.F. Anesthetic Implications of Concurrent Diseases. In: Miller, R.D., ed. *Anesthesia,* Vol. 1, 2nd edn. New York: Churchill Livingstone, 1986, p.278.

47. Prys-Roberts, C. Medical Problems of Surgical Patients. Hypertension and Ischaemic Heart Disease. *Ann. R. Coll. Surg. Engl.* 1976; 58: 465.

48. Magnusson, J., Thulin, T., Warner, O., Jarhult, J. and Thomson, D. Haemodynamic Effects of Pre-Treatment with

Metoprolol in Hypertensive Patients Undergoing Surgery. *Br. J. Anaesth.* 1986; **58**: 251.

49. Goldman, L. and Caldera, D.L. Risk of General Anesthesia and Elective Operation in the Hypertensive Patient. *Anesthesiology.* 1979; **50**: 285.

50. Bertrand, C.A., Steiner, N.V., Jameson, A.G. and Lopez, M. Disturbances of Cardiac Rhythm during Anesthesia and Surgery. *JAMA* 1971; **216**: 1615.

51. Atlee, J.L. Anaesthesia and Cardiac Electrophysiology. *Eur. J. Anaesthesiol.* 1985; **2**: 215.

52. Galloway, P.A. and Glass, P.S. Anesthetic Implications of Prolonged QT Interval Syndromes. *Anesth. Analg.* 1985; **64**: 612.

53. Liberman, B.A. and Teasdale, S.J. Anaesthesia and Amiodarone. *Can. Anesth. Soc. J.* 1985; **32**: 629.

54. Deutsch, L.S. and Dalen, J.E. Indications for Prophylactic Digitalization. *Anesthesiology* 1969; **30**: 648.

55. Rooney, S.M., Goldiner, P.L. and Muss, E. Relationship of Right Bundle Branch Block and Marked Left Axis Deviation to Complete Heart Block During General Anesthesia. *Anesthesiology* 1976; **44**: 64.

56. Bellocci, F., Santovelli, P., Di Genaro, M., Ansalone, G. and Fenici, R. The Risk of Cardiac Complications in Surgical Patients with Bifasicular Block. *Chest* 1980; **77**: 343.

57. Zaidan, J.R. Pacemakers. *Anesthesiology* 1984; **60**: 319.

58. Levine, P.A., Balady, G.J., Lazar, H.L., Belott, P.H. and Roberts, A.J. Electrocautery and Pacemakers: Management of the Paced Patient Subject to Electrocautery. *Ann. Thorac. Surg.* 1986; **41**: 313.

59. Simon, A.B. Perioperative Management of the Pacemaker Patient. *Anesthesiology* 1977; **46**: 127.

60. McShane, A.J. and Hone, R. Prevention of bacterial endocarditis: does nasal intubation warrant prophylaxis. *Br. Med. J.* 1986; **292**: 26.

61. Thompson, R.C., Liberthson, R.R. and Lowenstein, E. Perioperative Anesthetic Risk of Non-Cardiac Surgery in Hypertrophic Obstructive Cardiomyopathy. *JAMA* 1985; **254**: 2419.

62. Loubser, P., Suh, K. and Cohen, S. Adverse Effects of Spinal Anesthesia in a Patient with Idiopathic Hypertrophic Subaortic Stenosis. *Anesthesiology* 1984; **60**: 228.

63. Tinker, J.H. and Tarhan, S. Discontinuing Anticoagulant

Therapy in Surgical Patients with Cardiac Valve Prostheses. *JAMA* 1978; **239**: 738.

64. Katholi, R.E., Nolan, S.P. and McGuire, L.B. Living with Prosthetic Heart Valves: Subsequent Noncardiac Operations and the Risk of Thromboembolism or Hemorrhage. *Am. Heart J.* 1976; **92**: 162.

65. Michaels, L. Incidence of Thromboembolism After Stopping Anticoagulant Therapy. *JAMA* 1971; **215**: 595.

66. McIntyre, H. Management During Dental Surgery of Patients on Anticoagulants. *Lancet* 1966; **ii**: 99.

67. Merriman, E., Bell, W. and Long, D.M. Surgical Postoperative Bleeding Associated with Aspirin Ingestion: Report of Two Cases. *J. Neurosurg.* 1979; **50**: 682.

68. Jones, A. and Howitt, G. Eisenmenger syndrome in pregnancy. *Br. Med. J.* 1965; **1**: 1627.

69. Lumley, J., Whitwam, J.G. and Morgan, M. General Anesthesia in the Presence of Eisenmenger's Syndrome. *Anesth. Analg.* 1977; **56**: 543.

70. Foster, J.M.G. and Jones, R.M. The Anaesthetic Management of the Eisenmenger Syndrome. *Ann. R. Coll. Surg. Engl.* 1984; **66**: 353.

71. Bird, T.M. and Strunin, L. Anaesthesia for a Patient with Down's Syndrome and Eisenmenger's Complex. *Anaesthesia* 1984; **39**: 48.

72. Midwall, J., Jaffin, H., Herman, M.V. and Kupersmith, J. Shunt Flow and Pulmonary Hemodynamics During Labor and Delivery in the Eisenmenger Syndrome. *Am. J. Cardiol.* 1978; **42**: 299.

73. Spinnato, J.A., Kraynack, B.J. and Cooper, M.W. Eisenmenger's Syndrome in Pregnancy: Epidural Anesthesia for Elective Cesarean Section. *N. Engl. J. Med.* 1981; **304**: 1215.

74. Kanter, S.F. and Samuels, S.I. Anesthesia for Major Operations on Patients who have Transplanted Hearts: A Review of 29 Cases. *Anesthesiology* 1977; **46**: 65.

75. Grebenik, C.R. and Robinson, P.N. Cardiac Transplantation at Harefield: A Review from the Anaesthetist's Standpoint. *Anaesthesia.* 1985; **40**: 131.

76. Cooper, D.K., Becerra, E.A., Novitzky, D., Ozinksky, J., Horak, A. and Reichart, B. Surgery in Patients with Heart Transplants. Anaesthetic and Operative Considerations. *S. Afr. Med. J.* 1986; **79**: 137.

Chapter 75

The Principles of Cardiac Surgery

David J. Wheatley

Prior to the introduction of techniques for cardiopulmonary bypass in the mid 1950s, surgical procedures for heart disease were limited to those which could be performed without undue interference with the heart and circulation. Closure of patent ductus arteriosus, resection of aortic coarctation, construction of systemic to pulmonary shunts and closed mitral commissurotomy were the commonest operations in this era.

Successful complete heart–lung bypass was first reported in experimental animals in 1937 by Gibbon. Dennis attempted clinical application in 1951, but it was Gibbon in 1953 who first successfully used complete heart–lung bypass to repair an atrial septal defect.[1] Early techniques for cardiopulmonary bypass were applied to the correction of simpler congenital cardiac defects, such as atrial and ventricular septal defects and valvular stenosis. As cardiopulmonary bypass techniques became refined, more complex congenital lesions were corrected. In the early 1960s, heart valve prostheses became available, extending the scope of surgery for valvular heart disease. Coronary artery surgery became established in the late 1960s and a period of rapid expansion of cardiac surgical practice followed. Cardiac transplantation became a clinical prospect in the late 1960s and now has a well-established role in treating a relatively small number of patients who have end-stage cardiac disease.[2]

An indication of recent practice of cardiac surgery in the UK is given in a report of the period 1977–1982, during which there was a steady increase in the total number of cardiac operations, from 11 602 in 1977 to 15 890 in 1982. In 1977, coronary surgery accounted for 26% of all cardiac surgery performed in the UK; in 1982, 47% of cardiac operations were for coronary artery surgery. In 1982, the remainder of cardiac operations were for valvular heart disease (29%), congenital heart disease (21%), and miscellaneous procedures for acquired heart disease (3%).[3]

A report of thoracic and cardiovascular operations undertaken in the USA during the period 1979–1984[4] shows a similar pattern of increase in coronary surgery, although at a much higher level (114 000 operations for coronary artery disease alone in 1979 rising to 191 000 in 1983).

There is considerable variation in the level and nature of cardiac surgical practice between countries, and even within countries, reflecting the differing prevalence of disease and variations in the availability of resources. Care is required when applying experience from practice in one population to another. For example, the surgical management of valvular heart disease is very different in a country that has a high prevalence of rheumatic fever in a young population and poor access to medical supervision from that in a country in which there is little rheumatic fever and ready access to medical care.

Few cardiac surgical procedures remain in routine use for long without modification. The long-term outcome of many procedures is still uncertain, and there will always be the need for evaluation and critical review. Important lessons have been learned from randomized trials in coronary surgery,[5] and long-term follow-up has led to improved practice in congenital, valvular and coronary surgery. Other influences on the evolving practice and role of cardiac surgery include the advent of alternative methods of management, such as thrombolytic therapy[6] or percutaneous transluminal coronary angioplasty. The latter technique was applied in more than 60 000 patients in the USA alone in 1984,[7] usually as an alternative to coronary surgery. The optimal role for this procedure is not yet defined, emphasizing the need for continued critical follow-up and evaluation. Intervention in acute myocardial infarction is another area in which optimal management is not yet defined, and further advances are to be anticipated.[8]

SURGICAL ACCESS TO THE HEART

VERTICAL STERNOTOMY

Most cardiac operations are undertaken through a vertical incision, dividing skin, subcutaneous tissues and sternum in the midline. Powered sternal saws make the procedure rapid and simple. Blood loss is minimal and no muscle is divided. The pericardial cavity is opened to give good exposure of the ascending aorta and right atrium, allowing cannulation for cardiopulmonary bypass without interference with the heart or haemodynamic state (Fig.75.1).

When sternotomy is undertaken as a repeat procedure, adhesions between the heart and overlying pericardium or sternum may result in injury to the aorta, right ventricle or right atrium being sustained during the opening of the chest. This can cause

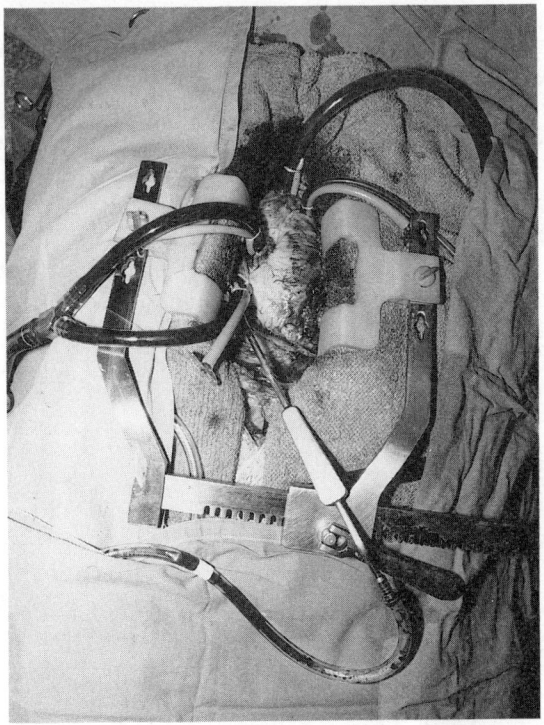

Fig.75.1. Vertical sternotomy. The divided sternum is held apart by a retractor. The ascending aorta and right atrium are exposed. At the top right of the picture the arterial cannula is shown entering the aorta. The two cannulas on the left are inserted into the venae cavae and the Y-connector joins them to the venous line draining to the pump oxygenator. The tube in the lower part of the picture is a suction tube for returning blood from the operating field to the extracorporeal circuit. The small tube on the right of the picture is a vent tube inserted into the pulmonary artery for decompression of the pulmonary circuit and left heart chambers.

profuse and life-threatening haemorrhage and accounts for at least part of the increased risk in repeat cardiac operations. Sharp dissection of the heart from the back of the sternum through an approach from the sub-xiphoid region allows gradual and safe division of the mobilized sternum from below upwards.[9]

Exposure of intracardiac structures is obtained by opening the great vessels, the atria or areas of myocardial scar. Incisions into normal myocardium are avoided as far as possible, in view of the scarring and loss of function caused by such incisions.

The aortic valve is approached via an incision in the root of the aorta made with the patient on cardiopulmonary bypass and with the ascending aorta cross-clamped as high as possible, just below the aortic perfusing cannula. Vertical sternotomy gives a good view of the aortic valve.

The mitral valve is exposed through an incision in the left atrium anterior to the right pulmonary veins. The tangential view obtained of the mitral valve is not always ideal from a sternotomy incision, but the safety of aortic cannulation and cross-clamping, and safety of cardiac de-airing from this incision, outweigh the difficulties of mitral exposure.

The right atrium is opened to give exposure of the tricuspid valve or for repair of atrial septal defects. Ventricular septal defects can often be repaired from this approach, working through the tricuspid orifice. If exposure of a ventricular septal defect is inadequate from this approach, the right ventricular infundibulum is opened. Infundibular incision is used particularly for correction of tetralogy of Fallot, because it allows closure of the ventricular septal defect, resection of trabecular obstructions or insertion of a right ventricular outflow tract enlarging patch as required.

LEFT THORACOTOMY

Left lateral thoracotomy requires division of chest wall muscles and retraction of lung. It gives good exposure of the descending thoracic aorta and left side of the heart and is used for closure of patent ductus arteriosus, repair of aortic coarctation and closed mitral commissurotomy. Establishment of cardiopulmonary bypass from this approach is most often achieved by cannulating a femoral artery and vein, supplementing drainage of venous blood by a cannula in the pulmonary artery or the right atrial appendage.

RIGHT THORACOTOMY

Exposure of the heart from a right lateral thoracotomy provides a good view of the atrial septum and the mitral valve. Access to the aorta is limited, making the approach less satisfactory than sternotomy when cardiopulmonary bypass is used.

CARDIOPULMONARY BYPASS

Most cardiac surgical procedures require that the heart be immobilized or opened. The function of the heart needs to be taken over by an artificial pump and, in practice, an extracorporeal circuit is used, with a pump and oxygenator providing an alternative for the heart and lungs–cardiopulmonary bypass.

PUMPS

Most pumps in current clinical practice are roller pumps, in which blood is propelled through flexible plastic tubing by rollers mounted on a rotating arm (Fig.75.2).[10] This simple pump is reliable, can be turned by hand in the event of a power failure and produces minimal injury to the blood in routine cardiopulmonary bypass. Prolonged procedures, as in left heart assistance, are complicated by significant haemolysis with roller pumps, and there are available centrifugal pumps that produce minimal haemolysis over a long period.[11] Such pumps can be used for routine cardiopulmonary bypass as well.

There have been many attempts to mimic the normal circulation more closely by imparting pulsatility to the arterial pressure. This is most simply achieved by a roller pump capable of rapid variation in speed and, hence, variable pulsatile output, which produces a close simulation of normal cardiac output. For routine cardiopulmonary bypass, there is little evidence of obvious superiority of such a pulsatile system, lack of pulsatility being well tolerated for several hours.[12] However, pulsatile flow does seem to ameliorate the progressive rise in systemic peripheral vascular resistance seen during cardiopulmonary bypass.

OXYGENATORS AND HEAT EXCHANGERS

Oxygenation of blood and removal of excess carbon dioxide is achieved in the extracorporeal circuit by the use of either a bubble oxygenator or a membrane oxygenator. There are a large number of commercially available, pre-sterilized, disposable oxygenators (Fig.75.3).[13]

Bubble oxygenators expose blood to a mixture of 95% oxygen and 5% carbon dioxide in the form of small bubbles. The systemic venous blood drains from the patient by gravity and runs through the oxygenator with little resistance. Gas exchange occurs at the surface of the bubbles, being most efficient for carbon dioxide, and equilibrates to give a blood P_{CO_2} of 40 mmHg and a blood P_{O_2} usually well in excess of physiological levels. The presence of gas bubbles in the blood is a hazard and their removal is accomplished by passing the blood over a defoaming section and allowing it to accumulate in a reservoir prior to being pumped back to the patient.

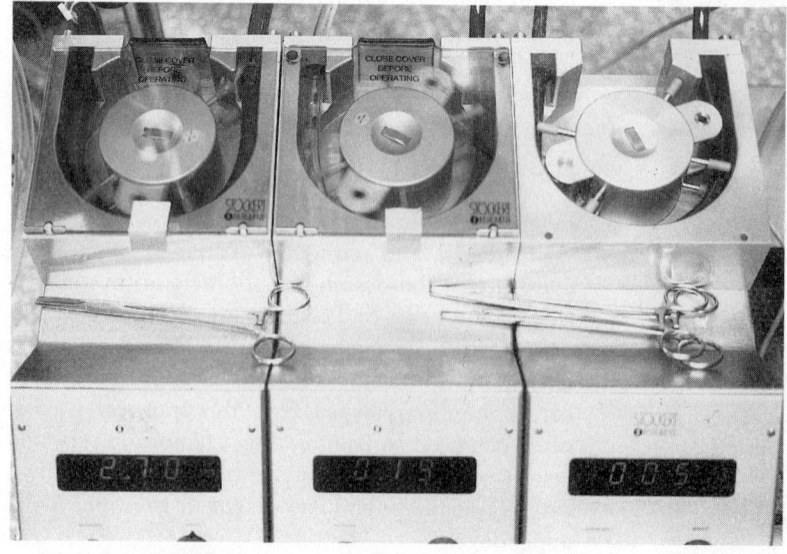

Fig.75.2. The pump console. Three roller pumps are used for the extracorporeal circuit. The pump on the left supports the extracorporeal circulation; the flow rate is indicated on the display. The centre pump is for return of blood from the operating field to the extracorporeal circuit. The pump on the right returns blood from the vent tube to the circuit.

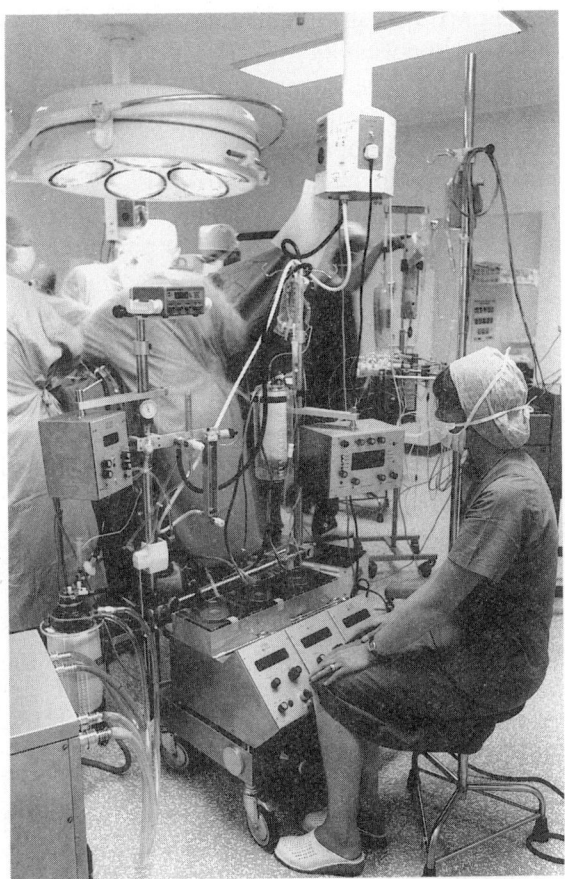

Fig.75.3. The extracorporeal circuit. In the foreground is the pump console under the control of a perfusionist. In the left foreground is the heater/cooler unit which circulates water to the bubble oxygenator to the left of the pump console.

In *membrane oxygenators*, blood and gas phases are separated by a gas-permeable membrane arranged either as a system of sheets or as a system of fine tubes designed to pass blood in thin films through the blood–gas interface region. This results in considerable haemodynamic resistance and it is necessary to pump the blood through membrane oxygenators, damping any pulsatility in the process. Membrane oxygenators cause less haemolysis than bubble oxygenators, and the reduction in the white cell and platelet counts is not as great. They are also less likely to allow the escape of microbubbles than are bubble oxygenators.[14] These advantages are less apparent with routine cardiopulmonary bypass than with prolonged circulatory support, where the use of membrane oxygenators is essential. Their cost has gradually become more competitive with that of bubble oxygenators, and their use for routine procedures is increasing.

Cooling of blood occurs inevitably in its extracorporeal transit. It is therefore necessary to warm the blood to prevent hypothermia from developing. This is achieved by a heat exchanger in which blood passes through a system of tubes surrounded by water circulating at a controlled temperature. Modern oxygenators incorporate a heat exchanger as part of an integral oxygenator/heat exchanger unit (Fig.75.3).

The heat exchanger is also used to lower blood temperature for the induction of systemic hypothermia as an adjunct to cardiopulmonary bypass. The same system returns body temperature to normothermic levels at the conclusion of the procedure.

THE CARDIOPULMONARY BYPASS CIRCUIT

Systemic venous blood is intercepted from the cavae, or from the right atrium, by plastic cannulae inserted via short incisions in the right atrial wall (a purse-string suture placed around such an incision helps to ensure a blood and air-tight seal, and closes the incision after removal of the cannula) (Fig.75.1). Blood drains by gravity through plastic tubing to the oxygenator and is returned to the arterial system by means of a plastic cannula inserted high up in the ascending aorta, or alternatively, into a major branch of the aorta (most commonly and conveniently a femoral artery).

The cannulae, tubing and oxygenator are sterile and require to be filled (or primed) with fluid prior to the institution of cardiopulmonary bypass. The extracorporeal circuit is primed with an isosmotic solution (5% dextrose water or balanced salt solutions form the basis of most priming solutions). The priming volume of approximately 1500 ml for an adult system results in haemodilution which is well tolerated. For infants, in whom priming volume forms a large proportion of total circulating volume during cardiopulmonary bypass, it is usually necessary to prime with blood.

Exposure of blood to foreign surfaces in the extracorporeal circuit activates clotting mechanisms. Thrombus formation is prevented by the administration of heparin to the patient (3 mg/kg) prior to cannulation for cardiopulmonary bypass. The level of heparin activity is checked by measurement of the activated clotting time and further heparin is given as necessary to maintain the activated clotting time at levels >400 s. Once the cannulae have been removed at the completion of the procedure, normal coagulation is restored by neutralizing circulating heparin with protamine.

MANAGEMENT OF BLOOD IN THE OPERATING FIELD

During the operation, there is usually an accumulation of blood in the operating field from the bronchial circulation, from non-coronary collateral flow to the myocardium, from the chest wall and from dissected areas around the heart. This blood is returned to the extracorporeal circuit by a separate sucker and pump (Fig.75.1). If improperly used, with excessive suction pressure, such suction systems contribute greatly to haemolysis and gaseous micro-emboli in the systemic arterial system.

It is important to avoid distension of the chambers of the heart and the pulmonary circulation. This is often achieved by insertion of a decompressing tube or 'vent' into the left atrium or pulmonary artery connected to the extracorporeal circuit for return of blood by a separate pump (Fig.75.1).

FLOW RATE, PRESSURE AND TEMPERATURE

The cardiopulmonary bypass circuit is required to deliver a flow of oxygenated blood at a rate sufficient to ensure adequate perfusion of the brain and other vital organs. The required flow rate is conventionally considered as 2.4 l/m²/min ('full flow'), corresponding to normal cardiac output in the anaesthetized state. A mean perfusion pressure of 50–70 mmHg is usually achieved at this flow rate. Many factors influence the pressure, including haemodilution (which reduces blood viscosity, and is seen particularly with blood-free priming), hypothermia (which increases blood viscosity), vasoconstriction (a response to hypothermia and to prolonged cardiopulmonary bypass), vasodilatation (often induced by anaesthetic agents or vasodilating drugs used to improve tissue perfusion) and pump flow rate (under the control of the perfusionist).

For nearly all cardiac surgical procedures, it is usual practice to induce systemic hypothermia, lowering the blood temperature to 20–28°C.[15–17] This allows the extracorporeal flow rate to be reduced to half to two-thirds of the normothermic 'full flow' level, thus minimizing blood damage and imparting a safety margin in the event of inadequate perfusion occurring. The lowered temperature and reduction in flow rate this permits also minimizes non-coronary collateral flow to the myocardium and is an important adjunct to cardioplegic techniques.

Prolonged periods of circulatory arrest can pro-vide optimal operating conditions for correction of congenital abnormalities in infants or for treatment of aortic arch aneurysms in adults. Induction of profound hypothermia (12–20°C) is achieved by cooling on cardiopulmonary bypass, following which periods of circulatory arrest of 45 min or longer may be safe. Cardiopulmonary bypass is then re-instituted for re-warming to normothermic levels.

TOTAL AND PARTIAL CARDIOPULMONARY BYPASS

Operations on the heart require diversion of all systemic return to the extracorporeal circuit, with a pump flow of 2.4 l/m²/min or more at normothermic levels – total cardiopulmonary bypass. Extracorporeal circulation may be used for part of the systemic venous return – partial bypass – and is most commonly applied to the treatment of descending aortic aneurysms. Venous blood is removed from the femoral vein or inferior vena cava, supplemented as necessary by drainage from the right atrium, pulmonary artery or left atrium. Blood is returned to the lower part of the body through a femoral arterial cannula. Safe cross-clamping of the descending aorta is possible with partial bypass— the upper part of the body being perfused by the heart and the lower part by the extracorporeal pump. Care is required to balance pump and heart outputs to maintain normal arterial pressure in the upper part of the body, and hypothermia is avoided as this would risk depression of the left ventricle and the possibility of ventricular fibrillation.

COMPLICATIONS OF CARDIOPULMONARY BYPASS

Perfusion accidents due to errors in the placement of cannulas or failure in the extracorporeal circuit are uncommon, but constant vigilance is required to ensure safety.

The arterial perfusion cannula must be positioned in a manner that allows unobstructed perfusion of the aortic arch, avoiding selective perfusion of the brachiocephalic artery. Dislodgement of atheromatous aortic plaque is a risk of cannulation, lessened by prior palpation to confirm normality of the chosen cannulation site. Venous cannulae may become kinked, or obstructed if inserted too far. Monitoring of jugular venous pressure and venous drainage give some warning of this event. Failure to remove air from the extracorporeal circuit, or entraining air by allowing the blood level in the oxygenator to fall too low, are obvious hazards, as are disconnection of tube connectors or rupture of flexible pump tubing.

Removal of air from the left-heart chambers is surprisingly difficult, and air embolism may complicate any procedure on the heart in which the left-sided chambers are opened to the air. Thrombus in the left atrial appendage or calcific debris on the aortic or mitral valves are other sources of embolus which may complicate cardiopulmonary bypass procedures.

Less obvious problems may arise from inadequacies of perfusion, whether this be due to inadequate flow rate, low arterial perfusing pressure, raised venous pressure, lack of pulsatility or inadequate oxygen-carrying capacity of the perfusing blood. There is a rapid fall in systemic vascular resistance at the onset of cardiopulmonary bypass, followed by a gradual increase over the course of the next hour or two (the usual duration of most procedures) and perfusing pressure may be low soon after the commencement of cardiopulmonary bypass. There is evidence that flow rate and arterial pressure can be safely reduced in the presence of hypothermia, although there is considerable difficulty in defining the minimum acceptable levels. In general, a reduction of flow rate to 1.2–1.6 l/m²/min with a blood temperature of 20–28°C appears to be safe.[17] A mean arterial pressure of more than 50 mmHg is desirable; if it is lower than this, flow rate should be increased.

Cardiopulmonary bypass may also be complicated by the occurrence of micro-embolization. Gaseous micro-emboli may arise from bubble oxygenators, from cardiotomy suction systems entraining large amounts of air, which may fail to be completely intercepted by the filter and defoaming systems, or from insertion of cannulae into the left-heart structures.[18] Micro-embolism of fat, platelet and fibrin aggregates, calcific debris and foreign material are all described.[19]

A further source of injury during cardiopulmonary bypass is the whole-body inflammatory response which occurs as a result of exposure of the blood to the foreign surfaces of the extracorporeal circuit. This results in activation of the kinin, clotting, fibrinolytic and complement systems. Widespread capillary endothelial damage occurs, with increased permeability, affecting particularly the pulmonary capillary beds. Other consequences include a possible increased susceptibility to infection as a result of depletion of complement.[20–24]

Although injury may occur to the lungs, the liver and kidneys, the brain is the most vulnerable organ and that which causes most concern. A high incidence of neurological and neuropsychological changes was described after cardiac surgery in early practice, but many of these problems could be ascribed to technical factors which may reasonably be expected to have been eliminated from more recent practice.[25] Nevertheless, there remains considerable concern about the incidence of diffuse neurological injury which may be manifested by neuropsychological abnormalities.

The incidence of neurological complications following cardiac surgery has been reported between 0%[26] and 100%,[27] depending on the study design, the timing and nature of neurological assessment, the diligence of the examiner and whether the information has been gathered in a retrospective or prospective fashion.[28] Furthermore, the application of sophisticated investigative techniques such as psychometric testing,[29,30] measurement of cerebral blood flow,[31] electroencephalography,[27] fluorescein retinal angiography[32] and examination of cerebrospinal fluid for biochemical markers of brain damage appear to demonstrate abnormalities in up to 100% of patients.

Approximately 1–2% of patients will develop obvious signs of cerebral injury following cardiac surgery.[33] Such injury is usually attributable to macro-embolization of air, calcium or thrombus from a variety of sources. The presence of asymptomatic carotid stenosis apparently does not increase the post-operative incidence of obvious cerebral deficit.[34]

Recent attention has focused on two reports indicating evidence of subtle cerebral impairment, as judged by psychometric testing, in 60% of patients following cardiopulmonary bypass.[29,30] The pathophysiology of such dysfunction is not known, although micro-embolization and impaired perfusion of the cerebral microcirculation during surgery are suspected. The clotting system is activated by the extracorporeal circuit and micro-embolization of platelets, fibrin and thrombus has been reported.[19] Such dysfunction appears to be transient in the majority of patients.[30] Indeed, the difficulty in interpretation of neuropsychiatric tests is illustrated by the finding that certain tests of intellectual function showed an improvement at 6 months' follow-up when compared with preoperative performance.

PROTECTION OF THE MYOCARDIUM DURING CARDIAC SURGERY

The myocardium is vulnerable to injury during cardiac surgical procedures, and failure of the heart to sustain adequate cardiac output following operation is one of the most important causes of hospital mortality.

Most patients undergoing cardiac surgery have disease in which the balance between myocardial perfusion and myocardial oxygen demand may be readily compromised during induction of anaesthesia and preparation for cardiopulmonary bypass. Patients with severe aortic valve disease or high-grade obstruction of the left main or proximal coronary arteries are the most vulnerable. Care in avoiding tachycardia, hypotension or hypertension does much to avoid peri-operative myocardial infarction in these patients.

Incisions in myocardium are deleterious to ventricular function, and are avoided whenever possible. Distension of the heart and handling or stretching of the myocardium during retraction of the ventricles may cause injury unless care is taken.

METHODS FOR IMMOBILIZING THE HEART

Immobility of the heart is necessary for operating on the coronary arteries, or when opening the chambers of the heart as this is much safer when the heart is immobile—frothing of blood and the risk of coronary air embolism are avoided. There are a number of methods for achieving a still heart, and all of these need to take account of the requirements for preserving myocardial integrity and function.

Induced ventricular fibrillation

The heart can be immobilized by the elective induction of ventricular fibrillation with an electrical fibrillator, a technique first proposed by Senning in 1952.[36] This technique was frequently used to prevent ejection from the heart during procedures to remove air prior to the conclusion of cardiopulmonary bypass. It was suggested that electrically maintained ventricular fibrillation, rather than spontaneous fibrillation, was deleterious to the heart, especially in the presence of left ventricular hypertrophy, by causing a decrease in subendocardial perfusion and, ultimately, subendocardial necrosis.[37,38] Cox et al.[39] showed induced ventricular fibrillation to be safe in non-hypertrophied hearts in an experimental study.

Akins[40] has described good results, comparable to those obtained with cardioplegia, for coronary surgery with the use of elective spontaneous ventricular fibrillation combined with systemic hypothermia to 28°C, cooling of the heart within the pericardial cavity using 4°C Ringer lactate solution, maintenance of systemic perfusion pressure between 80 and 100 mmHg, left ventricular venting and local vessel isolation during distal anastomoses without aortic occlusion. Using this technique, a hospital mortality of 0.4% has been reported in 1000 patients having elective coronary surgery, with a peri-operative myocardial infarction rate of 1.8.%[41] Akins has also reported[42] excellent results with the technique in patients undergoing emergency revascularization. As pointed out by Levitsky,[43] this technique produces very good results, although the need to apply a side-biting clamp to the ascending aorta with a high blood pressure is a drawback.

Intermittent ischaemic arrest

Cross-clamping of the ascending aorta may be used to produce ischaemic cardiac arrest during cardiopulmonary bypass. Myocardial ischaemia can be tolerated with reasonable safety for at least 15–20 min. This time is adequate for the construction of a coronary-to-graft anastomosis, and intermittent aortic cross-clamping is sometimes used for coronary surgery. The use of systemic cooling prior to aortic cross-clamping, or topical myocardial cooling, reduces the risk. This technique has been shown to produce results similar to those achieved with cardioplegia with St Thomas's Hospital solution.[44,45] A report of 500 patients having coronary surgery with this method,[46] showing a mortality rate of 1% and a peri-operative infarction rate of 3.6%, attests to the safety of the technique when properly applied. The drawback of the technique is the time limitation; it is less safe when total ischaemic time becomes prolonged.

Cardioplegic techniques

There are a very large number of methods for protecting the myocardium from the effects of ischaemia by infusing various fluids into the coronary tree; the literature on the subject is voluminous and bewildering.[47] The principles of cardioplegic techniques have been reviewed by Buckberg.[48] These include the rapid induction of electromechanical cardiac arrest to avoid energy depletion (usually by the use of potassium), and the reduction of metabolic rate by hypothermia (4–10°C). A substrate for continued energy production may be added (oxygen, glucose or precursors of Krebs cycle intermediates). Appropriate pH should be maintained with a buffer. Stabilization of the cell membranes may be aided by a number of additives, and myocardial oedema should be avoided by having an appropriate osmolarity for the cardioplegic solution.

Lowering of blood temperature prior to cross-clamping the aorta induces a degree of myocardial hypothermia, thus facilitating cardioplegic techniques. It also allows reduction in systemic pressure and flow during the period of aortic cross-clamping, and this reduces non-coronary collateral flow to the myocardium, which causes re-warming of the myocardium and washing out of cardioplegic solution.[49]

Buckberg has promoted the use of blood cardioplegia, and has refined the technique on the basis of extensive experimental work. An initial cold infusion (4–8°C) of blood containing a high potassium additive is used to induce cardioplegic arrest. Periodic re-infusion of blood cardioplegia with a lower potassium is required at about 20-min intervals. Buckberg also advocates the use of a brief re-infusion of normothermic substrate-enriched oxygenated blood cardioplegia to resuscitate energy-depleted hearts prior to administration of cold cardioplegia when a prolonged period of aortic cross-clamping is planned. Similarly, he recommends a brief normothermic infusion of oxygenated blood cardioplegia immediately prior to unclamping of the aorta to minimize post-ischaemic reperfusion injury.[48] Clinical application with good results has been reported.[50] Daggett et al.[51] have reported the use of cold oxygenated blood cardioplegia in 200 patients having a variety of cardiac operations, in whom a lower incidence of peri-operative myocardial infarction was seen when compared with a previous group of 200 patients having cold crystalloid cardioplegia. Mullen et al.[52] have shown that blood cardioplegia provided excellent protection for the left ventricle but that crystalloid cardioplegia produced colder right ventricular temperatures and better right ventricular function in a randomized study of 80 patients undergoing elective coronary surgery.

A variety of bloodless crystalloid cardioplegic solutions have been described. Some mimic intracellular fluid (Bretschneider's solution[53] and Kirsch's solution[54]); others mimic extracellular fluid with higher potassium concentration. Of the latter, St Thomas's Hospital cardioplegic solution[55,56] is probably the best designed and evaluated, and is in widespread clinical use. The solution is infused at 4°C into the aortic root or coronary ostia and repeated at intervals of 30–40 min, or earlier if electromechanical activity occurs.

At the conclusion of surgery on the heart itself, the aortic cross-clamp is released. This restores coronary flow and washes out cardioplegic solution. Spontaneous co-ordinated ventricular contractions may resume, but if ventricular fibrillation occurs and fails to revert to a spontaneous co-ordinated beat within a few minutes, a defibrillating countershock is applied directly to the ventricles. Re-warming to normothermic levels should be completed before weaning from cardiopulmonary bypass, and air should be evacuated from the heart before allowing ventricular ejection to occur. Suction on a short needle with side-hole close to its flange, inserted into the ascending aorta, provides an additional safeguard in removing air bubbles during the first few minutes after cardiac ejection begins.

Weaning from cardiopulmonary bypass is achieved by resuming ventilation of the lungs (which are not ventilated during the procedure), gradually restricting venous drainage to the extracorporeal circuit and reducing pump flow rate to allow filling of the heart and the restoration of physiological pressure in the left atrium. Measurement of left atrial pressure or pulmonary artery pressure at the stage of weaning from cardiopulmonary bypass provides a good guide to the adequacy of blood replacement and the function of the left ventricle. It is usually possible to return the entire blood content of the extracorporeal circuit to the patient; the excess fluid load of the original prime is lost in the ensuing few hours' urine output. Should a left atrial mean pressure of more than about 18–20 mmHg be required to achieve a normal blood pressure, inotropic support or intra-aortic balloon counterpulsation may be necessary.

BLOOD CONSERVATION

Modern cardiac surgical practice makes far fewer demands on transfusion services than in the earlier years of practice. The use of bloodless primes for the extracorporeal circuit, avoidance of unnecessary dissection and improved suture materials have all contributed.

Use of a cell-saver in routine cardiac surgery results in saving of homologous blood, although the amounts saved may not be great. In repeat operations, much greater blood salvage can be achieved. The cell-saver is a system in which shed blood is retrieved by suction and heparin is added close to the suction site. The system washes and centrifuges the retrieved red cells, and the resultant packed cells are available for re-infusion.[57]

During the first 12 h of the post-operative period, blood can be retrieved from the chest drainage tubes with an appropriate filter and collection system for re-infusion.[58,59] It is frequently possible to undertake cardiac surgical procedures without the use of donor blood,[60] particularly if a modest degree of early anaemia is accepted.

Platelet number and function, thrombosis and haemostasis are usually abnormal immediately after cardiopulmonary bypass, particularly in patients who have received pre-operative anticoagulants or those with longstanding hepatic congestion, as may be seen in advanced mitral valve disease. Attempts to conserve platelet function by infusion of prostacyclin during cardiopulmonary bypass have not shown a convincing benefit in modifying blood loss,[61,62] and there is a role at times for administration of specific clotting factors or platelets when abnormal bleeding is encountered post-operatively.

POST-OPERATIVE CARE

Post-operative care is concerned with maintaining haemodynamic stability while the patient recovers from anaesthesia and is weaned from the ventilator. Any complications are treated promptly, and potential problems are avoided by monitoring haemodynamic status, fluid and electrolyte balance and the electrocardiogram.[63,64]

Blood loss is measured and replaced as necessary. Efficient drainage of the pericardial and anterior mediastinal spaces reduces the risk of tamponade. Excessive blood loss or the suspicion of developing tamponade requires re-opening of the chest incision to control the source of bleeding and to empty the pericardial space.

Serum potassium levels should be checked; potassium is usually required by intravenous infusion to avoid excessively low levels, which often accompany the commonly seen diuresis in the early post-operative hours.

Measurement of blood gases and acid–base balance is a guide to the adequacy of cardiac output and ventilation; deviation from normal levels requires correction.

LOW CARDIAC OUTPUT STATE

Evidence of a low cardiac output state may be obtained from clinical observation of oliguria, cold, vasoconstricted extremities, reduced conscious level and hypotension. Early after hypothermic cardiopulmonary bypass, the patient still under the influence of anaesthesia may be very difficult to assess in this regard. Measurement of central venous pressure is of value in alerting to tamponade, and as a general guide to venous filling. Much more helpful is the left atrial or pulmonary arterial wedge pressure, which gives an indication of left ventricular performance. Measurement of cardiac output may be made where doubt exists: The performance of the heart in the early period following discontinuation of cardiopulmonary bypass is a good guide to the likely subsequent performance. Low output state due to myocardial failure can usually be predicted early on, and in these circumstances inotropic support or intra-aortic balloon counterpulsation is commenced in the operating room. When a low output state develops unexpectedly in the recovery room, there is frequently a different explanation, such as hypovolaemia, rapid heart rate with atrial fibrillation, severe bradycardia or tamponade.

INTRA-AORTIC BALLOON COUNTERPULSATION

The intra-aortic balloon has a capacity of 30–35 ml; it is a tube-like inflatable chamber located on a catheter intended for introduction into the descending thoracic aorta via a femoral artery by a percutaneous insertion technique. The balloon is rapidly inflated and deflated with carbon dioxide by a drive console. Inflation and deflation are synchronized with the cardiac cycle so that balloon deflation in the aorta reduces afterload during left ventricular systole, and balloon inflation during diastole augments diastolic pressure and increases coronary flow.

The intra-aortic balloon reduces left ventricular filling pressure and oxygen consumption, and allows inotropic support to be reduced. It is most commonly used to treat post-operative low output states, but it is also of value in supporting the circulation pre-operatively during investigation and induction of anaesthesia in those with severely compromised haemodynamic status, such as unstable angina or post-infarction ventricular septal defect. There is a risk of ischaemic complications in the leg as a consequence of introduction of the balloon through the femoral artery.[65,66]

INOTROPIC SUPPORT

When low cardiac output appears to be the consequence of myocardial failure, inotropic drugs are given by intravenous infusion. Dopamine and dobutamine are the commonest inotropic drugs used. Isoprenaline is useful if there is bradycardia.

Acidosis, hypoxia, low levels of serum calcium and high levels of serum potassium may contribute to low cardiac output states, and should be corrected.

HYPERTENSION

Hypertension is frequently seen in the early postoperative period following coronary surgery. It increases the work of the left ventricle and may be associated with poor tissue perfusion. Treatment is by intravenous infusion of sodium nitroprusside or by intravenous infusion of nitrate, provided that hypoxia, hypercarbia and inadequate analgesia have been excluded.

ANTIBIOTICS

Systemic broad spectrum antibiotic prophylaxis is used for about 48 h, commencing just before operation. This has been shown to reduce the risk of wound infection in the post-operative period.[67,68]

CONCLUSION

Although the principles of cardiac surgery are well established, refinements of technique and practice continue to be made. Advances in the past three decades have been spectacular, virtually all of current cardiac surgical practice having been developed within this period. Progress in the future is difficult to predict. Improvements in less invasive techniques may make inroads into some areas of traditional surgical practice, but present indications are that further expansion of the role of surgery in the treatment of heart disease can be expected.

REFERENCES

1. Hewitt, R.L. and Creech, O. Jr. History of the pump oxygenator. *Arch. Surg.* 1966; 93: 680.
2. Reitz, B.A. The current practice of heart transplantation. *Bull. Am. Coll. Surg.* 1985; 70: 11.
3. English, T.A.H., Bailey, A.R, Dark, J.F. and Williams, W.G. The UK cardiac surgical register, 1977–82. *Br. Med. J.* 1984; 289: 1205.
4. Rutkow, I.M. Thoracic and cardiovascular operations in the United States, 1979 to 1984. *J. Thorac. Cardiovasc. Surg.* 1986; 92: 181.
5. Julian, D.G. The practical implications of the coronary artery surgery trials. *Br. Heart J.* 1985; 54: 343.
6. Braunwald, E. The path to myocardial salvage by thrombolytic therapy. *Circulation* 1987; 76 (Suppl. II): II–2.
7. Loop, F.D. CASS continued. *Circulation* 1985; 72 (Suppl. II) II–1.
8. Braunwald, E. The aggressive treatment of acute myocardial infarction. *Circulation* 1985; 71: 1087.
9. Culliford, A.T. and Spencer, F.C. Guidelines for safely opening a previous sternotomy incision. *J. Thorac. Cardiovasc. Surg.* 1979; 78: 633.
10. Cooley, D.A. Development of the roller pump for use in the cardiopulmonary bypass circuit. *Texas Heart Inst. J.* 1987; 14: 113.
11. Sethia, B. and Wheatley, D.J. The current status of mechanical circulatory support. *Clin. Phys. Physiol. Meas.* 1986; 7: 101.
12. Hickey, P.R., Buckley, M.J. and Philbin, D.M. Pulsatile and nonpulsatile cardiopulmonary bypass: Review of a counterproductive controversy. *Ann. Thorac. Surg.* 1983; 36: 720.
13. Sethia, B., Wheatley, D.J. and Taylor, K.M. Short review: the current status of cardiopulmonary bypass. *Life Support Systems* 1983; 1: 271.
14. van Oeveren, W., Kazatchkine, M.D., Descamps-Latscha, B. *et al.* Deleterious effects of cardiopulmonary bypass. A prospective study of bubble versus membrane oxygenation. *J. Thorac. Cardiovasc. Surg.* 1985; 89: 888.
15. Kolkka, R. and Hilberman, M. Neurologic dysfunction following cardiac operation with low-flow, low-pressure cardiopulmonary bypass. *J. Thorac. Cardiovasc. Surg.* 1980; 79: 432.
16. Ellis, R.J., Wisniewski, A., Potts, R., Calhoun, C., Loucks, P. and Wells, M.R. Reduction of flow rate and arterial pressure at moderate hypothermia does not result in cerebral dysfunction. *J. Thorac. Cardiovasc. Surg.* 1980; 79: 173.
17. Fox, L.S., Blackstone, E.H., Kirklin, J.W., Stewart, R.W. and Samuelson, P.N. Relationship of whole body oxygen consumption to perfusion flow rate during hypothermic cardiopulmonary bypass. *J. Thorac. Cardiovasc. Surg.* 1982; 83: 239.
18. Pearson, D.T., Poslad, S.J., Murray, A. and Clayton, R. Extracorporeal circulation material evaluation: microemboli. *Life Support Systems* 1987; 5: 53.
19. Solis, R.T., Kennedy, P.S., Beall, A.C., Noon, G.P. and DeBakey, M.E. Cardiopulmonary bypass. Microembolization and platelet aggregation. *Circulation* 1975; 52:103.
20. Wildevuur, C.R.H. and van Oevern, W. Blood interactions in extracorporeal circulation: tests to evaluate the activation of proteins and formed blood elements. *Life Support Systems* 1987; 5: 85.
21. Fosse, E., Mollnes T.E. and Ingvaldsen, B. Complement activation during major operations with or without cardiopulmonary bypass. *J. Thorac. Cardiovasc. Surg.* 1987; 93: 860.
22. Cavarocchi, N.C., Pluth, J.R., Schaff, H.V. *et al.* Complement activation during cardiopulmonary bypass. Comparison of bubble and membrane oxygenators. *J.Thorac. Cardiovasc. Surg.* 1986; 91: 252.
23. Fleming, J.S., Royston, D., Westaby, S., Desai, J.B. and Taylor, K.M. Short communication: neutrophil malondialdehyde content as an indicator of activation during cardiopulmonary bypass. *Life Support Systems* 1986; 4: 257.

24. Utley, J.R., Wachtel, C., Cain, R.B., Spaw, E.A., Collins, J.C. and Stephens, D.B. Effects of hypothermia, haemodilution, and pump oxygenation on organ water content, blood flow and oxygen delivery, and renal function. *Ann. Thorac. Surg.* 1981; **31**: 121.

25. Aberg, T. and Kihlgren, M. Cerebral protection during open-heart surgery. *Thorax* 1977; **32**: 525.

26. Frank, K.A., Heller, S.S., Kornfeld, D.S. and Malm, J.R. Long-term effects of open-heart surgery on intellectual functioning. *J. Thorac. Cardiovasc. Surg.* 1972; **64**: 811.

27. Sachdev, N.S., Carter, C.C., Swank, R.L. and Blachly, P.H. Relationship between post-cardiotomy delirium, clinical neurological changes and EEG abnormalities. *J. Thorac. Cardiovasc. Surg.* 1967; **54**: 557.

28. Sotaniemi, K.A. Cerebral outcome after extracorporeal circulation. Comparison between prospective and retrospective evaluations. *Arch. Neurol.* 1983; **40**: 75.

29. Shaw, P.J., Bates, D., Cartlidge, N.E.F., Heaviside, D., Julian, D.G. and Shaw, D.A. Early neurological complications of coronary artery bypass surgery. *Br. Med. J.* 1985; **291**: 1384.

30. Smith, P.L.C., Treasure, T., Newman, S.P. *et al.* Cerebral consequences of cardiopulmonary bypass. *Lancet* 1986; **i**: 823.

31. Henriksen, L. and Hjelms, E. Cerebral blood flow during cardiopulmonary bypass in man: effect of arterial filtration. *Thorax* 1986; **41**: 386.

32. Blauth, C., Arnold, J., Kohner, E.M. and Taylor, K.M. Retinal microembolism during cardiopulmonary bypass demonstrated by fluorescein angiography. *Lancet* 1986; **ii**: 837.

33. Taggart, D.P., Reece, I.J. and Wheatley, D.J. Cerebral deficit after elective cardiac surgery (Letter). *Lancet* 1987; **i**: 47.

34. Ivey, T.D., Strandness, D.E., Williams, D.B., Langlois, Y., Misbach, G.A. and Kruse, A.P. Management of patients with carotid bruit undergoing cardiopulmonary bypass. *J. Thorac. Cardiovasc. Surg.* 1984; **87**: 183.

35. Shaw, P.J., Bates, D., Cartlidge, N.E.F., French, J.M., Heaviside, D., Julian, D.G. and Shaw, D.A. Long-term intellectual dysfunction following coronary artery bypass graft surgery: A six month follow-up study. *Q. J, Med.* 1987; **239**: 259.

36. Senning, A. Ventricular fibrillation during extracorporeal circulation. *Acta Chir. Scand.* 1952; **171** (Suppl.): 1.

37. Hottenrott, C., Towers, B., Kurkji, H., Maloney, J.V. and Buckberg, G. The hazard of ventricular fibrillation in hypertrophied ventricles during cardiopulmonary bypass. *J. Thorac. Cardiovasc. Surg.* 1973; **66**: 742.

38. Hottenrott, C., Maloney, J.V. and Buckberg, G. Studies of the effects of ventricular fibrillation on the adequacy of regional myocardial flow. 1. Electrical vs. spontaneous fibrillation. *J. Thorac. Cardiovasc. Surg.* 1974; **68**: 615.

39. Cox, J.L., Anderson, R.W., Pass, H.I. *et al.* The safety of induced ventricular fibrillation during cardiopulmonary bypass in non hypertrophied hearts. *J. Thorac. Cardiovasc. Surg.* 1977; **74**: 423.

40. Akins, C.W. Noncardioplegic myocardial preservation for coronary revascularisation. *J. Thorac. Cardiovasc. Surg.* 1984; **88**: 174.

41. Akins, C.W. and Carroll, D.L. Event-free survival following nonemergency myocardial revascularisation during hypothermic fibrillatory arrest. *Ann. Thorac. Surg.* 1987; **43**: 628.

42. Akins, C.W. Early and late results following emergency isolated myocardial revascularisation during hypothermic fibrillatory arrest. *Ann. Thorac. Surg.* 1987; **43**: 131.

43. Levitsky, S. Is hypothermic fibrillatory arrest a rational alternative to cardioplegic arrest? (Editorial). *Ann. Thorac. Surg.* 1987; **43**: 127.

44. Pepper, J.R., Lockey, E., Cankovic-Darracott, S. and Braimbridge, M.V. Cardioplegia versus intermittent ischaemic arrest in coronary bypass surgery. *Thorax* 1982; **37**: 887.

45. Flameng, W., Van der Vusse, G.J., de Mayers, R. *et al.* Intermittent aortic cross-clamping versus St Thomas' Hospital cardioplegia in extensive aortocoronary bypass grafting. *J. Thorac. Cardiovasc. Surg.* 1984; **88**: 164.

46. Bonchek, L.I. and Burlingame, M.W. Coronary artery bypass without cardioplegia. *J. Thorac. Cardiovasc. Surg.* 1987; **93**: 261.

47. McGoon, D.C. The ongoing quest for ideal myocardial protection. A catalog of the recent English literature. *J. Thorac. Cardiovasc. Surg.* 1985; **89**: 639.

48. Buckberg, G.D. Strategies and logic of cardioplegic delivery to prevent, avoid, and reverse ischemic and reperfusion damage. *J. Thorac. Cardiovasc. Surg.* 1987; **93**: 127.

49. Goor, D.A., Mohr, R. and Lavee, J. Enhanced protection of myocardial function by systemic deep hypothermia during cardioplegic arrest in multiple coronary bypass grafting. *J. Thorac. Cardiovasc. Surg.* 1982; **84**: 237.

50. Teoh, K.H., Christakis, G.T., Weisel, R.D. *et al.* Accelerated myocardial metabolic recovery with terminal warm blood cardioplegia. *J. Thorac. Cardiovasc. Surg.* 1986; **91**: 888.

51. Daggett, W.M. Jr, Randolph, J.D., Jacobs, M. *et al.* The superiority of cold oxygenated dilute blood cardioplegia. *Ann. Thorac. Surg.* 1987; **43**: 397.

52. Mullen, J.C., Fremes, S.E., Weisel, R.D. *et al.* Right ventricular function: A comparison between blood and crystalloid cardioplegia. *Ann. Thorac. Surg.* 1987; **43**: 17.

53. Bretschneider, H. J. Myocardial protection. *Thorac. Cardiovasc. Surg.* 1980; **28**: 295.

54. Bleese, N., Doring, V., Kalmar, P. *et al.* Clinical application of cardioplegia in aortic cross-clamping periods longer than 150 minutes. *Thorac. Cardiovasc. Surg.* 1979; **27**: 390.

55. Braimbridge, M.V., Chayen, J., Bitensky, L., Hearse, D.J., Jynge, P. and Cankovic-Darracott, S. Cold cardioplegia or continuous coronary perfusion. Report on preliminary clinical experience as assessed cytochemically. *J. Thorac. Cardiovasc. Surg.* 1977; **74**: 900.

56. Robinson, L.A., Braimbridge, M.V. and Hearse, D.J. Enhanced myocardial protection with high-energy phosphates in St Thomas' Hospital cardioplegic solution. *J. Thorac. Cardiovasc. Surg.* 1987; **93**: 415.

57. Cordell, A.R. and Lavender, S.W. An appraisal of blood salvage techniques in vascular and cardiac operations. *Ann. Thorac. Surg.* 1981; **31**: 421.

58. Cosgrove, D.M., Amiot, D.M. and Meserko, J.J. An improved technique for autotransfusion of shed mediastinal blood. *Ann. Thorac. Surg.* 1985; **40**: 519.

59. Schaff, H.V., Hauer, J.M., Bell, W.R. *et al.* Autotransfusion of shed mediastinal blood after cardiac surgery. A prospective study. *J. Thorac. Cardiovasc. Surg.* 1978; **75**: 632.

60. Carmichael, M.J., Cooley, D.A., Kuykendall, R.C. and Walker, W.E. Cardiac surgery in children of Jehovah's Witnesses. *Texas Heart Inst. J.* 1985; **12**: 57.

61. Fish, K.J., Sarnquist, F.H., van Steennis, C. *et al.* A prospective, randomized study of the effects of prostacyclin on platelets and blood loss during coronary bypass operations. *J. Thorac. Cardiovasc. Surg.* 1986; **91**: 436.

62. Faichney, A., Davidson, K.G., Wheatley, D.J., Davidson, J.F. and Walker, I.D. Prostacyclin in cardiopulmonary bypass operations. *J. Thorac. Cardiovasc. Surg.* 1982; **84**: 601.

63. Hinds, C.J. Current management of patients after cardiopulmonary bypass. *Anaesthesia* 1982; **37**: 170.

64. Kirklin, J.K. and Kirklin, J.W. Management of the cardiovascular subsystem after cardiac surgery. *Ann. Thorac. Surg.* 1981; **32**: 311.

65. Berg, G.A., Reece, I.J., Davidson, K.G. and Bain, W.H. Recent clinical experience with percutaneous intra-aortic balloon pumping. *Life Support Systems* 1986; **4**: 249.

66. Sanfelippo, P.M., Baker, N.H., Ewy, H.G. *et al.* Vascular

complications associated with the use of intraaortic balloon pumping. *Texas Heart Inst. J.* 1987; **14**: 178.
67. Fong, I.W., Baker, C.B. and McKee, D.C. The value of prophylactic antibiotics in aorta-coronary bypass operations. A double-blind randomized trial. *J. Thorac. Cardiovasc. Surg.* 1979; **78**: 908.
68. Myerowitz, P.D., Caswell, K., Lindsay, W.G. and Nicoloff, D.M. Antibiotic prophylaxis for open heart surgery. *J. Thorac. Cardiovasc. Surg.* 1977; 73: 625.

Chapter 76

Cardiovascular Fitness to Drive and to Fly: an Interface between Cardiology and Some Statutory Fitness Requirements*

Michael Joy

INTRODUCTION

GENERAL

Those individuals engaged in certain occupations and pastimes are required to undergo regular medical surveillance. The purpose of surveillance is severalfold: it may be directed at excluding those who should avoid working in a hostile environment, or at monitoring those exposed to potential biological hazard. In the field of transportation, it is directed at the protection of both the individual and the public, who may be innocent victims in the event of an accident.

Surveillance may be required by statute, or a code of practice may develop which is not backed by law. An example in the UK is the offshore oil industry. It is regulated by the Health and Safety at Work Act, 1974 (as amended 1977)[1] and the Offshore Installations (Operational Safety, Health and Welfare) Regulations, 1976 and 1987.[2,3] This legislation makes certain recommendations with regard to health of employees in the industry, but it is the medical advisory panel of the UK Offshore Operators Association that has laid down guidelines with regard to medical fitness standards and frequency of examination. These standards have been adopted and applied by all companies operating in the UK offshore environment.[4]

---

* Licensing requirements are constantly evolving, and medical fitness requirements also change to reflect in part progress in medicine. This chapter examines practice contemporary in the UK with respect to cardiovascular certification to drive and to fly. Opinions expressed are those of the author.

In civil aviation, fitness requirements are governed by international treaty which becomes effective when a state assumes membership of the International Civil Aviation Organisation (ICAO), although individual states have to enact the relevant legislation. In the UK, this is effected by the Air Navigation Order.[5] Motor vehicle driver licensing has no such international commonality of approach, but some countries such as the European Economic Community have taken steps to harmonize legislation[6] and individual states may recognize the licensing authority of others under reciprocal agreements.

There is inevitably variation worldwide in the approach of individual nations to the regulation of transportation. This also extends to medical fitness requirements and thus a comprehensive discussion is not possible within the confines of a single chapter. The contemporary UK approach to medical certification in the context of cardiovascular disease in relation to aviation and road transportation, therefore, has been examined in more detail. The principles involved should be applicable elsewhere.

RELATIVE RISK OF VARIOUS FORMS OF TRANSPORT

Transportation is not free of risk. Statutory authorities exist to regulate it in such a way as to attempt to achieve a high standard of safety, but the existing legislation does not attempt to render the transport industries completely safe.[7] The safest means of travel in Europe and North America is by railway. In the 5 years ending in 1985, approximately 70 people were killed each year on the railways in the

UK. Less than half of these were passengers who commonly fell out of a train.[8] Accidents occurred at a rate of < 1 in 1×10^6 miles (1.6×10^6 km) travelled, and no passenger or staff fatalities were recorded in train crashes in 1985.[8]

By comparison, there were 5165 fatalities in 4768 road traffic accidents in the UK in 1985; 70 980 people were injured seriously and 241 379 slightly in 245 645 reported accidents. There were 61 390 pedestrians involved in such accidents, of whom 1789 were killed.[9]

To obtain a meaningful assessment of the risks of air transportation, a worldwide view is necessary. In 1986, there were 836 fatalities in 38 accidents to scheduled and non-scheduled passenger, cargo and commuter aircraft in some 15×10^6 flying hours.[10] United Kingdom airlines flew 39 821 000 passengers in 999 400 fixed-wing flying hours the previous year,[11] a 50% increase in passengers and a 28% increase in hours flown over a 10-year period. The fatal accident rate to fixed-wing UK registered scheduled and non-scheduled passenger flights for 1976–1985 was 1.5 per million flights, 281 passengers and crew being lost over this period.[12] Rotary-wing airline operations accounted for 2 141 000 passengers and 122 400 flying hours in 1985; fixed-wing air-taxi operators flew 96 900 revenue hours, and in the General Aviation sector approximately 660 000 hours were flown in fixed-wing aircraft < 5700 kg with 105 000 hours being flown in rotary-wing aircraft. There were 41 fatalities in rotary wing operations in the period 1978–1985 and a fatal accident was recorded on air-taxi operations every 250 000 flying hours.[12] The fatal accident rate for general aviation aircraft was 2.5 (fixed wing) and 2.4 (rotary wing) per 100 000 flying hours, respectively.[12]

Direct comparisons of safety for the various modes of transport may be expressed as fatalities per 100×10^6 passenger/driver-kilometres. For the past 10 years, the fatal accident rate to aircraft flying worldwide on scheduled services (excluding the USSR) has been better than 0.1 fatality per 100×10^6 passenger-km travelled (Fig. 76.1).[13] This figure compares favourably with the overall death rate of road users in the UK of 1.8 per 100×10^6 km,[9] which may be broken down into pedal cyclists 6.2, motorcycle riders 12.0, car drivers 0.5, bus and coach drivers 0.0, and heavy goods vehicle drivers 0.2, all per 100×10^6 vehicle-km. Motorcycle riders are approximately 25 times more likely to be killed in a road accident than a car driver, who is at least 5 times more likely to be killed in a car than an aeroplane over the same distance. To some extent, the differing relative risk of accidents is acknowledged and reflected in differing licensing and medical fitness requirements.

As a knowledge of the environment is inseparable from informed licence decision-making, the different levels of operation in the differing modes of transport will be considered at some length.

THE AVIATION ENVIRONMENT

Although the first powered flight was made in December 1903 by Wilbur Wright at the Kill Devil Hills, North Carolina, 5 years were to elapse before his brother Orville carried the world's first passenger by air from the same spot for just under 4 min over a distance of 2.5 miles.[14] The intervening 80 years, given impetus by stategic needs, military conflict and the space programme, have witnessed remarkable developments in passenger air transportation. In 1986, worldwide, a total of almost 1 billion passengers were carried in some 15×10^6 flying hours and the International Air Transport Association (IATA) airlines alone flew 12.88×10^6 hours and made 7167×10^6 departures.[15]

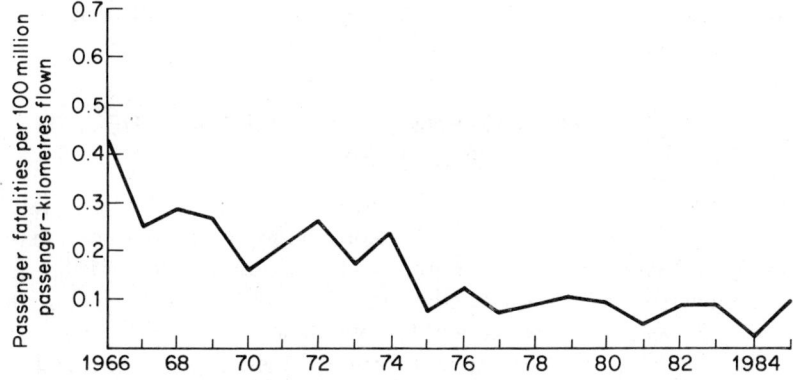

Fig. 76.1. Passenger fatalities per hundred million passenger-kilometres flown on world scheduled services excluding the USSR, 1966–1985. (By courtesy of Fritsch, O. and Santamaria, J. *ICAO Bulletin* 1987.)

AIRCRAFT CLASSIFICATION[5,16]

Aircraft are designated 'heavier-than-air' including aeroplanes, rotorcraft and gliders, or 'lighter-than-air' which includes airships and free balloons.[5]

1 Heavier-than-air machines are subdivided into those with a maximum all-up weight > 5700 kg (requiring a crew of at least two pilots), those with a maximum all-up weight between 2730 and 5700 kg in which single-crew operation may be permitted on public transport flights and those with a maximum all-up weight $<$ 2730 kg. This last category includes self-launching motorgliders and the majority of private aeroplanes. Microlite aeroplanes are heavier-than-air machines with a maximum empty weight < 150 kg which are designed to carry no more than 2 persons.[17]

   Rotorcraft are subdivided into helicopters and gyroplanes. Gliders are not normally covered by the Air Navigation Order and their regulation is the responsibility of the British Gliding Association.

2 Lighter-than-air aircraft include powered craft (airships either gas filled or hot air filled) and free balloons (gas filled, hot air filled or gas and hot air filled).

3 Hovercraft (ACV) certification is the responsibility of the UK Department of Transport, although hovercraft crew require a pilot's Class II medical certificate (see below) as an administrative convenience.

4 Hang-gliders do not come within most of the provisions of the Air Navigation Order and responsibility for their certification is vested in the British Hang-gliding Association.

TYPE OF OPERATION

Differing levels of operation exist.[12]

1 Public transport: this includes airline services (scheduled and non-scheduled passenger and cargo) and air-taxi operations. A scheduled service is regularly flown and is licensed by the CAA as such. Non-scheduled services include inclusive tours (IT) operations. Air taxis include public transport flights of irregular character, usually in aircraft < 15 tonnes.

   As of December 1986, there were 2441 (including 5 cargo) fixed- and rotary-wing aeroplanes of all weights in this category in the UK. Light aircraft (i.e. < 2730 kg) involved in instructional work require a public transport certificate of airworthiness.[16]

2 General aviation:
   i.   Commercial: experimental, test, agricultural, sales and survey flying. It may also include positioning of public transport aircraft.
   ii. Executive: company flying.
   iii. Club and group: all flying by members of a club or group, but not including instructional flying.
   iv. Private: business and pleasure flying, but not club or group flying.
   v.   Training: instructional flying, conversion, familiarization and training for various ratings.

   As of December 1986, there were 2406 private category aircraft and 103 aerial work aircraft (excluding hot air balloons) on the UK register.[16]

3 Other: In 1985, there were 478 registered hot air balloons, but no ballooning accidents; there were 4 fatal accidents involving microlite aircraft and 4 fatal accidents involving hang-gliders.[12]

THE ROAD TRANSPORT ENVIRONMENT IN THE UK

The development of the motor vehicle has been continuous for almost a century since the early work of Daimler and of Benz. In the UK, the Motor Car Act at 1903 introduced driving licences but 21 years were to elapse before the introduction of licences for heavy goods vehicles (see below).[9] In 1909, the first year for which statistics are available, there were 101 000 road vehicles in the UK. By 1950, this had risen to 4.4 million and by 1985 to 21.2 million. These vehicles operate in the main on a road network of 2838 km of motorway, 46 826 km of A roads, 28 952 km of B roads and 269 728 km of other roads.[9]

MOTOR VEHICLES CLASSIFICATION (BY TAXATION CLASS)[9]

1 Two-wheeled motor vehicles (TWMVs): this class includes motorcycles, motorcycle combinations, motor scooters and mopeds. In 1985, it contained a total of 1 148 000 road vehicles, of which 423 000 were mopeds.

2 Private motorcar and light goods vehicles: this

class includes cars and light vans. There were 16 453 000 cars and 1 708 000 other vehicles in this class in 1985.

3 Public transport vehicles: this class includes Public Services Vehicles (PSV) which are vehicles licensed for the carriage of passengers for hire or reward as defined by the Public Service Vehicle Act (1981).[18] There were 120 000 vehicles in this class in 1985.

4 Goods vehicles: this class includes farm goods vehicles. A heavy goods vehicle (HGV) is any goods vehicle whose maximum laden weight is > 7.5 metric tonnes. There were 582 000 in this category in 1985. Vehicles such as fire engines and some recovery vehicles may fall into this category.

5 Other goods vehicles: this class includes agricultural tractors and machinery, other motor vehicles such as cranes and diggers, together with crown-exempt vehicles. This category contained 1 155 000 vehicles in 1985.

PERSONNEL LICENSING

FLIGHT CREW LICENSING

Any pilot who flies for 'hire or reward' requires a professional licence.[5,19] The exceptions until 1 January 1988 were assistant and qualified flying instructors (AFI, QFI) who could instruct on a private flying licence, Chief Flying Instructors (CFI) who required a commercial licence. Pilots involved in aerial work (i.e. crop spraying, banner towing) require a basic commercial pilots licence (BCPL).

The commander of an aircraft with a maximum all-up weight > 20 000 kg must hold an airline transport pilot's licence (ATPL) while the commander of an aircraft 5700–20 000 kg requires at least a senior commercial pilot's licence (SCPL). Aircraft up to 5700 kg may be commanded by a commercial pilot (CPL) who may also co-pilot aircraft of any weight. After the age of 60 years, pilots may not fly as commander of aircraft > 20 000 kg maximum all-up weight, or on single-crew commercial operations. Flight engineers (FE), flight navigators (FN) and flight radio officers (FRO) also require licences, although the last two are becoming obsolete.

The medical certificate

A flying licence is not valid unless it contains a current medical certificate issued by a CAA

appointed authorized medical examiner (AME). Class I certificates are required by ALTP, SCPL, CPL, FN, FE and air traffic control officers (ATCO). Class II Certificates are required by CFI, QFI, AFI and hovercraft (ACV) pilots. A Class III medical certificate is required by student pilots (SPL) and private pilots (PPL). A declaration of health countersigned by an AME or the applicant's regular general practitioner is required for microlite aeroplanes (Group D) and balloons. The initial issue of all Class I certificates is ordinarily following examination at Medical Branch, CAA.

Validity of medical certificates[19]

The CAA is only required to assess fitness for a limited duration although it may give guidance informally for a longer period.

Class I certificates are renewed every 6 months (ALTP, SCPL; CPL > 40 years) or every 12 months (CPL < 40 years, FN, FE, ATCO). A Class I certificate-holder is permitted to engage in either single-crew or multicrew operations although he/she may never be involved in both.

Class II certificates are renewed every 12 months (QFI, AFI, ACV > 40 years) or every 24 months (QFI, AFI, ACV < 40 years).

Class III medical certificates are renewed every 60 months (SPL/PLL < 40 years), every 24 months (SPL/PPL > 40 years), every 12 months (SPL/PPL aged 50–69 years), every 6 months (SPL/PPL > 70 years).

The requirements for the Class II and Class III certificates are similar to those for Class I.

Responsibilities of airmen and of the civil aviation authority

An airman is required by law not to fly if medically unfit to do so, and to report any illness which is not self-limiting and of short duration to the CAA. The CAA employs medical officers and part-time medical consultants who are available to review problems and to give advice on certification. A limited number of other specialist opinions may be sought. In the event of significant difficulty, or disagreement, cases may be referred to the Medical Advisory Panel of the CAA which meets 3 or 4 times each year. This is a panel consisting of several consultants and industry medical advisers. There is no appeal against the final decision of the Chief Medical Officer, CAA.

In the UK, cardiovascular fitness to fly has also been reviewed extensively in two workshops.[20,21]

Cardiovascular aspects of fitness to fly

The ICAO based in Montreal, Canada, is responsible, *inter alia*, for standards of personnel licensing which are laid down in Annexe I to the Convention on International Civil Aviation as International Standards and Recommended Practices.[22] The fitness requirements in Chapter 6 of the Annexe are general statements only which are developed to some extent in the manual of Civil Aviation Medicine.[23] Any state, at its discretion, may require an increase, but not a decrease, in the stated fitness standards. The prevailing cardiovascular fitness requirements published by ICAO[22] are given in Table 76.1. In the UK, obligations to ICAO are promulgated and given the force of law in the Air Nagivation Order.[5]

Cardiologists have taken an almost obsessive interest in the cardiovascular health of pilots.[20,21,24–27] As aviation cardiology has developed, the early attitudes and recommendations have been superseded. It is interesting to reflect that it was not until 1965 that regular electrocardiographic scrutiny of professional aircrew was required in the UK.[28] The Eighth Bethesda Conference[26] and the Royal College of Physicians Report[27] were seen in the wake of the Trident disaster in Staines, Middlesex, in 1972.[29] This was the last recorded multicrew scheduled jet aircraft accident in which cardiovascular incapacitation of the captain of the aircraft was cited as a contributory cause. The Bethesda Conference[26] recommended routine exercise electrocardiography, a recommendation that was not accepted either by the Federal Aviation Administration (FAA) or the CAA. A better understanding of the theory of conditional probability[30] and improved operational training has rendered such a suggestion obsolete, although exercise electrocardiography may be desirable in certain circumstances.[31] For no clear reason, the Royal College of Physicians recommended exercise electrocardiography on admission to training, which is often at age 18 years. Some of the report was devoted to health maintenance and to appeal procedures against adverse medical decision.[27]

Table 76.1. Internationally agreed standards and recommended practices in relation to cardiovascular fitness to fly.[22] (Further official guidance is available.[23])

6.3.2.5 The applicant shall not possess any abnormality of the heart, congenital or acquired, which is likely to interfere with the safe exercise of the applicant's licence and rating privileges. A history of proven myocardial infarction shall be disqualifying.

Note: Such commonly occurring conditions as respiratory arrhythmia, occasional extrasystoles which disappear on exercise, increase of pulse rate from excitement or exercise, or a slow pulse not associated with auriculo-ventricular dissociation may be regarded as being within 'normal' limits.

6.3.2.5.1 Electrocardiography shall form part of the heart examination for the first issue of a licence and shall be included in re-examinations of applicants between the ages of 30 and 40 years no less frequently than every 2 years, and thereafter no less frequently than annually.

Note 1: The purpose of routine electrocardiography is case finding. It does not provide sufficient evidence to justify disqualification without further thorough cardiovascular investigation.

Note 2: Guidance on resting and exercise electrocardiography is published in the ICAO *Manual of Civil Aviation Medicine* (Doc 8984-AN1895).

6.3.2.6 The systolic and diastolic blood pressures shall be within normal limits.

Note 1: The use of drugs for control of high blood pressure is disqualifying, except for those drugs the use of which, according to accredited medical conclusion, is compatible with the safe exercise of the applicant's licence and rating privileges.

Note 2: Extensive guidance on the subject is published in the ICAO *Manual of Civil Aviation Medicine* (Doc 8984-AN1895).

6.3.2.7 There shall be no significant functional or structural abnormality of the circulatory tree.

DRIVER LICENSING IN THE UK

Ordinary driving licences (ODL)

An ordinary driving licence is required by any person conducting a motor vehicle on a road or in a public place.

The licensing authority is the Secretary of State for Transport. Licences are issued by the Driver and Vehicle Licensing Centre in Swansea (DVLC), where the Medical Advisory Branch is also situated.[32,33]

Subject to a satisfactory health declaration, ODLs are issued until the applicant's seventieth birthday or for 3 years, whichever is the longer. This is the Till-70 licence. After 70 years of age, the licence is renewed for 3 years at a time subject to a further health declaration and medical evidence of fitness, if required.

Vocational licences

Vocational licences include heavy goods vehicle licences (HGV) and public service vehicle licences (PSV) and are required in addition to an ODL. Traffic commissioners in the Traffic Areas which are independent authorities are responsible for issuing vocational driving licences. They are advised by the Medical Branch, DVLC, with regard to fitness requirements.

Heavy goods vehicle licences

Licences are valid for 3 years. An applicant for the initial issue of an HGV licence is required to make a fitness declaration and undergo a medical examination by a general practitioner. Subsequently, a health declaration is required on each renewal, but re-examination is not required until age 60 years. There is no requirement for routine electrocardiography.

Public service vehicle licences

Licences are valid for 5 years. An applicant for the initial issue of a PSV licence is required to make a fitness declaration and submit to medical examination, often by a medical officer of the company concerned, or by a general practitioner. Re-examination is required with renewals from age 46 years and annually above the age of 65 years. Ambulance, fire, police, taxi and car hire drivers should be advised as for vocational licences, which they may hold.[32]

Responsibilities of drivers and of the licensing authorities

A licence holder is required by law to give details to DVLC of any 'relevant' or 'prospective' disability[32] that may render him/her unfit to drive, unless it is likely to be self-limiting and of limited duration, such as a fractured limb. Failure to do so may have, *inter alia*, insurance consequences. It is the duty of a medical practitioner to advise a patient if he/she is unfit to drive, but not the licensing authority directly. A practitioner certifying a patient fit to drive contrary to the guidelines[32] may be considered negligent.[33]

The licensing authorities are empowered to call for further medical evidence if deemed necessary and they are also empowered to withdraw or suspend a licence on medical grounds. An applicant whose fitness is questioned may present to DVLC with specialist supporting evidence with regard to his/her medical status, for assessment. This is considered by full-time medical advisers. Exceptionally, a case may be referred to the Medical Advisory Panel which meets twice a year and is also responsible for updating the recommendations regarding fitness.[34] In the event of disagreement, an applicant may, together with an expert witness or witnesses, present his/her case to a magistrate where DVLC would be represented, together with expert witness or witnesses. Medical practitioners seeking guidance may contact a medical adviser at the DVLC at any time.

GENERAL PRINCIPLES OF STATUTORY FITNESS REQUIREMENTS

Fitness standards in the transportation industries have evolved in a largely empirical way. Conditions causing the abrupt onset of altered consciousness without warning, such as epilepsy, disbar from flying, although it may be possible to hold an ordinary driving licence in the UK subject to certain conditions.[35] Likewise insulin-dependent diabetes, significant hypertension and myocardial infarction may be viewed adversely in the context of aviation[22,23] whilst being permissible in ODL holders.[32] These differences to some extent reflect differences in the operational environment.

PRINCIPLES OF MEDICAL REVIEW

Any system of medical review should be mindful of the following guidelines:

1 It should be fair. This implies an evenness of approach. It is always administratively more easy to refuse certification than to arrive at a sound evaluation, based on the probability of an applicant's medical condition giving rise to acute illness which may place the applicant or other people at risk. An adverse decision may terminate a licence holder's employment or his/her employability, and at the least it will remove mobility. It is unsound, for example, to treat all applicants following myocardial infarction as though they had the *same prognosis* when all the evidence suggests that this is not the case. This does not necessarily imply that applicants should be certificated after myocardial infarction, only that a rigorous examination of the evidence is required to see if it is possible

to identify those who may be suitable. Vague statements suggesting 'that the risk is known and it seems right that other road users should be protected'[34] are unsatisfactory without relating the risk of an incapacitating event while driving, for example, to the overall accident experience, and taking into account the contribution of the condition concerned to this experience. It is evident that those who drive or fly professionally are likely to spend substantially more time 'at risk', an implication that bears with it the need for more stringent fitness requirements in those involved.

2   It should be scientific. There is increasing longitudinal evidence available on the natural history of several common conditions and, in particular, of cardiovascular conditions. Following proper evaluation, therefore, it should be possible to predict the likelihood or risk of a potentially incapacitating event. It is also necessary to take into account the frequency with which accidents are caused by medical incapacitation and for the licensing authorities to have some sort of theoretical target, expressing the allowable rate of accidents caused by a medical event as a percentage of the total accidents experienced. Accidents are inevitable, but it is not reasonable to require excessive standards of medical fitness if accidents from medical cause occur rarely or very rarely. Targets have recently been stated for the aviation environment of the UK,[7] and the concept of a risk-orientated approach to certification examined.[21,36]

Sometimes sufficient data are not available upon which to base a scientific judgement, and a reasonable approach is needed on the best evidence available. There is no place for a defensive approach on the part of medical advisers: 'If this man were to be certificated and there was an accident, I/we would be culpable.'

3   It should be practical. Medical review has to work within the confines of what is achievable. What may be possible in terms of investigation and supervision of the about 13 000 Class I and 26 000 Class III flying certificate holders in the UK is not likely to be applicable to the 250 000 PSV, 750 000 HGV and 24 × 10⁶ ODL holders. An unworkable system leads to evasion.

4   It should recognize the difficulties of follow-up. Many conditions are progressive and in particular diseases of the cardiovascular system. Recognition of the need for follow-up, which is as effective and yet as unobtrusive as possible is

required. It is not difficult to make a judgement on fitness the day following exercise evaluation and coronary angiography, although less easy to predict fitness 12 months hence. Coronary angiography cannot be repeated more than very infrequently and non-invasive investigations have limited sensitivity.

With the above premises in mind, the world accident experience from medical cause in aviation and road transportation is examined.

CARDIOVASCULAR CONDITIONS AS A CAUSE OF TRANSPORTATION ACCIDENTS

GENERAL CONSIDERATION

Cardiovascular causes of transportation accidents include such diverse conditions as stroke, transient ischaemic attacks, myocardial infarction, dissection of the aorta, arrhythmias and vasovagal episodes. Cardiovascular disease almost outnumbers all other causes of death taken together in the UK[37] and is the commonest cause of sudden death.[38] It is perhaps surprising that more accidents are not attributed to such events. Part of the reason relates to the elimination of high-risk individuals by medical scrutiny and part to the time-course for acutely incapacitating events in that their recognition, at least by a driver on the road, may give time for avoiding action to be taken. If a driver suffers chest pain which is sufficiently disabling, he or she may pull over and stop the vehicle. The symptoms may be relatively minor, however, before a fatal arrhythmic event. Raffle's[39] important study of 406 000 man-years of London Transport bus-driving over a 25-year period illustrated this point. Seventeen of 21 attacks of epilepsy led to a collision or other accident, whereas only 8 of 34 attacks of acute myocardial ischaemia led to such an outcome.

In an aircraft, the situation is different in the circumstances of a single-crew operation. Even in a light aircraft, it is likely that the time from onset of symptoms to the accomplishment of a safe landing, preferably at an airfield, will be considerably longer than in a motor vehicle. It will also involve more judgement over a longer period of time, especially if the pilot is required to fly by reference to the instruments. In this situation, symptoms that may not of themselves lead to complete incapacitation may impair function overall with equally serious results. In the Leeds–Bradford air-taxi accident,[40] it was concluded that the single pilot was incapacitated due to 'an acute myocardial episode' shortly after take-off and that the attempt by one of the passengers to retrieve the situation was unsuccessful. Within 1 year in the UK, there was a further single-crew accident in which there was 'a strong possibility that the pilot's ability to fly the aircraft became impaired by the onset of symptoms associated with coronary artery disease'.[41]

INCAPACITATION

Complete incapacitation

From the foregoing, it will have become clear that complete incapacitation implies loss of functional control, often without useful warning. Epilepsy and stroke are examples. In one review,[42] it was reported that 1 in 3 pilots had suffered temporary but complete incapacitation during their flying career and in 60% of these cases acute abdominal disorders such as gastro-enteritis and diarrhoea were the cause. Nevertheless, in a recent 10-year period with a review population of approximately 36 000 pilots, there were 10 cases of acute myocardial ischaemia, 7 epileptiform fits, 6 instances of syncope and 3 strokes.[43] None of these instances of incapacitation lead to an accident, underlining the inherent safety of multicrew operations. Since the accident to the Trident at Staines,[29] there has been no multicrew civil jet transport accident attributed to cardiovascular incapacitation of a crew member.

Incomplete and subtle incapacitation

More difficult to recognize, either by the subject or by a colleague in the cab of a vehicle, or on the flight deck of an aircraft, is incomplete or subtle incapacitation. Into this category fall some of the more nebulous complaints such as fatigue, 'illness', emotional distress and medication, which together were implicated by 14.2% of 2130 drivers involved in accidents assessed by the Road Research Laboratory.[44] Problems such as hypoglycaemia, vertigo and rhythm disturbances of the heart, either by direct distraction or by circulatory effect, may reduce critical task performance. Eighty per cent of all aircraft accidents and 60% of all fatal aircraft accidents are attributable to human error, thus the scope for interaction between impaired health and operational efficiency is evident.[45] Two-thirds of these accidents occur in the descent approach and landing phases of flight when any impairment of

performance may be additive to the problems of operation at night (Fig. 76.2) and adverse weather conditions.[43]

CARDIOVASCULAR DISEASE AND ROAD TRAFFIC ACCIDENTS

The economic impact of road traffic accidents is substantial. In 1975, road traffic injuries cost the USA $14.4 billion, slightly more than the cost of coronary artery disease at that time.[46] In the UK, in 1985, the cost of injury including a notional element for compensation was put at £2.82 billion ($4.5 billion).[9] In view of the economic considerations and that the great majority of road traffic accidents are due to human error,[47] it is perhaps surprising that the possible contribution of medical causes to the overall accident scene has not been more comprehensively evaluated, at least in the UK.

The possibility of driving as a provocative stress in the potentially ischaemic myocardium was first studied 20 years ago.[48] Of 76 subjects with known coronary artery disease, 16.7% developed significant electrocardiographic changes whereas none of the 65 younger control subjects did so. Taggart et al.[49], however, recorded significant ST-T changes in 3 of 32 normal drivers in London traffic and in 13 of 24 patients with known coronary artery disease. Similar observations have been made by other workers[50] and both normal subjects and patients with ischaemic heart disease demonstrate a substantial increase in catecholamine and adrenocortical excretion while driving in traffic.[51]

Age might be expected to have some impact on the accident rate overall. With youth, eyesight, health and reaction time are sharpest, but experience and judgement may be less well developed. In old age, infirmity and the risk of cardiovascular event are increased 100-fold or more.[52] The relationship of age to the incidence of road traffic accident mirrors that seen in the aviation environment. There are at least twice as many accidents occurring per 1000 drivers aged 20–29 than aged 50–59 years,[39] almost the same figure as applies to US commercial[43] and military airmen.[53] Nevertheless, drivers above the age of 60 years appear to have more accidents per unit mile, and more traffic violations,[54] although this may be confined to those members of this age-group with senility, with or without concomitant cardiovascular disease.[55]

Gerber[56] reviewed the autopsies of 168 drivers involved in single vehicle crashes. Severe coronary

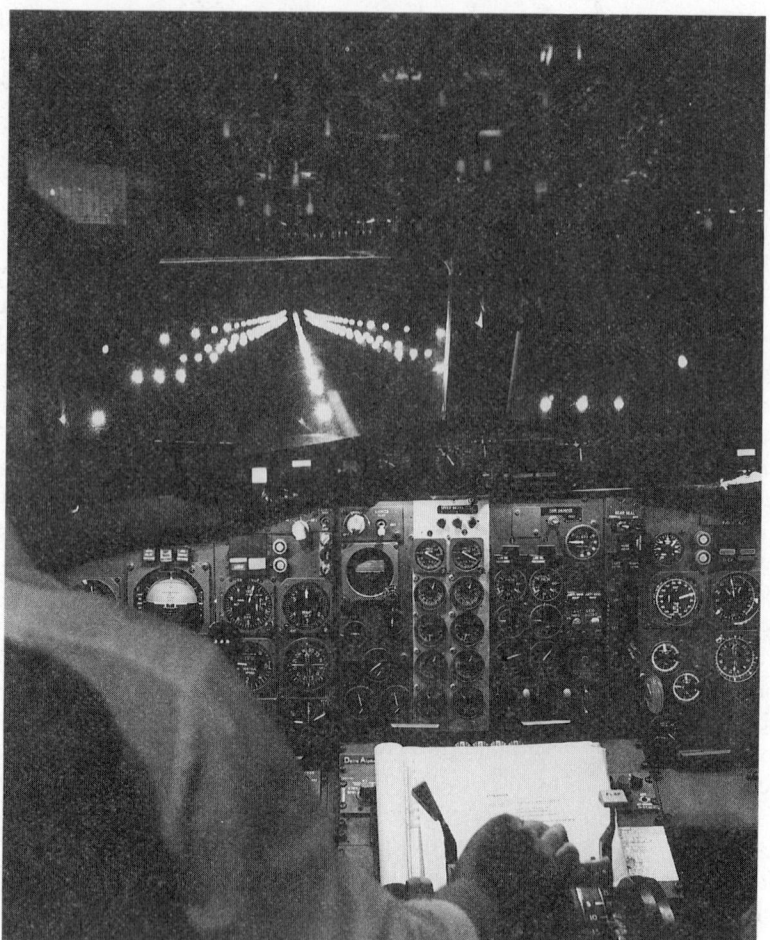

Fig. 76.2. Night departure. Flying at night and in poor visibility is by reference to instruments. Even minor impairment of function may contribute to the 'human factors' that are associated with 80% of all aviation accidents. (By courtesy of Siemens AG.)

disease was present in one-quarter overall and the prevalence of recent or remote myocardial infarction increased from 40% in those aged 45–54 years to 65% of those aged > 65 years. This is not an unexpected finding given the increased prevalence of coronary artery disease with age, although the co-existence of coronary artery disease in an unexplained accident does not necessarily imply a causal relationship.[57] Baker and Spitz[58] reviewed the autopsy and police reports of 328 drivers killed in road traffic accidents in the period 1964–1968 in Baltimore City. A similar frequency of arteriosclerotic heart disease was found in those drivers who were at fault as in those drivers not at fault. The fatality rate appeared to be higher in those above 60 years, probably due to the reduced ability of this age-group to survive trauma.[59] It seems likely that the expected increase in accident experience is not seen in healthy old age, probably due to advice by general practitioners and voluntary restriction by those involved to driving within the limits of their capability.[39]

It is not possible to be confident about the contribution of cardiovascular disease to road traffic accidents. Road accidents are common[9] and, although in the UK all fatal accidents come to the notice of the police and the coroner, the same in-depth investigation that follows a fatal aircraft accident is not carried out. Such data as are available are mostly derived from relatively small-scale studies, many of which are not very recent.

Herner *et al.*[60] analysed all accidents due to sudden illness on the part of the driver over a 5-year period in Göteborg, recording 41 out of a total of 44 255, an incidence approximating to 1 per 1000. About one-third were attributable to cardiovascular disease, including myocardial infarction (7), Adams–Stokes attacks (3), subarachnoid haemorrhage (2) and cerebrovascular accident (1). Grattan and Jeffcoate[61] in the UK concluded that the incidence of sudden illness-related accidents was low, about 1.5 per 1000 in a total of 9390 studied. This figure is of the same order of magnitude as the fatal accident rate due to natural death at the wheel estimated at 6 per 10 000.[62,63] But some of the evidence is conflicting. Waller[64] reported that drivers with known chronic medical conditions had twice as many accidents as their peers, whereas Ysander noted the reverse.[65] Washington DC drivers with licence restrictions by reason of 'heart disease' had significantly more accidents than matched controls although the 44 pacemaker patients in this study had no such increased risk.[66]

The opinion has been expressed that cardiovascular incapacitation of a driver usually gives sufficient warning for avoiding action to be taken[67–69] thereby reducing the risk of harm to the driver concerned and to others.[39,67] However, cerebrovascular insufficiency[70,71] and rhythm and conduction disturbances[60,72] may not afford this opportunity. Although bus drivers appear to be at relatively greater risk from coronary artery disease,[73,74] the risk to the public from road traffic accidents involving buses was remarkably low in the London Transport experience,[39] and the case for allowing some individuals to continue driving, subject to certain conditions and to cardiological review, may not be unreasonable.[75]

CARDIAC VASCULAR DISEASE AND AIRCRAFT ACCIDENTS

Aviation accidents are newsworthy and the death of a weekend flyer in a light aircraft is as likely to make the national newspapers as a multiple vehicle collision on a motorway. To some extent, this public awareness of air transportation has aided regulation of the industry. Accidents occurring in the Western world are investigated to determine cause.

Coronary artery disease is a common condition and it is to be expected that coronary atheroma is likely to be found in the victims of fatal aircraft accidents. Mason[57] reviewed autopsy material from 275 young men who died from trauma, 180 of whom were military or civilian professional pilots. The mean age of the group was 28.3 (18–42) years and 25% showed restriction ≥ 50% of at least one epicardial artery. The prevalence of coronary artery disease was related to age. These observations were broadly in agreement with those of Rigal[76] and of Catherman[77] who found significant coronary artery disease in approximately 21% of military personnel killed in aircraft accidents.

Scheinman[78] studied the coronary arteries of 206 military pilots and observed 'moderate or advanced'

atheroma in 55.4%, the age-range being 20–54. Again, the prevalence of atheroma appeared to be related to age and not to flying exposure. Similar figures were recorded by Booze et al.[79] who reviewed 764 fatal general aviation accidents in the period 1975–1977 and demonstrated at least some degree of coronary artery disease in 51%, although only 4.9% had 'severe disease'. The rate per thousand in whom severe (≥ 66%) stenosis in at least one major epicardial artery was demonstrated was 14.5 in those aged < 30 years, 22.1 in those aged 30–39 years, 63.6 in those aged 40–49 years and 89.9 in those aged ≥ 50 years; the prevalence of severe disease thus tripled between the age-intervals 30–39 and 40–49 years. Underwood-Ground[80] examined the coronary arteries of 288 aircrew, 135 military, 53 professional civilian and 100 private pilots, and found significant (≥ 50% stenosis) coronary artery disease in 17 (mean age 29.1 years), 24.5 (mean age 39.7) and 22% (mean age 37.2 years), respectively. But the discovery of significant coronary artery disease even in an otherwise unexplained aircraft accident should be treated with great caution and should not be taken to suggest a cause–effect relationship without corroborative data.[57,81–83]

The United Kingdom World Airline Accident Summary, 1946–1985,[84] records 29 accidents worldwide to aircraft ≥ 5700 kg which were or may have been due to incapacitation of one or more of the crew members. At least 4 accidents were ascribed to coronary artery disease which is probably an underestimate. Probably the first reported case of heart attack on the flight deck occurred half a century ago,[85] the 35-year-old military pilot nevertheless accomplished a successful landing, to the relief of his 9 passengers, only to die 1 h later. Orlady and Carter recorded 16 deaths due to coronary artery disease in civil pilots while on duty between 1952 and 1966 known to the United States Airline Pilots Association,[86] but only one apparently led to a fatal accident. Owing to the prevalence of coronary artery disease and the capriciousness of its manifestations, it is inevitable that some pilots will suffer a myocardial infarction while on duty. Routine electrocardiography at periodical medical examinations also uncovers clinically 'silent' myocardial infarctions that have occurred in the interval between examinations. In the United States Air Force, Caris[87] detected a rate of 1–2 cases of unrecognized myocardial infarction per 1000 pilots per year aged 40–50 years, while Joy[88] recorded a loss rate of UK professional flying licences of 1.5 per

1000 pilots per year from myocardial infarction or ischaemic heart disease in aircrew with a mean age of 48 ± 9.3 (SD) years uncovered at routine examination over a 30 month period.

The frequency of aircraft accidents due to cardiovascular cause in military pilots in the period 1958–1966 has been estimated at 0.4%, or 2.2.% if possible cardiovascular cause accidents are also included.[78] Between 1962 and 1971 at a time when the United States Air Force was flying $6–8 \times 10^6$ h per year, only 2 cases of confirmed and 5 cases of suspected inflight myocardial infarction leading to an accident were recorded. Nevertheless, of the remaining 199 accidents occurring during this period, 55 could not be explained although a cardiovascular cause seemed unlikely.[89]

Between 1959 and 1965, 37 US general aviation accidents were officially attributed as being due to cardiovascular cause,[90] from Canada, Hemming[91] described 6 cases of death of single crewmen in flight, which led to an accident in all but one case, over an 18 month period. Mohler and Booth[92] reported 13 per 1404 fatal accidents to general aviation aircraft following the death of the single pilot from myocardial infarction in the USA between 1974 and 1975, an incidence of 0.93%. Similar accidents were recorded at that time in the UK.[40,41]

In an international study,[42] with ICAO and the International Federation of Airline Pilots Associations (IFALPA) over the period 1961–1968, there were 5 cases in which death of an airman led directly to an accident and the loss of a total of 147 lives. Twelve more pilots died in multicrew operations without causing an accident, although in 5 further instances the margin between a successful and unsuccessful outcome of the flight was thought to be fine. A further 42 aircrew suffered non-fatal incapacitation. Based on the United States Airline Pilots Association experience over an 11-year period, Kulak et al.[93] predicted an annual rate of serious inflight incapacitation which spanned a range of 1 per 58 000 pilots aged 30–34 years to 1 per 3500 pilots aged 55–59 years. Assuming an average flying time each year of 600 h per pilot, this represents an incidence which spans 1 per 35×10^6 flying hours and 1 per 2.1×10^6 flying hours, respectively.

From the foregoing, it is evident that complete incapacitation or death will very likely, but not inevitably, lead to a fatal accident in a single-crew operation.[91] Owing to the recognition of the need[94] and requirement[5] for specific crew training in the possibility of sudden cardiovascular incapacitation of a member of a multicrew operation, there has not been a multicrew accident in which cardiovascular incapacitation has been implicated since 1972,[29] following which some 200×10^6 flying hours have been accumulated. Chapman[95] citing IATA medical statistics, noted an incapacitating event rate of 1 per 20×10^6 flying hours, but significant under-reporting is likely. He also reported his findings on 1300 simulator exercises in which sudden and/or subtle incapacitation was programmed to occur in a critical phase of flight, i.e. during or just after departure, or in the approach and landing phase. Eight 'crashes' resulted when there had already been another major system failure, but only two occurred in the absence of another major system failure—a risk of 1 accident in 400 events. Relating this to the incapacity occurrence rate observed by the IATA, he concluded that the probability of an accident occurring to a multicrew aircraft from this cause was of the order of 1 in 10^{10}. Bennett[96] criticized these data indicating that on each sortie the crew were alert to the possibility of incapacitation at a critical phase of flight, and a more realistic value is likely to be lower.

SPECIFIC PROBLEMS IN RELATION TO CARDIOVASCULAR CERTIFICATION TO FLY AND TO DRIVE

Tunstall Pedoe[97] in the First United Kingdom Workshop in Aviation Cardiology[20] introduced the concept of relating the fatal accident rate of passenger aircraft directly to the coronary heart attack rate in pilots. This was taken further in the Second Workshop.[21] Chaplin[7] has suggested an overall industry target for large jet aircraft should be better than 1 fatal accident per 10×10^6 flying hours. This has not yet been achieved. He also indicated that a fatal accident rate due to medical cause should not occur more often than 1 in 10^8–1 in 10^9 flying hours in such aircraft. This excludes the possibility of single-crew operation of such aircraft because cardiovascular mortality per year exceeds this assumption.[97] With an accident rate in single-crew commercial operations somewhere between 1 in every 100 000 flying hours[43] and 1 in every 250 000 flying hours,[12] it was further suggested that an accident rate from medical cause is acceptable at only perhaps 1 in every 100 accidents or 1 in $10–25 \times 10^6$ hours flown on these operations.[7] Only below 44 years of age in the average male in the UK does the risk of serious cardiovascular incapacitation achieve the industry target of 1 incident per 10×10^6 flying hours[93,36] although the overall risk is abated, as has been discussed earlier, by the better accident record of the older pilot.[43,53] No such targets are available in the UK for other modes of transport.

Industry-specific safety targets are required for all forms of transport in terms of the allowable accident rate due to medical cause if certification is to be scientific and fair. As good longitudinal data are not yet available for several conditions, an empirical approach may still be required. But it is unrealistic to require excessive standards of fitness if the overall accident experience and the contribution of physical incapacity to this experience does not warrant it. The subjects to be considered in this section will be discussed in terms of risk of occurrence and likely impact on the operational environment.

HYPERTENSION AND RISK FACTORS

Impact of hypertension and vascular risk factors

In the UK, 15–20% of the middle-aged population have a diastolic blood pressure of 90–109 mmHg, 4% a pressure of 110–129 mmHg and 0.5% a pressure > 130 mmHg.[98] About 10% of military aircrew may have a systolic and/or diastolic pressure $> 150/95$ mmHg although only 2% have both values above this level.[99] The consequences of hypertension are well known and include an increased risk of stroke, coronary artery disease, congestive heart failure and progressive renal impairment.[100] Treatment of hypertension lowers the risk of stroke and reduces the risk of development of renal impairment or congestive heart failure,[101] and it may reduce the risk of coronary artery disease.[102] The threshold at which treatment is thought to be indicated has been lowered progressively and the Hypertension Detection and Follow-up Programme has suggested a benefit in adults for treating fifth-phase diastolic blood pressure in adults at a level as low as 90 mmHg,[103] although treatment does not render the hypertensive patient an outlook similar to that accruing to a normal subject risk.[104]

Hypertension is easily detectable at routine medical examination, but the effect of co-existing risk factors is almost invariably forgotten. Familial hypercholesterolaemia (type IIa) is not common in the UK (2.5 per 1000 population), but half of the heterozygotes afflicted will have overt coronary disease by the age of 50 years.[105] Other lipid disorders are more common (i.e. type IIb), and the cardiovascular risk of a cholesterol level of 6.7 mmol/l in a patient with a systolic blood pressure of 140 mmHg who smokes is the same as that conferred by a cholesterol level of 10.4 mmol/l or a systolic pressure of 250 mmHg.[105] Substantial obesity ($> 130\%$ of optimum bodyweight) is an independent risk factor, and glucose intolerance doubles coronary heart disease mortality[106] or quadruples it if diabetes mellitus is overt.[107] In the Framingham study uric acid was not implicated as a risk factor,[108] but medication with thiazide diuretics[109] may increase plasma urate, cholesterol and triglycerides. Thiazides also have a diabetogenic effect, and they influence potassium metabolism with the attendant increased incidence of ventricular rhythm disturbances.[110] Contraceptive hormones increase the death rate from cardiovascular diseases fivefold when compared with those women who have never taken them and tenfold when taken for a period of 5 years or longer, although the relative risk from contraceptive hormone medication is small.[110] Smoking is probably a main cause of death from ischaemic heart disease below the age of 50 years;[111,112] thereafter its impact is diluted by other factors.

Pocock et al.,[113] using data from the British Regional Heart Study, predicted a median risk of major coronary event of 1 every 3×10^6 flying hours in middle-aged UK males, but the presence of hypertension, hypercholesterolaemia and smoking habit may increase this to 1 per 200 000 hours.[113] Nevertheless, membership of a high-risk group may not extend that risk to an individual in that group and, although the top quintile of any single risk factor distribution was found to carry a 1% risk of a major coronary event per year, only about three-fifths of subsequent heart attacks will occur in subjects in this quintile. Progressive intervention to reduce risk factors is likely to achieve a reduction in cardiovascular risk of only 30–50% when compared with age-matched control subjects.[113,114]

Such considerations are inseparable from proper judgement on fitness and have implications with regard to single-crew aircraft operations and possibly for vocational driving licence holders. The suggestion made in the First United Kingdom Workshop[20] that compulsory vascular risk profiling and exercise electrocardiography should be carried out at an appointed age, perhaps 50 years in pilots engaged in single crew operations, was not accepted by the CAA[96] on the grounds that the observed accident rate from cardiovascular cause did not support such an approach, even though there are insufficient aircrew in the UK flying such operations in this age-group to permit an adequate experience.

Acceptable levels

'The systolic and diastolic blood pressure shall be within normal limits' in aviators[22] and although hypotensive agents are 'disqualifying' their use is permitted subject to accredited medical opinion.[22] Perhaps 5% of adult hypertensive patients[100] have a potentially correctable cause for their blood pressure, and it is proper to attempt to identify any cause.[101] Severe hypertension would not be expected to occur in aircrew subject to regular medical scrutiny, although it does;[115] it is more likely to be seen in HGV drivers who undergo no routine medical examination between the initial issue of their licence and the age of 60 years. Non-pharmacological management of hypertension by means of weight reduction, reduction of alcohol intake and increased exercise is rational but of limited value on its own.[116] At present, treatment is probably indicated[31,101] when the systolic or fifth-phase diastolic pressure on routine examination exceeds 145/90 mmHg in those aged < 40 years, 155/95 mmHg in those aged 40–49 years and 160/100 mmHg in those aged > 50 years. Comparable figures in the USA span from 140/88 (aged 20–29 years) to 170/100 mmHg (aged > 50 years).[117]

Treatment

At present, ICAO,[22,23] the CAA[31] and the FAA[118] permit the use of diuretic agents and beta-adrenoreceptor blocking drugs in aviators; the CAA normally supervises those on treatment. Preferred beta-blocking agents include atenolol and propranolol. A simulator check is required following the initiation of therapy[31] to search for the possibility of unwanted central nervous effects of medication that might interfere with critical task performance. The problem of unwanted central nervous effects of hypotensive agents is well established[119,120] and for this reason agents such as methyldopa, clonidine and reserpine disbar individuals from flying[22,23] and from vocational driving.[32] The ganglionic and post-ganglionic blocking agents (bethanidine and guanethidine) are excluded because of possible risk of postural symptoms.[23,32] Recently, it has been

suggested that angiotensin converting enzyme inhibitors and the slow channel calcium blocking agents could be used in aircrew, subject to certain safeguards,[121] which should include a period during which treatment is established, perhaps of 1 month in duration, and an assessment in a flight simulator.[36] There seems no reason why these products should not also be used by vocational or other drivers. Any significant increase in the blood pressure (treated or untreated) should lead to temporary withdrawal of a licence to fly, a level of 200/110 mmHg also prohibiting holding a vocational driving licence.[32] The problem of an exaggerated alarm reaction, which is well known to those involved in the routine scrutiny of aircrew, may be overcome by ambulatory monitoring. This technique may give a better guide to prognosis.[102]

ISCHAEMIC HEART DISEASE

General

Diseases of the circulation cause more death in the USA than all other causes combined[122] despite a 30% decline in mortality rate over the last 3 decades. The situation in the UK is similar, and ischaemic heart disease accounted for 157 500 deaths in England and Wales in 1984[123] out of a total of 566 900 deaths from all causes. Total deaths from ischaemic heart disease in males below the age of 60 years (the normal age of retirement of airline pilots) was 14 500 and below the age of 65 years it was 26 000. Although there is evidence in North America that airmen as a whole suffer less from the consequences of coronary artery disease than their Framingham peers,[124] this advantage, the result of screening for significant risk factors such as severe hypertension and diabetes, is largely lost by the age of 50 years. It has been suggested in at least one study that the favourable trend in coronary artery disease mortality in the USA as a whole may not be reflected in the victims of military aircraft accidents[125] and United States Navy pilots appear to develop coronary artery disease on average 3 years before their non-flying peers.[126]

In England and Wales, in 1983, there were 168 000 deaths and discharges-from-hospital of patients diagnosed as having suffered or as suffering from ischaemic heart disease, a figure including some but not all of the certificated deaths from this cause.[127] An unknown number of subjects will have been undiagnosed, wrongly diagnosed or looked after at home by their family practitioners. More than 50% of professional aircrew losing their licences prematurely in the UK do so from cardiovascular cause[43,88] and one-third of these present spontaneously, i.e. with acute myocardial infarction,[88] rather than at routine screening. Vocational drivers undergo no routine medical examination until the age of 60 years, and electrocardiographic scrutiny is not required. It is likely that the removal of those at particular risk, i.e. in the year following myocardial infarction, will be haphazard and dependent on the inclination of the licence holder to declare a relevant 'disability'.[32] It is against this background that the substantial problem of coronary artery disease in this context is considered.

Minor electrocardiographic changes and exercise electrocardiography

Since 1965, routine resting electrocardiography has been a requirement in aircrew.[28] The frequency required is given in Table 76.1. Minor electrocardiographic changes involving the ST segments and T waves were seen in 2% of United States Air Force personnel[128,129] and in about 3% of symptom-free UK civilians[130] and Royal Air Force personnel,[131] raising the possibility of occult coronary artery disease. However, in a selected population of 103 asymptomatic airmen with minor ST-segment and T-waves changes, only 18% responded abnormally to symptom-limited exercise electrocardiography.[132] Not all of the subjects in that series underwent coronary angiography; in Froelicher's subgroup, all of the 111 symptom-free aircrew with abnormal exercise electrocardiograms underwent angiography[133] and only 31% were demonstrated to have significant coronary artery disease. Nevertheless, in a further group of 1390 asymptomatic aircrew,[134] the risk ratio (i.e. the percentage of those with an abnormal test in whom the disease developed versus the percentage of those with a normal test in whom it developed) was 14.3 over a mean of 6.3 years. This figure must be put into perspective by considering the effect of exercising a group of asymptomatic individuals. Exercise electrocardiography in such a group may be 75% sensitive (true positives versus true positives plus false negatives) and 95% specific (true negatives versus false positives plus true negatives), and the prevalence of significant coronary artery disease may be 2%. In that case, 50 aircrew out of every 1000 would have unnecessary doubt cast upon them; 15 of the 20 in whom the disease is present

will be detected. These figures may be enhanced by the use of thallium scintigraphy,[135,136] but such a test cannot be used for routine scrutiny. As exercise electrocardiography would be likely to generate many more 'false-positive' results than 'true positives' and multicrew operations have an excellent safety record from the cardiovascular viewpoint, the CAA and the FAA did not adopt the recommendations with regard to routine electrocardiography of the Eighth Bethesda Conference[26] or of the Royal College of Physicians.[27]

At present the Class I medical certificate permits single-crew operation up to the age of 60 years,[22] but it is not sensible to permit such operation when the combined cardiovascular risk of age, systolic blood pressure, cholesterol and smoking may impart a total risk that is unacceptably increased. Very many pilots with Class I certificates never fly other than as a member of a multicrew operation and the present ICAO recommendations allow a licensing authority to restrict an airman to fly only as a member of a multicrew operation.[22] A persuasive argument can be made for risk-profiling above a certain age, perhaps 50 years,[36] for those involved in single-crew operations in an attempt to maintain industry objectives in terms of accident rate from cardiovascular cause.[7] Such risk-profiling could include exercise electrocardiography. Exercise electrocardiography in this situation has a higher probability of detecting coronary artery disease.

There are no industry targets for the permissible rate of cardiovascular incapacitation in vocational drivers. In the UK, the accident rate, at least among London Transport drivers,[39] would seem to be acceptable and, although no operational restriction can be placed upon vocational driving licences in the sense that the licence is either granted or denied, it would seem appropriate to consider fitness standards required for vocational driving licences to be approximately those required by a Class I certificate holder who has been downgraded to fly as or with a co-pilot.[137] The usefulness and limitations of non-invasive investigation on asymptomatic subjects has recently been well and extensively reviewed in the context of aviation.[138]

Minor coronary artery disease

Significant coronary artery disease is likely to have been anticipated by evidence of a myocardial infarction or symptoms of angina pectoris. Minor disease may be discovered following investigation of electrocardiographic anomalies on routine electrocardiography, following exercise electrocardiography for whatever reason, or following investigation to elucidate symptoms of doubtful origin. The presence of minor disease is a predictor of future coronary events.[139]

Data from the London Chest Hospital[140] based on a heterogeneous group of 1514 patients followed for 12 years and treated medically disclosed an overall mortality of 2.4% per annum, although those patients who had distal vessel disease only had an annual mortality of 0.9%. Bruschke[141] recorded that the 5-year mortality rate for individuals with normal coronary arteriograms was 0.6%, for those with minor narrowing (< 30%) it was 2.0% and for those with moderate narrowing (30–50%) it was 5.3%. The mean age of his study population was 45 years. The mortality for subjects who had lesions causing a 30% narrowing was 3 times that experienced by those with normal coronary arteriograms.[141]

At present, the CAA will consider an airman for restricted certification on a case by case basis provided no single lesion of a distal vessel is > 50% and any more proximal lesion is > 30%.[31] Vocational drivers are denied a licence in the case of significant occlusive disease in the left main coronary artery, in the proximal left anterior descending coronary artery or when two or more vessels are involved. Non-proximal or single-vessel disease will not necessarily disbar a pilot, but he/she will be subject to annual review (Table 76.2d.)[32] The United States Air Force has been adopting a discretionary approach to the certification of asymptomatic individuals with minor coronary disease provided no single lesion is > 30% and the aggregate (sum) of lesions is not > 50%. Subjects with electrocardiographic or angiographic evidence of myocardial damage, serious arrhythmias or any degree of left main coronary disease are excluded: of a total of 12 pilots originally certificated, 5 have undergone further angiography at a mean interval of 30 months and 2 were disqualified due to progression of disease.[142] Although this experience is small, it underlines the need for regular follow-up of those with known coronary artery disease with at least exercise electrocardiography and/or thallium scintigraphy. It also underlines the inadvisability of certification of single-crew airmen in this situation.

Angina pectoris

The diagnosis of angina pectoris carries an annual mortality overall of about 4% per annum[143] but individual survival is dependent on several factors,[144,145] including the extent of the disease and overall left ventricular function. Of the 347 patients with chest pain and normal coronary arteries in Proudfit's series,[146] followed for 10 years, only 2 died from coronary artery disease (0.6%). Of the 101 patients with stenoses < 30%, 2 died (2.0%); of 63 who had 30–50% stenoses, 10 died (16.0%). This experience is similar to, perhaps better than, that of the general population, but current techniques tend to be better at identifying those with a poor prognosis than those with a good prognosis.[139] The presence of significant coronary disease with or without symptoms, i.e. 50% stenosis in the London Chest Hospital series,[140] reflects the findings of other studies—a survival at 5 years of 70% for significant two-vessel disease, of 50% for significant three-vessel disease and of 38% for significant left main stem disease.

The occurrence of angina pectoris in subjects in the population who are younger than retirement age is an indication for full non-invasive and invasive investigation. Distal and non-proximal single-vessel disease are likely to be treated with medication. Angina disbars individuals from any form of flying licence due to risk of sudden progression following plaque rupture,[147] irrespective of the modification or abolition of symptoms by medication. Stress-induced angina pectoris may lead to subtle incapacitation; plaque rupture may be associated with myocardial infarction and its attendant risks.

Vocational drivers are also disbarred from driving if they are symptomatic[32] (Table 76.2a) or in current need of treatment.[33] If in doubt, exercise electrocardiography should be performed and 2 mm of undefined ST-segment depression is felt to be diagnostic. Probably less significant changes would also disbar if the symptoms were typical. Convincing evidence of the detection of 'silent myocardial ischaemia' would be likely to lead to full investigation and loss of licence. An ordinary driving licence is permitted provided that symptoms are not 'easily provoked by driving or emotion' (Table 76.3b) unless medication causes symptoms of dizziness, faintness, loss of consciousness or fatigue (Table 76.3c).

Myocardial infarction

The prognosis following myocardial infarction may range from excellent to very poor. Left ventricular ejection fraction is the most discriminating variable in relation to survival.[148,149] The extent of coronary

Table 76.2. Summary of recommendations with regard to specific cardiac conditions in relation to fitness to drive a public service vehicle or a heavy goods vehicle.[32]

A person should be advised not to apply for or to hold a licence to drive a heavy goods or public service vehicle—including ambulance, fire, police, taxi and hire-car drivers—in the following circumstances.

a If subject to anginal pain, whether this is brought on by slight or energetic exercise or emotion, or meals, or if it awakens the individual from sleep. A maximum or submaximum electrocardiographic (ECG) test (Bruce or WHO protocols) should be carried out on a treadmill or bicycle ergometer when the identity of chest pain is in doubt and vocational driving should not be permitted if ST-segment depression of 2 mm or more develops.

b If a coronary attack or myocardial infarction has been documented in the past and the ECG shows persistent and typical Q waves of infarction.

c If a coronary attack or myocardial infarction has been documented in the past and the ECG shows persistent ST-segment and T-wave changes or has returned to normal but after recovery from the heart attack the maximum or submaximum exercise test is positive (more than 2 mm ST-segment depression). But, if the exercise test is negative, an individual might be licensed subject to the findings of coronary angiography (see (**d**) below).

d If, after a normal maximum or submaximum test, coronary angiography shows significant occlusive disease in the left main coronary artery, or the proximal part of the left anterior descending artery, or two or more affected coronary arteries. In other words, non-proximal or single artery disease is not necessarily a bar to holding a professional licence but the continued holding of such a licence must be reviewed annually and will depend on the maximum or submaximum exercise ECG remaining normal.

e If there has been more than one coronary heart attack or myocardial infarction, or one documented episode and also peripheral arterial disease.

f If the ECG is abnormal apart from the ischaemic abnormalities mentioned above, particularly if it shows left bundle branch block. Right bundle branch block should be regarded in the same light if it occurs after a previously recorded normal ECG or is detected for the first time after the age of 40 years, or when associated with chest pain, diabetes, or hypertension. Other non-specific abnormalities of the ST and T waves should be carefully appraised, using a maximum exercise test.

g If there is complete heart block or if a pacemaker has been implanted (except under exceptional circumstances when the case might be reviewed by the Honorary Medical Advisory Panel).

h If there is significant enlargement of the heart by X-ray examination, that is, if the cardiothoracic ratio is 0.55 or over.

i If there are any features, clinically or radiologically, to suggest aortic aneurysm.

j If there is a history of paroxysmal arrhythmia or if the ECG shows an arrhythmia. Occasional ectopic beats which disappear on exercise should not preclude licensing.

k If casual blood pressure readings are 200/110 mmHg or over. The comments on the drug treatment of hypertension in the section on private drivers (see above) are particularly applicable here. Persons whose hypertension is effectively controlled by diuretics or beta-blockers may be accepted but drivers undergoing treatment with more potent antihypertensive drugs, which may cause postural hypotension and syncope, should normally be rejected.

l If peripheral artery disease is disabling to the extent that it leads to sickness absence from work.

m If subject to vasovagal episodes or unexplained syncope.

n If 1 year after coronary artery bypass graft (CABG) surgery or coronary angioplasty, the individual is unable to meet the criteria listed under (**a**) to (**c**) and (**h**) above. A coronary arteriogram must be undertaken approximately 1 year after CABG to demonstrate patency of the grafts and after coronary angioplasty in order to conform with (**d**) above.

o If, after heart valve repair or replacement, single or multiple:
  i symptoms persist;
  ii the rhythm is not sinus;
  iii the individual is subject to paroxysmal arrhythmias;
  iv the heart is enlarged by X-ray (= 0.55);
  v the ECG is abnormal, particularly if it shows signs of ventricular enlargement, ischaemia or conduction defects;
  vi the blood pressure is abnormal;
  vii anticoagulants are prescribed;
  viii there are side-effects of medication.

p If complicated congenital heart disease is present. Those with minor congenital lesions, such as maladie de Roger, secundum type atrial septal defect, bicuspid aortic valve, a small patent ductus arteriosus or mild pulmonary stenosis may be accepted for holding a professional licence. When surgery has been undertaken for correction of the above minor lesions, the patient should be permitted to hold a professional licence provided other criteria set out in the recommendation, do not exclude him or her.

NB: If any part of the cardiovascular system is suspect in a driver who has been permitted to hold a heavy goods or public service licence, a yearly examination should be carried out.

disease present is also important,[148] as is the presence (or absence) of complex rhythm disturbance.[150] Angiography alone does not give an adequate guide to prognosis.[151] Chaitman *et al.*[152] identified a group of 2326 patients from the CASS registry who had a similar profile to that of average US airmen, i.e. they were < 60 years old at the time of surgery, without a previous history of heart surgery, congestive heart failure or insulin-dependent diabetes. Those who developed symptoms, heart failure or stroke within 12 months of surgery, who had hypertension or who had sustained a peri-operative myocardial infarction were also excluded. Those with normal left ventricular function, with or without a previous history of myocardial infarction, had a better than average survival when compared with their age-matched controls. The reverse was true in the presence of impaired left ventricular function. This subject has recently been reviewed in the context of certification to fly.[153]

Myocardial infarction disbars from certification to fly (Table 76.4), but airmen may regain certification subject to 'accredited medical opinion' under the so-called 'waiver clause' (I.2.4.8) of ICAO

Table 76.3. Recommendations relating to cardiac conditions which may prevent the holding of an ordinary licence.[32]

Patients with the following cardiac conditions should not drive a motor vehicle and should notify their condition to the Licensing Centre.

1 When a coronary heart attack or myocardial infarction has occurred within the last 2 months.
2 When angina is easily provoked during driving or by emotion
3 When medication for any cardiac condition, particularly anti-hypertensive drugs and beta-blockers for hypertension, angina or arrhythmias, has caused vertigo, transient faintness, loss of consciousness, postural hypotension, lack of alertness or easily induced fatigue
4 When there have been one or more episodes of unexplained syncope
5 When heart block exists

Annexe I.[22] In the UK, it is suggested that professional aircrew could be re-certified to fly as a member of a multicrew operation subject to the following conditions.[36]

1 Full review should take place no earlier than 9 months after the index event and re-certification should not be considered until 12 months had elapsed.
2 The subject should complete satisfactorily a symptom-limited exercise protocol (i.e. 4 stages of the Bruce protocol).
3 Radionuclide/contrast angiography should demonstrate a left ventricular ejection fraction > 50% without any significant abnormality of wall motion.
4 Ambulatory monitoring should show no significant rhythm disturbance.
5 Coronary angiography should detect no more than minor proximal disease in any vessel remote from the myocardial infarction and no more than 30% stenosis elsewhere without functional impairment in relation to any minor lesion.
6 Regular follow-up by a cardiologist with exercise electrocardiography/thallium-201 myocardial imaging.

Candidates completing the protocol satisfactorily should be restricted to multicrew operations. Private pilots may be considered for unrestricted operation, but, without coronary angiography, re-certification is likely to be delayed.

Q-Wave infarction disbars from a vocational driving licence (Table 76.2b). Non-Q-wave infarction, however, may carry a poorer prognosis at least at first,[154] but may be considered (Table 76.2c).

Following non-Q-wave infarction, if the exercise electrocardiogram demonstrates 2 mm of undefined ST-segment depression, licensing is likely to be denied. It might not be withheld in the presence of a 'normal exercise electrocardiogram' and 'satisfactory coronary angiogram' (i.e. non-proximal single-vessel disease). Satisfactory regular review would be required. More than one myocardial infarction evidently disbars (Table 76.2e), although single-vessel disease may progress to completion with little ventricular damage.

In the absence of regular routine medical examination and electrocardiographic scrutiny, there must be large numbers of HGV and smaller numbers of PSV drivers who continue to hold a licence either because symptoms of myocardial infarction pass unnoticed by them, or remain undiagnosed by their medical attendants, or they choose not to disclose an event for fear of loss of livelihood. Given such circumstances, and in the presence of an apparently very low rate of accidents caused by ischaemic heart disease, it would not seem unreasonable to suggest similar, or even less stringent, criteria to those outlined above for professional aircrew.

Coronary artery bypass grafting

The long-term prognosis following coronary artery bypass grafting was still being established at the time of the First United Kingdom Workshop in Aviation Cardiology. First-year graft attrition occurs at a rate of about 10% falling to 1–3% per annum thereafter. As time passes, disease in the native circulation progresses and atheroma builds up in the grafts.[155] Normal left ventricular function is associated with a much better 5-year survival (93% or greater),[149] regardless of the number of vessels involved. Severe symptoms in the presence of normal ventricular function, however, was associated with a 5-year survival of 74%. An internal mammary artery graft was associated with a 10-year survival of 86.6% after discharge from hospital in the Cleveland Clinic series,[157] with a lower risk of late myocardial infarction. Nevertheless, probably half of those undergoing coronary artery bypass grafting will experience angina within 6 or 7 years.

Both the CAA in the UK and the FAA in the USA currently re-certify professional airmen following coronary artery bypass grafting. The guidelines are broadly similar.[31,158,159]

Current CAA guidelines[36,158] require assessment

no sooner than 9 months after surgery and in the absence of myocardial infarction the following criteria are suggested.

1 The subject should complete a symptom-limited exercise electrocardiogram satisfactorily (usually to Bruce stage 4). Thallium scintigraphy may be indicated for future reference and in certain situations including the presence of a conduction disturbance.
2 Radionuclide/contrast ventriculography should demonstrate left ventricular ejection fraction > 50%.
3 Coronary angiography should show patent grafts, no significant proximal disease in any ungrafted vessel and no lesion > 30% in the remaining ungrafted native circulation.
4 In favourable cases, certification may be permitted no earlier than 9 months following surgery with annual follow-up by exercise electrocardiography/thallium scintigraphy. A further angiogram will usually be required no later than 5 years after surgery. Thereafter, repeat angiography should be at intervals of 2–3 years.

There have been one or two cases in the UK of civilian airmen who have undergone elective coronary artery bypass grafting for single-vessel disease in order to regain flying status.

Requirements for restoration of a vocational licence are broadly similar to the above, although at present (Table 76.2b and c) concomitant myocardial infarction appears to disbar.

Percutaneous transluminal coronary angioplasty

Percutaneous transluminal coronary angioplasty was not discussed in the First United Kingdom Workshop in Aviation Cardiology although guidelines were suggested.[31] Shiu reviewed the problem in the Second Workshop,[160] discussing background, selection of patients and results. He noted the overall success rate of coronary angioplasty was > 90% in established centres, but the mortality rate remains at around 1% and the incidence of major complications, such as myocardial infarction and emergency coronary artery bypass grafting is 4–6%. Patients with multivessel disease do not appear to fare as well. Restenosis occurred at a rate of 36.2% of men followed for a mean of 18 months, and only 51% were free of angina which would disbar from flying status. The consensus is that restenosis occurs in approximately 30% by 2

years.[161] Symptom recurrence is a strong predictor of angiographic restenosis. Late recurrence of angina suggests the emergence of new lesions.

Certification to fly as a member of a multicrew operation may be considered by the CAA no earlier than 9 months following the procedure subject to the following conditions.

1 Satisfactory completion of an exercise electrocardiogram (usually to Bruce stage 4) at 3 and 6 months following the procedure; thallium scintigraphy is recommended.
2 Radionuclide/contrast ventriculography should demonstrate a left ventricular ejection fraction > 50%.
3 A repeat coronary angiogram no earlier than 6 months following the procedure should demonstrate no lesion restricting the luminal diameter > 30% in any epicardial artery. Re-certification should be limited to multicrew operation and 6-monthly follow-up with exercise electrocardiography and annual follow-up with thallium scintigraphy is required. Repeat coronary angiography is probably indicated at 1, 3 and 5 years following re-certification. In the event of complicating myocardial infarction, the guidance given earlier would also apply. Private pilots may be granted full certification subject to convincing demonstration of the stability of the lesion.[36]

A vocational driver may regain a driving licence following coronary angioplasty (see Table 76.2n) providing there is no proximal disease. There is a requirement for annual review and exercise electrocardiography.

VALVULAR HEART DISEASE

Chronic rheumatic heart disease has been declining in incidence over many years in the Western world. Elsewhere, it is an important cause of cardiovascular mortality in children and young adults. In the UK, in 1984, there were 803 male and 2128 female certificated deaths from chronic rheumatic heart disease.[123] From the point of view of certification to fly or licensing to drive, other causes of valvular heart disease, such as bicuspid aortic valve and mitral leaflet prolapse, are much commoner, occurring in 1–2% and 5–8% of the population, respectively. Other causes of congenital abnormality of the heart valve will be considered separately.

Aortic valve disease

Severe aortic stenosis is a cause of sudden unexpected cardiac death and may be undiagnosed during life.[38] It is also associated with syncope, and cerebral embolism secondary to platelet accumulation on the closure line of the valve cusps. It may remain static for 10 or more years, or progress more rapidly.[162] A young person found to have an isolated aortic ejection sound is likely to have a good prognosis over the next 25 years,[163] radiographic evidence of calcification usually presaging deterioration.[162] Up to 2% of the male population may have a bicuspid aortic valve, only about two-thirds of which may be detectable on M-mode echocardiography.[164] Aortic regurgitation is well tolerated and may be present for very many years, the exception being the presence of a collagen dysgenesis, such as Marfan's syndrome. As with a bicuspid aortic valve in the absence of regurgitation, aortic regurgitation carries a risk of endocarditis.

Gravitational loading both in centrifuge and combat aircraft have demonstrated that minor aortic regurgitation is well tolerated under these conditions.

Flow murmurs

An innocent flow murmur may be detected in many young adults and on admission to a flying career they are best reviewed by a cardiologist. Brevity of the murmur and lack of an associated ejection sound and early diastolic murmur are favourable observations. A normal chest X-ray and electrocardiogram would be expected. Doppler echocardiography should be requested in cases of doubt, but, in only about 80% of subjects may it be possible to obtain high-resolution images. Sometimes, pulmonary outflow tract murmurs may confuse, but the time of onset is slightly later and often they are well localized to the left sternal edge tending not to radiate widely.

Bicuspid aortic valve

The identification of a bicuspid aortic valve should lead to regular occasional cardiological review, perhaps every 3 years, and advice with regard to antibiotics for dental or urinary tract manipulation. Its diagnosis is consistent with vocational driving and with unrestricted Class I certification to fly, subject to adequate review.

Aortic stenosis

The presence of mild aortic stenosis may be identified by continuous wave Doppler spectral analysis, which also provides a useful method for monitoring progression. Unrestricted certification may be possible if the heart is radiologically and electrocardiographically normal, if the valve orifice on two-dimensional echocardiography is > 15 mm in all views with normal left ventricular cavity size and fractional shortening, and if the peak systolic gradient is calculated to be < 20 mmHg. Exercise electrocardiography should be normal.[31,164] Cardiological review should be at least annual and any departure from these criteria should lead to restriction to multicrew operation only. Although not stated, such criteria would probably be acceptable for vocational driving. Moderate aortic stenosis, i.e. a pressure difference of 30–50 mmHg, is likely to lead to loss of a vocational licence or certification to fly.

Aortic regurgitation

Aortic regurgitation is often well tolerated and may be present for many years. Clinical examination should seek to identify the presence or absence of a high arched palate and if arachnodactyly is suspected the metacarpal index should be measured. Two-dimensional echocardiography is required to demonstrate the aortic root. Minor aortic regurgitation should be followed up regularly. Evidence of an increase in the cross-sectional end-systolic diameter of the left ventricle is likely to indicate at least moderate aortic regurgitation and it is unlikely it will be consistent with certification to fly or with vocational licensing.

Mitral valve disease

Acute rheumatic fever is now very rare in the UK and as a result chronic rheumatic heart disease is less common than it was. Diagnosis of mitral stenosis is on clinical grounds, confirmed by two-dimensional echocardiography. It is likely to be at least moderate in severity before it will be detected on routine examination. The abrupt onset of atrial fibrillation, whether paroxysmal or sustained, is part of the natural history of the condition and it is more prominently related to age than to the severity of the condition. The onset of atrial fibrillation may be at a very fast rate (i.e. > 200 beats/min) and this can be associated with a fall in cardiac output, or at least distraction by symptoms. Enlargement of the left atrium is associated with an increased risk of cerebral embolism, which may occur in sinus rhythm or, most frequently, following reversion to sinus rhythm. If mitral stenosis is moderate or severe, the onset of atrial fibrillation may precipitate pulmonary oedema. Amputation of the left atrial appendage at closed valvotomy appears to reduce the risk of cerebral embolism.

Mild mitral stenosis may be consistent, subject to close cardiological supervision (i.e. every 6 months), with restricted Class I certification, and with a vocational driving licence. Adverse factors are increasing age and left atrial enlargement (> 4.5 cm).[165]

Mitral regurgitation

Mitral regurgitation has several different causes which may be broadly classified into disorders of the leaflets (including rheumatic heart disease, infective endocarditis, systemic lupus erythematosus) and congenital defects, including atrioventricular cushion defects and isolated clefts. It may also complicate defects of connective tissue, including the syndromes of Marfan, Hurler and Ehlers–Danlos, disorders of the annulus, which may be degenerative and associated with calcification, and rheumatic heart disease; it may be secondary to left ventricular dilatation, chordal rupture, which may be idiopathic or secondary to bacterial endocarditis, rheumatic heart disease, Marfan's syndrome and the Ehlers–Danlos syndrome, and, finally, disorders of the papillary musculature secondary usually to ischaemic heart disease or, rarely, polyarteritis, sarcoidosis, amyloidosis and myocarditis. Diagnosis is on clinical grounds and confirmed by Doppler echocardiography. Mild mitral regurgitation, even when presenting with mild mitral stenosis, may impose no significant haemodynamic burden on the heart, and risk to the cardiovascular system relates to the onset of atrial fibrillation with the associated danger of cerebral embolus, which appears to increase substantially when the left atrial internal diameter is > 4.5 cm.

Mitral leaflet prolapse[168,169] may be present in up to 5% of males and 6–8% of females. It is frequently clinically silent and may remain undetected unless the subject is examined by a cardiologist. Mitral leaflet prolapse is not uncommonly associated with atypical chest pain, and there is a preponderance of both atrial and ventricular rhythm disturbances which may be both sustained and complex in form. None of the series is sufficiently large to identify the risk of its complications, which include cerebral embolus, endocarditis,

chordal rupture leading to significant mitral regurgitation, and sudden cardiac death. Schwartz et al.[170] reviewed 589 patients with the condition; ventricular tachycardia was recorded in 6% and sudden death in 1.4%. It is not possible to predict with confidence a group 'at risk' although those subjects who have a history of sudden death in the family, who have demonstrated ventricular tachycardia and who have infero-lateral abnormalities on the electrocardiogram may fall into this category.[171] Combat manoeuvres in military aircraft may precipitate ventricular tachycardia and/or frequent ventricular premature contractions,[172] but such gravitational forces are unlikely to be experienced in normal civilian air transportation. Nevertheless, of 253 cases of mitral leaflet prolapse under continuous review by the United States Air Force School of Aviation Medicine, 75 (30%) have been disqualified from flying duties, half because of rhythm disturbances.[173]

There will be very large numbers of undetected subjects with mitral leaflet prolapse holding vocational driving licences and smaller numbers flying as professional airmen, as both single crew and multicrew. In the event of the condition coming to the notice of a licensing authority, it is likely that the asymptomatic individual with no family history of sudden cardiac death or significant arrhythmia on Holter monitoring and with a normal resting and exercise electrocardiogram may continue with unrestricted certification provided the echocardiogram demonstrates no increase in size of the left atrial or left ventricular cavity.[31] Prolongation of the QT interval and unexplained ST-segment and T-wave changes are unfavourable findings. Any departure from the above may need careful consideration and restriction to multicrew operation in the case of aviators. No guidance is available in relation to vocational driving, but there seems to be no reason to disqualify vocational driving licence holders unless significant mitral regurgitation is present or significant rhythm disturbances have been demonstrated which may predispose to impairment of consciousness. After all, there must be many vocational drivers with the condition who have not been and will not be identified.

Mild mitral regurgitation, when not secondary to papillary muscle ischaemia, rheumatic heart disease, Marfan's syndrome or similar, and where left ventricular dimensions have been demonstrated to be normal, may be consistent with restricted certification to fly subject to regular cardiological review.

VALVE SURGERY

The majority of patients undergoing valve repair or replacement will be unfit to fly or hold a vocational licence by way of age, co-existent coronary artery disease, abnormality of ventricular function, rhythm or conduction disturbance, or the requirement for anticoagulants, which automatically disbar from certification to fly and from vocational driving.[23,32] It is evident that insertion of all currently available mechanical valves is likely to be inconsistent with continued flying, or vocational driving status. Consequently, these valves will not be considered.

Complications following valve replacement include embolism, 0.27% for a homograft valve, 1.59% for a Hancock prosthesis per annum,[174] endocarditis (0.5–1.5%),[175] peri-operative valve leak, valvar regurgitation[176] and valve failure (10% at 5 years, 28% at 10 years.[177] In the UK multicentre valve trial,[174] survival at 7 years following aortic valve replacement was 78–87% for prosthetic valves and 80–92% for tissue valves, the unmounted homograft valve performing most favourably. Other workers have reported similar data, and mitral valve replacement is associated with a poorer prognosis.[174,175,178]

Certification to fly following valve replacement was discussed at both Workshops in Aviation Cardiology[175,179] and, currently, certification is only likely to be permitted to individuals with an unmounted homograft valve in the aortic position. Requirements also include normal valve and normal or near-normal ventricular function as judged by Doppler echocardiography and resting and exercise electrocardiography. Coronary angiography at the time of surgery should have excluded the presence of significant coronary artery disease. If grafting was performed, the guidelines given previously apply.[36] Tissue valves fail at a greater rate in the first 5 years after implantation and heterograft valves carry a higher risk of embolism than homograft valves. Nevertheless, candidates whose risk is lowest might be considered those who have had Carpentier–Edwards or Ionescu–Shiley prostheses inserted into the aortic position. Regular cardiological follow-up and restriction to fly multicrew operations only is mandatory. Fairly similar, although less rigorous, recommendations have been suggested for vocational driving (Table 76.2o).

Reconstructive surgery for a floppy mitral valve from whatever cause may achieve good results with a low risk of embolism, particularly if the left appendage is resected.[179] Aortic valvotomy is unlikely to be performed in an adult patient before the age of retirement. Open valvotomy for mitral stenosis may obtain a good long-term result with relative freedom from cerebral embolus if the left atrial appendage is amputated. Following valvular heart surgery, no patient should be permitted to fly as pilot in sole command for 'hire or reward' although consideration could be given to the unrestricted certification of private flyers in the most favourable cases.

MYOCARDITIS

Many agents may cause myocarditis, perhaps the best known are the viruses of which the Coxsackie A and B are the most prominent. Other viruses, the *Rickettsia*, bacteria, fungi, protozoa and metazoa have all been implicated as causative agents. A variety of organic and inorganic compounds and physical agents may cause myocarditis, as may various allergic phenomena. Myocarditis, as a cause of death in England and Wales, is uncommon accounting for 75 certified deaths in 1984.[123] It is a cause of sudden cardiac death.[38] It has been described in association with aircraft accidents but does not appear to have been causally involved.[180] Probably some degree of 'myocarditis' is common in certain viral infections and it is almost certainly underdiagnosed.

Virus myocarditis usually resolves within a matter of weeks, although an unknown percentage of cases proceed to dilated cardiomyopathy (*vide infra*). The electrocardiographic changes may be prolonged, and evidence of complete resolution with return to normal myocardial function, as judged by echocardiography and exercise electrocardiography, and electrical stability, judged by Holter monitoring, is likely to be required before re-certification to fly could be considered. Similar requirements would be appropriate for vocational driving licence holders, although evidence of clinical recovery only may be sufficient in the case of the ordinary driving licence. Some myocarditides, such as Chagas' disease (*Trypanosoma cruzi*), run a protracted course leading to dilated myopathy and associated atrioventricular conduction disturbances which have appropriate licensing implications. Others are associated with acute infectious illness, or intoxication and, provided resolution occurs and the prognosis is good, licensing advice should be based on the evidence of myocardial integrity and electrical stability.

PERICARDITIS

Acute benign aseptic pericarditis is becoming more frequently recognized. It presents with chest pain and electrocardiographic changes and thus may be mistaken for acute myocardial ischaemia. It has recently been reviewed[181] in the context of aviation, and it is a benign condition. Nevertheless, in the acute condition, a subject is unfit to fly and to drive because systemic disturbance, including fever, pain and breathlessness due to tamponade, may occur. It has been suggested that an airman suffering from this condition should be considered unfit for a period of 6 months,[23] but, in the event of complete resolution with loss of symptoms and satisfactory evidence of the diagnosis (or demonstration of the absence of coronary heart disease, as an alternative diagnosis), this protracted period may not always be required. There is a tendency for the condition to relapse often after many years, but incapacitation following such an event is extremely unlikely.[181]

Other causes of pericarditis include other infections, neoplasia, auto-immune phenomena, metabolic abnormalities, trauma, myocardial infarction and drug hypersensitivity. Licensing advice should be based on the natural history of the underlying cause and the completeness of resolution. Satisfactory surgical treatment of constrictive pericarditis may permit restricted certification to fly but up to one-quarter of patients have atrial fibrillation and normal cardiac function is not always restored.[182]

CARDIOMYOPATHY

The description of a cardiomyopathy as a disorder of heart muscle of unknown cause or association[183] emphasized that the myocardial abnormality is a primary event. The term secondary cardiomyopathy, which for a while was unfashionable, may encompass such entities as 'ischaemic cardiomyopathy' and involvement of the myocardium, for instance, in sarcoidosis or amyloidosis.

Hypertrophic cardiomyopathy

Hypertrophic cardiomyopathy is associated with an increase in the right and/or left ventricular muscle mass and, in many subjects, asymmetric hypertrophy of the interventricular septum. It may be inherited as a dominant characteristic or present sporadically. It has been associated with phaeochromocytoma, neurofibroma, lentiginosis, hyperthyroidism, hyperinsulinism and Turner's syndrome.[184]

Its incidence is unknown partly due to difficulties of definition; isolated increase in thickness of the interventricular septum determined echocardiographically is not an uncommon finding. It has been estimated to cause 1 in 200 sudden cardiac deaths;[185] it was associated with an annual death rate of 3.4% in one series, in which 26 of the total of 49 deaths were sudden. Rhythm disturbances are common and may be supraventricular or ventricular; if such arrhythmias are fast and sustained, they are likely to be poorly tolerated in view of the loss of left ventricular compliance. Syncope via several mechanisms has been described. Systemic embolism is also common.

Hypertrophic myopathy has been reviewed in the context of aviation.[184] It was concluded that in view of the risk of sudden cardiac death, reduction of exercise performance, risk of rhythm disturbance, syncope and systemic embolism, patients with hypertrophic cardiomyopathy were unfit to fly. The performance of surgery which may bring about improvement in symptoms and possibly prognosis[186] does not alter this recommendation. No specific guidance is available for vocational drivers although on account of the foregoing they are likely to be disbarred as the condition may be a 'relevant disability'. The same should apply to symptomatic patients who hold ordinary driving licences.

Minor degrees of hypertrophy require careful review. Both asymmetric septal hypertrophy and systolic anterior motion of the mitral valve are non-specific findings and echocardiographic diagnosis is not necessarily accurate.[187] The electrocardiogram may be more specific if a pseudo-infarction pattern of QS waves (but with a discordant QRST angle) is present in the inferior or septal leads. Restricted certification to fly may be possible subject to satisfactory (usually to Bruce stage 4) exercise evaluation and Holter monitoring. Regular cardiological review is required. Vocational driving licence holders with the condition are unlikely to be detected but if they are there seems to be no reason to withhold licensing.

Dilated cardiomyopathy

Dilated cardiomyopathy is associated with right and/or left ventricular dilatation and reduced cardiac output. It may be idiopathic or related to previous viral encounter, alcohol abuse, hypertension[188] or a combination of these. Its incidence is about 10 cases per 100 000 population.[189] It has poor prognosis,[190] with about two-thirds of patients in one series dying within 2 years of diagnosis, although one-quarter survived a median of 11 years with no apparent deterioration and a small number recovered. In a second study, prognosis was better: mortality at 1 year was 23% and 48% at 2 years.[191] There is a risk of supraventricular and ventricular rhythm disturbances, of systemic embolism and of sudden cardiac death.[188,190] Arrhythmias, however, may be less important in determining prognosis in dilated cardiomyopathy than they are in hypertrophic cardiomyopathy.[188]

Established dilated myopathy requiring treatment is incompatible with fitness to fly and likely to be incompatible with vocational driving. In the small percentage of patients in whom recovery appears to take place, re-certification may be considered provided resting and exercise electrocardiography is satisfactory, and echocardiography confirms normal left ventricular dimensions and the absence of mural thrombus. Multiple gated acquisition study or contrast ventriculography should confirm the presence of normal left ventricular function, and Holter monitoring should fail to identify any significant rhythm disturbance. Any departure from these guidelines is likely to lead to denial of licensing status, although minor impairment of left ventricular performance in the absence of any other abnormality could be consistent with restricted flying status. There seems to be no reason to deny a vocational driving licence in this situation. The fitness of an ordinary driving licence holder will depend on the presence of symptoms, i.e. whether a 'relevant' or 'prospective' disability is present.

Obliterative and restrictive cardiomyopathies

Obliterative and restrictive cardiomyopathies have been comprehensively reviewed in the context of aviation.[192] The obliterative cardiomyopathies, both temperate and tropical in form, are now thought to be the result of eosinophilic heart disease. The prognosis is poor and associated with pulmonary and systemic emboli. In the established condition or in a patient in whom the presence of > 1×10^9/l circulating degranulated eosinophils has been identified, certification to hold a professional flying licence should be denied.[192] This is also likely to apply to a vocational driving licence.

Restrictive myopathies have the common feature of failure of diastolic function, usually due to a fibrotic or infiltrative process. Amyloidosis, sar-

coidosis (see below), non-specific hypertrophy/fibrosis and, rarely, connective tissue disorders are encountered as causes. The high incidence of arrhythmias and the often rapid onset of heart failure in amyloidosis and in non-specific fibrosis should disbar from certification to fly or holding a vocational driving licence. Restricted certification to fly might be considered for subjects with haemochromatosis provided the disease is well controlled by venesection, diabetes mellitus, if present, does not require therapy and two-dimensional echocardiography confirms normal myocardial appearance and function. Multiple gated acquisition scanning should be within normal limits, and Holter monitoring for 72 h should demonstrate no significant rhythm disturbance.[192] Regular follow-up by a cardiologist is essential. Patients with transfusion-dependent anaemias should not be considered for other than an ordinary driving licence.

SARCOIDOSIS

Sarcoidosis is a common multisystem granulomatous disorder occurring commonly in the second and third decade of life. It may be commoner in black subjects and has a prevalence in the UK of approximately 20 cases per 100 000 on radiographic survey.[193] Typically, the disease presents with fever, arthritis, erythema nodosum and uveitis, or at routine radiological examination of the chest when bilateral hilar lymphadenopathy may be detected. Systemic involvement occurs to an unknown extent; in about 5% of those with systemic involvement, there will be clinically overt cardiac involvement.

Any site in the heart may be involved in sarcoidosis, but presentation in complete heart block with Adams–Stokes attacks is frequent.[194,195] Ventricular rhythm disturbances are also frequent, and sudden cardiac death occurred in 15% of patients in one series, although in another review it was suggested it might be as high as 40–50%.[196] Congestive cardiac failure is one end-point in those with extensive myocardial infiltration. Aircrew with established sarcoidosis of the heart should be regarded as unfit.[194,196] Symptom-free individuals with bilateral hilar lymphadenopathy alone should undergo annual follow-up with a chest X-ray, resting and exercise electrocardiogram with thallium-201 myocardial imaging, Holter monitoring and lung function tests. Provided these investigations remain normal and there is evidence that the lymphadenopathy is static or retreating and there is no evidence of other organ or parenchymal lung involvement, flying status restricted to multicrew operation should be permissible.[36,194] Following a lapse of 2 years, unrestricted flying status may be possible although its desirability is more questionable. Patients without known cardiac involvement, who have normal lung function and who do not require steroid therapy may be considered for restricted certification subject to indefinite 6 monthly follow-up.[36,194]

THROMBO-EMBOLISM

Thrombo-embolism is rare in physically fit subjects,[197] but it may present in passengers flying on aircraft.[198,199] Other precipitating events include surgery, trauma, chronic thrombotic venous disease, pregnancy and possibly obesity.

The diagnosis of deep venous thrombosis, or of acute thrombo-embolic disease, in an airman needs to be established beyond doubt. Phlebography, pulmonary angiography and ventilation/perfusion (V/Q) scanning all contribute. Anticoagulant therapy disbars both flying and vocational driving,[23,32] thus its prescription interferes with employability. Isolated calf vein thrombosis is likely to lead to at least 3 months' treatment with warfarin, and the possibility of recurrence is low in the absence of an identifiable risk factor.[197]

In a physically fit subject who has an identifiable risk factor, the risk of recurrence of pulmonary embolism is probably < 0.25–0.5% per annum after the first few weeks.[197] In the absence of a defined risk factor, there is a twofold excess mortality over 5–9 years,[200] often due to occult malignancy. Subacute pulmonary embolism leading eventually to chronic thrombo-embolic pulmonary hypertension is rare, but established pulmonary hypertension (> 30 mmHg) is associated with a poorer prognosis.[197]

It has been suggested that aircrew may be recertificated following pulmonary embolism after discontinuation of warfarin provided they are restricted to fly as a member of a multicrew operation.[197] This applies to those who have an identifiable risk factor as well as to those in whom it was not possible to identify one, but only following a diligent search for the possibility of occult malignancy or abnormality of clotting function. Long-haul flying and driving are not ideal occupations following deep venous thrombosis because the risk of recurrence must be increased by prolonged

inactivity. Although the Second United Kingdom Workshop[37,197] did endorse re-certification to fly following a pulmonary embolus, in selected cases this may not be desirable.

CONGENITAL HEART DISEASE

Congenital heart disease in the context of aviation has been reviewed by McCartney.[201] Only conditions carrying a very low risk of complication before or after surgery were considered. These included atrial septal defect, ventricular septal defect, pulmonary stenosis, coarctation of the aorta and patent ductus arteriosus.

Atrial septal defect

Atrial septal defect accounts for about 28% of patients with congenital heart disease.[202] Ostium primum defects are associated with conduction disorders and progressive mitral regurgitation. Secondum defects should be recommended for closure if the heart is enlarged on chest X-ray or if the pulmonary to systemic flow ratio is > 1.5/1[201] in view of the low risk of surgery. There may be an excess risk of atrial rhythm disorders in later life. Surgery to a sinus venosus defect may carry an increased risk of sino-atrial nodal disease.[201] A small secundum atrial septal defect should be consistent with unrestricted certification to fly and to drive;[32,201] evidence of pulmonary hypertension would disbar. Ostium primum defects require careful consideration and, following correction, they appear to have a higher mortality. A sinus venosus defect carries an increased risk of arrhythmia following surgery but, provided an absence of significant rhythm disturbance can be demonstrated, it may be accepted for restricted certification to fly. Follow-up Holter monitoring is recommended.[201]

Ventricular septal defect

Ventricular septal defect comprises 31% of all congenital heart disease.[202] Subjects who have a heart of normal size on the chest X-ray, a pulmonary/systemic flow ratio < 2:1 and no evidence of pulmonary hypertension do not need intervention and their overall risk is probably only that occasioned by the possibility of endocarditis. Arrhythmias are uncommon. Subjects with a higher flow ratio should have the defect closed, but the subsequent increased risk of sudden unexpected death and arrhythmia should lead to caution in licensing decisions.

Pulmonary stenosis

Isolated pulmonary stenosis accounts for 10% of patients with congenital heart disease. It appears to have a good prognosis, and if the pressure gradient is < 30 mmHg the condition is very likely to be stable.[203] The condition is consistent at least with restricted certification to fly and with vocational driving. Clinical cardiological follow-up is required. The prognosis following surgery for isolated pulmonary stenosis is good, and such patients may be considered for certification provided the pulmonary gradient is < 30 mmHg.

Persistent patent ductus arteriosus

In the absence of any other abnormality, there would seem to be no other reason to withhold certification to fly or to drive from a patient who had undergone closure of a persistent patent ductus arterious, provided there is no evidence of pulmonary hypertension.[201] Up to one-third of patients will have an associated bicuspid aortic valve.

Coarctation of the aorta

There is evidence that repair of coarctation of the aorta after the age of 12 years is associated with a higher risk of sudden cardiac death and cerebrovascular accident.[204] If the condition is treated in infancy, the results appear excellent up to the age of 20 years and patients at risk appear to be those in whom there is persistent systemic hypertension after surgery. If a subject is normotensive, both at rest and on exercise, and correction was carried out before the age of 12 years, full certification to fly should be possible. Later surgical correction may lead to restriction of certification to fly but it should not interfere with a vocational driving licence.[31,201]

RHYTHM AND CONDUCTION DISTURBANCES

Atrioventricular block

First degree atrioventricular block is not uncommon amongst aircrew and a PR interval exceeding 0.20 s is seen in 1% or more. If there is no evidence of a bundle branch disturbance, the delay is usually proximal and the condition benign.[205] There are no licensing implications. More problematic in the author's experience is the problem of the very long PR interval, 0.4 s, which appears to have a preva-

lence of 0.01%. It shortens on exercise and treatment with atropine, although it may still be prolonged. It is likely to be a vagal phenomenon and may be associated with Mobitz type I atrioventricular block. It probably cannot be regarded as 'normal' and as such restriction of certification to fly is advised.

The presence of a bundle branch disturbance with first degree atrioventricular block suggests, but it is not diagnostic of, distal conducting tissue disease, particularly if left or right bundle branch block with left- or right-axis deviation co-exists. Such subjects have a higher incidence of disease in the distal conducting system and should be evaluated as for bundle branch disturbance (see below).

Asymptomatic Mobitz type I (Wenckebach) atrioventricular block of a short periodicity is not uncommon in normal individuals during sleep and appears to represent a vagal phenomenon. The presence of a narrow QRS complex almost always indicates atrioventricular nodal block, is likely to be benign and may be associated with first degree atrioventricular block.[206] However, in Shaw's group of 77 patients who had a higher mean age than the employed population (69 years), Mobitz type I block had a similar prognosis to that of Mobitz type II, irrespective of the presence of bundle branch block.[207] The results of at least two studies in young people suggest that it may progress to complete atrioventricular block[206] and such subjects require exercise electrocardiography, electrophysiological study to determine the site of the block and regular surface electrocardiography and 24-h ambulatory monitoring. Assuming a satisfactory outcome and no evidence of distal conducting tissue disease, restricted certification to fly may be considered.

The presence of Mobitz type II and 2:1 and 3:1 atrioventricular block carries a relatively high risk of progression to higher degrees of block; survival has been recorded in paced (78%) and unpaced (41%) subjects over a 5-year period,[207] although the mean age of the patients was much older than the pilot population. These conditions should disbar from certification to drive and to fly in an unpaced subject (see below).

Complete atrioventricular block

Congenital complete heart block

Congenital complete heart block is a rare condition which, although previously believed to carry a good prognosis and in the past has not disbarred from flying,[208] carries an unpredictable risk of impaired consciousness and sudden cardiac death. The presence of this condition is inconsistent with certification to fly or with the issuance of a vocational driving licence.

Intraventricular conduction disturbances

Right bundle branch block

Incomplete right bundle branch block is most commonly a normal variant and there is no evidence that it carries other than a normal prognosis in the asymptomatic subject.

Complete right bundle branch block

Complete right bundle branch block has a prevalence of approximately 0.2% among aircrew[128,129] and it does not appear to carry a significant risk developing syncope or high-grade atrioventricular block.[209] Recently acquired right bundle branch block probably also has a benign prognosis, at least for 5–6 years from the date of discovery.[210] In only one paper, from the Framingham study, was it suggested there is an increased risk of cardiovascular event, but most of the patients were older and the majority had systemic hypertension during the period of observation.[211] Nevertheless, it would seem prudent to perform full review including exercise electrocardiography, echocardiography and Holter monitoring in any such subject and to restrict licensing to multicrew operations only; this approach has been adopted elsewhere.[212] There seems to be no good reason to disqualify an individual from holding a vocational driving licence (Table 76.2f).

Left anterior hemiblock

Left anterior hemiblock in otherwise normal individuals is not uncommon and it is seen in 1.0–1.7% of aviators.[128–130] When isolated, it appears to carry no significant risk.[213] The same may not be true of recently acquired left anterior hemiblock, but data are scant. There seems to be no special risk of progression to left bundle branch block or to complete atrioventricular block.[209]

Left posterior hemiblock

Left posterior hemiblock has a prevalence in healthy airmen of 0.1%.[209] There are no adequate data on

the risk of progression to higher grades of atrioventricular block, or of sudden cardiac death.

Left bundle branch block

Left bundle branch block is less common than right bundle branch block and it is seen in 0.013% of healthy airmen.[128,209] Historically, left bundle branch block was thought to carry a poor prognosis, probably because much of the experience was derived from patients in whom coronary heart disease was common. Coronary artery disease was seen in only 24% of 34 airmen investigated by Froelicher,[133] and approximately 25% of asymptomatic aviators acquiring left bundle branch block will have evidence of co-existing organic heart disease.[214] Nevertheless, established complete left bundle branch block in subjects considered free of other cardiovascular disease carries a mortality risk ratio of between 1.26 and 1.38, according to data collected by two life insurance companies.[209] Recently acquired left bundle branch block does appear to be associated with 10 times the risk of sudden cardiac death after the age of 45 years although below this age the mortality risk was not increased.[215] In the Framingham study,[216] half of those subjects who acquired left bundle branch block had died within 10 years of its diagnosis of cardiovascular disease, 4 of whom died suddenly. The mean age of onset however was significantly older (62 years) than that in the pilot group.

Careful evaluation of pre-existing left bundle branch block by echocardiography, thallium-201 myocardial imaging and Holter monitoring, and probably coronary angiography, should permit the identification of a group at low risk who may be given restricted certification to fly subject to supervision. This group should also qualify for a vocational driving licence. Recently acquired left bundle branch block should disbar, but eventually the condition becomes established. There are no data with regard to the point at which reduction in risk occurs, but a QRS axis to the right of 0 and an absence of a left atrial conduction delay on the first electrocardiogram demonstrating left bundle branch block may be associated with a significantly better prognosis.[216] Reversible left bundle branch block has also been described in a pilot receiving chloroquine for malarial prophylaxis.[217]

Ventricular pre-excitation

The incidence of the Wolff–Parkinson–White syndrome, an example of ventricular pre-excitation, in a group of healthy individuals was 0.25%,[218] in whom the prevalence of documented tachyarrhythmias was 1.8% compared with 20% in patients who had been referred. Nevertheless, the pre-excitation syndromes are capricious. The development of a fast atrioventricular re-entrant tachycardia may cause hypotension, and the development or appearance of atrial fibrillation in the presence of a bypass pathway with a short effective refractory period may give rise to a very fast heart rate, syncope and possibly ventricular fibrillation.

It has been suggested that established aircrew with asymptomatic 'safe' Wolff–Parkinson–White syndrome, i.e. a long effective refractory period (> 500 ms), of the bypass pathway could be given restricted certification provided asymptomatic tachyarrhythmia cannot be identified on repeated Holter monitoring.[31,219] Successful surgical ablation of an accessory pathway may be acceptable for restricted certification to fly. Drug treatment of tachyarrhythmias is at present unacceptable. The issuance of an unrestricted Class I medical certificate would not be permitted, the same principles applying to the other pre-excitation syndromes. A pre-excitation pattern on the electrocardiogram should be consistent with holding a vocational driving licence provided there were no associated symptoms likely to cause impairment of consciousness.

Sinus node arrest and sino-atrial block

Sino-atrial disorders are not common in aircrew and the interface between the physiological and the pathological is not clear. Pauses > 2 s in duration are uncommon in normal subjects and those > 2.5 s are probably abnormal, although exaggerated vagal phenomena including sinus arrhythmia may be seen in athletes.[220] To some extent, the prevalence is age dependent and in young men it varies between 0.2 and 1.6 per 1000.[129] Progression of sinus node dysfunction may be very slow indeed and the condition is generally benign. It is best identified by Holter monitoring. Provocation by exercise or atropine administration may provoke a reduced heart rate response. Electrophysiology testing will reveal a prolonged sinus node recovery time in about 50% of those studied.[220]

Attacks of altered consciousness may not occur for years[221] or may present early.[220] Symptomatic pauses require pacemaking (see below). Subjects with asymptomatic pauses should be regularly monitored; airmen with asymptomatic pauses should be restricted to multicrew operation. If followed regularly, the condition should be consistent with vocational driving. Sino-atrial block has been described secondary to gravitational loading in a centrifuge, but significant g forces are unlikely to be encountered in civil aviation.[222]

Atrial fibrillation

Atrial fibrillation is a common rhythm disturbance. It has a prevalence of around 0.02%[223] in flying personnel but is commoner in the ageing population. Almost any cardiac condition may be associated with it, and many of these will disbar an individual from flying or driving.

'Lone' atrial fibrillation may be paroxysmal or established. There is no essential difference between the two and the prognosis may be normal.[224] No deaths were recorded in one series of 125 airmen.[225] With respect to certification, problems arise in the context of symptoms. Some people are unaware of repeated attacks of paroxysmal atrial fibrillation, whereas others may be prostrate due to symptoms of palpitation, dyspnoea, chest discomfort, clouding of the sensorium and, occasionally, polyuria. All these symptoms may be worsened by high levels of arousal and, although they do not lead to loss of consciousness, they may lead to distraction. This may not be important in vehicle driving because incapacitation is unlikely to be complete, but in the context of a single-crew aircraft operation the consequences could be profound.

Atrial fibrillation in the presence of mitral valve disease carried a 17-fold increased risk of stroke in the Framingham study, although in the absence of rheumatic heart disease the risk was only increased 5-fold.[226] Atrial fibrillation has been comprehensively reviewed in the context of aviation recently.[36,223,227] If present in an otherwise normal heart and well controlled with digoxin or a beta-blocking agent, restricted certification might be permissible. Paroxysmal atrial fibrillation should be considered only if completely suppressed or completely asymptomatic, as judged by multiple Holter recordings over a 6-month period.[36,227] Permissible agents include atenolol, verapamil at a dose not exceeding 40 mg t.d.s., quinidine as the long-acting preparation at a dose of 250 mg b.d. and sotalol 80 mg b.d. An additional requirement is the absence of unwanted effects and demonstration of satisfactory simulator performance. The institution of therapy with warfarin is disqualifying. Although such patients are at present advised that they should not hold a vocational driving licence, the overall risk in 'lone' atrial fibrillation is probably acceptable subject to regular review.

Other paroxysmal rhythm disturbances, such as atrial flutter and paroxysmal atrial tachycardia, disbar individuals from vocational driving (see Table 76.2j) and from certification to fly.[31,36,228]

Ventricular premature beats

Ventricular premature beats are a common finding in normal individuals.[229] As an isolated observation in the absence of other abnormality of the heart, they are of little importance although some subjects may be aware of them. Although more complex forms, including multiform complexes, R-on-T ectopic complexes and ventricular tachycardia, are more commonly seen in disease states, there is evidence[230] that such subjects if asymptomatic and otherwise healthy have a normal prognosis; however, frequent ectopic beats (60–100 per hour) appeared to have an adverse prognosis in subjects in the Busselton study, even when asymptomatic.[231] The definition of what is normal, therefore, is not clear; it has been suggested that ventricular premature beats occurring less often than 200 per 24 hours, of two or less morphologies and infrequently in pairs are 'normal' whereas others including R-on-T ectopic beats and salvos of ventricular tachycardia are 'abnormal'.[232,233]

Occasional ectopic beats, presumably atrial or ventricular, do not disqualify individuals from vocational driving (see Table 76.2j). In the context of aviation, it has been recommended that sustained ventricular tachycardia (> 5 s, > 120 min) should disbar aviators from flying duty. Non-sustained ventricular tachycardia and other complex forms in normal individuals free of symptoms may be consistent with restricted certification subject to full evaluation with echocardiography, Holter monitoring and exercise electrocardiography.[36,233] Slightly different recommendations have been made with regard to exercise-induced ventricular rhythm disturbances.[36,228]

Implantable devices and aviation

Up to 150 patients per million of the population in the UK will have a permanent endocardial pacemaker implanted; 25% of such individuals are below the age of retirement. To a large extent, subjects with an implanted pacemaker will be excluded from certification to fly or to drive by way of co-existing disease or age, but in a few the risk of pacemaker interference in the aviation environment, or of failure in either the aviation or road transport environment bears further consideration.

Toff and Camm[234] reviewed data available from 12 differing manufacturers and recorded a failure rate varying between 0.12 and 1.44% per year. They calculated a major failure rate of about 2.6 per 10^7 flying hours on a basis of 1200 hours flying each month, which is twice the normal number of hours flown. The possibility of electrical interference was also investigated in view of the multitude of direct current, alternating current and electromagnetic fields of a wide range of frequencies present in an aircraft.[235] That this could occur was demonstrated in the laboratory. The newer activity-sensing pacemakers using a piezo-electric crystal may also be upset by aircraft vibration,[236] notably in helicopters. Systems using impedance measurement techniques should be free of this complication.

Subjects with cardiac pacemakers may be permitted to hold a vocational licence subject to the agreement of the honorary Medical Advisory Panel to DVLC (Table 76.2g). It has been recommended that a subject may be considered for restricted certification to fly, provided there is no other disqualifying disorder, a period of 3 months has elapsed following insertion, pacemaker dependence is excluded as far as possible and follow-up by an approved cardiologist can be achieved on a 6-monthly basis.[36,234] Bipolar systems are to be preferred because of the smaller risk of electromagnetic interference, but the rate of major pacemaker failure in a dependent patient is too high to permit full Class III certification.

REFERENCES

1. The Health and Safety at Work Act 1974. Department of Employment. London: HMSO, 1974.
2. The Offshore Installations (Operational Safety, Health and Welfare) Regulations 1976. No. 1019. London: HMSO, 1976.
3. Health and Safety (Offshore Installation and Pipeline Works) First Aid Regulations. London: HMSO, 1987.
4. United Kingdom Offshore Operators Association. Recommended General Medical Standards of Fitness for Designated Offshore Employees. London: UK Offshore Operators Association, 1986.
5. Air Navigation. The Order and the Regulations. Civil Aviation Authority CAP 393. London: CAA, 1981.
6. First Council Directive of 4 September 1980. On the introduction of a community driving licence. *Official J. Eur. Comm.* 1980; 375: 1–15.
7. Chaplin, J. In perspective. The Safety of Aircraft Pilots and their Hearts. *Eur. Heart J.* 1988; 9 Suppl G: 17–20.

8. Henderson, M. *Living with Risk*. British Medical Association Guide. Chichester: John Wiley and Sons, 1987.

9. *Road Accidents Great Britain 1985. The Casualty Report*. London: HMSO, 1986.

10. Learmont, D. 1986: Safe but for Terrorism. *Flight International* 1987; **131**: 4046: 37–41.

11. UK Airlines. *Airline Operating Traffic and Financial Statistics 1986*, Civil Aviation Authority CAP 529. London: CAA, 1987.

12. UK Airlines. *Accidents to Aircraft on the British Register 1985*, Civil Aviation Authority CAP 525. London: CAA, 1986.

13. Fritsch, O. and Santamaria, J. Aviation Safety—a review of the 1985 record. Cited in *Flight Safety Focus* 1987; **1**: 1–6. Redhill, Flight Safety Committee.

14. Gibbs Smith, C.H. In: *The Rebirth of European Aviation*. London: HMSO, 1974.

15. International Air Transport Association. *World Air Transport Statistics 1986*. Geneva: IATA, 1987, p. 31.

16. Civil Aviation Authority. *International Register of Aircraft*. Cheltenham: CAA, 1986.

17. Civil Aviation Authority. *British Civil Airworthiness Requirements*, Section S, Civil Aviation Authority CAP 482. London: CAA, 1983.

18. The Public Service Vehicles Act (1981). London: HMSO, 1981.

19. Civil Aviation Authority. *Guidance Notes for Authorised Medical Examiners*. London: CAA, 1983.

20. The First UK Workshop in Aviation Cardiology, Eds Joy, M., Bennett, G. *Eur. Heart J*. 1984/5; (Suppl. A): 1–164.

21. The Second UK Workshop in Aviation Cardiology, eds Joy, M., Bennett, G. *Eur. Heart J*. 1988; **9** (Suppl. G): 1–179.

22. Personnel Licensing. International Standards and Recommended Practices. Annex I to the Convention on International Civil Aviation. Montreal: ICAO, 1982.

23. Manual of Civil Aviation Medicine. Second Ed. Montreal: ICAO, 1985.

24. First International Symposium on Cardiology and Aviation. Lamb L.K.E. (Ed.). School of Aviation Medicine, USAF Aerospace Medical Center (ATC), Brooks Air Force Base, Texas, 1959.

25. Standards of fitness of aircrew. First Bethesda Conference of the American College of Cardiology. *Am. J. Cardiol*. 1966; **18**: 630–636.

26. Cardiovascular problems associated with aviation safety. Eighth Bethesda Conference of the American College of Cardiology. *Am. J. Cardiol*. 1975; **36**: 573–620.

27. Cardiovascular fitness of airline pilots. Report of the working party of the Cardiology Committee of the Royal College of Physicians of London. *Br. Heart J*. 1978; **40**: 335–50.

28. Joy, M. The pilot and his heart. Development of a microspeciality. *St Thomas' Hosp. Gazette* 1980; **78**: 17–20.

29. Civil Aircraft Accident Report 4/73, Department of Trade and Industry 1973. Trident 1 G-ARPI. Report of the public enquiry into the causes and circumstances of the accident near Staines on 18 June 1972. London: HMSO, 1973.

30. Bayes, T. An essay towards solving a problem in the doctrine of chance. *Phil. Trans. R. Soc. Lond*. 1763; **53**: 370.

31. Joy, M. Introduction and summary of principal conclusions to the First UK Workshop in Aviation Cardiology 1984; **6** (Suppl. A): 1–7.

32. Medical Aspects of Fitness to Drive. A Guide for Medical Practiioners. Raffle, A. (Ed.). London: The Medical Commission on Accident Prevention, 1985.

33. Notes for Guidance of Doctors Completing Medical Certificates in Respect of Applicants for Heavy Goods Public Service Vehicle and Taxi Drivers licences. Fifth Edition. London: British Medical Association, 1983.

34. Petch, M.C. Cardiovascular aspects of fitness to drive. *Topics in Circulation* 1987; **2** (no. 3): 10–12.

35. Espir, M.L.E. The present regulations and their application. Royal Society of Medicine International Congress and Symposium Series 1982; **60**: 28–33.

36. Joy, M. A risk orientated approach to the problems of cardiovascular certification in aircrew. Summary of principal conclusions of the Second UK Workshop in Aviation Cardiology. *Eur. Heart J*. 1988 (Suppl. G); 1–8.

37. Office of Population Censuses and Surveyors. 1984 Mortality Statistics: Cause. Series DH2 no. 11 1985. London: HMSO.

38. Davies, M.J. Pathological Views of Sudden Death. *Br. Heart. J*. 1981; **45**: 88–96.

39. Raffle, P.A.B. The HGV/PSV driver and loss of impairment of consciousness. Royal Society of Medicine International Congress and Symposium Series 1982; **60**: 35–39.

40. Civil Aircraft Accident Report 15/75. Department of Trade Accident Investigation Branch 1975. Piper PA 31–350 Navajo Chieftan G-BBJG. Report on the accident at Horseforth near Leeds on 6 December 1974. London: HMSO, 1975.

41. Civil Aircraft Accident Report 15/76. Department of Trade Accident Investigation Branch 1976. Piper PA31-350 Navajo G-BBPV. Report on the accident at Little Sandhurst, Berkshire on 19 October 1975. London: HMSO 1976.

42. Buley, L.E. Incidence, causes and results of airline pilot incapacitation while on duty. *Aerospace Med*. 1969; **40**: 64–70.

43. Bennett, G. Aviation accident risk and aircraft licensing. *Eur. Heart. J*. 1984; **5** (Suppl. A): 9–13.

44. Transport and Road Research Laboratory. A preliminary survey of the role of drugs other than alcohol in road accidents. Leaflet LF 677. Taplow: Transport and Road Research Laboratory, 1977.

45. Cooper, L.E., White, M.D. and Lauber, J.K. Resource management on the flight deck. NASA Conference publication CP 2120. National Aeronautics and Space Administration. Government Printing Office, Washington DC, 1980.

46. Hartunian, N.S., Smart, C.N. and Thompson, M.S. The incidence and economic costs of cancer, motor vehicle injuries, coronary heart disease and stroke: a competitive analysis. *Am. J. Pub. Hlth* 1980; **70**: 1249–60.

47. Taylor, J. Medical fitness to drive. *In* Recent Advances in Occupational Health 3. Harrington, J.M. (Eds.). Edinburgh; Churchill, Livingstone, 1987.

48. Bellet, S., Roman, L., Kostis, J. and Slater, A. Continuous electrocardiographic monitoring during automobile driving. Studies in normal subjects and patients with coronary disease. *Am. J. Cardiol*. 1968; **22**: 856–62.

49. Taggart, P., Gibbons, D. and Somerville, W. Some effects of motor car driving on the normal and abnormal heart. *Br. Med. J*. 1969; **iv**: 130–34.

50. Lauwers, P., Aelvoet, W., Sneppe, R. and Remion, M. The effect of car driving on the electrocardiogram of patients with myocardial infarction and an ECG at rest devoid of dysrythmia and repolarisation abnormalities: Comparison with the ECG changes obtained during exercise. *Acta Cardiol. (Brux.)* 1973; **28**: 27–43.

51. Bellet, S., Roman, L. and Kostis, J. The effect of automobile driving on catecholamine and adrenocortical secretions. *Am. J. Cardiol*. 1969; **24**: 365–68.

52. Tunstall Pedoe, H. Risk of a coronary heart attack in the normal population and how it might be modified in flyers. *Eur. Heart J*. 1984; **5** (Suppl. A): 43–49.

53. Froom, P., Gross, N., Ribak, J. and Lewis, B. Accidents,

pilot experience, organic disease and inflight sudden incapacitation. *Aviat. Space Environ. Med.* 1987; **58**: 488.

54. McFarland, R.A., Tune, G.S. and Welford, A.T. On the driving of automobiles by older people. *J. Gerontol.* 1964; **19**: 190–97.

55. Waller, J.A. Cardiovascular disease, ageing and traffic accidents. *J. Chron. Dis.* 1967; **20**: 615–20.

56. Gerber, S.R., Joliet, P.V. and Feegel, J.R. Single vehicle accidents in Cuyahoga (Ohio) 1958–1963. *J. Forensic Sci.* 1966; **11**: 144–51.

57. Mason, J.K. Asymptomatic disease of coronary arteries of young men. *Br. Med. J.* 1963; **ii**: 1234–37.

58. Baker, S.P. and Spritz, W.A. Age effects on autopsy evidence of disease in fatally injured drivers. *Am. Med. Assoc.* 1970; **214**: 1079–88.

59. Haddon, W.J., Valien, P. McCarroll, J.R. *et al.* A controlled investigation of the characteristics of adult pedestrians fatally injured by motor vehicles in Manhattan. *J. Chron. Dis.* 1961; **14**: 655–78.

60. Herner, B., Smedley, B. and Ysander, L. Sudden illness as a cause of motor vehicle accidents. *Br. J. Industr. Med.* 1966; **23**: 37–41.

61. Grattan, E., Jeffcoate, G.O. Medical factors in road traffic accidents. *Br. Med. J.* 1968; **i**: 75–79.

62. Peterson, B.J. and Petty, C.S. Sudden natural death amongst automobile drivers. *J. Forensic Sci.* 1962; **7**: 274–285.

63. Baker, S.P. and Spitz, W.U. An evaluation of the hazard created by natural death at the wheel. *N. Engl. J. Med.* 1970; **283**: 405–409.

64. Waller, J.A. Chronic medical conditions and traffic safety. *N. Engl. J. Med.* 1965; **273**: 1413–20.

65. Ysander, L. The safety of drivers with chronic disease. *Br. J. Indust. Med.* 1966; **23**: 28–36.

66. Crancera, A.B. and O'Niel, P.A. A record analysis of Washington drivers with licence restrictions for heart disease. *North West Med.* 1970; **69**: 409–16.

67. Hosack, D.W. Death at the wheel. A consideration of cardiological diseases contributory factor to road accidents. *Med. J. Aus.* 1974; **1**: 164–66.

68. Hartman, H. The cardiovascular patient in traffic. *Helv. Med. Acta* 1965; **32**: 135–54.

69. Bowen, D.A.L. Deaths of drivers of automobiles due to trauma and ischaemic heart disease. *Forensic Sci.* 1973; **2**: 285–90.

70. Ferranti, E., Manfredi, M., Puoti, A. and Lauri, D. Traffic accidents due to indisposition during driving. Clinical–statistical study of cerebrovascular insufficiency. *Minerva Cardiol. Angiol.* 1974; **22**: 591–99.

71. Moze, S., Bank, H. and Wortreich, B. Subclavian steal syndrome and motor accidents. *Lancet* 1967; **ii**: 533–34.

72. Di Matteo, J. and Delarge, F. Role of cardiopathies in traffic accidents. *Bull. Acad. Natl. Med. (Paris)* 1982; **166**: 739–42.

73. Morris, J.N., Kagen, A., Patterson, D.C., Gardiner, M.J. and Raffle, P.A.B. Incidence and prediction of ischaemic heart disease in London busmen. *Lancet* 1966; **2**: 553–559.

74. Netterstrom, B. and Laursen, P. Incidence and prevalence of ischaemic heart disease among urban bus drivers in Copenhagen. *Scand. J. Soc. Med.* 1981; **9**: 75–79.

75. Robinson, K. and Mulcahy, R. Return to employment of professional drivers following myocardial infarction. *Ir. Med. J.* 1986; **79**: 31–34.

76. Rigal, D.R., Lovell, F.W. and Townsend, F.M. Pathologic findings in the cardiovascular system of military flying personnel. *Am. J. Cariol.* 1960; **6**: 19–25.

77. Catherman, R.L., Davidson, W.H. and Townsend, F.M. Coronary artery disease in military flying personnel. *Aerospace Med.* 1962; **33**: 1318–27.

78. Scheinman, H.Z. Coronary atherosclerosis in military pilots, 1. A Relationship to flying and aviation accidents. *Aerospace Med.* 1968; **39**: 1348–51.

79. Booze, C.F., Pidkowicz, J.K., Davis, A.K. and Bolding, F.A. Post mortem coronary atherosclerosis findings in general aviation accident pilot fatalities 1975–77. *Av. Space Environ. Med.* 1981; **52**: 24–27.

80. Underwood-Ground, K.E. Prevalence of coronary atherosclerosis in healthy United Kingdom aviators. *Av. Space Environ. Med.* 1981; **52**: 696–70.

81. Stevens, P.J. Aviation accident pathology, the search for the cause of an accident. *Proc. Roy. Soc. Med.* 1968; **61**: 1076–79.

82. Underwood-Ground, K.E. Interpretation of coronary disease in fatal aircraft accidents. *J.Roy. Soc. Med.* 1979; **72**: 377–81.

83. Jokl, E. and McLellan, J.T. Sudden cardiac death of pilots in flight with special consideration of syncope due to silent ischaemic heart disease and the differential diagnosis of other causes of episodes of incapacitation, unconsciousness, confusion and amnesia in flying personnel. *Cardiology* 1968; **52**: 210–34.

84. Civil Aviation Authority. World Airline Accident Summary CAP 479. Cheltenham, CAA, 1974.

85. Benson, O.O. Jr. Coronary artery disease. Report of a fatal cardiac attack in a pilot while flying. *J. Aviat. Med.* 1937; **8**: 81–84.

86. Orlady, H. and Carter, E.T. Medical disability in United States airline pilots. Proc XVI Int Cong Aviat Space Med. Lisbon, 1967.

87. Caris, T.N. Silent myocardial infarction in the United States Air Force flyers detected solely by annual required electrocardiograms. *Aerospace Med.* 1970; **41**: 669–71.

88. Joy, M. The impact of coronary vascular risk factors on professional aircrew licence loss in the United Kingdom. *In* Specific Findings in Cardiology and Pulmonary Function with Special Emphasis on Assessment Criteria for Flying. CPP 232, 1977, NATO AGARD, Neuilly-sur-Seine.

89. Rayman, R.B. Myocardial infarction; an inflight problem? *Aerospace Med.* 1974; **45**: 86–89.

90. Reighard, H.L. and Mohler, S.R. Some aspects of sudden incapacitation in airmen due to cardiovascular disease. *Aerospace Med.* 1967; **38**: 1273–75.

91. Hemming, F.O. Inflight coronary occlusions; a short series of cases. *Aerospace Med.* 1970; **41**: 773–75.

92. Mohler, S.R. and Booze, C.F. United States fatal general aviation accidents due to cardiovascular incapacitation 1974–75. *Aviat. Space Environ. Med.* 1978; 1225–28.

93. Kulak, L.L., Wick, R.L. and Billings, C.E. Epidemiological study of inflight airline incapacitation. *Aerospace Med.* 1971; **42**: 670–73.

94. Leighton-White, R.C. Airline pilot incapacitation training inflight. *Aerospace Med.* 1972; **43**: 661–64.

95. Chapman, P.J. The consequences of inflight incapacitation in civil aviation. *Aviat. Space Environ. Med.* 1984; **55**: 497–500.

96. Bennett, G. Pilot incapacitation and aircraft accidents. *Eur. Heart J.* 1988; **9** (Suppl. G): 21–24.

97. Tunstall-Pedoe, H. Risk of coronary heart attack in the normal population and how it might be modified in fliers. *Eur. Heart J.* 1984; **5** (Suppl. A): 43–49.

98. Beevers, D.G. The problem of hypertension in aviators. *Eur. Heart J.* 1985; **5** (Suppl. A): 29–32.

99. Schamroth, J.M. The role of military medical personnel in hypertension. *S. Afr. Med. J.* 1979; **56**: 362–64.

100. World Health Organization. Arterial hypertension; report of an expert committee. WHO Technical Report 1978; series no. 628: 1–57.

101. Robertson, J.I.S. The management of hypertension in aircrew. *Eur. Heart J.* 1988; **9** (Suppl. G): 41–44.

102. Ledingham, J.G.G. Section introduction: Hypertension and peripheral vascular disease in aircrew. *Eur. Heart J.* 1988; 9 (Suppl. G): 37–40.

103. Hypertension Detection and Follow-up Programme Co-operative Group. Five year findings I Reduction in mortality of persons with high blood pressure including mild hypertension. *J. Am. Med. Assoc.* 1979; 242: 2462–71.

104. Report by the management committee of the Australian therapeutic trial in mild hypertension. *Lancet* 1980; ii: 161–67.

105. Lewis, B. Risk factors for coronary heart disease—assessment in airline pilots. *Eur. Heart J.* 1984; 5 (Suppl. A): 17–24.

106. International Collaborative Group. Asymptomatic hypoglycaemia and coronary heart disease. *J. Chron. Dis.* 1979; 32: 683–837.

107. Keen, H. and Jarrett, J. (Eds). Complications of diabetes. London: Edward Arnold, 1980.

108. The Framingham Study: an epidemiological investigation of cardiovascular disease. Gordon T., Kannel, W.V., Sorlie, P.D. (Eds). Washington, US Government Printing Office, 1971.

109. Ames, R.P. and Hill, P. Raised serum lipid concentrations during diuretic treatment of hypertension: a study of predictive indexes. *Clin. Sci. Mol. Med.* 1978; 55: 311s–14s.

110. Beral, V. and Kay, C.R. Mortality amongst oral contraceptive users. *Lancet* 1977; ii: 727–31.

111. Townsend, J.L. and Meade, D.W. Ischaemic heart disease mortality risks for smokers and non-smokers. *J. Epidemiol. Comm. Hlth* 1979; 33: 243–27.

112. Meade, D.W. The prevention of ischaemic heart disease in flyers. *Eur. Heart J.* 1984; 5 (Suppl. A): 51–54.

113. Pocock, S.J., Shaper, A.G., Phillips, A.N. and Walker, M. Prediction of men at high risk of heart attack and its relevance to pilots. *Eur. Heart J.* 1988; 9 (Suppl. G): 25–30.

114. Tunstall-Pedoe, H. The concept of risk. *Eur. Heart J.* 1988; 9 (Suppl. G): 13–16.

115. Joy, M. and Cook, J.N.C. Hypertension in professional aircrew—a missed opportunity in preventative medicine? Proc 27 Int Cong Aviation Space Med London, 1978.

116. Swales, J.D. Non-pharmacological antihypertensive therapy. *Eur. Heart J.* 1988; 9 (Suppl. G): 45–52.

117. Engelberg, A.L. Gibbons, H.L. and Doege, T.C. A review of the medical standards for civilian airmen. Synopsis of a two year study. *J. Am. Med. Assoc.* 1986; 255: 1589–99.

118. Jordan, J. Federal Aviation Administration, Oaklahoma City, 1984. Personal communication.

119. Turner, P. The influence of anti-hypertensive drugs on psychosensory and psychomotor performance tests. *Eur. Heart J.* 1984; 5 (Suppl. A): 37–39.

120. Callender, J.S. Evaluation of the cerebral effects of antihypertensive medication. *Eur. Heart J.* 1988; 9 (Suppl. G): 59–64.

121. Ball, S.G. Newer antihypertensive agents and their use by aircrew. *Eur. Heart J.* 1988; 9 (Suppl. G): 53–58.

122. American Heart Association. Heart Facts. Dallas, Texas: AHA, 1978.

123. Office of Population Censuses and Surveys. Mortality statistics, cause. 1984. England and Wales. Series DH2 No. 11, London, HMSO, 1985.

124. Task Force I. Identification of ischaemic heart disease. *Am. J. Cardiol.* 1975; 36: 595–608.

125. Pettyjohn, F.S. and McMeekin, R.R. Joint Committee on Aviation Pathology XVI. Coronary Artery Disease and Preventative Cardiology in Aviation Medicine. *Av. Space Environ. Med.* 1985; 46: 1299–1304.

126. Hoiberg, A. Cardiovascular disease among United States Navy pilots. *Av. Space Environ. Med.* 1985: 397–402.

127. Office of Population Censuses and Surveys. Hospital Inpatient Enquiry. 1983. Series MB4 No. 22. London: HMSO, 1985.

128. Averill, K.H. and Lamb, L.E. Electrocardiographic findings in 67 375 asymptomatic subjects—I incidence of abnormalities. *Am. J. Cardiol.* 1960; 6: 76–83.

129. Hiss, R.G. and Lamb, L.E. Electrocardiographic findings in 122 043 individuals. *Circulation* 1962; 25: 947–83.

130. Joy, M.D. Contribution of the resting electrocardiograph to air transport safety. *Br. Heart J.* 1977; 39: 347.

131. Taggart, P., Carruthers, M., Joseph, S. *et al.* Electrocardiographic changes resembling myocardial ischaemia in asymptomatic men with normal coronary arteries. *Br. Heart J.* 1979; 41: 214–25.

132. Joy, M. and Trump, D.W. Significance of minor ST-segment and T wave changes in the resting electrocardiogram of asymptomatic subjects. *Br. Heart J.* 1981; 45: 48–55.

133. Froelicher, V.F., Thompson, A.J., Wolthurs, R. *et al.* Angiographic findings in asymptomatic aircrewmen with electrocardiographic abnormalities. *Am. J. Cardiol.* 1977; 39: 32–38.

134. Froelicher, V.F., Thomas, M.M., Pillow, C. and Lancaster, M.C. Epidemiologic study of asymptomatic men screened by maximal treadmill testing for latent coronary artery disease. *Am. J. Cardiol.* 1974; 770–76.

135. Youell, G.S., Kay, T.N. Hickman, J.R., Montgomery, M.A. and McGranahan, G.M. Detection of coronary artery disease in asymptomatic aircrew members with thallium 201 scintigraphy. *Av. Space Environ. Med.* 1980; 51: 1250–55.

136. Robinson, P. Radionuclide imaging. *Eur. Heart J.* 1984; 5 (Suppl. A): 65–68.

137. Joy, M. Fitness to drive and fitness to fly. *Update* 1988; 11: 3–10.

138. Dawkins, K. Critical review of the usefulness of non-invasive investigation of asymptomatic individuals. *Eur. Heart J.* 1988; 9 (Suppl. G): 83–90.

139. Poole Wilson, P.A. Natural history of minor coronary events. *Eur. Heart J.* 1984; 5(Suppl. A): 69–72.

140. Balcon, R. Prognostic significance of coronary angiography. *Eur. Heart J.* 1984; 5 (Suppl. A): 73–75.

141. Bruschke, A.V.G., Proudfit, N.L. and Sones, F.M. Clinical course of patients with normal and slightly or moderately abnormal coronary arteriograms, a follow up study on 500 patients. *Circulation* 1973; 47: 936–44.

142. McGranahan, G.M., Hickman, J.R., Youell, G.S., Montgomery, M.A. and Triebwasser, J.H. Minimal coronary artery disease and continuation of flying status. *Aviat. Space Environ. Med.* 1983; 54: 548–50.

143. Reid, R.C., Murphy, M.L. and Hultgren, H.N. Survival of men treated for chronic angina pectoris. A co-operative randomised study. *J. Thorac. Cardiovasc. Surg.* 1978; 75: 1–16.

144. Bruschke, A.V.G., Proudfit, N.L. and Sones, F.M. Progress study of 590 consecutive non surgical cases of coronary atery disease followed 5–9 years. I. Arteriographic correlation. *Circulation* 1973; 47: 1147–53.

145. Bruschke, A.V.G., Proudfit, N.L. and Sones, F.M. Progress study of 590 consecutive non surgical cases of coronary artery disease followed 5–9 years. II. Ventrilographic and other correlation. *Circulation* 1973; 47: 1154–64.

146. Proudfit, N.L., Bruschke, A.V.G. and Sones, F.M. Clinical course of patients with normal or slightly or moderately abnormal coronary angiograms. *Circulation* 1980; 62: 712–17.

147. Davies. M.J. and Thomas, A.C. Plaque fissuring—the cause of acute myocardial infarction, certain ischaemic death and crescendo angina. *Br. Heart J.* 1985; 53:

363–73.

148. Mock, M.B., Ringbest, I., Fisher, L.D. *et al.* Survival of medically treated patients in the coronary artery surgery (CASS) registry. *Circulation* 1982; **66**: 562–68.

149. Multicenter post-infarction research group. Risk stratification and survival after myocardial infarction. *N. Engl. J. Med.* 1983; **309**: 331–36.

150. Ruberman, W., Weinblatt, E., Goldberg, J.D., Frank, C.W., Chaudhray, B.S., and Shapiro, S. Ventricular premature complexes and sudden death after myocardial infarction. *Circulation* 1981; **64**: 297–302.

151. Julian, D.G. The practical implications of the coronary artery surgery studies. *Br. Heart J.* 1985; **54**: 343–50.

152. Chaitman, B.K., Davis, K.B., Dodge, H.T. *et al.* Should airline pilots be eligible to resume flight status after coronary artery bypass surgery? A CASS registry study. *J. Mol. Coll. Cardiol.* 1986; **A**: 1318–24.

153. Reid, J.M. and Dargie, H.J. Risk stratification after myocardial infarction with or without coronary artery bypass grafting. *Eur. Heart J.* 1988; **9** (Suppl. G): 91–100.

154. Marmor, A., Sobel, B.E. and Roberts, R. Factors presaging early recurrent myocardial infarction ('extension'). *Am. J. Cardiol.* 1981; **48**: 603–10.

155. Parker, D.J. The airline pilot after coronary artery bypass grafting. *Eur. Heart J.* 1984; **5** (Suppl. A): 77–79.

156. Wheatley, D.J. Coronary artery bypass graft surgery. Late survival and follow. *Eur. Heart J.* 1988; **9** (Suppl. G): 107–110.

157. Loop, F.D., Lytle, V.W., Cosgrove, D.M. *et al.* Influence of the mammary artery graft on ten year survival and other cardiac event. *N. Engl. J. Med.* 1986; **314**: 1–6.

158. Chamberlain, D.A. Introduction to section on ischaemic heart disease. *Eur. Heart J.* 1988; **9** (Suppl. G): 73–82.

159. Sams, J.M. Jr. Aviation medical certification after coronary artery surgery. *N. Engl. J. Med.* 1982; **307**: 52–54.

160. Shiu, M.F. Percutaneous transluminal coronary angioplasty and flying status. *Eur. Heart J.* 1988; **9** (Suppl. G): 101–106.

161. Cowley, M.J., Molin, S.M., Kelsey, S.F. *et al.* Sex differences in early and long term results in coronary angioplasty in the NHBLI PTCA registry. *Circulation* 1985; **71**: 90–97.

162. Frank, S., Johnson, A. and Ross, J. Natural history of valvular aortic stenosis. *Br. Heart J.* 1973; **35**: 249–59.

163. Mills, P., Leech, G., Davies, M. and Leatham, A. The natural history of a non-stenotic bicuspid aortic valve. *Br. Heart. J.* 1978; **40**: 951–57.

164. Hall, R.J.C. Aortic valve disease. *Eur. Heart J.* 1984; **5** (Suppl. A): 135–39.

165. Henry, W.L., Morgan Roth, J. and Pearlman, A.S. Relation between echocardiographically determined left atrial size and atrial fibrillation. *Circulation* 1976; **53**: 273–79.

166. Sherrid, M.V., Clark, R.D. and Cohn, K. Echocardiographic analysis of left atrial size before and after operation in mitral valve disease. *Am. J. Cardiol.* 1979; **43**: 171–78.

167. Shiu, M.F. Mitral valve disease. *Eur. Heart J.* 1984; **5** (Suppl. A): 131–34.

168. Engel. J.J. and Hickman, J.R. Mitral valve prolapse—a review. *Av. Space Environ. Med.* 1980; **51**: 273–86.

169. Malcolm, A.D. Mitral leaflet prolapse. *Eur. Heart J.* 1984; **5**: 127–30.

170. Schwartz, M.H., Teichholz, L.E. and Donoso, E. Mitral valve prolapse: a review of associated arrythmias. *Am. J. Med.* 1977; **62**: 377–382.

171. Campbell, R.W.F., Godman, M.G., Fidler, G.I., Marquis, R.M. and Julian, D.G. Ventricular arrhythmias a syndrome of balloon deformity of the mitral valve; definition of possible high risk group. *Br. Heart J.* 1976; **38**;

1053–57.

172. Brown, D.D., Stoop, D.R. and Stanton, K.C. Precipitation of cardiac symptoms in the midsystolic click—late systolic murmur syndrome by inflight plus Gz manoeuvers. *Aer. Space Med.* 1973; **44**: 1169–72.

173. Hickman, J.R. and McGranahan, G.M. Clinical aerospace cardiology. *In* Fundamentals of Aerospace Medicine, De Hart R. L. (Ed.). Philadelphia: Lea and Febiger, 1985.

174. Drury, P.J., Black, M.M., Lawford, P.V.K.R. *et al.* Multicentre valve trial—a report from the Department of Medical Physics and Clinical Engineering. University of Sheffield, 1986.

175. Parker, D.J. Long term morbidity and mortality after aortic and mitral valve replacement with tissue valves and certification to fly. *Eur. Heart J.* 1988; **9** (Suppl. G): 153–158.

176. Penta, A., Qureshi, S., Radley-Smith, R. *et al.* Patient status ten or more years after fresh homograft replacement of the aortic valve. *Circulation* 1984; **7** (Suppl. 1): 182–86.

177. Santinga, J.T., Kirsh, M.M., Flora, J.D. and Brymer, J.F. Factors relating to sudden cardiac death in patients having aortic valve replacement. *Am. Thorac. Surg.* 1980; **29**: 249–53.

178. Spencer, F.C, Grossie, A., Culliford, A.T. *et al.* Experience with 1643 porcine prosthetic valves in 1492 patients. *Ann. Surg.* 1986; **203**: 691–700.

179. Parker, D.J. The patient after cardiac valve surgery—risks and complications. *Eur. Heart J.* 1984; **5** (Suppl. A): 141–45.

180. Sopher, I.M. Myocarditis in the aircraft accident. *Aerospace Med.* 1974; **45**: 963–67.

181. Gold, R.G. Post-viral pericarditis. *Eur. Heart J.* 1988; **9** (Suppl. G): 175–79.

182. Hirshchmann, J.V. Pericardial constriction. *Am. Heart J.* 1978; **96**: 110–122.

183. Goodwin, J.F. and Oakley, C.M. Editorial. The cardiomyopathies. *Br. Heart J.* 1972; **34**: 545–532.

184. Gibson, D.G. Assessment of hypertrophic cardiomyopathy in potential aircrew. *Eur. Heart J.* 1984; **5** (Suppl. A): 155–59.

185. Marshall, T.K. *Med. Sci. Law* 1970; **10**: 3–6.

186. Shah, M.P., Adelman, H.E. and Douglas-Wigle, E. The natural (and unnatural) history of hypertrophic obstructive cardiomyopathy. *Circulation Res.* 1974; **34–35** (Suppl. II): 179–95.

187. Wei, J.Y., Weiss, J. and Bulkley, B.H. The heterogeneity of hypertrophic cardiomyopathy on autopsy and one dimensional echocardiograph study. *Am. J. Cardiol.* 1980; **45**: 24–32.

188. Webb-Peploe, M. Dilated cardiomyopathy. *Eur. Heart J.* 1984; **5** (Suppl. A): 161–64.

189. Torp, A. Incidence of congestive cardiomyopathy. *In* Goodwin, J.F., Hjalmarson, A. and Olsen, E.G.J. (Eds). *Congestive cardiomyopathy*. Molndal, Sweden; A.B. Hassle, 1981, pp. 18–22.

190. Fuster, V., Gersh, B.J., Guiliani, E.R., Tajik, A.J., Brandenburgh, R.O. and Fyre, R.L. The natural history of dilated cardiomyopathy. *Am. J. Cardiol.* 1981; **47**: 525–31.

191. Franciosa, J.A., Willen, M. Siesche, S. and Cohn, J. Survival in men with severe chronic left ventricular failure due to either coronary heart disease or idiopathic dilated cardiomyopathy. *Am. J. Cardiol.* 1983; **51**: 831–42.

192. Webb-Peploe, M.M. Obliterative and restrictive cardiomyopathies. *Eur. Heart J.* 1988; **9** (Suppl. G): 159–68.

193. Sharma, O.P. Sarcoidosis: clinical management. London: Butterworth, 1984. pp. 97–101.

194. Swanton, R.H. Sarcoidosis of the heart. *Eur. Heart J.* 1988 in press.

195. Fleming, H.A. Sarcoid heart disease. *Br. Med. J.* 1986; **292**: 1095–96.

196. Pettyjohn, F.S., Spoor, D.H. and Buckendorf, W.A. Sarcoid and the heart—an aeromedical risk. *Av. Space Environ. Med.* 1977; **48**: 955–58.

197. Hall. R. Thrombo-embolic disease. *Eur. Heart J.* 1988; **9** (Suppl. G): 147–52.

198. Lederman, J.A., Keshavarzian, A. Acute pulmonary embolism following air travel. *Postgrad. Med. J.* 1983; **59**: 104–05.

199. Thomas, J.E., Abson, C.P., Carins, N.J. Pulmonary embolism. A hazard of air travel. *Centr. African J. Med.* 1981; **27**: 85–87.

200. McIntyre, D., Moran, F. and Banham, S.W. Pulmonary embolism—a longterm follow up. *Postgrad. Med. J.* 1982; **58**: 222–25.

201. McCartney, F.J. Flying and congenital heart disease. *Eur. Heart J.* 1984; Suppl. A: 147–54.

202. Keith, J.D. Prevalence, incidence and epidemiology. *In* Keith, J.D., Rowe, R.D. and Vald, P. (Eds). Heart disease in infancy and childhood. New York: McMillan, 1978, pp. 4–5.

203. Nugent, E.W., Freedom, R.M., Nora, J.J., Ellison, R.G., Rowe, R.D. and Nadas, A.S. Clinical course in pulmonary stenosis. *Circulation* 1977; **56** I: 33–47.

204. Maron, B.J., Humphreys, J.O.N., Rowe, R.D. and Millits, E.D. Prognosis of surgically corrected coarctation of the aorta. A twenty year post-operative appraisal. *Circulation* 1973; **47**: 119–26.

205. Bexton, R.S. and Camm, R.J. First degree atrioventricular block. *Eur. Heart J.* 1984; **5** (Suppl. A): 107–09.

206. Bexton, R.S. and Camm, A.J. Second degree atrioventricular block. *Eur. Heart J.* 1984; **5**(Suppl. A): 111–14.

207. Shaw, D.B., Kerwick, C.A., Veale, D., Gowers, J. and Whistance, T. Survival in second degree atrioventricular block. *Br. Heart J.* 1985; **53**: 587–93.

208. Camm, A.J. and Bexton, R.S. Congenital complete heart block. *Eur. Heart J.* 1984; **5** (Suppl. A): 115–17.

209. Rowlands, D.J. Left and right bundle branch block, left anterior and left postrior hemiblock. *Eur. Heart J.* 1984; **5** (Suppl. A): 99–105.

210. Massing, G.K. and Lancaster, M.C. Clinical significance of acquired complete right bundle branch block in 52 patients without overt cardiac disease. *Aerospace Med.* 1969; **40**: 967–71.

211. Schneider, J.F., Thomas, H.E., Kreger, B.E., McNamara, P.M., Sorlie, P., Kannel, W.B. Newly acquired right bundle branch block. The Framingham Study. *Ann. Intern. Med.* 1980; **92**: 37–44.

212. Canaveris, G. Intraventricular conduction disturbances in flying personnel: right bundle branch block. *Aviat. Space. Environ. Med.* 1986; 591–96.

213. Rabkin, S.W., Mathewson, F.A.L. and Tate, R.B. Natural history of marked left axis deviation—left anterior hemiblock. *Am. J. Cardiol.* 1979; **43**: 605–11.

214. Wehrly, D.J. Historic aeromedical perspective on left bundle branch block. *Aviat. Space Environ. Med.* 1986; **57**: 462–65.

215. Rabkin, S.W., Mathewson, F.A.L. and Tate, R.B. Natural history of left bundle branch block. *Br. Heart J.* 1980; **43**: 164–69.

216. Schneider, J.F., Thomas, H.E., Kreger, B.E., McNamara, P.M. and Kannel, W.B. Clinical electrocardiographic correlates of newly acquired left bundle branch block. The Framingham Study. *Am. J. Cardiol.* 1985; **55**: 1332–38.

217. Boyce, J.B. and Beers, K. Aerospace medicine resident's teaching file. New left bundle branch block on screening examination. *Aviat. Space Environ. Med.* 1986; **57**: 381–83.

218. Davidoff, R., Schamroth, C.L. and Myburgh, D.P. The Wolff–Parkinson–White pattern in healthy aircrew. *Aviat. Space Environ. Med.* 1981; **52**: 554–55.

219. Ward, D. Ventricular pre-excitation. *Eur. Heart J.* 1984; **5** (Suppl. A): 119–124.

220. Shaw, D.B. and Southall, D.P. Sinus node arrest and sino-atrial block. *Eur. Heart J.* 1984; **5** (Suppl. A): 83–87.

221. Shaw, D.B. and Kekwick, C.A. Potential candidates for pacemakers. Survey of heart block and sino-atrial disorders (sick sinus syndrome).*Br. Heart J.* 1978; **40**: 99–105.

222. Whinnery, J.E., Laughlin, M.H. and Hickman, J.R. Concurrent loss of consciousness and sino-atrial block during +Gz stress. *Aviat. Space Environ. Med.* 1979; **50**: 635–38.

223. Bennett, D. Atrial fibrillation. *Eur. Heart J.* 1984; **5** (Suppl. A): 89–93.

224. Gajeuski, J. and Singer, R.B. Mortality in an insured population with atrial fibrillation. *J. Am. Med. Assoc.* 1981; **242**: 1504–05.

225. Busby, D.E. and Davids, A.W. Paroxysmal and chronic atrial fibrillation in airmen certification. *Aviat. Space Environ. Med.* 1976; **47**: 185–86.

226. Wolf, P.A., Dawber, T.R., Thomas, E. and Kannel, W.B. Epidemiologic assessment of chronic atrial fibrillation and risk of stroke: the Framingham study. *Neurology* 1978; **28**: 973–77.

227. Cobb, S.M. The implication of antiarrhythmic therapy in aviators. *Eur. Heart J.* 1988; **9** (Suppl. G): 127–32.

228. Toff, W.D., Joy, M. and Camm, A.J. Exercise induced arrhythmia. *Eur. Heart J.* 1988; **9** (Suppl. G): 129–136.

229. Campbell, R.W.F. Ventricular ectopic activity and its relevance to aircrew licensing. *Eur. Heart J.* 1984; **5** (Suppl. A): 95–98.

230. Kennedy, H.L. and Whitlock, W.H.I. Long term follow up of asymptomatic healthy subjects with frequent and complex ventricular ectopy. *N. Engl. J. Med.* 1985; **312**: 193–97.

231. Cullen, K., Wearne, K.L., Stenhous, N.S. and Cumpston, G.N. Q waves and ventricular extrasystoles in resting electrocardiogram. A 16 year follow up to the Busselton Study. *Br. Heart J.* 1983; **50**: 465–68.

232. Bjerregaard, P. Premature beats in healthy subjects 40–79 years of age. *Eur. Heart J.* 1982; **3**: 493–503.

233. Campbell, R.W.F. Ventricular arrhythmias in normal individuals and athletes. *Eur. Heart J.* 1988; **9** (Suppl. G.): 113–118.

234. Toff, W.D. and Camm, A.J. Implanted devices in aviation. *Eur. Heart J.* 1988; **9** (Suppl. G): 133–38.

235. Toff, W.D., Deller, A.G., McHobbs, R.A. *et al.* Electromagnetic interference with pacemaker function: hazard in the aviation environment. In press.

236. Toff, W.D., Leeks, C., Lau, C.P., Joy, M., Bennett, G. and Camm, A.J. The effect of aircraft vibration on the function of an activity sensing pacemaker. *Br. Heart J.* 1987; **57**: 573.

Appendix

A Brief Description of Some Commonly Used Cardiovascular Drugs

P.A. Poole-Wilson and L.H. Opie

This appendix is not an exhaustive guide to cardiovascular drugs. For further information on side-effects and current recommendations for dosage and prescribing, other authoritative texts should be consulted. Before prescribing an unfamiliar drug, the practitioner should consult the data sheet for that drug and other official texts.

BETA-ADRENOCEPTOR BLOCKING DRUGS (BETA-BLOCKERS)

Agent	Dose	Pharmacokinetics	Side-effects	Contra-indications and comments
Non-cardioselective beta-blockers				
Propranolol	40 mg o.d. to 120 mg t.d.s. Intravenously 0.1 mg/kg over 1 min preceded by atropine sulphate 1–2 mg. Maximum 10 mg. Long-acting preparation available	Half-life 1–6 h. Lipid soluble. Not cardioselective. First pass effect. No ISA[a]. Metabolized in liver. 90% protein bound. Reduce dose in liver or renal failure	Bradycardia, myocardial depression, heart failure, bronchoconstriction, heart block. Peripheral constriction, cold limbs, dreams, insomnia, intestinal disturbances, impaired intellectual activity	Late pregnancy, breast-feeding. Avoid abrupt withdrawal in angina. Asthma, bronchospasm, care if history of allergy. Heart failure, second or third degree heart block. Severe mental depression. Care in insulin-dependent diabetes
Sotalol	80–480 mg o.d. (can give in divided doses). Slow intravenous injection, 10–20 mg over 2–3 min, with ECG monitoring. Up to 100 mg in 10 min.	Half-life 15–17 h. Not lipid soluble. Not cardioselective. No first pass effect. No ISA. Loss from kidney. 5% protein bound	As for propranolol, may have fewer central side-effects. Can cause ventricular arrhythmias, notably torsades de pointes	As above. Avoid in hypokalaemia (risk of torsades). Not as co-therapy with agents increasing action potential duration, e.g. amiodarone, thiazide diuretics
Nadolol	80–240 mg o.d.	Half-life 16–24 h. Not lipid soluble. Not cardioselective. No first pass effect. No ISA. Loss from kidney. 20% protein bound	As for propranolol. May have fewer central side-effects	As for propranolol
Oxprenolol	40–160 mg t.d.s.	Half-life 2 h. Lipid soluble. Not cardioselective. First pass effect. Modest ISA. Loss from liver. 80% protein bound	As for propranolol	As for propranolol
Pindolol	5–30 mg o.d. (can give in divided doses)	Half-life 4 h. Small lipid solubility. Not cardioselective. Small first pass effect. Marked ISA. Loss from liver and kidney. 55% protein bound	As for propranolol	As for propranolol. May be safer in bronchospasm

[a]Intrinsic sympathomimetic activity.

Agent	Dose	Pharmacokinetics	Side-effects	Contra-indications and comments
Timolol	5 mg o.d. to 15 mg t.d.s.	Half-life 4–5 h. Small lipid solubility. Not cardioselective. Small first pass effect. No ISA. Loss from liver and kidney.	As for propranolol	As for propranolol
Cardioselective beta-blockers				
Atenolol	25–100 mg o.d.	Half-life 6–9 h. Not lipid soluble. Cardioselective. No first pass effect. No ISA. Loss by kidney. 10% protein bound	As for propranolol. Less risk of bronchoconstriction because cardioselective but avoid in asthma. Fewer cerebral side-effects	As for propranolol, except used in bronchospasm in a low dose, and fewer problems in insulin-dependent diabetes
Metoprolol	50 mg o.d. to 100 mg b.d. Intravenous 5 mg	Half-life 3 h. Partly lipid soluble. Cardioselective. First pass effect. No ISA. Metabolized in liver. 15% protein bound	As for atenolol	As for atenolol
Acebutolol	200–1200 mg o.d. (can give b.d.)	Half-life (diacetolol) 8–12 h. Not lipid soluble. Cardioselective. First pass effect. ISA. Loss from liver and kidney. 15% protein bound	As for atenolol	As for atenolol
Bisoprolol	5–10 mg daily, maximum 20 mg	Half-life 10–11 h. 50% metabolized in liver and remainder excreted unchanged	Lipophilicity between propranolol and atenolol, highly selective for beta$_1$-adrenoreceptor site—side-effects as for atenolol	Reduce dose in severe liver disease or renal impairment
Beta-blocker with vasodilator properties				
Labetalol	200–400 mg o.d. to 400 mg t.d.s. (1–2 ng/kg intravenously at 2 ng/min)	Half-life 3–4 h. High lipid solubility. Not cardioselective. Modest ISA. Vasodilator because of alpha blockade. Liver metabolism. 90% protein bound	As for propranolol. May be safer in presence of mild heart failure, asthma or bradycardia	As for propranolol with added vasodilator effect. Used for severe hypertension. Used for hypertension in pregnancy

BETA-ADRENOCEPTOR BLOCKING DRUGS WITH MARKED INTRINSIC SYMPATHOMIMETIC ACTIVITY

Agent	Dose	Pharmacokinetics	Side-effects	Contra-indications and comments
Xamoterol	200 mg b.d.	Half-life 5 h. Excreted by kidneys	As for propranolol. GI complaints. Headaches, dizziness. Rash, palpitations and muscle cramps	Avoid in severe heart failure. Great caution with obstructive airways disease. Not in pregnancy. Reduce dose if renal impairment

CARDIAC GLYCOSIDES

Agent	Dose	Pharmacokinetics	Side-effects	Contra-indications and comments
Digoxin	Maintenance 0.125 mg o.d. to 0.5 mg b.d. Rapid digitalization 1–1.5 mg over 24 h. Sometimes used acutely by infusion for control of atrial fibrillation. 0.75–1.0 mg in 50 ml over 2 h	Half-life 36 h. Most excreted by kidney. As a general guide, creatinine clearance < 25, 50, 80 ml/min reduce dose to 0.125, 0.01875, and 0.25 mg o.d. respectively. Therapeutic concentration 1–2 ng/ml (1.3–2.6 nmol/l). Toxic range > 2.5 ng/ml	Anorexia, nausea, vomiting, visual disturbance. Arrhythmias, ventricular ectopics, coupled beats, supraventricular tachycardia, heart block	Reduce dose in elderly and in renal failure. Beware hypokalaemia, hypothyroidism, hypertrophic cardiomyopathy, and Wolff–Parkinson–White (anterograde conduction). Increased blood levels with quinidine, verapamil, amiodarone. Increased sensitivity with diuretics if hypokalaemia. Absorption affected by cholestyramine, bran diet, antacid gels and gut motility. Antibiotics (erythromycin, tetracycline) can increase plasma concentration. Rifampicin can increase metabolism and lower blood level. May cause arrhythmias in patients with coronary artery disease and myocardial ischaemia

Agent	Dose	Pharmacokinetics	Side-effects	Contra-indications and comments
Digitoxin	Maintenance 0.05–0.2 mg o.d. Loading dose 0.8–1.2 mg in 24 h	Half-life 6–7 days. Largely metabolized or excreted in gut. Blood concentration only slightly affected by renal function. Therapeutic concentration 15–20 ng/ml. Toxic concentration > 35 ng/ml	As for digoxin	As for digoxin, problems in renal failure. Drug interactions may be fewer
Lanatoside C	Maintenance 0.25–1.0 mg o.d.	Less well absorbed than digoxin. Converted to digoxin. Dose depends on renal function	As for digoxin	As for digoxin

SYMPATHOMIMETICS

Agent	Dose	Pharmacokinetics	Side-effects	Contra-indications and comments
Dobutamine	Intravenous infusion 2.5–10 µg/kg/min depending on response	Half-life 2.4 min. Beta-1-adrenergic receptor agonist. Small beta-2 and alpha effect	Tachycardia, arrhythmias. Increase of systolic blood presure. Exacerbates myocardial ischaemia. Hypokalaemia	Arrhythmias. Care in myocardial ischaemia
Dopamine	Intravenous infusion 2–5 µg/kg/min depending on response, using long infusion line because of risk of local tissue necrosis.	Half-life 5 min. Stimulates dopaminergic receptors. High doses cause alpha-mediated vasoconstriction	Tachycardia, hypotension. Peripheral vasoconstriction and hypertension in high doses. Nausea and vomiting. Extravasation and sloughing. Hypokalaemia	Arrhythmias. Care in myocardial ischaemia. Low doses increase renal blood flow and stimulate dopaminergic receptors. Moderate doses have a positive inotropic effect on the heart. High doses cause vasoconstriction
Adrenaline	Subcutaneous or intramuscular 0.5 mg (0.5 ml of 1 in 1000). Central intravenous 0.5–1.0 mg. Intracardiac injection 0.1–0.2 mg	Half-life 2 min. Alpha- and beta-adrenergic receptor agonist. Beta-1 > beta-2	Tachycardia, arrhythmias. Anxiety, headache, cold extremities. Cerebral haemorrhage, pulmonary oedema. Hypokalaemia	Arrhythmias. Care in myocardial ischaemia

Agent	Dose	Pharmacokinetics	Side-effects	Contra-indications and comments
Isoprenaline	Intravenous infusion 0.5–10 μg/min	Half-life 2 min. Beta-adrenergic agonist. Beta-1 > beta-2.	Tachycardia, arrhythmias. Headache, tremor, sweating. Hypokalaemia	Arrhythmias. Care in myocardial ischaemia

Beta-2 Agonists sometimes used in cardiology

Agent	Dose	Pharmacokinetics	Side-effects	Contra-indications and comments
Salbutamol	2–4 mg t.d.s. Intravenous infusion 3–20 μg/min depending on response	Oral half-life 3 h. Intravenous half-life 5 min. Beta-2-adrenoceptor agonist. Small inotropic effect, mainly vasodilator	Tremor, headache, anxiety, peripheral vasodilatation, tachycardia, hypokalaemia	Care if myocardial ischaemia, tachycardia or arrhythmia. Care with hypertension, pregnancy, and elderly

Sympathomimetics causing vasoconstriction

Agent	Dose	Pharmacokinetics	Side-effects	Contra-indications and comments
Noradrenaline	Intravenous infusion 8–12 μg/min	Half-life 3 min. Alpha- and beta-adrenergic receptor agonist	Headache, tachycardia, palpitations, hypertension, bradycardia. Extravasation can cause necrosis.	Arrhythmias, myocardial ischaemia, pregnancy. Hypertension
Metaraminol	Subcutaneous or intramuscular 2–10 mg	Half-life 5 min. Alpha-adrenergic receptor agonist	Tachycardia, arrhythmias, reduced renal blood flow	Myocardial ischaemia, pregnancy. Hypertension
Phenylephrine	Slow intravenous injection 100–500 μg	Half-life 20 min. Alpha-adrenergic receptor agonist	Hypertension, headache, tachycardia, palpitations, vomiting, cold skin, arrhythmias	Hypertension, pregnancy, myocardial ischaemia

ANGIOTENSIN CONVERTING ENZYME INHIBITORS

Agent	Dose	Pharmacokinetics	Side-effects	Contra-indications and comments
Captopril	6.25 mg test dose to 12–25 mg b.d. Occasionally up to 50 mg t.d.s.	Half-life 6–8 h. Metabolized in liver and kidney. Contains sulphydryl group	Hypotension, loss of taste, cough, angioedema, rash, proteinuria, fatigue, hyperkalaemia, increased plasma urea, neutropenia	Pregnancy, bilateral renal artery stenosis. Beware renal failure and hypotension. Use low dose initially in heart failure. Care in patients on high doses of diuretics. Care if given with potassium-sparing diuretics, risk of hyperkalaemia

Agent	Dose	Pharmacokinetics	Side-effects	Contra-indications and comments
Enalapril	2.5–40 mg o.d. Starting dose 5 mg o.d. but if with diuretic 2.5 mg o.d.	Half-life 12/24 h, pro drug metabolized by liver and kidney to active compound enalapril. No sulphydryl group	Hypotension, hyperkalaemia, fatigue, dizziness, rash, angioedema, increased plasma urea, cough	As for captopril. Has longer half-life than captopril and usually given only once a day
Lisinopril	2.5–40 mg o.d. Starting dose 2.5 mg o.d.	Half-life 12 h. Cleared by kidney. No liver metabolism. Bioavailability 25%, 10% protein bound. No sulphydryl group	As for enalapril	As for enalapril. Long half-life. Reduce dose in severe renal failure

VASODILATORS

Agent	Dose	Pharmacokinetics	Side-effects	Contra-indications and comments
Nitroprusside	Intravenous infusion 10 µg/min increasing to 300 µg/min depending on response	Rapid action. Metabolized to thiocyanate and excreted by kidney. Degraded by light. Make fresh	Hypotension, cyanide or cyanate accumulation. Lactic acidosis. Hypoxia	Previous hypotension. Severe liver failure
Nitrates	See section on nitrates			
Diazoxide	100–150 mg intravenously over 5 min. Infusion 5 mg/kg at 15 mg/min	Rapid action	Hypotension, tachycardia, fluid retention, hyperglycaemia	Pregnancy, ischaemic heart disease, impaired renal function
Prazosin	0.5 mg o.d. to 10 mg b.d.	Half-life 3–4 h. Alpha-adrenergic receptor antagonist. First pass liver metabolism. Reduce dose in renal failure	Postural hypotension (first dose specially). Tachyphylaxis and tolerance	Care if co-therapy with nitrates
Hydralazine	25 mg o.d. to 50 mg b.d.	Half-life 2–8 h. Metabolized by acetylation in liver. Reduce dose in renal failure	Tachycardia. Fluid retention, nausea and vomiting. Lupus erythematosus-like syndrome, rare if dose < 100 mg/day	Angina, tachycardia

OPIOID ANALGESICS

Agent	Dose	Pharmacokinetics	Side-effects	Contra-indications and comments
Morphine	Intramuscular 10–15mg. Slow intravenous injection 5–20 mg (2 mg/min)			
Diamorphine	Intramuscular 5 mg. Slow intravenous injection 5–10 mg (1 mg/min)			

IONS

Agent	Dose	Pharmacokinetics	Side-effects	Contra-indications and comments
Calcium gluconate 10%	10 ml contains calcium 1.375 g or 0.23 mmol/ml. Slow intravenous injection	Rapid motion	Bradycardia, arrhythmias	Used during cardiac arrest or cardiac surgery as inotropic agent. Avoid adding to solutions containing bicarbonate, phosphates or sulphates
Calcium chloride 10%	0.68 mmol/ml. Slow intravenous injection	Rapid		As for calcium gluconate
Sodium bicarbonate	Continuous infusion (1.26% solution). Slow intravenous injection (8.4% solution)	1.26% solution contains 12.6 g/l. 150 mmol/l of sodium and bicarbonate		Avoid overuse early in cardiac resuscitation and ensure adequate ventilation of patient
Potassium salts	Varies with preparation		Nausea, vomiting, oesophageal or bowel stricture. Tablets can be difficult to swallow	Renal failure, plasma potassium above 5 mmol/l. Care if intestinal stricture or hiatus hernia
Potassium, effervescent tablets	Potassium bicarbonate 500 mg. Potassium acid titrate 300 mg. Equivalent to 6.5 mmol		As for potassium salts.	As for potassium salts
Potassium Sando K$^+$	Potassium bicarbonate and chloride equivalent to 12 mmol of potassium		As for potassium salts	As for potassium salts

Agent	Dose	Side-effects	Contra-indications and comments
Potassium slow K⁺	Potassium chloride equivalent to 8 mmol of potassium	As for potassium salts	As for potassium salts

NITRATES AND NITRATE-LIKE AGENTS

Agent	Route	Dose	Pharmacokinetics	Side-effects	Contra-indications and comments
Glyceryl trinitrate (nitroglycerin)	Sublingual (or buccal)	0.3–1.0 mg as needed; Tablets: usually 0.3, 0.5 or 0.6 mg	*Tablets* well absorbed from skin and oral mucosa, less so by gut. High first pass liver metabolism	Headaches, syncope, hypotension, tachycardia. Unexplained bradycardia occasionally in acute myocardial infarction. Prolonged high dosage can cause methaemoglobinaemia. Facial flushing. Halitosis. Tolerance to sustained high blood levels	Hypertrophic obstructive cardiomyopathy. Severe aortic stenosis. Cardiac tamponade. Constrictive pericarditis. Severe mitral stenosis. Relative contra-indications: Acute inferior myocardial infarction, cor pulmonale. Not glaucoma
	Spray	0.4 mg/metered dose as needed; onto oral mucosa especially tongue	*Sublingual*: peak blood level 2 min, half-life 7 min		
	Percutaneous	2% ointment 1–5 cm; or 12.5–40 mg (2.5 cm = 16.6 mg)	*Ointment*: slow onset of action effect lasts 4–6 h		
	Transdermal patches	16–25 mg per patch, releasing 5–25 mg/24 h	*Patches*: plasma levels constant for 2–24 h (risk of tolerance)		
	Oral sustained release	2.6, 6.4 or 10 mg. 1–2 tablets b.d.			
	Buccal sustained release	1.5 mg, between upper lip and gum			
	Intravenous	0.5–1.0 mg/ml. 0.3–0.6 mg/h up to 12.0 mg/h. 0.1 mg bolus (care, lower dose for new sets)			
Isosorbide dinitrate	Sublingual Oral (tablets 5, 10, 20 mg)	5–15 mg 5–80 mg 4–6 hourly (tolerance risk). 10–20 mg b.d.	Absorbed from oral mucosa and gut. Liver metabolism to active mononitrate, excreted by kidney. Half-life 10 h	As for nitroglycerin	As for nitroglycerin
	Chewable Oral; sustained release (20 or 40 mg)	5 mg as single dose 40 mg o.d. or b.d. (tolerance risk)			
	Intravenous	1 mg/ml. 1.25–5.0 mg/h (care; absorbed onto tubing)			
Isosorbide 5-mononitrate	Oral (tablets 10, 20, 40 mg). Oral sustained release	10–40 mg b.d., t.d.s. or q.d. (prefer b.d.) 40–100 mg o.d. (tolerance risk)	Peak plasma value 0.5–2 h. Active without liver metabolism. Excreted by kidneys partially unchanged and partially as inactive metabolite. Half-life 4–6 h	As for nitroglycerin	As for nitroglycerin
Pentaerythritol tetranitrate	Oral (tablets 30 mg). Oral sustained release	15–30 mg b.d., t.d.s. or q.d. 30 mg b.d. (tolerance risk)	Insufficient data	As for nitroglycerin	As for nitroglycerin
Molsidomine	Oral	2 mg t.d.s.	Vasodilatory intermediates formed by first pass liver metabolism	As for nitroglycerin, tolerance may not develop	As for nitroglycerin. Under evaluation

CALCIUM ANTAGONISTS

Agent	Indications	Dose	Pharmacokinetics	Side-effects	Contra-indications, precautions and drug interactions
Verapamil	Supraventricular tachycardia (SVT) narrow QRS complexes	1 Intravenous bolus 5–10 mg repeated after 10 min, then 0.005 mg/kg/min if needed to total of 10 mg 2 Intravenous infusion 1 mg/min to total of 10 mg 3 If myocardial disease, work up from 0.0001 mg/kg/min, titrating against heart rate	Good GI absorption, low bioavailability (10–20%), High first-pass liver metabolism. Elimination half-life 3–7 h, increased during chronic dosage, or liver or renal disease. 90% protein bound. Excretion of parent compound and active hepatic metabolite norverapamil (longer acting) is 75% renal, 25% gastro-intestinal	*Minor:* Constipation (frequent), headaches, dizziness, facial flushing. *Severe:* IV verapamil as a bolus given to patients with sick sinus syndrome, atrioventricular nodal disease or digitalis poisoning or excess beta-blockade can be fatal. Hypotension, especially if left ventricular failure	*Contra-indications:* Sick sinus syndrome, digitalis toxicity, excess beta-blockade, Wolff–Parkinson–White syndrome with anterograde conduction, myocardial failure. *Caution:* Combination with beta-blockade. *Drug interactions:* Digoxin levels increased; enhanced hypotensive effect with prazosin, nitrates, quinidine and disopyramide; excess nodal inhibition or hypotension with beta-blockade. Cimetidine increases half-life
	Atrial flutter/ fibrillation (control of ventricular rate)	Intravenous infusion, if needed (3 above); or 80–120 mg t.d.s. increasing to 80–120 mg q.d.			
	'Prophylaxis' of SVT	Orally 80–120 mg t.d.s. added to digoxin (watch digoxin level) Orally 80–120 mg t.d.s.			
	Angina of effort, angina at rest Prinzmetal's angina and hypertrophic cardiomyopathy	Orally 80–120 mg t.d.s. increasing to 80–120 mg q.d. (rarely higher doses). Later reduce dose to b.d.			
	Hypertension, mild-to-moderate	As for angina			
	Hypertension, severe	Oral: as for angina Intravenous: 25 mg over 10 min; adjust according to blood pressure			
	Hypertrophic cardiomyopathy	As for angina			
Nifedipine	Angina of effort	Capsules 10 mg t.d.s. to 20 mg q.d.	Nifedipine (capsule) is better absorbed after bite-and-swallow than sublingually. Hypotensive effect within 20 min of oral dose and 5 min of bite-and-swallow dose. Full GI absorption. Protein binding 95%. Almost complete hepatic oxidation to inactive metabolites, excreted in urine. Elimination half-life 2–4 h (capsule) and 6–11 h (tablet)	*Minor:* headache, tachycardia, facial flushing, ankle oedema. *Severe:* provocation of angina; rarely cerebral ischaemia, renal failure	*Contra-indications:* severe aortic stenosis, hypertrophic cardiomyopathy. Smoking decreases effect. *Caution:* myocardial failure, unstable angina with threatened infarction. *Drug interactions:* digoxin (small elevation), excess hypotension with prazosin or nitrates, quinidine, levels reduced. Cimetidine increases half-life and hypotensive effect
	Angina at rest and Prinzmetal's angina	Capsules 10 mg t.d.s. up to 20 mg every 4 h			
	Acute left ventricular failure (pulmonary oedema) in the setting of acute ischaemia or severe hypertension	10 mg sublingually 6 hourly			
	Hypertension, mild to moderate	Capsules 10 mg b.d., t.d.s. or q.d. Tablets 20–40 mg daily			
	Hypertension, severe or refractory	10 mg sublingually; repeat hourly to 40 mg; start with 5 mg in elderly patient			

Agent	Route	Dose	Pharmacokinetics	Side-effects	Contra-indications, precautions and drug interactions
Diltiazem	supraventricular tachycardia narrow QRS complexes	To abort attack: 120 mg plus propranolol 160 mg	90% absorbed from GI tract, first pass hepatic metabolism with 45% bioavailability. Onset of action within 30 min (oral), elimination half-life 4–7 h. Protein binding 83%. Liver metabolism to active deacyldiltiazem, which accumulates with chronic therapy.	Minor: (high dose) headaches, ankle oedema, constipation, bradycardia. Severe: rare skin rash. Adverse effects on sinus or atrioventricular node or myocardium can be expected in predisposed patients (see verapamil)	Contra-indications: as for verapamil. Caution: combination with beta-blockade. Drug interactions: Digoxin (small elevation), interactions with nitrates, quinidine, disopyramide, beta-blockade and cimetidine as for verapamil
	Atrial flutter/ fibrillation (control of ventricular rate)	Oral diltiazem added to digoxin			
	Angina of effort and angina at rest including Prinzmetal 'Prophylaxis' of SVT Hypertension, mild to moderate	Oral 60–90 mg t.d.s. increasing to q.d. as indicated			
		As for angina			
	Hypertrophic cardiomyopathy	As for angina			
Nicardipine	As for nifedipine	Oral 20–40 mg t.d.s. Intravenous use possible, not light-sensitive	Half-life 1–2 h. Extensive hepatic metabolism to inactive metabolites. Renal disease, no effect on kinetics	As for nifedipine	As for nifedipine

ANTI-ARRHYTHMIC DRUGS

Agent	Dose	Pharmacokinetics	Side-effects	Contra-indications, precautions and interactions
Quinidine (Class IA)	Orally 1.2–1.6 g/day in divided doses, 3–12 hourly depending on preparation. Not intravenous infusion	Half-life 7–9 h. Hepatic hydroxylation. Level[a]: 2.3–5 µg/ml.	Many side-effects including diarrhoea, nausea; rarely torsades de pointes and hypotension. Vagolytic	Monitor QRS, QT, plasma K^+. Increases digoxin levels. Care with drugs increasing hepatic metabolism (phenytoin, barbiturates, rifampicin) or decreasing metabolism (cimetidine). Hepatic interaction with warfarin
Procainamide (Class IA)	Intravenous infusion 100 mg bolus over 2 min up to 20 mg/min to 1 g in 1st h; then 2–6 mg/min. Oral 1 g, then up to 500 mg 3 hourly	Partially acetylated in liver to active N-acetyl procainamide. Half-life 3.5 h. Level 4–10 ≥ µg/ml. Toxic effects > 16 µg/ml. (Reduce dose in renal or cardiac failure). 15% protein bound	Hypotension with intravenous dose. Pro-arrhythmic effects. Agranulocytosis	Limit oral use to 6 months (lupus). Cimetidine inhibits renal clearance of procainamide

[a]'Level' stands for therapeutic blood level

Agent	Dose	Pharmacokinetics	Side-effects	Precautions and interactions
Disopyramide (Class IA)	Intravenous infusion 0.5 mg/kg over 5 min, repeat after 5 min (repeat twice more if needed), then 1 mg/kg/h from 0–3 h and 0.4 mg/kg/h for 3–18 h	Elimination: renal 50%, unchanged, bile 10%; rest metabolized to anticholinergic compound. Half-life 8 h, prolonged in renal failure and after myocardial infarction. Level 3–6 µg/ml; toxic > 7 µg/ml.	Hypotension, QRS or QT prolongation, torsades, congestive heart failure. Constipation. Visual disturbances. Hypoglycaemia. Cholestatic jaundice. Interference with therapy of myasthenia gravis. Prominent vagolytic and negative inotropic effects	Contra-indications: heart failure, urinary retention, glaucoma, hypotension. Relative contra-indications: sinus node dysfunction, therapy with beta-blockade or verapamil or other agents widening action potential duration. Precautions: monitor QRS, PR interval
Lignocaine (Class IB) (Lidocaine)	Intravenous infusion 100–200 mg; then 2–4 mg/min for 24–30 h	Hepatic metabolism (blood flow influences). Effect of single bolus lasts only few min, then half-life about 2 h. Level 1.4–5.0 µg/ml; toxic > 9 µg/ml	High-dose central nervous system effects	Contra-indications: none. Precautions: reduce dose by half if liver blood flow low (shock, beta-blockade, cirrhosis, cimetidine, severe heart failure)
Tocainide (Class IB)	Intravenous infusion 0.5–0.75 mg/kg min for 15 min. Oral loading 400–800 mg, then b.d. or t.d.s.	Peak plasma levels 1–2 h after oral dose. Up to 50% half excreted unchanged in urine. Half-life 13 h (increased in liver, renal disease). Level 4–10 µg/ml	CNS, GI side-effects. Sometimes immune-based problems. Contra-indication: pro-arrhythmic effect. Haemotological disorders including agranulocytosis and leucopaenia	Contra-indications: hypersensitivity, second or third degree heart block. Periodic blood counts: Drug interactions: few/none
Mexiletine (Class IB)	Intravenous infusion 100–250 mg at 12.5 mg/min, then 2.0 mg/kg/h for 3.5 h, then 0.5 mg/kg/h. Oral 100–400 mg 8 hourly; loading dose 400 mg	Good GI absorption. High bioavailability. 90% hepatic metabolism, 10% urinary excretion. Half-life 10–17 h. Level 1–2 µg/ml	CNS, GI side-effects. Bradycardia, hypotension. Tremor and nausea common	Contra-indications: cardiogenic shock, second or third degree heart block. Drug interactions: hepatic enzyme inducers reduce plasma levels. Concurrent disopyramide predisposes to negative inotropic effect. May combine with quinidine, beta-blockade, amiodarone
Phenytoin (Class IB)	Intravenous infusion 10–15 mg/kg over 1 h. Oral 1 g; 500 mg for 2 days; then 400–600 mg daily.	Erratic GI absorption. 90% protein bound. Hepatic hydroxylation, half-life 24 h. Level 10–18 µg/ml. Hepatic or renal disease requires reduced doses	Hypotension, drowsiness, vertigo, dysarthria, lethargy, gingivitis, macrocytic anaemia, lupus, pulmonary infiltrates	Contra-indications: anaemia, liver disease. Drug interactions: phenytoin induces hepatic enzymes and decreases doses required of quinidine, lidocaine and mexiletine

Agent	Dose	Pharmacokinetics	Side-effects	Contra-indications and comments
Flecainide (Class IC)	Intravenous infusion 1–2 mg/kg over 10 min, then 0.15–0.25 mg/kg/h. Oral 100–400 mg b.d.	No hepatic metabolism. Half-life 13–19 h. Keep trough level below 0.2–1.0 µg/ml	QRS prolongation. Pro-arrhythmic effect potentially serious. Depresses left ventricular function. CNS side-effects	Use only for life-threatening arrythmias. Contra-indications: significant conduction delay, sick sinus syndrome, myocardial depression. Drug interactions: additive inhibitory effects on sinus or atrioventricular node or added negative inotropic effects. Amiodarone increases flecainide levels. Slight increase in digoxin level
Encainide (Class IC)	25–75 mg t.d.s. daily	Half-life 1–2 h. Hepatic metabolism. Normal phenotype produces long-acting metabolites (3–12 h)	QRS prolongation. CNS side-effects. Pro-arrhythmic effect potentially serious	Use only for life-threatening arrythmias. Relative contra-indication: pre-existing inhibition of sinus atrioventricular node or conduction system
Amiodarone (Class III)	Oral loading dose 600–1600 mg daily; maintenance 200–400 mg daily. Occasional intravenous use (150–1000 mg over 15–60 min), in glucose not saline	Half-life 25–110 days. Level 1.0–2.5 µg/ml	Complex side-effects including pulmonary fibrosis, QT prolongation and thyroid dysfunction. Pro-arrhythmic effect. Corneal microdeposits. Blue discolouration of the skin	Precautions: consider side-effects, drug interactions. Drug interactions: pro-arrhythmic effect with drugs prolonging QT interval. Prolongs prothrombin time. Increases plasma digoxin
Bretylium tosylate (Class III)	Intravenous infusion 5–10 mg/kg, repeat to maximum 30 mg/kg, then 1–2 mg/min or intramuscularly 5–10 mg/kg 8 hourly at varying sites (local necrosis)	Half-life 7–9 h. Decrease dose in renal failure. Level 0.5–1.0 µg/ml	Hypotension, nausea, vomiting	Drug interactions: drug limited to recurrent ventricular fibrillation or tachycardia after lignocaine has failed

THIAZIDE DIURETICS

Agent	Dose		Pharmacokinetics	Side-effects	Contra-indications
Hydrochlorothiazide	12.5–50 mg	(BP)[a]	Incomplete but rapid GI absorption. Diuresis 1–12 h. Plasma half-life 3–4 h. Bound to red blood cells. Excreted unchanged in urine. 'Low ceiling'. Ineffective with glomerular filtration rate < 15–20 ml/min	Hypokalaemia, hyponatraemia, increased blood triglyceride, glucose intolerance, hyperuricaemia, impotence, lethargy, dizziness, sulphonamide-type side-effects (jaundice, rash, pancreatitis, blood dyscrasias, angiitis, pneumonitis, interstitial nephritis)	Renal oedema, severe renal failure, hypokalaemia, ventricular arrhythmias, co-therapy with pro-arrhythmic drugs. Relative contra-indication: pregnancy hypertension
	25–100 mg	(CHF)[b]			
Bendrofluazide (bendroflumethiazide)	2.5–5 mg	(BP)	Complete GI absorption, active hepatic metabolism, 30% excreted unchanged in urine. Plasma half-life 3–4 h.	As for hydrochlorothiazide	As for hydrochlorothiazide
	10 mg	(CHF)			
Chlorthalidone	12.5–50 mg		Half-life 4 h, increased in aged. 75% protein binding. 65% excreted in urine	As for hydrochlorothiazide	As for hydrochlorothiazide
Cyclopenthiazide	0.25 mg	(BP)	Diuresis 1–12 h	As for hydrochlorothiazide	As for hydrochlorothiazide
	0.5–1 mg	(CHF)			
Indapamide	2.5 mg	(BP)	Diuresis 1–36 h. Plasma protein binding 80%. Extensive metabolism, metabolites slowly excreted in urine	As for hydrochlorothiazide	As for hydrochlorothiazide
	2.5–5 mg	(CHF)			
Mefruside	25 mg	(BP)	Rapid GI absorption. Diuresis 2–24 h. Extensive metabolism to active metabolite. Two-thirds excreted in urine	As for hydrochlorothiazide	As for hydrochlorothiazide
	25–100 mg	(CHF)			

[a]BP = Use for blood pressure lowering.
[b]CHF = Use for congestive heart failure

Agent	Dose	Pharmacokinetics	Side-effects	Contra-indications
Metolazone	(BP) 1–5 mg (CHF) 5–20 mg	Plasma half-life 8 h. Diuresis 1–24 h. Excreted in urine chiefly unchanged. High protein binding	As for hydrochlorothiazide	As for hydrochlorothiazide, but may be more effective than thiazides in chronic renal failure; care in combination with frusemide
Xipamide	(BP) 20 mg (CHF) 20–40 mg	Complete GI absorption. 99% protein bound. Diuresis 1–12 h. Plasma half-life 5–8 h. Urinary excretion, unchanged or after metabolism. In renal failure, increased biliary excretion	As for hydrochlorothiazide	As for hydrochlorothiazide

POTASSIUM-SPARING DIURETICS

Agent	Dose	Pharmacokinetics	Side-effects	Contra-indications
Amiloride	2.5–20 mg	Secreted in proximal tubule. Acts on Na/K exchange distal tubule. Not metabolized. Not protein bound. Acts 4–5 days	Few. Hyperkalaemia and acidosis in renal disease. Mild uraemia. No diabetes nor gout as side-effect	Hyperkalaemia, renal failure. Generally combined with thiazide diuretic
Spironolactone	25–400 mg in divided doses; for hypertension, 50–100 mg in single dose	70% GI absorption. First pass hepatic metabolism to active canrenone. Dosage with meals increases canrenone formation. High protein binding. Acts 3–5 days	Gynaecomastia, impotence, menstrual dysfunction, GI disturbances. increases of blood K^+, creatinine, urate, triglyceride. Glucose unaltered. Blood Mg^{2+} falls.	Hyperkalaemia, renal failure, hypomagnaesimia. Relative contra-indication: co-therapy with ACE inhibitors or potassium-retaining diuretics. Caution: cirrhosis
Triamterene	25–200 mg	Secreted in proximal tubule. Acts on distal tubule Na^+/K^+ exchange. Highly metabolized in liver. 60% protein bound. Acts 8–12 h	As for amiloride. Also renal casts	As for amiloride. Caution: cirrhosis. Generally combined with thiazide diuretic

LOOP DIURETICS

Agent	Dose	Pharmacokinetics	Side-effects	Contra-indications and comments
Bumetanide	0.5–2 mg o.d. or b.d. oral; 1 mg intravenously; 2.5 mg intravenously (oliguria); maintenance: alternate days	Complete and rapid GI absorption. Duration of action 0.5–5 h. 90% protein bound. Renal excretion of unchanged and metabolized forms. Small faecal excretion. Elimination half-life 1.5 h.	As for frusemide, except less ototoxicity and more renal toxicity. Also myalgia, gynaecomastia	As for frusemide
Frusemide	20–40 mg (BP)[a]; 20–80 mg o.d. or b.d. (CHF)[b]; oral or intravenous 250–2000 mg (oliguria[c] or CHF)	Incomplete but rapid GI absorption. 99% protein bound. Renal excretion, largely unchanged. Non-renal (bile) elimination increased in renal failure. Duration of action 15 min to 5 h.	Chiefly electrolyte and volume disturbances especially hypokalaemia, hypovolaemia, oliguria. Hypernatremia. Hyperuricaemia. Skin eruptions, blood dyscrasias, ototoxicity, renal toxicity, gout, diabetes	Hypersensitivity to sulphonamides. Care with electrolyte imbalance, hypovolaemia. Enhanced nephrotoxicity with aminoglycosides
Piretanide	6–12 mg with breakfast (BP); higher doses for diuresis	Half-life similar to that of frusemide	As for frusemide, myalgia	As for frusemide

ANTI-THROMBOTICS AND THROMBOLYTICS

Agent	Dose	Pharmacokinetics	Side-effects	Contra-indications and comments
Anistreplase (anisoylated plasminogen streptokinase activator complex)	30 units over 5 min	Half-life 1.5 h. Fibrinolytic activity for 4–6 h. Acts by deacylation of plasminogen molecule	Bleeding. Allergy rare	As for streptokinase

[a]BP = Use for blood pressure lowering.
[b]CHF = Use for congestive heart failure
[c]Glomerular filtration rate < 20 ml/min; otherwise such high doses are contra-indicated, except in severe refractory congestive heart failure.

Agent	Dose	Pharmacokinetics	Side-effects	Contra-indications and comments
Aspirin	300 mg daily or alternate days or 150 mg daily. Up to 1300 mg daily	Pre-systemic hydrolysis to form salicylic acid with half-life 2–3 h. One dose of aspirin (325 mg) inhibits platelet aggregation for 4–7 days. Aspirin irreversibly acetylates cyclo-oxygenase	Dyspepsia, nausea, vomiting. GI bleeding	Aspirin intolerance, haemophilia, history of GI bleeding, renal disease, renal stones, liver disease. High dose aspirin exaggerates bleeding tendency
Dipyridamole	50–75 mg t.d.s. 1 h before meals	Ready GI absorption. Concentrated in liver, excreted in faeces. Vasodilator. Inhibits platelet adhesion. Anti-aggregatory	Rare. GI irritation; vasodilative and hypotensive effects; coronary steal	Few. Relative contra-indication severe aortic stenosis
Heparin	5000–10 000 units loading dose, repeat every 4–6 h or infuse. Ultra low dose: 1 unit/kg/h for 3–5 days. Subcutaneous: 15 000 units 12 hourly	Intravenous: onset of action within minutes, lasts 4–6 h. Metabolized in liver by heparinase to inactive metabolites. Inhibits thrombin and (in low doses) increases activity of antithrombin III. Increases activity of lipoprotein lipase	Occasional allergy. Haemorrhage, thrombocytopaenia, osteoporosis after prolonged use	Haemophilia and bleeding disorders, active peptic ulcer, cerebral aneurysm, severe liver disease, hypersensitivity
Phenindione	200 mg 1st day, 100 mg 2nd day, 50–150 mg daily. Check prothrombin time	Anticoagulant effect starts within 36–48 h and wanes 48–72 h after dose is stopped	As for warfarin with higher risk of renal or hepatic toxicity. Occasional skin necrosis	As for warfarin including pregnancy
Streptokinase	1.5 mU in 100 ml saline in 1 h	Activates plasminogen for as long as is infused	Minor and major bleeding. Allergic reactions, fever, rashes. Post surgical bleeding	Recent GI bleeding, cerebrovascular accident, coagulation defects, severe uncontrolled hypertension, recent streptococcal infections, haemorrhagic retinopathy, and high risk of left heart thrombus as in infective endocarditis. Pregnancy, menstruation

Agent	Dose	Pharmacokinetics	Side-effects	Contra-indications and comments
Sulfinpyrazone	200 mg b.d., t.d.s. or q.d.	Plasma half-life 3 h (after intravenous infusion). 25–50% excreted unchanged in urine within 24 h (reduce by probenecid). High plasma protein binding. Reversible inhibition of cyclo-oxygenase. Limits platelet adhesion to collagen. Uricosuric	GI. Occasional hypersensitivity or blood disorder	Peptic ulcer, renal failure, renal stones. After acute myocardial infarction, may cause renal failure. Warfarin displaced from plasma proteins to precipitate bleeding. Effects of sulphonylureas and insulin enhanced
Alteplase (Tissue-type plasminogen activator (tPA))	0.5 mg/kg over 90 min	Binds to fibrin-associated plasminogen to form plasmin, for as long as is infused	Bleeding	As for streptokinase except for streptococcal infections
Warfarin	Depends on prothrombin time. Initiate with 10–15 mg daily with maintenance dose of 1–20 mg according to prothrombin time	Hepatic metabolism. 99% protein bound. Peak plasma concentration 1 h after ingestion. Circulating half-life 36 h. Interferes with vitamin K-dependent clotting factors. K^+ salt less, bioavailable than Na^+ salt	Bleeding (treat with vitamin K) but few others. Occasional skin necrosis. Can damage fetus	Early pregnancy (6–12 weeks) – danger of abortion. Stroke, uncontrolled severe hypertension, cirrhosis, GI bleeding. Drug interactions: many potentiating and interfering drugs. Sulfinpyrazone displaces warfarin from blood proteins, so that very low dose is required

LIPID-LOWERING AGENTS

Agent	Dose	Pharmacokinetics	Side-effects	Contra-indications and comments
Bezafibrate	200 mg b.d. or t.d.s.	Does not enter liver cells. Activates lipoprotein lipase. Sterol excretion in bile enhanced	Myositis, renal failure, alopecia	Reduce dose during oral anticoagulant therapy

Agent	Dose	Pharmacokinetics	Side-effects	Contra-indications and comments
Cholestyramine	Up to 16–24 g daily	Anion exchange resin which binds bile acids with increased faecal loss compensated for by diversion of cholesterol	Nausea, constipation, diarrhoea, other GI symptoms, steatorrhoea	Complete biliary obstruction. Drug interactions: absorption of digitalis, chlorothiazide and warfarin reduced. Take such drugs 1 h before cholestyramine
Clofibrate	500 mg b.d. or t.d.s. after meals	Complete GI absorption to form a de-esterified compound in blood, plasma protein bound, urinary excretion. Half-life, second phase, 15 h. Does not enter liver cells. Activates lipoprotein lipase. Sterol excretion in bile enhanced.	Abdominal discomfort, muscle pains, cholesterol gallstones, pancreatitis. Potentiation of warfarin.	Biliary tract or hepatic disease, severe renal disease
Colestipol	5–10 g b.d. or t.d.s. in liquid	Similar to cholestyramine	See cholestyramine	See cholestyramine
Gemfibrozil	600 mg b.d. 30 min before meals	Complete GI absorption. Enterohepatic circulation. Ultimate renal excretion as glucuromide. Does not enter liver cells. Activates lipoprotein lipase. Sterol excretion in bile enhanced	Similar to clofibrate	Similar to clofibrate
Lovastatin	20–80 mg daily in 1 or 2 doses		GI, myalgia, skin rash, blurred vision. Corneal opacities	Liver disease. Pregnancy. Check blood transaminase and creatine phosphokinase levels
Nicotinic acid	100 mg t.d.s. up to 1–2 g t.d.s. with meals	Ready GI absorption. Short half-life. Metabolized in liver	GI, flushing, dizziness, palpitations, impaired glucose tolerance, increased blood urate, liver disorder, rashes	Relative contra-indication: diabetes. Aspirin 30 min before dose may reduce flushing

Agent	Dose	Pharmacokinetics	Side-effects	Contra-indications and comments
Probucol	500 mg b.d. with food	Highly lipophilic, persists in adipose tissue for 6 months. Low GI absorption, 10%. Eliminated by bile and faeces, not urine	Many, not serious. Nausea, vomiting, flatulence, diarrhoea, abdominal pain. Occasional QT prolongation. Substantially lower HDL cholesterol	Pregnancy – withdraw drug 6 months before. Hypokalaemia. Co-therapy with antiarrhythmics predisposing to QT prolongation

AGENTS FOR USE IN HYPERTENSIVE URGENCIES AND EMERGENCIES

Agent	Dose	Pharmacokinetics	Side-effects	Contra-indications and comments
Captopril	25 mg chewed	Hepatic, renal	Risk of renal failure especially in bilateral renal artery stenosis	Bilateral renal artery stenosis; not well tested. Sudden hypotension if high plasma renin
Diazoxide	100–150 mg IV every 5 min to total of 300 mg. Infusion: 5 mg/kg at 15 mg/min	Short-acting	Difficult to control hypotensive effect; risk of cerebral ischaemia. Prolonged use: diabetes	Avoid if possible
Dihydralazine	6.25–12.5 mg intravenous slowly or infuse. IV as 0.1 mg/min to total of 25 mg	See hydralazine	As for diazoxide, prefer infusion	Avoid if possible. Contra-indicated in tachycardia, angina, ischaemic strokes
Hydralazine	5–10 mg intravenous every 4–6 h	Half-life 2–8 h. Liver acetylation	Less danger of hypotension than diazoxide	Avoid if possible. As for dihydralazine
Labetalol	Infuse at 2 mg/min total of 1–2 mg/kg Pulsed doses 20–80 mg every 10 min. Oral 400 mg, then 200 mg 6-hourly	Half-life 3–4 h. Hepatic metabolism	Usually safe, may worsen cardiac failure or asthma	Smooth and rapid dose-related fall in blood pressure. Avoid tachycardia. Oral preparation under-used
Nifedipine	10–20 mg sublingually (bite-and-swallow) or orally	Short-acting 4–6 h. For most rapid absorption bite-and-swallow	Few unless excess hypotension. Risk of cerebral ischaemia	Aortic stenosis, hypertrophic cardiomyopathy. Caution: unstable angina. Needs further evaluation in presence of papilloedema and hypertensive encephalopathy

Agent	Dose	Pharmacokinetics	Side-effects	Contra-indications and comments
Nitroprusside	Infusion of 40–75 µg/min	Haemodynamic response rapid and stops rapidly. Converted free cyanide in red cells, thiocyanate formed in liver, and cleared by kidneys. Half-life 7 days	Hypotension, must monitor constantly. Fatigue, vomiting, disorientation wih prolonged infusion. Prolonged therapy, hypothyroidism	Especially useful if pulmonary oedema or encephalopathy or threatened stroke. Otherwise avoid
Phenoxybenzamine	10–100 mg daily orally (usually in divided doses). 15–40 mg slow intravenous infusion	Slow rate of onset of action due to formation of active hepatic metabolites	Postural hypotension, tachycardia, nasal congestion, retrograde ejaculation	Only indicated for phaeochromocytoma
Phentolamine	Intravenous 5–10 mg repeated as necessary. Intravenous infusion 10–20 µg/kg/min	Hepatic	Hypotension, tachycardia, nausea, diarrhoea, nasal congestion	Only indicated for hypertensive crises due to phaeochromocytoma, or other states of excess alpha-stimulation such as clonidine withdrawal, excess use of sympathomimetic agents, or hypertensive crisis associated with monoamine oxidase inhibitors
Reserpine	1 mg intramuscularly	Prolonged delayed effect. Hepatic metabolism	Drowsiness, hypotension	Avoid if possible. Delayed effect (1–4 h) with possible severe hypotension
Verapamil	160 mg orally. Intravenous 5–25 mg over 10–30 min	Half-life 4–6 h. Blood pressure fall starts within 0.5–1 h of oral dose	Sino-atrial, atrioventricular nodal inhibition. Negatively inotropic	Contra-indications as for nifedipine, plus sino-atrial, atrioventricular disease or inhibition; myocardial failure

DRUGS USED IN THE TREATMENT OF CHRONIC HYPERTENSION

Agent	Dose	Pharmacokinetics	Side-effects	Contra-indications and comments
Diuretics	Various	Hepatic metabolism, variable half-life	Metabolic, rash, haematological	Risk of gout, diabetes, hypokalaemia, ventricular arrhythmias. Keep dose low

Agent	Dose	Pharmacokinetics	Side-effects	Contra-indications and comments
Beta-blockers	Various	Lipophilic agents liver metabolized. Hydrophilic agents renal excreted	Cardiac, respiratory, central nervous system	Contra-indications: asthma, myocardial depression, heart block
Alpha-blockers				
Prazosin	1–10 mg b.d. Test dose 0.5 mg	Half-life 3–4 h. Hepatic metabolism. Decreased dose in renal failure	Postural hypotension. Palpitations. Drowsiness. Fatigue. Dry mouth. Blocked nose. Genito-urinary	First-dose syncope. Care during co-therapy with calcium antagonists (potentiating effects)
Terazosin	1–10 mg once daily sometimes b.d. First dose 1 mg	As for prazosin. Longer half-life	As for prazosin. May have less syncope	As for prazosin
Indoramin	25–100 mg b.d.	Half-life 4 h. Hepatic metabolism. Reduce dose in cirrhosis	May have less postural hypotension and tachycardia than prazosin. May have more dry mouth, drowsiness, sexual dysfunction than prazosin. Otherwise similar	As for prazosin. High-dose antihistaminic effect
Calcium antagonists				
Verapamil	120–240 mg b.d. (SR preparation 1–2 daily)	Hepatic metabolism. Active norverapamil metabolites	Constipation, dizziness	Contra-indication: conduction defects. Sick sinus syndrome, excess beta-blockade or digitalis, myocardial depression
Nifedipine	Capsules 5–20 mg t.d.s. Tablets 20–40 mg b.d.	Hepatic metabolism. Short half-life	Headaches, tachycardia, facial flushing, ankle oedema	Contra-indications: hypotension, severe aortic stenosis, obstructive cardiomyopathy
Diltiazem	60–120 mg t.d.s. (slow release form, b.d. dose)	Hepatic metabolism. Desacetyl metabolite probably active	Headaches, dizziness, ankle oedema	As for verapamil
Nicardipine	20–40 mg t.d.s.	As for nifedipine	As for nifedipine	As for nifedipine
Non-specific vasodilators				
Hydralazine	25–50 mg b.d. Occasionally 100 mg b.d.	Hepatic metabolism, depends on acetylator status. Half-life 2–8 h	Tachycardia, fluid retention, (give with beta-blocker, diuretic) high-dose lupus	Contra-indications: angina, ischaemic heart disease

Agent	Dose	Pharmacokinetics	Side-effects	Contra-indications and comments
Minoxidil	2.5 mg b.d. increased by 5–10 mg every 3 days or more. Maximum dose 50 mg once daily	Half-life 3 h, but may be sequestered in tissues, rapidly absorbed, with prolonged biological half-life metabolized mainly by conjugation to glucoronic acid in the liver. 12% excreted unchanged in urine	Hypertrichosis, fluid retention, tachycardia, gastro-intestinal disturbances, breast tenderness, very rarely myocardial fibrosis, Stevens–Johnson syndrome	Very effective vasodilator which will reduce blood pressure in resistant cases but requires combination with a drug, e.g. beta-antagonist/ACE inhibitor to block reflex tachycardia and large doses of loop diuretic, e.g. frusemide, are frequently needed to avoid fluid retention which related to dose, duration of administration and renal function. Hypertrichosis which occurs after 4 weeks' treatment in the majority is not acceptable to most women and alternative treatment should be considered. ST-segment depression and T-wave inversion have been reported. Rebound hypertension has been claimed to occur on withdrawal of drug. Care in congestive heart failure

Serotonin Antagonists

Agent	Dose	Pharmacokinetics	Side-effects	Contra-indications and comments
Ketanserin	20 mg b.d. max 40 mg b.d.	Half-life 15 h. Extensively metabolized in the liver. Metabolites excreted 68% in urine	Initially transient drowsiness, lack of concentration, lightheadedness, mainly in young patients. Most common side-effects: dizziness, fatigue, dry mouth, oedema. Dose-dependent prolongation of the QT interval (from 40 mg b.d. upwards)	Use with caution in patients with heart block grade II or III or concomitantly receiving anti-arrhythmics. Avoid hypokalemia; if combined with diuretics, a potassium-sparing diuretic should be included. Do not exceed 20 mg b.d. in severe liver disease

CENTRALLY ACTING DRUGS WHICH INTERFERE WITH ADRENERGIC NEURONAL FUNCTION

Agent	Dose	Pharmacokinetics	Side-effects	Contra-indications and comments
Methyldopa	250 mg b.d. to maximum total dose 3 g. Intravenous infusion 250–500 mg	Half-life 2 h. 30% excreted unchanged in urine and half-life prolonged when renal function impaired	Dry mouth, sedation, depression, drowziness, diarrhoea, fluid retention, failure of ejaculation, rarely haemolytic anaemia, lupus syndrome, liver impairment	Less frequently prescribed now with advent of newer drugs. Reduce initial dose in renal impairment. Up to 20% patients may have positive direct Coombs test (may affect cross-matching for blood transfusion). Care advised if history of depression or liver disease. May have extrapyramidal effects and potentiate lithium
Clonidine	0.1–0.3 mg as 2 or more doses to maximum 1.2 mg daily but rarely more than 0.3 mg b.d. 150–300 µg by slow IV injection. Slow release preparation available	Half-life 10 h. Rapidly absorbed, and 62% excreted unchanged in urine. Rest undergoes metabolism in liver	Dry mouth, sedation, depression, fluid retention, withdrawal hypertension, bradycardia, Raynaud's, central effects including vivid dreams and breathlessness. Impotence reported	Marked increases in pressure may occur if doses are omitted, 'Clonidine withdrawal' Reduce dose in renal impairment. Used in suppression tests for diagnosis of phaeochromocytoma (see Chapter 53)
Reserpine	Usually 0.05–0.25 mg daily in single dose (higher doses rarely used)	Half-life 4–5 h prolonged biological effect. Extensively metabolized after absorption	Dry mouth, sedation, nasal congestion, postural hypotension, fluid retention, depression, nightmares, abdominal cramp and diarrhoea	Less commonly used but side-effect profile acceptable if modest doses prescribed. Care in patients with depression or peptic ulceration. May worsen extrapyramidal side-effects of some drugs and care with monoamine oxidase inhibitors

Index

Page references in **bold typeface** indicate tables whereas those references in *italics* indicate figures.

VLDL, 1027
  increased number, *see*
      Hypertriglyceridaemia
  levels in familial
      hypercholesterolaemia, 1452
VMA (Vanilmandelic acid),
      measurement,
  phaeochromocytoma screening,
      1394
V_{max}, 474
Volume expansion therapy, use,
  acute circulatory failure, 42
  severe pre-eclampsia, 1381
Von Willebrand's syndrome,
  mitral valve prolapse in, **793**
Voodoo death, 1507
VVD pacemakers, 589
VVI pacemakers, 223, 587–588
VVT pacemakers, 587–588

W

Warfarin,
  contra-indications, 1624
  dosage, 1624
  drug interactions, 1624
      procainamide, 552
  pharmacokinetics, 1624
  side effects, 1624
  use,
      in pregnancy, 1368, 1624
      post-prosthetic heart valve
          surgery, 892
      laboratory control, 893
Water, drinking,
  and cardiovascular disease, *see*
      Drinking water
Water-hammer pulse, 102–103, **738**
Water retention,
  heart failure response, 51
  in chronic obstructive airways
      disease, 45
Waterstone's groove, location, 7–8
Weakness, causes, 95
Weather,
  and cardiovascular disease,
      cold weather, 1493–1494
      hot weather, 1494–1495
Wedensky phenomenon, 596
Wegener's syndrome,
  pericarditis in, 993
  pulmonary hypertension in, 1322
Weight, cardiac, **26**
Wenckebach point, 241
Wernicke-Korsakoff syndrome, 1515
Wheezing, occurrences, 1334, 1394
Whipple's disease,
  pericarditis in, 993
WHO MONICA study, 1004
Williams' syndrome, 684, 709, **1459**
Wolff-Parkinson-White pattern, 244
Wolff-Parkinson-White syndrome, 518,
      520, 521, 522
  ambulatory ECG appearance, *225*
  atrial fibrillation with, 245, 522–523
  classification, 522
  clinical electrophysiology study, 244
  clinical features, 519
      reversed S_2 splitting, 122

false-positive exercise testing cause,
      463
  incidence, 1600
  medical treatment, 523
      and transport certification, 1600
  normal PR interval mechanism, 521
  resting ECG appearance, 116, 186,
      527
      diagnostic criteria, 186, 188
  short PR interval mechanism, 521
  surgical treatment 523, 568–569
      and transport certification, 1600
  transport certification, 1600
  ventricular rate, 516
Work,
  post-infarction return to, 1196
  psychological stress in, 1500

X

X-linked disorders, 1453–1454, *see
      also* Hunter's syndrome
Xamoterol, 74
  contra-indications, 1610
  dosage, 1610
  pharmacokinetics, 1610
  side effects, 1610
  uses,
      chronic heart failure, 74
      sick sinus syndrome, 600
Xenon-127, use,
  ventilation imaging of lung, 452
Xenon-133, 440
  ventilation imaging of lung, 452
Xipamide,
  contra-indications, 1621
  dosage, 1621
  pharmacokinetics, 1621
  side effects, 1621
  uses, 1621

Z

Z-line, 27
Zone 4, 1343